SIXTH EDITION
VOLUME II

GLENN'S THORACIC AND CARDIOVASCULAR SURGERY

SIXTH EDITION
VOLUME II

GLENN'S THORACIC AND CARDIOVASCULAR SURGERY

Editor

Arthur E. Baue, MD
Professor of Surgery
Saint Louis University School of Medicine
St. Louis, Missouri

Coeditors

Alexander S. Geha, MD, MS
Chief, Division of Cardiothoracic Surgery
University Hospitals of Cleveland
The Jay L. Ankeney Professor and Director
Division of Cardiothoracic Surgery
Case Western Reserve University School
of Medicine
Cleveland, Ohio

Graeme L. Hammond, MD
Attending Surgeon
Yale-New Haven Hospital
Professor of Surgery
Yale University School of Medicine
New Haven, Connecticut

Hillel Laks, MD
Professor and Chief, Division of
Cardiothoracic Surgery
University of California, Los Angeles School
of Medicine
Los Angeles, California

Keith S. Naunheim, MD
Professor of Surgery
Saint Louis University School of Medicine
St. Louis, Missouri

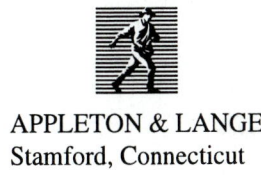

APPLETON & LANGE
Stamford, Connecticut

96 97 98 99 00 / 10 9 8 7 6 5 4 3 2 1

Prentice Hall International (UK) Limited, *London*
Prentice Hall of Australia Pty. Limited, *Sydney*
Prentice Hall Canada, Inc., *Toronto*
Prentice Hall Hispanoamericana, S.A., *Mexico*
Prentice Hall of India Private Limited, *New Delhi*
Prentice Hall of Japan, Inc., *Tokyo*
Simon & Schuster Asia Pte. Ltd., *Singapore*
Editora Prentice Hall do Brasil Ltda., *Rio de Janeiro*
Prentice Hall, *Englewood Cliffs, New Jersey*

Library of Congress Cataloging-in-Publication Data

Glenn's thoracic and cardiovascular surgery / [edited by] Arthur E.
  Baue . . . [et al.].—6th ed.
      p.   cm.
    Includes bibliographical references and index.
    ISBN 0–8385–3134–2 (set : casebound)
    1. Chest—Surgery.   2. Cardiovascular system—Surgery.   I. Glenn,
  William W. L.   II. Baue, Arthur.   III. Title: Thoracic and
  cardiovascular surgery.
    [DNLM: 1. Thoracic Surgery.   2. Cardiovascular System—surgery.
  WF 980 G5581G558   1995]
  RD536.G585   1995
  617.5′4—dc20
  DNLM/DLC
  for Library of Congress   95–14257
                                                      CIP

Acquisitions Editor: Edward Wickland
Managing Editor, Development: Kathleen McCullough
Production Coordinator: Jean Finn
Production Service: Spectrum Publisher Services, Blair Woodcock
Production Supervisor: Karen Davis
Designer: Elizabeth Schmitz
Cover Designer: Janice Barsevich Bielawa

ISBN 0-8385-3134-2

90000

9 780838 531341

PRINTED IN THE UNITED STATES OF AMERICA

This book, the Sixth Edition, bears the name of
William W.L. Glenn, MD, who carried the tradition of the original
book by Gustav E. Lindskog, MD, and the late Averill A. Liebow, MD.
We remember them as we dedicate this edition to those who have
supported us in these endeavors—to Rosemary Baue, Diane Geha,
Janet Hammond, and Rosanne Naunheim.

Little do such men know the toil, the pains,
the daily, nightly racking of the brains
to arrange the thoughts, the matter to digest
to cull fit phrases, and reject the rest.
Charles Churchill (1731–1764),
Gotham, Book II

Surgery is in large part a handicraft with
elaborate technics that may be grouped as
Technology . . . if one be honest . . . he cannot fail
to see that Surgery is seeded with ad hoc
hypotheses, or, in more frank terms, empiricisms,
and irrational beliefs.
Edward D. Churchill
Ann Surg 126:381, 1947

Contents

VOLUME II

**Section II: Surgery for Congenital
                Heart Disease** 953
*Hillel Laks, Section Editor,
and Lester C. Permut, Assistant
Section Editor*

Contributors

Michael A. Acker, MD
Attending Staff, Surgical Director Cardiac
  Transplantation Program
Hospital of the University of Pennsylvania
Assistant Professor of Surgery
University of Pennsylvania School of Medicine
Philadelphia, Pennsylvania

Lee P. Adler, MD
Director Cardiovascular MR
University Hospital of Cleveland
Associate Professor of Radiology
Case Western Reserve University School of Medicine
Cleveland, Ohio

Bradley S. Allen, MD
Attending Cardiothoracic Surgeon
University of Illinois Hospital
Assistant Professor of Surgery
Division of Cardiothoracic Surgery
University of Illinois College of Medicine
Chicago, Illinois

Mark S. Allen, MD
Consultant in General Thoracic Surgery
Mayo Clinic
Assistant Professor of Surgery
Mayo Graduate School of Medicine
Rochester, Minnesota

Nasser K. Altorki, MD
Associate Attending Cardiovascular–Thoracic Surgeon
The New York Hospital
Associate Professor, Cardiothoracic Surgery
Cornell University Medical College
New York, New York

Robert H. Anderson, BSc, MD, FRCPath
Honorary Consultant
Royal Brompton Hospital NHS Trust
Joseph Levy Professor of Paediatric Cardiac Morphology
National Heart & Lung Institute
London, United Kingdom

Joseph S. Auteri
Attending Cardiothoracic Surgeon
Arizona Heart Institute
Health West Regional Medical Center
Phoenix, Arizona

Carl L. Backer, MD
Attending Cardiovascular–Thoracic Surgeon
The Children's Memorial Hospital
Assistant Professor of Surgery
Northwestern University Medical School
Chicago, Illinois

Leonard L. Bailey, MD
Attending Surgeon—Cardiothoracic
Loma Linda University Medical Center
Professor and Chairman, Department of Surgery
Loma Linda University School of Medicine
Loma Linda, California

John C. Baldwin, MD
Chief of Surgical Services
The Methodist Hospital
Surgeon-in-Chief
Ben Taub General Hospital
DeBakey Professor and Chairman, Department of Surgery
Baylor College of Medicine
Houston, Texas

Paul G. Barash, MD
Attending Anesthesiologist
Yale New Haven Medical Center
Professor of Anesthesiology
Yale University School of Medicine
New Haven, Connecticut

Hendrick B. Barner, MD
Christian Hospital NE
Professor of Surgery
Washington University School of Medicine
St. Louis, Missouri

Arthur E. Baue, MD
Professor of Surgery
Saint Louis University School of Medicine
St. Louis, Missouri

Victor C. Baum, MD
Attending Physician
Departments of Anesthesiology & Pediatrics
University of Virginia Medical Center
Associate Professor of Anesthesiology and Pediatrics
University of Virginia
Charlottesville, Virginia

Carlos W.M. Bedrossian, MD
Chief of Cytopathology
Detroit Medical Center
Professor of Pathology
Wayne State University School of Medicine
Detroit, Michigan

Douglas M. Behrendt, MD
Professor and Chairman
Division of Cardiothoracic Surgery
The University of Iowa
Iowa City, Iowa

Ronald H.R. Belsey, MS, FRCS, FRCSI(Hon)
Emeritus Professor of Cardiothoracic Surgery
Bristol University
Bath, United Kingdom

John R. Benfield, MD
Chief of the Division of Cardiothoracic Surgery
University of California, Davis Medical Center
Professor of Surgery
University of California, Davis School of Medicine
Sacramento, California

Deborah A. Bishop, BS
Research Associate
The Children's Hospital
University of Colorado Health Sciences Center
Denver, Colorado

Edward L. Bove, MD
Director, Pediatric Cardiovascular Surgery
C.S. Mott Children's Hospital
Professor of Surgery
University of Michigan School of Medicine
Ann Arbor, Michigan

Carol M. Buchter, MD
Director, Heart Failure Evaluation
    and Treatment Program
University Hospitals of Cleveland
Assistant Professor of Medicine
Case Western Reserve University School of Medicine
Cleveland, Ohio

Gerald D. Buckberg, MD
Attending Staff
University of California, Los Angeles Medical Center
Professor of Surgery
University of California, Los Angeles School
    of Medicine
Los Angeles, California

Redmond P. Burke, MD
Associate in Cardiac Surgery
Childrens Hospital, Boston
Instructor in Surgery
Harvard Medical School
Boston, Massachusetts

Michael Burt, MD, PhD
Attending Surgeon
Memorial Sloan-Kettering Cancer Center
Associate Professor of Surgery
Cornell University Medical College
New York, New York

Alain Carpentier, MD, PhD
Chairman, Cardiovascular Surgery
    Department
Hospital Broussais
Professor of Cardiac Surgery
University of Paris
France

Bernard R. Chaitman, MD
Chief of Cardiology
Saint Louis University Health
    Sciences Center
Professor of Medicine
Saint Louis University School of Medicine
St. Louis, Missouri

Pauline W. Chen, MD
Medical Staff Fellow
Surgery Branch
National Cancer Institute
National Institutes of Health
Bethesda, Maryland

John S. Child, MD
Co-Chief, Clinical Cardiology
Department of Medicine
Professor of Medicine
University of California, Los Angeles Medical School
Los Angeles, California

Joseph M. Civetta, MD
Director, Surgical Trauma Intensive
    Care Units
Jackson Memorial Hospital
Professor and Chief
Division of Surgical Critical Care
Department of Surgery
University of Miami School of Medicine
Miami, Florida

David R. Clarke, MD
Chief, Pediatric Cardiothoracic Surgery
The Children's Hospital
Professor of Surgery
University of Colorado
Denver, Colorado

Brian L. Cmolik, MD
Veterans Administration Medical Center/University
  Hospitals
Assistant Professor of Surgery
Case Western Reserve University School
  of Medicine
Cleveland, Ohio

Lawrence H. Cohn, MD
Chief of Cardiac Surgery
Brigham & Women's Hospital
Professor of Surgery
Harvard Medical School
Boston, Massachusetts

Steven D. Colquhoun, MD
Chief, Liver Transplantation
University of California, Davis Medical Center
Assistant Professor of Surgery
University of California, Davis School of Medicine
Sacramento, California

John E. Connolly, MD
Professor of Surgery
University of California, Irvine School of Medicine
Irvine, California

Joseph S. Coselli, MD
Attending Surgeon
The Methodist Hospital
Associate Professor of Surgery
Baylor College of Medicine
Houston, Texas

John L. Cotton, MD
Fellow, Division of Pediatric Cardiology
University of California, Los Angeles School
  of Medicine
Los Angeles, California

James L. Cox, MD
Chief, Division of Cardiothoracic Surgery
Washington University Medical Center/
  Barnes Hospital
Evarts A. Graham Professor of Surgery
Washington University School of Medicine
St. Louis, Missouri

Willard M. Daggett, Jr., MD
Visiting Surgeon
Massachusetts General Hospital
Professor of Surgery
Harvard Medical School
Boston, Massachusetts

Harry J. D'Agostino, Jr., MD
Clinical Instructor
Division of Cardiothoracic Surgery
University of California, Los Angeles School
  of Medicine
Los Angeles, California

Gordon K. Danielson, MD
Consultant in Surgery
Mayo Medical Center
Roberts Professor of Surgery
Mayo Graduate School of Medicine Foundation
Rochester, Minnesota

Robert Duane Davis, MD
Surgical Director of Lung Transplantation
Duke University Medical Center
Assistant Professor of Surgery
Duke University School of Medicine
Durham, North Carolina

Jacob G. Davtyan, MD
Chief Resident, Cardiothoracic Surgery
Emory University School of Medicine
Atlanta, Georgia

Malcolm M. DeCamp, Jr., MD
Associate Thoracic Surgeon, Division
  of Thoracic Surgery
Brigham & Women's Hospital
Assistant Professor of Surgery
Harvard Medical School
Boston, Massachusetts

Marc R. de Leval, MD, FRCS
Consultant Cardiothoracic Surgeon
Great Ormond Street Hospital for Children NHS Trust
Institute of Child Health
London, United Kingdom

Michael del Rio, MD
Clinical Research Fellow in Cardiothoracic Pediatric
  Surgery
Loma Linda University Medical Center
Clinical Fellow
Division of Cardiothoracic Surgery, Department
  of Surgery
Loma Linda University School of Medicine
Loma Linda, California

Tom R. DeMeester, MD
Professor and Chairman
Department of Surgery
University of Southern California School of Medicine
Los Angeles, California

Davis C. Drinkwater, Jr., MD
Director, Pediatric Cardiac Transplant Program
University of California, Los Angeles Medical Center
Associate Professor of Surgery
University of California, Los Angeles School
    of Medicine
Los Angeles, California

Jeffrey L. Duerk, Ph.D.
Director, Physics Research
University Hospitals of Cleveland
Associate Professor, Radiology
    and Biomedical Engineering
Case Western Reserve University School of Medicine
Cleveland, Ohio

André Duranceau, MD
Professor of Surgery
University of Montreal
Division of Thoracic Surgery
Hôtel-Dieu de Montréal
Montreal, Quebec, Canada

Cornelius M. Dyke, MD
Fellow in Cardiothoracic Surgery
Medical College of Virginia/Virginia Commonwealth
    University
Richmond, Virginia

L. Henry Edmunds, Jr., MD
Active Staff, Division
    of Cardiothoracic Surgery
Hospital of the University of Pennsylvania
Julian Johnson Professor
    of Cardiothoracic Surgery
University of Pennsylvania School of Medicine
Philadelphia, Pennsylvania

John A. Elefteriades, MD
Attending Surgeon
Director of Adult Cardiac Procedures
Yale-New Haven Hospital
Professor of Surgery
Yale University Medical School
New Haven, Connecticut

F. Henry Ellis, Jr., MD, PhD
Chief Emeritus, Division
    of Cardiothoracic Surgery
Deaconess Hospital
Clinical Professor of Surgery Emeritus
Harvard Medical School
Boston, Massachusetts

Richard P. Embrey, MD
Director of Pediatric Cardiac Surgery
Medical College of Virginia Hospital
Assistant Professor of Surgery
Medical College of Virginia/Virginia Commonwealth
    University
Richmond, Virginia

M. Arisan Ergin, MD
Attending
Mount Sinai Hospital and Medical
    Center
Professor of Cardiac Surgery
Mount Sinai School of Medicine
New York, New York

L. Penfield Faber, MD
Director, Section General Thoracic Surgery
Presbyterian-St. Lukes Hospital
Professor of Surgery
Rush Medical College
Chicago, Illinois

James I. Fann, MD
Fellow, Cardiothoracic Surgery
    and Vascular Surgery
Stanford University Medical Center
Stanford, California

Mark K. Ferguson, MD
Chief, Section of Thoracic Surgery
University of Chicago Medical Center
Associate Professor of Surgery
University of Chicago Pritzker School
    of Medicine
Chicago, Illinois

T. Bruce Ferguson, Jr., MD
Associate Surgeon
Department of Surgery
Division of Cardiothoracic Surgery
Barnes Hospital
Associate Professor of Surgery
Washington University School of Medicine
St. Louis, Missouri

Peter F. Ferson, MD
University of Pittsburgh Medical Center and
    Veterans Administration Hospital
Professor of Surgery
University of Pittsburgh School of Medicine
Pittsburgh, Pennsylvania

Andrew C. Fiore, MD
Professor of Surgery
Saint Louis University School of Medicine
St. Louis, Missouri

Eric W. Fonkalsrud, MD
Professor of Surgery and
    Chief of Pediatric Surgery
University of California, Los Angeles School of Medicine
Los Angeles, California

Gregory P. Fontana, MD
Attending Cardiothoracic Surgeon
Cedars-Sinai Medical Center
Clinical Assistant Professor of Surgery
University of California, Los Angeles School of Medicine
Los Angeles, California

Kenneth L. Franco, MD
Yale-New Haven Hospital
Associate Professor of Surgery
Yale University School of Medicine
New Haven, Connecticut

Robert W.M. Frater, MD
Montefiore Medical Center
Jack D. Weiler Hospital of the Albert College of Medicine
Professor of Cardiothoracic Surgery
Albert Einstein College of Medicine
Bronx, New York

Timothy J. Gardner, MD
Chief, Division of Cardiothoracic Surgery
Hospital of the University of Pennsylvania
William M. Measey Professor of Surgery
University of Pennsylvania School of Medicine
Philadelphia, Pennsylvania

Richard N. Gates, MD
Congenital Heart Surgery/Transplant Fellow
University of California, Los Angeles Medical Center
University of California, Los Angeles School
    of Medicine
Los Angeles, California

J. William Gaynor, MD
Assistant Professor of Surgery
Duke University School of Medicine
Durham, North Carolina

Alexander S. Geha, MD, MS
Chief, Division of Cardiothoracic Surgery
University Hospitals of Cleveland
The Jay L. Ankeney Professor and Director
Division of Cardiothoracic Surgery
Case Western Reserve University School of Medicine
Cleveland, Ohio

Barbara George, MD
Associate Director, Cardiothoracic Intensive Care Unit
Center for the Health Sciences,
Associate Professor of Pediatrics
University of California, Los Angeles School
    of Medicine
Los Angeles, California

Robert J. Ginsberg, MD
Chief of Thoracic Service
Department of Surgery
Memorial Sloan-Kettering Cancer Center
Professor of Surgery
Cornell University Medical College
New York, New York

Paul Gordon, MD
Thoracic Surgery Resident
Southern Illinois University School of Medicine
Springfield, Illinois

William J. Greeley, MD
Division Chief, Division of Pediatric Cardiac
    Anesthesiology & Critical Care Medicine
Associate Professor of Anesthesiology & Pediatrics
Duke University School of Medicine
Durham, North Carolina

Randall B. Griepp, MD
Chairman, Department of Cardiothoracic Surgery
Mount Sinai Hospital
Professor of Cardiothoracic Surgery
Mount Sinai School of Medicine
New York, New York

Bartley P. Griffith, MD
Chief, Division of Cardiothoracic Surgery
Presbyterian University Hospital
Professor of Surgery
University of Pittsburgh
Pittsburgh, Pennsylvania

Hermes C. Grillo, MD
Visiting Surgeon, General Thoracic Surgery
Massachusetts General Hospital
Professor of Surgery
Harvard Medical School
Boston, Massachusetts

Claude M. Grondin, MD
Head, Division of Cardiothoracic Surgery
St. Luke's Hospital, Cleveland
Clinical Professor of Surgery
Case Western Reserve University School of Medicine
Cleveland, Ohio

Gary Haas, MD
Assistant Professor of Surgery and Pediatrics
University of California, San Francisco School of Medicine
San Francisco, California

Alden W. Hall, BA
Denver, Colorado

Graeme L. Hammond, MD
Attending Surgeon
Yale-New Haven Hospital
Professor of Surgery
Yale University School of Medicine
New Haven, Connecticut

John R. Handy, MD
Director of Lung Transplantation
Assistant Professor of Surgery
Assistant Professor of Clinical Services
Medical University of South Carolina
Charleston, South Carolina

Frank L. Hanley, MD
Chief, Division of Cardiothoracic Surgery
University of California, San Francisco Medical Center
Professor of Surgery
University of California, San Francisco
San Francisco, California

Alden H. Harken, MD
Professor and Chairman, Department of Surgery
University of Colorado
Denver, Colorado

Lynn H. Harrison, Jr., MD
Chief, Section of Cardiothoracic Surgery
University Hospital
Associate Professor of Surgery
Louisiana State University School of Medicine
New Orleans, Louisiana

Stephen R. Hazelrigg, MD
Chairman, Division of Cardiothoracic Surgery
Associate Professor
Southern Illinois University School of Medicine
Springfield, Illinois

Richard F. Heitmiller, MD
Chief, Division of General Thoracic Surgery
Johns Hopkins Hospital
Associate Professor of Surgery
Johns Hopkins University
Baltimore, Maryland

John Hennecken, MD
Director, Cardiac Cath Laboratories
Director Interventional Cardiology
Medical College of Georgia Hospital & Clinics
Augusta Veterans Affairs Medical Center
Associate Professor of Medicine
Medical College of Georgia
Augusta, Georgia

Clement A. Hiebert, MD
Chairman Emeritus
Department of Surgery
Maine Medical Center
Portland, Maine
Clinical Assistant in Surgery
Harvard Medical School
Boston, Massachusetts

Alan D. Hilgenberg, MD
Cardiac Surgeon
Massachusetts General Hospital
Associate Clinical Professor of Surgery
Harvard Medical School
Boston, Massachusetts

Lucius D. Hill, MD
Clinical Professor of Surgery
University of Washington School of Medicine
Seattle, Washington

George T. Hodakowski, MD
Resident in Cardiothoracic Surgery
The Emory University Hospital
Atlanta, Georgia

E. Carmack Holmes, MD
Chairman, Department of Surgery
University of California, Los Angeles Medical Center
Professor
University of California, Los Angeles School
   of Medicine
Los Angeles, California

Thomas M. Hyers, MD
Director, Division of Pulmonology & Pulmonary
   Occupational Medicine
Saint Louis University Health Sciences Center
James and Ethel Miller Professor of Internal Medicine
Saint Louis University School of Medicine
St. Louis, Missouri

Michel N. Ilbawi, MD
Director, Pediatric Cardiac Surgery
Heart Institute for Children
Associate Professor of Surgery
Northwestern University Medical School
Oak Lawn, Illinois

Josephine B. Isabel-Jones, MD
Professor of Pediatrics (Cardiology)
University of California, Los Angeles School of Medicine
Los Angeles, California

Marshall L. Jacobs, MD
Associate Cardiothoracic Surgeon
Children's Hospital of Philadelphia
Associate Professor of Surgery
University of Pennsylvania School of Medicine
Philadelphia, Pennsylvania

Stuart W. Jamieson, MD, FRCS.
Head of Cardiovascular and Thoracic Surgery
University of California, San Diego Medical Center
Professor of Surgery
University of California, San Diego School of Medicine
San Diego, California

Adib D. Jatene, MD
Director, Cardiovascular and Thoracic Surgery
Heart Institute
Professor of Surgery
University of Sao Paulo
Sao Paulo, Brazil

Ellis L. Jones, MD
Emory University Hospital
Professor of Cardiovascular Surgery
Emory University School of Medicine
Atlanta, Georgia

M.J. Jurkiewicz, MD
Attending Surgeon
Emory Affiliated Hospital
Professor of Surgery
Emory University School of Medicine
Atlanta, Georgia

George C. Kaiser, MD
Chief of Cardiothoracic Surgery
Saint Louis University Health Sciences Center
Professor of Surgery
Saint Louis University School of Medicine
St. Louis, Missouri

Larry R. Kaiser, MD
Chief, General Thoracic Surgery
Hospital of the University of Pennsylvania
Associate Professor of Surgery
University of Pennsylvania School of Medicine
Philadelphia, Pennsylvania

Tom R. Karl, MS, MD
Director, Cardiac Surgical Unit
Royal Children's Hospital
Melbourne, Australia

Robert J. Keenan, MD, FRCSC
Director, Lung Transplantation
University of Pittsburgh Medical Center
Assistant Professor of Surgery
University of Pittsburgh School of Medicine
Pittsburgh, Pennsylvania

David P. Kelsen, MD
Chief, Gastrointestinal Oncology Service
Memorial Sloan-Kettering Cancer Center
Professor of Medicine
Cornell University Medical College
New York, New York

Frank H. Kern, MD
Director, Pediatric Cardiac Anesthesia
   and Associate Director
Pediatric Intensive Care Unit
Duke University Medical Center
Associate Professor of Anesthesiology & Pediatrics
Duke University School of Medicine
Durham, North Carolina

Spencer B. King, III, MD
Director Cardiovascular Labs
Emory University Hospital
Professor of Medicine
Emory University School of Medicine
Atlanta, Georgia

Orlando C. Kirton, MD
Assistant Director, Surgical Intensive Care Unit
University of Miami/Jackson Memorial Medical Center
Assistant Professor of Clinical Surgery
University of Miami School of Medicine
Miami, Florida

Gary S. Kopf, MD
Chief, Pediatric Cardiac Surgery
Yale-New Haven Hospital
Professor of Surgery
Yale University School of Medicine
New Haven, Connecticut

Nicholas T. Kouchoukos, MD
Surgeon and Cardiothoracic Surgeon-in-Chief
The Jewish Hospital of St. Louis
John M. Shoenberg Professor of Cardiovascular Surgery
Washington University School of Medicine
St. Louis, Missouri

Jolene M. Kriett, MD
Attending Surgeon
Division of Cardiothoracic Surgery
University of California, San Diego Medical Center
Associate Professor of Surgery
University of California, San Diego School of Medicine
San Diego, California

Janine Krivokapich, MD
Director, UCLA Adult Cardiac Non-Invasive Laboratories
Professor of Medicine
University of California, Los Angeles School of Medicine
Los Angeles, California

Hillel Laks, MD
Professor and Chief, Division of Cardiothoracic Surgery
University of California, Los Angeles School
   of Medicine
Los Angeles, California

John J. Lamberti, MD
Chief of Cardiac Surgery
Children's Hospital—San Diego
Associate Clinical Professor
University of California, San Diego School
   of Medicine
San Diego, California

Rodney J. Landreneau, MD
Head, Section of Thoracic Surgery
University of Pittsburgh Medical Center
Associate Professor
University of Pittsburgh School of Medicine
Pittsburgh, Pennsylvania

Jai H. Lee, MD
Attending Cardiothoracic Surgeon
University Hospitals of Cleveland
Assistant Professor of Surgery
Case Western Reserve University School of Medicine
Cleveland, Ohio

K. Francis Lee, MD
Fellow in Cardiothoracic Surgery
Medical College of Virginia/Virginia Commonwealth
   University
Richmond, Virginia

Toni Lerut, MD
Chairman, Department of Thoracic
   Surgery
Catholic University Hospitals Leuven
Professor in Surgery
Catholic University Leuven
Leuven, Belgium

George V. Letsou, MD
Attending Surgeon
The Methodist Hospital
Associate Professor of Surgery
Baylor College of Medicine
Houston, Texas

James M. Lieberman, MD
Staff Radiologist
University Hospitals of Cleveland
Associate Professor of Radiology
Case Western Reserve University School of Medicine
Cleveland, Ohio

Wayne Lipson, MD
Cardiac Surgery Fellow
Brigham & Women's Hospital
Harvard Medical School
Boston, Massachusetts

Alex G. Little, MD
Chief of Surgery
University Medical Center
Professor and Chairman
University of Nevada School of Medicine
Las Vegas, Nevada

Joseph LoCicero, III, MD
Chief, General Thoracic Surgery
New England Deaconess Hospital
New England Baptist Hospital,
    Cambridge Hospital
Associate Professor
Harvard Medical School
Boston, Massachusetts

Gary K. Lofland, MD
Director, Congenital Heart Center
Columbia/HCA Henrico Doctors'
    Hospital
Clinical Professor of Surgery
Georgetown University School of Medicine
Richmond, Virginia

Donald E. Low, MD, FRCS(C)
Staff
Virginia Mason Clinic
Clinical Instructor
University of Washington School of Medicine
Seattle, Washington

Michael J. Mack, MD
Cardiothoracic Surgeon
Medical City Dallas Hospital
Clinical Assistant Professor of Thoracic Surgery
Southwestern Medical School
University of Texas
Dallas, Texas

Judith A. Mackall, MD
University Hospitals of Cleveland
Assistant Professor of Medicine
Case Western Reserve University School of Medicine
Cleveland, Ohio

James W. Mackenzie, MD
Chief of the Surgical Service
Robert Wood Johnson University Hospital
Professor and Chairman, Department of Surgery
University of Medicine & Dentistry of New Jersey
Robert Wood Johnson Medical School
New Brunswick, New Jersey

Joren C. Madsen, MD, DPhil
Assistant in Surgery
Massachusetts General Hospital
Assistant Professor of Surgery
Harvard Medical School
Boston, Massachusetts

Mitchell J. Magee, MD
Assistant Professor, Division of Cardiothoracic
    Surgery
Southern Illinois University School of Medicine
Springfield, Illinois

James A. Magovern, MD
Associate Attending Staff
Allegheny General Hospital
Associate Professor of Surgery
The Medical College of Pennsylvania
Pittsburgh, Pennsylvania

Richard D. Mainwaring, MD
Division of Cardiac Surgery
Children's Hospital—San Diego
San Diego, California

James B.D. Mark, MD
Head, Division of Thoracic Surgery
Stanford Medical Center
Johnson & Johnson Professor
    of Cardiothoracic Surgery
Stanford University School of Medicine
Stanford, California

Nael Martini, MD
Attending Thoracic Surgeon
Memorial Sloan-Kettering Cancer Center
Professor of Surgery
Cornell University Medical College
New York, New York

Joseph P. Mathew, MD
Attending Anesthesiologist
Yale New Haven Medical Center
Assistant Professor of Anesthesiology
Yale University School of Medicine
New Haven, Connecticut

Douglas J. Mathisen, MD
Visiting Surgeon and Chief,
  General Thoracic Surgery
Massachusetts General Hospital
Associate Professor of Surgery
Harvard Medical School
Boston, Massachusetts

Kenneth L. Mattox, MD
Chief of Staff
Ben Taub General Hospital
Professor of Surgery
Baylor College of Medicine
Houston, Texas

Constantine Mavroudis, MD
Division Head and A.C. Buehler Professor
  of Cardiovascular–Thoracic Surgery
The Children's Memorial Hospital
Professor of Surgery
Northwestern University Medical School
Chicago, Illinois

Lawrence R. McBride, MD
Director of Cardiac and Lung Transplantation
Saint Louis University Health Sciences Center
Professor of Surgery
Saint Louis University School of Medicine
St. Louis, Missouri

Charles J. McCabe, MD
Associate Chief, Emergency Services
Massachusetts General Hospital
Associate Professor of Surgery
Harvard Medical School
Boston, Massachusetts

Patricia M. McCormack, MD
Attending Surgeon, Thoracic Service,
  Department of Surgery
Memorial Sloan-Kettering
  Cancer Center
Associate Professor of Surgery
Cornell University Medical College
New York, New York

Richard Burr McElvein, MD
Chief, Thoracic Surgery
University Hospital and Birmingham Veterans
  Administration Hospital
Professor of Surgery, Retired
University of Alabama at Birmingham
Birmingham, Alabama

Joseph S. McLaughlin, MD
Head, Division of Thoracic & Cardiovascular Surgery
University of Maryland Medical Center
Professor of Surgery
University of Maryland School of Medicine
Baltimore, Maryland

D. Craig Miller, MD
Professor of Cardiovascular Surgery
Stanford University School of Medicine
Stanford, California

D. Douglas Miller, MD
Director, Nuclear Cardiology
Director, Cardiovascular Biology
Saint Louis University Health Sciences Center
Associate Professor of Medicine
Saint Louis University School of Medicine
St. Louis, Missouri

Joseph I. Miller, Jr., MD
Professor, Department of Surgery, Division
  of Cardiothoracic Surgery
The Emory Clinic
Emory University School of Medicine
Atlanta, Georgia

Bruce D. Minsky, MD
Associate Attending Physician
Memorial Sloan-Kettering Cancer Center
Associate Professor of Radiation Oncology
Cornell University Medical College
New York, New York

Ralph S. Mosca, MD
C.S. Mott Children's Hospital
Associate Professor of Surgery
University of Michigan School of Medicine
Ann Arbor, Michigan

Keith S. Naunheim, MD
Professor of Surgery
Saint Louis University School of Medicine
St. Louis, Missouri

Scott H. Norwood, MD
Director, Trauma Service
East Texas Medical Center
Tyler, Texas

William I. Norwood
Director, Division of Surgery
The Aldo Castañeda Institute
Clinique de Genolier
Genolier, Switzerland

Mark F. O'Brien, FRCS, FRACS
Cardiac Surgeon in Charge
Department of Cardiac Surgery
The Prince Charles Hospital
Brisbane, Australia

James A. O'Neil, Jr., MD
Surgeon-in-Chief
The Children's Hospital of Philadelphia
C. Everett Koop Professor of Pediatric Surgery
University of Pennsylvania School of Medicine
Philadelphia, Pennsylvania

Mark B. Orringer, MD
Professor and Head, Section of Thoracic Surgery
University of Michigan Medical Center
Ann Arbor, Michigan

Walter E. Pae, Jr., MD
Director of Cardiac Transplantation, Division
 of Cardiothoracic Surgery
University Hospital, The Milton S. Hershey
 Medical Center
Professor of Surgery
The Pennsylvania State University College
 of Medicine
Hershey, Pennsylvania

K. Michael Pagliero, MB, BS, FRCS
Consultant Thoracic Surgeon
Woodmill Hospital
Devon, United Kingdom

Peter C. Pairolero, MD
Chair, Department of Surgery
Mayo Medical Center
Professor of Surgery
Mayo Graduate School of Medicine
Rochester, Minnesota

Christian E. Paletta, MD, FACS
Associate Professor of Surgery
Division of Plastic and Reconstructive Surgery
Saint Louis University Health Sciences Center
Associate Professor of Surgery
Saint Louis University School of Medicine
St. Louis, Missouri

Harvey I. Pass, MD
Head, Thoracic Oncology Section
Senior Investigator, Surgery Branch
National Cancer Institute
National Institutes of Health
Bethesda, Maryland

G.A. Patterson, MD
Professor of Surgery
Washington University School of Medicine
St. Louis, Missouri

Jeffrey M. Pearl, MD
Chief Resident Cardiothoracic Surgery
University of California, Los Angeles School of Medicine
Los Angeles, California

Carlos A. Pellegrini, MD
Chairman, Department of Surgery
University of Washington Medical Center
Professor of Surgery
University School of Medicine
Seattle, Washington

D. Glenn Pennington, MD
Howard Holt Bradshaw Professor of Surgery
 and Chairman
Department of Cardiothoracic Surgery
Bowman Gray School of Medicine of Wake Forest
 University
Winston-Salem, North Carolina

Lester C. Permut, MD
Attending Surgeon
University of California, Los Angeles Medical Center
Assistant Professor of Surgery
University of California, Los Angeles School of Medicine
Los Angeles, California

Richard M. Peters, MD
Professor Emeritus Surgery
University of California at San Diego
Menlo Park, California

William S. Pierce, MD
Chief, Division of Cardiothoracic Surgery
University Hospital, The Pennsylvania State University
Professor, Cardiovascular & Thoracic Surgery
The Pennsylvania State University College of Medicine
Hershey, Pennsylvania

Marvin Pomerantz, MD
Professor of Surgery
Chief, Section of General Thoracic Surgery
University of Colorado
Denver, Colorado

Thomas W. Prendergast, MD
Fellow, Congenital Cardiothoracic Surgery
Children's Hospital of Los Angeles
University of California, Los Angeles School of Medicine
Los Angeles, California

Francisco J. Puga, MD
Chair, Division of Thoracic and Cardiovascular Surgery
Head, Section of Cardiovascular Surgery
Mayo Clinic
Professor of Surgery
Mayo Graduate School of Medicine
Rochester, Minnesota

Jan M. Quaegebeur, MD
Director of Pediatric Cardiac Surgery
Columbia Presbyterian Medical Center
Associate Professor of Surgery
Columbia University
New York, New York

Marlene Rabinovitch, MD
Staff Cardiologist, Department of Cardiology
Director, Cardiovascular Research
The Hospital For Sick Children
Professor of Pediatrics, Pathology and Medicine
University of Toronto
Toronto, Ontario, Canada

Vadiyala Mohan Reddy, MD
Fellow Pediatric Cardiac Surgery
University of California, San Francisco
    Medical Center
San Francisco, California

Carolyn E. Reed, MD
Associate Professor of Surgery
Medical University of South Carolina
Charleston, South Carolina

Michael S. Remetz, MD
Director, Goodyer Cardiology FIRM
Yale-New Haven Medical Center
Associate Professor of Medicine
Yale University School of Medicine
New Haven, Connecticut

Thomas W. Rice, MD
Head of the Section
    of General Thoracic Surgery
Department of Thoracic and Cardiovascular Surgery
The Cleveland Clinic Foundation
Cleveland, Ohio

David J. Riley, MD
Attending Staff
Robert Wood Johnson University Hospital
Professor of Medicine
University of Medicine & Dentistry of New Jersey
Robert Wood Johnson Medical School
New Brunswick, New Jersey

Norman W. Rizk, MD
Director of Clinical Services
Division of Pulmonary and Critical
    Care Medicine
Stanford University Hospital
Associate Professor of Medicine
Stanford University School of Medicine
Stanford, California

Eliot R. Rosenkranz, MD
Chief, Cardiothoracic Surgery
Children's Hospital of Buffalo
Associate Professor of Surgery
State University of New York at Buffalo
Buffalo, New York

Jack A. Roth, MD
Professor and Chairman
Department of Thoracic and Cardiovascular Surgery
University of Texas M.D. Anderson Cancer Center
Professor of Tumor Biology
University of Texas School of Medicine
Houston, Texas

Ehud Rudis, MD
Visiting Assistant Professor
University of California, Los Angeles School of Medicine
Los Angeles, California

Liisa A. Russell, MD
Associate Clinical Professor of Pathology
University of California, Davis School of Medicine
Sacramento, California

David H. Sachs, MD
Director, Transplantation Biology Research Center
Massachusetts General Hospital
Paul S. Russell/Warner-Lambert Professor
    of Surgery
Harvard Medical School
Boston, Massachusetts

Robert M. Sade, MD
Attending Surgeon
Medical University of South Carolina Medical Center
Professor of Surgery
Medical University of South Carolina
Charleston, South Carolina

Susheela Sangwan, MD
Assistant Clinical Professor of Anesthesiology
University of California, Los Angeles School
    of Medicine
Los Angeles, California

John S. Sapirstein, MD
Research Fellow
Division of Cardiothoracic Surgery
The Pennsylvania State University
Hershey, Pennsylvania

David S. Schrump, MD
University of Texas M.D. Anderson Cancer Center
Assistant Professor of Surgery
Department of Thoracic and Cardiovascular
    Surgery
University of Texas School of Medicine
Houston, Texas

Stewart M. Scott, MD
Chief, Surgical Service
Veterans Administration Medical Center
Consulting Professor of Surgery
Duke University Medical Center
Asheville, North Carolina

Thomas W. Shields, MD
Attending Surgeon Emeritus
Northwestern Memorial Hospital
Professor Emeritus of Surgery
Northwestern University
    Medical School
Chicago, Illinois

Dominique Shum-Tim, MD, MDCM, MSC, FRCS(C)
Chief Resident
Cardiovascular and Thoracic Surgery
McGill University
Montreal Children's Hospital
Montreal, Quebec, Canada

Mark L. Silen, MD
Attending Surgeon
Cardinal Glennon Children's Hospital
Assistant Professor
Saint Louis University School of Medicine
St. Louis, Missouri

Mika Sinanan, MD
Attending Surgeon and Co-Director
IFDR Endoscopy Surgery Center
Department of Surgery
University of Washington Medical Center
Assistant Professor
University of Washington
Seattle, Washington

David B. Skinner, MD
Attending Surgeon
The New York Hospital
Cornell Medical Center
Professor of Surgery
Cornell University Medical College
New York, New York

Philip C. Smith, MD, PhD
Attending, Pediatric Cardiovascular
  Surgery
The Heart Institute for Children
Assistant Professor
University of Illinois at Chicago
Oak Lawn, Illinois

Michael Sobel, MD
Chief, Vascular Surgery
H.H. McGuire Veterans Medical Center
Associate Professor of Surgery
Medical College of Virginia/Virginia Commonwealth
  University
Richmond, Virginia

Jonathan Somers, MD
Attending Cardiovascular Surgeon
Rush–Presbyterian–St. Luke's Medical Center
Assistant Professor of Surgery
Rush Medical College
Chicago, Illinois

Henry M. Spotnitz, MD
Attending Cardiothoracic Surgeon
Columbia–Presbyterian Medical Center
George H. Humphreys, II, Professor
  of Surgery
Columbia University
New York, New York

William D. Spotnitz, MD
Director TCV Postoperative Unit
University of Virginia Health Sciences Center
Professor of Surgery
University of Virginia
Charlottesville, Virginia

Thomas L. Spray, MD
Division Chief, Cardiothoracic Surgery
The Children's Hospital of Philadelphia
Professor of Surgery
University of Pennsylvania School of Medicine
Philadelphia, Pennsylvania

Jaroslav Stark, MD, FRCS
Consultant Cardiothoracic Surgeon
Great Ormond Street Hospital for Children
  NHS Trust
London, United Kingdom

Vaughn A. Starnes, MD
Director, Cardiopulmonary Transplantation
University of California, Los Angeles Medical Center
Professor of Surgery, Department of Surgery
University of California, Los Angeles School of Medicine
Los Angeles, California

David J. Sugarbaker, MD
Chief, Division of Thoracic Surgery
Brigham & Women's Hospital
Associate Professor of Medicine
Harvard Medical School
Boston, Massachusetts

R. Sudhir Sundaresan, MD
Assistant Professor of Surgery
Washington University School of Medicine
St. Louis, Missouri

Julie A. Swain, MD
Chief, Cardiovascular Surgery
Professor of Surgery
University of Nevada School of Medicine
Las Vegas, Nevada

Scott J. Swanson, MD
Associate Thoracic Surgeon
Brigham & Women's Hospital
Instructor of Surgery
Harvard Medical School
Boston, Massachusetts

Timothy Takaro, MD
Formerly Chief of Staff
Veterans Administration Medical Center
Formerly Clinical Professor of Surgery
Duke University School of Medicine
Asheville, North Carolina

Christo I. Tchervenkov, MD, FRCSC, FACS
Director, Cardiovascular Surgery
The Montreal Children's Hospital
Associate Professor of Surgery
McGill University
Montreal, Quebec, Canada

Marc D. Thames, MD
Chief, Division of Cardiology
University Hospitals of Cleveland
Joseph T. Wearn University Professor in Medicine
Case Western Reserve University School of Medicine
Cleveland, Ohio

Robert J. Touloukian, MD
Chief, Pediatric Surgery
Children's Hospital of Yale-New Haven
Professor of Surgery and Pediatrics
Yale University School of Medicine
New Haven, Connecticut

Thomas F. Tracy, Jr., MD
Attending Surgeon
Cardinal Glennon Children's Hospital
Associate Professor
Saint Louis University School of Medicine
St. Louis, Missouri

George A. Trusler, MD
Professor Emeritus, Department of Surgery
University of Toronto
Senior Surgeon
Hospital For Sick Children
Toronto, Ontario, Canada

Ross M. Ungerleider, MD
Chief, Pediatric Cardiac Surgery
Duke University Medical Center
Professor of Surgery
Duke University
Durham, North Carolina

Harold C. Urschel, Jr., MD
Professor Thoracic and Cardiovascular Surgery
Baylor College of Medicine
Dallas, Texas

Matthew Wall, Jr., MD
Deputy Chief of Surgery
Ben Taub General Hospital
Assistant Professor of Surgery
Baylor College of Medicine
Houston, Texas

Ralph L. Warren, MD
Clinical Director, Trauma Service
Department of Surgery
Massachusetts General Hospital
Assistant Surgeon
Harvard Medical School
Boston, Massachusetts

Paul F. Waters, MD
Director, General Thoracic Surgery
Director, Lung Transplant Program
University of California, Los Angeles Medical Center
Professor of Surgery
University of California, Los Angeles School of Medicine
Los Angeles, California

Thomas J. Watson, MD
Clinical Fellow, Cardiothoracic Surgery
University of California, Los Angeles School of Medicine
Los Angeles, California

Watts R. Webb, MD
Chief, Cardiac Surgery
New Orleans Veterans Administration Hospital
Professor of Clinical Surgery
Louisiana State University School of Medicine
New Orleans, Louisiana

Thomas R. Weber, MD
Director, Division of Pediatric Surgery
Cardinal Glennon Children's Hospital
Professor of Surgery
Saint Louis University School of Medicine
St. Louis, Missouri

Andrew S. Wechsler, MD
Chairman, Department of Surgery
Head, Division of Thoracic Surgery
Medical College of Virginia Hospitals
Stuart McGuire Professor of Surgery and Physiology
Medical College of Virginia/Virginia
    Commonwealth University
Richmond, Virginia

Debra E. Weese-Mayer, MD
Associate Professor of Pediatrics
Rush Medical College
Chicago, Illinois

Benson R. Wilcox, MD
Professor of Surgery and Chief
Division of Cardiothoracic Surgery
University of North Carolina School of Medicine
Chapel Hill, North Carolina

Roberta G. Williams, MD
Chief, Pediatric Cardiology
University of California, Los Angeles Medical Center
Professor of Pediatrics
University of California, Los Angeles School of Medicine
Los Angeles, California

Vallee L. Willman, MD
C. Rollins Hanlon Professor and Chairman, Department
    of Surgery
Saint Louis University School of Medicine
St. Louis, Missouri

Roger S. Wilson, MD
Chairman
Department of Anesthesiology and Critical
  Care Medicine
Memorial Sloan-Kettering Cancer Center
Professor of Anesthesiology
Cornell University Medical College
New York, New York

Michael K. Wolverson, MD
Attending Radiologist
Saint Louis University Health Sciences Center
Professor of Radiology
Saint Louis University School of Medicine
St. Louis, Missouri

James L. Zellner, MD
Resident in Cardiothoracic Surgery
Medical University of South Carolina
Charleston, South Carolina

Preface

The foundation for the sixth edition of *Glenn's Thoracic and Cardiovascular Surgery* was laid nearly 45 years ago by Drs. Gustav E. Lindskog, William H. Carmalt Professor of Surgery, and Averill A. Liebow, Professor of Pathology, both at the Yale University School of Medicine. They wrote a textbook entitled *Thoracic Surgery and Related Pathology* and included three contributing authors: Drs. Ralph D. Alley, William E. Bloomer, and Frederick C. Warring, Jr. Cardiovascular surgery was then in its infancy, and this subject was a very small part of the text.

Because of how well the first edition was received, a second edition was published in 1962. By that time, the fields of cardiac and vascular surgery had vastly expanded, and Dr. William W. Glenn, Professor of Surgery at Yale University School of Medicine, who had served as a consultant on the cardiovascular material in the first edition, was invited to be a coeditor and to write a section on cardiovascular surgery. The title of the book was expanded to *Thoracic and Cardiovascular Surgery with Related Pathology.* The three contributors to the first edition also participated in the second edition of the book.

In response to the favorable reception of the second edition of the book and the advances that had been made, especially in the surgical treatment of general thoracic and cardiovascular disease, a third edition was undertaken and published in 1975. The senior authors, who wrote portions of the text, were assisted by 11 contributing authors.

When the fourth edition was contemplated, it was evident that a simple revision would not suffice. The need was for a completely new book that involved a number of experts in the cardiothoracic field representing the basic sciences and clinical disciplines. Those of us who were at Yale University at that time joined Dr. Glenn as coeditors. The title was shortened to *Thoracic and Cardiovascular Surgery,* the text was completely rewritten, and there were 114 chapters contributed by 157 authors, more than 97% of whom were first-time contributors to the book. Broad-based

expertise was emphasized. Approximately one third of the authors were from disciplines other than surgery.

The fifth edition of the book, now entitled *Glenn's Thoracic and Cardiovascular Surgery,* represented another complete revision. The general format of the three main divisions of the book was retained. This edition too was well accepted by the cardiothoracic community. In recent years, many requests have been made for a new edition, which brings us to the sixth edition.

Although this sixth edition of *Glenn's Thoracic and Cardiovascular Surgery* evolved from five previous editions of a venerable textbook on cardiovascular surgery, it is truly a new book in that most of the 140 chapters are either new (13 chapters) to this edition, reflecting the many exciting developments in the field in the last five years, or have been rewritten or drastically revised.

We welcome 110 new authors to this edition. They represent a whole new generation of cardiothoracic surgeons. We also welcome back more than 100 of the same authors who contributed to the fifth edition.

All of the revised chapters have been updated, and many have a new organization of material and expanded content, with new illustrations and current and comprehensive references. Results, statistics, and recommendations have all been derived for the most current information.

The chapter authors were not required to adhere to a totally uniform format, because it was thought that full freedom of expression would be a refreshing change in a textbook. Only complete coverage and strict adherence to an assigned subject were requirements. They all complied with these requirements admirably, which has provided continuity of thought throughout each section of the book with minimal duplication or overlap of material. Where applicable, cross references are made in certain chapters to other chapter(s) for details of diagnosis, therapy, and other information.

Each section and most chapters in this new edition present general information on a subject beginning with the historical background, surgical anatomy and pathophysiology, diagnosis with particular emphasis on the newest technical aids, perioperative care, anesthesia, and supportive medical therapy. Following the general considerations, specific diseases or deformities susceptible to surgical treatment are described along with diagnosis, operations, management of complications, and the results of operations. The sixth edition of this book is meant to be encyclopedic, and we therefore have tried to include all the information that is currently known about a subject or field. In addition, the authors have provided the reader with the evidence for the best methods of therapy presently known and the ones they currently use.

The book is divided into three major sections. In Section I, General Thoracic Surgery, topics include the technological advances in the use of video-assisted thoracoscopy and laparoscopy for diagnostic and therapeutic pulmonary procedures and for surgery of the esophagus and diaphragm. The molecular biology and immunology of thoracic neoplasms (lung and esophagus) are now included in this section. Several chapters from the previous edition have been incorporated in other chapters in this edition. For example, the chapter on vena caval syndrome was combined with the one on the mediastinum; the chapter on tracheotomy is now part of the one on reconstruction of the trachea; and the chapter on esophageal perforation has been combined with the one on chemical burns, foreign bodies, and bleeding. The chapters describing the three methods most commonly used for prevention of reflux esophagitis have been retained in this edition, and once again have been written by the experts in or developers of these procedures. In addition, other techniques for managing esophageal reflux are included in the chapter on the surgical treatment of hiatal hernia and gastroesophageal reflux.

In Section II, Surgery for Congenital Heart Disease, major advances in the care of congenital heart disease are described, Heart–lung transplantation in children is included, as are cardiac-assist devices in infants. Discussions of the use of nitric oxide gas in anesthesia and adenosine for the diagnosis and management of arrhythmias make this book current and comprehensive.

In Section III, Surgery for Acquired Heart Disease, the major developments in adult cardiac surgery are described. Angioplasty is compared with coronary bypass grafting for the treatment of coronary artery disease. The reader is given a better understanding of ventricular support, cardiopulmonary bypass, and other aspects of the management of adult heart disease. New chapters in this section are those on the clinical/biologic interface of the basic science of the myocardial muscle and the coronary circulation; transplantation immunology; mitral valve repair; homografts and autografts of cardiac valves; and indications for percutaneous (nonsurgical) coronary revascularization. The increasing importance of echocardiography is described, as is the use

of intraoperative transesophageal echocardiography in both adults and infants.

New authors were selected on the basis of their contributions to the field of cardiothoracic surgery and their active involvement in operative surgery related to the subjects that they write about. In many instances, contributors who originally developed certain surgical operations or techniques and those who have popularized certain procedures continue their contributions in this edition. Thus, they know both the theoretical aspects of cardiothoracic surgery and what is practical in patients.

Indexing is a critical feature of a book such as this. Without an exhaustive index, vital information may not be readily apparent to the user of the book because it is buried within the text. We are very proud of the excellent and extensive index that has been compiled for this edition of the book.

The sixth edition of *Glenn's Thoracic and Cardiovascular Surgery* is truly international in scope in that it represents more than 100 medical schools worldwide. Therefore, it should serve as a reference source for practicing cardiothoracic surgeons and as a textbook and reference source for fellows in cardiothoracic surgery, particularly in preparation for the qualifying and certifying examinations of the American Board of Thoracic Surgery, and for students everywhere with an interest in cardiothoracic surgery. It should serve as the reference text of choice well into the twenty-first century.

A multiauthored textbook of this depth and breadth is not an easy undertaking for anyone involved in bringing it to fruition. Writing chapters for medical texts is a labor of love. Secretarial, medical illustration, and editorial costs must be borne in part or wholly by the departments or divisions of the institutions to which the participants belong. Authors have many other commitments for their time. They may be busy reporting the results of their work at national or international meetings, which require abstracts and manuscripts. Many others, because of their particular expertise, may be involved in the generation of material for several books at the same time. Acute and chronic overcommitment is characteristic of the capable surgeon. Thus, deadlines pass, chapters are not in, and months go by. As one of my senior colleagues once said, "There has been a certain amount of slippage in our editorial schedule." What he really meant was that the book was six months behind schedule. In spite of delays, the work eventually gets done. Overburdened authors come through and an excellent book such as this sixth edition of *Glenn's Thoracic and Cardiovascular Surgery* is produced. This book is the most comprehensive and complete work on cardiovascular surgery that I have ever seen.

We are grateful to many authors for their previous contributions and for helping to establish this textbook as a standard in the field. Many senior authors in previous editions, who have now retired, preferred not to continue as contributors in the sixth edition of the book. We are sad to report that two authors, Mr. Ian K. R. McMillan and Dr. E. Stanley Crawford, died in the years between the fifth and sixth editions.

We the editors are greatly indebted to all the contributors to this work for their participation and cooperation. It has been a most pleasant and stimulating experience to be associated with them in the vast effort to bring this sixth edition to publication.

I am particularly grateful to my coeditors, Drs. Keith S. Naunheim, Alexander S. Geha, Graeme L. Hammond, and Hillel Laks, and to their associates. Dr. Jai Lee has helped Dr. Geha with the work in Cleveland and has also contributed a chapter. Dr. Lester Permut has done yeoman service in developing Section II and helping to edit manuscripts and make suggestions for revisions and modifications.

I would also like to thank immensely those who have provided such excellent editorial assistance to us: My secretary Jean Finn, Delores Adams in Cleveland, Bambi Wojiechowski in Los Angeles, and Joan Batza in New Haven.

We would also like to acknowledge the fine photographic service and art work carried out in the divisions of medical illustrations from the many different universities from which contributors submitted original material for publication. We give special thanks to J. Anthony Stubblefield for his excellent medical illustrations prepared in the Department of Medical Illustrations at St. Louis University Health Sciences Center.

We greatly appreciate the help of Edward H. Wickland, Jr., Vice President and Publisher, and Kathleen McCullough, Managing Editor, Development, at Appleton & Lange.

We again salute Dr. William W. Glenn for his friendship, for his many contributions to this work, and for allowing us to continue this tradition in cardiothoracic education.

Finally, I want to again express my appreciation for the enormous effort put forth by the many people who contributed to this text. I am certain that the final product will be worthy of their trust in all of us who participated in the project.

Arthur E. Baue
with
Alexander S. Geha
Graeme L. Hammond
Hillel Laks
Keith S. Naunheim

SIXTH EDITION
VOLUME II

GLENN'S
THORACIC AND
CARDIOVASCULAR
SURGERY

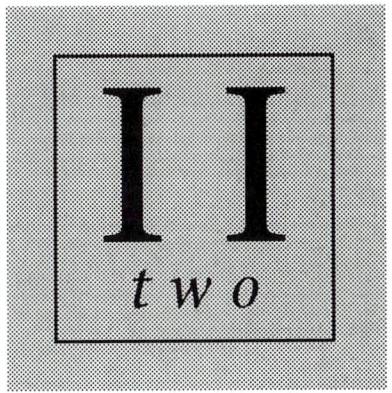

II
two

SURGERY FOR CONGENITAL
HEART DISEASE

CHAPTER

56

Normal and Abnormal Development of the Heart

Robert H. Anderson

The greater part of the controversy surrounding the nomenclature and description of cardiac malformations is a result of disagreements regarding concepts of modes of development that are difficult to substantiate. For cardiac surgeons, the observed anatomy must be paramount, and embryologic considerations should be subordinate to a detailed knowledge of the anatomy.[1] Others correctly point out that embryology in its own right is highly significant,[2] but this fact does not justify anatomic classifications based on embryologic theories. Concepts of embryology can facilitate the understanding of anatomy, particularly concerning the disposition of the vital but regrettably invisible atrioventricular (A-V) conduction tissues. In this chapter, the anatomy of congenitally malformed hearts will be described in terms of cardiac development. Many of the concepts are recognized as being simplistic. Some may prove to be inaccurate in the light of future detailed embryologic studies.[2]

BASIC PRINCIPLES

Knowledge of the early events that lead to the formation of the primary heart tube remains imprecise. Even the concept of a five-chambered heart tube existing at the start of recognizable chamber development has been questioned by experimental work in the developing chick heart.[3] Nonetheless, the five-chambered heart tube is so widely recognized, and proves such a useful platform for comprehension of subsequent development, that it will be taken as our starting point. In this tube (Fig. 56–1), there is evidence of bilateral symmetry at the venous and arterial poles. At the venous end, the chamber termed the *venous sinus* receives a sinus horn on each side, which, in turn, drains umbilical, vitelline,

and cardinal veins from placenta, yolk sac, and the embryo, respectively. At the arterial pole, the arterial chamber gives rise to the series of aortic arches that encircle the pharynx to drain into the descending aorta. Between these two chambers at the extremities of the cardiac tube are the three central chambers. The most cephalic, receiving the venous sinus, is the primordium of the atrial chambers. The next two chambers form the basis of the right and left ventricles. Different investigators have given these chambers many different names. For our purpose, to provide an understanding of definitive anatomy, the chambers will be termed the *atrium*, the *inlet component*, and the *outlet component* of the ventricular loop, respectively (Fig. 56–1). The junctions of these chambers are of utmost significance, since in lower animals there is evidence that the junctional myocardium is histologically specialized as the conduction tissues.[4] Junctional tissues in the human heart, however, can be identified with certainty only at the junction of the inlet and outlet components of the ventricular loop (Fig. 56–2).[5] As we will see, however, this ring is particularly important in explaining the morphogenesis of several malformations.

ATRIAL DEVELOPMENT AND MALDEVELOPMENT

Initially, bilaterally symmetrical systemic veins drain to the atrium. At the same time, a system of pulmonary veins is growing within the developing lung buds, which are formed by an outsprout from the foregut. Formation of the morphologically right and left atriums demands lateralization of the systemic venous return. This occurs by development of anastomotic channels in the head of the embryo, regression

955

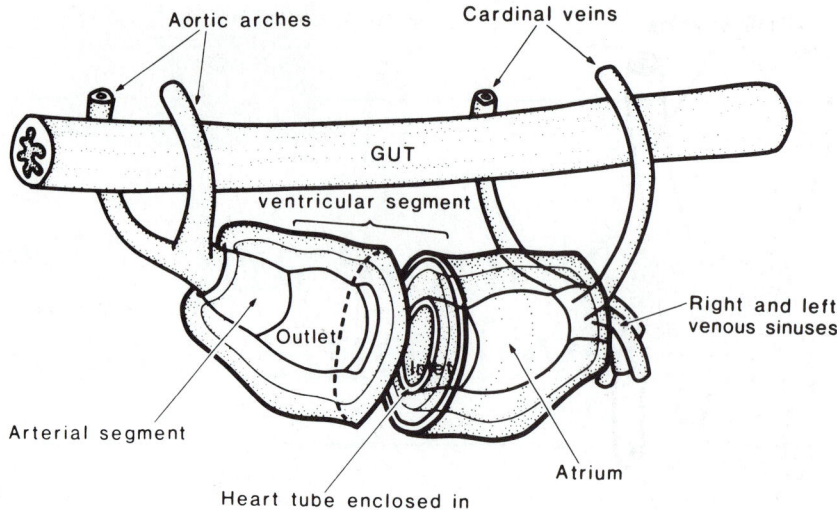

Figure 56–1. The shape of the initial heart tube showing evidence of bilateral symmetry at its arterial and venous poles. Simple descriptive terms are used to describe the different components of this tube. *(Modified from Anderson RH, Becker AE: Cardiac Anatomy—An Integrated Text and Colour Atlas, 1980. Courtesy of Gower Medical Publishing, London.)*

of the vitelline veins, and formation of the venous duct (*ductus venosus*), which channels umbilical venous blood to the right sinus horn (Fig. 56–3). As a consequence, the left sinus horn regresses, becoming the coronary sinus, and the venous sinus effectively comes to enter only the right side of the atrium. The primary pulmonary vein can then grow from the left posterior aspect of the atrium toward the growing lung buds (Fig. 56–4). Studies[6] suggest that this primary pulmonary vein develops concomitantly with the splanchnic venous plexus rather than growing actively from the heart as was previously believed. With normal development, the primary pulmonary vein fuses with the intrapulmonary veins. These lose their initial connection to the foregut splanchic veins, and the intrapulmonary veins are then cannibalized by the atrium to form the smooth-walled venous component of the morphologically left atrium (Fig. 56–4). During this development, pouches have grown forward from the atrium (the atrial appendages), to either side of the arterial pedicle, which has been placed anterior to the atrium as a consequence of ventricular looping. The stage is now set for atrial septation. Initially, a septum (the primary septum) grows down from the atrial roof between the left margin of the sinuatrial junction and the primary pulmonary vein (Fig. 56–5A). At the same time, the atrioventricular

canal is divided by formation and fusion of the atrioventricular cushions. The primary septum grows down to fuse with the upper edge of the cushions, but as it does so, its upper margin breaks down to form the secondary foramen (Fig. 56–5B). The primary foramen, the space between the leading edge of the primary septum and the cushions, is obliterated if atrial septation occurs normally. The atrial septal morphology is then prepared for subsequent postnatal closure of the interatrial communication by the atrial roof itself infolding to form the so-called secondary septum (Fig. 56–5C). These various changes convert the interatrial communication into the oval foramen. The superior rim is then the infolded interatrial fold, while the floor is the primary atrial septum. Initially, the sinuatrial junction is guarded by well-formed valves, but these regress during embryonic life, persisting as the eustachian valve (related to the inferior caval vein) and the thebesian valve (related to the coronary sinus).

Atrial anomalies can readily be explained on the basis of these embryologic events. Formation of discrete morphologically right and left atriums demands lateralization of systemic venous return (Fig. 56–3). Lateralization to the right produces normal atrial position (*situs solitus*) (Fig. 56–6A). Opposite lateralization would produce a left-sided

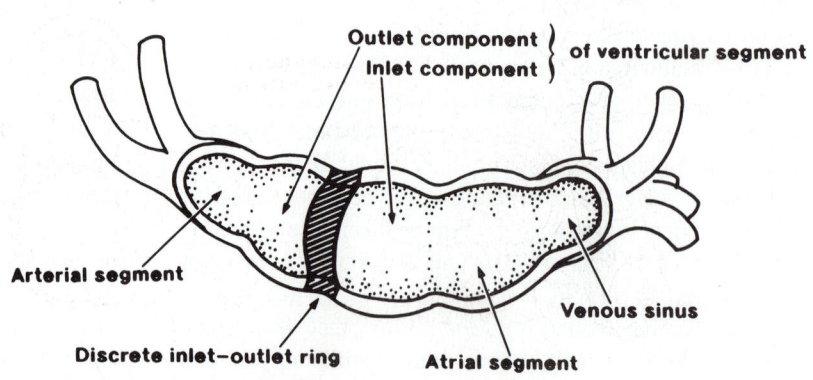

Figure 56–2. The concept of a five-segment heart tube is simplistic, but a useful starting point for a description of developmental events. It was previously thought that histologically discrete junctions existed between each of the segments. Recent evidence suggests[5] that the only discrete ring is at the junction of inlet and outlet components of the ventricular loop.

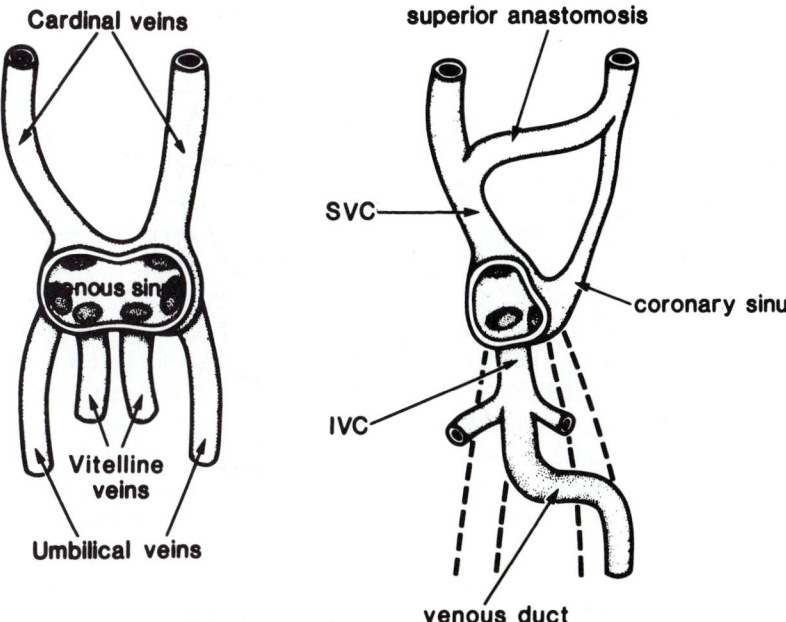

Figure 56–3. The processes of lateralization of systemic venous return, which are necessary for formation of the right and left atrial chambers. *(Modified from Anderson RH, Becker AE: Cardiac Anatomy—An Integrated Text and Colour Atlas, 1980. Courtesy of Gower Medical Publishing, London.)*

morphologically right atrium, that is, a mirror-image arrangement (*situs inversus*; see Fig. 56–6B). Failure of lateralization can also occur in both the heart and the thoracoabdominal organs. This failure results in the so-called splenic syndromes or visceral heterotaxy. The essence of these syndromes is symmetric development, which can take one of two forms: right or left isomerism. In terms of the atriums, right isomerism is associated with bilateral budding of morphologically right appendages, each with a terminal crest, and with retention of a midline venous sinus receiving bilaterally symmetrical systemic veins. The primary pulmonary vein, being a left-sided structure, is squeezed out so that totally anomalous pulmonary venous connection is the rule (Fig. 56–6C). Since the spleen is also a left-sided

structure, right isomerism is almost always associated with asplenia. Left isomerism involves formation of two morphologically left appendages, each lacking a terminal crest, but also involves formation of a symmetrical pulmonary venous atrial component, which sandwiches the venous sinus on each side between the pulmonary veins and the appendage (Fig. 56–6D). This venous component can either drain directly to the atrial roof, as in unroofed coronary sinus, or drain as a persistent caval vein via the coronary sinus. Left isomerism is usually associated with polysplenia.

The simplest and most common anomalous systemic venous connection is persistence of the left sinus horn as a left superior caval vein draining to the coronary sinus. Oc-

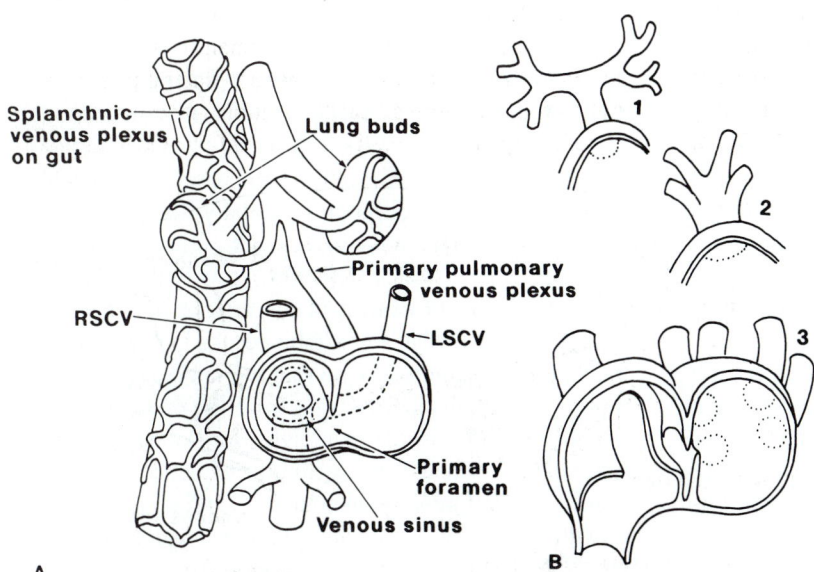

Figure 56–4. A, B. The primary pulmonary vein is developed at the same time as the splanchnic venous plexus related to the foregut.[6] These veins probably form at the same time, and establish concomitantly a connection with the developing left atrium (**A**). Conventional wisdom then holds that the connection with the splanchnic plexus breaks down (**B1**) and the left atrium "cannibalizes" the pulmonary veins (**B2, B3**).

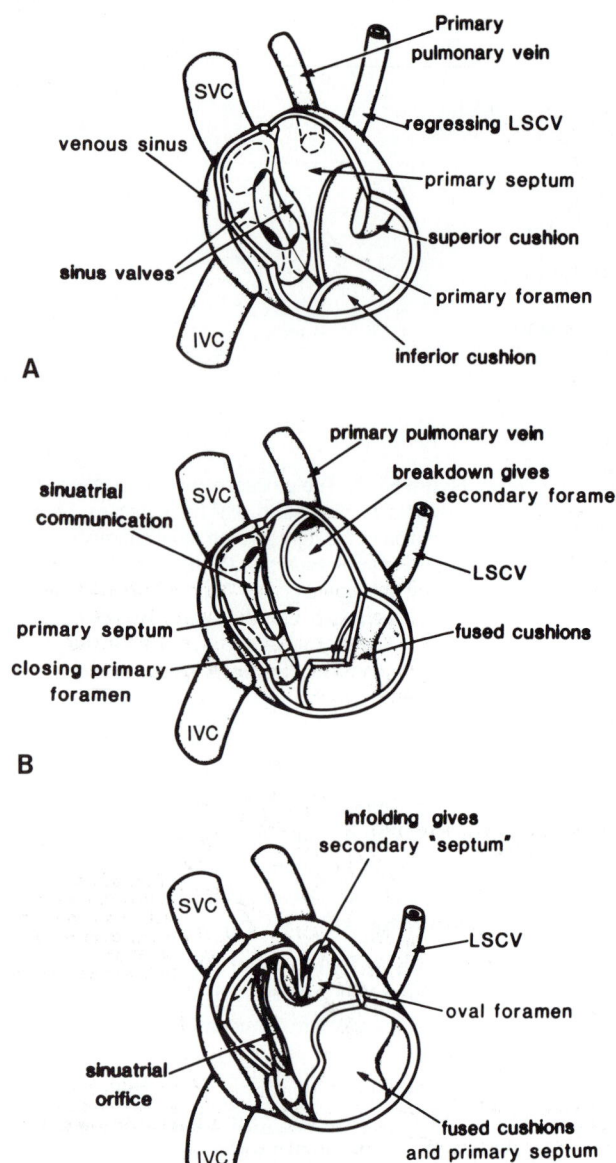

Figure 56–5. A–C. The steps involved in atrial septation. *(Modified from Anderson RH, Becker AE: Cardiac Anatomy—An Integrated Text and Colour Atlas, 1980. Courtesy of Gower Medical Publishing, London.)*

casionally, the walls between the left vein and the left atrium are absorbed so that the vein drains directly to the roof of the atrium between the appendage and the upper left pulmonary vein, while the orifice of the coronary sinus functions as an atrial septal defect. This arrangement is known as an *unroofed coronary sinus.*

Anomalous pulmonary venous connection is readily explained in all its variations by failure of formation of the veins connecting the intrapulmonary venous components with the developing left atrium.[6] The intrapulmonary veins drain to a suitable systemic vein, to which they were initially connected, while the morphologically left atrium lacks its pulmonary venous component.

Either of the atrial chambers can be divided (cor triatriatum). The morphologically right atrium is divided by persistence of the valves of the sinuatrial junction. The morphologically left atrium is divided by a membrane formed between its pulmonary venous and atrial components, probably as a consequence of entrapment of the primary pulmonary venous plexus during early development.[7]

Juxtaposition of the atrial appendages is a consequence of budding out of the appendages to the same rather than to either side of the arterial pedicle. It can occur to the right or to the left side.

Although various types of atrial septal defect are described, only defects at the site of the oval fossa (secundum defects) are true defects of the atrial septum. They occur because of deficiency of the primary septum, which can be unduly short or perforate. So-called ostium primum defects are caused by failure of the primary septum to fuse with the endocardial cushions. They involve a major maldevelopment of the A-V junction and are, in reality, an A-V septal defect. Sinus venosus defects, in my experience, have invariably been associated with partially anomalous pulmonary venous connection. The interatrial communication is produced above the rim of the oval fossa, in relation to either the superior or the inferior caval veins. It is a consequence of cannibalization of the interatrial fold by the ingrowing right pulmonary veins. The final type of atrial septal defect is associated with unroofed coronary sinus. It is the orifice of the left sinus horn.

The sinus node is phylogenetically a remnant of the sinuatrial junctional tissues. We have never found a complete ring at this junction in our studies.[8] Instead, the node is formed in its definitive position lateral to the site of the sinuatrial junction. No specialized internodal pathways are found at any time during embryologic development. In right isomerism, because of the bilateral sinuatrial junctions, there are bilateral sinus nodes.[9] In contrast, in left isomerism, the sinus node is grossly hypoplastic and is formed in unexpected situations close to the A-V junction.[10]

DEVELOPMENT OF THE VENTRICULAR MASS AND A-V CONNECTIONS

The development of the ventricular mass is intimately related to the process of looping. Initially, the primary heart tube is believed to be straight, with venous and arterial poles opposite to each other. With growth, the tube bends, which results in placement of the arterial pole anterior to the atrium and A-V junction. This results in reorientation of the ventricular component so that the inlet and outlet components are placed side by side, with the outlet component to the right. Following such rightward looping, the heart tube still has smooth walls, with little evidence of trabeculations, and is lined throughout by cardiac jelly. Further growth occurs by outpouching of trabecular pouches, one from the inlet and the other from the outlet component (Fig.

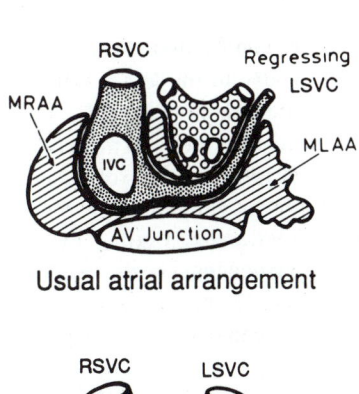
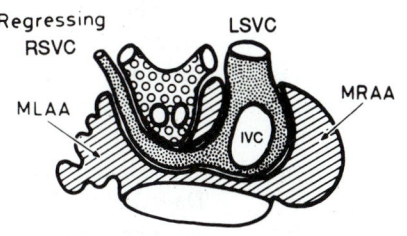
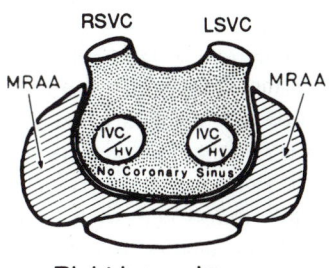
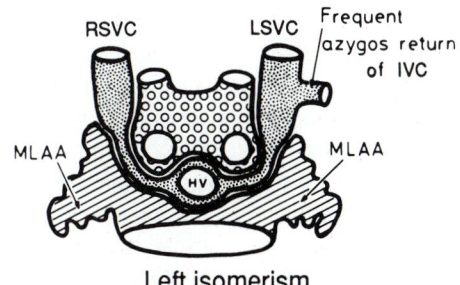

Usual atrial arrangement

Mirror-image atrial arrangement

Right isomerism

Left isomerism

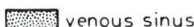

atrial segment   venous sinus   pulmonary venous component

Figure 56–6. The way in which the atrial segment, the venous sinus, and the pulmonary venous component interact to produce the different types of atrial arrangement.

56–7). The cardiac jelly persists in the A-V and ventriculoarterial junctions as the A-V and arterial cushions. It is the pouches that form the basis of the definitive ventricles. The trabecular component of the morphologically left ventricle grows from the inlet component, and that of the right ventricle from the outlet component of the primary tube. Following pouch formation, the atrial chambers still connect to the left ventricular pouch (via the ventricular inlet component), while the arterial component is connected exclusively to the right ventricular pouch (via the ventricular outlet component). Separating the A-V and ventriculoarterial junctions at this stage is the inner curvature of the primary heart tube. Normal development, therefore, requires effective transfer to the right ventricle of the A-V junctional component connected to the right atrium and transfer of the outlet component connected to the aorta to the left ventricular trabecular pouch. The precise mechanisms of these processes remain controversial,[2] but they are unimportant to the understanding. The significant point is that as these connections are produced (whether by active growth, by resorption, by differential growth, or by torsion is of little import to understanding of the anatomy), the developing muscular ventricular septum is brought into line with the outlet septum (Fig. 56–7). It is the outpouching of the trabecular components that produces the primary ventricular septum, which we call the *trabecular septum* because it separates the trabecular components. The inlet component is produced concomitant with the expansion of the right A-V junction.[5] Subsequent to this expansion, the septum fuses with the developing atrial septum, with the A-V endocardial cushions interposed between the two. The outlet septum, of minimal dimensions in the normal heart, is produced at the

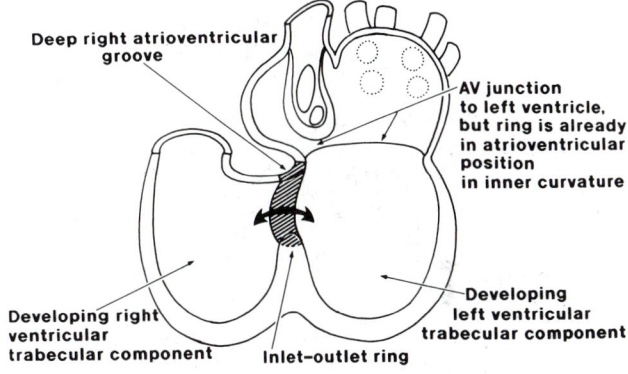

Figure 56–7. Evidence using immunocytochemistry[5] shows that the junction of the inlet and outlet components of the ventricular loop is marked by a ring of specialized tissue. After expansion of the right A-V junction, this inlet–outlet ring occupies the right A-V junction, showing that all components of the definitive right ventricle are derived from the outlet component of the initial ventricular loop (**B**).

site of the outlet endocardial cushions and it is brought into line with the primary septum only after the aorta has become connected to the left ventricle. The significant point is that ventricular septation can be successfully completed only after these transfers have occurred. The initial communication between inlet and outlet components of the ventricular loop is never closed. It becomes remodeled as the communication between the inlet and the remainder of the right ventricle and the outlet and the remainder of the left ventricle, respectively.[1] The precise origin of the tissue that eventually closes the intraventricular communication is also of relative unimportance in understanding morphology. What is important is to know that when the communication is closed, the septal leaflet of the tricuspid valve has yet to be formed. There is no way, therefore, that this tissue—which is the membranous part of the ventricular septum—can at its time of formation already have A-V and interventricular components.[11]

The normal A-V connections are established following these maneuvers. The mechanics readily permit understand-ing of formation of abnormal connections. Initially the atrial chambers were connected only to the left ventricular trabecular component. If this arrangement persisted, a double-inlet left ventricle would ensue, and the right ventricular trabecular component would then form the basis of an anterior rudimentary and incomplete right ventricle (Fig. 56–8). The A-V connections can then be guarded either by two valves or by a common valve, depending on the mode of septation of the A-V junction. This is the basis of the so-called single ventricle with outlet chamber, which is a heart with univentricular A-V connection to a left ventricle in the presence of a rudimentary right ventricle.[12] The right A-V junction could also fail to expand, so that the cushions formed at its right margin produced only a left A-V connection (Fig. 56–9). The left atrium would then be connected to a dominant left ventricle, with the right ventricular trabecular component again persisting as a rudimentary right ventricle. This is the morphology of classic tricuspid atresia, which is characterized by the absence of the right atrioventricular connection in the presence of univentricular A-V

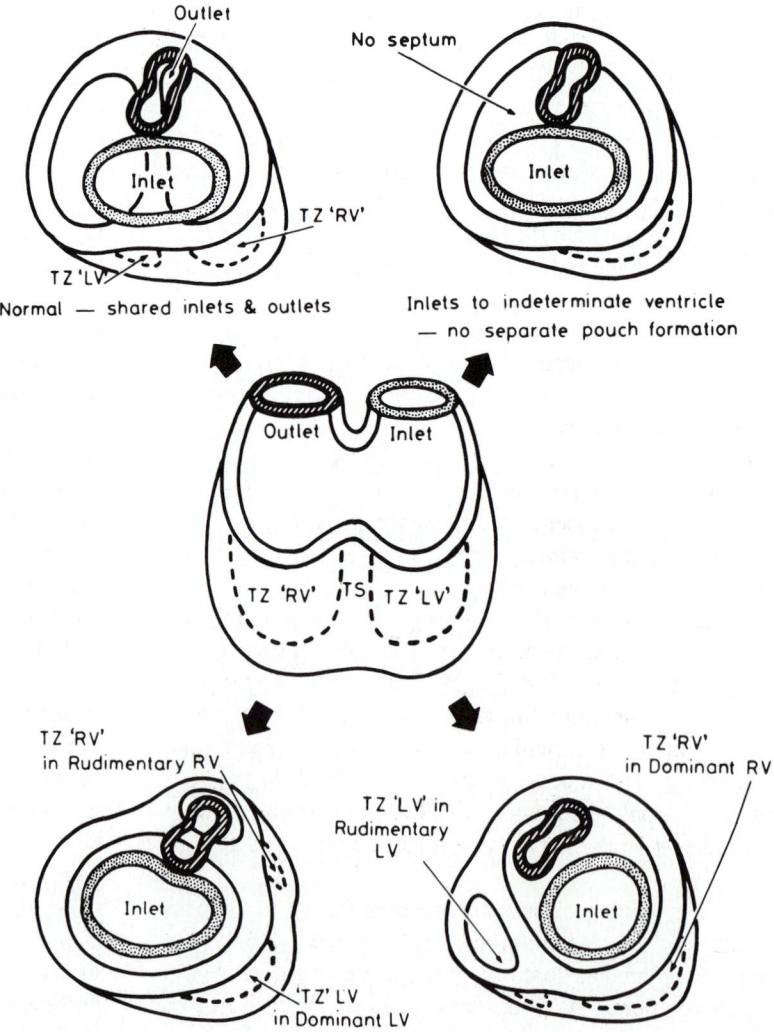

Figure 56–8. Diagrams illustrating the results of abnormal commitment of the ventricular inlet components to the trabecular pouches.

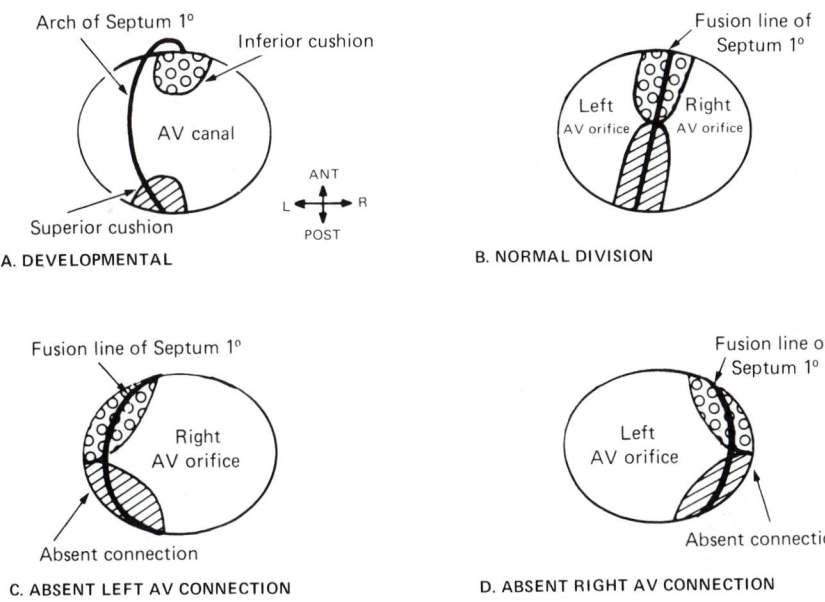

A. DEVELOPMENTAL

B. NORMAL DIVISION

C. ABSENT LEFT AV CONNECTION

D. ABSENT RIGHT AV CONNECTION

Figure 56–9. A concept of division of the A-V junction showing how eccentric fusion of the endocardial cushions and the primary atrial septum can produce absence of either the right or the left A-V connection. This normal division, or failure of division, when combined with formation of the various valvar morphologies illustrated in Figure 56–8, can account for all the known variations in valve morphology found in hearts with A-V connection apart from straddling and overriding valves. These are well explained on the basis of incomplete transfer or excessive transfer of the ventricular inlet portion to the trabecular components. *(From Becker AE, Wilkinson JL, Anderson RH: In Van Praagh R, Takao A (eds): Etiology and Morphogenesis of Congenital Heart Disease, 1980. Courtesy of Futura Publishing Company, Mount Kisco, NY.)*

connection to the dominant left ventricle.[13] Alternatively, the cushions could fuse at the left margin of the A-V junction, separating the left atrium from the ventricular mass. This results in absent left atrioventricular connection in the setting of a univentricular A-V connection to a dominant left ventricle. All the above has presumed retention of the initial connection of the ventricular inlet components to the left ventricular trabecular component.

The way in which the right part of the inlet component is transferred to the right ventricular pouch has already been described. It is reasonable to suppose that excessive transfer of the entire inlet component to the right ventricular trabecular pouch could occur.[14] This process, combined with equal or eccentric division of the A-V junction (Fig. 56–9), can then easily account for all the variability known to occur in hearts with univentricular A-V connection to a dominant right ventricle in the presence of a rudimentary left ventricle. The essence of these anomalies (Fig. 56–8) is that the trabecular (primary) ventricular septum is now posterior to the A-V connections.

Finally, it is possible to envisage the situation in which there is failure of excavation of the separate ventricular trabecular components (Fig. 56–8). Then the A-V and ventriculoarterial junctions would connect to and from an undivided solitary ventricular chamber of indeterminate morphology. The modes of division of the A-V junction (Fig. 56–9) could then produce this ventricular morphology with either double-inlet or absent right or absent left A-V connections.

The preceding discussion accounts for all the known variations in which the atriums are connected to only one ventricle, anomalies that we group collectively as hearts with univentricular A-V connections. There are then further variations possible in the majority of hearts in which each atrium is connected to its own ventricle, hearts that we

group as having biventricular A-V connections.[15] In the usual form of a heart with biventricular connections, the right atrium is connected to the right ventricle and the left atrium to the left ventricle, giving concordant A-V connections. This depends on there being atrial lateralization. If normal ventricular development occurred in the presence of isomeric appendages, with right isomerism, for example, one right atrium would be connected to a morphologically right ventricle and the other right atrium would be connected to a morphologically left ventricle. These are not concordant A-V connections but rather are biventricular and ambiguous A-V connections.[15]

In the preceding description of normal development, it was stated that the initial bending of the ventricular loop placed the outlet to the right of the inlet. It has been hypothesized[16,17] that bending can occur so that the outlet comes to lie to the left of the inlet connected to the atriums. If transfer then continued in the anticipated fashion, the left atrium would end up connected to the morphologically right ventricle and the right atrium connected to the morphologically left ventricle (Fig. 56–10). This produces discordant A-V connections. Recently, the whole concept of looping has been questioned; it has been suggested that the same pouch can, under different circumstances, develop either right or left trabecular characteristics.[18] This in no way negates the concept put forward in Figure 56–10 as an aid to understanding the anatomy of discordant A-V connections but if it is proven that leftward rather than rightward looping is an illusion, it calls into question the advisability of basing an entire nomenclature on the ventricular loop.[19] This is not to deny that there are two basic patterns of ventricular organization, which can be conveniently (although perhaps speciously) explained in terms of the development outlined above for concordant and discordant A-V connections, respectively. The patterns unequivocally exist. When

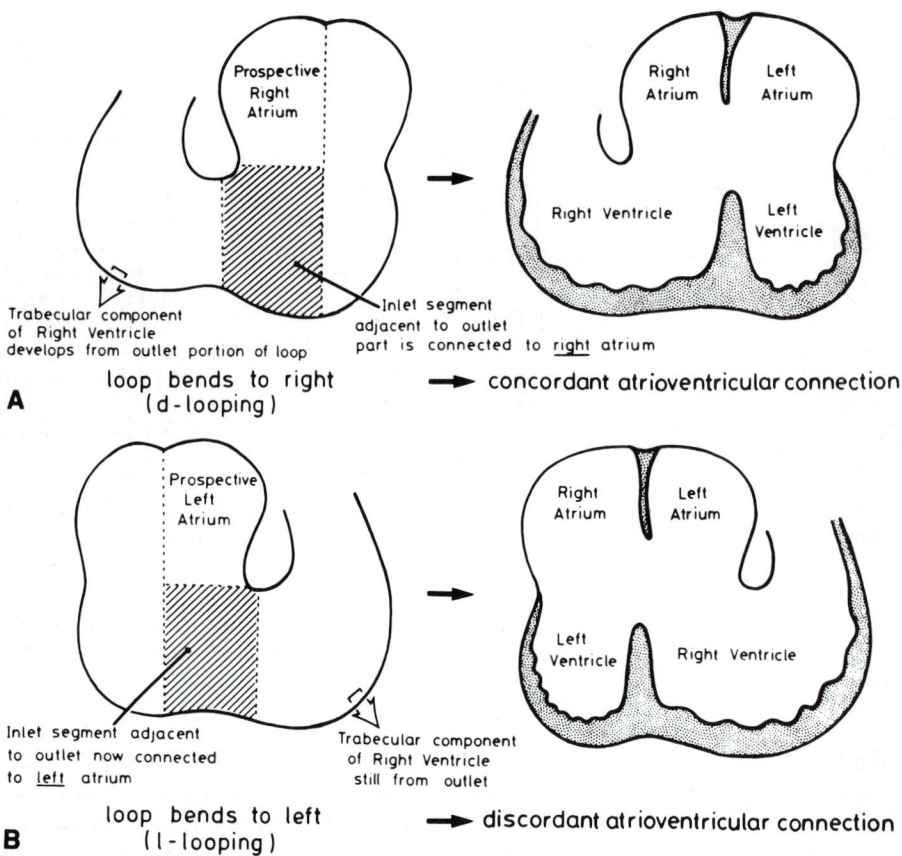

Figure 56–10. Diagrams illustrating how the presumed concept of leftward looping of the primary heart tube can result in discordant A-V connections.

describing definitive anatomy, it is perhaps more prudent to describe them using more evocative terms, such as "right-hand" and "left-hand" patterns of ventricular topology, rather than using the embryologically based terms "*d*-loop (right; dextro)" and "*l*-loop (left; levo)," which may ultimately be shown to be untenable. The importance of these ventricular patterns is illustrated in the setting of ambiguous A-V connections. The same ambiguous connection can be found when the ventricles have developed as for concordant or discordant patterns in cases where the atriums had been lateralized. It is then important to state whether the topology is that of a right-hand or left-hand pattern, since this affects conduction tissue disposition.

The concepts outlined above also permit an understanding of the intermediate anomalies that exist between hearts with univentricular atrioventricular connection, on one hand, and biventricular connections on the other hand. The essence of normal and abnormal development is sharing (whatever its mechanics) of the ventricular inlet components between the trabecular components. One has thus far considered only all-or-none transfer of the inlet components. It would be most unlikely if some hearts did not exhibit partial transfer. The hearts that have partial sharing are those with overriding atrioventricular valves. Cessation of such transfer could then occur either when the right inlet

portion was undergoing normal transfer or when the left inlet was undergoing abnormal transfer. A combination of incomplete transfer of either the right or left inlets combined with formation of a right-hand or left-hand ventricular topology and division or nondivision of the A-V junction can account for all the known variability in overriding A-V valves.[20] A significant point emerging from this knowledge is that a morphologically tricuspid valve overrides a septum that does not reach the crux (the point at which the plane of the atrial septum crosses the A-V junction), whereas the morphologically mitral valve overrides a septum that, although malaligned relative to the atrial septum, reaches to the crux.

DEVELOPMENT OF THE A-V CONDUCTION TISSUES

As already indicated, the conduction tissues have their origin in the junctional tissues between the initial components of the primary heart tube. From the standpoint of the A-V conduction tissues, the inlet–outlet junction is the significant junction.[5] A complete ring of tissue surrounds this junction, continuing as a drape of ventricular conduction tissue on the crest of the primary ventricular septum (Fig.

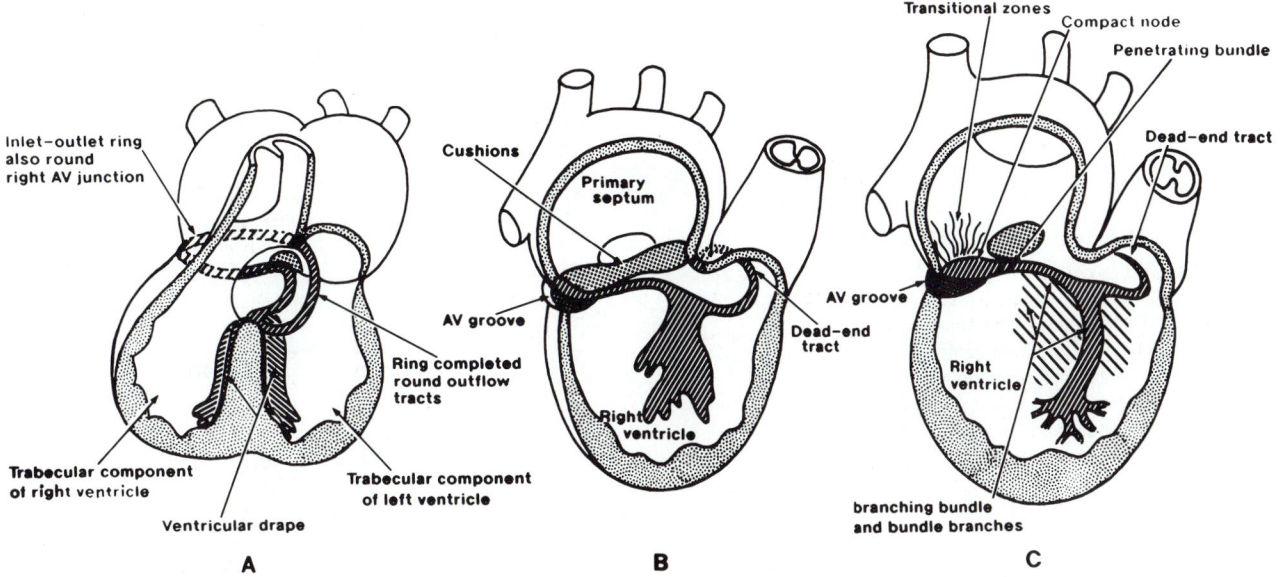

Figure 56–11. The A-V conduction system is derived from the ring of specialized tissue initially situated between the inlet and outlet components of the ventricular loop. These diagrams show the stages (**A** through **C**) required to transform the initial ring into the definitive A-V conduction system.[5]

56–11). Formation of a normal conduction tissue axis from these primordia depends on normal expansion of the right A-V junction. In its site of initial formation, the upper part of this ring, in the inner heart curvature, already produces an A-V connection. To bring this connection in line with the down-growing primary atrial septum, the right A-V junction must expand.[5] The septal component of this ring, covered by the A-V endocardial cushions, then forms the primordium of the compact A-V node and the penetrating A-V bundle (of His). Normal fusion of the atrial primary septum with the upper surface of the cushions produces the potential atrial transitional cell zone, and, as the cushion tissue recedes during subsequent development, the atrial component becomes the definitive atrioventricular node (Fig. 56–11B, C). The mechanics of normal conduction tissue development, therefore, demand appropriate alignment between the ventricular and atrial septums. Remnants of the initial ring of tissue persist around the orifice of the tricuspid valve, marking the sight of rightward expansion of the initial inlet–outlet ring.

In hearts in which the atriums connect only to a left ventricle, this alignment never occurs. The ventricular conduction tissues are formed in the anticipated position astride the primary ventricular septum. Because of the malalignment, these ventricular conduction tissues are unable to make contact with the regular atrial transitional cells. Because of the initial presence of a ring of conduction tissue around the inlet–outlet junction, an anomalous node is developed from this ring at the acute margin of the right A-V orifice. This is found by the rudimentary ventricle right-sided or left-sided. The only difference is that when the rudimentary ventricle is left-sided, an extensive nonbranching bundle encircles the outflow tract of the posterior great

artery (Fig. 56–12). When the right A-V orifice fails to form in a heart with a univentricular connection to a dominant left ventricle (classic tricuspid atresia), there is no anterior node. Instead, an extensive mass of nodal tissue is formed in the floor of the blind-ending right atrium. Otherwise, the disposition is as in double-inlet left ventricle.[21]

In hearts with a solitary and indeterminate ventricle, no trabecular or inlet septum is formed. The conduction tissues are somewhat randomly formed in the ventricular wall and originate from either an anterolateral node or a regular node via a free-running trabeculation.

In contrast, in hearts with the atriums connected only to a dominant right ventricle, the excessive transfer of the inlet components across the primary ventricular septum means that it is no longer an inlet septum in the definitive heart. Nonetheless, it still extends between atriums and trabecular conduction tissues. Because of this, there is a regular atrioventricular conduction tissue. The exception to this is the case where there is a left-hand pattern of ventricular topology. Then there may be a sling of conduction tissue between regular and anomalous anterior nodes.[22]

Anomalous conduction systems are the rule in hearts with discordant A-V connections; one feature of this connection with the usual atrial arrangement is gross malalignment between the atrial septum and the ventricular septum. This prevents formation of a regular penetrating bundle; instead, an anomalous anterior node is formed, as in hearts in which the atriums are connected to only a dominant left ventricle. The node is lateral to the outflow tract of the morphologically left ventricle, and a long, nonbranching bundle encircles the anterior quadrants of this outflow tract before descending onto the muscular septum. The bundle is consequently placed anterosuperiorly in relation to a perimem-

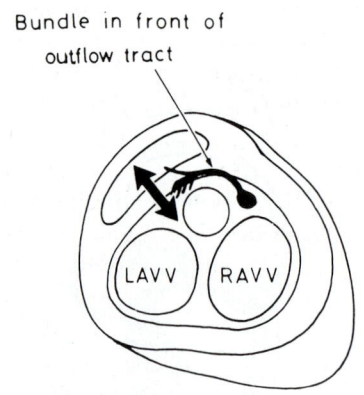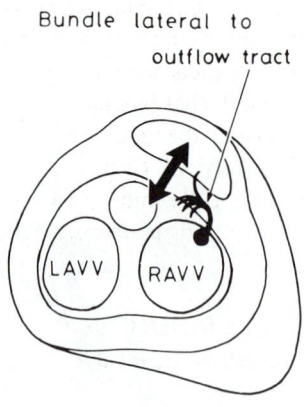

Figure 56–12. The position of the conduction tissues in hearts with double-inlet ventricle, showing how the location of the rudimentary right ventricle affects only the relation between the nonbranching bundle and the outflow tract from the dominant left ventricle.

A with left sided rudimentary RV   **B** with right sided rudimentary RV

branous ventricular septal defect.[23] When discordant A-V connections are found with mirror-image atrial arrangement, there is better alignment between atrial and inlet septums. Because of this, there is a regular node and bundle, although there exists the potential for formation of a sling. Slings have also been found in discordant A-V connections with the usual atrial arrangement when there is better alignment between atrial and inlet septums.[23]

There is also the potential to form anomalous conduction systems with ambiguous A-V connections. Here, the key is the ventricular topology. In our experience, in cases of both right and left isomerism, right-hand ventricular topology has been found with either an anterior conduction system or a sling between anterior and regular nodes.[10]

The final anomalous connection always found with an anomalous conduction system is overriding of the morphologically tricuspid valve in the presence of a right-hand ventricular topology. Here, the key is again the fact that the ventricular septum does not reach the crux and is consequently malaligned relative to the atrial septum. The anomalous node is formed at the point at which the ventricular septum reaches the A-V junction.[20,21]

FORMATION OF THE A-V VALVES

There is much misunderstanding concerning the development of the A-V valves. At the completion of septation of the atriums and ventricles, the greater part of the valvar leaflet tissue has not begun to develop. This is because the valves do not, as often presumed, differentiate entirely from A-V cushion tissue. Instead, part of the valve tissue is produced by delamination from the subendocardial layers of the developing myocardium; the latter process also produces the tension apparatus of the valves.[24,25] The A-V groove tissue at the hinge point of the leaflets separates the atrial from ventricular myocardium and produces the fibrous annulus.

The process of valvar formation is also pertinent to concepts regarding the formation of A-V septal defects (endocardial cushion defects). It is often presumed that the upper part of the atrial septum, together with the septal leaflets of the A-V valves, are derived from the A-V endocardial cushions. This is probably a fallacious concept. The cushions initially fuse together at the center of the A-V junction. This then permits the right and left A-V orifices to develop in spectacle fashion, and permits the aortic orifice to be transferred between the lenses of the spectacles to give a cloverleaf pattern. If the cushions do not fuse together, the junction will grow in ovoid fashion, and there will be no wedging of the aortic valve. In addition, there will be no platform for anchorage of the down-growing atrial primary septum to the muscular ventricular septum. The result is the characteristic ventricular morphology of the A-V septal defect, with its common A-V junction.[26–28] Whether the valve leaflets subsequently develop into a common orifice, or produce a connecting tongue of valvar tissue between the bridging valvar leaflets so as to produce separate right and left A-V orifices depends on subsequent events. What is certain is that if separate right and left valves are formed, they bear no resemblance to the tricuspid and mitral valves of the normal heart.

Another feature that warrants consideration is that occasionally a valve may be formed, but as an imperforate membrane. Such imperforate membranes can be found in either a tricuspid or mitral position. The difference between an imperforate valve and an absent A-V connection is significant. Occasionally, an imperforate tricuspid valve can be formed in a heart with concordant A-V connections, producing tricuspid atresia. This is the exception, seen most frequently with Ebstein's malformation. An imperforate tricuspid atresia does not always produce a univentricular A-V connection (although it may if found with double-inlet ventricle), but the commoner absent connection variety does. In contrast, imperforate mitral valves are probably the more common type of mitral atresia, but the univentricular connection variety of this anomaly certainly exists.

Ebstein's malformation is easy to understand in all its guises. It depends on failure of delamination of the septal and inferior leaflets from the walls of the right ventricular inlet portion.[24] That is why the valvar malformation never extends beyond the inlet–trabecular junction of the right ventricle. Rarely, an Ebstein-like malformation can affect the morphologically mitral valve, having the same developmental history. It then affects the mural leaflet of the valve.

MALDEVELOPMENT OF THE VENTRICULAR SEPTUM

As previously described, the normal ventricular septum has primary and outlet muscular components and is completed by the membranous septum. Normally, when the septum is closed, the septal leaflet of the tricuspid valve is unformed. Division of the membranous septum into A-V and interventricular components is, therefore, a late event. Ventricular septal defects cannot be explained on the basis of the ab-sence of the interventricular component of the membranous septum, although deficiencies in the embryologic structures forming the septum may potentiate to development of ventricular septal defects. From an anatomic stance, it seems that holes in the environs of the membranous septum result from deficiency or malalignment of the components of the muscular septum (Fig. 56–13). They are, in reality, perimembranous defects and can develop so as to open predominantly into the inlet, trabecular, or outlet parts of the right ventricle or a combination of these (Fig. 56–13).[29] Perimembranous defects are the most common ventricular septal defects. Because the conduction tissues are formed on the primary septum, they are always posteroinferior to perimembranous defects in hearts with concordant A-V connections (to the right hand as seen through the right atrium).[30]

Ventricular septal defects can also occur because of imperfect coalescence of the musculature of the septum. This can affect any part of the muscular septum. Defects of the muscular septum are frequently multiple, and the sep-

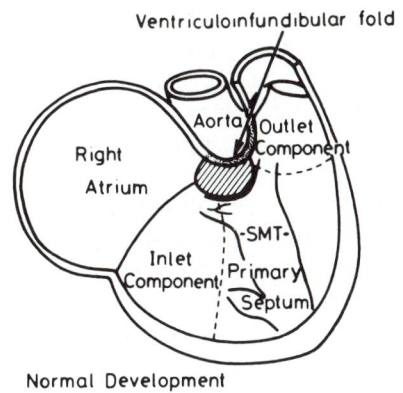

A Normal Development

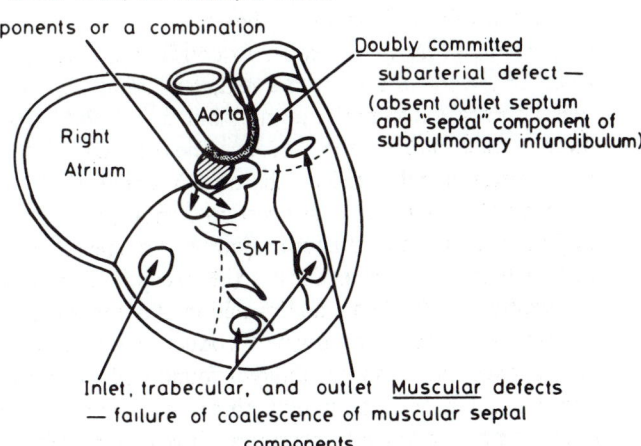

B Abnormal development

Figure 56–13. The abnormal development of the ventricular septum, which results in septal defects (**B**) interpreted in terms of the normal septal components (**A**).

tum may form in Swiss cheese fashion. Inlet muscular defects are important because the conduction tissue axis is anterosuperior relative to them (to the left hand as seen through the right atrium).[30]

The final type of ventricular septal defect results from complete absence of the outlet (infundibular) component of the muscular septum together with failure of formation of the septal component of the subpulmonary infundibulum. The resulting defect is roofed by the conjoined aortic and pulmonary valves and is in doubly committed subarterial position. Although frequently termed "supracristal," this term is not explicit since the doubly committed subarterial defect can extend to become perimembranous. More commonly, it has a muscular posterocaudal rim because the posterior limb of the septomarginal trabeculation fuses with the ventriculoinfundibular fold. This muscular rim is important because it protects the conduction tissues.

DEVELOPMENT AND MALDEVELOPMENT OF THE OUTFLOW TRACTS

As previously described, the arterial segment of the primary heart tube, connected to the ventricular outlet component, is initially supported in its entirety above the developing right ventricle. At this stage, the inner heart curvature separates the potential site of the arterial valves at the ventriculoarterial junction from the site of the A-V valves at the A-V junction. The arterial segment, together with the distal segment of the ventricular outlet component, is then divided by endocardial cushion tissue into subaortic and subpulmonary outflow tracts. These outlet cushions form little, if any, of the definitive muscular outlet septum. This is probably formed by coalescence of the walls of the outlet component as the outflow tracts grow out relative to their fused central portions.[1] Normal development, as already described, also necessitates effective transfer of the subaortic outlet component across the ventricular septum into the morphologically left ventricle. Again, the precise mechanics of this transfer remain uncertain. Indeed, "transfer" may itself be an imprecise word to use, as there is not necessarily any active movement of the aorta. It is possible that the rest of the heart grows around the subaortic outflow tract. Once more, this is of little significance to understanding outflow tract development. Initially, the developing aorta was positioned above the right ventricle. Finally, with normal development, it is positioned above, and is connected to, the left ventricle. In practical terms, it has been transferred to the left ventricle, although "become connected" might be a more appropriate description than "transferred." What is important is that the interventricular communication cannot be closed until this transfer, whatever its mechanics, is completed. Equally important, the developing aortic valve is separated initially from the developing mitral valve by the inner heart curvature. Usually, in the definitive heart after transfer, the aortic valve is in fibrous continuity with

the mitral valve. There has, therefore, been effective attenuation of the inner heart curve during development. Within the right ventricle, in contrast, the arterial valve remains separated from the A-V valve. The tissue separating the two valves is still the inner heart curvature, but in the definitive heart, we term this structure the *ventriculoinfundibular fold*.[31] The fold makes up the supraventricular crest, which inserts between the limbs of an extensive septal trabeculation of the right ventricle, often termed the "septal band," but, in our opinion, better referred to as the *septomarginal trabeculation*.

Another controversial topic is whether attenuation of the inner curve is an essential part of aortic transfer, or whether the two are independent events, if indeed absorption occurs at all.[32] Again, this is largely a problem of semantics, Certainly, complete attenuation is not essential for transfer, as it is known that normal hearts can exist with a muscular ventriculoinfundibular fold, albeit relatively small, separating the aortic and mitral valves. Be that as it may, normal or concordant ventriculoarterial connections require the subaortic outlet component, initially derived from the developing right ventricle, to become connected to the definitive morphologically left ventricle.

A series of anomalies is then easily understood on the basis of an incomplete connection of the subaortic outlet component. These anomalies all have overriding of the aortic valve. When aortic overriding is also associated with superocephalad deviation of the insertion of the outlet septum, the result is tetralogy of Fallot. The precise mechanics producing the deviation of outlet septal insertion remain uncertain. Tetralogy can be found with the aorta mostly connected to the right ventricle, depending on the degree of transfer that has occurred. When most of the aorta is connected to the right ventricle, we would categorize the ventriculoarterial connection as double-outlet from the right ventricle. In this respect, transfer of the aorta and attenuation of the ventriculoinfundibular fold certainly are separate events, as it is known that hearts with an unequivocal connection of both arteries to the right ventricle can have arterial–atrioventricular valve continuity resulting from attenuation of the ventriculoinfundibular fold.

The ventriculoarterial connection of double-outlet right ventricle is modified by the position of the ventricular septal defect. Although this can exist in a noncommitted position, the defect is usually related to one or other or both of the subarterial outflow tracts. The direction of the defect is determined by the position of the septal insertion of the outlet septum, although the morphogenetic cause of this is unknown. When the outlet septum is attached toward the anterior limb of the septomarginal trabeculation, the defect is beneath the posterior, right-sided great artery (almost always the aorta). When the outlet septum is attached to the posterior limb of the trabeculation, the defect opens beneath the left-sided great artery (almost always the pulmonary trunk). In terms of morphogenetic concepts, it is then surely significant that a series of anomalies can be observed between double-outlet right ventricle with subpulmonary ventricular septal defect and complete transposition with subpulmonary ventricular septal defect. This latter complex, frequently referred to as the *Taussig–Bing anomaly*, will be referred to again in relation to the development of discordant ventriculoarterial connections.

The outlet septum can be entirely deficient in double-outlet right ventricle. In such cases, the defect is in doubly committed subarterial position. The known existence of a series of malformations between this anomaly and double-outlet left ventricle[33] points strongly to transfer of both outlets as being the basis of double-outlet left ventricle. This anomaly can also exist with varying infundibular morphologies depending on the state of the ventriculoinfundibular fold.

Perhaps the most significant point with regard to the developmental aspects of the double-outlet right ventricle is the series of anomalies that exist between double-outlet right ventricle with subpulmonary defect and complete transposition.[34,35] This fact bears on both the development of the normal great arteries and the morphogenesis of discordant ventriculoarterial connections (aorta from morphologically right ventricle; pulmonary trunk from morphologically left ventricle). In the description of normal development, I have explained how the subaortic outflow tract becomes connected to the morphologically left ventricle. No consideration has been given to the way in which this particular outflow tract becomes connected to the aorta and the other outflow tract to the pulmonary trunk. This is related to the development of the arterial pole of the heart.

Initially, at least five pairs of aortic arches spring from the arterial segment of the primary heart tube. The fourth and sixth arches are primarily involved in formation of the great arteries; the left fourth arch becomes the aorta and the left sixth arch, the pulmonary trunk and the arterial duct (Fig. 56–14). It remains questionable if a fifth arch is ever formed during normal development. It is the way in which the pulmonary trunk and aorta become connected to the outflow tracts that is significant. At least two—and possibly three—structures are involved. The first is the septum of the ventricular outflow portions. Initially produced by cushion tissue, this subsequently becomes a muscular structure. Some argue that in early development these distal outflow cushions continue into the arterial septum.[36] Others argue that the outlet and arterial cushions are separate structures[37,38] and that they fuse in spiral fashion to divide the arterial segment.[37] All agree that a further component, the aortopulmonary septum, divides the aortic fourth and sixth arches, and that this septum grows toward the heart to fuse with the distal extent of the ventricular septum. This aortopulmonary septum is now known to be particularly important, as it is derived from cells that migrate from the neural crest.[39] In normal development, these septal structures fuse so as to connect the right ventricular outflow tract to the pulmonary trunk and the left ventricular outflow tract to the aorta.

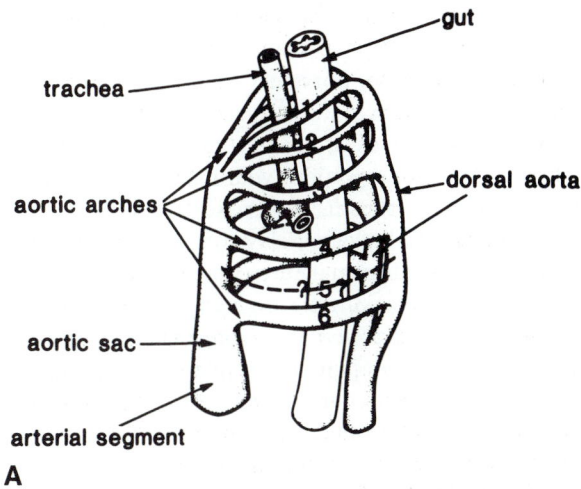

A

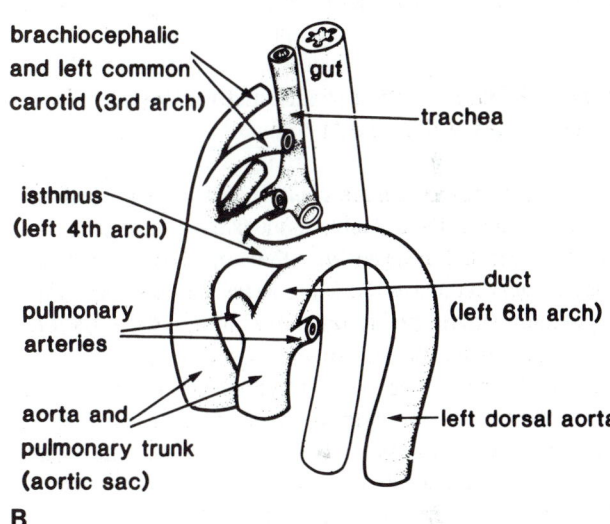

B

Figure 56–14. A, B. The steps involved in conversion of the bilaterally symmetric aortic arch system to the definitive great arteries. *(Modified from Anderson RH, Becker AE: Cardiac Anatomy— An Integrated Text and Colour Atlas, 1980. Courtesy of Gower Medical Publishing, London.)*

The different views concerning septation of the outflow tracts contribute to disagreements concerning the morphogenesis of discordant ventriculoarterial connections (*transposition*). The proponents of the spiral cushion hypothesis argue that fusion of these cushions in straight rather than spiral fashion will connect the arteries in inappropriate fashion.[37] Alternatively, those who contend that outlet and arterial segments are divided by separate cushions argue that inappropriate fusion of these two sets of cushions to each other will produce discordant connections.[38,40] If the outlet and arterial cushions are continuous structures, and if in the normal heart they fuse in straight fashion,[36] it is difficult to substantiate either of these hypotheses. Irrespective of the mode of division of the outlet and arterial segments, it is easy to envisage how the aortopulmonary septum could fuse with the ventricular septum so as to "plug" the great arteries into inappropriate outflow tracts (Fig. 56–15). From a conceptual stance, therefore, it is possible that discordant ventriculoarterial connections could result either from abnormal transfer of the subpulmonary outflow portion to the left ventricle with normal developmental connections of the great arteries or by normal formation of the outlet portions with reversed connections of the great arteries. Thus far, experiments designed to produce discordant ventriculoarterial connections have demonstrated only abnormal arterial development,[32] so that experimental evidence is lacking for the outlet maldevelopment hypothesis. Yet the evidence from congenitally malformed human hearts is, in my opinion, best interpreted in the light of this hypothesis. With our present state of knowledge, it seems fair to state that both disordered ventricular outlet development and abnormal formation of the aortopulmonary septum can independently result in discordant ventriculoarterial connections. To explain all the known variables of these connections encountered in human abnormalities, it is necessary to invoke both mechanisms and then to postulate further independent development and maldevelopment of the left ventricular ventriculoinfundibular fold, as these possibly indicate a secondary change within the framework postulated by Krediet and Klein.[41] In this way, it is possible to provide at least a plausible explanation not only for discordant ventriculoarterial connections in all their guises, but also for the known variations in double-outlet right ventricle and concordant ventriculoarterial connections with abnormal arterial relationships (anatomically corrected malposition).[42,43]

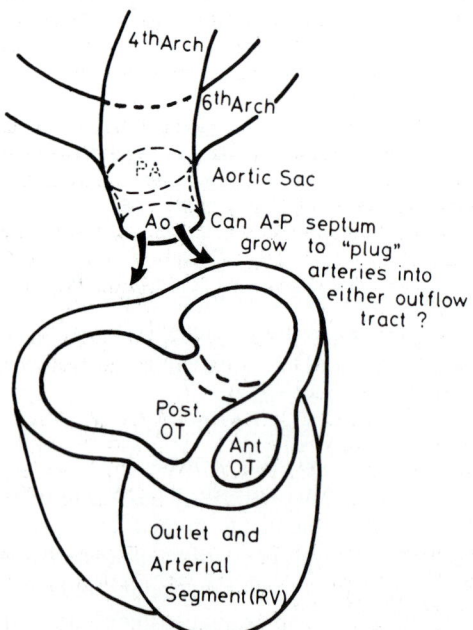

Figure 56–15. The way in which the direction of formation of the aortopulmonary septum and its fusion with the ventricular septum can connect the great arteries to either developing outflow tract. Either outflow tract could theoretically be transferred to the developing left ventricle. By combining abnormal transfer with abnormal plugging-in, it is possible to account for all known malformations of the ventricular outflow tracts and connections.

The final abnormal ventriculoarterial connection to be considered is single outlet of the heart. We divide single pulmonary trunk with aortic atresia, and single aortic trunk with pulmonary atresia. We classify aortic atresia and pulmonary atresia as single outlet only when it is not possible to trace the atretic trunk into contact with a ventricular chamber. As at the A-V junction, absent connection is a different type of defect from an imperforate valve. An absent connection either was never formed or was formed and became resorbed. Either way, an absent connection is underscored by a developmental process different from that which produces an imperforate valve. In the latter instance, there is disordered differentiation or, alternatively, subsequent fusion of the arterial valve leaflets that develop at the junction of the ventricular outlet and the arterial segment of the primary heart tube.[32] Common arterial trunk has a quite different cause. As indicated, usually the ventricular outlets are divided by the ventricular septum and the aortopulmonary septum. Common trunk results from failure of formation of the outlet septum and downward growth of the aortopulmonary septum. This produces the common arterial outlet guarded by a common truncal valve.[44] The commitment of the trunk to the ventricular mass depends on the degree of sharing the ventricular outlet components between the trabecular components. The form of the great arteries depends on the degree of aortopulmonary septation present.

Before leaving the subject of ventriculoarterial connections, it is pertinent to add a few comments on formation of the pulmonary arterial supply. Initially, the intrapulmonary arteries are themselves connected to the aortic arch system.[45] With normal growth, the sixth aortic arch subsumes the role of supplying the pulmonary arteries, as at this stage the sixth arch itself is connected via the arterial duct to the systemic circulation. These various connections form the basis for pulmonary arterial supply in the presence of pulmonary atresia. Thus, the lungs may be supplied by a pulmonary arterial confluence via the arterial duct (sixth-arch structures). Alternatively, the sixth-arch structures may not be formed if the lungs are supplied via the initial connections between the intrapulmonary arteries and the aortic arch system. Intermediate situations are rarely found in which the lungs are supplied via both the sixth-arch system and major aortopulmonary collateral arteries (Fig. 56–16). Finally, the bronchial arteries or intercostal arteries can themselves have a role in supplying the pulmonary arterial supply via acquired collateral branches.[46]

DEVELOPMENT OF THE CORONARY ARTERIES

Like the atrioventricular valves, the coronary arteries appear late in development. It is likely that three units are important. The first is the epicardial plexus of arteries, which communicates with intramyocardial plexuses derived from venous structures.[47] The second is a corona of potential arterial trunks, which develops around the pedicles of the great

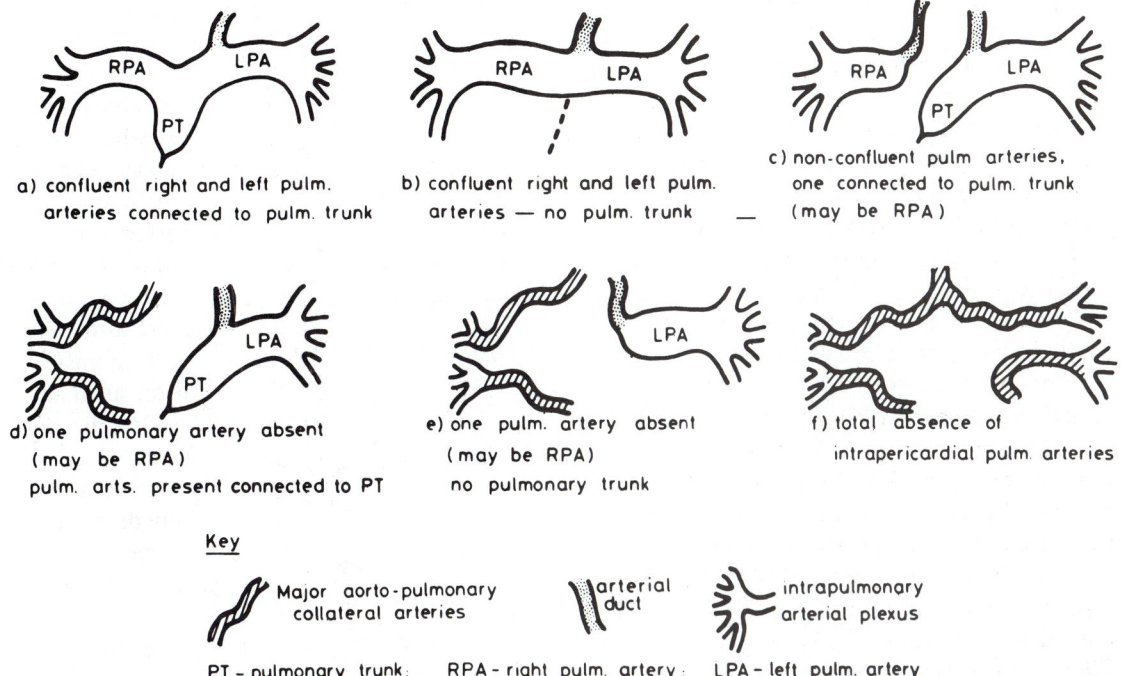

Figure 56–16. The embryologic segments that contribute to the pulmonary arteries, and the ways in which they can be interconnected in hearts with pulmonary atresia and ventricular septal defect. *(From Becker AE, Anderson RH: Pathology of Congenital Heart Disease, 1981. Courtesy of Butterworths, London.)*

arteries. The third is the buds of the coronary arteries themselves, which extend from the corona into the aorta.[48] All known coronary arterial malformations are readily explained according to the way in which these developmental units grow and connect relative to one another[49] (see Chap. 94).

ACKNOWLEDGMENTS

This chapter could not have been completed without the active collaboration of colleagues with whom the author discussed and refined at length the concepts expressed herein, notably James L. Wilkinson, Anton E. Becker, Michael Tynan, Fergus J. Macartney, Elliot A. Shinebourne, Tomas Pexieder, Wout Lamers, Nigel Brown, and Adri Gittenberger de Groot. The illustrations were splendidly drawn by Siew Yen Ho and Sharyn Wong.

REFERENCES

1. Anderson RH: Another look at cardiac embryology. *Prog Cardiol* **7:**1, 1978
2. Pexieder T: Mechanisms of cardiac morphogenesis and teratogenesis. *Perspect Cardiovasc Res* **5:**93, 1981
3. de la Cruz MV, Sanchez Gomez C, Manuel Arteaga M, Arguello C: Experimental study of the development of the truncus ad conus in the chick embryo. *J Anat* **123:**661, 1977
4. Keith A, Mackenzie I: Recent researches on the anatomy of the heart. *Lancet* **1:**101, 1910
5. Lamers WH, Wessels A, Verbeek FJ, et al: New findings concerning ventricular septation in the human heart: Implications for maldevelopment. *Circulation* **86:**1194–1205, 1992
6. De Ruiter MC, Gittenberger-de Groot AC, Poelman RE, et al: Development of the pharyngeal arch system related to the pulmonary and bronchial vessels in the avian embryo with a concept on systemic–pulmonary collateral artery formation. *Circulation* **87:**1306–1319, 1993
7. Van Praagh R, Corsini I: Cor triatriatum: Pathologic anatomy and a consideration of morphogenesis based on 13 postmortem cases and a study of normal development of the pulmonary vein and atrial septum in 83 human embryos. *Am Heart J* **78:**379, 1969
8. Anderson RH, Ho SY, Becker AE, Gosling JA: The development of the sinuatrial node. In Bonke FIM (ed): *The Sinus Node, Structure, Function, and Clinical Relevance.* The Hague, Martinus Nijhoff, 1978, pp 166–182
9. Van Mierop LHS, Patterson PR, Reynolds RW: Two cases of congenital asplenia with isomerism of the cardiac atria and the sinoatrial nodes. *Am J Cardiol* **13:**407, 1964
10. Dickinson DF, Wilkinson JL, Anderson KR, et al: The cardiac conduction system in situs ambiguus. *Circulation* **59:**879, 1979
11. Allwork SP, Anderson RH: Developmental anatomy of the membranous part of the ventricular septum in the human heart. *Br Heart J* **41:**275–280, 1979
12. Anderson RH, Becker AE, Tynan M, et al: The univentricular atrioventricular connection: Getting to the root of a thorny problem. *Am J Cardiol* **54:**822–828, 1984
13. Anderson RH, Rigby ML: The morphologic heterogeneity of "tricuspid atresia": Editorial note. *Int J Cardiol* **16:**67–73, 1987
14. Quero-Jimenez M, Perez Martinez VM, Maitre Azcarte MJ, et al: Exaggerated displacement of the atrioventricular canal towards the bulbis cordis (rightward displacement of the mitral valve). *Br Heart J* **35:**65, 1973
15. Anderson RH, Ho SY: Sequential segmental analysis of congenitally malformed hearts: Advances for the 1990's. *Australas J Cardiac Thorac Surg* **2:**10–17, 1993

16. Van Praagh R: The segmental approach to diagnosis in congenital heart disease. *Birth Defects* **8:**4, 1972

17. Van Praagh R: What is congenitally corrected transposition? *N Engl J Med* **282:**1097, 1970

18. Steding G, Seidl W: Contribution to the development of the heart. Part 2. Morphogenesis of congenital heart disease. *Thorac Cardiovasc Surg* **29:**1, 1981

19. Van Praagh R, Vlad P: Dextrocardia, mesocardia, and levocardia: The segmental approach to diagnosis in congenital heart disease. In Keith JD, Rowe RD, Vlad P (eds): *Heart Disease in Infancy and Childhood,* 3rd ed. New York, Macmillan, 1978, pp 638–697

20. Milo S, Ho SY, Macartney FJ, et al: Straddling and overriding atrioventricular valves, morphology and classification. *Am J Cardiol* **44:**1122, 1979

21. Becker AE, Wilkinson JL, Anderson RH: Atrioventricular conduction tissues: A guide in understanding the morphogenesis of the univentricular heart. In Van Praagh R, Takao A (eds): *Etiology and Morphogenesis of Congenital Heart Disease.* Mount Kisco, New York, Futura, 1980, pp 489–514

22. Essed CE, Ho SY, Hunter S, Anderson RH: Atrioventricular conduction system in univentricular heart of right ventricular type with right-sided rudimentary chamber. *Thorax* **35:**123, 1980

23. Anderson RH, Becker AE, Arnold R, Wilkinson JL: The conducting tissues in congenitally corrected transposition. *Circulation* **50:**911, 1974

24. Van Mierop LHS, Gessner IH: Pathogenetic mechanisms in congenital cardiovascular malformations. *Prog Cardiovasc Dis* **15:**67, 1972

25. Lamers WH, Viràgh S, Wessels A, et al: The formation of the tricuspid in the human heart. *Circulation* **91:**111–121, 1995

26. Van Mierop LHS: Personal communication, 1977

27. Penkoske PA, Neches WH, Anderson RH, Zuberbuhler JR: Further observations on the morphology of atrioventricular septal defects. *J Thorac Cardiovasc Surg* **90:**611–622, 1985

28. Anderson RH, Baker EJ, Ho SY, et al: The morphology and diagnosis of atrioventricular septal defects. *Cardiol Young* **1:**290–305, 1991

29. Soto B, Becker AE, Moulaert AJ, et al: Classification of ventricular septal defects. *Br Heart J* **43:**332, 1980

30. Milo S, Ho SY, Wilkinson JL, Anderson RH: The surgical anatomy and atrioventricular conduction tissues of hearts with isolated ventricular septal defects. *J Thorac Cardiovasc Surg* **79:**244, 1980

31. Anderson RH, Becker AE, Van Mierop LHS: What should we call the "crista"? *Br Heart J* **39:**856, 1977

32. Pexieder T: Development of the outflow tract of the embryonic heart. *Birth Defects* **14:**29, 1978

33. Brandt PWT, Calder AL, Barratt-Boyes BG, Neutze JM: Double outlet left ventricle. Morphology, cineangiography, diagnosis and surgical treatment. *Am J Cardiol* **38:**897, 1976

34. Goor DA, Edwards JE: The spectrum of transposition of the great arteries, with special reference to developmental anatomy of the conus. *Circulation* **48:**406, 1973

35. Anderson RH, Wilkinson JL, Arnold R, Becker AE, Lubkiewicz K: The morphogenesis of bulboventricular malformations. II. Observations on malformed hearts. *Br Heart J* **36:**948, 1974

36. Los JA: Embryology. In Watson H (ed): *Paediatric Cardiology.* London, Lloyd-Luke, 1968, pp 1–29

37. de la Cruz MV, Pio da Rocha J: An ontogenetic theory for the explanation of congenital malformations involving the truncus and conus. *Am Heart J* **51:**782, 1956

38. Van Mierop LHS, Alley RD, Kausel HW, Stranahan A: Pathogenesis of transposition complexes. I. Embryology of the ventricles and great arteries. *Am J Cardiol* **12:**216, 1963

39. Bartelings MM, Gittenberger-de Groot AC: The outflow tract of the heart: Embryologic and morphologic correlations. *Int J Cardiol* **22:**289–300, 1989

40. Van Mierop LHS, Wiglesworth FW: Pathogenesis of transposition complexes. III. True transposition of the great vessels. *Am J Cardiol* **12:**233, 1963

41. Krediet P, Klein HW: Synopsis of normal cardiac development. *Perspect Cardiovasc Res* **5:**7, 1981

42. Anderson RH, Pickering D, Brown R: Double outlet right ventricle with l-malposition and uncommitted ventricular septal defect. *Eur J Cardiol* **3:**133, 1975

43. Anderson RH: The morphogenesis of ventriculoarterial discordance. In Van Mierop LHS, Oppenheimer-Dekker A, Bruins C (eds): *Embryology and Teratology of the Heart and the Great Arteries* (Boerhaave Course 13). The Hague, Leiden University Press, 1978, pp 93–111

44. Van Mierop LHS, Patterson DF, Schnarr WR: Pathogenesis of persistent truncus arteriosus in light of observations made in a dog embryo with the anomaly. *Am J Cardiol* **41:**755, 1978

45. Congdon ED: Transformation of the aortic arch system during the development of the human embryo. *Contrib Embryol* **14:**65, 1922

46. Macartney FJ, Haworth SG: The pulmonary blood supply in pulmonary atresia with ventricular septal defect. In Godman MJ, Marquis RM (eds): *Paediatric Cardiology,* Vol 2. *Heart Disease in the Newborn.* Edinburgh, Churchill Livingstone, 1979, pp 314–338

47. Rychter Z, Rychterova V: Angio- and myoarchitecture of the heart wall under normal and experimentally changed morphogenesis. *Perspect Cardiovasc Res* **5:**431, 1981

48. Bogers AJJC, Gittenberger-de Groot AC, Dubbeldam JA, Huysmans HA: The inadequacy of existing theories on development of the proximal coronary arteries and their connexions with the arterial trunks. *Int J Cardiol* **20:**117, 1988

49. Anderson RH, Becker AE: Congenital anomalies of the endocardium, myocardium and epicardium and of the conduction tissues and coronary arteries. In Robertson WB (ed): *Systemic Pathology,* 3rd ed, Vol 10, Part A. *The Cardiovascular System.* Churchill Livingstone, Edinburgh, 1993, pp 287–302

CHAPTER

57

Structural and Functional Diagnosis of Congenital Heart Disease

John L. Cotton, Josephine B. Isabel-Jones, and Roberta G. Williams

The comprehensive anatomic and physiologic assessment of congenital heart disease is demanding because of the wide spectrum of anatomic variation, the evolving clinical picture imposed by physiologic changes after birth, and the demand for urgent medical and surgical management in the more critical forms of neonatal heart disease. Some fetuses and neonates may present with defects that are incompatible with life. In the older population, some patients with more complex and devastating cardiac lesions have been selected out by natural history or surgical intervention. Analysis of the entire cardiovascular system is required because in fetal life, anomalies often produce upstream or downstream defects by altering the early fetal blood flow pattern. Additionally, abnormal development or migration of the early cardiac primordia results in certain patterns of associated defects. In the newborn with critical obstructive heart disease, the presence of a low cardiac output state may mask an associated anomaly in series with the dominant obstructive defect. It is therefore imperative to define precisely all segments of the cardiovascular system: the systemic and pulmonary veins, the atria, the atrioventricular valves, the ventricles, the conotruncus, and the great arteries.

The goal of this chapter is to provide the reader with the criteria necessary to make clinical and surgical decisions about some specific diagnoses in patients with congenital heart disease. Clinical presentation, followed by pertinent clinical findings, will be described for most common lesions with emphasis on specific information needed in re-

lation to planning surgical intervention and the best diagnostic techniques to obtain this information. Finally, the relative contributions of the major invasive and noninvasive techniques will be elaborated.

ACYANOTIC LESIONS

Atrial Septal Defect

Guidelines for preoperative evaluation:

  I. Location and size
     A. Patent foramen ovale—fenestrated septum primum
     B. Ostium secundum defect
     C. Ostium primum defect
     D. Sinus venosus defect
     E. Coronary sinus—septal defect
 II. Chamber dilatation
III. Associated lesions
     A. Anomalous pulmonary venous return
     B. Atrioventricular valve abnormalities

Patients with an atrial septal defect generally have left-to-right shunting due to a more compliant right ventricle compared to the left ventricle. They usually present in early childhood with signs of right ventricular volume overload. On examination an increased right ventricular impulse is noted. The auscultatory hallmark is a widely split and fixed second heart sound and midsystolic murmur related to increased flow across the pulmonary valve. A loud first heart sound and early-to-middiastolic rumble at the tricuspid valve signify a left-to-right shunt of at least moderate proportions. Sinus venosus defects are often associated with partial anomalous pulmonary venous return. If the veins return near the septum they can be baffled to the left atrium across the defect, therefore it is important for the echocardiographic study to display the entrance of all of the pulmonary veins. A stretched foramen ovale will usually close spontaneously.

Echocardiography will reveal the size and location of the atrial septal defect[1] (Fig. 57–1). Pulsed and color Doppler identify the left-to-right shunt at the atrial level. Right ventricular volume overload produces diastolic bowing of the ventricular septum to the left during diastole with the left ventricle assuming an elliptical shape. Partial anomalous pulmonary veins can be determined by two-dimensional echocardiography. Their flow can be traced by color Doppler, which enhances the ability to trace the course of these veins. Transthoracic and subxiphoid echocardiography are usually sufficient to define the anatomy of the atrial septum and pulmonary veins in infants and in small children. Older children and adults may require transesophageal echocardiography to achieve full anatomic definition. Cardiac catheterization is not usually needed in the evaluation of atrial septal defects.

Ventricular Septal Defect

Guidelines for preoperative evaluation:

I. Anatomy
   A. Location
   B. Size
   C. Multiple defects

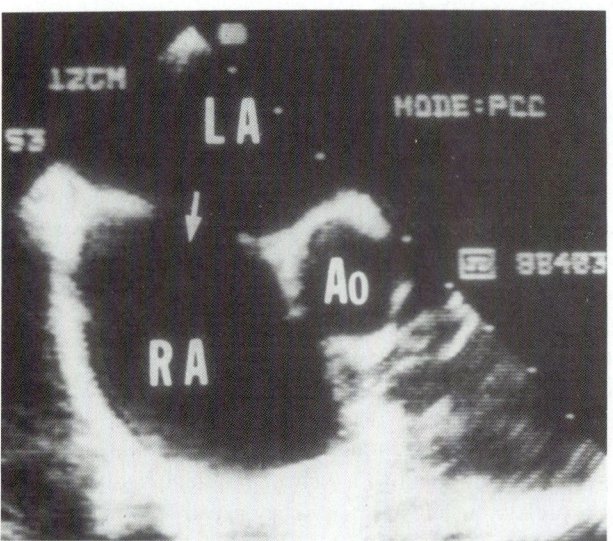

Figure 57–1. Transesophageal long axis view demonstrates a large secundum atrial septal defect (arrow) (LA, left atrium; RA, right atrium; Ao, aorta).

II. Hemodynamics
   A. Restrictive
   B. Nonrestrictive
   C. Pulmonary hypertension
III. Associated Defects
   A. Left ventricular/right ventricular outflow tract obstruction (posterior/anterior malalignment of the infundibular septum)
   B. Aortic insufficiency
   C. Tricuspid insufficiency
   D. Mitral insufficiency

In the absence of right heart obstruction, patients with a ventricular septal defect will usually develop left-to-right shunting coincident with reduction of pulmonary vascular resistance in the first weeks of life. The amount of shunting will then depend on the size of the defect and the balance between pulmonary and systemic vascular resistance. These patients are noted to have holosystolic murmurs that range from loud, high pitched in small muscular defects, to lower frequency in moderate-to-large defects. As the left ventricle becomes volume overloaded, congestive heart failure may ensue.

The surgical management of ventricular septal defects depends on their location, size, number, and associated lesions. Restrictive muscular septal defects have a 50% chance of spontaneous closure. Membranous ventricular septal defects, regardless of initial size, are likely (40%) to spontaneously close as well by 2 years of age.[2] Ventricular septal defects in other locations are not as likely to close, especially malaligned, inlet, or subarterial defects. A restrictive ventricular septal defect with no evidence of cardiomegaly can be followed without need for surgical intervention. Surgical intervention for ventricular septal defects with persistently large left-to-right shunts is indicated to prevent progressive pulmonary vascular obstructive disease. While closure of most ventricular septal defects can be accomplished through the tricuspid valve via a right atriotomy, the presence of defects in the anterior, posterior, or apical muscular septum may dictate an alternate approach. At the time of surgery, other associated lesions including aortic, mitral, or tricuspid insufficiency, and left or right ventricular outflow tract obstruction should be addressed.

The chest x-ray may be normal when the ventricular septal defect is small, but in the presence of a moderate or greater left-to-right shunt, radiographic findings of left ventricular dilatation and increased pulmonary vascular markings are found. At this point, the electrocardiogram may reveal left atrial enlargement and left or biventricular hypertrophy. Echocardiography plays an important role in the diagnosis of ventricular septal defects. Multiple views are needed to visualize the entire interventricular septum. Two-dimensional imaging can show the size and location of the interventricular communications[3] (Fig. 57–2). Color Doppler can evaluate the direction of shunting across the defect. By measuring the direction and velocity of flow

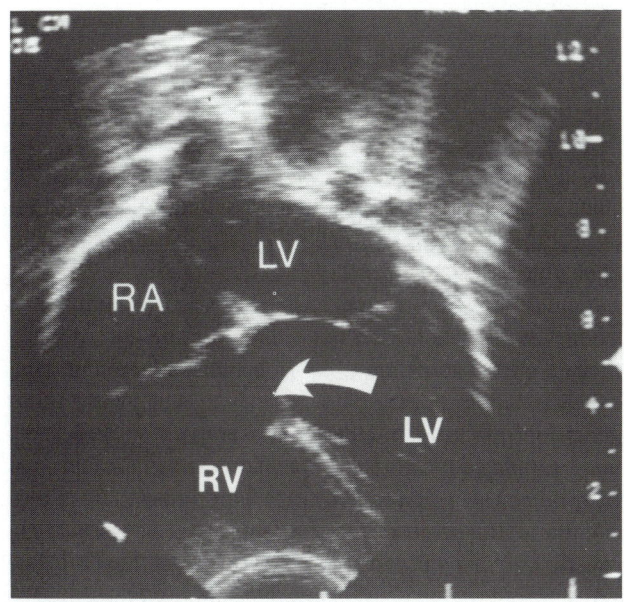
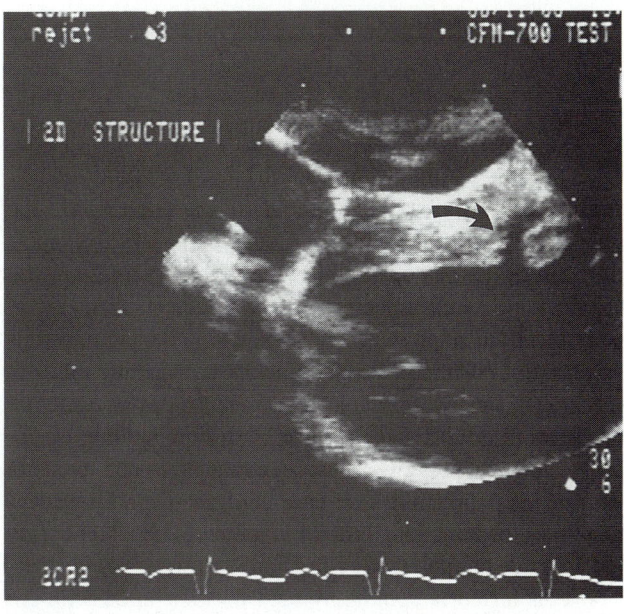

A   B

Figure 57–2. A. Subxiphoid view demonstrates a large ventricular septal defect (arrow) on the inflow portion of the interventricular septum, extending to the cardiac crux (RA, right atrium; LA, left atrium; RV, right ventricle; LV, left ventricle). **B.** Intraoperative echocardiogram with the transducer placed on the anterior ventricular surface displaying a tortuous midmuscular septal defect.

across the defect, pulsed and continuous wave Doppler can be utilized to estimate the pressure gradient across the defect.[4,5] Cardiac catheterization is not required prior to surgery unless physical and noninvasive findings are atypical or contradictory. Direct pressure and oxygen saturation recordings will define the size of the defect and will allow a calculation of the relative pulmonary to systemic blood flows and resistances. Angiography is especially useful in defining multiple ventricular septal defects.

Atrioventricular Septal Defect

Guidelines for preoperative evaluation:

I. Atrial septal defect component
II. Ventricular septal defect component
   A. Location (usually posterior/inlet)
   B. Extension
   C. Multiple
III. Atrioventricular valve anatomy
   A. Common atrioventricular valve
     1. Septal attachment (Rastelli classification)
      A. Type A—Superior bridging leaflet with appropriate septal attachments
      B. Type B—Superior bridging leaflet with straddling attachments
      C. Type C—Superior bridging leaflet with no attachment to septum
     2. Straddling mitral or tricuspid valve
   B. Intermediate type
     1. Cleft mitral valve

     2. Insufficiency/sufficiency of left atrioventricular valve tissue
   C. Double orifice mitral valve
   D. Atrioventricular valvular regurgitation/stenosis
   E. "Parachute" atrioventricular valve
   F. Unbalanced atrioventricular septal defect
     1. Ventricular hypoplasia
     2. Left ventricular outflow tract obstruction
IV. Pulmonary vascular resistance
V. Associated lesions

Complete atrioventricular septal defect is characterized by both an interatrial as well as interventricular communication via a single, centrally placed defect traversed by a common atrioventricular valve. The common valve has at least five leaflets and may provide equal (balanced) or unequal (unbalanced) flow to the ventricles. Partial or transitional (intermediate) forms can be seen with atrial or ventricular septal defects with or without significant atrioventricular valve anomalies. The timing of presentation will vary according to the size of the septal defect, amount of atrioventricular valve insufficiency, hypoplasia of either of the ventricles, or obstruction to the left ventricular outflow tract. Congestive heart failure ensues with the drop in pulmonary vascular resistance, which usually occurs in early infancy. Murmurs consistent with interventricular shunting appear during this time and may be initially nonspecific but gradually assume a holosystolic pattern as the pulmonary vascular resistance falls. The length and intensity of the murmur generally reflect the balance of the pulmonary vascular resistance and systemic vascular resistance across a nonrestrictive interventricular communication. The longer and louder the murmur, the lower the pulmonary vascular resistance is compared to the systemic vascular resistance. The absence or diminishing of a systolic murmur in the presence of a ventricular septal defect should raise concern for increased pulmonary vascular resistance. A prominent pulmonic component of the second heart sound (P2) would support that concern. With significant regurgitant flow, an early systolic murmur may be heard. Obstruction across the left ventricular outflow tract can give rise to an ejection murmur.

The electrocardiogram reveals a leftward or superior (northwest) frontal axis, depending on the completeness of the atrioventricular septal defect. Left, right, or biventricular hypertrophy may be seen depending on the completeness of the atrioventricular septal defect, site of predominant shunting, and presence of increased pulmonary vascular resistance.

This lesion is commonly seen in association with trisomy 21. Therefore a thorough cardiac evaluation should be routinely performed in infants with trisomy 21 even with minimal or no clinical symptoms. This is particularly important in these patients as they have a propensity for development of early pulmonary vascular disease.

The surgical repair of this lesion is based on whether there can be a biventricular or univentricular repair. A balanced atrioventricular septal defect with two adequate ventricles should be completely repaired in infancy prior to any evidence of fixed pulmonary vascular obstructive disease, ideally by 6 months of age. Patients with fixed pulmonary vascular obstructive disease are not candidates for surgical repair, therefore patients over the age of 9–12 months who exhibit clinical findings of increased pulmonary vascular resistance should be studied extensively to evaluate the effects of vasodilatory maneuvers and to rule out treatable causes such as upper airway obstruction. If there are complicating factors and a complete repair cannot be done, then pulmonary arterial banding is indicated to protect the lungs from unrestricted pulmonary blood flow. The exact anatomy and levels of obstruction will dictate the sequence of palliative operations.

Echocardiography is an important diagnostic tool for the preoperative assessment of atrioventricular septal defects. Two-dimensional imaging defines atrioventricular valve morphology. If the superior bridging leaflet (SBL) is divided and has attachments to the crest of the ventricular septum, it is considered a type A valve. Straddling of central SBL attachments to a papillary muscle in the right ventricle defines a type B valve. If there are no attachments of the SBL to the crest of the interventricular septum and the valve leaflet is free floating, it is considered a type C valve. The septal attachments of the SBL can obstruct the ventricular septal defect and restrict shunting or may cross the left ventricular outflow tract and cause obstruction to aortic blood flow. Anterolateral papillary muscle insertions tend to be rotated counterclockwise in atrioventricular septal de-

fects and sit in much closer proximity to the posteromedial papillary muscle, which may create a "parachute"-like deformity of the left portion of the atrioventricular valve if the superior and inferior leaflets are sutured to any significant length, creating stenosis. It is not uncommon in the intermediate form of atrioventricular septal defect to find shortened and immobile leaflets with thick, chordal attachments limiting the ability to properly fashion a functioning atrioventricular valve. This insufficiency of valvular tissue can sometimes be anticipated by echocardiographic findings.

Color, continuous wave, and pulsed Doppler echocardiography can assess potential gradients across the outflow tracts and show the direction of shunting across the septal defect. Color Doppler interrogation of the atrioventricular valve usually reveals some degree of insufficiency. A double orifice mitral valve can occur in approximately 5% of atrioventricular septal defects and can be identified by echocardiography. The usual ostium primum atrial septal defect can be well visualized with two-dimensional echocardiography. The ventricular septal defect component of atrioventricular septal defects is usually single and in the inlet position (Fig. 57–3). Multiple defects can be ruled out with close color Doppler interrogation of the septum.

Typically the left ventricular inlet is shortened and the left ventricular outflow tract is elongated in patients with atrioventricular septal defect. The outflow tract has potential for obstruction from several sources. These can be evaluated with echocardiography and/or cardiac catheterization. At catheterization, pulmonary vascular resistance can be calculated. With unbalanced atrioventricular septal defects, the volumes of the ventricles can be determined to help assess the feasibility of biventricular repair. The ventricular septum can be seen using angiography in the long axis oblique projection to evaluate for multiple defects. The hepatoclavicular projection can demonstrate the posterior/inlet position of the atrioventricular septal defect well.

Coarctation of the Aorta

Guidelines for preoperative evaluation:

I. Anatomy: Location of coarctation
   A. Juxtaductal
   B. Preductal
   C. Postductal
II. Severity of obstruction
   A. Aortic atresia
   B. Hemodynamically significant
   C. Insignificant
III. Associated lesions
   A. Ventricular septal defects
   B. Patent ductus arteriosus
   C. Bicuspid aortic valve
   D. Subaortic stenosis
   E. Mitral valve anomalies

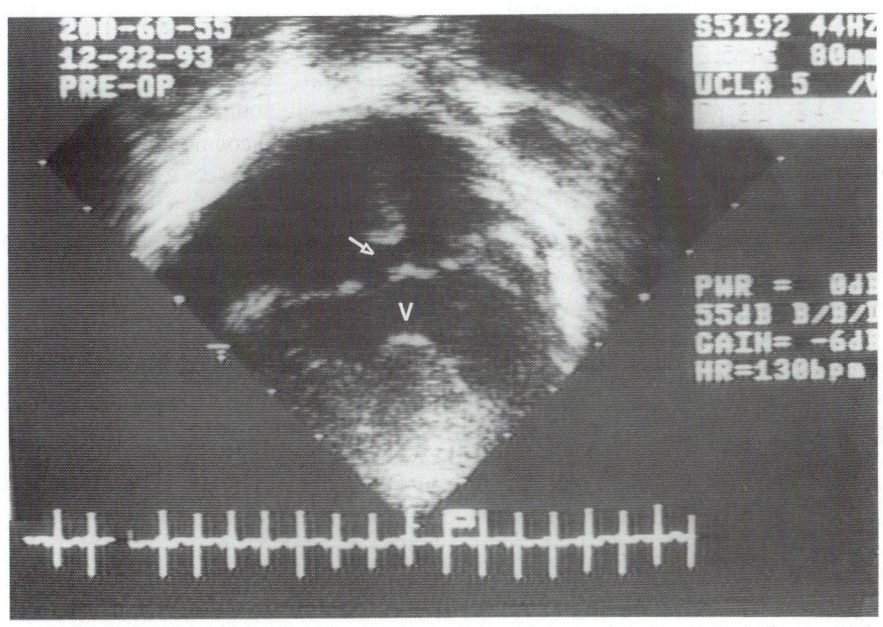

Figure 57–3. Apical four-chamber view of a patient with complete atrioventricular septal defect. An ostium primum atrial septal defect (arrow) and inlet ventricular septal defect (V) are seen. The relative portions of valve tissue overlying each ventricle are equal, indicating a balanced defect. There is unlikely to be inlet stenosis with complete surgical repair in this situation.

Coarctation of the aorta is characterized by a ledge along the outer curvature of the aorta, at the level of the ductus arteriosus. The narrowing causes a pressure gradient across the area. The presence of a patent ductus arteriosus usually abolishes this gradient, so the lesion is not usually diagnosed until the ductus closes.[6] A wide range of symptoms can be seen from moderate congestive heart failure to shock, depending upon the severity of the narrowing. If cardiac output is adequate, differential pulses and blood pressures may be noted between the upper and lower extremities. A late systolic ejection murmur may be heard in the interscapular area. With severe coarctation, no cardiac murmurs may be noted. Metabolic acidosis, upper extremity hypertension, and/or renal failure can be seen. Medical management is aimed toward improving the lower body perfusion by reopening the ductus arteriosus with prostaglandins.

The timing and technique of surgical repair for coarctation of the aorta are dictated by the severity of the coarctation, the adequacy of left ventricular compensation, and the presence of a ventricular septal defect or other associated anomalies. Simple coarctation without ventricular septal defect can be definitively addressed in different ways: resection of the area with end-to-end anastamosis, subclavian flap angioplasty, or patch aortoplasty. The anatomy of the distal transverse arch is important to the choice of surgical approach, therefore the initial echocardiogram is focused on the complete delineation of the aortic arch and branches in addition to the intracardiac anatomy.

The presence of a ventricular septal defect may alter the plan of repair. If the patient is stable, a definitive repair may be elected with concomitant closure of the ventricular septal defect. Complex lesions such as left ventricular inlet or outlet obstruction associated with coarctation and ventricular septal defect or significant left ventricular dysfunction may preclude complete repair of all associated lesions. In these cases, coarctation repair with pulmonary artery banding may be chosen as the initial palliation.

Associated anomalies may need to be addressed at the time of surgery, for example, other left-sided obstructive lesions. Shone's syndrome is a complex form of left heart obstructive lesions including coarctation of the aorta, supravalvar mitral ring, parachute mitral valve, and/or subaortic stenosis.

Echocardiography can be valuable in making the diagnosis of coarctation of the aorta.[7,8] The characteristic posterior ledge can be identified with two-dimensional imaging, but may be difficult to appreciate when the ductus arteriosus is patent[9] (Fig. 57–4). If a gradient is present at the time of the examination, a high-velocity jet will be present at the coarctation site. At the distal transverse arch, there is diastolic as well as systolic forward flow. Damped pulsatile flow is seen distal to the coarctation. There is often some degree of hypoplasia of the distal transverse aortic arch. Coarctation of the aorta can usually be distinguished from interrupted aortic arch by two-dimensional echocardiography (Fig. 57–5), but in the presence of ambiguous findings, angiography may be necessary. The presence and size of the ventricular septal defect can be well defined with echocardiography. Bicuspid aortic valve and mitral valve abnormalities can be closely interrogated by two-dimensional imaging, color flow, and pulsed Doppler probing. Finally, left ventricular outflow tract obstruction, as with ventricular septal defects with posterior infundibular malalignment, can be seen as well as other forms of subaortic obstruction.

Physical examination, chest radiographs, and the echocardiogram provide sufficient diagnostic information

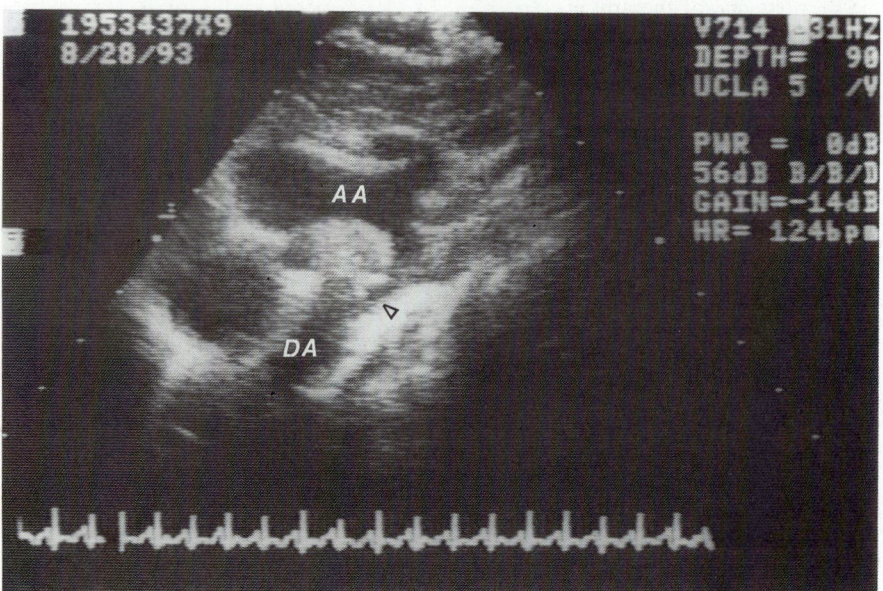

Figure 57–4. Suprasternal notch view of the aortic arch demonstrates a discrete narrowing at the site of coarctation (arrow) (AA, ascending aorta; DA, descending aorta).

for surgery without angiography in the majority of patients with coarctation of the aorta. Magnetic resonance imaging (MRI) also provides exquisite imaging of the aorta, but is subject to the problems of any "slice" imaging modality when the aorta is tortuous. Three-dimensional reconstruction MRI provides outstanding images and appreciation of spatial relationships, but the technique is not universally available and not currently well adapted for small and tachypneic infants.

Cardiac catheterization can further define the aortic anatomy and allow for direct pressure measurements at the coarctation site and is indicated whenever a diagnostic question is unanswered or there is conflicting data follow-ing a thorough physical examination and noninvasive testing. Contrast injection proximal to the coarctation or a descending aortogram with balloon occlusion in the left and right anterior oblique projection displays the position of the coarcted segment, the caliber of the distal transverse arch, and the relationship between the coarctation and the brachiocephalic vessels.

Semilunar Valve Stenosis

In general, semilunar valve stenosis is not considered a surgical problem. Intervention in the cardiac catheterization laboratory with percutaneous balloon valvuloplasty tends to

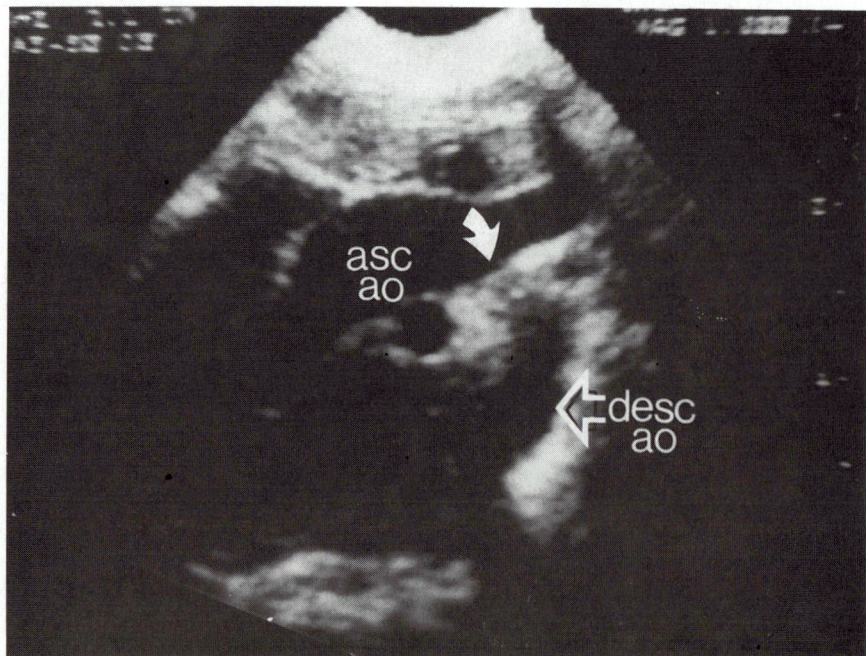

Figure 57–5. Suprasternal notch view of the aortic arch in a patient with interrupted aortic arch showing discontinuity (arrow) between the ascending aorta (asc ao) and descending aorta (desc ao) just distal to the takeoff of the first brachiocephalic branch.

be the first line of therapy in these patients. If the valve is found to be significantly dysplastic, then balloon valvuloplasty tends not to be as effective and surgery may be needed.

Anomalous Origin of the Left Coronary Artery

Guidelines for preoperative evaluation:

I. Coronary artery anatomy
II. Coronary collateral circulation
III. Left ventricular function
IV. Mitral valvular insufficiency

Anomalous origin of the left coronary artery from the pulmonary artery is usually undetectable until the pulmonary vascular resistance falls. With this event, flow in the left coronary artery will decrease, resulting in inadequate myocardial perfusion.[10] Shunting from the right coronary artery to the left coronary artery (via collateral circulation) to the main pulmonary artery may occur. The lower resistance of the pulmonary circulation may create a "steal" effect from the myocardium. In some cases, this is asymptomatic. In others, congestive heart failure from ventricular dysfunction may occur or acute coronary insufficiency may result in myocardial infarction, papillary muscle dysfunction, and mitral insufficiency. A later complication of left ventricular aneurysm formation may occur. On physical ex-

amination, a gallop rhythm is present and a blowing murmur of mitral insufficiency may be heard in some patients. The electrocardiogram shows a repolarization abnormality or frank anteroseptal myocardial infarction (Fig. 57–6). Chest x-ray reveals cardiac enlargement and pulmonary edema. This lesion must be differentiated from myocarditis or dilated cardiomyopathy.

Echocardiography demonstrates a dilated and poorly contractile left ventricle with areas of segmental wall motion abnormalities. Two dimensional interrogation of the coronary arteries must avoid the deception caused by the anomalous left coronary artery passing close to the left sinus of Valsalva of the aorta and appearing to arise from it. Once pulmonary vascular resistance has dropped, color and pulsed Doppler may demonstrate flow from the left coronary artery to the main pulmonary artery.

Cardiac catheterization is primarily indicated to precisely define the coronary anatomy when this diagnosis is suspected and in any infant presenting in congestive heart failure with dilated cardiomyopathy in whom the echocardiogram does not show anterograde flow in the left main coronary artery and proximal branches. Ascending aortic angiography can demonstrate retrograde flow from the right coronary artery through coronary collateral vessels to the left coronary artery and pulmonary artery (Fig. 57–7). The origin of the left coronary artery can often be demonstrated by a main pulmonary artery cineangiocardiogram. Any evidence of mitral regurgitation can be inves-

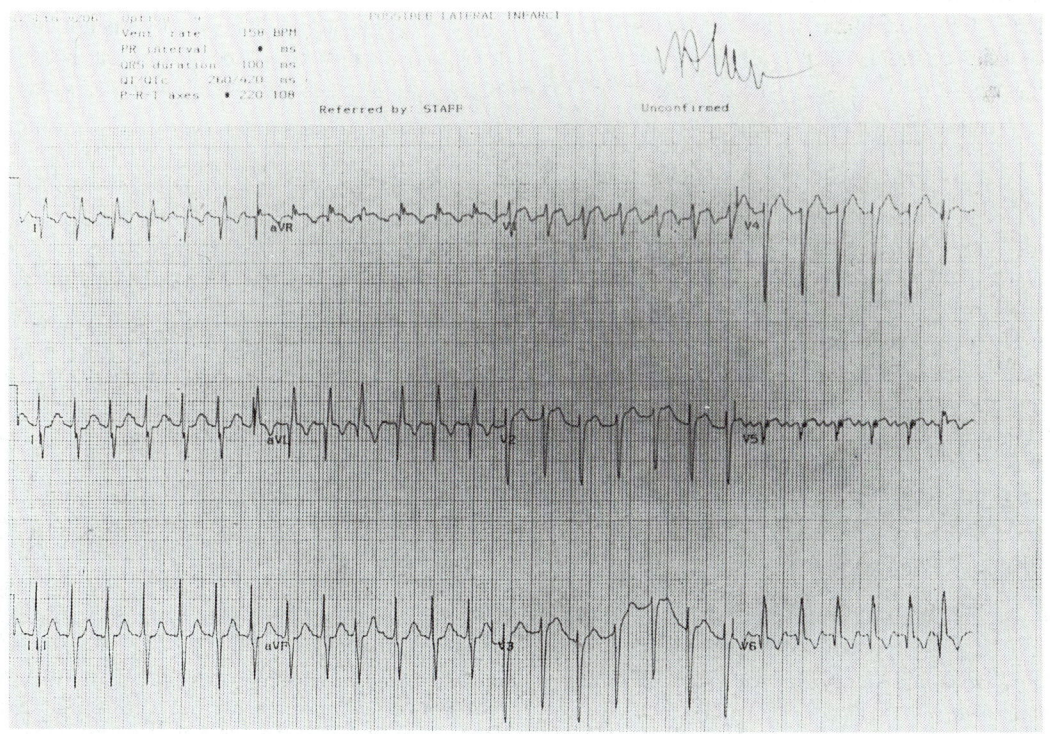

Figure 57–6. Electrocardiogram of a patient with anomalous origin of the left coronary artery. Note deep Q waves and inverted T waves in lead I, AVL, and the left precordial leads typically seen with this lesion.

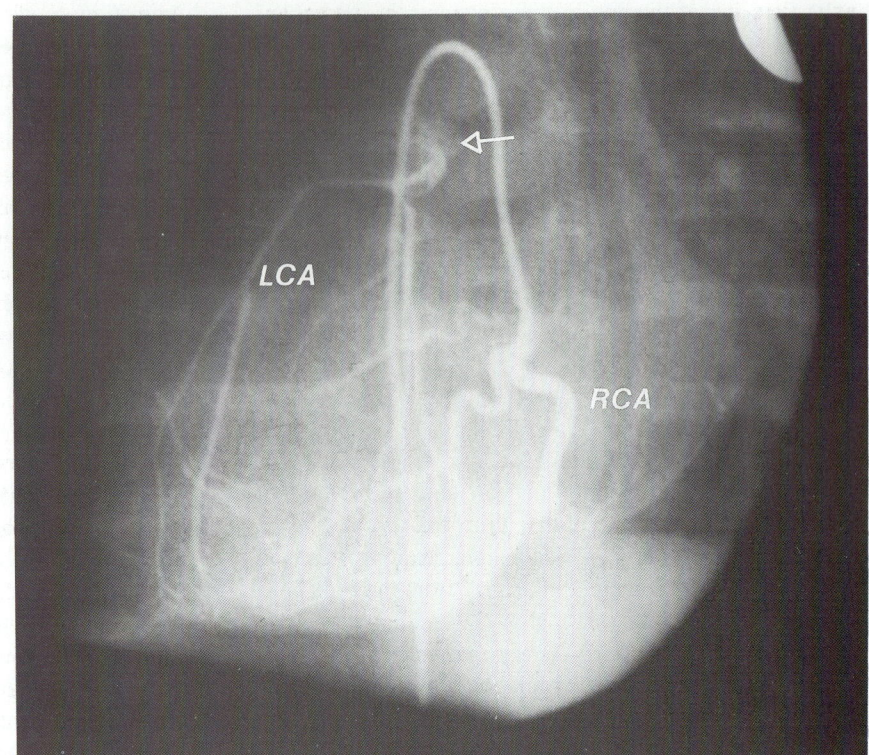

Figure 57–7. Lateral cineangiocardiogram of a patient with anomalous origin of the left coronary artery. A catheter is in the right coronary artery (RCA) and contrast is seen filling the left coronary artery (LCA) and a blush is seen in the pulmonary artery (arrow).

tigated and left ventricular function quantitated by a left ventriculogram.

CYANOTIC LESIONS

Transposition of the Great Arteries

Guidelines for preoperative evaluation:

I. Anatomy
  A. Vessel orientation: D-Transposition of the great arteries
  B. Coronary artery anatomy
  C. Associated lesions
    1. Ventricular septal defect
    2. Outflow tract obstruction
    3. Mitral/tricuspid anomalies
    4. Aortic arch anomalies
II. Hemodynamics
  A. Subaortic and subpulmonic obstruction
  B. Left ventricular volume, pressure, and mass
  C. Favorable/unfavorable streaming

Complete transposition of the great arteries (D-TGA) typically presents in the first hours of life with hypoxia in the absence of respiratory distress. Occasionally, there may be successful mixing due to left-to-right shunting at the foramen ovale and aorta to pulmonary shunting at the ductus arteriosus, so that cyanosis is not detected until spontaneous closure of the ductus occurs. As hypoxia pro-

gresses, hyperpnea becomes more evident and metabolic acidosis ensues. The clinical examination may be nonspecific, with only a loud single second heart sound noted, due to the anterior position of the aorta. A murmur may not be heard. On chest x-ray, a narrow mediastinum is usually seen, but this may be obscured by thymus early in the neonatal period. Initially pulmonary vascular markings are normal, but as the pulmonary vascular resistance falls the radiograph reveals pulmonary overcirculation (Fig. 57–8).

The initial management of transposition of the great arteries is aimed to ensure adequate pulmonary and systemic mixing. Prostaglandin is infused to maintain ductal patency. With a restrictive ventricular septal defect or intact ventricular septum, balloon atrial septostomy may be performed to increase mixing. Initial diagnostic work-up is therefore aimed at establishing the candidacy for early repair versus palliation and determining the adequacy of shunting or mixing at the atrial and ductal levels. The arterial switch operation for simple transposition is usually undertaken in the neonatal period prior to or soon after the normal fall in pulmonary vascular resistance. This will prevent a decrease in left ventricular mass, which would render the ventricle unable to support the systemic circulation. For this reason, in patients greater than 2–3 weeks of age with transposition and intact ventricular septum, it is important to direct echocardiographic study toward assessment of left ventricular pressure and mass.

In simple transposition of the great arteries, the arterial switch operation will require reimplantation of the coronary

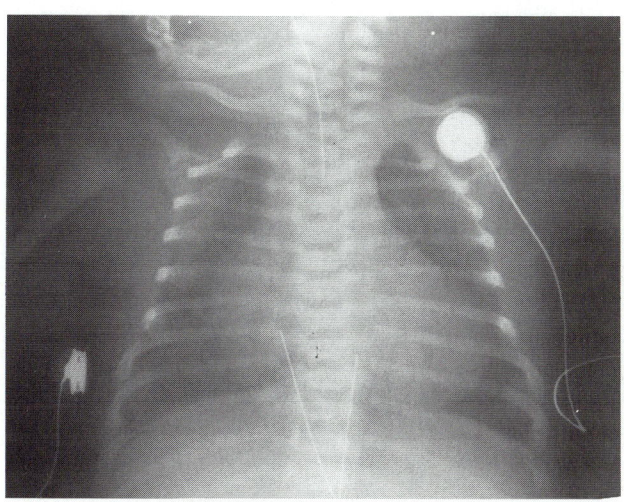

Figure 57–8. Chest radiograph demonstrating cardiomegaly, narrowed vascular pedicle, and increased pulmonary vascular marking typical of transposition of the great arteries.

arteries to the neoaorta. Rarely, the coronary anatomy may be unfavorable to reimplantation due to an intramural location or specific characteristics that may cause stretching or kinking of the vessel. In these cases an intra-atrial repair (venous switch) will be necessary.

In the presence of left ventricular outflow tract obstruction (LVOTO), an arterial switch may not be feasible. If the LVOTO can be successfully resected, then an attempt at a switch can be made. If the obstruction cannot be alleviated and the patient has a large ventricular septal defect, a Rastelli operation should be considered. This would entail tunneling through the septal defect from the left ventricle to the more anterior aorta with placement of a conduit from the right ventricle to the pulmonary artery. It is important, therefore, to completely define the size and position of ven-

tricular septal defects and the boundaries of the right and left ventricular outflow tracts.

Echocardiography can provide a definitive diagnosis by demonstrating the origin of the aorta from the right ventricle and the pulmonary artery from the left ventricle.[11] The size of the interatrial communication can be determined with cross-sectional imaging. The origins of the coronary arteries are usually clearly displayed by echocardiography, but considerable experience is needed to confidently define the branching patterns.[12–16] Pulsed and color flow Doppler will identify a patent ductus arteriosus and delineate the magnitude of shunting at the atrial and ventricular level. Ventricular mass and volumes can be quantitated with both two-dimensional and M-mode echocardiography. The shape of the interventricular septum in systole gives an indication of the differential pressures between the right and left ventricles, since the septum will bow toward the chamber with the least wall stress. Additionally, the left ventricular outflow tract can be closely interrogated for signs of obstruction (Fig. 57–9).

Cardiac catheterization may be used to complement echocardiography in the assessment of transposition of the great arteries. Biplane cineangiography of the aortic root in the left axial oblique and right anterior oblique projections with caudal angulation will help define the coronary artery anatomy. The imaging may be enhanced with balloon occlusion (Fig. 57–10). If further questions persist then selective injections into the coronaries should be considered (Fig. 57–11). Additionally, left ventricular angiography in the long axis oblique projection may be indicated to localize additional septal defects as well as to outline the left ventricular outflow area in cases of obstruction. Left ventricular pressure may be obtained directly during catheterization and left ventricular mass can be determined. If a diagnostic cardiac catheterization is not necessary, balloon atrial septostomy, if indicated, can be performed either in

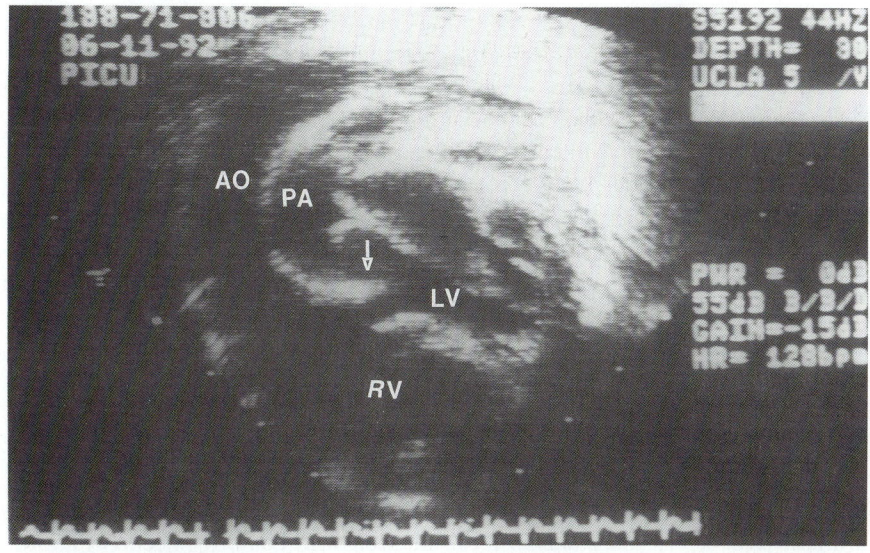

Figure 57–9. Subxiphoid short axis view of a patient with transposition of the great arteries and ventricular septal defect, with a posteriorly deviated infundibular septum (arrow) obstructing the left ventricular outflow tract. (LV, left ventricle; RV, right ventricle; PA, pulmonary artery; AO, aorta).

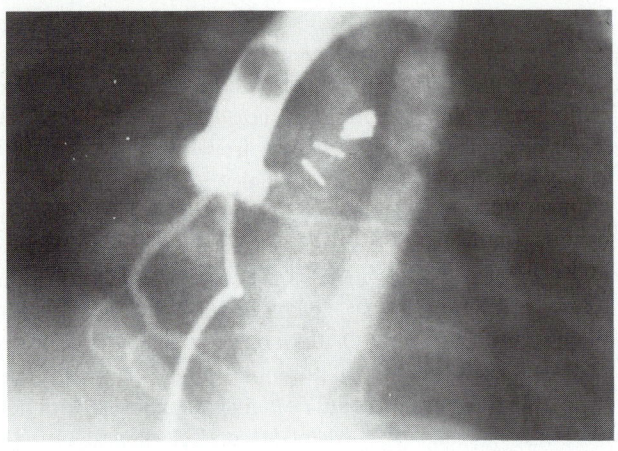

A

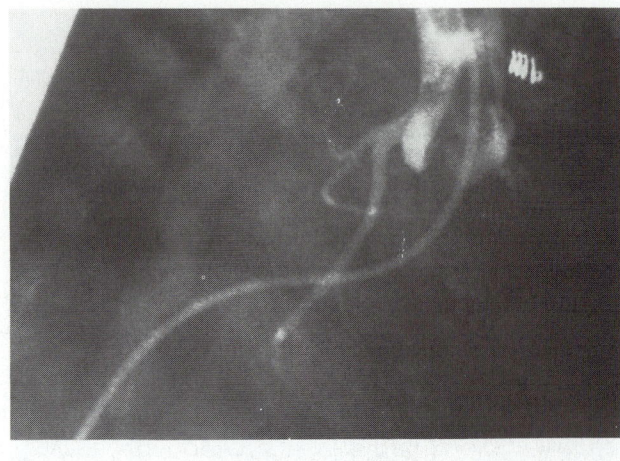

B

Figure 57–10. A, B. Balloon occlusion injection into the proximal ascending aorta of a child with transposition of the great arteries. Although both coronary systems are visualized, there is poor definition of the coronary ostia and proximal branching.

the catheterization laboratory or under echocardiographic guidance at the bedside.

Tetralogy of Fallot and Pulmonary Atresia with Ventricular Septal Defect

Guidelines for preoperative evaluation:

I. Right ventricular outflow tract obstruction
II. Pulmonary valve annulus size
III. Main pulmonary artery/branch pulmonary artery anatomy
   A. Size and continuity of main pulmonary artery and branches
   B. Collateral supply to each pulmonary segment (aortopulmonary, intercostal, and bronchial collaterals)
IV. Location, size, and number of ventricular septal defects
V. Coronary artery anatomy
VI. Aortic arch anatomy

The pathology of tetralogy of Fallot includes right ventricular outflow tract obstruction, a nonrestrictive ventricular septal defect with anterior malalignment of the infundibular septum, and an overriding aorta. Depending on the severity of the right ventricular outflow tract obstruction, these patients may present in the early neonatal period with severe hypoxemia after closure of the ductus arteriosus or later in infancy with progressive cyanosis. The intensity of the murmur correlates inversely with the amount of obstruction as the pressure gradient across the right ventricular outflow tract increases. A loud, harsh, midsystolic murmur with increased right ventricular impulse is typical of tetralogy of Fallot with moderate right ventricular outflow obstruction. When the obstruction is so severe that little or no flow crosses the right ventricular outflow tract, a soft, short murmur or no murmur may be heard. On chest x-ray, the heart is small with an upturned apex and a diminished or

concave main pulmonary artery segment ("boot-shaped heart") (Fig. 57–12).

The structures that need to be delineated prior to intervention include (1) the levels and severity of right ventricular outflow tract obstruction, (2) pulmonary valve annulus size, (3) main and branch pulmonary artery size, (4) ventricular septal defect (single vs. multiple), (5) origin of the left anterior descending coronary artery, (6) aortopulmonary collaterals, and (7) aortic arch anatomy. Most of these structures may be well visualized with echocardiography so that many infants do not need to undergo catheterization prior to repair of tetralogy of Fallot with a patent main pulmonary artery and continuity between the branches[17] (Fig. 57–13). The right ventricular outflow tract can be seen using a combination of echocardiographic planes[18] (Fig. 57–14). The diameter of the pulmonary valve annulus and the proximal pulmonary arteries can be measured from parasternal, subxiphoid, and suprasternal views. Close interrogation of the ventricular septum using both color flow and pulse Doppler techniques can reveal any additional septal defects, which are seen with greatest frequency in patients under 1 year of age. Both origins and proximal branches of the right and left coronary arteries must be visualized because the origin of the left anterior descending coronary from the right coronary or a prominent conal branch is an infrequent association that may significantly influence the surgical management of the right ventricular outflow tract in patients in whom an outflow patch may be required[19-21] (Fig. 57–15). There is an increased incidence of right aortic arch seen in patients with tetralogy of Fallot, and this should be noted prior to any staged shunt operation by a combination of plain chest radiography and echocardiography.

Cardiac angiography can elucidate any questions still remaining after echocardiographic examination. The coronary anatomy can be seen with contrast injection into the

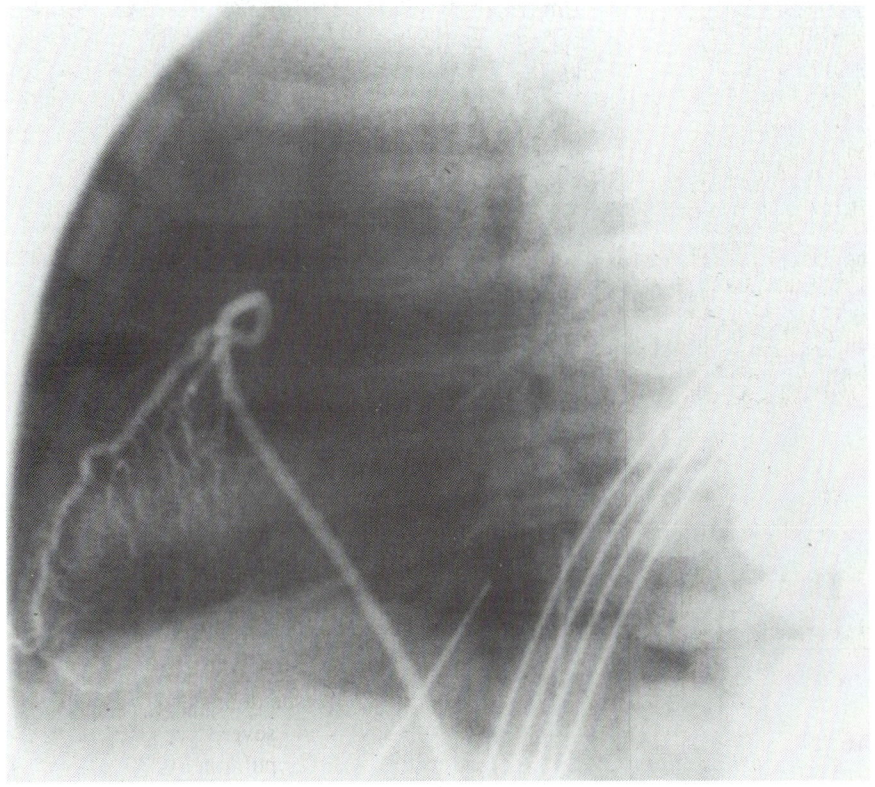

A

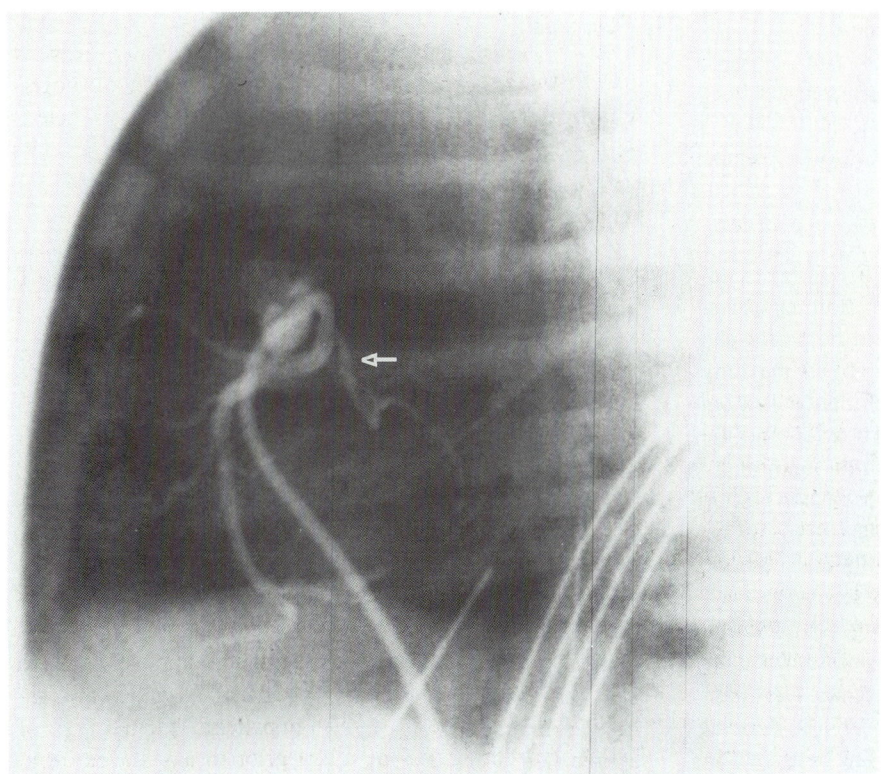

B

Figure 57–11. **A.** Selective left coronary artery injection filmed in the lateral view of a patient with transposition of the great arteries, demonstrating the left anterior descending artery as the sole branch. **B.** Selective right coronary artery injection in the same patient. A dominant right coronary system is seen arising posteriorly with the circumflex artery (arrow) branching very proximal to the coronary ostia.

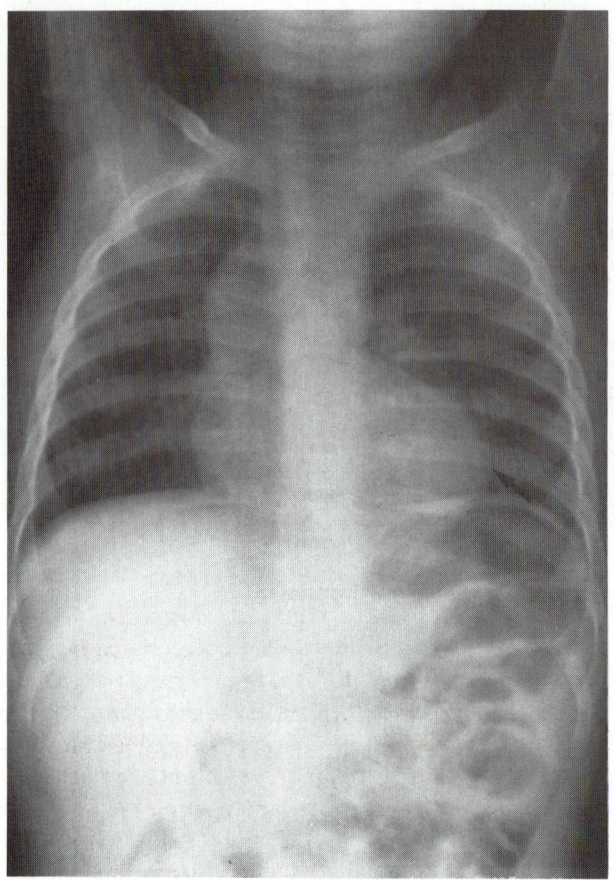

Figure 57–12. Typical radiographic findings in an infant with tetralogy of Fallot. The lung fields are oligemic. There is a prominent ascending aorta and absent pulmonary artery segment. The apex is typically upturned ("boot-shaped heart") (arrow).

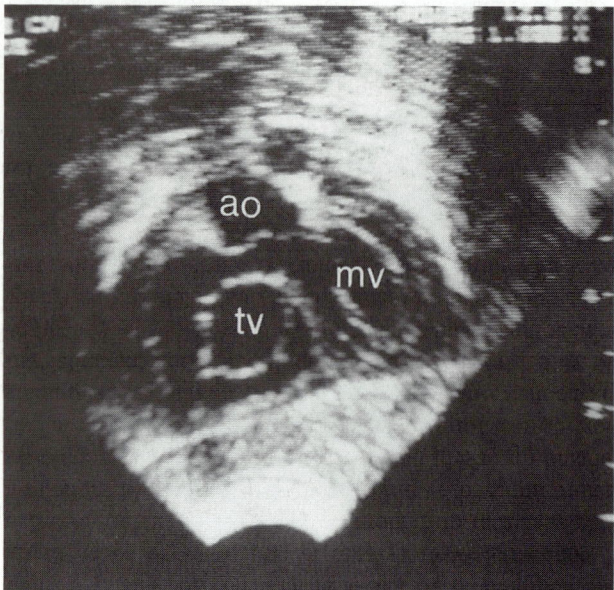

Figure 57–13. Subxiphoid view of a patient with tetralogy of Fallot demonstrates the aortic root (ao) overriding the interventricular septum. The orifices of the tricuspid (tv) and mitral (mv) are seen in cross section. The interventricular septum lies between these two structures.

aortic root using balloon occlusion in the left and right anterior oblique projections with caudal angulation. If necessary, selective coronary angiography should be performed for optimal definition. A left ventriculogram in the long axis oblique projection will define the ventricular septum and additional septal defects, if present. To determine the presence or absence of collateral arteries to the pulmonary bed, a descending aortogram with balloon occlusion can be performed (Fig. 57–16). If significant collateral vessels are demonstrated, coil embolization of the collaterals can be performed by retrograde entry into these vessels.

To assess growth of the pulmonary arteries in whom a shunt operation was performed, catheterization should be considered 3–6 months' post-palliation. Because the main and branch pulmonary arteries lie in a nearly horizontal plane, perpendicular to the sternum, they are best seen in the hepatoclavicular views (Fig. 57–17). By directly measuring the diameter of the branch pulmonary arteries at the takeoff of their lobar segments, adding them together, and dividing by the diameter of the descending aorta at the level of the diaphragm, a ratio can be calculated to predict right

ventricular to left ventricular pressure ratio following complete repair.[22]

Pulmonary Atresia with Intact Septum

Guidelines for preoperative evaluation:

I. Coronary artery anatomy
II. Right ventricular sinusoids to coronary artery connections
IV. Tricuspid valve size and structure
IV. Right ventricular volume, inflow and outflow length, outflow tract diameter
V. Interatrial communication
VI. Aortopulmonary collaterals

Patients with pulmonary atresia and intact ventricular septum (PA/IVS) present in the newborn period with cyanosis secondary to severe obstruction to pulmonary blood flow. Sudden increases in cyanosis may occur with the closing of the ductus arteriosus. The clinical examination is nonspecific: cyanosis without respiratory distress and little or no murmur. The lack of a normal right ventricular impulse at the lower left sternal border may be appreciated.

Surgical management of these patients is influenced by the presence or absence of right ventricular sinusoids to coronary artery fistulas (ventriculocoronary communications), coronary artery stenoses, tricuspid valve size, and the volume and morphology of the right ventricle. Right

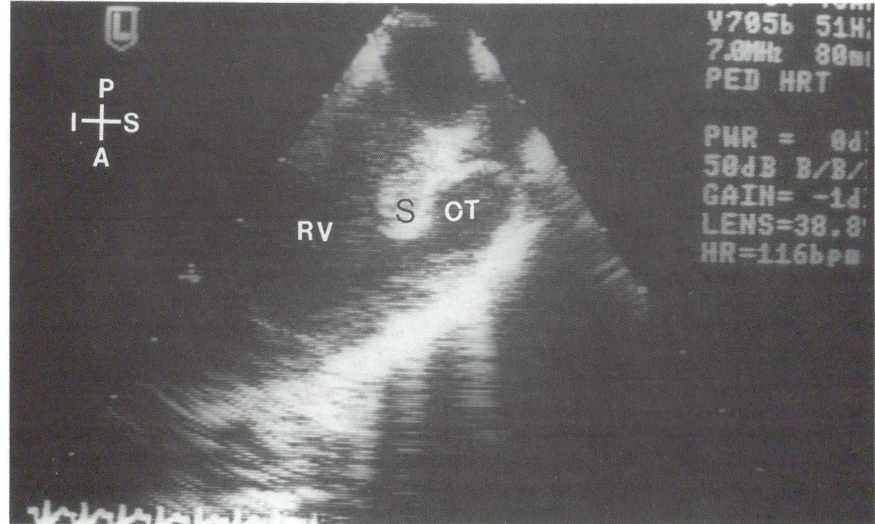

Figure 57–14. Transesophageal longitudinal view of the right ventricle (RV) and outflow tract (OT). The anterior deviation of infundibular septum (black S) is seen obstructing the right ventricular outflow tract which is characteristic of tetralogy of Fallot (S, superior; I, inferior; A, anterior; P, posterior).

ventricular to coronary fistulas in association with systemic or suprasystemic right ventricular pressures can result in right ventricular dependent coronary circulation.[23–25] Decompression of such a right ventricle to less than systemic levels may lead to coronary artery/myocardial steal with resultant ischemia. If right ventricular decompression cannot safely be achieved or if the right ventricle is severely hypoplastic, the surgical plan is altered toward a single ventricle-type palliation. If decompression can be achieved without compromise of the coronary circulation, and the tricusipid valve and right ventricular size are adequate, then the eventual repair should be biventricular. The staging procedures prior to the final repair will vary with the latter two variables.

An initial echocardiographic examination of these patients will yield much useful information by defining the principal anatomy, including the level of the right ventricular outflow tract obstruction and the right ventricular morphology identifying the three ventricular components: inlet, outlet, and trabecular.[26] The nature of the interatrial communication must be defined in order to rule out present or potential restriction to essential right-to-left shunting. Subxiphoid views of the interatrial septum demonstrate the size and position of the foramen ovale or septal defect. The flap valve of the foramen ovale is usually deviated toward the left atrium, but moves back and forth during the cardiac cycle unless there is an obstructive communication. The flow dynamics across the atrial septum can be further de-

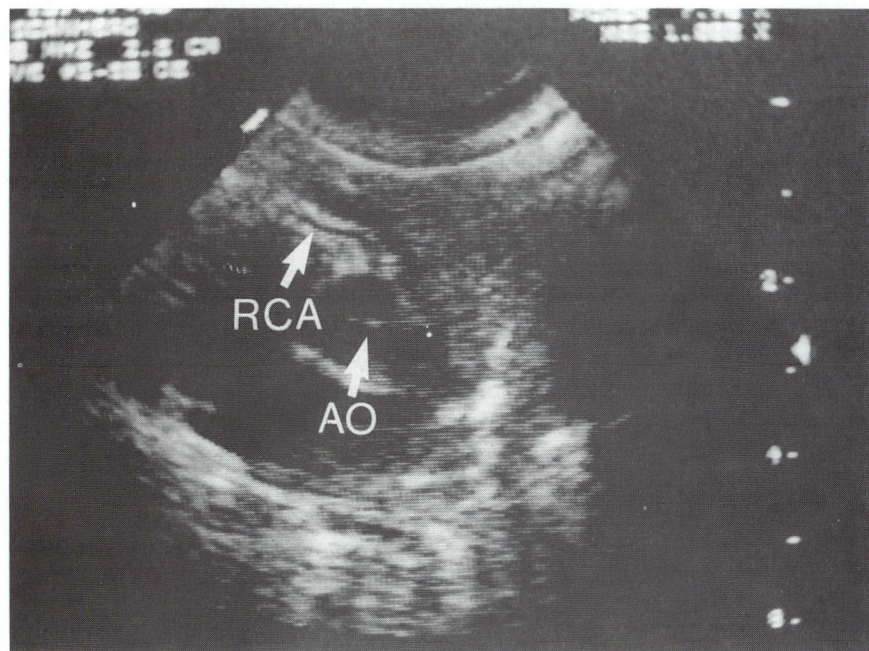

Figure 57–15. Parasternal short axis view of the aortic root in a patient with tetralogy of Fallot demonstrates the course of the right coronary artery (RCA), coursing from the aorta (AO) toward the atrioventricular groove without giving off major branches.

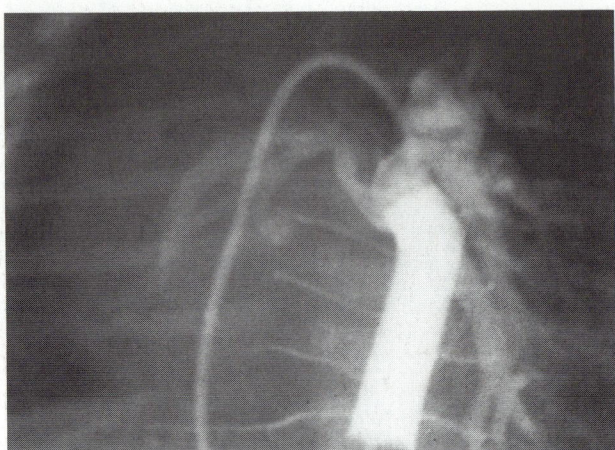

Figure 57–16. Anteroposterolateral projection of a balloon occlusion study in the descending aorta of a 3-wk-old female with tetralogy of Fallot and pulmonary atresia. There is filling of several large bronchial collateral vessels to both lungs. This patient required surgical banding of these collaterals to limit pulmonary blood flow and control intractable congestive heart failure.

fined by color flow and pulsed wave Doppler. The presence of nonpulsatile flow with a velocity in the range of 2 m/s is strongly suggestive of obstructive atrial communication, especially in the presence of hepatomegaly and low output state.

The tricuspid valve annulus size can be obtained and a Z-score calculated for comparison to normal[27] (Fig. 57–18). Pulmonary annulus and main pulmonary artery size can be measured by cross-sectional imaging from the parasternal and subxiphoid views. Suprasystemic right ventricular pressure, if present, may be indicated by systolic bulging of the

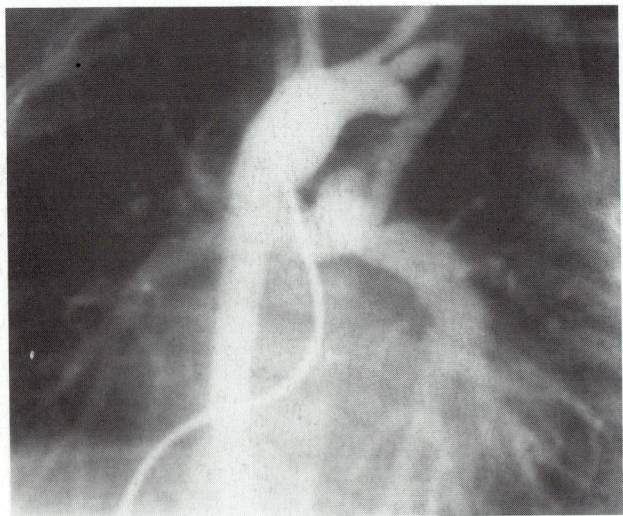

Figure 57–17. A 6-mo-old female with tetralogy of Fallot, right aortic arch, and pulmonary atresia, s/p left modified Blalock–Taussig shunt. There is mild narrowing of the left pulmonary artery at its anastomosis with the shunt.

interventricular septum into the left ventricle and by Doppler pressure assessment of tricuspid regurgitation.

Serial evaluation by echocardiography in the postoperative period is an essential monitoring tool in this patient population. Right ventricular function and growth can be evaluated and followed. In that coronary artery anomalies and stenoses are know to occur and progress in this lesion, evidence of hypokinetic or paradoxical segmental ventricular wall motion may indicate compromise of coronary perfusion. High frequency cross-sectional and color Doppler imaging can identify sinusoids in the right ventricular free wall and interventricular septum as well as demonstrate dilated coronary arteries. Pulsed Doppler and color M-mode can display the direction of flow in the sinusoids and coronary branches. To and fro flow in the coronary arteries denotes a connection between the coronary circulation and a suprasystemic right ventricle.

Cardiac catheterization in the newborn period is recommended to define the coronary artery anatomy and right ventricular sinusoids. Right ventricular and aortic root angiography will reveal sinusoidal communications between the right ventricle and coronary arteries and show any coronary stenoses (Fig. 57–19). Aortic root or selective coronary injections are required for definitive delineation of the coronary circulation (Fig. 57–20). Right ventricular pressure and volume measurements complement the echocardiographic findings. To define the presence of aortopulmonary collateral vessels, an angiogram in the descending aorta with balloon occlusion should be performed. Collateral arteries may also arise from the brachiocephalic vessels, so an injection into the transverse aortic arch or selectively in the subclavian arteries may be necessary.

After an initial palliative procedure, recatheterization is indicated to assess the adequacy of the initial intervention, to define the main and branch pulmonary artery anatomy and pressures, remeasure right ventricular volume and pressure, and obtain aortic oxygen saturation and pressure.

Anomalous Pulmonary Venous Return

Guidelines for preoperative evaluation:

I. Total anomalous pulmonary venous return
   A. Anatomy: Location of venous return
     1. Supracardiac
     2. Intracardiac
     3. Infradiaphragmatic
     4. Mixed
   B. Hemodynamics
     1. Obstructed
     2. Nonobstructed
II. Partial anomalous pulmonary venous return (PAPVR)
III. Associated lesions
   A. Atrial septal defect
   B. Patent ductus arteriosus

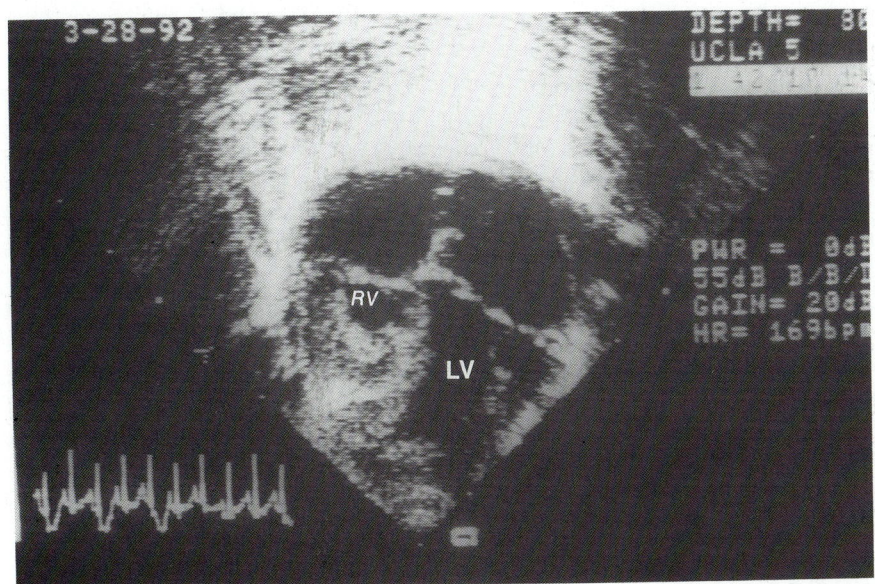

Figure 57–18. Apical four chamber view of a patient with pulmonary atresia and intact ventricular septum demonstrating relative right ventricle (RV) and left ventricle (LV) size. The size of the tricuspid valve annulus and mitral valve annulus can be measured in this view.

C. Asplenia/heterotaxy syndrome

D. Ventricular septal defect

In total anomalous pulmonary venous return, the pulmonary veins may drain to various sites of the systemic venous system or right atrium. Inflow to the left heart must then pass through the foramen ovale or atrial septal defect in such cases. The atrial communication is rarely obstructive in early life. The most common sites of drainage include (1) supracardiac drainage to the innominate or azygous vein through an ascending vertical vein (60–70%), (2) intracardiac drainage into the coronary sinus or right atrium (20–30%), and (3) infradiaphragmatic drainage into the in-

ferior vena cava, ductus venosus, hepatic veins, or portal system (10–12%). There may be mixed types of return seen (5%). Pulmonary venous obstruction, if present, usually occurs along the course of the vertical connecting vein as it ascends across a main stem bronchus or descends below the diaphragm or through the portal–caval venous system. Venous obstruction produces pulmonary edema and severe respiratory distress. This lesion may mimic respiratory distress syndrome and may be initially suspected when the expected clinical improvement does not occur within a few days of medical management. Severe obstruction produces such marked pulmonary vasoconstriction that right-to-left shunting occurs at the ductus arteriosus if patent. In such

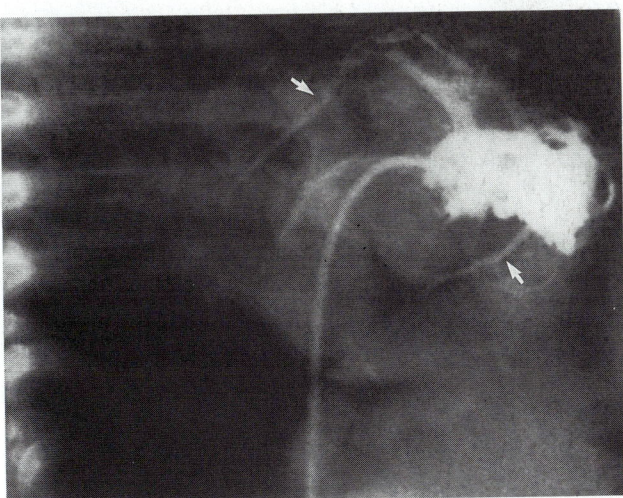

Figure 57–19. Lateral projection of an injection into the hypertensive right ventricle of a 6-mo-old with pulmonary atresia and intact ventricular septum, demonstrating a hypoplastic ventricle with fistulous communications with both right and left coronary artery systems (arrows). Minimal tricuspid regurgitation is noted.

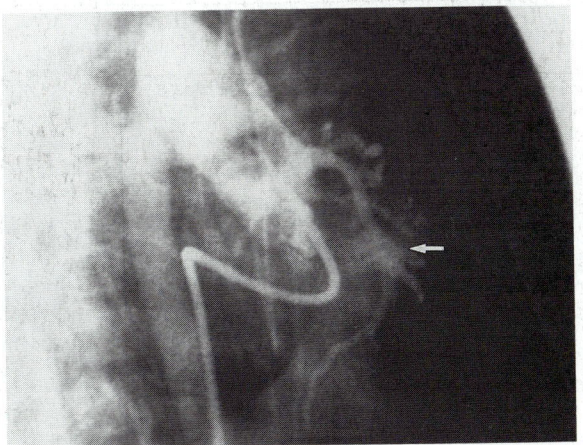

Figure 57–20. Balloon occlusion of the proximal ascending aorta demonstrating prominent right coronary artery with filling of an anterior right ventricle (arrow) via coronary artery fistulas in the same child with pulmonary atresia and intact ventricular septum.

patients, presentation is usually in the first hours of life with severe respiratory distress and acidosis. Depending on the degree of venous obstruction and the amount of pulmonary blood flow, cyanosis may vary from barely detectable to severe in patients with total anomalous pulmonary venous return.

Radiographic appearance of total anomalous pulmonary venous return with obstruction typically is that of a small to normal sized heart with pulmonary edema. If pulmonary return is to the superior vena cava, dilated veins in the superior mediastinum produce a "snowman" appearance (Fig. 57–21). With severe pulmonary vasoconstriction and right-to-left shunting at the ductus arteriosus, the pulmonary blood flow might look decreased.

Surgical repair of this lesion involves the connection of the common pulmonary venous channel to the left atrium, therefore it is important to note the position of the common pulmonary vein relative to the left atrium. If the left atrium or ventricle is somewhat small, an atrial septal defect or ascending vein may be left intact for decompression. It is important, therefore, to measure left atrial size and left ventricular volume.

Two-dimensional echocardiography has been shown to accurately delineate pulmonary venous anatomy[28] (Fig. 57–22). Color and pulsed Doppler examinations indicate the presence of obstruction. Turbulent nonpulsatile venous flow with a velocity equal to or greater than 2 m/s signifies hemodynamically significant obstruction. Definition of the intracardiac anatomy utilizing echocardiography will reveal that other significant congenital lesions occur approximately 30% of the time. These include patent ductus arteriosus, atrial isomerism, ventricular septal defect, single ventricle, transposition of the great arteries, and systemic venous anomalies. There is a strong association of total anomalous pulmonary venous return with complex congenital heart disease and asplenia.

Cardiac catheterization and angiography are employed in some institutions to confirm the echocardiographic findings. High oxygen saturations are found within the systemic veins at the site of the pulmonary venous connections and right atrium. The oxygen saturations in the four chambers rarely vary by more than 10%. Selective retrograde catheterization of the pulmonary venous channel is possible in some patients and may document the area of obstruction. Contrast agents are used sparingly, particularly in the case of pulmonary venous obstruction, because they are likely to worsen pulmonary vasoconstriction and edema.

Univentricular Hearts

Guidelines for preoperative evaluation:

I. Anatomy
    A. Visceral and atrial situs

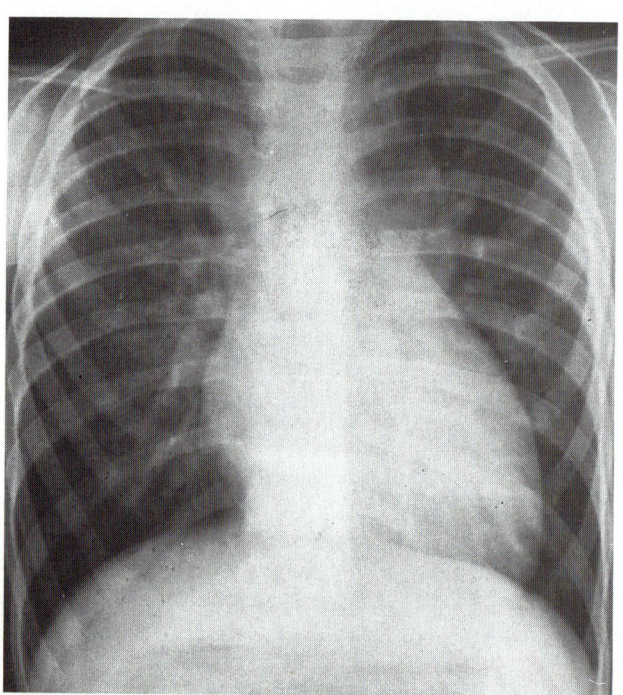

A

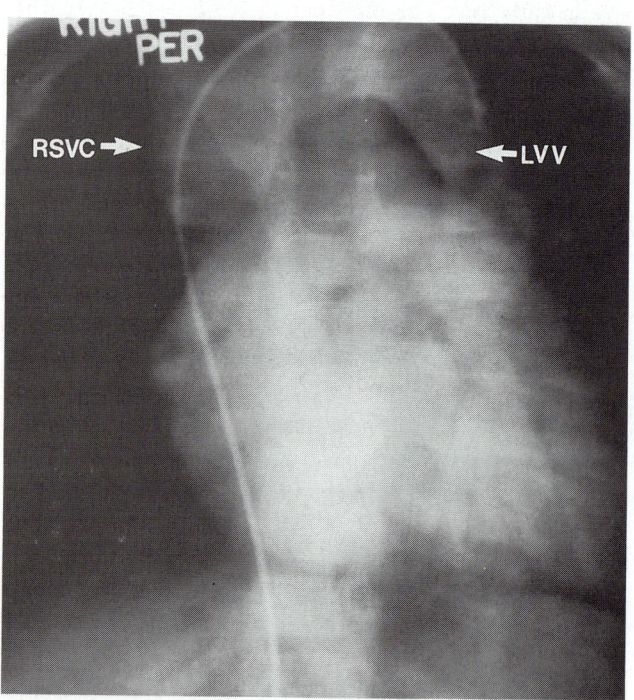

B

Figure 57–21. A. Classic "snowman" chest radiograph of a child with total anomalous pulmonary venous return to a vertical vein, left innominate vein, and dilated superior vena cava. **B.** Cineangiocardiogram obtained with the catheter in the left vertical vein (LVV) demonstrating the pulmonary venous return to a right superior vena cava (RSVC). Some retrograde filling of the pulmonary veins is seen.

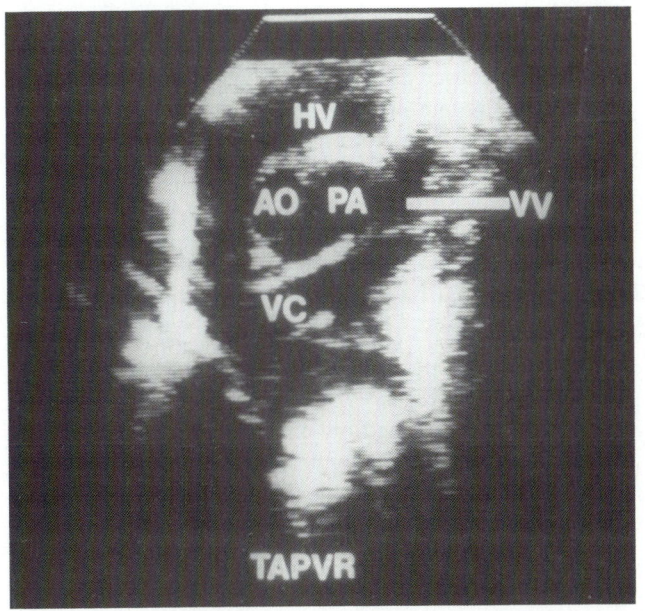

A

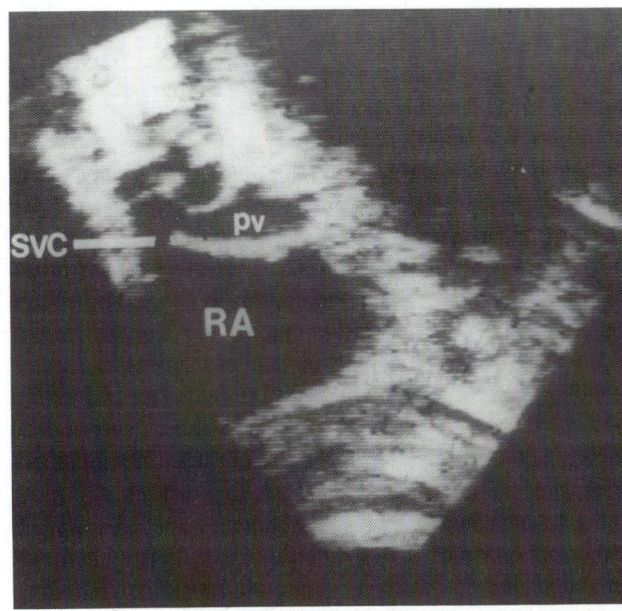

B

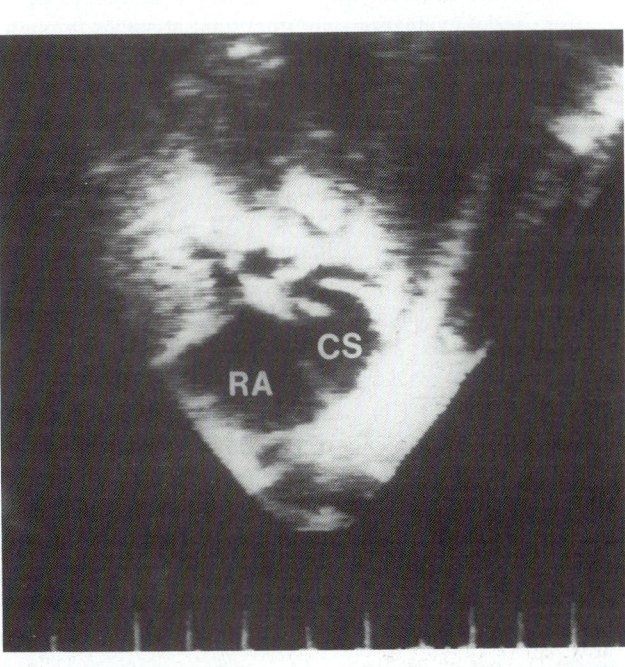

C

Figure 57–22. Types of total anomalous pulmonary venous return. **A.** Subxiphoid short axis view of a vertical vein (VV) draining to a horizontal vein (HV) which empties into the superior vena cava (VC) (AO, aorta; PA, pulmonary artery). **B.** Pulmonary veins (pv) seen connecting directly to the superior vena cava (SVC) (RA, right atrium). **C.** Subxiphoid long axis view demonstrating pulmonary veins entering a dilated coronary sinus (CS) (RA, right atrium).

B. Atrioventricular connection
  1. Tricuspid atresia
  2. Mitral atresia
  3. Double inlet
  4. Common atrioventricular valve
  5. Straddling valve
C. Ventricular morphology
  1. Right ventricle
  2. Left ventricle
  3. Biventricular: multiple ventricular septal defects
  4. Undifferentiated ventricular chamber

D. Ventriculoarterial connection
  1. Position of subarterial outlet chamber (hypoplastic ventricle or infundibulum)
  2. Patency, size, and gradient of subaortic and subpulmonic areas
  3. Position of great arteries relative to each other, the ventricles and the bulboventricular foramen or interventricular communication
E. Great arteries
  1. Presence of aortic coarctation or interrupted aortic arch

    2. Pulmonary artery branch stenosis or hypoplasia
II. Pulmonary circulation
    A. Sources of pulmonary blood flow
    B. Quantity of pulmonary blood flow
    C. Pulmonary vascular resistance
    D. Transpulmonary pressure gradient
III. Atrioventricular valve competence
IV. Ventricular function

The clinical presentation of patients with univentricular hearts is variable depending on the specific anatomy. With unrestricted pulmonary blood flow, tachypnea, respiratory distress, and other signs of congestive heart failure will dominate as the pulmonary vascular resistance drops. There will be little or no cyanosis noted. Patients with obstructed pulmonary blood flow may present with cyanosis and an outflow tract murmur. If there is atrioventricular valve obstruction, the exam will reflect both cyanosis and/or a low output state. Severe atrioventricular valve regurgitation will have characteristic auscultatory findings.

The ultimate goals of surgical repair of the univentricular heart are separation of the systemic and pulmonary circulations, decreasing the volume load on the ventricle, and preserving ventricular function. The path to achieving this goal varies with the specific cardiac lesion. Starting in the newborn period, palliation should be undertaken with a view toward a staged repair, with goals of maintaining low pulmonary arterial pressures and good ventricular function. The patients with excessive pulmonary blood flow benefit from pulmonary arterial banding as long as normal distal pulmonary pressure is documented postoperatively and the patient is followed carefully for signs of developing subaortic obstruction. This can be achieved by a combination of physical examination, chest radiography, and echocardiography.

Inadequate pulmonary blood flow in the neonatal period requires augmentation with a systemic to pulmonary shunt. These patients than need to be closely monitored for signs of increasing cyanosis, which may indicate decreasing pulmonary blood flow or pulmonary vascular obstructive disease. Patients with balanced pulmonary and systemic flow may receive a cavopulmonary shunt or Fontan procedure as their initial palliation.

The following key diagnostic points should be demonstrated during the course of medical and surgical management:

1. The nature and size of the interatrial communication should be known in all patients with right atrioventricular valve atresia or stenosis in whom a patent foramen ovale or atrial septal defect is the dominant pathway for right atrial outflow.
2. The course and connections of the pulmonary veins must be known and any obstruction evaluated. It is both important and difficult to pick up subtle signs of pulmonary venous obstruction in the face of diminished pulmonary blood flow.
3. The morphology and function of the atrioventricular

valves must be noted, particularly as they relate to the development of significant valvular regurgitation in the face of ventricular pressure and/or volume overload.
4. Ventricular morphology, position, and size must be initially defined and systolic and diastolic function must be evaluated on a periodic basis in patients with a single ventricle. These values should be evaluated in the context of volume and pressure loading conditions experienced by the single ventricle.
5. Aortic outflow must be assessed from the subaortic area to the distal systemic vascular bed. Signs of potential development of subaortic stenosis should be sought: the presence of an aorta arising from an anterior rudimentary outflow chamber or hypoplastic ventricle, an aorta much smaller than the pulmonary artery, or narrowing of the subaortic area between the infundibular septum and the right ventricular free wall. An anterior aorta is more likely to develop subaortic obstruction than a posterior one. Dynamic outflow obstruction may appear after any procedure or maneuver that would decrease the ventricular volume load, therefore serial evaluations are important at stages throughout life.
6. The size of the pulmonary arteries and severity of obstruction are important features in patients with pulmonary outflow obstruction. Conversely it is crucial to ascertain that patients have proper limitation to pulmonary blood flow by 4 to 6 months of age so as to prevent premature increased pulmonary vascular resistance.

Echocardiography is a powerful tool in the diagnosis of the univentricular heart. By its characteristic features, the specific ventricular anatomy is defined. Both the interatrial and interventricular communications are measured and obstructions noted with color directed pulsed Doppler. When there is an outflow chamber (hypoplastic ventricle) communicating with a dominant ventricle via a bulboventricular foramen (ventricular septal defect), the dimensions of the interventricular communication must be obtained by two orthogonal views and a prediction made about whether the connection may become obstructive in the future, based on its cross-sectional area, normalized to body surface area and its boundaries, muscular or membranous[29] (Fig. 57–23). Doppler examination of the subarterial outflow can detect even mild obstruction by an increase in velocity of blood flow. This is particularly important when the aorta arises from the hypoplastic chamber because of the danger of developing subaortic obstruction. For this reason, serial studies are necessary, particularly following interventions such as anticongestive medications or surgical procedures that reduce ventricular preload or afterload.

The atrioventricular valve anatomy is most clearly defined by echocardiographic imaging and any stenosis or regurgitation quantified via color and pulsed Doppler flow (Fig. 57–24). In the subset of patients with pulmonary artery band, echocardiography is utilized to evaluate the

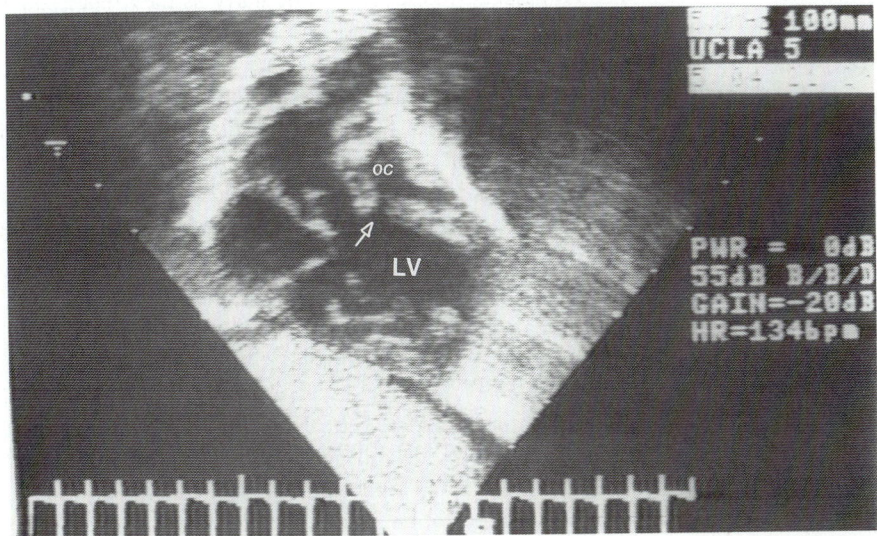

Figure 57–23. Subxiphoid long axis view of a patient with single left ventricle (LV), L-transposition of the great arteries, with an anterior outlet chamber (OC). The bulboventricular foramen (arrow) can be clearly seen.

band position, the morphology of the proximal pulmonary artery branches, and gradients at either level.

Finally, ventricular function can be estimated using echocardiography, but accuracy may be limited by nonuniform ventricular geometry, particularly in patients with a single morphologic right ventricle. Because of large differences in preload and afterload in patients with a single ventricle, load-independent measures of contractility, such as wall stress/velocity of circumferential fiber shortening (VCF) relation, are of greater value than a simple ejection fraction. However, such indices are not reliable in the face of subaortic obstruction or when ventricular geometry does not conform to a prolate ellipsoid. Such parameters can be followed after each stage of palliation to monitor cardiac function and help determine the timing for the next intervention.

Prior to each stage of palliation, catheterization will provide important information complimentary to echocardiography. Cardiac catheterization allows pressure measurements both in the pulmonary arteries and the left atrium for assessment of transpulmonary gradient. Pressure gradients across the interatrial or interventricular communications should also be measured for assessment of pulmonary vascular resistance. Biplane cineangiocardiograms are performed to assess the presence and degree of valvular regurgitation, the ventricular ejection fraction, and ventricular shape and to define alternative sources of pulmonary blood flow, including aortopulmonary collaterals. The collateral flow should be evaluated prior to a Glenn shunt or Fontan procedure and coil embolized if sufficient to cause a blush over the lung fields and apparent pulmonary venous return.

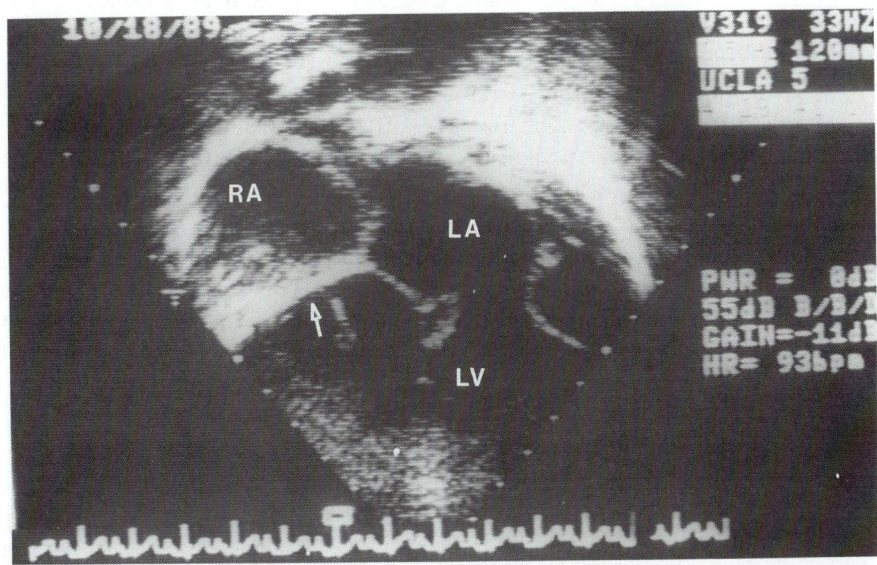

Figure 57–24. Apical four chamber view of a patient with tricuspid atresia. No tricuspid valve tissue (arrow) can be identified. The mitral valve is open (RA, right atrium; LA, left atrium; LV, left ventricle)

Truncus Arteriosus

Guidelines for preoperative evaluation:

I. Anatomy
   A. Pulmonary arterial connection
      1. Incompletely septated truncus arteriosus from which main pulmonary artery arises (Type I)
      2. Common truncus arteriosus with both pulmonary arteries arising close together (Type II)
      3. Common truncus arteriosus with pulmonary arteries arising separately, laterally (Type III)
   B. Truncal valve anatomy and function
   C. Size and position of the ventricular septal defect
   D. Aortic arch anomalies

Mild cyanosis, bounding peripheral pulses, a systolic ejection click followed by a long systolic murmur heard best in the mid left sternal border, and a loud single second heart sound characterize the clinical picture of truncus arteriosus. As the pulmonary vascular resistance drops, the pulmonary blood flow increases and congestive heart failure will ensue. The amount of truncal regurgitation and/or stenosis will affect the time of initial presentation, which is usually in the first weeks to months of life.

Surgical management of truncus arteriosus depends on the anatomy of the branch pulmonary arteries. In general, repair is done within the first few months of life to avoid high-pressure, high-volume, pulmonary blood flow and subsequent pulmonary vascular obstructive disease. Complete repair includes a right ventricular to pulmonary artery conduit and closure of the ventricular septal defect. Repair of the truncal valve may also be needed. Other aortic arch anomalies must be addressed prior to or during intracardiac repair.

Two-dimensional echocardiography plays an important role in defining the anatomy of this lesion. The large truncal root can be seen overlying a subarterial ventricular septal defect. The origin of the pulmonary arteries may be seen as a single trunk or separately arising from the proximal truncal root (Fig. 57–25). The number of truncal valve leaflets can be determined and Doppler echocardiography can reveal valvular regurgitation or stenosis. Stenoses at the pulmonary artery origin, if present, may be detected. The appearance of a small ascending aortic portion and a larger pulmonary portion of the common truncus should prompt a careful display of the aortic arch from the suprasternal, high parasternal, and subxiphoid transducer positions to detect an associated coarctation of the aorta or interrupted aortic arch.

In patients under 1 year of age, echocardiography alone usually provides all necessary preoperative information. In older infants and children with truncus arteriosus, cardiac catheterization is often employed to confirm the great vessel anatomy and to assess the pulmonary flow and resistance. A truncal root injection in the hepatoclavicular view will delineate the variable truncal and pulmonary anatomy. Pulmonary artery pressure can be measured directly. Assessment of pulmonary vascular resistance is especially important in the older patient with unobstructed pulmonary blood flow and suspected secondary pulmonary vascular obstructive disease. Aortic arch anomalies including interruption of the arch, coarctation of the aorta, or arch hypoplasia can be demonstrated usually with concomitant patent ductus arteriosus and often in association with a small ascending aorta and larger main pulmonary artery segment.

The Echocardiographic Diagnosis of Congenital Heart Disease

Multiple-plane imaging by two-dimensional echocardiography defines the anatomy of the heart and the great vessels.

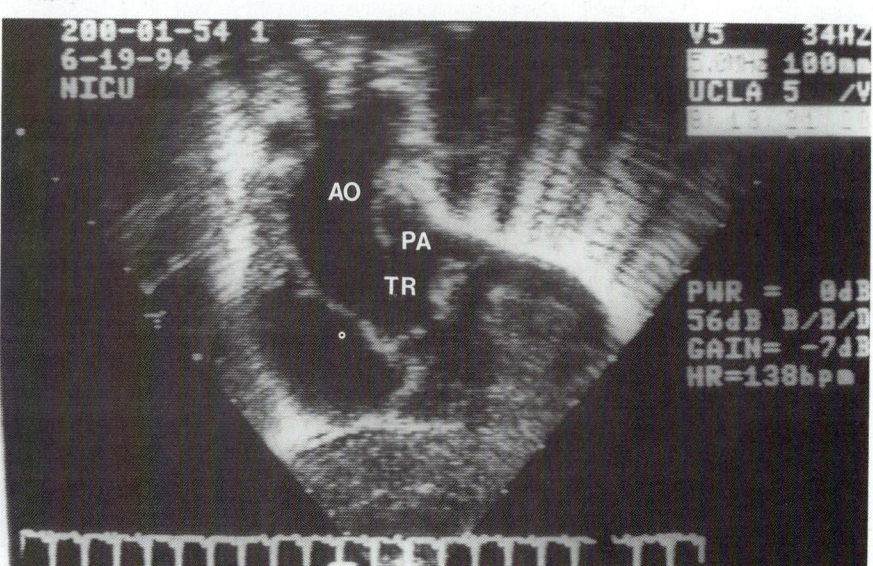

Figure 57–25. Subxiphoid long axis view of a patient with truncus arteriosus. A dilated ascending aorta (AO) is demonstrated with proximal takeoff of the pulmonary artery (PA) from the truncal root (TR).

Analysis of each cardiac segment allows complete definition of the configuration and position of the cardiac structures and their spatial interrelations. Cardiac chambers and intracardiac valves are imaged with superior definition, but tortuous vessels may be difficult to define by a "slice" technology such as echocardiogram or magnetic resonance imaging (MRI). Color Doppler provides a map of blood velocity and direction that complements the two-dimensional image. Small septal defects and fistulous connections may be recognized only by perturbations in blood flow when the anomaly is too small to visualize clearly. Pulsed and continuous-wave Doppler provide superior time resolution that allows precise quantification of blood velocity. Positional and velocity information are combined to assess the presence and severity of valvular obstruction or insufficiency, the position and size of jets associated with septal defects, and abnormal flow in large vessels in such lesions as anomalous systemic and pulmonary venous return, coarctation of the aorta, and patent ductus arteriosus.

Transesophageal echocardiography (TEE) allows different imaging planes than can be gained from a standard transthoracic study. Structures that are more posterior in the heart can be well visualized using this technology. Specific questions such as anomalous pulmonary venous return, pulmonary vein stenosis, and atrial baffle flow may be answered with intraoperative transesophagael echocardiography. In the older child or one in whom there are poor transthoracic windows, transesophageal echocardiography has a definite role in the evaluation of congenital heart disease. It should not substitute, however, for a complete preoperative transthoracic evaluation. Additionally, an immediate intraoperative or postoperative assessment of the adequacy of surgical repair can be obtained.

Pulmonary and aortic flow may be calculated from the mean velocity and the diameter of the vessel at the area of interest, utilizing the formula:

$$\text{blood flow} = (\text{mean flow velocity}) \times (\text{time}) \times (\text{cross-sectional area of vessel})$$

Peak instantaneous gradients may be calculated from a simplified Bernoulli equation, using peak flow velocity within the stenotic jet in the following formula:

$$\text{peak pressure gradient} = 4V^2$$

where V is the peak flow velocity.

Magnetic Resonance Imaging

The technologic advances in MRI now permit high-resolution imaging of the heart and great vessels with electrocardiographic gating to eliminate motion artifact. Echocardiographic imaging is somewhat limited by absorption of ultrasound energy in the lung and reflection (of energy) from bone. This limitation impedes visualization of vascular structures within the lung and sometimes even intracardiac structures in older patients or those with chest deformi-

ties. Magnetic resonance imaging has no such limitations. Cross-sectional images can be produced in any plane. Lesions in the pulmonary arteries and aorta are clearly displayed by this technique, but like echocardiography, tortuous vessels may not be displayed in any single plane.[30–33] Three-dimensional reconstructions using computer modeling may help alleviate this problem in the future. Echocardiography is more often used as a screening tool because data are acquired and displayed much more quickly and the equipment is portable. Magnetic resonance imaging is especially useful once specific anatomic areas have been targeted by echocardiographic examination.

Cardiac Catheterization in the Structural and Functional Diagnosis of Congenital Heart Disease

Cardiac catheterization continues to be an important tool in the structural and functional diagnosis of congenital heart disease. The role of this procedure has changed in recent years with the current sophistication of echocardiography and MRI as well as other essentially noninvasive techniques. Cardiac catheterization can now be focused to address specific questions limiting the requirement for extensive angiography. As a result, the risk of cardiac catheterization can be decreased, particularly in the young infant. Indications for cardiac catheterization in general include anatomic diagnosis as well as assessment of hemodynamic parameters, including measurement of pressures and calculations of shunts, vascular resistance, and ventricular function. Since anatomic diagnosis can accurately be determined in most cases by echocardiography, cardiac catheterization and cineangiography can complement the echocardiographic findings by further delineating lesions that are not clearly defined by echocardiography, particularly multiple small septal defects, the distal coronary circulation, and certain vascular abnormalities. Additionally, more interventional procedures are being done during cardiac catheterization including balloon valvuloplasty and angioplasty, balloon septostomy, coil embolization of collateral vessels, and stent placement in stenotic vessels.

Systemic (Q_s) and pulmonary (Q_p) flows are most often determined from oxygen consumption using the Fick principle indicated in the following formulas, where Vo_2 is the volume of oxygen consumed per minute.

$$Q_p = \frac{Vo_2}{(\text{pulm venous sat} - \text{pulm art sat}) \times (\text{Hgb}) \times (1.36) \times (10)}$$

$$Q_s = \frac{Vo_2}{(\text{aortic sat} - \text{superior vena cava sat}) \times (\text{Hgb}) \times (1.36) \times (10)}$$

From these flow determinations, left-to-right ($Q_{l>r}$) and/or right-to-left ($Q_{r>l}$) shunting can be determined by the following formulas:

$$Q_{l>r} = \frac{VO_2}{(\text{pulm art sat} - \text{superior vena cava sat}) \times (\text{Hgb}) \times (1.36) \times (10)}$$

$$Q_{r>l} = \frac{VO_2}{(\text{pulm venous sat} - \text{aortic sat}) \times (\text{Hgb}) \times (1.36) \times (10)}$$

$$Q_p/Q_s = \frac{\text{aortic sat} - \text{superior vena cava sat}}{\text{pulmonary venous sat} - \text{pulmonary arterial sat}}$$

In the absence of shunts, the cardiac output can be determined by the Fick principle or by thermodilution techniques. Pulmonary (R_p) and systemic (R_s) resistances are calculated on the basis of Poiseuille's law:

$$R_p = \frac{\text{mean pulmonary artery pressure} - \text{mean left atrium pressure}}{Q_p}$$

$$R_s = \frac{\text{mean aortic pressure} - \text{mean right atrium pressure}}{Q_s}$$

Cardiac catheters are selected according to purposes for use as well as the size of the patient. End-hole catheters or pressure tip transducers are more appropriate for determination of pressures and gradients. For cineangiocardiograms, side-hole catheters with large lumina and short lengths will allow safe and rapid delivery of contrast media. A large number of catheters of various types and sizes are usually needed in a pediatric catheterization laboratory.

SUMMARY

In patients with congenital heart disease, accurate and complete preoperative assessment of both cardiac anatomy and hemodynamics is essential prior to any surgical repair. Clinical information from history, physical examination, electrocardiography, chest radiography, echocardiography with Doppler, and sometimes cardiac catheterization and/or MRI can produce all the pertinent information needed to guide most management decisions.

The effect of refinements in noninvasive and catheterization techniques is to produce a highly accurate picture of the anatomy and evolving physiology of congenital cardiac lesions. Specifically focused invasive studies provide precise anatomic and hemodynamic information to help guide decision making. For many straightforward lesions, invasive studies may be eliminated entirely. In some lesions such as atrial septal defect, coarctation of the aorta, and patent ductus arteriosus, there is long experience with a purely noninvasive perioperative approach. A variety of complex lesions such as atrioventricular septal defects,

single ventricle, and complex conotruncal anomalies have been surgically palliated or repaired without cardiac catheterization. These conventions vary locally as a function of the experience of the diagnostic and surgical team with each specific abnormality. In other lesions, the number of cardiac catheterizations needed in the lifetime of a single patient is reduced. As echocardiography has become dominant in the preoperative evaluation of cardiac lesions, cardiac catheterization has moved to a more therapeutic role with closure of patent ductus arteriosus and septal defects, occlusion of vascular structures, and relief of outflow obstructions. These advances are closely interrelated with the evolution of cardiac surgery toward the repair of increasingly complex lesions at an increasingly earlier age.

REFERENCES

1. Bierman FZ, Williams RG: Subxiphoid two-dimensional imaging of the interatrial septum in infants and neonates with congenital heart disease. *Circulation* **60**(1):80–90, 1979
2. Ramaciotti C, Keren A, Silverman NH: Importance of (perimembranous) ventricular septal aneurysm in the natural history of isolated perimembranous ventricular septal defects. *Am J Cardiol* **57**: 268–272, 1986
3. Bierman FZ, Fellows K, Williams RG: Prospective identification of ventricular septal defects in infancy using subxiphoid two-dimensional echocardiography. *Circulation* **62**:4:807–817, 1980
4. Silbert DR, Brunson SC, Schiff R, et al: Determination of right ventricular pressure in the presence of a ventricular septal defect using continuous wave Doppler ultrasound. *J Am Coll Cardiol* **8**:379–384, 1986
5. Murphy DJ, Ludomirsky A, Huhta JC: Continuous wave Doppler in children with ventricular septal defect: Noninvasive estimation of intraventricular pressure gradient. *Am J Cardiol* **57**:428–432, 1986
6. Talner NS, Berman MA: Postnatal development of discrete coarctation of the aorta. *Pediatrics* **56**:562–569, 1975
7. Krabell KA, Ring WS, Foker JE, et al: Echocardiographic versus cardiac catheterization diagnosis of infants with congenital heart disease requiring cardiac surgery. *Am J Cardiol* **60**:351–354, 1987
8. George B, Disessa TG, Williams RG, et al: Coarctation repair without catheterization in infants. *Am Heart J* **114**(6):1421–1425, 1987
9. Nehoyannopoulos P, Karass S, Sapsford RN, et al: Accuracy of two-dimensional echocardiography in the diagnosis of aortic arch obstruction. *J Am Coll Cardiol* **10**:1072–1077, 1987
10. Edwards JE: Editorial: The direction of blood flow in coronary arteries arising from the pulmonary trunk. *Circulation* **29**:163–166, 1964
11. Bierman FZ, Williams RG: Prospective diagnosis of transposition of the great arteries in neonates by subxiphoid two-dimensional echocardiography. *Circulation* **60**:1496–1502, 1979
12. Pasquini L, Sanders SP, Parness IA, Colan SD: Diagnosis of coronary artery anatomy by two-dimensional echocardiography in patients with transposition of the great arteries. *Circulation* **75**:557–564, 1987
13. Shaher RM, Puddu GC: Coronary anatomy in complete transposition of the great vessels. *Am J Cardiol* **17**:355–361, 1966
14. Smith A, Arnold R, Wilkinson JL, et al: An anatomic study of the patterns of the coronary arteries and sinus node arteries in complete transposition. *Int J Cardiol* **12**:295–304, 1986
15. Elliot LP, Amplatz K, Edwards JF: Coronary arterial patterns in transposition complexes. *Am J Cardiol* **17**:362–378, 1966
16. Gittenberger-de Groot AC, Sauer U, Oppenheimer-Dekker A, Quaegebeur J: Coronary artery supply in transposition of the great ar-

teries: A morphometric study. *Pediatr Cardiol* **4**(suppl 1): 15–24, 1983

17. Sanders SP, Bierman FZ, Williams RG: Conotruncal malformation: Diagnosis in infancy using subxiphoid two dimensional echocardiography. *Am J Cardiol* **50**:1361–1367, 1982

18. Shimazaki Y, Maehara T, Blackstone EH, et al: The structure of the pulmonary circulation in tetralogy of Fallot with pulmonary atresia. *J Thorac Cardiovasc Surg* **95**:1048–1058, 1988

19. Dibizzi RP, Caprioli GC, Aiazzi L, et al: Distribution and anomalies of coronary arteries in tetralogy of Fallot. *Circulation* **61**:95–102, 1980

20. Fellows KE, Freed MD, Keane JF, et al: Results of routine pre-operative coronary angiography in tetralogy of Fallot. *Circulation* **51**: 561–566, 1975

21. Berry BE, McGoon DC: Total correction for tetralogy of Fallot with anomalous coronary artery. *Surgery* **74**:894–898, 1973

22. Blackstone EH, Kirklin JW, Bertranoa EG, et al: Preoperative prediction from cineangiograms of postrepair right ventricular pressure in tetralogy of Fallot. *J Thorac Cardiovasc Surg* **78**:542–552, 1979

23. Zuberbuhler JR, Anderson RH: Morphologic variations of pulmonary atresia and intact ventricular septum: Guidelines for surgical intervention. *Pediatr Cardiol* **4**:183–188, 1983

24. Calder AL, Co EE, Sage MD: Coronary arterial abnormalities in pulmonary atresia and intact ventricular septum. *Am J Cardiol* **59**:436–442, 1987

25. Kaszanica J, Ursell PC, Blanc WA, Gersony WM: Abnormalities of the coronary circulation in pulmonary atresia and intact ventricular septum. *Am Heart J* **114**:1415–1419, 1987

26. Leung MP, Mok CK, Hui PW: Echocardiographic assessment of neonates with pulmonary atresia and intact ventricular septum. *J Am Coll Cardiol* **12**:719–725, 1988

27. Hanley FL, Sade RM, Blackstone EH, et al: Outcomes in neonatal pulmonary atresia with intact ventricular septum: A multiinstitutional study. *J Thorac Cardiovasc Surg* **105**:406–427, 1993

28. Smallhorn JF, Freedom RM: Pulsed Doppler echocardiography in the pre-operative evaluation of total anomalous pulmonary venous connection. *J Am Coll Cardiol* **8**:1413–1420, 1986

29. Matitiau A, Geva T, Colan SD, et al. Bulboventricular foramen size in infants with double-inlet left ventricle or tricuspid atresia with transposed great arteries: Influence on initial palliative operation and rate of growth. *J Am Coll Cardiol* **19**:142–148, 1992

30. Gomes AS, Lois JF, George B, et al: Congenital abnormalities of the aortic arch: MR imaging. *Radiology* **165**:691–695, 1987

31. Kersting-Sommerhoff BA, Sechtem UP, Fisher MR, Higgins CB: MR imaging of congenital anomalies of the aortic arch. *Am J Radiol* **149**:9–13, 1987

32. Simpson IA, Chung KJ, Glass RF, et al: Cine magnetic resonance imaging for evaluation of anatomy and flow relations in infants with coarctation of the aorta. *Circulation* **78**:142–148, 1988

33. Boxer RA, LaCorte MA, Singh S, et al: Nuclear magnetic resonance imaging in the evaluation and follow-up of children treated for coarctation of the aorta. *J Am Coll Cardiol* **7**:1095–1098, 1986

58

Perioperative Care
of the Pediatric Patient

Barbara George and Lester C. Permut

The successful outcome of any pediatric cardiac operation (particularly in the neonate) depends on many factors; these include the accurate preoperative diagnosis and stabilization of the patient, the operative intervention itself (with close attention being paid to myocardial preservation), and meticulous postoperative care. Of these factors, the least well understood is postoperative care. This area remains the most controversial; the type of care given often varies widely from hospital to hospital. The advances that have occurred in surgical techniques are remarkable in that complex lesions can be repaired in infancy and sometimes even in the neonatal period. This places a tremendous burden on the perioperative care team to ensure an optimum outcome. Because of multiorgan dysfunction, these infants are often quite ill, both preoperatively and postoperatively. The purpose of this chapter is to provide general guidelines for the perioperative care of neonates, infants, and children who have undergone cardiac surgery and to mention specific circumstances in which the management requires a high degree of sophistication.

PREOPERATIVE EVALUATION AND CARE

For older infants and children, the preoperative evaluation usually involves a thorough discussion of the diagnosis and proposed surgical intervention prior to admission of the child to the hospital. Also, any discrepant information should be clarified, whenever possible, prior to the child's admission. Once the child has been admitted, the care is usually quite simple and should include meeting the family, examining the child, evaluating the laboratory data obtained on admission, discussing the proposed surgical intervention

and expected outcome, and then adjusting the doses of, or discontinuing, medications as appropriate. Digoxin and diuretics are usually discontinued the evening before surgery. The dose of propranolol is decreased depending on the indications for the medication, but is not stopped until approximately 4–6 hours before the start of the operation. Aspirin should be discontinued 10 days before surgery, unless the aspirin is being administered for prophylaxis in a patient who had a modified Blalock–Taussig shunt made of prosthetic material. In these circumstances, the aspirin should not be stopped until the day of admission. If a young patient is cyanotic, and will be made non per os (NPO) longer than his or her "usual" feeding schedule, an intravenous infusion should be started and fluids should be administered at a rate slightly above maintenance.

The preoperative evaluation and care of a neonate or an infant who will undergo cardiac surgery are frequently much more complicated than in the older child. While the diagnosis is being established, the cardiopulmonary status of the infant must also be stabilized. Close attention must be paid to maintaining body temperature, metabolic and fluid and electrolyte balance, respiratory stability, and myocardial function. This may require the use of mechanical ventilation, the institution of intravenous inotropic or vasoactive medications (or both), and, in certain neonates, the administration of prostaglandin E_1.[1] Prostaglandins play a very important role in stabilizing the condition of neonates with lesions in which the systemic or blood flow is ductus-dependent. When they are required, prostaglandins should be administered through a central line to ensure that the infusion will not be interrupted during transport of the baby either from an outlying hospital to the tertiary neonatal intensive care unit (ICU) or from this unit to the operating room. Supplemental oxygen may be appropriate, but should be used at the lowest possible levels. Oxygen should be avoided in lesions with excessive pulmonary blood flow, such as truncus arteriosus, since oxygen-mediated pulmonary vasodilation in these cases may lead to pulmonary flooding and acute left ventricular distension. If the neonate remains unstable, a pediatric cardiology member of the perioperative team should accompany the infant to the operating room and be available until the anesthesiologist is ready to accept the care of the child.

POSTOPERATIVE CARE

Postoperative care is divided into three parts: the immediate evaluation and stabilization of the patient on arrival in the postoperative ICU, the monitoring and complete assessment of the postoperative patient, and the early postoperative management (first 24–48 hours after surgery). Postoperative management after the initial 48 hours and late complications of surgery are not discussed.

Immediate Evaluation and Stabilization

Before the transport of the patient from the operating room to the ICU, it is extremely helpful for a member of the operating room team to notify the postoperative team (a direct telephone line is very useful) of the patient's general status, the type of monitoring lines in place, the type and dose of cardioactive medications being administered, and whether the patient requires an external cardiac pacemaker. It is also useful to give the expected time of transport of the patient from the operating room to the ICU. The expected respiratory parameters can also be communicated at this time. The postoperative team should check these parameters to ensure that they seem appropriate for the age and size of the patient and for the type of surgical intervention. This allows for adjustments to be made even before the patient arrives in the ICU. Once the patient arrives in the ICU, there may be a busy period during which the care of the patient is being transferred from the operating room team to the postoperative team. This is a very critical period in the patient's care; therefore, to avoid any major mishaps during this period, a very orderly but rapid approach to the assessment of the patient's status must take place. This initial evaluation can be very brief, and then time can be allowed for the nursing and respiratory therapy staffs to complete the transfer.

This brief, initial evaluation should include the cardiorespiratory systems and a gross estimate of the patient's blood loss since leaving the operating room. As soon as the patient is connected to the ventilator (assuming extubation has not taken place in the operating room), the chest should be observed for the presence of an adequate rise and bilaterally equal breath sounds; the oxygen saturation (easily and rapidly obtained from a pulse oximeter[2,3]) should be acceptable, and the oral or nasal endotracheal tube should be

secured. An arterial blood gas should be obtained as soon as possible. A brief evaluation of the circulatory system includes ascertaining that there is an adequate heart rate and rhythm, that pulses are palpable, and that the blood pressure is adequate. The amount of bleeding can be checked quickly and a rapid decision made as to whether additional blood or blood products will be required. Optimally, packed red blood cells and fresh frozen plasma should be brought from the operating room with the patient should they be needed urgently. This assessment should take no longer than a few minutes; the nursing staff can then proceed as noted above. While the patient is being secured and monitoring lines are being adjusted, an exchange of information between the operating team (surgeon and anesthesiologist) and the postoperative team should take place. In addition to the important details of the operation itself, it is vital that the operating team indicate to the ICU team the occurrence of any intraoperative complications, the final intracardiac pressures and saturations obtained, the aortic cross-clamp time, the cardiopulmonary bypass time, the types of intracardiac or other indwelling catheters that were placed, and any respiratory problems that occurred (either associated with intubation or subsequently). The doses of cardioactive agents should be confirmed, and any other important observations should be commented on. Mention should also be made of any coagulation promoting agents that have been given. A portable chest radiograph is obtained immediately after the patient arrives in the ICU. Once the patient is considered stable and care has been transferred to the postoperative team, a more lengthy, orderly assessment can take place.

Monitoring and Complete Assessment of the Postoperative Patient

Once the initial evaluation has taken place, a more complete assessment of all systems must occur to develop a rational plan for continued therapy. This section contains a description of the evaluation of the major organ systems that are likely to require attention in the immediate postoperative period. Each system is addressed separately; however, as will be noted, one system can, and usually does, have a major effect on the function of one or more other systems.

Cardiovascular System

The cardiovascular system remains the primary focus of attention during the early postoperative period. Perhaps more appropriately, this should be the cardiorespiratory system as the two are so closely linked, from a functional standpoint, during this time. However, for purposes of this discussion, they are separated.

Although most patients who have undergone cardiac surgery, particularly those who have required cardiopulmonary bypass, have at least one if not several monitoring devices present, the clinical examination remains the most important "monitoring device." The important clinical signs of inadequate cardiac output are tachycardia, cool periphery with slightly elevated central temperatures, decreased capillary refill, and inadequate urine output. If the child is awake, unexplained agitation can be an important physical sign.

However, as noted above, most patients have both invasive and noninvasive monitoring devices in place—the number and type depending on the age, size, and cardiac status of the patient, as well as the operation performed. However, even the simplest monitoring device must be in a proper location, be calibrated, and be checked periodically to ensure that the baselines have not drifted. Logical and appropriate management decisions can be made only if the data that form the basis for these decisions are accurate.

The comments that follow refer to the early postoperative period (first 24–48 hours) while the patient is still in the postoperative cardiac ICU. All patients should have continuous monitoring of their heart rates. Acute changes in heart rate must be evaluated in terms of the patient's waking state, volume status, estimated cardiac output, and cardiac rhythm. If a dysrhythmia is suspected, a multiple lead electrocardiogram should be obtained. Atrial electrograms, tracings obtained from atrial pacemaker leads,[4] can be very helpful in this regard. One should suspect a dysrhythmia if the heart rate is fixed (slow or fast), or shows very little variation with stimulation. Ventricular arrhythmias, although infrequent, are particularly worrisome in the immediate postoperative period. Most patients should have temporary atrial and ventricular pacing wires placed at the conclusion of the operation. These can serve as diagnostic tools (as noted above) or as therapeutic modalities.

All children should also have some measurement of blood pressure. Most patients arrive in the ICU with indwelling arterial catheters. These serve a dual purpose in that they can be used for blood sampling (they are flushed only with heparinized saline) as well as for blood pressure measurements. However, if the patient is vasoconstricted, and the catheter is in a small vessel, the blood pressure measurement may be inaccurate; hence, all patients should also have their blood pressures measured periodically by noninvasive devices. The combination of these two methods allows for a more accurate measurement of blood pressure and certainly allows for excellent tracking of trends. Arterial lines can result in complications, including infection and decreased perfusion distal to the insertion site; therefore, they should be removed as soon as is reasonable from a clinical standpoint.

Monitoring of the right- and left-sided filling pressures (preload)[5] is usually very important in patients who have undergone open heart surgery. Most patients return from the operating room with a right atrial line or a line that measures central venous pressure. This provides an estimate of the right ventricular end-diastolic (or filling) pressure. The right atrial or central venous line can also be used, when necessary, for infusion of cardioactive agents or drugs such as calcium chloride. Calcium chloride (and certain other agents) should only be given by infusion into a central vein

because it often results in sclerosis of peripheral veins. Whenever intracardiac or central venous lines are "entered," appropriate sterile techniques must be used. In addition, it is very important to clear the line of air bubbles as there may be residual right-to-left shunts in the immediate postoperative period; hence, failure to do so may result in cerebral air embolism. Changes in right-sided cardiac filling pressures can (and should) be estimated by liver size and fullness of the fontanelle in very young infants. The liver size in young infants and children, unlike the adult, changes very rapidly in response to changes in right-sided filling pressures. Left atrial catheters are very useful in estimating the filling pressures of the left ventricle, particularly in patients who have undergone extensive cardiac surgery. The right and left atrial pressures are usually very different from each other in the immediate postoperative period; hence, measurements of both provide valuable information as to the patient's status and therapy requirements. Infusion of inotropic or vasopressor agents via the left atrial line may occasionally be of benefit to avoid pulmonary vasoconstriction resulting from a "first-pass" effect in patients prone to pulmonary vasospasm. The concerns with regard to air embolism are even greater with left atrial lines; therefore, they should not be entered unless absolutely necessary. The use of right and left atrial lines for estimation of ventricular end-diastolic pressures again must be done with the notion that improper placement, pneumothorax, or pneumomediastinum can alter these readings such that the filling pressures no longer reflect the ventricular end-diastolic pressures.

Pulmonary arterial catheters can be of great value in patients with pulmonary hypertension.[6] When necessary, pulmonary vasoactive agents can be infused directly into these lines, thus ensuring that these agents exert their maximal effects directly on the pulmonary vasculature by avoiding any intracardiac right-to-left shunting that may be occurring. It should be noted, however, that there is not a single pressure value that is *the* correct pressure (i.e., right or left atrial) for all patients. Normal intracardiac pressures vary with age[7] and certainly vary with the primary cardiac lesion and subsequent surgical intervention; however, one can use the number to suggest trends, and the "best" left atrial pressure, for example, can be determined by trial and error. The goal is to achieve optimal cardiac output while minimizing negative effects of excessive volume administration. As a general guideline, one tries not to exceed a mean left atrial pressure of 15 mm Hg, as pressures higher than this may result in pulmonary edema. Intracardiac and pulmonary artery lines should be removed as soon as they are no longer considered essential for patient care. This is done most frequently during the first postoperative day. Before they are removed, the coagulation status of the patient (particularly the platelet count) must be normal and blood should be available should excessive bleeding occur with their removal.

The assessment of cardiac output is critical in the postoperative period. Although there are small thermistors available for measuring cardiac output by the thermodilution technique,[8] these may be inaccurate in the presence of residual left-to-right shunting or right-sided valvar regurgitation and, therefore, are rarely used. A fairly accurate way to evaluate the adequacy of perfusion, and thus cardiac output, is the measurement of toe temperature,[9] and comparison of this temperature to both the central body temperature and the ambient temperature. These measurements, in association with other clinical signs (i.e., heart rate, blood pressure, urine output), provide a very good estimate of cardiac output. The measurement of mixed venous oxygen saturations and the presence or absence of metabolic acidosis can also provide additional information in this regard. Once the adequacy of the cardiac output is determined, the other systems can then be evaluated. As mentioned above, the respiratory system may have required immediate attention, even before one takes the time to evaluate completely the cardiac system; similarly, the cardiovascular system may require urgent therapy before one can proceed with an evaluation of the other systems.

Respiratory System

Most patients arrive in the ICU with an oral or nasal endotracheal tube in place[10] and require mechanical ventilation. A pulse oximeter, which provides an excellent evaluation of major changes in oxygen saturation, is an extremely important and valuable tool.[2,3] After most cardiac operations, there is some atelectasis and frequently some pulmonary contusion present. Hence, most patients, particularly those who have required a prolonged period of cardiopulmonary bypass, require mechanical ventilation for at least several hours; however, if there are no major cardiac or respiratory complications, the majority of patients can be extubated within 6–8 hours after arrival in the ICU. There are specific contraindications to extubation that are discussed in the next section. As mentioned previously, upon arrival in the ICU, a rapid assessment of the patient's ventilatory status is performed. However, a more complete evaluation requires a chest radiograph and an arterial blood gas measurement to confirm the adequacy of ventilation. Patients under approximately 10 kg are placed on a pressure ventilator; whereas those over 10 kg are placed on a volume ventilator. The peak inspiratory pressure (PIP) is adjusted to obtain a good chest rise (usually a pressure of at least 20 cm H_2O is required). The positive end expiratory pressure (PEEP) is set at 3 cm H_2O for all patients initially (except those who have undergone a Fontan operation in which case no PEEP is used). The rate is usually set at the same rate that was required in the operating room. For those patients on a volume ventilator, the volume should be set to deliver approximately 10 mL/kg and then the adequacy of this should be judged initially by the chest rise. All patients are placed on intermittent mandatory ventilation. The PIP, PEEP, respiratory rate, tidal volume, and fraction of inspired oxygen

(FIO_2) are adjusted by the first blood gas measurements. If the PO_2 and saturation are appropriate for the FIO_2 and match the pulse oximeter, the FIO_2 is decreased to 0.40 or less. Of note, we have found that the measurement of transcutaneous PO_2 is very unreliable in this clinical setting. As opposed to the FIO_2, the PIP, PEEP, tidal volume, and respiratory rate are adjusted using measured arterial blood gases. As soon as the chest radiograph is available, it is examined for evidence of parenchymal lung disease, pleural effusions, endotracheal tube position, heart size, and location of intracardiac lines. If the infant is under 6 months of age, or if it is determined that the older infant will not be able to be extubated early, the oral endotracheal tube is sutured to a "moustache" fashioned from Elastoplast and taped firmly in place after the upper lip located with benzoin. This is performed only after the endotracheal tube position is confirmed by chest radiograph. This type of stabilization of the endotracheal tube is similar to what is done in most neonatal ICUs.[11,12] If a nasal endotracheal tube is in place, it is secured by firm taping to the nose and upper lip. In addition, all patients who require assisted ventilation should have a nasogastric tube inserted before the chest radiograph. This is done to prevent gastric distention that can result in respiratory compromise,[13] vomiting, and aspiration (the latter can be a major problem in patients who have uncuffed endotracheal tubes). The position of the gastric tube is confirmed by auscultation and by the chest radiograph, which always includes the upper abdomen.

Any unexpected arterial blood gas finding demands immediate investigation. Auscultation alone may be adequate to determine the etiology of the problem and dictate therapy; however, a repeat chest radiograph is frequently necessary. If hypoxemia is the problem, blood gas analysis from the right and left atria may localize the source to the lungs or to the heart. If intracardiac right-to-left shunting is suspected, two-dimensional echocardiography (with color flow or microbubble contrast) can be very valuable to identify the site of the right-to-left shunt. Two-dimensional echocardiography can also help localize pleural effusions for therapeutic thoracentesis, if needed. It is also important to note that a disordered cardiovascular system may, in itself, cause a disordered respiratory system (other than residual right-to-left shunts). Therefore, if no primary respiratory abnormality is found, a cardiac source must be considered (e.g., unsuspected low cardiac output). An inadequate cardiac output can result in hypoxemia, hypercapnea, and respiratory acidosis.

Hematologic System

The major hematologic problem that must be continuously evaluated during the immediate postoperative period is bleeding. Bleeding can occur secondary to a coagulopathy[14] or a surgical problem. A postoperative coagulopathy may be due to inadequate reversal of the heparin given during surgery, abnormal or inadequate clotting factors, poorly functioning or inadequate number of platelets, and occasionally secondary to fibrinolysis, or, rarely, excessive administration of protamine. Infants, and more commonly older children, who are profoundly cyanotic with marked polycythemia may have coagulation abnormalities preoperatively.[14,15] The routine coagulation studies that are performed preoperatively are rarely abnormal. Occasionally, when the hematocrit is 70% or greater, an exchange transfusion is performed. This hemodilution is performed 24–48 hours, at least, before surgery with the goal to bring hematocrit down to 60–65%. Further hemodilution may have serious side effects on the markedly cyanotic infant or child. Postoperatively, the quantity of bleeding is measured by the mediastinal and/or pleural tube output, and the severity of the bleeding is determined by comparing the quantity of blood loss per hour to an estimate of the patient's blood volume. An additional source of blood loss that is often overlooked is the amount of blood removed from the patient for various blood tests. This can represent a significant amount in the very young infant; hence, a meticulous blood balance record must be kept and the blood balance calculated on an hourly basis. To evaluate a patient for a bleeding problem, routine coagulation studies (prothrombin time, partial thromboplastin time, platelet count, and activated clotting time) are performed on all patients who have undergone open heart surgery and in any patient who is bleeding excessively postoperatively. Blood tests to evaluate clotting can be drawn from the arterial line if at least 5 mL of blood is withdrawn first. However, if serious unexplained derangements persist, it may be advisable to perform a venipuncture to obtain "uncontaminated" clotting studies. Routine amounts of blood loss are not replaced volume for volume unless there is evidence of hemodynamic need for blood volume replacement, and hematocrit is unacceptably low, or the bleeding is clearly substantial (~5–10 mL/kg per hr). If the patient appears to be losing a considerable amount of blood, the chest radiograph should be repeated in 4–6 hours to watch for mediastinal widening as an early sign of impending tamponade and to detect undrained blood which may collect in the pleural spaces.

Renal–Metabolic Systems

Although usually discussed separately, in the setting of the postoperative cardiac patient, the assessment of renal function, fluid and electrolyte balance, and metabolic homeostasis are best discussed together.

Any patient, particularly a young infant, who has undergone a cardiac surgical procedure that required cardiopulmonary bypass will invariably have some derangement of fluid balance and electrolyte homeostasis. All of these patients have excessive extravascular fluid, the exact amount of which is very difficult to estimate. However, close observation of ongoing losses (via nasogastric tube, urine output, and insensible losses particularly with elevated temperatures) and the presence of edema (usually facial) are reasonable indicators. In a manner similar to blood balance circulations (see below), fluid balance should be

monitored on an hourly basis. This allows for frequent adjustments of the amount of volume that should be administered. In addition, there are usually derangements in potassium[16] and glucose homeostasis.[17,18] Therefore, until the patient is stable, glucose, potassium, and other electrolytes must be monitored closely, usually every 4–6 hours in the immediate postoperative period; more frequent monitoring may be indicated if treatment is required. In extremely young infants (particularly neonates) and in cachectic patients, a rapid bedside "dipstick" test[19] may be used to monitor glucose levels on an hourly basis until the patient is stable. This reduces the need for frequent serum glucose determinations. Glucose levels are frequently high immediately postoperatively, but often drop precipitously within 6–12 hours postoperatively and can result in serious complications—seizures and myocardial dysfunction being two of the major problems. Serum potassium and calcium levels (ionized and total) also fluctuate widely in the immediate postoperative period, hence, the need for close observation on a routine basis.

As noted above, the estimation of the intravascular, as well as the extravascular, volume status of a patient who has undergone cardiopulmonary bypass is quite difficult. Hence, changes in urine output may be difficult to explain. The urine output can be affected by inadequate intravascular volume, by a direct insult to the kidneys during or after operation (as may occur with certain drugs), or can be a reflection of inadequate cardiac output. The response of the kidneys to inadequate perfusion secondary to poor cardiac output is salt and water retention, thus resulting in a decreased urine output.[20,21] In this fashion, the urine output can be used as a reflection of cardiac output; however, in the immediate postoperative period, there may be an osmotic diuresis either secondary to mannitol given at the conclusion of cardiopulmonary bypass or on the basis of glycosuria that is a reflection of hyperglycemia also known to occur after cardiopulmonary bypass. Thus, in the first few hours postoperatively, an apparently good urine output may not always be indicative of adequate cardiac output. With time, the osmotic diuresis will abate and the urine output will become a reasonable indicator of cardiac output. Because of this, the urine output must be monitored closely; therefore, all patients should have an indwelling bladder catheter in place for at least several hours postoperatively. If the serum creatinine is normal and the urine output is adequate (1 mL/kg per hour or greater than 15 mL/m^2), the renal perfusion (and hence cardiac output) is probably acceptable. However, the urine must be tested for glucose to ensure that the urine output is a reflection of adequate renal perfusion rather than an osmotic load. In addition, it is advisable to maintain a urine output that is closer to 2 mL/kg per hour (rather than 1 mL/h) during the early postoperative period both to preserve renal function as well as to mobilize the excessive extravascular volume that is always present. If the urine output is inadequate, it must be determined whether it is on the basis of primary renal dysfunction, on the basis of inadequate intravascular volume, or secondary to inappropriate antidiuretic hormone secretion.[21,22] Serum evaluations of serum creatinine, blood urea nitrogen, urine sediment, and specific gravity can be of some help in this regard. In addition, if diuretics have not been given recently, a comparison of serum and urine sodium, creatinine, and osmolality can be very useful.

Central Nervous System

Central nervous system function is extremely difficult to evaluate in the early postoperative period. It takes time for anesthetic agents to be excreted and, once they are, it is common for the patient to receive sedating agents. However, it is possible to note the fullness of the fontanelle in small infants, whether there are purposeful eye movements, whether the pupils react, whether the patient moves all extremities, and of course the presence or absence of seizures. As the patient awakens, a more complete neurologic evaluation can be done. The patients at the highest risk for neurologic sequelae are those with persistent intracardiac right-to-left shunts,[23] severe hypoxemia preoperatively or postoperatively, low cardiac output with hypotension or metabolic acidosis, or both, and those with profound electrolyte imbalance, particularly hypoglycemia. Intraoperative events may also have placed the patient at high risk for neurologic abnormalities.

Early Postoperative Management

In the previous section, a systematic approach to the evaluation of the early postoperative patient is presented. However, at any point during this assessment, it may become clear that one or more systems require immediate attention. When such an immediate problem has been dealt with, the rest of the evaluation can proceed as noted above. Once the assessment is complete, either "routine" postoperative care can be initiated or specific problems can be treated appropriately. This section deals with what one can consider to be routine postoperative care as well as suggested therapies for the most common, major problems or complications. It needs to be emphasized that although, for purposes of clarity, the various systems have been separated, major problems or complications occurring in any one system usually will have a significant effect on one or more other systems. Although the cardiovascular system remains the primary focus of interest, concerns regarding the respiratory, hematologic, and renal–metabolic systems are also of major importance.

Cardiovascular System

When the patient returns from the operating room with what would appear to be normal cardiac output (usually not measured directly, but inferred from various parameters as noted previously) and no evidence of significant damage to any other organ system, then the postoperative course is usually quite smooth. If the patient was on digoxin preoperatively, it should not be resumed until the first postoperative day because of the marked fluctuations in potassium that occur after cardiopulmonary bypass, and the need to avoid digoxin toxicity. In addition, digoxin can usually be resumed at maintenance doses (8–10 μg/kg per day) at this time, as the serum levels are usually still adequate.[24] However, should the cardiac output as reflected by blood pressure, perfusion, and urine output appear inadequate, then those variables that determine cardiac output (preload, afterload, contractility, and heart rate)[5,25] need to be examined and therapy chosen to address whichever of these variables are disordered.

Preload. Inadequate intravascular volume, hence inadequate preload, is one of the most common postoperative problems. Most pediatric patients who have been placed on cardiopulmonary bypass have undergone at least a mild degree of core cooling and some have undergone profound hypothermia (usually in association with very low pump flow or circulatory arrest). Hence, they are often severely vasoconstricted. Although they are "warmed up" before being removed from cardiopulmonary bypass, the operating room is usually cool and during the transport to the ICU there is usually some additional loss of body heat. As the patient warms up in the ICU (usually with the help of warming lights), a marked vasodilation occurs. This vasodilation, in association with ongoing volume losses of various sorts (blood loss, urine loss, etc.), usually results in an inadequate preload. If right and left atrial pressures are available, the detection of inadequate preload is easy (the optimal mean left atrial pressure probably varies between 5 and 12 mm Hg, depending on the original diagnosis and the type of surgical intervention). Treatment for inadequate preload is the administration of fluid. Colloid (in the form of 5% albumin, blood, or blood products) is the appropriate type of fluid to be used in the immediate postoperative period. It is desirable to maintain a hematocrit between 30 and 35% when the patient is acyanotic. Hence, packed red blood cells alone, red cells with fresh frozen plasma, or fresh frozen plasma alone are given to maintain the hematocrit in this range. If there is no evidence of a significant coagulopathy or bleeding problem, then 5% albumin administration is appropriate. There are only rare instances where crystalloid is the appropriate choice. The volume can be given in bolus form at a rate of 5–10 mL/kg per bolus. The response of the right and left atrial pressures must be watched closely. In addition, the liver size can provide an excellent guide as to the adequacy of therapy.

Excessive preload may be associated with an inadequate output. However, most commonly it results in circulatory congestion with a normal cardiac output. Under these circumstances, the use of preload reducing agents such as nitroglycerin (Table 58–1) and diuretics are indicated. It should also be noted that excessive left-sided filling pressures (e.g., a mean left atrial pressure of 18 mm Hg) may

TABLE 58–1. CARDIOACTIVE AGENTS

Drug	Dose	Comments
Amrinone	0.75 mg/kg IV[a] loading, then 5 µg/kg/min IV	May cause thrombocytopenia, hepatic, and GI disturbance,[b] fever, and arrhythmias; dosage schedule not well established for pediatric patients
Dobutamine	2–10 µg/kg/min IV (max. 40 µg/kg/min)	No direct effect on renal perfusion, some peripheral vasodilatation, little or no tachycardia usually
Dopamine	2–20 µg/kg/min IV (max. 50 µg/kg/min)	Lower doses: significant renal vasodilatation. Increasing doses have first dopaminergic then beta-adrenergic, and finally alpha-adrenergic effects. Dose/effect relations are speculative in neonates
Epinephrine	0.05–1.0 µg/kg/min IV	May cause hypertension and cardiac arrhythmias; inactivated in alkaline solution
Hydralazine	1.5–5 µg/kg/min IV (for afterload reduction)	May cause tachycardia, GI symptoms, neutropenia, lupuslike syndrome
Isoproterenol	0.05–0.5 µg/kg/min IV; usual 0.1 µg/kg/min (max. 1.5 µg/kg/min IV)	May decrease coronary blood flow, results in peripheral and pulmonary vasodilatation; often causes tachycardia
Nitroglycerin	0.5–2.0 µg/kg/min IV (max. 65 µg/kg/min IV)	Dosage not well established for infants and children
Nitroprusside	0.5–8 µg/kg/min IV	May result in thiocyanate (5–10 µg/dL) or cyanide (200 µg/dL) toxicity if used in high doses or for prolonged periods of time

[a]IV, intravenously.
[b]GI, gastrointestinal.

result in pulmonary edema and thereby have a profound effect on the respiratory system. This is discussed below.

Contractility. If the cardiac output still appears low despite correction of an inadequate preload, then the myocardial contractility or inotropic state of the heart should be assessed. A wide variety of inotropic agents (Table 58–1) are available for use. Note that digoxin has been excluded from this list. The use of intravenous, rapidly acting, and rapidly metabolized agents is highly desirable.[26] This allows for much better control. In addition, as noted previously, the serum potassium level varies so widely in the first 24–48 hours that digoxin toxicity can be a major problem that can easily be avoided by not using this agent in the early postoperative period. Because of its effectiveness in improving myocardial contractility, blood pressure, and renal blood flow, dopamine,[27,28] at a dose of 3 µg/kg per min, is chosen frequently as the first agent. Once an infusion rate of 10 µg/kg per min of dopamine is reached, and the inotropic state is still inadequate, an additional agent,[29] usually dobutamine, should begin at 3 µg/kg per min and be increased until the desired effect is achieved or untoward side effects, such as tachycardia, are encountered.[30–32] As the dobutamine dose is increased, the infusion of dopamine often may be decreased to 3–5 µg/kg per min to maintain the salutory renal effects of low-dose dopamine. If the heart rate is slow, isoproterenol may also be required. Neonates with profound myocardial dysfunction often respond best to epinephrine. In general, the addition of agents (rather than the replacement of one with another) is desirable; the goal is to keep all the inotropic agents at relatively low doses to avoid toxicity or untoward side effects. It should be noted that there is no such thing as the "perfect" inotropic agent. All inotropic agents increase the metabolic demands of the heart and all may have significant undesirable side effects. Therefore, the aim is to use the lowest effective dose. The use of nor-

epinephrine in these patients should be avoided because its potent vasoconstrictor effects may worsen organ perfusion. Amrinone is considered as a "second choice" agent in our unit because it has an unpredictable effect on the peripheral vasculature and may result in significant thrombocytopenia.

The effects of inotropic therapy are usually measured in indirect ways; however, echocardiography can be of some help in this regard. Although most experts usually institute inotropic therapy when preload augmentation appears to be inadequate in improving cardiac output, the other two determinants of cardiac function (heart rate and afterload) must be assessed and treated generally as it is always best to optimize the preload, afterload, and heart rate before beginning with inotropic agents.[5,25]

Pharmacologic therapy may be insufficient to maintain an adequate cardiac output in the presence of severe ventricular dysfunction. In these circumstances, mechanical support of cardiac function may be required. The results of intra-aortic balloon counterpulsation have been disappointing in the pediatric age range,[33] but use of the left ventricular assist device or extracorporeal membrane oxygenation can provide successful hemodynamic support and allow subsequent recovery.[34] A complete discussion of this topic is found in Chapters 35 and 93.

Heart Rate

Tachycardia. Normal heart rates vary with age; therefore it is important to know what the expected rate is before one can decide whether a specific rate represents a tachyarrhythmia. Heart rates of up to 180 beats/min in neonates and young infants, 160 beats/min in older infants, and 130–140 beats/min in young children are tolerated very well, and usually represent sinus tachycardias. However, most postoperative tachyarrhythmias in children are supraventricular. Therefore, it is important to decide whether one is dealing with a *sinus* tachycardia or a pathologic supraventricular tachycardia. As noted in the previous sections, this can be difficult and atrial electrograms may be very useful. IV administration of adenosine is safe in pediatric patients following cardiac surgery, and may aid in the diagnosis and management of paroxysmal supraventricular tachycardias.[35] It is important to recognize that sinus tachycardia almost invariably has an inciting cause. In neonates and young infants, the major response to an inadequate cardiac output is usually a marked sinus tachycardia. Sinus tachycardia can also be secondary to hypoxemia, hyperthermia, and a large variety of other metabolic abnormalities.[36] Factors such as pain or catecholamine administration must not be overlooked.[13] Hence, the treatment in these situations should be directed at the inciting cause rather than at the tachycardia itself. If the tachycardia is nonsinus, and cardiovascular collapse appears imminent, then cardioversion is indicated. Otherwise, a search for the etiology should again be undertaken; if cardiac output is compromised by a tachyarrhythmia, then appropriate pharmacologic intervention is warranted. It is in this setting that digoxin administration may be appropriate. Overdrive pacing in many of these patients may also be quite valuable. This involves pacing the heart at a slightly faster rate than the existing tachycardia and then slowly reducing the paced rate to a level that is tolerated by the patient (i.e., to a point at which the cardiac output improves).

Bradycardia

As with tachycardia, a bradycardia may be sinus in origin or, more frequently, may represent a nonsinus rhythm. A rhythm that is unacceptably slow may be the result of surgical manipulation in the area of the sinus or atrioventricular nodes, or may represent an electrolyte imbalance, hypoxemia, and, occasionally, low cardiac output. Hence, as for tachycardias, an etiology should be looked for and treated as well as treating the arrhythmia itself. Treatment most frequently can be accomplished by a combination of atrial and ventricular pacing.[37] It has been shown that a sinus mechanism in the normal heart can result in a 20% improvement in cardiac output compared with ventricular pacing. In the noncompliant heart it may result in a 50% improvement. For this reason, atrial or atrioventricular sequential pacing is preferred. If temporary pacing wires are not available or are nonfunctional, then very low dose isoproterenol (starting at 0.01 μg/kg per min, Table 58–1) is usually effective. The use of anticholinergic agents is not helpful because they cannot be titrated and are short acting. The ideal heart rate to optimize cardiac output varies with age. In the neonate or young infant, a rate of 140–160 beats/min is usually chosen. In the older infant, a rate of 120–140 beats/min is preferred; and, in the older child, a rate of 100–120 beats/min may be necessary to optimize cardiac output.

Afterload. Afterload cannot be measured directly at the bedside[5,25]; however, it can be estimated by an evaluation of the blood pressure and perfusion; toe temperature[9] is of

significant value in this regard. These measurements provide an estimate of the systemic vascular resistance that, in turn, is an estimate of afterload. If the blood pressure is normal or high, the toe temperature low (less than 32°C), and the cardiac output judged to be inadequate, it is appropriate to presume that the afterload is high and to use agents to decrease it. The most commonly used agent in the immediate postoperative period is sodium nitroprusside.[38,39] It may result in both pulmonary, as well as systemic, afterload reduction both of which are usually desirable. It is usually begun at a dose of 0.5 μg/kg per min (Table 58–1) and then increased until the desired effects have been achieved or untoward side effects are encountered. Both cyanide and thiocyanate levels must be monitored if this agent is used for more than 12 hours or at infusion rates greater than 5 μg/kg per min for even 3–6 hours. Both of these metabolites should be monitored as hepatic and renal dysfunction may be present postoperatively. If nitroprusside must be discontinued, nitroglycerin at high doses (greater than 10 μg/kg per min)[40] may achieve similar systemic effects. Hydralazine, as a continuous infusion, can also be used as a substitute for nitroprusside (Table 58–1). Most commonly, afterload reducing agents are used in conjunction with inotropic agents and preload reducing agents,[41,42] but occasionally they may be used alone, particularly if systemic hypertension is the major problem. These types of agents are preferred over any agent that is given by bolus or by mouth because they can be titrated easily and are generally metabolized quite rapidly.

The foregoing discussion has focused primarily on methods to reduce systemic afterload. Methods to reduce right ventricular afterload, or pulmonary hypertension, are discussed below.

Respiratory System

Because the respiratory management of patients with reactive pulmonary vascular disease is significantly different from those without, the following section on the management of the respiratory system is divided into two sections dealing with these two subsets of patients separately.

Patients Without Reactive Pulmonary Vascular Disease. The respiratory management of patients without pulmonary hypertension may be very straightforward, as noted in the previous section, and the patient may be prepared for extubation in the first 4–6 hours postoperatively. This is accomplished by lowering the FIO_2 to at least 0.4, the PIP to 20 cm H_2O, the PEEP to 3 cm H_2O, and the ventilatory rate to approximately 4 breaths/min. This does vary from patient to patient, however. Occasionally a patient may need a trial of constant positive airway pressure (CPAP) before extubation, but this is unusual. During the weaning process, the patient should be observed closely for evidence of excessive pulmonary secretions, inadequate respiratory effort, evidence of respiratory distress, and abnormalities of arterial blood gases. One aims to keep the blood fully saturated, the Pco_2 between 35 and 40 mm Hg, and the pH normal. If these parameters remain stable, one continues to prepare the patient for extubation. When it is judged that the patient is ready to be extubated, the airway should be suctioned well, the patient hand-ventilated with the appropriate Fio_2, and then extubated during an inspiratory effort. The patient is then given humidified, oxygenated air via a tent or mask. The percent of oxygen delivered is usually 10% higher than what was required while the patient was on the ventilator. Should stridor or bronchospasm occur with extubation, various types of inhalation therapy delivered via a hand-held nebulizer may be required. The patient must be watched very closely for the next 4–6 hours. Reintubation may be required, although this is unusual.

Contraindications to extubation may exist. These include low cardiac output (either on a primary myocardial basis or secondary to a residual cardiac defect), pulmonary hypertension with reactive pulmonary vascular disease,[6] primary pulmonary disease, major central nervous system pathology, excessive chest tube output, or whenever one believes that the patient will have to return to the operating room. Excessive preload resulting in pulmonary edema may also contraindicate removal of the patient from positive-pressure ventilation. In this situation, a forced diuresis in association with higher levels of PEEP may be required for at least a few hours. Once the chest radiograph is clearer and the other signs of excessive preload are gone, the preparation for extubation can continue as outlined above. A paralyzed diaphragm may make removal from the ventilator difficult. If this specific problem is suspected, ultrasound of the diaphragm using a portable machine can be diagnostic. It is common for neonates to require mechanical ventilation for at least 12–24 hours after an operation requiring cardiopulmonary bypass. Therefore, these patients are usually kept heavily sedated, often with a continuous infusion of fentanyl; in addition, they may require paralysis.

Patients With Reactive Pulmonary Vascular Disease (Pulmonary Hypertension). Patients with pulmonary hypertension and reactive pulmonary vasculature are deserving of special mention as the postoperative course of this type of patient is usually quite complicated and requires very specific care. In addition, this postoperative problem virtually always affects other systems, and these effects deserve special emphasis.

There are certain congenital lesions in which it can be anticipated that the patient is likely to have postoperative pulmonary hypertension crises. These include truncus arteriosus, complete atrioventricular canal defects, and total anomalous pulmonary venous return that is obstructed. Patients who have multiple ventricular septal defects (and hence were not candidates for early repair), and whose pulmonary vasculature has been inadequately protected (e.g., by loose or late pulmonary artery bands), are also at significant risk. When it is anticipated that the patient is at risk for pulmonary hypertensive crises, the placement in the operating room of a pulmonary artery line for pressure monitoring and drug infusion is extremely helpful. It is anticipated that these patients will not be extubated early; hence, they are given paralyzing agents such as pancuronium and continuous infusions of sedatives (usually fentanyl).[43,44] Their respiratory management is also quite different. These patients should be kept well oxygenated (Po_2 greater than 100 mm Hg, if possible) and hyperventilated to maintain the Pco_2 between 25 and 30 mm Hg, and the pH between 7.5 and 7.55. Periodic hand ventilation may be required during a hypertensive crisis. When suctioning of the airway is necessary, these patients again should be hand ventilated (hyperventilated) with 100% oxygen and then suctioned quickly while an assistant watches the pulse oximeter and the pulmonary artery pressures. If any significant drop in the oxygen saturation or significant increase in the pulmonary artery pressures is noted, the suctioning should be stopped. The same is true for any procedure that is done on the child; even loud noises should be avoided. It should be added that these patients should be manipulated or even touched only to the extent that it is absolutely necessary to do so and thus is mandated as appropriate patient care. Pharmacologic manipulation of the pulmonary vasculature is frequently required.[45] There is no perfect pulmonary vasodilator.[46] However, as has been documented in adults with pulmonary hypertension,[47] nitroglycerin may be quite helpful as it can often be used in doses that result in pulmonary vasodilatation but do not affect the systemic afterload (Table 58–1).[48,49] Other drugs that can be useful are prostaglandins[50] and low dose isoproterenol (beginning at 0.01 μg/kg per min and then increasing as tolerated). Prostaglandin E_1, while a patent pulmonary vasodilator, may cause systemic vasodilation, fever, and resultant increased capillary permeability with anasarca and intermittent pulmonary edema. Tolazoline is generally avoided as it is associated with a number of severe side effects and because it invariably decreases the systemic vascular resistance.[51] More than one of the aforementioned agents may be required to control the pulmonary reactivity. Direct infusion of these drugs into the pulmonary arteries by means of a pulmonary artery line may be beneficial.

More recently, inhaled nitric oxide gas has been employed as a treatment for pulmonary hypertension in a number of clinical settings, including perioperative congenital heart surgery. Endogenous nitric oxide is an endothelial-derived smooth muscle relaxation factor that appears to play an important role in the regulation of pulmonary vascular tone in normal children.[52] It is metabolized rapidly by red blood cells, resulting in an extremely short half-life in the bloodstream. When delivered directly to the lungs by inhalation, its potent vasodilator effects are therefore isolated to the pulmonary vascular bed without a concomitant decrease in systemic vascular resistance. Marked reduction of transpulmonary gradient and consequent improvement in arterial oxygen saturation have been described following delivery of nitric oxide gas at a dose of 10–30 ppm in infants undergoing cardiac surgery.[53,54] Randomized clinical trials are currently being performed, but the possibility of a potent, selective pulmonary vasodilator is promising.

If significant pulmonary reactivity is present, the patient is usually kept paralyzed and heavily sedated for at least 24 hours. As the patient improves, or at least stabilizes, the first thing to be withdrawn is the paralysis; however, any changes in therapy must be done very slowly as even small changes in a medication (nitroglycerin, for example) may trigger a crisis. Overall, these patients are extremely difficult to care for and require virtually constant bedside attention by both the nurse and the physician.

Hematologic System

The major postoperative hematologic problem is excessive bleeding. As noted previously, mild to major coagulopathies exist in virtually all patients who have undergone surgery that required cardiopulmonary bypass. These coagulopathies should be treated appropriately with protamine, packed red blood cells, fresh frozen plasma, platelets, cryoprecipitate, and occasionally ε-aminocaproic acid.[55,56] Hypothermia may exacerbate coagulopathy and effects should be made to achieve and maintain normothermia. Frequently, warming alone may substantially reduce bleeding, particularly in neonates and small infants. If the patient has persistent bleeding at a rate of approximately 5–10 mL of blood/kg per hour for 2–4 hours, and if the appropriate coagulation factors have been given, then strong consideration must be given to reexploration of the chest. The most serious consequence of excessive delay in reexploration is cardiac tamponade. Unfortunately, the classic signs of cardiac tamponade (excessive tachycardia, equal atrial filling pressures, widened mediastinum on chest radiograph, pulsus paradoxicus, and hypotension) may not be present. The only signs of impending tamponade may be oliguria, decreased peripheral perfusion, and mild metabolic acidosis. Excessive chest tube output that suddenly stops is particularly worrisome as it may indicate clotting of the tubes, which, if the source of bleeding continues, may lead to rapid tamponade. If the patient is unstable and there is any question as to whether there is cardiac tamponade, the chest should be reopened immediately in the ICU. If tamponade is suspected and the patient is reasonably stable, it may be ideal to return the patient to the operating room for reexploration.

Renal-Metabolic Systems

It is very difficult to calculate the exact fluid requirements of any young patient who has been on cardiopulmonary bypass. It is generally accepted that the total body fluid, particularly the extravascular volume, is increased in the first 24–48 hours. As a routine, these patients are placed on half-maintenance fluids calculated on an hourly basis. The fluid should consist of either a 5% dextrose solution (D_5W) or $D_{10}W$ (depending on the age and weight of the patient).

Higher concentrations of glucose may be required in neonates or very cachetic infants. The appropriate amount of sodium is provided either in the form of $D_5/0.2$ normal saline or sodium chloride is added to $D_{10}W$ as deemed appropriate. Monitoring lines all have sodium in them and, therefore, this must be taken into account when the sodium requirements are calculated. The fluid is continued at a half-maintenance rate (2 mL/kg per hour for the first 10 kg, 1 mL/kg per hour for the next 10 kg, etc.) until the patient is below his or her preoperative weight or there are obvious signs of intravascular free-water depletion. Patients whose operation did not require cardiopulmonary bypass are usually placed on full-maintenance fluids.

Potassium is never added as a routine infusion in the first 24 hours in patients who have undergone surgery that required cardiopulmonary bypass. If potassium is required, it is given as a bolus at a rate of 0.2 mEq of K^+/kg per hour. If renal function is normal, a maintenance amount of potassium is added after the first postoperative day. For patients who have not undergone a procedure requiring cardiopulmonary bypass, maintenance potassium can be added to their maintenance fluids as soon as it is determined that renal function is normal and adequate urine output has been established.

Routine infusion of calcium gluconate is usually not required until after the first 12–24 hours. However, whenever blood or blood products are administered, 1 mg of calcium chloride for every milliliter of blood or blood product administered should be given through a central line while the blood is being administered.[57,58] This counteracts the chelating effects of citrate and prevents sudden drops in ionized calcium that can be very detrimental to myocardial function. If urine output is inadequate, and the preload is excessive (as may be reflected by evidence of pulmonary edema on chest radiograph and increasing respiratory requirements), diuretics should be administered. Furosemide is the drug of choice. If the patient has not been on chronic diuretic therapy, one can begin with 0.5 mg/kg per dose. If this is ineffective, then doses of 1–2 mg/kg per dose may be required. Continuous furosemide infusion is gaining increasing popularity in the management of pediatric patients after cardiac surgery. Its advantages include more controlled and predictable urine output with less requirement and less urinary loss of sodium and chloride.[59] Ethacrynic acid is often quite helpful (1 mg/kg per dose) in patients who have been on chronic diuretic therapy prior to surgery. Low dose dopamine infusion (3–5 µg/kg per min) may improve glomerular blood flow and promote diuresis. If all measures of preload indicate that it is high and there is an inadequate response to diuretic therapy, renal dysfunction must then be considered and appropriate evaluation for acute renal failure must be undertaken as noted above. Therapy for acute renal failure will not be discussed in this chapter. Nitroglycerin and prostaglandin E_1 have both been used to decrease elevated filling pressures, particularly when the excessive preload is felt to be secondary to myocardial dysfunction. If the intravascular volume is considered to be low, but the extravascular volume is high, mannitol alone or mannitol plus a diuretic is very effective in promoting a diuresis that leads to a decrease in the extravascular volume. Care must be taken, however, if acute renal failure is suspected, as mannitol may produce a large osmolar load that cannot be excreted by the failing kidneys. This can be particularly detrimental in neonates who have a marked inability to deal with high osmolar loads.

Ongoing losses via mediastinal tubes, chest tubes, nasogastric tubes, and so forth, must be continuously evaluated. The replacement of chest tube losses volume for volume is not necessary, as noted previously. Rather one should give replacement as required by hemodynamic parameters such as tachycardia and low filling pressures. The routine replacement of chest tube output simply exacerbates the extravascular volume overload that is always present. Chest tube losses are replaced, when necessary, with whatever form of colloid is appropriate depending on the hematocrit and the patient's coagulation status.

After the patient has been extubated for 2–4 hours, and bowel sounds are present, oral feedings are begun if there are no signs of respiratory distress. If prolonged respiratory support is anticipated, hyperalimentation may be required, but is usually not instituted until 24–48 hours after surgery.

SUMMARY

This chapter has focused on the assessment and management of the early postoperative patient (first 24–48 hours). There are many complications that may occur several days later, but the complications that are most likely to be life threatening usually occur early in the postoperative period. Although this chapter has been divided into assessment of each major body system and then management of the routine patient, as well as patients with complications, it must be understood that the "routine" may have to be interrupted at any point to treat a serious complication or postoperative problem. Once this problem is dealt with, one can then proceed with the system-by-system evaluation and treatment. It should also be noted that to provide the best postoperative care for any patient, one must be familiar with the anatomic and hemodynamic problems preoperatively and be fully aware of what hemodynamic and anatomic problems are likely to occur postoperatively. Treatment based on anticipation of expected problems is most likely to result in a successful postoperative outcome.

REFERENCES

1. Freed MD, Heymann MA, Lewis AB, et al: Prostaglandin E_1 in infants with ductus arteriosus-dependent congenital heart disease. *Circulation* **64**:899, 1981

2. Fanconi S, Doherty P, Edmonds JF, et al: Pulse oximetry in pediatric intensive care: Comparison with measured saturations and transcutaneous oxygen tension. *J Pediatr* **107**:362, 1985

3. Fanconi S: Reliability of pulse oximetry in hypoxic infants. *J Pediatr* **112**:424, 1988

4. Yabek SM, Bechara FA, Berman W Jr, et al: Use of atrial epicardial electrodes to diagnose and treat postoperative arrhythmias in children. *Am J Cardiol* **46**:285, 1980

5. Friedman WF, George BL: Treatment of congestive heart failure by altering loading conditions of the heart. *J Pediatr* **106**:697, 1985

6. Wheller J, George BL, Mulder DG, Jarmakani JM: Diagnosis and management of postoperative pulmonary hypertensive crisis. *Circulation* **60**:1640, 1979

7. Rudolph AM: *Congenital Diseases of the Heart.* Chicago, Year Book, 1974, Chap 4, pp 49–167

8. Moodie DS, Feldt RH, Kaye MP, et al: Measurement of postoperative cardiac output by thermodilution in pediatric and adult patients. *J Thorac Cardiovasc Surg* **78**:796, 1979

9. Knight RW, Opie JC: The big toe in the recovery room: Peripheral warm-up of patterns of children after open-heart surgery. *Can J Surg* **24**:239, 1981

10. Spitzer AR, Fox WW: Post-extubation atelectasis—The role of oral versus nasal endotracheal tubes. *J Pediatr* **100**:806, 1982

11. McMillen DD, Rademaker AW, Buchan KA, et al: Benefits of orotracheal and nasotracheal intubation in neonates requiring ventilatory assistance. *Pediatrics* **77**:39, 1986

12. Gregory GA: Respiratory care of newborn infants. *Pediatr Clin N Am* **19**:311, 1972

13. Stark J: Postoperative Care. In Stark J, de Leval M (eds): *Surgery for Congenital Heart Defects.* New York, Grune & Stratton, 1983, Chap 9, pp 135–163

14. Bick RL: Alterations of hemostasis associated with cardiopulmonary bypass: Pathophysiology, prevention, diagnosis, and management. *Sem Thromb Hemost* **3**(2):59, 1976

15. Maurer HM: Hematologic effects of cardiac disease. *Pediatr Clin N Am* **19**:1083, 1972

16. Breckenridge IM, Deverall PB, Kirkin JW, Digerness SB: Potassium intake and balance after open intracardiac operations. *J Thorac Cardiovasc Surg* **63**:305, 1972

17. Baum D, Dillard DH, Porte D Jr: Inhibition of insulin release in infants undergoing deep hypothermic cardiovascular surgery. *N Engl J Med* **279**:1309, 1968

18. Benzing G III, Francis PD, Kaplan S, et al: Glucose and insulin changes in infants and children undergoing hypothermic open-heart surgery. *Am J Cardiol* **52**:133, 1983

19. Herrera AJ, Hsiang Y-H: Comparison of various methods of blood sugar screening in newborn infants. *J Pediatr* **102**:769, 1983

20. Cannon PJ: The kidney in heart failure. *N Engl J Med* **296**:26, 1977

21. Cohn JN, Levine TB, Francis GS, Goldsmith S: Neurohumoral control mechanisms in congestive heart failure. *Am Heart J* **102**:509, 1981

22. Szatalowicz VL, Arnold PE, Chaimovitz C, et al: Radioimmunoassay of plasma arginine vasopressin in hyponatremic patients with congestive heart failure. *N Engl J Med* **305**:263, 1981

23. Phornphutkul C, Rosenthal A, Nadas AS, Berenberg W: Cerebrovascular accidents in infants and children with cyanotic congenital heart disease. *Am J Cardiol* **32**:329, 1973

24. Holley FO, Ponganis KV, Stanski DR: Effect of cardiopulmonary bypass on the pharmacokinetics of drugs. *Clin Pharmacokinet* **7**:234, 1982

25. Friedman WF, George BL: New concepts and drugs in the treatment of congestive heart failure. *Pediatr Clin N Am* **31**:1197, 1984

26. Zaritsky A, Chernow B: Use of catecholamines in pediatrics. *J Pediatr* **105**:341, 1984

27. Lang P, William RG, Norwood WI, Castaneda AR: The hemodynamic effects of dopamine in infants after corrective cardiac surgery: *J Pediatr* **96**:630, 1980

28. Driscoll DJ, Gillette PC, McNamara DG: The use of dopamine in children. *J Pediatr* **92**:309, 1978

29. Richard C, Ricome JL, Rimailho A, et al: Combined hemodynamic effects of dopamine and dobutamine in cardiogenic shock. *Circulation* **67**:620, 1983

30. Schranz D, Stopfkuchen H, Jüngst BK, et al: Hemodynamic effects of dobutamine in children with cardiovascular failure. *Eur J Pediatr* **139**:4, 1982

31. Bohn DJ, Poirer CS, Edmonds JF, Barker GA: Hemodynamic effects of dobutamine after cardiopulmonary bypass in children. *Crit Care Med* **8**:367, 1980

32. Sonnenblick EH, Frishman WH, LeJemtel TH: Dobutamine: A new synthetic cardioactive sympathetic amine. *N Engl J Med* **300**:17, 1979

33. del Nido P, Swan P, Benson L, et al: Successful use of intraaortic balloon pumping in a 2-kilogram infant. *Ann Thorac Surg* **46**:574, 1988

34. Dalton HJ, Siewers RD, Fuhrman BP, et al: Extracorporeal membrane oxygenation for cardiac rescue in children with severe myocardial dysfunction. *Crit Care Med* **21**:(7) 1020, 1993

35. Rossi AF, Steinberg LG, Kipel G, et al: Use of adenosine in the management of perioperative arrhythmias in the pediatric cardiac intensive care unit. *Crit Care Med* **20**(8): 1107, 1992

36. Gelband M, Rosen MR: Pharmacologic basis for the treatment of cardiac arrhythmias. *Pediatrics* **55**:59, 1975

37. Hartzler GO, Maloney JD, Curtis JJ, Barnhost DA: Hemodynamic benefits of atrioventricular sequential pacing after cardiac surgery. *Am J Cardiol* **40**:232, 1977

38. Applebaum A, Blackstone EH, Kouchoukos NT, Kirklin JW: Afterload reduction and cardiac output in infants early after intracardiac surgery. *Am J Cardiol* **39**:445, 1977

39. Benzing G III, Helmsworth GA, Schrieber JT, et al: Nitroprusside after open-heart surgery. *Circulation* **54**:467, 1976

40. Benson LN, Bohn D, Edmonds JF, et al: Nitroglycerin therapy in children with low cardiac index after heart surgery. *Cardiovasc Med* **4**:207, 1979

41. Stemple DR, Kleiman JH, Harrison DC: Combined nitroprusside-dopamine therapy in severe chronic congestive heart failure. *Am J Cardiol* **42**:267, 1978

42. Stephenson LW, Edmunds LH, Raphaely R, et al: Effects of nitroprusside and dopamine on pulmonary arterial vasculature in children after cardiac surgery. *Cardiovasc Surg* **60**:I-104, 1979

43. Hickey PR, Hansen DD, Wessel D: Responses to high dose fentanyl in infants: I. Pulmonary and systemic hemodynamics. *Anesthesiology* **61**:A-445, 1984

44. Hickey PR, Hansen DD, Wessel D: Responses to high dose fentanyl in infants: II. Blunting of stress responses in the pulmonary circulation. *Anesthesiology* **61**:A-446, 1984

45. McGoon MD, Vlietstra RE: Vasodilator therapy for primary pulmonary hypertension. *Mayo Clin Proc* **59**:672, 1984

46. Drummond WH, Lock JE: Neonatal "pulmonary vasodilator" drugs. *Dev Pharmacol Ther* **7**:1, 1984

47. Pearl RG, Rosenthal MH, Schroeder JS, Ashton JPA: Acute hemodynamic effects of nitroglycerin in pulmonary hypertension. *Ann Intern Med* **99**:9, 1983

48. Damen J, Hitchcock JF: Reactive pulmonary hypertension after a switch operation. Successful treatment with glyceryl trinitrate. *Br Heart J* **53**:223, 1985

49. Ilbawi MN, Idriss FS, DeLeon SY, et al: Hemodynamic effects of intravenous nitroglycerin in pediatric patients after heart surgery. *Circulation* **72**:II-101, 1985

50. D'Ambra MN, LaRaia PJ, Philbin DM, et al: Prostaglandin E$_1$. A new therapy for refractory right heart failure and pulmonary hypertension after mitral valve replacement. *J Thorac Cardiovasc* **89**:567, 1985

51. Schranz D, Zepp F, Iversen S, et al: Effects of tolazoline and prostacyclin on pulmonary hypertension in infants after cardiac surgery. *Crit Care Med* **20**(9): 1243, 1992

52. Celermajer DS, Dollery C, Burch M, et al: Role of endothelium in the maintenance of low pulmonary vascular tone in normal children. *Circulation* **89**(5): 2041, 1994

53. Miller OI, Elliott MJ: Intraoperative use of inhaled low-dose nitric oxide. (Letters to the Editor) *J Thorac Cardiovasc Surg.* **105**:550, 1993

54. Selldén H, Winberg P, Gustafsson LE, et al: Inhalation of nitric oxide reduced pulmonary hypertension after cardiac surgery in a 3.2 kg infant. (Case Reports) *Anesthesiology* **78**:577, 1993

55. Lambert CJ, Marengo-Rowe AJ, Leveson JE, et al: The treatment of postperfusion bleeding using ε-aminocaproic acid, cryoprecipitate, fresh-frozen plasma, and protamine sulfate. *Ann Thorac Surg* **28**:440, 1979

56. McClure PD, Izsak J: The use of epsilon-aminocaproic acid to reduce bleeding during cardiac bypass in children with congenital heart disease. *Anesthesiology* **40**:604, 1974

57. Abbott TR: Changes in serum calcium fractions and citrate concentrations during massive blood transfusions and cardiopulmonary bypass. *Br J Anaesth* **55**:753, 1983

58. Olinger GN, Hottenrott C, Mulder DG, et al: Acute clinical hypocalcemic myocardial depression during rapid blood transfusion and postoperative hemodialysis. A preventable complication. *J Thorac Cardiovasc Surg* **72**:503, 1976

59. Singh NC, Kissoon N, Mofada SA, et al: Comparison of continuous versus intermittent furosemide administration in postoperative pediatric cardiac patients. *Crit Care Med* **20**(1): 17, 1992

59

Anesthesia for Pediatric Cardiac Surgery

Victor C. Baum and Susheela Sangwan

The development of pediatric cardiac anesthesia over the past decade as a special entity has made considerable strides as we have seen the application of advanced technology in cardiac monitoring, the availability of newer anesthetic, inotropic, and cardiovascular drugs, and perhaps a greater understanding of how best to utilize these for children. The anesthesiologist who wishes to practice in this field must have a knowledge of the anatomy and physiology of congenital heart disease in combination with training in pediatric anesthesia. This chapter assumes the reader already has an understanding of the pathophysiology of the various congenital heart defects.

PREOPERATIVE EVALUATION

Patients who present for cardiac surgery range from the newborn to young adults and this has important implications for the anesthesiologist, as there are anatomic and physiologic developmental differences. For instance the neonate has increased cardiac index, increased oxygen consumption, increased volume of distribution, lower functional residual capacity, slower drug metabolism, and requires a different pharmacologic and physiologic approach than the older children. The preoperative visit should be used to get all the pertinent information regarding the cardiac lesion and to prepare the child and his or her family for the perioperative events. It is also during this visit that the anesthesiologist can establish a rapport with the children and alleviate some if not all their fears regarding surgery.

History

It is necessary to obtain a history of previous anesthetic experience including any complications, and questions should be asked regarding any previous palliative surgery. For example, the presence of a systemic arterial to pulmonary arterial shunt can influence the placement of monitoring lines and also has implications for the ligation of the shunt prior to bypass (vide infra).

Physical Examination

During the routine physical examination it is important to look for loss or decrement in pulse amplitude in one arm in the presence of a Blalock–Taussig shunt, or there may be a difference of blood pressure in the extremities due to coarctation of the aorta. The assessment of airway is particularly important in children with Pierre Robin, Treacher Collins, or other dysmorphic syndromes. These children have a very difficult airway and in the presence of cyanotic lesions they may not have much respiratory reserve if there is a compromise of their airway during induction of anesthesia. Patients with Down syndrome can also have airway problems due to a large tongue and are also more prone to cervical spine dislocation.[1,2]

Laboratory Data

Blood

The determination of hemoglobin concentration is helpful in deciding whether the pump should be primed with blood.

This may be unnecessary in the presence of erythrocytosis. Hematocrit levels in these patients should be assessed only by automated techniques because determining hematocrit levels with microhematocrit tubes results in plasma trapping and falsely high measured levels.[3] Erythrocytosis in cyanotic heart disease can result in decreased tissue perfusion and care should be exercised regarding preoperative hydration orders. The level of hemoglobin can also have an effect on left-to-right and right-to-left shunting. In acyanotic patients with left-to-right shunting[4] a higher hematocrit improves the balance between pulmonary and systemic blood flow. In patients with cyanotic heart disease the optimal hematocrit is different for tetralogy of Fallot as compared to D-transposition. Studies[5] have found that by decreasing the hematocrit from 70 to 60% shunting increased between the pulmonary and systemic circulation in D-transposition, thus improving tissue oxygenation.

A variety of hemostatic abnormalities have been described in cyanotic, erythrocytotic patients.[6] Bleeding tendencies are usually absent or mild when hematocrit levels are less than 65%, although serious bleeding can occur with traumatic or surgical injury. The mechanisms of the hemostatic defects have not yet been fully defined. Generally, the degree of the bleeding diathesis tends to mirror the degree of erythrocytosis. Tests of coagulation may show a coagulopathy of polycythemia. This may be the result of a low-grade disseminated intravascular coagulation[7,8] with consumption of factors because of peripheral sludging. In patients with hematocrits greater than 70% an isovolemic exchange transfusion has been shown to be beneficial.[9] Abnormalities of the intrinsic and extrinsic coagulation systems with deficiencies of specific clotting factors have also been described in cyanotic patients.[10–14] The fibrinolytic pathways are normal.[15] Occasionally, patients with both cyanotic and acyanotic congenital heart diseases have deficiencies of the largest von Willebrand factor multimers,[16] which normalize after corrective surgery.[17] Neonates can have a decrease of coagulation factors due to immature hepatic function and may benefit from a dose of vitamin K. Platelet counts in cyanotic patients are typically in the low-normal range, but occasionally are significantly reduced.[10] Bleeding is, however, not related to thrombocytopenia per se. When corrected for red cell mass and blood volume, total platelet count is, with few exceptions, closer to normal. Abnormalities of platelet function have been reported.[11,18–20] Patients with synthetic vascular anastomoses are sometimes maintained on a platelet inhibitor (aspirin), which increases the risk of intraoperative bleeding. In addition to platelet counts, which are artificially reduced due to the decreased plasma volume, the prothrombin time and partial thromboplastin time may also be artificially elevated. Tubes for the determination of prothrombin time and partial thromboplastin time contain a fixed amount of citrate as anticoagulant. This volume of citrate assumes a normal hematocrit level, but is excessive for erythrocytotic blood, because each milliliter of blood contains more red

blood cells and therefore less plasma. Tubes with the correct amount of citrate can be prepared by the clinical laboratory if the patient's hematocrit level is known. This correction should be done when hematocrit levels are greater than 55%. Correcting to an idealized hematocrit level of 45% (plasma volume of 55%), the amount of citrate added to the tube can be calculated with the following formula.[21]

$$\text{ml of citrate} = (0.1 \times \text{blood volume collected})$$
$$\times \frac{(100 - \text{patient's hematocrit})}{55}$$

Serum Electrolytes

Infants are especially at risk for hypoglycemia and hypocalcemia, the effects of which will be masked under general anesthesia. Hence it is important to have a baseline evaluation and monitor these intraoperatively. Those children who are on diuretics should be evaluated for hypokalemia, which can be a particular problem if they are also on digoxin. Because of the diminished amount of plasma in each volume of erythrocytotic compared to normal blood, clinical laboratories may require larger samples of whole blood to obtain the required amounts of plasma or serum.

Blood Gas Tensions

In the past, preoperative measurement of arterial gas tensions has been found to be helpful in establishing the respiratory reserve of these children, in particular those with cyanotic disease. Cyanotic children will therefore not have much reserve if they become more hypoxic during induction of anesthesia and they require very careful management of their airway. However, presently oxygen saturation obtained by pulse oximetry has obviated the need to measure blood gas tensions.

Chest x-Ray and Electrocardiogram

The chest x-ray should be helpful in ruling out pulmonary edema in the presence of congestive heart failure. In children who present for repeat operations a lateral film can help determine the proximity of right heart and surgical conduits to the sternum and a decision may be made to electively expose/cannulate the femoral vessels. The greatest value of the ECG is to rule out preexisting dysrhythmias.

Echocardiographic and Catheterization Data

These data are essential in the formulation of appropriate anesthetic management. More patients are now presenting for surgery with echocardiography studies alone. Transthoracic Doppler echocardiography (TTE) is able to answer most but not all the questions regarding anatomy and flow in congenital heart disease. We have found it very useful to define the questions that need to be answered by intraoperative transesophageal echocardiography (TEE). This is discussed and decided for the individual cases during the preoperative clinical conference, which is held in conjunction with the cardiologist and surgeon. At our institution we have found it to be most useful for the pediatric cardiac anesthesia service to be an active participant in these conferences.

PREMEDICATION

Preoperative medication is used in children over 6 mo of age as an adjunct to alleviate anxiety, allow for comfortable removal from parents, and allow for gentle induction of anesthesia. A good preoperative visit may suffice for a cooperative older child and may help significantly to address and allay fears, while the very anxious younger child may require larger doses of preoperative medication. The goal is to have a lightly sedated anxiety-free child without producing respiratory depression. There are few if any disadvantages to appropriate premedication. In general, preoperative medication is not indicated or required in infants under 6 mo of age and should be used cautiously in patients with profound congestive failure. Ventilatory response to hypercarbia is normal in cyanotic patients and there is no need to avoid appropriate premedication. A variety of sedative medications have been used in pediatric patients given via oral, rectal, intramuscular, or intranasal routes. We have found it extraordinarily unusual for a patient to require a painful intramuscular premedication. Commonly used premedications are listed in Table 59–1. Adequate time (about 20 min) is required for onset of oral premedicants.

Most medications are given through to the morning of surgery. The two major exceptions to this rule are diuretics and digoxin. Most anesthetics are associated with some degree of vasodilatation, so diuretics are held to ensure that the patient is volume replete at the time of induction of anesthesia. Whether to continue digoxin depends on the indication for its use in each individual patient. It should be continued if it is indicated for control of atrial dysrhythmias, but we prefer to withhold it on the day of surgery if it is being given solely as an inotrope. This is because myocardium with significant digoxin levels is more likely to develop arrhythmias when stimulated by an intravascular wire or a surgeon's forceps. Digoxin itself is a relatively weak inotrope. If inotropic support is required there are numerous other more effective intravenous alternatives available.

PREOPERATIVE FASTING

Aspiration of gastric contents presents a potential danger during the induction of anesthesia when protective airway reflexes are no longer functional. Because of this anesthesiologists have insisted on delaying elective or urgent surgery for a period of time after the ingestion of food to allow for gastric emptying. This has typically been 8 hours for older children and 4 hours for younger children. Since these orders were usually written "npo after midnight" most children were often truly without fluids for 12 hours or more, as they would fall asleep after dinner and sleep through the night. This has proven problematic in erythrocytotic patients at risk for additional sludging of viscous blood and in young infants who become hungry, irritable, and potentially hypoglycemic. Data that have become available within the past few years have documented that a period of only 2

TABLE 59–1. DOSES OF COMMONLY USED PREMEDICANT DRUGS

Drug	Route	Dose	Comment
Atropine	Oral or intramuscular	0.01 mg/kg IM; 0.02 mg/kg Po	Added by some to reduce oral secretions and lessen chance of bradycardia on induction
Fentanyl	Oral lozenge[22]	As needed	"Lollipop" oral lozenge delivery system well tolerated; risk of respiratory depression; incidence of pruritus and emesis
Ketamine	Oral[23]	6 mg/kg	Dysphoria not a problem when given orally
Ketamine	Intramuscular	4 mg/kg	For preinduction; higher doses (10 mg/kg) are anesthetic
Midazolam (Versed®)	Oral[24]	0.5 mg/kg	Bitter taste needs to be disguised; some often spit out so dose may be 0.75 mg/kg
Midazolam (Versed®)	Rectal[25]	1 mg/kg	
Midazolam (Versed®)	Intranasal[26]	0.2 mg/kg	Stings on administration
Methohexital (Brevital®)	Rectal[27]	25 mg/kg	
Morphine	Intramuscular	0.1 mg/kg	Often combined with scopolamine 0.01 mg/kg; IM injection painful; primarily an analgesic, not an anxiolytic; risk of respiratory depression.
Pentobarbital (Nembutal®)	Rectal or oral	4 mg/kg	Delayed awakening from very brief nonbypass surgery
Sufentanil	Intranasal[26]	2 µg/kg	Risk of desaturation

hours is required after ingestion of clear fluids to allow for gastric emptying.[28–30] It should be stressed that this holds only for clear liquids and in the absence of other processes that may delay gastric emptying such as diabetes, trauma, and obesity.

MONITORS

The extent of monitoring depends to a large extent on the underlying clinical condition, the proposed operation, and the expected postoperative course. Children undergoing cardiac surgery require a variety of perioperative physiologic monitors as do adult patients. A major difference in pediatric patients is that placement of invasive monitors is often delayed until after the induction of anesthesia to prevent patient discomfort from pain or positioning. Depending on the patient's hemodynamic stability and cooperation, anesthesia may be elected to be induced with as little as a precordial stethoscope, with immediate addition of other monitors immediately following loss of consciousness. Routine monitors include the following.

Electrocardiogram

Pediatric patients should have placement of leads for monitoring multiple ECG leads. In addition to arrhythmia diagnosis, the ECG also serves as an ischemia monitor.[31,32] Pediatric patients may manifest myocardial ischemia as a direct result of their surgery (e.g., arterial switch procedure or truncus arteriosus) or may have ischemia unrelated directly to the structural abnormality (Fig. 59–1).

Respiration

Respiratory sounds should be monitored. Thoracic surgery usually precludes use of a precordial stethoscope beyond induction, and an esophageal stethoscope, usually combined with a thermistor to measure temperature, is used. In addition, expired carbon dioxide is now commonly measured intraoperatively. Not only does this confirm correct placement of the endotracheal tube, but confirms intratracheal positioning of the tube throughout surgery and allows noninvasive estimates of arterial P_{CO_2}. The precision of capnometry and end-tidal CO_2 as a measure of arterial P_{CO_2} varies with age and the type of anesthesia circuit.[33] In addition, end-tidal CO_2 underestimates arterial P_{CO_2} in cyanotic patients[34] and in patients with markedly diminished pulmonary blood flow.

Temperature

Profound hypothermia is often required during repair of complex congenital heart disease. While a single temperature probe is adequate for nonpump procedures, typically two separate thermistors are used for cases requiring car-

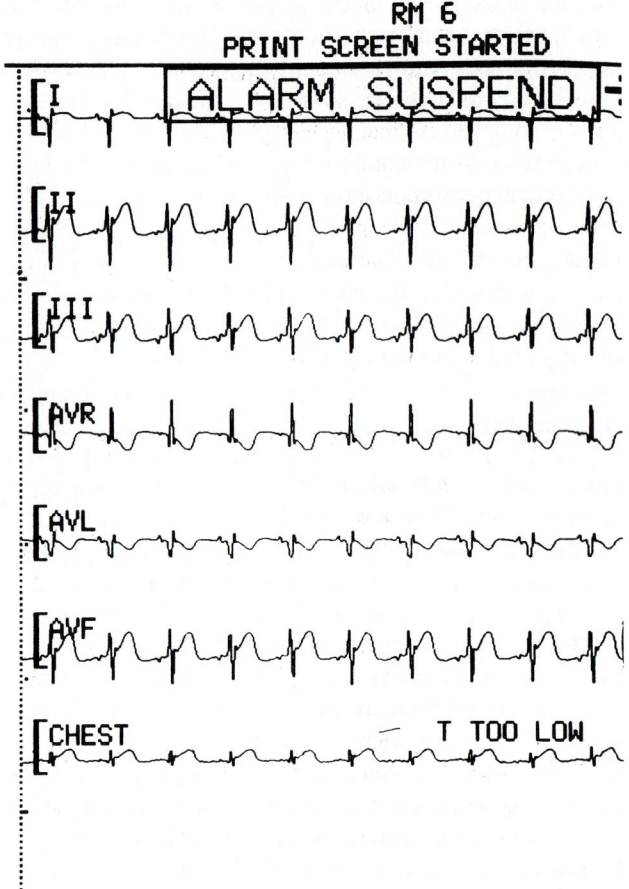

Figure 59–1. Multiple lead ECG in an infant. There were reproducible ST segment changes each time the suction tip irritated the diaphragmatic surface of the left ventricle.

diopulmonary bypass. An esophageal probe lies close to the aorta and reflects the temperature of blood returning through the aortic cannula. Rectal temperature tends to more closely reflect core temperature. Better measures of core temperature are obtained by placing thermistors in the bladder (in older children), in the external auditory canal to reflect tympanic temperature, or in the nasopharynx to more closely estimate brain temperature.

Pulse Oximetry

All patients should have placement of a pulse oximeter to measure intraoperative systemic arterial saturation. This is particularly useful during induction of anesthesia and in patients with cyanotic heart disease in whom the relative resistances in the pulmonary and systemic circulations are reflected in changes in systemic arterial oxygen saturation. This monitor may not function in the face of inadequate perfusion of the monitoring site, and can be used to ensure adequate perfusion of the dependent arm during operations in the lateral position. The response rate to changes in arterial oxygen saturation is faster in proximal locations. On occasion a probe placed on the tongue or the cheek will provide functional data in children when more routine sites on the extremities are nonfunctioning due to low flow states.[35,36] Although one normally assumes the role of the anesthesiologist is to maintain an oxygen saturation above a certain level, in premature infants retinopathy of prematurity (retrolental fibroplasia) is a risk of prolonged high oxygen levels, and in these infants the oxygen saturation should be kept below 95%. The exact degree and duration of hyperoxia responsible for retinopathy of prematurity remain unclear. There is little effect of fetal hemoglobin on the accuracy of pulse oximetry.

Systemic Arterial Catheter

Most patients will benefit from placement of a systemic arterial catheter. They are usually readily placed percutaneously even in the smallest patients. A variety of sites are available. Most routinely used are the radial and femoral arteries. The umbilical artery is also available in neonates during the first few days of life. Pressure obtained from radial arterial catheters is usually valid, but may underestimate aortic blood pressure postbypass in children as well as in adults.[37] Femoral artery catheterization does not carry an increased risk in pediatric patients.[38] Although catheters can be placed into the superficial temporal, dorsalis pedis, and posterior tibial arteries, these are less useful. The superficial temporal artery is contraindicated due to the risk of emboli passing to the nearby carotid artery and thence to the distribution of the ipsilateral middle cerebral artery.[39] Although the pedal arteries can provide a valid arterial pressure tracing prebypass and in nonbypass cases, these tracings are so often unacceptably dampened following bypass as to make them not useful. Placement of arterial catheters into an axillary artery may be required in children who have had multiple prior arterial catheters with no other patent superficial arteries.[40] Use of the brachial artery is contraindicated in children due to the risk of forearm ischemia. Although indwelling continuous measurement of blood gas tensions and pH is currently available using optode technology and can be placed in a catheter small enough to be introduced into the femoral artery of young infants, these catheters are currently quite expensive.

Central Venous Catheters

Catheters can be introduced either percutaneously into the central venous circulation or under direct vision into the right or left atrium. A variety of multilumen catheters is available for even the smallest patient. Catheters can be introduced percutaneously into the central circulation via the internal jugular, external jugular, subclavian or femoral veins, and umbilical vein in neonates. If placed preoperatively, the chest radiograph should be reviewed to document an intrathoracic position of the umbilical venous catheter tip to avoid infusion of caustic agents into the por-

tal vein and resultant hepatic damage. Venous pressure in the abdominal inferior vena cava reliably reflects right atrial pressure, in the absence of abdominal distension.[41,42] Femoral venous catheters can be placed and maintained safely in pediatric patients.[43] Specific arterial and venous vascular access considerations in pediatric cardiac surgery patients are listed in Table 59–2.

Pulmonary Arterial Catheters

Pulmonary arterial flotation (Swan-Ganz®) catheters are not routinely used in pediatric patients. Some centers place thermistor catheters into the pulmonary artery in young children under direct vision allowing for measurement of cardiac output by thermodilution postoperatively.[44] The use of a catheter in the pulmonary artery is of particular benefit in cases where postoperative changes in pulmonary vascular resistance and pulmonary arterial pressure are expected to be of major hemodynamic consequence.

Urine Output

Urine output is routinely measured by an indwelling bladder catheter in operations utilizing cardiopulmonary bypass, in even the smallest pediatric patients. Shorter, nonpump cases do not necessarily require placement of a bladder catheter.

Brain Metabolism and Blood Flow

Several centers are currently evaluating cerebral blood flow or metabolism by use of radiolabeled xenon,[45] near infrared spectroscopy to estimate brain high-energy phosphate concentrations,[46] jugular venous oxygen saturation,[47] or cerebral blood flow velocity as determined by transcranial

TABLE 59–2. VASCULAR ACCESS CONSIDERATIONS PARTICULAR TO PATIENTS WITH CONGENITAL HEART DISEASE

Potential for passage of air or other emboli right to left (even through a nominal left-to-right shunt)

Femoral vein thrombosis or ligation secondary to old catheterization

Anatomic discontinuity of inferior vena cava and right atrium (e.g., polysplenia)

Reduced lower extremity blood pressure with coarctation

Discontinuity of subclavian artery with Blalock–Taussig anastomosis during current or prior procedure, or subclavian artery stenosis with modified Blalock–Taussig anastomosis

Preductal vs postductal arterial sampling differences with right-to-left ductal level shunt

Umbilical vein catheter wedged into liver with risk of hepatic injury with injection of hypertonic fluids (e.g., bicarbonate)

Artifactually elevated right arm blood pressure with supravalvar aortic stenosis (Coanda effect)

Placement of an umbilical artery catheter tip into an aortic branch with consequent organ ischemia or thromboembolism

Doppler interrogation of the middle cerebral artery,[48–50] particularly during procedures requiring hypothermic circulatory arrest. Particulate and gaseous cerebral emboli are apparent on Doppler examination and inadvertent clamping of aortic arch vessels is also apparent by flow cessation. The use of these tools is currently experimental.

Transesophageal Echocardiography (TEE)

The initial application of TEE in the intraoperative setting was in adult cardiac surgery[51] but with the availability of pediatric transducers TEE has been found to be equally useful in the pediatric population.[52] TEE, when compared to epicardial echocardiography, does not interfere with surgery and allows for continuous monitoring of cardiac function. With the advent of small biplane transducers in combination with continuous wave Doppler, the use of epicardial echocardiography has declined but not disappeared, because there are regions of the heart such as the apical septum and the right ventricular outflow tract that are better seen with epicardial echocardiography. The indications for TEE include the need to answer questions not answered by external echocardiography in selecting the surgical approach, as an intraoperative monitor, and for evaluation of the surgical repair.

Intraoperative Diagnostic Indication

Anomalies of Pulmonary and Systemic Venous Return
TEE is superior to epicardial echocardiography[53] in the identification of abnormal systemic and venous connections including partial anomalous pulmonary venous drainage and the presence of a persistent left superior vena cava draining to the coronary sinus.

Sinus Venosus Defects
A diagnosis sometimes missed in older children by TTE, these are well seen by TEE.[54]

Atrioventricular Junction
TEE can provide detailed information concerning the morphology of the atrioventricular valves and chordal apparatus.[55] TEE is superior to TTE in assessment of chordal override.[56]

Ventricular Septal Defects
Most ventricular septal defects[57] are well seen by TEE, except small apical defects and anterior muscular defects, which remain difficult to see as they are in the far field.

Left Ventricular Outflow Tract
TEE is able to show both membranous and long segment tunnel obstruction[58] and their relationship to the mitral and aortic valves. With the availability of continuous wave Doppler it is now possible to calculate pressure gradients

across the left ventricular outflow tract from the transgastric view. The aortic valve is well seen in both planes and aortic regurgitation can be quantified using both planes.

Right Ventricular Outflow Tract
It is essential to have a longitudinal plane[59] to scan the right ventricular outflow tract, although sometimes far-field attenuation even with this plane can result in suboptimal definition of this area. The longitudinal plane is also useful in assessment of the degree of override of the aorta in patients with VSD, pulmonary atresia, or truncus arteriosus.

The Great Vessels
TEE is helpful in visualization of the distal pulmonary arteries although interposition of the left main bronchus may obscure a proximal part of the left pulmonary artery.

Intraoperative Monitoring of Function and Filling by TEE

This can help in the management of intraoperative hypotension either in the pre- or postbypass period. Left ventricular dysfunction due to intracardiac air is easy to diagnose and can be treated with appropriate measures such as increasing the blood pressure. Wall motion abnormalities are also well seen by TEE and if a new finding should necessitate a search for any reversible lesion such as coronary artery obstruction following the arterial switch procedure. We have found TEE to be almost indispensable in patients who are difficult to wean off bypass in the identification of the problem and its treatment, as it helps in distinguishing between functional and structural abnormalities. The management of structural abnormalities necessitates going back on bypass and correcting the problem, whereas functional problems can be managed with appropriate inotropic support.

Assessment of the Surgical Repair

VSD Repair
Residual patch leaks[60] have been noted in up to 55% of patients. Defects less than 3 mm in size are considered to be insignificant and those over 3 mm may be more important. Left-ventricle to right-atrium shunts even if small should be closed and are well seen by TEE.

Repair of Atrioventricular Valves
The degree of intraoperative atrioventricular valve regurgitation is similar to that obtained by TTE.[61] This was one of the first indications for intraoperative use of TEE. The hemodynamic loading conditions should be optimized before making assessments of the valvular repair to avoid underestimation or overestimation of the regurgitation.

Tetralogy of Fallot Repair
Assessment of right ventricular outflow tract obstruction is based on the minimum width of color flow Doppler in this

area during midsystole and the use of spectral Doppler distal to the pulmonary valve. TEE can be helpful in locating the size of obstruction[59] in the presence of a right ventricle to pulmonary artery gradient.

Fontan Procedure

TEE is helpful in localization of previously placed aortopulmonary shunts and in identification of aortopulmonary collaterals. It is used to confirm the patency of a surgically created adjustable atrial septal defect, its size, and the measurement of the gradient across the defect. Atriocavopulmonary anastomoses are clearly defined by TEE and can be useful to exclude any obstruction across the anastomosis. Nonpatency of the azygous vein can be looked for in patients undergoing a hemiFontan procedure.[62]

ANESTHETIC AGENTS

Successful anesthetic agents must not only provide the requisites of a good anesthetic, namely analgesia, akinesia, and amnesia with hemodynamic stability, but should prevent extremes of stress responses. In very young infants undergoing cardiac surgery major stress response has been associated with poorer outcomes.[63,64]

Inhalational Anesthetics

There are several inhalational anesthetics available for clinical use. These are the volatile agents halothane, isoflurane, and enflurane, the newer volatile agents desflurane and sevoflurane, and nitrous oxide. All of the inhalational agents should be used with caution because of cardiovascular depression. In any patient with marginal cardiac function, these agents may result in excessive cardiac depression. However, they can be very useful in inducing anesthesia in the absence of intravenous access and in supplementing intravenous anesthetics in controlling hypertensive responses. Halothane has a particular place in pediatric anesthesia. It is less pungent than the other volatile agents (save sevoflurane) and so is better tolerated by the patient during mask inductions of anesthesia. Although halothane (and the other volatile agents) are tolerated less well by neonates[65,66] and critically ill patients of all ages, it is used successfully, particularly in combination with nitrous oxide, as an induction agent. Atrial arrhythmias are not uncommon during induction with halothane. These are usually minor and of no consequence; however, the loss of p waves and the atrial component of ventricular filling may be significant in patients with poor ventricular function. "Halothane hepatitis" has not been a problem in children with or without heart disease.[67] Isoflurane and enflurane are sometimes used to supplement intravenous anesthesia following induction of anesthesia. In patients with good underlying cardiac function, they may even be used as the primary anesthetic with or without supplementation by intravenous agents. Isoflurane has vasodilatory properties not seen with the en-

flurane or halothane and is shorter acting, resulting in more rapid arousal once anesthetic is discontinued. These two qualities make it useful in particular circumstances. Enflurane is somewhat more of a myocardial depressant and is longer lasting. In all three cases, the concentration of anesthetic delivered to the patient is continuously modified based on the patient's hemodynamic responses. Because their advantage is primarily shorter duration, desflurane and sevoflurane may not become common in pediatric cardiac anesthesia.

Because of the potential of nitrous oxide to enlarge air emboli,[67–69] its use in pediatric cardiac anesthesia tends to be restricted to induction and emergence (if the trachea will be extubated in the operating room). This issue is of significance in pediatric cardiac surgery patients not only due to the increased risk of air entry via incisions in the heart and great vessels, but also to the increased risk of right-to-left passage of gas emboli if they do occur. The low solubility of nitrous oxide results in rapid uptake and elimination, making it particularly useful during induction and awakening. In adults nitrous oxide decreases cardiac output[70,71] and systemic arterial blood pressure, and increases pulmonary vascular resistance, particularly in patients in whom pulmonary vascular resistance is already elevated.[72–74] Such an increase in pulmonary vascular resistance would be problematic in children with already elevated pulmonary vascular resistance, or who required low pulmonary vascular resistance to ensure adequate pulmonary blood flow (such as following the Fontan procedure). However, in children, no increases in pulmonary vascular resistance were seen with the use of 50% nitrous oxide regardless of the preexisting pulmonary vascular resistance.[75] Nitrous oxide and halothane are routinely used to induce anesthesia in cyanotic pediatric patients, and systemic oxygen saturation routinely increases rather than decreases, suggesting again that nitrous oxide does not significantly increase pulmonary vascular resistance in these patients.[76,77] Although the use of nitrous oxide precludes the use of 100% oxygen, these children will still be receiving greater than the 21% oxygen they normally breathe, and increments or decrements in FIO_2 have only minimal effects on arterial PO_2 when arterial desaturation is caused by right-to-left shunting.[78] When added to halothane or isoflurane anesthesia in infants and young children, nitrous oxide decreases heart rate, cardiac output and pulmonary arterial pressure, while maintaining stroke volume and ejection fraction.[79]

The routine increase in oxygen saturation with the induction of anesthesia is felt due to the beneficial effect of anesthesia in decreasing oxygen consumption, thereby increasing the oxygen content of mixed venous (shunted) blood (Fig. 59–2).[77] The presence of intra- or extracardiac right-to-left or left-to-right shunts will theoretically affect the rapidity of uptake and distribution, and hence the rapidity of the induction of anesthesia, when using inhalational agents. These effects have been computer modeled[80] and are most pronounced for gases with low solubility such as

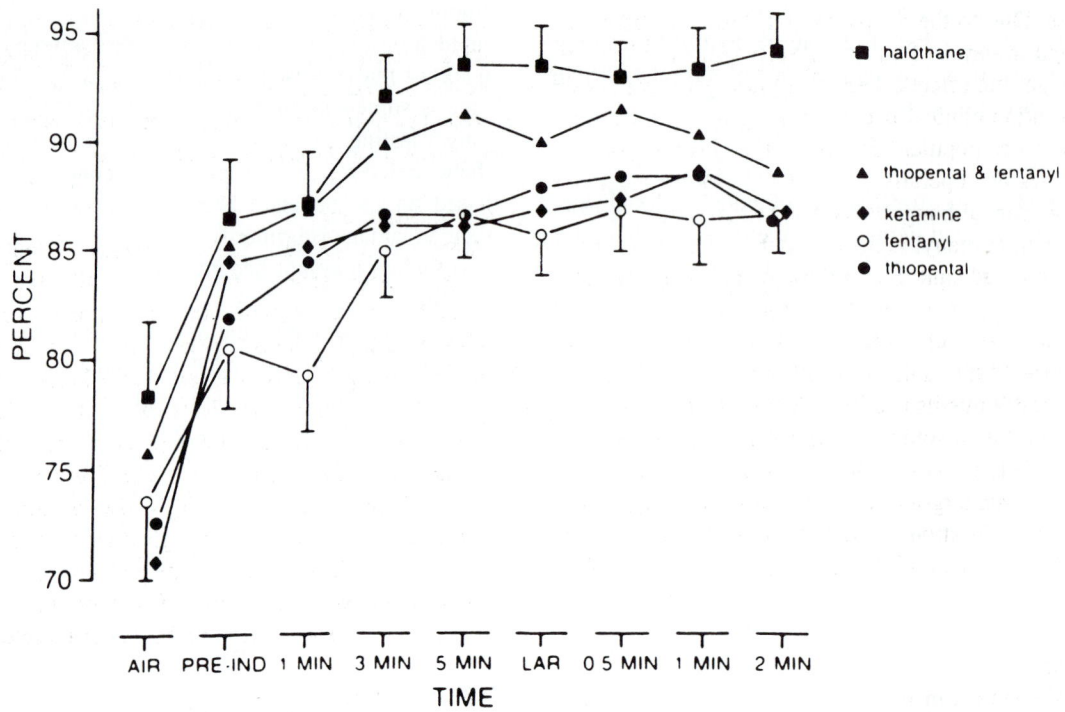

Figure 59–2. Effects of a variety of induction regimens on oxygen saturation in cyanotic children. AIR, breathing room air; PRE-IND, pre-induction breathing 100% oxygen; LAR, laryngoscopy. *(From Laishley RS, Burrows FA, Lerman J, et al: Anesthesiology 65:673, 1986, with permission.)*

nitrous oxide. The effects on gases of intermediate solubility such as halothane are less, and clinically these differences in the rapidity of induction are not of major import.

Intravenous Agents

Ketamine

Ketamine is often a useful anesthetic agent in pediatric cardiac anesthesia. Because of its effects to both increase central adrenergic activity and inhibit peripheral norepinephrine reuptake, it maintains myocardial function and is well tolerated in children with congestive heart failure or cyanosis.[76,77,81,82] It is particularly useful in cases in which maintenance of systemic vascular resistance is important in maintaining pulmonary blood flow, such as tetralogy of Fallot or patients who are dependent on an aortopulmonary shunt for pulmonary blood flow. The ability to use intramuscular ketamine as an anesthetic induction agent also increases its utility. Although ketamine has been reported to increase pulmonary vascular resistance in adults, in well-premedicated children ketamine produces no changes in pulmonary vascular resistance providing ventilation is supported and hypercarbia avoided.[83–85] Since ketamine is a sialogogue, concurrent use of an antisialogogue such as atropine or glycopyrrolate is useful. Simultaneous use of a benzodiazepine can blunt the dysphoric effects of ketamine, although this seems to be less pronounced in younger children. Ketamine is relatively contraindicated in situations

where hypertension, tachycardia, increased cardiac work, or elevated systemic vascular resistance would be poorly tolerated, such as critical aortic stenosis, anomalous left coronary artery, or hypoplastic left heart syndrome.

Narcotics

As in adults, anesthetic techniques based on high-dose narcotics have proven extremely safe in anesthetizing critically ill children and neonates, with hemodynamic stability and suppression of stress responses.[64,65] Anesthetic techniques consisting primarily of high-dose narcotics have become the standard for pediatric cardiac anesthesia. These agents can be safely used even in critically ill premature infants. Although narcotics are extremely safe, they do lack certain properties making them less-than-perfect anesthetics. In particular, they do not provide amnesia and there are cases of patient awareness during pure narcotic anesthesia. For these reasons supplementation with either a benzodiazepine or low doses of a volatile agent, if tolerated hemodynamically, is usual. As with the above anesthetics, oxygen saturation is usually increased following induction of anesthesia with a narcotic in cyanotic patients.[77,86] The hemodynamic stability of most of the narcotics is impressive. Changes in cardiac index, systemic vascular resistance, and pulmonary vascular resistance in neonates are minimal during induction with large doses of fentanyl.[87] Although the newer synthetic narcotics are extremely hemodynamically stable, high-dose morphine, no longer used as a primary cardiac anesthetic, can be associated with hypotension from histamine release. Due to the vagotonic properties of these narcotics, pancuronium is often the muscle relaxant of choice, due to its vagolytic effects. There are currently three potent opiates in routine clinical use as primary anesthetics. Fentanyl is the most popular. The use of high-dose fentanyl often mandates postoperative ventilatory support due to its duration of action, although this often needs to be only for a very few hours. Fentanyl is also available as an oral troche for use as a premedicant. Sufentanil and alfentanil are also currently available in parenteral formulations. Sufentanil provides little if any advantage over fentanyl, and at additional expense. Alfentanil is a shorter-acting opiate. Its shorter duration limits its use for routine cardiac anesthesia, although it may be of some use for shorter, nonbypass procedures. Remifentanil is an extremely short-duration potent opiate currently undergoing clinical trials. Again, because of its very brief duration of activity, it would not be expected to have a major place in routine pediatric cardiac anesthesia.

Barbiturates

Although thiopental can be used as an intravenous induction agent in children with good myocardial function, it is avoided in most cases due to myocardial depression. Myocardial depression is possible[88] and barbiturates are more lethal to neonatal than to mature animals.[89] Neonates have decreased ability to metabolize barbiturates[90] although this is not a practical problem with the shorter-acting barbiturates. Rectal methohexital can be used as an aid to induction in uncooperative children with good myocardial function.

Benzodiazepines

Midazolam (Versed®) is often used both as an effective premedicant and intraoperatively to supplement a base of narcotic anesthesia. Midazolam supplies an amnestic quality lacking in the narcotics. An anesthetic consisting of ketamine and midazolam has also been used in pediatric anesthesia.

Propofol

Because of its myocardial depressant effects, which approximate those of barbiturates, and its very short duration of activity, propofol (Diprivan®) is not used for routine pediatric cardiac anesthesia.

Muscle Relaxants

Succinylcholine

Because of its association with masseter spasm and malignant hyperthermia, the use of succinylcholine in pediatric anesthesiology is diminishing and it has recently been recommended that it not be used routinely in pediatric patients due to complications in patients with undiagnosed and unexpected myopathy. It is more and more being restricted to use when rapid onset of muscle relaxation is required. It

will likely be replaced in the next years with a nondepolarizing muscle relaxant of rapid onset. Succinylcholine may be associated with bradycardia in young infants and it is often accompanied by atropine in these patients. It may be given intramuscularly in the absence of intravenous access.

Pancuronium

Pancuronium (Pavulon®) has a relatively long duration of activity, with recovery from 95 to 50% block in approximately 45 min. Pancuronium has vagolytic activity and is associated with increases in heart rate. This is often beneficial in young infants who are more heart-rate dependent than older children and adults, is of little concern in children with no coronary artery disease and without severe aortic stenosis, and is often beneficial in that it counteracts the bradycardic effect of high-dose narcotic anesthesia. Pancuronium is excreted to a great (but not complete) degree by the kidneys, so its duration of action is prolonged in the face of renal insufficiency. Pancuronium is also significantly less expensive than are the newer muscle relaxants.

Vecuronium

This intermediate duration muscle relaxant has a duration of action approximately one-half that of pancuronium. It is metabolized by the liver. Vecuronium is not associated with hemodynamic changes even in large doses. The absence of heart rate changes may be of use in certain clinical circumstances. Combined with high-dose narcotics, there may be bradycardia.

Atracurium

Atracurium is also an intermediate duration muscle relaxant. It does not require either renal or hepatic excretion as it undergoes physicochemical degradation at body temperature. Atracurium is associated with histamine release, but this is rarely of hemodynamic consequence.

AIRWAY MANAGEMENT

The tracheas of young children are routinely intubated with uncuffed endotracheal tubes. These may be placed either nasally or orally. Children have less well-developed nasal capillary networks than do adults and significant bleeding after nasal intubation is not a major problem, even after systemic heparinization. Nasal intubation has the advantage of being easier to care for in the intensive care unit (no saliva) and being much more difficult for an unhappy toddler to dislodge. The correct sized endotracheal tube will be marked by a leak between the endotracheal tube and the trachea when airway pressure is increased to greater than about 20 cm H_2O. Following cardiopulmonary bypass pulmonary compliance decreases, so that a leak that was moderate but tolerable prior to bypass may become intolerably large following bypass, requiring intraoperative replacement of the endotracheal tube with one a size larger. The correct timing of safe extubation following surgery depends on the patient's preoperative condition, the type of surgery, the expectation for a prolonged period of postoperative hemodynamic or ventilatory support or manipulation, and the distance from the operating room to the intensive care unit or recovery room. It has been shown that neonates undergoing cardiac surgery benefit from a period of narcotic anesthesia continued into the intensive care unit.[64] Many children (not premature infants) can be safely extubated in the operating room following a thoracotomy. Similarly we routinely successfully extubate otherwise healthy children in the operating room following closure of an atrial septal defect, a small ventricular septal defect, or interruption of an abnormal conduction pathway. This presumes, of course, that an anesthetic plan was chosen that would not result in prolonged anesthesia. Many other children can be extubated within several hours of surgery. It is likely that over the next few years there will be a trend toward more early extubation of these patients in an effort to maximally utilize expensive intensive care resources.

INTRAOPERATIVE BLOOD USE

Blood components rather than whole blood are in almost universal use by blood banks. The appropriate use of blood products is similar in pediatric and adult patients; however, there are additional specific issues in pediatric patients. Manno found diminished blood loss when either fresh or 24- to 48-hour-old whole blood was used in young patients having complex repairs compared to "whole blood" reconstituted from banked constituents.[91] Since 24- to 48-hour-old blood is more practical to use than is fresh blood, these authors currently recommend that this be used in young infants with complicated repairs.[92] Blood which has been tested negative for cytomegalovirus (CMV) is supplied for small premature infants. Irradiated blood should be requested for patients who are immunoincompetent (such as children with DiGeorge syndrome). Blood is preserved with dextrose-containing fluid, and this partially accounts for the elevated blood glucose levels of children during cardiopulmonary bypass with a blood prime.[93] Neonatal myocardium is more reliant than is mature myocardium on extracellular calcium to support myocardial contraction. A rapid infusion of citrated fresh frozen plasma or platelets acutely decreases extracellular ionized calcium levels resulting in hypotension with maintained or elevated filling pressures. This can be reversed, and, more importantly, prevented, by infusions of calcium.

CONTROL OF BLEEDING DURING CARDIAC SURGERY

Several attempts have been made to reduce blood loss in children including the use of fresh whole blood and some prophylactic drugs such as aprotinin, desmopressin, ε-aminocaproic acid (Amicar®) and tranexamic acid. Aprotinin,[94] which is a basic polypeptide, acts on trypsin, tissue kallikrein, and, to a lesser extent, on plasma kallikrein. The clinical effect of aprotonin is based on the inhibition of the contact phase of coagulation and consequently reduced thrombotic and fibrinolytic activity during and after bypass. In addition it also appears to prevent platelet dysfunction[95] associated with cardiopulmonary bypass. The use of aprotinin in adult cardiac surgery[96] has been demonstrated to decrease postoperative bleeding significantly. Reports of its use in the pediatric population are few. In a study[97] looking at platelet function, blood loss, and the requirement of homologous blood the authors found that treatment with aprotinin did not lead to an improvement of platelet function nor did it reduce blood loss or transfusion of blood.

The use of desmopressin in children has also failed to reduce blood loss.[98] It is a synthetic vasopressin and increases factors VIII von Willebrand (VIIIvWF), factor VIII coagulant (VIIIc), and factor VIII-related antigen (VIIIr:Ag) activity by release from storage sites. The present indication for its use is in children with von Willebrand's disease and platelet dysfunction secondary to renal dysfunction.

ε-Aminocaproic acid is an inhibitor of the fibrinolysis that can accompany cardiopulmonary bypass. Studies in adults[99] have shown that it reduces postoperative bleeding after cardiac surgery. However, a study in cyanotic children by McClure et al[100] was unable to show a reduction in blood loss during cardiac surgery. Tranexamic acid,[101] also an inhibitor of fibrinolysis, provides more intense and sustained antifibrinolysis and has been shown to reduce blood loss in adults in cardiac surgery. Its use in children for cardiac surgery has not been reported.

ANESTHESIA FOR SPECIFIC LESIONS

There are numerous types of congenital heart disease, many with clinically significant subtypes, precluding a complete discussion of the specific anesthetic management of all. A brief discussion of the major classes follows. When the pathophysiology of the congenital defect and the pharmacologic and physiologic actions of administered medications and other manipulations are understood, an appropriate anesthetic approach naturally follows.

Large Left-to-Right Shunts (e.g., Nonrestrictive Ventriculoseptal Defect, Patent Ductus Arteriosus, or Atrioventricular Canal Defects)

In an effort to avoid major volume loading and distension of the left ventricle mild-to-moderate hypercarbia is tolerated and the F_{IO_2} is decreased to the lowest level which supports an adequate Pa_{O_2}.

Right-to-Left Shunt due to Fixed Obstruction (e.g., Valvar Pulmonary Stenosis or Pulmonary Atresia With Ventriculoseptal Defect, With or Without Aortopulmonary Shunt)

In these patients pulmonary vascular resistance is already low and not much will be gained from efforts at modulating pulmonary vascular resistance. Increases in systemic vascular resistance will, however, increase pulmonary blood flow, increasing PaO_2. FIO_2 should be kept at reasonably high levels. These patients are not at excessive risk of volume overload, and do better if volume repleted.

Right-to-Left Shunt due to Dynamic Obstruction (e.g., Tetralogy of Fallot)

Because of the risk of hypercyanotic "Tet" spells induced by anxiety, these patients require excellent preoperative sedation. Use of positive inotropic agents prior to bypass should be avoided as should hypovolemia as both will worsen right-to-left shunting. Decreases in systemic vascular resistance will also be reflected as systemic hypoxemia. β-Adrenergic antagonists have been used to decrease right ventricular outflow tract inotropy, but systemic vasoconstrictors (such as phenylephrine, 1–4 μg/kg) are usually more useful to minimize right-to-left shunting.[102]

D-Transposition of the Great Vessels (TGV)

The physiology, and hence anesthetic management, of TGV varies with the anatomical subtype, e.g., the presence of a ventricular septal defect, the presence of dynamic subpulmonary obstruction, or the presence of pulmonary vascular disease. For the neonate with TGV the anesthetic goals are to maintain intravascular volume to maintain bidirectional shunting, and to maintain ductal patency by continuing an infusion of alprostadil (prostaglandin E_1, PGE_1). Physicians must be particularly cognizant of ECG changes indicating myocardial ischemia following weaning from cardiopulmonary bypass in patients who have had repair by arterial switch with coronary reimplantation. Immediate postoperative blood pressure should be controlled to prevent excessive bleeding from long arterial suture lines.

Hypoplastic Left Heart Syndrome

Stage 1 Norwood Procedure

These neonates are in tenuous hemodynamic balance. Since all systemic blood flow derives from right ventricular output, these infants are ductal dependent and arrive in the operating room receiving an infusion of PGE_1 that must be continued until the onset of cardiopulmonary bypass. The goal of preoperative therapy is to maintain a pulmonary: systemic flow ratio (Q_p:Q_s) of close to 1:1. A ratio less than this results in significant hypoxemia. A ratio much greater than this results in systemic hypoperfusion and metabolic acidosis from pulmonary steal. Since all cardiac output derives from flow ejected into the pulmonary artery, if excessive blood flows to the lungs, an inadequate amount will supply the systemic tissues. The goal in patients with a Q_p:Q_s of approximately 1 (good peripheral perfusion and adequate arterial blood gas tensions without metabolic acidosis while breathing room air) is to maintain the current hemodynamic status. The anesthesiologist must be aware of changes that might occur with transport to the operating room, induction of anesthesia, and intubation that might serve to dilate the pulmonary circulation and increase pulmonary blood flow to the detriment of systemic blood flow (such as increases in FIO_2 or hyperventilation with respiratory alkalosis). Patients with profound hypoxemia due to inadequate pulmonary blood flow due to a restrictive atrial communication are uncommon. These patients should be managed with an effort to optimize oxygenation (FIO_2 1.0) and minimize pulmonary vascular resistance (hyperventilation). Infants with a widely patent atrial communication often have excessive pulmonary blood flow. Anything which dilates the pulmonary circulation or constricts the systemic circulation will worsen this situation. Efforts at modulating the pulmonary vascular resistance include maintaining a minimal FIO_2 and maintaining significant hypercarbia. Efforts at maintaining hypercarbia solely through manipulations in respiratory rate or tidal volume often result in unacceptably low PaO_2, felt likely to be due to an inability to maintain an adequate functional residual capacity (already low in neonates). Currently $PaCO_2$ is maintained by introducing carbon dioxide gas into the ventilator circuit under carefully controlled conditions.[103] In these infants, as in others with a common mixing lesion, pulmonary blood flow will be directly mirrored by changes in arterial blood oxygenation, as reflected by pulse oximetry. Should there be evidence of pulmonary overcirculation (systemic oxygen saturation >90% and low systemic blood pressure) a temporary snare can be placed around the right pulmonary artery after the chest is open.[104] Immediately postbypass following a stage 1 Norwood repair inadequate pulmonary blood flow is likely due to technical problems with the repair. However, factors that elevate pulmonary vascular resistance should be avoided.

Stage 2 and 3 Norwood Procedure

Variations in pulmonary flow related to changes in ventilation are less marked than in the neonate. A routine induction, intravenous or by mask, is tolerated. Following bypass the care is similar to other patients with a Glenn or Fontan procedure (vide infra).

Fontan Procedure

Following separation from cardiopulmonary bypass, these patients are dependent on passive perfusion of the pulmonary circulation. Thus adequate intravascular volume should be assured. In addition, all attempts should be made at minimizing pulmonary vascular resistance. These include avoiding cold, hypoxia, hypercarbia, metabolic acidosis, and high mean airway pressure.[105] Pulmonary vascular resistance is minimal at lung volumes around functional residual capacity, suggesting minimal levels of positive end expiratory pressure are beneficial.[106] Excessive PEEP, however, may overdistend alveoli and increase pulmonary vascular resistance.[107] Inotropes lacking significant α-adrenergic effects should be chosen to avoid pulmonary vasoconstriction. Pre-emptive use of pulmonary vasodilators, such as nitroglycerine, is often beneficial when weaning from bypass to decrease pulmonary vascular resistance. The approaches taken in assuring low pulmonary vascular resistance are similar to those taken in patients with elevated resistance and pulmonary arterial hypertension (vide infra).

Truncus Arteriosus

These infants are typically in some degree of congestive failure from pulmonary overcirculation at the time of operation. The large aortic runoff with low aortic diastolic pressure and the volume loaded left ventricle with elevated end-diastolic pressure conspire to decrease coronary perfusion pressure; at the same time increased left ventricular end-diastolic volume increases myocardial oxygen requirement. These infants are in tenuous hemodynamic balance. Changes related to anesthetic and surgical manipulation may allow for development of intraoperative coronary ischemia.[32] This is managed similarly to increased pulmonary flow with hypoplastic left heart syndrome with ventilatory manipulation and temporary snaring and constriction of the right pulmonary artery, which trade temporary decreases in oxygen saturation for increased systemic and coronary perfusion.

Pulmonary Arterial Hypertension

Although fixed pulmonary hypertension may be present in older children coming to the operating room for noncardiac surgery, essentially all children coming for cardiac surgery will have some degree of reversibility to their pulmonary vascular resistance. Factors known to contribute to elevations in pulmonary vascular resistance (cold, metabolic and respiratory acidosis, hypoxia, α-adrenergic agents) should be avoided. Hyperventilation with hypocapnia is commonly used to decrease pulmonary vascular resistance. It appears that the crucial effect is one of pH change, rather than hypocapnia per se.[108] In addition, the degree of right-to-left shunting will be increased by hypovolemia and systemic vasodilation. These children benefit from intraoperative placement of a pulmonary arterial catheter to allow close monitoring of postoperative pulmonary arterial pressure. Until recently there has been no pure pulmonary vasodilator and all drugs that were used to dilate the pulmonary vascu-

lature also had to some degree systemic effects. These included alprostadil (PGE$_1$, 0.02–2 µg/kg per min) and nitroglycerine (1–4 µg/kg per min) and amrinone (0.75 mg/kg loading dose, then 5–10 µg/kg per min). Because of its lack of α-adrenergic activity, isoproterenol has also been used (0.1 µg/kg per min). Recently there has been preliminary experience in patients using inhaled nitric oxide (10–80 ppm) as a selective pulmonary vasodilator in children undergoing cardiac surgery.[109,110] The preliminary results are extremely exciting and it is assumed that this drug will come into common clinical use over the next few years. However, its use requires specialized equipment for administration and monitoring. Children with pulmonary arterial hypertension particularly benefit from adequate postoperative pain relief to prevent increases in pulmonary vasoconstriction.

Valve Disease

The general anesthetic approach to the child with valve disease is similar to that taken with adults (see Chap. 100).

POSTOPERATIVE ANALGESIA

All children feel and react to pain. There is no child, no matter how young or infirm, who does not deserve, and who cannot tolerate, adequate postoperative analgesia. Postoperative pain has even been related to worse outcomes in neonatal cardiac surgery.[64] The management of postoperative pain in children following cardiac surgery can be challenging. It may be difficult to differentiate between discomfort from restraints or an endotracheal tube and incisional pain. Signs of pain in the preverbal or intubated child are nonspecific and may represent hemodynamic alterations secondary to the surgery or even hypoxia.

The mainstay of postoperative pain relief remains intravenous narcotics, given as a bolus or as an infusion. Children greater than about 6 years of age can often cooperate to operate patient-controlled analgesia (PCA) pumps. A good test is that if they can play video games, they can probably operate a PCA pump. The management of postoperative pain often begins in the operating room. Intercostal blocks with bupivacaine can be placed by the surgeon prior to the closure of a lateral thoracotomy. However, uptake is rapid and the duration of analgesia is shorter than in adults.[111]

Protracted intraoperative and postoperative analgesia is afforded to patients who have had thoracotomies by the placement of an epidural catheter that can be advanced to the thoracic region easily in children. In addition, epidural catheters can be introduced with minimal risk in children via the caudal space and these catheters can be advanced to the thoracic region.[112] Continuous infusion of local anesthetic (typically dilute solutions of bupivacaine) can be initiated. If instead epidural morphine is given[113] it can be given in the lumbar or caudal epidural space. There is a significant incidence of pruritus, nausea, and urinary retention with epidural morphine.

Close, complete, and timely communication between the cardiac surgical and cardiac anesthesia services allows the anesthesia service to provide extended periods of postoperative analgesia in appropriate patients. This often requires special preoperative consent, which is unavailable if the anesthesiologist is unaware of the type of incision planned until the patient arrives in the operating room.

REFERENCES

1. Moore RA, McNicholas KW, Warran SP: Atlantoaxial subluxation with symptomatic spinal cord compression in a child with Down's syndrome. Anesth Analg 66:89–90, 1987
2. Shaffer T, Dyment P, Luckstead E, et al: Atlantoaxial instability in Down's syndrome. Pediatrics 74:152–153, 1984
3. England JM, Walford DM, Waters DAW: Re-assessment of the reliability of the haematocrit. Br J Haematol 23:247–256, 1972
4. Lister G, Hellenbrand W, Kleinman C, et al: Physiologic effects of increasing hemoglobin concentration in left-to-right shunting in infants with ventricular septal defects. N Engl J Med 306:502–506, 1982
5. Rosenthal A, Fyler D: Effect of red cell volume reduction on pulmonary blood flow in polycythemia of cyanotic congenital heart disease. Am J Cardiol 33:410–414, 1974
6. Territo MC, Rosove MH, Rerloff JK: Cyanotic congenital heart disease: Hematologic management, renal function and urate metabolism. In Perloff JK, Child JS (eds): Congenital Heart Disease in Adults. Philadelphia, Saunders, 1991, pp 93–103
7. Ekert H, Sheers M: Preoperative and postoperative platelet function in cyanotic congenital heart disease. J Thorac Cardiovasc Surg 67:184–190, 1974
8. Komp D, Sparrow A: Polycythemia in cyanotic heart disease—A study of altered coagulation. J Pediatr 76:231–236, 1979
9. Maurer H, McCue C, Robertson L, et al: Correction of platelet dysfunction and bleeding in cyanotic congenital heart disease by simple red cell volume reduction. Am J Cardiol 35:831–835, 1975
10. Colon-Otero G, Gilchrist GS, Holcomb GR, et al: Preoperative evaluation of hemostasis in patients with congenital heart disease. Mayo Clin Proc 62:379–385, 1987
11. Ware JA, Reaves WH, Horak JK, Solis RT: Defective platelet aggregation in patients undergoing surgical repair of cyanotic congenital heart disease. Ann Thorac Surg 36:289–294, 1983
12. Ekert H, Gilchrist GS, Stanton R, Hammond D: Hemostasis in cyanotic congenital heart disease. J Pediatr 76:221–230, 1970
13. Suarez CR, Menendez CE, Griffin AJ, et al: Cyanotic congenital heart disease in children: Hemostatic disorders and relevance of molecular markers of hemostasis. Semin Thromb Hemost 10:285–289, 1984
14. Wedemeyer AL, Edson JR, Krivit W: Coagulation in cyanotic congenital heart disease. Am J Dis Child 124:656–660, 1972
15. Rosove MH, Hocking WG, Harwig SS, Perloff JK: Studies of β-thromboglobulin, platelet factor 4, and fibrinopeptide A in erythrocytosis due to cyanotic congenital heart disease. Thromb Res 29:225–235, 1983
16. Gill JC, Wilson AD, Endres-Brooks J, Montgomery RR: Loss of the largest von Willebrand factor multimers from the plasma of patients with congenital heart defects. Blood 67:758–761, 1986
17. Weinstein M, Ware JA, Troll J, Salzman E: Changes in von Willebrand factor during cardiac surgery: Effect of desmopressin acetate. Blood 71:1648–1655, 1988
18. Bhargava M, Sanyal SK, Thapar MD, et al: Impairment of platelet adhesiveness and platelet factor 3 activity in cyanotic congenital heart disease. Acta Haematol (Basel) 55:216–223, 1976
19. Ekert H, Dowling SV: Platelet release abnormality and reduced prothrombin levels in children with cyanotic congenital heart disease. Aust Paediatr J 13:17–21, 1977
20. Maurer HM, McCue CM, Caul J, Still WJS: Impairment of platelet aggregation in congenital heart disease. Blood 40:207–216, 1972
21. Perloff JK, Rosove MH, Child JS, Wright GB: Adults with cyanotic congenital heart disease: Hematologic management. Ann Int Med 109:406–413, 1988
22. Goldstein-Dresner MC, Davis PJ, Kretchman E, et al: Double-blind comparison of oral transmucosal fentanyl citrate with oral meperidine, diazepam and atropine as preanesthetic premedication in children with congenital heart disease. Anesthesiology 74:28–33, 1991
23. Gutstein HB, Johnson KL, Heard MB, Gregory GA: Oral ketamine preanesthetic medication in children. Anesthesiology 76:28–33, 1992
24. Parnis SJ, Foate JA, Van Der Walt JH, et al: Oral midazolam is an effective premedication for children having day-stay anaesthesia. Anaesth Intensive Care 20:9–14, 1992
25. Spear RM, Yaster M, Berkowitz ID, et al: Preinduction of anesthesia in children with rectally administered midazolam. Anesthesiology 74:670–674, 1991
26. Karl HW, Keifer AT, Rosenberger JL, et al: Comparison of the safety and efficacy of intranasal midazolam or sufentanil for preinduction of anesthesia in pediatric patients. Anesthesiology 76:209–215, 1992
27. Liu LMP, Goudsouzian NG, Liu P: Rectal methohexital premedication in children, a dose comparison study. Anesthesiology 53:343–345, 1980
28. Splinter WM, Schaffer JD, Zunder IH: Clear fluids three hours before surgery does not affect the gastric fluid contents of children. Can J Anaesth 37:498–501, 1990
29. Schreiner MS, Triebwasser A, Keon TP: Ingestion of liquids compared with preoperative fasting in pediatric outpatients. Anesthesiology 72:593–597, 1990
30. Nicolson SC, Dorsey AT, Schreiner MS: Shortened preanesthetic fasting interval in pediatric cardiac surgical patients. Anesth Analg 74:694–697, 1992
31. Bell C, Rimar S, Barash P: Intraoperative ST segment changes with myocardial ischemia in the neonate: Report of three cases. Anesthesiology 71:601–604, 1989
32. Wong RS, Baum VC, Sangwan S: Truncus arteriosus: Recognition and therapy of intraoperative cardiac ischemia. Anesthesiology 74:378–380, 1991
33. Badgwell JM: Respiratory gas monitoring in the pediatric patient. Int Anesth Clin 30:131–146, 1992
34. Burrows FA: Physiologic dead space, venous admixture, and the arterial to end-tidal carbon dioxide difference in infants and children undergoing cardiac surgery. Anesthesiology 70:219–225, 1989
35. Reynolds LM, Nicolson SC, Steven JM, et al: Influence of sensor site location on pulse oximetry kinetics in children. Anesth Analg 76:751–754, 1993
36. O'Leary RJ Jr, Landon M, Benumof JL: Buccal pulse oximeter is more accurate than finger pulse oximeter in measuring oxygen saturation. Anesth Analg 75:495–498, 1992
37. Gallagher JD, Moore RA, McNicholas KW, Jose AB: Comparison of radial and femoral arterial blood pressures in children after cardiopulmonary bypass. J Clin Monit 1:168–171, 1985
38. Glenski JA, Beynen FM, Brady J: A prospective evaluation of femoral artery monitoring in pediatric patients. Anesthesiology 66:227–229, 1987
39. Prian GW, Wright GB, Rumack CM, O'Meara OP: Apparent cerebral embolization after temporal artery catheterization. J Pediatr 93:115–118, 1978
40. Lawless S, Orr R: Axillary arterial monitoring of pediatric patients. Pediatrics 84:273–275, 1989

41. Chait HI, Kuhn MA, Baum VC: Inferior vena cava pressure reliably predicts right atrial pressure in pediatric cardiac surgery patients. *Crit Care Med* **22:**219–224, 1994

42. Reda ZY, Houri S, Davis AL, Baum VC: Airway pressure does not affect validity of inferior vena cava (IVC) pressure as a measure of central venous pressure (CVP). *Pediatr Res* (abstract, in press).

43. Stenzel JP, Green TP, Furhrman BP: Percutaneous femoral venous catheterizations: A prospective study of complications. *J Pediatr* **114:**411–415, 1989

44. Technique of intraoperative placement of thermodilution catheter for cardiac output measurement in children. *J Cardiovasc Surg* **21:**267–270, 1980

45. Greeley WJ, Ungerleider RM, Kern FH, et al: Effects of cardiopulmonary bypass on cerebral blood flow in neonates, infants and children. *Circulation* **80:**I209–I215, 1989

46. Greeley WJ, Bracey VA, Ungerleider RM, et al: Recovery of cerebral metabolism and mitochondrial oxidation state is delayed after hypothermic circulatory arrest. *Circulation* **84**(5 Suppl):III400–III406, 1991

47. Schell RM, Kern FH, Reves JG: The role of continuous jugular venous saturation during cardiac surgery with cardiopulmonary bypass. *Anesth Analg* **74:**627–629, 1992

48. van der Linden J, Priddy R, Ekroth R, et al: Cerebral perfusion and metabolism during profound hypothermia in children. A study of middle cerebral artery ultrasonic variables and cerebral extraction of oxygen. *J Thorac Cardiovasc Surg* **102:**103–114, 1991

49. Hillier SC, Burrows FA, Bissonnette B, Taylor RH: Cerebral hemodynamics in neonates and infants undergoing cardiopulmonary bypass and profound hypothermic circulatory arrest: Assessment by transcranial Doppler sonography. *Anesth Analg* **72:**723–728, 1991

50. Burrows FA, Bissonnette B: Cerebral blood flow velocity patterns during cardiac surgery utilizing profound hypothermia with low-flow cardiopulmonary bypass or circulatory arrest in neonates and infants. *Can J Anaesth* **40:**298–307, 1993

51. Kyo S, Takamoto S, Matsumura M, et al: Immediate and early postoperative evaluation of results of cardiac surgery by transesophageal two dimensional echocardiography. *Circulation* **76:**113–121, 1987

52. Cyran SE, Kimball TR, Mayer RA, et al: Efficacy of intraoperative transesophageal echocardiography in children with congenital heart disease. *Am J Cardiol* **63:**594–598, 1989

53. Stumper O, Vargas-Barron J, Rijlaarsdam M, et al: Assessment of anomalous systemic and pulmonary venous connections by transesophageal echocardiography in infants and children. *Br Heart J* **66:**411–418, 1991

54. Stumper O, Kaulitz R, Elzenga NJ, et al: The value of transesophageal echocardiography in children with congenital heart disease. *J Am Soc Echo* **4:**164–176, 1991

55. Roberson DA, Muihideen IA, Silverman NH, et al: Intraoperative transesophageal echocardiography of atrioventricular septal defects. *J Am Coll Cardiol* **18:**537–545, 1991

56. Sreeram N, Stumper OF, Kaulitz R: Comparative value of transthoracic and transesophageal echocardiography in the assessment of congenital abnormalities of the atrioventricular junction. *J Am Coll Cardiol* **16:**1205–1214, 1990

57. Roberson DA, Muihideen IA, Cahalan MK, et al: Intraoperative transesophageal echocardiography of ventricular septal defects. *Echocardiography* **8:**687–897, 1991

58. Stumper O, Elzenga NJ, Sutherland GR: Obstruction of the left ventricular outflow tract in childhood: Improved diagnosis by transesophageal echocardiography. *Int J Cardiol* **28:**107–109, 1990

59. Kobayashi T, Musewe NN, Smallhorn JF: Early postoperative transesophageal echocardiographic evaluation of results of right outflow tract reconstruction for congenital heart disease (abstract). *J Am Coll Cardiol* **17:**257A, 1991

60. Ritter SB: Transesophageal echocardiography in children: New peephole to the heart. *J Am Coll Cardiol* **16:**447–450, 1990

61. Muhiudeen IA, Roberson D, Silverman N, et al: Intraoperative trans-

esophageal echocardiography in infants and children with regurgitant valvular lesions (abstract). *J Am Soc Echo* **3:**213, 1990

62. Fyfe DA, Kline CH, Sade RM: The utility of transesophageal echocardiography during and after Fontan operations in small children. *Am Heart J* **122:**1403–1414, 1991

63. Anand KJS, Hansen DD, Hickey PR: Hormonal-metabolic stress responses in neonates undergoing cardiac surgery. *Anesthesiology* **73:**661–670, 1990

64. Anand KJS, Hickey PR: Halothane-morphine compared with high-dose sufentanil for anesthesia and postoperative analgesia in neonatal cardiac surgery. *N Engl J Med* **326:**1–9, 1992

65. Friesen RH, Henry DB: Cardiovascular changes in preterm infants receiving isoflurane, halothane, fentanyl and ketamine. *Anesthesiology* **64:**238–242, 1986

66. Friesen RH, Lichtor JL: Cardiovascular depression during halothane induction in infants: A study of three induction techniques. *Anesth Analg* **61:**42–45, 1982

67. Moore RA, McNicholas K, Gallagher JD, et al: Halothane metabolism in acyanotic and cyanotic patients undergoing open heart surgery. *Anesth Analg* **65:**1257–1262, 1986

68. Mehta M, Sokoll MD, Gergis SD: Effects of venous air embolism on the cardiovascular system and acid base balance in the presence and absence of nitrous oxide. *Acta Anaesthesiol Scand* **28:**226–231, 1984

69. Tuman KJ, McCarthy RJ, Sheikh KH, et al: Effects of nitrous oxide on coronary perfusion after coronary air embolism. *Anesthesiology* **67:**952–959, 1987

70. Siker D, Pagel PS, Pelc LR, et al: Nitrous oxide impairs functional recovery of stunned myocardium in barbiturate-anesthetized, acutely instrumented dogs. *Anesth Analg* **75:**539–548, 1992

71. Messina AG, Fun-Sun Y, Canning H, et al: The effect of nitrous oxide on left ventricular pump performance and contractility in patients with coronary artery disease: Effect of preoperative ejection fraction. *Anesth Analg* **77:**954–962, 1993

72. Hilgenberg JC, McCammon RL, Stoelting RK: Pulmonary and systemic vascular responses to nitrous oxide in patients with nitrous oxide and pulmonary hypertension. *Anesth Analg* **59:**323–326, 1980

73. Lappas DG, Buckley MJ, Laver MB, et al: Left ventricular performance and pulmonary circulation following addition of nitrous oxide to morphine during coronary-artery surgery. *Anesthesiology* **43:**61–69, 1975

74. Schulte-Sasse U, Hess W, Tarnow J: Pulmonary vascular responses to nitrous oxide in patients with normal and high pulmonary vascular resistance. *Anesthesiology* **57:**9–13, 1982

75. Hickey PR, Hansen DD, Strafford M, et al: Pulmonary and systemic hemodynamic effects of nitrous oxide in infants with normal and elevated pulmonary vascular resistance. *Anesthesiology* **65:**374–378, 1986

76. Greeley WJ, Bushman GA, Davis DP, et al: Comparative effects of halothane and ketamine on systemic arterial oxygen saturation in children with cyanotic congenital heart disease. *Anesthesiology* **65:**666–668, 1986

77. Laishley RS, Burrows FA, Lerman J, et al: Effect of anesthetic induction regimens on oxygen saturation in cyanotic congenital heart disease. *Anesthesiology* **65:**673–677, 1986

78. Lawler PGP, Nunn JF: A reassessment of the validity of the iso-shunt graph. *Br J Anaesth* **56:**1325–1335, 1984

79. Murray DJ, Forbes RB, Dull DL, Mahoney LT: Hemodynamic responses to nitrous oxide during inhalation anesthesia in pediatric patients. *J Clin Anesth* **3:**14–19, 1991

80. Tanner GE, Angers DG, Barash PG, et al: Effect of left-to-right mixed left-to-right, and right-to-left shunts on inhalational anesthetic inductions in children. *Anesth Analg* **64:**101–107, 1985

81. Levin RM, Seleny FL, Streczyn MV: Ketamine-pancuronium-narcotic technique for cardiovascular surgery in infants—a comparative study. *Anesth Analg* **54:**800–805, 1975

82. Vaughan RW, Stephen MD: Ketamine for corrective cardiac surgery in children. *South Med J* **66:**1226–1230, 1973

83. Gassner S, Cohen M, Aygen M, et al: The effect of ketamine on pulmonary artery pressure: An experimental and clinical study. *Anaesthesia* **29:**141–146, 1974

84. Hickey PR, Hansen DD, Cramolini MD: Pulmonary and systemic responses to ketamine in infants with normal and elevated pulmonary vascular resistance. *Anesthesiology* **62:**287–293, 1985

85. Morray JP, Lynn AM, Stamm SJ, et al: Hemodynamic effects of ketamine in children with congenital heart disease. *Anesth Analg* **63:**895–899, 1984

86. Hickey PR, Hansen DD: Fentanyl and sufentanyl-oxygen-pancuronium anesthesia for cardiac surgery in infants. *Anesth Analg* **63:**117–124, 1984

87. Hickey PR, Hansen DD, Wessel D, et al: Pulmonary and systemic hemodynamic responses of fentanyl in infants. *Anesth Analg* **64:**483–486, 1985

88. Forbes RB, Murray DJ, Dull DJ, et al: Hemodynamic effects of methohexitone for induction of anesthesia in children. *Can J Anaesth* **36:**526–529, 1989

89. Carmichael EB: The median lethal dose (LD_{50}) of pentothal sodium for both young and old guinea pigs and rats. *Anesthesiology* **8:**589–593, 1947

90. Mirkin BL: Perinatal pharmacology. *Anesthesiology* **43:**156–169, 1975

91. Manno CS, Hedberg KW, Kim HC, et al: Comparison of the hemostatic effects of fresh whole blood, stored whole blood, and components after open heart surgery in children. *Blood* **77:**930–936, 1991

92. Nicolson SC, Jobes DR: Hypoplastic left heart syndrome. In Lake CL (ed): *Pediatric Cardiac Anesthesia,* 2nd ed. Norwalk, Appleton & Lange, 1993, pp 275–280

93. Hosking MP, Beynem FM, Raimundo HS, et al: A comparison of washed red blood cells versus packed red blood cells (AS-1) for cardiopulmonary bypass prime and their effects on blood glucose concentration in children. *Anesthesiology* **72:**987–990, 1990

94. DeBakker A, DeHart S, Vlaeminck R: Effects of different forms of aprotinin during cardiopulmonary bypass. *Acta Anaesth Belg* **44:**45–51, 1993

95. Lavee J, Savion N, Smolinsky A: Platelet protection by aprotinin in cardiopulmonary bypass: Electron microscopic study. *Ann Thorac Surg* **53:**477–481, 1992

96. Bidstrup BP, Harrison J, Royston D: Aprotinin therapy in cardiac operation: A report on use in 41 cardiac centers in the United Kingdom. *Ann Thorac Surg* **55:**971–976, 1993

97. Boldt J, Knothe C, Zickmann B: Aprotinin in pediatric cardiac operations: Platelet function, blood loss and use of homologous blood. *Ann Thorac Surg* **55:**1460–1466, 1993

98. Reynolds LM, Nicolson SC, Jobes DR, et al: Desmopressin does not

99. Van der Salm TJ, Ansell JE, Okike ON, et al: The role of epsilon aminocaproic acid in reducing bleeding after cardiac operation: A double blind, randomized study. *J Thorac Cardiovasc Surg* **95:**538–540, 1988

100. McClure PD, Izsak L: The uses of epsilon aminocaproic acid to reduce bleeding during cardiac bypass in children with congenital heart disease. *Anesthesiology* **40:**604–608, 1974

101. Horrow JC, Hlavacek J, Strong MD, et al: Prophylactic tranexamic acid decreases bleeding after cardiac operations. *J Thorac Cardiovasc Surg* **99:**70–74, 1990

102. Nudel DB, Berman MA, Talner NS: Effects of acutely increasing systemic vascular resistance on oxygen saturation in tetralogy of Fallot. *Pediatrics* **58:**248–251, 1976

103. Jobes DR, Nicolson SC, Steven JM, et al: Carbon dioxide prevents pulmonary overcirculation in hypoplastic left heart syndrome. *Ann Thorac Surg* **54:**150–151, 1992

104. Hansen DD, Hickey PR: Anesthesia for hypoplastic left heart syndrome: Use of high-dose fentanyl in 30 neonates. *Anesth Analg* **65:**127–132, 1986

105. Fyman PN, Goodman K, Casthely PA, et al: Anesthetic management of patients undergoing Fontan procedure. *Anesth Analg* **65:**516–519, 1986

106. Jenkins J, Lynn A, Edmonds J, Barker G: Effects of mechanical ventilation on cardiopulmonary function in children after open-heart surgery. *Crit Care Med* **13:**77–80, 1985

107. Williams DB, Kiernan PD, Metke MP, et al: Hemodynamic response to positive end-expiratory pressure following right atrium-pulmonary artery bypass (Fontan procedure). *J Thorac Cardiovasc Surg* **87:**856–861, 1984

108. Schreiber MD, Heymann MA, Soifer SJ: Increased arterial pH, not decreased $PaCO_2$, attenuates hypoxia-induced pulmonary vasoconstriction in newborn lambs. *Pediatr Res* **20:**113–117, 1986

109. Wessel DL: Inhaled nitric oxide for the treatment of pulmonary hypertension before and after cardiopulmonary bypass. *Crit Care Med* **21:**S344–S345, 1993

110. Roberts JD Jr, Lang P, Bigatello LM, et al: Inhaled nitric oxide in congenital heart disease. *Circulation* **87:**447–453, 1993

111. Rothstein P, Arthur GR, Feldman HS, et al: Bupivacaine for intercostal nerve blocks in children: Blood concentrations and pharmacokinetics. *Anesth Analg* **65:**625–632, 1986

112. Gunter JB, Eng C: Thoracic epidural anesthesia via the caudal approach in children. *Anesthesiology* **76:**935–938, 1992

113. Rosen KR, Rosen DA: Caudal epidural morphine for control of pain following open heart surgery in children. *Anesthesiology* **70:**418–421, 1989

CHAPTER

60

Management of Cardiopulmonary Bypass in Infants and Children

Deep Hypothermia and Total Circulatory Arrest

J. William Gaynor, Frank H. Kern, William J. Greeley, and Ross M. Ungerleider

HISTORICAL ASPECTS

The application of hypothermia to cardiac surgery was first demonstrated by Bigelow in 1950 when he reported that dogs cooled to 20°C could survive 15 min of total circulatory arrest.[1,2] In 1952, Lewis and Taufic were the first to clinically apply the technique of hypothermia for repair of an atrial septal defect using surface cooling and inflow occlusion.[3] In 1951, Dennis and Varco unsuccessfully attempted closure of an atrial septal defect (later found to be an atrioventricular septal defect) using a pump-oxygenator.[4] The experimental work of Gibbon culminated in 1953 with the closure of an atrial septal defect in a patient supported by a pump-oxygenator.[5] In 1954, Lillehei and associates began to repair congenital heart lesions using "controlled cross-circulation" with an adult as the oxygenator.[6] This technique was later superseded by improved methods for cardiopulmonary bypass. Kirklin and colleagues at the Mayo Clinic began the first series of intracardiac repairs in 1955 using cardiopulmonary bypass.[7] In 1958, Sealy, Young, and Brown first reported the use of hypothermia in conjunction with cardiopulmonary bypass.[8] Young age and low weight have been considered risk factors for cardiopulmonary bypass.[9] Continued improvements in the techniques of cardiopulmonary bypass and deep hypothermic circulatory arrest, however, have made possible safe early repair of complex congenital heart disease, even in very small neonates.[10]

SYSTEMIC EFFECTS OF CARDIOPULMONARY BYPASS, HYPOTHERMIA, AND CIRCULATORY ARREST

Improvements in technology have greatly reduced the morbidity and mortality associated with cardiopulmonary bypass. The careful combination of hypothermia, cardiopulmonary bypass, and circulatory arrest allows for safe repair of complex heart disease. Ideal perfusion has been defined as cardiopulmonary bypass achieved without the body being aware of either the beginning or cessation of bypass.[11] However, cardiopulmonary bypass and circulatory arrest result in significant physiologic alterations that are particularly severe in the small infant and neonate.[11] Successful application of cardiopulmonary bypass for neonatal cardiac surgery requires careful planning and cooperation between the surgeon, anesthesiologist, and perfusionist. The conduct of bypass must be individualized for each patient and careful consideration must be given to circuit design, degree of hemodilution, choice of cannulae, flow rates, priming fluid, degree of hypothermia, and use of circulatory arrest.

The purpose of cardiopulmonary bypass is to maintain organ perfusion, meet the metabolic needs of the patient during the period of bypass, and provide optimal conditions for surgical repair. Hypothermia is usually utilized in conjunction with cardiopulmonary bypass to reduce the metabolic needs of the patient. Total circulatory arrest may be used to improve visualization of the operative field by allowing removal of cannulae and eliminating blood from the field and for procedures where continuation of bypass is technically difficult such as repair of an interrupted aortic arch. Variables that can be controlled during cardiopulmonary bypass include hematocrit and composition of the perfusate, temperature of the perfusate, pH of the perfusate, oxygen and carbon dioxide concentrations of the perfusate, pump flow rate, and characteristics of flow (i.e., pulsatile versus nonpulsatile).

Oxygen Consumption

During cardiopulmonary bypass at normothermia, oxygen consumption should be the same as for a patient under general anesthesia. However, during the period of bypass oxygen consumption is dependent upon oxygen delivery, which is primarily determined by the flow rate, hematocrit, and oxygen saturation of the perfusate. If portions of the microcirculation are not perfused, tissue ischemia may result and oxygen consumption may be less than normal. During normothermic bypass, whole body oxygen consumption is dependent on the flow rate until the flow rate reaches a level of 100–150 mL/kg per min at which point oxygen delivery exceeds oxygen consumption and oxygen consumption is at control levels. In neonates flow rates of 150–200 mL/kg per min may be necessary to provide adequate oxygen delivery at normothermia while in adults flow rates can be much lower (1.6 L/min per m^2) (Table 60–1). Perfusion of the microcirculation may be uneven, however, even during normothermic bypass. Activation of inflammatory mediators and endothelial injury during bypass may result in vasoconstriction and increased systemic vascular resistance with underperfusion of some capillary beds. Because of this uneven perfusion and tissue ischemia, lactic acid tends to ac-

cumulate during cardiopulmonary bypass even when adequate flows are maintained; however, the resulting metabolic acidosis is usually not severe. The mixed venous oxygen saturation should be maintained at normal levels (60–70%).[11]

Hypothermia is frequently utilized to decrease the metabolic rate and tissue oxygen consumption. Use of hypothermia allows utilization of decreased pump flow rates and total circulatory arrest. Adverse effects of hypothermia include vasoconstriction, endothelial cell dysfunction, and increased blood viscosity, which may further impair perfusion of the microvasculature.

Inflammatory Response to Cardiopulmonary Bypass

The interaction of blood with foreign material and nonendothelial surfaces during cardiopulmonary bypass initiates the release or activation of numerous substances resulting in a total body inflammatory response, which is likely to be responsible for many of the damaging effects of bypass.[12–14] Local and systemic effects include decreased or increased vascular resistance, increased vascular permeability, and activation of neutrophils, which may result in endothelial cell damage. Much of the morbidity of cardiopulmonary bypass results from the endothelial cell injury and resulting "capillary leak" induced by these substances and the process is exaggerated in neonates and small infants.[22]

With the onset of cardiopulmonary bypass, plasma levels of epinephrine and norepinephrine progressively increase and do not return to normal levels until 24 hours following bypass.[13] Factor XII (Hageman factor) is activated by contact of blood with the foreign surfaces of the oxygenator leading to activation of factor XI and conversion of prekallikrein to kallikrein. Kallikrein releases bradykinin from the precursor bradykininogen. Bradykinin is a vasodilator and increases vascular permeability.[13,15] Hypothermia also results in increased bradykinin levels. Bradykinin is degraded by a converting enzyme in the lungs and decreased pulmonary blood flow during bypass may result in a prolonged half-life.

The complement system is activated by the bypass circuit, particularly the oxygenator.[14,16] Both the classic and alternative pathways are activated leading to the formation of the anaphylatoxins C3a and C5a. There is evidence that heparin administration, hemodilution, and hypothermia may reduce the generation of C3a and C5a during bypass. Complement activation leads to neutrophil activation, aggregation, and sequestration in the microvasculature.[13,17–19]

Adhesion of activated neutrophils to endothelial cells occurs during bypass and may be responsible for endothelial damage.[20] The expression of neutrophil adhesion molecules increases following the initiation of cardiopulmonary bypass potentiating adhesion to endothelial surfaces. Release of superoxide radicals and lysosomal enzymes (elastase and myeloperoxidase) by activated neutrophils may injure endothelial cells.[21] Endothelial cell damage during

TABLE 60–1. PUMP FLOW RATES^a

Patient Weight (kg)	Calculated Flow (mL/kg per min)
0–7	120–200
7–10.0	100–150
10–20.0	80–120
>20	2.4 L/min per m^2

^{a}Flow rate must be adjusted from the calculated flow value to compensate for the effects of reservoir level, patient metabolism and venous saturation, temperature, hematocrit, use of ultrafiltration, surgeon requests, etc.

cardiopulmonary bypass possibly results from interaction with activated neutrophils leading to increased vascular permeability and accumulation of excess tissue water.[20,22] Leukocyte depletion during cardiopulmonary bypass may minimize endothelial cell injury and the use of monoclonal antibodies against neutrophil adhesion molecules may also diminish neutrophil-mediated injury.[23,24] Endothelin-1 is a vasoconstrictor produced by endothelial cells. Plasma concentrations of endothelin-1 increase progressively during bypass.[13,21,25,26] However, endothelin-1 is a locally active mediator and the significance of elevated circulating levels has not been demonstrated. Pulmonary vascular endothelial dysfunction with failure to release nitric oxide following cardiopulmonary bypass may also contribute to postbypass pulmonary dysfunction particularly in patients with preoperative pulmonary hypertension.[27,28]

Increased levels of prostanoids including prostaglandin E_2 and thromboxane A_2 occur during cardiopulmonary bypass.[13,29,30] The concentration of prostacyclin, a vasodilator produced by endothelial cells, increases at the start of bypass and thereafter progressively decreases during the period of bypass.[13] Concentrations of thromboxane A_2, which is a vasoconstrictor and an agonist for platelet aggregation, increase throughout the period of bypass.[13,21]

Elevated plasma cytokine levels during bypass have been reported including interleukin-6 (IL-6) and interleukin-8 (IL-8).[12,19,20,22] Increased levels of tumor necrosis factor (TNF) have not been reported.[13,19] Induction of interleukin-1 (IL-1) production by monocytes has been reported possibly secondary to the increased levels of C3a and C5a.[31] However, some investigators have not found increased levels of IL-1 during or after bypass.[19,22] IL-8 is a chemoattractant for neutrophils and may mediate neutrophil-induced endothelial cell injury.[20,22] It is important to remember that circulating levels of cytokines do not necessarily reflect the local concentrations which may be more important for adverse effects. The concentration of platelet activating factor, which amplifies platelet and leukocyte responses, increases during bypass and may remain elevated for 24 hours after surgery.[13]

Cardiopulmonary bypass results in a significant increase in total body water.[32–34] The increase in total body water is greatest in small neonates undergoing long periods of bypass with hemodilution.[33] Tissue edema and ultimately organ dysfunction result from this increase in total body water. Endothelial cell injury with increased vascular permeability secondary to the systemic inflammatory response to cardiopulmonary bypass and a decrease in the colloid oncotic pressure secondary to hemodilution are likely etiologic factors.

Coagulation and Fibrinolytic Cascade

Cardiopulmonary bypass results in activation of the coagulation system despite inhibition by heparinization. While consumption of coagulation factors may occur during bypass, hemodilution is responsible for most of the decrease in the levels of these factors. A 50% decrease in circulating coagulation factors and antithrombin III with a 70% reduction in platelet counts has been reported following initiation of cardiopulmonary bypass in neonates.[35] In this report, coagulation factor levels and platelet counts were not affected by cooling or exposure to the pump circuit, suggesting that the hemodilution utilized for cardiopulmonary bypass is responsible for the reduction of the circulating concentrations of these factors. While the coagulation cascade is inhibited by heparin during bypass, the fibrinolytic cascade is activated by cardiopulmonary bypass probably as a result of plasminogen activator expressed by endothelial cells stimulating the conversion of plasminogen to plasmin. Local activation of the clotting and fibrinolytic systems secondary to tissue factor and tissue plasminogen activator may also occur in shed blood in the pericardial cavity.[36]

The decrease in the platelet count immediately after the initiation of bypass is most likely due to hemodilution. More important, however, is bypass-induced platelet dysfunction with impaired aggregation and a prolonged bleeding time.[37,38] The interaction of platelets with the oxygenator and pump circuit leads to platelet aggregation and granule depletion.[37] The number of fibrinogen binding sites on the platelet surface as well as platelet membrane glycoprotein IIIa decrease during bypass.[39]

ORGAN DYSFUNCTION FOLLOWING CARDIOPULMONARY BYPASS AND CIRCULATORY ARREST

Brain

The brain has the lowest tolerance to ischemia of any organ. Maintenance of cerebral blood flow and prevention of cerebral injury is of utmost importance during cardiopulmonary bypass to minimize long-term neuropsychologic and developmental sequelae.[40–43] Assessment of neurologic injury following repair of congenital heart disease can be difficult. Developmental changes must be followed over time as acute neuropsychologic changes may be transient and early subtle changes may become significant over time. Postbypass neuropsychologic injury may be subtle and includes learning disabilities, behavioral problems, seizures, gross and some motor abnormalities, and choreoathetosis.[43–45] Risk factors for neuropsychologic injury following cardiopulmonary bypass have been incompletely defined but include use of circulatory arrest, the duration of arrest, and the brain temperature prior to and during the period of arrest. Factors that may contribute to the incidence of neurologic injury include the rate of cooling, arterial blood pressure and cerebral blood flow during cooling and rewarming, management of acid–base status, the level of arterial carbon dioxide during bypass, procedures on the systemic side of the heart (which increase the risk of embolization), and the presence of aortopulmonary collaterals or shunts.[42,44,45]

During normothermic cardiopulmonary bypass, cerebrovascular autoregulation maintains cerebral blood flow at a constant level despite variations in perfusion pressure (Fig. 60–1).[46] During moderately hypothermic cardiopulmonary bypass, cerebrovascular autoregulation is preserved in children; however, when deep hypothermia is utilized, cerebral pressure–flow autoregulation is lost and cerebral blood flow becomes dependent on the perfusion pressure.[40,41] Cerebral blood flow is also responsive to alterations in arterial Pco_2.[47] In awake adults, an increase in Pco_2 causes cerebral vasodilatation with increased cerebral blood flow. During hypothermic cardiopulmonary bypass in children, responsiveness to increased Pco_2 is present but is diminished at lower temperatures.[48] Use of an alpha-stat pH strategy (the arterial Pco_2 is not corrected for temperature) results in better maintenance of metabolism/flow coupling (i.e., less excessive cerebral blood flow for metabolic needs). However, the optimal choice of pH strategy during bypass (alpha-stat versus pH-stat) remains controversial.[49] The cerebral metabolic rate for oxygen ($CMRO_2$) is a measure of cerebral oxygen utilization. During cardiopulmonary bypass, $CMRO_2$ decreases exponentially with hypothermia (Fig. 60–2).[42,44,50]

Total circulatory arrest is frequently required during congenital heart surgery, and deep hypothermia is used to reduce cerebral metabolism (Fig. 60–2) in an effort to minimize neurologic injury. However even with deep hypothermia <20°C, the brain continues to utilize oxygen to maintain basal metabolism despite the absence of electrical activity on an electroencephalogram (EEG). Because of the brain's basal metabolic requirements, even at deep hypothermia, the use of circulatory arrest may result in neurologic injury even when substantial metabolic suppression is obtained. Measurements of $CMRO_2$ in infants on cardiopulmonary bypass before and after deep hypothermia circulatory arrest demonstrate a significant impairment in $CMRO_2$ during rewarming and after separation from bypass.[42] In comparison, infants undergoing deep hypothermia car-

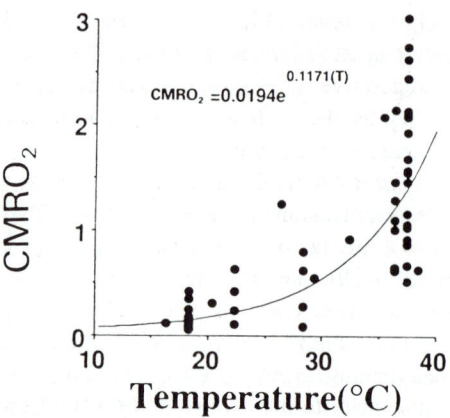

Figure 60–2. $CMRO_2$ decreases in an exponential fashion with temperature. The equation describing the exponential decrease in metabolism with temperature is shown in this figure. *(From Kern FH et al: The effects of bypass on the developing brain. Perfusion 8:49, 1993, with permission.)*

diopulmonary bypass without circulatory arrest demonstrated a return of $CMRO_2$ to baseline levels.[42] Many studies have attempted to define the safe duration of circulatory arrest. Experimental studies demonstrate a linear relationship between cerebral metabolic injury and duration of deep hypothermia circulatory arrest. Thirty minutes of total circulatory arrest at 15–20°C is well tolerated with a low incidence of neurologic injury. The risk of neurologic injury begins to rise for arrest periods between 45 and 60 min and after 60 min of circulatory arrest, there is a significant risk of developmental abnormalities. A variety of interventions have been utilized to increase the brain's tolerance to circulatory arrest. Topical hypothermia by packing the head in ice may enhance brain cooling, decrease regional differences in brain temperature, and decrease brain rewarming during the period of circulatory arrest.[50] The use of very low flow bypass ("trickle flow") at 10 mL/kg per min may provide improved cerebral protection compared to total circulatory arrest.[51] Intermittent reperfusion at 15–30-min intervals during the arrest period may also improve cerebral recovery.[52] A recent randomized trial of circulatory arrest versus low flow bypass during the repair of transposition of the great arteries demonstrated a greater incidence of seizures and a greater release of the brain isoenzymes of creatinine kinase in the group undergoing circulatory arrest suggesting a more significant cerebral injury.[43] There is also evidence that the brain remains vulnerable to injury in the immediate postbypass period and decreases in cerebral blood flow or oxygen delivery following separation from bypass may result in cerebral injury.[53]

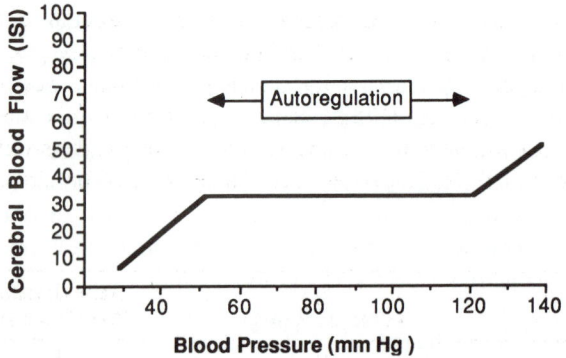

Figure 60–1. Relationship of cerebral blood flow and mean arterial pressure: autoregulation is maintained over a wide range of pressures encompassing the conventional physiological range. *(From Venn GE: Cerebral vascular autoregulation during cardiopulmonary bypass. Perfusion 4:105, 1989, with permission.)*

Kidney

Postoperative oliguria and renal failure may complicate the use of cardiopulmonary bypass and circulatory arrest.[54,55] Postoperative low cardiac output is the most important cause of oliguric renal failure. Preoperative renal failure and congestive heart failure are risk factors for the development of postoperative renal insufficiency. Young age at the time of surgery has been found to be a risk factor as well, possibly secondary to immaturity of the kidney. Hemodilution leads to increased renal blood flow, while hypothermia decreases renal perfusion.[54] Duration of cardiopulmonary bypass is also a risk factor for renal insufficiency. Hemolysis with release of free hemoglobin into the circulation may cause tubular damage. The effects of total circulatory arrest on renal function have not been fully delineated. Utilization of improved cooling techniques and maintenance of high pump flow rate prior to the period of circulatory arrest may decrease the incidence of postbypass renal insufficiency. The use of continuous low flow bypass with maintenance of an arterial pressure of at least 30 mm Hg may decrease the incidence of postoperative renal failure. The use of low-dose dopamine during the period of bypass does not appear to lower the incidence of postoperative renal failure in children.[56] In children with postoperative oliguric renal failure, peritoneal dialysis may be required.[55] Transient oliguria is common following circulatory arrest, however, dialysis is usually not necessary.

Lung

Postoperative pulmonary insufficiency is particularly common in neonates, infants, and children. Young age at the time of operation is a risk factor for postoperative pulmonary dysfunction.[57] The increased risk is probably secondary to an increased accumulation of total body water and endothelial cell injury during bypass. Pulmonary dysfunction following cardiopulmonary bypass is manifested by increased pulmonary vascular resistance, reduced pulmonary compliance, increased airway resistance, and an increased alveolar–arterial oxygen difference.[25,29,58] Neutrophil-mediated pulmonary endothelial injury leads to increased pulmonary vascular permeability with accumulation of lung water during the period of bypass.[25] The use of membrane oxygenators, arterial line filters, and heparin bonded tubing may minimize the incidence of postoperative pulmonary dysfunction while prolonged duration of bypass is a risk factor for pulmonary dysfunction. Patients who have pulmonary artery hypertension preoperatively are likely to have a reactive pulmonary vasculature and are at risk for the development of pulmonary hypertensive crises

secondary to arteriolar constriction in the postoperative period.[25] Down's syndrome and preoperative reactive airway disease are also risk factors for postoperative pulmonary dysfunction. Phrenic nerve injury, either from direct surgical trauma or secondary to iced slush used for topical hypothermia, may lead to atelectasis.

Thyroid

Plasma levels of triiodothyronine (T_3) and thyroxine (T_4) fall immediately after the initiation of bypass. In neonates and infants, thyroid hormone concentrations do not return to normal until 5–7 days following bypass.[59] Thyroid-stimulating hormone (TSH) levels increase during bypass.[59] The decrease in circulating thyroid levels may potentiate myocardial dysfunction. There is increasing evidence that the intravenous administration of T_3 following bypass is a useful method of inotropic support.

CIRCUIT DESIGN

The cardiopulmonary bypass circuit is constructed from multiple components each contributing to the performance characteristics of the circuit, the amount of priming volume required, and the potential ill-effects of bypass. While circuit design may vary considerably between centers, there are some common features. Blood drains via gravity from the right atrium or vena cavae to a cardiotomy reservoir and is pumped from the venous reservoir through a membrane oxygenator (usually incorporating a heat exchanger). Oxygenated blood is returned to the patient through a cannula in the aorta (or occasionally the femoral artery). A filter is positioned in the arterial line between the oxygenator and the patient to prevent microembolization. A hemofilter is sometimes placed in the circuit to allow ultrafiltration of the patient or circuit.

Circuit Tubing

Polyvinylchloride (PVC) tubing is used to construct the cardiopulmonary bypass circuit and the diameter of tubing utilized depends on the size of the patient. For infants weighing less than 6 kg, 1/4-in. internal diameter tubing is used for both the venous and arterial lines with progressively larger tubing for larger patients (Table 60–2). The circuit

TABLE 60–2. CIRCUIT TUBING[a]

Patient Weight (kg)	Arterial Line (in.)	Venous Line (in.)	Pump Boot (in.)	Approximate Total Volume
0–7	1/4	1/4	1/4	600
7–15	1/4	3/8	3/8	800
16–40	3/8	3/8	3/8	1500
>40	3/8	1/2	1/2	1650–2000

[a]The total volume for the adult circuit (>40 kg) is dependent on choice of oxygenators.

tubing should be kept as short as possible and the bypass circuit positioned as closely as possible to the patient to minimize the priming volume.[60] Heparin bonding of the tubing has been utilized in some centers and may decrease the need for anticoagulation and reduce the inflammatory response associated with bypass.[61,62]

Oxygenator

There are two major types of oxygenators: bubble oxygenators and membrane oxygenators.[63] Gas exchange in bubble oxygenators occurs at a blood–gas interface created by the introduction of air bubbles into the blood allowing oxygenation of the blood and removal of CO_2; however, precise control of PO_2 and PCO_2 is difficult. Before the blood leaves the oxygenator, the bubbles must be removed to prevent gaseous emboli. The large area of direct blood–gas contact results in damage to blood elements and activation of inflammatory mediators.[64] Bubble oxygenators have been shown to result in increased hemolysis and more severe thrombocytopenia when compared to membrane oxygenators. Because of concern over gaseous microemboli, damage to blood elements, and activation of inflammatory mediators, bubble oxygenators are rarely used and cannot be recommended for pediatric cardiopulmonary bypass.

Membrane oxygenators are commonly used for pediatric cardiopulmonary bypass. There are two major types of membrane oxygenators: hollow fiber oxygenators constructed from microporous polypropylene and Silastic semipermeable membrane oxygenators. In hollow fiber oxygenators, gas exchange occurs across tiny pores in the membrane and there is still a direct blood–gas interface, although much less than in bubble oxygenators. In the Silastic semipermeable membrane oxygenator, gas exchange occurs by diffusion across a semipermeable Silastic membrane and there is no direct blood–gas interface. The flow of ventilating gas can be regulated when membrane oxygenators are used allowing precise determination of the PO_2 and PCO_2 of the perfusate.

Pump

Most cardiopulmonary bypass circuits utilize a nonocclusive roller pump providing a nonpulsatile aortic flow. If the pump is occlusive, blood trauma is increased. The pump is placed in the circuit between the venous reservoir and the oxygenator. Some centers utilize a controlled Vortex (centrifugal pump) for adult cardiopulmonary bypass; however, experience with centrifugal pumps in pediatric bypass, particularly in neonatal bypass, is limited. Trauma to blood cells is similar for both types of pumps. However, in vitro evidence suggests that under conditions of high pressure and relatively low flow (such as neonatal bypass) use of centrifugal pumps results in more hemolysis than roller pumps.[65] In addition control of flow rates is less accurate

with centrifugal pumps particularly at flow rates less than 500 mL/min.

Suction Lines

Two or three suction lines are usually incorporated into the cardiopulmonary bypass system using separate roller pump heads. One line may be utilized as an intracardiac vent when there is increased venous return. The other suction lines may be used for intracardiac and pericardial suction for the removal of shed blood. While the use of intracardiac suction is often necessary to maintain adequate visualization of the operative field, it should be remembered that the suction devices may result in significant damage to the blood elements, especially platelets, and may cause significant hemolysis.[36,66]

Hemodilution and Composition of the Priming Fluid

Hemodilution is used during cardiopulmonary bypass to minimize the increase in blood viscosity occurring in conjunction with hypothermia.[14,54] Hemodilution prevents vascular sludging and improves perfusion of the microcirculation during the period of bypass. The use of hemodilution also minimizes the need for donor blood. Because of the small blood volume of neonates, the priming volume of the bypass circuit is much greater than the blood volume of the patient resulting in dilution of plasma proteins, decreased colloid oncotic pressure, and a greater increase in total body water (TBW) following bypass when compared with adults.[33] Blood must usually be added to the circuit to maintain an adequate hematocrit and oxygen-carrying capacity even when hemodilution is utilized. The level of acceptable hematocrit during cardiopulmonary bypass depends on the degree of hypothermia that is utilized. In general, the hematocrit is maintained at 18–22% when deep hypothermia (<22°C) is planned, at 22–25% during moderate hypothermia (22°–28°C), and at greater than 25% for lesser degrees of hypothermia.

The composition of the prime for the bypass circuit varies greatly between centers and remains controversial.[11] The prime usually consists of a balanced electrolyte solution with a variety of other additives (Table 60–3). Blood is added as necessary to achieve the desired hematocrit. Albumin is frequently added in order to minimize the reduction of plasma proteins and colloid oncotic pressure during bypass. A variety of other additives may be added to the perfusate including osmotic diuretics (Mannitol) and steroids. Bank blood contains citrate–phosphate–dextrose (CPD) as an anticoagulant, which binds calcium and results in a very low level of ionized calcium in the prime. Some institutions add additional calcium when CPD blood is utilized. However, a low level of ionized calcium in the perfusate may minimize the intracellular accumulation of calcium in the

TABLE 60–3. COMPOSITION OF PRIMING SOLUTION

	Neonate	Infant	Pediatric
Lactated Ringers (mL)	500	650	1000
Albumin—25% (mL)	50	100	100
$NaHCO_3$ (mEq)	10–25	15–30	40–50
Mannitol—25% (g/kg)	0.5	0.5	0.5
Solu-Medrol (mg/kg)	30 (10 kg max)	30 (10 kg max)	Consult surgeon
Packed RBCs	As needed	As needed	As needed
Heparin (units)	1000–1500	1000–2500	2000–4000

myocardium, which has been shown to be a mechanism for myocardial damage especially in neonates.

The amount of blood that must be added to the circuit to achieve the desired hematocrit can be estimated by the following formula:

$$donor\ blood\ (mL) = \frac{[(BV + PV) \times desired\ Hct] \ominus (BV \times Pt\ Hct)}{Hct\ of\ donor\ blood}$$

where BV is the patient blood volume (mL), PV is the circuit priming volume (mL), desired Hct is the desired hematocrit on bypass, Pt Hct is the patient's prebypass hematocrit, and Hct of donor blood is the hematocrit of the donor blood.[11] The blood volume of a neonate is assumed to be 85 mL/kg decreasing to 65 mL/kg by adolescence (Table 60–4).

MANAGEMENT DURING CARDIOPULMONARY BYPASS

Anticoagulation

With the current cardiopulmonary bypass circuits, anticoagulation with heparin must be utilized during the period of bypass. Prior to cannulation, a bolus of heparin (3 mg/kg) is given intravenously. The activated clotting time (ACT) is monitored following heparin administration and during bypass. Heparin is administered as necessary to maintain the ACT at greater than 400 seconds.[67] Because the response to heparin may vary significantly between patients and with different heparin preparations, the ACT should be monitored frequently during the period of bypass. Heparin resistance may occur in patients with low levels of antithrombin-III (AT-III). Administration of fresh frozen plasma

TABLE 60–4. ESTIMATED PATIENT BLOOD VOLUME

Patient Age	Blood Volume (mL/kg)
0–6 mo	85
6 mo–6 y	80
>6 y	70–75

restores AT-III levels and responsiveness to heparin. The use of heparin bonded circuits may decrease the need for systemic heparin.

Because cardiopulmonary bypass results in significant activation of the fibrinolytic system, a significant coagulopathy may develop during cardiopulmonary bypass. Aprotinin is a serine protease inhibitor (kallikrein, plasmin, trypsin, and other proteases) that blocks fibrinolysis and that may preserve platelet membrane glycoproteins during bypass. Aprotinin has been shown to decrease perioperative blood loss in adults; however, indications for use in children remain controversial.[68–70] Aprotinin interferes with the use of the ACT to monitor anticoagulation during bypass.[67,71] Heparin concentrations or heparin/protein titrate curves should be monitored rather than the ACT when aprotinin is used.

Cannulation

Most operations for repair of congenital heart disease are performed through a median sternotomy although occasionally a right or left thoracotomy may be utilized. Following sternotomy, the thymus is often resected to improve visualization and surgical access. The pericardium is opened and suspended with stay sutures. If necessary, a portion of the pericardium may be harvested for later use as a patch. Prior to heparinization, some dissection may be performed and previously placed shunts or a patent ductus arteriosus controlled. Failure to occlude aortopulmonary shunts or a patent ductus arteriosus may result in increased pulmonary blood flow following initiation of bypass with systemic hypoperfusion and distension of the heart. If shunts cannot be controlled prior to bypass, normothermia should be maintained until the shunts are occluded so the heart will continue to eject.

Most commonly the aorta is used for arterial inflow and the right atrium or both vena cavae for venous return. Cannula selection varies with the size of the patient and the procedure planned (Table 60–5). The size of the aortic cannula is of special importance. If the aortic cannula is too large, it may cause left ventricular outflow obstruction and severe hemodynamic instability. If the cannula is too small, the pressure gradient necessary for adequate flow will cre-

TABLE 60–5. CANNULAE[a]

Patient Weight (kg)	Arterial	Right Atrial
1–5	8–10 Fr	18–22 Fr single stage
5–10	10–12 Fr	22–24 Fr single stage
10–15	12–14 Fr	24–28 Fr single stage
15–20	14–16 Fr	28–32 Fr single stage
20–30	16–18 Fr	40–32 Fr two stage

[a]If separate SVC and IVC cannulation is planned appropriate sized metal right-angled cannulae are utilized.

ate turbulence and increased shear stress at the cannula tip that leads to increased hemolysis.

A single venous cannula is suitable for cases that are performed during deep hypothermic circulatory arrest and also in some cases when cardiac chambers are not entered. Direct cannulation of the superior and inferior vena cavae is performed in other situations to ensure a bloodless operative field. The inferior vena caval cannula must be carefully positioned to avoid obstruction of the hepatic veins, which may lead to ascites and hepatic dysfunction. Following cannulation of the superior vena cava, the central venous pressure must be monitored as superior vena caval obstruction can occur resulting in increased central venous pressure and decreased cerebral perfusion.

In some patients different techniques for cannulation are mandated by the anatomy. When an interrupted aortic arch is present, arterial cannulas may need to be placed in both the ascending aorta and the descending aorta (via the pulmonary artery and patent ductus) to provide total body perfusion. Similarly, anomalies of venous return such as a persistent left superior vena cava may require alternate techniques of venous cannulation.

After heparinization and cannulation, cardiopulmonary bypass is initiated and cooling begun. The venous line is unclamped and blood drains from the right atrium into the oxygenator by gravity. The arterial pump is started at a slow rate and gradually increased until full flow is reached. The rate at which venous blood drains from the patient is determined by the height difference between the patient and the oxygenator inlet, and the diameter of the venous cannula and line tubing. Venous drainage can be improved by increasing the height difference between the oxygenator and the patient. If venous return is diminished, arterial line pressure is high or mean arterial pressure excessive, pump flow rates must be reduced. High arterial line pressure and inadequate venous return are usually due to malposition or kinking of the arterial and venous cannulas, respectively. If a cold perfusate is used caution must be exercised in using the pump to infuse volume prior to initiating cardiopulmonary bypass. Infusion of cold perfusate prior to initiation of cardiopulmonary bypass may result in bradycardia and impaired cardiac contractility. Once bypass is initiated, it is essential to observe the heart as ineffective venous drainage can rapidly lead to ventricular distension. This is especially

true in infants and neonates where ventricular compliance is low and the heart is relatively intolerant of excessive preload augmentation. If ventricular distension occurs, the pump flow should be reduced and the venous cannula repositioned. Alternatively, the heart may be vented or a pump sucker placed into the right atrium. When circulatory arrest is planned the head vessels should be controlled so they can be occluded during the arrest period.

Hypothermia

Hypothermia is frequently utilized during cardiopulmonary bypass to decrease total body oxygen consumption and the adverse effects of bypass allowing use of lower flow rates.[18] The use of hypothermia reduces metabolic activity, allowing maintenance of cell viability during periods of low flow or total circulatory arrest. Nasopharyngeal and rectal temperatures are generally measured and represent cerebral and core temperatures, respectively. Bypass may be performed at either normothermia, moderate hypothermia (22°–28°C) or deep hypothermia (15°–22°C). Deep hypothermia is utilized when periods of low flow (25–50 mL/kg per min) or total circulatory arrest are anticipated for the surgical repair. The protective effects of hypothermia are especially important when pump flow must be reduced to improve visualization of the surgical field. Reductions in pump flow to less than 30–35 mL/kg per min at 28°C results in a cerebral oxygen debt while at 18°C flows of 5–30 mL/kg per min provide adequate cerebral oxygen delivery. In the early days of cardiopulmonary bypass, external surface cooling was frequently utilized. Currently, core cooling by perfusion with cold blood is most commonly performed. Regional differences in cooling are greater with core cooling than with surface cooling but can be minimized by using a prolonged cooling period (20 minutes). During cooling and rewarming the temperature gradient between the blood and water bath should be no more than 8–10°C. To minimize regional perfusion and temperature differences during cooling and rewarming, some centers administer vasodilators, phenoxybenzamine (1 mg/kg) or phentolamine (0.2 mg/kg), following the initiation of bypass. Isoflurane administered via the oxygenator is also a vasodilator that reduces systemic vascular resistance and regional differences in perfusion providing more homogeneous cooling. Surface cooling of the head may improve cerebral protection during periods of deep hypothermic total circulatory arrest.

Pump Flow Rate during Cardiopulmonary Bypass

Controversy still exists concerning the optimal flow rate during cardiopulmonary bypass (Table 60–1).[11] In neonates and infants a flow rate of 150–200 mL/kg per min should be utilized during normothermic cardiopulmonary bypass. As the patient is cooled, lower flow rates may be used to decrease the venous return to the heart and improve visualization of the surgical field. The mixed venous oxygen saturation of the blood returning to the bypass pump should be monitored and desaturation (<65–70%) suggests that pump flow is inadequate for metabolic needs. Metabolic demand can be lowered with hypothermia and anesthesia. When total circulatory arrest is utilized the patient is cooled to 15–18°C to decrease the metabolic rate and limit oxygen consumption. The use of deep hypothermic circulatory arrest, however, remains controversial because of the concern over cerebral injury. Circulatory arrest, however, is necessary for some procedures such as arch repair and greatly simplifies other procedures especially in very small infants. Use of circulatory arrest allows removal of cannulas and guarantees a bloodless field. For each patient the benefits and risks of circulatory arrest and continuous bypass must be carefully considered when planning the operation.

Following the initiation of bypass the systemic vascular resistance falls and then gradually increases. Pump flow rates are more important than the arterial pressure for maintenance of organ perfusion during bypass in children. However, when the arterial pressure is less than 30 mm Hg, cerebral perfusion may be compromised and it may be necessary to increase the pressure by pharmacologic methods. When the arterial pressure is greater than 100 mm Hg, vasodilators should be administered to decrease the systemic vascular resistance.

Acid–Base Monitoring

Acid–base monitoring and control of the arterial carbon dioxide concentration during bypass remain controversial. The alpha-stat method is based on the pH measured at 37°C. In this method, the pH is not corrected for the temperature of the blood and a normal level of arterial CO_2 is maintained. The pH-stat method is based on the pH measured at the temperature of the patient's blood. The pH is corrected by adding carbon dioxide resulting in hypercarbia and a respiratory acidosis. Cerebral blood flow is usually increased when the pH-stat method is used; however, cerebrovascular autoregulation is better maintained when the alpha-stat method is used.

Rewarming and Separation from Cardiopulmonary Bypass

Following completion of the intracardiac repair, cardiopulmonary bypass is reinstituted if total circulatory arrest has been utilized. The patient is rewarmed and the pump increased to full flow. Rewarming is continued until the nasopharyngeal and rectal temperatures are 37°C. Cardiac function is assessed and if necessary inotropic support initiated. In this period the use of epicardial or transesophageal echocardiography is especially useful to assess ventricular function and adequacy of the repair.[72] If necessary the repair may be revised or appropriate pharmacologic therapy

instituted prior to separation from bypass. When the patient is fully rewarmed, ventilation is begun and the pump flow rate gradually decreased and the patient separated from support. The heart is allowed to fill by partially clamping the venous return line and reducing the arterial inflow until adequate blood volume is achieved. Blood volume is assessed by direct visualization of the heart and measurement of right atrial or left atrial filling pressures. When filling pressures are adequate the venous cannula is clamped and the arterial inflow is stopped. The venous cannula is removed first and the arterial cannula left in place so that modified ultrafiltration may be utilized or a slow infusion of residual pump blood can be used to optimize filling pressures.[34,73] When the patient is stable, the arterial cannula may be removed.

Reversal of Anticoagulation and Treatment of Coagulopathy

After separation from bypass and decannulation, protamine sulfate is given to reverse the heparin effect. Protamine sulfate is a heparin antagonist with a rapid onset of action. The protamine dose for heparin reversal is usually 1.0 or 1.5 mg of protamine for each milligram or 100 units of circulating heparin.[67] Protamine administration often results in mild systemic vasodilatation. Occasionally a severe response with marked hypotension and hemodynamic instability may occur.[74] Protamine administration results in complement activation by the classic pathway, which may be the etiology of the hemodynamic changes.

The most common source of postoperative bleeding is inadequate surgical hemostasis; however, severe coagulation defects may develop during bypass. Hemodilution results in a significant decrease in circulatory coagulation factor levels. Consumption of coagulation factors may occur. Activation of the fibrinolytic system also leads to coagulopathy. Hypothermia following separation from bypass may impair clotting and platelet function. The use of fresh whole blood following neonatal heart surgery has been shown to significantly decrease perioperative blood loss.[75] However, fresh whole blood is frequently not available and component therapy must be utilized.

Modified Ultrafiltration following Cardiopulmonary Bypass

The increase in total body water following cardiopulmonary bypass may lead to tissue edema and multiple organ dysfunction. A variety of techniques have been developed to reverse tissue edema and hemodilution following cardiopulmonary bypass including ultrafiltration during cardiopulmonary bypass, postoperative peritoneal dialysis, postoperative continuous arterial-venous hemofiltration, and the aggressive use of diuretics.[32,55,76,77] Ultrafiltration during pediatric cardiopulmonary bypass is limited by the volume in the venous reservoir and may provide inadequate ability to remove excess tissue water. The technique of modified ultrafiltration was developed at the Hospital for Sick Children in London.[32,34] Modified ultrafiltration is performed in the immediate postbypass period. Blood from the aorta is pumped through a hemofilter and oxygenated concentrated blood is returned to the right atrium. A prospective randomized trial showed that modified ultrafiltration improved hemodynamics with a reduction of total body water and a decreased need for blood transfusion when compared to nonfiltered controls.[78] A separate trial documented increased systolic blood pressure and cardiac index with a decrease in pulmonary vascular resistance.[73] Modified ultrafiltration is also an effective method of salvaging circuit erythrocytes and raising the patient's hematocrit without transfusion of donor blood. Ultrafiltration following cardiopulmonary bypass has also been shown to reduce cytokine levels.[79] Plasma levels of C3a and C5a are reduced after hemofiltration.[80]

CONCLUSION

Rapid advances in technology, materials, and methods of cardiopulmonary bypass have made the safe repair of congenital heart lesions possible even in very small neonates. However, current bypass techniques are not ideal and significant physiologic alterations occur during bypass occasionally with long-term effects. Continued research is necessary to develop methods of bypass that will allow repair of congenital heart disease with minimal sequelae.

REFERENCES

1. Bigelow WG, Callaghan JC, Hopps JA: General hypothermia for experimental intracardiac surgery: the use of electrophrenic respirations, an artificial pacemaker for cardiac standstill, and radio-frequency rewarming in general hypothermia. *Ann Surg* **132**:531–539, 1950

2. Bigelow WG, Lindsay WK, Greenwood WF: Hypothermia: Its possible role in cardiac surgery: an investigation of factors governing survival in dogs at low body temperatures. *Ann Surg* **132**:849–866, 1950

3. Lewis FJ, Taufic M: Closure of atrial septal defects with the aid of hypothermia: Experimental accomplishments and the report of one successful case. *Surgery* **33**:52–59, 1953

4. Dennis C, Spring DS Jr, Nelson GE, et al: Development of a pump-oxygenator to replace the heart and lungs: An apparatus applicable to human patients, and application to one case. *Ann Surg* **134**:709–721, 1951

5. Gibbon JH: Application of a mechanical heart-lung apparatus to cardiac surgery. *Minn Med* **37**:171, 1954

6. Warden HE, Cohen M, Read RC, Lillehei CW: Controlled cross circulation for open intracardiac surgery: Physiologic studies and results of creation and closure of ventricular septal defects. *J Thorac Surg* **28**:331–343, 1954

7. Kirklin JW, DuShane JW, Patrick RT, et al: Intracardiac surgery with the aid of a mechanical pump-oxygenator system (Gibbon type): Report of eight cases. *Proc Staff Meet Mayo Clin* **30**:201–206, 1955

8. Sealy WC, Brown IW Jr, Young WG Jr: A report on the use of both extracorporeal circulation and hypothermia for open heart surgery. *Ann Surg* **147**:603–613, 1958

9. Kirklin JK, Blackstone EH, Kirklin JW, et al: Intracardiac surgery in infants under age 3 months: incremental risk factors for hospital mortality. *Am J Cardiol* **48**:500–506, 1981

10. Pawade A, Waterson K, Laussen P, et al: Cardiopulmonary bypass in neonates weighing less than 2.5 kg: Analysis of the risk factors for early and late mortality. *J Cardiovasc Surg* **8**:1–8, 1993

11. Elliott MJ: Perfusion for pediatric open heart surgery. *Semin Thorac Cardiovasc Surg* **2**:332–340, 1990

12. Butler J, Rocker GM, Westaby S: Inflammatory response to cardiopulmonary bypass. *Ann Thorac Surg* **55**:552–559, 1993

13. Downing SW, Edmunds LH, Jr: Release of vasoactive substances during cardiopulmonary bypass. *Ann Thorac Surg* **54**:1236–1243, 1992

14. Utley JR: Historical perspectives and basic pathophysiology. *Semin Thorac Cardiovasc Surg* **2**:292–299, 1990

15. Pang LM, Stalcup SA, Lipset JS, et al: Increased circulating bradykinin during hypothermia and cardiopulmonary bypass in children. *Circulation* **60**:1503–1507, 1979

16. Utley JR: Pathophysiology of cardiopulmonary bypass: Current issues. *J Card Surg* **5**:177, 1990

17. Kirklin JK, Westaby S, Blackstone EH, et al: Complement and the damaging effects of cardiopulmonary bypass. *J Thorac Cardiovasc Surg* **86**:845–857, 1983

18. Moore FD Jr, Warner KG, Assousa S, et al: The effects of complement activation during cardiopulmonary bypass: Attenuation by hypothermia, heparin, and hemodilution. *Ann Surg* **208**:95–103, 1988

19. Steinberg JB, Kapelanski DP, Olson JD, Weiler JM: Cytokine and complement levels in patients undergoing cardiopulmonary bypass. *J Thorac Cardiovasc Surg* **106**:1008–1016, 1993

20. Finn A, Naik S, Klein N, et al: Interleukin-8 release and neutrophil degranulation after pediatric cardiopulmonary bypass. *J Thorac Cardiovasc Surg* **105**:234–241, 1993

21. Hashimoto K, Miyamoto H, Suzuki K, et al: Evidence of organ damage after cardiopulmonary bypass: The role of elastase and vasoactive mediators. *J Thorac Cardiovasc Surg* **104**:666–673, 1992

22. Finn A, Rebuck N, Strobel S, et al: Systemic inflammation during paediatric cardiopulmonary bypass: Changes in neutrophil adhesive properties. *Perfusion* **8**:39–48, 1993

23. Wilson IC, DiNatale JM, Gillinov AM, et al: Leukocyte depletion in a neonatal model of cardiac surgery. *Ann Thorac Surg* **55**:9–12, 1993

24. Verrier ED, Shen I: Potential role of neutrophil anti-adhesion therapy in myocardial stunning, myocardial infarction, and organ dysfunction after cardiopulmonary bypass. *J Cardiovasc Surg* **8**:309–312, 1993

25. Komai H, Haworth SG: The effect of cardiopulmonary bypass on the lung: the injured pulmonary vascular endothelium. *Perfusion* **8**:55–62, 1993

26. Komai H, Adatia IT, Elliott MJ, et al: Increased plasma levels of endothelin-1 after cardiopulmonary bypass in patients with pulmonary hypertension and congenital heart disease. *J Thorac Cardiovasc Surg* **106**:473–478, 1993

27. Wessel DL: Inhaled nitric oxide for the treatment of pulmonary hypertension before and after cardiopulmonary bypass. *Crit Care Med* **21**:S344–S345, 1993

28. Wessel DL, Adatia I, Giglia TM, et al: Use of inhaled nitric oxide and acetylcholine in the evaluation of pulmonary hypertension and endothelial function after cardiopulmonary bypass. *Circulation* **88**(part 1):2128–2138, 1993

29. Cave AC, Manche A, Derias NW, Hearse DJ: Thromboxane A$_2$ mediates pulmonary hypertension after cardiopulmonary bypass in the rabbit. *J Thorac Cardiovasc Surg* **106**:959–967, 1993

30. Shafique T, Sellke FW, Thurer RL, et al: Cardiopulmonary bypass and pulmonary thromboxane generation. *Ann Thorac Surg* **55**:724–728, 1993

31. Haeffner-Cavaillon N, Roussellier N, Ponzio O, et al: Induction of interleukin-1 production in patients undergoing cardiopulmonary bypass. *J Thorac Cardiovasc Surg* **98**:1100–1106, 1989

32. Elliott MJ: Ultrafiltration and modified ultrafiltration in pediatric open heart operations. *Ann Thorac Surg* **56:**1518–1522, 1993

33. Maehara T, Novak I, Wyse RKH, Elliott MJ: Perioperative monitoring of total body water by bio-electrical impedance in children undergoing open heart surgery. *Eur J Cardiothorac Surg* **5:**258–265, 1991

34. Naik SK, Elliott MJ: Ultrafiltration and paediatric cardiopulmonary bypass. *Perfusion* **8:**101–112, 1993

35. Kern FH, Morana NJ, Sears JJ, Hickey PR: Coagulation defects in neonates during cardiopulmonary bypass. *Ann Thorac Surg* **54:**541–546, 1992

36. Tabuchi N, de Haan J, Boonstra PW, van Oeveren W: Activation of fibrinolysis in the pericardial cavity during cardiopulmonary bypass. *J Thorac Cardiovasc Surg* **106:**828–833, 1993

37. Woodman RC, Harker LA: Bleeding complications associated with cardiopulmonary bypass. *Blood* **76:**1680–1697, 1990

38. de Haan J, Schonberger J, Haan J, et al: Tissue-type plasminogen activator and fibrin monomers synergistically cause platelet dysfunction during retransfusion of shed blood after cardiopulmonary bypass. *J Thorac Cardiovasc Surg* **106:**1017–1023, 1993

39. Wenger RK, Lukasiewicz H, Mikuta BS, et al: Loss of platelet fibrinogen receptors during clinical cardiopulmonary bypass. *J Thorac Cardiovasc Surg* **97:**235–239, 1989

40. Greeley WJ, Ungerleider RM, Smith LR, Reves JG: The effects of deep hypothermic cardiopulmonary bypass and total circulatory arrest on cerebral blood flow in infants and children. *J Thorac Cardiovasc Surg* **97:**737–745, 1989

41. Greeley WJ, Ungerleider RM, Kern FH, et al: Effects of cardiopulmonary bypass on cerebral blood flow in neonates, infants, and children. *Circulation* 80 (suppl I):I-209–I-215, 1989

42. Greeley WJ, Kern FH, Ungerleider RM, et al: The effect of hypothermic cardiopulmonary bypass and total circulatory arrest on cerebral metabolism in neonates, infants, and children. *J Thorac Cardiovasc Surg* **101:**783–794, 1991

43. Newburger JW, Jonas RA, Wernovsky G, et al: A comparison of the perioperative neurologic effects of hypothermic circulatory arrest versus low-flow cardiopulmonary bypass in infant heart surgery. *N Engl J Med* **329:**1057–1064, 1993

44. Kern FH, Greeley WJ, Ungerleider R: The effects of bypass on the developing brain. *Perfusion* **8:**49–54, 1993

45. Wong PC, Barlow CF, Hickey PR, et al: Factors associated with choreoathetosis after cardiopulmonary bypass in children with congenital heart disease. *Circulation* 86(suppl II):II-118–II-126, 1992

46. Venn GE: Cerebral vascular autoregulation during cardiopulmonary bypass. *Perfusion* **4:**105, 1989

47. Kawaguchi M, Ohsumi H, Ohnishi Y, et al: Cerebral vascular reactivity to carbon dioxide before and after cardiopulmonary bypass in children with congenital heart disease. *J Thorac Cardiovasc Surg* **106:**823–827, 1993

48. Kern FH, Ungerleider RM, Quill TJ, et al: Cerebral blood flow response to changes in arterial carbon dioxide tension during hypothermic cardiopulmonary bypass in children. *J Thorac Cardiovasc Surg* **101:**618–622, 1991

49. Jonas RA, Bellinger DC, Rappaport LA, et al: Relation of pH strategy and developmental outcome after hypothermic circulatory arrest. *J Thorac Cardiovasc Surg* **106:**362–368, 1993

50. Greeley WJ, Kern FH, Meliones JN, Ungerleider RM: Effect of deep hypothermia and circulatory arrest on cerebral blood flow and metabolism. *Ann Thorac Surg* **56:**1464–1466, 1993

51. Mault JR, Ohtake S, Klingensmith ME, et al: Cerebral metabolism and circulatory arrest: Effects of duration and strategies for protection. *Ann Thorac Surg* **55:**57–64, 1993

52. Mault JR, Whitaker EG, Heinle JS, et al: Intermittent perfusion during hypothermic circulatory arrest: A new and effective technique for cerebral protection. *Am Coll Surg, Surg Forum* **43:**314–316, 1992

53. Mezrow CK, Midulla PS, Sadeghi AM, et al: A vulnerable interval for cerebral injury-comparison of hypothermic circulatory arrest and low flow cardiopulmonary bypass. *Cardiol Young* **3:**287–298, 1993

54. Utley R, Wachtel C, Cain RB, et al: Effects of hypothermia, hemodilution, and pump oxygenation on organ water content, blood flow and oxygen delivery, and renal function. *Ann Thorac Surg* **31:**121–133, 1981

55. Giuffre RM, Tam KH, Williams WW, Freedom RM: Acute renal failure complicating pediatric cardiac surgery: A comparison of survivors and nonsurvivors following acute peritoneal dialysis. *Pediatr Cardiol* **13:**208–213, 1992

56. Wenstone R, Campbell JM, Booker PD, McKay R: Renal function after cardiopulmonary bypass in children: Comparison of dopamine with dobutamine. *Br J Anaesth* **67:**591–594, 1991

57. Kanter RK, Bove EL, Tobin JR, Zimmerman JJ: Prolonged mechanical ventilation of infants after open heart surgery. *Crit Care Med* **14:**211–214, 1986

58. MacNaughton PD, Braude S, Hunter DN, et al: Changes in lung function and pulmonary capillary permeability after cardiopulmonary bypass. *Crit Care Med* **20:**1289–1294, 1992

59. Mitchell IM, Pollock JCS, Jamieson MPG, et al: The effects of cardiopulmonary bypass on thyroid function in infants weighing less than five kilograms. *J Thorac Cardiovasc Surg* **103:**800–805, 1992

60. Elliott M: Minimizing the bypass circuit: A rational step in the development of paediatric perfusion. *Perfusion* **8:**81–86, 1993

61. Jones DR, Hill RC, Hollingsed MJ, et al: Use of heparin-coated cardiopulmonary bypass. *Ann Thorac Surg* **56:**566–568, 1993

62. Redmond JM, Gillinov AM, Stuart RS, et al: Heparin-coated bypass circuits reduce pulmonary injury. *Ann Thorac Surg* **56:**474–479, 1993

63. Pearson DT: Gas exchange: Bubble and membrane oxygenators. *Semin Thorac Cardiovasc Surg* **2:**313–319, 1990

64. van Oeveren W, Kazatchkine MD, Descamps-Latscha B, et al: Deleterious effects of cardiopulmonary bypass: A prospective study of bubble versus membrane oxygenation. *J Thorac Cardiovasc Surg* **89:**888–899, 1985

65. Tamari Y, Lee-Sensiba K, Leonard EF, et al: The effects of pressure and flow on hemolysis caused by Bio-Medicus centrifugal pumps and roller pumps. *J Thorac Cardiovasc Surg* **106:**997–1007, 1993

66. Boonstra PW, van Imhoff GW, Eysman L, et al: Reduced platelet activation and improved hemostasis after controlled cardiotomy suction during clinical membrane oxygenator perfusions. *J Thorac Cardiovasc Surg* **89:**900–906, 1985

67. Kondo NI, Maddi R, Ewenstein BM, Goldhaber SZ: Anticoagulation and hemostasis in cardiac surgical patients. *J Card Surg* **9:**443–461, 1994

68. Blauhut B, Gross C, Necek S, et al: Effects of high-dose aprotinin on blood loss, platelet function, fibrinolysis, complement, and renal function after cardiopulmonary bypass. *J Thorac Cardiovasc Surg* **101:**958–967, 1991

69. Boldt J, Knothe C, Zickmann B, et al: Aprotinin in pediatric cardiac operations: platelet function, blood loss, and use of homologous blood. *Ann Thorac Surg* **55:**1460–1466, 1993

70. Edmunds LH Jr: Invitation letter concerning: aprotinin use in pediatric cardiac operations. *J Thorac Cardiovasc Surg* **105:**757–760, 1993

71. Najman DM, Walenga JM, Fareed J, Pifarre R: Effects of aprotinin on anticoagulant monitoring: Implications in cardiovascular surgery. *Ann Thorac Surg* **55:**662–666, 1993

72. Ungerleider RM, Greeley WJ, Kanter RJ, Kisslo JA: The learning curve for intraoperative echocardiography during congenital heart surgery. *Ann Thorac Surg* **54:**691–698, 1992

73. Naik S, Balaji S, Elliott M: Modified ultrafiltration improves hemodynamics after cardiopulmonary bypass in children. *JACC* **19:**37A, 1992

74. Kirklin JK, Chenoweth DE, Naftel DC, et al: Effects of protamine administration after cardiopulmonary bypass on complement, blood elements, and the hemodynamic state. *Ann Thorac Surg* **41:**193–199, 1986

75. Manno CS, Hedberg KW, Kim HC, et al: Comparison of the hemo-

static effects of fresh whole blood, stored whole blood, and components after open heart surgery in children. *Blood* 1991;77:930–936.

76. Paret G, Cohen AJ, Bohn DJ, et al: Continuous arteriovenous hemofiltration after cardiac operations in infants and children. *J Thorac Cardiovasc Surg* **104:**1225–1230, 1992

77. Zobel G, Stein JI, Kuttnig M, et al: Continuous extracorporeal fluid removal in children with low cardiac output after cardiac operations. *J Thorac Cardiovasc Surg* **101:**593–597, 1991

78. Naik SK, Knight A, Elliott M: A prospective randomized study of a modified technique of ultrafiltration during pediatric open-heart surgery. *Circulation* **84** (suppl III):422–431, 1991

79. Millar AB, Armstrong L, van der Linden J, et al: Cytokine production and hemofiltration in children undergoing cardiopulmonary bypass. *Ann Thorac Surg* **56:**1499–1502, 1993

80. Andreasson S, Gothberg S, Berggren H, et al: Hemofiltration modifies complement activation after extracorporeal circulation in infants. *Ann Thorac Surg* **56:**1515–1517, 1993

CHAPTER

61

Pediatric Myocardial Protection

Richard N. Gates, Davis C. Drinkwater, Jr., and Hillel Laks

The development of techniques for myocardial protection of the pediatric heart has greatly advanced the field of congenital heart surgery. Complex and lengthy procedures are now performed with an ever-decreasing morbidity and mortality. Nonetheless, the incidence of primary myocardial failure in the immediate postoperative period is proportionately greater in the pediatric population when compared to adults, and is responsible for up to 50% of early deaths.[1] This is no doubt due to the inherent structural and functional properties of the pediatric heart as well as the unique physiologic conditions under which operations are undertaken. When planning strategies for pediatric myocardial protection the surgeon must take these differences into account.

In this chapter we will discuss the structural and functional differences of the developing myocardium. In addition, the effects of abnormal physiologic conditions upon myocardial protection will be reviewed. The basic concepts of myocardial protection will be presented and synthesized into an integrated approach to myocardial protection of the pediatric heart.

STRUCTURAL, FUNCTIONAL, AND METABOLIC DIFFERENCES OF THE DEVELOPING MYOCARDIUM

There are numerous morphologic differences between the immature myocyte and the fully developed cell, the most obvious of which is smaller cell size. Rat myocytes increase in size by approximately 500% by full maturity.[2,3] The newborn's heart also represents a greater proportion of body mass at birth. A neonatal sheep heart comprises 0.73% of body mass as compared to 0.49% in the adult.[4]

This is primarily a result of increased right ventricular mass but is also a reflection of the higher water to collagen content of developing myocytes. There is also an increase in the ratio of type I to type III collagen in neonatal hearts.[5] Noncontractile structural elements comprise a greater percentage of cell mass in the developing heart.[6] Myofibrils are present in a more random orientation and may have incomplete sarcomeres.[7] Mitochondria to power these myofibrils are present in fewer numbers and lack well-developed cristae.[8,9] As such, the immature myocardium has a reduced oxidative capacity.[10]

These structural differences result in an immature myocardium that at any given point on a length–tension curve generates less force than its adult counterpart[4,11] (Fig. 61–1). Thus, myocardial compliance is reduced and the immature myocardium is unable to increase stroke volume to the same degree as adult myocardium per increase in preload. This relative lack of compliance is compensated for at baseline with increased contractility related to an elevated adrenergic state.[12] The immature myocardium also appears to be less tolerant to increases in afterload with a relatively greater decrease in stroke volume when compared to the adult.[13,14]

Essentially all fetal myocyte metabolism is based upon carbohydrate breakdown, in sharp contrast to the mature myocardium that relies primarily upon free fatty acid (FFA) metabolism.[15] The immature myocardium has greater glycogen stores and possesses superior anaerobic glycolytic ATP production.[16–18] As such, normal isolated immature myocardium tolerates warm or cold ischemia far better than mature myocardium with greater recovery of indices of myocardial function.[19–24] When anaerobic glycolysis is biochemically blocked in immature myocardium, a rapid functional decline during ischemia ensues.[25] Further, a direct

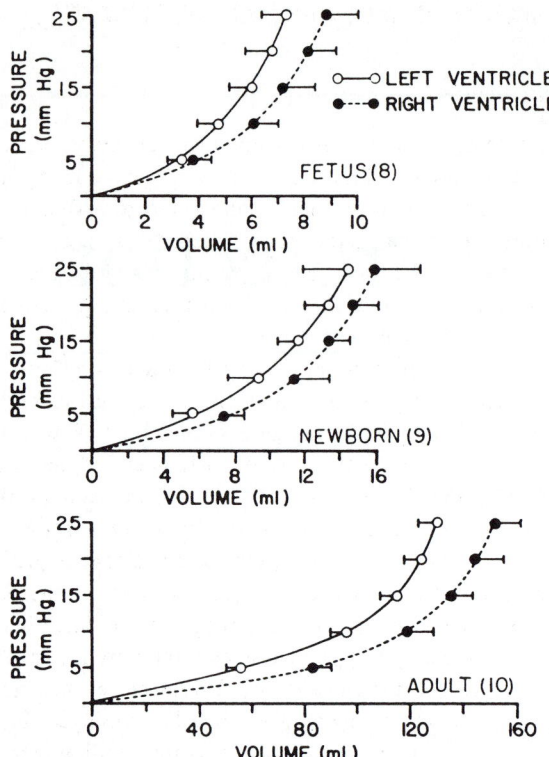

Figure 61–1. Left and right ventricular pressure–volume curves for fetal, newborn, and adult sheep. Notice the relatively greater compliance of the right ventricle at all ages and the increased compliance of both ventricles with maturation. *(From Romero T, Covell J, Friedman W: A comparison of pressure–volume relations of fetal, newborn, and adult hearts. Am J Physiol 222(5):1285, 1978, with permission.)*

correlation between myocardial glycogen content and survival after an ischemic insult has been documented.[26] These observations directly support the importance of anaerobic glycolysis in the neonatal heart during ischemia.[27] There is also evidence that the immature myocyte retains more ATP precursors after ischemia than its adult counterpart,[28] perhaps due to reduced nucleotidase levels in the immature myocardium.

There are significant differences between the immature and mature myocardium with regards to calcium-mediated processes. Calcium is critical in the myocyte and plays a role in membrane integrity,[29] excitation–contraction coupling,[30] and contraction.[31] The immature myocardium has a less well-developed sarcoplasmic reticulum and T-tubule system.[32,33] This is likely to account for the far greater dependency upon extracellular calcium demonstrated by the immature myocardium.[34]

These and other less well-described structural and metabolic properties of the immature myocardium are responsible for its differing functional and metabolic response to ischemia and to various cardioplegic solutions. When this knowledge is combined with an awareness of the unique physiologic conditions for which pediatric opera-

tions are undertaken it is easy to appreciate why a different approach to myocardial protection is needed in the pediatric population.

ABNORMAL PHYSIOLOGIC STATES

Congenital malformations of the heart frequently lead to physiologic abnormalities that affect all organ systems of the patient. Many of these physiologic conditions profoundly affect the heart itself. Acute or chronic hypoxia, pressure or volume overload, and increased noncoronary collateral flow all have significant effects upon the immature myocardium. These effects must be taken into account when planning a clinical approach to myocardial protection.

Experimentally, it has been frequently demonstrated that normal immature myocardium has a greater tolerance to hypoxia/ischemia when compared to normal mature myocardium.[21,35,36] Nonetheless, in clinical practice this is rarely observed and the immature myocardium is generally far more susceptible to injury during cardiac surgery.[1] This is almost certainly the result of the negative effects upon the myocardium of the various abnormal physiologic conditions for which operations are undertaken.

Acute Hypoxia and Acidosis

Acute hypoxia and acidosis may occur as a consequence of many congenital heart defects. In the neonatal period this is often associated with the partial or complete closure of the ductus arteriosus during the transition from a fetal to neonatal circulation. Prolonged severe hypoxia results in high-energy phosphate depletion and depressed myocardial function.[37,38] When acidosis is also present this further heightens the deleterious effects of hypoxemia.[39,40] Significant acute hypoxia forces the myocardium to rely upon anaerobic metabolism. Within an hour, glycogen, ATP, Kreb's cycle substrates, and intermediates may become depleted with associated myocardial dysfunction.[41] Such substrate and energy-depleted hearts are far less tolerant of future ischemic insults.

Chronic Hypoxia

Chronic hypoxia leads to cyanosis, a condition frequently encountered in infants and young children undergoing open heart surgery. Remarkably, such patients have no difference when compared to acyanotic children with regard to glucose uptake, free fatty acid (FFA) uptake, or oxygen consumption.[42] Nonetheless, cyanotic human hearts appear to have lower glycogen stores as well as other metabolic differences when compared to acyanotic hearts.[43] These differences result in a relatively greater intolerance to ischemia as more significant metabolic and functional impairment occurs in these hearts after a period of ischemic arrest.[44–46]

Pressure and Volume Overload

Volume overloading of the pediatric heart occurs in many conditions such as left-to-right shunts, single ventricle with mixed circulation, and severe atrioventricular valve insufficiency. The ability of the immature myocardium to compensate for this using the Frank–Starling mechanism is limited as these hearts normally function at a high diastolic volume and therefore have a limited diastolic reserve.[6,47,48] Further, neonatal animal studies have demonstrated that volume loading of one ventricle can severely effect the distensibility of the other ventricle.[4] A proposed mechanism of septal bowing probably explains why biventricular failure is a frequent clinical presentation in infants with large left-to-right shunts. As such ventricles hypertrophy and eventually dilate, their myocardial oxygen requirements increase and their structural and metabolic properties change. These changes have a significant effect upon the response of the myocardium to surgical stress or ischemia.

Congenital lesions that mechanically obstruct ventricular outflow or result in increased mean arterial pressure lead to ventricular hypertrophy. Ventricular hypertrophy quickly causes reduced diastolic compliance.[49] In mature myocardium ventricular hypertrophy results in lower high-energy phosphate levels and inefficient oxygen utilization.[50] As anticipated, studies of both adult and pediatric hypertrophied hearts have shown them to be more susceptible to ischemic insults.[51–53] Similar to the scenario with volume overloading, the hypertrophied and pressure overloaded ventricle may negatively influence the function of the remaining ventricle and its tolerance to ischemia.[54] Hypertrophy also effects regional myocardial blood flow with a relative hypoperfusion of the endocardium.[55] The structural and metabolic changes that occur within the hypertrophied immature myocardium make these hearts some of the most difficult to adequately protect.

Noncoronary Collateral Flow

In cyanotic congenital heart disease, collateral blood flow between the coronary, pericardial, and bronchial circulations is frequently significant. In conditions with reduced pulmonary blood flow bronchial collateral flow can represent up to 40% of total delivered flow on cardiopulmonary bypass.[56] Ventricular hypertrophy is also associated with an increase in noncoronary collateral flow.[57] The deleterious effects of noncoronary collateral flow include "washing out" of cardioplegia (with resumption of mechanical activity), rewarming of the heart (if there is a differential between myocardial and corporeal temperature), poor visualization, increased hemolysis and destruction of blood components (secondary to pump scavenger injury), and a "steal" of systemic flow (as the delivered perfusate is partially diverted to nonsystemic collaterals). As such, every effort should be made to preoperatively localize and angiographically embolize all large systemic to pulmonary collaterals.

CONCEPTS IN MYOCARDIAL PROTECTION

Basic Goals

Myocardial protection has become of great interest to most cardiac surgeons. While the significance of good myocardial protection should not be underestimated, it should also be remembered that myocardial protection is an adjunct to the operative procedure. The approach to myocardial protection should be individualized and facilitate the conduct of the operation, not the reverse.

In cardiac surgery excellent short- and long-term results demand surgical precision and a technically perfect procedure should be the surgeon's chief goal. Few would argue that this objective is not best achieved with an operative field where the heart is motionless and relaxed. Further, techniques to reduce the return of blood or cardioplegia onto the operative field are encouraged. These objectives are best achieved by electromechanical arrest of the heart using a potassium-based cardioplegic solution. Maintenance of a clear operative field is facilitated by intermittent cardioplegic techniques and good venting of the heart. However, continuous techniques may be employed during portions of the procedure where ongoing cardioplegic return is of minimal consequence.

The Five Phases of Myocardial Protection

It is generally accepted that myocardial function is negatively affected by two major events that may occur during the operative procedure. The first is the development of ischemia during the arrest period and the second is the infliction of a reperfusion injury at its conclusion. Strategies for myocardial protection have been developed primarily to address these two issues. It is useful when developing clinical strategies for myocardial protection to divide the process into five phases: (1) prearrest period, (2) induction of arrest, (3) maintenance of arrest, (4) reperfusion, and (5) postreperfusion period (Table 61–1).

The majority of clinical and research attention has been focused on phases 2 through 4, but, one should not overlook the importance of phases 1 and 5. Myocardium that enters a cardioplegic arrest in a state depleted of high-energy phosphates and/or glycogen is far more vulnerable to a reperfusion injury when the arrest is reversed.[42,58,59] The ability to reduce subsequent ischemic and reperfusion injury by judicious prearrest management has been demonstrated by Julia et al.[60] Using a model of energy-depleted hypoxic neonatal puppy hearts, these authors showed that a prearrest continuous infusion of glutamate, aspartate, glucose–insulin–potassium, mercaptopropionyl glycine, carnitine, and catalase reduced subsequent postischemic reperfusion damage. Preoperative maneuvers to improve hypoxia, decrease pressure or volume loads, and improve the metabolic and functional status of the myocardium prior to arrest are worthwhile and should be actively pursued. In the post-

TABLE 61–1. FIVE PHASES OF MYOCARDIAL PROTECTION AND SOME CLINICAL STRATEGIES TO IMPROVE MYOCARDIAL FUNCTION

Phase and Goals	Clinical Strategies
1. Prearrest; maximize oxygen supply and reduce demand by optimizing cardiopulmonary status	Optimize cardiopulmonary dynamics; optimize anesthetic induction; early institution of partial CPB
2. Arrest; replete myocardial substrate and energy stores if necessary; achieve complete electromechanical arrest of the decompressed heart	Warm substrate enhanced "resuscitation" cardioplegia if necessary; hyperkalemic arrest with maximum cardioplegic distribution
3. Maintenance; minimize the development of ischemia; provide optimal operative field	Hypothermic intermittent oxygenated cardioplegia with maximum distribution
4. Reperfusion; limit calcium and oxygen-free radical-mediated reperfusion injury	Warm substrate-enhanced, hypocalcemic cardioplegia; leukocyte depleting; free radical scavenging
5. Postarrest; maximize oxygen supply and reduce demand by optimizing cardiopulmonary status; reduce free water gain	Optimize cardiopulmonary dynamics; unload damaged myocardium (i.e., IABP, LVAD, ECMO); modified ultrafiltration

operative period, excessive functional demands in the presence of suboptimal hemodynamics hinder the ability of the myocyte to repair damage sustained during arrest and reperfusion. A low threshold for the appropriate use of ventricular assist devices should be maintained to avoid permanent and irreversible myocardial damage. Phases 2 through 4 have been studied extensively and will be presented below.

Induction Cardioplegia

The primary goals of the induction cardioplegic arrest dose are to achieve complete electromechanical quiescence of the heart and to reverse metabolic abnormalities within the myocardium. To achieve an optimal cardioplegic arrest, distribution of cardioplegia must be uniform and complete. The importance and theory of this concept are discussed in the distribution section below.

Antegrade infusion pressure during initial cardioplegic arrest is important as elevated pressures (> approx. 120 mm Hg) have been demonstrated to be injurious to the adult and neonatal heart.[61,62] It is therefore important to monitor both pressure and flow during cardioplegic administration. Initial arrest should be rapidly achieved with potassium concentrations between 15 and 30 mEq/L. Potassium concentrations should not exceed 30 mEq/L as this has been shown to be damaging to the endothelium and is associated with its subsequent dysfunction.[63] Decompression of the neonatal heart is also extremely important during initial arrest. Coronary perfusion pressure is related to pressure within the coronary ostia and pressure within the ventricular wall. Perfusion

pressure is thus maximized by emptying of the ventricular cavities. Neonatal and adult hearts that are distended during and after cardioplegic arrest have significant reductions in subsequent postarrest function.[64,65] Adequate ventricular decompression of the neonatal heart is usually easily accomplished by partial or complete cardiopulmonary bypass alone. However, the surgeon must be aware of aortic insufficiency or increased bronchial return, which may result in distension. If this occurs, the ventricle should be promptly decompressed.

One of the most significant developments in myocardial protection has been the conceptualization and clinical application of warm "induction" or "resuscitation" cardioplegia as proposed by Buckberg and colleagues.[58] The general theory suggests that metabolic abnormalities that may be present within the myocardium as a result of various stresses (i.e., ischemia, hypoxia, volume/pressure overload) prior to cardioplegia arrest may be reversed ("resuscitated") by an initial dose of normothermic substrate-enhanced blood cardioplegia. Critical to the theory is that the myocardium has a period to undergo reparative normothermic anaerobic metabolism when oxygen and substrate supply exceed demand. Clinically this is achieved by an initial cardioplegic dose of high-potassium, warm, substrate-enhanced blood cardioplegia delivered to the decompressed heart while on full cardiopulmonary bypass. Once "resuscitation" is complete, cardioplegia is switched to low-potassium, cold blood cardioplegia.

There is experimental evidence in both mature and immature myocardium that hearts that enter into a period of cold cardioplegic protection in an energy-depleted state have subsequently reduced myocardial function.[58–60] There is also abundant experimental evidence that a period of induction does improve the metabolic status of the energy-depleted heart. Warm blood substrate-enhanced cardioplegic induction enhances myocyte ATP levels, oxygen utilization, and subsequent ventricular function[60,66–69] (Fig. 61–2). Thus, in clinical situations where the pediatric heart is suspected of being energy depleted (acute hypoxia, chronic severe hypoxia, significant volume–pressure load, or ischemia) it is prudent to consider a period of warm induction cardioplegia at initial cardioplegic arrest. For elective pediatric procedures on non–energy-depleted hearts, warm induction is not necessary. Such patients should undergo arrest with a simple cold cardioplegic solution.

Maintenance Cardioplegia

The primary goal of maintenance cardioplegia is to prevent the development of ischemia during the arrest period. This is achieved by lowering myocardial oxygen demand and balancing this with oxygen supply. It is frequently stated that the cornerstone of myocardial protection is hypothermia. While hypothermia is an important element in myocardial protection, this is an overstatement of fact. As seen in Figure 61–3, the greatest reduction in oxygen requirement (90%) is achieved by electromechanical arrest and mechan-

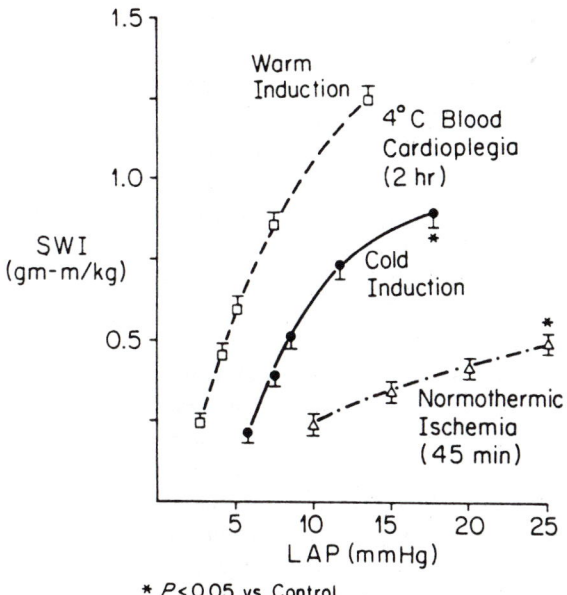

* $P < 0.05$ vs Control

Figure 61–2. Comparison of myocardial protection techniques in energy-depleted hearts. The figure plots SWI (stroke work index) versus LAP (left atrial pressure) 30 min after reperfusion and demonstrates the benefit of warm induction cardioplegia. *(From Rosenkranz E, Vinten-Johansen J, Buckberg GD, et al: Benefits of normothermic induction of cardioplegia in energy depleted hearts, with maintenance of arrest by multidose cold blood cardioplegic infusion. J Thorac Cardiovasc Surg 84:667, 1982, with permission.)*

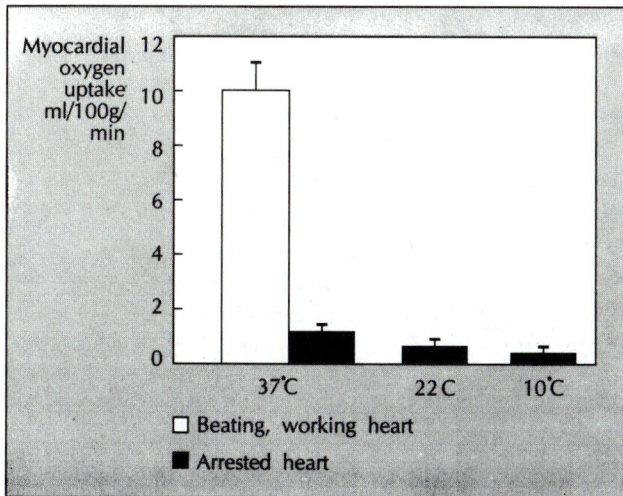

Figure 61–3. Myocardial oxygen uptake in the arrested heart compared with the beating, working heart (blood pressure 100 mm Hg, heart rate 100, cardiac output 100 mL/kg per min). Note that myocardial oxygen uptake is reduced 90% in the arrested, decompressed normothermic heart. Oxygen uptake is reduced another one-third as hypothermia is achieved. *(From Buckberg GD: Myocardial temperature management during aortic clamping for cardiac surgery. J Thorac Cardiovasc Surg 102:895–903, 1991, with permission.)*

ical decompression of the heart. Significant hypothermia does, however, further lower oxygen demands to one-third of arrested, decompressed, normothermic levels. With this in mind, the surgeon's primary interest during maintenance cardioplegia should be maintaining decompression and arrest of the heart.

Maintaining electromechanical arrest of the heart is complicated by noncoronary collateral flow. Such flow is present in all hearts to a variable degree, but is particularly great in those with cyanosis or ventricular hypertrophy.[70,71] Noncoronary collateral flow washes out cardioplegic solutions and leads to the recurrence of electromechanical activity. In normothermic hearts activity is obvious, however, in hypothermic hearts only microfibrillatory activity may be present and this may not be visually obvious.[72] Primary control of noncoronary collateral flow is gained by management of extracorporeal circulation as will be discussed below.

Intermittent delivery of oxygenated cardioplegic solutions at intervals of 15–20 min (or less if obvious electromechanical activity is present) ensures complete electromechanical arrest, allows for oxygen delivery, removes metabolic wastes, buffers accumulated acids, delivers metabolic substrates, and maintains the desired temperature of the heart. The continuous delivery of oxygenated cardioplegia may also achieve the above-described goals but without minor interval ischemia. From a theoretic standpoint this is optimal, however, as will be discussed later, other overriding technical issues negate this potential advantage.

Reperfusion

At the conclusion of the maintenance arrest period the aortic cross-clamp is released and reperfusion of the myocardium occurs. At this time energy and substrate-depleted ischemic myocardium may suffer a reperfusion injury. The consequences of this injury are structural and metabolic and may result in significantly depressed myocardial function.

When ischemia prior to reperfusion occurs, a cascade of negative reactions follow that includes increased cellular buildup of lactate and adenine nucleotide metabolites, activation of neutrophils and compliment, activation of proteolytic enzymes and phospholipases, and impaired cell membrane function.[73] When oxygen is reintroduced into this environment further cellular damage occurs predominantly through the production of oxygen-free radicals and intracellular calcium overload.[74] Oxygen-free radicals are injurious to myocytes as they cause denaturation of proteins and polyunsaturated fatty acids, enzyme and membrane dysfunction, and lipid peroxidation. Oxygen-free radicals are also believed to inappropriately increase intracellular calcium through their effects on the sarcoplasmic reticulum, sodium–calcium exchange pump, and cell membrane.[75,76] Intracellular calcium overload is believed to lead to functional depression of mitochondria and the sarcoplasmic reticulum, activation of phospholipases and proteolytic enzymes, and activation of neutrophils and compliment.[74]

The end result of reperfusion injuries is myocardial "stunning" or decreased myocardial function.[77] If minor, this may be clinically unnoticed; if major, reversible or nonreversible myocardial failure may ensue.

Strategies to reduce reperfusion injury have been developed. This has been accomplished using "controlled reperfusion" where reperfusion with warm modified blood cardioplegia is performed prior to release of the aortic cross-clamp. Variables of greatest significance that may be controlled are pressure and osmolality (to reduce edema formation), ionic calcium level (to reduce intracellular hypercalcemia), substrate enhancement (to replete energy in substrate-depleted myocytes), neutrophil content (to reduce neutrophil-mediated injury), and free radical scavengers (to reduce free radical mediated injury). The benefits of buffered, hypocalcemic, hyperosmolar, substrate-enhanced reperfusion of ischemic myocardium have been demonstrated in both mature and immature myocardium.[60,67,78–81] The addition of superoxide dismutase and catalase to reperfusates improves the subsequent ventricular function of immature hearts subjected to long-term preservation.[82,83] Mechanical leukocyte depletion with blood filters also significantly reduces reperfusion injury and improves ventricular function after long-term preservation.[84,85]

Distribution

The importance of uniform and complete cardioplegic distribution has only recently been appreciated. In studies of acute coronary artery occlusion, improved myocardial protection has been demonstrated when using retrograde as opposed to antegrade delivery techniques.[86,87] Analogous situations occur in pediatric patients with anomalous coronary arteries or right ventricular-dependant coronary circulations associated with pulmonary atresia and intact ventricular septum. In such instances cardioplegic infusion directly into a crossclamped pulmonary artery or into the body of the right ventricle with a competent tricuspid valve and crossclamped pulmonary artery, respectively, may be used to ensure antegrade delivery of cardioplegia. Alternatively, the retrograde approach may be used.

Fortunately, in the vast majority of pediatric procedures, excellent cardioplegic distribution may be achieved using the antegrade approach alone. Nonetheless, there is an increasing role for retrograde-delivered cardioplegia in pediatric patients. Retrograde cardioplegia is particularly useful in situations where there is significant aortic insufficiency and antegrade arrest cannot be achieved. It is also quite helpful in avoiding individual coronary ostial cannulation in procedures where the aortic root is opened. Furthermore, the combination of both antegrade and retrograde cardioplegia may maximize cardioplegic distribution.[88,89]

The distribution of retrograde cardioplegia has now become well documented in both animals and humans. In porcine and canine models the vast majority of capillary retrograde cardioplegia flow is to the anterior intraventricular septum and left ventricle. There is a pronounced lack of capillary flow to the right ventricle.[90–93] In humans, capillary flow/gram myocardium to the right ventricle is approximately one-fourth the amount that it is to the left ventricle during routine blind transatrial retrograde coronary sinus cannulation.[94,95] With direct coronary sinus cannulation and coronary sinus occlusion by pursestring application right ventricular perfusion is dramatically increased to one-half to near identical capillary flow/gram myocardium when compared to the left ventricle[96] (Table 61–2). Approximately one-third to two-thirds (depending on cannulation technique) of retrograde-delivered cardioplegia is shunted through thesbesian veins into the ventricular cavities.[96,97] Although thebesian veins are not known to provide capillary blood flow, these vessels (which traverse predominantly the musculature of the right ventricle and septum) are extremely effective in cooling the ventricles.

Topical hypothermia should be mentioned in its relation to distribution. While topical hypothermia alone may be used for myocardial protection,[98,99] the majority of experimental evidence has suggested that hypothermic cardioplegia is superior in its efficacy.[78,100–102] This logically follows as the conduction of hypothermia will be superior with its complete distribution through the capillary system as opposed to its application to the epicardium alone. Nonetheless, one should be aware of the potential for epicardial right ventricular warming during intermittent cardioplegia delivery as a result of the right ventricle's exposed position to the operating room lights. Topical ice packs easily eliminate this problem. An insulation sponge may also be useful

TABLE 61–2. RETROGRADE-DELIVERED CARDIOPLEGIC REGIONAL MYOCARDIAL BLOOD FLOW IN EXPLANTED HUMAN HEARTS AS MEASURED BY COLORED MICROSPHERES[a]

	Anterior	Lateral/Mid	Posterior
LV	.34 ± .32 vs. .25 ± .30	.20 ± .26 vs. .10 ± .07	.11 ± .13 vs. .26 ± .28
RV	.20 ± .21 vs. .21 ± .19	.05 ± .03 vs. .17 ± .13*	.04 ± .03 vs. .18 ± .13*
IVS	.12 ± .31 vs. .26 ± .20	.11 ± .08 vs. .24 ± .17	.02 ± .01 vs. .19 ± .10*
	RV	**IVS**	**LV**
Apex	.11 ± .07 vs. .23 ± .12*	.14 ± .12 vs. .35 ± .23*	.12 ± .18 vs. .30 ± .29

[a]The study compares the open versus occluded coronary sinus and demonstrates improved right ventricular flow when the coronary sinus is occluded. Clinically, coronary sinus occlusion is easily achieved in pediatric patients by placing a pursestring suture about the coronary sinus osteum and snaring the retrograde cannula in position. LV, left ventricle; RV, right ventricle; IVS, intraventricular septum; *P<0.05. All flows are expressed in mL/g myocardium. (From Rudis E, Gates RN, Laks H, et al: Coronary sinus osteal occlusion during retrograde cardioplegia delivery significantly improves cardioplegic distribution and efficiency. J Thorac Cardiovasc Surg (in press) with permission.)

in avoiding conductive loss of myocardial hypothermia to surrounding tissues. Such devices may further reduce the incidence of cold-related phrenic nerve paralysis as well.[103]

Warm and Cold Cardioplegia

Most simply put, warm conditions promote aerobic metabolism and should be used in scenarios where oxygened cardioplegia may be continuously delivered to meet ongoing metabolic demands. Cold conditions reduce metabolic demands and should be used in scenarios where oxygened cardioplegia is delivered intermittently. For induction and reperfusion, warm conditions are indicated and care should be taken to ensure adequate cardioplegic distribution to all regions of the myocardium. For maintenance cardioplegia, in theory, either warm continuous cardioplegia or cold intermittent cardioplegia may be used. However, several technical considerations favor the use of cold intermittent cardioplegia in the immature myocardium.

The first is the general preference of hypothermic cardiopulmonary bypass during congenital procedures. This reduces bronchial and noncoronary collateral return and improves visualization of intracardiac structures. It further allows for deep hypothermia with low flow cardiopulmonary bypass or circulatory arrest. During hypothermic cardiopulmonary bypass in small pediatric patients it is technically cumbersome to maintain myocardial normothermia for more than a short interval of time. The second major consideration is that continuous techniques result in a continuous effluent. Although this is easy to control during many adult procedures, this is a nuisance in pediatric procedures where the operation is frequently intracardiac. Nonetheless, when nearing the completion of many pediatric procedures (during rewarming and while incisions required for exposure are being closed) warm continuous techniques may often be used without disrupting the conduct of the procedure. A third consideration is that, as previously noted, the immature myocardium tolerates cold ischemia better than the mature myocardium.[21,24] This is likely related to the metabolic differences between immature and mature myocardium and the ability of immature myocardium to effectively perform anaerobic glycolysis for energy production. As such, cold intermittent maintenance cardioplegia is preferred for the immature myocardium.

EXTRACORPOREAL CIRCULATION AND ITS EFFECTS UPON MYOCARDIAL PROTECTION

Control of cardiopulmonary bypass plays a great role in pediatric myocardial protection. Bronchial blood flow and noncoronary collateral blood flow are frequently significant in the young, particularly in those with cyanotic congenital heart disease. Reduced systemic flow decreases bronchial and noncoronary collateral flow and is safely achieved by the addition of systemic hypothermia. Bronchial and non-

coronary collateral flow is eliminated entirely by the use of deep hypothermia and circulatory arrest. Thus, hypothermic cardiopulmonary bypass aids myocardial protection by reducing cardioplegic "wash-out" and helping to maintain myocardial hypothermia. Hypothermic cardiopulmonary bypass also helps improve visualization by decreasing the amount of blood returning to the heart, which requires venting or scavenging.

Interactions between the extracorporeal circuit and the patient's blood during cardiopulmonary bypass result in an inflammatory reaction. This reaction leads to the activation of complement, platelets, neutrophils, arachadonic acids, and other mediators of the inflammatory response.[104] The activation of these and other blood components may serve to heighten reperfusion injuries and is therefore of great relevance to myocardial protection. Advances in extracorporeal arachadonic circulation that serve to decrease the inflammatory response to cardiopulmonary bypass should also benefit myocardial protection.

In infants and neonates hypothermic cardiopulmonary bypass is frequently associated with a significant total body free water gain related to the "capillary leak" syndrome. This phenomenon is also seen in the heart and such myocardial edema may negatively affect myocardial function. Recently, postcardiopulmonary bypass-modified ultrafiltration has been introduced to help reverse free water gain.[105] This technique has been shown to reduce total body free water gain after cardiopulmonary bypass and to improve ventricular function.[106] Our experience with this technique has been very gratifying in achieving these goals.

AN INTEGRATED APPROACH TO PEDIATRIC MYOCARDIAL PROTECTION

In this section our approach at the UCLA Medical Center toward pediatric myocardial protection will be presented. These techniques are based upon a synthesis of the experimental and clinical material presented above. We employ blood cardioplegia for all procedures where a diastolic cardiac arrest is induced and maintained. The advantages of using blood as a vehicle for cardioplegia are numerous.[106,107] Briefly, blood cardioplegia allows for oxygen delivery, buffers, contains naturally occurring antioxidants, and delivers metabolic and structural substrates. Further, its use is uncomplicated and reduces the crystalloid volume load upon the extracorporeal circuit.

Blood cardioplegia may be produced by combining four parts blood from the extracorporeal circuit with one part crystalloid cardioplegic solution. We use four basic crystalloid solutions (standard arrest, warm arrest "resuscitation," standard maintenance, and modified reperfusion) for mixing with blood (Table 61–3). These solutions have a pH of 7.6–7.7, an osmolality of approximately 320 mosm, an ionized calcium of 0.6–0.8 mmol/L, and a potassium of 8–10 or 16–20 mmol/L. The calcium level may be con-

TABLE 61-3. CARDIOPLEGIA COMPOSITION[a]

Solution	Composition
Standard arrest	500 cm³ 0.2 mol/L NS
	200 cm³ 0.3 mol/L Tham
	50 cm³ CPD[b]
	60 mmol/L KCl
Warm arrest[c]	500 cm³ 0.2 mol/L NS
	200 cm³ 0.3 mol/L Tham
	50 cm³ CPD[b]
	60 mmol/L KCl
	250 cm³ 0.46 mol/L
	Monosodium glutamate/aspartate
Standard maintenance	500 cm³ 0.2 mol/L NS
	200 cm³ 0.3 mol/L Tham
	50 cm³ CPD[b]
	30 mmol/L KCl
Modified reperfusion[c]	500 cm³ 0.2 mol/L NS
	200 cm³ 0.3 mol/L Tham
	50 cm³ CPD[b]
	30 mmol/L KCl
	250 cm³ 0.46 mol/L
	Monosodium glutamate/aspartate

[a]CPD, citrate–phosphate–dextrose; NS, normal saline; Tham, tromethamine.
[b]Decreasing CPD amount will result in increased ionized calcium levels.
[c]When appropriate, mechanical leukocyte filtering may be added (see text).

trolled by adding or reducing citrate–phosphate–dextrose (CPD). Leukocyte-depleted cardioplegia is produced by leukocyte filtering of extracted extracorporeal circuit blood prior to mixing with the crystalloid component.

Standard arrest cold blood cardioplegia is used in procedures where ventricular function is good and the myocardium is not felt to be in an energy or substrate-depleted state. When ventricular function is decreased or the myocardium is judged to be in an energy or substrate-depleted state warm arrest or "resuscitation" blood cardioplegia is administered for 2–3 min. For neonates in severely compromised states we have included leukocyte depletion during this period of warm resuscitation. This has been based upon concerns that in such severely compromised hearts warm induction is analogous to warm reperfusion, and every attempt should be made to limit reperfusion injury at this time. After warm arrest cardioplegia an immediate dose of cold standard maintenance cardioplegia should be given to achieve uniform myocardial hypothermia. During the operative procedure we give intermittent doses of cold standard maintenance blood cardioplegia every 15–20 min. If activity is noted prior to interval replenishment short periods of standard arrest cardioplegia may be given while attempts to further systemically cool the patient and reduce extracorporeal flow rates are undertaken.

We use controlled warm reperfusion for every heart that has undergone cardioplegic arrest. Warm controlled reperfusion is performed prior to removal of the aortic cross-clamp at a time when all variables of reperfusion can be controlled. As reperfusion is always performed warm, reperfusion cardioplegia should be given continuously until the aortic crossclamp is removed. To reduce interval cold ischemia, warm reperfusion should be undertaken as soon as the continuous effluent that it produces is no longer a negative factor in the performance of the procedure. In pediatric operations this is generally at the conclusion of the intracardiac portion of the procedure. Approximately 2–5 min before cross-clamp removal is anticipated continuous warm standard maintenance blood cardioplegia may be discontinued and warm unmodified extracorporeal circuit blood infused with the cross-clamp remaining in place. This allows for a period of cardioplegia "wash-out" and the heart will generally regain a spontaneous rhythm during this time. Removal of the crossclamp when the heart is warm and in a spontaneous rhythm avoids problematic ventricular distension that may be encountered when the crossclamp is removed in asystolic cold hearts.

Initial warm reperfusion may be performed with either warm standard maintenance cardioplegia, modified reperfusion cardioplegia, or leukocyte-depleted modified reperfusion cardioplegia. In general, we have reperfused the myocardium with standard maintenance cardioplegia when the heart was arrested with standard arrest cardioplegia, modified reperfusion cardioplegia when arrested with warm arrest cardioplegia, and leukocyte-depleted modified reperfusion cardioplegia when arrested with leukocyte-depleted warm arrest cardioplegia (Table 61–4). The surgeon should use clinical judgment during reperfusion, however, and if there has been a prolonged crossclamp time or there is concern for inadequate intraoperative myocardial protection reperfusion should be performed with modified reperfusion or leukocyte-depleted modified reperfusion cardioplegia regardless of cardioplegia used to arrest the heart.

Cardioplegic distribution is extremely important. For warm aerobic techniques of blood cardioplegia to be effective, the cardioplegic solution must reach all microvascular beds lest there be regions of anaerobic warm metabolism. When using cold cardioplegic techniques a uniform distribution ensures even and effective cooling. As previously discussed, there is growing evidence that even in routine procedures cardioplegic distribution may be maximized by combining both antegrade and retrograde techniques. The surgeon can appreciate this by noting a routine clinical observation. After giving a dose of warm antegrade blood cardioplegia, if one immediately follows this with a dose of warm retrograde blood cardioplegia, the initial effluent emerging from the coronary ostea is dark and desaturated.

TABLE 61-4. GUIDELINES FOR REPERFUSION SOLUTIONS BASED UPON INITIAL ARRESTING SOLUTIONS

Arrest Cardioplegia	Reperfusion Cardioplegia
Cold standard arrest	Warm standard maintenance
Warm arrest cardioplegia	Warm modified reperfusion cardioplegia
Leukocyte-depleted warm arrest cardioplegia	Leukocyte-depleted warm modified reperfusion cardioplegia

Shortly thereafter the effluent will again become red and saturated. The implication of this clinical observation is obvious (the antegrade cardioplegia dose did not completely perfuse all capillary beds). As such, we have been combining either sequentially, or simultaneously, antegrade and retrograde blood cardioplegia on all but a few selected procedures. The selected procedures for the antegrade route alone are those cases where the following criteria are met: (1) The myocardium is not in an energy or substrate-depleted state, (2) there is no significant aortic insufficiency, (3) there is no ventricular hypertrophy, and (4) the procedure is of short duration.

The use of both the antegrade and retrograde approach to cardioplegia delivery is particularly important in cases where warm arrest cardioplegia is planned. In these procedures maximum cardioplegic distribution helps ensure that as much as possible of the myocardium is in fact resuscitated. Thus, both antegrade and retrograde delivery of cardioplegia should be used whenever employing warm arrest cardioplegia. During maintenance cardioplegia alternating doses of antegrade then retrograde standard maintenance cardioplegia or combined doses of antegrade–retrograde standard maintenance cardioplegia appear to be very effective. Periods of only sequential retrograde delivered cold standard maintenance cardioplegia without antegrade-delivered cardioplegia appear to be safe for several consecutive

doses. It may at times be beneficial to use this technique to facilitate procedures on small infant and neonates when the aortic root is opened. This avoids individual coronary osteal cannulation that is cumbersome and potentially injurious.

During the reperfusion period the antegrade alone approach may be used if only antegrade cardioplegia doses preceded reperfusion. However, if retrograde cardioplegia has been used during arrest or maintenance, it is important to use both the antegrade and retrograde approach during reperfusion. The use of both approaches (particularly at the end of reperfusion when unmodified extracorporeal circuit blood is given) ensures uniform rewarming and complete "wash-out" of cardioplegia that has been previously delivered. Failure to "wash-out" cardioplegia results in prolonged recovery of ventricular function and a delay in weaning from cardiopulmonary bypass as potassium levels fall within the myocardium and its functional capabilities resume.

We have been using the combined antegrade and retrograde approach for pediatric myocardial protection since early 1988. In 1992 we reported our results for the first 123

TABLE 61–5. OPERATIVE PROCEDURES AND OUTCOME FOR COMBINATION ANTEGRADE/RETROGRADE BLOOD CARDIOPLEGIA

Procedure	Number	Hospital Mortality
Fontan	20	
Aortic valve repair/replace	6+7	1
VSD closure	12	
Tetralogy of Fallot	10	
AV canal	10	1
Rastelli	10	
Konno/aortic root/Ross	4+4+1	
Subaortic membrane/myectomy	6+1	
Mitral repair/replace	5+1	
Coronary reimplant/fistula	3+3	
Truncus arteriosus	4	1
Conduit replacement	3	
Arterial switch	3	
Glenn Shunt	2	
Sinus venosus ASD	2	
DORV	1	
Aortopulmonary window	1	
Ebstein's anomaly	1	
Senning	1	
Interrupted arch	1	
Damus–Stansel–Kaye	1	
Total	123	3 (2.4%)

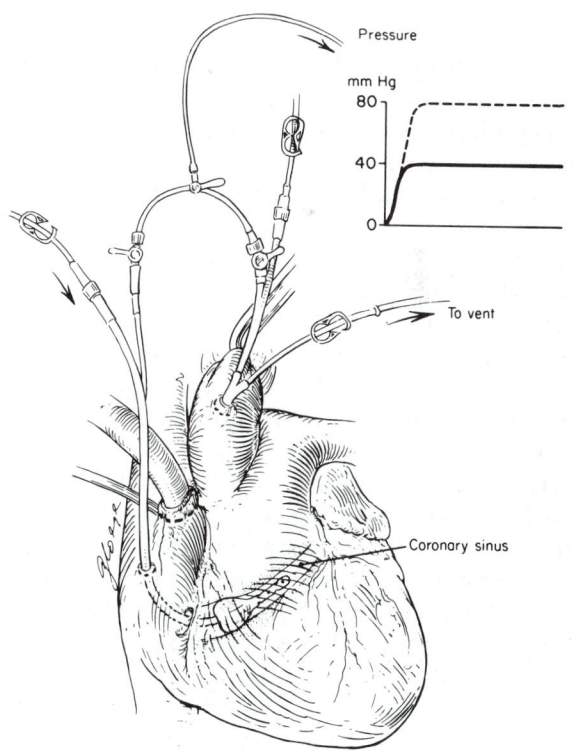

Figure 61–4. The clinical setup and infusion pressures for antegrade (aortic [dotted line]) and retrograde (coronary sinus [solid line]) combined technique of infusion of cardioplegic solution. During retrograde infusion, the aortic root vent is open for the effluent. Here the retroperfusion catheter has been placed transatrially through a pursestring in the right atrial wall. *(From Drinkwater DC, Cushin C, Laks H, et al: The use of combined antegrade-retrograde blood cardioplegia in pediatric open-heart surgery: The UCLA experience. J Thorac Cardiovasc Surg 104:1349–1355, 1992, with permission.)*

patients.[88] The approach was used for a wide variety of procedures with an overall mortality of 2.4% (Table 61–5), (Fig. 61–4). Ages ranged from 1 wk to 16 years with a mean of 4.5 years and the mean cross-clamp time was 87 min. There were no complications associated with the use of retrograde cardioplegia. In procedures where the right side of the heart was isolated and opened, direct coronary sinus cannulation with osteal pursestring occlusion was used. In cases where the right side of the heart was not isolated transatrial cannulation was performed as previously described.[106] We have found that integration of both antegrade and retrograde techniques of myocardial protection facilitate the conduct of the operation and appear to improve the overall efficacy of blood cardioplegia.

CONCLUSION

Improvements in extracorporeal circulation, cerebral protection, and myocardial protection underlie the recent advances in congenital heart surgery. Pediatric myocardial protection has benefited greatly from experimental work directed toward mature myocardium. However, one must be continually aware of the inherent structural, functional, and metabolic differences between the mature and immature myocardium. Further, an understanding of the unique physiologic states created by congenital heart lesions and their effects upon the immature myocardium should be appreciated. It is incumbent upon the surgeon to obtain a thorough appreciation of the basic concepts of myocardial protection along with an appropriate knowledge of currently available techniques for pediatric myocardial protection. With these skills in hand, the congenital heart surgeon may successfully plan an integrated approach to pediatric myocardial protection tailored to the individual patient.

REFERENCES

1. Bull C, Cooper J, Stark J: Cardioplegia protection of the child's heart. *J Thorac Cardiovasc Surg* **88**:287, 1984
2. Anversa P, Olivetti G, Loud A: Morphometeric study of early postnatal development in the left and right ventricular myocardium of the rat. *Circ Res* **46**:495, 1980
3. Korecky B, Rakusan K: Normal and hypertrophic growth of the rat heart: Changes in cell dimensions and number. *Am J Physiol* **234**:H123, 1978
4. Romero T, Covell J, Friedman W: A comparison of pressure-volume relations of fetal, newborn, and adult hearts. *Am J Physiol* **222**(5):1285, 1972
5. Marijianowski MM, van der Loos CM, Morrschladt MF, Becker AE: The neonatal heart has a relatively high content of total collagen and type I collagen, a condition that may explain the less compliant state. *J Am Coll Cardiol* **23**:1204, 1994
6. Romero T, Friedman W: Limited left ventricular response to volume overload in the neonatal period: A comparative study with the adult animal. *Pediatr Res* **13**:910, 1979
7. Legato M: Ultrastructural changes during normal growth in the dog and rat ventricular myofiber. In Lieberman M, Santo T (eds): *Developmental and Physiological Correlates of Cardiac Muscle.* New York, Raven Press 1975, p 249
8. Legato M: Cellular mechanisms of normal growth in the mammalian heart. II. A quantitative and qualitative comparison between the left and right ventricular myocyte in the dog from birth to five months. *Circ Res* **44**:263, 1979
9. Smith H, Page E: Ultrastructural changes in rabbit heart mitochondria during the perinatal period. Neonatal transition to aerobic metabolism. *Dev Biol* **57**:109, 1977
10. Tomec RJ, Hoppel CL: Carnitine palmitotransferase in bovine fetal heart mitochondria. *Arch Biochem Biophys* **170**:716, 1975
11. Friedman WF: The intrinsic physiologic properties of the developing heart. *Prog Cardiovasc Disc* **15**:87, 1972
12. Teitel DF, Sidi D, Chin T, et al: Developmental changes in myocardial contractile reserve in the lamb. *Pediatr Res* **19**(9):948, 1985
13. Berman W, Christensen D: Effects of acute preload and afterload stress on myocardial function in newborn and adult sheep. *Biol Neonate* **43**:61, 1983
14. Gilbert RD: Effects of afterload and baroreceptors on cardiac function in fetal sheep. *J Dev Physiol* **4**:299, 1980
15. Fisher DJ, Rudolph AM, Heymann MA: Myocardial oxygen and carbohydrate consumption in fetal lambs in utero and in adult sheep. *Am J Physiol* **238**:H399, 1980
16. Dawes GS, Mott JC, Shelley HF: The importance of cardiac glycogen for the maintenance of life in fetal lambs and newborn animals during anoxia. *J Physiol (London)* **146**:516, 1959
17. Rolph TP, Jones CT: Regulation of glycolytic flux in the heart of the fetal guinea pig. *J Dev Physiol* **5**:31, 1983
18. Hoerter JA, Opie LH: Perinatal changes in glycolytic function in response to hypoxia in the incubated or perfused rat heart. *Biol Neonate* **33**:144, 1978
19. Magovern JA, Pae WE Jr, Miller CA, et al: The mature and immature heart: response to normothermic ischemia. *J Surg Res* **46**:366, 1989
20. Nishioka K, Jarmakani JM: Effects of ischemia on mechanical function in the neonatal rabbit heart. *Pediatr Res* **25**:469, 1981
21. Grice WN, Konishi T, Apstein CS: Resistance of neonatal myocardium to injury during normothermic and hypothermic ischemic arrest and reperfusion. *Circulation* **76**(suppl 5):150, 1987
22. Gennser G: Influence of hypoxia and glucose on contractility of papillary muscles from adult and neonatal rabbits. *Biol Neonate* **21**:90, 1972
23. Bove EL, Stammers AH: Recovery of left ventricular function after hypothermic global ischemia: Age related differences in the isolated working rabbit heart. *J Thorac Cardiovasc Surg* **91**:115, 1986
24. Bove EL, Gallagher KP, Drake DH: The effect of hypothermic ischemia on recovery of left ventricular function and pre-load reserve in the neonatal heart. *J Thorac Cardiovasc Surg* **95**:814, 1988
25. Su JY, Friedman WF: Comparison of the responses of fetal and adult cardiac muscle to hypoxia. *Am J Physiol* **224**(6):1249, 1973
26. Gelli MG, Enhorning G, Hultman E, et al: Glucose infusion in pregnant rabbit and its effect on glycogen content and activity of fetal heart under anoxia. *Acta Paediatr Scand* **57**:209, 1968
27. Opie LH: The glucose hypothesis: Relation to acute myocardial ischemia. *J Mol Cell Cardiol* **1**:107, 1970
28. Grosso MA, Banerjee A, St Cyr JA, et al: Cardiac 5'-nucleotidase activity increases with age and inversely relates to recovery from ischemia. *J Thorac Cardiovasc Surg* **103**:206, 1992
29. Crevey BJ, Langer GA, Frank JS: Role of calcium in maintenance of rabbit myocardial cell membrane structural and functional integrity. *J Moll Cell Cardiol* **10**:1081, 1978
30. Bers DM, Langer GA: Uncoupling cation effects on cardiac contractility and sarcolemma CA++ binding. *Am J Physiol* **237**:H332, 1979
31. Nakanishi T, Seguchi M, Takao A: Development of the myocardial contractile system. *Experientia* **44**:936, 1988
32. Klitzner T: Maturational changes in excitation-contraction coupling in mammalian myocardium. *J Am Coll Cardiol* **17**:218, 1991

33. Mahony L: Maturation of calcium transport function in cardiac sarcoplasmic reticulum. *Pediatr Res* **24**:639, 1988

34. Boucek RJ, Shelton M, Artman M, et al: Comparative effects of verapamil, nifedipine, and diltiazem on contractile function in the isolated immature and adult rabbit heart. *Pediatr Res* **18**:948, 1984

35. Yano Y, Braimbridge M, Hearse D: Protection of the pediatric myocardium. Differential susceptibility to ischemic injury of the neonatal rat heart. *J Thorac Cardiovasc Surg* **94**:887, 1987

36. Baker J, Boerboom L, Olinger G: Age-related changes in the ability of hypothermia and cardioplegia to protect ischemic rabbit myocardium. *J Thorac Cardiovasc Surg* **96**:717, 1988

37. Jarmakani J, Nakazawa M, Nagatomo T, et al: Effect of hypoxia on mechanical function in the neonatal mammalian heart. *Am J Physiol* **235**:H469, 1978

38. Jarmakani J, Nakazawa M, Nagatomo T, et al: Effect of hypoxia on myocardial high energy phosphates in the neonatal mammalian heart. *Am J Physiol* **235**:475, 1978

39. Downing SE, Talner NS, Gardner TH: Influences of arterial oxygen tension and pH on cardiac function in the newborn lamb. *Am J Physiol* **211**(5):1203, 1966

40. Lee LC, Halloran KH, Taylor JFN, et al: Coronary flow and myocardial metabolism in newborn lambs: Effect of hypoxemia and acodosis. *Am J Physiol* **224**(6):1381, 1973

41. Julia P, Kofsky ER, Buckberg GD, et al: Studies of myocardial protection in the immature heart III. Models of ischemic and hypoxic/ischemic injury in the immature puppy heart. *J Thorac Cardiovasc Surg* **101**:14, 1991

42. Scheuer J, Shaver J, Kroetz F, et al: Myocardial metabolism in cyanotic congenital heart disease studied by artero-venous differences in lactase, phosphate, and potassium at rest and during atrial pacing. *Circulation* **55**:647, 1976

43. Scheurer J: Studies in the human heart exposed to chronic hypoxia. *Cardiology* **56**:215, 1972

44. Fujiwara T, Kurtts T, Anderson W, et al: Myocardial protection in cyanotic neonatal lambs. *J Thorac Cardiovasc Surg* **96**:700, 1988

45. Lupinetti FM, Wareing TH, Huddleston CB, et al: Pathophysiology of chronic cyanosis in a canine model. *J Thorac Cardiovasc Surg* **90**:291, 1985

46. Silverman NA, Kohler J, Levitsky S, et al: Chronic hypoxia depresses global ventricular function and predisposes to the depletion of high energy phosphates during cardioplegic arrest: Implications for repair of cyanotic congenital heart defects. *Ann Thorac Surg* **34**(4):304, 1984

47. Downing S, Talner N, Gardner T: Ventricular function in the newborn lamb. *Am J Physiol* **208**:931, 1965

48. Klopfenstein H, Rudolph A: Postnatal changes in the circulation and response to volume loading in the sheep. *Circ Res* **42**:839, 1978

49. Gaasch W, Levine H, Quinones M, et al: Left ventricular compliance: Mechanisms and clinical implications. *Am J Cardiol* **38**:645, 1976

50. Peyton RB, Hones RN, Attarian D, et al: Depressed high energy phosphate content in hypertrophied ventricles of animals and man. *Ann Surg* **196**:278, 1982

51. Buckberg GD: Left ventricular subendocardial necrosis. *Ann Thorac Surg* **24**:379, 1977

52. Sink J, Pellon G, Currie W, et al: Response of hypertrophied myocardium to ischemia. *J Thorac Cardiovasc Surg* **81**:865, 1981

53. Del Nido PJ, Mickle DAG, Wilson GJ, et al: Inadequate myocardial protection with cold cardioplegic arrest during repair of tetrology of fallot. *J Thorac Cardiovasc Surg* **95**:223, 1988

54. Del Nido PJ, Benson LM, Mickle DAG, et al: Impaired postischemic left ventricular function and metabolism in chronic right ventricular hypertrophy. *Circulation* **76**:168, 1987

55. Archie JP, Fixler DE, Ullyot DJ, et al: Regional myocardial blood flow in lambs with concentric right ventricular hypertrophy. *Circ Res* **34**:143, 1974

56. Hertzer R, Warnecke H, Wittock H, et al: Extra coronary collateral myocardial blood flow during cardioplegic arrest. *J Thorac Cardiovasc Surg* **28**:191, 1980

57. Brazier J, Hottenrott C, Buckberg G: *Ann Thorac Surg* **19**(4):426, 1975

58. Rosenkranz E, Vinten-Johansen J, Buckberg GD, et al: Benefits of normothermic induction of cardioplegia in energy-depleted hearts, with maintenance of arrest by multidose cold blood cardioplegic infusion. *J Thorac Cardiovasc Surg* **84**:667, 1982

59. Wittnich C, Maitland A, Vincente W, et al: Not all neonatal hearts are equally protected from ischemic damage during hypothermia. *Ann Thorac Surg* **52**:1000, 1991

60. Julia P, Kofsky ER, Buckberg GD, et al: Studies of myocardial protection in the immature heart: III. Models of ischemic and hypoxic/ischemic injury in the puppy heart. IV. Improved tolerance of immature myocardium to hypoxia and ischemia by intravenous support. *J Thorac Cardiovasc Surg* **101**:14, 1991

61. Author's unpublished data.

62. Brown A, Brainbridge M, Niles, M, et al: The effects of excessively high perfusion pressures on the histology, histochemistry, birefringence, and function of the myocardium. *J Thorac Cardiovasc Surg* **58**:655, 1969

63. Mankin PS, Chester AH, Yacoub MH: Role of potassium concentration in cardioplegic solutions mediating endothelial damage. *Ann Thorac Surg* **51**:89, 1991

64. Author's unpublished data.

65. Allen BS, Okamato F, Buckberg GD, et al: Studies of controlled reperfusion after ischemia. XIII. Reperfusate conditions: Critical importance of total ventricular decompression during regional reperfusion. *J Thorac Cardiovasc Surg* **92**(3)(suppl):605, 1986

66. Lazar HL, Buckberg GD, Manganaro AM, et al: Reversal of ischemic damage with aminoacid substrate enhancement during reperfusion. *Surgery* **88**(5):702, 1980

67. Lazar HL, Buckberg GD, Manganaro AM, et al: Myocardial energy replenishment and reversal of ischemic damage by substrate enhancement of secondary blood cardioplegia with amino-acids during reperfusion. *J Thorac Cardiovasc Surg* **80**:350, 1980

68. Rosenkranz E, Okamoto F, Buckberg GD, et al: Safety of prolonged aortic cross-clamping with blood cardioplegia. III. Aspartate enrichment of glutamate blood cardioplegia in energy-depleted hearts after ischemic and reperfusion injury. *J Thorac Cardiovasc Surg* **91**:428, 1986

69. Rosenkranz E, Okamoto F, Buckberg GD, et al: Safety of prolonged aortic cross-clamping with blood cardioplegia. II. Glutamate enrichment in energy-depleted hearts. *J Thorac Cardiovasc Surg* **88**:402, 1984

70. Brazier J, Hottenrott C, Buckberg G: Noncoronary collateral myocardial blood flow. *Ann Thorac Surg* **19**:426, 1975

71. Zureikat H: Collateral vessels between the coronary and bronchial arteries in patients with cyanotic congenital heart disease. *Am J Cardiol* **45**:599, 1980

72. Ferguson TB, Smith PK, Burhman WC, et al: Studies on the physiology of the conduction system during hyperkalemic, hypothermic cardioplegic arrest. *Surg Forum* **34**:302, 1983

73. Abd-Elfattah A, Wechsler AS: Myocardial protection in cardiac surgery: Subcellular basis for myocardial injury and protection. In Karp RB, Laks H, Wechsler AS (eds): *Advances in Cardiac Surgery*, Vol 3. St Louis, Mosby-Yearbook, 1992, p 73.

74. Opie LH: Reperfusion injury and its pharmacologic modification. *Circulation* **80a**:1049, 1989

75. Holmeberg SRM, Cummin DVE, Kusama Y, et al: Reactive oxygen species modify the structure and function of the cardiac sarcosmic reticulum calcium-release channel. *Cardioscience* **2**:19, 1991

76. Hearse DJ: Reperfusion induced injury: A possible role for oxidant stress and its manipulation. *Cardiovasc Drug Ther* **2**:623, 1988

77. Boli R: Mechanisms of myocardial "stunning." *Circulation* **82**:723, 1990

78. Milliken JC, Bhuta S, Laks H: Improved myocardial protection in neonatal lambs following hypoxia. *Surg Forum* **35**:336, 1984

79. Follete DM, Fey K, Livesay J, et al: Studies on myocardial reperfusion injury. Favorable modification by adjusting reperfusate pH. *Surgery* **82:**149, 1977

80. Allen BS, Okamoto F, Buckberg GD, et al: Reperfusate composition: Benefits of marked hypocalcemia and diltiazem on regional recovery. *J Thorac Cardiovasc Surg* **92:**564, 1986

81. Allen BS, Buckberg GD, Schwaiger M, et al: Studies of controlled reperfusion after ischemia. XVI. Consistent early recovery of regional wall motion following surgical revascularization after eight hours of acute coronary occlusion. *J Thorac Cardiovasc Surg* **92**(3)(suppl):636, 1986

82. Davatyan HG, Corno AF, Laks H, et al: Long term neonatal heart preservation. *J Thorac Cardiovasc Surg* **96:**44, 1988

83. Julia PL, Buckberg GD, Acar C, et al: Studies of controlled reperfusion after ischemia. XXI. Reperfusate composition: Superiority of blood cardioplegia over crystalloid cardioplegia in limiting reperfusion damage—importance of endogenous free radical scavengers in the red blood cell. *J Thorac Cardiovasc Surg* **101:**303, 1991

84. Breda M, Drinkwater DC, Laks H, et al: Prevention of reperfusion injury in the neonatal heart using leukocyte-depleted blood. *J Thorac Cardiovasc Surg* **97:**654, 1989

85. Stein D, Permut L, Drinkwater DC, et al: Complete functional recovery after 24 hour perservation with University of Wisconsin solution and modified reperfusion. *Circulation* **84**(suppl 3):III316, 1991

86. Gundry SR, Kirsh MM: A comparison of retrograde cardioplegia versus antegrade cardioplegia in the presence of coronary artery obstruction. *Ann Thorac Surg* **38:**125, 1984

87. Haan C, Lazr HL, Bernard S, et al: Superiority of retrograde cardioplegia after acute coronary artery occlusion. *Ann Thorac Surg* **51:**408, 1991

88. Drinkwater DC, Cushin C, Laks H, et al: The use of combined antegrade-retrograde blood cardioplegia in pediatric open-heart surgery: The UCLA experience. *J Thorac Cardiovasc Surg* **104:**1349, 1992

89. Aldea GS, Hou D, Fonger JD, Shemin RJ: Inhomogeneous and complementary antegrade and retrograde delivery of cardioplegic solution in the absence of coronary artery obstruction. *J Thorac Cardiovasc Surg* **107:**499, 1994

90. Gates RN, Laks H, Drinkwater DC, et al: The microvascular distribution of cardioplegic solution in the piglet heart: Retrograde versus antegrade delivery. *J Thorac Cardiovasc Surg* **105:**845, 1993

91. Crooke GA, Harris LJ, Grossi EA, et al: Biventricular distribution of cold blood cardioplegic solution administered by different retrograde techniques. *J Thorac Cardiovasc Surg* **102:**631, 1991

92. Partington MT, Acar C, Buckberg GD, et al: Studies of retrograde cardioplegia. I. Capillary blood flow distribution to myocardium supplied by open and occluded arteries. *J Thorac Cardiovasc Surg* **97:**605, 1989

93. Stirling MC, McClanahan TB, Schott RJ, et al: Distribution of cardioplegic solution infused antegradely and retrogradely in normal canine hearts. *J Thorac Cardiovasc Surg* **98:**1066, 1989

94. Ardehali A, Gates RN, Laks H, et al: The regional capillary distribution of retrograde blood cardioplegia in explanted human hearts (abstract). *74th Annual Meeting of the American Association for Thoracic Surgery,* New York, 1994

95. Allen BS, Hartz RS, Wiewall J, et al: Retrograde cardioplegia does not perfuse the right ventricle (abstract). *74th Annual Meeting of the American Association for Thoracic Surgery,* New York, 1994

96. Rudis E, Gates RN, Laks H, et al: Coronary sinus osteal occlusion during retrograde cardioplegia delivery significantly improves cardioplegic distribution and efficacy. *J Thorac Cardiovasc Surg* (in press).

97. Gates RN, Laks H, Drinkwater DC, et al: Gross and microvascular distribution of retrograde cardioplegia in explanted human hearts. *Ann Thorac Surg* **56:**410, 1993

98. Wisman CB, Waldhausen JA, Pierce WS, et al: Preservation of high-energy phosphates during ischemia in the isolated perfused neonatal pig heart: A comparison of hypothermic potassium cardioplegia with hypothermia alone. *Surg Forum* **33:**315, 1982

99. Lamberti JJ, Cohen LH, Laks H, et al: Local cardiac hypothermia for myocardial protection during correction of congenital heart disease. *Ann Thorac Surg* **20:**446, 1975

100. Kirklin JK, Blackstone EH, Kirklin JW, et al: Intracardiac surgery in infants under age 3 months: Incremental risk factors for hospital mortality. *Am J Cardiol* **48:**500, 1981

101. Bove EL, Stammers AH, Gallagher KP: Protection of the neonatal myocardium during hypothermic ischemia. *J Thorac Cardiovasc Surg* **94:**115, 1987

102. Lupinetti FM, Hammon JW, Huddleston CB, et al: Global ischemia in the immature canine ventricle. *J Thorac Cardiovasc Surg* **88:**287, 1984

103. Curtis JJ, Nawarawong W, Wall JT, et al: Elevated hemidiaphragm after cardiac operations: Incidence, prognosis, and relationship to the use of topical ice slush. *Ann Thorac Surg* **48:**764, 1989

104. Gates RN, Laks H, Drinkwater DC: Blood cardioplegia in adults and children. In Yacoub M, Pepper J (eds): *Annual of Cardiac Surgery 1992.* London, Current Science, 1992, p 59

105. Kirklin JW: Hypothermia, circulatory arrest, and cardiopulmonary bypass. In Kirklin JW, Barratt-Boyes BG (eds): *Cardiac Surgery,* 2nd ed. New York, Churchill Livingstone, 1992, p 61

106. Naik SK, Knight A, Elliot M: A successful modification of ultrafiltration for cardiopulmonary bypass in children. *Perfusion* **6:**41, 1991

107. Naik SK, Knight A, Elliot M: A prospective randomized study of a modified technique of ultrafiltration during pediatric open-heart surgery. *Circulation* **84**(suppl III):III423, 1991

108. Corno A, Bethencourt DM, Laks H, et al: Myocardial protection in the neonatal heart: A comparison of topical hypothermia and crystalloid and blood cardioplegic solutions. *J Thorac Cardiovasc Surg* **93:**163, 1987

109. Drinkwater DC, Laks H, Buckberg GD: A new simplified method of optimizing cardioplegia delivery without right heart isolation. *J Thorac Cardiovasc Surg* **100:**56, 1990

62

Pulmonary Vascular Disease

Marlene Rabinovitch

Congenital heart defects have three main effects on the pulmonary circulation: they increase or decrease pulmonary blood flow or increase pulmonary venous pressure. Each type of disturbance produces a different pattern of impaired growth and remodeling of the pulmonary vascular bed. There has been an explosion of new information concerning the cell and molecular biology of the vessel wall. Studies related to endothelial–smooth muscle interactions, degradation and synthesis of connective tissue proteins, smooth muscle differentiation, hyperplasia and hypertrophy, and angiogenesis may explain and, ultimately, lead to the control of pulmonary vascular disease. This chapter describes the nature of these pulmonary vascular changes and indicates how their presence and severity may influence the type and timing of surgical intervention. Recent clinical studies related to uncovering and treating the underlying mechanisms of heightened pulmonary vascular reactivity by inhaled nitric oxide will be presented. Moreover, advances in experimental studies will be discussed to show how this might lead to new and innovative therapies.

DEFECTS THAT INCREASE PULMONARY BLOOD FLOW

Victor Eisenmenger, in 1897, described a 32-year-old man with unexplained exercise intolerance and cyanosis who died in congestive heart failure after an episode of hemoptysis.[1] Postmortem examination revealed a large ventricular septal defect and more apparent-than-real overriding of the aorta. Many years later, it was observed that the symptoms this man had could also occur in patients with a variety of congenital heart defects, such as patent ductus arteriosus, atrial septal defect, or atrioventricular septal defect.[2–5] In these lesions, there is initially increased pulmonary blood flow secondary to left-to-right shunting, but later, in some

patients, a progressive elevation in pulmonary vascular resistance occurs, causing reversal of the shunt and cyanosis. The pathologic basis for this clinical entity, which came to be known as the Eisenmenger syndrome, was thought to be the development of endarteritis obliterans in very small abnormal peripheral arteries. Hence, the term *pulmonary vascular obstructive disease* was commonly applied to describe the functional state.[6] Natural history studies revealed that among the different congenital heart defects, the incidence of this complication and the rate of its development varied considerably.[7–20]

Natural History Studies

Approximately 15% of infants with large unrestrictive ventricular septal defects develop progressive elevation in pulmonary vascular resistance, and this will occur either in late infancy or in early childhood.[7] If surgical repair is carried out within the first 2 years of life, the increased pulmonary vascular resistance rarely persists. If correction is delayed longer, the degree of elevation either remains at levels observed preoperatively or progressively increases.[8,9] In addition, among the group repaired late, those patients who postoperatively have only slightly increased pulmonary vascular resistance at rest will usually exhibit an abnormal degree of elevation with exercise.[10] Patients with a large patent ductus arteriosus have a similar incidence and rate of development of pulmonary vascular disease.[5,11] Patients with a secundum atrial septal defect, however, usually have normal pulmonary arterial pressure in childhood, and the 20% who develop progressive pulmonary hypertension do so generally only after the third decade.[12] Even then, the pulmonary vascular disease is more slowly progressive, and it is for this reason, and also because of the relative technical ease of the operation, that some centers, including our own, have opted to repair secundum atrial septal defects in adult patients despite severe elevation in pulmonary vascular resistance and advanced vascular changes if there is a substantial net left-to-right shunt.[13] Rarely, infants with a secundum atrial septal defect will have rapidly progressive pulmonary vascular disease in the first year of life.[14] In some of these cases we have observed associated pulmonary vein stenosis, a condition that is frequently difficult to detect clinically.

Severe elevation in pulmonary vascular resistance will occur in the first year of life in 8% of patients with simple *d*-transposition of the great arteries[15] but in 40% of those who, in addition, have a ventricular septal defect or a patent ductus arteriosus.[16,17] In fact, by 2 years of age, 75% of the latter group are thus affected. There have been case reports of patients with simple *d*-transposition who developed progressive elevation in pulmonary vascular resistance after surgical repair, even though they had normal values preoperatively.[18]

Virtually all patients with common atrioventricular canal develop severe and irreversibly increased pulmonary vascular resistance in childhood. The majority will do so by 2 years of age, but, in some, this has been observed as early as the first year of life.[19] In patients with truncus arteriosus, a permanent increase in pulmonary vascular resistance may occur by the second year of life.[20,21]

The surgically created systemic-to-pulmonary artery shunts may also cause irreversible elevation in pulmonary vascular resistance. This occurs rarely with a Blalock–Taussig anastomosis, less than 10% of patients, but was common with a central shunt, where, after 5 years' duration, a 30% incidence was reported.[22]

Clinical and Hemodynamic Studies

Detecting the patient with a given congenital heart defect who will develop pulmonary vascular disease at all or who will do so particularly early is difficult. Clinical[23] and radiologic[24] manifestations are those of advanced disease. Electrocardiography,[25] vectorcardiography,[26] echocardiography,[27] and radionuclide studies[28] are relatively nonspecific. The use of Doppler echocardiography as described by Marx et al[29] to predict right ventricular pressure in patients with interventricular communications is certainly most promising but depends on the identification of a jet of tricuspid regurgitation which may not always be present. Studies of Musewe et al[30] have successfully applied pulsed Doppler to determine pulmonary artery pressure in the setting of a patient ductus arteriosus. Cardiac catheterization is still the most accurate way to determine and follow the level of pulmonary vascular resistance. Criteria have been suggested that distinguish patients in whom, even after repair, persistent severe elevation in pulmonary vascular resistance is likely[31,32]: a difference in oxygen saturation between pulmonary arteries and veins of greater than 2.5 vol% or an absolute level of pulmonary vascular resistance

of greater than 10 $\mu m \cdot m^2$. Values in the range between 8 and 10 are considered borderline but very promising if a decrease to 6 $\mu m \cdot m^2$ or less can be achieved with the inhalation of 100% oxygen or after the intravenous administration of nitric oxide or prostacyclin infusion. While the estimation of pulmonary vascular resistance by the Fick principle is most precise when oxygen consumption is measured,[33] the value obtained reflects the functional state at only one point in time. This measurement is influenced by the degree and type of sedation under which the patient is examined,[34] the presence of pulmonary disease,[35] the level of hematocrit,[36] and the amount of flow through systemic collateral vessels.[37] Thus, in certain cases in addition to the hemodynamic assessment, an evaluation of the structural state of the pulmonary vascular bed can provide useful information.

MORPHOLOGIC ASSESSMENT OF THE PULMONARY VASCULAR BED

As early as 1935, Brenner[38] recorded, from the study of autopsy material, different types of pulmonary vascular lesions occurring in patients with congenital heart defects. Heath and Edwards, in 1958,[39] suggested that there was a progression of structural changes—grades I through VI (Fig. 62–1). Grades I and II, medial hypertrophy and intimal hyperplasia, respectively, were considered mild and probably reversible. Grades III and IV are, respectively, lumen occlusion from intimal hyperplasia and early-to-advanced arterial dilatation. Grade III was thought to be probably still reversible, but grade IV was thought irreversible. Grades V and VI are terminal changes: V being angiomatoid formation and VI, fibrinoid necrosis.

The later changes indicating irreversible disease (grades IV, V, VI) seemed to take time to develop and were most frequently identified in older children. It was therefore more difficult to establish in infants and young children structural changes that correlated with severe and fixed elevation in pulmonary vascular resistance.[40] Several investigators tried to quantitate the degree of medial hypertrophy, but their measurements did not correlate closely with the preoperative level of pulmonary vascular resistance or with its change postoperatively.[41]

CONSIDERATION OF STRUCTURAL REMODELING AND GROWTH

Beginning in 1965, a new and quantitative method of analysis of the pulmonary vascular bed was developed by Elliot and Reid,[42] Davies and Reid,[43] and Hislop and Reid,[44] which was particularly applicable to the study of infants and young children, since it considered disturbances in the normal pattern of growth and structural remodeling. The method was worked out using the technique of arterial in-

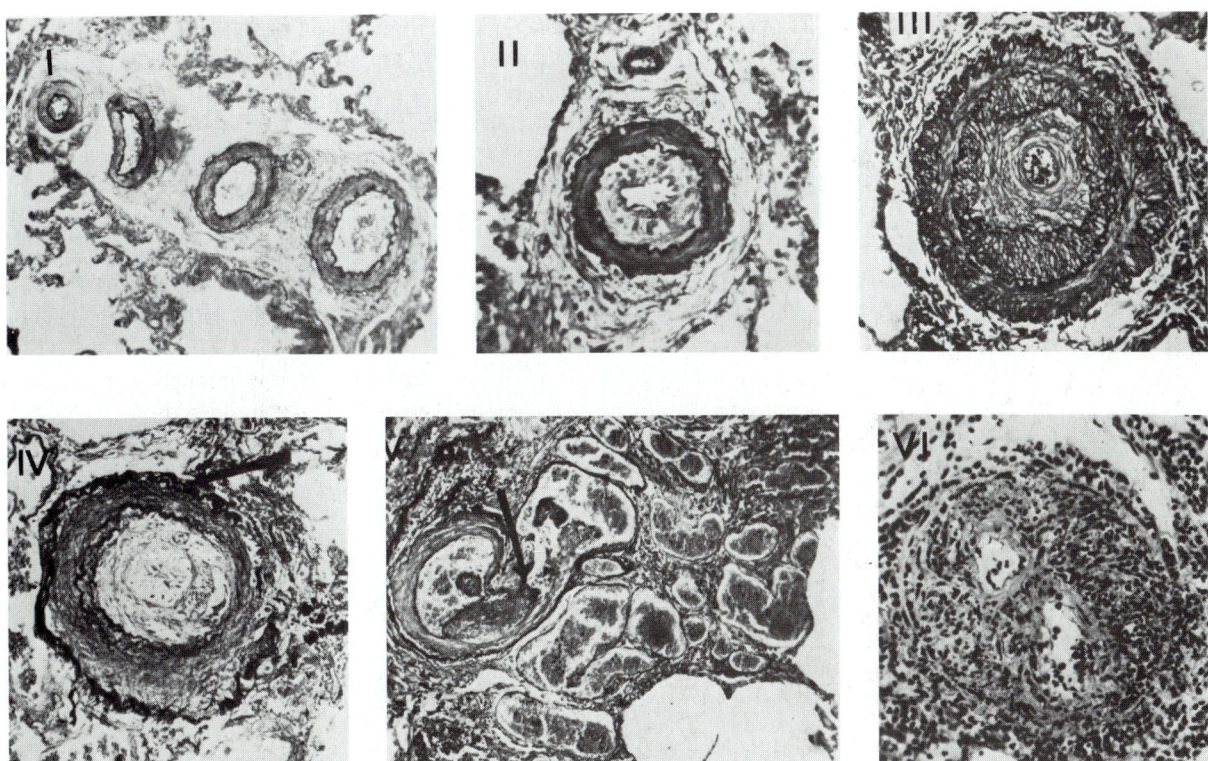

Figure 62–1. Heath–Edwards classification of pulmonary vascular changes. **I.** Grade I (medial hypertrophy): tortuous muscular pulmonary artery from a 2-year-old boy with truncus arteriosus and pulmonary hypertension. EVG ×94.5. **II.** Grade II: Cellular intimal proliferation in an abnormally muscular artery from the same patient. EVG, ×167. **III.** Grade III: occlusive changes: the media is thickened due to the development of fasciculi of longitudinal muscle both internal and external to the original media. The vessel is all but occluded by fibroelastic tissue (seen in a 41-year-old man with tetralogy of Fallot and a Blalock–Taussig anastomosis). EVG, ×94.5. **IV.** Grade IV: dilatation: the vessel is dilated, and the media is abnormally thin (*arrow*). The lumen is totally occluded by fibrous tissue (seen in a 26-year-old man with an aortopulmonary septal defect. EVG, ×94.5. **V.** Grade V: plexiform lesion: there is cellular intimal proliferation (*arrow*); clustered around this dilatation lesion are numerous thin-walled vessels of wide caliber that terminate as capillaries in the alveolar wall (seen in a 26-year-old woman with a patent ductus arteriosus). EVG, ×60. **VI.** Grade VI: acute necrotizing arteritis: a severe reactive acute inflammatory exudate is seen through all layers of the vessel (seen in a 26-year-old man with idiopathic pulmonary hypertension). HE, ×167. EVG, elastic Van Gieson stain; HE, hematoxylin–eosin stain. *(From Wagenvoort CA et al: The pathology of the pulmonary vasculature. Springfield, IL, 1964, Charles C Thomas, with permission.)*

jection of a postmortem lung specimen described by Short.[45] A radiopaque barium–gelatin mixture was injected at controlled constant temperature and the lung was subsequently inflated with formalin through the bronchial tree. By distending the arteries before fixation, measurement of their diameter and wall thickness was found to be consistent and precise.

It was observed from the postmortem arteriograms that, in the newborn, the vessels are prominent, whereas they are obscured in the adult by a dense background haze produced by the addition of many small intra-acinar arteries not present at birth (Fig. 62–2). On microscopic examination, three features of normal remodeling and growth of the pulmonary vascular bed were established. (1) With increasing age, muscle is observed in arteries located more peripherally within the acinus. At first, nonmuscular arteries become partially muscular and later they become fully muscularized. (2) At birth, the normally muscularized arter-

ies are very thick walled, but within a few days, the smallest muscular arteries ≤250 μm dilate and their walls thin to adult levels. By 4 mo of age, this process has included the largest elastic pulmonary arteries and is complete. (3) Arteries grow in both number and size and most rapidly in infancy. While alveoli also proliferate, the ratio of alveoli to arteries actually decreases from the newborn value of 20:1 to the value of 6–8:1 that is achieved first in early childhood and that persists (Fig. 62–3).

Morphometric analysis of the lungs from patients who had congenital heart defects revealed disturbed growth and remodeling of the pulmonary vascular bed (Table 62–1). On the postmortem arteriograms from infants with ventricular septal defect,[46] the axial arteries were dilated at the hilum but narrow peripherally. On microscopic examination of the pulmonary vascular bed, muscle extended precociously into normally nonmuscular peripheral intra-acinar arteries. In the normally muscular arteries, regression of the

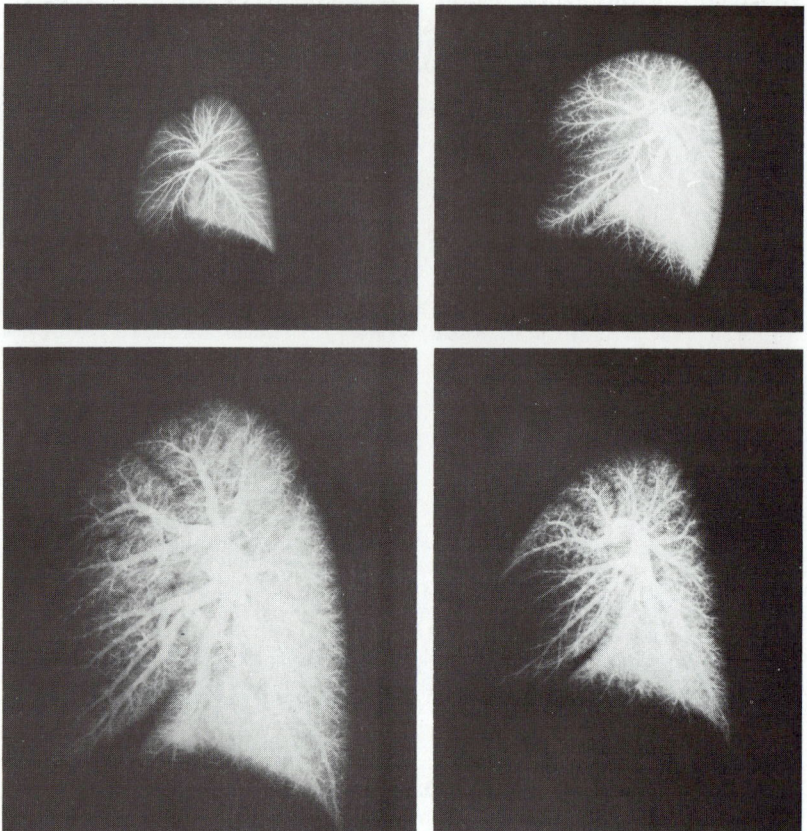

Figure 62–2. Arteriograms taken postmortem in a newborn (upper left), a 3-mo-old infant (upper right), a 1-year-old infant (lower right), and a 10-year-old child (lower left). The preacinar artery distribution is complete in the newborn, but with increasing age, the background becomes filled in by a dense haze due to the addition and growth of many small intra-acinar arteries.

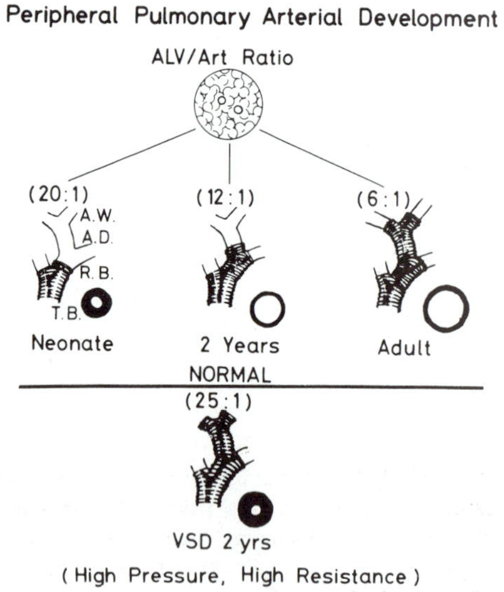

Peripheral Pulmonary Arterial Development

Figure 62–3. Schema showing morphometric changes: extension of muscle into peripheral arteries, percent wall thickness, and artery number (alveolar:arterial ratio) as they relate to age. **Upper panel.** Normal development. **Bottom panel.** Abnormalities in all three features in a 2-year-old child with a hypertensive ventricular septal defect. T.B., artery accompanying a terminal bronchiolus; R.B., artery accompanying a respiratory bronchiolus; A.D., artery accompanying an alveolar duct; A.W., artery accompanying an alveolar wall; ALV/Art, alveolar:arterial ratio. *(From Rabinovitch M et al: Circulation 58:1107, 1978, with permission.)*

perinatal musculature had not occurred and there was additional medial hypertrophy. In addition, the peripheral arteries had not grown normally in that they were small in size and few in number. Alveolar differentiation and multiplication, however, were normal. Since there were no regional variations in the lung, in the assessment of abnormal muscularity, or in the evaluation of arterial size or number,[47,48] application of the morphometric technique to analysis of lung biopsy tissue was feasible.

Lung Biopsy Studies

From lung biopsy studies, we were able to show that the severity of altered growth and development of the pulmonary vascular bed correlated with the hemodynamic state.[49] Three progressively severe stages were seen (Fig. 62–4). *Grade A:* There is either only abnormal extension of muscle into small peripheral arteries, or, in addition, a mild increase in wall thickness of the normally muscular arteries (less than 1.5 times normal). These patients have increased pulmonary blood flow but normal mean pulmonary arterial pressure. Meyrick and Reid[50] have shown from ultrastructural studies of lung biopsy tissue that the basis for this change is a differentiation to smooth muscle of the precursor cells, the pericyte in the nonmuscular region of the artery and the intermediate cell in the partially muscular region (Fig. 62–5). Since arteries become more muscular as

TABLE 62–1. STRUCTURAL FEATURES QUANTIFIED IN CONGENITAL HEART DEFECTS[a]

Congenital Heart Defect	Artery Size	Artery Number	Extension of Muscle	Medial Wall Thickness
Ventricular septal defect	↓	↓	↑	↑
Hypoplastic left heart	N	↑	↑	↑
Coarctation of the aorta	N	N	↑	↑
Total anomalous pulmonary venous connection	N	N	↑	↑
Tetralogy of Fallot	↓	N or ↑	N	↓ or ↑
Pulmonary atresia	↓	↓	N	↓

[a]↑, increased, above normal; ↓, decreased, below normal; N, normal.

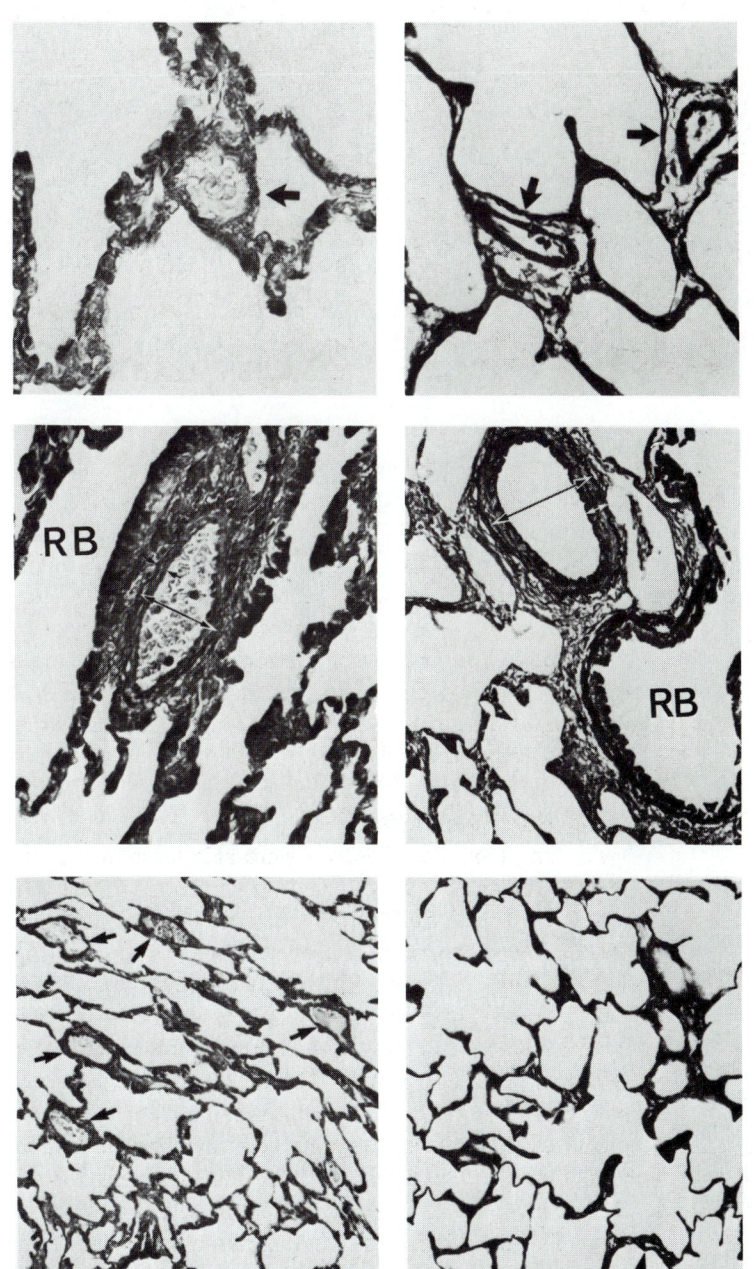

Figure 62–4. Morphometric features on lung biopsy tissue. **Left col.** A 2-year-old patient with ventricular septal defect and normal pulmonary arterial pressure. **Right col.** A 2-year-old with a defect of the atrioventricular canal, increased pressure and resistance. **Top.** Alveolar wall arteries (*arrows*) nonmuscularized on left and surrounded by a complete muscularized coat on right. ×175. **Middle.** Artery accompanying respiratory bronchiolus (RB) artery on left, with wall thickness only slightly increased, and on right, with wall thickness greatly increased. ×70. **Bottom.** An abundance of small arteries relative to alvioli (*arrows*) on left and only one small artery in a similar field on right. ×17.5. All from secions stained with elastic Van Gieson. *(From Rabinovitch M et al: Circulation 58:1107, 1978, with permission.)*

MUSCULAR   PARTIALLY   NON-MUSCULAR
                   MUSCULAR   & CAPILLARY

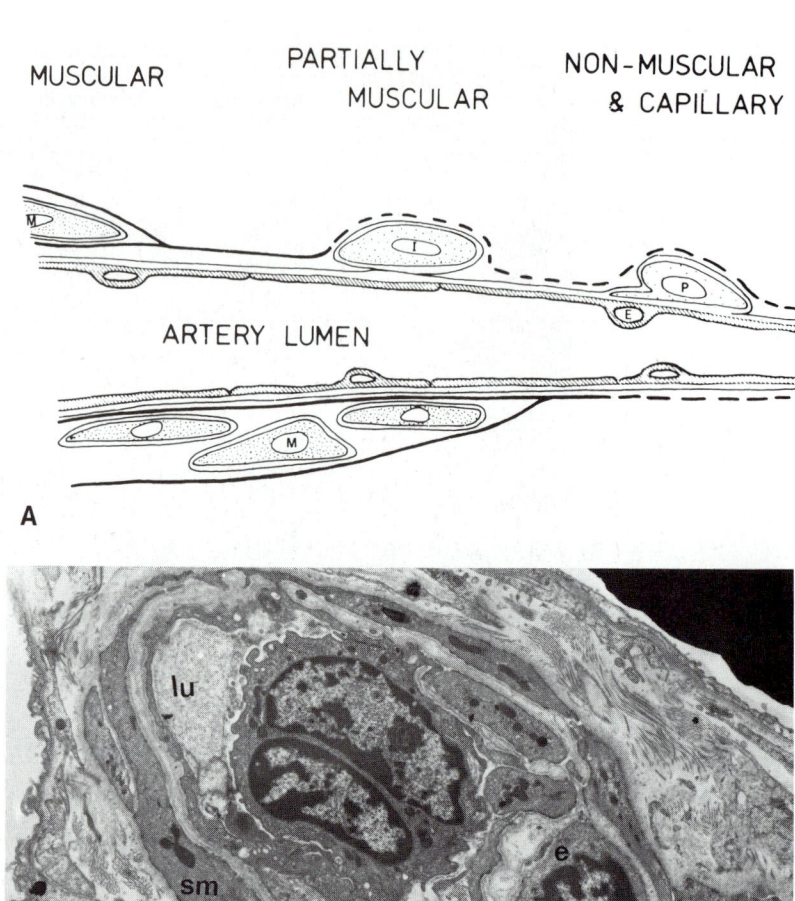

A

B

Figure 62–5. Diagrammatic representation of the cells in the wall of the distal part of a pulmonary artery. The smooth muscle cells (M) of the medial muscular coat are surrounded by a discrete basement membrane and situated between both an internal and external elastic lamina (*thick black lines*). In the nonmuscular region of the partially muscular artery, the intermediate cell (1) is seen. This cell is surrounded by a basement membrane that fuses in regions with that of the endothelial cell (E), and is situated internal to the single fragmented internal elastic lamina (*broken line*). In the wall of the nonmuscular artery and alveolar capillary, the pericyte (P) is found. This cell is ensheathed by a basement membrane that is continuous with and thereby shares that of the associated artery and like the intermediate cell, it is situated internal to the single elastic lamina. (*From Meyrick, Reid: Anat Rec 193:71, 1979.*) **B.** Electron micrograph of (a) an artery at the alveolar wall level with features suggesting abnormal extension. Plump endothelial cells (e) are surrounded by processes of smooth muscle cells (sm) containing myofilaments and dense bodies (db), lu, lumen. ×6070. (*From Meyrick B, Reid L: Am J Pathol 101:527, 1980, with permission.*)

they increase in size, it is tempting to speculate that, in the altered hemodynamic setting of chronic high flow and high pressure, "stretch" is the stimulus for smooth muscle cell differentiation from precursor cells. *Grade B:* As in grade A, there is increased extension of muscle, but, in addition, there is more severe medial hypertrophy of normally muscular arteries. When medial wall thickness is greater than 1.5 but less than 2 times normal (early grade B), mild pulmonary hypertension is usually present. When medial wall thickness is more than twice normal (late grade B), pulmonary hypertension is always present and often with pressure values greater than half systemic level. The medial thickness is due to hypertrophy rather than hyperplasia of preexisting smooth muscle cells and also an increase in the intracellular ground substance.[50] The mechanism causing medial hypertrophy is not known, but our recent ultrastructural studies have given us some clues.[51] It appears that with the development of pulmonary hypertension, there is

breakdown of the internal elastic lamina (Fig. 62–6) implicating an elastolytic process, the sequelae of which related to release of growth factors[52,53] will be discussed. *Grade C:* In addition to the findings of late grade B, arterial concentration is reduced and usually arterial size is also reduced. Patients with these changes have elevation in pulmonary vascular resistance of greater than 3.5 μm·m^2. When arterial number is less than half normal, pulmonary vascular resistance values are often in excess of 6 μm·m^2. The basis for grade C is likely the failure of new vessels to grow normally, although some loss of arteries may also occur.

Whether, and to what extent, abnormal growth and structural remodeling of the pulmonary vascular bed are permanent and result in functional impairment can best be determined by correlating these features with postoperative hemodynamic studies.[54,55] We correlated both the quantitative features and the qualitative changes described by Heath and Edwards with the hemodynamic behavior of the pul-

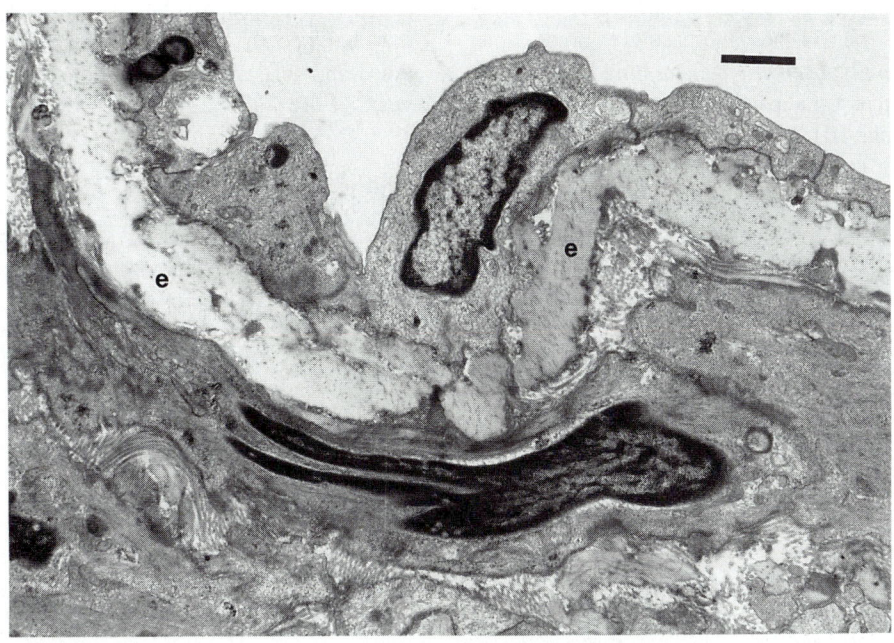

A

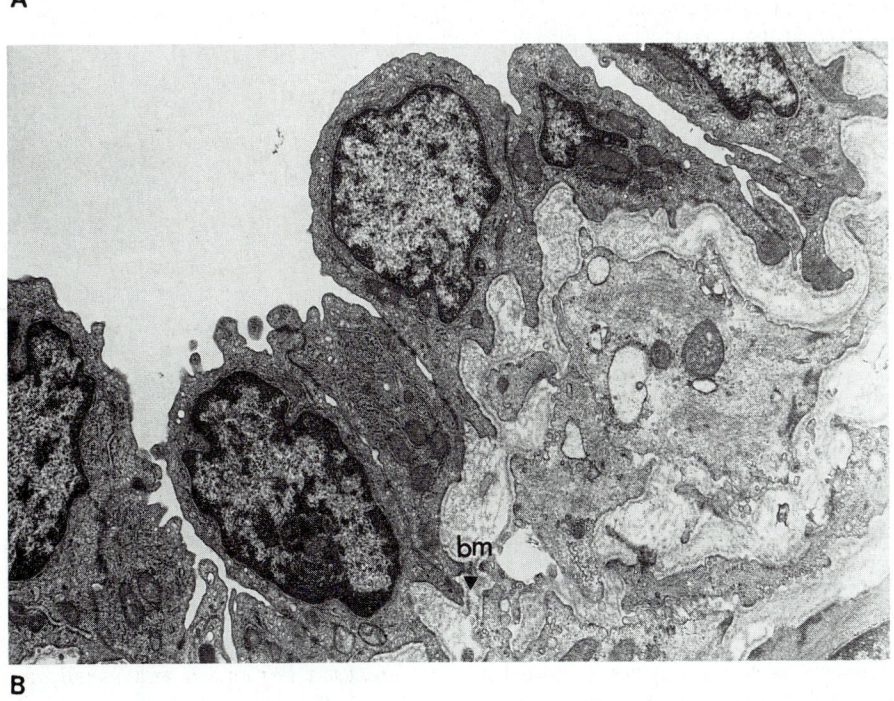

B

Figure 62–6. A. A section of a pulmonary artery 92 μm in diameter in a patient with normal pulmonary artery pressure shows an intact internal elastic lamina(e). **B.** In a section from a pulmonary artery 108 μm in diameter in a patient with increased pulmonary blood flow and pressure microfibrillar material is present in the subendothelial but no true internal elastic lamina. The endothelial and smooth muscle cells are separated by only a thick basement membrane(bm). Bar = 1 μm in both. *(From Rabinovitch M, et al: Lab Invest 55:632, 1986, with permission.)*

monary circulation observed in the Intensive Care Unit, 1 day after repair and at the time of routine cardiac catheter study, 1 year later.[55] Patients with grade A or mild grade B changes have normal pulmonary artery pressures in the early postoperative period or only a minimal degree of elevation. The majority of patients with more severe medial

hypertrophy, i.e., severe grade B and Heath–Edwards I, have elevated values. The pulmonary hypertension observed is frequently labile and almost always can be controlled. The nature of this increased pulmonary vascular reactivity resulting in "pulmonary hypertensive crises" and its therapeutic management will be addressed. Both the presence and the severity of pulmonary hypertension in the early postoperative period are increasingly predictable when there are more advanced changes on lung biopsy, i.e., reduced artery number (grade C) and intimal hyperplasia (Heath–Edwards II and III) (Fig. 62–7A).

One year after repair, however, patients operated within the first 8 mo of life tend to have normal pulmonary hemodynamics regardless of their age at repair. Patients surgically corrected between 9 mo and 2 years of life with

grade C and Heath–Edwards II and III structural changes may have persistent elevation in pulmonary vascular resistance and this appears inevitable in those operated after 2 years of life (Fig. 62–7B).

Analysis of the Frozen Section

Quantitative techniques have been successfully applied to the analysis of lung biopsy tissue prepared by frozen sec-

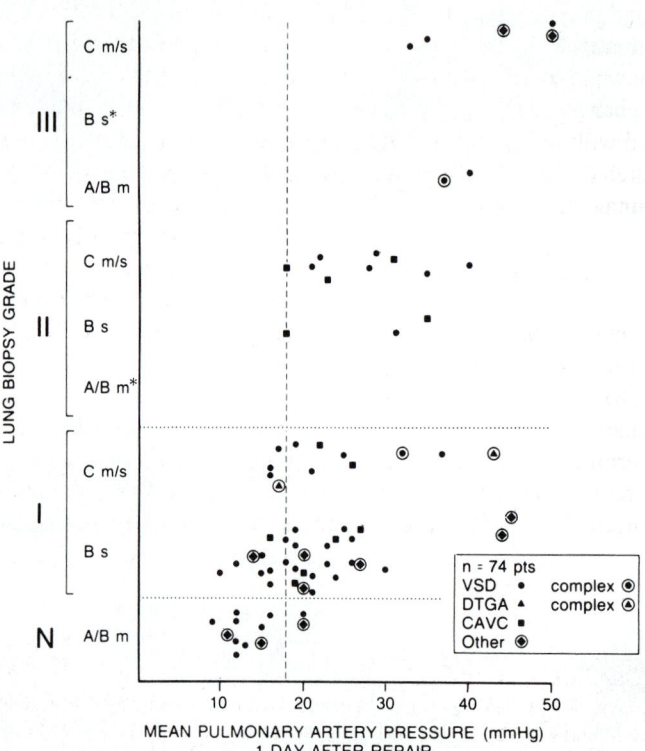

Figure 62–7. **A.** Lung biopsy grade is correlated with mean pulmonary arterial pressure recorded the day after surgical repair. The *dashed vertical lines* separate the normal from the abnormally elevated pressure values and the *dotted horizontal lines* separate the biopsy grades. Note that with the more severe Heath–Edwards changes on lung biopsy tissue there is a trend toward a greater proportion of patients with elevated pulmonary arterial pressures and higher values. A, B, C, morphometric grades; m, mild; s, severe. N, I, II, III, Heath–Edwards grades; N, normal; *, no patients in this group; VSD, ventricular septal defect; DTGA, *d*-transposition of the great arteries; CAVC, complete atrioventricular canal; complex, associated abnormality. **B.** Graph correlating lung biopsy grade with pulmonary vascular resistance 1 year after cardiac repair. Patients who underwent repair within the first 8 mo of life, but not those operated upon later had normal pulmonary vascular resistance regardless of the severity of their structural changes. *(From Rabinovitch M, et al: Vascular structure in lung biopsy tissue correlated with pulmonary hemodynamic findings after repair of congenital heart defects. Circulation 69:655–667, 1984, with permission.)*

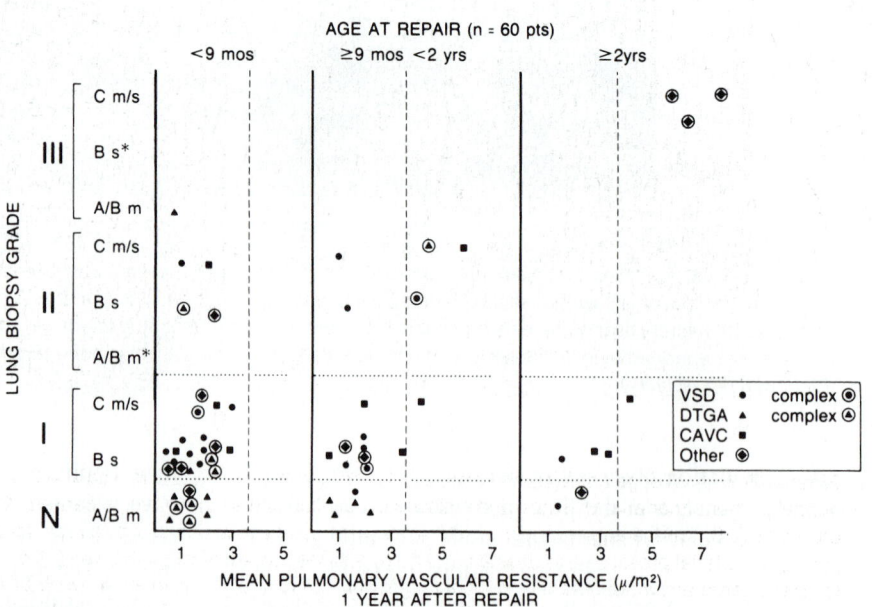

tion to help the surgeon decide between a palliative and a corrective procedure when preoperative hemodynamic data are borderline or difficult to obtain or interpret.[56] The ability to predict from biopsy tissue whether even mild elevation in pulmonary vascular resistance will be present postoperatively is of increasing importance in the consideration for surgery of patients who require a Fontan-type procedure, i.e., the placement of a right atrial-to-pulmonary arterial conduit.[57] Patients with tricuspid atresia who have had previous systemic-to-pulmonary arterial shunts and those with single ventricle and previous pulmonary arterial bands are particularly problematic.[58,59]

Studies have shown that after a Fontan procedure, even minor vascular changes on lung biopsy tissue (mild grade B) are associated with increased morbidity, including prolonged hospitalization due to the need for increased ventilator support and drainage from chest tubes.[59]

Wedge Angiography

Techniques of wedge angiography have been developed to assess preoperatively the structural state of the pulmonary vascular bed (Fig. 62–8).[60] Changes that can be evaluated quantitatively, i.e., sparsity of arborization of the pulmonary tree, abrupt termination, tortuosity and narrowing of small arteries, and reduced background capillary filling, generally reflect advanced changes in the preacinar arteries

of at least Heath–Edwards III severity. We described a technique that allows quantitative assessment of abnormalities in a pulmonary wedge angiogram.[61] A balloon catheter is directed to the origin of the axial artery of the posterior basal segment of the lower lobe (the right lung is usually chosen). Contrast material is injected and the injection is filmed on biplane cine. We evaluate the rate of tapering of the arteries by measuring the length of segment over which the lumen diameter narrows between 2.5 and 1.5 mm. The abruptness of tapering correlates in severity with the degree of abnormality in the intra-acinar arteries, assessed both morphometrically and by the Heath–Edwards classification (Table 62–2). However, there are several pitfalls and limitations in the interpretation of the pulmonary wedge angiogram. Pulmonary stenosis or previous placement of a pulmonary artery band will, because of poststenotic dilatation, give the impression of rapid tapering. With very advanced vascular disease, there is sometimes such extensive intimal hyperplasia that the vessel appears narrowed all the way from the hilum and so, abrupt tapering is no longer apparent. In that situation, however, the background haze is absent and the pulmonary circulation time is usually prolonged. Technical abnormalities can also result in difficulties in interpretation. If the injection of contrast fails to fill the vessels all the way out to the pleura, the background will appear dark and, if the balloon does not completely occlude the vessel, the false impression of a dense background

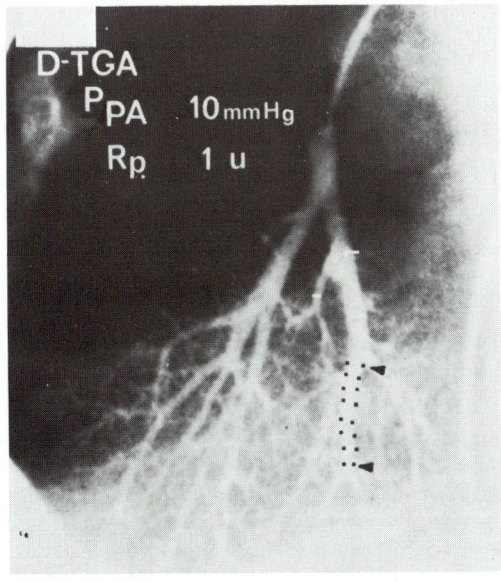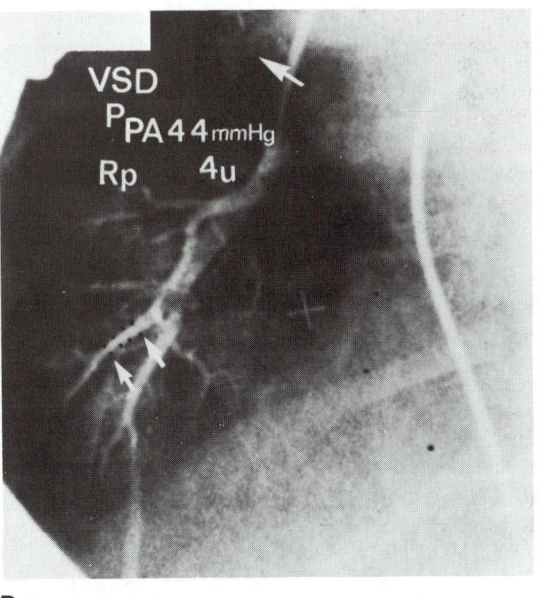

A **B**

Figure 62–8. A. Wedge angiogram shows slow tapering of the axial artery in a child with *d*-transposition of the great arteries and normal pulmonary arterial pressure and resistance. Approximate segment length between 2.5 and 1.5 mm internal diameter is marked off (*arrows*). **B.** Wedge angiogram in a child with a ventricular septal defect shows rapid tapering of the artery when there is increased pulmonary arterial pressure and resistance. An approximate segment length betwen 2.5 and 1.5 mm internal diameter is marked off (*arrows*). Large arrow denotes take-off to the right pulmonary artery. *(From Rabinovitch M, Reid L: Quantitative structural analysis of the pulmonary vascular bed. In Engle MA (ed): Pediatric Cardiovascular Disease. Philadelphia, FA Davis, 1981, 11/2:149, Cardiovascular Clinics, with permission.)*

TABLE 62–2. PATHOLOGIC, HEMODYNAMIC, RADIOGRAPHIC CORRELATION IN THE DEVELOPMENT OF PULMONARY VASCULAR DISEASE[a]

Grade	Pathology	Physiology			Wedge Angiogram
		$\dot{Q}p$	$\overline{P}pa$	Rp	
A	Abnormal extension of muscle	↑	N	N	Slow tapering of axial
	into small arteries	↑	N	N	arteries
	± mile medial hypertrophy				
B	A + severe medial hypertrophy	↑	↑	N	
C	B + ↓ arterial number and size	±↑	↑	↑	Abrupt tapering

[a]↑, increased, above normal; ↓, decreased, below normal; N, normal; $\overline{P}pa$, mean pulmonary arterial pressure; Qp pulmonary blood flow; Rp, pulmonary vascular resistance.

will be created owing to filling of capillaries and veins. The circulation time assessment depends on the exclusion of pulmonary vein stenosis and intrapulmonary shunting.

Control of the Reactive Pulmonary Circulation

A major challenge in pediatric cardiology has been to understand and control the mechanisms causing "pulmonary hypertensive crises" following intracardiac repair of congenital heart defects and left-to-right shunts and preoperative pulmonary hypertension. The mechanism causing heightened pulmonary vascular reactivity may reflect a decreased ratio of prostacyclin to thromboxane following cardiopulmonary bypass.[62] In addition, the production of platelet activating factor may play a role, although this has been difficult to confirm in clinical studies.[63] There is also controversy with regard to whether increased endothelin[64–66] release causes heightened pulmonary vasoreactivity or is involved in the pathophysiology of the structural changes, since endothelin is mitogenic for smooth muscle cells.[67]

Important clinical studies have shown that impaired endothelial function is the most likely cause of heightened pulmonary vascular reactivity following repair of a congenital heart defect.[68–70] On the preoperative heart catheter study in patients with congenital heart defects and left-to-right shunt lesions causing pulmonary hypertension, decreased responsivity to acetylcholine had been demonstrated. After intracardiac repair involving cardiopulmonary bypass, there is a greater decline or even an absence of acetylcholine responsivity, suggesting further impairment in endothelial-dependent relaxation.[70]

On the basis of these studies, postoperative pulmonary hypertensive crises have been successfully treated by administration of inhaled nitric oxide (Fig. 62–9). The efficacy of this therapy is currently being weighed against previous regimens that have included prolonged anesthesia with fentanyl,[71] infusion of prostacyclin,[72] or our own protocol that has involved hyperventilation followed by α-adrenoreceptor blockade with phenoxybenzamine (unpublished). The studies carried out thus far seem promising.[73]

There are, however, a few patients who maintain a high level of pulmonary vascular resistance and are refractory to vasodilator therapy despite what appears to be mild vascular changes on light microscopy (medial hypertrophy) and others who develop rapidly progressive pulmonary vascular disease despite early diagnosis and timely intervention.

Treatment of Fixed Pulmonary Hypertension

Prolonged home oxygen therapy has been shown to improve survival and symptoms in patients with Eisenmenger's syndrome,[74] and there may be a role for chronic

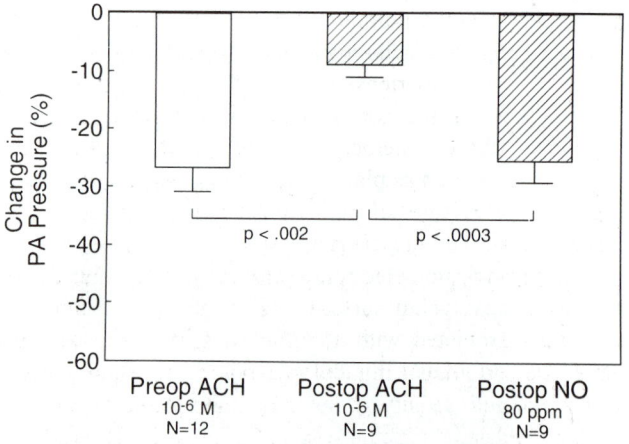

Figure 62–9. Among young children with elevated pulmonary vascular resistance associated with congenital heart disease, the endothelium-dependent vasodilator, acetycholine (ACH), elicits marked pulmonary artery (PA) vasodilation in preoperative (Preop) patients. This effect is attenuated during the immediate postoperative (Postop) period following surgical repair on cardiopulmonary bypass. However, these same postoperative patients fare fully responsive to the vasodilating effect of inhaled nitric oxide (NO) at a dose of 80 ppm. This suggests that the pulmonary vascular endothelium suffers from a transient ischemic injury during the immediate postoperative period. *(From Wessel DL, Adatia I, Giglia TM, et al: Use of inhaled nitric oxide and acetylcholine in the evaluation of pulmonary hypertension and endothelial function after cardiopulmonary bypass. Reproduced by permission. Circulation. 88:2128–2138. Copyright 1993 American Heart Association.)*

prostacyclin therapy[75] or other vasodilator agents, such as diltiazem,[76] although these measures may best serve to prolong life in anticipation of heart–lung transplantation. The use of antiplatelet aggregating agents or anticoagulants may be of value in the polycythemic patient and controlled trials need to be initiated, particularly since these patients are at risk for hemoptysis.[77] Single or double lung transplantation[78–82] may provide a more satisfactory alternative than heart–lung transplantation. This subject is extensively covered in Chapters 29, 92, and 114.

Clinical Studies Related to Mechanism of Pulmonary Vascular Changes

In lung biopsy studies from patients with congenital heart defects and pulmonary hypertension, we investigated altered endothelial–platelet, leukocyte, and endothelial–smooth muscle interactions that may be relevant to the mechanism of heightened pulmonary vascular reactivity and to the development of progressive pulmonary vascular disease.[51,63,83] Using scanning and transmission electron microscopy, we have identified structural changes in pulmonary vascular endothelial cells that suggest altered function and the potential for abnormal interaction with circulating blood elements, platelets, and leukocytes.[48] On scanning electron microscopy, the endothelial surface of normal thin-walled pulmonary arteries has a "corduroy-like" appearance in that the cells form narrow, even ridges (Fig. 62–10A). In contrast, the endothelial surface of hypertensive thick-walled pulmonary arteries has a "cable-like" texture in that the cells form deep twisted ridges (Fig. 62–10B). The hypertensive endothelium is, therefore, coarse relative to the normotensive endothelium and may be predisposed to interact abnormally with marginating blood elements such as platelets and leukocytes. This might result in the release of pulmonary vasoconstrictor substances and smooth muscle mitogens.

On transmission electron microscopy, it is evident that the altered endothelial surface of hypertensive pulmonary arteries is associated with abnormalities in the concentration of the endothelial intracytoplasmic components. There is an increased density of microfilament bundles and of rough endoplasmic reticulum (Fig. 62–11A, B). The former suggests an altered cytoskeleton that may serve to keep the endothelium wall anchored to the subendothelium, whereas the latter indicates increased protein synthesis and metabolic activity. Further observations on transmission electron microscopy suggested a potentially important underlying pathophysiologic mechanism that has been further addressed in experimental studies described below. We observed that the elastic lamina, which ordinarily separates the endothelial from the underlying smooth muscle cells, appeared fragmented. This suggested that an enzyme, having as one of its proteolytic properties the ability to degrade elastin, may be stimulating and perpetuating the disease process. We proposed that elastolysis might result in the re-

lease of growth factors from the matrix, as has been shown with other serine proteinases.[52] Another possibility is that peptides derived from elastin or other connective tissues susceptible to the proteolytic effects of this elastase enzyme might stimulate the neosynthesis of the connective tissue.[83]

Immunohistochemistry studies of the lungs of patients with advanced vascular disease awaiting lung transplantation (mostly with primary pulmonary hypertension but also including patients with congenital heart lesions) have provided insights into mechanisms of vascular disease. There is increased expression of the growth factor, transforming growth factor-β.[84] Transforming growth factor-β may be a smooth muscle cell mitogen under certain circumstances but is known to increase synthesis of a variety of connective tissue proteins, including elastin and collagen.[85] Moreover, even in advanced lesions, there is evidence by in situ hybridization, in addition to immunohistochemistry, of ongoing synthesis of elastin, collagen, and fibronectin.[86] It was also shown by immunohistochemistry, using an antibody that recognizes procollagen,[87] that intimal proliferation is associated with increased collagen synthesis (Fig. 62–12). The increase in fibronectin may be related to the influence of fibronectin in promoting smooth muscle cell migration.[88] Our most recent studies, however, suggest that fibronectin might also be important in the transendothelial migration and trafficking of inflammatory cells through interactions between certain peptide sequences in the fibronectin molecule and specific integrin receptors of the inflammatory cell surfaces.[89] Macrophages have been identified in advanced pulmonary vascular lesions.[90]

Other studies suggested what the products of increased endothelial metabolism might be. We hypothesized that since endothelial cells produce Factor VIII (von Willebrand), an increase in this protein may cause platelet adhesion and formation of microthrombi and this may also result in a release of pulmonary vasoconstrictor substances and smooth muscle mitogens.[51] Using an immunoperoxidase stain for Factor VIII, we observed that hypertensive pulmonary arteries stain densely, whereas nonhypertensive vessels do not (Fig. 62–13). Additional studies carried out in our laboratory[63] have shown that, in the early postoperative period, there is an increased synthesis of biologically active Factor VIII and this may induce platelet aggregation and release of vasoconstrictor substances, important in heightened pulmonary vascular reactivity (Fig. 62–14).

Experimental Studies

Experimental studies in animals have also shown that the effects of high flow and high pressure on the pulmonary vascular bed correlates with histologic changes. High pulmonary flow alone via pneumonectomy,[91] or pulmonary artery banding[92,93] or ligation results in minimal if any elevation in pulmonary artery pressure and structural changes in the vessels. Slight elevation in pulmonary artery pressure is accompanied by extension of muscle into peripheral ar-

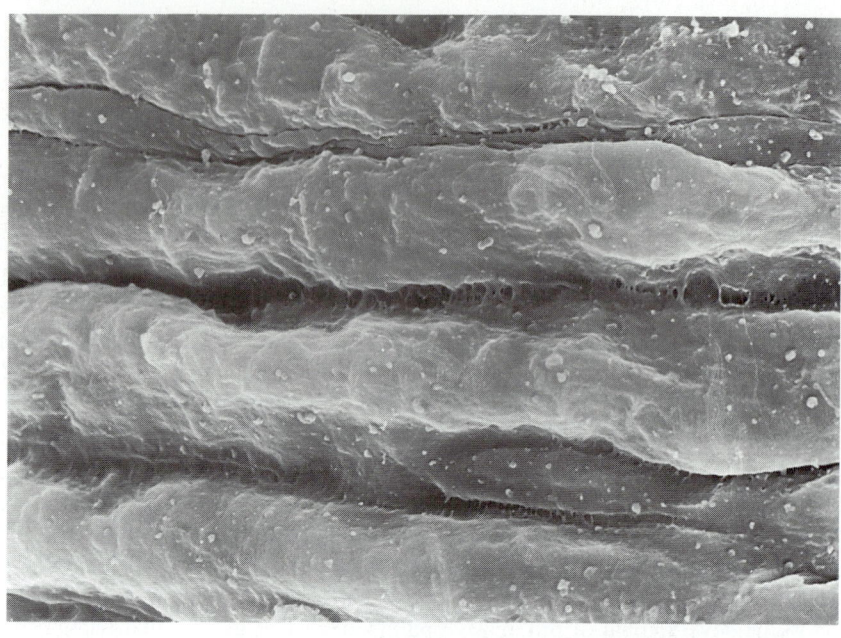

A

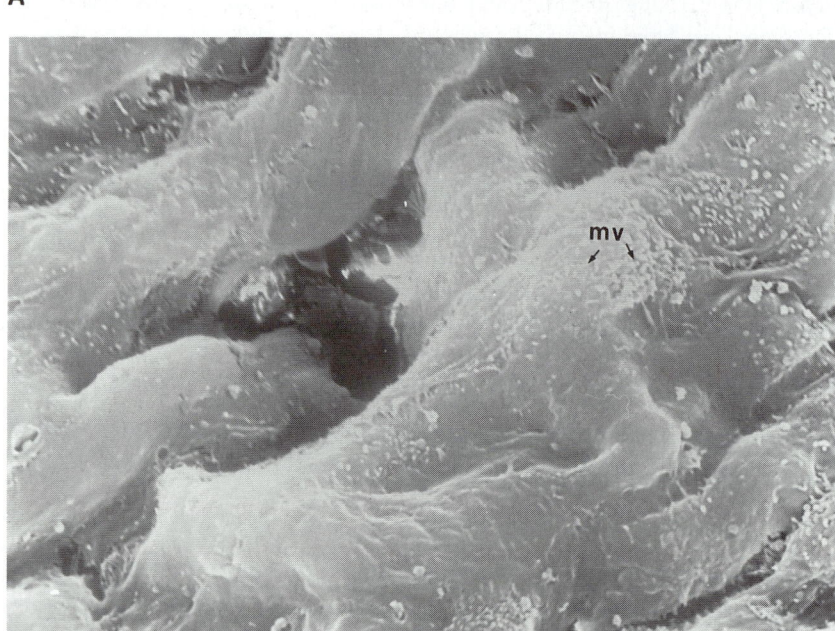

B

Figure 62–10. Scanning electron photomicrographs of pulmonary artery endothelial surfaces. **A.** Normal pulmonary artery shows "corduroy" pattern, neat closely aligned ridges. **B.** Hypertensive pulmonary artery shown "cable" pattern, deep knotted ridges, and numerous microvilli (mv). Magnification ×810. *(From Rabinovitch M, et al: Lab Invest 55:632, 1986, with permission.)*

teries, whereas larger shunts are associated with a progressive increase in pulmonary artery pressure and the extension of muscle into peripheral arteries, medial hypertrophy of muscular arteries, and reduced arterial number.[94] Takedown of the shunts during the period of rapid lung growth results in regression of the structural changes and pulmonary hypertension,[95] whereas persistence of a large aortopulmonary shunt results in rapidly progressive pulmonary vascular changes.[96] Increased elastin synthesis in the large central and hilar pulmonary arteries has been described in animal models of high pulmonary blood flow.[97] Stress–strain relationships in the isolated vessels, however, suggest

little elastin and morphometric analysis of ultrastructure reveals a decreased proportion of mature amorphous elastin and an altered distribution as islands rather than as laminae.[97] These changes in the large arteries precede evidence of abnormal muscularization of the peripheral vessels, suggesting that the increased distensibility of the central and hilar vessels may "absorb" some of the hemodynamic effect of the high flow and pressure.

Cell culture studies have further identified mechanisms whereby high flow might lead to vascular remodeling. For example, application of shear stress to cultured endothelial cells have shown release of prostacyclin[98] and

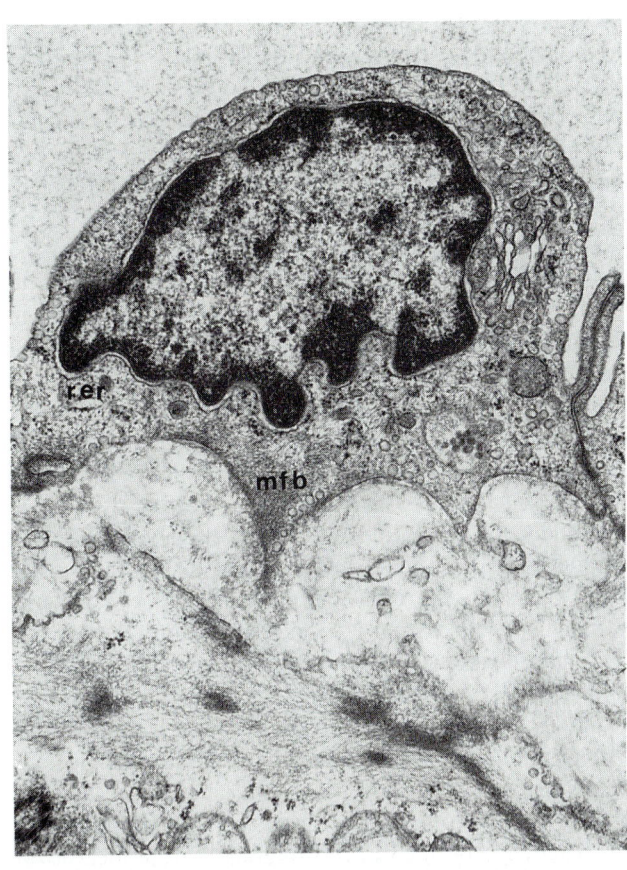
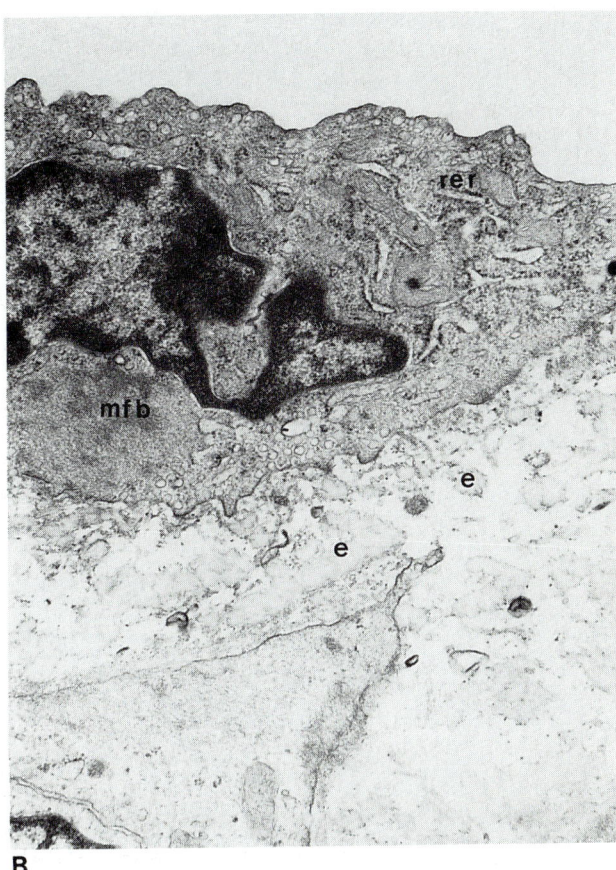

A

B

Figure 62–11. Transmission electron photomicrographs: **A.** An endothelial cell from a preacinar PA 320 μm in external diameter (group 1, no 4, 7 years of age); **B,** an endothelial cell from a preacinar PA 240 μm in external diameter (group 3, no 1, 8 mo of age). Observe the increased rough endoplasmic reticulum (rer) and microfilament bundles (mfb) in the latter patient, and the fragments of elastin (e) and microfibrillar material in the subendothelium; m, mitochondria; r, ribosomes. Bar = 1 μm in both. *(From Rabinovitch M, et al: Lab Invest 55:632, 1986, with permission.)*

endothelin.[99,100] Prostacyclin can inhibit smooth muscle cell proliferation, whereas endothelin is a mitogen. Expression of protooncogenes *(fos, jun,* and *myc)* is also stimulated by shear stress[101] and these early response genes direct induction of vascular smooth muscle cell migration and proliferation by growth factors.[102–104] Recently, progress has been made in identifying the sequence in the promoter–enhancer region of the platelet-derived growth factor gene PDGF[105] that is responsible for the induction of its transcription and subsequent protein expression. These are important studies as they will ultimately allow us to target genes specifically through only those elements that are abnormally "switched on." In some experimental models, such as the carotid balloon injury in rats, the use of antisense to protooncogenes c-*myb,*[106] antibodies to basic fibroblast growth factor,[107] or enzymes involved in proliferation such as cdc 2 kinase[108] have proven highly effective in preventing the subsequent smooth muscle cell proliferation and intimal lesions (Fig. 62–15). A variety of gene transfer technologies pioneered by the work of Nabel et al are proving efficacious in targeting mechanisms of induction of

smooth muscle cell migration and proliferation.[109] A novel mechanism related to p53 glycoprotein inhibition by a protein induced by the cytomegalovirus has also been suggested as a target to inhibit vascular smooth muscle cell proliferation.[110]

Intimal proliferation in pulmonary vascular pathobiology likely shares mechanistic features common to systemic arterial pathology. With this in mind, we used the ductus arteriosus as an experimental model to uncover important endothelial–smooth muscle cell–matrix interactions important in directing smooth muscle migration into the subendothelium.[111–116] The ductus develops intimal cushions in late gestation that ensures that it will close in the postnatal period following vasoconstriction with oxygenation. We have discovered that endothelial cells under the influence of transforming growth factor (TGF)-β produce and incorporate large amounts of hyaluronan and that the smooth muscle cells produced increased fibronectin by a non-TGF-β-mediated mechanism. The increased fibronectin is responsible for their switch from a contractile to a motile phenotype. The elongated appearance that they assume is

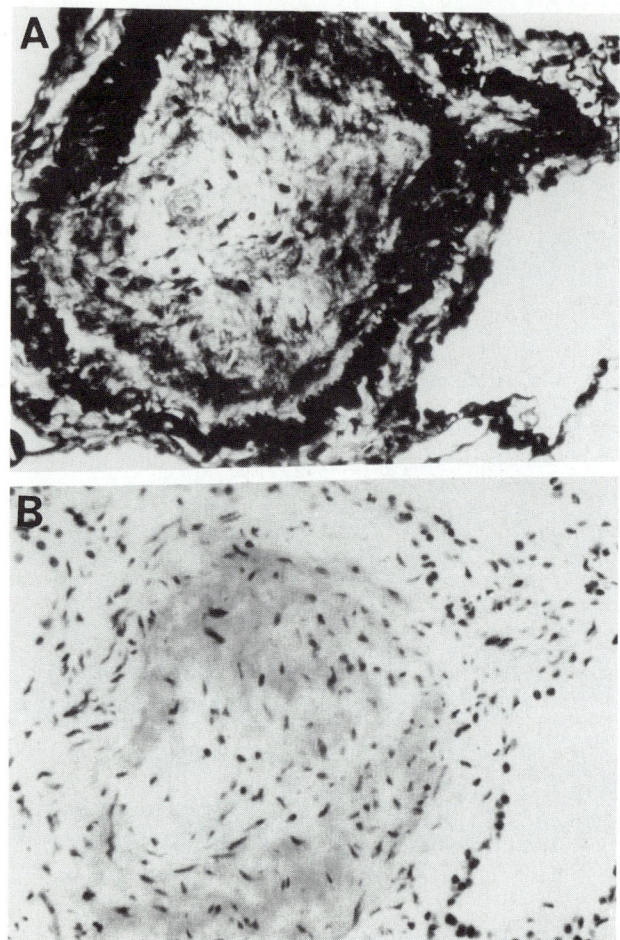

Figure 62–12. Immunohistochemistry was performed on formalin-fixed, paraffin-embedded parenchyma obtained from patients with severe primary pulmonary hypertension at the time of single-lung transplantation. Tissue sections were then stained with antibodies to the amino-terminal end of the procollagen type I propeptide (**B**). This antibody identifies newly synthesized αI(I) procollagen prior to cleavage of the amino-terminal propeptide following secretion and, therefore, can identify sites of active collagen deposition. An elastin-van Gieson stain demonstrates vascular structures (**A**). Procollagen immunoreactivity (**B**) is present only within the neointima of this occluded artery. Magnification ×100. *(From Botney M, et al: Active collagen synthesis by pulmonary arteries in human primary pulmonary hypertension. Am J Pathol 143:121–129, 1993, with permission.)*

associated with increased expression of receptors for hyaluronan, thereby directing their upward mobility (Fig. 62–16). At the same time, it appears that there is defective assembly of elastin that facilitates this process. It is of interest that neointimal formation in both experimental pulmonary hypertension[117–121] and in coronary artery disease[122] is associated with increased elastolytic activity. Using molecular techniques, we have shown that the elastase associated with pulmonary hypertension is related to the serine proteinase adipsin and is isolated on elastin substrate gel electrophoresis as a 20-kDa protein.[121] An anti-

body produced in our laboratory localized elastase largely to the smooth muscle cells of the arterial wall. A cause-and-effect relationship between increased elastase activity and pulmonary hypertension was demonstrated in experimental rat models of pulmonary hypertension in which elastase inhibitors were successfully used to prevent or retard the progression of both vascular and hemodynamic changes[118–120] (Fig. 62–17). We have evidence from in vitro studies that pulmonary artery smooth muscle elastase activity is induced by serum and endothelial factors that may gain increased access to the subendothelium when there is endothelial injury and loss of accompanying barrier function.[123] There appears to be an intracellular signaling mechanism related to binding of the serum factor to elastin and to the cell surface and subsequent induction of tyrosine kinase. Unpublished studies in our laboratory have shown that induction of pulmonary artery elastase releases the smooth muscle cell mitogen basic fibroblast growth factor from its bound state in the extracellular matrix to an active form. Elastase activity via release of elastin peptides may also induce fibronectin production. Figure 62–18 suggests hypothetically how induction of elastase might be important pathophysiologically if this leads to release of growth factors from the matrix and induction of fibronectin-mediated smooth muscle cell migration.

It is interesting that similar mechanisms of fibronectin-mediated smooth muscle cell migration are critical to the process of neointimal formation experimentally induced in coronary arteries of piglets following transplantation.[127] The induction of fibronectin appears to be mediated by a cytokine loop involving reciprocal coinduction of interleukin-1β and tumor necrosis factor-α.[128] In fact, we have recently shown that fibronectin plays a dual role in mediating rapidly progressive neointimal formation, first, in all likelihood, by inducing smooth muscle cell migration and also by inducing the transendothelial migration of T cells. We have shown that administration of the CS-1 peptide, which mimics the site on fibronectin that binds to the α4β1 integrin on T cells, will reduce by greater than 50% the incidence and severity of coronary artery intimal lesions following transplantation.[129]

DEFECTS THAT INCREASE PULMONARY VENOUS PRESSURE

Hemodynamic Studies

Congenital heart defects, such as mitral stenosis, cor triatriatum, or obstructed total anomalous pulmonary venous connection, have in common increased pulmonary vascular resistance secondary to elevated pulmonary venous pressure. Following surgical repair and relief of the pulmonary venous hypertension, pulmonary vascular resistance generally falls to normally values, but persistent elevation may occur in a small proportion of patients in whom these de-

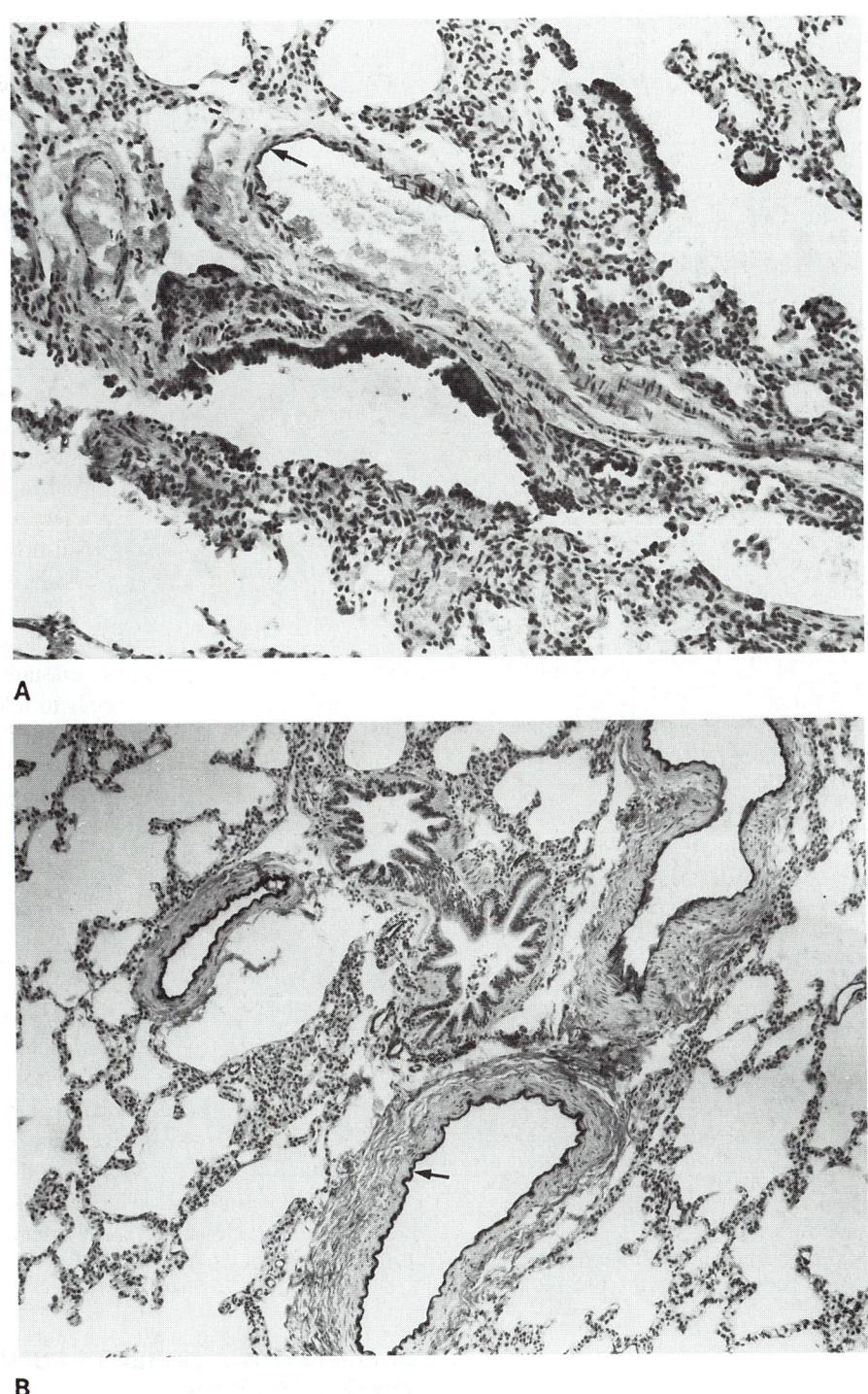

A

B

Figure 62–13. Lung biopsy section from a patient with normal pulmonary artery pressure (**A**) and with pulmonary hypertension (**B**). Note thin-walled pulmonary artery (**A**) with light rim of endothelial immunoperoxidase stain for Factor VII and thick walled pulmonary artery (**B**) with deeply positive endothelial stain (*arrows*). Magnification ×160.

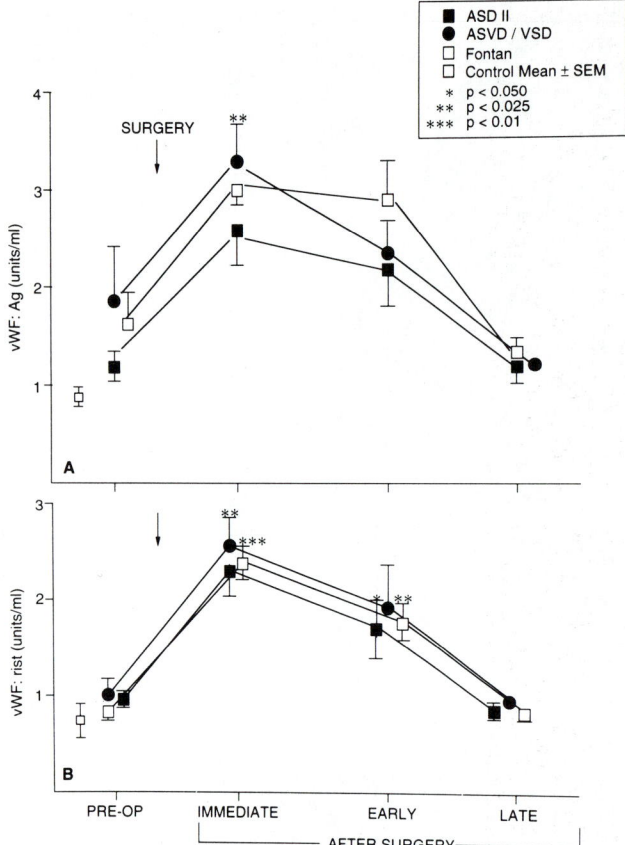

Figure 62–14. Changes in von Willebrand factor antigenic activity (vWF:Ag) (**A**) and von Willebrand factor biologic activity (vWF:rist) (**B**) after CPB in three CHD groups. Before operation there are no significant differences between the vWF:Ag and vWF:rist levels compared with the control group. After operation there is a marked increase in vWF:Ag ($p<0.025$, all groups) an in vWF:rist values [$p<0.025$ (ASD II, AVSD/VSD) and $p<0.01$ (Fontan)]. All values return to normal in the late postoperative period. Preoperative values are compared with control and postoperative values to the preceding time point. SEM, standard error of the mean. *(From Turner-Gomes SO, et al: J Thorac Cardiovasc Surg 103:87–97, 1992, with permission.)*

fects have been successfully corrected.[130–132] The latter group consists mostly of patients who had surgical repair after early infancy.

Morphologic Assessment of the Pulmonary Vascular Bed

Qualitative Studies

Collins-Nakai et al[130] reported greater than Heath–Edwards III changes in the majority of patients in their series with mitral stenosis. In patients with total anomalous pulmonary venous connection, abnormal muscularization of the small arteries and veins has been observed from birth and more severe structural changes of at least Heath–Edwards III

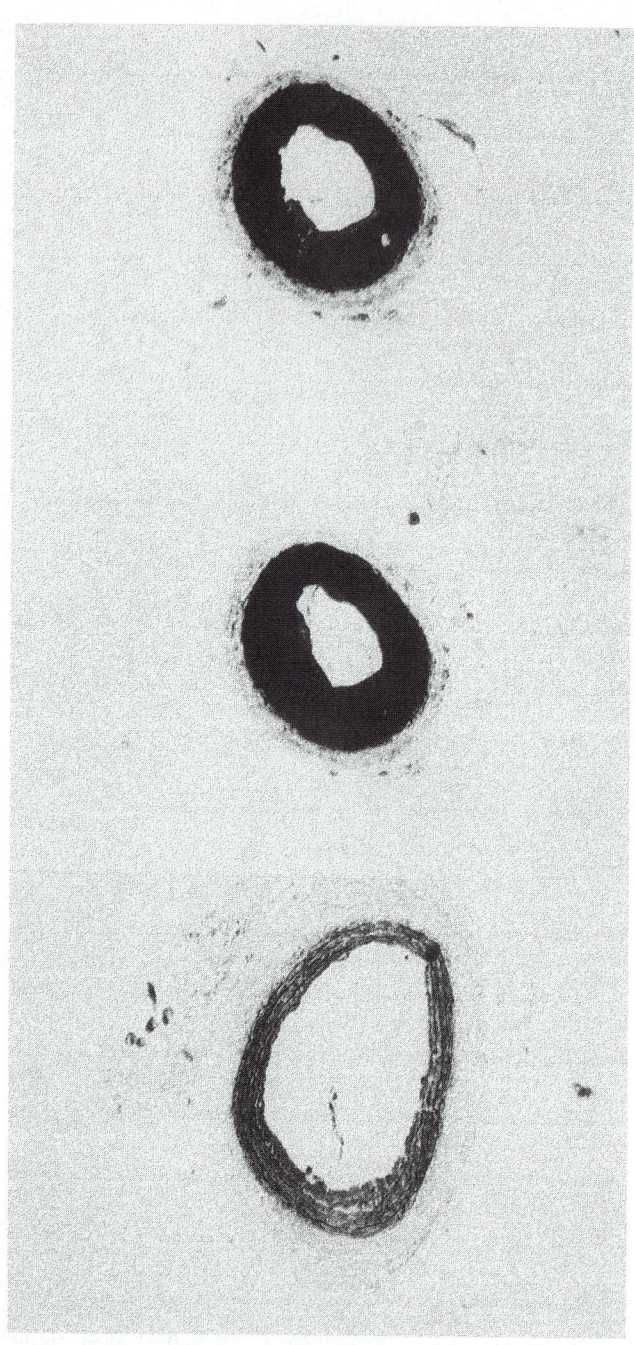

Figure 62–15. Effect of combination of antisense cdk 2 and cdc 2 kinase ODN (oligonucleotide) on neointima formation. Representative cross-sections: (*Top*) Injured carotid artery without any treatment; (*middle*) injured carotid artery treated with HVJ-sense ODN (15 μm each); (*bottom*) injured carotid artery treated with HVJ-antisense ODN (15 μm each) (×40). *(From Morishita R, et al: J Clin Invest 93:1458–1464, with permission.)*

have been described in infants as young as one month of age.[132] In infants with hypoplastic left heart syndrome, there is such severe medial hypertrophy of the small arteries and veins from birth that it must have developed in utero.[133]

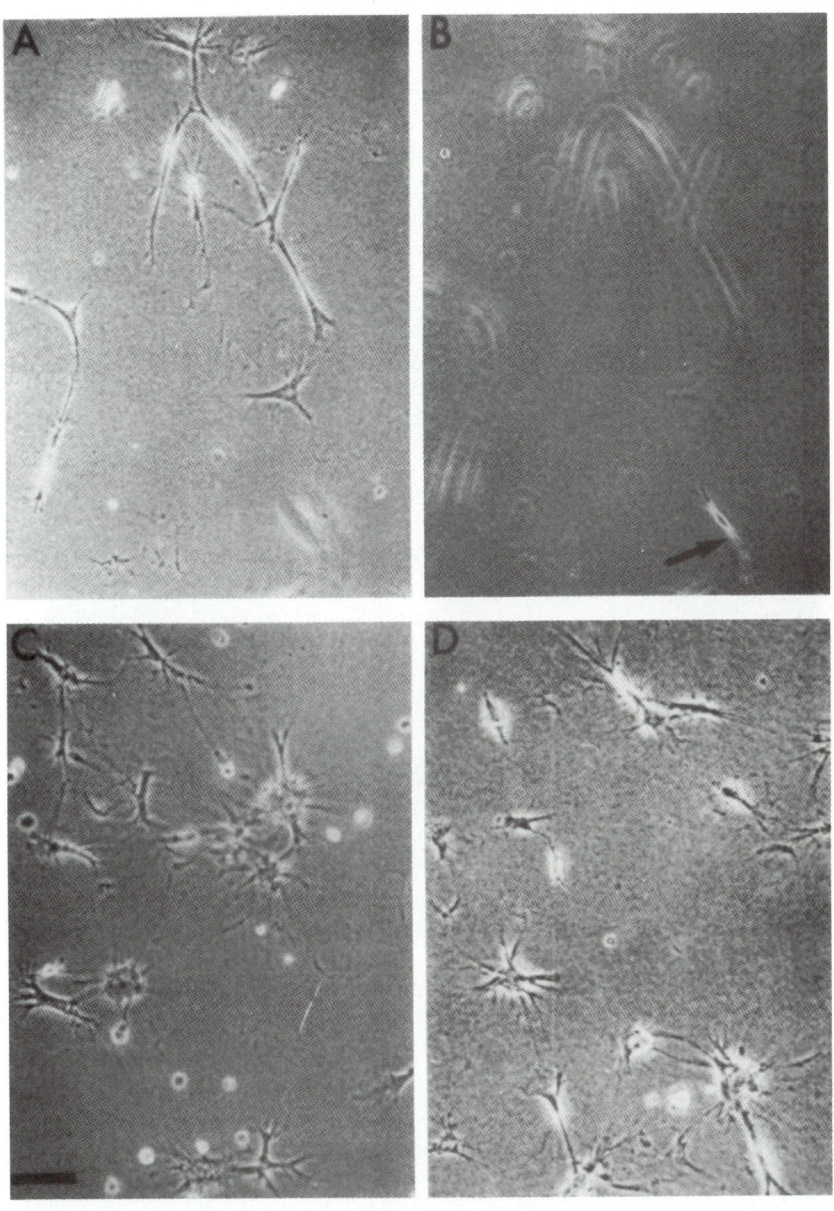

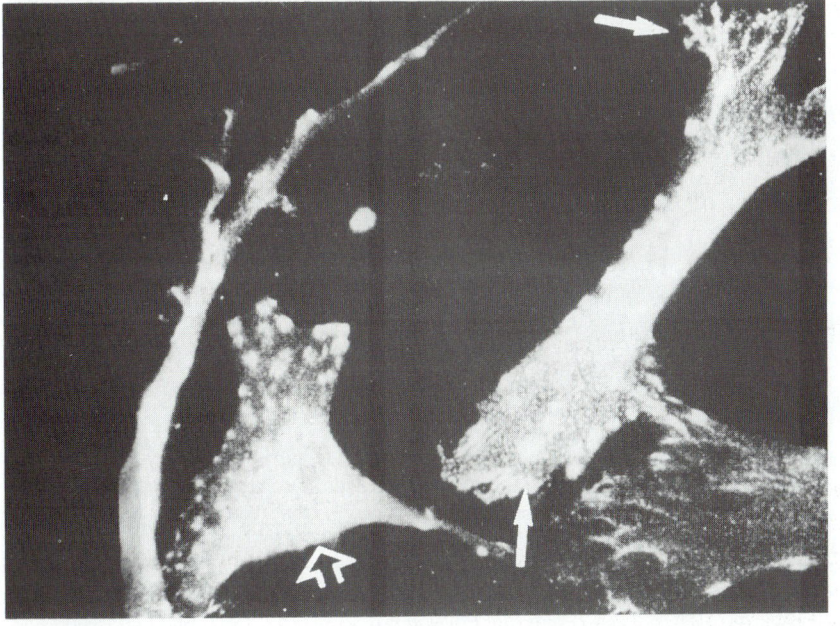

Figure 62–16. A–D. DA and Ao smooth muscle cells on collagen (2 mg/ml) gels.
(**A**) DA smooth muscle cells 2 days following seeding onto the surface of collagen gels. The cells exhibit a spindle-like elongated morphology and the majority of cells are visible on the surface of the gels. The arrow in (**B**) indicates the outline of a cell that has migrated below the surface of the gel. By focusing into the gel at a depth of 250 μm (**B**), this cell comes clearly into focus. (**C**) Ao cells, 2 days following seeding onto the surface of the gel, exhibit a flattened, stellate morphology. In the presence of antibodies against fibronectin (1:100) DA smooth muscle cells (**D**) also display a more flattened, stellate appearance (bar = 200 μm).
E. Immunofluorescent staining of receptor for hyaluronan-mediated mobility (RHAMM) on PA smooth muscle cells on glass coverslips using a 1:40 dilution of polyclonal antibodies to RHAMM and visualized by RITC goat anti-rabbit IgG. Positive staining for RHAMM was prominent in lamellipodia and leading edges as indicated by the closed arrows. *(From Boudreau N et al: Fibronectin, hyaluronan, and a hyaluronan binding protein contribute to increased ductus arteriosus smooth muscle cell migration. Dev Biol 143:235–247, 1991, with permission.)*

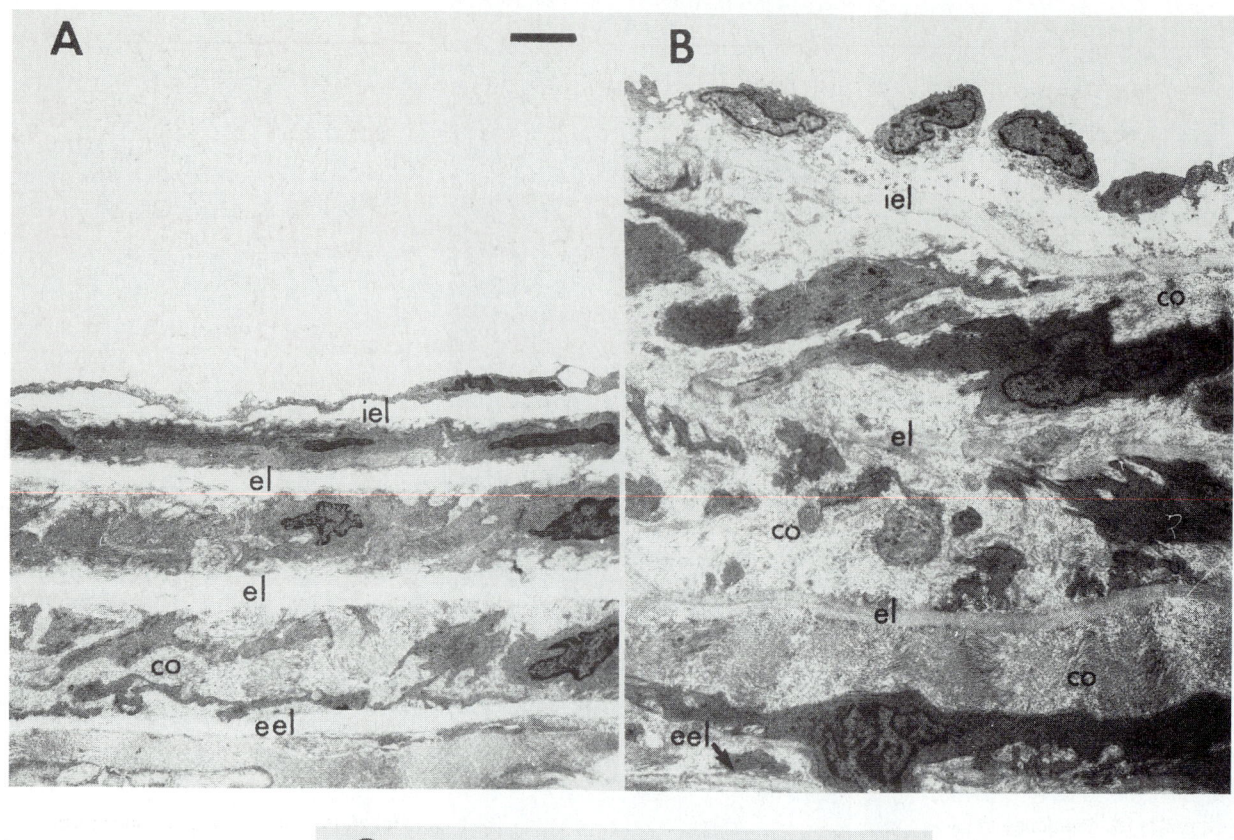

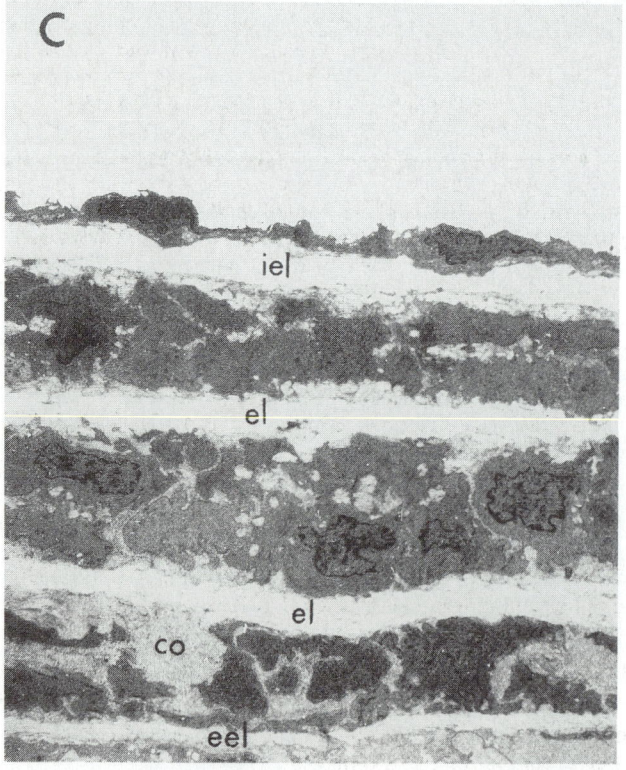

Figure 62–17. Representative electron photomicrographs of hilar arterial wall. **A.** Saline-injected rat hilar pulmonary artery showing internal elastic lamina (iel), 2 medial elastic laminae (el), and external elastic lamina (eel). Accumulation of collagen (co) is prominent in outer media. **B.** In monocrotaline/vehicle rat, 3 wk after injection of toxin, elastic laminae are reduced in proportion to increased thickness of vessel wall, and there is collagen in between smooth muscle cells. **C.** Monocrotaline/SC-37698 (elastase inhibitor) rat shows proportionately more elastin, and laminae appear more intact than in **B**. There is less intercellular collagen apparent. Original magnification ×3,670; bar, 1 μm. *(From Ye C, Rabinovitch M: Inhibition of elastolysis by SC-37698 reduces development and progression of monochrotaline pulmonary hypertension. Am J Physiol 261 (Heart Circ Physiol) H1255–H1267, 1991, with permission.)*

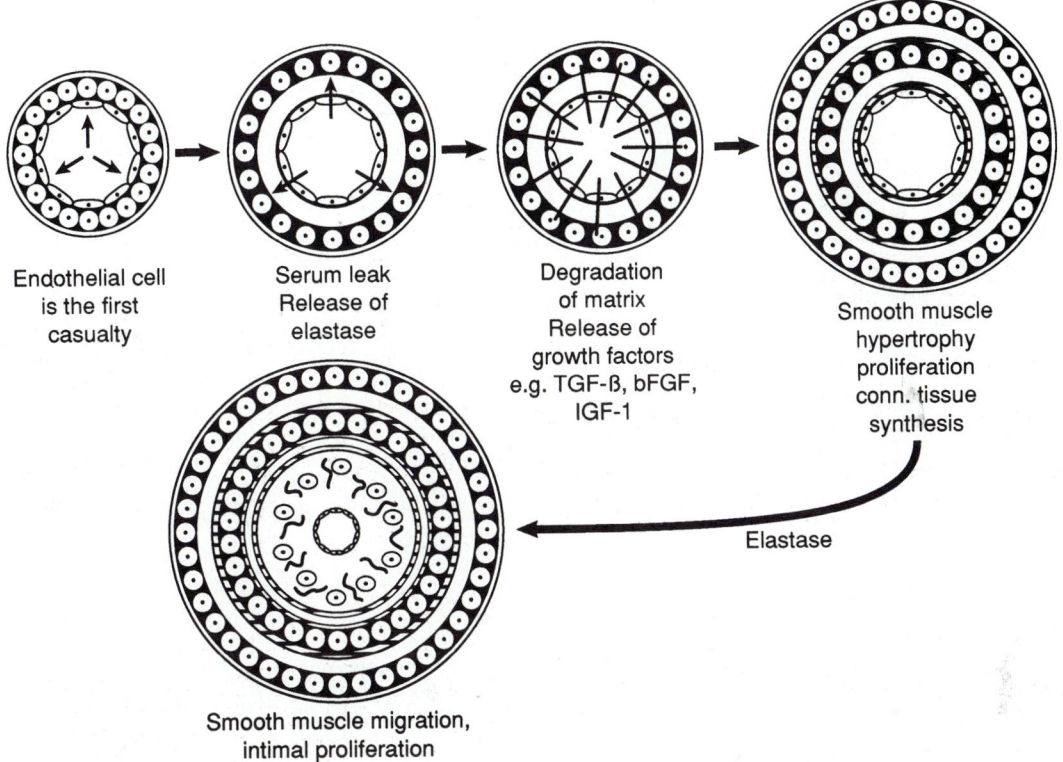

Endothelial cell
is the first
casualty

Serum leak
Release of
elastase

Degradation
of matrix
Release of
growth factors
e.g. TGF-ß, bFGF,
IGF-1

Smooth muscle
hypertrophy
proliferation
conn. tissue
synthesis

Elastase

Smooth muscle migration,
intimal proliferation

Figure 62–18. Response to injury in proximal muscular pulmonary arteries. We have speculated as to how a stimulus, such as the high flow and pressure of a congenital heart defect with a left-to-right shunt, might induce activity of an elastolytic enzyme and how this might initiate the remodeling process. The process of progressive pulmonary hypertension involves a series of switches in the smooth muscle cell phenotype, i.e., differentiation of muscle from nonmuscle precursor cells, smooth muscle cell hypertrophy, and proliferation accounting for medial hypertrophy and smooth muscle cell migration resulting in neointimal formation. We speculate that in response to a stimulus such as high flow and pressure, the first "casualty" would be the endothelial cell. As a result of structural and functional alterations in endothelial cells, some of the barrier function would be lost, allowing for leak into the subendothelium of a serum factor normally excluded from this region. The serum factor could induce activity of an elastolytic enzyme, as we have shown experimentally. This enzyme released from precursor or mature smooth muscle cells would activate growth factors normally stored in the extracellular matrix in a inactive form, such as basic fibroblast growth factor (bFGF) and transforming growth factor (TGF)-β and might also influence release of insulin-like growth factor (IGF-1). These growth factors are known to induce smooth muscle or precursor cell hypertrophy and proliferation and increases in connective (conn.) tissue protein (e.g., collagen and elastin) synthesis. This would result in the differentiation of precursor cells to mature smooth muscle related to the muscularization of normally nonmuscular small peripheral arteries and hypertrophy of the more proximal muscular arteries. Continued elastase activity would cause migration of smooth muscle cells in two ways, first, by removing a physical barrier and also by so changing the cell–extracellular matrix signaling processes that a new constellation of gene products would be produced, providing the smooth muscle cells with the machinery necessary to switch from the contractile to motile phenotype. Migration of smooth muscle cells and synthesis of extracellular matrix proteins would result in intimal proliferation.

Quantitative Studies

In the postmortem arteriograms in patients with elevated pulmonary venous pressure, the axial pulmonary arteries have a reduced lumen diameter all along their length.[134,135] The background haze is normal or slightly increased. On microscopic examination of the lung, there is severe extension of muscle into peripheral intra-acinar arteries and failure of regression of the fetal muscle of the normally muscular arteries. The vessels, however, appear normal in size and are normal or slightly increased in number.

The presence of pulmonary vascular changes in defects with high pulmonary venous pressure and the capacity for these abnormalities to regress with improvement in hemodynamics are of particular timely relevance, since the newly proposed staged surgical procedure for the treatment of hypoplastic left heart syndrome involves the eventual placement of a right atrial to pulmonary arterial conduit.[136]

DEFECTS THAT DECREASE PULMONARY BLOOD FLOW

Hemodynamic Studies

Congenital heart defects that cause decreased pulmonary blood flow, such as tetralogy of Fallot, pulmonary atresia, and tricuspid atresia, have been associated with increased pulmonary vascular resistance even after repair.[137] Pul-

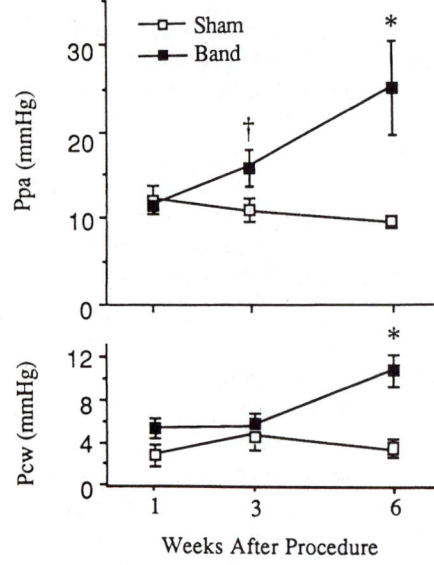

A

Figure 62–19. A. Pulmonary artery pressure (P$_{pa}$, upper panel) and pulmonary capillary wedge pressure (P$_{cw}$, lower panel) in banded and sham-operated piglets at 1, 3, and 6 wk after banding. Values are averages of mean ±SEM (n=6 piglets per group at each time point). At 1 wk there was no change. At 3 wk there was a significant increase in P$_{pa}$ that preceded the rise in P$_{cw}$ at 6 wk and the further increase in P$_{pa}$, *p<0.01;†p<0.05.

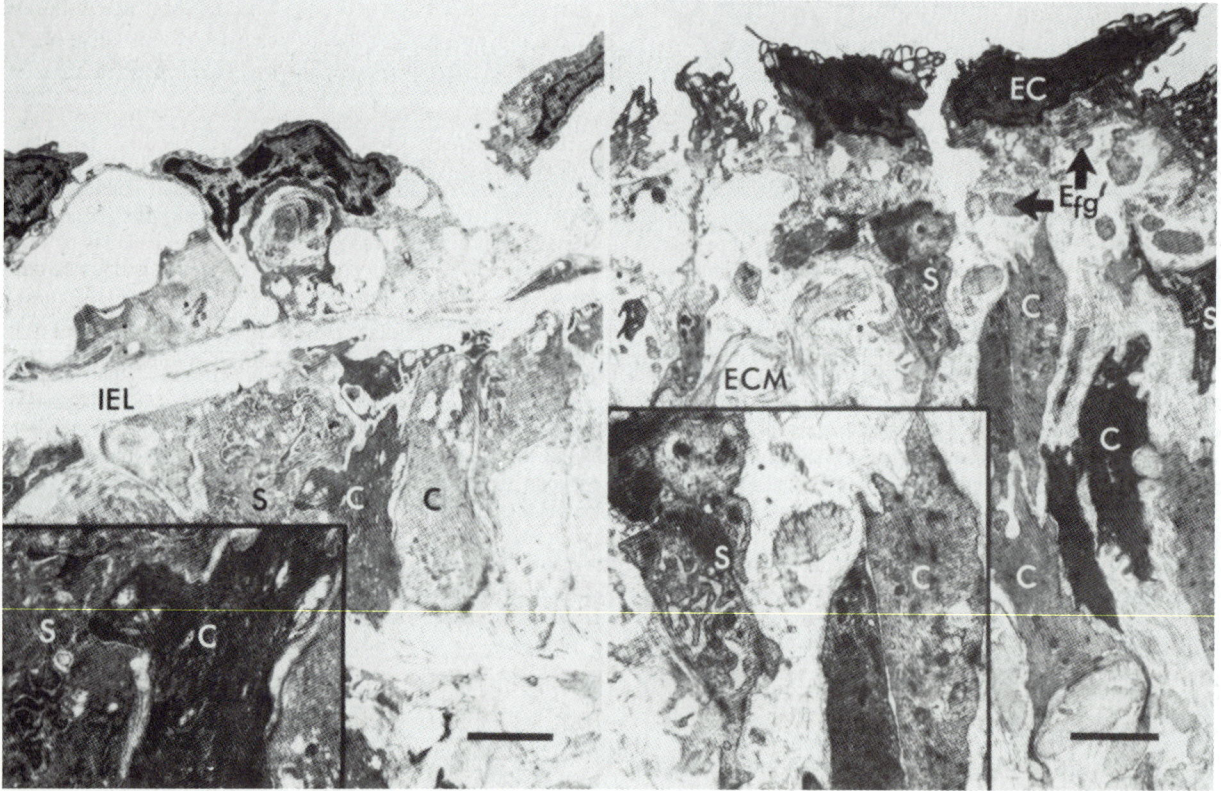

B

Figure 62–19. B. Transmission electron photomicro-graphs of representative pulmonary veins (PVs) from banded (**right panel**) and sham-operated (**left panel**) piglets at 3 wk after banding (magnification ×14,131) (inset magnification ×28,263). Both pulmonary veins show apparent injury and lifting of endothelial cells and subendothelial spaces due to poor preservation during handling. Sham-operated PV displays an intact internal elastic lamina (IEL) and predominantly contractile-appearing smooth muscle cells (C) in media. In contrast, PV from banded piglet depicts complete breakdown of IEL into elastin fragments (E$_{fg}$), a thickened subendothelium composed of collagen, extracellular matrix (ECM), and smooth muscle cells that appear to have migrated in from media, many of which have a synthetic-appearing phenotype (S) exemplified by large amount of endoplasmic reticulum and a corresponding paucity of contractile filaments. C and S smooth muscle cells are better appreciated in insets. Bar = 1 µm. *(From LaBourene JE et al: Alterations in elastic and collagen related to the mechanism of progressive pulmonary venous obstruction in a piglet model. Reproduced with permission. Circ Res 66:438–456. Copyright 1990 American Heart Association.)*

monary hypertension has been observed in patients who have had the creation of a large longstanding systemic to pulmonary artery anastomosis and also in those without shunts.

Morphologic Assessment of the Pulmonary Vascular Bed

Qualitative Studies

In patients with congenital heart defects causing low pulmonary blood flow, hypoplasia of the pulmonary arterial musculature is observed,[138] and in those in whom the hematocrit is particularly elevated, thromboembolic changes occur[139] (Fig. 62–19). The creation of systemic to pulmonary arterial shunts at first improves the hypoplasia, but secondary to abnormally high flow, medial hypertrophy and intimal hyperplasia soon occur.[140]

Quantitative Studies

On the postmortem arteriograms of all patients with decreased pulmonary blood flow, the axial arteries are abnormally narrow in lumen diameter,[141–143] and, in patients with pulmonary atresia, the background haze is also reduced. On microscopic examination of the lungs from patients with pulmonary atresia, the intra-acinar pulmonary arteries are abnormally thin-walled, small in size, and few in number. In patients with tetralogy of Fallot, these vessels are normal or decreased in muscularity, normal in number, and small in size. Alveolar development is impaired in patients with decreased pulmonary blood flow, and this is reflected mostly by reduction in alveolar number. Patients with tetralogy of Fallot and associated pulmonary atresia form a special subgroup in which the relative distribution of

central pulmonary arteries and aortopulmonary collaterals determines peripheral pulmonary vascular structure.[143–145] In patients with tricuspid atresia, the structural state of the pulmonary vascular bed is variable, depending on the degree of reduction in pulmonary blood flow.[146]

Studies suggest that the potential for growth of the central pulmonary arteries is correlated with the proportion of elastin in the media and the same may be true for the intrapulmonary vessels as well.[147] To study the abnormal development of the pulmonary vasculature, experimental models causing pulmonary vein, aorta, and pulmonary artery obstruction have been created.[148–152] It was interesting that, in our model of pulmonary venous obstruction,[133] mild hemodynamically imperceptible "injury" resulted in extensive fibrosis. In fact, elevated pulmonary arterial pressure preceded any detectable rise in pulmonary venous pressure and the latter, which occurred subsequently, was associated with fragmentation of elastin, increased collagen (fibrosis), and intimal proliferation (Fig. 62–20). Future studies need to be directed toward understanding the mechanism of vascular disease resulting from increased pulmonary venous pressure and low pulmonary blood.

CONCLUSION

There has been progress made in the diagnosis of patients at risk for developing progressive pulmonary vascular changes. This has led to early surgical intervention and improved postoperative management. New insights into the cellular and molecular mechanisms causing vascular changes will lead to better control of the reactive pulmonary circulation and new ideas about how to induce re-

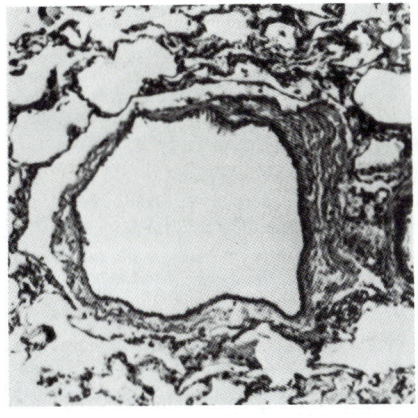
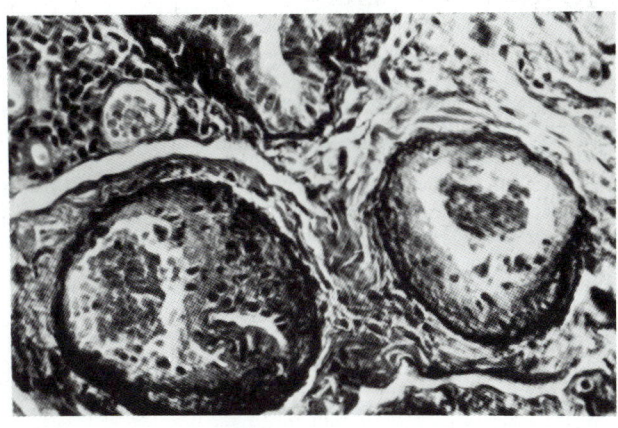

A   B

Figure 62–20. A. Muscular pulmonary artery in a 5-year-old boy with tetralogy of Fallot who was not subjected to any anastomotic or corrective operation. The arterial wall is extremely thin and contains hardly any muscle fibers. HE, ×65. **B.** Muscular pulmonary arteries in a 4-year-old boy with tetralogy of Fallot. The arteries show irregular thinning of the media and very marked intimal fibrosis, probably resulting from organized thrombi. The intimal fibrosis is eccentric and shows recanalization in one of the arteries. EVG, ×330. *(From Wagenvoort CA et al: The Pathology of the Pulmonary Vasculature, 1964. Courtesy of Charles C. Thomas.)*

gression of structural damage we now consider "permanent" are now being proposed.

REFERENCES

1. Eisenmenger V: Die angeborenen Defecte der Kammerscheidewand des Herzen. *Z Klin Med* [Suppl 32]:1, 1897
2. Bing RJ, Vandam LD, Gray FD: Physiological studies in congenital heart disease. *Bull Johns Hopkins Hosp* **80:**323, 1947
3. Bond VF Jr: Eisenmenger's complex. Report of two cases and review of cases with autopsy study. *Am Heart J* **42:**424, 1951
4. Wood P: The Eisenmenger syndrome of pulmonary hypertension with reversed central shunt. *Br Med J* **2:**701, 755, 1958
5. Rudolph AM, Nadas AS: The pulmonary circulation and congenital heart disease. Considerations of the role of the pulmonary circulation in certain systemic pulmonary communications. *N Engl J Med* **267:**96, 1022, 1962
6. Civin WH, Edwards JE: Pathology of the pulmonary vascular tree. *Circulation* **2:**545, 1950
7. Hoffman JIE, Rudolph AM: The natural history of ventricular septal defects in infancy. *Am J Cardiol* **16:**634, 1965
8. Castaneda AR, Zamora R, Nicoloff DM, et al: High pressure, high resistance ventricular septal defect: Surgical results of closure through right atrium. *Ann Thorac Surg* **12:**29, 1971
9. Friedli B, Kidd BS, Mustard WT, Keith JD: Ventricular septal defect with increased pulmonary vascular resistance. *Am J Cardiol* **33:**403, 1974
10. Maron BJ, Redwood DR, Hirschfeld FW Jr, et al: Postoperative assessment of patients with ventricular septal defect and pulmonary hypertension. Response to intense and upright exercise. *Circulation* **48:**864, 1973
11. Reid JM, Stevenson JG, Coleman EN, et al: Moderate to severe pulmonary hypertension accompanying patent ductus arteriosus. *Br Heart J* **26:**600, 1964
12. Besterman E: Atrial septal defect with pulmonary hypertension. *Br Heart J* **23:**587, 1961
13. DiSesa JV, Cohn LH, Grossman W: Management of adults with congenital bidirectional cardiac shunt, cyanosis and pulmonary vascular obstruction: Successful operative repair in 3 patients. *Am J Cardiol* **51:**1495, 1983
14. Haworth SG: Pulmonary vascular disease in secundum atrial septal defect in childhood. *Am J Cardiol* **51:**265, 1984
15. Viles P, Ongley P, Titus J: The spectrum of pulmonary vascular disease in transposition of the great arteries. *Circulation* **40:**31, 1969
16. Newfeld EA, Paul MH, Muster AJ, Idriss FS: Pulmonary vascular disease in complete transposition of the great arteries: A study of 200 patients. *Am J Cardiol* **34:**75, 1974
17. Waldman JD, Paul MH, Newfeld EA: Transposition of the great arteries with intact ventricular septum and patent ductus arteriosus. *Am J Cardiol* **39:**232, 1977
18. Berman W Jr, Whitman V, Pierce WS, Walhausen JA: The development of pulmonary vascular obstructive disease after successful Mustard operation in early infancy. *Circulation* **58:**181, 1978
19. Newfeld EA, Sher M, Paul MH: Pulmonary vascular disease in complete atrioventricular canal defect. *Am J Cardiol* **39:**721, 1977
20. Marcelleti C, McGoon DC, Mair DD: The natural history of truncus arteriosus. *Circulation* **54:**108, 1976
21. Juaneda E, Haworth SG: Pulmonary vascular disease in children with truncus arteriosus. *Br Heart J* **52:**1314, 1984
22. Paul MH, Miller RA, Potts WJ: Long-term results of aortic pulmonary anastomosis in tetralogy of Fallot: An analysis of the first 100 cases 11 to 13 years after operation. *Circulation* **23:**525, 1961
23. Weidman WH, DuShane JW, Kincaid OW: Observations concerning progressive pulmonary vascular obstruction in children with ventricular septal defects. *Am Heart J* **65:**148, 1963
24. Iverson RE, Linde LE, Kegel S: The diagnosis of progressive pulmonary vascular disease in children with ventricular septal defects. *Pediatrics* **68:**594, 1966
25. Johnson JB, Felter ML, West JR, Cournand A: The relation between electrocardiographic existence of right ventricular hypertrophy and pulmonary arterial pressure in patients with chronic pulmonary disease. *Circulation* **1:**536, 1940
26. Chou T, Masangkay MP, Young R, et al: Simple quantitative vectorcardiographic criteria for the diagnosis of right ventricular hypertrophy. *Circulation* **48:**1262, 1973
27. Silverman NH, Snider AR, Rudolph AM: Evaluation of pulmonary hypertension by M-mode echocardiography in children with ventricular septal defect. *Circulation* **61:**1125, 1980
28. Rabinovitch M, Fisher KC, Treves S: Quantitative thallium-201 myocardial imaging in assessing right ventricular pressure in patients with congenital heart defects. *Br Heart J* **45:**198, 1981
29. Marx GR, Allan HD, Goldberg SJ: Doppler echocardiographic estimation of systolic pulmonary artery pressure patients with interventricular communications. *J Am Coll Cardiol* **6:**1132, 1985
30. Musewe NN, Smallhorn JF, Benson LN, et al: Validation of Doppler-derived pulmonary arterial pressure in patients with ductus arteriosus under different hemodynamic states. *Circulation* **76:**1081, 1987
31. Mair DD, Ritter DG, Ongley PA, Helmholz HF Jr: Hemodynamics and evaluation for surgery of patients with complete transposition of the great arteries and ventricular septal defect. *Am J Cardiol* **28:**632, 1971
32. Vogel JHK, Grover RF, Jamieson G, Blount SG Jr: Long-term physiologic observation in patients with ventricular septal defect and increased pulmonary vascular resistance. *Adv Cardiol* **11:**108, 1974
33. Stocker FP, Wilkoss OS, Nadas AS: Oxygen consumption in infants with heart disease. *J Pediatr* **80:**43, 1972
34. Tarnow J, Hess W: Pulmonary hypertension and pulmonary edema caused by intravenous ketamine. *Anesthetist* **27:**486, 1978
35. Vogel JH, McNamara DC, Blount SG Jr: Role of hypoxia in determining pulmonary vascular resistance in infants with ventricular septal defect. *Am J Cardiol* **20:**346, 1967
36. Rosenthal A, Nathan DG, Marty AT, et al: Acute hemodynamic effects of red cell volume reduction in polycythemia of cyanotic congenital heart disease. *Circulation* **42:**297, 1970
37. Keane JF, Ellison RC, Rudd M, Nadas AS: Pulmonary blood flow and left ventricular volumes with transposition of the great arteries and intact ventricular septum. *Br Heart J* **35:**521, 1973
38. Brenner O: Pathology of the vessels of the pulmonary circulation. Part I. *Arch Intern Med* **56:**211, 1935
39. Heath D, Edwards J: The pathology of hypertensive pulmonary vascular disease. *Circulation* **18:**533, 1958
40. Heath D, Swan HJC, Dushane JW, Edwards JE: The relation to medial thickness of small muscular pulmonary arteries to immediate postnatal survival in patients with ventricular septal defect and patent ductus arteriosus. *Thorax* **13:**267, 1958
41. Naeye RL: The pulmonary arterial bed in ventricular septal defect. Anatomic features in childhood. *Circulation* **34:**962, 1966
42. Elliot FM, Reid L: Some new facts about the pulmonary artery and its branching pattern. *Clin Radiol* **6:**193, 1965
43. Davies G, Reid L: Growth of the alveoli and pulmonary arteries in childhood. *Thorax* **25:**669, 1970
44. Hislop A, Reid L: Pulmonary arterial development during childhood: Branching pattern and structure. *Thorax* **28:**129, 1973
45. Short DS: The application of arteriography to the pathological study of pulmonary hypertension. In Adams WR, Vieth I (eds): *Pulmonary Circulation.* New York, Grune & Stratton, 1959, p 233
46. Hislop A, Haworth SG, Reid L: Quantitative structural analysis of pulmonary vessels in isolated ventricular septal defects in infancy. *Br Heart J* **37:**1014, 1975
47. Haworth SG, Reid L: A morphometric study of regional variation in lung structure in infants with pulmonary hypertension and congeni-

tal heart defect. A justification of lung biopsy. *Br Heart J* **40**:825, 1978

48. Haworth SG, Hislop AA: Pulmonary vascular development: Normal values of peripheral vascular structure. *Am J Cardiol* **52**:578, 1983

49. Rabinovitch M, Haworth SG, Castaneda AR et al: Lung biopsy in congenital heart disease: a morphometric approach to pulmonary vascular disease. *Circulation* **58**:1107, 1978

50. Meyrick B, Reid L: Ultrastructural findings in lung biopsy material from children with congenital heart defects. *Am J Pathol* **101**:527, 1980

51. Rabinovitch M, Bothwell T, Hayakawa BN, et al: Pulmonary arterial endothelial abnormalities in patients with congenital heart defects and pulmonary hypertension: A correlation of light with scanning electron microscopy and transmission electron microscopy. *Lab Invest* **55**:632, 1986

52. Taipale J, Koli K, Keski-Oja J: Release of transforming factor-β1 from the pericellular matrix of cultured fibroblasts and fibrosarcoma cells by plasmin and thrombin. *J Biol Chem* **267**:25378, 1992

53. Sato Y, Rifkin DB: Inhibition of endothelial cell movement by pericytes and smooth muscle cells: Activation of a latent transforming growth factor-β1-like molecule by plasmin during co-culture. *J Cell Biol* **109**:309, 1989

54. Braulin EA, Moller JH, Patton C, et al: Predictive value of lung biopsy in ventricular septal defect: Long-term follow-up. *J Am Coll Cardiol* **8**:1113, 1986

55. Rabinovitch M, Keane JF, Norwood WI, et al: Vascular structure in lung biopsy tissue correlated with pulmonary hemodynamic findings after repair of congenital heart defects. *Circulation* **69**:655, 1984

56. Rabinovitch M, Castaneda AR, Reid L: Lung biopsy with frozen section as a diagnostic aid in patients wit congenital heart defects. *Am J Cardiol* **47**:77, 1981

57. Rabinovitch M, Sanders SP, Castaneda AR, et al: Morphometric analysis of lung biopsy tissue in candidates for Fontan-type surgical procedures (Abstr): *Am J Cardiol* **47**:947, 1981

58. Juaneda E, Haworth SG: Pulmonary vascular structure in patients dying after a Fontan procedure: The lung as a risk factor. *Br Heart J* **52**:575, 1984

59. Rosenberg H, Coles J, Williams WG, et al: An association between vascular changes on lung biopsy specimens and postoperative morbidity following the Fontan procedure. *J Am Coll Cardiol* **9**:204A, 1987

60. Nihill MR, McNamara DG: Magnification pulmonary wedge angiography in the evaluation of children with congenital heart disease and pulmonary hypertension. *Circulation* **58**:1094, 1978

61. Rabinovitch M, Keane JF, Fellows KE et al: Quantitative analysis of the pulmonary wedge angiogram in congenital heart defects: Correlation with hemodynamic data and morphometric findings in lung biopsy tissue. *Circulation* **63**:152, 1981

62. Christman BW, McPherson CD, Newman JH, et al: An imbalance between the excretion of thromboxane and prostacyclin metabolites in pulmonary hypertension. *N Engl J Med* **327**:70, 1992

63. Turner-Gomes SO, Andrew M, Coles J, et al: Abnormalities in von Willebrand factor and antithrombin III after cardiopulmonary bypass operations for congenital heart disease. *Thorac Cardiovasc Surg* **103**:87, 1992

64. Yoshibayashi M, Nishioka K, Nakao K et al: Plasma endothelin concentrations in patients with pulmonary hypertension associated with congenital heart defects. Evidence for increased production of endothelin in pulmonary circulation. *Circulation* **84**:2280, 1991

65. Chang H, Wu G-J, Wang S-M, Hung C-R: Plasma endothelin levels and surgically correctable pulmonary hypertension. *Ann Thorac Surg* **55**:450, 1993

66. Adatia I, Haworth SG: Circulating endothelin in children with congenital heart disease. *Br Heart J* **69**:233, 1993

67. Nakaki T, Nakayama M, Yamamoto S, Kato R: Endothelin-mediated stimulation of DNA synthesis in vascular smooth muscle cells. *Biochem Biophys Res Commun* **158**:880, 1989

68. Dinh Xuan AT, Higgenbottam TW, Clelland C, et al: Impairment of pulmonary endothelium-dependent relaxation in patients with Eisenmenger's syndrome. *Br J Pharmacol* **99**:9, 1990

69. Celermajor DS, Cullen S, Deanfield JE, et al: Impairment of endothelium-dependent pulmonary artery relaxation in children with congenital heart disease and abnormal pulmonary hemodynamics. *Circulation* **87**:440, 1993

70. Wessel DL, Adatia I, Giglia TM, et al: Use of inhaled nitric oxide and acetylcholine in the evaluation of pulmonary hypertension and endothelial function after cardiopulmonary bypass. *Circulation* **88**:2128, 1993

71. Hickey PR, Hansen DD, Wessel DL, et al: Blunting of stressing responses of the pulmonary circulation of infants by fentanyl. *Anesth Analg* **64**:1137, 1985

72. Bush A, Bust C, Knight WB, et al: Modification of pulmonary hypertension secondary to congenital heart disease with prostacyclin therapy. *Am Rev Respir Dis* **136**:767, 1987

73. Journois D, Pouard P, Mauriat P, et al: Inhaled nitric oxide as a therapy for pulmonary hypertension after operations for congenital heart defects. *J Thorac Cardiovasc Surg* **107**:1129, 1994

74. Bowyer JJ, Busst CM, Denison DM, et al: Effect of long-term oxygen treatment at home in children with pulmonary vascular disease. *Br Heart J* **55**:385, 1986

75. Bush A, Bust C, Knight WB, et al: Modification of pulmonary hypertension secondary to congenital heart disease with prostacyclin therapy. *Am Rev Respir Dis* **136**:767, 1987

76. Houde C, Bohn DJ, Freedom RM, Rabinovitch M: Profile of paediatric patients with pulmonary hypertension judged by responsiveness to vasodilators. *Br Heart J* **70**:461, 1993

77. Cohen M, Edwards WD, Fuster V: Regression in thromboembolic type of primary pulmonary hypertension during 2 1/2 years of antithrombotic therapy. *J Am Coll Cardiol* **7**:172, 1986

78. Dark JH, Patterson GA, Al-Jilaihawi AN, et al: Experimental en bloc double-lung transplantation. *Ann Thorac Surg* **42**:394, 1986

79. Starnes VA, Stinson EB, Oyer PE, et al: Single lung transplantation, a new therapeutic option for patients with pulmonary hypertension. *Transplant Proc* **23**:1209, 1991

80. Calhoon JH, Grover FL, Gibbons WJ, et al: Single lung transplantation: Alternative indications and technique. *J Thorac Cardiovasc Surg* **101**:816, 1991

81. Cooper JD: The evolution of techniques and indications for lung transplantation. *Ann Surg* **212**:249, 1990

82. Griffith BP: Heart and heart lung transplantation. In Welsh KJ (ed): *Pediatric Surgery*, ed. 4. Chicago, Year Book, 1986 pp 383–392

83. Foster JA, Rich CB, Miller MF: Pulmonary fibroblasts, an *in vitro* model of emphysema. Regulation of elastin gene expression. *J Biol Chem* **265**:14,444, 1990

84. Botney MD, Bahadori L, Gold LI: Vascular remodeling in primary pulmonary hypertension. Potential role for transforming growth factor-β. *Am J Pathol* **144**:286, 1994

85. Quaglino D, Nanney LB, Kennedy R, Davidson JM: Transforming growth factor-β stimulates wound healing and modulates extracellular matrix gene expression in pig skin. I. Excisional Wound Model. *Lab Invest* **63**:307, 1990

86. Botney MD, Kaiser LR, Cooper JD, et al: Extracellular matrix gene expression in atherosclerotic hypertensive pulmonary arteries. *Am J Pathol* **140**:357, 1992

87. Botney MD, Liptay MJ, Kaiser LR, et al: Active collagen synthesis by pulmonary arteries in human primary pulmonary hypertension. *Am J Pathol* **143**:121, 1993

88. Boudreau N, Turley E, Rabinovitch M: Fibronectin, hyaluronan and a hyaluronan binding protein contribute to increased ductus arteriosus smooth muscle cell migration. *Dev Biol* **143**:235, 1991

89. Molossi S, Elices M, Rabinovitch M: Blockade of interleukin-1-induced fibronectin/lymphocyte interaction in vitro inhibits lymphocyte transendothelial migration. *FASEB J* **8**(5):A1018, 1994

90. Liptay MJ, Parks WC, Mecham RP et al: Neointimal macrophages

colocalize with extracellular matrix gene expression in human atherosclerotic pulmonary arteries. *J Clin Invest* **91**:588, 1993

91. Davies P, McBride P, Murray GF, et al: Structural changes in the canine lung and pulmonary arteries after pneumonectomy. *Appl Physiol* **53**:859, 1982

92. Rabinovitch M, Konstam MA, Gamble WJ, et al: Changes in pulmonary blood flow effect vascular response to chronic hypoxia in rats. *Circ Res* **52**:432, 1983

93. Durmowicz AG, St Cyr JA, Clarke DR, et al: Unilateral pulmonary hypertension as a result of chronic high flow to one lung. *Am Rev Respir Dis* **142**:230, 1990

94. Rendas A, Lennox S, Reid L: Aortopulmonary shunts in growing pigs. *J Thorac Cardiovasc Surg* **77**:109, 1979

95. Rendas A, Reid L: Pulmonary vasculature after correction of aortopulmonary shunts. *J Thorac Cardiovasc Surg* **85**:911, 1983

96. Blank RH, Muller WH, Damman JF: Experimental pulmonary hypertension. *Am J Surg* **101**:143-153, 1961

97. Boucek MM, Chang R, Synhorst DP: Hemodynamic consequences in inotropic support with digoxin and amrinone in lambs with ventricular septal defect. *Pediatr Res* **19**:887, 1985

98. Frangos JA, Eskin S, McIntyre LV, et al: Flow effects on prostacyclin production by cultured human endothelial cells. *Science* **227**:1277, 1985

99. Sharefkin JB, Diamond SL, Eskin SG, et al: Fluid flow decreases preproendothelin mRNA levels and suppresses endothelin-1 peptide release in cultured human endothelial cells. *J Vasc Surg* **14**:1, 1991

100. Yoshizumi M, Kurihara H, Sugiyama T, et al: Hemodynamic shear stress stimulates endothelin production by cultured endothelial cells. *Biochem Biophys Res Commun* **161**:859, 1989

101. Hsieh H-J, Li N-Q, Frangos JA: Pulsatile and steady flow induces c-fos expression in human endothelial cells. *J Cell Physiol* **154**:143, 1993

102. Fox PL, DiCorleto PE: Regulation of production of a platelet-derived growth factor-like protein by cultured bovine aortic endothelial cells. *J Cell Physiol* **121**:298, 1984

103. Raines E, Dower S, Ross R: Interleukin-1 mitogenic activity for fibroblasts and smooth muscle cells is due to PDGF-AA. *Science* **243**:393, 1989

104. Taubman MB, Rollins BJ, Poon M, et al: JE mRNA accumulates rapidly in aortic injury and in platelet-derived growth factor-stimulated vascular smooth muscle cells. *Circ Res* **70**:314, 1992

105. Resnick N, Collins T, Atkinson W, et al: Platelet-derived growth factor β chain promoter contains a cis-acting fluid shear stress responsive element. *Proc Nat'l Acad Sci* **90**:4591–4595, 1993

106. Simons M, Rosenberg R: Antisense nonmuscle myosin heavy chain and c-myb oligonucleotides suppress smooth muscle cell proliferation *in vitro*. *Circ Res* **70**:835, 1992

107. Lindner V, Olson NE, Closes AW, et al: Inhibition of smooth muscle cell proliferation in injured rat arteries. Interaction of heparin with basic fibroblast growth factor. *J Clin Invest* **90**:2044, 1992

108. Morishita R, Gibbons GH, Ellison K, et al: Intimal hyperplasia after vascular injury is inhibited by antisense cdc 2 kinase oligonucleotides. *J Clin Invest* **93**:1458, 1994

109. Ohno T, Gordon D, San H, et al: Gene therapy for vascular smooth muscle cell proliferation after arterial injury. *Science* **265**:781, 1994

110. Speir E, Modali R, Huang E-S, et al: Potential role of human cytomegalovirus and p53 interaction in coronary restenosis. *Science* **265**:391, 1994

111. Boudreau N, Rabinovitch M: Developmentally regulated changes in extracellular matrix in endothelial and smooth muscle cells in the ductus arteriosus may be related to intimal proliferation. *Lab Invest* **64**:187, 1991

112. Boudreau N, Clausell N, Boyle J, Rabinovitch M: Transforming growth factor-β regulates increased ductus arteriosus endothelial glycosaminoglycan synthesis and a post-transcriptional mechanism controls increased smooth muscle fibronectin, features associated with intimal proliferation. *Lab Invest* **67**:350, 1992

113. Zhu L, Dagher E, Johnson DJ, et al: A developmentally regulated program restricting insolubilization of elastin and formation of laminae in the fetal lamb ductus arteriosus. *Lab Invest* **68**:321, 1993

114. Hinek A, Rabinovitch M, Keeley F, et al: The 67-kD elastin/laminin-binding protein is related to an enzymatically inactive, alternatively spliced form of β-galactosidase. *J Clin Invest* **91**:1198, 1993

115. Hinek A, Rabinovitch M: The ductus arteriosus migratory smooth muscle cell phenotype processes tropoelastin to a 52-kDa product associated with impaired assembly of elastic laminae. *J Biol Chem* **268**:1405, 1993

116. Hinek A, Boyle J, Rabinovitch M: Vascular smooth muscle cell detachment from elastin and migration through elastic laminae is promoted by chondroitin sulfate-induced "shedding" of the 67-kDa cell surface elastin binding protein. *Exp Cell Res* **203**:344, 1992

117. Todorovich-Hunter L, Dodo H, Ye C, et al: Increased pulmonary artery elastolytic activity in adult rats with monocrotaline-induced progressive hypertensive pulmonary vascular disease compared with infant rats with nonprogressive disease. *Am Rev Respir Dis* **146**:213, 1992

118. Maruyama K, Ye C, Woo M, et al: Chronic hypoxic pulmonary hypertension in rats and increased elastolytic activity. *Am J Physiol* **261**:H1716, 1991

119. Ye C, Rabinovitch M: Inhibition of elastolysis by SC-37698 reduces development and progression of monocrotaline pulmonary hypertension. *Am J Physiol* **261**:H1255–H1267, 1991

120. Shemie S, Rabinovitch M: Alpha-1 antitrypsin inhibits the early increase in elastase activity and delays progression of monocrotaline-induced pulmonary hypertension in rats. *Am J Resp Crit Care Med* (submitted)

121. Zhu L, Wigle D, Hinek A, et al: The endogenous vascular elastase that govern development and progression of monocrotaline-induced pulmonary hypertension in rats is a novel enzyme related to the serine proteinase adipsin. *J Clin Invest* **94**:1163–1171, 1994

122. Oho S, Rabinovitch M: Post-cardiac transplant arteriopathy in piglets is associated with fragmentation of elastin and increased activity of a serine elastase. *Am J Pathol* **145**:202, 1994

123. Kobayashi J, Wigle D, Childs T, et al: Serum-induced vascular smooth muscle cell elastolytic activity through tyrosine kinase intracellular signaling. *J Cell Physiol* **160**:121, 1994

124. Clausell N, Molossi S, Rabinovitch M: Increased interleukin-1β and fibronectin expression are early features of the development of the post-cardiac transplant coronary arteriopathy in piglets. *Am J Pathol* **142**:1772, 1993

125. Clausell N, Rabinovitch M: Upregulation of fibronectin synthesis by interleukin-1β in coronary artery smooth muscle cells is associated with the development of the post-cardiac transplant arteriopathy in piglets. *J Clin Invest* **92**:1850, 1992

126. Molossi S, Clausell N, Rabinovitch M: Coronary artery endothelial interleukin-1β mediates enhanced fibronectin production related to post-cardiac transplant arteriopathy in piglets. *Circulation* **88**:248, 1993

127. Clausell N, Molossi S, Sett S, Rabinovitch M: In vivo blockade of tumor necrosis factor-α in cholesterol-fed rabbits after cardiac transplant inhibits acute coronary artery neointimal formation. *Circulation* **89**:2768, 1994

128. Molossi S, Clausell N, Rabinovitch M: Reciprocal induction of tumor necrosis factor-α and interleukin-1β activity mediates fibronectin synthesis in coronary artery smooth muscle cells. *J Cell Physiol* **163**:19–29, 1995

129. Molossi S, Elices M, Arrhenius T, et al: Blockade of VLA-4 integrin binding to fibronectin with CS1 peptide reduces accelerated coronary arteriopathy in rabbit cardiac allografts. *J Clin Invest* (in press), 1995

130. Collins-Nakai RL, Rosenthal A, Castaneda AR, et al: A review of 20 years' experience. *Circulation* **56**:1039, 1977

131. Whight CM, Barratt-Boyes BG, Calder AL, et al: Total anomalous

pulmonary venous connection: Long-term results following repair in infancy. *J Thorac Cardiovasc Surg* **75**:52, 1978

132. Newfeld EA, Wilson A, Paul MH, Reisch JS: Pulmonary vascular disease in total anomalous pulmonary venous drainage. *Circulation* **61**:103, 1980

133. Naeye RL: Perinatal vascular changes associated with underdevelopment of the left heart. *Am J Pathol* **41**:287, 1962

134. Haworth SG, Reid L: Quantitative structural study of pulmonary circulation in the newborn with aortic atresia, stenosis or coarctation. *Thorax* **32**:121, 1977

135. Haworth SG, Reid L: Structural study of pulmonary circulation and of heart in total anomalous pulmonary venous return in early infancy. *Br Heart J* **39**:80, 1977

136. Norwood WI Jr, Kirklin JK, Sanders SP: Hypoplastic left heart syndrome: Experience with palliative surgery. *Am J Cardiol* **45**:87, 1980

137. Macartney FJ, Deverall PB, Scott O: Hemodynamic characteristics of systemic arterial blood supply to the lungs. *Br Heart J* **35**:28, 1973

138. Heath D, DuShane JW, Wood EH, Edwards JE: The aetiology of pulmonary thrombosis in cyanotic congenital heart with pulmonary stenosis. *Thorax* **13**:213, 1958

139. Wagenvoort CA, Edwards JE: The pulmonary arterial tree in pulmonic atresia. *Arch Pathol* **71**:646, 1961

140. Ferencz C: The pulmonary vascular bed in tetralogy of Fallot. I. Changes associated with pulmonary stenosis. II. Changes following a systemic-pulmonary arterial anastomosis. *Bull Johns Hopkins Hops* **106**:81, 100, 1960

141. Hislop A, Reid L: Structural changes in the pulmonary arteries and veins in tetralogy of Fallot. *Br Heart J* **35**:1178, 1973

142. Haworth SG, Reid L: Quantitative structural study of pulmonary circulation in the newborn with pulmonary atresia. *Thorax* **32**:129, 1977

143. Rabinovitch M, Herrera deLeon V, Castaneda AR, Reid L: The pulmonary vascular bed in patients with tetralogy of Fallot with and without pulmonary atresia. *Circulation* **64**:1234, 1981

144. Haworth SG, Macartney FJ: Growth and development of the pulmonary circulation in pulmonary atresia with ventricular septal defect and major aortopulmonary collateral arteries. *Br Heart J* **44**:14, 1980

145. Thiene G, Frescura C, Bini RM, et al: Histology of pulmonary arterial supply in pulmonary atresia with ventricular septal defect. *Circulation* **60**:1066, 1979

146. Rabinovitch M, Sanders SP, Castaneda AR, Reid L: Morphometric analysis of lung biopsy tissue in candidates for Fontan-type surgial procedures (Abstr). *Am J Cardiol* **47**:947, 1981

147. Rosenberg HC, Williams WG, Trusler GA, et al: Structural composition of central pulmonary artery shunts. *J Thorac Cardiovasc Surg* **94**:498, 1987

148. LaBourene JI, Coles JG, Johnson DJ, et al: Alterations in elastin and collagen related to the pathogenesis of pulmonary venous obstruction in a piglet model. *Circ Res* **66**:438, 1990

149. Silove ED, Tavernor WD, Berry CL: Reactive pulmonary arterial hypertension after pulmonary venous constriction in the calf. *Cardiovasc Res* **6**:36, 1972

150. Levin DL, Mills LJ, Parkey M: Morphological development of the pulmonary vascular bed in experimental coarctation of the aorta. *Circulation* **59**:349, 1979

151. Levin DL, Heymann MA, Rudolph AM: Morphological development of the pulmonary vascular bed in experimental pulmonic stenosis. *Circulation* **59**:179, 1979

152. Haworth SG, deLeval M, Macartney FJ: Hypo- and hypertension in the immature lung: Pulmonary arterial development following ligation of the left pulmonary artery in the newborn pig. *J Thorac Cardiovasc Surg* **82**:281, 1981

63

Palliative Procedures in Cyanotic Congenital Heart Disease

James L. Zellner and Robert M. Sade

Before 1945, infants with obstructive lesions of the right heart, reduced pulmonary blood flow, and right-to-left shunt usually had short lives characterized by progressive cyanosis, cerebrovascular or other vascular accidents, brain abscess, arrhythmias, or heart failure. The introduction of the subclavian artery-to-pulmonary artery shunt by Alfred Blalock and Helen Taussig in 1945[1] opened the door to palliation of tetralogy of Fallot and other cyanotic lesions. Other varieties of aortopulmonary shunts and the addition of the cavopulmonary anastomosis offered new alternatives for palliation. Palliative shunts that increase pulmonary blood flow are still widely used as life-saving procedures in infants who cannot undergo definitive repair until later in childhood, or, in rare cases, who cannot be offered repair at all. Prostaglandin E_1 can reopen or maintain patency of the ductus arteriosus in the neonate, reducing the urgency of performing shunts and allowing resuscitation of the patient preoperatively.[2]

The objective of a palliative shunt is to increase delivery of desaturated venous blood to the lungs. Patients with obstructive right heart defects may be severely symptomatic from cyanosis resulting from inadequate pulmonary blood flow. Symptoms and signs in the newborn may include severe hypoxia, metabolic acidosis, and respiratory distress. In the child, symptoms of chronic hypoxia may include failure to grow and develop normally, syncope during cyanotic spells, and easy fatigability. In older children, severe polycythemia resulting from cyanosis may be associated with vascular accidents, brain abscess, and cardiac arrhythmias. A successful shunt decreases cyanosis, polycythemia, and the symptoms with which they are associated. Increased pulmonary blood flow may also increase the size of hypoplastic pulmonary arteries. In addition, increased pul-

monary venous return may increase the capacity of the left atrium and ventricle. These benefits may be achieved by a systemic artery-to-pulmonary artery shunt or a cavopulmonary anastomosis. The choice of shunt depends on a number of anatomic and physiologic considerations.

SUBCLAVIAN ARTERY-TO-PULMONARY ARTERY SHUNT (BLALOCK–TAUSSIG)

The first subclavian artery-to-pulmonary artery anastomosis was performed in 1944 by Blalock on a severely cyanotic 15-mo-old girl.[1] By the early 1950s, he performed this operation on 779 patients with tetralogy of Fallot.[3] It rapidly became recognized as an excellent means of palliating cyanotic heart disease and is still, in one of its modifications, the most commonly performed operation to increase pulmonary blood flow. Its popularity is due to the predictability of blood flow through it: the diameter of the subclavian artery limits flow so that it is rarely excessive, yet the flow is great enough to provide good palliation.

Anastomosis of the end of the divided subclavian or innominate artery to the side of the pulmonary artery (Fig. 63–1) was the original or standard procedure. It is generally done on the side of the chest containing the innominate artery, contralateral to the side containing the aortic arch (because the aortic arch and the innominate artery are paired derivatives of the embryonic fourth aortic arch, they are always on opposite sides). The main advantage of using the subclavian artery that arises from the innominate artery is the extra vessel length that can be achieved by dissecting the innominate and carotid arteries. In contrast, kinking of the subclavian origin often occurs when it arises directly

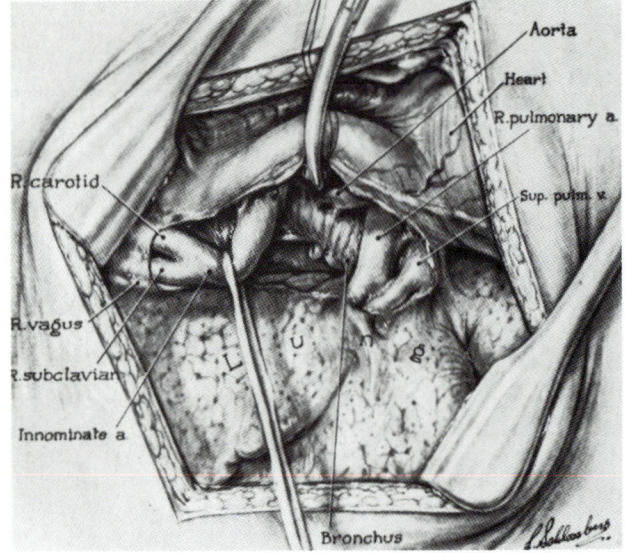

A

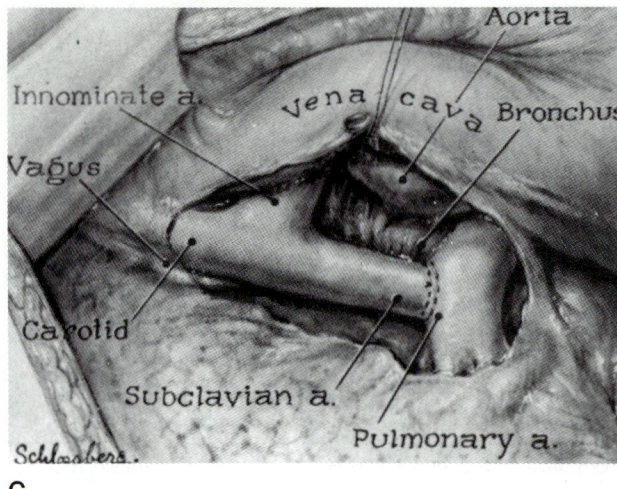

C

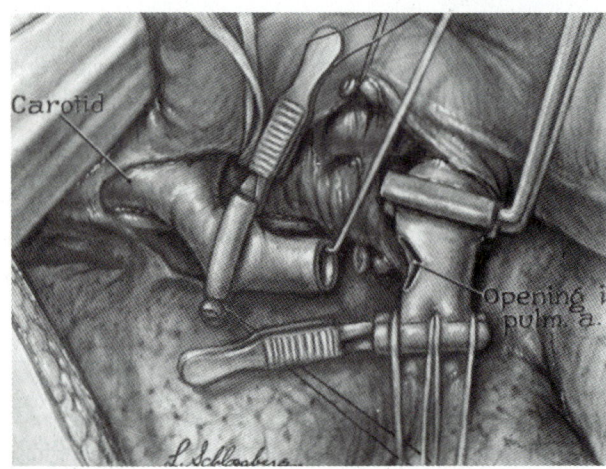

B

Figure 63–1. Technique of the standard Blalock–Taussig shunt.
A. This shunt is usually done on the side contralateral to the aortic
arch. The pulmonary artery and the innominate or subclavian artery
and its branches are mobilized, taking care to avoid injury to the
phrenic and recurrent laryngeal nerves. **B.** The subclavian artery
is clamped proximally and divided. It is pulled through the loop of the
recurrent laryngeal nerve (not shown in these drawings). Proximal
and distal control of the pulmonary artery is obtained and a
longitudinal arteriotomy is made. **C.** An end-to-side anastomosis is
completed using an averting continuous suture of silk, as depicted
here in one of Blalock's early papers, or with a simple continuous
absorbable suture like polydioxanone, as is our current practice.
*(From Blalock A: Surgical procedures employed and anatomical
variations encountered in the treatment of congenital pulmonic
stenosis. By permission of Surgery, Gynecology & Obstetrics
87:385, 1948.)*

from the aortic arch (i.e., on the side ipsilateral to the arch).
If the use of this vessel is necessary, as in a patient with a
previous standard Blalock–Taussig shunt, kinking can often
be prevented by subclavian arterioplasty.[4]

Most authors report excellent short- and long-term results with the Blalock–Taussig shunt.[3,5–7] The operation is
technically more difficult in the newborn due to shorter
length of the subclavian artery, smaller diameters of the
vessels involved, and more delicate structure of the small
vessels.[8] Some investigators have reported high morbidity
and mortality rates in infants operated on during the first
few weeks of life.[8] Additionally, smaller size makes distances from nearby nerves shorter, so injuries to the phrenic
nerve and the recurrent laryngeal nerve are more frequent in
newborns.[9] With improvements in anesthetic and microsurgical techniques, however, complications have become less
frequent and the safety and efficacy of the procedure have
been demonstrated even in newborns.[5–7,10,11]

The advantages of the Blalock–Taussig shunt are
many. Postoperative congestive heart failure is much less

common than with central aortopulmonary shunts. Shunt
flow, because it is limited by the diameter of the subclavian
artery, is seldom excessive. The shunt also may grow with
the child, often allowing many years of palliation.[3] Distortion of the pulmonary artery is uncommon and ligation of
the shunt is often easier than take-down of central aortopulmonary shunts at the time of the corrective procedure.

The Blalock–Taussig shunt also has several potential
complications. Shunt thrombosis or inadequate flow may
necessitate early or late reoperation. One cause of inadequate flow is stenosis of the anastomosis from tension on
the suture line or poor growth. A stenotic anastomosis may
be enlarged by use of a vein patch across the suture line.[12]
Injury to the phrenic nerve may cause serious respiratory
insufficiency, ventilator dependence, and need for diaphragmatic plication, especially in newborns in whom
phrenic nerve injury may be associated with a high mortality rate.[9] Other potential complications include Horner's
syndrome, hemorrhage from hilar collaterals, and lymphatic
leak with chylothorax. An intrapericardial approach to

avoid these complications has been proposed.[13] When the subclavian artery is divided, gangrene of the arm may rarely (0.2%) occur,[14] and many years after artery division a slight decrease in dimensions of the affected arm may be detected.[15] Pulmonary hypertension may develop after a Blalock–Taussig shunt, but this occurs much less commonly than after central aortopulmonary shunts.[16,17]

The technical difficulty of constructing a Blalock–Taussig shunt in small infants and the disadvantages of central aortopulmonary shunts (congestive heart failure, deformity of the pulmonary arteries) led to the use of prosthetic materials. Woven and knitted arterial grafts have not worked well because of early occlusion of small-diameter grafts by neointimal proliferation. Polytetrafluoroethylene tubes were introduced as vascular prostheses in 1972[18] and their use in vascular surgery became widespread, including implantation as aortopulmonary shunts for palliating cyanotic heart disease.[19] The modified Blalock–Taussig shunt consists of a polytetrafluoroethylene interposition graft between the side of the subclavian artery and the side of the pulmonary artery[20,21] (Fig. 63–2). The shunt is often constructed on the side ipsilateral to the aortic arch because the subclavian artery is usually longer before branching and there is less risk of recurrent laryngeal nerve injury.

Advantages over the standard shunt include less tendency to deform hypoplastic pulmonary arteries, less need for mediastinal dissection, preservation of subclavian arterial circulation to the upper extremity, and consistent shunt flow regardless of anatomic distances between aortic branches and pulmonary arteries.[22–26] In a series of 52 children undergoing modified or standard Blalock–Taussig shunts at our institution, several advantages of modified over standard shunts were found: greater pulmonary artery growth (increase in pulmonary artery index from 144 to 431 mm²/m² versus 118 to 189 mm²/m²), less frequent distortion of hypoplastic pulmonary arteries (4/11 versus 6/8), and less frequent early and late graft failure (4/24 versus 15/29).[27] Congestive heart failure is as uncommon after modified as after standard Blalock–Taussig shunt, as shunt flow is limited by subclavian arterial size.[19,28] To prevent congestive heart failure, care must be taken to avoid extending the graft anastomosis proximally onto a larger vessel (aorta or innominate artery), as the subclavian artery will then no longer limit flow. Graft thrombosis is uncommon, and has been successfully treated with low-dose streptokinase infusion.[29]

Although an important advantage of the modified Blalock–Taussig shunt is to preserve subclavian artery continuity, partial or complete obstruction of the artery distal to the graft has been reported.[24] Leakage of serous fluid through the polytetrafluoroethylene graft has been described[30] and may occur in the thorax, causing prolonged chest tube drainage and seroma formation.[31] We have not seen this complication, but others have reported that intraluminal fibrin glue at reoperation may control the serous leak.[32] Another rare but serious complication is false aneurysm formation,[33] which may present with fatal massive hemoptysis.

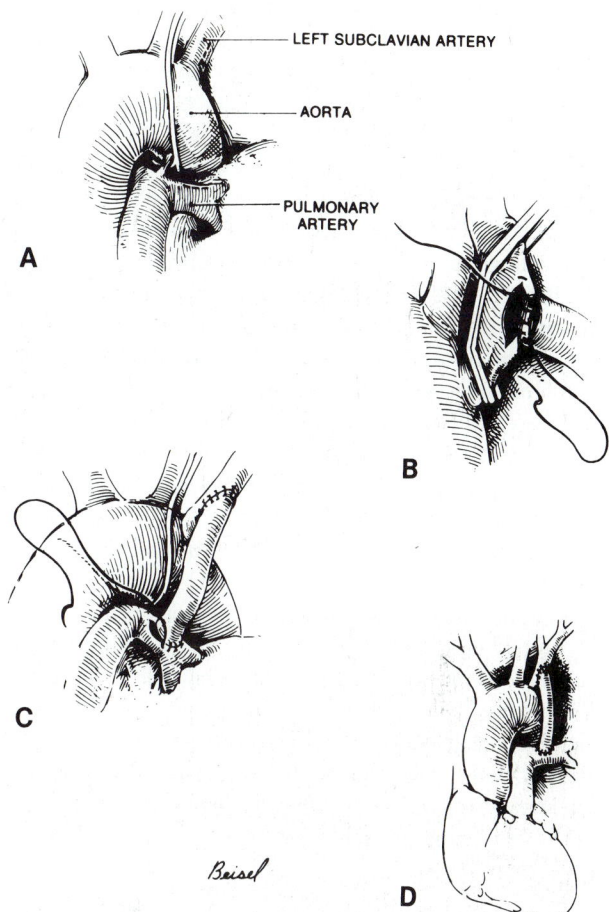

LEFT SUBCLAVIAN ARTERY

AORTA

PULMONARY ARTERY

Beisel

Figure 63–2. Technique of the modified Blalock–Taussig shunt. **A.** This shunt is usually performed on the side ipsilateral to the aortic arch. The subclavian artery and pulmonary artery are mobilized, carefully protecting the phrenic nerve from injury. Sites of incisions in the arteries are demonstrated. **B.** After vascular control is obtained, an incision in the subclavian artery and an end-to-end anastomosis completed between the artery and the Gore-Tex graft, with a continuous polypropylene suture. A 4- or 5-mm graft is used, depending on the size of the child. **C.** Vascular control of the pulmonary artery can be obtained with a vascular clamp proximally and encircling ligatures on distal branches, or with a single vascular C-clamp. A longitudinal arteriotomy is made in the pulmonary artery and an end-to-side anastomosis is performed with a continuous polypropylene suture. **D.** The completed shunt is demonstrated. Shunt flow is determined not by the diameter of the Gore-Tex graft, but by the subclavian artery size. *(From Waldhausen JA, Pierce WS: Johnson's Surgery of the Chest, 5th ed. Chicago, Year Book Medical Publisher, 1985, p 369, with permission.)*

DESCENDING AORTA-TO-LEFT PULMONARY ARTERY SHUNT (POTTS)

The success of the Blalock–Taussig shunt led other investigators to explore alternative methods of systemic-to-pulmonary shunts. In 1946, Potts and his co-workers described an anastomosis between the descending thoracic aorta and the left pulmonary artery.[34] It had been previously demonstrated that completely cross-clamping the aorta could cause paralysis in animals,[35,36] so a specially designed clamp was used to allow partial occlusion of the aorta while maintaining some distal flow. This was successful in preventing paralysis. Two years later, Potts reported the results of a series of 29 patients who had undergone this shunt for tetralogy of Fallot and tricuspid atresia.[37] Mortality was 13.8% and all the surviving children were described as improved.

Advantages of the shunt are its ease of construction and usual good palliation. Flow is dependent, however, upon the size of the anastomosis, and, unlike the subclavian diameter in the Blalock–Taussig shunt, there is no anatomic regulator of flow. Minor variations in the size of a Potts anastomosis may greatly affect shunt flow. For example, in a newborn, palliation will not be adequate if the anastomotic diameter is less than 2.5 mm, but congestive heart failure may develop due to too large a left-to-right shunt if the diameter is larger than 3.5 mm.[38,39] Pulmonary artery hypertension and pulmonary vascular obstructive disease may result from long-standing excessive flow.[40]

Another major disadvantage of the Potts shunt is difficulty in taking down the shunt at the time of definitive repair. Shunt occlusion is facilitated at the time of repair by use of deep hypothermia and circulatory arrest, during which the anastomosis is closed through a transpulmonary approach.[41] Because of difficulty in closing the shunt and the tendency for patients to develop congestive heart failure, the Potts shunt is rarely used.[42]

ASCENDING AORTA-TO-RIGHT PULMONARY ARTERY SHUNT (WATERSTON)

In 1955, Davidson[43] described an intrapericardial anastomosis of the ascending aorta to the main pulmonary artery that successfully palliated a severely symptomatic child with tetralogy of Fallot. He suggested that this shunt might be applicable to patients with branch pulmonary stenosis in whom a Blalock–Taussig shunt would be difficult, and proposed several advantages: the shunt provides balanced shunt flow to the two pulmonary arteries, is associated with little pulmonary artery distortion, and is easy to close through the main pulmonary artery at the time of definitive repair.

A similar ascending aorta-to-pulmonary artery shunt was reported by Waterston[44] in 1962 as an alternative to the standard Blalock–Taussig shunt. Ten years later, he and his colleagues[45] reported the results of the first 100 Waterston shunts. Hospital mortality was 26% overall, but was higher in infants (43%) than older children (12%). With careful preoperative evaluation and perioperative care, its safety in the neonate has been established.[46]

This shunt is relatively easy to construct in patients of all ages (Fig. 63–3). It has the advantage of a high patency rate, even when the right pulmonary artery is hypoplastic, as well as excellent palliation of cyanosis.

A common complication of the Waterston shunt is kinking of the pulmonary artery with resultant unequal flow distribution to the lungs and later, hypoplasia of the lower-flow pulmonary artery.[47–50] This problem is especially likely if the aortotomy is made in the posterolateral wall of the aorta rather than in the posterior midline.[51] It has also been suggested that kinking may develop due to differential growth and realignment of the great arteries, even when the shunt has initially been properly constructed.[49]

Difficulty of take-down of the anastomosis varies with the degree of pulmonary artery distortion and hypoplasia. In cases of minimal distortion, the anastomosis may be closed through an aortotomy with sutures or with a patch.[50,52] In cases of moderate distortion, a pulmonary arterioplasty may be performed by dissecting the pulmonary artery off the aorta and closing the enlarged pulmonary arteriotomy with a patch.[47] In severe cases, more extensive reconstruction of the pulmonary artery may be required.[48]

As with the Potts anastomosis, excessive flow may occur, even if the anastomosis is only slightly too large, causing congestive heart failure.[45,46] This can usually be managed with digitalis and diuretics, but such nonoperative therapy is usually less successful than with a Blalock–Taussig shunt and revision of the anastomosis is sometimes required to decrease shunt flow.[42] As with all other causes of prolonged excessive pulmonary blood flow, pulmonary vascular obstructive disease may be a late complication. The Waterston shunt has been used less frequently than the Blalock–Taussig shunt because of these potential complications.

SUPERIOR VENA CAVA-TO-PULMONARY ARTERY SHUNT (GLENN)

Anastomosis of the superior vena cava (SVC) to the right pulmonary artery as a means of palliating cyanotic heart disease was first proposed by Carlon and co-workers[54] in 1951 after experimenting on human cadavers and dogs. The clinical effectiveness of the cavopulmonary anastomosis was demonstrated by Glenn in 1958.[55] During the next several years the cavopulmonary anastomosis was used to palliate a variety of cyanotic congenital heart defects.[53,56]

The operation is performed through a right thoracotomy. The standard shunt consists of an anastomosis between the distal end of the divided right pulmonary artery and the side of the SVC. The SVC is ligated at the cavoatrial junction to direct all of its flow to the right lung.

The potential benefits are many. Pulmonary artery hypertension rarely develops, presumably because the shunted blood is at venous (low) pressure. The shunt does not increase the volume of work of the heart because venous return to the heart is unchanged by the shunt: the superior caval flow merely returns to the heart as saturated blood in the pulmonary veins rather than as desaturated blood in the caval orifice.[57]

There are several physiologic and anatomic limitations

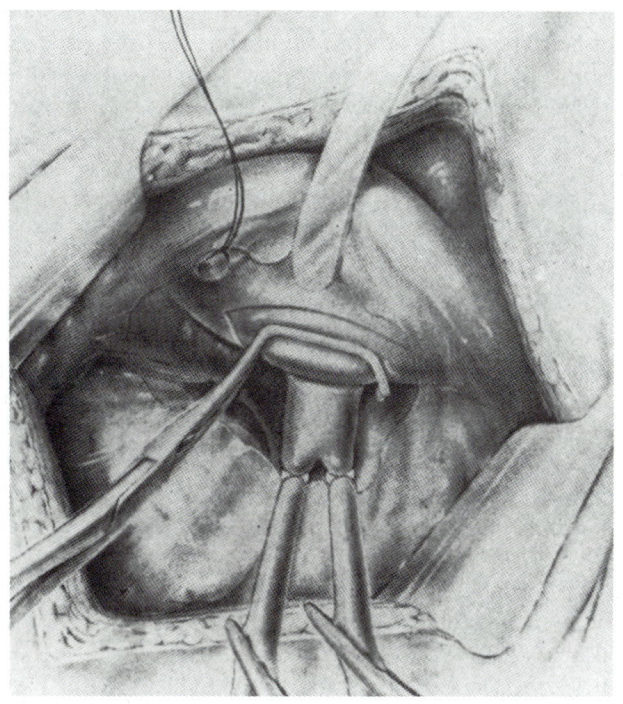

A

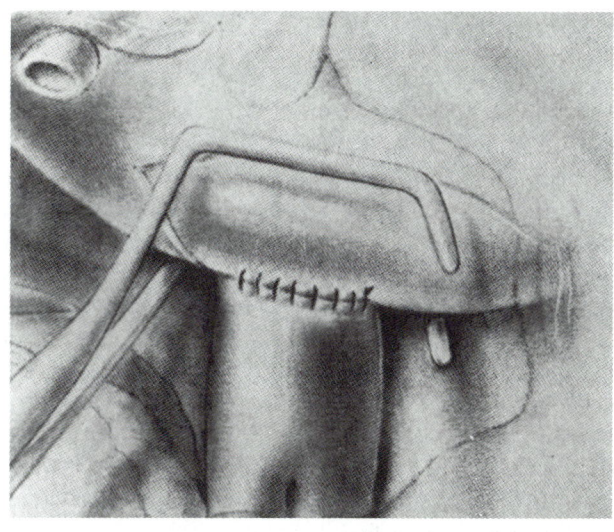

C

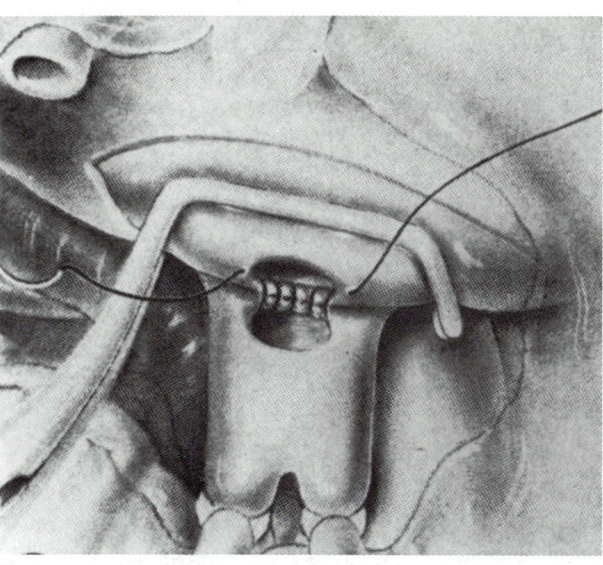

B

Figure 63–3. Technique of the Waterston shunt. **A.** Through a right thoracotomy, the aorta is approached posterior to the superior vena cava to ensure that the anastomosis is made directly posterior in the aorta. Division of the azygous vein is usually helpful. The right pulmonary artery and its branches are mobilized. After vascular control of the branches is obtained with encircling ligatures or tourniquets, a partial occlusion clamp is positioned so that one jaw lies behind the right pulmonary artery. Approximation of the jaws of the clamp completely occludes the proximal right pulmonary artery nd partially excludes the ascending aorta. The excluded portion of the aorta must include the posterior midline. **B.** Parallel incisions are made in the pulmonary artery and aorta. The size of the incisions must be accurate to avoid too large a shunt flow and yet provide adequate palliation. In a newborn, an anastomotic diameter of 3 mm is the goal, and can be achieved with incisions 4.5–5.0 mm long (9–10 mm circumference). A side-to-side anastomosis is performed using a continuous nonabsorbable suture. **C.** The anastomosis is completed and occlusion is released to establish flow through the shunt. *(From Waterston DJ et al: Surg 72:897, 1972, with permission.)*

to the operation, however. Pulmonary vascular resistance must be low, so small infants (under 3–6 mo of age) and patients with even mild pulmonary hypertension of any origin are not candidates.[58] Size of the right pulmonary artery is also critical: it must have a diameter of at least 50% of the SVC diameter or it will obstruct blood flow.[59,60] The consequence of obstruction to cavopulmonary blood flow, whether due to high pulmonary artery pressure, small pulmonary artery, or mechanical narrowing of the anastomosis, is superior venal caval hypertension, cerebral edema, and often, death.

A major late complication of cavopulmonary anasto-

mosis is increasing cyanosis, often caused by decreased perfusion of both the ipsilateral and contralateral lungs.[56,58] Decreased flow to the contralateral lung may be caused by progression of the original lesion obstructing blood flow from the ventricle to the pulmonary artery, or peripheral pulmonary vascular occlusion, usually caused by intravascular thrombosis. The ipsilateral lung may have decreased flow for several reasons. Polycythemia consequent to hypoxemia increases blood viscosity, which in turn diminishes flow through the pulmonary vascular bed. Connections between the SVC and the right atrium may either persist (e.g., a left SVC or azygous vein) or develop after the shunt (e.g., venous collaterals from superior to inferior vena cava). These connections allow venous blood to bypass the lungs and hypoxemia increases.

Another important cause of decreased shunt function 5–10 years after the operation has received much attention. Radioisotope studies have demonstrated maldistribution of SVC blood flow through the right lung.[61] Most of the blood perfuses the lower lobe and the flow to the upper and middle lobes is significantly decreased. This is thought to be caused by gravitational forces as well as the nonpulsatile nature of cavopulmonary flow. Furthermore, it has been documented by oximetry, contrast echocardiography, and angiography that arteriovenous malformations may develop in the hyperperfused lower lobe, which may contribute to shunt failure.[62] This complication has been treated in several different ways: embolization of the fistulas,[63] connecting the lower lobe veins to the right atrium,[62] lobectomy, and functional pneumonectomy (reconnection of the SVC to the right atrium and ligation of the right pulmonary artery).[64]

In patients who have undergone a cavopulmonary anastomosis and who are becoming more cyanotic from inadequate shunt flow, a corrective operation should be done if the patient is hemodynamically a candidate. If this is not feasible, a second shunt, such as a Blalock–Taussig or central aortopulmonary shunt, may be life saving. A right axillary arteriovenous fistula may be constructed to increase flow through the shunt.[65] This may lead a pulsatile character to blood flow through the shunt, improving flow through underperfused portions of the lung.[66]

The cavopulmonary anastomosis is infrequently used to augment pulmonary blood flow because of these late sequelae and because it is difficult to reconstruct the SVC and right pulmonary artery at corrective operation.

The indications for a cavopulmonary anastomosis at present are controversial.[67] The shunt may be useful in lesions like tricuspid atresia for which ultimate repair will be a right atrium-to-pulmonary artery connection (Fontan procedure).[65,68,69] An important disadvantage of the cavopulmonary anastomosis for initial palliation of tricuspid atresia is that this anastomosis commits the right pulmonary artery (normally containing about 55% of the pulmonary capillary bed) to the SVC drainage [only one-third (adults) to one-half (infants) of the systemic venous return].[70] While reconstruction of the cavoatrial junction at the time of definitive repair may be possible, it sometimes cannot be done, leaving a permanent mismatch between the volume of systemic venous return to each lung and available pulmonary capillary bed.

Our current practice seldom includes cavopulmonary anastomosis. We have used it occasionally, however, as the first step of a staged Fontan-like repair when right and left pulmonary arteries are discontinuous. In such cases, a cavopulmonary anastomosis may be performed using the right pulmonary artery, and at subsequent Fontan repair, the right atrium may be connected to the left pulmonary artery.

If cavoatrial continuity can be simultaneously re-established, both pulmonary arteries are open to the right atrium, allowing balanced distribution of systemic venous return to the two pulmonary arteries.

BIDIRECTIONAL CAVOPULMONARY ANASTOMOSIS AND HEMI-FONTAN PROCEDURE

The Fontan procedure and its variants, termed orthoterminal correction,[71] is the final goal for surgical treatment of patients with a single ventricle. However, certain anatomic and physiologic factors such as young age, poor ventricular function, small pulmonary arteries, and elevated pulmonary vascular resistance militate against the successful outcome of a Fontan procedure as the initial method of surgical management.

Recently, several methods have been introduced to achieve orthoterminal correction in stages, allowing gradual physiologic adjustment to dramatic changes acutely imposed by the Fontan operation. The bidirectional cavopulmonary anastomosis is a palliative procedure that provides adequate arterial oxygenation without increasing ventricular work, deforming the pulmonary arteries, or risking increases in pulmonary vascular resistance. In addition, other anatomical risk factors may be addressed at this setting. These include reconstruction of pulmonary artery deformities and resection of subaortic stenosis. A specific variant of the bidirectional cavopulmonary anastomosis, the hemi-Fontan operation, is described below.

Like the Glenn shunt, the bidirectional cavopulmonary anastomosis augments pulmonary flow without increasing ventricular work. In contrast to the classic shunt, however, the bidirectional cavopulmonary anastomosis directs SVC return to both lungs, providing bilateral pulmonary blood flow and avoiding the mismatch to flow to capillary bed seen in the classic shunt.[72]

Based on the work by Carlon in 1951, Haller and co-workers performed a bidirectional cavopulmonary anastomosis experimentally in 1966.[73] Hopkins later reported the utility of the bidirectional cavopulmonary shunt in congenital cyanotic heart disease.[72] In 1990 Lamberti et al reported a series of 17 infants and small children who underwent a bidirectional cavopulmonary anastomosis as palliation for single ventricle complex, hypoplastic right heart syndrome, and hypoplastic left ventricle.[74]

Typically, a right thoracotomy or median sternotomy can be used and the procedure may be performed with or without cardiopulmonary bypass. The pericardium is entered anterior to the phrenic nerve and the pulmonary artery is completely dissected. The azygous vein is ligated and divided. If cardiopulmonary bypass has not been used, the SVC may be shunted to the right atrium at this time to prevent venous hypertension. After heparinization, the SVC is divided a few millimeters above the right atrium. It is then anastomosed to the right pulmonary artery, avoiding kinking or twisting of either vessel.

Successful palliation of cyanotic congenital heart defects using the bidirectional cavopulmonary anastomosis has been reported by Pridjian, Albanese and others.[74–77] In a recent review, 50 patients aged 1 to 60 mo (median 12 mo) were palliated using the bidirectional cavopulmonary anastomosis.[75] Defects palliated included hypoplastic left heart, pulmonary atresia with intact ventricular septum, tricuspid atresia, double-inlet left ventricle, heterotaxy syndrome, and Ebstein's anomaly. Survival was 92% at 13 mo following the procedure. Significant risk factors for increased mortality included pulmonary vascular resistance greater than 3 Wood's units and the presence of significant pulmonary artery distortion requiring reconstruction. Albanese et al reported that heterotaxia syndrome and preoperative mean pulmonary artery pressure greater than 15 mm Hg were additional risk factors for increased mortality.[76] Complications of the bidirectional cavopulmonary anastomosis include prolonged pleural effusion, branch pulmonary artery stenosis. SVC syndrome, pulmonary arteriovenous malformations, and phrenic nerve injury.

Recently, bidirectional cavopulmonary anastomosis supplemented with a systemic-to-pulmonary artery shunt has been attempted to palliate those patients with cyanotic defects and increased pulmonary artery pressure. The safety and efficacy of adding pulsatile pulmonary flow to the bidirectional cavopulmonary anastomosis has been demonstrated by Matsuda.[76] A further modification of the bidirectional cavopulmonary anastomosis is the anastomosis of both ends of the divided SVC to the right pulmonary artery with placement of a prosthetic patch on the cardiac side of the SVC.[75,78] This modification makes the procedure similar in function to the hemi-Fontan operation.

The hemi-Fontan procedure is a refinement of the bidirectional cavopulmonary anastomosis: the ventricle is unloaded of all pulmonary work, deformity of the pulmonary artery is avoided, as is pulmonary vascular obstructive disease. In addition, however, all anatomically correctable risk factors for the Fontan procedure are repaired, and the Fontan anatomy is completely established, making the final stage a relatively simple procedure.

Cardiopulmonary bypass is established and deep hypothermia is used if needed. Aortopulmonary shunts are taken down and the azygous vein is ligated. The main pulmonary artery, if one is present, is divided and its proximal end closed. The opening in the main pulmonary artery is extended onto the right pulmonary artery behind the SVC, and also as far leftward as is needed to open any left pulmonary artery stenoses. The SVC is opened at the cavoatrial junction. The posterior aspect of the cavoatrial opening is then anastomosed to the inferior border of the right pulmonary arteriotomy. A prosthetic patch is sewn to the cavoatrial junction, thereby separating the right atrium from the cavoatriopulmonary anastomosis. A cryopreserved pulmonary artery homograft is then shaped and sewn to the remaining edges of the pulmonary artery and SVC, creating a widely open cavoatriopulmonary anastomosis (Figs. 63–4, 63–5).

The hemi-Fontan operation functions similarly to the bidirectional cavopulmonary anastomosis: unsaturated blood flowing through the shunt is not pumped by the ventricle,

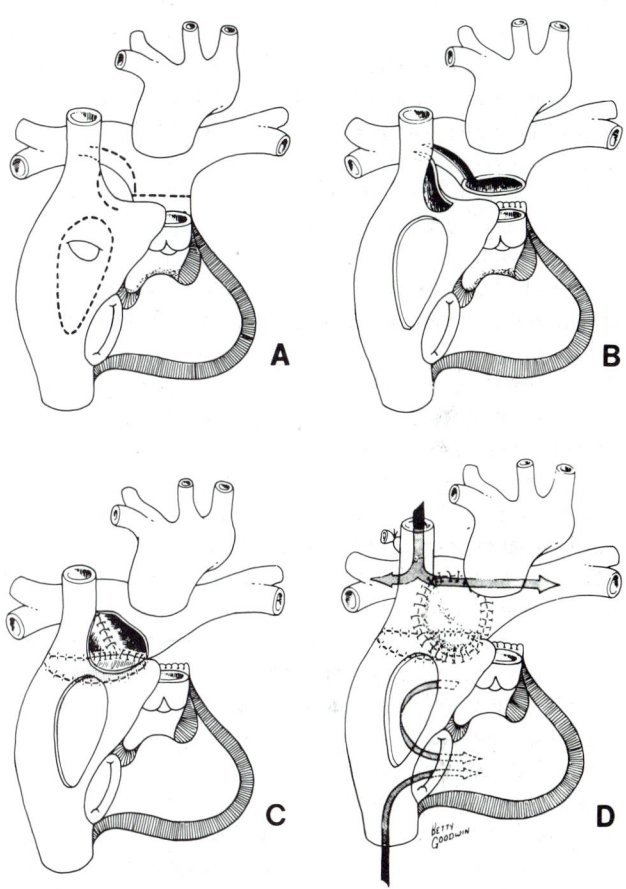

Figure 63–4. Technique of hemi-Fontan. **A.** A heart with a single ventricle and mitral atresia anatomy with the aorta cut away is illustrated. Incisions are indicated by dotted lines. **B.** A large atrial septal defect is created and the common pulmonary artery is transected and oversewn proximally. The incision in the open pulmonary artery is carried anteriorly onto the right pulmonary artery immediately posterior to the superior vena cave (SVC). The SVC is opened at the cavoatrial junction, and the incision spirals cephalad around the medial border of the SVC and ends posteriorly adjacent to the right pulmonary arteriotomy. It extends also into the base of the right atrial appendage. **C.** The posterior border of the cavotrial opening is sewn to the inferior edge of the pulmonary arteriotomy. A Gore-Tex patch is then sewn to the right atrium immediately below the cavoatrial junction through the open anastomosis, separating the atrium from the cavoatriopulmonary anastomosis. **D.** A patch of autogenous pericardium or (especially if deformed pulmonary arteries are being reconstructed) cryopreserved pulmonary artery homograft is cut to an appropriate shape and is sewn to the remaining edge of the pulmonary artery and carried onto the cavoatrial portion of the anastomosis. This patch lies lateral and posterior to the aorta. The SVC drainage goes into both pulmonary arteries, while the inferior vena caval drainage mixes with the pulmonary venous return in the single ventricle.

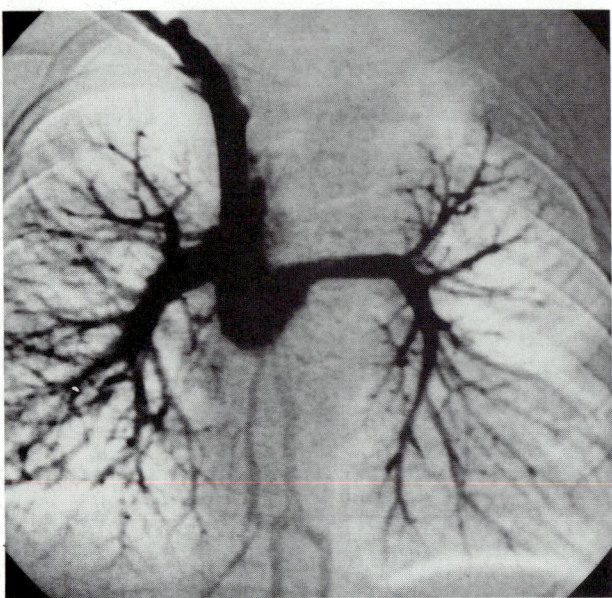

Figure 63–5. Pulmonary arteriogram in anterior posterior projection demonstrates flow of blood from the SVC to the pulmonary arteries through the cavoatriopulmonary anastomosis.

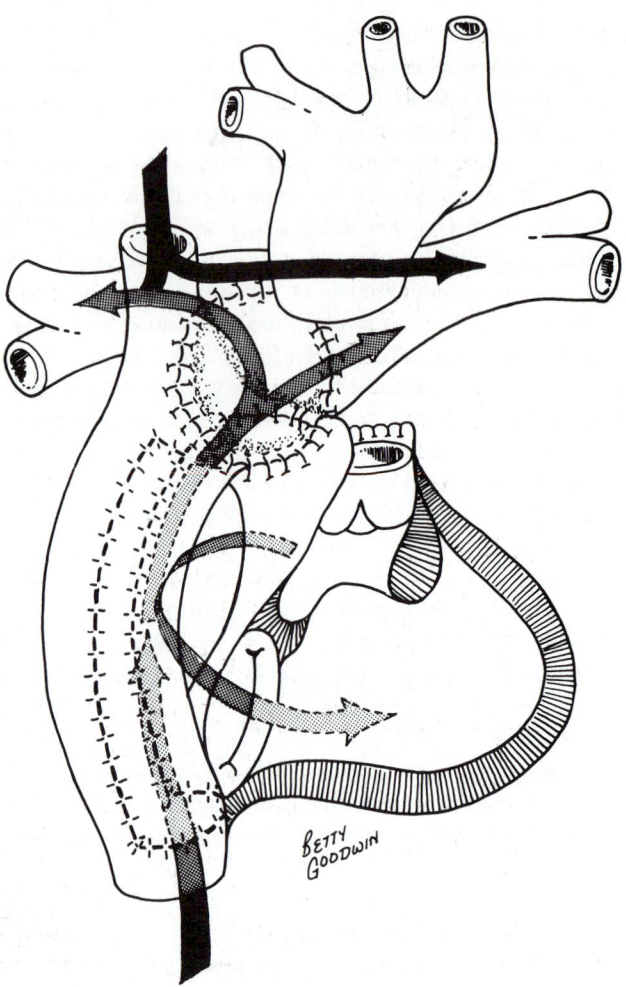

Figure 63–6. Conversion of hemi-Fontan to Fontan anatomy. The Fontan procedure is completed in the final stage by opening the right atrium, removing the atriopulmonary patch, and implanting a baffle from the inferior vena cava to the cavoatriopulmonary anastomosis. This directs all systemic venous return to the pulmonary arteries (arrows in the pulmonary arteries) and all pulmonary venous return to the ventricle (arrow in the ventricle).

thus relieving the ventricle of pulmonary volume work. However, it differs in that all sources of pulmonary blood flow other than the SVC and small peripheral aortopulmonary collaterals are interrupted. This unloads the ventricle of pulmonary volume work more completely. In addition, the Fontan reconstruction is virtually complete, requiring at subsequent operation only repositioning of the atriopulmonary patch to separate the systemic and pulmonary circulations (Fig. 63–6).

Three groups of patients with a single ventricle who may benefit from the hemi-Fontan operation have been described by Douville et al[79]: (1) children who are candidates for a Fontan operation but are at increased risk, such as patients with high pulmonary artery pressure or increased pulmonary vascular resistance, high end-diastolic pressure, significant pulmonary artery deformation, ventricular hypertrophy with subaortic obstruction; (2) children who may physiologically benefit from early unloading of ventricular volume, such as those with pulmonary atresia with intact ventricular septum; and (3) children who early after Fontan operation are experiencing low cardiac output with elevated pulmonary artery pressure.

CHOOSING A SHUNT

Choosing the most appropriate palliative shunt must be individualized, considering the patient's age and size, the underlying anatomy, the definitive operation that will be required, the anatomy of the pulmonary arteries, the patient's general condition, and the severity of cyanosis. Some general guidelines can be formulated, however, and the following schema reflects our current practice.

Newborns and older children with pulmonary stenosis or atresia (including tetralogy of Fallot) undergo a modified Blalock–Taussig shunt if the pulmonary arteries are normal or only moderately hypoplastic. This usually provides excellent palliation without significant complications until corrective surgery can be done.

If the pulmonary arteries are severely hypoplastic, a central aortopulmonary shunt may be preferred: a polytetrafluoroethylene interposition graft from the aorta to the main or branch pulmonary artery, though a Waterston shunt may be a reasonable alternative. These shunts can provide palliation while allowing the pulmonary arteries to grow as a consequence of increased flow. Concern about congestive heart failure due to increased pulmonary blood flow is minimal because severely hypoplastic pulmonary arteries will not usually permit large flow.

When an initial aortopulmonary shunt fails, the definitive corrective operation should be done. If this is not feasible, the original shunt may need to be revised or a second shunt performed.

Young infants who have tricuspid atresia or univentricular heart with anatomy ultimately amenable to a Fontan procedure are palliated with a modified Blalock–Taussig shunt. For patients 4 mo of age or older, bidirectional cavopulmonary anastomosis is the best choice for palliation. When the initial Blalock–Taussig shunt fails in a future Fontan candidate, we avoid a second shunt, proceeding instead directly to hemi-Fontan procedure in patients 4–12 mo of age, or to corrective operation in patients older than a year.

Patients with right and left pulmonary artery discontinuity may be best treated with a staged repair. If the pulmonary arteries are small, the initial stage can be a polytetrafluoroethylene graft from the side of the aorta to the divided end of one or both small pulmonary arteries. This shunt may induce sufficient growth of the small vessel to permit a subsequent Fontan repair. If discontinuous pulmonary arteries are of adequate size, a standard cavopulmonary anastomosis may allow later completion of Fontan repair by right atrium to left pulmonary artery anastomosis.

TRANSCATHETER MANAGEMENT OF CYANOTIC CONGENITAL HEART DEFECTS

Since the introduction of transluminal balloon dilation techniques in children by Kan et al[80] transcatheter methods have been utilized to augment pulmonary blood flow in children with cyanotic congenital heart defects. Lesions for which these techniques have been employed include pulmonary stenosis with ventricular septal defect, pulmonary stenosis and atresia with intact ventricular septum, stenotic aortopulmonary shunts, and postoperative stenosis of the pulmonary valve or arteries.

Labadidi and Wu first reported balloon pulmonary valvuloplasty in patients with tetralogy of Fallot in 1983.[81] The initial indication has been extended to other patients with pulmonary oligemia. It remains controversial whether growth or increase in the size of the pulmonary annulus or artery occurs following balloon dilation. Thus, only certain patients with diminished pulmonary flow and cyanosis may be candidates for balloon pulmonary valvuloplasty: (1) those who are not currently candidates for total surgical correction but need palliation and (2) those whose valvular obstruction contributes importantly to right ventricular outflow tract obstruction. Complications have included transient hypoxia and hypotension with balloon inflation, femoral vein occlusion, and pulmonary arterial laceration. Intermediate results after 12 mo of follow-up have been reported by Qureshi et al and Rao et al.[82,83] In these series, 4 of 15 and 2 of 11 children, respectively, required systemic to pulmonary shunts for significant hypoxia after pulmonary balloon valvuloplasty.

In patients with pulmonary stenosis and intact ventricular septum with atrial right-to-left shunt, pulmonary balloon valvuloplasty can increase pulmonary blood flow and relieve systemic hypoxia and right ventricular hypertension. Early and intermediate term results have been good; most patients experience relief of right ventricular hypertension and systemic arterial hypoxia. Rao et al reported 2 of 12 patients had significant residual pulmonary valvular gradients requiring repeat balloon pulmonary valvuloplasty with good results.[84]

Dilation of stenotic aortopulmonary shunts has been successful: standard Blalock–Taussig shunt,[84,85] modified Blalock–Taussig shunt,[86] and Waterston shunt.[87] These are done in patients with cyanotic heart defects not amenable to current surgical correction. Measurement of pulmonary artery pressure and visualization of pulmonary anatomy are additional benefits of this procedure.

Immediate improvement in oxygen saturation has been reported for nearly all patients undergoing this intervention. However, long-term follow-up data are lacking, and in the few patients who have undergone repeat catheterization, oxygen saturation was lower than immediately following initial dilation. No complications in these series were described; however, acute occlusion of Blalock–Taussig shunts following catheter manipulation has been reported.[88] Thus, heparinization and close monitoring of these children are recommended to ensure patency of the shunt following dilation.

Transcatheter approaches have been suggested in the management of pulmonary atresia with intact ventricular septum. Two strategies have been suggested. First, primary perforation of the atretic valve using transcatheter methods and laser has been followed immediately by balloon dilation.[89] Second, limited opening of the pulmonary valve at surgery (by knife or by laser) has been followed by balloon pulmonary valvuloplasty.[90]

Currently, the value of transcatheter methods has been firmly established in the palliation of certain cyanotic congenital heart defects. They may treat definitively or help to delay surgical intervention in children at high risk for early surgery. However, clarification of selection criteria and longer follow-up results are needed to define its role in the management of these patients.

REFERENCES

1. Blalock A, Taussig H: The surgical treatment of malformations of the heart in which there is pulmonary stenosis or pulmonary atresia. *JAMA* **128:**189, 1945
2. Browdie DA, Norberg W, Agnew R, et al: The use of prostaglandin E1 and Blalock-Taussig shunts in neonates with cyanotic congenital heart disease. *Ann Thorac Surg* **27**(6):508–513, 1979

3. Taussig HB, Crocetti A, Eshaghpour E, et al: Long-time observations on the Blalock-Taussig operation. I. Results of first operation. *Johns Hopkins Med J* **129**(5):243–257, 1971

4. Laks H, Castaneda AR: Subclavian arterioplasty for the ipsilateral Blalock-Taussig shunt. *Ann Thorac Surg* **19**(3):319–321, 1975

5. Chopra PS, Levy JM, Dacumos GJ, et al: The Blalock-Taussig operation: The procedure of choice in the hypoxic infant with tetralogy of Fallot. *Ann Thorac Surg* **22**(3):235–238, 1976

6. Guyton RA, Owens JE, Waumett JD, et al: The Blalock-Taussig shunt. Low risk, effective palliation, and pulmonary artery growth. *J Thorac Cardiovasc Surg* **85**(6):917–922, 1983

7. Laks H, Fagan L, Barner HB, Willman VL: The Blalock-Taussig shunt in the neonate. *Ann Thorac Surg* **25**(3):220–224, 1978

8. Daicoff GR, Aslami A, Victorica BE, Schiebler GL: Ascending aorta-to-pulmonary artery anastomosis for cyanotic congenital heart disease. *Ann Thorac Surg* **18**(3):260–268, 1974

9. Smith CD, Sade RM, Crawford FA, Othersen HB: Diaphragmatic paralysis and eventration in infants. *J Thorac Cardiovasc Surg* **91**(4):490–497, 1986

10. Tyson KR, Larrieu AJ, Kirchmer JJ: The Blalock-Taussig shunt in the first two years of life: A safe and effective procedure. *Ann Thorac Surg* **26**(1):38–41, 1978

11. Wells W, Lloyed D: Systemic-to-pulmonary artery shunts in the first month of life at Children's Hospital of Los Angeles. In Tucker B, Lindesmith G, Takahashi M (eds): *Obstructive Lesions of the Right Heart: Third Clinical Conference on Congenital Heart Disease.* Baltimore, University Park Press, 1984, p 95

12. Mills NL, Williams LC, Culpepper WS II: Technique and experience with azygos patch modified Blalock-Taussig anastomosis for congenital cyanotic heart disease. *Ann Thorac Surg* **39**(6):547–551, 1985

13. Pappas G, Hawes CR: Intrapericardial Blalock-Taussig shunt. *J Thorac Cardiovasc Surg* **83**(3):422–426, 1982

14. Geiss D, Williams WG, Lindsay WK, Rowe RD: Upper extremity gangrene: A complication of subclavian artery division. *Ann Thorac Surg* **30**(5):487–489, 1980

15. Currarino G, Engle M: The effects of ligation of the subclavian artery on the bones and soft tissues of the arm. *J Pediatr* **67**:808, 1965

16. Taussig H, Crocetti A, Eshaghpour E: Longtime observations on the Blalock-Taussig operation. III. Common complications. *Johns Hopkins Med J* **129**:274, 1971

17. Hofschire PJ, Rosenquist GC, Ruckerman RN, et al: Pulmonary vascular disease complicating the Blalock-Taussig anastomosis. *Circulation* **56**:124–126, 1977

18. Soyer T, Lempinen M, Cooper P, et al: A new venous prosthesis. *Surgery* **72**(6):864–872, 1972

19. Gazzaniga AB, Lamberti JJ, Siewers RD, et al: Arterial prosthesis of microporous expanded polytetrafluoroethylene for construction of aorta-pulmonary shunts. *J Thorac Cardiovasc Surg* **72**(3):357–363, 1976

20. de LM, McKay R, Jones M, et al: Modified Blalock-Taussig shunt. Use of subclavian artery orifice as flow regulator in prosthetic systemic-pulmonary artery shunts. *J Thorac Cardiovasc Surg* **81**(1):112–119, 1981

21. McKay R, de LM, Rees P, et al: Postoperative angiographic assessment of modified Blalock-Taussig shunts using expanded polytetrafluoroethylene (Gore-Tex). *Ann Thorac Surg* **30**(2):137–145, 1980

22. Bove EL, Sondheimer HM, Kavey RE, et al: Subclavian-pulmonary artery shunts with polytetrafluoroethylene interposition grafts. *Ann Thorac Surg* **37**(1):88–91, 1984

23. Donahoo JS, Gardner TJ, Zahka K, Kidd BS: Systemic-Pulmonary shunts inneonates and infants using microporous expanded polytetrafluoroethylene: Immediate and late results. *Ann Thorac Surg* **30**(2):146–150, 1980

24. Karpawich PP, Bush CP, Antillon JR, et al: Modified Blalock-Taussig shunt in infants and young children. Clinical and catheterization assessment. *J Thorac Cardiovasc Surg* **89**(2):275–279, 1985

25. Lamberti JJ, Carlisle J, Waldman JD, et al: Systemic-pulmonary shunts in infants and children. Early and late results. *J Thorac Cardiovasc Surg* **88**(1):76–81, 1984

26. Moulton AL, Brenner JI, Ringel R, et al: Classic versus modified Blalock-Taussig shunts in neonates and infants. *Circulation* **72**:(3 Pt 2):iI35–44, 1985

27. Ullom R, Sade R, Crawford F, Ross B: The Blalock-Taussig shunt in infants: Standard vs modified. *Ann Thorac Surg* **44**:539, 1987

28. McCabe JC: Modified subclavian-pulmonary artery shunts [letter]. *J Thorac Cardiovasc Surg* **91**(5):794–795, 1986

29. Le BJ, Culham JA, Chan KW, et al: Treatment of grafts and major vessel thrombosis with low-dose streptokinase in children. *Ann Thorac Surg* **41**(6):630–635, 1986

30. Martinez R, Vincente L, Ferrer F, et al: Perprosthetic cyst formation: An unusual complication of polytetrafluoroethylene prosthesis implantation. *Texas Heart Inst J* **9**:221, 1982

31. Le BJ, Albus R, Williams WG, et al: Serous fluid leakage: A complication following the modified Blalock-Taussig shunt. *J Thorac Cardiovasc Surg* **88**(2):259–262, 1984

32. Maitland A, Williams WG, Coles JG, et al: A method of treating serous fluid leak from a polytetrafluoroethylene Blalock-Taussig shunt. *J Thorac Cardiovasc Surg* **90**(5):791–793, 1985

33. Sethia B, Pollock JC: False aneurysm formation: A complication following the modified Blalock-Taussig shunt. *Ann Thorac Surg* **41**(6):667–668, 1986

34. Potts W, Smith S, Gibson S: Anastomosis of the aorta to a pulmonary artery: Certain types in congenital heart disease. *JAMA* **132**:627, 1946

35. Blalock A, Park E: The surgical treatment of experimental coarctation (atresia) of the aorta. *Ann Surg* **119**:445, 1944

36. Gross R, Hufnagel C: Coarctation of the aorta. *N Engl J Med* **233**:287, 1945

37. Potts W: Aortic-pulmonary anastomosis for pulmonary stenosis. *J Thorac Surg* **17**:223, 1948

38. Hallman GL, Stasney CR, Cooley DA: Surgical treatment of tricuspid atresia. *J Cardiovasc Surg (Torino)* **9**(2):154–160, 1968

39. Paul M, Miller R, Potts W: Long-term results of aortic-pulmonary anastomosis for tetralogy of Fallot: An analysis of the first 100 cases eleven to thirteen years after operation. *Circulation* **23**:525, 1961

40. Daoud G, Kaplan S, Helmsworth JA: Tetralogy of Fallot and pulmonary hypertension. Complication after systemic-to-pulmonary anastomosis. *Am J Dis Child* **111**(2):166–177, 1966

41. Kirklin J, Devloo R: Hypothermic perfusion and circulatory arrest for surgical correction of tetralogy of Fallot with previously constructed Potts' anastomosis. *Dis Chest* **39**:87, 1961

42. Arciniegas E, Farooki ZQ, Hakimi M, et al: Classic shunting operations for congenital cyanotic heart defects. *J Thorac Cardiovasc Surg* **84**(1):88–96, 1982

43. Davidson J: Anastomosis between the ascending aorta and the main pulmonary artery in the tetralogy of Fallot. *Thorax* **10**:348, 1955

44. Waterston D: The treatment of Fallot's tetralogy in children under one year of age. *Rozhl Chir* **41**:181, 1962

45. Waterston DJ, Stark J, Ashcraft KW: Ascending aorta-to-right pulmonary artery shunts: Experience with 100 patients. *Surgery* **72**(6):897–904, 1972

46. Stewart S, Mahoney EB, Manning J: The Waterston anastomosis with no deaths in the neonate. *J Thorac Cardiovasc Surg* **72**(4):588–592, 1976

47. Ebert PA, Gay WJ, Oldham HN: Management of aorta-right pulmonary artery anastomosis during total correction of tetralogy of Fallot. *Surgery* **71**(2):231–234, 1972

48. Gay WJ, Ebert PA: Aorta-to-right pulmonary artery anastomosis causing obstruction of the right pulmonary artery. Management during correction of tetralogy of Fallot. *Ann Thorac Surg* **16**(4):402–410, 1973

49. Rao PS, Ellison RG: The cause of kinking of the right pulmonary artery in the Waterston anastomosis. A growth phenomenon. *J Thorac Cardiovasc Surg* **76**(1):126–129, 1978

50. Sade RM, Sloss L, Treves S, et al: Repair of tetralogy of Fallot after aortopulmonary anastomosis. *Ann Thorac Surg* **23**(32):32–38, 1977

51. Reitman MJ, Galioto FJ, el SG, et al: Ascending aorta to right pulmonary artery anastomosis. Immediate results in 123 patients and one month to six year follow-up in 74 patients. *Circulation* **49**(5): 952–957, 1974

52. Clarke CP: Method of closure of the aorta-to-right pulmonary artery (Waterston) anastomosis during corrective operation. *Ann Thorac Surg* **16**(4):411–413, 1973

53. Young W, Sealy W, Houck W: Superior vena cava right pulmonary artery anastomosis in cyanotic heart disease. *Ann Surg* **157**:894, 1963

54. Carlon C, Mondini P, Marchi RD: Surgical treatment of some cardiovascular diseases (a new vascular anastomosis). *J Int Coll Surg* **16**:1, 1951

55. Glenn W: Circulatory bypass of the right side of the heart. IV. Shunt between superior vena cava and distal right pulmonary artery: Report of clinical application. *N Engl J Med* **259**:117, 1958

56. Mathur M, Glenn WW: Long-term evaluation of cava-pulmonary artery anastomosis. *Surgery* **74**(6):899–916, 1973

57. Robicsek F, Magistro R, Foti E: Vena cava-pulmonary artery anastomosis for vascularization of the lung. *J Thorac Surg* **35**:440, 1958

58. Glenn W, Browne M, Whittemore R: Circulatory bypass of the right side of the heart. Cava-pulmonary artery shunt-indications and results: Report of a collected series of 537 cases. In Cassels D (ed): *The Heart and Circulation in the Newborn and Infant.* New York, Grune & Stratton, 1966, p 245

59. Glenn W, Ordway N, Talner N, Call E: Circulatory bypass of the right side of the heart. VI. Shunt between superior vena cava and distal right pulmonary artery. Report of clinical application in thirty-eight cases. *Circulation* **31**:172, 1965

60. Trusler GA, Mac GD, Mustard WT: Cavopulmonary anastomosis for cyanotic congenital heart disease. *J Thorac Cardiovasc Surg* **62**(5):803–809, 1971

61. Samanek M, Oppelt A, Kasalicky J, Voriskova M: Distribution of pulmonary blood flow after cavopulmonary anastomosis (Glenn operation): *Br Heart J* **31**(4):511–516, 1969

62. McFaul RC, Tajik AJ, Mair DD, et al: Development of pulmonary arteriovenous shunt after superior vena cava-right pulmonary artery (Glenn) anastomosis. Report of four cases. *Circulation* **55**(1): 212–216, 1977

63. Gomes A, Benson L, George B, Laks H: Management of pulmonary arteriovenous fistulas after superior vena cava-right pulmonary artery (Glenn) anastomosis. *J Thorac Cardiovasc Surg* **87**:636, 1974

64. Van DBVHA, Derom F, Kunnen M, et al: Surgery for arteriovenous fistulas and dilated vessels in the right lung after the Glenn procedure. *J Thorac Cardiovasc Surg* **76**(2):195–197, 1978

65. Glenn WW, Fenn JE: Axillary arteriovenous fistula. A means of supplementing blood flow through a cava-pulmonary artery shunt. *Circulation* **46**(5):1013–1017, 1972

66. Furuse A, Brawley RK, Gott VL: Pulsatile cavo-pulmonary artery shunt. Surgical technique and hemodynamic characteristics. *J Thorac Cardiovasc Surg* **63**(3):495–500, 1972

67. Robicsek F: An epitaph for cavopulmonary anastomosis. *Ann Thorac Surg* **34**:208, 1982

68. Glenn WW: Superior vena cava-pulmonary artery anastomosis. *Ann Thorac Surg* **37**(1):9–11, 1984

69. Pennington D, Nouri S, Ho J: Glenn shunt: Long-term results and current role in congenital heart operations. *Ann Thorac Surg* **31**:532, 1981

70. Salim M, Case C, Sade RM, et al: Pulmonary/systemic flow ratio in children after cavopulmonary anastomosis. *J Am Coll Cardio* **25**:735–738, 1995

71. Sade R: Orthoterminal correction of congenital cardiovascular defects. *Ann Thorac Surg* **19**:105–107, 1975

72. Hopkins RA, Armstrong BE, Serwer GA, et al: Physiological rationale for a bidirectional cavopulmonary shunt. A versatile complement to the Fontan principle. *J Thorad Cardiovasc Surg* **90**(3): 391–398, 1985

73. Haller JJ, Adkins JC, Worthington M, Rauenhorst J: Experimetnal studies on permanent bypass of the right heart. *Surgery* **59**(6): 1128–1132, 1966

74. Lamberti JJ, Spicer RL, Waldman JD, et al: The bidirectional cavopulmonary shunt. *J Thorac Cardiovasc Surg* **100**(1):22–29, 1990

75. Pridjian AK, Mendelsohn AM, Lupinetti FM, et al: Usefulness of the bidirectional Glenn procedure as staged reconstruction for the functional single ventricle. *Am J Cardiol* **71**(11):959–962, 1993

76. Albanese SB, Carotti A, Di DR, et al: Bidirectional cavopulmonary anastomosis in patients under two years of age. *J Thorac Cardiovasc Surg* **104**(4):904–909, 1992

77. Chang AC, Hanley FL, Wernovsky G, et al: Early bidirectional cavopulmonary shunt in young infants. Postoperative course and early results. *Circulation* **88**(5 Pt 2):iI149–158, 1993

78. Seshadri M, Jagaannath BR, Koppula AS, et al: A new technique to simplify the Fontan procedure after a previous bidirectional Glenn shunt [letter]. *J Thorac Cardiovasc Surg* **106**(3):569–570, 1993

79. Douville EC, Sade RM, Fyfe DA: Hemi-Fontan operation in surgery for single ventricle: A preliminary report [see comments]. *Ann Thorac Surg* **51**(6):893–899, 1991

80. Kan JS, White RJ, Mitchell SE, Gardner TJ: Percutaneous balloon valvuloplasty: A new method for treating congenital pulmonary-valve stenosis. *N Engl J Med* **307**(9):540–542, 1982

81. Lababidi Z, Wu JR: Percutaneous balloon pulmonary valvuloplasty. *Am J Cardiol* **52**(5):560–562, 1983

82. Qureshi SA, Kirk CR, Lamb RK, et al: Balloon dilatation of the pulmonary valve in the first year of life in patients with tetralogy of Fallot: A preliminary study. *Br Heart J* **60**(3):232–235, 1988

83. Rao PS, Wilson AD, Thapar MK, Brais M: Balloon pulmonary valvuloplasty in the management of cyanotic congenital heart defects. *Cathet Cardiovasc Diagn* **25**(1):16–24, 1992

84. Rao PS, Levy JM, Chopra PS: Balloon angioplasty of stenosed Blalock-Taussig anastomosis: Role of balloon-on-a-wire in dilating occluded shunts. *Am Heart J* **120**(5):1173–1178, 1990

85. Marx GR, Allen HD, Ovitt TW, Hanson W: Balloon dilation angioplasty of Blalock-Taussig shunts. *Am J Cardiol* **62**(10 Pt 1):824–827, 1988

86. Parsons JM, Ladusans EJ, Qureshi SA: Balloon dilatation of a stenosed modified (polytetrafluoroethylene) Blalock-Taussig shunt. *Br Heart J* **62**(3):228–229, 1989

87. Gibbs JL, Wilson N, da CP: Balloon dilatation of a Waterston aortopulmonary anastomosis. *Br Heart J* **59**(5):596–597, 1988

88. Rajani RM, Dalvi BV, Kulkarni HL, Kale PA: Acutely blocked Blalock-Taussig shunt following cardiac catheterization: Successful recanalization with intravenous streptokinase. *Am Heart J* **120**(5):1238–1239, 1990

89. Qureshi SA, Rosenthal E, Tynan M, et al: Transcatheter laser-assisted balloon pulmonary valve dilation in pulmonic valve atresia. *Am J Cardiol* **67**(5):428–431, 1991

90. Latson LA, Fleming WH, Hofschire PJ, et al: Balloon valvuloplasty in pulmonary valve atresia. *Am Heart J* **121**(5):1567–1569, 1991

64

Pulmonary Artery Banding

Davis C. Drinkwater, Jr., and Hillel Laks

The first report of pulmonary artery banding was by Muller and Dammann in 1951, at which time a 5 mo old with a large ventricular septal defect (VSD) was palliated by "creation of pulmonic stenosis."[1] Their operation, made more complex than most present techniques because of the partial excision of the pulmonary artery, was recommended for patients with a functional single ventricle. Since that early experience, there have been great improvements in the medical and surgical management of complex congenital heart disease, and the indications for pulmonary artery banding (PAB) have been and will continue to be modified. The primary objective of PAB remains, however, similar to that of Muller and Dammann, namely reducing excessive blood flow to the pulmonary circulation.

PHYSIOLOGY

Placement of a pulmonary artery band decreases overperfusion of the pulmonary circulation by restricting pulmonary artery inflow. In patients with left-to-right shunting lesions, this reduces the shunt volume and consequently improves systemic blood pressure and overall forward cardiac output. The reduction of pulmonary blood flow also decreases the total blood volume returning to the systemic ventricle, thereby reducing volume overload and further improving ventricular function.

Decrease in pulmonary blood flow may not be tolerated in patients dependent on mixing of the systemic and pulmonary venous return to maintain systemic oxygen saturation, such as in single ventricle or transposition of the great arteries (TGA). It is, therefore, important to ensure that such patients have an unrestrictive interatrial communication prior to banding. Balloon atrial septostomy or atrial septectomy at the time of banding may be required.

With successful PAB, the physiologic effects de-

scribed above should result in clinical improvement. Signs and symptoms of congestive heart failure are improved, cardiac size decreases, and the development of irreversible pulmonary vascular disease is prevented.

INDICATIONS

The experience and the philosophy of the cardiology/surgery team will largely determine the types of patients who will require a staged repair with PAB. Early total intracardiac repair has replaced palliation with PAB in many patients, particularly those with VSDs and increased pulmonary blood flow, because of improved results with primary corrective surgery in the neonatal and infant age groups.[2]

There are, however, three groups of patients who continue to benefit from PAB. The largest group (Group I) are those patients with two ventricles and defects of septation who, because of the complexity of their cardiac and extracardiac anatomy, may have lower mortality with initial PAB and later staged operative repair of the septal defects or outflow tract anomalies.[3] Another group (Group II) are those patients with functionally single ventricles who will require a future Fontan procedure as "definitive" repair. These patients require a well-protected pulmonary vascular bed early in life to optimize their suitability for the Fontan operation.[4] A relatively recent and much smaller group (Group III) includes patients with TGA who require "training" of the left ventricle (LV) in preparation for the arterial switch procedure when this must be performed later than the first few weeks of life.[5]

Group I

In general, we perform complete repairs on patients with an isolated perimembranous VSD or with an uncomplicated atrioventricular (A-V) canal defect at the time of presentation for congestive heart failure not amenable to medical management. Patients in Group I more likely to require PAB and staged repair are those with complex VSDs, unbalanced complete A-V canal defects, or a need for a conduit or A-V valve repair or replacement.[6,7]

VSD

The group of complex VSDs includes patients with multiple VSDs (so-called "Swiss cheese septum") and younger patients with an apical muscular VSD that would likely require a left ventriculotomy for closure. When VSD is associated with coarctation of the aorta, complete repair may be carried out from a median sternotomy incision. However, staged repair of the coarctation with PAB followed subsequently by early closure of the VSD is an acceptable approach in the presence of significant congestive heart failure.

Complete A-V Canal Defect

PAB may be considered in certain patients with complete A-V canal defect. In the unbalanced type of complete A-V canal defect, excessive left-to-right shunting may result in right ventricular dominance while the left ventricle becomes relatively hypoplastic. Primary repair in such cases has been associated with higher mortality than in "balanced" defects. Also, complete A-V canal defect with deficient A-V valve tissue may be difficult to repair and consequently require valve replacement. This is generally best delayed to allow placement of a larger sized valve prosthesis. These subsets of patients with A-V canal defect might, therefore, benefit from PAB for palliation.

Conduit/Outflow Repairs

There is a group of patients who may require a conduit as part of the final repair, such as those with corrected TGA with VSD and some forms of double outlet right ventricle with mild or absent pulmonic stenosis. These patients have excessive pulmonary blood flow and may benefit from initial palliation with PAB to allow somatic growth prior to complete repair. Performing the definitive repair in an older, larger child will allow placement of a larger conduit, which should potentially increase conduit longevity. Additionally, patients in the first few years of life have been noted to develop an accelerated homograft stenosis relative to older age groups,[8] further supporting the advantage of delayed conduit placement.

In distinction, PAB is generally avoided in patients with truncus arteriosus. Although a main pulmonary artery is present in type I truncus, it is frequently so short that PAB may impinge on the right pulmonary artery, complicating subsequent complete repair. In types II and III, bilateral PABs would be required. Balancing left and right pulmonary blood flow to maintain acceptable arterial oxygen saturation without excessive pulmonary blood flow is extremely difficult in this situation. Even if successful, the resultant bilateral branch pulmonary artery stenosis is extremely difficult to repair at the time of subsequent conduit placement. For these reasons, patients with truncus arteriosus are best treated by early complete repair.[9]

Group II

Patients with single ventricles and unrestricted pulmonary blood flow require an early and adequately tight band to prevent the development of pulmonary vascular disease as well as ventricular dilatation and dysfunction. Common diagnoses for this group include tricuspid atresia with unrestrictive VSD, tricuspid atresia with TGA, and double inlet left ventricle. In one series, 9 of 20 patients with double inlet left ventricle under 1 year of age already demonstrated severe pulmonary artery medial hypertrophy on histologic examination.[10] Delay in placement of an adequate PAB early in infancy, generally before 2 to 3 mo, may result in irreversible pulmonary vascular disease, which may preclude subsequent Fontan operation.[11]

Single ventricle patients in whom the aorta arises from an outflow chamber such as with double inlet left ventricle or tricuspid atresia with TGA, particularly when associated with aortic arch anomalies, have the potential for development of subaortic obstruction. In the presence of such obstruction, or in patients who are at high risk for such obstruction, PAB is contraindicated. The ventricular hypertrophy that develops in response to banding causes rapid progression of subaortic stenosis. These patients are identified by careful preoperative assessment including cardiac catheterization with pullback pressure measurements across the subaortic region, angiography, and echocardiography. The presence of a gradient greater than 15–20 mm Hg or an echocardiographic outlet foramen area-index of less than 2 cm^2/m^2 precludes PAB. These patients instead undergo the Damus–Kaye–Stansel procedure and systemic-to-pulmonary artery shunt, which provides complete protection of the pulmonary vascular bed and bypasses the subaortic obstruction. If there is no evidence of obstruction and a low potential for later obstruction, patients undergo PAB with frequent interval echocardiographic follow-up. Later the Damus–Kaye–Stansel procedure or resection of subaortic stenosis (Fig. 64–1A,B) can be performed, if necessary, with a mortality rate of approximately 10%.[12,13]

PAB has been reported as a means of "radical" palliation in the presence of a hypoplastic ascending aorta in lieu of the more commonly applied Norwood procedure. This involves placement of a distal main pulmonary artery band in conjunction with a proximal pulmonary artery to descending aorta conduit, with best results in normally related great vessels.[14] While successful palliation can be achieved by this technique, the difficulty of the subsequent reconstructions makes this option less desirable than the Norwood approach. A similar palliation for hypoplastic left heart syndrome involving bilateral PABs and placement of a ductal stent had less favorable outcomes (50% early mortality), underscoring the difficulties of obtaining appropriate and balanced pulmonary blood flow after bilateral banding.[15]

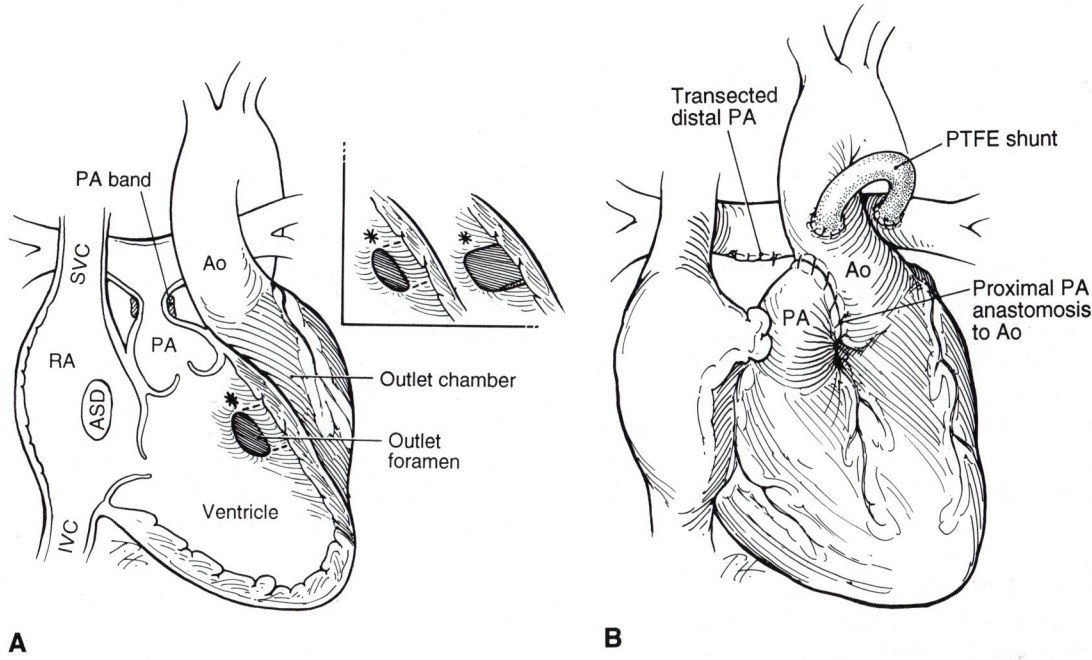

Figure 64–1. A. Example of a single ventricle with restrictive bulboventricular (outlet) foramen after pulmonary artery banding, with evidence of ventricular hypertrophy. Inset demonstrates the proper location away from the A-V conduction tissue for resection of subaortic stenosis and enlargement of the outlet foramen. Ao, aorta; ASD, atrial septal defect; IVC, inferior vena cava; PA, pulmonary artery; RA, right atrium; SVC, superior vena cava. **B.** Damus–Kaye–Stansel procedure with central shunt for subaortic stenosis that is not amenable to resection or enlargement of the outlet foramen. Ao, aorta; PA, pulmonary artery, PTFE, polytetrafluoroethylene.

Group III

Patients with TGA represent a recently evolved additional indication for PAB. Most patients with TGA undergo an arterial switch procedure in the neonatal period. Some newborn patients with TGA and intact ventricular septum, however, are not offered an arterial switch procedure due to active infection, coexistent noncardiac disease, or delay in diagnosis. Such patients were previously treated by later atrial switch, since arterial switch was precluded by rapid left ventricular involution consequent to the normal postnatal decrease in pulmonary vascular resistance. In the early experience with the arterial switch, neonatal PAB and concomitant systemic-to-pulmonary artery shunt resulted in preservation of the left ventricle to allow subsequent arterial switch later in infancy, thereby simplifying the technical aspects of the operation.[16] A similar approach has been applied to patients with TGA and intact ventricular septum older than 2 mo, and results indicate that the attenuation of left ventricular volume and muscle mass may be reversed. This is achieved by placement of a PAB to provide left ventricular afterload resistance in combination with a technique to increase arterial oxygen saturation and normalize ventricular volume loading.

PAB and Partial Senning

The first technique applied in such patients has been a partial atrial baffle in conjunction with PAB (Fig. 64–2A). Briefly, the inferior vena caval blood, representing the larger amount of desaturated blood, is directed toward the

pulmonary (left) ventricle through a pericardial baffle that can be easily taken down at the time of arterial switch. The larger amount of saturated blood from the right pulmonary veins is directed around the baffle to the systemic (right) ventricle. The improvements in saturation through redirected streaming allow placement of an adequately tight PAB with resultant left ventricular "preparation" for arterial switch. This procedure, which requires a short period of cardiopulmonary bypass, also provides long-term palliation for patients who may not be candidates for arterial switch.

PAB and Blalock–Taussig Shunt

PAB in conjunction with a modified Blalock–Taussig shunt is performed as a closed procedure without cardiopulmonary bypass, and therefore is a more desirable approach for short-term preparation compared with the partial Senning technique described above (Fig. 64–2B). After either technique, patients are followed with serial echocardiograms that allow quantitative measurements of left ventricular mass-index, as well as qualitative assessment of ventricular septal geometry. Left-to-right septal bowing is an indication that the left ventricle can generate near-systemic pressures. Left ventricular preparation is usually accomplished within 7–10 days, after which patients may undergo arterial switch, takedown of shunt, and removal of PAB. Early mortality rate is 4–5%, only slightly greater than that for a primary arterial switch.[17,18] This is despite the need for inotropic and ventilatory support in most patients during the preparatory period.

Figure 64–2. A. Partial Senning technique for improving saturation and providing both volume and afterload to the left ventricle after pulmonary artery banding in transposition of the great arteries. Autologous pericardium is used to baffle the inferior vena cava and left pulmonary veins across the mitral valve into the left (pulmonary) ventricle, with superior vena cava and right pulmonary vein drainage to the systemic ventricle. The band is best positioned distally to avoid valvar injury in anticipation of possible arterial switch operation. IVC, inferior vena cava; RPV, right pulmonary veins; TV, tricuspid valve. **B.** Pulmonary artery banding combined with modified Blalock–Taussig shunt for "rapid" preparation to arterial switch. This provides left ventricular volume and afterload and can be performed through a left lateral thoracotomy, avoiding the need for resternotomy at the time of arterial switch. Careful measurement of proximal pulmonary artery pressure is depicted to avoid overtightening the band. PA, pulmonary artery.

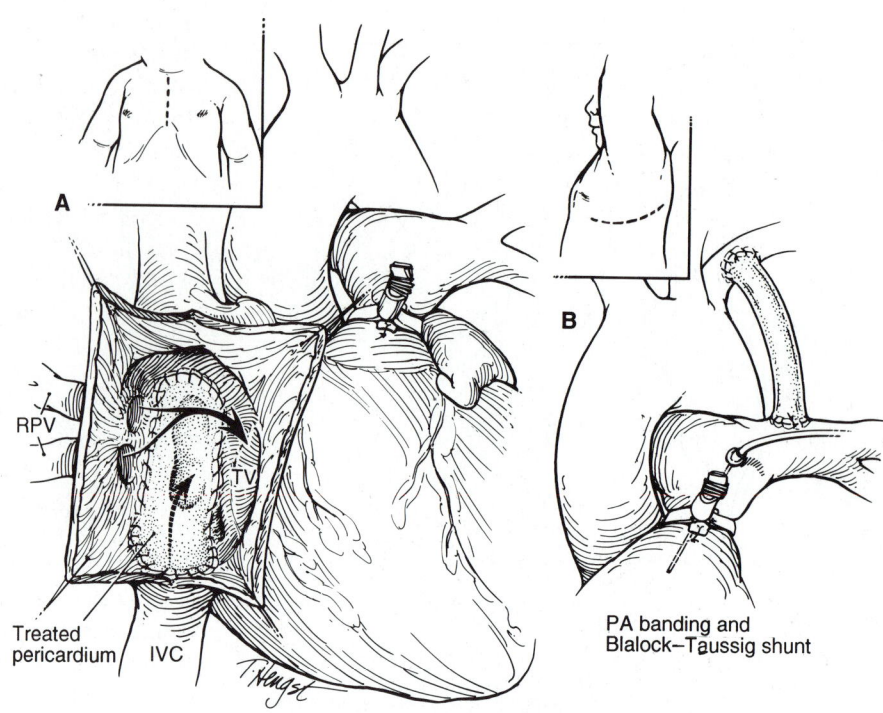

PA banding and Blalock–Taussig shunt

PAB for Right Ventricular Failure after Atrial Switch Procedures

PAB has been employed in a challenging group of patients in whom right ventricular dysfunction occurs later after the Senning or Mustard procedures. The PAB is maintained for a longer period of time compared with preparation in infancy, even up to 12 mo. While the overall early survival in this group approaches 90%, approximately one-half require transplantation due to coexisting left ventricular failure. In the group undergoing arterial switch, there is a high incidence of significant neoaortic valve insufficiency.[19]

SURGICAL PRINCIPLES AND TECHNIQUE

Incision

The surgical approach for PAB, if done as an isolated procedure, is through an anterior left thoracotomy in the second or third intercostal space (Fig. 64–3). If done in conjunction with a coarctation or interrupted aortic arch repair, a left lateral thoracotomy approach through the fourth intercostal space is utilized. In both cases, the pericardium is opened anterior to the phrenic nerve, retracting but not resecting thymic tissue superiorly. A third, infrequently used approach for PAB is through a median sternotomy incision. It is utilized for conditions in which intracardiac procedures (e.g., atrial septectomy, partial

Senning procedure) requiring cardiopulmonary bypass are to be performed.

Static vs. Adjustable Band

The pulmonary artery band may be constructed in a fixed or static manner such that once in place, no further adjustments in band tightness can be made. This may be adequate in the majority of cases, but there is a group of patients who may benefit from placement of a band that can be easily loosened or tightened at the initial or subsequent operations. The ability to readjust the band is particularly useful in patients in whom there are dynamic changes in cardiac output, pulmonary vascular resistance, and systemic vascular resistance. Additionally, it may be of benefit in patients with significant lung disease, e.g., pulmonary edema, pneumonia, and atelectasis. Such patients will develop severe arterial oxygen desaturation with PAB, but may tolerate gradually increasing band tightness as the pulmonary process improves. Adjustable banding is also helpful in patients with A-V valve regurgitation, in particular complex A-V canal. The acute increase in afterload that accompanies banding may exacerbate A-V valvar insufficiency. Gradual banding is usually well tolerated and allows improvement in regurgitation by decreasing ventricular volume overload.

Given the advantages of the adjustable band, this technique is used routinely at UCLA. Patients in whom adjustments of the PAB were made postoperatively are listed in Table 64–1. Eighteen percent of the patients underwent delayed tightening of the band, including 40% of patients in

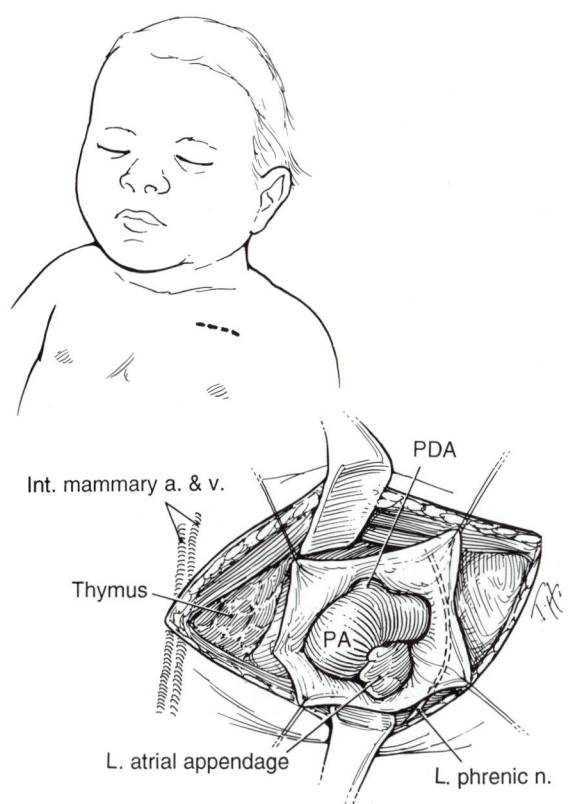

Figure 64–3. The left anterior thoracotomy approach through the second or third intercostal space gives excellent exposure for isolated pulmonary artery banding. Note anatomy of the adjacent structures with medial limits of the incision at the internal mammary vessels. The thymus is swept superiorly away from the phrenic nerve and the pericardium is opened over the main pulmonary artery. a. & v., artery and vein; Int., internal; L., left; n., nerve; PA, pulmonary artery; PDA, patent ductus arteriosus.

Group II. A small group of patients have undergone successful delayed loosening of the band carried out in the catheterization laboratory in conjunction with balloon pulmonary angioplasty at the band site.

Surgical Technique

Following exposure of the pulmonary artery and aorta, the band is prepared for placement. A variety of banding materials have been proposed, including plaited silk suture, umbilical tape, Dacron tube, Silastic tape, and Teflon tape. We prefer umbilical tape, which is broad enough to minimize the risk of "cutting through" the pulmonary artery wall, yet can be placed through a snare for use as an adjustable band. The estimated band circumference is marked on the umbilical tape with fine Tevdek suture according to the formula of Albus et al.[20] Circumference in patients with noncyanotic, nonmixing lesions (e.g., VSD) is 20 mm + 1 mm/kg body weight. For patients with mixing lesions (e.g., TGA with

VSD), the formula 24 + 1 mm/kg body weight is employed. In patients with single ventricles in whom the Fontan procedure is planned, an intermediate circumference of 22 mm + 1 mm/kg body weight is used. It should be noted that these estimates of band circumference are used simply as guidelines, and that the final tightness of the band is determined by physiologic assessment of the patient following band placement.

The site of band placement must be carefully selected in the midportion of the pulmonary trunk to avoid pulmonic valve injury proximally and branch pulmonary artery impingement distally. Dissection is begun in the adventitia between the aorta and pulmonary artery, and is limited to prevent proximal or distal band migration. The pulmonary artery is often dilated, thin-walled, and hypertensive, rendering it vulnerable to injury during band placement. The band is, therefore, first passed around the aorta and then through the transverse sinus to encircle the pulmonary artery. Fixed band construction is completed by suturing the premarked sites together anteriorly. The band is further fixed onto the pulmonary artery by adventitial or full-thickness sutures.

The initial technique for placement of an adjustable band, including mobilization of the pulmonary artery and premeasurement of band circumference according to Trusler's formula, is similar to that of the fixed type.[21] After encircling the pulmonary artery, however, the band is snared with a short segment of number 8 or 10 polyethylene tubing and fixed by medium hemoclips. A felt pledget is placed beneath the band between the end of the snare and the pulmonary artery wall to prevent injury to the pulmonary artery. The pledget and band material are then tacked to the pulmonary artery, similar to the fixed type, to prevent migration (Fig. 64–4). Tightening the band by the addition of one medium hemoclip is equivalent to a 1 mm decrease in band circumference. Wound closure is performed in standard fashion, and instruments for hemoclip removal accompany the patient to the intensive care unit to allow rapid loosening of the band if this becomes necessary. With this technique we have had no cases of device infection or erosion, and have retained the ability to perform readjustments perioperatively and as late as 36 mo after banding.

In selective cases, the snare is made longer, and the end of the device is left in the subcutaneous space. This technique is associated with a slightly increased infection rate (3–5%), but allows for simplified band readjustment, since the band can be retrieved from its superficial location under local anesthesia in the intensive care unit or catheterization laboratory. Readjustments are performed with echocardiogram guidance or direct catheter measurement of pulmonary artery pressure while monitoring systemic oxygen saturation and blood pressure. Investigation of completely implantable adjustable band devices has been limited to basic research and is without current clinical application.[22]

TABLE 64–1. PULMONARY ARTERY BANDING: UCLA 1986–1994[a] (n = 229)

Diagnosis	Number	Adjustment	Additional Surgery	(Overall 8%) Hospital Mortality
Group I				
VSD/Coart[b]	42	1		++
CAVC[c]	28	1	GS 1	++++
IAA/VSD[d]	24	2		+++
VSD(s)	24	1		
DORV	15	2	PS 1, GS 2, AS 1	
Truncus[e]	6	3		++
TGA/VSD	14	6	PS 5, GS 1	+
HLHS[f]	14	2	GS 2, AS 1, BTS 1	++++
TAPVR	4	2		
PA/VSD	2	1	GS 1	
Total	173	21 (12%)		16 (9%)
Group II				
SV(TGA,DILV)	37	16	GS 14, AS 5, CO 4	+
TA/VSD	10	3	GS 4	+
Total	47	19 (40%)		2 (4%)
Group III				
TGA/IVS	6		BTS 6	
TGA (s/p Sen)	2			
Total	8	0		0

[a]GS, Glenn shunt; PS, partial Senning; AS, atrial septectomy; Coart, coarctation; BTS, BT shunt; VSD, ventricular septal defect; CAVC, complete atrioventricular canal; IAA, interrupted aortic arch; DORV, double outlet right ventricle; Truncus, truncus arteriosus; PA, pulmonary atresia; SV, single ventricle; TA, tricuspid atresia; TGA/IVS, TGA/intra-ventricular septum; s/p Sen, s/p Senning; TGA, transposition of the great arteries; HLHS, hypoplastic left heart syndrome; TAPVR, total anomalous pulmonary venous return.
[b]Includes patients with TGA and DORV.
[c]Includes patients with pneumonia, unbalanced CAVC, PHT.
[d]Includes patients with SVs.
[e]Includes patients with IAA.
[f]Includes patients with subaortic stenosis, mitral and aortic atresia.

Physiologic Assessment

The goal of pulmonary artery banding is to produce a distal pulmonary artery pressure 30–50% of systemic pressure. This is achieved while simultaneously maintaining a satisfactory systemic oxygen saturation.[23] The definition of satisfactory saturation may vary from patient to patient. In general, we attempt to achieve saturations of approximately 85–90% with an inspired oxygen concentration of 50%. Lower saturations may be accepted, especially in patients with single ventricle physiology. Failure to achieve these levels in patients with mixed circulation suggests inadequacy of the interatrial communication. In such cases, the addition of an atrial sepectomy or septostomy may be necessary before or simultaneous with PAB.[24]

Physiologic assessment to determine the appropriate tightness of the PAB includes intraoperative measurement of proximal and distal pulmonary artery pressures, systemic blood pressure, and arterial oxygen saturation by pulse oximetry and by direct measurement from arterial blood gas sampling. In addition to the changes in pulmonary artery pressure and systemic oxygen saturation, one should ideally note a concomitant rise in systemic arterial pressure of 10–15 mm Hg.

The adequacy of banding is a multifactorial assessment that should be made under conditions of euvolemia and the absence of atelectasis. Although the measured pa-

rameters described above are helpful guides, overall clinical status is the most important assessment. This includes changes in systemic blood pressure, heart rate, and overall cardiac tolerance of the band. Hypotension, bradycardia, and ischemic electrocardiographic changes all indicate excessive band tightness. In all cases, final fixation should be delayed until a suitable period of time for assessment has passed, since rapid loosening may be required.

Postoperative assessment of PAB adequacy can be made by cardiac catheterization and direct measurement of pulmonary artery pressure, but this is not appropriate for frequent serial assessment. Color flow Doppler mapping[25] and, more recently, cinemagnetic resonance imaging[26] have been useful as noninvasive methods to evaluate band tightness and band placement after surgery.

RESULTS

Mortality

The mortality of PAB is clearly associated more with the complex cardiac anatomy and the overall condition of the patient than with the procedure itself. Patients who are selected for PAB and staged repair are often chosen because they are considered too ill to safely undergo definitive re-

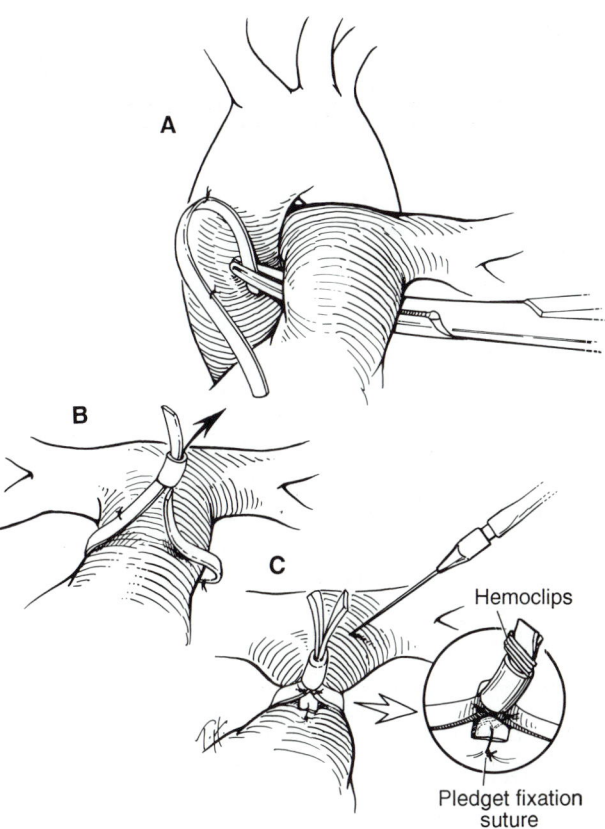

Figure 64–4. A–C. Pulmonary artery banding technique using pre-measured Trussler formula adjusted to the cardiac anatomy. An adjustable device is placed over a felt pledget with adventitial fixation sutures to prevent distal migration. Additional fixation sutures may be placed in the band itself. Each additional medium hemoclip causes a 1-mm change in band circumference. Distal pulmonary artery pressure is measured during tightening.

pair, thus selecting a higher risk group at the outset. The mortality rates from earlier series have therefore been as high as 25%.[27,28] Patients in Group II (single ventricle) in general have lower operative mortality for PAB than do patients in either Group I or III, although late mortality rate is equal among all groups.[29]

There have been modifications in the technique of PAB and, more importantly, improved patient selection and timing of surgery. This and a general improvement in perioperative management have resulted in a decreased mortality rate. Comparing their own experiences from the 1970s to that of a decade later, many groups have demonstrated dramatic decreases in overall mortality from 36 to 7.5% and indeed, as low as 3–5%.[30,31] The overall hospital mortality in 229 patients operated at UCLA from 1986 to 1994 is 8% (Table 64–1).

Morbidity

Nonlethal complications can occur in association with PAB, and these must be well recognized to avoid them when performing the procedure. The most common complication is distortion of the main and branch pulmonary arter-

ies. The right pulmonary artery is involved in most cases of branch stenosis. Indeed, one series reported a 37% incidence of branch pulmonary artery stenosis.[23] This particular complication may be limited, if not eliminated, by limiting dissection between the aorta and pulmonary trunk, and by fixing the band on the proximal pulmonary trunk. In selected cases in which the main pulmonary artery is markedly dilated (e.g., interrupted aortic arch or double outlet right ventricle), removing a segment of the main pulmonary artery may prevent distal migration and branch impingement. We have recently employed a simplified technique to accomplish this by longitudinal closure of a transverse pulmonary arteriotomy performed within a partial occluding clamp placed on the main pulmonary artery.

In general, distortion can be repaired quite readily at the time of definitive repair, but does add an element of morbidity both during the period of palliation and at the time of definitive repair (Fig. 64–5). The diagnosis is suggested by plain chest x-ray, which may show inequality of pulmonary blood flow between the left and right lungs. Definitive diagnosis may be made by Doppler echocardiography, radionuclide lung perfusion scan, MRI, and angiography prior to repair.[32] An unusual but important late complication of significant branch stenosis is underdevelopment of the ipsilateral lung with hypoplastic and decreased numbers of alveoli.[33] Early recognition of stenosis should allow band revision prior to development of this complication.

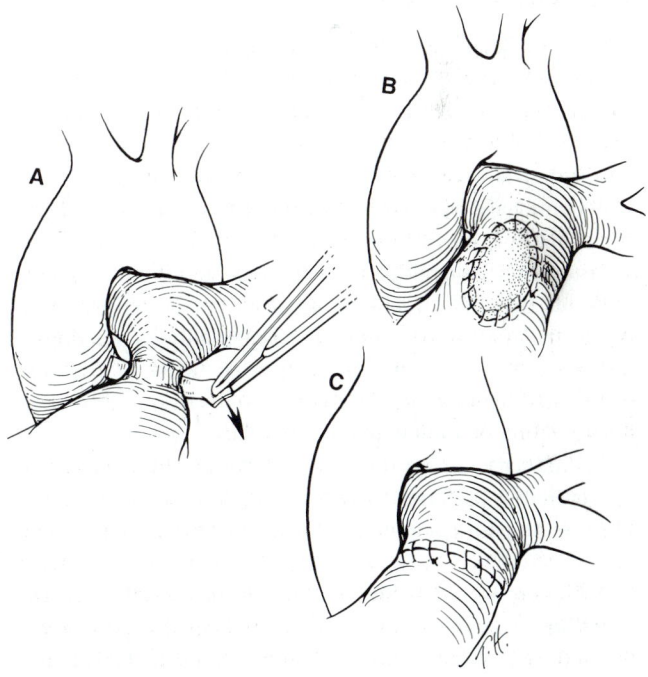

Figure 64–5. Reconstruction of the pulmonary artery after band removal (**A**) may be accomplished by patch arterioplasty using glutaraldehyde-treated autologous pericardium or PTFE material (**B**) or resection of the band site and end-to-end anastomosis using absorbable running sutures (**C**).

A second complication is ineffectual banding either from inadequate band tightness at the original procedure, or later disruption of the band or erosion of the pulmonary artery. Ineffectual banding may occur in as many as 15–20% of cases diagnosed by catheterization or by Doppler echo gradient.[34] The result of an ineffectual band is excessive pulmonary blood flow and early recurrence or continuation of congestive heart failure. In addition, there is the potential for development of pulmonary vascular disease in association with pulmonary arterial hypertension. Loss of the band murmur and recurrence of congestive heart failure after PAB suggest loosening or erosion of the band, and subsequent improvement may indicate the development of pulmonary vascular disease with decrease in left-to-right shunt volume.[35] Again, close follow-up and early detection should allow revision prior to development of such irreversible sequelae. In cases of band erosion, fibrosis around the band site generally prevents the occurrence of bleeding. Hemolytic anemia and/or thrombus formation have, however, been reported.[36] Erosion seems to occur with greater frequency when narrow banding material is used, although it may occur with any material including broad Silastic bands or umbilical tapes.

A third complication of PAB is the creation of dysplastic changes of the pulmonary valve leaflets, which occurs when the band is placed too proximally on the main pulmonary artery. This is particularly devastating when PAB is performed as preparation for arterial switch, since the pulmonic valve will become the neoaortic valve after the switch procedure. This complication can be avoided by placement of the PAB >15 mm distal to the pulmonic valve cusps.[23] In other circumstances, such as with single ventricle physiology, a more proximal band is desirable since the pulmonic valve will be oversewn at the time of the Fontan procedure and since branch stenosis from too distal placement is much more problematic in such patients.

Pulmonary artery pseudoaneurysm is a rare complication of PAB. It may be preceded by local infection and, like band erosion, is heralded by loss of the band murmur and gradient. Imaging studies demonstrate an enlarged mediastinal shadow on chest x-ray and a markedly enlarged pulmonary artery on echocardiogram or MRI.[37] Pseudoaneurysm formation requires urgent intervention. Repair is performed on cardiopulmonary bypass with patch repair of the pulmonary artery. Glutaraldehyde-treated autologous pericardium is preferred to synthetic material since this condition is sometimes associated with infection at the band site.

Another well-described complication of PAB is the development of subaortic obstruction from conal hypertrophy, particularly in patients with a single ventricle and a subaortic outflow chamber.[38] It may also result from hypertrophy of an abnormally positioned moderator band.[39] The development or persistence of subaortic stenosis post-PAB can adversely effect the outcome of future Fontan procedures through the development of ventricular hypertrophy and

consequent subendocardial ischemia.[40] Indeed, there are indications that the duration of PAB itself may be an independent risk factor for subsequent Fontan procedure.[41] If obstruction occurs later, we perform either a resection of the obstruction or, when this is not possible, a Damus–Kaye–Stansel procedure with or without concomitant Fontan operation.[42] Earlier cavopulmonary connection may be warranted when anatomy and pulmonary physiology are appropriate. The early operative mortality, when addressed early, is comparable to the overall group of Fontan patients (<5%).[43]

A final infrequent but significant complication of PAB is obstruction of coronary blood flow by direct impingement from the band. This occurs when the band is placed too proximally, and usually involves the circumflex coronary artery. Anomalous origin of a coronary artery may increase the risk of inadvertent occlusion.[44,45] Preoperative demonstration of coronary artery anatomy is helpful, but intraoperative vigilance during the banding procedure should safeguard against this potentially catastrophic complication.

SUMMARY

It is clear that although the role and frequency of pulmonary artery banding as originally postulated have decreased, the procedure continues to offer important palliation in certain patients. In particular, it may be useful in patients with a functional single ventricle not amenable to early repair and in whom a future Fontan procedure is anticipated. It may also be of benefit in patients with excessive pulmonary blood flow considered too ill to undergo complete repair of their cardiac defect. The ability to construct an adjustable band has been useful and may add a dimension to palliation that is of early benefit to a select group of patients. Finally, a new indication of preparing the left ventricle for arterial switch in older infants and children with transposition physiology appears to have expanded the role of this palliative procedure.

REFERENCES

1. Muller WH, Dammann JF: Treatment of certain congenital malformations of the heart by the creation of pulmonic stenosis to reduce pulmonary hypertension and excessive pulmonary blood flow: A preliminary report. *Surg Gynecol Obstet* **95**:213, 1952
2. Penkoske PA, Williams WG, Olley PM, et al: Subclavian arterioplasty: Repair of coarctation of the aorta in the first year of life. *J Thorac Cardiovasc Surg* **87**:894, 1984
3. Goldman S, Hernandez J, Pappas G: Results of surgical treatment of coarctation of the aorta in the critically ill neonate. *J Thorac Cardiovasc Surg* **91**:732, 1986
4. Moodie DS, Ritter DG, Tajik AH, et al: Long-term follow-up after palliative operation for univentricular heart. *Am J Cardiol* **53**:1648, 1984
5. Yacoub MH, Radley-Smith R, MacLaurin R: Two-stage operation for

anatomical correction of transposition of the great arteries with intact interventricular septum. *Lancet* **1**:1275, 1977

6. McNicholas K, DeLeval M, Stark J, et al: Surgical treatment of ventricular septal defect in infancy; Primary repair versus banding of pulmonary artery and later repair. *Br Heart J* **41**:133, 1979

7. Silverman N, Levitsky S, Fisher E, et al: Efficacy of pulmonary artery banding in infants with complete atrioventricular canal. *Circulation* **68**(Suppl II):11–48, 1983

8. Clarke DR, Campbell DN, Hayward AR, Bishop DA: Degeneration of aortic valve allografts in young recipients. *J Thorac Cardiovasc Surg* **105**:934–942, 1993

9. Pearl JM, Laks H, Drinkwater DC Jr, et al: Repair of truncus arteriosus in infancy. *Ann Thorac Surg* **52**(4):780–786, 1991

10. Juaneda E, Haworth SG: Double inlet ventricle: Lung biopsy finding and implications for management. *Br Heart J* **53**:515, 1985

11. Wagenvoort CA, Wagenvoort N, Draulans-Noë Y: Reversibility of plexogenic pulmonary arteriopathy following banding of the pulmonary artery. *J Thorac Cardiovasc Surg* **87**:876, 1984

12. Franklin RC, Sullivan ID, Anderson RH, et al: Is banding of the pulmonary trunk obsolete for infants with tricuspid aresia and double inlet ventricle with a discordant ventriculoarterial connection? Role of aortic arch obstruction and subaortic stenosis. *J Am Coll Cardiol* **16**(6):1455–1464, 1990

13. Huddleston CB, Canter CE, Spray TL: Damus-Kaye-Stansel with cavopulmonary connection for single ventricle and subaortic obstruction. *Ann Thorac Surg* **55**(2):339–345, 1993

14. Turley K: Growth of the hypoplastic ascending aorta after radical palliation. *Ann Thorac Surg* **52**(3):647–651, 1991

15. Gibbs JL, Wren C, Watterson KG, et al: Stenting of the arterial duct combined with banding of the pulmonary arteries and atrial septectomy or septostomy: A new approach to palliation for the hypoplastic left heart syndrome. *Br Heart J* **69**(6):479–480, 1993

16. Sievers HH, Lange PE, Arensman FW, et al: Influence of two-stage anatomic correction on size and distensibility of the anatomic pulmonary/functional aortic root in patients with simple transposition of the great arteries. *Circulation* **70**:202, 1984

17. Yasui H, Kado H, Yonenaga K, et al: Arterial switch operation for transposition of the great arteries, with special reference to left ventricle function. *J Thorac Cardiovasc Surg* **98**(4):601–610, 1989

18. Wernovsky G, Giglia TM, Mone SM, et al: Course in the intensive care unit after "preparatory" pulmonary artery banding and aortopulmonary shunt placement for transposition of the great arteries with low left ventricular pressure. *Circulation* **86**(5 Suppl):II133–139, 1992

19. Chang AC, Wenovsky G, Wessel DL, et al: Surgical management of late right ventricular failure after Mustard or Senning repair. *Circulation* **86**(5 Suppl):II140–149, 1992

20. Albus RA, Trusler GA, Izukawa T, et al: Pulmonary artery banding. *J Thorac Cardiovasc Surg* **88**:645, 1984

21. Dajee H, Benson L, Laks H: An improved method of pulmonary artery banding. *Ann Thorac Surg* **37**:254, 1984

22. Higgashidate M, Beppu T, Imai Y, Kurosawa H: Percutaneously adjustable pulmonary artery band. An experimental study. *J Thorac Cardiovasc Surg* **97**(6):864–869, 1989

23. Warnecke I, Bein G, Bucherl ES: The relevance of the intraoperative pressure and oxygen saturation monitoring during pulmonary artery banding in infancy. *J Cardiovasc Anesth* **3**(1):31–36, 1989

24. Rao PS, Julangara RJ, Moore HV, et al: Syndrome of single ventricle without pulmonary stenosis but with left atrioventricular valve atresia and interatrial obstruction. *J Thorac Cardiovasc Surg* **81**:127, 1981

25. Sutherland GR, Van Daele ME, Quaegebeur J: Intraoperative ultrasound monitoring of banding of the pulmonary trunk: A new technique? *Int J Cardiol* **22**(3):395–398, 1989

26. Simpson IA, Valdes-Cruz LM, Berthoty DP, et al: Cine magnetic resonance imaging and color doppler flow mapping in infants and children with pulmonary artery bands. *Am J Cardiol* **71**:1419–1426, 1993

27. Van Nooten G, Deuvaert FE, DePaepe J, Primo G: Pulmonary artery banding. Experience with 69 patients. *J Cardiovasc Surg* (*Torino*) **30**(3):334–337, 1989

28. Horowitz MD, Culpepper WS, Williams LC, et al: Pulmonary artery banding: Analysis of a 25-year experience. *Ann Thorac Surg* **48**(3):444–450, 1989

29. Kron IL, Nolan SP, Flanagan TL, et al: Pulmonary artery banding revisited. *Ann Surg* **209**(5):642–647, 1989

30. LeBlanc J, Ashmore T, Pineda E, et al: Pulmonary artery banding: Results and current indications in a pediatric surgery. *Ann Thorac Surg* **44**:628, 1987

31. Mahle S, Nicoloff DM, Knight L, et al: Pulmonary artery banding: Long-term results in 63 patients. *Ann Thorac Surg* **27**:216, 1979

32. Robertson MA, Penkoske PA, Duncan NF: Right pulmonary artery obstruction after pulmonary artery banding. *Ann Thorac Surg* **51**(1):73–75, 1991

33. Fletcher BD, Garcia EJ, Colenda C, et al: Reduced lung volume associated with acquired pulmonary artery obstruction in children. *AJR* **133**:47, 1979

34. Garcia EJ, Riggs T, Hirschfeld S, et al: Echocardiographic assessment of the adequacy of pulmonary arterial banding. *Am J Cardiol* **44**:487, 1979

35. Danilowicz D, Presti S, Colvin S: The disappearing pulmonary artery band. *Pediatric Cardiol* **11**(1):47–49, 1990

36. Kutsche LM, Alexander JA, Van Mierop LHS: Hemolytic anemia secondary to erosion of a silastic band into the lumen of the pulmonary trunk. *Am J Cardiol* **55**:1438, 1985

37. Lynch DA, Higgins CB: MR imaging of unilateral pulmonary artery anomalies. *J Comput Assist Tomogr* **14**(2):187–191, 1990

38. Freedom RM, Sondheimer H, Dische R, et al: Development of "subaortic stenosis" after pulmonary arterial banding for common ventricle. *Am J Cardiol* **39**:78, 1977

39. De Vivie R, Van Praagh S, Bein G, et al: Transposition of the great arteries with straddling tricuspid valve. Report of two rare cases with acquired subaortic stenosis after main pulmonary artery banding. *J Thorac Cardiovasc Surg* **98**(2):205–213, 1989

40. Caspi J, Coles JG, Rabinovich M, et al: Morphological findings contributing to a failed Fontan procedure. Twelve-year experience. *Circulation* **82**(5 Suppl):IV177–182, 1990

41. Malcic I, Sauer U, Stern H, et al: The influence of pulmonary artery banding on outcome after the Fontan operation. *J Thorac Cardiovasc Surg* **104**(3):743–747, 1992

42. Castenada AR, Lang P: Single ventricle (single or double inlet) complicated by subaortic stenosis: Surgical options in infancy. *Ann Thorac Surg* **39**:361, 1985

43. Stein DG, Laks H, Drinkwater DC, et al: Results of total cavopulmonary connection in the treatment of patients with a functional single ventricle. *J Thorac Cardiovasc Surg* **102**(2):280–286, 1991

44. Steussy HF, Caldwell RL, Wills ER, et al: High take-off of the left main coronary artery from the pulmonary trunk: Potentially fatal combination with pulmonary trunk banding. *Am Heart J* **108**:619, 1984

45. Daskalopoulos DA, Edwards WD, Driscoll DJ, et al: Fatal pulmonary artery banding in truncus arteriosus with anomalous origin of circumflex coronary artery from right pulmonary artery. *Am J Cardiol* **52**:1363, 1983

CHAPTER

65

Tracheoesophageal Compressive Syndromes of Vascular Origin

Rings and Slings

Richard D. Mainwaring and John J. Lamberti

Surgical management of vascular rings began in 1945 when Robert E. Gross repaired a double aortic arch.[1] Gross et al[2,3] and Willis J. Potts et al[4,5] subsequently defined the more common forms of vascular rings and the pulmonary artery sling. They proposed the operative management that is still utilized today. Thirty-four different forms of vascular ring are recognized, although most of these are exceedingly rare.

While much of the original attention focused on the aberrant course of vascular structures, it is evident that patient symptoms are related to the compressive effects on the trachea and/or esophagus. Surgery for vascular rings can be accomplished in a straightforward manner with little morbidity or mortality, but does not address damage to the trachea and esophagus that may already have occurred. It has become increasingly clear that both the short- and long-term success of operations directed at relief of tracheoesophageal compression depend on the integrity of these structures.

CLASSIFICATION

The term vascular ring describes abnormalities of the aortic arch that result in either complete or partial encirclement of the trachea or esophagus. Vascular sling refers to the condition in which the left pulmonary artery originates from the right pulmonary artery and passes between the trachea and esophagus. The tracheoesophageal compressive syndromes can be categorized into four groups: (1) double aortic arch,

(2) right aortic arch with left ligamentum arteriosum, (3) left aortic arch with arch vessel anomalies, and (4) pulmonary artery sling. Complete vascular rings occur in the first two groups.

EMBRYOLOGY AND PATHOLOGY

Our understanding of the embryology of vascular rings has been enhanced by many authors including Congdon,[6] Barry,[7] and Bahnson and Blalock.[8] Edwards[9] proposed a practical surgical classification based on a hypothetical model of paired segmental structures with a double aortic arch and bilateral ductus arteriosi (Fig. 65–1). The final configuration of the aortic arch depends on the preservation or involution of specific segments of this rudimentary aortic arch complex. A single left aortic arch is predicated upon involution of the primitive fourth right arch at 36–38 days' gestation.

Double aortic arch is the most common form of vascular ring necessitating surgical division. It is the result of a persistent right fourth arch. Two arches arise from the ascending aorta, pass on either side of the trachea and esophagus, and join the descending aorta to produce a true ring (Fig. 65–2). The right (posterior) arch gives origin to the right carotid and subclavian arteries. The left carotid and subclavian arteries arise from the left (anterior) arch, which is usually the smaller of the two arches.

Right aortic arch with left ligamentum is the second

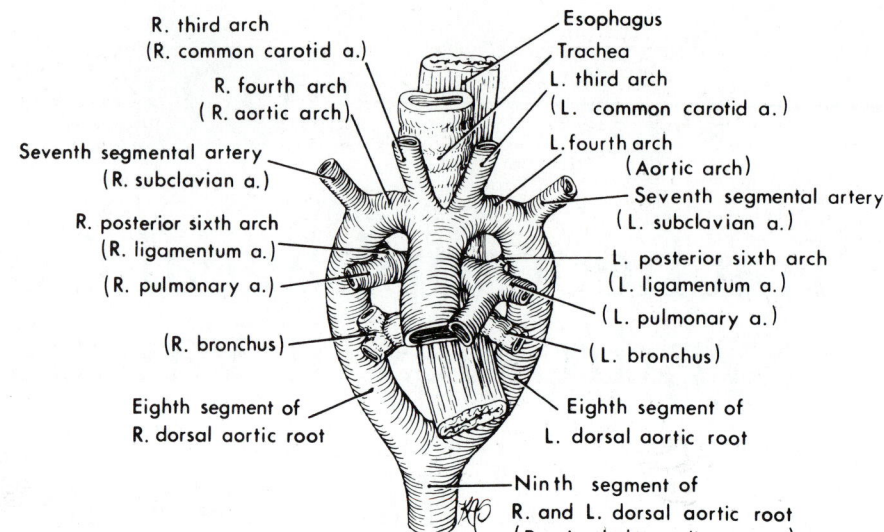

Figure 65–1. The embryonic aortic arch complex surrounding the trachea and the esophagus. The structures in the diagram are identified by their embryonic names—their eventual names are included in parentheses. *(From Idriss FS: Vascular ring. In Raffensperger JG (ed): Swendon's Pediatric Surgery. Norwalk, CT, Appleton and Lange, 1990, p 690.)*

most common vascular ring requiring surgical intervention. This anomaly is the result of a persistent right fourth arch and deletion of the left arch. A complete ring is formed by the ligamentum connecting the descending aorta to the left pulmonary artery (Fig. 65–3). The left subclavian artery may be associated with a diverticulum (termed Kommerell's diverticulum) at its origin from the aorta.

Right aortic arch with mirror image branching and left ligamentum arteriosum results from persistence of the right fourth aortic arch and involution of the left arch between the subclavian artery and the descending aorta. When the ligamentum originates from the descending aorta, a complete ring is formed, whereas if it originates from the innominate artery, a ring is not formed (Fig. 65–4).

Left aortic arch with aberrant right subclavian artery develops when the right fourth arch between the subclavian and carotid arteries regresses. The right subclavian artery persists as a branch from the descending aorta coursing posterior to the esophagus (Fig. 65–5). The path of this artery produces a posterior indentation of the esophagus, but does not form a complete vascular ring. This is the most common form of aortic arch anomaly, with an estimated incidence of 0.5%.[10]

The innominate artery may be responsible for anterior compression of the trachea. In this setting, the innominate compresses the trachea as the artery courses upward and to the right toward the thoracic outlet. It has been speculated that patients with this syndrome have an innominate artery

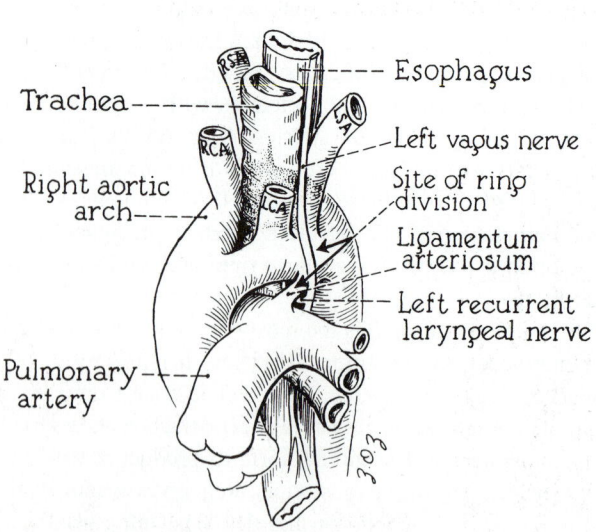

Figure 65–2. Double aortic arch, right arch dominant. The ring is divided where the lesser arch (left arch in this case) inserts into the descending aorta. The ligamentum arteriosum is also divided.

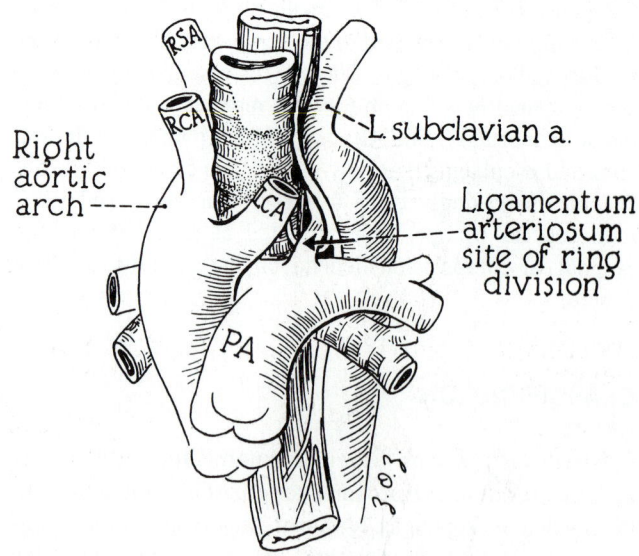

Figure 65–3. Right aortic arch with left ligamentum arteriosum and retroesophageal left subclavian artery. The ring is divided at the ligamentum arteriosum.

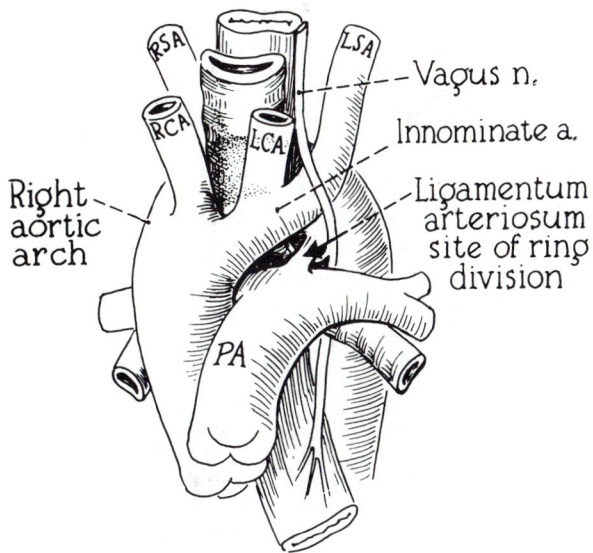

Figure 65–4. Right aortic arch with left ligamentum and mirror image left innominate. The ring is divided at the ligamentum arteriosum.

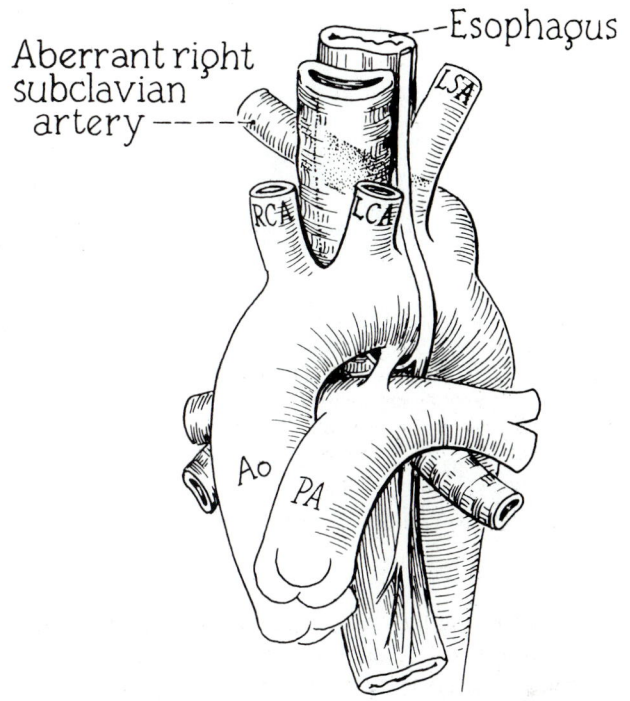

Figure 65–5. Left aortic arch with aberrant right subclavian artery arising from the descending aorta. This does not form a complete vascular ring.

origin somewhat more posterior and leftward than is seen in a normal aortic arch (Fig. 65–6). This problem is particularly common in patients who have previously undergone repair of a tracheoesophageal fistula.[11]

Pulmonary artery sling is a rare anomaly in which the left pulmonary artery originates from the right pulmonary artery instead of the main pulmonary artery. The left pulmonary artery then courses around the right main stem bronchus and passes between the trachea and esophagus (Fig. 65–7). The embryologic origin of a vascular sling is distinctly different from a vascular ring insofar as formation of a sling does not depend on preservation or involution of paired segmental structures. A pulmonary artery sling is the result of the left lung capturing its arterial supply from de-

rivatives of the right sixth arch instead of the left sixth arch. Pulmonary artery slings are associated with a variety of tracheobronchial anomalies such as accessory bronchi (Fig. 65–8) and bronchomalacia.[12] Complete tracheal rings may result in tracheal stenosis at sites remote from the aberrant pulmonary artery. These findings suggest an embryologic overlap with bronchopulmonary foregut malformations.[13] In contrast to vascular rings, pulmonary artery slings are often associated with intracardiac defects.[14]

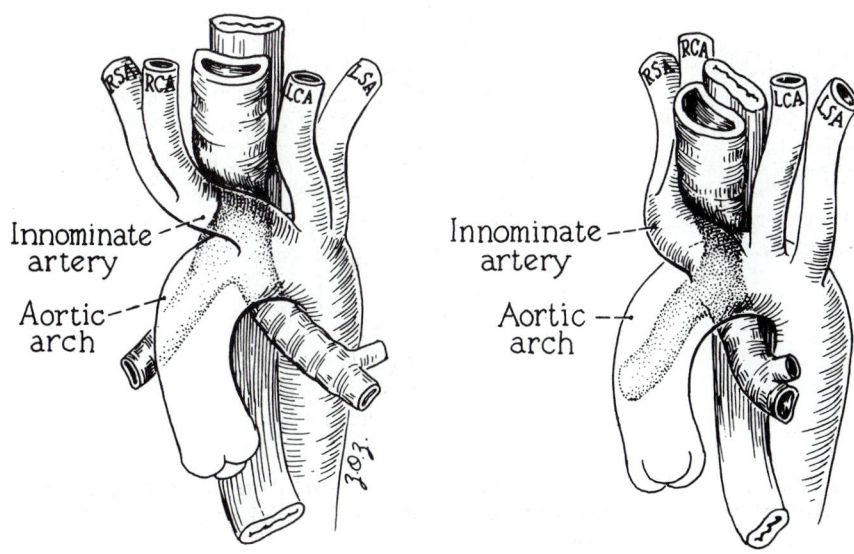

Figure 65–6. Anterior compression of the trachea caused by the innominate artery. The artery originates more posterior and leftward from the aortic arch than in the usual situation.

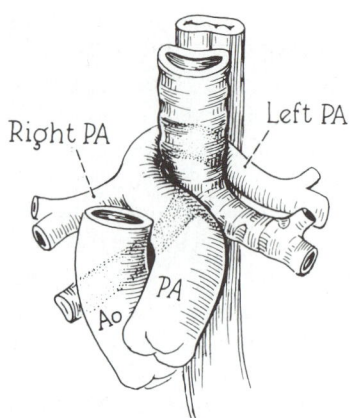

Figure 65–7. Pulmonary artery sling. The left pulmonary artery originates from the right pulmonary artery instead of the main pulmonary artery and compresses the trachea just above the carina.

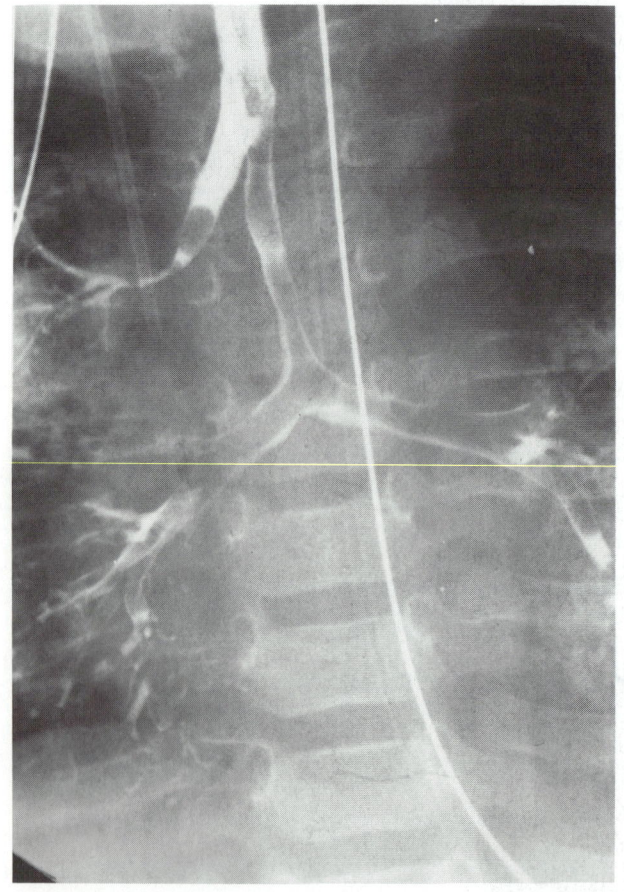

Figure 65–8. Tracheogram of a patient with pulmonary artery sling. The study demonstrates an accessory bronchus to the right upper lobe. A nasogastric tube indicates the position of the esophagus.

CLINICAL MANIFESTATIONS

The clinical manifestations of vascular rings and slings are the result of the compressive effects of the adjacent airway or esophagus. In general, the "tightness" of the ring will determine the age of presentation and clinical severity. For example, vascular slings that present in the neonatal age group are usually due to severe tracheobronchial narrowing, whereas some patients may remain asymptomatic for many years. Many patients are followed for extended periods of time before the proper diagnosis is made. This may be attributable to the relative rarity of tracheobronchial compressive syndromes as compared to more common problems such as asthma or bronchiolitis.

A thorough history is essential in the evaluation of these patients. Most parents retrospectively will recall symptoms of stridor and noisy respiration that they noticed since birth. These symptoms may be exacerbated by an upper respiratory illness, and some patients will have recurrent respiratory infections.[15] Many patients will have a chronic "brassy" cough related to irritation of the airway or difficulty in clearing secretions. Some infants will preferentially assume a hyperextended posture; this position places longitudinal traction on the trachea and effectively relieves the tracheal obstruction.

Dysphagia is a less common manifestation of tracheobronchial compressive syndromes, but on rare occasions may be caused by an aberrant right subclavian artery. The aberrant artery wraps posteriorly around the esophagus creating a spiral indentation (Fig. 65–9). This anatomy may result in solid food dysphagia, but is never severe enough to affect the swallowing of liquids. The vast majority of people with this anatomy are asymptomatic and require no treatment.[10] The phrase "dysphagia lusoria" [from the Latin *lusus naturae* meaning a sport (accident) of nature] was coined to describe the error of ascribing dysphagia to the radiologic finding of an aberrant right subclavian artery.

DIAGNOSIS

The diagnosis of a tracheoesophageal compressive syndrome is usually prompted by symptoms. Neonates may present with respiratory distress due to severe tracheobronchial narrowing. Infants and children usually have a history of chronic noisy breathing exacerbated by respiratory infections. The most important aspect in diagnosing tracheoesophageal compressive syndromes is to entertain aortic arch abnormalities as a possibility. Based on the typical symptoms, the preoperative workup logically proceeds to a chest radiograph to determine the position of the aortic arch (Fig. 65–10) and a barium swallow to demonstrate encroachment on the esophagus (Fig. 65–11).

An aortogram may occasionally be indicated in the workup of vascular rings. This study may be helpful in determining the position of the major and minor elements of

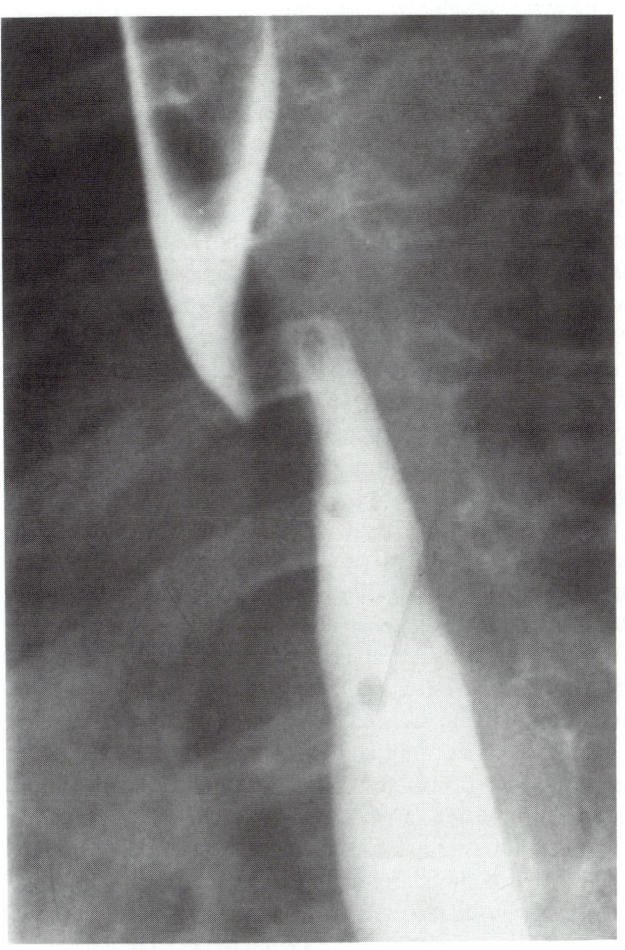

Figure 65–9. Barium swallow in a patient with an aberrant right subclavian artery. The aberrant artery results in a characteristic spiral indentation of the esophagus. This 5 year old had solid food dysphagia that was relieved following division of the subclavian artery.

the ring (double aortic arch) and the location of the arch vessels that contribute to tracheoesophageal compressive syndrome.[16] Other authors have suggested that patients should undergo endoscopy either prior to or at the time of surgery to determine the extent of airway compromise and identify coexistent airway abnormalities. This may be particularly true in cases of innominate artery compression or in the case of a vascular sling due to the higher incidence of associated tracheobronchial anomalies.[17] Both arteriography and endoscopy may be useful in selected cases where the information provided will impact the subsequent operation.

A number of noninvasive modalities have been proposed to assist in the delineation of vascular ring anatomy. Both magnetic resonance imaging (MRI) and computed tomography (CT) can provide detailed images of the relationship between the vascular structures and the trachea and esophagus[18,19] (Fig. 65–12). Both of these studies can be performed with computer-assisted three-dimensional reconstruction (Fig. 65–13). These studies provide exquisite demonstration of vascular ring anatomy, but the high cost is a significant disadvantage. Ultrasonography has also been espoused as a useful noninvasive test that can assist in delineating vascular ring anatomy.[20] Standard cardiac views may not be effective in demonstrating the aortic arch anatomy, and nonstandard views may be necessary when entertaining the diagnosis of a vascular ring.[21] Patients with pulmonary artery slings have a significant incidence of intracardiac defects and, therefore, this subset of patients should undergo echocardiography as a routine part of their evaluation. Although MRI, CT, and ultrasonography have all been shown to be effective in demonstrating vascular ring anatomy, a favorable influence on outcome has not been demonstrated.

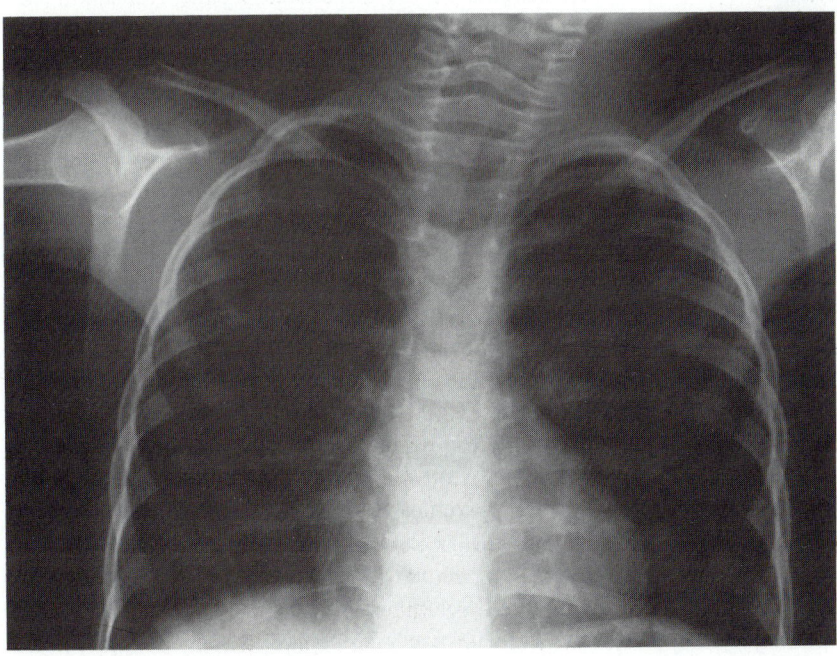

Figure 65–10. Chest radiograph of a child with a right arch with left ligamentum. The position of the arch to the right of the trachea is seen in this film.

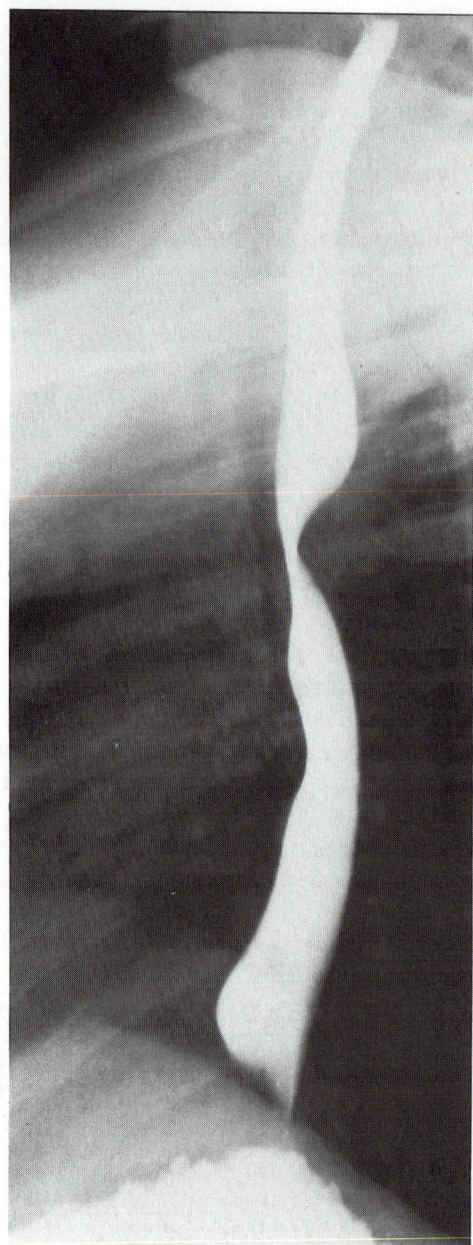

Figure 65–11. Esophagram of the right aortic arch with left ligamentum. The transverse indentation of the posterior esophagus is typical of complete vascular rings.

SURGICAL MANAGEMENT

Surgical intervention is indicated in all patients with *symptomatic* vascular rings. These patients may acutely decompensate from an upper respiratory infection, and thus should undergo surgery when they are clinically well. A chest radiograph may help in documenting the resolution of intercurrent illness. The management of *asymptomatic* vascular rings should be individualized. Patients who are asymptomatic but have a complete ring (double aortic arch or right aortic arch with left ligament) should undergo elective surgery. Although unproven, there is concern that injury to

the airway may be progressive in the case of complete rings. In contrast, patients with asymptomatic incomplete rings may be followed clinically.

The surgical approach to vascular rings may be through either a thoracotomy or sternotomy incision. A left posterolateral thoracotomy provides excellent exposure of double aortic arch or right arch/left ligament anatomy, and is the standard approach for these lesions. There are a few forms of vascular ring that may not be accessible from the left chest (right arch or left arch with a right ligamentum arteriosum) and necessitate right thoracotomy.[22] Surgeons accustomed to a median sternotomy approach may find this useful for vascular ring operations. A sternotomy incision is indicated when concomitant repair of intracardiac defects is planned or for the repair of pulmonary artery sling in which tracheal reconstruction is required.[23]

Repair of double aortic arch is accomplished by dividing the smaller of the two arches. The aorta and arch vessels are defined, and the smaller arch is temporarily occluded to ensure that there is no change in distal pressure. The vascular ring is divided in a manner that maintains continuity of the major arch vessels. In most cases, the anterior aorta is smaller and arch division is performed between the left carotid and descending aorta. This segment may be atretic in up to 40% of cases.[24] When the left (anterior) arch is dominant, division is performed between the right carotid and descending aorta. In addition, the ligament is divided and adventitial fibers freed around the trachea and esophagus. Injury to the recurrent laryngeal nerve has been reported to be more frequent following repair of double aortic arch.[25] Burke reported successful division of a double aortic arch using a video-assisted thoracoscopic (VAT) technique.[26]

Repair of right arch/left ligament can be readily accomplished through either a left thoracotomy or sternotomy approach. Division of the ductus usually results in wide separation of the divided ends and dramatic relief of compression. Debate exists regarding the significance of Kommerell's diverticulum. Some authors have advocated plication of this diverticulum or transection and reimplantation of the left subclavian artery when the diverticulum is of significant size.[27]

Repair of the left aortic arch anomalies must be individualized. It should be recalled that this group comprises incomplete rings. Surgical intervention is indicated only in the symptomatic patient where symptoms must be clearly attributable to the vascular anomaly and not a separate disease process. Repair of an aberrant right subclavian artery can be performed in younger children by dividing the subclavian at its origin through a left thoracotomy approach. Collateral blood flow is usually satisfactory to maintain viability of the extremity. In older patients, limb viability and subclavian steal are concerns that favor vascular reconstruction. This may be performed through either a sternotomy[28] or right thoracotomy[29] approach.

Innominate artery compression syndrome is repaired

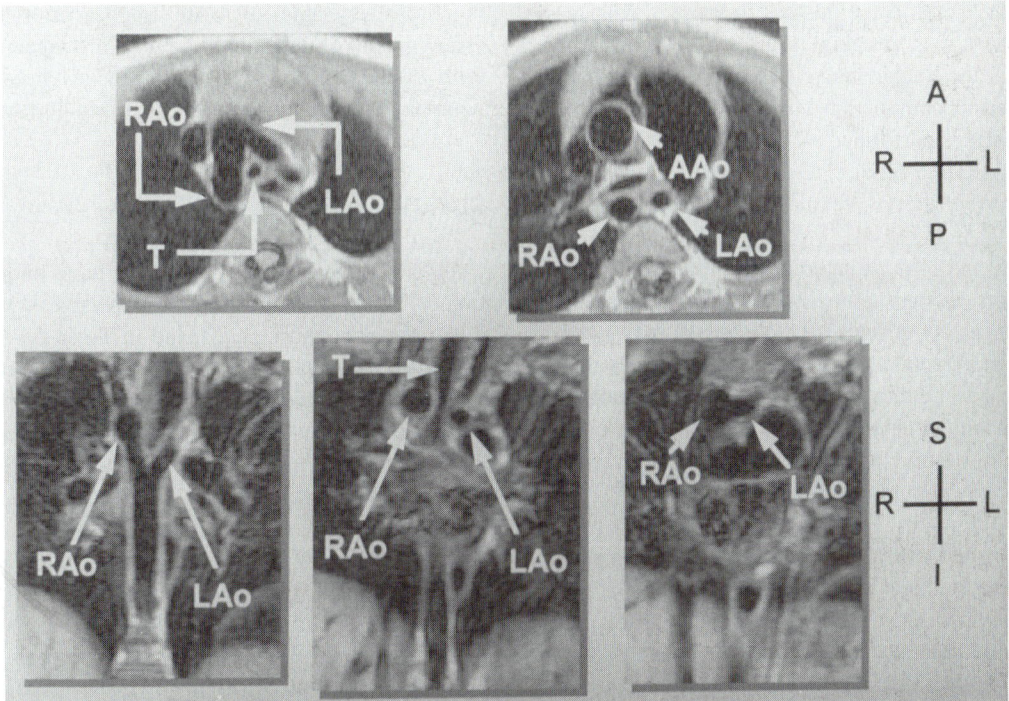

Figure 65–12. Magnetic resonance imaging (MRI) of a child with double aortic arch. The upper images are horizontal cross sections, whereas the lower images are coronal views. RAo, right aortic arch; LAo, left aortic arch; AAo, ascending aorta; T, trachea. *(Courtesy of Dr. Mark Fogel, Children's Hospital of Philadelphia.)*

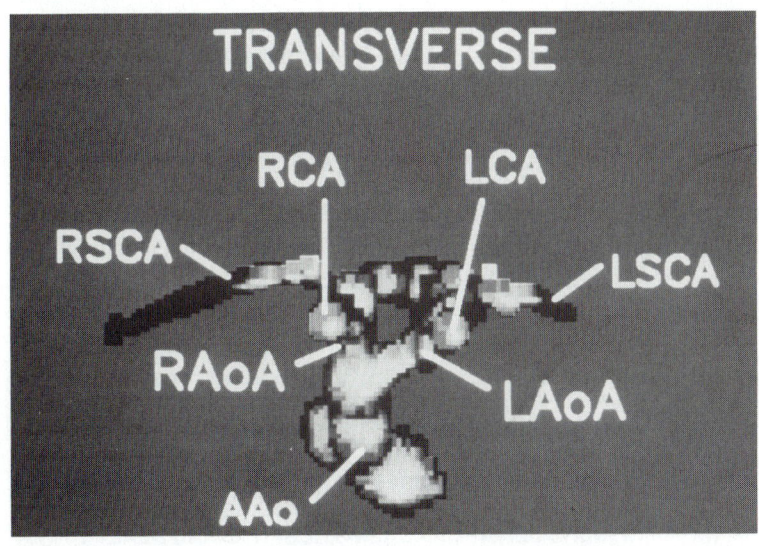

A

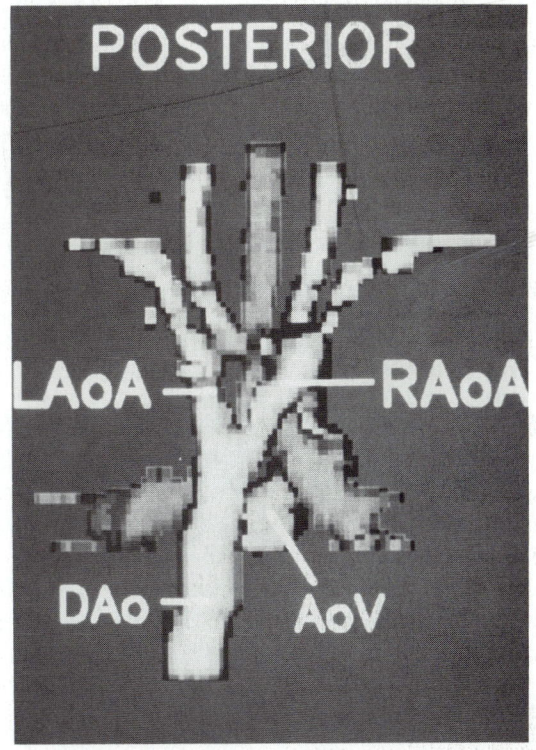

B

Figure 65–13. A,B. Computer-assisted three-dimensional reconstruction of the double aortic arch shown in Figure 65–12. LAoA, left aortic arch; RAoA, right aortic arch; AoV, aortic valve; DAo, descending aorta; AAo, ascending aorta; RSCA, right subclavian artery; RCA, right carotid artery; LCA, left carotid artery; LSCA, left subclavian artery. *(Courtesy of Dr. Mark Fogel, Children's Hospital of Philadelphia.)*

by suspending the aorta to the posterior aspect of the sternum. It was Dr. Gross' original premise that aortopexy would stent open the tracheomalacic segment.[3] The operation is performed in conjunction with bronchoscopy. Suspension of the aorta is performed while the airway is visualized to ensure adequate relief.[16] Occasionally, division of the innominate artery may be required to achieve adequate space for the airway.[30]

Between 15 and 30% of patients who have undergone repair of a tracheoesophageal fistula will demonstrate symptoms of airway compromise. Tracheomalacia typically develops where the trachea passes between the innominate artery anteriorly and the dilated (dysmotile) esophagus posteriorly. Patients who have undergone TEF repair should be followed with this in mind, and those who develop symptomatic airway disease should undergo aortopexy.[11]

Repair of pulmonary artery sling can be performed through either a left thoracotomy or sternotomy approach. Prior to surgery, patients should undergo either bronchoscopy or bronchography to identify associated tracheobronchial abnormalities. Patients with isolated pulmonary artery sling may undergo surgery through either a left thoracotomy or sternotomy approach. The left branch pulmonary artery, which may be hypoplastic, is divided at its origin and passed between the trachea and esophagus. The left pulmonary artery is then anastomosed to the main pulmonary artery (Fig. 65–14). Early reports suggested a high incidence of left pulmonary artery occlusion, but more recent series have demonstrated satisfactory results.[31] Patients with significant tracheal stenosis may present with respiratory distress in the neonatal period and may be ventilator dependent, as spontaneous ventilation results in tracheal collapse. These patients are minimally improved if only the aberrant pulmonary artery is addressed. Therefore, recent authors have proposed either tracheal resection utilizing cardiopulmonary bypass[32,33] (bringing the left pulmonary artery anterior to the trachea prior to tracheal reanastomosis) or pulmonary artery sling repair in association with tracheopexy.[34] These approaches hold promise for what had previously been an extremely high-risk group.

SURGICAL RESULTS

Over a 15-year period, 41 patients have undergone operations for tracheoesophageal compressive syndrome at our institution. Diagnoses are listed in Table 65–1. There were two operative deaths, both of which occurred in neonates with pulmonary artery sling and tracheal stenosis.

The majority of patients who undergo repair of vascular rings have prompt relief of symptoms. Some patients, however, will exhibit an exacerbation of symptoms. Presumably this is related to tissue dissection and edema adjacent to the airway as well as mucosal edema from intubation. Supportive care includes humidified oxygen, chest physiotherapy, diuretics, and racemic epinephrine treatments. Gradual improvement can be expected over a several day period.

LONG-TERM FOLLOW-UP

Little is known concerning the long-term follow-up of patients who have undergone repair of vascular ring. Most clinical series consider discharge from the hospital as a successful outcome. However, it is evident that many patients may not have complete relief of symptoms,[35] and it may take months or years until they "outgrow" the effects of tracheomalacia. In one study, pulmonary function tests were performed at a remote time from operative repair. More than half of the patients evaluated had abnormal flow volume loops indicative of central airway obstruction.[36] These findings suggest that tracheal or bronchial distortion persists in many patients despite their "asymptomatic" status.

It is conceivable that earlier repair could ameliorate the long-term effects of vascular ring on the tracheobronchial tree. If this proves to be the case, then the best treatment of airway malacia may be its prevention. Once damage to the airway has occurred, "pexy" procedures may be helpful.

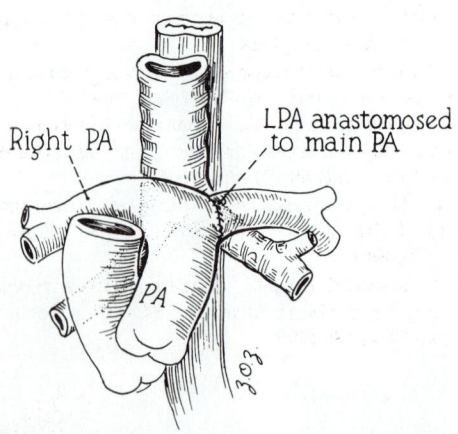

Figure 65–14. Repair of pulmonary artery sling. The left pulmonary artery has been divided from the right pulmonary artery, brought anterior to the trachea, and reanastomosed to the main pulmonary artery.

TABLE 65–1. DIAGNOSES OF PATIENTS UNDERGOING OPERATIONS FOR TRACHEOESOPHAGEAL COMPRESSIVE SYNDROMES AT CHILDREN'S HOSPITAL AND HEALTH CENTER OF SAN DIEGO, CALIFORNIA

Diagnoses	Number of Patients
Double aortic arch	13
Right arch/left ligament	13
Innominate artery compression	8
Aberrant right subclavian	3
Pulmonary artery sling	4

Other methods of treating tracheobronchial malacia are limited but do include resection or stenting.[37]

CONCLUSION

Vascular rings are an uncommon form of congenital heart problem. Although relatively sophisticated methods of diagnosis are now available, most patients can be adequately assessed based on their history, a chest x-ray, and a barium swallow. The operations for most vascular rings are straightforward and can be performed with little risk. Attention to the airway is of utmost importance, as this will determine the ultimate long-term status of these patients.

REFERENCES

1. Gross RE: Surgical relief of tracheal obstruction from a vascular ring. *N Engl J Med* **233:**586–590, 1945
2. Gross RE, Ware PF: Surgical significance of aortic arch anomalies. *Surg Gynecol Obstet* **83:**435, 1946
3. Gross RE, Neuhauser EB: Compression of the trachea by an anomalous innominate artery. An operation for its release. *Am J Dis Child* **75:**570–574, 1948
4. Potts WJ, Gibson S, Rothwell R: Double aortic arch: Report of two cases. *Arch Surg* **57:**227–233, 1948
5. Potts WJ, Holinger PH, Rosenblum AH: Anomalous left pulmonary artery causing obstruction to right main bronchus. Report of a case. *JAMA* **155:**1409, 1954
6. Congdon ED: Transformation of the aortic arch system during the development of a human embryo. *Contrib Embryol* **14:**47–110, 1922
7. Barry A: The aortic arch derivatives in the human adult. *Anat Rec* **111:**221, 1951
8. Bahnson HT, Blalock A: Aortic vascular rings encountered in surgical treatment of congenital pulmonic stenosis. *Ann Surg* **131:**356, 1950
9. Edwards JE: Malformations of the aortic arch system manifested as "vascular rings." *Lab Invest* **2:**56, 1953
10. Beabout JW, Stewart JR, Kincaid OW: Aberrant right subclavian artery, dispute of commonly accepted concepts. *Am J Roentgenol* **92:**855–864, 1964
11. Filler RM, Messineo A, Vinograd I: Severe tracheomalacia associated with esophageal atresia: Results of surgical treatment. *J Pediatr Surg* **27:**1136–1141, 1992
12. Sade RM, Rosenthal A, Fellows K, Castaneda AR: Pulmonary artery sling. *J Thorac Cardiovasc Surg* **69:**333–346, 1975
13. Rodgers BM, Harman PK, Johnson AM: Bronchopulmonary foregut malformations. *Ann Surg* **203:**517–524, 1986
14. Gikonyo BM, Jue KL, Edwards JE: Pulmonary vascular sling: Report of seven cases and review of the literature. *Pediatr Cardiol* **10:**81–89, 1989
15. Van Aalderen WMC, Hoekstra MO, Hess J, et al: Respiratory infections and vascular rings. *Acta Paediatr Scand* **79:**477–480, 1990
16. Smith RJH, Smith MCF, Glossop LP, et al: Congenital vascular anomalies causing tracheoesophageal compression. *Arch Otolaryngol* **110:**82–87, 1984
17. Ergin MA, Jayaram N, La Corte M: Left aortic arch and right descending aorta: Diagnostic and therapeutic implications of a rare type of vascular ring. *Ann Thorac Surg* **31:**82–85, 1980
18. Myer CM, Auringer ST, Wiatrak BJ, Bisset G: Magnetic resonance imaging in the diagnosis of innominate artery compression of the trachea. *Arch Otolaryngol Head Neck Surg* **116:**314–316, 1990
19. Azarow KS, Pearl RH, Hoffman MA, et al: Vascular ring: Does magnetic resonance imaging replace angiography? *Ann Thorac Surg* **53:**882–885, 1992
20. Lillehei CW, Colan S: Echocardiography in the preoperative evaluation of vascular rings. *J Pediatr Surg* **27:**1118–1121, 1992
21. Murdison KA, Andrews BAA, Chin HA: Ultrasonographic display of complex vascular rings. *J Am Coll Cardiol* **15:**1645–1653, 1990
22. McFaul R, Millard P, Nowicki E: Vascular rings necessitating right thoracotomy. *J Thorac Cardiovasc Surg* **82:**306–309, 1981
23. Backer CL, Idriss FS, Holinger LD, Mavroudis C: Pulmonary artery sling: Results of surgical repair in infancy. *J Thorac Cardiovasc Surg* **103:**683–691, 1992
24. Backer CL, Ilbawi MN, Idriss FS, DeLeon SY: Mediastinal vascular anomalies causing tracheoesophageal compression: Review of experience in children. *J Thorac Cardiovasc Surg* **97:**725–731, 1989
25. Nikaidoh H, Riker WL, Idriss FS: Surgical management of vascular rings. *Arch Surg* **105:**327–333, 1972
26. Burke RP, Chang AC: Video-assisted thoracoscopic division of a vascular ring in an infant. *J Cardiovasc Surg* **8:**537–540, 1993
27. van Son JAM, Julsrud PR, Hagler DJ, et al: Surgical treatment of vascular rings: The Mayo Clinic experience. *Mayo Clin Proc* **68:**1056–1063, 1993
28. Kalke BR, Magotra R, Doshi FM: A new surgical approach to the management of symptomatic aberrant right subclavian artery. *Ann Thorac Surg* **44:**86–89, 1987
29. van Son JAM, Vincent JG, van Oort A, Lacquet LK: Translocation of aberrant right subclavian artery in dysphagia lusoria in children through a right thoracotomy. *Thorac Cardiovasc Surg* **37:**52–54, 1989
30. Myer CM, Wiatrak BJ, Cotton RT, et al: Innominate artery compression of the trachea: Current concepts. *Laryngoscope* **99:**1030–1034, 1989
31. Dunn JM, Gordon I, Chrispin AR, et al: Early and late results of surgical correction of pulmonary artery sling. *Ann Thorac Surg* **28:**230–238, 1979
32. Hickey M St J, Wood AE: Pulmonary artery sling with tracheal stenosis: One-stage repair. *Ann Thorac Surg* **44:**416–417, 1987
33. Jonas RA, Spevak PJ, McGill T, Castaneda AR: Pulmonary artery sling: Primary repair by tracheal resection in infancy. *J Thorac Cardiovasc Surg* **97:**548–550, 1989
34. Conti VR, Lobe TE: Vascular sling with tracheomalacia: Surgical management. *Ann Thorac Surg* **47:**310–311, 1989
35. Thomson AH, Beardsmore CS, Firman R, et al: Airway function in infants with vascular rings: Preoperative and postoperative assessment. *Arch Dis Childh* **65:**171–174, 1990
36. Marmon LM, Bye MR, Haas JM, et al: Vascular rings and slings: Longterm follow up of pulmonary function. *J Pediatr Surg* **19:**683–692, 1984
37. Mair EA, Parsons DS, Lally KP: Treatment of severe bronchomalacia with expanding endobronchial stents. *Arch Otolaryngol Head Neck Surg* **116:**1087–1090, 1990

66

Anomalous Pulmonary and Systemic Venous Connections

Davis C. Drinkwater, Jr., and Harry J. D'Agostino, Jr.

Anomalous pulmonary and systemic venous connections represent one of the forms of congenital heart disease in which the embryologic origin of the defects is understood. Since the cardiac architecture itself is often normal, proper correction of these defects can have a profound influence on long-term prognosis.

EMBRYOLOGY

The lungs are derived from the embryologic foregut and their venous drainage is via the splanchnic plexus (cardinal and umbilicovitelline veins). There is no direct connection to the heart until the common pulmonary vein develops as an outpouching of the sinoatrial portion of the heart, to the left of the atrial septum primum. Once pulmonary connections are established, the splanchnic connections are lost and pulmonary venous drainage is to the left atrium. The cardinal veins eventually form the superior vena cava, innominate veins, coronary sinus (CS), and azygous and hemiazygous veins. The umbilicovitelline veins form the inferior vena cava, portal vein, and ductus venosus. Alterations in the developmental sequence account for the observed anomalous pulmonary and systemic venous connections.[1]

TOTAL ANOMALOUS PULMONARY VENOUS CONNECTIONS

Anomalous pulmonary venous connections are characterized by circulation of pulmonary venous return into systemic veins. This is an uncommon cardiac anomaly that

represents approximately 2% of the total congenital experience.[2] The term "connection" is preferred over "drainage" because the latter includes pulmonary venous drainage returning normally to the left atrium and flowing across an atrial septal defect.

Anomalous pulmonary venous connections almost always occur with an associated atrial septal defect. A patent ductus arteriosus is also present in many patients. In patients with visceral heterotaxy (atrial isomerism), the incidence of anomalous pulmonary venous connection can be as high as 50%, and its presence can greatly complicate patient management.[3]

History

In 1798, the first description of total anomalous pulmonary venous connection (TAPVC) was provided by Wilson.[4] Brody, in 1942, published a review of 37 cases.[5] In 1951, Muller at UCLA, performed the first partial correction, anastomosing the left pulmonary veins to the left atrial appendage.[6] In 1956 the first complete correction was performed by Lewis and Varco using moderate hypothermia and inflow occlusion in a patient with a cardiac connection.[7] The first corrections using cardiopulmonary bypass were reported in 1956–1957 by Burroughs and Kirklin[8] and by Cooley and Ochsner.[9]

Anatomy

Although wide variations in the anatomy of anomalous pulmonary venous connections exist, the classification by Darling and associates continues to be practical and is most commonly utilized.[10] The connections are divided into four types: supracardiac, cardiac, infracardiac, and mixed. With the exception of the mixed type, pulmonary venous effluent usually converges in a common pulmonary vein confluence located posterior to the left atrium. The route of the connection to the systemic circulation forms the basis of the anatomic classification. The frequency of various types of connections from several recent series is summarized in Table 66–1.

Supracardiac

The common pulmonary vein drains superiorly, most often through an ascending vertical vein, usually crossing anterior to the left pulmonary artery, into the left innominate vein (Fig. 66–1A). Blood then flows across the midline into the right superior vena cava and right atrium. On rare occasions, the ascending vertical vein will connect directly with the right superior vena cava or with the azygous system. Approximately 40% of patients have a supracardiac type of venous connection.

Cardiac

The common pulmonary vein connects most frequently to the coronary sinus (Fig. 66–2A). Often, an enlarged coronary sinus is the only clue to the presence of a cardiac connection. On occasion, individual pulmonary veins will connect directly with the right atrium. Approximately 25% of patients have a cardiac type of connection.

Infracardiac

Approximately 25% of patients have this anomaly in which the common pulmonary vein drains through the diaphragm into the portal vein or ductus venosus (Fig. 66–3A). This type has the greatest propensity for venous obstruction.

Mixed

This entity, accounting for 5% of patients, does not have a single common pulmonary venous confluence and may be a combination of any or all of the above three types.

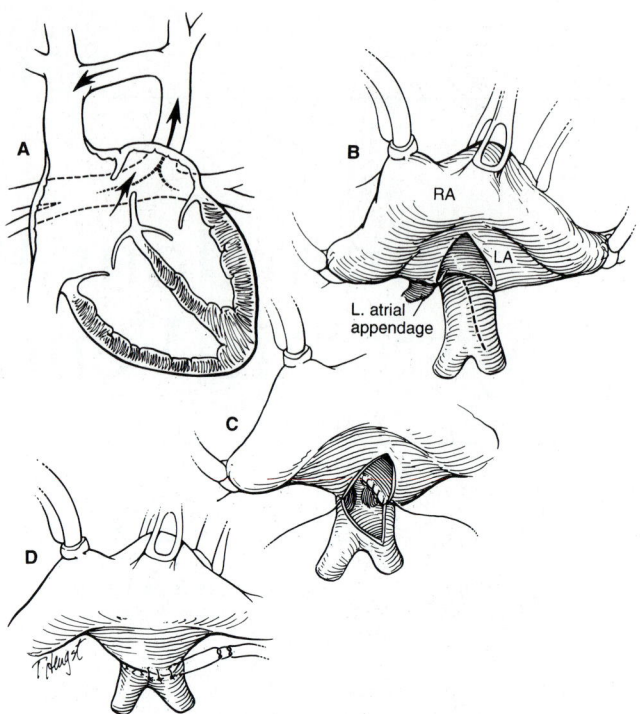

Figure 66–1. Supracardiac TAPVC. **A.** The common pulmonary vein connects via an ascending vertical vein to the left innominate vein. **B.** The right atrium is rotated to the left and a transverse atriotomy performed in the left atrium. The dashed line indicates the corresponding incision in the common pulmonary vein. **C.** The anastomosis is performed with running monofilament sutures taking care to avoid narrowing the pulmonary venous orifices. **D.** The suture line is completed with several interrupted sutures to avoid purse stringing and to permit growth.

Pulmonary Venous Obstruction

Anomalous pulmonary venous connection can also be classified by the presence or absence of venous obstruction. This is usually distal to the common pulmonary vein and may represent the impingement of adjacent structures or a functional obstruction in which the connecting veins have an aggregate caliber that is inadequate to accommodate the

TABLE 66–1. TOTAL ANOMALOUS PULMONARY VENOUS CONNECTION—TYPES

	Ann Arbor[14]	Boston[15]	Melbourne[16]	UCLA	Total
Supracardiac	19	8	16	21	64 (39%)
Cardiac	9	5	12	12	38 (23%)
Infracardiac	11	7	16	19	53 (33%)
Mixed	2	3	0	3	8 (5%)
Total	41	23	44	55	163

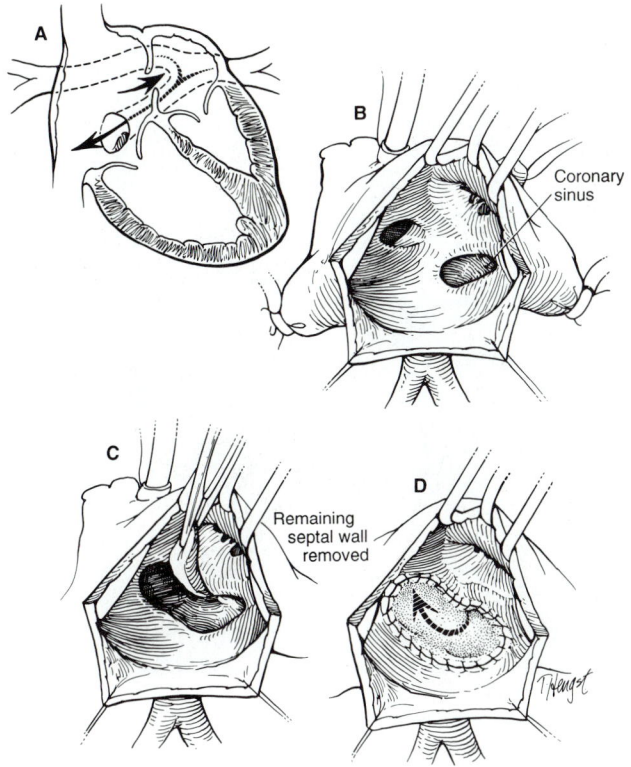

Figure 66–2. Cardiac TAPVC. **A.** The pulmonary venous confluence connects to the coronary sinus. **B.** An oblique right atriotomy gives excellent exposure of the anatomy. **C.** The coronary sinus is cut back into the left atrium and remaining tissue is removed. **D.** A large pericardial patch closes the defect, diverting coronary sinus and pulmonary venous blood to the left atrium.

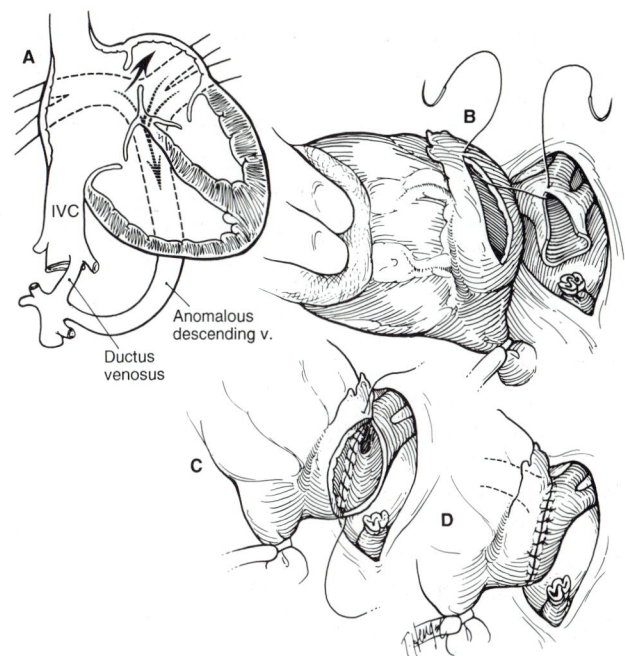

Figure 66–3. Infracardiac TAPVC. **A.** The descending vein connects to the ductus venosus. **B.** The heart is retracted superiorly and to the right. The posterior pericardium is incised and the descending vein is ligated at the diaphragm. A vertical incision is performed in the common pulmonary vein and a corresponding incision made in the left atrium, extending onto the appendage if needed. **C.** One side of the anastomosis has been completed. **D.** The completed anastomosis includes interrupted sutures.

venous return. Obstruction is most common in the infracardiac type, and is often functional. Obstruction in cardiac connections is uncommon, as the coronary sinus can enlarge over time. Obstruction in the supracardiac type can occur at the connection with the left innominate vein, or at any point along the course of the vertical vein. Data on the frequency and location of obstruction from several recent series are summarized in Table 66–2.

Pathophysiology

All pulmonary venous return is directed to systemic venous channels, which results in complete mixing within the right heart. Blood flow distribution depends on the size of the interatrial communication. If restrictive, there will be minimal blood flow to the left atrium, resulting in elevated right atrial pressures and decreased cardiac output. In most pa-

TABLE 66–2. TOTAL ANOMALOUS PULMONARY VENOUS CONNECTION—PRESENCE OF OBSTRUCTION

	Ann Arbor[14]	Boston[15]	Melbourne[16]	UCLA	Total
Supracardiac	10/19	2/8	5/16	15/21	32/64 (50%)
Cardiac	4/9	2/5	2/12	1/12	9/38 (23%)
Infracardiac	11/11	6/7	15/16	18/19	50/53 (94%)
Mixed	1/2	3/3	0/0	2/3	6/8 (75%)
Total	26/41	13/23	22/44	36/55	97/163 (60%)

tients the interatrial communication is large and nonrestrictive; blood flow depends on the relative compliance of each ventricle and the relative resistance of the pulmonary and systemic vasculature. During the neonatal period, as pulmonary vascular resistance decreases, more and more blood flows through the lungs. This can result in a pulmonary to systemic flow ratio (Q_p:Q_s) as high as 5:1. Continued exposure to massive pulmonary blood flow can cause pulmonary vascular changes and pulmonary hypertension. In patients with obstruction, elevated pulmonary venous pressures result in capillary leakage and pulmonary edema. Reflex pulmonary vasoconstriction occurs, causing pulmonary hypertension and suprasystemic right ventricular pressures. Such patients rapidly develop cyanosis, which can result in multiorgan dysfunction.

Diagnosis

Patient presentation will vary depending on the presence and level of obstruction. Patients with severe obstruction present in the newborn period with tachypnea and poor feeding. On examination there will be cyanosis, accessory muscle use, and hepatomegaly. Often there will be no murmur, only a loud second heart sound, consistent with pulmonary arterial hypertension. Electrocardiography will show right ventricular hypertrophy that, if persistent after the first 2 months of life, is abnormal. On occasion, an enlarged P wave in the right precordial or lead II tracings (P pulmonale) will be present. Chest x-ray will show florid pulmonary edema, but a normal heart size. Presence of these two should raise the clinical index of suspicion for total anomalous pulmonary venous connection with obstruction (Fig. 66–4). Also, an abnormally high oxygen saturation detected on umbilical vein catheterization is usually diagnostic of an infracardiac connection.[11]

Patients without significant obstruction often present beyond the newborn period. Symptoms are those of progressive congestive heart failure and include dyspnea on exertion, poor feeding, and failure to thrive. Older patients often note inability to keep up with peers and excessive fatigue at the end of the day. Respiratory infections may be more frequent. On examination, cyanosis is minimal. The precordium is hyperactive, the second heart sound is widely split, and a pulmonary outflow murmur may be noted. Electrocardiography shows right ventricular enlargement. The chest x-ray often shows cardiomegaly and increased pulmonary blood flow. In patients with supracardiac connection, the dilated vertical and innominate veins result in a widening of the superior mediastinum, giving a "snowman" appearance to the cardiothymic silhouette.

Echocardiography is the mainstay of diagnosis.[12] The common pulmonary vein is identified behind the left atrium (Fig. 66–5). The connection is also delineated as well as the atrial septal defect and any other associated abnormalities. Often right-to-left shunting through a patent ductus arteriosus can be demonstrated.

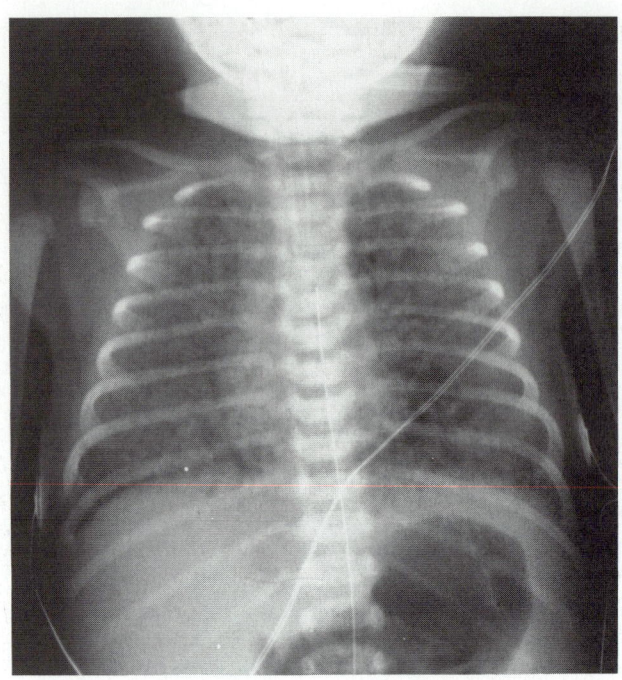

Figure 66–4. Neonate with TAPVC with obstruction. Note the extensive pulmonary edema pattern with a small cardiac silhouette.

With the refinement of echocardiographic techniques, cardiac catheterization is not routinely needed and often only serves to delay surgery. Also, the osmotic load induced by angiographic contrast may worsen the degree of pulmonary edema in severely ill infants. However, in older patients, catheterization may be useful in delineating other coexisting anomalies and in determining the degree of pulmonary hypertension.

Management

There is no satisfactory medical palliation for total anomalous pulmonary venous connection and, in most cases, surgery should proceed without delay. However, a brief period of medical stabilization including intubation, ventilation with 100% oxygen, and correction of metabolic acidosis may improve the patient's condition and impact favorably on outcome. Maintenance of ductal patency with prostaglandin E_1 may allow shunting of blood from right to left (i.e., the pulmonary artery to the aorta), helping to decompress the right heart and providing some improvement in cardiac output. However, this may decrease pulmonary blood flow and further impair oxygen saturation.

SURGICAL TECHNIQUE

Operative repair entails the creation of an anastomosis between the common pulmonary vein and the left atrium, interruption of the anomalous connection to the systemic ve-

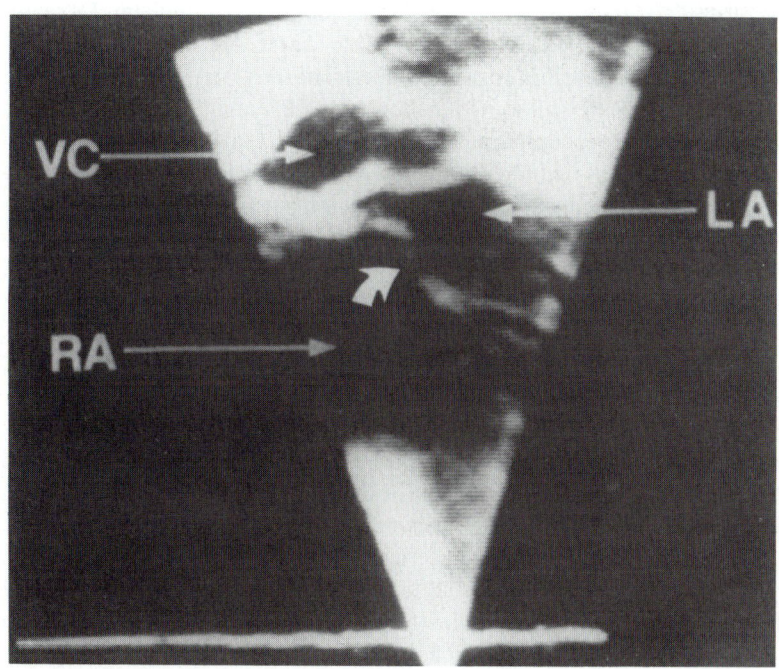

Figure 66–5. Echocardiogram of a patient with TAPVC showing the venous confluence (VC) posterior to the left atrium (LA). The arrow demonstrates the atrial septal defect. *(From Echocardiographic Diagnosis of Cardiac Malformations, Williams RG, Bierman FZ, Sanders SP, Boston, 1986, published by Little, Brown and Company.)*

nous system, and closure of the atrial septal defect. This is performed on cardiopulmonary bypass and may entail the use of hypothermic circulatory arrest or low flow perfusion.

In patients with supracardiac connections, the heart is rotated to the left and a transverse incision performed in the common pulmonary vein (Fig. 66–1). A parallel incision is made in the left atrium. The anastomosis is performed with running absorbable monofilament suture (e.g., Polydioxanone), taking care not to constrict the anastomosis or the orifices of the individual pulmonary veins. A portion of the anastomosis is usually done with interrupted sutures to avoid a "purse-string" constriction and to allow for growth. The vertical vein can be ligated at its exit from the pericardium or at its connection with the left innominate vein. Care should be taken to avoid the phrenic nerve, which courses on the lateral border of the vertical vein.

For cardiac connections, the repair is done from inside the atrium (Fig. 66–2). The coronary sinus is incised into the left atrium and the entire area is covered with a pericardial patch. The sutures are placed inside the orifice of the coronary sinus to avoid the conduction system. Both pulmonary venous and coronary sinus blood flow are directed into the left atrium, creating a small obligatory right-to-left shunt that is well tolerated.

In patients with infracardiac connections, the heart is elevated superiorly and a vertical incision performed in the common pulmonary vein (Fig. 66–3). A parallel incision is made in the left atrium and anastomosis completed with running and interrupted monofilament suture. The connection is usually ligated at the level of the diaphragm.

In the mixed type, repair represents a combination of the above techniques based on the individual anatomy.

POSTOPERATIVE MANAGEMENT

Postoperative care is directed toward optimization of cardiac output, peripheral perfusion, and respiratory function. Inotropes and afterload reduction are often required. In the early period following repair, left atrial and ventricular volumes may be small, compared to those on the right. Therefore, increases in cardiac output may be achievable only by increasing heart rate. Isoproterenol has been used for its inotropic and chronotopic effects. Fluid intake is usually restricted and diuretics used as well.

There is often residual pulmonary edema that may take several days to resolve and may require judicious ventilator adjustments including positive end expiratory pressure. Patients with preoperative pulmonary venous obstruction and elevated pulmonary artery pressures are especially prone to pulmonary hypertensive crises. These are usually manifested by sudden decreases in oxygen saturation followed by rapid development of metabolic acidosis and cardiovascular collapse, often precipitated by endotracheal suctioning. Interventions to maintain pulmonary vasodilation include hyperventilation to keep PCO_2 at approximately 30 torr, adequate oxygenation, deep sedation, and often paralysis.[13] Continuous fentanyl infusion, augmented with midazolam, has proved useful. Low-dose isoproterenol or nitroglycerin can also be used. In severe cases, nitric oxide has also been employed as a pulmonary vasodilator with some success.[19] Endotracheal suctioning should be performed carefully with additional sedation and hyperventilation as required. After 24–48 hours, the sedation may be discontinued. Several authors recommend a pulmonary artery pressure line for continuous monitoring of the efficacy of pulmonary vasodilator therapy.[14–16]

Results

Morbidity and mortality rates for repair of total anomalous pulmonary venous connection have decreased markedly in recent years. Improvements in preoperative preparation, anesthetic and surgical techniques, cardiopulmonary bypass, and postoperative management have resulted in mortality rates under 10% in most centers.

In a recent series from UCLA covering the period from 1982 to 1994, 55 patients presented with isolated total anomalous pulmonary venous connection. With a follow-up period of 1 mo to 12 years (mean 46 mo), early mortality was 7% (4/55) and late mortality was 4% (2/51). Comparative mortality rates for recent series are summarized in Table 66–3.

The UCLA series identified low birth weight and pulmonary venous obstruction as risk factors for early death. Patients with pulmonary venous obstruction tend to be more vulnerable to pulmonary hypertensive crises. Other series also implicate infracardiac connection as an incremental risk factor for hospital death, perhaps due to the strong association with pulmonary venous obstruction.[17] Poor preoperative condition has been suggested as a risk factor for early mortality. Often diagnosis is delayed and neonates may be moribund by the time the true nature of their condition is appreciated. Severe hypoxia, acidosis, and low cardiac output may not respond well to stabilization efforts and surgery with cardiopulmonary bypass in such infants is correspondingly hazardous. Two recent series have found that lack of a pulmonary artery pressure monitoring line was also a risk factor for early death.[15,16] Presence of associated complex defects such as heterotaxy syndrome (atrial isomerism) would be expected to increase mortality: in one recent series, the mortality rate for such patients undergoing repair was 33%.[3]

Most patients are corrected in the newborn period, and, following discharge, have a survival curve approaching that of the general population.[18] However, one significant problem identified in follow-up has been recurrent pulmonary venous obstruction. This occurs in 5–15% of patients and is usually detected in the first postoperative year.[16] The site of obstruction is at the anastomosis or within the pulmonary veins. In the case of anastomotic stricture, there is no correlation with the type of defect, surgical technique, or suture material used. The condition is correctable by reoperation. In the UCLA series, three patients (6%) required reoperation for this problem. Development of intrinsic pulmonary venous obstruction is more insidious. It is usually due to fibrosis and thickening of the vein wall at its junction with the common pulmonary vein. Reoperation has been attempted with generally poor success and high mortality.[16] Intraluminal stenting, balloon dilation, and lung transplantation have been proposed as alternative measures for this vexing problem.[20]

COR TRIATRIATUM

Cor triatriatum is a rare cardiac condition in which the pulmonary veins enter a left atrial chamber that is separated from the main body of the left atrium by a membrane that has one or more perforations. It occurs with a frequency of 0.4% in autopsy series.[21] It is currently believed that the malformation is accounted for by failure of incorporation of the common pulmonary vein into the left atrium. Multiple anatomic variations exist and include communication with the right atrium and connections to various systemic veins (Fig. 66–6).

Pathophysiology of cor triatriatum is based on the restrictive nature of the communication between the accessory chamber and the left atrium as well as the presence or absence of connections to the right atrium or other structures. In the classic form, physiology is similar to that found in mitral stenosis with elevated pulmonary venous pressure and pulmonary edema.

Patients present with respiratory symptoms including dyspnea and frequent respiratory infections. On occasion, patients can present beyond infancy, even in adulthood. On examination there is a loud second heart sound and a right ventricular heave. Rales are often present. Electrocardiography demonstrates typical findings of right ventricular overload with notched P waves in some cases. The chest x-ray often reflects pulmonary venous obstruction. Echocardiography is the diagnostic modality of choice. The membrane can be visualized within the left atrium and must be differentiated from a supravalvar mitral ring (Fig. 66–7). When the diagnosis is in doubt, cardiac catheterization can be performed. Hemodynamic data will demonstrate pulmonary hypertension and a gradient between the pulmonary capillary wedge pressure and the left atrial pressure. The levophase of pulmonary arteriography usually demonstrates the membrane and a delay in the passage of contrast is noted between the accessory left atrial chamber and the true left atrium.

TABLE 66–3. TOTAL ANOMALOUS PULMONARY VENOUS CONNECTION—MORTALITY

	Ann Arbor[14]	Boston[15]	Melbourne[16]	UCLA	Total
Number of deaths	2	0	1	4	7 (4%)
Total	41	23	44	55	163

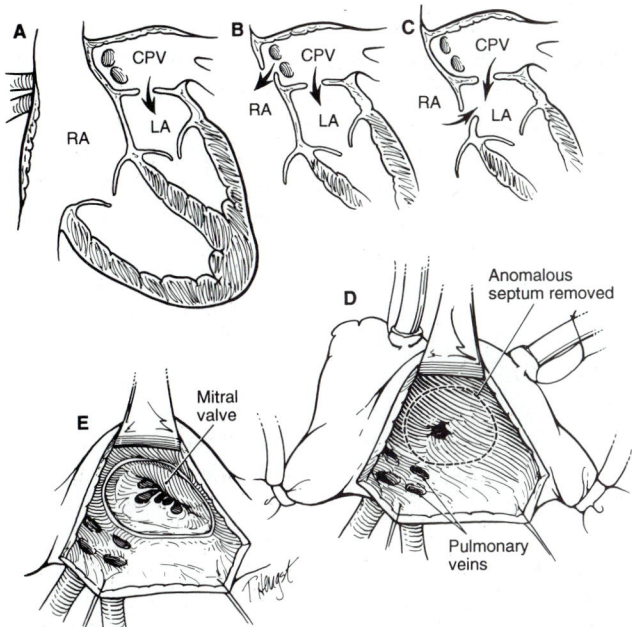

Figure 66–6. Various forms of cor triatriatum. **A.** In the classic form, the accessory chamber (common pulmonary vein, CPV) connects to the true left atrium through a perforation in the membrane. **B.** In this form, the ASD communicates with the accessory chamber. **C.** The ASD communicates with the true left atrium. **D.** The atrium is opened through the accessory chamber, exposing the membrane. **E.** Following membrane resection, the mitral valve is clearly visible.

Patients who present with pulmonary edema and right heart failure require initial stabilization after which surgery should proceed without delay. Correction of the classic form of cor triatriatum requires cardiopulmonary bypass. The membrane is approached through the enlarged accessory chamber that is opened through a vertical incision adjacent to the right pulmonary veins (Fig. 66–6E). The membrane is exposed and resected. When the accessory chamber communicates with the right atrium, the latter may be large because of the left-to-right shunt. In this case, the easiest approach is through the right atrium.[22] The atrial septal defect is enlarged to provide adequate exposure after which the membrane resection proceeds as before. The septum is reconstructed at the conclusion of the procedure, using autologous pericardium. Patients with other forms of cor triatriatum should have any anomalous connections identified and ligated. Correction proceeds then as before. Postoperative care is similar to that in patients with total anomalous pulmonary venous connection.

PARTIAL ANOMALOUS PULMONARY VENOUS CONNECTION

Partial anomalous pulmonary venous connection occurs when one or more, but not all, pulmonary veins connect to the right atrium or one of its tributaries. The condition is commonly associated with an atrial septal defect (ASD).

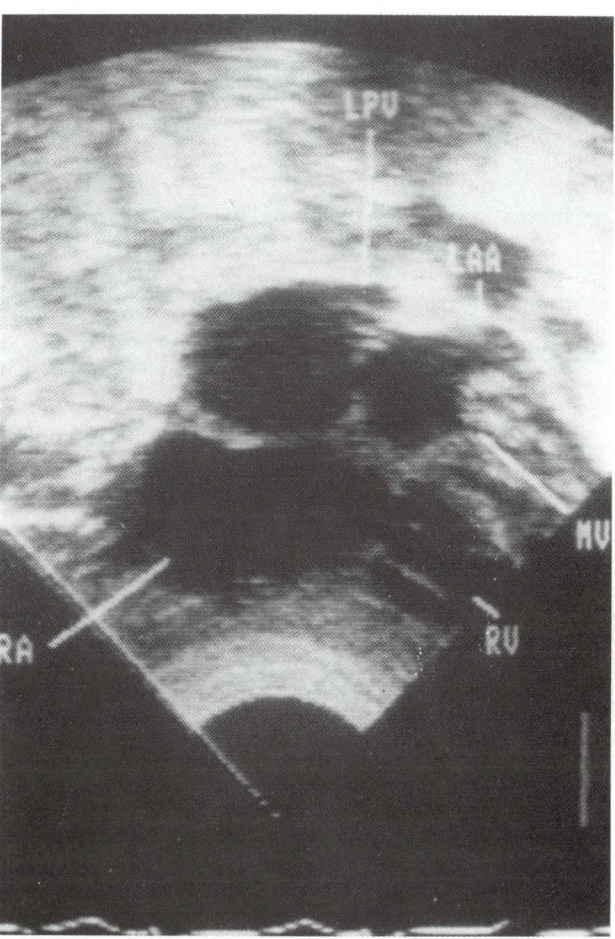

Figure 66–7. Echocardiogram of patient with cor triatriatum. The left pulmonary vein (LPV) enters the accessory chamber while the left atrial appendage (LAA) connects to the true left atrium. The membrane lies between and is remote from the mitral valve (MV). *(From Echocardiographic Diagnosis of Cardiac Malformations, Williams RG, Bierman FZ, Sanders SP, Boston, 1986 published by Little, Brown and Company.)*

Usually the right pulmonary veins connect to the right atrium or vena cavae. The left pulmonary veins connect to the coronary sinus or left innominate vein. Although numerous variations can occur, there are two specific syndromes.

Sinus Venosus Atrial Septal Defect

In patients with a sinus venosus atrial septal defect, the right upper and middle lobe veins connect to the superior vena cava at or below the azygous vein or to the cavoatrial junction. The septal defect itself may have no superior or lateral margin (Fig. 66–8).

Scimitar Syndrome

In rare cases, a right pulmonary vein, often representing the venous drainage of the entire right lung, connects to the inferior vena cava. The vein is frequently visible on a chest x-ray as a vertically oriented, crescent-shaped density adja-

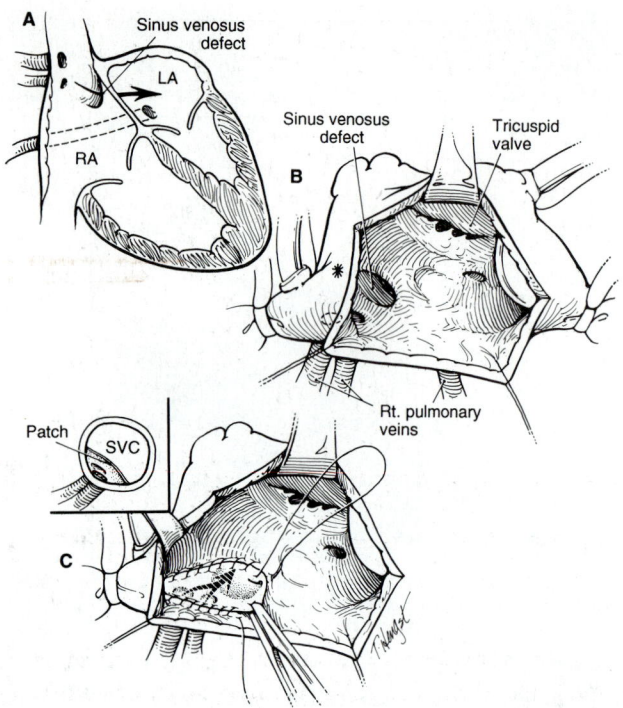

Figure 66–8. Sinus venous atrial septal defect. **A.** The right upper and middle lobe veins connect to the superior vena cava (SVC) near the atrial junction. **B.** The defect is exposed by an oblique right atriotomy. **C.** A patch of pericardium is sutured to the margin of the defect and over the pulmonary veins.

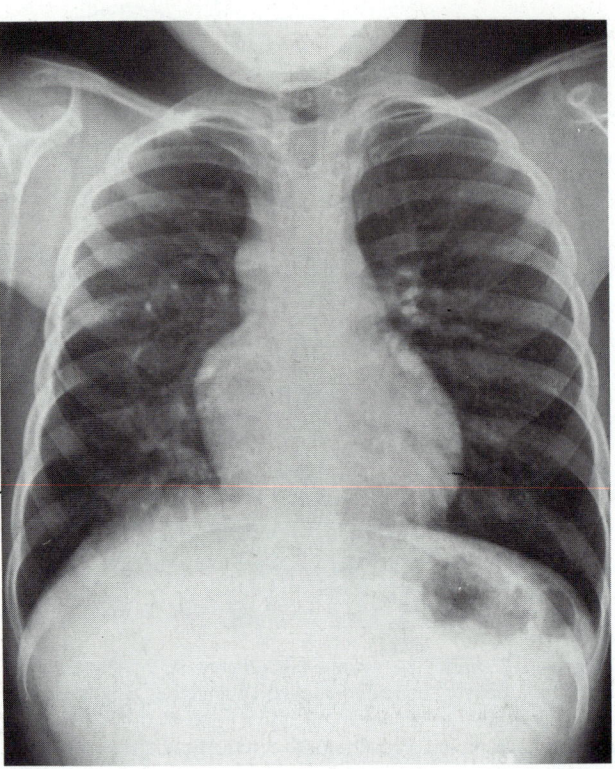

Figure 66–9. Partial anomalous venous connection to the inferior vena cava (Scimitar syndrome) in a 10-mo-old male. Note the crescentic shadow lateral to the right heart border, representing the right pulmonary vein.

cent to the right heart border. The shape of the density is reminiscent of a Turkish sword or "scimitar" (Fig. 66–9). The vein receives many tributaries, giving it a "fir tree" appearance on angiography. The abnormal development of the vein is accompanied by hypoplasia of the lung parenchyma and bronchi and by anomalies of arterial supply, either from the abdominal aorta or from a hypoplastic right pulmonary artery. When lung hypoplasia is severe, the mediastinal structures shift and the heart may occupy most of the right chest (dextroposition). In most cases of scimitar syndrome, an atrial septal defect is absent (Fig. 66–10A).

Physiologic effects of partial anomalous pulmonary venous connection depend on the number of veins involved, the sites of connection, and the size of the atrial septal defect. In patients with few connections, symptoms are similar to those in secundum atrial septal defect. With a greater number of connections, presentation is similar to that in total anomalous pulmonary venous connection. Diagnosis is by echocardiography; catheterization is usually not necessary unless other anomalies are present. In scimitar syndrome, catheterization can be very useful in determining the arterial blood supply to the right lung and in ruling out sequestration.

Repair of sinus venosus atrial septal defect involves placement of a patch anterior to the orifices of the associ-

ated pulmonary veins (Fig. 66–8). This directs the pulmonary venous blood flow under the patch and into the left atrium. Care is taken not to narrow the vein orifices or to obstruct the superior vena cava. Potential caval obstruction can be remedied by patch enlargement of the cavoatrial junction, performed posteriorly to avoid injury to the sinus node. When the pulmonary vein insertion is above the cavoatrial junction or the junction is narrow, superior vena caval obstruction is more likely. In this case, the superior vena cava is divided above the level of the pulmonary veins. The cardiac portion of the vena cava is baffled through the septal defect to the left atrium and the upper portion is anastomosed to the right atrial appendage (Warden procedure).[23]

Repair of a left pulmonary venous connection to the left innominate vein can be accomplished by ligation of the left vertical vein and anastomosis to the left atrial appendage. The atrial septal defect is closed in the usual manner. Anomalous connection to the coronary sinus is repaired as discussed previously.

In patients with scimitar syndrome, the anomalous connection is repaired by excising the atrial septum and baffling the pulmonary venous blood flow to the left atrium, taking care to avoid obstruction of the inferior vena cava (Fig. 66–10). In patients with severe lung hypoplasia, recur-

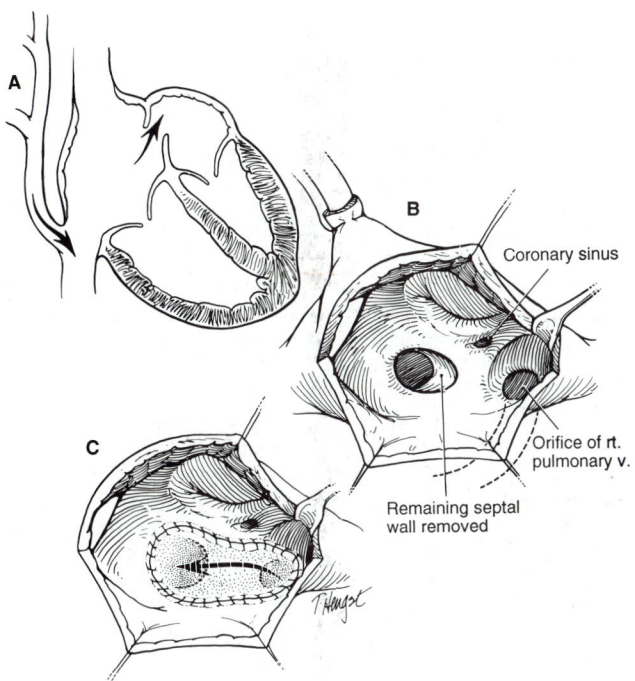

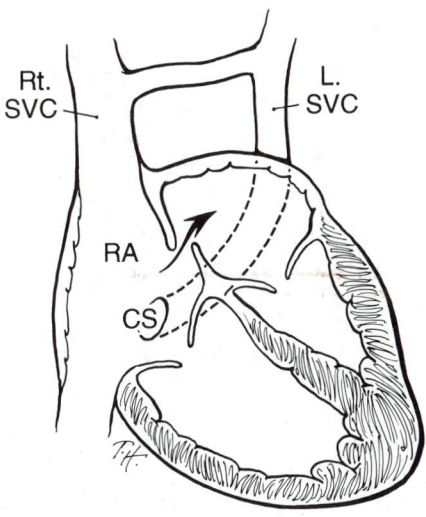

Figure 66–11. Persistent left superior vena cava (SVC).

Figure 66–10. Scimitar syndrome. **A.** A single right pulmonary vein connects to the inferior vena cava. **B.** The right atrium is opened by an oblique incision. **C.** A large pericardial patch directs pulmonary vein blood flow across the atrial septal defect. Care is taken to avoid obstruction of the inferior vena caval orifice.

rent pneumonia, or bronchiectasis, lobectomy, or pneumonectomy may be appropriate therapy.[24]

ANOMALOUS SYSTEMIC VENOUS CONNECTION

Anomalies of the systemic venous system encompass a wide range of abnormalities, but in general have few pathophysiologic effects. Anomalies that are of interest to the thoracic surgeon and may impact on the conduct of cardiac procedures include persistent left superior vena cava and inferior vena cava interruption with azygous continuation.

Persistent Left Superior Vena Cava

This is the most common anomaly of the superior vena caval system and in patients with other cardiac defects has a prevalence of 3–4%.[25] Usually the left superior vena cava courses anterior to the left pulmonary artery and posterior to the left atrial appendage where it enters the atrioventricular groove and joins the coronary sinus (Fig. 66–11). Presence of a left superior vena cava should be strongly suspected in patients with heterotaxy syndrome or enlarged coronary sinus visualized on echocardiography. Recognition of this anomaly is important because the surgeon should be prepared to deal with a large amount of systemic venous return entering the right atrium via the coronary sinus. Also, if administration of retrograde cardioplegia is contemplated, occlusion of the vein is mandatory lest the

majority of the dose be administered to the systemic venous circulation, thereby negating the myocardial protective effect.

Prior to cardiopulmonary bypass, the left superior vena cava (LSVC) is encircled with a silk tie or umbilical tape and snared. The pressure is measured above the level of the snare and if it is less than 15–20 mm Hg, the LSVC can be snared during cardiopulmonary bypass and ligated afterward if necessary. Otherwise cannulation of the LSVC can be performed directly or via the coronary sinus.

Occasionally a persistent left superior vena cava may be associated with an unroofed coronary sinus, thus allowing systemic venous return to the left atrium. Depending on the amount of systemic return and the size of the coronary sinus defect, the physiologic derangement may be mild or severe. In patients where the occlusion pressure of the left superior cava is less than 15 mm Hg, the structure can be ligated. Otherwise, repair can be performed either by closing the unroofed left atrial portion or, if this creates significant narrowing of the coronary sinus channel, a patch of pericardium can be used to direct the left superior vena caval blood to the right atrium. Following this the atrial septum can be reconstructed in the normal manner.

Interruption of the Inferior Vena Cava With Azygous Continuation

Interruption of the inferior vena cava with azygous continuation usually poses no physiologic abnormalities (Fig. 66–12). Although occasionally present in patients with normal cardiac architecture, it is more common in patients with congenital heart disease. Recognition is mandatory as inadvertent (or intended) ligation of the azygous vein can be disastrous. Variation in cannulation techniques may be required to provide adequate drainage of the hepatic veins, which converge at the inferior border of the right atrium,

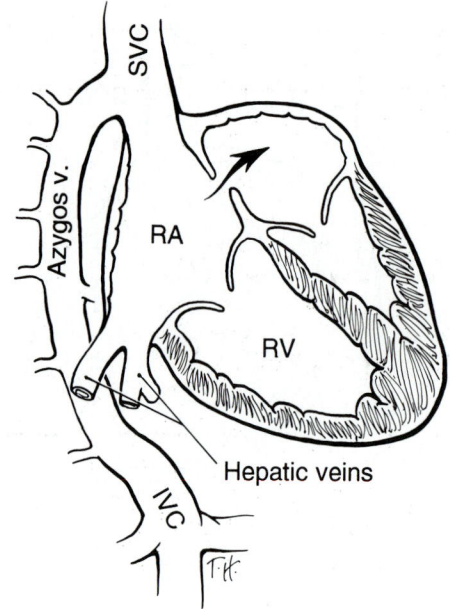

Figure 66–12. Interrupted inferior vena cava (IVC) with azygous continuation. Note the enlargement of the superior vena cava (SVC) and the convergence of the hepatic veins at the right atrium (RA).

and to accommodate the increased superior vena caval blood flow.

Patients with inferior vena caval interruption who are being considered for cavopulmonary connection pose a special problem. Placement of a classic Glenn shunt to the right pulmonary artery results in most of the cardiac output being directed to the right lung, which may not be tolerated. A bidirectional Glenn shunt provides more even pulmonary blood flow distribution, but is physiologically similar to a complete Fontan reconstruction. Therefore, such patients must be carefully assessed for their ability to tolerate such a procedure.

SUMMARY

Patients with anomalous pulmonary or systemic venous connections pose unique challenges for the thoracic surgeon. Careful identification of all abnormalities is important. Reconstruction can be performed in virtually all cases with low morbidity and mortality and with excellent long-term prognosis.

REFERENCES

1. Lucas RV Jr, Anderson RC, Amplatz K, et al: Congenital causes of pulmonary venous obstruction. *Pediatr Clin North Am* **10**:781, 1963

2. Mehrizi A, Hirsch MS, Taussig HB: Congenital heart disease in the neonatal period: Autopsy of 170 cases. *J Pediatr* **65**:721, 1964
3. Heinemann MK, Hanley FL, VanPraagh S, et al: Total anomalous pulmonary venous drainage in newborns with visceral heterotaxy. *Ann Thorac Surg* **57**:88, 1994
4. Wilson J: A description of a very unusual formation of the human heart. *Philos Trans R Soc London* **88**:346, 1798
5. Brody H: Drainage of the pulmonary veins into the right side of the heart. *Arch Pathol Lab Med* **33**:221, 1942
6. Muller WH: The surgical treatment of transposition of the pulmonary veins. *Ann Surg* **134**:683, 1951
7. Lewis FJ, Varco RL, Taufic M, Niazi SA: Direct vision repair of triatrial heart and total anomalous pulmonary venous drainage. *Surg Gynecol Obstet* **192**:713, 1956
8. Burroughs JT, Kirklin JW: Complete surgical correction of total anomalous pulmonary venous connection. Report of three cases. *Mayo Clin Proc* **31**:182, 1956
9. Cooley D, Ochsner A: Correction of total anomalous pulmonary venous drainage. *Surgery* **42**:1014, 1957
10. Darling RC, Rothney WB, Craig JM: Total pulmonary venous drainage into the right side of the heart. *Lab Invest* **6**:44, 1957
11. Tyler DC: Total anomalous pulmonary venous return. In Tyler DC (ed): *Nadas Pediatr Cardiology.* 1992, pp 683–691
12. Williams RG, Bierman FZ, Sanders SP: *Echocardiographic Diagnosis of Cardiac Malformations.* Boston, Little, Brown, 1986, p 74
13. Raisher BD, Grant JW, Martin TC, et al: Complete repair of total anomalous pulmonary venous connection in infancy. *J Thorac Cardiovasc Surg* **104**:443, 1992
14. Lupinetti FM, Kulik TJ, Beekman RH, et al: Correction of total anomalous pulmonary venous connection in infancy. *J Thorac Cardiovasc Surg* **106**:880, 1993
15. Van Der Velde ME, Parness IA, Colan SD, et al: Two-dimensional echocardiography in the pre- and postoperative management of totally anomalous pulmonary venous connection. *J Am Coll Cardiol* **18**:1746, 1991
16. Sano S, Brawn WJ, Mee RBB: Total anomalous pulmonary venous drainage. *J Thorac Cardiovas Surg* **97**:886, 1989
17. Hammon JW, Bender HW, Graham TP, et al: Total anomalous pulmonary venous connection in infancy: Ten years experience including studies of postoperative ventricular function. *J Thorac Cardiovas Surg* **80**:544, 1980
18. Kirklin JW, Barrett-Boyes BG: Total anomalous pulmonary venous connection. In Kirklin JW, Barrett-Boyes BG (eds): *Cardiac Surgery,* 2nd ed. New York, Churchill-Livingstone, 1993, pp 645–673
19. Girard C, Neidecker J, Laroux MC, et al: Inhaled nitric oxide in pulmonary hypertension after total repair of total anomalous pulmonary venous return. *J Thorac Cardiovasc Surg* **106**:369, 1993
20. O'Laughlin MP, Perry SB, Lock JE, Mullins CE: Use of endovascular stents in congenital heart disease. *Circulation* **83**:1923, 1991
21. Niwayama G: Cor Triatriatum. *Am Heart J* **59**:292, 1960
22. Van Son JAM, Danielson GK, Schaff HV, et al: Cor Triatriatum: Diagnosis, operative approach, and late results. *Mayo Clinic Proc* **68**:854, 1993
23. Warden HE, Gustafson RA, Tarnay TJ, Neil WA: An alternate method for repair of partial anomalous pulmonary venous connection to the superior vena cava. *Ann Thorac Surg* **38**:601, 1984
24. Dupuis C, Charaf LA, Abou CP, Breviere GM: Surgical treatment of the scimitar syndrome in children, adolescents and adults. A cooperative study of 37 cases. *Arch Mal Coeur* **86**:541, 1993
25. Campbell M, Deuchar DC: The left sided superior vena cava. *Br Heart J* **16**:423, 1954

CHAPTER

67

Atrial Septal Defects and Cor Triatriatum

Gary S. Kopf and Hillel Laks

ATRIAL SEPTAL DEFECT

Atrial septal defect (ASD) is one of the most common congenital cardiac anomalies, present in 10–15% of patients with congenital heart disease. It is the most common congenital cardiac lesion in the adult.[1] Primum ASD belongs to the group of lesions classified as *endocardial cushion defects* and is considered in Chapter 70. The present discussion pertains to the more common secundum-type ASD and its variations.

History

Atrial septal defect was the first cardiac lesion successfully corrected using extracorporeal circulation. Gibbon[2] performed this feat in 1953, thus beginning the modern era of open intracardiac surgery. Prior to this, several ingenious operations were successfully applied without the use of cardiopulmonary bypass. These included the purse-string suture described by Sondergard, the well technique of Gross, and direct suture closure during inflow occlusion combined with hypothermia, described by Lewis and Swan.

Embryology

The embryologic development of the atrial septum is described in Chapter 56. The usual form of secundum ASD is the result of underdevelopment of the primary septum, while defects near the inferior and superior cava are usually the result of regression of the interatrial fold. Many ASDs result from a combination of both abnormalities.

Anatomy

Approximately 20% of normal individuals will have a *patent foramen ovale* between the superior limbic septum and the septum ovale (Fig. 67–1). This is of no consequence clinically, as the flap mechanism between these structures will ordinarily prevent any significant left-to-right shunting. However, high right atrial pressures may result in significant right-to-left shunting, and if the atria are distended the foramen is widened and a significant interatrial communication will exist. This can result in significant desaturation, particularly after procedures involving reconstruction of the right side of the heart and elevated right atrial pressures. Therefore, a patent foramen ovale or ASD should routinely be closed during other cardiac procedures unless significant right heart failure is anticipated in which case a right-to-left shunt may be temporarily helpful in preserving cardiac output. Significant right-to-left shunting has also been reported with postural changes through a patent foramen ovale following pneumonectomy.

Several different varieties of interatrial communications come under the heading of *secundum type atrial septal defect,* and they can be classified according to their location. The most common form, accounting for approximately two-thirds of such defects, is the *foramen ovale type,* which is located in the midportion of the atrial septum (Fig. 67–2). This defect is the result of development failure of the septum primum. A variable-sized opening, usually oval shaped, 0.5–2 cm wide and 1–6 cm long, is present in the area of the fossa ovalis. In addition, the surrounding septal tissue is often thinned out and fenestrated, resulting in multiple small interatrial communications.

Approximately 10% of ASDs are of the *sinus venosus*

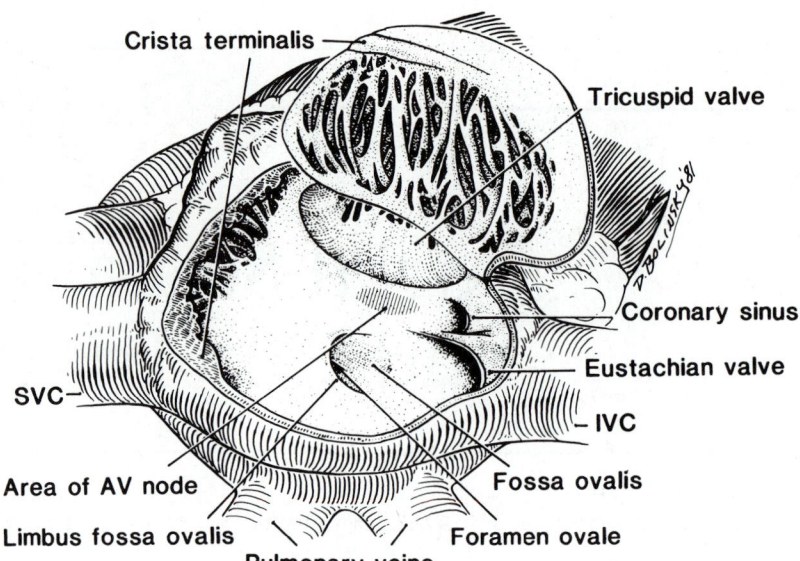

Figure 67–1. Surgical anatomy of the interior of the right atrium. SVC, superior vena cava; IVC, inferior vena cava.

or *superior vena cava* type. The interatrial communication is located at the junction of the superior vena cava (SVC) and the right atrium (Fig. 67–3). The inferior portion of the defect is the superior limbic septum, while superiorly the defect communicates with the lumen of the SVC. The orifice of the superior vena cava is malpositioned to the left, thus overriding the right and the left atrium. This lesion results from a complex developmental failure of the sinus venosus area. It is almost invariably associated with partial anomalous connection of the right upper and middle lobe pulmonary veins to the superior vena cava or right atrium.

A third type of secundum atrial septal defect, accounting for about 20%, is the *low or inferior vena caval defect,* which is located between the entrance of the inferior vena cava and the inferior limbic septum (Fig. 67–4). Anomalous connection of the right lower lobe vein to the inferior vena cava (IVC) or right atrium may be present but is much less

frequent than with the sinus venosus superior vena caval-type defect. The inferior vena cava is malpositioned to the left and opens into both the right and the left atrium. The defect has no inferior rim, and care must be taken to avoid compromise of the IVC orifice when closing such defects.

The *coronary sinus* may communicate through a defect in the coronary sinus tube with the left atrium, also termed an *unroofed* coronary sinus. It is usually associated with a persistent left superior vena cava and is believed to be a result of maldevelopment of the arteriosinus venosus fold. Occasionally, a low atrial septal defect will be associated with a coronary sinus draining directly into the left atrium (see Chap. 66).

Rarely, the entire atrial septum fails to develop, resulting in a *common* or *single atrium.* It is usually classified as an endocardial cushion defect if a primim ASD is present. Occasionally, a large secundum defect extending to the posterior wall of the atria and involving both the septum ovale and the limbic septum as well as parts of the sinus venosus area will appear as a common atrium but the defect does not extend to the atrioventricular valve tissue.

Associated Lesions

When ASD is the primary pathophysiologic problem it is often an isolated finding, but can be associated with pulmonary stenosis (10%), partial anomalous pulmonary venous return (7%), ventricular septal defect (VSD) (5%), patent ductus arteriosus (PDA) (3%), and mitral stenosis (2%).[3,4] A persistent left superior vena cava is present in approximately 2% of patients. An ASD can be present as an associated anomaly with almost any major type of congenital heart anomalies and is necessarily associated with certain entities such as tricuspid atresia, total anomalous pulmonary venous return, and mitral atresia.

Atrial septal defect associated with rheumatic mitral

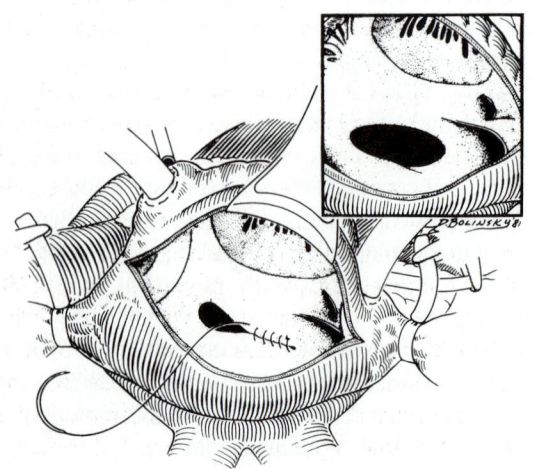

Figure 67–2. Primary closure of foramen ovale-type ASD (**inset**).

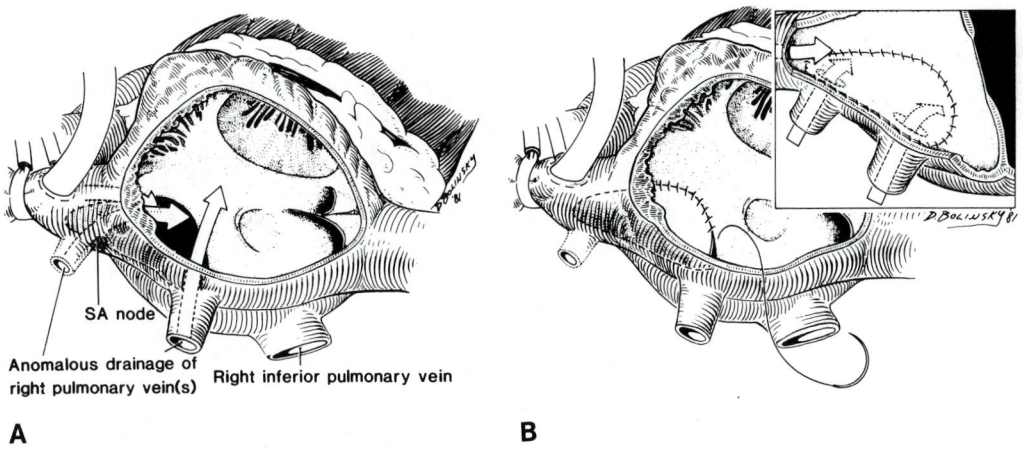

SA node

Anomalous drainage of
right pulmonary vein(s)   Right inferior pulmonary vein

A   **B**

Figure 67–3. A. Superior- or high-type ASD with anomalous connection of right superior pulmonary veins into SVC or right atrium.
B. Closure of high-type ASD. Note how patch reroutes anomalous pulmonary venous return into left atrium (**inset**).

stenosis is known as *Lutembacher syndrome.*[5] In rare instances, a secundum ASD can be associated with a cleft mitral valve.[6] Long-standing ASDs may result in hypertrophic changes in the mitral valve with increased susceptibility to rheumatic disease.[7] In the *Holt–Oram syndrome,* secundum-type ASD is associated with characteristic hand deformities.[8] Mitral insufficiency secondary to prolapsing mitral leaflets is being recognized more frequently in association with secundum ASD.[9]

Pathophysiology

The direction and amount of blood flow across an ASD depend on the size of the defect and the compliance of the left and right ventricles during diastole. Normally, the left ventricular compliance is higher than right ventricular compliance, and shunting is predominantly left to right with some right-to-left admixture. If the ASD is small, left-to-right shunting is limited. In defects larger than 1–2 cm^2, atrial pressures are equalized, and shunting will depend on the difference in compliance of the two ventricles. In the newborn period, left and right ventricular compliance are nearly equal, and shunting is mixed. In the first few weeks of life, as pulmonary vascular resistance decreases, right ventricular pressure drops and right ventricular compliance increases, resulting in increased left-to-right shunting. In the child with unrestrictive ASD, pulmonary blood flow is often two to four times systemic flow.

The limbus fossa ovalis, which may override the orifice of the inferior vena cava, tends to divert venous blood into the fossa ovalis septal defect. This may result in a small right-to-left shunt in spite of a large left-to-right shunt. As a result, there may be mild peripheral arterial desaturation, in the range of 5–10%.

Owing to its high compliance, the pulmonary vascular bed can accommodate large increases in flow with little or no rise in pulmonary arterial pressure. Although changes of medial hypertrophy and intimal proliferation are often present early in life, it is not until the third or fourth decade that more advanced and permanent changes may occur. In children, only 5–8% of individuals with an ASD will have an increase in pulmonary vascular resistance resulting in a pulmonary arterial pressure greater than 50 mm Hg. By age 40, however, as many as 35–50% will have developed significant pulmonary hypertension.[10,11] A small gradient, resulting from the increased flow associated with a large ASD, can be demonstrated frequently across the pulmonary outflow tract. This is a functional obstruction that disappears when the ASD is closed, as does the mild to moderately elevated right ventricular pressure. Systemic cardiac output is usually maintained despite the disproportionately large pulmonary blood flow. With severe exercise, however, these patients may have difficulty in maintaining the necessary high systemic cardiac output.

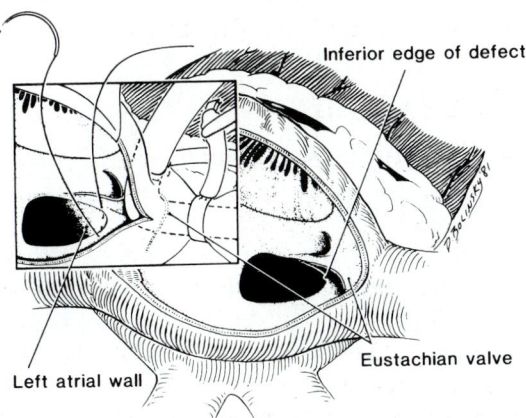

Inferior edge of defect

Left atrial wall   Eustachian valve

Figure 67–4. Low- or inferior-type ASD near mouth of inferior vena cava. **Inset.** Note how inferior edge of defect must not be confused with the eustachian valve.

Several studies of the natural history of ASDs indicate that the volume overload of the right ventricle and pulmonary vascular bed is well tolerated for long periods. However, by the third or fourth decade of life, there is a progressive rise in the incidence of pulmonary vascular disease, right ventricular failure, and atrial arrhythmias. The progression is usually slow, but certain individuals seem more prone to this process and develop severe pulmonary vascular disease at an earlier age. As these changes occur, right ventricular compliance falls, and left-to-right shunting will decrease. Eventually with severe pulmonary vascular disease and right ventricular failure, the shunt will reverse, producing cyanosis. At this stage, patients are no longer amenable to surgical therapy, since closure of the ASD will result in right ventricular overload and failure. Progression of pulmonary vascular disease will continue. The incidence of arrhythmias and the incidence of mitral valve disease rise with age. The estimated average life span of untreated patients with an ASD is approximately 50 years, with the majority dying of progressive congestive heart failure.[1,12,13]

Clinical Features

Secundum ASD typically appears in an asymptomatic child in whom a cardiac murmur is heard on a routine physical examination. Although children appear asymptomatic and lead relatively normal lives, careful study has shown that as many as 50–60% have easy fatigability and dyspnea with limited endurance, particularly those with large shunts. Patients are usually normal in height but may be thin, demonstrating the so-called gracile habitus. The male-to-female ratio is approximately 1:2. Although uncommon, infants sometimes exhibit severe cardiac failure, requiring early surgery. These patients often have associated partial anomalous pulmonary venous connection. Adults with this lesion may go undiagnosed or untreated until they present with decreased exercise tolerance, dyspnea or arrhythmias. Adults with other cardiac lesions, such as coronary artery disease, may be found at catheterization to have an unsuspected but hemodynamically significant ASD.

On physical examination, a prominent right ventricular impulse can be palpated along the lower left sternal border. A systolic ejection-type murmur of variable intensity, usually grade 2–3/6, is present in most children along the left sternal border, due to the increased flow across the pulmonary valve. A mid-diastolic murmur heard near the apex and sternum may be due to the rapid flow of blood across the tricuspid valve. The second heart sound is split and fixed, with the intensity of the pulmonary component normal or slightly increased.

The electrocardiogram typically shows evidence of right ventricular hypertrophy. A lengthened PR interval with incomplete right bundle branch block and with an RSR′ pattern in lead V_1 is characteristic. The mean QRS axis is usually between +95 and +150 degrees with a clockwise loop directed inferiorly and to the right. In addition, P

wave morphology may suggest atrial enlargement. Chest x-ray in patients with a large shunt will show cardiomegaly due to right ventricular dilation with a prominent proximal pulmonary arterial segment and increased pulmonary vascularity (Fig. 67–5). The heart size is, however, normal in a significant proportion of patients. Echocardiography reveals increased right ventricular and diastolic dimensions, and may also show reversed septal wall motion.

In most cases, diagnosis can be confirmed with echocardiography, and cardiac catheterization is not necessary. Occasionally catheterization is necessary to define associated anomalies or unusual anatomy. In adults, catheterization is sometimes needed to rule out coronary disease and to measure pulmonary vasculature changes. A step-up in oxygen saturation in the right atrium is the keystone to diagnosis. Right ventricular and pulmonary arterial pressures may be slightly elevated in the child but are often normal. Angiography with a catheter in the left atrium across the ASD or the levophase of a pulmonary arterial injection will reveal the position of the septal defect. Left ventriculography will indicate whether there is any significant mitral regurgitation. In a sinus venosus defect, injection in the right superior pulmonary vein will help locate the anomalous entrance of this vein in the superior vena cava or right atrium.

Differential Diagnosis

A septum primum ASD is distinguished by the typical clockwise QRS loop and the frequent presence of a mitral regurgitant murmur.[11,14] A gooseneck deformity will be seen on angiography. A rare VSD will shunt blood from the left ventricle to the right atrium, resulting in an oxygen step-up in the right atrium. However, this is accompanied by a typical harsh systolic murmur, which is quite distinc-

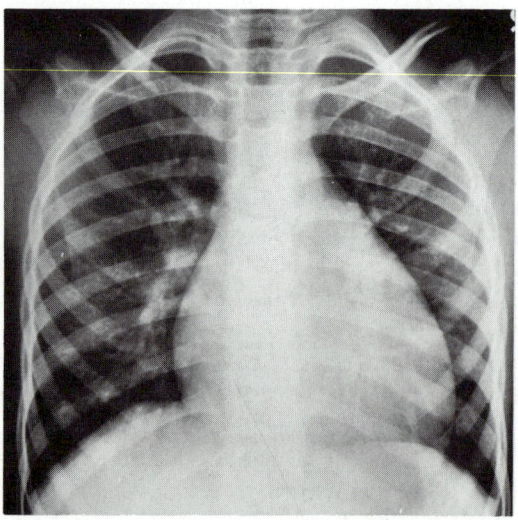

Figure 67–5. Chest x-ray of a 7-year-old child with ASD. Note the prominent proximal pulmonary arterial segment, increased pulmonary vascularity, and cardiomegaly.

tive. Other causes of oxygen step-up in the right atrium include anomalous pulmonary venous connection, a sinus of Valsalva aneurysm with rupture into the right atrium, coronary arterial fistulas into the right atrium, and other left-sided obstructive lesions that can cause left-to-right shunting through a patent foramen ovale.[14] These are distinguishable by physical findings, angiocardiography, and echocardiography.

Treatment

Indications for Operation

Atrial septal defect closure in an otherwise healthy individual is a safe, simple operation that carries an extremely low risk. Limited clinical trials on selected patients have demonstrated the feasibility of percutaneous transcatheter ASD closure utilizing catheter tipped umbrella devices as well as several other types of devices.[14a] This procedure may be particularly applicable in patients who are poor surgical candidates. Small-to-moderate sized defects, centrally located with good tissue margins all around, are ideal for this approach. Clinical trials are continuing to demonstrate the feasibility and safety of this technique.

Surgical closure remains the standard treatment of choice with low operative risk and excellent long-term results. All children with a significant ASD, as determined by clinical examination, ECG, echocardiography, and x-ray should undergo elective closure in childhood. The ideal time for closure is 3–5 years of age, before the child starts school. At an earlier age, psychologic trauma caused by separation from the parents is more likely. Spontaneous closure of an ASD is extremely rare after the age of 2 years. An occasional infant with ASD will have significant congestive heart failure. This will usually respond well to medical treatment, and surgical therapy can be delayed. However, if medical therapy fails, infants should undergo surgical closure.[15] Atrial septal defects may be closed safely in infancy.[16] Particular attention, however, should be paid to identify associated congenital defects that may be contributing to the congestive heart failure, such as patent ductus arteriosus, mitral stenosis, coarctation, or other left-sided obstructive lesions.[4]

Adults with a left-to-right shunt of greater than 1.5–2:1 should also be considered candidates for surgical closure. Age is not a contraindication to surgery.[17,18] Elderly patients with significant left-to-right shunt usually show symptomatic improvement, and the operative mortality although low, may be increased by the presence of cardiac failure, arrhythmias, pulmonary vascular disease, and other associated lesions.[19] The presence of severe pulmonary vascular disease, with pulmonary vascular resistance of one-half to two-thirds systemic, is a contraindication to surgery.[13] At this stage, the mortality rate is increased, and pulmonary vascular disease will continue to progress despite closure of the defect. Particular care must be taken in operating on adults with left-sided cardiac failure. In such patients, ASD closure can result in worsening congestive heart failure due to increased left atrial pressures following surgery.

Operative Management

Several ingenious closed methods were used before cardiopulmonary bypass was readily available and safe.[20–24] However, at the present time, ASD closure is safely and reliably performed on cardiopulmonary bypass.[25] A median sternotomy incision is used routinely. Some surgeons prefer a right submammary incision, entering the chest through the fourth intercostal space for simple ASDs. In the female patients, a transverse submammary skin incision is advocated by some surgeons for cosmetic purposes.[26] The ascending aorta and inferior and superior vena cavae are cannulated, with tapes placed around the cavae. The superior vena caval cannula is inserted via the right atrial appendage. The inferior vena caval cannula is placed through a purse-string suture low near the caval junction (Fig. 67–6), allowing for excellent intra-atrial exposure. Left ventricular venting is not necessary. If a high ASD is present, the right superior pulmonary vein is visualized, and the superior vena cava is cannulated at a point above the entrance of these veins to facilitate repair (Fig. 67–3B). A left superior vena cava may be cannulated directly in front of the left pulmonary artery, or through the coronary sinus after the right atriotomy is made. Mild systemic hypothermia to 30° to 32°C is employed. Prior to the cardioplegic era, repair was usually accomplished with the heart fibrillating without aortic cross-clamping.[25,27] With the patient turned to the left, the level of blood in the atria is kept near the rim of the defect to prevent air from entering the left side of the heart should it suddenly defibrillate and eject blood. Repair is now more often accomplished with aortic cross-clamping and cardioplegic infusion. This provides better visualization and prevents the possibility of air embolism during the repair.

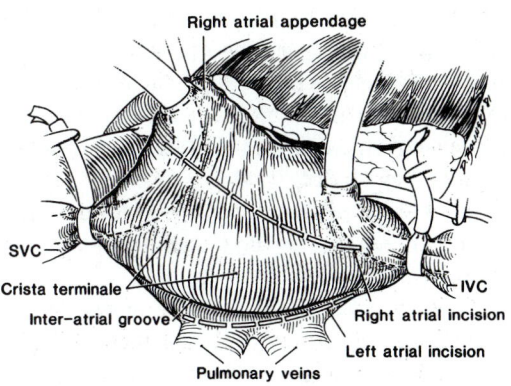

Figure 67–6. Cannulation and surgical incisions for approach to right and left atrium. IVC, inferior vena cava; SVC, superior vena cava.

A slightly oblique right atriotomy is made anterior to the crista terminalis (Fig. 67–6), avoiding the SA node area and preserving major internodal tracts. A careful exploration is carried out, taking particular care to identify the size and location of the ASD, the four pulmonary venous orifices, the atrioventricular (A-V) valves, the coronary sinus, the orifices of the superior and inferior vena cava, and the eustachian valve. The typical oval-shaped foramen ovale-type defect can be closed in most patients primarily with a continuous running suture or interrupted sutures (Fig. 67–2). If the edges cannot be approximated without tension or if the surrounding septal tissue appears insufficiently strong to hold sutures, it may be necessary to use a patch of pericardium or prosthetic material to close the defect. A large defect approaching the SA node region should be closed with a patch to avoid any tension that can result in conduction disturbances. In adults with larger defects the ASD is often closed with a patch to avoid tension on the suture line and thus minimize the development of atrial arrhythmias postoperatively.

When a high sinus venosus-type defect is present with concomitant right upper lobe anomalous pulmonary venous connection (Fig. 67–3), a pericardial or prosthetic baffle is sewn in place to close the defect at the superior vena caval orifice and, at the same time, direct the pulmonary venous flow from the right upper vein into the left atrium.[28] The atrial incision may be extended close to the entrance of the superior vena cava to facilitate insertion of the patch. However, care must be taken to avoid the area of the sinoatrial node. A combined transatrial and transcaval approach is sometimes utilized. Occasionally, a small pulmonary venous branch may enter the superior vena cava quite high. In such a case, it is often wise to close the atrial septal defect and leave this branch draining into the superior vena cava. The small resultant left-to-right shunt will be insignificant and the possible complication of superior vena caval obstruction, which can occur if a long baffle is placed inside the superior vena cava, will be avoided.

In closing an ASD that extends inferiorly, particular attention is taken to avoid compression of the inferior vena caval orifice, as the inferior vena cava is malpositioned to the left. The eustachian valve, which may be confused with the inferior rim of the defect, must be identified carefully.[29] In such cases, a patch is often used to avoid compromise of the IVS orifice (Fig. 67–4). Wide patency between the right atrium and IVC orifice must be confirmed after patch placement.

Before the last stitches are secured, the left side of the heart is filled with saline. Full insufflation of the lungs (Valsalva maneuver) will help to remove air from the pulmonary veins and the left atrium. The ascending aorta is vented. Any residual air is carefully removed from the left atrial roof and left ventricle by repeated needle aspirations. After removal of the aortic cross-clamp, aortic venting is continued until after the patient is off cardiopulmonary bypass for 5–10 min. A check for residual shunting is made by measuring the oxygen saturations in the superior vena cava and the right pulmonary artery. A significant right-to-left shunt may indicate a cava to left atrium shunt. Temporary pacing wires are not necessary in most cases. A single mediastinal chest tube is usually sufficient for drainage. Mechanical ventilatory support is usually discontinued in the operating room.

Results

The postoperative course is usually uneventful, and children are normally discharged approximately 4–5 days postoperatively. Most cardiac surgical centers report less than 1% mortality for elective closure of ASD. In a total series of 150 cases of ASD repair reported from Yale, deliberate ventricular fibrillation without cardioplegia or aortic cross-clamping was used to facilitate repair and prevent air embolism. There was no mortality or major complications.[25,27]

Complications

Occasional causes of significant morbidity include air embolism, which can cause stroke, or myocardial infarction due to right coronary embolism. If air is noted in the right coronary system during surgery with accompanying EKG changes, enough time must be taken on cardiopulmonary bypass to allow the air to flush through. Retrograde perfusion through the coronary sinus has been used in severe cases. Continuous flooding of the surgical field with carbon dioxide is used by some to ameliorate the effects of air embolism.

Supraventricular tachyarrhythmias are not uncommon and usually respond to the appropriate medications unless of long-standing duration. Heart block is prevented by avoiding undo suture line tension in the area of the A-V node.

Following repair of the sinus venosus defect, sick sinus syndrome may occur due to injury to the SA node. Adult patients with preoperative atrial fibrillation usually continue to have such arrhythmias postoperatively and require chronic anticoagulation to decrease the risk of embolization.[30] Mortality from closure of an ASD is more likely in the adult with long-standing right ventricular failure and pulmonary hypertension.[17,19,31–33]

After successful closure of an atrial septal defect, cardiomegaly usually regresses unless the operation was performed after the second decade of life.[34] Atrial arrhythmias, the presence of right interventricular conduction disturbances, and right ventricular hypertrophy by electrocardiogram usually persist.[17,18,30,35] Most adults will improve by at least one New York Heart Association (NYHA) classification, providing they have had a significant left-to-right shunt present preoperatively.[1,35–37] Life expectancy is probably normal and late problems are exceedingly rare in the child with successful closure of an ASD.[34]

In summary, surgical closure of a secundum ASD is a

low-risk operation with mortality under 1%. It should be carried out early in life before progression of disease leads to higher morbidity and mortality rates as well as permanent cardiovascular damage. The adult with an ASD can usually be significantly improved, providing severe pulmonary vascular disease and right ventricular failure have not intervened.

COR TRIATRIATUM

In contrast to ASD, cor triatriatum is a distinctly uncommon congenital anomaly. The lesion was first described by Church[38] in 1868, and since that time several hundred cases have been reported in the literature. In classic cor triatriatum, the pulmonary veins drain into an accessory atrial chamber, separated from the true atrial chamber by a fibromuscular membrane (Fig. 67–7). In the classic form, the proximal or upper chamber receives all pulmonary venous return. Blood must then pass through a variable-sized opening in the fibromuscular membrane into the distal or lower chamber, which contains the base of the left atrial appendage, as well as the atrioventricular valve apparatus.

Embryology

The lesion is thought to be a result of failure of incorporation of the embryonic common pulmonary vein into the left atrium, and, therefore, the lesion is embryologically linked with total and partial anomalous pulmonary venous return.[39] Van Praagh and Corsini[40] have theorized that entrapment of the common pulmonary vein in the right horn of the sinus venosus causes failure of incorporation of the common pulmonary vein into the left atrium. Thilenius and associates[41] have postulated that as the right horn of the sinus venosus develops into the septum primum and the left venosus valve, a cleft forms. The common pulmonary vein that lies close to this area may develop an abnormal communication with the sinus venosus. This explains those cases where the fossa ovalis communicates with the proximal chamber. Gharagozloo et al[42] have recently argued that

a persistent left superior vena cava might cause pressure indentation on the left atrial wall, leading to overgrowth and membrane formation. The left superior vena cava could then be absorbed after the abnormal membrane is induced. Several cases of cor triatriatum associated with left superior vena cava have been reported.

Pathology

Cor triatriatum is often associated with an atrial septal defect and some form of partial anomalous pulmonary venous connection (Fig. 67–8). A patent foramen ovale may allow communication between the proximal or distal chamber and the right atrium. An ASD between the proximal chamber and the right atrium will result in a large left-to-right shunt and may mimic total anomalous pulmonary venous connection. Less commonly, cor triatriatum is associated with more complex lesions, such as transposition and tetralogy of Fallot.[41]

The anomalous membrane consists of a fibromuscular structure with a rigid, sometimes calcified orifice 2–10 mm in diameter. This partition may be membranous, funnel-shaped, or, rarely, tubular in nature.[43] Thilenius has reported several rare types of cor triatriatum, wherein the anomalous accessory chamber communicates only with the right atrium, and another type where the proximal chamber located between the right and distal left atrium does not receive any pulmonary veins. Situations where the accessory chamber does not communicate directly with the true left atrial chamber are usually considered a variant of total anomalous pulmonary venous connection and are discussed in Chapter 66.

Pathophysiology

The pathophysiologic consequence of this lesion is obstruction to pulmonary venous return. This results in pulmonary congestion, pulmonary arterial hypertension, and eventually right ventricular hypertrophy and failure, mimicking other lesions producing mitral stenosis. Depending on the degree of obstruction, the results may be sudden decompensation in the newborn period or the insidious onset of congestive heart disease over many years.

A left-to-right shunt may be present due to an associated atrial septal defect or partial anomalous pulmonary venous connection (Fig. 67–8B,H). The increased pulmonary blood flow will exacerbate pulmonary congestion and compromise systemic output. Cyanosis may be present where an atrial septal defect between the right atrium and the low pressure true left atrium results in right-to-left shunting (Fig. 67–8D).

Clinical Presentation

The time of onset and severity of symptoms depend on the degree of obstruction to pulmonary venous return. Infants

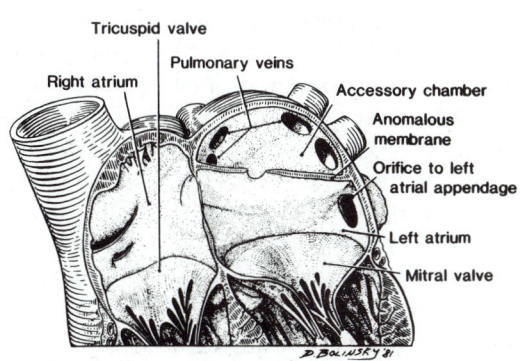

Figure 67–7. Surgical anatomy, classic form of cor triatriatum.

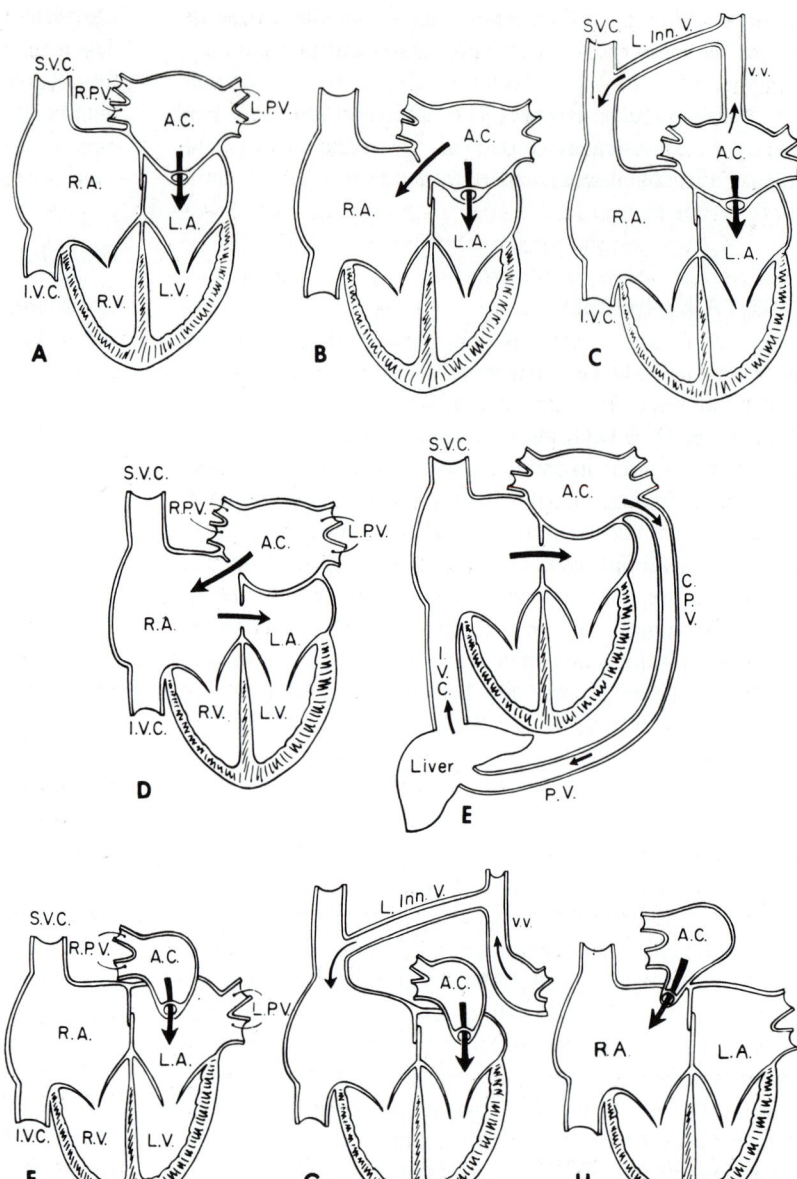

Figure 67–8. Some anatomic variations in cor triatriatum. AC, Accessory atrial chamber; CPN, Connor pulmonary vein; IVC, inferior vena cava; LA, left atrium; LInnV, left innominate vein; LPV, left pulmonary vein; LV, left ventricle; RA, right atrium; RPV, right pulmonary vein; RV, right ventricle; SVC, superior vena cava; VV, ventral vein. *(From Lucas RV Jr: In Moss et al (eds): Heart Disease in Infants, Children and Adolescents. 1977, p 455. Courtesy of Williams & Wilkins, Baltimore.)*

with high-grade obstruction present in the first week of life with severe pulmonary congestion, requiring emergency surgery.[44–46] On the other hand, patients with moderate obstruction may do well until the third or fourth decade of life, when the insidious progression of right-sided heart failure becomes apparent. Most patients have the onset of symptoms within the first few years of life, with dyspnea on exertion and frequent respiratory infections. On physical examination, signs of pulmonary hypertension are present, with a loud pulmonary component of the second heart sound and a prominent right ventricular heave. Right-sided heart failure with peripheral edema, liver enlargement, and ascites appears later. A diastolic or continuous murmur may be heard in the mitral area. The typical electrocardiogram shows a rightward axis between 120 and 160 degrees, peaked P waves suggestive of right atrial enlargement, and

evidence of right ventricular hypertrophy. The chest x-ray shows pulmonary venous obstruction with a reticular pulmonary pattern, venous engorgement, and enlargement of the main pulmonary artery. There may be moderate cardiac enlargement due to right ventricular enlargement. Echocardiography may be extremely helpful in identifying an anomalous membrane structure in the left atrial cavity.[47] Cardiac catheterization reveals pulmonary arterial hypertension with a high wedge pressure. Occasionally, a catheter can be passed into the distal left atrial chamber via the patent foramen ovale, revealing low pressures, which will help establish a diagnosis. A large left-to-right shunt may be detected in as many as 64% of patients if there is an associated ASD.[48] Selective angiocardiography from the pulmonary artery or the left atrium will demonstrate the abnormal accessory chamber. Angiography, with a catheter in the proximal or distal left atrial chamber, or the levophase of a pulmonary arterial injection, will reveal the anomalous membrane.[49]

Although surgical therapy is simple and effective, preoperative diagnosis may be difficult to make because of the rarity of this lesion and confusion with several other anomalies.[50–52] In the child with failure to thrive, severe dyspnea, evidence of pulmonary congestion, and right-sided heart failure, cardiac catheterization with high pulmonary arterial wedge pressure usually indicates a left-sided obstructive lesion. As many as 50% of surgical patients have incorrect preoperative diagnosis, including anomalous pulmonary venous drainage, mitral stenosis, ASD, and left atrial tumor.[48,53] Total anomalous pulmonary venous connection should be distinguishable based on angiographic and echocardiographic data. High wedge pressure with absence of left atrial enlargement is a strong clue to the diagnosis of cor triatriatum. Congenital mitral stenosis will present with a presystolic murmur and opening snap and left atrial enlargement on echocardiography. Congenital stenosis of individual pulmonary veins and supravalvular stenosing ring of the left atrium will give similar pathophysiologic consequences but should be distinguished on the basis of echocardiographic and angiographic findings.

Treatment

The first successful treatment of cor triatriatum was reported in 1956 by Lewis et al,[54] using inflow occlusion with excision of the membrane under direct vision, and by Vineberg and Giabretto,[55] using a closed finger-fracture technique. At the present time, the surgical treatment of cor triatriatum consists of the complete excision of the anomalous membrane with repair of any associated atrial septal defects or anomalous pulmonary venous return utilizing cardiopulmonary bypass. Symptomatic individuals in whom a diagnosis of cor triatriatum is made should undergo surgical repair.

Operative Technique

The ascending aorta and superior and inferior vena cava are cannulated. In the infant less than 8 kg, a single venous cannula may be used, with deep hypothermia and circulatory arrest. During the repair, the aorta is cross-clamped, and the heart is protected with cardioplegia infusion and topical hypothermia. The most popular approach to this lesion is through the right atrium and interatrial septum. This gives excellent exposure of both atria and both distal and proximal chambers, as well as the mitral valve and pulmonary vein orifices. In addition, it is easy to repair any associated defects in the interatrial septum and defects of pulmonary venous connection. In older children, a left atrial approach is possible.[48] A left atrial septal approach, as recommended by Brawley,[56] may also give excellent exposure.

The key to successful operation is complete excision of the anomalous membrane with relief of pulmonary venous obstruction. After an oblique incision is made in the right atrium (Fig. 67–6), an incision is made in the interatrial septum through the foramen ovale (Fig. 67–9A). The membrane is then completely excised back to the wall of the atrial septum, and the part of the atrial septum communicating with the membrane is also excised (Fig. 67–9B). The atrial septum can then be reconstructed with a Dacron or pericardial patch. In the left atrial approach (Fig. 67–10A), after incision is made in the left atrium posterior to the atrioventricular groove, the interatrial septum is retracted anteriorly, exposing the anomalous membrane, which is excised as fully as possible (Fig. 67–10B).

Results

Surgical deaths have been due to misdiagnosis with failure to recognize the obstructing membrane, residual pulmonary venous obstruction with low cardiac output, and associated congenital anomalies. Late results have shown excellent improvement in patients undergoing successful repair, with return of pulmonary arterial pressures to normal and relief

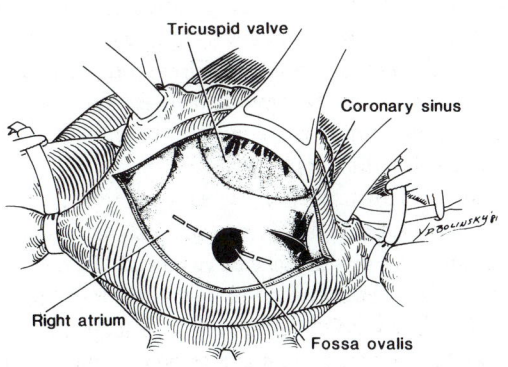
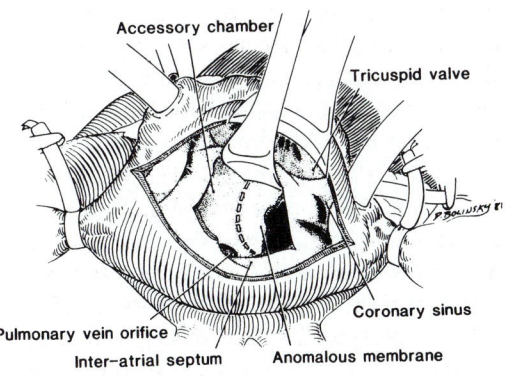

A   **B**

Figure 67–9. A. Right atrial approach to repair of cor triatriatum. **B.** View after excision of anomalous membrane.

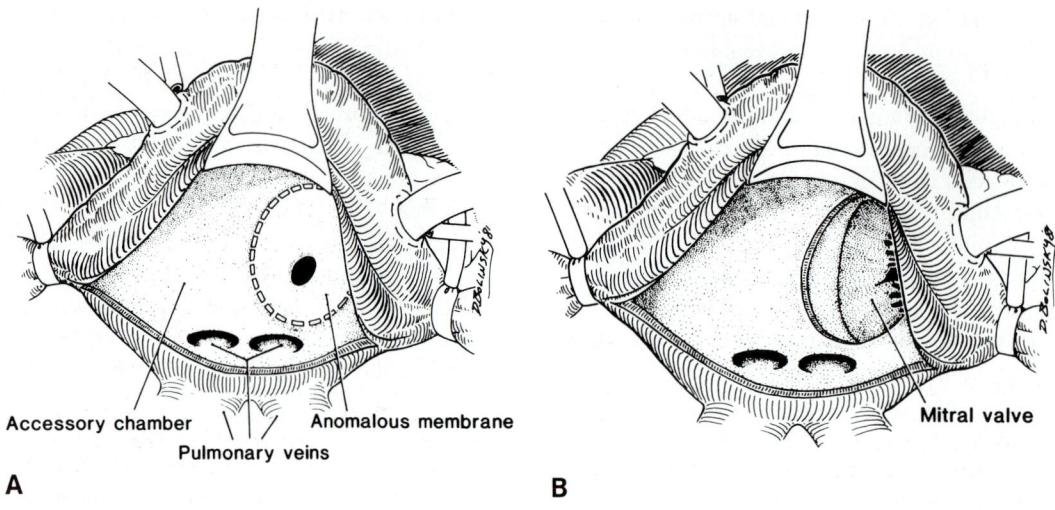

Accessory chamber   Anomalous membrane
Pulmonary veins

A   B

Mitral valve

Figure 67–10. A. Left atrial approach to cor triatriatum. **B.** View after excision of anomalous membrane.

of pulmonary venous congestion and right-sided heart failure.[48] An occasional patient will develop restenosis if the interatrial membrane is not completely excised, in which case a reoperation may be necessary. Lewis' first patient underwent successful reoperation 15 years later for recurrent pulmonary venous congestion.

In summary, cor triatriatum is a distinctly uncommon congenital anomaly that, despite very serious pathophysiologic consequences, is quite amenable to effective surgical therapy. The keys to successful treatment are a correct preoperative diagnosis of the lesion and any associated anomalies, and early surgical correction before permanent cardiovascular damage ensues.

REFERENCES

1. Hamilton WT, Haffajee CI, Dalen JE, et al: Atrial septal defect secundum: Clinical profile with physiologic correlates in children and adults. In Roberts WC (ed): *Congenital Heart Disease in Adults.* Philadelphia, Davis, 1979, pp 257–277
2. Gibbon JH Jr: Application of a mechanical heart and lung apparatus to cardiac surgery. *Min Med* **37:**171, 1954
3. Keith JD, Rowe RD, Vlad P: *Heart Disease in Infancy and Childhood,* 3rd ed. New York, Macmillan, 1978, Chap 22, p 380
4. Tandon R, Edwards JE: ASD in infancy. Common association with other defects. *Circulation* **49:**1005, 1974
5. Muller WH Jr, Littlefield JB, Beckwith JR: Surgical treatment of Lutembacher's syndrome. *J Thorac Cardiovasc Surg* **51:**66, 1966
6. Pifarre R, Dieter RA, Hoffman FG, et al: Atrial secundum septal defect and cleft mitral valve. *Ann Thorac Surg* **6:**373, 1968
7. John S, Munshi SC, Bhati BS, et al: Coexistent mitral valve disease with left-to-right shunt at the atrial level. Results of surgical treatment in 15 cases. *J Thorac Cardiovasc Surg* **60:**174, 1970
8. Holt M, Oram S: Familial heart disease with skeletal formations. *Br Heart J* **22:**236, 1960
9. Hynes KM, Fry RL, Brandenburg RO, et al: ASD (secundum) associated with mitral regurgitation. *Am J Cardiol* **34:**333, 1974
10. Blount SG, McCord MC, Swan H: Surgical closure of atrial septal

defect: The response in a patient with severe pulmonary hypertension. *Ann Surg* **20:**305, 1954
11. Bedford DE: The anatomical type of atrial septal defects, their incidence and clinical diagnosis. *Am J Cardiol* **6:**568, 1960
12. Craig RJ, Selzer A: Natural history and prognosis of atrial septal defect. *Circulation* **37:**805, 1968
13. Dalen JE, Haynes FW, Dexter L: Life expectancy with atrial septal defect. Influence of complicating pulmonary vascular disease. *JAMA* **200:**442, 1967
14. DuShane JW, Weidman WH, Brandenburg RO, et al: Differentiation of interatrial communications by clinical methods. Ostium secundum, ostium primum, common atrium and total anomalous pulmonary venous connection. *Circulation* **21:**363, 1960
14a. Hellenbrand WE, Mullins CE: Catheter closure of congenital cardiac defects. *Card Clin* **7:**351–368, 1989
15. Nakamura FF, Hauck AJ, Wadas AS: Atrial septal defects in infants. *Pediatrics* **34:**101, 1964
16. Spangler JF, Felot RH, Danielson GK: Secundum atrial septal defect encountered in infancy. *J Thorac Cardiovasc Surg* **71:**398, 1976
17. Ellis FH Jr, Brandenburg RO, Swan HJC: Defect of the atrial septum in the elderly. Report of successful surgical correction in 5 patients 60 years of age or older. *N Engl J Med* **262:**219, 1960
18. Gault JH, Morrow AG, Gay WA Jr, et al: Atrial septal defect in patients over the age of forty years: Clinical and hemodynamic studies and the effects of operation. *Circulation* **37:**261, 1968
19. Richmond DE, Lowe JB, Barratt-Boyes BG: Results of surgical repair of atrial and septal defects in the middle-aged and elderly. *Thorax* **24:**536, 1969
20. Lewis FJ, Taufic M, Varco RLL, et al: The surgical anatomy of atrial septal defects: Experience with repair under direct vision. *Ann Surg* **142:**401, 1955
21. Neptune WB, Bailey CP, Goldberg H: The surgical correction of atrial septal defects associated with transposition of the pulmonary veins. *J Thorac Surg* **26:**623, 1953
22. Disenhouse RB, Anderson RC, Adams P Jr, et al: Atrial septal defects in infants and children. *J Pediatr* **44:**269, 1954
23. Sellers RD, Ferlic RM, Sterns LP, Lillehei CW: Secundum type atrial septal defects: Early and late results of surgical repair using extracorporeal circulation in 275 patients. *Surgery* **59:**155, 1966
24. Kirklin JW, Weidman WH, Burroughs JT, et al: Hemodynamic results of surgical correction of atrial septal defect: Report of 33 cases. *Circulation* **13:**825, 1956
25. Stansel HC Jr, Talner NS, Deren M, et al: Surgical treatment of atrial

septal defect. Analysis of 150 corrective operations. *Am J Surg* **121:**485, 1971

26. Laks H, Hammond GL: A cosmetically acceptable incision for the median sternotomy. *J Thorac Cardiovasc Surg* **79:**146, 1980

27. Glenn WW, Toole AL, Longo E, et al: Induced fibrillatory arrest in open-heart surgery. *N Engl J Med* **262:**852, 1960

28. Kyger ER, Frazier OH, Cooley DA, et al: Sinus venosus atrial septal defects: Early and late results following closure in 109 patients. *Ann Thorac Surg* **25:**44, 1978

29. Ross JK, Johnson DC: Complications following closure of atrial septal defects of the inferior vena caval type. *Thorax* **27:**754, 1972

30. Hawe A, Rastelli GC, Brandenburg RO, et al: Embolic complications following repair of atrial septal defects. *Circulation* **39, 40** (Suppl 1):185, 1969

31. Nasrallah AT, Hall RJ, Garcia E, et al: Surgical repair of atrial septal defects in patients over 60 years of age. *Circulation* **41:**354, 1978

32. Yalav Z, Hedley Brown A, Braimbridge MV: Surgery for atrial septal defect in patients over 60 years of age. Report of surgical corrections in 12 patients. *J Thorac Cardiovasc Surg* **62:**788, 1971

33. Hairston P, Parker RF, Arravits JE, et al: The adult atrial septal defect: Results of surgical repair. *Ann Surg* **179:**799, 1974

34. Young D: Later results of closure of secundum atrial septal defect in children. *Am J Cardiol* **31:**14, 1973

35. Dave KS, Brojesh CP, Wooler GH, et al: Atrial septal defect in adults. Clinical and hemodynamic results of surgery. *Am J Cardiol* **31:**7, 1973

36. Hanlon CR, Barner HB, Willman VL, et al: Atrial septal defect: Results of repair in adults. *Arch Surg* **99:**275, 1969

37. Knight M, Lennox S: Results of surgery for atrial septal defect in patients of 40 years and over. *Thorax* **27:**577, 1972

38. Church WS: Congenital malformations of the heart. Abnormal septum in the left auricle. *Trans Pathol Soc London* **19:**188, 1868

39. Grondin C, Leonard AS, Anderson RC, et al: Cor triatriatum: A diagnostic surgical enigma. *J Thorac Cardiovasc Surg* **48:**527, 1964

40. Van Praagh R, Corsini J: Cor triatriatum: Pathologic anatomy and a consideration of morphogenesis based on 13 postmortem cases and a study of normal development of the pulmonary vein and atrial septum in 83 human embryos. *Am Heart J* **78:**379, 1969

41. Thilenius OG, Bharari S, Lev M: Subdivided left atrium—An ex-

panded concept of cor triatriatum sinistrum. *Am J Cardiol* **37:**743, 1976

42. Gharagozloo F, Bulkley BH, Hutchins GM: A proposed pathogenesis of cor triatriatum: Impingement of the left superior vena cava on the developing left atrium. *Am Heart J* **94:**618, 1977

43. Marin-Garcia J, Rojendra T, Lucas RV Jr, Edwards JE: Cor triatriatum: Study of 20 cases. *Am J Cardiol* **35:**59, 1975

44. Carpena C, Colokathis B, Subramanian S: Cor triatriatum: Successful correction in 4 patients including 2 under 1 year of age. *Ann Thorac Surg* **17:**325, 1974

45. Wolfe RR, Ruttenberg HD, Desilets DT, Mulder DE: Cor triatriatum: Total correction in an infant. *J Thorac Cardiovasc Surg* **66:**114, 1968

46. Jegier W, Gibbons JE, Wibleworth RW: Cor triatriatum: Clinical, hemodynamic and pathologic studies—Surgical correction in early life. *Pediatrics* **31:**255, 1967

47. Nimura Y, Matsumoto M, Beppu S, et al: Noninvasive reoperative diagnosis of cor triatriatum with ultrasonicardiotomogram and conventional echocardiogram. *Am Heart J* **88:**240, 1974

48. Richardson SV, Doty DB, Sievers RD, Zuberbuhler JR: Cor triatriatum (subdivided left atrium). *J Thorac Cardiovasc Surg* **81:**232, 1981

49. Millar GAH, Ongley PA, Anderson MW, et al: Cor triatriatum. *Am Heart J* **68:**298, 1964

50. Ahn C, Hosier DM, Sirak HD: Cor triatriatum: A case report and review of other operative cases. *J Thorac Cardiovasc Surg* **50:**177, 1968

51. Niwayama G: Cor triatriatum. *Am Heart J* **59:**291, 1960

52. Lam CR, Green G, Drake E: Diagnosis and surgical correction of two types of triatrial heart. *Surgery* **51:**127, 1962

53. Brickman RD, Wilson L, Zuberbuhler JR, Bahnson HT: Cor triatriatum: Clinical presentation and operative treatment. *J Thorac Cardiovasc Surg* **60:**523, 1970

54. Lewis FJ, Warco RL, Taufil M, Niazi SA: Direct vision repair of triatrial heart and total anomalous pulmonary venous drainage. *Surg Gynecol Obstet* **102:**713, 1956

55. Vineberg A, Giabretto O: Report of a successful operation for stenosis of common pulmonary vein (cor triatriatum). *Can Med Assoc J* **74:**719, 1956

56. Brawley RK: Improved exposure of the mitral valve in patients with a small left atrium. *Ann Thorac Surg* **29:**179, 1980

CHAPTER

68

Ventricular Septal Defect

Christo I. Tchervenkov and Dominique Shum-Tim

DEFINITION

A ventricular septal defect (VSD) is a hole in the interventricular septum. It may be congenital or acquired, single or multiple. It occurs in 1 in 1000 live births. Nearly 50% of patients with VSDs requiring surgical repair have additional major cardiovascular malformations. The most common of these are patent ductus arteriosus, aortic coarctation, and interrupted aortic arch. Alternatively, VSDs may be part of other congenital malformations such as tetralogy of Fallot, transposition of the great vessels, double outlet right ventricle, and tricuspid atresia. They may also occur in association with isolated atrial septal defects or as part of atrioventricular canals. This chapter will focus on isolated VSDs in a heart with concordant atrioventricular and ventriculoarterial connections, and normally positioned chambers and arteries.

HISTORICAL ASPECT

The first description of ventricular septal defects as a clinical entity was credited to Roger in 1879.[1] The term Roger's defect (maladie de Roger) is often used to indicate small VSDs. Eisenmenger, in 1897, described the end stage of the anomaly associated with severe pulmonary vascular obstructive disease in a 32-year-old patient who died with a VSD and overriding aorta.[2] The correlation between the clinical and pathologic findings was subsequently described by Abbott in 1932.[3] Further understanding of the natural history and pathophysiologic and hemodynamic effects of VSD was contributed by Lucas et al, Selzer, Fyler, and Heath and Edwards.[4–7] The principle of reducing excessive pulmonary blood flow with a pulmonary artery band and,

therefore, clinical improvement was reported by Mueller and Dammann in 1952.[8] The first successful intracardiac closure of a VSD under direct vision was reported by Lillehei et al in 1955, using the cross-circulation technique.[9] The development of extracorporeal circulation subsequently allowed successful closure of VSDs on a large scale as reported by Kirklin et al in 1957.[10]

ANATOMIC CLASSIFICATION

A thorough understanding of the anatomy of VSDs is a prerequisite for an accurate and safe repair avoiding potential hazard with respect to the conduction system. It is convenient to divide the interventricular septum into the following components[11]: (1) the membranous septum, (2) the outlet or conal septum, (3) the inlet or septum of the atrioventricular (A-V) canal, and (4) the muscular or trabecular septum (Fig. 68–1). VSDs can occur in any of these components and are therefore bordered by different structures. They can be divided into perimembranous, subarterial, A-V canal, and muscular types of defects. VSD repair patches are almost always placed within the morphological right ventricle. This avoids left ventriculotomy and minimizes the risk of heart block. It is therefore usual to focus on the septal anatomy as seen from the right ventricular side.

Perimembranous Ventricular Septal Defects

These defects (also known as conoventricular) comprise over 80% of all primary VSDs. The defect is usually located between the posterior and anterior divisions of the septal band and between the conal septum and the trabecu-

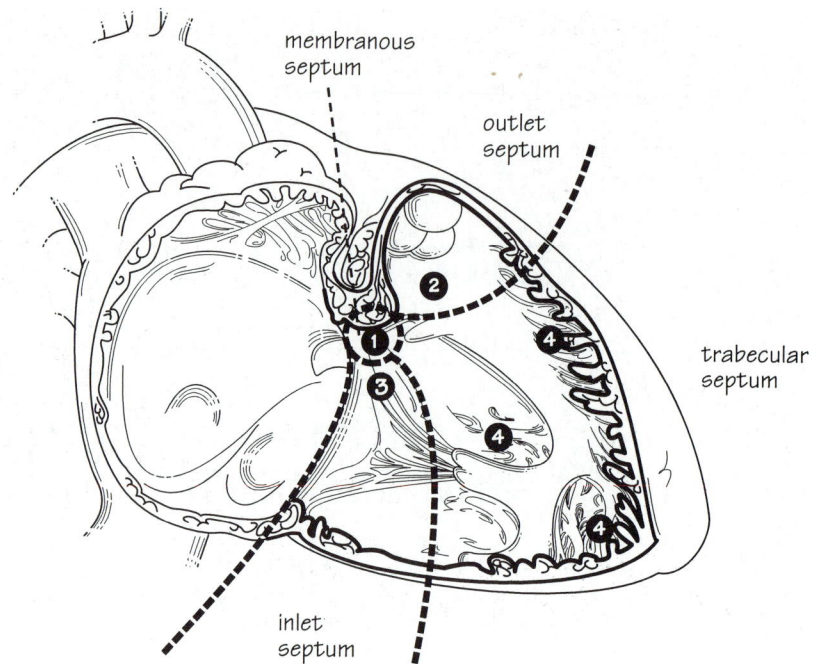

Figure 68–1. Anatomic locations of various types of ventricular septal defects. (1) Perimembranous (conoventricular) VSDs; (2) subarterial (outlet) VSDs; (3) atrioventricular canal-type (inlet) VSDs; (4) muscular (trabecular) VSDs.

lar interventricular septum[12–14] (Fig. 68–2). It is termed perimembranous because its margins include the membranous septum or its remnant. The VSD may extend into the inlet, trabecular, or outlet components of the interventricular septum.[15] Such VSDs can be seen in association with malalignment of the conal septum either anteriorly, as seen in tetralogy of Fallot, or posteriorly, causing left ventricular outflow tract obstruction and underdevelopment of the aortic arch.

The posteroinferior edge of perimembranous defects can extend to the annulus of the tricuspid valve in the region of the anteroseptal commissure. They may also extend to the base of the noncoronary leaflet of the aortic valve and may cause aortic regurgitation. Extension into the outlet, trabecular, and inlet regions of the interventricular septum is not unusual when the defect is large. The anterior leaflet of the tricuspid valve may bulge to the right during systole as blood passes beneath it. This gives the false impression of an aneurysm of the membranous septum on angiography. If the area of the commissure between the anterior and septal leaflets of the tricuspid valve becomes adherent to the edge of the VSD, blood may then course above the anterior tricuspid leaflet to create a left ventricle to right atrial shunt.[16,17] Rarely, a deficiency strictly in the atrioventricular septum may also result in a left ventricle to right atrium communication (Gerbode VSD).

Subarterial Ventricular Septal Defects

Various synonyms have been used to describe these defects. Outlet, conal, supracristal, or subpulmonary VSDs are lo-

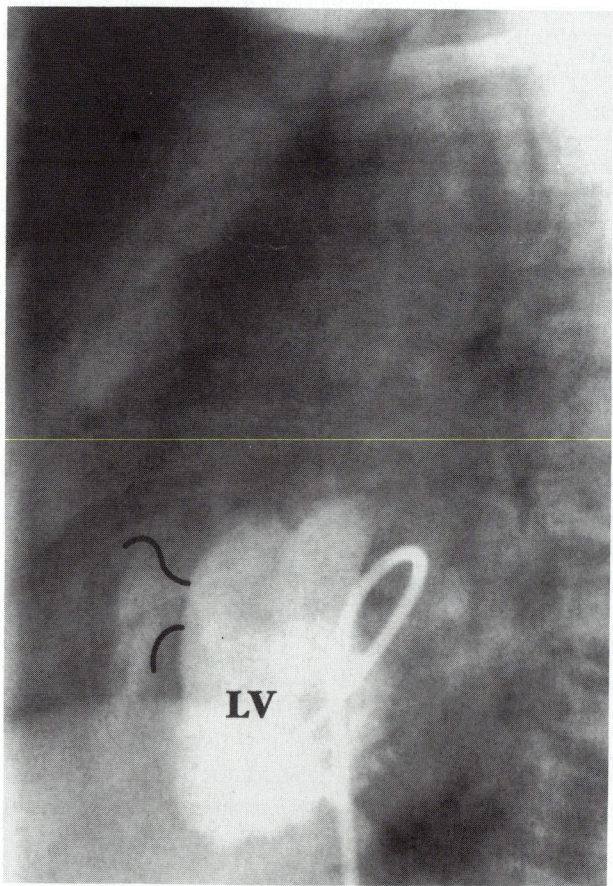

Figure 68–2. Left ventricular (LV) angiography demonstrating a perimembranous VSD.

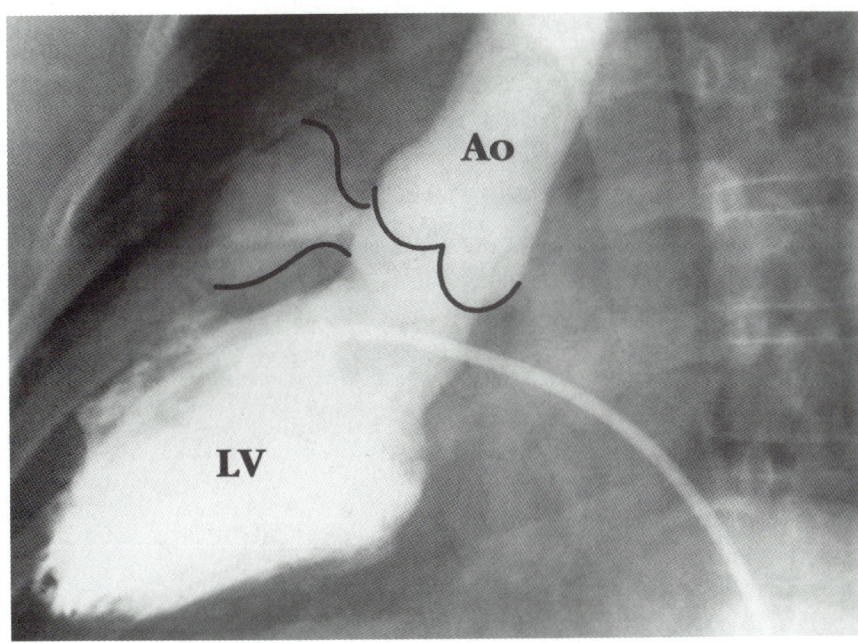

Figure 68–3. Left ventricular (LV) angiography of a subarterial VSD. Note its proximity to the aortic (Ao) valve.

cated in the outlet portion of both the right and left ventricles and comprise 5–10% of all VSDs (Fig. 68–3). The superior edge of the defect is the conjoined annuli of aortic and pulmonary valves.[18] This type of VSD is more common among Asians than among Caucasians or Blacks.[19]

Since the outlet septum is at least partly deficient, the adjacent portion of the aortic valve is relatively unsupported. Consequently, the right coronary cusp, or sometimes the noncoronary cusp, prolapses into the defect, causing various degrees of aortic insufficiency (Fig. 68–4). It is imperative to recognize this phenomenon commonly associated with subarterial VSD, because increasing prolapse of the aortic cusp may falsely occlude the defect and, thus, upon imaging, lead to underestimation of the size of the defect. Indeed, aortic insufficiency in this setting can be seen with either small or large defects since flow across small defects has a higher velocity causing greater deformity of the exposed aortic valve leaflet.[20]

Atrioventricular Canal-Type Ventricular Septal Defects

These VSDs are within the inlet part of the right ventricle spanning the length of the septal leaflet of the tricuspid valve. They make up less than 5% of surgically treated VSDs (Fig. 68–5). The posterior rim of this defect runs along the septal leaflet of the tricuspid valve to the central fibrous body and to the anterior leaflet of the mitral valve, which may have a cleft in association with this type of VSD. There is no intervening muscle between the VSD and the tricuspid valve. Superiorly, the defect usually extends to the membranous septum. The medial papillary muscle (of Lancisi) is attached to the anterior margin of the defect.

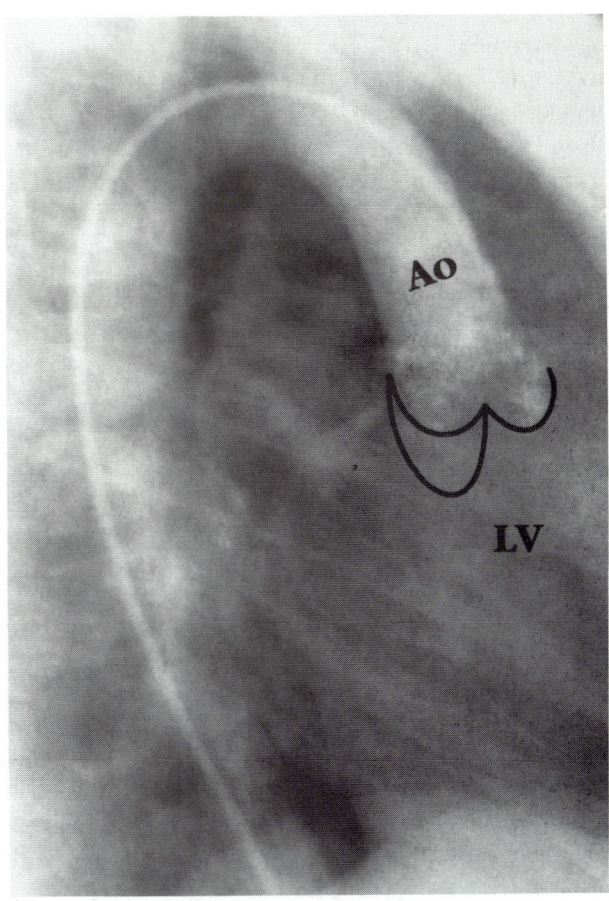

Figure 68–4. Aortogram demonstrating a prolapsed aortic (Ao) cusp obliterating the subarterial VSD. This was associated with a false closure of the interventricular septum and decrease in left-to-right shunting.

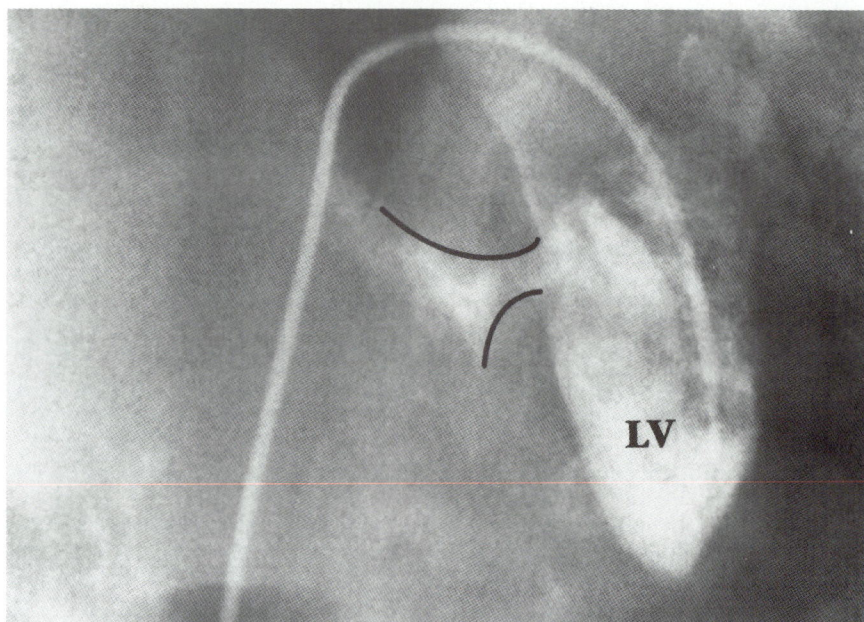

Figure 68–5. Left ventricular (LV) angiography of an A-V canal-type VSD.

Muscular Ventricular Septal Defects

Muscular VSDs are characterized by the presence of muscle tissue all the way around the defect. They are frequently multiple, and may exist anywhere within the muscular septum. According to their locations, they may be anterior, in the inlet septum, mid-muscular, or apical. It is important to note that inlet-type muscular VSDs are separated from the tricuspid valve and membranous septum by muscle tissue and are therefore different from A-V canal-type VSDs described above. This classification has surgical implications in that the inlet and midmuscular VSDs are closed by an approach through the tricuspid valve. The anterior VSDs are approached through a right ventriculotomy, while the apical VSDs are likely to require an apical left ventriculotomy. Infundibular (outlet) muscular VSDs are physiologically similar to subarterial VSDs, and, practically speaking, are considered with these. They differ from subarterial VSDs in that a small rim of muscle separates the VSD from the annuli of the semilunar valves.

Single or multiple muscular defects in the trabecular septum are more common in infants requiring surgical treatment than in older children. Sometimes, a large muscular defect may be partially covered by the septal band resulting in multiple openings when viewed from the RV side, yet being a single defect when viewed from the LV side. Rarely, true multiple defects may occur on both sides of the ventricular septum giving rise to the so-called "swiss-cheese"-type VSD (Fig. 68–6).

Atrioventricular Conduction System

The A-V node is located within the triangle of Koch and is the site of conduction of impulses from the SA node when the cardiac chambers are normally related. This area is bound

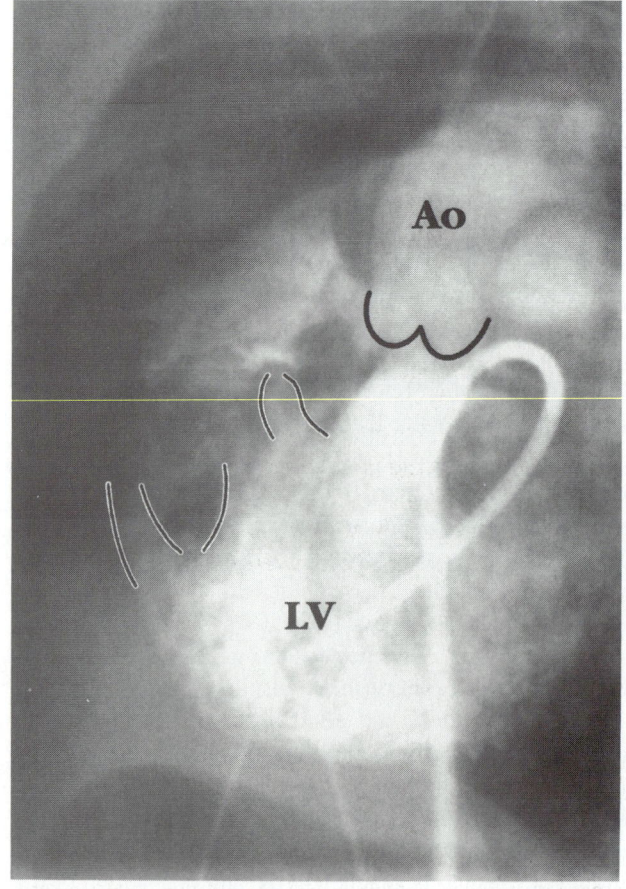

Figure 68–6. Left ventricular (LV) angiography of multiple muscular "swiss-cheese" VSD.

by the ligament of Todaro, the orifice of the coronary sinus, and the tricuspid septal leaflet. This is referred to as the posterior position. An additional anterior A-V node exists when there is atrioventricular discordance (see Chap. 95). When the inlet septum is deficient, the A-V node migrates posteriorly toward the crux of the heart (junction of the interventricular and atrioventricular grooves).[21]

The bundle of His normally traverses down to the interventricular septum through the central fibrous body in close relation to both the tricuspid and aortic valves. It first courses along the inferior margin of the membranous interventricular septum toward the left ventricle side of the muscular interventricular septum. Injury to this part of the conduction system is avoided during surgical repair of VSDs by suturing on the right ventricle side. The conduction tissue then divides into the left and right bundle branches.

The left bundle has several fascicles that travel subendocardially toward the anterolateral and posterolateral papillary muscles, respectively. The right bundle branch travels intramyocardially along the septal band and runs down to the apex traversing the base of the medial papillary muscle (of Lancisi), which itself is devoid of conduction tissue. It then travels to the right ventricular free wall via the moderator band and the apical muscular septum.

In the presence of a perimembranous VSD, the bundle of His passes along the posteroinferior rim of the defect. This area is to be avoided during surgery by placing the sutures superficially, a few millimeters below the edge of the VSD on the right ventricular side. Anterior to the muscle of Lancisi there is less danger of injuring the conduction tissue closer to the edge of the VSD.

In subarterial VSDs there is muscle tissue between the inferior rim of the VSD and the conduction system, decreasing the risk of injury during repair. The septal insertion of the ventriculoinfundibular fold (supraventricular crest) separates the conduction tissue from the edge of the defect.[21]

In A-V canal-type VSDs the conduction tissue runs along the *posteroinferior* rim of the VSD.

In muscular VSDs the conduction tissue lies in the normal anatomical position and is separated from the edge of the defect. It then follows that in the case of an inlet muscular VSD, in contrast to A-V canal-type VSDs, the conduction tissue will be along the *anterosuperior* (to the left) rim of the defect.[17,21]

PATHOPHYSIOLOGY

The pathophysiology of VSD is determined by the size of the defect and the pulmonary vascular resistance. An interaction of these variables will influence the pressure gradient and shunt volume across the defect. A VSD is considered nonrestrictive when it creates little resistance to flow, approximating at least the diameter of the aortic valve. The right ventricular (RV) systolic pressure nearly equals the left ventricular (LV) pressure and a large increase in pulmonary blood flow occurs. Multiple small VSDs may hemodynamically behave like a large defect.

In the early stages of the disease, the increase in pulmonary flow is inversely related to the pulmonary vascular resistance. For a large nonrestrictive VSD the RV pressure is systemic. Thus, during systole, the ventricular stroke volume is divided between the systemic bed and the pulmonary bed proportional to the resistance of these. Since the pulmonary vascular resistance falls after the neonatal period, blood is shunted left to right along this pathway of least resistance and blood flow through the lungs is markedly increased.

It is useful to consider the ratio of pulmonary to systemic blood flow (Q_p/Q_s) whenever assessing a VSD in clinical practice. This ratio is calculated from cardiac catheterization data. Flows are estimated from the oxygen saturation data using the Fick principal. The Q_p/Q_s ratio can be determined simply according to the following equation:

$$\frac{\text{aortic } O_2\% \text{ sat.} - \text{central venous } O_2\% \text{ sat.}}{\text{pulm. vein } O_2\% \text{ sat.} - \text{pulm. art. } O_2\% \text{ sat.}}$$

One can usually assume that aortic $O_2\%$ sat. is equal to pulmonary venous $O_2\%$ sat. This relation is also very useful when screening for residual VSDs in the operating room or in the ICU immediately following surgery.

The flow of blood across the defect (left to right shunt) and, subsequently, through the pulmonary vasculature causes elevation of the pulmonary artery pressure and blood return to the left side of the heart, leading to left atrial (LA) enlargement and LV overload. Pulmonary hypertension is reversible at this stage and there are no histologic changes early in the disease process. With time, progressive intimal proliferation and medial hypertrophy in the pulmonary arterioles will lead to a fixed irreversible pulmonary hypertension.[7]

Histologic severity of hypertensive pulmonary vascular disease is positively correlated with the pulmonary vascular resistance (PVR) and inversely related to the magnitude of shunting at the ventricular level. With a gradual increase in PVR, the pulmonary vascular tree replaces the left atrial pressure as the determinant of flow resistance across the lungs. The left-to-right shunt decreases, resulting in diminution of LV volume overload and resolution of congestive heart failure. This may be erroneously perceived as general improvement of the patient's clinical condition. If untreated, hypertensive pulmonary vascular disease eventually eliminates the left-to-right shunt. Cyanosis and cardiac failure (Eisenmenger's syndrome) ultimately lead to death due to a reversal of the shunt, which becomes right to left. Closing a VSD under these conditions would result in acute severe right heart failure since part of the RV blood volume could no longer be shunted into the pathway of least resistance, which at this stage is the systemic circulation. Pathologic features that comprise the Heath–Edwards grading and arterial density or number of vessels affected may help to predict the fall of pulmonary artery pressure after repair. Consequently, a histologic grading greater than 3 is unlikely to be associated with reversible hypertensive pulmonary vascular disease. On the other hand, a favorable outcome is expected as arterial density increases with growth.

A small VSD presents resistance to flow across the defect, which is of insufficient size to increase RV pressure. The Q_p/Q_s rarely exceeds 1.50. A small VSD does not significantly increase the pulmonary blood flow and does not impose an important hemodynamic burden on the left ventricle.

A moderate size VSD represents an intermediate group between the large and small defects and therefore can be restrictive. The Q_p/Q_s ranges between 1.5 and 2.5. It is less likely to cause fixed hypertensive pulmonary vascular disease.

NATURAL HISTORY

The clinical course of primary VSDs is influenced by several factors. Tendency for spontaneous closure is weighed against the development of hypertensive pulmonary vascular disease when deciding on surgical repair in the asymptomatic patient.

The severity of symptoms depends on the shunt volume across the VSD, which, in turn, is intimately related to the size of the defect and the magnitude of pulmonary vascular resistance. At birth, the newborn with a large VSD is usually asymptomatic. The shunt flow is limited by the elevated pulmonary vascular resistance normally present in the neonatal period. As the pulmonary resistance decreases during the first few weeks of life, the Q_p/Q_s becomes increasingly large. These infants have symptoms that reflect increased pulmonary blood flow and eventually heart failure. Recurrent respiratory infections, shortness of breath, and general failure to thrive are typical presentations. The pulmonary arteries may impose excessive pressure on the adjacent airways leading to air trapping.[17] If not properly treated, 10% of these patients will subsequently die from these complications during the first year of life. Irreversible pulmonary hypertension is uncommon in the first year of life.

Infants with persistent large VSDs who survive beyond the first year of life will eventually develop irreversible hypertensive pulmonary vascular disease and die of Eisenmenger's complex. They will have symptoms of hemoptysis, polycythemia, cerebral abscess, cerebral infarction, and right heart failure. This group of patients initially presents with excessive pulmonary blood flow and congestive heart failure. With evolution of the disease process, the pulmonary vascular resistance gradually increases, and the Q_p/Q_s decreases to levels seen in the early neonatal period. As discussed above, the ratio of pulmonary to systemic vascular resistance eventually increases to the point where the left-to-right shunt decreases. There is resolution of the pulmonary congestion, cardiomegaly, and the subsidence of

congestive heart failure. By the end of the first decade of life, cyanosis begins to occur. Premature death by the age of 35 years marks the eventual natural history of this group of patients with persistent large VSDs.[22]

It has been well documented that a VSD has a tendency to close spontaneously, which may explain the infrequent incidence in the adult population.[23] This is especially true for perimembranous VSDs but more unusual for A-V canal-type and subarterial VSDs. The probability of eventual spontaneous closure of congenital VSD is inversely related to the age of the patient.[22,24,25] Eighty percent of large VSDs seen at the age of 1 mo will eventually close spontaneously. On the other hand, only 50% of the large VSD present at the age of 6 mo and 25% of the VSD at 12 mo will close spontaneously. Nevertheless, spontaneous closure of VSD has been described even in adulthood.

Five to ten percent of patients with a VSD and nonrestrictive left-to-right shunt in infancy may develop subsequent infundibular pulmonary stenosis or right ventricular outflow tract obstruction secondary to myocardial hypertrophy.[22,25,26] When the right ventricular outflow tract obstruction becomes severe, a right-to-left shunt occurs, resulting in a clinical picture similar to tetralogy of Fallot. In this situation, the pulmonary vasculature is actually protected from excess blood flow.

Bacterial endocarditis represents a potentially serious complication for patients with VSD. The incidence is approximately 0.15–0.3% per year. It is more common in small and moderate size VSDs. The prognosis is good with antibiotic therapy.[27–29] VSDs should be closed following resolution of endocarditis.

Aortic valve insufficiency can occur in the presence of subarterial VSDs as described above or in perimembranous VSDs with subaortic extensions.[17] On a percentage basis this occurs more frequently with subarterial VSDs than with perimembranous ones. It is important, however, to recall that perimembranous VSDs are far more common. The right coronary cusp and/or uncommonly the noncoronary cusp may prolapse through the VSD. This must be addressed in the preoperative period and salvage of an aortic valve while it can still be repaired (vs. replacement) or before significant regurgitation occurs may become an indication for surgical treatment of both the VSD and the aortic valve. This line of reasoning is applied regardless of symptoms. If the aortic valve is bicuspid and insufficient but without cusp prolapse then the indication for surgery is dictated by symptoms as well as severity of aortic valve regurgitation rather than by the presence of the VSD.[17]

DIAGNOSIS

Clinical Features

The clinical presentation of patients with a VSD is a function of the relative pulmonary vascular resistance as well as the size of the ventricular septal defect at various stages of the disease process. Patients with small VSDs are usually asymptomatic and have no abnormal physical findings other than a harsh pansystolic murmur. Patients with large VSDs, on the other hand, have variable symptoms.[30] At one extreme, signs and symptoms of congestive heart failure predominate. These patients develop tachypnea, hepatomegaly, failure to thrive, as well as repeated pulmonary infections due to increased pulmonary blood flow. On physical examination, signs of a hyperactive heart are noted. A precordial pansystolic murmur is characteristic. When the pulmonary vascular resistance is not significantly elevated, there is a prominent third sound and a diastolic murmur is heard at the apex, reflecting increased blood flow across the mitral valve. With gradual spontaneous closure of a large VSD, these signs and symptoms may disappear. At the other extreme are patients who are less symptomatic and have elevated pulmonary vascular resistance. The shunt becomes bidirectional. The systolic murmur now becomes softer or absent, with no diastolic murmur. The heart is neither hyperactive nor volume overloaded at this stage. The pulmonary component of the second heart sound is loud and there is a palpable thrill over the left precordium. When the pulmonary vascular resistance advances, the patient becomes progressively cyanotic with fatigue, congestive heart failure, and other signs of Eisenmenger's complex.

Investigations

Electrocardiogram

The electrocardiogram reflects the hemodynamic alteration and the progression of cardiac chamber hypertrophy caused by the VSD. In patients with a small defect and no significant hemodynamic LV volume overload, the electrocardiogram is usually normal. When a large defect is associated with increased pulmonary blood flow but low pulmonary vascular resistance, the electrocardiogram reveals left atrial enlargement and isolated left ventricular hypertrophy. As the pulmonary vascular resistance increases, there is evidence of biventricular hypertrophy. As pulmonary vascular

resistance further increases and becomes fixed, right ventricular hypertrophy predominates.

Chest Roentgenogram

The chest roentgenogram also correlates well with the natural history of ventricular septal defect and the physiologic alteration it creates (Fig. 68–7). The roentgenogram is usually normal in patients with defects of minimal hemodynamic consequences. In patients with significant left-to-right shunting across the VSD, there is evidence of cardiomegaly due to left atrial dilatation, LV volume overload, and RV enlargement. Increasing vascular markings in the central and peripheral pulmonary arteries are also characteristics of increased pulmonary blood flow. As the pulmonary vascular resistance increases and the pulmonary blood flow decreases, the cardiac enlargement becomes less pronounced and the heart size is generally normal. In severe pulmonary hypertension, however, enlargement of the right ventricle and attenuation of the peripheral pulmonary vasculature become evident.

Two-Dimensional, Doppler, Color Echocardiography

With increasing experience, the two-dimensional echocardiogram can reliably assess the size and position of the defects. The echo Doppler interrogation is also useful to estimate the right ventricular pressure, the degree of pulmonary artery hypertension, the magnitude of shunting across the ventricles, and any gradient that may be present across the VSD itself. Color Doppler echocardiography is particularly helpful to visualize multiple ventricular septal defects. These techniques constitute important noninvasive methods for the evaluation and long-term follow-up of patients with VSDs.[31–33] In neonates with intractable symptomatic isolated VSD, one may proceed to surgery based on echocardiographic findings alone. As patients get older it is imperative to precisely identify VSDs with associated high fixed pulmonary vascular resistance using cardiac catheterization.

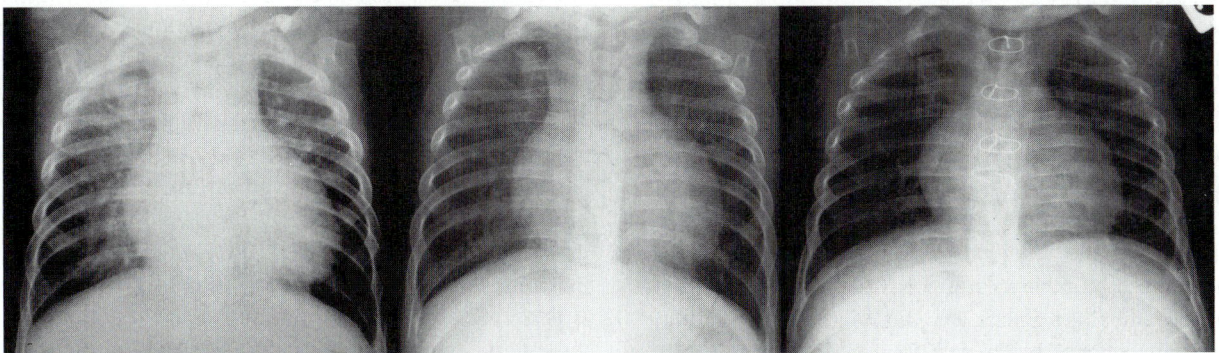

Figure 68–7. A term infant born with Down syndrome and symptoms of congestive heart failure at 1 mo of age with large A-V canal-type VSD. Left, anteroposterior chest radiograph demonstrates cardiomegaly, prominent pulmonary vascular markings, and pulmonary edema. Middle, pulmonary edema improved but there was persistent cardiomegaly after treatment with diuretics. Right, normal cardiac contour with normal pulmonary vascular markings following surgical closure.

Magnetic Resonance Imaging

The use of MRI to evaluate intracardiac ventricular defect seems promising, although more experience is required in many centers.

Cardiac Catheterization and Cineangiography

Cardiac catheterization and cineangiography are no longer used routinely to diagnose isolated VSDs. However, as stated above, in older children, it should be considered to more precisely document the pulmonary artery pressure and vascular resistance. Shunt volume, Q_p/Q_s, and the irreversible component of pulmonary hypertension may also be defined. The information obtained will help to decide if closure of the VSD can be safely undertaken. Left ventriculogram showing the interventricular septum allows the identification of the anatomy of various VSDs.

TREATMENT

The indication for treatment is dictated by the severity of symptoms attributed to the defect, the age at presentation, the magnitude of pulmonary vascular resistance, the size and type of a particular isolated VSD, and the presence of other coexisting malformations. Surgical repair in early life is indicated for infants with severe intractable CHF despite optimal medical therapy. Persistence of failure to thrive is the most common indication in infants. Associated cardiac anomalies should also be repaired at the same time when appropriate. In the remaining majority of patients with an isolated VSD, especially with low pulmonary vascular resistance, the operation is elective and can be delayed until 12 mo of age in hope of spontaneous closure. Afterward, the likelihood of spontaneous closure decreases and moderate-to-large VSDs should be closed. Infants older than 6 mo with elevated PVR should undergo prompt VSD closure. In addition, A-V canal-type and subarterial VSDs have no tendency to close spontaneously, and, therefore, should be repaired early.

In the young patient with a small defect, the natural tendency for the defect to become smaller and eventually close is sufficiently high that surgical intervention is not indicated. However, the management of a persistent small VSD beyond 10 years of age remains controversial. Although infective bacterial endocarditis can be avoided by surgical closure with minimal morbidity and mortality, the risk of these complications is, nevertheless, minimal with adequate antibiotic prophylaxis.

Single stage closure of a large isolated VSD rather than banding of the pulmonary artery is currently the treatment of choice for patients with VSD requiring surgical intervention. However, there are certain special situations where these general guidelines do not apply. Pulmonary artery banding is now recommended early only in symptomatic infants with multiple muscular VSDs of the "swiss cheese" variety and VSDs with a straddling AV valve. Because the risk of early primary intracardiac repair is significant in infants with large symptomatic VSDs and aortic coarctation, they were formerly treated by initial pulmonary artery banding and coarctation repair, followed by subsequent intracardiac repair and release of the band by the age of 5 years. Currently, we favor a single stage repair for a VSD associated with aortic coarctation or hypoplasia by a sternotomy if this can be done with acceptable risk.

Subarterial VSDs should be closed early because of the risk of damage to the aortic valve and subsequent development of aortic insufficiency. As already mentioned, the decrease in size of such a VSD may be misleading due to the prolapsing leaflet of the adjacent aortic valve, which may occlude the VSD.

OPERATIVE TECHNIQUE

Primary closure of all isolated VSDs has led to the virtual disappearance of patients with previous pulmonary artery banding and its associated complications. VSDs can be closed with standard cardiopulmonary bypass using bicaval cannulation. In young infants, especially those less than 8 kg, profound hypothermia down to 18°C and total circulatory arrest greatly facilitate the surgical repair. We routinely ligate the ductus arteriosus soon after the establishment of cardiopulmonary bypass to prevent air entry into the systemic circulation as well as excess blood in the operative field.[14] Myocardial protection consists of a single dose of cardioplegia solution with topical hypothermia in infants and multidose cardioplegia as well as topical myocardial hypothermia in patients beyond infancy.

Most VSDs, except for subarterial or muscular outlet defects, are repaired through the right atrium. Exposure of the defect is facilitated by retraction of the tricuspid valve. Detachment of the base of tricuspid septal leaflet has been advocated by some to improve exposure of a difficult VSD.[14,17,30] However, we have never had to use this technique. The VSD is closed with a prosthetic patch (Goretex) anchored with multiple pledgetted nonabsorbable sutures. As already discussed, the conduction system is avoided by placement of the sutures further away from the posteroinferior rim of the VSD. Occasionally, it is more convenient to use a continuous suture for the closure of the A-V canal-type VSD because it allows the weaving in and out between various tricuspid chordae and papillary muscles. The Goretex patch is usually sutured into the base of the annulus of the tricuspid septal leaflet. Extra care is necessary near the superior margin to avoid damage to the aortic valve.

The subarterial type VSDs are approached through the pulmonary valve without a ventriculotomy. The VSD patch is anchored superiorly by placement of pledgetted sutures through the annulus of the pulmonary valve with the pledgets lying inside the pulmonary valve sinus. When aortic insufficiency accompanies a subarterial VSD, patch closure of the defect may provide enough support to the prolapsing leaflet to improve or to eliminate the valvular regurgitation. Moderate-to-severe aortic insufficiency may require aortic valve repair through a concomitant aortotomy.

Closure of the muscular VSD depends on its location. The mid-muscular and inlet septal muscular defects can be closed with a single patch through the right atrium. Excessive trabeculations on the right ventricular surface may give the impression of multiple muscular VSDs, when in fact there is only one. Such trabeculations may have to be resected first, to properly visualize all the margins of the defect. A right ventriculotomy incision may be necessary to facilitate exposure of the anterior part of the muscular septum. Occasionally, one may also consider closure of anterior multiple muscular VSDs using buttressed sutures anchored in the interventricular septum and on the anterior right ventricular surface.[17,30]

Apical muscular defects can be extremely difficult to close by all conventional means, except through an apical LV incision. This approach is frequently complicated by global LV dyskinesia and the formation of an apical aneurysm. Operative or percutaneous transcatheter closure using an umbrella device has particular merit in dealing with this type of muscular VSD when the technical expertise is available.[34] Although this approach seems promising, more experience and long-term follow-up will be required.[14,30,35]

POSTOPERATIVE CARE

With the advent of modern anaesthesia, improved methods of myocardial protection and extracorporeal perfusion, and better understanding of the hemodynamic and natural history of the defects, the postoperative course following complete primary closure of a VSD is usually uneventful. Routine policies to insert right atrial, left atrial, and pulmonary artery catheters intraoperatively greatly facilitate the postoperative management and monitoring of these patients. The standard maintenance of adequate cardiac output and ventilation as well as monitoring of postoperative bleeding are similar to other postcardiotomy protocols. Potential complications associated with the primary repair of VSDs relate to the presence of residual left-to-right shunting. If the hemodynamic state remains poor early postoperatively, provided that preoperative pulmonary vascular hypertension is not significant, investigations should be performed to rule out the possibility of residual left-to-right shunt. A step-up of oxygen saturation at the PA level compared to the RA may easily rule out this possibility. Echocardiography may also be helpful to assess the degree of residual shunting during the immediate postoperative period.

Permanent, complete atrioventricular heart block is now rare but remains a potential complication following primary repair of VSD. The prevalence of these complications is slightly higher following the repair of multiple VSDs or major associated cardiac anomalies. Complete heart block persisting for more than 10–14 days after surgery should be treated by insertion of a permanent pacemaker.

RESULTS

Early mortality rate following repair of a large single VSD during early life approaches zero in most specialized centers.[14] It has been well documented that patients with high pulmonary vascular resistance operated on beyond infancy have a worse long-term outcome because of progression of their pulmonary vascular disease. Multiple VSDs and associated cardiac anomalies also increase the risk. In a recent large series, the hospital mortality rate of these high-risk patients was about 7%.[36]

Conduction disturbances are frequent after the repair of VSD. The prevalence of right bundle branch block after a right ventriculotomy is about 80%.[37] This decreases to 34% when the right atrial approach is used.[38] A smaller proportion of patients develops an electrocardiographic pattern of right bundle branch block and left anterior hemiblock following operation (8–17%).[37,38]

On the other hand, the incidence of surgically induced permanent heart block in isolated VSD currently approaches zero in most centers. The incidence of residual shunting due to an undiagnosed defect, incomplete closure, or patch dehiscence is also uncommon (0.7–2.0%) after patch closure with precise preoperative documentation of the cardiac anatomy.[24,38]

ACKNOWLEDGMENT

The authors would like to express their appreciation for the radiological advice and contribution of Dr. Bob Williams.

REFERENCES

1. Galen: *Opera Omnia* **IV**:243. Kuhn Edition. A translation from Dalton JC: *Doctrines of the Circulation.* Philadelphia, Lea's Son, 1884, p 68 Translated from the Greek, with an introduction and commentary by Mary Tallmadge May. Ithaca, NY, Cornell University Press, 1968, Vol 1, p 333
2. Wood O: The Eisenmenger syndrome or pulmonary hypertension with reversed central shunt. *Br Med J* **2**:701, 755, 1958
3. Abbott ME: Congenital cardiac disease. In Nelson T (ed): *Loose-leaf Medicine,* Vol 4. New York, Thomas Nelson, 1932, p 207
4. Lucas RV, Adams P, Anderson RC, et al: The natural history of isolated ventricular septal defect. *Circulation* **24**:1372, 1961
5. Selzer A: Defect of the ventricular septum. *Arch Intern Med* **84**:798, 1949
6. Fyler DC: Ventricular septal defects in children: A correlation of clinical, physiologic and autopsy data. *Circulation* **18**:833, 1958
7. Heath D, Edwards JE: The pathology of hypertensive pulmonary vascular disease. A description of six grades of structural changes in the pulmonary artery with reference to congenital cardiac septal defects. *Circulation* **18**:533, 1958

8. Mueller WH Jr., Dammann JF: The treatment of certain congenital malformations of the heart by creation of pulmonary stenosis to reduce pulmonary hypertension and excessive pulmonary blood flow. *Surg Gynecol Obstet* **95:**213, 1952

9. Lillehei CW, Cohen M, Warden HE, et al: The results of direct vision closure of ventricular septal defects in eight patients by means of controlled cross circulation. *Surg Gynecol Obstet* **101:**446, 1955

10. Kirklin JW, Harshbarger HG, Donald DE, et al: Surgical correction of ventricular septal defect: Anatomic and technical considerations. *J Thorac Cardiovasc Surg* **33:**45, 1957

11. Moulaert AJ: Anatomy of ventricular septal defect. In Anderson RH, Shinebourne EA (eds): *Pediatric Cardiology 1977*. Edinburg, Churchill Livingstone, 1978, p 113

12. Smolinsky A, Castaneda AR, Van Praagh R: Infundibular septal resection: Surgical anatomy of the superior approach. *J Thorac Cardiovasc Surg* **95:**486, 1988

13. Soto B, Ceballos R, Kirklin JW: Ventricular septal defects. A surgical viewpoint. *J Am Coll Cardiol* **14:**1291, 1989

14. Castaneda AR, Jonas RA, Mayer JE, Hanley F: Ventricular septal defect. In *Cardiac Surgery of the Neonate and Infant.* Philadelphia, Saunders, 1994, Chap 11, p 187–201

15. Becu LM, Fontana RS, DuShane JW, et al: Anatomy and pathologic studies in ventricular septal defect. *Circulation* **14:**349, 1956

16. Braunwald E, Morrow AG: Left-ventriculo-right atrial communication. Diagnosis by clinical, hemodynamic and angiographic methods. *Am J Med* **28:**913, 1960

17. Kirklin JW, Barratt-Boyes BG: Ventricular septal defect. In *Cardiac Surgery,* 2nd ed. New York, Churchill Livingstone, 1993, Chap 20, pp 749–786

18. Soto B, Becker AE, Moulaert AH, et al: Classification of ventricular septal defects. *Br Heart J* **43:**332, 1980

19. Tatsuno K, Ando M, Takao A, et al: Diagnostic importance of aortography in conal ventricular septal defect. *Am Heart J* **89:**171, 1975

20. de Leval MR, Pozzi M, Starnes V, et al: Surgical management of doubly committed subarterial VSDs. *Circulation* **78**(III):40, 1988

21. Anderson RH, Becker AE: The anatomy of VSDs and their conduction tissues. In Stark J, de Laval MR (eds): *Surgery for Congenital Heart Defects,* 2nd ed. Philadelphia, Saunders, 1994, Chap 7, pp 115–138

22. Keith JD, Collins RG, Kidd BSL: Ventricular septal defect: Incidence, morbidity and mortality in various age groups. *Br Heart J* **33** (Suppl):81, 1971

23. Collins G, Calder L, Rose V, et al: Ventricular septal defect: Clinical and hemodynamic change in the first five years of life. *Am Heart J* **84:**695, 1972

24. Blackstone EH, Kirklin JW, Bradley EL, et al: Optimal age and results in repair of large ventricular septal defects. *J Thorac Cardiovasc Surg* **72:**661, 1976

25. Hoffman JIE, Rudolph AM: The natural history of ventricular septal defects in infancy. *Am J Cardiol* **16:**634, 1965

26. Gasul BM, Dillon RF, Urla V, et al: Ventricular septal defects. Their natural transformation into those with infundibular stenosis or with the cyanotic or noncyanotic type of tetralogy of Fallot. *JAMA* **164:**857, 1957

27. Shah P, Singh WSA, Rose V, et al: Incidence of bacterial endocarditis in ventricular septal defects. *Circulation* **34:**127, 1966

28. Gersony WM, Hayes CJ: Bacterial endocarditis in patients with pulmonary stenosis, aortic stenosis, or ventricular septal defect. *Circulation* **56:**84, 1977

29. Campbell M: Natural history of ventricular septal defect. *Br Heart J* **33:**246, 1971

30. de Leval MR: Ventricular septal defects. Stark J, de Leval MR (eds): In *Surgery for Congenital Heart Defects* 2nd ed. Philadelphia, Saunders, 1994, Chap 23, pp 355–371

31. Bierman FZ, Fellows K, Williams RG: Prospective identification of ventricular septal defects in infancy using subxiphoid two-dimensional echocardiography. *Circulation* **62:**807, 1980

32. Ortiz E, Robinson PJ, Deanfield JE, et al: Localisation of ventricular septal defects by simultaneous display of superimposed colour Doppler and cross sectional echocardiographic images. *Br Heart J* **54:**53, 1985

33. Sutherland CA, Godman MJ, Smallhorn JF, et al: Ventricular septal defects. Two-dimensional echocardiography and morphological correlation. *Br Heart J* **437:**316, 1982

34. Castaneda AR, Jonas RA, Mayer JE, Hanley FA: Interventional cardiology. In *Cardiac Surgery of the Neonate and Infant.* Philadelphia, Saunders, 1994, Chap 7, pp 123–139

35. Bridges ND, Penny SB, Keane JF, et al: Preoperative transcatheter closure of congenital muscular ventricular septal defects. *N Engl J Med* **324:**1312, 1991

36. Rizzoli G, Blackstone EH, Kirklin JW, et al: Incremental risk factors in hospital mortality rate after repair of ventricular septal defect. *J Thorac Cardiovasc Surg* **80:**494, 1980

37. Barratt-Boyes BG, Neutze JM, Clarkson PM, et al: Repair of ventricular septal defect in the first two years of life using profound hypothermia—circulatory arrest techniques. *Ann Surg* **184:**376, 1976

38. Rein JG, Freed MD, Norwood WI, et al: Early and late results of closure of ventricular septal defect in infancy. *Ann Thorac Surg* **24:**19, 1977

69

Patent Ductus Arteriosus and Aortopulmonary Window

Gary Haas

Patent ductus arteriosus and aortopulmonary window are considered in this chapter as they both are extracardiac lesions that involve a direct, unguarded connection between the aorta and the pulmonary vasculature. They occur most commonly as isolated defects, but may also present in combination with other cardiovascular defects.

The physiological consequences of these defects result from the shunt that occurs between the systemic arterial and pulmonary circulations. This shunt, which is both systolic and diastolic, can often be characterized by the associated "machinery" murmur. The magnitude of the associated shunt is determined by the size of the defect and the difference in the systemic and arterial pressures. Small defects result in a small shunt with few consequences other than risk for subacute bacterial endocarditis (SBE). Large defects can result in a large shunt that can lead to severe congestive heart failure and rapid development of pulmonary vascular disease.

Although the pathophysiology, physical findings, and clinical presentation may be similar for both patent ductus arteriosus and aortopulmonary defect, their specific anatomy and reparative approaches differ greatly. Therefore, accurate definition of these lesions and clear differentiation between them and between other lesions with similar findings must be established before embarking on their surgical repair.

PATENT DUCTUS ARTERIOSUS

Definitions

Patent ductus arteriosus (ductus of Botalli) is an abnormality that results from persistence of the fetal ductus arterio-

sus in the postnatal period. It can be recognized in a variety of circumstances. Most often a patent ductus arteriosus presents as a simple shunt between the systemic arterial to pulmonary arterial circulations. As such, it may occur as a solitary lesion, or in association with other simple cardiac defects.

Alternatively, a patent ductus arteriosus may also present as a component of more complex forms of congenital heart disease. In these situations a patent ductus arteriosus may actually serve as a life-sustaining conduit. It may constitute the major source of pulmonary blood flow in patients with right-sided obstructive lesions, or as conduit for systemic arterial blood supply in patients with left-sided obstructive lesions.

This chapter will be primarily concerned with the patent ductus arteriosus as a simple arterial to pulmonary shunt. Patent ductus arteriosus as a component of more complicated cardiac lesions will be discussed in those chapters dealing with such lesions specifically.

Historical Background

Patent ductus arteriosus has a prominent place in the history, understanding, and treatment of congenital heart disease. The ductus arteriosus and its postnatal closure was described by Galen in 131 AD.[1] The physiologic importance of the ductus arteriosus was elucidated by Harvey in 1628,[2] and the classic auscultatory findings were described by Gibson in 1898.[3,4]

In 1907 Munro suggested the benefits of closure of the patent ductus arteriosus having demonstrated the feasibility of surgical closure in a cadaver.[5] The closure of a patent ductus arteriosus was first attempted by Strieder in 1937.[6]

Unfortunately the patient, a young woman with endocarditis, died of postoperative complications. A year later, the era of cardiac surgery was ushered in by the successful closure of a patent ductus arteriosus by Gross and Hubbard.[7]

Further innovations in the treatment of congenital heart disease are also related to closure of the patent ductus arteriosus. An important innovation includes the understanding of the role of prostaglandins in ductal patency and the use of inhibitors of PGE$_1$ synthesis to induce closure.[8] In addition, interventional catheterization techniques were developed in transarterial closure of a patent ductus arteriosus as reported by Portsmann and colleagues in 1971,[9] and Rashkind and Cuaso.[10] Finally, techniques for "thoracoscopic" closure of the patent ductus arteriosus are presently evolving.[11]

Anatomy and Physiology of the Fetal Ductus Arteriosus

The ductus arteriosus is a fetal vascular structure that connects the pulmonary and systemic vasculature. It is derived from the sixth aortic arch and is equal in diameter to the descending aorta (Fig. 69–1). It normally originates from the pulmonary confluence as a continuation of the main pulmonary artery and terminates in the left-sided descending aorta a few millimeters beyond the origin of the left subclavian artery.

The wall of the ductus arteriosus differs from that of other major vascular structures.[12,13] The medium is deficient of elastic fibers, and is instead composed primarily of smooth muscle cells. These are arranged in an outer poorly organized spiral configuration, and a longitudinal inner layer that may protrude centrally where intimal cushions are formed. A thickened wavy internal elastic lamina fragments into multiple layers adjacent to intimal cushions. Large gaps in the area of junction of medial structures and the intimal structures are filled with mucinous substances called "mucoid lakes." The smooth muscle in the wall of the ductus arteriosus is specifically sensitive to environmental factors, particularly prostaglandins (PGE$_2$ and PGI$_2$) that promote relaxation, and PO$_2$ that causes constriction.[14–16]

Physiology of the Ductus Arteriosus

During fetal development, the right and left ventricles function in parallel and share in systemic and placental perfusion. During this phase of development, the ductus arteriosus serves an important role as a conduit from the main pulmonary artery to the descending aorta. The distribution of fetal blood flow is shown in Figure 69–2.[17] The fetal pulmonary vascular resistance is high, and, as shown, most of the right ventricular output passes through the ductus arteriosus into the descending aorta.

Maintenance of fetal patency of the ductus arteriosus is the result of a series of factors. During fetal life, high levels of circulating and locally derived prostaglandin (PGE$_2$

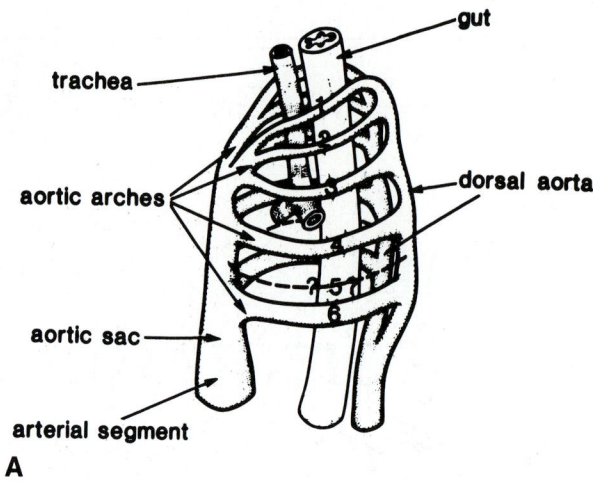

A

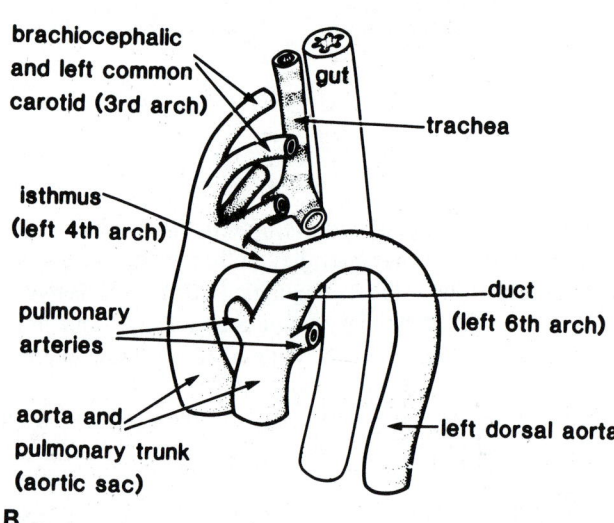

B

Figure 69–1. The steps involved in conversion of the bilaterally symmetric aortic arch system to the definitive great arteries. *(Modified from Anderson, Becker: Cardiac Anatomy—An Integrated Text and Colour Atlas, 1980. Courtesy of Gower Medical Publishing, London.)*

and PGI$_2$) cause relaxation of the ductal smooth muscle, and maintain ductal patency. As the fetus matures, the ductal smooth muscle becomes increasingly sensitive to the constrictive effect of O$_2$ (V), and thus the low PO$_2$ of the fetus is also a major factor maintaining ductal patency.[15,18,19] pH and levels of other factors also play a role.

Closure of the Ductus Arteriosus

At the time of birth, the fetus undergoes rapid circulatory and physiologic changes. Closure of the ductus arteriosus is an important component of these changes. Primarily, the right and left ventricles cease to function in parallel, and begin to function in series. The placenta is eliminated from the circulation, and, with ventilation of the lungs, the pulmonary resistance decreases rapidly and pulmonary flow increases. Venous return from the lungs fills the left atrium

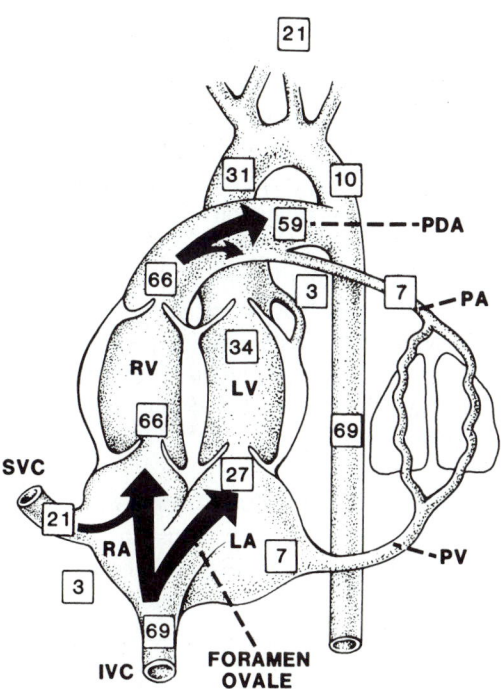

Figure 69–2. Diagram of the fetal circulation of the late gestation lamb. The numbers in squares indicate the percentage of the combined ventricular output that returns to the fetal heart and is ejected by each ventricle. *(From Rudolph: Congenital Diseases of the Heart. Chicago, Year Book, 1974.)*

and begins to close the foramen ovale. Concomitant closure of the ductus arteriosus commits the right ventricular output to the lungs, and prevents a reversal of fetal ductal flow pattern with the fall in pulmonary resistance.

Ductal closure occurs in two phases. The early "reversible" phase, which results from contraction of the smooth muscle in the wall of the ductus arteriosus, occurs in the first hours after birth. The late "irreversible" phase, which results from fibrosis of the ductus arteriosus, evolves over the next few weeks.[13,20]

Postnatal contraction of the ductal smooth muscle during the first phase of ductal closure is the consequence of events that, in essence, reverse those conditions present in fetal life that promote ductal patency. The most noted of these events include a marked increase in PO_2, and a rapid fall in prostaglandin levels.

Postnatal ventilation causes an increase in the PO_2. This increase in PO_2 is a strong direct stimulus for contraction of the ductal smooth muscle. Levels of prostaglandin decrease as a result of a number of factors including removal of the placenta, a source of circulating prostaglandin; and an increase in the blood flow to the lungs, which removes prostaglandin from the circulation. The reduction in levels of prostaglandin, which stimulate ductal smooth muscle relaxation, further promotes ductal smooth muscle contraction. Changes in pH, and the release of other vasoactive amines, also play a role in early contraction of ductal smooth muscle.

The contraction of ductal smooth muscle during the

first phase of closure shortens and narrows the circumference of the ductus. The intimal cushions protrude into the center of the ductus and plug the lumen. Smooth muscle constriction is greatest on the pulmonary side of the ductus arteriosus, and complete closure occurs first in this region of the ductus. Closure of the aortic side of the ductus follows shortly; however, incomplete closure may leave a "ductal ampulla" of the descending aorta. The early phase of ductal closure, usually completed in a matter of hours, can be reversed in the early postnatal period by intravenous infusion of prostaglandin.

Late and irreversible closure begins shortly thereafter. Hemorrhage and necrosis occurs in the medial layer, and fibrous proliferation occurs in the intimal layer.[21] As fibrous proliferation continues, the ductus arteriosus is converted to the "ligamentum" arteriosus.[22] These changes are usually completed by eight weeks of life, but on some occasions, closure may not be completed until two to three months of age.[13,20]

Persistent Patent Ductus Arteriosus

A ductus arteriosus that fails to close by the normal mechanisms before 3 months of age is considered a persistent or pathological patent ductus arteriosus. The ductus may remain widely patent leaving a nonrestrictive lumen, or it may close partially leaving a medium to small residual lumen. Rarely, an intermittently patent ductus may be observed.[23]

The incidence of a patent ductus arteriosus is estimated at 1 in 2000 in the general population,[24] but is much higher, 15%, in premature infants. The incidence of patent ductus arteriosus is twice as common in females as it is in males. Other etiologic factors include living at high altitudes, hypoxia, respiratory distress syndrome, maternal rubella, inheritance, low gestational age, and associated cardiac malformations.[25]

The histology of the persistent patent ductus arteriosus of the term infant can be differentiated from that of the normal ductus arteriosus, and it is thus considered a congenital malformation.[26] The media contains variable amounts of elastic lamina similar to the aorta, and the smooth muscle in the ductal wall is arranged in a fine helicoid spiral fashion. The intima is thick and is completely separated from media by a wavy, unfragmented internal elastic lamina. Mucoid deposits are variable and lie mostly in the media.[26]

Patent Ductus in the Premature Infant

The presences of a patent ductus arteriosus in the premature infant deserves special consideration. The incidence of patent ductus arteriosus in the premature infant is markedly increased in comparison to that of term infants, and is highest in premature infants of earlier gestational age and lower birth weights.[25] The overall incidence of a patent ductus arteriosus in the premature is 30% overall. The incidence is reported as 32% in premature infants less than 36 weeks gestational age and increases to 77% in patients of 28–30 weeks' gestational age.[27,28]

Evidence suggests the premature patent ductus arteriosus may not be histologically abnormal, but rather may simply be immature. The immature ductus is less sensitive to the constrictive effects of PO_2 and is more sensitive to the dilatory effects prostaglandin.[29] Thus it is less likely to respond to postnatal conditions that promote closure. Furthermore, many of the conditions associated with prematurity, particularly respiratory distress syndrome, and increased circulating levels of prostaglandin,[30] may give additional support to ductal patency. With pharmacologic inhibition of PGE synthesis, the premature ductus may be induced to close.[16] Often, with further maturation and resolution of other associated concerns, the premature ductus arteriosus may be capable of closing spontaneously.

Anatomic Considerations of the Patent Ductus Arteriosus

The patent ductus arteriosus usually exists as an extension of the main pulmonary artery continuing beyond the right and left branch pulmonary arteries. It curves leftward under the aortic arch often "hugging" the underside of the transverse and distal aortic arch. As it turns downward it joins the descending aorta at an acute angle a few millimeters beyond the origin of the subclavian artery. The segment of aorta between the subclavian artery and the ductal–aortic junction is termed the isthmus. The ductus arteriosus is intimately related to the recurrent laryngeal nerve. The recurrent laryngeal nerve separates from the vagus nerve lateral to the ductus, curves caudally around the underside of the ductus, and then courses medially and superiorly toward the tracheal esophageal groove.

Anatomic Variations of the Patent Ductus Arteriosus

Anatomic variations of the ductus arteriosus are usually associated with abnormalities of the aortic arch or intracardiac defects. The ductus, which is usually a unilateral left-sided structure, may be right sided, bilateral, or absent. The pulmonary end of the ductus may originate from the usual position at the pulmonary artery confluence or from either the right or left branch pulmonary arteries. The arterial end of the ductus arteries may join a right or left descending aorta, the innominate artery, the subclavian artery, or even a more distal artery. A right-sided aortic arch may be associated with a number of notable anatomic variations of the ductus arteriosus. These may include a ductus arteriosus that (1) originates from the pulmonary artery confluence and joins a mirror-image left innominate artery, (2) originates from the right pulmonary artery and joins the right descending aorta, (3) passes behind the esophagus from the pulmonary confluence to the right descending aorta, or (4) originates from the pulmonary confluence and connects to an aberrant retroesophageal left subclavian artery.[31,32] The latter abnor-

malities are considered elsewhere in a discussion of vascular rings.

Tetralogy of Fallot is frequently associated with absence of the ductus arteriosus. Tetralogy of Fallot and pulmonary atresia may be associated with a tortuous ductus arteriosus, which may originate from a varied arterial site and enter the pulmonary circulation via the branch pulmonary arteries. In some cases, it may be difficult to distinguish a "peripheral" ductus arteriosus from a major aortopulmonary collateral. When a ductus arteriosus enters a branch pulmonary artery, ductal tissue may be present in the wall of the pulmonary artery at the junction with the ductus arteriosus. This may produce a branch pulmonary artery stenosis analogous to a coarctation.

Aneurysms of the Ductus Arteriosus

Aneurysms of the ductus arteriosus are rare. They may occur as "spontaneous infantile ductal aneurysms" that present near birth,[33,34] or they may develop later in life. Infantile aneurysms usually involve the majority of the central portion of the ductus with closure of the pulmonary end and marked narrowing of the aortic end.[35] These aneurysms usually undergo spontaneous regression and resolve without therapy. On rare occasions, they may undergo progressive enlargement and require excision. The second form of ductal aneurysms usually occurs in later childhood or early adulthood. They are usually based on patency of the aortic end. They may undergo progressive enlargement and carry the potential for rupture and death.[36]

Pathophysiology

The pathophysiologic effects of an isolated patent ductus arteriosus are related to the associated left-to-right shunt, and these effects vary greatly, depending on the size of the shunt.

A patent ductus arteriosus is in essence a portal between the systemic and the pulmonary circulations. Its presence creates a shunt that diverts systemic blood flow back into the pulmonary circulation. Because the ductus creates a shunt beyond the aortic and pulmonary valves, shunt flow may occur during both systole and diastole.

The amount of blood flow diverted by this "left-to-right" shunt depends primarily on two factors, the size of the shunt, i.e., its diameter and length, and the difference between the pulmonary and systemic vascular resistances. As these two potential resistors are "in series," the controlling or "dominant resister" is the more restrictive one. Thus, if the ductus is small and/or the pulmonary resistance is high, the resulting shunt flow will be small. If the ductus is large and the pulmonary resistance low, a very large shunt can be the consequence.

At birth, pulmonary and systemic vascular resistances are usually similar, and so there is little flow across the patent ductus arteriosus regardless of its size. During the next few weeks, pulmonary resistance normally decreases, and, depending on the size of the patent ductus arteriosus, the left-to-right shunt across the patent ductus arteriosus tends to increase. As the difference between the pulmonary and systemic resistances increases, the size of the patent ductus arteriosus becomes the primary determinant of flow through the shunt.

Small Shunt

If the patent ductus arteriosus is small, the associated right-to-left shunt is severely restricted. With the postnatal fall in pulmonary resistance, a large pressure gradient develops between the aorta and the pulmonary artery. Flow across the small patent ductus arteriosus is limited to a low-volume, high-velocity jet. Hemodynamic effects of such a small shunt are minimal. However, turbulence caused by this high-velocity jet may compromise the integrity of the adjacent vascular endothelium and thus make the patient susceptible to endocarditis.

Large Shunt

A different scenario is associated with a large "nonrestrictive" ductus arteriosus. The large ductus presents minimal resistance to shunt flow. As a result, the pressure in the pulmonary arteries is equal to the pressure in the aorta, and the pulmonary blood flow increases according to the difference between the pulmonary vascular and systemic vascular resistances. Thus, as the pulmonary vascular resistance falls in the neonatal period, the left-to-right shunt across the ductus increases dramatically. This excessive shunt flow imposes a severe left ventricular volume overload with elevated left atrial pressures, limited systemic blood flow, and congestive heart failure. The combination of excessive pulmonary blood flow and elevated left atrial pressures leads to increased right-sided pressures, and pulmonary interstitial edema with compromised alveolar gas exchange.

A large ductus allows not only systolic but also a high degree of diastolic shunting. With a large diastolic shunt, blood flow in the descending aorta may reverse direction, and flow retrograde in late diastole. This results in a decrease in diastolic pressure and a dramatically widened systemic pulse pressure. This "diastolic runoff," in combination with the overall limited systemic flow, may impair organ perfusion and lead to compromised coronary circulation, renal dysfunction, and necrotizing enterocolitis.

Moderate Ductus

A moderately large ductus arteriosus allows enough shunting to cause hemodynamic changes, but restricts shunt flow sufficiently to allow pulmonary pressures to fall well below systemic levels. Hemodynamic sequelae include a moderate left ventricular volume overload, and a slight widening of the arterial pulse pressure. Systemic perfusion, while decreased, is usually adequate, and organ injury from hypoperfusion does not usually occur. Left ventricular volume overload and congestive heart failure can usually be overcome by left ventricular hypertrophy and other compen-

satory mechanisms. Pulmonary blood flow increases usually between two and three times normal, but pulmonary and other right-sided pressures fall to normal or near-normal levels. Pulmonary congestion occurs but rarely to the point of compromising alveolar gas exchange.

Persistent Fetal Circulation

In some circumstances, the neonatal pulmonary vascular resistance may actually remain at fetal levels and exceed that of the systemic circulation. In this condition, termed *persistent fetal circulation,* blood flow across a patent ductus arteriosus will occur in a right-to-left direction and cause systemic desaturation and hypoxia.

Clinical Presentation and Diagnosis

The signs, symptoms, and clinical presentation of a patient with an isolated patent ductus arteriosus are based on the pathophysiologic changes noted above. A small ductus has minimal hemodynamic or other effects, and thus a patient with a small ductus arteriosus may remain asymptomatic and undiscovered for many years. A patient with a small ductus usually presents with an incidental murmur noted on routine physical examination. A small ductus arteriosus may also be discovered during workup for subacute bacterial endocarditis.

Patients with a less restrictive ductus arteriosus and a moderate shunt usually present early in life with symptoms of congestive heart failure, respiratory difficulties, and/or pulmonary infection. Typical presenting symptoms include tachypnea, tachycardia, fevers, sweating, cough, irritability, poor feeding, poor weight gain, failure to thrive, etc.[37]

Symptoms and presentation may vary considerably during the course of development. In the early postnatal period, when the pulmonary resistance is still elevated, symptoms are often minimal, and the ductus arteriosus may not be apparent. Symptoms become most apparent during the ensuing few weeks as pulmonary resistance decreases and shunt flow increases. Symptoms, however, may again become less apparent as compensatory cardiac hypertrophy and other adaptive mechanisms bring about hemodynamic improvement.

In some instances, pulmonary resistance may not undergo the usual rapid fall in early life, but, instead it may remain elevated and significantly limit flow through the shunt. Under these circumstances, symptoms may be less pronounced and a significant patent ductus arteriosus may not be noticed.

Patients with elevated pulmonary resistance and/or compensated congestive heart failure may achieve a chronic "stabilized" state with minimal symptoms. These patients may present much later in life, usually the third or fourth decade of life, with a dilated cardiomyopathy and chronic heart failure, or Eisenmenger's syndrome.

Presenting symptoms in children with a large, nonrestrictive ductus arteriosus tend to be more dramatic, and, with the postnatal fall in pulmonary resistance, they tend to progress more rapidly. As the volume of the left-to-right shunt exceeds compensatory limits, patients may present with profound left ventricular failure, low cardiac output syndrome, pulmonary edema, and respiratory failure. Poor peripheral perfusion and associated multiorgan system compromise may accompany the large left-to-right shunt, and patients may present with renal failure, hepatic dysfunction, necrotizing enterocolitis, and/or seizures.

Excessive pulmonary blood flow may result in pulmonary infection, and patients with a large shunt may present with life-threatening pneumonia.[37] On occasion, patients with a nonrestrictive patent ductus arteriosus may achieve a compensated cardiac status and present later in childhood with pulmonary vascular disease and cyanosis.

Physical Findings

Physical findings are related to left ventricular volume overload and increased pulmonary blood flow. Typical findings include a hyperactive precordium with an in-

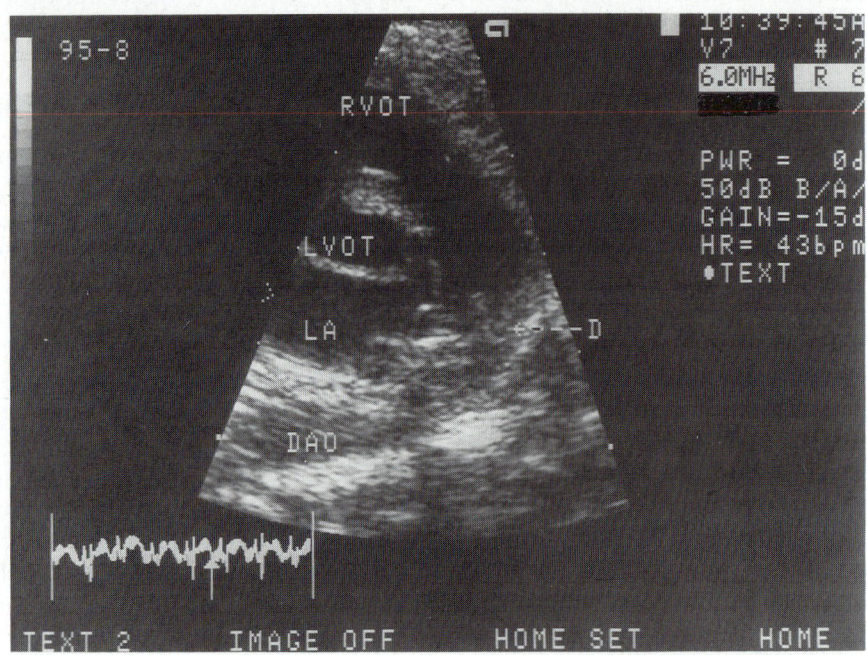

A

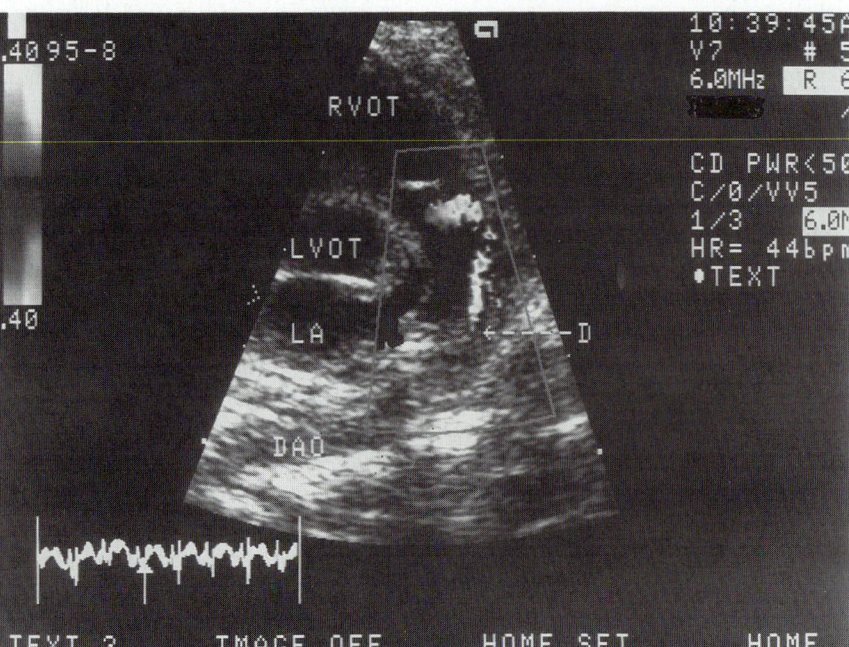

B

Figure 69–3. Echocardiograms of a small patent ductus arteriosus. A standard two-dimensional study is shown in **A,** and the typical wide systolic jet is shown by color flow Doppler in **B.** *(Continued.)*

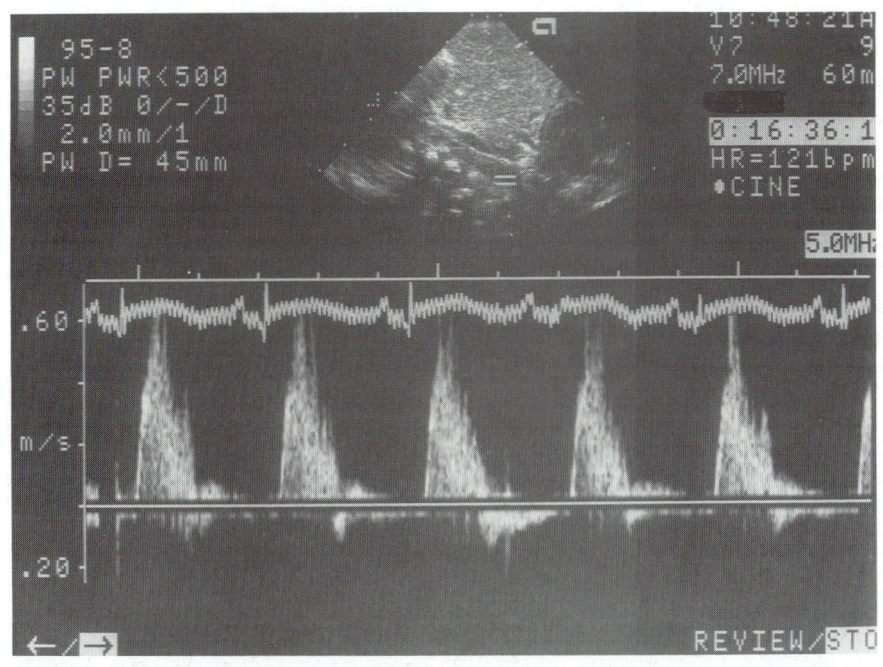

C

Figure 69–3. *(Continued.)* **C.** Pulsed Doppler showing antegrade systolic flow and retrograde diastolic flow (diastolic flow reversible). PDA, patent ductus arteriosus; Ao, aorta; RPA, right pulmonary artery; LPA, left pulmonary artery.

creased left ventricular impulse,[38] and a thrill palpable in the upper left sternal border. The peripheral pulses are bounding, sometimes "jerky," with a widened pulse pressure. Hepatomegaly and jugular venous distension may also present.

Auscultation usually reveals a systolic murmur that varies with the size of the shunt. The typical "machinery murmur" of a patent ductus arteriosus is a continuous murmur with systolic accentuation (crescendo) that trails off into diastole (decrescendo). The murmur of a very restrictive shunt may have a higher pitch and less of a diastolic component. The murmur of a large nonrestrictive ductus may be diminished or even absent. The second heart sound may be increased with little or no split and a third and a fourth heart sound may be appreciated.[39,40] Rales, rhonchi, and wheezing may be noted in all lung fields, and are usually most prominent at the bases.

Laboratory Tests

Electrocardiography
ECG findings usually show some degree of left ventricular hypertrophy. With larger shunts, left atrial hypertrophy may be indicated by a widened or biphasic P wave. Ventricular hypertrophy associated with pulmonary hypertension may be evidenced by increased right-sided forces across the precordial leads.

Roentgenography
Chest x-ray findings associated with a patent ductus arteriosus include varying degrees of cardiac enlargement and increased pulmonary vascular markings. With a small shunt, the chest x-ray may appear normal. With large shunts, left

atrial and left ventricular enlargement may become prominent, and pulmonary artery enlargement, increased vascular markings, and interstitial edema may be pronounced.

Echocardiography
Echocardiography is the diagnostic method of choice for evaluating the patient with a patent ductus arteriosus. Two-dimensional echocardiography and color Doppler can accurately define the anatomy of the patent ductus arteriosus and characterize the associated shunt flow (Figs. 69–3 and 69–4). Left atrial enlargement, ventricular function, and ventricular hypertrophy may be determined. The presence or absence of associated cardiac malformations may also be assessed. Pulsed-wave Doppler reveals additional important information. Examination of the shunt flow through the patent ductus arteriosus will reveal the pressure gradient between the aorta and pulmonary arteries, and the presence and degree of retrograde diastolic flow in the descending aorta may be used to estimate the size or volume of the shunt. Doppler evaluation of the velocity of tricuspid regurgitation will often determine further the level of increase in right ventricular and pulmonary artery pressures.[41,42]

Cardiac Catheterization
Cardiac catheterization provides the most accurate physiologic and anatomic evaluation of the patent ductus arteriosus. However, because most patients can be adequately evaluated by noninvasive methods, the role of cardiac catheterization in the present day is reserved primarily for the evaluation of patients suspected of having elevated pulmonary resistance (Eisenmenger's syndrome).

Pulmonary pressures and the gradient across the patent

ductus arteriosus can be directly measured. The extent of the left-to-right shunt can be defined at catheterization by the measured "step up" in pulmonary artery saturations, and the pulmonary resistance can be determined. Studies may also be undertaken to determine the response of the pulmonary vasculature to pharmacologic pulmonary vasodilator.

If pulmonary vascular resistance approaches systemic vascular resistance, flow across the ductus may be minimal and the patent ductus arteriosus may not be well described by techniques such as color flow echocardiography. In these circumstances passage of the catheter through the patent ductus arteriosus and/or the injection of radio-opaque dye adjacent to it can confirm its presence and define its anatomy.[43]

Magnetic Resonance Imaging

Magnetic resonance imaging, with phase contrast cine magnetic resonance (MR) and velocity-encoded magnetic resonance techniques, is becoming a more important diagnostic modality in the assessment of the patent ductus arteriosus. This is particularly important in the larger patients in whom echocardiographic studies may be more difficult. Sequential imaging in axial, coronal, and sagittal planes will accurately demonstrate the anatomy of the ductus arterio-

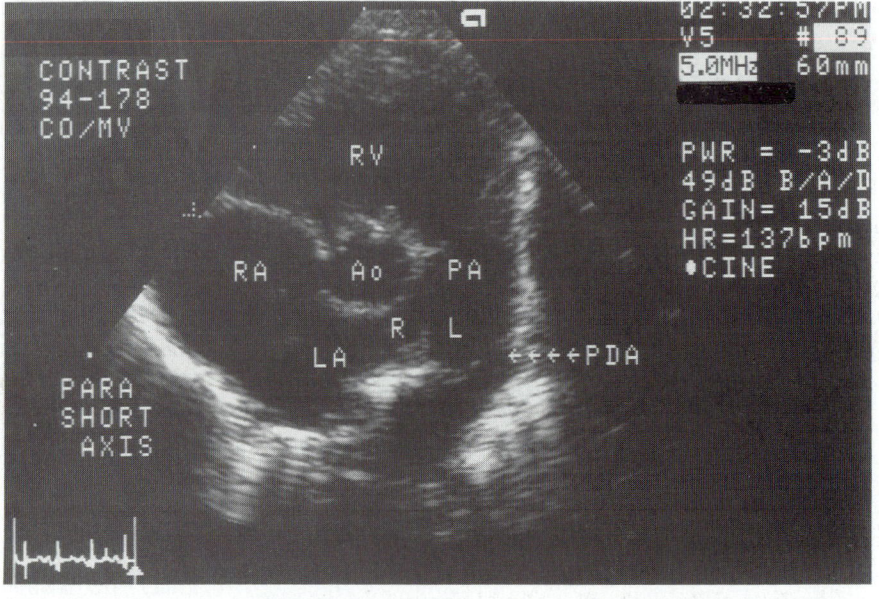

A

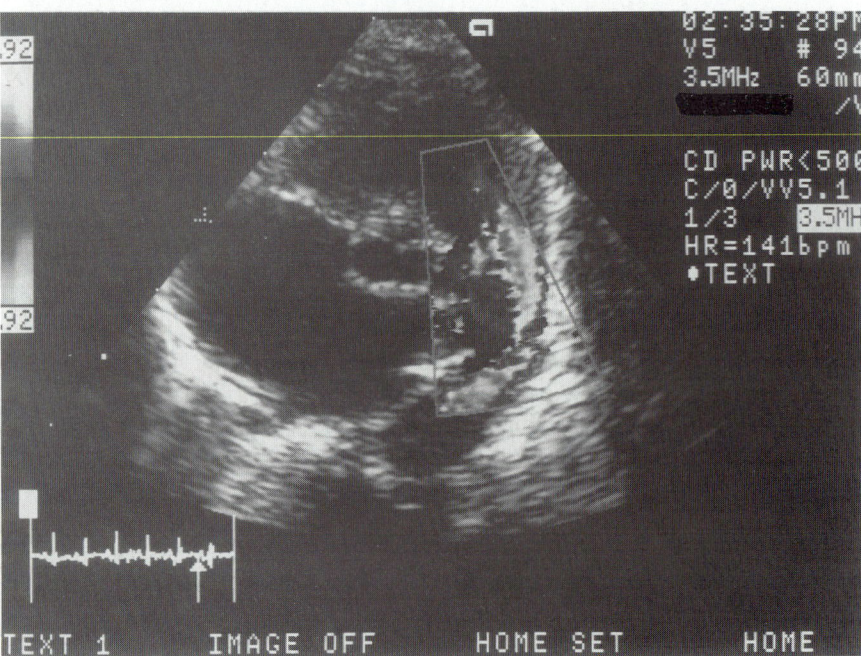

Figure 69–4. Echocardiograms of a large patent ductus arteriosus. A standard two-dimensional study is shown in **A**, and the narrow systolic jet is shown by color flow Doppler study in **B**. *(Continued.)*

B

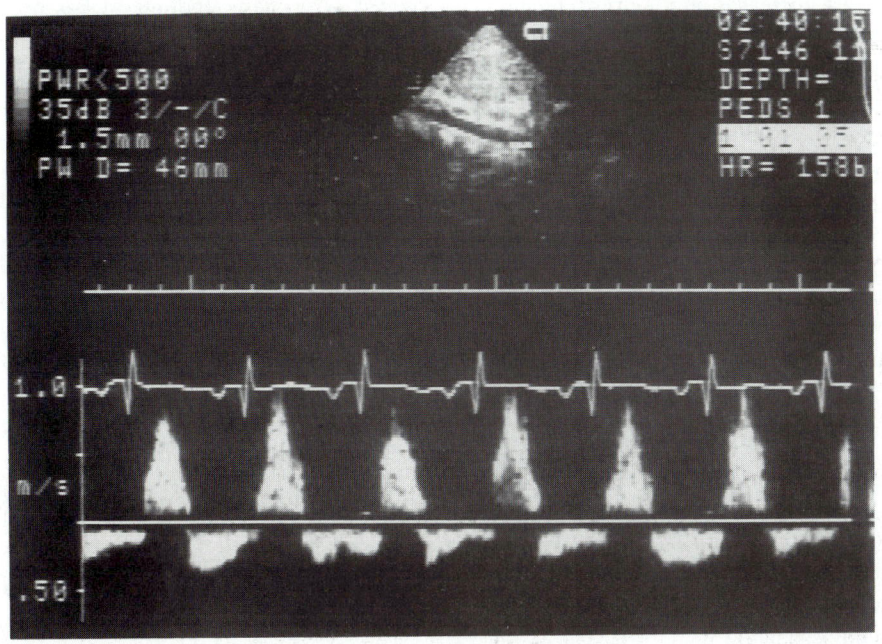

C

Figure 69–4. *(Continued.)* **C.** Pulsed showing antegrade systolic flow with a characteristically increased flow (high gradient) with little or no retrograde diastolic flow (reversible). PDA, patent ductus arteriosus; Ao, aorta; RA, right pulmonary artery; LA, left pulmonary artery.

sus. Flow techniques using phase contrast cine MR can be utilized to demonstrate and characterize the flow through the ductus, and velocity-encoded MR can be utilized to determine the pressure gradient across the patent ductus arteriosus.[44]

Natural History

The natural history depends largely on the size of the patent ductus arteriosus and the gestational age of the patient.

Spontaneous Closure

Spontaneous closure of a patent ductus arteriosus has been reported as occurring in 0.6% of term infants per year.[45] However, this estimate was based on clinical findings only and confirmed spontaneous closure of the ductus arteriosus is rare. Conversely, spontaneous closure of a ductus arteriosus in a premature infant is relatively common.

Subacute Bacterial Endocarditis

Subacute bacterial endocarditis (SBE) occurs primarily in children with a small ductus arteriosus. In the preantibiotic era, SBE was responsible for nearly one-half of the deaths due to patent ductus arteriosus.[46] Since the introduction of antibiotics, death due to SBE as a complication of a patent ductus arteriosus is rare. However, reinfection remains a concern.

Respiratory Infection

Repeated respiratory infections are common in infants with a patent ductus arteriosus. Death due to pneumonia may occur as a complication of a large shunt, but is uncommon in association with a restrictive ductus arteriosus.

Pulmonary Vascular Disease

The increased pulmonary blood flow associated with a patent ductus arteriosus causes pulmonary endothelial injury. This in turn leads to heightened pulmonary reactivity and an increase in pulmonary vascular resistance. Progression of these changes leads to irreversible pulmonary vascular disease and Eisenmenger's syndrome.

Pulmonary vascular changes occur rapidly in infants with a large patent ductus arteriosus. Increased pulmonary vascular resistance may develop in the first months of life and progress rapidly thereafter. Irreversible pulmonary vascular disease and Eisenmenger's syndrome may develop as early as 12 months of life.[25] Pulmonary vascular disease in patients with a moderate ductus arteriosus appears much later in life presenting, if at all, in the second to fourth decades of life. Pulmonary vascular disease does not occur with a small ductus arteriosus.

Congestive Heart Failure

Congestive heart failure may present early in infants with a large ductus arteriosus, and is usually poorly tolerated. Necrotizing enterocolitis, renal failure, pulmonary edema, as well as other organ system failure are associated with congestive heart failure in infants and children with a patent ductus arteriosus. It is estimated that congestive heart failure leads to death in 30% of children with an untreated patent ductus arteriosus.[25,45,46]

If compensatory mechanisms are sufficient, an infant with a large patent ductus arteriosus may survive beyond infancy and into childhood. If this occurs, the increased pulmonary vascular resistance that develops causes a decrease in shunt flow. The decrease in shunt flow reduces the volume load on the ventricle and may actually stabilize the patient's hemodynamics temporarily. However, increases in pulmonary vascular resistance to systemic levels in association with Eisenmenger's syndrome will eventually lead to right ventricular failure.[25]

Congestive heart failure in infants with a moderate-sized ductus is less severe, and is less likely to cause complications in infancy and childhood. Myocardial hypertrophy, along with other adaptive mechanisms, usually allows compensation for the moderate volume overload and allows hemodynamic stabilization. Death from heart failure in patients with a moderate-sized patent ductus arteriosus and chronic volume overload occurs most often in the third or fourth decade of life.

Treatment

Initial Therapy

Initial treatment of the patient with a patent ductus arteriosus is usually focused on the presenting symptoms. Medical management of congestive heart failure and associated increase pulmonary blood flow is based on the use of inotropic agents and diuretics. Patients with mild-to-moderate symptoms of congestive heart failure can usually be stabilized with the use of digoxin and diuretics. If the infant's symptoms are controlled with conservative medical therapy, it may be continued until 2–3 months of age to allow the ductus all opportunities to close.

Patients with more pronounced heart failure and pulmonary edema may require more aggressive support and stabilization in preparation for eminent closure of the ductus. Administration of intravenous inotropic agents such as dopamine may be necessary to improve cardiac failure, and positive pressure ventilatory support may be required for management of severe pulmonary edema and respiratory failure. Aggressive intravenous administration of diuretics may be of considerable benefit. In the presence of heart failure, oxygen administration is minimized as its pulmonary vasodilatory effects may lead to worsened cardiac failure and pulmonary edema.

Patients who present with endocarditis should receive a combination of antibiotic agents that cover a broad spectrum of bacteria. The antibiotic agents should be adjusted based on culture results, and a long-term, 4–6-week course of antibiotic therapy should be completed. Patients with associated pulmonary infections require antibiotics and supportive pulmonary care. Appropriate management of congestive heart failure may help in the treatment of pulmonary infections; however, pulmonary infections may be hard to eradicate in the presence of a large left-to-right shunt.

Pharmacologic Inducement of Ductal Closure in the Premature Infant

As noted above, patency of the ductus arteriosus in the premature infant has been related to a number of factors, most importantly the increased sensitivity of the immature ductus to prostaglandin and to the higher levels of circulating prostaglandin. In concert with these findings, it has been shown that the immature ductus arteriosus can be induced to close by pharmacological inhibition of prostaglandin synthesis.[47] Indomethacin is used in the clinical setting to induce closure of the premature infant patent ductus arteriosus. It is administered at a dose of 0.1–0.2 mg/kg body weight intravenously every 8 hours for three doses,[48] and may be repeated one or two more times.

Indomethacin is associated with renal, hepatic, and platelet dysfunction. Thus its use is contraindicated in the presence of renal dysfunction, hyperbilirubinemia, and bleeding disorders. In addition, the presence of severe congestive heart failure, poor tissue perfusion, sepsis, or compromise of other organ systems constitutes a strong relative contraindication to indomethacin therapy.

Interventional Management of a Ductus Arteriosus

Most term and many preterm patients with a patent ductus arteriosus require interventional methods for closure of their patent ductus arteriosus. Surgical therapy is the most definitive and proven therapy for a patent ductus arteriosus. It is, however, a major surgical procedure usually carried out through a posterior lateral thoracotomy or midline sternotomy. The procedure requires the use of general anesthesia, and there is a necessary convalescent recovery. Recently, an alternative surgical approach using thoracoscopic techniques has been described.[49] Experience with this technique is limited, and its role in clinical practice is being evaluated further. Interventional catheter techniques for ductal closure should also be given consideration. These techniques involving transarterial catheter closure with coils or other devices are being utilized clinically with greater frequency, and should be discussed as an alternative to the traditional surgical approach.

Indications for Surgery

The presence of a patent ductus arteriosus is in itself an indication for intervention and closure.[43,50,51] A small patent ductus arteriosus should be closed to prevent endocarditis. A moderate patent ductus arteriosus should be closed to control symptoms of congestive heart failure and to prevent the immediate and long-term cardiac and pulmonary complications discussed above.[52] A large patent ductus arteriosus, associated with a large left-to-right shunt, must be closed in response to immediately life-threatening cardiopulmonary failure and associated complications. Thus, upon recognition of a patent ductus arteriosus, the primary concerns are the timing and method of closure.

The term infant with a small or medically controlled shunt can be followed initially to allow for spontaneous closure. Indomethacin therapy is usually ineffective in the term infant, and if spontaneous closure has not occurred in 3 months time, surgical closure should be scheduled for the next convenient opportunity. When symptoms are present, but responsive to medical management, the patient's condition should be optimized medically, and surgery should be planned soon thereafter. However, should symptoms increase despite appropriate medical therapy, the patient's overall condition may deteriorate with increased associated risks, and closure should be accomplished in a more timely fashion.

If congestive heart failure is severe, accompanied by poor perfusion, pulmonary edema, respiratory compromise, and/or other organ dysfunction, the patient's life may be in imminent danger, and closure of the ductus arteriosus is a true surgical emergency. Under these circumstances, maximal supportive measures should be instituted immediately, and surgical closure undertaken as soon as possible.

Premature Infant

The indications for surgical intervention in the premature infant with a patent ductus arteriosus deserve special consideration because of the increased likelihood of spontaneous closure, and because of the possibility of pharmacological inducement of ductal closure. If the patent ductus arteriosus in a premature infant is small and asymptomatic, the infant may be followed in anticipation of spontaneous closure. If the ductus is larger, but the symptoms manageable, indomethacin may be used to induce closure.

Surgical therapy is indicated when symptoms are more threatening. If the severity of symptoms begin to increase, or heart failure is severe and life threatening, just as with the term infant, maximal supportive therapy and immediate surgical closure are indicated. Surgical therapy may also be required in the premature infant with moderate symptoms of congestive heart failure who has failed indomethacin therapy or presents with contraindications to the use of indomethacin.[52]

Operative Technique

In the vast majority of patients with an isolated patent ductus arteriosus, surgical closure is carried out through a left thoracotomy. Numerous techniques have been used for closure of a patent ductus arteriosus through this approach, and these can be considered in two general categories: ligation[53] and division.[54]

Techniques of ligation without division rely on circumferential ligatures tied around the ductus to completely obliterate the lumen of the patent ductus arteriosus. Techniques of division rely on closure and separation of the transected ends of the ductus to achieve the same. Either technique can be used successfully in most cases, and each one has some particular advantages in specific situations (which are discussed below). On rare occasions, it may be necessary to approach the patent ductus arteriosus through a midline sternotomy and using cardiopulmonary bypass, perform a direct closure of the patent ductus arteriosus through the opened pulmonary artery.[55–57]

General Considerations

In preparation for the procedure, the patient undergoing surgical closure of a patent ductus arteriosus is placed under general endotracheal anesthesia. Epidural administration of narcotics may be used in conjunction with the general anesthetic and may be used for pain control in the early postoperative period as well.

If the patient's condition is poor, arterial and central venous access may be needed for monitoring, blood sampling, and drug and fluid administration. In most cases, however, simple peripheral venous access and standard electrocardiogram (ECG) and blood pressure cuff monitoring are usually adequate.

The patient is positioned in the standard right side down, lateral thoracotomy position with the left arm raised above the head. The left chest is prepped and draped from the sternum anteriorly to the spine posteriorly, and from the base of the neck and shoulder superiorly to the lower rib cage inferiorly. The area of the groin vessels may be prepped and draped in older patients in whom aortic cross-clamping may be necessary in controlling and closing the patent ductus arteriosus.

Incision

The patient's chest is opened through a standard posterior lateral thoracotomy incision. For best exposure, the latissimus dorsi muscle is divided, and the posterior portion of the serratus anterior muscle may be divided as well. Complete division of the latissimus dorsi muscle may not be required in younger patients. In selected cases, skin flaps can be raised, and the serratus and latissimus muscles can be mobilized and retracted without being divided.

The pleural space may be entered through the third or fourth intercostal space. Some prefer entering the chest through the third interspace detaching the intercostal muscles from the superior aspect of the fourth rib. Although the anterior to posterior length of the third interspace is smaller, in most patients it opens directly over the ductus, and thus allows better exposure and access to the superior border of the ductus. If more room is needed interiorly, the fourth rib may be divided posteriorly or removed altogether.

Exposure

Once the pleural space is entered, the lungs are retracted anteriorly and medially. Prior to embarking on the dissection of the patent ductus arteriosus it is important to identify certain related structures such as the phrenic nerve, vagus nerve, left pulmonary artery, left subclavian artery, and distal aortic arch.

To expose the patent ductus arteriosus, a vertical incision is made in the parietal pleura over the descending aorta adjacent to the distal end of the patent ductus arteriosus. This incision is extended superiorly toward the base of the subclavian artery. At this point, the superior intercostal vein usually must be ligated and divided.

The edge of the pleura is dissected anteriorly and medially exposing the anterior medial aspect of the aorta and the distal aortic end of the ductus arteriosus. The vagus nerve and the origin of the recurrent laryngeal nerve lie just under the medial edge of the incised pleura (Fig. 69–5). They must be visualized and carefully pushed away from

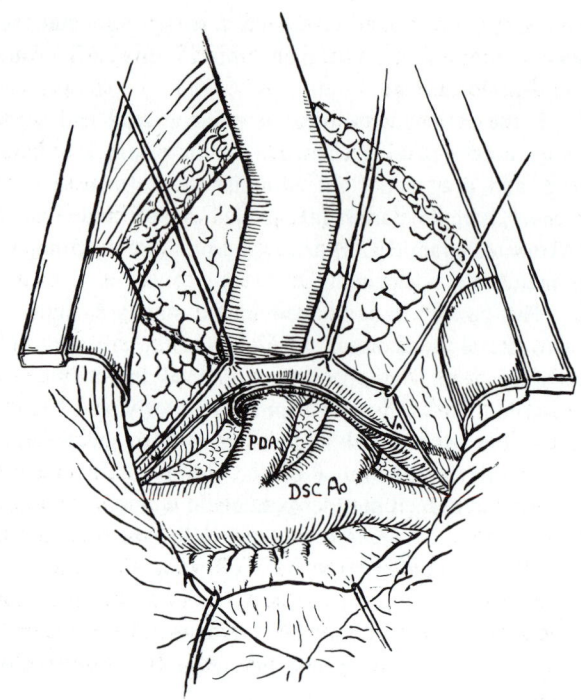

Figure 69–5. Anatomy of the patent ductus arteriosus (PDA) and related descending aorta (DSC Ao), pulmonary artery, vagus nerve (VA), and recurrent laryngeal nerve as they are viewed from the left thoracotomy.

the anterolateral and inferior aspects of the patent arteriosus. In patients with a short ductus these structures may require further mobilization to allow complete exposure of the pulmonary side of the patent ductus arteriosus. In most cases there is a reflection of the pericardial sac that extends onto the patent ductus arteriosus. This pericardial reflection must also be mobilized to achieve complete exposure of the entire length of the ductus.

In difficult situations, alternative access and exposure of the pulmonary side of the ductus arteriosus can be obtained by opening the pericardium anterior to the phrenic nerve and dissecting out the patent ductus arteriosus at its junction with the pulmonary artery confluence from inside the pericardial sac. Additional access to and control of the aortic side of the ductus arteriosus can be achieved by circumferentially mobilizing the aorta above and below the junction with the distal end of the patent ductus arteriosus, retracting the aorta anteriorly, and mobilizing the underside of the distal end of the patent ductus arteriosus from behind.

Closure of the Ductus

Preterm Infants. Closure of the patent ductus arteriosus in the premature infant can usually be accomplished with metal clips or a single ligature.[53,55] For these purposes, the patent ductus arteriosus need only be dissected free at the aortic or distal end, and the vagus and recurrent nerves retracted medially. Further dissection of the fragile tissues of the premature infant is unnecessary and may be associated with increased complications.

Another preference is to use two metal hemoclips to achieve a secure closure of the patent ductus arteriosus in the premature infant. After completion of the dissection, the first clip is placed gently on the patent ductus arteriosus at its junction with the aorta. With the pressure in the ductus reduced, a second clip is applied more securely to the patent ductus arteriosus a millimeter anterior and medially to the first clip.

Term Infants and Older Patients. As noted above, the patent ductus arteriosus exposed through a left thoracotomy may be closed either by ligation or by division.

Ligation

Double ligation of the patent ductus arteriosus at the aortic and pulmonary ends has been widely used. With this technique, the patent ductus arteriosus is dissected free on both the aortic and the pulmonary ends mobilizing and retracting the vagus and recurrent laryngeal nerves as needed. In most situations, the nerves need to be mobilized and retracted only slightly, and the pulmonary end does not need to be exposed extensively or all the way to the confluence of the pulmonary arteries. Using a right angle, ties are passed around the proximal and distal ends of the ductus arteriosus. The tie on the aortic side is tied down first and the knot is tightened carefully to avoid cutting into the sometimes fragile ductal tissue. Following this, the ligature on the pulmonary side is tied down under less pressure. Purse-string sutures may be used in place of simple ligatures. The purse-string sutures are placed circumferentially in the wall of the patent ductus arteriosus at both the aortic and pulmonary ends, and they are tied down in a similar fashion. This method is preferred as the purse-sting sutures do not tend to slide toward the same central point of the ductus as the un-fixed simple "tie" ligatures are prone to do.

The simple ligation technique has many added variations. The ligatures may be tied over felt pledgets, and additional ties or metal clips may be placed on the mid portion of the ductus, between the two initially placed ties, for additional security. A simple well established method is that of adding a third transfixing suture ligature in the midportion of the ductus (Fig. 69–6).[53] With this approach, purse-string sutures are placed into the pulmonary and aortic ends of the patent ductus arteriosus and tied down. A third suture is then placed in the middle of the ductus. It is first passed around the ductus arteriosus, after which it is placed through the center of the lumen of the patent ductus arteriosus, and then it is tied down.

Division

Techniques involving division of the patent ductus arteriosus are based on control of the aortic and pulmonary ends of the ductus, complete transection of the patent ductus arteriosus, and then closure of the two ends of the patent ductus arteriosus. The simplest technique is an extension of the technique of simple ligation. The ductus is dissected out for

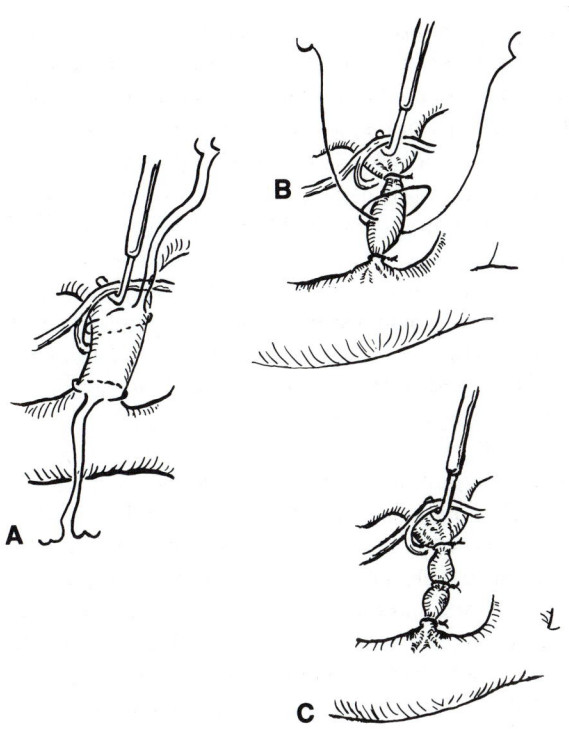

Figure 69–6. Classic method of ligation of the patent ductus arteriosus (PDA). Purse-string ligatures are placed around the PDA on both the pulmonary side and the aortic side (**A**). After the purse-string ligatures are tied, a third suture is placed around and then through the lumen of the central portion of the PDA (**B**), and then it is tied down (**C**).

the majority of its length. The aortic end is ligated with a purse-string suture placed in the aortic wall around the adjoining orifice of the patent ductus arteriosus. Alternatively, the aortic end may be closed with a plegetted mattress suture placed in the aortic wall and across the orifice of the patent ductus arteriosus. The pulmonary side of the ductus is ligated near the junction of the patent ductus arteriosus and the confluence of the pulmonary arteries. The ductus is then transected centrally and the ends closed with additional suture ligatures.

The more classic technique is the "clamp and divide" technique advocated by Gross.[57] For this approach, the ductus is mobilized for its entire length. We also advocate complete circumferential mobilization of the aorta around the area where it joins with the patent ductus arteriosus. The pulmonary side of the patent ductus arteriosus is mobilized as closely as possible to the pulmonary confluence. The pericardial lappet overlying the pulmonary side of the patent ductus arteriosus is dissected away, and if further exposure of the pulmonary side is needed, the vagus and recurrent nerves may be mobilized away from their medial attachments and retracted laterally. In some cases it may be necessary to open the pericardial sac and mobilize the pulmonary arteries and the junction with the proximal portion of the patent ductus arteriosus from inside the pericardium. If the tissue of the ductal wall appears adequate, vascular

clamps may be applied directly across the aortic and pulmonary ends of the patent ductus arteriosus. The ductus may then be transected between the clamps. The open ends of the transected patent ductus arteriosus are overseen, the clamps are removed, and the edges are inspected for hemostasis. If the tissue of the patent ductus arteriosus is too fragile, it may be necessary to place the vascular clamps directly onto the aorta (and/or rarely the pulmonary artery) including the junction with the patent ductus arteriosus. A "side biting" clamp is applied longitudinally to the aorta across the junction with the patent ductus arteriosus (Fig. 69–7A). If this cannot be accomplished, the aorta can be clamped transversely above and below its junction with patent ductus arteriosus completely excluding this region (Fig. 69–7B). Once the two ends of the patent ductus arteriosus are controlled with clamps, the patent ductus arteriosus is transected. The pulmonary side is overseen and the pulmonary clamp is removed. Following this, the aortic side is closed by oversewing the healthier tissue of the aorta at the base of the patent ductus arteriosus. The aortic end is usually closed primarily but may also be closed with a patch.

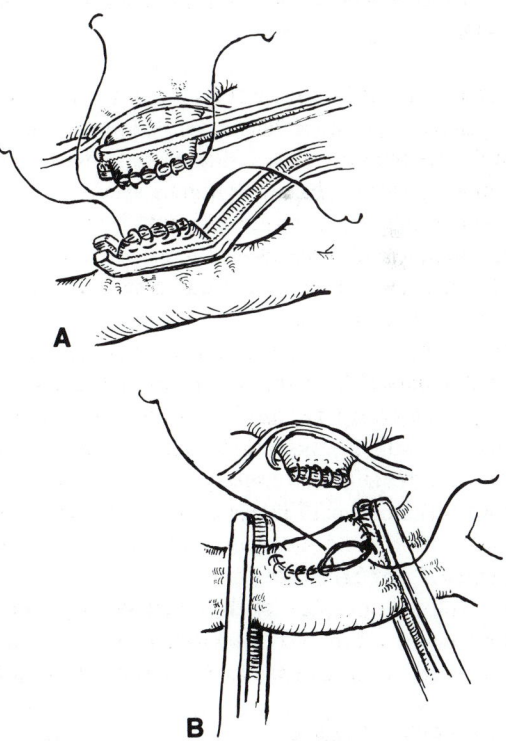

Figure 69–7. A. Classic clamp and divide methods of closure of the patent ductus arteriosus. The ductus clamped on both ends and divided with suture closure of both ends is depicted. The clamp on the aortic end is shown placed on the aorta at the base of the patent ductus arteriosus, as this may be safer than clamping the ductus itself. **B.** Cross-clamping of the aorta may be all that is required when the ductus is particularly brittle. The pulmonary end has been clamped and oversewn, and the aortic end has been excised and the healthier aortic wall is being closed with a patch.

Completion of the Left Thoracotomy

After closure of the ductus arteriosus, the bed of the dissection is inspected for bleeding and leakage of lymphatic fluid. It found, these are controlled surgically. Following the edges of the pleura overlying the aorta and ductus are closed with a fine running suture. A single straight chest tube is usually introduced into the pleural space through a separate site in the chest wall well below the incision. The intercostal space is closed by sequential figure-of-eight large dexon sutures. The transected muscles are closed individually in layers, and facial and skin layers are closed with fine absorbable sutures.

Open Method of Patent
Ductus Arteriosus Closure

This rarely used technique is reserved for special conditions. The patient is approached usually via a midline sternotomy. The aorta and pulmonary artery are separated and the left pulmonary artery and ductus arteriosus are dissected away from pericardial and mediastinal attachments. The patient's ascending aorta is cannulated in a standard fashion for arterial perfusion and the superior and inferior vena cava are cannulated individually for venous drainage. The patient is placed on cardiopulmonary bypass and the orifice of the patent ductus arteriosus is closed by digital pressure placed on the pulmonary artery wall over the ductus and left pulmonary artery. After the patient is cooled to 20–22°C, the bypass flow is decreased to 25–35% of normal. The patient is placed in slight trendelenburg position and the pulmonary artery is opened over the ductus arteriosus. External compression and low flow are used to control flow through the patent ductus arteriosus and allow visualization of the orifice in the wall of the pulmonary artery. The orifice of the patent ductus arteriosus is then closed either primarily or, as we prefer, with a cloth patch. The pulmonary artery is closed as the patent is warmed, and then bypass is weaned. Heparin is reversed with protamine, the cannulation sites are tied and reinforced, and chest tubes are place anteriorly and interiorly into the pericardial space. The sternum is closed with wires and the prepectoral fascia and skin are closed with running absorbable sutures.

Selection of Technique

The selection of a method for closure deserves consideration. Techniques of ligation without division are usually quicker and easier to complete. Generally, less dissection, mobilization, and retraction are required, and there is no concern for bleeding from the open ends of the transected ductus as there is when the patent ductus is divided. For these reasons, the technique of ligation without division is often preferred. However, there is some concern and controversy as to whether ligation without division carries increased risks of a residual patent ductus arteriosus and recanalization.[58] There certainly are conditions in which simple ligation of the ductus arteriosus is less applicable.

Ligation closes the patent ductus arteriosus by dimin-

ishing the circumference and crumpling the wall into may irregular folds that obliterate the lumen. Inherently, this technique causes significant distortion of the patent ductus arteriosus and its surrounding structures, and, in fact, often increases the local tissue stresses. Thus injury and disruption of the wall of the patent ductus arteriosus during ligation under pressure are issues of concern. With the associated pressures, stresses, and brittle nature of the wall of the patent ductus arteriosus, there is a tendency for a ligature to tear and/or cut into the patent ductus arteriosus wall as it is tied down. This can sometimes result in troublesome bleeding, or create the potential for late recanalization or pseudoaneurysm formation. The infolding of the ductal wall during ligation may also result in the creation of small tunnels within these mural folds. These small tunnels may persist resulting in a residual small patent ductus arteriosus. Consequently, characteristics of the patent ductus arteriosus of an infant or young child such as a smaller diameter, a longer length, and acceptable pliability greatly facilitate this method of closure. Conversely, characteristic of the ductus arteriosus of the older patient such as a brittle calcified ductal wall, an inflamed fragile ductal wall, and a large diameter-to-length ratio make simple ligation more difficult.

Techniques of division require more time and effort. Greater exposure and control are usually needed, and thus more dissection, mobilization, and retraction are necessary. Visualization and separation of the transected ends of the ductus, however, may provide greater assurance of complete closure, and this technique has been advocated as having a lower incidence of residual patency and recanalization.[57,58] The "clamp and divide" technique is often more suitable in patients having a patent ductus arteriosus with characteristics less suitable for the simple ligation technique. Greater control is achieved by increased mobilization and exposure, and with the use of vascular clamps, and this may be a great asset in difficult situations involving a short, inflamed, and/or brittle calcified patent ductus arteriosus.

The open technique is used only rarely, usually in patients of the fifth or sixth decade in whom the patent ductus is short, heavily calcified, and brittle, and in whom degenerative vascular disease makes clamping the aorta and pulmonary arteries through the left chest difficult.

Under present conditions, either approach, if done satisfactorily and under appropriate conditions, can be carried out with low risk and good long-term results. Thus, the choice of technique should be based on the judgment of surgeons given their experience and the individual situations encountered. It is our opinion that in an infant or young child with a relatively long patent ductus arteriosus with a typically compliant wall, the techniques of ligation without division are perfectly acceptable and likely to achieve an excellent result. Alternatively, we prefer the clamp and divide technique, placing the aortic side vascular clamp completely on the aortic wall in older patients and all patients with a ductus that is often relatively short, and/or has undergone degenerative changes of the wall, and has become calcified, brittle, inflamed, and/or fragile.

Complications

There are certain complications well known to be associated with ligation of the patent ductus arteriosus. Early complications include left vocal cord paralysis, phrenic nerve injury, Horners syndrome, and chylothorax. Left vocal cord paralysis results from injury to the upper vagus nerve or the recurrent laryngeal during mobilization and retraction. It usually recovers within a few months. Horner's syndrome results from dissection around the sympathetic nerves near or leading to the sympathetic trunk and the stellate ganglia. Phrenic nerve injury from traumatic manipulation is uncommon and results in paralysis of the diaphragm, which is usually resolved within weeks to months. Chylothorax is a rare complication of ligation of the patent ductus arteriosus. It usually results from excessive dissection away from the vascular structures and into areas of the lymphatic and thoracic duct. Chylothorax usually resolves spontaneously but may require surgical re-exploration and ligation of the thoracic duct on rare occasion.

Late complications after closure of a patent ductus arteriosus include recanalization and false aneurysm formation. Recanalization was considered a significant concern in earlier experiences[59-64] and was thought to occur in about 3–5% of patients in whom the ductus was ligated. In more recent series, the incidence of recanalization or residual patency approaches zero. A false aneurysm is a rare complication usually occurring after ligation, or in association with infection.[65-67]

Outcome

Most patients with an isolated patent ductus arteriosus face a normal life after its closure. Surgical risks are less than 1%[68] and subsequent difficulties are usually not related to complications of closure of the patent ductus arteriosus. The highest risks are associated with extremes of age and associated conditions. Premature infants who have had surgical closure of a patent ductus arteriosus may face problems associated with their prematurity, such as lung disease, and outcomes are related mostly to these other problems. Older patients do carry a higher risk of closure due to a combination of factors including their age, chronic heart failure, associated pulmonary hypertension,[69] and the increased surgical risk of rupture and bleeding from the older fragile patent ductus arteriosus during ligation.[70]

Alternative Procedures

Thoracoscopic Closure of a Patent Ductus Arteriosus. Limited experience has been reported using thoracoscopic techniques for closure of the ductus arteriosus without a major thoracotomy incision.[71-73] These techniques involve the use of surgical instruments in the pleural cavity introduced via trocars that are placed into the chest cavity through small stab wounds. The left lung is deflated by introducing air into the pleural space and creating a controlled tension pneumothorax. Trocars are then placed into the lateral left chest cavity through intercostal spaces anterior, superior, and inferior to the area of the patent ductus arteriosus. A video thoracoscope is passed through the trocar over the ductus for visualization of the dissection. Forceps, scissors, cautery forceps, and retractors can then be introduced through appropriately placed trocars, and used to mobilize the deflated lung and to dissect out the ductus. Once the patent ductus arteriosus is freed, a specialized clip applicator is introduced and the ductus is closed with the clips.

This technique is most applicable to younger patients with a small patent ductus arteriosus that is not at high risk for fragmentation and rupture. Early results in a small series suggest adequate closure of the patent ductus arteriosus and short hospital stays.[71-73] Experience is small and comparison to standard surgical approaches cannot be made at the present.

Transarterial Catheter Closure of the Patent Ductus Arteriosus. Transarterial catheter closure of the patent ductus arteriosus is a method gaining increasing interest and should be considered as an alternative to the surgical approach. Catheter "device" closure of the patent ductus arteriosus has been used since the early 1970s. Initial results using plugs and the early Rashkind occluder device were limited to about 60% successful closure.[9,10,74] Recently, enthusiasm has been raised with more current studies using the Rashkind PDA occluder device, the Lock clamshell occluder, and gianturco coils showing approximately 80% successful closure.[75-79] Recent results, using absence of demonstrable flow by doppler techniques as criteria of complete closure, suggest that there is 50% immediate complete closure rate, while 65–80% will be completely closed at 1 year, and 85–90% will be closed by 2.5 years. Results appear to be better in the small ductus arteriosus 3 mm or less in diameter, and acceptable in the patent ductus up to 10 mm in diameter.[80-83]

Currently none of the umbrella or clamshell devices is licensed for general use, and coils are the only devices actively in use. At this time there are no large long-term studies focused on the use of coils in occlusion of the patent ductus arteriosus, but results appear to be promising.[84-86] When the patent ductus is less than 3 mm in diameter, there is a 70% incidence of immediate complete closure, and 90% are closed at 6 months. Five percent are complicated by embolization of the coil into the pulmonary circulation, but retrieval of embolized coils is readily accomplished.

The advantages of transcatheter closure of the patent ductus arteriosus are primarily expediency and reduced morbidity. Patients do not require intubation or a general anesthetic for the procedure, and a major thoracic incision is avoided. Hospitalizations are short, and these procedures may in the future become outpatient procedures. On the down side, the efficacy does not approach that of surgery, which can be accomplished with a nearly zero percent mortality rate and a less than 1–2% early and late failure rate. Furthermore, transfusion is more often needed with the transcatheter approach than with an open surgical procedure. Currently we recommend transcatheter closure with coils in younger patients with a patent ductus arteriosus of 3 mm or less in diameter, and consider it with the family as a viable option to surgery when the patent ductus arteriosus is long, and up to 8–10 mm in diameter.

Summary

The patent ductus arteriosus is an important lesion that results from a persistence of the fetal ductus arteriosus beyond the newborn period. Depending on its size, the patent ductus can present with a wide range of symptoms and findings. Closure is indicated in nearly all patients with a patent ductus arteriosus regardless of size, and timing and method of closure are the primary concerns. The presence of advanced pulmonary vascular disease is the major contraindication. Direct surgical closure is the standard technique now achieving about 99% long-term success with nearly zero mortality, and few complications. Less invasive techniques that do not require a thoracotomy may be considered in selected cases but may not achieve as high a success rate.

AORTOPULMONARY SEPTAL DEFECT

Definition

Aortopulmonary septal defect or aortopulmonary window, as it is frequently called, is defect of conotruncal development in which there is incomplete separation of the aorta and pulmonary arteries. The result is a defect in their adjoining walls that creates a direct communication, or "window," between these two great vessels. Aortopulmonary septal defect is a very rare lesion occurring in about 0.2% of congenital heart lesions.[87–89] An aortopulmonary septal defect may occur as an isolated lesion, but it commonly occurs in conjunction with other cardiac lesions. It may occur in association with additional simple cardiac lesions or as an integral connection in a more complex combination of cardiovascular malformations. The physiological effects and clinical presentation are usually a consequence of the "left-to-right shunt" that occurs through the defect, and may be complicated further by the presence of additional defects. Clinical presentation is often dramatic, and clear definition of the lesion and associated defects is required in a timely fashion and specific intervention is often required.

History

Aortopulmonary septal defect was described first by Elliotson in 1830,[90] and again by Cotton[91] in 1899. Clinical presentation and diagnosis were described in the mid-1900s,[92,93] and the first successful repair was carried out shortly thereafter in 1952 by Gross.[94] Early attempts at closure were carried out by closed techniques.[95,96] However, difficulty in obtaining exposure and control rendered these methods susceptible to complications of bleeding and injury to nearby structures. The availability of cardiopulmonary bypass was an important advance in the surgical correction of these defects. The ability to take a direct open approach to these defects led to the development of safer and more effective techniques of closure.[97–99]

Embryology

Differentiation of the conotruncus into the aorta and pulmonary arteries begins during the fifth week of fetal life. Ingrowth of the left and right conotruncal ridges separates the truncal vessel into leftward (aortic) and rightward (pulmonary) components. The right and left sixth aortic arches, destined to become the branch pulmonary arteries, join with the rightward truncal vessel. Incomplete development of the conotruncal ridges is believed to be responsible for the more proximal and "simpler" form of aortopulmonary septal defect,[87] while the more complex distal forms of aortopulmonary septal defect, which usually involve the right branch pulmonary artery, are believed to result from malalignment of the conotruncal ridges.[100] Larger defects with poorly defined borders may result from complete absence of development of the conotruncal ridges.

Some believe that aortopulmonary septal defect is part of a spectrum of conotruncal malformations[101,102] ranging from anomalous origin of the right pulmonary artery, as the least severe form, through aortopulmonary septal defects as the intermediate forms, to truncus arteriosus as the most severe form.[103] However, this point is controversial. Kutsche and Van Mierop,[87] noting a very different spectrum of associated lesions, suggest that truncus arteriosus is a lesion developmentally unrelated to aortopulmonary septal defect.

Anatomy

Aortopulmonary septal defects create a direct opening in the adjacent walls of the central aorta and pulmonary arteries. They are bounded circumferentially by the conjoined, contiguous walls of the aorta and pulmonary arteries. The defects are usually relatively large in diameter, but the length of the internal aortopulmonary connection is minimal. Hence these lesions are often described by the term *aortopulmonary window*.

The shape and location of aortopulmonary septal defects vary. Three distinct anatomic patterns have been described that correspond to the three abnormalities of conotruncal development noted above (Fig. 69–8).[87,100] Type one defects are simple, nearly circular defects between the proximal ascending aorta and main pulmonary artery. The edges of these defects begin near, or even within, the upper region of the sinus of Valsalva, and end before the origin of the right branch pulmonary artery.[94]

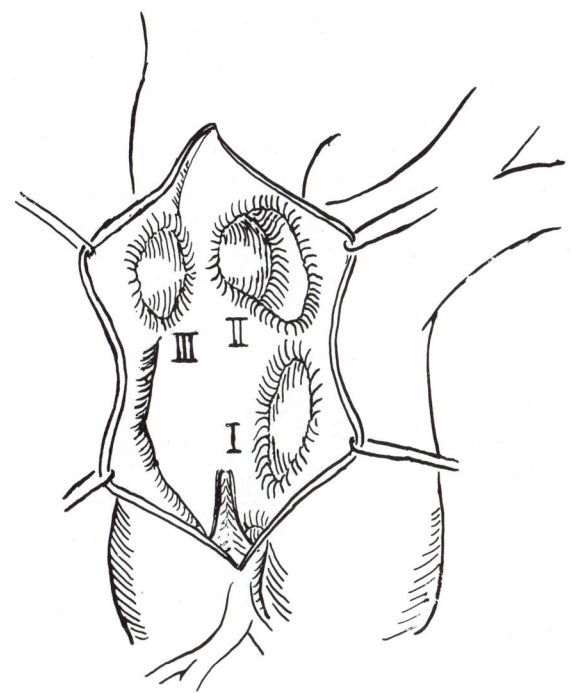

Figure 69–8. Figure showing the relative position of three basic varieties of aortopulmonary window. Type I is located inferiorly near the coronary artery ostia. Type II is more eccentric, is located higher, and involves the origin of the right pulmonary artery. Type III is distinguished by apparent relocation of the origin of the right pulmonary artery to an anomalous position on the right posterior lateral wall of the aorta.

The orifice of the right, or less commonly the left, coronary artery may be associated with the proximal rim of the defect, and in some cases may be located on the pulmonary side of the defect.[105–108] Type two defects are helicoid in shape and extend in a more cephalad direction. These defects frequently extend to the origin of the right pulmonary artery.[87,109,110] Type three defects may be larger, often without a discernible posterior rim, and can extend to involve the proximal right branch pulmonary artery and the posterior wall of the ascending aorta.[108,110] The "unroofed" proximal right pulmonary artery may appear to be incorporated into the posterior wall of the ascending aorta, and the right pulmonary artery may appear to originate from the right side of the ascending aorta.[108,110,111] In some lesions the defect does not involve the main pulmonary artery, and is limited to either an unroofed proximal right branch pulmonary artery,[108,110] or an isolated anomalous origin of the right pulmonary artery from the ascending aorta.[111]

Associated Defects

Aortopulmonary septal defects are associated with additional cardiovascular malformations in over half of the cases.[87,104,105,112] About 10% of patients with an aortopulmonary septal defect have minor associated anomalies including patent ductus arteriosus, atrial septal defect, and right aortic arch.[113–115] Major associated cardiovascular malformations occur in 30–50% of patients with an aortopulmonary septal defect.[104,105,112] The most commonly associated major cardiovascular malformations involve obstruction of the aortic arch, and include interruption of the aortic arch, usually type A, hypoplasia of the distal arch, and coarctation.[87,105,112,116–118] The combination of aortopulmonary septal defect and obstruction of the aortic arch is usually associated with a patent ductus arteriosus. Additional associated lesions include anomalous origin of one or both coronary arteries, ventricular septal defect, subaortic obstruction, and/or anomalous origin of the right pulmonary artery.[113,119] Aortopulmonary septal defect may also occur coincidentally with tetralogy of Fallot.[119,120]

Pathophysiology

The pathophysiologic changes that occur with an aortopulmonary septal defect are a consequence of the left-to-right shunt that occurs through the defect. Thus they are essentially the same as those in patent ductus arteriosus as discussed earlier in this chapter. As pulmonary vascular resistance decreases, systemic blood flow is diverted through the defect increasing pulmonary blood flow and placing a volume load on the left ventricle. Most aortopulmonary septal defects are large, allowing equalization of pressures within the aorta and pulmonary arteries. Thus, as pulmonary resistance decreases to lower levels, the left-to-right shunt becomes excessive and associated pathophysiologic changes progress to severe left ventricular failure, pulmonary interstitial edema, and low systemic output.

Special attention should be given to the association of an aortopulmonary septal defect with an obstructed aortic arch and patent ductus arteriosus. An aortic arch obstruction impedes systemic blood flow and promotes the shunting of systemic output to the pulmonary circulation, and thus may markedly increase the pathophysiologic effects of an associated aortopulmonary septal defect. Furthermore, lower body systemic perfusion in patients with an associated interruption of the aortic arch or coarctation of the aorta is accomplished via a patent ductus arteriosus. In essence, there is a left-to-right shunt through the aortopulmonary septal defect and a right-to-left shunt through the patent ductus, which is the source of blood flow to the distal systemic circulation. Spontaneous closure of the ductus arteriosus cuts off blood flow to the lower body, and forces more flow to the lungs, thus causing severe pulmonary edema and devastating hypoperfusion of lower body and organ systems. Consequently, the combination of these lesions can cause particularly life-threatening pathophysiologic consequences.[112]

Clinical Presentation

The clinical presentation of a patient with an aortopulmonary septal defect depends on the size of the defect, the pulmonary vascular resistance, and the presence of other associated malformations. The clinical presentation of a patient with an isolated aortopulmonary septal defect is like that of a patient with a patent ductus arteriosus. Patients may be asymptomatic if the defect is restrictive and/or the pulmonary resistance is high. However, these defects are usually larger, and more often infants with an isolated aortopulmonary septal defect present with tachypnea, tachycardia, feeding difficulties, poor weight gain, irritability, fever, cough, dyspnea, pneumonia, and other manifestations of left ventricular failure and excessive pulmonary blood flow. In the presence of low pulmonary vascular resistance and/or associated interruption of the aortic arch, patients may present with pulmonary edema, respiratory failure, left ventricular failure, and low cardiac output syndrome. Patients with an aortopulmonary septal defect and interrupted aortic arch may present with sudden closure of the ductus arteriosus, and under these conditions patients are usually in "extremis" with cardiovascular collapse and respiratory failure.

Pulmonary vascular disease progresses rapidly in children with aortopulmonary defects who survive infancy without repair. These children may present in the first few years of life with Eisenmenger's syndrome.[109]

Physical Examination

Physical examination will reveal the general status of the child and indicate the degree of cardiovascular compromise. The precordium is hyperactive, the second heart sound is accentuated without the characteristic splitting, and a murmur can be heard along the left sternal border. The murmur is systolic in most cases but may be continuous in patients with a restrictive defect.[104,115,121] With increased diastolic runoff, the peripheral pulses may be exaggerated and jerky and the pulse pressure is widened.

Pulmonary edema may be noted by auscultation of rales and rhonchi in the lung fields, and consolidation may indicate a pleural effusion or pneumonia.

Diagnosis

Chest radiography reveals an enlarged heart with prominent central and peripheral pulmonary vascular markings. Pulmonary interstitial fluid and cardiac enlargement may also be apparent.

ECG may reveal a tachycardia and other arrhythmias. Left and right ventricular hypertrophy are usually indicated by increased left- and rightward ventricular forces and left atrial enlargement may be suggested by widened, biphasic "P" waves.

Two-dimensional echocardiography can accurately demonstrate the anatomy of the lesion (Fig. 69–9).[122–125] The position and extent of the defect can be shown directly, and color flow doppler can accurately describe the shunt through the defect. Associated malformations can be described, and left and right ventricular function can be assessed. Pulsed doppler interrogation can be used to look for a gradient across the lesion, and to confirm right ventricular systolic pressures. Echocardiography can also rule out the presence of other lesions considered in the differential diagnosis such as truncus arteriosus, anomalous origin of the pulmonary artery, ventricular septal defect, and coronary artery fistulae.

Cardiac catheterization and cineangiography can accurately demonstrate the lesion, but usually these invasive techniques are not needed unless there is concern over pulmonary vascular disease and increased pulmonary vascular resistance.

Management

Indications

Spontaneous closure has not been reported with aortopulmonary septal defects and those few patients who survive early life with this lesion develop Eisenmenger's syndrome rapidly.[108,109] Thus, the management of patients with an aortopulmonary window is usually directed toward medical

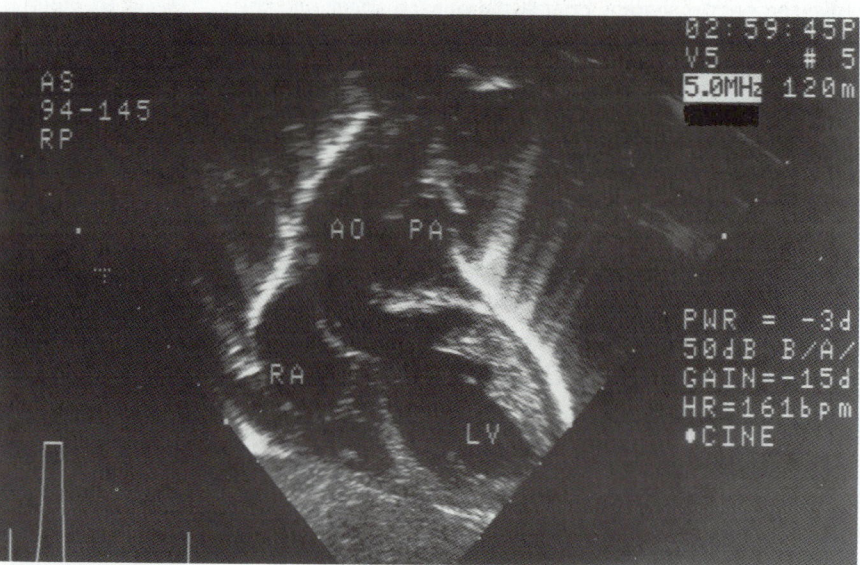

Figure 69–9. Typical echocardiogram showing a proximal aortopulmonary septal defect.

stabilization and management of presenting symptoms followed soon thereafter with surgical closure.

Medical Management

Medical management of patients who have mild-to-moderate symptoms of congestive heart failure consists primarily of digitalization and administration of diuretics. Transfusion should be carried out if the hematocrit is low, and oxygen administration should be avoided. Antibiotics should be administered for pneumonia.

Patients with severe congestive heart failure and pulmonary edema may require intubation and positive pressure ventilation, infusion of inotropic agents, and intravenous diuretic therapy. Prostaglandins infusion may be needed to open the patent ductus arteriosus in patients with associated obstructive lesions of the aortic arch. The administration of inspired CO_2 to raise pulmonary resistance may also be considered in the severely compromised patient.

Surgical Management

With the patient medically optimized surgical closure of the defect and repair of associated defects should be planned. Early surgical approaches used closed techniques including ligation[94] and clamping and division.[95] These techniques are difficult because the defects are usually large in diameter but have minimal length. The involved great vessels are large and important structures including valve commissures, and coronary artery origins are situated in close proximity. Troublesome bleeding and injury to surrounding structures frequently occurred.

The open approach accessing the defect directly through the aorta, pulmonary artery, or the wall of the defect itself is now preferred. This approach requires support of cardiopulmonary bypass and the defect is usually closed with a patch.

General Considerations

The patient is placed supine on the operating room table and placed under general endotracheal anesthesia. Arterial and venous access is established, and the entire anterior chest and upper abdomen are prepped and draped. The lesion is approached through a midline sternotomy, and the portion of the thymus inferior to the innominate vein is removed. The pericardium is opened with a leftward vertical incision, and the edges are sutured to the edges of the sternotomy incision.

The anterior, superior, and inferior borders of the defect can usually be discerned externally by visualizing the mural fusion of the aortic and pulmonary arteries. The aorta is dissected circumferentially above the lesion, and the branch pulmonary arteries, and if needed the patent ductus arteriosus, are surrounded with large sutures.

Cannulation and bypass in patients with an isolated aortopulmonary septal defect are straightforward. The aorta is cannulated distally near the origin of the innominate artery, and venous drainage cannulae can be placed directly in the right atrium. The patient is placed on bypass and cooled to between 26 and 28°C. The pulmonary arteries are snared closed to prevent flooding of the lungs and poor systemic perfusion on bypass. If open, the ductus arteriosus is tied closed.

The aorta is cross-clamped and cardioplegia is administered in the aortic root. If the arrested heart becomes distended, a left ventricular venting cannula may be placed via a stab incision in the right upper pulmonary vein.

Closure of the Defect

The defect is exposed and closed with a patch of either woven dacron, gortex, or glutaraldehyde-fixed pericardium. The patch is cut to fit the defect. In simple proximal type one defects, an oval patch is usually appropriate, and is sutured around the defect with a running 5-0 polypropylene suture (Fig. 69–10). Inferiorly the suture line may be carried to the right of the rim of the defect to avoid injury to the coronary ostia and if necessary may be carried further to the right around the origin of an anomalous coronary ostia. In more complicated lesions, the relationship of the superior edge of the defect to the origin of the right branch pulmonary artery must be clearly discerned.[126] In type two defects, the aortopulmonary septal defect may extend over the origin of the right pulmonary artery and tear a drop-shaped patch may be fashioned to facilitate closure (Fig. 69–11). Type three defects in which the further extension of the aortopulmonary septal defect may involve the proximal right branch pulmonary artery and/or displace the apparent origin of the right branch pulmonary artery to the right lateral wall of the aorta require a more complicated patch for repair (Fig. 69–12). The patch should be designed with a longer, wider extension that is sutured to the back wall of the aorta, around the unroofed portion of the right branch pulmonary artery and/or around the displaced (anomalous) origin of the right branch pulmonary artery.[127,128] This extension closes the central aortopulmonary septal defect in continuity with the right branch pulmonary artery and commits them to the pulmonary circulation. The extension should be large enough to create an unobstructed connection between the right branch pulmonary artery and the main pulmonary artery, and if necessary the aorta can be enlarged anteriorly with an additional patch to accommodate this.

The ideal approach to expose the aortopulmonary septal may vary depending on the type of defect encountered. The transpulmonary approach is convenient in accessing the simple, "low" type one defects.[97,109,115] Either a transverse or longitudinal incision allows excellent exposure of the rim of the defect and visualization of a coronary artery ostia. From this approach, the patch is easily placed to the right side of the defect and can readily be sutured around a coronary artery ostia that is anomalously positioned on the right side of the defect.

A transaortic approach also provides excellent expo-

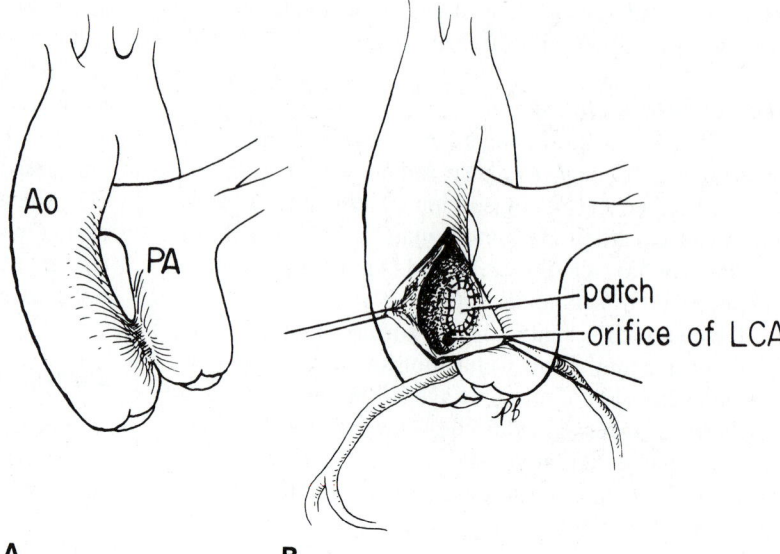

Figure 69–10. A. Surgical anatomy of type I defect. **B.** Transaortic closure using a dacron patch to close the defect. With this closure, the left coronary artery (LCA) orifice is identified and protected. *(From Richardson et al: J Thorac Cardiovasc Surg 78:21, 1979, with permission.)*

A   **B**

sure and may be preferred in the more distal type two defects.[98,129] This approach allows excellent assessment of the origin of the right pulmonary artery and facilitates placement of the patch to the left side of the defect in this region. If necessary, this incision can be extended superiorly and closed with a patch to enlarge the ascending aorta. The coronary ostia can be seen easily in their usual position but coronary ostia positioned anomalously on the right side of the defect may be more difficult to visualize from the aortic side.

The aortopulmonary septal defect may be accessed directly by opening the anterior wall of the defect between the aorta and pulmonary arteries.[131] This approach achieves good exposure of both sides of the defect. It allows access to the right side of the defect inferiorly in the region of the coronary artery ostia, and to the left side superiorly in the region of the origin of the right branch pulmonary artery. Using this method of exposure, the patch is sutured posteri-

orly, superiorly, and inferiorly about the rim of the defect. Anteriorly, where the wall of the defect has been incised, placement of the patch and closure of the incision are completed simultaneously by sandwiching the patch in between the wall of the pulmonary artery, and the wall of the aorta in the completed suture line.

An aortopulmonary defect isolated to the proximal right branch pulmonary artery is best approached anteriorly through the aorta. The patch is placed about this defect within the lumen of the aorta. The patch is sized generously to avoid creation of a stenosis in the proximal right branch pulmonary artery, and the aorta may need to be enlarged anteriorly to accommodate this.

Anomalous origin of the right pulmonary artery from the right side of the ascending aorta without an additional component of a central aortopulmonary septal defect can be repaired by excision of a cuff of aorta containing the origin of the right branch pulmonary artery followed by closure of

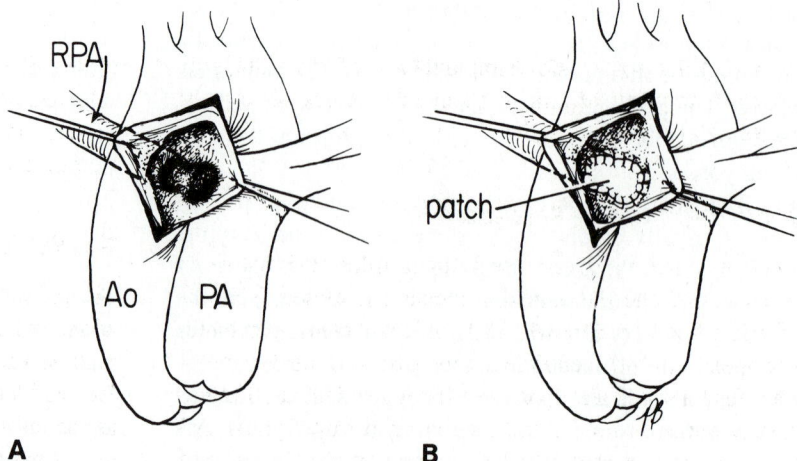

Figure 69–11. A. Surgical anatomy of type II defect. **B.** Use of a contoured dacron patch prevents stenosis of the proximal right pulmonary artery. *(From Richardson et al: J Thorac Cardiovasc Surg 78:21, 1979, with permission.)*

A   **B**

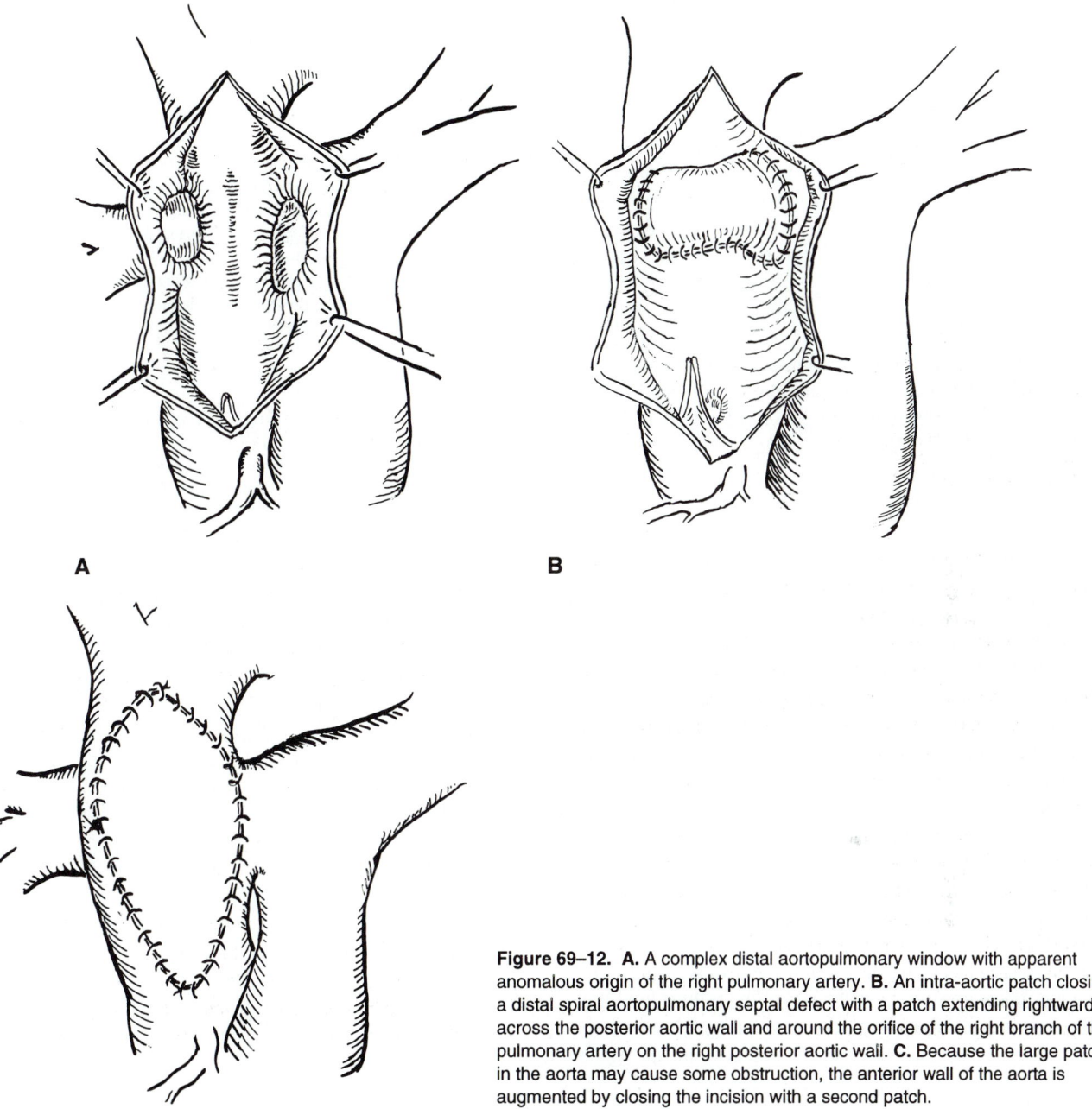

A

B

C

Figure 69–12. A. A complex distal aortopulmonary window with apparent anomalous origin of the right pulmonary artery. **B.** An intra-aortic patch closing a distal spiral aortopulmonary septal defect with a patch extending rightward across the posterior aortic wall and around the orifice of the right branch of the pulmonary artery on the right posterior aortic wall. **C.** Because the large patch in the aorta may cause some obstruction, the anterior wall of the aorta is augmented by closing the incision with a second patch.

the ascending aorta, and reimplantation of the right pulmonary artery into the main pulmonary artery directly or via a conduit.[127,128]

Completion of the Procedure

After the patch is placed, the heart is filled with saline to evacuate air, and the exposing incision is closed. The patient is placed head down, and the cross-clamp removed. The apex of the left ventricle is aspirated, and the cardioplegia infusion site is left open to vent any residual air. The patient is warmed to 37°C and then weaned from bypass. All cannulae are removed and the cannulation sites are snared

closed. Transthoracic central venous access and monitoring catheters are placed. The heparin is reversed and when hemostasis is completed, mediastinal drains are placed and the sternotomy is closed in a routine manner.

Special Modifications

The procedure may need to be modified in the presence of additional intracardiac malformations. Associated malformations such as an atrial septal defect, ventricular septal defect, and tetralogy of Fallot can be repaired at the same time as the aortopulmonary septal defect is closed. Cannulation may need to be modified to a bicaval technique and left ventricular venting may be more important in patients needing intracardiac repairs. Additional details regarding the repair of these associated malformations are covered in the respective chapters dealing with each of these malformations specifically.

Interruption of the aorta and hypoplastic abnormalities of the aortic arch may have a direct effect on the approach to the associated aortopulmonary septal defect. Usually aortic interruption is associated with a more complicated type of aortopulmonary septal defects involving the right branch pulmonary artery, and the size of the aorta may decrease abruptly just above the defect. Simultaneous repair of these malformations requires modifications of the usual techniques. Patients with these associated malformations are cannulated with two perfusion cannulae, one placed in the aorta above the defect and the other placed in the pulmonary artery for perfusion of the lower body, and the patent ductus arteriosus is left open during cooling. The patients are cooled to between 15 and 18°C and circulatory arrest is instituted for repair of the arch. Specific techniques for repair of the interrupted aortic arch are presented elsewhere in detail. In association with an aortopulmonary window, the interruption is repaired with an end-to-end anastomosis. In addition, the underside of the anastomosis is further augmented with a homograft patch that is continued proximally along the underside of the aortic arch ending at the superior aspect of the aortopulmonary septal defect where the aorta enlarges. The cross-clamp is placed a few millimeters beyond the proximal end of this patch well above the aortopulmonary septal defect. After removal of air from the aorta, perfusion is reinstituted for the remainder of the procedure through the ascending aorta cannulae. An anterior vertical incision is then made in the aorta and the aortopulmonary septal defect is closed from this approach. If the proximal right branch pulmonary artery is unroofed into the back wall of the aorta and/or the orifice of the right branch pulmonary artery is displaced to the right side of the aorta, a large intra-aortic extension of the aortopulmonary septal defect patch may be used to reconstitute the right branch pulmonary artery to the main pulmonary artery. This patch over the proximal right branch pulmonary artery may be large, and the potential for obstruction can be alleviated by closing the anterior, "exposing" incision in the ascending aorta with an additional patch that traverses the area of the reconstructed right branch pulmonary artery, and overlaps proximal extension of the patch on the underside of the aortic arch. The procedure then is completed as described above.

Results

Generally, present results with these lesions offer complete correction with low morbidity and a mortality. Early reports noted a mortality of 15–25%,[108,130,131] but more recently mortality rates for surgical repair are below 10%.[112] The risk of repair is also similar for patients with major associated malformations.[117,129,132,133]

REFERENCES

1. Galen: *Opera Omnia* **IV:**243. Kuhn Edition. A. Translation from Dalton JC: *Doctrines of the Circulation.* Philadelphia, Leas Son and Co., 1884, p 68. Translated from the Greek, with an Introduction and Commentary, Mary Tallmadge May. Ithaca, NY, Cornell University Press, 1968, Vol 1, p 333
2. Harvey W: *Exercitatio Anatomica de Muta Cordis et Sanguinis in Animalbus.* Francofurti, Sumptibus Gulielmi Fitzeri, 1628
3. Gibson GA: *Disease of the Heart and Aorta.* London, Pentland, 1898
4. Gibson GA: Persistence of the arterial duct and its diagnosis. *Edinb Med J* **8:**1, 1900
5. Munro JC: Surgery of the vascular system. Ligation of patent ductus arteriosus. *Ann Surg* **46:**335, 1907
6. Graybiel A, Strieder JW, Boyer NH: An attempt to obliterate the patent ductus arteriosus in a patient with subacute bacterial endarteritis. *Am Heart J* **15:**621, 1938
7. Gross RE, Hubbard JP: Surgical ligation of a patent ductus arteriosus. Report of first successful case. *JAMA* **112:**729, 1939
8. Ash R, Fisher D: Manifestations and results of treatment of patent ductus arteriosus in infancy and childhood. *Pediatrics* **16:**695, 1955
9. Portsmann W, Wierny L, Warnke H, et al: Catheter closure of patent ductus arteriosus, 62 cases treated without thoracotomy. *Radiol Clin North Am* **9:**203, 1971
10. Rashkind WJ, Cuaso CC: Transcatheter closure of patent ductus arteriosus. *Pediatr Cardiol* **1:**3, 1979
11. Ali Kahn MA, Mullins CE, Nihill MR, et al: Percutaneous catheter closure of the ductus arteriosus in children and young adults. *Am J Cardiol* **64:**218, 1989
12. Silver MM, Freedom RM, Silver MD, Oiley PM: The morphology of the human newborn ductus arteriosus: A reappraisal of its structure and function with special reference to prostaglandin E1 therapy. *Hum Pathol* **12:**1123, 1981
13. Jager BV, Wollenman OF Jr: An anatomical study of the closure of the ductus arteriosus. *Am J Pathol* **18:**595, 1942
14. Clyman RI, Heymann MA: Pharmacology of the ductus arteriosus. *Pediatr Clin North Am* **28:**77, 1981
15. Clyman RI: Ontogeny of the ductus arteriosus response to prostaglandins and inhibitors of their synthesis. *Semin Perinatol* **4:**115, 1980
16. Coceani F, Olley PM: Role of prostaglandin, prostacyclin, and thromboxanes in the control of prenatal patency and postnatal closure of the ductus arteriosus. *Semin Perinatol* **4:**109, 1980
17. Rudolph: *Congenital Diseases of the Heart.* Chicago, Yearbook Medical, 1974
18. Heymann MA, Rudolph AM: Control of the ductus arteriosus. *Physiol Rev* **55:**62, 1975
19. McMurphy DM, Heymann MA, Rudolph AM, et al: Developmental change in constriction of the ductus arteriosus: Response to oxygen and vasoactive substances in the isolated ductus arteriosus of the fetal lamb. *Pediatr Res* **6:**231, 1972
20. Gittenberger-DeGroot AC, Harnick ME, Becker AE: Histopathology of the ductus arteriosus after prostaglandin E1 administration in ductus dependent cardiac anomalies. *Br Heart J* **40:**215, 1978
21. Fay FS, Cooke PH: Guinea pig ductus arteriosus. 11. Irreversible closure after birth. *Am J Physiol* **222:**841, 1972
22. Christie A: Normal closing time of the foramen ovale and the ductus arteriosus. *Am J Dis Child* **40:**323, 1930
23. Dubrow IW, Fisher E, Hastreiter A: Intermittent functional closure of patent ductus arteriosus in a ten-month old infant: Hemodynamic documentation. *Chest* **68:**110, 1975

24. Coggin CJ, Parker KR, Keith JD: Natural history of isolated patent ductus arteriosus and the effect of surgical correction: Twenty years experience at the Hospital for Sick Children, Toronto. *Can Med Assoc J* **192**:718, 1970

25. Heymann MA: Patent ductus arteriosus. In Adams FA, Emmanoulides GC, Reimenschneider TA (eds): *Moss' Heart Disease in Infants, Children and Adolescents,* 4th ed. Baltimore, Williams & Wilkins, 1989

26. Gittenberger-De Groot AC: Persistent ductus arteriosus: Most probably a primary congenital malformation. *Br Heart J* **39**:610, 1977

27. Siassi B, Blanco C, Cabal LA, Coran AG: Incidence and clinical features of patent ductus arteriosus in low-birth weight infants. A prospective analysis of 150 consecutively born infants. *Pediatrics* **57**:347, 1976

28. Heymann MA, Rudolph AM, Silverman NH: Closure of the ductus arteriosus in premature infants by inhibition of prostaglandin synthesis. *N Engl J Med* **295**:530, 1976

29. Clyman RI, Heymann MA: Pharmacology of the ductus arteriosus. *Pediatr Clin North Am* **28**:77, 1981

30. Clyman RI, Murry F, Roman C, et al: Circulating prostaglandin E2 concentrations and patent ductus arteriosus in fetal and neonatal lambs. *J Pediatr* **97**:455, 1980

31. Arciniegas E, Hakimi M, Hertzler JH, et al: Surgical management of congenital vascular rings. *J Thorac Cardiovasc Surg* **77**:721, 1979

32. Shuford WH, Sybers RG: *The Aortic Arch and Its Malformations with Emphasis on the Angiographic Features.* Springfield, IL, Charles C Thomas, 1974

33. Heikkinen ES, Simila S, Laitinen J, Larmi T: Infantile aneurysm of the ductus arteriosus. *Acta Paediatr Scand* **63**:241, 1974

34. Das JB, Chesterman JT: Aneurysms of the patent ductus arteriosus. *Thorax* **11**:295, 1956

35. Falcone MW, Perloff JK, Roberts WC: Aneurysm of the non patent ductus arteriosus. *Am J Cardiol* **29**:422, 1972

36. Cruickshank B, Marquis RM: Spontaneous aneurysms of the ductus arteriosus. *Am J Med* **25**:140, 1958

37. Krovetz LJ, Warden HE: Patent ductus arteriosus. An analysis of 515 surgically proved cases. *Dis Ches* **42**:241, 1962

38. Ash R, Fischer D: Manifestations and results of treatment of patent ductus arteriosus in infancy and childhood. An analysis of 138 cases. *Pediatrics* **16**:695, 1955

39. Ravin A, Karley W: Apical diastolic murmur in patent ductus arteriosus. *Ann Intern Med* **33**:903, 1950

40. Ravin A, Karley W: Apical diastolic murmur in patent ductus arteriosus. *Ann Intern Med* **33**:903, 1950

41. Swemson RE, Maldes-Cruz LM, Sahn DJ, et al: Realtime Doppler color flow mapping for detection of patent ductus arteriosus. *J Am Coll Cardiol* **8**:1105, 1986

42. Silverman NH: Patent ductus arteriosus. In: *Pediatric Echocardiographer.* Baltimore, Williams & Wilkins, 1993, pp 167–177

43. Nadas AS, Tyler DC: *Pediatric Cardiology.* Philadelphia, Saunders, 1972, pp 405–426

44. Caputo GR, Kondo C, Higgin CB: Quantification of blood flow using magnetic resonance imaging. In Higgins CB (ed): *Magnetic Resonance Imaging.* New York, Raven Press, 1992

45. Campbell M: The natural history of persistent ductus arteriosus with untreated cases. *Br Heart J* **30**:4, 1968

46. Abbott M: *Atlas of Congenital Heart Disease.* New York, American Heart Association, 1936

47. Olly PM, Caceani F, Bodack E: E-Type prostaglandins: A new emergency therapy for certain cyanotic congenital heart malformations. *Circulation* **53**:728, 1976

48. Nadas AS: Indomethacin and the patent ductus arteriosus. *N Engl Med* **305**:97, 1981

49. LaBorde F, Noirhomme T, Karam K, et al: A new video thoracoscopy surgical technique for management of patent ductus arteriosus in infants and children. Abstract. Presented at the American Association of Thoracic Surgery Annual Meeting, Los Angeles, CA, 1992

50. Hutchkiss WS: Patent ductus arteriosus and the occasional cardiac surgeon. *JAMA* **173**:244, 1960

51. Levitsky S, Hastrieter AR: Cardiovascular surgical emergencies in the first year of life. *Surg Clin North Am* **52**:61, 1971

52. Hall GS, Helmsworth JA, Schreiber JT, et al: Premature infants with patent ductus arteriosus and respiratory distress: Selection for ductal ligation. *Ann Thorac Surg* **22**:146, 1976

53. Blalock A: Operative closure of the patent ductus arteriosus. *Surg Gynecol Obstet* **82**:113, 1946

54. Complete division for the patent ductus arteriosus. *J Thorac Surg* **16**:314, 1947

55. Levitsky S, Hastreiter AR: Cardiovascular surgical emergencies in the first year of life. *Surg Clin North Am* **52**:61, 1971

56. O'Donovan TG, Beck W: Closure of the complicated patent ductus arteriosus. *Ann Thorac Surg* **25**:463, 1978

57. Gross RE: Complete surgical division of the patent ductus arteriosus. *Surg Gynecol Obstet* **78**:36, 1944

58. Sorensen KE, Kristensen BO, Hansen OK: Frequency of occurrence of residual ductal flow after surgical ligation by color-flow mapping. *Am J Coll Cardiol* **67**:653, 1991

59. Daniels SR, Reller MD, Kaplan S: Recurrence of patency of the ductus arteriosus after surgical ligation in premature infants. *Pediatrics* **73**:56, 1984

60. Stark J, Jucin B, Aberdeen E, Waterston DJ: Cardiac surgery in the first year of life. Experience with 1049 operations. *Surgery* **69**:483, 1971

61. Gross RE, Longino LA: The patent ductus arteriosus. Observations from 412 surgically treated cases. *Circulation* **3**:125, 1951

62. Jones JC: Twenty-five years experience with the surgery of patent ductus arteriosus. *J Thorac Cardiovasc Surg* **50**:2, 1965

63. Panagopoulos PH, Tatooles CJ, Aberdeen E, Waterston DJ, et al: Patent ductus arteriosus in infants and children: A review of 936 operations. *Thorax* **26**:1937, 1971

64. Tutassaura H, Goldman B, Moes CAF, Mustard WT: Spontaneous aneurysm of the ductus arteriosus in childhood. *J Thorac Cardiovasc Surg* **57**:180, 1969

65. Punsar S, Scheinin T, Tala P, Telivuo L: Postoperative aneurysm of the patent ductus arteriosus. *Br J Radiol* **42**:858, 1968

66. Ross RJ, Feder FP, Spencer FC: Aneurysms of the previously ligated patent ductus arteriosus. *Circulation* **23**:350, 1961

67. Rosengrantz JG, Kelminson LL, Paton BC, Vogel JHK: False aneurysm after ligation of a patent ductus arteriosus. *Ann Thorac Surg* **3**:353, 1967

68. Ash R, Fischer D: Manifestations and results of treatment of patent ductus arteriosus in infancy and childhood. An analysis of 138 cases. *Pediatr* **16**:695, 1955

69. Ellis FH Jr, Kirklin JW, Callahan JA, Wood EH: Patent ductus arteriosus with pulmonary hypertension. *J Thorac Surg* **31**:268, 1956

70. Black LL, Goldman BS: Surgical treatment of the patent ductus arteriosus in the adult. *Ann Surg* **175**:290, 1972

71. Laborde F, Noirhomme P, Karam J, et al: A new video thoracoscopy surgical technique for interruption of patent ductus arteriosus in infants and children. *J Thorac Cardiovasc Surg*

72. McCarthy JF, Hurley JP, Wood AE: Imaged thoracoscopic surgery patent ductus arteriosus ligation. *Eur J CardioThorac Surg* **8**(2):108–109, 1994

73. Burke RP: Video-assisted thoracoscopic surgery for patent ductus arteriosus. *Pediatrics* **93**(5):823–825, 1994

74. Portsman W, Wierny L, Warnke H, et al: Catheter closure of the patent ductus arteriosus: 62 cases treated without thoracotomy. *Radiol Clin North Am* **9**:203, 1971

75. Ali Khan MA, Mullins CE, Nihill MR, et al: Percutaneous catheter closure of the ductus arteriosus in children and young adults. *Am J Cardiol* **64**:218, 1989

76. Rashkind WJ, Mullins CE, Hellenbrand WE, Tait MA: Nonsurgical closure of patent ductus arteriosus: Clinical application of the Rashkind PDA occluder system. *Circulation* **75**:583, 1987

77. Gianturco C, Anderson JW, Wallace S: Mechanical device for arterial occlusion. *Am J Radiol* **124**:428, 1975

78. Mullins CE: Pediatric and congenital therapeutic cardiac catheterization. *Circulation* **79**:1153, 1989

79. Musewe NN, Benson LN, Smallhorn JF, Freedom RM: Two-dimensional echocardiographic and color flow Doppler evaluation of ductal occlusion with the Rashkind prosthesis. *Circulation* **80**:1706, 1989

80. Wessel DI, Keane JF, Parness I, Lock JE: Outpatient closure of the patent ductus arteriosus. *Circulation* **77**:1068, 1988

81. Hosking MCK, Benson L, Musewe N, et al: Transcatheter occlusion of the persistently patent ductus arteriosus: Forty month follow-up and prevalence of residual shunting. *Circulation* **84**:2313, 1991

82. Gray DT, Fyler DC, Walker AM, et al: Clinical outcomes and costs of transcatheter as compared with surgical closure of the patent ductus arteriosus. *N Engl J Med* **329**:1517, 1993

83. Loyd TR, Fedderly R, Mendelsohn AM, et al: Transcatheter occlusion of the patent ductus arteriosus with gianturco coils. *Circulation* **88**(part 1):1412, 1993

84. Loyd TR, Fedderly R, Mendelsohn AM, et al: Transcatheter occlusion of the patent ductus arteriosus with gianturco coils. *Circulation* **88**(part 1):1412–1420, 1993

85. Cambier PA, Kirby WC, Wortham DC, Moore JW: Percutaneous closure of the small (<2.5) patent ductus arteriosus using coil embolization. *Am J Cardiol* **69**:815, 1992

86. Moore JW, George L, Kirkpatrick SE, et al: Percutaneous closure of the small patent ductus arteriosus using occluding spring coils. *J Am Coll Cardiol* **23**:759, 1994

87. Kutsche LM, Van Mierop LHS: Anatomy and pathogenesis of aorticopulmonary septal defects. *Am J Cardiol* **59**:443, 1987

88. Keith JD, Rowe RD, Vlad P: *Heart Disease in Infancy and Childhood,* 3rd ed. New York, Macmillan, 1978

89. Rowe RD: Aortopulmonary septal defect. In Keith JD, Rowe RD, Vlad P (eds): *Heart Disease in Infancy and Childhood,* 3rd ed. New York, Macmillan, 1978

90. Elliotson J: Case of malformation of the pulmonary artery and aorta. *Lancet* **1**:247, 1830

91. Cotton AC: Report of a case of anuria. *Arch Pediatr* **16**:774X, 1899

92. Dodds JH, Hoyle C: Congenital aortic septal defect. *Br Heart J* **11**:390, 1949

93. Gasul BM, Fell EH, Casas R: The diagnosis of aortic septal defect by retrograde aortography: Report of a case. *Circulation* **4**:251, 1951

94. Gross RE: Surgical closure of an aortic septal defect. *Circulation* **5**:858, 1952

95. Scott HW Jr, Sabiston DC Jr: Surgical treatment for congenital aorticopulmonary fistula. Experimental and clinical aspects. *J Thorac Surg* **25**:26, 1953

96. Fletcher G, DuShane JW, Kirklin JW, Wood EH: Aorticopulmonary septal defect. Report of a case with surgical division along with successful resuscitation from ventricular fibrillation. *Mayo Clin Proc* **29**:285, 1954

97. Putnam TC, Gross RE: Surgical management of aortopulmonary fenestration. *Surgery* **59**:727, 1966

98. Wright JS, Freeman R, Johnston JB: Aortopulmonary fenestration. A technique of surgical management. *J Thorac Cardiovasc Surg* **55**:280, 1968

99. Cooley DA, McNamara DG, Latson JR: Aorticopulmonary septal defect: Diagnosis and surgical treatment. *Surgery* **42**:101, 1957

100. Cucci CE, Doyle EF, Lewis EW: Absence of a primary division of the pulmonary trunk. An ontogenetic theory. *Circulation* **29**:124, 1964

101. Collett RW, Edwards JE: Persistent truncus arteriosus: Classification according to anatomic types. *Surg Clin North Am* **29**:1245, 1949

102. Van Praagh R, Van Praagh S: The anatomy of common aortopulmonary trunk (truncus arteriosus communis) and its embryologic implications. A study of 57 necropsy cases. *Am J Cardiol* **16**:406, 1965

103. Richardson JV, Doty DB, Rossi MP, Ehrenhaft JL: The spectrum of anomalies of aortopulmonary septation. *J Thorac Cardiovasc Surg* **78**:21, 1979

104. Neufeld HN, Lester RG, Adams P Jr, et al: Aorticopulmonary septal defect. *Am J Cardiol* **9**:12, 1962

105. Blieden LC, Moller JA: Aortopulmonary septal defect. An experience with 17 patients. *Br Heart J* **36**:630, 1974

106. Borroughs JT, Schumutzer KJ, Linder F, Neuhans G: Anomalous origin of the right coronary artery with aortico-pulmonary window and ventricular septal defect. *J Cardiovasc Surg* **3**:142, 1968

107. Luisi SV, Ashraf MH, Gula G, et al: Anomalous origin of the right coronary artery with aortopulmonary window: Functional and surgical considerations. *Thorax* **35**:446, 1980

108. Doty DB, Richardson JV, Falkovsky GE, et al: Aortopulmonary septal defect: Hemodynamics, angiography, and operation. *Ann Thorac Surg* **32**:244, 1981

109. Meisner H, Schmidt-Habelmann P, Sebening F, Klinner W: Surgical correction of aorto-pulmonary septal defects. A review of the literature and report of eight cases. *Dis Chest* **53**:750, 1968

110. Mori K, Ando M, Takao A, et al: Distal type of aortopulmonary window. Report of 4 cases. *Br Heart J* **40**:681, 1978

111. Berry TE, Bharati S, Muster AJ, et al: Distal aortopulmonary septal defect, aortic origin of the right pulmonary artery, intact ventricular septum, patent ductus arteriosus and hypoplasia of the aortic isthmus: A newly recognized syndrome. *Am J Cardiol* **49**:108, 1982

112. Tabak C, Moskowitz W, Wagner H, et al: Aortopulmonary window and aortic isthmic hypoplasia. *J Thorac Cardiovasc Surg* **86**:273, 1983

113. Faulkner SL, Oldham RR, Atwood GF, Graham TP: Aortopulmonary window, ventricular septal defect, and membranous pulmonary atresia with a diagnosis of truncus arteriosus. *Chest* **65**:3, 1974

114. Coleman EN, Barclay RS, Reid JM, Stevenson JG: Congenital aortopulmonary fistula combined with persistent ductus arteriosus. *Br Heart J* **29**:571, 1967

115. Deverall PB, Lincoln JCR, Aberdeen E, et al: Aortopulmonary window. *J Thorac Cardiovasc Surg* **57**:479, 1969

116. Chiemmongkoltip P, Moulder PV, Cassels DE: Interruption of the aortic arch with aorticopulmonary septal defect and intact ventricular septum in a teenage girl. *Chest* **60**:324, 1971

117. Ding W-X, Su Z-K, Cao D-F, Jonas RA: One-stage repair of absence of the aortopulmonary septum and interrupted aortic arch. *Ann Thorac Surg* **49**:664, 1990

118. Jacobson JG, Trusler GA, Izukawa T: Repair of interrupted aortic arch and aortopulmonary window in an infant. *Ann Thorac Surg* **28**:290, 1979

119. Tandon R, DaSilva V, Moller JH, Edwards JE: Aorticopulmonary septal defect coexisting with ventricular septal defect. *Circulation* **50**:188, 1974

120. Castaneda AR, Kirklin JW: Tetralogy of Fallot with aorticopulmonary window. Report of two surgical cases. *J Thorac Cardiovasc Surg* **74**:467, 1977

121. Morrow AG, Greenfield LJ, Braunwald E: Congenital aortopulmonary septal defect. Clinical and hemodynamic findings, surgical technique, and results of operative correction. *Circulation* **25**:463, 1962

122. Pieroni DR, Gingell RI, Roland J-MA, et al: Two-dimensional echocardiographic recognition and surgical management of aortopulmonary septal defect in the premature infant. *Thorac Cardiovasc Surg* **30**:180, 1982

123. Satomi G, Kakamus K, Imai Y, Takao A: Two-dimensional echocardiographic diagnosis of aorticopulmonary window. *Br Heart J* **43**:351, 1980

124. Rice MJ, Seward JB, Hagler DJ, et al: Visualization of aortopulmonary window by two-dimensional echocardiography. *May Clin Proc* **57**:482, 1982
125. Balaji S, Burch M, Sullivan ID: Accuracy of cross-sectional echocardiography in diagnosis of aortopulmonary window. *Am J Cardiol* **67**:650, 1991
126. Gula G, Chew C, Radley-Smith R, Yacoub M: Anomalous origin of the right pulmonary artery from the ascending aorta associated with aortopulmonary window. *Thorax* **33**:265, 1978
127. Armer RM, Schumacker HB, Klatta EC: Origin of the right pulmonary artery from the ascending aorta. Report of a surgically corrected case. *Circulation* **24**:662, 1961
128. Keane JF, Moltz D, Bernard WF, et al: Anomalous origin of one pulmonary artery from the ascending aorta. Diagnostic, physiological and surgical considerations. *Circulation* **50**:588, 1974

129. Clarke CP, Richardson JP: The management of aorticopulmonary window. Advantages of transaortic closure with a Dacron patch. *J Thorac Cardiovasc Surg* **72**:48, 1976
130. Tiraboschi R, Salomone G, Crupi G, et al: Aortopulmonary window in the first year of life: Report on 11 surgical cases. *Ann Thorac Surg* **46**:438, 1988
131. Johansson L, Michaelsson M, Westerholm CJ, Abert T: Aortopulmonary window: A new operative approach. *Ann Thorac Surg* **28**:290, 1979
132. Kitagawa T, Katoh I, Taki H, et al: New operative method for distal aortopulmonary septal defect. *Ann Thorac Surg* **51**:680, 1991
133. Prasad TR, Valiathan MS, Shyamakrishnan KG, Venkitachalam CG: Surgical management of aortopulmonary septal defect. *Ann Thorac Surg* **47**:877, 1989

70

Atrioventricular Septal Defects

Jaroslav Stark and Gary K. Lofland

Atrioventricular (A-V) septal defects form a spectrum of anomalies ranging from a primum atrial septal defect to a complete A-V septal defect involving the atrial septum, the ventricular septum, and both A-V valves. These entities have been variously described as endocardial cushion defects or A-V canal defects because the underlying defect is a deficiency of A-V septal structures.[1] While the embryogenesis of the defects within this spectrum is similar, the clinical manifestations and natural history are different. A thorough understanding of the anatomy and physiology of these defects is essential for successful diagnosis and correction.

EMBRYOLOGY

The primitive vertebrate heart begins as a simple cylindrical tube that, at approximately 21–25 days of gestation, begins to bend and twist to eventually form the four-chamber configuration in the 4–6 mm human embryo. At this stage, the posteriorly and inferiorly located right and left atriums communicate with the ventricles through an A-V canal. The anterior and posterior margins of this canal contain islands of mesenchymal tissue that enlarge to form the endocardial cushions. These cushions grow, meet, and fuse in the 10-mm embryo and ultimately result in septation of the primitive heart and development of left and right ventricular orifices. As further growth occurs, an additional pair of endocardial cushions develops on the right and left lateral aspects of the A-V canal, eventually closing the secondary interventricular foramen and forming the inlet portion of the ventricular septum. This occurs concurrently with the development of the conus septum and further defines the outflow channels of the left and right ventricles. A portion of the mesenchyma surrounding the newly developed (A-V) orifices becomes the anterior cusp of the mitral valve on one side, and the septal leaflet of the tricuspid valve on the

other. The remainder of the A-V valve cusps is formed from the muscular ventricular wall. Although the embryogenesis of A-V septal defects has never been directly observed, an understanding can be deduced by comparing the heart's normal and pathologic anatomy.

In all A-V septal defects, there is some failure of the major endocardial cushions to fuse and develop a normal arching. Consequently, the free borders of the septum primum find nothing with which to fuse, and an interatrial communication develops. The mechanism of development of a primum A-V septal defect thus differs from the development of secundum and sinus venosus-type atrial septal defect.

ANATOMY

Anatomically, A-V septal defects can be described as partial, complete, and complete with absent interatrial communication (Fig. 70–1). Because of abnormalities involving the endocardial cushions, hearts with A-V septal defects have absence of the usual "wedge" position of the aortic valve above the A-V valves. Instead, the aortic valve is elevated and deviated anteriorly.[2–4] The left ventricular inflow tract is shortened relative to the outflow portion[2–4,15] and there is a related reduction in the length of the diaphragmatic wall of the left ventricle. The left ventricular outflow tract is also narrowed, but rarely of sufficient degree to be hemodynamically significant, so that left ventricular outflow tract obstruction is uncommon.[5–10]

The concept of ventricular dominance was introduced by Bharati and Lev.[13] Usually the common A-V junction in A-V septal defects is more or less evenly shared between the morphologically right and left ventricles. This arrangement produces a so-called *balanced* defect.[13] On occasion, the sharing of the orifice between the ventricles is unequal

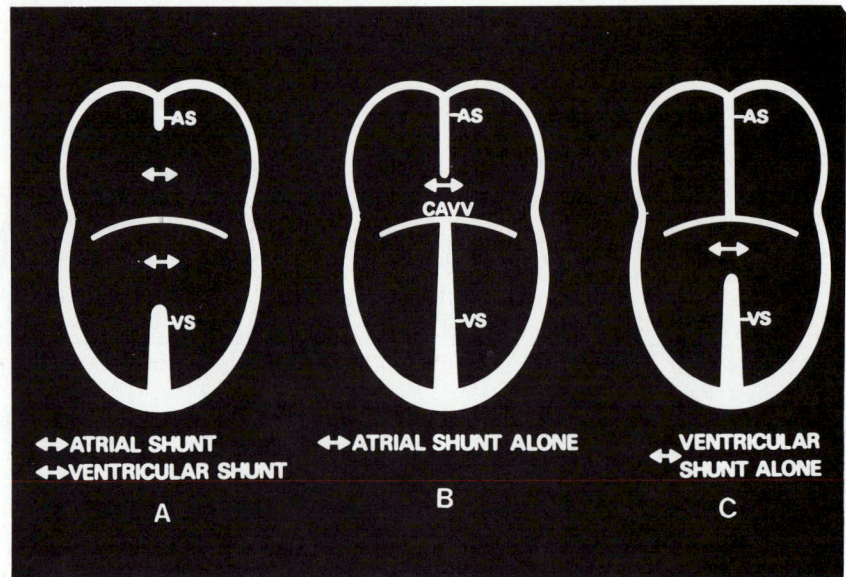

Figure 70–1. The diagram shows the physiology in patients with complete A-V septal defect (**A**), partial A-V septal defect (**B**), and complete A-V septal defect without atrial communication (**C**). AS, atrial septum; CAVV, common A-V valve; VS, ventricular septum.

and this has major prognostic significance. The inequality can favor either the right ventricle (right dominance) or the left ventricle (left dominance). When most of the junction is committed to the right ventricle, the left ventricle and the left component of the A-V valves are hypoplastic. This is associated with other left-sided abnormalities including coarctation of the aorta, hypoplastic aortic arch, and aortic stenosis. When the junction is predominantly committed to the left ventricle, the right ventricle becomes hypoplastic and may have associated pulmonary hypoplasia, pulmonary atresia, or tetralogy of Fallot.

Other anomalies are quite common with A-V septal defects.[11,12] Approximately 40–45% of patients with trisomy 21 will have an associated A-V septal anomaly.[43,44] In addition, other chromosomal anomalies may be present, and familial clustering has been reported.[15]

PARTIAL ATRIOVENTRICULAR SEPTAL DEFECT

In the partial form of A-V septal defect, the dominant anatomic features are an ostium primum type of atrial septal defect, and abnormalities of the left A-V valve. The ostium primum defect occupies the portion of the atrial septum immediately superior to the separately formed right and left A-V valves. The septal leaflets of the right A-V valves are fused to the crest of the ventricular septum and are displaced inferiorly. The left A-V valve was considered to have a cleft in the midportion of its anterior leaflet in earlier studies. The work of Carpentier,[16,17] Anderson et al,[18,19] and Ugarte et al,[20] however, has defined the left-sided valve in this defect as a three-leaflet structure. The three leaflets are more appropriately designated as left lateral, left superior, and left inferior. Consequently, there are anterolateral,

posterolateral, and septal commissures. The right-sided valve also has three leaflets that are named right superior, right lateral, and right inferior. Although in the partial A-V septal defect a ventricular component of the defect is not present, in some patients an additional ventricular septal defect unrelated to the A-V septal defect may be present.

Of obvious surgical significance is the anatomy of the conduction system. The defect in the A-V septum often displaces the coronary sinus ostium inferiorly. Consequently, the A-V node is displaced inferiorly and lies in the posterior right atrial wall over the crux of the heart, between the orifice of the coronary sinus and the ventricular crest in what has been termed the *nodal triangle*.[21] It, therefore, may not be at the tip of Koch's triangle.

Several cardiac anomalies are associated with partial A-V septal defect. Patent ductus arteriosus, complete or partial unroofed coronary sinus with a persistent left superior vena cava draining into the left atrium infrequently occur in combination with A-V canal defects. As mentioned previously, significant left ventricular outflow tract obstruction occurs rarely in A-V septal defect. Important left ventricular inflow obstruction may rarely occur from simple narrowing of the A-V valve orifice.

COMPLETE ATRIOVENTRICULAR SEPTAL DEFECT

A complete form of A-V septal defect also has a defect in the primum atrial septum. There is one A-V valve common to both right and left ventricular chambers. There are defects of the atrial septum above and ventricular septum below the common A-V valve. The common A-V valve usually has six leaflets that are termed left superior, left lateral, left inferior, right inferior, right lateral, and right superior. The left superior leaflets may form one common leaflet that bridges the crest of the ventricular septum. In 1966, Rastelli et al[22] classified the morphology of complete A-V septal defects into types A, B, and C. This typing was based on the anatomy of the left superior (anterior) bridging leaflet, and may be summarized as follows: type A, common leaflet but attached with chordae to the crest of the interventricular septum; type B, papillary muscular attachment to the left part of the common superior leaflet from the right of the septum; and type C, superior leaflet free floating without chordal attachments to the ventricular septal crest.

In complete A-V septal defect, the A-V valve orifice is always displaced apically. Occasionally, the displacement is extensive, resulting in a long, narrow left ventricular outflow tract. As in all forms of A-V septal defect, a discrepancy in the size ratio of the left and right ventricles may occur, with the left ventricle ordinarily appearing smaller than the right. In addition to the A-V nodal displacement described previously for partial A-V septal defects, there is also displacement of the His bundle and bundle branches in the complete form of A-V septal defect (Fig. 70–2). Electrophysiologic studies performed at the time of operation have demonstrated that the bundle of His passes anteriorly and superiorly from the node to the ventricular crest reaching it where the crest fuses posteriorly with the common

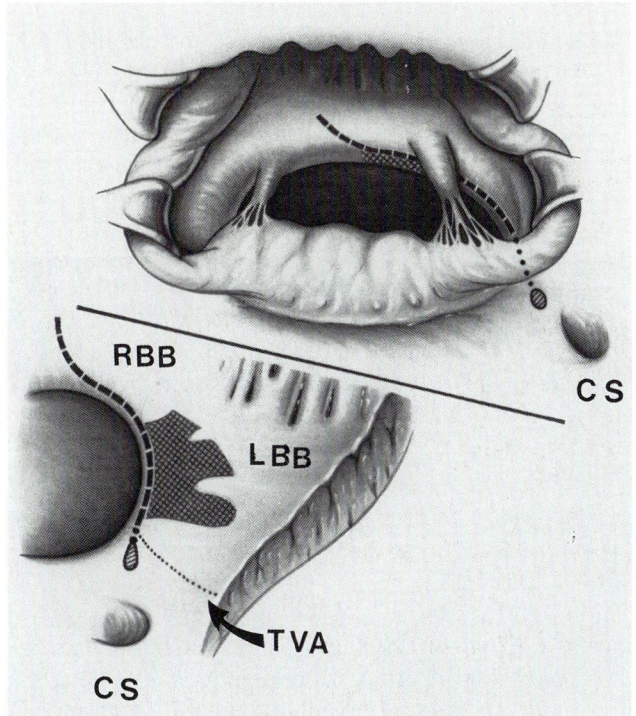

Figure 70–2. Position of conduction mechanism in A-V septal defect. Note the posterior displacement of the A-V node in relation to the coronary sinus. CS, coronary sinus; LBB, left bundle branch; RBB, right bundle branch; TVA, tricuspid (right A-V) valve annulus.

A-V valve annulus. It then travels along the crest of the ventricular septum, beneath the bridging portion of the left inferior leaflet, giving off the left bundle branches. Before it reaches the midportion of the crest of the ventricular septum it becomes the right bundle branch, which continues along the crest a bit further before it descends toward the muscle of Lancisi and moderator band. This morphology of the conduction system is a determinate of the electrocardiographic pattern usually seen in A-V septal defects.[23]

Anomalies associated with the complete form of A-V septal defect are identical to those seen in the partial form. Double outlet right ventricle with or without pulmonary stenosis uniquely complicates, however, complete A-V septal defect. Transposition of the great arteries is very rarely associated with complete A-V septal defects. Of special importance is the association of tetralogy of Fallot.[24–32] The displacement of the infundibular septum and severity of the mitral valve deformity with its associated prognostic significance will be described later in this chapter.

COMPLETE ATRIOVENTRICULAR SEPTAL DEFECT WITHOUT ATRIAL COMMUNICATION

Although rare, there exists a variant of complete A-V septal defect with all of the typical features of complete A-V septal defect with common valve orifice, but in which the primum septum is either intact or the relationship of the primum septum to the leaflets of the A-V valve is such that interatrial shunting does not occur. A well-formed atrial septum is present and is usually firmly attached to the atrial section of both the superior and inferior bridging leaflets. In addition, a secundum atrial septal defect or a patent foramen ovale may also be present. The interventricular communication is usually large and excavates the entire inlet septum. Valve morphology includes the entire spectrum of malformations known to afflict the superior bridging leaflet.[33]

DIAGNOSIS

The clinical presentation of patients with A-V septal defects is a function of the degree of left-to-right shunting and the degree of incompetence of the A-V valve. The degree of left-to-right shunt is in turn determined by the size of the atrial septal defect, the size of the ventricular septal defect, the relative compliance of the ventricles, and the relative resistances of the systemic and pulmonary vascular beds. A large left-to-right shunt is usually present with increased pulmonary blood flow. Left A-V valve regurgitation is frequently present. As a result, pulmonary vascular disease develops early. Since pressures are equal in the right and left ventricles if a large ventricular septal defect is present, pressure elevation in the pulmonary vascular bed is to be expected.

PARTIAL ATRIOVENTRICULAR SEPTAL DEFECT

The clinical manifestations of partial A-V septal defects include dyspnea, fatigue, failure to thrive, and repeated respiratory infections. If the defect is in the ostium primum alone, with no mitral regurgitation, the patient may be asymptomatic for years and show only signs of left-to-right shunt.

Physical examination in these patients reveals an active precordium with both right and left ventricular lifts or heaves. A prominent pulmonic flow murmur and wide fixed splitting of the second heart sound are present.

The *electrocardiogram* is often diagnostic, with left axis deviation, prominent P waves indicating atrial enlargement, and a prolonged PR interval. The *chest x-ray* reveals cardiac enlargement and an increased pulmonary vasculature. *Two-dimensional echocardiography* (Fig. 70–3) has proven useful in delineation of both atrial and ventricular septal defects.[34–36] Valve leaflet attachments in ostium primum defects can be distinguished easily from the complete form of A-V septal defects. Recently, transesophageal echocardiography has been demonstrated to be quite effective in the management of patients with atrioventricular septal defects, both preoperatively and intraoperatively.[37] Indeed, in patients in whom the physiology is not questioned and is consistent with physical examination (i.e., less than 6–9 months of age, large heart, and classic flow murmurs), the operation can be indicated and performed without any invasive investigation.[38]

In patients in whom the diagnosis is still questioned or who have physical and radiologic signs of increased pulmonary vascular resistance, *cardiac catheterization with angiography* is mandatory. The decreased pulmonary blood flow may be due to a high fixed pulmonary vascular resistance and thus be inoperable or due to a right-sided obstructive lesion. The exact anatomy and physiology must be precisely defined prior to attempted correction. The left ventricular angiogram is diagnostic demonstrating the characteristic "goose neck" deformity of the left ventricular outflow tract together with mitral regurgitation.[39] Although older patients have been reported,[40,41] survival is unusual beyond the age of 40 years. Dysrhythmias are common, a poor prognostic sign, and occur more frequently with advancing age.

COMPLETE ATRIOVENTRICULAR SEPTAL DEFECT

Patients with complete A-V septal defects present at an earlier age than patients with partial defects. These defects manifest themselves in early infancy, usually as severe congestive heart failure.

Patients with complete A-V septal defect also have characteristic findings on *physical examination*. These infants are usually thin, breathless, and exhibit marked precordial activity with a prominent thrill. Cyanosis is present in approximately 15%. Auscultatory findings include the following:

1. Split first heart sound due to pulmonary hypertension.
2. Holosystolic murmur along the left sternal border from the ventricular septal defect.
3. High pitched murmur from mitral insufficiency at the apex.
4. Mid-diastolic flow murmur across the common A-V valve.

Radiographically, four-chamber enlargement is present with marked pulmonary plethora. As in patients with

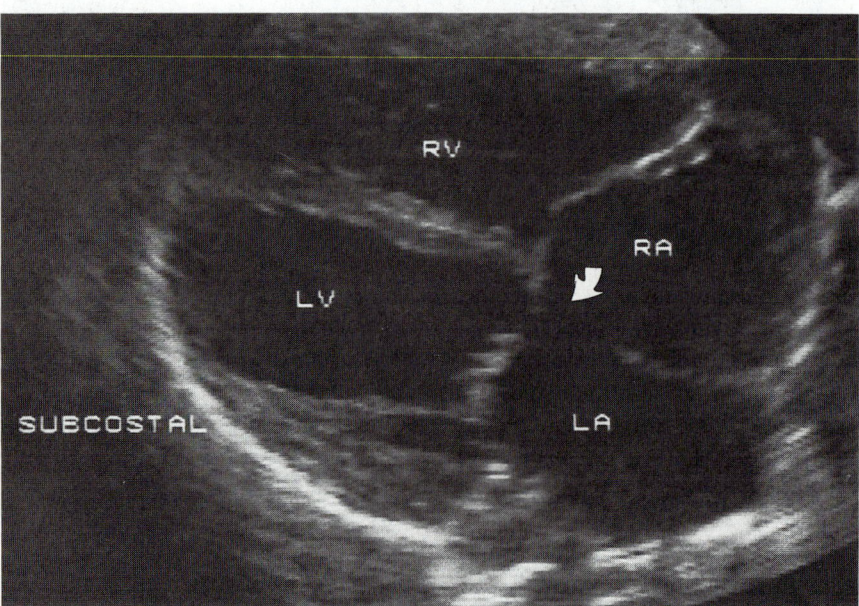

Figure 70–3. Echocardiogram (subcostal view) of partial A-V septal defect. *Arrow,* primum atrial septal defect; LA, left atrium; LV, left ventricle; RA, right atrium; RV, right ventricle.

atrial, ventricular, or A-V septal defect of all types, *two-dimensional echocardiography* has proven to be a useful diagnostic tool.[52] Two-dimensional echocardiography allows excellent visualization of septal and valve components (Fig. 70–4).[34,35,37] Of special importance is the attachment of the papillary muscles and the chordae. Two-dimensional echocardiography together with Doppler is usually sufficient for preoperative investigation of patients younger than 9–12 months. If we are concerned about the possibility of increased pulmonary arteriolar resistance, cardiac catheterization is mandatory. Some associated abnormalities may preclude biventricular repair and a Fontan-type operation may remain the only surgical option. Such patients usually require pulmonary artery banding in early infancy to protect the pulmonary vascular bed.

Cardiac catheterization demonstrates an oxygen step-up in the right atrium and the right ventricle, and pulmonary-to-systemic blood flow ratios that are usually greater than 1. *Angiography* shows a long, narrow left ventricular outflow tract with a scalloped right margin (Fig. 70–5).

Berger et al[42] quoted a 96% 5-year mortality without treatment. Their data were, however, based on necropsy material. Many patients with complete A-V septal defect have Down's syndrome. The life expectancy of a child with Down's syndrome is shorter than normal. When Down's syndrome is associated with complete A-V septal defect, survival at 10 and 15 years was 80% in the series by Bull et al.[43] There will be inevitable deterioration in exercise tolerance in late teens with the probability of premature death from pulmonary vascular disease in the third or fourth decade.

Although the suggestion that parents of children with A-V septal defect and Down's syndrome should be counseled differently from those with a chromosomally normal child with A-V septal defect contravenes the law in some countries, we believe that many parents may feel differently. We treat all patients with A-V septal defect the same way—irrespective of presence or absence of Down's syndrome.

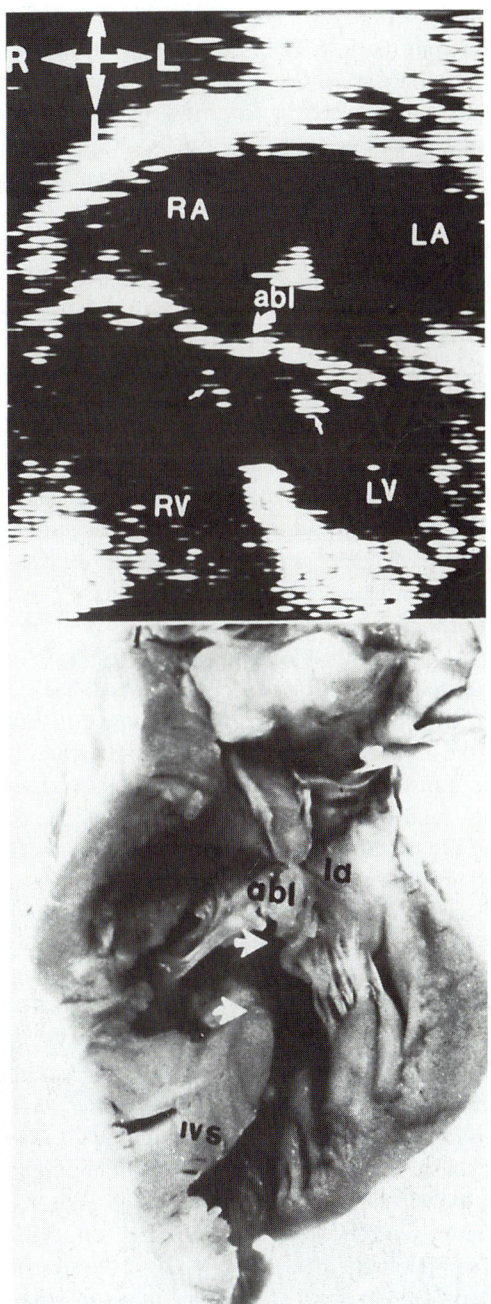

Figure 70–4. Echocardiogram and corresponding specimen from the patient with complete A-V septal defect. abl, anterior bridging leaflet; I, inferior; IVS, interventricular septum; L, left; LA, left atrium; LV, left ventricle; R, right; RA, right atrium; RV, right ventricle. The two arrows on the specimen point to the ventricular component.

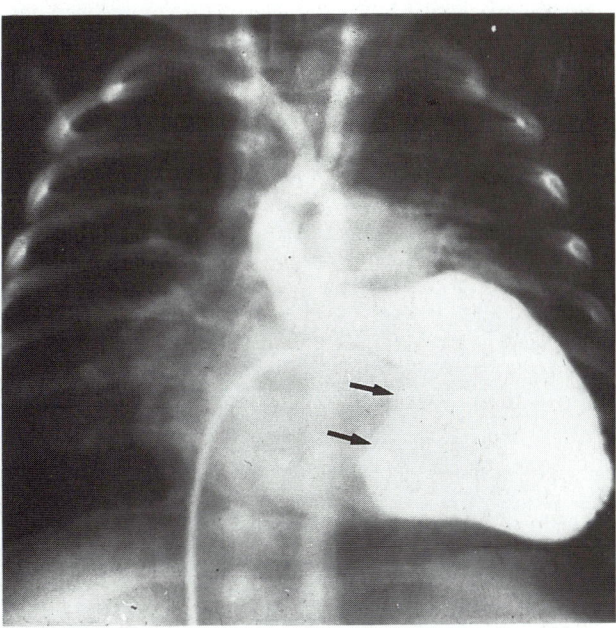

Figure 70–5. Left ventricular angiogram showing typical "goose neck" deformity of the left ventricular outflow tract.

If surgery is considered, it should be performed early before pulmonary vascular disease progresses. Currently, we recommend surgery at the age of 3–4 months. If severe symptoms are present we operate earlier. Pulmonary arteriolar resistance of more than 8–10 U/m^2 precludes surgical repair.

COMPLETE ATRIOVENTRICULAR SEPTAL DEFECT WITHOUT ATRIAL COMMUNICATION

The most accurate diagnosis is possible on *cross-sectional echocardiography* using the four-chamber view. At *cardiac catheterizaton* the diagnosis should be suspected when the atrial pressures are dissimilar or when the operator finds it difficult to enter the left atrium. Follow through of *angiogram* to the right ventricle may show an unusually good definition of the left atrium.

SURGICAL TECHNIQUE

The premedication, anesthesia, and preparation for operation do not differ from those used for other congenital heart defects. A median sternotomy is performed and a generous patch of pericardium removed and placed in heparinized saline. The ascending aorta is cannulated for arterial infusion; direct superior vena cava (SVC) and inferior vena cava (IVC) cannulation is used for venous drainage. We prefer specially designed metal venous cannulae (Fig. 70–6); alternatively, commercially available metal cannulae designed by Pacifico[45] are used. The advantage of direct cannulation is that it gives a totally unobstructed view of both atriums and the A-V valve. Bypass is commenced with cold perfusate at 25°C. Haemodilution is used; we aim for

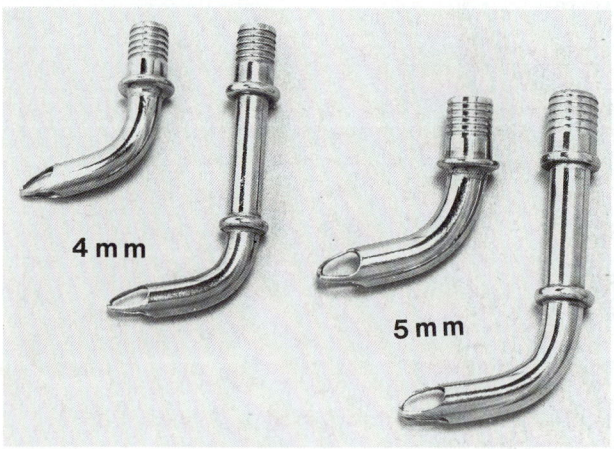

Figure 70–6. Metal venous cannulae (4 and 5 mm) used at Great Ormond Street Hospital. The longer ones are used for IVC, the shorter ones for SVC cannulation.

hematocrit of 20% on bypass. When full flow (2.4 L/m^2) is established, the perfusate is further cooled, the aim being to lower the patient's nasopharyngeal temperature to 19°–20°C. At this temperature the heart is better protected. It is also safe to reduce perfusion flow at this temperature to 1.0–1.6 L/m^2. If a persistent left SVC is present, it is advisable to place a monitoring line into the left internal jugular vein before operation. The left SVC may be occluded if the pressure in the left jugular vein does not increase above 25 mm Hg. It may be prudent to release the SVC once or twice for a short period during repair to ensure free venous drainage from the left SVC area. If the pressure after left SVC occlusion rises above 25 mm Hg, either total circulatory arrest can be used or low flow bypass with a sump sucker placed into or near the coronary sinus. Our other alternative, useful especially in older children, is the direct cannulation of the left SVC outside the heart. This is best achieved when the patient is already supported by cardiopulmonary bypass. A purse string is placed directly on the left SVC above the heart and the vein is cannulated with a short tip metal venous cannula (Fig. 70–6). When the desired flow is established, both SVC and IVC are occluded and ventilation stopped.

Alternatively, in young infants, the technique of deep hypothermia with circulatory arrest may be used. The right atrial appendage is cannulated with a venous cannula and the patient cooled on cardiopulmonary bypass to 18°–20°C (nasopharyngeal temperature). In addition, we use topical cooling, which is recommended by others.[46] Forty-five minutes of total circulatory arrest is then available for surgical repair. Some authors extend the time of "safe" circulatory arrest to 60 min but it is probably not advisable.

When the operation is performed on cardiopulmonary bypass, the aorta is cross-clamped and cold cardioplegic solution is infused into the aortic root. Various cardioplegic solutions, both crystalloid or blood, have been recommended. We use St Thomas' Hospital crystalloid cardioplegia at 20 mL/kg and repeat 10 mL/kg every 25–35 min. The right atrium is opened and cardioplegia is aspirated with a discard sucker. Technical details and rationale of our technique of cardioplegia have been described elsewhere.[47]

We open the right atrium close to the A-V groove. Inferiorly the incision extends in front of the IVC cannula. This provides an excellent approach to all structures to be visualized and repaired. Stay sutures buttressed with Teflon pledglets are placed; one is usually placed on the lateral edge of the atriotomy, the other two inside the right atrium close to the valve ring of the common A-V valve superiorly and inferiorly. The stitches are placed in rubber-shod clamps and put under gentle traction over the sternal retractor. It may also be useful to place another stay stitch on the edge of the secundum atrial septum. A sump sucker is placed into the left atrium through the ASD/PFO.

The anatomy of the A-V valve is then assessed. Cold saline is injected into the left ventricle or it is squirted from a large bulb syringe onto the valve. This will float the leaflets, show the appropriate places of coaptation, and any deficiency in the valve tissue or prolapse. Some surgeons prefer to test the valve as soon as the right atrium is opened, *before* cardioplegia is infused. More physiologic conditions with the ventricular muscle maintaining its tone may be obtained. If the heart does not fibrillate by this time, it should be fibrillated electrically to avoid air embolization during testing.

PARTIAL ATRIOVENTRICULAR SEPTAL DEFECT

The tips of the left superior and inferior leaflets are approximated with a fine monofilament suture that is not tied (Fig. 70–7). This identifies the septal commissure ("cleft"), which is then closed with interrupted sutures of 5-0 or 6-0 nonabsorbable material. In infants the sutures are buttressed with pericardial pledglets. Carpentier[16,17] has recommended that the left A-V valve should be treated as a three-leaflet valve; he does not close the septal commissure (cleft). We followed this principle for some time but several patients returned a few years later with severe left A-V valve incompetence after being well, on no medication, following initial repair. On subsequent investigation and at surgery the incompetence was entirely through the left A-V valve septal commissure (cleft). For this reason we now close the septal commissure (cleft) routinely. This is the current practice in many departments of pediatric cardiac surgery.[67,69] When the closure is completed, the size of the orifice of the left A-V valve is measured with Hegar dilators. A normal size orifice for age and weight should be created (Table 70–1). It is important to ensure that the repair of the septal commissure does not produce any valve stenosis.

TABLE 70–1. MEAN NORMAL DIAMETER OF ATRIOVENTRICULAR VALVES

BSD (m)	Mitral[a] (mm)	Tricuspid[a] (mm)
0.25	11.2	13.4
0.30	12.6	14.9
0.35	13.6	16.2
0.40	14.4	17.3
0.45	15.2	18.2
0.50	15.8	19.2
0.60	16.9	20.7
0.70	17.9	21.9
0.80	18.8	23.0
0.90	19.7	24.0
1.0	20.2	24.9
1.2	21.4	26.2
1.4	22.3	27.7
1.6	23.1	28.9
1.8	23.8	29.1
2.0	24.2	30.0

[a]The approximate standard deviations (±) are <0.3 m^2 = 1.9 mm, >0.3 m^2 = 1.6 mm; tricuspid <1.0 m^2 = 1.7 mm, >1.0 m^2 = 1.5 mm.
Data from Rowlatt et al: The quantitative anatomy of the child's heart. Pediatr Clin North Am 10:499, 1963.

The pericardial patch is then sutured to the raphe between the left and right A-V valves. Suturing with 4-0 or 5-0 monofilament material starts above the midpoint of the ventricular crest (Fig. 70–8). An over-and-over or continuous running mattress stitch is used. The first arm of the suture attaches the patch toward the annulus of the superior leaflet, the other one inferiorly toward the coronary sinus.

Inferiorly, two alternative techniques can be used. The

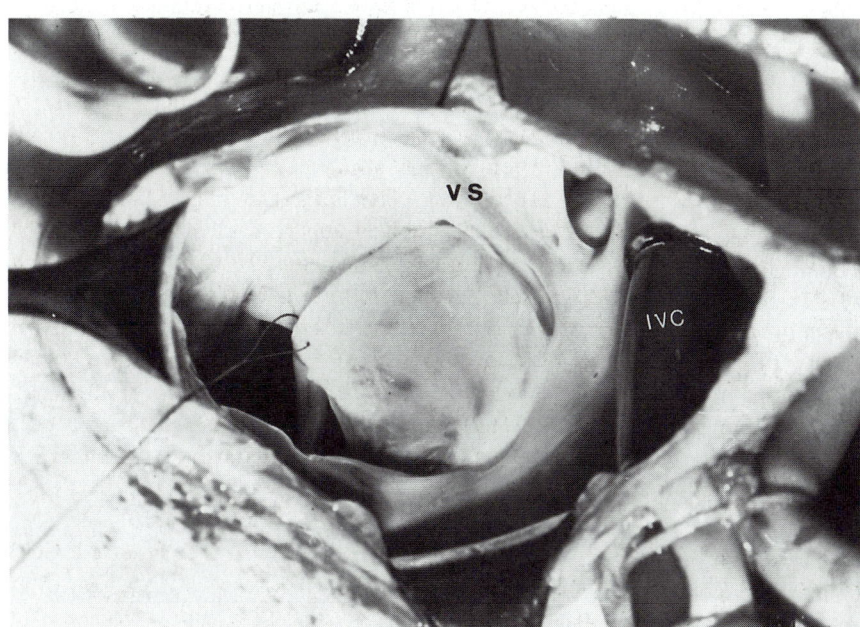

Figure 70–7. Operative view of a partial A-V septal defect. The stitch approximates the tip of the septal commissure (cleft). IVC, IVC cannulae; VS, ventricular septum.

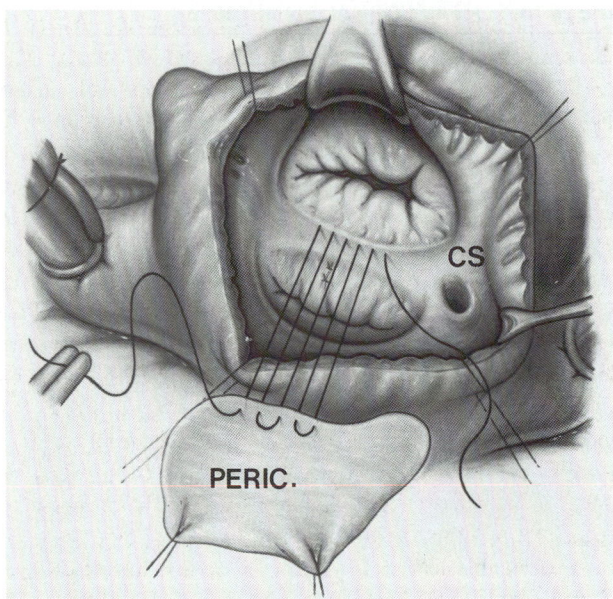

Figure 70–8. Septal commissure (cleft) is closed with two stitches. Pericardial patch is being attached with a running stitch of monofilament between the insertion of the right and left A-V valves. peric., pericardial patch; CS, coronary sinus.

suture line may be continued toward the right up onto the right atrial wall well behind the coronary sinus (between the orifice of the coronary sinus and the orifice of the IVC) until it reaches the edge of the interatrial septum. The coronary sinus is thus transferred into the left atrium; the minimal venous admixture is well tolerated and is not detected oximetrically on postoperative study. Using this technique the patch has to be tailored appropriately so that it balloons adequately over the orifice of the coronary sinus (Fig. 70–8).

Alternatively, the suture line attaching the pericardial patch to the crest between the right and left inferior leaflets moves to the left atrial wall and the patch is attached to the base of the left inferior leaflet. This suture line is to the left of the coronary sinus, which is left to drain into the right atrium. This is currently our technique of choice.

Both techniques described should safely avoid any damage to the conduction system. Simple running sutures complete the attachment of the patch to the atrial septum. Rewarming is now started. Before the patch is completed, the vent is removed from the left atrium, the foramen ovale is closed, and the air is removed from the left atrium. The aortic needle vent is placed on suction and the aortic clamp is removed. When the heart starts beating, the aorta is temporarily occluded and the lungs inflated while suction is maintained on the aortic needle vent. The right atrium is closed, caval tapes are released, and the right atrial pressure increased to 5 mm Hg. Routine deairing maneuvers are then repeated.

A left atrial pressure line may be inserted through a purse string at the base of the right upper pulmonary vein or through the right atrial appendage and through the atrial

septum. In most patients with partial A-V septal defect, monitoring the right atrial pressure or central venous pressure is adequate for postoperative management. When the patient is fully rewarmed, bypass is discontinued in the usual manner and intracardiac pressures are measured. Modified ultrafiltration is then carried out[48] to increase the hematocrit to 38–42%. Protamine is given, atrial and ventricular pacemaker wires are inserted, and pericardial and mediastinal drains are placed. The sternum is closed in the usual manner.

COMPLETE ATRIOVENTRICULAR SEPTAL DEFECT

Testing of the common A-V valve is the same as described in the previous section (Fig. 70–9). A fine suture is placed through the kissing edge of the tips of the left superior and left inferior leaflets. The size of the ventricular septal defect (VSD) is assessed. If we are not sure about the communication under the superior or inferior common leaflet, a fully curved dissector is passed from the left or the right side to see if the space under the leaflet is obliterated by fibrous tissue or dense chordae. Sometimes short secondary chordae obstruct the view of the VSD and make the attachment of the VSD patch difficult. Such chordae can be safely cut; the chordae attached to the margins of the leaflet must be preserved.

Two techniques have been used for the repair of complete A-V septal defect: a one-patch technique developed at

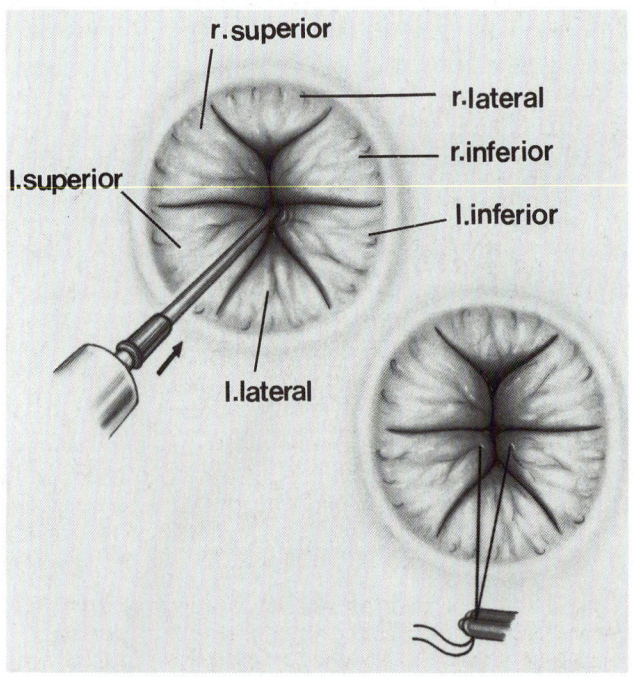

Figure 70–9. Testing the common A-V valve. A fine stay stitch approximates left superior and left inferior leaflet.

the Mayo Clinic[22] and the two-patch technique suggested by Carpentier.[17]

TWO-PATCH TECHNIQUE

This technique was proposed by Carpentier[17] and is currently our technique of choice. Its advantage is the fact that the superior bridging leaflet is not divided and that the pericardium is used for the atrial part of the repair. We use the technique as described by Pacifico.[45] After assessing the morphology of the common A-V valve, the superior bridging leaflet is retracted and the VSD is visualized (Fig. 70–10a). Retraction of the inferior bridging leaflet may be more difficult because often short dense chordae are present. If the chordae are very dense, a communication between them may be minimal; in such a case a small residual shunt in this area may be accepted in preference to difficult suturing that may damage the conduction system. Alterna-

tively, the inferior bridging leaflet is divided and treated in the same was as described in the one-patch technique. The VSD patch is tailored and attached to the right side of the interventricular septum (Fig. 70–10b,c). Interrupted mattress stitches buttressed with pledglets or a running stitch can be used. If a running stitch is used, each arm is placed in a rubber shod clamp when it comes through the annulus of the superior and inferior bridging leaflets. The exact position of suturing in the inferior corner is illustrated in Figure 70–11a,b. The top edge of the patch is then sutured to the middle of the bridging leaflets (Fig. 70–12). The suture is placed through the VSD patch, then the valve leaflet, and through the pericardial patch insert (Fig. 70–12). Either interrupted mattress sutures are used or, as illustrated in Figure 70–12a, a running suture with 5-0 or 6-0 prolene is used. If the inferior bridging leaflet was divided, the same technique as described for the one-patch technique is used to reattach this leaflet. The septal commissure ("cleft") is closed next. We use mattress sutures of 5-0 or 6-0 Ettibond, buttressed with pericardial pledglets. Two or three stitches are usually required. The valve orifice is then measured with Hegar dilators and compared to the tables for the appropriate size. One should always avoid creating a stenotic orifice. The valve is then tested. A small central leak is usu-

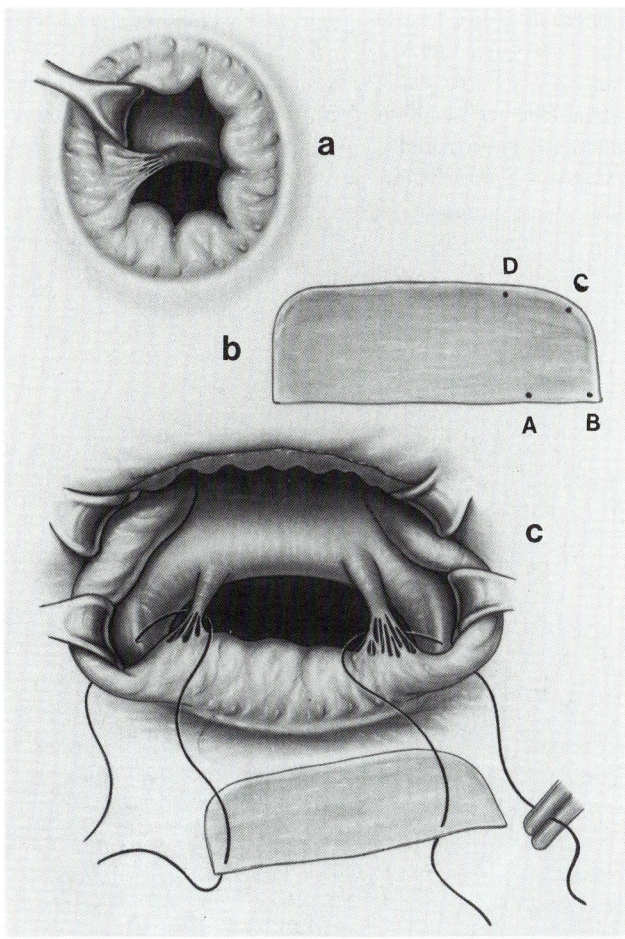

Figure 70–10. Insertion of a VSD patch. The anatomy is visualized (**A**) and patch measured and cut (**B**). One stitch is then passed through the edge of the patch and through the tip of the patch and through the annulus of the left-sided valve near the aorta. The other one is placed through the insertion of the left-sided valve in front of the coronary sinus (**C**).

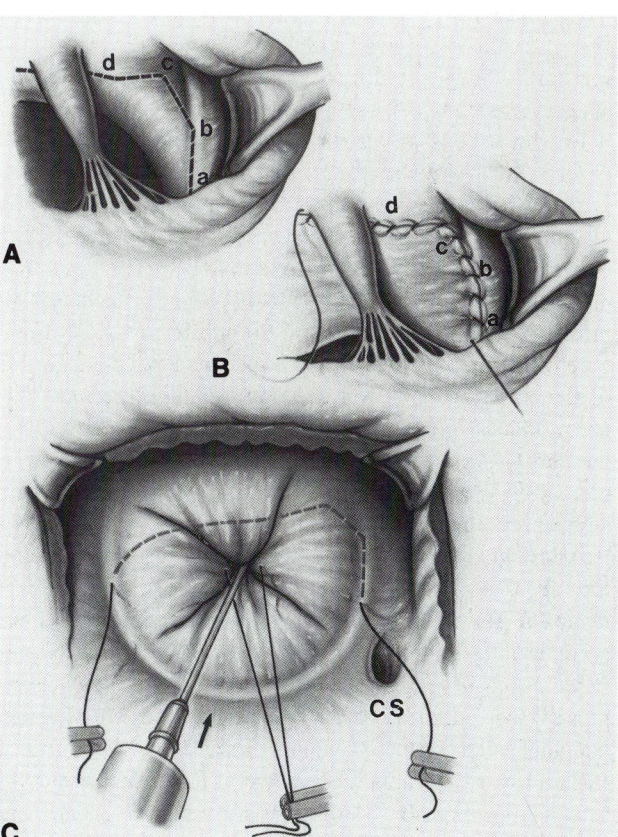

Figure 70–11. Suturing the VSD patch in the inferior corner. Position of the suture line is shown in **A;** patch completed in the inferior corner (**B**). **C** shows the testing of the valve.

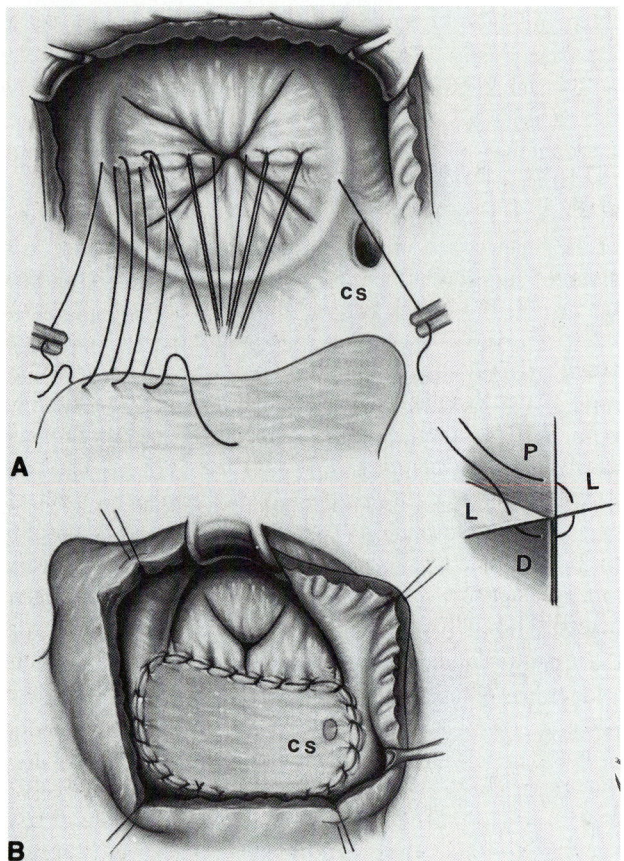

Figure 70–12. A. Closure of atrial septal defect with a pericardial patch. Mattress sutures are placed through the VSD patch, through the A-V valve leaflet, and then through the pericardial patch. **B.** Completion of the ASD patch leaving the coronary sinus (CS) to drain to the left atrium.

ally insignificant: it will disappear when the heart regains tone after removal of the aortic clamp.

The pericardial patch is now tailored according to the intended technique of suturing around the coronary sinus. One of the two techniques described under the section on partial A-V septal defect is used to close the atrial septal defect. Figure 70–12 illustrates the technique, which leaves the coronary sinus to drain into the left atrium. Currently, the author places the sutures through the base of the left-sided inferior leaflet. This leaves the coronary sinus to drain into the right atrium (Fig. 70–15). The aortic cross-clamp is then removed and rewarming is started. The heart is reperfused for 2–3 min and the aortic clamp is reapplied. At this point final testing of the left-sided A-V valve is carried out. If we are satisified with its repair, the aortic clamp is removed, the left atrial vent advanced into the left ventricle, and attachment of the atrial part of the patch is completed. If the heart action is very vigorous at this point, it may be safer to fibrillate the heart electrically or cross-clamp the aorta to avoid air embolization. The left atrium is filled with blood or saline, and the lungs are inflated to remove any residual left atrial air. The suture on the atrial patch is then tied. The aortic needle vent is placed on suction, the fibrilla-

tor (or aortic cross-clamp) removed, and deairing of the heart is repeated in the usual fashion. The patient is rewarmed and the right atriotomy closed. A left atrial pressure line is inserted, caval snares are released, and deairing is again repeated. Two atrial and two ventricular pacemaker wires are placed. When the patient is completely rewarmed and all air has been evacuated from the heart, perfusion is gradually discontinued. Modified ultrafiltration[48] is started, increasing the hematocrit to 38–40%. Intracardiac pressures are then measured; the cannulae are removed from the heart and protamine given. Insertion of chest drains and closure of the sternotomy complete the operation.

ONE-PATCH TECHNIQUE

The superior common leaflet (bridging leaflet) is divided in the middle to the annulus of the valve (Fig. 70–13). It may be advantageous to divide it 1–2 mm to the right; this provides slightly more tissue for the reconstruction of the left-sided valve. When the valve is eventually reattached onto the patch, it will not be deficient and good competence of the left A-V valve will be achieved. The inferior bridging leaflet is then cut in the same fashion. A patch of Gore-Tex is then measured and tailored. It is attached to the right side of the interventricular septum staying 3–5 mm away from the crest of the septum. A 4-0 or 5-0 monofilament suture buttressed with one Teflon pledglet is placed through the septum and the patch. One arm of this suture then attaches the patch with a continuous suture toward the aortic end of the septum; the other arm is used to attach the patch on the inferior side.

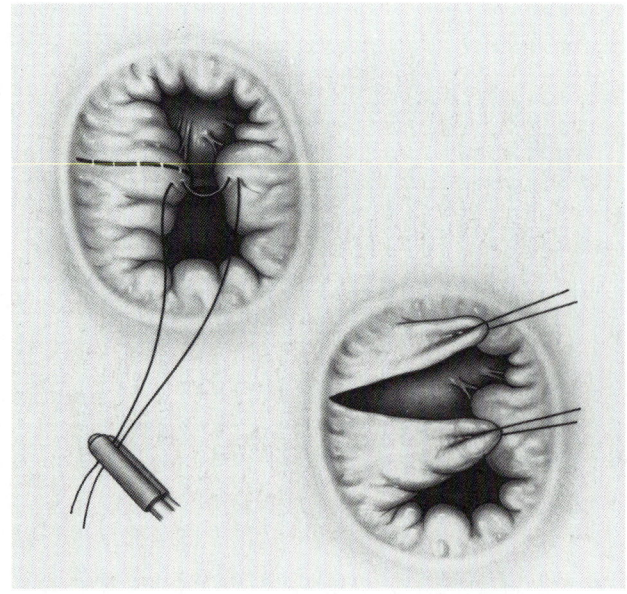

Figure 70–13. Superior leaflet is divided. Stay stitches are placed on both sides. *(From Stark J, de Leval M: Surgery for congenital heart defects, 2nd edition. Philadelphia, WB Saunders, 1994, p 384, with permission.)*

The valve is then reattached onto the patch. It is important to assess carefully the extent of the deficiency in the ventricular septum so that the valve is attached at an appropriate level (Fig. 70–14). Moving the valve with forceps and looking at the length of the chordae are helpful. Disruption of the suture attaching the valve to the patch has been described, especially when the valve tissue is very fine, as is the case in young infants. For this reason we prefer to reattach the valve with small pledglets. Currently, the authors prefer pledglets made from the patient's own pericardium. Fine 5-0 or 6-0 sutures are passed through the edge of the pericardium on the left side, through the edge of the left superior leaflet, the patch, the right superior leaflet, and the right-sided pericardium, the right superior leaflet, the patch, the left superior leaflet, and the edge of the left pericardium. Only then is a small piece of pericardium around the stitch on both sides cut to form a pledglet. Both superior and inferior leaflets are so reattached onto the patch.

The stay stitch placed previously on the edge of the left superior and inferior leaflets is now put on slight tension. This demonstrates clearly the extent of the septal commissure (cleft), which is then closed with interrupted sutures of 5-0 or 6-0 buttressed with pericardial pledglets. The valve is then tested by injecting saline into the left ventricle. A small amount of incompetence is accepted because it is likely that it will disappear when the heart regains its tone. Further testing may be done later after temporarily removing the aortic cross-clamp.

Closure of the primum ASD is then performed using the same technique as described for a two-patch technique. The coronary sinus is left usually on the right atrial side

(Fig. 70–15). Closure of the right atrium, deairing, termination of perfusion, and modified ultrafiltration do not differ from the technique described under "two-patch repair."

REPAIR OF TETRALOGY OF FALLOT WITH COMPLETE A-V SEPTAL DEFECT

Tetralogy of Fallot is present in nearly 10% of patients with A-V septal defect and is especially common in patients with Down's syndrome. The left superior leaflet markedly bridges the ventricular septal crest and the large interventricular communication beneath it extends anteriorly and superiorly into the subaortic position.[50] The right ventricular outflow tract has the typical tetralogy morphology with obstruction due to anterior–superior displacement of the infundibular septum. The latter differentiates it from cases of complete A-V septal defect with simple pulmonary valvular stenosis. The electrocardiogram characteristically demonstrates left anterior hemiblock in association with right ventricular hypertrophy. On two-dimensional echocardiography, the short-axis scans demonstrate clearly the tetralogy component, and the apical four-chamber scan shows the A-V septal defect portion with the bridging superior leaflet. Diagnosis may be confirmed by left and right heart cineangiography, which, in addition to the atrial and ventricular septal defects and right ventricular outflow tract obstruction, demonstrates the gooseneck deformity of the left ventricular outflow tract, and downward displacement of the superior leaflet of the common A-V valve. It also demonstrates any stenoses in the pulmonary artery and its peripheral branches.

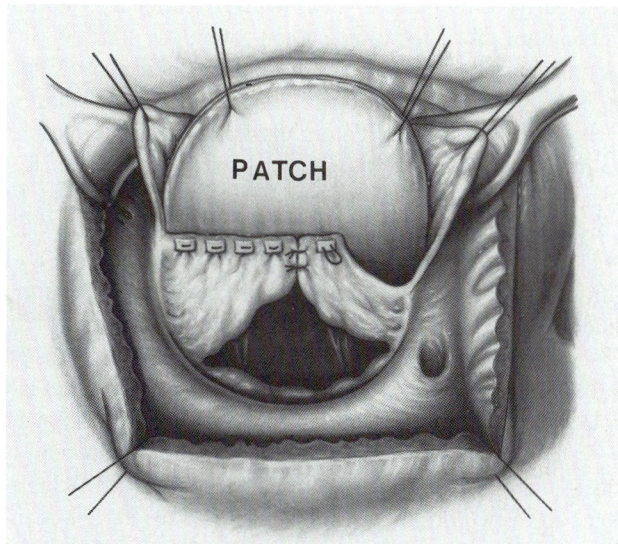

Figure 70–14. Reattachment of the valve onto the patch. Both the left- and right-sided part of the A-V valve are reattached. Small pericardial pledglets may be used to reinforce the sutures. *(From Stark J, de Leval M: Surgery for congenital heart defects, 2nd edition. Philadelphia, WB Saunders, 1994, p 385, with permission.)*

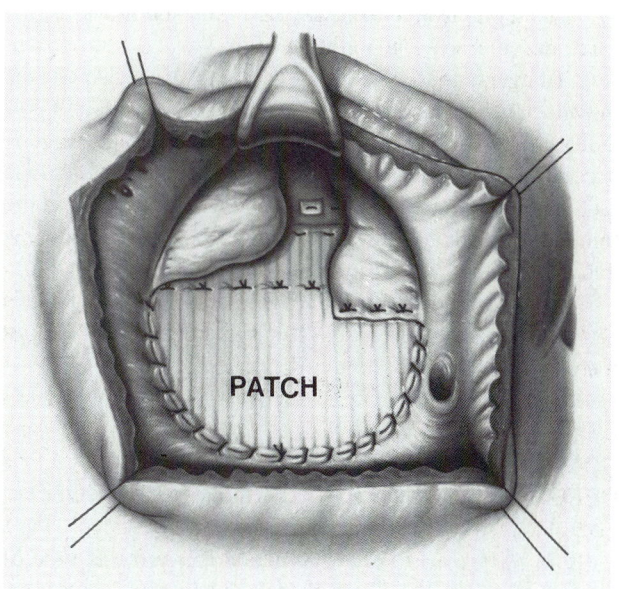

Figure 70–15. Operation using one-patch technique is completed. Note the position of the patch in front of the coronary sinus. *(From Stark J, de Leval M: Surgery for congenital heart defects, 2nd edition. Philadelphia, WB Saunders, 1994, p 385, with permission.)*

Precise preoperative diagnosis of this combination of anomalies is critical for careful planning of the surgical repair. From the cineangiogram, appropriate measurements must be made to determine that the right and left pulmonary arteries are of sufficient size. If they are small, a Blalock–Taussig shunt should be created to allow them to enlarge and total repair should be delayed until after 3–5 years of age.[46] Because the pulmonary vascular bed is protected by the pulmonary stenosis, there is no urgency to operate in infancy. If placement of a valved conduit is required, it is easier to perform the operation after the age of 2–3 years. Decisions for infundibulectomy, and pulmonary valvotomy, pulmonary artery patching (transannular or partial), and conduit placement are made preoperatively.

Complete repair is accomplished on cardiopulmonary bypass as previously described. After systemic to pulmonary shunts are closed, a right atriotomy is performed. The A-V valve is inspected and tested as described in the previous section. Infundibulectomy and techniques to relieve the pulmonary stenosis are performed as required. We prefer to close the VSD and relieve subpulmonary obstruction using a transatrial approach. Only occasionally is a short ventriculotomy required. The single or two-patch technique may be used to repair the atrial and ventricular septal defects.[24,26,28,49,53] In this combination of anomalies, however, the interventricular communication is larger and extends anteriorly up to the root of the dextraposed aorta. The ventricular septal defect patch, therefore, must be constructed differently from that used in complete A-V septal defect alone. The patch has to be enlarged in the superior part to have enough material to suture around the aortic valve annulus. Too small a patch may produce left ventricular outflow tract obstruction.

The septal leaflets are attached to the ventricular septal patch and the left- and right-sided A-V valves are reconstructed as previously described. The "cleft" is also closed. Incompetence of both right-sided valves (tricuspid and pulmonary) may be poorly tolerated. If the pulmonary valve is excised and the tricuspid valve is also incompetent, it is preferable to place an aortic or pulmonary homograft in the right ventricular outflow rather than to use a simple outflow tract patch.

After completion of the total repair, the patient is rewarmed, bypass is gradually discontinued, and the sternum is closed as described previously.

COMPLETE ATRIOVENTRICULAR SEPTAL DEFECT WITHOUT ATRIAL COMMUNICATION

Early in our experience when we encountered this type of A-V septal defect unexpectedly at operation, repair was attempted by resecting the atrial septum and thus converting the defect into a complete form of A-V septal defect. A standard one-patch technique was then used. Two of the three patients operated by this method required reoperation

for severe left A-V valve incompetence despite having had a competent valve before the operation.

The technique of repair was subsequently modified.[33] The left-sided components of the A-V valve are inspected, tested, and repaired through a secundum ASD when present, or through an incision in the fossa ovalis if the interatrial communication is absent. The superior and inferior bridging leaflets are retracted with stay sutures and the VSD is closed with a patch. The top edge of the VSD patch is then sutured to the bridging leaflet. Because the plane of the ventricular septum is to the right of the atrial septum, it is also necessary to obliterate the left ventricle to right atrial communication by approximation of the left superior and inferior bridging leaflets between their attachments to the atrial septum and the VSD patch.

Currently, we prefer the two-patch technique for complete A-V septal defect repair. If the visualization of the interventricular communication under the left superior bridging leaflet is difficult because of numerous chordae, we do not hesitate to divide the leaflet and use either one or two patches. Good results have been reported using a single patch[54–57,67] as well as the two-patch technique.[16,58,59,66,70]

POSTOPERATIVE CARE

The postoperative care of patients undergoing correction of A-V septal defect differs little from that of other patients undergoing intracardiac corrective procedures with one important exception. Patients with a complete form of A-V septal defect develop increased pulmonary arteriolar resistance early. Some have a very reactive pulmonary vascular bed and are prone to pulmonary hypertensive crises during the postoperative period. All patients with increased pulmonary arteriolar resistance receive phenoxybenzamine (1 mg/kg body weight) before cardiopulmonary bypass is started. The same dose is repeated during rewarming. Reduced dose (0.5 mg/kg) is then given intravenously at 12 hourly intervals until the extubation. If pulmonary hypertension persists or hypertensive crisis develops, infusion of nitroglycerin or prostacyclin is started. More recently nitric oxide has been used very successfully in this situation.[60]

All patients return to the intensive care unit intubated and ventilated. We monitor arterial, central venous, and left atrial pressures. In patients at risk of developing pulmonary hypertensive crises, a pulmonary artery monitoring line is placed through the right ventricular outflow tract. All patients have two atrial and two ventricular pacing wires inserted to allow sequential pacing.

Hemodynamically, the patients are managed at the lowest central venous or left atrial pressure consistent with good cardiac output. The adequacy of cardiac output is judged clinically by peripheral/central temperature, volume of peripheral pulses, urinary output, acid–base status, and arteriovenous oxygen difference. With the monitoring as described above, cardiac output can also be measured.

FIO_2 is gradually reduced to 0.4. The aim is to maintain an arterial PO_2 of over 100 mm Hg and a PCO_2 below 35 mm Hg. The exception to this principle is patients with reactive pulmonary vasculature. In such patients we aim to keep the PO_2 over 150 mm Hg because of the pulmonary vasodilatory effect of high oxygen concentrations. For this reason a higher FIO_2 is often used. If patients do not exhibit signs of pulmonary hypertensive crises, they are weaned off the ventilator and extubated when all organ subsystems are stable. This is usually after 12–24 hours.

Patients with reactive pulmonary vasculature constitute a special group. Pulmonary hypertensive crises are defined as a sudden increase in pulmonary artery and right ventricular pressures accompanied by a fall in systemic pressure. The pulmonary artery pressure may rise to suprasystemic levels.[61] Because of the high mortality associated with pulmonary hypertensive crises, the patients are carefully monitored and preventively treated with fentanyl anesthesia. Fentanyl infusion is continued in the intensive care unit. Phenoxybenzamine is also used routinely. If pulmonary hypertensive crises occur, the patient is immediately hyperventilated with 100% oxygen. This is usually the most effective step in reversing the rise in pulmonary artery pressure and drop in the systemic pressure. Other drugs include calcium chloride injection, nitroglycerin (2–8 mg/kg), and prostacyclin (10–20 mg/kg per min). If catecholamine support is required, isoprenaline and Dobutamine are preferred to dopamine; dopamine is used in low doses only (2–5 µg/kg per min). More recently, excellent results have been achieved with nitric oxide therapy.[60]

The fentanyl infusion is continued and the patient is usually paralyzed. When tolazoline and/or prostacyclin is used, H_2 receptor antagonists such as ranitidine or cimetidine are used to avoid gastrointestinal bleeding.

The treatment described above is usually continued for 48–72 hours. Paralyzing is then stopped, fentanyl reduced, and an attempt is made to wean the patient from the ventilator. Drugs are discontinued later.

RESULTS

Studer and colleagues[62] reviewed 310 patients who underwent repair of A-V septal defects between 1967 and 1982. Significant incremental risk factors for hospital death were earlier date of operation, younger age at operation, increase in severity of preoperative A-V valve incompetence, increased level of preoperative functional class, presence of interventricular communication, and presence of accessory valve orifices.

Because of detailed knowledge of the A-V conduction system, the risk of complete heart block has been minimized[51] although sinus and A-V nodal abnormalities have been noted on electrophysiologic studies.[63] Independent incremental risk factors for premature sudden death have been identified as severe preoperative left A-V valve incompetence, poor preoperative status, accessory A-V valve orifice, and Down's syndrome.[57]

In a series of 199 patients from the Mayo Clinic with partial A-V septal defect, late survival rates were 98% at 1 year and 96% at 20 years. Reoperation was necessary in 18 patients, one for left A-V valve incompetence and three for subaortic stenosis. The need for reoperation correlated with the severity of the postrepair mitral insufficiency.[64]

Because of the increased severity of the valvular involvement and earlier development of pulmonary vascular disease, patients with complete A-V septal defects have less gratifying results than patients with partial A-V septal defects.[71]

Hospital mortality of 16–30% was reported in earlier years (Berger et al,[42] 9/39, 20%; Chin et al,[55] 13/43, 40%; Merrill et al,[65] 17/103, 16%). Survival rates are not influenced by the presence of Down's syndrome (Rizzolli et al,[44] Hanley et al,[66] our own experience). Improving the techniques of perfusion, details of surgical technique, postoperative care, and operating earlier before severe increase in pulmonary resistance develops improved the results. We have compared 56 patients (Group A) operated during 1988–1991 to 68 patients (Group B) operated 1991–1994. Of patients in Group A 25% were younger than 6 months as opposed to 45% in Group B. Down's syndrome was present in 50 and 61% in Groups A and B, respectively. Hospital mortality was 13/56 (23%) in Group A compared to 1/68 (1.4%) in Group B. Late mortality was similar in both groups (4–2.9%). A similar trend was observed by Hanley et al.[66] Mortality rate was 35% before 1976 and 3% after 1987 in a group of 301 patients. Hospital mortality of 7.7% (6/78) during 1986–1990 was reported by Capouya et al.[67]

Repair of the left-sided A-V valve remains a problem. Hanley reported a 7% incidence of reoperations for valve-related problems. In our overall series (1988–1994) 7 patients out of 124 operated required left-sided valve replacement (6%). Three out of 7 died (42%). Kadoba et al[68] reported 12% replacement of left AV valve in patients with AV septal defect during the 1973–1987 period. There were 7 early and 4 late deaths.

Routine closure of the septal commissure (cleft) and frequent use of annuloplasty are recommended by Capouya et al[67] and Cobanaglu.[69] This is also our current practice.

In patients with A-V septal defects without an atrial component, operative mortality is higher compared to those with complete A-V septal defects. In the combined experience of our unit and the University of Alabama at Birmingham (1972–1982),[33] the diagnosis was made at operation in 10 patients. In three, the atrial septum was resected converting the anatomy into a complete A-V septal defect with interatrial communication. Two patients required reoperation for severe left A-V valve incompetence, and one of these died. Five patients operated on more recently had the defect repaired through the patent foramen ovale or through an incision in the atrial septum. One, who had additional muscular VSD, developed heart block and died in low cardiac output. Thus, 2 of 10 operated patients died.

In patients with unbalanced defects, surgical options are more limited. Patients with a small left ventricle are probably most appropriately treated as a variant of hypoplastic left heart syndrome. Other left-sided structures, including the subaortic region, aortic annulus, and ascending aorta, are frequently small, and there is also frequently a coarctation of the aorta. The possibility of ultimately building toward a Fontan-type circulation is guarded, primarily because of coexistent pulmonary vascular disease. Pulmonary artery banding has to be performed in early infancy to protect the pulmonary vascular bed.

REFERENCES

1. Wilcox BR, Anderson RH (eds): *Surgical Anatomy of the Heart.* New York, Raven Press, 1985
2. Goor DA, Lillehei CW: Atrioventricular canal malformations. In: Goor DA, Lillehei CW (eds): *Congenital Malformations of the Heart.* New York, Grune & Stratton, 1975, pp 132–153
3. Piccoli GP, Gerlis LM, Wilkinson JL, et al: Morphology and classification of complete atrioventricular defects. *Br Heart J* 42:633–639, 1979
4. Van Mierop LHS, Alley RD, Kausel HW, Stranahan A: The anatomy and embryology of endocardial cushion defects. *J Thorac Cardiovasc Surg* 43:71–83, 1962
5. Piccoli GA, Wilkinson JL, Macartney FJ, et al: Left-sided obstructive lesions in atrioventricular septal defects. *J Thorac Cardiovasc Surg* 83:453–460, 1982
6. DeBiase L, DiCionno C, Ballerini L, et al: Prevalence of left-sided obstruction in patients with atrioventricular canal without Down's syndrome. *J Thorac Cardiovasc Surg* 86:467, 1986
7. Ebels T, Ho SY, Anderson RH, et al: The surgical anatomy of the left ventricular outflow tract in atrioventricular septal defect. *Ann Thorac Surg* 41:483–488, 1985
8. Grow RM, Freedom RM, Williams WG, et al. Coarctation of the aorta or subaortic stenosis with atrioventricular septal defect. *Am J Cardiol* 53:1421–1428, 1984
9. Wright JS, Newman DC: Complete and intermediate atrioventricular canal in infants less than a year old: Observation of anatomic and pathologic variants in left ventricular outflow tract. *Ann Thorac Surg* 33:171, 1982
10. Heydavian M, Griffith BP, Zuberbuhler JR: Partial atrioventricular canal associated with discrete subaortic stenosis. *Am Heart J* 109:915, 1985
11. Alfieri O, Plokker M: Repair of common atrioventricular canal associated with transposition of the great arteries and left ventricular outflow obstruction. *J Thorac Cardiovasc Surg* 84:872–875, 1982
12. McGrath LB, Kirklin JW, Soto B, Bargaron LM: Secondary left atrioventricular valve replacement in atrioventricular septal (AV canal) defect: A method to avoid left ventricular outflow tract obstruction. *J Thorac Cardiovasc Surg* 89:632, 1985
13. Bharati S, Lev M: The spectrum of common atrioventricular orifice (canal). *Am Heart J* 86:553–561, 1973
14. Anderson RH, Ho SV, Rigby MC, Becker AE: A morphologic overview. In: Moulton AL (ed): *Congenital Heart Surgery—Current Techniques and Controversies.* Pasadena, CA, Appleton-Davies, 1984, pp 121–135
15. Tennant SN, Hammon JW Jr, Bender HW, et al: Familial clustering of atrioventricular canal defects. *Am Heart J* 108:175, 1984
16. Carpentier A: Mitral valve reconstruction in children. In: Anderson RH, Macartney FJ, Shinebourne EA, Tynan M (eds): *Paediatric Cardiology,* Vol 5. Edinburgh, Churchill Livingstone, 1983, pp 361–368
17. Carpentier A: Surgical anatomy and management of the mitral component of atrioventricular canal defects. In: Anderson RH, Shinebourne EA (eds): *Paediatric Cardiology,* Edinburgh, Churchill Livingstone, 1977, p 477
18. Anderson RH, Zuberbuhler JR, Penkoske PA, Neches WH: Of clefts, commissures and things. *J Thorac Cardiovasc Surg* 90:605–610, 1984
19. Penkoske PA, Neches WH, Anderson RH, Zuberbuhler JR: Further observations on the morphology of atrioventricular septal defects. *J Thorac Cardiovasc Surg* 90:611–622, 1985
20. Ugarte M, De Salamanca FE, Quero M: Endocardial cushion defects. An anatomical study of 54 specimens. *Br Heart J* 38:674–682, 1976
21. Thiene G, Wenink ACG, Frescura C, et al: The surgical anatomy of the conduction tissues in atrioventricular defects. *J Thorac Cardiovasc Surg* 82:923–937, 1981
22. Rastelli GC, Kirklin JW, Titus JL: Anatomic observations on complete form of persistent common atrioventricular canal with special reference to atrioventricular valves. *Mayo Clin Proc* 41:296–308, 1966
23. Feldt RH, DuShane JW, Titus JL: The atrioventricular conduction system in persistent common atrioventricular canal defect: Correlations with electrocardiogram. *Circulation* 42:437–444, 1970
24. Bastos P, de Leval M, Macartney F, Stark J: Correction of Type C atrioventricular canal associated with tetralogy of Fallot. *Thorax* 33:646–648, 1978
25. Guo-wei H, Mee RB: Complete atrioventricular canal associated with tetralogy of Fallot, or double-outlet right ventricle and right ventricular outflow tract obstruction: A report of successful surgical treatment. *Ann Thorac Surg* 41:612–616, 1986
26. Uretzky G, Puga FJ, Danielson GK, et al: Complete atrioventricular canal associated with tetralogy of Fallot. *J Thorac Cardiovasc Surg* 87:756–766, 1984
27. Vouhe PR, Neveux JY: Surgical repair of tetralogy of Fallot with complete atrioventricular canal. *Ann Thorac Surg* 41:342–344, 1986
28. Nath PH, Soto B, Bini RM, et al: Tetralogy of Fallot with atrioventricular canal. *J Thorac Cardiovasc Surg* 87:421–430, 1984
29. Bharati S, Kirklin JW, McAllister HA Jr, Lew M: The surgical anatomy of common atrioventricular orifice associated with tetralogy of Fallot, double outlet right ventricle and complete regular transposition. *Circulation* 61:6, 1980
30. Vargas FJ, Coto EO, Mayer JE, et al: Complete atrioventricular canal and tetralogy of Fallot: Surgical considerations. *Ann Thorac Surg* 42:258–263, 1986
31. Mack JW Jr, Rogers J, Wheller J: Early total repair of tetralogy of Fallot associated with complete atrioventricular canal. *J Cardiovasc Surg* 26:585–588, 1985
32. Westerman GR, Norton JB, Van Devanter SH: Double-outlet right atrium associated with tetralogy of Fallot and common atrioventricular valve. *J Thorac Cardiovasc Surg* 91:205–207, 1986
33. Stark J, McKay R, Anderson RH, et al: Atrioventricular septal defect with common valve orifice but without atrial component. In: Jiminez MQ, Martinez MS (eds): *Paediatric Cardiology.* Madrid, Ediciones Norma, 1987
34. Chin AJ, Bierman F, Sanders SP, et al: Subxiphoid 2-dimensional echocardiographic identification of left ventricular papillary muscle anomalies in complete common atrioventricular canal. *Am J Cardiol* 51:1695–1699, 1983
35. Smallhorn JF, de Leval M, Stark J, et al: Isolated anterior mitral cleft. Two dimensional echocardiographic assessment and differentiation from "clefts" associated with atrioventricular septal defect. *Br Heart J* 48:109–116, 1982
36. Cloez JL, Ravault MC, Worms AM, et al: Complete atrioventricular canal defect associated with congenitally corrected transposition of the great arteries: Two-dimensional echocardiographic identification. *J Am Coll Cardiol* 1:1123–1128, 1983

37. Smallhorn JF, Perrin D, Musewe N, et al: The role of transesophageal echocardiography in the evaluation of patients with atrioventricular septal defect. *Cardiol Young* **1**:324–333, 1991

38. Stark J, Smallhorn J, Huhta J, et al: Surgery for congenital heart defects diagnosed with cross-sectional echocardiography. *Circulation* **68**(Suppl II):II–129, 1983

39. Macartney FJ, Rees PG, Daly K, et al: Angiocardiographic appearances of atrioventricular defects with particular reference to distinction of ostium primum atrial septal defect from common atrioventricular orifice. *Br Heart J* **42**:640–656, 1979

40. Hynes JK, Tajik AJ, Seward JB, et al: Partial atrioventricular canal defect in adults. *Circulation* **66**:284, 1992

41. Hynes JK, Tajik AJ, Seward JB, et al: Partial atrioventricular canal defect in elderly patients (aged 60 years or older). *Am J Cardiol* **50**:59, 1982

42. Berger JJ, Blackstone EH, Kirklin JW, et al: Survival and probability of cure without and with operation in complete atrioventricular canal. *Ann Thorac Surg* **27**:104, 1979

43. Bull C, Rigby ML, Shinebourne EA: Should management of complete atrioventricular canal defect be influenced by coexistent Down syndrome? *Lancet* 1147–1149, 1985

44. Rizzoli G, Muzzacco A, Maizza F, et al: Does Down syndrome affect prognosis of surgically managed atrioventricular canal defects? *J Thorac Cardiovasc Surg* **104**:945–953, 1982

45. Pacifico AD: Atrio-ventricular septal defects. In Stark J, de Leval M (eds): *Surgery for Congenital Heart Defects,* 2nd Edition. Philadelphia, WB Saunders, 1994, pp 373–378

46. Kirklin JW, Barratt-Boyes BG (eds): *Cardiac Surgery.* New York, John Wiley, 1986

47. Bull C, Cooper J, Stark J: Cardioplegic protection of the child's heart. *J Thorac Cardiovasc Surg* **88**:287–293, 1984

48. Elliott MJ: Ultrafiltration and modified ultrafiltration in pediatric open heart operations. *Ann Thorac Surg* **56**:1518–1522, 1993

49. Pacifico AD, Kirklin JW, Bargeron LM Jr: Repair of complete atrioventricular canal associated with tetralogy of Fallot or double-outlet right ventricle: Report of 10 patients. *Ann Thorac Surg* **29**:351, 1980

50. Tandon R, Moller JH, Edwards JR: Tetralogy of Fallot associated with persistent common atrioventricular canal (endocardial cushion defect). *Br Heart J* **36**:197, 1974

51. Kirklin JW, Blackstone EH, Jonas RA, et al: Morphologic and surgical determinants of outcome events after repair of tetralogy of Fallot and pulmonary stenosis. *J Thorac Cardiovasc Surg* **103**:706–723, 1992

52. Hagler DJ, Tajik AJ, Seward JB, et al: Wide angle two-dimensional echocardiographic profiles of conotruncal abnormalities. *Mayo Clin Proc* **55**:73–82, 1980

53. Arciniegas E, Hakimi M, Farooki ZQ, et al: Results of total correction of tetralogy of Fallot with complete atrioventricular canal. *J Thorac Cardiovasc Surg* **81**:768, 1981

54. Bender HW, Hammon JW Jr, Hubbard SG, et al: Repair of atrioventricular canal malformation in the first year of life. *J Thorac Cardiovasc Surg* **84**:515–522, 1982

55. Chin AJ, Keane JF, Norwood WI, Castaneda AR: Repair of complete common atrioventricular canal in infancy. *J Thorac Cardiovasc Surg* **84**:437–445, 1982

56. Stewart S, Harris P, Manning J: Complete endocardial cushion defect. Operative technique and results. *J Thorac Cardiovasc Surg* **78**:914–919, 1979

57. Danielson GK: The "classic" (one-patch) operative approach. In Moulton AL (ed): *Congenital Heart Surgery—Current Techniques and Controversies.* Pasadena, CA, Appleton-Davies, 1984, pp 136–150

58. Moreno-Cabral RJ, Shumway NE: Double-patch technique for correction of complete atrioventricular canal. *Ann Thorac Surg* **33**:88–91, 1982

59. Ashraf HH, Amin Z, Sharma R, Subramanian S: Atrioventricular canal defect: Two-patch repair and tricuspidization of the mitral valve. *Ann Thorac Surg* **55**:347–351, 1993

60. Miller OI, Celeremajer DS, Deanfield JE, Macrae DJ: Very low dose inhaled nitric oxide: A selective pulmonary vasodilator after surgery for congenital heart disease. *J Thorac Cardiovasc Surg* **108**:487–494, 1994

61. Hopkins RA, Kostic I, Klages U, et al: Correction of coarctation of the aorta in neonates and young infants. An individualized surgical approach. *Eur J Cardio-thorac Surg* **2**:296–304, 1988

62. Studer M, Blackstone EH, Kirklin JW, et al: Determinants of early and late results of repair of atrioventricular septal (canal) defects. *J Thorac Cardiovasc Surg* **84**:523–542, 1982

63. Fournier A, Young M-L, Garcia OL, et al: Electrophysiologic cardiac function before and after surgery in children with atrioventricular canal. *Am J Cardiol* **57**:1137–1141, 1986

64. King RM, Puga FJ, Danielson GK, et al: Prognostic factors and surgical treatment of partial atrioventricular canal. *Circulation* **74** (Suppl 1):I42–I46, 1986

65. Merrill WH, Hammon JW, Graham TP, et al: Complete repair of atrioventricular septal defect. *Ann Thorac Surg* **52**:29–32, 1991

66. Hanley FL, Fenton KN, Jonas RA, et al: Surgical repair of complete atrioventricular canal defects in infancy. *J Thorac Cardiovasc Surg* **106**:387–397, 1993

67. Capouya ER, Laks H, Drinkwater DC, et al: Management of the left atrioventricular valve in the repair of complete atrioventricular septal defects. *J Thorac Cardiovasc Surg* **104**:196–203, 1992

68. Kadoba K, Jonas RA, Mayer JE, Castaneda AR: Mitral valve replacement in the first year of life. *J Thorac Cardiovasc Surg* **100**:762–768, 1990

69. Cobanaglou A: Discussion of Capouya et al. *J Thorac Cardiovasc Surg* **104**:202, 1992

70. Pozzi M, Remig J, Fimmers R, Urban AE: Atrioventricular septal defects. *J Thorac Cardiovasc Surg* **101**:138–142, 1991

71. McGrath LB, Gonzalez-Lavin L: Actuarial survival, freedom from reoperation, and other events after repair of atrioventricular septal defects. *J Thorac Cardiovasc Surg* **94**:582–590, 1987

Double Inlet Ventricle

Benson R. Wilcox and Robert H. Anderson

In this chapter, we discuss the cardiac morphology and diagnosis of patients in whom both atrial chambers are connected in their greater part to one ventricle, in other words those patients having a double inlet atrioventricular connection. In the past, it has been customary[1-3] to describe such patients as having a "single ventricle." Only rarely do such hearts truly possess a solitary ventricle.[4] Most patients have two ventricles: one (that connected to the atrial chambers) is dominant while the other (lacking an atrioventricular connection) is incomplete, rudimentary, and hypoplastic. The convention of using the term "single ventricle" to describe this group of hearts has led to problems regarding the assignation of varied patients into the entity by different investigators. It has also led to disagreements concerning the relationship between patients having so-called "single ventricle" and those with the variant of atrioventricular valve atresia due to complete absence of one atrioventricular connection.[5,6]

All these problems are resolved when it is appreciated that in a certain group of patients, the atrial chambers connect to only one ventricle, as opposed to the much larger group of patients in which each atrium is connected to its own ventricle. In other words, it is correct and justifiable to divide patients into those having univentricular and biventricular connections, but of much less value to distinguish those having univentricular and biventricular hearts.[7] Those patients with overriding atrioventricular valves fall between these groups and will not be discussed in this chapter. Others within the group having a univentricular atrioventricular connection will be described in Chapters 88 (Tricuspid Atresia) and 90 (Congenital Abnormalities of the Mitral Valve). Here, we are concerned only with those hearts having the more or less pure form of double inlet atrioventricular connection.

The surgical treatment of patients with double inlet ventricle has, like the anatomical considerations, undergone a radical evolution within the past decade. Although successful septation was achieved as long ago as 1957,[8] until recently most surgical treatment was palliative. Presently, the choice for subtotal correction must be made between the options of septation,[9,10] the Fontan procedure,[11,12] or total cavopulmonary anastomosis.[13] It is largely the anatomy discussed in this section that will determine the choice and potential success of these various options.

ANATOMY

Basic Definitions of the Condition

To prevent any confusion, we believe it is best from the outset to indicate precisely what we mean by a double inlet atrioventricular connection. In the normal heart, each atrium is connected to its own ventricle across separate and perforate atrioventricular junctions (Fig. 71-1A). At the margins of the perforate connections, the atrial myocardium becomes fused with the ventricular myocardium, although the two myocardial segments are separated anatomically and insulated electrically by the fibrofatty atrioventricular grooves at all points except the site of the penetrating atrioventricular bundle of His. These junctions can then be considered in terms of right- and left-sided parietal components and a septal component. In hearts having an atrioventricular septal defect,[14] the septal component is lacking. Hence, there is a common atrioventricular junction. Despite this, it is still an easy matter to recognize the separate right- and left-sided parietal junctions (Fig. 71-1B). The essence of hearts having biventricular atrioventricular connections, then, is the fact that each atrium is connected to its own ventricle across the right and left parietal junctions, irrespective of whether the junctions themselves are guarded by separate right and left atrioventricular valves or by a

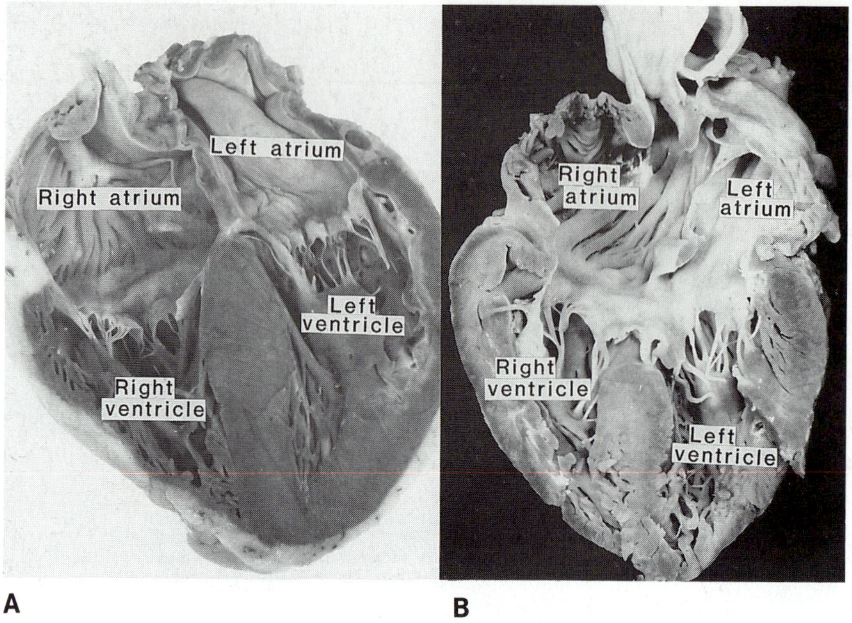

Figure 71–1. Simulated "four-chamber" cuts through two hearts with concordant atrioventricular connections showing that the arrangement of the atrioventricular valves does not alter the basic connection. **A.** A heart with two valves. **B.** An atrioventricular septal defect with a common valve. Irrespective of the valvar morphology, the atriums connect to appropriate ventricles in each example and, hence, there are concordant atrioventricular connections.

A

B

common atrioventricular valve. These biventricular atrioventricular connections can be concordant, discordant, or ambiguous depending on the morphology of the atriums and ventricles (see below).

The distinguishing feature of a double inlet atrioventricular connection is that both parietal segments of atrial myocardium (irrespective of their morphology) are connected to the same ventricle, which may be of left, right, or indeterminate morphology. The double inlet connection, therefore, defines the union of both atriums with one ventricle. It is unrelated to the arrangement of the atrioventricular valves guarding the junctions. Indeed, in these hearts, as in hearts with biventricular connections, the junctions may be guarded by separate valves or by a common valve without disguising the double inlet connection (Fig. 71–2). We have already indicated that some hearts, namely those with overriding atrioventricular valves, are in strictest terms intermediate between biventricular and double inlet atrioventricular connections. In terms of the connection itself, however, we recognize only the ends of this spectrum and categorize them one way or the other. Within that approach, it is possible to recognize double inlet ventricle in the setting of overriding and straddling valves.

Double inlet atrioventricular connection, therefore, can exist with any atrial arrangement (usual, mirror-image, or isomeric) and with the atriums connected to a left, right, or solitary and indeterminate ventricle (Fig. 71–3). When the atriums are connected to a dominant left or right ventricle, the complimentary ventricle is then incomplete and rudimentary. The position of the rudimentary ventricle is a further variable in categorization, as are the ventriculoarterial connections, the relationship of the arterial trunks, and the presence of associated malformations. All of these features can vary independently of one another, and the number of

possible combinations is so great that it may be wise to consider each individual case as being unique. Nonetheless, certain patterns stand out, and it is these patterns that we describe and illustrate further in this section devoted to anatomy. Before embarking on these descriptions, however, we consider it advisable to clarify the anatomical relationship between those hearts having biventricular and univentricular atrioventricular connections and those having double inlet connection and atrioventricular valve atresia. It is these features that condition the surgical options for treatment of a given case.

Biventricular Versus Univentricular Atrioventricular Connections

In terms of the atrioventricular junctions, all hearts can be placed into one of two groups. By far, the greater number fall into the group in which each atrium is connected to its own ventricle. Patients with such hearts, therefore, potentially have the systemic and pulmonary circuits in parallel, although this arrangement can itself be distorted by imperforateness occurring at any point along the two pathways.[15] Within the group of biventricular connections, three specific types of connection are described according to the morphology of the atriums and the ventricles. When morphologically right and left atriums are connected to morphologically appropriate ventricles, the connections are concordant, irrespective of the position of the chambers and irrespective of whether the valves guarding the atrioventricular junctions are perforate or imperforate. When the atrial chambers are each connected to morphologically inappropriate ventricles, the connections are discordant. When the atrial chambers are isomeric, then of necessity, the atrioventricular connection is biventricular but ambiguous.

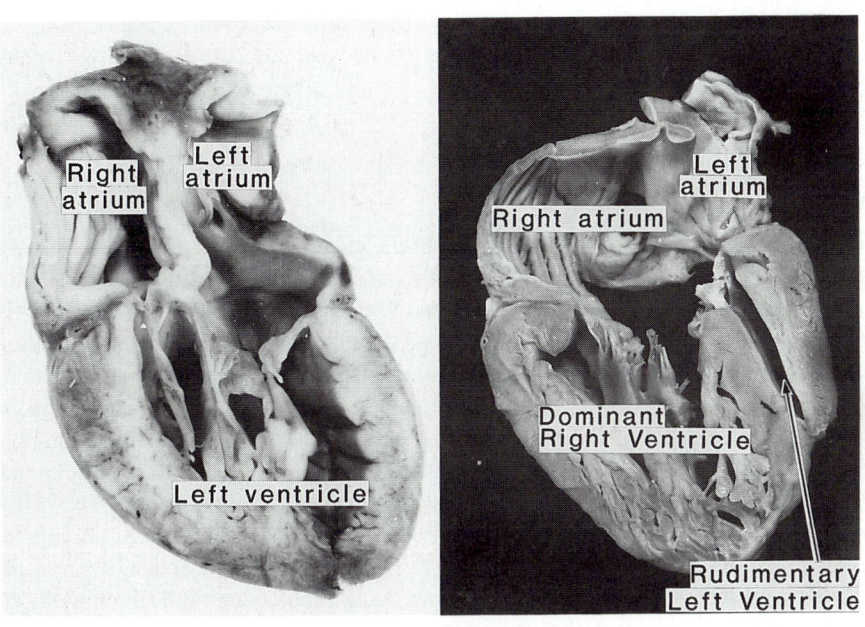

Figure 71-2. Similar "four-chamber" cuts to those shown in Figure 71-1 illustrating the same principle of mode versus type of connection in the setting of double inlet ventricle. **A.** A double inlet to a left ventricle through two atrioventricular valves. **B.** A double inlet right ventricle through a common valve. Again, the valve morphology simply modifies without changing the basic connection, which is double inlet ventricle.

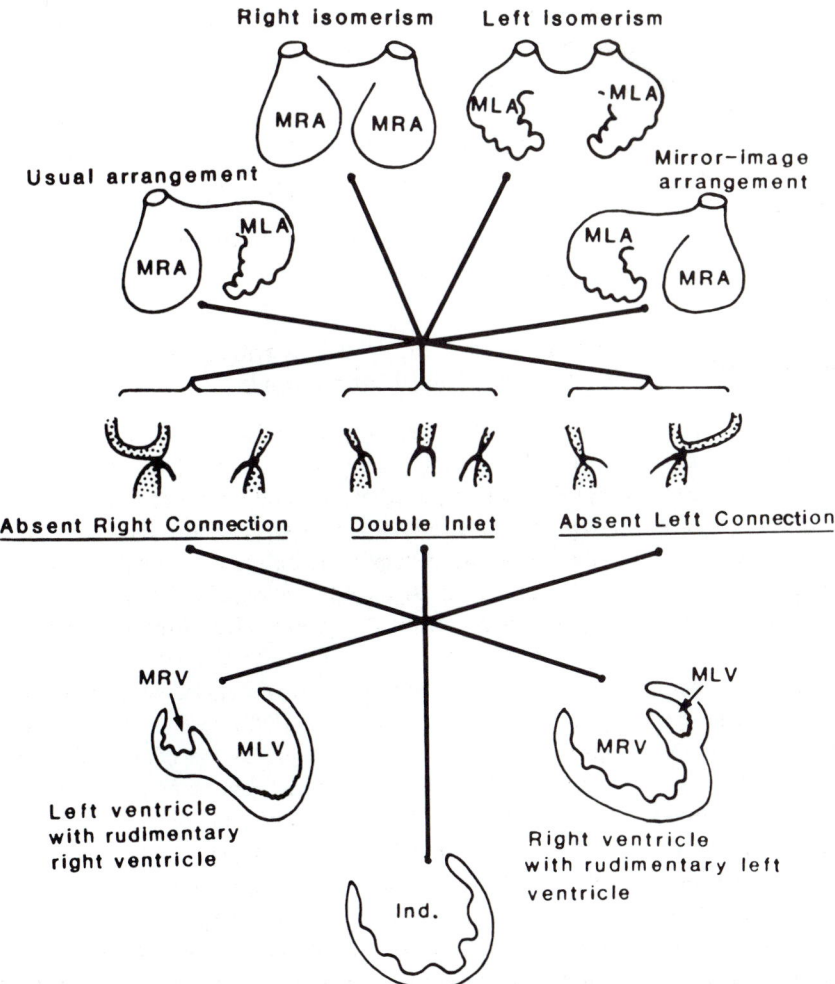

Figure 71-3. A diagram illustrating the basic principle of the univentricular atrioventricular connection. Heart with usual, mirror-image, or isometric atrial arrangements (*top panels*) can all exist with the atriums connected to only one ventricle because of double inlet, absent right or absent left atrioventricular connections (*middle panels*). The univentricular connection can be to a dominant left, a dominant right, or to a solitary and indeterminate ventricle (*lower panels*). These patterns can themselves vary further according to the relationships of dominant and rudimentary ventricles, the ventriculoarterial connections, the associated malformations, and so on. The point is that all the anomalies in this group differ from all those with biventricular atrioventricular connections because the atrial chambers are connected to only one instead of two ventricles. We would never, however, describe any individual heart in terms of its univentricular connection because we can be more precise, describing double inlet left ventricle and so on.

The second group of hearts are those with a univentricular atrioventricular connection. This means that, of necessity, the systemic and pulmonary circuits must be in series since all the blood flows through one ventricle. Two ventricles may be present, but the second ventricle will receive its blood from the first rather than through an atrioventricular junction. Double inlet ventricle, as defined above, is one type of univentricular atrioventricular connection. There are two further specific types of connection producing a similar arrangement. These are characterized by absence of either the right or the left atrioventricular connection, producing a type of atrioventricular valvar atresia that differs morphologically from that resulting from an imperforate valve. As with double inlet, it is usual for hearts with the type of atrioventricular valvar atresia produced by absence of one connection to have two ventricles, but one of the ventricles is again connected only to the dominant ventricle, having no direct junctional connection to an atrial chamber. We would never name any particular heart in terms of its *univentricular atrioventricular connection*, as this is a nonspecific term, serving only to distinguish the overall group of hearts from the larger number with biventricular connections. Thus, our preference now is to name the hearts discussed in this chapter as *double inlet ventricles*. They have a univentricular atrioventricular connection, but so do most hearts with *classic tricuspid atresia*. Very few in either group are *univentricular hearts* because almost all have two ventricles.

Double Inlet Versus Atrioventricular Valve Atresia

Double inlet ventricle, therefore, is a specific and precise anatomical term for one type of atrioventricular connection. The hearts within this grouping can vary in terms of the arrangement of their atriums and ventricles, but all have the same basic atrioventricular connection to only one ventricle, i.e., univentricular. Atrioventricular valvar atresia, in contrast, describes a clinical setting in which the blood entering one atrial chamber is unable to reach the ventricular mass without passing through the other atrium. The valvar atresia is most usually produced by complete absence of one atrioventricular connection, the muscular floor of the blind-ending atrium being separated by the fibrofatty tissue of the atrioventricular groove from the ventricular mass (Fig. 71–4). This type of atrioventricular connection, like double inlet, is univentricular. Atrioventricular valvar atresia, however, can also be produced by an imperforate valvar membrane blocking either the right-sided or left-sided atrioventricular junction (Fig. 71–5). This imperforate variant

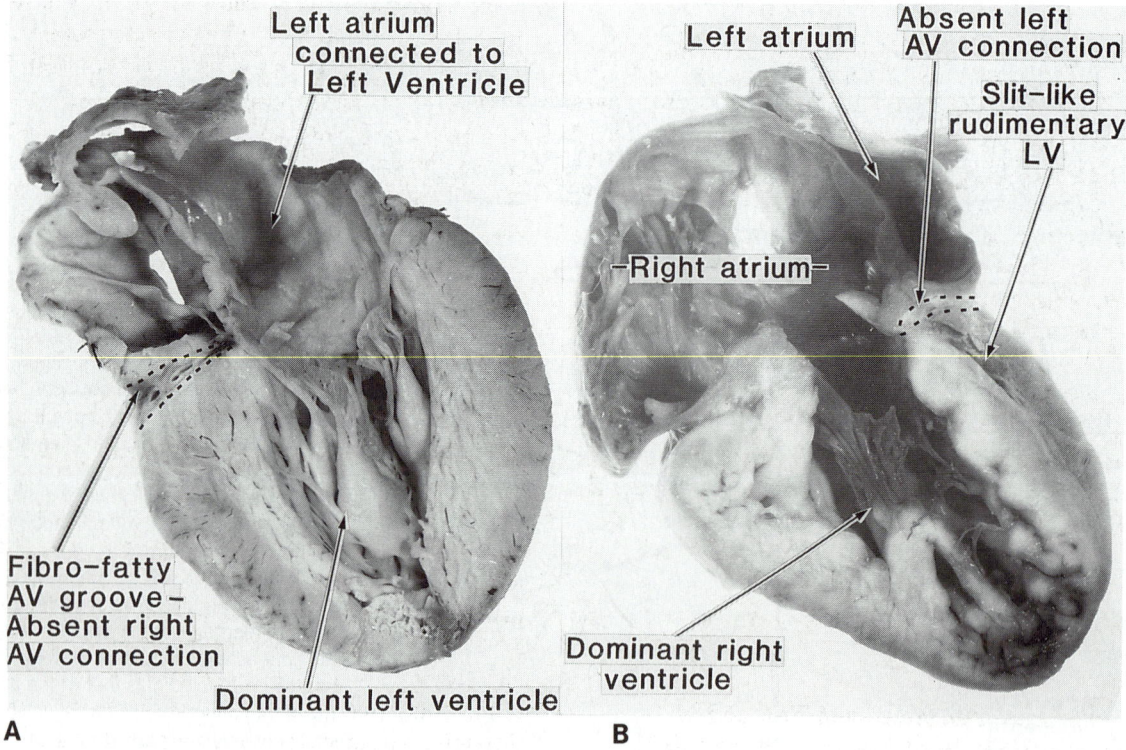

A Left atrium connected to Left Ventricle — Fibro-fatty AV groove - Absent right AV connection — Dominant left ventricle

B Left atrium — Absent left AV connection — Slit-like rudimentary LV — Right atrium — Dominant right ventricle

Figure 71–4. Simulated "four-chamber" sections showing the basic anatomy of absent right (**A**) and absent left (**B**) atrioventricular connections. Absent right connection is shown in the setting of a univentricular connection to a dominant left ventricle (classic tricuspid atresia). The rudimentary right ventricle is not visualized in this section because it is located anterosuperiorly within the ventricular mass. Absent left connection is shown with the right atrium connected to a dominant right ventricle, and the posteroinferior rudimentary left ventricle is also seen (an example of so-called hypoplastic left heart syndrome with mitral atresia).

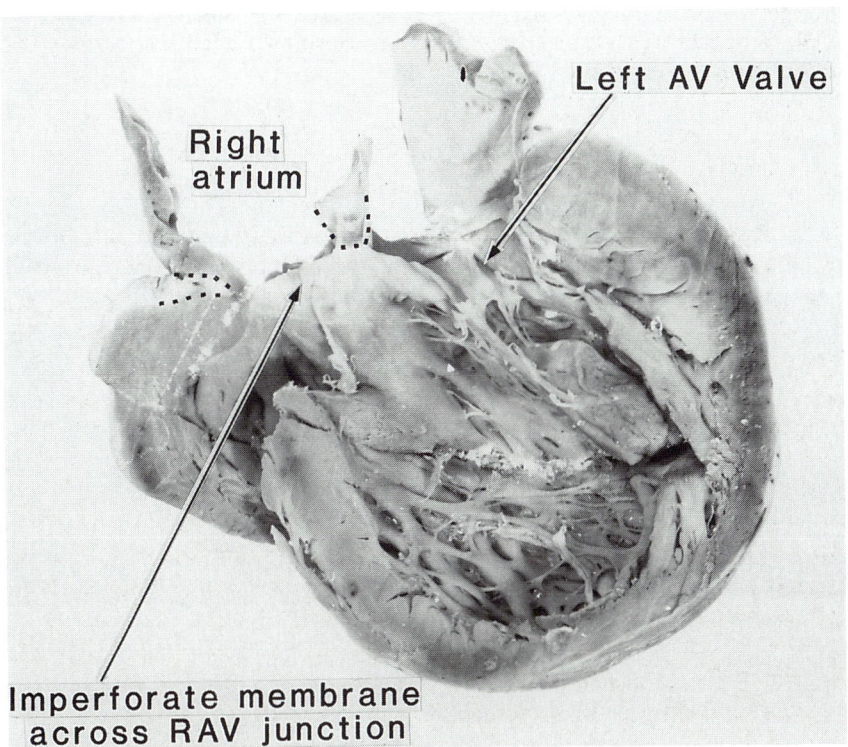

Figure 71–5. A rare example of a heart with concordant atrioventricular connections and an inperforate tricuspid valve shown by sectioning in the "four-chamber" plane. The arrangement produces tricuspid atresia, but the anatomy of the atrioventricular junction is fundamentally different from that usually found in the "classic" pattern, which exhibits absence of the right atrioventricular connection with the left atrium connected to a dominant left ventricle (see Fig. 71–4A). In the variant with an inperforate valve, the atrioventricular junction is well formed but blocked by the valvar membrane.

of atrioventricular valvar atresia modifies the type of atrioventricular connection. It can be encountered in the setting of concordant, discordant, ambiguous, or even double inlet atrioventricular connections. An imperforate valve in the setting of a double inlet connection, is, self-evidently, also univentricular. Imperforate valves in the other settings produce hearts with tricuspid or mitral atresia, but with biventricular atrioventricular connections. Atrioventricular valvar atresia, therefore, is usually due to the variant of univentricular atrioventricular connection produced by absence of one connection, but can exist in the setting of any of the biventricular connections or even, rarely, with double inlet itself. Hearts with either double inlet or atrioventricular valvar atresia are hardly ever univentricular in the sense that only one chamber exists in the ventricular mass. Rarely, they can exist in univentricular form, either when there is a solitary and indeterminate ventricle, or else when the clinician is unable to identify a very small rudimentary ventricle.

Anatomical Variants and Disposition of Conduction Tissues

Double Inlet Left Ventricle with Left-Sided Rudimentary Right Ventricle and Discordant Ventriculoarterial Connections

The commonest type of double inlet is that in which both atriums connect to a dominant left ventricle (Fig. 71–6). Within this subgroup, the most common variant is that in which the ventriculoarterial connections are discordant

(pulmonary trunk from dominant left ventricle and aorta from rudimentary right ventricle) and in which the rudimentary right ventricle is situated anterosuperiorly and to the left within the ventricular mass (Fig. 71–6B). This combination is usually found in patients with usual atrial arrangement and two atrioventricular valves, but can also be found in patients with right isomerism when there is usually a common atrioventricular valve (see Fig. 71–2B). In the usual variant, the apical trabecular septum is found anterosuperiorly to the atrioventricular valves and extends posteroinferiorly toward the obtuse margin of the ventricular mass. Its crest forms the floor of the usual ventricular septal defect (interventricular communication). The roof of the defect is the outlet septum. Its right border (the border toward the anterosuperior aspect of the heart) is a muscular ridge formed by fusion of the outlet and apical septal components. The atrioventricular conduction axis descends down this border, having encircled the semilunar attachments of the pulmonary valvar leaflets within the dominant left ventricle, the axis originating from an anterolateral node located within the right atrioventricular junction (Fig. 71–7). The posteroinferior border of the defect is much less well formed.[16] Indeed, in most instances, the defect extends to the obtuse marginal surface of the ventricular mass. If, therefore, the defect is to be enlarged, this is best achieved by resecting a wedge of apical trabecular septum next to the oblique marginal surface of the ventricles (Fig. 71–7). Restriction of the ventricular septal defect is a frequent occurrence and results in subaortic obstruction. It is usually associated with coarctation or interruption of the aortic arch.

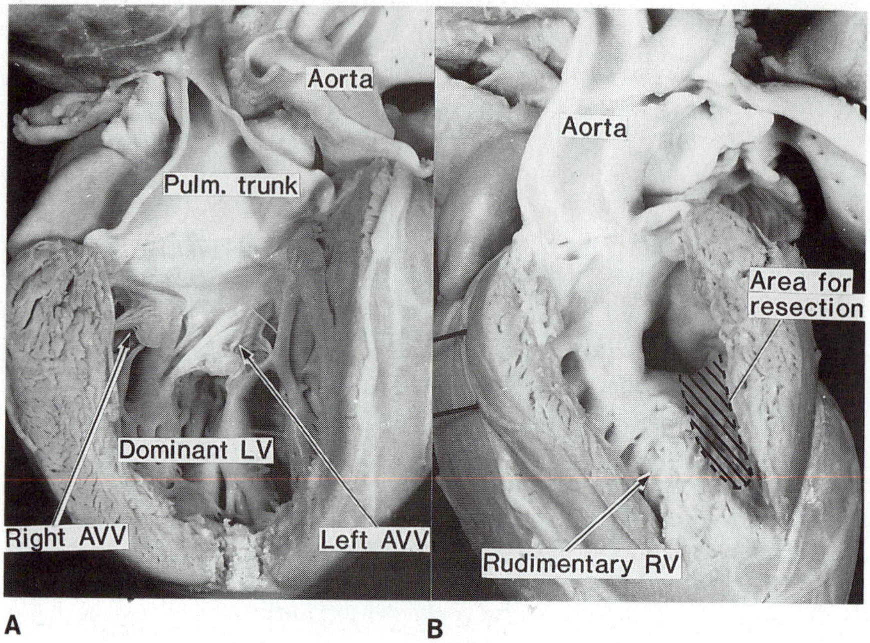

Figure 71–6. The typical anatomy of double inlet left ventricle with left-sided rudimentary right ventricle and discordant ventriculoarterial connections. **A.** The dominant ventricle opened through an anterior incision. The rudimentary ventricle is rotated away to the observer's right hand. Note the potential plane of cleavage between the atrioventricular valves. **B.** The rudimentary right ventricle opened from the front illustrating the area of apical trabecular septum that can be resected safely should it be necessary to enlarge the ventricular septal defect.

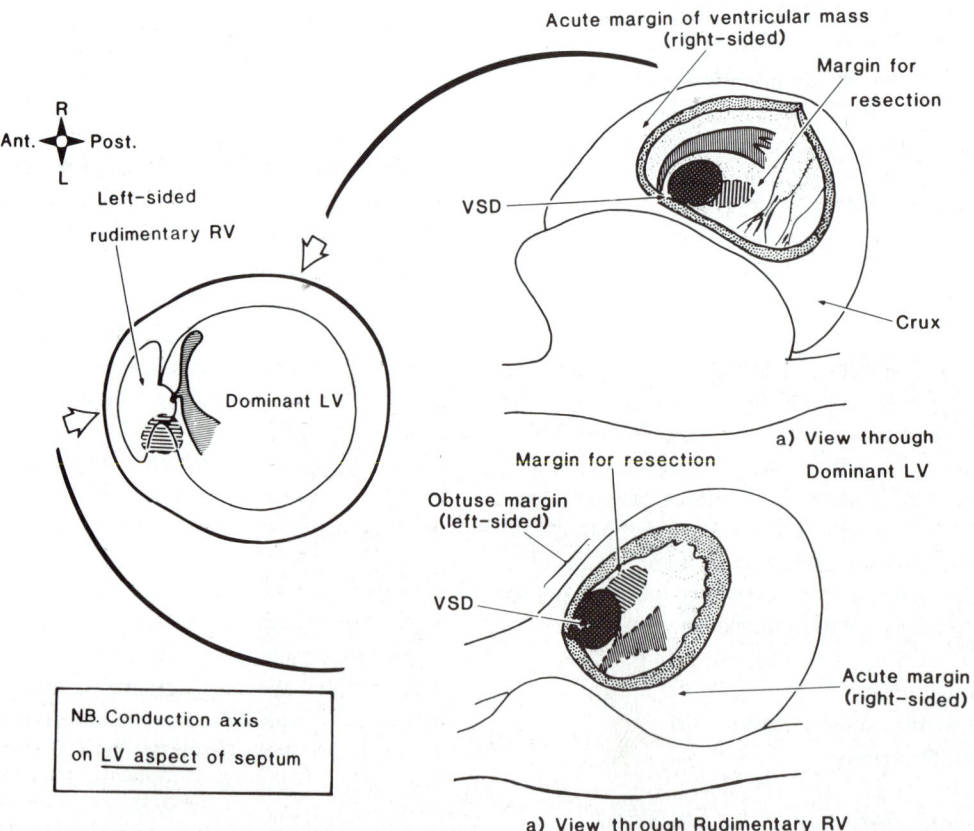

Figure 71–7. Diagram illustrating how the disposition of the conduction tissues in double inlet ventricle with left-sided rudimentary right ventricle can apparently vary according to the approach of the surgeon. The *left panel* shows the basic arrangement of the conduction axis as seen in short axis of the ventricular mass viewed from above. The "safe area" for excision of the apical trabecular septum is marked. The *upper right panel* shows how the surgeon would view the axis if approaching through the dominant left ventricle (or through the right atrioventricular valve). The *lower right panel* shows the view through the left-sided rudimentary right ventricle (compare with Fig. 71–6B).

Obstruction of the subpulmonary outflow from the dominant left ventricle is a much more favorable associated lesion. It is usually produced either by deviation of the outlet septum or by tissue tags derived from the leaflets of the atrioventricular valves. Usually there is a clear plane of cleavage between the atrioventricular valves in the dominant left ventricle, often marked by a posterior ridge that does not carry the atrioventricular conduction axis. Stenosis and hypoplasia of one or the other atrioventricular valve are frequent associated lesions.

Double Inlet Left Ventricle With Right-Sided Rudimentary Right Ventricle and Discordant Ventriculoarterial Connections

This variant is basically similar to the common pattern except that the rudimentary right ventricle sits on the right shoulder of the ventricular mass (Fig. 71–8). This distorts somewhat the orientation and anatomy of the ventricular septal defect, which remains, nonetheless, a muscular communication with apical trabecular septum as its floor and outlet septum as its roof.[16] It is the margin of the defect to the left that now is best formed, this separating the right-sided subaortic infundibulum from the posterior subpulmonary outlet. The border closest to the obtuse margin is less well formed, but the atrioventricular conduction axis descends onto this border as it penetrates the atrioventricular groove. In consequence, the axis has no relationship to the leaflets of the pulmonary valve (Fig. 71–9). It is the left border of the defect (toward the pulmonary trunk) that can be removed safely, along with the wedge of apical septum toward the obtuse margin of the ventricular mass. The asso-

ciated defects found are similar to those seen in the most common pattern.

Double Inlet Left Ventricle With Right-Sided Rudimentary Right Ventricle and Concordant Ventriculoarterial Connections

In this variant of double inlet left ventricle, the aorta arises from the dominant left ventricle while the rudimentary right ventricle supports the pulmonary trunk (Fig. 71–10). This pattern is found almost always with usual atrial arrangement but can have two atrioventricular valves or a common valve.[16] Often the right valve (or right component of a common valve) straddles and overrides the apical trabecular septum. The major feature is the morphology of the rudimentary right ventricle. The apical trabecular component is anterosuperior and right-sided but the outlet component is usually extensive, running across to a "normally related" pulmonary valve. The subarterial infundibulum in these hearts, therefore, is much more extensive than in those with discordant ventriculoarterial connections (Fig. 71–10B). The ventricular septal defect is again enclosed within the muscular septum and is usually restrictive. Either the roof (outlet septum) or the wedge of apical septum closest to the obtuse margin can be removed without damaging the conduction axis, which is disposed as in the cases with discordant ventriculoarterial connections and right-sided rudimentary right ventricle.

Double Inlet and Double Outlet Left Ventricle

The essential feature of this variant is that, in addition to both atrioventricular junctions, both ventriculoarterial junc-

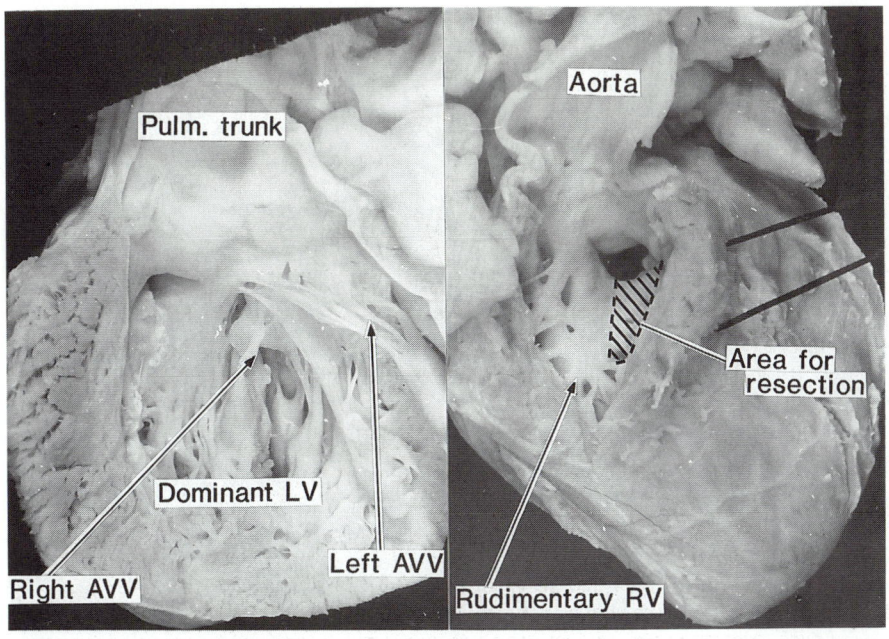

Figure 71–8. The typical anatomy of double inlet left ventricle with right-sided rudimentary right ventricle and discordant ventriculoarterial connections. **A.** The view of the dominant left ventricle opened through an anterior incision. The ventricular septal defect is to the left hand of the observer. **B.** The opened rudimentary right ventricle. As with Figure 71–6B, the safe area for enlargement of the septal defect has been marked.

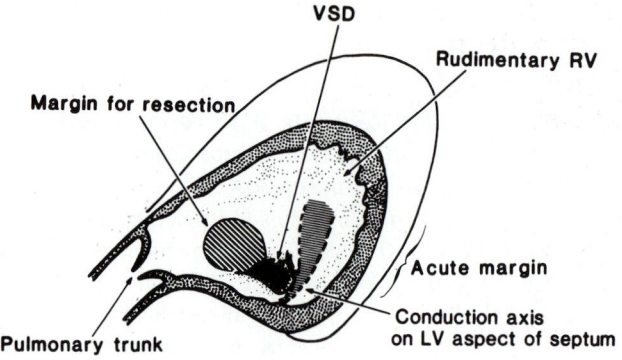

Concordant VA connections

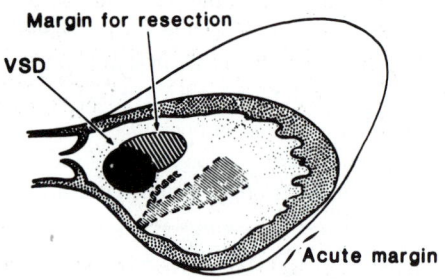

Discordant VA connections

Figure 71–9. Diagram illustrating the basic disposition of the conduction axis in double inlet left ventricle with right-sided rudimentary right ventricle (compare with Fig. 71–7). The "safe margin" for enlargement of the ventricular septal defect (VSD) varies according to whether the aorta (discordant ventriculoarterial [VA] connections) or the pulmonary trunk (concordant ventriculoarterial connections) arises from the rudimentary right ventricle.

tions are also connected to the dominant left ventricle.[4] This means that the apical component of the rudimentary right ventricle persists as a trabecular pouch in either a right-sided (Fig. 71–11) or a left-sided position. The right-sided border of the apical trabecular septum (closest to the acute margin of the ventricular mass) will carry the atrioventricular conduction axis from an anterior atrioventricular node within the right atrioventricular junction. The axis itself will be unrelated to the arterial valves when the rudimentary ventricle is right-sided but will encircle one or both valves when the right ventricle is left-sided. Subaortic obstruction is unlikely in this variant, but subpulmonary obstruction often exists because of a posterior deviation of the outlet septum, which is usually grossly hypoplastic or else represented only by a fibrous raphe between the leaflets of the aortic and pulmonary valves. Often the aortic valve overrides the septum. It may then be difficult to decide whether the ventriculoarterial connections are discordant or double outlet from the dominant left ventricle. Double outlet from the rudimentary right ventricle can occur but is rare. It tends to be associated with subarterial obstruction to one or both outlets.

Double Inlet and Double Outlet Right Ventricle

Double inlet right ventricle is much less common than double inlet left ventricle.[4] When found, most frequently there is also double outlet from the dominant right ventricle. The rudimentary left ventricle is then simply a trabecular pouch found most frequently in a left-sided position (Fig. 71–12A) but sometimes in a right-sided position (Fig. 71–12B). Irrespective of its sidedness, the rudimentary left ventricle is always located posteroinferiorly within the ventricular mass and is beneath and behind the atrioventricular valves. The

Figure 71–10. The typical anatomy of double inlet left ventricle with right-sided rudimentary right ventricle and concordant ventriculoarterial connections. This is the anomaly often termed the "Holmes heart." **A.** Double inlet to the dominant left ventricle. **B.** The rudimentary right ventricle with a restrictive ventricular septal defect (VSD). Note that the outlet component is much better formed when the pulmonary trunk rather than the aorta takes origin from the rudimentary right ventricle. Part of the outlet septum, therefore, is amenable to resection providing it does not give rise to the tension apparatus of either atrioventricular valve. Note also the similarity of the right ventricle to the comparable chamber seen in classic tricuspid atresia.

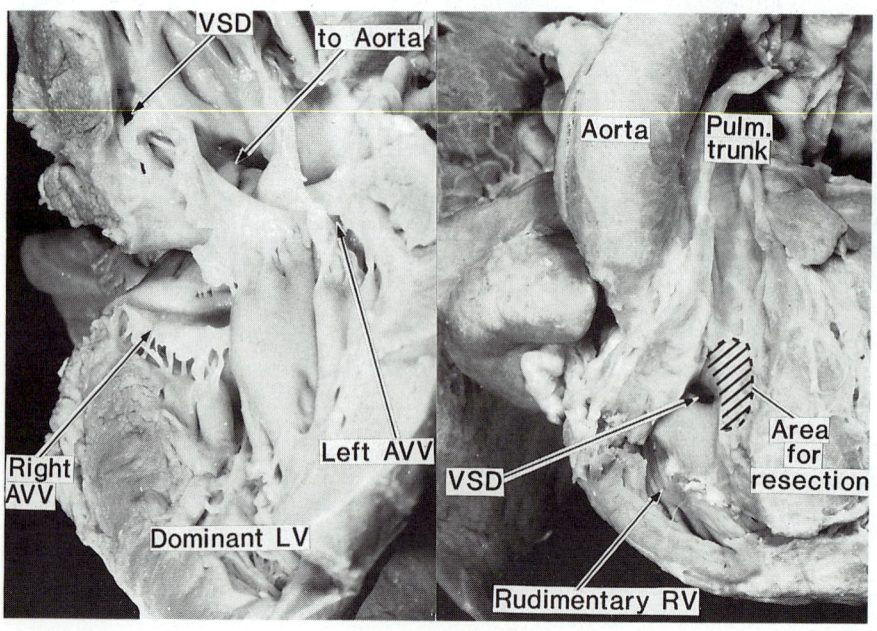

A   B

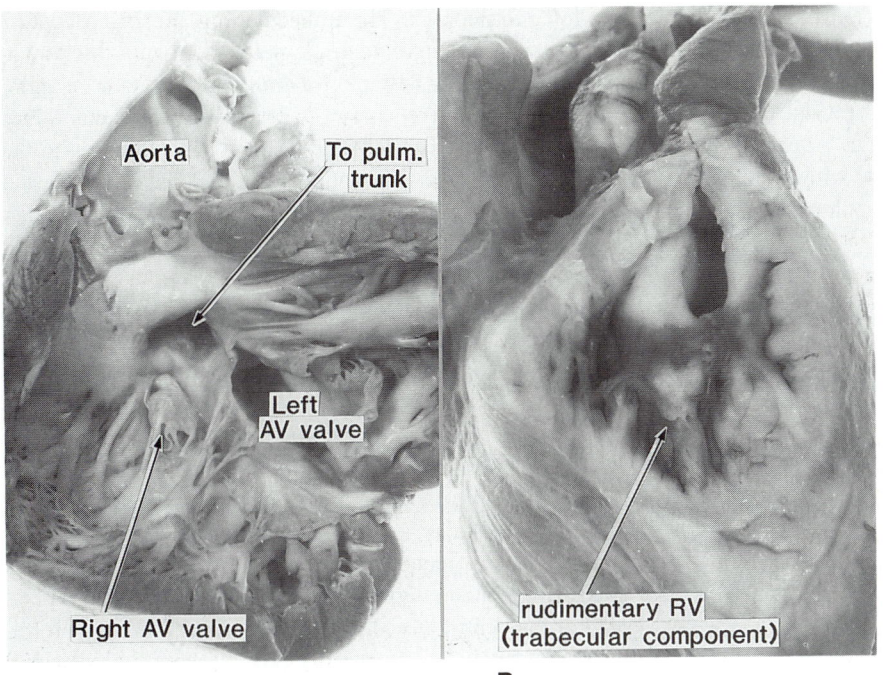

A   **B**

Figure 71–11. A. The cardiac anatomy seen when double inlet left ventricle is also associated with double outlet from the dominant ventricle. **B.** The rudimentary right ventricle is then simply an outpouching from the dominant ventricle and serves no useful function. It is still recognizable, however, as being of morphologically right ventricular pattern.

arrangement can be found with usual atrial arrangement and then there are often two atrioventricular valves, although a common valve can be found. Common valves, however, are more frequently encountered when this combination exists in the setting of right isomerism. Pulmonary atresia and stenosis together with totally anomalous pulmonary venous connection are then also to be expected. It is much rarer to find a clear cleavage plane between the atrioventricular valves in double inlet right ventricle. The site of the conduction axis depends on the atrial arrangement and the position of the rudimentary ventricle. With usual arrangement and left-sided rudimentary left ventricle, the conduction axis originates from a regular atrioventricular node and descends posteroinferiorly relative to the ventricular septal defect, which is usually perimembranous. When the rudimentary left ventricle is right-sided with usual atrial

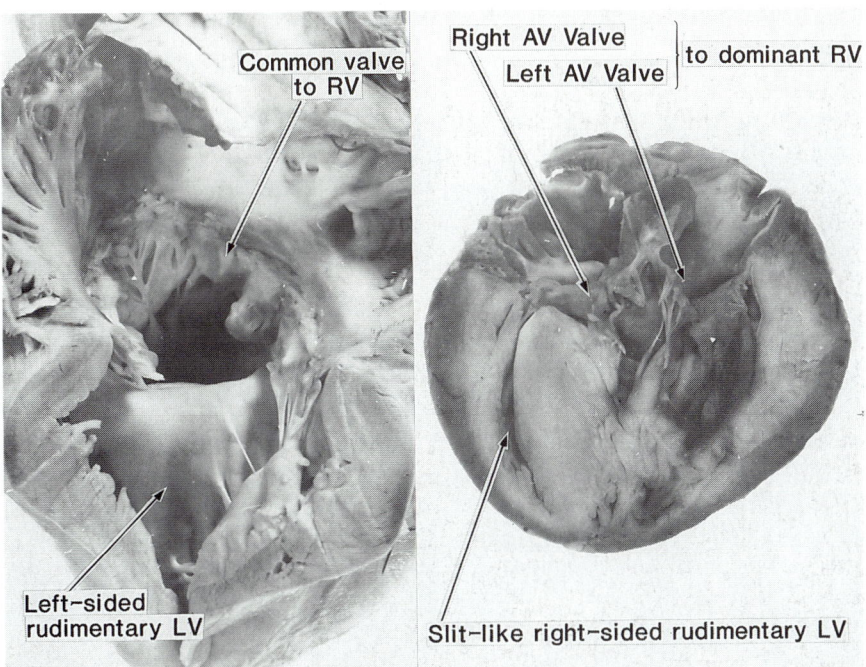

A   **B**

Figure 71–12. As with double inlet left ventricle, the rudimentary ventricle (now of left ventricular pattern) can be either left-sided (usual, **A**) or right-sided (rare, **B**) when both atriums are connected to a dominant right ventricle. **A.** The opened rudimentary left ventricle is then simply a pouch (double inlet and outlet from the dominant right ventricle). **B.** The "four-chamber" section showing the slitlike nature of the rudimentary left ventricle and double inlet to the dominant right ventricle.

arrangement, then there is almost always left hand pattern ventricular topology ("l-loop"). The conduction axis may descend from an anterolateral node in the right atrioventricular junction as in congenitally corrected transposition or double inlet left ventricle as described above. Alternatively, there may be a "sling" of conduction tissue within the ventricular mass connecting regular and anomalous anterolateral nodes.[17]

Double Inlet Right Ventricle With Concordant Ventriculoarterial Connections

A much rarer pattern of double inlet right ventricle exists when the atrioventricular junctions are connected to the dominant right ventricle, which also supports the pulmonary trunk, but the aorta is connected to the left-sided rudimentary left ventricle (Fig. 71–13). This variant usually occurs with usual atrial arrangement and with a common atrioventricular valve. It is the extreme form of an atrioventricular septal defect with right ventricular dominance and, most frequently, is also associated with hypoplasia or interruption of the aortic arch. The ventricular septal defect is perimembranous in position and the conduction axis descends posteroinferiorly from a regular atrioventricular node.

Double Inlet and Double Outlet from a Solitary Ventricle of Indeterminate Morphology

This is the rarest type of double inlet ventricle. It is also the only pattern that, logically, can be considered as a single ventricle. The distinguishing feature of these hearts, which, of necessity, must have either double outlet or single outlet from the solitary ventricle, is the indeterminate pattern of the apical trabecular component. The apical component is described as indeterminate insofar as it is of neither right

nor left morphology. The trabeculations are much coarser than those of the right ventricle and, often, very thick muscle columns cross the apex of the ventricle. One or more columns tend to give support to both atrioventricular valves so that there is no clear plane of cleavage extending to the crux (Fig. 71–14). This pattern is found either with usual atrial arrangement or with right isomerism. It must be distinguished from a huge ventricular septal defect where a rim of apical septum separates trabecular components of right and left ventricular morphology. The significance of this feature relates to the conduction tissue axis. Usually with a huge ventricular septal defect, the axis runs down the rim of ventricular septum from a regular atrioventricular node. We have seen only one case of this type where there was no remnant of the inlet septum and the conduction axis reached the apical rim along an anterior trabeculation running from a regular node. With a solitary and indeterminate ventricle, the conduction axis originates from an anomalous anterolateral node and either runs directly into the lateral wall of the ventricle or else descends along a prominent trabeculation.[18] In hearts of this type with right isomerism there are even more bizarre patterns, sometimes with a sling of conduction tissue formed from two nodes located on the posterior and lateral walls of the atrioventricular junction.[19]

NATURAL HISTORY

Most published studies have been devoted to the natural history of "single ventricle," which means that many cases of double inlet ventricle have been excluded. Furthermore, these experiences[20,21] tend to encompass those patients who have survived sufficiently long to reach centers of excellence, and do not provide information on what happens

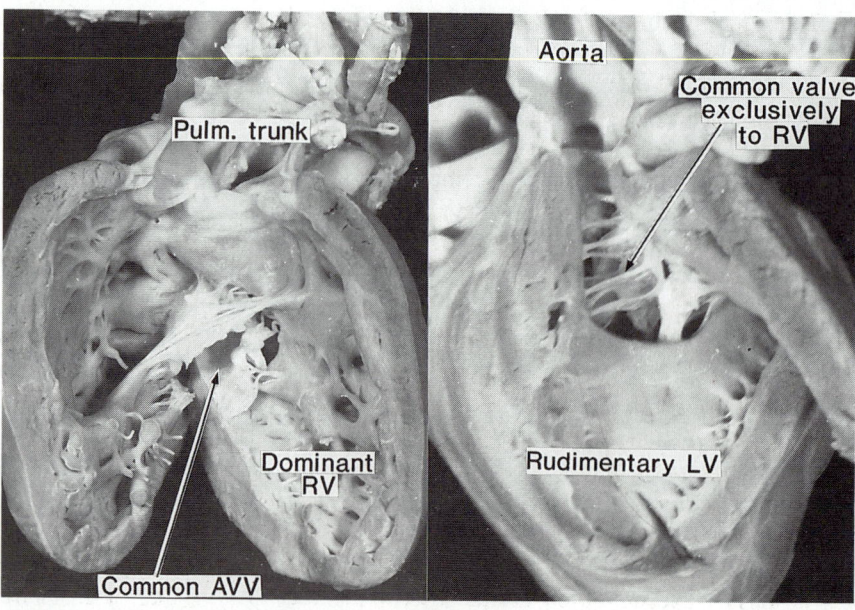

Figure 71–13. The typical anatomy of double inlet right ventricle through a common atrioventricular valve with concordant ventriculoarterial connections. **A.** The exclusive commitment of the common valve to the dominant right ventricle. **B.** The aorta taking origin from the left-sided rudimentary left ventricle.

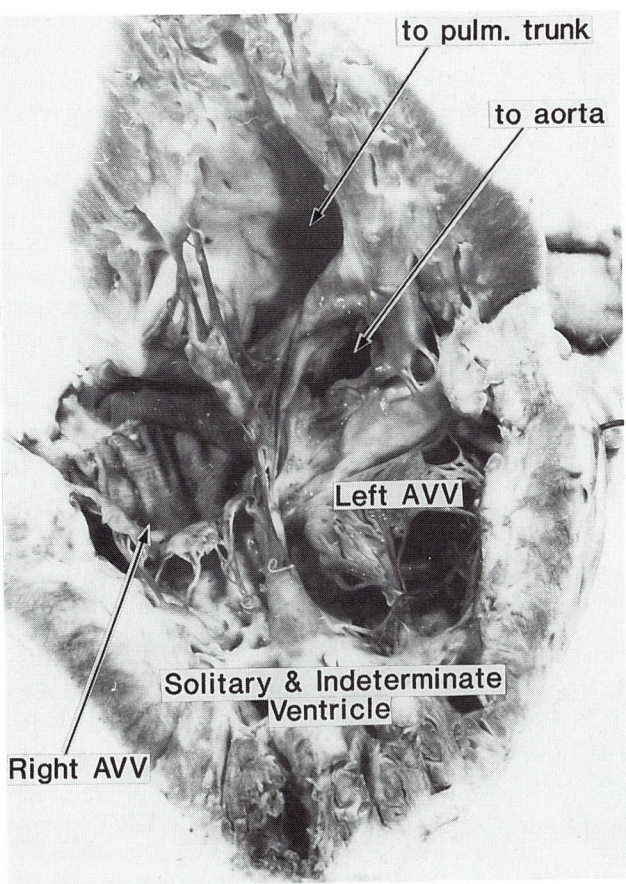

Figure 71–14. The typical anatomy of double inlet and double outlet from a solitary and indeterminate ventricle. The apical trabecular pattern is of neither right nor left ventricular pattern. It was not possible to discover a second chamber within the ventricular mass. AVV, atrioventricular valve.

to all those born with double inlet ventricle. Depressing as the results of these published series are, they still do not paint the true picture of the terrible prognosis of patients born with this atrioventricular connection. A picture much closer to the truth, but still not entirely accurate, is the one that comes from analysis of the combined patient referral of the Hospital for Sick Children and Brompton Hospital, London.[22–24] This study remains incomplete as it was devoted only to patients referred to these centers. Nonetheless, all patients studied were first seen within the first year of life, so a better indication is given of what happens to them. Most patients had double inlet left ventricle, but a good proportion had either a dominant right ventricle or a solitary and indeterminate ventricle. A surprisingly high proportion had right isomerism, and the prognosis for these patients was uniformly appalling. Furthermore, these patients did badly, irrespective of whether they were offered palliative surgery or left untreated. The wastage rate of those with usual atrial arrangement was also disappointingly high, although the recognized syndromes of associated lesions[25,26] account well for the observed mortality. The analysis of this study shows that, even with modern op-

erative treatment, less than half the patients born at present with double inlet ventricle survive to become candidates for subtotal correction.

PRESENTATION

The presentation and hence the clinical features of patients are governed by the associated lesions rather than the double inlet connection itself. Those patients with right isomerism have associated totally anomalous pulmonary venous connection and, usually, pulmonary atresia or severe stenosis. The pulmonary arterial supply is almost always via the arterial duct. These patients tend to present as cyanosed neonates and have a terribly poor prognosis. In the remaining patients, it is the volume of blood reaching the lungs that determines presentation. This tends to be inversely related to the integrity of the systemic circulation. In double inlet left ventricle, for example, an unobstructed pulmonary pathway is usually found with discordant ventriculoarterial connections. These patients present in heart failure that tends to be more severe and to occur earlier when there is coexisting coarctation or interruption of the aortic arch. A similar picture is seen in the patient with double inlet right ventricle and concordant ventriculoarterial connections. When there is obstruction to pulmonary flow, the patient presents with cyanosis. If severe, this will also bring the patient to attention during the neonatal period. A typical example of this presentation is the patient with double inlet left ventricle, concordant ventriculoarterial connections, and a severely restrictive ventricular septal defect. There is a small subset of patients, however, who have a relatively balanced circulatory pattern. Mostly found in those with double inlet left ventricle, these patients have unobstructed systemic flow and pulmonary stenosis of insufficient severity to produce marked cyanosis. Not surprisingly, these are the patients who do best in terms of survival and treatment.[22–24] As with tricuspid atresia, the presentation of patients can change during the course of the disease. The factor determining this feature is usually the state of the ventricular septal defect. In those with double inlet left ventricle, this structure is embedded within the musculature of the septum and has a tendency to decrease its caliber with the passage of time. The effects of this decrease will be determined by the ventriculoarterial connection and ventricular morphology. Thus, in double inlet left ventricle, reduction in size of the defect with concordant ventriculoarterial connections will produce increasing cyanosis but, with discordant connections, will simulate the effects of increasing aortic coarctation.

DIAGNOSIS

The precise diagnosis of double inlet ventricle is made either by cross-sectional echocardiography[15] or axial angiocardiography.[27] Clinical investigations, even with the help of chest radiography or electrocardiography, are insufficiently precise to permit the unequivocal diagnosis of double inlet. The chest radiograph is of great benefit in identifying those symptomatic neonates with atrial isomerism,[28] but the electrocardiogram provides very little new diagnostic information.[29] Cross-sectional echocardiography is now the technique of choice for unequivocal diagnosis. This permits the determination of atrial arrangement by inference from the relationship of the abdominal great vessels to the spine.[30] The technique then shows the presence of double inlet through two valves or a common valve and permits accurate recognition of the morphological nature of dominant, rudimentary, and solitary ventricles (Fig. 71–15). Ideally, ventricular identification is done according to the pattern of the apical trabeculations. This, however, is rarely feasible.

Instead, advantage is taken that, without exception, rudimentary right ventricles are found anterosuperiorly within the ventricular mass, whereas rudimentary left ventricles are located in the posteroinferior position. If it is not possible to find a rudimentary ventricle, then almost always the inference can be drawn that the solitary ventricle is of indeterminate morphology. Cross-sectional echocardiography is also ideal to determine the ventriculoarterial connections and identify associated lesions, particularly malformations of the atrioventricular valves. Axial angiocardiography provides the same precision in terms of identification of ventricular morphology. The position of the rudimentary ventricle is again the best guide to the pattern of the ventricular mass (Fig. 71–16). Angiographic studies are of less value in determining the precise arrangement of the atrioventricular

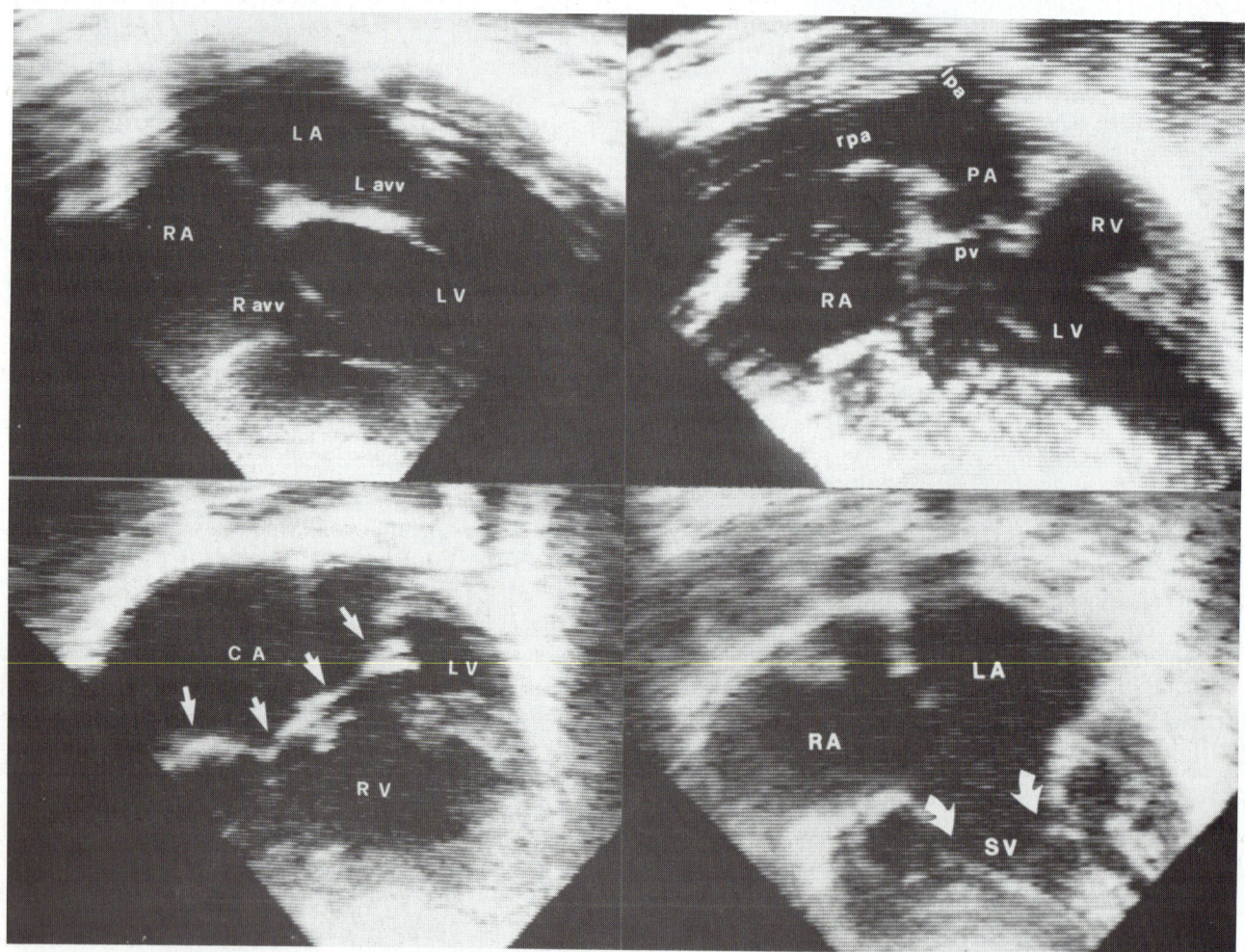

Figure 71–15. Cross-sectional echograms illustrating the value of this diagnostic technique to display the fundamental features of hearts with double inlet ventricle. The *upper panels* show double inlet to a dominant left ventricle (left hand) with an anterosuperior and left-sided rudimentary right ventricle (right hand). The *right panel* also shows the pulmonary trunk (PA) connected to the dominant left ventricle (LV). The *lower left panel* shows double inlet through a common valve from a common atrium (CA) to a dominant right ventricle (RV) with a left-sided posteroinferior rudimentary left ventricle. The *lower right panel* shows double inlet through a common valve to a solitary and indeterminate ventricle (SV). RA, right atrium; LA, left atrium; avv, atrioventricular valve; pa, pulmonary arteries; pv, pulmonary valve. *Arrows,* common atrioventricular valve. (*The echograms were taken by and are reproduced by kind permission of Dr. Michael Rigby, Brompton Hospital, London, and Dr. Mario Carminati, Ospedale Reuniti, Bergamo.*)

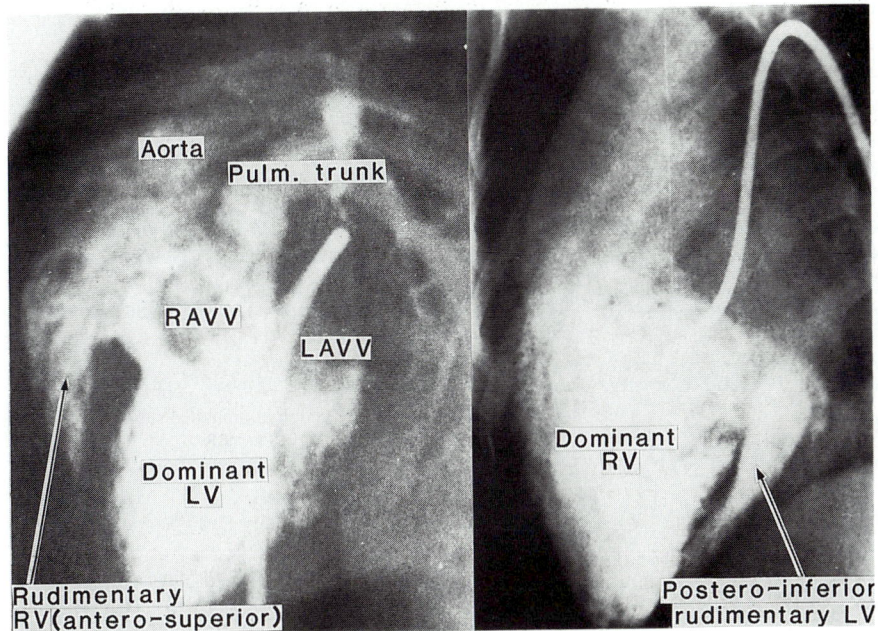

A   **B**

Figure 71–16. Representative angiograms showing how this technique helps in the identification of ventricular morphology. **A.** A double inlet through two atrioventricular valves (RAVV, LAVV) to a dominant left ventricle (LV). The rudimentary right ventricle (RV) is recognized both from its anterosuperior position and also because of its coarse apical trabeculations. There are discordant ventriculoarterial connections. **B.** A dominant right ventricle with a smooth-walled rudimentary left ventricle in the posteroinferior position. There is pulmonary atresia with the aorta arising from the dominant right ventricle. *(The angiograms were produced by and are printed with kind permission of Drs. L. M. Bargeron, Jr., and B. Soto, University of Birmingham in Alabama.)*

valves, but they delimit with greater ease the anatomy of the systemic and pulmonary arterial pathways. Catheter investigations also provide hemodynamic data. That of most value is the presence or absence of gradients across the ventricular outlets. Newer techniques, such as magnetic resonance imaging, demonstrate accurately the morphology of the ventricular mass, but it is questionable if they add any information over and above that provided by the skillful echocardiographer using cross-sectional techniques.

SUMMARY

Double inlet ventricle has a variety of anatomic variations with corresponding varied clinical presentations. Surgical correction follows one of two major courses. When possible, septation may be carried out by dividing the ventricle into two chambers, one dedicated to the pulmonary circulation and the other to the systemic circulation. Alternatively, the Fontan procedure may be used, which avoids attempts to divide the ventricular chamber, but rather separates the systemic and pulmonary circulation by directing systemic venous return away from the ventricle and directly to the pulmonary arteries. Each of these procedures has its place depending on the anatomy and physiology of the lesion and is discussed in detail in the next two chapters.

REFERENCES

1. Van Praagh R, Ongley PA, Swan HJC: Anatomic types of single or common ventricle in man: Morphologic and geometric aspects of sixty necropsied cases. *Am J Cardiol* **13**:367–386, 1964

2. Lev M, Liberthson RR, Kirkpatrick JR, et al: Single (primitive) ventricle. *Circulation* **39**:577–591, 1969

3. Edwards JE: Discussion. In Davila JC (ed): *2nd Henry Ford Hospital International Symposium on Cardiac Surgery.* New York, Appleton-Century-Crofts, 1977, p 242

4. Anderson RH, Tynan MJ, Freedom RM, et al: Ventricular morphology in the univentricular heart. *Herz* **4**:184–197, 1979

5. Anderson RH, Becker AE, Macartney FJ, et al: Is "tricuspid atresia" a univentricular heart? *Pediatr Cardiol* **1**:51–56, 1979

6. Bharati S, Lev M: The concept of tricuspid atresia complex as distinct from that of the single ventricle complex. *Pediatr Cardiol* **1**:57–62, 1979

7. Anderson RH, Becker AE, Tynan M, et al: The univentricular atrioventricular connection: Getting to the root of a thorny problem. *Am J Cardiol* **54**:822–828, 1984

8. McGoon DC, Danielson GK, Ritter DG, et al: Correction of the univentricular heart having two atrioventricular valves. *J Thorac Cardiovasc Surg* **74**:218–226, 1977

9. Pacifico AD, McKay R, Kirklin JW, Kirklin JK: Surgical management of the univentricular heart. In Anderson RH, Macartney FJ, Shinebourne EA, Tynan M (eds): *Paediatric Cardiology,* Vol 5. Edinburgh, Churchill Livingstone, 1982, pp 276–291

10. McKay R, Pacifico AD, Blackstone EH, et al: Septation of the univentricular heart with left anterior subaortic outlet chamber. *J Thorac Cardiovasc Surg* **84**:77–87, 1982

11. Gale AW, Danielson GK, McGoon DC, Mair DD: Modified Fontan operation for univentricular heart and complicated congenital lesions. *J Thorac Cardiovasc Surg* **78**:831–838, 1979

12. Danielson GK: The present role of the Fontan operation in the treatment of complex congenital heart disease. In Marcelletti C, Anderson RH, Becker AE, et al (eds): *Paediatric Cardiology,* Vol 6. Edinburgh, Churchill Livingstone, 1986, pp 307–313

13. Kawashima Y, Kitamura S, Matsuda H, et al: Total cavopulmonary shunt operation in complex cardiac anomalies: A new operation. *J Thorac Cardiovasc Surg* **87**:74–81, 1984

14. Becker AE, Anderson RH: Atrioventricular septal defects: What's in a name. *J Thorac Cardiovasc Surg* **83**:461–469, 1982

15. Rigby ML, Anderson RH, Gibson D, et al: Two-dimensional echocardiographic categorization of the univentricular heart: Ventric-

ular morphology, type, and mode of atrioventricular connection. *Br Heart J* **46:**603–612, 1981

16. Anderson RH, Penkoske PA, Zuberbuhler JR: Variable morphology of ventricular septal defect in double inlet left ventricle. *Am J Cardiol* **55:**1560–1565, 1985

17. Essed CE, Ho SY, Hunter S, Anderson RH: Atrioventricular conduction system in univentricular heart of right ventricular type with right-sided rudimentary chamber. *Thorax* **35:**123–127, 1980

18. Essed CE, Ho SY, Shinebourne EA, et al: Further observations on conduction tissues in univentricular hearts: Surgical implications. *Eur Heart J* **2:**87–96, 1981

19. Dickinson DF, Wilkinson JL, Anderson KR, et al: The cardiac conduction system in situs ambiguus. *Circulation* **59:**879–885, 1979

20. Moodie DS, Ritter DG, Tajik AJ, et al: Long-term follow-up after palliative operation for univentricular heart. *Am J Cardiol* **53:**1648–1651, 1984

21. Moodie DS, Ritter DG, Tajik AJ, O'Fallon WM: Long-term follow-up in the unoperated univentricular heart. *Am J Cardiol* **53:**1124–1128, 1984

22. Franklin RCG, Spiegelhalter DJ, Anderson RH, et al: Double-inlet ventricle presenting in infancy. I. Survival without definitive repair. *J Thorac Cardiovasc Surg* **101:**767–776, 1991

23. Franklin RCG, Spiegelhalter DJ, Anderson RH, et al: Double-inlet ventricle presenting in infancy. II. Results of palliative operations. *J Thorac Cardiovasc Surg* **101:**917–923, 1991

24. Franklin RCG, Spiegelhalter DJ, Anderson RH, et al: Double-inlet ventricle presenting in infancy. III. Outcome and potential for definitive repair. *J Thorac Cardiovasc Surg* **101:**924–934, 1991

25. Girod DA, Lima RC, Anderson RH, et al: Double inlet ventricle: Morphological analysis and surgical implications in 32 cases. *J Thorac Cardiovasc Surg* **88:**590–600, 1984

26. Quaegebeur J, Anderson RH: The anatomical potential for septation. In Anderson RH, Crupi G. Parenzan L (eds): *Double Inlet Ventricle.* Tunbridge Wells, Castle House Publications, 1986

27. Soto B, Bertranou EG, Bream PR, et al: Angiographic study of univentricular heart of right ventricular type. *Circulation* **60:**1325–1334, 1979

28. Deanfield J, Leanage R, Stroobant J, et al: Use of high kilovoltage filtered beam radiographs for detection of bronchial situs in infants and young children. *Br Heart J* **44:**577–583, 1980

29. Graham G, Kumpeng V, Antoniadis S: The electrocardiogram in double inlet ventricle. In Anderson RH, Crupi G, Parenzan L (eds): *Double Inlet Ventricle.* Tunbridge Wells, Castle House Publications, 1986

30. Huhta JC, Smallhorn JF, Macartney FJ: Two dimensional echocardiographic diagnosis of situs. *Br Heart J* **48:**97–108, 1982

72

Surgical Management of Complex Functional Single Ventricle

Gregory P. Fontana, Lester C. Permut, and Hillel Laks

A number of congenital heart defects share the common characteristic of a functionally single ventricle, including hypoplastic left heart syndrome (mitral atresia or stenosis; aortic atresia or stenosis), tricuspid atresia, double-inlet ventricles, and common ventricle. Several other anomalies also are grouped with these defects, because they currently do not permit a two-ventricle repair, e.g., double-outlet right ventricle with an uncommitted (inlet) ventricular septal defect, and the many forms of the heterotaxy syndrome. Associated abnormalities, such as pulmonary stenosis, restrictive bulboventricular foramen, coarctation of the aorta, interrupted aortic arch, atrial septal defect, patent ductus arteriosus, and atrioventricular valve anomalies are common in all of the aforementioned anomalies and generally determine the clinical presentation.

Therapy for these complex defects has markedly improved as the anatomy and physiology of the specific defects have been elucidated. Surgical therapy is divided into palliative and definitive procedures. Palliative procedures include pulmonary artery banding, systemic arterial to pulmonary arterial shunting, and relief outflow tract obstruction; their use and timing depend on the anatomic substrate and the potential for definitive repair. The Fontan procedure has emerged as the operation of choice for patients considered to be candidates for definitive repair of single ventricle. Ventricular septation is now rarely performed.

This chapter will present the anatomy and physiology of this complex spectrum of congenital malformations and describe the rationale for surgical therapy. Hypoplastic left heart syndrome and tricuspid atresia will be addressed in separate chapters.

TERMINOLOGY AND ANATOMY

Single ventricle is an imprecise term that refers to congenital cardiac abnormalities in which functionally there exists only a single ventricular chamber giving rise to the great vessels. A single ventricular chamber may occur from failure of ventricular septation and normal chamber development (as with a large ventricular septal defect), or from hypoplasia of the left or right ventricle. A number of classification systems have been developed to characterize and classify single ventricle abnormalities. While these systems have improved the understanding of anatomic variations, the lack of a standard nomenclature has proved problematic. The following reviews the major classifications and their terminology.

Van Praagh et al referred to the terms *single ventricle* and *common ventricle* when defining one ventricular chamber receiving flow from either both the tricuspid and mitral valves, or from a common atrioventricular (A-V) valve.[1] *Common ventricle* is distinguished by the presence of right and left ventricle morphology with a rudimentary ventricular septum. Tricuspid and mitral atresia were excluded from Van Praagh's description. Hearts were categorized according to morphology of the main ventricle and positional relation of the great arteries. More recently, further distinction has been made denoting morphologically single left ventricles and morphologically single right ventricles.[2]

Van Praagh now employs the segmental approach to assist further in clarifying the anatomy.[3] The segmental approach describes the three major cardiac segments in venoarterial sequence (atria, ventricles, great arteries). The letters in braces {X,X,X} refer to the visceroatrial situs (situs solitus=S, situs inversus=I, situs ambiguous=A), the ventricular loop or chirality (D-loop=D, L-loop=L), and the position of the great arteries (normally related=S, inverted normally related great arteries=I, D-transposition or D-malposition=D, L-transposition or L-malposition=L), respectively. An example of the system's application is {S,L,L}, which represents situs solitus with an L-loop ventricle, and L-transposition of the great arteries.

Anderson et al defined univentricular heart as the commitment of A-V valves to only one chamber in the ventricular mass, exclusive of tricuspid and mitral atresia.[4] Morphology was described in three subsets: a left ventricular pattern with rudimentary right ventricle, a right ventricular pattern with a rudimentary left ventricle, and an indeterminate pattern of ventricular mass. Common ventricle, a very rare defect, was defined as a heart with evidence of both right and left ventricles, but with an absent or rudimentary interventricular septum.

The term single ventricle with double-inlet atrioventricular connection, or double-inlet ventricle, is applied to hearts in which the inflow from two anatomically distinct atria enter into a single ventricular chamber via two atrioventricular valves. Double-inlet ventricles are distinguished from hearts with straddling and overriding atrioventricular valves by having a greater than 50% override of the atrioventricular connection (see Fig. 73–2, Chap. 73). Double-inlet ventricle encompasses a variety of anatomic anomalies that share the physiologic characteristics of a single ventricle. While these are generally termed single ventricular hearts, the literal existence of a single ventricle is rarely the case, because the majority of these hearts have an additional incomplete, rudimentary, or hypoplastic ventricle.[5] The single functional ventricle is composed of an inlet portion, supporting the subvalvular tensor apparatus, a trabecular zone extending to the apex, and an outlet (infundibulum) portion to a great artery. Ventricular outflow is either directly to an attached great artery, or through an outlet chamber composed of rudiments of the opposite ventricle to the *other* great artery. The connection between the main ventricular chamber and the outlet chamber through the trabecular septum has been given a variety of names, including outlet foramen, trabecular septal defect, ventricular septal defect, bulboventricular foramen, and interventricular communication. If the rudimentary ventricle, or chamber, gives rise to more than half of a great artery, it is designated an outlet chamber. Otherwise, it is called a trabecular pouch.

Because of variations in cardiac position (dextrocardia, levocardia, mesocardia), situs (solitus, inversus, ambiguous) and ventricular looping (chirality), separate atrioventricular valves are designated as right-sided or left-sided, instead of tricuspid or mitral. In some single ventricles, a common atrioventricular valve is present as a component of complete atrioventricular septal defect (complete A-V canal).

Another aspect of surgical anatomy deserving special attention is the position of the conduction system. In the normal heart, the atrioventricular node is positioned in the triangle of Koch (delineated by the tendon of Todaro, the orifice of the coronary sinus, and the septal leaflet of the tricuspid valve). The inlet portion of the ventricular septum extends to the crux of the heart and carries the penetrating bundle of His connecting the A-V node in the atrial septum with the bundle branches on the trabecular septum. Because of the variable presence of the inlet septum, the course of the conduction tissue is frequently abnormal.[6] For example, the hallmark of double-inlet left ventricle is the absence of the inlet septum in which the septum does not extend to the crux. As a result, the conduction system carried on the trabecular septum does not make contact with the normal A-V node, but instead communicates with the anterolateral expansion of a ring of nodelike tissue that is formed around the tricuspid orifice and is present in all developing human hearts. With a left-sided rudimentary right ventricle, the bundle takes a course bringing it into proximity with the ostium of the posterior great artery (pulmonary artery) before reaching the septum. It proceeds over the top of the origin of the pulmonary artery and descends along the superior aspect of the outlet foramen (Fig. 72–1). In a right-sided rudimentary right ventricle, the penetrating bundle courses along the rim of the outlet foramen away from the ostium of the posterior great artery[7] (Fig. 72–2). Atrioventricular conduction tissue in double-inlet ventricle with a straddling atrioventricular valve is not much different (see Chapter 73). With a straddling right atrioventricular valve, a posterolateral-positioned node is most likely, and with a straddling left atrioventricular valve, the most likely site for the node is anterolateral.[7] Although most forms of complex single ventricle have predictable patterns of conduction, the incidence of heart block remains significant. In the more ambiguous forms of single ventricle, the conduction pathways are unpredictable without electrophysiologic mapping.

The anatomy of the coronary arteries also varies significantly.[8] Keeton et al studied the coronary arteries as they relate to the outlet chamber and rudimentary pouches in univentricular hearts.[8] When the main chamber was of left ventricular morphology and the outlet chamber was anterior, the left anterior cusp was the noncoronary cusp, with the right and left posterior sinuses giving rise to the right and left coronary arteries, respectively. A major branch termed the *delimiting artery* arose from each of the two vessels outlining the surface boundaries of the outlet chamber in the majority of cases. The right delimiting artery was invariably larger than the left. The right coronary artery gave off a number of large anterior branches parallel to the right delimiting artery in the area where a ventriculotomy would be placed. Therefore, the optimal site of a ventriculotomy in this subset of patients is as far apically as possible. Because of the significant anatomical variations, a preoperative angiogram should be routinely performed as well as careful intraoperative assessment.

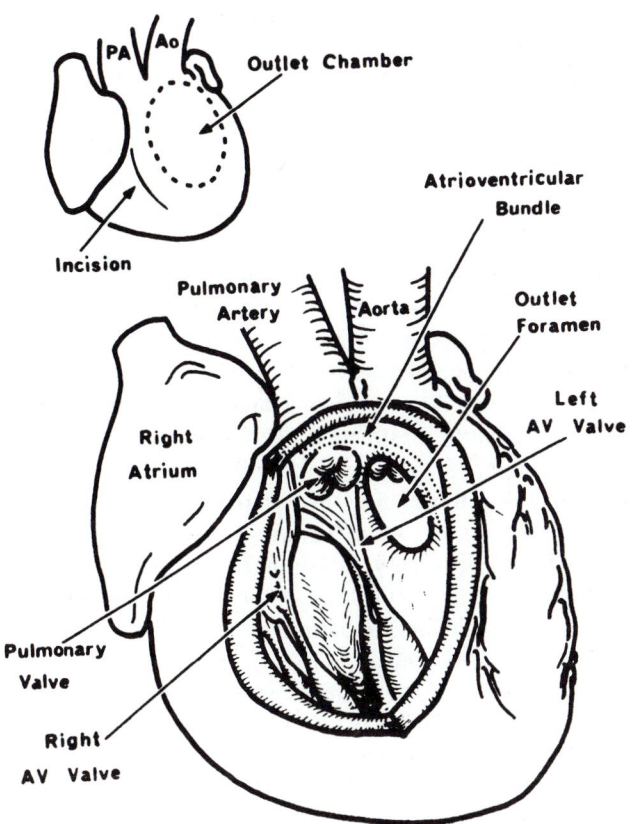

Figure 72–1. The disposition of the conduction tissue in double-inlet left ventricle with left-sided rudimentary right ventricle.[7] *(From Becker AE, Wilkinson JL, Anderson RH: Atrioventriventricular conduction tissues in the univentricular hearts of the left ventricular type. Herz 4:166, 1979.)*

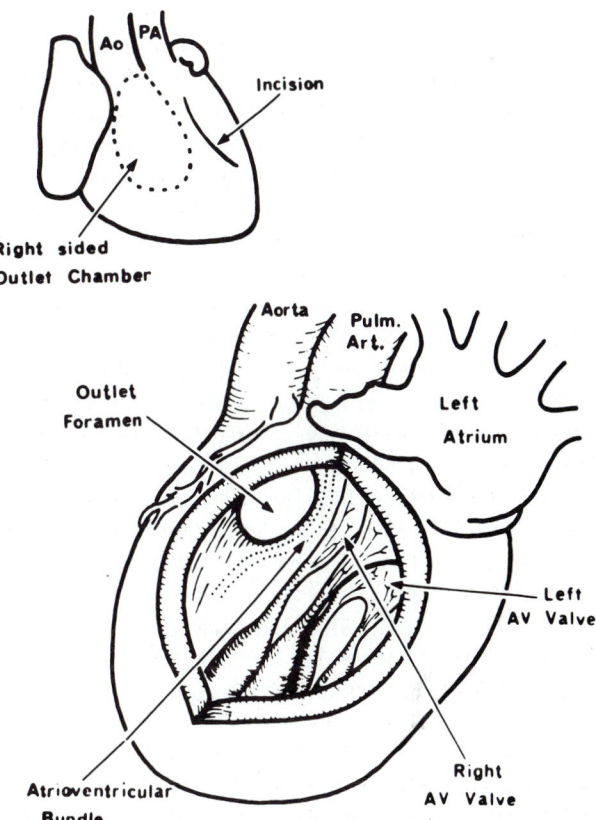

Figure 72–2. The disposition of the conduction tissue in double-inlet left ventricle with a right-sided rudimentary right ventricle.[7] *(From Becker AE, Wilkinson JL, Anderson RH: Atrioventricular conduction tissues in the univentricular hearts of the left ventricular type. Herz 4:166, 1979.)*

NATURAL HISTORY

In unoperated patients with univentricular heart, Moodie et al found a 50% mortality 14 years after diagnosis. The most common causes of death were congestive heart failure (20%), dysrhythmia (20%), and sudden and unexplained death (10%).[9] Franklin et al reviewed the survival without definitive repair in 191 patients presenting with double inlet ventricle before 1 year of age. The actuarial survival was 57% at 1 year, 43% at 5 years, and 42% at 10 years.[10] The poor long-term survival in unoperated and palliated patients justifies an aggressive surgical approach.

CLINICAL PRESENTATION

The clinical presentation is most dependent on the associated lesions and the degree of pulmonary blood flow. With unobstructed pulmonary blood flow, the large left-to-right shunt will lead to congestive heart failure. This condition may be more severe or present earlier in life when there is a coincident coarctation or aortic arch interruption. The typical appearance of such a patient is a small, underdeveloped,

diaphoretic, tachypneic infant who may be mildly cyanotic. In contradistinction, the patient with obstruction to pulmonary flow will exhibit a more marked cyanosis without signs or symptoms of congestive heart failure. The rare patient with a well-balanced circulation due to unobstructed systemic blood flow and sufficient pulmonary stenosis to control pulmonary blood flow has the best survival and treatment outcome.

Oxygen saturation in complex single ventricles can also be affected by the streaming effect. Mixing of systemic and pulmonary venous blood occurs in the main chamber and may result in nearly identical aortic and pulmonary arterial oxygen saturations. However, streaming patterns within the ventricle may lead to significant differences in oxygen saturations between the great vessels.

PREOPERATIVE EVALUATION

A precise preoperative diagnosis is essential to proper surgical planning and successful definitive repair. The history, physical examination, chest radiograph, and electrocardiogram will not lead to a specific diagnosis. The history and physical examination will be helpful in identifying the presence of congenital heart disease, the position of the heart, the presence of a cyanotic lesion, and signs and symptoms of congestive heart failure. The chest radiograph aids in determination of cardiac position and whether pulmonary blood flow is increased, decreased, or normal. The electrocardiogram may be helpful in identifying the presence of heart disease, abnormal conduction patterns, and cardiac position but, again, is nonspecific.

Two-dimensional echocardiography most accurately identifies which variation of complex single ventricle is present, and identifies ventricular morphology.[11–13] In addition, two-dimensional echocardiography provides important morphologic details such as atrial situs, anatomy of the atrioventricular valves, ventriculoarterial connections, position of the bulboventricular foramen and semilunar valve, and anatomy of the great vessels. Utilizing Doppler techniques, it also offers hemodynamic information, such as atrioventricular valve competency or stenosis, and degree of obstruction across a bulboventricular foramen or semilunar valve. Finally, it identifies associated defects.

Axial angiocardiography also accurately identifies the presence of complex single ventricle and the ventricular morphology.[14] Its advantages over two-dimensional echocardiography are better delineation of the great vessel anatomy, more precise measurement of pressure gradients across ventricular outlets, and elucidation of the coronary artery pattern. However, with angiography, the precise arrangement of the atrioventricular valves cannot be well established.

SURGICAL THERAPY

Palliative Procedures

The majority of patients with complex single ventricle will ultimately be candidates for a Fontan-type procedure. Patients must undergo early appropriate palliation to avoid the effects of excessive pulmonary blood flow, i.e., pulmonary hypertension, ventricular dilatation, and ventricular outlet obstruction. The palliative procedures include pulmonary artery banding for excessive pulmonary blood flow, systemic to pulmonary artery shunts for inadequate pulmonary blood flow, and procedures to relieve systemic ventricular outflow obstruction. In addition, associated defects, such as coarctation of the aorta, aortic arch interruption, and patent ductus arteriosus, must be addressed.

Patients with unrestricted pulmonary blood flow will develop pulmonary vascular obstructive disease without surgical intervention. In addition, their ventricular volume load will result in ventricular dilatation and ventricular dysfunction. Attenuation of pulmonary blood flow is achieved by placement of a pulmonary artery band. This technique was first described by Muller and Damman in 1952 for palliation of infants with severe left-to-right shunting.[15]

Pulmonary artery banding effectively limits excessive pulmonary blood flow, thereby protecting the patient from pulmonary vascular disease and ventricular dysfunction. The operative mortality has decreased significantly in recent years ranging from 0 to 24%.[16,20,21] Complications of pulmonary artery banding include erosion of the band into the pulmonary artery lumen, distal migration with obstruction of the right or left pulmonary arteries, and pulmonary insufficiency secondary to dilatation of the pulmonary annulus.

In the case of neonates with double-inlet left ventricle with minimal (<30 mm Hg) or no obstruction of the bulboventricular foramen and unrestricted pulmonary blood flow, pulmonary artery banding may hasten the development of subaortic obstruction by reduction of ventricular volume and progressive ventricular hypertrophy. Hypertrophy may also impair diastolic ventricular function, potentially worsening the result after subsequent Fontan procedure. Since pulmonary artery banding has become an increasingly short-term palliation, the feared adverse effects are not so significant, because subaortic obstruction does not develop immediately. These patients should be followed closely with two-dimensional echocardiography to assess both the adequacy of the pulmonary artery band and the development of subaortic obstruction. If subaortic stenosis occurs, the patient may proceed to a Damus–Stansel–Kaye procedure and a bidirectional cavopulmonary shunt as a stage toward a Fontan procedure.[17] The optimal timing for this step is not known; however, it may be performed as early as 2–3 months.[18]

Relief of systemic outflow tract obstruction may be required in some patients with complex single ventricle. Subaortic stenosis develops in up to 84% of patients with double-inlet left ventricle with discordant ventriculoarterial connection.[19] The bulboventricular foramen may be restrictive in the neonatal period or may become restrictive in infancy or early childhood.[20] A restrictive bulboventricular foramen is more commonly associated with obstructive anomalies of the aortic arch, such as coarctation and interruption. As discussed above, the obstruction may be dynamic and respond to isoprenalin.[19] Application of a PA band may hasten the development of subaortic stenosis in this subset of patients.[18,19,21]

Neonates with a restrictive bulboventricular foramen may be treated with a palliative arterial switch procedure and a central shunt.[22,23] Older children who present with mild to moderate subaortic stenosis (<50 mm Hg) may undergo a combined Fontan procedure with associated relief of subaortic obstruction by muscle resection or a Damus–Stansel–Kaye procedure. Those who present with severe subaortic obstruction (gradient >50 mm Hg) have a high mortality rate if a Fontan procedure is performed in the presence of severe left ventricular hypertrophy.[19] These patients should undergo instead a procedure to relieve the subaortic stenosis and stage toward a Fontan arrangement with a bidirectional cavopulmonary anastomosis. The safest approach to the treatment of subaortic stenosis is with the

Damus–Stansel–Kaye procedure because it avoids damage to the conduction system by obviating the need for a ventriculotomy. It may, however, result in distortion of the pulmonary or aortic valves, thereby causing regurgitation. This can usually be avoided by assuring the great vessel connection does not distort the semilunar valves.[17] If the pulmonary valve is insufficient, a muscular resection of the outflow obstruction is preferred. Improved knowledge of the conduction tissue and its relationship to the bulboventricular foramen has allowed resection with a reduced incidence (5–10%) of heart block. The bulboventricular foramen may be exposed by an incision in the bulboventricular chamber,[24] or the resection can be performed via an aortotomy and avoid a ventriculotomy.[25]

Patients with inadequate pulmonary blood flow and arterial oxygen desaturation may require a palliative procedure to improve blood flow to the lungs. Inadequate pulmonary blood flow is a consequence of pulmonary atresia, valvular pulmonary stenosis, or subvalvular pulmonary stenosis. A variety of palliative systemic to pulmonary shunts may be used, including the classical Blalock–Taussig (B-T) shunt with direct subclavian artery to pulmonary artery anastomosis, a modified B-T shunt using an interposition Gore-Tex graft, a central Gore-Tex shunt, and a Glenn shunt (superior vena cava to pulmonary artery anastomosis). Appropriate shunt selection is based on patient age, hemodynamics, and anatomic factors.

In neonates and young infants, pulmonary vascular resistance and pulmonary vasoreactivity generally preclude construction of a systemic *venous* to pulmonary artery shunt (Glenn shunt). Instead, a systemic arterial to pulmonary artery shunt (B-T, modified B-T, central) is the palliative procedure of choice. The modified B-T shunt has the patency of the classical B-T shunt and the advantage of preserving the subclavian artery. An older infant may be a candidate for a bidirectional cavopulmonary anastomosis (modified Glenn shunt) as the first shunt if the pulmonary vasculature has been protected by pulmonic stenosis or a previously placed pulmonary artery band. If the pulmonary resistance is elevated, a systemic arterial to pulmonary shunt may be required. An excessively large shunt must be avoided in any patient considered a future candidate for a Fontan procedure.

In appropriately selected patients, a Glenn shunt provides excellent pulmonary blood flow and reduces the systemic ventricular volume loading. Because the pulmonary flow occurs at lower pressures, the development of pulmonary vascular disease is avoided. The lower age limit for performing the Glenn shunt has not been established, but patients in their second month of life have successfully undergone this procedure.[18,25]

The classic Glenn shunt (superior vena cava to right pulmonary artery) is now rarely performed and has largely been replaced by the bidirectional cavopulmonary anastomosis (modified Glenn shunt), which provides pulmonary blood flow to both lungs and maintenance of pulmonary

artery continuity. The bidirectional Glenn shunt can be created using a temporary superior vena cava (SVC) to right atrial shunt, obviating the need for cardiopulmonary bypass.[26] The deleterious effects of cardiopulmonary bypass, increased pulmonary vascular resistance and ventricular dysfunction, thereby are avoided. If concomitant intracardiac procedures are required (e.g., relief of subaortic obstruction, repair of an atrioventricular valve, and enlargement of an atrial septal defect), then cardiopulmonary bypass is utilized.

The SVC carries between 40 and 50% of the systemic venous return in infants. In older children the SVC carries 33% of the systemic venous return. Therefore, as the patient grows, pulmonary blood flow decreases. However, flow through the shunt does not increase with exercise. Therefore, some centers add an additional small source of pulmonary blood flow to a bidirectional Glenn shunt in older children.[25] This may be accomplished by placing a small central Gore-Tex shunt or by allowing and limiting flow from the ventricle by placing a tight pulmonary artery band. Either technique will provide an increase in pulmonary blood flow during exercise. In patients with poor ventricular function, definitive repair with the Fontan procedure may be precluded; however, a bidirectional Glenn shunt combined with a small systemic source of pulmonary blood flow may provide excellent long-term palliation.

Definitive Procedures

Ventricular septation was first successfully performed by Kirklin in 1956 and reintroduced by McGoon as an attractive approach to creating a biventricular circulation.[27] Experience with this procedure, however, demonstrated significant associated mortality and morbidity, including postoperative complete heart block requiring permanent pacing, late residual VSD, incompetent A-V valve requiring reoperation, and a high incidence of sudden death.[16] The success with ventricular septation has been largely with double inlet left ventricle with ventriculoarterial discordance and left-sided rudimentary right ventricle with absent or mild pulmonary stenosis.[27,28] The important surgical considerations include the anatomy of the A-V valves and the presence or absence of pulmonary and subaortic stenosis. The competence and precise morphology of the A-V valves need to be assessed preoperatively by Doppler echocardiography and intraoperative direct inspection. A-V valve repair or replacement is associated with increased risk and morbidity, but may be necessary.[16] For example, the presence of a common A-V valve or straddling A-V valve may not allow successful septation without valve repair or replacement.

Patients with subvalvular PA stenosis or a hypoplastic valve annulus may require an extracardiac conduit, which is also associated with increased morbidity and mortality.[28,29] The presence of subaortic stenosis due to a restrictive outlet foramen has been treated with concurrent subarterial resection; however, when septation is attempted in such patients, it is associated with a prohibitive mortality.[16,30]

Ebert has proposed a modification to this technique in performing the septation in two stages.[31] In the first year of life, two septation patches are loosely tacked into place with several sutures. Fibrosis occurs near the border of the patch and allows a safe second stage to close the residual defects and minimize the risk of heart block.

Imai et al has reported 19 patients who were considered poor candidates for Fontan physiology and underwent ventricular septation.[32] An incidence of third degree heart block of 26% with one early and three late deaths was reported. This marked improvement in outcome was attributed to performing partitioning at an early age (1 year) and utilizing a transatrial approach.

Ventricular septation is performed through a median sternotomy using cardiopulmonary bypass and moderate hypothermia. Mapping of the bundle of His should be considered before administration of cardioplegia. The anatomy of the coronary arteries is determined to plan the proper incision. A right atriotomy is made; ventricular morphology, size and location of VSD, and subpulmonic stenosis are assessed. With a discordant ventriculoarterial connection and left-sided rudimentary right ventricle, a straight patch can be placed. However, if the aorta is anterior or right-sided, a spiral patch is required.

Septation can be performed either transatrially or through an inferior fish-mouthed ventriculotomy (Fig. 72–3), making sure the incision does not interfere with the origin of a papillary muscle and that it remains to the right or directly at the side of the septal patch. Generally, a transatrial approach is preferred in an attempt to preserve ventricular function. The patch must be inserted between the atrioventricular valves, which carries a risk of heart

block in patients with double-inlet left ventricle and discordant ventriculoarterial connection. This risk may be reduced with the aforementioned two-stage partitioning technique. Both arterial outlets may be placed on the left side of the patch, creating a double-outlet left ventricle, which requires an external conduit from the right side of the patch to the pulmonary artery. The patch is secured in place with multiple pledgeted sutures placed along the charted location (Fig. 72–4). The area between the anterior and posterior sutures along the base of the heart is closed with a continuous running polypropylene suture. If a ventriculotomy was performed, it then is closed over Teflon felt strips. Finally, the atrial septal defect is closed followed by the atriotomy. Permanent epicardial pacing leads are placed due to the high incidence of heart block.[30]

If patients have a subaortic chamber to the left, no previous congestive heart failure, and no prior palliative procedures, late survival after the septation procedure has been reported as high as 70 to 80%.[16,29,32] However, in unselected cases, operative mortality approaches 50%.[31] Therefore, with improved results with the modified Fontan procedure, ventricular septation has been limited to patients with complex single ventricle who are poor candidates for a Fontan circulation.

The Fontan procedure is now established as an effective definitive procedure in selected patients. Since Fontan first described the operation in 1971[33] for tricuspid atresia, the indications for this procedure have been significantly broadened to include many forms of complex single ventricle. In addition, some defects which have two well-developed ventricles and cannot be repaired have been successfully treated with the Fontan procedure. The selection criteria have also been repeatedly redefined. Since Choussat's selection criteria were published in 1977,[34] many cen-

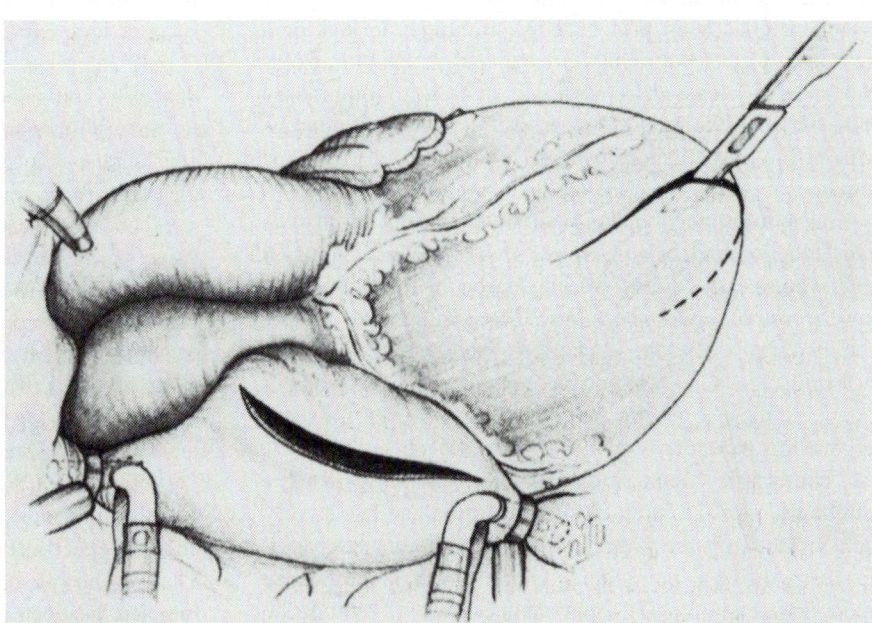

Figure 72–3. The position of the atriotomy and ventriculotomy incisions for ventricular septation.[29] *(From Pacifico AD, Kirklin JK, Kirklin JW: Surgical management of double inlet ventricle, World J Surg 9:579, 1985.)*

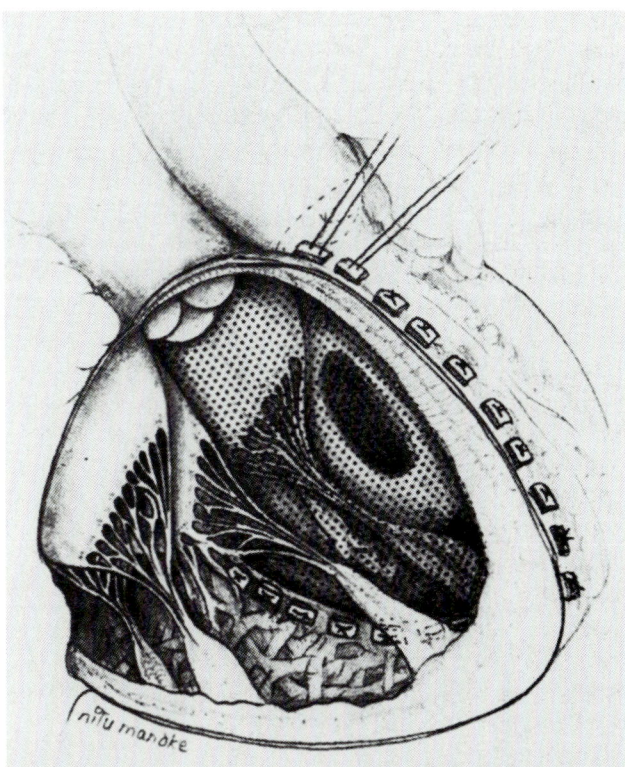

Figure 72–4. The position of the septation patch is shown inserted between the atrioventricular valves creating a right and left component.[29] *(From Pacifico AD, Kirklin JK, Kirklin JW: Surgical management of double inlet ventricle, World J Surg 9:579, 1985.)*

TABLE 72–1. RISK STRATIFICATION FOR FONTAN PROCEDURE[a]

	Risk		
	Low	*Medium*	*High*
PVR (Wood units/m^2)	<2.0	2–3	>3
Mean PA pressure (mm Hg)	<12	13–15	>15
Transpulmonary gradient (mm Hg)	5	5–10	>10

[a]PVR, pulmonary vascular resistance; PA, pulmonary artery.

ters have attempted to refine his recommendations by trying to determine which combination of criteria can be ignored without compromising a successful outcome.[35]

The optimal age for the Fontan procedure has not been fully established and an individualized approach is warranted. Although the early recommendations of Choussat included age greater than 4 years, recent reports have contradicted this age limit.[36–38] Excessive delay can result in progressive ventricular dysfunction due to volume loading.

Many of the anatomic factors contraindicated for the Fontan procedure are often amenable to repair.[39] For example, distorted or stenotic pulmonary arteries may be dilated, stented, or patched. Anomalies of pulmonary and systemic venous drainage may be corrected surgically. A regurgitant atrioventricular valve may be repaired or replaced. Ventricular outflow obstruction may be treated with muscular resection or a Damus–Stansel–Kaye procedure.

The most important criteria for the Fontan procedure are pulmonary vascular resistance and ventricular function. Risk has been stratified accordingly and is illustrated in Table 72–1.[25,40] Low- and medium-risk patients should be considered for an early (< 2 years) and/or primary Fontan procedure (depending on their other risk factors), while high-risk patients should be staged with a bidirectional Glenn shunt. Ventricular dysfunction is more difficult to assess than is pulmonary artery resistance, and a combination

of parameters are used. Ejection fraction less than 45%, left ventricular end-diastolic pressure >16 mm Hg, increased systemic ventricular diastolic dimension, and severe hypertrophy secondary to outflow tract obstruction all place patients at increased risk.[36–38] Generally, these high-risk patients would undergo a preliminary bidirectional Glenn shunt to reduce excessive pulmonary blood flow. In addition, concomitant procedures to repair a regurgitant atrioventricular valve and relieve ventricular outflow obstruction should be performed in an attempt to improve ventricular function and to optimize the chances for future completion of the Fontan procedure.

The original technique of the Fontan procedure has undergone several modifications. Currently, most utilize the total cavopulmonary connection or a combination of the bidirectional cavopulmonary anastomosis with an extracardiac conduit. These techniques minimize the exposure of the right atrial myocardium to high right atrial pressures, and may, therefore, reduce the incidence of arrhythmias. In addition, there may be a hemodynamic advantage by eliminating the turbulence associated with a contracting, dilated atrium.[41] Generally included in these procedures is the creation of a communication between the systemic venous tunnel, or conduit, and the atrial chamber (Fig. 72–5). This communication is either a fixed or a snare-controlled adjustable fenestration (Fig. 72–6) which creates a right-to-left shunt at the atrial level, allowing cardiac output to be maintained at the expense of oxygenation in the presence of any condition that transiently retards pulmonary blood flow during the early postoperative period.[42–44] By limiting the postoperative increase in right-sided pressures, the incidence and/or duration of postoperative pleuropericardial effusions have been reduced.[36] This technique has not only reduced perioperative morbidity and mortality, but is credited for allowing higher risk patients to successfully undergo definitive therapy with a Fontan procedure. For the technical details of the Fontan procedure and postoperative management, see Chapter 88.

The early results after modified Fontan procedures have dramatically improved over the past 25 years with operative mortality less than 10% in many reports.[40,45–48] Mortality is clearly related to preoperative risk factors, with pulmonary vascular resistance and ventricular function of greatest importance. Results have improved with the appli-

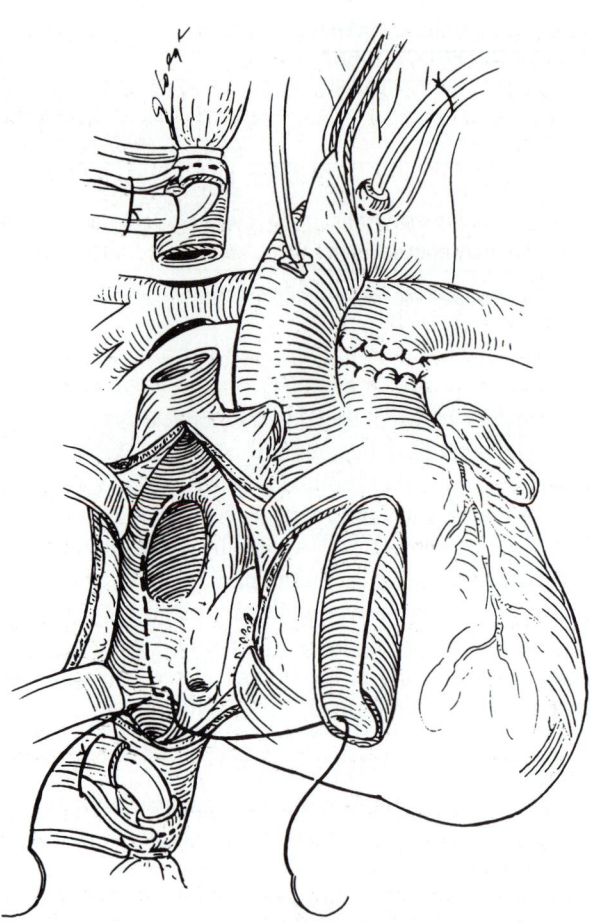

Figure 72–5. Creation of the lateral tunnel with PTFE tube graft.[40] *(From Pearl JM et al: Ann Thorac Surg 52:189, 1991.)*

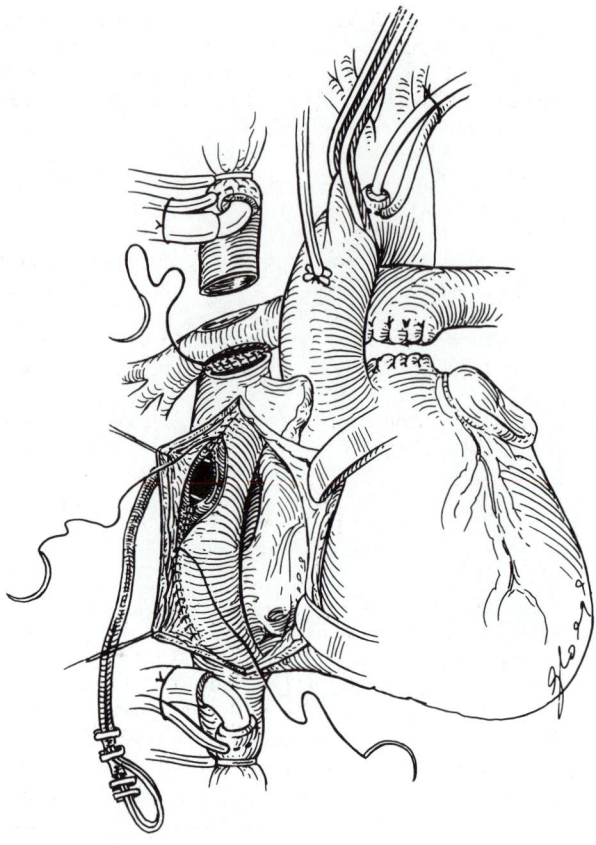

Figure 72–6. Snare-controlled atrial septal defect as a component of a lateral tunnel procedure.[42] *(From Laks H et al: Ann Thorac Surg 52:1084, 1991.)*

cation of more liberal use of staging with the bidirectional Glenn shunt and the inclusion of either a fixed or adjustable fenestration between the systemic and pulmonary venous chambers. The incidence of postoperative pleuropericardial effusions has been markedly reduced to approximately 10%.[36]

The late results after a Fontan procedure are also influenced by preoperative risk factors.[35] Ten-year survival has been reported to be 90% or greater in some subgroups, e.g., double-inlet ventricle and tricuspid atresia.[45,47] However, overall 10-year rates have been reported between 60 and 81%.[48,49] In addition, functional capacity has decreased over time in many patients. A correlation of this decrease exists in patients who had a Fontan procedure performed at an older age.[48] Late deaths are secondary to persistent or progressive systemic venous hypertension, dysrrhythmias, chronic systemic ventricular failure, and protein-losing enteropathy.[40,45–48] Careful follow-up is warranted to detect surgically correctable causes of deterioration including progressive atrioventricular valve dysfunction, systemic ventricular outflow obstruction, pulmonary artery stenosis, and obstruction of systemic venous drainage. In patients who

continue to decline in the absence of surgically correctable lesions, cardiac transplantation should be considered.

REFERENCES

1. Van Praagh R, Ongley PA, Swan HJC: Anatomic types of single or common ventricle in man: Morphologic and geometric aspects of 60 necropsied cases. *Am J Cardiol* **13**:367, 1964
2. Van Praagh R, Plett JA, Van Praagh ST: Single ventricle: pathology, embryology, terminology, and classification. *Herz* **4**:113, 1979
3. Van Praagh R: Terminology of congenital heart disease. *Circulation* **56**:139, 1977
4. Anderson RH, Tynan M, Freedom RM, et al: Ventricular morphology of the univentricular heart. *Herz* **4**:184, 1979
6. Anderson RH, Becker AE, Wenink, ACG: The development of the conducting tissues. In Roberts NK, Gelband H (eds): *Cardiac Arrhythmias in the Neonate, Infant, and Children.* New York, Appleton and Crofts, 1977
7. Becker AE, Wilkinson JL, Anderson RH: Atrioventricular conduction tissues in the univentricular hearts of the left ventricular type. *Herz* **4**:166, 1979
8. Keeton BR, Lie JT, McGoon DW, et al: Anatomy of coronary arteries in univentricular hearts and its surgical implications. *Am J Cardiol* **43**:569, 1979

9. Moodie DS, Ritter DG, Tajik AJ, et al: Long-term follow-up in the unoperated univentricular heart. *Am J Cardiol* **53:**1124, 1984

10. Franklin RCG, Spielgelhalter DJ, Anderson RH, et al: Double-inlet ventricle presenting in infancy. I. Survival without definitive repair. *J Thorac Cardiovasc Surg* **101:**767, 1991

11. Bevilacqua M, Sanders SP, Van Praagh S, et al: Double-inlet single left ventricle: Echocardiographic anatomy with emphasis on the morphology of the atrioventricular valves and ventricular septal defect. *J Am Coll Cardiol* **18:**559, 1991

12. Rice MJ, Seward JB, Edwards WD, et al: Straddling atrioventricular valve: Two-dimensional echocardiographic diagnosis, classification, and surgical implications. *Am J Cardiol* **55:**505, 1985

13. Shiraishi H, Silverman NH: Echocardiographic spectrum of double-inlet ventricle: Evaluation of the interventricular communication. *J Am Coll Cardiol* **15:**1401, 1990

14. Macartney FJ, Partridge JB, Scott O, et al: Common or single ventricle: An angiocardiographic and hemodynamic study of 42 patients. *Circulation* **53:**5434, 1976

15. Muller WH, Damman JF: The surgical significance of pulmonary hypertension. *Ann Surg* **136:**495, 1952

16. Stefanelli G, Kirklin JW, Naftel DC, et al: Early and intermediate-term (10-year) results of surgery for univentricular atrioventricular connection ("single ventricle"). *Am J Cardiol* **54:**811, 1984

17. Laks H, Gates RN, Elami A, et al: The Damus-Stansel-Kaye procedure: Technical modifications. *Ann Thorac Surg* **54:**169, 1992

18. Jonas RA: Indications and timing for the bidirectional Glenn shunt versus the fenestrated Fontan circulation. *J Thorac Cardiovasc Surg* **108:**522, 1994

19. Freedom RM, Benson LN, Smallhorn JF, et al: Subaortic stenosis, the univentricular heart, and banding of the pulmonary artery: An analysis of 43 patients with univentricular heart palliated by pulmonary artery banding. *Circulation* **73:**758, 1986

20. Franklin RCG, Spiegelhalter DJ, Anderson RH, et al: Double-inlet ventricle presenting in infancy. II. Results of palliative operations. *J Thorac Cardiovasc Surg* **101:**917, 1991

21. Nooten GB, Deuvaert FE, De Paepe P, Primo G: Pulmonary artery banding: Experience with 69 patients. *J Cardiovasc Surg* **30:**334, 1989

22. Karl TR, Watterson KG, Sano S, et al: Operation of subaortic stenosis in univentricular hearts. *Ann Thorac Surg* **52:**420, 1991

23. Freedom RM, Trusler GA: Arterial switch for palliation of subaortic stenosis in single ventricle and transposition: No mean feat! *Ann Thorac Surg* **52:**415, 1991

24. Cheung HC, Lincoln C, Anderson RH, et al: Options for surgical repair in hearts with univentricular atrioventricular connection and subaortic stenosis. *J Thorac Cardiovasc Surg* **100:**672, 1990

25. Esmailian F, Permut LC, Gates RN, Laks H: Single ventricle with double inlet atrioventricular connection. In Mavroudis C, Backer C (eds): *Pediatric Cardiac Surgery,* 2nd ed 1994, p 401

26. Stein DG, Laks H, Drinkwater DC, et al: Results of total cavopulmonary connection in the treatment of patients with a functional single ventricle. *J Thorac Cardiovasc Surg* **102:**280, 1991

27. McGoon DC, Danielson GK, Ritter DG, et al: Correction of univentricular heart having two atrioventricular valves. *J Thorac Cardiovasc Surg* **74:**218, 1977

28. McKay R, Pacifico AD, Blackstone EH, et al: Septation of the univentricular heart with left anterior subaortic outlet chamber. *J Thorac Cardiovasc Surg* **84:**77, 1982

29. Pacifico AD, Kirklin JK, Kirklin JW: Surgical management of double inlet ventricle. *World J Surg* **9:**579, 1985

30. Feldt RH, Mair DD, Danielson GK, et al: Current status of the septation procedure for univentricular heart. *J Thorac Cardiovasc Surg* **82:**97, 1981

31. Ebert PA: Staged partitioning of the single ventricle. *J Thorac Cardiovasc Surg* **88:**908, 1984

32. Imai Y, Hoshino S, Koh YS, et al: Ventricular septation for univentricular connection of the left ventricular type. *Sem Cardiovasc Surg* **6:**48, 1994

33. Fontan F, Baudet E: Surgical repair of tricuspid atresia. *Thorax* **26:**240, 1971

34. Choussat A, Fontan F, Besse P, et al: Selection criteria for Fontan's procedure. In Anderson RH, Shinebourne EA (eds): *Pediatric Cardiology,* Edinburgh, Churchill Livingstone, 1977

35. Gewillig M: The Fontan circulation: Late functional results. *Sem Thorac Cardiovasc Surg* **6:**56, 1994

36. Castaneda AR: From Glenn to Fontan: A continuing evolution. *Circulation* **86**(suppl II):II-80, 1992

37. Mayer JE, Bridges ND, Lock JE, et al: Factors associated with marked reduction in mortality for Fontan operations in patients with single ventricle. *J Thorac Cardiovasc Surg* **103:**444, 1992

38. Esmailian F, Permut LC, Gates RN, Laks H: Single ventricle with double-inlet atrioventricular connection. In Mavroudis C, Backer CL (eds): *Pediatric Cardiac Surgery,* 2nd ed. St. Louis, Mosby Year Book, 1994, p 401

39. Mayer JE, Helgason H, Jonas RA, et al: Extending the limits for modified Fontan procedures. *J Thorac Cardiovasc Surg* **92:**1021, 1986

40. Pearl JM, Laks H, Stein DG, et al: Total cavopulmonary anastomosis versus conventional modified Fontan procedure. *Ann Thorac Surg* **52:**189, 1991

41. de Leval MR, Kilner P, Gewillig M, et al: Total cavopulmonary connection: A logical alternative to atriopulmonary connection for complex Fontan operation-experimental studies and early clinical experience. *J Thorac Cardiovasc Surg* **96:**682, 1988

42. Laks H, Pearl JM, Haas GS, et al: Partial Fontan: The advantages of an adjustable interatrial communication. *Ann Thorac Surg* **52:**1084, 1991

43. Billinsly AM, Laks H, Boyce SW, et al: Definitive repair in patients with pulmonary atresia and intact ventricular septum. *J Thorac Cardiovasc Surg* **97:**746, 1989

44. Bridges ND, Lock JE, Castaneda AR, et al: Baffle fenestration with subsequent transcatheter closure: Modification of the Fontan operation for patients at increased risk. *Circulation* **82:**1681, 1990

45. Mair DD, Hagler DH, Julsrud PR, et al: Early and late results of the modified Fontan procedure for double-inlet left ventricle: the Mayo Clinic experience. *J Am Coll Cardiol* **18:**1727, 1991

46. Laks H, Milliken JC, Perloff JK, et al: Experience with the Fontan procedure. *J Thorac Cardiovasc Surg* **88:**939, 1984

47. Mair DD, Hagler DJ, Puga FJ, et al: Fontan operation in 176 patients with tricuspid atresia-results and a proposed new index for patient selection. *Circulation* **82**(Suppl IV):164, 1990

48. Fontan F, Kirklin JW, Fernandez G, et al: Outcome after a "perfect" Fontan operation. *Circulation* **81:**1529, 1990

49. Driscoll DJ, Offord KP, Feldt RH, et al: Five- to fifteen-year follow-up after Fontan operation. *Circulation* **85:**469, 1992

CHAPTER

73

Straddling and Overriding Atrioventricular Valves

Gregory P. Fontana and Redmond P. Burke

Atrioventricular (A-V) valvular abnormalities are often difficult to correct and can substantially complicate the repair of coexisting congenital heart defects. The predominant defects are stenosis and insufficiency of A-V valves aligned to either the left or right ventricle. Rarely, the mitral or tricuspid valves have chordal attachments to the opposite, or improper, ventricle. These valves are *straddling,* and always occur in conjunction with a ventricular septal defect (VSD), with chordae crossing through and finding attachment directly to the septum or to a papillary muscle either on the septum or on the ventricular free wall. An A-V valve is considered *overriding* when the atrioventricular junction to which the A-V valve leaflets attach is connected to both the right and left ventricles (Fig. 73–1). This anomaly similarly occurs exclusively in the presence of a VSD. If the override exceeds 50% of the A-V valve diameter, the defect is called a *double inlet ventricle,* either right or left (Fig. 73–2), and is discussed in Chapters 71 and 72.

Other congenital heart defects associated with straddling and/or overriding A-V valves include complete transposition of the great arteries, double outlet ventricles, pulmonic stenosis, and ventricular hypoplasia. Generally, straddling *and* overriding occur; however, one may be present without the other. The more severe the override and/or the straddle, the more severe the ventricular hypoplasia.

Surgical strategy is based on the degree of override and/or straddle, the severity of ventricular hypoplasia, and the associated defects, any or all of which may limit the possibility of complete correction.

HISTORICAL

The anatomic features of straddling A-V valves were first described by Lambert in 1952.[1] Many others described A-V valves that either straddled, overrode, or both.[2–4] However, it was not until 1979 that Milo et al first outlined a complete system of classification.[5] Pacifico et al and Danielson et al first published the surgical management of this phenomenon that same year.[6–8] Once the morphologic variations were identified and two-dimensional echocardiography allowed accurate preoperative diagnosis, surgical techniques and strategy quickly evolved.

MORPHOLOGY

Normally, each ventricle is associated with a particular atrioventricular valve that identifies ventricular morphology as left or right, irrespective of situs or position. The tricuspid valve is associated with the morphologic right ventricle, except for the case of the double inlet left ventricle. The mitral valve is associated with the morphologic left ventricle, except for the case of double inlet right ventricle. These atrioventricular valves may override, straddle, or both (Fig. 73–1). Because the ventricular arrangement may be abnormal, the A-V valves are generally described as left or right, rather than as tricuspid or mitral.

Several anatomic syndromes have been identified to include straddling and/or overriding atrioventricular

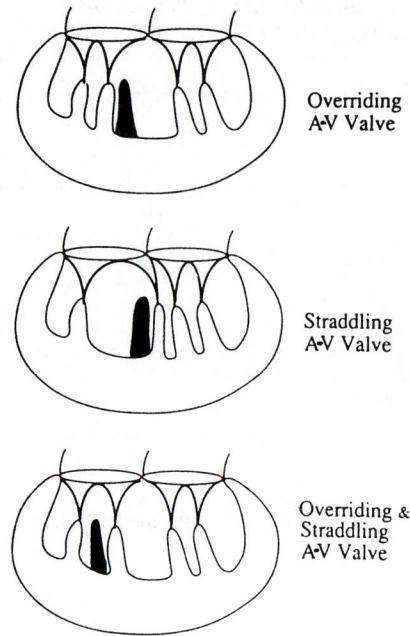

Figure 73–1. Diagram illustrating the terms overriding and straddling. The solid area is the ventricular septum. Overriding describes the relationship of the valve annulus to the ventricular septum; straddling describes valve tensor apparatus that is attached to both sides of the septum. *(From Lambert.[1])*

valves.[9] These syndromes, including their segmental anatomy, are listed below. The segmental approach describes the three major cardiac segments in a venoarterial sequence {atria, ventricles, great arteries}. The letters in braces ({X,X,X}) refer to the visceroatrial situs (situs solitus=S, situs inversus=I, situs ambiguous=A), the ventricular

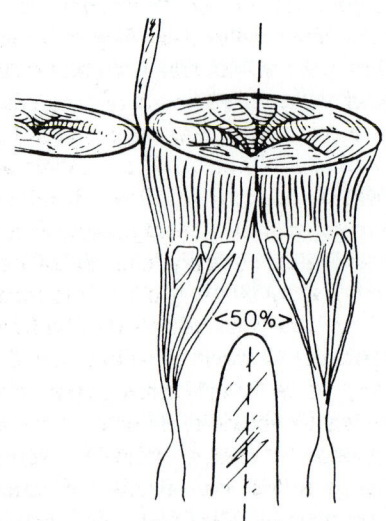

Figure 73–2. Overriding atrioventricular valve indicating biventricular commitment of the annulus. Less than or equal to 50% commitment of the annulus is considered a minor or major override, respectively, whereas greater than 50% denotes a double inlet ventricle. *(From Rice et al.[11])*

loop (D-loop=D, L-loop=L), and the position of the great arteries (normally related great arteries=S, inverted normally related great arteries=I, D-transposition or D-malposition=D, L-transposition or L-malposition=L), respectively.[10]

Anatomic Variations

1. Atrial situs solitus, right-handed ventricular loop (D-loop), atrioventricular and ventriculoarterial concordance {S,D,S}: the right A-V valve may override and/or straddle in association with a juxtacrucial (posteriorly placed) inlet VSD. The right ventricle is generally hypoplastic to varying degrees depending on the severity of the overriding A-V valve. The interventricular septum does not attach to the crux.

2. Atrial situs solitus, right-handed ventricular loop, atrioventricular and ventriculoarterial concordance {S,D,D} with double outlet right ventricle: when the VSD is juxta-aortic (and usually perimembranous and juxtacrucial) the right AV valve may override and usually straddle. Conversely, the VSD may be juxtapulmonary and anterior (not extending to the crux) with an overriding and straddling left A-V valve (Taussig–Bing variant) {S,L,L}.

3. Atrial situs solitus, ventricular right-handedness, AV concordant connection, ventriculoarterial discordance {S,D,D}(complete transposition of the great arteries): an overriding left A-V valve is in association with an anterior VSD.

4. Atrial situs solitus, left-handed ventricular loop, A-V discordant connection, ventriculoarterial discordance {S,L,D}(corrected transposition of the great arteries): a right A-V valve overrides an anterior VSD where the ventricular septum does extend to the crux. If override exceeds 50%, then this defect is termed double inlet right ventricle. Conversely, a left A-V valve may override a posterior VSD when the ventricular septum does *not* reach the crux {S,L,L}. Again, if the override exceeds 50%, this lesion is termed a double inlet left ventricle.

5. "Criss-Cross Heart," i.e., those with A-V discordance, a juxtacrucial VSD that coincides with straddling and overriding of one or both A-V valves: the ventricles are usually positioned "upstairs-downstairs" or "over-and-under" and commonly are associated with double outlet right ventricle.

All of the above may occur, more rarely, in the setting of atrial situs inversus {I,X,X} or atrial situs ambiguous {A,X,X}. Common A-V valves (atrioventricular septal defects, complete A-V canal defects) also may straddle and/or override and occasionally are associated with some of the above complex variations.

Overriding A-V valves exceeding 50% of the valve diameter are classified as double inlet ventricles (Fig. 73–2). Some authors have distinguished between minor and major overriding as those less than and approximating 50%, respectively.[11]

Straddling A-V valves are also classified according to their severity.[11,12] Type A valves include those that have chordae crossing a VSD and attaching on the septum within 1 cm of the defect (Fig. 73–3). In type B valves, chordal attachments are greater than 1 cm from the VSD crest, but still are on the septum. Type C valves have chordae that insert into the free wall or the papillary muscles of the contralateral ventricle. The degree of override tends to correlate with the severity of the straddle (Table 73–1).[11] There is an equal distribution of overriding right and left A-V valves in clinical reports from both the Mayo Clinic[11] and the University of Alabama at Birmingham[9]; however, several pathologic reports show a prevalence of overriding right A-V valves.[11]

Conduction System

Milo et al examined cadaveric hearts with straddling and/or overriding A-V valves in an effort to define the conduction system of the various groups.[5] They found the position of the conduction system unaffected when the VSD did not reach the crux of the heart. In corrected transposition of the great arteries with an overriding tricuspid valve, the atrioventricular node was anterolateral and conduction continued along the anterior aspect of the VSD (Fig. 73–4). When there was atrioventricular concordance and the septum did not extend to the crux, the atrioventricular node was positioned posterolaterally. Despite this knowledge, surgically

TABLE 73–1. ASSOCIATION OF OVERRIDING WITH ATRIOVENTRICULAR VALVE[a]

| Type of Straddling | Overriding | | | |
| | Minor (<50%) | | Major (≈50%) | |
	n	%	n	%
A	21[b]	78	6	22
B	10	77	3	23
C	3	27	8	73
Total	34	67	17	33

[a] Ten patients (19%) with double inlet ventricle not included.
[b] Two patients (4%) had no overriding.
(From Rice et al.[11])

created heart block remains a significant source of postoperative morbidity.

INCIDENCE

Straddling and overriding AV valves are rare, occurring in approximately one in 4200 live-births (3% of congenital heart defects).[9] They occur most commonly in association with complex congenital heart defects such as double outlet right ventricle and transposition of the great arteries. A-V discordant connections are more common than concordant.

DIAGNOSIS

The coexisting cardiac anomalies, not the straddling and/or overriding A-V valve, generally determine the clinical syndrome, the natural history, and the diagnostic features in patients with straddling and/or overriding A-V valves.[9,13] Although history, physical examination, chest radiograph, and ECT may lead to the identification of congenital heart disease, there are no specific identifying criteria for straddling and/or overriding A-V valves. These valves are typically competent and do not restrict inflow; therefore, diagnosis may not be made until the patient undergoes a two-dimensional echocardiogram or cardiac catheterization.

No other imaging modality permits as accurate a visualization of the atrioventricular valve leaflets and their support apparatus as does two-dimensional echocardiography.[11] In general, the echocardiographic distinction between a double inlet ventricle and other forms of A-V connection associated with minor or major overriding is not difficult. The presence and severity of straddling A-V valves are accurately identified with two-dimensional echocardiography.[11]

Angiography will demonstrate overriding A-V valves, particularly in the axial view.[14,15] It does not always, however, accurately delineate chordal insertions in valves which straddle.[11] Magnetic resonance imaging has been

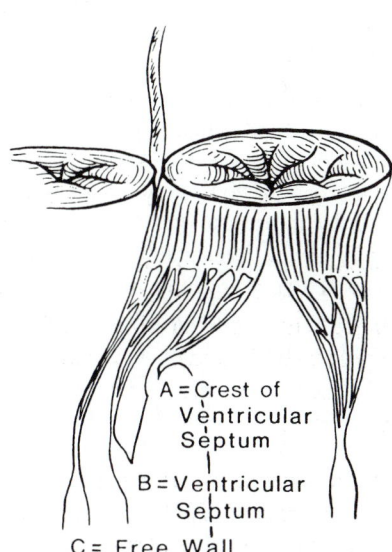

A = Crest of Ventricular Septum
B = Ventricular Septum
C = Free Wall

Figure 73–3. Classification of straddling atrioventricular valves. In type A, the chordae insert into the contralateral ventricle within 1 cm of the crest; in type B, the chordae insert into the contralateral ventricular septum greater than 1 cm from the crest; in type C, the chordae insert onto the free wall or papillary muscle of the contralateral ventricle. *(From Rice et al.[11])*

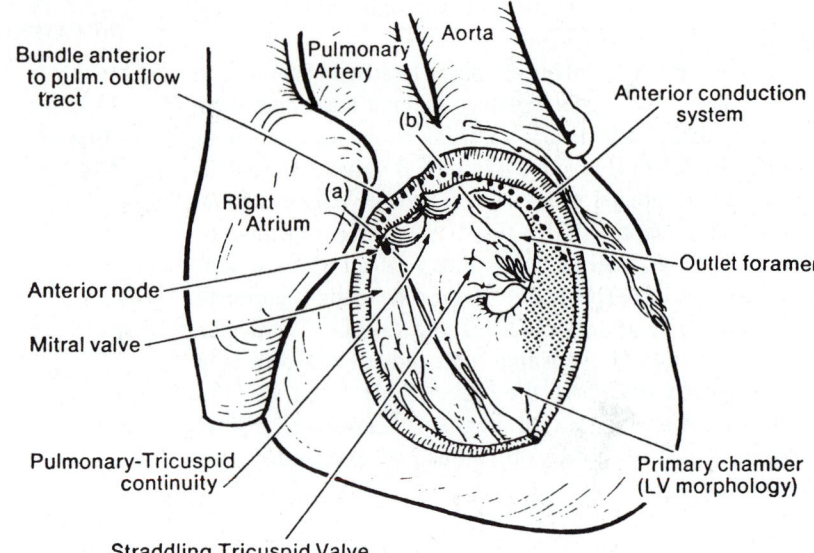

Figure 73–4. The course of the conduction pathways in a heart with corrected transposition of the great arteries {S,D,L} is along the anterior aspect of the VSD. (a), anterior atrioventricular node; (b), anterior nonbranching bundle. (*From Milo et al.*[5])

successfully utilized to diagnose complex cardiac disease and may be useful in some cases.[13]

SURGICAL TREATMENT

A number of techniques have been described to successfully treat straddling and/or overriding atrioventricular valves.[6–9,16] The primary consideration is in determining whether or not a two-ventricle repair is possible. When the straddle and/or override is minimal, a two ventricle repair is generally achieved. Only minor alterations to a VSD closure, such as deviation of the suture-line to accommodate the override or straddle, are necessary. When the override and/or straddle are severe and associated with significant ventricular hypoplasia, palliative procedures or staging toward a Fontan-type physiology may be required. In the rare case of severe straddling and/or overriding A-V valves with a cardiomyopathy, cardiac transplantation may be the only option. Whether a single- or two-ventricle repair is performed, every effort should be made to preserve a normally functioning A-V valve. Infrequently, valve replacement is required.

The approach to symptomatic neonates with straddling and/or overriding A-V valves is initial palliation by limiting or providing pulmonary blood flow, as appropriate, by means of a pulmonary artery band, or systemic to pulmonary artery shunt, respectively. Asymptomatic patients whose pulmonary arterial blood flow is appropriate can be managed medically until a two-ventricle repair is possible or staging toward a Fontan-type repair is feasible.

TECHNIQUES

Minor septation entails closing a VSD or creating an intraventricular tunnel with a patch altering the suture line to allow the straddling A-V valve to lie within the appropriate ventricle. This technique is most easily performed when the valve straddles into the ventricle in which the surgeon is working. A more challenging technique is placing a patch through the VSD (Fig. 73–5). A less desirable approach through a ventriculotomy may be used to perform a minor septation (Fig. 73–6).

Sectioning of straddling chordae can be performed if leaflet support is not compromised. This technique is relevant only in mild degrees of straddling.

Slotting of the VSD patch has been described by incising the patch along the course of the chordae, allowing closure of the VSD with maintenance of the leaflet support. The slot is then closed around the chordae. There may be some question as to the mobility of the chordae after this procedure. This technique is suitable for mild, or possibly for moderate override, and may be combined with minor septation.

Reattachment of sectioned tensor apparatus is employed in cases of mild and moderate straddling where the straddling chordae insert into one papillary muscle or an accessible region of the ventricular septum. The sectioned chordae are moved as a group to the appropriate ventricle. The VSD is closed and the chordae are reattached to the patch. If practical, the muscular insertion site of the chordae, i.e., papillary muscle or muscular septum, may be resected and moved with the chordae to maintain their orientation. The chordae or muscular insertion site is then sutured to the VSD patch.

Valve replacement or repair is rarely required because straddling and overriding A-V valves are usually competent. A-V valve replacement can be employed in complex and severe straddling to allow a two-ventricle repair.[7]

Fontan procedure is indicated when moderate-to-severe ventricular hypoplasia is present, or when a two-ventricle repair is not possible due to the anatomy of the valvular apparati and/or position of the ventricular septal defect.[16]

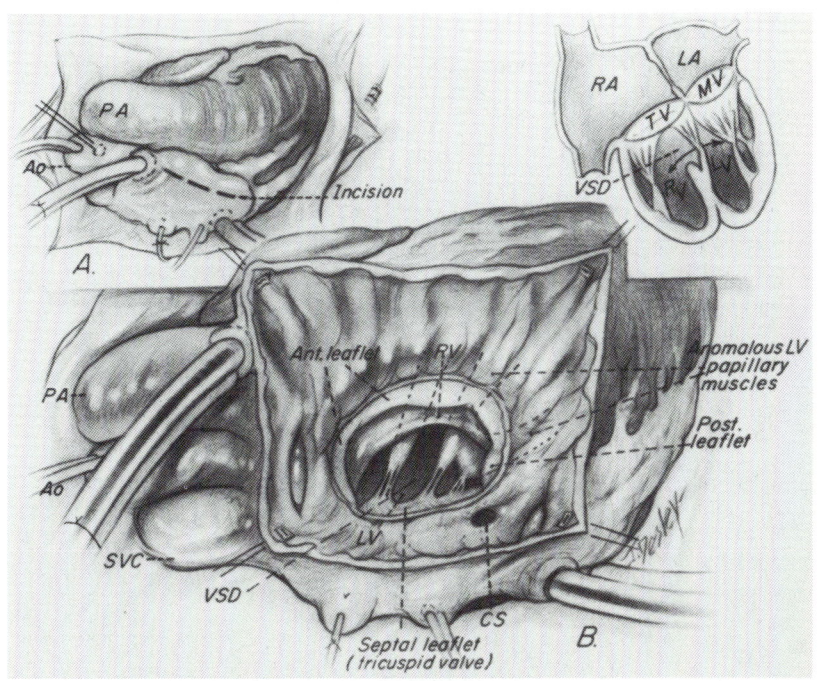

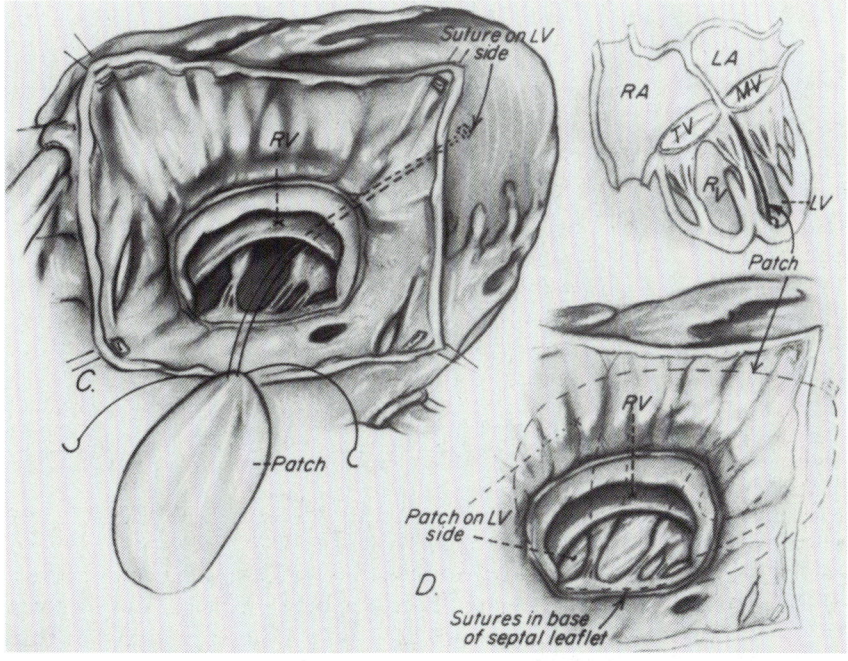

Figure 73–5. Technique for minor septation. **A.** The approach is through a right atriotomy. **B.** Cords of the septal leaflet straddle across the VSD to attach anomalously to contraventricular papillary muscles. **C.** The repair is performed through the tricuspid valve placing the patch on the left ventricular side of the septum to the left of the insertion site of the straddling right atrioventricular valve. **D.** Completed repair. Ao, aorta; CS, coronary sinus; LA, left atrium; LV, left ventricle; MV, mitral valve; PA, pulmonary artery; RA, right atrium; RV, right ventricle; SVC, superior vena cava; TV, tricuspid valve. *(From Pacifico et al.[6])*

An initial palliative procedure may be required, because neonatal pulmonary resistance is too great to allow pulmonary blood flow to depend on systemic pressure alone. A staged approach is generally used, with early palliation, if indicated, followed by an interval bidirectional cavopulmonary anastomosis, then completion Fontan procedure. The optimal timing of the various stages is not well defined; however, a bidirectional cavopulmonary anastomosis at 3–6 months of age and a completion Fontan procedure at 12–24 months of age are currently recommended.[17]

Cardiac transplantation has rarely been performed as

a primary procedure and is indicated only if severe cardiomyopathy is present.

RESULTS

The early and intermediate outcome after surgery for straddling and for overriding A-V valves is dependent on the anatomy as well as the type of repair performed. Those patients with A-V concordance and mild degrees of straddle or override where the repair of a VSD is minimally altered

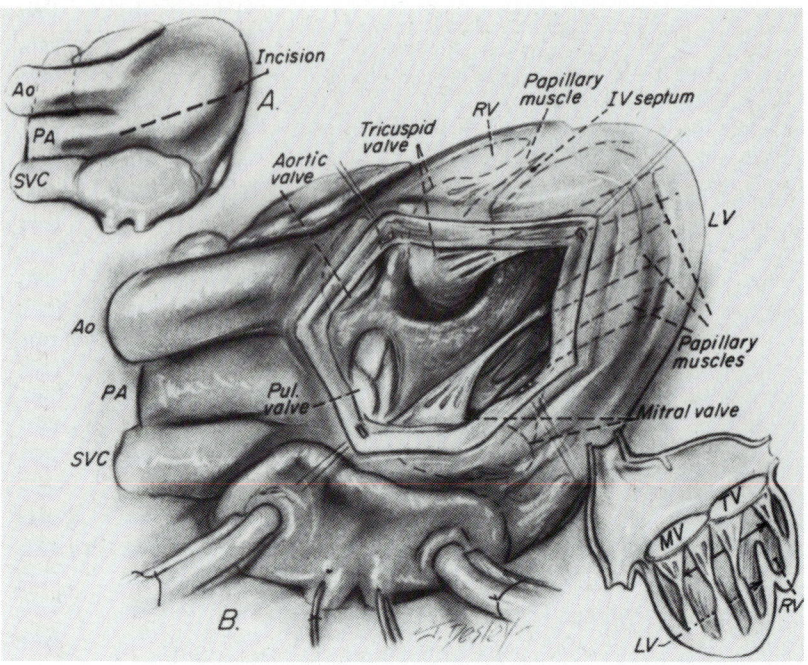

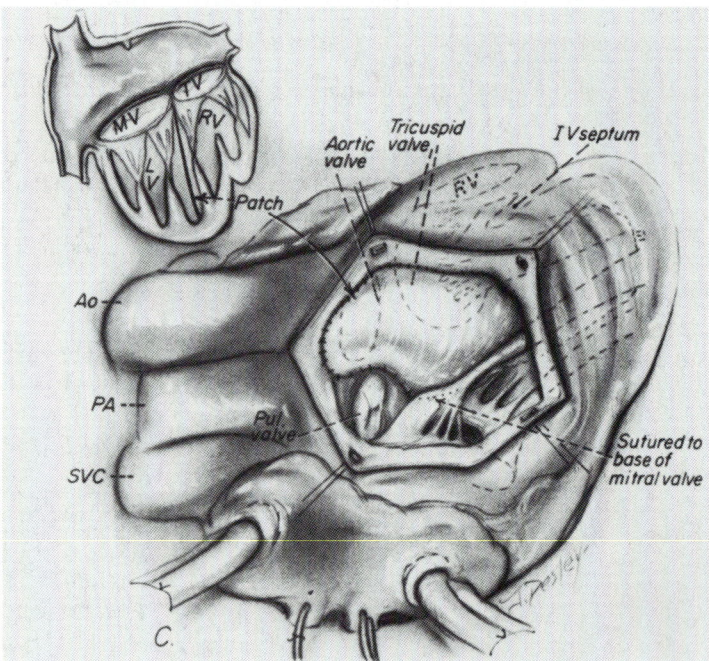

Figure 73–6. Transventricular tunnel repair incorporating a minor septation for the straddling and overriding left A-V valve in a patient with anatomically corrected transposition of the great arteries and approximately 40% overriding of the aorta onto the right-sided left ventricle. **A.** A vertical left (right-sided) ventriculotomy is performed. **B.** The straddling and overriding left A-V valve is exposed as well as the overriding aorta. **C.** Creation of an intraventricular tunnel allowing blood flow from the left-sided right ventricle to the aorta and keeping the left AV valve apparatus on the appropriate side. See Figure 73–5 for abbreviations. *(From Pacifico et al.[6])*

should have a low operative mortality (<3%) and excellent long-term survival.[9] If a complex reconstruction is required and there is A-V discordance, the operative risk increases. Heart block remains a significant source of morbidity, especially in A-V discordance or A-V concordance when the VSD extends to the crux leading to abnormal conduction pathways.[9,13]

Survival after Fontan-type procedures continues to improve, utilizing multiple modifications, including the lateral tunnel,[18] the total cavopulmonary anastomosis,[19] and baffle fenestration techniques.[20] Although the short and interme-

diate results are excellent, long-term morbidity and mortality data are not yet available.

SUMMARY

Straddling and overriding atrioventricular valves represent a rare anomaly that always occurs in the presence of a ventricular septal defect. The valves are usually competent and their defects vary from mild to severe. One may choose from several techniques to attempt to repair this defect while maintaining a two-ventricle arrangement. When a two-ventricle arrangement is not possible, a Fontan-type procedure is effective palliation.

REFERENCES

1. Lambert EC: Single ventricle with a rudimentary outlet chamber. Case report. *Bull Johns Hopkins Hosp* **88:**231–238, 1952
2. Van Praagh R, Ongley PA, Swan HJC: Anatomic types of single or common ventricle in man: Morphologic and geometric aspects of 60 necropsied cases. *Am J Cardiol* **13:**367–386, 1964
3. Mehrizi A, McMurphy DM, Ottesen OE, Rowe RD: Syndrome of double inlet left ventricle. Angiographic differentiation from single ventricle with rudimentary outlet chamber. *Bull Johns Hopkins Hosp* **119:**255, 1966
4. Liberthson RR, Paul MH, Muster AJ, et al: Straddling and displaced atrioventricular orifices and valves with primitive ventricles. *Circulation* **43:**213–226, 1971
5. Milo S, Ho SY, Macartney FJ, et al: Straddling and overriding atrioventricular valves: Morphology and classification. *Am J Cardiol* **44:**1122, 1979
6. Pacifico AD, Soto B, Bargeron LM Jr: Surgical treatment of straddling atrioventricular valves. *Circulation* **60:**655–664, 1979
7. Danielson GK, Tabry IF, Fulton RE, et al: Successful repair of straddling atrioventricular valve by technique used for septation of univentricular heart. *Ann Thorac Surg* **28:**554–560, 1979
8. Tabry IF, McGoon DC, Danielson GK, et al: Surgical management of straddling atrioventricular valve. *J Thorac Cardiovasc Surg* **77:**191–201, 1979
9. Kirklin JW, Barratt-Boyes BG: Ventricular septal defects. In Kirklin JW, Barratt-Boyes BG (eds): *Cardiac Surgery,* 2nd ed. New York, Churchill Livingstone, 1993, pp 749–824
10. Van Praagh R: Terminology of congenital heart disease: Glossary and commentary. *Circulation* **56:**139–143, 1977
11. Rice MJ, Seward JB, Edwards WD, et al: Straddling atrioventricular valve: Two-dimensional echocardiographic diagnosis, classification, and surgical implications. *Am J Cardiol* **55:**505–513, 1985
12. Seward JB, Tajik AJ, Hagler DJ, Mair RG: Straddling atrioventricular valve. Diagnostic two-dimensional echocardiographic features (abstr). *Am J Cardiol* **41:**354, 1978
13. Watson DC Jr: Straddling and overriding atrioventricular valves. In Mavroudis C, Backer CL (eds): *Pediatric Cardiac Surgery,* 2nd ed. St. Louis, Mosby-Year Book, 1994, pp 474–478
14. LaCorte MA, Fellows KE, Williams RG: Overriding tricuspid valve: Echocardiographic and angiographic features. *Am J Cardiol* **37:**911–919, 1976
15. Soto B, Ceballos R, Nath PH, et al: Overriding atrioventricular valves. An angiographic-anatomical correlate. *Int J Cardiol* **9:**327–339, 1985
16. Russo P, Danielson GK, Puga FJ, et al: Modified Fontan procedure for biventricular hearts with complex forms of double-outlet right ventricle. *Circulation* (suppl III):III-20–III-25, 1988
17. Jonas RA: Indications and timing for the bidirectional Glenn shunt versus the fenestrated Fontan circulation. *J Thorac Cardiovasc Surg* **108:**522–524, 1994
18. Jonas RA, Castañeda AR: Modified Fontan procedure: Atrial baffle and systemic venous to pulmonary artery anastomotic techniques. *J Cardiac Surg* **3:**91–96, 1988
19. de Leval MR, Kilner P, Gewillig M, et al: Total cavopulmonary connection: A logical alternative to atriopulmonary connection for complex Fontan operations. *J Thorac Cardiovasc Surg* **96:**683, 1988
20. Bridges ND, Mayer JE, Lock JE, et al: Effect of fenestration on outcome of Fontan repair. *Circulation* **86:**1762–1769, 1992

CHAPTER

74

Truncus Arteriosus

Ralph S. Mosca and Edward L. Bove

Truncus arteriosus is a rare anomaly that accounts for 0.4–4.0%[1-3] of all cases of congenital heart disease. A single arterial vessel arises from the heart, overriding the ventricular septum and giving rise to the systemic, coronary, and pulmonary circulations. In 1798 Wilson first described this unusual cardiac malformation,[4] and its basic morphology was outlined by Lev and Saphir in 1942.[5] Two classification schemes have been proposed, one by Collett and Edwards in 1949[6] and the other by Van Praagh and Van Praagh in 1965[7] (Fig. 74–1). The classification of Collett and Edwards focused on the origin of the pulmonary arteries from the common arterial trunk (Table 74–1). The system offered by Van Praagh and Van Praagh, a somewhat more surgically oriented scheme, is based on the degree of formation of the aorticopulmonary septum, the presence or absence of a ventricular septal defect (VSD), and the status of the aortic arch (Table 74–2). In addition, they required that at least one of the pulmonary arteries arise from the trunk eliminating "pseudotruncus" from the spectrum of truncus arteriosus and including it instead as a form of pulmonary atresia with aortopulmonary collaterals.

EMBRYOLOGY

Persistent truncus arteriosus occurs as a result of the failure of development of the aorticopulmonary septum and subpulmonary infundibulum (conal septum). Normal septation leads to both pulmonary and systemic outflow tracts, the division of the semilunar valves, and aorta and pulmonary arteries. Failure of septation results in a VSD (absence of the infundibular septum), single semilunar valve, and single arterial trunk. The deficiency in septation of the truncus accounts for the variability in the origin of the pulmonary arteries and the association with interrupted aortic arch.

MORPHOLOGIC ANATOMY

In truncus arteriosus, a single artery larger in size than the normal aorta arises from the base of the heart. It is usually associated with normal atrial situs and d-ventricular loop arrangement. In the vast majority of cases, it is associated with a VSD. The VSD is reminiscent of that found in tetralogy of Fallot being nonrestrictive and cradled by the two limbs of the septal band. In approximately two-thirds of cases, the posterior limb of the VSD is formed by the posterior radiation of the septal band and the conduction system is remote from the VSD margin. In one-third of cases the defect extends to the tricuspid valve annulus (perimembranous) and the conduction system is vulnerable during closure. Unlike the typical VSD in tetralogy of Fallot, the superior margin of the defect is formed by the truncal valve.

The truncal root overrides the ventricular septum equally in approximately 60% of cases, the remaining cases having either a predominant right or less often left ventricular override. The truncal valve annulus is in the normal position and truncal to mitral fibrous continuity is preserved. The leaflets are often dysmorphic being thickened, fleshy, and often restricted in their motion. Leaflet number is highly variable with approximately 65% being tricuspid, 25% quadricuspid, and 9% bicuspid. The remaining 1–2% of cases may have greater than five leaflets.[2,8] As a result of these abnormally developed valve leaflets, approximately half of the patients present with some degree of truncal valve regurgitation. Truncal valve stenosis can be seen alone or in combination with regurgitation and is present in about one-third of cases of truncus arteriosus. Significant obstruction is predicted by gradients of greater than 30 mm Hg in the presence of normal cardiac output.

The pulmonary arteries are usually of normal size and most often arise from the left posterolateral aspect of the

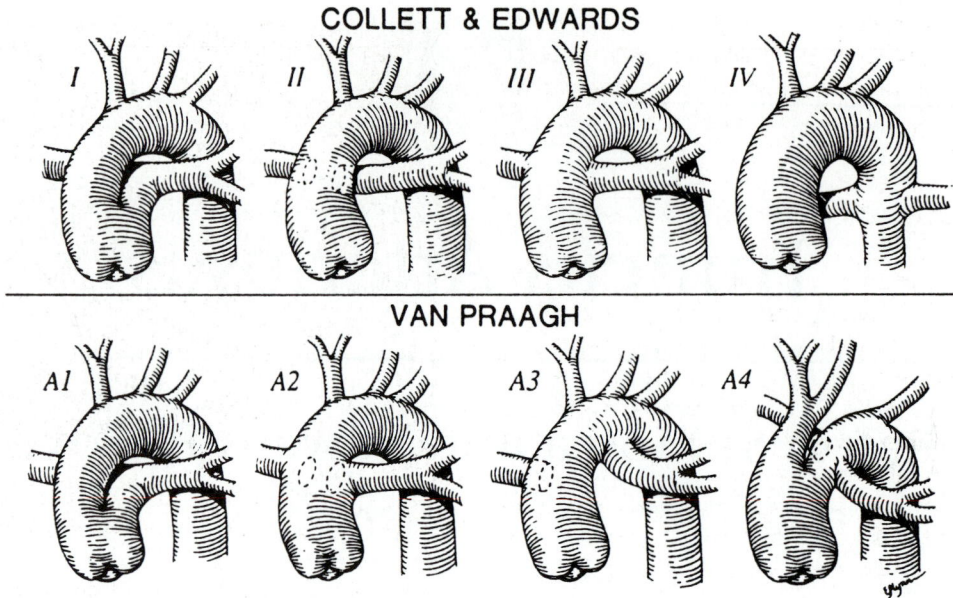

COLLETT & EDWARDS

I *II* *III* *IV*

VAN PRAAGH

A1 *A2* *A3* *A4*

Figure 74–1. Truncus arteriosus: Classification schemes as described by Collett and Edwards[6] as well as Van Praagh and Van Praagh.[7] *(Taken with permission from Hernanz-Schulman M, Fellows KE: Persistent truncus arteriosus: Pathologic, diagnostic and therapeutic considerations. Semin Roentgenol 20:121–129, 1985.)*

truncal artery, in close proximity to the truncal valve and left coronary artery. Collett and Edwards defined Type I truncus as that situation in which the main pulmonary artery is distinct and quickly bifurcates into a left and right pulmonary artery. Type II truncus referred to those cases in which the pulmonary arteries arise separately from the posterolateral aspect of the truncus. In fact, many cases appear to fall into a Type I $\frac{1}{2}$ category in which the left pulmonary artery appears to take origin from a short main pulmonary artery segment and the right pulmonary artery arises from the posterolateral aspect of the truncus. In Type III truncus the two pulmonary arteries also take origin from the posterior truncus, but their orifices are widely separated. Rarely, one of the pulmonary arteries is absent and the affected lung is supplied by aortopulmonary collaterals (Type A3 Van Praagh classification.)

ASSOCIATED ANOMALIES

A patent foramen ovale is very common, and a true atrial septal defect is present in about 10% of cases. A persistent left superior vena cava has been reported to occur with similar frequency and is often associated with partial anomalous pulmonary venous return. Various mitral valve anomalies have been reported to occur with a frequency of 5–10%. Tricuspid stenosis, atresia, and atrioventricular (A-V) canal defects are rare.

Approximately 10–20% of patients with truncus arteriosus have associated aortic arch anomalies, either coarctation or interrupted arch (usually Type B). A right aortic arch is present 25–35% of the time. In addition there may be associated anomalous origin of the brachiocephalic vessels, usually the subclavian arteries (10%).

Coronary artery abnormalities are quite common (50%) and include abnormal and stenotic coronary ostia, close proximity of the ostia to the commissures, an usually high and angled takeoff of the coronary arteries, unusual courses of the LAD and large conal and diagonal branches of the RCA that crosses the right ventricular outflow tract.[9] These abnormalities have led to a continued finite prevalence of coronary arterial injury during repair of truncus arteriosus.[10]

TABLE 74–1. CLASSIFICATION OF TRUNCUS ARTERIOSUS ACCORDING TO COLLETT AND EDWARDS[6]

Type I	Common arterial trunk gives rise to a main pulmonary artery and the aorta
Type II	Right and left pulmonary arteries arise directly and in close proximity from the posterior wall of the truncus
Type III	Right and left pulmonary arteries arise from more widely separate orifices on the posterior truncal wall
Type IV	Absence of branch pulmonary arteries: pulmonary blood flow is derived from aortopulmonary collaterals

TABLE 74–2. CLASSIFICATION OF TRUNCUS ARTERIOSUS ACCORDING TO VAN PRAAGH AND VAN PRAAGH[7]

Type A	With a VSD
Type B	Without a VSD

1. The aorticopulmonary septum is partially developed (partially separate main pulmonary artery)
2. The aorticopulmonary septum is absent (no main pulmonary artery segment) both branch PAs arise from the common trunk[a]
3. Absence of either branch PA
4. Hypoplasia, coarctation, atresia, or absence of the aortic isthmus in association with a large PDA[a]

[a]PA, pulmonary artery; PDA, patent ductus arteriosus.

Noncardiac anomalies are present in about 20% of cases and may contribute to death. In particular, the DiGeorge syndrome is often associated with truncus arteriosus and screening of these infants has become routine.

PATHOPHYSIOLOGY

The morphologic anatomy of truncus arteriosus results in obligatory mixing of the systemic and pulmonary venous blood at the level of the VSD and truncal valve. Most commonly this produces systemic arterial saturations of approximately 85–90%. Normally, due to preferential streaming of the saturated blood into the systemic portion of the truncus the pulmonary arterial saturation may be 10–15% lower than that in the peripheral systemic circuit. The systemic arterial saturation depends upon the volume of pulmonary blood flow, which in turn is determined by the pulmonary vascular resistance (PVR). In the first few days of life, the pulmonary flow is restricted by the relatively high pulmonary vascular resistance of the neonate. As the PVR begins to fall, pulmonary overcirculation ensues leading to pulmonary congestion with minimal cyanosis. However, this nonrestrictive left-to-right shunt at the level of the truncus may lead to the early development of irreversible pulmonary vascular obstructive disease.

The presence of truncal valve abnormalities poses further hemodynamic burdens. Truncal valve regurgitation leads to ventricular dilatation and low diastolic coronary perfusion pressures and can result in myocardial ischemia. Truncal valve stenosis promotes ventricular hypertrophy, increases myocardial oxygen demand, and limits coronary and systemic perfusion, especially in the face of the large volume runoff into the pulmonary vascular bed.

DIAGNOSIS

Neonates with truncus arteriosus present with signs of congestive heart failure and collapsing peripheral pulses due to the high-volume pulmonary artery runoff. Chest radiography shows marked cardiomegaly, pulmonary plethora, often with minimal thymus shadow and a right aortic arch. The electrocardiogram most often depicts biventricular hypertrophy. Echocardiography is the diagnostic procedure of choice. In the parasternal long axis view, a single great vessel is seen emanating from the heart, overriding the ventricular septum and with fibrous continuity with the mitral valve (Fig. 74–2). Echocardiography can also demonstrate the pulmonary arterial anatomy in the majority of cases. Lastly, it provides valuable information concerning the structure and degree of stenosis or regurgitation of the truncal valve. Cardiac catheterization is reserved for those cases in which the anatomy is unclear, further information is needed concerning the status of the truncal valve, or in those patients in whom the status of the pulmonary vascula-

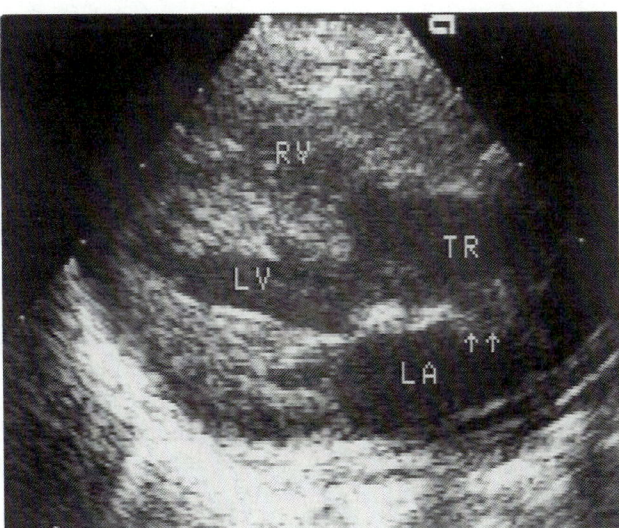

Figure 74–2. Modified parasternal long axis view in a patient with truncus arteriosus. The large truncal root (TR) overrides the ventricular septum and gives rise to the aorta (AO) and the pulmonary artery (arrows). LV, left ventricle; LA, left atrium; RV, right ventricle.

ture is unclear, i.e., infants greater than 3 months of age at diagnosis.

CLINICAL COURSE

The natural history of patients born with truncus arteriosus is that of early demise. One-half of the infants die within the first month of life, 70% by 3 mo, and over 80% by a year.[11] Early death is due to congestive heart failure. Those patients who survive beyond the first year of life may fair well until they develop irreversible pulmonary vascular obstructive disease. These patients ultimately die during the third to fourth decades of life with Eisenmenger's syndrome. Patients with pulmonary stenosis may have a more prolonged course due to the protection of their pulmonary vasculature. Infants born with truncal valve stenosis or regurgitation as well as interrupted aortic arch or coarctation have a worse prognosis.[2,12,13]

TREATMENT

The ultimate treatment of truncus arteriosus is surgical therapy. Medical treatment is directed toward the control of congestive heart failure by fluid restriction, diuretics, digitalis, and afterload reduction. In the absence of significant pulmonary stenosis, as the pulmonary vascular resistance decreases congestive failure will ultimately occur. In fact, now that repair of truncus arteriosus in the neonate is well accepted, the onset of tachypnea can be used as a marker to identify declining pulmonary vascular resistance and the optimal timing for repair.

Initial treatment of truncus arteriosus consisted of banding of one or both pulmonary arteries.[14,15] However, this approach was plagued by high perioperative mortality, lack of reliability of the banding procedure in preventing pulmonary hypertension, as well as distortion of the pulmonary arteries, which increased the risk for subsequent repair. In 1975, Poirier and colleagues reported that 43 of 76 patients who underwent PA banding for truncus arteriosus ultimately succumbed.[16] In view of the high mortality and morbidity of the banding procedure and improving results with complete repair in infancy, pulmonary artery banding for truncus arteriosus has been abandoned in most centers.

The first intracardiac repair was reported from The University of Michigan in 1962 using a nonvalved Teflon conduit.[17] In 1968, McGoon et al described the repair of truncus arteriosus utilizing an aortic valve homograft conduit.[18] In 1973, Bowman and colleagues successfully used a gluteraldehyde-treated porcine valve implanted in a Dacron tube to re-establish RV to PA continuity.[19] Due to the difficulties encountered during the removal of the pulmonary arteries in Types II and III truncus arteriosus, various attempts at intraluminal partitioning of the aorta and pulmonary artery were described such as that by Smith and Cooley in 1979 and Young et al in 1988.[20,21] The first successful surgical series of the treatment of truncus arteriosus in infants was published by Ebert et al in 1984.[22] Although the approach to the repair has changed little since the initial report by McGoon, the improved pre- and postoperative care of neonates and better intraoperative myocardial protection has made the routine repair of truncus arteriosus in neonates possible with good results.[23,24]

SURGICAL TECHNIQUE

Complete repair of truncus arteriosus entails separation of the pulmonary arteries from the truncus, repair of the resultant defect in the aorta, ventricular septal defect closure, and restoration of RV outflow tract continuity utilizing an extra cardiac conduit.

Repair is via a median sternotomy utilizing standard techniques of deep hypothermia and low flow bypass with periods of circulatory arrest. Pericardium is harvested and placed in 0.6% gluteraldehyde solution for approximately 7 mins. The thymus is inspected and excised. The aorta is cannulated as high as possible. Venous return is provided by a single right angle DLP cannula placed in the right atrial appendage (12F, DLP Corporation, Grand Rapids, MI). The patient's head is topically cooled with ice and a bolus dose of steroids is administered. The aorta and pulmonary arteries are widely mobilized, cardiopulmonary bypass is established, and the pulmonary arteries are snared as cooling to 18°C is instituted. During this time, any further mobilization is accomplished and the exact anatomy is identified. In particular, one must be wary of the possible existence of nonconfluent pulmonary arteries (9%) and

coronary arterial abnormalities. An unusual course of the LAD and large conal or diagonal branches that traverse the right ventricular outflow tract has been described and potentially complicates the repair. These variations as well as coronary ostial lesions and intramural coronary arteries have been described by Lenox et al[9] and should be well known to the surgeon addressing the repair of truncus arteriosus. The existence of an interrupted aortic arch requires full mobilization of the ascending aorta, head vessels, arch, and descending aorta well past the insertion of the ductus arteriosus to allow for a tension-free end-to-end repair.

A dose of 20 mL/kg of cold blood cardioplegia is utilized in all patients and generally repeated when the cross-clamp time exceeds 45–60 min. In the presence of significant truncal valve regurgitation, the valve may be made competent by digital compression of the left ventricular outflow tract, temporary aortic cusp apposition,[25] or cardioplegia given directly into the coronary ostia or retrograde into the coronary sinus.[26]

The pulmonary arteries are excised from the truncus with a generous cuff of arterial wall whenever possible. Removal of the pulmonary arteries must be done carefully because the distance from the pulmonary artery origin to the ostium of the left coronary artery and to the attachment of the truncal valve may be quite short. It may be necessary to tailor the incision around the coronary artery ostia or truncal valve commissures to avoid injuring these structures. Removal of the pulmonary arteries can often be approached posteriorly beginning over the superior aspect of the left pulmonary artery; however, in Types II and III truncus arteriosus, a small counter incision over the anterior wall of the truncus is helpful in precisely locating these structures (Fig. 74–3). On occasion, division of the ascending aorta can greatly facilitate exposure. Any significant defect in the ascending aorta is then repaired with a patch of homograft or pericardial tissue to prevent distortion of the truncal valve or coronary arteries. The distal anastomosis of the conduit to pulmonary artery is then performed. The RV to PA conduit can be an aortic or pulmonary homograft as well as a valved heterograft. If a valved heterograft is chosen the distal anastomosis is performed as close as possible to the heterograft valve to place the rigid sewing ring well below the shoulder of the ventricle and avoid later compression between the sternum and the heart.

Utilizing a period of circulatory arrest, the VSD is closed with a Gore-Tex patch via a right ventriculotomy. Any obstructing right ventricular muscle bundles are resected and large atrial septal defects are closed. The proximal anastomosis of the conduit is constructed during systemic rewarming. The posterior conduit wall is anastomosed directly to the ventriculotomy and the anterior aspect is augmented with excess homograft tissue or Gore-Tex material (Fig. 74–4). When moderate truncal valve regurgitation is present the cross-clamp is left in place until sufficient rewarming has occurred to allow for immediate cardiac contraction to prevent LV distension. Alternatively,

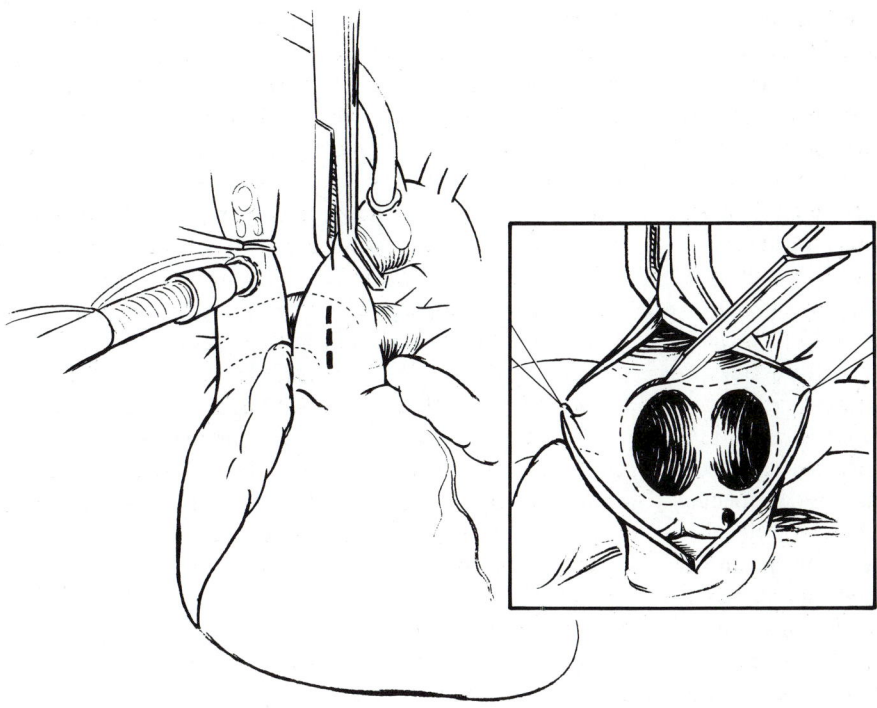

Figure 74–3. Patient with Type II truncus arteriosus. An incision can be made in the anterior wall of the truncal vessel to allow the accurate removal of the pulmonary artery bifurcation without damaging the valve or left coronary artery.

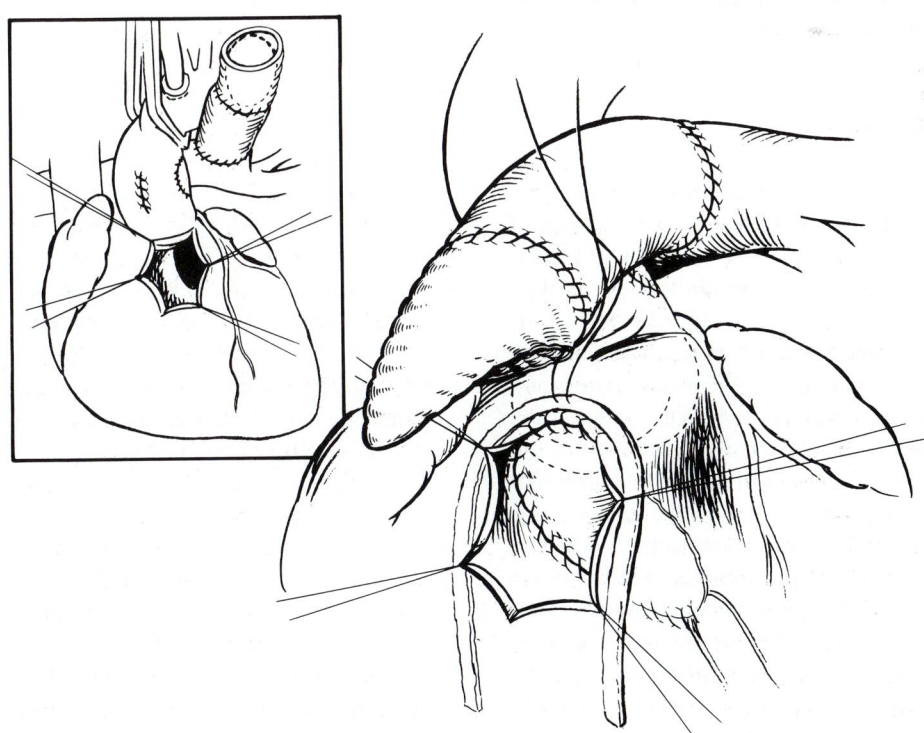

Figure 74–4. Right ventricle to pulmonary artery reconstruction. The homograft is attached to the pulmonary artery distally. The proximal aspect of the homograft is attached to the margin of the ventriculotomy and augmented on its anterior aspect with a Gore-Tex or dacron hood.

the heart may be rewarmed with a dose of warm substrate-enriched cardioplegia.

Cardiopulmonary bypass is discontinued at a rectal temperature of >36°C often with low-dose inotropic support consisting of amrinone or dobutamine. Respiratory parameters are adjusted to provide mild-to-moderate degrees of alkalosis and a fentanyl infusion begun to prevent any catecholamine-induced swings in pulmonary vascular resistance.

SPECIAL OPERATIVE CONSIDERATIONS

Truncal Valve Regurgitation

Severe truncal valve regurgitation prognosticates decreased long-term survival[25] and necessitates valve replacement. Moderate truncal valve regurgitation can often be well tolerated in the perioperative period and may improve postoperatively as the cardiac output traversing the truncal valve is markedly reduced. Truncal valve repair has been attempted in a small number of patients with reasonable results.[27] However, the valve substrate, numerous abnormal cusps, along with annular dilation can present some formidable difficulties and an overzealous attempt can lead to significant aortic insufficiency. The ideal replacement is a cylinder of cryopreserved aortic or pulmonary homograft in sizes ranging from 10 to 15 mm. The coronary arteries are excised from the truncal arterial wall and reimplanted on the homograft using absorbable suture (7-0 maxon). The replacement of the truncal route adds significant complexity to the procedure and will require later reoperation on the aorta and should be done only in cases of hemodynamically severe regurgitation.[28]

Interrupted Aortic Arch

The repair of truncus arteriosus associated with interruption of the aortic arch requires some technical modifications (Fig. 74–5). The aortic cannula is positioned in the noncoronary sinus of Valsalva, and wide mobilization of the ascending aorta, head vessels, and descending aorta is accomplished during cooling. The branch right and left pulmonary arteries are snared at the onset of bypass. The innominate, left carotid, and left subclavian arteries are fully mobilized and encircled with snares for occlusion during circulatory arrest. Once the circulation is arrested, the branch pulmonary arteries are excised and the ductus is divided and all residual ductal tissue is removed from the descending aorta (Fig. 74–6). Beginning at the base of the left carotid artery, a primary end-to-end anastomosis is performed using absorbable suture partially reconstructing the aortic arch. The remaining defect in the undersurface of the aortic arch is then repaired using a portion of allograft tissue (Fig. 74–7). This technique augments the ascending aorta eliminating any residual hypoplasia between the truncal valve and the aortic arch anastomosis and avoids placing the descending

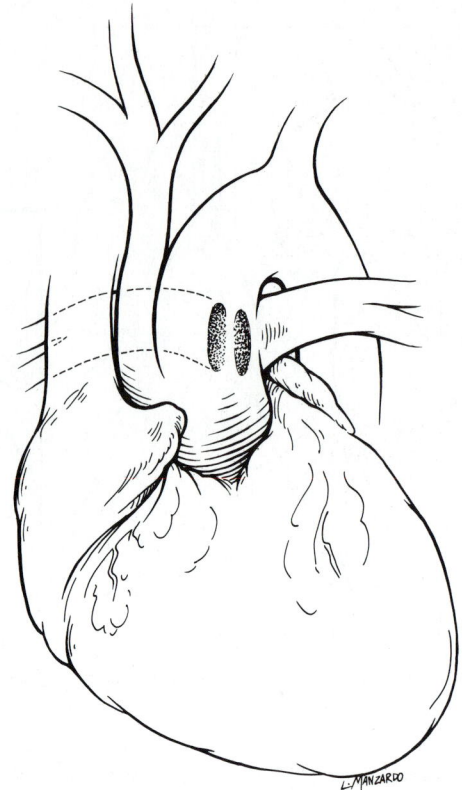

Figure 74–5. Truncus arteriosus with interrupted aortic arch Type B.

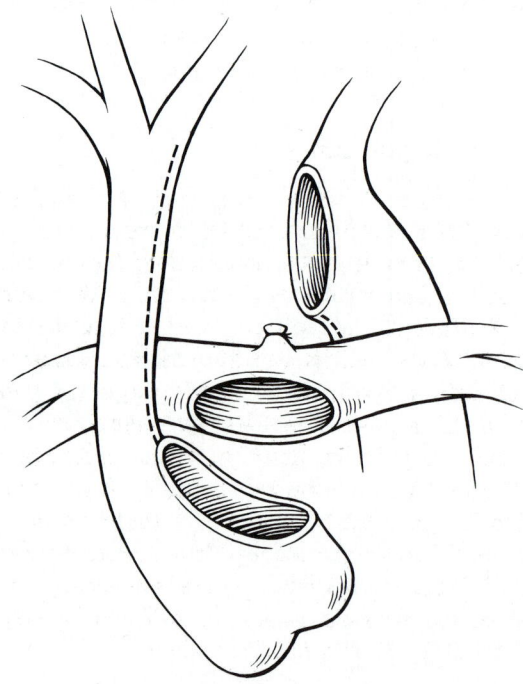

Figure 74–6. Truncus arteriosus with interrupted aortic arch Type B. The branch pulmonary arteries are excised as is the ductus arteriosus. The remainder of the ascending aorta is opened along its medial surface.

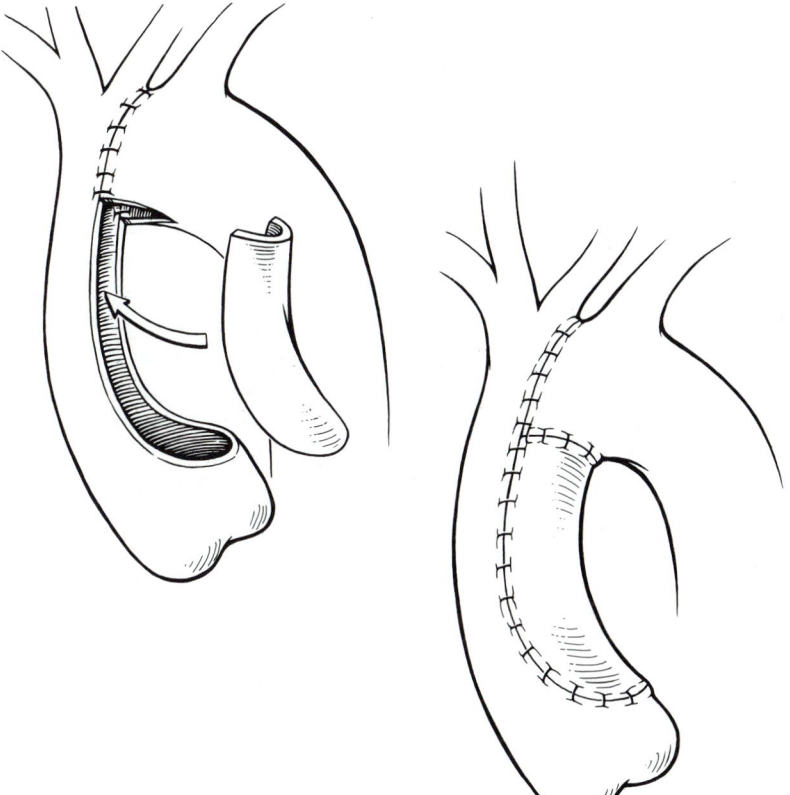

Figure 74–7. Truncus arteriosus with interrupted aortic arch. Primary end-to-end anastomosis of the ascending and descending aorta along with allograft augmentation of the ascending aorta.

aorta too far proximally on the ascending aorta, which can result in compression of the left pulmonary artery or left main stem bronchus. The ventricular septal defect is then repaired, cardiopulmonary bypass is resumed, and the homograft conduit placed as previously described.

Ventricular Septal Defect Closure

The VSD in truncus arteriosus is located high and anterior in the ventricular septum and the truncal valve forms its superior border. The inferior border of the VSD is bounded by the septal band and posteriorly it is rimmed by the ventriculoinfundibular fold. The conduction system is related to the position of the VSD and its relation to the membranous septum. In the majority of cases, the VSD margin is separated from the membranous septum by a rim of muscle distancing it from the tricuspid valve and right fibrous trigone placing the A-V bundle posterior on the anatomic left side and unrelated to the rim of the VSD. However, the branching bundle may be closed to the VSD margin and susceptible to injury. If the VSD extends into the membranous septum and approaches the tricuspid valve, the A-V bundle may be close to the VSD and susceptible to injury.[29]

RV Outflow Tract Reconstruction

Right ventricular to pulmonary artery continuity can be restored in a variety of ways. Most surgeons favor the insertion of a valved homograft or heterograft conduit, especially in the neonate.[30] However, the use of a nonvalved conduit[31] and direct suture of the pulmonary artery to the right ventriculotomy with or without a modified Lecompte maneuver have been reported.[32,33] Assuming a valved conduit may offer potential benefits in the neonate with labile pulmonary vascular resistance[34] and help to prevent against late right ventricular failure the issue becomes that of ease of use and longevity of the conduit.

Porcine valve heterograft conduits are available in limited sizes, are more difficult to handle, and can lead to distortion of the pulmonary arteries or compression of underlying coronary arteries. Porcine conduits implanted in neonates tend to fail at approximately 2–3 years' postinsertion and require replacement due to obstruction caused by calcific valve dysfunction and/or pseudointimal formation.[35]

Fresh antibiotic sterilized and cryopreserved aortic or pulmonary valve homografts are easier to handle, more hemostatic, less prone to compression of adjacent structures, and although limited in supply are available in smaller sizes than the valved heterografts. Although the longevity of adult-sized cryopreserved homografts appears much improved over radiation-sterilized aortic homografts and valved heterografts,[36,37] the fate of small homografts in neonates still needs to be elucidated.

It is our experience that aortic homografts especially in the smaller sizes, i.e., 8–12 mm diameter, tend to fail earlier than do the pulmonary homografts. This is supported by the observations of Heinemann et al.[38] At a mean observation period of 31 mo they found that all patients receiving small aortic homografts required intervention versus 64% of those in whom pulmonary homografts were implanted. Conversely, Hawkins et al[39] found conduit failure was similar between aortic and pulmonary homografts. Of note, however, is that the actuarial freedom from reoperation for conduit dysfunction at 5 years was 94% for those patients operated on at greater than 1 year of age and 0% for those implanted in infancy. Sharma et al[40] reported that 5% of conduits required replacement at 40 mo follow-up. Again, this was a much older patient population (mean age 9.1 +/– 1.1 years) utilizing predominantly adult-sized homografts. Solution to these questions awaits a larger series of infants and neonates repaired with aortic or pulmonary homografts and followed up until they require reoperation.

POSTOPERATIVE MANAGEMENT

Left and right atrial lines as well as atrial and ventricular pacing wires are inserted. Older infants with truncus arteriosus can develop episodes of pulmonary hypereactivity triggered by hypercarbia, hypoxia, acidosis, temperature instability, and low cardiac output. For these reasons patients are kept paralyzed and heavily sedated for 24–72 hours. Neonates and infants operated upon before 3 mo of age rarely develop these crises and this has been a benefit of early repair. Initially a fentanyl drip of 3 μg/kg per min is utilized and after 24 hours switched to a morphine sulfate drip of between 10 and 30 μg/kg per min. An arterial PO_2 of 100 mm Hg and a PCO_2 of 30 mm Hg are considered ideal. The infant's temperature is well regulated and any metabolic derangements are quickly corrected. Most infants require some form of inotropic support (dopamine or dobutamine) for a period of approximately 48 hours. High doses of inotropes and pulmonary vasoconstriction are avoided. Weaning from the ventilator is begun at about 48 hours if the postoperative course has been smooth. Episodes of pulmonary hypertension are treated by hyperventilation and oxygenation as well as pulmonary vasodilators, i.e., nitroglycerin, nitroprusside, or PGE_1. On occasion, a pulmonary arterial line is placed intraoperatively to allow both monitoring of pressure and the direct infusion of vasodilators into the pulmonary circulation. Lastly, nitric oxide (NO) may be very useful in the treatment of infants with refractory pulmonary hypertensive episodes.

RESULTS

The results of repair of truncus arteriosus have improved greatly over the last two decades. Before the importance of early operation to avoid pulmonary vascular obstructive disease was recognized, most institutions were repairing pa-

tients at an average of 2 to 5 years of age. Most patients had pulmonary hypertension and the mortality rates ranged from 25 to 88%.[41–42] Ebert et al showed that repair in the first 6 mo of life was not only possible but preferable and reported a mortality of 9%.[22] Recent reports from Bove et al,[24] McKay et al,[43] Pearl et al,[44] and Hanley et al[23] demonstrate improving results with mortality rates for complicated neonatal repairs ranging from 8 to 30%. In their most recent review Hanley et al found that the presence of aortic arch interruption, severe truncal valve regurgitation, coronary artery anomalies, or age greater than 100 days were important risks factors for perioperative death. Repair is now recommended in the first month of life before the development of critical congestive heart failure or irreversible pulmonary vascular disease.

At the C.S. Mott Children's Hospital of the University of Michigan, between January 1986 and January 1992, 46 neonates and infants underwent repair of truncus arteriosus. Their ages ranged from 1 day to 7 mo (median 13 days) and weights from 1.8 to 5.4 kg (mean 3.1 kg). Associated cardiac anomalies were frequent and included, interrupted aortic arch (n=5), nonconfluent pulmonary arteries (n=4), hypoplastic pulmonary arteries (n=4), and major coronary artery anomalies (n=3). Truncal valve replacement was performed in five patients with severe regurgitation, three of whom had truncal valve systolic pressure gradients of 30 mm Hg or more. Actuarial survival was 81 +/– 6% at 90 days and beyond. Multivariate and univariate analyses failed to demonstrate a relationship between hospital mortality and age, weight, or associated cardiac anomalies. Despite this, it remains our impression that these risk factors do complicate the perioperative course. Primary repair promptly after presentation has become the standard of therapy in truncus arteriosus.

REFERENCES

1. Tandon R, Hanck AJ, Nadas AS: Persistent truncus arteriosus: A clinical, hemodynamic, and autopsy study of 19 cases. *Circulation* **28:**1050, 1963
2. Calder L, Van Praagh R, Van Praagh S, et al: Truncus arteriosus communis: Clinical angiocardiographic and pathologic findings in 100 patients. *Am Heart J* **92:**23, 1976
3. Rowe RD, Freedom RM, Mehrizi A, et al: *The Neonate with Congenital Heart Disease.* Philadelphia, PA, W. B. Saunders, 1981
4. Wilson J: A description of a very unusual malformation of the human heart. *Phil Trans R Soc London (Biol)* **18:**346, 1798
5. Lev M, Saphir O: Truncus arteriosus communis persistens. *J Pediatr* **20:**74, 1943
6. Collett RW, Edwards JE: Persistent truncus arteriosus: A classification according to anatomic types. *Surg Clin North Am* **29:**1245, 1949
7. Van Praagh R, Van Praagh S: The anatomy of common aorticopulmonary trunk (truncus arteriosus communis) and its embryologic implications: A study of 57 necropsy cases. *Am J Cardiol* **16:**406, 1965
8. Butto F, Lucas RV, Edwards JE: Persistent truncus arteriosus: Pathologic anatomy in 54 cases. *Pediatr Cardiol* **7:**95–101, 1986
9. Lenox CC, Detrich DE, Zuberbuhler JR: Role of coronary artery abnormalities in the prognosis of truncus arteriosus. *J Thorac Cardiovasc Surg* **104:**1728–1742, 1992

10. Anderson KR, McGoon DC, Lie JT: Surgical significance of the coronary arterial anatomy in truncus arteriosus communis. *Am J Cardiol* **41:**76–81, 1978

11. Kirklin JW, Barratt-Boye BG (eds): Truncus arteriosus. In *Cardiac Surgery*. New York, Churchill Livingstone, 1992, pp 1131–1151

12. Ebert PA: Truncus arteriosus. In Parenzan L, Crupi G, Graham (eds): *Congenital Heart Disease in the First Three Weeks of Life*. Bologna, Italy, Paxon Editore, 1981

13. Gelband H, Van Meter S, Gersony WM: Truncal valve abnormalities in infants with persistent truncus arteriosus: A clinicopathologic study. *Circulation* **45:**397, 1972

14. Heilbrunn A, Kittle CF, Diehl AM: Pulmonary arterial banding in the treatment of truncus arteriosus. *Circulation* **29**(1):102, 1964

15. Smith GW, Thompson WM, Damman JF, Muller WH: Use of pulmonary artery banding procedure in treating Type II truncus arteriosus. *Circulation* **29**(suppl):1–108, 1964

16. Poirier RA, Berman MA, Stansel HC Jr: Current status of the surgical treatment of truncus arteriosus. *J Thorac Cardiovasc Surg* **69:**169, 1975

17. Behrendt DM, Kirsh MM, Stern A, et al: The surgical therapy for pulmonary artery–right ventricle discontinuity. *Ann Thorac Surg* **18:**122, 1974

18. McGoon DC, Rastelli GC, Ongley PA: An operation for the correction of truncus arteriosus. *JAMA* **205:**59, 1968

19. Bowman FOG, Hancock WD, Malm JR: A valve containing dacron prosthesis: Its use in restoring pulmonary artery–right ventricular continuity. *Arch Surg* **107:**724, 1973

20. Smith MJ, Cooley DA: Modified procedure for correction of truncus arteriosus, Types II and III. *Ann Thorac Surg* **29**(4):387–389, 1980

21. Young NJ, Piascastelli C, Harell J, et al: Internal banding for palliation of truncus arteriosus in the neonate. *Ann Thorac Surg* **47:**420–422, 1989

22. Ebert PA, Turley K, Stanger P, et al: Surgical treatment of truncus arteriosus in the first six months of life. *Ann Thorac Surg* **200:**451–456, 1984

23. Hanley FL, Heinemann MK, Jonas RA, et al: Repair of truncus arteriosus in the neonate. *J Thorac Cardiovasc Surg* **105:**1047–1056, 1993

24. Bove EL, Lupinetti FM, Pridjian AK, et al: Results of a policy of primary repair of truncus arteriosus in the neonate. *J Thorac Cardiovasc Surg* **105:**1057–1066, 1993

25. DeLeval MR, McGoon DC, Wallace RB, et al: Management of truncal valvular regurgitation. *Ann Surg* **180:**427–432, 1974

26. Drinkwater DC Jr, Cushen CK, Laks H, Buckberg GD: The use of combined antegrade-retrograde blood cardioplegia in pediatric open heart surgery—the UCLA experience. *J Thorac Cardiovasc Surg* **104:**1349–1355, 1992

27. Elami A, Laks H, Pearl JM: Truncal valve repair: Initial experience with infants and children. *Ann Thorac Surg* **57**(2):397–402, 1994

28. Elkins RC, Steinberg JB, Raxook JD, et al: Correction of truncus arteriosus with truncal valvar stenosis or insufficiency using two homografts. *Ann Thorac Surg* **50:**728–733, 1990

29. Bharati S, Karp R, Lev M: The conduction system in truncus arteriosus and its surgical significance. *J Thorac Cardiovasc Surg* **1204:**954–960, 1992

30. Castaneda AR, Jonas RA, Mayer JE, Hanley FL: In *Truncus Arteriosus in Cardiac Surgery of the Neonate and Infant*. Philadelphia, PA, W. B. Saunders, 1994, pp 281–294

31. Spicer RL, Behrendt D, Crowley DC: Repair of truncus arteriosus in neonates with the use of a valveless conduit. *Circulation* **70** (suppl I):26–29, 1984

32. LeCompte Y, Neveus JY, Leca F, et al: Reconstruction of the pulmonary outflow tract without prosthetic conduit. *J Thorac Cardiovasc Surg* **84:**727–733, 1982

33. Barbero-Marcial M, Riso A, Atik E, et al: A technique for correction of truncus arteriosus type I and II without extracardiac conduits. *J Thorac Cardiovasc Surg* **99:**364, 1990

34. Boyce SW, Turley K, Yee ES, et al: The fate of the 12mm porcine valved conduit from the right ventricle to the pulmonary artery: A ten year experience. *J Thorac Cardiovasc Surg* **95:**201–207, 1988

35. Agarwal KC, Edwards WD, Feldt RH, et al: Pathogenesis of nonobstructive peels in right-sided procine-valved extracardiac conduits. *J Thorac Cardiovasc Surg* **83:**584–589, 1982

36. Moodie DS, Mair DD, Fulton RE, et al: Aortic homograft obstruction. *J Thorac Cardiovasc Surg* **72:**553–561, 1976

37. Kay PH, Ross DN: Fifteen year's experience with the aortic homograft: The conduit of choice for right ventricle outflow tract reconstruction. *Ann Thorac Surg* **40:**360–364, 1985

38. Heinemann MK, Hanley FL, Fenton KN, et al: Fate of small homograft conduits after early repair of truncus arteriosus. *Ann Thorac Surg* **55:**1409–1412, 1993

39. Hawkins JA, Bailey WW, Dillon T, Schwartz DC: Midterm results with cryopreserved allograft valved conduits from the right ventricle to the pulmonary arteries. *J Thorac Cardiovasc Surg* **104:**910–916, 1992

40. Sharma S, Cobanoglu A, Dobbs J, Rice M: Clinical results of cryopreserved valved conduits in the pulmonary ventricle to pulmonary artery position. *Am J Surg* **165:**587–591, 1993

41. Stark J, Gandhi D, DeLeval M: Surgical treatment of truncas arteriosus in the first year of life. *Br Heart J* **40:**1280–1287, 1978

42. Parenzan L, Crupi G, Alfieri O, et al: Surgical repair of persistent truncus arteriosus in infancy. *Thorac Cardiovasc Surg* **28:**18–20, 1980

43. McKay R, Miyamoto S, Peart I, et al: Truncus arteriosus with interrupted arch: Successful correction in a neonate. *Ann Thorac Surg* **48:**587, 1989

44. Pearl JM, Laks H, Drinkwater DC, et al: Repair of truncus arteriosus in infancy. *Ann Thorac Surg* **52:**780–786, 1991

Congenital Malformations of the Aortic Valve and Left Ventricular Outflow Tract

David R. Clarke and Deborah A. Bishop

Congenital anomalies of the left ventricular outflow tract encompass a variety of lesions that produce isolated or combined obstruction and/or regurgitation. The combined forms of aortic stenosis are one of the five most prevalent types of congenital heart disease and occur in 3 to 8% of children with congenital cardiac anomalies.[1,2]

HISTORY

The existence of aortic stenosis as a cardiac abnormality has been acknowledged since the 1600s. In 1679, death in an otherwise healthy male was attributed to aortic stenosis when the only abnormal autopsy finding was calcified aortic valve cusps. In the mid-nineteenth century, sudden death as a result of aortic stenosis was documented multiple times and bicuspid valves were known to be susceptible to disease processes. Aortic stenosis in children and young adults was recognized as congenital by the early 1900s.[3] Clinical symptoms and natural history of the disease have been well defined since 1940.[4]

As early as 1913, Jeger and Tuffier independently published methods for surgically dealing with aortic valve stenosis in an animal model.[5] Jeger devised a method for bypassing the aortic valve with a graft conduit. Tuffier attempted to dilate the aortic valve by invagination of the aortic wall. Interest in surgical correction of aortic stenosis was then dormant until the mid-1950s.

Attempts to surgically palliate a stenotic aortic valve were based on techniques used to repair pulmonary steno-

sis. Marquis et al[4] first reported attempts to dilate stenotic aortic valves in 1954. A special dilating instrument was inserted through the ventricular apex to perform the valvotomy. Results were unpredictable and not solely beneficial due to the creation or exacerbation of aortic insufficiency in every patient. The surgical objective was to make as large an orifice as possible thus avoiding the necessity for reoperation.

Swan and Kortz, in Denver, reported the first successful open heart surgery to palliate aortic stenosis in 1956.[5] Hypothermia and a transaortic approach were used. Their primary concern was avoidance of air embolism that could result from exposure of the coronary ostia to air. To accommodate the situation, patient position was emphasized and it was the cardinal principle that the incision into the heart or great vessel be the most superior point. Because the production or exacerbation of aortic insufficiency was already known to be a nagging problem, Swan and Kortz emphasized the importance of erring on the side of incomplete relief of stenosis to avoid creating insufficiency.

Later in 1956, Lewis et al[6] reported the Minnesota results in three patients using a method of surgical aortic valvotomy that incorporated direct vision, hypothermia, and inflow occlusion. Like the Denver surgeons, Lewis and colleagues were concerned with the potential for air embolus. To avoid such an occurrence, saline was injected, under pressure, into the heart to displace air.

As cardiopulmonary bypass developed in the 1950s through 1970s, the performance of many cardiac surgical procedures was facilitated. Aortic valvotomy and valve replacement were no exception. The luxury of additional time greatly increased technical precision and reduced morbidity and mortality.

The next major development in the palliative management of congenital aortic stenosis was not until the early 1980s when Lababidi and his associates published their experience with percutaneous balloon aortic valvuloplasty.[7] In 23 consecutive patients, the mean transvalvar aortic gradient was decreased from 113 to 32 mm Hg. No sign of insufficiency was observed in 13 children and mild regurgitation was produced in 10 children. Multiple studies have been conducted to document optimal techniques, common complications, and results.[8–10] In the interest of avoiding iliofemoral artery complications and retrograde crossing of the aortic valve, anterograde balloon valvuloplasty was proposed by Hausdorf in 1993.[11] Residual gradients were comparable to those seen with retrograde valvuloplasty.

Aortic valve replacement in children has been practiced widely since the 1960s. Many types of bioprosthetic valves were preferentially implanted in children initially, but by the early 1980s bioprostheses had proven themselves unsuitable for use in children due to accelerated calcification and degeneration.[12,13] Mechanical valve replacements had demonstrated two inherent drawbacks with respect to pediatric application. Concomitant anticoagulation was required and they were unavailable in sizes that were small enough to be useful in infants and young children.[14] In the United States, cryopreserved allografts became available for aortic valve replacement in the mid-1980s.[15] At present, many centers consider allografts as the "gold standard" for pediatric aortic valve replacement.

EMBRYOLOGY

The aortic root, aortic valve, and left ventricular outflow tract are derived from primitive bulbar structures.[16,17] Via a process called cardiac looping, the initially straight, primitive heart tube begins to fold to the right at the caudal end. The bulbus cordis is positioned most cephalad followed by the ventricular and atrial areas, respectively (Fig. 75–1). During cardiac looping, the bulboventricular flange is formed within the heart tube (Fig. 75–2). The embryonic ventricle forms inferior to the bulboventricular flange and the superior portion becomes the bulbus cordis.

Localized areas of development eventually create the four cardiac chambers. The conus cordis is the middle section of the bulbus cordis (Fig. 75–3) and becomes the right and left ventricular outflow tracts. The superior aspect of the bulbus cordis forms the aortic roots and pulmonary artery. By processes of cell proliferation, extracellular matrix production, and cell migration, the conotruncal cushions enlarge to separate the aortic and pulmonary outflow tracts (Fig. 75–4). Septation continues as trabeculated tissue from two apposed sides grows together to separate left and right ventricles. A narrow opening is left between the approaching walls and eventually is closed by tissue prolifera-

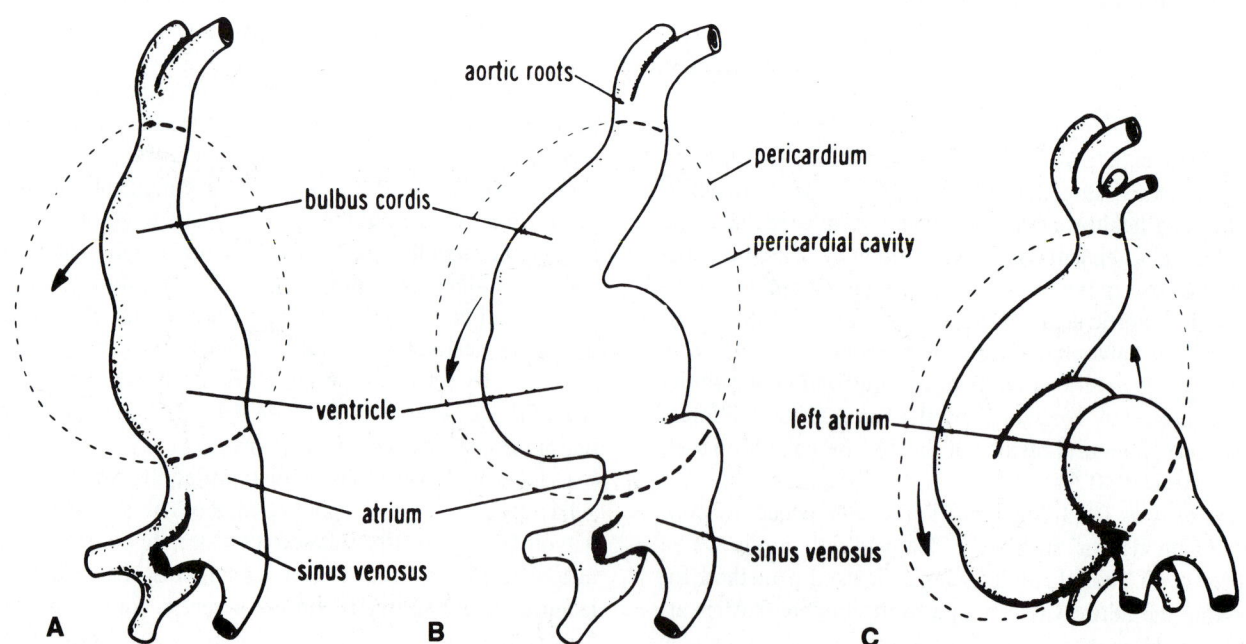

Figure 75–1. Cardiac looping of the heart tube at the embryologic stages of (**A**) 8 somites, (**B**) 11 somites, and (**C**) 16 somites. Dashed line, parietal pericardium. *(From Clark EB, Van Mierop LHS: Development of the cardiovascular system. In Adams FH, Emmanouilides GC, Riemenschneider TA (eds): Heart Disease in Infants, Children, and Adolescents, 4th ed. Baltimore, Williams & Wilkins, 1989, p 2.)*

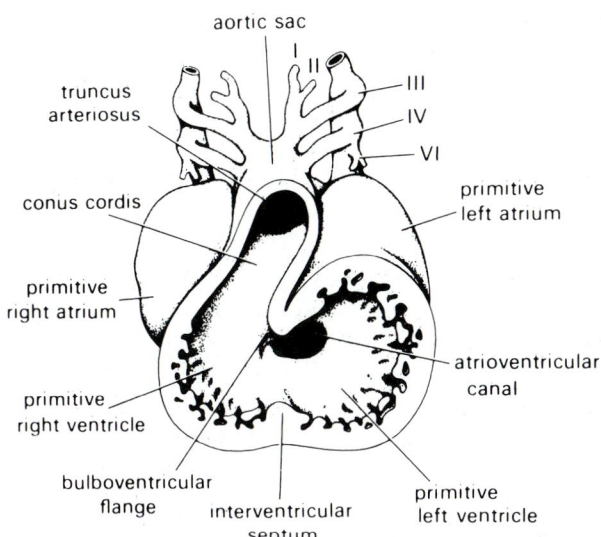

Figure 75–2. Frontal section of a 5-mm embryonic heart. *(From Clark EB, Van Mierop LHS: Development of the cardiovascular system. In Adams FH, Emmanouilides GC, Riemenschneider TA (eds): Heart Disease in Infants, Children, and Adolescents, 4th ed, Baltimore, Williams & Wilkins, 1989, p 2.)*

tion from surrounding structures. Failure of the tissues to close the foramen will result in a ventricular septal defect.

The aortic valve forms along with the pulmonary valve, where the truncal cushions meet the aortopulmonary septum. Both valve channels first appear as small paired tubercles. A third tubercle forms in each channel and the

three tubercles progressively thin from the top to form valve leaflets and sinuses.

Aberrations in these important developmental steps can result in a variety of isolated or combined anomalies of the aortic valve, aortic root, or left ventricular outflow tract. Abnormal aortic leaflet development or fusion of leaflet commissures can result in a bicuspid or unicuspid valve. Faulty transfer of the posterior conal segment in combination with a lack of absorption of conal elements results in persistence of the interventricular foramen in a vertical plane and becomes the egress route from the left ventricle. Postnatally, it may be restrictive and produce subvalvar aortic stenosis. Similarly, faulty transfer that places the primary interventricular foramen in a subpulmonic rather than a subaortic position produces an infundibulum beneath the aorta with a connection to the right ventricle either in the form of transposition of the great arteries or double outlet right ventricle. Subaortic infundibula can also be restrictive and produce subvalvar aortic stenosis.

In the presence of proper transfer of the primary interventricular foramen, unabsorbed or malaligned conal masses can persist and produce real or potential muscular obstruction in a formed left ventricular outflow tract. Fibrous union between the mitral and aortic valves can leave adhesions with subsequent reactive proliferation from mitral valve structures that also become a subaortic obstruction in an otherwise well-formed left ventricular outflow tract.

The fact that structural abnormalities within the left heart are frequently associated with abnormalities of the aorta such as coarctation, arch interruption, and hypoplasia

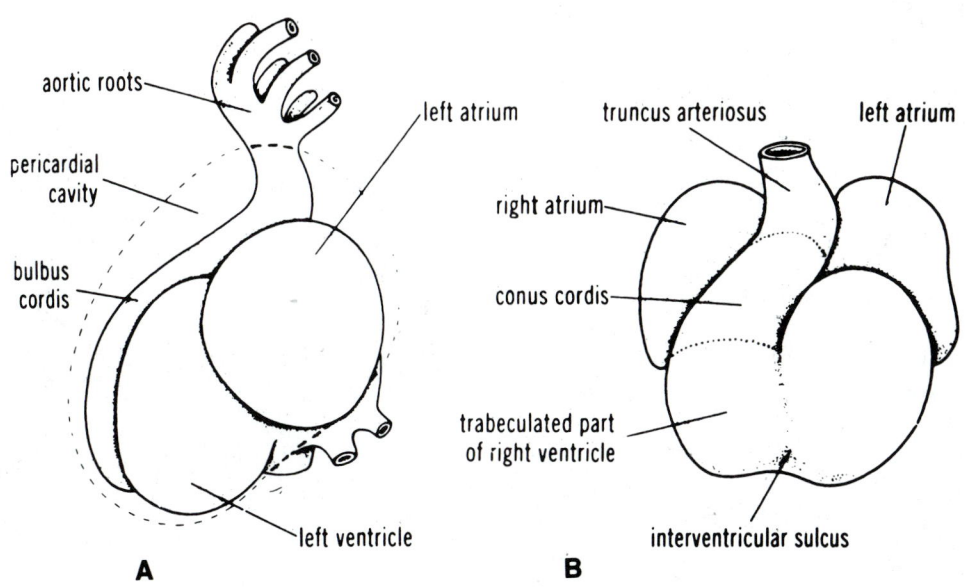

Figure 75–3. A 5-mm embryonic heart (**A**) from the left and (**B**) from the front. *(From Clark EB, Van Mierop LHS: Development of the cardiovascular system. In Adams FH, Emmanouilides GC, Riemenschneider TA (eds): Heart Disease in Infants, Children, and Adolescents, 4th ed, Baltimore, Williams & Wilkins, 1989, p 2.)*

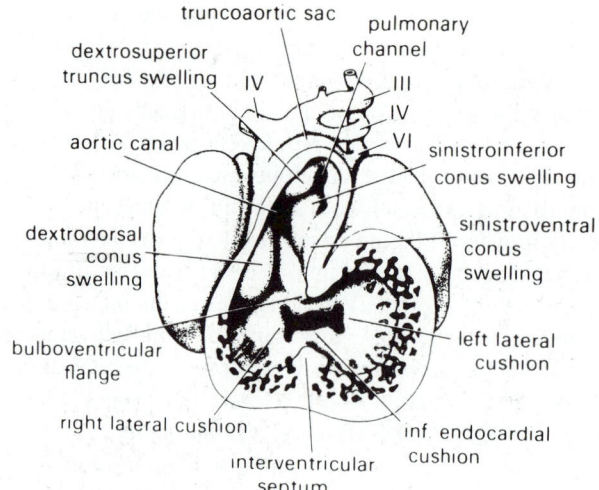

Figure 75–4. Frontal section of a 9-mm embryonic heart. *(From Clark EB, Van Mierop LHS: Development of the cardiovascular system. In Adams FH, Emmanouilides GC, Riemenschneider TA (eds): Heart Disease in Infants, Children, and Adolescents, 4th ed, Baltimore, Williams & Wilkins, 1989, p 2.)*

has led to a theory of hemodynamic molding. The theory postulates that during development, size of structures in the central circulation is related to the volume of blood passing through them and that configuration is related to the profile of the flowing blood.[18] For example, the developing right and left fetal heart handles approximately one-half of the blood flow destined for the fetal aorta. Impediments to blood flow through the left side of the heart result in augmentation of ductal flow and a diminution of transaortic valve flow. Rudolf and associates[19] first suggested that such a disturbance would diminish flow through the isthmic portion of the aorta and thereby diminish its developed size resulting in a preductal narrowing or coarctation of the aorta. Hutchins[20] expanded upon the idea and suggested that further decrease in flow would create a branch point opposite the ductus with bidirectional flow into the aorta, and that such an arrangement could initiate the development of a juxtaductal coarctation. In more extreme cases of decreased left ventricular output and increased right ventricular output, disturbances in relationship of ductal and transaortic flow could produce a null point of flow in the aortic arch. This might account for the development of arch interruptions. The complete absence of left ventricular output and total dependence on right ventricular output and ductal flow would result in the progressively decreasing size of the more proximal aortic arch and ascending aorta as seen in hypoplastic left heart syndrome. The unproven theory of hemodynamic molding is supported by circumstantial evidence such as the observation that aortic coarctation and interruption are often associated with frank obstructive lesions in the left heart. These lesions are often associated with hypoplastic left ventricle, abnormalities of the mitral

valve, and a restrictive foramen ovale during fetal development.[18]

Formation of the aortic valve, the left ventricular outflow tract, and associated structures is the result of multifactorial and often related embryologic events. There are a variety of developmental abnormalities that can affect the aortic valve and left ventricular outflow tract to produce isolated lesions or extremely complex abnormalities. The subsequent discussion will focus on more common lesions that involve the aortic root, aortic valve, and left ventricular outflow tract. Surgical therapy is directed toward correction of the lesion. The frequently associated anomalies of the aortic arch as well as more complex syndromes that include such lesions are discussed in Chapters 76 and 77.

ANATOMY

The normal aortic valve (Fig. 75–5) consists of three equally sized pouch-like cusps with semilunar shaped free margins. The cusps or leaflets are normally thin, smooth, and compliant and should open flush with the aortic wall during cardiac systole. The sinuses of Valsalva are dilated pockets between the cusps and the aortic wall. A fibrous swelling called the nodulus Arantii is at the center of the free margin of each leaflet. The cusps are designated left coronary, right coronary, and noncoronary cusps and are named according to the coronary artery that does or does not originate from each sinus of Valsalva.

The aortic root is the most proximal part of the ascending aorta and is contiguous with the aortic valve annulus.

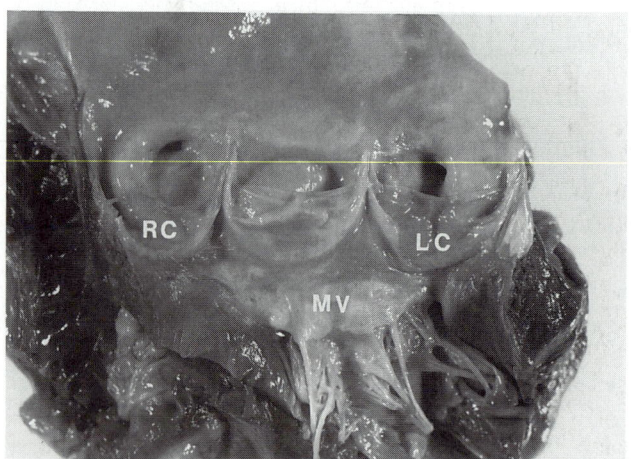

Figure 75–5. A normal aortic valve: Three semilunar cusps are within a circular fibrous annulus. The midportion of each cusp is marked by the corpora Arantii. The valve cusps are designated according to the coronary artery arising from the respective sinus of Valsalva; left coronary cusp, right coronary cusp, and noncoronary cusp. The anterior leaflet of the mitral valve is in continuity with portions of the left and noncoronary cusps. LC, left coronary cusp; RC, right coronary cusp; MV, mitral valve.

The three sinuses of Valsalva lie above and opposite the three aortic valve leaflets and are separated by the attachments of the valve cusps at each commissural support. A small indentation of the aortic root is often present, but significant narrowing of the lumen is abnormal.

The outflow tract of the left ventricle supports the aortic valve. Its posterior half is fibrous and the anterior half is muscular. There is an intimate relationship between the left ventricular outflow tract and adjacent structures. The muscular portion consists primarily of the infundibular or conal septum. The posterior fibrous portion is principally the fusion of the anterior leaflet of the mitral and aortic valves. A much smaller part of the posterior fibrous portion of the left ventricular outflow tract is made up by the central fibrous body, which is a small triangular structure interposed anteriorly and medially between the anterior (aortic) leaflet of the mitral valve and the muscular portion of the outflow tract.

In a normal heart, the relationship of the three aortic valve cusps to underlying supportive structures of the left ventricular outflow tract is relatively constant. Parts of the noncoronary and left coronary cusps are usually in fibrous continuity with the anterior leaflet of the mitral valve. The posterior part of the noncoronary cusp is also in fibrous continuity with the central fibrous body. Relatively poor support by the fibrous body might represent a weak point that could contribute to development of sinus of Valsalva aneurysms. Usually the anterior portion of the noncoronary cusp along with the entire right coronary and a portion of the left coronary cusps are attached to the muscular ventricular outlet and are additionally supported by a fibrous skeleton. The membranous ventricular septum lies directly anterior, immediately underneath the commissure between the right and noncoronary cusps. The bundle of His lies just beneath the membranous septum and therefore is situated only a few millimeters inferior to the aortic annulus.

The anomaly that is known as valvar aortic stenosis is comprised of varying degrees of thickening and rigidity of the valve tissue and varied levels of diminished separation of commissures. Most often, the anomalous aortic valve is bicuspid. The leaflets are usually of unequal size with a raphe or false commissure apparent in the larger of the leaflets.[21,22] The leaflets are usually oriented right and left (Fig. 75–6) with the true commissures oriented anterior and posterior. Most commonly, the right and left coronary leaflets comprise the larger, fused leaflet and the noncoronary leaflet is separate with true commissures. The free edges of a bicuspid valve are more straight than rounded producing limited mobility. Fusion of all three leaflets of the aortic valve produces a unicuspid valve. It may have a central opening without a true commissure or an eccentric, narrow opening that extends to the annulus. Occurrence of a quadricuspid valve is extremely rare except in association with truncus arteriosus, which is discussed in Chapter 74.

Subvalvar aortic stenosis anatomy can take one of several forms: a discrete ridge, a hypertrophied septal muscle

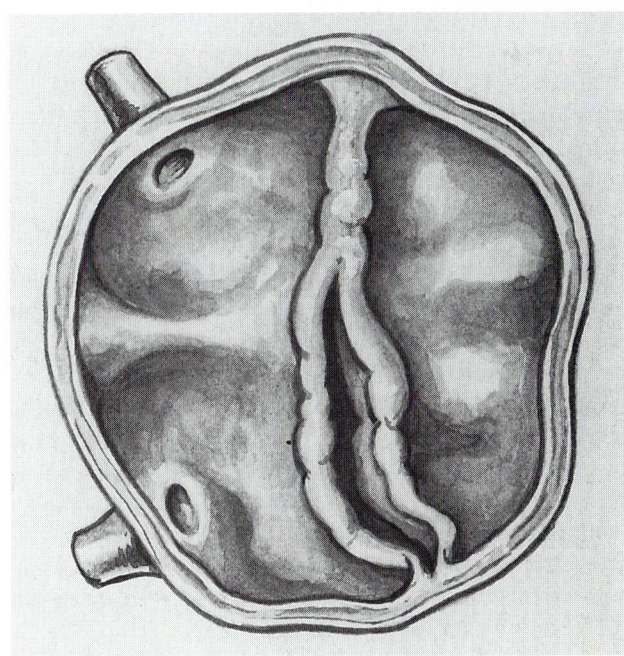

Figure 75–6. A congenitally bicuspid aortic valve with left and right leaflets and fusion of the anterior commissure.

that causes dynamic narrowing, or a rigid, fibromuscular, tunnel obstruction.[23,24] The discrete type of obstruction is most common and occurs in 75 to 85% of patients. Most recently, it has been postulated that discrete subvalvar aortic stenosis is not purely a fibrous ridge but is partially fibromuscular, often with coexistent septal muscle hypertrophy.[25]

There are three morphologic forms of supravalvar aortic stenosis. Fifty to 75 percent of patients have an hourglass shaped deformity,[26,27] approximately 25% have more diffuse narrowing of the ascending aorta of variable length,[27] and a small percentage of patients have a discrete obstruction above the aortic valve.[26,28] Branches of the aortic arch are often involved at their origins.[29] Concurrent minor abnormalities of the aortic valve itself are also common.[27,29]

VALVAR AORTIC STENOSIS

Valvar aortic stenosis presents at one extreme, within the first few weeks after birth as a medical emergency. At the other extreme, aortic stenosis is diagnosed in an asymptomatic child after a murmur is detected during routine clinical examination. Infants with critical aortic stenosis whose systemic circulations are dependent on flow across the patent ductus arteriosus present abruptly with hypotension and shock as the ductus closes within the first few days or weeks of life. Children in whom a reasonable cardiac output is maintained following ductal closure have mild or no symptoms of congestive heart failure.

The incidence of valvar aortic stenosis in males is three to five times higher than in females.[30–32] Other cardiac defects are present in up to 20% of children whose primary diagnosis is valvar aortic stenosis. The most commonly associated anomalies are patent ductus arteriosus, coarctation of the aorta, and ventricular septal defect.[2,33]

Infantile Aortic Stenosis

Infants with valvar aortic stenosis severe enough to initiate symptoms of congestive heart failure by definition have critical infantile aortic stenosis. Symptoms result from changes that occur during the transition from the fetal to neonatal circulatory pattern. Reduced pulmonary vascular resistance leads to an increased blood volume delivered to the left ventricle. If there is obstruction to left ventricular outflow, the ventricle can neither fill nor eject a normal volume of blood. When the ductus arteriosus constricts, systemic cardiac output cannot be maintained and the infant becomes hypotensive and presents a shocky appearance with poor peripheral perfusion and obvious cyanosis. By 2 mo of age, approximately two-thirds of patients with infantile aortic stenosis become symptomatic. A small percentage of these children develop symptoms after 6 mo of age.[34–37] Tachypnea, feeding problems, and failure to thrive are the most common symptoms displayed by infants in congestive heart failure. Hepatomegaly and peripheral edema are not common but can be present.

Critical aortic stenosis patients can deteriorate rapidly and present a medical emergency. Neonates or infants who exhibit severe cardiac failure and poor perfusion should be treated with aggressive inotropic support and mechanical ventilation if necessary. Initial palliative therapy is often directed toward support of the systemic circulation by maintenance or restoration of fetal shunts. Prostaglandin E_1 is used to maintain ductal patency and tissue perfusion[38–40] and can reverse acidosis and shock. Due to the potential for sudden deterioration and almost uniform inability to resolve signs of congestive heart failure, prolonged medical management is contraindicated and noninvasive evaluation should be performed immediately.[34,35,41]

Clinical Evaluation

Upon physical examination, the most prominent findings in infants with critical aortic stenosis are poor pulses and a hyperactive precordium. Although the typical aortic stenosis murmur is present in less than 20% of younger infants,[34] the majority exhibit at least a soft ejection murmur along the left upper sternal border that radiates to the neck. The murmur can be subtle in younger patients with severe cardiac failure. The typical resting electrocardiogram in infantile aortic stenosis is neither normal nor diagnostic. Arrhythmias are rare and other than first degree atrioventricular block, atrioventricular conduction defects are also rare.[41] In the majority of neonates, chest roentgenogram reveals cardiomegaly. Pulmonary vascular markings are usu-

ally normal but pulmonary congestion is diagnosed in 30 to 50% of cases.[42] In most infants, echocardiography is sufficiently specific diagnostically to eliminate the need for cardiac catheterization.[43–45] Catheterization is necessary if there is any doubt about a complete or accurate diagnosis, if associated defects cannot be sufficiently evaluated with noninvasive techniques, or if transcatheter therapy is contemplated.

Treatment

Size of the left ventricle and condition of the left ventricular myocardium are often the determining factors in selection of surgical management and in outcome for infants with critical aortic stenosis. In the extreme form of aortic atresia, a hypoplastic left ventricle or the presence of endocardial fibroelastosis is common. When the left ventricle is not functional, a Norwood procedure that converts cardiac anatomy to that of a single right ventricle is one surgical option.[46,47] Cardiac transplantation is also appropriate for these infants.[48,49] Hypoplastic left ventricle and cardiac transplantation are discussed thoroughly in Chapters 77 and 91, respectively. For infants without obvious hypoplastic left heart syndrome or endocardial fibroelastosis, evaluation of left ventricular size is extremely important to the determination of appropriate patient management. Operative mortality is lower in patients whose left ventricular cavity size is adequate.[50] Although the final determination of competence is left to the surgeon's judgment, the potential for adequate left ventricular function should be evaluated echocardiographically.[51–53] Unfavorable surgical outcome is correlated with a left ventricular inflow dimension of less than 25 mm when measured from the apex to the posterior mitral annulus, a ventriculoaortic junction less than 5 mm, and a mitral valve orifice diameter less than 9 mm.[53] If the left ventricle is determined unable to support systemic circulation, a Rashkind balloon atrial septostomy should be performed,[54] which reduces pulmonary venous hypertension and, along with prostaglandin E_1, can provide palliation while awaiting a Norwood procedure or cardiac transplant.

The only sustained resolution of symptoms is obtained from procedures that relieve the mechanical obstruction to the aortic valve. Transcatheter balloon dilation of the valve is sometimes the first interventional procedure undertaken for infantile aortic stenosis.[7,10,55] When limited vascular access or difficulty crossing the valve is encountered, balloon valvuloplasty is not possible. Dysplastic valves with an associated small annulus also are not usually amenable to balloon dilation. Early results are similar to those with surgical valvotomy with an approximate 50% gradient reduction in most patients. Development of new or slightly increased aortic regurgitation is common.[56,57]

Surgical aortic valvotomy remains the standard surgical approach to critical aortic stenosis in the newborn. Historically, neonatal aortic valvotomies were performed with moderate hypothermia and caval occlusion[37,58] or with cardiopulmonary bypass[59] with only sporadic success. In retrospect, the high failure rate was likely not related to operative technique, but to the infant's compromised condition with profound systemic hypoperfusion, acidemia, and myocardial ischemia. Somerville[60] and Edmunds and associates[61] have suggested the poor operative results might be better explained by left ventricular dysfunction rather than unrelieved obstruction. Prostaglandin therapy now allows the surgeon the luxury of operating on neonates and young infants with more stable hemodynamics after appropriate resuscitation.

Surgical approach to infantile aortic stenosis currently differs from institution to institution. Controversy continues concerning the use of cardiopulmonary bypass versus inflow occlusion. Many surgeons prefer to implement cardiopulmonary bypass for infant aortic valvotomy.[62,63] Through a midline sternotomy, an aortic infusion cannula is placed in the distal ascending aorta and a single venous drainage cannula is inserted into the right atrial appendage. After the patient is cooled and the aorta is cross-clamped, cardioplegia is infused into the aortic root. The valvotomy is initiated by exposing the aortic valve with a vertical aortotomy directed toward the noncoronary cusp. Edges of the opposing leaflet are grasped and separated to expose the area of leaflet fusion (Fig. 75–7). Taking care not to cut into either leaflet, the fused portion of the leaflets is separated with a scalpel. A conservative approach that reduces transvalvar gradient but does not create aortic insufficiency is recommended as an operative strategy. Because cardiopulmonary bypass is often poorly tolerated in infants, and a

valvotomy can be performed easily in 1.5 to 2 min, some surgeons prefer mild hypothermia with inflow occlusion.[40,64,65]

Infants who survive aortic valvotomy in the newborn period show marked clinical improvement but there is a high surgical mortality rate. Early series quoted operative mortalities greater than 50%;[34,66] more recently 25 to 50% has been reported.[35,37,65,67] It has been postulated that the high mortality is due to associated abnormalities such as mitral regurgitation,[68] small mitral annulus,[69] small left ventricle,[35,70] or the presence of endocardial fibroelastosis.

Valvotomy performed in infancy should be considered palliative and not curative.[71] Many infants who undergo surgery for critical aortic stenosis will develop recurrent aortic stenosis, aortic stenosis with regurgitation, or isolated regurgitation within 1 year of their initial procedure. Repeat aortic valvotomy is rarely effective and valve replacement is usually necessary. Placement of a left ventricular apical to aortic conduit has been attempted in children with stenosis but without significant aortic regurgitation.[72] It has since become evident that this extra-anatomic technique creates late complications related to left ventricular mechanical damage, valved conduit failure, and the inappropriate physiology of retrograde ejection.[73]

Infants who require aortic valve replacement usually require substantial annulus enlargement before implantation can be accomplished. While experience suggests the annulus diameter of these patients is usually no more than 10 mm, the smallest prosthetic valve currently available has a minimum implantation diameter of 16 mm. An aortoventriculoplasty or Konno procedure[74,75] that enlarges the aortic annulus anteriorly and can effectively double the implantation diameter can be incorporated into the repair. A variation on annulus enlargement is the extended aortic root replacement procedure that uses an aortic allograft, the anterior mitral leaflet of which is used to patch the infundibular septum and enlarge the entire left ventricular outflow tract (Fig. 75–8).[76] Cryopreserved aortic valve allografts ranging from 10 to 17 mm internal diameter have been implanted in infants.[77]

The majority of infants who present with critical aortic stenosis beyond the neonatal period can usually be surgically treated with an aortic valvotomy using cardiopulmonary bypass. As in the neonatal aortic stenosis population, the policy for older infant valvotomies is conservative. The surgery should provide symptomatic relief and avoid creation or aggravation of aortic insufficiency. The procedure is palliative due to a high incidence of residual or recurrent aortic stenosis and significant regurgitation.[35,37,65]

Aortic Stenosis in Children Greater Than One Year of Age

In contrast to infants with critical aortic stenosis, 95% of older children with valvar aortic stenosis are asymptomatic with normal growth and development.[78] The children nor-

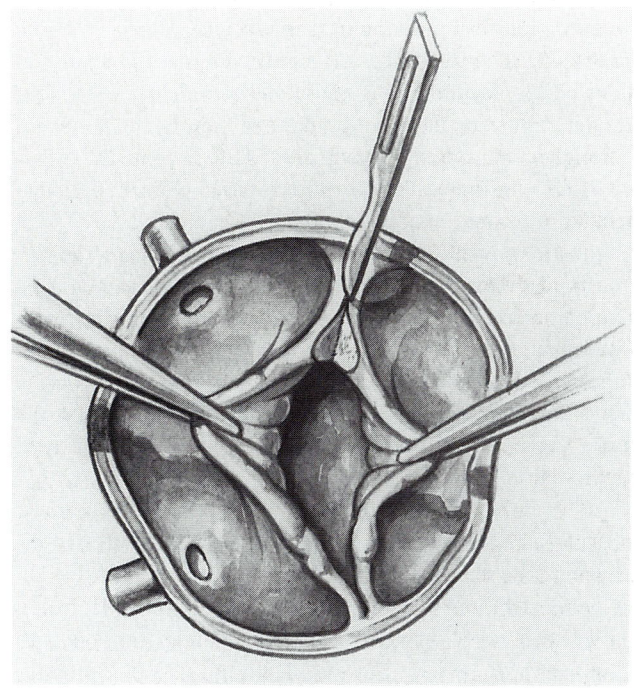

Figure 75–7. Aortic valvotomy for congenital aortic stenosis.

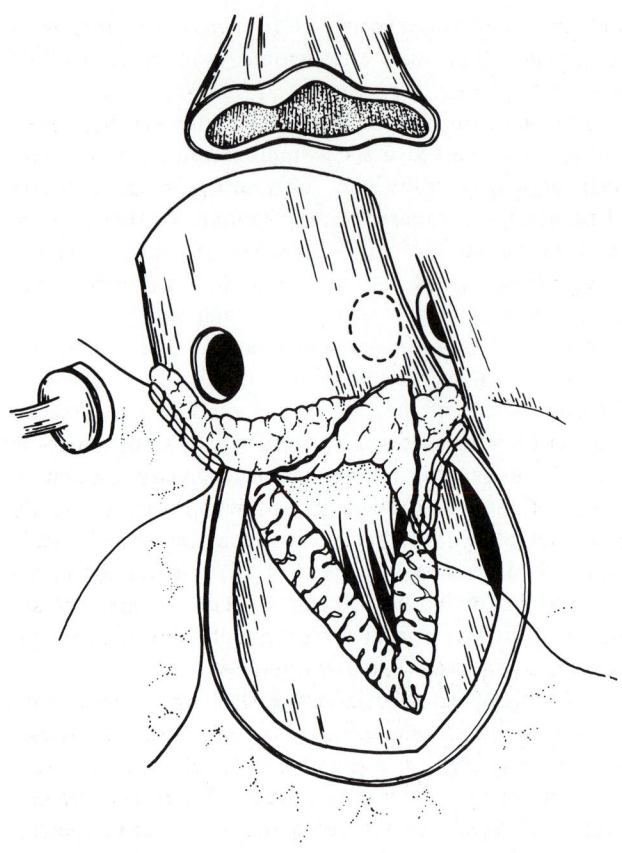

Figure 75–8. The anterior mitral leaflet of the donor allograft aortic valve is used to enlarge the left ventricular outflow tract. *(From Clarke DR: Extended aortic root replacement for treatment of left ventricular outflow tract obstruction. J Cardiac Surg 2(suppl 1):121 1987.)*

mally receive attention when a murmur is detected on routine physical examination. When symptoms do occur, the most common is fatigue followed by exertional dyspnea, angina pectoris, and syncope.[33] Approximately three children per 1000 patient-years develop endocarditis[79]; its occurrence cannot be correlated to lesion severity. There is also the potential for sudden death that is reported to strike from 1.2 to 19% per year of children with this lesion.[30,80–82] Children who experience sudden death are usually those with more severe obstruction who are symptomatic. Approximately 50% of sudden deaths in aortic valvar stenosis occur during or immediately after exercise.[83] Ventricular dysrhythmia initiated by acute subendocardial ischemia seems to be the most plausible explanation for the deaths.

Valvar aortic stenosis is the most commonly encountered form of congenital aortic stenosis. Hypoplasia of the aortic annulus is one form of aortic stenosis, but in the majority of cases, stenosis presenting after 1 year of age occurs as a result of abnormally formed valve leaflets. A bicuspid valve with one fused commissure is present in 70% of cases.[33]

Congenital valvar aortic stenosis is a progressive

anomaly and clinical deterioration should be expected. The stenotic aortic valve orifice is of relatively fixed diameter in the pediatric population and does not grow with increasing body size.[84–86] Appearance or intensification of symptoms results from an increase in the severity of obstruction or the development of significant aortic insufficiency. Because a malformed aortic valve is a potential site for bacterial infection, all patients with aortic stenosis should observe SBE prophylaxis regardless of the severity of the lesion.

Clinical Evaluation

Physical examination of children with valvar aortic stenosis is normally characteristic enough to make an accurate diagnosis. With the exception of extremely severe cases, vital signs are normal.[87] The murmur of aortic valve stenosis is a classic systolic ejection murmur with maximum intensity at the upper right sternal border. An ejection click also can be present.

There is no electrocardiographic parameter that is sensitive enough to estimate stenotic severity in children less than 2 years of age.[88] In patients greater than 2 years old, a resting electrocardiogram is moderately helpful in determining the degree of aortic valve stenosis. An abnormal T wave in lead V_6 indicates the presence of a large aortic transvalvar gradient. An exercise electrocardiogram can improve sensitivity for detecting severe stenosis in children who are old enough to cooperate. A typical left ventricular strain pattern along with a stable or decreased systolic blood pressure during monitored exercise signifies the presence of severe aortic obstruction. However, even severe aortic stenosis is often accompanied by normal exercising cardiac function.[89]

On chest roentgenogram, there is little correlation between degree of cardiac enlargement and degree of aortic stenosis.[33] The presence of significant cardiomegaly in older children with valvar aortic stenosis denotes left ventricular failure or the development of significant aortic insufficiency and implies a poor immediate prognosis.[4]

Echocardiographic diagnostic parameters can reveal detailed information about an abnormal aortic valve. As the diagnostic powers of echocardiography improve, an increasing number of children are sent to surgery without cardiac catheterization. For these patients, thorough echocardiographic examination of the heart and great vessels is imperative to rule out associated lesions. M-mode echocardiography demonstrates multiple diastolic echoes of the aortic valve as opposed to the normal single closure line. Asymmetric valve leaflet opening and closing is evident,[90,91] left ventricular size and wall thickness can be measured, and ventricular function estimated. With two-dimensional echocardiography, aortic valve morphology can be delineated and the symmetry of opening and closing leaflets can be observed.[92] Restricted leaflet motion with "doming" appears in systole and leaflet prolapse, if present, is evident in diastole.[93] Color Doppler echocardiography identifies disturbed blood flow patterns[94] and continuous-wave Doppler is used to measure systolic blood flow velocities in the central jet for calculation of transvalvar pressure gradients.[95,96]

If necessary to determine the need for intervention, the final step in the medical examination of a child with valvar aortic stenosis is cardiac catheterization. Cardiac catheterization is useful for establishing the site and severity rather than the presence of left ventricular outflow obstruction since aortic stenosis is normally diagnosed by clinical examination and noninvasive study. Children with valvar aortic stenosis are catheterized when they are borderline surgical candidates. If there are any diagnostic questions or uncertainties, catheterization is invaluable in resolving them. Left ventricular and aortic root angiograms should be performed. Transvalvar aortic gradient is measured by simultaneously recording the left ventricular and ascending aortic pressures or by pulling back an end hole catheter from left ventricle to aorta with continuous pressure recordings. Angiographically, a stenotic aortic valve appears thick and domes in systole (Fig. 75–9).[97] Right heart catheterization is useful for detecting or excluding associated defects such as patent ductus arteriosus, ventricular septal defect, or pulmonic stenosis. Extensive myocardial sinusoids suggests the presence of endocardial fibroelastosis.[70] Left ventricular volume and ejection fraction can be compared to normal values for age.

Because older children are rarely symptomatic and indications for operation are more obscure, appropriate timing of surgical intervention is not obvious beyond the infant stage. Mild or moderate aortic transvalvar gradients of less than 40 to 50 mm Hg are usually well tolerated for several years in children with normal cardiac output. They should undergo noninvasive cardiologic workup every 1 to 2 years depending upon the specifics of each situation.[98,99] Echocardiographic and exercise tests can be especially informative. Arrhythmias or left ventricular strain with exercise are indications for intervention. Absolute transvalvar gradients greater than 70 or 75 mm Hg constitute severe aortic stenosis and require intervention even when symptoms are not present. Angina, syncope, and progressive left ventricular hypertrophy also provide indications for invasive therapy.

Treatment

Balloon dilation of the stenotic aortic valve is often possible in older children because catheter access is simpler than in newborns. If the valve can be crossed, it is usually amenable to balloon dilation due to the presence of pliable valve leaflets and a general absence of calcification in patients less than 18 years of age.[9,33] Balloon valvuloplasty produces no greater incidence or severity of aortic regurgitation than does surgical valvotomy.[10,56]

The standard surgical procedure for children with valvar aortic stenosis is open aortic valvotomy. Total cardiopulmonary bypass with aortic cross-clamping is used. For myocardial preservation, blood cardioplegia is administered in a single dose into the aortic root prior to opening the aorta. Retrograde administration of cardioplegia via the coronary sinus can be used and is preferable if significant aortic regurgitation is present. Because the leaflets are usually pliable, the commissures can be incised easily with dramatic relief of obstruction (Fig. 75–10). Incision of the raphe is possible only if it is suspended high enough to pre-

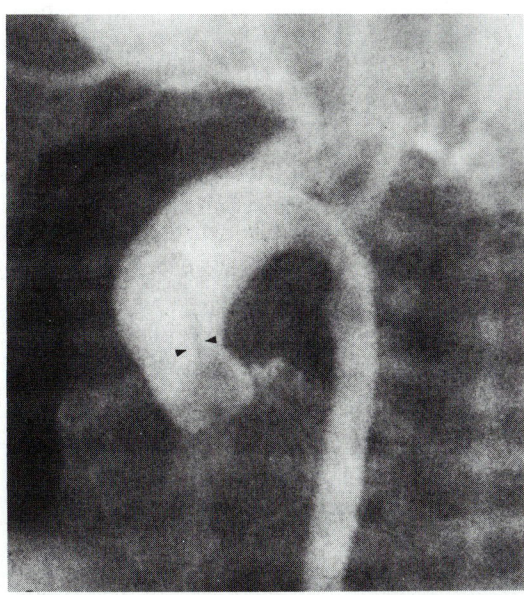

Figure 75–9. Aortogram demonstrating valvar aortic stenosis: The domed appearance of the aortic valve and the jet of blood through the narrow valve ostium (small arrows) are evident.

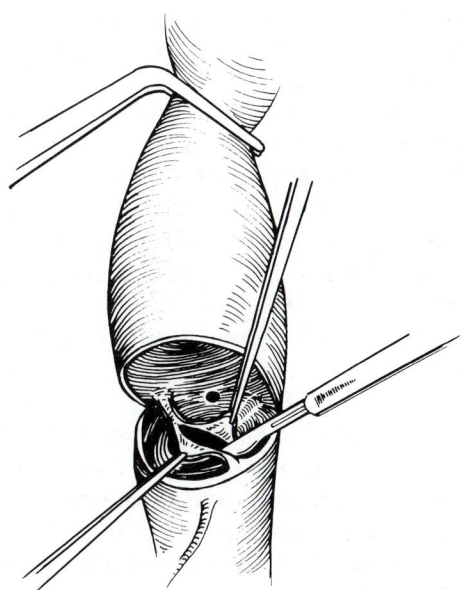

Figure 75–10. Surgical aortic valvotomy is used to palliate congenital valvar aortic stenosis.

vent leaflet prolapse. If the leaflets are thick and dysplastic, they can be thinned to produce additional relief of obstruction. A warm dose of cardioplegia can be injected after the aortotomy is closed.

Operative mortality in children beyond the infant age group is approximately 2%.[100–102] The majority of surviving patients show a significant reduction in transvalvar gradient and symptomatic improvement. Since the valve is by no means normal, antibiotic prophylaxis is necessary in the postoperative child even if the gradient is virtually eliminated.

Although aortic valvotomy can provide years of palliation, most children will require valve replacement at some point later in life. Since the valve leaflets remain deformed, further degeneration, including calcification, leads to recurrent stenosis and/or insufficiency in later years. By 10 years postoperatively, 50% of children will suffer from residual stenosis of a moderate-to-severe degree, moderate-to-severe aortic insufficiency, reoperation, bacterial endocarditis, or late death.[100,102]

Reoperative surgical intervention should be considered for children who develop a recurrent obstruction or significant aortic regurgitation diagnosed clinically or by echocardiography. Left ventricular dysfunction, progressive left ventricular dilation, or symptoms of decreased exercise tolerance are late indicators of recurrence. For patients with recurrent aortic stenosis, repeat valvotomy is not usually effective[103] and aortic valve replacement is therefore often required for stenosis as well as progressive aortic insufficiency.

Valve replacement in a child almost always includes annulus enlargement. The Manouguian procedure[104] en-

larges the aortic annulus posteriorly with the use of a patch that extends into the anterior mitral leaflet. The technique allows implantation of a prosthesis that is one to two sizes larger than the original annulus dimension or a maximum increase in implantation diameter of 4 mm. An aortoventriculoplasty[74,75] or extended aortic root replacement[76] procedure can double the implantation diameter and is necessary if further enlargement is required.

Options for Aortic Valve Replacement

The decision concerning the best choice for aortic valve replacement in the pediatric population is difficult. Bioprostheses, mechanical valves, and allografts are currently available but each valve type has inherent drawbacks. Currently available porcine bioprostheses are contraindicated in children because they calcify and degenerate quickly.[13,105,106] As little as 2 years after implantation, calcification can lead to restenosis and/or regurgitation. With the aortoventriculoplasty technique, a mechanical prosthesis can be implanted but the child is then burdened with requisite anticoagulation that is often poorly tolerated and difficult to regulate. Allograft valves do not readily calcify in older children nor do they require anticoagulation and therefore avoid related complications as well as incidents of thromboembolus. In children who were 3 years of age or older at operation, follow-up of 29 survivors of extended aortic root replacement reveals that 80% are free from death or valve explantation at over 6.5 years of follow-up (Fig. 75–11).[107] Allografts are often the only available surgical option for neonates and small infants who have extremely small aortic annuli. However, it is in this same patient

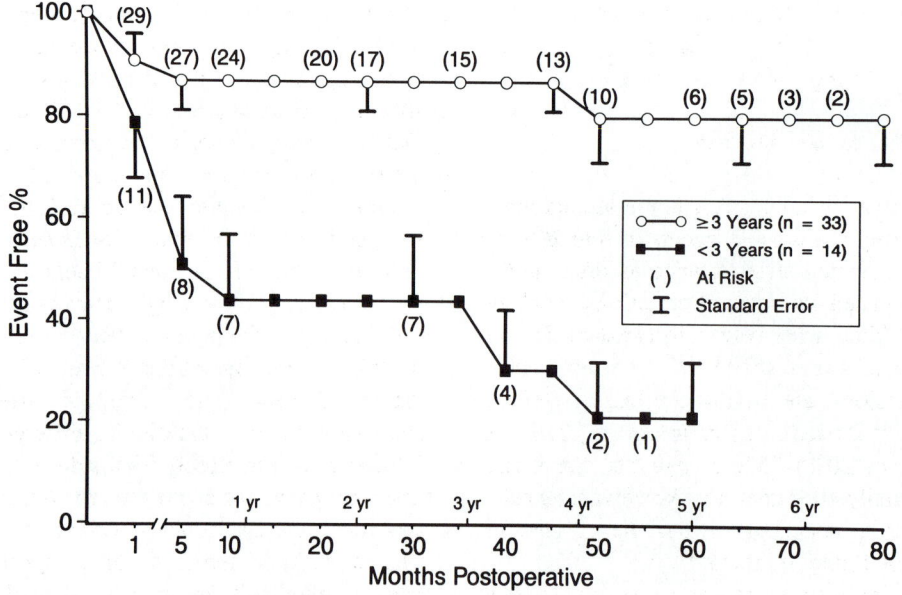

Figure 75–11. Actuarial event-free curve that illustrates freedom from death or allograft explanation in patients less than 3 years of age at operation versus patients greater than or equal to 3 years of age. *(From Clarke DR, Campbell DN, Hayward AR, Bishop DA: Degeneration of aortic valve allografts in young recipients. J Thorac Cardiovasc Surg 105:934, 1993.)*

group that allografts have been shown to exhibit an accelerated rate of fibrocalcification and degeneration.[107,108] As was the case with porcine bioprostheses, the specific mechanism of allograft failure is a mystery. One theory proposes that degeneration might be caused by an immunologically mediated host response to the allograft, but investigation is in preliminary stages.

Use of the pulmonary autograft for placement in the left ventricular outflow tract presents another surgical option for children with aortic stenosis.[109–111] The pulmonary autograft technique transfers the patient's native pulmonary valve to the left ventricular outflow tract and reconstructs the sacrificed right ventricular outflow tract with a pulmonary valve allograft. The advantages and disadvantages must be weighed seriously before such a repair is attempted. To credit the procedure, the autograft is without question immunologically compatible and clinical follow-up suggests the potential for growth in its new position.[109] However, the operation itself is a relatively long procedure that is technically challenging. Excision of the autograft is difficult and can be hazardous in an infant or small child because the left main and left anterior descending coronary arteries are at risk during the dissection. Follow-up is not without complication. In 19 years of pulmonary autograft follow-up reported by Matsuki and colleagues, the incidence of late endocarditis is 1.2% per patient-year.[110]

Follow-up of children who have undergone aortic valve replacement is crucial. Patients who receive mechanical valves must maintain adequate anticoagulation. In aortic allograft recipients, early detection of degeneration that manifests as calcification and/or progressive insufficiency is important. If these conditions develop, low-dose cyclosporine therapy might be appropriate. Although experience with such situations is limited, cyclosporine has prevented the progression of allograft degeneration in two patients.[40]

SUBVALVAR AORTIC STENOSIS

Fibromuscular subvalvar aortic stenosis is the second most common form of aortic stenosis and occurs in 8 to 20% of all cases. Males are affected at least twice as often as females.[24,112,113] Associated cardiac malformations are more common than in children with valvar aortic stenosis and occur in 50 to 65% of patients.[24,114,115] The most commonly associated lesions are ventricular septal defect, coarctation of the aorta, patent ductus arteriosus, and left superior vena cava. In 20 to 25% of patients, the aortic valve is also congenitally abnormal. Unlike valvar stenosis, severe subvalvar aortic stenosis is almost never seen in newborns and is rarely found in infants.[116,117]

The physiology of isolated subvalvar aortic stenosis appears to be similar to that of aortic valvar stenosis. Left ventricular hypertrophy develops in response to high systolic pressures. The aortic valve frequently is thickened in

patients with subvalvar aortic stenosis but is usually tricuspid. Trauma to the valve from the subaortic jet may be the etiology of the 30 to 50% incidence of aortic insufficiency seen in these patients.[23,113]

Clinical Evaluation

Subvalvar aortic stenosis in children is often masked by the presence of associated lesions. In over 50% of patients, a murmur is noted by the age of 1 year.[24] The murmur of isolated subvalvar aortic stenosis is typical of left ventricular outflow tract obstruction. In association with other anomalies, the murmur is often misconstrued as functional or caused by a small ventricular septal defect, but becomes more typical of left ventricular outflow tract obstruction as the child grows older.[24,118] The diastolic murmur of aortic insufficiency is heard more often than with valvar aortic stenosis.

Although the electrocardiogram is usually abnormal in patients with subvalvar aortic stenosis, even children with severe obstruction can occasionally have a normal study.[24,119] Varying degrees of left ventricular hypertrophy are seen in 65 to 85% of all children with subvalvar aortic stenosis and in approximately half of children with only mild stenosis.[120] Similar to patients with valvar aortic stenosis, the chest roentgenogram in children with subvalvar obstruction most often shows normal heart size but can reveal mild cardiomegaly or left ventricular prominence.

A narrowed left ventricular outflow tract is seen on M-mode echocardiography. Abnormal fluttering of the aortic valve leaflets and early systolic partial closure caused by turbulence distal to the obstruction are present.[121] Visualization via two-dimensional echocardiography differentiates the forms of subvalvar aortic stenosis.[122,123] With recent technical innovations, echocardiography is felt to be superior to angiography in its ability to recognize and distinguish subvalvar stenoses.[115,124] The severity of obstruction, however, cannot be determined accurately based on the echocardiographic appearance of the lesion.[125,126] Continuous-wave Doppler quantitates left ventricular outflow tract gradients[126–128] and color Doppler verifies the presence or absence of aortic insufficiency.

Combined left and right heart catheterization is recommended due to the high incidence of associated cardiac abnormalities. Position of the subvalvar lesion is often immediately adjacent to the valve and difficult to distinguish from valvar aortic stenosis. To differentiate the two, it is important to look closely for the discrete ridge (Fig. 75–12) and the presence of contrast medium trapped between ridge and valve. The aortic valve cusps are often thickened and in systole attain a more pyramidal appearance with straight edges as opposed to the rounded, domed appearance associated with valvar stenosis.[129]

Subvalvar aortic stenosis is a progressive lesion in most patients, especially in children with tunnel-type steno-

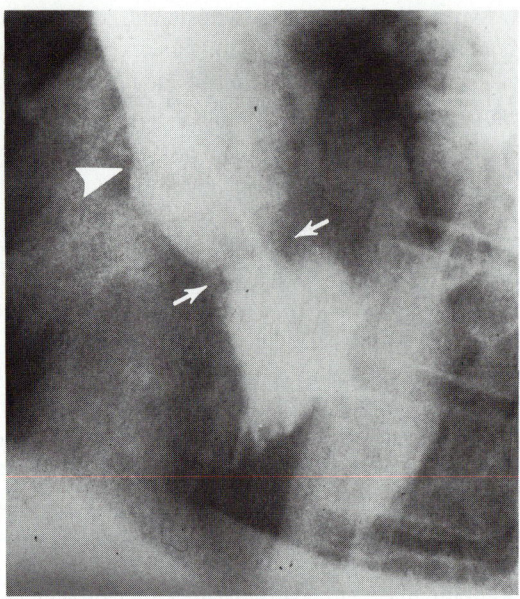

Figure 75–12. A left ventriculogram that demonstrates discrete subvalvar aortic stenosis. The large arrow points to an anatomically normal aortic valve. The small arrows point out a discrete ridge that is 1 cm below the aortic valve.

sis. The incidence of aortic insufficiency also increases with age.[115,120] The mechanism that creates or aggravates aortic insufficiency associated with subvalvar stenosis is most likely repetitive trauma caused by the high velocity jet that traverses an unresected or incompletely resected subvalvar lesion and strikes the aortic valve during systole.[121,130] Due to the rapid progression of the subvalvar aortic lesion, children less than 3 years of age should be followed clinically every 6 mo and annually after the age of 3 years. Sudden death has been reported but is not as prevalent as it is with valvar aortic stenosis.[24]

Treatment

Even in the presence of relatively mild subvalvar aortic obstruction, surgery appears to be the best option to prevent permanent damage to the aortic valve by unrelenting turbulent blood flow. Using cardiopulmonary bypass, resection of a subvalvar aortic fibrous ridge[131] involves determination of the plane that exists between the ridge and the endocardium of the left ventricular outflow tract. With blunt and sharp dissection, a spiral-shaped ledge of fibrous tissue can be removed. Complete relief of left ventricular outflow tract obstruction cannot be obtained by enucleation alone in most cases. The technique temporarily eliminates the fibrous tissue deposited on the interior of the left ventricular outflow tract. The muscular component that has been most recently hypothesized as part of discrete obstruction remains intact. Combined fibrous resection and myectomy realizes more effective long-term relief of subvalvar gradient than does resection alone or with myotomy.[25,132–134] The myectomy

is similar to a Morrow procedure[135] but is less extensive (Figs. 75–13 and 75–14). It includes one deep septal incision at the base of the right aortic cusp, another behind the commissure between the right and left aortic cusps, and a third connecting incision beginning at the superior end of the first two incisions. Excess tissue is resected toward the mitral valve anterior leaflet and the papillary muscles. In addition to gradient relief, the technique carries a low risk of operative mortality, complete heart block, or iatrogenic ventricular septal defect. Geometry of the left ventricular outflow tract is often significantly altered such that the risk of recurrent subvalvar obstruction is reduced as is the incidence of late aortic insufficiency.

Even when myectomy is performed, discrete subvalvar aortic stenosis recurs within 5 to 10 years postoperatively in approximately 16% of patients.[25,134] The anatomy is often identical to the original lesion and repeat resection is usually ineffective with a recurrence rate of almost 90% within 5 years after reoperation.[40] Recurrence might be attributed to an inadequate modification of left ventricular outflow geometry and a more extensive procedure is required. The aortoseptal approach suggested by Vouhe can relieve the obstruction without sacrificing the native aortic valve (Fig. 75–15).[136] The septum is incised as in aortoventriculoplasty and the aortic annulus is divided at the commissure between left and right aortic leaflets. The septotomy edges are trimmed of excess muscle to enlarge the subvalvar area and the septum is closed primarily.

An alternative surgical reoperative repair is the conal enlargement technique. Transatrially or through a right ventriculotomy sometimes using an existing ventricular septal defect, the conal septum is incised up to the aortic valve followed by patch closure of the ventricular septum to enlarge the left ventricular outflow tract (Fig. 75–16).[137] Because conduction tissue often shifts leftward after initial myectomy, there is a small but definite risk of complete heart block in addition to the ever-present risk of inadvertently creating a ventricular septal defect.

In tunnel-type subvalvar aortic stenosis and in recurrent muscular obstruction, the aortic valve is often severely deformed and dysfunctional, the mitral valve anterior leaflet is often involved, and surgery becomes a significantly greater challenge. Aortic valve replacement is usually required, which often mandates the use of aortoventriculoplasty, or simple or extended aortic root replacement.

Idiopathic hypertrophic subaortic stenosis (IHSS) is caused by muscular hypertrophy in the left ventricular outflow tract that can result in obstruction. It is usually associated with a global or concentric left ventricular hypertrophic cardiomyopathy and the obstructive component represents a small fraction of the disease process. The Morrow procedure[135] has proven effective in some children with idiopathic hypertrophic subaortic stenosis (Figs. 75–13 and 75–14). Extensive resection of hypertrophied muscle from beneath the aortic valve right coronary leaflet that extends to the border of the anterior mitral leaflet is required.

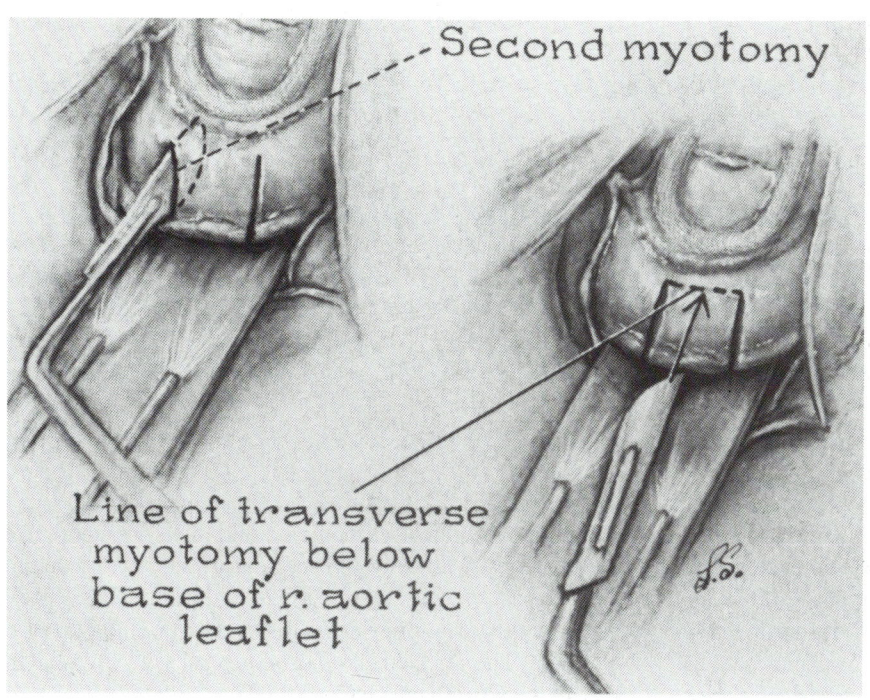

Figure 75–13. The first septal incision is made at the base of the right aortic cusp and the second incision is made approximately 1 cm to the left of and parallel to the first incision. A transverse incision at the base of the valve leaflet connects the two vertical incisions. *(From Morrow AG: Hypertrophic subaortic stenosis: Operative methods utilized to relieve left ventricular outflow obstruction. J Thorac Cardiovasc Surg 76:427; 1978.)*

Injury to conduction tissue that produces complete heart block and due to inability to judge the thickness of the resection, iatrogenic ventricular septal defects can occur. When the Morrow procedure is performed through the aortic valve, injury to the fragile aortic valve leaflets should be avoided during retraction and resection of the muscle block. Removal of the muscle block is facilitated with the use of skin hooks. Myocardial resection does not reverse the hypertrophy and is associated with increased operative mortality and high recurrence rate.

SUPRAVALVAR AORTIC STENOSIS

Supravalvar aortic stenosis occurs less frequently than valvar or subvalvar anomalies. Approximately 30 to 50% of

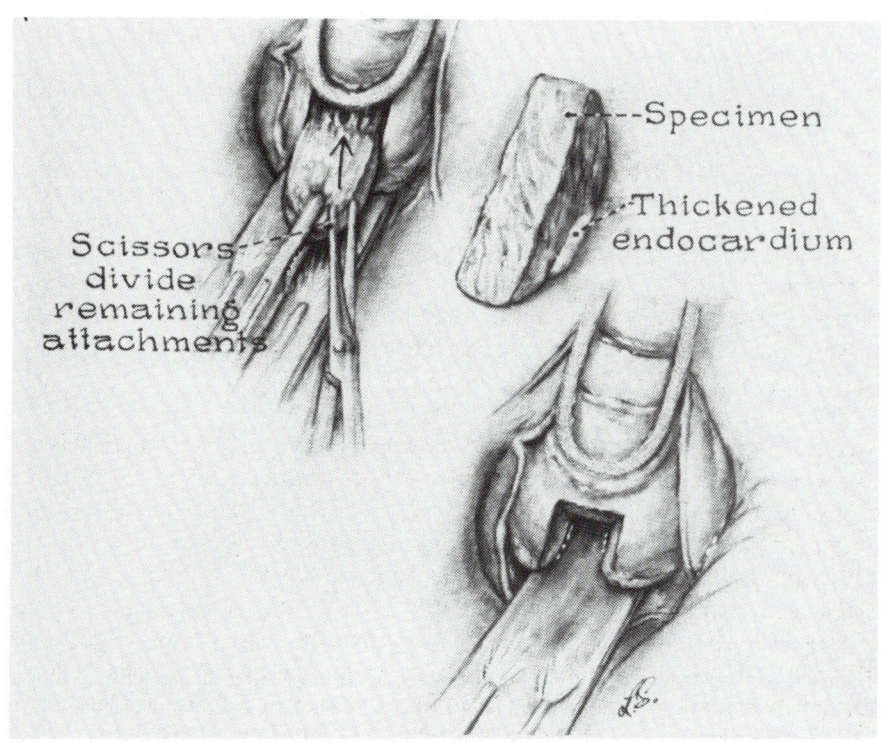

Figure 75–14. Excess muscle is resected toward the anterior leaflet of the mitral valve and the papillary muscles. *(From Morrow AG: Hypertrophic subaortic stenosis: Operative methods utilized to relieve left ventricular outflow obstruction. J Thorac Cardiovasc Surg 76:427; 1978.)*

Figure 75–15. (**A**) The subvalvar aortic outflow tract is opened and (**B**) diffuse, stenotic segments are resected from the edges of the septal incision. (**C**) The left ventricular outflow tract is sutured closed. RV, right ventricle; IVS, interventricular septum; LVOT, left ventricular outflow tract; MV, anterior mitral leaflet; lc, left coronary aortic annulus; rc, right coronary aortic annulus; nc, noncoronary aortic annulus; arrows, conduction pathways. *(From Vouhe PR, Poulain H, Bloch G, et al: Aortoseptal approach for optimal resection of diffuse subvalvular aortic stenosis. J Thorac Cardiovasc Surg 87:890; 1984.)*

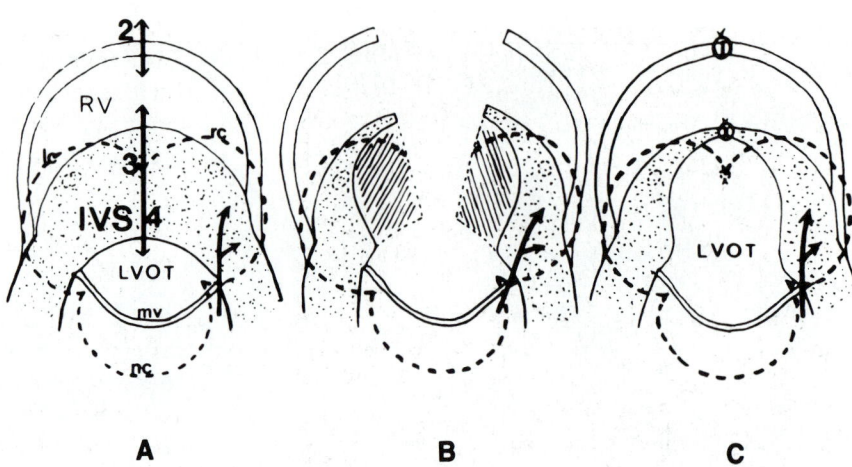

children with supravalvar stenosis have Williams syndrome.[26,27] Incidence in males and females is evenly distributed. Major branches of the aortic arch are often affected[29] and at least minor abnormalities of the aortic valve are common. Supravalvar aortic stenosis can also present as an isolated lesion secondary to previous ascending aortic or aortic valve surgery.

There are three morphologic variations of supravalvar aortic stenosis. Seventy-five percent of supravalvar anomalies consist of a discrete hourglass deformity (Fig. 75–17) with a constricting ridge at the distal extent of the sinuses of Valsalva. The affected tissue is abnormal with little potential for growth. Ostial stenoses of the sinuses of Valsalva is common and must be relieved at the time of surgery to pre-

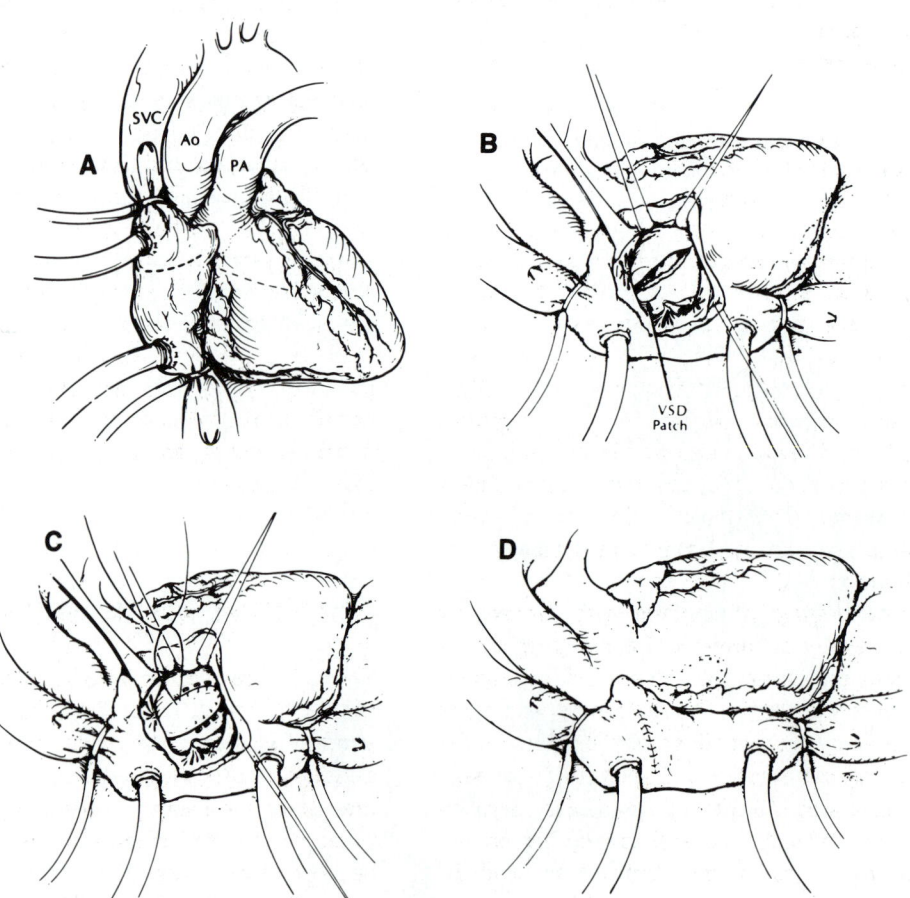

Figure 75–16. A, B. Through a right atriotomy, an incision is extended downward through the body of the left ventricle and the obstruction. **C, D.** A patch is used to enlarge the outflow tract. *(From DeLeon SY, Ilbawi MN, Roberson DA, et al: Conal enlargement for diffuse subaortic stenosis. J Thorac Cardiovasc Surg 102:814; 1991.)*

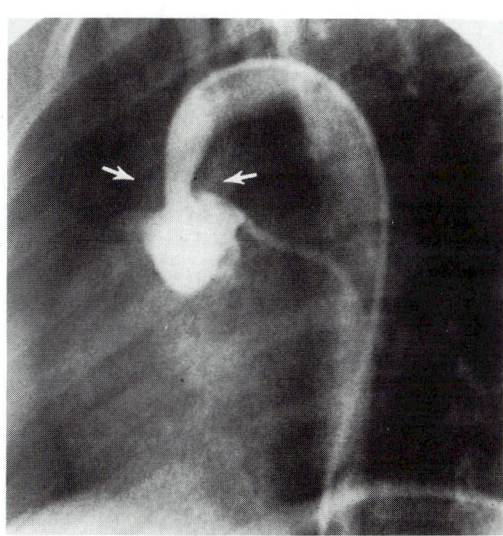

Figure 75–17. An aortogram that shows supravalvar aortic stenosis of the hourglass variety.

vent compromised coronary blood flow.[40] More diffuse narrowing along the ascending aorta is detected in 25% of children with supravalvar stenosis. The additional presence of a localized membrane immediately above the valve is reported rarely and might be a form of the discrete hourglass anomaly.

Clinical Evaluation

Children with supravalvar aortic stenosis present with clinical symptoms similar to those of valvar aortic stenosis. A systolic murmur is usually the first sign that cardiologic evaluation is necessary. Bilateral extremity blood pressures are discrepant by 5 to 10 mm Hg in up to 86% of patients.[138] The majority of children are symptomatic. Angina and exertional dyspnea are common. Associated cardiac anomalies are present in two-thirds of patients and include pulmonary stenosis, coarctation of the aorta, patent ductus arteriosus, and mitral regurgitation. Concurrent valvar and/or subvalvar stenosis are evident in approximately one-third of the children.[139]

The electrocardiogram of children with supravalvar aortic stenosis is usually abnormal and exhibits right ventricular hypertrophy in younger patients and left ventricular hypertrophy in older patients.[29,139] Chest roentgenogram is usually normal. M-mode echocardiography is helpful in determining degree of left ventricular hypertrophy but normally underestimates the severity of supravalvar narrowing.[140,141] Two-dimensional echocardiography has proven an accurate means of estimating supravalvar stenosis. Doppler echocardiography demonstrates turbulence and high velocity blood flow in the stenotic area, but the determination of an accurate gradient is not possible with less discrete lesions. Magnetic resonance imaging is also used to

illustrate anatomy of the ascending aorta and the area immediately distal to the valve.[142] Left and right heart catheterization is usually part of routine work-up in a child with supravalvar aortic stenosis due to the prevalence of associated anomalies.

Treatment

Surgical repair of supravalvar aortic stenosis usually consists of patching the ascending aorta. In general, the best results are obtained in children with more discrete lesions. It is usually necessary to incise not only across the narrowed segment of the aorta, but to continue the incision into the noncoronary sinus of Valsalva and to the aortic valve by separating the commissural tips of the valve. The standard approach is a lateral aortotomy, resection of the obstruction, and insertion of a dacron patch over the aortotomy.[27,139] Anatomy usually dictates whether the patch will extend into one, two, or all three sinuses of Valsalva. One oval patch that extends into the noncoronary sinus is usually sufficient for the repair of stenosis caused by prior surgery on the left ventricular outflow tract. For most cases of primary supravalvar stenosis,[40] it is necessary to use a horseshoe-shaped patch that extends, in addition, into the right coronary sinus.[143] The patch enlarges an inverted Y-shaped incision in the anterior ascending aorta and straddles the right coronary ostium (Fig. 75–18). If the orifice of the left coronary sinus of Valsalva is small, the surrounding fibrous tissue should be resected. If resection is unsuccessful, a three-prong patch technique proposed by Szarnicki is an option (Fig. 75–19).[144] Allograft ascending aortic replacement or simple or extended aortic root replacement can be the best alternative when the supravalvar aortic stenosis is severe with a deformed valve or is accompanied by obstruction at multiple levels. When the aorta is markedly hypoplastic, the patch technique does not eliminate the obstruction but merely displaces the gradient distally. In this situation, the entire hypoplastic aorta must be replaced with an appropriate prosthesis.

CONGENITAL AORTIC INSUFFICIENCY

The incidence of aortic insufficiency as an isolated lesion in children is much lower than that of any form of aortic stenosis. However, congenital aortic insufficiency can be associated with congenital aortic stenosis at all levels. Progressive or acute aortic insufficiency can develop as a complication of infective endocarditis, rheumatic fever, previous operative intervention, or natural history of a left ventricular outflow lesion. The aortic valve can also become regurgitant secondary to congenital connective tissue disorders that affect the aortic root such as Marfan's syndrome or Ehlers–Danlos syndrome.

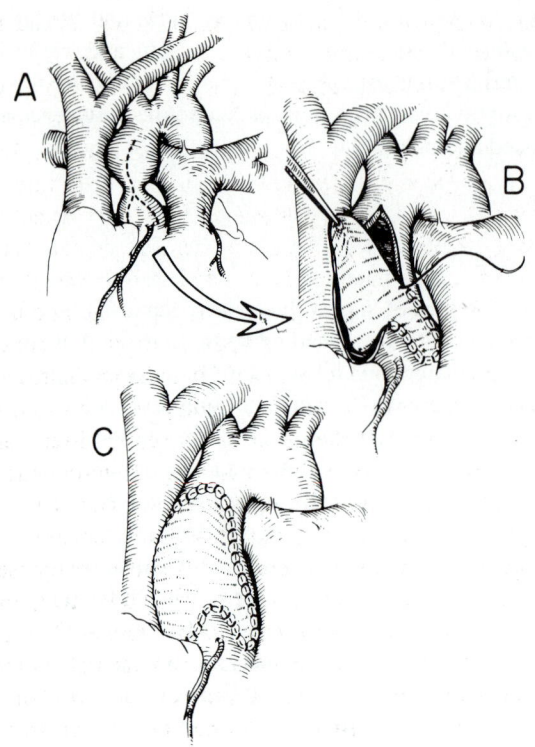

Figure 75–18. A surgical technique for the repair of supravalvar aortic stenosis. **A.** An inverted Y-shaped incision is used to open the aorta. **B.** A horseshoe-shaped patch straddles the right coronary ostium. **C.** The anterior ascending aorta has been enlarged with completion of the patch.

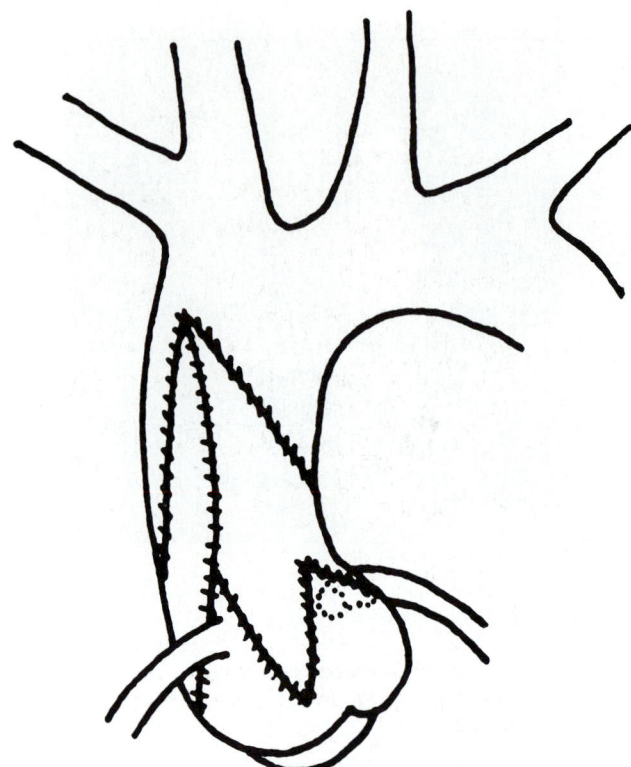

Figure 75–19. Repair of supravalvar aortic stenosis using a three-prong patch.

Clinical Evaluation

Children with aortic insufficiency are normally asymptomatic unless the regurgitation is severe. Chronic insufficiency, if untreated, results in increased left ventricular end diastolic volume, left ventricular dysfunction, and eventually the clinical features of dyspnea on exertion, pulmonary edema, and congestive heart failure. Diastolic blood pressure is inversely related to the severity of aortic insufficiency. Severity and duration of regurgitation are also reflected in electrocardiographic changes that indicate left ventricular enlargement. Chest roentgenogram exhibits cardiomegaly, sometimes with atrial dilation. Echocardiography can detect anatomical aortic valve leaflet abnormalities such as perforation or prolapse. Location and direction of the regurgitant blood flow jet can be viewed with Doppler imaging. Cardiac catheterization is useful in assessing left ventricular function, and ruling out other cardiac anomalies.

Aortic Insufficiency with Associated Cardiac Lesions

Congenital aortic insufficiency can be associated with ventricular septal defect, aortico-left ventricular tunnel, and sinus of Valsalva aneurysms. Aortic insufficiency associ-

ated with an underlying ventricular septal defect is caused by prolapse of the valve leaflets into the ventricular septal opening.[145] Aortic insufficiency occurs most commonly in association with an outlet or supracristal ventricular septal defect and only occasionally with a membranous defect. The right coronary cusp is usually involved, although the noncoronary cusp can be affected. Leaflet prolapse is caused by loss of underlying leaflet support in the septal defect area and by high velocity flow through the ventricular septal defect that pulls the leaflet downward. The chronically prolapsed state causes the leaflet's free edges to elongate such that normal coaptation is impossible (Fig. 75–20).

Aortico-left ventricular tunnel is the most common cause of severe aortic insufficiency that presents in children who are less than 2 years of age.[146] The anomaly was first described as a congenital defect by Levy et al, in 1963.[147] Aortico-left ventricular tunnel consists of an aberrant endothelialized communication from the anterior aspect of the ascending aorta to the left ventricle. The tunnel arises distal to or near the right coronary artery ostium, passes anterior to the aortic valve through the interventricular septum, and opens immediately beneath the aortic valve. The tunnel is often aneurysmal and bulges anteriorly. Unrestricted regurgitation from aorta to left ventricle results in sinus of Valsalva dilation, left ventricular dilation, and widening of the

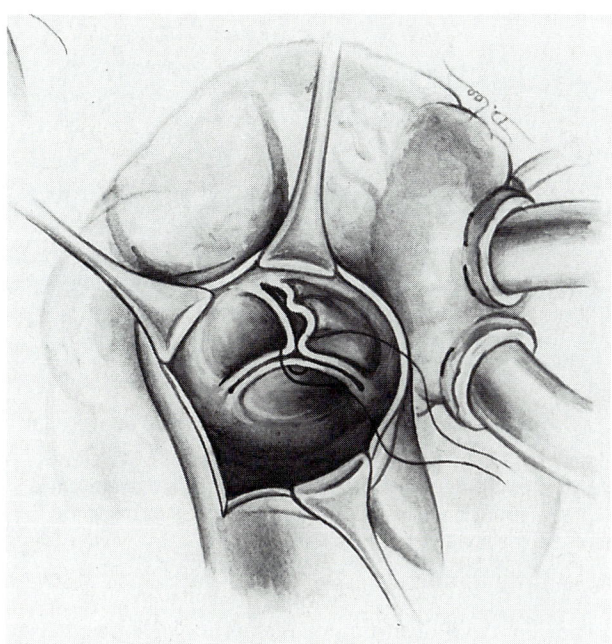

Figure 75–20. Redundant aortic valve leaflet associated with an underlying ventricular septal defect.

ascending aorta. The expanding diameter of the aortic annulus eventually precludes proper coaptation of the aortic valve leaflets.

The most prevalent symptom of aortico-left ventricular tunnel results from left ventricular failure as a result of the severe aortic regurgitation. The presence of a dicrotic notch in the aortic pressure pulse in the setting of severe regurgitation is diagnostically supportive. Chest roentgenography usually reveals dilation of the ascending aorta and the sinus of Valsalva. Aortico-left ventricular tunnel can often be documented using noninvasive techniques. If necessary, aortography confirms the diagnosis.

Aneurysms of the sinus of Valsalva and the fistulas that result from their expansion against and rupture into neighboring structures are rare malformations. They most commonly are associated with ventricular septal defect or coarctation of the aorta.[148] The etiology of such aneurysms has been debated extensively without conclusion. Sinus of Valsalva aneurysms are postulated to evolve from incomplete fusion of proximal and distal bulbus cordis structures,[149] or from a defect in elastic tissues between the base of the aorta and the annulus fibrosis.[150]

Aneurysms that arise from the right coronary sinus rupture into the right ventricle or right atrium, those arising in the noncoronary sinus impinge upon and rupture into the right atrium, and aneurysms of the left coronary sinus are extremely rare but expand and rupture into the left atrium. Instances of aneurysmal rupture generally occur during the second to fourth decades of life. Rupture of sinus of Valsalva aneurysms occurring in childhood was associated only with bacterial endocarditis[151] until the early 1990s

when Breviere et al[152] and Perry et al[153] documented separate cases of rupture in neonates.

Patients with unruptured sinus of Valsalva aneurysms are usually asymptomatic. The presence of a fistula can be diagnosed in asymptomatic children when cardiologic follow-up is incited by detection of a murmur. Detection of an unruptured, uninfected sinus aneurysm is rare. Attention is drawn to the patient only when a coexisting cardiac anomaly is present or when an unexpected cardiac event occurs as a consequence of aneurysmal encroachment on other intracardiac structures. The so-called classic picture of aneurysmal rupture does not occur in most patients. It consists of sudden severe chest pain associated with a loud continuous murmur and the onset of congestive heart failure due to massive left-to-right shunting. Two-dimensional transthoracic echocardiography with color Doppler allows noninvasive detection of sinus of Valsalva aneurysms.[154] Echocardiography easily excludes differential diagnoses of tetralogy of Fallot with absent pulmonary valve, mitral stenosis, and aortico-left ventricular tunnel.[153] Transesophageal echocardiography has proven accurate in the localization and hemodynamic assessment of sinus of Valsalva aneurysms, particularly unruptured aneurysms left undetected by transthoracic echocardiography.[155] Definitive diagnosis of sinus of Valsalva fistula is made by retrograde aortic root angiography that demonstrates the anatomy of the aneurysm and the fistula site (Fig. 75–21).

Treatment

Indications for operation are more obscure with aortic insufficiency than with aortic stenosis. With the exception of a prolapsing leaflet and underlying ventricular septal defect, the surgical repair of aortic valvar insufficiency often requires valve replacement. Patients are treated medically until there is clinical evidence of progressive cardiomegaly, symptoms, or decreased ejection fraction at rest or during exercise. Patients with aortic root involvement such as those with Marfan's syndrome usually require combined aortic valve and root replacement.

When aortic insufficiency is caused by a prolapsing cusp and associated ventricular septal defect, early surgical intervention is recommended in an attempt to halt progression of the lesion. Degree of redundancy of each half of the prolapsing cusp is estimated by suturing the three corpora Arantii together. Several pledgetted sutures are then used to plicate the redundant leaflet tissue against the aortic wall at the commissure (Fig. 75–22).[156] A figure-eight stitch or small hood of pericardium is sutured across the commissure to close any gap between the two leaflets adjacent to the aortic wall. The ventricular septal defect is then closed with a patch in the standard fashion.

Even in the absence of symptoms, aortico-left ventricular tunnel should be repaired soon after diagnosis to prevent progression of left ventricular dilation or damage to the aortic valve and root.[157] Surgical repair must not distort

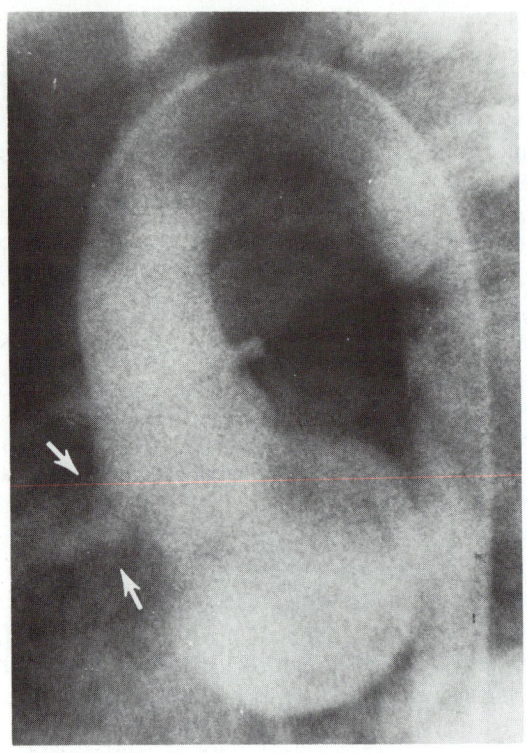

Figure 75–21. A transaortic left ventriculogram that demonstrates a ruptured sinus of Valsalva aneurysm. The resultant fistula originates in the right noncoronary sinus of Valsalva and empties into the right atrium. Arrows mark the fistula tract.

the aortic valve or leaflets, nor compromise the right coronary orifice or conduction system. Several technical variations are available for surgical repair of aortico-left ventricular tunnel.[158] When the aortic opening is a narrow slit, direct suture closure of the aortic end of the tunnel is appro-

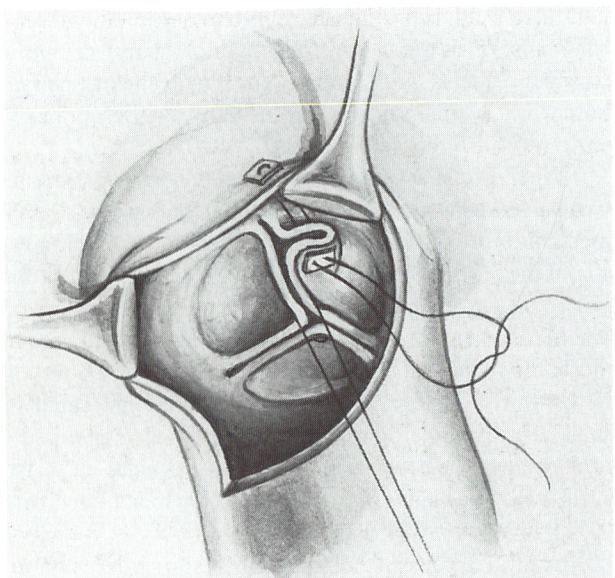

Figure 75–22. Surgical repair of a redundant aortic valve leaflet associated with an underlying ventricular septal defect.

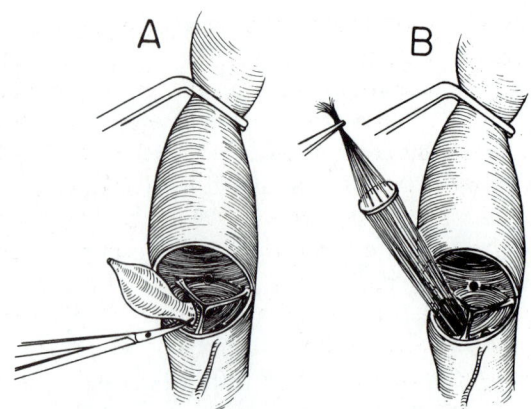

Figure 75–23. Surgical repair of a ruptured sinus of Valsalva aneurysm: **A.** Following an aortotomy, the ruptured aneurysm is withdrawn from the right atrium and is excised at its origin. **B.** The ostium of the aneurysm is patched.

priate. To avoid distortion of the aortic valve cusps, patch material should be used to close the aortic end of the tunnel when the opening is oval shaped. Obliteration of the tunnel via patch closure of the aortic and ventricular ends is advocated to avoid potential obstruction to the right ventricular outflow tract.[159] However, the technique can become complicated in extremely small patients and when a coronary artery arises from within the tunnel. When an intracardiac tunnel aneurysm is present, use of a reinforcing patch that includes the subvalvar septum and aortic annulus is recommended.

Progressive aortic insufficiency is common in patients who have undergone patch repair of aortico-left ventricular tunnel.[160] Regurgitation results from associated aortic valve abnormalities and changes in valve mechanics created by the presence of the tunnel anomaly. Approximately 50% of patients eventually will require aortic valve replacement.

Surgical repair of a ruptured or unruptured sinus of Valsalva aneurysm[161–163] is indicated electively or upon observance of the earliest symptoms of failure. In pediatric patients, it is important to maintain aortic valvar competence. The technique (Fig. 75–23) is relatively simple and can be performed via the aortic root, the chamber into which the aneurysm has ruptured, or both. It is sometimes possible to withdraw the aneurysm from the cardiac chamber into the aorta, excise its elongate structure, and repair the mouth of the fistula. Direct suture of the mouth of the fistula can distort the valve leaflets and produce aortic insufficiency making patch closure of the opening necessary in many cases.

SUMMARY

Unfortunately, many children currently are born with infinite variations on the theme of congenital aortic stenosis. Surgery to palliate valvar aortic stenosis whether with balloon or open valvuloplasty continues to be plagued by the potential for creation of aortic insufficiency. Significant advances have occurred in the area of aortic valve replacement, however, development of valve replacement options that approach the ideal of unlimited availability and durability and avoidance of anticoagulants still fall short. Future research likely will be devoted to the immunology of allograft degeneration, manipulation of coagulation, and development of improved prosthetic materials.

Isolated obstruction at other levels of the left ventricular outflow tract is invariably associated with progressive secondary effects. Since valve replacement is not required routinely, aggressive management of discrete sub- and supravalvar stenoses is recommended.

ACKNOWLEDGMENTS

The authors would like to thank Dr. Lilliam Valdez-Cruz and her associate Dr. Raul Cayre for their editorial assistance.

REFERENCES

1. Hoffman JI, Christianson R: Congenital heart disease in a cohort of 19,502 births with long-term follow-up. *Am J Cardiol* **42**:641, 1978
2. Serratto M, Hastreiter AR, Miller RA: Management of congenital aortic stenosis in children and young adults. *Prog Cardiovasc Dis* **8**:78, 1965
3. Campbell M: Calcific aortic stenosis and congenital bicuspid aortic valves. *Br Heart J* **30**:606, 1968
4. Marquis RM, Logan A: Congenital aortic stenosis and its surgical treatment. *Br Heart J* **17**:373, 1955
5. Swan H, Kortz A: Direct vision trans-aortic approach to the aortic valve during hypothermia: Experimental observations and report of a successful clinical case. *Ann Surg* **144**:205, 1956
6. Lewis FJ, Shumway NE, Niazi SA: Aortic valvulotomy under direct vision during hypothermia. *J Thorac Cardiovasc Surg* **32**:481, 1956
7. Lababidi Z, Wu JR, Walls JT: Percutaneous balloon aortic valvuloplasty: Results in 23 patients. *Am J Cardiol* **53**:194, 1984
8. Sholler GF, Keane JF, Perry SB, et al: Balloon dilation of congenital aortic valve stenosis. Results and influence of technical and morphological features on outcome. *Circulation* **78**:351, 1988
9. Shaddy RE, Boucek MM, Sturtevant JE, et al: Gradient reduction, aortic valve regurgitation and prolapse after balloon aortic valvuloplasty in 32 consecutive patients with congenital aortic stenosis. *J Am Coll Cardiol* **16**:451, 1990
10. O'Connor BK, Beekman RH, Rocchini AP, Rosenthal A: Intermediate-term effectiveness of balloon valvuloplasty for congenital aortic stenosis. A prospective follow-up study. *Circulation* **84**:732, 1991
11. Hausdorf G, Schneider M, Schirmer KR, et al: Anterograde balloon valvuloplasty of aortic stenosis in children. *Am J Cardiol* **71**:460, 1993
12. Geha AS, Laks H, Stansel HC Jr, et al: Late failure of porcine valve heterografts in children. *J Thorac Cardiovasc Surg* **78**:351, 1979
13. Sanders SP, Levy RJ, Freed MD, et al: Use of Hancock porcine xenografts in children and adolescents. *Am J Cardiol* **46**:429, 1980
14. Emery RW, Nicoloff DM: St. Jude Medical cardiac valve prosthesis: In vitro studies. *J Thorac Cardiovasc Surg* **78**:269, 1979
15. McKowen RL, Campbell DN, Woelfel GF, et al: Extended aortic root replacement with aortic allografts. *J Thorac Cardiovasc Surg* **93**:366, 1987
16. Van Mierop LHS, Alley RD, Kausel HW, Stranahan A: Pathogenesis of transposition complexes. I. Embryology of the ventricles and great arteries. *Am J Cardiol* **12**:216, 1963
17. Clark EB, Van Mierop LHS: Development of the cardiovascular system. In Adams FH, Emmanouilides GC, Riemenschneider TA (eds): *Heart Disease in Infants, Children, and Adolescents*, 4th ed, Baltimore, Williams & Wilkins, 1989, p 2
18. Weldon CS: Congenital obstruction to left ventricular outflow. In Aberdeen E, Benson CD, Randolph J, et al (eds): *Pediatric Surgery*, 3rd ed., Vol 1. Chicago, Year Book, 1978, p 633
19. Rudolph AM, Heymann MA, Spitznas U: Hemodynamic considerations in the development of narrowing of the aorta. *Am J Cardiol* **30**:514, 1972
20. Hutchins GM: Coarctation of the aorta explained as a branch point of the ductus arteriosus. *Am J Pathol* **63**:203, 1971
21. Roberts WC: The congenitally bicuspid aortic valve. A study of 85 autopsy cases. *Am J Cardiol* **26**:72, 1970
22. Osler W: The bicuspid condition of the aortic valves. *Trans Assoc Am Physicians* **2**:185, 1886
23. Roberts WC: Valvular, subvalvular and supravalvular aortic stenosis: Morphologic features. *Cardiovasc Clin* **5**:97, 1973
24. Newfeld EA, Muster AJ, Paul MH, et al: Discrete subvalvular aortic stenosis in childhood. Study of 51 patients. *Am J Cardiol* **38**:53, 1976
25. van Son JA, Hoffman D, Puga FJ, Hagler DJ: Surgery for membranous subaortic stenosis. Long-term follow-up. (letter) *Eur J Cardiothorac Surg* **8**:110, 1994
26. O'Connor WN, Davis JB Jr, Geissler R, et al: Supravalvular aortic stenosis. Clinical and pathological observations in six patients. *Arch Pathol Lab Med* **109**:179, 1985
27. Flaker G, Teske D, Kilman J, et al: Supravalvular aortic stenosis. A 20-year clinical perspective and experience with patch aortoplasty. *Am J Cardiol* **51**:256,1983
28. Peterson TA, Todd DB, Edwards JE: Supravalvular aortic stenosis. *J Thorac Cardiovasc Surg* **50**:734, 1965
29. Blieden LC, Lucas RV Jr, Carter JB, et al: A developmental complex including supravalvular stenosis of the aorta and pulmonary trunk. *Circulation* **49**:585, 1974
30. Campbell M: The natural history of congenital aortic stenosis. *Br Heart J* **30**:514, 1968
31. Frank S, Johnson A, Ross J Jr: Natural history of valvular aortic stenosis. *Br Heart J* **35**:41, 1973
32. Mody MR, Mody GT: Serial hemodynamic observations in congenital valvular and subvalvular aortic stenosis. *Am Heart J* **89**:137, 1975
33. Braunwald E, Goldblatt A, Aygen MM, et al: Congenital aortic stenosis. I. Clinical and hemodynamic findings in 100 patients. II. Surgical treatment and the results of operation. *Circulation* **27**:426, 1963
34. Moller JH, Nakib A, Eliot RS, Edwards JE: Symptomatic congenital aortic stenosis in the first year of life. *J Pediatr* **69**:728, 1966
35. Kugler JD, Campbell E, Vargo TA, et al: Results of aortic valvotomy in infants with isolated aortic valvular stenosis. *J Thorac Cardiovasc Surg* **78**:553, 1979
36. Olley PM, Bloom KR, Rowe RD: Aortic stenosis: Valvular, subaortic, and supravalvular. In Rowe RD (ed): *Heart Disease in Infancy and Childhood,* 3rd ed. New York, Macmillan, 1978, p 698
37. Keane JF, Bernhard WF, Nadas AS: Aortic stenosis surgery in infancy. *Circulation* **52**:1138, 1975
38. Artman M, Boucek RJ Jr, Hammon J, Graham TP Jr: Emergency palliation of critical valvular aortic stenosis. A new application of prostaglandin E1. *Am J Dis Child* **137**:339, 1983
39. Weldon CS: Obstructions to left ventricular outflow. *World J Surg* **9**:522, 1985
40. Clarke DR: Left ventricular outflow tract obstruction in children. In

Karp RB (ed): *Advances in Cardiac Surgery.* St. Louis, Mosby-Year Book, 1990, p 159

41. Hastreiter AR, et al: Congenital aortic stenosis syndrome in infancy. *Circulation* 28:1084, 1963

42. Latson LA: Aortic stenosis: Valvular, supravalvular, and fibromuscular subvalvular. In Garson A Jr, Bricker JT, McNamara DG (eds): *The Science and Practice of Pediatric Cardiology.* Philadelphia, Lea & Febiger, 1990, p 1334

43. Huhta JC, Glasow P, Murphy DJ Jr, et al: Surgery without catheterization for congenital heart defects: management of 100 patients. *J Am Coll Cardiol* 9:823, 1987

44. Hagler DJ, Tajik AJ, Seward JB, Ritter DG: Noninvasive assessment of pulmonary valve stenosis, aortic valve stenosis and coarctation of the aorta in critically ill neonates. *Am J Cardiol* 57:369, 1986

45. Krabill KA, Ring WS, Foker JE, et al: Echocardiographic versus cardiac catheterization diagnosis of infants with congenital heart disease requiring cardiac surgery. *Am J Cardiol* 60:351, 1987

46. Norwood WI, Kirklin JK, Sanders SP: Hypoplastic left heart syndrome: experience with palliative surgery. *Am J Cardiol* 45:87, 1980

47. Norwood WI, Lang P, Castaneda AR, Campbell DN: Experience with operations for hypoplastic left heart syndrome. *J Thorac Cardiovasc Surg* 82:511, 1981

48. Bailey LL, Nehlsen-Cannarella SL, Doroshow RW, et al: Cardiac allotransplantation in newborns as therapy for hypoplastic left heart syndrome. *N Engl J Med* 315:949, 1986

49. Bailey LL, Assaad AN, Trimm RF, et al: Orthotropic transplantation during early infancy as therapy for incurable congenital heart disease. *Ann Surg* 208:279, 1988

50. Hammon JW Jr, Lupinetti FM, Maples MD, et al: Predictors of operative mortality in critical valvular aortic stenosis presenting in infancy. *Ann Thorac Surg* 45:537, 1988

51. Edmunds LH Jr, Wagner HR, Heymann MA: Aortic valvulotomy in neonates. *Circulation* 61:421, 1980

52. Latson LA, Cheatham JP, Gutgesell HP: Relation of the echocardiographic estimate of left ventricular size to mortality in infants with severe left ventricular outflow obstruction. *Am J Cardiol* 48:887, 1981

53. Leung MP, McKay R, Smith A, et al: Critical aortic stenosis in early infancy. Anatomic and echocardiographic substrates of successful open valvotomy. *J Thorac Cardiovasc Surg* 101:526, 1991

54. Rashkind WJ, Miller WW: Creation of an atrial septal defect without thoracotomy: A palliative approach to complete transposition of the great arteries. *JAMA* 196:991, 1966

55. Lababidi Z, Weinhaus L: Successful balloon valvuloplasty for neonatal critical aortic stenosis. *Am Heart J* 112:913, 1986

56. Rocchini AP, Beekman RH, Ben Shachar G, et al: Balloon aortic valvuloplasty: Results of the Valvuloplasty and Angioplasty of Congenital Anomalies registry. *Am J Cardiol* 65:784, 1990

57. Kasten-Sportes CH, Piechaud JF, Sidi D, Kachaner J: Percutaneous balloon valvuloplasty in neonates with critical aortic stenosis. *J Am Coll Cardiol* 13:1101, 1989

58. Coran AG, Bernhard WF: The surgical management of valvular aortic stenosis during infancy. *J Thorac Cardiovasc Surg* 58:401, 1969

59. Idriss FS, Dieter R, Riker WL, Paul MH: Left ventricular outflow obstruction in infancy and childhood. *Arch Surg* 99:257, 1969

60. Somerville J: Variant of congenital aortic valve disease (letter). *Am J Cardiol* 44:578, 1979

61. Edmunds LH Jr, Wagner HR, Heymann MA: Aortic valvulotomy in neonates. *Circulation* 61:421, 1980

62. Sandor GG, Olley PM, Trusler GA, et al: Long-term follow-up of patients after valvotomy for congenital valvular aortic stenosis in children: A clinical and actuarial follow-up. *J Thorac Cardiovasc Surg* 80:171, 1980

63. Edmunds LH Jr, Wagner HR, Heymann MA: Aortic valvulotomy in neonates. *Circulation* 61:421, 1980

64. Keane JF, Bernhard WF, Nadas AS: Aortic stenosis surgery in infancy. *Circulation* 52:1138, 1975

65. Sink JD, Smallhorn JF, Macartney FJ, et al: Management of critical aortic stenosis in infancy. *J Thorac Cardiovasc Surg* 87:82, 1984

66. Lakier JB, Lewis AB, Heymann MA, et al: Isolated aortic stenosis in the neonate. Natural history and hemodynamic considerations. *Circulation* 50:801, 1974

67. Gundry SR, Behrendt DM: Prognostic factors in valvotomy for critical aortic stenosis in infancy. *J Thorac Cardiovasc Surg* 92:747, 1986

68. Moller JH, Nakib A, Edwards JE: Infarction of papillary muscles and mitral insufficiency associated with congenital aortic stenosis. *Circulation* 34:87, 1966

69. Pelech AN, Dyck JF, Trusler GA, et al: Critical aortic stenosis. Survival and management. *J Thorac Cardiovasc Surg* 94:510, 1987

70. Mocellin R, Sauer U, Simon B, et al: Reduced left ventricular size and endocardial fibroelastosis as correlates of mortality in newborns and young infants with severe aortic valve stenosis. *Pediatr Cardiol* 4:265, 1983

71. Ettedgui JA, Tallman-Eddy T, Neches WH, et al: Long-term results of survivors of surgical valvotomy for severe aortic stenosis in early infancy. *J Thorac Cardiovasc Surg* 104:1714, 1992

72. Bernhard WF, Poirier V, LaFarge CG: Relief of congenital obstruction to left ventricular outflow with a ventricular-aortic prosthesis. *J Thorac Cardiovasc Surg* 69:223, 1975

73. DiDonato RM, Danielson GK, McGoon DC, et al: Left ventricle-aortic conduits in pediatric patients. *J Thorac Cardiovasc Surg* 88:82, 1984

74. Konno S, Imai Y, Iida Y, et al: A new method for prosthetic valve replacement in congenital aortic stenosis associated with hypoplasia of the aortic valve ring. *J Thorac Cardiovasc Surg* 70:909, 1975

75. Rastan H, Koncz J: Aortoventriculoplasty: A new technique for the treatment of left ventricular outflow tract obstruction. *J Thorac Cardiovasc Surg* 71:920, 1976

76. Clarke DR: Extended aortic root replacement in 12 patients with complex left ventricular outflow tract obstruction. In Yankah AC, Hetzer R, Miller DC, et al (eds): *Cardiac Valve Allografts 1962–1987: Current Concepts on the Use of Aortic and Pulmonary Allografts for Heart Valve Substitutes.* New York, Springer-Verlag, 1988, p 157

77. Clarke DR: Invited letter concerning: Accelerated degeneration of aortic allografts in infants and young children. *J Thorac Cardiovasc Surg* 107:1162, 1994

78. Cohen LS, Friedman WF, Braunwald E: Natural history of mild congenital aortic stenosis elucidated by serial hemodynamic studies. *Am J Cardiol* 30:1, 1972

79. Hossack KF, Neutze JM, Lowe JB, et al: Congenital valvular aortic stenosis. Natural history and assessment for operation. *Br Heart J* 43:561, 1980

80. Friedman WF: Congenital aortic valve disease: Natural history, indications and results of surgery. In Morse D (ed): *New Aspects in Congenital Valvular and Coronary Artery Disease.* New York, Futura Publishing, 1975, p 43

81. Gamboa R, Hugenholtz PG, Nadas AS: Comparison of electrocardiograms and vectorcardiograms in congenital aortic stenosis. *Br Heart J* 27:344, 1965

82. Johnson AM: Aortic stenosis, sudden death, and the left ventricular baroreceptors. *Br Heart J* 33:1, 1971

83. Lambert EC, Menon VA, Wagner HR, Vlad P: Sudden unexpected death from cardiovascular disease in children. A cooperative international study. *Am J Cardiol* 34:89, 1974

84. Friedman WF: Aortic stenosis. In Adams FH, Ammanouilides GC, Riemenschneider TA (eds): *Heart Disease in Infants, Children, and Adolescents,* 4th ed. Baltimore, Williams & Wilkins, 1989, p 224

85. el-Said G, Galioto FM Jr, Mullins CE, McNamara DG: Natural hemodynamic history of congenital aortic stenosis in childhood. *Am J Cardiol* 30:6, 1972

86. Gersony WM, Krongrad E: Evaluation and management of patients

after surgical repair of congenital heart diseases. *Cardiovasc Dis* **18**:39, 1975

87. Ellison RC, Wagner HR, Weidman WH, Miettinen OS: Congenital valvular aortic stenosis: Clinical detection of small pressure gradient. Prepared for the Joint Study on the Natural History of Congenital Heart Defects. *Am J Cardiol* **37**:757, 1976

88. Wagner HR, Weidman WH, Ellison RC, Miettinen OS: Indirect assessment of severity in aortic stenosis. *Circulation* **56**(Suppl 1):I–20, 1977

89. Orsmond GS, Bessinger FB Jr, Moller JH: Rest and exercise hemodynamics in children before and after aortic valvotomy. *Am Heart J* **99**:76, 1980

90. Fowles RE, Martin RP, Abrams JM, et al: Two-dimensional echocardiographic featues of bicuspid aortic valve. *Chest* **75**:434, 1979

91. Schapira JN, Davidson RM, Charuzi Y: Valvular heart disease. In Schapira JN (ed). *Two-Dimensional Echocardiography.* Baltimore, Williams & Wilkins, 1982, p 267

92. Huhta JC, Gutgesell HP, Latson LA, Huffines FD: Two-dimensional echocardiographic assessment of the aorta in infants and children with congenital heart disease. *Circulation* **70**:417, 1984

93. Schapira JN, Davidson RM, Charuzi Y: Valvular heart disease. In Schapira JN (ed). *Two-Dimensional Echocardiography.* Baltimore, Williams & Wilkins, 1982, p 249

94. Goldberg SJ, Kececioglu-Draelos Z, Sahn DJ, et al: Range gaited echo-Doppler velocity and turbulence mapping in patients with valvular aortic stenosis. *Am Heart J* **103**:858, 1982

95. Currie PJ, Hagler DJ, Seward JB, et al: Instantaneous pressure gradient: a simultaneous Doppler and dual catheter correlative study. *J Am Coll Cardiol* **7**:800, 1986

96. Bengur AR, Snider AR, Serwer GA, et al: Usefulness of the Doppler mean gradient in evaluation of children with aortic valve stenosis and comparison to gradient at catheterization. *Am J Cardiol* **64**:756, 1989

97. Glanz S, Hellenbrand WE, Berman MA, Talner NS: Echocardiographic assessment of the severity of aortic stenosis in children and adolescents. *Am J Cardiol* **38**:620, 1976

98. Gutgesell HP, et al: Recreational and occupational recommendations for young patients with heart disease. A statement for physicians by the Committee on Congenital Cardiac Defects of the Council on Cardiovascular Disease in the Young. *Am Heart Assoc* **74**:1195A, 1986

99. Freed MD: Recreational and sports recommendations for the child with heart disease. *Pediatr Clin N Am* **31**:1307, 1984

100. Jones M, Barnhart GR, Morrow AG: Late results after operations for left ventricular outflow tract obstruction. *Am J Cardiol* **50**:569, 1982

101. Friedman WF: Indications for and results of surgery in congenital aortic stenosis. *Adv Cardiol* **17**:2, 1976

102. Hsieh KS, Keane JF, Nadas AS, et al: Long-term follow-up of valvotomy before 1968 for congenital aortic stenosis. *Am J Cardiol* **58**:338, 1986

103. Fulton DR, Hougen TJ, Keane JF, et al: Repeat aortic valvotomy in children. *Am Heart J* **106**:60, 1983

104. Manouguian S, Seybold-Epting W: Patch enlargement of the aortic valve ring by extending the aortic incision into the anterior mitral leaflet. *J Thorac Cardiovasc Surg* **78**:402, 1979

105. Gallo I, Nistal F, Blasquez R, et al: Incidence of primary tissue valve failure in porcine bioprosthetic heart valves. *Ann Thorac Surg* **45**:66, 1988

106. Kutsche LM, Oyer P, Shumway N, Baum D: An important complication of Hancock mitral valve replacement in children. *Circulation* **60**(suppl 1): I98, 1979

107. Clarke DR, Campbell DN, Hayward AR, Bishop DA: Degeneration of aortic valve allografts in young recipients. *J Thorac Cardiovasc Surg* **105**:934, 1993

108. Clarke DR: Extended aortic root replacement with cryopreserved allografts: Do they hold up? *Ann Thorac Surg* **52**:669, 1991

109. Gerosa G, McKay R, Ross DN: Replacement of the aortic valve or root with a pulmonary autograft in children. *Ann Thorac Surg* **51**:424, 1991

110. Matsuki O, Okita Y, Almeida RS, et al: Two decades' experience with aortic valve replacement with pulmonary autograft. *J Thorac Cardiovasc Surg* **95**:705, 1988

111. Stelzer P, Jones DJ, Elkins RC: Aortic root replacement with pulmonary autograft. *Circulation* **80**(suppl 3): 209, 1989

112. Doty DB, Polansky DB, Jenson CB: Supravalvular aortic stenosis. Repair by extended aortoplasty. *J Thorac Cardiovasc Surg* **74**:362, 1977

113. Champsaur G, Trusler GA, Mustard WT: Congenital discrete subvalvar aortic stenosis. Surgical experience and long-term follow-up in 20 paediatric patients. *Br Heart J* **35**:443, 1973

114. Reis RL, Peterson LM, Mason DT, et al: Congenital fixed subvalvular aortic stenosis. An anatomical classification and correlations with operative results. *Circulation* **43**(suppl 1):I11, 1971

115. Freedom RM, Pelech A, Brand A, et al: The progressive nature of subaortic stenosis in congenital heart disease. *Int J Cardiol* **8**:137, 1985

116. Freedom RM, Fowler RS, Duncan WJ: Rapid evolution from "normal" left ventricular outflow tract to fatal subaortic stenosis in infancy. *Br Heart J* **45**:605, 1981

117. Freedom RM, Dische MR, Rowe RD: Pathologic anatomy of subaortic stenosis and atresia in the first year of life. *Am J Cardiol* **39**:1035, 1977

118. Vogel M, Freedom RM, Brand A, et al: Ventricular septal defect and subaortic stenosis: An analysis of 41 patients. *Am J Cardiol* **52**:1258, 1983

119. Kelly DT, Wulfsberg E, Rowe RD: Discrete subaortic stenosis. *Circulation* **46**:309, 1972

120. Shem-Tov A, Schneeweiss A, Motro M, Neufeld HN: Clinical presentation and natural history of mild discrete subaortic stenosis. Follow-up of 1–17 years. *Circulation* **66**:509, 1982

121. Sabbah HN, Stein PD: Mechanism of early systolic closure of the aortic valve in discrete membranous subaortic stenosis. *Circulation* **65**:399, 1982

122. Weyman AE, Feigenbaum H, Hurwitz RA, et al: Cross-sectional echocardiography in evaluating patients with discrete subaortic stenosis. *Am J Cardiol* **37**:358, 1976

123. Vogt J, Rupprath G, de Vivie R, Beuren AJ: Discrete subaortic stenosis: The value of cross-sectional sector echocardiography in evaluating different types of obstruction. *Pediatr Cardiol* **4**:253, 1983

124. Wilcox WD, Seward JB, Hagler DJ, et al: Discrete subaortic stenosis. Two-dimensional echocardiographic features with angiographic and surgical correlation. *Mayo Clin Proc* **55**:425, 1980

125. Vered Z, Schneeweiss A, Meltzer RS, Neufeld HN: Echocardiographic assessment of left ventricular outflow tract obstruction. *Am Heart J* **106**:177, 1983

126. Lima CO, Sahn DJ, Valdes-Cruz LM, et al: Prediction of the severity of left ventricular outflow tract obstruction by quantitative two-dimensional echocardiographic Doppler studies. *Circulation* **68**:348, 1983

127. Yoganathan AP, Valdes-Cruz LM, Schmidt-Dohna J, et al: Continuous-wave Doppler velocities and gradients across fixed tunnel obstructions: Studies in vitro and in vivo. *Circulation* **76**:657, 1987

128. Kinney EL, Machado H, Cortada X, Galbut DL: Diagnosis of discrete subaortic stenosis by pulsed and continuous wave echocardiography. *Am Heart J* **110**:1069, 1985

129. Allen HD, Moller JH, Formanek A, Nicoloff D: Atresia of the proximal left coronary artery associated with supravalvar aortic stenosis. *J Thorac Cardiovasc Surg* **67**:266, 1974

130. Gewillig M, Daenen W, DuMoulin M, van der Hauwaert L: Rheologic genesis of discrete subvalvular aortic stenosis: A Doppler echocardiographic study. *J Am Coll Cardiol* **19**:818, 1992

131. McKay R, Ross DM: Technique for the relief of discrete subaortic stenosis. *J Thorac Cardiovasc Surg* **84**:917, 1982

132. Cain T, Campbell D, Paton B, Clarke D: Operation for discrete subvalvular aortic stenosis. *J Thorac Cardiovasc Surg* **87**:366, 1984

133. Lavee J, Porat L, Smolinsky A, et al: Myectomy versus myotomy as an adjunct to membranectomy in the surgical repair of discrete and tunnel subaortic stenosis. *J Thorac Cardiovasc Surg* **92**:944, 1986

134. Lupinetti FM, Pridjian AK, Callow LB, et al: Optimum treatment of discrete subaortic stenosis. *Ann Thorac Surg* **54**:467, 1992

135. Morrow AG: Hypertrophic subaortic stenosis. Operative methods utilized to relieve left ventricular outflow obstruction. *J Thorac Cardiovasc Surg* **76**:423, 1978

136. Vouhe PR, Poulain H, Bloch G, et al: Aortoseptal approach for optimal resection of diffuse subvalvular aortic stenosis. *J Thorac Cardiovasc Surg* **87**:887, 1984

137. DeLeon SY, Ilbawi MN, Roberson DA, et al: Conal enlargement for diffuse subaortic stenosis. *J Thorac Cardiovasc Surg* **102**:814, 1991

138. French JW, Guntheroth WG: An explanation of asymmetric upper extremity blood pressures in supravalvular aortic stenosis: The Coanda effect. *Circulation* **42**:31, 1970

139. Keane JF, Fellows KE, LaFarge CG, et al: The surgical management of discrete and diffuse supravalvular aortic stenosis. *Circulation* **54**:112, 1976

140. Bolen JL, Popp RL, French JW: Echocardiographic features of supravalvular aortic stenosis. *Circulation* **52**:817, 1975

141. Nasrallah AT, Nihill M: Supravalvular aortic stenosis. Echocardiographic features. *Br Heart J* **37**:662, 1975

142. Boxer RA, Fishman MC, LaCorte MA, et al: Diagnosis and postoperative evaluation of supravalvular aortic stenosis by magnetic resonance imaging. *Am J Cardiol* **58**:367, 1986

143. Doty DB, Polansky DB, Jenson CB: Supravalvular aortic stenoses. Repair by extended aortoplasty. *J Thorac Cardiovasc Surg* **74**:362, 1977

144. Szarnicki RJ: personal communication

145. Keane JF, Plauth WH Jr, Nadas AS: Ventricular septal defect with aortic regurgitation. *Circulation* **56**(suppl 1):I172, 1977

146. Somerville J: Aortic stenosis and incompetence. In Anderson RH, Macartney FJ, Shinebourne EA, Tynan M (eds): *Pediatric Cardiology*. New York, Churchill Livingstone, 1987, p 977

147. Levy MJ, Lillehei CW, Anderson MD, et al: Aortico-left ventricular tunnel. *Circulation* **27**:841, 1963

148. Sakakibara S, Konno S: Congenital aneurysm of the sinus of Valsalva. Anatomy and classification. *Am Heart J* **63**:405, 1962

149. Mall FP: Aneurysms of the membranous septum projecting into the right atrium. *Anat Rec* **6**:219, 1912

150. Edwards JE, Burchell HB: The pathological anatomy of deficiencies between the aortic root and the heart. *Thorax* **12**:125, 1957

151. Gleason MM, Hardy C, Chin AJ, Pigott JD: Ruptured sinus of Valsalva aneurysm in childhood. *Am Heart J* **114**:1235, 1987

152. Breviere GM, Vaksmann G, Francart C: Rupture of a sinus of Valsalva aneurysm in a neonate. *Eur J Pediatr* **149**:603, 1990

153. Perry LW, Martin GR, Galioto FM Jr, Midgley FM: Rupture of congenital sinus of Valsalva aneurysm in a newborn. *Am J Cardiol* **68**:1255, 1991

154. Rubin DC, Carliner NH, Salter DR, et al: Unruptured sinus of Valsalva aneurysm diagnosed by transesophageal echocardiography. *Am Heart J* **124**:225, 1992

155. McKenney PA, Shemin RJ, Wiegers SE: Role of transesophageal echocardiography in sinus of Valsalva aneurysm. *Am Heart J* **123**:228, 1992

156. Frater RW: The prolapsing aortic cusp. Experimental and clinical observations. *Ann Thorac Surg* **3**:63, 1967

157. Sreeram N, Franks R, Arnold R, Walsh K: Aortico-left ventricular tunnel: Long-term outcome after surgical repair. *J Am Coll Cardiol* **17**:950, 1991

158. Hovaguimian H, Cobanoglu A, Starr A: Aortico-left ventricular tunnel: a clinical review and new surgical classification. *Ann Thorac Surg* **45**:106, 1988

159. Knott-Craig CJ, van der Merwe PL, Kalis NN, Hunter J: Repair of aortico-left ventricular tunnel associated with subpulmonary obstruction. *Ann Thorac Surg* **54**:557, 1992

160. Meldrum-Hanna W, Schroff R, Ross DN: Aortico-left ventricular tunnel: late follow-up. *Ann Thorac Surg* **42**:304, 1986

161. Howard RJ, Moller J, Castaneda AR, et al: Surgical correction of sinus of Valsalva aneurysm. *J Thorac Cardiovasc Surg* **66**:420, 1973

162. Sanchez HE, Barnard CN, Barnard MS: Fistula of the sinus of Valsalva. *J Thorac Cardiovasc Surg* **73**:877, 1977

163. Meyer J, Wukasch DC, Hallman GL, Cooley DA: Aneurysm and fistula of the sinus of Valsalva. Clinical considerations and surgical treatment in 45 patients. *Ann Thorac Surg* **19**:170, 1975

CHAPTER

76

Coarctation of the Aorta and Interrupted Aortic Arch

Carl L. Backer and Constantine Mavroudis

Coarctation of the aorta (from the Latin *coarctere,* to contract) is a congenital narrowing of the descending thoracic aorta usually occurring just distal to the left subclavian artery adjacent to the site of insertion of the ductus arteriosus (Fig. 76–1). Interrupted aortic arch is a lesion morphologically and physiologically more severe and is characterized by loss of luminal continuity between the ascending and descending aorta, with blood flow into the descending aorta directly from the ductus arteriosus (Fig. 76–2). The occurrence rate of coarctation of the aorta is 0.2–0.6 per 1000 live births and this represents 5 to 8% of all cases of congenital heart disease.[1,2] By itself, coarctation is the eighth most common congenital heart defect. It is often associated with other congenital heart defects including patent ductus arteriosus, ventricular septal defect, bicuspid aortic valve, and mitral valve abnormalities.[3] Interrupted aortic arch occurs much less frequently, accounting for only 0.5 to 1.3% of patients with congenital heart disease.[4,5] Interrupted aortic arch is nearly always associated with a large ventricular septal defect and is commonly associated with bicuspid aortic valve, left ventricular outflow obstruction, and DiGeorge syndrome. The clinical presentation of coarctation varies from cardiovascular collapse in infancy to asymptomatic hypertension in an adult. Interrupted aortic arch nearly always presents in the first few days of life when the ductus arteriosus begins to close.

The history of the surgical management of both of these lesions is fascinating and parallels technical advances in congenital heart surgery (Table 76–1). Robert Gross[6] initiated experimental procedures directed at repair of coarcta-

tion in 1938. He documented in animals the possible complications of hemorrhage and paraplegia. The first successful resection and repair of coarctation of the aorta in a human was performed in Stockholm, Sweden by Clarence Crafoord[7] on October 19, 1944 in a 12-year-old boy. This was the third true historical landmark in congenital heart surgery, following ligation of a patent ductus arteriosus by Gross and Hubbard[8] in 1938 and the Blalock-Taussig shunt[9] from 1944. Crafoord's patient had no complications, relief of hypertension, and normalization of lower extremity blood pressure. The surgical management of coarctation of the aorta since then has truly gone full circle as the procedure of choice has evolved from resection and end-to-end anastomosis[7] to prosthetic patch aortoplasty[10] to subclavian flap aortoplasty[11] back to resection with *extended* end-to-end anastomosis.[12] Interrupted aortic arch mirrors other complex congenital heart lesions in that the original approach involved staged correction with initial palliation followed by intracardiac repair when the child was older.[13] The first procedure was ductus ligation and arch repair with a prosthetic graft and placement of a pulmonary artery band and the second stage was intracardiac repair with removal of the pulmonary artery band.[14] Single-stage complete repair in infancy was first reported by Barratt-Boyes et al[15] using a Dacron graft in 1972 and without the use of prosthetic material by Trusler and Izukawa[16] in 1975. This is now the standard of care at many centers. The embryology, anatomy, natural history, pathophysiology, diagnostic techniques, surgical alternatives, and postoperative considerations for coarctation of the aorta and interrupted aortic arch will be considered separately.

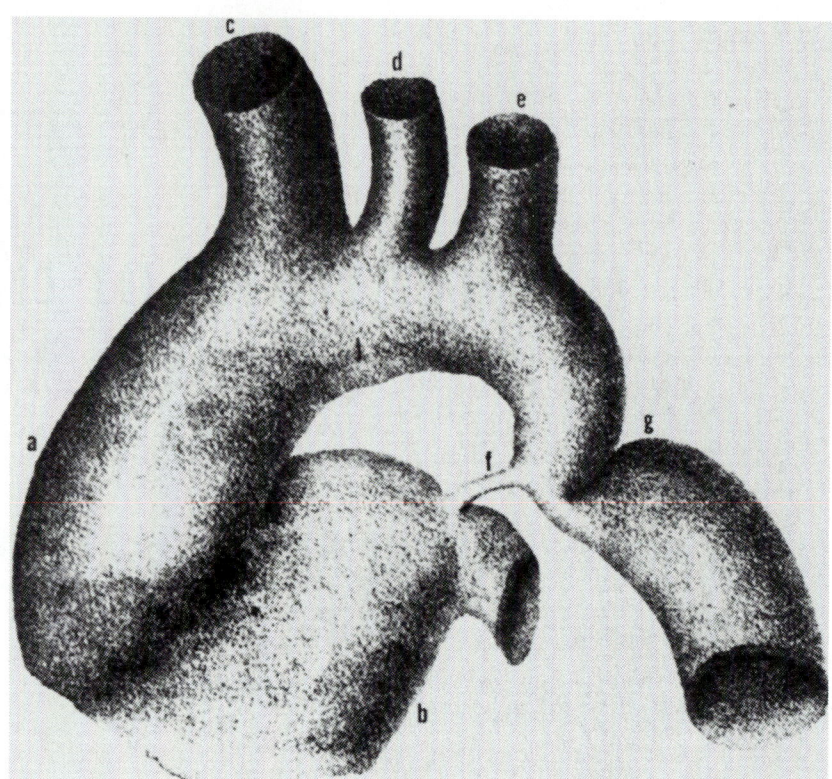

Figure 76–1. Illustration of coarctation of the aorta from *The Dublin Medical Journal,* 1834. (a) The aorta; (b) the pulmonary artery; (c) the innominate artery; (d) the left carotid artery; (e) the left subclavian artery; (f) the ligamentum arteriosum; (g) "the constriction" or coarctation of the aorta. *(Reproduced with permission from Jarcho S: Historical milestones: Aortic coarctation and aortic stenosis (Nixon 1834). Am J Cardiol 11:239, 1963. Reprinted with permission from American Journal of Cardiology.)*

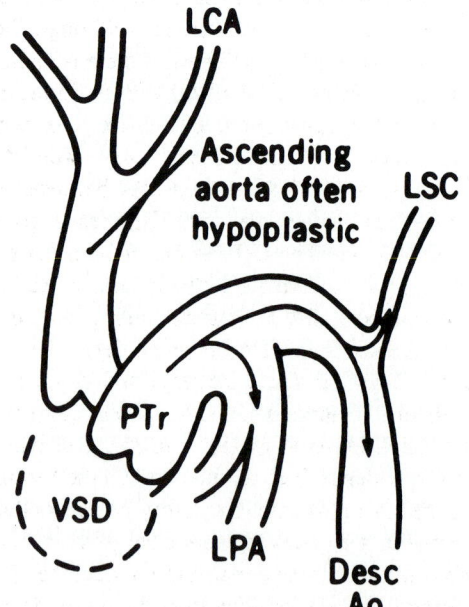

Figure 76–2. Interrupted aortic arch. There no continuity between the ascending and descending aorta. All blood flow to the descending aorta is from the patent ductus arteriosus. Desc Ao, descending aorta; LCA, left carotid artery; LPA, left pulmonary artery; LSC, left subclavian artery; PTr, pulmonary trunk; VSD, ventricular septal defect.

COARCTATION OF THE AORTA

Embryology and Anatomy

Coarctation of the aorta, first noted as an autopsy finding by Morgagni in 1760, was described as a localized constriction of the descending aorta.[17] In 1903, Bonnet suggested divid-

TABLE 76–1. SURGICAL MILESTONES

Surgical Procedure	Author	Year
Coarctation of the Aorta		
Resection with end-to-end anastomosis	Crafoord and Nylin[7]	1944
Prosthetic patch augmentation	Vossschulte[10]	1957
Subclavian flap aortoplasty	Waldhausen and Nahrwold[11]	1966
Resection with *extended* end-to-end anastomosis	Lansman et al[12]	1986
Interrupted Aortic Arch		
Arch repair (homograft)	Chamberlin[168]	1954
Arch repair—first stage, VSD closure—second stage	Samson et al[13]	1955
Simultaneous arch repair, VSD closure		
Dacron graft	Barratt-Boyes et al[15]	1972
No prosthetic material	Trusler and Izukawa[16]	1975

ing patients with coarctation of the aorta into two groups, infantile and adult.[18] In the infantile group, there is a preductal coarctation of the aorta with tubular narrowing of the isthmus of the aorta proximal to a patent ductus arteriosus, which supplies the blood flow to the descending aorta (Fig. 76–3). The adult type of coarctation is characterized by a shelf-like narrowing within the lumen of the aorta with the ductus, now closed, forming a ligamentum arteriosum (Fig. 76–4). This classification is somewhat superficial as infants with "adult-type" coarctation may have profound life-threatening cardiac failure and the "infantile" or preductal type may be encountered in older children. The critical factors that determine the hemodynamic burden are the size of the transverse arch and the degree of narrowing at the coarctation site. The unifying view of Van Praagh and associates[19] that the site of discrete coarctation of the aorta is always juxtaductal, with or without an associated isthmic hypoplasia, appears to be sensible. In surgical series, particularly for evaluating outcome, a classification system of three groups has held up fairly well over time. Based on the presence or absence of associated anomalies, they are as follows: Group I, patients with isolated coarctation; Group II, patients with coarctation and ventricular septal defect; and Group III, patients with coarctation and complex intracardiac anomalies other than isolated ventricular septal defect.

Embryology

There are two primary theories explaining the development of coarctation of the aorta: (1) the flow theory and (2) the ductal sling theory. These theories and their relationship to the development of coarctation of the aorta are not neces-

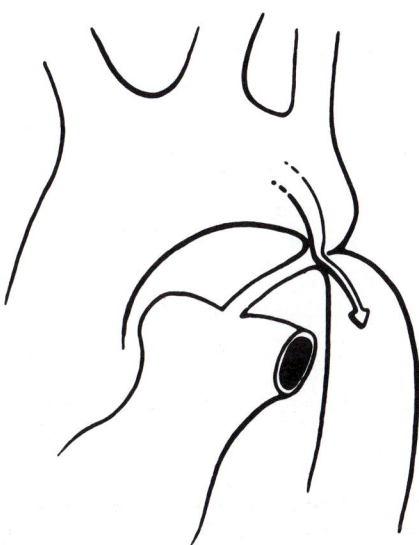

Figure 76–4. "Adult"-type coarctation of the aorta. The area of narrowing is juxtaductal and consists of a prominent posterior ridge projecting into the lumen. The ductus arteriosus has closed and is a ligamentum arteriosum.

sarily independent of each other. The flow theory rests on the hypothesis that blood flow through the cardiac chambers and great arteries during fetal growth determines their size at birth. The flow theory explains coarctation of the aorta as occurring secondary to disturbances in the balance of fetal blood flow through the aorta and pulmonary artery.[20] In a normal fetus, the left and right ventricles have approximately equal stroke volumes, although they function in parallel rather than in series. If there is an increase in flow through the right heart because of an intracardiac defect or left-sided obstruction, then there is a decrease in flow through the left heart and hence the aortic isthmus. In essence, coarctation of the aorta forms because of lack of fetal blood flow across the aortic isthmus—"no flow, no grow!" The intracardiac defects that would cause coarctation on the basis of the flow theory are in fact clinically commonly associated with patients with coarctation of the aorta. These include ventricular septal defect, bicuspid aortic valve, congenital aortic stenosis, and congenital mitral valve stenosis.[3] Although the development of coarctation of the aorta secondary to these rather dramatic lesions is easily understood, it should be remembered that the hemodynamic disturbances in embryonic circulatory pathways that lead to reduced aortic arch flow need not be gross.[21] The role of the limbus of the foramen ovale is to deflect the appropriate proportion of the inferior vena caval blood to the ascending aorta. Prenatal narrowing of the foramen ovale or an improper angulation of its limbus can lead to variable degrees of hypoplasia of the left-sided structures. This may explain Shone's syndrome[22] (coarctation of the aorta, parachute mitral valve, supravalvar mitral ring of the left atrium, and subaortic stenosis) and hypoplastic left heart syndrome.[23]

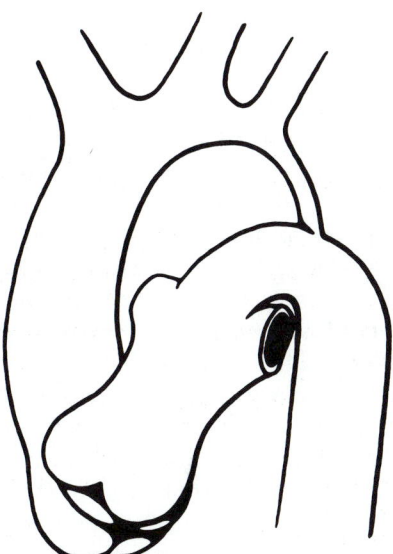

Figure 76–3. "Preductal" coarctation of the aorta. The ductus arteriosus provides the majority of blood flow to the descending aorta. There is tubular narrowing of the transverse arch and a small aortic isthmus.

In sharp contrast, lesions that reduce right heart output such as tetralogy of Fallot, pulmonary stenosis, and tricuspid atresia are almost never associated with coarctation of the aorta.[20]

The flow theory, however, is not very convincing for patients with no intracardiac defect (aside from a patent ductus arteriosus). This is referred to as primary, pure, or isolated coarctation of the aorta. For these patients the ductal sling theory is more appealing. More than 100 years ago Skoda postulated that abnormal extension of contractile ductal tissue into the aorta is a significant factor in the pathogenesis of coarctation of the aorta.[24] More recently it has been microscopically shown that the obstructing shelf can be composed of tissue similar to that found in the ductus arteriosus.[25] Careful histological examination of resected coarctation specimens has demonstrated extension of ductal tissue in a circumferential sling extending from the ductus arteriosus and surrounding the aorta at the level of the coarctation shelf.[26] Contraction and fibrosis of this "ductal sling" at the time of ductal closure would lead to constriction of the aorta and a primary coarctation (Fig. 76–5). This may more accurately explain the origin of coarctation of the aorta without associated intracardiac lesions, which occurs in approximately half of patients with coarctation of the aorta.[4] In addition to these two principal theories, other authors have advanced ideas that may also play some role in the formation of coarctation of the aorta. Kappetein and colleagues believe that an abnormality of neural crest development plays a role in the pathogenesis of coarctation of the aorta.[27] Clagett speculated that proximal movement of the left seventh intersegmental artery (left subclavian artery) beyond the junction of the sixth aortic arch (the ductus) with the aorta was involved.[28] There may also be genetic factors given the increased incidence of coarctation of the aorta in females with Turner's syndrome.[29] The syndrome was originally described in adult karyotype XO female patients having sexual infantilism, webbed neck, and cubitus valgus; 15 to 36% of these patients have associated coarctation of the aorta.

Once there is an obstruction to aortic flow at the coarctation site, there is progressive enlargement of collateral blood vessels around the narrowed segment. The collateral flow around the coarctation is predominantly from the subclavian artery and its branches; the internal mammary, intercostals, scapular, cervical, vertebral, epigastric, and spinal arteries (Fig. 76–6).[28] These vessels enlarge steadily and in older children (more than 4 years of age) and adults the chest roentgenogram will show the characteristic "notching" of the inferior aspect of the ribs due to the presence of dilated and tortuous collaterals. The scapular vessels may be easily palpated. Large collateral vessels often provide enough flow to the lower body to maintain organ function and growth.

The anatomic features of coarctation depend on the age of the patient, whether there is an associated patent ductus arteriosus, and the degree of hypoplasia of the trans-

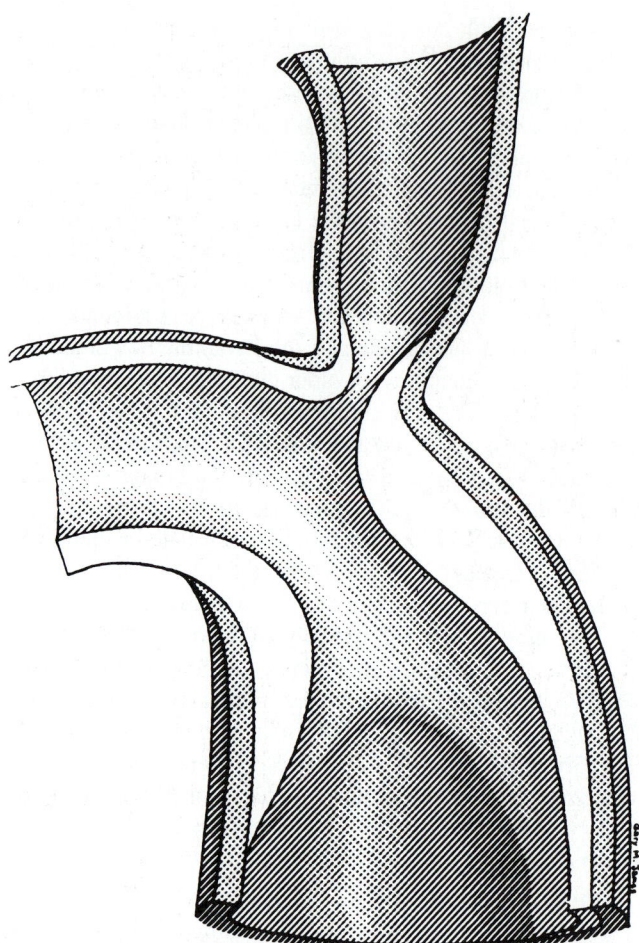

Figure 76–5. Schematic illustration of the extent of ductal tissue present in a coarctation of the aorta specimen. The white areas show the coarctation shelf, circumferential sling, and the prolongations distally in the aorta. *(Reproduced with permission from Russell GA, Berry PJ, Watterson K et al: Patterns of ductal tissue in coarctation in the first three months of life. J Thorac Cardiovasc Surg 102:596–601, 1991.)*

verse arch. In a typical infant with coarctation of the aorta and patent ductus arteriosus, there is a diffuse narrowing of the aorta distal to the left common carotid artery and below the left subclavian artery. A large patent ductus arteriosus the size of the descending aorta connects the descending aorta to the pulmonary artery. The opened aorta reveals a coarctation membrane proximal to the entrance of the ductus. There is minimal poststenotic dilatation of the descending aorta and only minor enlargement of the intercostal arteries. In an older child with a juxtaductal coarctation and ligamentum arteriosum, there is a visible external narrowing of the descending aorta at the level of the ligamentum. The degree of external narrowing, however, has no relation to the inner lumen of the aorta, which will contain a shelf-like concentric narrowing that may result in a pin-point lumen. The aorta proximal and distal to the coarctation is often dilated with enlargement of the proximal subclavian artery. The aortic wall may be very thin in the region of

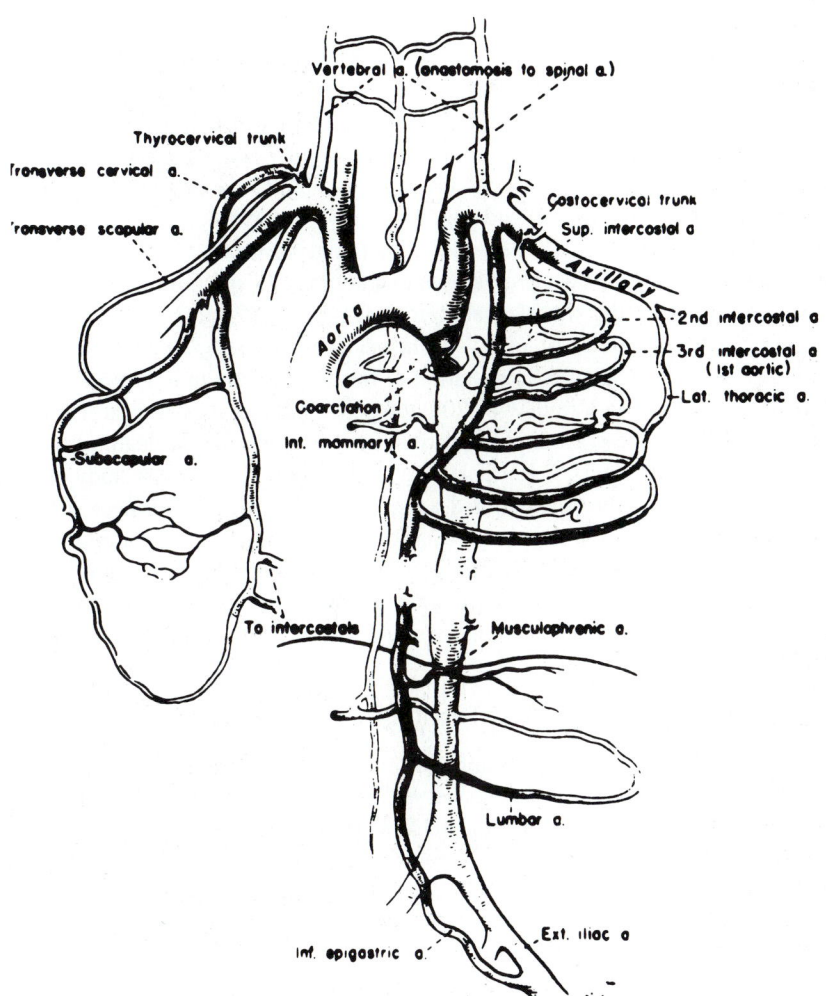

Figure 76–6. The collateral circulation in coarctation of the aorta. *(Reproduced with permission from Edwards JE: Congenital malformations of the heart and great vessels. Malformations of the thoracic aorta. In Gould SE (ed): Pathology of the Heart and Blood Vessels, 4th ed. 1968. Courtesy of Charles C. Thomas, Publisher, Springfield, Illinois.)*

poststenotic dilatation. The intercostal vessels entering the descending aorta are large, thin-walled, and may even become aneurysmal.

Pseudocoarctation of the aorta is a rare condition presumably resulting from a congenital elongation of the aortic arch.[30] The elongation leads to redundancy and kinking of the aorta, which may appear similar to a coarctation of the aorta but has no obstruction to blood flow (Fig. 76–7). There is usually little or no demonstrable pressure gradient present in pseudocoarctation.[31] Because of the tortuous nature of the aorta, however, there is a tendency for dilatation and aneurysm formation presumably related to turbulent flow beyond the kink.[32] These patients should be followed closely and surgical intervention is required only if dilatation compresses surrounding structures (i.e., esophagus) or aneurysm formation is discovered.[33]

Coarctation of the abdominal aorta occurs in only 0.5 to 2% of all coarctations.[1] The embryology of abdominal coarctation may be congenital or related to congenital rubella, Takayasu's arteritis, or von Recklinghausen's disease.[34] In two-thirds of cases the narrowing is circumscribed, and in one-third there is a long diffuse hypoplasia.

Diagnosis is confirmed by angiography. It is important to establish the condition of the renal arteries in these patients. Effective surgical therapy has included patch aortoplasty and local bypass grafts.[35–37]

Natural History and Pathophysiology

The presentation of coarctation of the aorta tends to occur in a bimodal distribution. The first group of patients includes those infants with associated cardiac anomalies and severe coarctation with blood flow to the lower extremities dependent on a patent ductus arteriosus. These patients present in infancy, sometimes with cardiovascular collapse, at the time of ductus closure. At that time collateral flow is inadequate and ischemia of organs distal to the coarctation results in renal failure and acidosis. At the same time the sudden increased afterload on the left ventricle results in acute congestive heart failure. The management of these symptomatic neonates was greatly improved by the introduction of prostaglandin E_1 (PGE_1), which opens and maintains the patency of the ductus arteriosus. PGE_1 was initially used (1975) successfully for infants with cyanotic heart disease

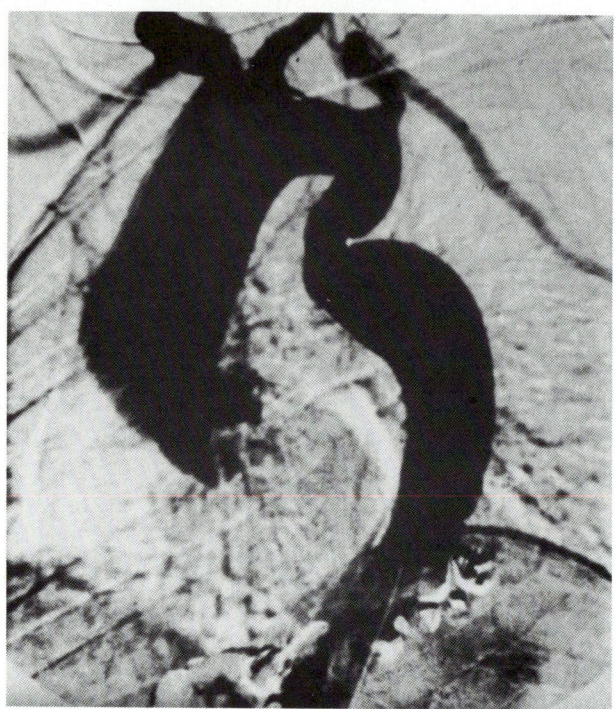

Figure 76–7. Pseudocoarctation. Aortogram showing a dilated ascending aorta, elongation of the arch, and kinking of the descending thoracic aorta in the region of the ligamentum. There was only a 20 mm Hg systolic pressure gradient across the pseudocoarctation, but marked poststenotic dilatation of the descending thoracic aorta. Resection with interposition graft was performed to relieve dysphagia. *(From Kessler RM, Miller KB, Pett S, Wernly JA: Pseudocoarctation of the aorta presenting as a mediastinal mass with dysphagia. Reprinted with permission from the Society of Thoracic Surgeons, the Annals of Thoracic Surgery 55:1993, 1003–1005.)*

(pulmonary atresia, transposition of the great arteries),[38,39] and later (1979) applied to infants with aortic arch interruption and coarctation of the aorta.[40] Intravenous infusion of prostaglandin E_1 dilates and maintains the patency of the ductus arteriosus, which augments perfusion to the lower body and improves left ventricular failure. The use of PGE_1 combined with intubation and ventilation, intravenous inotropic support (dopamine and dobutamine), and intravenous sodium bicarbonate acts to correct the low output state and reverse metabolic acidosis and renal failure. Surgical intervention can then be planned on a semielective basis at a time when the function of the various organ systems has been optimized.

Another group of patients remains essentially asymptomatic and presents usually with subtle findings later in life or with a catastrophic event such as rupture of an aneurysm of the circle of Willis.[41] The main cause of symptoms in these patients is the proximal systemic hypertension, which may cause headaches or epistaxis. They may also have claudication from inadequate lower extremity perfusion with exercise. Alterations in renal, adrenal, and baroreceptor function all contribute to the development of

this proximal systemic hypertension. This may lead to circle of Willis aneurysms, aortic aneurysm proximal or distal to the coarctation, aortic dissection, and increased coronary atherosclerotic heart disease with associated myocardial infarction.[42] The following diagnoses are the cause of death in patients with coarctation: congestive heart failure (26%), bacterial endocarditis (25%), spontaneous rupture of the aorta (21%), and intracranial hemorrhage (13%).[43] Intercostal aneurysms may rupture and infection may occur at the site of coarctation, at a bicuspid aortic valve, or in the circle of Willis.[44] The survival curve of patients with an unoperated coarctation of the aorta is shown in Figure 76–8.[45] In a review of 200 autopsies in patients with coarctation of the aorta, Abbott found the average age at death was 33.5 years.[46] Reifenstein and associates in a similar study of 104 autopsies quoted a figure of 35.0 years.[43] In these patients pregnancy increases the risk of associated complications. There is essentially no medical therapy for an older child or adult with coarctation and they should be referred for elective surgical intervention in a timely fashion.

Diagnostic Techniques

Physical examination of the infant with critical coarctation and ductus closure will reveal a patient in shock. The child will be tachypneic and tachycardic, and will appear pale. Upper extremity pulses may be thready and lower extremity pulses absent. The child may be hypotensive and the liver will be enlarged. Chest radiograph will demonstrate cardiomegaly and evidence of congestive heart failure. Electrocardiogram may reveal a left ventricular strain pattern. Two-dimensional echocardiography with color Doppler interrogation should be diagnostic in most instances.[47–50] The echocardiogram will demonstrate lack of pulsatile flow in the descending aorta, the actual coarctation site, the size of the transverse arch, and any other associated intracardiac anomalies. The study continues to be useful after the administration of prostaglandin and reopening the ductus, and should demonstrate right-to-left shunting at the ductal level into the descending aorta. In many instances a comprehensive echocardiogram is all that is required to prepare a patient for preoperative medical management followed by surgical intervention after stabilization of organ systems. However, if there are complex associated cardiac anomalies cardiac catheterization can safely be performed in a stable baby who is being maintained on prostaglandin infusion. This will reveal the precise great vessel morphology, significant hemodynamic parameters, and intracardiac anatomy.[21]

Physical examination of an older child with no symptoms should reveal upper extremity hypertension and absent or greatly diminished femoral pulses. Electrocardiogram will demonstrate left ventricular hypertrophy and left ventricular strain. Chest radiograph will demonstrate "notching" of the ribs if the patient is over 4 years of age. In addition, the classic "3" sign is caused by dilatation of the

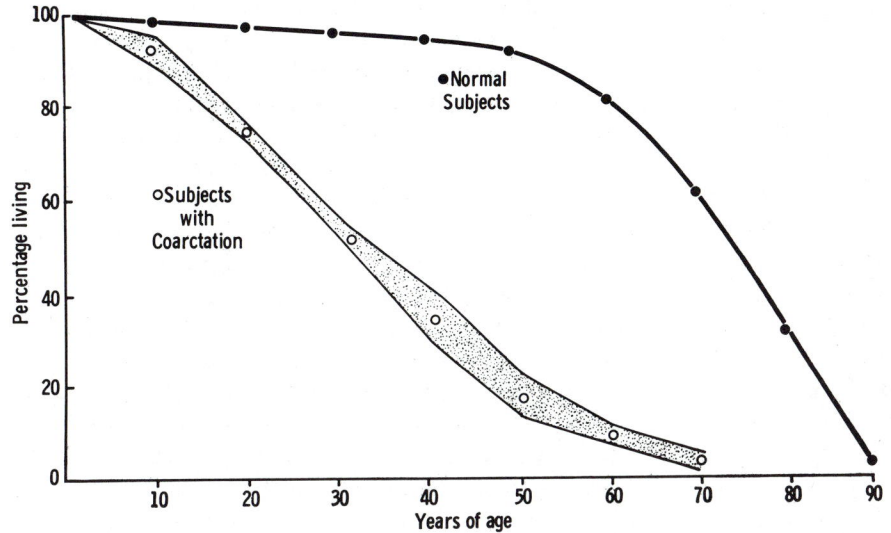

Figure 76–8. Survival curve of patients with coarctation of the aorta surviving the first year of life as compared with normal subjects. *(Reproduced with permission from Campbell M: Natural history of coarctation of the aorta. Br Heart J 32: 633–640, 1970.)*

subclavian artery, the narrowing of the coarctation site, and poststenotic dilatation of the descending aorta. The echocardiogram in most instances of simple coarctation in older children, adolescents, and adults will provide the diagnosis without requiring cardiac catheterization.[51] Cardiac catheterization is required for these patients only if there are associated intracardiac anomalies or a question with regard to the size of the collateral vessels. In addition to these standard studies, other modalities that may be useful for the noninvasive assessment of aortic coarctation include computed tomography (CT), cine CT, magnetic resonance imaging (MRI), cine MRI, transesophageal echocardiography, and computerized three-dimensional reconstruction of the heart with MRI or echocardiography.[52–57] In summary, assessment of aortic coarctation can be accomplished accurately and comprehensively in most instances by using the combined methodologies of two-dimensional and Doppler echocardiography. In the critically ill infant echocardiographic diagnosis may obviate the need for a preoperative emergent cardiac catheterization. In all cases a complete two-dimensional and Doppler echocardiographic examination of intracardiac anatomy is mandatory to reach appropriate therapeutic and surgical recommendations.

Surgical Techniques

General Considerations

The surgical approach in most instances is through a left posterolateral thoracotomy incision entering the thorax through the fourth intercostal space. The exception to this is a transmediastinal approach for patients with associated cardiac anomalies that are repaired simultaneously. The arterial blood pressure is monitored in the right radial artery. Should the right subclavian artery arise anomalously below the coarctation the temporal artery provides a useful site for monitoring the proximal aortic pressure. In early reports the

latissimus dorsi and serratus anterior muscles were both divided. More recently the serratus anterior muscle has been spared dividing only the latissimus muscle. In older children the multiple chest wall collateral vessels should be individually ligated and divided to prevent hemorrhage either during the operation or postoperatively. The lung is retracted anteriorly and the mediastinal pleura overlying the coarctation site is incised. Any large lymphatic channels are either preserved or ligated and divided. The vagus nerve and recurrent laryngeal nerve are carefully preserved by retracting and dissecting these structures with the mediastinal pleura anteriorly. The descending aorta, left subclavian artery, ductus (or ligamentum) arteriosus, and transverse aortic arch distal to the left carotid artery should be mobilized. An anomalous artery originally described by Abbott is an infrequently encountered collateral vessel originating from the posterior wall of the aortic arch or subclavian artery.[58] This vessel is not found in normal subjects or described in standard anatomy textbooks (Fig. 76–9). If present it should be either controlled with a vessel loop or ligated and divided. Oversewing and division or ligation and division of the ductus (or ligamentum) arteriosus will increase the mobility of the aorta. In older children there are large collateral intercostal vessels entering the descending aorta distal to the coarctation. These should be carefully mobilized and encircled with vessel loops and may require ligation and division in order to fully mobilize the area of the coarctation. Unlike adult vascular procedures, heparin is generally not administered and vascular clamps are applied to the proximal and distal aorta.

It is very important that the proximal aortic pressure be allowed to stay quite high (160–200 mm Hg) during the time of the aortic cross-clamp to provide adequate mean aortic arterial blood pressure distal to the clamp and prevent the dreaded complication of paraplegia. In contrast to adult aortic surgery, sodium nitroprusside should never be used during the time of cross-clamping for coarctation repair.

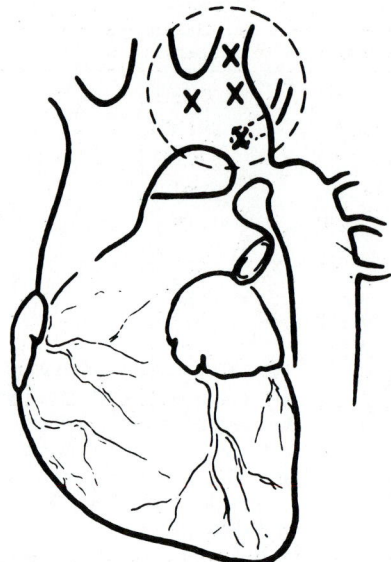

Figure 76–9. Abbott's artery. Drawing outlines the area on the posterior wall of the aortic arch or subclavian artery from which a blood vessel, which Gross chose to call Abbott's artery, may take its origin. X, possible sites of origin. *(Reproduced with permission from Schuster SR, Gross RE: Surgery for coarctation of the aorta. A review of 500 cases. J Thorac Cardiovasc Surg 43:54–70, 1962.)*

The use of nipride while the aorta is clamped has actually been shown to increase the incidence of paraplegia postoperatively.[59] A distal aortic pressure monitoring line can be placed in older children either in the posterior tibial, dorsalis pedis, or femoral artery location. In these older children the mean distal aortic pressure should be maintained above 45 mm Hg during the period of aortic cross-clamp.[60] During the first 10 min of cross-clamping the mean distal aortic pressure usually increases 5 mm Hg. Maintaining the distal aortic pressure can be done by the administration of volume expanders, use of inotropes such as dopamine or dobutamine, or reduced anesthetic during the time period of the cross-clamp. Another useful maneuver is to readjust the clamps to allow flow in the left subclavian artery or to allow more intercostal arteries to remain open. Should the mean pressure drop below 45 mm Hg, alternative techniques such as the use of cardiopulmonary bypass with left atrial and descending aortic cannulation or various shunts, both extraluminal and intraluminal, should be considered.[61–64] However, in almost all cases of primary coarctation repair this is unnecessary. The various techniques of repair are now reviewed separately (Table 76–1).

Resection and End-to-End Anastomosis

Cradoord and Nylin[7] reported the first successful resection of coarctation of the aorta with end-to-end anastomosis. Their two patients were a 12-year-old boy and a 27-year-old man operated on in October 1944. Gross'[65] first patient was operated on in June 1945. Kirklin et al[66] described the

successful surgical treatment of coarctation of the aorta in an infant when they operated on a 10-week-old child performing successful coarctation resection with end-to-end anastomosis (and ligation of the left subclavian artery) in 1951.

The original technique of resection and end-to-end anastomosis as described by Willis Potts is shown in Figure 76–10. The obviously narrowed coarctation segment was excised with a direct end-to-end circumferential anastomosis of the aorta. Note that the aorta must be mobilized to a significant degree to have a successful anastomosis without tension. Early repairs utilized silk suture in a continuous fashion posteriorly and interrupted everting horizontal mattress sutures anteriorly. The mortality and recoarctation rates using resection and end-to-end anastomosis in several series[63,67–75] are shown in Table 76–2. Although the mor-

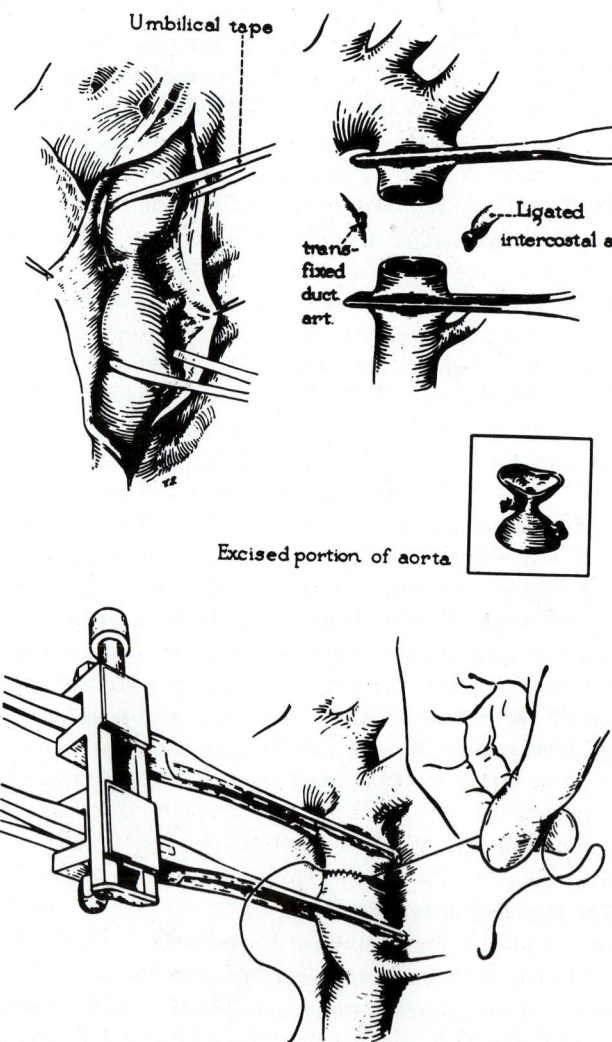

Figure 76–10. Resection of coarctation with end-to-end anastomosis using toothed coarctation clamps and a vise to bring the ends of the aorta into apposition. *(Reproduced with permission from Potts WJ: Coarctation of the aorta. In The Surgeon and the Child. Philadelphia, W. B. Saunders, 1959, pp 103–108.)*

TABLE 76–2. RESULTS OF RESECTION WITH END-TO-END ANASTOMOSIS

Author	Age	Year	Patients	Mortality	Recoarctation
Hartmann[67]	<2 yr	1970	20	—	4 (20%)
Williams[68]	<1 yr	1980	176	66 (38%)	39 (33%)
Cobanoglu[69]	<3 mo	1985	55	16 (29%)	3 (8%)
Körfer[70]	<4 mo	1985	55	2 (4%)	3 (6%)
Pennington[63]	<1 yr	1985	19	4 (21%)	27%
Ziemer[71]	<1 mo	1986	24	8 (33%)	4 (25%)
Brouwer[72]	<2 yr	1991	32	—	4 (13%)
Kappetein[73]	<3 yr	1994	48	5 (10%)	86%[a]
Van Heurn[74]	<3 mo	1994	42	5 (12%)	11 (30%)
CHSS[75b]	<1 mo	1994	139	20 (14%)	6 (4%)

[a]Kaplan–Meier estimate at 30 years.
[b]CHSS, Congenital Heart Surgeon's Society.

tality rate was very acceptable in large series[76] several institutions reported a relatively high recoarctation rate (20 to 86%) particularly in the age group <1 year.[63,67,68,73,74] This high rate of stenosis in retrospect is attributed to (1) the use of silk sutures instead of the currently available fine monofilament suture,[77] (2) inadequate resection of all ductal tissue, which may extend into areas of normal-appearing aorta,[71] (3) lack of growth at a circumferential suture line,[67] and (4) lack of growth of a hypoplastic transverse arch. More recent series tend to indicate that with modern microvascular suture and techniques, the recoarctation rate is less than previously thought.[70,72,75] In particular, the use of absorbable polydioxanone suture may help prevent residual coarctation formation.[78]

Prosthetic Patch Aortoplasty

Chiefly because of the high rate of recoarctation with the classic end-to-end anastomosis technique, the technique of prosthetic patch aortoplasty was introduced. Vossschulte[10] in 1957 described an "isthmusplastic" procedure that developed into the prosthetic patch aortoplasty. As discussed earlier under general considerations, this operation is performed through a left thoracotomy and fourth intercostal space incision. After vessel dissection and ductus ligation, the aorta can either be occluded with two separate vascular clamps or in some instances with a single clamp encompassing the extent of the patch placement. The aorta is then incised longitudinally through the site of the coarctation with the incision being extended well beyond the level of the coarctation both distally and proximally. Proximally this means that the patch often extends up onto the left subclavian artery. If the isthmus is hypoplastic with stenosis between the left subclavian and left carotid artery, the patch may be extended up into this area by placing the proximal clamp proximal to the left carotid artery. In the initial descriptions of this procedure, the posterior coarctation membrane or fibrous shelf was excised. This maneuver, however, may contribute to disruption of the intima and later

aortic aneurysm formation and is no longer recommended. A circular prosthetic patch (slightly elliptical) made of polytetrafluoroethylene is sutured in place longitudinally along the aortotomy edge. An effort is made to use the largest patch feasible and place the widest portion of the patch at the level of the aortic constriction (see Fig. 76–11). The pleura should be closed as completely as possible over the patch.

The prosthetic patch technique offers several advantages. (1) It avoids extensive dissection and prolonged cross-clamp time, which may be required for the end-to-end technique. (2) The collateral vessels are all preserved and do not require ligation and division. (3) The technique allows simultaneous enlargement of isthmic hypoplasia if necessary. (4) The anastomosis is always tension free and quite easy to perform. (5) The posterior aortic wall and even a hypoplastic aortic arch will grow after prosthetic patch repair.[79] The chief reported late complication of this technique is aneurysm formation on the posterior aortic wall opposite the patch.[80,81] This may be explained by several different factors. One theory attributes the aneurysm formation to the resection of the coarctation site with violation of the intimal layer.[82,83] Another theory for aneurysm formation is the altered hemodynamics arising from the different tensile strengths of the prosthetic patch and the posterior aortic wall, and the pulsatile waveform being completely directed to the posterior aortic wall by the inflexible anterior patch.[84,85] Another theory is a congenital abnormality of the aortic wall at the coarctation site.[86] Mortality, recoarctation rates, and incidence of aneurysm formation in several series[75,79,83–85,87–91] of patch aortoplasty are shown in Table 76–3. The issue of aneurysm formation is addressed in greater detail in the section on postoperative complications.

At the Children's Memorial Hospital in Chicago we have used polytetrafluoroethylene (PTFE) patch aortoplasty for infants and children older than 1 year of age at the time of diagnosis of their coarctation. Between 1979 and 1993, 125 infants and children underwent PTFE patch aortoplasty

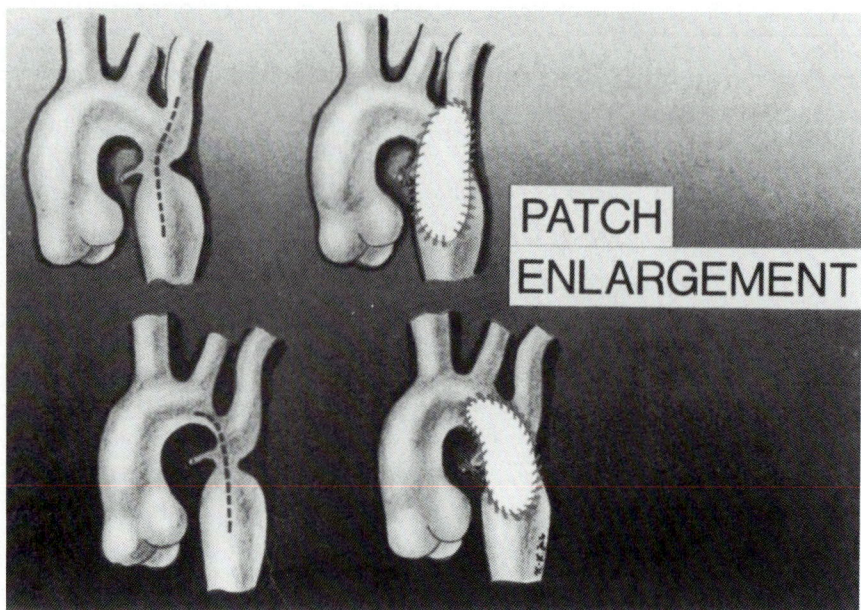

Figure 76–11. Patch aortoplasty. A large elliptical PTFE patch forms a roof over the coarctation ridge. The ridge should *not* be excised. As illustrated here, the patch may extend onto the left subclavian artery or a hypoplastic transverse arch. *(From Messmer BJ, Minale C, Mühler E, v Bernuth G: Surgical correction of coarctation in early infancy: Does surgical technique influence the result? Reprinted with permission from the Society of Thoracic Surgeons, The Annals of Thoracic Surgery 1991, 52: 594–603.)*

for coarctation of the aorta; 111 were primary repairs, 14 were reoperations following subclavian flap aortoplasty (7), resection with end-to-end anastomosis (6), and Dacron patch (1). The posterior coarctation ridge was not excised. The mean age at the time of surgery in this series was 5.1 years. There were no instances of intraoperative mortality or paraplegia. There were four deaths (3% mortality) at 10 to 40 days postoperatively, all in neonates having additional intracardiac procedures for complex lesions. In intensive follow-up with echocardiography and chest radiographs, only one patient has developed an aneurysm and this was a false aneurysm detected 4 mo after the surgery. No patient has developed a late true aneurysm. In this series 10 patients (8%) having PTFE aortoplasty as their original procedure have a residual or recurrent coarctation (defined as a residual gradient greater than 20 mm Hg). Other surgeons

have also reported excellent results utilizing the patch aortoplasty.[87,91] At our institution PTFE patch aortoplasty remains the procedure of choice for children whose coarctation is diagnosed at more than 1 year of age. We do not recommend use of this technique in neonates because of the often associated long segment arch hypoplasia, which in our experience and others'[75,90] have had a higher incidence of restenosis or recoarctation.

Prosthetic Interposition Graft

The use of a prosthetic interposition graft was first described by Robert Gross in 1951 when he used an aortic homograft as a replacement for a coarctation in a child with a long narrowed coarctation segment.[92] In 1960 Morris, Cooley, DeBakey, and Crawford described the use of a Dacron

TABLE 76–3. RESULTS OF PATCH AORTOPLASTY[a]

Author	Age	Year	Patients	Operative Mortality	Recoarctation	Aneurysm	Patch
Yee[87]	<1 yr	1984	100	0	10 (12%)	0	PTFE
Sade[79]	<2 yr	1984	21	2 (10%)	2 (11%)	0	PTFE
Clarkson[85]	>15 yr	1985	38	NS	6 (16%)	5 (13%)	Dacron
Hehrlein[83]	2 d–64 yrs	1986	317	16 (5%)	4 (1.3%)	18 (6%)	Dacron
Rheuban[84]	8.5 yr (mean)	1986	45	NS	NS	8 (17%)	Dacron
Del Nido[88]	3 d–32 yr	1986	63	1 (2%)	8 (13%)	3 (5%)	Dacron
Ala-Kulju[89]	15–54 yr	1989	67	NS	NS	22 (33%)	Dacron
Messmer[90]	<1 mo	1991	8	NS	4 (50%)	0	NS
Ungerleider[91]	NS	1991	54	0	2 (5%)	0	PTFE
CMH	5.1 yr (mean)	1994	125	4 (3%)	10 (8%)	0	PTFE
CHSS[75]	<1 mo	1994	38	11 (29%)	8 (21%)	NS	NS

[a]CMH, Children's Memorial Hospital; CHSS, Congenital Heart Surgeon's Society; NS, not specified.

prosthetic interposition graft in 3% of 171 patients undergoing coarctation repair.[93] Currently prosthetic interposition grafts are most useful in adults with an associated aneurysm or complex long-segment coarctation, or a recurrent coarctation following one of the other techniques of repair. It is also a useful technique if during resection and end-to-end anastomosis it appears that the anastomosis will be under tension or the aorta requires further resection because of poor, thinned aortic wall secondary to poststenotic dilatation. The obvious disadvantage of the interposition graft is the developmental size discrepancy in the growing child, making the operation more applicable for adult patients. Another consideration is the longer aortic cross-clamp time taken to perform two circular anastomoses.

Subclavian Flap Aortoplasty

The subclavian flap aortoplasty technique was introduced by Waldhausen and Nahrwold[11] in 1966. Successful coarctation repair was reported in three patients aged 4 mo, 6 mo, and 3 years (see Fig. 76–12). The operation is performed through the left fourth intercostal space as described earlier under general considerations. The aortic arch, subclavian artery, isthmus, and descending aorta are exposed and dissected. The ligamentum or ductus arteriosus is ligated. The aorta is clamped proximal to the left subclavian artery as well as distal to the coarctation. The left subclavian artery is ligated at the origin of the vertebral artery, which may or may not be included in the ligature. The subclavian artery is

then opened along its lateral margin and divided. The incision is extended through the isthmus across the coarctation into the area of poststenotic dilatation. The diaphragm of the coarctation in the original procedure was excised, although concern about aneurysm formation has led us to currently leave the ridge in place. The subclavian artery is folded down onto the incision in the aorta and then the subclavian "flap" is sutured in place with continuous fine polypropylene suture. The clamps are released and the appearance is usually that of an excellent expanse of autogenous tissue creating a "roof" over the area of the previous coarctation. The issue of ligation of the vertebral artery is still unresolved, as leaving it intact provides collateral circulation to the arm but may possibly cause subclavian steal syndrome as the child grows.[94] If possible, the internal mammary artery and the thyrocervical trunk are left intact to provide collateral circulation to the left arm. Occasionally more length is required to span the coarctation site and sacrifice of these vessels is required. Failure to extend the incision far enough downstream across the coarctation and onto the area of poststenotic dilatation may contribute to restenosis at a later date. Several variations of this technique have been described for complex coarctations. In 1983 Hart and Waldhausen[95] described the reversed subclavian flap technique for repair of a coarctation proximal to the left subclavian artery. Brown et al[96] introduced an isthmus flap aortoplasty as an alternative to subclavian flap for long-segment coarctation of the aorta in infants. This allowed the subclavian artery not to be sacrificed. Meier et

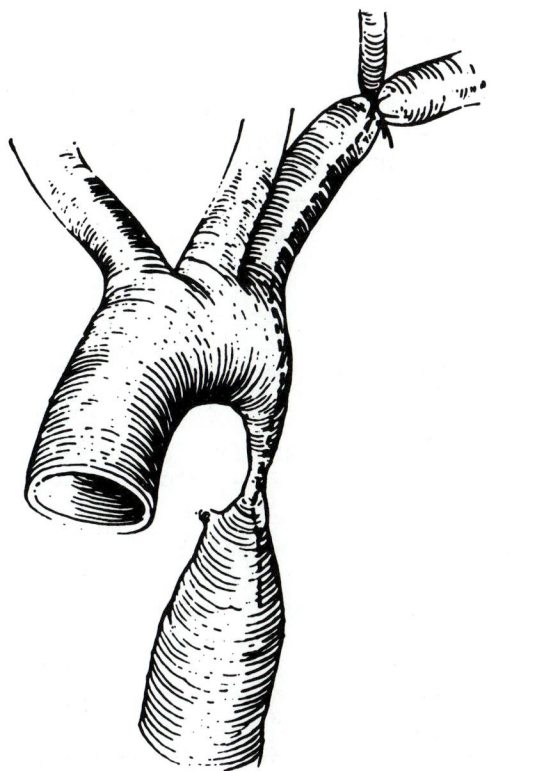
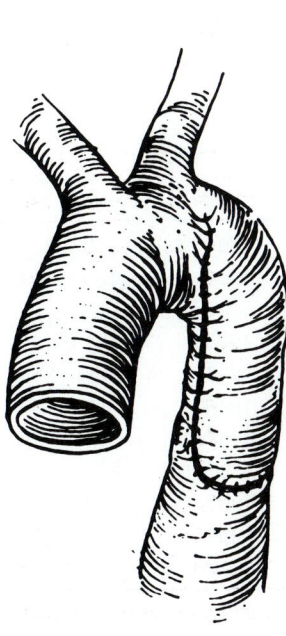

Figure 76–12. Subclavian flap aortoplasty. The subclavian artery is ligated, divided, and opened longitudinally (see dotted line). It is then turned down as a flap over the coarctation site, carrying the flap as far distal as is possible. *(Reproduced with permission from Waldhausen JA, Nahrwold DL: Repair of coarctation of the aorta with a subclavian flap. J Thorac Cardiovascular Surg 51:532–533, 1966.)*

al[97] also described a technique for subclavian reimplantation in 1986 to preserve the arterial blood flow to the left arm. Dietl et al[98] used a combined technique of coarctation resection and subclavian flap aortoplasty.

The advantage of the subclavian flap technique includes its simplicity, short cross-clamp time, avoidance of prosthetic material, easy anastomotic hemostatic control, and increased anastomotic growth owing to the use of an autogenous noncircumferential flap.[99] Until recently the subclavian flap repair was widely utilized as the method of choice for repair of coarctation of the aorta in infants and children under 1 year of age.[100,101] We are hesitant to perform it in older children mainly for fear of left arm ischemia following ligation of the subclavian artery.[102] In addition, sacrifice of the left subclavian artery may affect long-term growth and function in the left upper limb.[103] Aneurysm occurrence has been described after subclavian flap aortoplasty[104] and in our institution we had one child who developed a false aneurysm following a subclavian flap aortoplasty utilizing absorbable suture. Subclavian flap aortoplasty was widely used from the mid-1970s to the mid-1980s.[105] As the long-term follow-up was continued it appeared that the incidence of recoarctation, initially thought to be low, was higher than expected ranging up to 42% in some series (Table 76–4).[71,72,74,75,101,105–109] It was particularly in the smaller infant less than 2 mo in age that the subclavian flap aortoplasty appeared to have a high recurrence rate.[107] Because of this surgeons became interested again in the resection with end-to-end anastomosis technique, this time, however, with more extensive dissection and resection. Some surgeons continue to feel that subclavian flap aortoplasty is the procedure of choice for neonatal coarctation of the aorta.[101,106]

Resection with Extended End-to-End Anastomosis

In 1986 Lansman and associates[12] reported a modification of the classic resection and end-to-end anastomosis utilizing an extended technique. The technique was applied in 17 infants (mean weight 3.5 kg) operated on between 1977 and 1985. Forty-seven percent of these patients had a hypoplastic distal aortic arch and isthmus. The initial exposure is as described earlier for the other techniques. The ductus arteriosus is ligated and divided. The descending aorta is mobilized almost to the diaphragm and often at least the first set of intercostal vessels is ligated and divided. However, the proximal aortic clamp is positioned either between the left carotid and the left subclavian or in some circumstances between the innominate artery and the left carotid artery. The distal cross-clamp is placed well below the coarctation. The entire coarctation segment is completely excised, including a portion of the undersurface of the aortic arch. Proximally a long incision is made on the inferior surface of the arch up to the proximal cross-clamp. Distally the descending aorta is incised laterally and the anastomosis is then performed with polypropylene suture. In Lansman's review mean cross-clamp time was 17 min. There was one in-hospital death in a child with associated atrioventricular canal, and there were two late recoarctations (12%). Zannini et al[110] described a similar technique in the Italian literature. Elliott[111] modified the technique to address transverse arch hypoplasia utilizing a clamp proximally to occlude the left subclavian artery, the left carotid artery, and even part of the right innominate artery (Fig. 76–13). This allowed extension of the aortic arch incision more proximally than in Lansman's technique; the "radically extended end-to-end anastomosis." Zannini et al described another modification of this technique using a median sternotomy approach, with resection of the isthmic portion and side-to-side anastomosis of the ascending and descending thoracic aorta.[112] Because of the length of the resection and anastomosis, the technique requires a steady assistant to carefully hold the clamps together during the time of the anastomosis. Although an interrupted suture technique would be theoretically attractive to promote growth of the anastomosis, Lansman proposes a running suture technique to decrease cross-clamp time. Growth of the anastomosis will occur be-

TABLE 76–4. RESULTS OF SUBCLAVIAN FLAP AORTOPLASTY

Author	Age	Year	Patients	Mortality	Recoarctation
Campbell[106]	<1 yr	1984	53	2 (4%)	2 (4%)
Penkoske[105]	<1 yr	1984	106	25 (23%)	5 (6%)
Moulton[99]	<1 yr	1984	29	4 (14%)	1 (3%)
Metzdorff[107]	<2 mo	1985	60	11 (18%)	10 (17%)
Sanchez[108]	<3 mo	1986	26	3 (12%)	5 (22%)
Ziemer[71]	<1 mo	1986	70	8 (11.4%)	9 (15%)
Ehrhardt[109]	<1 mo	1989	45	14 (31%)	7 (23%)
Milliken[101]	<1 mo	1990	123	11 (9%)	20 (16%)
Brouwer[72]	<2 yr	1991	19	NS	7 (33%)
Van Heurn[74]	<3 mo	1994	15	1 (7%)	6 (42%)
CHSS[75]	<1 mo	1994	112	9 (8%)	12 (12%)

[b]CHSS, Congenital Heart Surgeon's Society; NS, not specified.

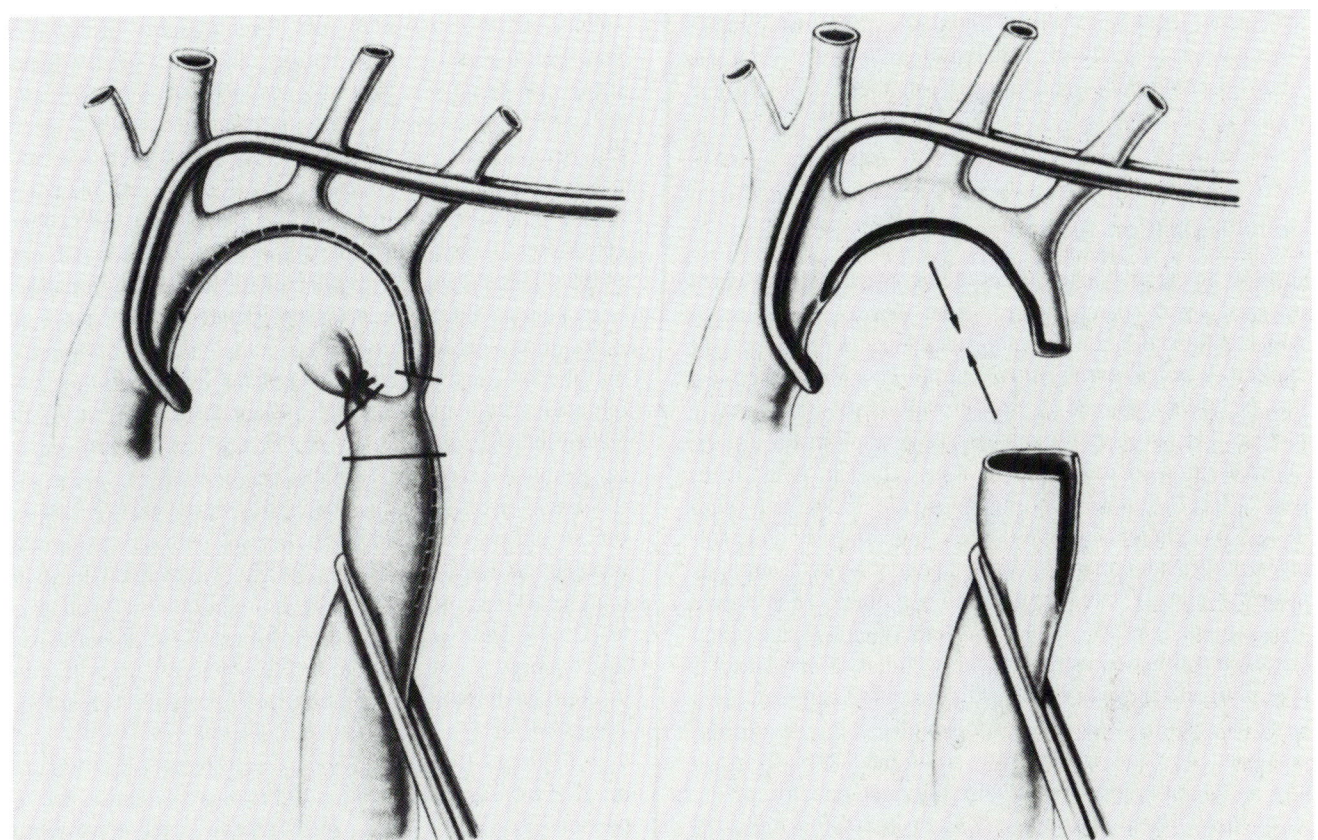

Figure 76–13. Resection with extended end-to-end anastomosis. The proximal clamp is partially occluding the innominate artery. The proximal arch incision is extended proximal to the left carotid artery. The distal arch incision is carried laterally to allow accurate approximation and a wide anastomosis. *(From Elliott MJ: Coarctation of the aorta with arch hypoplasia: Improvements on a new technique. Reprinted with permission from the Society of Thoracic Surgeons, The Annals of Thoracic Surgery, 1987, 44:321–323.)*

cause of eventual disruption of the suture line as the anastomotic site matures. This appears to be substantiated by indirect evidence of growth of a circumferential suture line following the arterial switch procedure.[113] Since the original reports using this technique several surgeons have now described excellent results with the extended end-to-end repair in the neonatal population (Table 76–5).[73,74,112,114,115]

Many surgeons now feel that this is the procedure of choice for the infant with symptomatic coarctation. The obvious advantage of the technique is that all coarctation tissue with uncertain potential for future growth is completely resected. The left subclavian artery is preserved, avoiding

potential arm growth disorders. The aorta is left widely patent providing maximal relief of systemic afterload. The procedure addresses and corrects hypoplasia of the distal aortic arch, the aortic isthmus, and the transverse arch. The technique avoids prosthetic material, limits the potential for aneurysm formation, and preserves normal vascular anatomy. When applied to the infant with complex associated cardiac lesions, one-stage total repair with this technique through a median sternotomy is an alternative that may reduce mortality.[116] It should be noted that some surgeons feel that a hypoplastic arch will grow with increased flow across a patent standard end-to-end anastomosis[117] or

TABLE 76–5. RESULTS OF RESECTION WITH "EXTENDED" END-TO-END ANASTOMOSIS

Author	Age	Year	Patients	Operative Mortality	Recoarctation
Lansman[12]	<6 mo	1986	17	1 (6%)	2 (12%)
Vouhe[114]	<3 mo	1988	80	21 (26%)	6 (10%)
LaCour-Gayet[115]	<1 mo	1990	66	9 (14%)	7 (12%)
Zannini[112]	<3 mo	1993	21	4 (19%)	4 (23%)
Van Heurn[74]	<3 mo	1994	77	5 (6%)	8 (11%)
Kappetein[73]	<3 yr	1994	26	4 (15%)	0%

subclavian flap aortoplasty[118] and that extended arch repair should be reserved for the small group of infants with transverse aortic arch-to-ascending aorta diameter ratios of less than 0.25.[119]

Balloon Dilation Angioplasty

In 1979 Sos et al[120] demonstrated that a surgically resected neonatal aortic coarctation could be successfully enlarged with a balloon dilation catheter. Lock et al[121] performed dilatation on seven resected coarctation segments and showed that eight atmospheres of pressure produced considerable increase in internal aortic diameter as a result of linear intimal tearing with medial extension. Lababidi et al[122] reported successful balloon angioplasty in 27 patients with native coarctation in 1984. In 1986 Marvin and colleagues[123] first reported the development of aortic aneurysms near the site of balloon dilation angioplasty for native coarctation. Four of 11 patients undergoing dilation had aneurysm formation at the previously dilated site within 1 year. Surgical excision of the coarctation segments revealed an absence of muscle and elastic lamella in the area of the aneurysms.[124] This report led to an immediate suspension of the technique in patients with native coarctation of the aorta at all but a few centers. Cooper et al[125] reported

aneurysm formation in three of seven patients. Microscopy revealed disruption of the intima and elastic media, which resulted in thinning of the intact adventitial wall of the vessel.

In 1989 the Valvuloplasty and Angioplasty of Congenital Anomalies (VACA) Registry reported data from 140 patients for native coarctation of the aorta. A residual gradient of more than 20 mm Hg was detected in 23 patients (16%) and late aneurysms were detected in 6 patients (4%).[126] The study group concluded that although balloon angioplasty reduced the pressure gradient and increased the coarctation diameter, concerns about femoral artery injury and the late appearance of aneurysms called into question inclusion of the technique in the armamentarium of the interventional cardiologist.[127] Controversy continues to exist regarding the safety and efficacy of balloon angioplasty in the management of native coarctation of the aorta.[128] Based on our experience we limit the use of balloon angioplasty for native coarctation of the aorta to selected infants with complex intracardiac anatomy who require initial palliation, to patients with major systemic illness that increases the risk of surgical intervention, and to older patients with mild discrete coarctation of the aorta and poorly developed collaterals.

In contrast to the above described results with balloon dilation for native coarctation the results of dilation for *recurrent* coarctation (Fig. 76–14) have been consistently

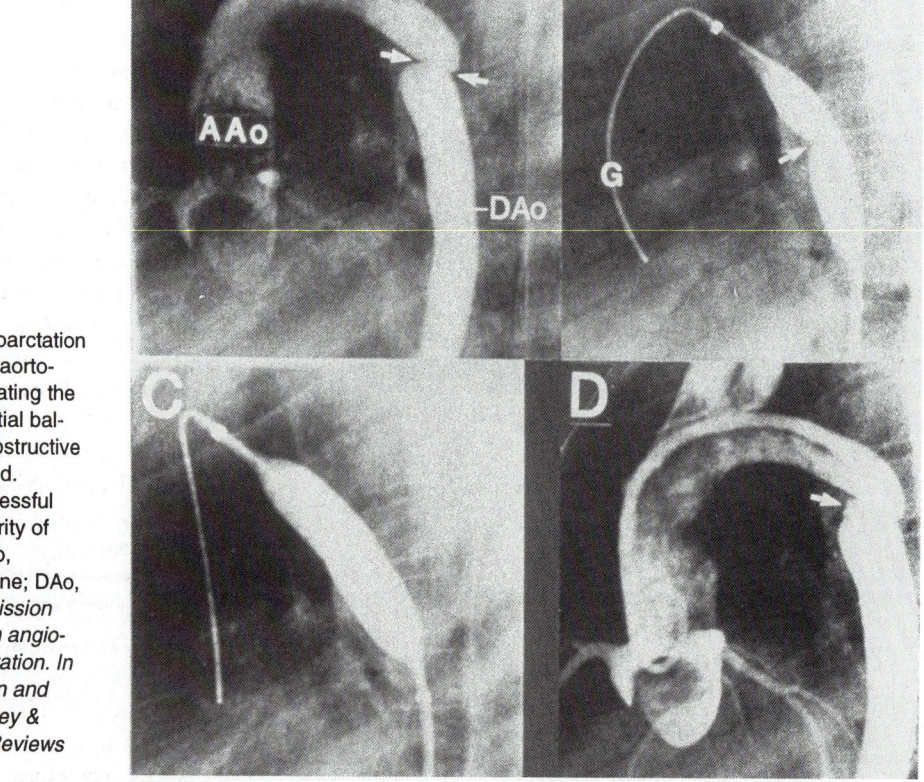

Figure 76–14. Balloon angioplasty of recoarctation after surgical repair with subclavian patch aortoplasty. **A.** Predilation aortogram demonstrating the narrowed recoarct segment *(arrow)*. **B.** Initial balloon inflation with creation of waist from obstructive shelf. **C.** Upon full inflation, waist is relieved. **D.** Postangioplasty aortogram shows successful dilation of recoarct segment. Note irregularity of vessel wall in the dilated area *(arrow)*. AAo, ascending aorta; Ar, aortic arch; G, guideline; DAo, descending aorta. *(Reproduced with permission from Zales VR, Muster AJ: Balloon dilation angioplasty for the management of aortic coarctation. In Mavroudis C, Backer CL (eds): Coarctation and Interrupted Aortic Arch. Philadelphia, Hanley & Belfus; Cardiac Surgery: State of the Art Reviews 7:133–146, 1993.)*

more successful with an apparent lower incidence of aneurysm formation.[129,130] Saul and colleagues[131] reported a 90% success rate in a large series of patients with recurrent coarctation. The fibrous perivascular postsurgical scar appears to allow safe use of this technique for recoarctation in contrast to the danger of aneurysm formation when balloon dilation is used for native coarctation of the aorta. A multicenter prospective study[132] of balloon angioplasty for recurrent coarctation of the aorta reported 200 patients from 26 institutions. The prior method of surgical repair did not affect the postangioplasty gradient relief or diameter. A residual gradient of more than 21 mm Hg was present in 41 patients (20%). There were five deaths (2.5%) from aortic rupture (1), unexplained sudden death (2), cerebrovascular accident (1), and left heart failure (1). One patient had a cerebrovascular accident, another aortic dissection requiring urgent surgical intervention. There were no late aneurysms. Hijazi et al[130] reported 27 patients undergoing balloon angioplasty for recurrent coarctation of the aorta. One patient was undilatable, one patient developed a stable aneurysm, and two patients developed restenosis. It would appear that balloon angioplasty is the initial procedure of choice for recurrent coarctation of the aorta following initial surgical repair.

Complications

The list of possible complications both during and following coarctation repair is extensive and their prevention requires careful attention to all details of the technique (Table 76–6).

Hemorrhage

During the time period that the aortic clamps are in place and following their removal, the anesthesiologist should have blood available and prepared for administration so that it is immediately accessible in the event of excessive suture line hemorrhage after clamp release. Even though none of the techniques utilized requires intravenous heparin (except if cardiopulmonary bypass is used) the suture lines nearly always have an initial moderate degree of bleeding until clots form within the needle holes. This can be particularly

TABLE 76–6. POTENTIAL COMPLICATIONS

Hemorrhage
Recurrent laryngeal nerve injury
Phrenic nerve injury
Homer's syndrome
Chylothorax
Hypertension
Paraplegia
Stroke
Aneurysm formation
Recoarctation
Left arm ischemia

dramatic after PTFE patch aortoplasty. At the termination of the procedure, chest tubes should be left in position to monitor and evacuate postoperative blood loss. Any sudden increase in the amount of bleeding from the chest tube should result in the patient's immediate return to the operating room for control of bleeding.

Paradoxical Postoperative Hypertension

That the correction of a coarctation of the aorta, an apparently straightforward cause of hypertension, can provoke a postoperative increase in blood pressure is unexpected and illogical, hence the name paradoxical hypertension.[133] The etiology of the postoperative hypertension is felt to occur secondary to two hypertensive responses.[134] The first response occurs immediately and subsides in most patients within 24 hours and is due to the release of the stretch on the baroreceptors in the carotid arteries and aortic arch after removal of the aortic obstruction. An increase in blood pressure occurs for a few hours after operation until the baroreceptors are set at a lower level. The best evidence for this is the marked increase in sympathetic activity indicated by elevations in norepinephrine level after operation.[135] This occurs in slightly over half of patients and in most cases subsides within 24 hours.[136] The second phase (which is more pronounced in diastole) appears within 48 to 72 hours and occurs in about one-third of those experiencing the first phase of hypertension. It is associated with elevated levels of renin and angiotensin, which may be stimulated by the first phase of paradoxical hypertension.[137,138] This second response may be the adaptation gone awry that ensures adequate flow to exercising muscles below the coarctation, above and beyond that delivered by increasing the systolic pressure.

Unchecked hypertension in either postoperative phase can have disastrous results. Because the mesenteric arteries have been accustomed to a very low blood pressure, the sudden increase of the mean arterial pressure in these arterioles may lead to severe reactive acute inflammatory changes. This may result in mesenteric arteritis and subsequent evolution to mesenteric ischemia.[139,140] The child then develops severe abdominal pain, distension, and tenderness. On occasion this will cause severe gastrointestinal bleeding and may require laparotomy with bowel resection. Thus postoperative hypertension must be very carefully monitored and managed. In the immediate postoperative period the administration of sodium nitroprusside intravenously can be used to titrate the blood pressure. We have also found it useful to use intravenous enalapril (angiotensin converting enzyme inhibitor) beginning shortly after the procedure with eventual conversion to oral captopril after several days. Oral propranolol is also quite useful in blunting the sympathetic response and managing the hypertensive response.[141] Gidding and co-workers showed that *preoperative* administration of propranolol helped prevent the postoperative hypertensive response.[142] Because of the risk of mesenteric arteritis, even in patients with well-controlled blood pressure, we usually keep our patients NPO for the first 48 hours following coarctation repair. The hypertension usually resolves within 2 to 4 wk after surgical correction although long-standing hypertension may occasionally occur following successful coarctation repair. The tendency to have persistence of the hypertension is proportional to the age of the child at the time of the operative repair.[143] Of course persistent hypertension following repair of coarctation of the aorta despite medical intervention merits investigation to rule out a recurrent coarctation.

Paraplegia

Paraplegia was first reported by Gross and Hufnagel[6] as a possible complication following coarctation of the aorta repair and to this day remains a serious and feared complication. Bing et al[144] reported the first human to develop paraplegia after coarctation repair in 1948. In a landmark review from 1972, Brewer et al[145] surveyed 12,532 cases of coarctation of the aorta repair and found an incidence of 0.41% spinal cord complications (1 in 250 patients). He was unable to correlate these complications with any specific factor such as number of intercostals divided or length of cross-clamp time. Lerberg et al[146] more recently reported an incidence of paraplegia of 1.5% (5/334). Paraplegia correlated with the length of aortic cross-clamping (mean cross-clamp time in those patients with paraplegia was 49 minutes) and the presence of an aberrant origin of the right subclavian artery below the coarctation (one of eight patients). Crawford and Sade[147] reported three patients in whom intraoperative hyperthermia appeared (temperature maximum 38.7°, 39.8°, 40°C) to play a significant role in the development of postoperative spinal cord injury. As previously discussed under operative technique, the distal aortic pressure would appear to be very important and should be kept over 40 to 45 mm Hg.[60] In younger infants where distal aortic pressure is not monitored, it is important that the proximal aortic pressure be kept high (150 to 200 mm Hg). Acidosis should be avoided during the time of the aortic cross-clamp as this may contribute to low cardiac output and hypotension.[63] Cerebrospinal fluid drainage has been reported to provide spinal cord protection.[148] Somatosensory evoked potentials (SSEP) are a possible method of assessing reversible spinal cord ischemia.[149]

In summary, to avoid paraplegia we recommend (1) aortic cross-clamp time as short as possible, (2) careful technical anastomosis so reapplication of clamps is not necessary, (3) moderate hypothermia (34° to 35°C), (4) high proximal blood pressure, (5) no acidosis, and (6) adequate distal mean blood pressure (> 40 mm Hg).

Aneurysm Formation

Both true and false aneurysms have been reported as complications after all types of coarctation of the aorta repair. Aneurysms are also known to occur in patients *not* undergoing surgical treatment.[81] However, there have been significantly more reports of true aneurysm formation following prosthetic patch aortoplasty. In 1980 Bergdahl and Ljungqvist[80] reported four adult patients with aneurysm formation in the aortic wall opposite a Dacron patch. Two of the patients had the patch placed at the time of reoperation after prior resection with end-to-end anastomosis. Microscopy revealed degenerative changes in the aortic wall opposite the patch. They postulated that the reason for the aneurysm formation was that part of the circumference of the aorta was replaced by a material with tensile characteristics differing from those of the aorta itself. In 1986 Rheuban and associates[84] reported eight aneurysms in a follow-up of 45 patients who had Dacron patch aortoplasty at a mean age of 8.5 years. In this series if a significant coarctation ridge was noted it was excised, even though the authors state this did not increase the incidence of aneurysm formation. Clarkson et al[85] reported "aneurysm" formation in 5 of 38 patients (13%) in whom a Dacron patch aortoplasty was performed. In 20 of these patients the intimal ridge was excised. Only one patient had a true aneurysm after primary coarctation repair without excision of the intima, four patients had false aneurysms. Del Nido et al[88] reported a 5% incidence of aneurysm formation after 63 patch aortoplasties. Two of the three patients developing an aneurysm had the patch placed as a repair of recoarctation following primary resection of coarctation with end-to-end anastomosis during infancy. These were repaired using partial left heart bypass with a left atrial-to-descending aorta or femoral bypass. Interposition of a Dacron tube graft with resection of the aneurysm was the procedure of choice.

In one of the largest series reported, starting with the patients originally operated on by Vossschulte, Hehrlein et al[83] reported 18 aneurysms occurring in 317 patients (6%). Of the 14 patients for whom detailed information was available, 12 of 14 had an extensive resection of the fibrous coarctation membrane. Hehrlein and associates concluded that resection of a fibrous membrane of the aortic isthmus at the first intervention seemed to be an essential predisposing factor for development of aneurysms and the posterior ridge should not be excised. Experimental evidence confirming this observation was provided by DeSanto et al,[82] who studied Dacron and PTFE patches in dogs with and without concomitant intimal excision opposite the patch. Aneurysms formed in 8 of 12 dogs undergoing intimal excision and none of the control animals. Heikkinen et al[86] reported histopathological studies of aneurysms and found medionecrosis in 13 of 14 patients and foreign body reaction in 11 patients. They concluded that these patients have an inherent weakness of the segment of the aortic wall owing to medial cystic degeneration. The same group reported successful management of such patients with aneurysm resection and insertion of a tubular prosthesis using femorofemoral or left atriofemoral bypass.[89] This group, which has the highest reported incidence of aneurysm formation (33%), speculated that this might reflect the fact that most of the patients were adults when the primary repair was done. Acquired components and prolonged hemodynamic stress may have weakened the aortic wall of these patients. Recent series using PTFE for the patch have not reported any aneurysms although the follow-up period is short.[87,91] The risk of aneurysm formation would appear to be higher for patients operated on at >15 years of age or operated on as a recoarctation following resection with end-to-end anastomosis.

Recoarctation and Reoperation

Recurrent or residual coarctation has been reported after every type of coarctation repair. The rate of recurrence for each procedure from different institutions can vary widely because there are so many variables affecting the recoarctation rate. These include associated lesions contributing to mortality, actual morphology of the coarctation, age and condition of the child at the time of surgery, and the definition of recoarctation itself. Numerous factors have been shown to increase the risk of recoarctation including age less than 2 to 3 mo,[73,107,108] weight less than 5 kg,[72] the morphology of the coarctation,[90] silk suture material instead of polypropylene,[77] and residual ductal tissue.[150]

Recoarctation is usually defined as a postoperative arm-to-leg peak systolic pressure gradient exceeding 20 mm Hg across the repaired area.[151] The resting gradient is not necessarily sensitive enough to "rule out" significant hypertension seen with exercise. Simultaneous arm/leg pressure measurements after exercise are the best way to exclude the possibility of residual obstruction at the coarctation repair site.[152] Magnetic resonance imaging, digital subtraction angiography, and bicycle exercise testing may also be useful in detecting residual coarctation of the aorta.[153]

It seems clear that the initial reports of resection and end-to-end anastomosis had a high recoarctation rate.[68] This was probably secondary to the use of silk sutures instead of the currently available fine monofilament suture, inadequate resection of all ductal tissue that may extend into areas of normal-appearing aorta, lack of growth at a circumferential suture line, and lack of growth of a hypoplastic transverse arch. Recent reports of resection and end-to-end anastomosis using microvascular technique appear to have a much lower recoarctation rate.[75] The subclavian flap aortoplasty, although originally felt to nearly eliminate recoarctation,[105] definitely has a rate of recoarctation higher than initially thought.[69] The patch aortoplasty is excellent for older children, but probably should not be used in infants because of the high recoarctation rate. Resection with extended end-to-end anastomosis appears to have the lowest recoarctation rate,[73,74] but may not necessarily be required for *all* neonates. Also, the follow-up of these patients is short. Our current approach is to use either subclavian flap aortoplasty or resection with extended end-to-end anastomosis for neonates on prostaglandin E_1, based on the arch morphology. For older children we use patch aorto-

plasty, but continue to monitor these patients for aneurysm formation.

As discussed in the section on balloon angioplasty, this procedure is now considered the initial procedure of choice for most children with recurrent coarctation of the aorta.[126,132] The initial success rate is high with a low incidence of complications. If balloon dilation is not successful or for some reason is not felt to be indicated, reoperation may be required. In most cases reoperation is considerably more difficult owing to dense scarring in the region of the previous repair. The gradient is usually not high, decreasing the impetus for collateral formation and increasing the risk of spinal cord complications.[154] The previously discussed indications for partial left atriofemoral bypass or temporary aortic shunts to maintain adequate distal aortic perfusion pressure should be seriously considered for every reoperation. No single technique of reoperation is applicable to all patients but the majority of patients can be managed by either patch graft angioplasty, resection and interposition graft, or a local bypass graft technique.[155] Reresection and primary end-to-end anastomosis may be difficult secondary to adhesions and the amount of mobilization required to avoid tension on the suture line of what is usually a very friable aorta.

Sweeney et al[155] reported 53 patients who underwent reoperation for aortic coarctation. Interestingly, no temporary shunts or left heart bypass was used, all patients survived, and there were no instances of paraplegia. Twenty-six patients had Dacron patch angioplasty, 16 had bypass grafts around the coarctation, 8 had resection and interposition grafting, and 3 had resection and end-to-end anastomosis. Only three patients had a postoperative gradient more than 10 mm Hg and none more than 20 mm Hg. Kron et al[156] reported 24 reinterventions in 23 patients with recoarctation with one death and no paraplegia. Techniques employed included patch aortoplasty (13), balloon dilation (6), end-to-end anastomosis (2), interposition graft (2), and subclavian flap (1). He recommends balloon dilation as primary therapy for restenosis. For patients with a long segment recoarctation, very dense adhesions, or requiring a cardiac operation, Jacob et al[157] has reported success in 10 patients using an ascending aorta-to-descending aorta bypass graft placed with a combined left thoracotomy, median sternotomy approach. Moderate-to-severe hemodynamic abnormalities may persist during exercise after reoperation for coarctation of the aorta.[158] Diligent efforts to repair all hemodynamically significant residual and recurrent coarctations are necessary if the natural fate of premature death is to be avoided for patients with these lesions.

Conclusion

The management of both the infant and child with coarctation of the aorta remains controversial. PGE_1 has dramatically improved the outcome for neonates with critical coarctation. We recommend either subclavian flap aortoplasty or resection with extended end-to-end anastomosis for neonates based on the morphology of the transverse arch. The smaller the arch, the more we lean toward resection with extended end-to-end anastomosis. For complex coarctation of the aorta, transmediastinal repair of the cardiac defect and resection with extended end-to-end anastomosis may prove to provide the best outcome. We continue to utilize patch aortoplasty with PTFE for children over 1 year of age; however, the risk of aneurysm formation has led some groups to prefer resection with end-to-end anastomosis. Balloon dilatation is the initial procedure of choice for recoarctation. If this is unsuccessful, reoperation with patch aortoplasty or graft interposition has good results.

INTERRUPTED AORTIC ARCH

Interrupted aortic arch is a rare, severe congenital cardiac lesion in which there is loss of luminal continuity between the ascending and descending aorta. Blood flow into the descending aorta is provided by a large ductus arteriosus. This uncommon lesion was first described by Steidele[159] in 1778 and was later classified into three types of Celoria and Patton.[160] If interrupted aortic arch is untreated, the median age at death is 4 days in 90% of infants, usually following closure of the ductus arteriosus.[5] Interrupted aortic arch is rarely an isolated lesion and in 70 to 90% of cases there is an associated large, isolated ventricular septal defect.[5] Other commonly associated anomalies include bicuspid aortic valve, left ventricular outflow tract obstruction, DiGeorge syndrome, truncus arteriosus, single ventricle, transposition of the great arteries, and aortopulmonary window.[4] The incidence of each of these associated anomalies is shown in Table 76–7.

Anatomy and Embryology

The classification system first designed and now most commonly used for interrupted aortic arch is that of Celoria and Patton (Fig. 76–15).[160] Type A interruption occurs distal to the left subclavian artery at the level of the aortic isthmus.

TABLE 76–7. ASSOCIATED ANOMALIES IN INTERRUPTED AORTIC ARCH

Anomaly	Frequency Rate (%)
VSD (malalignment)	70–90
Bicuspid aortic valve	30–50
Left ventricular outflow obstruction	25–40
DiGeorge syndrome	15–30
Truncus arteriosus	10
Single ventricle	5
Aortopulmonary window	4
Transposition of the great arteries	3

The innominate, left carotid, and left subclavian arteries all originate from the ascending aorta. The descending aorta is supplied with blood flow exclusively from the patent ductus arteriosus. This accounts for 25 to 35% of patients with interrupted aortic arch.[185] Type B interruption occurs between the left common carotid artery and the left subclavian artery. This is the most common form of interrupted aortic arch and accounts for 60 to 70% of all cases. The type B interruption is frequently associated with aberrant origin of the right subclavian artery from the descending aorta. There is an increased risk of left ventricular outflow tract obstruction secondary to subaortic stenosis with aberrant origin of the right subclavian artery. Type C interruption is the most rare occurring in less than 5% of these patients. Type C interruption occurs between the innominate artery takeoff and the left common carotid.

Embryology

The embryologic etiology of interrupted aortic arch is multifactorial in nature. The large ventricular septal defect causes preferential shunting of blood into the pulmonary artery and ductus arteriosus in utero, leading to a reduction of flow in the ascending aorta and the potential for aortic arch interruption.[20] Embryologically the different segments of the arch of the aorta are derived from different components. Interrupted aortic arch may be the result of a disappearance of the normally persisting connection between the left fourth and sixth arches as a result of flow imbalance in early cardiogenesis.[161] The proximal aortic arch is derived from the aortic sac, the distal aortic arch from the fourth embryonic arch, and the isthmus from the junction of the sixth embryonic arch (ductus) with the left dorsal aorta and fourth embryonic arch.[162] Celoria and Patton[160] postulated that type A interrupted aortic arch resulted from regression or atrophy of the segment of the aortic arch between the ductus arteriosus and the left subclavian artery. Type B represented a failure of formation of the left fourth arch since the left subclavian remains with the descending aorta. Finally, type C was attributed to partial or complete failure of formation of the left third and fourth arches and persistence of the segment of the dorsal aorta between these arches as the left common carotid artery. The high incidence of DiGeorge syndrome and anomalous origin of the right subclavian artery in interrupted aortic arch type B have aided in the understanding of the embryology of this lesion. Neonatal hypocalcemia and defective thymic dependent cellular immunity (the DiGeorge syndrome) are related to abnormal development of the thymus and parathyroid glands, which are derived embryologically from the third and fourth pharyngeal pouches, and many of these patients have anomalies of the aortic arch.[163] The importance of the neural crest in the development of the pharyngeal arch derivatives has been demonstrated by removing or cauterizing premigratory neural crest in chick embryos, creating anomalies of

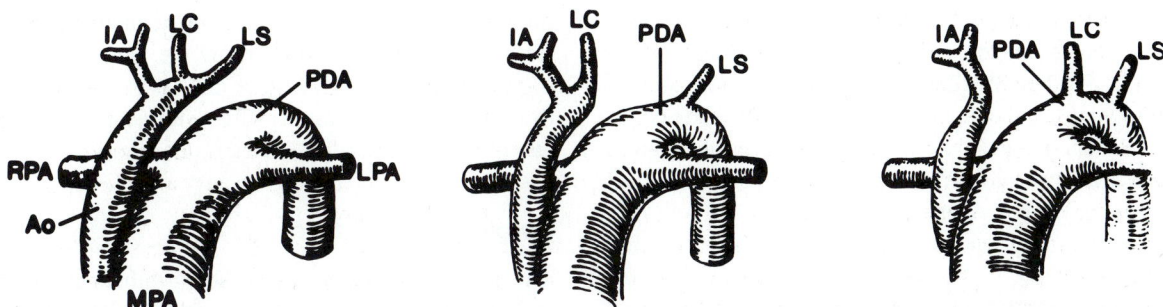

Figure 76–15. Interrupted aortic arch. The three types A, B, and C as originally described by Celoria and Patton, as based on the origin of the brachiocephalic vessels. **Left.** Type A, interruption distal to the left subclavian artery. **Center.** Type B, interruption between the left subclavian and left carotid arteries. **Right.** Type C, interruption between the left carotid and innominate arteries. The percentages listed below each illustration are the incidence of each type as found in a review of the literature by Van Praagh et al[185] in 1971. AO, aorta; IA, innominate artery; LC, left carotid artery; LPA, MPA, RPA, left, main, and right pulmonary arteries; LS, left subclavian artery; PDA, patent ductus arteriosus. *(Reproduced with permission from Jonas RA: Interrupted aortic arch. In Mavroudis C, Backer CL (eds): Pediatric Cardiac Surgery, ed. 2. St. Louis, Mosby–Year Book, 1994, p 184.)*

both the truncal conal regions of the heart and the aortic arch system.[164,165]

Pathophysiology and Clinical Presentation

Most infants with interrupted aortic arch present within the first few days of life, generally at the time of ductus closure. When the ductus begins to close the reduction or loss of systemic blood flow to the lower extremities causes acidosis, anuria, necrotizing enterocolitis, and hepatic ischemia. In addition to the poor peripheral perfusion of the lower body, the pulmonary circulation is flooded as the pulmonary vascular resistance drops, causing severe congestive heart failure. Cardiac decompensation rapidly ensues with tachypnea, tachycardia, and possibly cardiac arrest. The infant will appear gray, listless, and cyanotic. Examination for pulses will reveal usually only a right radial pulse in the common type B interrupted aortic arch, or in some cases with type A interrupted aortic arch only a right and left radial pulse. A patient with type B interruption and aberrant origin of the right subclavian artery may have no pulses palpable in any of the extremities. Rapid resuscitation is required.

The most important contribution to the medical management of interrupted aortic arch was the introduction of prostaglandin E_1. Use of prostaglandin E_1 specifically for interrupted aortic arch was confirmed by Heymann and associates[40] in 1979. Careful resuscitation of the neonate with prostaglandin E_1 over a timespan of several days is associated with a dramatic improvement in surgical outcome. Prostaglandin E_1 opens the ductus arteriosus and allows perfusion of the lower extremities, including the kidney, liver, and gut.

After the child has had successful establishment of ductal patency, attention should be directed to the technique of ventilation. It is important that the elevated pulmonary vascular resistance is maintained to increase the amount of blood flowing to the systemic circulation and decrease the amount of blood passing through the pulmonary circulation. This can be achieved by avoiding a high level of inspired oxygen, as well as avoiding respiratory alkalosis caused by hyperventilation. Control of ventilation is best achieved by intubation, sedation, and paralysis with pancuronium. The pCO_2 should be maintained at a level between 40 and 50 mm Hg. Metabolic acidosis must be aggressively treated with sodium bicarbonate, although care must be taken to avoid producing an overall alkalotic pH. Myocardial function is, in almost all cases, depressed because of the acidosis and time necessary for resuscitation and this will respond to an inotropic agent such as dopamine or dobutamine. Dopamine also maximizes renal perfusion in the context of the ischemic renal insult. Most infants who are intubated, ventilated, placed on prostaglandin E_1, administered sodium bicarbonate, and given inotropic support will have excellent organ function recovery and may be taken to the operating room on a more elective basis. Of note, the DiGeorge syndrome with absent thymus and associated hypocalcemia and immunologic deficiency occurs in 15 to 30% of infants with interrupted aortic arch.[4] These neonates require treatment for hypocalcemia and should receive only irradiated blood. This syndrome should be pursued routinely and the presence or absence of thymic tissue should be noted at the time of surgery.

Diagnostic Techniques

Historically, angiography has been used to assess the hemodynamics, intracardiac morphology, and precise arch anatomy of interrupted aortic arch.[21] The ascending aorta is usually about half the normal diameter; it has no arch curvature but ascends straight toward the head, generally with two branches of equal size, the angiographic "V" sign. The main pulmonary artery is very large with the descending aorta a direct continuation of the ductus arteriosus from the pulmonary artery. More recently, echocardiography has been used alone to make the diagnosis of interrupted aortic arch[166] (Fig. 76–16). The combination of two-dimensional echocardiography and color Doppler, along with increasing experience, has enabled this in many instances to be the only study used prior to surgical intervention.[167] Echocar-

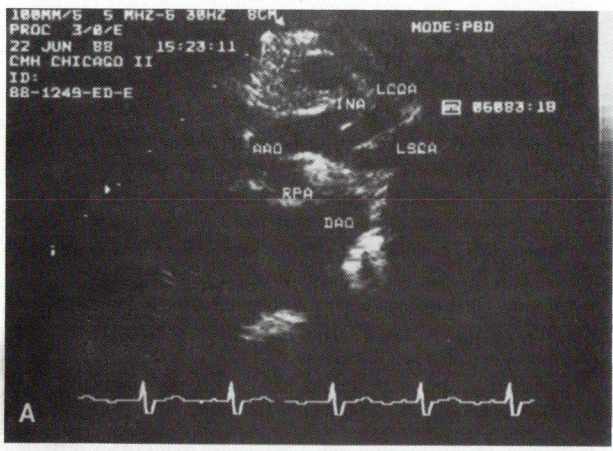

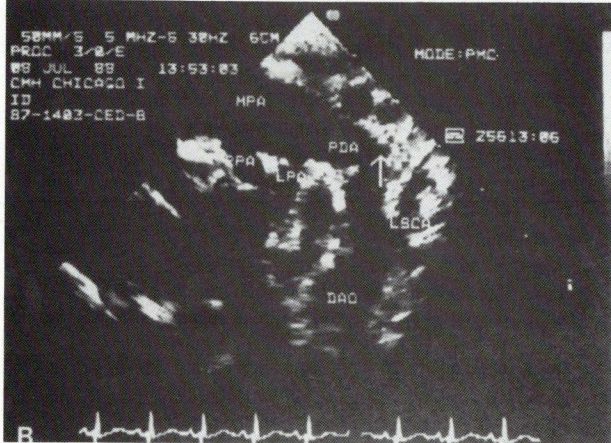

Figure 76–16. Two-dimensional echocardiographic images of aortic arch interruption. **A.** Type A interrupted aortic arch as viewed from the suprasternal notch long-axis plane. Note the interruption distal to the left subclavian artery. **B.** Type B interruption as seen from the high left parasternal view. The patent ductus arteriosus enters the descending aorta near the left subclavian artery and the interruption occurs proximal to the left subclavian artery *(arrow)*. The more proximal aortic arch is not visualized in this view. Care should be taken not to mistake the "ductus arch," i.e., the arch formed by the main pulmonary artery, patent ductus arteriosus, and descending aorta, as seen here, for the true aortic arch, which gives rise to the brachiocephalic vessels. AAO, ascending aorta; DAO, descending aorta; INA, innominate artery; LCCA, left common carotid artery; LPA, left pulmonary artery; LSCA, left subclavian artery; MPA, main pulmonary artery; PDA, patent ductus arteriosus; RPA, right pulmonary artery. *(Reproduced with permission from Webb CL, Berdusis K: Echocardiographic diagnosis of coarctation of the aorta and aortic arch interruption. In Mavroudis C, Backer CL (eds): Coarctation and Interrupted Aortic Arch. Philadelphia, Hanley & Belfus; Cardiac Surgery: State of the Art Reviews 7:47–71, 1993.)*

diography should localize the site of interruption, tell the length of the discontinuity, show the narrowest dimension of the left ventricular outflow tract as related to the posterior displacement of the conal septum, and reveal the diameter of the aortic anulus and ascending aorta.

Surgical Management

The surgical approach for children with interrupted aortic arch remains controversial. The first successful correction of interrupted aortic arch was apparently performed by J. Maxwell Chamberlin in 1954 and reported by Gokcebay et al[168] in 1972. This patient had no associated cardiac defects and the interrupted aortic arch was repaired with an aortic homograft through a left thoracotomy. Samson described a successful surgical repair in 1955 in a patient with a short segment type A interrupted aortic arch utilizing a direct anastomosis.[13] The associated ventricular septal defects were successfully closed 4 years later. Single-stage complete repair from a median sternotomy approach using a Teflon graft was first reported by Barratt-Boyes et al[15] in 1972. In 1975 Trusler and Izukawa[16] reported the first anatomically complete correction without prosthetic material. Even today there is controversy within the literature with regard to the best approach, staged correction versus single-stage complete repair.[169,170] Both methods continue to have advocates and the advantages and disadvantages of both are reviewed.

Staged Correction

Prior to the widespread use of cardiopulmonary bypass techniques in neonates, this approach was really the only safe alternative (see Fig. 76–17). The classic first operation is through a left posterolateral thoracotomy. Arterial monitoring is achieved through the right radial artery unless the right subclavian artery originates distal to the interruption in which case the temporal artery is used. The ascending and descending aorta, along with the patent ductus arteriosus and the aortic arch branches, are dissected. The patent ductus arteriosus is ligated. From that point the operation must progress swiftly because of minimal blood flow to the lower extremities. The aortic arch may be reconstructed directly without prosthetic material using endogenous vessels as described by Tyson et al.[171] Alternatively, a PTFE interposition graft may be used as described by Sturm et al.[172] An 8- or 10-mm PTFE graft is anastomosed between the ascending and descending aorta with 7-0 polypropylene suture. The graft is kept as short as possible and beveled to prevent kinking. In either case the clamps are released to reestablish blood flow to the descending aorta within 30 min. Next the pericardium is opened anterior to the phrenic nerve to gain access to the great vessels. A Teflon-impregnated Dacron band is placed around the pulmonary artery using a subtraction technique with the aorta. The band is then sequentially tightened until the pressure distal to the

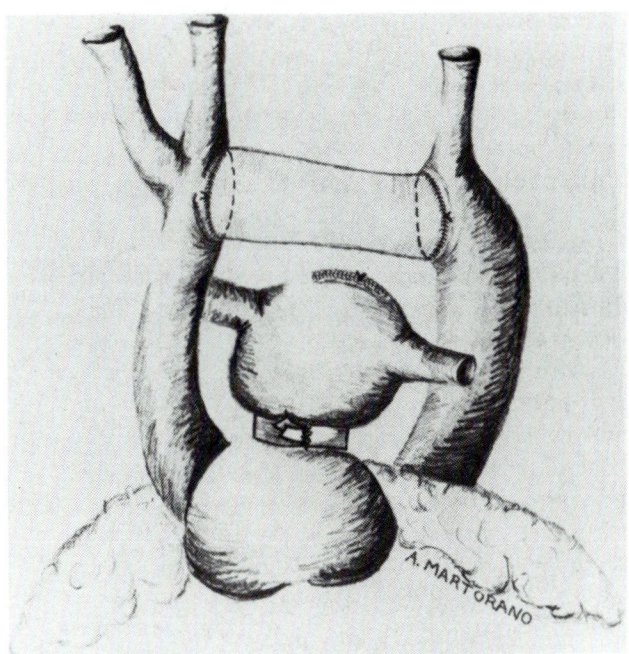

Figure 76–17. Staged correction of interrupted aortic arch. Illustration shows first stage with PTFE interposition graft between the ascending and descending aorta and pulmonary artery band. *(Reproduced with permission from Backer CL, Mavroudis C: Interrupted aortic arch. In Mavroudis C, Backer CL (eds): Coarctation and Interrupted Aortic Arch. Philadelphia, Hanley & Belfus; Cardiac Surgery: State of the Art Reviews 7:105–117, 1993.)*

band is 40% or less of systemic systolic blood pressure. The banding should increase the peripheral arterial pressure by 10 to 15 mm Hg but should not be so tight as to produce peripheral oxygen arterial desaturation below 85%. After the child has recovered from the first stage, elective cardiac catheterization is performed to prepare for the second stage. The timing of the second stage has changed over the years, but the ideal time is now thought to be only 2 to 3 mo after the initial palliation.[14] Through a median sternotomy and using extracorporeal circulation the ventricular septal defect is closed (usually through the right atrium) with a prosthetic patch and the pulmonary artery band is removed. Reconstruction of the pulmonary artery in the area of the prior pulmonary artery band is required. If a PTFE graft is used in the initial repair the child is subject to multiple revisions as somatic growth occurs. In most cases a third operation (stage 3) is required when the child is 8 to 12 years of age and begins to develop a significant gradient across the PTFE graft. Often a second conduit, preferably 16 to 20 mm in size, can be placed between the ascending and descending aorta to augment flow through the neonatal graft. The results of staged repair of interrupted aortic arch in recent series are shown in Table 76–8.[14,173–178] Although the survival in some series[14,176] is quite good, others[174,175] have reported no or few long-term survivors using a staged approach.

Single Stage Complete Repair

Theoretically, a single reparative operation is preferable to a staged approach in which two or more operations are required to obtain a complete repair. This is now the accepted standard for many other congenital heart defects. Early reports[179] of primary repair utilized a graft interposition with ventricular septal defect closure, while more recent series[180] have emphasized direct anastomosis of the arch. Primary definitive repair avoids the potential problems of a prosthetic graft that does not grow and the complications associated with pulmonary artery banding.[181] The complexity of the single reparative operation must, however, be kept in perspective in considering the one-stage repair. In addition there are two complications associated with the one-stage repair including compression of the right pulmonary artery or the left main bronchus, neither of which occurs with the two-stage approach.[14] The technique of single-stage complete repair is performed as follows and illustrated in Figure 76–18.

Through a median sternotomy the head vessels, right

TABLE 76–8. RESULTS WITH STAGED REPAIR OF INTERRUPTED AORTIC ARCH[a]

Series	Year	Technique (First Stage)	Patients	Survival (%) Stage I	Stage II	Overall Survival (%)
Fowler[173]	1984	PTFE graft, PAB	12	75	60	67
Hammon[174]	1986	End-to-end, PAB	7	14	—	0
Scott[175]	1988	PTFE graft, PAB	7	71	—	28
		End-to-side, PAB	3	100	100	100
Lamberti[176]	1991	PTFE graft, PAB	19	95	88	79
Irwin[14]	1991	PTFE graft, PAB	20	100	83	75
Griffin[177]	1992	Direct aortoplasty, no PAB	11	100	80	73
CHSS[178]	1994	Repair IAA, PAB	40	65	NS	—

[a]CHSS, Congenital Heart Surgeon's Society; IAA, interrupted aortic arch; PAB, pulmonary artery band.

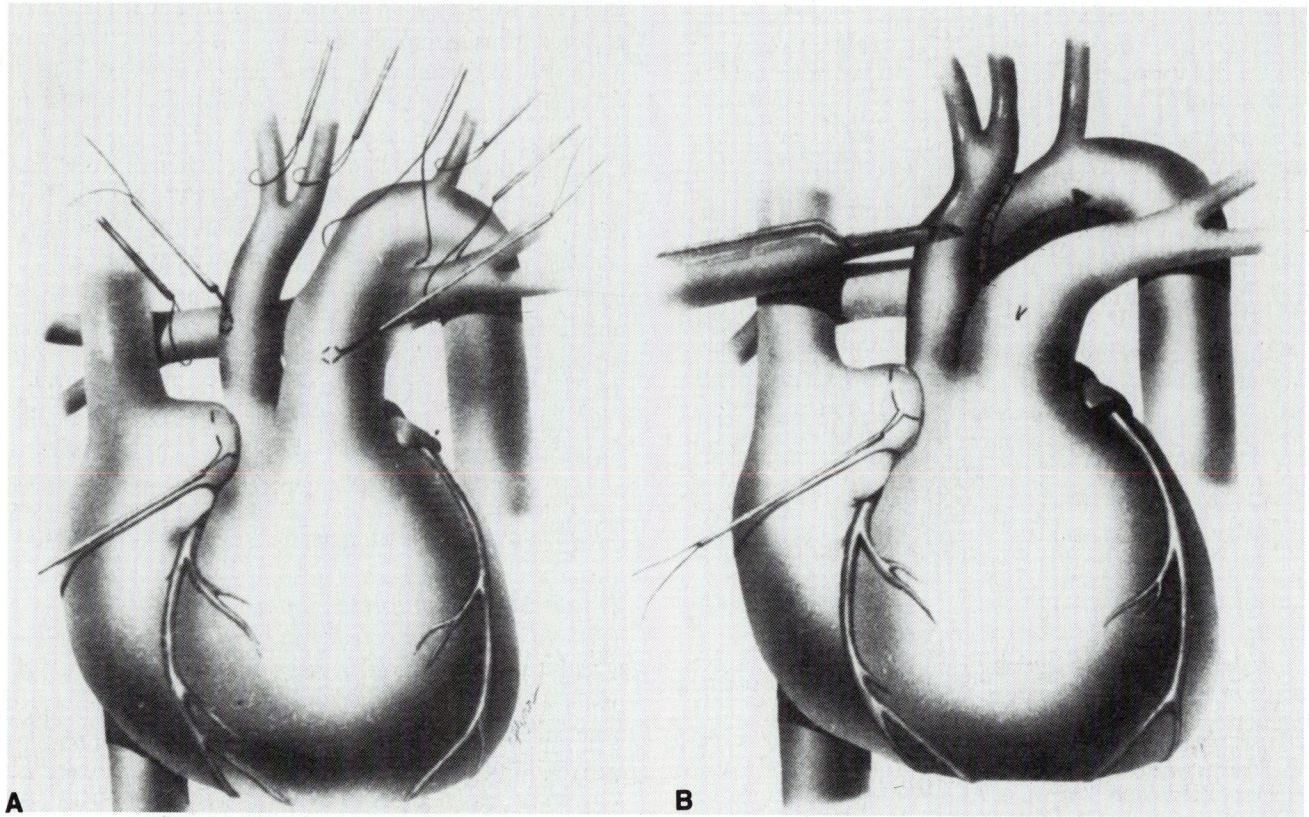

Figure 76–18. Complete one-stage repair of interrupted aortic arch. **A.** Purse strings on the aorta and pulmonary arteries indicate the siting of the two arterial cannulas. Before cannulation, all of the vessels are thoroughly dissected to maximize their mobility and minimize tension on the anastomosis. **B.** The completed anastomosis is shown. *(Reproduced with permission from: Sell JE, Jonas RA, Mayer JE et al: The results of a surgical program for interrupted aortic arch. J Thorac Cardiovasc Surg 96:864–877, 1988.)*

and left pulmonary arteries, and ductus arteriosus are encircled with vessel loops. Cannulation of both the ascending and descending aorta (via the pulmonary artery and ductus arteriosus) may be employed to facilitate cooling to 18°C. During cardiopulmonary bypass the right and left pulmonary arteries are occluded with tourniquets to prevent flooding of the lungs and to maintain systemic pressure. Circulatory arrest is used for resection of all ductal tissue followed by end-to-side anastomosis of the ascending and descending aorta. The ventricular septal defect is closed through the pulmonary trunk or the right atrium. Results with single-stage complete repair are illustrated in Table 76–9.[174,175,178,180,182–184] In a large series of neonates with interrupted aortic arch that underwent single-stage complete repair at Boston Children's Hospital, mortality rate declined strikingly over time as experience was gained.[180] The two chief complications following complete repair were development of left ventricular outflow tract obstruction and persistent or recurrent aortic arch obstruction. Left ventricular outflow tract obstruction developed in 8 of 33 patients (24%) and recurrent or persistent aortic arch obstruction became evident after repair in 15 patients. When direct anas-

tomosis was used, treatment of recurrent aortic arch obstruction with percutaneous balloon aortoplasty was successful.[131]

The largest series of infants with interrupted aortic arch to date is the multiinstitutional report from the Congenital Heart Surgeon's Society et al.[178] The study entered 183 neonates between 1987 and 1992. Of these, 116 under-

TABLE 76–9. RESULTS OF SINGLE-STAGE COMPLETE REPAIR OF INTERRUPTED AORTIC ARCH[a]

Series	Year	Patients	Survival (%)	Reoperation (%)
Moulton[182]	1981	5	80	NS
Hammon[174]	1986	8	88	12
Scott[175]	1988	11	73	NS
Sell[180]	1988	14	71	29
Menahem[183]	1992	26	77	NS
Yasui[184]	1993	20	90	17
CHSS[178]	1994	116	62	NS

[a]CHSS, Congenital Heart Surgeon's Society.

went single-stage repair with 44 deaths (38%). Forty underwent repair of interrupted aortic arch and pulmonary artery band with 14 deaths (35%). Risk factors for death were low birth weight, younger age at repair, interrupted arch type B, outlet and trabecular ventricular septal defects, smaller size of the ventricular septal defect, and subaortic narrowing.

Interrupted Aortic Arch with Severe Subaortic Stenosis

Some infants with interrupted aortic arch will have severe subaortic stenosis requiring attention in the neonatal time period. The infundibular septum is displaced posteriorly, the opposite to the anteriorly displaced infundibular septum seen in Fallot's tetralogy. For these patients Van Praagh et al[185] described a palliative procedure in 1972 creating an "artificial ductus" (prosthetic tube graft) from the proximal pulmonary artery to the distal aorta along with ligation of the native patent ductus arteriosus and distal banding of the main pulmonary artery. Other authors[186] reported survivors with this technique. More recently, Menahem et al[187] recommended complete single-stage repair of this lesion with resection of the infundibular septum and closure of the ventricular septal defect with either a transpulmonary artery or trans-right atrial approach. Bove et al[188] recently reported a similar technique in 7 patients with 1 late death and no residual subaortic gradients.

Interrupted Aortic Arch With Transposition of the Great Arteries

Transposition of the great arteries occurs in 3% of infants with interrupted aortic arch and among infants with transposition of the great arteries 1.5% have interrupted aortic arch. First attempts at repair of transposition of the great arteries with interrupted aortic arch focused on initial arch repair and pulmonary artery banding followed by remote Mustard/Senning operation with removal of the pulmonary artery band. Because of the advances in the arterial switch procedure the current approach to this combination of lesions is complete primary repair in the neonatal period with arterial switch and simultaneous aortic arch reconstruction and ventricular septal defect closure. Planché and associates[189] recently reported a comparison between single and two-stage repair of transposition of the great arteries with ventricular septal defect and aortic arch obstruction. Overall early mortality with a staged approach (26 patients) was 31% with 11 of the patients requiring a reoperation. With a single-stage procedure (14 patients) early mortality was 14% with only 2 patients requiring reoperation. They concluded that the single-stage procedure (1) allows complete repair in neonates without the need for multiple reoperations and (2) may decrease early mortality, length of intensive care unit stay, and reoperation rate.

Interrupted Aortic Arch With Truncus Arteriosus

Type A4 truncus arteriosus is defined by Van Praagh and Van Praagh[190] as interrupted aortic arch (usually type B) with truncus arteriosus. The truncus gives rise to an ascending aorta with brachiocephalic vessels and a pulmonary artery that in turn gives rise to the right and left pulmonary arteries as well as a patent ductus arteriosus that feeds the descending aorta. The first successful repair of this anomaly was reported by Gomes and McGoon[191] in 1971. The largest series of infants with truncus arteriosus and interrupted aortic arch was reported by Sano et al[192] in 1990. Seven patients with this lesion underwent repair through a median sternotomy with cardiopulmonary bypass, hypothermia, cardioplegia, and circulatory arrest. The aortic arch was reconstructed by direct anastomosis with total excision of ductal tissue. Right ventricle-to-pulmonary artery continuity was established with a valved conduit. There were no early or late deaths in this series.

Conclusions

Surgical management of the infant with interrupted aortic arch continues to have a mortality rate higher than that for many other congenital lesions because of the commonly associated defects such as DiGeorge syndrome, subaortic stenosis, truncus arteriosus, and transposition of the great arteries. The initial medical management has been greatly improved by the administration of prostaglandin E_1, which stabilizes the neonate prior to diagnostic and therapeutic interventions. Controversy still exists with regard to optimal surgical management. Historically the two-stage repair with initial arch repair and pulmonary artery banding followed by remote repair of the associated cardiac defects, was the first successful technique and has now been perfected to a high degree at several institutions. Primary complete repair is a more complex innovative technique requiring circulatory arrest but having the advantage of complete correction with a single operation early in life. The optimal technique for repair of these critically ill neonates must be individualized to the institution and surgeon, but the trend seems to be toward that of complete early definitive primary repair in the neonatal period.

REFERENCES

1. Keith JD: Coarctation of the aorta. In Keith JD, Rowe RD, Vlad P (eds): *Heart Disease in Infancy and Childhood,* 3rd ed. New York, Macmillan, 1978, pp 736–760
2. Rudolph AM: *Congenital Disease of the Heart.* Chicago, Year-Book, 1974
3. Tawes RL Jr, Aberdeen E, Waterston DJ, Bonham-Carter RE: Coarctation of the aorta in infants and children: A review of 333 operative cases, including 179 infants. *Circulation* **39–40**(suppl I):I-173–I-184, 1969
4. Van Mierop LHS, Kutsche LM: Development of the aortic arch sys-

tem and pathogenesis of coarctation of the aorta and interrupted aortic arch. In Mavroudis C, Backer CL (eds): *Coarctation and Interrupted Aortic Arch*. Philadelphia, Hanley and Belfus; *Cardiac Surgery: State of the Art Reviews* 7:1–22, 1993

5. Collins-Nakai RL, Dick M, Parisi-Buckley L, et al: Interrupted aortic arch in infancy. *J Pediatr* 88:959–962, 1976

6. Gross RE, Hufnagel CA: Coarctation of the aorta. Experimental studies regarding its surgical correction. *N Engl J Med* 233:287–293, 1945

7. Crafoord C, Nylin G: Congenital coarctation of the aorta and its surgical treatment. *J Thorac Surg* 14:347–361, 1945

8. Gross RE, Hubbard JP: Surgical ligation of a patent ductus arteriosus. *JAMA* 112:729–731, 1939

9. Blalock A, Taussig HB: The surgical treatment of malformations of the heart in which there is pulmonary stenosis or atresia. *JAMA* 128:189–202, 1945

10. Vossschulte K: Surgical correction of coarctation of the aorta by an "isthmusplastic" operation. *Thorax* 16:338–345, 1961

11. Waldhausen JA, Nahrwold DL: Repair of coarctation of the aorta with a subclavian flap. *J Thorac Cardiovasc Surg* 51:532–533, 1966

12. Lansman S, Shapiro AJ, Schiller MS, et al: Extended aortic arch anastomoses for repair of coarctation in infancy. *Circulation* 74(Suppl I):I-37–I-41, 1986

13. Merrill DL, Webster CA, Samson PC: Congenital absence of the aortic isthmus: Report of a case with successful surgical repair. *J Thorac Surg* 33:311–320, 1957

14. Irwin ED, Braunlin EA, Foker JE: Staged repair of interrupted aortic arch and ventricular septal defect in infancy. *Ann Thorac Surg* 52:632–639, 1991

15. Barratt-Boyes BG, Nicholls TT, Brandt PWT, Neutze JM: Aortic arch interruption associated with patent ductus arteriosus, ventricular septal defect, and total anomalous pulmonary venous connection. *J Thorac Cardiovasc Surg* 63:367–373, 1972

16. Trusler GA, Izukawa T: Interrupted aortic arch and ventricular septal defect. *J Thorac Cardiovasc Surg* 69:126–131, 1975

17. Morgagni JB: De sedibus et causis morborum. *Epist* **XVIII**:Article 6, 1760

18. Bonnet LM: Stenose congenitale de l'aorte. *Rev Med Paris* 23:108, 1903

19. Van Praagh R, O'Connor B, Chacko KA: Aortic coarctation. Pathology of the malformation. First World Congress of Pediatric Cardiac Surgery, Bergamo, June 1988, p 5 (abstract)

20. Rudolph AM, Heymann MA, Spitznas U: Hemodynamic considerations in the development of narrowing of the aorta. *Am J Cardiol* 30:514–525, 1972

21. Muster AJ: Angiographic anatomy of aortic coarctation: A classification based on the associated morphology of the aortic arch. In Mavroudis C, Backer CL (eds): *Coarctation and Interrupted Aortic Arch*. Philadelphia, Hanley and Belfus; *Cardiac Surgery: State of the Art Reviews* 7:23–45, 1993

22. Shone JD, Sellers RD, Anderson RC, et al: The developmental complex of "parachute mitral valve," supravalvular ring of left atrium, subaortic stenosis, and coarctation of aorta. *Am J Cardiol* 11:714–725, 1963

23. Lev M: Pathologic anatomy and interrelationship of hypoplasia of the aortic tract complexes. *Lab Invest* 1:61, 1952

24. Skoda J: Demonstration eines Falles von Obliteration der Aorta. *Wochenblatt der Zeitschrift der Kaiserlichen-Königliche Gesellschaft der Aertze zur Wein* 1:710–720, 1855

25. Elzenga NJ, Gittenberger-de Groot AC, Oppenheimer-Dekker A: Coarctation and other obstructive aortic arch anomalies: Their relationship to the ductus arteriosus. *Int J Cardiol* 13:289–308, 1986

26. Russell GA, Berry PJ, Watterson K, et al: Patterns of ductal tissue in coarctation in the first three months of life. *J Thorac Cardiovasc Surg* 102:596–601, 1991

27. Kappetein AP, Gittenberger-de Groot AC, Zinderman AH, et al: The neural crest as a possible pathogenic factor in coarctation of the

aorta and bicuspid aortic valve. *J Thorac Cardiovasc Surg* 102:830–836, 1991

28. Clagett OT, Kirklin JW, Edwards JE: Anatomic variations and pathologic changes in coarctation of the aorta. *Surg Gynecol Obstet* 98:103–114, 1954

29. Ravelo HR, Stephenson LW, Freidman S, et al: Coarctation resection in children with Turner's syndrome. *J Thorac Cardiovasc Surg* 80:427–430, 1980

30. Hoeffel JC, Henry M, Mentre B, et al: Pseudo-coarctation or congenital kinking of the aorta: Radiologic considerations. *Am Heart J* 89:428–436, 1975

31. Gay WA, Young WG: Pseudocoarctation of the aorta, a reappraisal. *J Thorac Cardiovasc Surg* 58:739–745, 1969

32. Bahabozorgui S, Bernstein RG, Frater RWM: Pseudocoarctation of the aorta associated with aneurysm formation. *Chest* 60:616–617, 1971

33. Kessler RM, Miller KB, Pett S, Wernly JA: Pseudocoarctation of the aorta presenting as a mediastinal mass with dysphagia. *Ann Thorac Surg* 55:1003–1005, 1993

34. Riemenschneider TA, Emmanouilides GC, Hirose F, Linde LM: Coarctation of the abdominal aorta in children: Report of three cases and review of the literature. *Pediatrics* 44:716–726, 1969

35. Rees AH, Elbl F, Villafane J, et al: Surgical repair of atypical coarctation of the abdominal aorta in an infant. *Kentucky Med* 62–65, 1990

36. Scott HW Jr, Dean RH, Boerth R, et al: Coarctation of the abdominal aorta: Pathophysiologic and therapeutic considerations. *Ann Surg* 189:746–757, 1979

37. Pierce WS, Vincent WR, Fitzgerald E, Miller FJ: Coarctation of the abdominal aorta with multiple aneurysms. *Ann Thorac Surg* 20:687–693, 1975

38. Elliott RB, Starling MB, Neutze JM: Medical manipulation of the ductus arteriosus. *Lancet* 1:140, 1975

39. Neutze JM, Starling MB, Elliott RB, Barratt-Boyes BG: Palliation of cyanotic congenital heart disease in infancy with E-type prostaglandins. *Circulation* 55:238–241, 1977

40. Heymann MA, Berman W Jr, Rudolph AM, Whitman V: Dilatation of the ductus arteriosus by prostaglandin E_1 in aortic arch abnormalities. *Circulation* 59:169–173, 1979

41. Shearer WT, Rutman JY, Weinberg WA, Goldring D: Coarctation of the aorta and cerebrovascular accident. A proposal for early corrective surgery. *J Pediatr* 77:1004–1009, 1970

42. Cokkinos DV, Leachman RD, Cooley DA: Increased mortality rate from coronary artery disease following operation for coarctation of the aorta at a late age. *J Thorac Cardiovasc Surg* 77:315–318, 1979

43. Reifenstein GH, Levine SA, Gross RE: Coarctation of the aorta. A review of 104 autopsied cases of the adult type. *Am Heart J* 33:146–168, 1947

44. Landtman B, Tauteri L: Vascular complications in coarctation of the aorta. *Acta Paediatr* 48:329–334, 1959

45. Campbell M: Natural history of coarctation of the aorta. *Br Heart J* 32:633–640, 1970

46. Abbott ME: Coarctation of the aorta of the adult type II. *Am Heart J* 3:574, 1928

47. Weyman AE, Caldwell RL, Hurwitz RA, et al: Cross-sectional echocardiographic detection of aortic obstruction: coarctation of the aorta. *Circulation* 57:498–502, 1978

48. Shaddy RE, Snider AR, Silverman NH, Lutin W: Pulsed Doppler findings in patients with coarctation of the aorta. *Circulation* 73:82–88, 1986

49. Marx GR, Allen HD: Accuracy and pitfalls of Doppler evaluation of the pressure gradient in aortic coarctation. *J Am Coll Cardiol* 7:1379–1385, 1986

50. Simpson IA, Sahn DJ, Valdes-Cruz LM, et al: Color Doppler flow mapping in patients with coarctation of the aorta: new observations and improved evaluations with color flow diameter and proximal acceleration as predictors of severity. *Circulation* 77:736–744, 1988

51. Fyler DC: Coarctation of the aorta. In Fyler DC (ed): *Nadas' Pediatric Cardiology*. St. Louis, Mosby-Year Book, 1992, pp 536–556

52. Predey TA, McDonald V, Demos TC, Moncada R: CT of congenital anomalies of the aortic arch. *Semin Roent* 24:96–111, 1989

53. Holt WW, Wong E, Lipton EJ: Conventional and ultrafast cine-computed tomography in cardiac imaging. *Curr Opin Radiol* 2:159–165, 1989

54. Stern HC, Locher D, Wallnofer K, et al: Noninvasive assessment of coarctation of the aorta: Comparative measurements by two-dimensional echocardiography, magnetic resonance, and angiography. *Pediatr Cardiol* 12:1–5, 1991

55. Simpson IA, Chung KJ, Glass RF, et al: Cine magnetic resonance imaging for evaluation of anatomy and flow relations in infants and children with coarctation of the aorta. *Circulation* 78:142–148, 1988

56. Stern H, Erbel R, Schreiner G, et al: Coarctation of the aorta: Quantitative analysis by transesophageal echocardiography. *Echocardiography* 4:387–395, 1987

57. Laschinger JC, Vannier MW, Gutierrez F, et al: Preoperative three-dimensional reconstruction of the heart and great vessels in patients with congenital heart disease. *J Thorac Cardiovasc Surg* 96:464–473, 1988

58. Lerberg DB: Abbott's artery. *Ann Thorac Surg* 33:415–416, 1981

59. Marini CP, Grubbs PE, Toporoff B, et al: Effect of sodium nitroprusside on spinal cord perfusion and paraplegia during aortic cross-clamping. *Ann Thorac Surg* 47:379–383, 1989

60. Watterson KG, Dhasmana JP, O'Higgins JW, Wisheart JD: Distal aortic pressure during coarctation operation. *Ann Thorac Surg* 49:987–990, 1990

61. Buckels NJ, Willetts RG, Roberts KD: Left heart bypass in the surgery of aortic coarctation in children. *Thorax* 43:1003–1006, 1988

62. Alexander JC Jr: Maintenance of distal aortic perfusion by a Heparin-bonded shunt during repair of coarctation of the aorta with minimal collateral circulation. *Ann Thorac Surg* 32:304–306, 1981

63. Pennington DG, Dennis HM, Swartz MT, et al: Repair of aortic coarctation in infants: Experience with an intraluminal shunt. *Ann Thorac Surg* 40:35–40, 1985

64. Lam CR, Arciniegas E: Surgical management of coarctation of the aorta with minimal collateral circulation. *Ann Surg* 178:693, 1973

65. Gross RE: Surgical correction for coarctation of the aorta. *Surgery* 18:673, 1945

66. Kirklin JW, Burchell HB, Pugh DG, et al: Surgical treatment of coarctation of the aorta in a ten week old infant: Report of a case. *Circulation* 6:411–414, 1952

67. Hartmann AF Jr, Goldring D, Hernandez A, et al: Recurrent coarctation of the aorta after successful repair in infancy. *Am J Cardiol* 25:405–410, 1970

68. Williams WG, Shindo G, Trusler GA, et al: Results of repair of coarctation of the aorta during infancy. *J Thorac Cardiovasc Surg* 79:603–608, 1980

69. Cobanoglu A, Teply JF, Grunkemeier GL, et al: Coarctation of the aorta in patients younger than three months. A critique of the subclavian flap operation. *J Thorac Cardiovasc Surg* 89:128–135, 1985

70. Körfer R, Meyer H, Kleikamp G, Bircks W: Early and late results after resection and end-to-end anastomosis of coarctation of the thoracic aorta in early infancy. *J Thorac Cardiovasc Surg* 89:616–622, 1985

71. Ziemer G, Jonas RA, Perry SB, et al: Surgery for coarctation of the aorta in the neonate. *Circulation* 74(suppl I):25–31, 1986

72. Brouwer MHJ, Kuntze CEE, Ebels T, et al: Repair of aortic coarctation in infants. *J Thorac Cardiovasc Surg* 101:1093–1098, 1991

73. Kappetein AP, Zwinderman AH, Bogers AJJC, et al: More than thirty-five years of coarctation repair. An unexpected high relapse rate. *J Thorac Cardiovasc Surg* 107:87–95, 1994

74. Van Heurn LWE, Wong CM, Spiegelhalter OJ, et al: Surgical treatment of coarctation of aorta in infants younger than 3 months: 1985–1990. Success of extended end-to-end arch aortoplasty. *J Thorac Cardiovasc Surg* 107:74–86, 1994

75. Quaegebeur JM, Jonas RA, Weinberg AD, et al: Congenital Heart Surgeons Society: Outcomes in seriously ill neonates with coarctation of the aorta: a multiinstitutional study. *J Thorac Cardiovasc Surg* 108:841–854, 1994

76. Schuster SR, Gross RE: Surgery for coarctation of the aorta. A review of 500 cases. *J Thorac Cardiovasc Surg* 43:54–70, 1962

77. Harlan JL, Doty DB, Brandt B III, et al: Coarctation of the aorta in infants. *J Thorac Cardiovasc Surg* 88:1012–1019, 1984

78. Arenas JD, Myers JL, Gleason MM, et al: End-to-end repair of aortic coarctation using absorbable polydioxanone suture. *Ann Thorac Surg* 51:413–417, 1991

79. Sade RM, Crawford FA, Hohn AR, et al: Growth of the aorta after prosthetic patch aortoplasty for coarctation in infants. *Ann Thorac Surg* 38:21–25, 1984

80. Bergdahl L, Ljungqvist A: Long-term results after repair of coarctation of the aorta by patch grafting. *J Thorac Cardiovasc Surg* 80:177–181, 1980

81. Ala-Kulju K, Järvinen A, Maamies T, et al: Late aneurysms after patch aortoplasty for coarctation of the aorta in adults. *Thorac Cardiovasc Surg* 31:301–305, 1983

82. DeSanto A, Bills RG, King H, et al: Pathogenesis of aneurysm formation opposite prosthetic patches used for coarctation repair. *J Thorac Cardiovasc Surg* 94:720–723, 1987

83. Hehrlein FW, Mulch J, Rautenburg HW, et al: Incidence and pathogenesis of late aneurysm after patch graft aortoplasty for coarctation. *J Thorac Cardiovasc Surg* 92:226–230, 1986

84. Rheuban KS, Gutgesell HP, Carpenter MA, et al: Aortic aneurysm after patch angioplasty for aortic isthmic coarctation in childhood. *Am J Cardiol* 58:178–180, 1986

85. Clarkson PM, Brandt PWT, Barratt-Boyes BG, et al: Prosthetic repair of coarctation of the aorta with particular reference to dacron onlay patch grafts and late aneurysm formation. *Am J Cardiol* 56:342–346, 1985

86. Heikkinen L, Sariola H, Sala J, Ala-Kulja K: Morphological and histopathological aspects of aneurysms after patch aortoplasty for coarctation. *Ann Thorac Surg* 50:946–948, 1990

87. Yee ES, Soifer SJ, Turley K, et al: Infant coarctation: A spectrum in clinical presentation and treatment. *Ann Thorac Surg* 42:488–493, 1986

88. Del Nido PJ, Williams WG, Wilson GJ, et al: Synthetic patch angioplasty for repair of coarctation of the aorta: Experience with aneurysm formation. *Circulation* 74(suppl I):32–36, 1986

89. Ala-Kulju K, Heikkenen L: Aneurysms after patch graft aortoplasty for coarctation of the aorta: Long-term results of surgical management. *Ann Thorac Surg* 47:853–856, 1989

90. Messmer BJ, Minale C, Mühler E, v Bernuth G: Surgical correction of coarctation in early infancy: Does surgical techniques influence the result? *Ann Thorac Surg* 52:594–603, 1991

91. Ungerleider RM: Commentary: Is there a role for prosthetic patch aortoplasty in the repair of coarctation? *Ann Thorac Surg* 52:601–602, 1991

92. Gross RE: Treatment of certain aortic coarctations by homologous grafts. *Ann Surg* 134:753–768, 1951

93. Morris GC, Cooley DA, DeBakey ME, Crawford ES: Coarctation of the aorta with particular emphasis upon improved techniques of surgical repair. *J Thorac Cardiovasc Surg* 40:705–722, 1960

94. Folges GM Jr, Shah KD: Subclavian steal in patients with Blalock-Taussig anastomosis. *Circulation* 31:241–246, 1965

95. Hart JC, Waldhausen JA: Reversed subclavian flap for arch coarctation of the aorta. *Ann Thorac Surg* 36:715, 1983

96. Brown JW, Fiore AC, King H: Isthmus flap aortoplasty: An alternative to subclavian flap aortoplasty for long-segment coarctation of the aorta in infants. *Ann Thorac Surg* 40:274–279, 1985

97. Meier MA, Lucchese FA, Jazbik W, et al: A new technique for repair of aortic coarctation. Subclavian flap aortoplasty with preservation of arterial blood flow to the left arm. *J Thorac Cardiovasc Surg* 92:1005–1012, 1986

98. Dietl CA, Torres AR, Favaloro RG, et al: Risk of recoarctation in neonates and infants after repair with patch aortoplasty, subclavian flap, and the combined resection-flap procedure. *J Thorac Cardiovasc Surg* **103:**724–732, 1992

99. Moulton AL, Roberts G, Ali S, et al: Subclavian flap repair of coarctation of the aorta in neonates: Realization of growth potential? *J Thorac Cardiovasc Surg* **87:**220–235, 1984

100. Bergdahl LAL, Blackstone EH, Kirklin JW, et al: Determinants of early success in repair of aortic coarctation in infants. *J Thorac Cardiovasc Surg* **83:**736–742, 1982

101. Milliken JC, Brawn WJ, Mee RB: Neonatal coarctation: Clinical spectrum and improved results. *J Am Coll Cardiol* **15:**78A, 1990

102. Geiss D, Williams WG, Lindsey WK, Rowe RD: Upper extremity gangrene. A complication of subclavian artery division. *Ann Thorac Surg* **30:**487–489, 1980

103. Todd PJ, Dangerfield PH, Hamilton DI, Wilkinson JL: Late effects on the left upper limb of subclavian flap aortoplasty. *J Thorac Cardiovasc Surg* **85:**678–681, 1983

104. Martin MM, Beekman RH, Rocchini AP, et al: Aortic aneurysms after subclavian angioplasty repair of coarctation of the aorta. *Am J Cardiol* **61:**951–953, 1988

105. Penkoske PA, Williams WG, Olley PM, et al: Subclavian arterioplasty. Repair of coarctation of the aorta in the first year of life. *J Thorac Cardiovasc Surg* **87:**894–900, 1984

106. Campbell DB, Waldhausen JA, Pierce WS, et al: Should elective repair of coarctation of the aorta be done in infancy? *J Thorac Cardiovasc Surg* **88:**929–938, 1984

107. Metzdorff MT, Cobanoglu A, Grunkemeier GL, et al: Influence of age at operation on late results with subclavian flap aortoplasty. *J Thorac Cardiovasc Surg* **89:**235–241, 1985

108. Sanchez GR, Balsara RK, Dunn JM, et al: Recurrent obstruction after subclavian flap repair of coarctation of the aorta in infants. *J Thorac Cardiovasc Surg* **91:**738–746, 1986

109. Ehrhardt P, Walker DR: Coarctation of the aorta corrected during the first month of life. *Arch Dis Child* **64:**330–332, 1989

110. Zannini L, Lecompte Y, Galli R, et al: Aortic coarctation with arch hypoplasia: A new surgical technique. *G Ital Cardiol* **15:**1045, 1985

111. Elliott MJ: Coarctation of the aorta with arch hypoplasia: Improvements on a new technique. *Ann Thorac Surg* **44:**321–323, 1987

112. Zannini L, Gargiulo G, Albanese SB, et al: Aortic coarctation with hypoplastic arch in neonates: A spectrum of anatomic lesions requiring different surgical options. *Ann Thorac Surg* **56:**288–294, 1993

113. Jonas RA: Coarctation: Do we need to resect ductal tissue? *Ann Thorac Surg* **52:**604–607, 1991

114. Vouhe PR, Trinquet F, Lecompte Y, et al: Aortic coarctation with hypoplastic aortic arch. Results of extended end-to-end aortic arch anastomosis. *J Thorac Cardiovasc Surg* **96:**557–563, 1988

115. Lacour-Gayet F, Bruniaux J, Serraf A, et al: Hypoplastic transverse arch and coarctation in neonates. Surgical reconstruction of the aortic arch: A study of sixty-six patients. *J Thorac Cardiovasc Surg* **100:**808–816, 1990

116. Lacour-Gayet F, Planché C: Commentary: Indications for extended aortic arch reconstruction. *Ann Thorac Surg* **52:**608–614, 1991

117. Brouwer MHJ, Cromme-Dijkhuis AH, Ebels T, Eijgelaar A: Growth of the hypoplastic aortic arch after simple coarctation resection and end-to-end anastomosis. *J Thorac Cardiovasc Surg* **104:**426–433, 1992

118. Myers JL, McConnel BA, Waldhausen JA: Coarctation of the aorta in infants: Does the aortic arch grow after repair? *Ann Thorac Surg* **54:**869–875, 1992

119. Siewers RD, Ettedgui J, Pahl E, et al: Coarctation and hypoplasia of the aortic arch: Will the arch grow? *Ann Thorac Surg* **52:**608–614, 1991

120. Sos T, Sniderman KW, Rettek-Sos B, et al: Percutaneous transluminal dilatation of coarctation of thoracic aorta post mortem. *Lancet* **2:**970, 1979

121. Lock JE, Castaneda-Zuniga WR, Bass JL, et al: Balloon dilation of excised aortic coarctations. *Radiology* **143:**689–691, 1982

122. Lababidi ZA, Daskalopoulos DA, Stoeckle H: Transluminal balloon coarctation angioplasty: Experience with 27 patients. *Am J Cardiol* **54:**1288–1291, 1984

123. Marvin WJ, Mahoney LT, Rose EF: Pathologic sequelae of balloon dilation angioplasty for unoperated coarctation of the aorta in children. *J Am Coll Cardiol* **7:**117A, 1986

124. Brandt B, Marvin WJ, Rose EF, Mahoney LT: Surgical treatment of coarctation of the aorta after balloon angioplasty. *J Thorac Cardiovasc Surg* **94:**715–719, 1987

125. Cooper RS, Ritter SB, Rothe WB, et al: Angioplasty for coarctation of the aorta: Long-term results. *Circulation* **75:**600–604, 1987

126. Tynan M, Finley JP, Fontes V, et al: Balloon angioplasty for the treatment of native coarctation: Results of valvuloplasty and angioplasty of congenital anomalies registry. *Am J Cardiol* **65:**790–792, 1990

127. Lock JE: Now that we can dilate, should we? *Am J Cardiol* **54:**1360, 1984

128. Zales VR, Muster AJ: Balloon dilation angioplasty for the management of aortic coarctation. In Mavroudis C, Backer CL (eds): *Coarctation and Interrupted Aortic Arch.* Philadelphia, Haney & Belfus; *Cardiac Surgery: State of the Art Reviews* **7:**133–146, 1993

129. Hess J, Mooyaart EL, Busch HJ, et al: Percutaneous transluminal balloon angioplasty in restenosis of coarctation of the aorta. *Br Heart J* **55:**459–461, 1986

130. Hijazi ZM, Fahey JT, Kleinman CS, et al: Balloon angioplasty for recurrent coarctation of the aorta: Immediate and long-term results. *Circulation* **84:**1150–1156, 1991

131. Saul JP, Keane JF, Fellows KE, Lock JE: Balloon dilation angioplasty of postoperative aortic obstructions. *Am J Cardiol* **59:**943–948, 1987

132. Hellenbrand WE, Allen HD, Golinko RJ, et al: Balloon angioplasty for aortic recoarctation: Results of valvuloplasty and angioplasty of congenital anomalies registry. *Am J Cardiol* **65:**793–797, 1990

133. Sealy WC, Harris JS, Young WG, et al: Paradoxical hypertension following resection of coarctation of the aorta. *Surgery* **42:**135–147, 1957

134. Sealy WC: Paradoxical hypertension after repair of coarctation of the aorta: A review of its causes. *Ann Thorac Surg* **50:**323–529, 1990

135. Goodall McC, Sealy WC: Increased sympathetic nerve activity following resection of coarctation of the thoracic aorta. *Circulation* **39:**345–351, 1969

136. Sealy WC: Coarctation of the aorta and hypertension. *Ann Thorac Surg* **3:**15–28, 1967

137. Rocchini AP, Rosenthal A, Barger C, et al: Pathogenesis of paradoxical hypertension after coarctation resection. *Circulation* **54:**382–387, 1976

138. Fox S, Pierce WS, Waldhausen JA: Pathogenesis of paradoxical hypertension after coarctation repair. *Ann Thorac Surg* **2:**135–141, 1980

139. Lober PH, Lillehei CW: Necrotizing panarteritis following repair of coarctation of aorta: Report of two cases. *Surgery* **35:**950, 1954

140. Benson WR, Sealy WC: Arterial necrosis following resection of coarctation of the aorta. *Lab Invest* **5:**359, 1956

141. Leenen FHH, Balfe JA, Pelech AN, et al: Postoperative hypertension after repair of coarctation of aorta in children: Protective effect of propranolol. *Am Heart J* **113:**1164, 1987

142. Gidding SS, Rocchini AP, Beekman R, et al: Therapeutic effect of propranolol on paradoxical hypertension after repair of coarctation of the aorta. *N Engl J Med* **312:**1224, 1985

143. Presbitero P, Demarie D, Villani M, et al: Long term results (15–30 years) of surgical repair of aortic coarctation. *Br Heart J* **57:**462–467, 1987

144. Bing RJ, Handelsman JC, Campbell JA, et al: The surgical treatment and physiopathology of coarctation of the aorta. *Ann Surg* **128:**803–824, 1948

145. Brewer LA, Fosberg RG, Mulder GA, et al: Spinal cord complica-

tions following surgery for coarctation of the aora. *Ann Thorac Cardiovasc Surg* **64:**368–381, 1972

146. Lerberg DB, Hardesty RL, Siewers RD, et al: Coarctation of the aorta in infants and children: 25 years of experience. *Ann Thorac Surg* **33:**159–170, 1982

147. Crawford FA Jr, Sade RM: Spinal cord injury associated with hyperthermia during aortic coarctation repair. *J Thorac Cardiovasc Surg* **87:**616–618, 1984

148. McCullough JL, Hollier LH, Nugent M: Paraplegia after thoracic aortic occlusion: Influence of cerebrospinal fluid drainage. *J Vasc Surg* **7:**153, 1988

149. Pollock JC, Jamieson MP, McWilliam R: Somatosensory evoked potentials in the detection of spinal cord ischemia in aortic coarctation repair. *Ann Thorac Surg* **41:**251–254, 1986

150. Goldman S, Hernandez J, Pappas G: Results of surgical treatment of coarctation of the aorta in the critically ill neonate. *J Thorac Cardiovasc Surg* **91:**732–737, 1986

151. Kirklin JW, Barratt-Boyes BG: *Cardiac Surgery.* New York, John Wiley, 1986, p 1061

152. Freed MD, Rocchini A, Rosenthal A, et al: Exercise-induced hypertension after surgical repair of coarctation of the aorta. *Am J Cardiol* **43:**253–258, 1979

153. Kappetein PA, Guit GL, Bogers AJJC, et al: Noninvasive long-term follow-up after coarctation repair. *Ann Thorac Surg* **55:**1153–1159, 1993

154. Foster ED: Reoperation for aortic coarctaion. *Ann Thorac Surg* **38:**81–89, 1984

155. Sweeney MS, Walker WE, Duncan JM, et al: Reoperation for aortic coarctation: Techniques, results, and indications for various approaches. *Ann Thorac Surg* **40:**46–49, 1985

156. Kron IL, Flanagan TL, Rheuban KS, et al: Incidence and risk of reintervention after coarctation repair. *Ann Thorac Surg* **49:**920–926, 1990

157. Jacob T, Cobanoglu A, Starr A: Late results of ascending aorta-descending aorta bypass grafts for recurrent coarctation of the aorta. *J Thorac Cardiovasc Surg* **95:**782–787, 1988

158. Beekman RH, Rocchini AP, Behrendt DM, Rosenthal A: Reoperation for coarctation of the aorta. *Am J Cardiol* **48:**1108–1114, 1981

159. Steidele RJ: Verschiedener in der chirug. 'prakt. *Lehrschule Gemachten Beobb* **2:**114, 1777–1778

160. Celoria GC, Patton RP: Congenital absence of the aortic arch. *Am Heart J* **58:**407–413, 1959

161. Moore GW, Hutchins GM: Association of interrupted aortic arch with malformations producing reduced blood flow to the fourth aortic arches. *Am J Cardiol* **42:**467–472, 1978

162. Jonas RA: Interrupted aortic arch. In Mavroudis C, Backer CL (eds): *Pediatric Cardiac Surgery,* ed. 2. St. Louis, Mosby-Year Book, 1994, pp 183–192

163. Freedom RM, Rosen FS, Nadas AS: Congenital cardiovascular disease and anomalies of the third and fourth pharyngeal pouch. *Circulation* **46:**165–172, 1972

164. Kirby ML, Gale TF, Stewart DE: Neural crest cells contribute to normal aortopulmonary septation. *Science* **220:**1059–1061, 1983

165. Bockman DE, Redmond ME, Kirby ML: Alterations of early vascular development after ablation of cranial neural crest. *Anat Rec* **225:**209–217, 1989

166. Riggs TW, Berry TE, Aziz KU, Paul MH: Two-dimensional echocardiographic features of interruption of the aortic arch. *Am J Cardiol* **50:**1385–1390, 1982

167. Quereshi S, Mazuszewski B, Mckay R: Determinants of survival following repair of interrupted arch in infancy. *Int J Cardiol* **26:**303–312, 1990

168. Gokcebay TM, Batillas J, Pinck RL: Complete interruption of the aorta at the arch. *Am J Roentgenol* **114:**362–370, 1972

169. Jonas RA: Commentary: The argument for one-stage repair. *Ann Thorac Surg* **52:**638–639, 1991

170. Kron IL, Rheubanm KS, Carpenter MS, Nolan ST: Interrupted aortic arch: A conservative approach for the sick neonate. *J Thorac Cardiovasc Surg* **86:**37–40, 1983

171. Tyson KRT, Harris LC, Nghiem QX: Repair of aortic arch interruption in the neonate. *Surgery* **67:**1006–1010, 1970

172. Sturm JT, van Heeckeren DW, Borkat G: Surgical treatment of interrupted aortic arch in infancy with expanded polytetrafluoroethylene grafts. *J Thorac Cardiovasc Surg* **81:**245–250, 1981

173. Fowler BN, Lucas SK, Razook JD, et al: Interruption of the aorta arch: Experience in 17 infants. *Ann Thorac Surg* **37:**25–32, 1984

174. Hammon JW, Merrill WH, Prager RL, et al: Repair of interrupted aortic arch and associated malformations in infancy: Indications for complete or partial repair. *Ann Thorac Surg* **42:**17–21, 1986

175. Scott WA, Rocchini AP, Bove EL, et al: Repair of interrupted aortic arch in infancy. *J Thorac Cardiovasc Surg* **96:**564–568, 1988

176. Lamberti JJ: Commentary: Staged repair of interrupted aortic arch. *Ann Thorac Surg* **52:**637, 1991

177. Griffin S, Richens D, Behl R: Early results of direct repair of aortic interruption by the lateral approach. *Ann Thorac Surg* **53:**430–434, 1992

178. Jonas RA, Quaegebeur JM, Kirklin JW, et al, and the Congenital Heart Surgeon's Society: Outcomes in patients with interrupted aortic arch and ventricular septal defect: A multiinstitutional study. *J Thorac Cardiovasc Surg* **107:**1099–1113, 1994

179. Norwood WI, Lang P, Castaneda AR, Hougen TJ: Reparative operations for interrupted aortic arch with ventricular septal defect. *J Thorac Cardiovasc Surg* **86:**832–837, 1983

180. Sell JE, Jonas RA, Mayer JE, et al: The results of a surgical program for interrupted aortic arch. *J Thorac Cardiovasc Surg* **96:**864–877, 1988

181. Jonas RA: Modified arch anastomosis for interrupted aortic arch. *Ann Thorac Surg* **56:**5–6, 1993

182. Moulton AL, Bowman FO Jr: Primary definitive repair of type B interrupted aortic arch, ventricular septal defect and patent ductus arteriosus. *J Thorac Cardiovasc Surg* **82:**501–510, 1981

183. Menahem S, Rahayoe AU, Brawn WJ, Mee RBB: Interrupted aortic arch in infancy: A 10-year experience. *Pediatr Cardiol* **13:**214–221, 1992

184. Yasui H, Kado H, Yonenaga K, et al: Revised technique of cardiopulmonary bypass in one-stage repair of interrupted aortic arch complex. *Ann Thorac Surg* **55:**1166–1171, 1993

185. Van Praagh R, Bernhard WF, Rosenthal A, et al: Interrupted aortic arch: Surgical treatment. *Am J Cardiol* **27:**200–211, 1971

186. Ilbawi MN, Idriss FS, DeLeon SY, et al: Surgical management of patients with interrupted aortic arch and severe subaortic stenosis. *Ann Thorac Surg* **45:**174–180, 1988

187. Menahem S, Brawn WJ, Mee RBB: Severe subaortic stenosis in interrupted aortic arch in infancy and childhood. *J Cardiac Surg* **6:**373–380, 1991

188. Bove EL, Minich LL, Pridjian AK, et al: The management of severe subaortic stenosis, ventricular septal defect, and aortic arch obstruction in the neonate. *J Thorac Cardiovasc Surg* **105:**289–296, 1993

189. Planché C, Serraf A, Comas JV, et al: Anatomic repair of transposition of great arteries with ventricular septal devect and aortic arch obstruction: One-statge versus two-stage procedure. *J Thorac Cardiovasc Surg* **105:**925–933, 1993

190. Van Praagh R, Van Praagh S: The anatomy of common aorticopulmonary trunk (truncus arteriosus communis) and its embryologic implications. A study of 57 necropsy cases. *Am J Cardiol* **16:**406–425, 1965

191. Gomes MMR, McGoon DC: Truncus arteriosus with interruption of the aortic arch: Report of a case successfully repaired. *Mayo Clin Proc* **46:**40, 1971

192. Sano S, Brawn WJ, Mee RBB: Repair of truncus arateriosus and interrupted aortic arch. *J Cardiac Surg* **5:**157–162, 1990

77

Hypoplastic Left Heart Syndrome

Marshall L. Jacobs and William I. Norwood

Hypoplastic left heart syndrome is an anatomic constellation of cardiac malformations with the central feature of marked hypoplasia or absence of the left ventricle and hypoplasia of the ascending aorta. As a consequence, the newborn with hypoplastic left heart syndrome has a systemic circulation dependent upon patency of the ductus arteriosus and obligatory admixture of pulmonary venous and systemic venous blood in the right atrium and ventricle. Among congenital cardiac malformations where there is only one effective ventricle such as tricuspid atresia, "univentricular" heart or double-outlet right ventricle with mitral atresia, hypoplastic left heart syndrome is the most common form.[1] As such, physiologic correction is possible by reconstructive surgical techniques initially advanced for the treatment of tricuspid atresia by Fontan and colleagues and Kreutzer and colleagues.

The term hypoplastic left heart syndrome was initially coined by Noonan and Nadas in 1958 to encompass a variety of cardiac malformations consisting of developmental abnormalities of the left heart structures.[2,3] Although the diagnosis has subsequently become more focused, the anatomic associates that are currently categorized as hypoplastic left heart syndrome are varied. However, the physiologic similarity of this collection of lesions has resulted in acceptance of the term. Moreover, the advent of surgical management has stimulated interest in a more precise definition to better understand the anatomic implications on physiology, diagnosis, therapy, and prognosis.[1-16] This malformation is not uncommon. The recorded incidence of 7% of infants presenting in the first year of life in the New England Regional Infant Cardiac Program ranks it with coarctation and patent ductus arteriosus in incidence. The majority of newborns with hypoplastic left heart syn-

drome are otherwise well-developed babies with no associated extracardiac developmental abnormalities. Although initially felt to have a low incidence of associated genetic and congenital malformations, the true incidence is only now being appreciated as interest in therapy has increased. Without surgical intervention, hypoplastic left heart syndrome is universally lethal, accounting for 25% of cardiac mortality in the first week of life.[17]

ANATOMY

In general, the collective term hypoplastic left heart syndrome encompasses those cardiac malformations in which there is severe aortic valve hypoplasia, stenosis or atresia, and hypoplasia or absence of the left ventricle. Hypoplasia of the ascending aorta always coexists. In association with a hypoplastic or absent left ventricle, there is severe mitral hypoplasia or mitral atresia. Ten percent of patients seen at The Children's Hospital of Philadelphia with hypoplastic left heart syndrome have double-outlet right ventricle with severe aortic valve hypoplasia or atresia. The remainder have normally related great arteries.[14] Approximately 15% of patients have malalignment of the common atrioventricular canal with regard to the muscular ventricular septum and associated aortic valve stenosis or atresia. Cases involving transposition of the great arteries with hypoplasia of the left ventricle and pulmonary artery, or hypoplasia of the right ventricle and aorta, are not considered hypoplastic left heart syndrome.

The most likely embryologic cause of hypoplastic left heart syndrome is severe underdevelopment of the left ventricular outflow in the form of isolated aortic valve atresia or the conotruncal abnormality of double-outlet right ventricle with aortic valve atresia. In a smaller percentage, the progenitor may be a limitation of left ventricular inflow in the form of severe malalignment of the atrioventricular canal. The abnormal development of the remaining cardiac structures results primarily from the blood flow patterns associated with atresia or marked hypoplasia of the aortic valve. When the ventricular septum is intact, the left ventricle is markedly hypoplastic or absent. In approximately 3% of patients with aortic valve atresia, there is an associated unrestrictive ventricular septal defect and almost always there is normal left ventricular and mitral valve development. Therefore, a primary myocardial abnormality does not appear to be a likely cause of hypoplastic left heart syndrome. Although a congenitally small or absent foramen ovale has been postulated as a cause of hypoplastic left heart syndrome, the atrial septal anatomy is probably not primary but rather a consequence of altered flow patterns secondary to left ventricular hypoplasia.[18,19]

The pathologic anatomy of hypoplastic left heart syndrome has been detailed.[13,17,20-33] Since the entire cardiac output passes through the right atrium, right ventricle, and main pulmonary artery, these structures are generally dilated and the tricuspid orifice and right ventricle are enlarged (Fig. 77–1). The inferior and right superior venae cavae are connected to the right atrium normally. Occasionally there is a persistent left superior vena cava draining to

the coronary sinus.[1,18] Although Bharati reported three patients with thickened nodular pulmonary valve leaflets, the pulmonary valve is usually normal, albeit enlarged.[34] The right pulmonary arterial orifice arises just distal to the pulmonary valve apparatus from the posterior aspect of the main pulmonary artery and the left pulmonary artery branch orifice is somewhat distal to the right pulmonary arterial orifice. In patients dying before 2 weeks of age, there is no significant difference from normal in the size and character of the small and medium-sized pulmonary artery branches.[16]

Occasionally, there is anomalous pulmonary venous connection or normal connection with anomalous pulmonary venous drainage through a persistent left vertical vein, but the pulmonary venous connections are usually normal.[17] In those with common atrioventricular canal defect, there may be an associated atrial septal defect of the ostium primum type. Most commonly, however, there is a patent foramen ovale.[17,22] Two percent of patients present with severe cyanosis and limited pulmonary venous drainage secondary to a virtually intact atrial septum, in which case the septum primum is muscular and thicker than normal. Sixty-five percent of patients with aortic valve atresia have posterior leftward displacement of the right lateral attachment of septum primum vis-à-vis the septum secundum.[32] It is important for the surgeon to understand this anatomy when performing an atrial septectomy.

In those with malaligned atrioventricular canal, the inlet portion of the ventricular septum may be absent and the development of the left ventricle depends on the degree of malalignment of the atrioventricular valve. An intermediate-sized left ventricle can exist when the common atrioventricular valve partially enters the left ventricle. However, this ventricle still does not form the apex of the heart. Approximately 60% of patients with aortic valve atresia have marked hypoplasia of the mitral valve. The remaining patients have associated mitral valve atresia. When a patent left ventricular inflow exists, there is frequently endocardial fibroelastosis and myofibril disarray has been noted in this circumstance. The ascending aorta and transverse aortic arch are hypoplastic. In those with aortic valve atresia, the ascending aorta generally measures 1–3 mm in diameter while those with aortic valve hypoplasia have an ascending aorta that is somewhat larger but usually measures less than 5 mm in diameter. The coronary arteries generally originate normally from the aortic root with a normal distribution pattern. Freedom and Zaurer have suggested that in those with patent left ventricular inflow, the coronary arteries may have intimal and medial thickening in the subendocardial region.[28] The prognostic implications of this finding are not apparent from the clinical information of patients undergoing reconstructive surgical management.[14]

Although there are reports to the contrary, true coarctation of the aorta is not a common finding.[22,24,45] There is, however, a prominent posterior lateral intimal ridge at the junction of the aortic isthmus, ductus arteriosus, and tho-

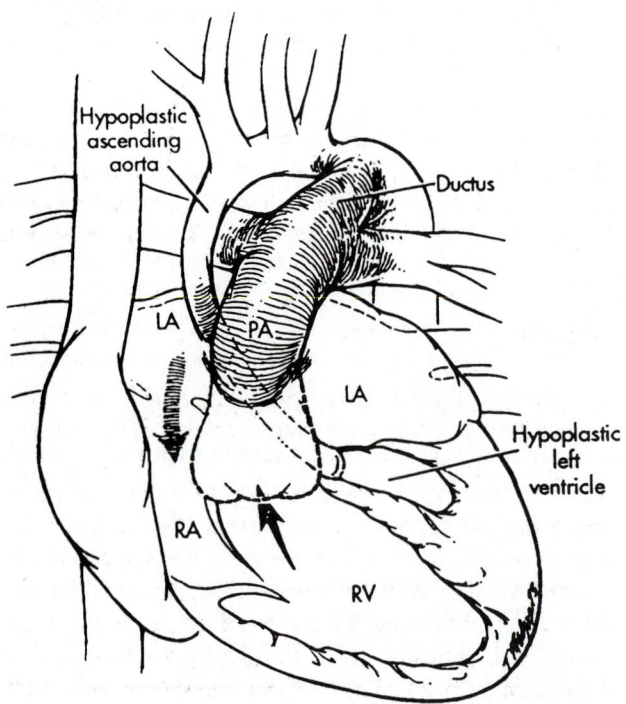

Figure 77–1. An artist's representation of the anatomy of hypoplastic left heart syndrome, showing the diminutive ascending aorta and left ventricle, and the large main pulmonary artery and ductus arteriosus (shaded). LA, left atrium; RA, right atrium; RV, right ventricle; PA, pulmonary artery.

racic aorta in the majority of patients. This architecture is seen with any natural branch point in the arterial circulation and is probably a consequence of the isthmus functioning as a branch of the main pulmonary artery–ductus–thoracic aorta continuum with retrograde flow in the isthmus of the aorta, aortic arch, and ascending aorta.

PHYSIOLOGY

Physiologically, the left ventricle is essentially a nonfunctional structure and the systemic circulation is dependent upon output from the right ventricle through the ductus arteriosus. Pulmonary venous return must eventually reach the right atrium. In utero, the right ventricle is able to maintain systemic output through the ductus arteriosus with oxygenation via the placenta, and the fetus develops otherwise normally. Postnatally, oxygenated pulmonary venous return must pass through an interatrial communication to mix with systemic venous blood and provide systemic oxygenation. The lungs are usually normal and the degree of hypoxemia is determined by the relative ratio of pulmonary and systemic blood flow. This is dependent upon the delicate balance between pulmonary and systemic vascular resistance. At birth, pulmonary vascular resistance is nearly systemic but decreases naturally thereafter.

Anatomically, the two major determinants of neonatal physiology in hypoplastic left heart syndrome are the nature of the interatrial communication and the degree of patency of the ductus arteriosus. The patent foramen ovale is usually somewhat restrictive of pulmonary venous return in these patients and this contributes importantly to the balance of systemic and pulmonary blood flow. In the absence of lung disease, a PaO_2 less than 25 mm Hg is usually associated with limited pulmonary blood flow secondary to a very restrictive interatrial communication. In most cases, the ductus arteriosus begins to close shortly after birth and systemic blood flow decreases with a corresponding increase in pulmonary blood flow. The PaO_2, therefore, is increased but there may be marked metabolic acidosis as a consequence of inadequate systemic perfusion.

An appreciation of the anatomy of hypoplastic left heart syndrome and its consequential physiology allows the clinical features and preoperative management strategy of these patients to be easily understood. Typically, Apgar scores are normal at birth but within 24 to 48 hours most patients develop dusky cyanosis with associated tachypnea.[3,17,22,26] When the ductus arteriosus begins to close, the patient develops metabolic acidosis and evidence of markedly diminished systemic perfusion, pallor, and lethargy. Depending on the degree of ductal patency at the time of initial evaluation, peripheral pulses may be normal, diminished, or absent. Occasionally, the ductus arteriosus remains patent and recognition of heart disease by respiratory distress or cyanosis is delayed.[17]

On examination, there is usually a dominant right ventricular impulse on palpation with decreased impulse at the apex.[35] S2 is single and increased in intensity. One-third of patients have a gallop rhythm at the apex and about two-thirds have a nonspecific soft systolic murmur at the left sternal border. An apical middiastolic flow murmur can be heard in some patients.[22] Right atrial enlargement is apparent on electrocardiogram in approximately one-third of patients and right ventricular hypertrophy is present in the majority.[16] Cardiomegaly on chest film is reported in 75% of patients and the pulmonary vascular markings are generally increased in appearance.[16] A patient with a reticular pattern on chest film reminiscent of total anomalous pulmonary venous connection usually has a very restrictive interatrial communication.

Two-dimensional echocardiography is diagnostic of this congenital malformation and cardiac catheterization is usually not indicated either for acquisition of diagnostic information or therapy.[25,36–38] The anatomy of the ascending aorta, aortic arch, and upper descending thoracic aorta is readily assessed by suprasternal imaging. A very diminutive ascending aorta is characteristic of this malformation. Usually the atrial septum is bowed from left to right, and, if not, anomalous pulmonary venous connection should be suspected. In approximately two-thirds of patients with aortic valve atresia, the septum primum will be noted to have posterior deviation of its right lateral and superior attachment as much as 1 cm from the superior limbic band. The anatomy and function of the tricuspid valve can be appreciated using color flow imaging, pulsed Doppler, and continuous-wave Doppler. Approximately half of patients with hypoplastic left heart syndrome have some degree of tricuspid regurgitation (35% mild, 16% moderate, and 5% severe). Cardiac catheterization is rarely indicated in neonates with hypoplastic left heart syndrome. Moreover, balloon atrial septotomy should be avoided as it may contribute to hemodynamic deterioration as a consequence of increasing pulmonary blood flow at the expense of systemic perfusion.

THERAPY

Two surgical strategies have been advanced for the management of hypoplastic left heart syndrome. Staged reconstructive surgery leading to a modification of the Fontan procedure has evolved over the last 15 years.[39] More recently, heart replacement in the neonatal period by cardiac transplantation has been advanced.[4] The advantage of cardiac transplantation is replacement of an abnormal circulation with a normal four-chambered heart, ideally in one operation. The effectiveness of this strategy is hampered by current limited availability of size and tissue-matched donor hearts, within the time constraints dictated by the fragile nonpalliated physiology of the newborn with hypoplastic left heart syndrome. In addition, this approach is associated with requirement for lifelong immunosuppressive therapy and the inherent chronic management of rejection versus infection. How these two modalities will be applied to this congenital cardiac malformation will become apparent only as continued refinements of both strategies develop.

The preoperative care of the newborn with hypoplastic left heart syndrome is the same regardless of the surgical approach chosen. When the diagnosis is made, continuous infusion of prostaglandin E_1 intravenously at a dose of 0.05 µg/kg per m^2 should be instituted in all patients. This therapy is begun electively in those in whom the diagnosis is made by physical findings and emergently in those who develop circulatory collapse and metabolic acidosis with closure of the ductus arteriosus. An arterial line is inserted for monitoring arterial oxygen saturation and acid–base status. To preserve peripheral arterial access, placement of an umbilical arterial catheter is preferable.

The goal in the preoperative period is to ensure adequate systemic perfusion and oxygenation to meet metabolic demands. Usually the pulmonary vascular resistance is less than the systemic vascular resistance, and care must be taken not to further decrease pulmonary resistance and increase pulmonary blood flow at the expense of systemic perfusion. Thus, even in the neonate who is being resuscitated from circulatory collapse, ventilation with high concentration of oxygen should be avoided as supplemental oxygen serves only to decrease pulmonary vascular resistance. The principal metabolic factor that appears to influence the pulmonary vascular resistance is PCO_2, and, thus, ventilation can be manipulated to establish a satisfactory balance between pulmonary and systemic blood flow. PCO_2 in the range of 40 to 50 mm Hg is associated with an increase in pulmonary vascular resistance, whereas PCO_2 below 40 mm Hg is associated with a diminution in pulmonary vascular resistance. Thus, both in neonates breathing spontaneously through a natural airway and in those with mechanical ventilation via an endotracheal tube, addition of carbon dioxide to the inspired gases is an effective strategy to influence the ratio of pulmonary vascular resistance to systemic vascular resistance, and avoid the circumstance of excessive pulmonary blood flow at the expense of peripheral perfusion.[40] Catecholamine infusions should generally be avoided. While these agents may be useful in cases with underlying abnormalities such as sepsis, inotropic agents are usually unnecessary and may have the harmful effect of increasing systemic vascular resistance resulting in excessive pulmonary blood flow.

Emergency surgery is necessary only in the rare circumstance where there is a virtually intact interatrial septum. These patients usually have a septum primum that is thick and muscular and it does not lend itself to balloon or even blade septotomy. These children have severe hypoxemia, which results in metabolic acidosis. In virtually all other patients, hemodynamic stability can be maintained by simple infusion of prostaglandin E_1 and appropriate adjustment of arterial blood gases. In those who have had a period of hemodynamic instability associated with sepsis or closure of the ductus arteriosus, observation until renal and he-

patic insufficiency has largely resolved is appropriate. Due to the occasional association of partial chromosomal deletion, a karyotype analysis may be felt to be appropriate in patients with hypoplastic left heart syndrome.

RECONSTRUCTIVE SURGERY

Reconstructive surgical management of hypoplastic left heart syndrome is directed at eventual application of the Fontan procedure to this complex malformation with a single ventricle. At birth, the systemic circulation is dependent upon continued patency of the ductus arteriosus, and thus early surgical intervention is mandated. However, the pulmonary vasculature is immature and the pulmonary vascular resistance is prohibitively high in the newborn, thus preventing the application of the Fontan operation as initial surgical therapy. Therefore, staged surgical intervention is necessary.

Initial Palliative Surgery (Stage I)

The goals of the first stage are to achieve a stable physiology for normal growth, development, and maturation of the pulmonary vasculature as well as preservation of right ventricular function. A surgical technique designed to use in large measure native cardiovascular tissue to palliate this lesion was first described in 1980 and this approach has undergone several modifications to minimize the development of abnormalities of the aorta, pulmonary vasculature, and right ventricle prior to the eventual Fontan procedure.[14] The first stage of surgical palliation is initiated by induction of general anesthesia with Fentanyl and Pancuronium. A midline sternotomy incision is made exposing the thymus in the superior mediastinum, which is largely excised to gain exposure of the aortic arch and upper thoracic aorta. Cardiopulmonary bypass is instituted by cannulation of the main pulmonary artery with the arterial cannula placed just distal to the sinuses of Valsalva. No effort is made to manipulate the cannula through the ductus arteriosus. Venous return to the oxygenator is established with a single venous cannula placed in the right atrial appendage. When cardiopulmonary bypass has been initiated, the right and left branch pulmonary arteries are independently occluded with suture tourniquets to ensure adequate systemic perfusion through the ductus arteriosus, and the core temperature is reduced to 20°C. During cooling, the brachiocephalic vessels are exposed in preparation for occlusion with suture tourniquets during aortic arch reconstruction. The circulation is then discontinued. The brachiocephalic vessels are occluded and the arterial and venous cannulae are removed. Cardioplegia solution is infused through the cannulation site in the main pulmonary artery, while the thoracic aorta is temporarily occluded with forceps. This ensures retrograde perfusion of the coronary arteries via the ascending aorta. The septum primum is then excised to create as large an interatrial communication as possible. Careful examination of the septum is necessary as the position of the septum primum is unusual in the majority of the patients with hypoplastic left heart syndrome. These maneuvers can usually be accomplished through the right atrial cannulation site, but occasionally a separate atriotomy incision is required to facilitate exposure. The main pulmonary artery is transected just proximal to the origin of the right branch pulmonary artery (Fig. 77–2A). The distal main pulmonary artery is closed with a patch to minimize the likelihood of stenosis or discontinuity between the right and left pulmonary artery branches (Fig. 77–2B). The ductus arteriosus is then ligated and divided at its entrance into the thoracic aorta. An incision is made in the aorta extending into the thoracic aorta approximately 1 to 2 cm distal to the entrance of the ductus arteriosus. This aortotomy is then extended proximally on the inferior aspect of the aortic arch and down the left lateral aspect of the diminutive ascending aorta to a level adjacent to the transected proximal main pulmonary artery. The entire aortic arch complex is then augmented with a gusset designed to create a uniform ascending aorta, aortic arch, and thoracic aorta when the aortic reconstruction is completed (Fig. 77–2C). The elastic and hemostatic properties of cryopreserved pulmonary artery homograft make this an ideal tissue for use in the aortic reconstruction. The shelf of intimal tissue at the junction of the isthmus with the thoracic aorta is excised to minimize the likelihood of acquired aortic arch obstruction postoperatively. Once the gusset has been sutured to the thoracic aorta, aortic arch, and ascending aorta, the reconstruction is completed by anastomosis of the proximal main pulmonary artery to the adjacent ascending aorta and the most proximal portion of the gusset (Fig. 77–2D). Although a continuous monofilament suture technique is used in the major portion of this reconstruction, in those patients with the most diminutive ascending aortas, a few interrupted sutures are appropriate to initiate the anastomosis between the proximal main pulmonary artery and the ascending aorta. This strategy is designed to avoid obstruction of the entrance into the tiny aortic root and thus the coronary arteries. Pulmonary blood flow is provided by the placement of an interposition graft of PTFE between the systemic circulation and the pulmonary arteries. This is most often accomplished by interposition of a short segment of 4 mm PTFE graft between the innominate artery and the superior aspect of the proximal right branch pul-

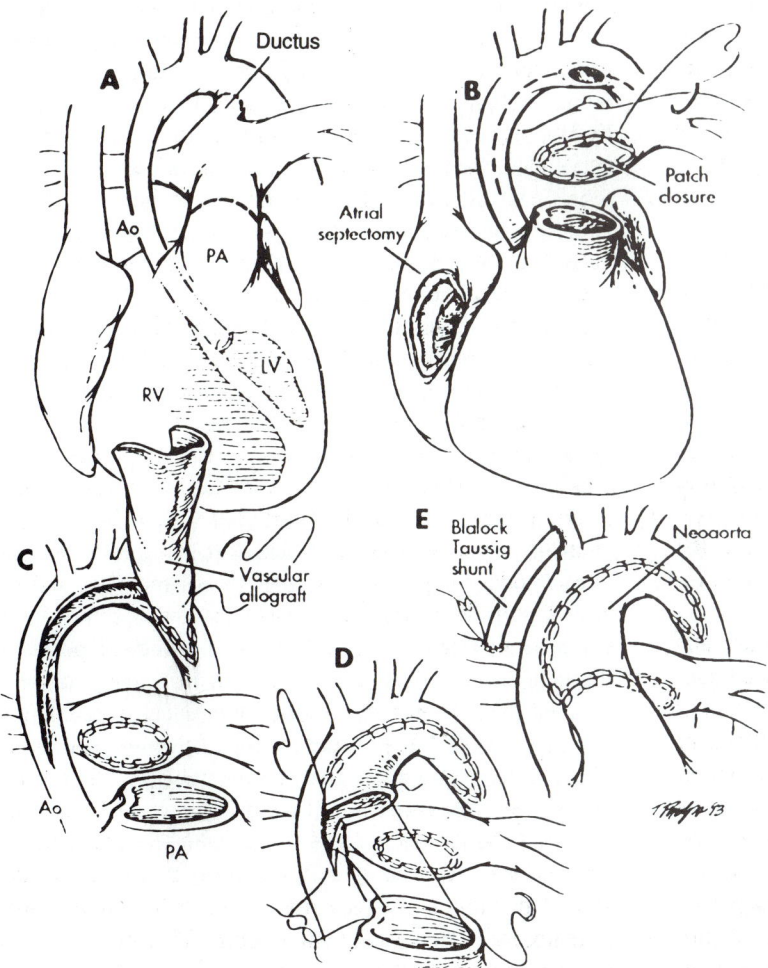

Figure 77–2. Stage I palliation for hypoplastic left heart syndrome. **A.** The proposed site of transection of the main pulmonary artery immediately proximal to the origin of the right branch pulmonary artery. **B.** Excision of septum primum (atrial septectomy) is accomplished either through the right atrial cannulation site or through a separate atriotomy incision. After transection of the main pulmonary artery, the distal main pulmonary artery is closed with a patch of cryopreserved pulmonary artery homograft. The ductus arteriosus is ligated and transected at its entrance into the thoracic aorta. The incision is carried distally for 1 or 2 cm on the medial aspect of the thoracic aorta and proximally along the underside of the aortic arch and the medial aspect of the diminutive ascending aorta (dotted line). **C.** The entire aortic arch complex is augmented with a gusset of cryopreserved pulmonary artery homograft. **D.** Proximally the transected main pulmonary artery is anastomosed to the ascending aorta and to the proximal portion of the homograft gusset. **E.** An interposition graft of PTFE is constructed between the innominate artery and the right pulmonary artery.

monary artery (Fig. 77–2E). Occasionally, as in instances when the innominate artery is diminutive, or when there is aberrant origin of the right subclavian artery from the thoracic aorta, it is appropriate to construct a short central shunt by interposition of a segment of 3.5-mm or 4-mm PTFE graft between the underside of the reconstructed aortic arch and the confluence of the pulmonary arteries. After completing the reconstruction, cardiopulmonary bypass is reinstituted and the patient is rewarmed to 37°C. During this time, the systemic to pulmonary artery shunt remains occluded. After the completion of rewarming, the shunt is opened and cardiopulmonary bypass is discontinued. Arterial and venous cannulae are removed, pressure monitoring catheters are placed in the right atrium, and heparin is reversed with Protamine. The use of inotropic infusions is rarely necessary, and can in fact adversely influence the balance of systemic vascular resistance and pulmonary vascular resistance.

In the early postoperative period, the goal is to maintain a balance between systemic and pulmonary vascular resistances, which results in a ratio of pulmonary blood flow to systemic blood flow ($Q_p:Q_s$) of approximately 1. This results in a level of systemic arterial oxygen saturation that is sufficient to meet metabolic needs, while minimizing the excessive volume work of the single ventricle that must provide both the systemic and pulmonary blood flow. In the early postoperative period, systemic and pulmonary vascular resistances are very dynamic, resulting in significant fluctuations of the systemic arterial oxygenation and systemic perfusion. This physiologic lability was thought to account for a considerable proportion of the early mortality in previous years. As mentioned earlier, it is clear that pulmonary vascular tone is extremely sensitive to carbon dioxide, with increased tone as P_{CO_2} increases. While an increase in P_{CO_2} and thus pulmonary vascular tone could be accomplished by reduction of the minute ventilation, such a strategy can be quite destabilizing during the early postoperative phase, which includes emergence from general anesthesia and alterations in airway resistance and chest wall compliance. On the other hand, a strategy involving the maintenance of a generous minute ventilation combined with the addition of carbon dioxide to the inspired gas mixture to ensure a level of P_{CO_2} consistent with a favorable ratio of pulmonary to systemic vascular resistance has been associated with a marked stabilization of the early postoperative physiology and salutatory reduction in early postoperative mortality.[36] Thus, in recent years, ventilatory management of the patient in the early postoperative period includes positive pressure ventilation with a volume preset ventilator set at an IMV rate of 20, a tidal volume of approximately 30 mL/kg, and F_{IO_2} of 0.21 to 0.30, and a partial pressure of carbon dioxide in the inspired gas mixture of 14 to 21 torr. The patient should be weaned from mechanical ventilation and extubated as soon as tolerated; this can frequently be accomplished within 24 hours of surgery but occasionally several days of ventilatory support are re-

quired. Nutritional support should be instituted early after surgery with a goal of achieving intake of approximately 150 kcal/kg per day through a combination of enteral and intravenous nutrition. At present, all patients are routinely administered digoxin and furosemide following initial palliative reconstructive surgery up until such time as the volume work of the single ventricle can be reduced by means of a second stage reconstructive procedure.

After the infant is released from the hospital, regular cardiovascular evaluations are important for monitoring anatomic and physiologic development. The incidence of aortic arch obstruction is low following augmentation of the distal aortic arch, but when it develops, its immediate recognition is critical. Concurrent right ventricular volume and pressure load can result in rapid deterioration of ventricular function. Two-dimensional echocardiography with suprasternal imaging of the arch and the sequential pulse Doppler interrogation of multiple points along the reconstructed aorta has proved reliable in detecting arch obstruction. If echocardiography suggests aortic abnormalities, cardiac catheterization should be performed to confirm the anatomy and physiology. In most instances, localized aortic arch obstruction can be satisfactorily managed by balloon angioplasty. Evaluation should assess for rapidly progressing cyanosis. This may be due to limited flow through the systemic to pulmonary artery shunt, or in some instances may occur secondary to a restrictive interatrial communication. Mild regurgitation of the native pulmonary valve (neoaortic valve) has been detected in some postoperatively by Doppler echocardiography but has not proved clinically significant. Tricuspid regurgitation can develop or persist. Significant tricuspid regurgitation is poorly tolerated by the already volume loaded right ventricle. Annuloplasty or valve replacement may be required in cases with severe tricuspid regurgitation. This has occurred in approximately 2% of our patients. The chest roentenogram usually reveals cardiomegaly following the palliative surgery and pulmonary vascular markings generally appear normal.

Second Stage—The Hemi-Fontan

Up to 1990, initial surgical palliation was followed by a modified Fontan operation, which was usually accomplished between the age of 18 and 24 months. Based on the recognition that some interval attrition was inevitable owing to the physiology of the palliated state wherein the single ventricle was required to handle the volume work of both the systemic circulation and the pulmonary circulation, and that conversion from this volume loaded state to the post-Fontan circulation was sometimes accompanied by marked alterations in ventricular geometry resulting in diminished ventricular compliance and potentially life threatening low cardiac output, a strategy of dividing Fontan's procedure into two stages has been systemically applied since 1989.[12] Thus, with a goal of early reduction of the volume work of the single ventricle, the first stage of

Fontan's procedure (the hemi-Fontan) is undertaken at approximately 6 months of age, the pulmonary vasculature having undergone a physiologic process of maturation with diminution of the pulmonary vascular resistance. The essential features of the hemi-Fontan operation are closure of the systemic to pulmonary artery shunt, association of the superior vena cava(e) with the branch pulmonary arteries, and augmentation of the confluence of the pulmonary arteries to address any potential areas of distortion or obstruction.[11]

The hemi-Fontan procedure is accomplished through a median sternotomy. Cardiopulmonary bypass is established following placement of the perfusion cannula in the ascending aorta and a single venous cannula in the appendage of the right atrium. With the initiation of bypass, the previously constructed systemic to pulmonary artery shunt is occluded. After achieving core cooling to a temperature of 20°C, the aorta is cross-clamped and a single dose cardioplegia solution is infused into the aortic root. The circulation is temporarily discontinued and the cannulae are removed. The confluence of the pulmonary arteries is dissected free from behind the reconstructed aorta. The con-

fluence of the pulmonary arteries is opened with a single longitudinal anterior incision that extends from a point just medial to the origin of the upper lobe branch of the right pulmonary artery to a corresponding point just medial to the origin of the upper lobe branch of the left pulmonary artery (Fig. 77–3A). An incision is made in the most superior aspect of the right atrium and carried onto the medial aspect of the right superior vena cava. Through the atriotomy, the interatrial communication is inspected and if necessary is enlarged. The right pulmonary artery is then anastomosed to the posterior lip of the right superior vena cava utilizing continuous fine monofilament suture (Fig. 77–3B). A gusset of cryopreserved pulmonary artery homograft is used to augment anteriorly the confluence of the pulmonary arteries and to create a roof over the patulous anastomosis of the pulmonary arteries to the right atrium and right superior vena cava (Fig. 77–3C). A portion of the same homograft is used as a dam to close the enlarged junction of the right atrium with the right superior vena cava (Fig. 77–3D). When bilateral superior vena cava are present, the left superior vena cava is associated in similar fashion with the left

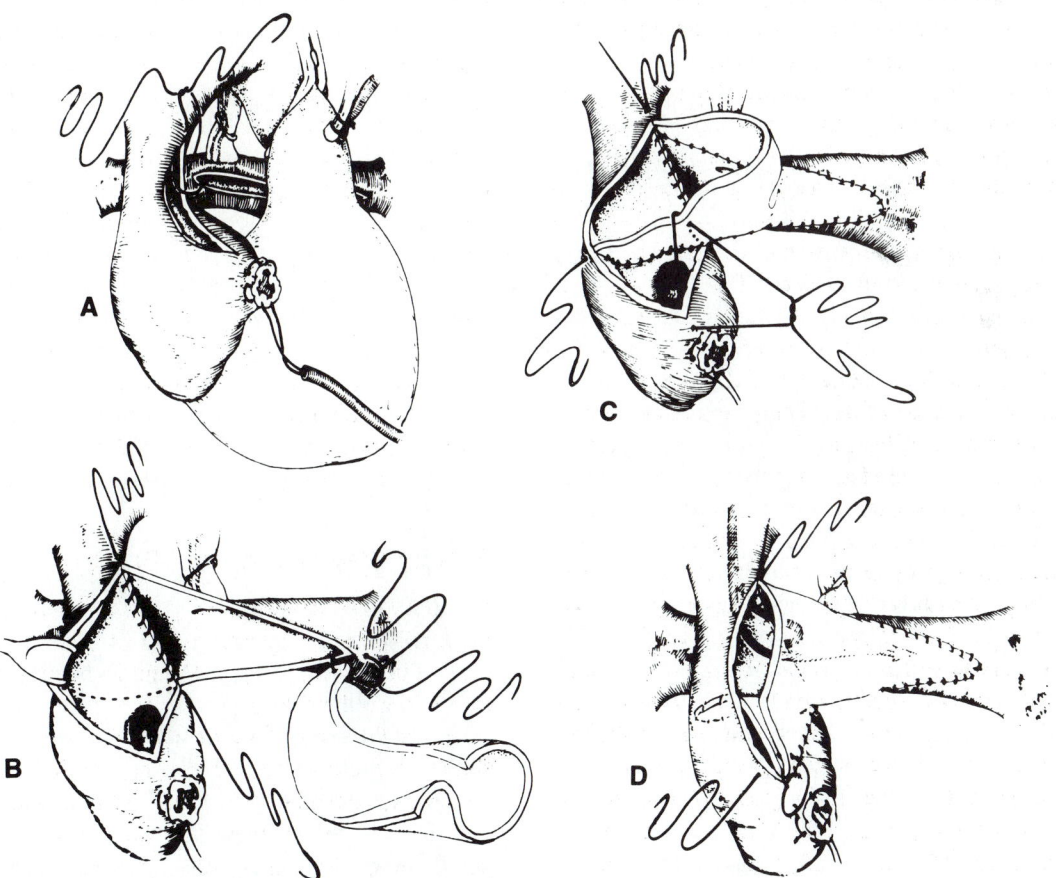

Figure 77–3. The hemi-Fontan procedure. **A.** The systemic to pulmonary artery shunt is occluded. The confluence of the pulmonary arteries is opened anteriorly. An incision is made in the superior aspect of the right atrium and extended onto the medial aspect of the right superior vena cava where the right pulmonary artery is anastomosed to the posterior lip of the superior vena cava. **B.** The confluence of the pulmonary arteries is augmented anteriorly with a gusset of cryopreserved pulmonary artery homograft. **C.** This is used to create a roof over the patulous anastomosis of the right superior vena cava to the pulmonary arteries. **D.** A portion of the same homograft is used as a dam to close the junction of the right atrium with the right superior vena cava.

branch pulmonary artery. Cannulae are reinserted and by-pass is resumed. The patient is rewarmed to 37°C, and then cardiopulmonary bypass is discontinued. The circulatory physiology after a hemi-Fontan operation is similar to that following a bidirectional Glenn shunt (Fig. 77–4A), usually resulting in a level of systemic arterial saturation of 82 to 84%. The unique technical features of the hemi-Fontan operation make it a more appropriate preparatory step in antic-ipation of an eventual completion Fontan procedure. The majority of patients are maintained on no cardiac medica-tions after the hemi-Fontan procedure.

Third Stage Reconstruction—
The Completion Fontan

Approximately 6 to 12 mo after the hemi-Fontan procedure, the patient undergoes full hemodynamic evaluation in antic-ipation of completion of Fontan's procedure. This time pe-riod allows for remodeling of the single ventricle after the reduction of volume work that results from the hemi Fontan procedure. Thus the completion Fontan operation can be undertaken when the relationship of ventricular mass to volume has normalized and it is anticipated that ventricular

compliance would be optimal. The unique preparatory na-ture of the hemi-Fontan operation makes the completion Fontan procedure a very straightforward technical exercise. Following median sternotomy, bypass is established with an arterial perfusion cannula in the ascending aorta and a single venous cannula in the appendage of the right atrium. After cooling to a core temperature of 20°C, the aorta is cross-clamped and a single dose of cardioplegia solution is infused into the aortic root. The circulation is temporarily discontinued. A longitudinal incision is made in the free wall of the right atrium anterior and parallel to the sulcus terminalis. The homograft dam which had been used to close the junction of the right atrium with the right superior vena cava and pulmonary arteries is widely excised (Fig. 77–4B). Care is taken to ensure that the resulting orifice is as large or larger than the inferior vena cava. A gusset of appropriate length is then cut from a portion of a PTFE tube graft that has been opened longitudinally. This is used to create a lateral atrial tunnel by which inferior vena caval flow is directed to the pulmonary arteries (Fig. 77–5). A portion of the tunnel is comprised of the free wall of the right atrium, thus having the potential for growth. This par-titioning of the atrium is fundamentally similar to tech-niques previously described by de Leval et al,[41] Puga et

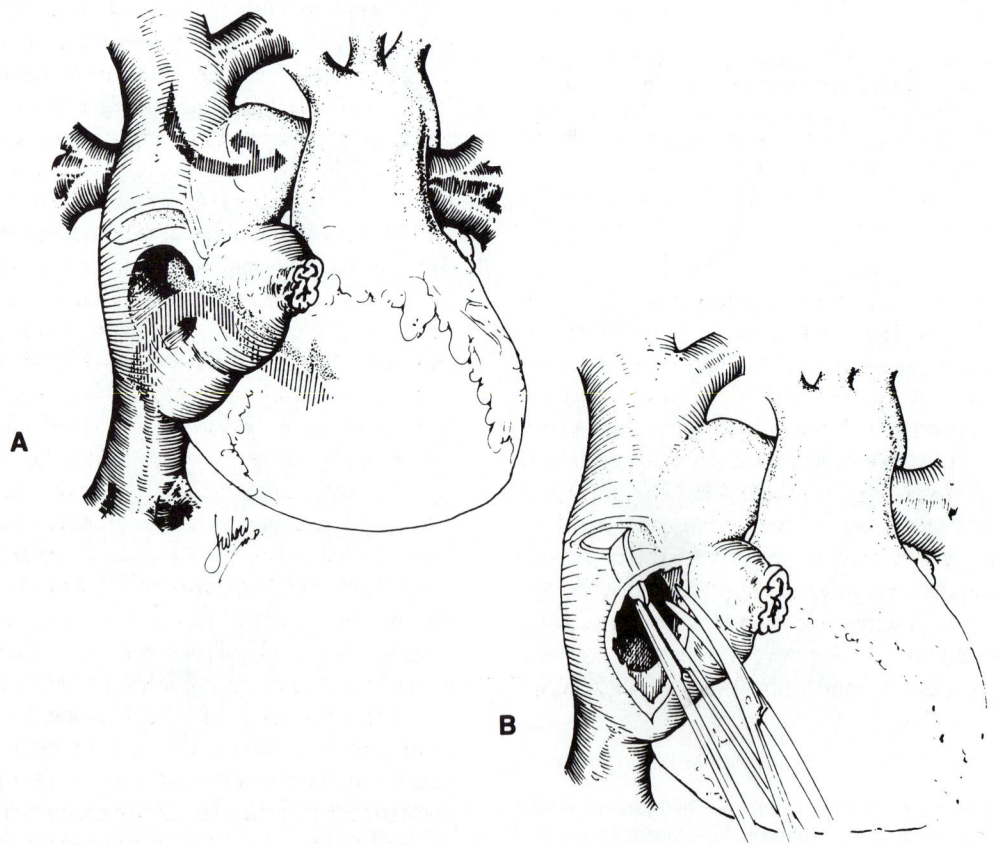

Figure 77–4. A. An artist's depiction of the circulatory pattern following the hemi-Fontan procedure. All superior vena caval return is obligated to flow into the right and left branch pulmonary arteries. **B.** The initial steps of the completion Fontan procedure include wide excision of the homograft dam, which had been used to close the junction of the right atrium with the right superior vena cava.

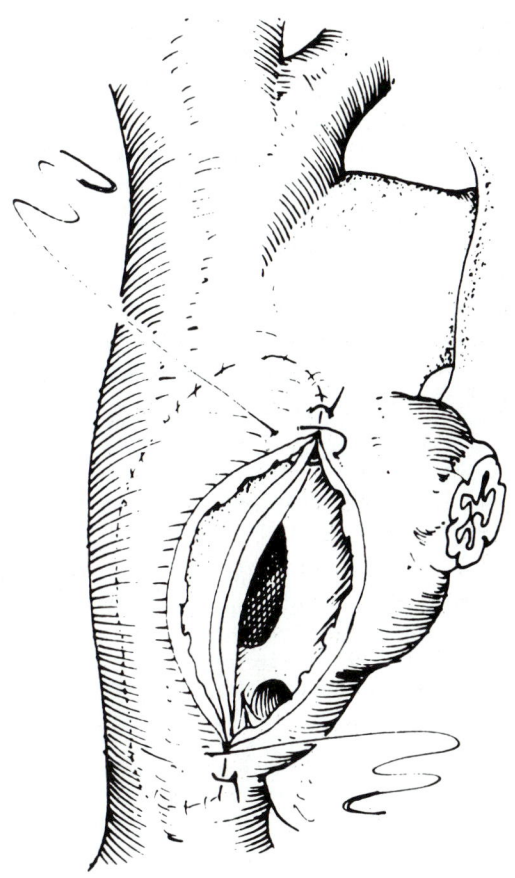

Figure 77–5. The completion Fontan consists of the construction of a lateral atrial tunnel to direct inferior vena caval return to the confluence of the pulmonary arteries and superior vena cava. The pathway is created using a baffle of PTFE and the wall of the right atrium, thus ensuring the potential for growth of the systemic venous pathway.

al,[42] Norwood et al[43] and others. After closure of the atriotomy incision, reperfusion and rewarming and separation from bypass are accomplished. Catheters are inserted for the postoperative measurement of pressures within the atrium and the systemic venous pathway. The authors have achieved a significant reduction in the mortality associated with Fontan's procedure by accomplishing the process in two stages as described here.[44] Further technical modifications have been introduced in an effort to minimize the morbidity associated with pleural and pericardial effusions and ascites following Fontan's procedure. These include the creation of fenestrations in the interatrial baffle or the exclusion of one or more hepatic veins from the systemic venous pathway.

RESULTS

The results for initial surgical palliation for hypoplastic left heart syndrome at the Children's Hospital of Philadelphia from January 1984 through May 1993 include 406 patients.

There were 125 (27%) early deaths and 35 (10%) late deaths in the total group of patients. Early in this experience, it became clear that survival was dependent not solely on a surgical exercise but most critically upon management of the physiology of a single ventricle providing combined systemic and pulmonary outputs with the circulations connected in parallel. Thus, not only has the surgical technique undergone progressive refinement but the perioperative management has been modified with a goal of minimizing the impact of the dynamic alterations in pulmonary and systemic resistance on the infants' hemodynamic well-being. The concept of addition of carbon dioxide to the inspired gas mixture has been an important adjunct to the perioperative management and has resulted in a significant diminution in early postoperative mortality.[45] Thus, contemporary results of initial surgical palliation for hypoplastic left heart syndrome at The Children's Hospital of Philadelphia include 63 patients operated between May 1992 and May 1993 with an early mortality of 10% (6 patients) and late mortality of 3% (2 patients).

As described, the hemi-Fontan procedure is undertaken early within the first year of life to achieve early reduction of the volume work of the single ventricle. It also serves to attenuate the adverse effects of geometric changes that may occur in the early postoperative period following reduction of ventricular volume work, which contributes significantly to the morbidity and mortality associated with a primary Fontan operation. From May 1989 to May 1993, 200 patients have undergone hemi-Fontan operation at The Children's Hospital of Philadelphia in the management of hypoplastic left heart syndrome. There have been 21 early deaths (10%) and 6 late deaths (3%). The majority of the mortality was related to those patients who underwent hemi-Fontan operation emergently at less than 6 months of age because of severe hemodynamic disturbances such as limited pulmonary blood flow or important ventricular dysfunction. Contemporary results are represented by the 45 patients with hypoplastic left heart syndrome who underwent hemi-Fontan procedure between May 1992 and May 1993, with one early death and no late deaths.

From January 1990 to May 1993, 127 patients with hypoplastic left heart syndrome who had undergone a previous hemi-Fontan procedure had a completion Fontan procedure at The Children's Hospital of Philadelphia with six early deaths (5%) and two late deaths (1.5%). Contemporary results are represented by 40 patients who from May 1992 to May 1993 underwent a completion Fontan for hypoplastic left heart syndrome with no early or late mortality.

The results of heart transplantation for hypoplastic left heart syndrome reflect not only the outcome of heart replacement, but the impact of donor availability as well. The Pediatric Heart Transplant Study group[46] recently reviewed the experience of the 21 member institutions with transplantation for hypoplastic left heart syndrome. Between January 1, 1993 and December 31 1993, 69 infants with hypoplastic left heart syndrome were listed for transplantation. Of the 69 infants, 24 died before transplantation. Two were removed from the transplant list following successful reconstructive surgery. As of June 30, 1994, 28 infants had undergone transplantation and were alive at follow-up. Twelve had undergone transplantation and had died, and three were still awaiting transplantation.

In conclusion, the management of hypoplastic left heart syndrome has evolved progressively over the last 15 years culminating in either heart replacement or a strategy of reconstructive surgery in three stages: initial palliation being undertaken shortly after birth, a hemi-Fontan procedure planned at about 6 months, and a completion Fontan operation at 1 to 2 years of age. It is clear that with an increased understanding of the physiology associated with each of the various operated states, reconstructive surgical therapy for hypoplastic left heart syndrome can be achieved with low mortality and with a long-term prognosis essentially comparable to that for other heart malformations where there is a single ventricle and where treatment is based upon the principles of Fontan's procedure.[47]

REFERENCES

1. Fyler DC: Report of the New England Regional Infant Cardiac Program. *Pediatrics* **65**(suppl):463, 1980
2. Lev M: Pathologic anatomy and interrelationship of hypoplasia of the aortic tract complexes. *Lab Invest* **1**:61–70, 1952
3. Noonan JA, Nadas AS: The hypoplastic left heart syndrome. *Pediatr Clin North Am* **5**:1029–1056, 1958
4. Bailey LL, et al: Cardiac allotransplantation in newborns as therapy for hypoplastic left heart syndrome. *N Engl J Med* **315**:949–951, 1986
5. Bailey L, Conception W, Shattuck H, Huang L: Method of heart transplantation for hypoplastic left heart syndrome. *J Thorac Cardiovasc Surg* **92**:105, 1986
6. Bailey L, Nehlsen-Cannarella SL, Conception W, Jolly WB: Baboon-to-human xenotransplantation in a neonate. *JAMA* **254**:3321–3329, 1985
7. Doty DB, Knott HW: Hypoplastic left heart syndrome. Experience with an operation to establish functionally normal circulation. *J Thorac Cardiovasc Surg* **74**:624–630, 1977
8. Jonas RA, et al: First-stage palliation of hypoplastic left heart syndrome. *J Thorac Cardiovasc Surg* **92**:6–13, 1986
9. Milo S, Ho SY, Anderson RH: Hypoplastic left heart syndrome. Can this malformation be treated surgically? *Thorax* **35**:351–354, 1980
10. Moodie DS, Gallen WJ, Friedberg DZ: Congenital aortic atresia. Report of long survival and some speculation about surgical approaches. *J Thorac Cardiovasc Surg* **63**:726–731, 1972
11. Norwood WI, Kirklin JK, Sanders SP: Hypoplastic left heart syndrome. Experience with palliative surgery. *Am J Cardiol* **45**:87–91, 1980
12. Norwood WI, Lang P, Hansen D: Physiologic repair of aortic atresia-hypoplastic left heart syndrome. *N Engl J Med* **308**:23–26, 1983
13. Norwood WI, Lang P, Castaneda AR, Campbell DN: Experience with operations for hypoplastic left heart syndrome. *J Thorac Cardiovasc Surg* **82**:511–519, 1981
14. Pigott JD, Murphy JD, Barber G, Norwood WI: Palliative reconstructive surgery for hypoplastic left heart syndrome. *Ann Thorac Surg* **45**:122–128, 1988
15. Sade RM, Fyfe D, Alpert CC: Hypoplastic left heart syndrome: A simplified palliative operation. *Ann Thorac Surg* **43**:309–312, 1987
16. Sinha SN, et al: Hypoplastic left ventricle syndrome. Analysis of thirty autopsy cases in infants with surgical consideration. *Am J Cardiol* **21**:166–173, 1968
17. Watson DG, Rowe RD: Aortic-valve atresia report of 43 cases. *JAMA* **179**:14–18, 1962
18. Bharati S, Lev M: The surgical anatomy of hypoplasia of aortic tract complex. *J Thorac Cardiovasc Surg* **88**:97–101, 1984
19. Lehman E: Congenital atresia of the foramen ovale. *Am J Dis Child* **33**:585–589, 1927
20. Bjerregaard P, Laursen HB: Persistent left superior vena cava. *Acta Paediatr Scand* **69**:105–108, 1980
21. Bulkley BH, D'Amico B, Taylor AL: Extensive myocardial fiber disarray in aortic and pulmonary atresia. *Circulation* **67**:191–198, 1983
22. Elliot RS, et al: Mitral atresia. A study of 32 cases. *Am Heart J* **71**:6–22, 1965
23. Elzenga NJ, Gittenberger de Grott AC: Coarctation and related aortic arch anomalies in hypoplastic left heart syndrome. *Int J Cardiol* **8**:379–393, 1985
24. Hawkins JA, Doty DB: Aortic atresia: Morphologic characteristics affecting survival and operative palliation. *J Thorac Cardiovasc Surg* **88**:620–626, 1984
25. Jonas RA, et al: First-stage palliation of hypoplastic left heart syndrome. The importance of coarctation and shunt size. *J Thorac Cardiovasc Surg* **92**:6–13, 1986
26. Kanjuh VI, Elliot RS, Edwards JE: Coexistent mitral and aortic valvular atresia. A pathologic study of 14 cases. *Am J Cardiol* **15**:611–621, 1965
27. Moodie DS, et al: The hypoplastic left heart syndrome: Evidence of preoperative myocardial and hepatic infarction in spite of prostaglandin therapy. *Ann Thorac Surg* **42**:307–311, 1986
28. O'Connor WN, et al: Ventriculocoronary connections in hypoplastic left heart syndrome: An autopsy microscopic study. *Circulation* **66**:1078–1085, 1982
29. Roberts WC, et al: Aortic valve atresia: A new classification based on necropsy study of 73 cases. *Am J Cardiol* **37**:753–756, 1976
30. van der Horst RL, Hastreiter AR, DuBrow IW, Eckner FAO: Pathologic measurements in aortic atresia. *Am Heart J* **106**:1411–1415, 1983
31. Von Reuden TJ, Knight L, Moller JH, Edwards JE: Coarctation of the aorta associated with aortic valve atresia. *Circulation* **52**:951–954, 1975
32. Weinberg PM, et al: Postmortem echocardiography and tomographic anatomy of hypoplastic left heart syndrome after palliative surgery. *Am J Cardiol* **58**:1228–1232, 1986
33. Weinberg PM, Peyser K, Hackney JR: Fetal hydrops in a newborn with hypoplastic left heart syndrome: Tricuspid valve stopper. *J Am Coll Cardiol* **6**:1365–1369, 1985
34. Bharati S, Nordenberg A, Brock RR, Lev M: Hypoplastic left heart syndrome with dyplastic pulmonary valve with stenosis. *Pediatr Cardiol* **5**:127–130, 1984
35. Barber G, et al: The significance of preoperative tricuspid regurgitation in hypoplastic left heart syndrome. *Circulation* **74**(suppl II):II-36, 1986
36. Helton JG, et al: Analysis of potential anatomic or physiologic determinants of outcome of palliative surgery for hypoplastic left heart syndrome. *Circulation* **74**(suppl I):I-70–I-76, 1986
37. Mandorla S, et al: Fetal echocardiography. Prenatal diagnosis of hypoplastic left heart syndrome. *G Ital Cardiol* **14**:517–520, 1984
38. Sahn DJ, et al: Prenatal ultrasound in utero association with hydrops fetalis. *Am Heart J* **104**:1368–1372, 1982
39. Norwood WI, Jacobs ML: Fontan's operation in two stages. *Am J Surg* **166**:548–551, 1993
40. Jacobs ML, Murphy JD, Nicolson SC, et al: Manipulation of inspired carbon dioxide in neonates with one ventricle and systemic-to-pulmonary artery shunt. *Circulation* **84**(suppl II):238, 1991
41. de Leval MR, Kilner P, Gewillig M, Bull C: Total cavopulmonary connection: A logical alternative to atriopulmonary connection for

complex Fontan operations. *J Thorac Cardiovasc Surg* **96:**908–913, 1988

42. Puga FJ, Chiavarelli M, Hagler DJ: Modifications of the Fontan operation applicable to patients with left atrioventricular valve atresia or single atrioventricular valve. *Circulation* **76:**(Suppl 3):53–59, 1987

43. Norwood WI Jr: Hypoplastic left heart syndrome. *Ann Thorac Surg* **52:**688–695, 1991

44. Jacobs ML, Norwood WI: Fontan's operation: Influence of modifications on morbidity and mortality. *Ann Thorac Surg* 1994 (in press)

45. Gullquist S, Schmitz ML, Hannon GD, et al: Carbon dioxide in the inspired gas improves early postoperative survival in neonates with congenital heart disease following stage I palliation (Norwood). *Circulation* **86:**(suppl I):1435, 1992

46. Pediatric Heart Transplant Study: *Multi-institutional Data Analysis, November 1994.* Prepared by the PHTS Data Collection and Analysis Center at the University of Alabama at Birmingham (unpublished)

47. Norwood WI, Jacobs ML, Murphy JD: Fontan operation for hypoplastic left heart syndrome. *Ann Thorac Surg* **54:**1025–1030, 1992

78

Pulmonary Stenosis with Intact Ventricular Septum

Single Pulmonary Artery and Aneurysms of the Pulmonary Arteries

Eliot R. Rosenkranz

This chapter covers three separate problems involving the right ventricular outflow tract and the pulmonary arteries: (1) pulmonary stenosis (including valvar pulmonary stenosis and double chamber right ventricle), (2) aneurysms of the pulmonary arteries, and (3) single and/or absent pulmonary artery (Fig. 78–1). Although obstructive lesions of the right ventricular outflow tract are seen in 25–30% of all patients with congenital heart defects,[1] isolated pulmonary stenosis with intact ventricular septum is less common, comprising approximately 8–10% of all congenital heart defects.[2] Single or absent pulmonary arteries and pulmonary artery aneurysms are quite rare, in comparison.

PULMONARY STENOSIS WITH INTACT VENTRICULAR SEPTUM

Pulmonary stenosis with intact ventricular septum is the most common cause of right ventricular outflow tract obstruction, comprising 8–10% of all congenital heart lesions as noted above. First described by Morgagni in 1761,[3] pulmonary stenosis was first approached surgically by Doyen[4] who in 1913 attempted an unsuccessful transventricular valvotomy with a tenotomy knife. Sellors[5] and Brock[6] in 1948 applied the concept of blunt valve dilatation described earlier by Tuffier,[6] Souttar,[6] and Cutler and Beck[6] for treatment of aortic and mitral valve stenosis. These procedures opened the era of surgical management of valvar pulmonic stenosis that continues to be applied at many centers worldwide. Swan et al in 1953[7] successfully employed a direct, open approach for repair of a stenotic pulmonary valve in 15 patients using systemic hypothermia and a brief period of unsupported circulatory arrest (ventricular fibrillation). The application of cardiopulmonary bypass support during open pulmonary valvotomy was introduced in 1953[8] and remains the favored approach by most centers today. Open repair by brief normothermic inflow occlusion has also been employed with good clinical results.

The modern era of management of valvar pulmonary stenosis was opened by Semb et al[9] in 1979 and Kan et al[10] in 1982 who introduced balloon pulmonary valvotomy, which has since been widely applied to all pathologic entities of valvar pulmonic stenosis, in all age groups. As will be discussed subsequently, this has become the favored initial therapeutic intervention in many centers. It is, therefore, ironic that valvar pulmonic stenosis is the lesion that historically brought management of a congenital heart defect into the surgeon's hands and was also the first lesion to largely be removed from the surgical arena by "less invasive" balloon dilatation techniques.

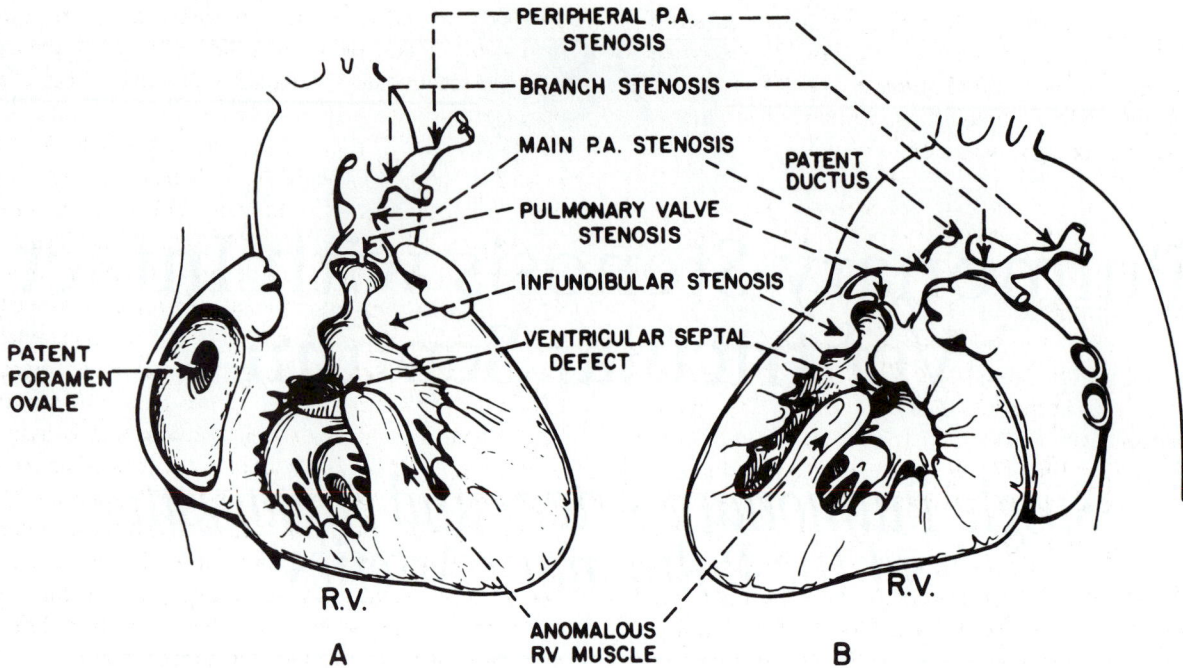

Figure 78–1. Levels of obstruction to right ventricular outflow at ventricular, valvar and pulmonary artery levels. **A.** Anterior view. **B.** Lateral view. R.V., right ventricle.

PULMONARY VALVE PATHOLOGY

Gikonyo and associates[11] described six subgroups of pulmonary valve morphology in patients with valvar pulmonary stenosis: tricuspid, bicuspid, unicommissural, domed (acommissural), hypoplastic annulus and valve, and dysplastic valve. In isolated pulmonary stenosis, tricuspid or domed (acommissural) valves account for approximately 70% of surgical specimens[12] in contrast to tetralogy of Fallot where bicuspid and unicommissural valves predominate. In tricuspid valves, the valve commissures are usually well defined, although fused, and are often adherent to the adjacent pulmonary artery wall resulting in supravalvar stenosis as well. Poststenotic pulmonary artery dilatation is seen in approximately 70% of patients outside the neonatal age group.[13]

Pulmonary valve dysplasia represents a distinct pathological entity found in 10–20% of patients with isolated valvar pulmonic stenosis[14] and was defined by Koretzky and associates in 1969.[15] The dysplastic valve is typically tricuspid with nonfused leaflets, characterized by marked thickening due to an accumulation of primitive mesodermal tissue in the spongiosa layer of the valve leaflets, resulting in severe immobility of the leaflets themselves. Pads of excess tissue are also present in the valve sinuses, which inhibit lateral motion of the valve leaflets during ventricular systole.[15] The valve annulus is hypoplastic in 10–20% of cases[16] and supravalvar pulmonary artery narrowing may be caused by commissural tethering of the adjacent pulmonary artery wall. Pulmonary valve dysplasia is found more commonly in patients with Noonans syndrome[17] and cardiofacial syndrome.[18] Due to these characteristic pathologic features (thickened, nonfused leaflets and narrowed annulus), a particular surgical or balloon dilatation strategy must be employed as will be discussed subsequently.

The associated pathologic changes of right-sided cardiac structures in patients with pulmonary valvar stenosis is strongly linked to the clinical presentation (age) and, as such, these aspects of pathological morphology will be discussed in conjunction with these individual categories.

CRITICAL PULMONARY STENOSIS OF THE NEONATE

Clinical Presentation

Whereas the majority of patients with pulmonary stenosis and intact ventricular septum are minimally symptomatic, neonates with critical pulmonary stenosis generally present within the first week of life,[19,20] critically ill, with tachypnea and moderately severe cyanosis due to atrial level right-to-left shunt and variable patency of the arterial duct. Survival beyond the first month of life is unlikely without surgical intervention. Physical examination may suggest the diagnosis of valvar pulmonary stenosis when a systolic murmur is heard at the base along with an ejection click on cardiac auscultation in association with hepatomegaly due to tricuspid regurgitation. Diminished pulmonary vascular markings and moderate cardiomegaly are characteristically seen on the frontal chest x-ray examination. The electrocardiogram may show a predominance of left ventricular forces despite right ventricular hypertrophy, due to the relative hypoplasia of right ventricular mass.

Diagnosis

Echocardiography

Two-dimensional echocardiography and color flow Doppler studies should provide the diagnosis of critical pulmonary stenosis in the majority of neonates. The stenotic, thickened, and often mildly hypoplastic pulmonary valve is easily identified (Fig. 78–2) and the valve gradient estimated by continuous wave Doppler. Pulmonary valve gradient and right ventricular pressure can be estimated from the transpulmonary valve and tricuspid valve flow velocities utilizing the modified Bernoulli equation (valve gradient = $4 \times V_{MAX}^2$)[21] (Figs. 78–3 and 78–4). The true degree of pulmonary valve obstruction may be underestimated, however, due to a low cardiac output state, severe tricuspid regurgitation, as well as significant right-to-left shunt at the atrial level.

Morphologically, the pulmonary valve may have the characteristics described earlier in the section on pulmonary valve pathology. Hanley and associates,[20] in a series of 101 neonates with critical pulmonary stenosis, noted mild pulmonary annular hypoplasia in most patients (median Z score = −1.6) and severe hypoplasia in 15% (Fig. 78–5). The tricuspid valve was similarly mildly stenotic (median Z score = −1.0) in most patients and significantly stenotic in 15% of patients. In contrast, moderate-to-severe tricuspid incompetence is noted in over 90% of patients due both to right ventricular failure (dilatation) and right ventricular hypertension.

The right ventricle was mildly to moderately reduced in volume in 49% of patients in Hanley's series[20] and severely hypoplastic in 4%. Similar findings are reported by other studies,[19,22–24] and right ventricular size does not significantly impact on postintervention survival in contrast to that seen in patients with pulmonary atresia with intact ventricular septum.[20,22,24,25] The exception to this is when extremes of right ventricular hypoplasia or severe right ventricular enlargement are found. Concentric right ventricular hypertrophy is characteristically present and is associated with a variable degree of endocardial fibrosis that increases in patients with severe right ventricular hypoplasia. The degree of right ventricular hypertrophy and the resultant decrease in right ventricular end diastolic volume and right ventricular diastolic compliance influence the early hemodynamics and the amount of residual right-to-left shunt after pulmonary valve intervention (see below).

The proximal pulmonary arteries in the neonate are typically normal in size, being significantly hypoplastic in less than 4%.[22] However, they may appear relatively underfilled preoperatively depending upon the amount of pulmonary blood flow provided by the ductus arteriosus at the time of study. Poststenotic dilatation is not seen in the neonate.

The right atrium is always enlarged in critical pulmonary stenosis, particularly when tricuspid valve regurgitation is severe in magnitude. A patent foramen ovale or true atrial septal defect is also always present, allowing a variable degree of right-to-left shunt and resultant mainte-

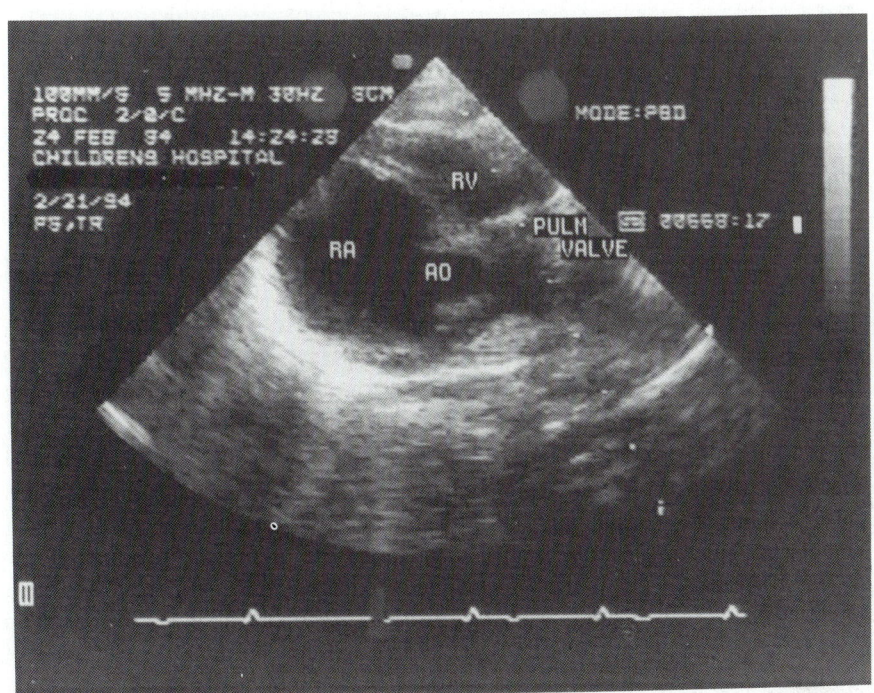

Figure 78–2. Parasternal short axis two-dimensional echocardiogram of 3-day-old neonate with critical pulmonary stenosis. Note thickened echodense pulmonary valve (pulm valve); RA, right atrium; AO, aorta; RV, right ventricle.

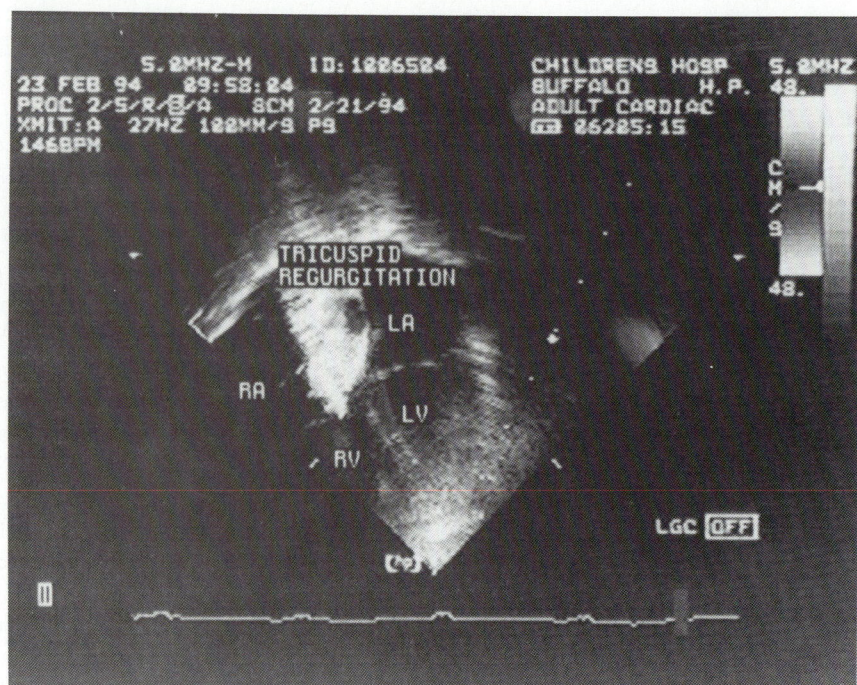

Figure 78–3. Apical four chamber two-dimensional echocardiogram and color Doppler study of same patient in Figure 78–2. Note severe tricuspid regurgitation. See abbreviations in Figure 78–2; LV, left ventricle.

nance of systemic cardiac output despite severe right ventricular outflow tract obstruction at the time of clinical presentation. Coexisting cardiac anomalies, except for patent ductus arteriosus, are rarely found.

Cardiac Catheterization and Angiography

Routine diagnostic cardiac catheterization and angiography have largely been replaced by noninvasive two-dimensional echocardiography and color-directed Doppler studies. Invasive preoperative studies have largely been limited to situa-

tions where the diagnosis is equivocal or the presence of an associated anomaly is suspected. Most often, invasive diagnostic studies are performed in association with a therapeutic intervention such as balloon pulmonary valvotomy. Right heart catheterization documents systemic or suprasystemic right ventricular pressure. Right heart angiography confirms the anatomy and degree of pulmonary valvar obstruction (Fig. 78–6), the pulmonary artery anatomy, the right ventricular dimension, the tricuspid valve size, and its competence (Fig. 78–7).

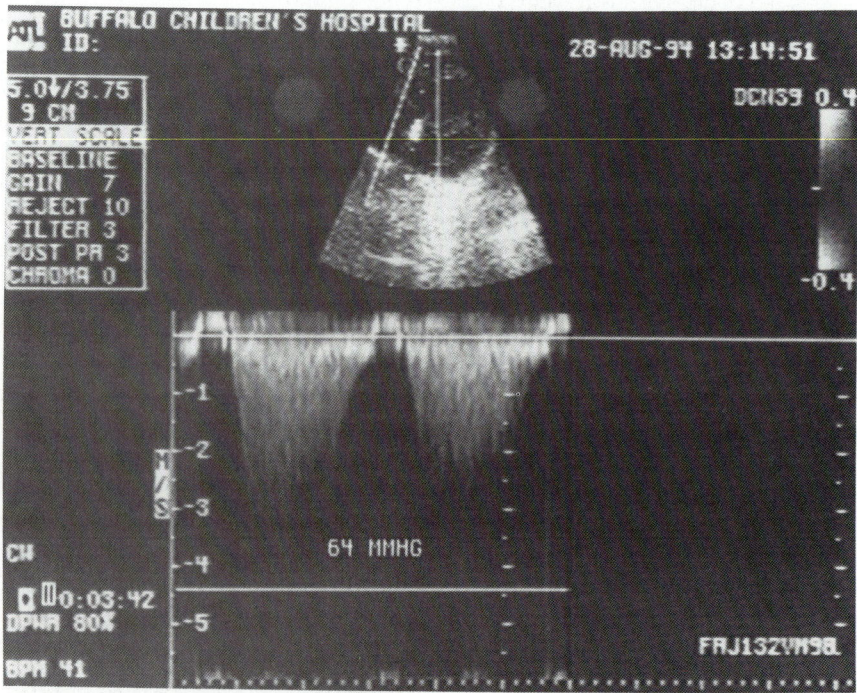

Figure 78–4. Continuous-wave Doppler velocity of tricuspid regurgitant jet used to estimate right ventricular systolic pressure (64 mm Hg) in 1 day old with critical pulmonary stenosis.

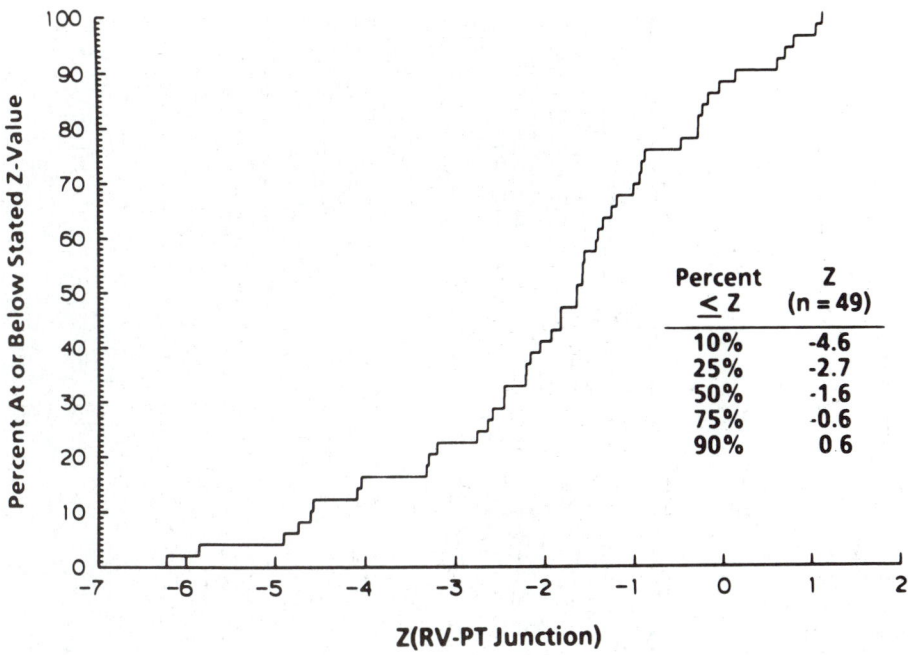

Percent ≤ Z	Z (n = 49)
10%	-4.6
25%	-2.7
50%	-1.6
75%	-0.6
90%	0 6

Figure 78–5. Distribution of dimensions of pulmonary valve annulus (RV–PT junction) in neonate with critical pulmonary stenosis. Note that median dimension was 1.6 standard deviation below the mean normal dimension. (*From: Hanley et al.[20] Reprinted with permission from the American College of Cardiology (Journal of the American College of Cardiology, 1993, 22:183–192.).*)

Management and Intervention

Preintervention Stabilization

Most neonates with critical pulmonary stenosis present within the first week of life critically ill, as noted earlier, and often require resuscitation in parallel with diagnostic studies. Insertion of umbilical artery and vein cannulae will allow arterial blood gas assessment and correction of acid–base abnormalities. Prostaglandin E_1 infusion is initiated to reestablish or maintain ductal patency. Intubation with mechanical ventilation reduces the risk of prostaglandin associated apnea and decreases the cardiac work load. Inotropic support may be initiated according to physical and laboratory assessment of the adequacy of cardiac output.

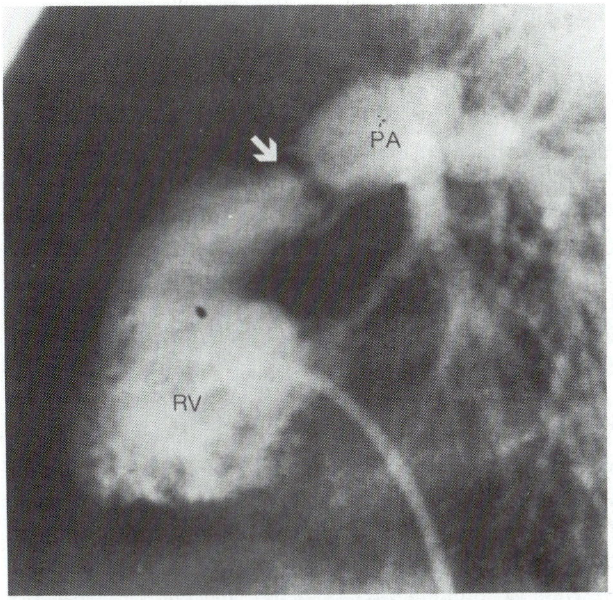

Balloon Pulmonary Valvotomy

Balloon pulmonary valvotomy has become the preferred initial treatment for moderately severe pulmonary valvar stenosis in infants, children, and adults. Balloon pulmonary valvotomy is also rapidly replacing surgical intervention as the preferred initial modality in neonates.[20,26,27] It is of note that the initial transcatheter treatment of pulmonary valvar stenosis performed by Semb et al[9] in 1979 was carried out in a neonate with critical pulmonary stenosis.

Technique. Balloon pulmonary valvotomy in neonates is significantly more difficult than in infants and older patients due to the neonates clinical instability and the difficulty in positioning the catheter guidewires.[27] Balloon pulmonary valvotomy is performed after medical stabilization with prostaglandin E_1 infusion as outlined earlier. Percutaneous transfemoral vein right heart catheterization is performed to calibrate the size of the pulmonary valve annulus and the infundibulum to help choose the correct balloon size and to rule out significant infundibular hypertrophy which is a risk factor for failure of balloon pulmonary valvotomy (Fig. 78–8A). A soft guidewire is positioned

Figure 78–6. Lateral right ventriculogram in a 3 day old with critical pulmonary stenosis. Note severely thickened, immobile pulmonary valve (white arrow). RV, right ventricle; PA, pulmonary artery.

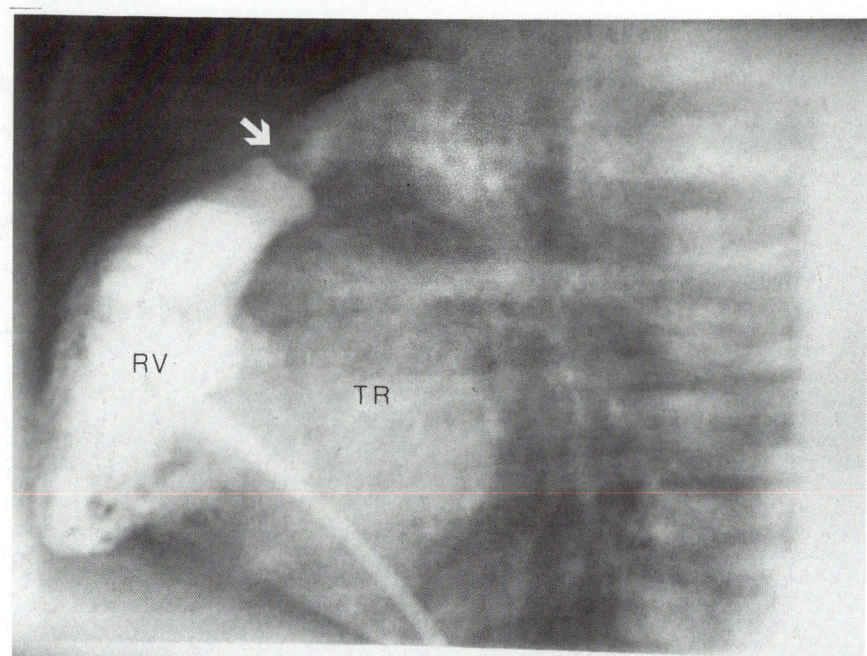

Figure 78–7. Lateral right ventriculogram in a 5 day old with critical pulmonary stenosis. Note severe tricuspid regurgitation (TR) and severely thickened pulmonary valve (white arrow). RV, right ventricle.

across the stenotic pulmonary valve and across the patent ductus arteriosus into the descending aorta. Sequentially graduated balloons (2 mm up to 120–130% of annulus size) are placed and inflated until the balloon waist (representing the stenotic valve) disappears (Fig. 78–8B). A repeat right ventriculogram is performed to evaluate the infundibulum and catheterization is carried out, anticipating a residual gradient of less than 30 mm Hg with a $P_{RV/LV}$ of 0.4–0.6.

Results. No large long-term follow-up series is available following balloon pulmonary valvotomy in neonates with critical pulmonary stenosis. However, several short and intermediate term studies have been reported. On average, balloon pulmonary valvotomy is successful in 50–90% of cases of patients with critical pulmonary stenosis. More than 50% of the procedural failures are due to the inability to pass the stenotic pulmonary valve with a guidewire or the inability to stabilize the guidewire across the pulmonary valve in the patent ductus arteriosus.[19,20,26–32] In patients successfully balloon dilated, restenosis is reported in approximately 25% of patients by 1-year follow-up and has been associated with the use of a dilating balloon that is less than 120% of the predilation pulmonary valve annulus diameter.[26–32] Redilation of these recurrent stenotic valves is associated with approximately 20% late restenosis. Morbidity following balloon pulmonary valve dilation occurs in approximately 5–7% of neonates (principally blood loss, iliofemoral vein thrombosis, and transient infundibular obstruction). Mortality averages 5–10% (usually not directly procedure related).[27,30]

Recognized risk factors for failure of balloon pulmonary valvotomy in critical pulmonary stenosis and, therefore, relative contraindications to the procedure include (1) a small pulmonary valve annulus ($Z \leq -3$), (2) significant right ventricular and/or infundibular hypoplasia, (3) use of a balloon-to-annulus ratio of less than 100%, and (4) significant tricuspid regurgitation. Overall, the short-term results of balloon pulmonary valvotomy in patients with critical pulmonary stenosis compare favorably with surgical intervention. Postprocedural evaluation demonstrates a significantly lower incidence of pulmonary valve regurgitation and a lower periprocedure mortality when compared to older surgical series [94% 6-mo survival (Fig. 78–9), 91% event-free survival (Fig. 78–10)].[20,27,32]

Surgical Valvotomy

Surgical intervention by any of several techniques is indicated at institutions where balloon pulmonary valvotomy in neonates is not available, in patients in whom balloon pulmonary valvotomy was not possible or successful (severe persistent hypoxemia), or in patients with associated large atrial septal defects. Although several surgical procedures have been reported with good results, Hanley and associates[20] have reported superior results with open valvotomy on cardiopulmonary bypass with brief cardioplegic arrest, which is also our preferred surgical approach (Fig. 78–11). Similar results have been reported by others utilizing open valvotomy with brief inflow occlusion[33–36] or closed valvotomy either via transventricular[5,6,20,23,24,37,38] or transpulmonary artery[19] approaches. Prior to any surgical procedure, medical stabilization including prostaglandin E_1 infusion to maintain ductal patency, mechanical ventilation, and selective use of inotropic agents is indicated. After adequate venous and arterial accesses are established, general anesthesia is induced with administration of adequate intra-

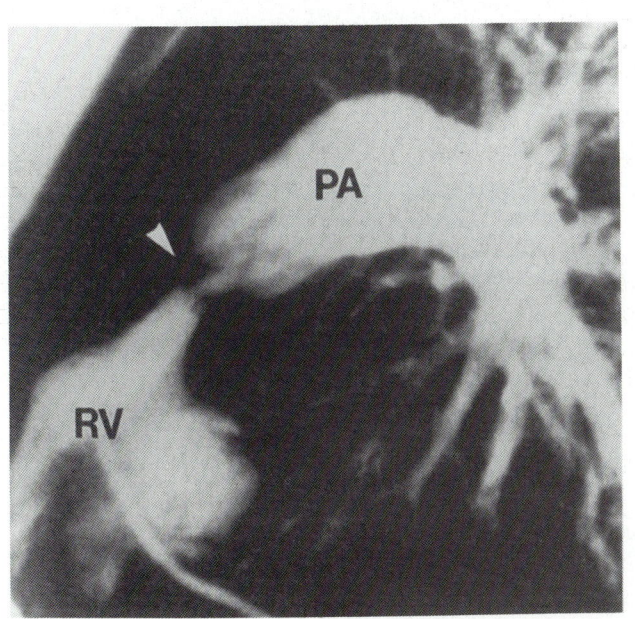

A

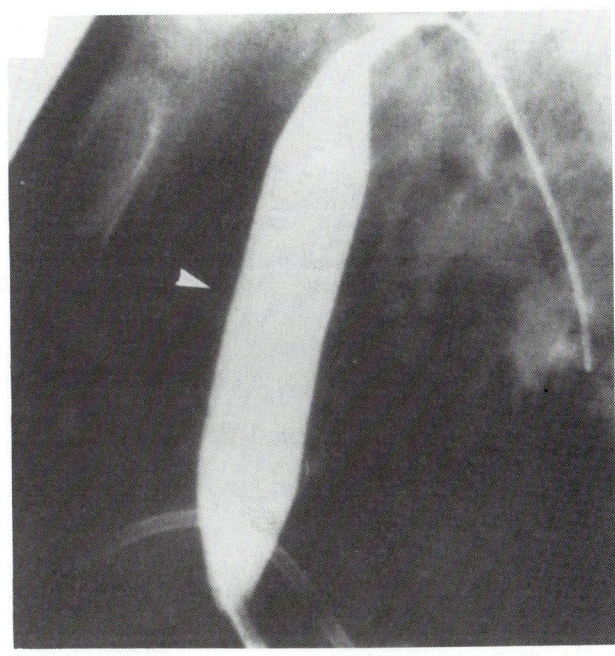

B

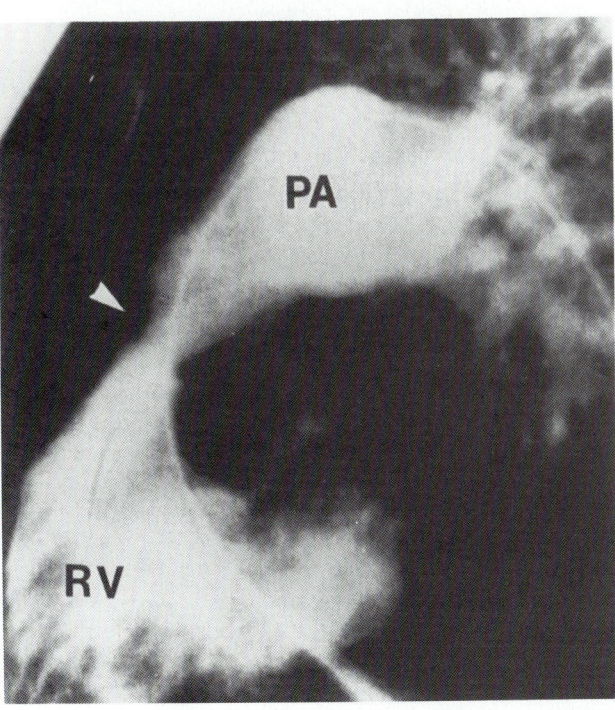

C

Figure 78–8. A. Lateral right ventriculogram of patient with severe valvar pulmonary stenosis. Note severely thickened pulmonary valve (arrowhead). RV, right ventricle; PA, pulmonary artery. **B.** Valvuloplasty balloon has been placed across the balloon and inflated. Note the absence of a residual "waist" at pulmonary valve level (arrowhead). **C.** Postdilation ventriculogram. Note minimal residual valvar stenosis (arrowhead).

venous volume to maintain filling of the hypertrophied and poorly compliant right ventricle.

Open Pulmonary Valvotomy on Cardiopulmonary Bypass With Cardioplegic Arrest. Via a median sternotomy, bicaval venous and aortic arterial cardiopulmonary bypass is established with mild hypothermia (32°C) (Fig. 78–12). Intraoperative epicardial two-dimensional echocardiography and color-directed Doppler interrogation are useful

adjuncts to confirm the preoperative anatomy and pathophysiology. The previously isolated ductus arteriosus is temporarily controlled with a snare to allow subsequent reopening if postvalvotomy arterial blood gas saturations are inadequate (pO$_2$ < 35 mm Hg). The aorta is cross-clamped and cold blood cardioplegia is administered into the aortic root to obtain diastolic arrest[39] (an alternative approach is the use of warm blood cardioplegic induction followed by cold blood cardioplegic maintenance infusion[40]). A longitu-

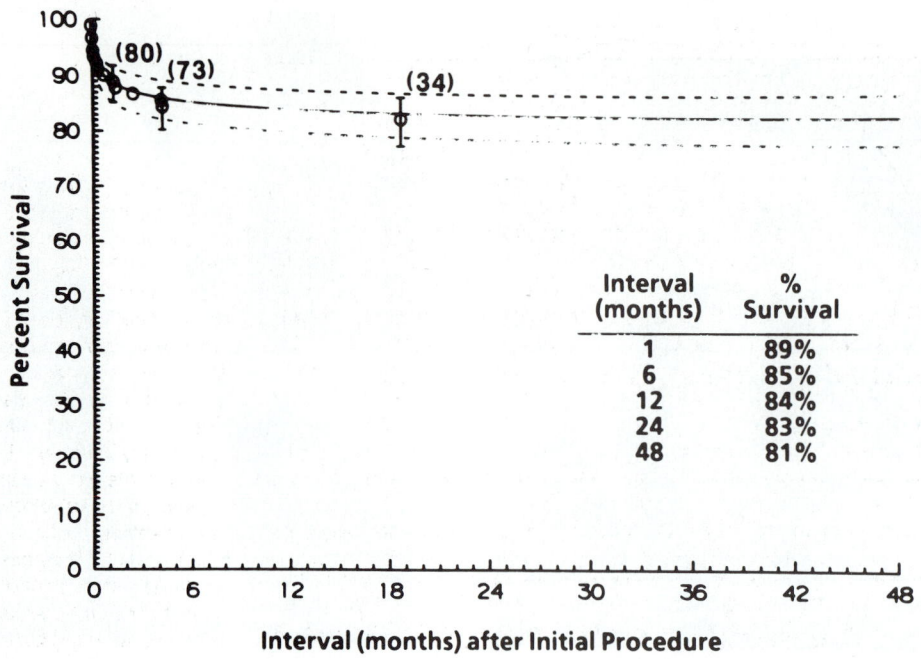

Figure 78–9. Actuarial survival after intervention for critical pulmonary stenosis by Kaplan–Meier analysis. Dashed lines represent 70% confidence intervals. *(From Hanley et al.[20] Reprinted with permission from the American College of Cardiology (Journal of the American College of Cardiology, 1993, 22:183–192).)*

dinal pulmonary arteriotomy is performed, the valve examined, the fused commissures widely incised with an 11 scalpel blade, and the valve gently dilated with a fine mosquito clamp. The annulus is then calibrated with a Hegar dilator and compared to the normal valve diameters based

on the patient's preoperative body surface area[41,42] (Table 78–1). Valve excision is infrequently required, limited to cases where severe pulmonary valve dysplasia is apparent. The pulmonary artery is then closed with running 6-0 polypropylene suture. The right atrium is then opened and

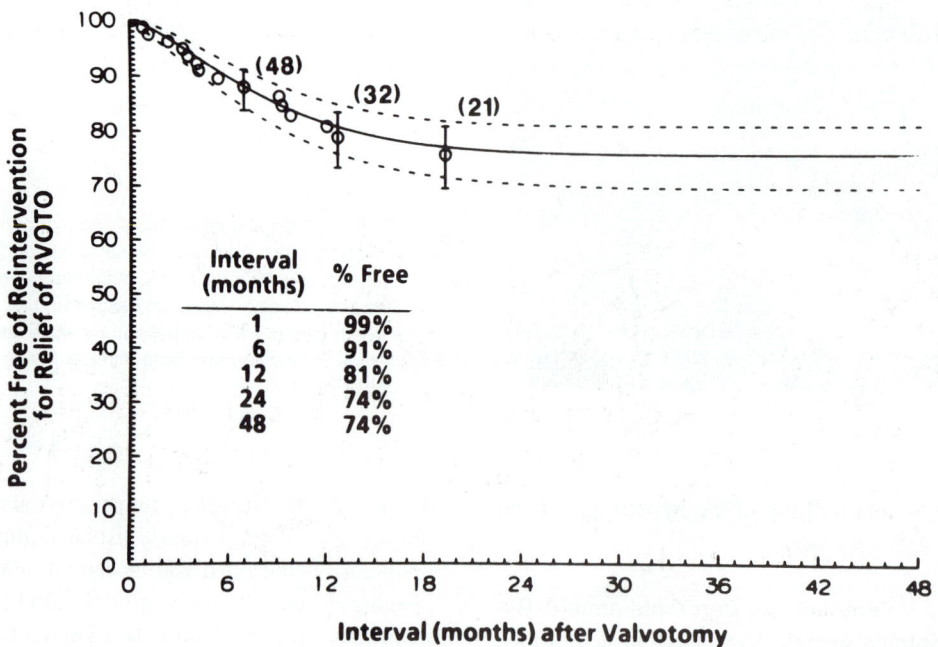

Figure 78–10. Freedom from reintervention for relief of right ventricular outflow tract obstruction and after initial procedure in patients with critical pulmonary stenosis. Dashed lines represent 70% confidence intervals. Note increasing need for reintervention beyond 6 months follow-up reaching 26% 2 years after the initial procedure. *(From Hanley et al.[20] Reprinted with permission from the American College of Cardiology (Journal of the American College of Cardiology, 1993, 22:183–192).)*

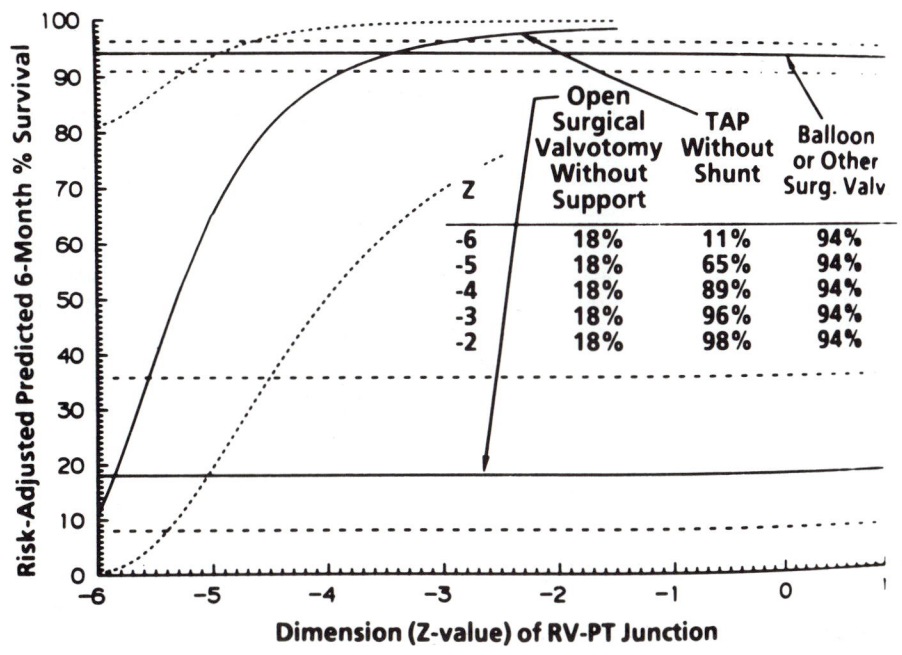

Z	Open Surgical Valvotomy Without Support	TAP Without Shunt	Balloon or Other Surg. Valv
-6	18%	11%	94%
-5	18%	65%	94%
-4	18%	89%	94%
-3	18%	96%	94%
-2	18%	98%	94%

Figure 78–11. Nomogram showing risk-adjusted survival at or beyond 6 mo after the initial procedure according to the dimension (*Z* value) of the pulmonary valve annulus (RV–PT junction). Note high mortality rate for open valvotomy without bypass support irrespective of annulus size, increasing survival for patients with larger annulus size when a transannular patch was done without a simultaneous aorto-pulmonary shunt, and lower periopera-tive and late mortality after balloon val-votomy, open valvotomy on bypass, or transventricular closed valvotomy. *(From Hanley et al.[20] Reprinted with permission from the American College of Cardiology (Journal of the American College of Cardiology, 1993,22:183–192).)*

the patent foramen ovale or atrial septal defect partially closed, leaving a small residual orifice to allow a controlled right-to-left atrial level shunt during the perioperative period. This assures maintenance of cardiac output at lower right atrial pressures in the face of poor early right ventricu-lar diastolic function. The right atriotomy is then closed, warm blood cardioplegic reperfusate administered, and the aorta unclamped. A left atrial pressure monitoring catheter is placed, and the patient is weaned from cardiopulmonary bypass. A postrepair epicardial two-dimensional echocar-diogram with color-directed Doppler interrogation is used

to assess the residual gradient across the right ventricular outflow tract and to determine the degree of residual tricus-pid regurgitation and the direction of atrial level shunt. If the pO_2 is greater than or equal to 35 mm Hg, the ductus ar-teriosus is ligated. If the pO_2 is less than 35 mm Hg, the ductus snare is released and prostaglandin infusion is con-tinued and ductal patency confirmed by a rise in the arterial pO_2. In addition, a color disturbance in the pulmonary artery may be detectable on epicardial echo study. A con-comitant systemic to pulmonary artery Gore-Tex shunt is reserved for situations where the pO_2 remains less than 35

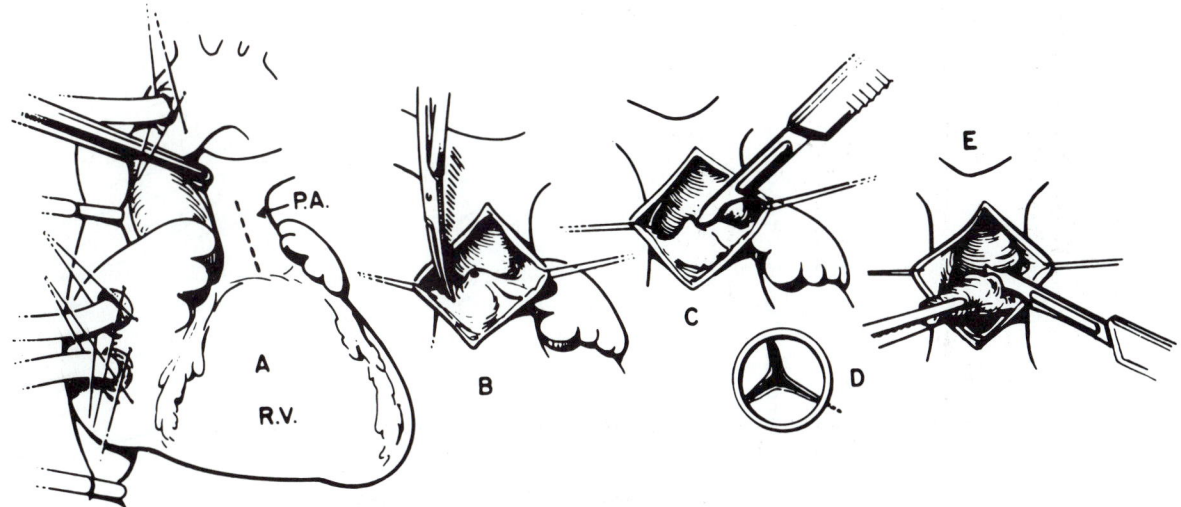

Figure 78–12. Technique for open pulmonary valvotomy on cardiopulmonary bypass. See text for full description. **A.** Standard and bicaval cannulation for bypass. Dashed line denotes site for pulmonary valvotomy. **B.** Pulmonary valve commissures are mobilized from the wall of the pulmonary artery. **C., D.** Fused commissures are incised to the hinge points at the valve annulus. **E.** Valve debridement or valve excision for thickened or dysplastic valves.

TABLE 78–1. MEAN NORMAL DIAMETER OF PULMONARY VALVE

BSA (m²)	Pulmonary Annulus
0.25	8.4
0.30	9.3
0.35	10.1
0.40	10.7
0.45	11.3
0.50	11.9
0.60	12.8
0.70	13.5
0.80	14.2
0.90	14.8
1.0	15.3
1.2	16.2
1.4	17.0
1.6	17.6
1.8	18.2
2.0	19.0

Data from Rowlatt et al.[41]

mm Hg despite adjunctive measures and documentation of adequate relief of the right ventricular outflow tract obstruction.

As noted earlier, significant pulmonary valve annular hypoplasia is uncommon (less than 10% of cases) and placement of a transannular patch during the primary operation should be limited to situations where the pulmonary valve annulus Z score is less than −3[20] (Fig. 78–13) on the preoperative echocardiogram and confirmed by intraoperative Hegar dilator calibration (Table 78–1). Patients with small right ventricular cavities may also have residual right ventricular outflow tract obstruction due to hypertrophied muscle bundles despite an adequate pulmonary valve annulus size. Localized resection with or without placement of a transannular patch may be beneficial in these settings. Progressive resolution of right ventricular outflow tract muscle hypertrophy, however, is anticipated in most situations. When a transannular patch is indicated, the pulmonary artery incision is continued proximally into the right ventricular outflow tract until an adequate sized Hegar dilator can pass into the right ventricular body. An autologous pericardial patch is the preferred material, and this is sized with the guidance of the Hegar dilator.

Open Pulmonary Valvotomy During Normothermic Inflow Occlusion. Varco,[43] Mistrot et al,[33] Sade et al,[34] and Jonas et al,[35,36] have reported excellent results with pulmonary valvotomy performed during a brief period of normothermic inflow occlusion. This technique necessitates coordinated anesthesia and surgical teams to maximize perioperative hemodynamic stability and provide adequate exposure to allow meticulous surgical technique in the limited time frame available during inflow occlusion. The patient is prepared as outlined for open pulmonary valvotomy on cardiopulmonary bypass. Retraction sutures of 6-0 polypropylene are placed at the pulmonary valve annulus and 1.5–2 cm distally on the anterior wall of the pulmonary artery to allow placement of a fine partial occlusion clamp. Caval snares are positioned and the patient ventilated with 100% oxygen for 5 min and sodium bicarbonate (1 mEq/kg) is administered intravenously prior to caval occlusion. The heart

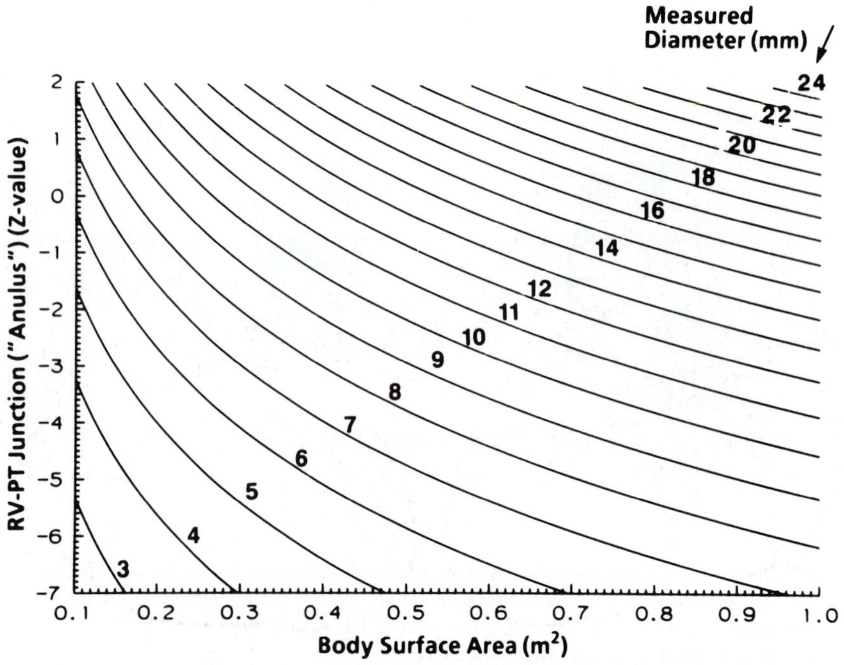

Figure 78–13. Nomogram for determining *Z* value of pulmonary valve annulus (RV–PT junction) from measured diameter of valve and body surface area. Note that measured diameter of valve annulus is from the echocardiogram or magnification corrected angiogram. (From Hanley et al.[20] Reprinted with permission from the American College of Cardiology (Journal of the American College of Cardiology, 1993, 22:183–192).)

is allowed to beat 2–3 times to empty the right ventricle after the caval snares are secured, and the main pulmonary artery is occluded by placement of a fine vascular clamp proximal to the ductus arteriosus. A 1–1.5 cm pulmonary arteriotomy is performed and pulmonary valvotomy is carried out. The pulmonary valve annulus is calibrated with Hegar dilators as described earlier. The inferior caval snare is then released, the right ventricle and pulmonary artery deaired via the pulmonary arteriotomy, and the arteriotomy controlled with a fine partial occlusion clamp with the assistance of the previous placed traction sutures. The entire procedure should be limited to 2–3 min.

The pulmonary arteriotomy is then closed with 6-0 polypropylene suture. The ductus arteriosus is generally left open and maintenance of prostaglandin E_1 infusion is guided by arterial oxygen saturations as described for open pulmonary valvotomy.

Brief inflow occlusion allows open pulmonary valvotomy plus the advantage of avoiding the morbidity and financial expense of cardiopulmonary bypass. Significant disadvantages include (1) limited procedural time frame, (2) inability to simultaneously close an atrial septal defect, (3) the inability to place a transannular patch in patients with significant annular hypoplasia or subpulmonic obstruction, and (4) inadequate time to perform an adequate pulmonary valvectomy in patients with severe pulmonary valve dysplasia. As such, the latter situations are contraindications for the use of inflow occlusion and mandate open pulmonary valvotomy with the assistance of cardiopulmonary bypass.

Closed Valvotomy. Doyen,[4] Sellors,[5] and Brock[6] provided the original techniques of transventricular closed pulmonary valvotomy that, with minor variation, are still utilized at many centers[20,23,24,37,38] (Fig. 78–14). After

preparation as described under open pulmonary valvotomy on cardiopulmonary bypass, a pericardial pledget-reinforced 5-0 polypropylene purse-string suture is placed in the right ventricular infundibulum and is controlled with a tourniquet. A small stab incision is placed in the center of the purse string, the incision dilated with a fine mosquito clamp, and graduated Hegar dilators passed across the right ventricular outflow tract and pulmonary valve guided with an index finger adjacent to the pulmonary artery. After passage of a 6–7 French Hegar dilator, the purse string is secured and the residual gradient assessed by direct pressure measurement or epicardial two-dimensional echocardiography with color-guided continuous-wave Doppler. Further dilatation is possible through the purse string. Closed valvotomy has the advantages of not requiring cardiopulmonary bypass and can be performed quite expeditiously. Its principal disadvantages are the higher rate of perioperative mortality (10–20% in a current series[19,38]) and a higher need for reintervention (25–50% reoperation rate[19,20,38]) including repeat valvotomy, transannular patch, and/or shunt placement due to persistent hypoxemia or recurrent pulmonary valve stenosis. It is of note that a similar experience is now being reported in the mid to late follow-up after balloon pulmonary valvotomy.

Surgical Results. The multi-institutional study by Hanley and associates[20] reported a 30-day survival of 89% and a 4-year survival of 81% including all modes of intervention in patients with critical pulmonary stenosis (Fig. 78–9). For patients undergoing either balloon pulmonary valvotomy, open valvectomy on cardiopulmonary bypass or with inflow occlusion, as well as closed surgical valvotomy, perioperative survival was 94% (Fig. 78–11), which demonstrates the improved current results compared to those of 5–10 years ago.[19,44] Event-free survival, however, was sig-

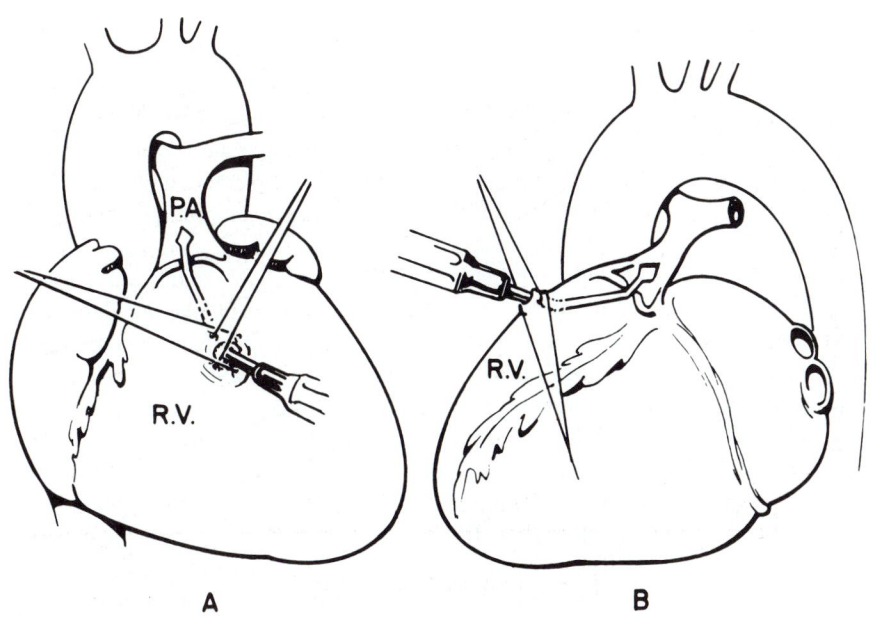

A   B

Figure 78–14. Technique for closed transventricular pulmonary valvotomy. See text for full description. Heart is exposed in a standard median sternotomy. **A.** Pledget-reinforced mattress sutures or purse strings are placed in the right ventricular outflow tract, a stab incision made, and graduated Hegar dilators or valvulotomes passed across the stenotic valve. **B.** Lateral view of passage of valvulotome across valve. R.V., right ventricle; P.A., pulmonary artery.

nificantly less favorable; 26% of patients required reintervention within 2 years due to residual or recurrent pulmonary valvar stenosis defined as a gradient of greater than or equal to 30 mm Hg (Fig. 78–10). The greatest incidence of reintervention occurred during the first week following the primary valve operation due to persistent hypoxemia, which necessitated insertion of an aortopulmonary shunt. Factors associated with the need for reintervention were higher initial right ventricular to left ventricular pressure ratio (i.e., more severe right ventricular outflow tract obstruction), small initial right ventricular cavity size (higher incidence of infundibular obstruction necessitating a transannular patch), and closed surgical valvotomy as the initial procedure. Similar results for closed valvotomy have been reported by earlier series as well.[10] Smaller balloon-to-annulus-size ratio (< 110–130%) has similarly been identified as a risk factor for early recurrence of pulmonary valvar stenosis following balloon pulmonary valvotomy.[26–32]

After successful valvotomy (either after initial procedure or reintervention), right ventricular size approaches normal in over 90% of patients,[22] suggesting significant growth potential even for the hypoplastic right ventricle. By 4 years of follow-up, Hanley reports that 85% of patients had completed a biventricular repair although several had required reintervention.

PULMONARY VALVE STENOSIS IN INFANTS, CHILDREN, AND ADULTS

Pulmonary valvar stenosis outside the neonatal age group is generally a more indolent and benign clinical lesion. Morphologically, the pulmonary valve is more normally developed with commissural fusion being the most common mechanism for valve stenosis. Annular hypoplasia is uncommon in children and adults except in cases of pulmonary valve dysplasia. In contrast to the neonate, poststenotic dilatation of the proximal main pulmonary artery is common[45,46] in children and adults with pulmonary valvar stenosis. The branch and distal pulmonary arteries are usually normal.

Progressive infundibular subpulmonary obstruction is associated with increasing age in previously untreated patients with pulmonary valvar stenosis outside of infancy, due to progressive right ventricular hypertrophy. Right ventricular systolic and diastolic volume are typically normal. Progressive right ventricular hypertrophy leads to decreasing right ventricular diastolic compliance and, hence, increasing right-to-left atrial level shunt when a patent foramen ovale or atrial septal defect is present. The latter may lead to presentation with new onset or increasing cyanosis. In contrast to the neonate with critical pulmonary stenosis, significant tricuspid regurgitation is uncommon in the older age groups.

Progressive right atrial enlargement and hypetrophy also parallel increasing age. Thirty to 40% of patients have an atrial level communication, either a patent foramen ovale or a small atrial septal defect, allowing a variable degree of right-to-left shunt.[45,46]

Clinical Presentation

The category and severity of symptoms in patients presenting with isolated pulmonary valvar stenosis often follow the degree of valvar obstruction, which, in turn, dictates the age at which initial presentation occurs.[47] As such, the frequency of cardiovascular or respiratory symptoms tends to decrease in patients outside of infancy until patients reach mid to late adulthood when secondary symptoms due to right ventricular hypertrophy, atrial arrhythmias, and right heart failure lead to clinical presentation. It is of note, however, that some patients with severe pulmonary stenosis may remain asymptomatic until they present with significant right heart failure symptoms.[45] In most series, 25–35% of patients are asymptomatic at the time they present (usually undergoing evaluation of a detected systolic heart murmur).[47–50] When symptoms do occur, dyspnea on exertion and fatigue are most common (50–70% of patients)[46,47,51] followed by cyanosis with exercise or at rest (30–50% of patients).[46,47,51] The presence of cyanosis confirms the coexistence of an atrial communication, severe right ventricular hypertrophy, and probable suprasystemic right ventricular pressures. Chest pain (angina), syncope, and congestive heart failure are uncommon until adulthood.

A harsh Grade III–IV/VI systolic ejection-type murmur and thrill are typically present at the second or third intercostal space on physical examination, often associated with an ejection click in late systole unless severe stenosis or pulmonary valve dysplasia limits valve excursion. The P2 component of the second heart sound may be split, diminished, or absent. Right ventricular hypertrophy may be appreciated on physical examination by prominence of the left chest border and the presence of a right ventricular heave. Diastolic murmurs are absent prior to interventional procedures. Right axis deviation on the electrocardiogram parallels the degree of valvar stenosis. Electrocardiographic evidence for right atrial enlargement and right ventricular hypertrophy is present in nearly all patients with pulmonary valvar stenosis[46,47,51] and R-wave amplitude in lead V1 parallels the degree of right ventricular hypertension.[47,51,52] A right ventricular strain pattern of ST- and T-wave inversion in the precordial leads also parallels the degree of valve obstruction. The resolution of these characteristic findings on the preoperative electrocardiogram is a useful indication for the resolution of obstruction postoperatively.

The chest x-ray may be normal or may show mild cardiomegaly when valve stenosis is mild. With increasing obstruction, prominence of the pulmonary artery knob may be visible on the frontal film (due to poststenotic dilatation), and progressive right ventricular hypertrophy may be noted on the lateral film as evidenced by filling of the retrosternal space. Significant right ventricular enlargement is uncommon outside of infancy.

Diagnosis

The diagnosis of pulmonary valvar stenosis is strongly suspected by the clinical presentation of symptoms (or lack thereof) and findings on physical examination as outlined above. Confirmation of the diagnosis is most commonly obtained by two-dimensional echocardiography and color-directed Doppler interrogation (Fig. 78–15A,B). This can be carried out by surface transthoracic or transesophageal windows.[53,54] As discussed earlier, features of pulmonary valve morphology and annular dimension, associated in-

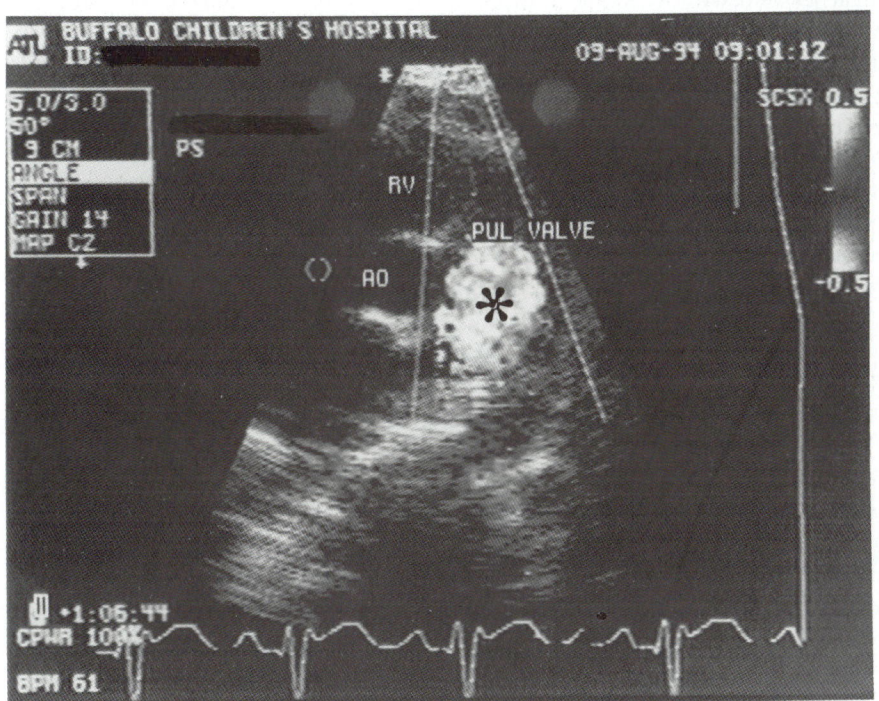

A

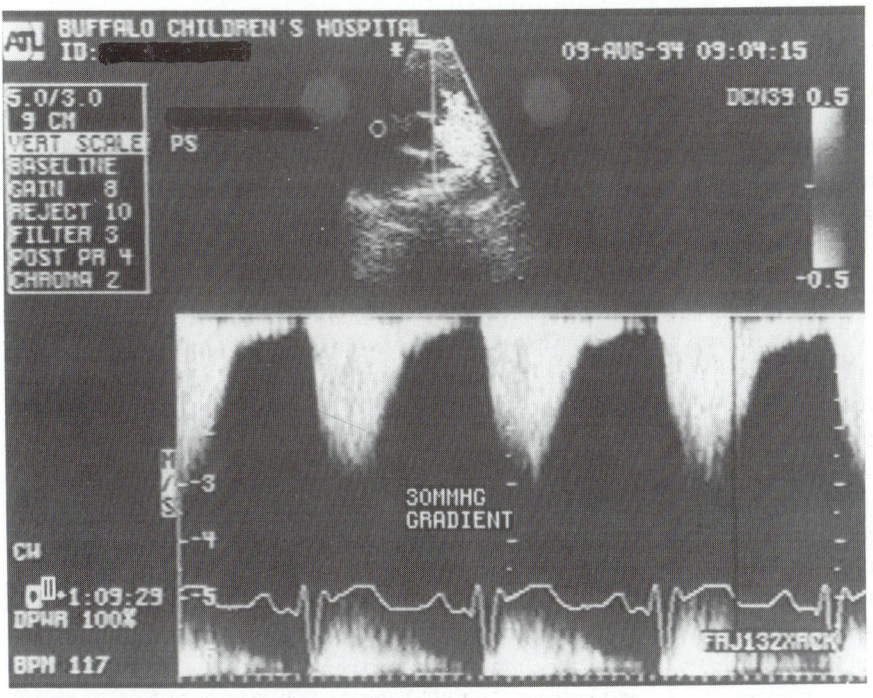

B

Figure 78–15. A. Parasternal short axis two-dimensional echocardiogram and color flow Doppler study of 5 year old with mild pulmonary valvar stenosis. Note broad color jet (*) beyond pulmonary valve (PUL VALVE). RV, right ventricle; AO, aorta. **B.** Continuous-wave Doppler velocity reveals transvalvar gradient of 30 mm Hg.

fundibular obstruction due to hypertrophied right ventricular muscle, tricuspid valve regurgitation, and atrial level shunt due to the coexistence of a patent foramen ovale or atrial septal defect can be accurately obtained noninvasively. The transvalvar gradient can be estimated from the Doppler velocity measured across the right ventricular outflow tract as calculated by the modified Bernoulli equation[21,55] (Fig. 78–15B). Right ventricular pressure can also be estimated from tricuspid valve regurgitant jet velocity. Serial noninvasive estimates of transvalvar gradient, right ventricular pressure, and right ventricular hypertrophy by two-dimensional echo and Doppler studies can help determine the appropriate timing for intervention, particularly in the absence of significant clinical symptoms. Invasive cardiac catheterization and angiography strictly for diagnostic purposes are limited to situations where the diagnosis is otherwise equivocal or when associated cardiac lesions are suspected. Diagnostic catheterization is most commonly performed as a prelude to intervention by balloon pulmonary valvotomy.

Interventions

Indications

A number of patients with isolated pulmonary valvar stenosis will present with mild, if any, symptoms despite a significant degree of obstruction across the pulmonary valve. The timing of intervention, therefore, must be dictated either by the presence of symptoms or, more commonly now, by the development of a transvalvar gradient in excess of 50 mm Hg. Hayes et al,[56] of the Second Natural History Study of Congenital Heart Defects, reported that patients with a pulmonary valve gradient less than 25 mm Hg had a less than 5% chance of needing intervention (valvotomy) through adulthood and had an anticipated survival equivalent to that of the general population. These findings confirm earlier studies.[46,49] In contrast, most patients with gradients greater than 50 mm Hg required intervention due to the progression of the transvalvar gradient.[56] The likelihood of requiring intervention increased by 10.6% for each 1 mm Hg increase in gradient above 50 mm Hg. Patients with gradients between 25 and 50 mm Hg had a 20% chance of needing intervention during the follow-up period with the caveat that age at presentation appeared to influence the likelihood of subsequent progression of the outflow tract obstruction. Children less than 2 years of age at presentation were more likely to present initially with cardiomegaly and right ventricular hypertrophy.[47] Patients less than 1 year of age who present with even mild pulmonary valvar stenosis were significantly more likely to progress to moderate or severe stenosis over a subsequent 5-year follow-up period compared to patients above age 1 year.[49,50] As such, younger patients with mild obstruction (i.e., a gradient of 25–49 mm Hg) warrant careful serial observation with Doppler estimates of transvalvar gradient to identify gradient progression as an indication for intervention.

Methods

As noted earlier, isolated pulmonary valvar stenosis without an associated atrial septal defect has largely become a nonsurgical lesion. Balloon pulmonary valvotomy has replaced surgical valvotomy as the primary treatment of choice for infants, children, and adults. Surgical intervention is indicated when balloon pulmonary valvotomy is not technically possible or yields incomplete relief of obstruction or when an atrial septal defect is present necessitating surgical closure.[57] The relative contraindications for balloon pulmonary valvotomy versus surgical valvotomy are less well defined for patients with pulmonary valve dysplasia.

Balloon Pulmonary Valvotomy

Balloon pulmonary valvotomy is performed in infants in the same manner as described earlier for neonates with critical pulmonary stenosis. For children, cardiac catheterization and angiography are performed to confirm the site of obstruction and to calibrate the pulmonary valve annulus size to allow appropriate balloon selection (Fig. 78–16). Use of a balloon 110–130% of the predilated pulmonary valve annulus has been reported to decrease the chances of residual gradient or early gradient recurrences.[27,30,58,59]

The balloon is positioned across the valve and multiple inflations carried out until the waist is eliminated, denoting dilatation of the valve. Acute reduction of right ventricular pressure to less than 50 mm Hg and pulmonary valve gradient to less than 30 mm Hg is anticipated by current techniques.[27,32,57,58,60,61] Further reduction in residual gradient is generally observed during the immediate follow-up period[57,59,62] (Fig. 78–17). Procedure-related mortality is less than 2%. The incidence of pulmonary valve insufficiency after balloon pulmonary valvotomy is substantially less than that seen after open surgical valvotomy.[62]

The freedom from late reintervention after balloon pulmonary valvotomy in infants and children ranges from 15 to 33%.[27,61,62] Recurrent valve stenosis is correlated with failure to use oversized balloons during the initial procedure. Repeat balloon pulmonary valvotomy with oversized balloons is an effective treatment in these patients.[63,64]

Balloon pulmonary valvotomy is equally effective in adolescents and adults as it is in infants and children.[65–68] Technically, double balloon dilatation is often required due to the small size of commercially available single balloons (20 mm) in comparison to the larger adult pulmonary valve annulus.[69,71] The immediate relief of pulmonary transvalvar gradient may be less effective in adolescents and adults due to their higher incidence of residual infundibular obstruction. This can be managed acutely pharmacologically utilizing β-blocker therapy with the anticipation of resolution of infundibular hypertrophy within the subsequent 6–12 mo.[67,71,72]

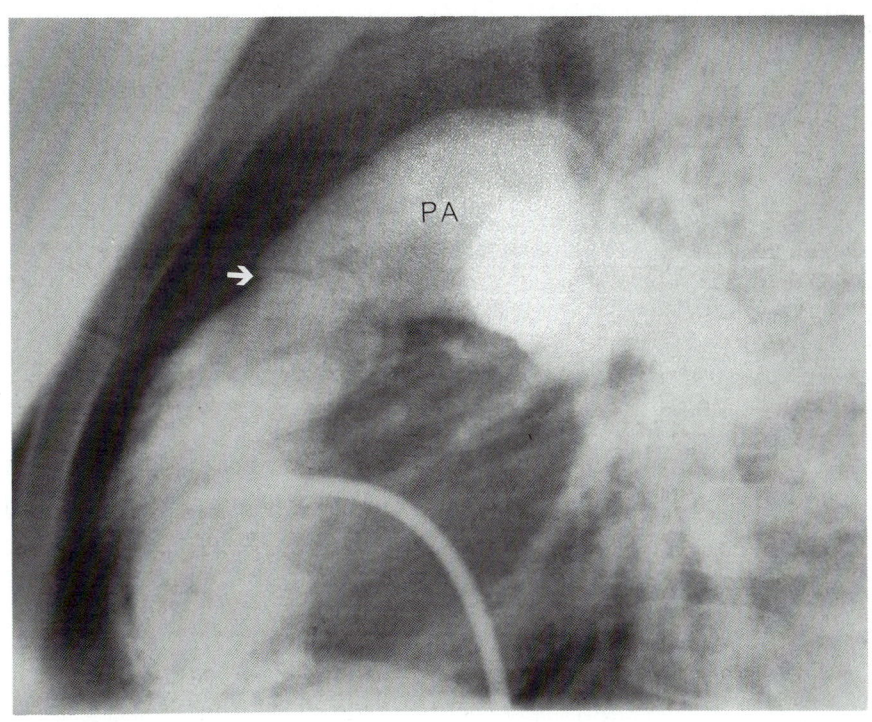

Figure 78–16. Lateral right ventriculogram from patient in Figure 78–15. Note characteristic "doming" of pulmonary valve (white arrow) and poststenotic dilation of main pulmonary artery (PA).

Surgery

The preferred method of surgical valvotomy is the open technique on cardiopulmonary bypass at normothermia or with mild hypothermia[45,51] and cold blood cardioplegic myocardial protection. Closed transventricular valvotomy should be avoided or limited to neonates and infants. The use of intraoperative two-dimensional echocardiography and color-directed Doppler interrogation by epicardial or transesophageal techniques allows precise preoperative definition of the pulmonary valve anatomy, annular size, and detection of significant infundibular subvalvar stenosis. Open valvotomy allows precise commissural incision and valve remodeling by cusp debridement and thinning.

Valvectomy may be opted when severe malformation or dysplasia of the valve leaflets is present. Annular and outflow tract calibration with Hegar dilators is carried out with reference to standard tables to determine the need for transannular outflow patch augmentation and/or infundibular muscle resection (Table 78–1).[41,42] Simultaneous closure of a patent foremen ovale or atrial septal defect is carried out by standard technique.

Perioperative mortality risk is low, approaching 0%, in current series,[46,56] and acute relief of right ventricular hypertension and transvalvar gradient is excellent. Long-term actuarial survival for patients undergoing surgical valvotomy before age 21 is equivalent to the general population.

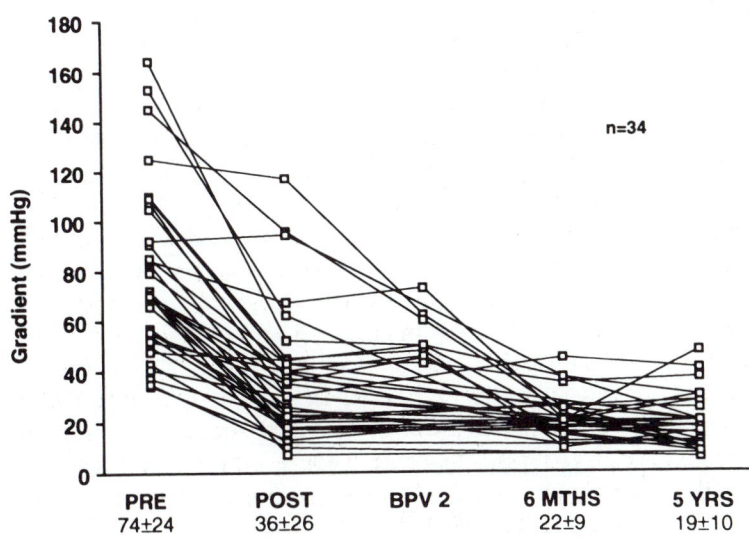

Figure 78–17. Transpulmonary valve gradient before (pre) and after (post) balloon pulmonary valvotomy. Note eight patients underwent a second balloon pulmonary valvotomy procedure (BPV 2) and progressive decline in gradient during follow-up in most patients. *(From Masura et al.[59] Reprinted with permission from the American College of Cardiology (Journal of the American College of Cardiology, 1993, 21:132–136).)*

In contrast, patients undergoing valvotomy in the third decade of life or later have an expected survival significantly below an age- and sex-matched population[46,56] (Fig. 78–18).

Postintervention Natural History

The Second Natural History Study of Congenital Heart Defects[56] and other studies[46] provide evidence that the probability for survival by medical management for patients with mild pulmonary stenosis (gradient of < 25 mm Hg) or successful intervention by a balloon pulmonary valvotomy or surgery for patients with moderate or severe pulmonary stenosis is equivalent to that of the normal population (25-year survival 95.7 ± 0.9% versus 96.6 ± 0.3%). Risk factors for death during follow-up were older age at intervention and the presence of cardiomegaly. The need for a transannular patch as a part of the intervention decreased long-term survival, although postoperative pulmonary insufficiency did not affect long-term outcome.[46]

The incidence of pulmonary insufficiency is significantly greater in surgical patients (approximately 100%) versus patients undergoing balloon pulmonary valvotomy (10–15%). The importance of postintervention pulmonary insufficiency remains controversial. Although late mortality is not significantly affected,[46,73] right ventricular enlargement, right ventricular arrhythmias, and abnormal right ventricular response to exercise have been documented.[74,75] Surgical patients with successful valvotomy had a freedom from reintervention of 96% at 10-year follow-up. Late reintervention was most likely due to residual infundibular obstruction[46] that had failed to resolve within 6–20 mo after valvotomy.[76] Risk factors for late cardiac

events (death and reoperation) were older age at the time of operation and a higher right ventricular systolic pressure before operation and after valvotomy. A reduction in right ventricular mass (hypertrophy) is generally seen after successful relief of right ventricular outflow obstruction.

PULMONARY VALVE DYSPLASIA

The characteristic pulmonary valve morphology associated with the entity pulmonary valve dysplasia has been discussed earlier (see pulmonary valve pathology).

Clinical Presentation

Patients with pulmonary valve dysplasia frequently present with mild or no symptoms and may present for evaluation due to the presence of a systolic heart murmur and/or the physical stigmata of Noonans syndrome. Some patients present with mild dyspnea or cyanosis as detailed in the discussion of patients with simple pulmonary valve stenosis.

In the original description of pulmonary valve dysplasia, Koretzky and associates[15] noted the following physical features that distinguish them from patients with simple pulmonary valve stenosis: (1) small physical stature due to retarded growth in height and weight, (2) abnormal facies as described by Noonan[17] and Linde et al,[18] (3) a harsh Grade III–IV/VI systolic ejection murmur at the base of the heart with the absence of a systolic ejection click on cardiac examination, and (4) a higher incidence of a familial pulmonary stenosis. The electrocardiogram in patients with pulmonary valve dysplasia typically shows a more extreme degree of right axis deviation with a QRS axis greater than

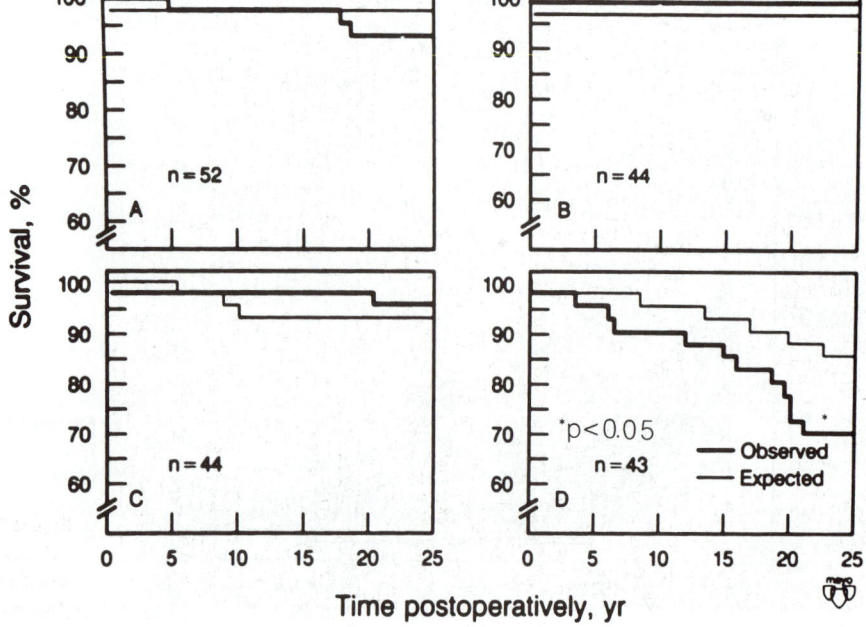

Figure 78–18. Long-term survival after open pulmonary valvotomy separated by age at the time of operation. **A.** Age 0–4 years. **B.** Age 5–10 years. **C.** Age 11–20 years. **D.** Age 21–68 years. Heavy line (observed) is survival of operated patients. Thin line (expected) is survival of an age and sex-matched control population. Note significant difference in long-term survival observed only in oldest cohort of patients. **D.** *(From Kopecky et al.[46])*

170° in most patients. The classic angiographic features include the absence of the classical doming of the pulmonary valve and the presence of thickened pulmonary valve leaflets. Despite the strong association of pulmonary valve dysplasia in patients with Noonans syndrome, it is clearly apparent that pulmonary valve dysplasia may be present in from 10 to 20% of patients with pulmonary valve stenosis[14,77] and, of those patients, only 10–30% have the true features of Noonans syndrome.

Diagnosis

The diagnosis of pulmonary valve dysplasia, in contrast to simple pulmonary valve stenosis, is often made by the co-existence of features of Noonans syndrome as noted above. In other patients, the absence of a systolic ejection click in the presence of the classical physical findings of pulmonary valve stenosis is a suggestive feature. Confirmation of the diagnosis is currently made by two-dimensional echocardiography and color-directed Doppler as described earlier for simple pulmonary valve stenosis. The distinguishing pathological features including thickened, immobile valve leaflets, annular and supraannular narrowing pulmonary artery narrowing, and the absence of poststenotic dilatation of the main pulmonary artery can be identified echocardiographically.[78,79] The indications for invasive catheterization and angiography are the same as those discussed earlier in reference to simple pulmonary valve stenosis (Fig. 78–19).

Intervention

Indications

The indications for and the timing of intervention are the same for patients with pulmonary valve dysplasia as those discussed earlier for patients with simple pulmonary valve stenosis. The preferred method of intervention remains controversial. Earlier reports on series of balloon pulmonary valvotomies reported poor results in patients with pulmonary valve dysplasia.[78,79] In contrast, more recent series have demonstrated an important role for balloon pulmonary valvotomy in patients with dysplastic pulmonary valves.

Balloon Pulmonary Valvotomy

The preparation for and the methods of balloon pulmonary valvotomy in patients with pulmonary valve dysplasia are the same as those described earlier. The only important difference is that the use of oversized balloons appears to be even more important in patients with dysplastic valves to avoid early restenosis.[78,80] Although the early and late success of balloon pulmonary valvotomy in dysplastic valves is less than that noted in pulmonary valve stenosis, many patients will have sustained hemodynamic benefit, whereas others will obtain initial palliation for which repeated balloon valvotomy or surgical intervention are options if recurrent stenosis occurs.

Surgical Intervention

Surgical intervention is indicated as discussed earlier for simple pulmonary valve stenosis (inability to perform bal-

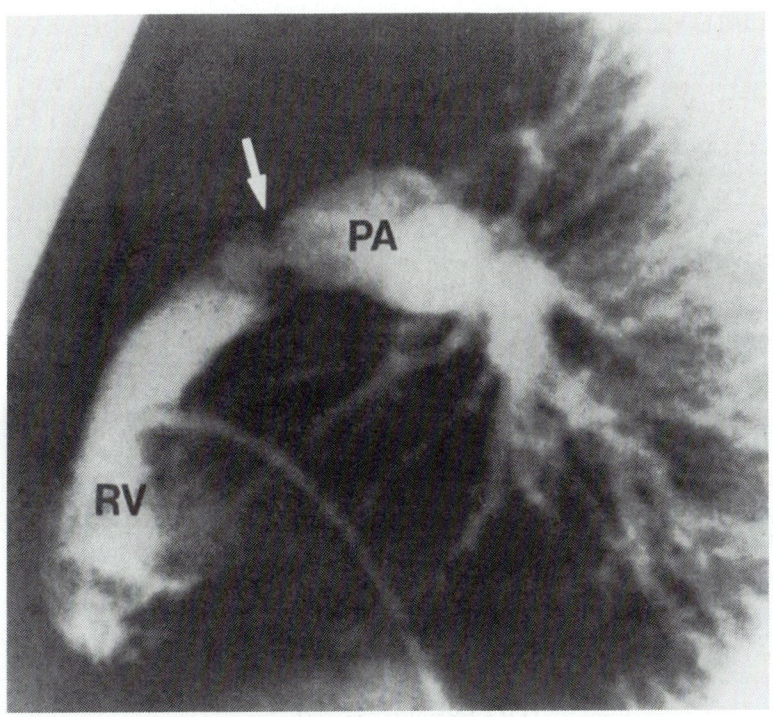

Figure 78–19. Lateral right ventriculogram of patient with pulmonary valve dysplasia. Note thickened, "nondoming" pulmonary valve (arrow). RV, right ventricle; PA, pulmonary artery.

loon pulmonary valvotomy, incomplete relief of stenosis or early recurrence of stenosis following prior valvotomy, the presence of an atrial septal defect) as well as when significant annular or supraannular hypoplasia is present necessitating outflow tract enlargement. In contrast to simple pulmonary valve stenosis, open pulmonary valvectomy is the procedure of choice in patients with pulmonary valve dysplasia.[14,77,81] The preparation for and conduct of the operation are the same as those described for simple pulmonary valve stenosis. Hegar dilator calibration of the pulmonary valve annulus, subannular region, and supraannular region of the main pulmonary artery is carried out to determine the need for a transannular patch and/or pericardial patch augmentation of the proximal main pulmonary artery. Right ventricular outflow tract reconstruction is required more frequently in patients with pulmonary valve dysplasia with a 43–100% incidence reported in recent series.[77,81–83]

Postoperatively, there is a higher tendency for moderate residual right ventricular outflow tract obstruction in the subpulmonic region, due principally to the presence of hypertrophied infundibular muscle bundles.[71] Patients treated with pulmonary valvectomy (compared to pulmonary valvotomy or partial valvectomy) have an early and late result and freedom from recurrence similar to that observed in patients with pulmonary valve stenosis.[14,82]

DOUBLE CHAMBER RIGHT VENTRICLE

Double chamber right ventricle is an uncommon form of right ventricular outflow tract obstruction (1–1.5% of congenital heart lesions[84]) that is characterized by hypertrophied, anomalous muscle bundles causing right ventricular outflow tract obstruction at the junction between the trabecular and outlet portions of the right ventricle (Fig. 78–20). This results in a hypertensive proximal right ventricular chamber and a normotensive distal (infundibular) right ventricular chamber. The presence of a normal, nonstenotic right ventricular infundibulum and normal pulmonary valve annulus distinguishes this type of right ventricular outflow tract obstruction from that associated with tetralogy of Fallot.

Lucas and associates[85] clarified the pathophysiology of this lesion and described its surgical correction. This and subsequent early surgical series[85–89] suggested that the obstructing muscle bundles were separate from the moderator band, taking origin as anomalous bands or wedges of muscle from the septoparietal complex in distinction from the normal moderator band itself. More recent series[90–94] suggest that superior and posteromedial malposition and subsequent hypertrophy of the moderator band are the principal morphologies of this lesion.

An associated membranous ventricular septal defect is found in at least 80% of patients.[85,90–92, 95] It has been suggested that a ventricular septal defect is present in all cases with spontaneous closure in some patients prior to their clinical presentation.[90] Pulmonary valvar stenosis, atrial septal defect, discrete subaortic stenosis, aortic insufficiency, double right ventricle, and total anomalous pulmonary venous connection have also been reported in association with double chamber right ventricle.[84,90,92,96–98] Hypertrophy of the proximal (hypertensive) chamber is

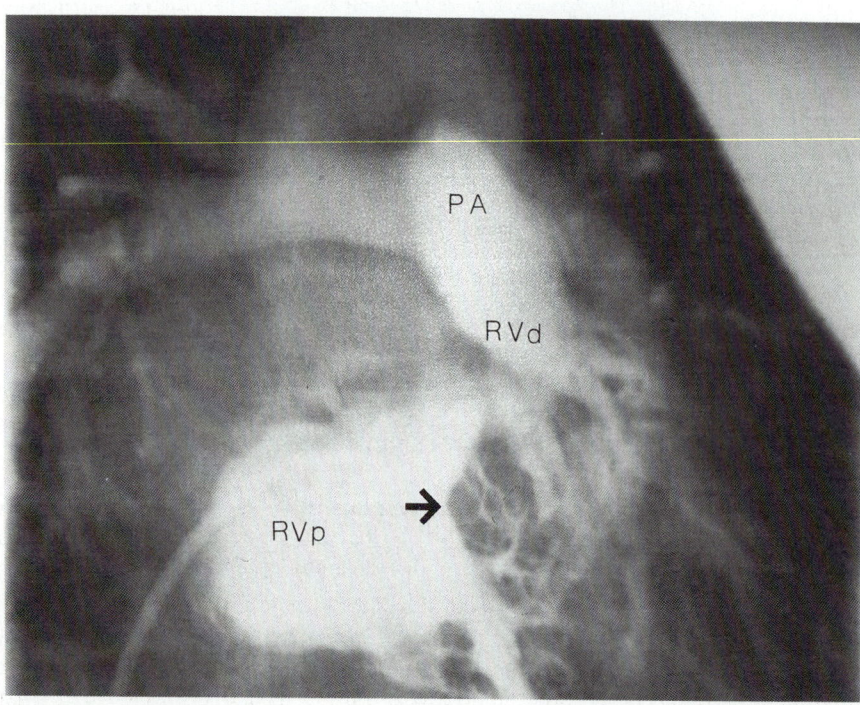

Figure 78–20. Anterior right ventriculogram in 2 year old with double chamber right ventricle and ventricular septal defect. Note hypertrophied, obstructing anomalous muscle bundle (arrow), hypertensive proximal right ventricular chamber (RVp), normotensive distal right ventricular chamber (RVd). PA, pulmonary artery.

found in cases where the anomalous muscle bundle causes moderate-to-severe obstruction.

Clinical Presentation

Patients with double chamber right ventricle may come to clinical attention in early infancy due to the presence of a Grade II–IV/VI systolic ejection murmur, which is often attributed clinically to a ventricular septal defect. In older patients, clinical presentation is determined by the presence of a ventricular septal defect and the initial degree of or progression of right ventricular outflow tract obstruction.[86,88,90,97] Patients with intact ventricular septum or a very restrictive ventricular septal defect will present clinically much like patients with pulmonary valve stenosis with intact ventricular septum, having few if any symptoms. Patients with a large ventricular septal defect and mild right ventricular outflow tract obstruction present like patients with an isolated ventricular septal defect with a variable degree of congestive heart failure due to left-to-right shunt. Patients with a ventricular septal defect and severe right ventricular outflow tract obstruction present in a manner that is difficult to distinguish clinically from tetralogy of Fallot. It is important to note that right ventricular outflow tract obstruction may be a progressive lesion and, as such, may alter the natural history and presentation of patients prior to surgical correction.[91,98]

In the absence of clinical cyanosis or congestive heart failure, the physical examination is suggestive of pulmonary valvar stenosis with a harsh Grade III–IV/VI systolic ejection murmur and thrill on cardiac examination. Distinguishing auscultatory findings in some patients with double chamber right ventricle compared to those with pulmonary valvar stenosis include a peak intensity of the systolic murmur and thrill located lower on the left sternal border of the chest wall and a normal intensity and split of the pulmonary component of the second heart sound.[88] Mild cardiomegaly with right ventricular prominence on chest x-ray and right ventricular hypertrophy (prominent R-wave in V3R and V1) as well as right axis deviation on electrocardiogram do not distinguish these patients clinically from others with pulmonary valvar stenosis.

Diagnosis

As is the case for pulmonary valve stenosis, two-dimensional echocardiography with color-directed Doppler interrogation has largely replaced invasive catheterization for defining double chamber right ventricle and distinguishing it from pulmonary valvar stenosis, simple ventricular septal defect, and tetralogy of Fallot.[89,92,93,99] Subxiphoid and subcostal right ventricular inflow–apex–outflow views on two-dimensional echocardiography have been most helpful in demonstrating the superior and medial malposition of the obstructing moderator band as well as the absence of infundibular hypoplasia or septal malposition seen in tetral-

ogy of Fallot. In addition, pulmonary valvar annular hypoplasia and pulmonary valve doming can easily be identified from this view. Measurements of pulmonary valve to moderator band distance, indexed to the tricuspid valve diameter, have been proposed as a means of predicting the potential for development of significant right ventricular outflow tract obstruction in infants with double chamber right ventricle.[93] Serial estimates of the degree of obstruction can be determined by Doppler measurement of right ventricular outflow tract velocity across the anomalous muscle bundles.[21] Associated lesions (ventricular septal defect, subaortic stenosis, aortic insufficiency, atrial septal defect, etc.) can also be detected noninvasively.

Cardiac catheterization and angiography are reserved for situations where the diagnosis is equivocal or associated lesions may be present. Angiographically,[91] the obstructing muscle bundles can be profiled crossing the right ventricular outflow tract in the region of the septoparietal bands and moderator band with obstruction occurring during systole (Fig. 78–20). A normal distal chamber (infundibulum) distinguishes this lesion from tetralogy of Fallot. Left-sided cardiac catheterization and angiography are indicated to exclude associated subaortic stenosis and ventricular septal defect. Catheterization demonstrates the presence of a gradient between the proximal trabecular (hypertensive) and the distal outlet (normotensive) chambers. The magnitude of this pressure gradient is directly proportional to the degree of obstruction caused by the anomalous muscle bundles.

Intervention

The indications and timing of surgical intervention for patients with double chamber right ventricle are dictated by the manner of clinical presentation as described earlier. Patients presenting like isolated pulmonary valvar stenosis with intact ventricular septum or restrictive ventricular septal defect should be referred for surgical correction if symptomatic or if the right ventricular outflow tract gradient exceeds 50 mm Hg. Patients with lower gradients require careful follow-up since progression of the obstruction is commonly observed. Patients presenting with symptoms comparable to a simple ventricular septal defect (left-to-right shunt and mild right ventricular outflow tract obstruction) warrant intervention when the Q_p/Q_s exceeds 1.1:5. Patients presenting with symptoms like tetralogy of Fallot undergo surgical correction at the onset of cyanosis.

Methods

Surgical correction is carried out via median sternotomy on cardiopulmonary bypass with bicaval cannulation utilizing mild hypothermia (32°C) and cold blood cardioplegic arrest. Warden et al[87] reported the presence of a "dimple" and a thrill in the proximal right ventricular outflow tract as distinguishing clinical features notable after opening the pericardium and examining the external anatomy of the heart. Currently, intraoperative epicardial or transesophageal two-dimensional echocardiography and color Doppler are useful adjuncts in the preoperative and postoperative assessment of intracardiac anatomy as well as the adequacy of the surgical correction. Although transventricular resection has been the classical surgical approach for the relief of right ventricular outflow tract obstruction in this lesion, we and others[85,87,98,100–102] have exclusively used the transatrial and transpulmonary artery approach for the resection of obstructing anomalous muscle bundles, mobilization of the septal and parietal bands, and patch closure of the ventricular septal defect. Early and late mortality approaches 0%, and freedom from reoperation (ventricular septal defect, recurrent or residual right ventricular outflow tract obstruction) is greater than 90% in current series.[100–102] Late follow-up suggests excellent symptom relief. Late development of subaortic stenosis due to a subaortic membrane warrants periodic reevaluation by two-dimensional echocardiography.[103]

PULMONARY ARTERY STENOSIS

Pulmonary artery stenosis is found as a pathologic component in approximately 2–3% of patients with congenital heart defects.[27,104,105] Significant stenoses play an even more prominent role in patients with tetralogy of Fallot with pulmonary stenosis or pulmonary atresia, Williams syndrome,[105–108] and Noonans syndrome.[17,109] Peripheral pulmonary stenoses are also found in association with congenital Rubella syndrome,[110] Ehlers–Danlos syndrome,[111] and Cutis Laxa.[112] Series reporting results of interventional procedures for treatment of pulmonary stenoses also have reported a nearly equal incidence of native and postsurgical stenoses (i.e., from shunts, bands, anastomoses, etc.).

McCue and associates[113] classified native pulmonary artery stenoses in the following manner: (1) stenosis of the main pulmonary artery or proximal right or left branch pulmonary arteries (Fig. 78–21), (2) coarctation of the pulmonary artery bifurcation (Fig. 78–22), (3) multiple peripheral pulmonary artery stenoses (beyond the pericardial reflection) (Fig. 78–23), and (4) presence of proximal main or branch pulmonary stenoses plus multiple peripheral pulmonary artery stenoses. Multiple peripheral stenoses is the most common entity, followed by a combined presence of both proximal and peripheral pulmonary artery stenoses.

Clinical Presentation

Pulmonary artery stenoses may remain benign clinically, particularly when right ventricular pressure remains less than 50% systemic.[108] Patients with Williams syndrome and multiple peripheral pulmonary artery stenoses may show a decrease in right ventricular pressure over time. As

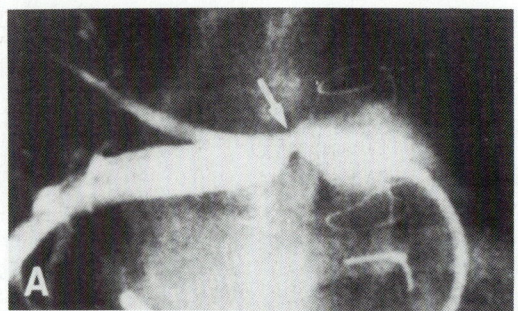
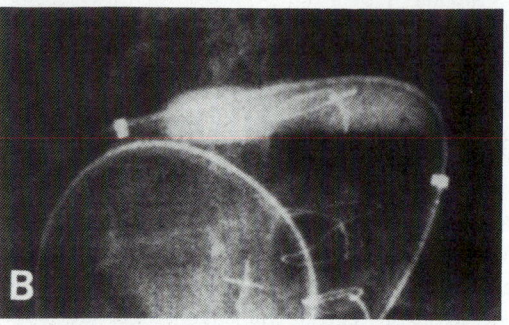
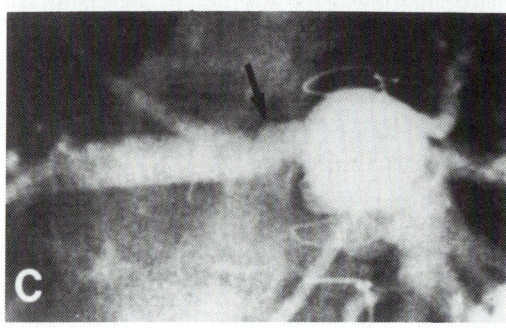

Figure 78–21. Balloon angioplasty of proximal right pulmonary artery stenosis in postoperative patient. **A.** Predilation angiogram showing location of discrete stenosis (white arrow). **B.** Inflated angioplasty balloon. **C.** Postangioplasty angiogram showing near complete relief of stenosis. Black arrow shows area of probable intimal tear. *(From Rothman et al.[105])*

right ventricular pressure increases to near systemic or suprasystemic levels, symptoms including dyspnea on exertion, poor growth, frequent respiratory tract infections, cyanosis, precordial chest pain, and effort syncope occur in most patients.[113]

On physical examination, a systolic murmur and an increased pulmonary component of the second heart sound are often present at the second intercostal space. Continuous murmurs are often present throughout both of the lung fields in patients with multiple peripheral pulmonary artery stenoses. Nonspecific patterns of right ventricular hypertrophy and strain are seen in the electrocardiogram and diminished peripheral vascular lung markings are seen in the affected lung fields on chest x-ray.

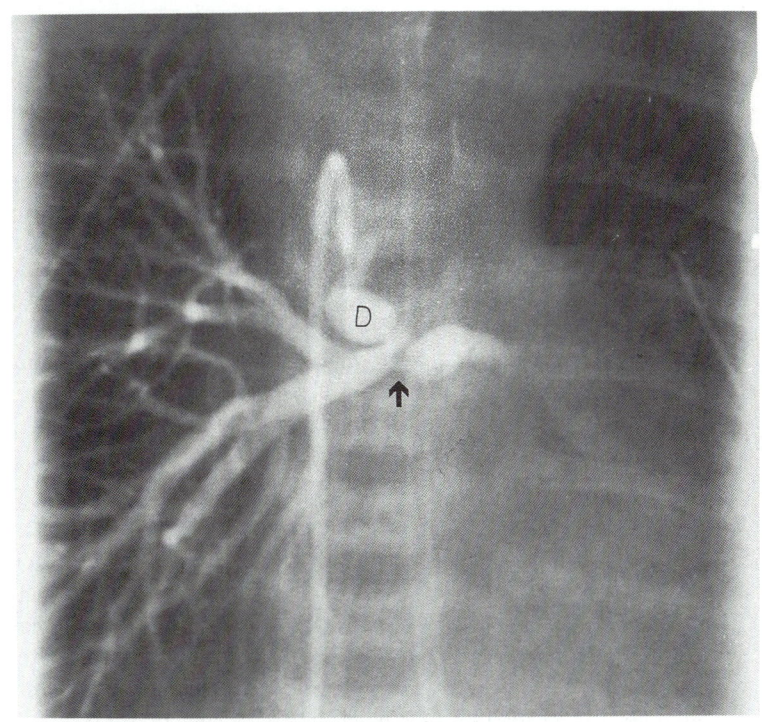

Figure 78–22. Anterior pulmonary angiogram via ductus arteriosus (D) in 8 day old with complex pulmonary atresia and coarctation of the pulmonary arteries. Note complex stenosis of confluence of pulmonary arteries at the insertion site of the ductus arteriosus (arrow).

Diagnosis

Transthoracic or transesophageal two-dimensional echocardiography with color-directed Doppler may demonstrate main pulmonary artery or proximal branch pulmonary artery stenoses. Right heart cardiac catheterization with se-

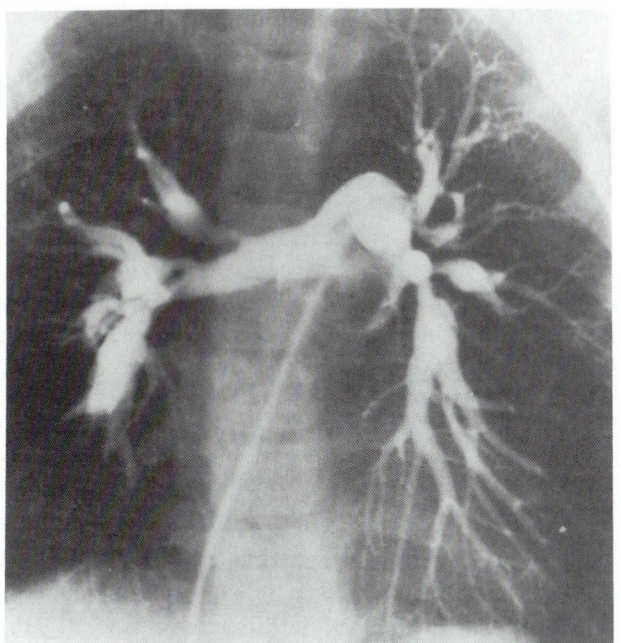

Figure 78–23. Anterior pulmonary angiogram demonstrating multiple peripheral pulmonary artery stenoses.

lective pulmonary angiography is necessary to fully define the sites of stenoses (main pulmonary artery, branch pulmonary artery, peripheral pulmonary arteries) (Figs. 78–21 to 78–23) and to quantify the degree of obstruction by measurements of gradients across these stenoses and measurement of the right ventricular pressure relative to systemic aortic pressure. Currently, diagnostic catheterization is often done in association with therapeutic balloon angioplasty and/or insertion of pulmonary artery stents (see below). Nuclear medicine scintigraphic lung scans provide useful quantification of the relative diminution of regional blood flow beyond the stenotic pulmonary arteries.[114]

Intervention

As is the case of pulmonary valve stenosis, surgical intervention for pulmonary artery stenosis is rapidly being replaced by balloon pulmonary angioplasty, often combined with the deployment of a wire mesh stent. This change in therapeutic approach has particularly been employed in the management of peripheral pulmonary artery stenoses, which often are beyond the realm of surgical reconstruction.

The general indications for intervention by any modality, either surgery or balloon angioplasty include[104,105,115] (1) systemic or suprasystemic systolic blood pressure in the right ventricle, (2) segmental pulmonary artery hypertension, (3) evidence for significantly decreased blood flow to the affected pulmonary vascular bed as demonstrated by scintigraphic lung scan,[114] or (4) the presence of symptoms as outlined earlier.

Surgery

McCue et al[113] and Smith et al[116] reported early surgical approaches for the management of branch pulmonary artery stenoses utilizing vein patch angioplasty. Currently, main pulmonary artery and branch pulmonary artery stenoses are most often repaired in conjunction with the correction of an associated congenital cardiac defect (i.e., tetralogy of Fallot with pulmonary atresia, univentricular heart palliation, truncus arteriosus, etc.). Cardiopulmonary bypass with moderate or deep hypothermia and cold blood cardioplegic arrest are employed. Intermittent low-flow cardiopulmonary bypass and/or brief periods of deep hypothermia with circulatory arrest are often required for the control of bronchial collateral blood return and to optimize conditions for reconstruction. Autologus pericardium as an onlay patch, flap, or even tube interposition are the preferred materials,[117] when they are available (Fig. 78–24). Pulmonary artery homograft tissue provides a very satisfactory alternative.

The short-term results of pulmonary artery reconstruction have been good, although intermediate and late-term restenosis is common. Several recent reports describe limited experience with intraoperative use of balloon pulmonary artery dilatation and stent deployment for treatment of more peripherally located pulmonary artery stenoses.[104,105,118]

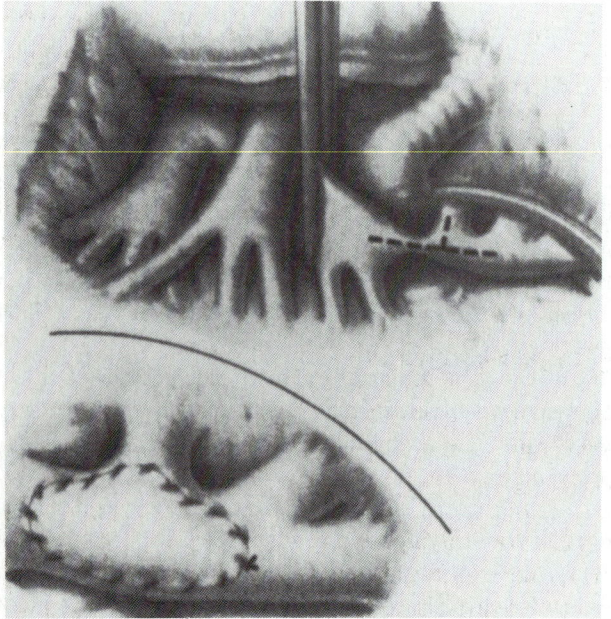

Figure 78–24. Technique for surgical repair of peripheral stenosis of right lower lobe pulmonary artery using a pericardial patch.

Balloon Pulmonary Artery Angioplasty and/or Stent Deployment

Balloon dilatation has been increasingly employed for central and peripheral pulmonary artery stenoses in parallel with its development and application for the treatment of coronary artery and peripheral systemic arterial stenoses (Fig. 78–21). In comparison to the high success rate for balloon dilatation of pulmonary valvar stenosis, balloon dilatation of pulmonary artery stenosis has been less efficacious. Acute success in most series is reported in the range of 50–60% of cases.[104,105,115,119–121] Increased success has been associated with the use of balloons 3 1/2 to 4 times the diameter of the arterial stenosis, measured on diagnostic angiography.[105,120–122] Balloon dilatation has been most successful for cases of idiopathic peripheral pulmonary artery stenoses (75% success[104]) and tetralogy of Fallot (78% success[104]). Most recent series have found that stenoses associated with prior surgical procedures (shunts, bands, patch angioplasties, anastomoses, etc.) are quite amenable to balloon pulmonary artery dilatation,[104,105,120,121] whereas others have noted early restenosis in such cases.[115,123] Results with peripheral pulmonary artery stenosis in Williams syndrome and Alagille syndrome have been poor.[104,123]

The overall complication rate associated with balloon dilatation of pulmonary artery stenoses (artery perforation or occlusion, aneurysm formation, segmental pulmonary edema) is significantly greater in occurrence than that reported for pulmonary valve dilatation, ranging from 3 to 10%.[104,124] Procedure-related mortality is reported to occur in from 1.8 to 4%[115,120,124] of cases.

A major deficit of balloon dilatation of pulmonary stenoses is the rate of early and intermediate term restenosis, which occurs in 16–25% of cases,[120,124] due to elastic recoil of the lesion and/or early intimal hyperplasia at the site of the dilatation.[119,125] To address these problems, deployment of wire mesh stents has been added in some cases of balloon dilatation with excellent early and intermediate term results in small series.[119,125,126] This has been applied both for discrete short stenoses as well as longer segment stenoses. Stent deployment has been particularly useful in association with postsurgical stenoses in conjunction with definitive repairs of tetralogy of Fallot, Fontan procedures, etc. Longer term results are needed to determine the late incidence of restenosis and to explore the success of stent redilatation in the growing child.

Coarctation of the Pulmonary Arteries

Coarctation of the pulmonary arteries refers to a specific entity resulting in narrowing of the proximal branch pulmonary arteries or the pulmonary artery bifurcation in the region of insertion of the ductus arteriosus[127,128] (Fig. 78–22). This lesion is more commonly found in patients with tetralogy of Fallot with pulmonary stenosis or pulmonary atresia as well as patients with complex univentricular heart anatomy in association with pulmonary atresia.

Morphologically, this lesion is similar to coarctation of the aorta in that ductal tissue in the wall of the pulmonary arteries is associated with the pathologic development of central or branch pulmonary artery stenosis.[128] The overall outcome of patients with coarctation of the pulmonary artery is poor, especially in patients with pulmonary atresia, due to the need for extensive pulmonary artery reconstruction in association with palliative shunt or complex intracardiac repair.[127] As such, careful definition of the patency of the pulmonary artery bifurcation and the proximal right and left branch pulmonary arteries is mandatory in infants prior to initial palliative shunt so that simultaneous resection or patch augmentation of a coarcted segment can be carried out if found. The latter must be performed on cardiopulmonary bypass.

ANEURYSMS OF THE PULMONARY ARTERIES

Aneurysms of the main pulmonary artery and its peripheral branches are rare lesions. Autopsy series report an incidence of 1:14,000 necropsies[129,130] and pulmonary artery aneurysms represent less than 1% of all thoracic artery aneurysms.[129]

Pathology

Deterling and Clagett[129] and Bartter et al[131] have reported complimentary classifications of pulmonary artery aneurysms.

Aneurysms With Structural Cardiac Defects

From 40 to 50% of pulmonary artery aneurysms are seen in patients with structural heart lesions,[131–135] which can be divided into those with congenital heart defects versus those with acquired heart defects. The majority of patients with pulmonary artery aneurysms associated with congenital heart disease have significant pulmonary hypertension as an associated etiologic factor. Patent ductus arteriosus,[131–135] truncus arteriosus, and tetralogy of Fallot are the lesions most frequently associated with aneurysms of the main pulmonary artery. Branch pulmonary artery aneurysms are seen more frequently in association with Blalock–Taussig[136] and Waterston shunts.[137] Pulmonary artery aneurysms occur less frequently in patients with acquired heart lesions such as mitral stenosis and in patients with secondary pulmonary hypertension due to pulmonary fibrosis or chronic pulmonary emboli.[129]

Infections

Extravascular infections including tuberculosis (Rasmussen's aneurysm), syphilis, and fungal cavitary lesions (aspergillosis, etc.) were commonly associated with development of pulmonary artery aneurysms in older series in the literature.[129] Endovascular infections due to bacterial emboli (*Staphylococcus aureus, Streptococcus pneumonia, Candida albicans, Aspergillosis*) predominate in the more recent series. This group of infections most frequently results in peripheral artery aneurysms that are often multiple in number.[131] Aneurysms of this type are commonly seen in intravenous drug abusers and in patients with subacute bacterial endocarditis due to congenital or acquired cardiac defects.[138]

Structural Pulmonary Vascular Lesions

Marfan's syndrome and other causes of cystic medial necrosis may rarely affect the main pulmonary artery causing aneurysmal enlargement. Inflammatory lesions such as giant cell arteritis, Bechets disease,[139,140] and Hughes–Stovin syndrome[140] are rare inflammatory disorders associated with the development of peripheral artery aneurysms. Bechets disease is characterized by oral and genital ulcerations, uveitis, arthralgias, and periodic fevers with multiple peripheral pulmonary artery aneurysms. Hughes–Stovin syndrome is similar in many respects to Bechets disease, although male predominance and multiple superficial and deep venous thromboses characterize the former. Both syndromes may be heralded by massive hemoptysis due to endobronchial rupture of the peripheral pulmonary artery aneurysm.

Trauma

Penetrating and blunt trauma may result in pulmonary artery aneurysm formation, frequently due to the development of arteriovenous communications.[131] Peripheral pulmonary artery aneurysm is an increasing complication of use of Swan–Ganz flotation catheters due to an excessively peripheral position while obtaining a wedge reading, prolonged balloon inflation, or balloon hyperinflation. These lesions are characteristically nodular in shape and are well circumscribed radiographically (Fig. 78–25). They are often times inadvertently interpreted as metastatic lesions[133,141,142] and may present clinically with episodic hemoptysis.

Clinical Presentation

The most common symptoms associated with pulmonary artery aneurysm are dyspnea on exertion, cough with hemoptysis, chest pain, and cyanosis. Patients with pulmonary artery aneurysms associated with systemic illness or syndromes (endocarditis, Bechets syndrome, Hughes–Stovin syndrome, etc.) may present with symptoms attributable to the underlying disorder. Physical examination is nonspecific in most cases. A harsh Grade II–III/VI systolic ejection murmur at the second or third intercostal space is frequently present. Sudden death due to aneurysm dissection

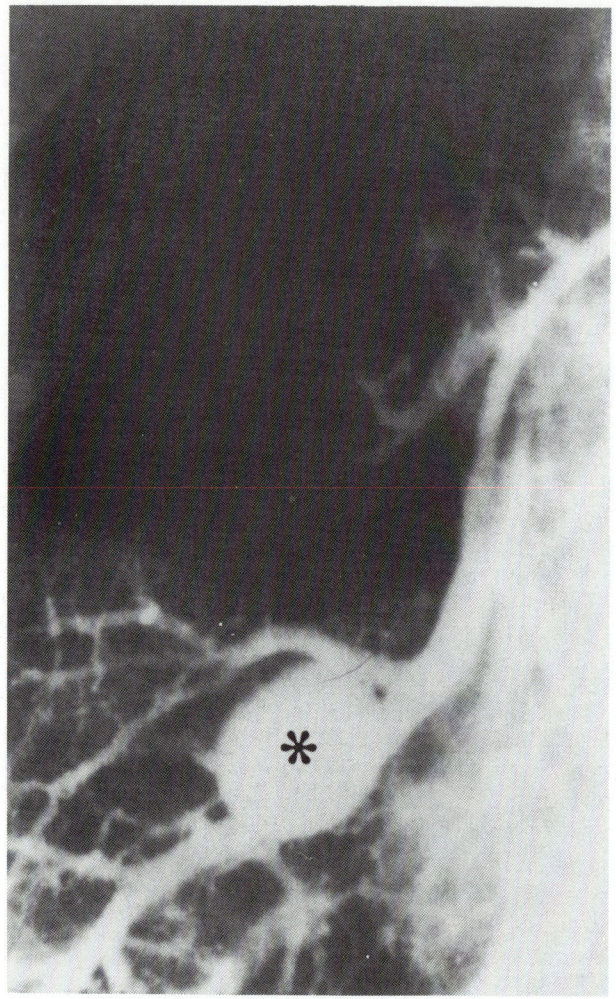

Figure 78–25. Selective pulmonary angiogram demonstrating a 2-cm false aneurysm (*) of the anterior basal branch of the right descending pulmonary artery. *(From Dieden et al.[143])*

and/or rupture resulting in cardiac tamponade or massive hemoptysis has been reported in up to 50% of patients with previously unrecognized and asymptomatic pulmonary artery aneurysms.[132,135,139,142,143]

Diagnosis

Frontal chest x-ray may reveal enlargement of the pulmonary component of the cardiac silhouette in cases of main or branch pulmonary artery aneurysm. Lateral x-ray may demonstrate filling of the retrosternal space due to pulmonary artery enlargement. Peripheral pulmonary artery aneurysms may appear as nodular round densities similar to primary or metastatic malignancy. Pulmonary angiography remains the gold standard for definite diagnosis, although transthoracic or transesophageal echocardiography[134,144] and magnetic resonance imaging[131] are gaining increasing utility, particularly as a means for serial evaluation of patients with small aneurysms.

Intervention

Due to the infrequent nature of pulmonary artery aneurysms, most reports in the literature contain only small clinical experiences. No longitudinal natural history studies are available. As such, indications for and timing of intervention are based on small series and case reports.

Pulmonary artery aneurysms appear to pose a significant risk for mediastinal or endobronchial rupture,[130,131,145] although isolated reports of long-term survival occasionally appear.[146] Pulmonary artery dissection is most commonly seen in patients with concomitant pulmonary hypertension, especially in association with Eisenmenger's syndrome due to patent ductus arteriosus, truncus arteriosus, tetralogy of Fallot, or atrial or ventricular septal defect.[132,141,147] Due to the inherent instability of these lesions, intervention is usually indicated once the diagnosis is made in large aneurysms or in situations where enlargement of a small aneurysm is documented on serial follow-up study.

Central pulmonary artery aneurysms are most frequently repaired by resection and graft interposition or aneurysmorrhaphy.[131,148,149] Peripheral aneurysms have traditionally been treated by pulmonary lobectomy or pneumonectomy.[150] More recently, limited segmental resection[151] or transvenous coil embolization[152] have gained favor as the treatments of choice.

Emergency operation for treatment of dissection or rupture of a pulmonary aneurysm carries a 33–50% perioperative mortality in small series.[131,145,147] In contrast, elective lobar resection or embolization therapy carries a low morbidity and mortality in most series.[131]

ABSENT OR SINGLE PULMONARY ARTERY

Unilateral absence of the pulmonary artery is a rare lesion that may occur in isolation or in combination with other congenital heart defects.[153–155] Initially described by Fraentzel in 1868,[156] absent pulmonary artery has since been the subject of several comprehensive reviews.[153–155,157]

It is useful clinically to classify unilateral absence of the pulmonary artery into two categories[153]: (1) origin of the right or left pulmonary artery from the ascending aorta, and (2) unilateral absence of the proximal right or left pulmonary artery with perfusion of the distal left or right pulmonary artery by a patent ductus arteriosus or aortopulmonary collateral vessel.

ORIGIN OF THE PULMONARY ARTERY FROM THE ASCENDING AORTA

Origin of either the left or right pulmonary artery from the ascending aorta results in a large left-to-right shunt via the anomalous pulmonary artery and overperfusion of the contralateral lung with the entire cardiac output of the right ventricle plus any additional flow due to the presence of an intracardiac shunt from a coexisting atrial septal defect, patent ductus arteriosus, ventricular septal defect, etc. As a result, congestive heart failure and early development of pulmonary hypertension are characteristic clinical features that often become evident in early infancy. Anomalous origin of the right pulmonary artery from the ascending aorta is more common than anomalous origin of the left pulmonary artery and is most frequently associated with left aortic arch, patent ductus arteriosus, aortopulmonary window, hypoplastic or interrupted aortic arch, or atrial septal defect.[153] In contrast, anomalous origin of the left pulmonary artery from the ascending aorta is most frequently associated with a right aortic arch and tetralogy of Fallot.[153,158,159]

There are two major hypotheses concerning the embryologic origin of this defect. The most commonly held theory states that reabsorption of the proximal segment of the left or right sixth aortic arch (ventral bud) results in absence of the respective proximal pulmonary artery segment. Incomplete migration of the distal pulmonary artery segment to join the truncus arteriosus results in the aortic origin of the anomalous pulmonary artery.[153,155] Alternatively, the second hypothesis states that truncal malseptation results in asymmetric division of the truncus arteriosus and may lead to its anomalous fusion with the left or right pulmonary artery.

Clinical Presentation

Patients with anomalous origin of the right pulmonary artery from the ascending aorta typically present in infancy with congestive heart failure, tachypnea, failure to thrive, and mild cyanosis.[153] Pulmonary vascular occlusive disease may develop early in life with resultant biventricular failure.[153,155,160] Associated intracardiac defects resulting in left-to-right shunt (i.e., patent ductus arteriosus, ventricular septal defect, atrial septal defect, aortopulmonary window) accelerate the development of symptoms. Physical examination is nonspecific, although a harsh Grade II–III/VI systolic ejection murmur is characteristically present on physical examination.[161]

Patients with anomalous origin of the left pulmonary artery from the ascending aorta present with predominantly congestive symptoms due to excessive left lung pulmonary blood flow, and a patent right-sided ductus arteriosus is often additionally present (with a right aortic arch). Similar clinical presentation is seen in patients with associated tetralogy of Fallot.[158,159,162]

Diagnosis

Chest x-rays may reveal a unilateral or bilateral increase in pulmonary vascular markings. Electrocardiogram may reveal left, right, or biventricular hypertrophy depending upon the presence of an associated structural cardiac defect. Selective pulmonary angiography has traditionally been the definitive test for diagnosis, although two-dimensional echocardiography with color-guided Doppler interrogation may provide adequate anatomic definition to determine this diagnosis.[153] Magnetic resonance imaging, computerized tomography, and radionuclide angiography are useful adjunctive studies.[163,164]

Intervention

Due to the early and progressive development of pulmonary vascular obstructive changes, surgical intervention is advocated after the definitive diagnosis has been made. In 1961, Armer and associates[165] reported the first successful surgical correction of this defect in a 10-month-old boy with anomalous origin of the right pulmonary artery from the ascending aorta with an associated patent ductus arteriosus. Right pulmonary artery continuity with the main pulmonary artery was established with a 13-mm Dacron tube graft (Fig. 78–26). Alternatively, primary correction by direct reanastomosis of the anomalous right pulmonary artery to the main pulmonary artery has been reported.[160,161] Case reports of surgical correction of anomalous origin of the left pulmonary artery with associated tetralogy of Fallot have been associated with high surgical mortality.[158,159,162]

UNILATERAL ABSENCE OF THE PROXIMAL RIGHT OR LEFT PULMONARY ARTERY

The pathophysiology of unilateral absence of the right or left pulmonary artery is dependent upon the presence of associated intracardiac defects.[154] Pulmonary overcirculation and congestive symptoms may be present if a left-to-right shunt secondary to an associated cardiac defect (i.e., patent ductus arteriosus, ventricular septal defect, atrial septal defect) is present.[154,157] In contrast, patients with isolated unilateral absence of the pulmonary artery may remain asymptomatic and present later in life with hemoptysis.[154,166–168] Pulmonary hypertension is present in from 19 to 26% of patients[167] and is more likely to be reversible after surgical correction than pulmonary hypertension found in patients with anomalous origin of the pulmonary artery from the ascending aorta.

Unilateral absence and aortic origin of the pulmonary artery share the common embryologic feature of malabsorption of the proximal sixth aortic arch (ventral bud of the aortic sac).[154] From there, however, the embryology of these two lesions differs in that in the former, the affected lung may derive its blood supply from either the dorsal bud of the aortic sac (the precursor of the ductus arteriosus) or from vessels of the dorsal aorta below the sixth aortic arch, which are precursors to bronchial vessels (i.e., bronchial collateral vessels). Alternatively, the distal pulmonary artery of the affected lung may connect to the distal ascend-

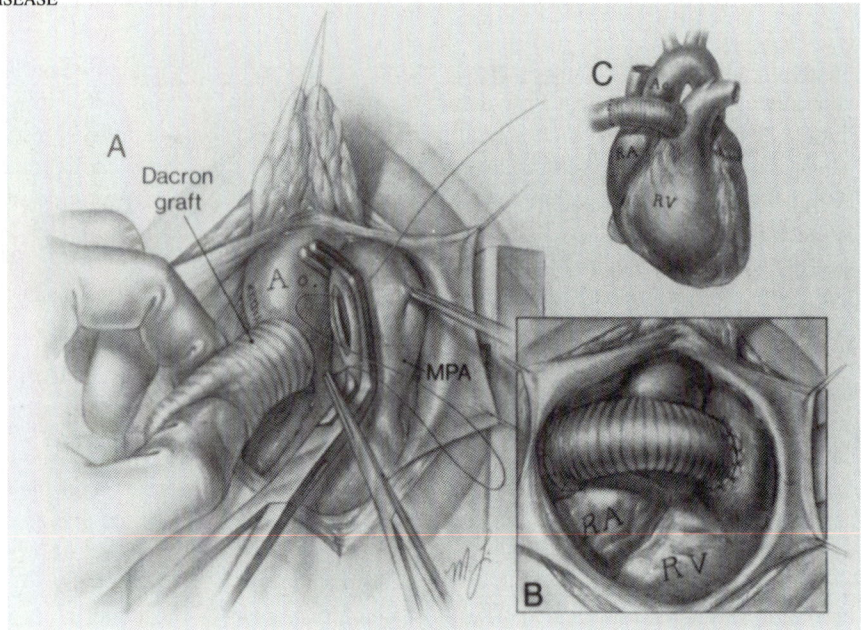

Figure 78–26. Technique for repair of anomalous origin of right pulmonary artery from the ascending aorta. **A.** Right pulmonary artery has been detached from the aorta (Ao). A Dacron graft is anastomosed to the main pulmonary artery (MPA). **B.** The distal end of the graft has been anastomosed to the proximal right pulmonary artery (RA) in the hilum. **C.** Complete repair. *(From Fontana GP, Spach MS, Effmann EL, Sabiston DC: Origin of the right pulmonary artery from the ascending aorta. Ann Surg 206:100–113, 1987[153].)*

ing aorta and migrate to the right innominate artery.[169] Others have speculated that abnormal truncal septation plays a role in the embryology of this lesion as described earlier for aortic origin of the pulmonary artery.[154]

Unilateral absence of the pulmonary artery occurs with nearly equal frequency as an isolated lesion as it does in conjunction with other congenital defects. Patent ductus arteriosus is predominantly associated with absent right pulmonary artery. Atrial septal defect or ventricular septal defect is found in equal distribution with either absent right or left pulmonary artery. Tetralogy of Fallot is primarily found in association with absent left pulmonary artery in patients with left aortic arch. Finally, unilateral absence of the pulmonary artery has been found in 12% of patients with truncus arteriosus in whom 65% have concordance between the side of the aortic arch and the affected pulmonary artery.[170,171]

Clinical Presentation

Due to the more heterogeneous degree of pulmonary blood supply to the affected lung, clinical presentation of patients with absent pulmonary artery may mimic aortic origin of the pulmonary artery with predominant symptoms of congestive heart failure. Conversely, few symptoms may be present early in life despite total perfusion of the unaffected lung by the complete cardiac output from the right ventricle. The latter situation may result in severe pulmonary hypertension, which presents as cough and hemoptysis in 10–20% of patients who were previously asymptomatic.[167] Coexistent lesions (i.e., tetralogy of Fallot or truncus arteriosus) may dictate the features of clinical presentation.

Diagnosis

The most common radiologic feature of unilateral absence of the pulmonary artery is decreased vascularity and decreased lung volume on the affected side.[154,172] Although a characteristic x-ray finding, it must be differentiated from patients with coarctation of the pulmonary arteries, pulmonary embolus, and agenesis of the lung. Angiography remains the most specific diagnostic intervention, although magnetic resonance scan[163] and cine computerized tomography[164] may be useful to confirm the presence of hilar pulmonary arteries on the affected side.

Intervention

Early intervention after diagnosis is warranted to avoid the development of pulmonary vascular obstructive disease, particularly in patients who present with symptoms of congestive heart failure. Exploring the pulmonary hilum will generally yield a pulmonary artery amenable to establishment of a connection with the main pulmonary artery by placement of an interposition graft[173–175] (Fig. 78–27). This will likely reduce the contralateral lung pulmonary hypertension. Correction of tetralogy of Fallot in association with absent left pulmonary artery has been carried out in general without unifocalization of the pulmonary arteries. Surgical risk is significantly greater than in cases with normal pulmonary arborization due to persistently elevated pulmonary vascular resistance and elevated ratio between the right and left systolic ventricular pressures. Earlier surgical correction and the use of a valved right ventricle to pulmonary artery conduit have been advocated to reduce perioperative morbidity and mortality.[176] A similar incremental surgical risk has been associated with the repair of

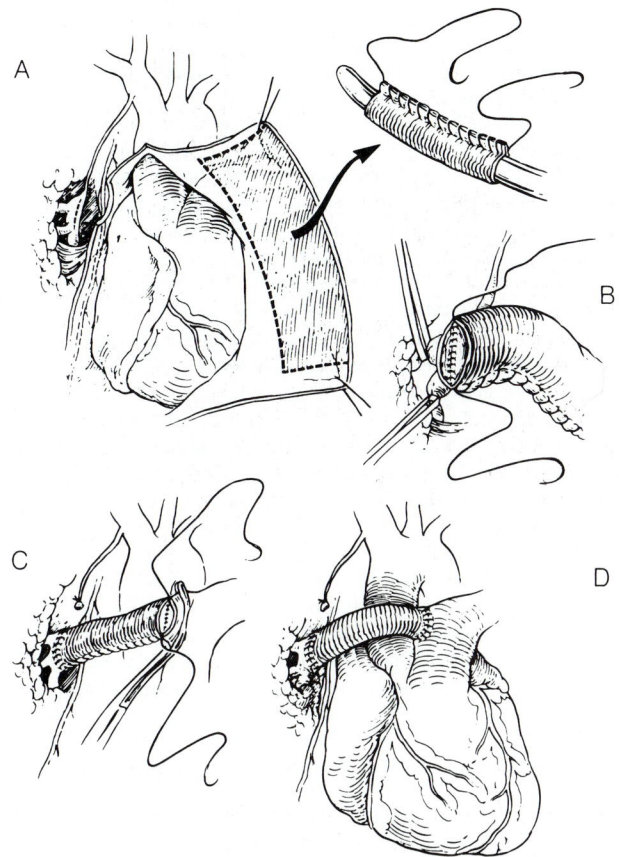

Figure 78–27. Technique for repair of unilateral absence of the pulmonary artery. **A.** A pericardial interposition graft is fashioned over a Hegar dilator. **B.** The distal end is anastomosed to the right pulmonary artery in the hilum. **C.** The proximal end is anastomosed to the main pulmonary artery. **D.** Completed repair. *(From Moreno-Cabral RJ, MacNamara JJ, Reddy VJ, Caldwell P: Unilateral absent pulmonary artery: Surgical repair with a new technique. J Thorac Cardiovasc Surg 102:463–464, 1991.)*

truncus arteriosus in patients with unilateral absence of the pulmonary artery.[170,171]

From 10 to 20% of patients with unilateral absence of the pulmonary artery will present later in life with hemoptysis as their primary symptom. This is due either to pulmonary hypertension in the contralateral lung or the development of large aortopulmonary collateral vessels with endobronchial rupture in the affected lung. Some patients will benefit from anatomic correction with a relief of the hemoptysis. Alternatively, pneumonectomy has been advocated in some patients with excessive bronchial collateral flow to the lung with absent pulmonary artery.[168] Conservative management has been advocated in other series.[167]

REFERENCES

1. Emmanouilides GC: Obstructive lesions of the right ventricle and pulmonary arterial tree. In Moss AJ, Adams FH, Emmanouilides GC (eds): *Heart Disease in Infants, Children and Adolescents,* 2nd ed. Baltimore, Williams & Wilkens, 1977

2. Mitchell SM, Korones SB, Berendes HW: Congenital heart disease in 56, 109 births. Incidence and natural history. *Circulation* **43:**323–332, 1971

3. Morgagni JB: De sedibus et causis morborum. *Epist* **17:**435, 1761

4. Doyen E: Chrugie des malformations congenitals ou acquises du coeur. *Presse Med* **21:**860–863, 1913

5. Sellors TH: Surgery of pulmonary stenosis. A case in which the pulmonary valve was successfully divided. *Lancet* **1:**988–989, 1948

6. Brock RC: Pulmonary valvotomy for the relief of congenital pulmonary stenosis. Report of three cases. *Br Med J* **1:**1121–1126, 1948

7. Swan H, Zeavin I, Blount SG, Virtue RW: Surgery by direct vision in the open heart during hypothermia. *JAMA* **153:**1081–1085, 1953

8. Kirklin JW: Open-heart surgery at the Mayo Clinic. The 25th anniversary. *Mayo Clinic Proc* **55:**339–345, 1980

9. Semb BKH, Tjonneland S, Stake G, Aabyholm G: "Balloon valvotomy" of congenital pulmonary valve stenosis with tricuspid valve insufficiency. *Cardiovasc Radiol* **2:**239–241, 1979

10. Kan JS, White RI, Mitchell SE, Gardner TJ: Percutaneous balloon valvuloplasty: A new method for treating congenital pulmonary valve stenosis. *N Engl J Med* **307:**540–542, 1982

11. Gikonyo BM, Lucas RV, Edwards JE: Anatomic features of congenital pulmonary valvar stenosis. *Pediatr Cardiol* **8:**109–115, 1987

12. Altrichter PM, Olson LJ, Edwards WD, et al: Surgical pathology of the pulmonary valve: A study of 116 cases spanning 15 years. *Mayo Clin Proc* **64:**1352–1360, 1989

13. Greene DG, Baldwin ED, Baldwin JS, et al: Pure congenital pulmonary stenosis and idiopathic congenital dilatation of the pulmonary artery. *Am J Med* **6:**24–31, 1949

14. Watkins Jr L, Donahoo JS, Harrington D, et al: Surgical management of congenital pulmonary valve dysplasia. *Ann Thorac Surg* **24:**498–507, 1977

15. Koretzky ED, Moller JH, Korus ME, et al: Congenital pulmonary stenosis resulting from dysplasia of valve. *Circulation* **40:**43–53, 1969

16. Freedom RM: Pulmonary Valve Stenosis with intact ventricular septum and congenital pulmonary valve stenosis. In Freedom RM, et al (eds): *Angiocardiography of Congenital Heart Disease.* New York, Macmillan, 1984, pp 343–377

17. Noonan JA: Hypertelorism, with Turners phenotype. A new syndrome with associated congenital heart disease. *Am J Dis Child* **62:**995–1002, 1983

18. Linde L, Turner SW, Sparkes RS: Pulmonary valvular dysplasia. The cardiofacial syndrome. *Br Heart J* **35:**301–304, 1973

19. Caspi J, Coles JG, Benson LN, et al: Management of neonatal critical pulmonary stenosis in the balloon valvotomy era. *Ann Thorac Surg* **49:**273–278, 1990

20. Hanley FL, Sade RM, Freedom RM, et al: Outcomes in critically ill neonates with pulmonary stenosis and intact ventricular septum: A multiinstitutional study. *J Am Coll Cardiol* **22:**183–192, 1993

21. Hatle L, Angelsen B: *Doppler Ultrasound in Cardiology.* Philadelphia, Lea & Febiger, 1985, pp 108–110

22. Freed MD, Rosenthal A, Bernhard WF, et al: Critical pulmonary stenosis with a diminutive right ventricle in neonates. *Circulation* **48:**875–881, 1973

23. Weldon CS, Hartmann AF Jr, McKnight RC: Surgical management of hypoplastic right ventricle with pulmonary atresia or arterial pulmonary stenosis and intact ventricular septum. *Ann Thorac Surg* **37:**12–24, 1984

24. Merrill WH, Shuman TA, Graham Jr TP, et al: Surgical intervention in neonates with critical pulmonary stenosis. *Ann Surg* **205:**712–717, 1987

25. Schmidt KG, Cloez J-L, Silverman NH: Changes of right ventricular size and function in neonates after valvectomy for pulmonary atresia or critical pulmonary stenosis and intact ventricular septum. *J Am Coll Cardiol* **19:**1032–1037, 1992

26. Zeevi B, Keane JF, Fellows KE, Lock JE: Balloon dilation of critical pulmonary stenosis in the first week of life. *J Am Coll Cardiol* **11**:821–824

27. Beekman RH, Lloyd TR: Balloon valvuloplasty and stenting for congenital heart disease. In Topol EJ (ed): *Textbook of Interventional Cardiology,* 2nd ed. Philadelphia, W.B. Saunders, 1994, pp 1277–1297

28. Burzynski JB, Kveselis DA, Byrum CJ, et al: Modified technique for balloon valvuloplasty of critical pulmonary stenosis in the newborn. *J Am Coll Cardiol* **22**:1944–1947, 1993

29. Rey C, Marache P, Francart C, Dupuis C: Percutaneous transluminal balloon valvuloplasty of congenital pulmonary valve stenosis with a special report on infants and neonates. *J Am Coll Cardiol* **11**:815–820, 1988

30. Stanger P, Cassidy SC, Girod DA, et al: Balloon pulmonary valvuloplasty: Results of the valvuloplasty and angioplasty of congenital anomalies registry. *Am J Cardiol* **65**:775–783, 1990

31. Ladusans EJ, Qureshi SA, Parsons JM, et al: Balloon dilatation of critical stenosis of the pulmonary valve in neonates. *Br Heart J* **63**:362–367, 1990

32. McCrindle BW, Kan JS: Long-term results after balloon pulmonary valvuloplasty. *Circulation* **83**:1915–1922, 1991

33. Mistrot J, Neal W, Lyons G, et al: Pulmonary valvuloplasty under inflow stasis for isolated pulmonary stenosis. *Ann Thorac Surg* **21**:30–37, 1971

34. Sade RM, Crawford FA, Hohn AR: Inflow occlusion for semilunar valve stenosis. *Ann Thorac Surg* **33**:570–575, 1982

35. Jonas RA, Castaneda AR, Norwood WI, Freed MD: Pulmonary valvotomy under normothermia caval inflow occlusion. *Aust NZ J Surg* **55**:39–44, 1985

36. Jonas RA, Castaneda AR, Freed MD: Normothermic caval inflow occlusion. Application to operations for congenital heart disease. *J Thorac Cardiovasc Surg* **89**:780–786, 1985

37. Milo S, Yellin A, Smolinsky A, et al: Closed pulmonary valvotomy in infants under 6 months of age: Report of 14 consecutive cases without mortality. *Thorax* **35**:814–818, 1980

38. Smolinsky A, Arav R, Hegesh J, et al: Surgical closed pulmonary valvotomy for critical pulmonary stenosis: Implications for the balloon valvuloplasty era. *Thorax* **47**:179–183, 1992

39. Buckberg GD, Steed D, Becker H, Rosenkranz ER: Myocardial protection during pediatric cardiac surgery. In Marcelletti C, Anderson R, Becker A, et al (eds): *Pediatric Cardiology.* London, Churchill Livingston, 1986, pp 39–52

40. Rosenkranz ER, Vinten-Johansen J, Buckberg GD, et al: Benefits of normothermic induction of blood cardioplegia in energy-depleted hearts with maintenance of arrest by multidose cold blood cardioplegic infusions. *J Thorac Cardiovasc Surg* **84**:667–676, 1982

41. Rowlatt UF, Rimoldi HJA, Lev M: The quantitative anatomy of the childs heart. *Pediatr Clin North Am* **10**:499, 1963

42. Mercer JL: Acceptable size of the pulmonary valve ring in congenital cardiac defects. *Ann Thorac Surg* **20**:567–570, 1975

43. Varco RL: In discussion of WH Muller Jr, WP Longmire Jr, The surgical treatment of cardiac valvular stenosis. *Surgery* **30**:41, 1951

44. Coles JG, Freedom RM, Olley PM, et al: Surgical management of critical pulmonary stenosis in the neonate. *Ann Thorac Surg* **38**:458–465, 1984

45. Danielson GK, Exarhos ND, Weidman WH, McGoon DC: Pulmonic stenosis with intact ventricular septum. Surgical consideration and results of operation. *J Thorac Cardiovasc Surg* **61**:228–234, 1971

46. Kopecky SL, Gersh BJ, McGoon MD, et al: Long term outcome of patients undergoing surgical repair of isolated pulmonary valve stenosis. Follow up at 20–30 years. *Circulation* **78**:1150–1156, 1988

47. Nugent EW, Freedom RM, Nora JJ, et al: Clinical course in pulmonary stenosis. *Circulation* **62**(Suppl I):I-38–I-47, 1977

48. Moller I, Wennevold A, Lynborg KE: The natural history of pulmonary stenosis. Long-term follow up with serial heart catheterization. *Cardiology* **58**:193–202, 1973

49. Mody M: The natural history of uncomplicated valvular pulmonic stenosis. *Am Heart J* **90**:317–321, 1975

50. Wennevold A, Jacobsen JR: Natural history of valvular pulmonary stenosis in children below the age of two years. Long-term follow up with serial heart catheterizations. *Eur J Cardiol* **8**:371–378, 1978

51. Tandon R, Nadas AS, Gross RE: Results of open-heart surgery in patients with pulmonic stenosis and intact ventricular septum. A report of 108 cases. *Circulation* **31**:190–210, 1965

52. Brock R: The surgical treatment of pulmonary stenosis. *Br Heart J* **23**:337–356, 1961

53. Frantz EG, Silverman NH: Doppler ultrasound evaluation of valvar pulmonary stenosis from multiple transducer positions in children requiring pulmonary valvuloplasty. *Am J Cardiol* **61**:844–849, 1988

54. Nishimura RA, Pieroni DR, Bierman FZ, et al: Second natural history study of congenital heart defects. Pulmonary stenosis: Echocardiography. *Circulation* **87** (Suppl I):I–73–I–79, 1993

55. Murphy DJ, Ludemirsky A, Danford DA, Huhta JC: Doppler echocardiography in pulmonary stenosis. *Echocardiography* **4**:187–202, 1987

56. Hayes CJ, Gersony WM, Driscoll DJ, et al: Second natural history of congenital heart defects. Results of treatment of patients with pulmonary valvar stenosis. *Circulation* **87** (Suppl I):I–28–I–37, 1993

57. Sullivan ID, Robinson PJ, Macartney FJ, et al: Percutaneous balloon valvuloplasty for pulmonary valve stenosis in infants and children. *Br Heart J* **54**:435–441, 1985

58. Radtke W, Keane JF, Fellows KE, et al: Percutaneous balloon valvotomy of congenital pulmonary stenosis using oversized balloons. *J Am Coll Cardiol* **8**:909–915, 1986

59. Masura J, Burch M, Deanfield JE, Sullivan ID: Five-year follow up after balloon pulmonary valvuloplasty. *J Am Coll Cardiol* **21**:132–136, 1993

60. Rocchini AP, Beekman RH: Balloon angioplasty in the treatment of pulmonary valve stenosis and coarctation of the aorta. *Texas H Inst J* **13**:337–385, 1986

61. Ballerini L, Mullins CE, Cifarelli A, et al: Percutaneous balloon valvuloplasty of pulmonary valve stenosis, dysplasia and residual stenosis after surgical valvotomy for pulmonary atresia with intact ventricular septum: Long-term results. *Cath Cardiovasc Diag* **19**:165–169, 1990

62. O'Conner BK, Beekman RH, Lindauer A, Rocchini A: Intermediate-term outcome after pulmonary balloon valvuloplasty: Comparison with a matched surgical control group. *J Am Coll Cardiol* **20**:169–173, 1992

63. Rao PS, Thapar MK, Kutryli F: Causes of restenosis after balloon valvuloplasty for valvular pulmonary stenosis. *Am J Cardiol* **62**:979–982, 1988

64. Alikhan MA, Al-Josef S, Moore JW, Sawyer W: Results of repeat percutaneous balloon valvuloplasty for pulmonary valvar restenosis. *Am Heart J* **120**:878–881, 1990

65. Pepine CJ, Gessner IH, Feldman RL: Percutaneous balloon valvuloplasty for pulmonic valve stenosis in the adult. *Am J Cardiol* **50**:1442–1445, 1982

66. Al Kasab S, Ribeiro PA, Zaibag MA, et al: Percutaneous double balloon pulmonary valvotomy in adults: One- to two-year follow up. *Am J Cardiol* **62**:822–824, 1988

67. Fawzy ME, Galal D, Dunn B, et al: Regression of infundibular pulmonary stenosis after successful balloon pulmonary valvuloplasty in adults. *Cath Cardiovasc Diag* **21**:77–81, 1990

68. Herrmann HC, Hill JA, Krol J, et al: Effectiveness of percutaneous balloon valvuloplasty in adults with pulmonary valve stenosis. *Am J Cardiol* **68**:1111–1113, 1991

69. Mullins CE, Nikill MR, Vick GW, et al: Double balloon technique for dilation of valvular or vessel stenosis in congenital and acquired heart disease. *J Am Coll Cardiol* **10**:107–114, 1987

70. Alikhan MA, Al Josef S, Mullins CE: Percutaneous transluminal balloon pulmonary valvuloplasty for the relief of pulmonary valve stenosis with special reference to double-balloon technique. *Am Heart J* **112**:158–166, 1986

71. Fawzy ME, Mercer EN, Dunn B: Late results of pulmonary balloon valvuloplasty in adults using double balloon technique. *J Interven Cardiol* **1**:35–42, 1988

72. Thapar MK, Rao PS: Significance of infundibular obstruction following balloon valvuloplasty for valvar pulmonic stenosis. *Am Heart J* **118**:99–103, 1989

73. Talbert JL, Morrow AG, Collins NP, Gilbert JW: The incidence and significance of pulmonic regurgitation after pulmonary valvulotomy. *Am Heart J* **65**:590–596, 1963

74. Mara GR, Hicks RW, Allen HD, Goldberg SJ: Noninvasive assessment of hemodynamic responses to exercise in pulmonary regurgitation after operations to correct pulmonary outflow obstruction. *Am J Cardiol* **61**:595–610, 1988

75. Gutgesell HP: Pulmonary valve insufficiency: Malignant or benign? *J Am Coll Cardiol* **20**:174–175, 1992

76. Engle MA, Holswade GR, Goldberg HP, et al: Regression after open valvotomy of infundibular stenosis accompanying severe valvular pulmonic stenosis. *Circulation* **17**:862–873, 1958

77. Milo S, Mohr R, Goor DA: Right ventricular pressure dynamics after operation for pulmonary stenosis. *Ann Thorac Surg* **48**:572–574, 1989

78. Marantz PM, Huhta JC, Mullins CF, et al: Results of balloon valvuloplasty in typical and dysplastic pulmonary valve stenosis: Doppler echocardiographic follow-up. *J Am Coll Cardiol* **12**:476–479, 1988

79. Musewe N, Robertson MA, Benson LN, et al: The dysplastic pulmonary valve: Echocardiographic features and results of balloon dilatation. *Br Heart J* **57**:364–370, 1987

80. Rao PS: Balloon dilatation in infants and children with dysplastic pulmonary valve with short-term and intermediate-term results. *Am Heart J* **116**:1168–1173, 1988

81. Polansky DB, Clark EB, Doty DB: Pulmonary stenosis in infants and young children. *Ann Thorac Surg* **39**:159–164, 1985

82. Merrill WH, Stewart JR, Hammon Jr JW, et al: Surgical management of patients with pulmonary valve dysplasia. *Ann Thorac Surg* **42**:264–268, 1986

83. Vancini M, Roberts KP, Silove ED, Singh SP: Surgical treatment of congenital pulmonary stenosis due to dysplastic leaflets and small valve annulus. *J Thorac Cardiovasc Surg* **79**:464–468, 1980

84. Hartmann Jr AF, Goldring D, Furgeson TB, et al: The course of children with the two-chambered right ventricle. *J Thorac Cardiovasc Surg* **60**:72–83, 1970

85. Lucas Jr RV, Varco RL, Lillehei RW, et al: Anomalous muscle bundle of the right ventricle. Hemodynamic consequences and surgical consideration. *Circulation* **25**:443–455, 1962

86. Hartmann AF Jr, Goldring D, Carlson E: Development of right ventricular obstruction by aberrant muscular bands. *Circulation* **30**:679–685, 1964

87. Warden HE, Lucas RV Jr, Varco RL: Right ventricular obstruction resulting from anomalous muscle bundles. *J Thorac Cardiovasc Surg* **51**:53–65, 1966

88. Forster JW, Humphries JO: Right ventricular anomalous muscle bundles. Clinical and laboratory presentation and natural history. *Circulation* **43**:115–127, 1971

89. Shimada R, Tajimi T, Koyanagi S, et al: Two-dimensional echocardiographic findings in double chamber right ventricle. *Am Heart J* **108**:1059–1061, 1984

90. Rowland TW, Rosenthal A, Castaneda AR: Double-chamber right ventricle: Experience with 17 cases. *Am Heart J* **89**:455–462, 1975

91. Fellows KE, Martin EC, Rosenthal A: Angiocardiography of obstructing muscle bands of the right ventricle. *Am J Roentgenol* **128**:249–256, 1977

92. Martin D, Van Doesburg NH, Fouran J-C, et al: Subxiphoid two-dimensional echocardiographic diagnosis of double-chambered right ventricle. *Circulation* **67**:885–888, 1983

93. Wang PC, Sanders SP, Jonas RA, et al: Pulmonary valve-moderator band distance and association with development of double-chambered right ventricle. *Am J Cardiol* **68**:1681–1686, 1991

94. Pongiglione G, Freedom RD, Cook D, Rowe RD: Mechanism of acquired right ventricular outflow tract obstruction in patients with ventricular septal defect: An angiographic study. *Am J Cardiol* **50**:776–780, 1982

95. Danilowicz D, Ishmael R: Anomalous right ventricular muscle bundle: Clinical pitfalls and extracardiac anomalies. *Clin Cardiol* **4**:146–150, 1981

96. Brimstock A, Fellows KE, Rosenthal A: Combined double chamber right ventricle and discrete subaortic stenosis. *Circulation* **57**:299–310, 1978

97. Simpson Jr WF, Sade RM, Crawford FA, et al: Double-chambered right ventricle. *Ann Thorac Surg* **44**:7–10, 1987

98. Coates JR, McClenathan JE, Scott III LP: The double-chambered right ventricle. A diagnostic and operative pitfall. *Am J Cardiol* **14**:561–567, 1964

99. Von Doenhoff LJ, Nanda NC: Obstruction with the right ventricular body: Two-dimensional echocardiographic features. *Am J Cardiol* **51**:1498–1501, 1983

100. Ford DK, Bullaboy CA, Derkac WM, et al: Transatrial repair of double-chambered right ventricle. *Ann Thorac Surg* **45**:412–415, 1988

101. McGrath LB, Joyce DH: Transatrial repair of double-chambered right ventricle. *J Cardiac Surg* **4**:291–298, 1989

102. Penkoske PA, Duncan N, Collins-Nakai RL: Surgical repair of double-chambered right ventricle with or without ventriculotomy. *J Thorac Cardiovasc Surg* **93**:385–393, 1987

103. Keveselis D, Rosenthal A, Ferguson P, et al: Long-term prognosis after repair of double-chamber right ventricle with ventricular septal defect. *Am J Cardiol* **54**:1292–1295, 1984

104. Beekman RH, Rocchini AP, Rosenthal A: Therapeutic cardiac catheterization for pulmonary valve and pulmonary artery stenosis. *Cardiol Clin* **7**:331–340, 1989

105. Rothman A, Perry SB, Keane JF, Lock JF: Balloon dilation of branch pulmonary artery stenosis. *Sem Thorac Surg* **2**:46–54, 1990

106. Roberts N, Moes CAF: Supravalvar pulmonary stenosis. *J Pediatr* **82**:838–844, 1973

107. D'Orsonga L, Sandor GGS, Culhan JAG, Patterson M: Successful balloon angioplasty of peripheral pulmonary stenosis in Williams syndrome. *Am Heart J* **114**:647–648, 1987

108. Wren C, Oslizlok P, Bull C: Natural history of supravalvar aortic stenosis and pulmonary artery stenosis. *J Am Coll Cardiol* **15**:1625–1630, 1990

109. Noonan JA, Ehmke DA: Associated noncardiac malformations in children with congenital heart disease. *Am J Cardiol* **63**:468–470, 1963

110. Rowe RD: Cardiovascular disease in the rubella syndrome. *Cardiovasc Clin* **5**:61–80, 1973

111. Lee MV, Menasche VD, Sunderland CO: Ehlers-Danlos syndrome associated with multiple pulmonary artery stenoses and tortuous systemic arteries. *J Pediatr* **75**:1031–1036, 1969

112. Hayden JG, Talner NS, Klaus SV: Cutis laxa associated with pulmonary artery stenosis. *J Pediatr* **72**:506–509, 1969

113. McCue CM, Robertson LW, Lester RG, Mauch Jr HP: Pulmonary artery coarctations. A report of 20 cases with review of 139 cases from the literature. *J Pediatr* **67**:222–238, 1965

114. Agrons GA, Muslack MM, Parry CE, Latour MGN: Multiple coarctations of the pulmonary artery: Scintigraphic appearance. *Clin Nuc Med* **1**:19–21, 1990

115. Ring JC, Bass JL, Marvin W, et al: Management of congenital stenosis of a branch pulmonary artery with balloon dilation angioplasty. Report of 52 procedures. *J Thorac Cardiovasc Surg* **90**:35–44, 1985

116. Smith GW, Thompson Jr WM, Muller Jr WH: Surgical treatment of pulmonary hypertension secondary to multiple bilateal pulmonary artery stenosis. *Circulation* 29:152–156, 1964

117. Hvass U, Khoury W, Pansard Y, Videcog M: Repair of pulmonary artery branches with broadly based autologous pericardial flaps. *J Thorac Cardiovasc Surg* 95:738, 1988

118. Mendesohn AM, Bove EL, Lupinetti FM, et al: Intraoperative and percutaneous stenting of congenital pulmonary artery and vein stenosis. *Circulation* 86:I 359, 1991

119. O'Laughlin M, Perry SP, Lock JE, Mullins CE: Use of endovascular stents in congenital heart disease. *Circulation* 83:1923–1939, 1991

120. Rothman A, Perry SB, Keane JF, Lock JE: Early results and follow-up of balloon angioplasty for branch pulmonary artery stenosis. *J Am Coll Cardiol* 15:1109–1117, 1990

121. Lock JE, Castaneda-Zuniga WR, Fuhrman BP, Bass JL: Balloon dilation angioplasty of hypoplastic and stenotic pulmonary arteries. *Circulation* 67:962–967, 1983

122. Rao PS: Transcatheter treatment of pulmonary outflow tract obstruction: A review. *Prog Cardiovasc Dis* 35:119–158, 1992

123. Rocchini AP, Kveselis D, Dick M, et al: Use of balloon angioplasty to treat peripheral pulmonary stenosis. *Am J Cardiol* 54:1069–1073, 1984

124. Kan JS, Marvin Jr WJ, Bass JL, et al: Balloon angioplasty-branch pulmonary artery stenosis: Results from the valvuloplasty and angioplasty of congenital anomalies registry. *Am J Cardiol* 65:798–801, 1990

125. Hosking MK, Benson LN, Nakanishi T, et al: Intravascular stent prosthesis for right ventricular outflow obstruction. *J Am Coll Cardiol* 20:373–380, 1992

126. Mullins CE, O'Laughlin MP, Vick III WG, et al: Implantation of balloon-expandable intravascular grafts by catheterization in pulmonary arteries and systemic veins. *Circulation* 77:188–199, 1988

127. Elzenga NJ, Suyler RJ, Frohn-Mulder I, et al: Juxtaductal pulmonary artery coarctation. An underestimated cause of branch pulmonary artery stenosis in patients with pulmonary atresia or stenosis and a ventricular septal defect. *J Thorac Cardiovasc Surg* 100:416–424, 1990

128. Elzenga NJ, Gittenberger-de Groot AC: The ductus arteriosus and stenoses of the pulmonary arteries in pulmonary atresia. *Int J Cardiol* 11:195–208, 1986

129. Deterling Jr RA, Clagett T: Aneurysm of the pulmonary artery: Review of the literature and report of a case. *Am Heart J* 34:471–497, 1947

130. Arom KV, Richardson JD, Grover FL, et al: Pulmonary artery aneurysm. *Am Surg* 46:688–692, 1978

131. Bartter T, Irwin RS, Nash G: Aneurysms of the pulmonary arteries. *Chest* 94:1065–1075, 1988

132. Butto F, Lucas Jr RV, Edwards JE: Pulmonary artery aneurysm. A pathologic study of five cases. *Chest* 91:237–241, 1987

133. Coard KCM, Martin MP: Ruptured saccular pulmonary artery aneurysm associated with patent ductus arateriosus. *Arch Pathol Lab Med* 116:159–161, 1992

134. Vargas-Barron J, Avila-Rosales L, Romero-Cardras A, et al: Echocardiographic diagnosis of a mycotic aneurysm of the main pulmonary artery and patent ductus arteriosus. *Am Heart J* 123:1707–1709, 1992

135. Caralps JM, Bonin JO, Oter R, Aris A: True aneurysm of the main pulmonary artery: Surgical correction. *Ann Thorac Surg* 25:561–563, 1978

136. Donahue BC, Binder SW, Perloff JK, Child JS: Rupture of an aneurysmal pulmonary artery trunk 40 years after Blalock-Taussig anastomosis. *Am J Cardiol* 61:477–478, 1988

137. Monarrez CN, Rao PS, Moore HV, Strang WB: False aneurysm of the right pulmonary artery. New complication of aorta-right pulmonary artery anastomosis. *J Thorac Cardiovasc* 77:738–741, 1979

138. Navarro C, Dickinson PCT, Kondapoodi P, Hagstrom JWC: Mycotic aneurysms of the pulmonary arteries in intravenous drug addicts. *Am J Med* 76:1124–1131, 1984

139. Kohno S, Fujikawa M, Kanda T, et al: A case of Bechets syndrome with rupture of a pulmonary artery aneurysm: Autopsy findings and literature review. *Japn J Med* 25:293–300, 1986

140. Durieux P, Bletry O, Huchon G, et al: Multiple pulmonary arterial aneurysms of Bechets disease and Hughes-Stovin syndrome. *Am J Med* 71:736–741, 1981

141. Nagelsmith MJ, Eulderick F: Dissecting aneurysm of the pulmonary trunk. *Am J Cardiol* 58:660–661, 1986

142. Feng WC, Singh AK, Drew T, Donat W: Swan-Ganz catheter-induced massive hemoptysis and pulmonary artery false aneurysm. *Ann Thorac Surg* 50:644–645, 1992

143. Dieden JD, Friloux LA, Renner JW: Pulmonary artery false aneurysms secondary to Swan-Ganz pulmonary artery catheters. *Am J Rad* 149:901–906, 1987

144. Bhandari AK, Nanda NC: Pulmonary artery aneurysms: Echocardiographic features in 5 patients. *Am J Cardiol* 53:1438–1441, 1984

145. Thomason PA, Krach KR: Spontaneous rupture of the pulmonary artery. *Ann Emerg Med* 63:115–117, 1988

146. Gould L, Reddy CVR, Yang CS: Aneurysms of the pulmonary arteries. *Angiology* 28:119–124, 1977

147. Rosenson RS, Sutton MS: Dissecting aneurysm of the pulmonary trunk in mitral stenosis. *Am J Cardiol* 58:1140–1141, 1986

148. Finch EL, Mitchell RS, Guthaner DF, et al: Pulmonary artery surgical aneurysmorrhaphy: Where do we go from here? *Am Heart J* 106:614–618, 1983

149. Garcia-Rinaldi R, Howell J: Aneurysm of the main pulmonary artery: Long-term survival after aneurysmorrhaphy and closure of a ventricular septal defect. *Ann Thorac Surg* 22:180–183, 1975

150. Ungaro R, Saab S, Almond CH, Kumar S: Solitary peripheral pulmonary artery aneurysms. Pathogenesis and surgical treatment. *J Thorac Cardiovasc Surg* 4:566–571, 1976

151. Murphy JP, Adyanthaya AV, Adams PR, et al: Peripheral pulmonary artery aneurysm in a patient with limited respiratory reserve: Controlled resection using cardiopulmonary bypass. *Ann Thorac Surg* 43:323–325, 1987

152. Taylor BG, Cockerill EM, Manfredi F, Klatte EC: Therapeutic embolization of the pulmonary artery in pulmonary arteriovenous fistula. *Am J Med* 64:360–365, 1978

153. Fontana GP, Spach MS, Effmann EL, Sabiston DC: Origin of the right pulmonary artery from the ascending aorta. *Ann Surg* 206:100–113, 1987

154. Pool PE, Vogel JHK, Blount SG Jr: Congenital unilateal absence of a pulmonary artery. The importance of flow in pulmonary hypertension. *Am J Cardiol* 10:706–731, 1962

155. Sotomora RF, Edwards JE: Anatomic identification of so-called absent pulmonary artery. *Circulation* 57:624–633, 1978

156. Fraentzel O: Ein Fall von abnormer communication der aorta wit der arteria pulmonalis. *Virchow's Arch Pathol Anat* 43:420–428, 1868

157. Shakibi JG, Rastan H, Nazarian I, et al: Isolated unilateral absence of pulmonary artery. Review of the world's literature and guidelines for surgical repair. *Jpn Heart J* 19:439–451, 1978

158. Calder L, Brandt PWT, Barrett-Boyes BG, Neutze JM: Variant of tetralogy of Fallot with absent pulmonary valve leaflets and origin of one pulmonary artery from the ascending aorta. *Am J Cardiol* 46:106–116, 1980

159. Saxena A, Shrivastava S, Sharma S: Anomalous origin of the left pulmonary artery from the ascending aorta in a patient with tetralogy of Fallot and "absent pulmonary valve". *Int J Cardiol* 33:315–317, 1991

160. Matsuda H, Zavanella C, Lee P, Subramanian S: Aortic origin of the right pulmonary artery. *Ann Thorac Surg* 24:374–378, 1977

161. Kirkpatrick SE, Girod DA, King H: Aortic origin of the right pulmonary artery. Surgical repair without a graft. *Circulation* 36:777–782, 1967

162. Buchler JR, Jatene AD, Andrade J: Congenital unilateral absence of the right pulmonary artery and complex of Fallot. A rare association. *Jpn Heart J* **27**:885–892, 1986

163. Debatin JF, Moon RF, Spritzer C, et al: MRI of absent left pulmonary artery. *J Comp Assist Tomogr* **16**:641–645, 1992

164. Sondheimer HM, Oliphant M, Schneider B, et al: Computerized axial tomography of the chest for visualization of "absent" pulmonary arteries. *Circulation* **65**:1020–1025, 1982

165. Armer RM, Shumacker HB, Klatte EC: Origin of the right pulmonary artery from the ascending aorta. Report of a surgically corrected case. *Circulation* **24**:662–668, 1961

166. Mehta AC, Livingston DR, Kawalek W, et al: Pulmonary artery agenesis presenting as massive hemoptysis—a case report. *Angiology* **38**:67–71, 1987

167. Cogswell T, Singh S: Agenesis of the left pulmonary artery as a cause of hemoptysis. *Angiology* **37**:154–159, 1986

168. Byrne RJR, Bloom DL: Absence of the right pulmonary artery as a cause of hemoptysis. *J Thorac Cardiovasc Surg* **59**:264–268, 1970

169. Pfefferkorn JR, Loser H, Peck G, et al: Absent pulmonary artery. A hint to its embryogenesis. *Pediatr Cardiol* **3**:283–286, 1982

170. Mair DD, Ritter DG, Danielson GK, et al: Truncus arteriosus with unilateral absence of a pulmonary artery. Criteria for operability and surgical results. *Circulation* **55**:641–647, 1974

171. Fyfe DA, Driscoll DJ, DiDonato RM, et al: Truncus arteriosus with single pulmonary artery: Influence of pulmonary vascular obstructive disease early and late operative results. *J Am Coll Cardiol* **5**:1168–1172, 1985

172. Kieffer SA, Amplatz K, Anderson RC, Lillehei CW: Proximal interruption of a pulmonary artery. Roentgen features and surgical correction. *Am J Radiol* **95**:592–597, 1965

173. Toews WH, Pappas G: Surgical management of absent right pulmonary artery with associated pulmonary hypertension. *Chest* **84**:497–499, 1983

174. Cobanoglu A, Abbruzzese P, Brauner D, et al: Therapeutic consideration in congenital absence of the right pulmonary artery. Use of the internal mammary artery as a preparatory shunt. *J Cardiovasc Surg* **25**:241–245, 1984

175. Moreno-Cabral RJ, MacNamara JJ, Reddy VJ, Caldwell P: Unilateral absent pulmonary artery: Surgical repair with a new technique. *J Thorac Cardiovasc Surg* **102**:463–464, 1991

176. Mistrot JJ, Bernhard WF, Rosenthal A, Castaneda AR: Tetralogy of Fallot with a single pulmonary artery: Operative repair. *Ann Thorac Surg* **23**:249–253, 1977

79

Pulmonary Atresia with Intact Ventricular Septum

Early Palliation, Subsequent Management, and Possible Role of Fetal Surgical Intervention

Vadiyala Mohan Reddy and Frank L. Hanley

Pulmonary atresia with intact ventricular septum (PA.IVS) is a rare lesion accounting for about 1–1.5% of all congenital heart defects.[1,2] In the New England registry it comprised 3% of all critically ill infants with congenital heart disease.[3] The lesion is much more complex than implied by its name, since significant associated morphologic abnormalities of the tricuspid valve, right ventricle, coronary arteries, and left heart are common.[1,4] PA.IVS may be considered as the most severe lesion along the spectrum which also includes critical pulmonary stenosis in the neonate, and isolated pulmonary stenosis in children. The benefit of such a perspective is that it emphasizes certain similarities of morphology and therapy between milder forms of PA.IVS and the more severe forms of critical pulmonary stenosis. It may also be beneficial to perceive PA.IVS as a lesion distinct from pulmonary stenosis because of the common occurrence and severity of associated pathology involving the right ventricle, tricuspid valve, myocardium, and coronary arteries. It is not only the pulmonary atresia itself, but, more importantly, the associated lesions that dictate the surgical strategies. The present theory regarding development of these associated lesions is that severe obstruction at the right ventricular outlet during fetal life is the primary event causing hemodynamic changes which secondarily induce the more complex and clinically troublesome right sided lesions. The notion that very early intervention to relieve the

pulmonary atresia might result in fewer and less severe secondary changes is a persuasive argument for considering fetal intervention as a unique and effective form of primary therapy for management of this lesion.

ETIOLOGY

The exact cause of this lesion is not known. Though definitive proof is lacking, PA.IVS is thought to result from an insult occurring relatively late in embryologic development, often following primary cardiac morphogenesis.[5] It seems logical to assume that the spectrum of severity of morphologic lesions at the pulmonary valve, tricuspid valve, right ventricular myocardium, and coronary arteries is affected by the timing of the initial insult in utero. Presumably, atresia occurring very early would result in a completely undeveloped pulmonary valve, a diminutive right ventricle, small tricuspid valve, and extensive right ventricular to coronary artery communications. However, atresia occurring later in gestation would probably result in a pulmonary valve that has three developed sinuses of Valsalva and three developed valve leaflets that are completely fused, a good sized right ventricle, and absence of coronary anomalies. The exact nature of the insult that induces the pulmonary valve atresia is speculative. An inflammatory or infectious etiology has been invoked[5,6]; however, a primary hemodynamic alteration resulting secondarily in pulmonary valve atresia is possible. Subtle alterations in the tricuspid valve, foramen ovale, and patent ductus arteriosus during early development might encourage left heart loading, which might result in left-to-right ductal flow and failure of generated right ventricular systolic pressure to reach pulmonary artery pressure, such that the pulmonary valve would fail to open. This could lead to fusion of the pulmonary valve leaflets as development proceeds. Rarely genetic factors may be the cause of pulmonary atresia.[7,8]

MORPHOLOGY

PA.IVS with rare exceptions[9] occurs with situs solitus and normal atrioventricular and ventriculoarterial connections. Marked morphologic heterogeneity (Table 79–1) is the hallmark of this lesion.[1,4,10] All of these morphologic abnormalities occur proximal to the right ventriculoarterial junction, in contrast to pulmonary atresia with ventricular septal defect, where the major abnormalities occur distal to this junction.

An *interatrial communication* is virtually always present. A true secundum atrial septal defect (ASD) is present in about 20% of cases,[11] and a sprung foramen ovale (PFO) in the rest. In about 5–10% of cases the interatrial communication is restrictive with the septum primum bulging into the left atrium.[12] The *right atrium* is quite often dilated (Fig. 79–1), with the degree of dilation often being proportional to the severity of tricuspid regurgitation.

Varying degrees of *tricuspid valve* (TV) abnormality are present in most cases. Typically, the valve is smaller than normal (Fig. 79–1), but it may range from Ebstein's anomaly with an enlarged dilated annulus on the one hand, to an extremely stenotic valve on the other.[10,13] In the Congenital Heart Surgeons Society (CHSS) study the median Z value of the tricuspid annulus was −2.2 (Z value represents the normalized tricuspid annulus diameter with 0 being normal[14] and the values above and below it representing the number of standard deviations from the normal).[10] The size of the tricuspid valve correlates well with the right ventricular cavity size.[4,10,13,15] Stenotic valves exhibit varying degrees of dysplasia. The valve margins may attach directly to the papillary muscles without chordal development.[13] Some of these dysplastic valves are verrucous without any evidence of commissural development.[16] Unguarded tricuspid orifice is associated with extreme dysplasia and deficiency of the valve tissue.[17] In about 5–10% of cases Ebstein's deformity of the tricuspid valve is present.[10,18] Occasionally, parachute deformity of the tricuspid valve has been described.[13] Functionally the tricuspid valve may be regurgitant, stenotic, or both. Some degree of tricuspid regurgitation is present in most cases—with severe tricuspid regurgitation present in 25% of cases.[10] Hypoplastic valves are inherently stenotic but may have varying degrees of regurgitation. Rarely severe stenosis may be present with Ebstein's anomaly with a tiny tricuspid orifice.[19]

TABLE 79–1. MORPHOLOGY OF PA.IVS[a]

Category	Subcategory	Percentage
Pulmonary atresia (*n* = 50)	Membranous	10
	Probably membranous	24
	Muscular	10
	Probably muscular	26
	indeterminable	20
RV cavity size (*n* = 144)	−4 to −5	54
	−2 to −3	29
	0 to −1	11
	+1 to +3	0.2
	+4 to +5	3
Tricuspid valve (*n* = 144)	<−2	52
	<−4	26
Sinusoids-coronary anomalies	No RV sinusoids	49
	RV sinusoids	51
(*n* = 149)	Without RV-coronary fistulas	5
	With RV-coronary fistulas	44
	Without RVDCC	35
	With RVDCC	8
	Unknown	1
	Unknown regards fistulas	2
Pulmonary arteries	Normal in most	
	Hypoplastic in 6 patients	

[a]*Based on the data from the congenital heart surgeons society.*[42]

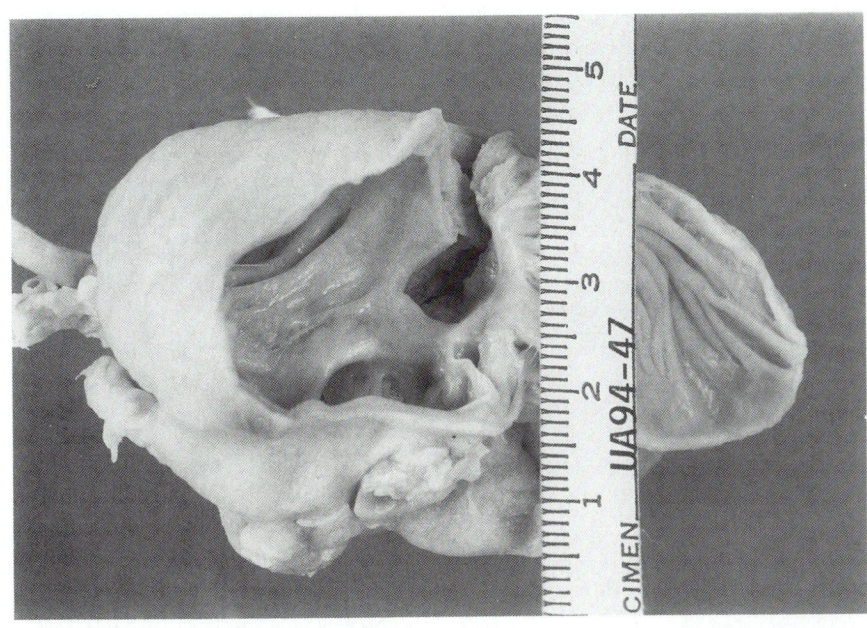

Figure 79–1. Pathologic heart specimen of pulmonary atresia with intact ventricular septum. Note the dilated large right atrium and hypoplastic tricuspid valve.

The *right ventricle* (RV) is hypertrophied (Fig. 79–2) with a reduced cavity in 90% of cases, severely so in about 60% of cases.[10] Less commonly, in about 5–10% of cases an enlarged and dilated right ventricle is found in association with more severe degrees of tricuspid regurgitation and with Ebstein's anomaly.[10] Rarely Uhl's anomaly (parchment RV) may be present. The "tripartite" concept of right ventricular organization[20] has been used to categorize the right ventricular morphology in this lesion.[15] The right ventricle may be unipartite (inlet part only), bipartite (inlet and outlet parts), or tripartite (inlet, outlet, and trabecular parts).[15] The validity of these distinctions, at least on an embryologic or developmental level, has been questioned by some, more recently. Even the smallest right ventricles are thought to have all three components; however, the massive hypertrophy may obliterate the trabecular and/or outlet parts.[1] Associated diffuse fibrosis of the hypertrophied ventricular muscle may be present and in severe cases varying degrees of endocardial fibroelastosis are seen.[4,21–23] These may be due to chronic myocardial ischemia. In the majority of cases myocardial fiber disarray is typical.[24]

Coronary artery abnormalities and right ventricular myocardial sinusoids are common in PA.IVS[1,4,10,25,26] (Fig. 79–3A and B). Right ventricular sinusoids, defined as endothelial lined blind channels within the substance of the right ventricular mass, which communicate with the right ventricular cavity, are present in about 50% of cases.[10] The myocardial sinusoids are remnants of sinusoidal spaces that nourish the myocardium before the development of coronary arteries. These may persist and may be the site of communications with the coronary arteries following pulmonary atresia.[15,27,28] These coronary artery to right ventricular fistulae are present in the majority of cases in which sinusoids are present and the prevalence of these le-

sions correlates inversely with tricuspid valve diameter, right ventricular cavity size, and degree of tricuspid incompetence.[10] Right ventricular systolic pressure is directly related to their prevalence.[1,10,25,29] These fistulae may be of relatively minor consequence, i.e., providing right ventricu-

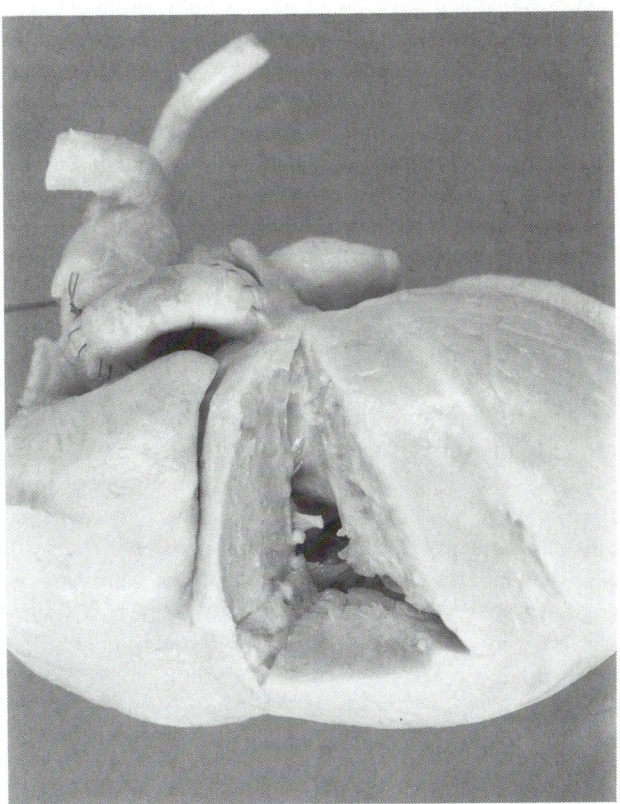

Figure 79–2. Pathologic heart specimen of pulmonary atresia (muscular) with intact ventricular septum. Note the hypertrophied right ventricle with reduced cavity size.

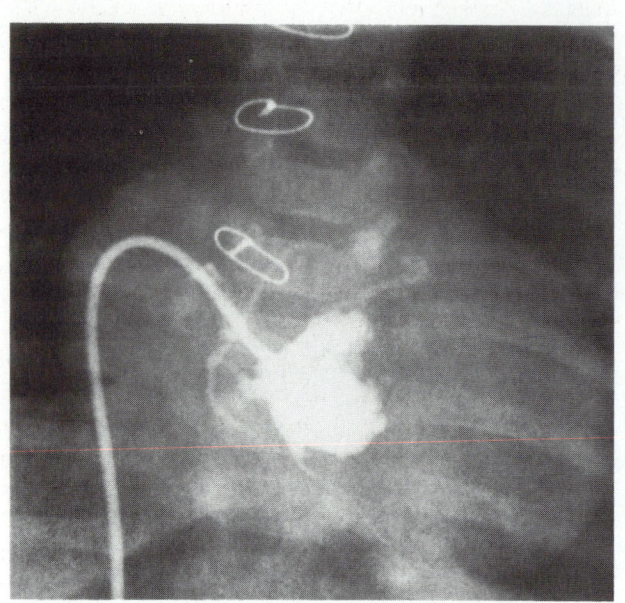

A

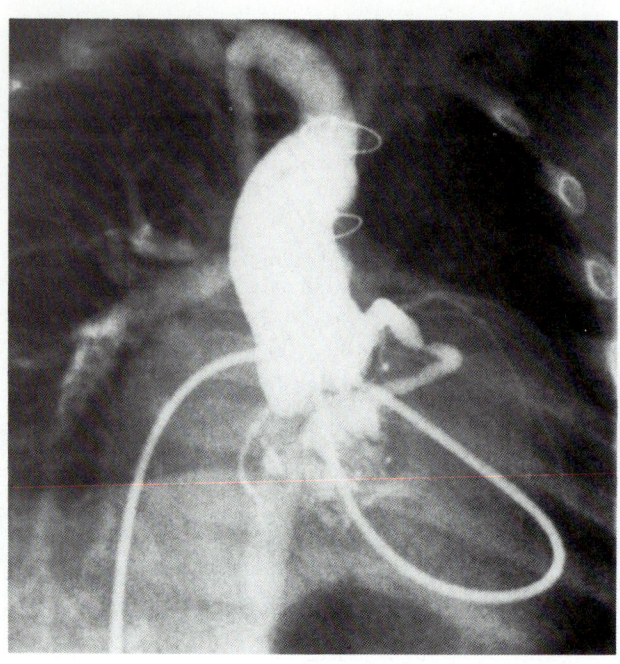

B

Figure 79–3. A. Angiogram—right ventricular injection showing myocardial sinusoids with retrograde filling of the coronary arteries. **B.** Angiogram—aortic injection showing coronary artery to ventricular communication with a stenotic segment in the coronary artery.

lar blood to relatively small areas of myocardium with dual supply from the normal aortocoronary route, or they may be of profound consequence with absence of antegrade aortocoronary flow. In about 20% of these cases the coronary circulation or some important part of it is solely derived from the right ventricle.[10] This is described as right ventricular-dependent coronary circulation. Intermediate degrees of right ventricular-dependent flow are common with some segments of myocardium receiving bloodflow only from the right ventricle via the fistulous connections. This dependency of myocardial blood flow on the right ventricle is due to the development of stenosis or occlusion in the proximal coronary arteries supplying that segment. The coronary stenoses are characterized by myointimal hyperplasia with changes ranging from simple thickening of the intima and media to marked replacement of the arterial wall with fibrous tissue.[25] The pathogenesis of these coronary obstructive lesions in fetal life is thought to be secondary to the turbulent competitive flow conditions between antegrade aortocoronary flow and flow through the high-pressure right ventricular to coronary artery fistulae.[30] These lesions generally progress after birth. Sinusoids and right ventricular to coronary artery fistulae are generally not present in cases of Ebstein's anomaly or a dilated tricuspid valve annulus with severe tricuspid regurgitation.[10,25]

The *pulmonary valve* may be well formed with definable but fused commissures, however, in most cases, the *ventriculoarterial junction* is fibrous. Some argue that this fibrous remnant is pulmonary valvar tissue and others presume it to be imperforate fibrous tissue overlying muscular infundibular atresia.

The *pulmonary arteries* (PA) nearly always branch normally and are of normal size with significant hypoplasia present in only about 6% of cases.[10] The *ductus arteriosus* is almost always present.

Left heart abnormalities have not received proper attention until recently; however, a number of these abnormalities have now been characterized.[4] The *left atrium* is enlarged and the *left ventricle* (LV) shows varying degrees of hypertrophy and sometimes manifests endocardial fibroelastosis. Ventricular myocardial ischemia of varying degrees is often seen.[31,32] Subaortic obstruction due to abnormal positioning of the hypertrophied ventricular septum bulging into the left ventricle has been identified, presumably related to the RV hypertension.[33]

NATURAL HISTORY

Pulmonary atresia with intact septum is a lesion with dismal prognosis if untreated. Within 2 wk of birth, 50% of patients die and by 6 mo of age 85% succumb.[34] The most common mode of death is severe metabolic acidosis from hypoxia resulting from ductal closure. Rarely patients with an alternate source of pulmonary bloodflow or in whom the ductus stays open have survived to the second or third decade of life.[35,36]

With the advent of fetal echocardiography the in utero natural history can be closely followed. Cases have now been documented in which forward flow across the pulmonary valve has been observed, but on serial fetal studies and at birth, pulmonary atresia is present.[37,38] This supports the concept that PA.IVS is, at least in some cases, not a lesion of primary morphogenesis. Fetuses with small hypertrophied right ventricles are not usually compromised during fetal life. The incidence of a dilated right ventricle plus severe tricuspid regurgitation appears to be more common in fetal life than in the neonatal period.[39] With severe tricuspid regurgitation and a dilated right ventricle, fetal hydrops can result causing fetal demise. This natural selection during fetal life reduces the incidence of this variant seen at birth. Fetal intervention has the potential to salvage these cases.

PATHOPHYSIOLOGY

Once pulmonary atresia develops in the fetus the stage is set for abnormal hemodynamics and altered fetal circulation. Having no forward egress across the outflow tract, blood in the right ventricle may be ejected across the tricuspid valve or the right ventricle may develop an isovolumic contraction with no forward ejection. If significant tricuspid regurgitation develops, the right ventricular pressure remains low and sinusoids and coronary fistulae do not develop. In cases of very severe tricuspid regurgitation the right ventricle may dilate. If the tricuspid regurgitation is mild or absent, the right ventricle remains small and hypertrophies, and right ventricular systolic hypertension develops. If this process develops early enough in gestation, myocardial sinusoids and coronary fistulae may develop. Since there is very little antegrade flow across the tricuspid valve in this case the valve may become hypoplastic. In all instances of PA.IVS the venous return has to cross the foramen ovale into the left side of the heart to reach the systemic circulation and the placenta. This relative volume overload on the left ventricle results in some degree of hypertrophy and dilatation. Also the aortic root may enlarge. The severity of the atresia (membranous or long segment) and the development of the secondary consequences (RV hypoplasia, coronary sinusoids, etc.) are probably dependent upon the gestational age at which the primary lesion (pulmonary atresia) develops. In theory, fetal intervention to correct the primary lesion would correct the abnormal hemodynamics, thereby, preventing or minimizing the secondary morphologic consequences.

The infant born with PA.IVS is compromised physiologically almost immediately. The atretic pulmonary valve causes an obligatory dependance on patency of the ductus arteriosus for pulmonary bloodflow. Closure of the ductus arteriosus results in profound hypoxia; therefore, resuscitation with prostaglandin E_1 (PGE$_1$) is critical within hours to days of birth. Assuming ductal patency, these infants usually maintain adequate cardiac output because the left sided structures are relatively normal. However, septal hypertrophy causing left ventricular outflow tract obstruction and left ventricular myocardial ischemia secondary to coronary fistulae can compromise function. Complete mixing of oxygenated and unoxygenated blood occurs, since most of the

systemic venous return must cross the atrial septal defect to enter the left atrium. The left ventricle is volume loaded since it must maintain a full normal systemic cardiac output, as well as the equivalent of one to three additional outputs to the lungs via the patent ductus arteriosus. The volume load will depend on the size of the ductus itself and the pulmonary vascular to systemic vascular resistance ratio.

Systemic oxygen saturation is usually mildly to moderately depressed, depending on pulmonary blood flow, ranging from 70 to 95%. Systemic arterial blood pressure usually shows a somewhat widened pulse pressure, secondary to runoff through the ductus arteriosus into the pulmonary circuit. Right ventricular pressure is typically systemic or suprasystemic in the small hypoplastic right ventricle, but may be lower in a completely decompensated dilated right ventricle with profound tricuspid regurgitation.[34]

The pathophysiology of coronary bloodflow can be a critical issue in patients who have right ventricular to coronary artery fistulae. In the most severe case of a completely right ventricular-dependent coronary blood supply, i.e., absence of antegrade aortocoronary flow, the myocardium is supplied by desaturated blood at systemic to suprasystemic systolic pressures and relatively low diastolic pressures. These physiologic alterations clearly reduce coronary reserve since it is well-established that under normal conditions myocardial bloodflow occurs primarily in diastole and myocardial oxygen extraction is almost maximal. The extremely marginal coronary reserve in these patients can be easily compromised if right ventricular systolic pressure is reduced by any means (relief of right ventricular outflow tract obstruction, balloon disruption of tricuspid valve, significant hypovolemia). This can result in irreversible left ventricular myocardial ischemia. Varying configurations of coronary fistulae and proximal coronary stenoses may result in lesser degrees of myocardial dependence on right ventricle to coronary bloodflow, with important, but less severe consequences if right ventricular pressure is reduced.

Tricuspid valve dysfunction is common, with some degree of valve insufficiency present in most cases. The insufficiency may be moderate or severe, its extent being correlated directly with right ventricular cavity size and inversely with right ventricular pressure.[10] The etiology of tricuspid regurgitation is partly physiologic, i.e., secondary to right ventricular outflow tract obstruction (RVOTO), and partly morphologic since about one-third of patients with this lesion have morphologic abnormalities.[13]

CLINICAL FEATURES, DIAGNOSIS, AND INDICATIONS FOR SURGERY

The majority (over 90%) of patients with PA.IVS present in the first 3 days of life.[10] Moderate cyanosis and a systolic murmur of ductal flow are evident on physical examination of the neonate. In infants with severe tricuspid regurgitation an additional systolic murmur may be present. The second heart sound is single. As the ductus arteriosus constricts, cyanosis becomes more marked. The electrocardiogram will usually lack the typical dominant right ventricular forces found in the neonate. A prominent P wave may be present indicating right atrial enlargement. Chest radiography will show a normal cardiac silhouette unless severe tricuspid regurgitation and right atrial and ventricular enlargement are present. Pulmonary vascular markings are diminished or normal but may be variable, depending on the degree of ductal patency.

A definitive and detailed diagnosis is usually made by echocardiography. Morphologic details of the right ventricular outflow tract (RVOT), right ventricular cavity, tricuspid valve, atrial septum, and the patency of ductus arteriosus can be evaluated thoroughly and accurately. Tricuspid regurgitation, right to left atrial flow, and ductal flow can be assessed. Echocardiography can also document coronary artery fistulae[40,41] and give a reliable estimate of right ventricular pressure derived from the tricuspid regurgitation flow velocity. Ventricular function and regional wall motion can also be evaluated. However, right ventricular dependency of coronary bloodflow cannot be reliably assessed by echocardiography. Echocardiography is the only technique currently capable of diagnosing PA.IVS in utero accurately (Fig. 79–4A and B).

Cardiac catheterization and angiography are recommended in essentially all cases, primarily to define the coronary anatomy, specifically, major stenoses and fistulae. By a combination of aortic root and right ventricular injections, the extent of right ventricular dependency of the coronary circulation can be accurately estimated (Fig. 79–3A and B). This is of utmost importance in initiating an appropriate surgical plan of management.

Surgical intervention within the neonatal period is indicated in all cases of PA.IVS immediately following diagnosis, based on the natural history of this lesion.

MANAGEMENT

Historical Perspective and Overview

Surgical therapy by PA.IVS began in the early 1960s. In 1967 a review of literature by Gersony et al,[42] revealed that only 2.5% of patients with PA.IVS were alive at 3 years of age. In the early reports palliative shunts or closed pulmonary valvotomies were performed. Bowman et al in 1971[43] and later Trusler and colleagues in 1976[44] described the combination of a right ventricular outflow tract procedure with a systemic to pulmonary artery shunt. This approach, combined with many other reports[15,45–63] recognizing the right ventricular and coronary arterial variations in this lesion, represent important contributions that have led to the present concept of morphology-specific management of this lesion in the neonatal period. In spite of this recognition, a consensus regarding the specifics of initial manage-

ment has not emerged. This is because individual institutional experiences generally are small and vary widely in terms of the morphologic spectrum encountered and the surgical procedures performed. These factors contribute both to institutional/physician bias in choosing the initial operative procedure and to variable outcomes.

Numerous approaches have been suggested, however, none of these have been universally accepted. Steinberger et al[61] pursued an aggressive decompression of the right ventricular outflow tract in the neonatal period using outflow tract patches. Realizing the need for an additional source of blood flow in the immediate postoperative period they have maintained ductal patency by PGE_1 infusion for an average of 6 days, but occassionally up to 3 weeks. They reported an 80% success rate in achieving a biventricular repair regardless of the initial RV morphology. Following a similar strategy McCaffrey et al[57] reported failure of the outflow tract patch approach in patients with tricuspid valve diameter measuring less than 0.75 cm and with tricuspid valve/mitral valve ratio less than 0.7. As described above some have followed the strategy of adding a systemic to pulmonary artery shunt at the time of outflow tract patch procedure in the neonatal period.[10] One disadvantage of this approach is that it requires an additional intervention to close the shunt later. This must be weighed against the risks, costs, and benefits of continuing PGE_1 for prolonged periods of time.

Still others have performed pulmonary valvotomy (closed/open) and some form of systemic to pulmonary artery shunt (Blalock–Taussig/central) with success in achieving biventricular repair.[46,52,53,59,60,64] Shaddy et al[60] have applied this strategy to patients with a patent infundibulum regardless of the tricuspid valve size. They reported 91% of their patients either had or were awaiting a biventricular repair. Pawade et al,[64] using a similar strategy, reported the actuarial probability of achieving a biventricular repair as 60% at 40 months. Likewise Hawkins et al[53] accomplished biventricular in about 60% of their patients. Some others have performed pulmonary valvotomy alone as the initial procedure, using various indices of adequacy of the right ventricle and tricuspid valve to guide this choice.[46,52,54,59,65]

In patients with complete dependency of the myocardial blood supply on the RV, there is a consensus to avoid RV decompression and to perform a shunt alone as the initial procedure.[10,66] However, there is no consensus in patients with lesser degree of RV dependency. At what level of RV dependency it is safe to decompress the RVOT has not been determined with certainty, although recommendations have been made.[66] With lesser degrees of RV dependency, regional wall motion abnormalities of the LV have been documented to increase after RV decompression.[67,68] A number of other suggestions appear in the literature for managing the very small hypertensive RV, including tricuspid valve excision or balloon disruption, closure of the tricuspid valve, and thrombo-occlusion of the RV.[53,56,69,70]

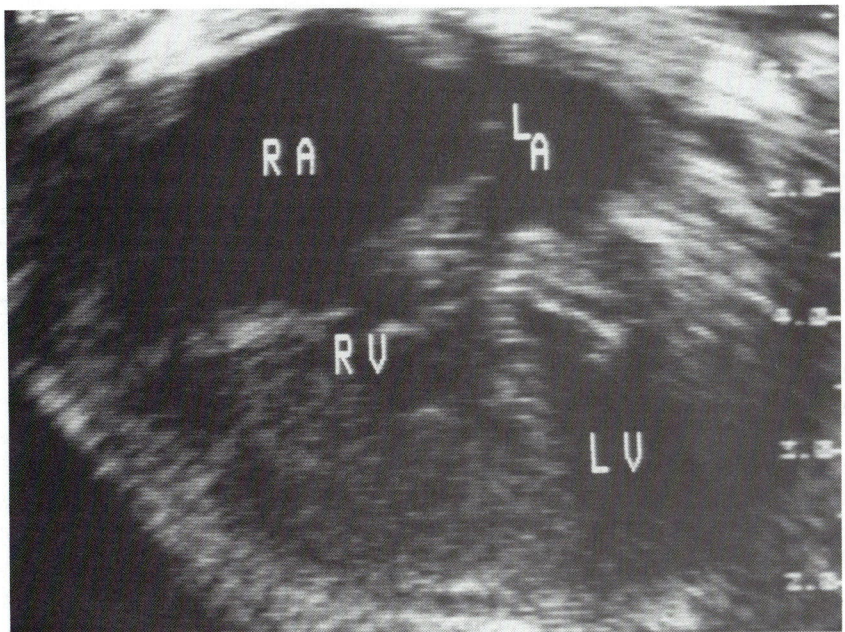

A

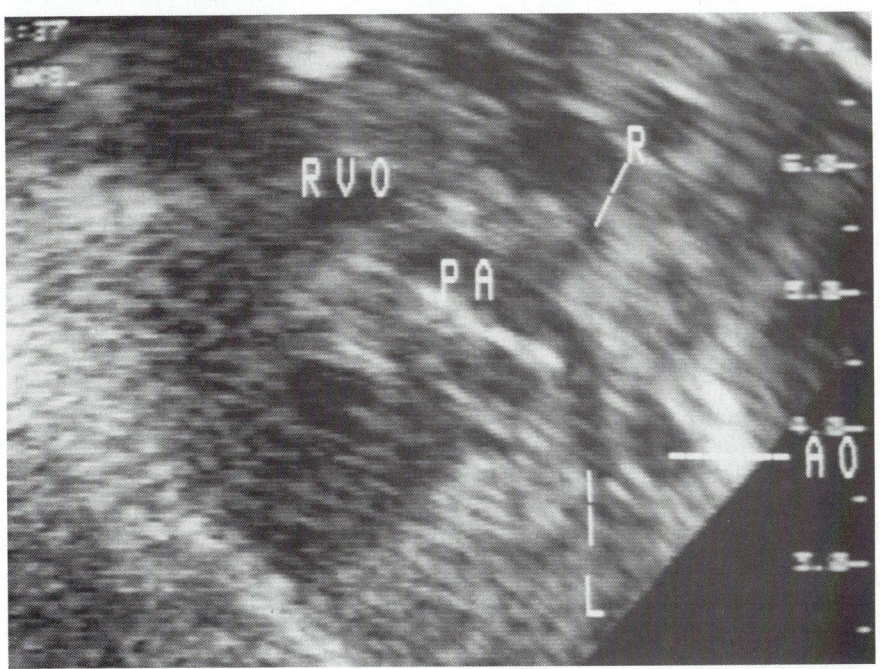

B

Figure 79–4. Echocardiogram of 24-week-old fetus. **A.** Note the severely hypertrophied right ventricle. LA, left atrium; LV, left ventricle; RA, right atrium; RV, right ventricle. **B.** Note the atretic segment between the right ventricle and the pulmonary artery. RVO, right ventricular outflow; PA, main pulmonary artery; R, right pulmonary artery; L, left pulmonary artery.

The subsequent surgical management of PA.IVS is also complex. It is generally accepted that a two ventricle circulation with completely separated pulmonary and systemic circuits is ideal. But it is also realized that some patients can never achieve this. There has been a distinct evolution of thought away from the position that all patients should have as their definitive physiology either a complete two ventricle circulation or a Fontan circulation. The interatrial communication (ASD or PFO) is generally not closed during initial surgical management. If at a later evaluation the right ventricle is deemed adequate, the interatrial communication is closed (if still patent) and any other source of pulmonary bloodflow, i.e., shunt or ductus arteriosus is removed. On the other hand if the RV is inadequate to sustain the entire cardiac output, rather than opting for a Fontan procedure in all cases, some degree of mixing is accepted at the atrial level while still utilizing the RV to pump blood into the lungs. The ASD may be left open, or a surgically adjustable ASD may be created.[71] In other cases, creation of a bidirectional superior cavopulmonary shunt that results in a reduced preload on the right ventricle has been used with success by some.[72,73] This procedure is appealing in the case of an inadequate RV because the interatrial communication may then be closed allowing the circulations to be separated completely. In patients with severely hypoplastic RVs, some modification of the Fontan procedure is considered definitive.[10,50,64,72] Cardiac transplantation is a last resort procedure, generally reserved for patients with associated left heart compromise.

Current Recommendations

Preoperative Management

If the diagnosis is made shortly following birth, it is likely that unrestricted ductal patency will be present. Initiation of therapy with PGE_1 to maintain ductal patency will usually ensure preoperative stability; however, mechanical ventilation and inotropic support may be required in about one-third of patients. If the diagnosis is delayed, profound cyanosis secondary to ductal constriction may be the mode of patient presentation. In this case aggressive resuscitation with PGE_1, sodium bicarbonate, inotropic support, and mechanical ventilation may be necessary. Following stabilization, arterial oxygen saturations over 90% suggest excessive pulmonary bloodflow. Ventilation and inspired oxygen should be reduced, and inspired CO_2 may be used accordingly to prevent pulmonary edema and systemic acidosis. Patients should be adequately stabilized whenever possible and thoroughly evaluated before performing the initial surgical procedure.

Initial Surgical Management

In an effort to overcome the anecdotal nature of most reports, inconsistencies in morphologic characterization, individual institutional bias, and selection variability, a prospective multicenter study involving over 40 centers was initiated by the Congenital Heart Surgeon's Society (CHSS) in 1987. This study focused on defining the complete morphologic spectrum of and the optimal management approaches to PA.IVS in the neonatal period. In the initial report from the CHSS 171 neonates seen between 1987 and 1991 were evaluated.[10] The spectrum of morphologic findings is summarized in Table 79–1. Many of these important morphologic findings have been discussed in the morphology section. Overall survival in this study was 81% at 1 mo and 64% at 4 years. Numerous initial procedures were performed in these 171 patients; however, these procedures can be categorized into three general types: relief of RVOTO alone, relief of RVOTO plus a systemic to PA shunt, and systemic to PA shunt alone. An extensive multivariable analysis was performed to identify morphology-specific, procedure-specific, and experience-specific risk factors for death. This analysis showed small diameter of tricuspid valve and marked right ventricular coronary artery dependency to be important morphologic risk factors for

death. It should be remembered that the size of the TV correlated closely with the size of the RV cavity, therefore TV can be considered a measure of RV size. A smaller tricuspid valve was an important risk factor only when the initial operative procedure included some form of RVOTO relief, either a valvotomy or a transannular patch, but not when it was a shunt alone. In other words, if a shunt alone was performed the size of the TV (RV) did not effect survival. Figure 79–5 shows these important relationships among the types of initial procedures, the size of tricuspid valve, and survival.

It should be emphasized that the CHSS study is an ongoing project. In a more recent interim analysis of the CHSS data performed in 1993, the patient population has increased to 306 and 2 years further follow-up was available.[74] This analysis (Fig. 79–6) identified some important changes. Although the general relationships shown in Figure 79–5 are still valid, many patients who had undergone an RVOT procedure plus a concomitant shunt were doing more poorly than anticipated. As a result, the present recommendations (see below) have narrowed the morphologic spectrum for which an RVOT procedure plus shunt is the initial operation of choice.

In the original CHSS report a number of issues other than risk-adjusted survival were examined.[10] One of these was the need for a second but nondefinitive procedure following the initial procedure. Subsequent procedures were required in 51% of these 171 patients. These procedures fell into two categories. One category involved only patients whose initial RVOT procedure had been a pulmonary valvotomy. A subsequent outflow tract patch was needed in 55% of these patients, in some as late as 3 years following the initial operation (Fig. 79–7). The other category involved patients whose initial procedure did not include a shunt. Over half of them required a shunt within a month of the initial procedure (Fig. 79–8). This suggests that the majority of patients with PA.IVS will not be able to avoid, either initially or subsequently, both a shunt and a transannular patch. These findings are at variance with many of the historical studies reviewed in the overview portion of this section. The unselected nature of the population and large number of patients in the CHSS study argue convincingly for the validity of this study.

Recommendations for Choosing the Initial Procedure. Based on the CHSS data, recommendations were made for choosing the initial surgical procedure for PA.IVS. It should be emphasized that the data from the CHSS study continue to evolve, as underscored by the 1993 interim analysis[74] mentioned above. Recommendations for management will likely evolve as well.

The ideal outcome for a patient with pulmonary atresia with intact ventricular septum is a completely separated in series two ventricle circulation. The central issue in achieving this is whether the right ventricle can function as the sole provider of pulmonary bloodflow at normal filling

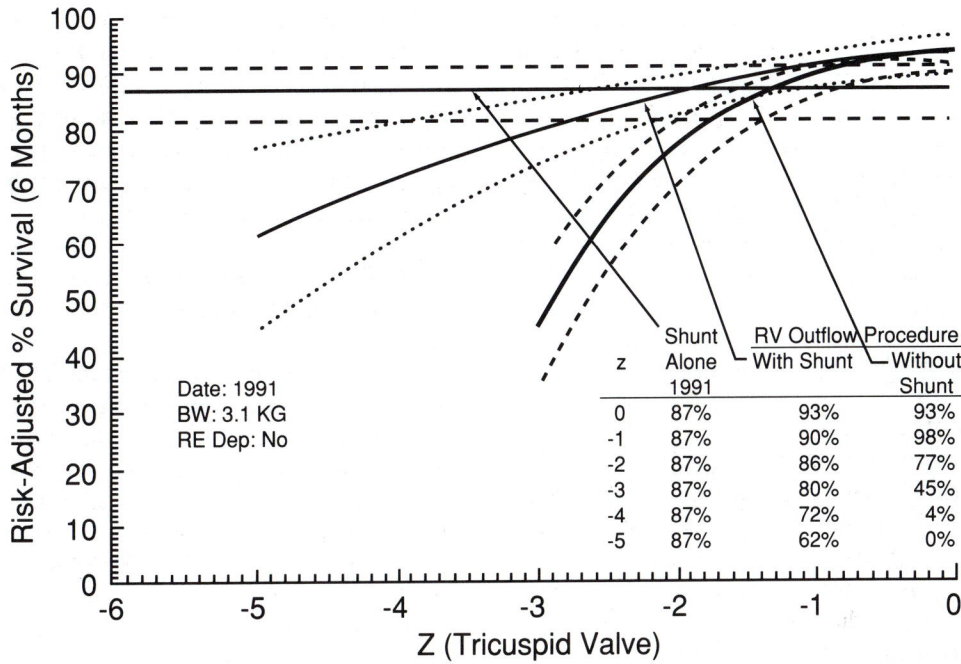

Figure 79–5. The effect of the diameter (*Z*-value) of the tricuspid valve and the type of initial procedure on survival in neonates with pulmonary atresia with intact ventricular septum. The phrase "right ventricular outflow procedure" includes both valvotomy and transannular patching. *(From Hanely FL, et al: Outcomes in neonatal pulmonary atresia with intact ventricular septum: A multiinstitutional study. J Thorac Cardiovasc Surg 105:406–427, 1993. Reproduced with permission.)*

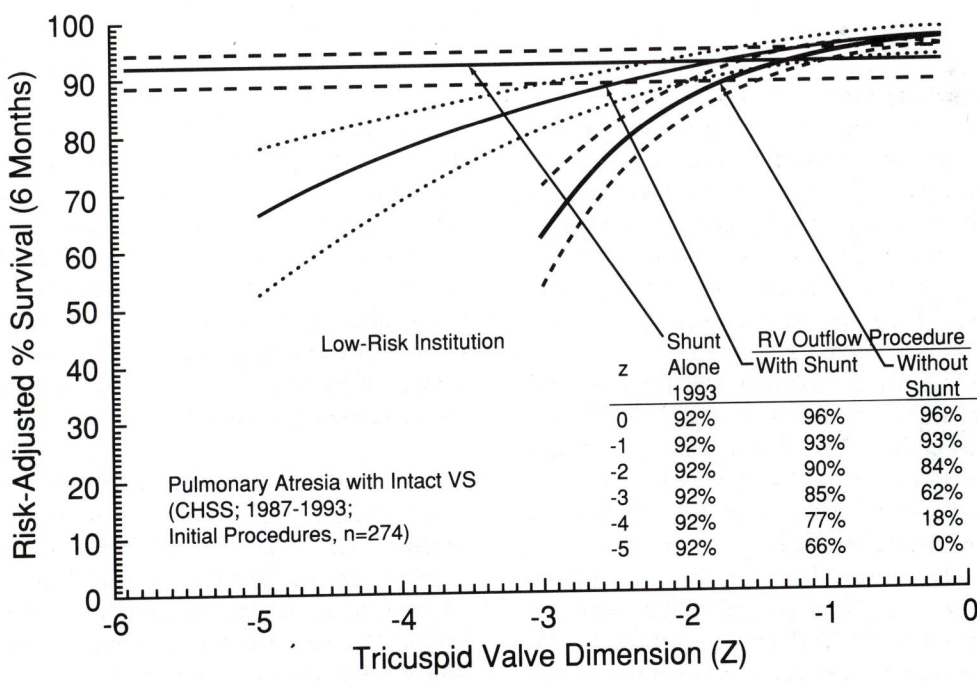

Figure 79–6. The effect of the diameter (*Z*-value) of the tricuspid valve and the type of initial procedure on survival in neonates with pulmonary atresia with intact ventricular septum. The phrase "right ventricular outflow procedure" includes both valvotomy and transannular patching. The confidence limits of RV outflow procedure and shunt alone stop overlapping at a *Z*-value of –3. Note the difference when compared the similar graph in Figure 79–5 where the confidence limits stop overlapping at a *Z*-value of –4. *(From Kirklin JW and the Congenital Heart Surgeons Society: Unpublished observations. Reproduced with permission.)*

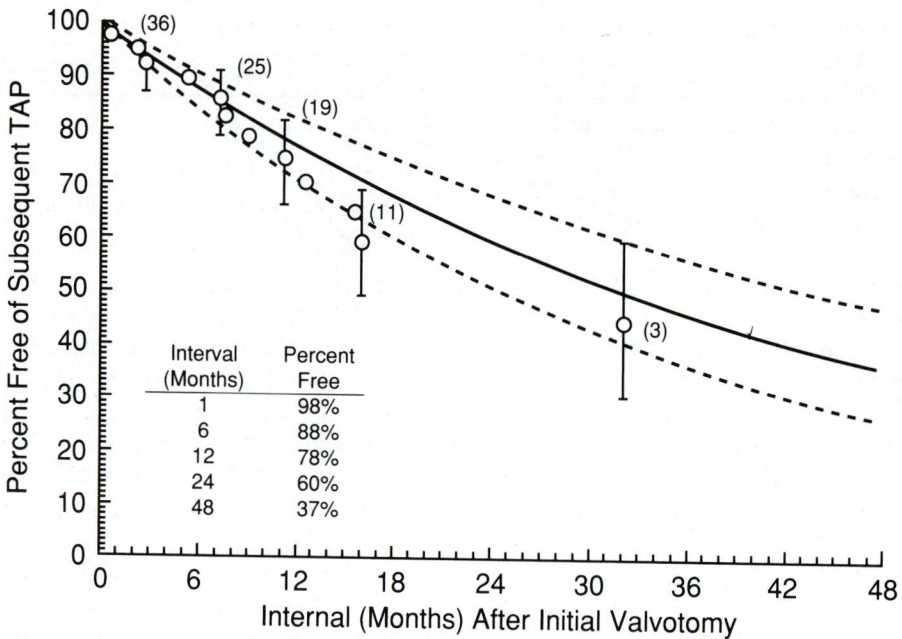

Figure 79–7. Freedom from a transannular patch as a subsequent procedure after initial pulmonary valvotomy (with or without shunt) in 46 patients who did not have Ebstein's malformation and/or right ventricular cavity size greater than normal. Multivariable anaylsis did not reveal any risk factors for this event. *(From Hanley FL, et al: Outcomes in neonatal pulmonary atresia with intact ventricular septum: A multiinstitutional study. J Thorac Cardiovasc Surg 105:406–427, 1993. Reproduced with permission.)*

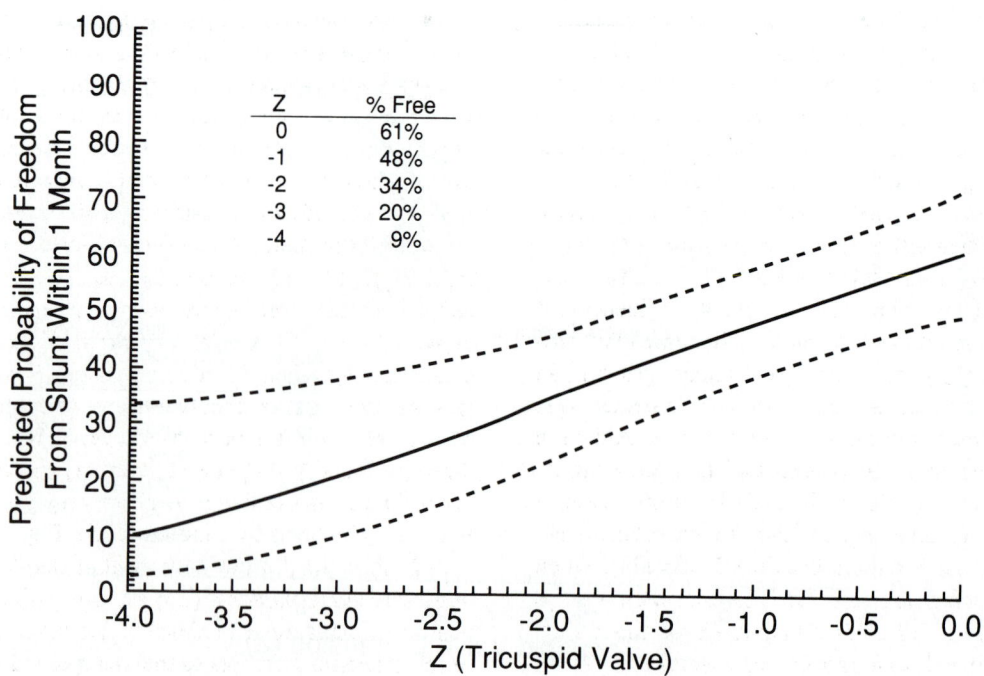

Figure 79–8. The probability of being free of a subsequent shunt procedure after an initial pulmonary valvotomy, or placement of a transannular patch without a concomitant shunt. Diameter (*Z*-value) of the tricuspid valve was the only risk factor identified (*p* = 0.04). All shunt procedures were performed in the first month after the initial procedure. *(From Hanley FL, et al: Outcomes in neonatal pulmonary atresia with intact ventricular septum: A multiinstitutional study. J Thorac Cardiovasc Surg 105:406–427, 1993. Reproduced with permission.)*

pressures. Before discussing the recommended approach to the neonate with PA.IVS, a clear appreciation of the goals of initial surgical therapy should exist. The primary goal is to minimize mortality. The second goal should be to promote growth of the right ventricle, thereby optimizing the chances of a two ventricle circulation. The final goal should be to minimize the need for nondefinitive subsequent surgical procedures.

Although these goals are intuitively sensible, there are several hidden assumptions that should be clarified. Data from the CHSS suggest that survival after a systemic to pulmonary shunt alone is equal to or better than any other initial procedure, regardless of right ventricular morphologic variation (Figs. 79–5 and 79–6).[10] Therefore, if low mortality alone is the goal, then shunt alone can be viewed as the initial procedure of choice in all patients of PA.IVS. However, if the right ventricle is not decompressed, it will not grow. The result is an intractably small right ventricle. Therefore, shunt alone is likely to commit many patients unnecessarily to one ventricle repairs. There is a substantial amount of evidence to support this position. Right ventricular growth has been documented with procedures that relieve the outflow tract obstruction especially when these are performed as the initial procedure in the neonatal period.[29,61,75–82] Late decompression or no decompression is not attended by right ventricular growth, thereby compromising the chances of a two ventricle circulation. Although definitive proof is lacking that early relief of pulmonary atresia will convert patients with an inadequate RV to patients with RVs that will ultimately support the entire circulation in all cases, a review of the literature indicates that this process does occur in a significant number of cases. Therefore, there is a generally recognized incentive for relieving the RVOTO, if such a procedure is deemed safe.

The fact remains that at birth the ultimate functional potential of the right ventricle in many of these patients is unclear. Therefore, the specific morphology of the right ventricle may influence the surgeon to consider an individual patient as able (or unable) to eventually have a two ventricle circulation. This perception may then influence the choice of the initial procedure, which, in turn, may profoundly influence further right ventricular growth. In essence, the initial procedure that is chosen (whether right or wrong) may determine the ultimate outcome. Although this uncertainty regarding the potential of the right ventricle cannot be removed completely in each individual case, a logical approach to each patient can be undertaken. No clear guidelines exist at the present time for deciding when a neonatal right ventricle is too small to have the potential to ultimately carry a full cardiac output. Given this uncertainty, it seems logical to approach each individual patient with an initial procedure, which is most likely to promote an ultimate two ventricle repair, as long as this approach does not expose the patient to increased mortality.

The following morphology-specific treatment guidelines seem to give the best chances of fulfilling the three goals mentioned above. These guidelines are based on the more recent interim analysis (Fig. 79–6) of the data from the CHSS study.[74] In general, surgical treatment will involve one of the following:

1. Relief of RVOTO: valvotomy or transannular patch.
2. Creation of a systemic to pulmonary artery shunt.
3. Relief of RVOTO plus shunt.

The choice of procedure would be based on the morphology of the right heart and the coronary circulation (Fig. 79–9):

1. *In a small subset of patients where the tricuspid valve diameter ($Z = 0$ to -2) and right ventricular cavity approach normal size*, it may be ideal to perform a right ventricular outflow tract procedure alone. There is no increased mortality (Fig. 79–6) and the establishment of right ventricular forward flow will encourage growth of the tricuspid valve and right ventricle. The need for a subsequent shunt in this setting is relatively low (Fig. 79–8).[10] The options for the right ventricular outflow tract procedure itself are either a pulmonary valvotomy or a transannular patch. Ideally, the procedure should be a pulmonary valvotomy; however, this choice is likely to increase the need for a subsequent transannular patch (Fig. 79–7).[10] It seems logical, but nevertheless speculative, that morphologic features of the atresia itself, i.e., presence of muscular obstruction, thickness and pliability of the atretic valve tissue, and annular dimensions of the atretic valve, will influence the need for a subsequent transannular patch. If in the future it is possible to predict which patients are more likely to need a subsequent outflow tract patch, the decision making will be easier. Additionally, the technique used for the valvotomy may be important. On the other hand, an initial transannular patch alone will establish forward flow as effectively as a valvotomy, and may reduce the need for a subsequent right ventricular outflow tract procedure. It seems logical but, again, speculative, that the accompanying pulmonary insufficiency may cause increased right ventricular failure, increased right-to-left atrial shunting, cyanosis, and, therefore, an increased likelihood for the need for a subsequent shunt. Whether valvotomy alone or transannular patch alone is chosen as the initial procedure, careful ongoing evaluation is critical. If valvotomy alone is performed, further relief of right ventricular outflow tract obstruction may be necessary over the next several years. With either procedure, profound postoperative cyanosis indicates the need for a shunt. This is likely to be necessary in slightly less than half of patients by 1 month of life (Fig. 79–8).

2. *For the patient with mild to moderate tricuspid valve annular hypoplasia ($Z = -2$ to -3)*, the goal of a two ventricle circulation is achievable. However, the likelihood of this outcome decreases as the tricuspid valve annular size decreases. For this morphologic subset, the risk of death is similar for shunt alone and right ventricular outflow tract procedure with a concomitant shunt (Fig. 79–6). The right ventricular outflow tract procedure with concomitant shunt is favored, however, for several reasons. This procedure

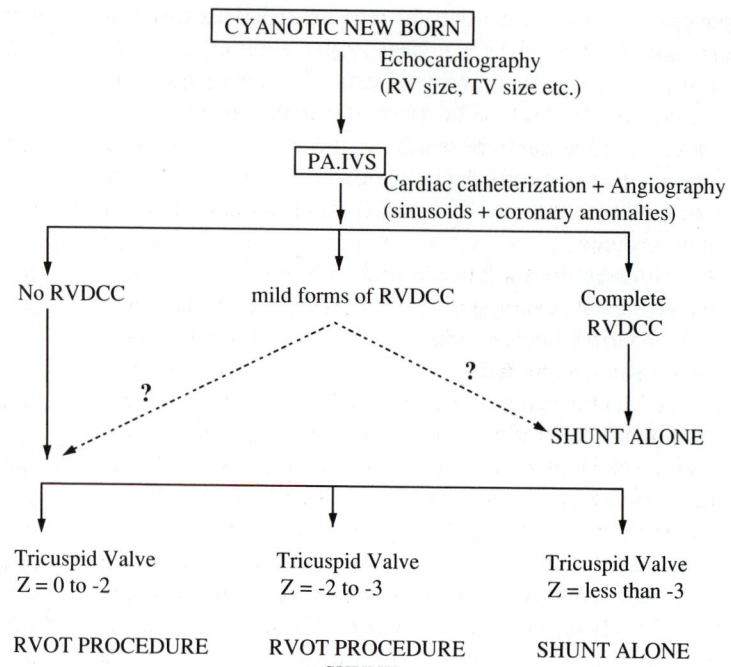

Figure 79–9. Morphology-based scheme of initial management of neonates with pulmonary atresia with intact ventricular septum.

promotes forward flow and encourages right ventricular growth, and it has the lowest risk of requiring subsequent procedures.[10] The right ventricular outflow tract part of the procedure may be either a valvotomy or a transannular patch; however, a transannular patch is less likely to require subsequent right ventricular outflow tract procedures, for the reasons previously mentioned above in (1). On the other hand, a transannular patch will cause insufficiency and this may result in unfavorable physiology in the presence of a shunt. Retrograde shunt flow across the patch and across the regurgitant tricuspid valve into the RV has been observed.

3. *For the subset of patients with severe tricuspid valve annular hypoplasia (Z = −3 or less),* the preferred procedure is a shunt alone. Mortality is lower than for any of the procedures that include relief of the right ventricular outflow obstruction (Fig. 79–6). In addition, the incentive for establishing forward flow across the right ventricular outflow tract is markedly diminished, because an ultimate two ventricle repair is quite unlikely in this subset. In the CHSS study, no patient with a tricuspid valve annulus size less than three standard deviations below normal (Z = ≤−3) has achieved a two ventricle repair.[10] Additionally, the likelihood of right ventricular-dependent coronary circulation or extensive right ventricular to coronary artery fistulae is quite high in this patient subset with severely hypoplastic tricuspid valves,[10,74] a finding that contraindicates right ventricular decompression.

4. *Any patient with right ventricular-dependent coronary circulation to a large segment of ventricular myocardium* should undergo shunt alone, regardless of the size of the right ventricle or tricuspid valve. The survival fol-

lowing shunt alone has improved in this high risk patient group, with a 70% survival at 6 months.[10] Since right ventricular-dependent coronary circulation correlates closely with small tricuspid valve and right ventricular size, the decision to perform a shunt alone will usually be made on the basis of the tricuspid valve hypoplasia itself. However, in the unusual case in which a right ventricular-dependent coronary circulation is present with a larger right ventricle, a right ventricular outflow tract procedure is still contraindicated. Decompression of the right ventricle under these circumstances will most likely result in severe myocardial ischemia. It must be emphasized that varying degrees of right ventricular-dependent coronary circulation exist, ranging from complete dependence with absence of antegrade aortocoronary flow, across a spectrum of combinations of coronary artery stenoses with fistulae, to fistulae alone without proximal coronary stenoses. Again, it seems logical, although speculative, that ventricular compromise, and, therefore, outcome, will correlate closely with the amount of myocardium at risk if right ventricular pressure is lowered by an outflow tract procedure.

Subsequent Management

Close follow-up is indicated in all patients irrespective of the initial procedure.

1. *Patients who received a shunt alone* and are expected to ultimately undergo a single ventricle repair should have a follow-up catheterization within 3 to 6 mo, with the plan of initiating the process of separating the two circulations. Subsequent systemic to pulmonary artery shunts should be avoided if at all possible. Depending on the hemodynamics at this evaluation, a bidirectional superior

cavopulmonary shunt (i.e., bidirectional Glenn anastomosis) may be performed between 3 and 12 mo of age. Between 1 and 4 years of age, consideration should be given to converting this to one of the modifications of the Fontan procedure. In patients who have extensive coronary artery fistulae or right ventricular-dependent coronary circulation, the modification of the Fontan procedure should involve a total cavopulmonary reconstruction, such that oxygenated blood is delivered to the right ventricle and coronary fistulae, and the coronary sinus is drained to the low-pressure atrial chamber, thereby maximizing coronary perfusion and myocardial oxygen delivery.

2. *Patients with a shunt plus RVOT procedure as the initial procedure* should have follow-up catheterization and echocardiography at 3 to 6 mo of age to evaluate the differential growth of the right ventricle and tricuspid valve. If these structures are judged to be adequate for a two ventricle repair, then temporary closure of the shunt should be performed in the catheterization laboratory at about 6 mo of age. If systemic oxygen saturation remains adequate, the shunt should be closed permanently, either with coils in the catheterization laboratory or in the operation room. At the same time, the interatrial communication should also be temporarily occluded, and hemodynamics evaluated by measuring the increase in right atrial pressure and the decrease in mixed venous oxygen saturation and mean systemic arterial pressure. If these values are acceptable, the atrial septum should be also closed. An alternative approach would be to evaluate the possibility of device closure of the interatrial communication at a subsequent catheterization, approximately 6 mo after closure of the systemic to pulmonary artery shunt.

In patients where there has been little or no growth of the right ventricle at follow-up, despite an initial right ventricular outflow tract procedure, intractable hypoplasia of the right heart may be present, and a single ventricle repair plan should be undertaken, as described above.

In cases of borderline adequacy of the right ventricle at follow-up, reevaluation with a subsequent catheterization and echocardiography should be done at about 1 year of age. If the right ventricle still appears to be borderline at this stage, there are still a number of options. Follow-up may be continued to evaluate for a possible two ventricle repair in the future or the patient may be committed to a single ventricle repair. Alternatively, at this time a definitive "one and a half ventricle repair" may be performed, which involves creation of a superior cavopulmonary shunt, takedown of the systemic to pulmonary artery shunt, and closure of the atrial septal defect, thereby achieving permanently reduced preloading of the small right ventricle by inferior vena caval blood only. Another alternative is to leave the patient with a right to left atrial shunt, allowing the RV to pump less than a full cardiac output to the pulmonary circuit.

3. *In patients with tricuspid valve annular sizes that approach normal and who have received only an outflow tract procedure* the follow-up is similar to the group who initially received an outflow tract procedure with concomitant shunt. It is likely, however, that a higher percentage of these patients will have a right ventricle capable of sustaining a two ventricle circulation. Some of these patients may still have a patent interatrial communication that needs to be closed.

Surgical Technique

Relief of Right Ventricular Outflow Tract Obstruction. A midline sternotomy approach is used. A patch of pericardium is harvested and treated with glutaraldehyde. Cardiopulmonary bypass is strongly recommended. This is instituted by cannulating the ascending aorta with an arterial cannula and the right atrial appendage with a single venous drainage cannula. The heart is allowed to remain beating by using a normothermic calcium supplemented blood pump prime, and allowing temperatures to drift only to approximately 32°C. At the initiation of bypass, the ductus arteriosus is dissected and ligated. In the unusual case with an adequate pulmonary annulus, a longitudinal pulmonary arteriotomy is made and the valve is inspected. Valvotomy is performed using a surgical knife to open the three identifiable commissures. The commissural incisions are extended up to the annulus. The arteriotomy is subsequently closed with a running monofilament absorbable suture. In the more usual case, inspection of the valve will reveal inadequate valve tissue and annulus. The longitudinal arteriotomy incision is extended across the annulus onto the right ventricular outflow region until a clear opening into the right ventricular cavity is established. Hypertrophied muscle bundles in the outflow tract are resected. An oval pericardial patch that was previously treated with glutaraldehyde is then tailored and sewn to the two edges of the incision, to create a right ventricular outflow tract with a diameter that is slightly smaller than normal.

Following this, the patient is rewarmed fully. A systemic to pulmonary artery shunt is then created, if one is deemed necessary, or the patient is weaned off bypass in standard fashion.

Creation of Systemic Artery to Pulmonary Artery Shunt. Regardless of whether the shunt is performed alone or as a supplement to RVOT procedure, a midline sternotomy approach for creating a modified Blalock–Taussig shunt has many advantages. A 3.0- to 4.0-mm ePTFE tube graft (size dependent on patient size) is used. In the case of a shunt procedure alone, cardiopulmonary bypass is not used. However, if a right ventricular outflow tract procedure has been performed, the patient will be on cardiopulmonary bypass at the time of creation of the shunt. In either case, the innominate artery is identified and dissected, exposing its bifurcation into the right carotid and right subclavian artery. A segment of the right subclavian artery adequate enough to place a side biting vascular clamp is exposed. Similarly the right pulmonary artery is dissected in the space between the ascending aorta and the superior vena cava. If a shunt alone is the procedure, heparin is given (1 mg/kg) intravenously. The exposed right pulmonary artery is then partially side clamped, and the PTFE tube graft is anastomosed end-to-side to a longitudinal incision on the cephalad aspect of the right pulmonary artery, with 7-0 Gore-Tex suture material using a continuous suture technique. The length and bevel of the graft are then tailored to reach the under surface of the right subclavian artery. The graft is then anastomosed end-to-side to a longitudinal incision on the caudad aspect of the right subclavian artery using the same suture and technique as before. In the case of a shunt alone procedure, following establishment of flow through the shunt, oxygen saturations and hemodynamics are monitored carefully to assess the adequacy of the shunt. The ductus arteriosus is permanently ligated once adequate shunt flow is demonstrated. In the case of a shunt that accompanies a right ventricular outflow tract procedure, once the patient is fully rewarmed on bypass, shunt flow is established and the patient is weaned from cardiopulmonary bypass.

FUTURE DIRECTIONS: FETAL INTERVENTION FOR PA.IVS

In considering fetal intervention for congenital heart defects three essential criteria should be fulfilled: (1) ability to diagnose the defects accurately in utero, (2) potential benefit of correcting the lesion in utero as opposed to neonatal correction (otherwise there would be little reason for fetal intervention), and (3) ability to safely perform the surgical procedure in utero. Fetal echocardiography can accurately diagnose many congenital heart defects between 12 and 18 wk of gestation.[39,83] The potential benefit of correcting some heart defects in utero can be convincingly argued, based on their in utero pathogenesis and relatively poor outcome following neonatal intervention. According to the flow-related theory of cardiac development,[84] a relatively simple primary defect that occurs during primary morphogenesis may lead, in the developing heart, to altered pressure and flow patterns, which then gradually induce secondary hypoplasia or maldevelopment of major cardiac structures such as heart chambers or great vessels. For example, in PA.IVS many of the important morphologic abnormalities including hypoplasia of the right ventricle and tricuspid valve, ventricular hypertrophy, myocardial sinusoids, and coronary abnormalities develop secondary to the primary lesion of right ventricular outflow tract atresia. As cited earlier in this chapter, relief of outflow tract obstruction, especially in the neonatal period (when there is still potential for myocyte hyperplasia), allows for the growth of the hypoplastic right ventricle. The earlier this is achieved the greater is the benefit. If this concept is extrapolated to fetal life, it is logical to assume that with fetal relief of right ventricular outflow tract obstruction, the secondary morphologic consequences could be minimized, prevented, or even allowed to regress. Similar arguments based on flow-related theory of cardiac development can be used for other lesions as well, as outlined in Table 79–2.

Having established that fetal diagnosis is possible, and that fetal intervention is potentially beneficial, it is necessary to focus on the last criterion, i.e., ability to safely perform the necessary cardiac surgical procedure in utero. From Table 79–2 it is clear that the surgical procedures that are anticipated to be performed in the fetus are technically simple such as pulmonary valvotomy, aortic valvotomy, and atrial septectomy. Based on clinical experience with corrective surgery in premature and low-birthweight babies frequently weighing less than 1500 g, it is obvious that the limitations to fetal cardiac surgery would not likely be technical issues. This was confirmed in the early attempts at experimental cardiac surgery in the sheep fetus.[85,86] Technical issues were easily mastered, however, and it became clear that important physiologic road blocks existed based on the responses of the fetus to the stress of intervention, and to the response of the placenta to extracorporeal circulation.[87] These initial studies in experimental fetal cardiac surgery demonstrated very dramatically that the present status of fetal intervention for cardiac defects is reminiscent of the overall field of cardiac surgery in the late 1940s and early 1950s. It was obvious at that time that relatively simple and easily achieved procedures like closure of an atrial septal defect or a ventricular septal defect would have great clinical benefit. However, the major obstacle was a lack of a safe and effective method of gaining intracardiac access. Subsequent development of clinically applicable cardiopul-

TABLE 79–2. PATHOGENESIS OF CARDIAC DEFECTS IN UTERO

Primary Lesion	PA.IVS	Critical AS	TOF + APVS	Absent/Restrictive PFO
↓				
Altered flow	RVOTO	LVOTO	Free PR/absent PDA	Reduced LV inflow
↓				
Secondary lesion	Hypoplastic RV	Hypoplastic LV	Aneurysmal PAs	Hypoplastic LV/aorta
↓				
Fetal intervention	Pulmonary valvotomy	Aortic valvotomy	Ligate MPA + shunt	Atrial septectomy

TABLE 79–3. EFFECT OF FETAL CARDIAC BYPASS ON CATECHOLAMINE LEVELS IN SHEEP

Catecholamine	Normal	Prebypass (Mean ± SD)	On bypass (Mean ± SD)	Postbypass (Mean ± SD)
Epinephrine (pg/mL)	<80	21 ± 37	178 ± 128	311 ± 166
Norepinephrine (pg/mL)	750	3789 ± 1349	2138 ± 912	2229 ± 650
Vasopressin (pg/mL)	11	432 ± 179	807 ± 278	797 ± 248

monary bypass and myocardial protection techniques allowed a reliable way to achieve intracardiac access and has resulted in rapid progress in cardiac surgery. The rapid accumulation of knowledge regarding the physiologic responses of the organism to extracorporeal circulation allowed development of techniques that minimized these pathophysiologic responses and, as a result, the use of extracorporeal circulation soon became the technique of choice, quickly outperforming other ingenious but much more limited techniques for gaining intracardiac access.

At present, lack of sufficient understanding of the fetal responses to stress, intervention, and extracorporeal circulation limits clinical application of fetal cardiac intervention. Early models of fetal extracorporeal circulation suggested that progressive metabolic acidosis causing fetal death during fetal bypass might be due to depressed or redirected cardiac output.[88,89] Subsequent studies indicated that several factors are probably responsible for this. Mid to late gestation fetuses are capable of mounting an immense stress response. Catecholamine levels increase by over 50-fold during fetal exposure and during fetal bypass (Table 79–3).[87] This results in significant elevation of the total fetal vascular resistance, presenting the fetal heart with an increased afterload, which is not tolerated by the immature contractile

apparatus of the fetal myocardium. Additionally, previously used fetal anesthetics (inhalational agents given to the mother such as halothane) not only are ineffective in blunting fetal stress response but also cause myocardial depression (Fig. 79–10).[90] Total spinal anesthesia, which does not have the aforementioned detrimental effects, has been shown to improve fetal hemodynamics and placental gas exchange function before, during, and after fetal bypass.[91] Although total spinal anesthesia is very effective as a research tool, this technique of anesthesia is not practical in the human fetus. Further studies in a more appropriate primate animal model using clinically applicable anesthetics such as high dose narcotics are needed.

It was also evident from early studies of fetal bypass that placental vascular resistance rises (Fig. 79–11) and placental gas exchange function deteriorates during and after fetal bypass resulting in early fetal death from hypercarbia, acidosis, and ventricular fibrillation. Studies addressing the mechanism of this placental dysfunction have suggested that vasoactive products of the arachidonic acid cascade have an important role in this dysfunction. Using indomethacin and methylprednisolone to block the synthesis of prostaglandins, an improvement in placental function has been observed during and after bypass (Fig. 79–12).[92] Sim-

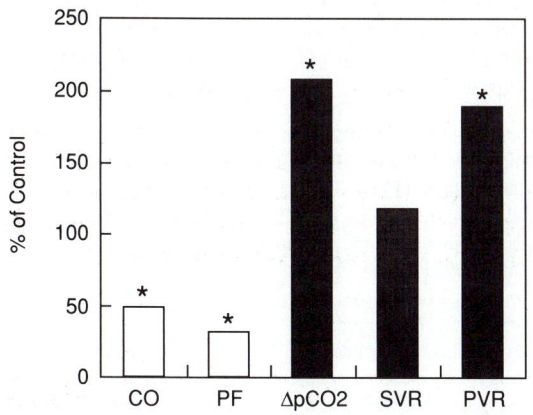

Figure 79–10. Effect of halothane anesthesia on hemodynamics and PCO_2 in fetal lambs. The normal values were taken from chronic resting fetal lamb preparations at 120 days of gestation. CO, cardiac output; PCO_2, arterial carbon dioxide tension; PF, placental bloodflow; PVR, pulmonary vascular resistance; SVR, systemic vascular resistance. *(From Hanley FL: Fetal responses to extracorporeal circulatory support. Cardiol Young 3:263–272, 1993. Reproduced with permission.)*

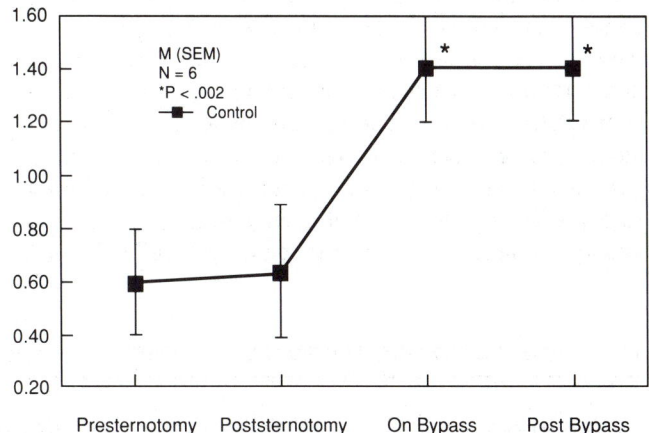

Figure 79–11. Effect of fetal cardiac bypass on placental vascular resistance in fetal lambs at 120 days of gestation. Since the fetal blood pressure remained unchanged the placental bloodflow decreased reciprocally with increasing placental vascular resistance. *(From Hanley FL: Fetal responses to extracorporeal circulatory support. Cardiol Young 3:263–272, 1993. Reproduced with permission.)*

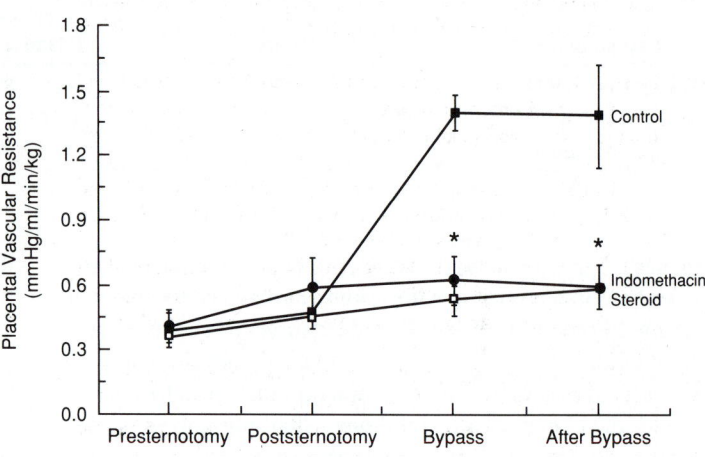

Figure 79–12. Placental vascular resistance (PVR) in the control and indomethacin- and methylprednisolone-treated groups. The rise in PVR seen in control group is prevented by the administration of indomethacin or methylprednisolone, both of which are blockers in the arachidonic acid pathway. *(From Sabik JF, Heinemann MK, Assad RS, et al: High dose steroids prevent placental dysfunction after fetal cardiac bypass. J Thorac Cardiovasc Surg 107:116–125, 1994. Reproduced with permission.)*

ilar beneficial effects have also been observed with the exclusion of the placenta from the bypass circuitry and use of an oxygenator.[93] The inclusion of an artificial oxygenator in the bypass circuit has the disadvantage of the need for large priming volumes and exposure to large foreign surfaces, which may be deleterious to the fetus. In spite of these recent advances, at the present time the ideal method of handling the placenta during fetal bypass remains uncertain.

With a growing appreciation of the negative effects of fetal stress and the mechanisms of placental dysfunction during fetal intervention and extracorporeal circulation, future studies are likely to enable successful use of extracorporeal circulation in the fetus. Recent experimental protocols using this knowledge have resulted in survival of 90% of fetuses to full term following fetal bypass without any deleterious effects.[94] Give those advances it seems likely that fetal cardiac surgery will take its place as a useful form of therapy for certain forms of congenital heart defects.

REFERENCES

1. Freedom RM: *Pulmonary Atresia and Intact Ventricular Septum.* New York, Futura, 1989, p 262
2. Mitchell SC, Korones SB, Berends HW: Congenital heart disease in 56, 109 births. *Circulation* **43**:323, 1971
3. Buckley LP, Dooley KJ, Fyler DC: Pulmonary atresia and intact ventricular septum in New England. *Am J Cardiol* **37**:124, 1976
4. Zuberbuhler JR, Anderson RH: Morphological variations in pulmonary atresia with intact ventricular septum. *Br Heart J* **41**:281–228, 1979
5. Kutsche LM, Van Mierop LHS: Pulmonary atresia with and without ventricular septal defect: A different etiology and pathogenesis for the atresia in the 2 types? *Am J Cardiol* **51**:932–935, 1983
6. Oka M, Angrist GM: Mechanism of cardiac valvular fusion and stenosis. *Am Heart J* **74**:37, 1967
7. Chitayat D, McIntosh N, Fouron JC: Pulmonary atresia with intact ventricular septum: A single gene disorder. *Am J Med Genet* **42**:304–306, 1992
8. Eriksen NL, Buttino LJ, Juberg RC: Congenital pulmonary atresia

and patent ductus arteriosus in two sibs. *Am J Med Genet* **32**:187–188, 1989
9. Steeg CN, Ellis K, Bransilver B, Gersony WM: Pulmonary atresia and intact ventricular septum complicating corrected transposition of great arteries. *Am Heart J* **82**:382, 1971
10. Hanley FL, Sade RM, Blackstone EH, et al: Outcomes in neonatal pulmonary atresia with intact ventricular septum. A multiinstitutional study. *J Thorac Cardiovasc Surg* **105**:406–423, 1993
11. Elliot LP, Adams P, Edwards JE: Pulmonary atresia with intact ventricular septum. *Br Heart J* **25**:489, 1963
12. Sahn DJ, Alleu HD, Anderson R, Goldberg SJ: Echocardiographic diagnosis of atrial septal aneurysm in an infant with hypoplastic right heart syndrome. *Chest* **73**:727, 1978
13. Freedom RM, Dische MR, Rowe RD: The tricuspid valve in pulmonary atresia and intact ventricular septum. *Arch Pathol Lab Med* **102**:28–31, 1978
14. Rowlatt UF, Rimoldi HJA, Lev M: The quantitative anatomy of the normal child's heart. *Pediatr Clin North Am* **10**:499–588, 1963
15. Bull C, de Leval MR, Mercanti C, et al: Pulmonary atresia and intact ventricular septum: A revised classification. *Circulation* **66**:266–272, 1982
16. Becker AE, Becker MJ, Edwards JE: Pathologic spectrum of dysplasia of the tricuspid valve. *Arch Pathol* **91**:167, 1971
17. Cole RB, Muster AJ, Leu M, Paul MH: Pulmonary atresia with intact ventricular septum. *Am J Cardiol* **21**:23, 1968
18. Stellin G, Santini F, Thiene G, et al: Pulmonary atresia, intact ventricular septum, and Ebstein's anomaly of the tricuspid valve. Anatomic and surgical considerations. *J Thorac Cardiovasc Surg* **106**:255–261, 1993
19. Zuberbuhler JR, Allwork SP, Anderson RH: The spectrum of Ebsteins anamoly of the tricuspid valve. *J Thorac Cardiovasc Surg* **77**:202, 1979
20. Goor DA, Lillehei CW: *Congenital Malformations of the Heart.* New York, Grune & Stratton, 1975
21. Bryan CS, Oppenheimer EH: Ventricular endocardial fibroelastosis. Basis for its presence or absence in cases of pulmonic or aortic atresia. *Arch Pathol* **87**:82, 1969
22. Essed CE, Klein HW, Kredict P: Coronary and endocardial fibroelastosis of the ventricles in the hypoplastic left and right heart syndromes. *Virchows Arch [A]* **368**:87–97, 1975
23. O'Connor WN, Cottril CM, Johnson CL, et al: Pulmonary atresia with intact ventricular septum and ventriculocoronary communications: Surgical significance. *Circulation* **65**:805, 1982
24. Bulkley BH, D'Amico B, Taylor AL, et al: Extensive myocardial fiber disarray in aortic and pulmonary atresia. Relevance to hypertrophic cardiomyopathy. *Circulation* **67**:191, 1983

25. Freedom RM, Benson LN, Trusler GA: Pulmonary atresia and intact ventricular septum: A consideration of the coronary circulation and ventriculocoronary artery connections. *Ann Cardiac Surg* 38–44, 1989

26. Lauer RM, Fink HP, Petry EL, et al: Angiographic demonstration of intramyocardial sinusoids in pulmonary valve atresia with intact ventricular septum and hypoplastic right ventricle. *N Engl J Med* **271**:68, 1964

27. Freedom RM, Harrington DP: Contributions of intramyocardial sinusoids in pulmonary atresia and intact ventricular septum to a right sided circular shunt. *Br Heart J* **36**:1061, 1974

28. Williams RR, Kent GB Jr, Edwards JE: Anomalous cardiac blood vessels communicating with the right ventricle: Observations in a case of pulmonary atresia with intact ventricular septum. *Arch Pathol* **52**:480, 1951

29. Patel RG, Freedom RM, Moes CAF, et al: Right ventricular volume determinations in 18 patients with pulmonary atresia and intact ventricular septum. Analysis of factors influencing right ventricular growth. *Circulation* **61**:428, 1980

30. Gittenberger-De Groot AC, Sauer U, Bindl L, et al: Competition of coronary arteries and ventriculocoronary arterial communications in pulmonary atresia with intact ventricular septum. *Int J Cardiol* **18**:243–258, 1988

31. Fyfe DA, Edwards WD, Driscoll DJ: Myocardial ischemia in patients with pulmonary atresia and intact ventricular septum. *J Am Coll Cardiol* **8**:402, 1986

32. Hausdorf G, Gravinghoff L, Keck EW: Effects of persisting myocardial sinusoids on LV performance in pulmonary atresia with intact ventricular septum. *Eur Heart J* **8**:291, 1987

33. Sholler GF, Colan SD, Sanders SP: Effect of isolated right ventricular outflow obstruction on left ventricular function in infants. *Am J Cardiol* **62**:778, 1988

34. Kirklin JW, Barratt-Boyes BG: *Cardiac Surgery,* ed 2. New York, Churchill Livingstone, 1993, Chap 25

35. McArthur JD, Munsi SC, Sukumar IP, Cherian G: Pulmonary valve atresia with intact ventricular septum. *Circulation* **44**:740, 1971

36. Robicsek F, Bostoen H, Sander PW: Atresia of pulmonary valve with normal pulmonary artery and intact ventricular septum in a 21 year old woman. *Angiology* **17**:896, 1966

37. Allan LD: Development of congenital heart lesions in mid to late gestation. *Int J Cardiol* **19**:36, 1988

38. Allan LD, Crawford DC, Tynan MJ: Pulmonary atresia in prenatal life. *J Am Coll Cardiol* **8**:1131, 1986

39. Allan LD: Fetal echocardiography. 7th Charleston symposium on congenital heart diseases. Charleston, SC, March 9–11, 1994

40. Sanders SP, Parness IA, Colan SD: Recognition of abnormal connections of coronary arteries with the use of doppler color flow mapping. *J Am Coll Cardiol* **13**:922–926, 1989

41. Velvis H, Schmidt KG, Silverman NH, Turley K: Diagnosis of coronary artery fistula by two dimensional echocardiography, pulsed doppler ultrasound and color flow mapping. *J Am Coll Cardiol* **14**:968, 1989

42. Gersony WM, Bernhard WF, Nadas AS, et al: Diagnosis and surgical treatment in infants of critical pulmonary outflow obstruction. *Circulation* **35**:765, 1967

43. Bowman FO Jr, Malm JR, Hayes CJ, et al: Pulmonary atresia with intact ventricular septum. *J Thorac Cardiovasc Surg* **61**:85–95, 1971

44. Trussler GA, Yamamoto N, Williams WG, et al: Surgical treatment of pulmonary atresia with intact ventricular septum. *Br Heart J* **38**:957, 1976

45. Ajiki H, Nakamura M, Baba M, et al: Surgical treatment of pulmonary atresia with intact ventricular septum in infancy-analysis of right ventricle growth potential after pulmonary valvotomy. *Nippon Kyobu Geka Gakkai Zasshi* **39**:1049–1054, 1991

46. Amodeo A, Keeton BR, Sutherland GR, Monro JL: Pulmonary atresia with intact ventricular septum: Is neonatal repair advisable? *Eur J Cardiothorac Surg* **5**:17–21, 1991

47. Bull C, Kostelka M, Sorensen K, et al: Outcome measures for the neonatal management of pulmonary atresia with intact ventricular septum. *J Thorac Cardiovasc Surg* **107**:359–366, 1994

48. Coles JG, Freedom RM, Lightfoot NE, et al: Long-term results in neonates with pulmonary atresia and intact ventricular septum. *Ann Thorac Surg* **47**:213–217, 1989

49. de Leval M, Bull C, Stark J, et al: Pulmonary atresia and intact ventricular septum: Surgical management based on a revised classification. *Circulation* **66**:272–280, 1982

50. de Leval M, Bull C, Hopkins R, et al: Decision making in the definitive repair of the heart with a small right ventricle. *Circulation* **72**[suppl II]: II52–60, 1985

51. Giglia TM, Jenkins KJ, Matitiau A, et al: Influence of right heart size on outcome in pulmonary atresia with intact ventricular septum. *Circulation* **88**(suppl I): I2248–2256, 1993

52. Hartyanszky IL, Kadar K, Faller K, Lozsadi K: Surgical management of pulmonary atresia with intact ventricular septum. Right ventricular size as guide line for surgical intervention. *Acta Paediatr Hung* **31**:443–456, 1991

53. Hawkins JA, Thorne JK, Boucek MM, et al: Early and late results in pulmonary atresia and intact ventricular septum. *J Thorac Cardiovasc Surg* **100**:492–497, 1990

54. Leung MP, Mok CK, Lee J, et al: Management evolution of pulmonary atresia and intact ventricular septum. *Am J Cardiol* **71**:1331–1336, 1993

55. Lewis AB, Wells W, Lindesmith GG: Evaluation and surgical treatment of pulmonary atresia and intact ventricular septum in infancy. *Circulation* **67**:1318–1323, 1983

56. Mainwarning RD, Lamberti JJ: Pulmonary atresia with intact ventricular septum. Surgical approach based on ventricular size and coronary anatomy. *J Thorac Cardiovasc Surg* **106**:733–738, 1993

57. McCaffrey FM, Leatherbury L, Moore HV: Pulmonary atresia and intact ventricular septum. Definitive repair in the neonatal period. *J Thorac Cardiovasc Surg* **102**:617–623, 1991

58. Milliken JC, Laks H, Hellenbrand W, et al: Early and late results in the treatment of patients with pulmonary atresia and intact ventricular septum. *Circulation* **72**[suppl]:61–69, 1985

59. Niederhauser U, Bauer EP, von Segesser LK, et al: Early and late results after surgical treatment of pulmonary atresia with intact ventricular septum. *Helv Chir Acta* **57**:551–556, 1991

60. Shaddy RE, Stuetevant JE, Judd VE, McGough EC: Right ventricular growth after transventricular pulmonary valvotomy and central aortopulmonary shunt for pulmonary atresia and intact ventricular septum. *Circulation* **82**(suppl IV):IV157–163, 1990

61. Steinberger J, Berry JM, Bass JE, et al: Results of right ventricular outflow patch for pulmonary atresia with intact ventricular septum. *Circulation* **86**(suppl III):III67–75, 1992

62. Subramanian S: Surgical treatment of complex cyanotic anomalies in infants: Pulmonary atresia with intact ventricular septum. In Davila JC (ed): *Second Henry Ford Hospital International Symposium on Cardiac Surgery,* New York, Appleton-Century Crofts, 1977, p 316

63. Weldon CS, Hartman AF Jr, McKnight RC: Surgical management of hypoplastic right ventricle with pulmonary atresia or critical pulmonary stenosis and intact ventricular septum. *Ann Thorac Surg* **37**:12–24, 1984

64. Pawade A, Capuani A, Penny DJ, et al: Pulmonary atresia with intact ventricular septum. Surgical management based on right ventricular infundibulum. *J Cardiac Surg* **8**:371–383, 1993

65. Latson LA: Nonsurgical treatment of a neonate with pulmonary atresia and intact ventricular septum by transcatheter puncture and balloon dilation of the atretic valve membrane. *Am J Cariol* **68**:277–279, 1991

66. Giglia TM, Mandell VS, Connor AR, et al: Diagnosis and management of right ventricle-dependent coronary circulation in pulmonary atresia with intact ventricular septum. *Circulation* **86**:1516–1528, 1992

67. Akagi T, Benson LN, Williams WG, et al: Ventriculocoronary arter-

ial connections in pulmonary atresia with intact ventricular septum, and their influence on ventricular performance and clinical course. *Am J Cardiol* **72**:586–590, 1993

68. Gentles TL, Colan SD, Giglia TM, et al: Right ventricular decompression and left ventricular function in pulmonary atresia with intact ventricular septum. The influence of less extensive coronary anomalies. *Circulation* **88**(suppl II):II183–188, 1993

69. Squittieri C, di Carlo C, Giannico S, et al: Tricuspid avulsion or excision for right ventricular decompression in pulmonary atresia with intact ventricular septum. *J Thorac Cardiovasc Surg* **97**:779–784, 1989

70. Williams WG, Burrows P, Freedom RM, et al: Thromboexclusion of the right ventricle in children with pulmonary atresia and intact ventricular septum. *J Thorac Cardiovasc Surg* **101**:222–229, 1991

71. Laks H, Pearl JM, Drinkwater DC, et al: Partial biventricular repair of pulmonary atresia with intact ventricular septum. Use of an adjustable atrial septal defect. *Circulation* **86**(suppl III):III59–66, 1992

72. Billingsley AM, Laks H, Boyce SW, et al: Definitive repair in patients with pulmonary atresia and intact ventricular septum. *J Thorac Cardiovasc Surg* **97**:746–754, 1989

73. Muster AJ, Zales VR, Ilbawi MN, et al: Biventricular repair of hypoplastic right ventricle assisted by pulsatile bidirectional cavopulmonary anastamosis. *J Thorac Cardiovasc Surg* **105**:112–119, 1993

74. Kirklin JW: Congenital Heart Surgeons Society, personal communication, 1994

75. Graham TP, Bender HW, Atwood GF, et al: Increase in right ventricular volume following valvulotomy for pulmonary atresia or stenosis with intact ventricular septum. *Circulation* **50**[suppl II]:II69, 1974

76. Hanseus, Bjorkhem G, Lundstrome NR, Laurin S: Cross-sectional echocardiographic measurements of right ventricular size and growth in patients with pulmonary atresia and intact ventricular septum. *Pediatr Cardiol* **12**:135–142, 1991

77. Ishizawa E, Horiuchi T, Tadokora M, et al: Surgical management of pulmonary atresia and critical pulmonary stenosis with intact ventricular septum. *Tohoku J Exp Med* **150**:135–144, 1986

78. Lewis AB, Wells W, Lindesmith GG: Right ventricular growth potential in neonates with pulmonary atresia and intact ventricular septum. *J Thorac Cardiovasc Surg* **91**:835–840, 1986

79. Luckstead EF, Mattioli L, Crosby IK, et al: Two-stage palliative surgical approach for pulmonary atresia with intact ventricular septum (Type 1). *Am J Cardiol* **29**:490, 1972

80. Mansfield PB, Hall DG, Rittenhouse EA, et al: Surgical treatment of pulmonary atresia with right ventricular hypoplasia and intact septum. *Mod Prob Pediatr* **22**:167, 1983

81. Metzdorff MT, Pinson CW, Grunkemeir GL, et al: Late right ventricular reconstruction following valvotomy in pulmonary atresia with intact ventricular septum. *Ann Thorac Surg* **42**:45–51, 1986

82. Moller JH, Girod D, Amplatz K, et al: Pulmonary valvotomy in pulmonary atresia with hypoplastic right ventricle. *Surgery* **68**:630, 1970

83. Dolkart LA, Reimers FT: Transvaginal echocardiography in early pregnancy. Normative data. *Am J Obstet Gynecol* **165**:688, 1991

84. Rose V, Clark LE: Etiology of congenital heart diseases. In Freedom RM, Benson LN, Smallhorn JF (eds): *Neonatal Heart Disease*. New York, Springer-Verlag, 1992, pp 3–13

85. Bical O, Gallix P, Toussaint M, et al: Intrauterine creation and repair of pulmonary stenosis in fetal lambs. *J Thorac Cardiovasc Surg* **93**:761–766, 1987

86. Slate RK, Verrier ED, Stevens MR, et al: Intrauterine repair of pulmonary stenosis in fetal lambs. *Surg Forum* **36**:246–247, 1985

87. Hanley FL: Fetal responses to extracorporeal circulatory support. *Cardiol Young* **3**:263–272, 1993

88. Bradley SM, Hanley FL, Duncan BW, et al: Fetal cardiac bypass alters regional blood flows, arterial blood gases and hemodynamics in sheep. *Am J Physiol* **263**:H919–928, 1992

89. Bradley SM, Hanley FL, Jennings RW, et al: Regional blood flows during cardiopulmonary bypass in fetal lambs: Effect of nitroprusside. *Circulation* **82**(suppl III):III413, 1990

90. Sabik JF, Assad RS, Hanley FL: Halothane as an anesthetic for fetal surgery. *Pedeatr Surg* **28**:542–547, 1993

91. Fenton KM, Heineman MK, Hickey PR, et al: Inhibition of fetal stress response improves cardiac output and gas exchange after fetal cardiac bypass. *J Thorac Cardiovasc Surg* **107**:1416–1423, 1994

92. Sabik JF, Heinemann MK, Assad RS, et al: High dose steriods prevent placental dysfunction after fetal cardiac bypass. *J Thorac Cardiovasc Surg* **107**:116–125, 1994

93. Fenton KM, Heineman MK, Hanley FL: Exclusion of the placenta during fetal cardiac bypass allows improved systemic perfusion and provides important information about the mechanism of placental injury. *J Thorac Cardiovasc Surg* **105**:502–512, 1992

94. Reddy VM, Liddicoat JR, Hanley FL: Chronic survival to term after cardiac bypass from midline sternotomy using hemopump in fetal lambs. 1994 (to be published)

CHAPTER

80

Surgical Management of Pulmonary Atresia with Ventricular Septal Defect

Lester C. Permut and Hillel Laks

Pulmonary atresia with ventricular septal defect is a complex congenital heart defect that is the subject of continued controversy. In its simplest form, with normal pulmonary vascular architecture, management is relatively uncomplicated, and the defect can be considered an extreme form of tetralogy of Fallot. However, in the presence of multiple aortopulmonary collateral vessels, disagreement exists regarding the appropriateness of surgical therapy, the timing of operation, and the optimal techniques for repair.[1,2] The reason for these differences centers around the diversity of morphologic and consequent physiologic forms with which this defect presents. The relatively small number of patients and large number of subgroups make meaningful comparison between differing treatment strategies difficult. The current approach utilized at the UCLA Medical Center will be described in detail, with emphasis on the management of patients with multiple aortopulmonary collaterals.

MORPHOLOGY

Pulmonary atresia with ventricular septal defect can present with a variety of morphologic findings.[3] The defining anatomic features include concordant atrioventricular and ventriculoarterial connections with ventricular septal defect and absence of continuity between the right ventricle and the pulmonary trunk. The ventricular septal defect is usually large, and results from anterior malalignment of the infundibular septum. As with simple tetralogy of Fallot, the

defect may extend posteriorly to the fibrous trigone or may have a completely muscular rim. The cardiac conduction system is located in its usual position, relating to the posteroinferior aspect of the ventricular septal defect. Coronary artery anomalies are uncommon, but may be present.

The pulmonary blood supply is derived from "true" pulmonary arteries and aortopulmonary collateral vessels (Fig. 80–1). True pulmonary arteries are located in the anterior hilum. They may be adequate in size, or may exhibit varying degrees of hypoplasia. The left and right pulmonary arteries, when present, may be confluent or nonconfluent. Systemic-to-pulmonary collateral vessels have been categorized into three groups by Rabinovitch et al.[4] Enlarged bronchial arteries constitute the first type, and typically anastamose with the true pulmonary arteries within the lung parenchyma. The second group consists of collaterals that arise directly from the descending thoracic or, rarely, abdominal aorta. They enter the hilum posteriorly to anastamose with the true pulmonary arteries or intraacinar vessels. The third type of collateral arises from branches of the aorta, most frequently from the brachiocephalic, internal mammary, and intercostal arteries. These tend to be smaller vessels that anastamose to the true central pulmonary arteries or spread out over the surface of the visceral pleura. Stenoses occur frequently in the second and third types, most often at their origin but occasionally within the hilum of the lung. These stenoses are due to intimal proliferation thought to result from turbulent bloodflow.[5] While such classification systems may be useful for anatomic discus-

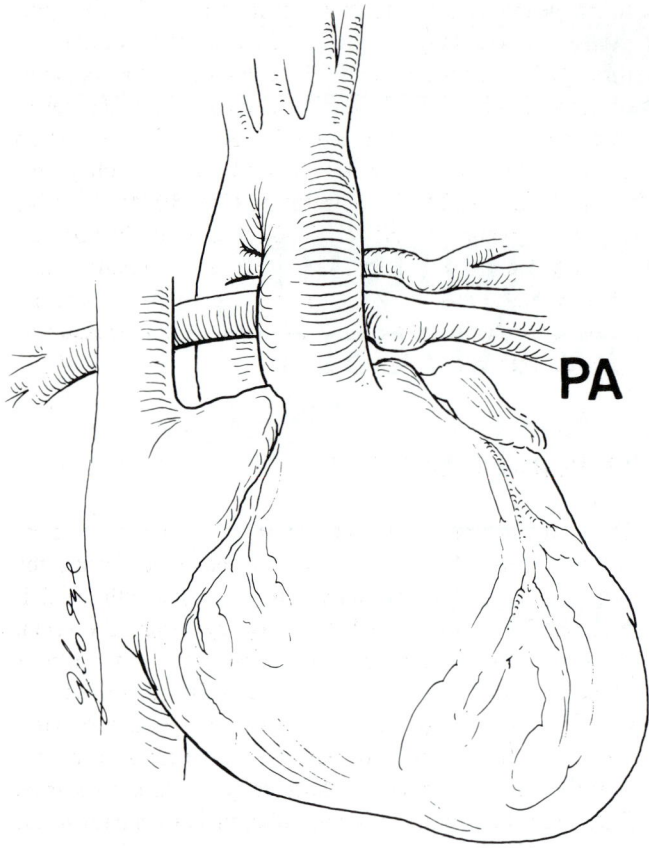

Figure 80–1. Anatomy of pulmonary atresia with ventricular septal defect demonstrating true pulmonary arteries in the anterior hilum and an aortopulmonary collateral in the posterior hilum. PA, true pulmonary artery. *(From Permut LC, Laks HL: Surgical management of pulmonary atresia with ventricular septal defect and multiple aortopulmonary collaterals. Adv Card Surg 5:75–95, 1994. Reproduced with permission from Mosby-Year Book, Inc.)*

sion, the relevance of morphologic classification to surgical decision making is questionable.[6] All three types may exist in patients with pulmonary atresia and ventricular septal defect, but major collaterals arising from the aorta and its branches, when present, comprise an important morphologic and physiologic component of the defect that must be addressed in the planning of complete repair.

Distribution of pulmonary bloodflow to individual bronchopulmonary segments may be via the true pulmonary arteries, collateral vessels, or both. The collaterals may be the only source of bloodflow in certain bronchopulmonary segments or may coexist with true pulmonary arteries. Such collateral vessels may nevertheless be important sources of pulmonary bloodflow when the true pulmonary arteries in these segments are hypoplastic. "Essential collaterals" are those that are either the only blood supply to a portion of the lung or are so large that they are essential to the size of the pulmonary vascular bed. "Redundant collaterals" are those that are small and overlap with the true pulmonary artery distribution.

NATURAL HISTORY

The natural history of pulmonary atresia with ventricular septal defect is dependent on the nature of the pulmonary bloodflow. At birth, true pulmonary artery bloodflow is ductus dependent. In the presence of adequate sized pulmonary arteries, minimal cyanosis may be present. After ductal closure, or in the presence of hypoplastic pulmonary arteries, pulmonary bloodflow is dependent on the presence of collateral vessels. Patients may present in one of three ways. Bloodflow through the collaterals may be excessive with resultant large left-to-right shunt, pulmonary congestion, only mild cyanosis, and left ventricular volume overload. Moderate stenosis of the collateral vessels may result in a balanced pulmonary bloodflow and minimal symptoms, while severe collateral stenosis produces inadequate pulmonary bloodflow and consequent severe cyanosis.

Poor early survival is expected in patients with excessive or inadequate pulmonary bloodflow, and operative therapy in these patients is generally accepted as appropriate. There is disagreement, however, regarding the need for surgical intervention in those patients with balanced pulmonary bloodflow. A number of these patients will survive to adulthood without surgical intervention or with palliative shunts alone. While data are not available to directly compare the results of operative and nonoperative therapy, studies of the natural history of these patients show that they develop decreased left ventricular function as a result of chronic left-to-right shunting and left ventricular volume overload. Further, aortic annular dilatation develops commonly since all right and left ventricular bloodflow exits the heart via the aorta. Nearly 80% of unoperated or palliated adults in our series had significant aortic insufficiency, further impairing left ventricular function.[7] Based on these findings, we recommend operative therapy for all patients whose general condition and anatomic findings are amenable to surgical repair.

DIAGNOSIS

History and Physical Examination

As described above, the presentation will vary depending on the patency of the ductus arteriosus and the presence and degree of obstruction of aortopulmonary collateral vessels. Most commonly, pulmonary bloodflow is inadequate, and cyanosis is the main presenting feature. Infants with excessive pulmonary bloodflow via a large ductus and unobstructed collaterals may present with symptoms of congestive heart failure including dyspnea, tachypnea, diaphoresis, and difficulty feeding. Those with balanced pulmonary bloodflow may be asymptomatic or have mild cyanosis.

Physical examination reveals a normal first heart sound and single second heart sound. A loud, systolic murmur is audible at the lower sternal border and represents flow across the ventricular septal defect. Absence of a pulmonic ejection murmur distinguishes pulmonary atresia from tetralogy of Fallot with pulmonic stenosis. A continuous murmur is present in patients with patent ductus or large aortopulmonary collaterals. The murmur from collateral vessels is best heard posteriorly.

Electrocardiogram

Electrocardiographic findings are nondiagnostic and consist primarily of right axis deviation and right ventricular hypertrophy. Infants with excessive pulmonary blood flow may demonstrate combined left and right ventricular hypertrophy.

Echocardiography

Two-dimensional echocardiography is diagnostic of pulmonary atresia with ventricular septal defect. Accurate definition of the intracardiac anatomy, including demonstration of right ventricle–pulmonary artery discontinuity and malalignment ventricular septal defect, can be accomplished easily at the bedside. Some assessment of central pulmonary artery size and morphology can be made, but visualization of the more distal branch pulmonary arteries and of aortopulmonary collaterals is suboptimal.

Cardiac Catheterization

Detailed knowledge of the true pulmonary artery and collateral distribution is essential for planning the surgical approach in each patient. Cardiac catheterization is the primary means of obtaining this information. The true pulmonary arteries may be visualized by injection of contrast through the ductus arteriosus or via collaterals that communicate with them (Fig. 80–2). Pulmonary vein wedge injections may be necessary as well (Fig. 80–3). Demonstration of collateral vessels is best obtained by a descending aortogram with distal balloon occlusion (Fig. 80–4). Selective contrast injections in individual collaterals can then be performed. Occasionally, magnetic resonance imaging may provide additional information about pulmonary vascular architecture; its role compliments but does not replace cardiac catheterization.

SURGICAL TREATMENT

The principles of surgical management of pulmonary atresia and ventricular septal defect are the same despite the wide spectrum of pulmonary vascular patterns with which it presents. The ultimate goal is to close the ventricular septal defect and establish continuity between the right ventricle and pulmonary artery. Successful definitive repair requires the presence of an adequate pulmonary vascular bed, without which right ventricular failure will occur as a consequence of the high resulting pulmonary vascular resistance. To prevent this, early efforts must be made to maximize the size and distribution of the pulmonary arteries. Preparation for definitive repair should provide adequate pulmonary bloodflow to maintain an adequate arterial oxygen saturation while avoiding excessive pulmonary bloodflow with resultant pulmonary congestion and left ventricular volume overload.

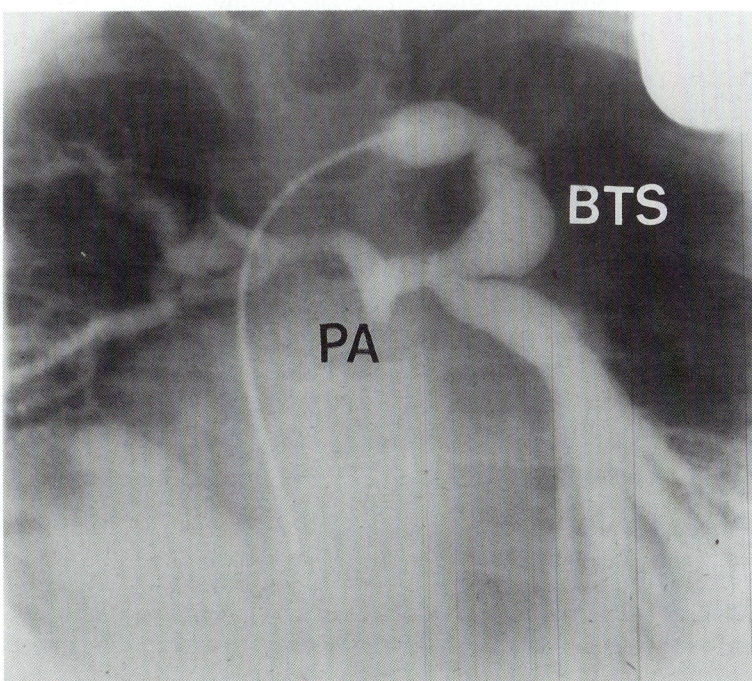

Figure 80–2. Cineangiogram demonstrating hypoplastic true pulmonary arteries filling through a Blalock–Taussig shunt. PA, pulmonary artery; BTS, Blalock–Taussig shunt. *(From Permut LC, Laks HL: Surgical management of pulmonary atresia with ventricular septal defect and multiple aortopulmonary collaterals. Adv Card Surg 5:75–95, 1994. Reproduced with permission from Mosby–Year Book, Inc.)*

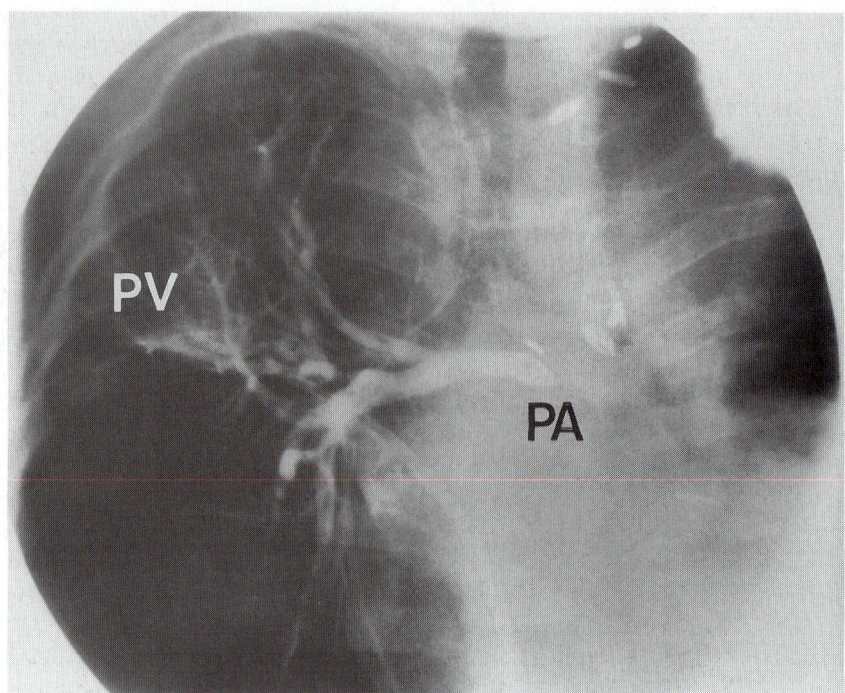

Figure 80–3. Pulmonary vein wedge angiogram demonstrating the true pulmonary artery. PA, pulmonary artery; PV, pulmonary vein. *(From Permut LC, Laks HL: Surgical management of pulmonary atresia with ventricular septal defect and multiple aortopulmonary collaterals. Adv Card Surg 5:75–95, 1994. Reproduced with permission from Mosby-Year Book, Inc.)*

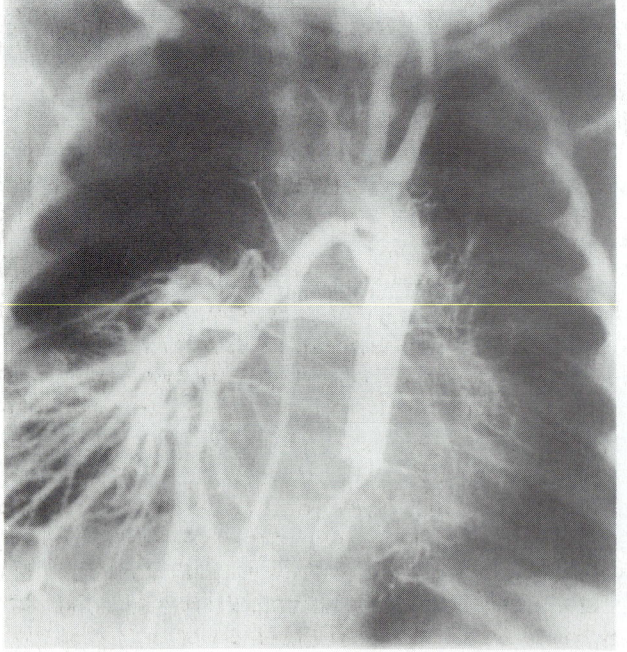

Figure 80–4. Balloon occlusion descending aortogram demonstrating large aortopulmonary collateral vessels. *(From Permut LC, Laks HL: Surgical management of pulmonary atresia with ventricular septal defect and multiple aortopulmonary collaterals. Adv Card Surg 5:75–95, 1994. Reproduced with permission from Mosby-Year Book, Inc.)*

EARLY PALLIATIVE PROCEDURES

Palliative procedures are usually performed in the neonatal period or early infancy. The goal of these procedures is to create a balanced pulmonary bloodflow and to promote growth of the true pulmonary arteries. Palliation is required in patients with excessive or inadequate pulmonary bloodflow.

Excessive Pulmonary Bloodflow

Stenoses at the origin of the collateral vessels usually develop due to intimal proliferation in the first few months of life. Patients may occasionally present with multiple, large, unobstructed aortopulmonary collaterals and excessive pulmonary bloodflow. While redundant collateral vessels may be ligated or embolized,[8] some collaterals may be the sole sources of bloodflow to specific segments of the lungs. Flow may be decreased by creating stenoses at the origin of these collaterals. This is accomplished by placing pledgetted mattress sutures in the aortic wall immediately adjacent to the origin of the collateral vessel (Fig. 80–5). The degree of stenosis can be adjusted according to the distal collateral blood pressure, the arterial oxygen saturation, and the rise in arterial diastolic pressure.

Inadequate Pulmonary Bloodflow

In the simplest cases, the true pulmonary arteries are of adequate size and distribution, and the collateral vessels are re-

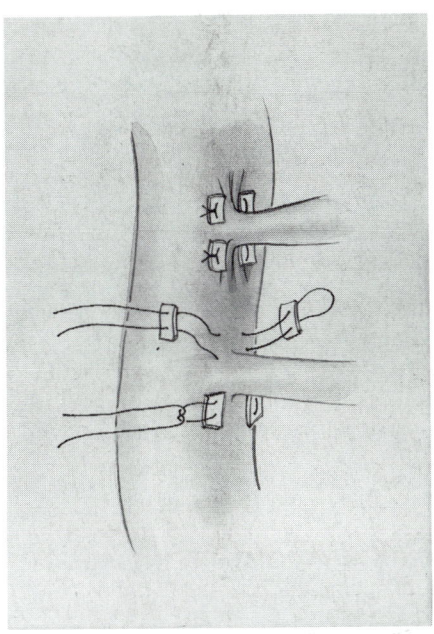

Figure 80–5. Technique of banding aortopulmonary collateral vessels with excessive pulmonary bloodflow. Pledgetted mattress sutures are placed in the aortic wall on either side of the collateral vessel. *(From Permut LC, Laks HL: Surgical management of pulmonary atresia with ventricular septal defect and multiple aortopulmonary collaterals. Adv Card Surg 5:75–95, 1994. Reproduced with permission from Mosby-Year Book, Inc.)*

dundant. Palliation with a systemic-to-pulmonary shunt procedure is performed in the neonatal period to maintain arterial oxygen saturation in an acceptable range (80–85% on room air). We prefer construction of a modified Blalock–Taussig shunt using a 3- or 4-mm Gore-Tex graft. Such shunts avoid a median sternotomy and are relatively easy to take down at the time of definitive repair. The patient may eventually outgrow the shunt and develop worsening cyanosis. Repeat shunting may be necessary on the contralateral side, or, if the child is large enough, definitive repair may be considered at 3 or 4 years of age. Redundant collaterals may be ligated surgically at the time of shunting, or embolized during cardiac catheterization. In some patients, maintaining flow through redundant collaterals may be desirable to maintain an adequate arterial oxygen saturation. Snares may be placed loosely around such vessels and positioned to be accessible from the anterior mediastinum. Closure of these collaterals is then accomplished by tightening the snares at the time of definitive repair.

Hypoplastic pulmonary arteries are found in 25–30% of patients with pulmonary atresia and ventricular septal defect with major aortopulmonary collaterals.[9] When present, they pose a greater therapeutic challenge. The primary goal in these cases is augmentation of central pulmonary bloodflow to promote bilateral pulmonary artery growth and maintain adequate oxygenation. Previously, initial pallia-

tion was achieved by placement of a central (ascending aorta to pulmonary artery) Gore-Tex shunt. More recently, we and others prefer construction of a right ventricle to pulmonary artery conduit without ventricular septal defect closure in the neonatal period.[10,11] When the right ventricular infundibulum is in close proximity to the pulmonary trunk, an outflow tract patch of pericardium or synthetic material can be used. More frequently, the distance between the right ventricle and pulmonary artery must be bridged with a conduit. This can be accomplished with a simple Gore-Tex tube graft or with a valved aortic or pulmonary homograft. In most cases, these procedures can be performed without cardiopulmonary bypass (Fig. 80–6 and 80–7).[12,13] Occasionally, cardiopulmonary bypass with hypothermic low flow or circulatory arrest is required.

The advantages of this approach over central shunting include reduction of left ventricular volume overload and exposure of the hypoplastic pulmonary vasculature to more pulsatile blood flow, which has been shown to enhance growth. Additionally, such a connection provides catheter access to the pulmonary arteries, facilitating subsequent evaluation and intervention, e.g., balloon dilatation of stenotic segments.[14] The growth potential of hypoplastic pulmonary arteries, which appears related to the amount of elastin in the vessel wall,[15] declines with age, so early intervention provides the best chance of an optimal outcome. Redundant collaterals should be ligated or embolized. Collaterals that provide the only source of bloodflow to specific bronchopulmonary segments should be preserved for subsequent incorporation prior to definitive repair.

UNIFOCALIZATION

Patients with nonredundant aortopulmonary collaterals can be described as having multifocal sources of bloodflow to one or both lungs. Unifocalization refers broadly to those procedures that join the multifocal sources (true pulmonary artery and one or more collaterals) into a single source. A variety of procedures has been reported, most of which entail direct anastomosis of collaterals to the true pulmonary arteries[16–18] or placement of interposition grafts (synthetic,[16,18,19] autologous artery or vein,[17,18] xenograft pericardium,[20] or autologous pericardium[17]) between collateral vessels and the true pulmonary arteries. In our experience, such procedures are suboptimal. The ideal unifocalization procedure should (1) allow incorporation of all nonredundant collaterals and the true pulmonary artery to each lung without distortion, (2) utilize conduits that will either grow or be large enough to supply adequate bloodflow in adulthood without replacement, (3) minimize the risk of thrombosis, and (4) be easily accessible from the mediastinum at the time of definitive repair. We have described a technique of pericardial tube unifocalization that fulfills these criteria.[21]

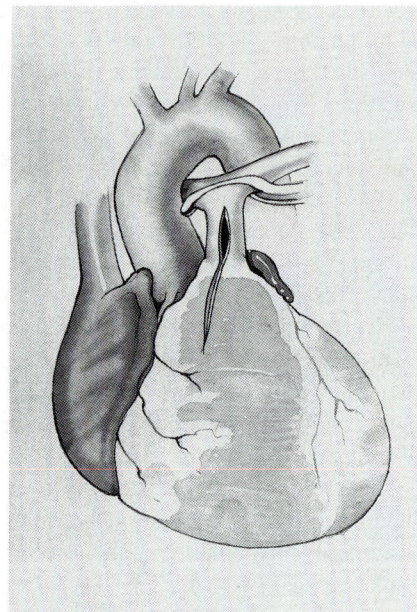

A

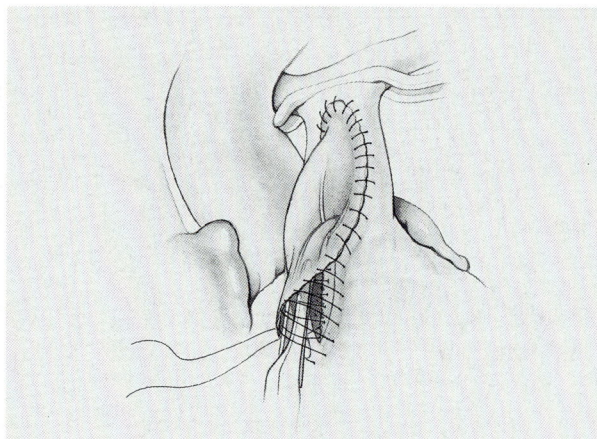

B

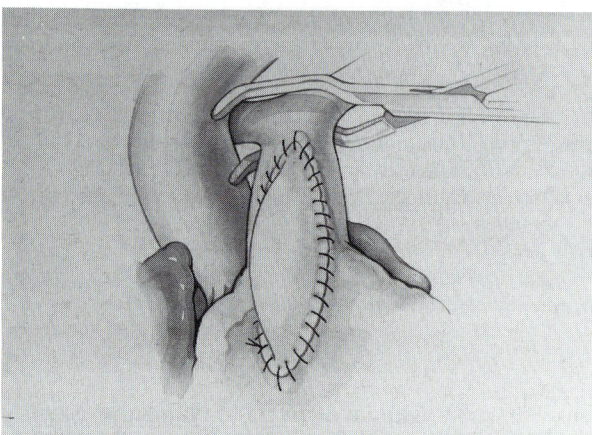

C

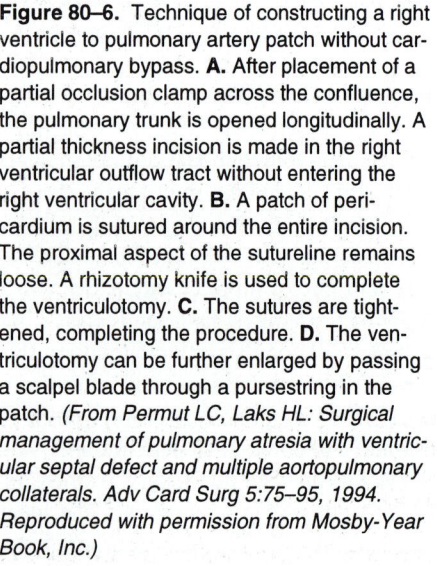

Figure 80–6. Technique of constructing a right ventricle to pulmonary artery patch without cardiopulmonary bypass. **A.** After placement of a partial occlusion clamp across the confluence, the pulmonary trunk is opened longitudinally. A partial thickness incision is made in the right ventricular outflow tract without entering the right ventricular cavity. **B.** A patch of pericardium is sutured around the entire incision. The proximal aspect of the sutureline remains loose. A rhizotomy knife is used to complete the ventriculotomy. **C.** The sutures are tightened, completing the procedure. **D.** The ventriculotomy can be further enlarged by passing a scalpel blade through a pursestring in the patch. *(From Permut LC, Laks HL: Surgical management of pulmonary atresia with ventricular septal defect and multiple aortopulmonary collaterals. Adv Card Surg 5:75–95, 1994. Reproduced with permission from Mosby-Year Book, Inc.)*

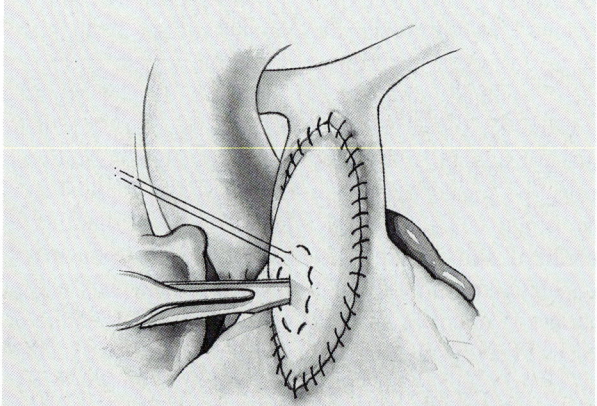

D

Pericardial Tube Unifocalization

Unifocalization is performed through a posterolateral thoracotomy incision. A double-lumen endotracheal tube should be employed, when possible, in larger children and adults.

Single lung ventilation of the contralateral lung, when tolerated, greatly facilitates exposure. The apex of the lung is retracted inferiorly and posteriorly to allow identification and dissection of the true pulmonary artery in the anterosuperior aspect of the hilum (Fig. 80–8). Retraction of the lung ante-

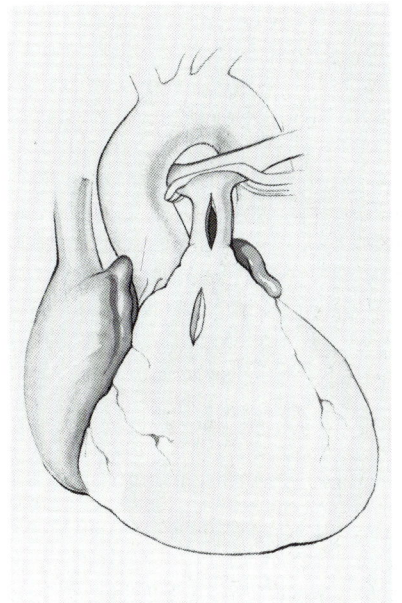

A

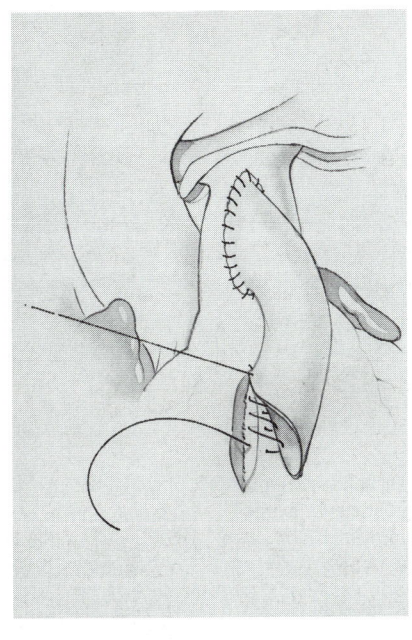

C

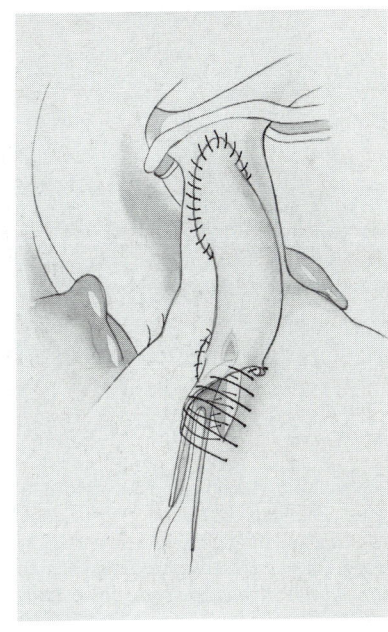

D

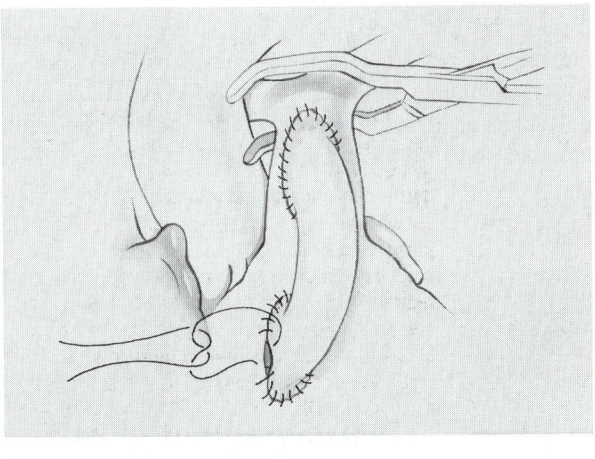

B

E

Figure 80–7. Technique of constructing a right ventricle to pulmonary artery conduit without cardiopulmonary bypass. **A.** After placement of a partial occlusion clamp across the confluence, a pulmonary arteriotomy is made. A partial thickness incision is made in the right ventricular outflow tract without entering the right ventricular cavity. **B.** The distal anastomosis is constructed. **C.** The proximal end of the Gore-Tex tube is sutured to the epicardium around the planned ventriculotomy site. The proximal aspect of the sutureline remains loose. **D.** A rhizotomy knife is used to complete the ventriculotomy. **E.** The sutures are tightened, completing the repair. *(From Permut LC, Laks HL: Surgical management of pulmonary atresia with ventricular septal defect and multiple aortopulmonary collaterals. Adv Card Surg 5:75–95, 1994. Reproduced with permission from Mosby-Year Book, Inc.)*

riorly allows identification of aortopulmonary collaterals that enter the hilum posteriorly. Redundant collaterals are carefully ligated and divided.

A large patch of pericardium is harvested anterior or posterior to the phrenic nerve. The patch is then draped, with serous aspect facing upward, over the posterior and superior hilum. It is aligned so that its midportion overlies each collateral and the true pulmonary artery to be incorporated in the unifocalization. A sterile pen is used to precisely mark the sites of anastomosis on the pericardial

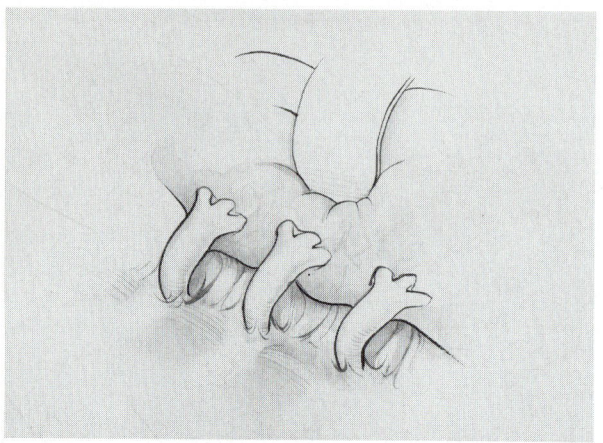

Figure 80–8. Technique of pericardial tube unifocalization of right sided collaterals. Collateral vessels identified in the posterior hilum, as visualized through a right posterolateral thoractomy incision. *(From Permut LC, Laks HL: Surgical management of pulmonary atresia with ventricular septal defect and multiple aortopulmonary collaterals. Adv Card Surg 5:75–95, 1994. Reproduced with permission from Mosby-Year Book, Inc.)*

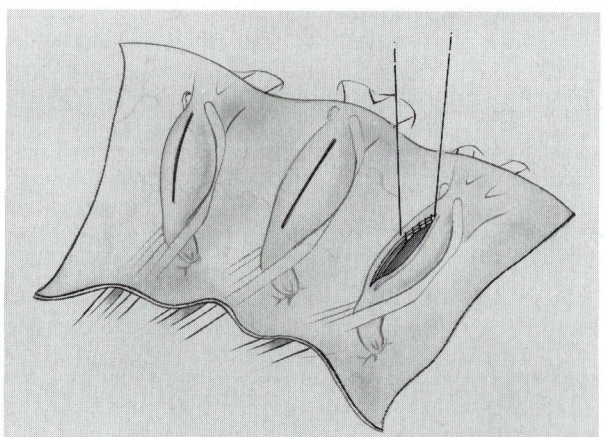

Figure 80–10. Technique of pericardial tube unifocalization. The pericardium is draped over the collaterals and incisions are made in the most inferior collateral and overlying pericardium. A side-to-side anastomosis is constructed using 6-0 or 7-0 PDS suture. *(From Permut LC, Laks HL: Surgical management of pulmonary atresia with ventricular septal defect and multiple aortopulmonary collaterals. Adv Card Surg 5:75–95, 1994. Reproduced with permission from Mosby-Year Book, Inc.)*

patch. The collaterals are individually clamped with shallow U-shaped vascular clamps (Fig. 80–9). An incision is made in the most inferiorly located collateral. The pericardium is again draped over it and incised at the previously marked site. A side-to-side anastomosis is then constructed with a continuous suture of 6-0 or 7-0 PDS. The remaining collaterals and true pulmonary artery are then sequentially anastomosed to the pericardial patch in a similar fashion

(Fig. 80–10). The edges of the pericardium are folded over and sutured with a continuous suture of 6-0 prolene to create a closed tube 1.5–2 cm in diameter (Fig. 80–11). The tube is constructed so that its superior aspect extends over the hilum toward the anterior mediastinum. If the tube does not reach the anterior mediastium, an adult sized (16-, 18-, or 20-mm) interposition Gore-Tex graft is added to the pericardial tube. Inflow to the tube is then provided either by a

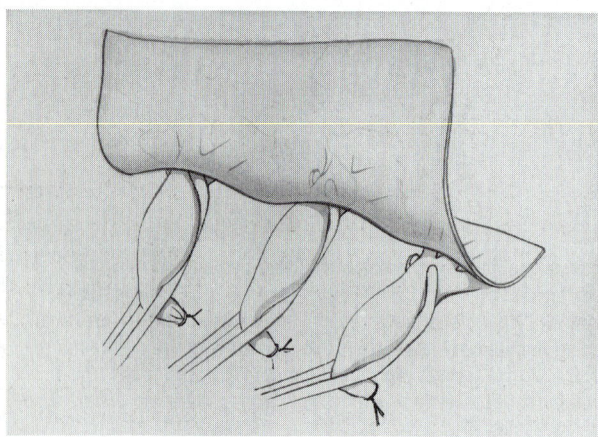

Figure 80–9. Technique of pericardial tube unifocalization. Collaterals are ligated at their origin and individually clamped. The pericardium has been harvested and fixed in glutaraldehyde. The position of the collaterals has been marked on the pericardium with a sterile marker. *(From Permut LC, Laks HL: Surgical management of pulmonary atresia with ventricular septal defect and multiple aortopulmonary collaterals. Adv Card Surg 5:75–95, 1994. Reproduced with permission from Mosby-Year Book, Inc.)*

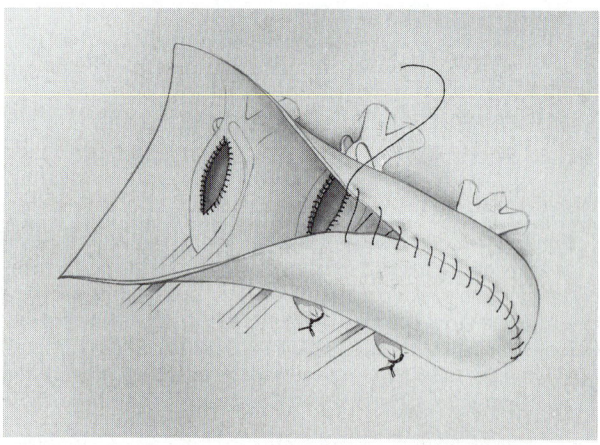

Figure 80–11. Technique of pericardial tube unifocalization. Following completion of all anastomoses, the pericardium is furled anteriorly and sutured to create a tube. *(From Permut LC, Laks HL: Surgical management of pulmonary atresia with ventricular septal defect and multiple aortopulmonary collaterals. Adv Card Surg 5:75–95, 1994. Reproduced with permission from Mosby-Year Book, Inc.)*

side-to-side anastomosis to the ascending aorta or by a suitable sized Gore-Tex graft from the subclavian artery to the tube (Fig. 80–12). In the case of a subclavian artery shunt, a snare is placed around the Gore-Tex shunt and positioned in the anterior mediastinum to allow occlusion of the shunt at the time of definitive repair. The clamps are removed, air is vented from the pericardial tube, and blood flow is restored to the lung. The proximal end of each collateral is ligated. Prior to chest closure, the pericardial defect is replaced with Gore-Tex membrane.

Gore-Tex Tube Unifocalization

In patients with a single large collateral supplying the entire blood flow to a lung, an "adult-sized" (16-, 18-, or 20-mm) Gore-Tex graft may be placed between the collateral and the ascending aorta. A suitable sized ascending aorta to Gore-Tex graft anastomosis is constructed. The graft is positioned to be accessible at the time of definitive repair through a median sternotomy incision (Fig. 80–13).

Timing of Unifocalization

Unifocalization should be undertaken at an age when the collateral vessels are large enough to allow a large anastamosis that is less likely to become stenotic with growth. Although this may vary between patients depending on collateral size, unifocalization can usually be performed without difficulty in patients greater than 3 years old. We have, however, performed unifocalization procedures in children as young as 8 months of age. Staged procedures may be required for bilateral multiple aortopulmonary collateral vessels. Bilateral unifocalization as a single operation may be

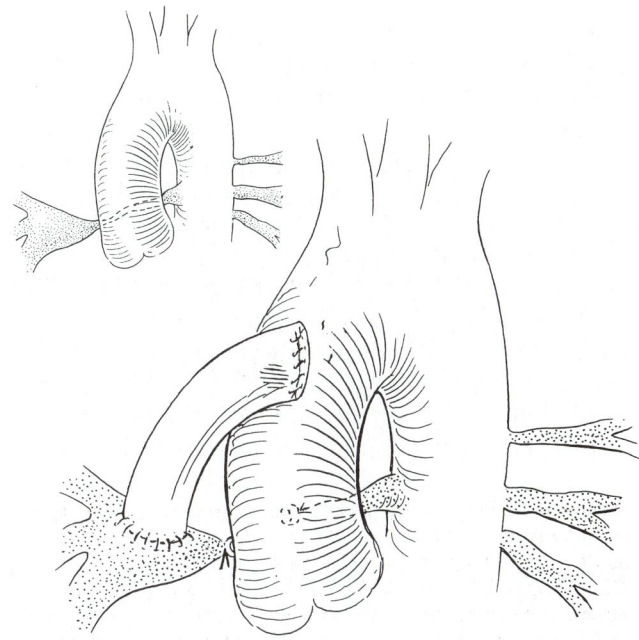

Figure 80–13. Unifocalization in a patient with a large collateral supplying the entire lung. An "adult-sized" (16- to 20-mm) Gore-Tex graft is used. *(From Permut LC, Laks HL: Surgical management of pulmonary atresia with ventricular septal defect and multiple aortopulmonary collaterals. Adv Card Surg 5:75–95, 1994. Reproduced with permission from Mosby-Year Book, Inc.)*

considered, but the magnitude of the operation, especially the pulmonary contusion and congestion seen in the immediate postoperative period, usually prohibits this. The size of the shunt is adjusted to achieve an arterial oxygen saturation of 80% in room air. This usually correlates with an intraoperative arterial oxygen saturation of 88% to 90% when $FIO_2 = 100\%$.

DEFINITIVE REPAIR

Definitive repair in pulmonary atresia and ventricular septal defect entails patch closure of the ventricular septal defect and establishment of continuity between the right ventricle and the pulmonary arteries. All systemic-to-pulmonary shunts, including redundant collaterals and surgically created shunts, should have been previously occluded or be retrievable from a median sternotomy incision to allow occlusion at the time of complete repair. Successful definitive repair, as discussed above, is dependent on the adequacy of the pulmonary vascular bed. A number of methods are available to predict this preoperatively, based on pulmonary artery size and an estimate of the pulmonary vascular resistance. The McGoon ratio calculates the sum of the diameters of the left and right pulmonary arteries at the origin of the upper lobe branch, normalizing the value by dividing the sum by the descending aortic diameter measured at the

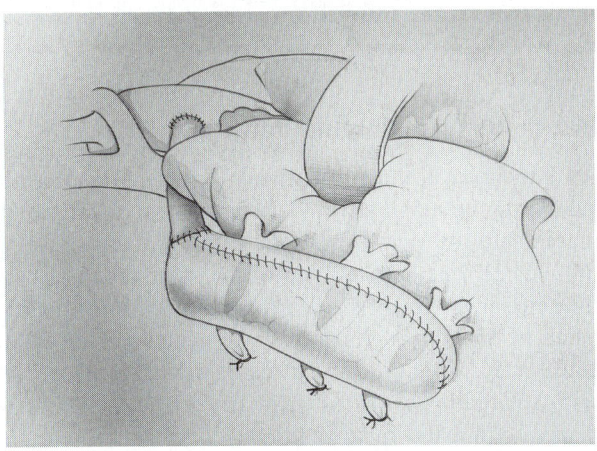

Figure 80–12. Technique of pericardial tube unifocalization. The pericardial tube is anastomosed to the aorta by interposition of a Gore-Tex graft. *(From Permut LC, Laks HL: Surgical management of pulmonary atresia with ventricular septal defect and multiple aortopulmonary collaterals. Adv Card Surg 5:75–95, 1994. Reproduced with permission from Mosby-Year Book, Inc.)*

level of the diaphragm.[22] A ratio greater than 1 predicts successful definitive repair. Nakata and colleagues refined this method by calculating the sum of the cross-sectional areas of the left and right pulmonary arteries, indexed to body surface area.[23] An index of 150 mm^2/m^2 or more is considered adequate for definitive repair. Kirklin, Blackstone, and colleagues have demonstrated that the McGoon ratio and number of aortopulmonary collaterals were important predictors of high right ventricle/left ventricle pressure ratio and death within 6 mo of operation.[24,25] While such predictive indices are valuable as guidelines for repair, they are not without shortcomings. Underestimation of pulmonary artery size may occur in conditions of low pulmonary bloodflow. In addition, measurement of distal pulmonary artery pressure may be difficult and, as flow cannot be measured accurately, the pulmonary vascular resistance may be difficult to determine with accuracy. Predicted postrepair right ventricular pressure greater than 2/3 systemic is associated with prohibitive risk for early and late morbidity and mortality following definitive repair.

Conduit Repair

Definitive repair is deferred until the patient is approximately 4–5 years old so that an adult-sized conduit can be used, reducing the number of conduit replacements which will be required subsequently. A longitudinal incision is made in the right ventricular infundibulum, with care taken to identify and avoid any coronary arteries that may be present. We utilize a double velour Dacron patch for closure of the ventricular septal defect through the right ventriculotomy which will be used for anastomosis of the proximal end of the conduit. A composite conduit is constructed by anastamosing a woven Dacron tube to a valved aortic or pulmonic homograft. If adequate sized confluent true pulmonary arteries are present, the distal anastomosis is made to the pulmonary artery to the left of the aorta. The pericardial tube unifocalization grafts are taken down from the aorta and the resulting aortic defects are oversewn (Fig. 80–14). When hypoplastic or nonconfluent pulmonary arteries are present, the bilateral pericardial tubes (or unilateral tube and contralateral true pulmonary artery) are made confluent by placing a reinforced 16- to 20-mm Gore-Tex tube graft between them. This graft may be placed behind the ascending aorta to follow the normal course of the right pulmonary artery. The distal anastomosis of the right ventricle-to-pulmonary artery conduit is then made to this transverse reinforced Gore-Tex graft to the left of the aorta (Fig. 80–15). Alternatively, the distal end of the homograft is anastomosed to the left pulmonary artery and a reinforced Gore-Tex graft is placed between the side of the homograft and the right pulmonary artery either in front of or behind the aorta. Following completion of the distal anastomosis, the Dacron graft is bevelled and sutured to the right ventriculotomy. Creating the anastomoses in this fashion places

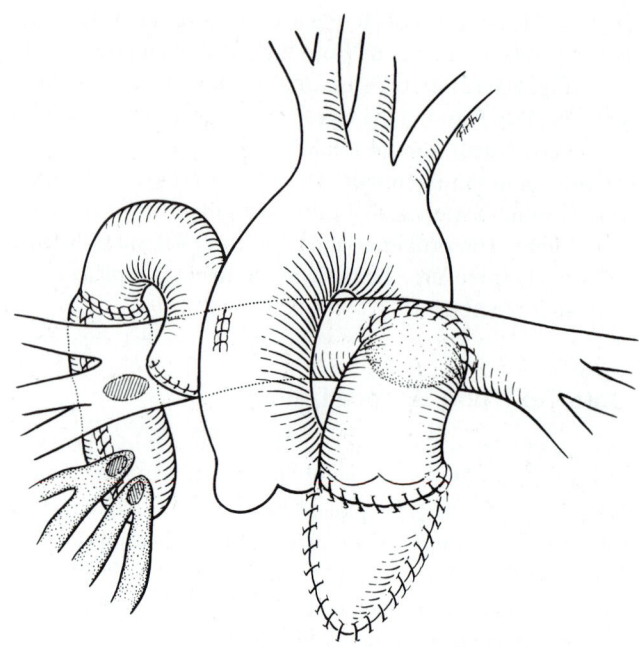

Figure 80–14. Completed definitive repair in a patient with confluent pulmonary arteries. A composite homograft conduit establishes continuity between the right ventricle and pulmonary artery. The anastomosis between the unifocalized collaterals and aorta has been taken down and oversewn. The ventricular septal defect has been closed with a double velour Dacron patch prior to conduit construction. *(From Permut LC, Laks HL: Surgical management of pulmonary atresia with ventricular septal defect and multiple aortopulmonary collaterals. Adv Card Surg 5:75–95, 1994. Reproduced with permission from Mosby-Year Book, Inc.)*

the conduit to the left of the sternum and the homograft valve distal to the shoulder of the right ventricule. This reduces the possibility of compression of the conduit by the sternum. Placing the conduit to the left of the sternum and using a Gore-Tex membrane pericardial substitute greatly facilitates reoperation.

Repair Using a Porcine Valve and Patch

An alternative technique utilizing a porcine bioprosthetic valve may be employed in selected patients. The valve is placed into the right ventricular outflow tract so that approximately one-half or more of the valve area lies below the anterior surface of the heart. A right ventricular outflow patch of Dacron or glutaraldehyde-treated pericardium is constructed. The portion of patch overlying the bioprosthesis is sutured to the valve sewing ring. Because the valve is placed within the right ventricular outflow tract it has a lower profile and a large valve may be inserted. The rigid sewing ring is less susceptible to compression compared with an extracardiac conduit. While there is some concern regarding the durability of the porcine bioprosthesis in the pediatric age group, it is usually possible to use a much larger valve than conduit, and on the low-pressure right side

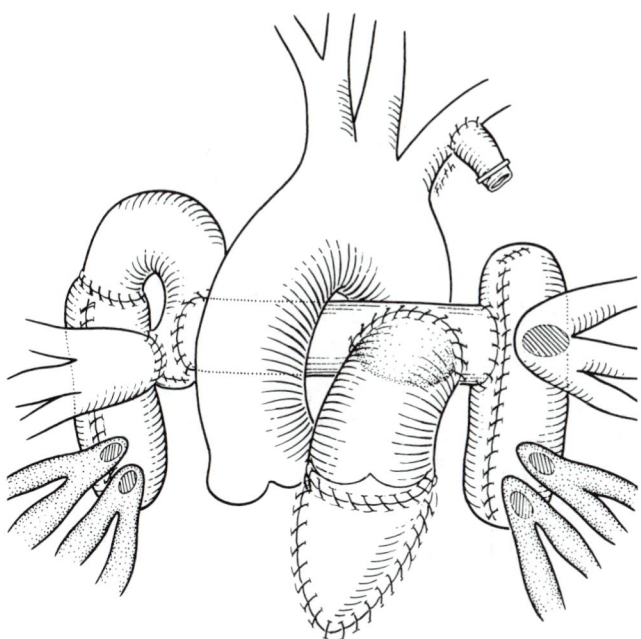

Figure 80–15. Completed definitive repair in a patient with nonconfluent pulmonary arteries. A reinforced Gore-Tex graft is passed behind the ascending aorta to connect the right and left unifocalizations. *(From Permut LC, Laks HL: Surgical management of pulmonary atresia with ventricular septal defect and multiple aortopulmonary collaterals. Adv Card Surg 5:75–95, 1994. Reproduced with permission from Mosby-Year Book, Inc.)*

the long-term durability is excellent.[26] This technique is possible only when the main pulmonary artery is contiguous with the right ventricle, and is particularly suitable for conduit replacement where the posterior bed of the conduit can be used as the posterior wall and a patch may be placed anteriorly.

Measurement of the ratio of right ventricle to left ventricle systolic pressure allows intraoperative assessment of the repair. A ratio of 0.75 or less immediately after termination of cardiopulmonary bypass is acceptable, and the ratio can be expected to decrease to 0.66 or less in the first few days after operation. Higher ratios suggest inadequate pulmonary runoff, and will likely result in eventual right ventricular failure. If the pressure on the right side is near systemic or suprasystemic, perforation of the ventricular septal defect patch may provide reasonable palliation. Patients who are not candidates for definitive repair, usually due to inadequate pulmonary runoff, or who fail definitive repair due to high right ventricular pressure, may be candidates for heart–lung transplantation.[27]

RESULTS

From 1989 to 1993, 18 patients have undergone 21 pericardial tube unifocalization procedures at UCLA Medical Center. An average of 2.7 vessels were unifocalized at each

procedure. There were no early deaths and one late death. Morbidity included bleeding requiring reexploration in 1 patient (5%) and pulmonary contusion requiring prolonged intubation (> 48 hours) in 2 patients (10%). Angiography in all patients prior to definitive repair disclosed patent anastomoses with no significant stenoses. To date, 6 patients have had definitive repair. RV/LV pressure ratio was measured intraoperatively following definitive repair in 4 patients with a mean value of 0.45 (0.33–0.53). There was a single early death secondary to a perioperative cerebral hemorrhage in a 4 year old who had a hemodynamically successful repair. There have been no late deaths, but one patient required heart–lung transplant for right ventricular failure and pulmonary hypertension 3 years after definitive repair. The remaining 4 patients are asymptomatic, or minimally limited in activity. Eleven patients await either contralateral unifocalization or definitive repair.

CONCLUSIONS

Pulmonary atresia and ventricular septal defect is a complex form of congenital heart disease that presents with a wide spectrum of morphologic findings. A staged approach to treatment, individualized for each patient, is required for optimal outcome. The essential features of this approach, as employed at the UCLA Medical Center, are (1) early establishment of right ventricle to pulmonary artery flow to maximize pulmonary artery growth, (2) ligation or embolization of redundant collaterals, (3) unifocalization using the pericardial tube technique, and (4) biventricular repair using a valved conduit. While final assessment of this approach requires analysis of long-term results, we believe that the low morbidity and mortality as well as the inevitable worsening cyanosis and left ventricular volume overload without operation warrant surgical management in all patients whose anatomic findings are amenable to repair.

REFERENCES

1. Sullivan ID, Wren C, Stark J, et al: Surgical unifocalization in pulmonary atresia and ventricular septal defect: A realistic goal? *Circulation* **78**(Suppl III):III5–III13, 1988
2. Stark J: The surgical anatomy of tetralogy of Fallot with pulmonary atresia rather than pulmonary stenosis (Editorial comment). *J Cardiac Surg* **6**:58–59, 1991
3. Anderson RH, Devine WA, DelNido P: The surgical anatomy of tetralogy of Fallot with pulmonary atresia rather than pulmonary stenosis. *J Cardiac Surg* **6**:41–58, 1991
4. Rabinovitch M, Herrera-de Leon V, Castaneda AR, et al: Growth and development of the pulmonary vascular bed in patients with tetralogy of Fallot with or without pulmonary atresia. *Circulation,* **64**:1234–1249, 1981
5. Rabinovitch M: Pathology and anatomy of pulmonary atresia and ventricular septal defect. *Prog Pediatr Cardiol* **1**:9–17, 1992
6. DeRuiter MC, Gittenberger-de Groot AC, Bogers AJJC, Elzenga NJ: The restricted surgical relevance of morphologic criteria to classify

systemic-pulmonary collaterals in pulmonary atresia with ventricular septal defect. *J Thorac Cardiovasc Surg* **108:**692–699, 1994.

7. Marelli AJ, Perloff JK, Child JS, Laks H: Pulmonary atresia and ventricular septal defect in the cyanotic adult. *Circulation* **89:**243–251, 1994

8. Perry SB, Radtke W, Fellows KE, et al: Coil embolization to occlude aortopulmonary collaterals and shunts in patients with congenital heart disease. *J Am Coll Cardiol* **13:**100–108, 1989

9. Puga FJ, Danielson GK: Surgical treatment of pulmonary atresia with a ventricular septal defect. In Arcinegas E (ed): *Pediatric Cardiac Surgery.* Chicago, Year Book Medical, 1985

10. Castaneda AR, Mayer JE, Lock JE: Tetralogy of Fallot, pulmonary atresia, and diminutive pulmonary arteries. *Prog Pediatr Cardiol* **1:**50–60, 1992

11. Rome JJ, Mayer JE, Cartanedo AR, Lock JE: Tetralogy of Fallot with pulmonary atresia: rehabilitation of dimunitive pulmonary arteries. *Circulation* **88** (part I):1691–1698, 1993

12. Puga FG, Uretzky G, McGoon DC: Establishment of right ventricular and hypoplastic pulmonary artery continuity without the use of extracorporeal circulation. *J Thorac Cardiovasc Surg* **83:**74–80, 1982

13. Haas GS, Laks H, Milgalter E: Pulmonary atresia with ventricular septal defect. *Cardiac Surg: State of the Art Reviews* **3:**425–443, 1989

14. Lock JE, Castaneda-Zuniga WR, Fuhrman BP, et al: Balloon dilation angioplasty of hypoplastic and stenotic pulmonary arteries. *Circulation* **67:**962–967, 1983

15. Rosenberg HG, Williams WG, Trusler GA, et al: Structural composition of central pulmonary arteries: Growth potential afer surgical shunts. *J Thorac Cardiovasc Surg* **94:**498–503, 1987

16. Puga FJ, Leoni FE, Julsrud PR, Mair DD: Complete repair of pulmonary atresia, ventricular septal defect, and severe arborization abnormalities of the central pulmonary arteries: Experience with preliminary unifocalization procedures in 38 patients. *J Thorac Cardiovasc Surg* **98:**1018–1029, 1989

17. Barbero-Marcial M, Jatene AD: Surgical management of the anomalies of the pulmonary arteries in the tetralogy of Fallot with pulmonary atresia. *Sem Thorac Cardiovasc Surg* **2:**93–107, 1990

18. Iyer KS, Mee RBBB: Staged repair of pulmonary atresia with ventricular septal defect and major systemic to pulmonary collaterals. *Ann Thorac Surg* **51:**65–72, 1991

19. Benson LN, Laks H, Lois J, et al: Surgical correction of pulmonary atresia and ventricular septal defect with large systemic-pulmonary collaterals. *Ann Thorac Surg* **38:**522–525, 1984

20. Sawatari K, Imai Y, Kurosawa H, et al: Staged operation for pulmonary atresia and ventricular septal defect with major aortopulmonary collaterals: New technique for unifocalization. *J Thorac Cardiovasc Surg* **98:**738–750, 1989

21. Permut LC, Laks H, Haas G, et al: Surgical management of pulmonary atresia and ventricular septal defect with major systemic-pulmonary collaterals. *J Am Coll Cardiol* **15:**79A (abstract), 1990

22. Nakata S, Imai Y, Takanashi Y, et al: A new method for the quantitative standardization of cross-sectional areas of the pulmonary arteries in congenital heart diseases with decreased pulmonary blood flow. *J Thorac Cardiovasc Surg* **88:**610–619, 1984

23. McGoon DC, Baird DK, Davis GD: Surgical management of large bronchial collateral arteries with pulmonary stenosis or atresia. *Circulation* **52:**109–118, 1975

24. Blackstone EH, Shimazaki Y, Maehara T, et al: Prediction of severe obstruction to right ventricular outflow after repair of tetralogy of Fallot and pulmonary atresia. *J Thorac Cardiovasc Surg* **96:**288–293, 1988

25. Kirklin JW, Blackstone EH, Shimazaki Y, et al: Survival, functional status, and reoperations after repair of tetralogy of Fallot with pulmonary atresia. *J Thorac Cardiovasc Surg* **96:**102–116, 1988

26. Razzouk AJ, Williams WG, Cleveland DC, et al: Surgical connections from ventricle to pulmonary artery: Comparison of four types of valved implants. *Circulation* **86**(Suppl II):II154–II158, 1992

27. Kriet JM, Jamieson JW: Transplantation for congenital heart disease with special observations on pulmonary atresia with ventricular septal defect. *Prog Ped Cardiol* **1:**61, 1992

81

Tetralogy of Fallot

Tom R. Karl

Tetralogy of Fallot (TOF) has both historical and immediate relevance for the cardiothoracic surgeon. To place TOF in its proper prospective, one might consider the following points:

1. TOF was the first cyanotic cardiac lesion to be formally described, and much information about its nature had accumulated long before other less complex lesions were well characterized.
2. The first palliative *and* definitive operations for complex congenital heart disease were performed for children with TOF, and the refinements in surgical treatment have run parallel to the development of open heart surgery. TOF is thus the prototype for treatment of complex pediatric cardiac disorders.
3. In the modern era, open heart surgery has converted this lesion from one with an almost uniformly fatal outcome to one with excellent prospects for long-term palliation (if not cure).
4. Treatment of this highly variable and sometimes unpredictable lesion can still be challenging for the cardiac surgical team. Despite decades of study and analysis, issues such as optimal surgical technique, timing of operation, and myocardial protection remain controversial.
5. TOF has played a central role in analysis of the molecular biology of genetic transmission of congenital heart defects.
6. TOF is the first complex cardiac lesion in which large numbers of children have survived to adult life. As such, it has become a model for the study of the "unnatural" history of surgically treated congenital heart disease.

For all of these reasons, TOF has assumed an important role as a benchmark in the treatment of congenital heart disease.

HISTORY

Descriptions of what is now known as TOF appeared as early as the seventeenth century.[1,2] A remarkable description of the clinical features and pathological findings of the malformation, including such phenomena as clubbing, squatting, cyanotic spells, and cerebral abscess and a review of the available literature up to that time, was included in the monograph written by John Farre in 1814, who considered this combination of defects to be the commonest cause of cyanosis. Some 70 years later the comprehensive account of tetralogy, by Fallot himself, appeared in Marseille Medicale in 1888.[3,4] In this pathologic study of 55 patients with "la maladie bleue," Fallot noted the consistently appearing anatomic features of pulmonary stenosis, ventricular septal defect (VSD), rightward position of the aorta relative to the interventricular septum, and hypertrophy of the right ventricle (RV) (Fig. 81–1). Detailed observations of the clinical features and natural history of the lesion appeared over the next century and provided a major stimulus to the development of pediatric cardiology as an independent discipline.

TOF became a surgically important lesion in 1944, when Blalock, Taussig, and Thomas collaborated to conceive and perform the first systemic to pulmonary artery (PA) shunt at Johns Hopkins University (Fig. 81–2). In doing so, they opened the modern era of pediatric cardiac surgery.[5] Other palliative operations to augment pulmonary blood flow were soon developed by Potts, Glenn, Waterston, and other.[6–9] In 1954, Lillehei and co-workers at the University of Minnesota performed the first successful open correction of TOF, initially using cross-circulation between parent and child, and later their own bubble oxygenator.[10] This TOF group included the first patients to undergo patch VSD closure, RV outflow tract reconstruction, correction of pulmonary atresia, ischemic cardiac arrest, and temporary

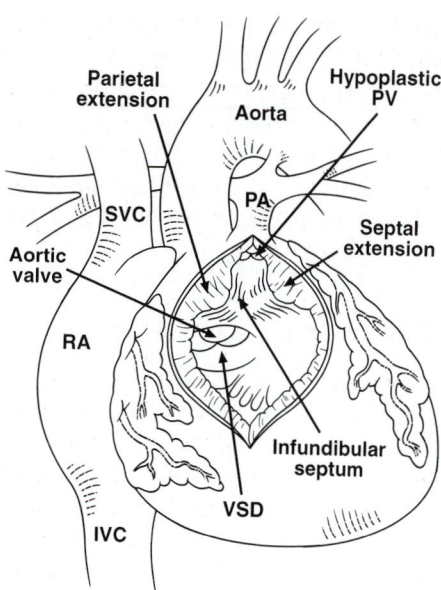

Figure 81–1. Anterior and cephalad displacement of the infundibular septum in tetralogy of Fallot results in malalignment VSD, RVOTO, and right ventricular hypertrophy. The pulmonary arterial tree may show any degree of hypoplasia.

external pacing.[11] The majority of Lillehei's original cohort of TOF patients survive to this day,[11] and have enjoyed good quality of life and freedom from reoperation.

The importance of Dr. Lillehei's pioneering work to all cardiac surgeons and to children with congenital heart disease cannot be overstated. Other major innovators in open correction of TOF include Kirklin, Kay, Ross, Hudspeth, Barratt-Boyes, Castaneda, and others,[12–15] all of whose contributions have been critical to current good results worldwide.

ANATOMIC FEATURES

Developmental Events

Although Fallot's original concept included a combination of four lesions, current thinking implicates anterocephalad deviation of the outlet septum as the primary "cause." The four classical lesions, right ventricular outflow tract obstruction (RVOTO), overriding aorta, malalignment ventricular septal defect (VSD), and right ventricle (RV) hypertrophy can then be explained as consequences. From a surgical viewpoint, such a unifying concept is attractive.

Embryologically, the Fallot complex has been explained by primary malalignment of the conotruncal ridges,[16] "underdevelopment" of the distal RV infundibulum,[17] and anterior displacement of the columns of the aortopulmonary septum relative to the RV outlet.[18] Recently, in studies of the ventriculoarterial junction in human embryos (Carnegie stages 15–19), a similarity between postnatal TOF hearts and stage 18 embryos has been noted.[19] Thus, there is evidence that TOF results from an arrest in rotation of the outflow septum, as compared to the normal heart.

After a century of speculation, it is fair to say that the embryologic events leading to TOF are still somewhat controversial, and the reader is referred to the extensive literature on this subject for further details. In any case, it is the postnatal morphology that is of prime importance to the cardiac surgeon. From this perspective, a description of the most critical features follows.

VSD

The VSD in TOF is typically large (similar in size to the aortic valve) and in 75–80% of cases perimembranous in

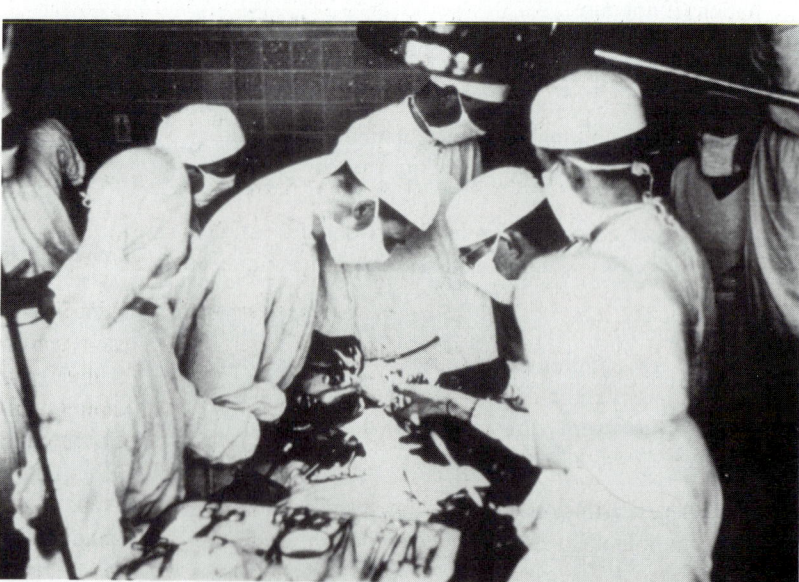

Figure 81–2. Dr. Alfred Blalock performs the first systemic to pulmonary shunt on a 15-month-old girl with tetralogy of Fallot. This procedure took place on November 29, 1944, at Johns Hopkins University. By 1949 over 1000 shunt operations had been performed at that institution. *(Photograph courtesy of Professor Vincent L. Gott.)*

location. The VSD is situated between the infundibular septum and the two limbs of the septomarginal trabecula. The upper border is formed by the aortic valve, which is usually visible to the surgeon looking through the VSD at operation. Inferiorly, the border is formed by the crest of the trabecular septum (Fig. 81–1). Unlike the perimembranous VSD in non-TOF hearts, the VSD in TOF is not in the septal plane, but nearly perpendicular to it (as a consequence of "malalignment"). Consequently, when the VSD has been repaired via the tricuspid valve, the patch usually disappears from the surgeon's view upon removal of the valve leaflet retractors.

In 20% of cases, there may be a muscular ridge separating the VSD from the central fibrous body, protecting the AV conduction tissue from suture injury during VSD closure (see below). Rarely, the VSD may be partly occluded by a flap of accessory leaflet tissue, resulting in a pressure-restrictive interventricular communication. Additional muscular VSDs may be encountered in 3–15% of cases of TOF.[20] Another 10% of patients may have complete absence of the infundibular septum, with a doubly committed subarterial VSD. This lesion is probably most common in Asia and Central America, and, depending on which definition one uses, might be excluded from the TOF group by virtue of absent rather than anterocephalad displacement of the infundibular septum. In such cases, the pulmonary valve annulus is invariably hypoplastic.

Aorta

As in all lesions with restricted pulmonary blood flow, the aorta tends to be quite large. The aortic arch courses to the right of the trachea (but descends in the left hemi thorax) in 25% of TOF patients, most of whom also have mirror image branching of the head vessels. The aorta overrides the VSD, i.e., has a biventricular origin, and is rotated clockwise. The degree of aortic commitment to the RV varies from 15 to 95%.[21] Cardiologists and surgeons who define double outlet right ventricle (DORV) on the basis of the so-called "50% rule" frequently include those examples with more marked overriding of the aorta within the category of DORV, though this does not necessarily exclude them from the TOF group, as the two categories (DORV and TOF) overlap. Some morphologists prefer to use the presence of discontinuity between the aortic and mitral valves ("double conus"), even though such hearts resemble TOF in other respects, as the main determinant of double outlet right ventricle.[22,23] Such hearts have a greater tendency toward having a small LV and mitral valve, restrictive VSD, and multiple VSDs.

Conduction Tissue

As in other hearts with concordant AV connections and perimembranous VSD, the His bundle in TOF emerges posteriorly from the right fibrous trigone, beneath the noncoronary aortic cusp. The fibers run around the inferior margin of the VSD, toward the left side of the septum. In patients with a muscle bar running between the VSD and the central fibrous body, the main bundle courses posterior to the VSD and on the leftward side of the septum. Although this theoretically affords some protection during VSD suture placement, in practice the technique does not vary from that used in closure of a perimembranous VSD.

Right Ventricle and Outflow Tract

The hypertrophic RV wall is similar in thickness to that of the left ventricle (LV) and the RV end diastolic volume may be reduced. The leftward (septal) end of the infundibular septum inserts more anteriorly and leftward than in a normal heart, in front of the septal band (septomarginal trabeculum), rather than between its divisions.[17,24] The rightward (parietal) end is rotated anteriorly so that the infundibular septum and its parietal extensions are in a nearly sagittal plane. Secondary hypertrophy of muscle bands adds to the degree of RVOTO, and is age related. These muscle bands include the outlet septum itself, the anterior limb of the septomarginal trabecula, and connections between the RV free wall and infundibular septum, in addition to various anomalous muscle bundles within the RV cavity. Occasionally, a localized prominent low lying muscle band creates a discrete outlet chamber (double chambered RV) with a fibrotic "os infundibulum." The latter can be mistaken for a VSD at operation.

Further along the RVOT, most TOF hearts will have obstruction at the pulmonary valve level as well. Approximately 75% of cases have some degree of valvar pulmonary stenosis, and two-thirds have a bicuspid valve.[25,26] The pulmonary valve "ring" is a largely muscular rather than fibrous structure and is usually hypoplastic relative to aortic annulus size and body weight. In assessing the annulus size, it should be borne in mind that the pulmonary annulus diameter varies during the cardiac cycle. In 15–20% of cases the pulmonary valve and/or the infundibulum is congenitally atretic. Pulmonary atresia in TOF may also be acquired, typically following systemic-pulmonary shunt procedures.[27,28] The distribution of sites of obstruction varies with age, but by the second decade 96% have subvalvar, 84% valvar, and 33% supravalvar RVOTO.[29]

Pulmonary Arterial Tree

Pulmonary artery hypoplasia is the rule in TOF (Fig. 81–3). The hypoplasia tends to be central rather than peripheral, and is extremely variable in degree. Discrete stenoses may complicate the picture, occurring, in order of frequency, at the bifurcation, main pulmonary artery (PA), right or left PA, centrally and peripherally together, and peripherally only. The main PA or either branch may be atretic or discontinuous, most commonly on the left side. Bronchial arteries can contribute significant flow to the pulmonary arte-

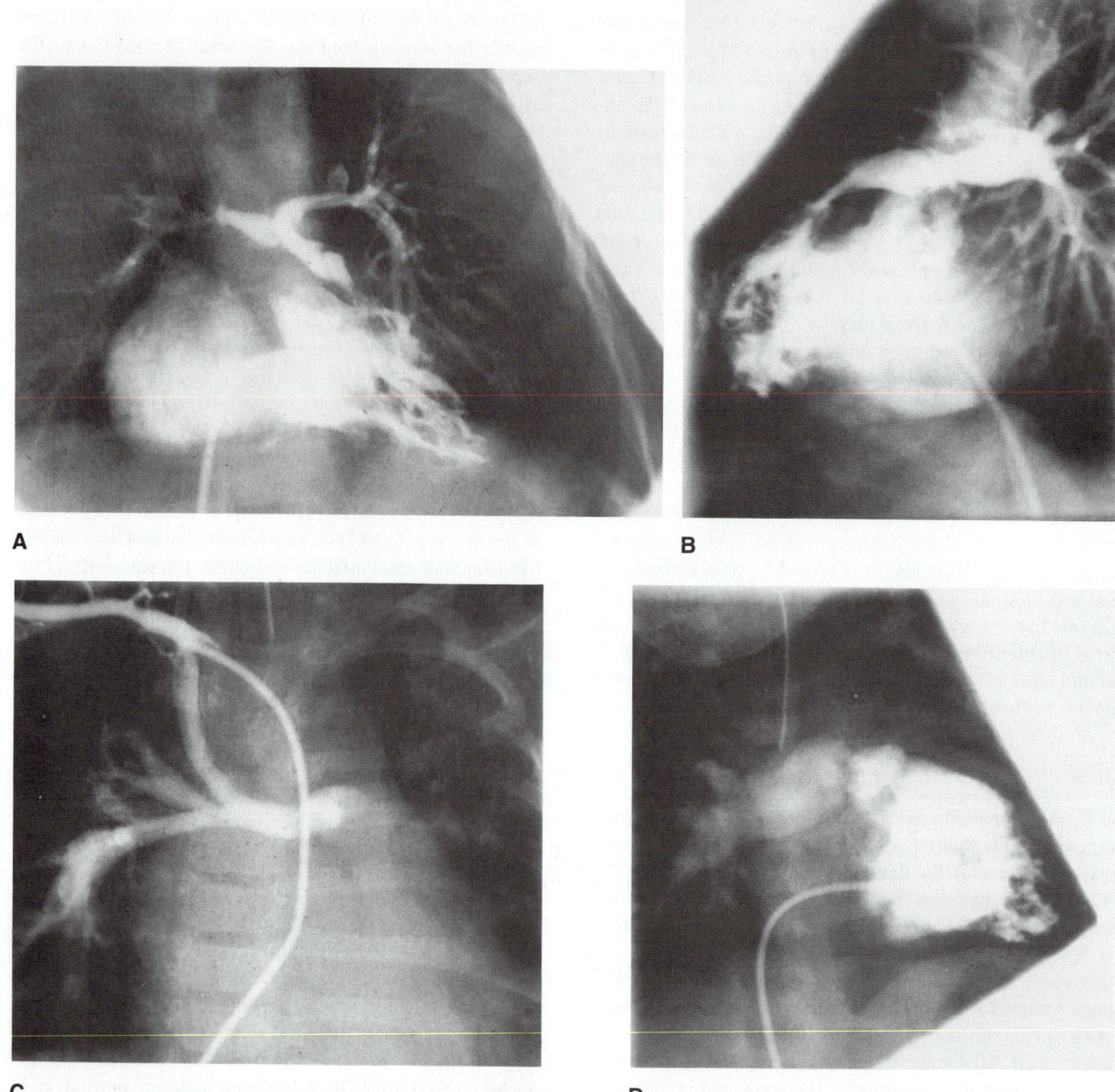

A

B

C

D

Figure 81–3. Cineangiography in tetralogy of Fallot. **A.** Hypoplastic main and branch PAs. The pulmonary valve is small, and the subvalvar outflow tract is likewise severely stenotic. **B.** Severe hypertrophy of infundibular septum, with near-obliteration of RVOT in systole. The pulmonary valve itself is not severely stenotic. **C.** Moderately hypoplastic RPA filled by a modified Blalock–Taussig shunt. Proximal shunt placement on the RPA reduces the changes of branch stenosis. **D.** Absent pulmonary valve syndrome, with moderate RVOTO, free pulmonary regurgitation, and marked dilation of main and branch PAs.

rial tree in TOF, but are to be distinguished from major aortopulmonary collateral arteries (MAPCAs). The latter vessels are most commonly encountered in pulmonary atresia with VSD, hypoplastic central PAs, and major PA arborization defects (this topic is discussed in detail in Chap. 79). MAPCAs are persistent segmental arteries rather than part of the bronchial arterial network, the latter vessels not being strongly associated with arborization defects (see below). In older TOF patients, additional collateral arterial supply is derived from intercostal and other chest wall arterial branches. Collateral circulation of this type presents problems during operation, as maintenance of perfusion pressure and left heart decompression can be difficult.

The pre- and intra-acinar PAs in TOF are small compared to normal, and have a thinner media.[30–33] ^{99m}Tc-labeled albumin scans have demonstrated abnormalities of distribution of pulmonary blood flow in TOF (pre- and postoperatively), both in right versus left and within each lung.[34] Total lung volume, alveolar size, and alveolar number are all reduced as compared to normal. The fact that most alveolar and PA growth is complete by 2 years of age has been used in arguments favoring early repair of TOF,[36,38] as a means to maximize alveolar and PA development by increasing antegrade pulmonary blood flow.

Left Ventricle

The LV in TOF varies in end diastolic volume, and there is a tendency toward hypoplasia in severe cases.[25,35–37] This can be of surgical significance, as biventricular repair may be inadvisable under circumstances of extreme LV hypoplasia. For clinical purposes, the LV may be considered hypoplastic if the cardiac apex is formed by the RV rather than LV and if the mitral annulus (normalized to the patient's body surface area) is more than 2 standard deviations below mean normal.

Coronary Arteries

Coronary artery anomalies are found in 5–12% of patients with TOF.[38] Most frequently, the left anterior descending artery arises from the right coronary artery and crosses the RVOT inferiorly to the pulmonary valve. This anomaly is of great importance to the surgeon, as, during repair, the safe inferior extension of a transannular incision in the RVOT will be limited. Other coronary anomalies encountered in TOF include right coronary artery from left coronary artery, left coronary artery from PA, single coronary from the left sinus, and accessory left anterior descending from the right coronary artery.[38] "Acquired" anomalies, such as an enlarged conus branch of right coronary artery and coronary-bronchial collaterals, may be encountered, and will also have implications for conduct of cardiopulmonary bypass and myocardial protection during corrective surgery.

Associated Anomalies and Fallot Variants

Coexisting cardiac lesions noted at the time of complete repair of "classical" TOF with pulmonary stenosis in the Royal Children's Hospital (RCH) series,[39] in order of frequency, include the following: left superior vena cava (SVC) (7%), atrioventricular (A-V) septal defect (5%), patent ductus arteriosus (PDA) (3.3%), atrial septal defect (ASD) (2.7%), anomalous course of a coronary artery (2.4%), discontinuous left PA (1%), interrupted inferior vena cava (IVC) (0.8%), and aorticopulmonary (AP) window, common atrium, mitral stenosis, straddling mitral valve, PAPVD, and TAPVD (all 0.2%). None of these lesions precludes successful repair, although operative risk and long-term prognosis may be affected.

Pulmonary atresia with VSD is characterized by hy-

poplasia of the central and peripheral PAs, often with MAPCAs and arborization defects. The main PA may be absent (approximately 5%) or the branches may be nonconfluent or stenotic (20–30%). Cases with ductus rather than MAPCA-dependent PA supply are anatomically similar to TOF, although timing and technique of surgery may be quite different. The subject of pulmonary atresia with VSD is covered in detail in Chapter 79.

Atrioventricular septal defect may complicate TOF in 5–6.5% of cases, and is more likely to be found in patients with Down's syndrome.[40] Atrioventricular valve anatomy is similar to that of non-TOF A-V septal defects, but the inlet VSD extends far into the outlet septum, with a varying degree of RVOTO. Features of DORV may be present. Timing and technique of repair are discussed below.

The *absent pulmonary valve syndrome* (APVS) is a Fallot variant characterized by combined pulmonary stenosis and incompetence with aneurysmal dilation of the main and branch PAs, usually including the main lobar branches at the lung hilum. The pulmonary valve leaflets are rudimentary, and moderate RVOTO, with hypoplasia of the pulmonary valve annulus, is usually present (Fig. 81-4). Characteristically, the ductus arteriosus is absent in this group and the gross dilatation of the central pulmonary arteries may be related to pulmonary insufficiency in the absence of the ductus, which would otherwise allow runoff into the descending aorta during fetal life.[41,42]

Intrinsic abnormalities of the PA wall and the ventriculoarterial junction are also found in APVS.[42–45] In the symptomatic infants, the central feature is usually airway compression and tracheobronchomalacia, affecting the major lobar bronchi.[41] Intrinsic airway problems as well as vascular abnormalities may persist out to the level of small bronchi. Reduction of the central PA diameter, in an attempt to decompress the major bronchi, may therefore not completely relieve the respiratory problems.

Cellular and Ultrastructure Abnormalities

Multiple ultrastructural abnormalities in the myocardium of children with TOF have been described, independent of secondary hypertrophy or hypoxic damage.[46] LV myocytes are abnormally sized and have an increased number of large mitochondria, ribosomes, and Golgi complexes, and lysosomes.[47] T-tubules may be dilated and tortuous, with abnormal folding and convolution of nuclear membranes.[48] Older individuals with TOF may have variable degrees of myofibrillar degeneration, with alterations in surface membrane integrity in both myocytes and capillaries.[48]

RV myocardium, as compared to that of normal children, has similar adrenergic fiber and β-receptor content, but a significantly greater number of α-receptors.[49] Acetylcholine and calcitonin gene-related polypeptide containing neurons are decreased in number. Abnormalities of temporal expression of myosin light chain isotypes have also been described in TOF myocardium.[46] While the complete clini-

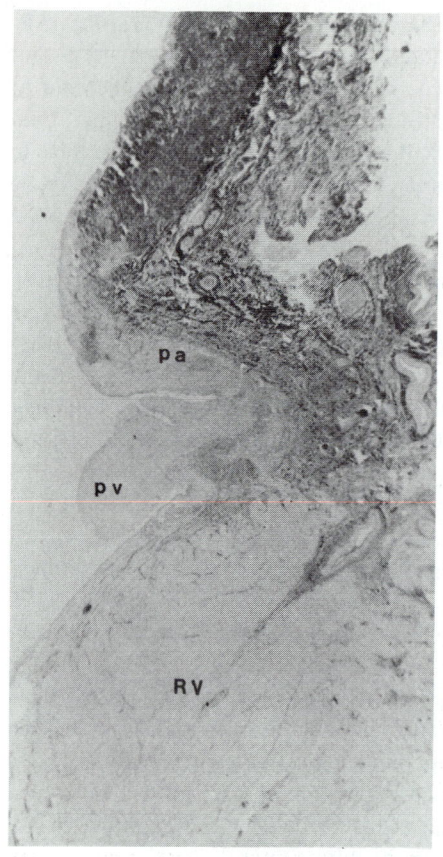

A

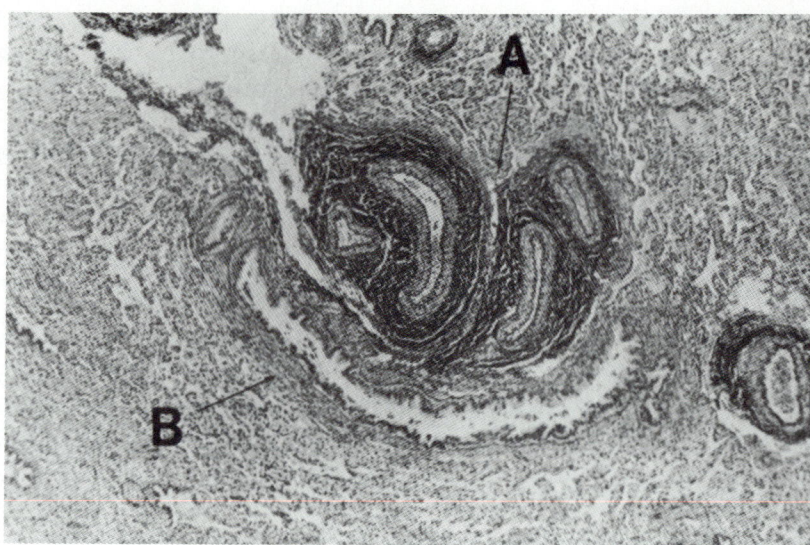

B

Figure 81–4. Absent pulmonary valve syndrome (APVS). **A.** Section (×12) taken through ventriculoarterial junction of an infant with APVS. The valve tissue (pv) is represented by rudimentary nodules. The pulmonary artery (pa) lacks the normal RV myocardial support, and the proximal PA portion is deficient in elastin. **B.** Cross section of lung from an infant with APVS showing distortion of the bronchus by a leash of abnormal muscular arteries. Tracheobronchial compression in APVS is encountered more proximally as well, consequent to aneurysmal dilation of the main and branch PAs.

cal ramifications of such findings remain uncertain at this writing, the evidence for abnormalities in both RV and LV myocardium in TOF continues to accumulate.

Of extreme importance to the surgeon are the implications of chronic hypoxemia for reperfusion injury following ischemic arrest. Reduced myocardial activity of superoxide dismutase, catalase, and glutathione peroxidase (the myocardial "antioxidant" enzymes) has been observed in TOF,[50] as well as in myocyte cultures grown at low pO_2.[51] Levels of these enzymes appear to correlate with preoperation pO_2. In cell culture, myocytes grown at reduced pO_2 (40 mm) are more sensitive to hypoxanthine–guanine oxidase-mediated free radical injury than are those cultured at 150 mm.[51] Glutathione peroxidase mRNA levels were lower in TOF myocytes cultured at 40 mm pO_2 than were those cultured at 150 mm, suggesting that production of this enzyme may be regulated by O_2 tension at the RNA transcription level.[54] Finally, myocardial biopsy analysis in patients undergoing TOF repair would suggest that despite cardioplegic hypothermic arrest, a drop in ATP levels is seen after reperfusion, accompanied by increased lactate levels. Both are correlates of a defect in oxidative metabolism, with subsequent postischemic reperfusion injury.[53] Right ventricular failure following TOF repair may occur due to acute volume loading following damage caused by resection, ventriculotomy, suture placement, and new pul-

monary and/or tricuspid incompetence. In this context, these cellular and ultrastructural abnormalities may be of critical importance in influencing the course of recovery.

EPIDEMIOLOGY AND GENETICS

TOF is found in 6% of infants with congenital heart disease, and the prevalence is 3.9–8.6%, depending on how TOF is defined. TOF also occurs in horses, rats, cattle, dogs, and probably other mammals as well.

TOF is sporadic and nonfamilial in 95% of cases, but occurs with greater frequency (3%) in sibs of patients with TOF than in the general population.[54,55] Also, there is a recurrence risk of 4% if 1 parent has TOF.[54] The incidence of *congenital heart disease* in offspring of a parent affected with TOF is 7.3%.[11] These latter figures may be revised, as we see larger numbers of children with TOF surviving through child-bearing age.

Irrefutable evidence of a genetic basis for TOF is lacking. WKY/NCr rats develop a TOF-like syndrome spontaneously, and the inheritance appears to be autosomal recessive (or dominant with incomplete penetrance). The genetic syndrome has variable expression and may therefore be polygenic. Inheritance of conotruncal defects (including TOF) in Keeshond dogs suggests a defect at a single autosomal locus, interfering with myocardial growth in the conotruncus and resulting in failure of formation of the conotruncal septum in homozygotes.

In humans, a weak familial tendency has been demonstrated, as noted above. Rarely, stronger familial clustering has been noted in children of nonconsanguineous parents (e.g., multiple sibs with TOF).[56,57] It is likely that in *non-syndromal* TOF, inheritance and expression are polygenic and multifactorial, with the possible existence of a rare autosomal recessive form.

TOF, more than other congenital heart defects, is likely to be associated with major extracardiac anomalies.[58,59] The associated defects may be severe, including cleft lip and palate, hypospadias, and skeletal and craniofacial abnormalities. A partial list of known TOF associations is given in Table 81–1. Many of these syndromes have a stronger genetic pattern than isolated TOF, supporting a hereditary basis, at least in this context. The strongest association may be the San Luis Valley recombinant chromosome 8 syndrome, in which 93.3% of afflicted infants have congenital heart disease, 40.5% of which is TOF.[60]

Facial dysmorphism, whether associated with a named syndrome or not, is a prominent feature in conotruncal abnormalities, TOF included.[61] Features may include hypertelorism, low set ears, small mouth, short philtrum, and micrognathia.[62] In the embryo, the cardiac outflow tracts, aortic arches, face, and thymus develop together, and all receive migrating neural crest cells. It is not surprising, therefore, that in conotruncal malformations, including TOF, immunocompetence may be affected. Although clinical DiGeorge syndrome is rare in TOF, low levels of T-lymphocytes, complement and immunoglobulins may frequently be found, especially in patients with facial anomalies.[63] Among patients with DiGeorge syndrome, 20% have TOF.[64] There is a strong phenotypic overlap of DiGeorge syndrome and velocardiofacial syndrome (VCFS).[65,66] In the latter syndrome, there is an 85% incidence of congenital heart disease, and a strong TOF association. Both syndromes are now known to be consequences of 22q11 monosomy or interstitial deletion.[67–70] Because surgical correction and prolonged survival will increase the likelihood of transmission of a chromosomal deletion, the incidence of syndromic (and heritable) TOF is likely to increase.

Environmental factors may also be associated with TOF. The administration of bis-diamine to pregnant rats causes TOF in the fetus. Thalidomide has been similarly implicated in humans.[71]

Physiology and Clinical Presentation

Most children with TOF have equalization of RV and LV pressure, the exception being cases in which an accessory leaflet or membranous flap partially obstructs the VSD (allowing RV pressure to become suprasystemic). The subset of patients with minimal RV outflow tract obstruction may have no net shunt or even a left-to-right shunt, and not develop cyanosis during infancy or early childhood (acyanotic or pink tetralogy). Such children may present in congestive heart failure if a large left-to-right shunt is present. The majority of children with unrestrictive VSD will have enough obstruction at one or more levels in the RVOT to result in a net right-to-left shunt at the ventricular level, though this may not be sufficient to produce clinically apparent cyanosis early in infancy. With the resultant limitation of pulmonary blood flow, pulmonary pressure is usually normal or low. Cyanosis is a central feature of TOF, the degree varying with the ratio of total pulmonary resistance to systemic resistance. In TOF, total pulmonary resistance may be considered to be the resistance of the obstructed RVOT plus that of the distal pulmonary bed. The degree of cyanosis is also affected by presence of alternate sources of pulmonary blood flow (e.g., bronchial collaterals, MAPCAs).

The RVOTO in TOF is usually progressive and dynamic, and the shunt characteristics may change with time, due both to gradual increase in obstruction and to acute changes related to other factors that may affect the dynamics from hour to hour, day to day, or even within a given cardiac cycle. Cyanosis tends to increase with activity, because fixed or increasing RVOTO prevents a pulmonary bloodflow increase with increasing systemic flow (the latter responding to a drop in peripheral vascular resistance). In cases with pulmonary atresia, RVOTO is fixed and pulmonary bloodflow varies only with the amount of collateral flow to the lungs (and therefore with systemic arterial pressure and pulmonary vascular resistance). $HbSO_2$ in TOF also varies directly with mean arterial pressure, even in the absence of pulmonary atresia.

TABLE 81–1. FACTORS AND SYNDROMES ASSOCIATED WITH TOF

DiGeorge syndrome
VACTERL syndrome
Down's syndrome
Turner's syndrome
Noonan's syndrome
XXX syndrome
Velocardiofacial syndrome
Diabetic embryopathy
Goldenhar syndrome
Facial dysmorphism (nonsyndromic)
Klippel–Feil syndrome
Cornelia de Lange syndrome
Low birthweight
CHARGE association
Maternal thalidomide administration
Fetal alcohol syndrome
Maternal antiepileptic drugs
San Luis Valley Recombinant chromosome 8 syndrome

Cyanosis in TOF is usually present by 6 weeks to 6 months of age. If seen in the newborn, pulmonary atresia with duct dependency might be suspected. Hypercyanotic "spells" have long been recognized as being associated with TOF, but in fact may occur with other cyanotic lesions as well. Spells vary in severity and duration, and may occur spontaneously or in response to activity, fright, injury, sepsis, a general anesthetic, or other stimuli. Spells are characterized by profound cyanosis, hyperventilation, and metabolic acidosis. The "cause" is probably increased cardiac contractility due to endogenous catecholamine production and changes in sympathetic tone. The resultant exacerbation of RVOTO often coupled with a coinciding fall in systemic vascular resistance associated with factors such as muscle activity, increasing hypoxia, and acidosis. Tachycardia and decreased blood volume may also acutely increase the right-to-left shunt, and contribute to the severity of spells. Equally important is the acute reduction in end diastolic ventricular volume seen with hypovolemia (due to dehydration or vasodilation), tachycardia, loss of atrioventricular synchrony, and other factors. Improvement is seen with treatment aimed at increasing ventricular preload or slowing the heart rate to allow increased diastolic filling time. The hyperpnea associated with spells is a manifestation of the acute hypoxia and discomfort of the situation, which itself exacerbates the catecholamine and sympathetic surge, augmenting the right-to-left shunt, and contributing further to acidosis by increasing the work of breathing.

Children with TOF instinctively squat or assume the knee chest position to increase $HbSO_2$. By increasing the intra-abdominal pressure, a brief but nonsustained rise in venous return to the heart is produced. At the same time, an increase in systemic arterial resistance favors pulmonary rather than systemic bloodflow.

Factors that may exacerbate cyanosis in TOF are summarized in Table 81–2.

Natural History

Without specific surgical treatment, 25–35% of children with TOF will die in the first year of life, 40–50% by year

TABLE 81–2. SOME FACTORS THAT MAY INCREASE CYANOSIS IN TOF

Anemia
Exercise
Acidosis
Increased cardiac contractility
β-Adrenergic drugs
Systemic hypotension/vasodilation
General anaesthesia
Decreased blood volume/dehydration
Ductal closure in the newborn
Infection
Stress
Posture

3, 70–76% by year 10, 90% by year 21, and 95% by year 40.[72,73] Survival without treatment, while rare, has been documented into the seventh and eighth decades. Surgical treatment of TOF in some of these older patients has been surprisingly successful. The natural history is worse for patients with Fallot variants such as pulmonary atresia and absent pulmonary valve syndrome, the majority of whom will die in the neonatal or infant period without treatment.

Children with TOF have delayed somatic growth and development compared to their peers, even with effective palliation.[74,75] Two-thirds remain below the 16th percentile for height and weight. Undoubtedly, some of these problems are attributable to associated noncardiac conditions.

The ongoing morbidity and mortality in TOF is primarily due to consequences of chronically low pO_2. In naturally balanced or palliated TOF, the Hb level usually runs in the 15–17 g/dl range, which is well tolerated. When the Hb rises above that level, increasing blood viscosity is associated with an escalating risk of neurologic complications. Intravascular thrombosis, systemic embolization, bacteremia, and brain abscess all may contribute to severe and permanent cerebral damage, either spontaneously or as a complication of invasive procedures. Delayed intellectual and motor development and seizures may also result.[76] EEG abnormalities have been found in 50% of patients with TOF.[77] A relative anemia can also contribute to some of these neurologic sequelae.

Another correlate of chronic hypoxemia is coagulopathy, especially at Hb levels above 18 g/dl. Prolonged prothrombin time, and low platelet counts and fibrinogen levels are of particular concern to the surgeon planning an operation involving cardiopulmonary bypass. These abnormalities are probably due to subclinical disseminated intravascular coagulation.[78,79] Hyperuricemia may occur as a consequence of polycythemia and increased RBC turnover, with clinical sequelae of gout and urate nephropathy.

Congestive heart failure is uncommon in infancy or early childhood, but may develop late in the course of TOF, due to the progressive myocardial changes outlined above. The risk of surgical treatment, when carried out at a stage when such deterioration is already well established, will increase accordingly. Infectious endocarditis occurs in TOF (as in any other complex lesion), but the true incidence is probably unknown. Ten percent of patients surviving 10 years after a Blalock shunt have developed this complication.[80]

Finally, life threatening hemoptysis may develop spontaneously in TOF due to rupture of enlarged bronchial collateral arteries, with bleeding into the airway.

The unnatural history of TOF (i.e., following early repair) is so superior to the natural history that it is somewhat rare to encounter an older patient with TOF today in parts of the world where access to medical care is available for all children. Hence, the problems noted above have been greatly attenuated, but continue to challenge surgeons working in less developed areas of the world.

Diagnosis

Physical findings are not specific for TOF, but may be helpful in the differential diagnosis of cyanosis. As mentioned above, the degree of cyanosis varies with anatomy and age. Because cyanosis is impossible to quantitate visually, and highly subjective, confirmation of low $HbSO_2$ with pulse oximetry is highly desirable for initial diagnosis. It should be noted, however, that the true $HbSO_2$ may be overestimated at values < 0.8.[81] Clubbing may be present after infancy. The features peculiar to a given associated syndrome may be the predominant findings for TOF occurring in that context. Cardiac auscultation usually reveals a crescendo–decrescendo systolic murmur, loudest at the upper left sternal border. The intensity varies with the degree of RVOTO and the cardiac output to the PA, and the murmur may be diminished during a cyanotic spell. The pulmonary component of the second heart sound is usually absent in cyanotic TOF. The presence of a continuous to-and-fro murmur may suggest the presence of collaterals. The chest x-ray shows a normal cardiothoracic ratio with a concave pulmonary segment and, in some cases, an uptilted apex, which may give the cardiac silhouette a resemblance to a Dutch clog (coeur en sabot), often referred to as a "boot shaped" heart (Fig. 81–5). This x-ray silhouette reflects RV hypertrophy and a concave upper left heart border due to a small or absent main PA. Additionally there are usually diminished pulmonary vascular markings (pulmonary oligemia). Characteristically this x-ray picture (coeur en sabot) is seen with the extreme forms of TOF, especially with pulmonary atre-

sia. In the more common variants of TOF the cardiac contour is often not dramatically abnormal. The ECG usually shows RV hypertrophy and right axis deviation, the former more obvious in older patients.

The "gold standard" for quick and accurate noninvasive diagnosis is two-dimensional (2D) echocardiography. The accuracy of echo diagnosis has been confirmed at surgery.[82] Currently, prenatal echo diagnosis of TOF is possible as early as 16–18 wk gestation. Caution is advisable, however, as the prognosis offered for TOF in early pregnancy may not be accurate for extrauterine life, due to evolution of the lesion.[83] A higher surgical mortality has been noted for infants and children whose initial diagnosis was made prenatally, probably due to the higher incidence of related chromosomal and extracardiac anomalies in that group.[85]

Echocardiography in TOF can be used to delineate many of the fine points of pathologic anatomy (Fig. 81–6). Aortic override of the septum, enlargement of the aortic root, and aortic-mitral continuity are apparent in the parasternal long axis view, while the hallmark anterocephalad displacement of the outlet septum can be seen in the short axis. Other points, which can be outlined in many cases with 2D echo/Doppler studies, include the level and severity of RVOTO, location, type, and number of VSDs, size and shape of both ventricles, anatomy of the pulmonary valve, main, and branch PAs, collateral sources of pulmonary blood flow, A-V valve anatomy and function, caval connections, and aortic arch anatomy. In some cases, coronary artery configuration can be outlined with echo as

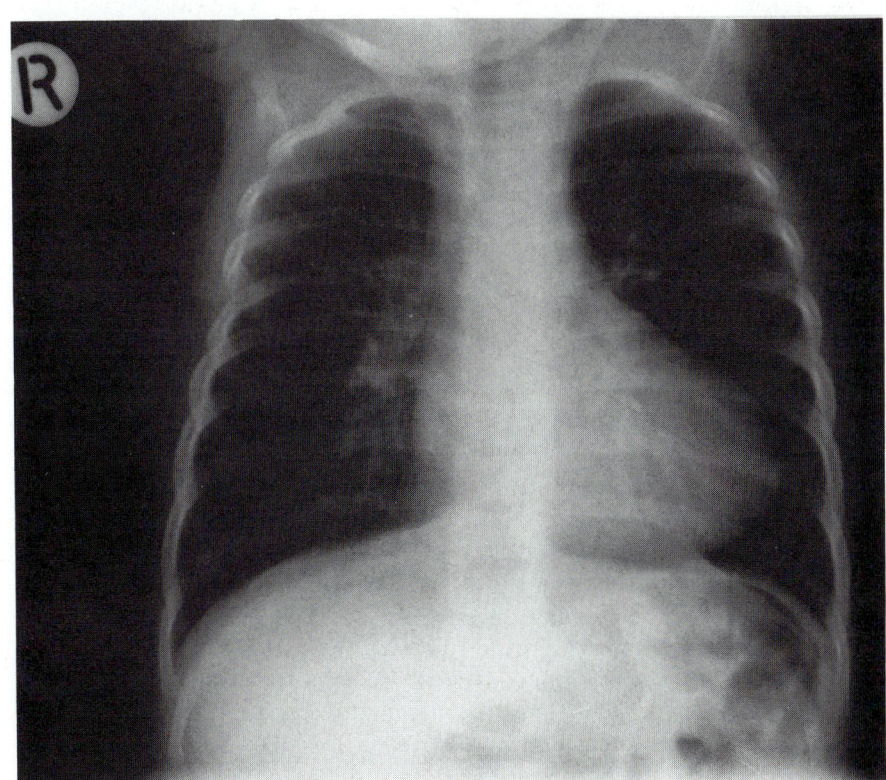

Figure 81–5. *"Coeur en sabot"* cardiac silhouette in tetralogy of Fallot. The upturned apex and concave left heart border reflect RV hypertrophy and a small main PA. Pulmonary vascular markings are diminished.

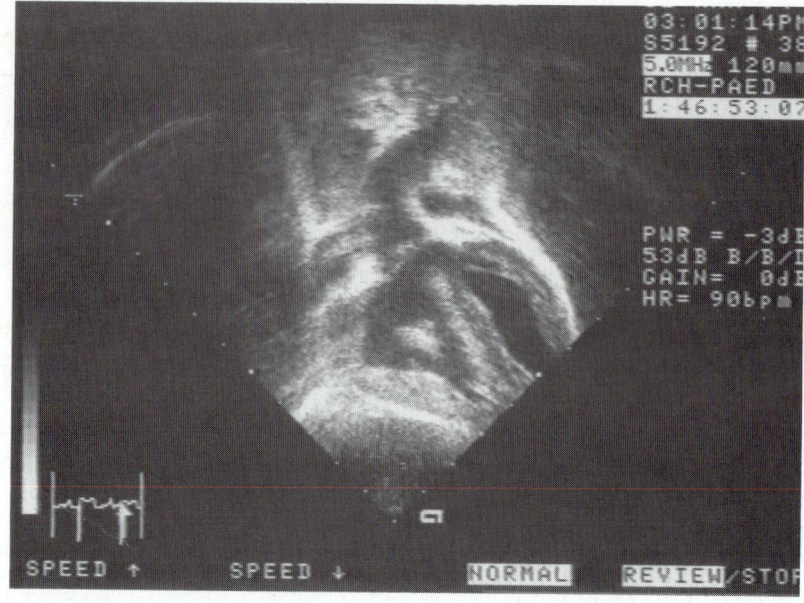

A

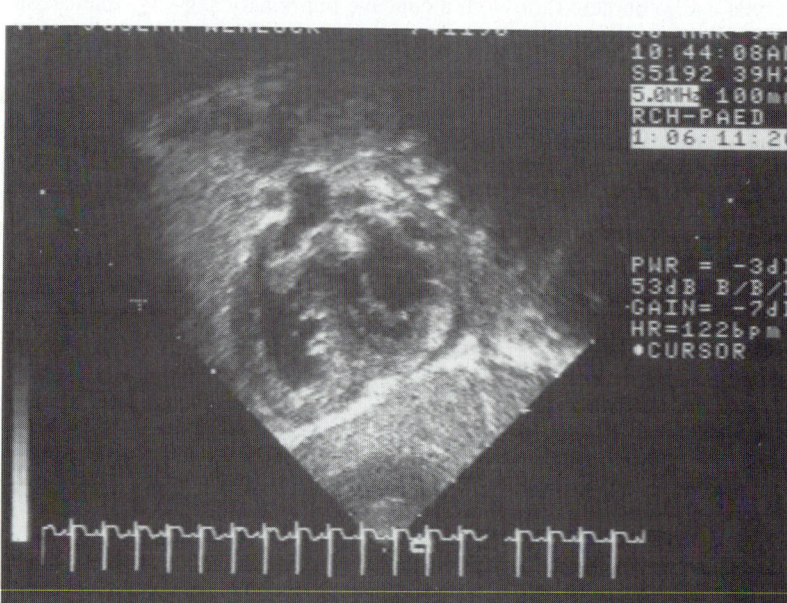

B

Figure 81–6. Echocardiographic features of tetralogy of Fallot. **A.** Subcostal coronal view demonstrating >50% override of aorta (relative to ventricular septum), as well as RV hypertrophy. The large aorta is also typical for tetralogy. **B.** Subcostal sagittal view showing anterior and cephalad deviation of outlet septum relative to inferior septum, with consequent narrowing of the RVOTO.

well.[84] Transgastric views obtained with the transesophageal probe may provide additional information.

Whether echo diagnosis provides adequate information to allow the surgeon to plan a palliative or definitive operation remains a point of debate. The resolution depends heavily on local experience, expertise, and the availability of high quality equipment. The weak points of echo diagnosis include the presence of additional VSDs and coronary artery anomalies. Anatomy of the pulmonary arteries, beyond the proximal branches, cannot be adequately assessed and this is particularly a problem with those forms of extreme TOF or pulmonary atresia where arborization anomalies exist. At the Royal Children's Hospital, 2D echo diag-

nosis is considered adequate for most palliative operations (i.e., modified Blalock shunts), but cardiac catheterization is generally performed prior to making decisions about definitive repair.[39] This approach varies worldwide, and currently about 25% of major pediatric centers perform TOF correction without cardiac catheter studies in the majority of their patients.

Magnetic resonance imaging (MRI) can provide good delineation of aortic and RVOT anatomy, VSD, RV hypertrophy, PAs, and in some cases, collateral circulation and shunt patency[85] (Fig. 81–7). Such MRI information has also correlated well with catheter and surgical findings.[86] Hemodynamic information may also be obtained with MRI

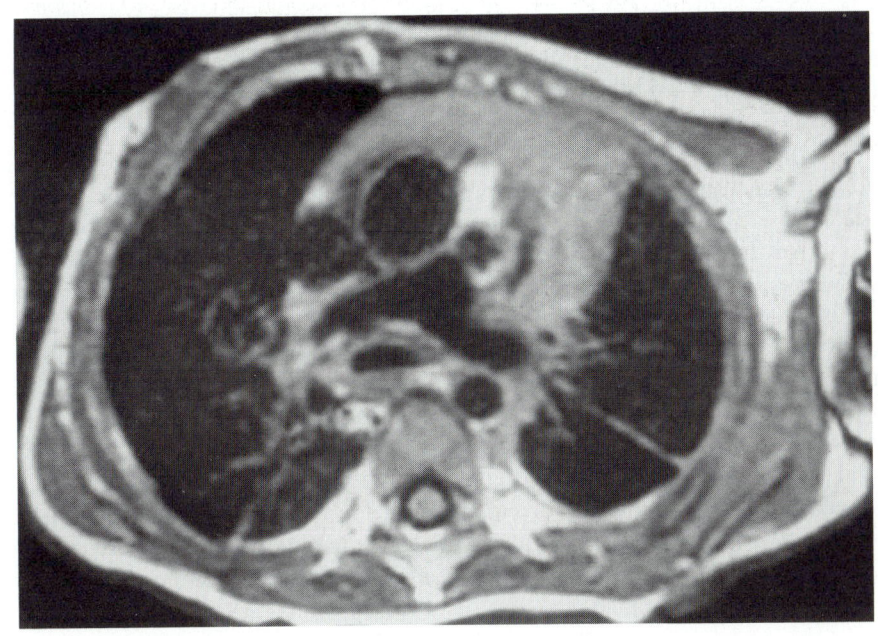

Figure 81–7. Magnetic resonance imaging in tetralogy of Fallot: This cardiac gated T-1 weighted spin echo sequence demonstrates confluent branch PAs with a severe stenosis just proximal to the bifurcation of the LPA. This area could not be imaged on angiography, as contrast selectively filled the RPA. Also evident are valvar pulmonary stenosis and aortic enlargement.

blood flow velocity mapping.[87] The disadvantages of MRI are the long imaging times, and requirement for a general anesthetic in small children, which is made more difficult by the inability to observe the patient when enclosed in the MRI tunnel and the necessity to use special nonmetallic equipment.

For a detailed elective diagnosis, cardiac catheterization and cineangiography will provide good information. The procedure is not risk free, however, and one cannot overemphasize the value of having an experienced cardiac anesthetist present. A child who is at risk of spells needs to be well sedated (usually with morphine) prior to induction of anesthesia and to be kept well asleep and pain free throughout the procedure. Hemodynamic data to be obtained include atrial, ventricular, and pulmonary artery pressures, cardiac output, and shunt quantification. Generally, a 20–30° (from the AP) RAO view, with 15° craniocaudal tilt, gives the best view of the RVOT obstruction, while a left anterior oblique view, with 20–30° craniocaudal tilt, is optimal for the VSD. Details of levels of stenosis, additional VSDs, coronary anatomy, ventricular function, PA anatomy, arch and head vessels, and collateral circulation (including MAPCAs) should be obtainable in nearly every case. Such information is extremely useful in making decisions about timing of complete repair and surgical approach, but as mentioned above, much of it can be obtained with 2D echo.

SURGICAL TREATMENT

The timing of complete repair remains a controversial subject and varies from center to center. It is clear that good early results can be achieved in selected patients in all age groups, newborn to septagenarians. We currently perform elective repair of TOF when a child is about 1 year of age. The timing represents an attempt to balance the time-related detrimental effects of cyanosis against technical suitability for repair without a major ventriculotomy (transatrial–transpulmonary approach). Although thousands of patients have had a successful operation using a transventricular approach, we have been concerned about the poor hemodynamic status of some long-term survivors of this type of procedure. Late RV dysfunction and arrythmias may be related, in part, to the presence of a large right ventriculotomy, and the transatrial approach has therefore been the method of choice over the past decade in our unit and many others as well.[13,37,88–91] This approach has a risk similar to or lower than a transventricular approach, and should result in better preservation of RV function.[92–96] The main problem with this strategy occurs when younger, smaller infants (especially neonates) become symptomatic with either spells or continual unacceptably low HbSO$_2$ (<80%). A decision must then be made regarding suitability for complete repair by a transatrial approach, versus a transventricular approach or a palliative operation. We would perform repair in most symptomatic infants over 6 kg whose branch pulmonary arteries are of adequate caliber (within 1 mm of normal, based on data of Rowlatt).[97] Other criteria include absence of multiple VSDs, A-V septal defect, pulmonary atresia, or other complicating features, and a degree of aortic override that does not require a large intraventricular baffle for septation (DORV). The presence of an anomalous coronary artery crossing the RVOT might lead to deferral of surgery to about 2 years of age, as would the presence of AVSD. The presence of other severe noncardiac anomalies should also be taken into account. Symptomatic infants who are judged to be unsuitable for complete repair are usually treated with a modified Blalock–Taussig shunt. Others may be considered for complete repair. This policy has provided very satisfactory results in our own hands,[39] although many centers currently advocate complete repair in infancy for symptomatic (and in some cases asymptomatic) patients. This is usually in the context of a transventricular approach to both VSD and RVOTO relief.[98,99] The need for a transannular patch has not in itself been considered a contraindication to repair in early infancy.[100–102] A careful ongoing evaluation of early and late results will be necessary to see if this latter approach is justified. In our practice we are tending toward earlier elective repair as well, although we feel that very small infants may not be the best candidates for the transatrial transpulmonary approach, which is likely to have some long-term advantages over the transventricular approach.

Modified Blalock–Taussig Shunt

A number of palliative operations have been used for tetralogy of Fallot, but most are currently of historical interest only. The modified Blalock–Taussig shunt (MBTS) is currently the procedure of choice.[103,104] This operation involves interposition of a small polytetrafluorethane (PTFE) graft between a subclavian artery and the ipsilateral branch PA. The MBTS has several advantages over other previously used shunts, including

1. Preservation of subclavian artery.
2. Suitability for use on either side, irrespective of the course of the ascending aorta relative to trachea.
3. Good relief of cyanosis without excessive pulmonary bloodflow (in most cases) when proper size prosthesis is selected.
4. Ease of control and closure at time of complete repair.
5. Excellent early patency rate, usually allowing elective repair after 1 year of age.[105–109]
6. Low incidence on iatrogenic pulmonary or systemic artery problems.[105]

Technique of Modified Blalock–Taussig Shunt

We prefer to perform the shunt on the right side, irrespective of the side of the arch. The pulmonary end of the shunt can be placed more medially on the right than on the left, and subsequent closure via median sternotomy is therefore easier and safer. The thorax is opened posterolaterally through the third or fourth intercostal space. The lung is retracted inferiorly and posteriorly, exposing the PA at the superior aspect of the hilum. Diathermy is used to isolate the PA and its lobar branches. Medially, the dissection is carried posterior to the SVC on the right, or intrapericardially on the left. Branches are looped with Silastic snares. Retraction is shifted to the anterior and inferior direction, and

the pleura overlying the subclavian artery (SCA) is opened. Only a limited SCA dissection is needed to place a loop around the vessel and pull it into the operative field. Care is taken to avoid the recurrent laryngeal nerve as well as surrounding lymphatic channels. Heparin (1 mg/kg) is administered systemically, and a small Castañeda clamp is placed on the SCA. A PTFE prosthesis (thin walled PTFE, 4 or 5 mm) is tapered and anastomosed to the SCA with a 7-0 polypropylene suture (Fig. 81–8). The clamp is released for 2 heartbeats to assess proximal patency and flow, and then reapplied to the artery. The PA is exposed again and controlled with loops distally and a cross clamp is placed as proximally as possible. A second end-to-side anastomosis is constructed, and the snares and clamps are removed. A thrill is usually palpable on a functioning shunt, and a rise in $HbSO_2$ is noted immediately. Chest closure is performed over an intercostal catheter. Patency of the shunt can be verified after chest closure and in the ICU by auscultation of the endotracheal tube (using the bell of the stethoscope)

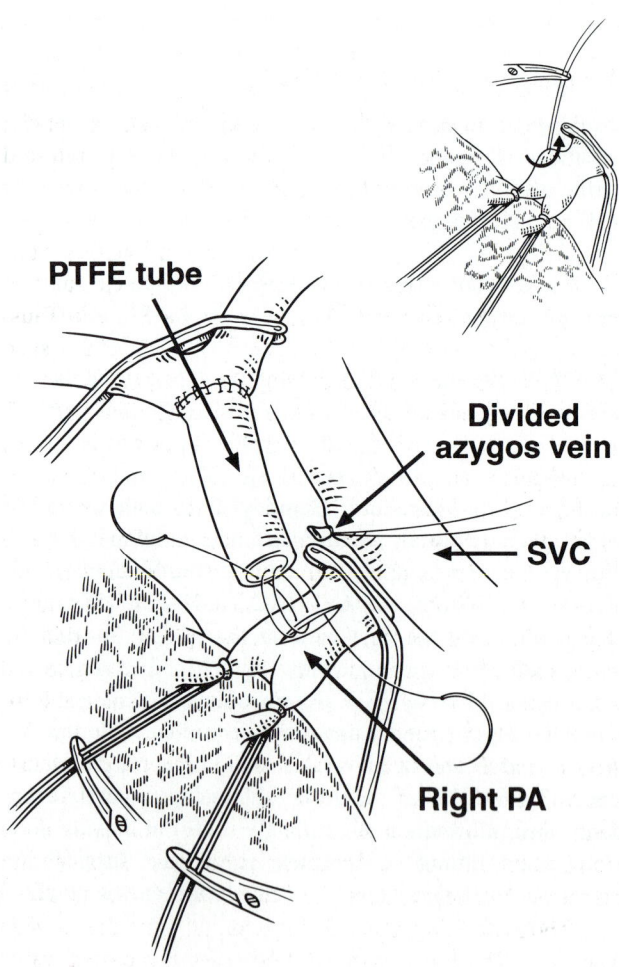

Figure 81–8. The modified Blalock–Taussig shunt: A 4- or 5-mm PTFE tube is interposed between the subclavian artery and branch PA. This operation is generally performed on the right side, irrespective of arch anatomy, to facilitate closure at subsequent repair.

while the apneic patient is briefly disconnected from the ventilator (as the shunt lies in proximity to the bronchus, the continuous murmur is well transmitted).

Postoperatively, infants undergoing modified Blalock–Taussig shunts are kept paralyzed and ventilated for 12–24 hours. The main early complications are consequences of an acute increase in pulmonary blood flow, including diastolic hypotension, metabolic acidosis, and hemorrhagic pulmonary edema. Most of these problems will resolve within 24–48 hours of operation with supportive care and ventilation. Other complications include chylothorax, Horner's syndrome (usually temporary), shunt thrombosis, and serous leak through the PTFE graft. The latter complication can be avoided by not exposing the occluded graft to systemic arterial pressure prior to establishing outflow. Nonresolving serous leak may require graft replacement. Heparin is maintained at 10 units/kg per hour until oral aspirin (5 mg/kg daily) can be started, the latter being maintained until 5 days prior to complete repair.

Operative mortality for MBTS is low, approaching zero even for neonates.[105,107,110–112]

Technique of Complete Repair

Anesthetic management for open repair of TOF is critical, but beyond the scope of this chapter. The reader is referred to the section on anesthetic management as well as to other reviews of the subject.[113,114]

Complete repair is performed via a median sternotomy, with full invasive monitoring. Prior to cannulation for CPB, a previously constructed modified Blalock–Taussig shunt is dissected using diathermy. CPB is established using ascending aortic and direct bicaval cannulation with right angle metal tipped cannulas. During cooling to 25°C, the shunt is doubly ligated and usually divided. It is critical that the shunt be controlled while cardiac contractions remain forceful, otherwise distension of the LV can occur, with rapid irreversible damage to the myocardium. Either a right or left MBTS is best dissected by following the respective branch PA. Following shunt control, the aortic clamp is applied, and crystalloid cardioplegia is administered via a small ascending aortic needle, and augmented with topical cold saline. During initial cardioplegia infusion, the RA is opened longitudinally posterior to the AV groove, and a cardiotomy sucker is placed through the natural (or surgically created) ASD. Especially in older patients, there may be a significant amount of collateral blood return to the LA via the bronchial circulation. This venting maneuver will help to keep the field relatively bloodless.

The main PA is opened longitudinally and the valve is inspected. The most frequent finding is a bicuspid valve with fusion at both commissures. An incision is made exactly through the points of fusion, right back to the annulus (Fig. 81–9). A small Hegar dilator is inserted through the valve into the RV cavity and left in place. Retractors are then placed in the RA, through the TV, to expose the

RVOT. The proximal extent of the obstruction is located by the position of the Hegar dilator. The parietal extension of the infundibular septum is grasped with forceps, pulled into the operative field, and excised with scissors as a large single wedge of tissue (Fig. 81–10). Accessory muscle bands that tether the infundibular septum to the RV free wall are divided on both ends of the infundibular septum. One should avoid cutting major muscle bands that are not obstructive, in an attempt to preserve RV function. Fibrous tissue in the outflow tract is also excised, the end point being visualization of the inferior aspect of the pulmonary valve leaflets.

Hegar dilators are then passed through the TV into the PA to calibrate the RVOT. Under cardioplegia, we aim to pass a dilator 2–3 mm larger than the mean normal sized pulmonary annulus. This method of sizing predicts an acceptable RV/PA pressure ratio at postoperative catheterization.[39] In TOF with absent infundibular septum, the annulus is almost invariably hypoplastic and will require placement of a transannular patch.[115] In such cases, the VSD can sometimes be closed using the transpulmonary approach. If a dilator of adequate caliber cannot be passed through the RVOT and PV, then the PA incision is extended across the annulus, exactly through the anterior commissure (in an attempt to preserve some PV function), for 5–10 mm onto the RV free wall. Other methods for assessing the need for transannular patching are available based on either preoperative or intraoperative measurements.[20]

The VSD is exposed through the RA, with retractors placed through the TV annulus. Plegetted polypropylene sutures are placed through the base of the septal leaflet of the TV (Fig. 81–11) and retracted to facilitate exposure of the muscular portion of the VSD. Around the inferior rim of the VSD, sutures are placed 1–2 mm from the defect to avoid conduction tissue, and the process is continued in an anticlockwise direction. The transected end of the parietal extension of the infundibular septum now comes into view, and sutures are placed with pledgets behind it, the needle exiting through the aortic annulus. Suture placement continues around the aortic annulus until the first suture placed through the septal TV leaflet is met. All sutures are then placed through a Dacron patch, which will approximate the size of the aortic annulus. The patch is seated and sutures are tied gently to avoid tearing the delicate myocardium, especially in the area of RVOT resection. The TV leaflets are mobilized with forceps to be sure that they are not distorted by the patch. The ASD is closed and the heart is deaired via the ascending aorta and ASD. Some surgeons prefer to leave a small ASD to avoid high RA pressure in patients expected to have postoperative RV dysfunction (especially small infants). In practice, this may lead to severe hypoxemia, and we avoid it. The aortic clamp is removed during a brief period of reduced pump flow, which is increased to full flow over 1–2 min. The patient is then warmed to 37°C, and the RA is closed.

During warming, the branch PAs are calibrated with

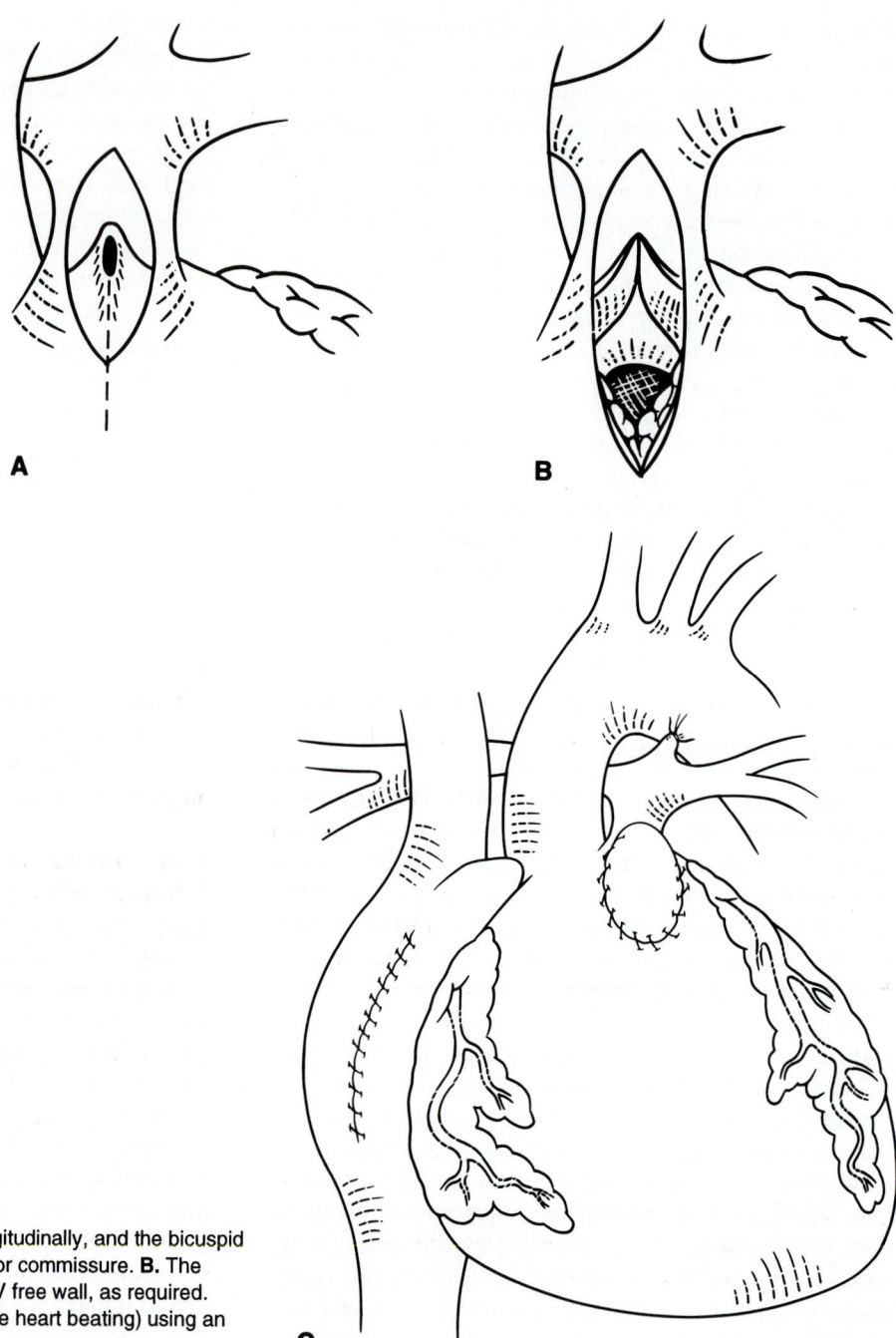

Figure 81–9. A. The main PA is opened longitudinally, and the bicuspid pulmonary valve is incised through the anterior commissure. **B.** The incision is continued for 1–10 mm onto the RV free wall, as required. **C.** RVOT reconstruction is completed (with the heart beating) using an autologous pericardial patch.

Hegar dilators to assess the need for patch enlargement. The main PA, branch PAs (if necessary), and RV incision (if used) are closed with an untreated autologous pericardial patch sutured in place on the beating heart, using running polypropylene suture (Fig. 81–9). If severe bifurcation stenosis is present, a bifurcated pulmonary allograft may be a better solution than direct reconstruction with pericardium, especially in older patients.[116] The right branch PA can be exposed by retracting the aorta to the right or left using a vessel loop. The width of the oval RVOT patch is tailored according to the fraction of Hegar dilator circumference exposed at the annulus during RVOT calibration.

Care is taken to avoid injury to the left coronary artery, which is in proximity at the top of the RVOT incision. If the distal PAs are small and a large patch is required, we have employed a monocusp onlay using part of an aortic allograft.[117]

A pressure monitoring catheter is placed through the LA appendage, and atrial and ventricular pacing wires are fixed to the epicardium. The patient is gradually separated from CPB, usually receiving a dopamine infusion (2–5 μg/kg per minute). Protamine is administered, followed by decannulation. Because the RV/LV pressure ratio at this point is not predictive of the ratio observed at postoperative

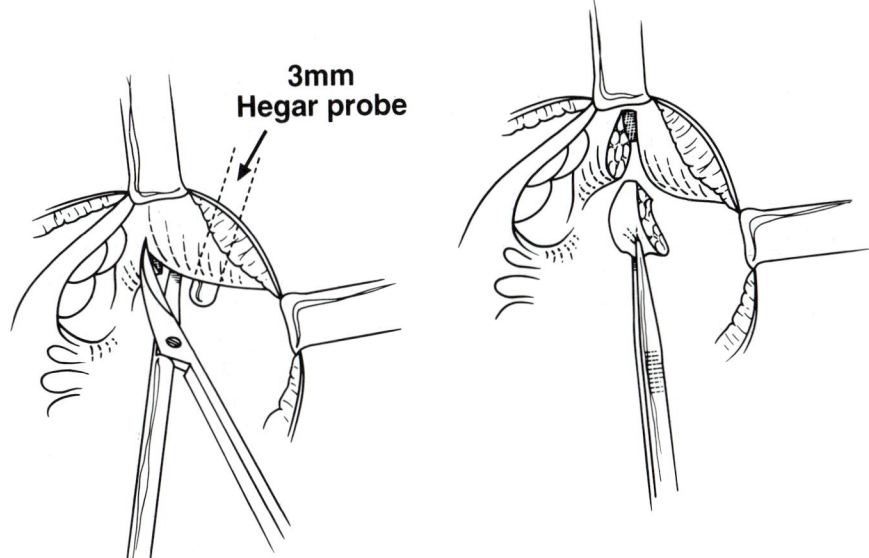

3mm Hegar probe

Figure 81–10. RVOT muscle resection. With a small probe passed retrogradely from the PA, the RVOT is enlarged by excising a large wedge of muscle from the parietal extension of the infundibular septum. Additional muscle bands may also be resected, the end point being visualization of the PV. Care is taken to avoid the VSD rim and aortic valve.

follow-up, it is not routinely measured. An exception would be cases in which poor hemodynamics are noted immediately following CPB. Intraoperative transesophageal echocardiography, caval and PA oximetry data, and direct pressure measurements are all useful in this latter situation to detect residual severe RVOTO, residual VSDs, or other problems that might require further surgical attention. After hemostasis is achieved, the operation is completed by insertion of a single chest drain and a peritoneal dialysis catheter, followed by sternotomy closure.

Postoperative Care

Patients are usually kept sedated, paralyzed, and ventilated for 6–12 hours postoperatively, and low dose inotropic support (dopamine) is used for 24–72 hours. Systemic arterial and right and left atrial pressures are monitored. Most patients can be extubated within 24 hours of operation. Intravenous antibiotics are continued for 24 hours after opera-

tion, and fluid restriction is enforced for 5 days. Most children will be discharged on diuretics, which are continued for 2–4 wk. The following specific postoperative problems might be encountered:

Low Cardiac Output

Following TOF repair, patients occasionally show signs of tachycardia, poor peripheral perfusion, hypotension, low urinary output (< 1 mL/kg per hour), metabolic acidosis, and generalized capillary leak. Right-sided filling pressures are usually elevated, and an LA pressure rise is often seen concurrently in patients with a small LV. Echocardiography or oximetry may identify a residual anatomic lesion, which can be treated with prompt reoperation, but usually this is not the case. RV dilation/hypocontractility is the more common finding. Severe edema may further complicate the picture, due to the abnormal capillary fragility found in some children with cyanotic congenital heart disease.

In such patients the strategy should be to support the

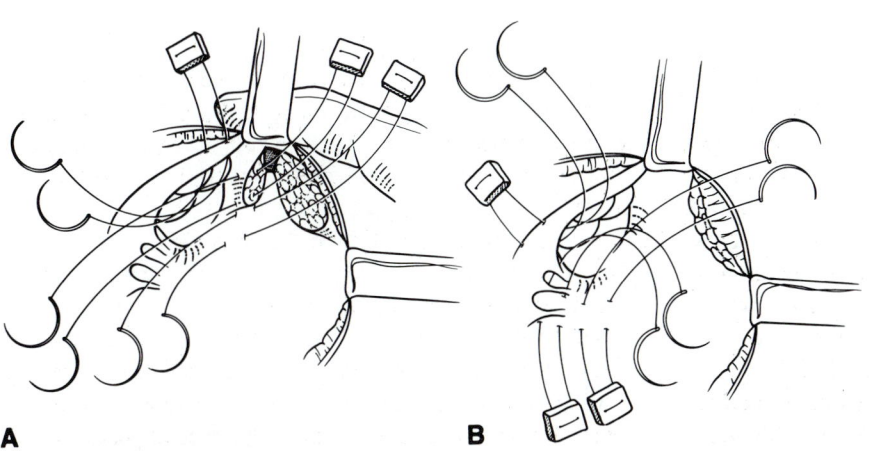

A   **B**

Figure 81–11. VSD closure. **A.** Working through the RA and tricuspid valve, pledgetted sutures are placed through the transected parietal extension and aortic valve annulus. **B.** In the area of conduction tissue (inferior–posterior border of VSD), sutures are placed through the base of the tricuspid septal leaflet and through myocardium 3–4 mm away from the defect.

systemic circulation and metabolism until spontaneous improvement occurs, usually within 24–48 hours. Prompt initiation of peritoneal dialysis is extremely useful in this situation, as repeated doses of diuretics are usually ineffective and only result in further metabolic derangement. In severely compromised patients, core cooling to 34°C with cold dialysate for 12–24 hours may decrease metabolic needs to the point where low output is tolerated without significant acidosis. Beyond this time period, however, the risk of infection probably outweighs the benefits.

In our experience, patients in low cardiac output often respond favorably to noradrenaline. There may be minimal β-adrenergic effect at this dose, and the drug probably serves to support the central arterial circulation without exacerbating residual RVOTO. One must be aware of the potential for vasoconstriction and reduced peripheral tissue perfusion, especially at higher doses.

Arrhythmias

Even with the transatrial approach, right bundle branch block is common following TOF repair. At least acutely, the clinical consequences of this type of conduction defect are minimal, even in the presence of left anterior hemiblock.[118] Complete heart block is rare, but may require pacemaker insertion if it persists longer than 5 days. The most troublesome electrical problem in the early postoperative period is supraventricular tachycardia, which may be very poorly tolerated hemodynamically. Junctional ectopic tachycardia (JET) is the most difficult to control. Causative factors, additive to surgical trauma, include inadequate sedation, muscle relaxants (especially pancuronium), inotropes (especially dopamine and dobutamine), fever, and low cardiac output. Reduction in β-adrenergic drugs, the use of vecuronium rather than pancuronium, and core cooling with cold peritoneal dialysate are all important therapeutic measures. Intravenous amiodarone is our drug of choice for most supraventricular arrhythmias, but it is usually ineffective in JET. Propafenone may prove to be a superior drug for JET as more experience accumulates.

RESULTS

At the Royal Children's Hospital, we have performed 456 consecutive tetralogy of Fallot repairs (including patients with AVSD and DORV with subaortic VSD and RVOTO) using the transatrial transpulmonary approach.[39] Thirty-seven percent had palliative procedures prior to repair (MBTS). Median age over the past 2 years has been 12 mo. Hospital mortality for complete repair was 1.1% (CL 0.4–2.5%). Similar results have been reported in other centers worldwide.[118,120–122] After more than 1500 patient years follow up, we have had 5 late deaths, possibly related to coexisting noncardiac problems. Actuarial survival probability for our first 369 patients, is shown in Figure 81–12, approximating 97.5% (CL = 95–99%) at 42 months. Postrepair survival reported by Kirklin and associates has been 94, 92, 91, 90, and 87% at 1 mo, 1 year, 5 years, 10 years, and 20 years, respectively.[123] Twenty-year survival has exceeded 90% in some reports.[124,125] Late follow-up of large cohorts of patients from institutions with an early and large TOF experience suggests that there is a constant phase of hazard for late death, which is low but higher than that of the general population. A late rising phase has not been observed, however.[11,20,123,126,127]

A number of incremental risk factors for early and late death following TOF repair have been identified. While not all of them will apply within a given institution, it is generally accepted that the following are important:

1. Young age, probably less than 3 mo, or more recently less than 1 mo.[128–132]
2. Old age, probably beyond 4 years: This may be due to effects of chronic cyanosis on ventricular function as

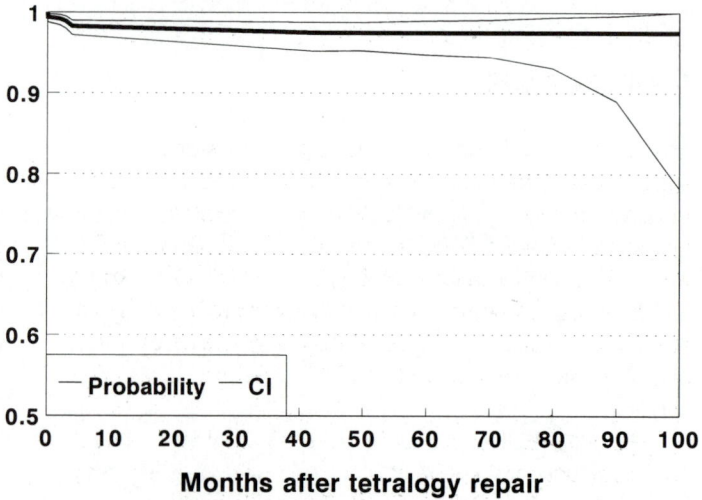

Probability (95% confidence intervals)

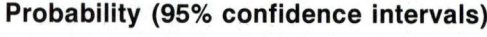

Figure 81–12. Kaplan–Meier survival probability for patients undergoing transatrial–transpulmonary TOF repair at the Royal Children's Hospital. The estimates include both hospital and late mortality.

well as various organ systems.[133] However, operations performed later in life may still yield good results,[134–136] and the age effect remains debatable. Much of the current experience with late repair has been reported from developing nations.

3. Postoperative pRV/LV, especially if > 0.7: This has been predictive of both early and late mortality in various series.[12,137–139] The ratio at 24 hours probably carries more predictive value than that obtained immediately following cessation of CPB.

4. High hematocrit[139]: This itself may relate to age at operation.

5. LV volume (if LV end diastolic volume is less than 55–65% of predicted value for body surface area).[139]

Late outcome for survivors finds most patients in the pediatric equivalent of NYHA class I,[39,91,101] although maximal exercise capacity may be reduced in some. Late repair, high pRL/LV, and severe PI are more likely to be found in patients with abnormal responses to exercise.[140–148]

Much has been written regarding late death due to arrhythmia. Sudden death from ventricular arrhythmia has been reported in 0.5–5% of patients within 10 years of repair.[94,95,149,150] In our own patients, routine Holter monitoring is employed, although we have rarely detected ventricular arrhythmias requiring treatment. From the world literature, it would appear that arrhythmic events occur in <1% of patients having an early operation.[150–154] Map guided ablative surgery may be possible for macroreentry-induced ventricular tachycardia related to RVOT resection.[12] The likelihood of arrhythmia probably increases significantly in patients undergoing operation after the first few years of life[155,156] and also in patients with residual hemodynamic problems.[141,157,158] At present we lack firm data that a transatrial approach decreases the incidence of late arrhythmias, however, it is likely that it will if ventricular function is preserved.[159] As with most repaired heart defects, the risk of endocarditis is probably present for life, but significantly lower than in uncorrected cases.

REOPERATIONS

Postoperative catheter data from our own patients would suggest that a favorable hemodynamic situation exists for the great majority of patients.[39] Actuarial freedom from reoperation following TOF repair at the RCH is shown in Figure 81–13, approximating 95% (CL = 92–97%) at both 5 and 10 years follow-up. Reoperations were either for residual VSD or residual/recurrent RVOTO. Some cases would currently be treatable with balloon dilation rather than surgery.

Residual VSD is poorly tolerated in tetralogy of Fallot, as such hearts may not be able to cope with an acutely imposed volume load. While small, echocardiographically de-

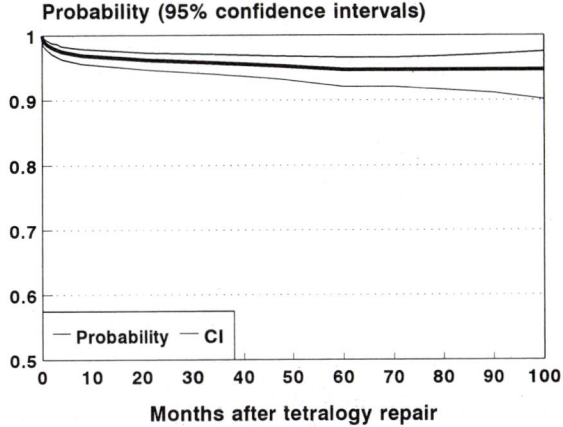

Figure 81–13. Kaplan–Meier probability of freedom from reoperation following transatrial–transpulmonary TOF repair at the Royal Children's Hospital.

tected residual VSDs are quite common after tetralogy repair and of no significance to the patient, larger defects (Q_p/Q_s > 1.5) may require reoperation, ideally within a week of the primary procedure. The residual defect usually occurs in the superior corner of the VSD patch, just below the aortic valve, which is sometimes a difficult area to see at the time of repair. Closure through the atrium is usually still possible, using pledgetted sutures or an additional small patch. This type of surgery can be performed at very low risk to the patient early in the postoperative period, and may result in dramatic improvement.

Residual right ventricular outflow obstruction causing right heart failure should also be repaired earlier rather than later. Such RVOTO may be due to muscle bundles that have been overlooked at the initial operation. Reoperation through the transatrial approach is still likely to be effective. Extension of the transannular patch may be required, although it should still be kept as small as possible (consistent with relief of the obstruction). Reoperation for RVOT in the early postoperative period is also well tolerated and may convert a difficult postoperative course into quite a smooth one. The ischemic time should be short, and the patient will generally have had normal oxygenation in the interval since the first operation, as compared to preoperatively.

Late reoperations for TOF may be required for recurrent RVOTO, or the effects of chronic pulmonary insufficiency. Recurrent RVOTO is usually due to continued muscular hypertrophy or fibrosis. Although rarely symptomatic, patients with RVOTO should be reoperated upon to preserve ventricular function in cases with an RV to PA systolic pressure ratio greater than 2/3. Repair through the transatrial approach may or may not be possible, depending on the technique used for the original operation.

Patients with severe chronic pulmonary insufficiency have usually had a transventricular repair. In the absence of a high pRV/LV or other residual hemodynamic problems, the insufficiency may well be tolerated for 1–2 decades. Deleterious effects on ventricular function and exercise capacity have been documented, however, especially when additional lesions are present.[160,161] Valve interposition improves functional status as well as ventricular function.[162–166] The decision to reoperate requires some judgment on the part of the physician following the patient. While the development of new symptoms of congestive heart failure would be considered a good indication, decision making for patients who remain asymptomatic is more complicated. We have looked for an increasing cardiothoracic ratio on chest x-ray, and a change in ventricular function on serial radionuclide studies in this later group. Although each patient must be considered on his or her own merits, we would suggest that reoperation for valve interposition is appropriate for patients who demonstrate such changes. We take into account the patient's age, as those who have completed most somatic growth will be better candidates for valve interposition than smaller children.

The technique of reoperation is straightforward. Cardiopulmonary bypass may be established with a single venous cannula, and the entire operation can be performed on the beating heart employing mild hypothermia. The main pulmonary artery is transected just proximal to the bifurcation, and a suitably sized cryopreserved pulmonary or aortic homograft is sutured as an interposition graft between the main pulmonary artery and the RV outflow tract. Posteriorly, the sutures may be placed at the level of the pulmonary annulus, or the infundibular septum. The original transventricular patch, if still in good condition, may be used to augment the anterior portion. In practice this patch is often heavily calcified or aneurysmal, and should be removed completely and replaced with a new one made of homograft wall or autologous pericardium. Hemodynamic improvement following late pulmonary allograft insertion has been documented by ourselves and others, especially for patients with a high pRV/LV.[162,167] There have been no operative deaths in a group of 25 patients so treated at the RCH (0%, CL=0–13.7%). Evaluation of the results of pulmonary valve interposition is difficult, especially in patients who are asymptomatic preoperatively.

ANATOMIC SUBSETS: SPECIAL CONSIDERATIONS

Absent Pulmonary Valve Syndrome (TOF With Absent Pulmonary Valve)

Repair may be required within the first few months of life if airway compression is severe. In less symptomatic patients timing of surgery is similar to that for TOF. Basic operative strategy consists of transatrial repair as outlined for TOF. The RVOTO is usually not severe. The size of the enlarged branch PAs is reduced by resection of the main PA and the anterior wall of both primary PA branches. A short homograft valved conduit is then used to reconstruct the RVOT,

as continued PI may induce further aneurysmal dilation of the abnormal PAs[42,168] (Fig. 81–14). Some surgeons rely on PA aneurysm reduction, and repair is performed with direct valveless RVOT reconstruction.[41] With either approach, the postoperative course may be difficult in patients with APVS, with requirements for prolonged ventilator support. The outcome is related primarily to the degree of preexisting tracheobronchomalacia. In 19 infants operated upon at the RCH for airway obstruction, hospital mortality was 16% (CL 7–29%).[41] There has been a 25% incidence of reoperation for PA problems within 5 years of the initial procedure.

Tetralogy of Fallot With Atrioventricular Septal Defect

The surgical procedure for TOF and AVSD is an extensive one. The main operative consideration is maintenance of A-V and pulmonary valve competence. We currently prefer to delay this operation until a child is about 10 kg, as we have found that the valve repair is more reliable in larger patients. A preliminary modified Blalock–Taussig shunt is therefore usually required for patients with significant right ventricular outflow tract obstruction and cyanosis. The operative strategy for repair is a combination of that used for isolated A-V septal defect and tetralogy of Fallot.[40] Initial steps of the operation are similar to isolated TOF, up to the point of VSD closure. For this part of the operation, a large comma-shaped patch is employed. Pledgetted sutures are placed around the aortic valve and the inlet portion of the VSD, and then through the patch, which is seated beneath the tricuspid chordae (Fig. 81–15). Sutures are then placed through the crest of the Dacron VSD patch, through the A-V valve leaflets, and through one edge of an autologous pericardial patch, to partition the single large A-V valve into 2 nonstenotic orifices. The left ventricle is then inflated with cold saline to assess competence. Sutures are then placed in the accessory septal commissure as required. Other valvuloplasty techniques may also be employed. A similar exercise is employed for the right ventricle and tricuspid portion of the partitioned A-V valve, with the pulmonary artery temporarily occluded. The ostium primum is then closed with the autologous pericardial patch, leaving the coronary sinus in the left or right ventricle, depending on the amount of fibrous tissue present between the coronary sinus and A-V valve tissue. The heart is deaired and the cross clamp is removed. RV outflow reconstruction is then performed as for isolated TOF. Recently, we have employed homograft RV to PA conduits as an in situ pulmonary valve replacement in patients who would have severe pulmonary incompetence due to lack of leaflet tissue or extent of right ventriculotomy. The haemodynamic burden of severe tricuspid and pulmonary valve incompetence may result in an unstable postoperative course.

The risk of repair for children with TOF and AVSD does not differ significantly from that of isolated TOF or AVSD.[40,169] We have, however, observed a significantly

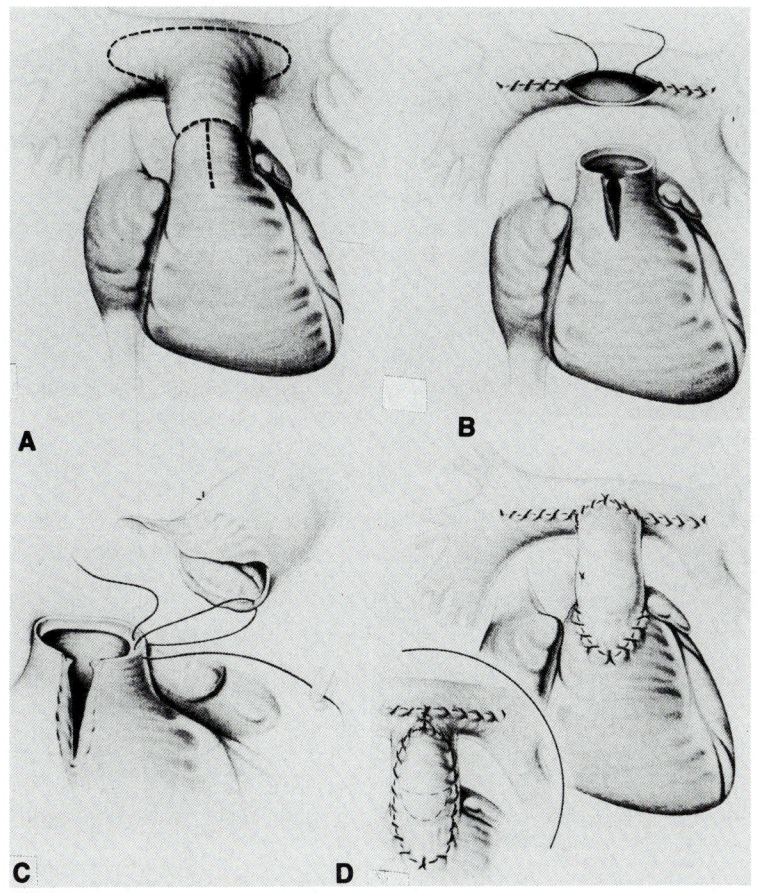

Figure 81–14. Repair of absent pulmonary valve syndrome. **A.** The main PA and an ellipse of branch PA anterior wall are excised. **B.** The lateral portion of the PA branches is closed directly and a short incision is made in the RVOT. **C.** A cryopreserved aortic homograft is sutured to the annulus. **D.** The homograft anterior mitral leaflet is used to augment the RVOT. A homograft monocusp patch (inset) can also be used.

lower actuarial freedom from reoperation, primarily due to residual VSD and AV valve insufficiency.

Tetralogy of Fallot With Anomalous Course of a Coronary Artery

If a coronary artery has an abnormal course and crosses the RVOT (i.e., LAD or LCA from RCA), then the extent of ventriculotomy will be limited. The transatrial transpulmonary approach is usually effective in this situation, still allowing short transannular incision (if required) to relieve RVOTO. This is combined with an extensive transatrial muscle resection. In rare cases an RV–PA conduit may be required. Mobilization of the coronary artery with patch placement beneath it is not recommended. We have performed transatrial–transpulmonary repair in 14 patients with TOF and anomalous coronary artery.[39] There has been no mortality (0% CL = 0–23%). Transannular patches were employed in 7 patients, and the remainder had supraannular PA reconstruction plus pulmonary valvotomy.

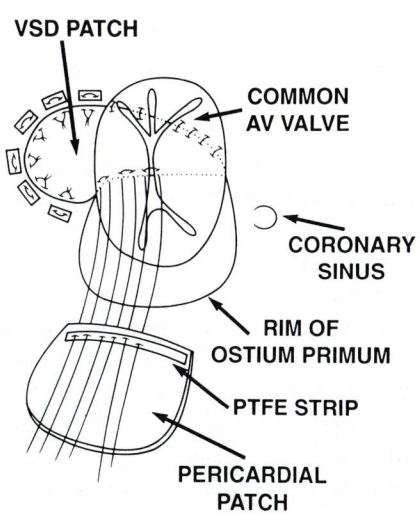

Figure 81–15. Tetralogy of Fallot with atrioventricular septal defect. The VSD is closed using a large comma-shaped patch. The left-hand rounded edge is sutured around the aortic annulus. The upper edge of the patch is sutured to bridging leaflet tissue to create two separate A-V valves. The ostium primum is repaired with an autologous pericardial patch reinforced with a PTFE strip. The coronary sinus usually remains on the left side of the patch, thereby avoiding injury to the conduction tissue.

VSD PATCH

COMMON AV VALVE

CORONARY SINUS

RIM OF OSTIUM PRIMUM

PTFE STRIP

PERICARDIAL PATCH

Tetralogy of Fallot With Pulmonary Atresia (Pulmonary Atresia With VSD)

This subject is covered in detail in Chapter 79.

SUMMARY

In the current era, children with uncomplicated forms of TOF are expected, in the absence of limiting noncardiac problems, to enjoy long-term survival with a good quality of life. The surgical procedures are not curative, however, and continued cardiologic surveillance into adult life is recommended.

REFERENCES

1. Willus FA: Cardiac clinics: An unusually early description of the so-called tetralogy of Fallot. *Meet Mayo Clin Proc* **23:**316, 1948
2. Sandifort E: *Observations Anatomico-Pathologicae Ludg.* Batt P.v.d, Eukl et D. Vygh, 1777, Chap 1, Fig 1
3. Fallot EAL: Contribution à l'anatomie pathologique de la maldie bleue (cyanose cardiaque). *Marseille Med* **25:**77,138,207,270,341, 403, 1888
4. Allwork SP: Tetralogy of Fallot: The centenary of the name. A new translation of the first of Fallot's papers. *Eur J Cardiothorac Surg* **2**(6):386–392, 1988
5. Blalock A, Taussig HB: The surgical treatment of malformations of the heart in which there is pulmonary stenosis or pulmonary atresia. *JAMA* **128:**189, 1945
6. Potts WJ, Smith S, Gibson S: Anastomosis of the aorta to a pulmonary atery. Certain types in congenital heart disease. *JAMA* **132:**627, 1946
7. Glenn WWL: Circulatory bypass of the right side of the heart. IV. Shunt between superior vena cava and distal right pulmonary artery - Report of clinical application. *N Engl J Med* **259:**117, 1958
8. Waterston DJ: Treatment of Fallot's tetralogy in children under one year of age. *Rozhl Chir* **41:**181, 1962
9. Brock RC, Campbell M: Infundibular resection or dilatation for infundibular stenosis. *Br Heart J* **12:**403, 1950
10. Lillehei CW, et al: Direct vision intracardial surgical correlation of the tetralogy of Fallot, pentalogy of Fallot, and pulmonary atresia defects: Report of the first ten cases. *Ann Surg* **142:**418, 1955
11. Lillehei CW, Varco RL, Cohen M, et al: The first open heart corrections of tetralogy of Fallot. A 26–31 year follow-up of 106 patients. *Ann Surg* **204:**490–502, 1986
12. Kirklin JW, Ellis FH, McGoon DC, et al: Surgical treatment for the tetralogy of Fallot by open intracardiac repair. *J Thorac Surg* **37:**22, 1959
13. Kay JH, Anderson RM, Lewis RR, et al: Complete correction of the tetralogy of Fallot by open heart surgery. *JAMA* **170:**792, 1959
14. Hudspeth AS, Cordell AR, Johnston FR: Transatrial approach to total correction of tetralogy of Fallot. *Circulation* **27:**796–800, 1963
15. Ross DN, Somerville J: Correction of pulmonary atresia with a homograft aortic valve. *Lancet* **2:**1446–1447, 1966
16. Edwards JE, Bulbulian A, Rogers HM: Pathologic and embryologic considerations in tetralogy of Fallot. *Proc Staff Meet, Mayo Clin* **22:**166, 1947
17. Van Praagh R, Van Praagh S, Nebessar RA, et al: Tetralogy of Fallot: Underdevelopment of the pulmonary infundibulum and its sequelae. *Am J Cardiol* **26:**25, 1970
18. Bartelings MM, Gittenberger de Groot AC: Morphogenetic considerations on congenital malformations of the outflow tract. Part 1: Common arterial trunk and tetralogy of Fallot. *Int J Cardiol* **32:**213–230, 1991
19. Lomonico MP, Bostrom MP, Moore GW, Hutchins GM: Arrested rotation of the outflow tract may explain tetralogy of Fallot and transposition of the great arteries. *Pediatr Pathol* **8:**267–281, 1988
20. Kirklin JW, Baratt-Boyes BG: Ventricular septal defect and pulmonary stenosis or atresia. In: *Cardiac Surgery.* New York, John Wiley, 1986, pp 669–819
21. Anderson RH, et al: Surgical anatomy of tetralogy of Fallot. *J Thorac Cardiovasc Surg* **81:**887, 1981
22. Edwards WE: Double outlet right ventricle and tetralogy of Fallot. Two distinct but not mutually exclusive entities. *J Thorac Cardiovasc Surg* **82:**418, 1981
23. Wilcox BR, et al: Surgical anatomy of double outlet right ventricle with situs solitus and atrioventricular concordance. *J Thorac Cardiovasc Surg* **82:**405, 1981
24. Anderson RH, Allwork SP, Ho SY, et al: Surgical anatomy of tetralogy of Fallot. *J Thorac Cardiovasc Surg* **81:**887, 1981
25. Lev M, Eckner FAO: The pathologic anatomy of tetralogy of Fallot and its variations. *Dis Chest* **45:**251, 1964
26. Nagao GI, Daoud GI, McAdams AJ, et al: Cardiovascular anomalies associated with tetralogy of Fallot. *Am J Cardiol* **20:**206, 1967
27. Sabiston DC Jr, Cornell WP, Criley JM, et al: The diagnosis and surgical correction of total obstruction of the right ventricle. An acquired condition developing after systemic artery-pulmonary artery anastomosis for tetralogy of Fallot. *J Thorac Surg* **48:**577, 1964
28. Casta A: Acquired pulmonary atresia following placement of modified Blalock-Taussig shunt in tetralogy of Fallot. *Int J Cardiol* **15:**244, 1987
29. Agrawal S, Soni D, Dhawan S, et al: Sites of right ventricular outflow tract obstruction in tetralogy of Fallot—a retrospective study. *Indian Heart J* **43:**455–459, 1991
30. Johnson RJ, Haworth SG: Pulmonary vascular and alveolar development in tetralogy of Fallot: A recommendation for early corection. *Thorax* **37:**893, 1982
31. Rabinovitch M, Herrera-DeLeon V, Castaneda A, Reid L: Growth and development of the pulmonary vascular bed in patients with tetralogy of Fallot with or without pulmonary aresia. *Circulation* **64:**1234, 1981
32. Hislop A, Reid L: Structural changes in the pulmonary arteries and veins in tetralogy of Fallot. *Br Heart J* **35:**1178, 1973
33. Johnson RJ, Sauer U, Buhlmeyer K, Haworth SG: Hypoplasia of the intrapulmonary arteries in children with right ventricular outflow tract obstruction, ventricular septal defect and major aortopulmonary collateral arteries. *Pediatr Cardiol* **6:**137, 1985
34. Hashimoto K, Nakamura Y, Matsui M, et al: Alteration of pulmonary blood flow in tetralogy of Fallot: Pre-and postoperative study with macroaggregates of 99mTc-labeled human serum albumin. *Jpn Circ J* **56:**992–997, 1992
35. Jarmakani JM, Graham TP Jr, Canent RV Jr: Left heart function in children with tetralogy of Fallot before and after palliative or corrective surgery. *Circulation* **46:**478, 1973
36. Lev M, Rimoldi HJA, Rowlatt DF: Quantitative anatomy of cyanotic tetralogy of Fallot. *Circulation* **30:**531, 1964
37. Miller GAH, Kirklin JW, Rahimtoola S, Swan HFC: Volume of the left ventricle in tetralogy of Fallot. *Am J Cardiol* **16:**488, 1965
38. Shrivastava S, Mohan JC, Mukhopadhyay S, et al: Coronary artery anomalies in tetralogy of Fallot. *Cardiovasc Intervent Radiol* **10:**215–218, 1987
39. Karl TR, Sano S, Pornvilawan S, Mee RBB. Transatrial transpulmonary repair of tetralogy of Fallot: Favourable outcome of non-neonatal repair. *Ann Thorac Surg* **54:**903–907, 1992
40. Malm T, Karl TR, Mee RBB: Transatrial-transpulmonary repair of atrioventricular septal defect with right ventricular outflow tract obstruction. *J Card Surg* **8:**622–627, 1993
41. Watterson K, Malm T, Karl TR, Mee RBB: Absent pulmonary valve sysdrome: Treatment in infants with airway obstruction. *Ann Thorac Surg* **54:**1116–1119, 1992
42. Karl TR, Musumeci F, de Leval M, et al: Surgical treatment of absent pulmonary valve syndrome. *J Thorac Cardiovasc Surg* **91:**590–597, 1986
43. Rabinovitch M, Grady S, David I, et al: Compression of intrapulmonary bronchi by abnormally branching pulmonary arteries associated with absent pulmonary valves. *Am J Cardiol* **50:**804–813, 1983
44. Miller RA, Lev M, Paul MH: Congenital absence of the pulmonary

valve. The clinical syndrome of tetralogy of Fallot with pulmonary regurgitation. *Circulation* **26**:266–278, 1962

45. Macartney FJ, Miller GAH: Congenital absence of the pulmonary valve. *Br Heart J* **32**:483–490, 1970

46. Toussaint M, Planché C, Duboc D, et al: Left venricular ultrastructure in pulmonary stenosis and in tetralogy of Fallot. *Virchows Arch A* **411**:33, 1987

47. Isomura T, Hisatomi K, Inuzuka H, et al: Ultrastructural alterations of right and left ventricular myocytes in tetralogy of Fallot. *Kurume Med J* **37**:177–183, 1990

48. Lee YS, Chen YC: Alterations of ultrastructures and anionic sites in basement membranes of myocardial cells and capillaries in patients with cyanotic congenital heart disease due to tetralogy of Fallot. *Jpn Heart J* **28**:333–347, 1987

49. McGrath LB, Chen C, Gu J, et al: Determination of infundibular innervation and amine receptor content in cyanotic and acyanotic myocardium: relation to clinical events in tetralogy of Fallot. *Pediatr Cardiol* **12**:155–160, 1991

50. Teoh KH, Mickle DA, Weisel RD, et al: Effect of oxygen tension and cardiovascular operations on the myocardial antioxidant enzyme activities in patients with tetralogy of Fallot and aorta-coronary bypass. *J Thorac Cardiovasc Surg* **104**:159–164, 1992

51. Li RK, Mickle DA, Weisel RD, et al: Effect of oxygen tension on the anti-oxidant enzyme activities of tetralogy of Fallot ventricular myocytes. *J Mol Cell Cardiol* **21**:567–575, 1989

52. Cowan DB, Weisel RD, Williams WG, Mickle DA: The regulation of glutathione peroxidase gene expression by oxygen tension in cultured human cardiomyocytes. *J Mol Cell Cardiol* **24**:423–433, 1992

53. del Nido PJ, Mickle DA, Wilson GJ, et al: Inadequate myocardial protection with cold cardioplegic arrest during repair of tetralogy of Fallot. *J Thorac Cardiovasc Surg* **95**:223–229, 1988

54. Nora JJ, Nora AH: The evolution of specific genetic and environmental counseling in congenital heart disease. *Circulation* **57L**:205, 1978

55. Guntheroth WG, Morgan BC, Mullins GL: Physiologic studies of paroxysmal hyperpnea in cyanotic congenital heart disease. *Circulation* **31**:70, 1965

56. Pankau R, Siekmeyer W, Stoffregen R: Tetralogy of Fallot in three sibs. *Am J Med Genet* **37**:532–533, 1990

57. Pacileo G, Musewe NN, Calabro R: Tetralogy of Fallot in three siblings: A familial study and review of the literature. *Eur J Pediatr* **151**:726–727, 1992

58. Voisin M, Doan B, Elboury S, et al: Malformations extracardiaques dans la tetralogie de Fallot. *Arch Mal Coeur Vaiss* **82**:689–692, 1989

59. Kramer H, et al: Malformation patterns in children with congenital heart disease. *Am J Dis Child* **141**:789, 1987

60. Gelb BD, Towbin JA, McCabe ER, Sujansky E: San Luis Valley recombinant chromosome 8 and tetralogy of Fallot: A review of chromosome 8 anomalies and congenital heart disease. *Am J Med Genet* **40**:471–476, 1991

61. Bell RA, Arensman FW, Flannery DB, et al: Facial dysmorphologic and skeletal cephalometric findings associated with conotruncal cardiac anomalies. *Pediatr Dent* **12**:152–156, 1990

62. Radford DJ, Thong YH: Facial and immunological anomalies associated with tetralogy of Fallot. *Int J Cardiol* **22**:229–239, 1989

63. Radford DJ, Lachman R, Thong YH: The immunocompetence of children with congenital heart disease. *Int Arch Allergy Appl Immunol* **81**:331–336, 1986

64. Van Mierop LHS, Kutsche LM: Cardiovascular anomalies in DiGeorge syndrome and importance of neural crest as a possible pathogenic factor. *Am J Cardiol* **58**:133–137, 1986

65. Goldberg R, Marion R, Morderon M, et al: Phenotypic overlap between velocardiofacial syndrome (VCF) and the DiGeorge syndrome (DGS) (Abstract). *Am J Hum Genet* **37**:A54, 1985

66. Stevens CA, Carey JC, Shigeoka AO: DiGeorge anomaly and velocardiofacial syndrome. *Pediatrics* **85**:526–530, 1990

67. Carey AH, Roach S, Williamson R, et al: Localisation of 27 DNA

68. markers to region of human chromosome 22q11-pter deleted in patients with DiGeorge syndrome and duplicated in the der22 syndrome. *Genomics* **7**:299–306, 1990

68. Scambler PJ, Carey AH, Wyse RKJ, et al: Microdeletions within 22q11 associated with sporadic and familial DiGeorge syndrome. *Genomics* **10**:201–206, 1991

69. Carey AH, Kelly D, Halford S, et al: Molecular genetic study of the frequency of monosomy 22q11 in DiGeorge syndrome. *Am J Hum Genet* **51**:964–970, 1992

70. Driscoll DA, Budarf ML, Emanuel B: A genetic etiology for DiGeorge syndrome. Consistent deletions and microdeletions of 22q11. *Am J Hum Genet* **50**:924–933, 1992

71. Vickers TH: The thalidomide embryopathy in hybrid rabbits. *Br J Exp Pathol* **48**:107, 1967

72. Bertranou EG, Blackstone EH, Hazelrig JV, et al: Life expectancy

73. Campbell M, Deuchar DC, Brock R: Results of pulmonary valvotomy and infundibular resection in 100 cases of Fallot's tetralogy. *Br Med J* **2**:111, 1954

74. Silbert A, et al: Cyanotic heart disease and psychological development. *Pediatrics* **43**:192, 1969

75. Mehrizi A, Drash A: Growth disturbance in congenital heart size. *J Pediatr* **61**:418, 1962

76. Phornphutkul C, Rosenthal A, Nadas AS, Berenberg W: Cerebrovascular accidents in infants and children with cyanotic congenital heart disease. *Am J Cardiol* **32**:329, 1973

77. Wasser S, Schneider P, Henne B: Das EEG bei Patienten mit Fallotscher Tetralogie mit und ohne hypoxamische Anfalle. *SO Kinderarztl-Prax* **60**:297–301, 1992

78. Komp DM, Sparrow AW: Polycythermia in cyanotic heart disease: A study of altered coagulation. *J Pediatr* **76**:231, 1970

79. Kontras SB, Bedenbender JG, Craenen J, Hosier DM: Hyperviscosity in congenital heart disease. *J Pediatr* **76**:214, 1970

80. Taussig HB, Crawford H, Pelargonio S, et al: Ten to thirteen year follow-up on patients after a Blalock–Taussig operation. *Circulation* **25**:630, 1962

81. Schmitt HJ, Scheutz WH, Proeschel PA, Jaklin C: Accuracy of pulse oximetry in children with cyanotic congenital heart disease. *J Cardiothorac Vasc Anesth* **7**:61–65, 1993

82. Saraclar M, Ozkutlu S, Ozme S, et al: Surgical treatment in tetralogy of Fallot diagnosed by echocardiography. *Int J Cardiol* **37**:329–335, discussion 337–338, 1992

83. Allan LD, Sharland GK: Prognosis in fetal tetralogy of Fallot. *Pediatr Cardiol* **13**:1–4, 1992

84. Jureidini SB, Appleton RS, Nouri S: Detection of coronary artery abnormalities in tetralogy of Fallot by two-dimensional echocardiography. *J Am Coll Cardiol* **14**:960–967, 1989

85. Stark P, Agness M, Holshouser B, Hinshaw D Jr: Kernspintomographie der Fallot-Tetralogie. *Radiologe* **31**:375–377, 1991

86. Mirowitz SA, Gutierrez FR, Canter CE, Vannier MW: Tetralogy of Fallot: MR findings. *Radiology* **171**:207–212, 1989

87. Martinez JE, Mohiaddin RH, Kilner PJ, et al: Obstruction in extracardiac ventriculopulmonary conduits: Value of nuclear magnetic resonance imaging with velocity mapping and Doppler echocardiography. *J Am Coll Cardiol* **20**:338–344, 1992

88. Edmunds LH, Saxena NC, Friedman S, et al: Transatrial resection of the obstructed right ventricular infundibulum. *Circulation* **54**:117, 1976

89. Edmunds LH, Saxena NC, Friedman S, et al: Transatrial repair of tetralogy of Fallot. *Surgery* **80**:681, 1976

90. Hudspeth AS, Cordell AR, Johnston FR: Transatrial approach to total correction of tetralogy of Fallot. *Circulation* **27**:796, 1963

91. Katz NM, Blackstone EH, Kirklin JW, et al: Late survival and symptoms after repair of tetralogy of Fallot. *Circulation* **65**:403, 1982

92. Horowitz LN, Vetter VL, Harken AH, Josephson ME: Electrophysiologic characteristics of sustained ventricular tachycardia occurring after repair of tetralogy of Fallot. *Am J Cardiol* **46**:446–452, 1980

93. Harkin AH, Horowitz LN, Josephson ME: Surgical correction of re-

current sustained ventricular tachycardia following complete repair of tetralogy of Fallot. *J Thorac Cardiovasc Surg* **80:**779–781, 1980

94. Foster V, McGoon DC, Kennedy MA, et al: Long term evaluation (12–22 years) of open heart surgery for tetralogy of Fallot. *Am J Cardiol* **46:**625–682, 1980

95. Rosing DR, Borer JS, Kent KM, et al: Long term hemodynamic and electrocardiographic assessment following operative repair of tetralogy of Fallot. *Circulation* **58:**209–217, 1978

96. Zimmermann M, Friedli B, Adamec R, Oberhansli I: Ventricular late potentials and induced ventricular tachycardia after surgical repair of tetralogy of Fallot. *Am J Cardiol* **67:**873–878, 1991

97. Rowlatt UF, Rimoldi JH, Lev M: The quantitative anatomy of the normal child's heart. *Pediatr Clin North Am* **10:**499–506, 1963

98. Groh MA, Meliones JN, Bove EL, et al: Repair of tetralogy of Fallot in infancy. Effect of pulmonary artery size on outcome. *Circulation* **84:**206–212, 1991

99. Uva MS, Lacour-Gayet F, Komiya T, et al: Surgery for tetralogy of Fallot at less than six months of age. *J Thorac Cardiovasc Surg* **107:**1291–1300, 1994

100. Kirklin JK, Kirklin JW, Blackstone EH, et al: Effect of transannular patching on outcome after repair of tetralogy of Fallot. *Ann Thorac Surg* **48:**783, 1989

101. Kirklin JW, Blackstone EH, Jonas RA, et al: Morphologic and surgical determinants of outcome events after repair of tetralogy of Fallot and pulmonary stenosis. *J Thorac Cardiovasc Surg* **103:**706, 1992

102. Kirklin JW, Blackstone EH, Kirklin JK, et al: Surgical results and protocols in the spectrum of tetralogy of Fallot. *Ann Surg* **198:**251, 1983

103. Gazzaniga AB, Elliott MP, Sperling DR, et al: Microporous expanded polytetrafluoroethylene arterial prosthesis for construction of aortopulmonary shunts. Experimental and clinical results. *Ann Thorac Surg* **21:**322, 1976

104. de Leval MR, McKay R, Jones M, et al: Modified Blalock–Taussig shunt. Use of subclavian artery orifice as flow regulator in prosthetic systemic-pulmonary artery shunts. *J Thorac Cardiovasc Surg* **81:**112, 1981

105. Bove EL, Kohman L, Sereika S, et al: The modified Blalock–Taussig shunt: Analysis of adequacy and duration of palliation. *Circulation* **76:**19, 1987

106. Donahoo JS, Gardner TJ, Zahka K, et al: Systemic pulmonary shunts in neonates and infants using microporous expanded polytetrafluoroethylene: Immediate and late results. *Ann Thorac Surg* **30:**146, 1980

107. Kay PH, Capuani A, Franks R, Lincoln C: Experience with the modified Blalock–Taussig operation using polytetrafluoroethylene (Impra) grafts. *Br Heart J* **49:**359, 1983

108. McKay R, de Leval MR, Rees P, et al: Postoperative angiographic assessment of modified Blalock–Taussig shunts using expanded polytetrafluoroethylene (Gore-Tex). *Ann Thorac Surg* **30:**137, 1980

109. Honda J: Growth of the pulmonary arteries and morphological assessment after Blalock–Taussig shunts. *Nippon Kyobu Geka Gakkai Zasshi* **41:**569–577, 1993

110. Guyton RA, Owens JE, Waumett JD, et al: The Blalock–Taussig shunt: Low risk, effective palliation, and pulmonary artery growth. *J Thorac Cardiovasc Surg* **85:**917, 1983

111. Lamberti JJ, Carlisle J, Waldman JD, et al: Systemic-pulmonary shunts in infants and children. *J Thorac Cardiovasc Surg* **88:**76, 1984

112. Tyson KRT, Larrieu AJ, Dirchmer JR Jr: The Blalock–Taussig shunt in the first two years of life: A safe and effective procedure. *Ann Thorac Surg* **26:**38, 1978

113. Lake CL: *Pediatric Cardiac Anesthesia.* Norwalk, Appleton & Lange, 1988

114. Brown TCK, Fisk GC: *Anaesthesia for Children,* 2nd ed. Oxford, Blackwell Scientific, 1992, pp 183–205

115. Vargas FJ, Kreutzer GO, Pedrini M, et al: Tetralogy of Fallot with subarterial ventricular septal defect. Diagnostic and surgical considerations. *J Thorac Cardiovasc Surg* **92:**908, 1986

116. Burczynski PL, McKay R, Arnold R, et al: Homograft replacement of the pulmonary artery bifurcation. *J Thorac Cardiovasc Surg* **98:**623, 1989

117. Marchand P: The use of a cusp-bearing homograft patch to the outflow tract and pulmonary artery in Fallot's tetralogy and pulmonary valvular stenosis. *Thorax* **22:**497, 1967

118. Cairns JA, Dobell ARC, Gibbons JE, Tessler I: Benign prognosis of right bundle branch block and left anterior hemiblock after intracardiac repair of tetralogy of Fallot. *Am Heart J* **90:**549, 1975

119. Arcinegas E, Farooki ZQ, Hakimi M, et al: Early and late results of total correction of tetralogy of Fallot. *J Thorac Cardiovasc Surg* **80:**770, 1980

120. Gustafson RA, Murray GF, Warden HE, et al: Early primary repair of tetralogy of Fallot. *Ann Thorac Surg* **45:**235, 1988

121. Pacifico AD, Sand ME, Bargeron LM Jr, Colvin EC: Transatrial-transpulmonary repair of tetralogy of Fallot. *J Thorac Cardiovasc Surg* **93:**919, 1987

122. Pacifico AD, Kirklin JK, Colvin EV, et al: Transatrial-transpulmonary repair of tetralogy of Fallot. *Semin Thorac Cardiovasc Surg* **2:**76, 1990

123. Fuster V, McCoon DC, Kennedy MA, et al: Long-term evaluation (12 to 22 years) of open heart surgery for tetralogy of Fallot. *Am J Cardiol* **46:**635, 1980

124. Kawashima Y, Kobayashi J, Matsuda A: Long term evaluation after correction of tetralogy of Fallot. *Kyobu Geka* **43:**660–665, 1990

125. Miyamura H, Eguchi S: Long term follow-up (20–25 years) of tetralogy of Fallot after correction. *Kyobu Geka* **43:**640–644, 1990

126. Horneffer PJ, Zahka KG, Rowe SA, et al: Long-term results of total repair of tetralogy of Fallot in childhood. *Ann Thorac Surg* **50:**179, 1990

127. Lillehei CW: Discussion of paper by Horneffer and colleagues. *Ann Thorac Surg* **50:**184, 1990

128. Chiariello L, Meyer J, Wukasch DC, et al: Intracardiac repair of tetralogy of Fallot. Five-year review of 403 patients. *J Thorac Cardiovasc Surg* **70:**529, 1975

129. Clayman JA, Ankeney JL, Leibman J: Results of complete repair of tetralogy of Fallot in 156 consecutive patients. *Am J Surg* **130:**601, 1975

130. Hamilton DI, Di Eusanio G, Piccoli GP, Dickinson DF: Eight years experience with intracardiac repair of tetralogy of Fallot. Early and late results in 175 consecutive patients. *Br Heart J* **46:**144, 1981

131. Puga FJ, DuShane JW, McGoon DC: Treatment of tetralogy of Fallot in children less than 4 years of age. *J Thorac Cardiovasc Surg* **64:**247, 1972

132. Villani M, Gamba A, Tiraboschi R, et al: Surgical treatment of tetralogy of Fallot. Recent experience using a prospective protocol. *Thorac Cardiovasc Surg* **31:**151, 1983

133. Borow KM, Green LH, Castaneda AR, Keane JF: Left ventricular function after repair of tetralogy of Fallot and its relationship to age at surgery. *Circulation* **61:**1150, 1980

134. Lukacs L, Kassai I, Arvay A: Total correction of tetralogy of Fallot in adolescents and adults. *Thorac Cardiovasc Surg* **40:**261–265, 1992

135. Podzolkov VP, Plotnikov LR, Ngvenia L: Neposredstvennye rezul'taty radikal'noi korrektsii tetrady Fallo u vzroslykh. *Grud Serdechnososudistaia Khir* (2):8–10, 1993

136. Wu QY: Corrective surgery for tetralogy of Fallot. Analysis of 156 cases. *Chung-Hua-Wai-Ko-Tsa-Chih* **30:**207–209, 254, 1992

137. Kirklin JW, Payne WS, Theye RA, DuShane JW: Factors affecting survival after open operation for tetralogy of Fallot. *Ann Surg* **152:**485, 1960

138. Kirklin JW, Wallace RB, McGoon DC, DuShane JW: Early and late results after intracardiac repair of tetralogy of Fallot: 5-year review of 337 patients. *Ann Surg* **162:**578, 1965

139. Richardson JP, Clarke CP: Tetralogy of Fallot. Risk factors associated with complete repair. *Br Heart J* **38:**926, 1976

140. Delisle G, Olley PM: Epreuve d'effort sous-axial chez les enfants atteints de tetralogie de Fallot: Avant et après correction chirurgicale. *Union Med Can* **103:**886, 1974

141. Wessels HU, Cunningham WJ, Paul MH, et al: Exercise performance in tetralogy of Fallot after intracardiac repair. *J Thorac Cardiovasc Surg* **80:**582, 1980

142. Perrault H, Drblik SP, Montigny M, et al: Comparison of cardiovascular adjustments to exercise in adolescents 8 to 15 years of age after correction of tetralogy of Fallot, ventricular septal defect of atrial septal defect. *Am J Cardiol* **64:**213, 1989

143. Oku H: Operative results and postoperative hemodynamic results in total correction of tetralogy of Fallot. *Arch Jpn Chir* **45:**87, 1976

144. d'Allaines C, Sover R, Rioux C, et al: Tetralogies de Fallot: Resultats à distance de la correction complète. *Nouv Presse Med* **2:**961, 1973

145. Marx GR, Hicks RW, Allen HD, Goldberg SJ: Non-invasive assessment of hemodynamic responses to exercise in pulmonary regurgitation after operations to correct pulmonary outflow obstruction. *Am J Cardiol* **61:**595, 1988

146. Rowe SA, Zahka KG, Manolio TA, et al: Lung function and pulmonary regurgitation limit exercise capacity in postoperative tetralogy of Fallot. *J Am Coll Cardiol* **17:**461, 1991

147. Vetter HO, Reichart B, Seidel P, et al: Non-invasive assessment of right and left ventricular volumes of 11 to 24 years after corrective surgery on patients with tetralogy of Fallot. *Eur J Cardiothorac Surg* **4:**24, 1990

148. Carvalho JS, Shinebourne EA, Busst C, et al: Exercise capacity after complete repair of tetralogy of Fallot: Deleterious effects of residual pulmonary regurgitation. *Br Heart J* **67:**470–473, 1992

149. Katz NM, Blackstone EH, Kirklin JW, et al: Late survival and symptoms after repair of tetralogy of Fallot. *Circulation* **65:**403–410, 1982

150. Kirklin JK, Kirklin JW, Blackstone EH, et al: Sudden death and arrhythmic events after repair of tetralogy of Fallot. In Crupi G, Parenzan L, Anderson RH (eds): *Perspectives in Paediatric Cardiology,* Vol 2. *Pediatric Cardiac Surgery,* Part 1. Mt. Kisco, NY, Futura, 1989, p 204

151. Castaneda AR, Mayer J, Jonas R, et al: Tetralogy of Fallot: Repair in infancy. In Crupi G, Parenzan L, Anderson RH (eds): *Perspectives in Pediatric Cardiology,* Vol. 2 *Pediatric Cardiac Surgery,* Part 1. Mt. Kisco, NY, 1989

152. Walsh EP, Rockenmacher S, Keane JF, et al: Late results in patients with tetralogy of Fallot repaired during infancy. *Circulation* **77:**1062, 1988

153. Kavey REW, Blackman MS, Sondheimer HM: Incidence and severity of chronic ventricular dysrhythmias after repair of tetralogy of Fallot. *Am Heart J* **103:**342, 1982

154. Kobayashi J, Hirose H, Nakano S, et al: Ambulatory electrocardiographic study of the frequency and cause of ventricular arrhythmia after correction of tetralogy of Fallot. *Am J Cardiol* **54:**1310, 1984

155. Sullivan ID, Presbitero P, Gooch VM, et al: Is ventricular arrhythmia in repaired tetralogy of Fallot an effect of operation or a consequence of the course of the disease? A prospective study. *Br Heart J* **58:**40, 1987

156. Touati GD, Vouhe PR, Amodeo A, et al: Primary repair of tetralogy of Fallot in infancy. *J Thorac Cardiovasc Surg* **99:**396, 1990

157. Wessel HU, Bastanier CK, Paul MH, et al: Prognostic significance of arrythmia in tetralogy of Fallot after intracardiac repair. *Am J Cardiol* **46:**843, 1980

158. Kavey REW, Thomas FD, Byrum CJ, et al: Ventricular arrhythmias and biventricular dysfunction after repair of tetralogy of Fallot. *J Am Coll Cardiol* **4:**126, 1984

159. Miura T, Nakano S, Shimazaki Y, et al: Evaluation of right ventricular function by regional wall motion analysis in patients after correction of tetralogy of Fallot. Comparison of transventricular and non-transventricular repairs [see comments]. *J Thorac Cardiovasc Surg* **104**(4):1173–1174, 1992; *J Thorac Cardiovasc Surg* **104:**917–923, 1992

160. Bove EL, Byrum CJ, Thomas FD, et al: The influence of pulmonary insufficiency on ventricular function following repair of tetralogy of Fallot. *J Thorac Cardiovasc Surg* **85:**691, 1983

161. Finck SJ, Puga FJ, Danielson GK: Pulmonary valve insertion during reoperation for tetralogy of Fallot. *Ann Thorac Surg* **45:**610, 1988

162. Bove EL, Kavey REW, Byrum CJ, et al: Improved right ventricular function following late pulmonary valve replacement for residual pulmonary insufficiency or stenosis. *J Thorac Cardiovasc Surg* **90:**50, 1985

163. Shaher RM, Foster E, Farina M, et al: Right heart reconstruction following repair of tetralogy of Fallot. *Ann Thorac Surg* **35:**421, 1983

164. Ilbawi MN, Idriss FS, DeLeon SY, et al: Long-term results of porcine valve insertion for pulmonary regurgitation following repair of tetralogy of Fallot. *Ann Thorac Surg* **41:**478, 1986

165. Laks H, Hellenbrandt WE, Kleinman CS, et al: Patch reconstruction of the right ventricular outflow tract with pulmonary valve insertion. *Circulation* **64:**154, 1981

166. Misbach GA, Turley K, Ebert PA: Pulmonary valve replacement for regurgitation after repair of tetralogy of Fallot. *Ann Thorac Surg* **36:**684, 1981

167. Finck SJ, Puga FJ, Danielson GK: Pulmonary valve insertion during reoperation for tetralogy of Fallot. *Ann Thorac Surg,* **45:**610, 1988

168. Ilbawi M, Idriss F, Muster A, et al: Tetralogy of Fallot with absent pulmonary valve. *J Thorac Cardiovasc Surg* **81:**906–915, 1981

169. Pacifico AD, Ricchi A, Bargeron LM Jr, et al: Corrective repair of complete atrioventricular canal defects and major associated cardiac anomalies. *Ann Thorac Surg* **46:**645, 1988

82

The Mustard Procedure

George A. Trusler

Although predated by the Senning operation as a successful repair of transposition of the great arteries (TGA), the Mustard procedure was the first to find widespread success. This stimulated a surge of interest in all aspects of the management of transposition, which has continued unabated since.

HISTORY

In 1955, Albert first suggested rearranging venous inflow at the atrial level for repair of TGA.[1] Subsequently, this was attempted clinically by Merendino et al,[2] Kay and Cross,[3] Creech et al,[4] and Wilson et al.[5] They used a variety of materials within the atria but all were unsuccessful. Senning did the first successful atrial repair in 1959 using flaps of atrial wall and septum to partition the atria.[6] Kirklin et al[7] performed a small series of Senning operations with success but relatively high mortality. The operation seemed complicated and enthusiasm was restrained. Using a large, crimped tube of Teflon to connect the pulmonary veins to the tricuspid valve, Barnard et al[8] reported a successful repair.

Mustard attempted repair of TGA as early as 1951 and also attempted a partial venous repair at that time.[9] His interest was increased by the success of the Senning procedure and focused by the chance occurrence of inferior vena cava to left atrial shunts following atrial septal defect repair. Rather than the artificial materials employed by Albert, Merendino, and others, Mustard partitioned the atriums with a large patch of pericardium, redirecting caval venous return to the left ventricle and pulmonary venous return to the right ventricle.[10] The operation proved simple, safe, and reproducible; it met with immediate, widespread acceptance.

INDICATIONS

Whereas initially the Mustard repair became the basis for management of TGA, the occurrence of baffle complications and dysrhythmias stimulated a number of surgeons to rediscover and employ the Senning atrial repair. There appears to be little difference between the results of the Mustard and Senning operations, except that the latter, using living tissue, may be preferable if repair is necessary in the first month of life. However, excellent results have been reported using the Mustard procedure in neonates.[11] Both atrial repairs have since been largely superseded by the Jatene et al[12] arterial repair.

In most centers, simple TGA [TGA in patients with intact ventricular septum as well as in patients with small insignificant ventricular septal defects (VSDs) and minor forms of pulmonary stenosis] is presently best managed by arterial repair and usually in the first 2 weeks of life. Indications for atrial repair in this group of patients have been restricted to a few special situations. The presence of a single coronary artery particularly if running an intramural course was considered an indication, but techniques[13] have been developed to manage the coronary artery and arterial repair is now preferred by many surgeons. Severe incorrectable pulmonary stenosis is still an indication for atrial repair but is seen less frequently now that arterial repair is done in early infancy. This suggests that much of the pulmonary stenosis is an acquired condition which develops with time. Older age (more than 3 or 4 wks of age) is a risk factor for death after arterial repair because the left ventricle (LV) is no longer conditioned to accept systemic pressures. Most surgeons will employ atrial repair in this circumstance but some[14] would still do an arterial repair up to 2 mo of age and others[15] would recondition the ventricle with a pulmonary artery band followed by a later arterial repair. In some parts of the world many infants with TGA are not identified until older and they are usually managed with atrial repair. Other rare indications for atrial repair are isolated atrioventricular discordance and the presence of a small LV. In the latter a bidirectional cavopulmonary shunt is done in association with the Mustard repair to reduce the load on the small LV.

In complex TGA with large VSD, results are clearly best with arterial repair. An atrial repair, however, is the best form of palliation for a child with TGA, VSD, and severe pulmonary vascular disease in that the initial operative mortality is lower and the long term palliation possibly better.

Most infants with the complex of TGA, VSD, and pulmonary stenosis (PS) have palliative Blalock–Taussig shunts in infancy and later a Rastelli repair. In some children, the pulmonary stenosis is mild or can be relieved directly, while the VSD is relatively small or not suited for a Rastelli repair. In these cases, simultaneous direct repair of the PS and VSD can be accomplished at the same time as atrial repair of the transposition. If, as is frequently the case in infancy, the pulmonary valve is normal and the stenosis can be managed surgically, an arterial switch repair is generally preferred.

Where TGA, intact ventricular septum is combined with a fixed severe form of left ventricular outflow tract obstruction (PS), infants are managed best by atrial repair (Mustard or Senning) along with direct relief of the PS. If the PS can be permanently relieved and the pulmonary valve is essentially normal an arterial repair is preferred. In some cases where the PS is particularly severe or difficult, possibly requiring an LV–PA conduit, palliation with a Blalock–Taussig shunt is appropriate while postponing the repair until the child is older. It would appear, however, that in many cases the PS is an acquired lesion for it is seen less frequently since the advent of neonatal arterial repair.

TECHNIQUES

The Mustard operation can be performed at any age but postoperative complications, both early and late, seem more common when operating on infants younger than about 6 weeks. All infants have a balloon atrial septostomy (BAS) at initial cardiac catheterization. Those requiring more help before 6 wks will have a Blalock–Hanlon atrial septectomy at our institution. The Mustard operation is performed sometime after 6 weeks and usually when the infant is 6 to 12 mo old.

Through a median sternotomy incision, the anterior surface of the pericardial sac is cleared from the diaphragm to the great arteries. The thymus is mobilized, and often one lobe is excised for exposure. A large patch of pericardium is excised for use as the future atrial baffle. The pericardium is roughly dumbbell shaped with two bulbous ends and a waist that is 2.5 to 3.0 cm wide (Fig. 82–1). For an infant of 10 kg body weight, the long side is 7 cm and the

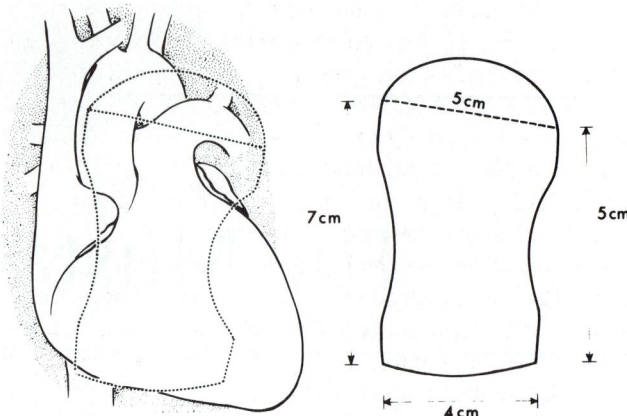

Figure 82–1. Excision of anterior pericardium for atrial baffle. For a child weighing 10 kg, the sides are 7, 5, 5, and 4 cm long. *(From Trusler GA, Freedom RM: Complete transposition of the great arteries. In Arciniegas (ed): Pediatric Cardiac Surgery. Chicago, Year Book Medical Publishers, 1985, p 257.)*

short side 5 cm long. The superior vena cava (SVC) end is 4 cm, and the inferior vena cava (IVC) end is 5 cm. For a child weighing 5 kg, the margins are all 0.5 cm shorter. Both ends are rounded, particularly the IVC to provide flexibility in choosing the most appropriate suture line. The long axis of the pericardium is usually taken longitudinally, but it can be harvested transversely between the phrenic nerves. This size of pericardial patch provides a baffle that is always ample. Other surgeons use different shapes and sizes. Brom and his colleagues have used a baffle shaped like a pair of trousers where the two limbs are sized according to the diameter of the superior and inferior caval veins.[16]

In children weighing over 9 or 10 kg, both venae cavae are cannulated. The SVC is cannulated directly, and the IVC is cannulated through the atriocaval junction. The repair is done on cardiopulmonary bypass with moderate hypothermia and, where necessary, low flow perfusion. If the aorta is cross-clamped, cardioplegia is given, the heart is kept cold, and the time short.

Most infants and children weigh less than 9 kg at repair and deep hypothermic circulatory arrest is used. The aorta and right atrial appendage are cannulated directly. Core cooling on cardiopulmonary bypass is continued until the rectal temperature is below 18°C (esophageal 12° to 14°C). Vasodilator drugs are given to assist cooling, which empirically is continued for at least 3 min for every kilogram of body weight to ensure adequate hypothermia of vital organs. During cooling, the aorta is dissected and the caval veins encircled with tourniquets. At the appropriate temperature, the aorta is clamped, blood cardioplegia given, the caval tourniquets tightened, and the venous cannula clamped and removed. A small "cooling pad" placed around the ventricles will maintain the myocardia temperature at 10° to 12°C. The total circulatory arrest and aortic cross clamp time is usually less than 50 min.

A longitudinal incision in the right atrium gives ample exposure (Fig. 82–2A). After inspecting the interior of the atrium, the residual atrial septum is partially excised (Fig. 82–2B). An initial incision is made from the center of the fossa ovales superiorly toward the center of the SVC until the top of the atrial septum is reached. The septum medial to this cut is saved, for it may contain the artery to the sinoatrial (S-A) node and have the potential to conduct impulses from the S-A node to the atrioventricular (A-V) node. The septum lateral to the cut is excised. The coronary sinus wall is cut from its orifice down into the left atrium for a distance of approximately 10 to 15 mm. All thick, raw edges of septum are oversewn to reduce contracture and adhesion to the baffle (Fig. 82–2C).

The pericardial baffle is now inserted into the common atrial chamber with a double ended 3-0 braided synthetic suture (Fig. 82–2D). The middle of the long border of the baffle is sutured anterior to the left pulmonary veins. The suture lines runs around the orifice of the left superior pulmonary vein, across the posterior wall of the left atrium dipping slightly inferiorly to enlarge the SVC channel and then up to the region of the right superior pulmonary vein. The first corner of the baffle should reach the right atrial wall. The SVC end of the baffle is sutured to the internal orifice of the SVC using small bites and gathering up the baffle to produce a moderate redundancy. The suture line is then carried across the roof of the right atrium so that the second corner of the baffle ends halfway between the SVC orifice and the tricuspid valve.

At this point, we start the other end of the original stitch and suture the baffle around the left inferior pulmonary vein and across the posterior wall of LA toward the

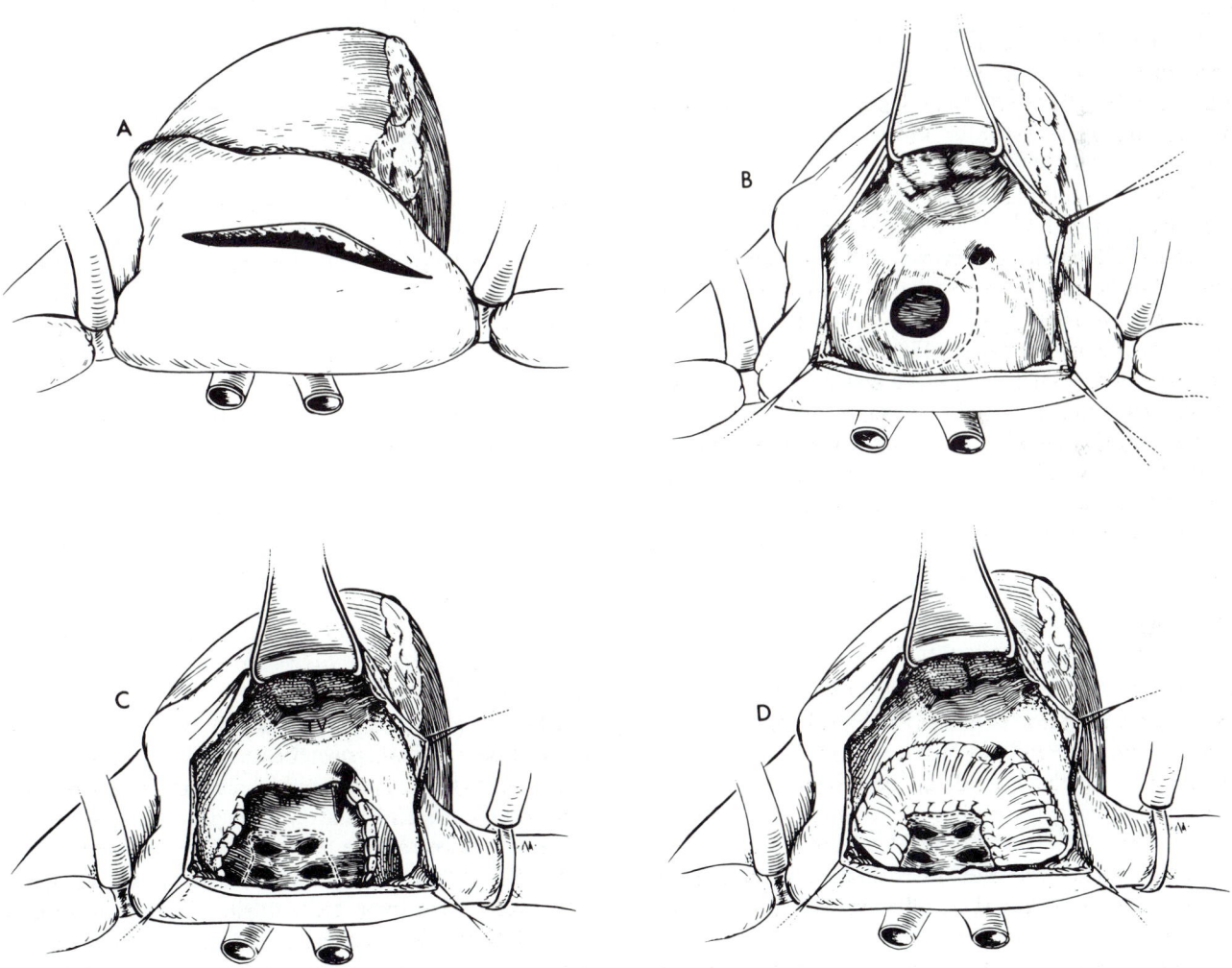

Figure 82–2. The Mustard operation. **A.** The right atrium is opened with a longitudinal incision well away from the sinoatrial node. **B.** The atrial septum is incised from the midpoint on the superior border of the atrial septal defect to the middle of the superior vena caval orifice. All the septum lateral to this incision is excised, avoiding the orifices of the right pulmonary veins. The ridge of septum medially is preserved. **C.** The coronary sinus is cut back into the left atrium and all raw margins of atrial septum are oversewn. The dotted line indicates where the baffle will be sutured. **D.** The suture starts at the anterior lip of the left pulmonary vein orifices and when completed diverts the caval venous return to the mitral valve and the pulmonary venous return to the tricuspid valve. *(From Trusler GA, Freedom RM: Transposition of the great arteries: The Mustard procedure. In Sabiston, Spencer (eds): Gibbon's Surgery of the Chest. Philadelphia, W.B. Saunders, 1983, p 1138.)*

right inferior pulmonary vein. Between the left and right veins, the suture lines may curve up slightly to enlarge the IVC channel but should not be closer than 10 to 15 mm to the upper suture line. Near the right inferior pulmonary vein, the suture line angles down toward the IVC to widen the channel for the pulmonary veins. The third corner of the baffle should reach the right atrial wall.

During circulatory arrest, suturing the IVC end is simplified by removing the tourniquet from the IVC so that the best suture line can be chosen. This may be the eustachian valve if it is strong, the base of the eustachian valve if convenient, or more often some ridge of atrial tissue near the IVC orifice. The baffle is tailored accordingly so that it is ample without excess redundancy. After passing around the IVC, the suture line is directed to the cut orifice of the coronary sinus where the final corner of the baffle is sutured. Within the coronary sinus, small bites are taken about 5 mm deep or to the left of the actual orifice until the other cut margin of sinus wall is reached. The baffle is sutured to this margin and then to the residual flap of atrial septum adjacent to the tricuspid valve continuing up to the upper suture line. Saline is injected into the left side to fill out the baffle and check its shape and fit.

From below, the aortic valve is frustrated momentarily while a final amount of cardioplegia is started. After half a dose the cardioplegia is reduced to low flow while the right atrium is closed, the venous cannula reinserted in the right atrial appendage, and the infant placed back on bypass for rewarming. The remaining caval tourniquet is removed. As the aortic clamp is removed, cardioplegia is stopped. The tip of the right atrial cannula is gently inserted through the tricuspid valve momentarily to evacuate air in the right ventricle. Since the venous cannula is now in the pulmonary atrium, the lungs are ventilated and the heart gently massaged to promote flow of blood through the lungs. Usually the heart beats in 2 or 3 min and then the systemic venous pressures return toward normal. Two atrial and two ventricular temporary pacemaker wires are inserted and connected to an A-V sequential pacemaker. Once the infant has rewarmed (rectal temperature over 34°C) bypass is discontinued. When stable, the right atrial venous cannula is removed and replaced by a small line to monitor atrial pressure postoperatively. The chest is closed in a standard way.

If there is associated VSD or PS requiring treatment, part of the repair is done on bypass to avoid an excessively long circulatory arrest. During a brief period of circulatory arrest, the atrium is opened and the single atrial cannula replaced by two curved metal caval cannulas. Now on complete bypass, the atrial septum is excised and the posterior part of the baffle suture lines inserted. Then at an appropriately low temperature, circulation is arrested once more, the caval cannulas removed, the baffle completed, and the associated defect, VSD or PS, repaired. In larger infants, the presence of the associated defects encourages the use of bypass rather than circulatory arrest.

In the presence of left juxtaposition of the right atrial appendage or mesocardia, the right atrium is small, and should be enlarged with a patch of pericardium.

The postoperative course is usually uncomplicated without need for inotropic support except where repair is carried out in the first 2 mo of life. Most infants are extubated within 24 to 48 hours. Occasionally, postoperative bleeding will require return to the operating room, particularly in infants with adhesions from previous surgery. Temporary phrenic nerve paralysis, which prolongs the need for ventilatory assistance, occurs in about 5% of infants but is more frequent in those with previous surgery.

RESULTS

Early Mortality

The mortality for Mustard repair of simple TGA has improved greatly. In our series of 358 children with simple TGA operated on before January 1994, there were 13 (3.6%) early deaths. Since 1973, the mortality rate has been 0.8%, and there have been no deaths in the last 190 operations since early 1978. Others have achieved a similar low mortality.[17,18] Mortality is increased if significant associated lesions such as VSD or PS require repair. The most common causes of early death were myocardial failure and dysrhythmia.

Complications

The fate of the baffle is very important. Soon after operation, the baffle becomes coated with fibrin, which organizes into a layer of fibrous tissue that subsequently contracts.[19] The final shape seems to depend less on the size of the baffle than on the integrity and position of the suture lines. Dacron baffles shrink more than pericardium. Atrial volume is maintained by growth of normal atrial wall.

Baffle Leaks

Baffle leaks are common but usually not identified until postoperative cardiac catheterization.[20] In total, we have done 529 Mustard operations on both simple and complex transposition malformation. Two hundred and seven of the 480 early survivors have had a catheter study with baffle leaks identified in 48 (23%). Most leaks are small, but seven were significant L–R shunts with a pulmonary/systemic flow ratio of 1.5 to 2.2:1. Two children had right-to-left shunts of 1.5:1. One child already mentioned died from a major baffle detachment. Seven had reoperation for repair of the leak.

Superior Vena Cava Obstruction

Narrowing of the SVC channel, a moderately common problem[21,22] was found in 40 (19%) of the 207 children who had postoperative cardiac catheterization. Twenty children had a moderate or severe degree of stenosis, but only five of them had sufficient symptoms to require operative repair. Balloon dilatation and stenting provided effective relief of stenosis in three children.[23] Much of the narrowing was related to the residual ridge of septum between the SVC and tricuspid valve, however, in some cases, it was due to a small baffle that is flattened across the SVC channel or to some of the sutures pulling out, and causing both a leak and stenosis.

Inferior Vena Cava Obstruction

The large IVC channel provides a greater margin of safety against critical stenosis so that narrowing is much less common. We encountered this in 6 of the 480 early surviving children: 3 were mild and 3 severe. One caused late death and two required repair. If several baffle sutures pull out, a combination of a leak and a stenosis may be produced.

Pulmonary Venous Obstruction

This dangerous complication occurred usually at the level of the original atrial septum just anterior to the right pulmonary vein orifices. It seems to result from a progressive adhesion of the baffle to the raw edge of excised septum. Oversewing the raw margins and keeping the upper and lower baffle suture lines wide apart by the right pulmonary veins and the lateral wall of the RA help prevent this complication. Seven of the 480 (1.5%) early surviving children in our total series developed this complication. Despite attempted repair in five children, all but one died eventually. Like caval stenosis, this complication was noted more frequently when Dacron baffles were used.[24,25]

Stenosis of the Left Pulmonary Venous Channel

Narrowing of the left pulmonary venous channel in the posterior LA, near the orifices of the left pulmonary veins, has also occurred in 6 (1.2%) patients. We believe this occurs if the upper and lower baffle sutures lines on the LA are too close together. One child died before the diagnosis. The other five were repaired: one died and the other four have little or no flow from the left lung by Doppler echocardiography. At reoperation in these cases, there is secondary pulmonary venous ostial stenosis with associated narrowing or hypoplasia of the whole vein so that treatment is difficult. We have also encountered stenosis in the left pulmonary vein ostia at the time of the Mustard repair on two occasions, perhaps related to imbalance in perfusion of right and left lungs.

Dysrhythmias

The most common late complication is usually a result of sinus node dysfunction, emphasizing the importance of avoiding injury to the S-A node and its artery.[26,27] Preserving a ridge of atrial septum between the SVC and tricuspid

valve appeared to reduce the incidence of dysrhythmias.[28] A-V node problems seem uncommon if reasonable care is taken and the baffle suture line kept a short distance away. VSD repair in complex TGA increases the risk of A-V node problems, right bundle branch block, and dysrhythmia.

In recent years, 91% of infants and children have been in sinus rhythm on their discharge ECG. Only 51% of the patients with simple TGA that we operated on in the first decade (1963 to 1973) were in sinus rhythm on their last ECG, whereas 73% of patients operated on later (1974 to 1985) were in sinus rhythm.[29] We hoped, as did others,[30,31] that the incidence of dysrhythmia had been reduced by technical modifications, and we believe it has to some extent, but 24 hour ambulatory monitoring reveals a still high incidence of sinus node dysfunction. Perioperative electrophysiologic studies suggested that this dysfunction existed from the time of operation but only became clinically apparent later with an increasing incidence of dysrhythmia. Dysrhythmias increase with time[32] and in a small group of our earliest patients repaired in the first decade who are now adults only 6 of 24 are in sinus rhythm.

Right Ventricular Dysfunction and Tricuspid Incompetence

There is general concern that the right ventricle and tricuspid valve will not support systemic pressures indefinitely. Right ventricular dysfunction and tricuspid incompetence occurred more frequently following repair of complex TGA with closure of a VSD. This is partly related to the occurrence of right bundle branch block (RBBB) and at times some distortion of the tricuspid valve. Consequently, arterial switch repair is now favored in this group of children.

The main question centers about the extent of the problem in simple TGA. Subjective interpretation of postoperative RV angiograms by our radiologists and cardiologists revealed that RV contractility was possibly reduced in up to one-third of patients following repair of simple TGA but only 11% of angiograms showed moderate or severe diminution in RV contractility, and even these patients were asymptomatic. A few (4 of 126 catheterizations) also had some tricuspid regurgitation, and 9 had tricuspid incompetence without obvious RV dysfunction. Careful comprehensive studies by a number of authors[33-35] showed that the RV end diastolic volume is frequently increased and RV ejection fraction decreased after atrial repair. Benson et al found an abnormal response to exercise stress in over 50% of children.[36] Others found similar results.[37-39] Graham et al[40] recently found that patients operated on after 1974 had better postoperative RV ejection fractions than did those repaired earlier, perhaps due to a younger age at repair. Certainly this emphasizes the importance of meticulous perioperative myocardial care, which includes efficient cardiopulmonary bypass, good myocardial protection, a reasonably short ischemic time with effective myocardial hypothermia, adequate postoperative cardiac outputs, and the avoidance

TABLE 82–1. RESULTS OF MUSTARD OPERATION FOR TGA

Type	May 1963–Dec 1973			Jan 1974–Dec 1993		
	No.	Early Death	Late Death	No.	Early Death	Late Death
Simple TGA	106	11	23	252	2	13
TGA, VSD	35	14	7	42	8	6
TGA, VSD, PS	13	6	4	32	0	6
TGA, intact septum, PS	9	3	1	40	5	3
Total	163	34	35	366	15	28

of serious dysrhythmias at all times to avoid hypoperfusion and tricuspid incompetence.

Despite the anxiety regarding late RV function, surviving children are well. They generally grow at close to normal rates.[41] In our recent review of patients who had repair of simple TGA before 1981, we found that 76% were in NYHA Class I and 24% in Class II. None was in Class III or IV. Seventy-eight percent were on no medication, while the other 22% were taking medication, largely for dysrhythmia control. Of a group of 24 of our earliest patients, both simple and complex followed at the adult clinic, 11 are in Class I, 12 Class II, and 1 Class III.

Late Mortality

Thirty-six of the 345 early surviving infants and children following Mustard repair of simple TGA died late. The common causes of death were dysrhythmia, pulmonary venous obstruction, and cardiac failure. Actuarial analysis shows a 10- and 15-year survival of 85.8 and 81.5% for all children with simple TGA but 93 and 91% for those repaired since 1973.

The risk of late mortality was increased in children with complex TGA when the associated defects required repair (Table 82–1). Most late deaths occurred within 4 years of operation, suggesting a relationship to surgery and stressing the need for a careful operation with good myocardial protection and avoidance of dysrhythmia.

Therefore, in general terms, patients with simple transposition, treated with a Mustard procedure, seem to be doing better than expected with very few symptoms despite the potential concern about RV function. Although the continuing incidence of dysrhythmia, the greatest long-term problem, has led many to prefer arterial repair, there are still indications for the Mustard operation.

REFERENCES

1. Albert HM: Surgical correction of transposition of the great vessels. *Surg Forum* **5**:74, 1955
2. Merendino KA, Jesseph JE, Herron PW, et al: Interatrial venous transposition—a one stage intracardiac operation for the conversion of complete transposition of the aorta and pulmonary artery to corrected transposition: Theory and clinical experience. *Surgery* **42**:898, 1957
3. Kay EB, and Cross FS: Transposition of the great vessels corrected by means of atrial transposition. *Surgery* **41**:938, 1957
4. Creech O Jr, Maffey DE, Sayegh SF, Sailors EL: Complete transposition of the great vessels: A technique for intracardiac correction. *Surgery* **43**:349, 1958
5. Wilson HE, Nafrawi AG, Cardozo RH, Aguillon A: Rational approach to surgery for complete transposition of the great vessels. *Ann Thorac Surg* **155**:258, 1962
6. Senning A: Surgical correction of transposition of the great vessels. *Surgery* **45**:966, 1959
7. Kirklin JW, Devloo RA, Weldman WH: Open intracardiac repair for transposition of the great vessels: 11 cases. *Surgery* **50**:58, 1961
8. Barnard CN, Schrire V, Beck W: Complete transposition of the great vessels: A successful complete correction. *J Thorac Cardiovasc Surg* **43**:768, 1962
9. Mustard WT, Chute AL, Keith JD, et al: A surgical approach to transposition of the great vessels with extracorporeal circuit. *Surgery* **36**:39, 1954
10. Mustard WT: Successful two-stage correction of transposition of the great vessels. *Surgery* **55**:469, 1964
11. de Begona JA, Kawauchi M, Fullerton D, et al: The Mustard procedure for correction of simple transposition of the great arteries before one month of age. *J Thorac Cardiovasc Surg* **104**:1218, 1992
12. Jatene AD, Fontes VF, Paulista PP, et al: Successful anatomic correction of transposition of the great vessels. A preliminary report. *Arq Bras Cardiol* **28**:461, 1975
13. Takeuchi S, Katogi T: New technique for the arterial switch operation in difficult situations. *Ann Thorac Surg* **50**:1000, 1990
14. Davis AM, Wilkinson JL, Karl TR, Mee RBB: Transposition of the great arteries with intact ventricular septum. *J Thorac Cardiovasc Surg* **106**:111, 1993
15. Jonas RA, Giglia TM, Sanders SP, et al: Rapid, two stage arterial switch for transposition of the great arteries and intact ventricular septal beyond the neonatal period. *Circulation* **80**(Suppl I):I203, 1989
16. Brom GA: Technique of Mustard operation. In Hahn C (ed): *Thorax Chirurgie*, Leiden 1950, p 75; Leiden, Netherlands, Drukkerij Bedrijf BC, 1975
17. Piccoli GP, Wilkinson JL, Arnold R, et al: Appraisal of the Mustard procedure for the physiological correction of "simple" transposition of the great arteries. *J Thorac Cardiovasc Surg* **82**:436, 1981
18. Ebert PA, Gay WA Jr, Engle MA: Correction of transposition of the great arteries: Relationship of the coronary sinus and postoperative arrhythmias. *Ann Surg* **180**:433, 1974
19. Mohri H, Barnes RW, Rittenhouse EA, et al: Fate of autologous pericardium and Dacron fabric used as substitutes for total atrial septum in growing animals. *J Thorac Cardiovasc Surg* **59**:501, 1970
20. Park SC, Neches WH, Mathew RA, et al: Hemodynamic function after the Mustard operation for transposition of the great arteries. *Am J Cardiol* **51**:1514, 1983

21. Hagler DJ, Ritter DG, Mair DD, et al: Clinical angiographic and hemodynamic assessment of late results after the Mustard operation. *Circulation* **57**:1214, 1978

22. Arciniegas E, Farooki ZQ, Hakimi M, et al: Results of the Mustard operation for dextro-transposition of the great arteries. *J Thorac Cardiovasc Surg* **81**:580, 1981

23. Chatelain P, Meier B, Friedli B: Stenting of superior vena cava and inferior vena cava for symptomatic narrowing after repeated atrial surgery for D-transposition of the great arteries. *Br Heart J* **66**:466, 1991

24. Silverman NH, Snider AR, Colo J, et al: Superior vena caval obstruction after Mustard's operation by two-dimensional contrast echocardiography. *Circulation* **64**:392, 1981

25. Driscoll DJ, Nihill MR, Vargo TA, et al: Late development of pulmonary venous obstruction following Mustard's operation using a Dacron baffle. *Circulation* **55**:484, 1977

26. Gillette PC, Kugler JD, Garson A Jr, et al: Mechanisms of cardiac arrhythmias after the Mustard operation for transposition of the great arteries. *Am J Cardiol* **45**:1225, 1980

27. Henglein D, Mocellin R, Brodherr S, et al: Electrocardiographic and electrophysiologic studies after the Senning procedure in patients with complete transposition of the great arteries. *Herz* **6**:352, 1981

28. Trusler GA, Williams WG, Izukawa T, Olley PM: Current results with the Mustard operation in isolated transposition of the great arteries. *J Thorac Cardiovasc Surg* **80**:381, 1980

29. Trusler GA, Williams WG, Duncan KF, et al: Results with the Mustard operation in simple transposition of the great arteries. *Ann Surg* **206**:251, 1987

30. Southall DP, Keton BR, Leanage R, et al: Cardiac rhythm and conduction before and after Mustard's operation for complete transposition of the great arteries. *Br Heart J* **43**:21, 1980

31. Turley K, Ebert PA: Total correction of transposition of the great arteries: Conduction disturbances in infants younger than three months of age. *J Thorac Cardiovasc Surg* **76**:312, 1980

32. Deanfield JE, Camm J, Macartney F, et al: Arrhythmia and late mortality after Mustard and Senning operation for transposition of the great arteries: An eight-year prospective study. *J Thorac Cardiovasc Surg* **96**:569, 1988

33. Graham TP Jr, Atwood GF, Boucek RJ Jr, et al: Abnormalities of right ventricular function following Mustard's operation for transposition of the great arteries. *Circulation* **52**:678, 1975

34. Jarmakani JMM, Canent RV Jr: Preoperative and postoperative right ventricular function in children with transposition of the great vessels. *Circulation* **49, 50**(II):II39, 1974

35. Hagler DJ, Ritter DG, Mair DD, et al: Right and left ventricular function after the Mustard procedure in transposition of the great arteries. *Am J Cardiol* **44**:276, 1979

36. Benson LN, Bonet J, McLaughlin P, et al: Assessment of right ventricular function during supine bicycle exercise after Mustard's operation. *Circulation* **65**:1052, 1982

37. Murphy JH, Barlai-Kovach MM, Mathews RA, et al: Rest and exercise right and left ventricular function late after the Mustard operation: Assessment by radionuclide ventriculography. *Am J Cardiol* **57**:1142, 1986

38. Parrish MD, Graham TP Jr, Bender HW, et al: Radionuclide angiographic evaluation of right and left ventricular function during exercise after repair of transposition of the great arteries. *Circulation* **67**(1):178, 1983

39. Ramsay JM, Venables AW, Kelly MJ, Kalff V: Right and left ventricular function at rest and with exercise after the Mustard operation for transposition of the great arteries. *Br Heart J* **51**:364, 1984

40. Graham TP Jr, Burgery J, Bender HW, et al: Improved right ventricular function after intra-atrial repair of transposition of the great arteries. *Circulation* **72**(II):II45, 1985

41. Levy RJ, Rosenthal A, Castaneda AR, Nadas NS: Growth after surgical repair of simple d-transposition of the great arteries. *Ann Thorac Surg* **25**:225, 1978

83

The Senning Operation

Marc R. de Leval

The concept of transposing the entire venous return using an intracardiac approach as a treatment for ventricular arterial discordance [concordant transposition of the great arteries (TGA)] was suggested and experimentally performed by Albert in 1954.[1] In 1959, Senning[2] described an ingenuous technique of complete intra-atrial redirection of the venous return. Probably because of its apparent technical complexity the procedure was not widely used at first. The less complicated baffle operation suggested by Mustard et al[3] in 1964 became immediately more popular. In 1975 the Leiden group[4] revived the Senning procedure, which, in subsequent years, became the operation of choice for the treatment of simple transposition in many centers. In retrospect, the higher mortality rate originally reported with the Senning operation compared to the Mustard operation was probably related to associated anomalies such as ventricular septal defects and pulmonary vascular changes in the two patients populations that were compared.[4,5]

The main advantage of the Senning over the Mustard procedure is the very small amount of foreign material required in the former technique with, therefore, a greater potential for growth.

INDICATIONS

With the advent of the arterial switch procedure that is becoming more and more widely accepted as the treatment of choice for simple transposition of the great arteries, the indications for the Senning procedure have largely decreased over recent years. Our current indications are as follows:

1. Simple transposition of the great arteries in patients who are too old for a primary arterial switch. Currently we would do a primary arterial switch up to the age of 2 months for a transposition of the great arteries with intact ventricular septum. An alternative approach for those patients who are too old is to band the pulmonary artery and do a systemic to pulmonary artery shunt to prepare the left ventricle for an arterial switch operation.

2. Transposition of the great arteries with intact ventricular septum and organic left ventricular outflow tract obstruction other than resectable subvalvar obstruction.

3. Transposition of the great arteries, ventricular septal defect, and severe pulmonary vascular obstructive disease for which a "palliative" Senning is performed without closing the ventricular septal defect. (We prefer the Senning to the arterial switch, mainly because of the major size discrepancy between the pulmonary artery and the aorta and because there is no advantage in connecting the pulmonary artery to the right ventricle as both ventricles function at the same pressure.)

4. Patients with double-inlet ventricles, pulmonary vascular disease, and transposition physiology (pulmonary arterial saturation higher than the aortic saturation) in whom a palliative Senning can occasionally be helpful.

5. Atrioventricular discordance and ventriculoarterial concordance (ventricular inversion) are rare conditions for which the Senning operation constitutes a "complete repair."

6. An atrial (Senning) and arterial switch has been recently advocated as a treatment of atrioventricular and ventriculoarterial discordance with ventricular septal defect.[6] In the presence of ventricular septal defect and pulmonary stenosis, the Senning operation can be combined with a Rastelli-type procedure consisting of closing the ventricular septal defect so as to connect the left ventricle to the aorta in the setting of ventriculoarterial discordance.

Left juxtaposition of the atrial appendages is a contra-indication for the Senning technique whereas a left superior cava to the coronary sinus or the left atrium and a previous atrial septectomy are not contraindications.

SURGICAL TECHNIQUES

Except for very small infants in which we would use the technique of profound hypothermia and total circulatory arrest, we routinely perform the Senning repair on cardiopulmonary bypass, with profound hypothermia and cold cardioplegia.

The ductus arteriosus is routinely dissected and ligated to prevent systemic embolization during the period of circulatory arrest. The pursestring sutures are placed for arterial and venous cannulation. The aorta is routinely cannulated immediately below the origin of the innominate artery. To minimize cardiac manipulations prior to going on bypass, we recommend a staged cannulation of the venae cavae. The first pursestring is placed caudad to the tip of the right atrial appendage. A second oval-shaped pursestring suture is placed on the anterior aspect of the superior vena cava well away from the cavoatrial junction. We currently use the thin-walled right-angled metal tip venous cannulas designed by Pacifico (DLP Inc., Walker, MI). The cannula, which will eventually be placed in the inferior vena cava, is first introduced through the pursestring in the tip of the right atrial appendage while the superior caval cannula is filled and ready for immediate insertion. Cardiopulmonary bypass is initiated with the atrial cannula. the superior vena caval cannula is then inserted and the patient is cooled to 22°C. The junction between the inferior vena cava and the diaphragm is then dissected so as to place the pursestring suture below the eustachian valve (cavoatrial junction). The first venous cannula is now removed from the right atrium and placed into the inferior vena cava. Snares are placed around both cavae and tightened with tourniquets before the right atrium is opened. While going around the inferior vena cava, we try to preserve the pericardial reflection between the inferior vena cava and the right lower pulmonary vein, which can be used to sew the atrial flap at the end of the procedure.

If the technique of total circulatory arrest is used, a single venous cannula is introduced in the right atrial appendage and the patient cooled to 17 or 18°C.

The interatrial groove on the right side (Waterston groove) is dissected as deeply as possible without entering the left atrium (Fig. 83–1). This provides additional length for the construction of the pulmonary venous pathway. The aorta is then cross-clamped and the cold cardioplegic solution is infused. A small vent sucker is introduced into the left atrium through a stab wound in the interatrial groove.

The right atrium is then opened anterior and parallel to the crista terminalis, thus anterior to the sinus node. The distance between the atrioventricular groove and the right atriotomy incision should correspond to approximately two-thirds of the circumference of the superior vena cava.[7] Prac-

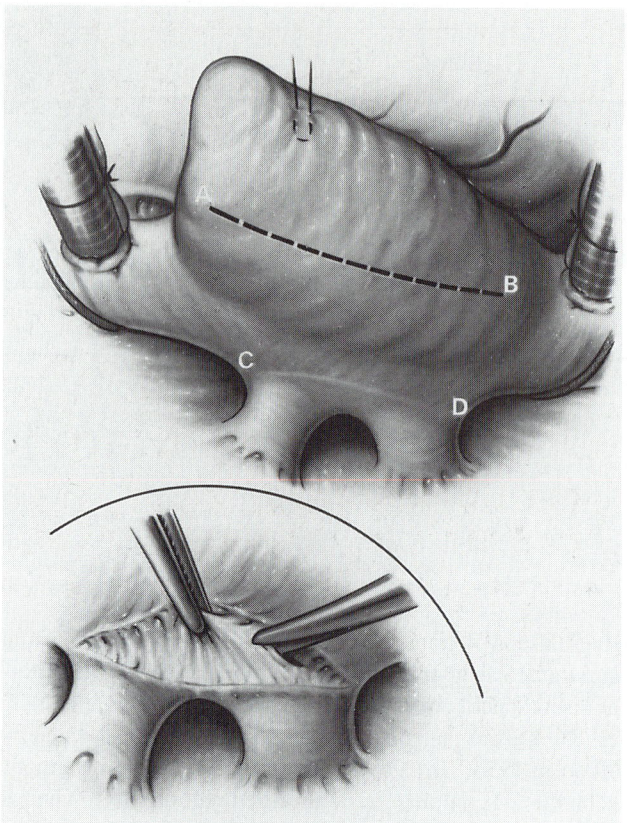

Figure 83–1. See discussion in text.

tically, the incision is made 5 to 10 mm anterior to the crista terminalis. The incision is completed inferiorly at a later stage when the anatomy of the eustachian valve has been assessed (Fig. 83–1).

Next the atrial septal flap is developed. When the foramen ovale is small, it is closed and the septal flap is created. When there is a large atrial septal defect, only the superior and posterior aspects of the limbus are available for this atrial flap. Superiorly, the incision of the limbic tissue must be done toward and within the superior vena caval orifice. If the incision is carried more to the right, there is a risk of opening the roof of the right atrium into the transverse sinus and damaging the sinus node artery. A ridge of limbic tissue left in place at the cavoatrial junction can contribute to superior vena caval obstruction later. The atrial flap remains hinged to the interatrial groove. When there is a large septal defect, we personally extend the atrial flap with a small triangular patch of Dacron or pericardium (Fig. 83–2). However, alternative measures are used by others to augment the atrial septal flap without using foreign material. They include the imbrication of the left atrial appendage or the anterior incision of the coronary sinus, which leaves a posterior lip to make the inferior part of the septal flap. The atrial flap is then sutured between the left pulmonary veins and the left atrial appendage. The flap is sutured superiorly within the left atrium to the junction between the su-

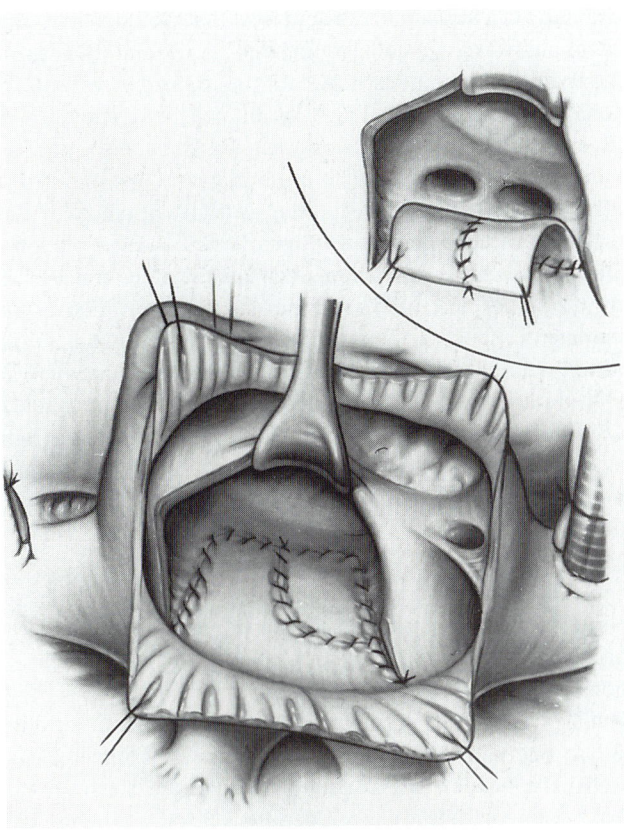

Figure 83–2. See discussion in text.

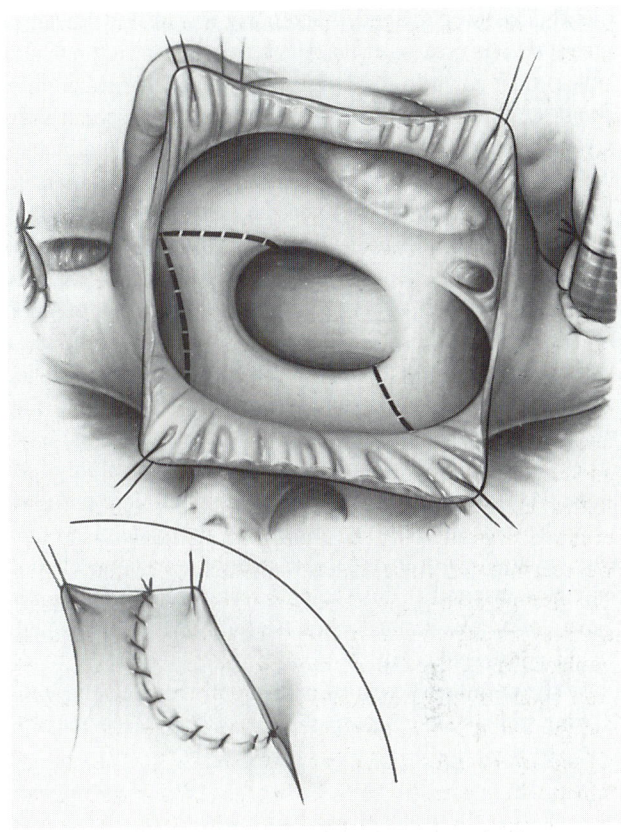

Figure 83–3. See discussion in text.

perior vena cava and the right upper pulmonary vein, inferiorly to the junction between the inferior vena cava and the right lower pulmonary vein. This makes the floor of the tunnel that will connect the caval orifices with the mitral valve (Fig. 83–3).

Next the left atrium is incised deep into the interatrial groove enlarging the stab wound made earlier to introduce the left atrial vent. The incision is extended superiorly to the junction between the superior vena cava and the right upper pulmonary vein and inferiorly to the junction between the inferior vena cava and the right lower pulmonary vein. The dissection is carried up to the sutures at the corners of the interatrial flap and care must be taken not to cut them. Superiorly, the incision should not be carried beneath the superior vena cava, which would otherwise be constricted while completing the pulmonary venous pathway.

The opening in the left atrium is usually further enlarged by incising one or both right pulmonary veins or, alternatively, between the two veins (Fig. 83–4).

At this stage, we usually establish total circulatory arrest and remove the inferior vena caval cannula to inspect the cavoatrial junction and the eustachian valve. If the eustachian valve is well developed, it can be used to construct the inferior vena caval pathway and the right atriotomy incision is extended posteriorly toward the cavoatrial junction. If the eustachian valve is not well developed, the atri-

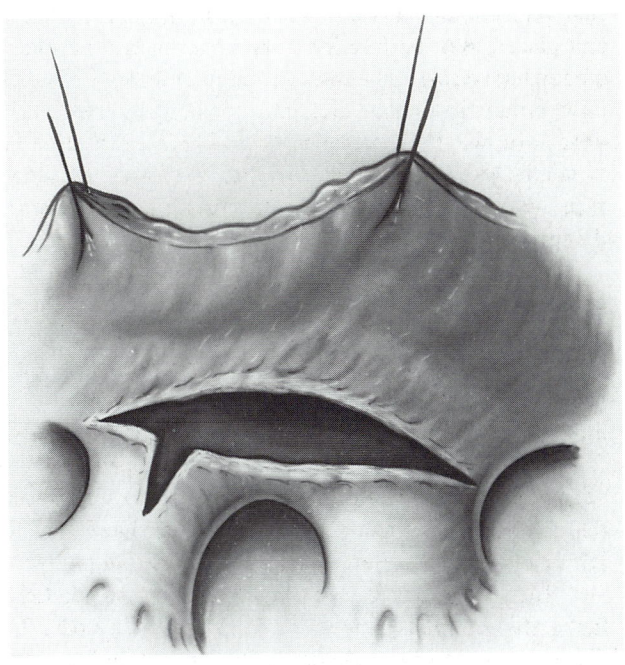

Figure 83–4. See discussion in text.

otomy incision is extended anteriorly toward the cavoatrial junction. The posterior margin of the right atriotomy incision is then sewn to the atrial wall or the eustachian valve about the inferior vena cava orifice. If the eustachian valve is not used, the first step in completing this caval pathway is the placement of a half pursestring suture that gathers together the right atrial wall and the posterior aspect of the atriotomy incision. The suture line is then carried out toward the coronary sinus, which is left opening into the new pulmonary venous atrium, and along the anterior remnant of the limbus tissue, staying away from the atrioventricular node area. Similarly, around the superior vena caval orifice, a half pursestring suture gathers together the muscular ridge made by the crista terminalis, which is guarding the caval orifice and the posterior margin of the right atriotomy incision. The suture line is then carried on the limbic tissue toward the first suture, thus completing the systemic venous pathway to the mitral valve. The inferior vena caval cannula may be reinserted at this stage, to resume cardiopulmonary bypass or at a later stage when the pulmonary venous pathway is constructed (Fig. 83–5).

The pulmonary venous pathway to the tricuspid valve is now completed. During this procedure, care must be taken to (1) avoid a pursestring effect that would narrow the caval pathways, (2) damage the sinus node, and (3) restrict the pulmonary venous flow to the tricuspid valve. To achieve this, the original right atrial incision is extended at its extremities by two relaxing anterior incisions that augment the perimeter of the atrial flap. Two 5-0 or 6-0 monofilament sutures are placed at each extremity of the original atriotomy incision (points A and B in Fig. 83–6). One arm is used as a traction stitch and the other one is used for the suture line. Inferiorly, the flap is sewn obliquely on the lateral aspect of the inferior vena cava (and sometimes the pericardial reflection). Superiorly, the suture line is placed on the superior vena cava in front of the sinus node and the cavoatrial junction (Fig. 83–7). Posteriorly, the flap is sewn to the widely opened orifice made in the right pulmonary veins. To obtain as large an opening as possible, one takes epicardial bites without approximating the endocardial edges.

The rewarming of the patient is initiated before the completion of this last suture line if cardiopulmonary bypass is used. If total circulatory arrest is employed, the venous cannula is reinserted into the morphologic right appendage (new left atrium) after the completion of this suture line and cardiopulmonary bypass is resumed to rewarm the patient. We routinely remove the air from the heart, using an aortic needle vent and placing a large-bore needle into the anterior aspect of the right (systemic) ventricle. Temporary atrial and ventricular pacing wires are routinely inserted to be able to pace sequentially if needed in the postoperative period.

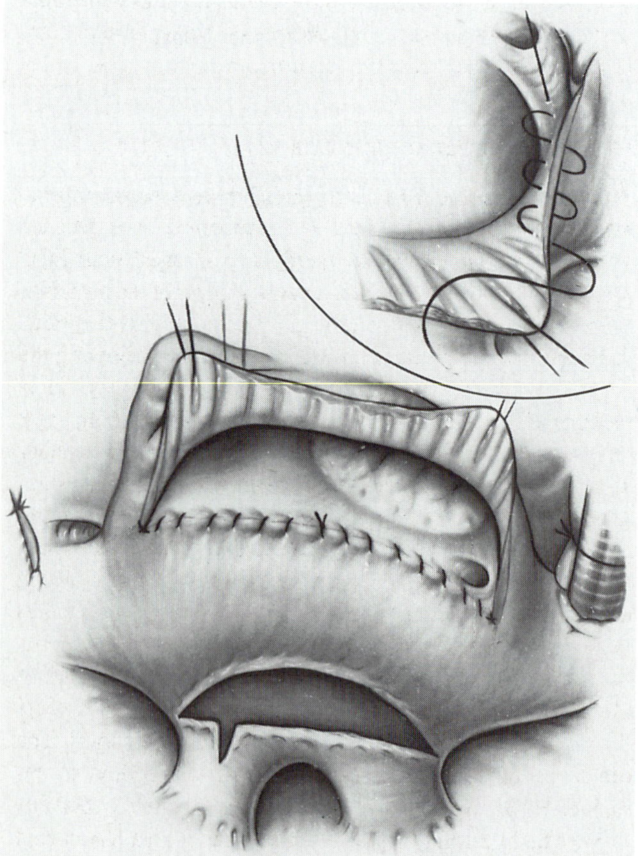

Figure 83–5. See discussion in text.

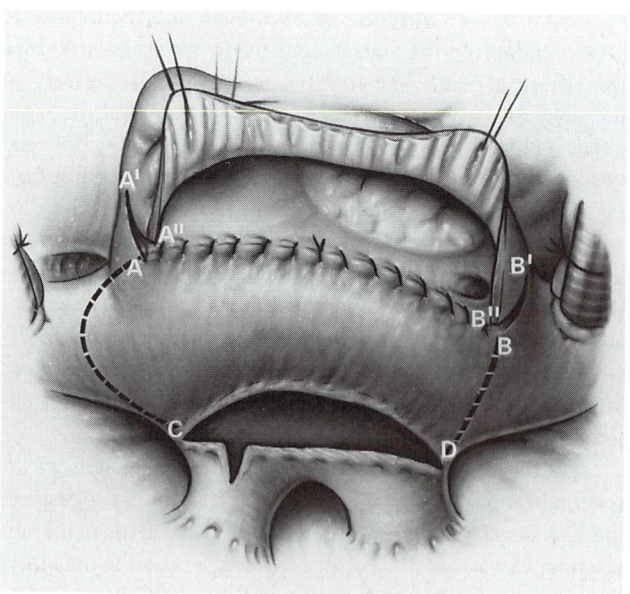

Figure 83–6. See discussion in text.

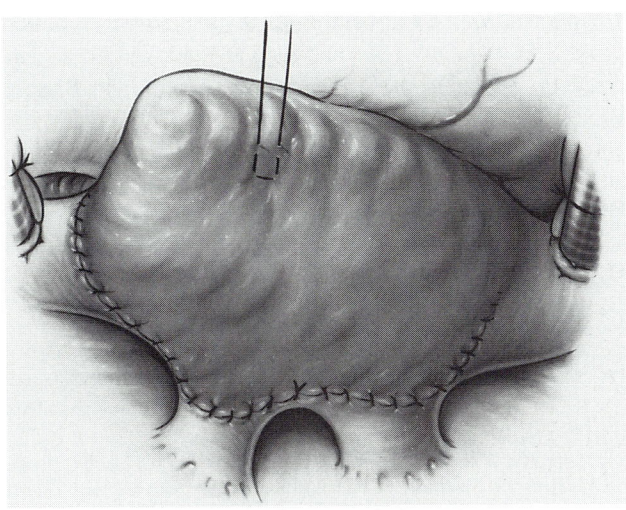

Figure 83–7. See discussion in text.

RESULTS

Morbidity

Early and late post-Senning complications include systemic and/or pulmonary venous hypertension, electrophysiologic disturbances, right ventricular dysfunction, tricuspid valve incompetence, and left ventricular outflow tract obstruction.

Venous Hypertension

Some degree of venous hypertension is very common following the Senning repair. The mechanisms include pathway obstructions, atrial dysfunction, ventricular dysfunction, atrioventricular valve incompetence, and arrhythmias.

Pathway obstructions are less common following the Senning repair than the Mustard repair. Furthermore, when they occur following the Senning, it is always an early complication, thus indicating that it relates to the surgical techniques rather than the growth of the patient. Thus far, we have never reoperated on a Senning patient for acquired late venous pathway obstruction.

Superior vena caval obstruction can occur if the superior aspect of the limbus tissue is not excised well within the superior vena cava, if the atrial incision (A, B) is too posterior, if the suturing of the atrial flap on the lateral aspect of the superior vena cava has a pursestring effect, or as a complication of direct caval cannulation (stricture or thrombus formation).

Pulmonary venous pathway obstruction can occur if the atrial septal flap is sewn too posteriorly, thus interfering with the drainage of the left pulmonary veins, if the opening within the interatrial groove is too small, or if there is excessive tension of the atrial flap that would impair pulmonary venous flow to the tricuspid valve.

Atrial dysfunction may occur because the geometry of

the atrial chambers is profoundly altered by the Senning procedure. Their roughly spherical cavity is transformed into a tubular pathway whose efficiency as a pump and a reservoir is reduced. Filling pressures are consequently higher.

Ventricular dysfunction and atrioventricular valve incompetence may lead to elevated diastolic pressure and atrioventricular valve regurgitation, which inevitably increase the corresponding venous pressures. In our experience, patients with more than mild left ventricular outflow-tract obstruction often have an elevated systemic venous pressure postoperatively, thus indicating that those patients have probably some degree of diastolic dysfunction as well as systolic dysfunction.

Arrhythmias may occur as a result of the extensive atrial suture line, and the loss of sinus rhythm may cause an increased venous pressure in the post-Senning repair patient. Generalized swelling, hepatomegaly, ascites, and pleural effusions (occasionally a chylothorax) are signs of significant systemic venous hypertension requiring postoperative cardiac catheterization and reoperation if they are related to a surgically correctable problem.

Some degree of pulmonary congestion is very common following the Senning repair. In addition to the above described impairment to the venous return, some patients have an excessive bronchial flow that also contributes to this congestion. Pulmonary edema with a small heart on a plain chest x-ray is also indication for postoperative reinvestigation and possible reoperation.

Electrophysiologic Disturbances

The true incidence of surgically related arrhythmias following a Senning repair is difficult to determine as it depends on the methods of detection (surface ECG or 24 hour ECG monitoring),[7] on the presence or absence of arrhythmias preoperatively, and on the criteria of normality of the ECG. A prospective analysis of the late arrhythmias following the Senning procedure in our institution[8] has shown that most patients are in sinus rhythm on the 24-hour recording 2 wk postoperatively (84%). Most of the remainder had either sinus rhythm with intermittent junctional escape or established junctional rhythm. Supraventricular tachycardia and atrial flutter were observed in 2% and 4% of the patients, respectively. Serial 24-hour Holter monitoring revealed a decrease in sinus rhythm during follow-up. At 5–8 (mean 7) years after the operation only 56% of the Senning patients had stable sinus rhythm. The maximum heart rate during the 24-hour period was significantly lower at 5 to 8 years than during the early postoperative monitoring period. The incidence of active arrhythmias during the follow-up remained relatively low: 12% showed paraoxysmal supraventricular tachycardias at 5 to 8 years. Sudden death occurred in two patients (4.5% of hospital survivors). Both patients were in sinus rhythm at hospital discharge and at last surface ECG. The Holter monitoring during follow-up had revealed only intermittent junctional rhythm in one of them. Surgical damage to the sinus node and/or its blood supply must be responsible for some of these postoperative arrhythmias.[9] The surgical maneuvers responsible for such injury include cannulation of the superior vena cava or suturing the atrial flap too close to the sinus node, direct trauma with forceps, and overzealous excision of the limbus tissue that can damage the sinus node artery.[10] In addition, early and late electrophysiological abnormalities are probably inevitable consequences of extensive atrial surgery involved in the procedure.[11]

Right Ventricular Dysfunction

Right ventricular function is often reduced following the Senning repair.[7] However, right ventricular failure with symptoms of congestive heart failure following the Senning repair of simple transposition of the great arteries is rare.[12] It is more common in patients who, in addition, had a large ventricular septal defect closed.[13]

Tricuspid Valve Incompetence

This is a rare complication of the Senning procedure for simple transposition of the great arteries. It can be either secondary to right ventricular dilatation or a primary tricuspid valve anomaly. The latter is more common in patients who also had a ventricular septal defect.

Left Ventricular Outflow Tract Obstruction

Dynamic types of left ventricular outflow-tract obstruction rarely progress after the atrial switch procedure.[7,14]

Mortality

Hospital mortality following the Senning repair for simple transposition of the great arteries is less than 10% in most centers. It was 4.6% in a series of 87 patients who were admitted as neonates in our unit between 1978 and 1986 and who were managed according to the Senning protocol. Including the pre-Senning mortality, the actuarial survival of

100 patients with transposition of the great arteries is anticipated to be 84% at 5 years and 81% at 9 years.[15] These data are very similar to those reported by Kirklin and Barratt-Boyes.[7]

REFERENCES

1. Albert HM: Surgical correction of transposition of the great vessels. *Surg Forum* **5**:74, 1954
2. Senning A: Surgical correction of transposition of the great vessels. *Surgery* **45**:966, 1959
3. Mustard WT, Keith JD, Trusler GA, et al: The surgical management of transposition of the great vessels. *J Thorac Cardiovasc Surg* **48**:953, 1964
4. Quaegebeur JH, Rohmer J, Brom AG: Revival of the Senning operation in the treatment of transposition of the great arteries. *Thorax* **32**:517, 1 1977
5. Pacifico AD: Concordant transposition. Senning operation. In Stark J, de Leval M (eds): *Surgery for Congenital Heart Defects.* London, Grune & Stratton, 1983, p 345
6. Imai Y, Sawatari K, Hoshino S, et al: Ventricular function after anatomic repair in patients with atrioventricular discordance. *J Thorac Cardiovasc Surg* **107**:1272–1283, 1994
7. Kirklin JW, Barratt-Boyes BG: *Cardiac Surgery.* New York, John Wiley, 1986, p 1129
8. Deanfield J, Camm J, Macartney F, et al: Arrhythmia and late mortality after Mustard and Senning operations for transposition of the great arteries. An eight year prospective study. *J Thorac Cardiovascv Surg* **96**:569, 1988
9. Edwards WD, Edwards JE: Pathology of the sinus node in d-transposition following the Mustard operation. *J Thorac Cardiovasc Surg* **75**:213, 1978
10. Smith A, Arnold R, Wilkinson J, et al: An anatomical study of the patterns of the coronary arteries and sinus nodal artery in complete transposition. *Int J Cardiol* **12**:295, 1986
11. Wittig JH, de Leval M, Stark J: Intraoperative mapping of atrial activation before, during and after the Mustard operation. *J Thorac Cardiovasc Surg* **73**:1, 1977
12. Graham TP, Burger J, Bender HW, et al: Improved right ventricular function after intra-atrial repair for transposition of the great arteries. *Circulation* **72** (suppl II):45, 1985
13. Mee RB: Severe right ventricular failure after Mustard or Senning operations. Two stage repair: Pulmonary artery banding and switch. *J Thorac Cardiovasc Surg* **92**:385, 1986
14. Park SC, Neches WH, Mathews RA, et al: Hemodynamic function after the Mustard operation for transposition of the great arteries. *Am J Cardiol* **41**:1514, 1983
15. Rubay J, de Leval M, Bull C: To switch or not to switch? The Senning alternative. *Circulation* **78** (suppl III):1, 1988

84

The Rastelli Procedure for Transposition of the Great Vessels, Pulmonary Stenosis, and Ventricular Septal Defect

Francisco J. Puga

Those forms of transposition of the great vessels associated with "fixed" obstruction of the left ventricular (pulmonary) outflow tract are not candidates for arterial correction (Jatene procedure).[1] For these patients, the Rastelli operation, introduced in 1969 continues to be the preferred method for surgical reconstruction.[2] This procedure restores ventriculoarterial concordance and relieves the obstruction to pulmonary flow. "Dynamic" subpulmonary stenosis resulting from leftward deviation of the ventricular septum in patients with transposition and intact ventricular septum and with a "hypotensive" left ventricle can be managed with the Jatene procedure, which results in an increase of the afterload of the left ventricle with restoration of the normal alignment of the ventricular septum and resolution of the left ventricular outflow obstruction.[3]

Preoperative assessment of candidates for the Rastelli operation requires echocardiography, cardiac catheterization, and angiography. The objectives of the preoperative evaluation include assessment of ventricular and valvular function, the position and size of the ventricular septal defect and its spatial relationship to the subaortic area, the central and peripheral pulmonary arterial morphology, the patency of surgical shunts, the coronary arterial distribution, and the pressure and resistance of the pulmonary arterial circulation. The best candidates for the Rastelli procedure are those patients with D-transposition of the great arteries and a perimembranous *subaortic ventricular septal defect.* Less desirable candidates are those in whom the ventricular septal defect occupies the inlet or muscular portion of the septum (uncommitted or distant).[4] Finally, a "two-ventricle repair" is possible only when there are two normal sized ventricles and two normal sized atrioventricular valves committed to their respective ventricles. In general terms, significant *straddling* of either atrioventricular valve over the ventricular septal defect precludes or increases the risk of the Rastelli procedure.[5]

As described by Rastelli et al,[2] the procedure involves construction of an intracardiac tunnel that results in closure of the ventricular septal defect in such a way as to direct left ventricular outflow through the ventricular septal defect toward the aortic valve. Enlargement of a "restrictive" ventricular septal defect is necessary in up to 45% of patients. This maneuver requires resection of the infundibular septum so as to avoid damage of the conduction tissue.[6,7] The connection between the left ventricle and the pulmonary artery is interrupted by division of the main pulmonary artery with suture closure of the proximal end or by patch closure of the pulmonary valve; finally, the procedure is completed by connecting the right ventricle with the distal pulmonary arterial confluence with a valved extracardiac conduit, such as a pulmonary or aortic cryopreserved homograft (Fig. 84–1). The procedure requires extracorporeal circulation, using ascending aortic cannulation for arterial inflow and bicaval cannulation for venous outflow. We prefer the use of cold blood cardioplegic arrest of the heart during periods of aortic cross-clamp for myocardial protection.

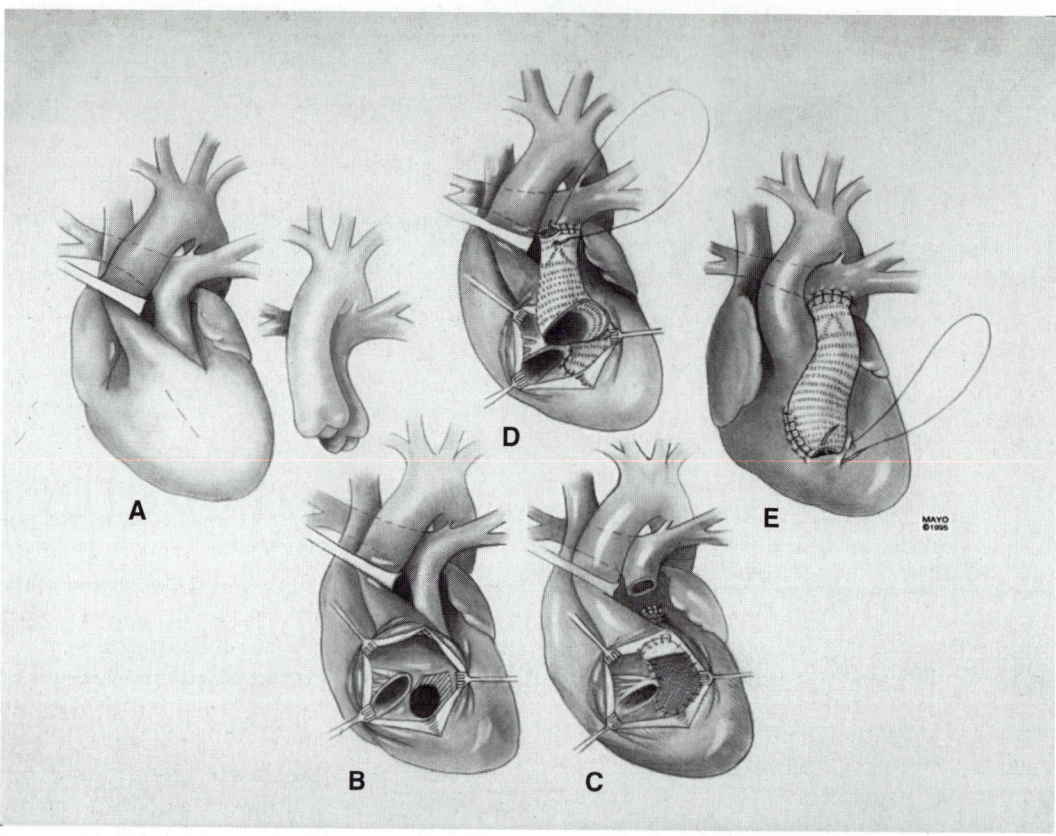

Figure 84–1. The Rastelli procedure for transposition of the great arteries, ventricular septal defect, and pulmonary stenosis. **A.** Site of right ventricular outflow tract incision. **B.** Enlargement of a ventricular septal defect by resection of its anterior and superior margins. **C.** Septating baffle directing left ventricular outflow through the ventricular septal defect toward the aortic valve. The main pulmonary artery has been transected and the proximal end oversewn. **D.** Insertion of a valved extracardiac conduit between the right ventricle and the distal pulmonary arterial confluence. **E.** The completed procedure.

At the present time patients considered for the Rastelli procedure are beyond infancy or early childhood so most have undergone previous palliative procedures for relief of cyanosis and hypoxemia. Thus, most patients present with a patent systemic-pulmonary artery shunt of which the modified Blalock–Taussig shunt or a central shunt (ascending aorta to pulmonary artery graft) is most common.[8] In addition, patients may have undergone balloon septostomy at birth and/or palliation by balloon dilatation of a stenotic pulmonary valve. Prior to undertaking the intracardiac repair, the surgeon must gain control of all patent systemic-pulmonary connections so that they can be interrupted at the time of institution of cardiopulmonary bypass. Pulmonary arterial distortion resulting from previous surgical shunts or from native stenotic lesions must be corrected at the time of definitive repair so as to minimize right ventricular outflow obstruction.

The Mayo Clinic experience with the Rastelli procedure was last reported in 1976.[9] We have recently updated this experience, which now includes 117 patients who have undergone the Rastelli procedure during the period ending in 1990. This population of patients excluded any other car-

diac morphology than those patients with D-transposition of the great arteries (TGA), ventricular septal defect (VSD), and pulmonary stenosis (PS). Age at operation ranged from 4 months to 29 years (mean = 6 years). Previous palliative surgical procedures had been done in 80 patients (68%) as shown in Table 84–1. A typical high, paramembranous, subaortic ventricular septal defect was present in 95 (81%) patients. Other types of ventricular septal defects included posterior (inlet), supracristal (subarterial), and/or muscular. The atrioventricular valves were committed to their respective ventricles in 97 patients and there were varying degrees of straddling of either atrioventricular valve in the remaining patients. Enlargement of the ventricular septal defect by resection of the infundibular septum was required in 53 patients (45%). This maneuver was required because of the small size of the defect or because of atypical location and/or abnormal chordal attachments. Follow-up information was available in 94% of patients and extended from 7 mo to 22.6 years (mean = 13.2 years). Overall surgical mortality in this series was 16% (19 patients). As shown in Table 84–2, operative mortality was strongly influenced by young age and small size of patients. Hospital mortality was

TABLE 84–1. RASTELLI PROCEDURE FOR TGA, VSD, AND PS: PREVIOUS SURGICAL PROCEDURES

Procedure	Number of patients
Systemic-pulmonary artery shunt	65
Atrial septectomy	25
Anastomosis of atrial appendages	1
PDA ligation	5
Baffes procedure	1
Edwards procedure	1
Coarctation repair	1
Pulmonary valvotomy	1
Pulmonary debanding	1
LPA angioplasty	1
Exploratory thoracotomy	2

TGA, transposition of the great arteries; VSD, ventricular septal defect; PS, pulmonary stenosis.

also influenced by the position of the ventricular septal defects with the best results obtained in those patients with "typical defects" located in the perimembranous area and spatially related to the subaortic area. Hospital mortality for patients with "typical" defects was 15%, while it was 43% for those patients with "atypical" defects. Mortality for patients with multiple ventricular septal defects was high (36%). Hospital mortality was also high (25%) in patients with straddling or abnormal chordal insertion of either atrioventricular valve. The causes for hospital mortality are listed in Table 84–3. Mortality during the follow-up period was 27.5% (27 of the 98 early survivors). Causes of late deaths are shown in Table 84–4. Actuarial survival for all patients is shown in Figure 84–2. Ten-year survival was 61% and 18-year survival was 58%. Survival probability improved for those patients having "ideal" anatomy for the Rastelli procedure (single ventricular septal defect in the perimembranous, subaortic position and no straddling of either of the atrioventricular valves). For this group, survival after 10 years was 69% and after 18 years, 66%. For those patients not meeting these qualifications, survival was 50 and 47%, respectively. While the operative risk was higher for those patients operated at a younger age (<5 years), they experienced better long-term survival than patients operated after 5 years of age (Fig. 84–3). Survival also favored those

TABLE 84–2. RASTELLI PROCEDURE FOR TGA, VSD: PS: AGE AND OPERATIVE MORTALITY

Age (years)	Number of Patients (%)	Number of Operative Deaths (%)	Chi-square Test (p)
<5	52 (44)	13 (25)	0.022
>5	65 (56)	6 (9)	
<4	32 (27)	9 (28)	0.034
5–12	60 (51)	8 (13)	
>13	25 (21)	2 (8)	

TABLE 84–3. RASTELLI PROCEDURE FOR TGA, VSD, AND PS: CAUSES FOR HOSPITAL MORTALITY

Cause	Number of Patients
Low cardiac output	9
Myocardial infarction	3
Pulmonary hypertension	2
Respiratory failure (ARDS)	1
Residual LV–PA shunt	1
Right heart failure	1
Residual LV–RA Communication	1
Tamponade	1
Total	**19/117 (16%)**

patients with lower postrepair right ventricular pressures (PRV/LV systolic pressure ratio <0.5) (Fig. 84–4).

The need for further surgical procedures has been common after the Rastelli operation. Thirty-one percent of patients operated on at the Mayo Clinic required reoperation after 5 years, 70% after 10 years, and 84% after 18 years. The most common cause for reoperation has been obstruction of the extracardiac conduit used to connect the right ventricle with the pulmonary arterial confluence. Obstruction of the extracardiac conduit continues to be a problem of all prostheses used for this type of reconstruction.[10–12] Aside from the inherent limitation imposed by the behavior of the implanted prosthesis,[13] obstruction of these conduits after the Rastelli procedure has also resulted from anterior compression by the chest wall, a problem exacerbated by the fact that the ventricular anastomosis of these conduits is located in the most anterior part of the heart and is very susceptible to compression at the time of sternal closure (Fig. 84–5). In our experience, the only solution to this problem has been resection of the bony components of the chest wall overlying the conduit. The probability of having a conduit replacement procedure in our population of surviving patients was 62% after 10 years and 80% after 15 years. Other causes for reoperation have included recur-

TABLE 84–4. RASTELLI PROCEDURE FOR TGA, VSD, AND PS: CAUSES FOR LATE DEATH

Cause	Number of Patients
Sudden death	8
Pulmonary hypertension	4
Left ventricular dysfunction	3
Mitral insufficiency	3
Bacterial endocarditis	3
Subaortic obstruction	2
Myocardial infarction	1
Reoperation	1
Non cardiac death	1
Unknown	1
Total	**27/98 (27%)**

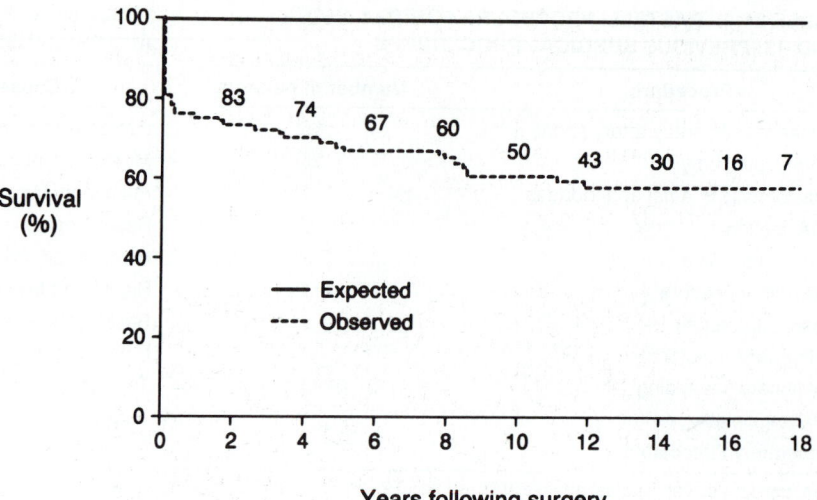

Figure 84–2. The Rastelli procedure. Actuarial survival for all patients.

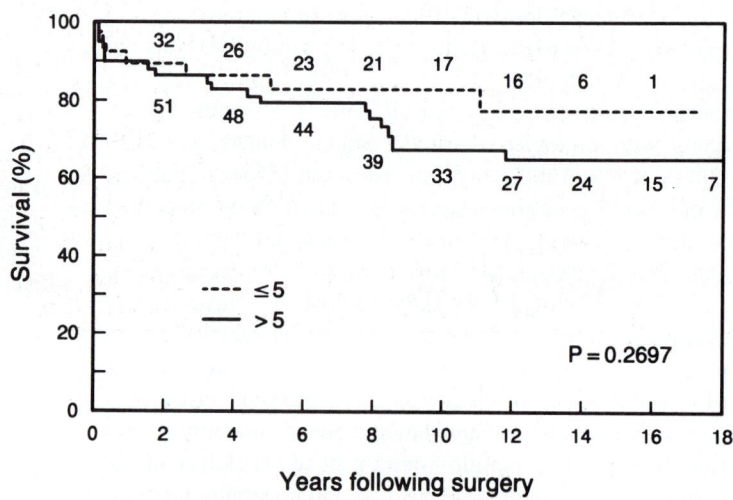

Figure 84–3. The Rastelli procedure. Actuarial survival according to age at operation. Based on patients with >30 days of follow-up.

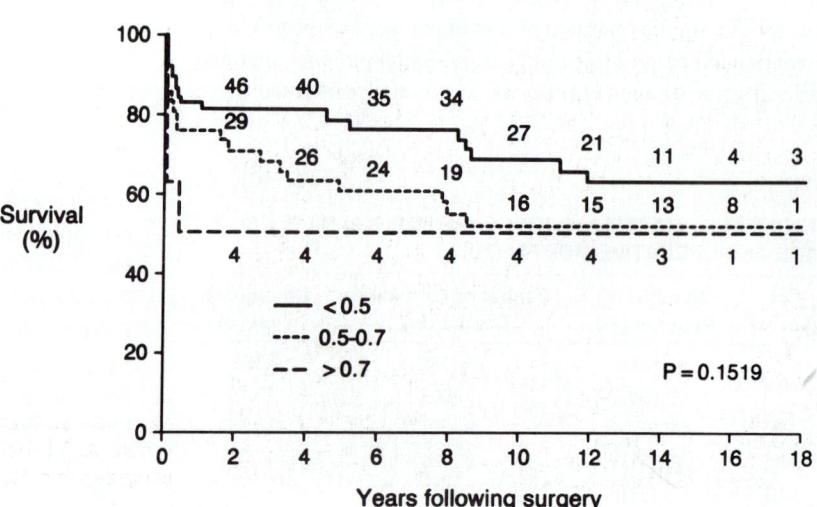

Figure 84–4. The Rastelli procedure. Actuarial survival according to postrepair peak RV–LV systolic pressure ratio.

rent/residual ventricular septal defect, residual left ventricle-to-pulmonary artery connection, and subaortic obstruction.

Other significant late complications included atrial and/or ventricular arrhythmias requiring medical treatment and/or insertion of permanent pacemakers, bacterial endocarditis, myocardial infarction, etc. Nevertheless, the quality of life of most patients has been significantly improved by the Rastelli procedure. In our group of patients, more than 90% were in functional Class I or II, and 73% were taking no cardiac medications. Six patients had successful pregnancies.

Similar results with the Rastelli procedure for transposition with ventricular septal defect and pulmonary stenosis

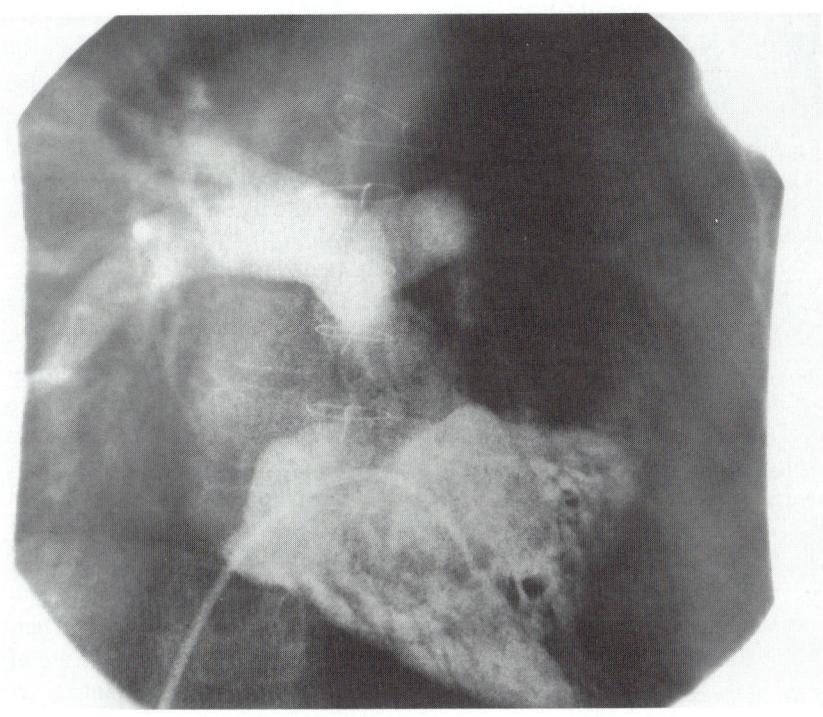

A

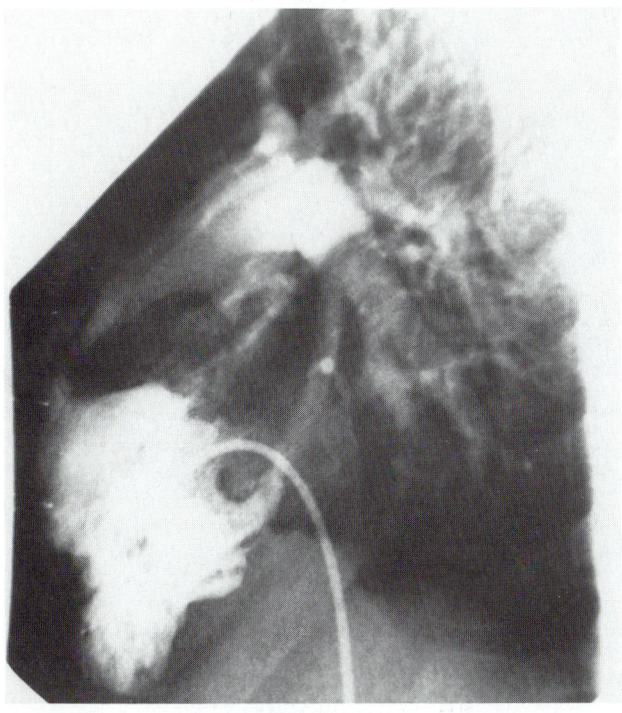

B

Figure 84–5. Obstruction of extracardiac conduit after the Rastelli procedure. **A.** A-P view of right ventriculogram. **B.** Lateral view shows compression of RV conduit anastomosis.

have been reported by other authors.[14,15] Although the procedure restores ventriculoarterial concordance by connecting the left ventricle with the aorta, there appear to be persistent abnormalities of ventricular function. Graham et al[16] studied left ventricular wall stress and contractile function after the Rastelli procedure in transposition patients, and concluded that left ventricular function remained abnormal with persistent left ventricular dilatation and hypertrophy. Palik et al[17] found the abnormal right ventricular function and hypertrophy persisted because of the proclivity to obstruction evidenced by the extracardiac conduits.

As indicated before, the type and position of the ventricular septal defect play important roles in the feasibility and success of the procedure. Defects that are not placed in the perimembranous subaortic region, or those that are straddled by either of the atrioventricular valves, are less than ideal for the Rastelli procedure, and results in these patients are less favorable.[18] Furthermore, attempts at complex intracardiac tunneling in an effort to connect distant or noncommitted ventricular septal defects with the subaortic region may result in distortion and compromised function of the tricuspid valve.[19,20] Postoperative stenosis in the subaortic region may occur as a result of improper position of the intracardiac baffle, inadequate enlargement of a restrictive ventricular septal defect, patient growth, or scarring and contraction of the repaired area. Flow restriction by the intracardiac tunnel may be easily uncovered by echocardiography.[21]

The major problem affecting the late result of the Rastelli procedure is the behavior of the extracardiac conduit used to restore continuity between the right ventricle and the pulmonary arterial confluence. Traditionally, a valved conduit has been chosen for restoration of right ventricle to pulmonary artery continuity. The irradiated aortic homografts used in the early Mayo Clinic experience failed because of early calcification and obstruction. Anterior compression may have also played a role in the premature failure of these conduits.[22] Dacron conduits containing glutaraldehyde-preserved porcine valves were used after the initial experience, and although durability was improved over the irradiated homografts,[22] these conduits tend to fail because of calcification of the valve and/or formation of an obstructive fibrous endoluminal peel as shown by Agarwal et al.[23] While reoperation for replacement of these obstructed conduits can be carried out safely,[24] the search for more permanent conduits continues. In recent years, cryopreserved aortic and especially pulmonary valved homografts have become the conduit of choice for these types of reconstructions.[25,26]

There have been two important technical modifications to the Rastelli procedure. One makes it applicable to small infants and children, and the other allows patients with transposition of the great vessels, *intact ventricular septum*, and pulmonary stenosis to undergo reconstruction with this technique.

LeCompte and co-authors have reported on the use of a modified Rastelli procedure in small infants with transposition of the great vessels, ventricular septal defect, and pulmonary stenosis.[27] They have proposed avoiding the use of an extracardiac conduit by anastomosing the pulmonary ar-

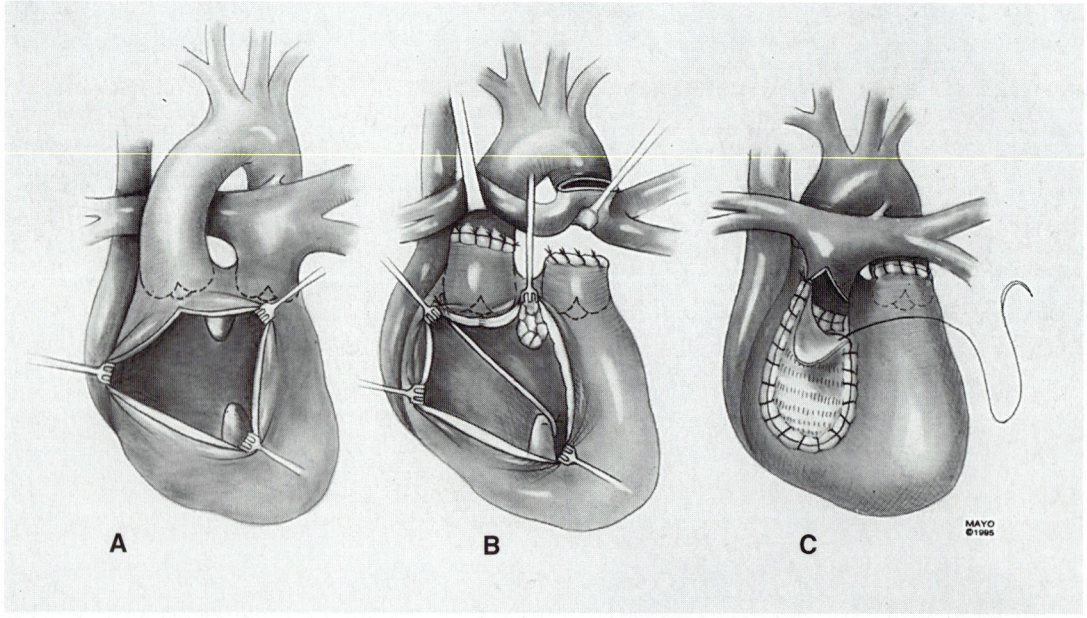

Figure 84–6. LeCompte's modification of the Rastelli procedure. **A.** Right ventricular incision. **B.** Intracardiac septation and resection of infundibular septum. Division of main pulmonary artery and closure of proximal end. Transplantation of pulmonary arterial confluence anterior to the ascending aorta. **C.** Right ventricular outflow tract reconstruction without a valved conduit.

teries directly to the right ventriculotomy. To accomplish this, the aorta is transected, the main pulmonary is also transected, and the proximal (cardiac) end is oversewn. The distal pulmonary arterial confluence is then transplanted anterior to the ascending aorta, which is reanastomosed (LeCompte maneuver). The infundibular septum is widely resected and the intracardiac tunnel constructed establishing left ventricle to aorta continuity. The procedure is completed by anastomosing the pulmonary arterial confluence to the right ventricular incision using a patch of autologous pericardium to complete the anterior portion of the anasto-

mosis (Fig. 84–6). Eliminating the need for an extracardiac conduit allows the application of the procedure to small infants and children who might otherwise require interim palliative procedures. Borromee et al[28] reported on 50 patients who underwent this procedure. Twenty-six had transposition with ventricular septal defect and pulmonary stenosis. Ages at operation ranged from 4 mo to 13 years (mean = 3.5 years). Hospital mortality was 18% (9 patients). While follow-up was short, four patients exhibited significant pressure gradients in the right ventricular outflow tract. Other authors have also reported on the use of this proce-

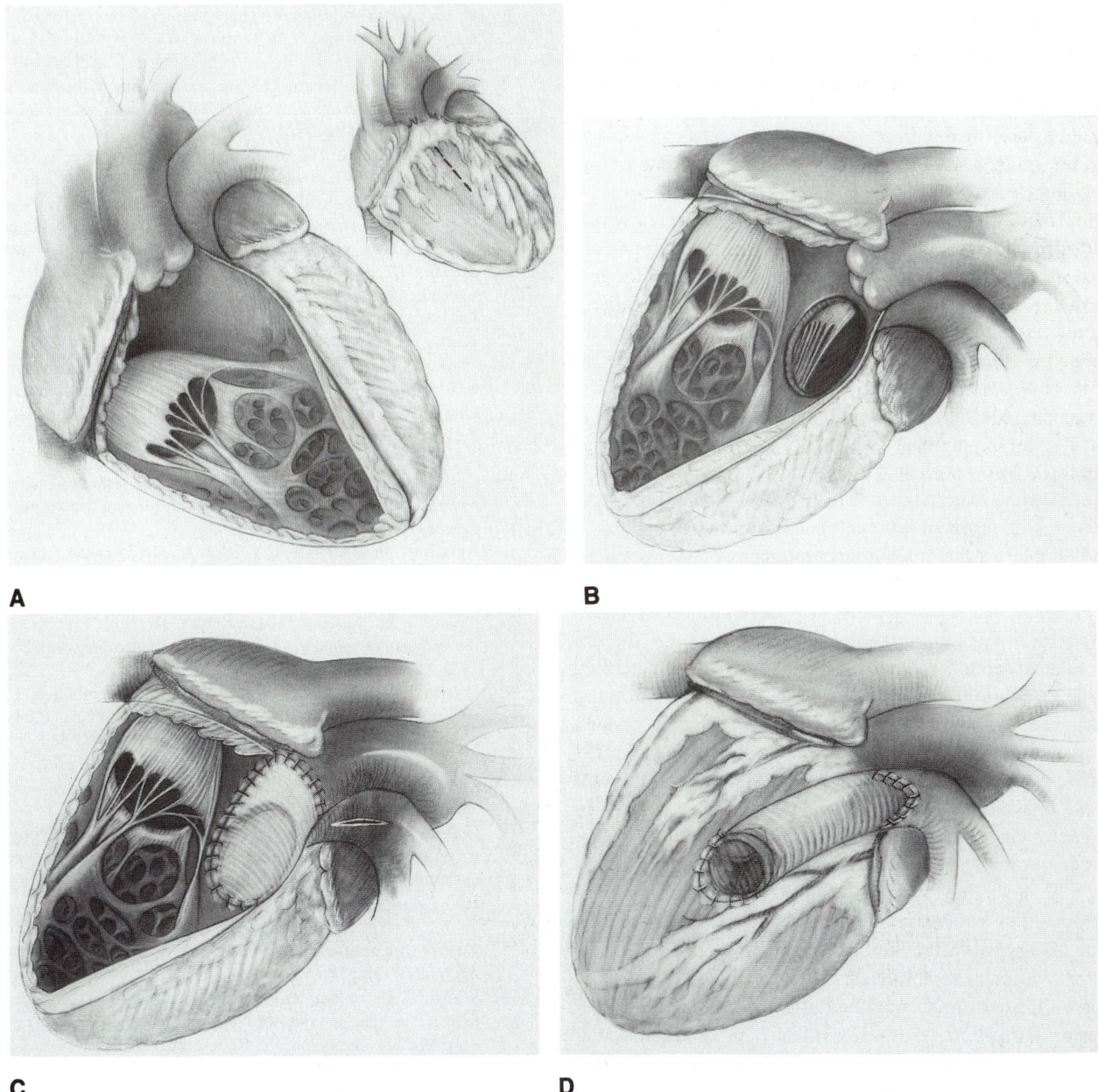

Figure 84–7. The modified Rastelli procedure for transposition of the great arteries, intact ventricular septum and pulmonary stenosis. **A.** Right ventricular incision. **B.** Creation of a ventricular septal defect in the infundibular septum. **C.** Intracardiac baffle directing left ventricular outflow through the newly created ventricular septal defect toward the aorta. **D.** Right ventricular outflow reconstruction with valved extracardiac conduit.

dure.[29,30] Singh et al[31] did a retrospective comparison of results obtained in patients with transposition of the great vessels, ventricular septal defect, and pulmonary stenosis when treated with the Rastelli procedure or with LeCompte's modification. Their patient population included 62 patients of whom 22 underwent the conventional Rastelli operation and the rest were treated with the modified procedure. Mortality for the Rastelli procedure was 9%, and for the modified Rastelli 12.5%. The probability of surviving 5 years was equal at about 84%. The late need for reoperation and the presence of residual right ventricular outflow tract obstruction was similar for both groups, but the follow-up was yet short for the modified procedure. It is not clear whether the absence of a competent pulmonary valve will have an impact in the long-term results of LeCompte's modification of the Rastelli operation. Additionally, it is not clear yet whether this procedure can indeed be performed with consistent good results in infants or young children, thus obviating the need for interim palliative procedures.

The lack of a ventricular septal defect has traditionally excluded patients with transposition of the great arteries, intact ventricular septum, and pulmonary stenosis for any form of reconstruction that achieved restoration of ventricular arterial concordance. Thus, these patients were not candidates for the Jatene or the Rastelli procedures. Traditionally, these patients have been treated with an inflow procedure (Mustard or Senning) associated with attempts at direct relief of pulmonary stenosis or the concomitant insertion of a left ventricle to pulmonary artery conduit.[31,32] Based on the experience afforded by the Konno procedure for complex forms of left ventricular outflow obstruction,[33] and on the fact that a significant number of patients undergoing the Rastelli operation require surgical enlargement of their ventricular septal defects, we[34] have proposed *the creation of a ventricular septal defect* located on the infundibular septum so that these patients can be corrected using the Rastelli approach (Fig. 84–7). This operation has been used for those patients with *fixed* valvular or subvalvular pulmonary stenosis who are not amenable for the Jatene procedure. In these patients, the left ventricular outflow obstruction should have resulted in preservation of the left ventricular muscle mass and the capacity of this ventricle to sustain systemic pressures. This modification to the Rastelli technique allows inclusion of this subgroup of transposition patients into the anatomic (arterial) correction type of surgical techniques. Furthermore, the ability to create a ventricular septal defect in the ideal (subaortic) position for the performance of the Rastelli procedure allows inclusion of patients with less ideally placed ventricular septal defects (noncommitted inlet or muscular ventricular septal defects) who in the past were high risk candidates for the procedure. These patients should undergo closure of the less favorable defects and creation or enlargement of defects suitable for the creation of the left ventricular-aorta tunnel.

REFERENCES

1. Jatene AD, Fontes VF, Paulista PP, et al: Anatomic correction of transposition of the great vessels. *J Cardiovasc Surg* **72**:364–370, 1976

2. Rastelli GC, McGoon DC, Wallace RB: Anatomic correction of transposition of the great arteries with ventricular septal defect and subpulmonary stenosis. *J Thorac Cardiovasc Surg* **58**:545–552, 1969

3. Serraf A, Comas JV, Lacour Gayet F, et al: Neonatal anatomic repair of transposition of the great arteries and ventricular septal defect. *Eur J Cardiothorac Surg* **6**:630–634, 1992

4. Imamura S, Morikawa T, Tatsuno K, et al: Surgical considerations of ventricular septal defect associated with complete transposition of the great arteries and pulmonary stenosis. *Circulation* **44**:914–923, 1971

5. Huhta JC, Edwards WD, Danielson GK, Feldt RH: Abnormalities of the tricuspid valve in complete transposition of the great arteries with ventricular septal defect. *J Thorac Cardiovasc Surg* **83**:569–576, 1982

6. Kurosawa H, Van Mierop LH: Surgical anatomy of the infundibular septum in Transposition of the great arteries with ventricular septal defect. *J Thorac Cardiovasc Surg* **91**:123–132, 1986

7. Bharati S, Lev M: The conduction system in simple, regular (D), complete transposition with ventricular septal defect. *J Thorac Cardiovasc Surg* **72**:194–201, 1976

8. Bachet J, Chetochine FL, Neveux JY, et al: Palliative surgery of transposition of great vessels associated with pulmonary stenosis. *Arch Mal Coeur Vaiss* **68**:353–362, 1975

9. Marcelletti C, Mair DD, McGoon DC, et al: The Rastelli operation for transposition of the great arteries. Early and late results. *J Thorac Cardiovasc Surg* **72**:427–434, 1976

10. Chun PK, Rocchini AP, Gibbs HR, et al: Pannus formation in a Hancock valved conduit resulting in proximal intraconduit obstruction: Late complication of Rastelli procedure for complete transposition of the great vessels with ventricular septal defect and pulmonic stenosis. *Am Heart J* **101**:855–857, 1981

11. Corno A, Giamber A, Giannico S, et al: Long-term results after extracardiac valved conduits implanted for complex congenital heart disease. *J Card Surg* **3**:495–500, 1988

12. Ishihara K, Imai Y, Misumi Y, et al: A valved conduit replacement for a calcified homograft 12 years following a Rastelli operation: A case report. *Nippon Geka Gakkai Zasshi* **89**:957–961, 1988

13. Ciaravella JM, McGoon DC, Danielson GK, et al: Experience with the extracardiac conduit. *J Thorac Cardiovasc Surg* **78**:920–930, 1979

14. Daenen W, de Leval M, Stark J: Proceedings: Transposition of great arteries, ventricular septal defect, and left ventricular outflow tract obstruction: Results of 23 Rastelli operations. *B Heart J* **38**:878, 1976

15. Imamura E, Morikawa T, Tatsuno K, et al: Conduit repairs of transposition complexes. A report of 14 cases. *J Thorac Cardiovasc Surg* **73**:570–577, 1977

16. Graham TP Jr, Franklin RC, Wyse RK, et al: Left ventricular wall stress and contractile function in transposition of the great arteries after the Rastelli operation. *J Thorac Cardiovasc Surg* **93**:775–784, 1987

17. Palik I, Graham TP Jr, Burger J: Ventricular pump performance in patients with obstructed right ventricular pulmonary artery conduits. *Am Heart J* **112**:1271–1278, 1986

18. Villagra F, Quero Jimenez M, Maitre Azcarate MJ, et al: Transposition of the great arteries with ventricular septal defects. Surgical considerations concerning the Rastelli operation. *J Thorac Cardiovasc Surg* **88**:1004–1011, 1984

19. Dubost C, Brunet A, Chvd S, et al: Transposition of the great vessels with ventricular septal defect, pulmonary stenosis and tricuspid valvular insufficiency. Surgical treatment with Rastelli procedure and tricuspid valve replacement. *Ann Chir* **34**:581–584, 1980

20. Deanfield JE, Gundry SR, Stark J: Surgical creation of a double out-

let right atrium for tricuspid valve stenosis after a Rastelli operation. *Br Heart J* **60:**172–174, 1988

21. Rocchini AP, Rosenthal A, Castaneda AR, et al: Subaortic obstruction after the use of an intracardiac baffle to tunnel the left ventricle to the aorta. *Circulation* **54:**597–960, 1976

22. McGoon DC, Danielson GK, Puga FJ, et al: Late results after extracardiac conduit repair for congenital heart defects. *Am J Cardiol* **49:**1741–1749, 1982

23. Agarwal KC, Edwards WD, Feldt RH, et al: Clinicopathologic correlates of obstructed porcine-valved extracardiac conduits. *J Thorac Cardiovasc Surg* **81:**591–601, 1981

24. Schaff HV, DiDonato RM, Danielson GK, et al: Reoperation for obstructed pulmonary ventricle-pulmonary artery conduits. *J Thorac Cardiovasc Surg* **88:**334–343, 1984

25. Livi U, Kay P, Ross D: The pulmonary homograft: An improved conduit for RVOT reconstruction. *Circulation* **74**(Suppl II):II–250 (abstract), 1986

26. McGrath LB, Gonzalez-Lavin L, Graf D: Pulmonary homograft implantation for ventricular outflow tract reconstruction: Early phase results. *Ann Thorac Surg* **45:**273–277, 1988

27. LeCompte Y, Neveux JY, Leca F, et al: Reconstruction of the pulmonary outflow tract without prosthetic conduit. *J Thorac Cardiovasc Surg* **84:**727–733, 1982

28. Borromee L, LeCompte Y, Basse A, et al: Anatomic repair of anomalies of ventriculoarterial connection associated with ventricular septal defect. II. Clinical results in patients with pulmonary outflow tract obstruction. *J Thorac Cardiovasc Surg* **95:**96–102, 1988

29. Zannini L, Santorelli MC, Gargiulo G, et al: Transposition of the great vessels with interventricular defect and stenosis of the left ventricular efflux channel: Anatomical correction by the intraventricular repair technique. *G Ital Cardiol* **17:**300–305, 1987

30. Aoki M, Imai Y, Kurosawa H, et al: Successful LeCompte's operation of transposition of great arteries with ventricular septal defect and pulmonary stenosis. *Nippon Kyobu Geka Gakkai Zasshi* **35:**1066–1071, 1987

31. Singh AK, Stark J, Taylor JFN: Left ventricle to pulmonary artery conduit in the treatment of transposition of the great arteries, restrictive ventricular septal defect, and acquired pulmonary atresia. *Br Heart J* **38:**1213–1216, 1976

32. Ilbawi MN, Quinn K, Idriss FS, et al: The surgical management of left ventricular outflow tract obstruction due to tricuspid valve pouch in complete transposition of the great arteries. *J Thorac Cardiovasc Surg* **87:**66–73, 1984

33. Konno S, Imai Y, Iida Y, et al: A new method for prosthetic valve replacement in congenital aortic stenosis associated with hypoplasia of the aortic valve ring. *J Thorac Cardiovasc Surg* **70:**909–917, 1975

34. Jex RK, Puga FJ, Julsrud PR, Weidman WH: Repair of transposition of the great arteries with intact ventricular septum and left ventricular outflow obstruction. *J Thorac Cardiovasc Surg* **100:**682–686, 1990

85

Transposition of the Great Arteries

The Arterial Switch Operation

Jan M. Quaegebeur and Joseph S. Auteri

INTRODUCTION AND HISTORY

The first description of transposition of the great arteries (TGA) is credited to Baillie in 1797,[1] and the use of the term "transposition of aorta and pulmonary artery" to Farre[2] in 1814. In the years that followed confusion arose around the term transposition since it was applied to any condition in which the aorta occupied an abnormal position relative to the pulmonary artery. This situation lasted until Van Praag et al in 1971[3] clarified the definition of transposition and introduced the term "malposition" to indicate positional anomalies of the great vessels.

The term *transposition of the great arteries* describes a cardiac anomaly with atrioventricular concordant and ventriculoarterial discordant connection; in this chapter the term is not applicable to patients with TGA and double inlet atrioventricular or discordant atrioventricular connection. A number of patients with TGA will also have a ventricular septal defect (VSD). These defects are classified according to their number and location in the ventricular septum,[4,5] and the right ventricular components of the ventricular septum bordering the defects are named with the usual terms.[6,7] In addition, the defects can also be subdivided according to their commitment to the great arteries as described by Lev and colleagues.[8] This subdivision is useful both in TGA and in double outlet right ventricle (DORV).

The surgery of TGA started in 1950, when Blalock and Hanlon,[9] working at the Johns Hopkins Hospital, described a palliative operation during which a part of the atrial septum was excised (atrial septectomy) in order to improve the mixing of pulmonary and systemic venous blood. A modification of this procedure was proposed by Edwards, Bargeron, and Lyons[10] at the University of Alabama in Birmingham where the atrial septum was shifted so that the right pulmonary veins were connected with the right atrium. The Blalock-Hanlon operation remained popular until the introduction of balloon atrial septostomy by Rashkind and Miller in Philadelphia.[11]

Surgical procedures were also devised during which the pulmonary and systemic veins were reconnected at the atrial level (partial atrial switch). Lillehei and Varco[12] in 1953 anastomosed the right pulmonary veins to the right atrium and then the inferior caval vein (IVC) to the left atrium. Baffes[13] popularized the same procedure but used a homograft to connect the IVC to the left atrium.

The first attempts of total correction of TGA were directed at the atrial level. In 1954 Mustard et al in Toronto[14] tried to perform an arterial switch operation, while using a monkey lung as oxygenator, in 7 patients with TGA. The youngest of these patients was 19 days old. The transfer of the aorta included the left coronary artery. Mustard noticed that the coronary arteries always arose "in a position that is relatively close to the pulmonary artery" and described the three most commonly encountered coronary arterial branching patterns.

Bjork and Bouckaert[15] at Karolinska described an experimental technique for "switch-over anastomosis" of the great arteries in TGA, using segments of homografts to reconnect the aorta and pulmonary artery, which were then interrupted between the homografts. The coronary arteries were left in situ on the right ventricle (RV). They were probably the first to introduce the term "switch" for this concept. They also realized that a systemic left ventricular pressure was necessary before a switch operation could be undertaken. Also in 1954, Bailey[16] attempted to switch the great arteries in 3 children (one of whom was 11 days old) using hypothermia, but without coronary artery transfer. One 7-month-old child with TGA and VSD survived the operation, but developed cardiac arrest 30 hours later during bronchoscopy for retained secretions.

Idriss et al at the Children's Hospital in Chicago[17] developed a technique of switching the great arteries including coronary transfer. After transecting the aorta and pulmonary artery, an aortic segment containing both coronary ostia was excised, was turned over 180°, and was reanastomosed above the pulmonary root. The great arteries were then switched and were connected to the appropriate ventricles. Idriss et al also emphasized that the operation could only be successful if associated conditions had maintained a systemic pressure in the left ventricle (LV), or if it is done early in the life of the patient.

The concept of a physiological repair by redirecting the venous inflow in the atria was first proposed by Albert[18] in 1954 in a meeting of the American College of Surgeons. He indicated that atrial inflow correction could by achieved by using the patient's own atrial septal tissue or by inserting a prosthetic patch. The first successful atrial switch was accomplished by Senning[19] in 1958 and was reported in 1959. Senning formed an intraatrial baffle using the tissue of the right atrial wall and atrial septum. Modifications were suggested quickly, including those of Barnard et al[20] in 1962 and Shumacker[21] in 1961. The original Senning operation was used at the Mayo Clinic, University Hospital in Bordeaux, and in Leiden, but its success was limited primarily because of unsolved problems around the use of extracorporeal circulation and the presence of pulmonary vascular disease.

The Mustard operation[22] was introduced in 1963 at the Toronto Children's Hospital. The atrial inflow switch was achieved with a pericardial baffle. This technique became accepted in almost all surgical centers, although the size and shape of the baffle underwent many modifications, including Brom's "trouser patch."[23] The introduction of the balloon atrial septostomy (BAS) by Rashkind and Miller in 1966[11] dramatically improved the results of initial palliation by "buying time" until surgical repair was considered possible. Because of persisting problems with baffle obstructions, arrhythmia, and the increasing tendency to perform these operations in infants, the Senning operation was reintroduced in 1977 by Brom and colleagues[24] with good results; the operation was subsequently successfully adopted in many centers.

Within 8 years, however, McGoon[25] and others[26]

began to question the durability of these atrial level repairs despite satisfactory early operative results. Rastelli et al[27] suggested an operation for TGA with VSD and subpulmonary stenosis that involved construction of an intracardiac tunnel, which would divert blood from the left ventricle across the VSD and into the aorta, thus making the left ventricle the systemic ventricle. A right ventricle-to-pulmonary artery conduit was then placed to provide pulmonary blood flow. Subsequently, Damus,[28] Kaye,[29] and Stansel[30] (DKS) described operative approaches in which the proximal pulmonary artery (arising from the left ventricle) was sewn to the ascending aorta. The right ventricle was then connected to the pulmonary artery by a conduit. In this DKS repair, the left ventricle again became the systemic ventricle and a physiologic arterial switch was accomplished without coronary artery transfer. However, an artificial conduit was used, which would require replacement as growth occurred. Finally, Jatene reported his initial successful experience with the arterial switch operation, including coronary transfer, for transposition with ventricular septal defect at the 1975 Henry Ford Symposium,[31] and then at the American Association for Thoracic Surgery meeting.[32] At the latter meeting, several others reported their initial experiences with arterial switch procedures as well. However, Jatene expressed concern that in patients with TGA and an intact ventricular septum (TGA/IVS), the left ventricle would be accustomed to a low pressure pulmonary circuit and might be unable to generate sufficient force to function in the systemic circulation. Since 70% of patients with TGA have an intact ventricular septum (IVS), the next step was to apply the arterial switch concept to this group as well. Two different approaches were undertaken for the TGA/IVS patients. Yacoub and coworkers placed pulmonary artery bands to narrow the pulmonary artery and increase the afterload on the left ventricle.[33] This procedure "prepared" the left ventricle by forcing it to generate higher pressure and the arterial switch procedure was then performed several months later.

In 1983 our group in Leiden,[34] and Castañeda at the Children's Hospital in Boston,[35] independent of each other started to use the arterial switch operation as the primary procedure for neonates with simple TGA, taking advantage of the window of opportunity before the left ventricle loses its capacity to carry the systemic workload. This approach is now routinely employed worldwide for patients with TGA with or without VSD.

RATIONALE FOR ARTERIAL SWITCH OPERATION

Theoretical Consideration

The fact that the left ventricle becomes the systemic ventricle has been the primary impetus for surgeons to develop the arterial switch procedure. Indeed, the right ventricle might not possess the intrinsic structural properties to pump against a high resistance circuit for a lifetime. The inflow portion is perpendicular to its outflow tract and therefore conveys a commalike shape to its cavity. Its contraction propagates much like a peristaltic wave from its inflow to its outflow portion, in contrast to the twistlike contraction of the more ellipsoid left ventricle, providing for a rapid and more forceful ejection of blood. Moreover, the location of the papillary muscle insertion points of the tricuspid valve inside the right ventricular cavity is triangular. The septal insertion point is opposite to the ones on the ventricular free wall. Therefore, any degree of right ventricular dilatation will increase the distance between these insertion points rapidly. This phenomenon could easily pull away the tricuspid valve leaflets from each other and could result in tricuspid valve incompetence. Furthermore, the right ventricle might be hypoplastic to some degree in patients with transposition and, not infrequently, tricuspid valve anomalies are present, especially in the presence of a VSD.

Mortality

The current hospital mortality after atrial switch operations for simple TGA varies between 0% and 15%.[36-44] Tynan[49] in 1971 showed that BAS did not allow all babies with TGA to survive until repair. In addition, mortality before and after BAS must be taken into account in order to present a comprehensive mortality assessment of the atrial switch repair.[42,50,51] Efforts have been made to perform the atrial switch procedure in the first months of life[45-51] in order to decrease the possibly deleterious effects of hypoxia while awaiting surgical repair. Survival after atrial switch in neonates is excellent.

Late mortality after atrial switch is by no means negligible and all series are marked by a significant and continuous decrease in survival rate for as long as the follow-up extends. Generally the cumulative survival at ten years, including hospital deaths, varies between 75% and 85%. The main causes for this late mortality are: sudden death probably caused by arrhythmia, mechanical problems with the intraatrial baffle (including mortality associated with reoperations for this complication), and right ventricular dysfunction.

In TGA with VSD, the risk of atrial switch is substantially higher with a published early mortality rate between 10% and 60%[52-54] even in the 1980s.[55,56] The presence of a VSD in TGA has remained an incremental risk factor for death after atrial switch even when the VSD is closed transatrially. Although the operation can be performed on young patients without increasing the risk any further,[55] the expected late survival remains significantly less than in TGA with intact septum.

The primary reason that the atrial switch operation was developed as a surgical treatment[18] was the lack of survival associated with attempts at correction on the arterial level. Until recently, when discussing the advantages of either the atrial or arterial switch operations, higher hospital mortality associated with the arterial operation remained an important obstacle to the procedure's widespread acceptance. In the current era, at least in institutions properly prepared to perform neonatal cardiac surgery, the immediate survival after the arterial switch operation is 96% or higher, which refutes the previous argument.

Postoperative Rhythm

Although there is a significant incidence of arrhythmia following the atrial switch operation, the analysis of arrhythmia is difficult, in part because its reported incidence depends on whether 24-hour Holter monitoring has been performed. In normal children it has been established that abrupt changes in heart rate occur relatively frequently[57,58] over a 24-hour period, and it is also known that a small number of children with TGA have arrhythmia preoperatively.[59,60] Holter monitoring studies that fail to recognize these probably normal variations overrate the incidence of arrhythmia. Therefore the reported incidence of arrhythmia after atrial switch varies between 13% and 100%[46,59,61–65] The incidence includes sinus node dysfunction, different degrees of atrioventricular (A-V) block, supraventricular ectopic beats, supraventricular tachycardia, atrial flutter, junctional rhythm and premature ventricular contractions, and tachy-bradycardia. The cause of these arrhythmias is not clear, but may be the result of injury to the sinus node or its blood supply, the presence of suture material close to the node, extensive incisions in the atrial septum, and the presence of long suture lines creating pockets of delayed conduction predisposing to re-entrant tachycardias. It has also been shown that although the patient is in sinus rhythm immediately after the atrial switch operation, he continues to be at risk for losing his sinus rhythm, since the incidence of arrhythmia increases with the length of the follow-up period.[66,67] In a study of 95 patients who had undergone Mustard's operation, new rhythm disturbances were detected during each year of follow-up, so that by the sixth year 75% of the patients had atrial rhythm disorders.[68]

Sudden death is reputed to occur after atrial switch operations and has been associated with these arrhythmias, but unfortunately even patients who are known to be in sinus rhythm are still at risk of this feared complication.

Modifications of the surgical technique[43,62,69] and special care taken by the surgeon to preserve the sinus node and its artery have decreased but have not eliminated the incidence of arrhythmias. Incidentally, there is no significant difference in the postoperative cardiac rhythm occurring after the Mustard or the Senning operations.[67,70,71]

Right Ventricular Dysfunction

Despite the anatomical and physiological characteristics of the right ventricle, which are unfavorable in terms of their capacity for systemic workload, most of the patients do not have signs of congestive heart failure. However, abnormal RV function has been demonstrated by angiography, video-densitometric determination of ejection fraction and RV volume, and radionuclide angiography.[72–76] Right ventricular dysfunction more frequently occurs when there is an associated VSD or patent ductus arteriosus than in simple TGA. Hagler et al.[73] reported severe depression of RV function after the Mustard operation in 33 asymptomatic patients, with relatively preserved LV function. There is no significant difference in RV performance after the Mustard or the Senning operation.[74] At least some of these patients have reduced ejection fraction preoperatively.[76] The abnormal function of the RV, as well as the LV function, can be further decreased by exercise[77,78] in these patients, even though exercise capacity and LV function can be normal. The reported reduction in ejection fraction is remarkably similar in these patients and could not be explained by changes in preload, afterload, and heart rate. Furthermore, Borrow and colleagues[80] demonstrated a significant depression of the (systemic) RV function in response to afterload stress (methoxamine infusion) after atrial switch as compared with the (systemic) LV response in patients after repair of VSD or Tetralogy of Fallot. Parrish et al.[77] found a similar impairment of systemic (RV) ventricular function in patients with congenitally corrected transposition. Clinical congestive heart failure was rare in these patients before the age of 35 years, but in older patients the incidence of congestive heart failure increased significantly.[79] Although progressive deterioration is still uncommon, late death caused by RV failure in patients who had been asymptomatic until shortly before death, has been reported.[81,82] The reasons that RV dysfunction occurs in some patients and not in others are unknown. Although preoperative hypoxia could play a role, there is no increased incidence of RV dysfunction in patients operated on later in life, having been exposed to longer periods of hypoxia. Moreover, LV function, although not always normal, was relatively preserved. Right ventricle dysfunction may be accompanied or precipitated by the presence of tricuspid incompetence. This was first reported by Tynan and colleagues[83] and its incidence is higher in patients with TGA and VSD.[84] Thus the tricuspid valve might not be suited anatomically to sustain systemic pressure throughout life.

Although these abnormal findings are only of direct clinical importance in a minority of patients, the findings strongly suggest the abnormal systemic RV function may become a significant long-term problem over time in an unknown number of patients with a previous atrial switch.

Systemic Venous Obstruction

Although systemic venous obstruction is potentially associated with premature late death,[85,86] patients with complete obstruction of the superior limb of the intraatrial baffle may be completely asymptomatic. Caval obstruction has been differently defined by various authors, ranging from purely qualitative methods describing obstruction as mild, moderate, or severe, to obstruction defined by pullback pressure measurements at catheterization. Therefore the true incidence of caval obstruction may not be known. An estimate of the incidence of caval obstruction can only be based on hemodynamic data reported in the literature. Postoperative data after Mustard's operation for TGA from the accumulated experience of 12 different institutions[41,42,47,86–94] were available on 471 patients. Various degrees of caval obstruction were diagnosed in 147 patients (31%) with an incidence ranging from 0–67%. From these observations and from the experience of Stark et al.[85,95] it would appear that caval obstruction occurred more frequently when a Dacron baffle was used. Others believe that the shape and the mode of the baffle's insertion are of greater importance than the actual material used.[23,88,91] The introduction of a "trouser-shaped" baffle by Quagebeur and Brom,[23] with a carefully measured size, has reduced but not eliminated completely the incidence of this complication. The incidence of caval obstruction after atrial switch procedures has since been reduced to 5–10%.[96] Ullal et al[43] reported 6 superior caval obstructions in 106 patients and Buis-Liem[64] measured a 5–6 mm Hg pressure gradient between the superior caval vein and the right atrium in 6 patients late postoperatively after Mustard's operation with the Brom patch. Young age at operation is probably a risk factor for baffle obstruction, even when the baffle has been correctly shaped.[88] The revival of the Senning operation has dramatically reduced the incidence of caval obstruction.[24] In the combined series of Bergamo (Italy), the Hospital for Sick Children in London, and Leiden, caval obstruction did not develop in any of the 146 surviving patients,[97] but Marx and colleagues[47] found superior caval obstruction present in 6 of 57 recatheterized patients after the Senning operation.

Pulmonary Venous Obstruction

In contrast to caval obstruction, pulmonary venous obstruction is a less common but more lethal complication. It is usually symptomatic and therefore its real incidence should be better known. Among 433 patients, in whom post-Mustard catheterization data were available,[41,42,47,87–94] forty-one (9%, range 7.5–11%) had pulmonary venous obstruction. Using the trouser-shaped patch, pulmonary venous obstruction was absent in Ullal's series of 106 patients[43] and occurred in 2 of 49 patients in the Leiden series.[64] This complication has been reported after the Senning operation as well,[47,98,99] but the insertion of a patch to enlarge the pulmonary venous atrium in some of these patients[39] may have contributed to this incidence. Pulmonary venous obstruction should occur infrequently after the Senning operation.

Miscellaneous

A few other complications may occur after atrial switch operations, including residual intraatrial shunts,[87,91] selective perfusion of the right lung,[100,101] decreased atrial volume and compliance partially compromising atrial function,[102,103] and persistent left ventricular outflow tract obstruction.[87,89,92,104–106] These complications are mentioned here for the sake of completeness.

SPECIAL PHYSIOLOGIC AND ANATOMIC CONSIDERATIONS IN ARTERIAL SWITCH REPAIRS

The feasibility of the arterial switch operation is primarily dependent upon the status of the LV since the LV must pump against the systemic vascular resistance. The risk of failure increases with higher wall stress, which is proportional to intracavitary pressure and dimension and is inversely proportional to wall thickness. In neonates with TGA and intact ventricular septums and no significant pulmonary stenosis, the left ventricular wall thickness is normal, but will decrease in response to the fall of pulmonary vascular resistance. By 2 to 4 months of age, the left ventricular dimension and wall thickness have adapted themselves to the pulmonary circulation and will no longer be able to sustain systemic workload. These findings were substantiated by anatomical[112,113] and echocardiographic[115] studies that implied that the probability for acute LV failure after the arterial switch increases the longer the operation is postponed after birth. Therefore it is recommended that the operation be performed in the first days or in at least the first two weeks of life.

When a VSD is present, the LV wall thickness remains normal during the first year of life and theoretically the operation can be postponed.

Other anatomic considerations are important when an arterial switch operation is undertaken. Left ventricular outflow-tract obstruction may occur in up to 10% of all patients with transposition (including those with VSD) and the obstruction can be caused by subpulmonary membrane,[116,117] an anomalous mitral valve attachment to the septum,[117] pulmonary valve abnormalities,[117] prolapsing tricuspid valve tissue,[117,118] or "dynamic" septal displacement.[111] Since the left ventricular outflow tract will function as the outlet for the systemic ventricle following an arterial switch, these abnormalities have obvious importance. Abnormalities of the mitral valve may also exist in up to 10% of TGA hearts from autopsy series.[119] Anomalies include cleft anterior leaflet, parachute mitral valve and A-V canal defects, and abnormal attachments of chordae to the septum. These anomalies may result in mitral valve stenosis or regurgitation, which may become more significant when this valve becomes the systemic A-V valve.[119] In clinical practice, however, it is rare to encounter mitral valve abnormalities that would preclude the arterial switch procedure. The dynamic form of LV outflow-tract obstruction is of less concern since septal displacement is relieved when the relationship between RV and LV pressure is reversed following the arterial switch procedure.[120] A final anatomic consideration is the morphology of the pulmonary root and semilu-

nar valve, which functions as the systemic semilunar valve after arterial switch. Anatomically, the pulmonary valve closely resembles the normal aortic valve, although the pulmonary root in hearts with TGA is less wedged between the atrioventricular valve rings than the aortic root in normal hearts. Usually there is good alignment of the commissures between the facing aortic and pulmonary sinuses. Major malalignment, implying that the commissures between the two facing sinuses of the aorta are opposed to the middle of the corresponding pulmonary sinus, is present in about 10% of the cases.

CORONARY ARTERIAL ANATOMY IN TRANSPOSITION OF THE GREAT ARTERIES

The origin and distribution of the coronary arteries in TGA were documented before the first successful arterial switch operation was performed.[121,122,123] Since the transfer of the coronary arteries during the arterial switch operation is the most technically demanding part of the procedure, simple and precise documentation of the origin and branching pattern of the coronaries is essential. A correct description of the anatomy of the coronary arteries in TGA requires a precise knowledge of the position of the aorta relative to the pulmonary artery. The aortic position among patients can vary from right posterior to right side-by-side, right anterior, directly anterior, and the leftward position. This variable position of the aorta in turn influences the position of the sinuses of Valsalva. Right, left, and posterior does not clarify the origin of the coronary arteries. In order to overcome the confusion around the terminology of the aortic sinuses, we use an enumerative system that is independent of the spatial relationship of the aorta and pulmonary artery. The system is based upon the observation that the coronary arteries arise from the sinuses that face the pulmonary root, which we have found to be the case during our entire clinical experience since 1977 and in the cases published in the literature, except for perhaps two observations. The observer is positioned in the nonfacing sinus, looking toward the pulmonary artery. The sinus on the right side is called sinus 1 and the sinus on the left side is sinus 2. The three main coronary arteries are considered separately (right coronary artery, R; left anterior descending, L; circumflex coronary artery, Cx). The different branching patterns are then specified by assigning each coronary to its sinus, starting with the first coronary artery originating from sinus 1, and enumerating all three of them in a counterclockwise fashion. This enables the observer to construct a purely descriptive code for each branching pattern without enforcing a rigid categorical system. Neither the presence nor absence of a main stem, branching later into two major arteries, nor the existence of multiple ostia within the same sinus is used in this coding system since these do not significantly alter the operative procedure. For example, when the left anterior descending (LAD) and Cx originate from sinus 1 and RCA from sinus 2, the code will be 1 LCx-2 R. When all three major coronary arteries arise from the same sinus (from a single or double ostium) only that particular sinus is named with the three major arteries in a sequence corresponding to their epicardial distribution pattern, observed in a counterclockwise manner.

In 94% of the observations there exists a dual coronary artery system, where both coronary arteries arise from the two aortic sinuses facing the pulmonary artery; there are four different branching patterns in this situation. The LAD and Cx arise from sinus 1 as a branching coronary artery, and the right coronary artery (RCA) from sinus 2 (1 LCx-2 R) in 70% of the cases. In 14% of cases the LAD arises as a nonbranching artery from sinus 1 and the Cx arises in conjunction with the RCA from sinus 2 (1 L-2 CxR). Less frequently (6% of cases) the RCA and the LAD arise from sinus 1, whereas the Cx arises from sinus 2 (1 RL-2 Cx). Rarer still (3% of cases), the RCA arises from sinus 1 as a solitary branch and the LAD with the Cx from sinus 2 (1 R-2 LCx,). The most common patterns of dual coronary artery systems are shown in Figure 85–1, and those with a single coronary system in Figure 85–2.

In all categories considered there is a striking relationship between the type of coronary branching pattern and the position of the aorta relative to the pulmonary artery. When the aorta is either directly anterior, right anterior, or left anterior, the most common type (1 LCx-2 R) is extremely prevalent. This is especially true with transposition of the great arteries with ventricular septal defect (TGA/VSD) where this type seems to be an exclusive occurrence. On the other hand, when the aorta is in a right side-by-side position relative to the pulmonary artery, relatively rarer types of coronary branching patterns are almost always found.

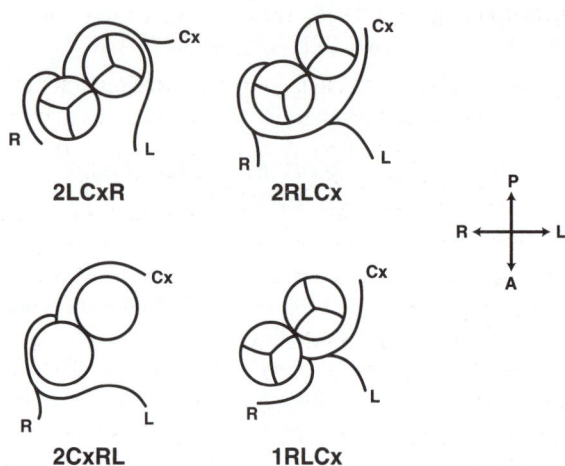

Figure 85–2. Origins of all 3 major coronary arteries from a single sinus in hearts with TGA.

Coronary Ostia

In the vast majority of clinical cases, the orifice of the coronary artery is situated approximately in the middle of the sinus of Valsalva, just below the sinutubular junction. Whereas minor deviations from this central position are frequently found, attention is drawn to this eccentric position of the ostium only when it is located close to one of the valve commissures, which occurs in approximately 10% of the cases. Ostia can rarely be located above the level of the valve commissures in the tubular portion of the aorta. Occasionally two ostia will arise from the same sinus (usually sinus 2).

A small right ventricular branch, arising from a small separate ostium within sinus 1, is occasionally encountered in patients possessing a single or dual coronary system.

Intramural Coronary Artery

The proximal portion of the coronary artery can rarely course aberrantly between the aortic and pulmonary roots.[135] In our experience this has always involved the LAD (usually in conjunction with the Cx, rarely with the RCA). Upon outward inspection of the heart, the LAD seems to originate from sinus 1. In fact, the proximal coronary artery takes an intramural course of a few millimeters where it is inseparable from the aortic wall itself. Its ostium is located just behind the valve commissure in either sinus 1 or 2 or occasionally more distally in the tubular portion of the aorta above the commissure. This situation has been called an "in between course" of the left coronary artery,[133,134] however, this description does not conform with reality since the proximal portion of the coronary artery does not simply run between the aorta and pulmonary artery, but is completely embedded in the wall of the aorta and cannot be dissected from it.[120]

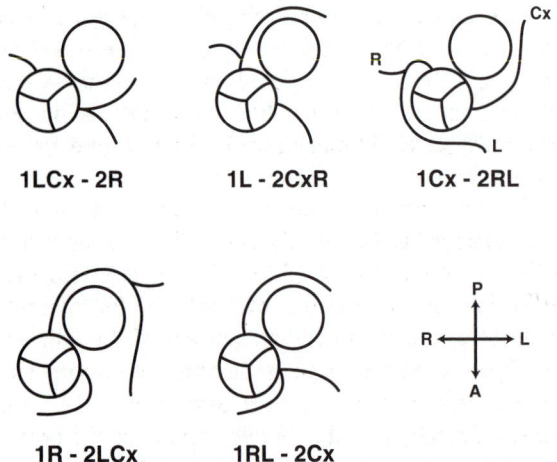

Figure 85–1. The most common patterns of dual coronary artery systems in transposition of the great arteries. Cx, Circumflex; R, right coronary artery; L, left anterior descending.

CURRENT MANAGEMENT

High quality 2-dimensional (2-D) echocardiography can aid in the diagnosis of transposition and echocardiography provides detailed information about associated lesions in all instances. The presence of a ventricular septal defect and its size and location can almost always be determined, particularly with the use of color-Doppler. The 2-D echocardiogram also yields important anatomic details about mitral valve morphology and the anatomy of the left ventricular outflow tract. Frequently the proximal portions of the coronary arteries can be visualized, predicting the type of branching pattern to be encountered in the operating room.[126] Details of semilunar valve anatomy can also be determined. Finally the position of the ventricular septum and the left ventricular shape can be determined and these are an accurate reflection of the relative right and left ventricular pressures.[127] If the ventricular septum bows into the left ventricle, it is likely that the LV pressure is less than half of the RV pressure. In the presence of precise echocardiographic diagnosis, cardiac catheterization and angiography usually do not yield additional important information. In the current era, babies with TGA with or without VSD undergo the arterial switch operation on the basis of echocardiography alone. Cardiac catheterization is performed when uncertainty exists about left ventricular outflow tract obstruction or aortic arch anomalies, or to exclude multiple VSDs. Although coronary artery patterns can be determined by a balloon occlusion aortic root angiogram, precise preoperative knowledge about the coronary artery anatomy does not improve the safety of the operation. The presence of an intramural coronary artery is usually better diagnosed with echocardiography than with angiography.

Patients with TGA and intact ventricular septum or with a small VSD are offered the arterial switch operation as primary treatment. If the foramen ovale is restrictive and the operation cannot be performed promptly, a balloon atrial septostomy is indicated since this will improve oxygenation and will stabilize the condition of the neonate coming to repair. This can be performed under echo guidance in the intensive care unit and does not necessarily require cardiac catheterization.

Beyond the age of 2–3 weeks, the status of the left ventricle seems less certain. The limits of older age, left ventricular wall thickness, the lower LV pressure are not established and each patient will need individual evaluation. When there is leftward septal bulging upon echocardiography and the LV to RV pressure ratio is <0.6, there is an increased probability for LV failure after primary arterial switch. These patients can undergo pulmonary artery banding in association with systemic to pulmonary shunt to recondition the left ventricle. There is a rapid increase in LV mass, usually 30–35% within one week, and the arterial switch operation can then be performed.

In patients with a nonrestrictive VSD, the arterial switch operation can be performed safely beyond the neonatal period. However, congestive heart failure usually develops early. In the current era patients with TGA and VSD undergo the arterial switch operation in the neonatal period, or as soon as the diagnosis is made.

Fixed LV outflow tract obstruction or significant pulmonary valve stenosis continue to be contraindications to the arterial switch operation. Patients with bicuspid nonstenotic pulmonary valves are good candidates for the arterial switch operation.

SURGICAL TECHNIQUE

Technique of Operation

The technique of the arterial switch operation has evolved since the original description by Yacoub et al[128] (Fig. 85–3). Through a median sternotomy, the aorta and pulmonary artery are dissected from surrounding structures as much as possible before establishing cardiopulmonary bypass. The ligamentum or ductus arteriosus is dissected and the branches of the right and left pulmonary arteries are mobilized into the hilum of the lung on either side. The area superior to the bifurcation of the pulmonary artery is completely cleared. The aorta is cannulated at the anteromedial aspect of the junction between the ascending aorta and the transverse aortic arch. The superior and inferior vena cavae are cannulated directly with right-angled cannulae. Cardiopulmonary bypass is established at a flow of 2.4 L/min per m^2. The patient is cooled to 18°C and the perfusion flow rate is then further reduced to 0.7–1.0 L/min per m^2. When necessary to improve exposure, the flow is reduced to 0.5 L/min per m^2 or lower for brief periods. On infrequent occasions, short periods of total circulatory arrest are used. Alternatively, a single venous cannula with its tip positioned at the entrance of the inferior caval vein can be used in combination with continuous low-flow perfusion. The dissection is completed during cooling, the ductus arteriosus is divided between ligatures, and both ends are oversewn. The right atrium is opened and a small sump sucker is placed into the left atrium through a naturally occurring or surgically created foramen ovale. This is not done when a single venous cannula is used.

After the patient is moderately cooled, the ascending aorta is clamped as far distally as possible and the cold cardioplegic solution is injected through a needle temporarily inserted into the aorta at the level selected for transection. This level is usually in the midportion of the aorta or is more distal when the surgeon chooses not to perform the Lecompte maneuver (see further discussion). The aorta is retracted caudally and the anterior aspect of the proximal pulmonary artery is completely cleared down to its base. The pulmonary artery is then transected a few millimeters proximal to the bifurcation, taking care not to deviate the incision into the origin of the left pulmonary artery. The

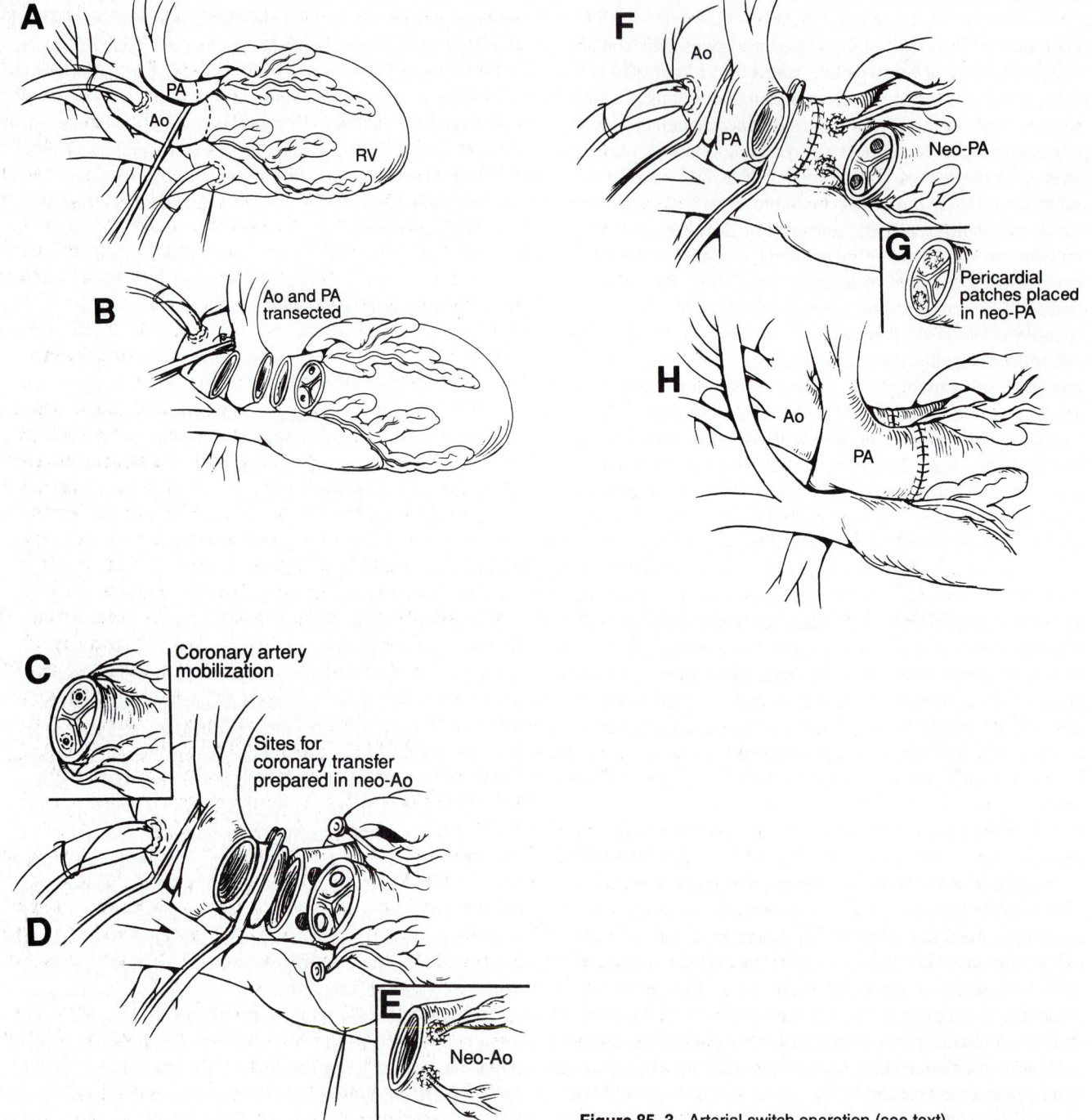

Figure 85–3. Arterial switch operation (see text).

bases of both great arteries are stabilized using stay sutures. The sutures are placed above each commissure of the semilunar valves and they improve exposure both for excision and reimplantation of the coronary arteries.

The coronary artery arising from sinus 1 is typically excised first. The incision is begun at the aortic transection site, is carried down towards the coronary ostium, and then around the ostium to create as large a button of sinus wall tissue as is possible without damage to the valve leaflets. During this process, the anatomy is viewed primarily from

within so as to allow good visualization of the ostium and leaflets. The exact course of the coronary arteries originating from the button is defined by gently probing from within using a 1 mm coronary probe, and then only the very proximal portion of the artery is mobilized, allowing the periarterial tissue around it to remain, which decreases the risk of kinking. No attempt is ever made to dissect the coronary arteries from outside. The dissection is performed enough to allow the coronary artery to "fall upon" a point on the extended proximal segment of the neoaorta. With stay sutures in the proximal neoaortic segment to facilitate this, a stab wound is made in the proximal neoaorta at this point and, while looking from within to protect the valve leaflets, a ±5 mm opening is made. A simple incision is made in the neoaortic sinus. The coronary button is then anastomosed to this orifice with a continuous 7-0 or 8-0 polypropylene suture. With the stay sutures holding the aortic root open, the second coronary ostium with its button is excised circumferentially. This is performed from within the aortic root, beginning with a small stab wound above the coronary ostium and then completing the excision with small sharp pointed scissors. The course of the arteries coming from this coronary ostium is determined similarly by probing; a limited dissection of the initial portion of the coronary artery is performed until this button also falls upon a point at the base of the extended neoaorta. A stab wound is made at the selected point and the second button is similarly anastomosed to the neoaorta. When both the circumflex and right coronary artery arise from sinus 2 (1L–2CxR), the standard transfer could kink the circumflex coronary artery. Extensive dissection of the coronary artery only increases the risk of kinking. Anastomosing the coronary button at a more downstream level elongates the curve made by the circumflex branch during its transfer, preventing its kinking. Moreover, an L-shaped incision is made from the transection site, which produces a medially hinged flap of neoaortic wall that, much like a "trap-door," rotates outward. This incision alters favorably the angle of attachment of the button to the neoaortic sinus, which prevents kinking. When two ostia emerge from the same sinus, both ostia are included within the same button of sinus of Valsalva tissue.

The neoaorta is then constructed. Unless the great arteries are truly side by side, the Lecompte maneuver is performed by threading the aorta beneath the bifurcation of the pulmonary artery, its end grasped with a tissue forceps, and the aortic clamp released and replaced on the aorta inferior to the pulmonary artery bifurcation.[129] This keeps the distal aortic segment in proper position for the anastomosis. When the distal aorta is considerably smaller than the proximal neoaortic segment, the anterior wall of the distal aorta is incised to create a large orifice and occasionally a triangular patch of pericardium is inserted into the defect thus created. Any discrepancy in the circumferences of the two segments is taken up in the posterior part of the suture line; if taken up anteriorly, the coronary ostia can be distorted.

In preparation for the construction of the neopulmonary artery, the defects left by the button excision of the coronary ostia are filled by suturing into place pieces of autologous pericardium. Handling of these patches can be facilitated by fixation in glutaraldehyde (5 min in 1.5% glutaraldehyde). The patch used to repair sinus 1 can have an extended tongue that can be sized appropriately in order to match the discrepancy in diameter between the neopulmonary root and the native pulmonary bifurcation. The technique of closing the left side of the pulmonary bifurca-

tion and enlarging the orifice by incising the orifice of the right pulmonary artery is no longer used. Generally, the aortic clamp is released and rewarming is begun during the construction of the neopulmonary artery. The sump sucker is brought back into the right atrium and the left atrium is allowed to fill with blood before the clamp is removed.

When the aorta is severely deviated to the right of the pulmonary artery, or is in a right side-by-side position to it, the Lecompte maneuver is not used because the fully distended aorta would compress the left pulmonary artery. In this situation the pulmonary bifurcation is slipped behind the aorta and to the right for a direct anastomosis with the neopulmonary artery. Only under these circumstances is it sometimes necessary to close the origin of the left PA, using a small patch of pericardium, and to extend the incision into the right pulmonary artery.

When a VSD is present in the perimembranous position, it is usually repaired by the transatrial approach before commencing the actual arterial switch operation. Alternatively, particularly with VSDs in other locations, after the great arteries have been transected the VSD can be viewed through the proximal aortic or pulmonary artery and, if easier, it can be repaired using this approach. If the repair is performed through the proximal aortic segment (neopulmonary artery), it is done after excision of the coronary buttons; if repair is performed through the pulmonary artery (neoaorta), it is done before the coronary reimplantation. When the VSD is subpulmonary, the pulmonary trunk usually overrides the crest of the ventricular septum, and sutures can easily be placed on the morphologic right side of the ventricular septum, thus avoiding the conduction system. The VSD is rarely repaired by an approach through the right ventricle.

Aortic arch anomalies, such as coarctation with or without aortic arch hypoplasia or interrupted aortic arch, are repaired under deep hypothermic circulatory arrest at the beginning of the procedure. Our practice has been to repair these lesions during a single procedure performed through the midline sternotomy.

Atrial septal defects are usually repaired by direct suture, but a patch is used if a Blalock-Hanlon operation has previously been performed. Associated anomalies are managed in the usual manner. During the rewarming phase, a left atrial pressure monitoring line is inserted through a purse-string suture in the right superior pulmonary vein or the left atrial appendage, and a temporary ventricular and atrial pacing wire are placed.

SURGICAL IMPLICATIONS OF CORONARY ARTERY ANATOMY

Although different coronary arterial branching patterns are seen in TGA, consistently both in autopsy and clinical series, only 5 variations with dual coronary artery system are possible and 4 of them account for approximately 92% of the patterns found. In the rare cases with single coronary artery system, 4 different branching patterns have been described. All the basic types of patterns have been encountered during the operation and methods have evolved enabling the surgeon to excise and transfer the coronary arteries to the pulmonary root in all types, irrespective of the aortopulmonary relationship[130,131] (see Surgical Technique). For this reason we believe that all types of coronary artery branching patterns are amenable to the arterial switch procedure.

Variations in the origin of the coronary arteries do need to receive special attention. A double coronary ostium should be treated surgically as if it was a branching coronary artery with a single ostium. The complete wall of the aortic sinus should be excised together with both ostia. No attempt should be made to separate the ostia, because the wall of the coronary artery can be thin in this area and anastomotic difficulties with potential narrowing may occur.[132]

Eccentric position of the orifice occurs in about 10% of cases, but the artery can be excised with the same size cuff of sinus by placing the ostium eccentrically within the cuff.

Accessory right ventricular branches arising from sinus 1 in conjunction with a major coronary artery are occasionally seen and are excised within the same cuff. In the rare case of a single coronary artery system arising from sinus 2 and an accessory branch from sinus 1, this accessory branch has been left untouched. However, fistulous communication between the neoaorta and the neopulmonary artery may develop later on (personal communication). It might be preferable to close the ostium of that small RV-branch.

A coronary artery with a high (distal) orifice may be inadvertently transected upon opening the aorta. This can be safely avoided by opening the anterior aspect of the aorta first, and locating the coronary ostia before proceeding with the aortic transection.

Intramural coronary arteries do pose a problem during the arterial switch operation. In all known cases, the LAD is involved, usually with the Cx and in some cases in conjunction with the RCA. The orifice and intramural portion of the coronary artery have to be excised en bloc from the aortic wall. When the intramural portion courses behind the valve commissure, the commissure should be detached and resuspended later during the reconstruction of the neopulmonary artery to allow a proper excision of the origin of the coronary artery. In addition, one cannot usually make the orifice face the pulmonary root without twisting the coronary artery. Instead, it should be allowed to fall upon the anterior wall of the pulmonary artery keeping its original orientation. A superiorly hinged U-flap incision is then made into the pulmonary artery, exactly behind the position of the coronary button, and the flap of pulmonary wall that is produced will cover the origin of the excised coronary, usually with the extension of a small autologous pericardial patch.

RESULTS

Survival

In a multi-institutional study of 513 patients with TGA ± VSD, the 1-month and 1-year survival was 84% and 82% respectively.[144] At Babies and Children's Hospital in New York, the hospital mortality in 132 consecutive patients undergoing the arterial switch since 1990 was 1.5%.

As of the mid-1990s, in institutions properly prepared for the arterial switch procedure for TGA ± VSD, the risk of dying postoperatively was less than 5%. Typically the hazard function for death after this repair has a single, rapidly declining phase, so that by 6 to 12 months postoperatively, the survivorship after the arterial switch operation is the same as that for an age-, race-, and sex-matched population.[34,144]

Risk Factors

Several incremental risk factors for death after the arterial switch operation for TGA ± VSD, and other associated conditions, have been identified. The factors are related to the morbid morphology of the disease, the procedure itself, the intraoperative support system, and the institution performing the arterial switch procedure.

Significant differences between institutions do exist and in a single institution the prevalence of different risk factors changes as time passes. Certain risk factors that were active in the early phase, when a particular institution (or surgeon) adopted the arterial switch protocol, can be neutralized by growing experience.

After 18 years of experience with the arterial switch operation, the only persistent risk factor in our institution is the presence of an intramural coronary artery, although its importance has decreased. No specific coronary branching patterns could ever be identified as risk factors. In the CHSS study, the retropulmonary course of the entire left coronary artery, or one branch of it (Cx), was a risk factor. Other risk factors include earlier date of operation, older age at repair in patients with simple TGA, longer periods of circulatory arrest, multiple VSDs, augmentation of the aortic arch, and a number of "high-risk" institutions.[144,145]

Ventricular Function

Intermediate term follow-up data strongly suggest that left ventricular function and mechanics remain within normal limits in patients with TGA ± VSD undergoing the arterial switch operation in the neonatal period. Borow and associates found normal contractility and dimensions in 10 of 12 patients studied between 2 and 7 years postoperatively.[107] The group at Tokyo Women's Medical College reported better systemic ventricular function after the arterial switch operation than those having Senning operations.[108] Our data and those from Boston Children's Hospital[109,146] indicate that with longer follow-up, left ventricular size and function continue to be normal. All the evidence available about long-term survival and left ventricular function after the arterial switch for TGA ± VSD strongly support the notion that in relation to LV function, these children will have a normal life expectancy. In contrast, in the rapid two-stage arterial switch the echocardiographic indices of LV function seem to be mildly but significantly reduced as compared with normal subjects.[146]

Rhythm Disturbances

The incidence of arrhythmia has been remarkably low in patients after the arterial switch operation. Lange and coworkers[110] reported that 33 of 34 patients were in sinus rhythm with normal A-V conduction during follow-up intervals of up to 7 years. Some premature atrial and ventricular beats were noted and one patient had sinus bradycardia with junctional escape.

A report from the Boston Children's Hospital studying 364 patients surviving the arterial switch operation for TGA ± VSD showed that 96% were in sinus rhythm on surface ECG and 99% were in sinus rhythm during 24-hour Holter monitoring. In contrast to atrial switch operations, sinus node function was preserved in a majority of patients and there was no evidence of atrial flutter or fibrillation.[147]

Aortic and Pulmonary Anastomosis

Since the use of conduits for reconstruction of the right ventricular outflow tract was abandoned, the need for surgical reintervention has decreased dramatically. But even with the surgical modification, including the Lecompte maneuver, RV outflow obstruction occurs in 5–10% of patients, usually within 6 to 9 months after repair. In our experience using two generous autologous pericardial patches, and in the experience of C. Planche using a single pantaloon-shaped pericardal patch, the frequency of this complication has remained lower than 5%. Usually, the obstruction is localized within the pulmonary trunk, presumably secondary to inadequate growth. Occasionally the stenosis is at the level of the neopulmonary valve and/or annulus and sometimes the stenosis is farther upstream at the origin of the pulmonary branches. Treatment for post-switch pulmonary stenosis includes both reoperation and balloon angioplasty, although the latter treatment has been less successful than in other types of RV obstructive lesions. Surgical patch angioplasty of the main pulmonary artery and bifurcation is usually effective. In rare instances, a transannular patch may be required; in this case it is important to know the coronary artery distribution. Left ventricular outflow obstruction is extremely uncommon after arterial switch procedures.

Neoaortic Valve Incompetence

When the arterial switch operation began to be used for the treatment of TGA, the fate of the neoartic valve and annulus was the subject of controversy and speculation about whether it would withstand the increased pressure load. Initial experience, particularly in those patients undergoing preliminary pulmonary artery banding, suggested that a significant incidence of valve regurgitation might be expected.[124,125] However, experimental data demonstrated that diastolic pressure loading of the pulmonary root in a fresh pig model had an inelastic phase between 50 and 200 mm Hg without dilatation or rupture.[142] Our own clinical experience demonstrates that mild or trivial aortic regurgitation is present in about 30% of the patients after the arterial switch operation. This regurgitation is often detectable by Echo-Doppler only, and only 5% have more than moderate incompetence. Patients with a large pulmonary root before the switch procedure (Taussig-Bing, large VSD, preswitch banding of the pulmonary artery) are more likely to develop incompetence than patients with normal pulmonary root preoperatively. Moreover Hourihan et al demonstrated growth of the neoaortic annulus and root after arterial switch in neonates, which was proportional to somatic growth,[143] with a 32% incidence of mild aortic regurgitation. Reports on reoperation for neoaortic valve incompetence are extremely rare.

REFERENCES

1. Baillie M: *The morbid anatomy of some of the more important parts of the human body.* London, Johnson and Nichol, 1797, p 38
2. Farre JR: Pathological researches. Essay 1: *On malformations of the human heart.* London, Longman, Hurst, Rees, Orme, Brown, 1814, p 28
3. Van Praag R, Perez-Trevino C, Lopez-Cuellar M, et al: Transposition of the great arteries with posterior aorta, anterior pulmonary artery, subpulmonary conus and fibrous continuity between aortic and atrioventricular valves. *Am J Cardiol* **28:**621, 1971
4. Soto B, Becker AE, Moulaert AJ, et al: Classification of ventricular septal defects. *Br Heart J* **43:**332, 1980
5. Moene RJ, Oppenheimer-Dekker A, Wenink ACG, et al: Morphology of ventricular septal defects in complete transposition of the great arteries. *Am J Cardiol* **55:**1566, 1985
6. Wenink ACG, Oppenheimer-Dekker A, Moulaert AJ (Eds.): *The ventricular septum of the heart. Boerhaave series, vol. 21.* The Hague, Leiden University Press, 1981
7. Oppenheimer-Dekker A, Gittenberger-de Groot AC, Bartelings MM, et al: Abnormal architecture of the ventricles in hearts with an overriding aortic valve and a perimembranous ventricular septal defect ("Eisenmenger VSD"). *Int J Cardiol* **9:**341, 1985
8. Lev M, Bharati S, Meng CCL, et al: A concept of double-outlet right ventricle. *J Thorac Cardiovasc Surg* **64:**271, 1972
9. Blalock A, Hanlon CR: The surgical treatment of complete transposition of the aorta and pulmonary artery. *Surg Gynecol Obstet* **90:**1, 1950
10. Edwards WS, Bargeron LM, Lyons C: Reposition of right pulmonary vein in transposition of the great vessels. *JAMA* **188:**522, 1964
11. Rashkind WJ, Miller WW: Creation of an atrial septal defect without thoracotomy: a palliative approach to complete transposition of the great arteries. *JAMA* **196:**991, 1966
12. Lillehei CW, Varco RL: Certain physiologic, pathologic, and surgical features of complete transposition of the great vessels. *Surgery* **34:**376, 1953

13. Baffes TG: A new method for surgical correction of transposition of the aorta and pulmonary artery. *Surg Gynecol Obstetr* **102:**227, 1956

14. Mustard WT, Chute AL, Keith JD, et al: A surgical approach to transposition of the great vessels with extracorporeal circuit. *Surgery* **36:**39, 1954

15. Bjork VO, Bouckaert L: Complete transposition of the aorta and the pulmonary artery. An experimental study of the surgical possibilities for its treatment. *J Thorac Surg* **28:**632, 1954

16. Bailey CP, Cookson BA, Downing DF, Neptune WB: Cardiac surgery under hypothermia. *J Thorac Surg* **27:**73, 1954

17. Idriss FS, Goldstein IR, Grana L, et al: A new technique for complete correction of transposition of the great vessels. An experimental study with a preliminary clinical report. *Circulation* **24:**5, 1961

18. Albert HM: Surgical correction of transposition of the great vessels. *Surg Forum* **5:**74, 1954

19. Senning A: Surgical correction of transposition of the great vessels. *Surgery* **45:**966, 1959

20. Barnard CN, Schrire V, Beck W: Complete transposition of the great vessels: successful complete correction. *J Thorac Cardiovasc Surg* **43:**768, 1962

21. Shumacker HB: A new operation for the transposition of the great vessels. *Surgery* **50:**773, 1961

22. Mustard WT: Successful two-stage correction of transposition of the great vessels. *Surgery* **55:**469, 1964

23. Quaegebeur JM, Brom AG: The truser-shape baffle for use in the Mustard operation. *Ann Thorac Surg* **25:**240, 1978

24. Quaegebeur JM, Rohmer J, Brom AG, Tinkelenberg J: Revival of the Senning operation in the treatment of transposition of the great arteries. Preliminary report on recent experience. *Thorax* **32:**517, 1977

25. McGoon DC: Surgery for transposition of the great arteries (editorial). *Circulation* **45:**1147, 1972

26. Anagnostopoulos CE, Athanasuless AB, Arcilla RA: Toward a rational operation for transposition of the great arteries. *Ann Thorac Surg* **16:**458, 1973

27. Rastelli CG, McGoon DC, Wallace RB: Anatomic correction of transposition of the great arteries with ventricular septal defect and subpulmonary stenosis. *J Thorac Cardiovasc Surg* **58:**545, 1969

28. Damus PG: Letter to the editor. *Ann Thorac Surg* **20:**724, 1975

29. Kaye MP: Anatomic correction of transposition of the great arteries. *Mayo Clin Proc* **50:**638, 1975

30. Stansel HC: A new operation for D-loop transposition of the great arteries. *Ann Thorac Surg* **19:**565, 1977

31. Jatene AD: Discussion of transposition of the great arteries with ventricular septal defect: Surgical experience with the Mustard operation and transatrial closure of the ventricular septal defect. In Davila JC (ed): *Second Henry Ford Hospital International Symposium on Cardiac Surgery.* New York, Appleton-Century-Crofts, 1977, p 335

32. Jatene AD, Fontes VF, Paulesta PP, et al: Anatomic correction of transposition of the great vessels. *J Thorac Cardiovasc Surg* **72:**364, 1976

33. Yacoub MH, Radley-Smith R, MacLaurin R: Two-stage operation for anatomical correction of transposition of the great arteries with intact ventricular septum. *Lancet* **1:**275, 1977

34. Quaegebeur JM, Rohmer J, Ottenkamp J, et al: The arterial switch operation: An eight year experience. *J Thorac Cardiovasc Surg* **92:**361, 1986

35. Castañeda AR, Norwood WI, Jones RA, et al: Tansposition of the great arteries and intact ventricular septum: Anatomical repair in the neonate. *Ann Thorac Surg* **38:**438, 1981

36. Parenzan L, Locatelli G, Alfieri O, et al: The Senning operation for transposition of the great arteries. *J Thorac Cardiovasc Surg* **76:**305, 1978

37. Brom AG, Quaegebeur JM: Venous versus arterial switch for repair

of transposition of the great arteries. Data presented at the Symposium on Arterial Switch for Transposition of the Great Arteries. Bergamo, 1981

38. Egloff L, Freed M, Dick M, et al: Early and late results with the mustard operation in infancy. *Ann Thorac Surg* **26:**474, 1978

39. Otero-Coto E, Norwood WI, Lang P, Castañeda AR: Modified Senning procedure for transposition of the great arteries. *J Thorac Cardiovasc Surg* **78:**721, 1979

40. Bender HW, Graham TP, Bovcek RJ, et al: Comparative operative results of the Senning and Mustard procedures for transposition of the great arteries. *Circulation* **62:**197, 1980

41. Arciniegas E, Farooki ZQ, Hakimi M, et al: Results of the Mustard operation for dextro-transposition of the great arteries. *J Thorac Cardiovasc Surg* **81:**580, 1981

42. Meisner H, Feder E, Struck E, et al: Mustard versus Senning procedure: A comparison of primary atrial inversion procedures in 108 patients with transposition of the great arteries. *Herz* **4:**259, 1982

43. Ullal RR, Anderson RH, Lincoln C: Mustard's operation modified to avoid dysrhythmias and pulmonary and systemic venous obstruction. *J Thorac Cardiovasc Surg* **78:**431, 1979

44. Trusler GA, Williams WG, Izukawa T, Olley PM: Current results with the Mustard operation in isolated transposition of the great arteries. *J Thorac Cardiovasc Surg* **80:**381, 1980

45. Matherne GP, Razook JD, Thompson WM, et al: Senning repair for transposition of the great arteries in the first week of life. *Circulation* **72:**840, 1985

46. Turley K, Ebert PA: Total correction of transposition of the great arteries. Conduction disturbances in infants younger than three months of age. *J Thorac Cardiovasc Surg* **74:**312, 1978

47. Marx GR, Hougen TJ, Norwood WI, et al: Transposition of the great arteries with intact ventricular septum: Results of Mustard and Senning operations in 123 consecutive patients. *J Am Coll Cardiol* **2:**476, 1983

48. Bailey LL, Jacobson IG, Merrit WH, et al: Mustard operation in the first month of life. *Am J Cardiol* **49:**766, 1982

49. Tynan M: Survival of infants with transposition of the great arteries after balloon atrial septostomy. *Lancet* **1:**612, 1971

50. Trusler GA, Gonsalves J, Williams WG, et al: Isolated transposition of the great arteries: The present unnatural history. In: Doyle EF, et al (eds): *Second World Congress of Pediatric Cardiology June 2–6, 1985. Abstracts 2.* New York, Springer-Verlag, 1985, p 25

51. Kirklin JK, Blackstone EH, Pacifico AD, et al: Current comprehensive 5-year survival rates using a protocol of balloon atrial septostomy and atrial switching in simple TGA. In: Doyle EF, et al (eds): *Second World Congress of Pediatric Cardiology June 2–6, 1985. Abstracts 2.* New York, Springer-Verlag, 1985, p 157

52. Castañeda AR, Metras D, Williams RG: Transposition of the great arteries with ventricular septal defect: Surgical experience with Mustard operation and transatrial closure of ventricular septal defect. In: Davila IC (ed): *Second Henry Ford International Symposium on Cardiac Surgery.* New York, Appleton-Century-Crofts, 1977, p 321

53. Mahoney L, Turley K, Ebert P, Hegmann M: Long-term results after atrial repair of transposition of the great arteries in early infancy. *Circulation* **66:**253, 1982

54. Stark J, de Leval MR, Waterston D: Corrective surgery of transposition of the great arteries in the first year of life. *J Thorac Cardiovasc Surg* **67:**673, 1974

55. Kirklin JW, Barratt-Boyes BG: *Cardiac Surgery, 1st ed,* New York, John Wiley & Sons: 1985, pp 1194–1195

56. Penkoske PA, Westerman GR, Marx GR, et al: Transposition of the great arteries and ventricular septal defect: Results with the Senning operation and closure of the ventricular septal defect in infants. *Ann Thorac Surg* **36:**281, 1983

57. Dickinson DF, Scott O: Ambulatory electrocardiographic monitoring in 100 healthy teenage boys. *Br Heart J* **51:**179, 1984

58. Southall DP, Johnston F, Shinebourne EA, Johnston PG: Twenty-four hours electrocardiographic study of heart rate and rhythm patterns in a population of healthy children. *Br Heart J* **45:**281, 1981

59. Southall DP, Keeton BR, Leanage R, et al: Cardiac rhythm and conduction before and after Mustard's operation for complete transposition of the great arteries. *Br Heart J* **43:**21, 1980

60. Moene RJ, Ross JP, Eygelaar A: Cardiac arrhythmia following the creation of an atrial septal defect in patients with transposition of the great arteries. *Thorax* **28:**147, 1973

61. Clarkson PM, Barratt-Boyes BG, Neutze JM: Late dysrhythmias and disturbances of conduction following Mustard operation for complete transposition of the great arteries. *Circulation* **53:**519, 1976

62. Lewis AB, Lindesmith GG, Takahashi M, et al: Cardiac rhythm following the Mustard procedure for transposition of the great vessels. *J Thorac Cardiovasc Surg* **73:**919, 1977

63. El-Said G, Rosenberg HS, Mullins CE, et al: Dysrhythmias after Mustard's operation for transposition of the great arteries. *Am J Cardiol* **30:**526, 1972

64. Buis-Liem TN: Mustard operatie bij transposition van de grote arterien. *Thesis,* Leiden, 1982

65. Gillette PC, El-Said GM, Sivarajan N, et al: Electrophysiological abnormalities after Mustard's operation for transposition of the great arteries. *Br Heart J* **36:**186, 1974

66. Beerman CB, Neches WH, Fricker FJ, et al: Arrhythmias in transposition of the great arteries after the Mustard operation. *Am J Cardiol* **51:**1530, 1983

67. Van Veen EC, Rohmer J, Quaegebeur JM: Long-term results of the Senning operation for simple transposition. In: Doyle EF et al (eds): *Second World Congress of Pediatric Cardiology, June 2–6, 1985. Abstracts 2.* New York, Springer-Verlag, 1985, p 90

68. Hajes CJ, Gersony WM: Arrhythmia after the Mustard operation for transposition of the great arteries: A long-term study. *JACC* **7:**133, 1986

69. El-Said GM, Gillette PC, Cooley DA, et al: Protection of the sinus node in Mustard's operation. *Circulation* **53:**788, 1976

70. Stark J: Evaluations of inflow-type repairs for transposition of the great arteries. *Ped Cardiol* **4**(suppl I):159, 1983

71. Martin TC, Smith L, Hernandez A, Weldon CS: Dysrhythmias following the Senning operation for dextro-transposition of the great arteries. *J Thorac Cardiovasc Surg* **85:**928, 1983

72. Louhimo I, Kala R, Tuuteri L: Postoperative studies in transposition. In: Doyle EF, et al (eds): *Second World Congress of Pediatric Cardiology, June 2–6, 1985. Abstract 2.* New York, Springer-Verlag, 1985, p 90

73. Hagler DJ, Ritter DG, Mair DD, et al: Right and left ventricular function after the Mustard procedure in transposition of the great arteries. *Am J Cardiol* **44:**276, 1979

74. Bender HW, Graham TP, Boucek RJ, et al: Comparative results of the Senning and Mustard procedures for transposition of the great arteries. *Circulation* **62**(suppl I):I–197, 1980

75. Jarmakani JM, Canent RN: Preoperative and postoperative right ventricular function in children with transposition of the great vessels. *Circulation* **53**(suppl II):II–39, 1974

76. Graham TP, Atwood GF, Boucek RJ, et al: Abnormalities of right ventricular function following Mustard's operation for transposition of the great arteries. *Circulation* **52:**678, 1975

77. Parrish MD, Graham TP, Bender HW, et al: Radionuclide angiographic evaluation of right and left ventricular function during exercise after repair of transposition of the great arteries. Comparison with normal subjects and patients with congenitally corrected transposition. *Circulation* **67:**178, 1983

78. Murphy JH, Barlai-Kovach MM, Mathew RA, et al: Rest and exercise right and left ventricular function late after the Mustard operation: Assessment by radionuclide ventriculography. *Am J Cardiol* **51:**1520, 1983

79. Masden RR, Franch RH: Isolated congenitally corrected transposi-

80. Borrow KM, Keane JF, Castañeda AR, Freed MD: Systemic ventricular function in patients with tetralogy of Fallot, VSD and transposition of the great arteries repaired during infancy. *Circulation* **64:**878, 1981

81. Mair DD, Hagler DJ: Late results of the Mustard operation for transposition of the great arteries. *Proc 8th World Congress of Cardiology,* Tokyo, 1978, p 515

82. Lemoine G, Lacour-Gayet F, Zannini L, et al: Mid-term results of the Senning operation for simple transposition of the great vessels (TGV). 74 patients. In: Doyle EF, et al (eds): *Second World Congress of Pediatric Cardiology, June 2–6, 1985. Abstracts 2.* New York, Springer-Verlag, 1985, p 5

83. Tynan M, Aberdeen E, Stark J: Tricuspid incompetence after the Mustard operation for transposition of the great arteries. *Circulation* **46**(suppl I):I–III, 1972

84. Huhta JC, Edwards WD, Danielson GK, Feldt RH: Abnormalities of the tricuspid valve in complete transposition of the great arteries with ventricular septal defect. *J Thorac Cardiovasc Surg* **83:**569, 1982

85. Stark J, Silove ED, Taylor JF, Graham GR: Obstruction to systemic venous return following the Mustard operation for transposition of the great arteries. *J Thorac Cardiovasc Surg* **68:**742, 1974

86. Venables AW, Edis B, Clarke CP: Vena caval obstruction complicating the Mustard operation for complete transposition of the great arteries. *Eur J Cardiol* **1:**401, 1974

87. Park SC, Neches WH, Mathews RA, et al: Hemodynamic function after the Mustard operation for transposition of the great arteries. *Am J Cardiol* **51:**1514, 1983

88. Cobanoglu A, Abbruzzese PA, Freimanis I, et al: Pericardial baffle complication following the Mustard operation. Age-related incidence and ease of management. *J Thorac Cardiovasc Surg* **87:**371, 1984

89. Clarkson PM, Neutze JM, Barratt-Boyes BG, Brandt PW: Late postoperative hemodynamic results and cineangiographic findings after Mustard atrial baffle repair for transposition of the great arteries. *Circulation* **53:**525, 1976

90. Takahashi M, Lindesmith GG, Lewis AB, et al: Long-term results of the Mustard procedure. *Circulation* **56**(suppl II):II–85, 1977

91. Graham TP: Hemodynamic residua and sequelae following intra-atrial repair of transposition of the great arteries: A review. *Ped Cardiol* **2:**203, 1982

92. Hagler DJ, Ritter DG, Mair DD, et al: Clinical angiographic and hemodynamic assessment of late results after Mustard's operation. *Circulation* **57:**1214, 1978

93. Morgan JR, Miller BL, Daicoff GR, Andrews EJ: Hemodynamic and angiographic evaluation after Mustard procedure for transposition of the great arteries. *J Thorac Cardiovasc Surg* **64:**878, 1972

94. Godman MJ, Friedli B, Pasternac A, et al: Hemodynamic studies in children four to ten years after the Mustard operation for transposition of the great arteries. *Circulation* **53:**532, 1976

95. Stark J, de Leval MR, Waterston DJ, et al: Corrective surgery for transposition of the great arteries in the first year of life. Results in 63 infants. *J Thorac Cardiovasc Surg* **67:**673, 1974

96. Kirklin JW, Baratt-Boyes BG: *Cardiac Surgery, 1st ed,* New York, John Wiley & Sons, 1985, p 1184

97. Stark J: Evaluation of inflow-type repairs for transposition of the great arteries. *Ped Cardiol* **4**(suppl I):159, 1983

98. Satomi G, Nakamura K, Takao A, Imai Y: Two-dimensional echocardiographic detection of pulmonary venous channel stenosis after Senning's operation. *Diagn Meth Surg* **68:**545, 1983

99. Chin AJ, Sanders SP, Williams RG, et al: Two dimensional echocardiographic assessment of caval and pulmonary venous pathway after the Senning operation. *Am J Cardiol* **52:**118, 1983

100. Muster AJ, Paul MH, Van Grondelle A, Conway JJ: Asymetrical

distribution of pulmonary blood flow between the right and left lungs in D-transposition of the great arteries. *Am J Cardiol* **38**:352, 1976

101. Vidne BA, Duszynski D, Subramanian S: Pulmonary blood flow distribution in transposition of the great arteries. *Am J Cardiol* **38**:62, 1976

102. Wyse RK, Macarthney FJ, Rohmer J, et al: Differential atrial filling after Mustard and Senning repairs. *Br Heart J* **44**:692, 1980

103. Smallhorn JF, Gow R, Freedom RM, et al: Pulsed doppler echocardiographic assessment of the pulmonary venous pathway after the Mustard or Senning procedure for transposition of the great arteries. *Circulation* **73**:765, 1986

104. Silverman NH, Payot M, Stanger P, Randolph AM: Echocardiographic profile of patients after Mustard operation. *Circulation* **58**:1083, 1978

105. Aziz KU, Paul MH, Idriss FS, et al: Clinical manifestations of dynamic left ventricular outflow tract stenosis in infants with D-transposition of the great arteries with intact ventricular septum. *Am J Cardiol* **44**:290, 1979

106. Yacoub MH, Arensman FW, Keck E, Radley-Smith R: Fate of dynamic left ventricular outflow tract obstruction after anatomic correction of transposition of the great arteries. *Circulation* **68**(suppl II):II–56, 1983

107. Borow KM, Arensman FE, Webb C, et al: Assessment of left ventricular contractile state after anatomic correction of transposition of the great arteries. *Circulation* **69**:106, 1984

108. Okuda H, Kakezawa M, Imai Y, et al: Comparison of ventricular function after Senning and Jantene procedures for complete transposition of the great arteries. *Am J Cardiol* **55**:530, 1985

109. Helgason H, Hougen TJ, Jacobs M, et al: Hemodynamic results of primary anatomic repair of transposition of the great arteries. In Doyle EF: Engle MA, Gersony WM, et al (eds): *Pediatric Cardiology: Proceedings of the 2nd World Congress.* New York, Springer-Verlag, 1985, p 558

110. Lange PE, Sievers HH, Onnasch D, et al: Up to 7 years of follow-up after two-stage anatomic correction of simple transposition of the great arteries. *Circulation* **74**(suppl I):I–47, 1986

111. Paul MH: Transposition of the great arteries. In Adams FH, Emmanouildes GC, (eds): *Heart Disease in Infants, Children, and Adolescents.* Baltimore, Williams & Wilkins, 1983, p 311

112. Bano-Rodrigo A, Quero-Jimenez M, Moreno-Granada F, Gamalto-Anat C: Wall thickness of ventricular chambers in transposition of the great arteries. *J Thorac Cardiovasc Surg* **79**:592, 1980

113. Huhta JC, Edwards WD, Feldt RH, Puga FJ: Left ventricular wall thickness in complete transposition of the great arteries. *J Thorac Cardiovasc Surg* **84**:97, 1982

114. Smith A, Wilkinson JC, Arnold R, et al: Growth and development of ventricular walls in complete transposition of the great arteries with intact septum (simple transposition). *Am J Cardiol* **49**:362, 1982

115. Danford DA, Huhta JC, Gutgesell HP: Left ventricular wall stress and thickness in complete transposition of the great arteries. *J Thorac Cardiovasc Surg* **89**:610, 1985

116. Chui I, Anderson RH, McCarthy FJ, et al: Morphologic features of an intact ventricular septum susceptible to subpulmonary obstruction in complete transposition. *Am J Cardiol* **53**:1633, 1984

117. Shrivastava J, Tadavarthy SM, Fukuda T, Edwards JE: Anatomic causes of pulmonary stenosis in complete transposition. *Circulation* **54**:154, 1976

118. Ilbawi MN, Quinn K, Riggs TW, et al: The surgical management of left ventricular outflow tract obstruction due to tricuspid valve pouch in complete transposition of the great arteries. *J Thorac Cardiovasc Surg* **87**:66, 1984

119. Layman TE, Edwards JE: Anomalies of the cardiac valves associated with complete transposition of the great vessels. *Am J Cardiol* **19**:247, 1967

120. Yacoub MH, Arensman FW, Keck E, Radley-Smith R: Fate of dynamic left ventricular outflow tract obstruction after anatomic cor-

rection of transposition of the great arteries. *Circulation* **68**(suppl II):II–56, 1983

121. Elliott LP, Amplatz K, Edwards JE: Coronary arterial pattern in transposition complexes. Anatomic and angiographic studies. *Am J Cardiol* **17**:362, 1966

122. Rowlatt VF: Coronary artery distribution in complete transposition. *JAMA* **179**:269, 1961

123. Vlodaver HD, Neufeld HN, Edwards JE: Patterns of origin and distribution of coronary arteries in transposition complexes and tetralogy of Fallot. In: *Coronary Arterial Variations in the Normal Heart and in Congenital Heart Disease.* San Diego, Academic Press, 1975, p 111

124. Williams WG, Freedom RM, Culham G, et al: Early experience with arterial repair of transposition. *Ann Thorac Surg* **32**:8, 1981

125. Lange PE, Sievers HH, Onnasch D, et al: Up to 7 years of followup after two-stage anatomic correction of simple transposition of the great arteries. *Circulation* **74**(suppl I):I–47, 1986

126. Pasquini L, Sanders SP, Parness I, Colan SD: Diagnosis of coronary artery anatomy by two-dimensional echocardiography in patients with transposition of the great arteries. *Circulation* **75**:557, 1987

127. King ME, Braun H, Goldblatt A, et al: Interventricular septal configuration as a predictor of right ventricular systolic hypertension in children: A cross sectional echocardiographic study. *Circulation* **68**:68, 1982

128. Yacoub MH, Radley-Smith R, Maclaurin R: Two-stage operation for anatomical correction of transposition of the great arteries with intact interventricular septum. *Lancet* **1**:1275–1278, 1977

129. Lecompte Y, Zannini L, Hazan E, et al: Anatomic correction of transposition of the great arteries. *J Thorac Cardiovasc Surg* **82**:629–631, 1981

130. Yacoub MH: Personal communication, 1985

131. Jatene AD: Personal communication, 1985

132. Firmin RL, Lima R, Anderson RH, et al: Anatomic problems associated with arterial switch procedures for double outlet right ventricle with subpulmonary VSD. *Thorac Cardiovasc Sugeon* **31**:365, 1983

133. Smith A, Arnold R, Wilkinson JL, et al: An anatomical study of the patterns of the coronary arteries and sinus nodal artery in complete transposition. *Int J Cardiol:* 1996 (in press).

134. Kirklin JW, Barratt-Boyes BG: Cardiac Surgery, Chapter 39: *Transposition of the great arteries.* New York, John Wiley & Sons, 1985, p 1136

135. Gittenberger-de Groot AC, Sauer V, Quaegebeur JM: Aortic intramural coronary artery in three hearts with transposition of the great arteries. *J Thorac Cardiovasc Surg* 1986

136. Radley-Smith R, Yacoub MH: Ten year experience of anatomic correction of simple transposition of the great arteries (abstract). *Circulation* **74**(suppl):II–50, 1986

137. Kanter KR, Anderson RH, Lincoln CR, et al: Anatomic correction for complete transposition and double outlet right ventricle. *J Thorac Cardiovasc Surg* **90**:690, 1985

138. Becal O, Hagan E, LeCompte Y, et al: Anatomic correction of transposition of the great arteries associated with ventricular septal defect: Midterm results in 50 patients. *Circulation* **70**:891, 1984

139. Arensman FW, Sievers H, Lange P, et al: Assessment of coronary and aortic anastomoses after anatomic correction of transposition of the great arteries. *J Thorac Cardiovasc Surg* **90**:597, 1985

140. Yacoub MH, Bernhard A, Radley-Smith R, et al: Supravalvular pulmonary stenosis after anatomic correction of transposition of the great arteries: Causes and prevention. *Circulation* **66**(suppl I):I–193, 1982

141. Mee RH: Severe right ventricular failure after Mustard or Senning operation: Two-stage repair: Pulmonary artery banding and switch. *J Thorac Cardiovasc Surg* **92**:385, 1986

142. Sievers HH, Leyh R, Loose R, et al: Time course of dimension and function of the autologous pulmonary root in the aortic position. *J Thoracic Cardiovasc Surg* **105**:775–780, 1993

143. Hourihan M, Colan SD, Wernovsky G, et al: Growth of the aortic

anastomosis, annulus, and root after the arterial switch procedure performed in infancy. *Circulation* **88:**615–620, 1993

144. Kirklin JW, Blackstone EH, Tchervenkov CI, et al: Clinical outcomes after the arterial switch operation for transposition. Patient, support, procedural, and institutional risk factors. *Circulation* **86:**1501–1515, 1992

145. Wernovsky G, Mayer JE, Jonas RA, et al: Factors influencing early and late outcome of the arterial switch operation for transposition of the great arteries. *Circulation* **109:**289–302, 1995

146. Colan SD, Boutin C, Castañeda AR, Wernovsky G: Status of the left ventricle after arterial switch operation for transposition of the great arteries. *Circulation* **109:**311–321, 1995

147. Rhodes LA, Wernovsky G, Keane JF, et al: Arrhythmias and intracardiac conduction after the arterial switch operation. *Circulation* **109:**303–310, 1995

86

Congenitally Corrected Transposition of the Great Arteries

Michel N. Ilbawi and Philip C. Smith

The term *physiologically corrected transposition of the great arteries* refers to a congenital cardiac lesion with malposition of the great arteries where the aorta arises from the right ventricle and the pulmonary artery from the left ventricle. Unlike the more common form of simple transposition, this ventriculoarterial discordance is associated with atrioventricular discordance where the right atrium empties into the left ventricle and the left atrium empties into the right ventricle. In situs solitus, the embryogenesis of this malformation is abnormal folding of the cardiac tube to the left (*l*-loop) instead of the normal folding to the right (*d*-loop) resulting in a left-sided right ventricle and a right-sided left ventricle, so-called ventricular inversion. The division of the conotruncus, which embryologically is related to the right ventricle, gives rise to an anterior and left-sided aorta arising from the right ventricle and a posterior right-sided pulmonary artery arising from the left ventricle (*l*-malposition).[1] In situs inversus, the end result is a mirror image. The physiologic sequence of this double "anatomic error" is normal circulatory pathways in series regardless of the position of the great arteries.

The terminologies used to describe this malformation have varied and could be a source of confusion. Commonly, it is referred to as *l*-TGA to imply a left-sided location of the aorta in relation to the pulmonary artery and to distinguish it from the more common classic complete transposition of the great arteries (*d*-TGA). However, this term could be misleading in the presence of dextrocardia or reversal of visceral orientation present in around 25% of the cases. In this situation, the aorta is far to the right of the pulmonary

artery, and therefore does not fulfill the *l*-malposition definition. Furthermore, leftward aorta is not pathognomonic of physiologically corrected malposition of the great arteries and could be present in other malformations. The segmental anatomy described by Van Praagh, using a three-letter code definition of situs, ventricular loop, and great arteries position, may best describe the lesion. Thus, a congenitally corrected transposition would be referred to as S,L,L in situs solitus and I,D,D in situs inversus.

NATURAL HISTORY

The natural history of congenitally corrected transposition is extremely important as it influences the surgical decision making. In the absence of associated lesions this condition may go unrecognized until the third or fourth decade of life where 40% of patients may present with left-sided (anatomically tricuspid, functionally mitral) valve dysfunction. In another 40%, spontaneous onset of complete atrioventricular block occurs at a rate of 2%/pt year.[2] Most importantly, however, a high percent of patients may present with heart failure due to a progressive decrease in systemic right ventricular function with time.[3,4]

In the majority of patients, the associated lesions dictate the natural history and outcome. The presence of ventricular septal defect, if untreated, leads to onset of congestive heart failure and progressive pulmonary vascular disease. The more common combination of ventricular septal defect and pulmonary stenosis may result in balanced circulation with no early symptoms, but progressive cyanosis later in life when the degree of stenosis becomes severe.

SURGICAL ANATOMY

In congenitally corrected transposition of the great arteries, the coronary anatomy is a mirror image of normal. The left anterior descending artery comes off the right-sided and rather anterior artery. The left coronary artery is single and gives rise to the circumflex vessel.[5]

Ventricular septal defect is present in 75–85% of cases, and is due to characteristic malalignment of the atrial and ventricular septa. Most defects are large, subpulmonary, and perimembranous, but could be in any part of the septum.[6,7] The pulmonary valve commonly overrides the defect. Pulmonary stenosis occurs in 45–60% of patients. Obstruction to pulmonary blood flow is usually subannular and is either fibrous or muscular. It results from the pulmonary outflow tract being low and wedged between the right and left atrioventricular valve.[8]

The location of the atrioventricular node and bundle of His differs from normal. There are two atrioventricular nodes in patients with situs solitus; a posterior one, normally located in front of the coronary sinus at the tip of Koch's triangle, and an anterior one at the junction of the anterior horn of the limbus with the atrioventricular ring. The latter gives rise to the penetrating bundle of His. The long bundle perforates the ventricular septum at the anterior aspect of the pulmonary annulus and encircles its superior quadrant before it descends on the septum's anterior right border (anatomically the left side) in a mirror image fashion to that of patients with atrioventricular concordance.[9] If ventricular septal defect is present, the bundle passes along the anterior and superior border of the defect on the anatomic left side of the septum (Fig. 86–1).

The tricuspid valve is left-sided and has the normal three leaflet configuration. The septal and posterior leaflets, however, are more medial and anterior, and frequently dysplastic with abnormal chordal attachments. Occasionally, there might be downward, albeit not significant, Ebstein-like displacement of the anterior leaflet toward the apex, but the abnormally located leaflet is not enlarged.[10]

CLINICAL PRESENTATION AND DIAGNOSIS

The clinical picture in patients with corrected transposition reflects the pathophysiology of associated lesions. In patients with isolated ventricular septal defect, presentation is that of left-to-right shunt and increased pulmonary blood flow. Severe congestive heart failure is less likely than in patients with normally related vessels due to restriction to blood flow by the abnormally located pulmonary outflow tract, even in the absence of recognizable anatomic obstruction. In contrast, patients with associated valvar or subvalvar pulmonary stenosis may be asymptomatic in infancy, or may present with progressive cyanosis. Physical examination is not diagnostic. Chest x-ray reveals the characteristic straight left side border produced by the anterior leftward position of the ascending aorta (Fig. 86–2). ECG may show a Q wave in the right precordial leads.

Definitive diagnosis is established by echocardiography.[11] A tricuspid valve connects the left atrium to a trabeculated left-sided right ventricle, which gives rise to the aorta (Fig. 86–3). Angiography is also helpful.[12] A left atrial injection opacifies a trabeculated right ventricle and an anterior aorta, while injection in the right atrium, identified by its blunt-end appendage, fills a smooth-walled left ventricular chamber and a posterior pulmonary artery (Fig. 86–4).

MEDICAL TREATMENT

Medical and surgical management is dictated by associated lesions and onset of symptoms. Patients with a large ven-

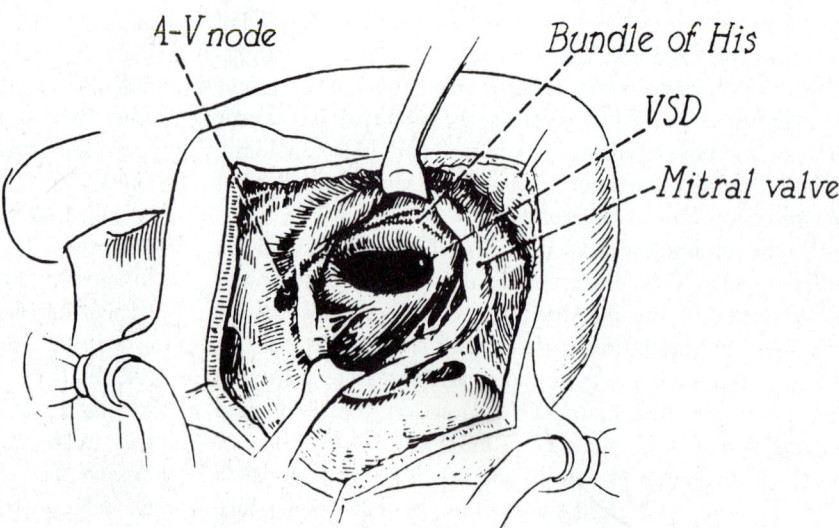

Figure 86–1. Relationship of the conduction system to pulmonary valve and ventricular septal defect in corrected transposition of the great arteries. The bundle passes anterior and superior on the left side of the septum.

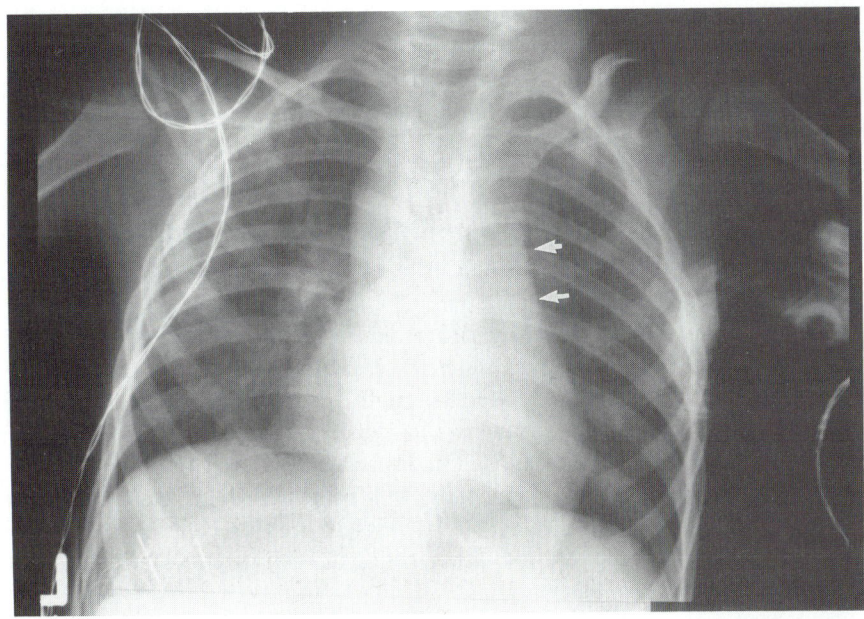

Figure 86–2. Typical chest x-ray appearance. The characteristic straight left heart border (arrows) is produced by the anterior and left-sided ascending aorta.

tricular septal defect and increased pulmonary bloodflow require treatment with digoxin and diuretics in early infancy. Cardiac catheterization is indicated before 1 year of age to monitor changes in pulmonary vascular resistance. Failure of symptoms to respond to medical treatment or evidence of progressive increase in pulmonary vascular resistance are indications for surgery.

Patients with ventricular septal defect and pulmonary stenosis may not require treatment in early infancy. Onset of progressive cyanosis with arterial desaturation below 80% and rising hemoglobin level are indications for systemic to pulmonary artery shunt or complete correction depending on the age of the patient.

Heart failure secondary to left-sided atrioventricular valve (tricuspid valve) regurgitation requires early treatment using digoxin, diuretics, and afterload reduction. Prolonged medical treatment was recommended in the past and valve surgery was postponed until onset of significant signs and symptoms. Recent reports have indicated significant and fast onset of ventricular failure in these patients, in spite of optimal medical treatment, probably due to the inherent anatomic abnormalities of the valve and the subopti-

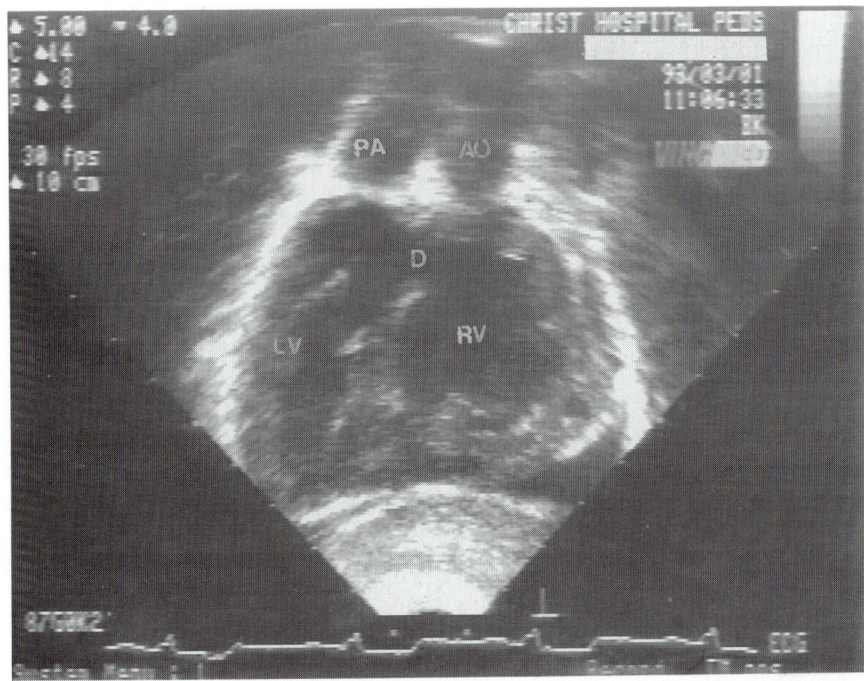

Figure 86–3. Echocardiographic findings in congenitally corrected transposition. Note the left-sided trabeculated right ventricle (RV) giving rise to aorta (Ao). The left ventricle (LV) gives rise to the pulmonary artery (PA). D, VSD.

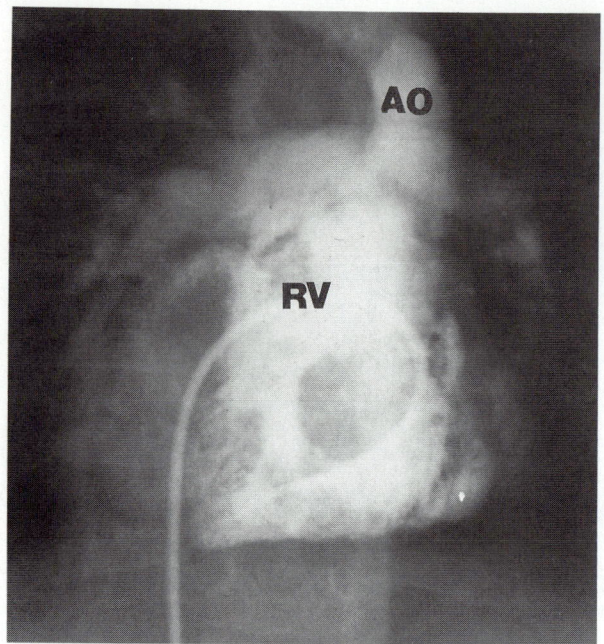

Figure 86–4. Angiographic findings in situs solitus. The right ventricle (RV) gives rise to left-sided anterior aorta (Ao).

mal performance of the systemic right ventricle. Therefore, aggressive surgical treatment of this condition is indicated early in the course to avoid onset of irreversible ventricular dysfunction.

Complete atrioventricular block rarely requires treatment. Implantation of a permanent pacemaker is indicated in symptomatic patients with significant bradycardia.[13] Epicardial ventricular lead is preferred in patients less than 3 years of age. However, transvenous approach could also be used in small children. A rate-responsive pacemaker provides an adequate physiologic response to exercise. Atrioventricular pacing may be needed in patients with associated myocardial dysfunction in whom synchronized atrioventricular contractions improve cardiac output.

SURGICAL TREATMENT

Palliative Approach

Palliative surgery for corrected transposition of the great arteries, like other congenital cardiac malformations, is being used less and less frequently. In patients with associated ventricular septal defect initial medical treatment provides adequate relief of symptoms in the majority of cases until definitive surgery is performed. Palliative pulmonary artery banding is rarely needed and total repair is indicated if symptoms persist in spite of treatment or if pulmonary vascular resistance increases. In cyanotic young infants, however, palliation is advisable, as total correction in this age group requires placement of ventriculopulmonary artery

conduit and subsequent need for early replacement. The preferred palliation for these patients is a modified Blalock–Taussig shunt (5–6 mm graft) constructed on the side of the right pulmonary artery for ease of future takedown.

Definitive Treatment

The principles underlying surgical repair have evolved through the years. This evolution has been prompted by several major concerns: disappointment with the short- and long-term results of previously used approaches, concern over the fate of the right ventricle as a systemic pumping chamber, the high incidence of reoperation following repair of intracardiac lesions, and the higher perioperative mortality when compared with patients with atrioventricular concordance.[13,14] As a result, there is a continued interest in and effort to find a better alternative to previously used approaches.

Repair of Ventricular Septal Defect

Several techniques have been described for the closure of ventricular septal defect. All aim at decreasing the high incidence of postsurgical atrioventricular block, to which the anomalous location of the conduction system predisposes, and at avoiding the need for an incision in the systemic right ventricle.

The Transaortic Approach. Closure through the aortic valve is best used in patients with situs inversus because the ventricles partially overlie the right atrium and preclude transatrial exposure of the defect.[15] Following bicaval cannulation and establishment of cardiopulmonary bypass cardioplegia is given. The use of retrograde cardioplegia in combination with antegrade cardioplegia into the coronary ostia provides adequate myocardial protection. The aorta is opened and valve leaflets are retracted. The ventricular septal defect is visualized and sutures are placed on the side of the septum facing the morphologic right ventricle, to avoid the conduction system. Exposure might be difficult in the presence of a long subaortic infundibulum. The technique has the advantage of minimizing injury to the His bundle and avoiding a ventriculotomy.

Right Atrial Approach. This is the most frequently used approach. The ventricular septal defect is visualized through the mitral valve (right-sided atrioventricular valve). The leaflets are retracted to provide exposure of the defect edges. Care should be taken to avoid excessive pull on the valve as that might result in complete heart block. The anterior leaflet may be detached from the annulus to improve exposure to the superior and anterior quadrants of the defect. Sutures for patch closure of the defect are placed on the right septal side through the defect in an attempt to minimize the incidence of atrioventricular block (Fig. 86–5).[16] The repair of an isolated defect using this approach is best

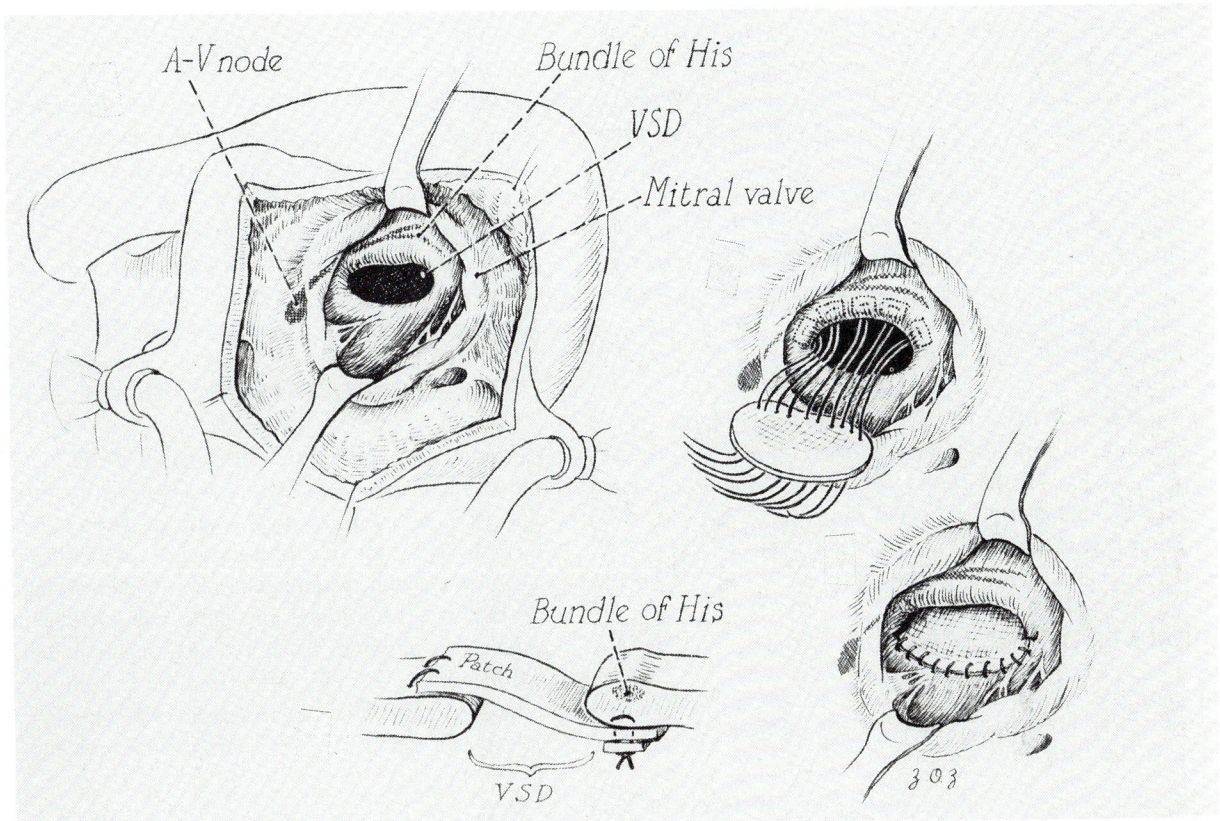

Figure 86–5. A–D. Transatrial approach to closure of ventricular septal defect. The sutures are placed on the right side of the septum in the superior and anterior border of the defect to avoid the conduction system.

postponed until 2–4 years of age to allow better exposure through the right-sided atrioventricular valve and placement of sutures on the right side of the septum.

Left Ventricular Approach. This approach could be used whenever a ventriculotomy is needed for placement of a ventriculopulmonary artery conduit. It is especially advantageous when the ventricles overlie the right atrium, precluding optimal atrial approach. Exposure and technique of suture placement are similar to those of the right atrial approach.

Other Approaches. These are rarely used at present. The transpulmonic valve approach is fraught with a high incidence of complete atrioventricular block.[17] The transaortic root approach has been discussed but not reported.[18] A right ventriculotomy for exposure is rarely indicated, as it may result in myocardial dysfunction of the systemic pumping chamber.

Repair of Pulmonary Outflow Tract Stenosis

The posterior location of the outflow tract and its close proximity to the conduction tissue increase considerably the incidence of complete atrioventricular block and injury to the atrioventricular valves if direct resection of the obstructing tissue is attempted. Relief of the stenosis is best

achieved by placement of ventriculopulmonary artery external conduit in the majority of cases.[18] Homograft conduits are most commonly used because they conform to available space and are easy to handle. The long-term results of these homografts in this location are not available, although it is becoming apparent that early failure and calcification are likely to occur necessitating repeated operations.[19] An alternative approach to the management of subpulmonary stenosis is the use of a spiral incision extending from the pulmonary artery through the valve annulus into the posterior subvalvar myocardium. This technique minimizes the need for conduit insertion with its attendant need for replacement, and allows enlargement of the subvalvar area, or even valve replacement if needed.[20] It could, however, result in atrioventricular block and damage to the atrioventricular valves. In isolated cases, obstruction is localized to the valve and simple valvotomy is sufficient.

Repair of Left-sided (Tricuspid) Valve

Tricuspid regurgitation is frequently present and could result in progressive right ventricular dysfunction, especially when Ebstein-like malformation is present. Traditionally, management of this valve abnormality has been conservative with attempts at delaying surgery until the patient is quite symptomatic. This has been due to lack of successful valvuloplasty techniques, and difficulties associated with valve replacement in young children, further exaggerated by the anterior location of the tricuspid valve and the relatively small right ventricle.[21,22] Recent advances in valvuloplasty techniques, especially those applicable to right-sided Ebstein's anomaly and the use of a transeptal approach, have allowed early surgical control of regurgitation and preservation of ventricular function.[23] If the regurgitation is severe and the valve is not amenable to repair, replacement may be needed. The modified Medtronic Hall or St. Jude prostheses may be used in these young patients with good results.

Management of Other Associated Lesions

Hypoplasia of the right ventricle, or straddling atrioventricular valve may result, and are approached like other single ventricle equivalents. Modified Fontan has been used to treat these patients.

RESULTS OF TRADITIONAL SURGICAL TREATMENT

Early Results

The most common complication of surgical closure of ventricular septal defect in physiologically corrected transposition is iatrogenic complete atrioventricular block. The incidence varies between 10 and 40%, although it has decreased in the past few years due to better understanding of the anatomy and improvement in techniques.[15,16] Advances in pacing technology have minimized the deleterious side effects of this complication, especially in the immediate postoperative period where synchronized atrioventricular contractions are most helpful in the recovering heart.[13]

When pulmonary stenosis is present, the resultant balanced circulation protects the pulmonary vascular bed, and allows a delay in the surgical treatment. As a result, operative risk in this situation is quite low (less than 4%) and immediate outcome is good. However, the problem of iatrogenic complete atrioventricular block remains unchanged.

Operative risk of traditional valve repair or replacement has been high (14%). Experience with newer valvuloplasty techniques is limited, but early results are encouraging.

Late Results

Late results of patients with corrected transposition and other associated lesions have been disappointing. The poor outcome is related to persistent residual lesions, progression of complete atrioventricular block, poor right ventricular function, and development of tricuspid valve regurgitation.[14] Actuarial survival at 15 years varies between 50 and 80% depending on the functional status of the right ventricle and the tricuspid valve at the time of initial repair. The

incidence of late right ventricular dysfunction is not clear, although there is compelling evidence that given enough time, most right ventricles in the systemic side of circulation are bound to fail, especially if associated with abnormalities in the tricuspid valve. Need for reoperation also has been a problem with up to 40% of patients requiring additional surgery, such as pacemaker change, conduit changes, and valve replacement by 8 years following initial procedure.

THE NEW ALTERNATIVE SURGICAL APPROACH

Prompted by the multiple drawbacks of the traditional surgical management for associated lesions in corrected transposition, an alternative approach has been introduced.[24–27] The basis for the new operation is to use the right-sided left ventricle as the systemic chamber, and close the ventricular septal defect from the right septal side. This technique eliminates the problem of short- and long-term failure of systemic right ventricle, minimizes the hemodynamic significance of the left-sided tricuspid valve regurgitation, and decreases the incidence of iatrogenic atrioventricular block.

Technique

Using direct bicaval cannulation, cardiopulmonary bypass with moderate hypothermia (25°C) is initiated. Antegrade cardioplegic protection is used and the right atrium is opened in appropriate fashion and a Mustard or Senning procedure is performed. Following the venous switch procedure, a right ventriculotomy is made and the ventricular septal defect is closed using multiple interrupted pledgeted sutures placed on the right side of the septum and around the aortic root to direct the left ventricular output toward the aorta. In most cases, the subaortic conus is attenuated or even absent, facilitating the tunnelling procedure. Occasionally, enlargement of the ventricular septal defect might be needed. In patients with pulmonary stenosis, a valved conduit is then placed between the pulmonary artery and right ventricle on the right side of the aorta with care taken to avoid compression of the right coronary artery by the conduit (Fig. 86–6). In the absence of any pulmonary outflow tract stenosis, ventricular septal defect closure tunnels the left ventricle to the aorta as mentioned, but the venous switch operation is followed by an arterial switch operation, the so-called double switch. The coronary arteries are transferred to the pulmonary side with a cuff of aortic wall in the usual manner and the great arteries are then switched.[24,25]

Results of the New Approach

Experience with this double switch operation is still limited and long-term results are not available. We have performed this procedure on eight patients with ventricular septal defect and pulmonary stenosis. There was no operative mor-

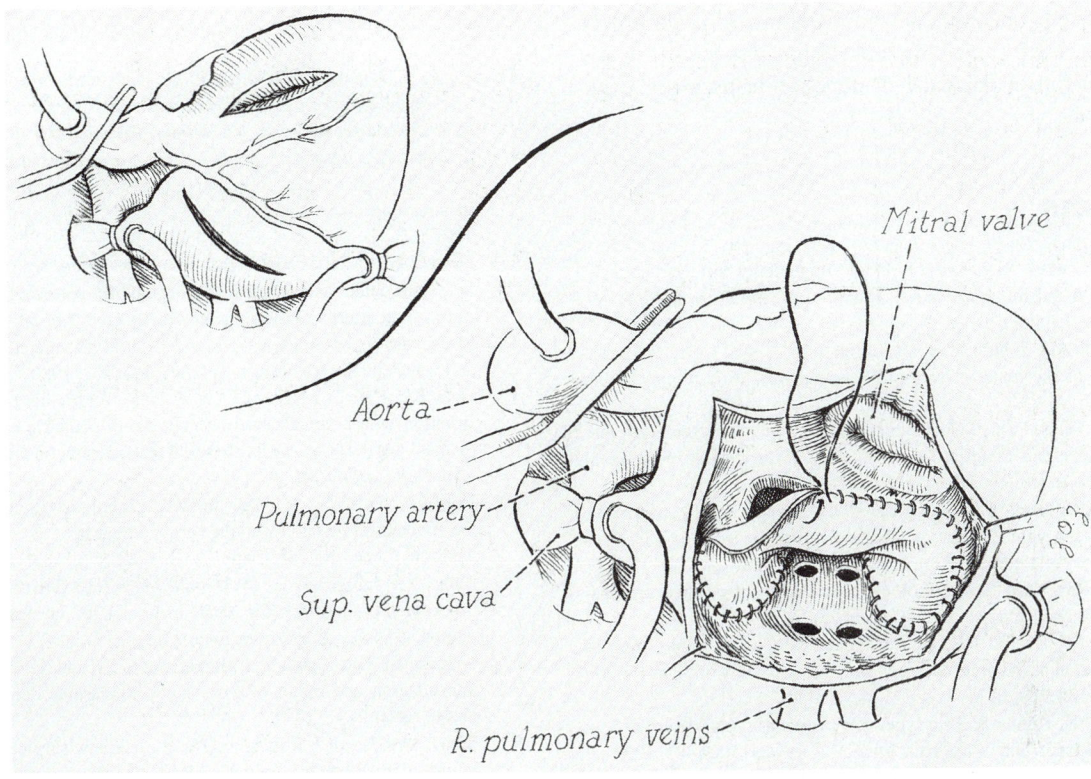

A

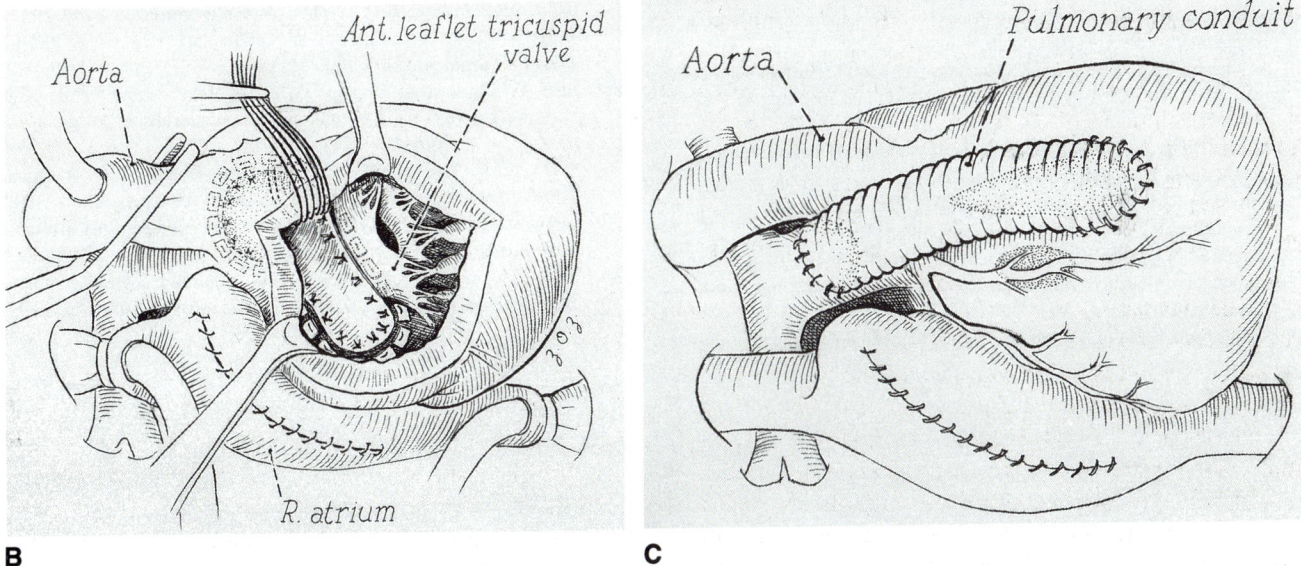

B   **C**

Figure 86–6. Details of the double switch operation. **A.** The right atrium is opened and a venous switch operation is performed. **B.** Through a right ventriculotomy, the tunnel patch is inserted to direct the blood from the right-sided left ventricle into the aorta. Sutures are placed around the ventricular septal defect inferiorly and the aortic root superiorly. **C.** A conduit is placed between the right ventricle and pulmonary artery after closing the pulmonary valve.

tality and no iatrogenic heart block. At a follow-up of 6 years, one patient developed tachybrady atrial arrhythmia and needed a pacemaker, and two required replacement of their conduits. Imoi et al reported similar experience with 18 patients under 15 years of age. Operative mortality was 11%. Follow-up revealed normal right and left ventricular

volumes and ejection fractions. No patients required pacemaker insertion on a mean follow-up of 23 months.[25]

The drawbacks of this procedure when compared with conventional treatment are the potential complications of the venous switch operation, which include venous obstruction and dysrhythmias. However, its advantages outweigh these relatively uncommon complications. It is definitely the procedure of choice for this lesion, especially in the presence of right ventricular dysfunction or tricuspid valve regurgitation.

REFERENCES

1. Attie F, Cerda J, Richheimer R, et al: Congenitally corrected transposition with mirror image atrial arrangement. *Int J Cardiol* **14:**169, 1987

2. Lieberson AD, Schumacher RR, Childress RH, et al: Corrected transposition of the great vessels in 73 yr old man. *Circulation* **39:**96, 1976

3. Graham TP Jr, Parrish MD, Boucek RJ Jr, et al: Assessment of ventricular size and function in congenitally corrected transposition of the great arteries. *Am J Cardiol* **51:**245, 1983

4. Dimas AP, Moodie DS, Sterba R, Gill CC: Long-term function of the morphologic right ventricle in adult patients with corrected transposition of the great arteries. *Am Heart J* **118:**526, 1989

5. Lev M, Rowlatt F: The pathologic anatomy of mixed levocardia. A review of thirteen cases. *Am J Cardiol* **25:**216, 1961

6. Allwork SP, Bentall HH, Becker AE, et al: Congenitally corrected transposition of the great arteries: Morphologic study of 32 cases. *Am J Cardiol* **38:**910, 1976

7. Okamura K, Konno S: Two types of ventricular septal defect in corrected transposition of the great arteries. *Am Heart J* **85:**483, 1993

8. Anderson RH, Becker AE, Gerlis LM: The pulmonary outflow tract in classically corrected transposition. *J Thorac Cardiovasc Surg* **69:**747, 1975

9. Anderson RH, Arnold R, Wilkinson JL: The conduction tissue in congenitally corrected transposition. *Lancet* **1:**1286, 1973

10. Anderson KR, Danielson GK, McGoon DC, Lie JT: Ebstein's anomaly of the left-sided tricuspid valve. *Circulation* **58:**(Supp I) I–87, 1978

11. Duncan WJ: *Atlas of Pediatric Two-Dimensional Echocardiography.* Springfield, IL, Charles C Thomas, 1981

12. Freedom RM, Culham JAG, Moes CAF: *The Angiography of Congenital Heart Disease.* New York, Macmillan, 1984

13. Williams WG, Suri R, Shindo G, et al: Repair of major intracardiac anomalies associated with atrioventricular discordance. *Ann Thorac Surg* **31:**527, 1981

14. Lundstrom V, Ball C, Wyse RK, et al: The natural and unnatural history of congenitally corrected transposition. *Am J Cardiol* **65:**1222, 1990

15. Russo P, Danielson GK, Driscoll DJ: Trans-aortic closure of ventricular septal defect in patients with corrected transposition with pulmonary stenosis or atresia. *Circulation* **76:**(Supp III) 88, 1987

16. deLeval MR, Bastros P, Stark J, et al: Surgical technique to reduce the risks of heart block following closure of ventricular septal defect in atrioventricular discordance. *J Thorac Cardiovasc Surg* **73:**353, 1977

17. Olinger GN, Maloney JV: Transpulmonary artery repair of ventricular septal defect associated with congenitally corrected transposition of the great arteries. *J Thorac Cardiovasc Surg* **73:**353, 1977

18. Marcellatti C, Maloney JD, Ritter DG, et al: Corrected transposition and ventricular septal defect. *Am Surg* **191:**751, 1980

19. Chan KC, Fyfe D, McKay CD, et al: Right ventricular outflow reconstruction with cryopreserved homografts in pediatric patients: Intermediate term follow-up with serial echocardiographic assessment. *J Am Coll Cardiol* **24:**483, 1994

20. Doty DB, Trusedell SC, Marvin WY: Techniques to avoid injury of the conduction tissue during the surgical treatment of corrected transposition. *Circulation* **68:**(Supp II) 63, 1983

21. Bailey LL, Laughlin LL, McDonald ML, et al: Corrected transposition: Another approach for repair of associated intracardiac malformation. *J Thorac Cardiovasc Surg* **75:**815, 1978

22. Westerman GR, Lang P, Castaneda AR, Norwood WI: Corrected transposition and repair of associated intracardiac defects. *Circulation* **66**(pt 2) I:197, 1982

23. Ilbawi MN, Caspi J, Roberson DA, et al: A new surgical approach in infants with Ebstein's anomaly. Poster Presentation. ACC, March, 1993, Anaheim, CA

24. Ilbawi MN, DeLeon SY, Backer CL, et al: An alternative approach to the surgical management of physiologically corrected transposition with ventricular septal defect and pulmonary stenosis or atresia. *J Thorac Cardiovasc Surg* **100:**410, 1990

25. Imai Y, Sawatari K, Hoshino S, et al: Ventricular function after anatomic repair in patients with atrioventricular discordance. *J Thorac Cardiovasc Surg* **107:**1272, 1994

26. DiDonato R, Troconis C, Marino B, et al: Combined Mustard and Rastelli operations: An alternative approach for repair of associated anomalies in congenitally corrected transposition in situs inversus. *J Thorac Cardiovasc Surg* **105:**1067, 1993

27. Yamagishi Y, Imai Y, Hoshino S, et al: Anatomic correction of atrioventricular discordance. *J Thorac Cardiovasc Surg* **105:**1067, 1993

87

Double-Outlet Right Ventricle and Double-Outlet Left Ventricle

Vaughn A. Starnes and Thomas W. Prendergast

DOUBLE-OUTLET RIGHT VENTRICLE

Double-outlet right ventricle (DORV) encompasses a spectrum of congenital cardiac anomalies in which both great arteries take their origin from the right ventricle (RV). The exact definition of the anatomy constituting a true DORV is controversial; similarly the embryology is a matter of debate.[1] The important anatomic variants that delineate this diagnosis are the relationship of the great arteries to each other and the relationship of the ventricular septal defect (VSD) to the great arteries. Numerous other anomalies are found in association with DORV, especially pulmonary stenosis (PS) and atrioventricular valve (A-V) anomalies.[1] Fortunately, DORV is relatively uncommon, occurring in only 0.09 in 1000 births.[2] The physiology may range from congestive heart failure to deep cyanosis. The diagnosis is made on the basis of conventional evaluations and testing, which usually require cardiac catheterization. The differential diagnosis includes VSD, tetralogy of Fallot, and transposition of the great arteries. The natural history of untreated children with DORV is generally poor. Surgical treatments of the various forms of DORV are varied and encompass a vast array of operative options, especially for the subpulmonic form of DORV.

Definition

The anatomic substrate that represents a DORV varies with regard to the degree to which the arterial trunks emerge from the right ventricle (RV), and the continuity between the A-V and semilunar valves. Neufeld et al describe DORV as both arterial trunks arising entirely from the RV, with the aorta lying to the right of the pulmonary trunk, and typically having discontinuity of mitral and aortic valve tissue.[3] Lev defines DORV as a condition in which both arterial trunks emerge completely or almostly completely from the RV with or without mitral-aortic or mitral-pulmonic continuity.[1] It is now generally accepted that DORV represents a situation in which more than half of the circumference of both arterial valves are in continuity with the RV,[4] which usually has a persistent subaortic conus with some muscle interposed between the aortic and mitral valves.[5]

Embryology

Like the definition, the embryology of DORV is not universally agreed upon. The essential embryologic derangement lies in abnormal development of the bulboventricular loop, namely with conal rotation and conal absorption (Fig. 87–1).[4] This abnormal developmental loop and the final abnormal anatomy probably represent a spectrum from Tetralogy of Fallot (TOF) to DORV to transposition of the great arteries (TGA). For instance, TOF is typified by counterclockwise rotation of the aortic conus, looking from above, while DORV results from further counterclockwise rotation of the aortic conus.[5] TGA results if there is a counterclockwise shift of the pulmonary conus.[6] In TOF, conal absorption occurs in the mid-portion of the bulboatrioventricular ledge (BAL), allowing mitral-aortic continuity; in DORV absence of absorption occurs in the BAL between the aortic valve and mitral valve, allowing no continuity between the A-V and semilunar valves.[5] In complete TGA, absorption of the left margin of the BAL has occurred allowing mitral-pulmonary continuity.[5]

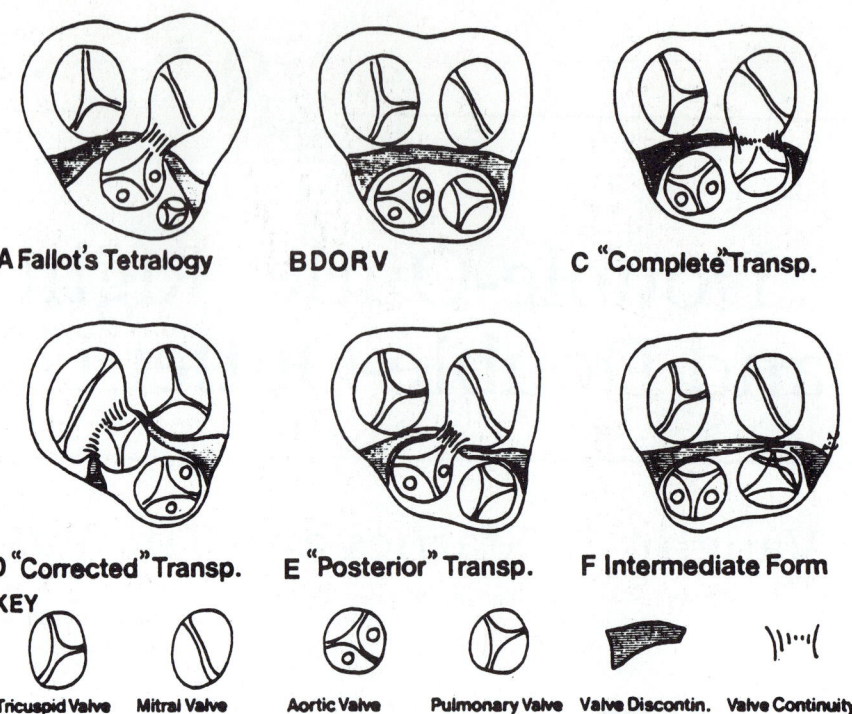

Figure 87–1. A–F. Essential features of development that differentiate TOF, DORV, and TGA are in the conal rotation, conal absorption, and bulboatrioventricular ledge (BAL). The final position of the great arteries, their relationship with each other, and mitral-aortic continuity are ultimately determined by these embryologic events. *(From Anderson et al: Br Heart J 36:949, 1974, with permission.)*

Pathology and Anatomy

From an anatomic standpoint, DORV is described in terms of the relationships of the great arteries and relationship of the associated VSD. The four relationships of the great arteries are side-by-side, dextromalposition, levomalposition, and normal. Side-by-side is the most common and normal arrangement is rare.[7] The four types of VSD are subaortic, subpulmonary, doubly-committed, and noncommitted (Fig. 87–2). Subaortic VSD is the most common and the doubly-committed and noncommitted types are uncommon.[7] DORV hearts with subpulmonary VSD and double conus can be referred to as Taussig–Bing malformation.[8] The relationships of the great arteries and associated VSDs are seen in various combinations (Table 87–1).[9] These anatomic variations reflect differences in physiology, but must also be considered in the context of other associated conditions. Associated conditions include PS, pulmonary vascular obstructive disease (PVOD), atrial septal defect (ASD), A-V canal, patent ductus arteriosus (PDA), subaortic stenosis, left ventricular outlet tract obstruction (LVOTO), mitral valve anomalies, and others (Table 87–2).[7,10] Other important anatomic considerations include size of the VSD, coronary artery anatomy, and A-V concordance or discordance.

Pulmonic stenosis is commonly associated with DORV, especially with subaortic VSD. Forty percent of all patients with DORV in Lev's series and 70% of the patients with DORV and malposition of the great arteries had PS associated.[1] The obstruction can be at the level of the subpulmonary or the pulmonary valve level or both.[9]

PVOD without PS is also associated with DORV,

being present in 35% in one large series.[7] In the absence of anatomic PS, excessive pulmonary bloodflow could lead to high pulmonary vascular resistance, especially in younger patients.[7]

ASDs can be of varying size and location. They may be the only outlet for the left side of the heart for DORV associated with intact ventricular septum or mitral atresia.[7] ASDs reported range from defects at the fossa ovalis to Rastelli Type C A-V canal.[7] A-V canals were present in 8% of patients in two series.[1,7]

Multiple levels of left ventricular outflow tract obstruction occur. Subaortic stenosis most often occurs in association with subaortic and subpulmonary VSD.[10] It appears to result from hypertrophy of the parietal limb of the crista supraventricularis.[7] Obstruction to systemic flow also occurs at the level of the aorta, with reports of hypoplasia of the aortic arch, interrupted aortic arch, and coarctation of the aorta.[10,11] These aortic obstructions may be associated with each other or with subaortic stenosis. They are usually associated with subpulmonary VSD, and in one series was the coexistent malformation most commonly associated with DORV (Table 87–2).[10,11]

Anomalies of the mitral valve that occur in patients with DORV include straddling mitral valve, supravalvular mitral ring, parachute mitral valve, and mitral atresia.[7,10] There is a tendency for these anomalies to be associated with subaortic VSD.[7,10]

Coronary artery anatomic variations are particularly important, as arterial switch operation (ASO) with coronary artery reimplantation is becoming the favored operation for many Taussing–Bing hearts.[12–14] Although coronary

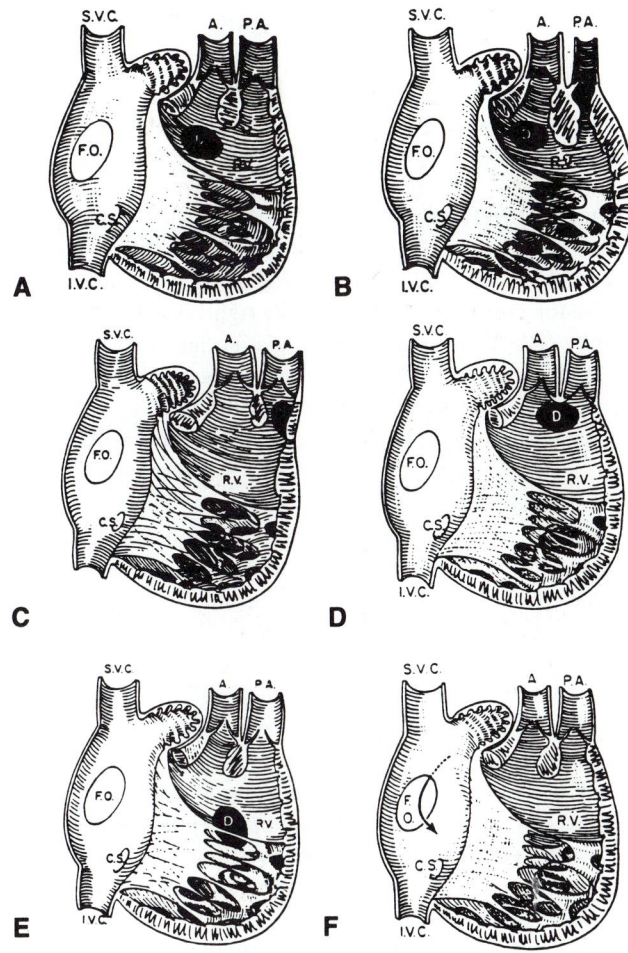

Figure 87–2. Diagrammatic representation of the various positions of VSD in relation to the great arteries. **A.** Subaortic VSD without pulmonic stenosis (PS); **B.** suboaortic VSD with PS; **C.** subpulmonary VSD; **D.** doubly committed VSD; **E.** noncommitted VSD; **F.** DORV with intact ventricular septum. S.V.C., superior vena cava; I.V.C., inferior vena cava; A, aorta; P.A. pulmonary artery; D, VSD; F.O., fossa ovalis; C.S., coronary sinus; R.V., right ventricle. *(From Zamora et al Chest 68:675, 1975, with permission.)*

anatomy in DORV is most often normal,[15,16] there is a tendency for coronary abnormalities due to the rotational changes of the great vessels during development.[1] Earlier descriptions of coronary anatomy reported the origin of the left anterior descending (LAD) from the right coronary artery (RCA) as being one of the most common coronary artery anomalies,[7,15] similar to that observed in tetralogy of Fallot. Since the arterial switch has been used for some forms of DORV, anomalies in coronary arteries have been better documented. In general, normal coronary artery predominates in patients with subaortic VSD (77%) and doubly committed VSD (60%) and in the majority of patients with side-by-side great vessels (63%) and those in which the aorta is in a right posterior oblique position (83%).[14] Thus, diverse coronary artery patterns were present in those with subpulmonary and noncommitted VSD and those in whom the aorta was in the right anterior oblique position.[14] Coronary arterial patterns resemble those for TGA when the aorta is directly anterior or in the left anterior oblique position.[13,14]

Physiology

The wide spectrum of anatomic combinations of DORV and the many associated conditions lead to a similar wide spectrum of physiology, ranging from pulmonary undercirculation to pulmonary overcirculation. The pulmonary and systemic bloodflow are determined by the great artery relationships, the position and size of the VSD, and the specific associated conditions. These anatomic combinations result in physiology ranging from cyanosis to congestive heart failure (CHF) with pulmonary edema, which have important implications for medical and surgical management.

Of the numerous variables investigated by measuring systemic and pulmonary arterial oxygen saturation, it is recognized that location of the VSD has a greater influence on intracardiac streaming than great artery relationship, PS, PVOD, or associated anomalies (Table 87–3).[9] Certain important generalizations have been realized from these physiologic data.[7,9] For instance, all subpulmonary VSDs had pulmonary oxygen saturation (PA) > systemic arterial oxy-

TABLE 87–1. ANATOMIC RELATIONSHIP OF THE GREAT VESSELS AND VSD IN 70 PATIENTS WITH DORV

	Location of VSD[a]				
	Subaortic	Subpulmonary	Doubly Committed	Noncommitted	Total
Side-by-Side	32	6	2	5	45
D-MGA[b]	11	7	0	0	18
L-MGA	2	3	0	0	3
Normal	2	0	0	0	2
Total	47	16	2	5	70

[a]Not included in this table are two adolescent patients with intact ventricular septum.
[b]MGA, malposition of the great arteries.
Modified from Sridaromont S, et al: Mayo Clinic Proc 53:555, 1978 with permission.

TABLE 87–2. CARDIOVASCULAR CONDITIONS ASSOCIATED WITH DOUBLE-OUTLET RIGHT VENTRICLE[a]

Condition	Percent of Cases of DORV (n = 62)[b]	Percent of Cases of DORV (n = 33)[c]
PS	47	21
ASD	26	21
PDA	16	—
AV Canal	8	—
Subaortic stenosis	3	30
Coarctation of aorta, IAA, hypoplastic arch	2	45
Mitral valve anomalies	—	30

[a]PS, pulmonic stenosis; ASD, atrial septal defect; PDA, patent ductus arteriosus; IAA, interrupted aortic arch.
[b]Data from Sridaromont S, et al: Am J Cardiol 38:85, 1976 with permission.
[c]Data from Zamora R, et al: Chest 68(5):672, 1975 with permission.

gen saturation (SA), regardless of the presence or absence of PS or PVOD.[7,9] Also, all subaortic VSDs with malposition of the great arteries have SA > PA and when the SA > PA, the VSD is likely to be subaortic (24 of 27 cases).[7,9] While these generalizations are helpful, physiology in DORV is not entirely predictable based on anatomy alone.

Diagnosis

The diagnosis of DORV is based on history, physical examination, electrocardiogram (ECG), echocardiogram (ECHO), and cardiac catheterization. The median age at diagnosis is less than 2 mo.[11] The spectrum of presenting symptoms and physical findings depends on the patient's specific anatomy, particularly the location of the VSD and presence or absence of PS.[11] The most common group has subaortic VSD and PS and presents with cyanosis similar to patients with TOF; the next most common group has subpulmonary VSD without PS and presents as a child with TGA and VSD with

CHF.[10] Another group presenting with CHF has subaortic VSD without PS, and these patients may go on to develop PVOD.[10] This presenting constellation of symptoms is strongly influenced by the associated conditions, such as aortic and subaortic obstructions and A-V canal.[6]

Physical findings depend on anatomy, and do not distinguish DORV from other forms of congenital heart disease; in fact, the first diagnosis of DORV prior to necropsy was not reported until 1962.[17] ECG has a low predictive value for the diagnosis of DORV; right ventricular hypertrophy (RVH) and right axis deviation are the most common features.[3,18] Left ventricular hypertrophy (LVH) is also observed at times, particularly if the VSD or surgical systemic-to-pulmonary shunt adds to the work load of the left ventricle (LV).[18] Radiographic appearance usually reveals cardiomegaly. Lung fields are oligemic when cyanosis is the predominant symptom complex, particularly when PS is present. On the other hand, increased pulmonary vascularity will be observed when CHF is the predominant pathophysiologic problem.

Echocardiogram provides the most helpful information regarding location of the VSD, which provides information necessary for planning surgical management (Fig. 87–3).[19] Different conotruncal malformations are now generally differentiated on the basis of echocardiogram, with the ability to arrive at an accurate diagnosis in approximately 95% of cases.[20] Typically, M-mode or two-dimensional echocardiography delineates mitral-semilunar valve discontinuity reasonably well. Two-dimensional echocardiographic findings demonstrate the origin and orientation of the great arteries found on the RV and the absence of LV outflow other than that from the VSD.[21,22] Echocardiogram is beneficial in assessing VSD to great artery relationship. Additional problems can also be assessed, such as straddling A-V valves, cleft valves, or complete A-V canals.[21] While echocardiogram is excellent at arriving at the diagnosis of DORV along with some anatomic details, the 16 variations

TABLE 87–3. RELATION OF VSD, OXYGEN SATURATION, PULMONARY STENOSIS, AND PULMONARY VASCULAR OBSTRUCTIVE DISEASE IN DOUBLE-OUTLET RIGHT VENTRICLE[a]

Location of VSD	Number of Cases	Oxygen Saturation	With PS	Without PVOD	No PVOD	Total
Subpulmonary	13	PA > SA	5	3	5	13
Subaortic	40	PA > SA	1	7	1	9
		SA > PA	16	5	3	24
		PA = SA	5	1	1	7
Subaortic and subpulmonary	2	PA > SA	0	2	0	2
Remote (A-V canal)	5	PA > SA	0	0	1	1
		SA > PA	2	1	0	3
		PA = SA	0	1	0	1
Intact septum	2	PA = SA	0	1	1	2
Total	62		29	21	12	62

[a]PA, pulmonary arterial; PS, pulmonary stenosis; PVOD, pulmonary vascular obstructive disease; SA, systolic arteria.
from Sridaromont S, et al: Am J Cardiol 38:85, 1976 with permission.

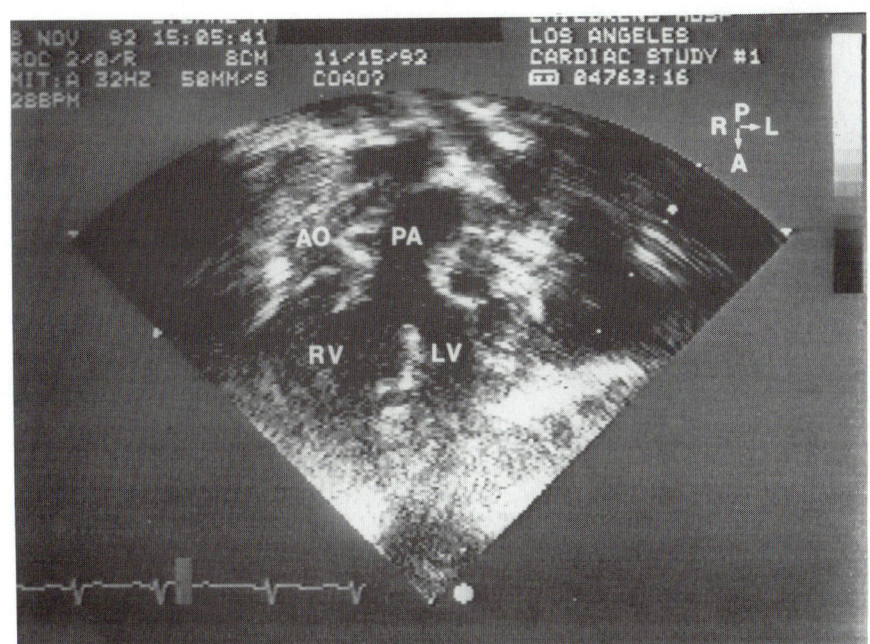

Figure 87–3. Echocardiogram of DORV with subpulmonary VSD. Both great arteries can be seen originating from the RV, and the position of the VSD is demonstrated. AO, aorta; PA, pulmonary artery; RV, right ventricle; LV, left ventricle. *(Courtesy of Barry Marcus, MD, Childrens Hospital Los Angeles.)*

of DORV regarding VSD location and relationship of the great arteries are often nicely supplemented by cardiac catheterization.[7,9]

Because of some of the limitations of echocardiogram, cardiac catherterization is preferred in most surgical patients. It supplements information gained from echocardiogram, and amplifies details already assessed by echocardiogram, particularly regarding VSD location. Cardiac catheterization sometimes achieves greater detail about relationship and orientation of the great arteries to each other and with the ventriculoarterial connection (Figs. 87–4, 87–5, and 87–6).[9] Atrioventricular concordance is perhaps better evaluated by cardiac catheterization.[23] Coronary artery anatomy is well characterized by cardiac catheterization in DORV,[15] which has particular relevance because repair often involves coronary artery translocation or anomalous branches across a right ventricular outflow tract (RVOT), which may require outflow tract patch or conduit based on coronary artery anatomy. Most VSDs are accurately described by echocardiogram,[21] however, complex details of multiple small VSDs, remote VSD, or absence of VSD may be better characterized by cardiac catheterization. Hemodynamic measurements and peripheral PA anatomy are much better assessed by cardiac catheterization as well. Thus echocardiogram and cardiac catheterization should both be performed prior to surgical correction of DORV.

Operation

Operations for DORV depend on the anatomic subtype, particularly the location of the VSD, and the associated anomalies. The type and timing of early palliative procedures before definitive repair must also be considered, al-

though there is a trend toward early total biventricular repair as a neonate or infant when possible.[14]

Early Palliative Operations

Most early palliative operations are done for cyanosis or congestive heart failure and consist of systemic-to-pulmonary shunts (SPS) or pulmonary artery banding (PAB), respectively. Other early palliative procedures include balloon or open atrial septostomy, repair of coarctation of the aorta, or other anomalies of the aorta and ligation of PDA.[12,14] Table 87–4 lists the previous palliative procedures that have been performed prior to total corrections of DORV in 33 of 73 patients in a recently reported series.[14]

In older series, total correction was done after 1–2 years of age in the majority of cases, and children were treated with SPS or PAB if DORV was discovered at an early age.[11] Another option is to perform selective early palliation, depending on the patient's specific anatomy and physiology. For instance, one group uses preliminary palliation in all patients with subaortic or doubly committed VSDs, and performs early definitive repair in patients with subpulmonary VSD.[12] Because of the sequelae of long-term palliation, many surgeons now prefer early definitive repair for all types of DORV, in the majority of cases.[14]

Subaortic VSD

Subaortic VSD with AV concordance is the most common variant of DORV. It is repaired by creating an intraventricular tunnel from the VSD to the aorta, posterior to the pulmonary outflow tract (Fig. 87–7).[24] This diverts blood from the LV into the aorta. It can be done via a right atriotomy in about one quarter of cases, but requires a right ventriculotomy in the majority.[14] RV outflow patches or external

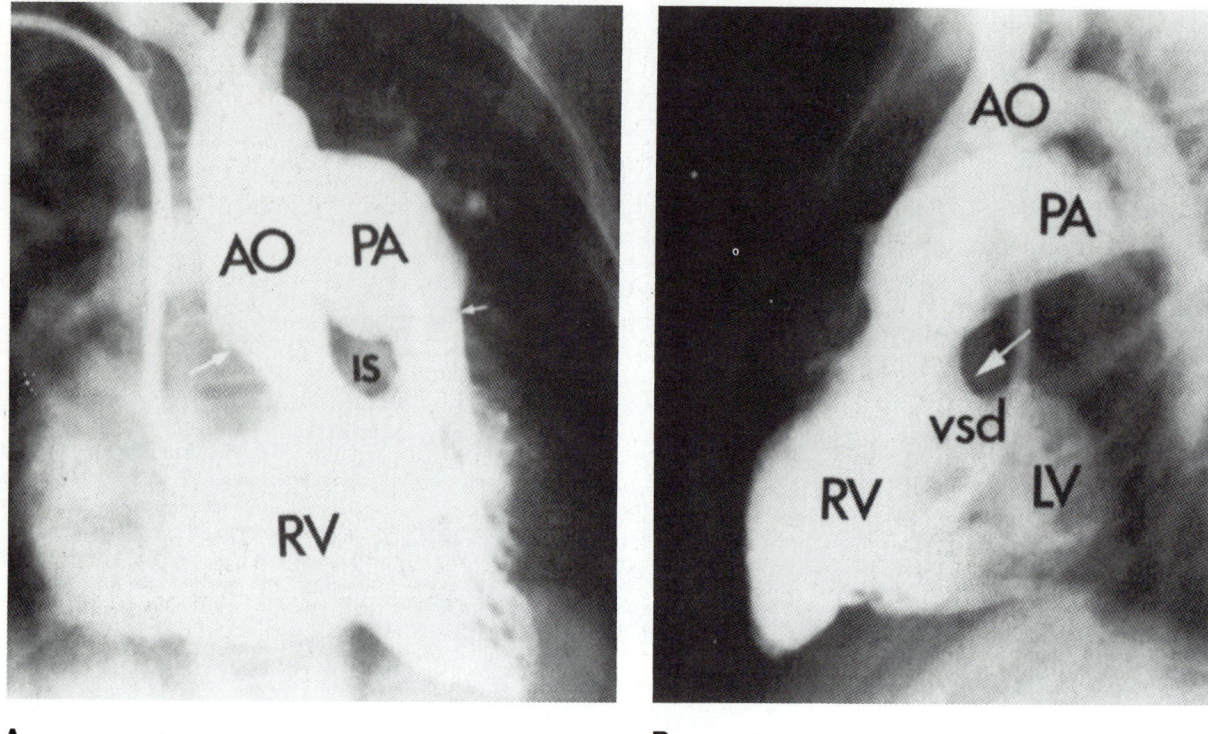

Figure 87–4. DORV, side-by-side great arteries, and subaortic VSD. **A.** Frontal right ventriculogram. **B.** Lateral right ventriculogram. The lateral right ventriculogram shows both great arteries originating from the anatomic RV, and the posterior anatomic LV filled via the subaortic VSD. AO, aorta; PA, pulmonary artery; IS, infundibular septum; RV, right ventricle; LV, left ventricle; VSD, ventricular septal defect. *(From Freedom RM, et al: Angiocardiography of Congenital Heart Disease. New York, Macmillan, 1984, with permission.)*

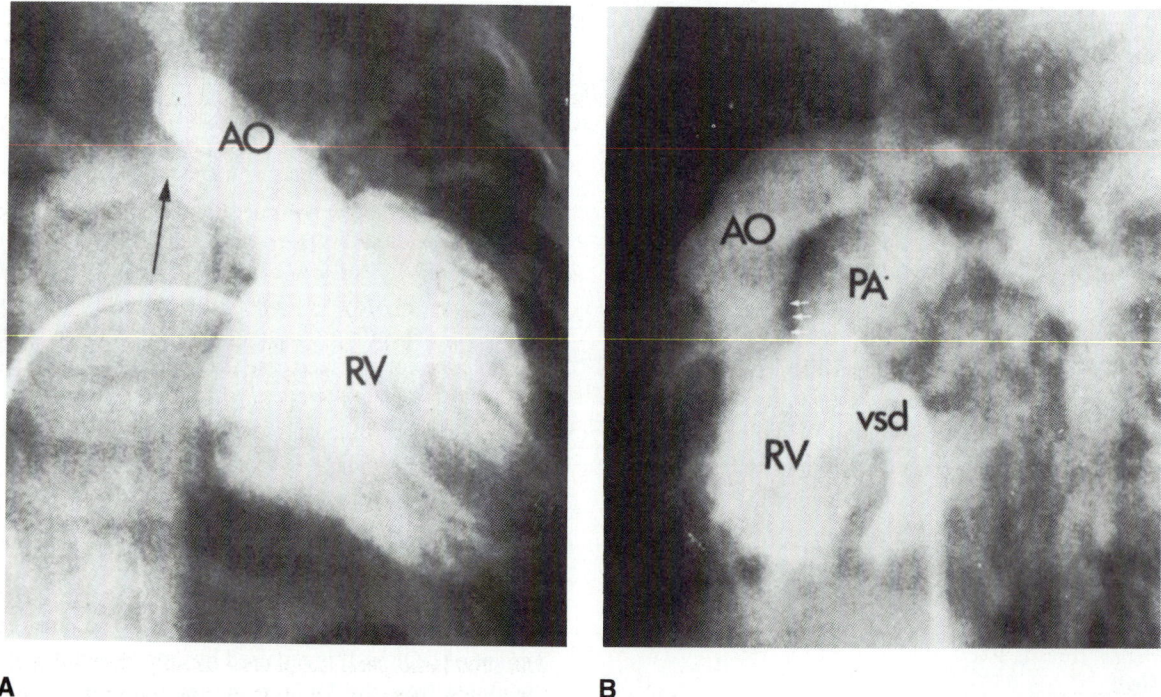

Figure 87–5. DORV, levopositioned aorta, and subpulmonary VSD. **A.** Frontal right ventriculogram. **B.** Lateral right ventriculogram. The lateral right ventriculogram shows both great arteries originating from the anatomic RV, with a subpulmonary VSD. The infundibular septum is represented by the white arrows. AO, aorta; PA, pulmonary artery; RV, right ventricle; vsd, ventricular septal defect. *(From Freedom RM, et al: Angiocardiograpy of Congenital Heart Disease. New York, Macmillan, 1984, with permission.)*

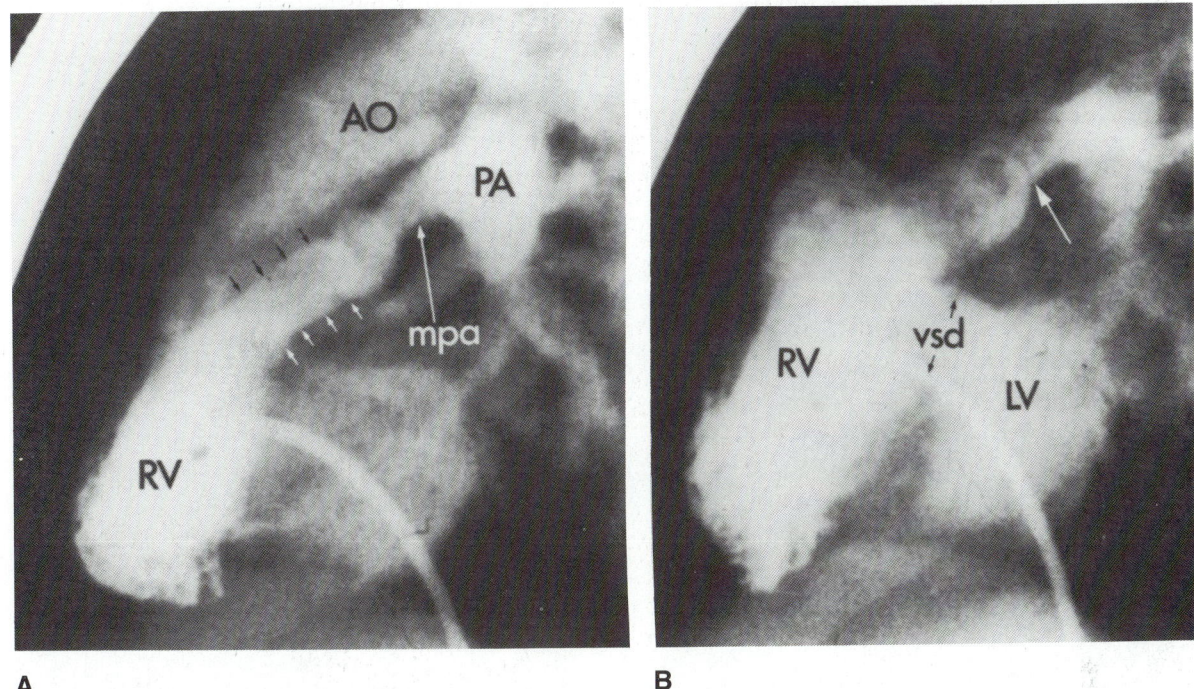

A   **B**

Figure 87–6. DORV and doubly committed VSD, with valvular and subvalvular pulmonary stenosis. **A.** Early frame of lateral right ventriculogram. **B.** Later frame of right ventriculogram. The aorta and pulmonary artery both originate from this anatomic RV and the LV is opacified via the VSD. There is subpulmonary infundibular stenosis represented by the arrows, and proximal main pulmonary artery stenosis. AO, aorta; PA, pulmonary artery; RV, right ventricle; mpa, main pulmonary artery; LV, left ventricle; vsd, ventricular septal defect. *(From Freedom RM, et al: Angiocardiography of Congenital Heart Disease. New York, Macmillan, 1984, with permission.)*

conduits to the PA are often necessary even in patients without known preoperative PS, because of encroachment from the tunnel on the RV outflow tract (Fig. 87–8).[25] The tunnel material is a section of woven Dacron arterial prosthesis.[26] When the defect is significantly smaller than the aortic annulus, it must be enlarged to the size of the aortic

TABLE 87–4. PREVIOUS PALLIATIVE PROCEDURES PRIOR TO TOTAL CORRECTION OF DOUBLE-OUTLET RIGHT VENTRICLE[a]

Procedure	Number
BTS	9
BTS then second BTS with pectus repair	1
PAB	9
PAB with ectopia cordia repair	1
PAB then BTS	1
AAR	13
Simultaneous AAR/PAB	6
AAR followed by PAB	1
Simultaneous AAR/PAB then BTS	2
Blalock–Hanlon procedure	1
Repair of vascular ring	1
Total (%)	33 (45%)

BTS, Blalock–Taussig shunt; PAB, pulmonary artery band; AAR, aortic arch repair.
Modified from Aoki M, et al: J Thorac Cardiovasc Surg 107(2):338, 1994 with permission.

annulus by incising the part of the septum anterior to the defect.[24,25,27] The relationship of the conal septum with regard to the projected baffle position is of utmost importance. The baffle must be created such that left ventricular outflow obstruction does not result from the position of the patch. This complication may occur in approximately 5% of cases of DORV repair.[14]

Results of repair of subaortic VSD with DORV are generally good with early survival ranging from 85 to 90%.[14,28] Early deaths are predominately due to low cardiac output syndrome and RV failure.[28] Late mortality ranges from 3 to 21%, and is most often due to arrhythmias.[14,28] Arrhythmias occur in approximately one-third of survivors of repair.[28,29] Other morbidities from this operation include recurrent VSD, aortic valve regurgitation, RV aneurysm, and problems associated with conduits.[28] As mentioned above, late development of left ventricular outflow obstruction has also been described.[14,30] The vast majority of survivors are in NYHA Class I.

Repair of subaortic VSD with DORV and A-V discordance follows similar principles as in A-V concordance. The prosthetic patch is placed usually through a morphologic right ventriculotomy such that the aorta arises exclusively from the systemic (morphologic right) ventricle and the PA arises exclusively from the pulmonary (morphologic left) ventricle (Fig. 87–9).[23] Another technique describes morphologic left ventriculotomy with closure of VSD to

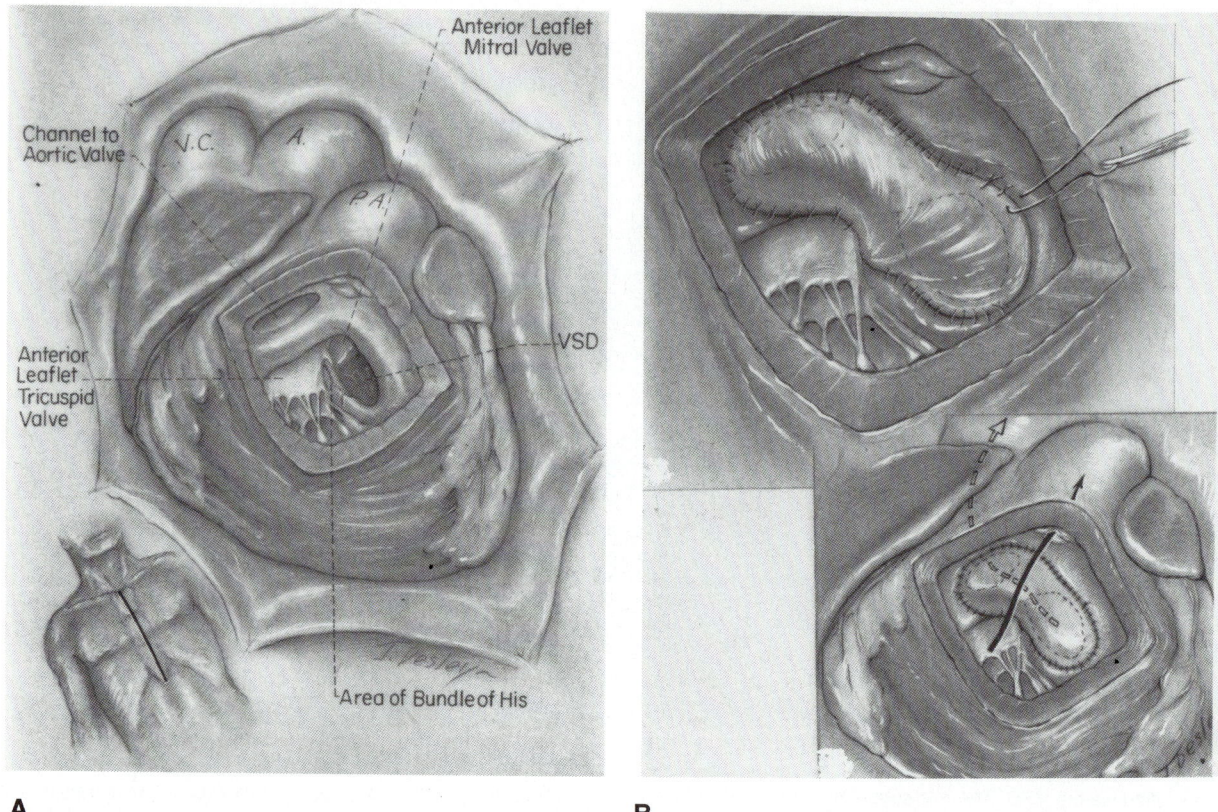

A   **B**

Figure 87–7. Intraventricular tunnel repair of a subaortic VSD. **A.** Through a median sternotomy, a transverse right ventriculotomy is made, exposing the subaortic VSD. **B.** The VSD is closed with a patch, such that LV blood is directed into the aorta. RV blood is now directed into the PA. Simple closure of the right ventriculotomy may result in RVOT obstruction, necessitating patch closure or RV–PA conduit. (This repair may also be done via vertical right ventriculotomy or right atrial incision). *(From Kirklin, et al: J Thorac Cardiovasc Surg 48:1033–1035, 1964, with permission.)*

leave both great arteries emptying the systemic ventricle, with conduit placed between the ventriculotomy and the proximally oversewn PA.[23] Results are similar to those for repair in A-V concordant hearts.[23]

Subpulmonary VSD

Subpulmonic VSD with bilateral conus and side-by-side semilunar valves is one of the most complex of DORV hearts.[8] Numerous forms of repair have been applied to this subtype of DORV, which most surgeons understand to be the Taussig–Bing heart.[31] Surgical options used with reasonable success include creating a tunnel posterior to the pulmonary outflow tract,[32] using a tubular prosthesis as a conduit,[33] tubular prosthesis anterior to the PA,[34] spiral tunnel coursing to the left of the PA,[35] Senning or Mustard operation,[36] Danus–Kaye–Stansel (DKS) procedure,[37–39] and arterial switch operation (ASO).[40] Many surgeons are now performing the ASO for repair when the VSD is baffled to the pulmonary trunk during the course of closing the subpulmonary VSD, as described below.[12–14,31,40–42] These other options for repair of Taussig–Bing hearts are still important, as each is still favored as the best option by some surgeons rather than the ASO.

The technique described by Kawashima et al consists of resection of the distal conal septum along with patch repair of the subpulmonary VSD, in such a manner as to make the LV communicate with the aorta.[32] This is done using a prosthetic tunnel posterior to the pulmonary outflow tract.[32] Abe et al described an operation that excises the subaortic conal septum and implants a nonvalved conduit between the VSD and aortic conus.[33] This requires a large RV so that RV blood can course around the prosthesis and into the PA.[33]

When the VSD is subpulmonary and the aorta anterior to the PA, repair becomes more complex. The choices then encompass closing the VSD to the aorta by a long passageway or closing the VSD to the PA and thus creating complete TGA. A long pathway from VSD to aorta can be created with an intraventricular conduit, in which the VSD is brought into continuity with the aorta, via a tubular prosthesis, described by Doty.[34] This prosthesis runs transversely from VSD to subaortic conus and the transverse ventriculotomy is sutured to the external surface of the conduit.[34] Alternatively, the VSD may be tunnelled into the aorta by joining the VSD via a long oval patch coursing to the left of the PA and joining the aorta anterior to the PA.[35] This

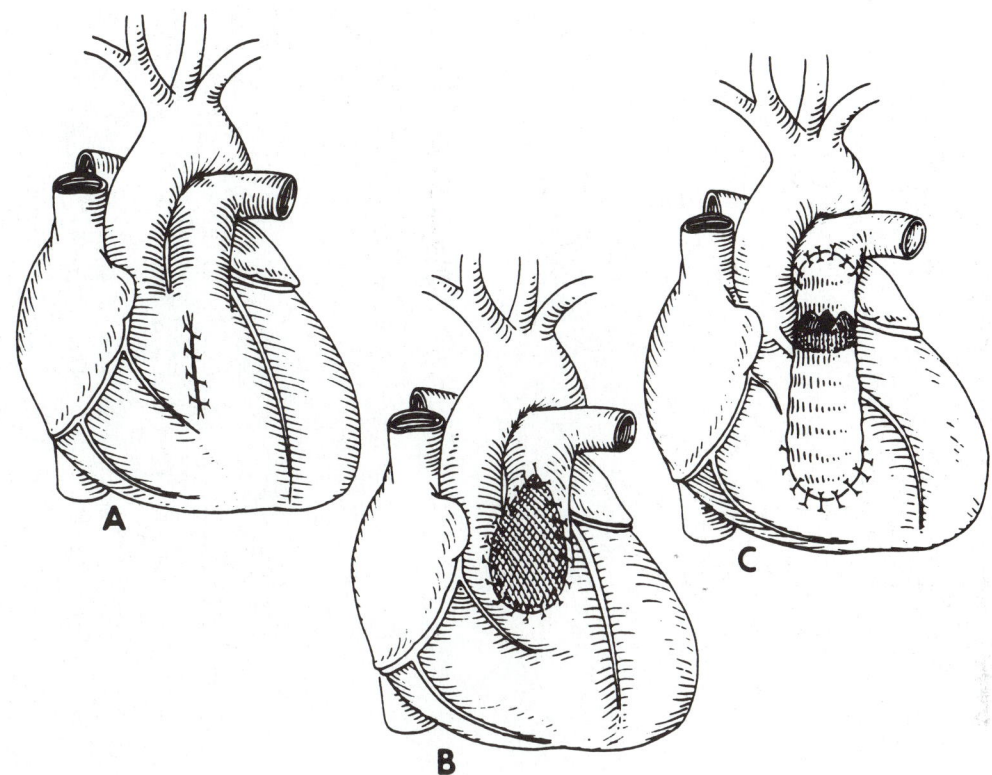

Figure 87–8. Strategies for reconstruction of RVOT for native RVOT obstruction or for obstruction that results after creation of the intraventricular tunnel. **A.** At times, the right ventriculotomy may be directly closed without need for any augmentation. **B.** Pericardial patch augmentation of RVOT, which may extend into the main pulmonary artery. **C.** A valved or nonvalved RV–PA conduit. Not pictured here is an RV–PA homograft, which is another option. *(From Judson et al: J Thorac Cardiovasc Surg 85:37, 1983, with permission.)*

operation, described by Patrick and McGoon, also requires a large RV to prevent pulmonary outflow tract obstruction.[35]

In some instances of Taussig–Bing anomalies, the location of the subpulmonary VSD renders it optimally closed to the PA, which then results in complete TGA. The transposition is then corrected by Senning or Mustard operation,[36] DKS procedure,[37] or ASO. The Senning or Mustard operation with this anatomy creates intra-atrial transposition of venous blood after separating ventricular outflow with the VSD closure, as described first by Hightower et al.[36] Anatomic arterial switch is now generally favored over atrial switch, as intra-atrial repair has a variable incidence of systemic and pulmonary venous obstruction, supraventricular arrhythmias, tricuspid valve incompetence, and RV dysfunction as well as substantial early and late mortality.[40] DKS operation for DORV is performed by closing the VSD such that the PA and aorta arise from the LV; the transected PA is then anastomosed to the RV with an extracardiac conduit.[39] Coronary artery translocation is thus avoided.[38] DKS is preferred by some surgeons over ASO, particularly when coronary anatomy precludes ASO, or in the presence of aortic or subaortic obstruction.[14,39] Because of substantial improvements in survival and functional results in patients undergoing ASO, it is now preferred by many sur-

geons when closure of the subpulmonary VSD in Taussig–Bing hearts creates TGA. Early survival after ASO for Taussig–Bing anomaly ranges from 84 to 95%.[12,14,15] Although not quite as good as survival for ASO in TGA with intact ventricular septum, survival rates after ASO for Taussig–Bing anomaly compare most favorably over nonanatomic repair.[40,42] An additional operation described for this anomaly tunnels the LV blood to the aorta, and the pulmonary trunk origin is translocated onto the RV anterior to the aorta.[43] This is referred to as réparation à l'etage ventriculare (REV), as reported by Lecompte et al[43] REV and ASO are both feasible only in the absence of left ventricular outflow tract obstruction. REV results in pulmonary valve insufficiency and therefore ASO is preferred in patients with increased pulmonary artery pressure.[43]

In summary, a reasonable approach to Taussig–Bing anomaly is simple intraventricular tunnel, which is possible in approximately one-quarter of cases.[13,14] ASO is performed in the remainder unless anatomy necessitates DKS repair.[14]

Tabry's series of DORV with A-V discordance included 14 of 20 patients with subpulmonary VSD.[23] Despite A-V discordance, 6 of the 14 were able to undergo an entirely intracardiac repair; the remainder underwent VSD closure with placement of an extracardiac conduit between

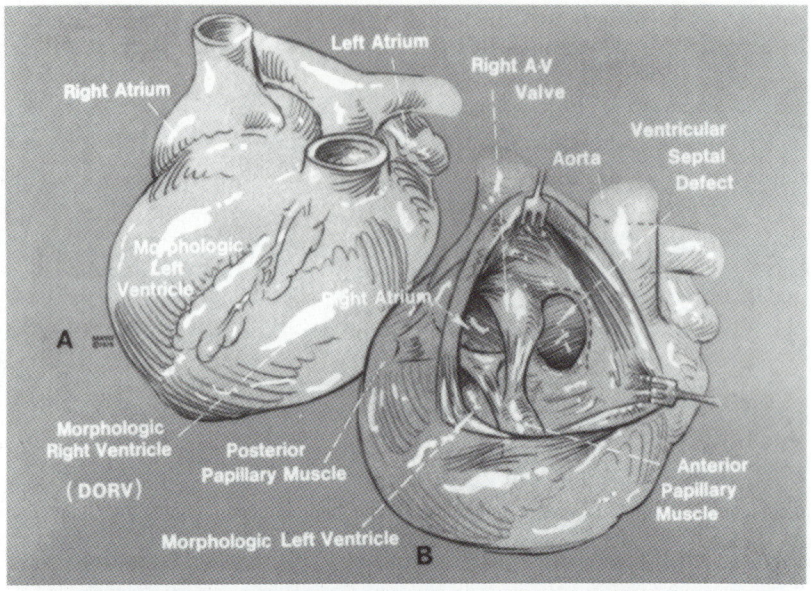

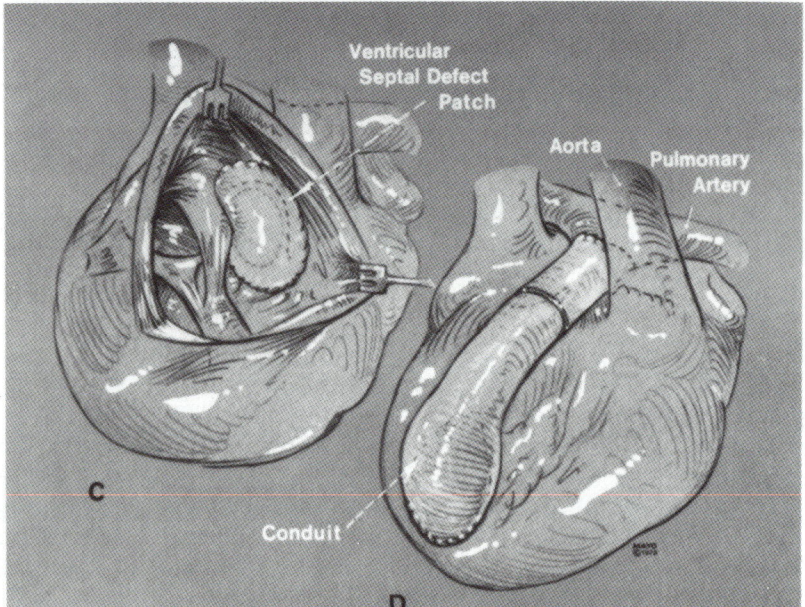

Figure 87–9. Repair of DORV in AV discordance. **A.** DORV with A-V discordance. **B.** Incision through right-sided pulmonary (morphologic left) ventricle, exposing VSD. **C.** Patch closure of VSD. **D.** Extracardiac conduit between ventriculotomy and distal end of pulmonary artery. *(From Tabry et al: J Thorac Cardiovasc Surg 76:340, 1978, with permission.)*

a ventriculotomy in the morphologic LV and the distal end of the proximally oversewn PA.[23]

Doubly Committed VSD

Doubly committed VSD in association with DORV are relatively uncommon. This represented 3% of all DORV hearts in the Stewart et al series[44] and 8% in the Kirklin et al series.[45] The surgical management and results from this surgery for this anomaly do not differ significantly from those for subaortic VSD.[28,44] That is, a tunnel is created with a patch from the VSD to the aorta and the RVOT is reconstructed when necessary with an outflow or transannular patch or by an external RV–PA conduit.[44]

Doubly committed VSD in DORV with A-V discordance was not present in the 20 patients with A-V discordance described by Tabry et al.[23] Surgical management of

this combination should be similar to that for subaortic VSD with A-V discordance as described above.

Noncommitted VSD

DORV with noncommitted VSD is a challenging problem and numerous types of repairs are reported. There is a higher prevalence of severe associated lesions, especially subaortic stenosis and aortic arch obstruction,[10,14,46] and results of surgery are generally worse, when compared to other types of VSDs associated with DORV.[14]

Noncommitted VSD is not uncommon among DORV series, representing approximately 15–20% of the reported VSD associated with DORV.[14,45] Intraventricular repair with an internal baffle connecting the LV to the aorta is possible in approximately one-third of cases.[14,46] This most often necessitates some form of RVOT augmentation or external conduit.[14,46] Double external conduits from the LV to the aorta and from the RV to PA after VSD repair has been reported for this anomaly.[47] Conversion to TGA by VSD closure followed by atrial switch[44] or anatomic arterial switch has also been applied to this form of DORV.[14,44] Intraventricular baffle is probably associated with the best results.

Results from surgical correction are worse when compared with subaortic or doubly committed VSD repairs.[14] Two of three patients in one series died after repair of this lesion[12] and 3 of 10 in another series.[14] Kirklin et al reported only 22% survival rate 10 years after repair of DORV with noncommitted VSD.[45] Also, need for reoperation after repair of this anomaly is generally higher than that for other types of VSDs in DORV.[14] Should noncommitted VSD associated with A-V discordance be encountered, a similar approach could be used.

Complex Forms of DORV

DORV is associated with numerous complex anomalies that preclude biventricular repair, for irreparable anatomy or anatomy resulting in repairs with generally poor outcomes. Wilcox et al examined 63 DORV hearts from clinicopathologic specimens and determined that 36% would not have been operable during life.[25] Some anatomic associations that prevent reasonable results from biventricular repair include some noncommitted VSDs,[12,45,48] some complete A-V canals,[44,45,48,49] some cases of multiple VSDs,[14] univentricular hearts, hypoplastic ventricles, straddling tricuspid valves, and straddling mitral valves.[49] In these instances, if PS is present at birth, aortopulmonary shunt may be necessary early in life to treat cyanosis; alternatively, if there is no PS, then a PA band may be required to protect the pulmonary circulation for eventual Fontan circulation.[49] A bidirectional cavopulmonary anastomosis can then be performed at 6 mo of age, followed by completion Fontan procedure at 1–2 years of age. In a series of 23 patients treated in this manner, there were six hospital deaths and another death at 9 mo postoperatively for a cumulative mortality of 30%.[49] There does not yet appear to be any explicit reports on cardiac transplantation for these particularly difficult forms of DORV.

DOUBLE-OUTLET LEFT VENTRICLE

The first report of a clinically diagnosed and autopsyproved case of origin of both arteries from the morphologic left ventricle was in 1970.[50] However, a case in which both arteries arose from the morphologic LV was first repaired in 1964.[51]

Definition

Double-outlet left ventricle (DOLV) is a condition in which both arterial trunks emerge completely or mostly from the morphologic LV. The existence of this anomaly was originally doubted on embryologic grounds, but now is a recognized congenital cardiac malformation.[52]

Embryology

Clinical and autopsy data imply that the developmental problem lies in the differential conal growth hypothesis, concerning the morphogenesis of the great arteries.[50] Differential conal absorption and counterclockwise conotruncal inversion may continue to the point that both coni are absorbed above the primitive LV and thus both great arteries emerge from the LV.[53]

Pathology and Anatomy

Like DORV, DOLV is described anatomically by the relationship of the great vessels and position of the VSD. Peculiarities of DOLV, compared to DORV, are that there are two interrelations of the great arteries (aorta to right of PA and aorta anterior to PA), and there are tricuspid valve abnormalities in one-third of the cases.[54] The relative frequency of position of the VSD is similar to that for DORV: subaortic 70%, subpulmonary 18%, doubly committed 9%, and the remainder noncommitted.[54] Absence of VSD is rarely described for DOLV, as for DORV.[54] The vast majority of DOLV hearts are associated with pulmonary stenosis.[54,55] Other associated anomalies include abnormalities of the tricuspid valve, namely Ebstein's anomaly, tricuspid stenosis, tricuspid atresia, and RV hypoplasia.[54,55]

Physiology

Most patients with DOLV are cyanotic, because of either coexisting PS or because of the relation of the VSD and great arteries resulting in parallel systemic and pulmonic circulation.[54,55] The physiology most closely resembles TOF or TGA. Associated lesions also influence the pathophysiology, as for DORV.

Diagnosis

Presenting symptoms usually are from cyanosis, and most patients present with systolic murmur.[55] ECG most often demonstrates right axis deviation and right ventricular hypertrophy while chest radiograph may range from oligemia to plethora.[55] As for DORV, ECHO and cardiac catheterization are both preferred prior to surgical intervention.

Operations

Initial palliation in infancy is most often accomplished by systemic-to-pulmonary shunt, as most of these patients are cyanotic. However, when the physiology mimics TGA with VSD, pulmonary overcirculation may necessitate PA banding. Systemic-to-pulmonary shunt is particularly favored in children who will eventually require an extracardiac conduit for PS, to reduce the number of conduit changes the child will need as he or she grows. Otherwise, total primary repair in infancy is favored, as for DORV, to avoid the sequelae of long-term palliation.[14]

Numerous operations for total repair exist, and the choice depends on the anatomy. In the absence of PS, closure of the VSD with an intraventricular tunnel directs RV blood into the PA and LV blood into the aorta, and is the operation of choice. Any subpulmonic obstruction can be resected through the RA, PA, or right ventriculotomy. If the patient has associated PS, or if PS is created by the intraventricular patch VSD closure, it is necessary to create a valved conduit between the RV and PA,[56,57] a Dacron tube conduit,[58] or homograft[59] after creation of the intraventricular tunnel.

Another surgical option is PA translocation, which is used when subpulmonic obstruction is present with DOLV.[60] The technique does not involve an RVOT patch so that coronary artery anatomy about the RVOT is undisturbed; it does not involve an extracardiac conduit with its attendant morbidity.[60] The technique involves a right ventriculotomy, through which the subpulmonary area and VSD is closed. The main PA is dissected free from the base of the LV, and the posterior portion of the pulmonary valve ring is inserted into the superior RV wall through the ventriculotomy. Pericardium is then used to patch the anterior pulmonary valve ring and patch close the right ventriculotomy.[60]

DOLV has a frequent association with abnormalities of the tricuspid valve and hypoplasia of the RV.[54,55] These and other abnormalities may be severe enough to necessitate univentricular repair.[61] In these cases, bidirectional cavopulmonary anastomosis can be performed at 6 mo of age, followed by total cavopulmonary connection at 1–2 years of age.

Results from this rare anomaly are scanty. Four different reports describe four different patients with a good surgical result,[58,59,62,63] and another paper with two good results.[59] In a series of five cases, one child was inoperable and died without surgery, one died in the early postoperative period, and another died 2 years after surgery.[55] The largest surgical series reports eight patients, with 88% survival rate.[54] A single reoperation after repair of DOLV is reported in the literature, having been performed 13 years after original repair, using a new Dacron graft and aortic valve homograft to replace the old nonvalved Dacron conduit.[64]

REFERENCES

1. Lev M, Bharati S, Meng CCL, et al: A concept of double-outlet right ventricle. *J Thorac Cardiovasc Surg* **64**:271, 1972
2. Mitchell SC, Korones SB, Berendes HW: Congenital heart disease in 56,109 births: Incidence and natural history. *Circulation* **43**:323, 1971
3. Neufeld HN, Lucas RV, Lester RG, et al: Origin of both great vessels from the right ventricle without pulmonary stenosis. *Br Heart J* **24**:393, 1962
4. Anderson RH, Becker AE, Wilcox BR, et al: Surgical anatomy of double-outlet right ventricle: A reappraisal. *Am J Cardiol* **52**:555, 1983
5. Anderson RH, Wilkinson JL, Arnold R, et al: Morphogenesis of bulboventricular malformations II: Observations on malformed hearts. *Br Heart J* **36**:948, 1974
6. Goor DA, Edwards JE: The spectrum of transposition of the great arteries: With special reference to developmental anatomy of the conus. *Circulation* **48**:406, 1973
7. Sridaromont S, Feldt RH, Ritter DG, et al: Double-outlet right ventricle: Hemodynamic and anatomic correlations. *Am J Cardiol* **38**:85, 1976
8. Van Praagh R: What is the Taussig–Bing Malformation? (editorial) *Circulation* **38**:445, 1968
9. Sridaromont S, Ritter DG, Feldt RH, et al: Double-outlet ventricle: Anatomic and angiocardiographic correlations. *May Clin Proc* **53**:555, 1978
10. Zamora R, Moller JH, Edwards JE: Double-outlet right ventricle: Anatomic types and associated anomalies. *Chest* **68**:672, 1975
11. Sondheimer HM, Freedom RM, Olley PM: Double-outlet right ventricle: Clinical spectrum and prognosis. *Am J Cardiol* **39**:709, 1977
12. Musumeci F, Shumway S, Lincoln C, Anderson RH: Surgical treatment for double-outlet right ventricle at the Brompton Hospital, 1973 to 1986. *J Thorac Cardiovasc Surg* **96**:278, 1988
13. Serraf A, Lacour-Gayet F, Bruniaux J, et al: Anatomic repair of Taussig–Bing hearts. *Circulation* **84**(Suppl III): III–200, 1991
14. Aoki M, Forbess JM, Jonas RA, et al: Result of biventricular repair for double-outlet right ventricle. *J Thorac Cardiovasc Surg* **107**:338, 1994
15. Elliott LP, Amplatz K, Edwards JE: Coronary arterial patterns in transposition complexes: Anatomic and angiocardiographic studies. *Am J Cardiol* **17**:362, 1966
16. Gordillo L, Faye-Petersen O, de la Cruz MV, Soto B: Coronary arterial patterns in double-outlet right ventricle. *Am J Cardiol* **71**:1108, 1993
17. Cheng TO: Double-outlet right ventricle: Diagnosis during life. *Am J Med* **32**:637, 1962
18. Krongrad E, Ritter DG, Weidman WH, DuShane JW: Hemodynamic and anatomic correlation of electrocardiogram in double-outlet right ventricle. *Circulation* **46**:995, 1972
19. Macartney FJ, Rigby ML, Anderson RH, et al: Double-outlet right ventricle: Cross sectional echocardiographic findings, their anatomical explanation, and surgical relevance. *Br Heart J* **52**:164, 1984
20. Sanders SP, Bierman FZ, Williams RG: Conotruncal malformations: Diagnosis in infancy using subxiphoid 2-dimensional echocardiography. *Am J Cardiol* **50**:1361, 1982
21. Hagler DJ, Tajik AJ, Seward JB, et al: Double-outlet right ventricle: Wide-angle two-dimensional echocardiographic observations. *Circulation* **63**:419, 1981
22. DiSessa TG, Hagan AD, Pope C, et al: Two dimensional echocardiographic characteristics of double outlet right ventricle. *Am J Cardiol* **44**:1146, 1979
23. Tabry IF, McGoon DC, Danielson GK, et al: Surgical management of double-outlet right ventricle associated with atrioventricular discordance. *J Thorac Cardiovasc Surg* **76**:336, 1978
24. Kirklin JW, Harp RA, McGoon DC: Surgical treatment of origin of both vessels from right ventricle including cases of pulmonary stenosis. *J Thorac Cardiovasc Surg* **48**:1026, 1964
25. Wilcox BR, Ho SY, Macartney FJ, et al: Surgical anatomy of double-outlet right ventricle with situs solitus and atrioventricular concordance. *J Thorac Cardiovasc Surg* **82**:405, 1981
26. Marin-Garcia J, Neches WH, Park SC, et al: Double-outlet right ventricle with restrictive ventricular septal defect. *J Thorac Cardiovasc Surg* **76**:853, 1978
27. Stewart S: Double-outlet right ventricle: A collective review with a surgical viewpoint. *J Thorac Cardiovasc Surg* **71**:355, 1976
28. Judson JP, Danielson GK, Puga FJ, et al: Double-outlet right ventri-

cle: Surgical results, 1970–1980. *J Thorac Cardiovasc Surg* **85**:32, 1983

29. Shen WK, Holmes DR, Porter CJ, et al: Sudden death after repair of double-outlet right ventricle. *Circulation* **81**:128, 1990

30. Chaitman BR, Crondin CM, Theroux P, Bourassa MG: Late development of left ventricular outflow tract obstruction after repair of double-outlet right ventricle. *J Thorac Cardiovasc Surg* **72**:265, 1976

31. Quaegebeur JM: The optimal repair for the Taussig–Bing heart (editorial). *J Thorac Cardiovasc Surg* **85**:276, 1983

32. Kawashima Y, Fujita T, Miyamoto T, Manabe H: Intraventricular rerouting of blood for the correction of Taussig–Bing malformation. *J Thorac Cardiovasc Surg* **62**:825, 1971

33. Abe T, Sugiki K, Izumiyama O, Komatsu S: A successful procedure for correction of the Taussig–Bing malformation. *J Thorac Cardiovasc Surg* **87**:403, 1984

34. Doty DB: Correction of Taussig–Bing malformation by intraventricular conduit. *J Thorac Cardiovasc Surg* **91**:133, 1986

35. Patrick DL, McGoon DC: An operation for double-outlet right ventricle with transposition of the great arteries. *J Thorac Cardiovasc Surg* **6**:537, 1968

36. Hightower BM, Barcia A, Bargeron LM, Kirklin JW: Double-outlet right ventricle with transposed great arteries and subpulmonary ventricular septal defect: The Taussig–Bing malformation. *Circulation* **39**(Suppl I):I–207, 1969

37. Smith EEJ, Pucci JJ, Walesby RK, et al: A new technique for correction of the Taussig–Bing anomaly. *J Thorac Cardiovasc Surg* **83**:901, 1982

38. Binet JP, Lacour-Gayet F, Conso JF, et al: Complete repair of the Taussig–Bing type of double-outlet right ventricle using the arterial switch operation without coronary translocation: Report of one successful case. *J Thorac Cardiovasc Surg* **85**:272, 1983

39. Lui RC, Williams WG, Trusler GA, et al: Experience with the Damus-Kaye-Stansel procedure for children with Taussig-Bing hearts or univentricular hearts with subaortic stenosis. *Circulation* **88**:11–170, 1993

40. Kanter KR, Anderson RH, Lincoln C, et al: Anatomic correction for complete transposition and double-outlet right ventricle. *J Thorac Cardiovasc Surg* **90**:690, 1985

41. Yacoub MH, Radley-Smith R: Anatomic correction of the Taussig-Bing anomaly. *J Thorac Cardiovasc Surg* **88**:380, 1984

42. Brawn WJ, Mee RBB: Early results for anatomic correction of transposition of the great arteies and for double-outlet right ventricle with subpulmonary ventricular septal defect. *J Thorac Cardiovasc Surg* **95**:230, 1988

43. Lecompte Y, Batisse A, Di Carlo D: Double-outlet right ventricle: A surgical synthesis. In *Advances in Cardiac Surgery,* Vol. 4. St. Louis, Mosby, 1993, p 109

44. Stewart RW, Kirklin JW, Pacifico AD: Repair of double-outlet right ventricle: An analysis of 62 cases. *J Thorac Cardiovasc Surg* **78**:502, 1979

45. Kirklin JW, Pacifico AD, Blackstone EH, et al: Current risks and protocols for operations for double-outlet right ventricle: Derivation from an 18 year experience. *J Thorac Cardiovasc Surg* **92**:913, 1986

46. Kirklin JK, Castaneda AR: Surgical correction of double-outlet right ventricle with noncommitted ventricular septal defect. *J Thorac Cardiovasc Surg* **73**:399, 1977

47. McGoon DC: Left ventricular and biventricular extracardiac conduits. *J Thorac Cardiovasc Surg* **72**:7, 1976

48. Luber JM, Castaneda AR, Lang P, Norwood WI: Repair of double-outlet right ventricle: Early and late results. *Circulation* **68**(Suppl II), II–144, 1983

49. Russo P, Danielson GK, Puga FJ, et al: Modified Fontan Procedure for biventricular hearts with complex forms of double-outlet right ventricle. *Circulation* **78**(Suppl III):III–20, 1988

50. Paul MH, Muster AJ, Sinha SN, et al: Double-outlet right ventricle with an intact ventricular septum: Clinical and autopsy diagnosis and developmental implications. *Circulation* **41**:129, 1970

51. Sahahibara S, Takao A, Arai T, et al: Both great vessels arising from the left ventricle. *Bull Heart Inst Jpn* 66–86, 1967

52. Anderson R, Galbraith R, Miller G: Double outlet left ventricle. *Br Heart J* **36**:554, 1974

53. Goor DA, Dische R, Lillehei CW: The conotruncus: I. Its normal inversion and conus absorption. *Circulation* **56**:375, 1972

54. Bharati S, Lev M, Stewart R, et al: The morphologic spectrum of double outlet left ventricle and its surgical significance. *Circulation* **58**:558, 1978

55. Brandt PW, Calder AL, Barrat-Boyes BG, Neutze JM: Double outlet left ventricle: Morphology, cineangiocardiographic diagnosis and surgical treatment. *Am J Cardiol* **38**:897, 1976

56. Kerr AR, Barcia A, Bargeron LM, Kirklin JW: Double-outlet left ventricle with ventricular septal defect and pulmonary stenosis: Report of surgical repair. *Am Heart J* **81**:688, 1971

57. Pacifico AD, Kirklin JW, Bargeron LM, Soto B: Surgical treatment of double outlet left ventricle: Report of four cases. *Circulation* **47,48**(Suppl III):III–19, 1973

58. Conti V, Adams F, Mulder DG: Double outlet left ventricle. *Ann Thorac Surg* **18**:402, 1974

59. Villani M, Lipscombe S, Ross DN: Double outlet left ventricle: How should we repair it? Anatomic details and report of two successful surgical cases. *J Cardiovasc Surg* **20**:413, 1979

60. Chiavarelli M, Boucek MM, Bailey LL: Arterial correction of double outlet left ventricle by pulmonary artery translocation. *Ann Thorac Surg* **53**:1098, 1992

61. Fontan F, Baudet E: Surgical repair of tricuspid atresia. *Thorax* **26**:240, 1971

62. Murphy DA, Gillis DA, Sridhara KS: Intraventricular repair of double outlet left ventricle. *Ann Thorac Surg* **31**:364, 1981

63. Rivera R, Infantes C, de la Pena MG: Double outlet left ventricle: Report of a case with intraventricular surgical repair. *J Cardiovasc Surg* **21**:361, 1980

64. Dadourian BJ, Perloff JK, Drinkwater DC, et al: Double outlet left ventricle: Long survival after surgical correction (correspondence) *Ann Thorac Surg* **51**:159, 1991

CHAPTER

88

Tricuspid Atresia

Jeffrey M. Pearl, Lester C. Permut,
and Hillel Laks

INTRODUCTION

Tricuspid atresia is a congenital malformation characterized by lack of a communication between the right atrium and the right ventricle. Accompanying this malformation are an interatrial communication, enlargement of the mitral valve and left ventricle, and a varying degree of right ventricular hypoplasia.[1]

Tricuspid atresia is the third most common cyanotic heart lesion, occurring in approximately 3% of postmortem[2–4] and clinical congenital heart disease series.[2]

Van Praagh[5] postulated that tricuspid atresia is due to a combination of defects: (1) malalignment of the ventricular septum with the atrioventricular canal, (2) absence of the right ventricular sinus resulting in shifting of the ventricular septum to the right, and (3) obliteration of the right atrioventricular orifice. Tricuspid atresia may also be associated with complete atrioventricular canal.

ANATOMY

Tricuspid Valve

There are five forms of valvular atresia.[4] The most common (76%) is muscular, in which often there is a dimple on the muscular floor of the atrium directly opposite the morphologic left ventricle.[6] In one autopsy series, however, only 33 of 97 hearts (34%) with classic tricuspid atresia had a dimple.[7] The dimple probably represents the atrial portion of the membranous septum and not the atretic tricuspid valve. It is significant because of its close proximity to the atrioventricular (A-V) node.[7] A membranous type of valvular atresia, in which a portion of the membranous septum

between the right atrium and left ventricle appears in the location of the atretic tricuspid valve, occurs in 12%. A valvular type (6%) has a thin membrane of fused valve tissue, which may also have attached rudimentary chordae and lies between the right atrium and the rudimentary right ventricle.[8] An Ebstein type (6%) has obstructing leaflet tissue attached to the walls of the small right ventricular cavity. A fifth type, reported by Van Praagh,[5] occurs with common atrioventricular canal and consists of a leaflet of the common valve sealing the entrance to the right ventricle.

Interatrial Communication

Some type of atrial defect must be present to allow blood to exit from the right atrium. Two-thirds of patients have a patent foramen ovale of variable size,[1] while one-third of patients have a ostium secundum type of atrial septal defect. In one autopsy series, 85% of the atrial septal defects were nonrestrictive.[7] Less commonly, complete absence of the atrial septum may occur. The right atrial wall is usually markedly hypertrophied in tricuspid atresia.

Right Ventricle

In most patients, the right ventricular cavity is small and the infundibulum is the only portion consistently present. There may also be a trabeculated lower portion containing rudimentary papillary muscles. The ventricular septal defect (VSD) usually communicates with the upper, outflow (infundibular) portion of the right ventricle, although it may occur more toward the apex as well. The ventricular septal defect is generally restrictive, producing some obstruction to pulmonary flow. The infundibular portion of the right ventricle may also be narrow, resulting in obstruction to

1431

pulmonary bloodflow. Occasionally, neither the ventricular septal defect nor the infundibular chamber is appreciably restrictive, with consequent excessive pulmonary bloodflow.[1,7]

Mitral Valve and Left Ventricle

The mitral valve is usually larger than normal, and although of normal shape, may have three or more leaflets.[9–10] The valve is usually competent, but may become regurgitant over time secondary to continued volume overload. There may be overriding of the ventricular septum.[11] The left ventricle is hypertrophied and the mass/volume ratio markedly increased.[12] Both systolic and diastolic function may be depressed.[13–15]

Position of the Great Arteries

The great arteries may be normally related, *d*-transposed, or *l*-transposed in tricuspid atresia (Fig. 88–1). The aorta may be either anterior or posterior to the pulmonary artery, or the two vessels may be side-by-side. When the aorta arises from the right ventricle (*d*-transposition), a pressure gradient may exist between the left ventricle and the aorta if the ventricular septal defect becomes restrictive, or the infundibular right ventricle is narrowed. In *l*-transposition, subaortic stenosis may also exist.

Pulmonary Artery

Valvular pulmonary stenosis or atresia is common in tricuspid atresia. Stenosis or hypoplasia of the pulmonary artery may also be present in those patients with obstruction at the valvular level.

CLASSIFICATION

Tricuspid atresia has been classified into three types, depending on ventriculoarterial concordance. Type I (69–83%) refers to hearts in which the great arteries are in concordance with the ventricles. Type II (17–27%) comprises hearts with *d*-transposition, and Type III (3%) includes hearts with *l*-transposition.

Subgroups are defined depending on the degree of obstruction to pulmonary bloodflow and the size of the ventricular septal defect. In type a, pulmonary atresia is present. Type b refers to hearts with pulmonary stenosis, and type c hearts have no restriction of pulmonary bloodflow[1,16] (Fig. 88–1A–C).

PATHOPHYSIOLOGY

The pathophysiology, and subsequent early management, of tricuspid atresia is based primarily on the degree of obstruc-

tion to pulmonary bloodflow. The majority of patients, 71%, have reduced pulmonary bloodflow resulting in cyanosis.[3] Depending on the degree of obstruction, cyanosis may be present in the neonatal period, or develop later as the ventricular septal defect starts to close or infundibular stenosis develops. Neonates with pulmonary atresia (type Ia or IIa) are ductus dependent for pulmonary bloodflow and will develop severe cyanosis if the ductus is allowed to close. Generally, those patients with obstruction to pulmonary bloodflow have unobstructed systemic flow.

Alternatively, patients with unobstructed pulmonary flow tend to have some obstruction to systemic flow. In this smaller group of tricuspid atresia patients with unobstructed pulmonary flow, cyanosis is mild or absent, and congestive heart failure is often present. These patients present with dyspnea, poor feeding, and recurrent respiratory infections. If not palliated early with pulmonary artery banding, subsequent irreversible pulmonary vascular disease may develop preventing future definitive repair.[17] Cardiac failure may progress rapidly, resulting in early death, particularly when *d*-transposition of the great arteries (TGA) associated with a large pulmonary artery and coarctation or hypoplasia of the aorta is present.[18]

Patients with increased pulmonary bloodflow in early life may develop cyanosis later in life as the ventricular septal defect closes or narrowing of the infundibular outflow occurs.[18–19] Conversely, in patients with *d*-transposition, in whom the aorta arises from the small right ventricle, restriction to systemic flow and worsening of pulmonary plethora can develop as the VSD closes or infundibular obstruction worsens.[20]

Most infants with tricuspid atresia and a restrictive atrial septal defect (ASD) undergo balloon atrial septostomy early in life. However, if left with a restrictive ASD, systemic venous hypertension develops, complicated by pulsatile hepatomegaly, ascites, and peripheral edema.

Chronic volume overload of the left ventricle affects both systolic and diastolic function. This results in a progressive decrease in the ejection fraction and an increase in the end-diastolic volume and pressure.[12–14,21] Mitral valve regurgitation frequently develops as the left ventricle dilates. These hearts typically demonstrate an increased mass/volume ratio, which has an inverse correlation with the long-term success of a Fontan repair.[12,14,22] The presence of subaortic stenosis also has a negative impact on ventricular function, significantly increasing the mass/volume ratio.[23]

DIAGNOSTIC PROCEDURES

Auscultation

A harsh systolic ejection murmur is present along the left sternal border in most patients.[24] This murmur may be absent in those with pulmonary atresia in which the character-

Tricuspid Atresia with No Transposition (69 - 83%)

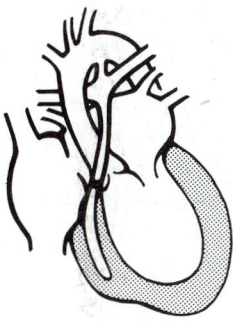 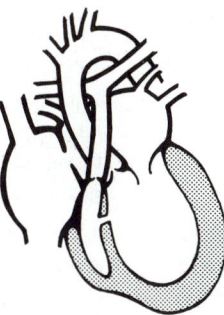 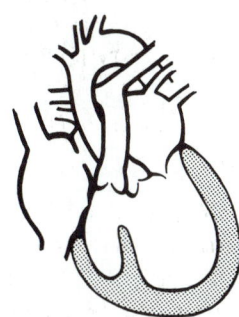

I(a)
Pulmonary atresia

I(b)
Pulmonary hypoplasia,
small ventricular
septal defect

I(c)
No pulmonary
hypoplasia, large
ventricular septal
defect

A

Tricuspid Atresia with D Transposition (17 - 27%)

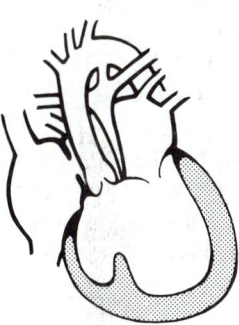 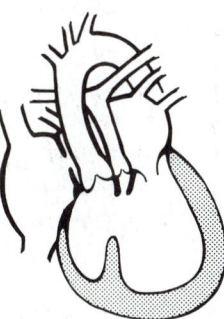 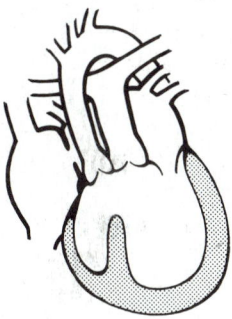

II(a)
Pulmonary atresia

II(b)
Pulmonary or
subpulmonary stenosis

II(c)
Large pulmonary
artery

B

Tricuspid Atresia with L Transposition (3%)

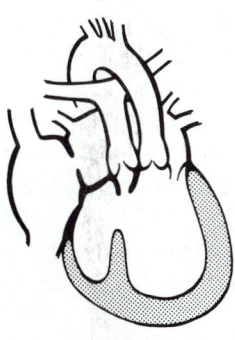 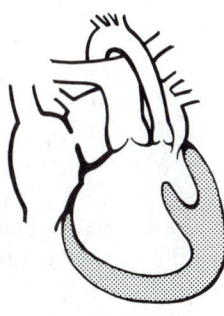

III(a)
Pulmonary or
subpulmonary stenosis

III(b)
Subaortic stenosis

Figure 88–1. A–C. The anatomic classification of tricuspid atresia. Percentages given as ranges from both clinical and autopsy series. Type Ib is most common occurring in 63.5% of tricuspid atresia patients.

C

istic murmur of a patent ductus arteriosus is heard. When pulmonary blood flow is increased, a mid-diastolic rumble may be present. While tricuspid atresia can be suspected based on physical exam, it may be difficult to distinguish it from other cyanotic congenital heart defects such as transposition, or tetrology of Fallot.

Electrocardiography

The electrocardiogram usually shows a prominent, notched P wave with a taller initial peak (P tricuspidale).[25] Left axis deviation is usually present unless TGA with a large pulmonary artery is present, in which case right axis deviation will be demonstrated. Evidence of left ventricular hypertrophy is commonly present.

Chest Radiograph

Although a "classic" radiographic appearance of tricuspid atresia has been described, the x-ray pattern is actually quite variable.[26] The characteristic findings are a flattened right heart border, a tall, blunt left heart border with a high apex, and a concave middle arc at the junction of the aorta and lower segment (Fig. 88–2). The x-ray may demonstrate the "coeur-en-sabot" or "boot-shaped" configuration as in tetralogy of Fallot. If transposition is present the heart may appear as "an egg on a string."

The pulmonary vasculature usually appears oligemic, but may appear normal or increased in patients with unobstructed pulmonary bloodflow.

Echocardiography

The quality, and hence the usefulness, of echocardiography has increased markedly over the past several years. The diagnosis of tricuspid atresia can routinely be made by this noninvasive modality. The gradient across the atrial septal defect, the pulmonary valve, or the infundibulum can be determined using m-mode and color-flow Doppler. Mitral valve incompetence and subaortic stenosis can also be accurately diagnosed. Ventricular function can be quantified by measuring the fractional shortening, and ejection fraction can be estimated (Fig. 88–3). For uncomplicated tricuspid atresia, cardiac catheterization is not necessary prior to palliation, although is generally done prior to Fontan repair.

MRI

The usefulness of magnetic resonance imaging (MRI) in diagnosis of congenital heart disease is presently unknown. Accurate depiction of many lesions can be obtained with MRI[27] (Fig. 88–4). Whether this offers a significant advantage over other modalities and is a cost-effective modality is still being investigated.

Cardiac Catheterization

Despite the ability to accurately diagnose tricuspid atresia with echocardiography, cardiac catheterization is still necessary to define the anatomy of the pulmonary arteries, search for aortic collaterals, and measure the left ventricular end-diastolic pressure, pulmonary artery pressure, and pulmonary venous wedge pressures prior to consideration for a Fontan. The pulmonary vascular resistance and shunt fraction can be calculated from the data obtained.

Angiography confirms the diagnosis and identifies the source of pulmonary bloodflow. Contrast injected into the right atrium passes entirely to the left atrium. Failure to opacify a right ventricular inflow causes a triangular-shaped "right ventricular window," which is bordered by the right atrium, the left ventricle, and the diaphragm[28–30] (Fig. 88–5). The sizes of the ventricular septal defect, right ventricular cavity, and outflow tract are delineated, as well as the anatomy and relationship of the great vessels. Left ven-

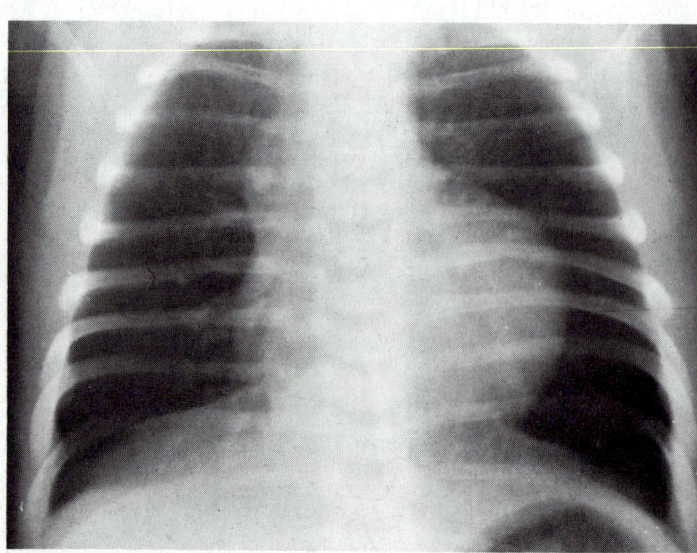

Figure 88–2. Chest radiograph in an infant with tricuspid atresia demonstrates decreased pulmonary vascularity, left ventricular enlargement, and prominence of the ascending aorta.

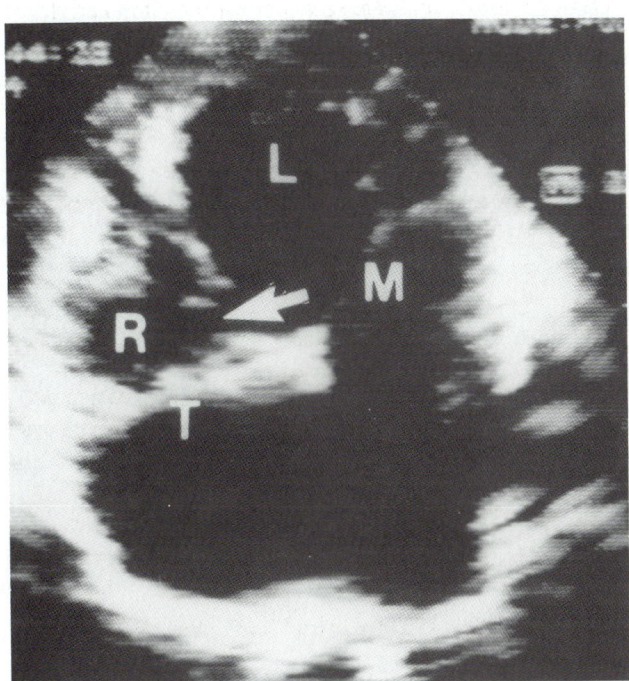

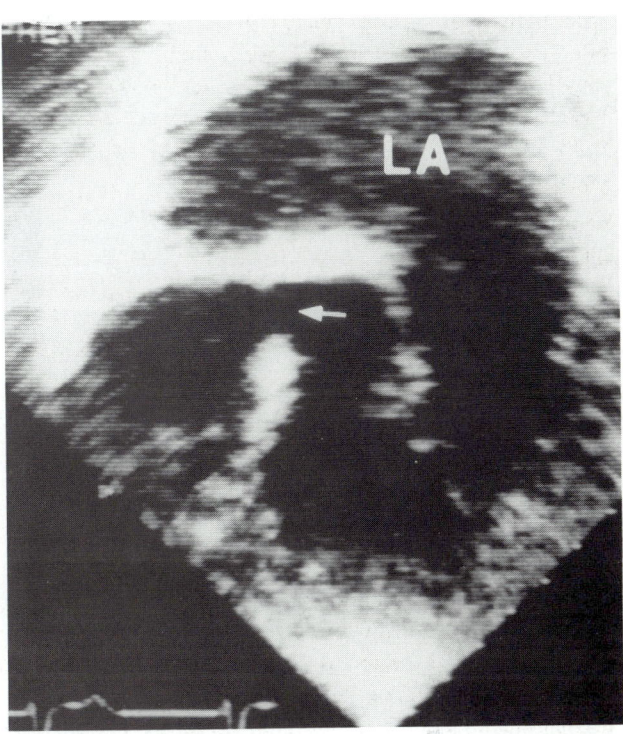

A   **B**

Figure 88–3. **A.** A two-dimensional echocardiogram in tricuspid atresia demonstrates absence of the tricuspid valve (T), mitral valve anatomy (M), the size of the interatrial communication (arrow), and the venous drainage to the left (L) and right (R) atria. **B.** A long-access view demonstrates right ventricular hypoplasia, left ventricular enlargement, and the size and position of the ventricular septal defect (arrow).

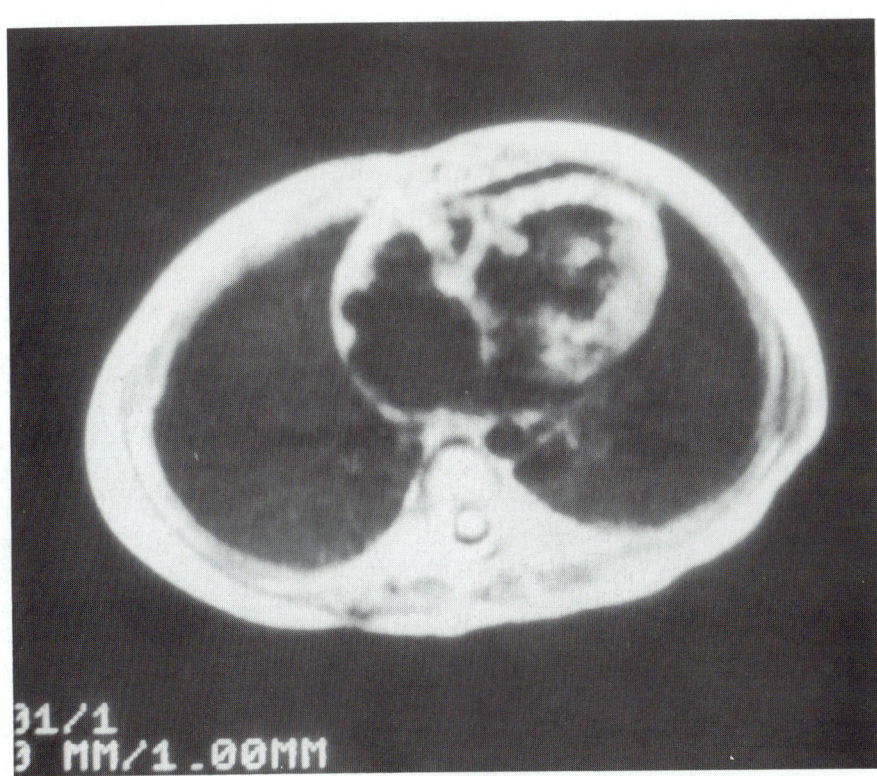

Figure 88–4. Magnetic resonance image demonstrating enlarged left ventricle, right ventricular hypoplasia, and an enlarged right atrium in tricuspid atresia.

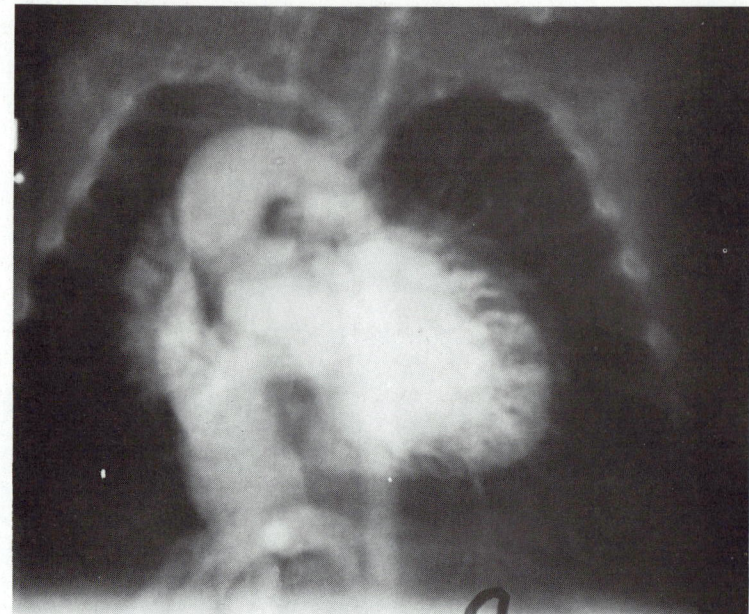

Figure 88–5. Cardiac catheterization in a neonate with tricuspid atresia. Right atrial injection demonstrates passage of contrast from the right atrium to the left atrium, and then to the left ventricle and out the aorta. Significant pulmonic stenosis is present and the pulmonary arteries are fed via a patent ductus arteriosus. The right ventricle is not visualized and the characteristic triangular "right ventricular window" formed by the right atrium, left ventricle, and diaphragm is demonstrated.

tricular injection demonstrates both ventricles, systolic ventricular function, and the presence of mitral regurgitation.[31] A balloon occlusion descending aortogram should be performed to look for systemic-to-pulmonary collaterals.

Cardiac catheterization often shows a prominent A wave in the right atrium, and may demonstrate a pressure gradient across the atrial septum if the communication is restrictive. An accurate left ventricular end-diastolic pressure and pulmonary artery or pulmonary venous wedge pressure are critical. The pulmonary vascular resistance can be calculated based on the pressures obtained. Measurement of the different chamber oxygen saturations will permit calculation of a shunt ratio.

Nuclear Perfusion Scan

There may be some role for preoperative lung perfusion scanning prior to Fontan. Specifically, the percent flow to each lung is determined. This is of particular importance if a unidirectional Fontan is being considered, or a prior Glenn shunt has been placed. In addition to raising the possibility of A-V fistula, discovery of abnormal distribution patterns may influence the type of Fontan connection performed.

NATURAL HISTORY

The natural history of tricuspid atresia is influenced greatly by the degree of obstruction to pulmonary bloodflow. Patients with unimpeded, high pulmonary bloodflow (type IIc) do poorly and usually die by the third month of life. The prognosis is best for patients with more balanced pulmonary flow as in type Ic and IIb who have a mean survival

of approximately 8 years.[3,32] Most patients, however, have a prognosis somewhere between these two extremes, with children with reduced flow (type Ia, Ib, or IIa) having an intermediate survival. The earlier the onset of cyanosis, the worse the long-term prognosis. Overall, 50% of infants born with tricuspid atresia die by 6 months, 60% by 1 year, and 90% by 10 years.[3] Therefore, without surgical intervention, only 10% of infants will be alive at 10 years.

Of 26 adults with tricuspid atresia enrolled in the UCLA adult congenital heart disease registry, only two have remained unoperated upon and remain relatively asymptomatic. Even the rare patient that survives to adulthood without surgical intervention is not guaranteed a long-term survival. Progressive ventricular failure remains a concern in all of these patients, and undoubtly some may eventually require cardiac transplantation.

TREATMENT

Until the advent of the Blalock–Taussig shunt in 1945, patients with tricuspid atresia had a dismal long-term prognosis with less than 10% survival to 10 years.[3] While palliation has improved the bleak prognosis, its main impact has been to extend the mortality curve; ultimately, the same late outcome occurs.[33–37] Long-term survival greater than 10 to 20 years is uncommon with palliation alone. The advent of partial right heart bypass (Glenn shunt),[38–41] and shortly thereafter complete right heart bypass (Fontan), provided a means of physiologic correction. Although not an anatomic correction, the Fontan procedure[42–43] has significantly improved both the early and the late survival and functional capacity for many tricuspid atresia patients.[12,44–48] Under ideal conditions, Fontan repair provides essentially a normal survival curve and functional outcome.

Presently, medical therapy and surgical palliation of patients with tricuspid atresia must be undertaken with the ultimate goal of Fontan repair. Protection of the pulmonary vasculature and preservation of left ventricular function are critical for a successful long-term outcome.

Medical Management

Nonsurgical treatment of tricuspid atresia in infancy is applicable to those few patients presenting in the neonatal period and beyond who have adequate but not excessive bloodflow to the lungs. Continued medical therapy is warranted until an age at which definitive repair can be safely instituted, usually after 12–18 mo of age for the Fontan or after 6–12 mo for a Glenn shunt. Continued medical therapy despite apparent good clinical status is not justified beyond 4–5 years of age due to the progressive damage to ventricular function that occurs from chronic hypoxia and volume overload.

In many neonates, cardiac catheterization is done early in life. In those with signs of a restrictive interatrial communication, balloon septostomy should be done.[49,50] If restriction to interatrial flow develops beyond the first few months of life, blade septostomy may be required.

SURGICAL PROCEDURES

Palliative Operations

The goals of palliative surgery for tricuspid atresia are to (1) improve clinical symptoms, which usually involves relief of cyanosis; (2) prevent damage to ventricular function and the pulmonary vasculature; (3) facilitate future definitive repair by preserving physiologic parameters and preventing anatomic distortion; and (4) correct associated abnormalities, such as atrioventricular valve regurgitation or subaortic stenosis. While associated with an increase in short- and mid-term survival, palliative procedures in general do not provide adequate long-term functional results and are used primarily in anticipation of eventual right heart bypass.[35–37,51–54]

Atrial septectomy is performed in those cases in which there is a restrictive interatrial communication that cannot be opened by either balloon septostomy or, in older children, blade septostomy with balloon dilatation. The Blalock–Hanlon procedure is the preferred method of closed atrial septectomy[55]; however, in some cases direct atrial septectomy is necessary. For these procedures we prefer cardiopulmonary bypass over inflow occlusion due to the concern of air embolism.[56]

Systemic-to-pulmonary artery shunts remain the most common palliative procedure done for patients with tricuspid atresia. When appropriately sized, these shunts increase

pulmonary bloodflow and improve oxygen saturation. The goal is to obtain a saturation of around 85%. A saturation above 87% indicates too large a shunt with an increased risk of developing pulmonary vascular disease and excessive ventricular volume load. Conversely, an inappropriately small shunt will inadequately relieve cyanosis and fail to provide adequate symptomatic palliation.

For this reason, the Blalock–Taussig shunt is preferred by most surgeons as there is less tendency for excessive pulmonary flow with this approach.[33,34,57] Furthermore, its performance via a lateral thoracotomy preserves the anterior mediastinum for a midline transternal approach for eventual definitive repair. Construction of the Blalock–Taussig shunt is performed on the left side, when feasible, to preserve the right side for a possible Glenn shunt. Subclavian arterioplasty[34] or a polytetrafluoroethylene interposition graft may be used. Our current preference is to use a polytetrafluoroethylene interposition graft. A graft of 4 mm is usually adequate for most infants.

Series reporting on the experience with the Potts[53] or Waterston[58] shunts have shown that although effective at lessening cyanosis these shunts are less reliable and are more prone to cause kinking and distortion of the pulmonary artery.[59,60] They are also more likely to result in excessive pulmonary flow.[24,56] While a Blalock–Taussig shunt is less likely to produce these complications, meticulous attention must be paid to proper sizing and technique, as pulmonary artery distortion and adverse pulmonary vascular changes have been reported in up to 23% of patients.

There is a wide range of mortality rates reported for the Blalock–Taussig shunt, with even recent series reporting a mortality rate of up to 17% (2–17%).[32,35–37] Lamberti et al reported a 2.3% early mortality in 44 tricuspid atresia patients undergoing placement of a Blalock–Taussig shunt.[59] Our own results with the Blalock–Taussig shunt are quite similar, with operative mortality quite uncommon.

Glenn Shunt

While technically a palliative procedure, the Glenn shunt provides partial physiologic correction. Its main advantage is that it provides obligatory pulmonary bloodflow and avoids the left ventricular volume overload accompanying systemic-to-pulmonary artery shunts.[41,60–63] Furthermore, good long-term results have been obtained with the Glenn shunt, although eventual Fontan repair should be carried out in those considered acceptable candidates.[53,60,64,65] For high-risk patients, a Glenn shunt may be possible when a Fontan is not, as venous hypertension is better tolerated in the head, neck, and upper extremities than it is in the inferior vena caval system.[66,67] The Glenn shunt may be particularly applicable to patients considered to be at increased risk for a Fontan procedure, or those in whom additional defects require correction prior to Fontan repair. Stansel procedure combined with a Glenn is not an uncommon approach to patients with subaortic stenosis in whom ventricular function is impaired.[68,69] As mentioned, the Glenn shunt is also applicable to patients less than 12–18 mo of age who require further palliation, but may be too young for Fontan repair.

If no intracardiac repairs are planned, a bidirectional Glenn shunt can be performed without cardiopulmonary bypass by using a high superior vena caval (SVC) to right atrial shunt. The classic end-to-end Glenn shunt is associated with distortion of the pulmonary artery, loss of the right upper lobe pulmonary artery, and the development of pulmonary arteriovenous fistula, and, therefore, is no longer routinely used. The bidirectional Glenn shunt avoids some of the problems associated with the classic Glenn, and may not require takedown at the time of Fontan repair. Operative mortality for a Glenn shunt varies according to indications and diagnoses but is approximately 5%.[53,60] The operative mortality in over 100 Glenn shunts performed at UCLA is 4%. Improvement in mean arterial saturation from 69 to 83% with creation of a Glenn shunt has been documented in two different series.[60,62]

Experience with the Glenn shunt for tricuspid atresia has demonstrated it to be a good short- and mid-term therapy.[53] Despite some reports of 100% actuarial survival at 9 years,[53] most patients experience 5–7 years of palliation, followed by rapid deterioration with progressive cyanosis and cardiac failure.[54,70–72] A Glenn shunt should be reserved for those patients who are not Fontan candidates, or as an interim stage prior to Fontan repair. Long-term results do not support it as the sole procedure in otherwise acceptable Fontan candidates.[53,54,70–72]

Disadvantages of the Glenn shunt include the development of venous collaterals from the SVC to the inferior vena cava (IVC) with subsequent shunting of blood resulting in worsening of cyanosis. Arteriovenous fistula development in the lung, especially in the right lower lobe, is a known complication of the classic Glenn procedure but is unusual with the bidirectional Glenn shunt.[64,66,73] The A-V fistulae may be managed by transcatheter embolization, but on occasion lobectomy has been required prior to or concomitant with the Fontan procedure.[12]

Pulmonary Artery Banding

Palliative pulmonary artery banding is reserved for the small number of tricuspid atresia patients with excessive pulmonary flow in whom it is used to treat congestive cardiac failure and to prevent the development of pulmonary vascular disease. Almost all children requiring this procedure have transposition of the great arteries and a large ventricular septal defect (type IIc). Pulmonary artery banding is rarely required in children without transposition and a large ventricular septal defect (type Ic). Medical management is usually sufficient until progressive closure of the ventricular septal defect or infundibular obstruction results in cyanosis and the possible need for a shunt procedure.[18,19]

Strategy of Palliative Surgery

In addition to the operative mortality for a palliative shunt, the additive mortality of multiple palliative procedures and late deaths needs to be considered when comparing palliation to early Fontan repair.[35–37,52,59,74] Fontan candidacy may be lost secondary to improper or multiple palliative procedures.[52] Even well-palliated patients should be referred for definitive repair by 4–5 years of age or earlier. Patients over 12 mo of age with progressive cyanosis should be strongly considered for Fontan repair rather than additional palliative procedure. However, many would still prefer a staged approach with a preliminary Glenn shunt in these younger patients. Those with increased symptoms between 6 and 12 mo of age should undergo a palliative procedure, preferably a Glenn shunt, rather than Fontan repair, as Fontan repair is associated with an increased mortality in patients less than 1 year.[44,75] Glenn shunts are technically difficult and are associated with an increased mortality in patients less than 6 mo of age.[64,66] Therefore, in symptomatic patients less than 6 mo of age, traditional palliation with a systemic-to-pulmonary artery shunt should still be the mainstay of surgical treatment.

Fontan Repair and Its Modifications

The concept of total right heart bypass became a reality in 1971 with the first successful Fontan procedure. Concomitantly, Kreutzer introduced his version of right heart bypass. The Fontan–Kreutzer procedure and its numerous modifications are based on the concept that an elevated systemic venous pressure is an adequate driving force for pulmonary bloodflow, and that a pumping right ventricle is unnecessary. Separation of the pulmonary and systemic venous circulation is achieved, resulting in an improved systemic arterial oxygen saturation and a reduced volume load on the left ventricle.[42] The majority of right heart bypass procedures in current practice bear little anatomic similarity to the original procedure, yet the physiologic basis is the same. The use of valves in the inferior IVC or in the various conduits has since been abandoned. The incorporation of the right ventricle, initially thought to be critical, has also been abandoned except in certain instances.

Most patients now undergo a total cavopulmonary connection, often with either an adjustable ASD or fenestration, a partial Fontan.[76–80] In addition, the operative mortality for the modified Fontan procedure has decreased significantly with most centers reporting an early mortality of around 5% for tricuspid atresia, and 5–10% for other forms of single ventricle.[81]

Patient Selection

Due to the unique physiology accompanying a Fontan procedure, proper patient selection remains crucial. A low pulmonary vascular resistance and good systemic ventricular function are the critical elements for a successful Fontan. All preceding palliative procedures must be undertaken with the goal of preserving these two parameters for future Fontan repair.

The initial selection criteria by Choussat et al for acceptable Fontan patients were quite stringent.[82] Although the principles remain valid, most of the criteria are no longer relevant. Improved understanding of Fontan physiology, more coordinated treatment algorithms including appropriate preliminary palliation, increased operative experience, and increased experience with postoperative management have continued to improve the early and late outcome following Fontan repair.[44,75,81,84–87,89] Increased use of a staged approach with a preliminary Glenn shunt and/or the introduction of the partial Fontan have allowed many patients thought previously to be at increased risk by Choussats criteria to undergo successful Fontan repair.[83] Despite these improvements, there are still criteria that permit risk stratification.[14,23,81,88,89] Treatment plans are determined by classification of patients into low, medium, and high-risk categories (Table 88–1).

Age is no longer considered to be an independent risk factor for Fontan repair with good results obtained in young patients (less than 4 years of age),[75,83,87,90,91] as well as in the adult population.[92] Obviously, when possible, Fontan repair should be done prior to adulthood. Although early operative mortality remains comparable for repair at older ages, late mortality and the occurrence of a poor functional status are increased due to progressive ventricular failure in patients with long-standing cyanosis and volume overload.[92–94, 95] Late sudden death secondary to arrhythmias or myocardial failure has been associated with older age at the time of Fontan repair.[93,96–98]

Recent data suggest that, especially in tricuspid atresia, Fontan repair between 1 year and 4 years may be preferable, especially if worsening cyanosis is present and there is consideration for performing a second palliative shunt.[75,83,87] The mortality for Fontan repair for a combined group of diagnoses at UCLA was 8.9% for those less than 4 years of age, and 6.7% for those less than 2 years of age.[75] The mortality for 25 patients undergoing Fontan repair between 12 and 24 mo was only 4%. In the 36 tricuspid atresia patients in this series there was only one early death, giving an operative mortality of 2.7%. In 13 tricuspid atresia patients under 2 years of age there were no operative deaths.[75] Myers et al[87] have also reported a zero mortality in 13 patients less than 3 years of age who underwent Fontan repair. In comparison, following age restriction criteria, de Brux et al reported a 53% incidence of second palliative procedures, a second palliation operative mortality of 13.2%, and 22% mortality while awaiting Fontan repair. Hence, the mortality for either a second palliative procedure or for delaying Fontan repair was more than twice the early mortality for a Fontan procedure itself.[16]

In addition to avoiding the cumulative mortality and morbidity of multiple palliative procedures, a major advantage of early repair includes relief of ventricular volume overload and chronic cyanosis with preservation of ventricular function. The preservation of ventricular function is of paramount importance, as most late Fontan failures and late deaths are secondary to ventricular failure.[93,95] Prolonged cyanosis and volume overload are associated with an inappropriately hypertrophied LV myocardium and impaired diastolic function. An elevated LV mass/volume ratio is inversely related to Fontan outcome.[14]

Arrhythmias are a second cause of late Fontan failure. A report from the Netherlands found that arrhythmias did not develop in patients who underwent Fontan repair at age 4 years compared with those undergoing Fontan repair at a mean of 7.6 years of age.[12] In addition to the preservation of ventricular function, early relief of cyanosis and a mixed circulation decrease the likelihood of developing paradoxical emboli, cerebral abscesses, and developmental delay.

As seen in Table 88–1, systolic ventricular function as measured by echocardiography and/or angiography is an important predictor of Fontan outcome. Ventricular diastolic function is probably of equal importance, as achieving an adequate preload pressure for the left ventricle may be difficult in a Fontan circulation. Obtaining an accurate measurement of the left ventricular end-diastolic pressure (LVEDP), before contrast injection, is of paramount importance in the pre-Fontan evaluation. A pulmonary venous wedge pressure may suffice as an indirect indicator of left ventricular diastolic function when LVEDP cannot be measured directly. When ventricular function is significantly impaired, correction of contributing conditions such as A-V valve regurgitation or subaortic stenosis should be undertaken, usually concomitant with placement of a Glenn shunt. When ventricular impairment is less severe, Fontan

TABLE 88–1. PATIENT CLASSIFICATION

	Low Risk	Medium Risk	High Risk
Mean pulmonary artery pressure (mm Hg)	<15	15–20	>20
Pulmonary vascular resistance (Woods Units)	<2	2–3	>3
Transpulmonary gradient (mm Hg)	<7	7–12	>12
Ejection fraction	>60%	45–60%	<45%
Left ventricular end-diastolic pressure (mm Hg)	<6	6–12	>12
Outflow gradient (mm Hg)	<30	30–50	>50
A-V valve regurgitation	Mild	Moderate	Severe
Options	Fontan or partial Fontan	Partial Fontan	Glenn, correct associated anomalies

repair with concomitant Stansel or A-V valve repair may be considered.

Pulmonary artery pressure and pulmonary vascular resistance are also important predictors of Fontan outcome and are critical parts of the preoperative evaluation. Preoperative pulmonary vascular resistance above 3–4 Woods Units predicts excessive venous hypertension and early Fontan failure, and is therefore a contraindication to Fontan repair. Care must be taken to distinguish reversible elevated pulmonary artery pressures secondary to excessive pulmonary bloodflow from fixed pulmonary hypertension secondary to pulmonary vascular disease. In the absence of a Glenn shunt, increased arterial oxygen saturations associated with high pulmonary artery pressures indicate increased pulmonary flow and reversible pulmonary hypertension. Decreased arterial saturations associated with elevated pulmonary artery pressures suggest decreased pulmonary bloodflow and irreversible pulmonary hypertension.

The transpulmonary gradient is also a useful criterion, as it translates the pulmonary artery pressures and the ventricular end-diastolic pressure into a useful value, roughly correlating with the pulmonary vascular resistance. The guidelines listed in Table 88–1 have proven helpful in determining the appropriate surgical approach.

Surgical Technique

The Fontan procedure is performed via a median sternotomy. Systemic-to-pulmonary artery shunts and collaterals are isolated and occluded prior to cardiopulmonary bypass. Alternatively, collaterals may be coil embolized preoperatively. Bicaval cannulation is used. The SVC dissection needs to be carried out quite high with cannulation almost at the SVC/inominate junction. Cardiopulmonary bypass with hypothermia to 24°C is instituted. Myocardial protection includes intermittent cold blood cardioplegia and topical hypothermia. Retrograde cardioplegic infusion may be carried out intermittently when the coronary sinus ostium is accessible. Warm reperfusion is also utilized.

Techniques for creation of a classic right atrial to pulmonary artery Fontan are well known.[99,100] A posterior atriopulmonary anastomosis is preferred to avoid sternal compression. However, if the anatomy is unsuitable because of a previously placed Glenn shunt or a posteriorly positioned aorta in patients with normally related great arteries, an anterior connection is used. A nonvalved direct right atrial to pulmonary artery connection is generally performed (Fig. 88–6). The pulmonary artery is transected and the proximal end oversewn. With transposition of the great arteries, the pulmonary artery does not need to be repositioned and the pulmonary valve is simply oversewn. A large incision is made in the roof of the right atrium and the trapdoor-shaped atrial flap is flipped on itself to create the posterior wall of the connection. Pericardial or prosthetic material may be required as a patch anteriorly. If an adjustable

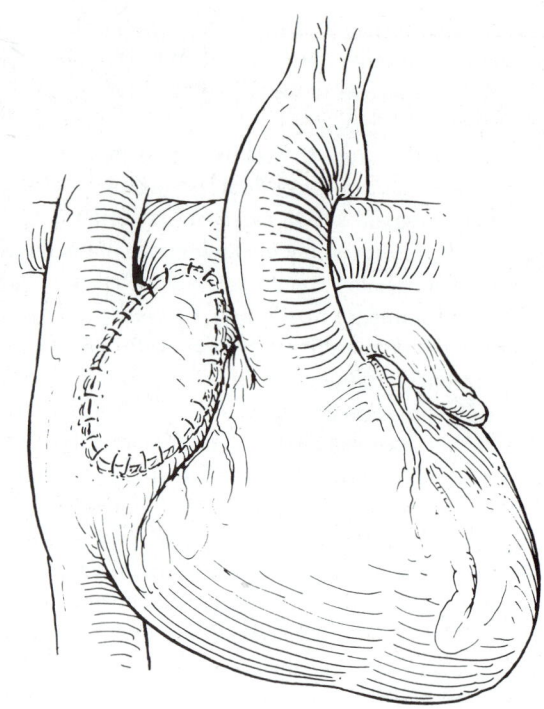

Figure 88–6. A direct right atrium to pulmonary artery connection. The anterior portion of the connection is augmented with pericardium, the atrial appendage, and atrial wall making up the posterior wall.

ASD is to be placed it can be incorporated into primary closure of the native ASD, if small, or placed in the edge of a prosthetic patch when used for a large secundum ASD (Figs. 88–7 and 88–8).

Right Atrial to Right Ventricle Connection

This connection is applicable to Fontan repair only in patients with tricuspid atresia without pulmonary obstruction who have a well-developed right ventricle, usually greater than 30% of normal size. These are usually patients who have had a nonrestrictive ventricular septal defect. Right atrial to right ventricle connection is warranted under specific conditions in which pulsatile flow is expected to result from incorporation of the small right ventricle. This needs to be weighed against the potential for worse hemodynamics secondary to turbulence created by less streamlined bloodflow. While some series have suggested improved survival when the right ventricle is incorporated in the circulation,[101,102] this was when compared to the traditional right atrial to pulmonary artery connection rather than to the currently preferred total cavopulmonary connection.[103–105] The decision to incorporate the right ventricle in the Fontan circulation should be made on an individual basis among the select group of tricuspid atresia patients whose anatomy is amenable to this approach.

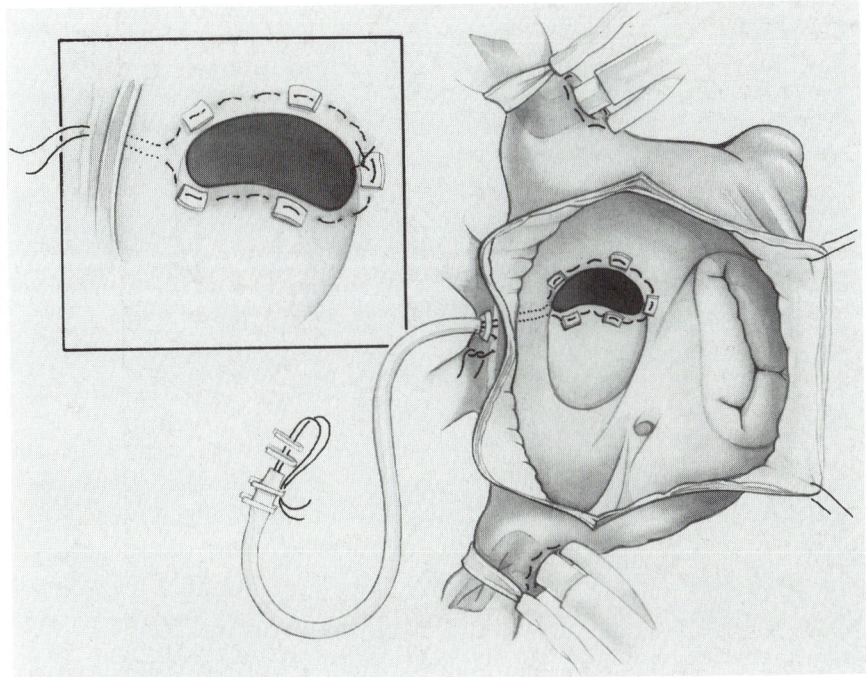

A

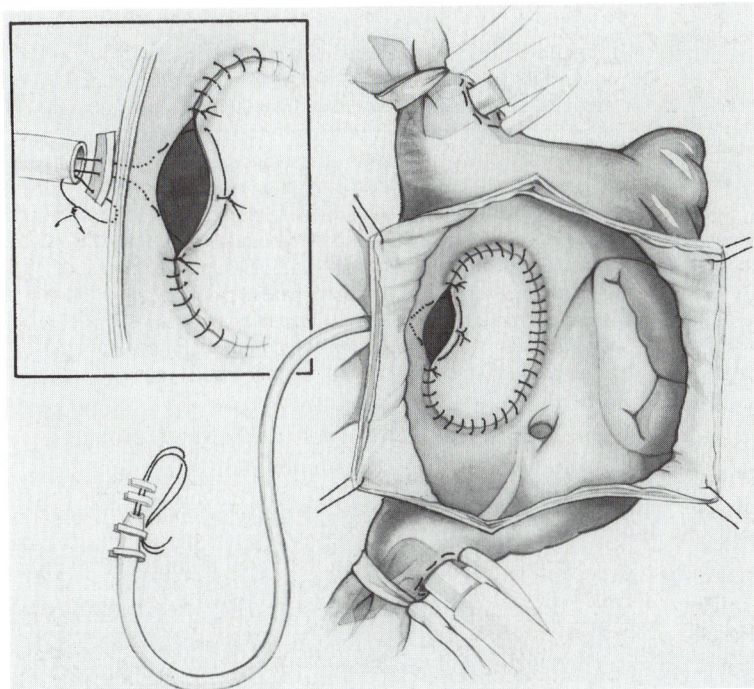

B

Figure 88–7. Technique for construction of an adjustable ASD when a classic right atrial to pulmonary artery or right atrial to right ventricle Fontan is performed. **A.** A pursestring is sewn around the border of an enlarged ASD and brought out through the interatrial septum and through the snare device. Pledgets may be used to reinforce the pursestring. **B.** If a large secundum ASD is present, it may be closed with a prosthetic patch and a defect left in the lateral wall. The heavy prolene suture is brought through the interatrial septum and placed as a horizontal mattress stitch through the edge of the patch. This is anchored to the patch with a 5–0 chromic suture.

Technique of Right Atrium to Right Ventricle Connection

The ventricular septal defect is closed with a prosthetic patch.[106] The right ventricular chamber can be enlarged by resection of some of the trabeculae and muscle bands. For a valved connection, an aortic homograft augmented with a Dacron tube graft is sutured in place (Fig. 88–9). To create a nonvalved connection, a trapdoor incision in the right atrial appendage is made, through which the ASD is closed, or an adjustable ASD placed.[76,107] The atrial flap created by the three-sided incision is then sutured to the right side of the ventricular incision, creating the posterior wall of the anastomosis. The anterior wall is completed with a pericardial or Dacron patch, allowing a generous anterior bulge to avoid obstruction. If pericardium is used it is first treated with 3% gluteraldehyde to increase strength.

The choice of a valved versus a nonvalved conduit

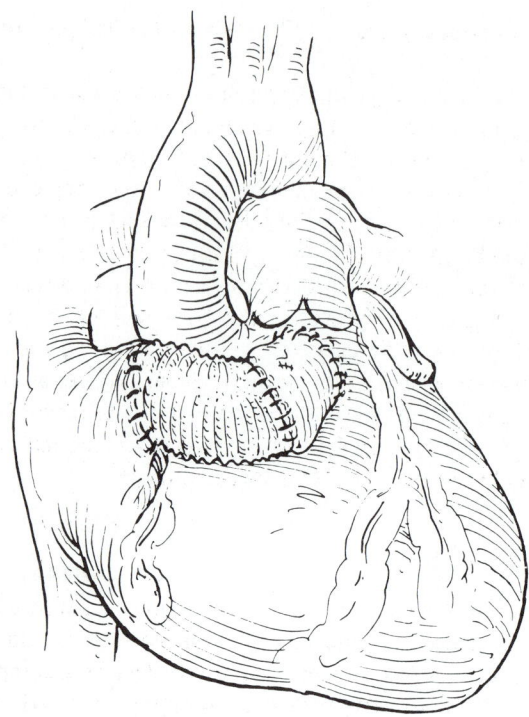

Figure 88–8. A right atrium to right ventricle Fontan utilizing a conduit composed of an aortic homograft with a Dacron tube extension.

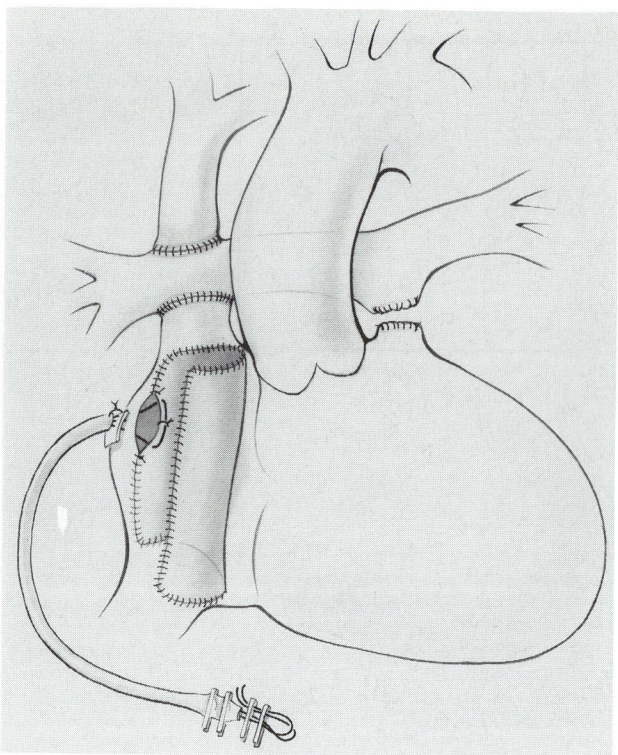

Figure 88–9. A total cavopulmonary connection (lateral tunnel Fontan) with an adjustable ASD. A tunnel of uniform caliber is created by suturing a piece of an 18-mm Gore-Tex tube graft or Gore-Tex cardiovascular patch to the orifice of the inferior and superior vena cavae and to the sinus venosus portion of the lateral atrial wall. The adjustable ASD is created by passing a #1 polypropylene suture through the lateral portion of the interatrial septum and secured to the edge of the Gore-Tex tunnel with a 5–0 polypropylene suture. The suture is then brought back out through the interatrial groove, through a pericardial pledget, and through a snare constructed of an 8F pediatric suction catheter. The snare is anchored to the heart by placing a suture through the end of the snare, through the pledget, and through the atrial wall.

versus a direct connection is not clear. It would seem that a valved connection would give more favorable hemodynamics, especially if significant ventricular contraction was present. However, use of valved conduits has been complicated with a significant incidence of conduit obstruction resulting in the need for reoperation. In one series,[51] there was a 17% incidence of reoperation for conduit obstruction for right atrial to right ventricular valved and nonvalved conduits, versus a 2% incidence for direct right atrial to right ventricular connections. The reoperative mortality for conduit replacement in this large series was 24%.

Total Cavopulmonary Connection (Lateral Tunnel Fontan)

Increased knowledge of post-Fontan physiology has demonstrated not only that the right ventricle is unnecessary in the Fontan circulation, but that the right atrium is unnecessary as well.[77,108] In detailed flow experiments, de Leval et al demonstrated increased turbulence associated with flow through a round chamber compared with a straight tube.[63] This turbulence resulted in decreased effective forward flow, and a pressure gradient. In a clinical model this would translate into a higher central venous pressure necessary to maintain pulmonary flow. Right atrial contraction has not been shown to be helpful, even when the right atrium is hypertrophied. In fact, contraction of the right atrium may be detrimental by creating more turbulence. Presently, direct right atrial to pulmonary artery con-

nections are done at our institution only in tricuspid atresia patients with small right atriums that preclude construction of a lateral tunnel.

Creation of a lateral tunnel Fontan is somewhat simplified from earlier techniques, and is applicable to almost any anatomic configuration. With the heart arrested, an oblique incision is made in the right atrium anterior to the crista terminalis. After excision of the medial portion of the atrial septum, a composite tunnel is created by suturing either a piece of 18-mm Gore-Tex (W.L. Gore & Associates, Flagstaff, AZ) tube graft or Gore-Tex Cardiovascular Patch around the orifices of the superior and inferior vena cavae and to the sinus venosus portion of the lateral atrial wall. We prefer the tube graft over the cardiovascular patch because it is thicker, stiffer, and easier to handle, and has a natural curve that creates a tubular-shaped tunnel (Fig. 88–10). The tunnel is fashioned to create a pathway of uniform size from the IVC to the SVC orifice.[77,100]

If an adjustable interatrial communication is to be in-

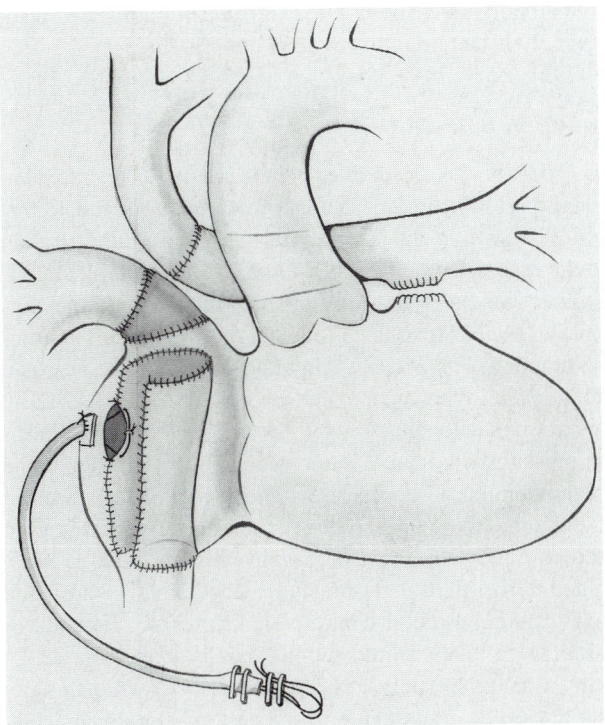

Figure 88–10. A unidirectional Fontan in which the IVC flow is directed entirely to the larger right lung, and the SVC flow to the relatively smaller left lung. An intra-atrial lateral tunnel is created in the usual fashion. An adjustable ASD is incorporated into the IVC tunnel, thus committing the full benefit of decompression entirely to the inferior vena cava system where lower venous pressures are more critical.

corporated, a 1 cm gap is left between the lateral atrial wall and the Gore-Tex patch with the suture lines ending at the inferior and superior edge of this defect. A #1 polypropylene suture is placed as a horizontal mattress stitch through the edge of the Gore-Tex patch at this site and brought out through the lateral atrial wall at the level of the interatrial groove. The suture is passed through a Silastic snare, which is anchored to the heart by a chromic stitch passed first through the edge of the snare, second through a pledget, and third through the lateral atrial wall. This prevents migration of the snare and allows for opening as well as closure of the interatrial defect.[76]

Following creation of the tunnel, the main pulmonary artery is transected and ligated. Pulmonary artery reconstruction is carried out if necessary. The superior vena cava is transected proximal to the cavoatrial junction and an end-to-side anastomosis is performed between the distal end of the SVC and the inferior aspect of the right pulmonary artery. The proximal end of the SVC is anastomosed to the superior aspect of the right pulmonary artery. To limit turbulence, these anastomoses are staggered so they are not entering the pulmonary artery directly opposite each other. If a unidirectional Fontan is to be performed, end-to-end anastomoses are performed directing the IVC to the right

pulmonary artery and the SVC toward the left pulmonary artery.

The total cavopulmonary connection, or lateral tunnel Fontan procedure, creates a streamlined pathway for pulmonary bloodflow. Although a slightly lower mean right atrial pressure has been demonstrated,[77] the incidence of postoperative pleural effusions has not been shown to be influenced by the lateral tunnel Fontan. The avoidance of extensive atrial suture lines decreases the extent of atrial scarring and fibrosis. This is a major advantage of the lateral tunnel Fontan and along with a lower atrial wall tension may be responsible for the lower incidence of late atrial arrhythmias and pacemaker requirements.[77] The reader is referred to several excellent discussions of the lateral tunnel Fontan for a more in-depth understanding.[63,77]

Partial Fontan

The partial Fontan operation refers to procedures in which some interatrial communication is allowed to remain following completion of what would otherwise be a complete Fontan procedure. It was devised to improve the early outcome of high risk Fontan patients.[76,79,80,99] We developed an adjustable ASD that allows for a restrictive interatrial communication that can be narrowed or closed postoperatively via a snaring device. The concept is based on retaining a right-to-left shunt that reduces right atrial pressure and improves LV filling and cardiac output while maintaining an acceptable oxygen saturation. Up to one-third of the venous return can be shunted through the interatrial communication while maintaining an oxygen saturation of around 85%, which should be well tolerated in a chronically cyanotic child. As the pulmonary vascular resistance drops and ventricular function improves, the communication can be narrowed or closed completely by means of a snare left under the linea alba. This adjustment can be done in the intensive care unit using local anesthesia. Concurrent echocardiography may be helpful to document changes in hemodynamics as well as to confirm complete closure of the shunt. The adjustable ASD is applied to all medium and high-risk candidates, in addition to being routinely used in any child less than 2 years of age (and usually most less than 4 years of age). It is also placed in children in whom the pulmonary vascular pressures and resistance are not known.

Since the introduction of the adjustable ASD in 1987, other techniques to achieve a similar effect have been devised.[78,109] Alternative techniques usually involve creation of single or multiple fenestrations in the interatrial baffle or lateral tunnel wall. These fenestrations require transcatheter closure with a clam shell device in the catheterization laboratory.[78,108] No provision for partial closure or adjustment is possible with this technique. With continued experience and documentation of the safety and benefits of the partial Fontan, its use has been liberalized and is currently applied to most Fontan patients at our institution. Although we favor the adjustable ASD due to the precise postoperative control it allows, the fenestration technique has also proven useful. Both techniques are associated with a lower central venous pressure, increased cardiac output, decreased fluid requirements, and a decreased incidence of pleural effusions. The need for a venous assist device has become rare since the introduction of the adjustable ASD.[110] The hemodynamic benefits of a partial Fontan and the changes accompanying the closure of the adjustable ASD or fenestration(s) have been documented in several recent studies.[111,112]

Unidirectional Fontan

The authors have begun utilizing a unidirectional approach to Fontan repair in which the superior vena cava is diverted solely to the left lung via an end-to-end Glenn anastomosis, and the inferior vena caval return is directed solely to the right lung. An adjustable ASD is always used in this modification (Fig. 88–11). This approach has several potential advantages compared to total cavopulmonary anastomosis. First, improved pulmonary bloodflow may occur due to better streaming and avoidance of turbulence. In addition, the larger portion of venous return (60%) is directed to the larger right lung, and the smaller portion of venous return from the superior vena cava to the smaller left lung. Presumably, improved V/Q matching would be obtained with such an approach. Furthermore, in high-risk patients with excessive postoperative venous pressures, superior vena caval hypertension is better tolerated than inferior vena caval hypertension, which can be relieved by means of a restrictive, adjustable interatrial communication placed in the interatrial tunnel. Thus the entire benefit of the right-to-left shunt can be applied to the inferior vena cava where lowering pressure is more critical. Finally, the Glenn shunt provides obligatory pulmonary bloodflow, which maintains arterial saturation despite the interatrial shunt (Fig. 88–11A and B).

A nuclear lung scan is performed preoperatively in these patients to determine the percent ventilation and perfusion to each lung. Potential disadvantages of this approach include the need to take down a preexistent bidirectional Glenn, which often requires reconstruction with pericardium or prosthetic material to connect the SVC to the left pulmonary artery. In addition, postoperative pulmonary complications such as pneumonia in the right lung could have a significant impact on oxygenation and inferior vena caval pressures. Further experience with this approach is necessary before determining whether its theoretical advantages significantly outweigh the potential difficulties. So far, our unidirectional Fontan experience in over 20 patients has been quite good with only one death. At completion of bypass, the mean SVC pressure has been 15.7 ± 3.5 mm Hg, and mean IVC pressure has been 10.3 ± 2.8 mm Hg with a mean sat of 93 ± 3%. Most of these patients were single ventricle diagnoses other than tricuspid atresia, but

this technique is easily applied to tricuspid atresia as well, especially if increased risk factors are present.

Postoperative Care

The goal of postoperative management is to maintain enough preload (central venous pressure) for adequate forward flow, while avoiding excessive fluid administration and the associated peripheral edema, ascites, and pleural effusions. This is best accomplished by keeping the pulmonary vascular resistance low and optimizing left ventricular function. Factors that stimulate pulmonary vasospasm such as pain, hypercapnea, and hypoxia are avoided. Early extubation is desirable to avoid the negative effects of positive pressure ventilation. Inotropic support with dopamine and dobutamine in doses of 5 µg/kg/per minute is used in the postoperative period. Intravenous nitroglycerin is used routinely, and other pulmonary vasodilators such as prostaglandin E$_1$ (PGE$_1$) or inhaled nitric oxide[113] are used when the right atrial or central venous pressure rises above 15 mm Hg. Fluid is administered liberally in the first 12–24 hours to maintain right atrial pressure. Following this period, once the patient has warmed and is hemodynamically stable, fluid administration is restricted and diuretics are used liberally. Careful attention is paid to indirect measures of cardiac output such as toe temperature, base deficit, and urine output, and appropriate intervention is carried out when these parameters change.

In patients with an adjustable ASD, narrowing may be required in the first 24 hours if excessive shunting occurs. The closure of the atrial septal defect or fenestration usually is accompanied by an increase in the right atrial pressure and a mild decrease in cardiac output. However, due to the increased oxygen saturation, oxygen delivery is unaffected.[109,111]

COMPLICATIONS

Pleural effusions in the early postoperative period require aggressive treatment. Repeated thoracentesis, chest tube placement and sclerosant therapy may be required. Previously, approximately 30% of patients developed pleural effusions persisting greater than 7–10 days. However, with the expanded use of the partial Fontan, the incidence of serious effusions has dropped to around 10–15%.[76,78] The volume of pleural drainage is also less in patients who have had a previous Glenn shunt, presumably because of a compensatory expansion of pleural lymphatic channels. Ascites and protein losing enteropathy are two additional abnormalities seen in some patients after the Fontan procedure. Generally effusion and ascites do not persist past 6 mo unless the patient remains with elevated CVP and in poor clinical condition. However, protein losing enteropathy and liver dysfunction may persist. Cronne-Dijkhus et al[96] looked at 66 Fontan patients (including 21 with tricuspid atresia) and

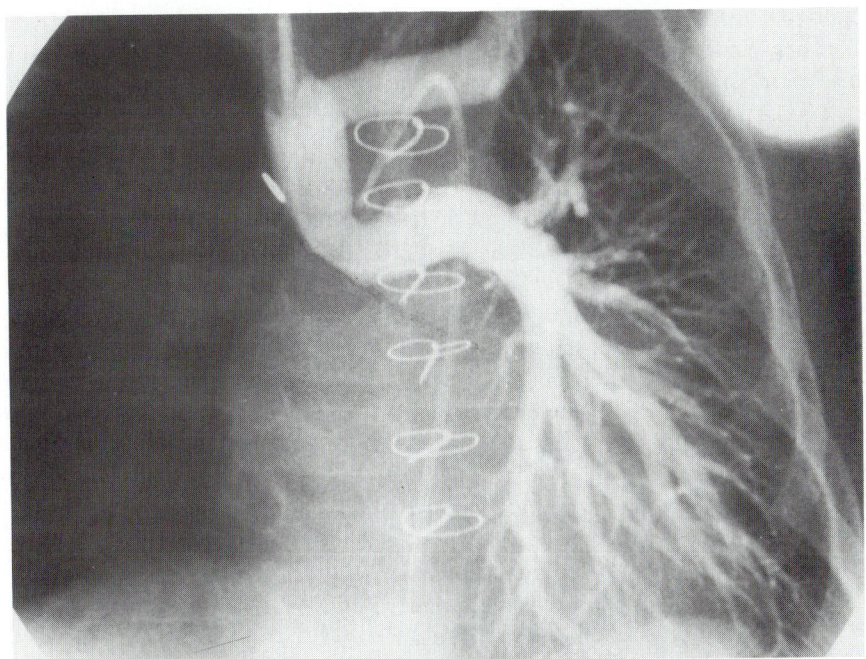

A

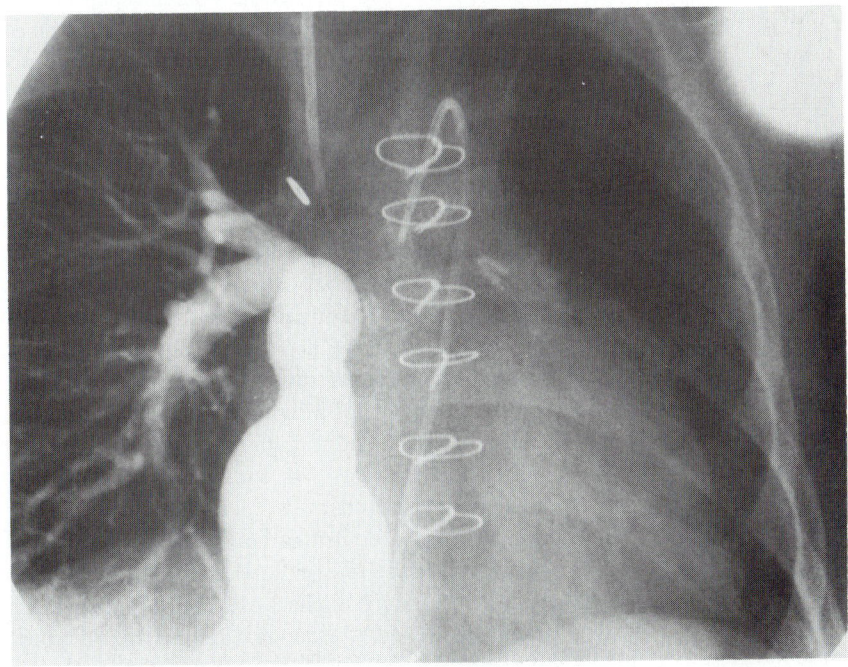

B

Figure 88–11. A,B. Postoperative angiogram following a unidirectional Fontan. The streamline flow pattern can be appreciated.

found that 61% had abnormal liver function tests and 41/66 (62%) had protein C deficiency despite good functional status in the majority of patients.

Arrhythmias

The incidence of atrial arrhythmias following the Fontan procedure is a serious concern, as synchronous left atrial contraction is vital.[114] A loss of atrial contraction or con-

traction against a closed mitral valve may increase the left atrial pressure and pulmonary venous pressure, and, hence, increase systemic venous pressures. This can result in a significant decrease in cardiac output secondary to inadequate flow across the pulmonary vascular bed. There is a bimodal distribution of atrial arrhythmias following Fontan repair.[46,77,96–98,113] Early postoperative arrhythmias are related to increased atrial pressures, fresh suture lines, and the general irritability of the myocardium following cardiopulmonary bypass with intracardiac repair. Porter reported a 15% incidence of in-hospital supraventricular tachycardia in 134 patients undergoing Fontan procedure for tricuspid atresia.[113]

The second phase occurs late and continues to increase over time. This is characterized by conduction delays as well as recalcitrant supraventricular arrhythmias. This phase is probably related to scarring at suture lines and chronic venous hypertension. While the method of repair does not appear to affect the incidence of early arrhythmias, the lateral tunnel technique is associated with a lower incidence of late arrhythmias and need for pacemakers.[77] In Porter's series,[114] the risk of supraventricular arrhythmias (SVT) in 120 hospital survivors was 25% at 5 years and 37% at 7.5 years. In those patients experiencing in-hospital SVT, the incidence of SVT after discharge was 66% by 5 years. This study was performed from 1973–1985, prior to the introduction of the lateral tunnel Fontan and the partial Fontan. Chen et al[97] reported a 35% incidence of supraventricular arrhythmias during a similar time period. This high incidence of supraventricular arrhythmias is somewhat discouraging as many of these are difficult to control medically, and can lead to late death. Perhaps, as early evidence supports,[76] the incidence of late arrhythmias will remain low with the lateral tunnel technique.

Late Outcome

In 1989, Fontan published an article entitled "Outcome after a 'Perfect' Fontan Operation" in which he stated: "The premature decline in survival and functional status and the late rise in hazard function are not from the Fontan state per se and that the Fontan operation is, therefore, palliative but not curative."[94] Whether this statement is accurate for all modifications of the Fontan procedure is certainly questionable, but clearly for patients in whom a "Perfect Fontan" operation is not performed, premature decline in survival and functional status can be expected.

In properly selected patients undergoing early Fontan repair with the newer modified technique, however, long-term survival and functional status are quite good.[45–48,75,115] In 28 Fontan patients followed 11–16 years, Mair et al[46] found that 50% were on no medication, 23/27 had excellent or good functional status, and 76% were employed full-time or were full-time students. In 42 patients evaluated by Gewillig et al[47] after the Fontan procedure, resting CI, SWI, and SBP were comparable to controls, but the increase in these parameters with exercise was blunted. When the 10 best performers were evaluated, however, no difference at any level of exercise was found compared with age matched controls.

It is clear that outcome may be quite variable.[116] Some patients may go on to lead completely normal lives with excellent functional capacity. In fact, successful pregnancies and deliveries have been reported in women after Fontan repair. Conversely, some patients will go on to develop pro-

gressive ventricular failure with a poor clinical outcome, arrhythmias, and sudden death. Some of these patients will require cardiac transplantation, which can improve overall longevity.[117,118]

CURRENT STATUS AND OUTCOME OF TRICUSPID ATRESIA

As mentioned, the prognosis for untreated tricuspid atresia is dismal with only 10% survival at 10 years. Surgical palliation has significantly improved the early and mid-term outcome of these patients, but has not provided a means for long-term survival with adequate functional status. Furthermore, repeated palliative procedures carry with them a significant and cumulative mortality, morbidity, and cost. In addition, a number of patients will die secondary to ventricular failure, arrhythmias, or other complications related to chronic cyanosis and volume overload prior to being referred for Fontan repair.

Experience has shown that for most patients, needless delays prior to Fontan repair negatively impact the overall long-term results for tricuspid atresia. Fontan repair can be safely undertaken in children over 1 year of age and is superior to additional palliative procedures in otherwise acceptable Fontan patients. In those not yet ready for a Fontan who require additional palliation, a bidirectional Glenn shunt has significant advantage over a second systemic-to-pulmonary artery shunt and can be safely performed after 6 mo of age.

Most tricuspid atresia patients do not have an adequate right ventricle for a right atrial to right ventricular connection, and the high incidence of conduit obstruction may outweigh the slight survival or functional advantage associated with a biventricular type of repair. Earlier Fontan repair may negate the advantage of a right ventricle by preserving left ventricular function and maintaining a low pulmonary vascular resistance. Only patients with a small right atrium are candidates for direct right atrial to pulmonary artery connection. With the documented advantages of the lateral tunnel Fontan, there is little indication for a direct right atrial to pulmonary artery connection. Early Fontan repair with a lateral tunnel and adjustable ASD provides the best means for improved long-term survival with a good functional status for patients with tricuspid atresia. The role of the unidirectional Fontan is still being evaluated.

REFERENCES

1. Vlad P: Tricuspid Atresia. In Keith JD, Rowe RD, Vlad P (eds): *Heart Disease in Infancy and Childhood,* 3rd ed. New York, Macmillan, 1978
2. Nadas AS, Fyler DC: *Pediatric Cardiology,* 3rd ed. Philadelphia, Saunders, 1972
3. Keith JD, Rower RD, Vlad P: *Heart Disease in Infancy and Childhood.* New York, Macmillan, 1967

4. Weinberg PM: Anatomy of tricuspid atresia and its relevance to current forms of surgical therapy. *Ann Thorac Surg* **29**:306, 1980

5. Van Praagh R: In Barratt-Boyes BG, Neutze JM, Harris EA (eds): *Heart Disease in Infancy. Diagnosis and Surgical Treatment.* London, Churchill Livingstone, 1973, p 246

6. Rosenquist GC, Levy RJ, Rower RD: Right atrial and left ventricular relationships in tricuspid atresia—position of the presumed site of the atretic valve as determined by transillumination. *Am Heart J* **80**:493, 1970

7. Thoele DG, Ursell PC, Ho SY, et al: Atrial morphologic features in tricuspid atresia. *J Thorac Cardiovasc Surg* **102**:606–610, 1991

8. Cliche P: Etude anatomique et clinique des atresies tricuspidiennes. *Arch Mal Coeur* **44**:981, 1952

9. Thomas HM: Congenital cardiac malformations. *Bull Int AM Museums* **21**:58, 1941

10. Ross CF: A case of tricuspid atresia with transposition of the great vessels. *Arch Dis Child* **27**:89, 1952

11. Fragoyannis S, Kardalinos A: Transposition of the great vessels, both arising from the left ventricle (juxtaposition of pulmonary artery). Tricuspid atresia, atrial septal defect and ventricular septal defect. *Am J Cardiol* **10**:601, 1962

12. Gewillig MH, Lundstrom UR, Deanfield JE, et al: Impact of Fontan operation on left ventricular size and contractility in tricuspid atresia. *Circulation* **81**:118–127, 1990

13. Akagi T, Benson LN, Green M, et al: Ventricular performance before and after repair for univentricular atrioventricular connection. Angiographic and radionuclide assessment. *J Am Coll Cardiol* **20**:920–926, 1992

14. Seleim M, Muster AJ, Paul MH, Benson W: Relation between preoperative left ventricular muscle mass and outcome of the Fontan procedure in patients with tricuspid atresia. *J Am Coll Cardiol* **14**:750–755, 1989

15. Sandor GS, Patterson MWH, LeBlanc JG: Systolic and diastolic function in tricuspid valve atresia before the Fontan operation. *Am J Cardiol* **73**:292–297, 1994

16. de Brux JL, Zannini L, Binet JP, et al: Tricuspid atresia: Results of treatment in 115 children. *J Thorac Cardiovasc Surg* **85**:440–446, 1983

17. Dick M, Fyler DC, Nadas AS: Tricuspid atresia: THe clinical course in 96 patients. *Am J Cardiol* **33**:135, 1974

18. Marcano BA, Riemenschneider TA, Ruttenberg HD, et al: Tricuspid atresia with increased pulmonary blood flow. Analysis of 13 cases. *Circulation* **40**:339, 1969

19. Gallagher ME, Fyler DC: Observations on changing hemodynamics in tricuspid atresia without associated transposition of the great vessels. *Circulation* **35**:381, 1967

20. Neches WH, Park SC, Lenox CC, et al: Tricuspid atresia with transposition of the great arteries and closing ventricular septal defect. Successful palliation by banding of the pulmonary artery and creation of an aorticopulmonary window. *J Thorac Cardiovasc Surg* **65**:538, 1973

21. Akagi T, Lee B, Williams WG, Freedom RM: Regional ventricular wall motion abnormalities in tricuspid atresia after the Fontan procedure. *J Am Coll Cardiol* **22**:1182–1188, 1993

22. Kirklin JK, Blackstone EH, Kirklin JW, et al. The Fontan operation. Ventricular hypertrophy, age, and date of operation as risk factors. *J Thorac Cardiovasc Surg* **92**:1049–1064, 1986

23. Caspi J, Coles JG, Rabionovich M, et al: Morphologic findings contributing to a failed Fontan procedure: Twelve-year experience. *Circulation* **82**(suppl IV):IV-177–IV-182, 1990

24. Paul MH: Tricuspid atresia. In Watson H (ed): *Pediatric Cardiology.* St Louis, Mosby, 1968

25. Gamboa R, Gersony NM, Nadas AS: The electrocardiogram in tricuspid atresia and pulmonary atresia with intact ventricular septum. *Circulation* **34**:24, 1966

26. Wittenborg MN, Neuhauser EBD, Spung WH: Roentgenographic findings in congenital tricuspid atresia with hypoplasia of the right ventricle. *AJR* **66**:712, 1951

27. Fletcher BD, Jaconstein MD, Abramowsky CR, et al: Right atrioventricular valve atresia: Anatomic evaluation with MR imaging. *AJR* **148**:671, 1987

28. Campbell M, Gardner FE: Radiological features of enlarged bronchial arteries. *Br Heart J* **12**:183, 1950

29. Cooley RN, Sloan RD, Hanlon CR, Bahnson HT: Angiocardiography in congenital heart disease of cyanotic type II. Observations on tricuspid stenosis or atresia with hypoplasia of the right ventricle. *Radiology* **54**:848, 1950

30. Campbell M, Hills TH: Angiocardiography in cyanotic congenital heart disease. *Br Heart J* **12**:650, 1950

31. Lacorte MA, Dick M, Scheer G, et al: Left ventricular function in tricuspid atresia. Angiographic analysis in 28 patients. *Circulation* **52**:996, 1975

32. Patel MM, Overy DC, Kozonis MC, et al: Long-term survival in tricuspid atresia. *J Am Coll Cardiol* **9**:338, 1987

33. Taussig HB, Keinonen R, Momberger N, Kirk H: Long-time observations on the Blalock-Taussig operation. IV. Tricuspid atresia. *Johns Hopkins Med J* **132**:135, 1973

34. Laks H, Williams W, Trusler G, et al: The subclavian arterioplasty for the ipsilateral subclavian to pulmonary artery shunt. *Circulation* **60**(suppl 2):115, 1979

35. Cleveland DC, Kirklin JK, Naftel DC, et al: Surgical treatment of tricuspid atresia. *Ann Thorac Surg* **38**(5):447–457, 1984

36. Fesslova V, Hunter S, Stark J, Taylor JFN: The long-term clinical outcome of patients with tricuspid atresia. *J Cardiovasc Surg* **32**:225–232, 1991

37. Tam CK, Lightfoot NE, Finlay CD, et al: Course of tricuspid atresia in the Fontan era. *Am J Cardiol* **63**:589–593, 1989

38. Glenn WWL, Patino JF: Circulatory bypass of the right heart. I. Preliminary observations on the direct delivery of vena caval blood into the pulmonary arterial circulation. Azygous vein-pulmonary artery shunt. *Yale J Biol Med* **27**:147, 1954

39. Nuland SB, Glenn WWL, Guilfoil PH: Circulatory bypass of the right heart. III. Some observations on the long term survivors. *Surgery* **43**:184, 1958

40. Glenn WWL: Circulatory bypass of the right side of the heart IV. Shunt between the superior vena cava and distal right pulmonary artery. Report of clinical application. *N Engl J Med* **259**:117, 1958

41. Glenn WWL, Brown M, Whittemore R: Circulatory bypass of the right side of the heart. Cavo-pulmonary artery shunt—Indications and results: Report of a collected series of 537 cases. In Cassels DE (ed): *The Heart and Circulation in the Newborn and Infant.* New York, Grune & Stratton, 1966, p 345

42. Fontan F, Baudet E: Surgical repair of tricuspid atresia. *Thorax* **36**:240, 1971

43. Kreutzer G, Galindez E, Bono H, et al: An operation for the correction of tricuspid atresia. *J Thorac Cardiovasc Surg* **66**:613, 1973

44. Humes RA, Porter CJ, Mair DD, et al: Intermediate follow-up and predicted survival after the modified Fontan procedure for tricuspid atresia and double-inlet ventricle. *Circulation* **76**(supplIII):III67–III71, 1987

45. Driscoll DJ, Offord KP, Feldt RH, et al: Five-to-fifteen year follow-up after Fontan operation. *Circulation* **85**:469–496, 1992

46. Mair DD, Puga FJ, Danielson GK: Late functional status of survivors of the Fontan procedure performed during the 1970's. *Circulation* **86**(suppl II):II-106–II-109, 1992

47. Gewillig MH, Lundstrom UR, Bull C, et al: Exercise responses in patients with congenital heart disease after Fontan repair. Patterns and determinants of performance. *J Am Coll Cardiol* **15**:1424–1432, 1990

48. Fontan F, Deville C, Quaegebeur J, et al: Repair of tricuspid atresia in 100 patients. *J Thorac Cardiovasc Surg* **85**:647–660, 1983

49. Rashkind W, Waldhausen J, Miller W, Freidman S: Palliative treatment in tricuspid atresia. Combined balloon atrioseptostomy and surgical alteration of pulmonary blood flow. *J Thorac Cardiovasc Surg* **57**:812, 1969

50. Lenox CC, Zuberbuhler JR: Balloon septostomy in tricuspid atresia after infancy. *Am J Cardiol* **25:**723, 1970

51. Fernandez G, Costa F, Fontan F, et al: Prevalence of reoperation for pathway obstruction after Fontan operation. *Ann Thorac Surg* **48:**654–659, 1989

52. Franklin RCG, Spiegelhalter DJ, Sullivan ID, et al: Tricuspid atresia presenting in infancy. Survival and suitability for the Fontan operation. *Circulation* **87:**427–439, 1993

53. Trusler GA, Williams WG: Long-term results of shunt procedures for tricuspid atresia. *Ann Thorac Surg* **29:**213, 1980

54. Trusler GA, Williams WG: Long-term results of shunt procedures for tricuspid atresia. *Ann Thorac Surg* **29:**312–316, 1980

55. Blalock A, Hanlon CR: The surgical treatment of transposition of the aorta and pulmonary artery. *Surg Gynecol Obstet* **90:**1, 1950

56. Hallman GL, Stasney CR, Cooley DA: Surgical treatment of tricuspid atresia. *J Cardiovasc Surg* **9:**154, 1968

57. Deverall PB, Lincoln JCR, Aberdeen E, et al: Surgical management of tricuspid atresia. *Thorax* **24:**239, 1969

58. Edmunds LH Jr, Fishman NH, Heymann MA, Rudolph AM: Anastomosis between aorta and right pulmonary artery (Waterston) in neonates. *N Engl J Med* **284:**464, 1971

59. Lamberti JJ, Carlisle J, Waldman JD, et al: Systemic-pulmonary shunts in infants and children. Early and late results. *J Thorac Cardiovasc Surg* **88:**76–81, 1984

60. Lamberti JL, Spicer RL, Waldman JD, et al: The bidirectional cavopulmonary shunt. *JTCVS* **100:**22–30, 1990

61. Somerville J, Yacoub M, Ross DN, Ross K: Aorta to right pulmonary artery anastomosis (Waterston's operation) for cyanotic congenital heart disease. *Circulation* **39:**593, 1969

62. Di Carlo D, Williams WG, Freedom RM, et al: The role of cava-pulmonary (Glenn) anastomosis in the palliative treatment of congenital heart disease. *J Thorac Cardiovasc Surg* **83:**437–442, 1982

63. de Leval MR, Kilner P, Gewillig M, Bull C: Total cavopulmonary connection: A logical alternative to atriopulmonary connection for complex Fontan operations. *J Thorac Cardiovasc Surg* **96:**682–695, 1988

64. Laks H, Mudd JG, Standeven JW, et al: Long-term effect of the superior vena cava-pulmonary aratery anastomosis on pulmonary blood flow. *J Thorac Cardiovasc Surg* **74:**253, 1977

65. Mazzera E, Corno A, Picardo S, et al: Bidirectional cavopulmonary shunts: Clinical applications as staged or definitive palliation. *Ann Thorac Surg* **47:**415–420, 1989

66. Mather M, Glenn WWL: Long-term evaluation of cava-pulmonary artery anastomosis. *Surg* **74:**899, 1973

67. Ishikawa T, Neutze JM, Brandt PW, Barratt-Boyes BG: Hemodynamics following the Kreutzer procedure for tricuspid atresia in patients under two years of age. *J Thorac Cardiovasc Surg* **88:**373–379, 1984

68. Cheung HC, Lincoln C, Anderson RH, et al: Options for surgical repair in hearts with univentricular atrioventricular connection and subaortic stenosis. *J Thorac Cardiovasc Surg* **100:**672–681, 1990

69. Gates RN, Laks H, Elami A, et al: Damus-Stansel-Kaye procedure: Current indications and results. *Ann Thorac Surg* **56:**111–119, 1993

70. Bargeron LM Jr, Karp RB, Barcia A. Late deterioration of patients after superior vena cava-right pulmonary artery anastomosis. *J Thorac Cardiovasc Surg* **60:**531–539, 1970

71. Williams WG, Rubis L, Fowler RS, et al: Tricuspid atresia (results of palliation in 160 children). *Am J Cardiol* **38:**235–240, 1976

72. Martin SP, Anabtawi IN, Selmonosky CA, et al: Long-term followup after superior vena cava-right pulmonary artery anastomosis. *Ann Thorac Surg* **9:**339–346, 1970

73. McFaul RC, Tajik AJ, Mair DD, et al: Development of pulmonary arteriovenous shunt after superior vena cava-right pulmonary artery (Glenn) anastomosis. *Circulation* **54**(suppl 2):101, 1976

74. Mietus-Snyder M, Lang P, Mayer JE, et al: Childhood systemic-pulmonary shunts: Subsequent suitability for Fontan operation. *Circulation* **76**(suppl III):III–39, 1987

75. Pearl JM, Laks H, Drinkwater DC, et al: Modified Fontan procedure in patients less than 4 years of age. *Circulation* **86**(suppl II):II-100–II-105, 1992

76. Laks H, Pearl JM, Haas GS, et al: Partial Fontan: Advantages of an adjustable interatrial communication. *Ann Thorac Surg* **52:**1084–1095, 1991

77. Pearl RM, Laks H, Stein DG, et al: Total cavopulmonary anastomosis versus conventional modified Fontan procedure. *Ann Thorac Surg* **52:**189–196, 1991

78. Bridges ND, Lock JE, Castaneda AR: Baffle fenestration with subsequent transcatheter closure: Modifications of the Fontan operation for patients at increased risk. *Circulation* **82:**1681–1689, 1990

79. Laks H, Haas GS, Pearl JM, et al: The use of an adjustable interatrial communication in patients undergoing Fontan and other definitive right heart procedures. *Circulation* **78**(suppl 2):II–357, 1987

80. Laks H, Pearl J, Wu A, et al: Experience with the Fontan procedure including use of an adjustable intraatrial communication. In *Perspectives in Pediatric Cardiology: Pediatric Cardiac Surgery,* Part 2. New York, Futura, 1989

81. Stellin G, Mazzucco A, Bortolotti U, et al: Tricuspid atresia versus other complex lesions: Comparison of results with a modified Fontan procedure. *J Thorac Cardiovasc Surg* **96:**204–211, 1988

82. Choussat A, Fontan F, Besse P, et al: Selection criteria for Fontan's procedure. In Anderson RH, Shinebourne EA (eds): *Paediatric Cardiology* 1977, Edinburgh, Churchill Livingstone, 1978, pp 559–566

83. Mayer JE, Helgason H, Jonas RA, et al: Extending the limits for modified Fontan procedures. *J Thorac Cardiovasc Surg* **92:**1021–1028, 1986

84. Abrams LD: Side-to-side cavo-pulmonary anastomosis for the palliation of primitive ventricle (abstract). *Br Heart J* **39:**926, 1977

85. Shemin RJ, Merrill WH, Pfeifer JS, et al: Evaluation of right atrial-pulmonary artery conduits for tricuspid atresia. *J Thorac Cardiovasc Surg* **77:**685–690, 1979

86. Mair DD, Rice JM, Hagler DJ, et al: Outcome of the Fontan procedure in patients with tricuspid atresia. *Circulation* **72**(supp II):88–92, 1985

87. Myers JL, Waldhausen JA, Weber HS, et al: A reconsideration of risk factors for the Fontan operation. *Ann Surg* **221**(6):738–744, 1990

88. Fontan F, Fernandez G, Costa F, et al: The size of the pulmonary arteries and the results of the Fontan operation. *J Thorac Cardiovasc Surg* **98:**711–724, 1989

89. Mair DD, Hagler DJ, Puga FJ, et al: Fontan operation in 176 patients with tricuspid atresia. Results and a proposed new index for patient selection. *Circulation* **82**(suppl IV):IV-164–IV-169, 1990

90. Bartmus DA, Driscoll DJ, Offord KP, et al: The modified Fontan operation for children less than 4 years old. *J Am Coll Cardiol* **15**(2):429–435, 1990

91. Nakazawa M, Nakanishi T, Okuda H, et al: Dynamics of right heart flow in patients after Fontan procedure. *Circulation* **69:**306–312, 1984

92. Humes RA, Mair DD, Porter CBJ, et al: Results of the modified Fontan operation in adults. *Am J Cardiol* **61:**602–604, 1988

93. Fontan F, Kirklin JW, Fernandez G, et al: Outcome after a "perfect" Fontan operation. *Circulation* **81:**1520–1536, 1990

94. Jones M, Ferrans VJ: Myocardial degeneration in congenital heart disease: Comparisons of morphological findings in young and old patients with congenital heart disease associated with muscular obstruction to the right ventricular outflow. *Am J Cardiol* **39:**1051–1063, 1977

95. Parikh SR, Hurwitz RA, Caldwell RL, Girod DA: Ventricular function in the single ventricle before and after Fontan surgery. *Am J Cardiol* **67:**1390–1395, 1991

96. Cromme-Dijkhuis AH, Hess J, Hahlen K, et al: Specific sequelae after Fontan operation at mid- and long-term followup. Arrhythmia, liver dysfunction, and coagulation disorders. *J Thorac Cardiovasc Surg* **106:**1126–1132, 1993

97. Chen S, Nouri S, Pennington DG: Dysrhythmias after the modified Fontan procedure. *Pediatr Cardiol* **9:**215–219, 1988

98. Weber HS, Hellenbrand WE, Kleinman CS, et al: Predictors of rhythm disturbances and subsequent morbidity after the Fontan operation. *Am J Cardiol* **64:**762–767, 1989

99. Haas G, Laks H, Pearl JM: Modified Fontan procedure. In *Advances in Cardiac Surgery.*

100. Pearl JM, Laks H: Current status of the modified Fontan procedure. *1990–91 Annual of Cardiac Surgery,* Vol 1. Chicago, Year Book Medical Publishers, 1990

101. Coles JG, Leung M, Kielmanowicz, et al: Repair of tricuspid atresia: Utility of right ventricular incorporation. *Ann Thorac Surg* **45:**384–389, 1988

102. Kurosawa H, Imai Y, Fukuchi S, et al: Septation and Fontan repair of univentricular atrioventricular connection. *J Thorac Cardiovasc Surg* **99:**314–319, 1990

103. Bowman FO, Malm JR, Hayes CJ, et al: Physiologic approach to surgery for tricuspid atresia. *Circulation* **58**(suppl 1):2978, 1978

104. Otternkamp J, Rohmer J, Quaegebeur JM, et al: Nine years experience of physiologic correction of tricuspid atresia: Long-term results and current surgical approach. *Thorax* **37:**718, 1982

105. Bull C, de Leval MR, Stark, et al: Use of a subpulmonic ventricular chamber in the Fontan circulation. *J Thorac Cardiovasc Surg* **85:**21, 1983

106. Kirklin JW, Barratt-Boyes BG: Tricuspid atresia. In *Cardiac Surgery.* New York, John Wiley, 1993

107. Laks H, Pearl JM, Wu A, et al: Experience with the Fontan procedure including the use of the adjustable interatrial communication. In Crupi G, Parenzan L, Anderson RH (eds): *Perspectives in Pediatric Cardiac Surgery.* Mt. Kisco, NY, Futura, 1989

108. Stein DG, Laks H, Drinkwater DC, et al: Results of total cavopulmonary connection in the treatment of patients with a functional single ventricle. *J Thorac Cardiovasc Surg* **102:**280–287, 1991

109. Kopf GS, Kleinman CS, Hijazi ZM, et al: Fenestrated Fontan operation with delayed transcatheter closure of atrial septal defect: Improved results in high-risk patients. *J Thorac Cardiovasc Surg* **103:**1039–1048, 1992

110. Milliken JC, Laks H, George B: Use of a venous assist device after repair of complex lesions of the right heart. *J Am Coll Cardiol* **8:**922, 1986

111. Hijazi ZM, Fahey JT, Kleinman CS, et al: Hemodynamic evaluation before and after closure of fenestrated Fontan: An acute study of changes in oxygen delivery. *Circulation* **86:**196–202, 1992

112. Harake B, Elami A, Pearl J, et al: Hemodynamic effects of closure of the adjustable interatrial communication after the Fontan procedure. *J Am Coll Cardiol* **23:**1671–1676, 1994

113. Roberts JD, Lang P, Bigatello LM, et al: Inhaled nitric oxide in congenital heart disease. *Circulation* **87:**447–453, 1993

114. Porter J, Garson A: Incidence and management of dysrhythmias after Fontan procedure. *Herz* **18:**318–327, 1993

115. Parikh SR, Hurwitz RA, Caldwell RL, Girod DA: Ventricular function in the single ventricle before and after Fontan surgery. *Am J Cardiol* **67:**1390–1395, 1991

116. Sanders SP, Wright GB, Keane JF, et al: Clinical and hemodynamic results of the Fontan operation for tricuspid atresia. *Am J Cardiol* **49:**1733–1740, 1982

117. Menkis AH, McKenzie FN, Novick RJ, et al: Special considerations for heart transplantation in congenital heart disease. *J Heart Transplant* **9:**602–607, 1990

118. Pearl JM, Laks H, Drinkwater DC: Cardiac transplantation following the modified Fontan procedure. *Transplant Sci* **1:**1–3, 1992

Ebstein's Anomaly

Gordon K. Danielson

The rare malformation of the tricuspid valve that was first described by Ebstein in 1866[1] is characterized by a deformity of the valve leaflets with a coexisting malformation of the ventricle and usually, but not always, by displacement of the septal and posterior leaflets to a position below the annulus fibrosus (Fig. 89–1).[2,3] These leaflets are thickened, shortened, and adherent to the wall of the ventricle. Their downward displacement reduces the distal chamber of the right ventricle, leaving a portion of the ventricle above the valve as an integral part of the right atrium (atrialized ventricle). The entire wall of the right ventricle, both proximal and distal to the abnormal insertion of the tricuspid leaflets and including the infundibulum, is dilated. Morphometric histopathologic studies demonstrate that dilatation of the right ventricle is associated not only with thinning of the wall, but also with an absolute decrease in the number of myocardial fibers.[4]

The anterior leaflet in Ebstein's anomaly is usually large and billowy; attached to the annulus fibrosus, and fused to the posterior and septal leaflets, it may extend in "basket" fashion into the right ventricle. There it is secured, as are the other leaflets, by short chordae tendineae and papillary muscles, many of which are abnormal in number and position. The leaflets may be fenestrated, partially fused to the underlying endocardium (failure of delamination), or absent (especially the posterior leaflet). The malformed tricuspid valve is usually incompetent, but may occasionally be stenotic or, rarely, imperforate. Frequently, there are associated anomalies.[3]

The atrioventricular (A-V) conduction system is normally situated, beginning in the A-V node, penetrating the membranous septum, and dividing into right and left bundle branches in the usual manner. The right bundle typically courses beneath the dysplastic and displaced septal leaflet which attaches on its left side to the annulus near the membranous septum and descends on the septum rightward and toward the apex.

Left-sided Ebstein's anomaly is a common finding in patients having A-V discordance with ventriculoarterial discordance (corrected transposition).[5] In this condition, the nature of the displacement of the septal and posterior leaflets is similar to that in right-sided Ebstein's anomaly; however, the anterior leaflet is smaller and anatomically quite different. There is less thinning of the wall of the atrialized ventricle, and rarely is the functional portion of the morphologically right ventricle dilated. The atrioventricular conduction tissue in corrected transposition is right-sided and anterior, well removed from the left-sided tricuspid valve.[6]

The functional impairment of the right ventricle and the incompetence of the deformed valve retard blood flow from the right atrium.[7] Moreover, during contraction of the atrium, the atrialized portion of the right ventricle is in diastole and may balloon out, taking up a portion of the blood volume to be ejected. During ventricular systole, this ballooned section contracts, creating a pressure wave in the otherwise relaxed right atrium. In most cases, the atrial septum is deficient owing to patency or fenestration of the foramen ovale or to a separate atrial defect. The movement of blood through the septal opening is predominantly from right to left, but may be bidirectional or exclusively left to right. The overall effect of these structural abnormalities upon the right atrium is gross dilatation, which frequently reaches enormous proportions. This dilatation begets further incompetence of the tricuspid valve and further widening of the interatrial communication.

Ebstein's anomaly occurs in about 1 in every 210,000 births, accounts for less than 1% of all congenital heart disease, and is evenly distributed between the sexes. The life expectancy of affected persons is usually severely limited,

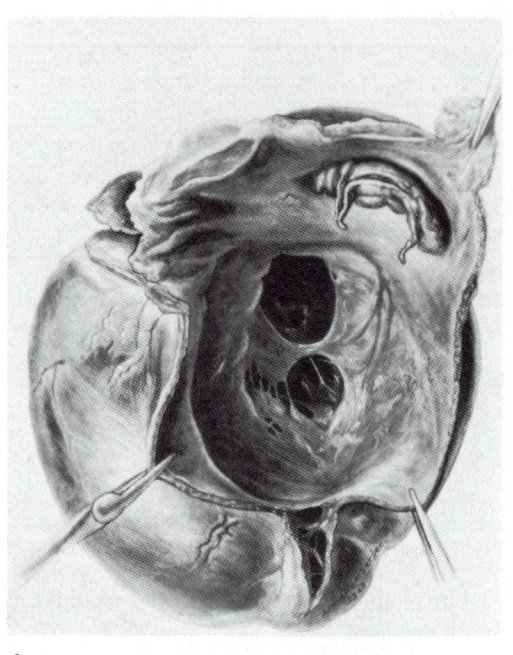

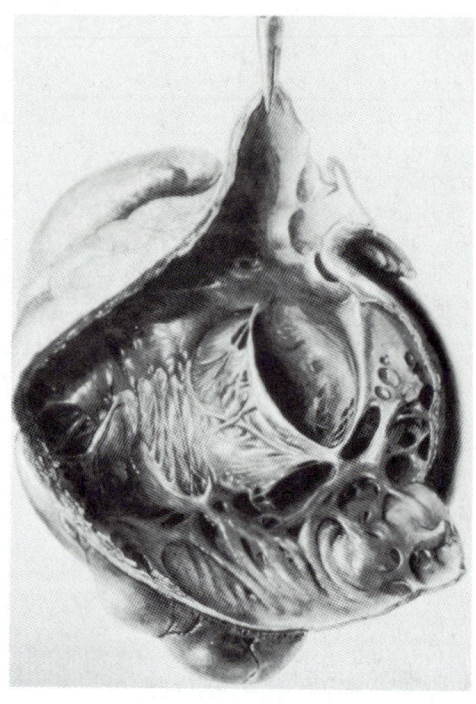

A   **B**

Figure 89–1. Ebstein's malformation with a widely patent foramen ovale in a 16-year-old male. **A.** Atrial surface of an anomalous and fenestrated tricuspid valve. Displacement of the ring posteriorly toward the apex. **B.** Ventricular surface of the anomalous and defective tricuspid valve. Bizarre papillary muscle attachments to all parts of the ventricular wall. *(From Krongrad E, Malm JR, Bowman FO Jr: J Thorac Cardiovasc Surg 67:875, 1974, with permission.)*

although rare patients reach advanced age.[8] The most common causes of death are congestive heart failure, hypoxia, and cardiac arrhythmias. When the diagnosis of Ebstein's anomaly is made in infancy, the prognosis is worse; from one third to one half of all patients will die before 2 years of age.[9,10] Intrauterine (fetal) diagnosis of Ebstein's anomaly carries an appalling outlook, as 1-year survival is only 15%.[11]

DIAGNOSIS

Clinical Features

Because of the broad spectrum of pathologic changes in Ebstein's anomaly, the hemodynamic alteration is variable. Symptoms are related to the severity of the incompetence of the tricuspid valve, the presence or absence of an associated atrial septal defect, and the impairment of right ventricular function.

In the early neonatal period, any tricuspid incompetence is accentuated by the normally increased pulmonary arteriolar resistance at this time, and infants with a severe valve deformity may present very early with congestive heart failure. Because the foramen ovale is patent in early infancy, severe tricuspid incompetence, with its resultant elevation in right atrial pressure, will produce a right-to-left atrial-level shunt, and such infants may be markedly cyan-

otic. If the infant survives this critical period, the degree of cyanosis and the symptoms will often diminish as the pulmonary arterioles gradually involute from the fetal state and pulmonary resistance decreases.

In patients beyond infancy, the predominant symptoms of Ebstein's anomaly are fatigability, dyspnea on exertion, and cyanosis. Peripheral edema and palpitations, in the form of paroxysmal atrial arrhythmias and premature ventricular beats, are less frequent.

Accessory conduction pathways were present in 14.8% of patients in our surgical series, and such pathways may be responsible for paroxysmal supraventricular tachycardia or paroxysmal atrial fibrillation at any age.

In an experience with 67 patients who had a mean follow-up of 12 years, Giuliani[10] found that 39% remained in functional Class I or II, and 61% progressed at some time into Class III or IV. Death occurred in 21% of the patients, and these were characterized by one or more of the following features: (1) they were in functional Class III or IV, (2) the cardiothoracic ratio was greater than 0.65, (3) they had cyanosis or an arterial oxygen saturation of less than 90%, or (4) they were infants when the diagnosis was made.

Physical Signs

The heart sounds in cases of Ebstein's anomaly are usually soft, and there is often a multiplicity of sounds and murmurs, all originating from the right heart. A systolic murmur of tricuspid regurgitation is heard along the left sternal border. Frequently, there are also diastolic and presystolic murmurs of low intensity, which are due to anatomic or functional tricuspid stenosis. These murmurs all become louder with inspiration. The first and second heart sounds are widely split. Both atrial and ventricular filling sounds are relatively common and contribute to the cadence quality that is so often heard in patients with Ebstein's anomaly. Because of frequent prolongation of atrioventricular conduction, there is often summation of these gallop sounds.

The arterial and jugular venous pulse forms are usually normal. A large V wave can sometimes be seen in the jugular venous pulse, but usually this is not prominent. The liver may be palpably enlarged, but is almost never pulsatile.

Electrocardiography

The electrocardiogram typically indicates right complete or incomplete bundle branch block and right axis deviation. The P waves are large and the R waves in leads V_1–V_4 are small. Often the P-R interval is prolonged and the QRS complex is slurred. Arrhythmias are common. Ventricular pre-excitation via accessory conduction pathways (Wolff–Parkinson–White syndrome) is usually of the right ventricular free-wall type, sometimes combined with a second pathway in the posterior septum.

Roentgenography

The cardiac silhouette in Ebstein's anomaly may vary from near normal to a configuration that is typical for this disease. The typical contour consists of a globular-shaped heart with a narrow waist similar to that seen in cases of pericardial effusion. This appearance is produced by enlargement of the right atrium and displacement of the right ventricular outflow tract outwards and upwards. Vascularity of the pulmonary fields is either normal or decreased (Fig. 89–2A).

Angiography

Injection of contrast medium into the right atrium demonstrates enlargement of this chamber, but with the tricuspid annulus located in its normal position. An impression ("notch") on the inferior wall of the right ventricle may be seen some distance to the left of the tricuspid annulus; this represents the site of origin of the displaced leaflets of the tricuspid valve (Fig. 89–2B). The leaflets sometimes appear as lines within the body of the right ventricle, the functioning portion of which is displaced laterally and superiorly. In cineangiograms, there may be shunting of contrast medium back and forth between the right atrium and the atrialized portion of the right ventricle. Right-to-left or left-to-right shunting at the atrial level may be found in the presence of

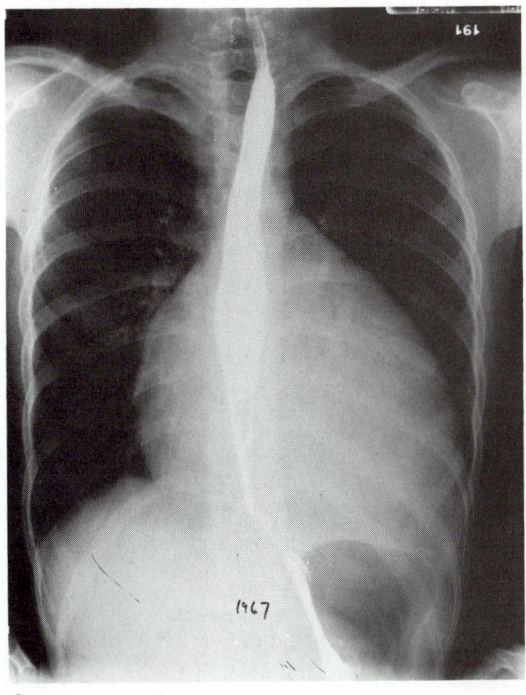 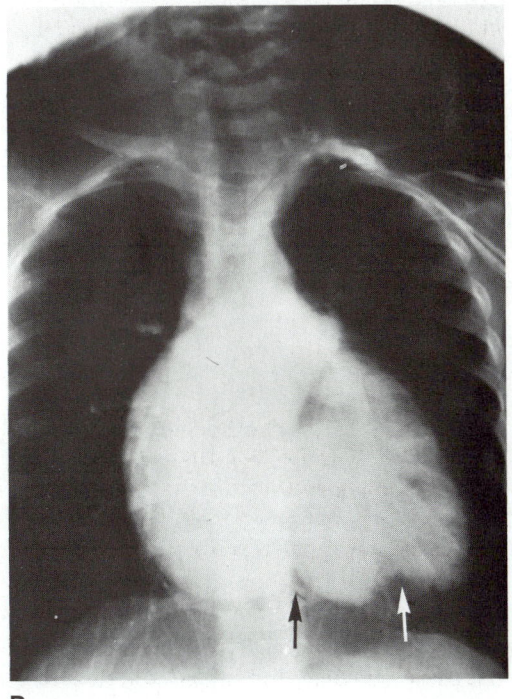

A   B

Figure 89–2. **A.** Plain films reveal marked cardiomegaly with prominence of the right atrium and the right ventricular outflow tract in this patient with Ebstein's malformation of the tricuspid valve. Vascularity is decreased. **B.** Angiography with injection in the left antecubital vein reveals marked enlargement of the right atrium. The tricuspid annulus is indicated by the black arrow. An indentation in the floor of the right ventricle (*white arrow*) indicates the position of attachment of the displaced leaflets of the tricuspid valve.

an atrial septal defect or foramen ovale. Blood flow through the lungs is usually slow.

Cardiac Catheterization

In the majority of patients with Ebstein's anomaly, the right atrial pressure is found to be moderately elevated and the pulse contour most often shows a dominant V wave with a steep Y descent. However, in patients with a markedly dilated right atrium, the atrial pressure pulse may be normal despite the presence of severe tricuspid incompetence. The right ventricular pressure is most often normal, although the end-diastolic pressure may be elevated. The pulmonary artery pressure is normal or decreased. In patients with an associated atrial septal defect and a right-to-left shunt, oximetry will demonstrate systemic arterial desaturation, and intracardiac dye dilution curves from the venae cavae will show the shunt. In some cases, there is an additional or exclusive left-to-right shunt through an atrial septal defect; this will also be shown by oximetry and dye dilution curves.

Echocardiography

The M-mode echocardiogram is abnormal. The most reliable single criterion is the relationship of mitral valve closure to tricuspid valve closure.[10]

Two-dimensional ultrasonic imaging of the heart has become the definitive method for diagnosis of Ebstein's anomaly (Fig. 89–3). Cardiac catheterization is rarely done today unless associated lesions are present or a previous shunt has been performed. Two-dimensional echocardiography allows accurate evaluation of the anatomic relationships of the tricuspid leaflets to the right heart, the size of the right atrium including the atrialized portion of the right ventricle, and the size and function of the right ventricle. It also gives us the best method for assessing which patients will be amenable to a valve reconstruction procedure and which will require tricuspid valve replacement.[12]

Doppler echocardiography and color flow imaging effectively establish the presence of an atrial septal defect and the direction of shunt flow. In addition, color flow imaging allows excellent assessment of the site and degree of tricuspid valve regurgitation.[13]

TREATMENT

Medical management succeeds in keeping about 50% of patients born with Ebstein's anomaly alive to the age of 13. The prognosis is poorest in those who have congestive heart failure, marked cyanosis, associated cardiac anomalies, extreme cardiomegaly (cardiothoracic ratio greater than 0.65),

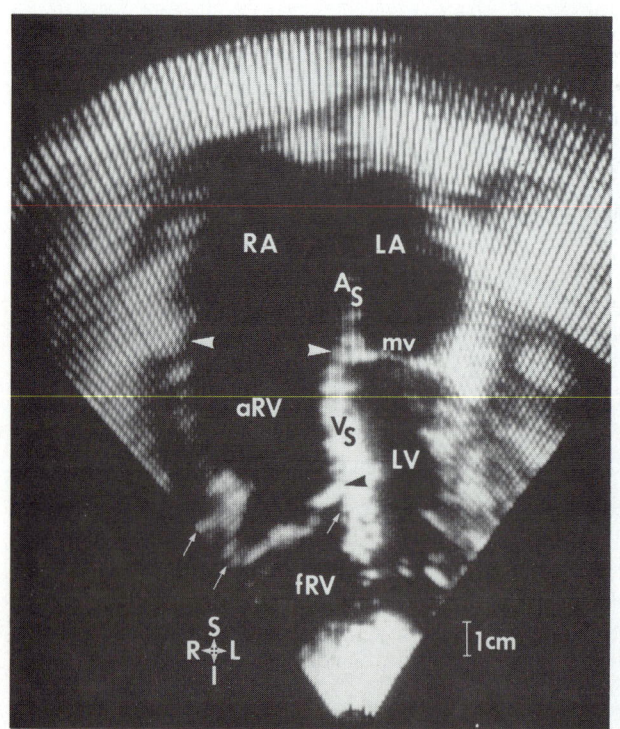

A

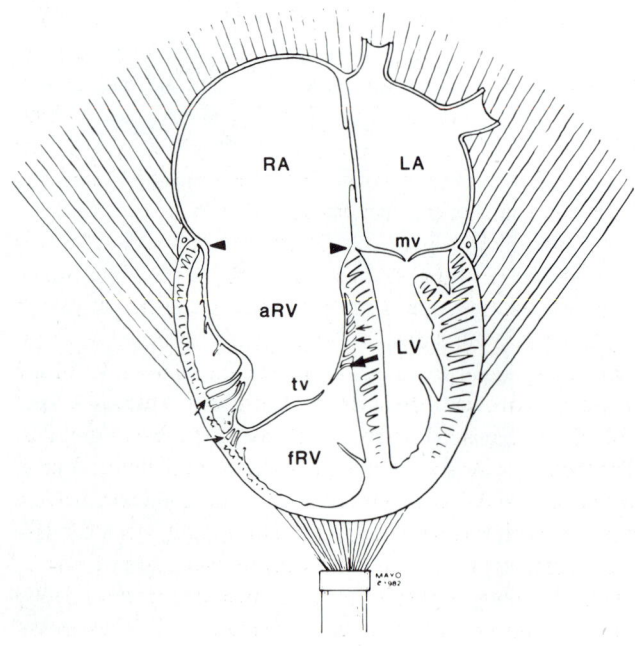

B

Figure 89–3. Two-dimensional echocardiogram (four-chamber view) and interpretive diagram, showing features typical of Ebstein's anomaly. RA, right atrium; LA, left atrium, mv, mitral valve; LV, left ventricle; fRV, functional right ventricle; tv, tricuspid valve; aRV, atrialized right ventricle; A_s, atrial septum; V_s, ventricular septum; arrows, tethering of leaflets. *(Reprinted with permission from the American College of Cardiology. Shiina A, Seward JB, Edwards WD, et al: Two-dimensional echocardiographic spectrum of Ebstein's anomaly: Detailed anatomic assessment. Journal of the American College of Cardiology, 1984, 3:356-370.)*

and diagnosis of the condition in infancy.[9,10] Serious cardiac arrhythmias without congestive failure or hypoxemia may also be life threatening.

Medical management alone is advised for only mildly symptomatic pediatric patients. Those patients who have survived infancy generally do well for a number of years, and correction can thus be postponed in such cases until deterioration is evident. However, since all patients with Ebstein's anomaly will ultimately show progressive deterioration, all will sooner or later become possible candidates for surgical correction.

The surgical management of Ebstein's anomaly has evolved during the past three decades. In the 1950s, palliative procedures were tried. For those patients with obstruction of blood flow through the right heart caused by pulmonary valvular or subvalvular stenosis or a stenotic or imperforate tricuspid valve, a systemic-pulmonary shunt in infancy may be lifesaving. In the absence of obstructing lesions, systemic-pulmonary shunts have usually not benefited patients or have ended fatally. A superior vena cava-pulmonary artery shunt was proposed as a more physiologic means of improving oxygenation; with this, one-half to one-third of the unoxygenated venous return would be diverted away from the right side of the heart and directly into the pulmonary system.[14] However, the caval shunt is of limited usefulness in Ebstein's anomaly. In a collected series of 36 cases of vena cava-pulmonary artery shunts performed for this anomaly, 17 patients survived the operation and 14 were benefited by it.[15]

Reconstruction or replacement of the deformed tricuspid valve, directed toward total correction of the hemodynamic abnormality, began in 1958, when Hunter and Lillehei attempted to create a competent valve by repositioning the displaced posterior and septal leaflets.[16] Their method, employed in two patients, also entailed excluding the atrialized ventricular chamber and closing the atrial septal defect when the latter was present. Both patients had complete heart block and neither patient survived.

Later, Hardy and his colleagues[17] revived and modified the Hunter–Lillehei operation. They placed interrupted sutures close together on the spiral line of the displaced posterior and septal cusp bases and wider apart in the annulus. The tying of the sutures created multiple tucks in the leaflets, narrowed the tricuspid orifice somewhat, and pulled the displaced leaflets back to the tricuspid annulus. The technique was subsequently used in six patients, four of whom survived. However, although some good results were reported with this technique, it is not effective in establishing a competent valve in the moderate and severe forms of Ebstein's anomaly. With the suture placement as originally shown, heart block has occurred. Moreover, it is not possible to transpose the septal leaflet and medial portions of the posterior leaflet to the tricuspid annulus, as the ventricular septum cannot be plicated in the same way as the free wall of the right ventricle. Finally, direct approximation of the displaced leaflets to the tricuspid annulus along the free

wall does not obliterate the atrialized ventricle, which protrudes below the heart as an aneurysmal sac and, despite efforts to the contrary, usually remains in communication with the right ventricle.

Replacement of the deformed tricuspid valve with a mechanical prosthetic valve was done successfully by Barnard and Schrire in 1963.[18] They used a mechanical valve in two other patients; one succumbed during the operation and the other later required reoperation because of thrombosis in the atrium. In their technique, the sutures for anchoring the prosthesis were deviated cephalad to the coronary sinus and atrioventricular node in order to avoid injuring the node and the conduction bundle. With the sutures thus placed, blood from the coronary sinus drained directly into the right ventricle. The atrialized portion of the ventricle was not obliterated.

In 1967, Lillehei and his co-workers reported the tricuspid valve with a Starr-Edwards ball valve in five patients.[19] In two patients, the prosthetic valve was sutured to the true annulus, causing complete atrioventricular dissociation. One of the two died; in the remaining three patients, attachment of the prosthesis according to the Barnard and Schrire technique avoided heart block.

Other surgical techniques used for Ebstein's anomaly include ventricular plication combined with tricuspid valve replacement,[20] and replacement of the tricuspid valve with a tissue valve along with obliteration of the atrialized portion of the right ventricle and closure of the atrial septal defect.[21] For neonates, closure of the tricuspid valve, atrial septectomy, and an aorta-pulmonary shunt have been advocated.[22]

Prosthetic valve replacement, although remaining the most popular way to repair Ebstein's anomaly, has given less than ideal results for some patients. Valve replacement in the tricuspid area is associated with a higher frequency of valve malfunction and thrombotic complications than is replacement of the other cardiac valves.[23] Tissue valves do not have the thromboembolic complications of mechanical valves, but they do have a limited life expectancy, particularly in infants and children. In our experience, the failure-free rate of porcine heterograft valves in children is only 58.5% at 5 years.[24] In addition, a prosthetic valve is undesirable in a small patient, since reoperation will be required for replacement of the valve because of growth.

In 1972, the author developed a new method of valve repair, which is described in the following section.[25] More recently, other types of valve reconstruction have been proposed,[26–28] (Fig. 89–4) but the number of patients reported is small and late results are not available.

Operative Management

Our operative management of patients with Ebstein's malformation consists of (1) electrophysiologic mapping for the localization of accessory conduction pathways in those patients having ventricular pre-excitation, (2) closure of the

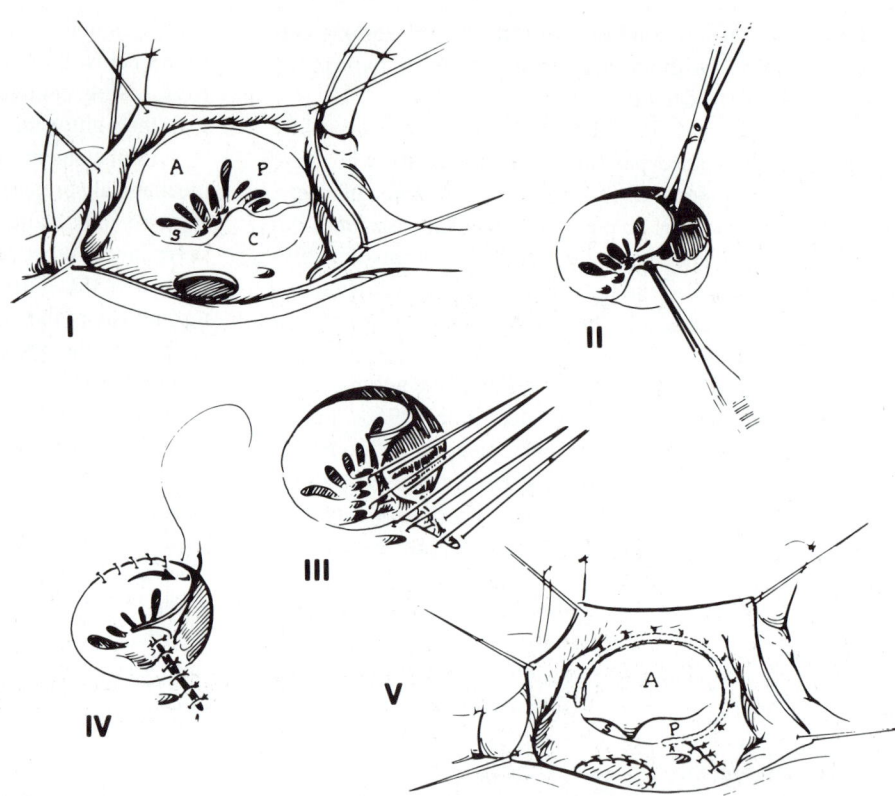

Figure 89–4. Carpentier technique of repair. **I.** Operative view. *A,* Anterior leaflet; *P,* posterior leaflet; *S,* septal leaflet; *C,* atrialized chamber. **II.** Anterior leaflet and adjacent portion of posterior leaflet are detached from anulus. Leaflet time is mobilized by cutting fibrous bands attached to ventricular wall. Interchordal spaces are fenestrated if obliterated. **III.** Longitudinal plication of right ventricle by simple sutures passed through septal and posterior leaflet remnants. Tricuspid annulus and right atrium are plicated. **IV.** Anterior and posterior leaflets are sutured to tricuspid annulus after clockwise rotation (*arrow*) to cover entire orifice area. **V.** Prosthetic ring is inserted to remodel orifice and to reinforce repair. Atrial septal defect is closed. *(From Carpentier, et al: A new reconstructive operation for Ebstein's anomaly of the tricuspid valve. J Thorac Cardiovasc Surg 96:92, 1988, with permission.)*

atrial septal defect or patent foramen ovale, (3) plication of the atrialized portion of the right ventricle, (4) tricuspid valve repair, if feasible, or replacement with a prosthetic valve, and (5) correction of any associated anomalies, such as the relief of pulmonary stenosis or the division of accessory conduction pathways (see Chap. 131).

Technique of Plication

The repair we have employed—plication of the free wall of the atrialized portion of the right ventricle, posterior tricuspid annuloplasty, and right reduction atrioplasty—has been used since 1972[25,29,30] (Fig. 89–5). This repair is based on the construction of a monocusp valve by the use of the anterior leaflet of the tricuspid valve, which, as noted earlier, is usually enlarged in Ebstein's anomaly.

The ventricular plication sutures are placed so as to avoid the posterior descending coronary artery and obvious large branches of the right coronary artery. Occasionally, the right coronary artery does not run in the atrioventricular groove, but courses laterally across the atrialized portion of the right ventricle. When all plication sutures have been placed, and again when they have been tied, the anterior and posterior aspects of the right ventricle are inspected to ascertain that no injury has occurred to the major coronary arteries.

The posterior annuloplasty (Fig. 89–5D and E) is a critical part of the procedure. The posterior aspect of the annulus is first narrowed with the annuloplasty suture and then further obliterated by additional interrupted mattress sutures passed through felt pledgets from the free wall an-

nulus to the septum as needed to provide complete competence of the reconstructed valve. After the reconstruction is completed, the tricuspid valve is tested by temporarily clamping the pulmonary artery and injecting saline under pressure into the right ventricle with a bulb syringe and large catheter (Fig. 89–5, continued).

Because this repair is based on the presence of a satisfactory anterior leaflet, significant abnormalities of the leaflet may compromise the result. For most patients with fenestrations or perforations in the anterior leaflet, the defects can be satisfactorily repaired with fine running sutures. Small anterior leaflets may permit construction of a competent tricuspid valve, but at the expense of creating some (usually acceptable) degree of tricuspid stenosis. Anterior leaflets with linear or hyphenated attachment of the leading edge to the right ventricular endocardium, a condition associated with absence of the papillary muscles and chordae, are currently not considered appropriate for reconstruction. The presence of short papillary muscles and chordae does not preclude a satisfactory repair if the remaining leaflet tissue is well formed. A few patients will have enough posterior leaflet tissue present to permit a bileaflet repair, and rarely, all three leaflets will be moderately well formed but displaced, permitting a trileaflet repair.

Following venous decannulation, the surgeon's finger may be introduced into the right atrium for direct palpation of the tricuspid valve in the beating heart. The results have also been assessed by intraoperative transesophageal echocardiography since 1985. Temporary pacemaker wires

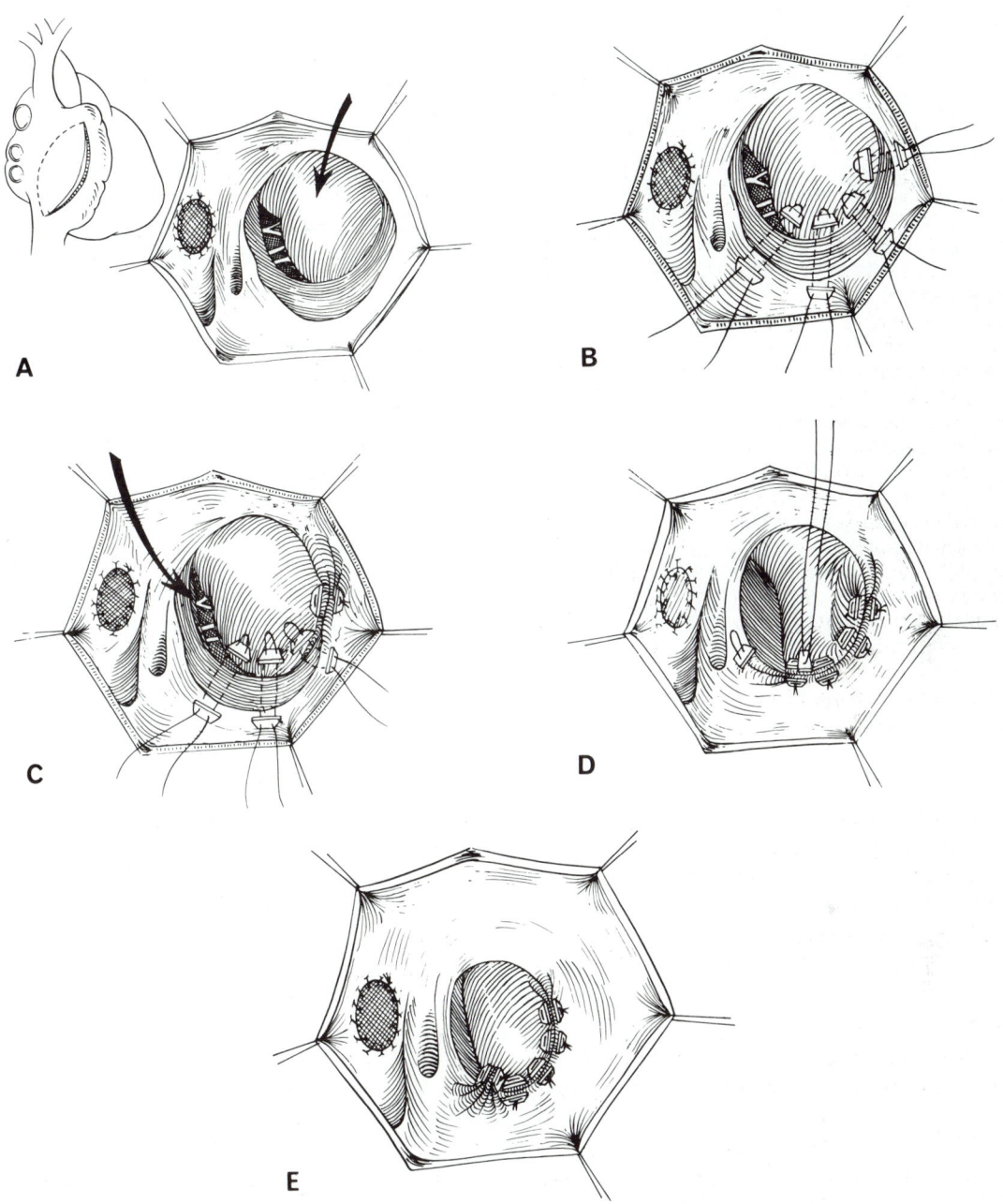

Figure 89–5. Diagram of repair. **A. Left.** The right atrium is incised from the atrial appendage to the inferior vena cava. During closure of the right atriotomy, the redundant portion of right atrium is excised (*dotted line*) so that the final size of the right atrium is normal. **Right.** The atrial septal defect is closed with a pericardial patch. The large anterior leaflet is indicated by the arrow. The posterior leaflet is displaced down from the annulus. The septal leaflet is hypoplastic and is not seen in this view. **B.** Mattress sutures passed through pledgets of Teflon felt are used to pull the tricuspid annulus and tricuspid valve together. Sutures are placed in the atrialized portion of the right ventricle as shown, so that when they are subsequently tied, the atrialized ventricle is plicated and the aneurysmal cavity is obliterated. **C.** The sutures are tied down sequentially. The hypoplastic, markedly displaced septal leaflet is now visible (*arrow*). **D.** Posterior annuloplasty is performed to narrow the diameter of the tricuspid anulus. The coronary sinus marks the postero-leftward extent of the annuloplasty, which is terminated there to avoid injury to the conduction bundle. Occasionally, one or two additional mattress sutures are required to obliterate the posterior aspect of the annuloplasty repair in order to render the valve totally competent. The tricuspid annulus at this time will admit two or more fingers in adult patients. **E.** Completed repair, which allows anterior leaflet to function as a monocusp valve. *(Continued.)*

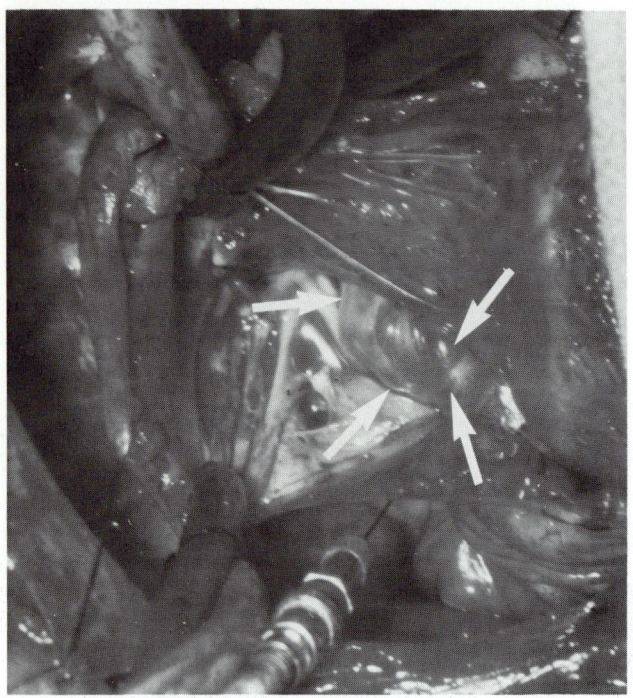

F

Figure 89–5. *(Continued.)* **F.** Operative photograph of completed repair. Large anterior leaflet forms competent monocusp valve (*arrows*). *(From Danielson GK, Maloney JD, Devloo RAE: Mayo Clin Proc 54:185, 1979, with permission.)*

are attached to the right atrium and right ventricle for postoperative monitoring of rhythm and for pacing in selected cases. The basic techniques of repair have not changed since the original successful case in 1972. However, the anatomy in no two patients is exactly alike, so each repair is tailored appropriately until the valve is competent.

Technique of Valve Replacement

When the tricuspid valve cannot be reconstructed, the valve is excised and a prosthetic valve is inserted. The suture line is placed on the atrial side of the coronary sinus and A-V node to avoid injury to the conduction mechanism (Fig. 89–6). In patients with normal hearts, mechanical prostheses in the tricuspid position have a higher incidence of malfunction and thrombotic complications than they do in either the aortic or mitral position.[23] However, mechanical valves have functioned better in patients with Ebstein's anomaly, perhaps because the right ventricles are larger and there is less tendency for fibrous tissue ingrowth into the prostheses. In our experience, bioprosthetic valves also last longer in the tricuspid position in Ebstein's anomaly compared with their performance in hearts with normal ventricular anatomy.

RESULTS

Between April 1972 and May 1995, 288 consecutive patients underwent operation for Ebstein's anomaly. The pa-

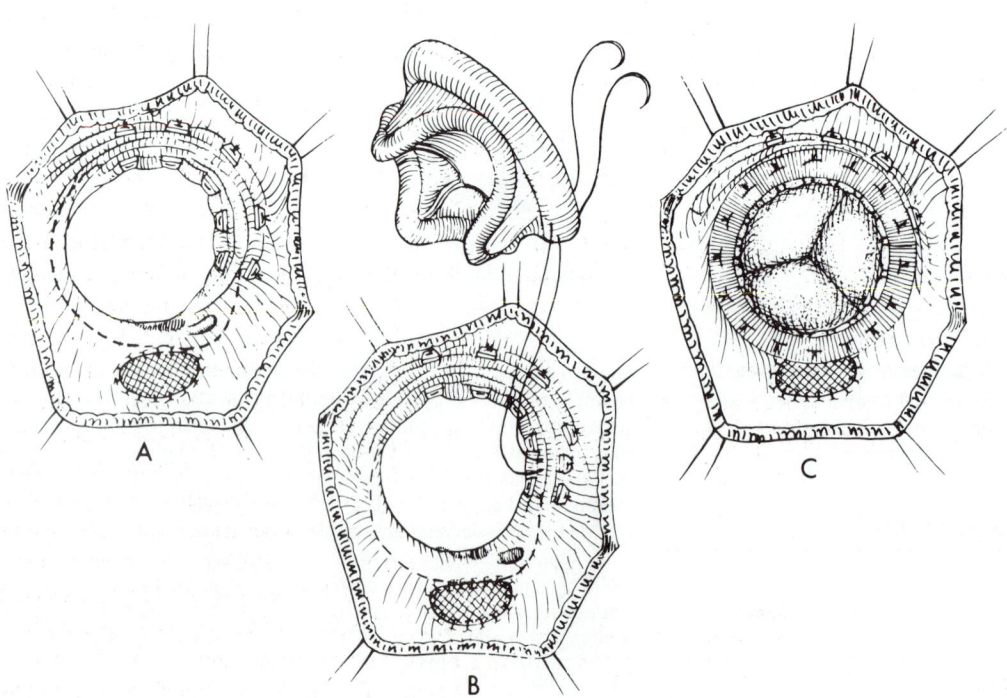

Figure 89–6. Diagram of technique for tricuspid valve replacement in Ebstein's anomaly. **A.** If the atrialized right ventricle is dilated, thin, and noncontractile, it is plicated. **B.** The suture line is placed on the atrial side of the coronary sinus and A-V node to avoid injury to the conduction mechanism. **C.** The sutures are tied with the heart perfused and beating to ensure that a conducted rhythm is preserved.

tient's ages ranged from 9 mo to 71 years. The results of the first 189 patients have been analyzed.[30] Hemoglobin values ranged between 10.8 and 23.4 g/dL, cardiothoracic ratios ranged between 0.49 and 0.96, and arterial oxygen saturations ranged between 65 and 98%. Forty-nine previous cardiac operations had been performed, including 15 systemic-pulmonary shunts, 8 closures of atrial septal defect, 6 Glenn procedures, 6 pacemaker insertions, 5 attempted repairs elsewhere (including the use of a rigid ring), and 2 pericardiectomies.

Valve repair by plication of the atrialized right ventricle and valvuloplasty was accomplished in 110 of the 189 consecutive patients (58.2%) (Table 89–1). Tricuspid valve replacement was required in 69 patients (36.5%). Right ventricular plication was added to the valve replacement if the atrialized ventricle was dilated, thin, and noncontractile. Porcine bioprostheses were used in 50 patients; 19 received mechanical prostheses. Two patients (1.1%) with a prior Glenn anastomosis who had unrepairable valves underwent plication of the atrialized right ventricle and resection of their tricuspid valves without valve replacement, a type of modified Fontan procedure. Eight other patients (4.2%) who had hemodynamically mild tricuspid insufficiency underwent repair of other significant anomalies without a procedure on the tricuspid valve.

Associated procedures are shown in Table 89–2. In all 28 patients, the accessory conduction pathways were successfully ablated, and the four patients with A-V nodal reentry tachycardia underwent successful ablation of their arrhythmia. There were no instances of permanent complete heart block in the entire series except for one patient who had paroxysmal atrial flutter and fibrillation who underwent planned cryoablation of the A-V node and implantation of a permanent pacemaker for control of the arrhythmias.

Twelve deaths (6.3%) occurred within 30 days or during the initial hospitalization (Table 89–1). Four deaths were caused by sudden ventricular fibrillation in patients who were otherwise doing well but who had massive cardiomegaly. Other causes of death included low cardiac output ($n = 5$), postoperative hemorrhage ($n = 1$), respiratory arrest ($n = 1$), and coagulopathy ($n = 1$).

Postoperative cardiac catheterizations, when performed, have shown satisfactory tricuspid valve function in most patients. (Fig. 89–7). When two-dimensional echocar-

TABLE 89–2. ASSOCIATED PROCEDURES

Operation	Number of Patients
Repair of atrial septal defect	169
Ablation of accessory pathway(s)	28
Repair of pulmonary stenosis	16
Closure of shunt	13
Repair of ventricular septal defect	7
Repair of partial A-V canal	4
Ablation of A-V nodal reentry tachycardia	4
Closure of patent ductus arteriosus	2
Repair of partial anomalous pulmonary venous connection	2
Other	9

diography and Doppler and color-flow imaging became available, all patients were studied by these modalities before hospital discharge. The vast majority of patients had tricuspid insufficiency rated as trivial or mild. The atrial septum was intact in all patients.

There have been 10 late deaths; causes of death were sudden (presumably arrhythmic) in four patients, congestive heart failure in three, automobile accident (passenger) in one, abdominal abscess in one, and unknown in one. Because of the high incidence of both early and late sudden deaths in our initial experience, presumably related to ventricular arrhythmias, we now administer intravenous lidocaine prophylactically for the first 48 hours, then discontinue the lidocaine and observe the patient for ventricular ectopy. If ventricular ectopy or other risk factors are present such as giant cardiomegaly or history of ventricular arrhythmias, procainamide is instituted with an initial intravenous loading dose and subsequent oral doses. We advise the continuation of procainamide administration for 3 mo, at which time its use can be tapered and discontinued if no further tendency to development of ventricular ectopy is seen in the patient. Twenty-four-hour ambulatory monitoring is then suggested for rhythm assessment.

Reoperations for tricuspid valve replacement were required in 4 of the 110 patients who had undergone tricuspid valve repair. This represents a total incidence of 3.6% in a follow-up extending to 19 years. In the first patient, who was 1 year old, a less-than-ideal repair was accepted as an alternative to valve replacement, in the hope that the child would grow further before a valve prosthesis would be required. The child developed for 6 1/2 years before valve replacement was necessary, at which time she received a 31-mm (adult size) porcine bioprosthesis. The second patient sustained an inferior wall myocardial infarction from kinking of the distal right coronary artery at the time of operation. This produced enough distortion of the right ventricle that the valve became insufficient and required replacement 1 year later. The other two patients required valve replacement 6 to 14 years after initial repair, respectively, because of progressive dilatation of the tricuspid annulus

TABLE 89–1. OPERATIONS

Procedure	Number of Patients	Early Death n	Early Death %
Plication and valvuloplasty	110	8	7.3
Tricuspid valve replacement	69	4	5.8
Plication and Fontan procedure	2	0	0
Other	8	0	0
Total	189	12	6.3

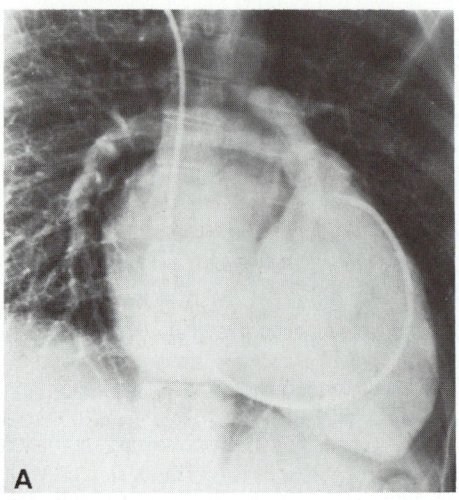
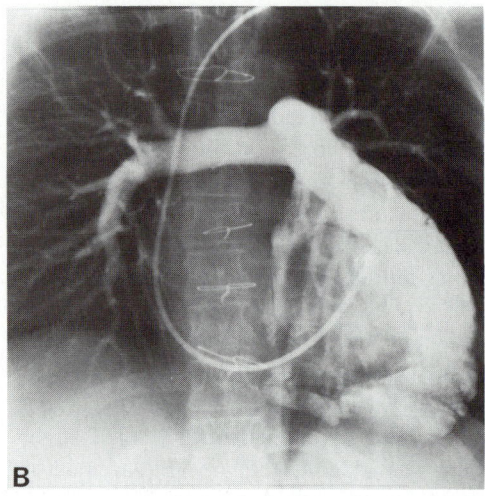

Figure 89–7. Angiogram from right ventricle of a 20-year-old woman with Ebstein's anomaly. **A.** Preoperative. Note massive tricuspid insufficiency into enlarged right atrium. **B.** Two years postoperatively. Tricuspid valve remains competent. Filling defect created by large anterior leaflet is shown. The patient is asymptomatic and off all medications 20 years after operation. *(From Danielson GK, Maloney JD, Devloo RAE: Mayo Clin Proc 54:185, 1979, with permission.)*

and right ventricle. All four patients survived reoperation and are now in New York Heart Association Class I or II. Two additional patients required reoperation for replacement of a mechanical valve and both survived. Only one patient has returned for replacement of a porcine valve (stenotic).

Of survivors more than 1 year after surgery, 92.9% were in New York Heart Association Class I or II. Postoperative reduction in heart size was usual and occasionally

considerable (Fig. 89–8). Nine female patients have undergone a total of 12 successful pregnancies with delivery of normal children.

In a study of cardiac arrhythmias in some of these patients, Oh and associates[31] found that of patients with preoperative paroxysmal supraventricular tachycardia and paroxysmal atrial fibrillation or flutter, only 33% continued to have symptomatic tachycardia after operation.

Maximum exercise testing shows a significant increase

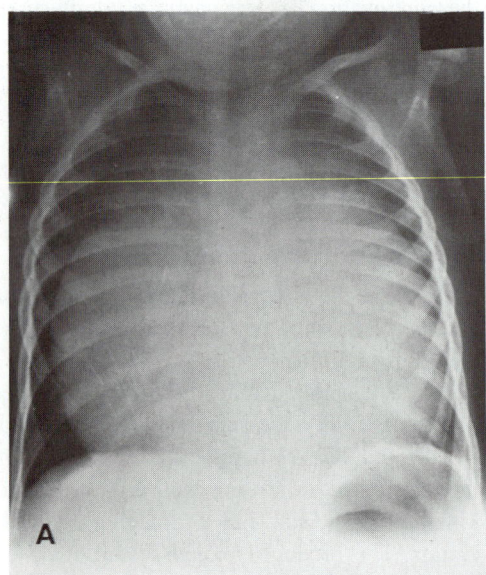
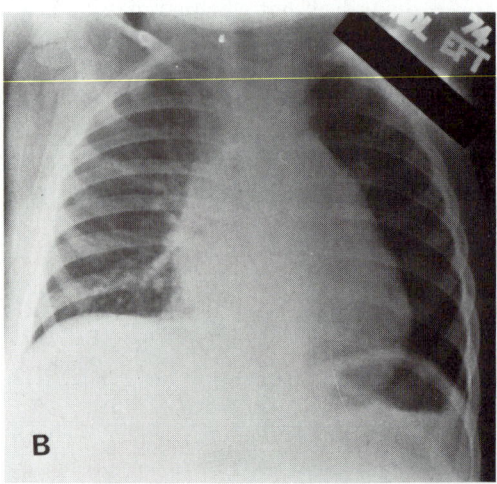

Figure 89–8. Chest x-ray films of a 2-year-old girl with Ebstein's anomaly. **A.** Preoperative (cardiothoracic ratio 0.9). **B.** Thirteen days postoperatively (cardiothoracic ratio 0.55). The patient remains well and off all medications 19 years after operation. *(From Danielson GK, Maloney JD, Devloo RAE: Mayo Clin Proc 54:185, 1979, with permission.)*

in work performance, exercise duration, and maximum oxygen uptake after operation.[32] Maximal oxygen consumption in our patients increased from a mean of 47% of predicted value before operation to a mean of 72% of predicted value after operation. Operative treatment of Ebstein's anomaly also favorably affects cardiac output, particularly in response to exercise, normalizes systemic arterial oxygen saturation, and reduces excess ventilation at rest and during exercise. These results are very favorable when compared with the natural history of patients having Ebstein's anomaly who are in functional Class III or IV.[10,33]

REFERENCES

1. Mann RJ, Lie JT: The life story of Wilhelm Ebstein (1836–1912) and his almost overlooked description of a congenital heart disease. *Mayo Clin Proc* **54**:197, 1979
2. Anderson KR, Züberbuhler JR, Anderson RH, et al: Morphologic spectrum of Ebstein's anomaly of the heart: A review. *Mayo Clin Proc* **54**:174, 1979
3. Lev M, Liberthson RR, Joseph RH, et al: The pathologic anatomy of Ebstein's disease. *Arch Pathol* **90**:334, 1970
4. Anderson KR, Lie JT: The right ventricular myocardium in Ebstein's anomaly. A morphometric histopathologic study. *Mayo Clin Proc* **54**:181, 1979
5. Anderson KR, Danielson GK, McGoon DC, Lie JT: Ebstein's anomaly of the left-sided tricuspid valve: Pathological anatomy of the valvular malformation. *Circulation* **58**(suppl 1):87, 1978
6. Anderson RH, Becker AE, Arnold R, Wilkinson JL: The conduction tissues in congenitally corrected transposition. *Circulation* **50**:911, 1974
7. Gasul BM, Weinberg M Jr, Luan L, et al: Superior vena cava-right main pulmonary artery anastomosis. Surgical correction for patients with Ebstein's anomaly and for congenital hypoplastic right ventricle. *JAMA* **171**:1797, 1959
8. Seward JB, Tajik AJ, Feist DJ, Smith HC: Ebstein's anomaly in an 85-year-old man. *Mayo Clin Proc* **54**:193–196, 1979
9. Kumar AE, Fyler DC, Miettinen OS, et al: Ebstein's anomaly. *Am J Cardiol* **28**:84, 1971
10. Guiliani ER, Fuster V, Brandenburg RO, Mair DD: The clinical features and natural history of Ebstein's anomaly of the tricuspid valve. *Mayo Clin Proc* **54**:163, 1979
11. Celermajer DS, Bull C, Till JA, et al: Ebstein's anomaly: Presentation and outcome from fetus to adult. *J Am Coll Cardiol* **23**:170–176, 1994
12. Shiina A, Seward JB, Tajik AJ, et al: Two-dimensional echocardiographic-surgical correlation in Ebstein's anomaly: Preoperative determination of patients requiring tricuspid valve plication vs replacement. *Circulation* **68**:534–544, 1983
13. Reeder GS, Currie PJ, Hagler DJ, et al: Use of Doppler techniques (continuous-wave, pulsed-wave, and color flow imaging) in the noninvasive hemodynamic assessment of congenital heart disease. *Mayo Clin Proc* **61**:725–744, 1986
14. Glenn WWL, Patiño JF: Circulatory bypass of the right heart. I. Preliminary observations on the direct delivery of vena caval blood into the pulmonary arterial circulation. Azygos vein-pulmonary artery shunt. *Yale J Biol Med* **27**:147, 1954
15. Glenn WWL, Browne M, Whittemore R: Circulatory bypass of the right side of the heart: Cava-pulmonary artery shunt—Indications and results (report of a collected series of 537 cases). In Cassels DE (ed): *The Heart and Circulation in the Newborn and Infant.* New York, Grune & Stratton, 1966, pp 345–357
16. Hunter SW, Lillehei CW: Ebstein's malformation of the tricuspid valve: Study of a case, together with suggestions of a new form of surgical therapy. *Dis Chest* **33**:297, 1958
17. Hardy KL, May IA, Webster CA, et al: Ebstein's anomaly: A functional concept and successful definitive repair. *J Thorac Cardiovasc Surg* **48**:927, 1964
18. Barnard CN, Schrire U: Surgical correction of Ebstein's malformation with prosthetic tricuspid valve. *Surgery* **54**:302, 1963
19. Lillehei CW, Kalke BR, Carlson, RG: Evolution of corrective surgery for Ebstein's anomaly. *Circulation* **35, 36**(suppl 1):111, 1967
20. Timmis HH, Hardy JD, Watson DG: The surgical management of Ebstein's anomaly. The combined use of tricuspid valve replacement, atrioventricular plication, and atrioplasty. *J Thorac Cardiovasc Surg* **53**:385, 1967
21. Ross D, Somerville J: Surgical correction of Ebstein's anomaly. *Lancet* **2**:280, 1970
22. Starnes VA, Pitlick PT, Bernstein D, et al: Ebstein's anomaly appearing in the neonate. *J Thorac Cardiovasc Surg* **101**:1082–1087, 1991
23. Sanfelippo PM, Giuliani ER, Danielson GK, et al: Tricuspid valve prosthetic replacement: Early and late results with the Starr-Edwards prosthesis. *J Thorac Cardiovasc Surg* **71**:441, 1976
24. Williams DB, Danielson GK, McGoon DC, et al: Hancock porcine heterograft valve replacement in children. *J Thorac Cardiovasc Surg* **84**:446–450, 1982
25. Danielson GK, Maloney JD, Devloo RAE: Surgical repair of Ebstein's anomaly. *Mayo Clin Proc* **54**:185, 1979
26. Schmidt-Habelmann P, Meisner H, Struck E, Sebening F: Results of valvuloplasty for Ebstein's anomaly. *Thorac Cardiovasc Surg* **29**:155, 1981
27. Carpentier A, Chauvaud S, Mace L, et al: A new reconstructive operation for Ebstein's anomaly of the tricuspid valve. *J Thorac Cardiovasc Surg* **96**:92–101, 1988
28. Quaegebeur JM, Sreeram N, Fraser AG, et al: Surgery for Ebstein's anomaly: The clinical and echocardiographic evaluation of a new technique. *J Am Coll Cardiol* **17**:722–728, 1991
29. Danielson GK: Ebstein's anomaly: Surgical treatment. In Jamieson SW, Shumway NE (eds): *Rob & Smith's Operative Surgery—Cardiac Surgery,* 4th ed. London, England, Butterworths, 1986, pp 208–214
30. Danielson GK, Driscoll DJ, Mair DD, et al: Operative treatment of Ebstein's anomaly. *J Thorac Cardiovasc Surg* **104**:1195–1202, 1992
31. Oh JK, Holmes DR Jr, Hayes DL, et al: Cardiac arrhythmias in patients with surgical repair of Ebstein's anomaly. *J Am Coll Cardiol* **6**:1351–1357, 1985
32. Driscoll DJ, Mottram CD, Danielson GK: Spectrum of exercise intolerance in 45 patients with Ebstein's anomaly and observations on exercise tolerance in 11 patients after surgical repair. *J Am Coll Cardiol* **11**:831–836, 1988
33. Mair DD, Danielson GK: Ebstein's malformation. In Fortuin NJ (ed): *Current Therapy in Cardiovascular Disease,* Vol 2. Philadelphia, B.C. Decker, 1986, pp 131–134

CHAPTER

90

Congenital Abnormalities of the Mitral Valve

Richard P. Embrey and Douglas M. Behrendt

Congenital anomalies of the mitral valve are a diverse group of malformations that are particularly vexatious for the thoracic surgeon. These malformations typically occur in combination with other cardiac lesions, often involve more than one component of the mitral apparatus, and tend to cause symptoms in small infants. Because repair is often difficult and prosthetic valve replacement in children has inherent difficulties, management of congenital mitral valve abnormalities is often problematic. Fortunately, these malformations are relatively rare, with isolated congenital mitral stenosis or insufficiency affecting less than 1% of patients with congenital heart defects.[1,2] More commonly, mitral valve abnormalities are associated with other cardiac lesions (Table 90–1), such as partial atrioventricular septal defects or left ventricular outflow tract obstruction and coarctation of the aorta (in the so-called Shone's complex).[3]

The structural mitral valve lesions discussed in this chapter are those that are found in association with a morphologic left ventricle supporting the systemic circulation, i.e., in atrioventricular and ventriculoarterial concordance. Discussed elsewhere are atrioventricular valve abnormalities in the setting of a single ventricle (Chaps. 71 and 72), atrioventricular septal defects (Chap. 70), corrected transposition (Chap. 86), and straddling or overriding atrioventricular valves (Chap. 73). The treatment of anatomically normal mitral valves rendered incompetent by congenital disease, such as Marfan's, is covered in Chapters 118 and 119.

HISTORY

Interestingly, the first successful operation for mitral stenosis was performed on a pediatric patient, although the etiol-ogy of the stenosis was acquired rather than congenital. On May 20, 1923, Elliot Cutler of the Peter Bent Brigham Hospital operated on an 11-year-old girl suffering from rheumatic mitral stenosis, performing a closed, transventricular valvotomy of the anterior mitral leaflet.[4] The patient survived more than 4 years, but with significant mitral insufficiency. Closed commissurotomy of a congenitally stenotic mitral valve was first attempted unsuccessfully by Clarence Crafoord in 1951,[5] and a year later Bower et al reported a similar procedure with a successful outcome.[6] In 1954 Braudo et al performed a successful digital commissurotomy of a mitral valve in a 3-mo-old infant.[7]

The advent of cardiopulmonary bypass brought with it a heightened interest in the surgical treatment of congenital mitral lesions. In 1959, George Starkey at the Children's Hospital in Boston reported using a pump-oxygenator to perform a commissurotomy under direct vision in a 2-year-old boy. The child could not be weaned from bypass, however, and postmortem examination of the heart revealed fused chordae and papillary muscles, hypoplasia of the left ventricle, and subaortic obstruction suggestive of Shone's complex, an association which would not be formally described for another 4 years.[3,8] Levy, Varco, Lillehei and Edwards presented a series of 17 patients ranging in age from 3 to 20 years who were operated on for mitral insufficiency between 1955 and 1960.[9] Four of six patients with congenital mitral insufficiency survived. The valves were repaired by a variety of methods, including annular plication, annuloplasty, and posterior leaflet extension with a prosthetic patch, an extraordinarily complex technique for that era. In 1976, Alain Carpentier and colleagues from Leiden and Bergamo reported a group of 47 patients operated on for congenital malformations of the mitral valve.[10] Valve repair was possible in 80% of the patients. Carpen-

TABLE 90–1. CARDIAC ANOMALIES ASSOCIATED WITH MITRAL VALVE DISEASE

Congenital Mitral Stenosis	Congenital Mitral Insufficiency
Ventricular septal defect	Complete atrioventricular septal defects
Aortic stenosis	
Patent ductus arteriosus	Partial atrioventricular septal defects
Coarctation	
Tetralogy of Fallot	Secundum atrial septal defects
Tricuspid stenosis, insufficiency	Endocardial fibroelastosis
Atrial septal defect	Anomalous coronary artery
Subaortic stenosis	Coarctation
	Marfan syndrome
	Cardiomyopathy
	Pulmonary stenosis

tier's classification of congenital mitral valve malformations has served as the basis for a systematic surgical approach to these lesions.

ANATOMY AND FUNCTION

The mitral valve is complex in both structure and function. The mitral apparatus consists of an annulus, leaflets, chordae tendinae, and papillary muscles. The mitral annulus is an integral part of the fibrous skeleton of the heart. Anteromedially, the mitral annulus lies directly beneath the aortic valve, between the right and left fibrous trigones. Posteriorly, the mitral annulus follows the atrioventricular sulcus, but is structurally less well defined than anteriorly.

The mitral valve has two major leaflets. The larger anterior or septal leaflet is roughly triangular in shape and attaches to approximately 150° of the annulus beneath the aortic-mitral curtain from posterior to the left fibrous trigone to a point beyond the right trigone. Thus it forms the posterior boundary of the left ventricular outflow tract. The shallow posterior or mural leaflet occupies the remainder of the annular circumference. The combined area of the two leaflets approaches twice that of the mitral orifice.[11] This contributes to the large area of coaptation between the leaflets. The posterior leaflet edge is scalloped, often giving this leaflet a trilobulated appearance, but these divisions have no apparent functional significance. The atrial surface of both the anterior and posterior leaflets is rough along the areas of closure. The remainder of the leaflet surfaces is smooth and is termed the clear zone. Near the annulus, the leaflets thicken into a basal zone.

The anterior and posterior mitral leaflets are separated at the annulus by the well-defined anterolateral and posteromedial commissures. Small amounts of leaflet tissue within the commissures are occasionally present. These are referred to as commissural leaflets. Beneath these commissures are two corresponding papillary muscles. They are ex-

tensions of the subendocardial ventricular myocardium, rendering them notably prone to ischemia. Chordae tendinae from the papillary muscles insert on both sides of the corresponding commissures so each leaflet receives chordae from both papillary muscles. This is not true of congenital "clefts" within the valve leaflets, each side of which receives chordae from different papillary muscles. Considerable variation is found in the morphology of the papillary muscles between individuals, with many being elongated, conical structures with only two heads and others short and broad with four or five distinct heads, thus resembling a baseball mitt.

Although the majority of chordae tendinae arise from the papillary muscles and merge imperceptibly with the edge of the leaflets, some chordae arise from the ventricular wall as well. The chordae are conveniently categorized into three groups.[12] First-order chordae insert on the free edge of the leaflets. Second-order chordae originate from the papillary muscles and insert in the rough zone of the leaflets a few millimeters away from the edge, and third-order chordae are thick bands which extend from the posterior ventricular endocardium to the basal zone of the mural leaflet.

Normal closure of the mitral valve results from a combination of both active and passive processes. The leaflets float posteriorly toward the plane of the mitral annulus during late ventricular diastole, pushed upward by eddy currents within the ventricle. During subsequent atrial contraction, the leaflets briefly reopen. Annular contraction, which may reduce the mitral orifice area by as much as 30%, begins at the onset of atrial systole and continues throughout ventricular contraction.[13] At the onset of ventricular depolarization, the sail-like anterior mitral leaflet swings into apposition with the crescent-shaped posterior leaflet. Firm closure of the two leaflets is enhanced the by large area of coaptation between the leaflets, which is predominantly in an orthogonal plane to the valve annulus. This allows intracavitary pressure within the ventricle to contribute to a tight seal between the leaflets during systole. With the end of isovolumic contraction of the ventricle and ejection of blood into the aorta, the aortic annulus enlarges, compressing the mitral annulus into a concave shape. Although the chordae tendinae and papillary muscles do not shorten during ventricular systole, isometric contraction of these muscles serves to stabilize the mitral leaflets during ejection.

CONGENITAL MALFORMATIONS OBSTRUCTING INFLOW TO THE LEFT VENTRICLE (MITRAL STENOSIS)

Limitation to left ventricular inflow may be caused by a supravalvular mitral ring, hypoplasia of the mitral annulus, or malformation of the leaflets, chordae tendinae, or papillary muscles themselves. Commonly, obstruction is due to abnormalities at multiple levels within the mitral apparatus.

Supravalvular Ring

This lesion consists of a circumferential fibrous ring of tissue that usually attaches to the anterior mitral leaflet just distal to the annulus and the atrial wall immediately above the posterior leaflet. The opening within the ring may be eccentric, and its size determines the degree of obstruction. Stenosing supravalvular mitral ring is distinguished from cor triatriatum sinister by the location and histology of the ring. In cor triatriatum, an obstructing trilaminar fibromuscular septum is found distal to the pulmonary veins but proximal to the left atrial appendage. Supravalvular rings, however, are located distal to the appendage, which may be dilated when the ring is highly obstructive. Microscopically, the ring is very similar in appearance to normal valvular tissue. When it is the cause of hemodynamically important mitral stenosis, supravalvular mitral ring occurs as an isolated lesion in approximately 50% of cases.[14] Usually, the underlying mitral valve is abnormal and often stenotic.

Mitral Annulus and Leaflets

Only very rarely is the mitral annulus sufficiently small to cause stenosis unless there is concomitant hypoplasia of the left ventricle. Although the mitral annulus is quite often smaller than normal in patients with ventricular septal defects and coarctation of the aorta, this is rarely important.[15] There may be congenital absence of the valve commissures, typically in association with shortened and thickened chordae as well as papillary muscle abnormalities. Occasionally, the leaflets are thickened and immobile in the presence of normally formed commissures. A double-orifice mitral valve may be formed by a persistent bridge of valve tissue connecting the two leaflets (Fig. 90–1). This may cause obstruction, particularly if the anterolateral commissure is absent as well.

Chordae and Papillary Muscles

Malformations of the chordae tendinae are a common cause of congenital mitral stenosis. There may be persistence of interchordal tissue, and this in and of itself may limit flow through the mitral apparatus. In the most severe form, the fused chordae are continuous with abnormally thickened leaflets forming a so-called "funnel valve." Chordae may be absent altogether, with thick, obstructive papillary muscles inserting directly onto the valve commissures. Carpentier has used the term "hammock valve" to describe a group of malformations in which the two normal papillary muscles are replaced with multiple short muscles located just beneath the posterior leaflet and connected to the valve leaflets by very short, broad chordae.[10] The thick chordae crossing the mitral orifice from the posterior ventricular wall to the anterior leaflet produce the characteristic hammock appearance as well as the stenosis. The leaflets themselves are often normal.

Perhaps the most severe malformation of the papillary muscles occurs with the parachute mitral valve, a term introduced by Schiebler et al.[16] Typically, the anterior papillary muscle is absent and the chordae converge on a single, large posterior muscle, limiting the orifice of the valve (Fig. 90–2).[17,18] The leaflets and chordae may be grossly normal, and the cause of the stenosis inapparent when the valve is viewed from the left atrium until the leaflets are retracted and the subvalvar apparatus inspected.

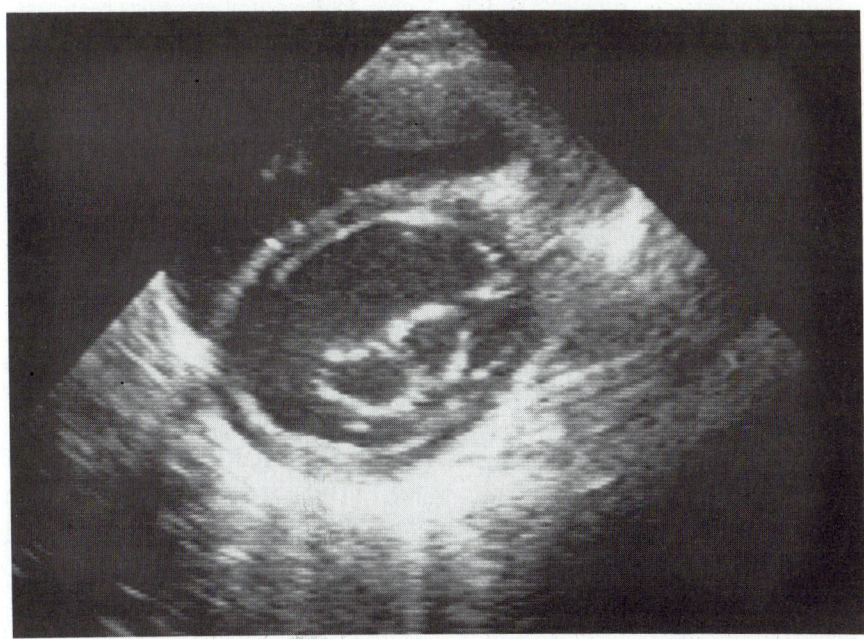

Figure 90–1. Transthoracic echocardiogram from a patient with double-orifice mitral valve. The two openings in the valve are easily seen in this short axis taken just below the level of the mitral annulus.

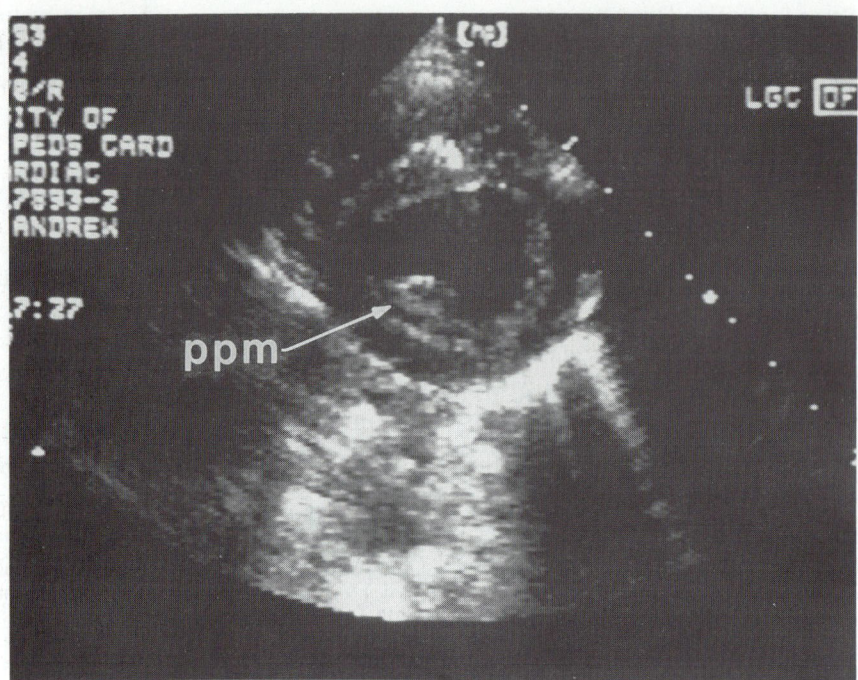

Figure 90–2. Transthoracic echocardiogram from a patient with parachute mitral valve. This short axis view of the left ventricle shows absence of the anterior papillary muscle and a large, single posterior papillary muscle (ppm).

CONGENITAL MALFORMATIONS LEADING TO MITRAL INSUFFICIENCY

Mitral insufficiency may be seen with any of the stenotic malformations described in the previous section. Annular dilation may lead to insufficiency even in the presence of an otherwise normal valve. This is the mechanism of mitral incompetence associated with diseases that produce left ventricular dilation, such as cardiomyopathy, endomyocardial fibrosis, and anomalous left coronary arising from the pulmonary trunk.[19] A few cases of primary annular dilation leading to mitral insufficiency have been described in newborn infants who develop congestive heart failure in the first few days of life, without associated left ventricular outflow tract obstruction or coarctation. Primary annular dilation may be asymmetric, most often affecting the posterior commissure and posterior leaflet. This lesion has been seen in association with ostium secundum atrial septal defects, ventricular septal defect, and coronary artery fistula to the right ventricle.[10]

Hypoplasia of the posterior leaflet is an uncommon cause of congenital mitral insufficiency. Mitral valve prolapse with severe chordal elongation and/or rupture has been found to be a cause of mitral incompetence even in very young children.[20] Chordal agenesis has been described by Carpentier, with the unsupported segment of the leaflet being poorly formed.[10]

Clefts in the anterior mitral leaflet are one of the most common causes of congenital mitral incompetence. Such clefts may be found with or without ostium primum atrial septal defects or other evidence of atrioventricular septal defect. The anteroposterior diameter of the valve annulus is also increased with anterior mitral clefts. Posterior clefts are exceedingly rare.[21]

CONGENITAL MALFORMATIONS ASSOCIATED WITH LEFT VENTRICULAR OUTFLOW TRACT OBSTRUCTION

Because the mitral valve complex and outflow tract of the left ventricle are contiguous, forming the posteromedial and superior portion of the ventricle, it is not surprising that malformations of the mitral apparatus may affect the subaortic region. Double-orifice mitral valve has been associated with discrete fibromuscular subaortic stenosis.[22] Also, anomalous chordae may traverse the outflow tract, causing obstruction.[23] Accessory mitral valve tissue may be a source of progressive outflow stenosis (Fig. 90–3).[24] Perimembranous ventricular septal defects, which are virtually always present, may mask the severity of the subaortic obstruction, particularly if the accessory tissue protrudes into the defect during systole.[25]

The constellation of supravalvular mitral ring, parachute mitral valve, subaortic stenosis, and coarctation of the aorta deserves special note because of the pivotal role of the mitral valve in this complex anomaly. When Shone first described this entity in 1963, he noted that the most critical element in the malformation appeared to be the severity of the mitral valve lesion.[3] Bolling reported on a group of 30 patients with Shone's complex, of whom 26 had mitral valve abnormalities.[26] Eleven of the 26 patients required repair or replacement of the mitral valve. Operative mortality for replacement was 67%. Those patients with elevated pul-

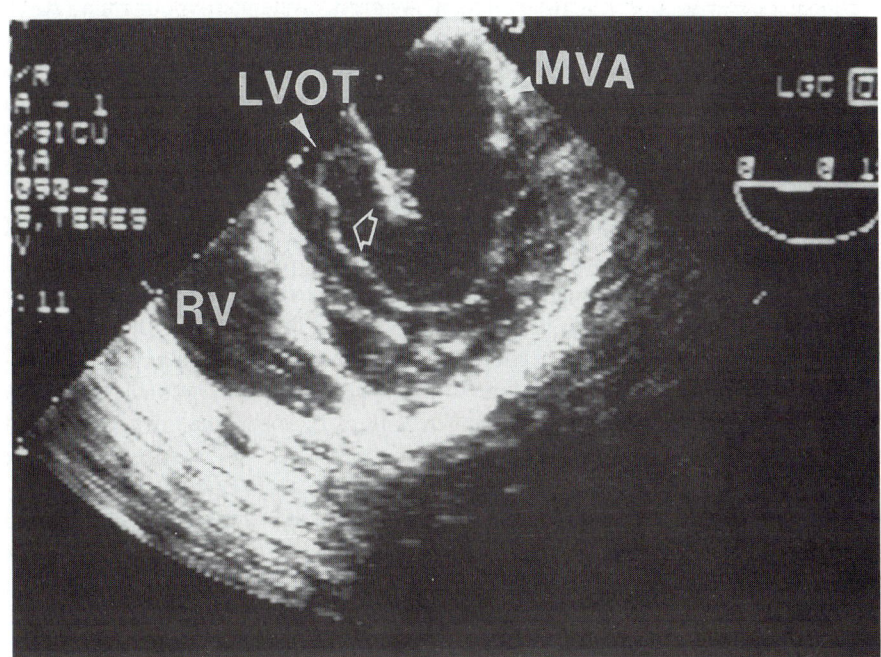

Figure 90–3. Four-chamber view from an intraoperative transesophageal echocardiogram of a patient with ventricular septal defect, double-orifice mitral valve, and accessory mitral tissue obstructing the left ventricular outflow tract. Note the accessory mitral tissue (open arrow) filling the outflow tract (LVOT). MVA, mitral annulus; RV, right ventricle.

monary artery pressures were noted to have a poorer outcome overall. Because most of these patients were found to have severe left ventricular outflow obstruction, Bolling and associates postulated that elevation of pulmonary artery pressures secondary to the mitral stenosis caused reversed ventricular septal curvature, and that this contributed to outflow obstruction.

CLINICAL PRESENTATION

Because the systemic circulation may be supplied through a large ductus arteriosus, even severe mitral stenosis or atresia does not hemodynamically compromise the fetus. The onset and intensity of symptoms in the infant are related to the severity of the stenosis and presence of associated lesions, which in turn affect the growth rate and nutritional state of the infant.[27] Poor weight gain, difficulty feeding, tachypnea, and recurrent pulmonary infections are typical presenting symptoms of older infants with mitral valve obstruction. Newborns with more severe mitral stenosis may develop symptoms earlier, with frank pulmonary edema, poor peripheral perfusion, and hepatosplenomegaly, a clinical picture that is predictive of a poor outcome.[27]

On physical examination, infants and children with congenital mitral stenosis may have a prominent right ventricular impulse and an accentuated second heart sound if pulmonary hypertension is present. A mid-diastolic murmur is present, but the relatively immobile mitral leaflets lead to a soft or absent first heart sound, a finding that may help differentiate congenital from rheumatic mitral stenosis in older children.[28] If important mitral insufficiency is pres-

ent, the left ventricular apical impulse will be displaced laterally, and an apical pansystolic murmur will be heard on auscultation.

Chest radiography in congenital mitral stenosis shows left atrial enlargement. Left atrial dilation out of proportion to that expected from coexisting malformations is an important finding that points to the presence of mitral stenosis.[29] The left mainstem bronchus may be elevated and occasionally complete atelectasis of the left lower lobe is observed when the left atrial pressure is high. The findings of pulmonary venous congestion are typically present. Left ventricular enlargement is noted in patients with mitral insufficiency, and right ventricular enlargement may be seen in the lateral radiograph of patients with pulmonary hypertension. Electrocardiography usually shows left atrial hypertrophy, and the presence of right ventricular hypertrophy indicates pulmonary hypertension.

Two-dimensional echocardiography is invaluable in the evaluation of patients with congenital mitral valve abnormalities. Coupled with Doppler flow interrogation, transthoracic and transesophageal echocardiography facilitate examination of annulus size, leaflet morphology, and mobility, presence of anomalous chordae, and papillary muscle configuration.[30] Transvalvular gradients and chamber pressure estimations by echocardiography are reliable and reproducible, but may be operator-dependent. Cardiac catheterization is required when the diagnosis is in question, in complex cases or when severe pulmonary hypertension is suspected. Magnetic resonance imaging (MRI) is particularly helpful in evaluating congenital malformations involving the left atrium, such as supravalvular mitral ring and cor triatriatum.

TREATMENT

Unfortunately, therapeutic options for infants and small children presenting with symptomatic mitral valve disease are limited. Congenital stenosis often is quite severe, and death usually occurs within the first 5 years of life without treatment.[30] Isolated mitral insufficiency commonly causes symptoms later in childhood, and these may be medically controlled, delaying surgical intervention.

Only about 40% of patients diagnosed with congenital mitral stenosis have obstruction severe enough to require intervention. Nonetheless, because of associated cardiac lesions, a 30% mortality during infancy has been observed in children with less severe mitral stenosis.[31] However, surviving children have not exhibited a progression in the severity of stenosis when followed over time. Thus, medical management is prudent, followed by valve repair when symptoms become severe or uncontrollable. Valve replacement should be undertaken only in those patients in whom repair has failed to make symptoms medically manageable.

Balloon Dilation for Congenital Mitral Stenosis

Although percutaneous balloon dilation of the mitral valve has been a successful treatment for rheumatic mitral stenosis in children, the rarity of congenital mitral stenosis has limited the evaluation of this technique in these patients. The best results appear to be obtained in children with stenosis confined to the valve leaflets, and the poorest results in children with concomitant papillary muscle abnormalities.[32] Mortality for the procedure has varied from 0 to 15%.[33] In a series of 18 infants reported by Moore, improvement in transmitral gradient was obtained in 15 of 18 patients who received balloon dilation.[31] However, symptomatic improvement persisted in less than half of patients, and 2 of 3 infants undergoing repeat dilation died during the procedure.

OPERATIVE TECHNIQUES FOR CONGENITAL MITRAL VALVE DISEASE

Because congenital anomalies of the mitral valve are such a heterogeneous group of malformations, the specific techniques utilized to repair these lesions are likewise varied and must be tailored to the findings in each individual patient. Many of these techniques are identical to those employed for acquired diseases of the mitral valve in adults. These are described in further detail in Chapter 119. Those which are of particular importance to congenital mitral valve disease are discussed here.

Operations for mitral valve disease in infants and children are generally best performed via median sternotomy, which also allows treatment of most coexisting cardiac lesions. Bicaval cannulation for cardiopulmonary bypass is necessary unless the procedure is to be performed under hy-

pothermic circulatory arrest. Systemic hypothermia (20°C) permits low-flow cardiopulmonary bypass during the repair, reducing troublesome pulmonary venous return. The mitral valve is usually exposed through the right atrium and interatrial septum, although an approach anterior to the right pulmonary veins can be employed in older children and adolescents. For stenotic lesions involving the subvalvar apparatus, an apical left ventriculotomy has been reported to afford excellent exposure.[34] To minimize air embolization and facilitate exposure, aortic cross-clamping and cardioplegic arrest should be employed. Before any repair is begun, careful examination and analysis of all components of the mitral apparatus should be undertaken in a systematic manner. The orifice size should be calibrated with Hegar dilators or prosthetic valve sizers. With the heart open, mitral valve competence can be assessed by insufflation of saline into the left ventricle directly through the valve, via a catheter inserted into the left ventricular apex, or by administration of cardioplegia into the aorta while the root is compressed to induce aortic incompetence.

After termination of cardiopulmonary bypass, adequacy of the surgical repair should be assessed by intraoperative transesophageal echocardiography (TEE) whenever possible. Alternatively, surface echocardiography can be employed but is less satisfactory. Technological improvements have produced dual-frequency biplane TEE probes with 64-element sensors contained in a 9.1-mm tip, with color-flow, pulsed-wave, and continuous-wave Doppler capability. Such probes can provide high-resolution images and can be used safety in infants weighing as little as 3 kg. If significant mitral incompetence remains after repair, TEE may localize the site of leakage and direct additional repairs. Prebypass TEE examination of the mitral valve can often be helpful in guiding the repair as well. To assess the hemodynamic adequacy of procedures on stenotic valves, a small polyethylene catheter may be placed across the mitral valve and a direct pull-back gradient measured once the patient has stabilized following the termination of bypass.

PROCEDURES FOR MITRAL INSUFFICIENCY

When adequate anterior leaflet without elongated or ruptured chordae is present, such as with isolated annular dilation or hypoplasia of the posterior leaflet, annuloplasty may be sufficient for adequate repair. Annuloplasty is always necessary when there has been secondary annular dilation. In infants and children, a prosthetic ring should be avoided because it does not allow normal annular growth.

Wooler (Eccentric) Annuloplasty

With this procedure, dilation of the posterior mitral annulus is reduced by two heavy sutures placed beginning just anterior to each commissure and directed a variable distance along the mural annulus. The amount of posterior annulus to be included can be judged by placing a nerve hook or forceps under each commissure and gently pulling in opposite directions.[35] This prevents the elongated posterior leaflet from dropping below the plane of the annulus. Sutures are placed so that this prolapse is eliminated (Fig. 90–4). This technique has provided excellent short- and long-term results, with over 70% of patients becoming asymptomatic following the repair and the vast majority remaining so for follow-up periods of over 10 years (Fig. 90–5).[36]

Modified De Vega Annuloplasty

The circumference of the posterior annulus is reduced by horizontal mattress sutures placed in the atrial wall around the annulus and tightened until the valve becomes competent (Fig. 90–6). Interrupting the annuloplasty at one or two points permits annular growth. Aharon and associates have reported superb results using this technique for reduction of annular dilation in children, with 82% of patients having minimal or no regurgitation postoperatively, and 98% of patients being asymptomatic up to 10 years following operation.[37]

Leaflet Resection and Plication

If chordal agenesis or rupture has rendered the valve incompetent, resection of the unsupported portion of the leaflet is appropriate. Between one-third and one-half of the posterior leaflet may be resected, however, only a very small wedge of the anterior leaflet should be excised or, alternatively, plicated (Fig. 90–7). Larger areas of unsupported anterior leaflet should be repaired by chordal shortening, transfer, or replacement. Because any leaflet resection increases the disparity between mitral orifice size and leaflet area, concomitant annuloplasty is mandatory.

Repair of Clefts and Double-Orifice Valves

Clefts in the anterior leaflet may be repaired with interrupted sutures placed from the annulus to the point where primary chordae support the leaflet edges. To maximize leaflet area, sutures should be placed in the unrolled, free edge of the leaflet on either side of the cleft (Fig. 90–8). The suture line should not extend centrally beyond the chordal insertion, so as not to limit proper opening of the valve. Posterior clefts are remedied by quadrangular resection. If there is associated annular dilation, simultaneous annuloplasty should be performed. When one opening of a double-orifice valve is incompetent, suture closure can be undertaken if the remaining valve orifice is of sufficient size. In the rare instance where a double-orifice valve is stenotic, the bridging tissue should not be divided because of the high likelihood of resulting incompetence.

Chordal Repair

Leaflet prolapse and incompetence due to chordal elongation can be treated by chordal shortening. With this technique, an incision is made into the tip of the papillary muscle, and a small suture is then passed through each side of the groove and around the elongated chordae. The chordal length is thus reduced by twice the distance between its insertion on the tip of the papillary muscle and the level where the suture is placed into the muscle. Alternatively, an unsupported portion of the anterior leaflet can be repaired with quadrangular excision of the opposing segment of the posterior leaflet and transfer of the primary chordae by suturing the segment to the atrial surface of the anterior leaflet. Although chordal replacement with polytetrafluoroethylene (PTFE) suture has been used in adults with good early results, there is only anecdotal experience in infants and children.

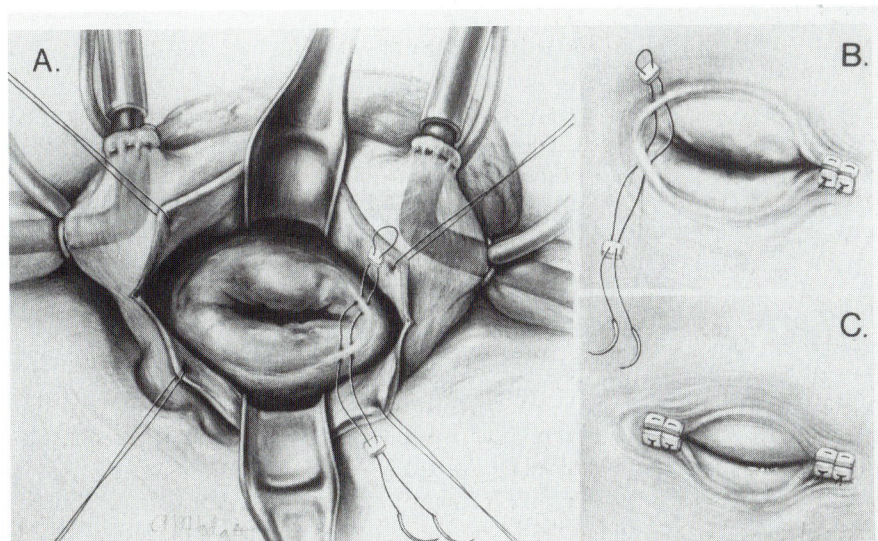

Figure 90–4. Wooler or eccentric annuloplasty. **A.** The initial pledgetted suture is placed just anterior to the posteromedial commissure and then through the posterior annulus, away from the commisure. **B.** Suture passed through the anterolateral commissure. Note that the annuloplasty may be accomplished with a single suture or, alternatively, several smaller sutures at each commissure. **C.** Completed repair which has preserved the length of the anterior leaflet and shortened the posterior leaflet.

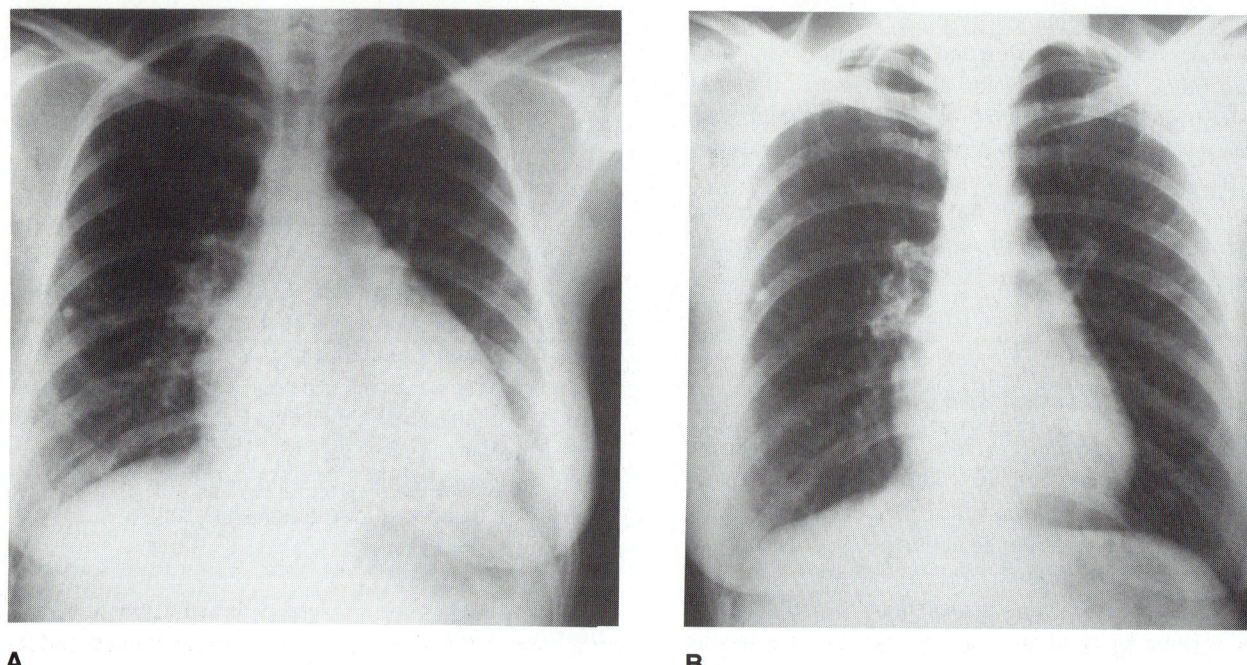

Figure 90–5. Chest radiograph preoperatively (**A**) and 12 years after eccentric annuloplasty (**B**) for congenital mitral insufficiency.

PROCEDURES FOR MITRAL STENOSIS

Resection of Supravalvular Mitral Ring

Although care must be taken not to injure the underlying mitral valve, the supravalvular ring is easily separated from the valve. Resection is started posteriorly, where there is often more distance between the ring and valve, and then extended anteriorly. Because isolated supravalvular mitral ring is unusual, the mitral valve apparatus should be carefully inspected for coexisting lesions after the ring has been excised.

Commissurotomy

When the commissures are absent or fused, commissurotomy can restore considerable mobility to leaflets that are otherwise pliable. Inspection of the subvalvar apparatus and

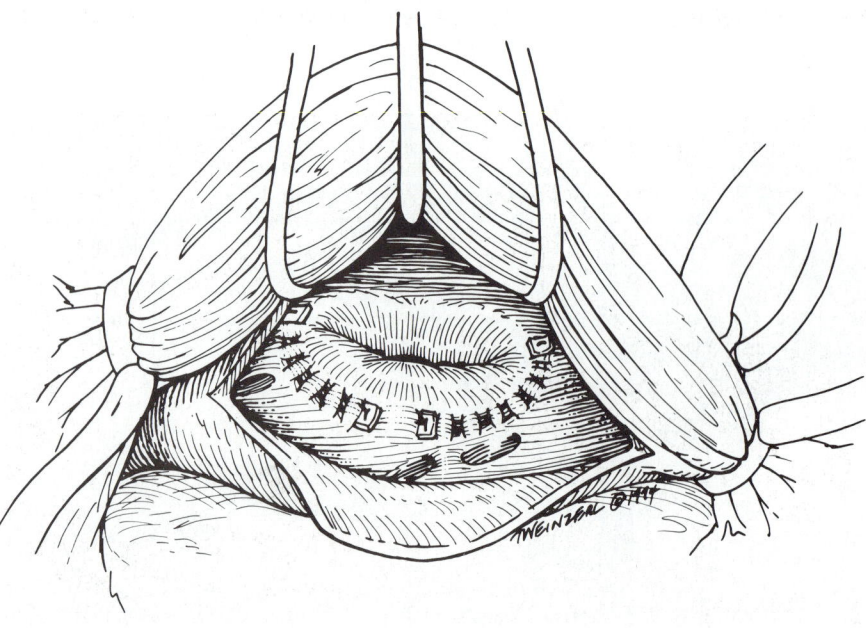

Figure 90–6. Modified DeVega annuloplasty of the mitral valve. Two sutures have been placed from the commissures toward the middle of the mural leaflet, reducing the posterior annular circumference. Interrupting the annuloplasty permits growth.

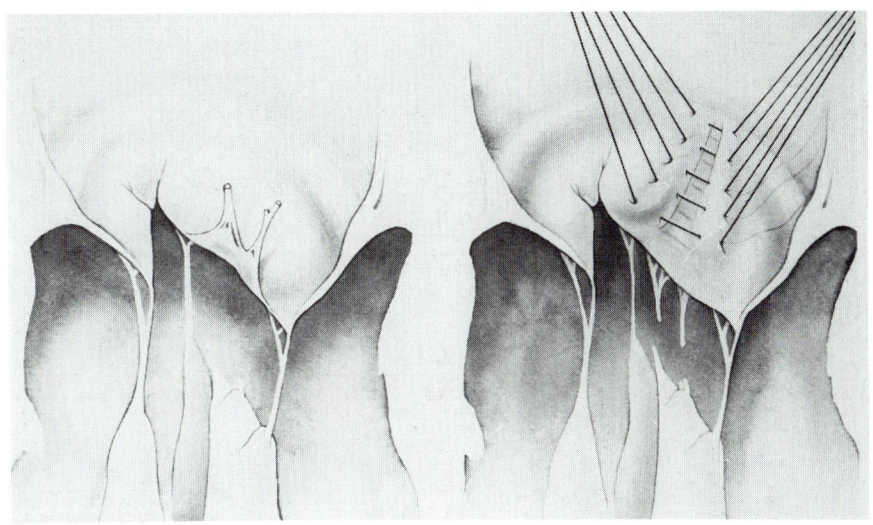

Figure 90–7. Method of plication for flail anterior leaflet. Note that the interrupted suture line narrows toward the annulus, imbricating a wedge-shaped segment of the leaflet. The suture line should be extended onto the atrial wall for a short distance to minimize distortion of the valve.

gentle traction on the leaflets may be helpful in demonstrating the line of division between the leaflets. Incision is begun medially and extended toward the annulus. The annulus itself should not be incised or incompetence may result. Often there is underlying chordal and papillary muscle fusion. Careful incision and separation of these structures will maximize the effective mitral orifice (Fig. 90–9).

Chordal Fenestration and Papillary Muscle Splitting

Often, persistence of interchordal tissue presents a major impediment to left ventricular inflow in congenital mitral stenosis. Removal of the tissue between primary chordae and resection of secondary chordae can greatly increase the effective mitral orifice. When leaflet mobility is limited by abnormally short chordae or malformed papillary muscles (as in parachute and hammock valves) splitting the papillary muscles may improve leaflet excursion. Unfortunately,

when such severe malformations of the subvalvar apparatus are present, relief of obstruction is often incomplete and resulting insufficiency the rule.[18]

Extracardiac Valved Conduit

In those rare cases when the mitral valve is irreparable and prosthetic mitral replacement is not possible because of annular hypoplasia or a small atrium, extracardiac porcine-valved conduits may be used to preserve a biventricular system. This technique has been successfully employed in a handful of patients.[39] Proximally, the conduit is attached to the left atrium via an incision between the base of the appendage and the left pulmonary veins. The distal end of the graft is connected to the apex of the left ventricle just lateral to the left anterior descending coronary. If the native mitral valve has been rendered incompetent by repair attempts, it may be necessary to suture the leaflets closed. Suture obliteration of the annulus itself should be avoided if possible,

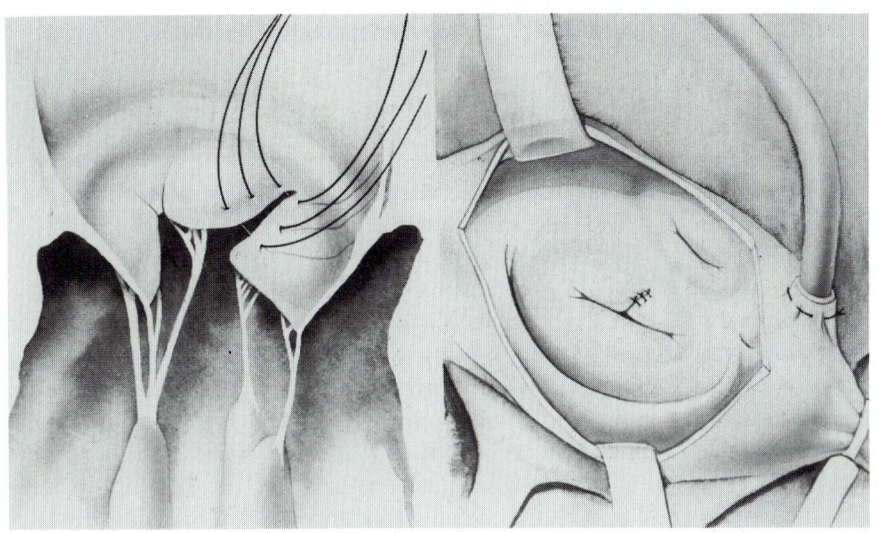

Figure 90–8. Suture of cleft anterior mitral leaflet in a patient with a partial atrioventricular septal defect. The interrupted sutures are placed through the unrolled edge of the leaflet on either side of the cleft to maximize leaflet area.

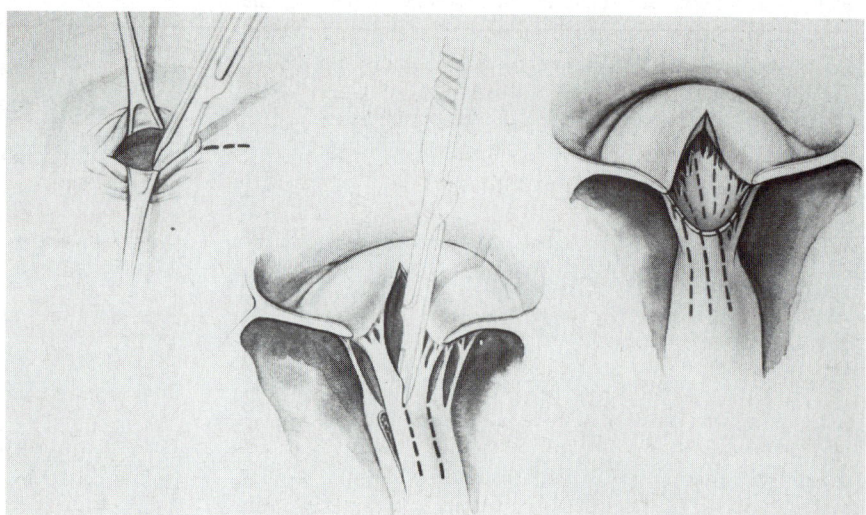

Figure 90–9. Commissurotomy for congenital mitral stenosis. After the valve leaflets are mobilized, the underlying chordae and papillary muscles are inspected and may be split if necessary.

to allow for annular growth and permit future orthotopic valve replacement.

MITRAL VALVE REPLACEMENT IN INFANTS AND CHILDREN

With the reparative techniques available to the surgeon, satisfactory repair of incompetent mitral valves can be accomplished in upward of 80% of cases.[10,40] Unfortunately, the results of repair for stenotic valves and those with mixed lesions are less favorable. When obstructive lesions of the submitral apparatus such as parachute and hammock deformities are operated upon, severe mitral stenosis is often supplemented by florid insufficiency. In such instances, it is not uncommon for mitral valve replacement to be required because of unacceptable hemodynamics following attempted repair.

In older children with an annulus measuring 20 mm or larger, the technique of mitral valve replacement is identical to that used in adults. Preservation of chordal attachments is usually not possible due to malformations of the subvalvar apparatus. Even in adolescents, the rigid mitral prosthesis can cause some degree of left ventricular outflow obstruction, so it is helpful to measure the left ventricular pressure following termination of cardiopulmonary bypass.

When the annulus is not large enough to accept a prosthesis in the orthotopic position, the valve may be placed in a supraannular position within the left atrium. The suture line is begun inferolaterally between the orifice of the left atrial appendage and the true annulus. Special care must be taken not to allow the prosthesis to obstruct the inferior pulmonary veins, a fatal complication.[41] Anteriorly along the interatrial septum, the suture line may be angled superiorly to allow the largest possible prosthesis to be inserted.

The most appropriate type of prosthesis for mitral replacement in children appears to be a low-profile, bileaflet mechanical prosthesis. Heterograft valves exhibit trans-

valvular gradients that are prohibitively high in the smaller sizes and degenerate at an accelerated rate when implanted in the mitral position in children under age 5.[42] Because valve orientation can be critical in young patients with small ventricular cavity size, a rotatable prosthesis may be advantageous.

Although anticoagulation with aspirin and dipyridamole has been employed with satisfactory short-term results,[43] the risk of catastrophic thrombosis and embolization is high in children with mechanical mitral prostheses.[44] Therefore, long-term anticoagulation with Warfarin is optimal for patients with mitral prostheses, and prothrombin time international normalized ratios (INR) of 2.5 to 3.5 should be maintained. However, an antiplatelet regimen may be substituted for Warfarin if bleeding complications are a major concern.

The operative mortality for mitral replacement in children is now quite low, the rate approaching zero.[45] However, repeat valve replacement is common, with nearly 50% of patients requiring reoperation within 3 years. Despite improved early results, long-term survival following mitral valve replacement in young children remains poor, with an actuarial 5-year survival rate of approximately 50%.[42,45]

SUMMARY

Congenital abnormalities of the mitral valve represent a wide spectrum of malformations that cause obstruction, insufficiency, or both. Any or all of the components of the mitral apparatus may be affected. Surgical intervention is reserved for those patients with hemodynamic compromise or whose symptoms cannot be medically controlled. Using a variety of techniques borrowed from surgery for acquired mitral disease (modified to permit annular growth), valve repair is accomplished whenever possible. Prosthetic valve replacement is often necessary for complex or severe deformities. The operative mortality and hemodynamic results of valve replacement are initially satisfactory, however, the risk of thromboembolism and endocarditis, the requirement for long-term anticoagulation, the need for multiple valve replacements in the growing child, and the poor 5-year actuarial survival are of concern with prosthetic replacement of the mitral valve is required.

REFERENCES

1. Davachi F, Moller JH, Edwards JE: Diseases of the mitral valve in infancy. *Circulation* **43**:565, 1971

2. Gausal BM, Arcilla RA, Lev M: *Heart Disease in Children.* Philadelphia, J.B. Lippincott, 1966

3. Shone JD, Sellers RD, Anderson RC, et al: The developmental complex of "parachute mitral valve," supravalvular ring of the left atrium, subaortic stenosis and coarctation of the aorta. *Am J Cardiol* **11**:714, 1963

4. Cutler EC, Levine SA: Cardiotomy and valvotomy for mitral stenosis, experimental observations and clinical notes concerning an operated case with recovery. *Boston Med Surg J* **188**:1022, 1923

5. Mannheimer E, Bengtsson E, Weinberg J; Pure congenital mitral stenosis due to fibroelastosis. *Cardiologia* **21**:574, 1952

6. Bower BD, Gerrard JW, D'Abreu AL, et al: Two cases of congenital mitral stenosis treated by valvotomy. *Arch Dis Child* **28**:91, 1953

7. Braudo JL, Javett SN, Adler DI, Kessel I: Isolated congenital mitral stenosis. Report of two cases with valvotomy in one. *Circulation* **15**:358, 1957

8. Starkey GWB: Surgical experiences in the treatment of congenital mitral stenosis and mitral insufficiency. *J Thorac Cardiovasc Surg* **38**:336, 1959

9. Levy MJ, Varco RL, Lillehei CW, Edwards JE: Mitral insufficiency in infants, children and adolescents. *J Thorac Cardiovasc Surg* **45**:434, 1963

10. Carpentier A, Branchini B, Cour C, et al: Congenital malformations of the mitral valve. Pathology and surgical treatment. *J Thorac Cardiovasc Surg* **72**:854, 1976

11. Ranganathan N, Lam JHC, Wigle ED, Silver MD: Morphology of the human mitral valve, II. The valve leaflets. *Circulation* **41**:459, 1970

12. Tandler J: *Anatomie des Herzens: Handbuch des Anatomie des Mensihen,* Vol 3, Pt 1. Jena, Gustav Fischer, 1913

13. Little RC: The mechanism of closure of the mitral valve: A continuing controversy. *Circulation* **49**:615, 1974

14. Sullivan ID, Robinson PJ, de Leval M, Stark J: Congenital supravalvular mitral stenosis: A treatable form of congenital heart disease. *J Am Coll Cardiol* **8**:159, 1968

15. Rosenquist GC: Congenital mitral valve disease associated with coarctation of the aorta. A spectrum that includes parachute deformity of the mitral valve. *Circulation* **49**:985, 1974

16. Schiebler GL, Edwards JE, Burchell HB, et al: Congenital corrected transposition of the great vessels. A study of 33 cases. *Pediatrics* **27**(suppl.):851, 1961

17. Terzaki AK, Leachman RD, Ali MK, et al: Successful surgical treatment for "parachute mitral valve" complex. *J Thorac Cardiovasc Surg* **56**:1, 1968

18. Schachner A, Varsano I, Levy MJ: The parachute mitral valve complex. Case report and review of the literature. *J Thorac Cardiovasc Surg* **70**:451, 1975

19. Wood AE, Boyle D, O'Hara MD, Leland J: Mitral annuloplasty in endomyocardial fibrosis: An alternative to valve replacement. *Ann Thorac Surg* **34**:446, 1982

20. Freed MD, Keane JF, Van Praagh R, et al: Coarctation of the aorta with congenital mitral regurgitation. *Circulation* **49**:1175, 1974

21. McEnany MT, English TA, Ross DN: The congenitally cleft posterior mitral valve leaflet. An antecedent to mitral regurgitation. *Ann Thorac Surg* **16**:281, 1973

22. Mercer FL, Tubbs OS: Successful surgical management of double mitral valve with subaortic stenosis. *J Thorac Cardiovasc Surg* **67**:440, 1974

23. Johnson TB, Fyfe DA, Swanger SJ: Double orifice mitral valve associated with subaortic stenosis— echocardiographic and anatomic findings. *Cardiol Young* **4**:168, 1994

24. Knight-Mathis V, Cottrill CM, Salley RK: Accessory tissue tags arising from the mitral valve—an unusual cause of ventricular flow obstruction. *Cardiol Young* **4**:175, 1994

25. Yasui H, Kado H, Tokunaga S, et al: Trans-ventricular septal defect approach for resection of accessory mitral valve tissue. *Ann Thorac Surg* **55**:950, 1993

26. Bolling SF, Iannettoni MD, Dick M, et al: Shone's anomaly: Operative results and late outcome. *Ann Thorac Surg* **49**:887, 1990

27. Daoud G, Kaplan S, Perrin EV, et al: Congenital mitral stenosis. *Circulation* **27**:185, 1963

28. Anabtawi IN, Ellison RG: Congenital stenosing ring of the left atrioventricular canal (supravalvular mitral stenosis). *J Thorac Cardiovasc Surg* **49**:994, 1965

29. Kirklin JW, Barrett-Boyes BG: *Cardiac Surgery,* 2nd ed. New York, John Wiley, 1993

30. Collins-Nakai RL, Rosenthal A, Castaneda AR, et al: Congenital mitral stenosis. A review of 20 years' experience. *Circulation* **56**:1039, 1977

31. Moore P, Adatia I, Spevak PJ, et al: Severe congenital mitral stenosis in infants. *Circulation* **89**:2099, 1994

32. Spevak PJ, Bass JL, Ben-Shachar G, et al: Balloon angioplasty for congenital mitral stenosis. *Am J Cardiol* **66**:472, 1992

33. Alday LE, Juaneda E, Spillman A, Ruiz E: Early and late results of balloon dilation for congenital mitral stenosis. *Cardiol Young* **4**:122, 1994

34. Barbero-Marcial M, Riso A, De Alberquerque AT, et al: Left ventricular apical approach for the surgical treatment of congenital mitral stenosis. *J Thorac Cardiovasc Surg* **106**:105, 1993

35. Wooler GH, Nixon PGF, Grimshaw VA: Experiences with the repair of the mitral valve in mitral incompetence. *Thorax* **17**:49, 1962

36. Kahn DR, Stern AM, Sigmann JM, et al: Long-term results of valvuloplasty for mitral insufficiency in children. *J Thorac Cardiovasc Surg* **53**:1, 1967

37. Aharon AS, Laks H, Drinkwater DC, et al: Early and late results of mitral valve repair in children. *J Thorac Cardiovasc Surg* **107**:1262, 1994

38. David TE, Bos J, Rakowski H: Mitral valve repair by replacement of chordae tendinae and polytetraflouroethylene sutures. *J Thorac Cardiovasc Surg* **101**:495, 1991

39. Mazzera E, Corno A, Di Donato R, et al: Surgical bypass of the systemic atrioventricular valve in children by means of a valved conduit. *Ann Thorac Surg* **49**:887, 1990

40. Stellin G, Bortolotti U, Mazzucco A, et al: Repair of congenitally malformed mitral valve in children. *J Thorac Cardiovasc Surg* **95**:480, 1988

41. Adiatia I, Jonas RA, Moore P, Keane JF: Supraannular mitral valve replacement in early childhood. *J Am Coll Cardiol* **24**(suppl):484A, 1994

42. Zweng TN, Bluett MK, Mosca R, et al: Mitral valve replacement in the first five years of life. *Ann Thorac Surg* **47**:720, 1989

43. Pass HI, Sade RM, Crawford FA, Hohm AR: Cardiac valve prostheses in children without anticoagulation. *J Thorac Cardiovasc Surg* **87**:832, 1984

44. McGrath LB, Gonzalez-Lavin L, Eldredge WJ, et al: Thromboemboli and other events following valve replacement in a pediatric population without anticoagulation. *Circulation* **71**(suppl III):148, 1985

45. Kadoba K, Jonas RA, Mayer JE, Castaneda AR: Mitral valve replacement in the first year of life. *J Thorac Cardiovasc Surg* **100**:762, 1990

91

Heart Transplantation for Congenital Heart Disease

Michael del Rio and Leonard L. Bailey

The last decade has ushered in a new era of orthotopic heart transplantation specifically oriented toward the pediatric population. Congenital heart disease has essentially replaced cardiomyopathy as the major indication for transplantation. Included in this new cohort of recipients are newborns and infants with the most severe forms of congenital cardiac anomalies for whom transplantation represents primary surgical therapy. Additional candidates arise from a large population of children whose lives have been extended by various palliative operations, but who have begun to fail. These potential recipients are characterized by deepening cyanosis, worsening congestive heart failure, ascites, enteropathy, or dysrhythmia. Risk of further palliative intervention greatly exceeds any realistic benefits for them. Like children with severe cardiomyopathic illness, heart transplantation represents their last reasonable avenue of hope. It seems appropriate, therefore, to review pediatric heart transplantation in a separate chapter devoted to those aspects of care that are unique to infants and children with congenital heart disease.

Kantrowitz performed the first newborn heart transplant procedure in 1967 at Maimonides Hospital in New York.[1] The infant, who was being treated for Ebstein's anomaly, died several hours postoperatively. Thereafter, beginning in the late 1970s, an occasional youngster with cardiomyopathy had heart transplantation, but little momentum developed that would expand indications for pediatric heart transplantation or nurture public interest in pediatric heart donation. The advent of cyclosporine, a unique and powerful immunosuppressant, rekindled investigation of heart transplantation in newborn laboratory animals.[2] Survival and maturation data from these experimental animals were compelling,[3] and led to the first successful heart trans-

plantation procedure in a newborn baby with hypoplastic left heart syndrome. This was accomplished in 1985 by Bailey and associates at Loma Linda University in California.[4] Since then, 135 centers worldwide have performed nearly 2000 heart transplantation procedures in children 0–17 years of age. One-quarter of these procedures has been accomplished in newborn babies.[5] Children account for approximately 9% of all cardiac transplant operations performed annually, and infant heart transplantation represents the predominant growth area in the field.

The objectives of this chapter are to outline current indications, perioperative management, and specific technical aspects of transplantation as they pertain to the infant or child with congenital heart disease. Immunoregulation and its complications are reviewed. Diagnosis and control of graft rejection are also emphasized. Finally, outcomes of pediatric heart transplantation and future directions in this field are briefly discussed.

INDICATIONS AND PREOPERATIVE ISSUES

Today, the majority of infants and children who present for cardiac transplantation have severe congenital heart disease. The most common indication is hypoplastic left heart syndrome or its equivalent. Specific indications for heart transplantation during early life are listed in Table 91–1. Some children are referred for treatment of cardiomyopathy, but since they are analogous in technical and perioperative management to the adult population, they will not be considered in this chapter.

The single most prevalent risk factor for death immediately following heart transplantation is high pulmonary

TABLE 91–1. CARDIAC ABNORMALITIES FOR WHICH TRANSPLANTATION MAY BE CONSIDERED[a]

HLHS
   With bilateral TAPVC
   With unilateral TAPVC
   With IAA

Hypoplastic LV with hypoplastic AscAo

AS with severe LV EFE, s/p valvotomy

AVSD unbalanced (hypoplastic LV)

MA, DORV, severe subAS, and/or hypoplastic arch

PTA with truncal valve stenosis

Double inlet ventricle with TGA

IAA type B with severe AS

SubAS with multiple VSDs or tricuspid valve straddling

PA, IVS, with Ebstein's anomaly or RV-dependent coronary
   circulation

TA with TGA or double orifice mitral valve

Corrected TGA with hypoplastic RV (systemic), complete heart
   block

Left atrial isomerism

Right atrial isomerism

Anomalous origin of left coronary artery

CHD and CMP with biventricular outflow obstruction

CMP, dilated

CMP, restrictive, hypoplastic RV

Cardiac tumor

[a] The list of indications is dominated by complex forms of single ventricle. HLHS, hypoplastic left heart syndrome; TAPVC, total anomalous pulmonary venous connection; IAA, interrupted aortic arch; LV, left ventricle; AscAo, ascending aorta; AS, aortic stenosis; EFE, endocardial fibroelastosis; s/p, status post; AVSD, atrioventricular septal defect; MA, mitral atresia; DORV, double-outlet right ventricle; subAS, subaortic stenosis; PTA, persistent truncus arteriosus; TGA, transposition of the great arteries; VSD, ventricular septal defect; PA, pulmonary atresia; IVS, intact ventricular septum; RV, right ventricle; TA, tricuspid atresia; CHD, congenital heart disease; CMP, cardiomyopathy.
From Bailey et al.,[39] with permission of Mosby-Year Book.

vascular resistance that is unresponsive to vasodilator therapy.[6] Hence, significant elevation in fixed pulmonary vascular resistance (>4 Wood Units) is a contraindication to isolated orthotopic transplantation. Multiorgan failure, immune deficiency, active infection, and neurologic or chromosomal abnormalities that impair survival are additional exclusion criteria. There are very few anatomic contraindications for heart transplantation in infancy and childhood.

Preoperative mortality among infants listed for transplantation may reach 25%. This mortality relates almost exclusively to infants with single ventricle pathology, whose balance between systemic and pulmonary circulation relies upon patency of both the ductus arteriosus and the atrial septum.[7] Pretransplant mortality may be reduced significantly by aggressive early resuscitative efforts, maintenance of ductus and atrial septal patency, and measures that balance pulmonary resistance to that of the systemic circulation. In practical terms, this demands close observation of individual pretransplant recipients in a tertiary intensive care unit with interventional capability. Ductus-dependent

infants are maintained on a constant intravenous infusion of prostaglandin E_1. Investigators have recently reported stenting of the ductus arteriosus in waiting recipients resistant to prostaglandin E_1 therapy.[8] Balancing of circulatory resistance between the pulmonary and systemic circuit is most responsive to measures aimed at preventing hypocarbia and excessive inspired oxygen. Experience at Loma Linda University and elsewhere suggests that pCO_2 will autoregulate appropriately if inspired oxygen levels are kept between 18 and 20%. Maintenance mechanical ventilation is seldom required. The potential recipient's atrial septum is regularly observed using echocardiography. Should the septal communication become too restrictive, prompt balloon or blade septostomy is accomplished. If this fails, urgent surgical septectomy or more extensive palliative reconstruction, as advocated by Norwood, is required.[9] Beyond these interesting physiologic imperatives of pretransplant care, nutritional support and control of infectious complications become more important as the waiting period for a donor organ becomes prolonged. Table 91–2 outlines pretransplant measures utilized routinely for ductus-dependent infants at Loma Linda University. An occasional infant with unrestricted pulmonary blood flow may require pulmonary artery banding prior to transplantation. This is accomplished if no donor has become available, between the third and fourth month of life in an effort to prevent development of pulmonary vascular obstructive disease during the waiting period.

ANESTHESIA

With the induction of anesthesia, pulmonary and systemic vascular resistances are balanced through changes in ventilation, acid-base, and inotropic support.[10] Negative inotropic anesthesics are avoided as well as nitrous oxide, which has pulmonary vasoconstrictive properties. Fentanyl is used because of its cardiovascular stability in infants, particularly those with hypoplastic left heart syndrome. Pul-

TABLE 91–2. PRETRANSPLANT MANAGEMENT TECHNIQUES FOR YOUNG INFANTS WITH COMPLEX CONGENITAL HEART DISEASE[a]

Ductus-Dependent Circulation		Pulmonary Overcirculation
Pulmonary	Systemic	
PGE_1	PGE_1	Pulmonary arterial band
S/P shunt	FIO_2 (18%)	
Ductus stent	$FICO_2$	
	Controlled Ventilation	
	Ensure atrial mix	
	Ductus stent	
	Norwood's OMNI procedure	

[a] PGE_1, prostaglandin E_1; S/P, systemic/pulmonary; FIO_2, inspired oxygen concentration; $FICO_2$, inspired carbon dioxide concentration.

monary vasodilators are not used before the onset of extracorporeal circulation. Surface cooling is initiated after all catheters are placed and surgical preparation is started. Inotropic and vasoactive agents are utilized to aid separation from cardiopulmonary bypass. All blood products are irradiated or filtered and are negative for cytomegalovirus.

ORGAN DONOR ISSUES

Transplantation is the only rational surgical therapy for end-stage pediatric cardiomyopathic disease. It may also be the best surgical option for many young patients with univentricular congenital heart disease. What keeps heart transplantation out of the mainstream of surgical options for treatment of structural heart disease is the limitation in donor organ supply. Pediatric organ donation is based on a clear declaration of brain death.[11] Aside from this, donation is limited by social and emotional issues relating to families of infants and children declared dead, and by the skills and willingness of health care providers to effect organ donation. Given 40,000 annual deaths from all causes among infants in the first year of life alone in the United States, it might be reasonable to expect improvement in the supply of donor organs as more families and pediatric providers embrace and facilitate the concept of organ transplantation.

Organ donation and procurement are fundamental to a successful pediatric heart transplantation program. A decade of experience by the Loma Linda University program suggests that virtually all hearts offered for donation can be utilized. At least two factors are responsible for this unique situation. As a rule, pediatric donors have been reasonably healthy until very near the time death was declared. In addition, most procurement agencies have become quite skillful at managing potential pediatric donors until the hour of procurement. Donor cardiopulmonary resuscitation, inotropic support, treated infection, geographic distance (graft cold ischemic time), and donor-recipient size mismatch (up to 4:1) now rarely limit successful heart transplantation.[14,15] Very clear contraindications should exist before a donor heart is rejected.

Contraindications for use of a pediatric donor heart might include complex congenital heart disease, severe global dysfunction of the heart (shortening fraction <25% with adequate preload and inotropic support), genetic myopathic disease, uncontrolled infectious disease, or cancer (other than primary brain tumors). Since the majority of pediatric donors derive from an acute process such as trauma, birth asphyxia, sudden death, or some other event limited to the brain, these contraindications seldom apply.

THE DONOR OPERATION

Heart procurement is based upon specific recipient requirements. It ranges from removal of only the heart, to en bloc removal of the heart, systemic veins, and great vessels. Because multiorgan donation is the rule, advanced planning for individual organ requirements is vital. A recipient with surgically distorted or atretic central pulmonary arteries may require donor pulmonary arteries extending from lung to lung to facilitate transplantation reconstruction. The same donor cannot easily provide lungs as separate organs. A recipient with situs inversus, as another example of extended procurement, will require en bloc removal of systemic veins to complete engraftment of a heart with atrial situs solitus.

Graft procurement, even with extended requirements, need not be difficult. Donors are given antibiotics, methylprednisolone, and dextrose intravenously. The donor's chest is fully extended prior to preparation and draping. Through a midline incision, the thymus is removed and the veins and great vessels required for transplant reconstruction are dissected free of surrounding tissue. The ductus arteriosus (or ligamentum) is doubly ligated and divided. Unnecessary tributaries and branches are ligated and divided. A cardioplegic delivery catheter is inserted into the root of the aorta after the donor is heparinized in concert with other procurement teams. The pericardium is opened widely into both pleural spaces, following which the inferior vena cava and at least one pulmonary vein are transected. The heart is permitted to empty, the aorta is clamped just beyond the cardioplegia catheter, and cold cardioplegic infusion is commenced. Many solutions are useful for this purpose. The Loma Linda University group utilizes 5% dextrose in water containing 27 mEq/L of sodium, 20 mEq/L of potassium, 250 mg/L of methylprednisolone, and 3 mEq/L of magnesium. The solution is buffered with sodium bicarbonate to a normal pH. It contains no calcium.

The remaining pulmonary and systemic veins are divided, followed by division of branch pulmonary arteries and the aorta, The collapsed heart, still being perfused with cold cardioplegic solution, is transferred into a basin of cold saline for additional trimming and closure of any septal defects. The graft is then packaged in simple 5% dextrose in saline solution, placed in a plastic cooler in which it is surrounded by ice, and made ready for transport. Hearts prepared in this way have been successfully transplanted following more than 8 hours of cold ischemic time.[14] The donor procurement process is illustrated in Figures 91–1 to 91–4. Figures 91–5 and 91–6 illustrate the final graft appearance based upon individual recipient requirement for transplant reconstruction.

RECIPIENT OPERATIONS

Neonatal and very young infant recipients with complex structural anomalies are referred for heart transplantation as primary surgical intervention. Older infants and children have usually had one or more previous palliative procedures, and heart transplantation is an exercise in reoperative

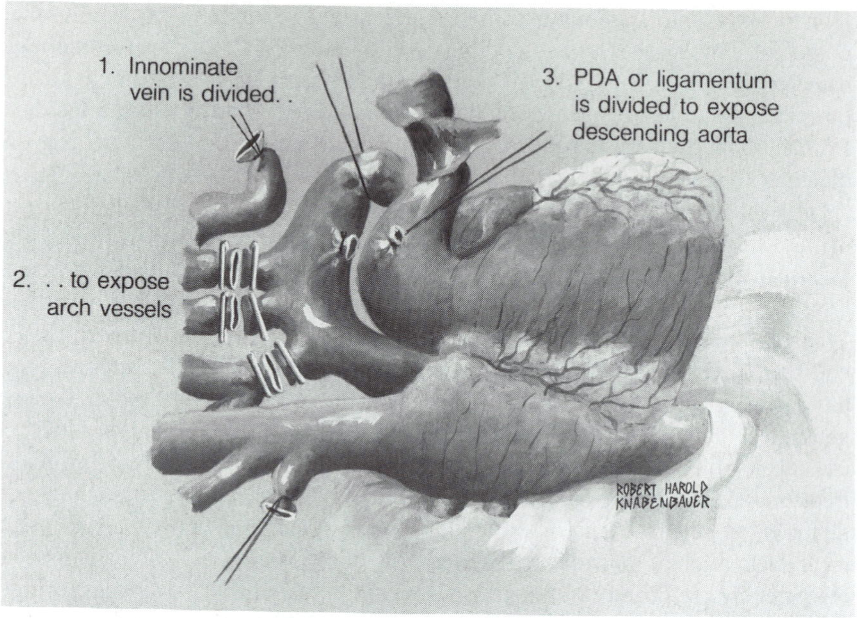

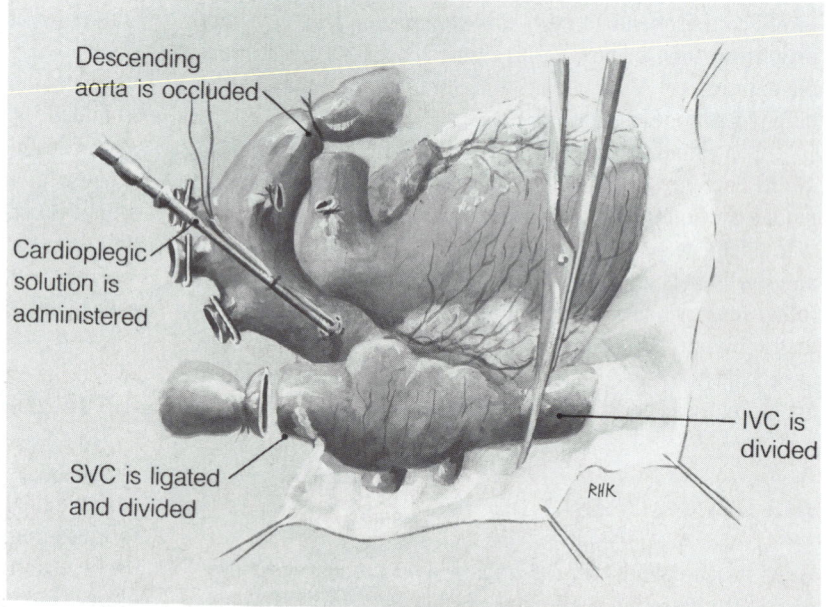

Figure 91–1. Donor heart procurement for an infant recipient with hypoplastic left heart syndrome is illustrated. The thymus is removed and the innominate vein divided. Exposed aortic arch vessels are clipped or ligated and divided. The ductus (or ligamentum) is doubly ligated and divided. The entire aortic arch and proximal descending aorta are mobilized. *(From Chiavarelli M, Gundry S, Razzouk A, Bailey L: Operative procedures for infant cardiac transplantation. In Kapoor A, Laks H (eds): Atlas of Heart-Lung Transplantation. New York, McGraw-Hill, 1994, with permission.)*

reconstruction.[15] Some recipients with complicated iatrogenic and native structural anomalies, such as those with visceral heterotaxia, atrial situs inversus, hypoplastic or interrupted aortic arch, or complex pulmonary venous drainage patterns, require quite tedious reconstruction. Nevertheless, with rare exception (notably, absence or marked hypoplasia of intrahilar pulmonary arteries or veins), successful heart transplantation has been achieved.[18–20]

Neonatal and infant heart transplant procedures are accomplished using simple cannulation techniques, profound systemic hypothermia, low flow perfusion, and intermittent periods of circulatory arrest. These same techniques apply to older and larger children when complicated reoperative anatomy is an issue. Standard perfusion techniques utilized for heart transplantation among older children and young adults with normal anatomy are described elsewhere in this volume. In keeping with the pediatric focus of this chapter, the following operative descriptions are directed toward recipients whose indication for heart transplantation is complex congenital heart disease.

HYPOPLASTIC LEFT HEART SYNDROME OR EQUIVALENT

Through a median sternotomy, the thymus is removed and the pericardium opened widely. A silk suture is placed

Figure 91–2. After heparinization of the donor, a cardioplegia perfusion catheter is inserted into the ascending aorta and attached to a gravity-fed cold cardioplegia delivery system. The pericardium is opened widely into both pleural spaces. The superior vena cava (SVC) is ligated. The inferior vena cava (IVC) and at least one pulmonary vein are divided. The superior vena cava is then divided and the graft is permitted a few seconds during which to empty. The descending aorta is then ligated and cold cardioplegia is delivered. *(From Chiavarelli M, Gundry S, Razzouk A, Bailey L: Operative procedures for infant cardiac transplantation. In Kapoor A, Laks H (eds): Atlas of Heart-Lung Transplantation. New York, McGraw-Hill, 1994, with permission.)*

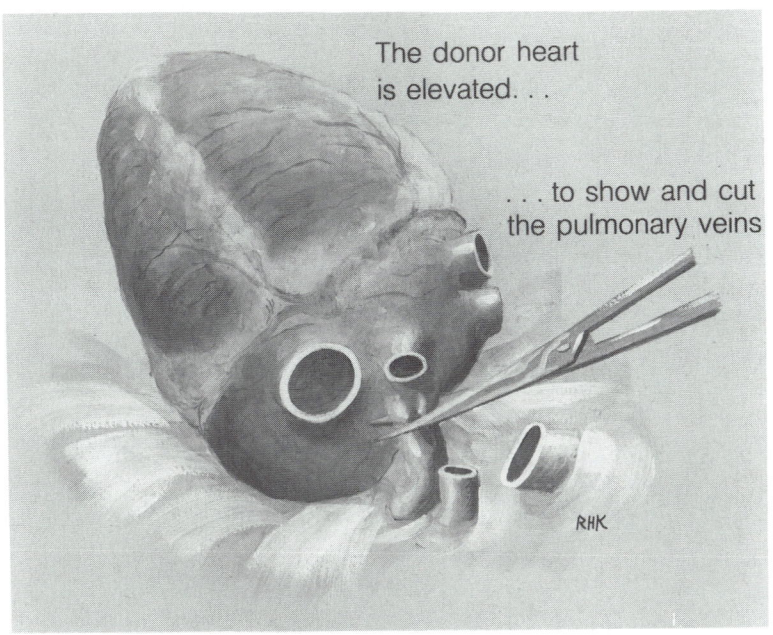

Figure 91–3. The donor graft is retracted and the remaining atrial and pulmonary artery attachments are divided. The ascending aorta is then clamped and the distal aortic arch is divided, releasing the graft for transfer into a basin of cold saline. The cardioplegia catheter is removed, any septal defect is repaired, and the graft is trimmed for implantation. *(From Chiavarelli M, Gundry S, Razzouk A, Bailey L: Operative procedures for infant cardiac transplantation. In Kapoor A, Laks H (eds): Atlas of Heart-Lung Transplantation. New York, McGraw-Hill, 1994, with permission.)*

loosely about the ductus arteriosus to be used later as a tourniquet, and thereafter as a ligature and retraction device. Heparin is administered. An arterial cannula is inserted into the large main pulmonary artery, the tip of which is directed into the ductus arteriosus. A venous return cannula is placed into the right atrium, and extracorporeal circulation is begun to induce systemic hypothermia to a core temperature of 18°–20°C. Arterial flow is directed exclusively to systemic circulation by tightening the ductus tourniquet. During this period of time, aortic arch vessels are isolated and looped with silk sutures, which later become tourniquet retractors during open aortic arch reconstruction. The small ascending aorta is ligated and divided to facilitate exposure and dissection of the entire aortic arch, ductus arteriosus,

and proximal descending aorta. The left recurrent laryngeal and phrenic nerves are vulnerable during this dissection, but injury to these structures can be avoided by careful and patient dissection.

After 12–20 min of systemic cooling to the desired level of hypothermia, aortic arch vessels are occluded, extracorporeal circulation is discontinued, and perfusion cannulae are removed. The ductus arteriosus is ligated at its pulmonary artery end. It is then divided, and the ligature is used to retract the pulmonary arteries away from the distal aortic arch and proximal descending aorta. Additional ductus tissue is excised off the aortic wall and the aorta is opened distally and proximally along its lesser curvature. The heart is removed, leaving right and left native atrial components be-

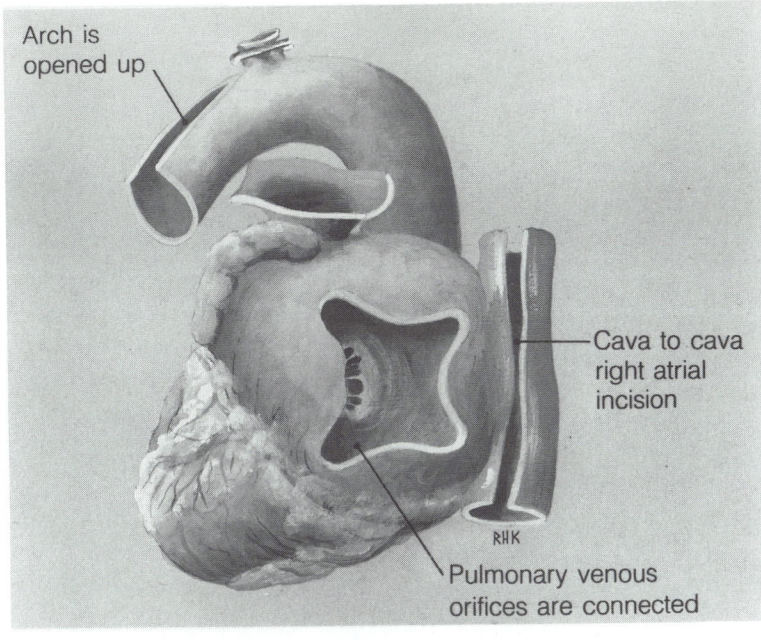

Figure 91–4. Final appearance of the donor heart intended for implantation into an infant recipient with hypoplastic left heart syndrome or its univentricular equivalent. The graft is ready for cold storage and transport. *(From Chiavarelli M, Gundry S, Razzouk A, Bailey L: Operative procedures for infant cardiac transplantation. In Kapoor A, Laks H (eds): Atlas of Heart-Lung Transplantation. New York, McGraw-Hill, 1994, with permission.)*

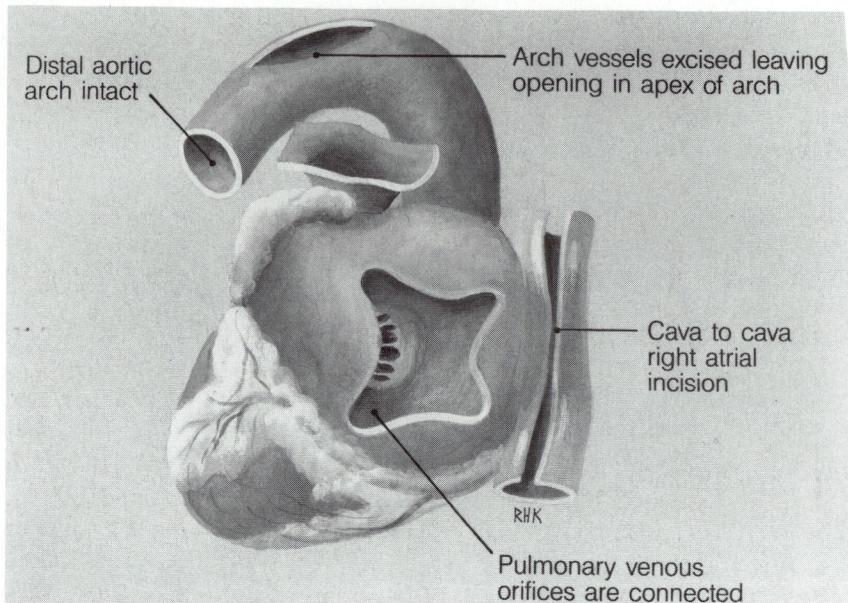

Figure 91–5. Final appearance of a donor heart destined for transplantation reconstruction in an infant with interruption of the aortic arch. The distal aortic arch is intact and the arch vessels are excised en bloc, leaving a site for onlay of the recipient's cluster of aortic arch vessels. *(Reprinted with permission from The International Society for Heart and Lung Transplantation. From Bailey.[20])*

hind as with any heart transplant procedure. The left pericardium, anterior to the left phrenic nerve, is removed.

Donor graft implantation is accomplished by continuous suturing of interatrial septum, right atrium, and left atrium in sequence. The left side of the heart is filled with cold saline just before completion of the left atrial suture line. The donor aortic arch is transected immediately proximal to the ductus insertion. The ligated stumps of left carotid and subclavian arteries are excised and the greater curvature of the donor aortic arch is opened from the left carotid to the transected distal end. Arch reconstruction is begun at the distal end of the recipient incision, completing the posterior 7-0 continuous suture line first. The anterior row of sutures completes aortic reconstruction. Next, the

ligature is removed from the brachiocephalic arterial stump. The previous cardioplegic infusion site is dilated (as a vent site), air is displaced out of the aorta with cold saline, and the arterial cannula is inserted through the stump of the brachiocephalic artery. The cannula is secured with a tourniquet suture. The new right atrium is cannulated and extracorporeal circulation is gently recommenced. Tourniquets are removed from the recipient's aortic arch vessels to permit head reperfusion. Circulatory arrest seldom exceeds 45 min using this operative approach. Rewarming is begun, and the rate of perfusion gradually increased. Rhythmic cardiac contractions tend to recover spontaneously and rhythm evolves to normal sinus as the infant and donor heart are rewarmed. The pulmonary artery anastomosis is accom-

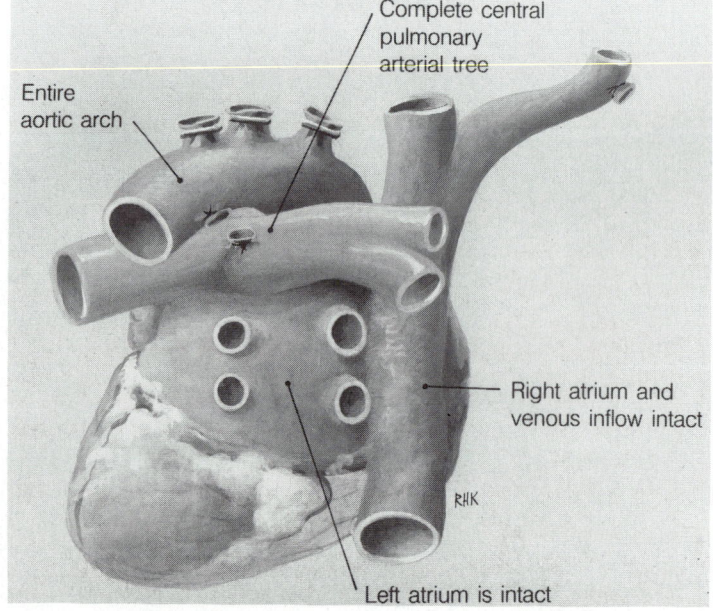

Figure 91–6. Final appearance of a donor heart graft intended for transplant reconstruction in an infant or child with previous cavopulmonary shunts, absent or destroyed central pulmonary arteries, and visceral heterotaxia. The right atrium is intact with attached lengths of systemic veins. The left atrium is also left intact since the location of the left atrial incision may vary, depending on the recipient's anatomy. This heart would also accomodate a recipient with atrial situs inversus. *(Reprinted with permission from The International Society for Heart and Lung Transplantation. From Bailey.[20])*

plished during this phase of operation. Graft reperfusion with extracorporeal support is extended to 60 min or more to ensure adequate recovery. During the last half of reperfusion, calcium and potassium levels are corrected. Drug infusions, instituted by the anesthiologists, consist of (1) dopamine, 2μg/kg per minute, (2) tolazoline, 1 mg/kg per hour, (3) prostaglandin E_1, 0.05 μg/kg per minute, and, occasionally, (4) isoproterenol, 0.01–0.02 μg/kg per minute. Dopamine and tolazoline are continued for the initial 24–48 posttransplant hours. Prostaglandin E_1 is slowly tapered during 5–7 days, and then discontinued.

After an hour or more of reperfusion, extracorporeal circulation is discontinued. Protamine and blood products are administered, and surgical hemostasis is verified. Chest drains are inserted, optional temporary pacer wires applied, and, in most instances, the chest is closed primarily. The decision for or against primary closure is based on experience and judgment. This decision is no different for heart transplantation than for any other heart operation during early infancy. The goal is to avoid mechanical hemodynamic compromise during the early recovery phase.

Transplantation for hypoplastic left heart syndrome and equivalent malformations is illustrated in Figures 91–7 to 91–12. Variation in techniques for infants who have interruption of the aortic arch and/or total anomalous pulmonary venous connection complicating hypoplastic left heart syndrome is illustrated in Figures 91–13 to 91–15.

OTHER COMPLEX MALFORMATIONS

Older infants and children with complex variations of single ventricle and one or more previous palliative cardiac operations present for transplantation because of failed physiology and increasing cyanosis. Infants with reconstructive procedures for hypoplastic left heart syndrome sometimes fall into this category. Scores of older children with single ventricle, whose history includes palliative systemic-pulmonary shunts or atriopulmonary connection, may also become candidates for transplantation as a final, definitive procedure. These children represent a formidable technical challenge. Several examples of transplant reconstruction of complex anatomic variations are illustrated in Figures 91–16 to 91–18.

The Loma Linda University approach to infants and children in this category is to re-explore the chest with an eye to simple isolation and cannulation of the distal ascending aorta, and either the right or left atrium. Rarely, the arterial system is approached by groin cannulation. Extracorporeal circulation is established early during re-exploration. Hypothermia is induced to permit the options of low flow perfusion and intermittent circulatory arrest. The vast majority of dissection is achieved during the cooling phase of extracorporeal circulation. Despite the complex nature of recipient pathology, a minimum of operative morbidity has been encountered. A more detailed description of alternatives for transplant reconstruction among these complicated recipients may be found among the references provided.[19–21] Important considerations in the surgical management of these infants and children include the following: (1) avoid transplanting a child with fixed pulmonary vascular disease, (2) understand and patiently dissect out the anatomic features, (3) utilize graft procurement that includes adequate donor veins and arteries with which to effect reconstruction in the recipient, and (4) use systemic hypothermia with perfusion options that facilitate transplant reconstruction.

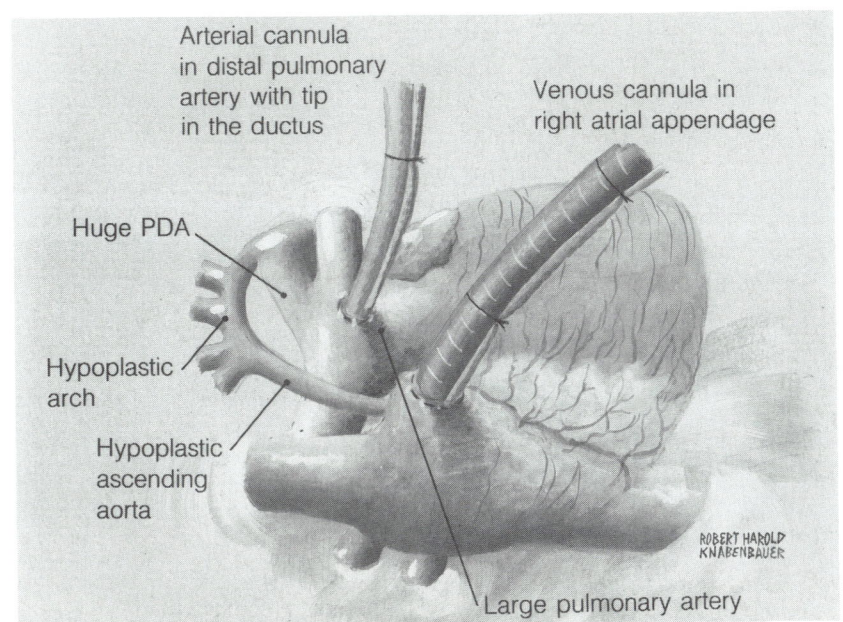

Arterial cannula in distal pulmonary artery with tip in the ductus

Venous cannula in right atrial appendage

Huge PDA

Hypoplastic arch

Hypoplastic ascending aorta

ROBERT HAROLD KNABENBAUER

Large pulmonary artery

Figure 91–7. Perfusion techniques used to achieve heart transplantation in an infant with hypoplastic left heart syndrome. Systemic arterial perfusion is achieved by way of the patent ductus arteriosus (PDA). *(From Chiavarelli M, Gundry S, Razzouk A, Bailey L: Operative procedures for infant cardiac transplantation. In Kapoor A, Laks H (eds): Atlas of Heart-Lung Transplantation. New York, McGraw-Hill, 1994, with permission.)*

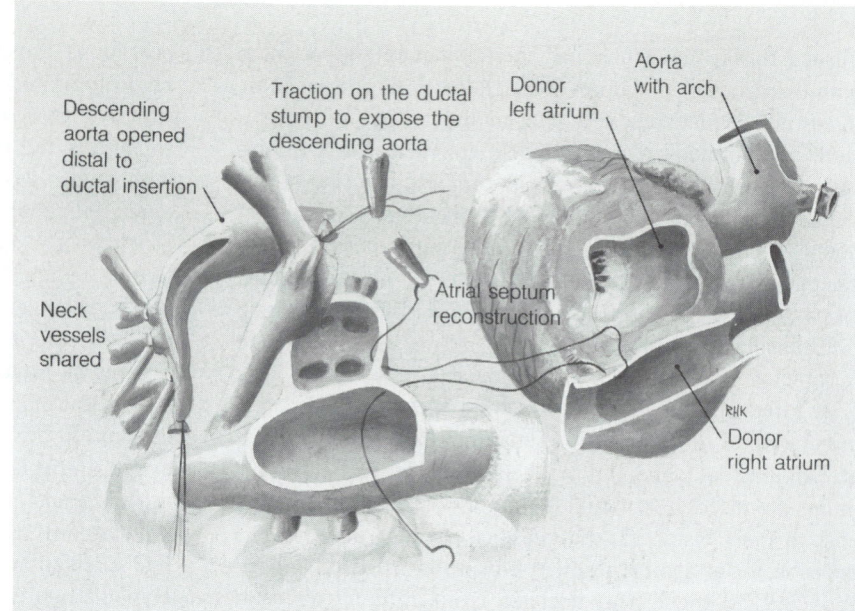

Figure 91–8. After excision of the native heart, the recipient's aortic arch is opened widely along the lesser curvature to a point well below the ductus arteriosus. Implantation of the heart graft commences at the base of the atrial septum. *(From Chiavarelli M, Gundry S, Razzouk A, Bailey L: Operative procedures for infant cardiac transplantation. In Kapoor A, Laks H (eds): Atlas of Heart-Lung Transplantation. New York, McGraw-Hill, 1994, with permission.)*

Postoperative Support

Early perioperative management is typically uneventful. Cyclosporine is started intravenously, preoperatively, withheld during extracorporeal circulation, and restarted in a dose of 0.1 mg/kg per hour. Methylprednisolone is administered intraoperatively and continued postoperatively at a dose of 25 mg/kg given intravenously every 12 hours for two days. Maintenance steroids are used by many groups, but steroids have not been part of the Loma Linda University immunomodulation protocol. Rabbit antithymocyte globulin has been used as induction therapy for all non-newborn recipients (0.5 mL/kg × 5 days). Prospective randomized trials have confirmed decreased rejection rates

with this induction protocol.[22] Azathioprine is initiated at 3 mg/kg per day and adjusted to maintain a white blood count >4000/mL.[3]

Infection prophylaxis includes use of cephalosporin and standard isolation techniques. Four to six doses of immunoglobulin (400 mg/kg per dose) are administered intravenously during the first postoperative week. Acyclovir is given prophylactically during the first three posttransplant months to help prevent systemic cytomegalovirus infection.

Routine blood analyses, chest roentgenogram, and electrocardiogram are monitored daily during the first posttransplant week, and twice per week thereafter during hospitalization. Noninvasive surveillance with echocardiography is performed twice per week. Older children are

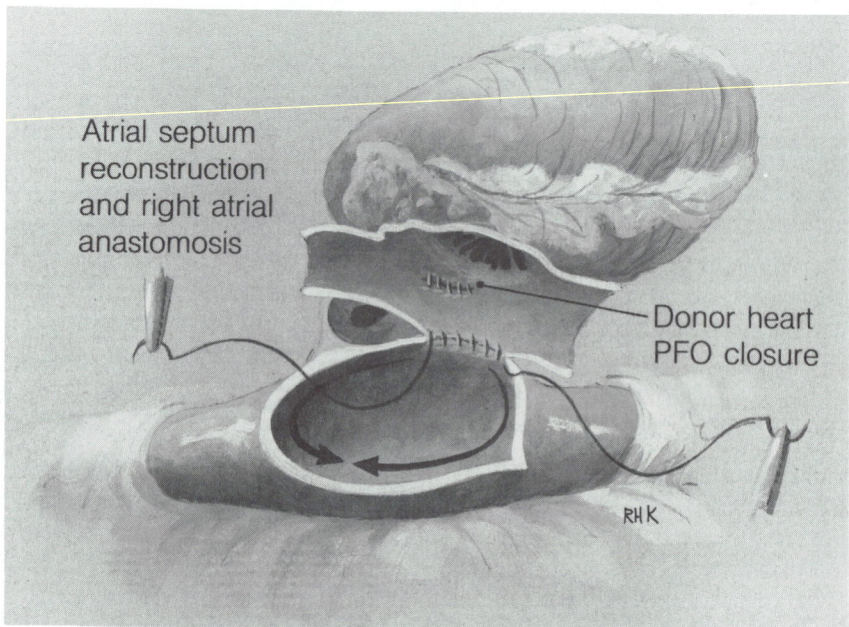

Figure 91–9. The atrial septal and right atrial anastomoses are completed first. Any defect in the donor atrial septum is repaired. PFO, patent foremen ovale. *(From Chiavarelli M, Gundry S, Razzouk A, Bailey L: Operative procedures for infant cardiac transplantation. In Kapoor A, Laks H (eds): Atlas of Heart-Lung Transplantation. New York, McGraw-Hill, 1994, with permission.)*

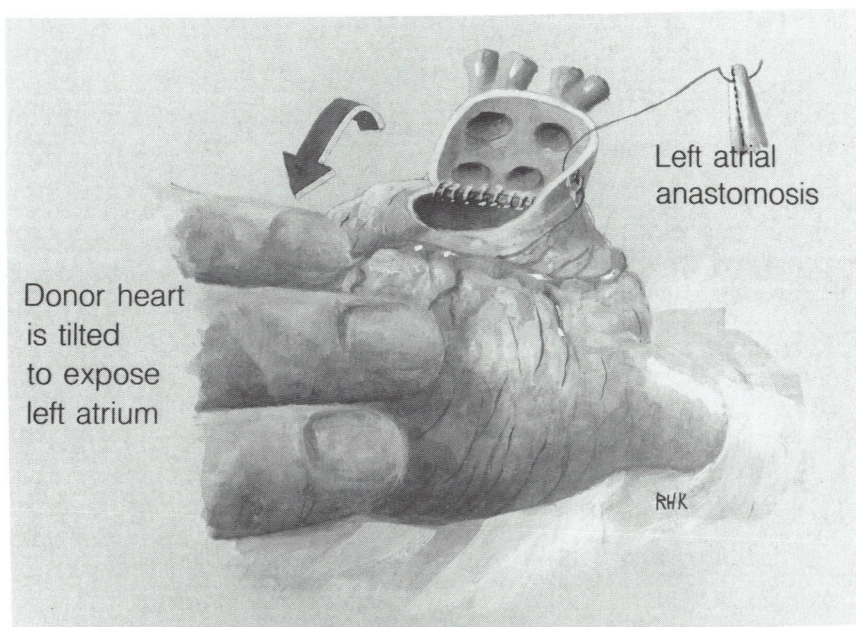

Figure 91–10. The donor heart is retracted toward the operating surgeon and the left atrial anastomosis is completed. The left heart is filled with cold saline before final closure of the left atrial suture line. *(From Chiavarelli M, Gundry S, Razzouk A, Bailey L: Operative procedures for infant cardiac transplantation. In Kapoor A, Laks H (eds): Atlas of Heart-Lung Transplantation. New York, McGraw-Hill, 1994, with permission.)*

subjected to one or two screening endomyocardial biopsies during perioperative surveillance.

IMMUNOSUPPRESSION

Many centers performing pediatric heart transplant procedures utilize triple drug therapy consisting of cyclosporine, azathioprine, and prednisone.[23] Some use antithymocyte induction, while others choose to reserve T cell antibody therapy for treatment of rejection episodes.[24] Programs with maintenance protocols that include corticosteroid make every effort to minimize the dose or gradually withdraw recipients from steroid maintenance during the late follow-up period.[25] Double drug therapy, which eliminates steroid from maintenance immunoregulation, is employed by the Loma Linda University and Harefield Hospital (England) groups.[26] This steroid-free protocol is aimed at avoiding the well-known side effects of chronic administration of corticosteroid and its possible contribution to graft coronary artery disease. Double drug therapy consists of cyclosporine and either azathioprine or methotrexate. The Pittsburgh group is noteworthy for its experimental maintenance therapy using a newer agent called FK-506. This drug, similar in action to cyclosporine, is thought to be somewhat more efficacious, permitting FK-506 monother-

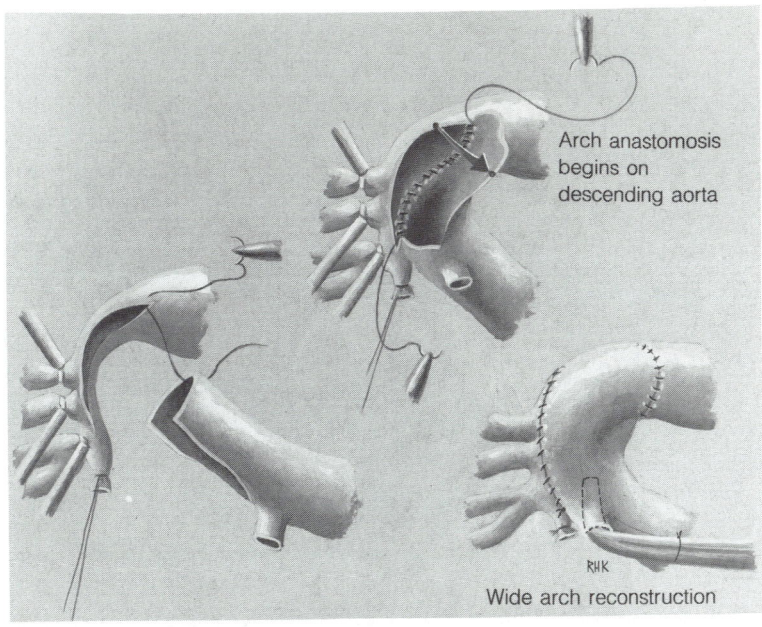

Figure 91–11. Aortic arch reconstruction begins on the descending aorta using a posterior, then an anterior running suture line to complete the repair. The aortic perfusion cannula is inserted into the newly constructed aortic arch by way of the donor brachiocephalic arterial stump. *(From Chiavarelli M, Gundry S, Razzouk A, Bailey L: Operative procedures for infant cardiac transplantation. In Kapoor A, Laks H (eds): Atlas of Heart-Lung Transplantation. New York, McGraw-Hill, 1994, with permission.)*

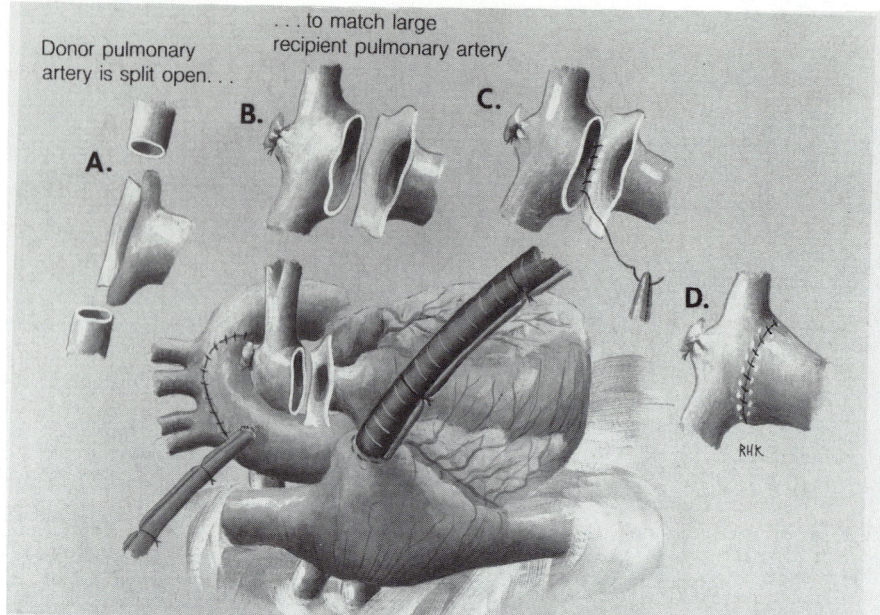

Figure 91–12. A–D. During extracorporeal reperfusion, the pulmonary artery anastomosis is completed. *(From Chiavarelli M, Gundry S, Razzouk A, Bailey L: Operative procedures for infant cardiac transplantation. In Kapoor A, Laks H (eds): Atlas of Heart-Lung Transplantation. New York, McGraw-Hill, 1994, with permission.)*

apy for some pediatric recipients.[27] The Loma Linda University protocol uses oral cyclosporine in a dose of 20 mg/kg per 24 hours. That dose is regulated to obtain blood levels in the range of 250–300 ng/mL during the first six posttransplant months, 150–200 ng/mL during the second 6 mo, and 100–150 ng/mL thereafter. A monoclonal antibody assay is utilized for measurement of blood cyclosporine levels. Azathioprine is tapered to 1 mg/kg per day during the first posttransplant year, and is discontinued among neonatal recipients at 1 year if graft rejection has not been an issue.

REJECTION DIAGNOSIS AND TREATMENT

Surveillance is accomplished noninvasively by utilizing the echocardiogram, electrocardiogram, chest roentgenogram, blood analyses, and clinical evaluation. Echocardiographic findings of a new pericardial effusion, thickening of the posterior and septal left ventricular wall, new mitral regurgitation, or decreasing left ventricular shortening fraction are consistent with rejection.[28] In addition, R-wave summation electrocardiography, cyclosporine levels, and immune activation assays aid analysis. Endomyocardial biopsies are performed routinely in some centers, but are reserved for ambiguous situations in the Loma Linda University surveillance protocol. For example, the average number of endomyocardial biopsies performed at Loma Linda University is 0.26/pediatric patient per year during the first posttransplant year.

The most active period of rejection appears to be the first three posttransplant months when surveillance visits are coordinated twice weekly. After 6 months if no signifi-

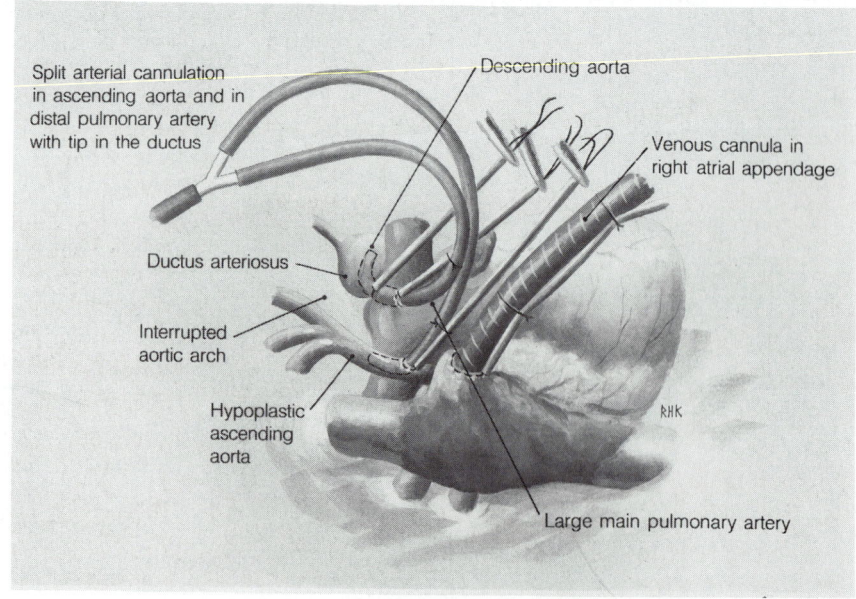

Figure 91–13. Orientation of extracorporeal perfusion in an infant with hypoplastic left heart syndrome and aortic arch interruption. A split arterial cannula ensures perfusion of both head and body. *(Reprinted with permission from The International Society for Heart and Lung Transplantation. From Bailey.[20])*

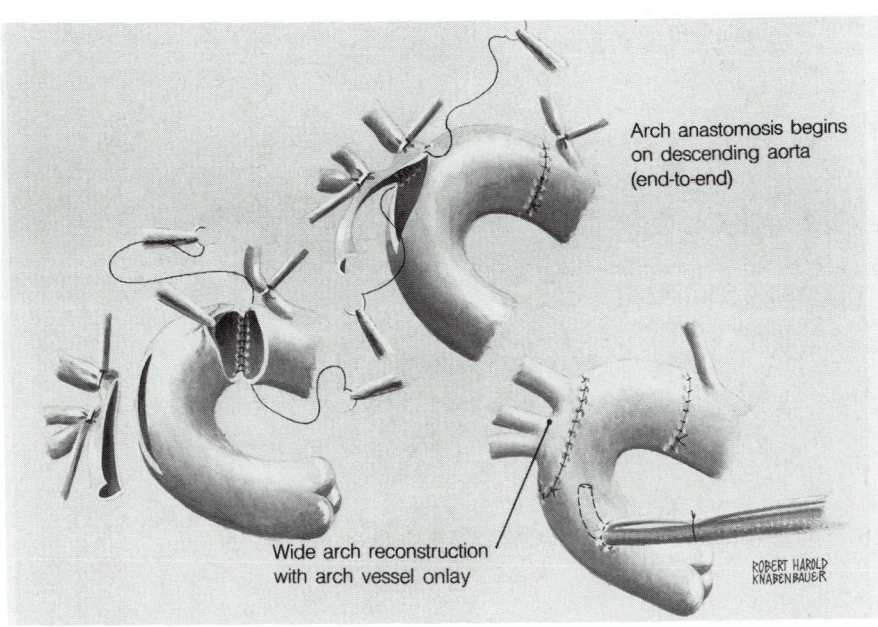

Figure 91–14. Aortic arch reconstruction in an infant with arch interruption. A distal end to end anastomosis is created followed by onlay of the arch vessels. *(Reprinted with permission from The International Society for Heart and Lung Transplantation. From Bailey.[20])*

cant rejection episode has occurred, visits are arranged monthly. All children are subjected to complete cardiac catheterization, which includes endomyocardial biopsy at 1 year. Surveillance visits decrease to once every 3 months if findings suggest immune quiescence.

High dose methylprednisolone is used as initial treatment for a diagnosed rejection episode. It is administered intravenously twice daily for 4 days (25 mg/kg per dose). If response is poor (delayed) or rejection appears very early after transplantation or is particularly severe, a 7–10 day course of antithymocyte globulin is used. Methotrexate is added to the treatment regimen if there is recurrent rejection that seems unresponsive to steroid or antithymocyte treatment. Methotrexate is also used if rejection has caused he-

modynamic compromise.[29] It is administered in a dose of 10 mg/m^2 per week, divided into three doses. Total lymphoid irradiation has been advocated for management of difficult immune responders.[30] Two of four recipients treated with total lymphoid irradiation for recalcitrant rejection at Loma Linda University are surviving.

Rejection has correlated with age at transplantation and with active cytomegalovirus infection. Long-term freedom from rejection was 19% for newborns, 42% for infants, and 25% for children/adolescents.[31] HLA mismatching has not predicted early rejection or increased rejection episodes in the Loma Linda University series. Only 32% of patients have had any HLA-DR match.[32] Rejection is influenced by the seasonal variation in risk of infection, with

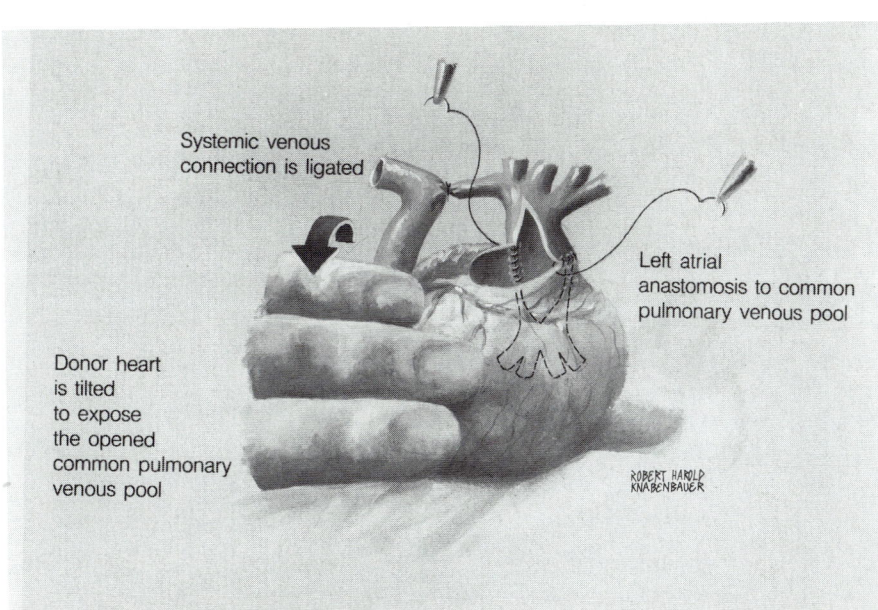

Figure 91–15. Total anomalous pulmonary venous connection complicates transplantation in this infant with hypoplastic left heart syndrome. The donor left atrium is anastomosed to the recipient common pulmonary venous channel. The anomalous left vertical vein is ligated. *(Reprinted with permission from The International Society for Heart and Lung Transplantation. From Bailey.[20])*

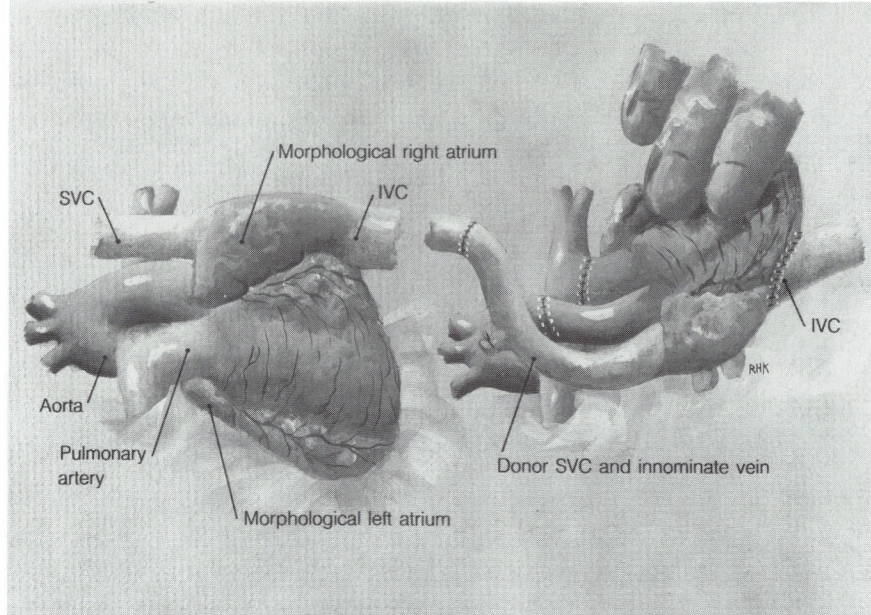

Figure 91–16. Cardiac transplant reconstruction in a recipient with atrial situs inversus using a donor heart with atrial situs solitus. The native inferior vena cave (IVC) is extended using native right atrial tissue. The left atrium is attached first, followed in sequence by inferior vena cava (IVC), pulmonary artery, aorta, and, finally, the superior vena cava. The great vessels are widely mobilized and the donor main pulmonary artery is anastomosed to the recipients left pulmonary artery.

winter having the greater number of both infection and rejection episodes. Graft coronary artery disease has been strongly linked to recipients with higher rejection rates.[33]

COMPLICATIONS

Graft failure due to pulmonary hypertension during the immediate postoperative period has become the exception. Objective recipient selection and vigorous use of postoperative pulmonary vasodilator and respiratory therapy should virtually eliminate this regrettable source of transplantation grief.

Most complications relate to the use of immunosuppressive agents and their side effects. Infection has accounted for 15–20% of postoperative deaths.[34] The major-

ity of serious infections occur during periods of maximal immunosuppression. Hence, they occur during the first 3 months after transplantation or after a significant rejection episode. In the early postoperative period, infecting organisms are frequently Gram-negative rods, reflective of a nosocomial source. During long-term follow-up, community-acquired organisms are more commonly seen. Respiratory syncytial virus is an important source of infection for infants less than 1 year of age. This potentially lethal infection has responded well, however, to ribovarin and bronchodilator therapy. Cytomegalovirus infection continues to be a problem in transplantation because of its frequency, and its potential chronic consequences. Treatment consists of intravenous gancyclovir for 2–3 weeks and oral acyclovir prophylaxis. Forty percent of young infant survivors become seropositive for cytomegalovirus, but a much

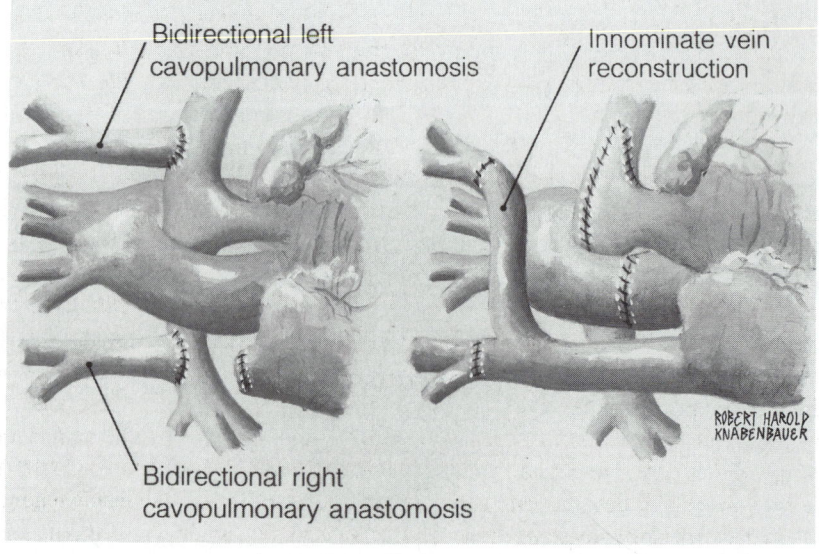

Figure 91–17. Transplant reconstruction in a recipient who has had bilateral, bidirectional cavopulmonary shunts for palliation of single ventricle-pulmonary stenosis complex. Donor veins and pulmonary arteries facilitate remote connections and pulmonary artery reconstruction. *(From Chiavarelli M, Gundry S, Razzouk A, Bailey L: Operative procedures for infant cardiac transplantation. In Kapoor A, Laks H (eds): Atlas of Heart-Lung Transplantation. New York, McGraw-Hill, 1994, with permission.)*

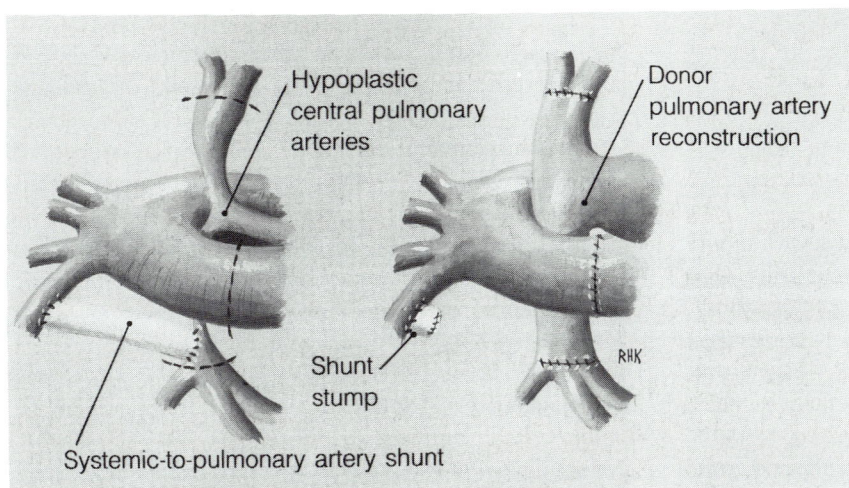

Figure 91–18. Transplantation reconstruction in a recipient with hypoplastic central pulmonary arteries and a previous interposition systemic-pulmonary shunt. The entire central pulmonary artery tree is replaced. Pulmonary artery anastomoses are accomplished in the hilum of each lung. *(From Chiavarelli M, Gundry S, Razzouk A, Bailey L: Operative procedures for infant cardiac transplantation. In Kapoor A, Laks H (eds): Atlas of Heart-Lung Transplantation. New York, McGraw-Hill, 1994, with permission.)*

smaller cohort developed cytomegalovirus disease requiring treatment with gancyclovir and immunoglobulin. Respiratory syncytial virus and symptomatic cytomegalovirus infections are often preludes to a rejection episode. Hence, these infections signal the need for increased rejection surveillance. Despite its ubiquitous nature, cytomegalovirus infection has directly caused only one late death in the Loma Linda University series. Pneumocystis pneumonia has been an unusual infection, but should be considered in the differential of any respiratory illness in a transplanted child. Pneumocystis pneumonia responds well to specific medical management and has produced no serious late sequellae. Prophylactic therapy for this relatively unusual infection may not be particularly efficacious. Fungal infections have been extremely uncommon among recipients on double drug protocols. When diagnosis has been confirmed, fungal infections have been responsive to specific therapy.

Renal dysfunction in the neonate is not unusual and may be multifactorial, secondary to preoperative hypoperfusion, to high cyclosporine levels, or to some catastrophic perioperative hemodynamic event. An aggressive approach to perioperative acute renal failure, which includes early peritoneal dialysis, has resulted in improved outcomes.[35] A small number of long-term survivors (<3% in the Loma Linda University series) have had evidence of chronic renal failure. None has required late dialysis therapy, and all are either stable or improving.

Systemic hypertension has been observed in a small percentage of pediatric heart transplant recipients. Etiology is multifactorial, and may relate to markedly oversized donors, high cyclosporine levels, residual coarctation, or perioperative renal failure. Medical therapy with calcium channel blockers or angiotensin-converting enzyme inhibitors is usually effective. Need for specific antihypertensive therapy has rarely been required, however, beyond the first post-transplant year. Some children, particularly those in a chronic low cardiac output state prior to transplantation, will develop a so-called hyperperfusion syndrome during the first 7–10 days after transplantation. The syndrome is characterized by hypertension, headache, seizure, and even coma. Recovery is not always assured, and the syndrome is better anticipated and avoided than it is managed after the fact. Immediate control of hypertension, including use of β-blockade, at the earliest sign or symptom will prevent the syndrome. Newborns and infants do not appear to be at risk for this complication.

Perioperative anticonvulsant therapy has been required for 10–15% of heart transplant recipients. Intermittent perioperative seizure activity is also multifactorial, and has not related, per se, to a poor neurodevelopmental outcome. Nevertheless, neurodevelopmental delay has been observed in 11% of long-term survivors of heart transplantation during early infancy.[35] Growth of infants and children following heart transplantation has been normal among those requiring little or no corticosteroid therapy. Neoplastic disease has occurred rarely among pediatric heart transplant recipients and appears to relate to that cohort of recipients requiring maximal immunoregulation to maintain cardiac engraftment.

The most significant late complication following heart transplantation is development of graft coronary artery disease. This unique form of coronary disease is characterized by diffuse narrowing or obstruction of coronary arteries, which occurs as a result of exuberant proliferation of endothelial cells. Incidence ranges between 6 and 20% among late survivors. Etiology remains obscure, but the process clearly relates to frequency and intensity of rejection episodes.[36] A link with cytomegalovirus disease has also been postulated. Unfortunately, graft coronary artery disease is not always apparent from coronary angiography and diagnosis is left to the autopsy pathologist. Late sudden mortality is almost entirely a result of graft vasculopathy. Intravascular ultrasound may become a useful tool with which to confirm or rule out significant coronary occlusive disease. However, better understanding and prevention of this dreaded complication will be worth far more than all the diagnostic measures combined.

Other transplant-related complications stem from residual abnormalities requiring repair. These have included recurrent coarctation and late pulmonary venous obstruction, along with scattered noncardiac congenital anomalies.[37]

OUTCOME

Figures 91–19 and 91–20 illustrate current worldwide outcomes following pediatric heart transplantation. Thirty-day mortality for recipients 0–17 years of age is 16.6% and actuarial survival at 36 mo is 72% for children 1–18 years of age and 66% for infants under a year of age. Eighty-one percent of recipients in the first year of life have been treated for congenital heart disease compared to 30% among older children. Worldwide data are collected from 233 participating institutions and compiled by the Registry of the International Society for Heart and Lung Transplantation.[38]

Two hundred fifty-one pediatric patients have undergone heart transplantation at Loma Linda University, of whom 185 were infants during their first year of life. Actuarial survival of the neonatal (age 0–30 days) group of recipients (*n*=71) is 85% at 2 years and 79% at 3 years and beyond.[39] Actual numbers of infants surviving late after heart transplantation are still small, but several recipients are now living between 8 and 10 years after their heart transplantation procedure, including the first neonatal recipient. Five-year actuarial survival exceeds 60% of all infants with hypoplastic left heart syndrome who were listed for transplantation in the Loma Linda University system.[40] This compares favorably with results of palliative surgery for this malformation. Some recipients were registered for heart transplantation while in utero. Fifteen of 20 babies in this subgroup achieved transplantation (75%), and 13 of these are chronic survivors. Actuarial survival at 5 years is 87% for these fortunate infants. Late deaths from rejection or infection appear to cluster during the first 12–15 post-transplant months. The occasional very late death has usually resulted from graft coronary disease, malignancy,

questionable compliance with the immunotherapy and surveillance program, or some issue unrelated to transplantation.

Retransplantation remains a controversial issue, given the problem of scarce donor organs. Emergency retransplantation has resulted in dismal outcomes and appears to be a poor use of the limited donor resource. Elective retransplantation may be more efficacious, but late outcomes are much inferior to initial procedures.[41]

FUTURE DIRECTION

Pediatric heart transplantation is confronted by several significant challenges. These relate to donor organ supply, reliable diagnosis of early graft rejection, and the potential for immune tolerance induction. In 1984, a baboon heart (xenograft) was transplanted experimentally into a human newborn girl with hypoplastic left heart syndrome.[42] The baby lived for 20 days, and although she died, the experience demonstrated that a newborn with severe congenital heart disease could survive the operative procedure of cardiac transplantation. More importantly, the event stimulated pediatric organ donation. Now, 10 years after that experimental operation, heart transplantation has become an accepted procedure for infants and children with complex, incurable congenital heart disease. Pediatric heart transplantation is, nevertheless, limited in scope and usefulness because its application depends on the capricious nature of organ donation. Currently, only abut 300 pediatric donor hearts become available in the United States annually. Supplementing this limited donor organ resource is the major objective of continuing research in cross-species transplantation.[43]

Reanimation and transplantation of heart grafts from donors whose death resulted from cessation of cardiac activity are other fruitful areas of laboratory research. Experimental data obtained from animal models suggest the num-

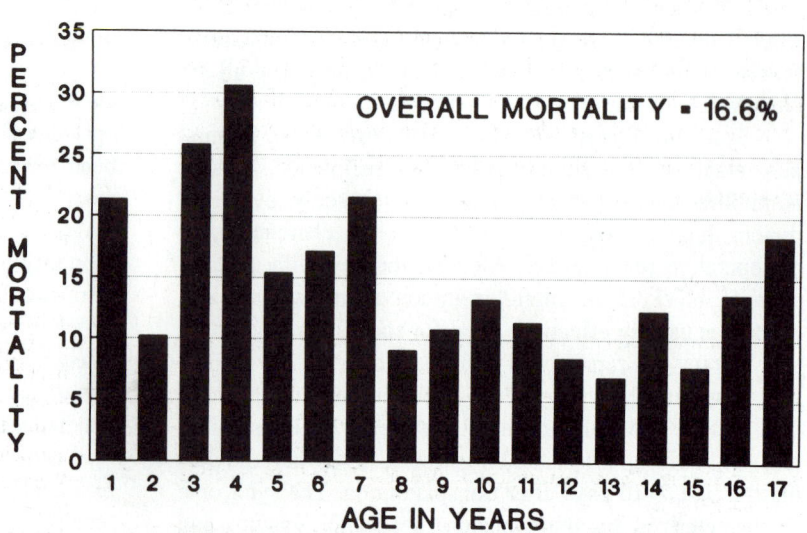

Figure 91–19. Pediatric heart transplantation: 30 day mortality. *(Reprinted with permission from The International Society for Heart and Lung Transplantation. From Kaye.[5])*

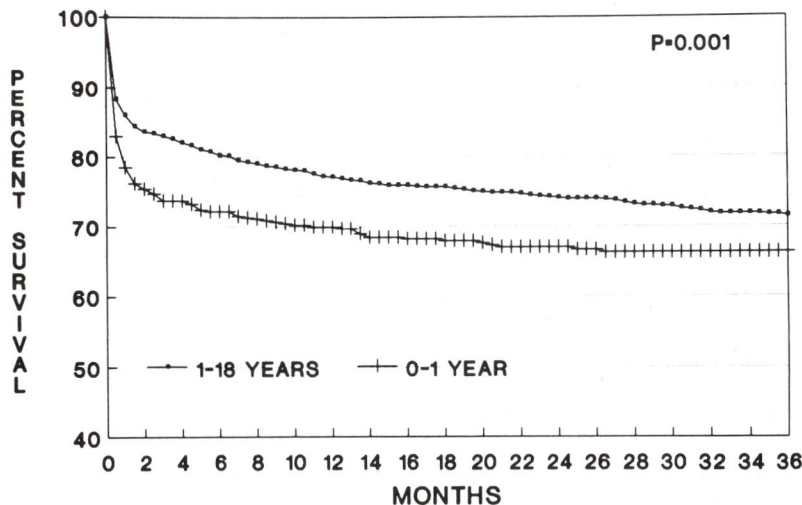

Figure 91–20. Actuarial survival of infants and children following heart transplantation. *(Reprinted with permission from The International Society for Heart and Lung Transplantation. From Kaye.[5])*

ber of donor hearts could be vastly increased by utilizing "dead heart" donors.[44] Long-term outcome studies are needed before this potential new donor resource is investigated clinically.

Reliable, noninvasive means to diagnose early acute graft rejection are not well-developed. Techniques described in this chapter are very useful, but they are cumbersome and inconvenient for recipient families. They occasionally lead to confusion about the actual etiology of a significant host immune response. Ambiguity may sometimes be clarified by endomyocardial biopsy, but not always. In the final analysis, transplantation physicians and surgeons must still rely heavily upon their experience and intuitive clinical skills to help them make the diagnosis of cardiac graft rejection. Someday, the early diagnosis of graft rejection will be made simply and with assurance. Perhaps the concerns about graft rejection will be eliminated altogether by something called organ-specific host immune tolerance.

Induction of immune tolerance in pediatric heart transplant recipients is a viable goal. Immunologists and molecular biologists continue to investigate the potential for tolerance induction. Their data stimulate optimism that a baby might someday have a heart transplantation without the concerns relating to immunosuppression. Until then pediatric heart transplantation, even in its present form, is remarkably effective, albeit exceptional therapy for complex congenital heart disease.

REFERENCES

1. Kantrowitz A, Haller JD, Joos H, et al: Transplantation of the heart in an infant and an adult. *Am J Cardiol* **22:**782–790, 1968
2. Bailey LL, Lacour-Gayet F, Perier P, et al: Orthotopic cardiac transplantation in the neonate: Survival studies in a goat model. *Proceedings of Beijing Symposium on Cardiothoracic Surgery.* Co-published by Beijing, China Academic and New York, John Wiley, 1982, pp 350–352
3. Bailey LL, Ze-Jian L, Jolley WB: Host maturation after orthotopic cardiac transplantation during neonatal life. *Heart Transplant* **3:**265–267, 1984
4. Bailey LL, Nehlsen-Cannarella SL, Doroshow RW, et al: Cardiac allotransplantation in newborns as therapy for hypoplastic left heart syndrome. *N Engl J Med* **315:**949–951, 1986
5. Kaye MP: Pediatric thoracic transplantation: The world experience. *J Heart Lung Transpl* **12:**S344–350, 1993
6. Bando K, Konishi H, Komatsu K, et al: Improved survival following pediatric cardiac transplantation in high-risk patients. *Circulation* **88**(part 2):218–223, 1993
7. Boucek MM, Mathis CM, Razzouk AJ, et al: Indications and contraindications for heart transplantation in infancy. *J Heart Lung Transplant* **12:**S154–S158, 1993
8. Ruiz CE, Gaura H, Zhang HP, et al: Stenting of the ductus arteriosus as a bridge to cardiac transplantation in infants with hypoplastic left heart syndrome. *N Engl J Med* **328:**1605–1608, 1993
9. Starnes VA, Griffin ML, Pitlick PT, et al: Current approach to hypoplastic heart syndrome—Palliation, transplantation, or both? *J Thorac Cardiovasc Surg* **164:**189–195, 1992
10. Martin RD, Parisi F, Robinson TW, Bailey LL: Anesthetic management of neonatal cardiac transplantation. *J Cardiothorac Anesth* **3**(4):465–469, 1989
11. Ashwal S, Schneider S: Pediatric brain death: Current perspectives. In Barnes LA, (ed): *Advances in Pediatrics.* Chicago, Mosby-Year Book, 1991, pp 181–202
12. Boucek MM, Mathis CM, Kanakriyeh MS, et al: Donor shortage: Use of the dysfunctional donor heart. *J Heart Lung Transplant* **12:**S186–S190, 1993
13. Fullerton DA, Gundry SR, Alonso de Begona J, et al: The effects of donor-recipient size disparity in infant and pediatric heart transplantation. *J Thorac Cardiovasc Surg* **104:**1314–1319, 1992
14. Kawauchi M, Gundry SR, Alonso de Begona J, et al: Prolonged preservation of human pediatric hearts for transplantation: Correlation of ischemic time and subsequent function. *J Heart Lung Transplant* **12:**55–58, 1993
15. Menkis AH, McKenzie FN, Novick RJ, et al: Expanding applicability of transplantation after multiple prior palliative procedures. *Ann Thorac Surg* **52:**722–726, 1991
16. Backer CL, Zales VR, Idriss FS, et al: Heart transplantation in neonates and in children. *J Heart Lung Transplant* **11:**311–319, 1992
17. Turrentine MW, Kesler KA, Caldwell R, et al: Cardiac transplantation in infants and children. *Ann Thorac Surg* **57:**546–554, 1994
18. Vouhe PR, Tamisier D, Le Bidois J, et al: Pediatric cardiac transplantation for congenital heart defects surgical considerations and results. *Ann Thorac Surg* **56:**1239–1247, 1993

19. Chartrand C: Pediatric cardiac transplantation despite atrial and venous return anomalies. *Ann Thorac Surg* **52:**716–721, 1991

20. Bailey LL: Heart transplantation techniques in complex congenital heart disease. *J Heart Lung Transplant* **12:**S168–S175, 1993

21. Mayer JE Jr, Petty S, O'Brien P, et al: Orthotopic heart transplantation for complex congenital heart disease. *J Thorac Cardiovasc Surg* **99:**484–492, 1990

22. Boucek MM, Mathis CM, Lebeck LK, et al: Prophylactic antithymocyte series reduces rejection frequency after pediatric heart transplantation (abstract). *J Heart Lung Transplant* **11:**203, 1992

23. Canter CE, Saffitz JE, Moorhead S, et al: Early results after pediatric cardiac transplant with triple immunosuppression therapy. *Am J Cardiol* **71:**971–975, 1993

24. Brown JW, Tirrentine MW, Kesler KA, et al: Triple-drug immunosuppression for heart transplantation in infants and children. *J Heart Lung Transplant* **12:**S265–S274, 1993

25. Canter CE, Moorhead S, Saffitz JE, et al: Steroid withdrawal in the pediatric heart transplant recipient initially treated with triple immunosuppression. *J Heart Lung Transplant* **13:**74–80, 1994

26. Radley-Smith RC, Yacoub MH: Long term results of pediatric heart transplantation. *J Heart Lung Transplant* **11:**5277–5281, 1992

27. Armitage JM, Fricker FJ, del Nido P, et al: A decade (1982 to 1992) of pediatric cardiac transplantation and the impact of FK 506 immunosuppression. *J Thorac Cardiovasc Surg* **105:**464–473, 1993

28. Tantengco MV, Dodd D, Frist WH, et al: Echocardiographic abnormalities with acute cardiac allograft rejection in children: Correlation with endomyocardial biopsy. *J Heart Lung Transplant* **12:**S203–S210, 1993

29. Bouchart F, Gundry SR, VanSchaack-Gonzales J, et al: Methotrexate as rescue/adjunctive immunotherapy in infant and adult heart transplantation. *J Heart Lung Transplant* **12:**427–433, 1993

30. Kirklin JK, George JF, McGiffin DC, et al: Total lymphoid irradiation: Is there a role in pediatric heart transplantation. *J Heart Lung Transplant* **12:**S293–S300, 1993

31. Chinnock RE, Baum MF, Larsen R, Bailey LL: Rejection management and long-term surveillance of the pediatric heart transplant recipient: The Loma Linda experience. *J Heart Lung Transplant* **12:**S255–S264, 1993

32. Alonso de Begona J, Gundry SR, Nehlsen-Cannarella SL, et al: HLA matching and its effect on infant and pediatric cardiac graft survival. *Transpl Proc* **23**(1),1139–1141, 1991

33. Bork J, Chinnock RE, Ogata K, Baum MF: Infectious complications in infant heart transplantation. *J Heart Lung Transplant* **12:**S199–S202, 1993

34. Vricella LA, Alonso de Begona A, Gundry SR, et al: Aggressive peritoneal dialysis for treatment of acute kidney failure after neonatal heart transplantation. *J Heart Lung Transplant* **11:**320–329, 1992

35. Baum ME, Chinnock RE, Ashwal S, et al: Growth and neurodevelopmental outcome of infants undergoing heart transplantation. *J Heart Lung Transplant* **12:**S211–S217, 1993

36. Bailey LL, Zuppan CW, Chinnock RE, et al: *Graft Vasculopathy Among Recipients of Heart Transplantation During the First 12 Years of Life.* Amsterdam, Elsevier, 1994 (in press)

37. Razzouk AJ: Surgical intervention in children after heart transplantation. *J Heart Lung Transplant* **12:**S195–S198, 1993

38. Kaye MP: The Registry of the International Society for Heart and Lung Transplantation Tenth official report—1993. *J Heart Lung Transplant* **12:**541–548, 1993

39. Bailey LL, Gundry SR, Razzouk AJ, et al: Bless the babies: One hundred fifteen late survivors of heart transplantation during the first year of life. *J Thorac Cardiovasc Surg* **105:**805–815, 1993

40. Chiavarelli M, Gundry SR, Razzouk AJ, Bailey LL: Cardiac transplantation for infants with hypoplastic left-heart syndrome. *JAMA* **22/29 270:**2944–2947, 1993

41. Michler RE, Edwards NM, Hsu D, et al: Pediatric retransplantation. *J Heart Lung Transplant* **12:**S319–S327, 1993

42. Bailey LL, Nehlsen-Cannarella SL, Conception W, et al: Baboon to human cardiac xenotransplantation in a neonate. *JAMA* **254:**3321–3329, 1985

43. Kawauchi M, Gundry SR, Alonso de Begona J, et al: Prolonged orthotopic xenoheart transplantation in infant baboons. *J Thorac Cardiovasc Surg* **106:**779–786, 1993

44. Gundry SR, Alonso de Begona J, Bailey LL: Transplantation and reanimation of hearts 30 minutes after warm, asystolic "death". *Arch Surg* **128:**989–993, 1993

CHAPTER

92

Heart–Lung and Lung Transplantation in Children

Thomas L. Spray

Since the clinical introduction of heart–lung and lung transplantation more than 10 years ago, thousands of patients have benefitted from these surgical interventions. As in the field of heart transplantation, the use of heart–lung and lung transplantation in children lagged behind the widespread use of these techniques in adults. Although improving results in heart–lung and lung transplantation led to eventual application of these techniques to the pediatric population, less than 5% of the total transplants have been performed in the pediatric age group.[1]

Heart–lung transplantation has been by far the most frequent operative procedure utilized for lung transplantation in children and the majority of these procedures have been performed for pulmonary hypertension or cystic fibrosis.[1] However, over the past 5 years, increasing experience in lung transplantation with preservation of the native heart has been gained in children, although the number of procedures remains relatively small.[2]

Although the early results of heart–lung and lung transplantation in children have gradually improved and now equal the results seen in adult patients, the difficulties of management of children with end-stage cardiopulmonary disease and uncertainties about long-term outcomes for the transplanted lungs continue to limit the application of these techniques. In spite of many potential problems and significant technical complications, the numbers of pediatric pulmonary and cardiopulmonary transplants have gradually increased and the intermediate term results suggest that pulmonary transplantation will become more widely used for treatment of end-stage pulmonary and cardiopulmonary disease in children.

HISTORY

Early experimental experience in heart–lung transplantation was obtained with heterotopic heart–lung transplantation by Carrel and Guthrie in 1905 and orthotopic heart–lung transplantation by Demikhov in 1946.[3,4] Experimental studies by Castaneda and others showed that the use of primates for autotransplantation of the heart and lungs resulted in normal pulmonary function as compared to the very abnormal function of the denervated heart and lungs in dog experiments.[5] Clinical heart–lung transplantation began in the late 1960s and, in fact, the first clinical heart–lung transplant was performed in a 2.5-mo-old child with atrioventricular canal defect and pulmonary hypertension who died of pulmonary insufficiency 14 hours after the operation.[6] The first clinical success in heart–lung transplantation, however, did not occur until 1981 when Reitz performed a heart–lung transplant in a 45-year-old patient with pulmonary hypertension.[7] Since the initial success, there has been a gradual increase in the number of heart–lung transplants performed and as success was demonstrated in the adult population, a gradual increase occurred in the number of pediatric heart–lung transplants, from only a few in 1984 to as many as 40 per year in 1988.[1]

The success of clinical lung transplantation by Cooper in 1984 established the possibility of isolated lung transplantation for certain forms of cardiopulmonary disease.[8] The technique of single lung transplantation and the evolution of bilateral lung transplantation from en-bloc heart–lung transplantation to en-bloc double lung transplantation and, ultimately, to bilateral sequential lung transplantation

1491

occurred over the 10 years since the introduction of clinical lung transplantation. As noted in heart–lung transplantation, the extension of these techniques to the pediatric population has lagged behind the adult experience, such that by September 1994 only approximately 250 lung transplants had been performed in patients under 20 years of age worldwide.[9] As the use of heart–lung transplantation has gradually been restricted to those patients with irreparable cardiac defects associated with pulmonary disease, the number of heart–lung transplantations done annually has gradually decreased while the number of lung transplants, either single or bilateral, has increased proportionately.[1]

INDICATIONS FOR PEDIATRIC HEART–LUNG OR LUNG TRANSPLANTATION

The general indications for heart–lung or lung transplantation in pediatric patients are similar to those in adults, that is, end-stage restrictive or obstructive pulmonary disease or primary or secondary end-stage pulmonary vascular disease. Secondary pulmonary vascular disease associated with correctable congenital cardiac defects can be considered an indication for potential lung transplantation if cardiac repair can be undertaken at the time of the transplant. Significant left ventricular dysfunction or cardiopulmonary defects that are either uncorrectable or correctable only with the high likelihood of a need for future surgical intervention may best be treated by combined heart–lung transplantation. A general requirement for consideration for transplantation is severe functional limitation and an anticipated life expectancy of only 12 to 18 mo without transplantation.

Although the general requirements for consideration for lung transplantation are similar in adults and children, the types of pulmonary disease seen in children that require transplantation early in life are markedly different from those noted in adults. The indications for lung transplantation or heart–lung transplantation in children are listed in Table 92–1. Emphysema and chronic obstructive lung disease, which are common indications for pulmonary transplantation in adults, are very infrequent causes of end-stage lung disease in children. The various forms of pulmonary fibrosis that become severe enough to require transplantation in the first 16 to 18 years of life are extremely rare; however, small numbers of children with unusual types of fibrotic pulmonary disease and congenital surfactant protein deficiencies may have severe enough ventilatory dysfunction to require transplantation even in infancy. The majority of primary and secondary pulmonary vascular diseases and fibrotic pulmonary diseases permit reasonable function and survival to beyond the pediatric age range and, thus, require transplantation only in adulthood.

Primary pulmonary vascular disease with pulmonary hypertension is rarely severe enough to cause deterioration and death in patients under the age of 16 years.[10–12] For this reason, a relatively small proportion of children will

TABLE 92–1. PEDIATRIC INDICATIONS FOR LUNG OR HEART-LUNG TRANSPLANTATION

Pulmonary Fibrosis
Usual interstitial fibrosis (UIP)
Desquamative interstitial fibrosis (DIP)
Pulmonary alveolar proteinosis
Idiopathic pulmonary alveolar microlithiasis
Cystic fibrosis
Radiation-induced pulmonary fibrosis
Obliterative bronchiolitis
Bronchopulmonary dysplasia
Congenital surfactant deficiencies
Collagen vascular disease

Pulmonary Vascular Disease
Primary pulmonary hypertension
Pulmonary hypertension after corrected congenital heart disease
Pulmonary hypertension and correctable congenital heart disease (Eisenmenger's syndrome)
Pulmonary hypertension and uncorrectable congenital heart disease
"Inadequate" pulmonary vascular bed
    Pulmonary atresia, ventricular septal defect, no central pulmonary arteries
    Congenital diaphragmatic hernia

present with progressive dilatation of the right ventricle, syncope, or other complications of pulmonary vascular disease including low cardiac output such that pulmonary transplantation is required. A larger subgroup of patients, however, includes those with secondary pulmonary vascular disease coexisting with significant corrected or uncorrected congenital heart disease. The combination of pulmonary hypertension and congenital heart disease may result in progressive right ventricular dysfunction and cyanosis and if palliative surgical procedures are exhausted and progressive disability is noted, pulmonary transplantation and repair of the cardiac defect may be indicated in childhood.[12] In addition, those patients who have uncorrectable cardiac defects such as single ventricle, or those with biventricular dysfunction after previous cardiac repair or congenital cardiac defects that have a high likelihood of requiring repeated intervention over a few years may best be treated by combined heart–lung transplantation.

A specific pediatric population of patients that may require cardiopulmonary transplantation or pulmonary transplantation involves children with cystic fibrosis.[14,15] Although the majority of cystic fibrosis patients will survive to adulthood with intensive medical management, a small proportion of children may require transplant before 16 to 18 years of age. Indications for consideration for pulmonary transplantation in the cystic fibrosis population include an increasing frequency of hospitalizations for antibiotic therapy, progressive weight loss in older patients, or a persistent lack of weight gain in younger patients despite adequate nutritional supplementation, an increase in oxygen dependence, or hypercarbia with gradual deterioration of pulmonary function to an FEV_1 of less than 30% of predicted values.[2] Children with cystic fibrosis who meet indications for lung transplantation are in most cases quite debilitated and, in addition, multiple antibiotic-resistant organisms may colonize the tracheobronchial tree complicating transplantation and increasing the possibility of posttransplantation septic complications. Some potential indications for pulmonary or cardiopulmonary transplantation in infancy include congenital diaphragmatic hernia, surfactant protein deficiencies, pulmonary vein stenosis or venoocclusive disease, or primary pulmonary hypoplasia.[2]

Because the natural history of patients with pulmonary hypertension (either primary or secondary) remains poorly defined, the indications for transplantation in this group of children are more subjective. General indications for consideration for transplant include progressive exercise deterioration with a Heart Association clinical class of III to IV, the onset of syncope, hemoptysis, angina pectoris, or right ventricular failure.[16] Hemodynamic considerations include an elevation of the right atrial pressure to greater than 8 mm Hg with a cardiac index of less than 2.2 L/min per m^2 and a total pulmonary vascular resistance index of greater than 20 Woods Units/m^2 either at initial evaluation in patients who do not respond to pulmonary vasodilators or at follow-up on vasodilator therapy.[11] In patients with Eisenmenger's syndrome with the presence of a right-to-left cardiac shunt, the onset of progressively severe polycythemia in association with right ventricular failure, hemoptysis, or progressive symptoms may be considered indications for intervention.[17]

As in all medical procedures in children, it is of primary importance for the family of the pediatric patient to be committed to long-term health care and to be willing and able to comply with medical interventions before, during, and after the transplant procedure to ensure the long-term success of the transplant and a favorable outcome for the child.

CONTRAINDICATIONS TO TRANSPLANTATION

Contraindications to pulmonary transplantation include the presence of severe scoliosis or other chest wall mechanical defects that would restrict chest wall compliance and pulmonary function despite a successful transplant procedure. Significant renal insufficiency or uncontrolled diabetes mellitus with associated renal complications are a relative contraindication to transplant. In addition, patients with significant portal hypertension or biliary cirrhosis associated with longstanding primary or secondary pulmonary hypertension may be considered unsuitable for cardiopulmonary or pulmonary transplant alone and may require additional transplant procedures. Prior surgical procedures, especially when multiple and involving both pleural spaces, complicate the transplant procedure due to dense adhesions and bleeding, especially in chronically cyanotic patients. Thus, the presence of cyanosis and multiple previous thoracic operations may be considered a relative contraindication to transplant because bleeding complications may be severe

and potentially fatal. Steroid dependence in high doses may be associated with poor bronchial healing or sepsis following transplant and is also considered a relative contraindication, although small to moderate doses of steroids are not associated with significant healing complications and, therefore, the consideration of patients for transplant must be individualized. A longstanding history of noncompliance of the patient or the family with medical interventions may also be considered a contraindication to undertaking a procedure of this magnitude. As in adults, children with uncontrolled collagen vascular disease or ongoing malignancy must be excluded from consideration for transplantation.

SELECTION OF OPERATIVE PROCEDURE

Combined en-bloc heart and lung transplantation was the first successful clinical procedure for pulmonary replacement in children and, therefore, the majority of transplants to date have been done by this technique.[1] Nevertheless, the evolution of indications for cardiopulmonary transplantation as opposed to pulmonary transplant alone in children has followed the evolution of these procedures in adult patients. Whereas it is clear that comparable results can be obtained with heart–lung and lung transplantation, the need to maximize the availability of scarce donor organs and utilize the heart for additional patients has led to a gradual decrease in the use of combined heart–lung transplantation for primary pulmonary diseases.[1] Therefore, combined heart–lung transplantation is now reserved for patients who have uncorrectable congenital heart defects in association with pulmonary vascular disease that precludes cardiac transplant alone. In addition, heterotopic heart transplantation may be utilized in some children with elevated pulmonary vascular resistance in whom some gradual improvement in pulmonary resistance might be anticipated, but in whom the magnitude of pulmonary resistance would severely limit the function of a primary orthotopic cardiac transplant.[18] Thus, combined heart–lung transplantation may now be reserved for those children with congenital heart disease who have a poor chance of long-term correction and those patients with severe left or biventricular dysfunction. Pulmonary transplantation with preservation of the native heart may be considered in patients with cystic fibrosis or other septic lung diseases, pulmonary fibrosis and primary or secondary pulmonary vascular disease associated with normal left ventricular function, the absence of coronary artery disease, a simple or correctable congenital heart defect with a high likelihood of long-term correction, and those patients with a right ventricular ejection fraction greater than 10% and less than severe tricuspid and pulmonary insufficiency. Some cardiac defects that have been associated with successful repair and pulmonary transplantation are listed in Table 92–2.

An additional consideration in children is the use of single or bilateral sequential lung transplantation in patients with pulmonary fibrosis or pulmonary vascular disease. The

TABLE 92–2. REPARABLE CARDIAC DEFECTS WITH LUNG TRANSPLANTATION

Atrial septal defect

Ventricular septal defect—single

Patent ductus arteriosus

Vascular rings

Atrioventricular canal defects

Pulmonary vein stenosis

Peripheral pulmonary stenosis

Pulmonary atresia with nonconfluent pulmonary arteries

selection of bilateral sequential lung transplantation in patients with cystic fibrosis is based on the need to remove the infected lungs to prevent contamination of the newly transplanted lungs. In addition, patients with other septic lung diseases including chronic bronchiectasis must be considered best served by bilateral sequential transplantation. Single lung transplantation, however, may be considered in patients with pulmonary fibrosis and in those with pulmonary vascular disease. Although successful series of single lung transplants for primary or secondary pulmonary hypertension have been reported, the postoperative course is more complicated in these patients due to the entire cardiac output being delivered to the transplanted lung and, in addition, there are potential concerns with the instability of patients should complications of infection, rejection, or bronchiolitis obliterans occur in the only transplanted lung.[19–21] Therefore, the trend has been toward bilateral sequential lung transplant in these patients. However, single lung transplantation may still be considered for patients with primary pulmonary hypertension in whom there is a relative contraindication to transplant of the other lung, such as patients who have had multiple previous thoracotomies on one pleural space. The selection of operation for each child must therefore be individualized based on the patient's cardiac and pulmonary anatomy and previous surgical history. In addition, bilateral sequential transplantation has been preferred in younger children and infants to allow for the maximum possible growth and development of the lungs.

DONOR SELECTION

Donors for both cardiopulmonary and pulmonary transplantation are relatively rare compared to donors for other organs. It has been estimated that only 10 to 15% of cardiac donors may be suitable for heart–lung or lung donation.[22] The reason for the unsuitability of many potential donors includes the high possibility of gastric aspiration during trauma or a sudden neurologic event. In addition, the presence of severe pulmonary edema, either neurogenic or cardiac related, can significantly affect the oxygen exchange of potential donor lungs and preclude their use. In general, criteria for pulmonary donors include the presence of normal

gas exchange with a pAO_2 of greater than 100 mm Hg on 40% FIO_2 and 5 cm of PEEP. Normal lung compliance with a peak airway pressure of less than 30 cm of water, clear chest x-ray, age less than 45 years, and normal electrocardiogram and echocardiogram are considered criteria for cardiopulmonary and pulmonary donors. A history of pulmonary disease or prolonged smoking or asthma is considered a contraindication for donation. In addition, heavy contamination of the tracheobronchial tree with bacteria or fungus or the presence of severe lung contusion, penetrating chest injuries, or demonstrated aspiration of gastric contents is considered a contraindication to donor lung suitability. For the cardiopulmonary donor, a large dose of inotropic drugs after suitable fluid management or evidence for significant ventricular hypertrophy or dysfunction on echocardiogram is considered a contraindication to use of the heart in the combined heart–lung bloc.

While donor criteria may often be unsuitable, with aggressive donor management many previously unsuitable organs may be rendered suitable for transplantation. It is possible in patients with poor gas exchange of both lungs to selectively intubate each mainstem bronchus, and in patients with unilateral pulmonary dysfunction the contralateral lung may be quite suitable for use in pulmonary transplantation. Thus, careful evaluation of each potential donor is important to maximize the availability of suitable donor organs.[23]

The presence of HIV or hepatitis A, B, or C is also considered a contraindication for organ donation.

The presence of positive serology for cytomegalo-virus does not preclude organ donation; however, donor and recipient CMV status matching should be considered where possible. Nevertheless, the scarcity of potential donor organs has now led to the crossing of CMV mismatches between donor and recipient in many centers with acceptable long-term results.[9] Thus, while it is generally advisable to match CMV positive donors with CMV positive recipients, successful transplantation is not precluded and complications of CMV infection can usually be adequately treated.

Size matching between donor and recipient is important in pediatric lung transplantation. For heart–lung transplantation it is generally desirable to have the weight of the donor within 20 to 30% of the weight of the recipient. While it is possible to use hearts of several times the body weight of the recipient in isolated cardiac transplantation in infants and young children, the combination of the heart and lung bloc limits the size discrepancy that may be permissible in the heart portion of the combined procedure since the transplanted lungs, if significantly larger than the recipient, may produce pulmonary tamponade of the heart.

The donor–recipient size matching is more liberal when double lung or single lung transplant is contemplated. The lungs have the capacity to expand to fill the chest cavity in significantly larger recipients. In addition, it is possible to use significantly larger donor lungs than the recipient and to perform lobectomies or trim portions of the parenchyma of the lungs to allow for the lungs to fill the chest without impinging on cardiac function.[24] In general, bronchial size between donor and recipient has been correlated better with height and age of the donor and recipient rather than weight. Measurement of the chest dimensions on plain chest radiograph of the vertical height from the diaphragm to the chest apex bilaterally and the transverse measurement horizontally at the level of the diaphragm between donor and recipient have been used to assure suitability of size-match between donor and recipient.

ORGAN PROCUREMENT

All donors undergo bronchoscopy and inspection of the lungs at the time of procurement. The presence of pulmonary contusions or direct trauma to the lungs by chest tube insertion must be evaluated prior to acceptance of the donor. The donor receives methylprednisolone and antibiotics and is fully heparinized prior to organ procurement. The technique of organ procurement is described in other chapters. The technique of organ procurement from pediatric donors is similar to that in adults except that the volumes of cardioplegia and pulmonoplegic solutions are adjusted for the weight of the donor. In general, cardioplegia is administered for a total dose of approximately 20 mL/kg of donor weight and pulmonoplegia from 25 to 40 mL/kg of donor weight. Crystalloid cardioplegia and either Euro-Collins or University of Wisconsin pulmonoplegia have been utilized in most centers for organ preservation. If harvesting of the heart and lung bloc is to be performed as a single organ, the cardioplegia is administered into the aorta and pulmonoplegia administered directly into the pulmonary artery with venting of the heart by division of the left atrial appendage. In addition, division of the inferior vena cava at the diaphragm permits evacuation of cardioplegia without ventricular distension. The trachea is mobilized above the level of the carina and minimal dissection of the carina performed and the lungs gently inflated and the trachea stapled with the lungs in mild inflation. The superior vena cava is ligated and divided and the esophagus mobilized in the superior mediastinum and stapled and divided. The aorta is then transected at the level of the innominate artery and the distal aorta in the posterior pericardial space mobilized and ligated and divided. With incision of the pleura at the paraspinal region bilaterally the entire heart–lung bloc can then be excised in toto and the esophagus removed from the combined heart–lung bloc out of the operative field.[25]

For separate heart and lung explantation, cardioplegia is administered and pulmoplegia simultaneously administered as in the heart and lung en-bloc excision. The interatrial groove is developed and then the heart is excised by division of the aorta and pulmonary artery, leaving the bifurcation of the pulmonary artery for the lung bloc. The left atrium is then excised with a limited left atrial cuff leaving

as much of the pulmonary venous confluence bilaterally as possible for lung implantation. The right atrium is excised by division of the superior vena cava and inferior vena cava at the pericardial reflection. The lung bloc is then excised as in the heart lung bloc by division of the trachea with the lungs in gentle inflation after stapling and the esophagus stapled proximally and distally and removed in toto with the double lung bloc for dissection away from the operative field. The heart–lung bloc or lung blocs are then placed in iced saline solution in sterile bags and transported to the recipient center in ice.

In some centers, cooling of the donor with cardiopulmonary bypass has been utilized; however, in most cases this is a cumbersome technique and is not widely utilized. For details of organ procurement and preservation see Chapter 112. Preservation of up to 9 hours for lung transplantation has been satisfactory with the use of these techniques.

RECIPIENT OPERATION

Great care must be taken in the removal of recipient organs for heart–lung or lung transplantation to obtain perfect hemostasis in areas of pleural adhesions or large bronchial collateral vessels and to avoid injury to the phrenic, recurrent laryngeal and vagus nerves. Although median sternotomy has typically been utilized for heart–lung transplantation in several centers, the use of the bilateral thoracosternotomy (clam-shell) incision has permitted excellent access to the pleural spaces for take-down of adhesions and obtaining hemostasis prior to implantation of the donor organs.[26]

HEART–LUNG TRANSPLANTATION

The technical aspects of heart–lung implantation in children are similar to those described in adult heart–lung transplantation in Chapter 114. The recipient is supported on cardiopulmonary bypass while the lungs are sequentially excised and then the heart excised leaving a cuff of right atrium and distal aorta for implantation. The phrenic nerves are carefully protected on a pedicle of pericardium. The donor heart–lung bloc is then passed behind the phrenic pedicles and anastomoses between donor and recipient trachea, aorta, and right atrium accomplished on cardiopulmonary bypass. In small children the use of absorbable sutures may permit better growth of the anastomoses. A vent may be inserted through the amputated left atrial appendage or through the right superior pulmonary vein of the heart–lung bloc to decompress the heart while reperfusion is permitted prior to weaning from cardiopulmonary bypass.

BILATERAL SEQUENTIAL LUNG TRANSPLANTATION

The patient is placed in the supine position and the shoulders either elevated on a rolled towel or the arms secured to an ether screen. A bilateral transverse incision is made in the fourth intercostal space and across the sternum transversely in the midline (Fig. 92–1A). The internal mammary pedicles are divided bilaterally. Chest retractors are then placed and the thymus divided in the midline or resected completely in small children. The pericardium is opened and the heart may be suspended with stay sutures. Heparinization of the patient is then performed and the patient cannulated in the ascending aorta and in the body of the right atrium with a single venous cannula if isolated lung implantation is contemplated or separate caval cannulation utilized if cardiac repair is contemplated in addition to lung implantation. After the patient is placed on cardiopulmonary bypass the lungs are removed bilaterally by ligation of the pulmonary artery, pulmonary venous drainage, and stapling of the right and left mainstem bronchi (Fig. 92–1B). Because of the small size of some infants and children and the lack of double lumen endotracheal tubes for use in infants and small children, cardiopulmonary bypass has routinely been utilized for lung transplantation.[2] After removal of the lungs in patients with cystic fibrosis, the blind trachea and bronchi can be irrigated with antibiotic solution and cleansed of purulent material prior to implan-

tation of the donor lungs. Donor lung implantation then proceeds with the patient on cardiopulmonary bypass by anastomosis of the bronchus, cut within 2 rings of the take-off of the upper lobe orifice. Running absorbable suture is utilized for the membranous bronchus and interrupted absorbable suture for the cartilaginous bronchus in hopes of maximizing long-term growth. End-to-end anastomosis of the bronchus without telescoping is utilized in small children to prevent stenosis or malacia of the anastomotic area. In older children and adults, however, telescoping bronchial anastomoses have been utilized with good success.[27] The pulmonary arterial anastomosis is then created between donor and recipient using running absorbable suture and the pulmonary venous confluence of the recipient opened widely and an anastomosis created with absorbable suture. Just prior to completion of the venous anastomosis, venous return is permitted to the heart and the arterial clamp released and air aspirated from the pulmonary veins prior to opening of each lung sequentially for reperfusion.

If cardiac repair is performed in association with bilateral sequential lung transplantation the patient is cooled on bypass and the aorta cross-clamped and cardioplegia administered and the cardiac repair performed prior to lung implantation to permit the maximum reperfusion time of the heart after ischemia while the lungs are implanted. Closure of intracardiac defects is performed through the right atrium if possible to prevent incisions in the right ventricle in patients with pre-existing significant pulmonary hyper-

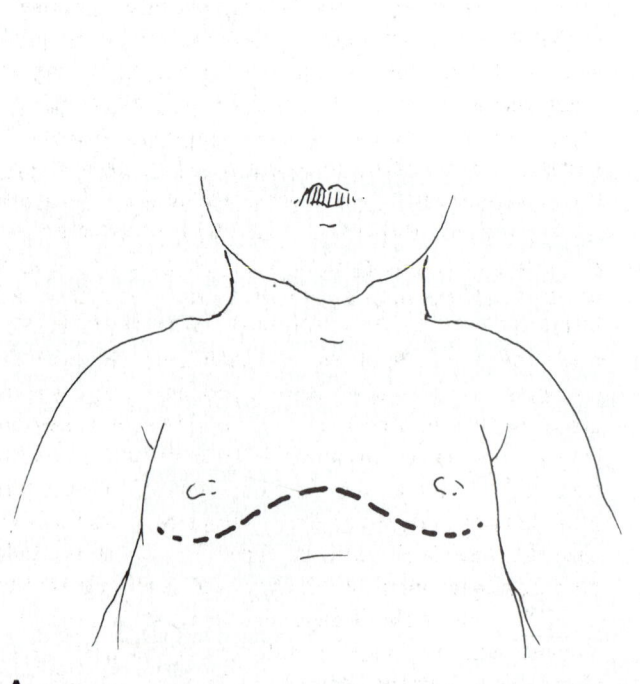

A

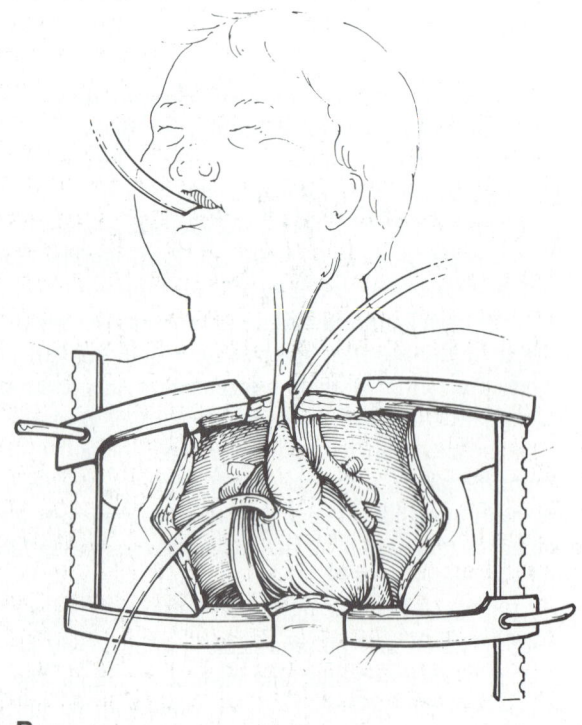

B

Figure 92–1. A. Transverse bilateral thoracosternotomy incision for lung transplantation in children. **B.** Diagram of the chest after excision of both lungs with the child on cardiopulmonary bypass and with the aorta clamped for repair of an intracardiac defect.

tension in whom right ventricular function may be depressed.

SINGLE LUNG TRANSPLANTATION

For patients in whom only a single lung is required operation is performed either through a posterolateral thoracotomy on the transplant side or with the patient in a supine position and a partial thoracosternotomy crossing the sternum in the midline, but leaving one pleural space essentially closed. With this technique, access to the heart for cannulation for cardiopulmonary bypass is simplified. Explantation of the lung and implantation of the donor lung then proceeds as in bilateral sequential lung transplantation.

POSTOPERATIVE MANAGEMENT

Restriction of postoperative fluid administration is important early after heart–lung and lung transplantation to decrease the magnitude of reperfusion edema of the transplanted lungs, which may be exacerbated by the affects of cardiopulmonary bypass. In addition, the affects of cyclosporine on renal function may require the administration of diuretics and the use of low dose dopamine for renal perfusion to maximize urine output during this period. In patients who have undergone heart–lung transplantation, the use of isoproterenol to maintain the cardiac rate at 110 to 115 bpm is useful. In addition, the isoproterenol may effectively lower pulmonary vascular resistance early in the transplant period. The FIO_2 is weaned rapidly to as low an inspired oxygen concentration as possible to maintain a pAO_2 of greater than 70 mm Hg. PEEP is added to 3 to 5 cm of water to aid in prevention of atelectasis. Attempts are made to wean the patient from the ventilator over the first 24 to 48 hours post-transplant in children. We generally do a fiberoptic bronchoscopy to examine the anastomoses 12 to 24 hours after lung transplantation and to suction any bronchial secretions prior to weaning to extubate the patient. In children who undergo lung transplantation (either single or double) for pulmonary hypertension or in patients with associated significant congenital heart disease, prolonged weaning to extubation may be necessary and it may be advisable to keep the patient paralyzed and sedated early after transplant to decrease the risk of hemodynamic instability and pulmonary hypertensive events. Patients with cystic fibrosis who have had chronic hypercarbia prior to transplant may require prolonged weaning from the ventilator due to a tendency to retain carbon dioxide. Chest radiographs are performed every 12 hours for the first 2 days following the transplant and then daily thereafter. Perihilar fluffiness and infiltrates or diffuse pulmonary infiltrates may be noted early after transplant and have been associated with the so-called reperfusion or reimplantation response.[28] The etiology of this response has been attributed to denervation of the transplanted lungs, ischemic injury of the donor organs, fluid volume overload, loss of lymphatic drainage, and possibly neutrophil-mediated vascular pulmonary capillary injury.[28–30] Such early reperfusion damage, which is manifested by diffuse alveolar damage on histologic examination, generally resolves over the first 5 to 7 days following the transplant. Although chest tubes are rarely removed early following transplant due to often copious amounts of drainage from the chest wall in patients who have had significant adhesions requiring lysis, or from transudative fluid loss across the visceral pleura of the transplanted lungs in other patients, early mobilization of the children is encouraged. Surveillance cultures of sputum, urine, and blood are routinely performed and recently bronchoalveolar lavage for viral cultures and immunologic staining of samples of the donor and recipient lungs at transplant for common viruses have been performed in hopes of identifying early potential viral infections of the transplanted lungs.

IMMUNOSUPPRESSION

The immunosuppression utilized for heart–lung and lung transplantation in most institutions is similar to that used for infant and pediatric heart transplants. There is, however, no single standardized regimen of immunosuppression utilized at present. In our own institution, triple immunosuppression with azathioprine, cyclosporine, and steroids is utilized with the initiation of steroids immediately following the transplant procedure. Azathioprine is begun at 2 mg/kg and given intravenously both before and after the transplant procedure until oral intake is assured. Cyclosporine is begun at 0.25 to 0.5 mg/kg intravenously over the first 3 hours following the implantation of the lungs and the dosage is then decreased to 1.5 to 2.5 mg/h and adjusted to maintain whole blood cyclosporine levels at 300 to 350 ng/mL in the immediate postoperative period. Steroids have been utilized in the form of methylprednisolone at 1 mg/kg per day intravenously following the transplant and azathioprine added at 3 mg/kg per day orally or intravenously. Antiviral agents are administered for documented cytomegalic inclusion virus (CMV infection or when donor/recipient CMV mismatch has occurred). Other immunosuppressive protocols have been described for pediatric lung transplantation utilizing either FK506 and azathioprine rather than cyclosporine or cyclosporine and azathioprine without steroids.[31,32] From the limited number of pediatric heart–lung and lung transplants performed to date it is unclear that there is a significant superiority of one particular immunosuppression protocol, however, newer agents such as FK506 may make dosage and administration easier in children who may require multiple divided doses of cyclosporine to maintain adequate cyclosporine levels and for patients with cystic fibrosis who may have difficulty with gastrointestinal cyclosporine absorption. In addition, the common complications of cyclosporine administration such as hirsutism, seizures, and gum hyperplasia in addition to renal dysfunction may be diminished somewhat with the use of FK506 and other agents. Steroid use may be associated with onset of diabetes mellitus or fluid retention, although an increased incidence of infection has not been documented. Although weight gain has been appropriate in small children who have undergone lung transplantation, bone growth may be diminished somewhat by the use of immunosuppression regimens that include steroids.

REJECTION SURVEILLANCE: DIAGNOSIS AND MANAGEMENT

Bronchoscopy is performed early in the postoperative period in heart–lung and lung transplant recipients to assess the bronchial anastomoses for blood supply and healing and to improve evacuation of pulmonary secretions. Rigid bronchoscopy may be necessary in small infants and children in whom fiberoptic bronchoscopes do not have adequate suction ports for clearing of secretions. Biopsies are obtained through the bronchoscope with sampling of at least two areas of the transplanted lungs under fluoroscopic guidance for monitoring of rejection. Three to six biopsy specimens are taken at each biopsy session. A routine surveillance transbronchial biopsy is obtained approximately 1 week after the transplant procedure and then 1 to 3 additional biopsies performed in the first 3 months or more frequently if there have been more significant changes in the clinical status of the child or to evaluate the resolution of documented rejection episodes. After the first year post-transplant, biopsies are performed every 6 months for surveillance for bronchiolitis obliterans or chronic mild rejection. In association with biopsy, bronchioalveolar lavage for infection diagnosis and management, including viral cultures and buffy coat cultures for CMV, are performed.

If inadequate tissue is obtained on transbronchial biopsy and in the presence of suspected rejection episodes, pulse steroids are administered and if there is no objective improvement in the patients clinical status, open lung biopsy may be necessary. Although inadequate specimens may be obtained from transbronchial biopsies for the diagnosis of bronchiolitis obliterans, a late, sudden, or progressive decrease in FEV_1 and vital capacity in the absence of documented rejection is considered evidence for obliterative bronchiolitis and treated with an increase in immunosuppression therapy with antithymocyte globulin, antilymphoblast globulin, or other cytolytic agents such as OKT3 if the patient does not rapidly respond to an increase in steroid dosage.

Surveillance pulmonary function tests are performed 2 weeks after the transplant procedure and weekly thereafter and the children perform home spirometry and oximetry and report these data to the transplant center. Changes in daily values are monitored to detect early rejection episodes or the onset of obliterative bronchiolitis. Daily rehabilitation therapy for the first 3 mo after the transplant is considered important to obtain the optimal return to full activity in children. In small infants and young children who cannot cooperate with pulmonary function testing, pulse oximetry is monitored to detect early changes in lung function.

Acute rejection episodes are often diagnosed clinically by the presence of a dry cough, increased inspiratory crackles at the bases on auscultation, pyrexia, a decrease in oxygen saturation, or the onset of new pleural effusions on chest radiograph. In the absence of evidence of infectious problems, pulse steroid therapy can be utilized in such circumstances with biopsy obtained if there is not a rapid clinical response.

Children with heart–lung transplantation require echocardiography to evaluate cardiac function. The onset of differential rejection of the heart and lungs has been well documented, however, cardiac rejection appears rare in the absence of pulmonary rejection and the incidence of cardiac rejection in cardiopulmonary transplantation seems lower than in cardiac transplantation alone.[33–35].

Manifestations of organ rejection after lung transplantation include acute rejection, which is a perivascular lymphocytic infiltration of the lung, which may extend into interstitial airways. Acute rejection is labeled with grades 1 to 4 and is generally reversible. Chronic rejection or bronchiolitis obliterans is defined as a presumably immune mediated injury of the small airways with inflammatory, fibrotic, and proliferative manifestations and is generally considered irreversible. The diagnosis of rejection can be made on clinical grounds including pyrexia, malaise, dyspnea, and chest tightness or physical signs including late inspiratory crackles, pleural effusion, friction rubs, decreased oxygen saturation, or a decrease in pulmonary function tests with a decrease in the FEV_1 or $FEF^{25–75}$. Radiologic features of rejection include hilar infiltrates, pulmonary edema, or pleural effusions, but the chest x-ray may also be normal.[36] Usually infiltrates, when present, are symmetrical. Refractory rejection is treated with antithymocyte globulin at 10 to 15 mm/kg over 4 hours for 7 to 10 days and B1 or B2 lymphocytic bronchitis treated with methotrexate 0.1 to 0.2 mg/kg once per week and occasionally immunoglobulin 100 mg/kg IV.

INFECTIOUS COMPLICATIONS OF PULMONARY TRANSPLANTATION

Infection is common following cardiopulmonary or pulmonary transplantation.[37] Predisposing factors to infection after lung transplantation include a lower respiratory infection of the donor lungs, the effects of surgery and cardiopulmonary bypass, or lower respiratory infection in the recipient prior to transplant. The presence of an indwelling endotracheal tube and central venous catheters, defective mucociliary function of the transplanted lungs, and an absent cough reflex beyond anastomoses also contribute to sources of infection. The effects of immunosuppression and continued exposure to potential pathogens in children cannot be minimized. To attempt to limit the effects of early infection following lung transplantation, broad spectrum antimicrobials are utilized for the first 7 to 10 days following transplant and in cystic fibrosis patients IV anti-*Pseudomonas* antibiotics are continued for 7 to 10 days followed by aerosolized colistin or tobramycin for 1 to 2 mo. In addition, nystatin mouth wash is given for 3 to 6 mo

post-transplant. Trimethoprim-sulfa is given 3 days each week to decrease the risk of pneumocystis infection. Gancyclovir at 5 mg/kg IV daily is given for 6 to 9 wk if the donor or recipient is CMV positive.

In the first week following transplantation the most common infectious complications are acute pneumonias or bacteremias from central lines and intravenous access. After ICU discharge lower respiratory infection is a common cause of infectious complications in the transplanted lung. Central line bacteremia in patients with long-term in-

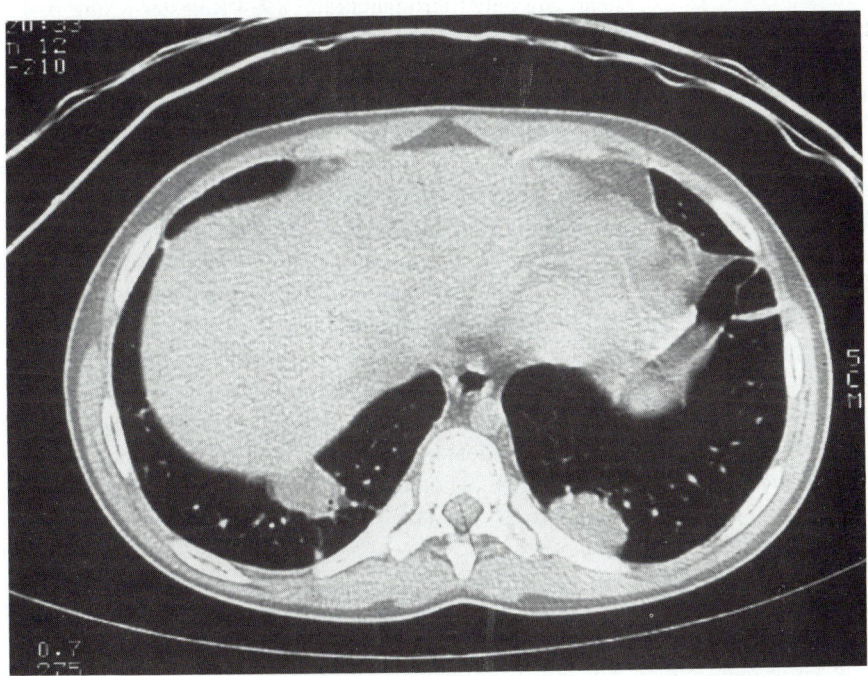

A

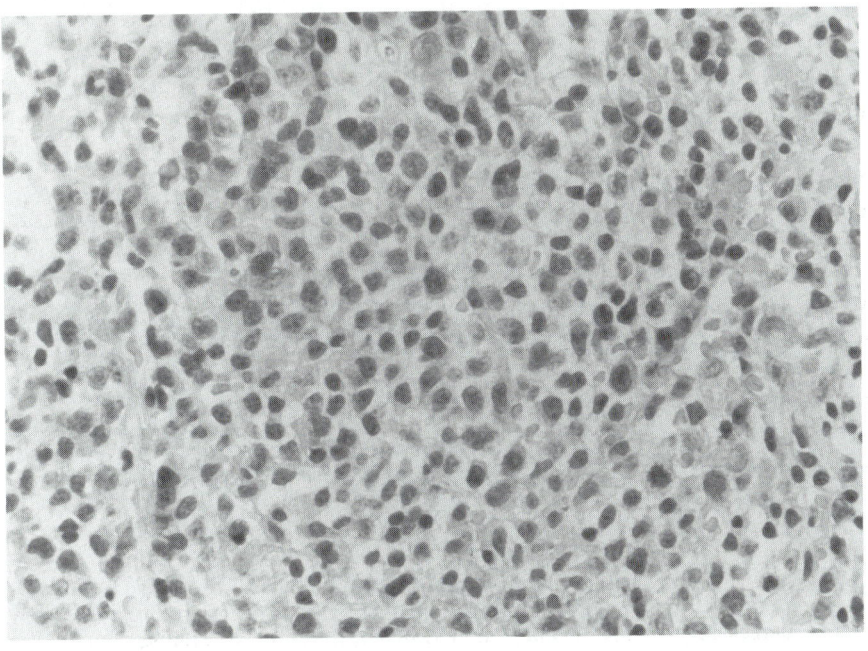

B

Figure 92–2. A. Transplant lymphoproliferative disease. This CT scan was taken 2 mo following bilateral sequential lung transplantation in a 9-year-old child who underwent transplantation for peripheral pulmonary stenosis. The onset of disease was associated with seropositivity for Epstein–Barr virus. The CT scan showed nodular densities in the pulmonary parenchyma bilaterally. **B.** Photomicrograph of specimen taken from a different patient with post-transplant lymphoproliferative disease showing multiple sheets of mononuclear cells consistent with a lymphoproliferative disorder.

dwelling central lines used for venous access for blood drawing in small infants and children may be associated with transient infection. Sepsis can occur from any of the above sources and sinusitis and otitis media are common in cystic fibrosis patients and otitis media common in young infants and children after lung transplantation as in the normal pediatric population. The most common fungal infections following lung transplantation include *Aspergillus*, which may either be localized in the lung or systemic. It is not uncommon for tracheal colonization with *Aspergillus* to be present in cystic fibrosis patients. When present, aspergillus is treated with itraconazole or amphotericin B. Candida infections can occur, although colonization is more common than actual pulmonary infection. Documented infection is treated with itraconazole, fluconazole, or amphotericin B as appropriate.

Viral infections are common after lung transplantation, especially in children where viral challenges may be frequent. Herpes simplex infection is treated with oral or IV Acyclovir, and varicella infections with IV acyclovir as promptly as the diagnosis is made. There is a higher incidence of seronegativity for varicella in children than in adults and there is a significant ongoing exposure after transplant due to exposure to other children. Early diagnosis and prompt initiation of acyclovir therapy can limit this potentially devastating viral infection. Documented CMV infection in the lung or positive buffy coat cultures from bronchial washings are treated with acyclovir or foscarnet with hyperimmune globulin reserved for severe cases. Respiratory syncytial virus is treated with ribavirin, influenza A with amantadine, and influenza B, parainfluenza, and measles with ribavirin. An additional virus common in children, unlike adults following transplant, is Epstein–Barr (EB) virus. There is a higher incidence of seronegativity for this viral pathogen in children than in adults and there is a subtlety of EB virus infection in early childhood that may make diagnosis difficult. An increased risk for post-transplant lymphoproliferative disease in patients who have sustained an EB virus infection following transplant has been noted that may respond to decreasing immunosuppression, or in polyclonal types of lymphoproliferative disease, may progress despite decreased immunosuppression (Fig. 97–2).

RESULTS

Although combined heart and lung transplantation has been performed in several centers and the world experience with this technique in pediatric patients is considerable, relatively few pediatric series of cardiopulmonary or pulmonary transplantation have been reported.[2,13,14,38–45] The largest series of combined heart and lung transplantation has been reported from Yacoub at Harefield Hospital in England. A series of 303 consecutive patients was reported in 1992, of whom 70 were in the pediatric age range

(23%).[39] Of the patients 57% were transplanted for pulmonary vascular disease and 43% for parenchymal lung disease. In this group, the survival of pediatric patients was not broken down; however, the actuarial survival for the total group at 1 and 2 years after surgery was 61 and 51%, respectively. The cumulative probabilities of developing bronchiolitis obliterans in these patients at 1, 2, 3, and 4 years were 13, 32, 40, and 40% respectively.[39]

The Registry of the International Society for Heart and Lung Transplantation offers the opportunity to evaluate survival in the combined series from several institutions of heart and lung transplantation.[1] 1994 Registry results reveal a total of 255 heart–lung transplants performed in children under 18 years of age. Actuarial survival was related to patient age at transplant with an approximately 45% survival at 3 years in patients older than 6 years of age and only 25 to 30% at 3 years in patients transplanted at under 5 years of age.[1] The age distribution for pediatric heart–lung transplantation over the years is described in Figure 92–3.

Results with pediatric lung transplantation have been similar to the result noted in heart–lung transplantation in children reflecting perhaps the use of lung transplant techniques in the patients who may have parenchymal lung disease and more correctable forms of congenital heart disease. The age distribution for pediatric lung transplantation over time is noted in Figure 92–4. The indications for pediatric transplantation (heart–lung vs lung or heart) are shown in Figure 92–5. Actuarial pediatric lung survival of the patients in the 6 to 18 year age range is approximately 40% at 36 mo, quite comparable to the heart–lung transplant survival statistics in the same age group.[1]

An additional Registry of lung transplant recipients, which does not include heart–lung recipients, is kept by the St. Louis International Lung Transplant Registry. As seen in Figure 92–6, the survival for pediatric lung transplantation reported to this Registry is similar to that noted in heart–lung transplant patients (approximately 51% at 2 years). By September 1994, however, a total of only 133

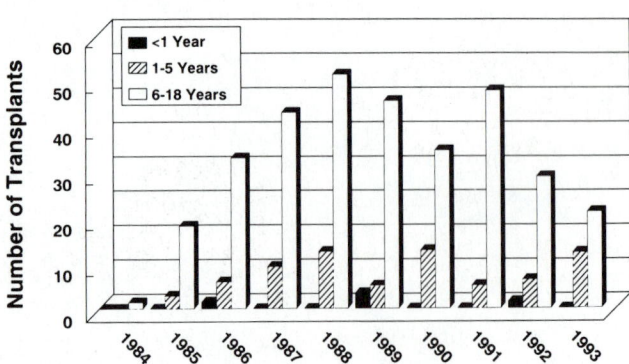

Figure 92–3. Age distribution for pediatric heart–lung transplantation over time.[1] *(From the Registry of the International Society for Heart and Lung Transplantation, 11th Official Report 1994, Mosby–Year Book, with permission.)*

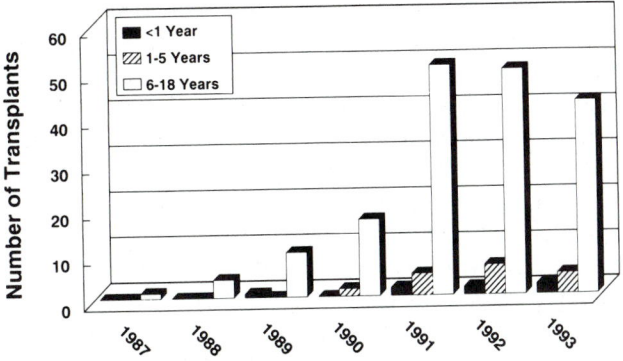

Figure 92–4. Age distribution of pediatric lung transplantation over time.[1] *(From the Registry of the International Society for Heart and Lung Transplantation, 11th Official Report 1994, Mosby–Year Book, with permission.)*

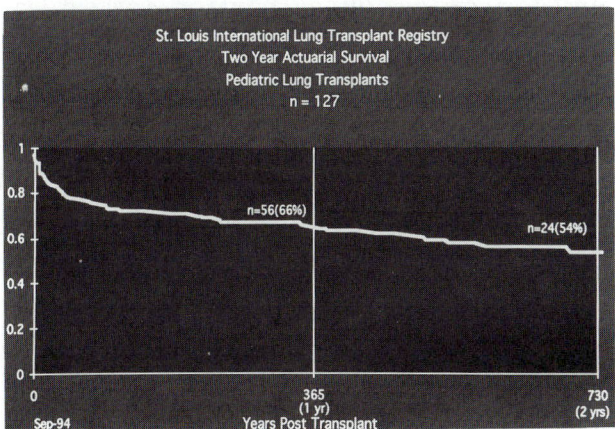

Figure 92–6. Survival from the St. Louis Pediatric Lung Transplant Registry in children under 16 years of age.

pediatric lung transplants in children less than 16 years of age had been reported to the Registry. The indication for the majority of the transplants was cystic fibrosis with primary pulmonary hypertension as the second most common identifiable cause for transplant. The diagnoses for pediatric transplants are shown in Table 92–3.

In our own experience at St. Louis Children's Hospital from July of 1990 through September of 1994, 66 pediatric lung transplants have been performed in 71 patients. Age ranged from 3 mo to 24 years with a mean age of 9.8 years. Survival was 47 of the 66 patients or 71%. Actuarial survival of the total population is shown in Figure 92–7. The follow-up has been from 1 to 47 mo with a mean of 13 mo. Fifty of the transplants were bilateral, 6 single, 4 lobar, and 2 heart–single lungs, 3 heart–lungs, and 1 living-related bilateral lobar transplant. Five patients underwent redo bilateral transplantation. As expected in a pediatric lung transplant population, 12 of the 66 patients were on a ventilator from 3 days to 4.5 years in duration prior to the transplant procedure. Of this group, 9 or 75% survived. The diagnoses

for which transplantation was performed are shown in Tables 92–4 and 92–5. Forty-one patients were transplanted for a diagnosis of pulmonary fibrosis and 25 underwent lung transplantation and cardiac repair or heart–lung transplantation. Mortality was 13 of 66 (20%) early (less than 3 mo post-transplant) and 6 (9%) children died late (greater than 3 mo post-transplant). The survival by diagnosis of the transplant patients is shown in Figure 92–8.

Other reported groups of pediatric lung transplant patients have had excellent results. One series of cystic fibrosis patients had an 80% early and late survival up to 2 years following transplant.[42] Another series from Pittsburgh has shown excellent early results with a 75% survival at 1 year.[44] An additional series of heart–lung and lung transplantation in children from Pittsburgh reported a 78% survival with a perioperative mortality rate of 15%.[45] No late deaths up to 7 years post-transplant were recorded in this series.

Although only relatively early results are presently available on pediatric lung transplantation, comparison of

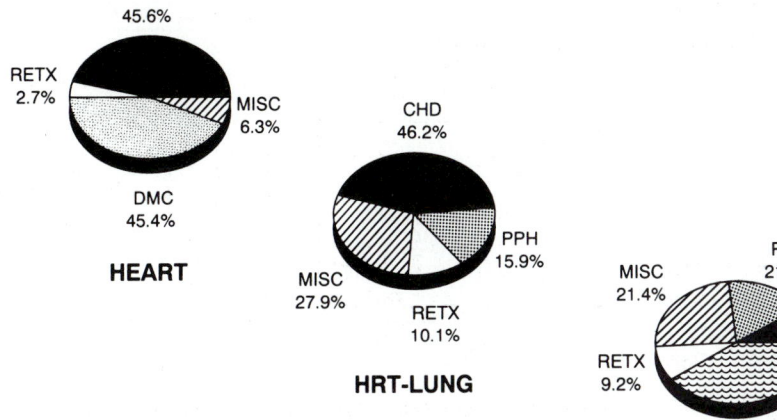

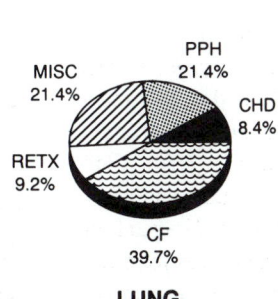

Figure 92–5. Indications for heart-lung versus lung transplantation in children as compared to indications for heart transplantation.[1] *(From the Registry of the International Society for Heart and Lung Transplantation, 11th Official Report 1994, Mosby–Year Book, with permission.)*

TABLE 92–3. ST. LOUIS INTERNATIONAL TRANSPLANT REGISTRY—SEPTEMBER 1994 REPORT: PEDIATRIC TRANSPLANTS (0–16 YEARS)

Diagnosis	Age (Years)			
	0–5 (n=19)	6–10 (n=31)	11–16 (n=83)	Total (n=133)
Cystic fibrosis	0	16	48	64
Pulmonary fibrosis	2	1	7	10
Primary pulmonary hypertension	8	2	10	20
Eisenmenger's	1	1	3	5
Bronchiolitis obliterans	0	5	3	8
Retransplant	0	1	5	6
Other	8	5	7	20

the lung transplant results in the International Registries and the reported series of heart–lung transplants suggests that results are comparable with these two types of treatment in the majority of patients.

LOBAR TRANSPLANTATION

Lobar transplantation has been performed in a very small number of children at the present time.[2,24,46] Down-sizing of adult lungs with use of isolated lobes for transplantation into children offers an attractive option in the very ill patients who would not be likely to live long enough for otherwise suitable donor lungs. However, the scarcity of donors and the large waiting list for adult organs suggests that few adult donor lungs will be available for down-sizing for use in children. Living-related lobar lung transplantation may offer an attractive alternative for selected patients who present late in the course of their illness. The use of living-

related lobar transplant and bilateral lobar transplantation in children and young adults with cystic fibrosis has been pioneered by Starnes.[47] The use of lower lobes from separate adult donors has been performed in several patients with cystic fibrosis, including one patient at our center. The short ischemic times of the donor lungs and the ability to obtain lungs rapidly in children who otherwise have rapid deterioration while awaiting suitable donor organs make lobar transplantation attractive. Nevertheless, the wisdom of this approach will await longer term follow-up. While the immune advantage of living-related transplantation has not been documented, there is evidence that differential rejection of the donated lobes from different individuals may occur (Fig. 97–9A,B,C). Down-sizing of small pediatric

TABLE 92–4. PEDIATRIC LUNG TRANSPLANTATION: PULMONARY FIBROSIS, 7/90–9/94[a]

Cystic fibrosis		26
Pulmonary fibrosis		11
AML, BM TX, RAD fibrosis	3	
Bronchiolitis obliterans (OB)	2	
PF/Stevens–Johnson	1	
BPD with PF	1	
Chronic aspiration with PF	1	
Interstitial pneumonitis with PF	2	
Histiocystosis X-RAD fibrosis	1	
Surfactant protein B deficiency		2
ARDS		1
Redo bilateral		5
Acute graft failure	1	
ARDS	2	
OB	2	
Total		40

[a]AMI, acute leukemia; BM TX, bone marrow transplant; RAD, radiation; PF, pulmonary stenosis; BPD, bronchopulmonary dysplasia; ARDS, respiratory distress syndrome.

TABLE 92–5. PEDIATRIC LUNG TRANSPLANTATION: LUNG TRANSPLANTATION AND CARDIAC REPAIR 7/90–9/94[a]

Pulmonary atresia/VSD	4
VSD, Eisenmerger's	1
VSD, PDA, Eisenmerger's	1
PDA, PHTN	3
ASD, PHTN	4
Pulmonary vein stenosis	3
Heart Tx, left LTX, reconstruct PA	1
Heart Tx, right LTX, reconstruct SVC	1
Heart–lung TX	3
PHTN after heart repair	3
Peripheral PS, ASD	1
Total	25

[a]VSD, ventricular septal defect; PDA, patent ductus arteriosus; PHTN, pulmonary hypertension; TX, transplant; LTX, lung transplant; PS, pulmonary stenosis; ASD, atrial septal defect.

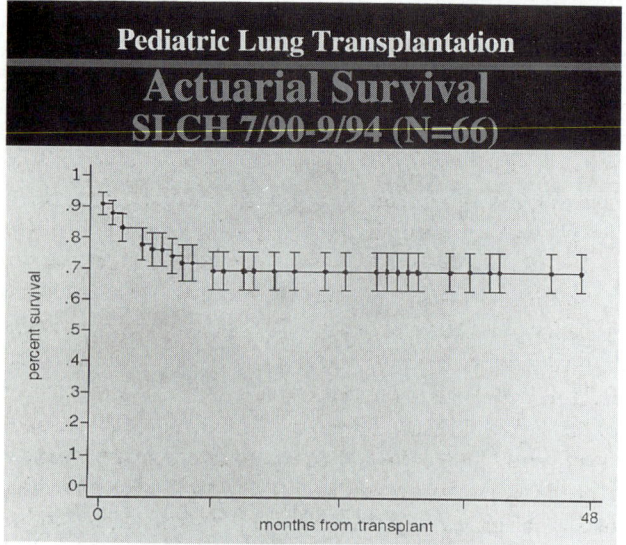

Figure 92–7. Actuarial survival for pediatric lung transplants performed at St Louis Children's Hospital through September 1994.

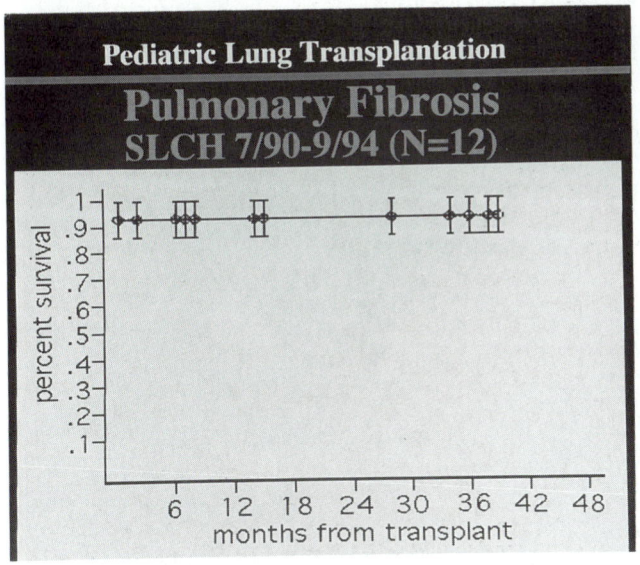

A

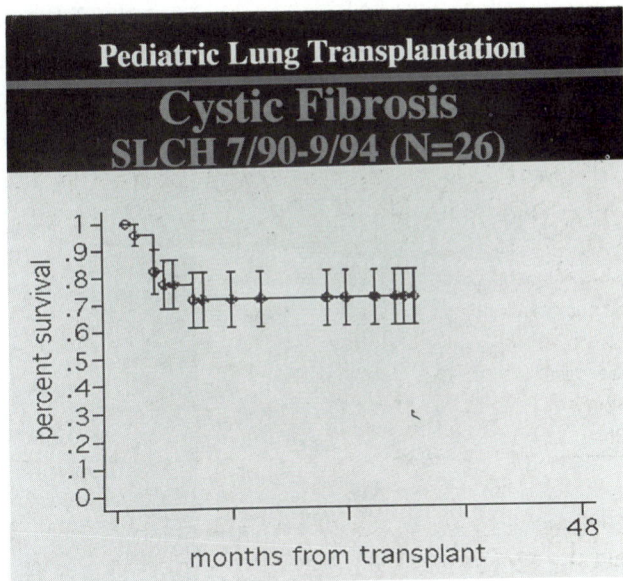

B

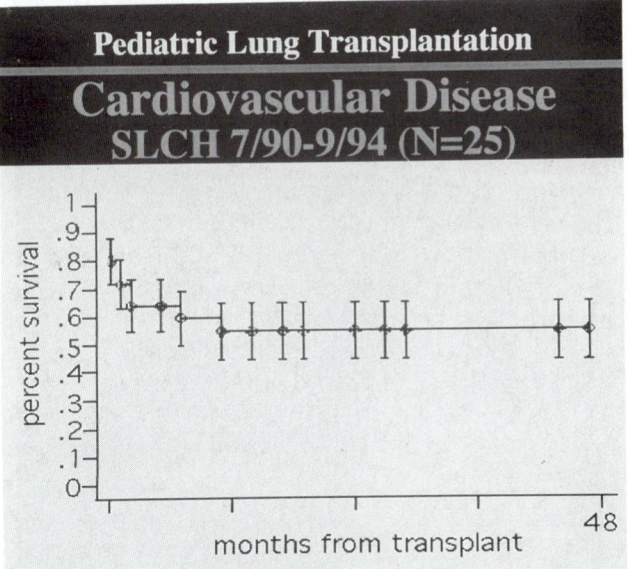

C

Figure 92–8. A. Actuarial survival of St. Louis Children's Hospital Pediatric Lung Transplants performed for pulmonary fibrosis through September 1994. **B.** Actuarial survival of children transplanted for cystic fibrosis at St Louis Children's Hospital through September 1994. **C.** Actuarial survival for children transplanted for pulmonary hypertension or congenital heart disease through September 1994.

lungs may provide the opportunity to implant a single lobe in very small infants with severe progressive respiratory insufficiency such as the surfactant protein deficiencies, isolated pulmonary hypertension, significant pulmonary fibrosis or bronchopulmonary dysplasia, or congenital diaphragmatic hernia.

LONG-TERM RESULTS

The major limitation to long-term survival following lung transplantation in children is the development of bronchiolitis obliterans. Although this entity may be a manifestation of chronic rejection, other possible factors such as repeated viral infections may be important in its etiology.[48–52] The

onset of bronchiolitis obliterans is associated with progressive dyspnea and a reduction in oxygen saturation on room air. In addition, the child may have a documented decrease in forced expiratory volume in 1 sec on spirometry as the initial sign of development of this problem. The chest x-ray in patients with bronchiolitis obliterans may be remarkably normal although occasionally hyperinflation of the lung fields is noted and in the late stages contraction and scarring of the upper lobes may be present (Fig. 92–10). The diagnosis of bronchiolitis obliterans may be entertained on clinical grounds if there is evidence for a sudden decrease of FEV_1 of 20% or greater of the maximum post-transplant baseline level unassociated with evidence for infection or bronchial complication or other etiology. Histologic confirmation can be obtained on transbronchial biopsy if an adequate speci-

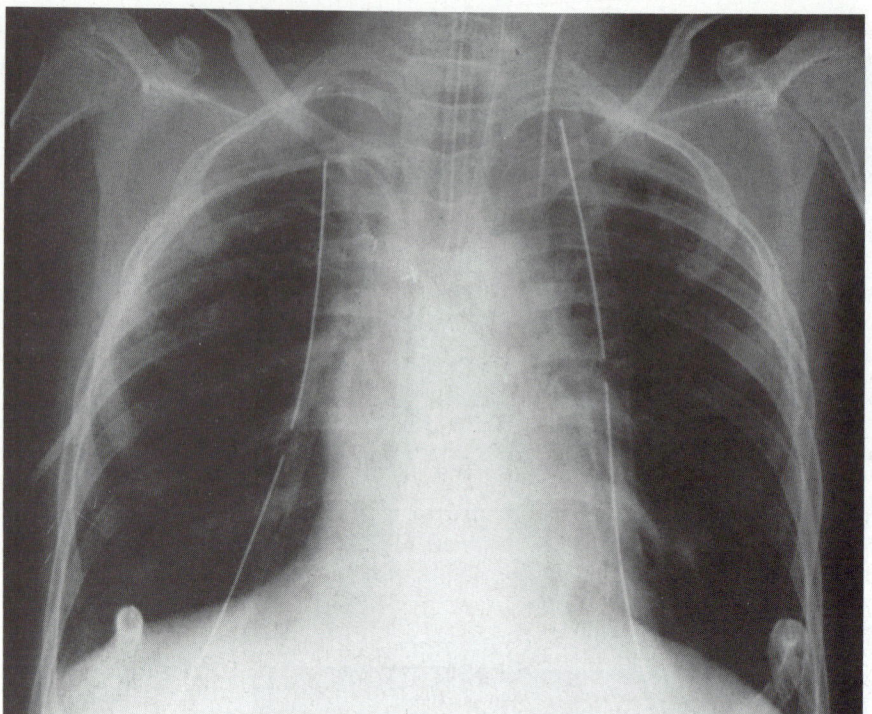

A

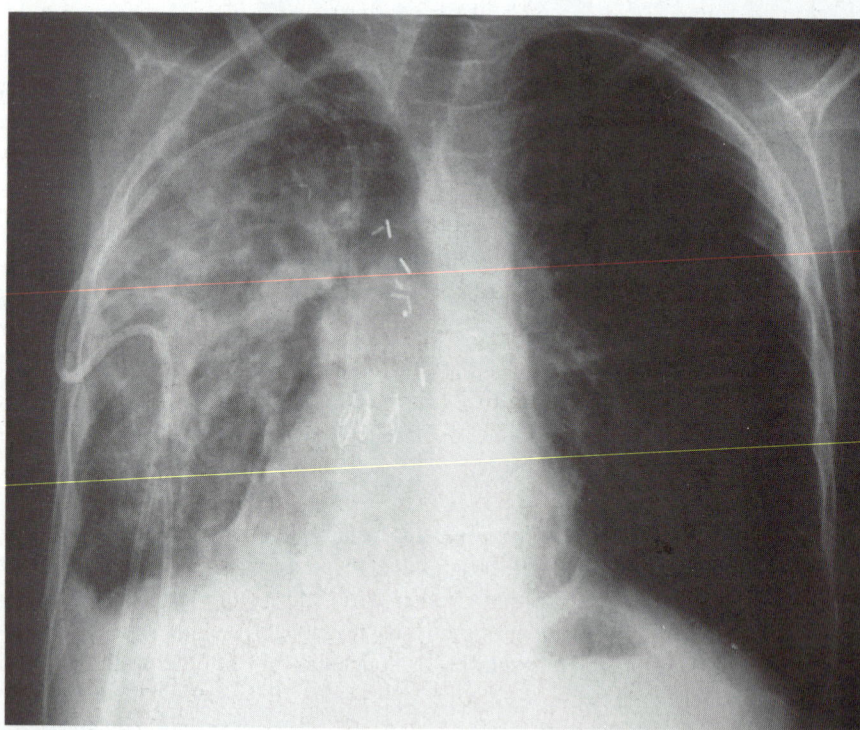

B

Figure 92–9. Chest radiographs in a 12-year-old child with cystic fibrosis who underwent living-related bilateral lobar transplantation from his parents. **A.** Initial post-transplant chest radiograph showing clear lungs bilaterally. **B.** Chest radiograph taken 1 week posttransplant with evidence for clear lung on the left (maternal) side and diffuse infiltrates in the right (paternal) lung. Biopsy of the right lung revealed evidence of a Grade 2 rejection. *(Continued.)*

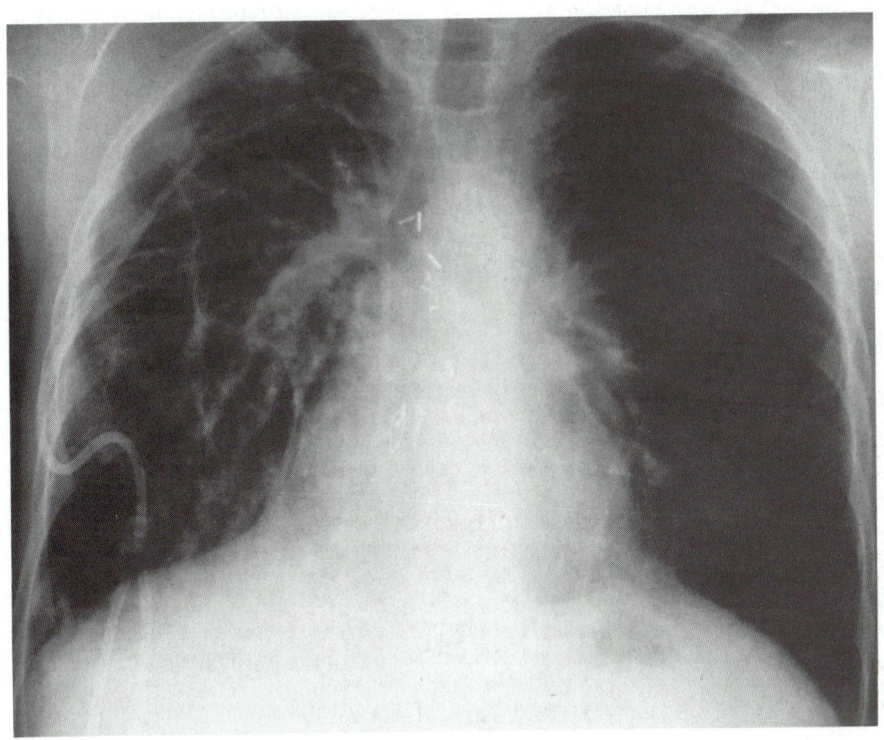

C

Figure 92–9. *(Continued.)* **C.** Chest radiograph after treatment with pulse steroids for acute rejection showing resolution of infiltrates in the right (paternal) lobe.

men is obtained or on open lung biopsy if required to confirm the diagnosis in the absence of other diagnostic modalities. Although lung function has stabilized in occasional patients with the onset of bronchiolitis obliterans with increased immunosuppression including steroids and occasionally methotrexate, in many patients there is rapid progression of respiratory deterioration. Retransplantation has been considered for some of these children, although the results of retransplantation have been poor with only a few retransplants done in the pediatric population.[1] Results in

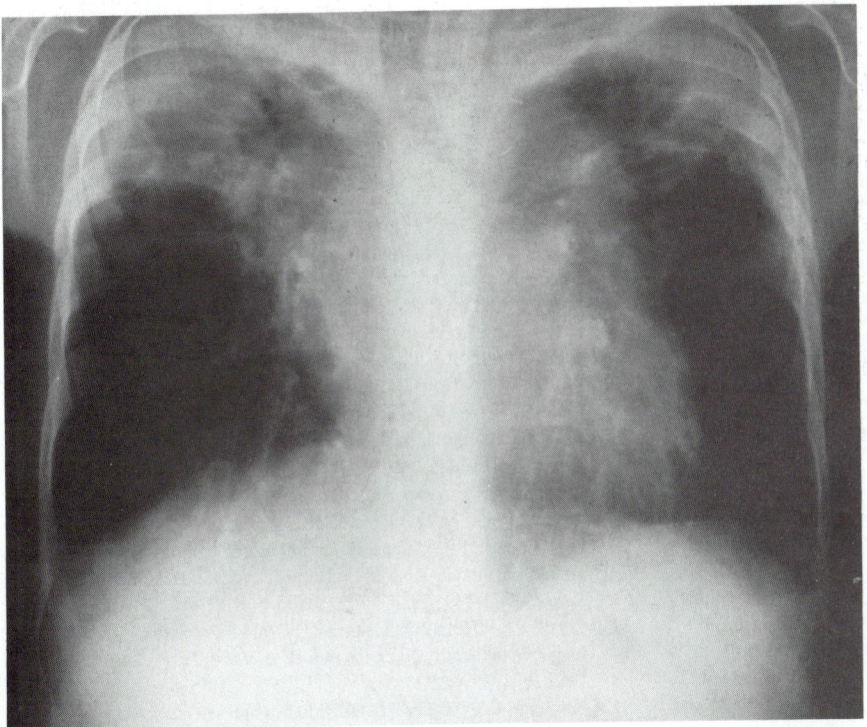

Figure 92–10. Chest radiograph of an 11-year-old child who underwent bilateral sequential lung transplantation at 9 years of age for severe cystic fibrosis. She developed progressive bronchiolitis obliterans with severe restrictive pulmonary disease. The chest radiograph showed destruction of the upper lobes of the transplanted lungs with severe pleural scarring and contraction. She underwent redo bilateral lung transplantation 23 months after the initial transplant procedure.

adults with retransplantation for bronchiolitis obliterans have shown a decreased long-term survival with an approximately 40% survival at 1 year.[53]

In heart–lung transplant recipients the onset of bronchiolitis obliterans can occur independent of the development of coronary graft atherosclerosis.

SUMMARY

The majority of pediatric heart–lung and lung transplants to date have been performed in patients with cystic fibrosis and relatively few children have had transplantation of these organs for Eisenmenger's syndrome, primary pulmonary hypertension, or forms of pulmonary fibrosis. This small experience in pediatric patients coupled with the variation in indications for transplantation make comparisons difficult between pediatric and adult populations. Pediatric cardiopulmonary and pulmonary transplantation has only relatively recently been performed and long-term follow-up data are not yet available on a significant number of patients. The medium and intermediate term results of pediatric cardiopulmonary transplantation, however, appear similar to the results noted in adults for whom there is a somewhat longer follow-up available. The results are encouraging, however obliterative bronchiolitis remains a serious problem that must be addressed for the future success of cardiopulmonary transplantation in children. Whether lung transplantation or combined heart–lung transplantation becomes the preferred technique in pediatric patients, it is apparent that children represent a particularly difficult patient group and careful selection coupled with attention to multiple medical conditions relating to the underlying disease process are required for achievement of optimal results.

REFERENCES

1. Hosenpud JD, Novick RJ, Breen TJ, Daily OP: The Registry of the International Society for Heart and Lung Transplantation: Eleventh Official Report—1994. *J Heart Lung Transplant* **13**:561–570, 1994

2. Spray TL, Mallory GB, Canter CE, Huddleston CB: Pediatric lung transplantation. Indications, techniques, and early results. *J Thorac Cardiovasc Surg* **107**:990–1000, 1994

3. Carrel A: The surgery of blood vessels. *Johns Hopkins Bull* **18**:18, 1907

4. Demikhov VP: Some essential points of the techniques of transplantation of the heart, lungs and other organs. In Haigh B (transl): *Experimental Transplantation of Vital Organs*. New York, Consultants Bureau, 1962; Moscow, Medgiz, 1960, p 29

5. Castaneda AR, Arnar O, Schmidt-Habelman P, et al: Cardiopulmonary autotransplantation in primates. *J Thorac Cardiovasc Surg* **37**:523–531, 1972

6. Cooley DA, Bloodwell RD, Hallman GL, et al: Organ transplantation for advanced cardiopulmonary disease. *Ann Thorac Surg* **8**:30, 1969

7. Reitz BA, Wallwork J, Hunt SA, et al: Heart-lung transplantation: A successful therapy for patients with pulmonary vascular disease. *N Engl J Med* **806**:557–563, 1982

8. Cooper JD: The evolution of techniques and indications for lung transplantation. *Ann Surg* **212**:249–256, 1990

9. St. Louis International Lung Transplant Registry: September 1994 Report. 3108 Queeny Tower, 4989 Barnes Hospital Plaza, St. Louis, MO 63110.

10. D'Alonzo GE, Barst RJ, Ayres SM, et al: Survival in patients with primary pulmonary hypertension. Results from a national prospective registry. *Ann Intern Med* **115**:343–349, 1991

11. Houde C, Bohn DJ, Freedom RM, et al: Profile of pediatric patients with pulmonary hypertension judged by responsiveness to vasodilators. *Br Heart J* **70**:461–468, 1993

12. Glanville AR, Burke CM, Theodore J, et al: Primary pulmonary hypertension: Length of survival in patients referred for heart–lung transplantation. *Chest* **91**:675–680, 1987

13. Spray TL, Mallory GB, Canter CE, et al: Pediatric lung transplantation for pulmonary hypertension and congenital heart disease. *Ann Thorac Surg* **54**:216–225, 1992

14. Smyth RL, Scott JP, Whitehead B, et al: Heart lung transplantation in children. *Transplant Proc* **22**:1470–1471, 1990

15. Smyth RL, Scott JP, Higgenbottom TW, et al: The use of heart-lung transplantation in management of terminal respiratory complications of cystic fibrosis. *Transplant Proc* **22**:1472–1473, 1990

16. Dantzker DR: Primary pulmonary hypertension. The American experience. *Chest* **105**(Suppl.):26S–28S, 1994

17. Young D, Mark H: Fate of the patient with Eisenmenger's syndrome. *Am J Cardiol* **28**:658–669, 1971

18. Radley-Smith R, Adams D, Yacoub M: Heart-lung versus heterotropic heart transplantation for children with cardiomyopathy and severe pulmonary hypertension. *J Heart Lung Transplant* **13**:S35 [Abstract], 1994

19. Pasque MK, Kaiser LR, Dresler CM, et al: Single lung transplantation for pulmonary hypertension: Technical aspects and immediate hemodynamic results. *J Thorac Cardiovasc Surg* **103**:475–482, 1992

20. Shumway SJ, Hertz MI, Jessurun J, et al: Obliterative bronchiolitis after lung or heart-lung transplantation for pulmonary hypertension (abstract). Meeting of the 72nd American Association for Thoracic Surgery, Los Angeles, CA, 1992

21. Lupinetti FM, Bolling SF, Bove EL, et al: Selective lung or heart-lung transplantation for pulmonary hypertension associated with congenital cardiac anomalies. *Ann Thorac Surg* **57**:1545–1549, 1994

22. Harjula A, Baldwin JC, Starnes VA, et al: Proper donor selection for heart-lung transplantation. The Stanford experience. *J Heart Transplant* **4**:234, 1985

23. Shumway SJ, Hertz MI, Petty MG, Liberalization of donor criteria in lung and heart-lung transplantation. *Ann Thorac Surg* **57**:92–95, 1994

24. Bisson A, Bonnette P, Ben El Kadi N, et al: Bilateral pulmonary lobe transplantation: Left lower and right middle and lower lobes. *Ann Thorac Surg* **57**:219–221, 1994

25. Sundaresan S, Trachtiotis GD, Aoe M, et al: Donor lung procurement: Assessment and operative technique. *Ann Thorac Surg* **56**:1409–1413, 1993

26. Pasque MK, Cooper JD, Kaiser LR, et al: Improved technique for bilateral lung transplantation: rationale and initial clinical experience. *Ann Thorac Surg* **49**:785–791, 1990

27. Calhoon JH, Grover FL, Gibbons WJ, et al: Single lung transplantation: Alternative indications and technique. *J Thorac Cardiovasc Surg* **101**:816–825, 1991

28. Siegelman SS, Sinha SB, Veith FJ: Pulmonary reimplantation response. *Ann Surg* **177**:30–36, 1973

29. Prop J, Ehrie MG, Crapo JD, et al: Reimplantation response in inografted rat lungs: Analysis of causal factors. *J Thorac Cardiovasc Surg* **87**:702–711, 1984

30. Corris PA, Odom NJ, Jackson G, et al: Reimplantation injury after lung transplantation in a rat model. *J Heart Transplant* **6**:234–237, 1987

31. Armitage JM, Fricker FJ, del Nido P, et al: A decade (1982–1992) of

pediatric cardiac transplantation and the impact of FK506 immuno-suppression. *J Thorac Cardiovasc Surg* **105**:464–473, 1993

32. Tsang V, Hodson ME, Yacoub MH: Lung transplantation for cystic fibrosis. *Br Med Bull* **48**:949–971, 1992

33. Cooper DTC, Novitzky D, Rose AG, et al: Acute pulmonary rejection precedes cardiac rejection following heart-lung transplantation in a primate model. *J Heart Transplant* **5**:279–285, 1986

34. Higgenbottom TW, Hanter JA, Stewart S, et al: Transbronchial biopsy has eliminated the need for endomyocardial biopsy in heart-lung recipients. *J Heart Transplant* **7**:435–439, 1988

35. Joshi A, Oyer PE, Billingham ME: Pathology of the heart in heart-lung transplantation (abstract). *J Heart Lung Transplant* **13**:S34, 1994

36. Kirby TJ, Mehta A, Rice TW, Gephardt GN: Diagnosis and management of acute and chronic lung rejection. *Sem Thorac Cardiovasc Surg* **4**:126–131, 1992

37. DeHoyos A, Maurer JR: Complications following lung transplantation. *Sem Thorac Cardiovasc Surg* **4**:132–146,1992

38. Madden B, Radley-Smith R, Hodson M, et al: Medium-term results of heart and lung transplantation. *J Heart Lung Transplant* **11**:S241–S243, 1992

39. Bolman RM III, Braunlin E, Shumway SJ, et al: Pediatric lung and heart-lung Transplantation at the University of Minnesota. *Transplant Proc* **26**:203–204, 1994

40. Metras D, Kreitmann B, Shennib H, Noirclerc M: Lung transplantation in children. *J Heart Lung Transplant* **11**:S282–285, 1992

41. Starnes VA, Marshall SE, Lewiston NJ, et al: Heart-lung transplantation in infants, children, and adolescents. *J Pediatr Surg* **26**:434–438, 1991

42. Metras D, Shennib, Kreitmann B, et al: Double-lung transplantation in children: A report of 20 cases. *Ann Thorac Surg* **55**:352–357, 1993

43. Spray TL, Huddleston GB: Pediatric lung transplantation. *Chest Surg Clin NA* **3**:123–143, 1993

44. Noyes BE, Kurland G, Orenstein DM, et al: Experience with pediatric lung transplantation. *J Pediatr* **124**:261–269, 1994

45. Armitage JM, Fricker FJ, Kurland G, et al: Pediatric lung transplantation: Expanding indications 1985 to 1993. *J Heart Lung Transplant* **12**:S246–254, 1993

46. Starnes VA, Barr ML, Cohen RG: Lobar transplantation: Indications, technique, and outcome. *J Thorac Cardiovasc Surg* **108**:403–411, 1994

47. Cohen RG, Barr ML, Schenkel FA, et al: Living-related donor lobectomy for bilateral lobar transplantation in patients with cystic fibrosis. *Ann Thorac Surg* **57**:1423–1428, 1994

48. Maurer JR, Morrison D, Winton TL, et al: Late pulmonary complications of isolated lung transplantation. *Transplant Proc* **23**:1224–1225, 1991

49. Scott JP, Sharples L, Mullins P, et al: Further studies on the natural history of obliterative bronchiolitis following heart-lung transplantation. *Transplant Proc* **23**:1201–1202, 1991

50. Burke C, Glanville AR, Theodore J, et al: Lung immunogenicity, rejection, and obliterative bronchiolitis. *Chest* **92**:547–549, 1987

51. John R, Hertz M, Savik K, et al: Multivariate analysis of risk factors for obliterative bronchiolitis in lung allograft recipients (abstract). *J Heart Lung Transplant* **13**:S53, 1994

52. Winter J, Groen M, Prop J: Bronchiolitis obliterans is caused by nonspecific inflammation after respiratory viral infections in rat lung allografts with chronic rejection. *J Heart Lung Transplant* **13**:S47, 1994

53. Miller J, Patterson GA: Retransplantation following isolated lung transplantation. *Sem Thorac Cardiovasc Surg* **4**:122–125, 1992

CHAPTER

93

Circulatory Support in Infants and Children

Ehud Rudis and Davis C. Drinkwater, Jr.

HISTORICAL PERSPECTIVE

Although the last decade has brought dramatic improvements in the technology of mechanical circulatory support, these advances have been largely limited to the adult population. The first report of mechanical support in children was by Spencer in 1963 in a 6-year-old girl who developed severe heart failure with pulmonary hypertension after closure of a ventricular septal defect.[1] Venoarterial bypass was used for several hours until lethal arrhythmias developed. In 1967, DeBakey successfully used an atrial–axillary artery ventricular assist device for acute cardiac failure after mitral valve replacement in a 16-year-old patient.[2] The experience with mechanical assist devices to support the failing heart in the pediatric population has been limited almost exclusively to patients with cardiac failure after surgery for congenital heart disease.[3–5] However, there are reports of supporting children with acute myocarditis,[6] as well as a bridge to cardiac transplantation.[7]

Ventricular assist devices (VADs) have been available in a limited way for the pediatric group of patients since the late 1970s. Recent experience with postcardiotomy VADs, from both Melbourne Children's Hospital and Children's Hospital in Boston, have been encouraging with survival rates around 50%.[8,9] The other area in which VADs have been useful in the pediatric population is in association with cardiac transplantation, with successful bridging to transplantation reported in 60%.[10]

The mechanical support of the failing heart of a child should be tailored according to many parameters. Recognizing the indications, contraindications, and understanding the mechanisms, as well as potential complications, will help to achieve better overall results and survival rates.

To this end, modifications have been made in both the intra-aortic balloon pump and VADs, predominantly in size, which allow expanded use in pediatric patients. Their use (and usefulness) requires a close appreciation of the anatomic defect and method of correction to allow selection of the type of assist and an early focus toward recovery or replacement of the native myocardium.

INTRA-AORTIC BALLOON PUMPS (IABP)

An intra-aortic balloon pump (IABP), is a balloon catheter device placed into the descending aorta via the femoral artery that provides hemodynamic augmentation and is synchronized to the diastolic phase of the cardiac cycle (Fig. 93–1). This device has had a limited role in pediatric patients because of their relatively small arterial size, with the vascular problems of insertion, and the elasticity of their aortic wall whereby the counterpulsation effect is partially lost. The rapid heart rate (>150/min) also interferes with complete inflation–deflation with 1:1 tracking. Additionally, with a patent coronary vascular system, such as is present in most pediatric patients, there is little added benefit from diastolic augmentation on the coronary perfusion.[11,12]

In 1979 Pollock reported the use of an intra-aortic balloon pump in a series of infants and children undergoing open heart surgery.[12] The ages in this group ranged from 1.5 to 1.8 years. There were only six long-term survivors, none of whom was under 5 years of age. They inserted the balloon surgically via a side arm Dacron graft on the common femoral artery. Inadequate augmentation was reported, and was felt to be due to the relatively compliant aortic wall of children. Several major complications related to the large

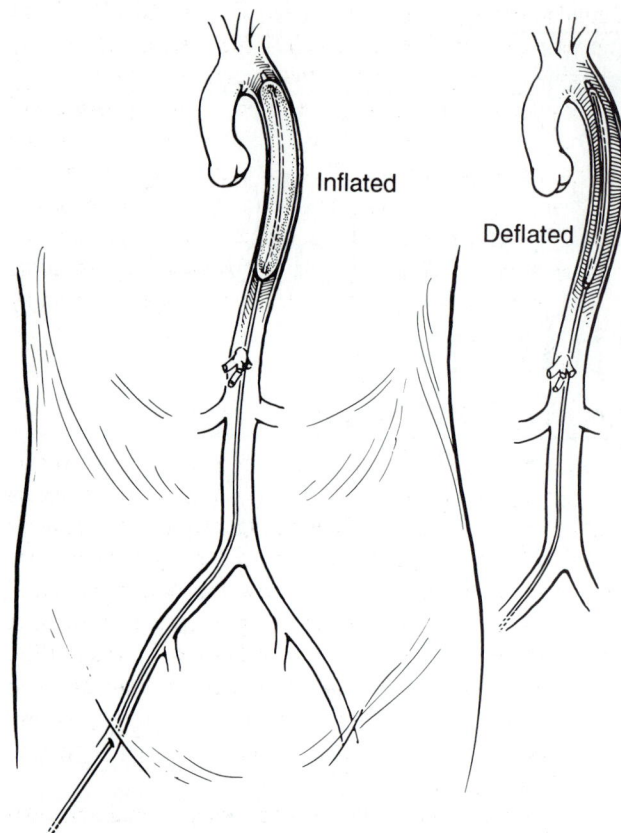

Figure 93–1. Intra-aortic balloon pump (IABP). The catheter is inserted through the common femoral artery, and the balloon positioned in the descending aorta just distal to the left subclavian artery and proximal to the celiac arteries. The inflation during diastole provides augmented coronary blood flow, and deflation during systole decreased afterload for the LV.

size of the balloon catheter were noted including superior mesenteric and renal artery occlusions and severe limb ischemia.

In 1981 Veasy developed pediatric balloons ranging in size from 0.75 to 5 mL attached to 4 and 5 Fr catheters.[13] These catheters achieved the desired hemodynamic effect of afterload reduction and augmentation of diastolic pressure. To obtain optimal augmentation, the balloon volume should be equal to at least 50% of the stroke volume formulated by the following equation.[14]

$$\frac{2000 \times (\text{cardiac index}) \times (\text{body surface area})}{\text{heart rate}}$$

$$\times\ 0.5\ =\ \text{balloon volume}$$

In the pediatric patient poor IABP augmentation is generally the result of a very elastic aorta as well as a high resting heart rate, which makes the timing of the balloon difficult. This can be partially resolved by converting to a 1:2 mode when heart rates exceed 150–160/min. Veasy reported a low incidence of complications with a reasonable survival of 50% of patients so treated.[14] Although successful IABP

augmentation has been reported in infants as small as 2 kg,[14] present restrictions in size continue to limit the use of IABP in smaller children and infants, mainly because of introducer size and subsequent arterial jeopardy.

EXTRACORPOREAL MEMBRANE OXYGENATION (ECMO)

Introduction

The use of venoarterial bypass with an oxygenator for prolonged circulatory (or pulmonary) support is known as "extracorporeal membrane oxygenation" or ECMO. The pioneering usage of this technique in patients with severe cardiac failure was first reported in 1957 but was not commonly used until the 1980s.[15] The prior experience of Bartlett and colleagues had shown that while this technique is successful for infants with severe respiratory failure, their early results in postoperative cardiac failure were disappointing. However, later experience demonstrated the effectiveness of ECMO in some postcardiotomy patients. The most recent data published by experienced groups report a survival rate that exceeds 50%. Current considerations for ECMO include the complexity of the heart defects, the need for continued heparinization to prevent clotting in the circuit, and the incidence of infection related to the surgical implantation of the system.[16–20]

The indications for ECMO are well established in the treatment of selected patients with respiratory failure. Its use has also been extended to cardiac and pulmonary support after cardiac surgery in children and infants.[21,22] The first successful application of ECMO in postcardiotomy failure was reported by Soeter in 1973.[23] The effect of ECMO on the heart includes a decrease in preload, a slight increase in afterload, and a concomitant elevation in left ventricular wall stress.[24] The advantages of ECMO (over VAD alone) include support of both right and left ventricles, improvement of systemic oxygenation, and ease of placement. ECMO support in postcardiotomy patients may be provided with either venoarterial or venovenous cannulation. Venoarterial cannulation provides the optimal cardiac support when ventricular dysfunction predominates the clinical picture. However, studies have also shown that venovenous bypass, primarily by improving venous oxygenation, may improve myocardial oxygenation and decrease pulmonary vascular resistance in selected patients, thus providing adequate cardiac recovery and support.[25,26] Cases of ventricular dysfunction caused by acute cyanosis and hypoxia may respond to improving systemic arterial saturation using this technique.

Cannulation Technique

Venoarterial ECMO may be performed by extrathoracic cannulation (carotid artery and jugular vein, or femoral artery and femoral vein), or more commonly transthoracic cannulation through the median sternotomy incision (the aorta and the right atrium) (Fig. 93–2). Carotid–jugular cannulation may best be used in patients who are weaned from cardiopulmonary bypass in the operating room and develop myocardial dysfunction with cardiogenic shock after operation. Advantages of this approach are a separate incision site remote from the median sternotomy wound and a lower incidence of bleeding from the mediastinal wound. Both of these factors may contribute to a decreased risk of mediastinal infection.[27]

In patients with a cavopulmonary connection (Glenn or Fontan circulation), direct access from the jugular vein to the right atrium is not feasible. A transthoracic approach is therefore needed in these cases. Femoral arteriovenous cannulation can be used in certain older children, with placement of intravascular catheters into the inferior vena cava or right atrium through the femoral vein and into the common femoral or iliac artery for arterial return (Fig. 93–3). The venous return with this type of cannulation may be restrictive unless a centrifugal type pump is used that provides active venous drainage. The advantage of this peripheral technique includes the noninvasive surgical approach and the more secure cannula fixation.

We believe transthoracic cannulation (right atrium to aorta) is preferable in patients who cannot be weaned from cardiopulmonary bypass in the operating room or in those circumstances where the chest was opened for the purpose of resuscitation in the postoperative period. The standard

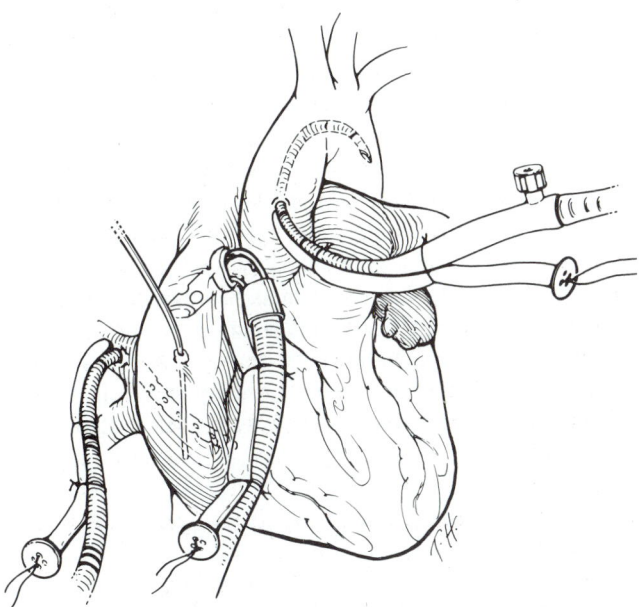

Figure 93–2. ECMO cannulation. Through a median sternotomy an angled cannula is placed in the right atrium to drain systemic venous return. The blood is oxygenated in a membrane oxygenator and returned via a cannula in the ascending aorta. A long aortic catheter is placed through the transverse arch, distal of the head vessels. A left atrial venting cannula can be inserted through the right superior pulmonary vein to unload the left ventricle.

cannulae for bypass can be converted to the ECMO circuit and brought out through or below the median sternotomy incision. Whenever possible, the sternum should be closed unless edema of the myocardium prevents this. Closure will help to decrease the incidence of infection and bleeding during this support phase. The goal of ECMO support in patients after cardiac surgery differs from that in neonates with hypoxemia resulting from pulmonary dysfunction. Maintenance of adequate tissue perfusion while providing complete or nearly complete cardiac bypass is the primary goal.

Conduct of ECMO Support

The prevention of cardiac distension, minimizing myocardial energy expenditure and maximizing potential myocardial recovery through mechanical support, is vital. Flows as high as 150 mL/kg per minute are frequently needed to reduce both right and left atrial pressure. When left atrial (LA) pressures remain elevated despite optimal flow, it is critical to vent the LA to the venous drainage system (Fig. 93–2). This scenario is frequently found in patients with multiple aortopulmonary collaterals (Fig. 93–2). High flows should be maintained for 48–72 hours before attempting to wean from ECMO.

During ECMO support it is important to maintain adequate pulmonary ventilation to prevent atelectasis while recognizing that this may also create hypocarbia and excessive PaO_2. This should be controlled by reducing ventilatory rate (not tidal volume) and adjusting the O_2 and CO_2 flow to the membrane. Adequate tidal volume and extracorporeal flow rates should never be altered to manage PaO_2 or PcO_2.

Anticoagulation and Bleeding

The major disadvantage of the transthoracic approach includes the potential risks of mediastinal hemorrhage, infection, and cannula dislodgment during repositioning or transport. Control of hemorrhage on ECMO is of great importance[28] as it is a frequent cause of death, and because massive transfusion may lead to ARDS and irrevocable pulmonary impairment. Anticoagulation is monitored by keeping the activated clotting time (ACT) around 200 seconds with a continuous IV heparin infusion. If bleeding persists, the ACT can be lowered temporarily to 180 seconds. The prothrombin time is maintained as near normal as possible, by transfusing 10 mL/kg of fresh frozen plasma every 6 hours as necessary. The platelet count is preferred over 100,000/mm^3 with platelet transfusions given as needed. All transfusions are leukofiltered and/or irradiated if transplantation is at all likely to occur. This avoids further presensitization and antibody development that might promote allograft rejection, and also restricts cytomegalovirous (CMV) exposure. The development of heparin bonded circuits may greatly aid the field of ECMO by reducing the

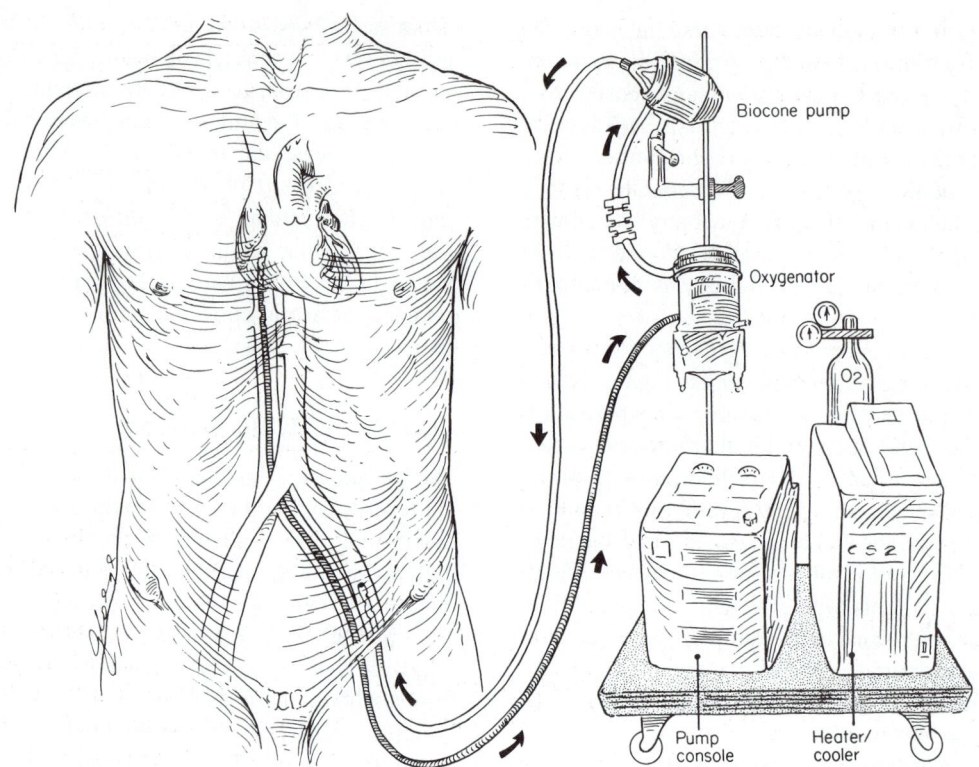

Figure 93–3. Peripheral ECMO circuit. In larger children, peripheral cannulation may be adequate to give both pulmonary and cardiac support. The centrifugal pump is able to obtain more complete flows through active venous sumping. The oxygenator is placed into the circuit as well as the heater/cooler to maintain normothermia. This avoids a median sternotomy and possible bleeding and/or infection.

need for significant anticoagulation and its attendant risks. Indeed, closed circuits (ECMO) with tip-to-tip heparin coating appear to have the most favorable results in this new field.[29]

Venovenous cannulation (jugular and femoral veins, femoral and femoral veins, or a double lumen catheter in femoral or jugular vein) provides oxygenation support to venous blood. When myocardial dysfunction is primarily due to inadequate oxygenation or elevated pulmonary vascular resistance improvement may be accomplished by increasing the saturation of the venous blood. Such situations are uncommon in pediatric cardiac surgery and as such venovenous ECMO has infrequently been used in this patient population.

Indications for ECMO Placement

The *preoperative* use of ECMO in infants with congenital heart disease is controversial (Table 93–1). The group from St. Louis Children's Hospital has published their experience with patients who had unoperated cyanotic heart disease and cardiopulmonary collapse associated with hypercyanotic spells, pulmonary hypertension, or sepsis.[27] Their indications for ECMO included arterial oxygen saturation <60% on maximal medical therapy, with hypotension and metabolic acidosis despite maximal support including hyperventilation with 100% oxygen, inotropes, vasodilators,

or both. The duration of ECMO support ranged from 1 to 38 days (mean 18 days). Seven of the eight patients underwent corrective or palliative surgery while on ECMO or within 48 hours after decannulation. The survival rate was 62%, and the survivors had normal growth and development. Other groups have described the successful use of ECMO as a bridge to transplant in pediatric patients.[30]

Intraoperative ECMO is used when the child cannot be weaned from cardiopulmonary bypass despite maximal inotropic therapy and optimal operative repair. Decisions about venting of the left ventricle at the time of initiation of ECMO in the operating room depend on the measurement of left atrial pressure on full ECMO support. If the left ventricle distends or left atrial pressure rises above 10 mm Hg despite adequate flow rates, the left atrium should be

TABLE 93–1. INDICATIONS FOR ECMO CARDIAC SUPPORT

Preoperative: Arterial O_2 sat. <60% on 100% FIO_2, maximal medical therapy support with inotropes, vasodilators, and pharmacologic paralysis and sedation, associated with hypotension and metabolic acidosis

Intraoperative: Inability to wean from CPB despite maximal inotropic therapy and/or IABP

Postoperative: Low cardiac output as defined by progressive decrease in urine output, elevated RA and LA filling pressures despite maximal inotropic support, widened A-V O_2 difference

vented. In the majority of patients placed on ECMO for inability to wean from cardiopulmonary bypass, ECMO is maintained via the original bypass cannulae. To improve and simplify venous return, bicaval cannulation should be converted to a single venous cannula. The patient is then converted to a closed ECMO system with brief clamping of the cannulae and connection of sterile lines on the operative field. In patients with systemic-to-pulmonary shunts, pulmonary blood flow can be limited by partial occlusion of the shunt. This may be opened gradually to provide pulmonary blood flow and possible pulmonary parenchymal nutrition prior to weaning from ECMO.[31]

The development of *postoperative* low cardiac output which requires ECMO support represents a unique group of patients with favorable results (Table 93–2.). Those patients usually present with decreased urine output (less than 1 mL/kg per hour), poor peripheral perfusion, low systemic venous saturation (a wide AVo_2 difference), and elevated filling pressures despite maximal inotropic and diuretic support. The myocardial injury in those patients is usually less than in those who cannot be weaned from CPB. The interval between surgery and initiation of the ECMO may give sufficient time for the recovery of relatively normal coagulation, an important factor which may positively affect the outcome of these infants and children.[19]

Weaning

The ability to decrease inotropic support along with an improvement in renal function and diuresis of retained fluid are initial indicators of myocardial recovery. After a period of time in which the myocardial contractility is permitted to improve, as assessed by serial echocardiograms, an attempt is made to wean from ECMO. With reasonable inotropic support (dopamine at 5 µg/kg per minute and epinephrine at 0.05 µg/kg per minute) ECMO flow is gradually lowered to 100–200 mL/min. If myocardial contractility remains satisfactory, and the filling pressures are low, decannulation may be accomplished.

Complications

Mechanical support of infants and children with ECMO results in several possible complications (Table 93–3). The

TABLE 93–2. DIAGNOSES FOR WHICH ECMO IS MORE COMMONLY USED AFTER CARDIAC SURGERY

Atrioventricular septal defect
Truncus arteriosus
Total anomalous pulmonary venous return
Tetralogy of Fallot
Anomalous coronary artery
Ebstein's malformation of the tricuspid valve
Heart and/or lung transplantation
Fontan procedure

TABLE 93–3. COMPLICATIONS OF ECMO SUPPORT

Bleeding (50–60%)
  Mediastinal
  Groin
  Hemothorax
  Retroperitoneal hematoma
Renal insufficiency (30–40%)
  Ultrafiltration
  Hemodialysis
Neurologic injury (15–20%)
  Embolic
  Seizures
Infection (20–25%)
  Mediastinitis
  Sepsis

major complication of postcardiotomy ECMO in pediatric patients is hemorrhage. A large proportion of children (40–50%) require reexploration for hemorrhage during the time of support. To minimize the magnitude of bleeding, the activated clotting time (ACT) is maintained in the 200 second range by continuous heparin infusion, and the platelet count is kept >100,000/mm[3]. The primary determinant of significant hemorrhage is the duration of ECMO.[28] Keeping the chest open is sometimes necessary to facilitate reexploration and to prevent periods of cardiac tamponade. The use of heparin-coated circuits and oxygenators presents promising possibilities that include avoidance of heparin, improved biocompatibility, and less complement activation.[32] When ECMO is initiated before the development of anuria, a rapid renal recovery without the need for ultrafiltration or dialysis frequently occurs. Conversely, when ECMO is begun in the presence of anuria, renal failure often ensues. An additional important complication of prolonged ECMO support is mediastinal infection and sepsis. This is a result of many factors such as continued bleeding from mediastinal structures, multiple cannulae and catheters in the mediastinal cavity with exit through the skin, low cardiac and renal output, and multiple transfusions. To decrease the incidence of infection, broad-spectrum coverage with antibiotics, aseptic technique, together with attempts to minimize the time on support are encouraged.

Clinical Results

In 1992 Spray summarized the results of ECMO for pediatric cardiac support,[33] based on the available published information[5,14,20,31,34] and on the cumulative information in the Registry of the Extracorporeal Life Support Organization[36] (Table 93–4). In this report the early survival was 40–44%, with somewhat better survival (43–54%) when the lesion was either tetralogy of Fallot, truncus arteriosus, atrioventricular canal, or total anomalous pulmonary venous return. Lower survival rates (14%) were reported for patients with the diagnosis of single ventricle, hypoplastic left

TABLE 93–4. CLINICAL RESULTS WITH ECMO SUPPORT

	Number of Patients	Age (Year)	Duration of Support (Days)	Wean (%)	Survival (%)
Children's Hospital, St. Louis, Missouri	14	1.4	11.4	64	36
Children's Hospital, Detroit, Michigan	36	1.1	4.9	61	58
University of Michigan, Ann Arbor, Michigan	16	5.5	6.0	25	25
University of Pittsburgh, Pittsburgh, Pennsylvania	10	1.8	3.7	80	70
Total (mean)	76	2.2	3.9	57	49

heart syndrome, and other malformations that required a Fontan procedure. The difference in the survival rates between these two groups suggests that a complete biventricular operative repair is associated with improved survival, while an operation with shunt dependent pulmonary blood flow is associated with lower overall recovery rates. A consistent finding in all the reports is a decreased survival rate (0–27%) when ECMO is needed because the patient could not be weaned from CPB, suggesting perhaps a greater degree of myocardial damage in such patients. In the Registry of the ECMO Support Organization (Table 93–4), the mean age was 2.1 years (range 2 days to 18 years) and the mean time of support was 94 hours (range 1 to 160 hours). Forty-three patients (56.6%) were weaned of whom 37 patients (48.7%) were discharged from the hospital.

VENTRICULAR ASSIST DEVICES (VAD)

The left ventricular assist device (LVAD) has proven to be effective in selected adult patients with postcardiotomy failure,[35–38] but its application to infants and children has been limited and has generally been less successful.[40–43] In distinction to the adult patients with ischemic heart disease, who constitute the main adult LVAD group, the pediatric group with congenital heart disease and severe left ventricular dysfunction is much less likely to have preserved right ventricular and pulmonary function. As such, these patients may not benefit from LVAD support alone.

Right ventricular failure without the presence of pulmonary dysfunction, which is uncommon in the pediatric group of patients, can be supported by right ventricular assist device (RVAD).

Failure of both ventricles without pulmonary dysfunction is rare in this group of patients but potentially can be supported by biventricular assist device (BVAD). The use of BVAD in children is technically demanding and associated with many complications.

Indication for LVAD

Indications for LVAD are evolving in the pediatric age group. The ideal candidate has isolated life-threatening LV dysfunction that is likely reversible, and does not have multiorgan failure, severe coagulopathy, or intracranial bleeding. Although active infection may present serious prob-

lems during and after LVAD support, it is not an absolute contraindication.

There are several potential advantages in using the LVAD in the clinical setting of myocardial failure either postoperatively or in the presence of acute myocarditis. The LVAD reduces both preload and wall stress, which can lead to reductions in inotropic and afterload medication, with a decrease in the side effects such as sinus tachycardia, arrhythmias, and increased myocardial oxygen consumption. Ratcliffe et al have shown that ventricular assist devices acutely improve myocardial performance in dilated poorly contractile hearts by reducing both end-systolic and end-diastolic volumes, as well as ventricular wall stress.[44] Reducing the left atrial and pulmonary capillary pressures prevents the development, or progression of pulmonary edema and facilitates ventilatory support, and thus may avoid further right heart failure. By providing circulatory support, increasing cardiac output, and decreasing systemic venous pressure, the LVAD may prevent the development of end-organ ischemic injury such as renal failure, cerebral edema, hepatic necrosis, or mesenteric ischemia.[45] Patients not showing early myocardial recovery with LVAD support should be considered for heart transplantation, if they are appropriate candidates. Good survival after VAD bridge to transplantation (60–70%) has been reported by a number of centers.[46,47]

Pump Types

Previous studies have shown an advantage of centrifugal pumps over the roller-pumps, with a lower index of hemolysis.[48,49] (Fig. 93–4) They are more responsive to changes in the peripheral circulation due to their constrained vortex design. This permits fine adjustments of vasodilator and inotropic therapy during LVAD support in anticipation of weaning. The centrifugal pump has been used as an LVAD in the adult population for up to 1 mo and in pediatric patients for up to 2 wk.[8] For larger individuals more long-term devices are available that are semi-implantable with drive line or power source transiting the skin. A number of devices are presently undergoing clinical testing of portable (wearable) more long-term device modifications.

Technique of Cannulation and LVAD Support

All patients are supported with left atrial or common atrial to ascending aortic partial or complete left heart bypass

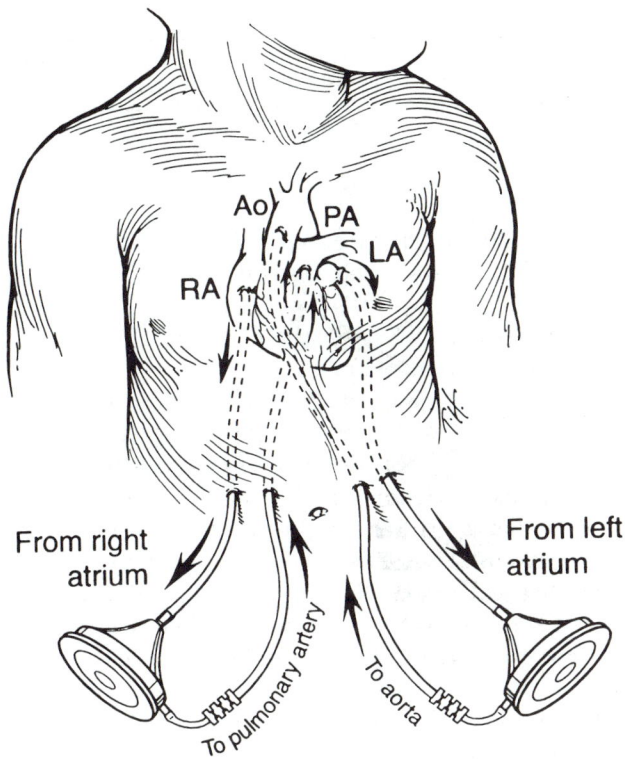

Figure 93–4. Biventricular assist device (BVAD). The right heart is drained through a cannula in the right atrium (RA) and the inflow return into the main pulmonary artery (PA). The left heart is drained through a cannula located in the left atrial (LA) appendage or (via the right superior pulmonary vein) and the inflow returned to the ascending aorta (Ao). All the cannulae are brought through separate skin incisions if possible.

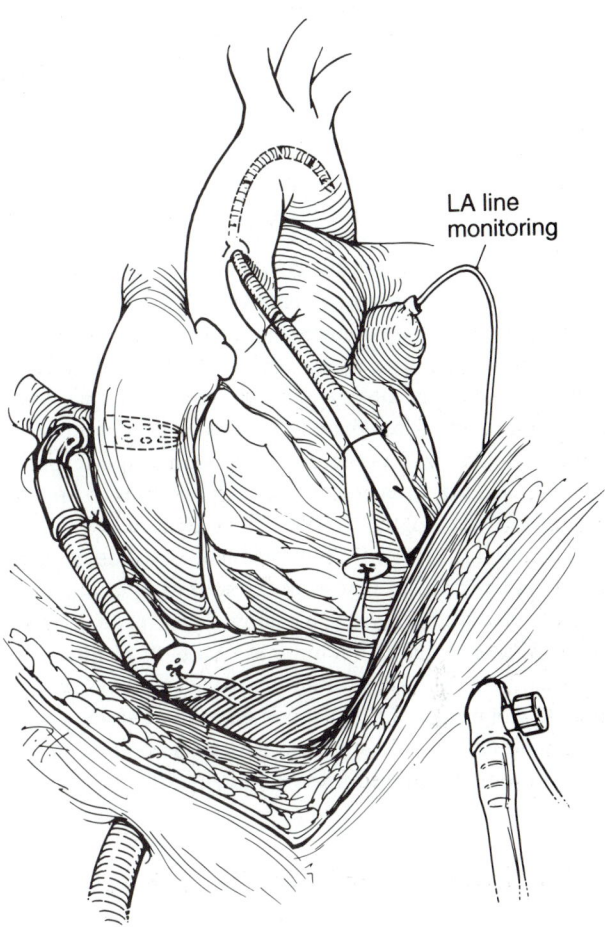

Figure 93–5. Left ventricular assist device (LVAD) cannulation. The left atrium (LA) is drained through an angled cannula placed via the right superior pulmonary vein. The inflow cannula is inserted through the transverse arch beyond the takeoff of the head vessels. Both lines are brought out through separate skin incisions, thus giving better stabilization and allowing chest closure.

(Fig. 93–5). The left atrium is usually cannulated just posterior to the interatrial groove near the origin of the right upper pulmonary vein. A right-angle atrial cannula is used and secured with one or two pursestring sutures made fast with silicone rubber tourniquets.

The venous cannulae used are generally one size smaller than those required for full CPB, as based on the child's weight. The standard size aortic cannula is used and secured in the ascending aorta in similar fashion. The venous cannulae exit the mediastinum via either a subcostal or intercostal incision, or through the operative incision if the chest remains open. The aortic cannula can exit either the upper or the lower portion of the sternotomy incision, as well as a separate skin incision.

VAD Initiation

The aortic and atrial cannulae are connected to a closed centrifugal pump circuit. CPB flow is discontinued, and VAD left heart bypass is commenced at minimal flow and quickly increased to >2.5 L/min per m². In this technique the left atrium is allowed to fill before full LVAD support begins, thus preventing air entry associated with cavitation around the inflow cannulae. Right ventricular and pul-

monary function are considered adequate to continue isolated LVAD support if oxygenation remains stable (pO₂ > 80–90 mm Hg), right atrial pressures remain below 12 mm Hg, and the right ventricle is not distended. Inotropes, particularly isoproterenol (Isuprel) as well as PGE₁ for the vasodilator effect, may be helpful in aiding RV function.

The LVAD circuit consists of a remote pump head on a flexible drive cable with inlet and outlet pressure monitors and inline arterial flow probe. The circuit length is kept to a minimum needed to reach the pump head to avoid larger resistance and hemodilution as well as to decrease contact activation and heat loss. An ultrafiltration circuit may also be placed in circuit to allow removal of intravascular volume. After an initial stabilization period with the LVAD, heparin is partially reversed with protamine (0.5 mg protamine per 1 mg of heparin). After hemostasis is obtained, chest tubes are inserted in the regular fashion, and the skin, if not the sternum, is closed if possible.

Anticoagulation is achieved with a continuous intravenous infusion of heparin (starting dose of 10 units/kg per hour), which is titrated to an activated clotting time (ACT) of around 150 seconds. Normothermia is maintained with a heating/cooling blanket as well as the intrinsic heat produced by the centrifugal pump. Patients are kept sedated and paralyzed during the assistance. The inotropic support is reduced to a minimal level sufficient for adequate right heart function. During the period of mechanical support the patient receives vasodilators, parenteral or enteral (if possible) nutrition, and periodic infusions of fresh frozen plasma and platelets as needed to maintain hemostasis.

After a period of recovery (24–48 hours), flows are reduced if possible, to allow some left ventricular ejection at left atrial pressures less than 8 to 10 mm Hg. For weaning from the LVAD, left ventricular contractility and response to volume loading are evaluated serially by clinical impression and echocardiography while flows are reduced in 10% increments. If a functional improvement is sustained, with satisfactory peripheral perfusion, as well as systemic, pulmonary, and atrial pressures, weaning is continued. Patients are finally observed on a minimal safe flow (150–200 mL/min) for 1 to 2 hours, after which decannulation is carried out. Delayed sternal closure is generally chosen, unless under unusual circumstances the patient is completely stable and the myocardium is not compressed by mediastinal structures.

Clinical Results

The data accumulated by the American Society of Artificial Internal Organs (ASAIO) recently presented the results of 66 pediatric patients supported by a ventricular assist device (Table 93–5). The mean age of the patients was 10 years (range from 1 mo to 18 years) and the mean time of support was 9 days (range from 1 to 146 days). Fifty-six percent of the patients were weaned from the VAD support. In 34 patients (51%) the VAD was used as a bridge to transplantation, of whom 24 patients (70%) were successfully transplanted. The successful weaning rates in patients supported with biventricular assist device (BVAD) or total artificial heart (TAH) are somewhat higher than in patients supported solely by left ventricular (LVAD) or right ventricular (RVAD) assist devices.

The results reported by the cardiac surgical unit at the Royal Children's Hospital in Melbourne, Australia show that the weaning rate can be as high as 76% (22/29) by this experienced group.[33] Our own results at UCLA Medical Center with a mean follow-up of greater than 2 years in 15 patients are an 80% weaning rate and 70% survival rate at 25 mo after VAD removal.

General Management of Patients on a Ventricular Assist Device

Anticoagulation: Bleeding and Thromboembolism

Bleeding is the most frequent complication reported in every series of VAD implantation.[50,51] The need for massive blood product transfusion because of coagulopathy is the single most important cause of morbidity and mortality in VAD patients.[47] Severely ill patients, especially those with congestive heart failure or cyanosis, may have limited hemostatis reserve. Baseline coagulation studies (prothrombin time, partial thromboplastin time, platelet count, and bleeding time) may not detect hepatic or bone-marrow dysfunction. When coupled with surgery, anesthesia, cardiopulmonary bypass, and possible multiple transfusions this limited reserve often results in postoperative coagulopathy. Thrombocytopenia, altered platelet aggregation, reduced soluble coagulation factors, fibrinolysis, and disseminated intravascular coagulation have been frequently documented in these postoperative patients with low cardiac output.

To reduce bleeding and the development of a coagulopathy perioperatively one should attempt to minimize CPB time, reduce the usage of blood sump suction, and limit flows to 2.5 L/min per m_2. Meticulous surgical technique and hemostasis, administration of fresh frozen plasma and platelets, cryoprecipitate if fibrinogen is low, topical agents such as surgical glue or Gelfoam, and systemic agents such as ε-carpoic acid (Amicar) or aprotinin, can help reduce the magnitude of bleeding.[52,53]

Several factors influence which anticoagulation regimen is used in a particular patient. For example, the expected duration of support as well as the type of device can influence the anticoagulation regimen. In general, anticoagulation should not be initiated until bleeding after device insertion has decreased to less than 1 mL/kg body weight/hour. Maintaining the ACT or the heparin levels in

TABLE 93–5. CLINICAL RESULTS WITH VENTRICULAR ASSIST DEVICES[a]

	Number of Patients	Age (Year)	Duration of Support (Days)	Wean (%)	Bridge to Tx (%)	Tx Done (%)
LVAD	30	13	8.6	46	46	43
RVAD	5	4.2	2.4	20	20	20
BVAD	25	11.2	10.8	72	52	44
TAH	6	16	9.6	0	100	66

[a]ASAIO report, September 1994

the recommended range may both limit the tendency for bleeding and the chance for thromboembolism. Reducing the length of tubing within the circuit and increasing the usage of heparin coated circuits may allow a much lower anticoagulation level. During the first 12–24 hours after placement we use low molecular weight dextran at 5 mL/h as the initial anticoagulant, to be followed by heparin infusion once the bleeding has stabilized.

Ventilation: Pulmonary Dysfunction

Pulmonary dysfunction is common in patients undergoing VAD placement. Mild transient dysfunction manifested as hypoxemia may be attributed to preexistent lung disease, postoperative atelectasis, the pulmonary effects of CPB and hypothermia, as well as the effects of volume overload and poor left ventricular function. The use of diuretics, renal dose of dopamine, or PGE_1 may improve fluid balance within 24–48 hours as well as improve pulmonary blood flow.

Moderate pulmonary insufficiency characterized by more severe hypoxemia and a reduction in pulmonary compliance is very common in the VAD patient. Multiple blood transfusions, sepsis, pulmonary infection, with or without aspiration of gastric contents, along with a period of shock may contribute to the development of this insufficiency. In order to permit tissue repair, the FIO_2 and the peak airway pressure should be minimized, and the fluid and electrolyte balance achieved. Proper antibiotic treatment should be instituted based on sputum cultures. Nutritional support should also be maintained preferably by the enteral route to potentially offset the translocation of gastrointestinal bacteria, as well as to satisfy caloric needs and requirements.

In a limited number of VAD patients, severe pulmonary insufficiency develops and is manifested as severe hypoxemia and poor compliance. If not treated vigorously, this may lead to irreversible pulmonary fibrosis, which is associated with a very high mortality rate. Conversion of a VAD to ECMO support may give the lung an opportunity to recover and regain the ability to support the respiratory needs of the patient.

Fluid Balance: Renal Dysfunction

Profound hypo- or hypervolemia often complicates the postoperative management of VAD patients. With hypervolemia, renal function is usually inadequate to permit rapid diuresis as desired. Neuroendocrine changes secondary to shock as well as low oncotic pressure contribute to fluid retention. Use of a combination of different diuretics may improve diuresis. Continuous arteriovenous hemofiltration permits gradual fluid removal and helps mobilize third-space fluids without the hemodynamic instability that may accompany acute hemodialysis.[54] Indeed, there are good data that ultrafiltration may remove not only water, but also soluble mediators that result in lower inotrope needs and improve hemodynamics.[55] We include this capability in each circuit setup (Fig. 93–6).

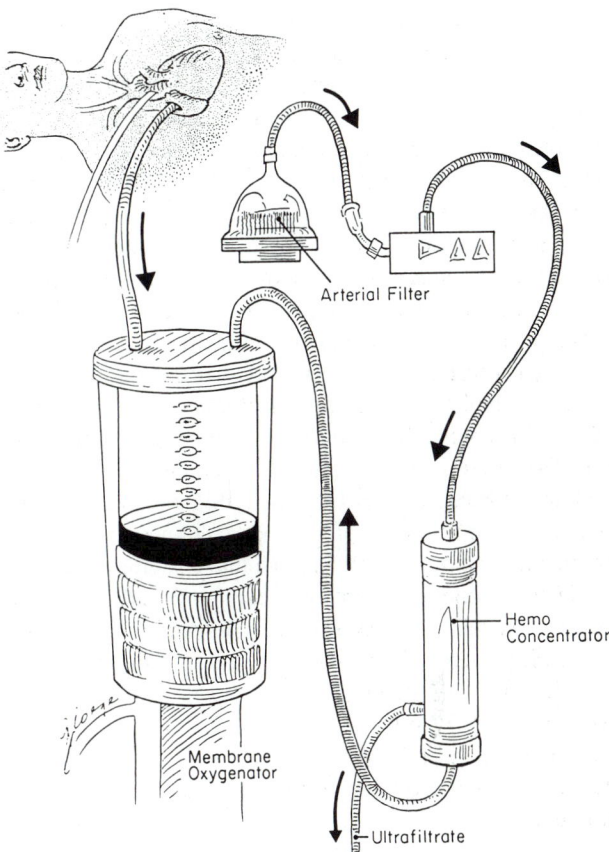

Figure 93–6. ECMO circuit and ultrafiltration. The addition of in line ultrafiltration can be made in both ECMO and VAD circuits. The removal of a predictable volume of free water as well as soluble factors such as inflammatory mediators facilitates fluid balance and pulmonary function and recovery.

Infections

Infection is a major limiting factor to the long-term use of assist devices. A widely ranging incidence of 17–80% of infectious complications has been reported either in the setting of postcardiotomy failure or as a bridge to transplantation.[56]

Open heart surgical procedures have been reported to cause immunologic depression. They reduce the absolute numbers of T-lymphocytes and natural killer cells as well as alter the normal helper/suppressor cell ratio.[57,58] Cardiopulmonary bypass provokes activation of the complement system, pulmonary sequestration, and degranulation of leukocytes, and activates the fibrinolytic cascade.[59] Changes in the cellular immune response may lead to decreased immunocompetence, and expression of interleukins during long-term support.

The risk of an infectious complication increases according to the severity of illness, duration of support, and duration of hospital stay prior to implantation. Pulmonary congestion, prolonged intubation, and a postoperative opened chest all contribute to the risk of infection, the most common of which is pulmonic.

Infection Prophylaxis

The prevention of infectious complications starts early in the preimplantation period where vigilance is needed to rule out potential contamination of any indwelling catheters. Pulmonary and limb physiotherapy is particularly important in bedridden patients to help maintain fitness and prevent pulmonary infection.

During the time of surgery and implantation of the device, aseptic technique in preparation of the skin is very important, along with the use of broad-spectrum intravenous antibiotic coverage (particularly staphylococcal coverage). Antibiotic irrigation of the surgical site, meticulous hemostasis to prevent hematoma formation, and adequate drainage of blood and fluids from the mediastinum and pleural cavities are important anti-infection practices. Intravenous antibiotics are continued during the perioperative period and adjusted for any positive culture that appears during the time of support. Routine line changes and culturing of the intravenous catheters, sputum, and urine may help to provide early detection of infections, preventing septic complications while awaiting transplantation.

SUMMARY

Although the field of pediatric cardiac support is rather new, there is some evidence that the outcomes may be at least as good, if not better than, those for the adult population. The proper selection of the device to match the individual patient and their physiology is vital. The selection of device (single or biventricular, with or without membrane oxygenation) may change with the patient's condition over time. Building in flexibility may allow rapid transition from ECMO to VAD support, for example. Finally, the use of more biocompatible material (heparin-bonded) in these closed systems is advantageous and should be used throughout the entire setup.

REFERENCES

1. Spencer FC, Eiseman B, Trinkle JK, et al: Assisted circulation for cardiac failure following intracardiac surgery with cardiopulmonary bypass. *J Thorac Cardiovasc Surg* **49:**65, 1965
2. DeBakey ME: Left ventricular bypass pump for cardiac assistance: Clinical experience. *Am J Cardiol* **27:**3, 1971
3. Mee RB: Retraining of the left ventricule with a left ventricular assist device after the arterial switch operation. *J Thorac Cardiovasc Surg* **101:**171, 1991
4. Moat NE, Pawade A, Lewis BC, et al: Circulatory support in infants with postcardiopulmonary bypass left ventricular dysfunction using left ventricular assist device. *Eur J Cardiothorac Surg* **4:**649, 1990
5. Rogers AJ, Trento A, Siewers RD, et al: Extracorporeal membrane oxygenation for postcardiotomy shock in children. *Ann Thorac Surg* **47:**903, 1989
6. Chang AC, Hanley FL, Wiendling SN, et al: Left heart support with ventricular assist device in an infant with acute myocarditis. *Crit Care Med* **20:**712, 1992

7. Warnecke H, Berdjis F, Henning E, et al: Mechanical left ventricular support as a bridge to cardiac transplantation in childhood. *Eur J Cardio-Thorac Surg* **5:**330, 1991
8. Kark TR, Sano S, Horton S, et al: Centrifugal pump left heart assist in pediatric cardiac operation. Indication, technique, and results. *J Thorac Cardiovasc Surg* **102:**624, 1991
9. Castaneda AR, Jonas RA, Mayer JE, Hanley FL: Postcardiotomy mechanical ventricular assistance. In *Cardiac Surgery of the Neonate and Infant,* Philadelphia, W.B. Saunders, 1994, p 104
10. Delius RE, Zwishenberger JB, Gilley R, et al: Prolonged extracorporeal life support of pediatric and adolescent cardiac transplant patients. *Ann Thorac Surg* **50:**791, 1990
11. Veasy LG, Webster HW, Bonchek MM, et al: Pediatric use of intra-aortic balloon pumping. In Doyle EF, Engle MA, Gersony WM, et al (eds): *Pediatric Cardiology.* New York, Springer-Verlag, 1986, pp 600–602
12. Pollack JC, Charlton MC, Williams WG, et al: Intra-aortic balloon pumping in children. *Ann Thorac Surg* **29:**522, 1980
13. Veasy LG, Blaybock N, Fukamasu H, et al: Preclinical evaluation of intra-aortic balloon pumping for pediatric use. *Trans Am Soc Art Intern Organs* **27:**490, 1981
14. Veasy LG, Webster H: Intra-aortic balloon pumping in infants and children. *Cardiac Assists* **2:**1, 1985
15. Bartlett RH, Gazzaniga AB, Fong SW, et al: Extracorporeal membrane oxygenator (ECMO) for cardiorespiratory failure: Experience with 28 cases. *J Thorac Cardiovasc Surg* **73:**375, 1977
16. Anderson HL, Attorri RJ, Custer JR, et al: Extracorporeal membrane oxygenation for pediatric cardiopulmonary failure. *J Thorac Cardiovasc Surg* **99:**1011, 1990
17. Raithel SC, Boegner E, Fiore A, et al: Extracorporeal membrane oxygenation in children following cardiac surgery. *Circulation* **84** (suppl 2): 240, 1991
18. Zapol WM, Snider MT, Hill JD, et al: Extracorporeal membrane oxygenation in severe respiratory failure. *JAMA* **242:**2193, 1979
19. Weihaus L, Carter C, Noetzel M, et al: Extracorporeal membrane oxygenation for circulatory support after repair of congenital heart defects. *Ann Thorac Surg* **48:**206, 1989
20. Klein MD, Shaheen KW, Whittlesey GC, et al: Extracorporeal membrane oxygenation for the circulatory support of children after repair of congenital heart disease. *J Thorac Cardiovasc Surg* **100:**498, 1990
21. Kanger KR, Pennington DG, Weber TR, et al: Extracorporeal membrane oxygenation for postoperative cardiac support in children. *J Thorac Cardiovasc Surg* **93:**27, 1987
22. Bavaria JE, Ratcliff MB, Gupta KB, et al: Changes in left ventricular systolic wall stress during biventricular circulatory assistance. *Ann Thorac Surg* **45:**526, 1988
23. Soeter RJ, Mamiya RT, Sprague AY, et al: Prolonged extracorporeal oxygenation for cardiorespiratory failure after tetralogy correction. *J Thorac Cardiovasc Surg* **66:**214, 1973
24. Cornish JD, Hiess KF, Clark RH, et al: Preferential use of venovenous ECMO for neonates with significant circulatory compromise. 8th Annual CNMC ECMO Symposium. Breckenridge, CO (Abstract), 1992
25. Strieper MJ, Sharma S, Clark RH, et al: Effects of venovenous extracorporeal membrane oxygenation on cardiac performance as determined by echocardiographic measurement. 8th Annual CNMC ECMO Symposium. Breckenridge, CO (Abstract), 1992
26. Hankeler NM, Canter CE, Donze A, et al: Extracorporeal life support in cyanotic congenital heart disease before cardiovascular operation. *Am J Cardiol* **69:**790, 1992
27. Karl TR, Lyer KS, Mee RBB: Infant ECMO cannulation technique allowing preservation of carotid and jugular vessels. *Ann Thorac Surg* **50:**105, 1990
28. Sell LL, Cullen ML, Lerner GR, et al: Hemorrhagic complications during extracorporeal membrane oxygenation: Prevention and treatment. *J Pediatr Surg* **21:**1087, 1986

29. Fosse E, Moen O, Johnson E, et al: Reduced complement and grannulocyte activation with heparin-coated cardiopulmonary bypass. *Ann Thorac Surg* **58:**472–474, 1994

30. Jurmann MJ, Haverich A, Demertizis S, et al: Extracorporeal membrane oxygenation as a bridge to lung transplantation. *Eur J Cardiothorac Surg* **5:**94, 1991

31. Ziomek S, Harrell JE, Fasules JW, et al: Cardiopulmonary failure after congenital heart surgery: Results of treatment with extracorporeal membrane oxygenation. Society of Thoracic Surgeons, Orlando, FL, November 1991 (abstract)

32. Karl TR: Extracorporeal circulatory support in infants and children. *Seminars Thorac Cardiovasc Surg* **6:**154, 1994

33. Spray TL: Extracorporeal membrane oxygenation for pediatric cardiac support. *Cardiac Surg State of Art Reviews* **7**(2), 1993

34. Zwischenberger JB, Bartlett RH: Extracorporeal circulation for respiratory or cardiac failure. *Semin Thorac Cardiovasc Surg* **2:**320, 1990

35. *Extracorporeal Membrane Oxygenation Registry Report:* Ann Arbor, MI, Extracorporeal Life Support Organization, 1991

36. Park SB, Liebler GA, Burkholder JA, et al: Mechanical support of the failing heart. *Ann Thorac Surg* **42:**627, 1986

37. Pennington DG, McBride LR, Swartz MT, et al: Use of the Pierce-Donachy ventricular assist device in patients with cardiogenic shock after cardiac operation. *Ann Thorac Surg* **47:**130, 1989

38. Rose DM, Connolly JN, Cunningham JN, et al: Technique and results with roller pump left and right heart assist device. *Ann Thorac Surg* **47:**124, 1989

39. Kauber KR, Pennington DG, Ruzevich SA, et al: Failure of isolated left ventricular support in children (abstract). American Society for Artificial Internal Organs, 34th Annual Meeting, 1988

40. Bolman RM, Cox JL, Marshall W, et al: Circulatory support with centrifugal pump as a bridge to cardiac transplantation. *Ann Thorac Surg* **47:**108, 1989

41. Drinkwater DC, Laks H: Clinical experience with centrifugal pump ventricular support at UCLA Medical Center. *ASAIO Trans* **34:**505, 1988

42. Frazier OH, Bricker JT, Macris MP, et al: Use of left ventricular assist device as a bridge to transplant in a pediatric patient. *Tex Heart Inst J* **16:**46, 1989

43. Karl TR, Horton SB, Mee RBB: Left heart assist for ischemic postoperative ventricular dysfunction in an infant with anomalous left coronary artery. *J Cardiac Surg* **4:**352, 1989

44. Ratcliffe MB, Bavaria JE, Wenger RK, et al: Left ventricular mechanics of ejecting postischemic hearts during left ventricular circulatory assistance. *J Thorac Cardiovasc Surg* **101:**245, 1991

45. Daily BB, Pierce WS: Management of secondary organ dysfunction *Cardiac Surg State of the Art Reviews.* **7:**413, 1993

46. Schiessler A, Warnecke H, Friedel N, et al: Clinical use of the Berlin biventricular assist device as a bridge to transplantation. *ASAIO Trans* **36:**706, 1990

47. Miller CA, Pae WE, Pierce WS: Combined registry for the clinical use of mechanical assist pumps and the total artificial heart in conjunction with heart transplantation. Fourth official report. *J Heart Transplant* **9:**453, 1989

48. Hoerr HR, Kraemer MF, Williams JL, et al: In vitro human blood heart assist model: Roller versus centrifugal. *J Extracorp Technol* **19:**316, 1987

49. Oku T, Harasaki H, Smith W, et al: Hemolysis: A comparative study of four nonpulsatile pumps. *ASAIO Trans* **34:**500, 1988

50. Kormos RL, Borovetz HS, Gasior T, et al: Experience with univentricular support in mortally ill cardiac transplant candidate. *Ann Thorac Surg* **49:**261, 1990

51. McCarthy PM, Portner PM, Tobler HG, et al: Clinical experience with the Novacor ventricular assist system. *J Thorac Cardiovasc Surg* **102:**578, 1991

52. Blauhut B, Gross C, Necek S, et al: Effect of high-dose aprotinin on blood loss, platelet function, fibrinolysis, complement, and renal function after cardiopulmonary bypass. *J Thorac Cardiovasc Surg* **101:**958, 1991

53. Havel M, Teufelsbauer H, Knobel P, et al: Effect of intraoperative aprotinin administration on postoperative bleeding in patients undergoing cardiopulmonary bypass operations. *J Thorac Cardiovasc Surg* **101:**968, 1991

54. Macris MP, Barcenas CG, Parnis SM, et al: Simplified method of hemofiltration in ventricular assist device patients. *ASAIO Trans* **34:**708, 1988

55. Elliot MJ: Ultrafiltration and modified ultrafiltration in pediatric open heart operations. *Ann Thorac Surg* **56:**1518–1522, 1993

56. Kawai A, Kormos RL, Griffith BP: Management of infections in mechanical circulatory support devices. *Cardiac Surg State of the Art Reviews.* **7:**413, 1993

57. Stelzer GT, Ward RA, Wellhausen SR, et al: Alterations in select immunologic parameters following total artificial heart implantation. *Artif Organs* **11:**52, 1987

58. Tajima K, Yamamoto F, Kawazoe K, et al: Cardiopulmonary bypass and cellular immunity: Changes in lymphocyte subsets and natural killer cell activity. *Ann Thorac Surg* **55:**625–630, 1993

59. Van Oeveren W, Kazatchkine MD, Bescamps-Latsha B, et al: Deleterious effects of cardiopulmonary bypass: A prospective study of bubble versus membrane oxygenator. *J Thorac Cardiovasc Surg* **89:**888, 1985

94

Anomalies of the Coronary Vessels

D. Glenn Pennington and Vallee L. Willman

Anomalies of the coronary arteries vary widely in importance, from those that strikingly limit survival to those that are of concern only because of the risk presented by injuring them during cardiac operations. The normal anatomy of the coronary arteries is described in Chapters 95 and 123. For the purpose of systematic discussion, we will consider significant anomalies in terms of the origin, termination, and course of the coronary arteries. (Table 94–1).

ANOMALOUS ORIGIN OF THE CORONARY ARTERIES

Coronary arteries of anomalous origin arise most commonly from the aorta and the pulmonary artery. Rare instances of the origin of coronary arteries from the carotid artery and the innominate artery[1] have been reported, but were associated with severe cardiac malformations, which were incompatible with life. An exhaustive summary of anomalies of coronary origin is offered by Roberts,[2] from a review of adults without other cardiac defects.

Origin From the Pulmonary Artery

Coronary arteries arising from the pulmonary artery represent the most common coronary artery anomalies and present some of the most serious threats to survival as well as the most interesting challenges for correction. Origin of a coronary artery from the pulmonary artery was first described by Brooks in 1885.[3] Soloff[4] described four conditions in which the anomalous artery was a left coronary artery, a right coronary artery, both coronary arteries, or an accessory artery. Figure 94–1 depicts these four conditions,

as well as the anomalous origin of a circumflex artery from the pulmonary artery.[5]

Origin of both coronary arteries from the pulmonary artery is infrequent and usually incompatible with life for more than a short time following birth.[6] There have been occasional instances of survival beyond the first month of life, when associated anomalies kept pulmonary artery pressure high, but no long-term survivors of attempted correction.[7,8]

Origin of the Left Coronary Artery from the Pulmonary Artery

Although it occurs in only one of every 300,000 live births,[9] origin of the left coronary artery from the pulmonary artery is the most common congenital coronary artery anomaly. The altered hemodynamics resulting from this condition are variable. Brooks,[3] working from pathologic studies, reasoned that in cases of coronary arteries originating from the pulmonary artery, blood would flow from the coronary artery of normal aortic origin through communicating collateral vessels into the thin-walled anomalous coronary artery, and would drain into the pulmonary artery. However, it is now apparent that the direction and extent of this bloodflow depend upon the degree of development of the intercoronary collaterals. The following classifications is useful:[10] (1) minimal or no collateral development, providing no left-to-right flow and resulting in forward flow from the pulmonary artery to the coronary artery and myocardium; (2) moderate collateral development, in which left-to-right shunting is detectable only by angiography or indicator-dilution methods, and not by oximetry; and (3) profuse collateral development with left-

**TABLE 94–1. CONGENITAL MALFORMATION
OF THE CORONARY ARTERIES**

I. Anomalous origin
   A. Origin from the pulmonary artery
      1. Left or right coronary artery
      2. Both coronary arteries
      3. Accessory (conus) artery
      4. Left circumflex artery
   B. Origin from the aorta
      1. Single coronary artery
         a. One artery supplies entire heart
         b. Single coronary divides into two branches
            Left coronary from right aortic sinus
            Right coronary from left aortic sinus
      2. Anomalous left circumflex coronary artery
      3. Anomalous left anterior descending artery
      4. Fusion of aortic cusp to aortic wall
      5. Atresia of coronary ostium
   C. Origin from carotid artery
   D. Origin from innominate artery
II. Anomalous termination
   Right, left, both, or single coronary artery fistula with:
   A. Left-to-right shunt
   B. Left-to-left shunt
III. Anomalous course
   A. Branch from single coronary artery passes
      1. Anterior to great vessels
      2. Between great vessels
      3. Posterior to great vessels
   B. Variable left anterior descending artery and other variations
      in tetralogy of Fallot
   C. Variations in truncus arteriosus
   D. Variations in transposition of the great vessels
   E. Mural coronary (myocardial bridging)
IV. Coronary arterial aneurysm

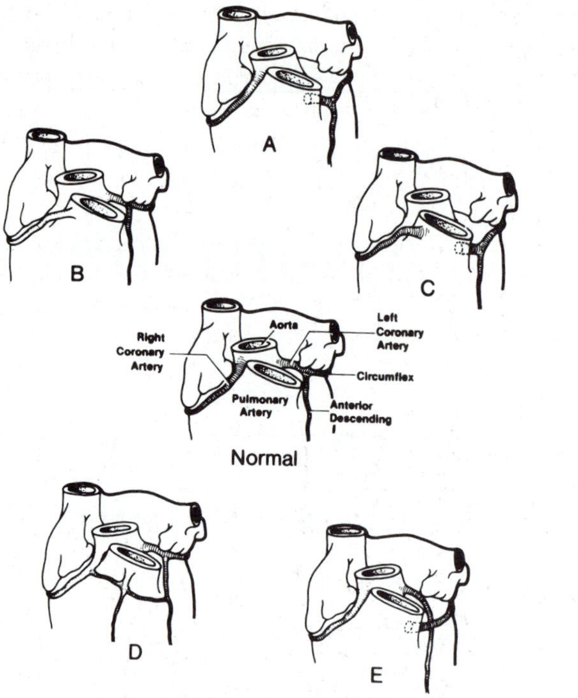

Figure 94–1. Artist's conception of anomalous origins of coronary arteries from the pulmonary artery. **A.** Origin of the left coronary artery from the pulmonary artery. **B.** Origin of the right coronary artery from the pulmonary artery. **C.** Origin of both coronary arteries from the pulmonary artery. **D.** Origin of an accessory coronary artery from the pulmonary artery. **E.** Origin of a circumflex artery from the pulmonary artery.

to-right shunting, resulting in an oxygen stepup in the pulmonary arterial blood. Although patients with well-established collaterals have been classified as the "adult type" of collateral and those with no collaterals as the "infantile type," Edwards[11] believes that these functional states actually represent different phases in collateral circulation occurring in the same patient, and that the changes engendered by each phase determine the patient's clinical course.

Clinical Features

Origin of the left coronary artery from the pulmonary artery is perfectly compatible with life in utero, in which both the pulmonary artery pressure and oxygen content are relatively high. During neonatal life, the pulmonary artery pressure is initially high, and even though there is a subnormal oxygen supply in the myocardium served by the anomalous artery, this supply is sufficient to prevent myocardial ischemia. However, as the pulmonary vascular resistance decreases (between 1 and 3 months of age), forward flow in the anomalous coronary artery decreases and there is a strong stimulus to the development of collateral circulation. A critical transitional phase occurs in which flow reverses in the

anomalous coronary artery and most infants suffer myocardial ischemia or infarction, resulting in myocardial or endocardial fibrosis or mitral insufficiency. The mortality in 60 infants reported by Wesselhoeft et al[12] was 80% before the end of the first year of life. Even if there is full development of collateral vessels, myocardial ischemia may still result from "coronary steal" of blood into the low pressure pulmonary artery.[13] In untreated individuals who survive infancy, there is an 80–90% incidence of sudden death.[14] Rarely, patients may survive to the sixth or seventh decades of life.[15]

Bland et al[16] described the clinical features of angina during infancy in cases of pulmonary artery origin of the left coronary artery, a symptom complex often referred to as the "Bland–White–Garland syndrome." Beginning at 1 to 3 mos, feeding or crying induces dyspnea, profuse sweating, pallor, fatigue, and a semblance of pain. Between attacks, the physical examination is frequently normal. Signs of heart failure and failure to thrive are common. A mitral insufficiency murmur is frequently heard, and, when there is a well-developed collateral circulation, a precordial murmur may be heard. The diagnosis is aided by the finding of an electrocardiographic pattern of anterolateral myocardial infarction in infants,[12] and by cardiac enlargement on the roentgenogram. The anomalous coronary artery can be di-agnosed reliably by the combined use of two-dimensional echocardiography, pulsed Doppler, and Doppler color-flow mapping.[17–19] Criteria for diagnosis are direct visualization of the anomalous left coronary artery from the pulmonary trunk and demonstration of retrograde flow of the anom-alous left coronary artery through collateral from the dilated right coronary artery into the pulmonary trunk.[18,19] Antero-lateral perfusion defects have been detected by thallium-201 myocardial imaging.[20] The diagnosis can usually be made by left ventriculography, aortography, and coronary arteriography. There is usually a poorly contracting left

ventricle with hypokinesis of the anterior wall. An enlarged right coronary artery, arising normally from the aorta and filling the left coronary artery in a retrograde fashion, is seen following aortic root injection or selective right coro-nary injection. On late films, the left coronary artery can be seen emptying into and opacifying the pulmonary artery. (Fig. 94–2). The left coronary artery may at times be opaci-fied following injection into the pulmonary artery. There are occasional cases in which contrast angiography is not diagnostic,[21] and angiography is no longer considered es-sential prior to repair, especially in very ill infants.[18] Re-gional wall motion patterns in infants with this lesion are

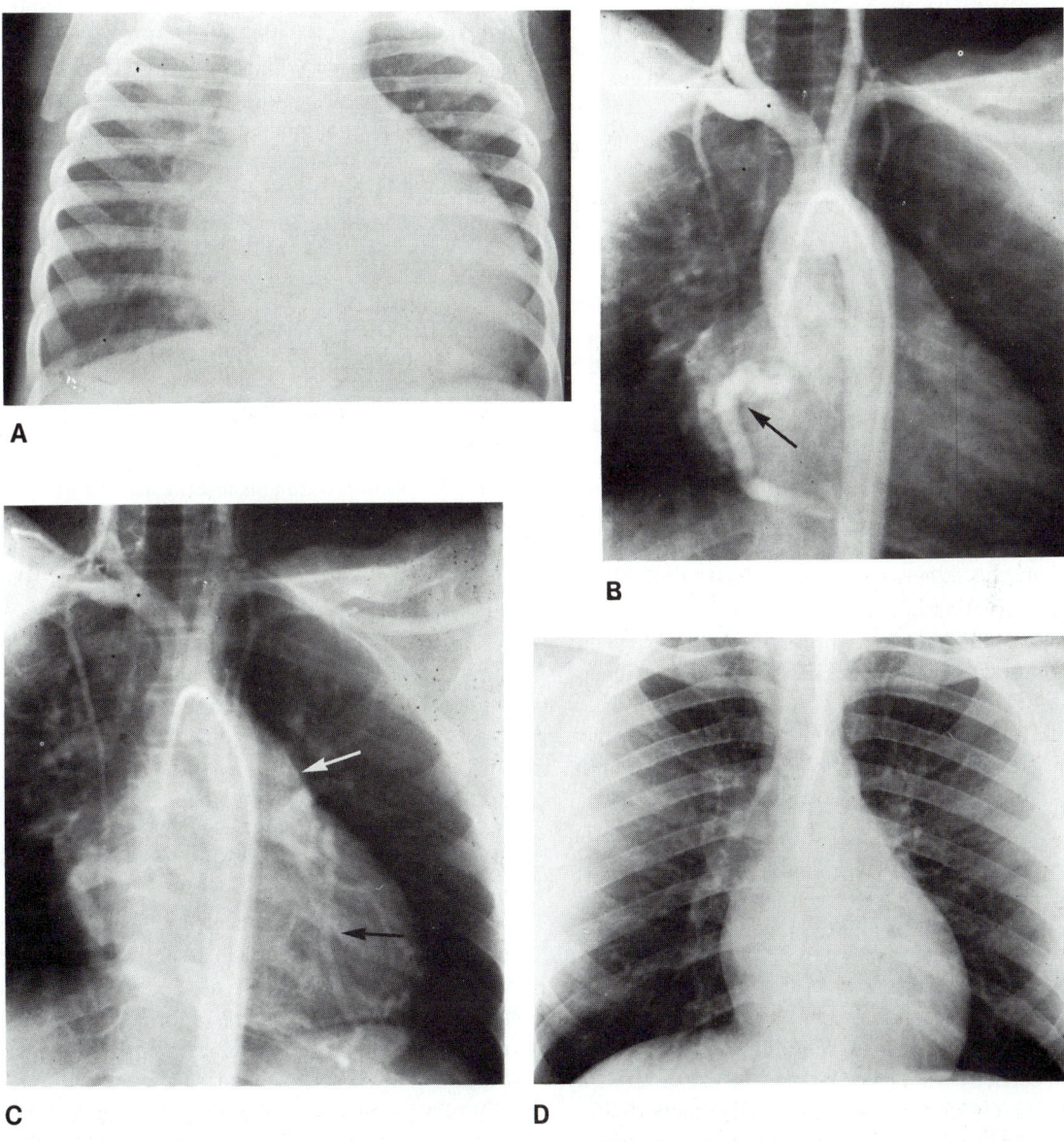

Figure 94–2. Anomalous left coronary artery. **A.** Plain films of 8-mo-old patient demonstrate cardiomegaly with enlargement of the left atrium and left ventricle, and some vascular congestion. **B.** Injection of contrast medium into the aorta opacifies a large right coronary artery (arrow), but the left coronary artery is not opacified. **C.** A film obtained one and one-third seconds after injection reveals the left coronary artery to be opacified by collaterals from the right coronary artery (black arrow). There is faint opacification of the main pulmonary artery (white arrow). **D.** Chest film of the patient at the age of 14 years demonstrates relatively normal heart size, although there is still some prominence of the left ventricle and the left atrium.

not useful in distinguishing this problem from other causes of congestive cardiomyopathy.[22]

Treatment

Because of the high mortality in untreated infants, operation should be performed as soon as the diagnosis is established. In earlier series, ligation of the anomalous left coronary artery eliminated the "coronary steal" into the pulmonary artery if there were significant collaterals. Some patients were long-term survivors,[23,24] but the mortality rate with ligation alone was 50%[12,25] The establishment of a two coronary artery system is clearly preferable, and several ingenious techniques have been employed. Aortocoronary bypass grafting with reversed autogenous saphenous vein[24] or internal mammary artery[26] has been successful in adults and children, but is more difficult in infants. Furthermore, saphenous veins have a high rate of failure.[27]

In 1968, Meyer reported the use of left subclavian artery–coronary artery anastomosis,[28] which can be accomplished without ischemic cardiac arrest[29–32] and has provided long-term survivors.[29,30,32,33] with graft patency.[29] Disadvantages of this technique are inadequate length of the graft, kinking at its origin, late stenosis, and arm ischemia. However, the technical aspects of the operation are facilitated by use of a bilateral transverse thoracic incision.[29]

Aortic reimplantation of the anomalous left coronary artery into the aorta has now been used successfully in several series.[24,31,34–37] A simplified technique, recently described by Laks et al, is illustrated in Figure 94–3.[38] The advantages are that no conduit is required so it can be done at any age and short-term patency rates are high.[24,31,36] The need to clamp the aorta in an ischemic myocardium probably contributes to the mortality with this procedure,[31,36] but results are improving.[37] The occasional problem of inadequate length of the anomalous artery to reach the aorta can usually be solved by dividing the pulmonary artery, or performing an elongation procedure.[39] The intrapulmonary tunnel technique designed by Takeuchi et al[40] is another solution, but has the potential disadvantages of pulmonary artery stenosis, aortic regurgitation, or tunnel stenosis.[27] Aortic reimplantation seems to be the most favored method to establish a two coronary system but will require long-term (20 years) follow-up to prove its effectiveness.

Recent survival rates after establishment of a two coronary system range from 0 to 30%. It is encouraging that the severely damaged infant myocardium has tremendous regenerative capacity, which encourages the use of all measures including prolonged cardiopulmonary support after surgical repair.[41,42] When a two-coronary artery system is established, there is usually apparent reversal of ischemic changes, improved contractility and reasonable hope for long-term graft patency and survival. However, postrepair evaluation of the chronically hypoperfused myocardium suggests that there are delayed subcellular adaptive responses[43] and persistent perfusion defects by stress thallium-201 myocardial imaging.[44] Although mitral regurgitation is common in infants, it is rarely necessary to replace the mitral valve.[21,27,36] Only rarely has cardiac transplantation been performed in infants with origin of the left coronary artery from the pulmonary artery.[45]

Origin of the Right Coronary Artery from the Pulmonary Artery

This rare anomaly has been reported in less than 50 cases in the literature,[46] and contributed to cardiac arrest or death in only a few.[47] The anomaly is more benign than anomalous left coronary artery, perhaps because the low-pressure right ventricle allows for better myocardial bloodflow. The diagnosis can be made with echocardiography and may be enhanced by Doppler color-flow mapping.[48] The operation of choice is direct implantation of the right coronary artery into the aorta, which has been accomplished in at least 15 cases, and is facilitated by the anterior origin of the right coronary artery from the pulmonary artery.

ANOMALOUS ORIGIN FROM THE AORTA

Single Coronary Artery

In rare instances, a single coronary ostium may develop from the primitive truncus arteriosus, and give rise to a single coronary artery; alternatively, the absence of one proximal coronary artery may be associated with two or three ostia in the other aortic sinus.[49] Smith [50] divided cases of single coronary artery into those in which there is only one artery supplying the entire heart (type 1), those in which the single coronary artery divides into two branches with a normal distribution (type 2), and those in which the criteria for types 1 and 2 are not met (type 3). Using a modification of this classification (Fig. 94–4), Sharbaugh and White[51] reported that of 164 cases studied, 41 were of type 1, 79 were of type 2, and 44 were of type 3. The single artery was a left artery in 75 cases, a right artery in 66, and of indeterminate nature in 23 cases.

The clinical importance of single coronary artery has been emphasized by Cheitlin et al,[52] Liberthson et al,[53] and others, who have described cases of coronary insufficiency and sudden death in patients with an anomalous left coronary artery arising from the right aortic sinus. Roberts and Shirani[54] described four subsets of anomalous left main coronary artery from the right. If the anomalous artery coursed anterior to the great vessels, behind the right ventricular outflow tract or dorsal to the ascending aorta, symptoms of cardiac dysfunction or myocardial ischemia did not result. However, if the anomalously arising left main coronary artery courses between the pulmonary trunk and ascending aorta, symptoms of myocardial ischemia usually

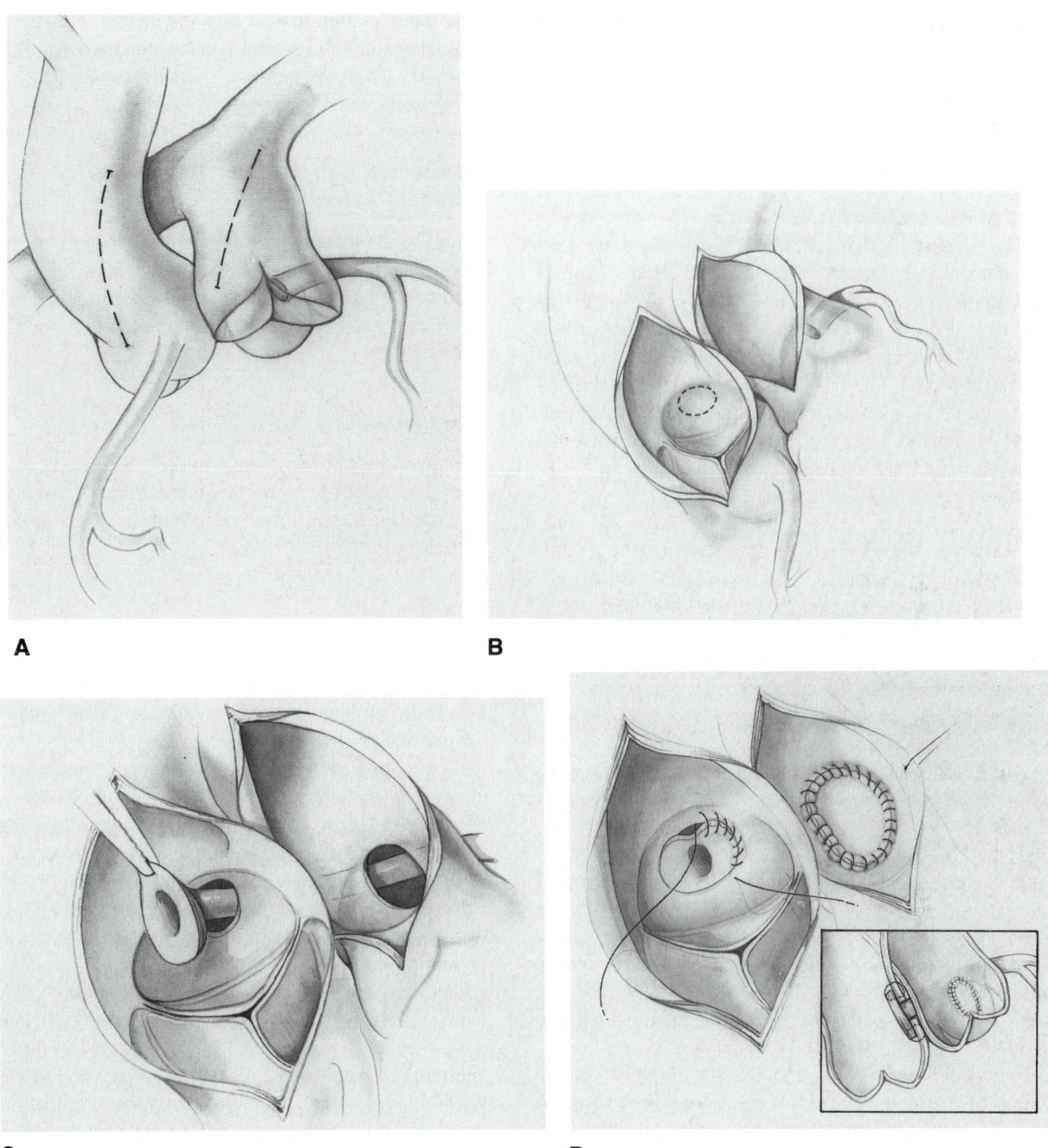

Figure 94–3. Technique of anterior coronary reimplantation. **A.** Incision sites in aorta and pulmonary artery. **B.** Site of reimplantation in the left sinus of Valsalva. **C.** The left coronary artery and a cuff of pulmonary artery wall are excised as a button and transferred to the aorta. **D.** The defect in the pulmonary artery is replaced with a pericardial patch. The coronary anastomosis is performed from within the aorta. Inset demonstrates completed repair. *(From Laks et al: Aortic implantation of anomalous left coronary artery: An improved surgical approach. J Thorac Cardiovasc Surg 109:519–523,1995, with permission.)*

occur, and death is a frequent consequence.[54] Liberthson et al,[53] delineated two patient subgroups, the first composed of 20 young males one to 36 years (mean 16 years), all of whom died suddenly after physical exertion. The second was made up of older patients who did not die suddenly or have syncope. In contrast to the older patients, all members of the younger group had proximal anatomic or physiologic

obstruction of the left coronary artery. The mechanism of death with this anomaly has been attributed to compression of the artery between the aorta and pulmonary artery, or to acute angulation and kinking of the coronary artery at the anomalous site of origin.[54]

In most early reports, the diagnosis of an anomalously originating left coronary artery was made at autopsy. More

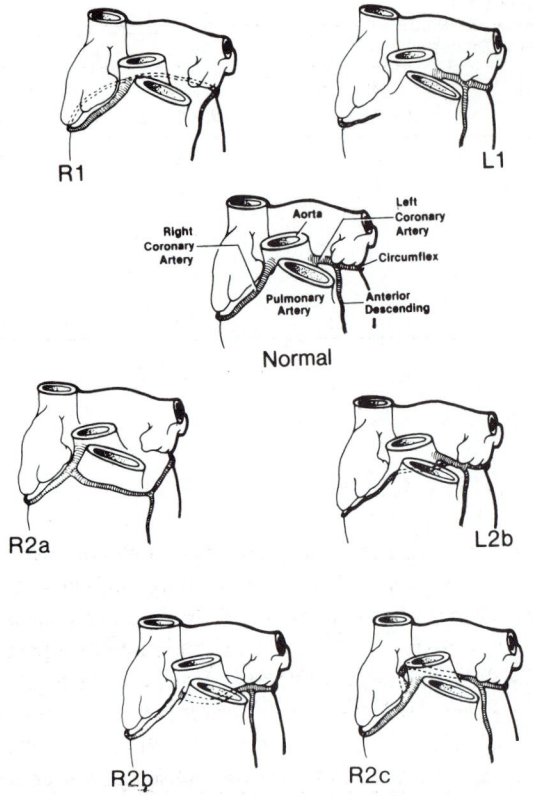

Figure 94–4. Artist's modification of Sharbaugh and White's classification[51] of patterns of distribution of single coronary artery. R is
right artery; L, left. Type is indicated by 1, 2 or 3. Subdivisions of
type 2 are as follows: (**a**) branch corresponding to missing artery
passes anterior to great vessels; (**b**) branch passes between great
vessels; and (**c**) branch passes posterior to great vessels.

recently, it has been made by coronary angiography[53,55,56]
and transesophageal echocardiography,[57] making it possible to consider operative treatment. Arterioplasty[52] has not
been successful. Coronary bypass grafting[58,59] is preferred
for symptomatic patients.

Anomalous origin of the right coronary artery from the
left sinus of Valsalva or from the left coronary artery was
previously thought to be a benign lesion.[60,55] However, recent studies have documented both symptomatology and
death due to this lesion,[60] and surgical correction has been
accomplished.[61]

Anomalous Left Circumflex Coronary Artery

Origin of the left circumflex coronary from the right sinus
of Valsalva is the most common anomaly of aortic origin
and occurs with a frequency of 0.37[62]–0.6%[63] in patients
undergoing coronary angiography. While there has been
general agreement that this anomaly of itself is not associated with functional disability, there are reports of severe
atherosclerotic involvement of the proximal anomalous
coronary artery, making the recognition and angiographic
definition of such abnormalities imperative.[62,63] Saphenous

vein grafting from the aorta to the proximal portion of the
anomalous circumflex artery has been successfully accomplished.[64] Complete absence of the left circumflex coronary
artery has been rarely reported.[65]

Anomalous Left Anterior Descending Coronary Artery

Origin of the left anterior descending artery from the right
coronary artery or sinus of Valsalva is relatively rare, and,
in the absence of congenital heart disease, has no clinical
significance.[35,62] It is present in up to 5% of cases of tetralogy of Fallot.

Anomalous Left Aortic Cusp

Fusion of the left aortic cusp to the aortic wall[66] and congenital atresia of the left coronary ostium[67] have been corrected surgically by aortic valve replacement[66] or coronary
bypass grafting.[67]

ANOMALOUS TERMINATION OF THE CORONARY ARTERIES

Fistulous communication between a coronary artery and a
cardiac chamber was reported by Krause[68] in 1865 and further described by Abbot in 1906.[69] The right or left coronary artery, or a branch of one of these arteries, may terminate directly in a cardiac chamber, the pulmonary artery or
vein, the bronchial circulation, the coronary sinus or veins,
or in the venae cavae. Oldham et al[70] collected 200 cases of
coronary artery fistulas from the literature (Table 94–2). A
right coronary artery–right ventricle fistula was the most
common such lesion, while left heart fistulas are rare. Since
Oldham's summary, several interesting studies of anomalous termination of the coronary arteries have been reported, including additional cases of coronary artery–left
ventricular fistula and coronary artery–left atrial fistula.[24,71] Additional cases of fistulous termination of a
coronary artery in the coronary sinus have been reported by
Ogden et al,[72] with a plea that because of their unique
pathophysiology, these cases be considered separately from
those with termination in the right atrium.

With the widespread use of coronary angiography,
coronary arteriovenous fistulas have become more frequently reported as incidental findings in patients with
coronary arterial obstruction.[73,74] Involvement of more
than one coronary artery with arteriovenous fistulas may
occur,[70,71,73] and, rarely, all three major coronary arteries
were involved.[75]

Clinical Features

In most reviews, the incidence of symptoms in patients with
anomalously terminating coronary arteries ranged from 30

TABLE 94–2. ORIGIN AND TERMINATION OF 200 CORONARY ARTERY FISTULAS

Coronary Artery	Recipient Chamber					
	Right Atrium[a]	*Right Ventricle*	*Pulmonary Artery*	*Left Atrium[b]*	*Left Ventricle*	*Total*
Right	41	49	13	4	3	110
Left	18	23	19	8	2	70
Both	3	2	5			10
Single		4	2			6
Not stated	4					4
Total	66	78	39	12	5	200

[a]Includes fistulas entering the coronary sinus and venae cavae.
[b]Includes fistulas entering the pulmonary veins.
From Oldham HN, et al: Ann Thorac Surg 12:503, 1971 with permission.[70]

to 55%.[70,71,76,77] However, in a recent survey by Fernandes, 73% of patients with isolated coronary fistula were symptomatic.[24] The most frequent symptoms were angina on exertion, palpitations, and symptoms of congestive heart failure. In a review of 174 patients,[77] fistula-related complications such as congestive heart failure (12%), myocardial infarction (4%), rupture (1%), bacterial endocarditis (3%), and death (6%) occurred in 327 patients; an overall complication incidence of only 21% occurred. Age was an important determinant of the frequency of both symptoms[24,77] and fistula-related complications, which occurred in 19% of patients less than 20 years old but in 63% of those over 20 years of age.[77]

The diagnosis of anomalously terminating coronary artery is most often made by the detection of a continuous murmur, characteristically heard along the left sternal border and at the apex, and easily confused with the murmur of patent ductus arteriosus. Occasionally a to-and-fro murmur or only a systolic murmur is heard. Electrocardiographic abnormalities were found in 54% of patients reviewed by Rittenhouse et al,[76] but were nonspecific, and only 3% of the patients had evidence of myocardial infarction. About 50% of all patients with anomalously terminating coronary arteries have cardiomegaly or increased pulmonary vascular markings on a chest roentgenogram,[76] and aortic dilation occurs in some cases.

Recently, two-dimensional and Doppler echocardiography have been helpful in the diagnosis of coronary artery fistula.[17] Aortography will often demonstrate an enlarged, tortuous vessel, frequently aneurysmal, which ends by opening into a cardiac chamber (Fig. 94–5). However, cardiac catheterization and coronary angiography are advised to precisely define the anatomic features of the anomalous vessel,[24] coexisting cardiac abnormalities, or the presence of coronary arterial obstruction. Left-to-right shunt flow in 73 patients averaged 1.6:1 (Q_p/Q_s), with no correlation between clinical symptoms and the degree of shunting. However, in older patients (over 20 years of age) there seemed to be an increased incidence of complications related to the size of the shunt.[77] Pulmonary arterial hypertension due to a coronary arteriovenous fistula is extremely rare.[78]

Treatment

There has been general agreement that all symptomatic patients with an anomalously terminating coronary artery should undergo closure of the fistula, perhaps as soon as the diagnosis is made.[24,71,77] In symptomatic infants, operation may be delayed until childhood. However, Jaffe et al[79] question the advisability of operating on patients with small-to-moderate shunts, since little functional or anatomic change occurred in six patients they observed for an average of 10 years, and there are rare cases of spontaneous closure.[79,80] Although overall morbidity and mortality from anomalously terminating coronary arteries are low, most patients who are not operated upon develop symptoms and fistula-related complications with increasing age, and incur increased morbidity and mortality when ligation is performed later in life. Therefore, ligation of a coronary arteriovenous fistula in childhood is advised, even in the asymptomatic patient.[24,71,77]

The first ligation of coronary arteriovenous fistula was reported by Bjorck and Crafoord in 1947.[81] Direct ligation has been the most commonly used technique.[76] Since ligation of the fistula proximal to its entrance into the cardiac chamber has in some cases resulted in myocardial ischemia or infarction,[82] the fistula should be ligated just at its entrance into the cardiac chamber during electrocardiographic monitoring. Tangential arteriorrhaphy has been employed successfully in fistula closure.[24] In a recently reported experience, there were no operative deaths in 56 patients undergoing repair of isolated coronary artery fistula(s).[24] For fistulous drainage into the right atrium or pulmonary artery, cardiopulmonary bypass was used to close the distal opening under direct vision from within the recipient cavity. For right ventricular fistulas, closure was accomplished by tangential arteriorrhaphy and by distal ligation of the feeding artery on the surface of the heart, often without cardiopulmonary bypass. Coronary artery fistula to the left ventricle was closed by ligation during cardiopulmonary bypass.[24] Others have recommended cardiopulmonary bypass for all coronary artery fistulas to avoid ligating the wrong artery or failing to close all fistulous orifices. The cumulative results

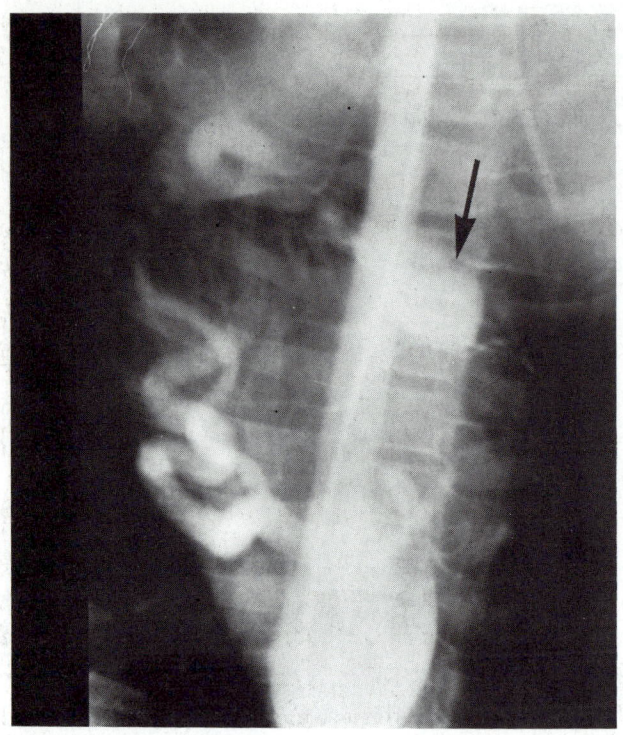

A

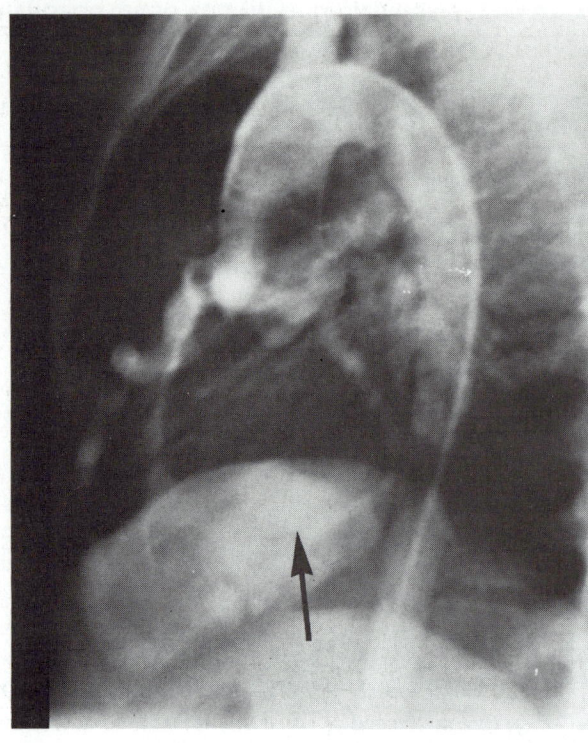

B

Figure 94–5. Coronary artery fistula in 4-year-old girl with a continuous murmur. Frontal (**A**) and lateral (**B**) films from the aortogram demonstrate opacification of an enlarged, tortuous left coronary artery. The left anterior descending coronary artery is continuous with the posterior descending coronary artery, which opens into the right atrium. At the site of the fistula (arrows), there is aneurysmal dilation of the vessel.

of recent operations have been excellent, with an early mortality of 0 to 2%[24,71,76] and a 3.6% incidence of postoperative myocardial infarction.[76] Nonoperative closure of coronary artery fistulas has been accomplished in some cases by transcatheter embolization of detachable balloons, platinum microcoils, and steel coils.[83]

ANOMALOUS COURSE OF THE CORONARY ARTERIES

Abnormal origin of a coronary artery is commonly associated with an abnormal course of the distal vessel. The occurrence and significance of the anomalous courses of single coronary arteries and coronary arteries that take origin from the pulmonary artery have been discussed above.

The importance of anomalies of coronary course relates primarily to the frequency with which they complicate the repair of complex congenital heart defects. Several coronary artery anomalies have been reported in patients with tetralogy of Fallot.[84] In the most common anomaly, the left anterior descending artery takes origin from the right coronary artery and courses across the right ventricular outflow tract. Injury to the anomalous artery can be avoided by modifying the usual operative repair to include transverse right ventriculotomy, dissection and elevation of

the anomalous vessel, saphenous vein grafting, or construction of a right ventricle–pulmonary artery conduit.[85,86] Anomalies of coronary artery origin and course also complicate the repair of truncus arteriosus[87] and transposition of the great arteries.[88,89] Since injury to anomalous coronary arteries can best be avoided by their preoperative recognition, preoperative aortography[90] or selective coronary angiography[91] should be performed in all patients with complex congenital heart defects. If a major coronary artery is inadvertently injured, the surgeon must be prepared to perform meticulous repair by end-to-end anastomosis,[86] saphenous vein, or internal mammary artery grafting.[92] Such repairs are possible even in infants and small children.[86,92]

One of the most common variants of anomalous coronary artery course encountered by cardiac surgeons is the "mural coronary,"[93] a vessel covered by a bridge of myocardium and difficult to expose for coronary bypass grafting. However, in most cases, it is possible to incise the vessel near the apex, where it is visible, and to pass a probe retrogradely, thus allowing an incision to be made through the myocardium directly over the obscure coronary artery. In rare instances, the myocardial bridge overlying the "mural coronary" may obstruct the vessel during systole. Although myocardial bridges were noted in from 5.4 to 85.5% of all autopsied hearts in two studies,[94] the evidence of systolic constriction of a coronary artery by a myocardial bridge was found in only 0.5 to 1.6% of patients undergoing coronary arteriography.[95,96] Sudden death has been attributed to this condition. However, the significance of contracting myocardial bridges remains controversial.[97] A recent study suggests that deep intramural tunnels may be more likely to lead to sudden death.[98]

ANEURYSMS OF THE CORONARY ARTERIES

Although once considered rare, aneurysms of the coronary arteries have now been reported in over 140 cases, including 1.4% of 644 autopsies,[99] 1.5% of 742 patients undergoing coronary angiography,[100] and 2.24% of 1654 patients who had coronary bypass grafting.[101] Coronary artery aneurysms occur as a result of atherosclerosis, infection, trauma, syphilis, and vasculitis, and are rarely of congenital origin.[95] The mucocutaneous lymph node syndrome described by Kawasaki et al[102] is the most common cause of coronary aneurysms in Japan, and has been recognized with increasing frequency in the United States.[103] Indeed, some of the coronary aneurysms in infants and children that were previously assumed to be of congenital origin may have resulted from Kawasaki's syndrome.[104] Since there are no specific diagnostic criteria for congenital aneurysms of the coronary arteries, the diagnosis is made by exclusion, and the true incidence of these defects is not known.

Although many patients with coronary artery aneurysms are asymptomatic, those with symptoms usually have angina or myocardial infarction. There are usually no consistent physical findings related to the aneurysms, but systolic and diastolic murmurs have been reported. The diagnosis is usually made at the time of coronary angiography, but recent reports indicate that coronary aneurysms can be defined noninvasively by echocardiography. The threats of thrombosis and rupture of coronary aneurysms have led to the recommendation that aneurysmectomy and saphenous bypass grafts be performed for all but small or diffuse aneurysms. However, infants in the acute phase of mucocutaneous lymph node syndrome should not be operated on because of the technical difficulties of saphenous vein grafts in infants and the incidence of spontaneous regression of many of these aneurysms. Older children with Kawasaki's disease have undergone successful saphenous vein bypass grafting.[105]

ANOMALIES OF THE CORONARY SINUS

Seven anomalies of the coronary sinus are of concern to the cardiac surgeon: (1) Persistent left superior vena cava, (2) anomalous pulmonary venous connection to the coronary sinus, (3) coronary artery–coronary sinus fistula, (4) absence of the coronary sinus,[72,106,107] atresia of the coronary sinus orifice,[108] coronary sinus diverticulum,[109] and coronary sinus septal defect.[110] The first two of these are discussed in detail in other sections of this book (see Chapter 66); coronary artery–coronary sinus fistula has been discussed in this chapter. Absence of the coronary sinus is a rare anomaly of importance to the cardiac surgeon who normally uses the ostium as a landmark for locating the positions of the atrioventricular node and conduction bundle. Atresia of the coronary sinus is usually associated with a left superior vena cava, which is the only outlet for coronary venous flow.[108] Coronary sinus diverticula have been associated with the Wolff–Parkinson–White syndrome, and division of the neck of the diverticulum may be necessary to interrupt the accessory pathway.[109] Coronary sinus septal defect should be repaired[110] if it is diagnosed.[111]

REFERENCES

1. Davis JS, Lie JT: Anomalous origin of a single coronary artery from the innominate artery. *Angiology* **28:**(11):775, 1977
2. Roberts WC: Major anomalies of coronary arterial origin seen in adulthood. *Am Heart J* **111:**841, 1985
3. Brooks H St JL Two cases of an abnormal coronary artery of the heart arising from the pulmonary artery. *J Anat Phsyiol* **20:**26, 1985
4. Soloff LA: Anomalous coronary arteries arising from the pulmonary artery. *Am Hear J* **24:**118, 1942
5. Ott DA, Cooley DA, Pinsky W, Mullins CE: Anomalous origin of circumflex coronary artery from pulmonary artery. Report of a rare anomaly. *J Thorac Cardiovasc Surg* **76:**190, 1978
6. Tedschi CG, Helbern MM: Heterotopic origin of both coronary arteries from the pulmonary artery. *Pediatrics* **14:**53, 1954
7. Keeton BR, Keenan DJM, Monro JL: Anomalous origin of both coronary arteries from the pulmonary trunk. *Br Heart J* **39:**397, 1983
8. Feldt RH, Ongley PA, Titus JL: Total coronary arterial circulation from pulmonary artery with survival to age of seven. Report of a case. *Mayo Clin Proc* **40:**539, 1965
9. Keith JD: The anomalous origin of the left coronary artery from the pulmonary artery. *Br Heart J* **21:**149, 1959
10. Perry LW, Scott LP: Anomalous left coronary artery from pulmonary artery. Report of 11 cases: Review of indications for and results of surgery. *Circulation* **41:**1043, 1970
11. Edwards JE: The direction of blood flow in coronary arteries arising from the pulmonary trunk (editorial). *Circulation* **29:**163, 1964
12. Wesselhoeft H, Fawcett, JS, Johnson AL: Anomalous origin of the left coronary artery from the pulmonary trunk. Its clinical spectrum, pathology, and pathophysiology, based on a review of 140 cases with seven further cases. *Circulation* **38:**403, 1968
13. Wright NL, Baue AE, Baum S, et al: Coronary artery steal due to an anomalous left coronary artery originating from the pulmonary artery. *J Thorac Cardiovasc Surg* **59:**461, 1970
14. George JM, Knowlan DM: Anomalous origin of the left coronary artery from the pulmonary artery in an adult. *N Engl J Med* **261:**933, 1959
15. Purut CM, Sabiston DC Jr: Origin of the left coronary artery from the pulmonary artery in older adults. *J Thorac Caridovasc Surg* **102:**566, 1991
16. Bland EF, White PD, Garland J: Congenital anomalies of the coronary arteries: Report of an unusual case associated with cardiac hypertrophy. *Am Heart J* **8:**787, 1933
17. Chu E, Cheitlin MD: Diagnostic considerations in patients with suspected coronary artery anomalies. *Am Heart J* **126:**1427, 1993
18. Jureidini SB, Nouri S, Crawford C, et al: Reliability of echocardiog-

raphy in the diagnosis of anomalous origin of the left coronary artery from the pulmonary trunk. *Am Heart J* **122:**61, 1991

19. Karr SS, Parness IA, Spevak PJ, et al: Diagnosis of anomalous left coronary artery by doppler color flow mapping: Distinction from other causes of dilated cardiomyopathy. *Pediatr Cardiol* **19:**1271, 1992

20. Finley, JP, Howman-Giles, R, Gilday DL, et al: Thallium-201 myocardial imaging in anomalous left coronary artery arising from the pulmonary artery. *Am J Cardiol* **42:**675, 1978

21. Menahem S, Venables AW: Anomalous left coronary artery from the pulmonary artery: A 15 year sample. *Br Heart J* **58:**378, 1987

22. Rein AJJT, Colan SD, Parness IA, Sanders SP: Regional and global left ventricular function in infants with anomalous origin of the left coronary artery from the pulmonary trunk: Preoperative and postoperative assessment. *Circulation* **75:**115, 1987

23. Shrivastava S, Castenada AR, Moller JH: Anomalous left coronary artery from pulmonary trunk. *J Thorac Cardiovasc Surg* **76:**130, 1978

24. Fernandes ED, Kadivar H, Hallman GL, et al: Congenital malformations of the coronary arteries: The Texas Heart Institute experience. *Ann Thorac Surg* **54:**732, 1992

25. Arciniegas E, Farooki ZQ, Hakimi M, Green EW: Management of anomalous left coronary artery from the pulmonary artery. *Circulation* **62**(suppl 1)**:** 180, 1980

26. Kitamura S, Kawachi K, Nishii T, et al: Internal thoracic artery grafting for congenital coronary malformations. *Ann Thorac Surg* **53:**513, 1992

27. Bunton R, Jonas RA, Lang P, et al: Anomalous origin of the left coronary artery from pulmonary artery. *J Thorac Cardiovasc Surg* **93:** 103, 1987

28. Meyer BW, Stefanik G, Stiles QR, et al: A method of definitive surgical treatment of anomalous origin of left coronary artery: A case report. *J Thorac Cardiovasc Surg* **56:**104, 1968

29. Kesler KA, Pennington DG, Nouri S, et al: Left subclavian to left coronary artery anastomosis for anomalous origin of the left coronary artery: Long-term follow-up. *J Thorac Cardiovasc Surg* **98:**25, 1989

30. Stephenson LW, Edmunds LH, Friedman S, et al: Subclavian-left coronary artery anastomosis (Meyer operation) for anomalous origin of left coronary artery from the pulmonary artery. *Circulation* **64**(Suppl II):II 130, 1981

31. Sauer U, Stern H, Meisner H, et al: Risk factors for perioperative mortality in children with anomalous origin of the left coronary artery from the pulmonary artery. *J Thorac Cardiovasc Surg* **104:**696, 1992

32. Backer CL, Stout MJ, Zales VR, et al: Anomalous origin of the left coronary artery: A twenty-year review of surgical management. *J Thorac Cardiovasc Surg* **103:**1049, 1992

33. Berdjis F, Takahashi M, Wells WJ, et al: Anomalous left coronary artery from the pulmonary artery: Significance of intercoronary collaterals. *J Thorac Cardiovasc Surg* **108:**17, 1994

34. Grace RR, Angelini P, Cooley D: Aortic implantation of anomalous left coronary artery arising from pulmonary artery. *Am J Cardiol* **39:**608, 1977

35. Richardson JV, Doty DB: Correction of anomalous origin of the left coronary artery. *J Thorac Cardiovasc Surg* **77:**669, 1979

36. Vouhé PR, Tamisier D, Sidi D, et al: Anomalous left coronary artery from the pulmonary artery: Results of isolated aortic reimplantation. *Ann Thorac Surg* **54:**621, 1992

37. Alex-Meskishvili V, Hetzer R, Weng, Y: Anomalous origin of the left coronary artery from the pulmonary artery: Early results with direct reimplantation. *J Thorac Cardiovasc Surg* **108:**354, 1994

38. Laks H, Ardehali A, Grant PW, Allada V: Aortic implantation of anomalous left coronary artery: An improved surgical approach. *J Thorac Cardiovasc Surg* **109:**519–523, 1995

39. Sese A, Imoto Y: New technique in the transfer of an anomalously originated left coronary artery to the aorta. *Ann Thorac Surg* **53:**527, 1992

40. Takeuchi S, Imamura H, Katsumoto J, et al: New surgical method for repair of anomalous left coronary artery form the pulmonary artery. *J Thorac Cardiovasc Surg* **78:**7, 1979

41. Raithel S, Pennington DG, Boegner E, et al: Extracorporeal membrane oxygenation in children following cardiac surgery. *Circulation* **86**(supp):II 305, 1992

42. Taub JO, Klinedienst WJ, Pennington DG. Case Report: Left ventricular assistance in a two month old following repair of an anomalous left coronary artery. *Proc Acad Cardiopul Perfusion* **9:**162, 1988

43. Shivalkar B, Borgers M, Daenen W, et al: ALCAPA Syndrome: An example of chronic myocardial hypoperfusion? *J Am Coll Cardiol* **23:**772, 1994

44. Seguchi M, Nakanishi T, Kakazawa M, et al: Myocardial perfusion after aortic implantation for anomalous origin of the left coronary artery from the pulmonary artery. *Eur Heart J* **11:**213, 1990

45. Mavroudis C, Harrison H, Klein JB, et al: Infant orthotopic cardiac transplantation. *J Thorac Cardiovasc Surgery* **96:**912, 1988

46. Vairo U, Marion B, De Simone G, Marcelletti C: Early congestive heart failure due to origin of the right coronary artery from the pulmonary artery. *Chest* **102:**1610, 1992

47. Lerberg DB, Ogden JA, Zuberbuhler JR, Bahnson HT: Anamalous origin of the right coronary artery from the pulmonary artery. *Ann Thorac Surg* **27:**87, 1979

48. Shah RM, Nanda NC, Hsiung MC, et al: Identification of anomalous origin of the right coronary artery from pulmonary trunk by Doppler color flow mapping. *Am J Card* **57:**366, 1986

49. Ogden JA: Congenital anomalies of the coronary artery. *Am J Cardiol* **25:**474, 1970

50. Smith J: Review of single coronary artery with report of two cases. *Circulation* **1:**168, 1950

51. Sharbaugh AH, White RS: Single coronary artery. Analysis of the anatomic variation, clinical importance, and report of five cases. *JAMA* **230:**243, 1974

52. Cheitlin MD, DeCastro CM, McAllister HA: Sudden death as a complication of anomalous left coronary origin from the anterior sinus of Valsalva. A Not-so-minor congenital anomaly. *Circulation* **50:**780, 1974

53. Liberthson RR, Dinsmore RE, Fallon JT: Aberrant coronary artery origin from the aorta. Report of 18 patients, review of literature and delineation of natural history and management. *Circulation* **59:**748, 1979

54. Roberts WC, Chirani J: The four subtypes of anomalous origin of the left main coronary artery from the right aortic sinus (or from the right coronary artery). *Am J Cardiol* **70:**119, 1992

55. Chaitman BR, Lesperance J, Saltiel J, Bourassa MG: Clinical, angiographic, and hemodynamic findings in patients with anomalous origin of the coronary arteries. *Circulation* **53:**122, 1976

56. Serota H, Barth CW III, Seuc CA, et al: Rapid identification of the course of anomalous coronary arteries in adults: The "Dot and Eye" method. *Am J Cardiol* **65:**891, 1990

57. Fernandes F, Alam M, Smith S, Khaja F: The role of transeosophageal echocardiography in identifying anomalous coronary arteries. *Circulation* **88:**2532, 1993

58. Moodie DS, Gill C, Loop FD, Sheldon WC: Anomalous left main coronary artery originating from the right sinus of Valsalva. *J Thorac Cardiovasc Surg* **80:**198, 1980

59. Thomas D, Salloum J, Montalescot G, et al: Anomalous coronary arteries coursing between the aorta and pulmonary trunk: Clinical indications for coronary artery bypass. *Eur Heart J* **12:**832, 1991

60. Roberts WC, Siegal RJ, Zipes DP: Origin of the right coronary artery from the left sinus of Valsalva and its functional consequences: Analysis of 10 necropsy patients. *Am J Cardiol* **49:**863, 1982

61. Nelson-Piercy C, Rickards AF, Yacoub MH: Aberrant origin of the right coronary artery as a potential cause of sudden death: Successful anatomical correction. *Br Heart J* **64**:208, 1990

62. Kimbiris D, Iskandrian AS, Segal BL, Bemis CE: Anomalous aortic origin of coronary arteries. *Circulation* **58**:606, 1978

63. Page HL, Engel HJ, Campbell WB, Thomas CS: Anomalous origin of the left circumflex coronary artery. *Circulation* **50**:768, 1974

64. Killen DA, Wathanacharoen S: Proximal bypass to anomalous circumflex coronary artery. *J Thorac Cardiovasc Surg* **107**:447, 1994

65. Barresi V, Susmano A, Colandrea MA, et al: Congenial absence of the circumflex coronary artery. Clinical and cinearteriographic observations. *Am Heart J* **86**:811, 1973

66. Line DE, Babb JD, Pierce WS: Congenital aortic valve anomaly-Aortic regurgitation with left coronary isolation. *J Thorac Cardiovasc Surg* **77**:533, 1979

67. Mullins CE, El-Said G, McNamara DG, et al: Artesia of the left coronary artery ostium—Repair by saphenous vein graft. *Circulation* **46**:989, 1972

68. Krause W; Uber den Ursprung einer accessorischen A. coronaria cordis aus der A. pulmonalis. *Zeit Rationelle Med* **24**:225, 1865

69. Abbott ME: Anomalies of the coronary arteries. In McCrae T (ed): *Osler's Modern Medicine*. Philadelphia, Lea & Febiger, 1906, p. 420

70. Oldham HN, Ebert PA, Young WG, Sabiston DC: Surgical management of congenital coronary artery fistula. *Ann Thorac Surg* **12**:503, 1971

71. Bogers AJJC, Quaegebeur JM, Huysmans HA: Early and late results of surgical treatment of congenital coronary artery fistula. *Thorax* **42**:396, 1987

72. Ogden JA, Stansel HC Jr: Coronary arterial fistulas terminating in the coronary venous system. *J Thorac Cardiovasc Surg* **63**:172, 1972

73. Hobbs RE, Millit HD, Raghavan PV, et al: Coronary artery fistulae: A 10-year review. *Cleveland Clinic Quart* **49**:191, 1982

74. Iskandrian AS, Kimbiris D, Bemis CE, Segal BL: Coronary artery to pulmonary artery fistulas. *Am Heart J* **94**:605, 1978

75. Rose AG: Multiple coronary arteriovenous fistulae. *Circulation* **58**:178, 1978

76. Rittenhouse EA, Doty DB, Ehrenaft JL: Congenital coronary artery-cardiac chamber fistula. Review of operative management. *Ann Thorac Surg* **20**:468, 1975

77. Liberthson RR, Sagar K, Berkoben JP, et al: Congenital coronary arteriovenous fistula. Report of 13 patients, review of the literature and delineation of management. *Circulation* **59**:849, 1979

78. McNamara JJ, Gross RE: Congenital coronary artery fistula. *Surgery* **65**:59, 1969

79. Jaffe RB, Glancy DL, Epstein SE, et al: Coronary arterial-right heart fistulae. Long-term observations in seven patients. *Circulation* **47**:133, 1973

80. Griffiths SP, Ellis K, Hordof AJ, et al: Spontaneous complete closure of a congenital coronary artery fistula. *J Am Coll Cardiol* **2**:1169, 1983

81. Bjorck G, Crafoord C: Arteriovenous aneurysm on the pulmonary artery simulating patent ductus arteriosus Botalli. *Thorax* **2**:65, 1947

82. Liotta D, Hallman GL, Hall RJ, Cooley DA: Surgical treatment of congenital coronary artery fistula. *Surgery* **70**:856, 1971

83. Reidy JF, Anjos RT, Quershi SA, et al: Transcatheter embolization in the treatment of coronary artery fistulas. *J Am Coll Cardiol* **18**:187, 1991

84. Dabizzi RP, Caprioli G, Aiazzi L, et al: Distribution and anomalies of coronary arteries in tetralogy of Fallot. *Circulation* **61**:95, 1980

85. Humes RA, Driscoll DJ, Danielson GK, Puga FK: Tetralogy of Fallot with anomalous origin of left anterior descending coronary artery. *J Thorac Cardiovasc Surg* **94**:784, 1987.

86. Landolt CC, Anderson JE, Zorn-Chelton S, et al: Importance of coronary artery anomalies in operations for congenital heart disease. *Ann Thorac Surg* **41**:351, 1986

87. Lenox CC, Debich DE, Zuberbuhler JR: The role of coronary artery abnormalities in the prognosis of truncus arteriosus. *J Thorac Cardiovasc Surg* **104**:1728, 1992

88. Yacoub MH, Radley-Smith R: Anatomy of coronary arteries in transposition of the great arteries and methods for their transfer in anatomical correction. *Thorax* **33**:418, 1978

89. Wernovsky G, Sanders SP: Coronary artery anatomy and transposition of the great arteries. *Coronary Artery Dis* **4**:148, 1993

90. O'Sullivan J, Bain H, Hunter S, Wren C: End-on aortogram: Improved identification of important coronary artery anomalies in tetralogy of Fallot. *Br Heart J* **71**:102, 1994

91. Fellows KE, Freed MD, Keane JF, et al: Results of routine preoperative coronary angiography in tetralogy of Fallot. *Circulation* **51**:561, 1975

92. Cooley DA, Dunean JM, Gillette PC, McNamara DG: Reconstruction of coronary artery anomaly in an infant using the internal mammary artery. *Pediatr Cardiol* **8**:257, 1987

93. Geiringer E: The mural coronary. *Am Heart J* **41**:359, 1951

94. Edwards JC, Burnaides C, Swarm RL, Lansing AI: Arteriosclerosis in the intramural and extramural portion of coronary arteries in the human heart. Circulation **13**:235, 1956

95. Nobole J, Bourassa MG, Petitclerc R, Dyrda I: Myocardial bridging and milking effect of the left anterior descending coronary artery: Normal variant or obstruction? *Am J Cardiol* **37**:993, 1976

96. Ishimori T, Raizner AE, Chachine RA, et al: Myocardial bridges in man: Clinical correlation and angiographic accentuation with nitroglycerin. *Cathet Cardiovasc Diagn* **3**:39, 1977

97. Cheitlin MD: The intramural coronary artery: Another cause for sudden death with exercise? (editorial) *Circulation* **62**:238, 1980

98. Morales AR, Romanelli R, Tate LG, et al: Intramural left anterior descending coronary artery: Significance of the depth of the muscular tunnel. *Human Pathol* **24**:693, 1993

99. Daoud AS, Pankin D, Tulgan H, Florentin RA: Aneurysms of the coronary artery. *Am J Cardiol* **11**:228, 1963

100. Falsetti HL, Carroll RJ: Coronary artery aneurysm. A review of the literature with a report of 11 new cases. *Chest* **69**:630, 1976

101. Alford WC, Stoney WS, Burrus GR, et al: Recognition and operative management of patients with arteriosclerotic coronary artery aneurysms. *Ann Thorac Surg* **22**:317, 1976

102. Kawasaki T, Kosai F, Okawa S, et al: A new infantile acute febrile mucocutaneous lymph node syndrome (MLNS) prevailing in Japan. *Pediatrics* **54**:271, 1974

103. Morens DM, Anderson LJ, Hurwitz ES: National surveillance of Kawasaki Disease. *Pediatrics* **65**:21, 1980

104. Neufeld HN, Schneeweiss A: Congenital coronary aneurysm. In Neufeld HN, Schneeweiss A (eds): *Coronary Artery Disease in Infants and Children*. Philadelphia, Lea & Febiger, 1983, pp 59–64.

105. Takeuchi Y, Suma K, Shiroma K, et al: Coronary artery changes in Kawasaki disease and its surgical treatment by aorto-coronary bypass grafting. *Jpn J Thorac Surg* **31**:356, 1978

106. Mantini F, Grondin CM, Lillehei CW, et al: Congenital anomalies involving the coronary sinus. *Circulation* **33**:317, 1966

107. Frank CG, Maloney JV Jr: Surgical significance of congenital anomalies of the coronary sinus. *J Cardiovasc Surg* **9**:420, 1968

108. Watson GH: Artesia of the coronary sinus orifice. *Pediatr Cardiol* **6**:99, 1985

109. Guiraudon GM, Guiraudon CM, Klein GJ, et al: The coronary sinus diverticulum: A pathologic entity associated with the Wolf-Parkinson-White Syndrome. *Am J Cardiol* **62**:733, 1988

110. Quaegebeur J, Kirklin JW, Pacifico AD, Bargero LM Jr: Surgical experience with unroofed coronary sinus. *Ann Thorac Surg* **27**:418, 1979

111. Chin AJ, Murphy JD: Identification of coronary sinus septal defect (unroofed coronary sinus) by color Doppler echocardiography. *Am Heart J* **124**:1655, 1992

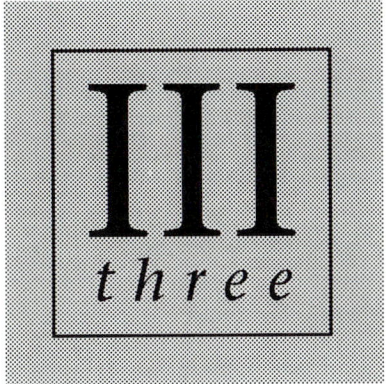

III
three

SURGERY FOR ACQUIRED HEART DISEASE

CHAPTER

95

Surgical Anatomy of the Heart

Benson R. Wilcox and Robert H. Anderson

There have been few attempts to describe the nuances of cardiac anatomy as perceived by the surgeon.[1,2] In this chapter we will describe the significant features of the normal position of the heart and its relation to the other thoracic organs, paying particular attention to the course of the important nerve trunks around the heart. Then we will describe chamber, septal, and valvar anatomy as seen through various approaches used by the cardiac surgeon. We will emphasize the position of the all-important but surgically invisible conduction tissues, basing this vital consideration on our previous experience using histologic and reconstruction techniques.[3-5]

CARDIAC POSITION AND RELATIONSHIPS

Although usually described in terms of a triangle, the heart is actually more akin to a four-sided pyramid, and its shape when projected to the chest wall is trapezoidal. Its overall mass when viewed relative to the thorax is positioned so that one-third is to the right of the midline and two-thirds is to the left. The long axis of the heart is oriented from the left hypochondrium to the right shoulder. Its short axis corresponds to the plane of the atrioventricular (A-V) groove and is oblique, being closer to the vertical than to the horizontal plane (Fig. 95-1). The heart is a mediastinal structure, and its anterior sternocostal surface abuts directly on the chest wall. Its right and left surfaces are flanked by the lungs and are formed by the vessels of the lung hila posteriorly. The right lung extends over the right surface of the heart to reach the midline, whereas the left lung retracts away from the midline in the area of its cardiac notch.

Inferiorly the heart has an extensive diaphragmatic surface, while posteriorly it lies directly on the esophagus and, slightly superiorly, on the bifurcation of the trachea into the lung hila. When viewed from its apex the three

sides of the pyramidal ventricular mass are readily seen. Two of the edges are named: the inferior edge is characteristically sharp and is the acute margin; the superior margin is much more diffuse and is the obtuse margin. The posterior margin is not named as such but it, too, is a gentle transition.

The vagus (tenth cranial) and phrenic nerves descend through the mediastinum and cross the lung hila in relation to the heart. Both enter through the thoracic inlet—the vagus along the carotid arteries and the phrenic on the surface of the anterior scalene muscle covered by the prevertebral fascia. The phrenic nerve is anterior to the vagus on both sides. The internal thoracic artery (internal mammary artery) is found anterior to the phrenic nerve at the thoracic inlet, separated from it by the internal thoracic vein. On the right side, the vagus branches high to give off the right recurrent laryngeal nerve, which then passes around the right subclavian artery before ascending out of the thoracic cavity. The right vagus continues posteriorly into the hilum, ramifying to form the right pulmonary plexus, and then reconstituting to exit from the thorax along the esophagus. In contrast, the right phrenic swings forward anteriorly to the hilum, crossing the right border of the heart to reach the dome of the right diaphragm (Fig. 95-2). On the left side, the phrenic and vagus nerves course forward across the aortic arch toward the heart. As they cross the arch, the superior intercostal vein insinuates itself between them to drain into the brachiocephalic vein. Having crossed the arch, the vagus gives off its recurrent laryngeal branch, which passes around the arterial ligament between the aorta and the left pulmonary artery before running up to the larynx. The vagus continues posteriorly into the lung hilum as on the right. The left phrenic nerve swings forward onto the ventricular mass and skirts over its left posterior border, anterior to the lung hilum, to reach the left dome of the diaphragm (Fig. 95-2). On both sides a further significant

1535

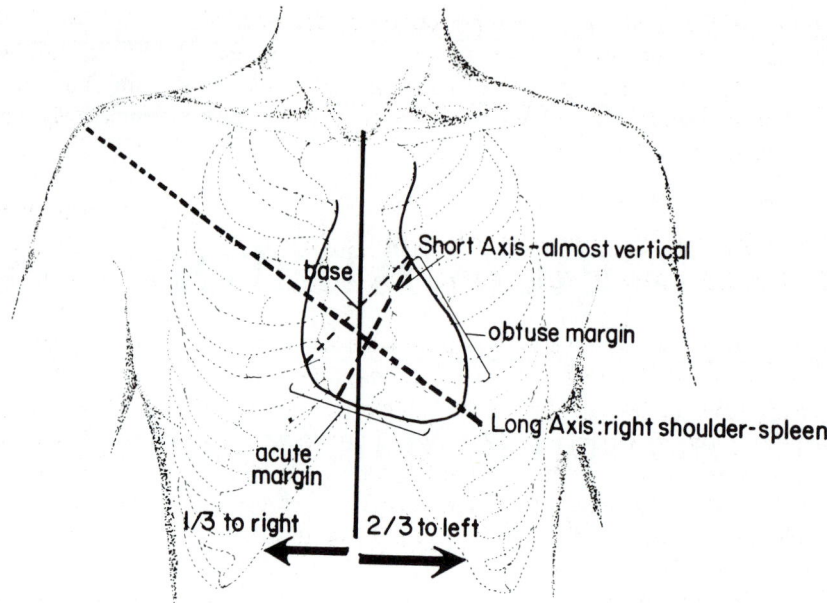

Figure 95–1. Diagram showing position of the heart in the chest and the salient features of the surface anatomy of the heart.

nervous structure is found around the subclavian arteries. This is the subclavian loop, a small nerve trunk that carries fibers from the stellate ganglion to the iris and head. Injudicious liberation of the subclavian arteries during shunt procedures can injure the delicate nerve roots and result in Horner's syndrome.

The heart is firmly enclosed within the pericardium, which adheres to the walls of the great vessels at their entry to and exit from the heart, and to the diaphragm along the inferior margin of the cardiac pyramid. Pericardial anatomy is best considered in terms of a double-layered bag into

which the heart has been placed apex foremost. The inner layer, a fine serous membrane, is then invaginated by the heart to form two further layers. The innermost of these is adherent to the surface of the heart and is the epicardium. The outer layer of the serous pericardium is adherent to the outer pericardial sac, the two together forming the fibrous pericardium with its serous parietal lining. The pericardial cavity functionally is then the space between the fibrous pericardium and the epicardium. There are two recesses within it that are lined by serous pericardium. The first is the transverse sinus, bounded anteriorly by the posterior

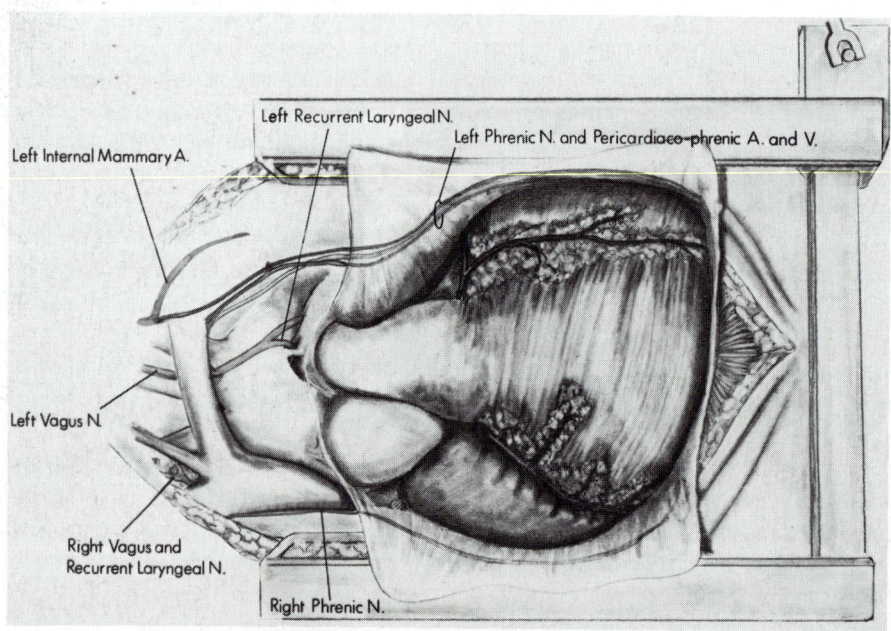

Figure 95–2. The relationship of the important major nerve trunks to the heart and the usual pericardial incision.

surface of the great arteries and posteriorly by the anterior surface of the interatrial groove. The second is the oblique sinus, a cul-de-sac behind the left atrium limited by the reflection of serous pericardium from the pulmonary veins and the inferior caval vein.[6]

SPATIAL RELATIONSHIPS OF THE CARDIAC CHAMBERS AND GREAT ARTERIES

The surgical anatomy and approaches to the heart can be understood fully only when the positioning of these structures is known relative to the cardiac silhouette. As already indicated, the A-V junction is obliquely oriented, being closer to the vertical than to the horizontal plane. If the atrial mass and the great arteries are removed by a cut just parallel to the junction, the plane can be viewed from above (Fig. 95–3). Then it can be seen that the A-V and arterial valves of the right side of the heart are widely separated by the inner heart curvature, lined by the transverse sinus. In contrast, the A-V and arterial valves of the left heart are closely adjacent to one another; indeed, their leaflets are in fibrous continuity. But the aortic valve also interposes in part between the tricuspid and pulmonary valves, and, as will be seen, there is fibrous continuity between leaflets of the aortic and tricuspid valves via the substance of the central fibrous body. From study of this short-axis view of the A-V junction, and the overview of the heart illustrated in Figure 95–18, it is then possible to deduce the basic rules of cardiac anatomy. First, the atrial chambers lie to the right relative to their corresponding ventricles. Second, the right atrium and ventricle are anterior relative to their left-sided counterparts, and the septal structures between them are very much obliquely oriented. Third, by virtue of its "wedge" position, the aortic valve is directly related to all the cardiac chambers.

Other significant features of cardiac anatomy can be culled by further dissection of the short-axis view of the

A-V junction. Because of the wedge position of the aortic valve, there is only a short area of the septum where the mitral and tricuspid valves are attached directly opposite each other (Fig. 95–4). Furthermore, because the tricuspid valve is attached to the septum further toward the ventricular apex than is the mitral valve, this part of the septum, interposed between the right atrium and the left ventricle, is the A-V muscular septum (Fig. 95–5). Cephalad and anterior to this area is the keystone of the fibrous skeleton of the heart where the leaflets of the aortic, mitral, and tricuspid valves meet. This is the so-called *central fibrous body*. It is made up in part of the right fibrous trigone, a thickening of the right side of the area of aortic-mitral fibrous continuity (Fig. 95–6). The remainder is the fibrous partition between the left ventricular outflow tract and the right heart chambers. This so-called membranous septum is itself divided into two because the septal leaflet of the tricuspid valve is directly attached across it (Fig. 95–7). Thus, the membranous septum has an A-V component between right atrium and left ventricular outflow tract, and an interventricular component between the two ventricles (Fig. 95–8). Removal of the noncoronary leaflet of the aortic valve then demonstrates the full significance of the wedge position of the left ventricular outflow tract on chamber relationships. The subaortic region separates the greater part of the mitral ori-

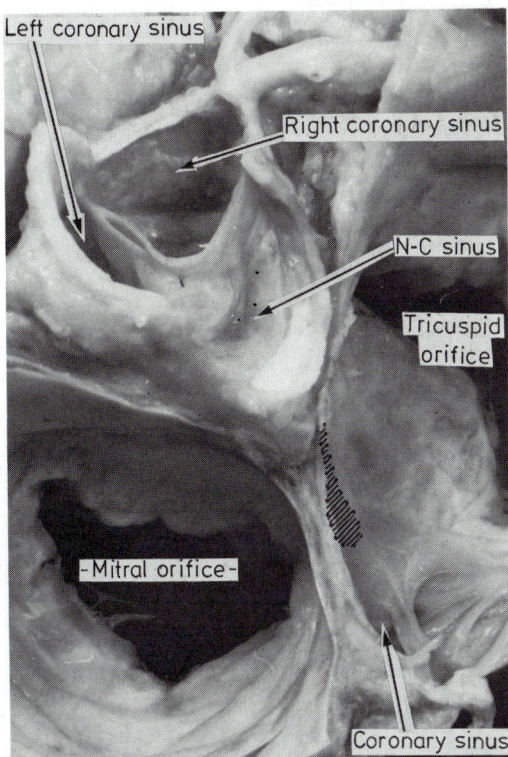

Figure 95–4. A dissection of the short-axis of the heart showing the relationships of the aortic, mitral, and tricuspid valves. The position of the atrioventricular node has been superimposed. N-C, noncoronary.

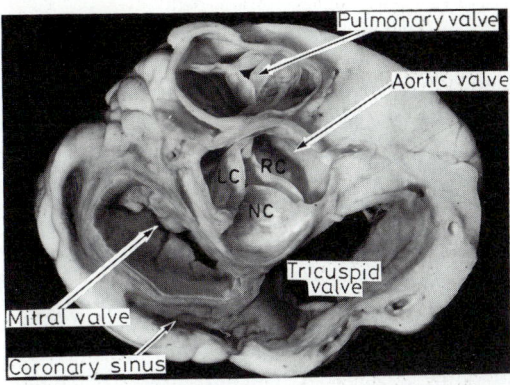

Figure 95–3. A short-axis section of the heart viewed from above following removal of the atriums and great arteries. *(Specimen photographed and reproduced by kind permission of Professor Anton E. Becker, Wilhelmina Gasthuis, Amsterdam.)*

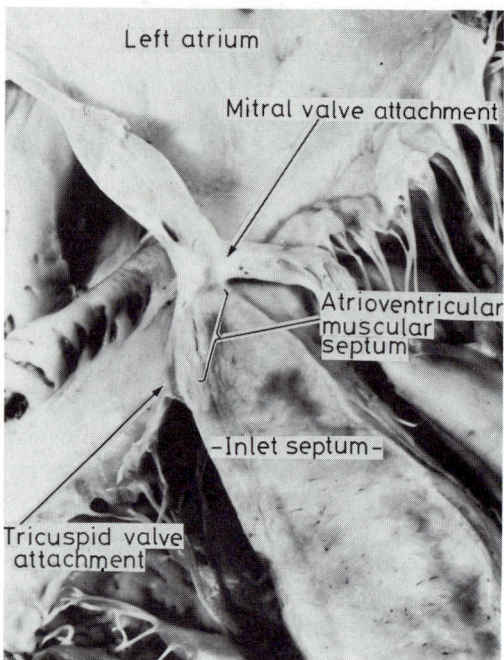

Figure 95–5. A coronal section (four-chamber cut) of the heart showing how the different levels of attachment of the tricuspid and mitral valves to the septum make a muscular atrioventricular structure.

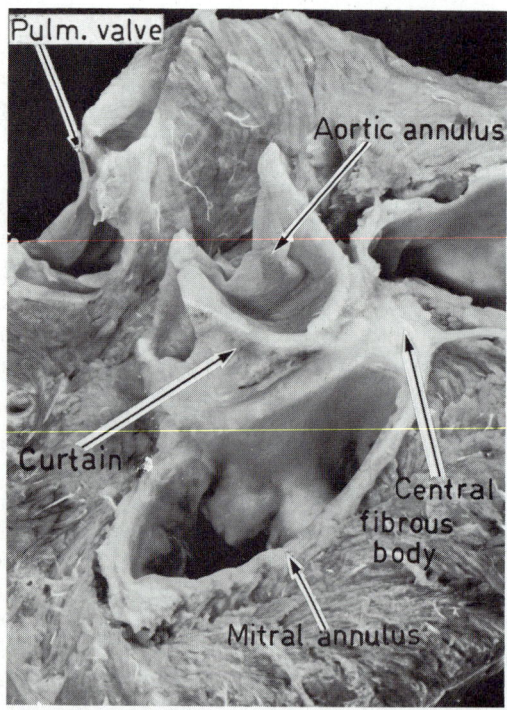

Figure 95–6. A dissection showing the fibrous skeleton of the heart, also illustrating how the aortic valve leaflets are attached to the skeleton in tented-up coronet fashion. The aortic-mitral curtain is directly related to the transverse sinus of the pericardium. *(From Anderson RH, Becker AE: Cardiac anatomy for the surgeon. In Danielson GK (ed): Practice of Surgery. Hagerstown, MD, Harper & Row, 1979 with permission.)*

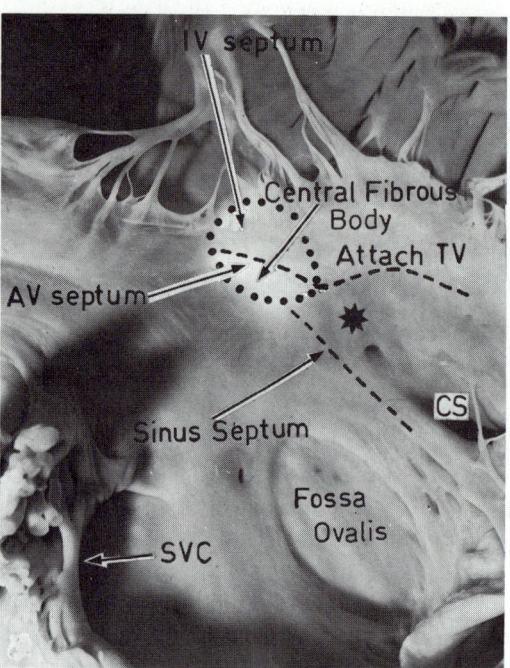

Figure 95–7. A transilluminated view of the membranous septum viewed from the right atrium showing how the attachment of the tricuspid valve divides the septum into atrioventricular and interventricular components. AV, atrioventricular; CS, coronary sinus; IV, interventricular; SVC, superior vena cava; asterisk, triangle of Koch. *(From Anderson RH, Becker AE: Cardiac anatomy for the surgeon. In Danielson GK (ed): Practice of Surgery. Hagerstown, MD, Harper & Row, 1979 with permission.)*

fice from the septum (Fig. 95–9). This feature is significant not only to the position of the A-V conduction tissues but also to the positional anatomy of the leaflets and tension apparatus of the mitral valve.

DETAILED ANATOMY OF THE CARDIAC CHAMBERS AND VALVES

The Morphologically Right Atrium

The right atrium has three basic parts: the appendage, the vestibule, and the venous component, the latter receiving the systemic venous return. Externally, the junction of the appendage and the venous component is identified by the presence of a prominent groove, the terminal groove (Fig. 95–10), which matches the internal location of the terminal crest. The appendage is an extensive structure shaped as a blunt triangle. It has a wide junction with the venous sinus across the terminal groove. The appendage, with its walls marked by the parallel pectinate muscles originating at right angles from the terminal crest, also has an extensive junction with the vestibule of the right atrium, which is a smooth-walled fringe of atrial myocardium inserting into the leaflets of the tricuspid valve at the A-V junction. The

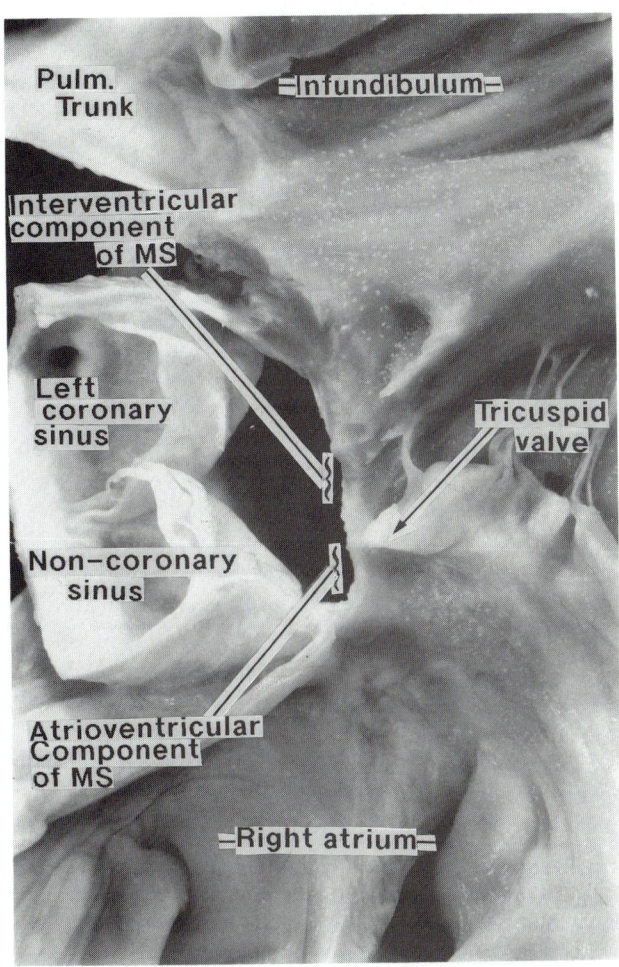

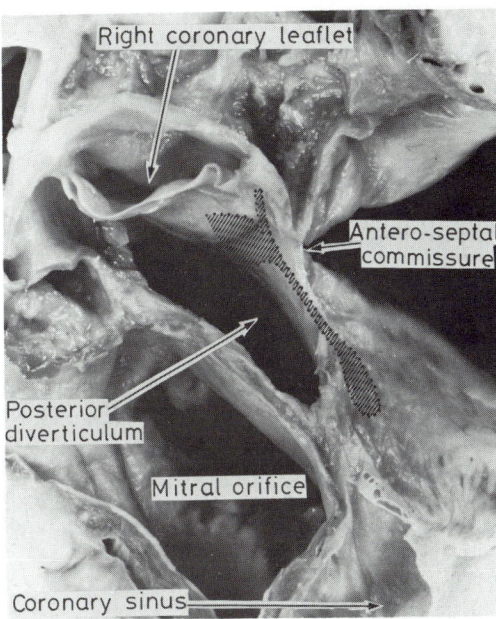

Figure 95–9. Further dissection of the short-axis view illustrated in Fig. 95–4 showing the extensive posterior diverticulum of the aortic outflow tract. The position of the conduction tissues has been marked.

Figure 95–8. This dissection has been made by removing the right coronary sinus and leaflet of the aortic valve. It shows the membranous component of the ventricular septum and demonstrates how the attachment of the tricuspid valve divides this membranous septum (MS) into interventricular and atrioventricular components. Pulm, pulmonary.

most characteristic and constant feature of the morphologically right atrium is that the pectinate muscles within the appendage extend all the way round the parietal margins of the A-V junction (Fig. 95–11). The venous component of the right atrium is small when viewed externally, extending between the terminal groove and the interatrial groove (Waterston's groove). It receives the superior and inferior caval veins at its cephalic and caudal extremities. Cephalad and anteriorly, the appendage has a further important relation with the superior caval vein. Here the appendage terminates in a prominent crest that forms the summit of the terminal groove and is continuous behind the aorta with the interatrial groove. The major surgical significance of this anatomy is that the sinus node lies within the terminal groove in a subepicardial position (Fig. 95–10). Almost always the node is a spindle-shaped structure lying in the groove to the right of the appendage crest, that is, lateral to the superior cavoatrial junction. In about one-tenth of cases,

however, the node extends across the crest into the interatrial groove, being draped across the cavoatrial junction in horseshoe fashion.[7]

Also of significance is the course of the important artery to the sinus node. This is an initial branch of the right coronary artery in about 55% of individuals, and of the circumflex artery in most of the remainder. Irrespective of its origin, it usually courses through the anterior interatrial groove toward the superior cavoatrial junction, frequently running within the atrial myocardium. Having reached the crest of the appendage, its course is variable. In some hearts it crosses over the crest to enter the node at its cephalic end. In others, it courses behind the cavoatrial junction and enters the caudal end of the node. In yet other hearts there is a complete arterial circle formed around the cavoatrial junction. In a small minority of individuals, the artery to the sinus node arises more distally from either the right or the circumflex arteries (Fig. 95–12). When arising distally from the right coronary artery, the sinus node artery courses laterally across the atrial appendage. This position places it very much at risk during a standard right atriotomy (Fig. 95–12B). When the artery arises distally from the circumflex artery, it crosses the dome of the left atrium as it ascends toward the cavoatrial junction. This places it at major risk during some approaches to the mitral valve (see below). In our experience this variability, if carefully sought, can be judged by gross inspection. Taken together with the variable position of the node itself, it serves to show that the entire superior cavoatrial junction is a potential surgical danger area. Incisions made to gain access to either right or left atrial chambers should always be made

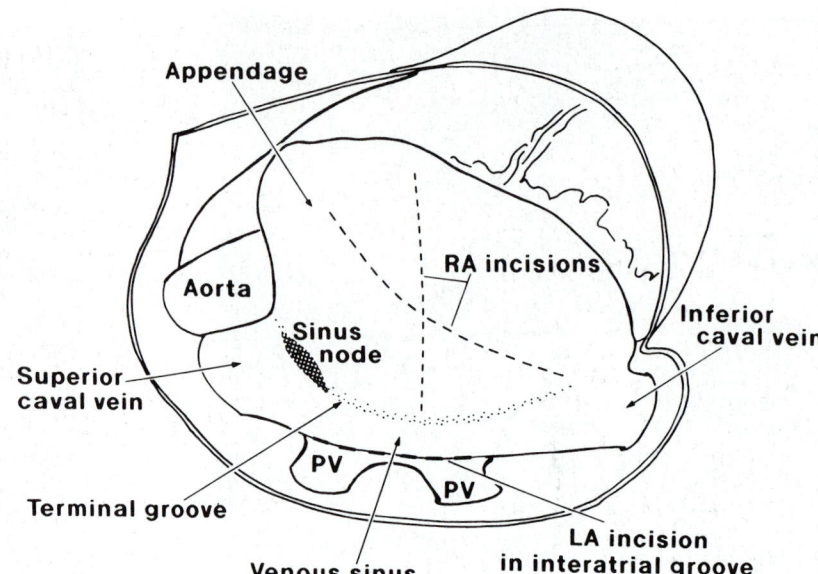

Figure 95–10. The surface features of the right atrium showing the sinus node and the best anatomical sites of "safe" incisions into the right and left atrial chambers. PV, pulmonary veins; RA, right atrial; LA, left atrial.

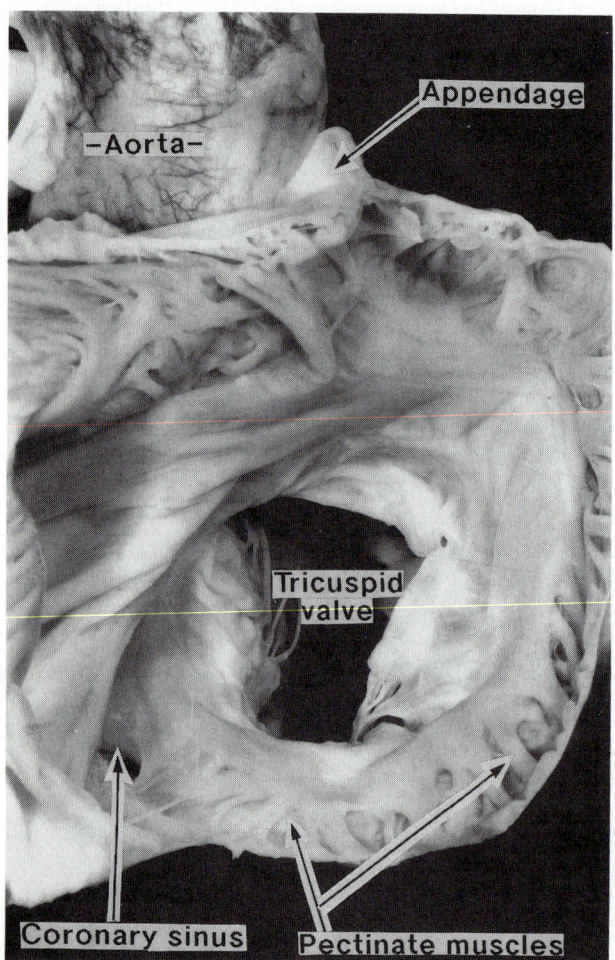

Figure 95–11. Dissection of the right atrium showing how the pectinate muscles of the appendage extend all the way round the margins of the atrioventricular junction. Compare with Figure 95–15.

with this anatomic variability firmly in mind. They will need to be modified if certain patterns are encountered.

The safest incision into the right atrium is probably one made into the atrial appendage more or less parallel with, but some distance away from, the terminal groove (Fig. 95–10). This incision, nonetheless, would place at risk a right lateral sinus node artery. Opening the atrium through such an incision shows that the terminal groove is the external marking of a prominent muscle bundle, the terminal crest, which separates the pectinate muscles of the appendage from the smooth walls of the venous component. Anteriorly the crest curves in front of the orifice of the superior caval vein to become continuous with the so-called septum secundum, in reality the superior rim of the oval fossa. On first sight, when inspecting the right atrium through this incision, there appears to be an extensive septal surface between the orifices of the caval veins and the orifice of the tricuspid valve (Fig. 95–13). Opening into and from this "septal" surface are the oval fossa and the orifice of the coronary sinus. But the apparent extent of this septum is spurious.[2,8] The true septum between right and left atrial chambers is confined to the immediate environs of the fossa, as shown by the dissection illustrated in Figure 95–14. The extensive superior rim of the fossa, although usually called the septum secundum, is produced by the extensive infolding of the interatrial groove between the venous component of the right atrium and the pulmonary veins.

The area around the coronary sinus is where the right atrial wall overlies the A-V muscular septum (Figs. 95–4 and 95–9). The upper margin of this wall between the oval fossa and the coronary sinus is where another important muscle bundle, the sinus septum or inferior rim of the oval fossa, swings in from the terminal crest. This septum separates the orifices of the inferior caval vein and the coronary

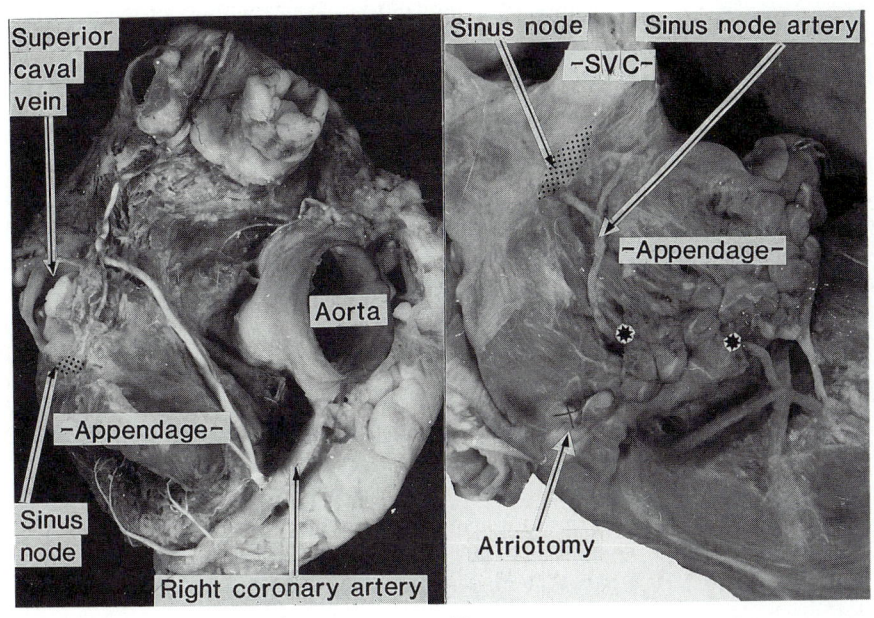

A   **B**

Figure 95–12. A. Sinus nodal artery passing medial to the right atrial appendage and superior vena cava. **B.** The lateral course of this sinus nodal artery was interrupted by the right atriotomy (*—*).

sinus. Only a small part of the extensive anterior rim of the fossa is a septal structure. Its larger part is the anterior atrial wall overlying the aortic root. These limited margins of the septum are of major surgical importance, because it is an easy matter to pass outside the heart when attempting to gain access to the left atrium via a right atrial incision.

In addition to the position of the sinus node and the extent of the atrial septum, the other major area of surgical significance is the site of the A-V node.[3] This is contained within the triangle of Koch (Figs. 95–7 and 95–13). This important landmark area is bounded by the tendon of Todaro, the attachment of the septal leaflet of the tricuspid valve, and the orifice of the coronary sinus. The tendon of Todaro is a fibrous structure formed by the junction of the eustachian valve (valve of the inferior caval vein) and the thebesian valve (valve of the coronary sinus). The commissure of these two valvar structures buries itself in the sinus septum and runs forward as the tendon of Todaro to insert into the central fibrous body (Figs. 95–7 and 95–13). The entire atrial component of the A-V conduction tissues is

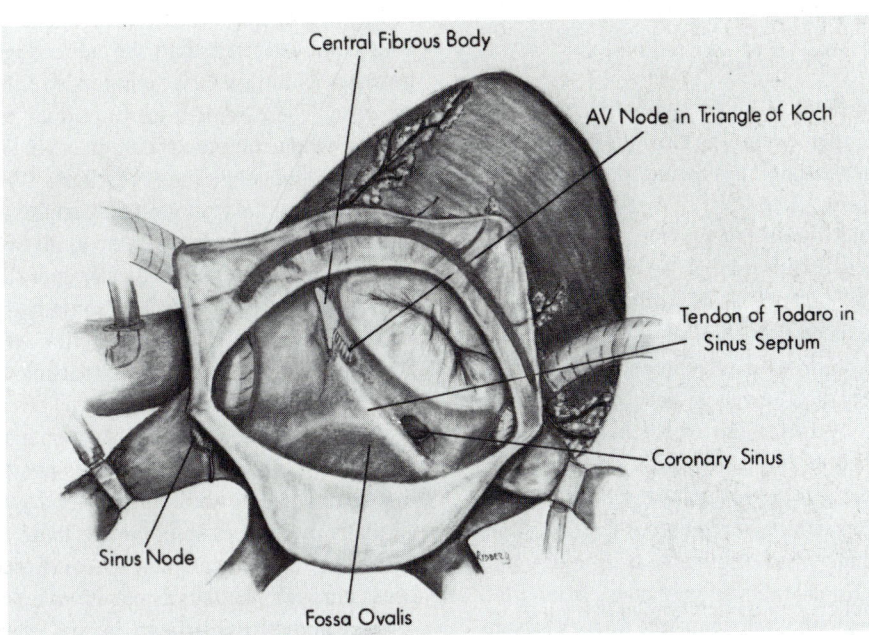

Figure 95–13. The surgeon's view of the right atrium showing the position of the atrioventricular node in the triangle of Koch (see also Fig. 95–7) and the site of the right coronary artery and the sinus node. Artistic license has been used in making a generous incision.

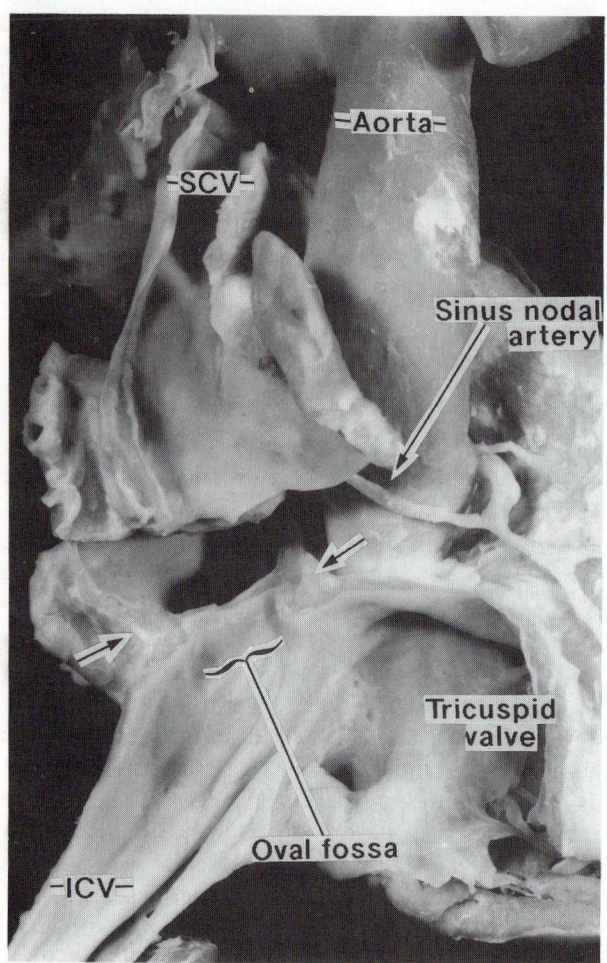

Figure 95–14. This heart has been sectioned through the mid-portion of the oval fossa to show the limited extent of the true septum, confined in essence to the floor of the fossa. The run of the fossa (so-called "septum secundum") is simply the infolded atrial wall (*arrows*). SCV, superior caval vein; ICV, inferior caval vein.

contained within the confines of the triangle of Koch. If this area is scrupulously avoided during surgical procedures, the A-V conduction tissues cannot be damaged. Should the node need to be precisely identified, it should be remembered that the tricuspid valvar attachment is some way down the surface of the septum relative to the mitral valve attachment (Fig. 95–5). The node itself, sitting in interatrial position on the sloping face of the A-V muscular septum, is therefore some distance above the attachment of the tricuspid valve. The A-V bundle, however, penetrates more or less directly at the apex of the triangle of Koch, so this point serves as a landmark should one need to divide the bundle in the treatment of intractable supraventricular tachycardia.

The key to avoiding atrial arrhythmias is the fastidious preservation of the sinus and atrioventricular nodes and their blood supplies. No advantage is gained from time spent in attempting to preserve nonexistent tracts of "specialized atrial conduction tissues."

Although it is not always easy, it is generally possible

to distinguish three leaflets in the vestibule of the tricuspid valve: the anterosuperior, the septal, and the inferior or mural leaflets. They join together at their zones of apposition, or commissures, and are tethered by the fan-shaped commissural chords arising atop the prominent papillary muscles of the valve. Thus, the anteroseptal commissure is supported by the medial papillary muscle and lies "round the corner" from the area of the central fibrous body and the membranous septum. The major leaflets of the valve extend from this position in anterosuperior and septal direction. The third (mural or inferior) leaflet is less well defined. The anteroinferior commissure is usually supported by the prominent anterior papillary muscle, but this muscle can also be attached directly to the midpoint of the anterosuperior leaflet. Then the inferior (mural) leaflet may seem to be duplicated, as it is often not possible to nominate one specific inferior papillary muscle supporting an inferoseptal commissure. This distinction is of minimal surgical significance, and almost always the leaflets meet in trifoliate fashion. The entire parietal attachment of the tricuspid valve is usually encircled by the right coronary artery running around the vestibule in the A-V groove (Fig. 95–13). There is no well-formed collagenous "annulus" for the tricuspid valve. Instead, the groove more or less folds itself directly into the tricuspid valvar leaflets at the vestibule, and the atrial and ventricular myocardial masses are separated almost exclusively by the fibrofatty tissue of the groove.

The Morphologically Left Atrium

Owing to its position, only the appendage of the left atrium is immediately evident to the surgeon on exposing the heart. Like the right atrium, the left atrium has a venous component in addition to its appendage and vestibule. Unlike the right atrium, the venous component of the left atrium is considerably larger than the appendage and has a narrow junction with it that is unmarked by either a terminal groove or crest. There is also an important difference in the left atrium, when compared with the right, between the relationship of appendage and vestibule. As shown in Figure 95–12, in the morphologically right atrium the pectinate muscles of the appendage extend all round the vestibule. In contrast, in the morphologically left atrium the appendage, with the pectinate muscles contained almost exclusively within it, has a very limited junction with the vestibule. The larger part of the vestibule, supporting and inserting into the mural leaflet of the mitral valve, is directly continuous with the smooth-walled pulmonary venous component of the atrium (Fig. 95–15). Owing to its posterior position and its firm anchorage by the four pulmonary veins, the left atrium is relatively inaccessible, though there are various routes by which the surgeon can gain access. Probably the most popular is through the interatrial groove (Fig. 95–10). As described above, the groove is the extensive infolding between the right pulmonary veins and the venous component of the right atrium, this groove producing the so-called sep-

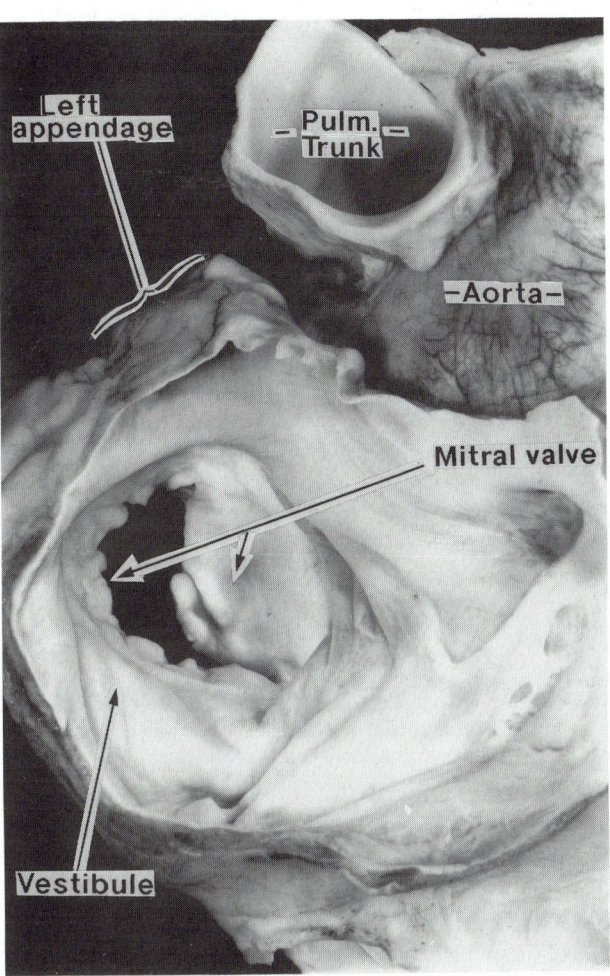

Figure 95–15. Dissection of left atrium showing the limited junction between the appendage and the vestibule, with the wall of the vestibule merging with the pulmonary venous component. Compare with Figure 95–12.

the circumflex artery. Also, in some instances, this artery passes through the interatrial groove to reach the terminal groove. As discussed, in even rarer cases the artery may cross the dome of the left atrium itself when it has a distal origin from the circumflex artery.

When access is gained to the left atrium, the small size of the mouth of the appendage is immediately apparent, lying to the left of the mitral orifice as viewed by the surgeon. The greater part of the pulmonary venous atrium will usually be located inferiorly away from the operative field. It is the vestibule of the mitral orifice that dominates the picture (Fig. 95–16). The septal aspect will be anterior, and the true septum will be in a relatively inferior position, exhibiting the typically roughened flap valve aspect of its left side. The large sweep of tissue between the flap valve of the septum and the mouth of the appendage is the internal aspect of the deep anterior interatrial groove. The mitral valve itself is supported by two prominent papillary muscles and their commissural cords. These muscles are positioned in anteromedial and posterolateral positions. The two leaflets delineated by the solitary zone of apposition between them have widely different appearances. The anterosuperior leaflet is short, squat, and relatively square. This is the leaflet that is in fibrous continuity with the aortic valve (Figs. 95–3, 95–4, 95–9, and 95–16). It is best termed the *aortic leaflet,* as it is not strictly in either anterior or superior position. The other leaflet is narrower, but its annular attachment is more extensive, being connected to the parietal part of the mitral annulus. It is accurately termed the *mural leaflet* and is divided into a number of subunits that fold against the aortic leaflet when the valve is closed. Usually three in number, it is sometimes possible to find up to five or six of these scallops in the mural leaflet. Unlike the tricuspid valve, the leaflets of the mitral valve are supported to various extent by a rather dense collagenous annulus. It is rare, however, for the annulus to be a complete ring. The parts best formed differ from heart to heart. They usually extend parietally from the fibrous trigones, the greatly thickened areas at either end of the area of fibrous continuity between the leaflets of the aortic and mitral valves. The area of the valvar orifice and septum related to the right fibrous trigone and central fibrous body is most vulnerable in terms of conduction tissue, because the A-V node and penetrating bundle lie here (Figs. 95–9 and 95–16). The area of mitral orifice between the two trigones (more or less the midportion of the aortic leaflet) is directly related to the commissure between the noncoronary and left coronary leaflets of the aortic valve. Here the aortic root "tents" itself up (see below). An incision apparently through the atrial wall in this area can be extended into the subaortic outflow tract. The deep inner curvature of the heart, lined by the transverse sinus, overlies and runs to either side of the curtain between the leaflets of the mitral and aortic valves. Encircling the mural leaflet of the mitral valve are the circumflex coronary artery from below and to the left and the coronary sinus from below and to the right (Fig. 95–16).

tum secundum. A leftward-directed incision along this groove, or parallel between it and the right pulmonary veins, takes the surgeon directly into the left atrium. Because the infolding also forms the superior rim of the oval fossa, much the same access can be gained by approaching via the right atrium and incising just cephalad in the fossa. It must then be remembered that an extensive incision will take the surgeon out of the confines of the septum. If accurately repaired, this is unlikely to produce complications. A further approach to the left atrium is the superior approach through the so-called dome. We have already indicated how the crest of the right atrial appendage turns medially into the interatrial groove. If the aorta is pulled forward and to the left, it can be shown that this groove is an extensive trough between the two atrial appendages. An incision through the roof of this trough, between the pulmonary veins from the upper lobes, provides direct access to the left atrium. When making such incisions to enter the left atrium, it must always be remembered that in 45% percent of cases the sinus node artery courses upward through this area from

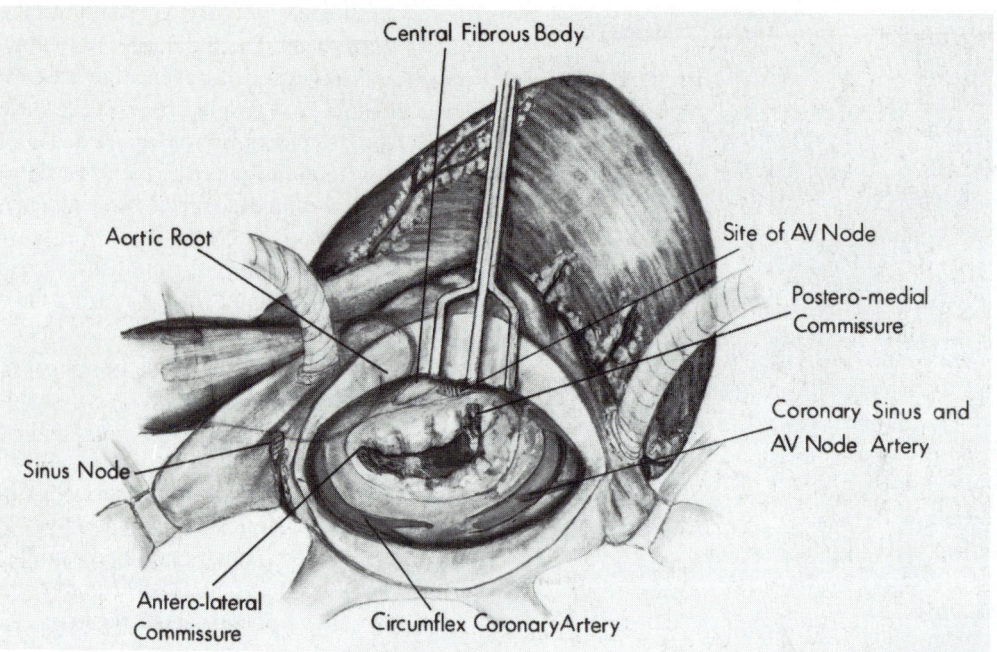

Figure 95–16. A surgeon's view of the left atrium as entered through an incision in the interatrial groove. The sites of the left coronary artery, central fibrous body, atrioventricular node, coronary sinus, artery to the atrioventricular node, and the sinus node with its artery have all been superimposed. The mitral valve is drawn in open position showing the sites of the papillary muscles with the heart somewhat distorted by the atrial retractor.

Also, in about 45% of cases, the A-V nodal artery will run in close proximity to the right side of the mitral orifice—arising either from the circumflex or right coronary artery.[6] The margin directly related to the circumflex artery is somewhat variable. When the left coronary artery is dominant, however, the entire mural leaflet attachment can be intimately related to the coronary artery (see Wilcox and Anderson,[2] p 3.5, Fig. 3.7).

The Morphologically Right Ventricle

The understanding of both the ventricles, morphologically right and left, is greatly aided by considering their morphology in terms of three components rather than the traditional "sinus" and "conus" parts. The three portions are the inlet, apical trabecular, and outlet portions, respectively.[2] The inlet portion of the right ventricle contains and is limited by the tricuspid valve and its tension apparatus. A distinguishing feature of the tricuspid valve is the direct septal attachments of its septal leaflet. The apical trabecular component of the right ventricle extends out to the apex, where its wall is particularly thin and especially vulnerable to perforation by cardiac catheters and pacemaker electrodes. The outlet component of the right ventricle is a complete muscular structure, the infundibulum, which supports the leaflets of the pulmonary valve (Fig. 95–17A). The three leaflets of the pulmonary valve do not have ring-like attachments. Instead, they are attached to the infundibular musculature in semilunar fashion. The pulmonary attachments are, there-

fore, much higher at the peripheral margin of the zones of apposition between the adjacent leaflets (the commissures) than at the basal level within the ventricle. As a consequence, these attachments, marking the hemodynamic ventriculoarterial junction, cross the anatomic ventriculoarterial junction where the fibroelastic wall of the pulmonary trunk is supported by the infundibular musculature of the right ventricle. Anatomically, it is this circular junction that forms a true annulus, or else the prominent ring at the junction of the sinuses of the pulmonary trunk with the tubular component. Alternatively, a third ring can be constructed by joining together the basal attachments of the three leaflets to the infundibular musculature. None of these rings, however, corresponds to the attachments of the leaflets, which need to be semilunar so as to permit the valve to open and close in competent fashion (Fig. 95–18). A distinguishing feature of the right ventricle is the prominent muscular shelf separating the tricuspid and pulmonary valves, called the supraventricular crest. Although, at first sight, it has the appearance of a large muscle bundle, in reality it is the posterior aspect of the subpulmonary muscular infundibulum supporting the leaflets of the pulmonary valve. In other words, it is part of the inner heart curvature. Incisions through this part run into the transverse septum and jeopardize the right coronary artery. It is often thought that the area is the "outlet" component of the interventricular septum. In fact, the entire subpulmonary infundibulum, including the ventriculoinfundibular fold, can be removed without entering the cavity of the left ventricle (Fig.

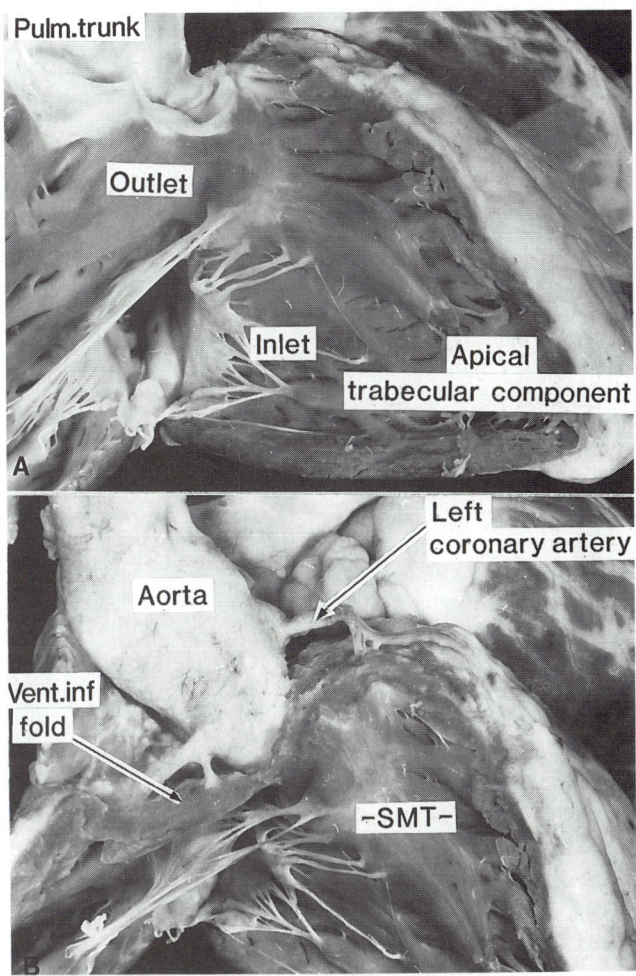

Pulm.trunk

Outlet

Inlet

Apical trabecular component

A

Left coronary artery

Aorta

Vent.inf fold

–SMT–

Figure 95–17. A. Opened right ventricle showing inlet, apical trabecular, and outlet portions. The pulmonary valve is supported by the muscular infundibulum. **B.** The subpulmonary infundibulum has been excised revealing the aorta and coronary arteries. The left ventricle is intact. SMT, septomarginal trabeculation.

95–17B). This is because the leaflets of the pulmonary valve, and the "facing" leaflets of the aortic valve (see below), are supported on separate sleeves of right and left ventricular outlet musculature, respectively. There is an extensive external tissue plane between the walls of the aorta and pulmonary trunk, the valve leaflets having markedly different levels of attachment within the ventricles (Fig. 95–19). Once the subpulmonary infundibulum has been removed from the right ventricle, however, it can be seen that its component, which is described as the supraventricular crest, inserts between the limbs of another prominent right ventricular muscle column, the septomarginal trabeculation (Fig. 95–17B). This trabeculation has a body that divides superiorly into anterior and posterior limbs. The anterior limb runs up into the infundibulum and supports the leaflets of the pulmonary valve. The posterior limb extends backward beneath the interventricular membranous septum to run into the inlet component of the ventricle. The medial

papillary muscle arises from this posterior limb. The body of the septomarginal trabeculation runs to the apex of the ventricle, breaking up into a sheath of smaller trabeculations. Some of these mingle into the apical trabecular portion while some support tension apparatus of the tricuspid valve. Two trabeculations can be particularly prominent. One becomes the anterior papillary muscle, while the other crosses the ventricular cavity as the moderator band.

The Morphologically Left Ventricle

Just as with the right ventricle, the left ventricle can conveniently be considered in terms of inlet, apical trabecular, and outlet components. The inlet component surrounds, and is limited by, the mitral valve and its tension apparatus. The papillary muscles of the valve, although basically in anterolateral and posteromedial position, are positioned rather close to each other. Unlike the tricuspid valve, the leaflets of the mitral valve have no direct septal attachments. This is because the deep posterior diverticulum of the left ventricular outflow tract displaces the aortic leaflet of the mitral valve away from the inlet septum (see Fig. 95–9). The trabecular component of the left ventricle has characteristically fine trabeculations and extends out to the ventricular apex. As in the right ventricle, the apical myocardium is surprisingly thin (see Wilcox and Anderson,[2] p 2.17). The outlet component of the left ventricle supports the aortic valve. Unlike its right ventricular counterpart, it is not a complete muscular structure. The septal wall is largely composed of muscle, but the fibrous membranous septum is also part of the subaortic outflow tract. The deep posterior diverticulum of the outflow tract is that space extending from the fibrous septum across to the aortic leaflet of the mitral valve, and this extensive fibrous curtain supports the leaflets of the aortic valve. The lateral quadrant around to the septum is then a muscular structure, namely, the left lateral margin of the inner heart curvature lined externally by transverse sinus. The septal surface of the outflow tract is characteristically smooth, and down this smooth surface cascades the fanlike left bundle. The landmark to the descent of the left bundle branch is the membranous septum immediately beneath the commissure between right coronary and noncoronary leaflets of the aortic valve. The left bundle descends initially as a relatively narrow solitary fascicle but soon divides into three interconnected fascicles that radiate into anterior, septal, and posterior divisions. The interconnecting radiations do not fan out to any degree until the bundle itself has descended to between one-third and one-half the length of the septum. As with the pulmonary valve, the aortic valve does not have a discrete annulus. Rather, the leaflets are attached to the outflow tract in semilunar fashion (Fig. 95–20). Because this valve forms the keystone of the heart, and because it is related to each of the other cardiac chambers and valves, we will describe its detailed morphology in a separate section.

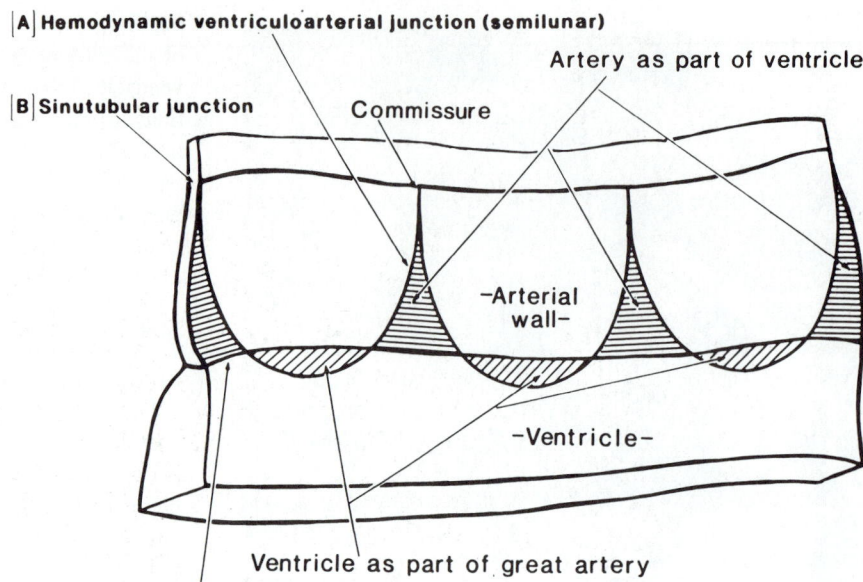

Figure 95–18. Diagram showing the semilunar arrangement of attachment of the leaflets of the pulmonary valve, and how this incorporates crescents of infundibular musculature within the sinuses and triangles of arterial wall within the ventricular outflow tract.

The Aortic Valve

The aortic outflow tract is in part muscular and in part fibrous. The three semilunar leaflets (or cusps) of the aortic valve also therefore have attachments that are in part fibrous and in part muscular. The leaflets themselves are attached within the expanded aortic sinuses. Because two of these sinuses give rise to coronary arteries and one does not, the aortic leaflets can conveniently be named after their sinuses as right coronary, left coronary, and noncoronary (Fig. 95–21). When the aortic wall is removed, the attachments of the valve can be seen to be in the form of a three-piece coronet, with the three commissures being the zenith of the valve attachment (Fig. 95–6). The commissure between the noncoronary and the left coronary leaflets is positioned along the area of aortic-mitral valve continuity. Beneath this commissure is the so-called fibrous subaortic curtain (Fig. 95–6). To the right relative to this commissure, the noncoronary leaflet is attached above the extensive posterior diverticulum of the outflow tract. This is the part of the valve directly related to the right atrial wall (Fig. 95–21). From the inferior attachment of the noncoronary leaflet in relation to the right atrium, the valve tents up again to the commissure between the noncoronary and right

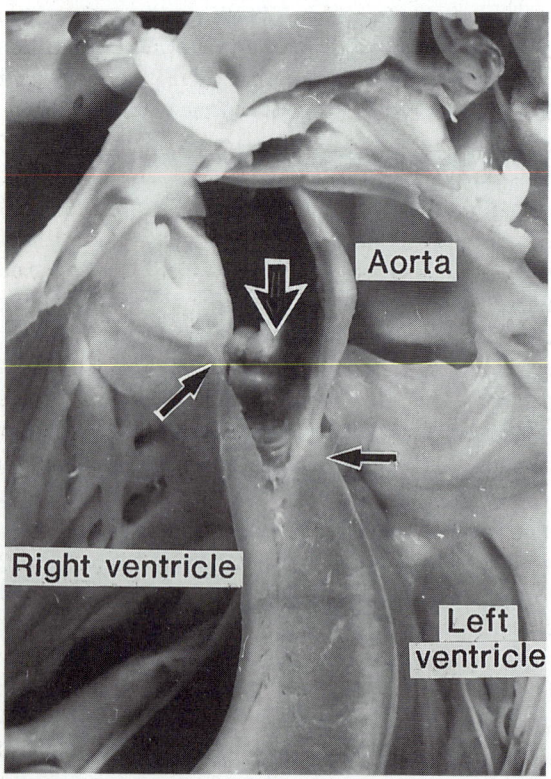

Figure 95–19. The decided difference in the level of attachments of the aortic and pulmonary valves is demonstrated.

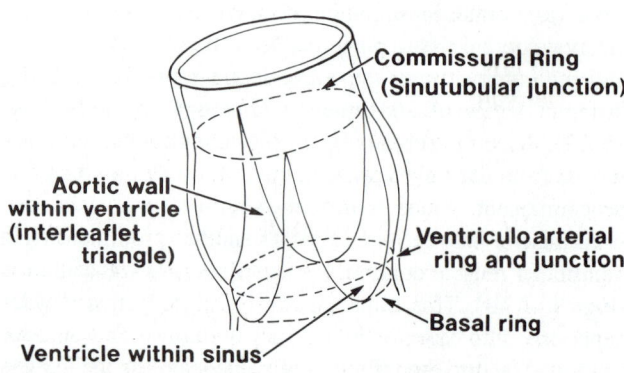

Figure 95–20. Idealized view of the aortic valve showing the semilunar arrangement of the attachment of the leaflets and the different rings within the valvar complex, none of which corresponds to the hinge points of the leaflets.

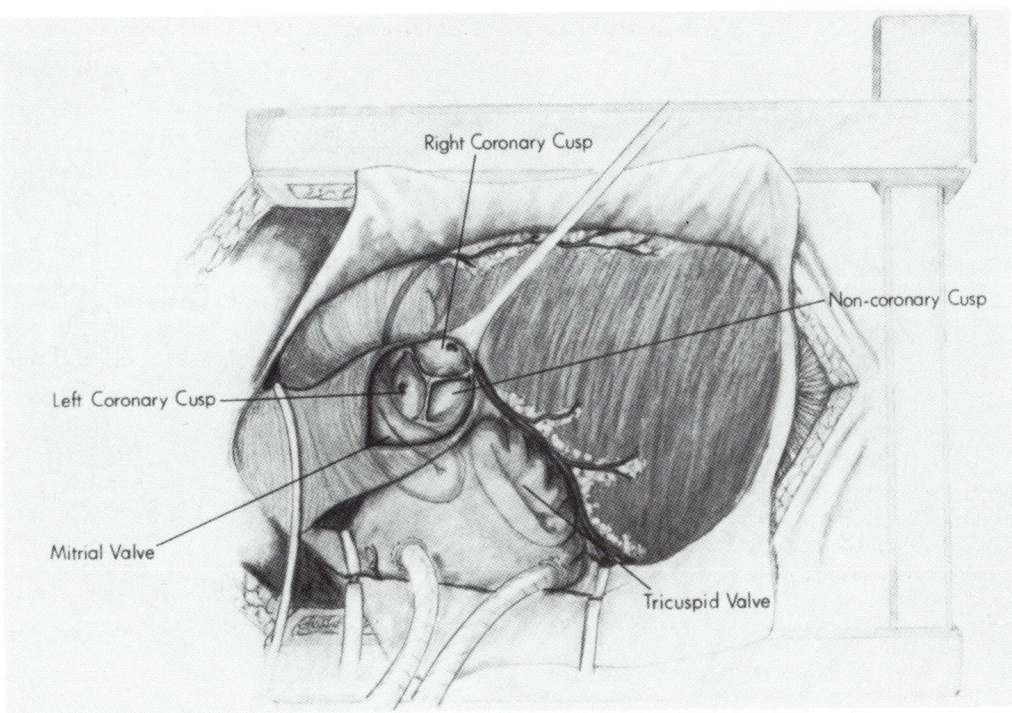

Figure 95–21. A surgeon's view of the aortic valve as seen through an aortic incision and illustrating its relationship to the other valves and cardiac chambers.

coronary leaflets. The ascending part of the noncoronary leaflet is then positioned directly above the part of the atrial septum containing the A-V node, while the commissure itself is above the penetrating atrioventricular bundle and the membranous septum (Fig. 95–22A). When seen from the right side, the site of this commissure is outside the heart, being related to the transverse sinus of the pericardium and, less immediately, to the right coronary artery. The attachment of the right coronary leaflet then dips down across the central fibrous body before ascending to the commissure between the right coronary and left coronary leaflets, which is also supported high on the aortic wall. Immediately beneath this commissure, the uppermost part of the subaortic outflow tract is formed by the wall of the aorta itself. An incision through this area passes into the space between the facing surfaces of the aorta and the pulmonary trunk (Fig. 95–18). As the facing leaflets descend from the commissure, they then take origin from the outlet muscular component of the left ventricle. As described above, only a very small part of this area in the normal heart is a true outlet septum, as both arterial valves are supported on their own sleeves of myocardium. Thus, although the outlet components face each other, an incision below the aortic valve enters low into the infundibulum of the right ventricle. As the lateral part of the left coronary leaflet descends from the facing commissure toward the base of the sinus, it becomes the only part of the aortic valve not intimately related to another cardiac chamber, this being the part of the valve that

takes origin from the lateral margin of the inner heart curvature.

The anatomy described is significant not only to the routine replacement of the aortic valve but also to operations devised to enlarge the aortic root. Two of these demand intimate knowledge of the anatomy. The Konno–Rastan operation depends on opening and enlarging the outer part of the subaortic region (Fig. 95–22B).[9,10] Approached from the right ventricle, the incision must be made from the most medial part of the supraventricular crest into the left ventricular outflow tract. When making this incision, the marked difference in level of attachment of aortic and pulmonary leaflets must be borne in mind. To avoid the left bundle branch, the incision must then be continued in a leftward direction away from the ventricular septum. The second type of operation involves incising the outflow tract in the region of aortic-mitral valvar continuity.[11] Use can be made here of the tent of subaortic outflow tract beneath the commissure between the noncoronary and left coronary leaflets, because the triangle of subaortic curtain immediately beneath the commissure can be safely incised before damaging the aortic leaflet of the mitral valve.

The critical importance of knowing the anatomy of this region is demonstrated in one additional circumstance.[12,13] With the aortic valve occupying this keystone position in relation to the other valves and cardiac chambers, endocarditis involving the aortic valve can be particularly devastating, especially when accompanied by forma-

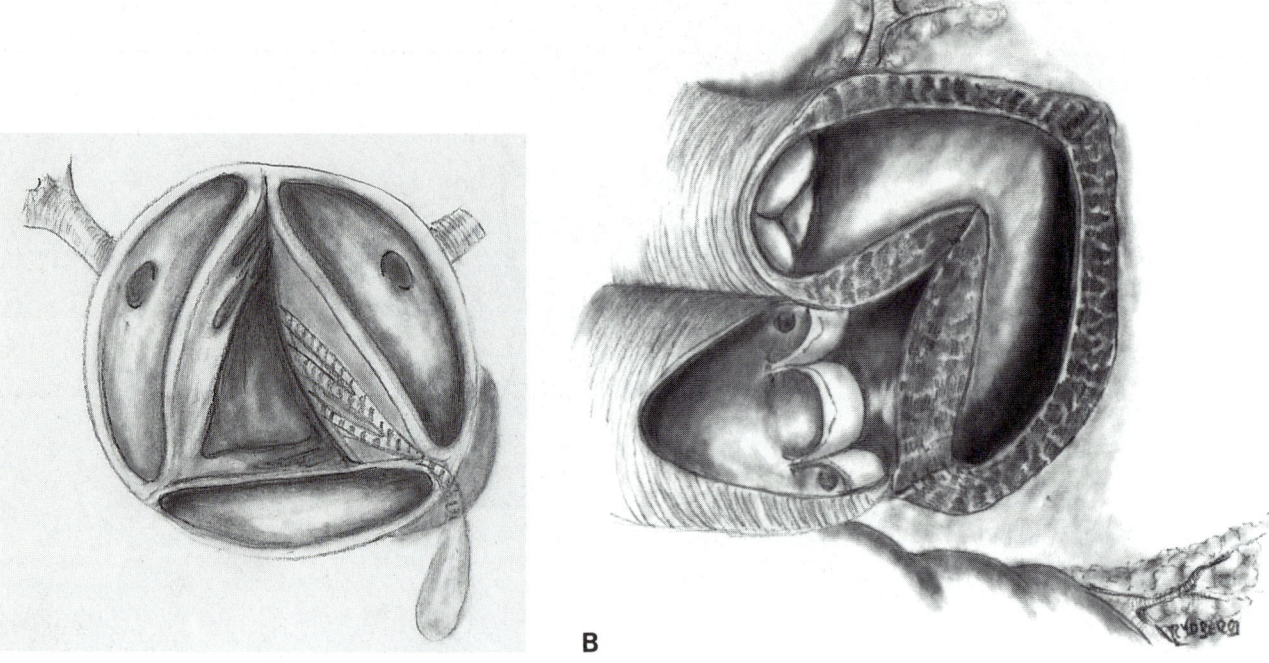

Figure 95–22. **A.** A view of the left ventricular outflow tract as seen through the aortic valve and showing the position of the atrioventricular conduction tissues. **B.** The interventricular septum can be incised to gain access to the aortic root. This incision will allow enlargement of the aortic root.[9,10]

tion of an abscess. With an eroding abscess, a fistula can form between the aorta and any of the four chambers of the heart. Thus, the clinical presentation in such patients can be quite complex, with findings of left heart failure, and/or left-to-right shunting, or complete heart block in addition to the usual signs of sepsis. Surgical management can be very difficult and self-evidently requires a detailed knowledge of the anatomy of the aortic valve discussed above and in Chapter 120.

THE CORONARY CIRCULATION

Coronary circulatory anatomy will be described in Chapter 123.

REFERENCES

1. Anderson RH, Becker AE: Cardiac anatomy for the surgeon. In Danielson GK (ed): *Practice of Surgery.* Hagerstown, MD, Harper & Row, 1979, Chap 16
2. Wilcox BR, Anderson RH: *Surgical Anatomy of the Heart.* New York, Raven Press, 1985
3. Anderson RH, Becker AE, Brechenmacher C, et al: The human atrioventricular junctional area. A morphological study of the atrioventricular node and bundle. *Eur J Cardiol* **3:**11, 1975
4. Becker AE, Anderson RH: Morphology of the human atrioventricular junctional area. In Wellens HJJ, Lie KI, Janse MJ (eds): *The Conduction System of the Heart—Structure, Function and Clinical Implications.* New York, Lea & Febiger, 1976, pp 263–286
5. Anderson RH, Becker AE, Tranum-Jensen J, Janse MJ: Anatomico-electrophysiological correlations in the conduction system. A review. *Br Heart J* **45:**67, 1981
6. McAlpine WA: *Heart and Coronary Arteries.* New York, Springer-Verlag, 1975
7. Anderson KR, Ho SY, Anderson RH: The location and vascular supply of the sinus node in the human heart. *Br Heart J* **41**(1):28, 1979
8. Sweeney LJ, Rosenquist GC: The normal anatomy of the atrial septum in the human heart. *Am Heart J* **98**(2):194, 1979
9. Konno S, Imai Y, Iida Y, et al: A new method for prosthetic valve replacement in congenital aortic stenosis associated with hypoplasia of the aortic valve ring. *J Thorac Cardiovasc Surg* **70:**909, 1975
10. Rastan H, Koncz J: Aortoventriculoplasty. A new technique for the treatment of left ventricular outflow tract obstruction. *J Thorac Cardiovasc Surg* **71:**920, 1976
11. Blank RH, Pupello DF, Bessone LN, et al: Method of managing the small aortic annulus during valve replacement. *Ann Thorac Surg* **22:**356, 1976
12. Wilcox BR, Murray GF, Starek PJK: The long-term outlook for valve replacement in active endocarditis. *J Thorac Cardiovasc Surg* **74:**860, 1977
13. Frantz PT, Murray GF, Wilcox BR: Surgical management of left ventricular-aortic discontinuity complicating bacterial endocarditis. *Ann Thorac Surg* **29:**1, 1980

96

Cardiovascular Function and Physiology

Hendrick B. Barner

INTRODUCTION

It is imperative that the surgeon operating on the adult heart have an acute awareness of cardiovascular function and physiology. All aspects of a cardiac intervention may be influenced by circulatory dynamics or may alter the cardiovascular system, whether it is normal or abnormal.

HISTORY

Our understanding of circulatory physiology has gradually unfolded since William Harvey reported the circulation of blood in 1628. Starling contributed the concept of the heart responding to increased filling with greater ejection.[1] Skeletal muscle mechanisms have been applied to the myocardium[2] but do not consider the unique cross-fiber orientation of the myocardium. Newer techniques such as transesophageal echocardiography, three-dimensional echocardiography, nuclear magnetic resonance tagging, three-dimensional magnetic resonance imaging, and on-line continuous measurements of ventricular performance using computer interfacing provide the tools to better assess the heart and its workings.

THE MUSCLE

The study of isolated muscle strips or papillary muscle has provided us with an understanding of muscle mechanisms that can be applied to the globular left ventricle of the mammalian heart. The model proposed for skeletal muscle by Hill[2] has been applied to cardiac muscle and consists of a contractile element in series, an elastic element in series, and an elastic component in parallel with the contractile element and the series elastic element (Maxwell model) or an elastic component in the parallel with the contractile element only (Voight model). The elastic components are functional in nature and do not have a definable anatomic basis.

Length-Tension Relationship

The basic unit of the contractile apparatus is the sarcomere with a maximum resting length[3] of 2.2 μm and a contracted length of 1.9 μm or 13.6% shortening.[4] Sarcomere length (up to its maximum of 2.2 μm) in the intact heart is determined by the degree of stretch on the myocardium or the end-diastolic volume, which determines the point on the length-active tension curve at which the muscle operates and so determines the force of the subsequent systole (Fig. 96–1). This relationship was recognized by Starling,[1] who stated that if the filling of the heart is increased, it contracts more forcefully (Starling's law of the heart, Frank–Starling mechanism).[5] This dependence of the stroke volume on the degree of filling is the primary mechanism for ensuring that the two sides of the heart remain in balance.

The empty left ventricle has an average sarcomere length of 1.9 μm; as the ventricle is filled, sarcomere lengths increase so that at a filling pressure of 12 mm Hg (upper normal filling pressure) sarcomere length averages 2.2 μm. With further ventricular distention, filling pressure rises markedly for small increments in ventricle volume; only small increases in sarcomere length accompany large increases in intraventricular pressure (Fig. 96–1).

Geometric considerations dictate some variability in sarcomere length. Sarcomeres tend to be longest in the mid-

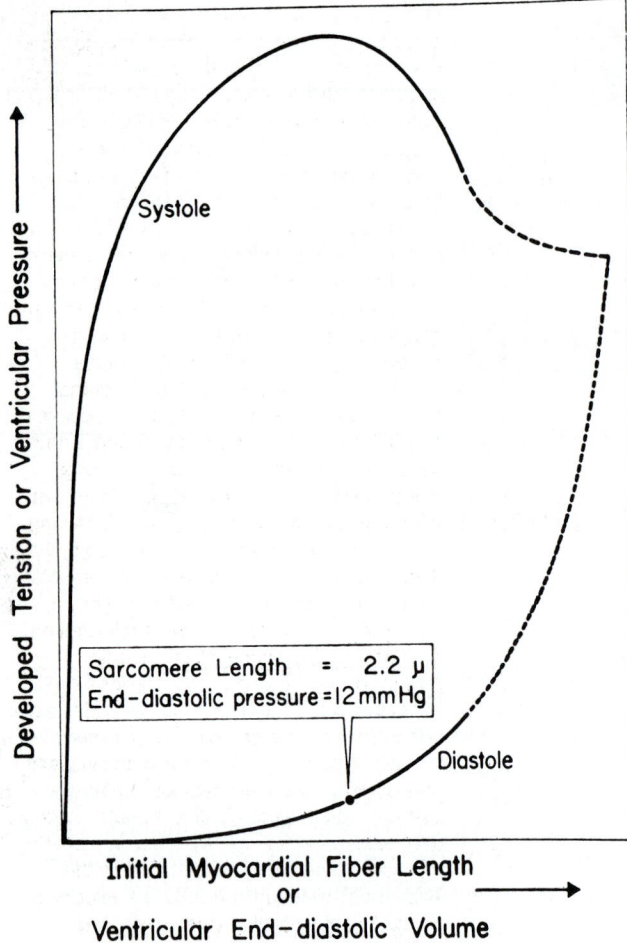

Figure 96–1. Relationship of myocardial fiber length or end-diastolic volume to developed tension or peak systolic pressure in the intact dog heart. Maximal ventricular systolic pressure is developed at an average sarcomere length of 2.2 μm, which corresponds closely with a filling pressure of 12 mm Hg. *(From Berne RM, Levy MN: Cardiovascular Physiology. St. Louis, Mosby, 1967, p 61, with permission.)*

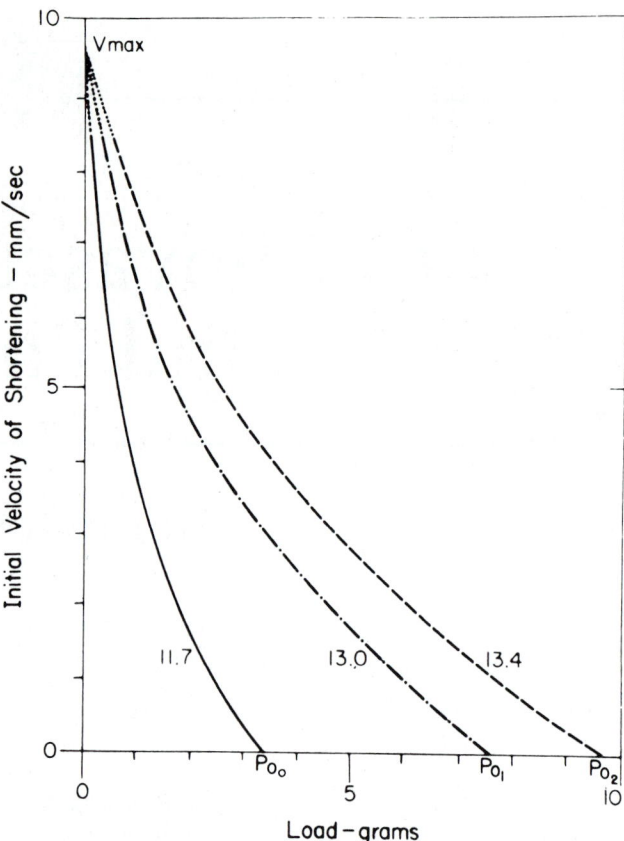

Figure 96–2. Force-velocity curves for a papillary muscle at three different initial fiber lengths (preloads). Increase in initial length from 11.7 to 13.0 and 13.4 mm produced increases in maximum developed tension (Po_0, Po_1, and Po_2, respectively). Extrapolation of the three curves back to zero yields a single value for maximum velocity of shortening (V_{max}). *(From Berne RM, Levy MN: Cardiovascular Physiology. St. Louis, Mosby, 1967, p 66, with permission.)*

wall of ventricle and reach a maximal length (2.25 μm) at filling pressures of 10 mm Hg, when subendocardial and subepicardial sarcomeres are shorter.[6] As filling pressure is raised further, sarcomere length increases across the entire wall; this recruitment of shorter sarcomeres from across the wall may constitute one of the principal functional reserves of the Frank–Starling mechanism.[7]

Force-Velocity Relation

A papillary muscle is loaded or stretched (*preload*) and after the onset of contraction, the muscles sense any additional load (*afterload*). The inverse relations between the tension (force) developed and the velocity of contraction constitutes the force–velocity curve (Fig. 96–2). The maximum velocity of shortening (V_{max}) is obtained by extrapolation of the force–velocity curve back to zero load and represents the peak intensity (contractility) of the active state.[8]

As initial fiber length is increased, the force–velocity curve is shifted to the right and more forceful contractions results, but V_{max} (contractility) is unchanged (see Fig. 96–2).

Inotropic interventions (addition of norepinephrine, calcium ions, or cardiac glycosides) enhance contractility and result in a new family of force–velocity curves in which the rate of tension development, velocity of shortening, and extent of shortening with a given load are increased so that the force–velocity curve is shifted upward and to the right.[9] Thus, a change in contractility may be defined in terms of change in V_{max} or a change in force at the same resting fiber length.

Force-Velocity-Length

The interdependence among force, velocity, and muscle length can be plotted as a force–velocity–length diagram (Fig. 96–3). This relation is relatively independent of time

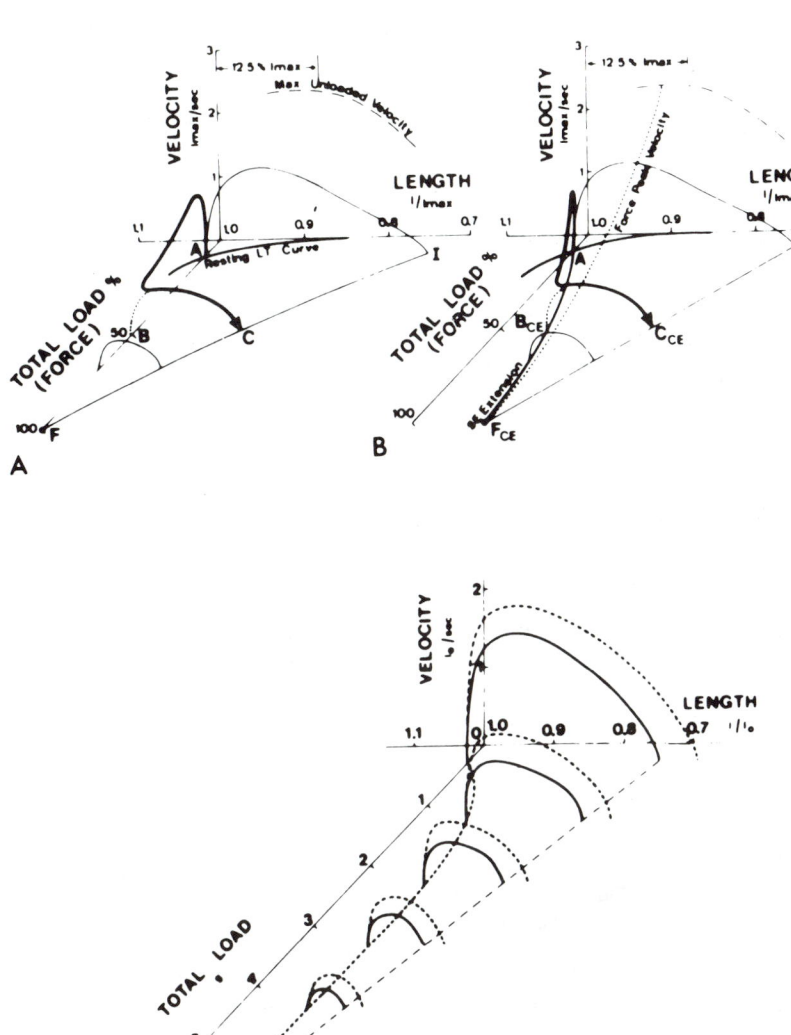

Figure 96–3. A. The length–velocity relations of isotonic contractions obtained at L_{max} have been replotted as a function of total load. The course of velocity of a hypothetical afterloaded isotonic contraction is superimposed (darker line). The velocity of shortening during the isometric phase of the contractions has been theoretically derived from a two-component muscle model. Velocity rises rapidly to the level appropriate for the plane of this three-dimensional composite. During isometric contraction V_{ce} falls as force rises. This velocity is not seen but is expressed in terms of the rate of force development (*dp/dt*). At point B the force development equals the load, and external shortening can then proceed between points B and C. Velocity of shortening between B and C depends on the level of the force–velocity–length plane. The velocity–length relation and the maximum unloaded velocity of shortening (V_{max}) is shown on the right. Projection to the right of the plane of the force–velocity–length relation provides the force–velocity relation, while the length–tension curve is reflected on the base. **B.** The force–velocity–length relations of the same muscle as shown in **A** after correction for extension of the series elastic component. The entire curve is moved to the right. The dashed line shown on the plane created by the force–velocity–length represents the force–velocity curve as obtained from afterloaded contractions. **C.** Effect of a positive inotropic intervention (dashed line) on the force–velocity–length relation. The velocity of shortening at any given muscle length is augmented, so that the entire surface relating force–velocity and length is increased and the extent of shortening is augmented. The projection of this surface to the right would be characterized by an increase in V_{max}. *(From Brutsaert DL, Sonnenblick EH: Cardiac muscle mechanics in the evaluation of myocardial contractility and pump function: Problems, concepts and directions. Prog Cardiovasc Dis 16:337, 1973, with permission.)*

during a major portion of muscle shortening, but late in the course of contraction shortening diverges from the velocity–length phase planes indicating that the active state is declining.[10]

The full active state of cardiac muscle commences rapidly after stimulation. The duration of the active state is sufficient to allow shortening to the same end-systolic length, regardless of the initial length if afterload and contractility remain constant. This property of cardiac muscle is critical to the use of end-systolic cardiac dimensions or volume for the assessment of contractility.[11]

In the past it has been commonly assumed that changes in muscle length and inotropic interventions are independent regulators of myocardial performance. However, it has been recognized that inotropic interventions and changes of muscle length may both act through processes that involve Ca^{2+} activation.[12] Decreasing sarcomere lengths below the optimum results in a partial inhibition of Ca^{2+}-triggered release of Ca^{2+} from the sarcoplasmic reticulum of cardiac cells.[13] Decreasing muscle length does not decrease the Ca^{2+} signal;[14] but the inotropic effect of extracellular changes in Ca^{2+} is dependent on muscle length, and the mechanical performance of cardiac muscle is more sensitive to changes in extracellular Ca^{2+} at shorter than at longer muscle lengths.[15] Thus, there is evidence that all changes in contractile behavior may occur primarily from alterations in the degree of activation of the contractile system and that muscle length (preload) and contractility should not be regarded as totally independent regulators of myocardial performance.[16] The total amount of Ca^{2+} released in the myofibril relates to a change in contractility while the length of the sarcomere appears to alter its sensitivity to Ca^{2+}. Despite these considerations and regardless of the fundamental molecular mechanisms involved, the consideration of preload (fiber length) and contractile state as separate determinants of myocardial performance remains an extremely useful concept.

The Heart

Preload, afterload, and contractile state determine performance of isolated muscle and the intact ventricle. Heart rate is a fourth determinant of the heart's performance per unit of time.

In comparing the heart to isolated muscle, heart volume and pressure are analogous to muscle length and tension. In a sphere, volume is defined by the equation, $V = 4/3\pi r^3$, where V = volume and r = radius. Because the circumference is $2\pi r$, volume is also related to the third power of circumference, so that a 50% reduction of the circumference of a sphere is accompanied by a reduction in volume to one-eighth its initial volume. The relationship between ventricular pressure and tension in the wall is defined by the law of LaPlace, which in its simplest form is stated as $T = P \times r$ where T = wall tension (dyn/cm), P = pressure (dyn/cm^2), and r = radius (cm). Thus, wall tension at any pressure increases as the radius increases. Thickness of the ventricular wall is considered by the relation $T = Pr/2h$, where h = wall thickness (cm). Because the ventricle is not a simple sphere, more complex formulas have been used to calculate these relationships.

During left ventricular ejection, the minor (transverse) axis of the inner wall shortens by 27–37% while the major (apex-to-base) axis shortens by 9%.[17] Therefore, shortening of the minor axis accounts for 85–90% of the stroke volume.[17] Casts of canine left ventricles arrested at end-diastolic and end-systole have given similar values and, in addition, have shown that the ratio of the major-to-major axis changed from an average 1.49 in diastole to 1.93 in systole.[18] Left ventricular wall thickness increases by 25–35% during systole in animals[17] and humans[19]; however, prediction of wall thickening (about 8%) from sarcomere shortening and simple geometric considerations is inconsistent with this but can be explained on the basis of structural morphology. Fibers of the left ventricular wall change from an oblique orientation at the epicardium to a circumferential orientation at the midwall to reverse oblique direction at the endocardium.[20] Interaction with differently aligned fibers at a distance appears to be the mechanism for amplifying small amounts of fiber shortening into extensive myocardial thickening.[21]

The Cardiac Cycle

The temporal relationship of the events of the cardiac cycle are shown diagramatically in Figure 96–4. The initial phase of ventricular contraction is isovolumetric with the maxi-

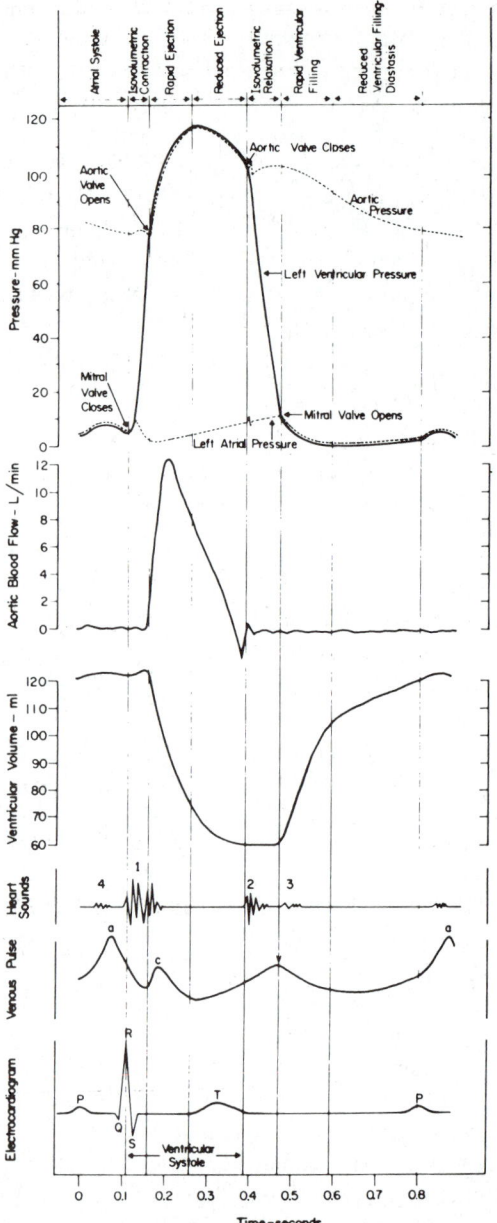

Figure 96–4. Left atrial, aortic, and left ventricular pressure traces correlated in time with aortic flow, ventricular volume, heart sounds, venous pulse, and electrocardiogram during a complete cardiac cycle. *(From Berne RM, Levy MN: Cardiovascular Physiology. St. Louis, Mosby, 1967, p 78, with permission.)*

mum rate of pressure change (peak *dp/dt*) occurring just prior to the onset of ejection. The *rapid ejection* phase begins with opening of the semilunar valves and is characterized by a sharpened rise in ventricular and aortic pressure, a more abrupt decrease in ventricular volume, and a greater aortic bloodflow. It is followed by the *reduced ejection phase,* which is of longer duration and ends with closure of the semilunar valves, which produce the incisura on the aortic pressure tracing. The interval between closure of the semilunar valves and opening of the atrioventricular (A-V) valves is termed *isovolumetric relaxation* and is marked by a precipitous fall in ventricular pressure without a change in ventricular volume. As ventricular pressure falls below atrial pressure, the A-V valves open and the *rapid filling phase* begins with the major part of ventricular filling occurring followed by a slow filling period and then a second rapid filling phase as a consequence of atrial systole. At slow heart rates, the atrial contribution to ventricular filling is minimal. At more rapid rates or with stenosis of the A-V valves, the contribution of atrial systole to ventricular filling becomes increasingly important. In the failing heart, the contribution by atrial systole can result in a 20–30% increase in cardiac output.

Preload

In the normal heart, most changes in cardiac output can be accounted for by return of blood to the heart from the venous system, which in turn alters filling pressure (preload) and determines ventricular end-diastolic volume, wall tension, or stress, and therefore sarcomere length. In heart failure, the heart is operating in the region of the pressure–volume curve where sarcomere length is maximal. Thus, end-diastolic cardiac dimensions cannot be increased as a means to enhance performance, which requires an increase in contractility and heart rate if cardiac performance is to be enhanced.[22]

It has been debated whether there is a descending limb of cardiac function for the Frank–Starling curve.[23] When end-diastolic pressure was increased to 60 mm Hg in the isovolumetrically contracting isolated canine left ventricle, there was no reduction of developed wall stress or systolic pressure; raising end-diastolic to 100 mm Hg resulted in only a 7.5% decline in developed pressure. At these high end-diastolic pressures, sarcomere lengths[24] averaged 2.27–2.30 μm. Thus, there does not appear to be a descending limb of the sarcomere length–tension curve. A descending limb of function could be demonstrated in dogs when volume loading was carried out to achieve an end-diastolic pressure exceeding 30 mm Hg after mean aortic pressure had initially been elevated.[25] In this setting, slight further increases in aortic pressure occurred with volume loading, and it was concluded that the descending limb of function results from reduced myocardial shortening due to an increased afterload, when the ventricle is unable to compensate by further increases in sarcomere lengths. A similar descending limb of function has been described in the failing human heart when afterload was augmented by vasopressor infusion[26] in the face of absent preload reserve.[27]

Reduction of blood volume or impairment of venous return to the heart will reduce cardiac output correspondingly. Gravitational pooling, positive-pressure ventilation, and particularly positive end-expiratory pressure (PEEP) reduce venous return. Acute elevation of intrapericardial pressure (uremic effusion, postoperative bleeding) or

chronic constrictive pericarditis limits ventricular filling, despite normal or elevated right atrial pressure.

Afterload

As applied to the ventricle, *afterload* may be defined as the tension, force, or stress (force per unit cross-sectional area) in the ventricular wall. In the organism, afterload is determined largely by the peripheral vascular resistance, the physical characteristics of the arterial system, and the volume of blood that it contains at the onset of ejection.

Afterload elevation in the intact organism frequently results in a compensatory rise of ventricular end-diastolic volume and radius (*preload*). LaPlace's law dictates that myocardial wall tension will rise further and, as a consequence, fiber shortening will be reduced. However, geometric considerations indicate that stroke volume may remain constant even though myocardial fiber shortening declines, assuming that venous inflow is not limited and preload can rise. The cardiac response to increased aortic pressure is dependent on both the level of myocardial contractility and the preload so that the normal heart responds to a moderate pressor stress by maintaining or increasing stroke volume,[26] while in the failing heart, with impaired contractility and already elevated preload, stroke volume will decline.[27] As a corollary, a reduction in afterload will not greatly alter stroke volume in the normal heart, but will increase it in the failing heart.

Afterload becomes an increasingly important determinant of cardiac performance when muscle function is impaired. Recognition of this relationship in the past decade has resulted in the adaptation of vasodilator therapy for the management of myocardial failure,[28] mitral[29] and aortic[30] insufficiency, intraoperative hypertension with left ventricular dysfunction,[31] and low cardiac output after cardiac operations[32] using sodium nitroprusside,[33] hydralazine,[34] and occasionally nitroglycerin.

A positive inotropic effect following abrupt elevation of systolic aortic pressure was described by Von Anrep[35] in 1912 and has been termed the *Anrep effect* or homeometric autoregulation.

CONTRACTILITY

Myocardial contractility indicates the inotropic state of the muscle independent of loading conditions. The maximum rate or rise of ventricular pressure (max *dp/dt*) is highly sensitive to changes in contractility.[36] When measured before aortic valve opening, it is independent of afterload;[37] but it may be altered by fluctuations in preload and ventricular volume and it cannot be corrected for changes in muscle mass secondary to hypertrophy.[38]

Contractility may be measured as velocity of the contractile element (V_{ce}) and calculated as *dp/dt/KP* where *K* is a stiffness constant for the elastic series element and *P* is simultaneous intraventricular pressure. When extrapolated to zero pressure, V_{ce} becomes V_{max}, which is relatively independent of acute changes in preload at low left ventricular pressures[39] but declines at end-diastolic pressures[40] exceeding 10 mm Hg. The V_{max} extrapolated relation is also influenced by the model chosen (total pressure is used in the Voight model and developed pressure in the Maxwell model).

The mean velocity of circumferential fiber shortening (V_{cf}) in circumference/s is calculated as the quotient of circumferential fiber shortening during ejection (in circumferences) and ejection time (in seconds).[41] Afterload and contractility codetermine V_{cf} so that this measurement cannot be used to estimate contractility in conditions of extraordinary afterload.[42]

The end-systolic pressure–volume relationship (ESPVR) is one of three relatively load-insensitive indices of contractility.[43] To define this relationship left ventricular end-systolic pressure (P_{es}) and volume (V_{es}) points are determined through each cardiac cycle during abrupt preload reduction (caval occlusion) and a straight line fitted to these points [$P_{es} = E_{es} (V_{es} - V_0)$] where E_{es} and V_0 are the slope and volume–axis intercept, respectively. Linear extrapolation of this line would misrepresent a curvilinear relationship beyond the range of measured data. Calculation of the left ventricular end-systolic volume required to generate an end-systolic pressure of 100 mm Hg ($E_{es\,100}$), which incorporates changes in both the slope and the volume–axis intercept of the LV ESPVR, allows it to be reliably used as a single variable to quantify left ventricular contractility.[44] An increase in $E_{es\,100}$ indicates that a greater end-diastolic volume is required to obtained an end-systolic pressure of 100 mm Hg (impaired contractility) and a decrease in $E_{es\,100}$ reflects a smaller EDV and improved contractility.

The other two indices are preload recruitable stroke work (PRSW)[45] and the dP/dt_{max}–end-diastolic volume (EDV) relationship.[46] The external pressure–volume left ventricular stroke work (SW) is computed as the area within each left ventricular pressure–volume loop throughout the cardiac cycle:

$$SW = \int P \cdot dV$$

The left ventricular PRSW and dP/dt_{max}–EDV relationships are obtained by the following linear regressions: $SW = M_w (\text{EDV} - V_w)$ and $dP/dt_{max} = M_{dP/dt} (\text{EDV} - V_{dP/dt})$, where M_w, V_w, $M_{dP/dt}$, and $V_{dP/dt}$ represent the slope and volume–axis intercepts for each relationship, respectively. As above, to avoid linear extrapolation beyond the range of acquired data, the EDV required to obtain an SW of 1000 mm Hg/mL (PRSW$_{1000}$) and EDV required to obtain a dP/dt_{max} of 1500 mm Hg/s (dP/dt_{1500}) are calculated and used to characterize global left ventricular systolic function.[44]

Release of norepinephrine by intramyocardial sympathetic nerve endings is probably the most important regulator of myocardial contractility.[47] Release of norepinephrine and epinephrine from the nerve-stimulated adrenal medulla results in blood-borne catecholamine stimulation of the heart. Exogenous inotropic agents include cardiac glycosides, isoproterenol, dopamine, dobutamine, and Ca^{2+}.

Negative inotropic influences include β-adrenergic receptor-blocking agents, norepinephrine-depleting agents (reserpine, guanethidine), calcium channel-blocking agents (nifedipine, diltiazem), anoxia,[48] and acidosis.[49]

Heart Rate

At a constant stroke volume, cardiac output is a linear function of heart rate, so that this a critical mechanism for the adjustment of cardiac output. The importance of this mechanism is reflected in the inability of the patient with third-degree heart block to elevate cardiac output appropriately even when the myocardium is normal. Thus, this is the most important mechanism for adjustment of cardiac output during exercise, and it is obviously dependent on increasing venous return as heart rate is augmented to achieve an increased cardiac output. If heart rate is artificially varied between 60 and 160 beats/min in the resting state, there is little effect on cardiac output because venous return is stable.[47] Ultimately, the augmented cardiac output achieved by tachycardia is limited by the increasing proportion of the cardiac cycle occupied by systole and the reduction of time for diastolic filling.

Increasing the heart rate also improves myocardial contractility in isolated cardiac muscle and in the anesthetized dog.[48] In humans, the positive inotropic effect is less than in the anesthetized animal, the depressed heart, and isolated cardiac muscle.[48]

CARDIAC PERFORMANCE

Determination of cardiac performance is important to the surgeon from the standpoint of assessing operative risk and for management of the patient intraoperatively and postoperatively. When myocardial contractility is normal, cardiac output is dependent on peripheral factors that regulate preload and afterload. In myocardial failure, enhancement of contractility with digitalis or catecholamines may elevate cardiac output significantly, but a suboptimal preload, or, more likely, an elevated afterload (secondary to heightened sympathetic activity) may significantly limit the improvement in cardiac output. Thus, assessment of cardiac performance requires measurement of cardiac output, loading conditions, and contractility. It is the latter determinant of function that has proven most elusive to determine, and the many indices of contractility that have been proposed attest to this lack.

Measurement of cardiac output (L/min) is readily accomplished by thermodilution and, when divided by the body surface area (m^2), gives the cardiac index. The normal range for cardiac index (2.5–4.2 L/min per m^2) is so broad that it becomes an insensitive parameter of cardiac function. Nevertheless, this measurement is particularly valuable in the care of the patient having open heart surgery where the cardiac index is frequently below normal following operation and directional changes to therapeutic endeavors, when combined with measurement of preload and afterload, indicate the appropriateness of interventions.

Left ventricular end-diastolic pressure can be measured as mean left atrial pressure, mean pulmonary wedge pressure, and, in the absence of pulmonary vascular disease, as pulmonary diastolic pressure. The finding of a normal cardiac index and left ventricular filling pressure (6–12 mm Hg) is a more accurate indicator of normal contractility than is either measurement alone. An elevation of filling pressure and a depressed cardiac index indicate that contractility is probably impaired. Elevation of left ventricular filling pressure does not necessarily mean an increased diastolic volume because ventricular compliance may be reduced by pericardial disease, restrictive myocardial disease, myocardial hypertrophy, and myocardial ischemia so that end-diastolic volume remains normal, despite elevated filling pressures.

Cardiac chamber volume can be measured with single or biplane contrast ventriculography,[50] by radionuclide cardioangiography,[51] or by two-dimensional echocardiography.[52] From these data, it is possible to determine left ventricular end-diastolic and end-systole volumes, muscle mass, and segmental wall motion. The normal left ventricle has a volume of 70 ± 20 mL/m^2 SD (standard deviation).[3,53] The thickness of the left ventricular wall averages 10.9 ± 2.0 m^2 (SD) and the muscle mass 92 ± 16 g/m^2 (SD) of body surface area.[54]

The ratio of stroke volume (the amount ejected in one cardiac cycle) to end-diastolic volume is the *ejection fraction* (EF), which is an index of ventricular fiber shortening and is one of the most useful measures of pump function. The EF averages 0.67 ± 0.08 (SD) in normal subjects.[55] The EF is closely related to and can be predicted from the percentage of shortening (fractional shortening) during systole of the left ventricular minor axis, which can also be determined by echocardiography.[56] The *fractional shortening* (FS = $32 \pm 5\%$) is calculated from the diameter perpendicular to the midpoint of the long axis of the left ventricle. Visual assessment of segmental wall motion from the contrast ventriculogram provides a useful and simple way to quantitate ventricular function.[57]

Ejection phase indices of ventricular performance (EF, FS, V_{cf}) decline when end-diastolic volume (preload) is acutely reduced or aortic pressure (afterload) is acutely elevated. Conversely, ejection phase indices may be normal in conditions of reduced afterload (e.g., mitral regurgitation, arteriovenous fistula) even though contractility is depressed. Thus, these indices do not simply reflect changes in contractility, but they are useful in determining the level of contractility in the basal state in the presence of chronic heart disease in which the influence of changes in preload and afterload tends to be corrected for by compensatory dilatation and hypertrophy.[58–60]

Accurate measurement of *dp/dt* is not possible with usual catheter-manometer systems, and catheter-tip micromanometers are needed. Measurements of contractile element velocity are likewise limited by the difficulties in determining *dp/dt*. The isovolumetric phase indices (peak *dp/dt*, V_{ce}, V_{max}) are of limited value clinically and have had little application in the management of patients related to operation, although they have been employed in clinical research.

Management of the patient during and after cardiac operations relies on measurements of preload (left atrial pressure, pulmonary wedge, or diastolic pressure), afterload (aortic pressure), heart rate, and cardiac output. Suboptimal preload is altered by transfusion or infusion. Excessive preload can be reduced by vasodilating drugs (nitroprusside, nitroglycerin), which increase venous capacitance and thereby sequester a portion of the blood volume and decrease preload. Afterload is related primarily to cardiac output and systemic (peripheral) vascular resistance, which can be calculated as

$$SVRI = \frac{MAP - RAP}{CI} \times 80$$

where SVRI is systemic vascular resistance index, MAP is mean arterial pressure, RAP is right atrial pressure, and CI is cardiac index. Most commonly, the SVRI is elevated (normal range = 1700–2400 dyn/s per cm^{-5}) and can be lowered with vasodilating drugs (above), which in turn will reduce mean arterial pressure, facilitate ventricular emptying, and increase cardiac output. The major limitation to vasodilator therapy is maintaining an adequate mean arterial pressure (60 mm Hg) for coronary perfusion. Vasodilator therapy is frequently helpful and should be considered in all patients with reduced cardiac output after calculation of systemic vascular resistance. An occasional patient has excessive vasodilation with a low arterial pressure and requires vasoconstrictor therapy (norepinephrine or epinephrine). Contractility is assessed by inference, and the use of inotropic agents is based on failure of optimal preload and afterload to achieve an adequate cardiac index (2.2 L/min per m^2).

The pulmonary artery balloon-tipped, thermistor catheter is commonly introduced percutaneously via the right internal jugular vein at the time of induction of anesthesia to measure pulmonary artery pressure, wedge pressure, and thermodilution cardiac output.[61] This catheter has a proximal opening positioned in the right atrium with an associated thermistor to record the temperature of a 10-mL bolus of normal saline, which mixes with and cools the blood in the right side of the heart; the final temperature is recorded by a second thermistor at the tip of the catheter and is related to the flow rate. This catheter has been modified by adding an oxygen sensing electrode for continuous measurement of pulmonary artery oxygen saturation (PaO$_2$), which represents mixed venous oxygen[62] (PvO$_2$).

When the heart is exposed, a left atrial catheter may be introduced for direct measurement of left atrial pressure in the instance of pulmonary hypertension or to assess mitral valve function when there is associated mitral valve disease. Left ventricular function may also be monitored intraoperatively by means of transesophageal two-dimensional echocardiography.[63] Operatively implanted ultrasonic dimension gauges (sonomicrometry) have been used to measure wall thickening, segmental wall motion, and the minor axis of the left ventricle to permit determination of systolic and diastolic properties of the left ventricle.[64–66]

CORONARY FLOW AND MYOCARDIAL OXYGEN CONSUMPTION

Just as the heart provides for the circulatory needs of the body, it also supplies its own metabolic requirements through the coronary circulation. Because of the limited capacity for anaerobic metabolism to support cardiac work, its metabolism can be considered to be essentially aerobic from the standpoint of function, although anaerobic metabolism is highly important from the viewpoint of ischemic injury and myocardial preservation.

A unique feature to the coronary circulation is the high degree of oxygen extraction under basal conditions (coronary venous oxygen saturation is 20–30%) so that the heart can adjust to changing oxygen needs by only a small increment in oxygen extraction. Accordingly, increasing oxygen requirements must be met by proportionate increases in coronary flow.

CORONARY FLOW

Coronary Hemodynamics

Coronary flow, as in any vascular bed, is a function of driving pressure and resistance as stated in the equation $Q = P/R$, where Q is coronary flow, P is the driving pressure across the coronary vascular bed, and R is total coronary resistance.

Viscous resistance (R_1) can be defined as the impedance to flow offered by the entire coronary vascular bed during diastole when fully dilated and can be considered to be relatively static.

Autoregulatory resistance (R_2) is a major component of resistance (being four to five times greater than R_1) and is thought to result from tonic contraction of vascular smooth muscle at the arteriolar level. Control of this autoregulatory resistance has been and continues to be intensely investigated. Of the three mechanisms for adjusting arteriolar tone (metabolic, neurohumoral, and myogenic) the first is thought to be most important.

Although numerous agents have been proposed as metabolic regulators of coronary resistance, the role of

adenosine is pivotal in current thinking.[67] With the onset of myocardial hypoxia, adenosine is formed from 5′-adenosine monophosphate (5′-AMP) and released into the interstitial space where it produces vasodilation by an unexplained action on resistance vessels. Adenosine is removed by (1) conversion to inosine and hypoxanthine in red cells and vascular endothelium, (2) transport across the sarcolemma into the myocyte, and (3) intravascular transport. Adenosine is found in very small concentrations (10^{-9} M) in myocardial perfusates, tissue homegenates, and coronary sinus blood.[68–71] Others believe that adenosine is not the primary metabolic controller of coronary resistance and that this is a role for prostaglandins.[72]

Coronary vascular smooth muscle is known to be responsive to neurohumoral stimuli including adrenergic constrictor and dilator mechanisms.[73,74] A vagal cholinergic dilator mechanism has also been described.[75]

Compressive resistance (R_3) arises from compression of vascular channels by intramyocardial pressure as it varies through the cardiac cycle. There is an intramyocardial systolic pressure gradient that varies from 20 to 40 mm Hg in the outer third of the myocardium to 100 mg Hg or more in the inner third.[76–80] Diastolic intramyocardial pressures have been measured at 4 to 20 mm Hg without a transmural gradient.[73,75,81] In the empty beating (on cardiopulmonary bypass) normal or hypertrophic heart the gradient in myocardial tissue pressure persists.[76–78] Ventricular fibrillation is associated with a continuous gradient across the ventricular wall and a subendocardial pressure of 50 mm Hg in the normal heart and 67 mm Hg in the hypertrophic heart.[82–84]

The transmural gradient in intramyocardial pressure during systole is primarily responsible for the normal phasic coronary flow in which 70–80% of flow occurs during diastole.[85,86] Thus, little or no coronary flow reaches the middle and deep myocardium during systole when flow is limited to more superficial layers of the myocardium.[87] To compensate for this systolic maldistribution, a correspondingly greater proportion of diastolic flow must be delivered to the inner myocardium. This is accomplished by reduction of autoregulatory tone in the deeper myocardium so that resistance is lower than in the more superficial myocardium permitting greater subendocardial perfusion.[88] With maximal subendocardial vasodilation, bloodflow is dependent on mean diastolic aortic pressure (driving pressure) minus left ventricular diastolic pressure and the duration of diastole, which can be defined by the superimposed aortic and left ventricular pressure tracings and the subtended area.[89] This area (Fig. 96–5) was designated the *diastolic pressure time index* (DPTI), and when multiplied by heart rate, it represents the driving pressure and time available for perfusing the subendocardial muscle every minute. The area under the left ventricular pressure curve in systole was termed the *systolic pressure time index* (SPTI) and was used as a measure of left ventricular oxygen needs. This area has been traditionally termed the *tension–time index*[90]

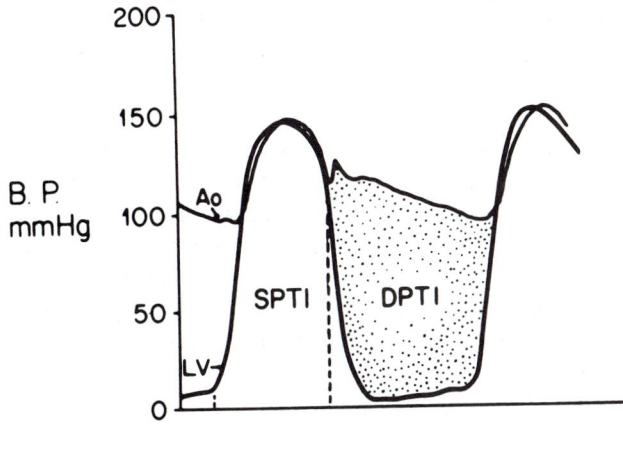

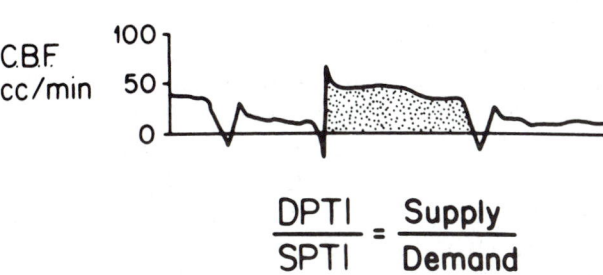

$$\frac{DPTI}{SPTI} = \frac{Supply}{Demand}$$

Figure 96–5. Superimposed left ventricular and central aortic pressure tracings (above) and simultaneous recording of coronary flow in the anesthetized dog. The importance of diastole (stippled areas) when approximately 80% of coronary flow occurs is emphasized. SPTI (estimate of left ventricular myocardial oxygen need, or demand) is measured as the area under the systolic portion of the left ventricular pressure curve from the onset of systole to closure of the aortic valve (excludes period of isometric relaxation). DPTI (estimate of potential flow to the left ventricular subendocardium, or supply) is measured as the area between the aortic and left ventricular pressure curves from the closure of the aortic valve until the next upstroke of aortic pressure (includes period of isometric contraction of next systole). The ratio of these areas, DPTI:SPTI, describes the theoretical supply–demand relationship of the subendocardial layer of the left ventricle. Ao, aortic; CBF, coronary blood flow; DPTI, diastolic pressure time index; LV, left ventricle; SPTI, systolic pressure time index. *(From Vincent WR, Buckberg GD, Hoffman JIE: Left ventricular subendocardial ischemia in severe valvular and supravalvular aortic stenosis. Circulation 49:326, 1974, with permission.)*

and has been shown to relate to oxygen consumption of the left ventricle.[90,91] Therefore, the ratio of DPTI:SPTI reflects blood supply and oxygen demand, and a reduction in the ratio to a critical level may be associated with subendocardial ischemia. To assess ischemia, the ratio of subendocardial to subepicardial flow per gram (determined with radioactive microspheres) was used with the assumption that subepicardial flow represents the flow needed by the myocardium because it is unrestricted (or minimally so) by intramyocardial pressure.[88] When the DPTI:SPTI ratio was lowered, the ratio of subendocardial to subepicardial flow per gram remained about 1 until a critical supply–demand

ratio of about 0.7 was reached, after which both ratios fell together.[89] Relative subendocardial ischemia occurred only after maximal vasodilation had been attained as shown by minimal or absent reactive hyperemia.[89,90]

This model relating myocardial supply/demand to the ratio of subendocardial/subepicardial flow is important because it brings to focus the transmural variation in coronary flow and the vulnerability of the subendocardium to ischemic injury. Not only is subendocardial injury frequently secondary to coronary disease,[92] which reduces driving pressure below that defined by the DPTI, but it is a common complication of cardiac operations.[93–95] Intraoperative and postoperative conditions of ventricular fibrillation, ventricular hypertrophy, aortic stenosis, aortic regurgitation, anemia, arterial desaturation, hypotension, tachycardia, catecholamine excess, coronary stenosis or occlusion, and elevated left ventricular and diastolic pressure may unfavorably alter the supply/demand relationship and result in subendocardial ischemia, injury, and secondary pump failure.[87]

Coronary Microcirculation

The coronary microcirculation is highly important but less well studied than other aspects of the coronary circulation. The concept of capillary recruitment to increase capillary density and decrease intercapillary distance is basic with regard to delivery of oxygen to the subendocardium and the balance between myocardial oxygen demand and supply. During arterial hypoxemia, mean intercapillary distance decreased from 17 to 11 μm, which corresponds to doubling of the number of open capillaries.[96] Measurements of tissue oxygen with O_2 electrodes, although problematic, seem to show a lower level of interstitial partial pressure of oxygen, arterial (P_{O_2}) in the subendocardium than in the subepicardium. This finding suggests that oxygen extraction is greater in the subendocardium than in the subepicardium, and this concept is supported by direct measurements of regional venous oxygen saturation in isolated hearts developing normal left ventricular pressures.[97] Since flow per gram of myocardium is the same in the inner and outer layers of the heart,[98,99] it follows that oxygen uptake may normally be greater in the subendocardium than in the subepicardium. This may reflect greater oxygen demands in the inner layer of the heart, which is consistent with models of transmural variations in developed stress[84,100] and in vivo measures of transmural variations in diastolic sarcomere length.[7] Although interstitial P_{O_2} may be less in the inner than outer myocardium, oxygen tension at the mitochondrial level can be maintained by capillary recruitment and reduction of intercapillary distances so that diffusion distances are reduced and intracellular P_{O_2} is maintained despite increased arteriovenous O_2 extraction.[101] Intracellular measurements of P_{O_2} have revealed very low levels (4–6 mm Hg) with little change when arterial O_2 saturation was reduced to as low as 40–50%.[102]

MYOCARDIAL OXYGEN CONSUMPTION

Carefully controlled animal studies have delineated factors that govern oxygen requirements of the myocardium. Although mean myocardial oxygen consumption (MVO$_2$) is difficult to measure, clinical studies have been consistent with laboratory data. The normal heart has sufficient coronary reserve to meet myocardial oxygen needs, but knowledge of the determinants of myocardial oxygen demand is critical to the management of patients with cardiac disease.

The oxygen cost of pressure development or "pressure work" as opposed to "volume work" was demonstrated by Sarnoff et al.[90] Although their tension–time index correlated with oxygen consumption better than other parameters of aortic pressure or systolic duration alone, subsequent studies revealed the dominant effect of pressure development alone.[103] Oxygen consumption correlated with the tension–time index only until the peak systolic pressure had been attained, at which point 91% of oxygen consumption per beat had occurred.[103] Thus, myocardial oxygen consumption is not a uniform function of the duration of systole (tension–time index) because it is insensitive to the duration of pressure maintenance between peak systolic pressure and the end of relaxation. Wall stress is more fundamentally related to MVO$_2$ than is pressure development.[104] This fact explains how digitalis may increase oxygen requirements of the normal heart (through its inotropic effect) and not change oxygen requirements of the failing heart by virtue of reduced dimensions and diminished wall stress according to LaPlace's law.[105] External work requires only a small portion of the total oxygen consumed by the heart (6% in a depressed preparation,[106] which may be extrapolated to 15–20% in a more normal heart).

Myocardial contractility or inotropic state is the second major determinant of MVO$_2$. Inotropic interventions (norepinephrine, calcium, or paired electrical stimulation) that increase V_{max} by 50% result in a 40% increase in MVO$_2$.[107] Myocardial contractility is as important as pressure development as a determinant of MVO$_2$.[108]

The fairly direct relationship between heart rate and myocardial oxygen consumption is well known.[90] When oxygen consumption per beat is measured, it did not exceed that which could be accounted for on the basis of the concomitant increase in the velocity of the contractile element.[109]

Basal oxygen requirements of the potassium plegic heart (2.0 mL/100 g per minute) are about 20% of the oxygen consumption of the working heart.[110] Catecholamine stimulation of the working and arrested heart indicated that 20% of the total increased oxygen demand in the contracting heart could be measured in the arrested heart, which represents enhanced basal cell metabolism.[111]

Finally, the oxygen cost of electrical activation of the heart has been determined to be less than 1% of the oxygen need of the normal working heart.[112]

Knowing that pressure development is costly in my-

ocardial oxygen demand, the surgeon will be alert to vigorously treat hypertension occurring perioperatively or in the patient awaiting coronary bypass. This is best accomplished with continuous intravenous infusion of vasodilating drugs such as nitroglycerin, nitroprusside, and hydralazine. β-Blocking drugs reduce contractility and heart rate, but must be used cautiously when these compensatory mechanisms are critical to adequate myocardial performance in the face of lesions such as aortic stenosis. Calcium channel-blocking agents are similarly useful and limited, but have a more favorable effect on peripheral vascular resistance than β-blockers.

COMMENT

The function and physiology of the cardiovascular system do not change. Our understanding of the system advances as we gain new insights through continued experimental and clinical observations, which derive in part from new tools that provide information not attainable or imprecise in the past. These new insights and data may then enhance our understanding of older data, modify original conclusions, or permit the emergence of new concepts and principles.

REFERENCES

1. Starling EH: *Linacre Lecture on the Law of the Heart (1915)*. London, Longmans, Green, 1918
2. Hill AV: The heat of shortening and the dynamic constants of muscle. *Proc R Soc London Ser B* **126**:136, 1938
3. Sonnenblick EH, Spino D, Cottrell JS: Fine structural changes in heart muscle in relation to the length-tension curve. *Proc Natl Acad Sci USA* **49**:193, 1963
4. Pollack AH, Huntsman LL: Sarcomere length-active force relations in living mammalian cardiac muscle. *Am J Physiol* **227**:383, 1974
5. Frank O: On the dynamics of cardiac muscle (Chaporan CB, Wasserman E, trans). *Am Heart J* **58**:282, 1959
6. Sponitz HM, Sonnenblick EH, Spiro D: Relation of ultrastructure and function in the intact heart: Sarcomere structure relative to pressure-volume curves of the intact left ventricles of dog and cat. *Circ Res* **18**:49, 1966
7. Yoran C, Covell JW, Ross J Jr: Structural basis for ascending limb of left ventricular function. *Circ Res* **32**:297, 1973
8. Abbott BC, Mommaerts WFHM: A study of inotropic mechanisms in the papillary muscle preparation. *J Gen Physiol* **42**:533, 1959
9. Sommenblick EH: Force-velocity relations in mammalian heart muscle. *Am J Physiol* **202**:931, 1962
10. Henderson AH, Van Ocken E, Brutsaert DL: A reappraisal of force-velocity measurements in isolated heart muscle preparation. *Eur J Cardiol* **1**:105, 1973
11. Grossman W, Braunwald E, Mann T, et al: Contractile state of the left ventricle in man as evaluated from end-systolic pressure-volume relations. *Circulation* **56**:845, 1977
12. Jewell BR: A reexamination of the influence of muscle length on myocardial performance. *Circ Res* **40**:366, 1977
13. Fabiato A, Fabiato F: Dependence of the contractile activation of skinned cardiac cells on the sarcomere length. *Nature (London)* **256**:54, 1975

14. Allen DG, Blinks JR: Calcium transients in aequorin-injected frog cardiac muscle. *Nature (London)* **273**:509, 1978

15. Huntsman LL, Stewart DK: Length-dependent calcium inotropism in cat papillary muscle. *Circ Res* **40**:366, 1977

16. Jewell BR: The physiology of cardiac muscle contraction. In Dickinson CJ, Marks J (eds): *Developments in Cardiovascular Medicine.* Cambridge, MA, MIT Press, 1978, pp 129–144

17. Rankin JS, McHale PA, Arentzen CE, et al: The three dimensional geometry of the left ventricle in the conscious dog. *Circ Res* **39**:304, 1976

18. Ross J Jr, Sonnenblick EH, Covell JW, et al: The architecture of the hearts in systole and diastole: Technique of rapid fixation and the analysis of the left ventricular geometry. *Circ Res* **21**:409, 1967

19. Sandler H, Alderman E: Determination of left ventricular size and shape. *Circ Res* **34**:1, 1974

20. Greenbaum RA, Ho SY, Gibson DG, et al: Left ventricular fibre architecture in man. *Br Heart J* **45**:248–263, 1981

21. Rademakers FE, Rogers WJ, Guier WH, et al: Relation of regional cross-fiber shortening to wall thickening in the intact heart. *Circulation* **89**:1174–1182, 1994

22. Parker JO, Case RB: Normal left ventricular function. *Circulation* **60**:4, 1979

23. Katz AM: The descending limb of the Starling curve and the failing heart (Editorial). *Circulation* **32**:871, 1965

24. Monroe RA, Gamble WJ, LaFarge CG, et al: Left ventricular performance at high end diastolic pressures in isolated, perfused dog hearts. *Circ Res* **26**:85, 1970

25. MacGregor DC, Covell JW, Mahler F, et al: Relation between afterload, stroke volume and the descending limb of Starling's curve. *Am J Physiol* **227**:884, 1974

26. Ross J Jr, Braunwald E: The study of left ventricular function in man by increasing resistance to ventricular ejection with angiotension. *Circulation* **29**:739, 1964

27. Ross J Jr: Afterload mismatch and preload reserve: A conceptual framework for the analysis of ventricular function. *Prog Cardiovasc Dis* **18**:255, 1976

28. Chatterjee K, Parmley WW, Massie B, et al: Oral hydralazine therapy for chronic refractory heart failure. *Circulation* **54**:879, 1976

29. Chatterjee K, Parmely WW, Swan HJC, et al: Beneficial effects of vasodilator agents in severe mitral regurgitation due to dysfunction of subvalvular apparatus. *Circulation* **48**:684, 1973

30. Greenberg BH, Demots H, Murphy E, Rahimtoola S: Beneficial effects of hydralazine on rest and exercise hemodynamics in patients with chronic severe aortic sufficiency. *Circulation* **62**:49, 1980

31. Lappas DG, Lowenstein E, Waller J, et al: Hemodynamic effects of nitroprusside infusion during coronary artery operation in man. *Circulation* **54**(Suppl 3):4, 1976

32. Kouchoukos NT, Sheppard LC, Kirklin JW: Effect of alterations in arterial pressure on cardiac performance early after open cardiac operations. *J Thorac Cardiovasc Surg* **64**:563, 1972

33. Stinson ED, Holloway EL, Derby A, et al: Comparative hemodynamic responses to chlorpromazine, nitroprusside, nitroglycerin and trimethaphan immediately after open-heart operations. *Circulation* **51–52**(Suppl 2):26, 1975

34. Swartz MJ, Kaiser GC, Willman VL, et al: Continuous hydralazine infusion for afterload reduction. *Ann Thorac Surg* **31**:549, 1981

35. Von Anrep G: On the part played by the supra-renals in the normal vascular reactions of the body. *J Physiol (London)* **45**:307, 1912

36. Mason DT: Usefulness and limitations of the rate of rise of intraventricular pressure (dp/dt) in the evaluation of myocardial contractility in man. *Am J Cardiol* **23**:516, 1969

37. Wallace AG, Skinner NS Jr, Mitchell JH: Hemodynamic determinants of the maximal rate of left ventricular pressure. *Am J Physiol* **205**:30, 1963

38. Mason DT, Spann JF Jr, Zelis R: Quantification of the contractile state of the intact human heart. Maximal velocity of contractile element shortening determined by the instantaneous relation between the rate of pressure rise and pressure in the left ventricle during isovolumic systole. *Am J Cardiol* **26**:248, 1970

39. Wolk MJ, Keefe FJ, Bing OHL, et al: Estimation of V_{max} is isotonic systoles from the rate of relative increase of isovolumic pressures (dp/dt)dp. *J Clin Invest* **50**:1276, 1971

40. Grossman W, Haynes G, Paraskos JA, et al: Alterations in preload and myocardial mechanics in dog and in man. *Circ Res* **31**:83, 1972

41. Stack RS, Sohn YH, Weissler AM: Accuracy of systolic time intervals in detecting abnormal left ventricular performance in coronary artery disease. *Am J Cardiol* **47**:603, 1981

42. Mahler F, Ross J Jr, O'Rourke RA: Effects of changes in preload, afterload and inotropic state on ejection and isovolumic phase measures of contractility in the conscious dog. *Am J Cardiol* **35**:626, 1975

43. Sagawa K, Suga H, Shoukas AA, et al: End-systolic pressure-volume ratio: A new index of contractility. *Am J Cardiol* **40**:748–753, 1977

44. Toombs CF, Vinten-Johansen J, Yokoyama H, et al: Nonlinearity of indexes of left ventricular performance: Effects on estimation of slope and diameter axis intercepts. *Am J Physiol* **260**:H1802–1809, 1991

45. Glower DD, Spratt JA, Snow ND, et al: Linearity of the Frank-Starling relationship in the intact heart: The concept of preload recruitable stroke work. *Circulation* **71**:994–1009, 1985

46. Little WC: The left ventricular dP/dt$_{max}$–end diastolic volume relation in closed-chest dogs. *Circ Res* **56**:808–815, 1985

47. Yamogouchie N, deChamplain J, Nadeau R: Correlation between the response of the heart to sympathetic stimulation and the release of endogenous catecholamines into the coronary sinus of the dog. *Circ Res* **36**:662, 1975

48. Beierholm EA, Grantham RN, O'Keefe DD, et al: Effects of acid-base changes, hypoxia and catecholamines on ventricular performance. *Am J Physiol* **228**:1555, 1975

49. Williamson JR, Shaffer SW, Ford C, Safen B: Contribution of tissue acidosis to ischemic injury in the perfused rate heart. *Circulation* **53**(Suppl 1):3, 1976

50. Dodge HT, Sandler H, Ballew DW, Lord JD Jr: The use of biplane angiocardiography for the measurement of left ventricular volume in man. *Am Heart J* **60**:762, 1960

51. Upton MT, Rerych SK, Newman GE, et al: The reproducibility of radionuclide, angiographic measurements of left ventricular function in normal subjects at rest and during exercise. *Circulation* **62**:126, 1980

52. Schiller NB, Acquatella H, Ports TA, et al: Left ventricular volume from paired biplane two-dimensional echocardiography. *Circulation* **60**:760, 1979

53. Milnor WR: Arterial impedance as ventricular afterload. *Circ Res* **36**:965, 1975

54. Rackley CE: Quantitative evaluation of left ventricular function by radiologic techniques. *Circulation* **54**:862, 1976

55. Dodge HT: Hemodynamic aspects of cardiac failure. In Braunwald E (ed): *The Myocardium: Failure and Infarction.* New York, H.P. Publishing, 1974, pp 70–79

56. Fortuin NJ, Hood WP Jr, Sherman ME: Determination of left ventricular volumes by ultrasound. *Circulation* **44**:575, 1971

57. Griffith LSC, Achaff SC, Conti CR: Changes in intrinsic coronary circulation and segmental ventricular motion after saphenous vein coronary bypass graft surgery. *N Engl J Med* **288**:589, 1979

58. Dodge HT, Baxley WA: Left ventricular volume and mass and their significance in heart disease. *Am J Cardiol* **23**:528, 1969

59. Ross J Jr, McCullogh WH: The nature of enhanced performance of the dilated left ventricle during chronic volume overloading. *Circ Res* **30**:549, 1972

60. Sasayama S, Theroux P, Romero M, et al: Adaption of the left ventricle to chronic pressure overload. *Am J Cardiol* **35**:167, 1975

61. Swan HJC, Ganz W, Forrester JW, et al: Catheterization of the heart in man with use of a flow-directed balloon-tipped catheter. *N Engl J Med* **283**:447, 1970

62. Schweiss JF: Mixed venous hemoglobin saturation; theory and application. *Int Anestesiol Clin* **25**:113, 1987

63. Cahalan MK, Kremer P, Schiller NB, et al: Intraoperative monitoring with two-dimensional transesophageal echocardiography. *Anesthesiology* **57**:A153, 1982

64. Chitwood WR, Hill RC, Sink JD, et al: Measurement of global ventricular function in patients during cardiac operations using sonomicrometry. *J Thorac Cardiovasc Surg* **80**:724, 1980

65. Chitwood WR, Hill RC, Sink JD, Wechsler AJ: Diastolic ventricular properties in patients during coronary revascularization. *J Thorac Cardiovasc Surg* **85**:595, 1983

66. Moores WY, LeWinter MM, Long WB, et al: Sonomicrometry: Its application as a routine monitoring technique in cardiac surgery. *Ann Thorac Surg* **38**:117, 1984

67. Rubio R, Berne RM: Regulation of coronary blood flow. *Prog Cardiovasc Dis* **18**:105, 1975

68. Rubio R, Berne RM, Katori M: Release of adenosine in restrictive hyperemia of the dog heart. *Am J Physiol* **216**:56, 1969

69. Rubio R, Berne RM: Release of adenosine by the normal myocardium in dogs and its relationship to the regulation of coronary resistance. *Circ Res* **25**:407, 1969

70. Fox AC, Reed GE, Glassman E: Release of adenosine from human hearts during angina induced by rapid atrial pacing. *J Clin Invest* **53**:1447, 1974

71. Olsson RA: Changes in content of purine nucleoside in canine myocardium during coronary occlusion. *Circ Res* **26**:301, 1970

72. Block AJ, Feinberg H, Herbaczynska-Cedro K: Anoxia-induces release of prostaglandins in rabbit isolated hearts. *Circ Res* **36**:34, 1975

73. Berne RM, DeGeest H, Levy MN: Influence of the cardiac nerves on coronary resistance. *Am J Physiol* **208**:763, 1965

74. Pitt B, Elliot EC, Gregg DE: Adrenergic receptor activity in the coronary arteries of the unanesthetized dog. *Circ Res* **21**:75, 1967

75. Fiegl EO: Parasympathetic control of coronary blood flow in dogs. *Circ Res* **25**:509, 1969

76. Johnson JR, DiPalma JR: Intramyocardial pressure and its relationships to aortic blood pressure. *Am J Physiol* **125**:234, 1939

77. Gregg DE, Eckstein RW: Measurements of intramyocardial pressure. *Am J Physiol* **132**:781, 1941

78. Amour JA, Randall WC: Canine left ventricular intramyocardial pressures. *Am J Physiol* **220**:1833, 1971

79. Baird RJ, Manktelow RT, Shah PA, Ameli FM: Intramyocardial pressure: A study of its regional variations and its relationship to intraventricular pressure. *J Thorac Cardiovasc Surg* **59**:810, 1970

80. Archie JP Jr: Intramyocardial pressure: Effect of preload on transmural distribution of systolic coronary flow. *Am J Cardiol* **35**:904, 1975

81. D'Silva JL, Mendel D, Winterton MC: Determinants of intramyocardial pressure in the cat. *Am J Physiol* **207**:1117, 1964

82. Baird RJ, Goldbach MM, DeLaRocha A: Intramyocardial pressure: The persistence of its transmural gradient in the empty heart and its relationship to myocardial oxygen consumption. *J Thorac Cardiovasc Surg* **64**:635, 1972

83. Baird RJ, Dutka F, Okumori M, et al: Surgical aspects of regional myocardial blood flow and myocardial pressure. *J Thorac Cardiovasc Surg* **69**:17, 1976

84. Archie JP: Determinants of intramyocardial pressure. *J Surg Res* **19**:338, 1973

85. Gregg DE, Lowenshohn HS, Rayford CR: Systemic and coronary energetics in the resting unanesthetized dog. *Circ Res* **16**:102, 1965

86. Khouri EM, Gregg DE, Rayford CR: Effect of exercise on cardiac output, left coronary flow and myocardial metabolism in the unanesthetized dog. *Circ Res* **17**:427, 1965

87. Hoffman JIE, Buckberg GD: Transmural variations in myocardial perfusion. In Yu PN, Goodwin JF (eds): *Progress in Cardiology,* Vol 5. Philadelphia, Lea & Febiger, 1976, pp 37–89

88. Griggs DM Jr, Nakamura Y: Effects of coronary constriction on myocardial distribution of iodoantipyrine-131 I. *Am J Physiol* **215**:1082, 1968

89. Buckberg GD, Fixler DE, Archie JC, Hoffman JIE: Experimental subendocardial ischemia in dogs with normal coronary arteries. *Circ Res* **30**:67, 1972

90. Sarnoff SJ, Braunwald E, Welch GH Jr, et al: Hemodynamic determinants of oxygen consumption of the heart with special reference to the tension time index. *Am J Physiol* **192**: 148, 1958

91. McDonald RH, Taylor RR, Cingolani HE: Measurement of myocardial developed tension and its relationship to oxygen consumption. *Am J Physiol* **211**:667, 1966

92. Edwards JE: Correlations in coronary arterial disease. *Bull NY Acad Med* **33**:199, 1957

93. Taber RE, Morales AR, Fine G: Myocardial necrosis and the postoperative low cardiac output syndrome. *Ann Thorac Surg* **4**:12, 1967

94. Najafi H, Henson D, Dye WS, et al: Left ventricular hemorrhagic necrosis. *Ann Thorac Surg* **7**:550, 1969

95. Buckberg GD, Towers B, Paglia DE, et al: Subendocardial ischemia after cardiopulmonary bypass. *J Thorac Cardiovasc Surg* **64**:669, 1972

96. Bourdear-Martini J, Odoroff CL, Honig CR: Dual effect of oxygen on magnitude and uniformity of coronary intercapillary distance. *Am J Physiol* **226**:800, 1974

97. Gamble WJ: Regional coronary venous oxygen saturation and myocardial oxygen tension following abrupt changes in ventricular pressure in the isolated dog heart. *Circ Res* **34**:672, 1974

98. Kirk ES, Honig CR: Non-uniform distribution of blood flow and gradients of oxygen tension within the heart. *Am J Physiol* **207**:661, 1964

99. Moir TW: Subendocardial distribution of coronary blood flow and the effect of antianginal drugs. *Circ Res* **30**:621, 1972

100. Mirsky J: Left ventricular stresses in the intact human heart. *Biophys J* **8**:189, 1969

101. Meyers WW, Honig CR: Number and distribution of capillaries as determinants of myocardial oxygen tension. *Am J Physiol* **207**:653, 1965

102. Coburn RF: Myocardial myoglobin oxygen tension. *Am J Physiol* **224**:870, 1973

103. Monroe RG: Myocardial oxygen consumption during ventricular contraction and relaxation. *Circ Res* **14**:294, 1964

104. Rodbard S, Williams F, Williams C: Spherical dynamics of the heart (myocardial tension, oxygen consumption, coronary blood flow and efficiency). *Am Heart J* **57**:348, 1959

105. Covell JW, Braunwald E, Ross J Jr, Sonnenblick EH: Studies on digitalis. XVI. Effects on myocardial oxygen consumption. *J Clin Invest* **45**:1535, 1966

106. Burns JW, Covell JW: Myocardial oxygen consumption during isotonic and isovolumetric contractions in the intact heart. *Am J Physiol* **225**:1491, 1972

107. Sonnenblick EH: Velocity of contraction as a determinant of myocardial oxygen consumption. *Am J Physiol* **209**:919, 1965

108. Graham TP Jr, Covell JW, Sonnenblick EH, et al: Control of myocardial oxygen consumption: Relative influence of contractile state and tension development. *J Clin Invest* **47**:375, 1968

109. Boerth RC, Covell JW, Pool PE, Ross J Jr: Increased myocardial oxygen consumption and contractile state associated with increased heart rate in dogs. *Circ Res* **24**:725, 1969

110. McKeever WP, Gregg DE, Canney PC: Oxygen uptake of the nonworking left ventricle. *Circ Res* **6**:612, 1958

111. Klocke FJ, Kaiser GA, Ross J Jr, Braunwald E: Mechanism of increase of myocardial oxygen uptake produced by catecholamines. *Am J Physiol* **209**:913, 1965

112. Klocke FJ, Braunwald E, Ross J Jr: Oxygen cost of electrical activation of the heart. *Circ Res* **18**:357, 1966

C H A P T E R
97

The Clinical–Biological Interface

Graeme L. Hammond

The revolution in cardiac surgery that occurred 25 years ago with the development of coronary artery surgery was paralleled by another revolution in the basic sciences—the development of molecular biology. The added burden of patients with coronary artery disease all but precluded the entry of surgeons into this new and powerful area of investigation. As a consequence, a generation of surgeons came of age in almost total isolation from the advances that were occurring in the basic sciences. What surgeons conceived and brought forth as a technically brilliant solution to a serious problem has in retrospect, however, changed cardiac surgery's image and put its future in serious jeopardy.

Laboratory techniques familiar to surgeons, carried out primarily in the dog laboratory, led to the development of cardiothoracic surgery as we know it today. Nevertheless, these techniques are from the past and will no longer hold in today's competitive funding environment. Unfortunately, most surgeons are ill equipped to work at the cellular or subcellular level where advances in cancer therapy, transplantation, organ preservation, ischemia, reperfusion injuries, ARDS, shock, and so forth must be made. Does this mean that surgery, against its tradition, will become scientifically irrelevant? Can surgery maintain influence at the NIH? Considering the time and attention to detail required for research, will interested surgeons lose clinical credibility and stature? These are difficult questions, and the answers are not in sight.

Before time and events reveal the answers, it is helpful to examine where surgeons fit into the larger picture of advancing fundamental knowledge. Although grappling with modern science can be a daunting experience, the problem for surgeons is more one of language and point of view than of insight or interest. Through its entire history, surgeons have dealt with the large, generally intact organs and structures of sick patients. We are the only individuals that, on a daily basis, see and handle living, diseased tissues that are a part of an integrated, functioning organism. Sensory input from the eyes and hands provide surgeons with an unusual perspective on biology that is shared with no one else. This in itself places surgeons in a powerful position for making observations and asking questions. The surgeon also has an understanding of physiology that is sharpened by the ever-present specter of failure and death. What happens in the patient is only a magnification of what is happening in the cells. But to function in today's environment, surgeons must be armed with the language of molecular biology, cell biology, and protein chemistry. This requires thinking in terms of counts per minute and spots on a gel in addition to flow, pressure, and saturation.

Happily, solutions are readily available for the thoughtfully led, financed, and motivated department of surgery. One week hands-on courses in molecular techniques are provided by community colleges in virtually every city in the country and an industry for everyone's use has sprung up around molecular biology. This includes cell lines and hybridomas from American Type Culture Collection, restriction enzymes, cloning kits, translation kits, polemerase chain reaction kits, and myriad other components that, for the beginner, only require an idea, then opening the kit and following the directions. As experience is gained, and clinical and scientific scope is focused, the combination of a surgeon's perspective on biology and heightened understanding of physiology can place the specialty in an authoritative position for facing the challenges of the twenty-first century.

For this reason, this chapter is included in a clinical textbook. Initially discussed is the first structure to be damaged in reperfusion injuries, the plasma membrane. This is followed by an analysis of the new discipline of cell stress, the eventual outcome of which is growth, but the immediate outcome, because of the requirement for energy conservation, may underlie the clinical syndrome loosely described as failure to thrive. The biology of cell stress provides the basis for understanding complications and deaths in critically ill patients that may undergo a technically perfect operation.

MUSCLE MEMBRANE MORPHOLOGY

Before one can comprehend the significance of surgically relevant plasma membrane disorders, one must first understand normal plasma membrane architecture and function, particularly as it relates to cardiac contraction.

Biochemically, the muscle plasma membrane is composed of a phospholipid bilayer consisting of the P (or protoplasmic) face and E (or extracellular) face. Each face is composed of a hydrophilic choline–phosphate–glycerol head facing outward, toward the extracellular space, or inward, toward the cytoplasm, and a hydrophobic fatty acid tail facing the cleavage plain between the two faces. Morphologically, the plasma membrane, or sarcolemma, of muscle differs significantly from the plasma membrane of other cells. In muscle, numerous invaginations project deeply into, and even through, the cell substance. These invaginations, or transverse tubules (T tubules), are a continuum of the plasma membrane and do not directly communicate with cellular organelles. Attached closely to the outer side of the plasma membrane is a negatively charged, amorphous ground substance that forms the basement membrane or glycocalyx. The glycocalyx is significant in muscle cell function as it specifically binds cations, the most important of which is Ca^{2+}. In this sense, the glycocalyx serves as a cation-exchange resin.[1]

The internal cellular membrane, or sarcoplasmic reticulum, is an intricate, calcium-containing sac that forms a lace-like network around the myofibrils. It does not communicate with the extracellular space or T tubules. However, foot-like projections extend from the sarcoplasmic reticulum and are closely adherent to the T tubules and plasma membrane.[2] The significance of these projections is unknown, but they probably serve to communicate the depolarization wave from the plasma membrane to the sarcoplasmic reticulum (Fig. 97–1).[3]

THE MYOFIBRILS AND CONTRACTION

Considerable research has been undertaken in the past 15 years to elucidate the ultrastructure of the myofibrils and to explain contraction on a molecular basis. The proteins that structurally compose the myofibril and those that are required for contraction are

- Actin: In its functioning state, this protein, with a molecular weight of 42,000 exists in long strands of double helical globular polymers.
- Myosin: This is a golf-club-shaped hybrid of heavy and light chains with an aggregate molecular weight of

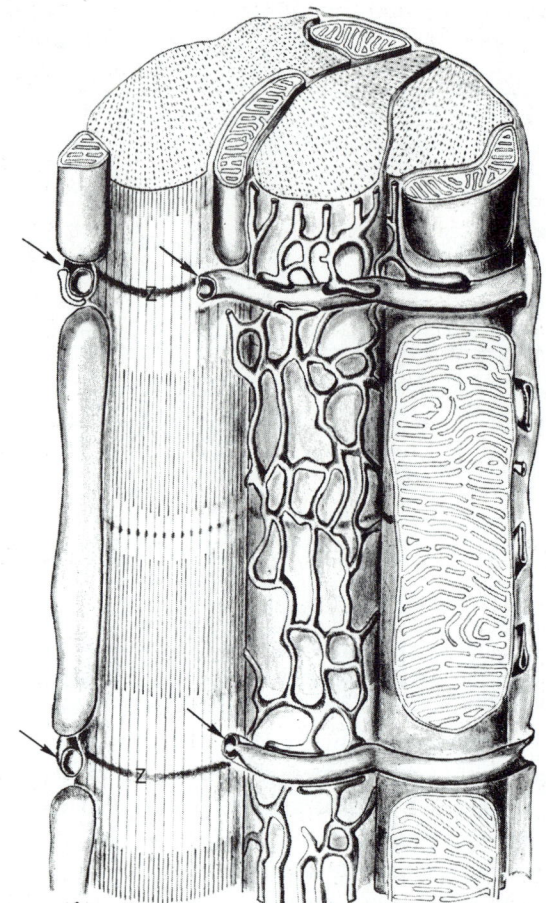

Figure 97–1. Diagram of heart muscle cell showing T tubules (arrow) as a continuation of the plasma membrane and the foot-like projection from the sarcoplasmic reticulum making contact with the T tubule. *(From Smith DS: Muscle. New York, Academic Press, 1972, with permission.)*

460,000. In addition to being a contractile element, myosin is also an enzyme that hydrolyzes ATP to ADP and inorganic phosphate.[4]

- Tropomyosin: This protein fits into the groove of the actin double helix. Its function is unknown, although it could play a role in Ca^{2+} binding or adjust the pitch of the actin double helix.[4]
- Troponin: This is a regulatory protein complex composed of three separate and distinct subunits—troponin C, I, and T. Their aggregate molecular weight is 74,000. These proteins reside on the actin filament and are spaced at every seventh actin globular subunit.[5] The function of troponin C is to form a temporary bond with Ca^{2+}. The binding of Ca^{2+} to troponin C rearranges the molecular configuration of troponin I and T, thereby exposing binding sites on the actin molecule for its interaction with myosin.[5]
- Calmodulin: This protein, widely found in all cells, is activated when it forms a temporary bond with Ca^{2+}. In the active form, it initiates the enzymatic properties of myosin resulting in its phosphorylation.[4,6] The energy re-

leased by this reaction produces a 45° change in angle of the myosin head in relation to its shaft.[7] The myosin head, having engaged actin, produces fiber shortening (Fig. 97–2).

Accordingly, Ca^{2+} is essential to muscle contraction because it (1) exposes myosin binding sites on the actin fiber, and (2) initiates the hydrolysis of ATP on the myosin molecule.

Relaxation results only when Ca^{2+} is removed from the contractile elements. This is achieved by actively pumping Ca^{2+} into the sarcoplasmic reticulum.[8] It is an energy-dependent process and requires phosphorylation of the membrane protein phospholambane.[9] As will be discussed later, this reaction is indirectly mediated by cyclic AMP.

THE PLASMA MEMBRANE AND CONTRACTION

The cells of all excitable tissues require the ability to transfer an electrical charge rapidly from one side of their plasma membrane to the other. This has been demonstrated in numerous voltage clamp studies.[10,11] In muscle tissue, the depolarization wave must then initiate, i.e., be coupled with, contraction. The steps in which the plasma membrane is involved in coupling are as follows:

1. A rapid shift of Na^+ ions from outside the cell to the inside and K^+ ions from inside to outside results in depolarization. The T tubules conduct the depolarization wave to the center of the cell much faster than could occur by simple diffusion alone.[3]

2. A slower influx of Ca^{2+} ions from the glycocalyx occurs simultaneously. The depolarization wave carried by the T tubules also initiates Ca^{2+} release from the sarcoplasmic reticulum.[12]
3. Ca^{2+} initiates contraction as previously described.
4. Na^+ and K^+ are pumped back across the cell membrane in opposite directions, resulting in repolarization.
5. Ca^{2+} is transported back into the sarcoplasmic reticulum and glycocalyx, resulting in relaxation.

Although simple in design, it is a complicated system. The rapid cyclical shifts of cations necessary for contraction, the necessity to vary the baseline concentration of intracellular Ca^{2+} so that muscle tone can be regulated, and the governance of inotropic and chronotropic responses must be managed simultaneously. To accomplish this, the plasma membrane contains a complex set of channels, pumps, and receptors classified as follows.

PASSIVE CHANNELS

Passive channels work in the direction of ionic gradients and hence are not energy dependent, i.e., they are passive. The concept of passive channels helps explain excitation–contraction. However, they have not been identified as distinct anatomic entities, and most of the experiments that have elucidated their function have been carried out in isolated organ experiments that, of course, are far removed from the normal situation. Nevertheless, abundant experimental evidence gives strong support to their existence (Fig. 97–3).[13,14]

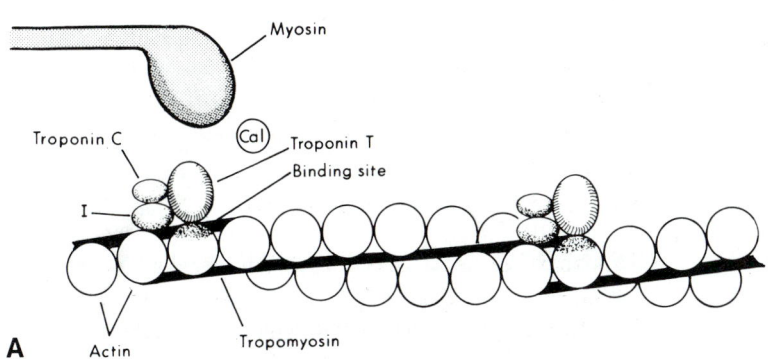

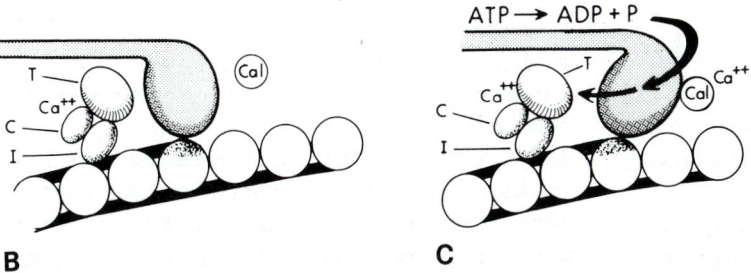

Figure 97–2. A. Contractile proteins in resting state. Binding site on actin is covered by troponin complex, calmodulin (Cal) is unbound, and there is no cross-bridging between actin and myosin. **B.** Ca^{2+} has bound with troponin C, thereby exposing binding site on actin. Actin–myosin cross-bridging has occurred. **C.** Ca^{2+} has activated calmodulin, which in turn initiates the hydrolysis of ATP on the myosin molecule resulting in a change of angulation of the myosin head and fiber shortening.

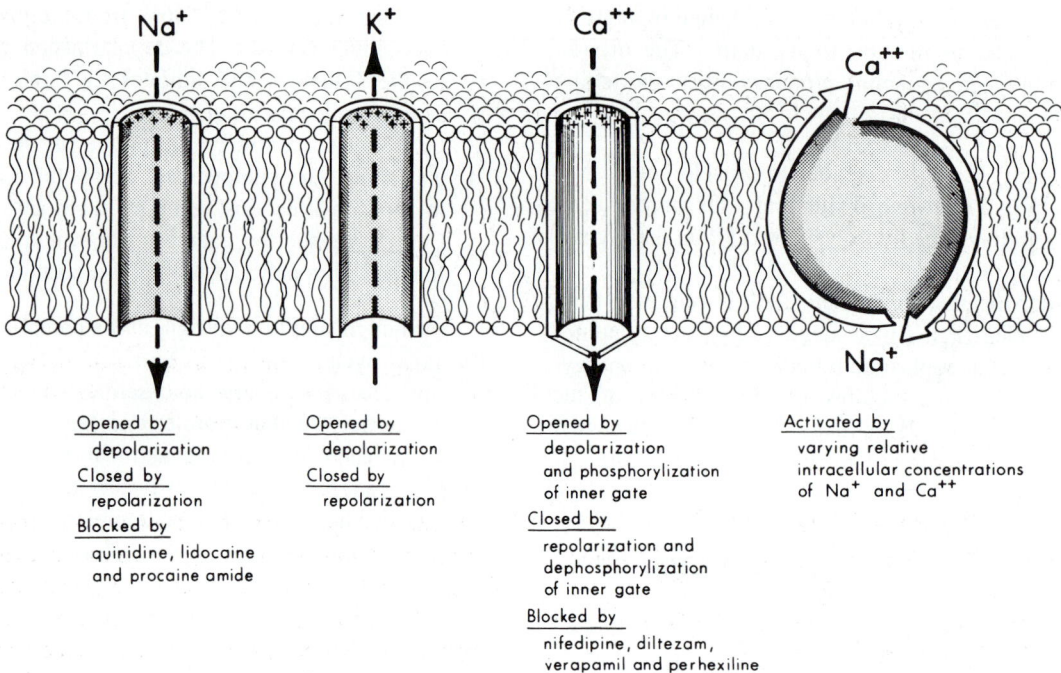

Figure 97–3. Passive channels showing outer ionic gate on Na$^+$, K$^+$, and Ca^{2+} channels and inner, energy-dependent gate on Ca^{2+} channel. The Na$^+$, Ca^{2+} exchange diffusion channel is not controlled by a gate mechanism.

1. Na$^+$ channel: This is a relatively simple channel. Whether it is opened or closed depends only upon a voltage-dependent gate. This is initially opened by a local change in voltage arising from the nodal or conducting system. It is opened by depolarization and closed by repolarization. The depolarization wave is carried by this channel, and since depolarization occurs rapidly, it is also referred to as the fast channel.
2. K$^+$ channel: Opened by depolarization, closed by repolarization.
3. Ca^{2+} channel: This is more complicated than the Na$^+$ channel. Although it is classified as passive, the moment-to-moment regulation of Ca^{2+} flow through the channel is energy dependent. This is accomplished by two sets of gates. The outer gate, like the Na$^+$ channel, is passive and voltage dependent. It is opened by depolarization and closed by repolarization. Unlike the Na$^+$ channel, there is an inner gate that requires phosphorylation for opening.[15,16] As discussed under adrenergic receptors, the degree to which the inner gate is opened is mediated by cyclic AMP.[17] Whether this channel provides the Ca^{2+} for coupling or triggers the release of Ca^{2+} for coupling from the sarcoplasmic reticulum is not well understood.[18,19] Contraction occurs more slowly than, and after, depolarization. Since Ca^{2+} moves across its channel more slowly than Na$^+$, it is also referred to as the slow channel.
4. Na$^+$, Ca^{2+} exchange diffusion channel: This is a rotary channel that expels either Na$^+$ or Ca^{2+} from the cell depending on the intracellular concentration of Na$^+$ in relation to its extracellular concentration. For every Na$^+$ ion expelled, a Ca^{2+} ion enters, or vice versa.

ACTIVE PUMPS

Active pumps work against gradients and hence are energy dependent, i.e., they are active (Fig. 97–4).

1. The Na$^+$–K$^+$ pump restores resting concentration of intracellular Na$^+$ and K$^+$ following depolarization.
2. The Ca^{2+} pump returns Ca^{2+} to the glycocalyx following contraction and maintains baseline intracellular Ca^{2+} concentration.

ADRENERGIC AND CHOLINERGIC RECEPTORS

The adrenergic or sympathetic receptor is a composite of three proteins arranged in such a way that the outer protein, or that facing the extracellular space, has the molecular configuration to recognize and accept vasoactive amines. The second or coupler protein resides in the middle of the phospholipid bilayer and, when activated by the acceptor protein, initiates the conversion of guanidine triphosphate (GTP) to guanidine monophosphate (GMP). The third protein, that facing the cytoplasm, is the enzyme adenylate cyclase. When activated by the coupler protein, this enzyme converts ATP to cyclic AMP. Cyclic AMP, in turn, plays a major role in regulating intracellular Ca^{2+} concentra-

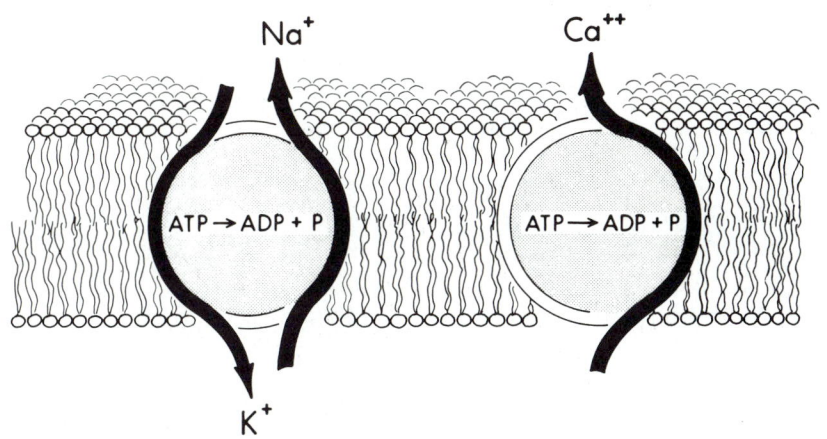

Figure 97–4. Active pumps require ATP and ATPase for movement of Na^+, K^+, and Ca^{2+} against gradients.

tion.[20,21] The specific action of cyclic AMP is to activate the protein A-kinase, possibly by removing an inhibitory subunit. This is an extremely important protein that phosphorylates other proteins. As pointed out by Watanabe in his review of autonomic receptors,[22] phosphorylation of proteins by this kinase could be a universal mechanism by which cyclic AMP modifies proteins and thus the function of cellular organelles. For example, in its active form A-kinase phosphorylates (1) Ca^{2+} channels allowing more Ca^{2+} to enter the cell, (2) the Ca^{2+} pump on the plasma membrane, thus speeding the removal of Ca^{2+} from the cell, (3) the Ca^{2+} pump on the sarcoplasmic reticulum, thus hastening the removal of Ca^{2+} from the contractile elements,and (4) the regulatory proteins of the actin–myosin complex. Consequently, stimulating a β-receptor increases both the force of contraction by increasing the intracellular Ca^{2+} concentration, thereby enhancing sensitivity of the Ca^{2+}/dependent contractile proteins, and the rate of contraction by increasing the rapidity of Ca^{2+} removal from the contractile elements (Fig. 97–5).

The cholinergic or parasympathetic receptors are perhaps less important from a clinical standpoint. Nevertheless, the onset of a sudden, severe bradycardia in the operating room can require blockade of these receptors. Unlike the adrenergic receptors, they are composed of a complex of two rather than three proteins. The outer protein again is designed to recognize and to bind acetylcholine. The inner protein is guanylate cyclase, i.e., the enzyme that converts GTP to cyclic GMP. When stimulated, the action of this receptor is (1) to block the action of the coupler protein in the adrenergic receptor and (2) to block the formation of active A-kinase by interfering with the cyclic AMP-inactive A-kinase reaction (Fig. 97–6).[23]

PHARMACOLOGIC BLOCKERS AND STIMULATORS

The previous description of membrane physiology and muscle contraction pertains to all muscle types. The chan-nels, pumps, and receptors of the plasma membrane are also present in cardiac-conducting tissue as well. However, discrete differences between tissues can permit drugs to act effectively on one type of muscle or nerve but not on another. Digitalis, which increases the force of cardiac muscle contraction but not skeletal muscle contraction, is an example of this phenomenon. Generally speaking, any agent that blocks Na^+ entry into the cell will depress electrical activity, while any agent that blocks Ca^{2+} entry into the cell will depress contractility. Drugs that enhance Ca^{2+} entry into the cell will increase contractility.

The action of epinephrine, norepinephrine, dopamine, and isuprel, of course, is to activate the sequence controlled by adrenergic or β-receptors in the cardiac plasma membrane. The action of inderal, of course, blocks this response by occupying the acceptor portion of the β-receptor complex. Atropine occupies a similar position in the cholinergic receptor complex and produces a tachycardia, though only indirectly, by allowing an unmodulated β response to occur.

Digitalis acts by blocking the ATPase system in the Na^+–K^+ pump. The inactivated pump, no longer able to pump Na^+ out of the cell, causes the intracellular Na^+ concentration to rise, which in turn reverses the normal action of the Na^+–Ca^{2+} exchange diffusion channel so that Na^+ is passively removed from the cell by passively moving Ca^{2+} into the cell (Fig. 97–7). The increased Ca^{2+} concentration produces a positive inotropic response. Since digitalis does not enter the cell or act on the sarcoplasmic reticulum, the rate of Ca^{2+} removal from the contractile proteins is not affected, and therefore a chronotropic response does not occur.

The Na^+ channel is blocked by lidocaine, procaine amide, quinidine, the experimental drug tetrodotoxin, and elevated extracellular K^+ concentration.[24] Blockade of this channel delays or inhibits depolarization and hence suppresses arrhythmias.

The Ca^{2+} channel blockers include nifedipine, diltiazem, verapamil, and perhexiline. Present information about these drugs suggests that they are extremely effective on the smooth muscle of coronary and peripheral arteries and the

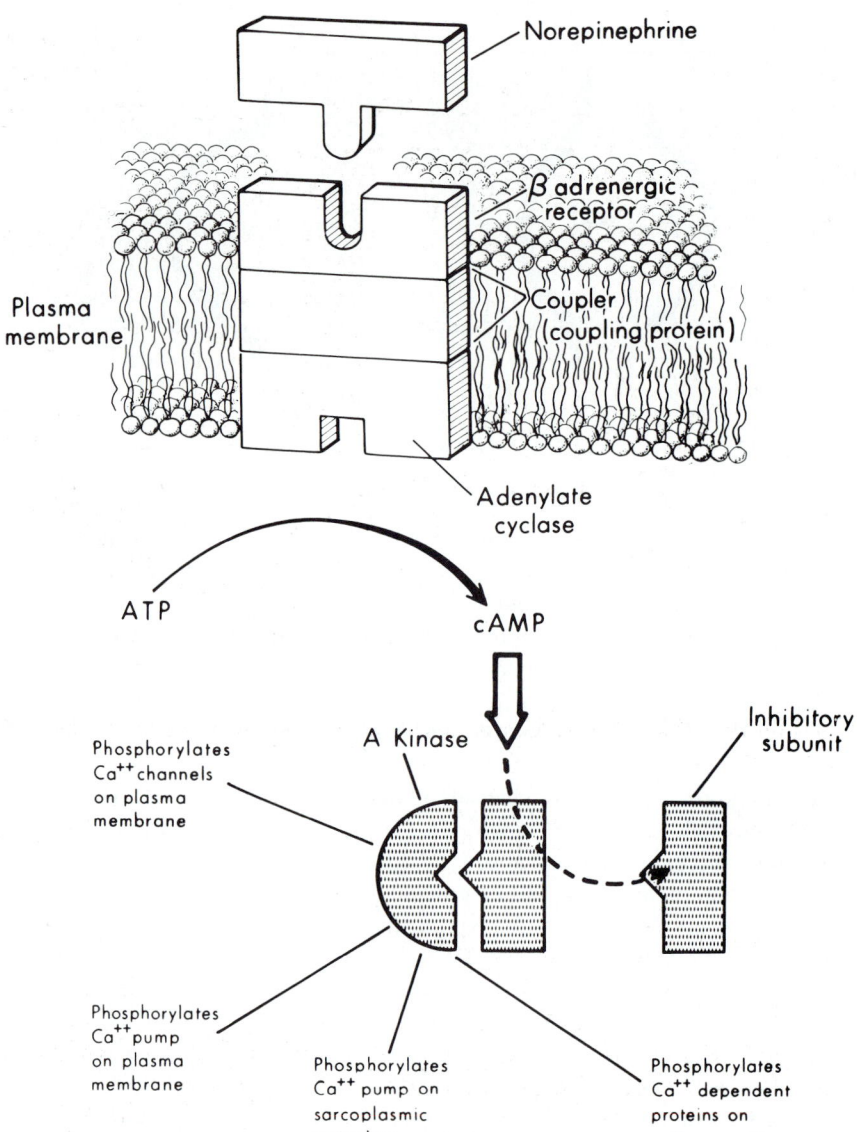

Figure 97–5. β-Adrenergic receptor mechanism, when activated, creates cAMP, active A kinase, and phosphorylization of proteins.

His–Purkinje system.[25] Nifedipine, for example, is particularly effective for treating coronary spasm[26] or for dilating small coronary vessels that may be too small to graft in the operating room. Verapamil has a profound effect on supraventricular arrhythmias that are primarily the result of reentry through the sinus or atrioventricular node.

The pharmacologic management of membrane disorders is a rapidly advancing science and one that may be of great future benefit to cardiac surgeons. For example, aneurysmectomy and coronary artery bypass grafting are presently quite unsuccessful for treating ventricular arrhythmias,[27] and unless this surgery is carried out at institutions where experienced clinicians are present to map aberrant conduction pathways and carry out their excision, the operative mortality remains extremely high.

Verapamil can reduce primary pulmonary hypertension in patients.[28] This could have implications for treating the sudden, intense pulmonary hypertension that occasion-

ally develops when coming off cardiopulmonary bypass. It has also been shown that pretreatment with nifedipine or verapamil protects the myocardium from reperfusion injuries following global ischemia[29] and that nifedipine preserves ventricular function during cardiopulmonary bypass with 1 to 2 hours of total myocardial ischemia.[30] On the other hand, if rapid-acting drugs can be found that specifically keep cardiac Ca^{2+} channels open or block the Ca^{2+} pump, then low cardiac output following surgery might no longer require the intra-aortic balloon or more exotic devices to maintain peripheral perfusion.

SURGICALLY RELEVANT PLASMA MEMBRANE DISORDERS

Scanning electron photomicrographs of freeze-fractured cardiac plasma membrane provide some idea of the total

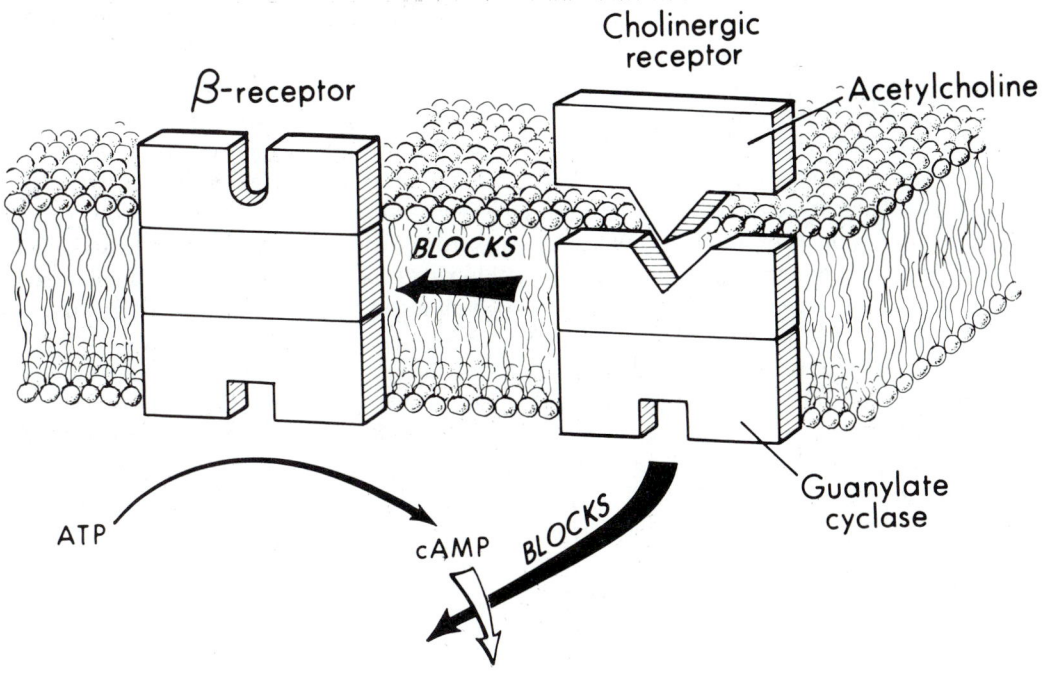

Figure 97–6. Cholinergic receptor mechanism; when stimulated blocks conversion of GTP to GMP in coupler protein of β-receptor and blocks formation of active A kinase.

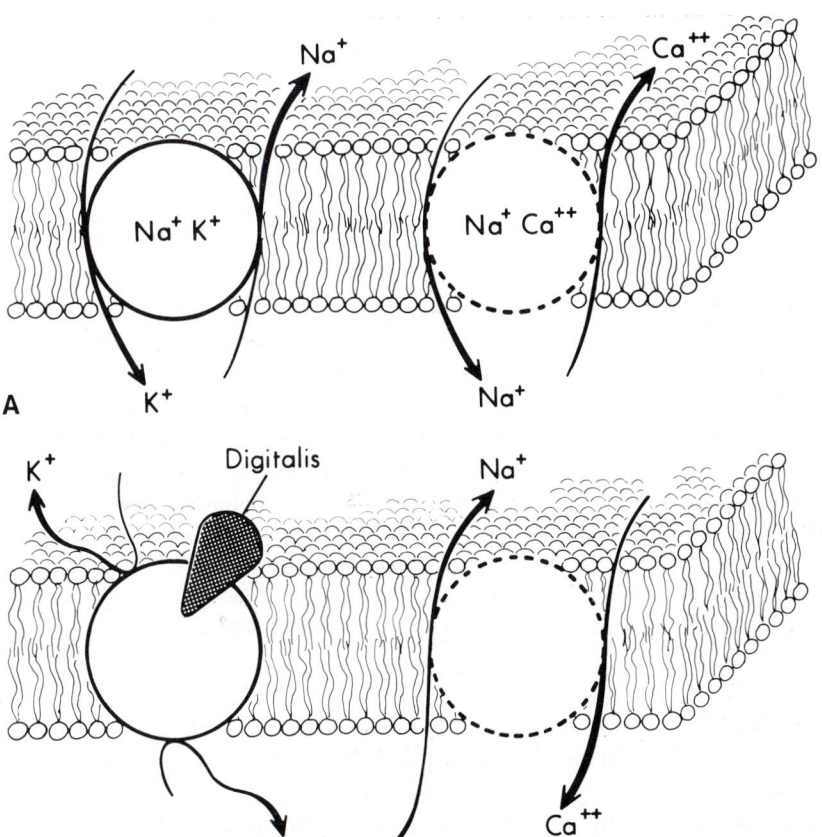

Figure 97–7. Normal relationship between the Na+–K+ pump and Na+–Ca2+ exchange diffusion channel (**A**) and the effect digitalis has on this relationship (**B**). The net effect is to increase intracellula Ca2+ concentration.

population of P face particles, i.e., channels, carriers, and receptors that traverse the bilayer of ventricular myocytes.[31] The average diameter of a P face particle is 6.86 nm, their average density is $4680/\mu m^2$, and they occupy approximately 17% of the plasma membrane surface area.[32]

Several conditions with which cardiac surgeons must deal are related to plasma membrane disorders. For example, hypertrophic cardiomyopathies are associated with increased intracellular Ca^{2+} concentration. This, in turn, is associated with decreased ATPase activity of the Ca^{2+} pump[33] and an increase in the number of Ca^{2+} channels.[33,34] This phenomenon, it is suggested, is directly responsible for the increase in myocyte necrosis associated with hypertrophic cardiomyopathies.[33] While concentric hypertrophic cardiomyopathy is not a surgical disease, idiopathic hypertrophic subaortic stenosis (IHSS) often is (see Chap. 120). Understanding the Ca^{2+} fluxes that may occur with hypertrophic cardiomyopathies suggest that Ca^{2+} should not be used, and β-agonists should be used carefully, as weaning agents from cardiopulmonary bypass following septal myomectomy for IHSS.

Primary systemic hypertension seems to be associated with either a decrease in number or activity in β-adrenergic receptors.[35] This may be one of the explanations as to why the ventricles of hypertensive patients are slow to recover following declamping and are relatively insensitive to catecholamine administration during attempts to wean from cardiopulmonary bypass.

A similar situation also occurs in diabetes. The occurrence of congestive heart failure in diabetic patients is twice as common as in those without the disease.[36] Although there are many explanations for this observation, the plasma membrane of hearts from diabetic experimental animals contains approximately half the number of β-adrenergic receptors as those from controls.[37]

REPERFUSION INJURIES AND PLASMA MEMBRANE LIPID PEROXIDATION

By far the most common and serious plasma membrane disorder that surgeons must face is iatrogenically produced lipid peroxidation. The P and E faces of the lipid bilayer are held together by hydrophobic interactions rather than covalent bonding. Although this arrangement allows rapid resealing should the membrane be breached or lacerated, it also permits P and E face distraction with far less energy than would be required to disrupt covalent forces. This is an important consideration when one analyzes the cascade of events that can result from aortic cross-clamping and subsequent reperfusion.

During ischemia, energy substrates cannot reach the cell. The cell responds by shutting down all nonimminently essential cell functions.[38] The ion pumps on the plasma membrane are usually one of the first energy-dependent processes to cease functioning. Extracellular sodium either

from vascular space blood or cardioplegic solutions enters the cell by osmotic gradients producing cell swelling. Even minor degrees of cell swelling that are undetectable morphologically can cause plasma membrane separation. Ischemia also has a direct effect on the energy delivery system by degrading ATP to its end-stage purine base hypoxanthine and, through proteolytic degradation, converting xanthine dehydrogenase to xanthine oxidase.[39] Following declamping, the vasculature is immediately flooded with blood, usually with a partial pressure of oxygen (PO_2) ≥ 200 mm Hg. The blood may also be warm, thereby shifting the oxygen dissociation curve to the right. Cardiac cells are usually still cold at this point resulting in depressed superoxide dismutase and catalase kinetics. Even worse, the overabundance of oxygen cannot be immediately converted into carbon dioxide and water through the cytochrome system because the heart's requirement for energy is so low. The following reactions now occur:

$$\text{Hypoxanthine} + O_2 + H_2O \xrightarrow{\text{xanthine oxidase}} \text{xanthine} + H_2O_2$$

$$\text{Xanthine} + O_2 + H_2O \xrightarrow{\text{xanthine oxidase}} \text{uric acid} + H_2O_2$$

$$\text{Uric acid} + 2H_2O + O_2 \rightarrow \text{allantoin} + CO_2 + H_2O_2$$

Note that the degradation of 1 mole of ATP can produce 3 moles of H_2O_2. All remaining unutilizable O_2 then reacts as follows:

$$O_2 \xrightarrow{H} HO_2^{\bullet} \xrightarrow{H} H_2O_2 \xrightarrow{H} H_2O + {}^{\bullet}OH \xrightarrow{H} 2H_2O$$

Or put another way, the successive reduction of oxygen proceeds as

$$\text{oxide} \xrightarrow{H} \text{superoxide} \xrightarrow{H} \text{peroxide} \xrightarrow{H} \text{hydroxide} \xrightarrow{H} \text{water}$$

Accordingly, to reduce one molecule of oxygen, four hydrogen ions are required.

Oxygen, with two unoccupied valence slots only two orbitals from an eight proton nucleus, possesses formidable oxidizing power. With dismutase and catalase systems overwhelmed and little need for aerobic energy, oxygen starts to oxidize whatever is available. Any exposed hydrophobic group then becomes a substrate for the reduction of molecular oxygen. For these reductions to occur, oxygen must form covalent attachments to extraneous hydrogen atoms. Following 1–2 hours of ischemia these atoms become readily accessible from lipid groups of distracted plasma membranes. Oxygen free radicals have sufficient energy to abstract a hydrogen atom from a methyl carbon of an unsaturated fatty acid, which then has the potential for initiating a chain reaction in the entire membrane.[40]

As the attack proceeds, plasma membrane fluidity decreases, and the transmembrane receptors, channels, pumps, enzymes, and messenger pathways that are involved in regulating cell function cease to work.[41] These fluidity changes are closely associated with membrane lipid breakdown.[42]

Even under normal working conditions, when oxygen has a temporary home in the cytochrome system and the PO_2 of blood reaching the cell is in the physiologic range, oxygen free radical formation still occurs due to the leakage of 1–5% of oxygen from the cytochrome pathway.[43] However, free radicals from this source can usually be handled by the superoxide dismutase and catalase enzymes as follows:

$$HO_2^{\bullet} + HO_2^{\bullet} \xrightarrow{\substack{\text{superoxide} \\ \text{dismutase}}} H_2O_2 + O_2$$

$$H_2O_2 + H_2O_2 \xrightarrow{\text{catalase}} 2H_2O + O_2$$

Superoxide dismutase (SOD) has the affect of transferring hydrogen atoms from one molecule of superoxide to another. One molecule is therefore reduced as the other is oxidized. Catalase removes atomic oxygen from hydrogen peroxide to form molecular oxygen and water. Both arrangements allow the formation of water from superoxide without requiring additional hydrogen. At 37°C and normal PO_2, both enzymes act instantaneously and in concert. The redox reaction approaches the theoretical limit set by diffusion,[44] thereby preventing oxygen from cannibalizing hydrogen atoms from adjacent biologic molecules.

Several reports in the literature propose adding superoxide dismutase and catalase to cardioplegic or preservation solutions. Although some experimental studies show that these enzymes may be beneficial,[45,46] the effects, in general, of enzyme or other antioxidant therapy have been conflicting and at present a firm position regarding their use cannot be made.[47] However, there are restricted areas in which antioxidants do help and there are innovative methods now under study as possible preventive or therapeutic measures for dealing with oxygen toxicity. For example, preservation solutions containing the xanthine oxidase inhibitor allopurinol along with glutathione, which, in its enzymatic form of glutathione peroxidase, converts hydrogen peroxide to water has reduced the incidents of renal failure following kidney transplantion.[47] There have been no carefully analyzed studies showing a beneficial effect in heart or lung transplant patients or as an additive to cardioplegic solutions in patients undergoing routine cardiac surgery.

There may be a serious flaw in the rationale for using SOD and catalase in cardioplegic or preservation solutions. These enzymes are large molecules that do not enter cells and are needed only after declamping when oxygenated blood re-enters the organ. At this point, they are quickly swept away and cleared from the circulation.[48] To overcome this difficulty, a group from Kumamoto University in Japan covalently linked fatty acids to the lysyl residues of SOD. Because of the amphipathic nature of the synthetic molecule, i.e., the hydrophobic property of the fatty acid and the hydrophilic property of the enzyme, the hybrid molecule could bind, by hydrophobic interactions, to the plasma membrane while leaving the SOD group free to interact with superoxides. The efficacy of this approach has been shown in cell culture and the corneal epithelium of laboratory animals, but it has not been used clinically.[48] Another innovative approach was proposed by a group from the University of Alberta. They prepared erythocyte ghosts by rupturing the cell membrane and removing hemoglobin in hypotonic buffer. The ghosts were then incubated in SOD and resealed with buffer of normal tonicity. Oxygen free radicals were then generated by adding xanthine and xanthine oxidase to the cells and the scavenging of radicals by the SOD laden cells determined by electron spin resonance. Again, these studies have shown effective elimination of oxygen free radicals in culture but have not been used clinically.[49]

As always, the best technique for preventing lipid peroxidation is careful and expeditious surgical technique that keeps cross-clamp time to a minimum and reperfusion of the ischemic myocardium with blood at physiologic PO_2 levels.

CELL STRESS AND THE PHYSIOLOGY OF SURVIVAL

Cardiac cells must function in a universe whose very fabric favors disorder over order, disarray over structure. Natural forces, true to the second law of thermodynamics, constantly drive the ordered structure of cells to the disordered, random collection of their component elements.[50] Order cannot be maintained, or arise out of chaos, without help. In all systems, physical or biological, this help comes only in the form of energy. Consequently cellular structure and function are interwoven in an inseparable relationship with energy. The energy required to maintain cellular order, however, cannot be used to perform work, and, as nature will have it, the more work that is performed, the more energy must then be diverted to maintain cellular order.

The energy–structure relationship is exemplified by the appearance and disappearance of water. When hydrogen and oxygen are ignited, for example in a rocket engine or joined as the end product of the electron transport chain, energy is liberated as covalent bonds are formed. If the same amount of energy is driven back into the newly formed water molecules, covalent bonds are broken and hydrogen and oxygen reappear. Variations of this simple principle form the basis for all biological energy transfers and explain not only how a cell derives energy but also how and why cellular structures yield and degrade. For example, an energy equivalent of approximately 80 K cal/mol is required to rupture a carbon—carbon (C–C) bond. Although it is difficult to precisely measure the energy absorbed by cardiac proteins during contraction, force generation can be converted into mcal/g,[51] as can the energy derived from oxidative metabolism. At an O_2 consumption of 9 mL/min per 100 g of heart muscle, approximately 8 kcal/h of energy is generated by the average adult human heart. Although much of this energy is used to eject blood, some is absorbed by the contractile proteins and other cellular structures. This may seem like a manageable amount of wear and tear, but it is well to remember that there is a minimum of 6×10^{23} C–C linkages per mole of any substance containing two or more carbon atoms, and the rupture of only one linkage renders any protein functionally useless. As a result, the half-life of cardiac proteins is only 4 to 6 days for just the normal maintenance of physiologic activity.[52] Random degradation of proteins, including those at or near the breaking point, provides room for newly synthesized proteins and ensures a steady state configuration of healthy cellular components. Accordingly, protein degradation is the counterpart to protein synthesis that forms the essential symmetry permeating most, if not all, natural phenomena. On their way from cradle to grave, the contractile protein's short life span consists of performing work, absorbing energy, and becoming the substrate for enzymatic degradation.

Under normal operating conditions, cardiac cells direct energy into work production and order maintenance by adjusting coronary blood flow so that oxidation proceeds aerobically. The key to understanding cardiac stress is to recognize that the heart must adapt to a prolonged alteration in the normal balance between aerobic energy supply and energy expenditure per cell while, simultaneously, maintaining critical cell function and cellular order. When the demand for work energy increases abnormally, these requirements can be met only by temporarily turning off, or throttling down, many nonimminently essential cell functions. This is where troubles arise for cardiac and transplant surgeons. Because all cells must have a mechanism for adjusting to stress, the resulting response is not unique to the heart.

In general, the long-term response to a sublethal stress in any organ is growth. For example, a physiologic, or pathophysiologic, stimulus provokes increased heart size after aortic banding, kidney size after unilateral nephrectomy, or restoration of liver size after hepatic lobectomy. Whether the imposed stress is an increase in mechanical work, in active transport of sodium, or in synthesis of albumin, the end result is the same, and all are related to changes in cellular energy requirements induced by altered environmental situations.

Bear in mind, however, that end-stage growth, or hypertrophy, is only the final visible result of a sequence of complex and precisely programmed events that are extremely difficult to unravel. A deeper level of understanding is possible when one analyzes the immediate cellular events that are produced by stress before cellular changes—such as polyploidization of nuclei, mitochondrial multiplication, and fibroblast proliferation—occur. In this regard, the heart plays a unique role, as its need for energy is so clearly tied to mechanical work, which, in turn, can be precisely monitored and easily observed.

EARLY RESPONSES TO STRESS OCCUR IN THE NUCLEUS

If the eventual outcome of cell stress is growth, then an overall increase in protein synthesis must occur. However, quantifying protein synthesis is not simple and the rate at which labeled amino acids are incorporated into protein can be interpreted in many ways.

Less controversial is the observation that messenger ribonucleic acid (mRNA) synthesis increases in response to stress. It is less controversial, however, only if

1. measurements do not depend upon scintillation counting of labeled nucleotides administered to intact cells (which raise the same problems that plague interpretation of data from protein synthesis).
2. data are obtained from in vivo experiments, thereby avoiding the uncertainty of whether metabolic changes are related to the experimental conditions one wishes to study or to the trauma of extirpation for experiments conducted in vitro. In our experience, the conditions required for retention of normal metabolic function are extremely exacting and it is impossible to reproduce these conditions in any in vitro system.

These problems can be avoided by analyzing translational activity of RNA, extracted from intact, in situ, hearts subjected to various forms of stress. Translational activity provides an extremely accurate measurement of the proportion of mRNA in any particular sample of total RNA extracted from cells. Because it is not necessary to extract all mRNA from tissues, one is freed from the errors involved in total extraction. Translational activity therefore represents the ratio between mRNA to other RNA species in the portion of RNA being examined. The disadvantage of this technique is that mRNAs that synthesize proteins of over 80 kD do not translate well in in vitro systems. It should be kept in mind that the biochemical changes that occur in the cell cultures, or hearts of experimental animals, described below also occur, to one degree or another, in the hearts of patients, or heart donors, whenever the aorta is cross-clamped.

Shown in Figure 97–8 are sodium dodecyl sulfate (SDS) gels of proteins translated in vitro by equal amounts of RNA extracted from the right and left ventricle of a dog 1 hour after producing an 80 mm Hg gradient across the ascending aorta. The increased translational activity of the stressed left ventricle is obvious in comparison to the nonstressed right ventricle.

An alteration in the rate of RNA synthesis, produced by stress, may occur either by changes in chromatin template activity or RNA polymerase activity. This question was addressed by Cutilletta, from Johns Hopkins, who used homologous RNA polymerase II to measure chromatin tem-

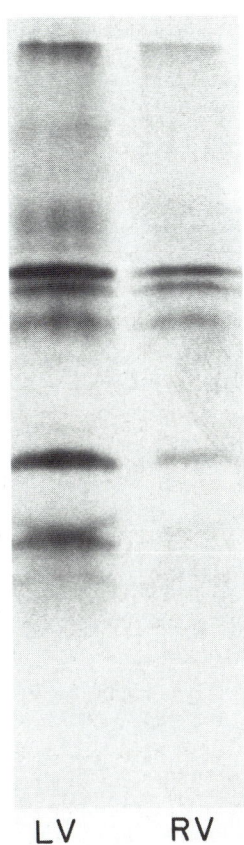

LV   RV

Figure 97–8. Translation products produced by 5 μg of RNA from normal right ventricle and acutely stressed left ventricle of a canine heart. *(From Hammond GL, Weiben E, Markert CL: Molecular signals for initiating protein synthesis in organ hypertrophy. Proc Natl Acad Sci USA 76:2455–2459, 1979.)*

plate activity. He found that template activity increased 1 day after aortic constriction, that is, enhanced local separation of the complimentary DNA strands provided greater template exposure for transcription initiation but the RNA polymerase activity itself did not increase. However, 3 days after aortic constriction, RNA polymerase activity did increase.[53] Therefore, it appears that the initial and immediate increase in mRNA is due to a change in DNA template activity, but the sustained increase in RNA synthesis is due to increased polymerase activity.

AN IMMEDIATE AND UNIVERSAL RESPONSE TO SEVERE STRESS IS STRESS PROTEIN SYNTHESIS

Stress proteins should not be confused with the acute phase proteins that are released from cells (primarily hepatocytes and immune system cells) during less severe, although potentially life-threatening, periods of stress. Acute phase proteins include C-reactive protein, complement, interferon γ, fibrinogens, and α-trypsin, etc. that combat the systemic effects of stress. Stress proteins, on the other hand, are synthesized by cells of all organs and remain in the cell.

A considerable volume of literature describes the stress response in a variety of organisms and cells in culture that have been subjected to heat shock. These systems all produce the so-called heat shock proteins (or, more properly, stress proteins) that have been found in species from bacteria to humans and are produced by many varieties of cellular stress.[54] Studies of cell cultures showed that stress proteins are synthesized following hypoxia,[55] uncouplers of oxidative phosphorylation, inhibitors of electron transport, and blockers of hydrogen receptors such as actinomycin A,[56] arsenate,[56] and cyanide.[57]

Figure 97–9 shows two-dimensional autoradiograms of translation products directed by RNA extracted from tissue samples of canine right ventricle before and after 1 hour of heat shock.[58] Four newly synthesized stress protein mRNAs (and hence stress proteins) can be seen following stress induction. Otherwise, the autoradiograms are indistinguishable. Numerous stress proteins (sp's) have been reported, but by far the most common is the sp 70.

The biological significance of stress proteins is an evolving science, but the following statements can now be made with a reasonable degree of certainty:

1. The proteins are absolutely essential for growth, both in response to stress and for differentiation and development.[59]
2. Stress proteins entail a major redirection of the activities of the cell. During hyperthermia in *Escherichia coli,* for example, stress proteins constitute nearly a quarter of the protein mass of the cell.[60]
3. The general pattern and time course of heat shock response are similar from bacteria to humans.

The finding of such strong homology from species to species of the stress proteins themselves is truly unprecedented. Preliminary data of our own give some idea of the unifying effect stress proteins have had on understanding the stress responses in all species so far studied. Figure 97–10 shows hybridization experiments conducted in our laboratory by P. Havre, Ph.D., using the nick-translated sp 70 DNA from *Drosophila* (cloned by Schedl)[61] as a probe for identifying sp 70 gene activity in dog organs. A high degree of homology between the *Drosophila* sp 70 gene and human sp 70 gene has also been demonstrated.[62]

Conservation to this extent portends an importance of these genes, the magnitude of which is still unknown. Understanding the regulation of stress protein synthesis, how these proteins function, and the role they may play in adaptation will doubtless provide deep insights into the nature of cellular organization and clarify our understanding of how cells respond to stress.

STRESS RECOGNITION

A fundamental question is: How does the heart recognize stress or, in other words, how does the heart translate a physiological impulse such as pressure overload or is-

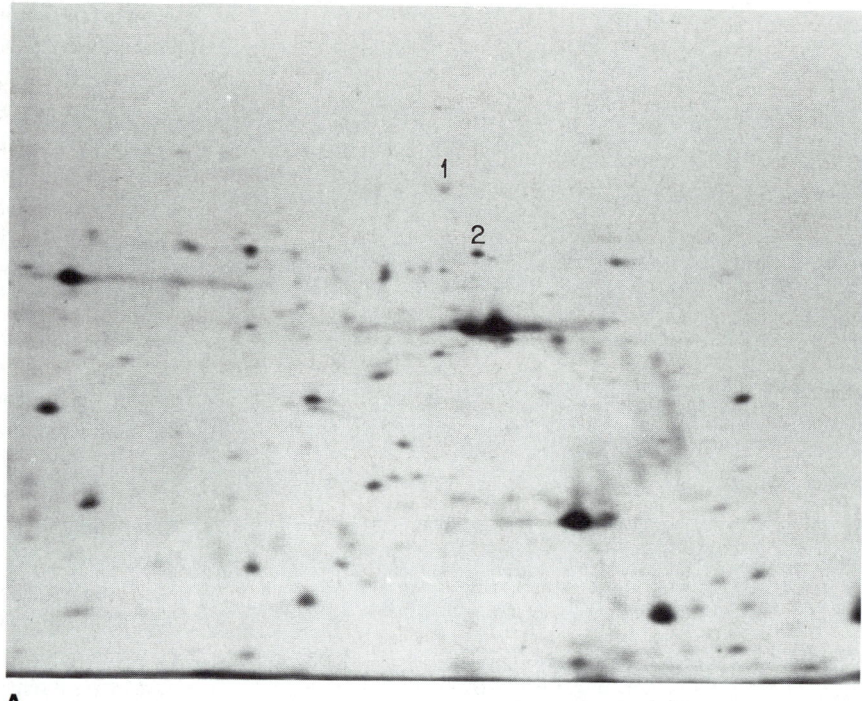

A

B

Figure 97–9. **A.** Two-dimensional autoradiograms of translation products directed by
mRNA extracted from canine ventricle
before dog was subjected to 1 hour of heat
shock. Normal occurring reference proteins
1 and 2 labeled. **B.** Two-dimensional autoradiograms of translation products from same
heart as in **A** after 1 hour of heat shock.
Newly synthesized 71-kD stress proteins A,
B, C, and D appear to the left of reference
proteins. Other than the presence of stress
proteins, the pre- and post-stress patterns
are indistinguishable. *(From Lai Y-K, Havre
PA, Hammond GL: Heat shock stress
initiates simultaneous transcriptional and
translational changes in the dog heart.
Biochem Biophys Res Commun
134:166–171, 1986, with permission.)*

chemia into a biochemical signal that initiates stress protein
synthesis?

There are two clinical observations that may provide a
clue. First is the association of angina with both aortic
stenosis and coronary artery disease, and second is the observation that the ventricles of patients with aortic stenosis
often resemble those of patients with advanced triple-coro-
nary artery disease. Provided there are no large areas of

transmural infarction, the hearts in both clinical conditions
may develop fibrotic, noncompliant, hypertrophied ventricles. The observation that ventricular hypertrophy occurs
with coronary artery disease, often in the absence of etio-
logical factors such as hypertension, is well documented.[63,64]

The common denominator for both pathologic conditions, whether produced by decreased blood supply or in-

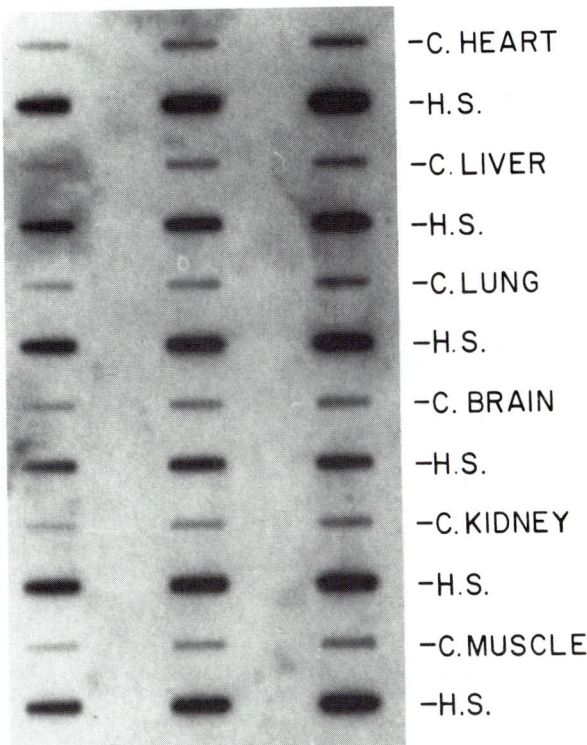

Figure 97–10. *Drosophila* hsp 70 cDNA and canine sp 70 mRNA hybridization. RNA was extracted from control and heat shocked dog organs and mRNA isolated following oligo dT cellulose chromatography. Hybridization can clearly be seen between the probe and canine sp 70 mRNA.

creased cardiac work, is a prolonged discordance between energy requirements and energy expenditure per cell. If this discordance is severe, the cell dies; but if intermittent or less severe, the difference between energy requirement and aerobic energy production is made up by glycolysis, resulting in lactic acid formation. Alterations in the balance between energy supply and energy expenditure may be the universal mechanism by which cells recognize stress and respond in ways that compensate for environmental changes. We studied the association between cellular acidosis and stress protein synthesis in several ways.

First, we applied four different forms of stress to intact rats, and then analyzed the cardiac RNA-translation products.[65] One group underwent aortic banding for 1 hour, a second group underwent core hyperthermia to 42°C for 1 hour, a third group was slowly cooled over 90 min to 18°C, and a fourth group swam to exhaustion, which required approximately 1 hour. In all cases, the cardiac metabolic rate was increased either by swimming, shivering, pressure overload, or hyperthermia. Following termination of the experiments, the RNA was extracted and translated, and the proteins resolved by two-dimensional electrophoresis and visualized by autoradiography. Only two stresses provoked cardiac stress protein synthesis: aortic banding and heat shock. Autoradiograms from control hearts and hearts responding to stress are shown in Figure 97–11. Two salient

features are apparent: first, like those obtained from the dog heart in Figure 97–9, the protein patterns are indistinguishable except for the presence of stress proteins in stressed hearts; and second, hearts stressed by heat shock synthesized stress proteins in greater abundance than those stressed by aortic banding.

To determine if there was a relationship between these findings and the utilization of energy, we analyzed cardiac lactic acid concentration as an indicator of the metabolic condition of the heart muscle after the four stresses. The findings from these experiments are shown in Table 97–1. Not only was there an association between lactic acid content and stress protein synthesis, but the greater the concentration of lactic acid, the greater the concentration of stress protein.

In a second group of experiments, the correlation between stress protein synthesis, arterial pH, and lactic acidosis was studied. Dogs were heated to 42°C with a heat exchanger placed between the femoral vessels. At approximately 5-min intervals, samples of lung were removed, RNA extracted and translated, and proteins visualized by autoradiography. Arterial pH and lactate analyses were simultaneously performed. Figure 97–12 shows pH and lactic acid changes in relation to time at 42°C and the point at which stress proteins were synthesized. Autoradiograms from the serial lung samples show that a progressive increase in sp 70 mRNA translation products occurs quickly as the pH falls (Fig. 97–13). The critical point at which stress protein synthesis occurred was at a temperature-corrected pH of 7.24 and lactic acid content of 60 mg%. Figure 97–14 (a subset from Fig. 97–13) shows that other stress protein mRNAs appear as pH decreases, and also reveals that the synthesis of at least one normally occurring mRNA is inhibited.

Therefore evidence is accumulating that, as in the common occurrence of angina and hypertrophy with both aortic stenosis and coronary artery disease, the underlying trigger that initiates stress protein synthesis, and subsequently growth, may be related to pH changes produced by an alteration between energy requirements and expenditure. Whether the workload has increased beyond oxidative capacity, or the blood supply is so diminished that oxidative metabolism is hindered, may make little difference. As far as the cell is concerned, the end result is the same.

Because stress protein synthesis occurs in cells in culture as well as extirpated organs, and individually stressed organs of intact animals, another difficult question is posed. How are the stress protein genes induced to transcribe? Gene activation by the common transduction pathway of hormone binding to membrane receptors as, for example, induction of the MHC genes by interferon γ,[66] cannot occur. Induction of stress protein genes must be a purely postreceptor binding event and therefore likely acts through pathways not associated with the plasma membrane. At the present time the pathway for stress protein gene induction is unknown. However, because alterations in energy metabo-

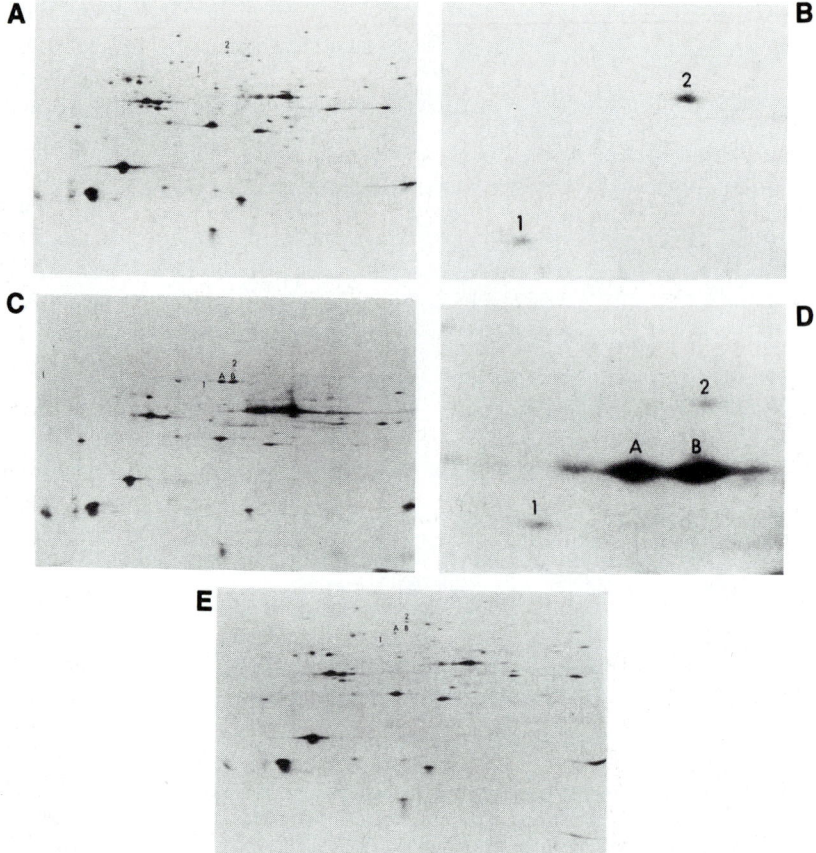

Figure 97–11. Two-dimensional autoradiograms of translation products. **A.** From a control heart, proteins 1 and 2 occur normally and are labeled for reference purposes. This autoradiogram is indistinguishable from those from hearts of swimmers or chilled rats. **B.** Magnified view of area of reference proteins 1 and 2 in **A. C.** From a heat-shocked heart. New proteins A and B can be seen between reference proteins 1 and 2. **D.** Magnified view of area of reference proteins 1 and 2 in **C.** There was relatively greater synthesis of proteins A and B in hearts from heat-shocked rats than in hearts from rats with banded aortas. This increase corresponds with the increased lactic acid concentration in heat-shocked hearts, which was five times that in hearts from rats with banded aortas. **E.** From a heart after aorta banding. Two distinct new proteins, A and B, can be seen between reference proteins 1 and 2. *(From Hammond GL, Lai Y-K, Markert CL: Diverse forms of stress lead to new patterns of gene expression through a common and essential metabolic pathway. Proc Natl Acad Sci USA 79:3488, 1982.)*

lism are so tightly linked to stress protein synthesis, the mitochondria become prime candidates for involvement in the stress response.

In the intact cell, many stress proteins are transported to the mitochondria.[67] Therefore, to determine if mitochondria can independently recognize stress and respond by synthesizing stress proteins from its own DNA, the mitochondria must be isolated to establish with certainty the origin of mitochondrial stress proteins (msp). These studies were performed by heat shocking-isolated mitochondria, labeling newly synthesized proteins, and then comparing the autoradiograms with unstressed mitochondria and the stressed whole cells of the type from which the mitochondria were isolated. We discovered that the mitochondria synthesize a stress protein of 18 kDa (Fig. 97–15). However, the concentration of the mitochondrial stress protein is so low that it cannot be seen on autoradiograms from whole cell lysates. We calculated that there were only 2.5×10^{-9} g of mitochondrial stress protein per gram of tissue.[68]

Although it may be too simplistic to suggest that an msp acts directly on the genome, cells also contain specific "stat" proteins that are preformed molecules, always present in cells that act as signal transducers as well as activators of transcription.[69] A potential avenue for investigation, therefore, is to determine if the msp 18 can bind to, or phosphorylate, a stat protein. An interesting experiment performed in 1965, before stress proteins had been discovered, demonstrated that when extracts from mitochondria were injected into cells, changes characteristic of transcription initiation occurred in the chromosomes.[70]

WHAT ARE THE PURPOSES OF STRESS PROTEINS?

Knowledge about the biological significance of stress proteins is evolving rapidly (reviewed by Welch[71]). Although the molecular biology of the phenomenon is unknown, increased expression of cardiac stress proteins by hyperther-

TABLE 97–1. LACTIC ACID CONTENT OF CONTROL AND STIMULATED RAT HEARTS

Treatment	n	Lactic acid (mg/g)
Control	8	0.696 ± 0.090^a
Banded	4	$1.440 \pm 0.180^*$
Heat shock	4	$7.348 \pm 0.510^*$
Cold shock	4	0.861 ± 0.125
Swimming	4	0.690 ± 0.191

^{a}Results are shown as mean ± SEM.
$^*p < 0.01$.
From Hammond GL, Lai Y-K, Markert CL: Diverse forms of stress lead to new patterns of gene expression through a common and essential metabolic pathway. Proc Natl Acad Sci USA 79:3485–3488, 1982.

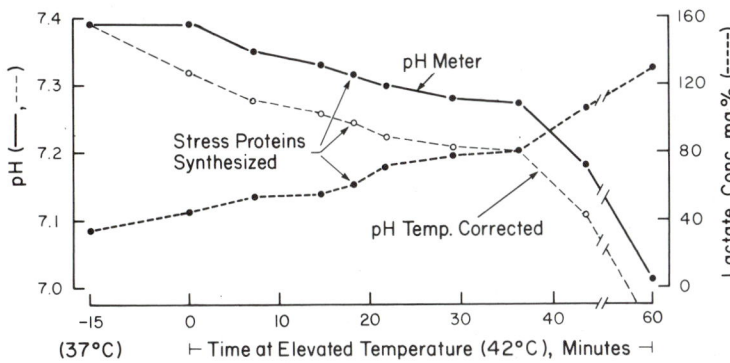

Figure 97–12. Lactate and pH curves in relation to time at 42° C. Stress proteins are synthesized at pH 7.24 and lactate concentration of 60 mg%. *(From Hammond GL: Cell stress and the initiation of growth. In Legato MJ (ed): The Stressed Heart. Boston, Martinus Nijhoff, 1987, pp 21–47.)*

mia of the whole animal seems to confer a protective effect to the heart upon subsequent ischemic stress.[72]

The metallothionine gene appears to be a stress gene and is activated in the liver during hypovolemic shock.[73] This stress protein may serve a role in protecting cells against free radical injury as metallothionine reacts to detoxify hydroxyl radicals.[74] Another function that is now well recognized is the capacity of stress proteins to maintain tertiary conformation of other proteins. Applied stress, such as heat shock, hypertrophy induction, traumatic injury,

LUNG

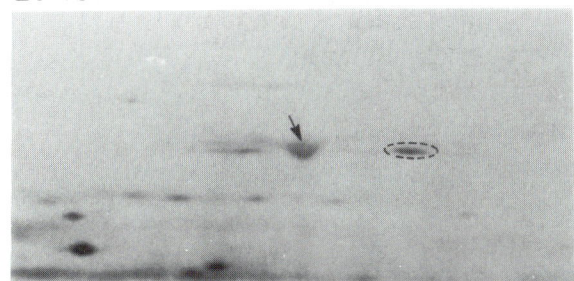

Time 11 min   pH 7.26   Lactate 55 mg %

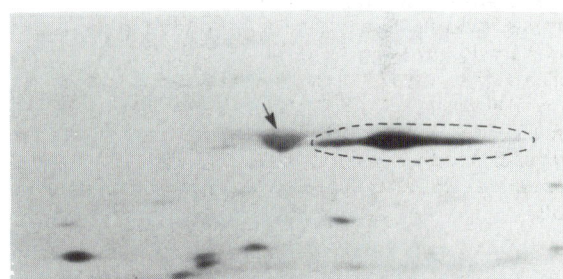

Time 24 min   pH 7.21   Lactate 74 mg %

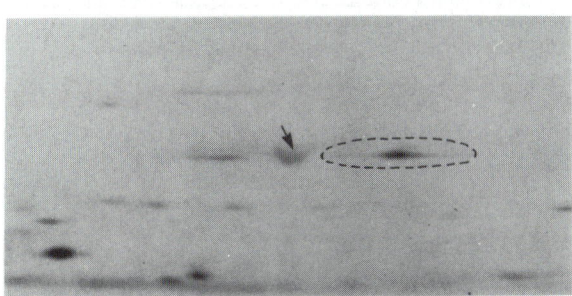

Time 18 min   pH 7.24   Lactate 60 mg %

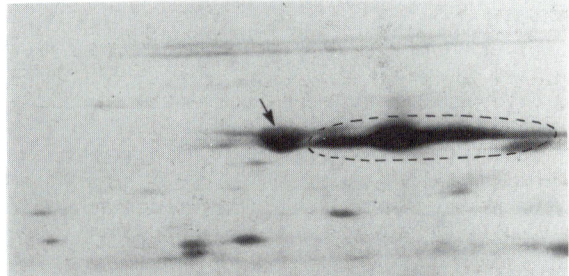

Time 34 min   pH 7.19   Lactate 78 mg %

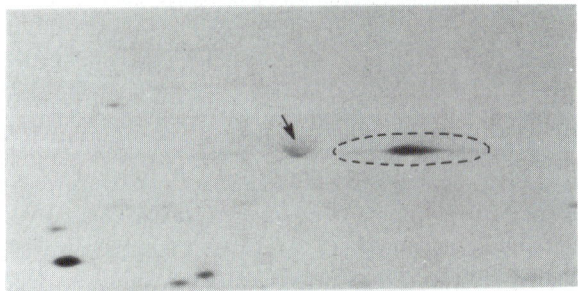

Time 22 min   pH 7.22   Lactate 68 mg %

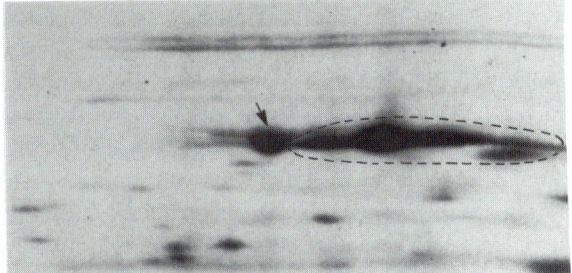

Time 39 min   pH 7.18   Lactate 80 mg %

Figure 97–13. Serial examinations of translation products from the lung as the dog becomes progressively acidotic points to normally occurring proteins (NOP 70) (representing NOP 70 mRNA). Most obvious change is ever-increasing quantity of sp 70 mRNA; sp 70 is circled. *(From Hammond GL: Cell stress and the initiation of growth. In Legato MJ (ed): The Stressed Heart. Boston, Martinus Nijhoff, 1987, pp 21–47.)*

LUNG

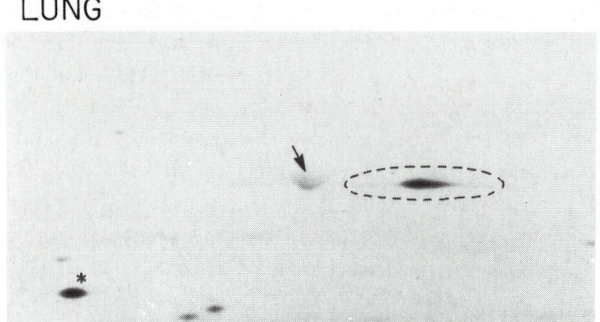

Time 22 min   pH 7.22   Lactate 68 mg %

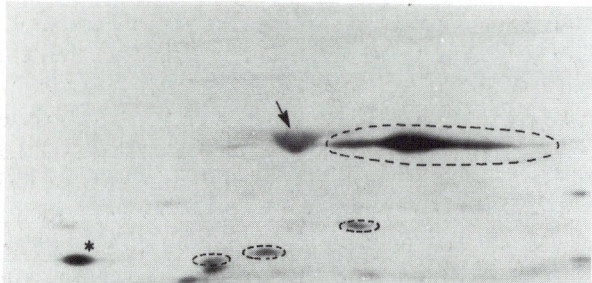

Time 24 min   pH 7.21   Lactate 74 mg %

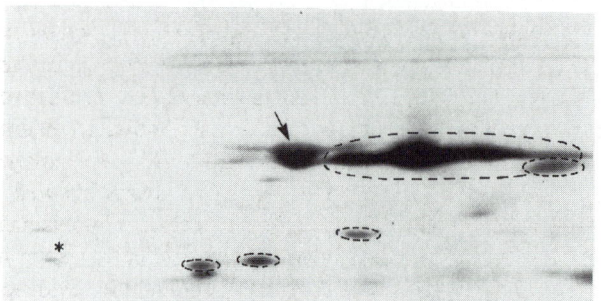

Time 34 min   pH 7.19   Lactate 78 mg %

Figure 97–14. Subtle changes also occur in the lung with acidosis. These are three of the same panels that appear in Figure 97–13. With increasing acidosis, more genes are activated as other sp mRNAs appear (stress proteins circled) while at least one gene (*) is inhibited. *(From Hammond GL: Cell stress and the initiation of growth. In Legato MJ (ed): The Stressed Heart. Boston, Martinus Nijhoff, 1987, pp 21–47.)*

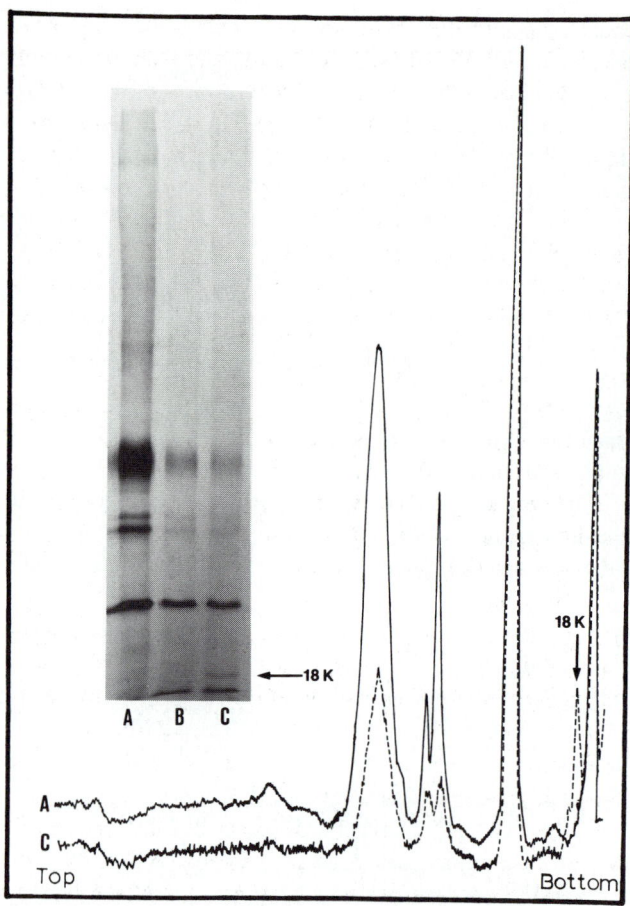

Figure 97–15. Autoradiograms with densitometric scans obtained from proteins synthesized by isolated mitochondria and resolved by SDS-polyacrylamide gel electrophoresis. **A.** (——) Unheated control; mitochondrial protein synthesis was carried out at 37°C and labeled for 2 hours. **B.** The sample was labeled at 41°C for 2 hours. **C.** (----) The sample was labeled at 43°C for 2 hours. Arrows indicate position of the msp 18. *(From Lai Y-K, Lee W-C, Hu C-H, Hammond GL: The Mitochondria Are Sensory Organelles for Cell Stress Recognition. J Surg Res 1995, submitted.)*

or other physical or chemical conditions that are severe enough to produce anaerobiosis will result in rapid and excessive energy absorption by proteins that maintain the structural and functional integrity of the cell. The function of any protein, of course, is dictated by its shape, which in turn is determined by its tertiary conformation; and tertiary conformation is largely maintained by noncovalent forces. These forces are weaker than covalent bonds by a factor of 10 and are only slightly stronger than the average energy of thermal collision at 37°C.[75] Accordingly, as stress increases, tertiary conformation and therefore function is lost. A critical role of the most commonly identified stress proteins, i.e., the sp 70 group, is to function as splints for cellu-

lar proteins to help maintain their tertiary conformation.[67,76] Nowhere is this more important than in the energy delivery systems of the cell, i.e., the mitochondria where both the sp 60 and sp 70 groups are present in abundance.

Once synthesized in the cytoplasm, some species of the sp 70 group, and perhaps other stress proteins, return to the nucleus.[77,78] In the nucleus, they appear in areas where chromatin is uncondensed and where transcription may be initiated. If in fact stress proteins play a role in gene regulation, many other findings associated with the stress response could be explained, particularly isozyme shifts. For example, cardiac myosin exists in isozymic forms.[79] Each molecule is composed of two heavy chains and four light chains. Two different types of heavy chains, α and β, have been found in the ventricles of mammalian laboratory animals. The heavy chains form dimers of αα, αβ, and ββ.[80] These correspond to the V_1, V_2, and V_3 forms predominant in fetal hearts, while adult hearts are composed primarily of the V_1 form.[81] In left-ventricular pressure overload, however, the isozymic pattern in adult animals shifts to the V_3 form, which is adapted for slow tension development.[82] The shift is beneficial for energetic contraction economy since slower shortening velocity improves the efficiency of contraction for equivalent work in much the same way that β-blockade lowers myocardial oxygen consumption. There has been some difficulty, however, in showing similar shifts in hypertrophied hearts from human postmortem specimens.[80]

We have examined LDH isozymes and have shown that increased right ventricular work, produced by pulmonary artery banding, produces a shift in the pattern toward a distribution rich in A-subunits, or those that are associated with anaerobic metabolism. We have also shown the identical response in ventricular muscle biopsies of angina patients, undergoing coronary artery bypass grafting.[83] Creatine kinase activity has been analyzed[84] and similar distribution changes in creatine kinase isozymes also appear in hypertrophied hearts.

Changes in myosin, LDH, and creatine kinase isozymic distribution indicate genetic regulation of these proteins in response to stress. There are undoubtedly many other changes in protein patterns yet to be discovered during the course of stress induction and subsequent hypertrophy. It is conceivable that the role of stress proteins is to modulate the genome in a way that specifically initiates or represses transcription so that proteins specifically needed to meet the stress are synthesized.

AN INITIAL RESPONSE TO STRESS IS ALSO TRANSLATIONAL INHIBITION

The end result of prolonged stress is the process of growth and hypertrophy, a heavy consumer of energy. This poses a fundamental question regarding metabolic control during the initial response to stress. How can an energy-dependent process of this magnitude be initiated, when the organ itself must function more vigorously? The acutely banded heart is relatively ischemic and the acutely harvested or cross-clamped heart is totally ischemic, consequently they are operating, partially or totally, by anaerobiosis. Therefore, energy must be saved everywhere possible to maintain viability of the heart so that function can be maintained while the heart is adapting to the stress or when perfusion is reinstituted.

A possible answer to his question was published in 1981 by Currie and White from the University of Newfoundland.[85] They were the first group to demonstrate con-

clusively that protein synthesis in cardiac tissue comes almost to a standstill during periods of acute stress. Their observations were made from two-dimensional autoradiograms of cardiac proteins translated and labeled in vivo by hearts stressed by heat shock or by extirpation and slicing. These experiments showed that a powerful control mechanism was at work in mammalian tissue to inhibit protein synthesis during the acute-stress response. Our studies, shown in Figure 97–16, confirm their findings.

Comparison of the autoradiograms in Figures 97–9 and 97–11 with those in figure 97–16 raises an important point. When examining products of RNA, translated in vitro from stressed and control hearts, the only discernible difference is the presence of stress proteins. On the other hand, autoradiograms of proteins, synthesized in vivo by the cardiac cells themselves, show not only the presence of stress proteins in stressed hearts, but also that the synthesis of many normally occurring proteins has ceased. The evidence suggests that the control site for the generalized suppression of protein synthesis operates predominantly at the translational, rather than the transcriptional, level, while the control site for stress protein synthesis is clearly at the transcriptional level.

To test these observations, we analyzed polysomes extracted from the right ventricle of dogs before and after heat shock.[58] Sucrose gradient sedimentation profiles of polysomes from control myocardial tissue showed a distribution with the peak at four to five ribosomes per message. The profile obtained from heat-shocked hearts showed a larger monosomal peak and a sharp decline of polysomal material toward the heavier polysomal region as shown in Figure 97–17. This and the autoradiographic evidence strongly support the contention that stress-induced suppression of protein synthesis operates through translational inhibition. There are at least three advantages that accrue to the cell by inhibiting protein synthesis:

1. Available energy can be diverted to areas more imminently vital to cell function.
2. Free ribosomes are available for the rapid synthesis of stress proteins.
3. Free ribosome accumulation may inhibit transcription of rRNA genes, thereby saving more energy (shown in eukaryotes).[86]

There are numerous disadvantages that accrue to the surgeon and patient by inhibiting protein synthesis:

1. hypoproteinemia
2. hemorrhagic disorders
3. wound dehiscences
4. anastomotic dehiscence
5. multiorgan systems failure
6. compromised immune system, etc

Unfortunately, even though an acute stress may be of short duration, the response itself, i.e., stress protein synthe-

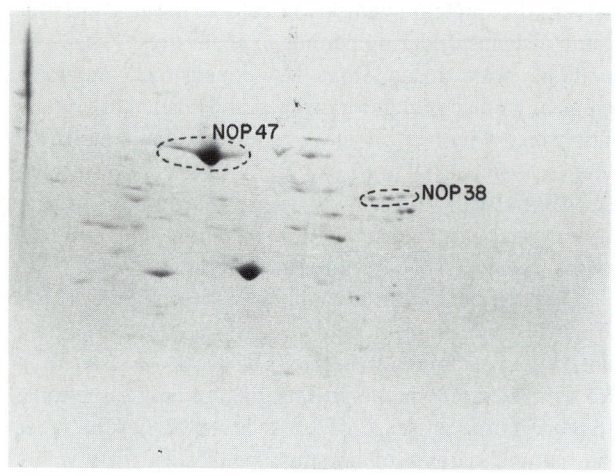

A

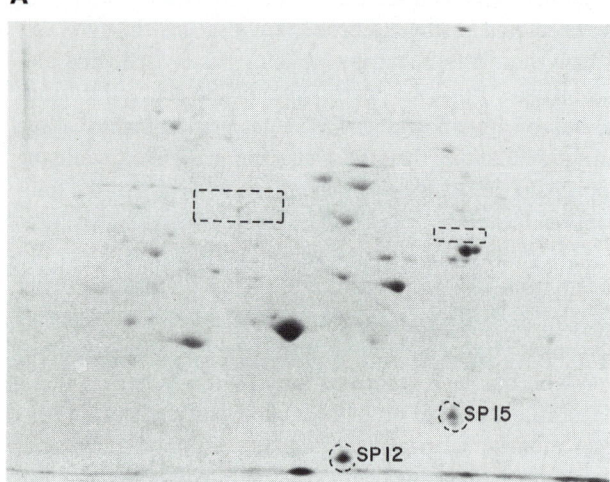

B

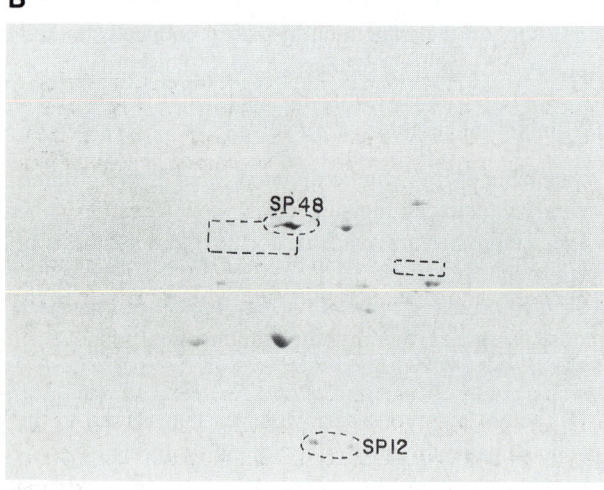

C

Figure 97–16. Two-dimensional autoradiogram of proteins extracted from rat hearts. **A.** Control; normally occurring proteins (NOPs) 47 and 38 are circled. **B.** Heart that underwent aortic banding for 1 hour; rectangular boxes show where NOPs 47 and 38 have disappeared while SPs have been synthesized; **C.** Heart from a rat that was heat shocked at 42° C for 1 h; rectangular boxes again show where NOPs 47 and 38 have disappeared while sps have been synthesized. *(From Lai Y-K, Havre PA, Hammond GL: Cardiac hypertrophy cannot proceed without initial suppression of protein synthesis. Biochem Biophys Res Commun 135:857–863, 1986, with permission.)*

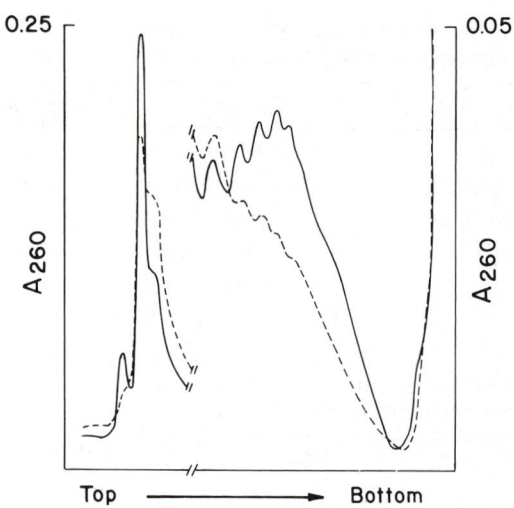

Figure 97–17. Sedimentation distribution of polysomes isolated from control (——) and heat-shocked (– – –) canine heart tissue. The ordinate scale is expanded 5-fold after the monosome peak. *(From Lai Y-K, Havre PA, Hammond GL: Heat shock stress initiates simultaneous transcriptional and translational changes in the dog heart. Biochem Biophys Res Commun 134:166–171, 1986.)*

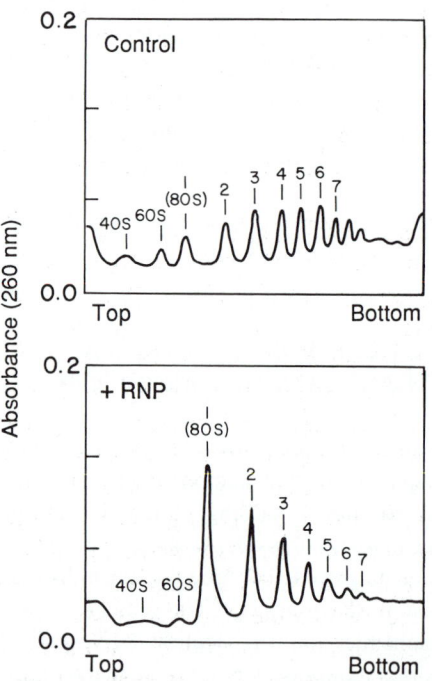

Figure 97–18. Cardiac polysomes isolated from control tissue were incubated for 80 min with water (control) or 5 ng of RNP (ribonuclease-like peptide). Treated polysomes were centrifuged for 100 min on 0.4–1.2 *M* sucrose gradients. Gradients were fractionated by pumping sucrose from the bottom of the tube and absorbance monitored at 260 nm. Each peak (after 60 S) is labeled as to number of ribosomes/message. See Table 97–2 for quantitation of number of ribosomes/message. *(From Havre PA, Hammond GL: Isolation of a translation inhibiting peptide from myocardium. Am J Physiol 255(Part II):H1024–H1031, 1988.)*

TABLE 97–2. PERCENTAGE OF RIBOSOMES IN MONOSOMES AND POLYSOMES

Ribosomes/mRNA[a]	Control (%)	RNP[b] Treated (%)
1	9.7	32.6
2	11.6	20.0
3	13.3	16.9
4	11.2	9.7
5	9.8	7.4
6	10.8	4.5
7	6.15	3.1

[a]1, monosomes; 2, disomes; 3, trisomes, etc.
[b]RNP (ribonuclease-like peptide).
From Havre PA, Hammond GL: Isolation of a translation inhibiting peptide from myocardium. Am J Physiol 255(Part II):H1024–H1031, 1988.

sis and translational inhibition, once initiated, continues for an as yet unknown period of time even though resuscitation may have reversed the acidotic trigger that set the response in motion. No matter how quickly we extirpated hearts, placed them in iced saline, and commenced normoxic Krebs solution perfusion (approximately 5 min), the stress response was initiated.[87] Because suppression of protein synthesis has such dire clinical consequences, we examined the molecular biology of the response.

We noted previously, as shown in Figure 97–17, that the suppression was associated with a shift in the polysome profile toward the monosome region. That is to say, each mRNA strand that normally has an average of two to seven attached ribosomes, under stress conditions, had only one to three attached ribosomes. This configuration, of course, would sharply decrease the amount of protein synthesized by each polysome.

Using an in vitro translation assay to follow activity, we developed a purification scheme that led to the purification, from cardiac tissue, of a ribonuclease-like peptide that produced translational inhibition. The peptide caused the polysome profile to shift toward the monosome region when added to polysome preparations (Fig. 97–18, Table 97–2) and produced marked suppression of translational activity when added to the in vitro assay system. The peptide appeared to act by preventing formation of the 80 S initiation complex.[88] That is, by keeping separate the two components, 40 S and 60 S, of ribosomes (Fig. 97–19).

Why translational inhibition occurs in most cellular mRNAs, but not stress protein mRNA, is unknown. The inhibitory effect of stress on transcription and translation can have severe clinical effects. Bulkley et al from the Department of Surgery at Johns Hopkins examined the effect of hemorrhagic shock and resuscitation on transcription of heat shock and acute phase protein genes in liver and found that if the stress was severe enough, the heat shock genes would be transcribed, but not the acute phase protein genes.[89] Taken together, generalized suppressed translation and suppressed transcription of the acute phase protein genes would leave a patient completely unable to mount a systemic defence. These findings help explain why micro-

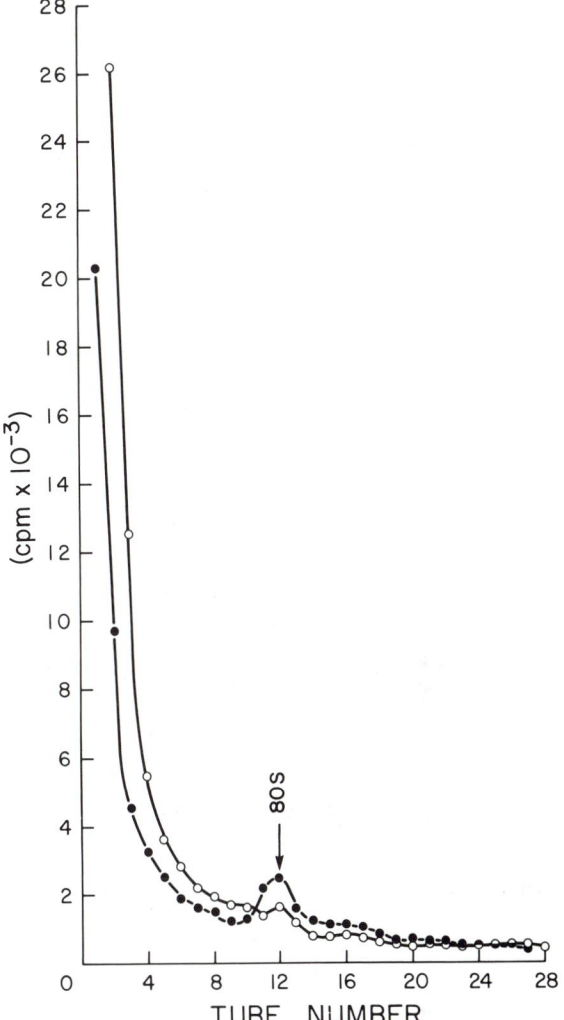

Figure 97–19. Effect of ribonuclease-like peptide on formation of the 80 S initiation complex. Initiation in the presence or (●—●) or absence (○—○) of peptide. *(From Havre PA, Hammond GL: Isolation of a translation inhibiting peptide from myocardium. Am J Physiol 255(Part II):H1024–H1031, 1988.)*

scopic evidence of massive cell death is not a common finding in patients dying from multisystem failure. The cells are viable but cannot function. For the future, it will be important to separate the stress response so that the beneficial effect conferred by stress proteins on subsequent stresses, i.e., preserving tertiary conformation of other proteins, possible induction of adaptive genes, and possible generation of free radical scavengers, can be maintained while the translation inhibitory effects can be limited to the time of the stress itself with no extension into the postresuscitive period. Figure 97–20 illustrates the possible pathways involved in the cell stress response.

Understanding cell stress provides a sound biological rationale for reinforcing surgical principles. Pre-, intra-, and postoperative homeostasis must be maintained. Ischemic times must be kept to a minimum. Hypoxia, acidosis, and shock must be treated immediately.

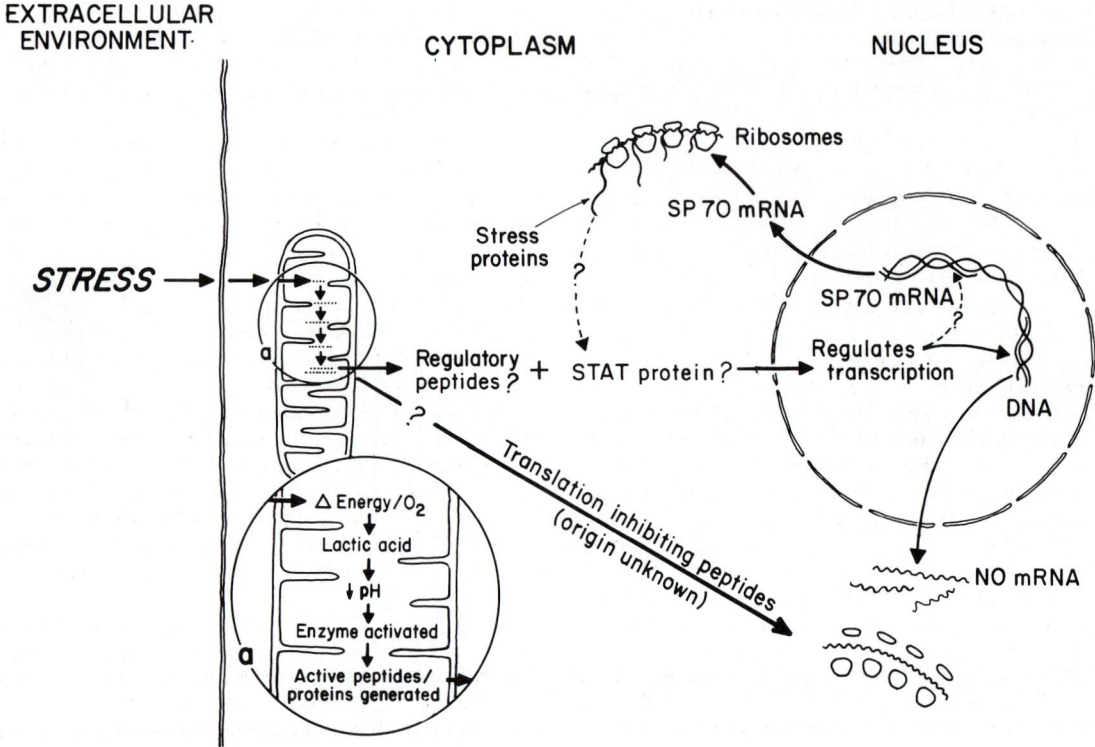

Figure 97–20. Theoretical pathway for the conversion of physiological stimuli into biochemical signals that initiate the stress response. mRNA is shown as either translating sp 70, separated from ribosomes, or normally occurring (NO) but not in polysomal configuration.

REFERENCES

1. Shine KI, Langer GA: Control of ion movement by cardiac sarcolemma. *Rec Adv Stud Cardiac Struct Metab* **9**:21–31, 1976
2. Smith DS: *Muscle.* New York, Academic Press, 1972
3. Stephenson EW: Activation of fast skeletal muscle: Contributions of studies on skinned fibers. *Am J Physiol* **240**(Cell Physiol 9):C1–C19, 1981
4. Adelstein RS, Hathaway DR: Role of calcium and cyclic adenosine 3′:5′ monophosphate in regulating smooth muscle contraction. *Am J Cardiol* **44**:783–787, 1979
5. Perry SV: The contractile and regulatory proteins of the myocardium. In Nayler WG (ed): *Contraction and Relaxation in the Myocardium.* London, Academic Press, 1975, pp 29–77
6. Hathaway DR, Eaton CR, Adelstein RS: Regulation of human platelet myosin kinase by calcium-calmodulin and cyclic AMP. In Mann KG, Fletcher FB (eds): *The Regulation of Coagulation.* New York, Elsevier North-Holland, 1980
7. Noble MIM, Pollack GH: Cardiac contraction. In Nayler WG (ed): *Contraction and Relaxation in the Myocardium.* London, Academic Press, 1975, p 79–112
8. Internal membranes and the synthesis of macromolecules. In Alberts B, Bray D, Lewis J, et al (eds): *Molecular Biology of the Cell.* New York, Garland, 1983, p 339
9. Tada M, Kirchberger MA, Katz AM: Regulation of calcium transport in cardiac sarcoplasmic reticulum by cyclic AMP-dependent protein kinase. *Rec Adv Stud Cardiac Struct Metab* **9**:225–239, 1976
10. Fozzard HA, Beeler GW: The voltage clamp and cardiac electrophysiology. *Circ Res* **37**:403, 1980
11. Hauswirth O, Singh BN: Ionic mechanisms in heart muscle in relation to the genesis and the pharmacological control of cardiac arrhythmias. *Pharmacol Rev* **30**:5, 1978
12. Fabiato A, Fabiato F: Techniques of skinned cardiac cells and of isolated cardiac fibers with disrupted sarcolemmas with reference to the effects of catecholamines and of caffeine. *Rec Adv Stud Cardiac Struc Metab* **9**:81–94, 1976
13. Coraboeuf E: Ionic basis of electrical activity in cardiac tissues. *Am J Physiol* **23**:H101–116, 1978
14. Noble E: *The Initiation of the Heartbeat.* Oxford, Clarendon Press, 1975
15. Sperelakis N, Schneider JA: A metabolic control mechanism for calcium ion influx that may protect the ventricular myocardial cell. *Am J Cardiol* **37**:1079–1085, 1976
16. Tsien RW: Cyclic AMP and contractile activity in heart. *Adv Cyclic Nucleotide Res* **8**:363–420, 1977
17. Tsien RW, Giles WR, Greengard P: Cyclic AMP mediates the effects of adrenaline on cardiac Purkinje fibres. *Nature (New Biol)* **240**:181–183, 1972
18. Golenhofen K, Weston AH: Differentiation of calcium activation systems in vascular smooth muscle. In Betz E (ed): *Ionic Actions on Vascular Smooth Muscle.* New York, Springer-Verlag, 1976, pp 21–25
19. Fabiato A, Fabiato F: Calcium and cardiac excitation-contraction coupling. *Annu Rev Physiol* **41**:473–484, 1979
20. Krebs EG, Beavo JA: Phosphorylation-dephosphorylation enzymes. *Annu Rev Biochem* **48**:923–959, 1979
21. Kuo JB, Greengard P: Cyclic nucleotide-dependent protein kinases. IV. Widespread occurrence of adenosine 3′,5′-monophosphate dependent protein kinase in various tissues and phyla of the animal kingdom. *Proc Natl Acad Sci USA* **64**:1349–1355, 1969
22. Watanabe AM, Lindemann JP, Jones LR, et al: Biochemical mechanisms mediating neural control of the heart. In Abboud FM, Fozzard HA (eds): *Disturbances in Neurogenic Control of the Circulation.* Baltimore, Waverly Press, 1981, pp 189–203
23. Antman EM, Stone PH, Muller JE: Calcium channels blocking agents in the treatment of cardiovascular disorders. Part I: Basic and clinical electrophysiologic effects. *Ann Intern Med* **93**:875–885, 1980

24. Reuter H: Properties of two inward membrane currents in the heart. *Annu Rev Physiol* **41**:413–424, 1979

25. Ellrodt G, Chew CYC, Singh BN: Therapeutic implications of slow-channel blockade in cardiocirculatory disorders. *Circulation* **62**:669–679, 1980

26. Stone PH, Antman EM, Muller JE, et al: Calcium channel blocking agents in the treatment of cardiovascular disorders. Part II: Hemodynamic effects and clinical applications. *Ann Intern Med* **93**:886–904, 1980

27. Harken AH, Horowitz LN, Josephson ME: Comparison of standard aneurysmectomy with directed endocardial resection for the treatment of recurrent sustained ventricular tachycardia. *J Thorac Cardiovasc Surg* **80**:527–534, 1980

28. Landmark K, Refsum AM, Simonsen S, et al: Verapamil and pulmonary hypertension. *Acta Med Scand* **204**:299–302, 1978

29. Nayler WG, Ferrari R, Williams A: Protective effect of pretreatment with verapamil, nifedipine and propranolol on mitochondrial function in the ischemic and reperfused myocardium. *Am J Cardiol* **46**:242–248, 1980

30. Clark RE, Christlieb IY, Henry PD, et al: Reduction of consequences of ischemia and preservation of myocardium with nifedipine. *Am J Cardiol* **43**:361, 1979

31. Kordylewski L, Karrison T, Page E: P-face particle density of freeze-fractured vertebrate cardiac plasma membrane. *Am J Physiol* **245**:H992, 1983

32. Kordylewski L, Karrison T, Page E: Measurements on the internal structure of freeze-fractured cardiac plasma membrane. *Am J Physiol* **28**:H297, 1985

33. Kuo TH, Tsang W, Wiener J: Defective Ca^{2+}-pumping ATPase of heart sarcolemma from cardiomyopathic hamster. *Biochim Biophys Acta* **900**:10, 1987

34. Wagner JA, Reynolds IJ, Weisman HF, et al: Calcium antagonist receptors in cardiomyopathic hamster: Selective increases in heart, muscle, brain. *Science* **25**:515, 1986

35. Sharma RV, Gupta RC, Ramanadham M, et al: Reduced cAMP levels and glycogen phosphorylase activation in isoproterenol perfused SHR myocardium. *Basic Res Cardiol* **78**:695, 1983

36. Kannel WB, Hjoltland M, Castelli WP: Role of diabetes in congestive heart failure: The Framingham study. *Am J Cardiol* **34**:29, 1974

37. Nishio Y, Kashiwagi A, Kida Y, et al: Deficiency of cardiac β-adrenergic receptor in streptozocin-induced diabetic rats. *Diabetes* **37**:1181, 1988

38. Havre PA, Hammond GL: Isolation of a translation-inhibiting peptide from myocardium. *Am J Physiol* **255**(Part II):H1024, 1988

39. Rangan U, Bulkley GB: Prospects for treatment of free radical-mediated tissue injury. *Br Med Bull* **49**:700–718, 1993

40. Gutteridge JMC: Lipid Peroxidation: Some problems and concepts. In Halliwell B (ed): *Oxygen Radicals and Tissue Injury: Proceedings of an Upjohn Symposium.* Bethesda, MD, Federation of American Societies for Experimental Biology, 1988, pp 9–19

41. Sawada M, Carlson JC: Rapid plasma membrane changes in superoxide radical formation, fluidity, an phospholipase A_2 activity in the corpus luteum of the rat during induction of luteolysis. *Endo* **128**:2992–2998, 1991

42. Wu X, Yao K, Carlson JC: Plasma membrane changes in the rat corpus luteum induced by oxygen radical generation. *Endo* **133**:491–495, 1993

43. Reilly PM, Bulkley GB: Tissue injury by free radicals and other toxic oxygen metabolites. *Br J Surg* **77**:1324–1325, 1990

44. McGilvery RW: *Biochemistry: A Functional Approach.* Philadelphia, PA, W.B. Saunders, 1983, p 418

45. Gharagozloo F, Melendez FJ, Hein RA, et al: Superoxide dismutase and catalase preserve right and left ventricular function and compliance in the ex vivo sheep heart preserved for eight hours. *Surg Forum* **37**:243, 1986

46. Gharagozloo F, Melendez FJ, Hein RA, et al: The effect of oxygen free radical scavengers on the recovery of regional myocardial function after acute coronary occlusion and surgical reperfusion. *J Thorac Cardiovasc Surg* **95**:631, 1988

47. Bulkley GB: Free radicals and other reactive oxygen metabolites: Clinical relevance and the therapeutic efficacy of antioxidant therapy. *Surgery* **113**:479–483, 1993

48. Ando Y, Inoue M, Utsumi T, et al: Synthesis of acylated SOD derivatives which bind to the biomembrane lipid surface and dismutate extracellular superoxide radicals. *FEBS Lett* **240**:216–220, 1988

49. Mao GD, Poznansky MJ: Electron spin resonance study on the permeability of superoxide radicals in lipid bilayers and biological membranes. **305**:233–236, 1992

50. De Duve C: *A Guided Tour of the Living Cell,* Vol. 2. New York, Scientific American Books, 1994

51. Alpert NR, Mulieri LA: Increased myothermal economy of isometric force generation in compensated cardiac hypertrophy induced by pulmonary artery constriction in the rabbit. *Circ Res* **50**:491–500, 1982

52. Morgan HE, Rannels DE, McKee EE: Protein metabolism of the heart. In Berne RM, Sperelakis N, Geiger SR (eds): *The Handbook of Physiology—Section 2, The Cardiovascular System.* Bethesda, MD, American Physiological Society, 1979, pp 845–868

53. Cutiletta AF: Muscle and nonmuscle cell RNA polymerase activities in early myocardial hypertrophy. *Am J Physiol Soc* H901–H907, 1981

54. Schlesinger MJ, Ashburner M, Tissieres A: *Heat Shock—From Bacteria to Man.* New York, Cold Spring Harbor Laboratory, 1982

55. Ashburner M, Bonner JJ: The induction of gene activity in Drosophila by heat shock. *Cell* **17**:241–254, 1971

56. Leenders HJ, Berendes HD: The effect of changes in the respiratory metabolism upon genome activity in Drosophila. I. The induction of gene activity. *Chromosoma* **37**:433–444, 1972

57. Leenders HJ, Kemp A, Koninkx JG, Rosing J: Changes in cellular ATP, ADP, and AMP levels following treatments affecting cellular respiration and the activity of certain nuclear genes in Drosophila salivary glands. *Exp Cell Res* **86**:25–30, 1974

58. Lai Y-K, Havre PA, Hammond GL: Heat shock stress initiates simultaneous transcriptional and translational changes in the dog heart. *Biochem Biophys Res Commun* **134**:166–171, 1986

59. Van de Ploeg LHT, Giannini SH, Cantor CR: Heat shock genes: Regulatory role for differentiation in parasitic protozoa. *Science* **228**:1443–1446, 1985

60. Neidhardt FC, Van Bogelen RA, Vaughn V: The genetics and regulation of heat-shock proteins. *Annu Rev Genet* **18**:295–329, 1984

61. Schedl P, Artavenis-Tsakonas S, Steward R, et al: Two hybrid plasmics with D. melanogaster DNA sequences complementary to mRNA coding for the major heat shock protein. *Cell* **14**:921–929, 1978

62. Hunt C, Morimoto RI: Conserved features of eukaryotic hsp 70 genes revealed by comparison with the nucleotide sequence of human hsp70. *Proc Natl Acad Sci USA* **81**:6455–6459, 1985

63. Gudbjamason S, Brasch W, Bing RJ: Protein synthesis in cardiac hypertrophy and heart failure. In *Herzinsuffiziena.* Symposium in Hintzerzarten (Schwarzwald). Stuttgart, Georg Thieme Verlag, 1968, pp 184–189

64. Meerson FZ: Development of modern components of the mechanisms of cardiac hypertrophy. *Circ Res* Suppl **II,** 35–58, 1974

65. Hammond GL, Lai Y-K, Markert CL: Diverse forms of stress lead to new patterns of gene expression through a common and essential metabolic pathway. *Proc Natl Acad Sci USA* **79**:3485–3488, 1982

66. Peyman JA, Hammond GL: Localization of interferon-γ receptor in first trimester placenta to trophoblasts but lack of stimulation of HLA-DRA, -DRB or invarient chain mRNA expression by interferon-γ *J Immunol* **149**:2675–2680, 1992

67. Welch WJ: How cells respond to stress. *Sci Am* **268**:56–62, 1993

68. Lai Y-K, Lee W-C, Hu C-H, Hammond GL: The mitochondria are sensory organelles for cell stress recognition. *J Surg Res,* 1995 (submitted)

69. Johnson HM, Bazer FW, Szente BE, Jarpe MA: How interferons fight disease. *Sci Am* **270**:68–75, 1994

70. Sin YT: Induction of puffs in Drosophila salivary gland cells by mitochondrial factor(s). *Nature (London)* **258**:159–160, 1975

71. Welch WJ: Mammalian stress response: Cell physiology, structure/function of stress proteins, and implications for medicine and disease. *Physiol Reviews* **72**:1063–1081, 1992

72. Karmazyn M, Masler K, Currie RW: Acquisition and decay of heat shock-enhanced postischemic ventricular recovery. *Am J Physiol* **259**(Heart Cir Physiol 28):H421–431, 1990

73. Buchman TG, Cabin DE, Porter JM, Bulkley GB: Change in hepatic gene expression after shock/resuscitation. *Surgery* **106**:283–291, 1989

74. Thornalley PJ, Vasak M: Possible role for metallothionein in protection against radiation-induced oxidative stress. Kinetics and mechanism of its reaction with superoxide and hydroxyl radicals. *Biochim Biophys Acta* **827**:36–44, 1985

75. Alberts B, Bray D, Lewis J, et al (eds): *Molecula Biology of the Cell*, 2nd ed. New York, Garland, 1989, p 88

76. Koll H, Guiard B, Hartl FU: Antifolding activity of hsp 60 couples protein import into the mitochondrial matrix with export to the intermembrane space. *Cell* **68**:1163–1175, 1992

77. Welch WJ, Feramisco JR: Rapid purification of mammalian 70,000-dalton stress proteins: Affinity of the proteins for nucleotides. *Mol Cell Biol* **5**:1229–1237, 1985

78. Velazquez JM, DiDomenico BJ, Lindquist S: Intracellular localization of heat shock proteins in Drosophila. *Cell* **20**:679–689, 1980

79. Hoh JF, McGrath PA, Hale PT: Electrophoretic analysis of multiple forms of rat cardiac myosin: Effect of hypophysectomy and thyroxine replacement. *J Mol Cell Cardiol* **10**:1053–1076, 1978

80. Mercadier J-J, Bouveret P, Gorza L, et al: Myosin isoenzymes in normal and hypertrophied human ventricular myocardium. *Circ Res* **53**:52–62, 1983

81. Hoh JFY, Yeoh GPS, Thomas MAW, Higginbottom L: Structural differences in the heavy chains of rat ventricular myosin isozymes. *FEBS Lett* **97**:330–334, 1979

82. Litten III RZ, Martin BJ, Low RB, Alpert NR: Altered myosin isozyme patterns from pressure-overloaded and thyrotoxic-hypertrophied rabbit hearts. *Circ Res* **50**:856–864, 1982

83. Hammond GL, Nadal-Ginard B, Talner NS, Markert CL: Myocardial LDH isozyme distribution in the ischemic and hypoxic heart. *Circulation* **53**:637–643, 1976

84. Vatner DE, Ingwall JS: Effects of moderate pressure overload in cardiac hypertrophy on the distribution of creatinine kinase isozymes. *Proc Soc Exp Biol Med* **175**(1):5–9, 1984

85. Currie RW, White FP: Trauma-induced protein in rat tissues: A physiological role for a "heat shock" protein? *Science* **214**:72–73, 1981

86. Nomura M: The control of ribosome synthesis. *Sci Am* **250**:102–114, 1984

87. Hammond GL, Lai Y-K, Markert CL: Preliminary characterization of molecules that increase cell free translational activity of cardiac cytoplasmic RNA. *Eur Heart J* Suppl **F**:225–229, 1984

88. Havre PA, Hammond GL: Isolation of a translation inhibiting peptide from myocardium. *Am J Physiol* **255**(Part II):H1024–H1031, 1988

89. Schoeniger LO, Reilly PM, Bulkley GB, Buchman TG: Heat-shock gene expression excludes hepatic acute-phase gene expression after resuscitation from hemorrhagic shock. *Surgery* **112**:355–363, 1992

98

Transplantation Immunology

Joren C. Madsen and David H. Sachs

INTRODUCTION

Graft reduction is a complex immunological process resulting from the recognition of allogeneic histocompatibility antigens of the grafted tissue. To effectively prevent rejection, most transplant recipients require indefinite immunosuppressive therapy after transplantation. Though remarkably effective, current immunosuppressive regimens including cyclosporine or FK506, prednisolone, and azathioprine, are, for the most part, immunologically nonspecific in their mode of action. While diminishing the immune response to antigens presented by the graft, they also decrease the host's resistance to infection and malignancy. In addition, these agents have detrimental tissue-specific side effects such as cyclosporine-induced nephropathy, steroid-induced peptic ulceration, and azathioprine-induced hepatic dysfunction. If it were possible to induce a state of immunological unresponsiveness or tolerance in the recipient that was specific for the alloantigens of the organ donor, the complications of rejection and its treatment could be potentially eliminated. Thus, a major goal of clinical transplantation is to achieve a state of tolerance to alloantigen or xenoantigen, such that the long-term use of immunosuppressive drugs is no longer required.

In this chapter an overview is provided of (1) the immune mechanisms mediating graft rejection, (2) clinical and experimental methods of suppressing the rejection response, (3) chronic rejection, and (4) xenotransplantation.

MECHANISMS OF ALLOGRAFT REJECTION

The Major Histocompatibility Complex

Transplants are rejected due to recognition by the immune system of histocompatibility antigens on the surface of cells of the donor that are not present on cells of the recipient. If there are no such disparate antigens, such as in the case of identical twins, then no rejection response occurs. However, in all other cases, there are numerous antigenic differences between members of the same species that can provide sufficient stimulus to cause rejection. In general, histocompatibility antigens are inherited as Mendelian dominant characteristics and are codominantly expressed, so that if an individual has the genes for such an antigen, that antigen will be expressed on the individual's tissues. The most important histocompatibility antigens are those of the major histocompatibility complex (MHC), known in human beings as the HLA system. It is generally believed that the prime physiological role of MHC antigens is to distinguish "self" from "nonself." Therefore, it is not surprising that MHC antigens provide a formidable barrier to a transplant. There are numerous other antigens capable of causing rejection, termed minor histocompatibility antigens. The response to these minor antigens is weaker and can be overcome with relatively small doses of immunosuppressive agents.

The genetic region coding HLA antigens can be divided into a series of genes coding for class I (HLA-A, B, C) and class II (DP, DQ, DR) antigens (Fig. 98–1), which differ in tissue distribution and function. Class I antigens are expressed on almost all cells of an organism while Class II antigens show a limited tissue distribution, being expressed on antigen presenting cells, including B lymphocytes, activated T lymphocytes, macrophages, dendritic cells, and endothelium in some species, including man. Functionally, Class I molecules present antigenic peptides primarily to T lymphocytes expressing the CD8 surface antigen, while Class II molecules present peptides to T cell expressing the CD4 phenotype. This restriction is due to the fact that the CD8 and CD4 molecular complexes bind to monomorphic determinants on Class I and Class II molecules, respectively.

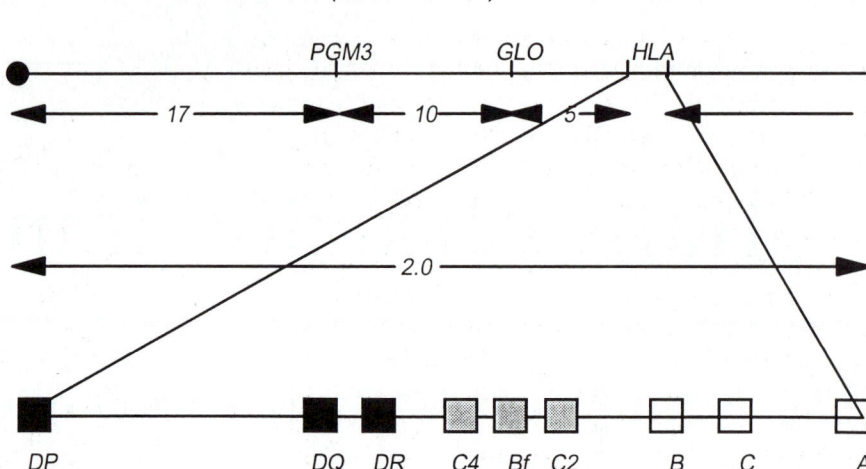

Figure 98–1. A linear map of the HLA complex.

Genetics of the MHC

HLA antigens are among the most polymorphic molecules within the species. That is, within each class of HLA molecules, a large number of variants (alleles) exist in the population as a whole. Thus, if a large number of individuals from the population were examined, many genes for each type of product would be found, each coding for a separate MHC allele or variant. However, it is important to remember that each individual has only a very small set of different MHC genes and expresses a maximum of two alleles at each locus. While polymorphism presumably conveys a survival advantage to the species by ensuring a broad capacity to respond to a large number of foreign antigens, it also makes the likelihood of achieving a MHC match in two unrelated humans extremely small.

For instance, in bone marrow transplantation, living *un*related donors may be used. Thus, large banks of potential unrelated donors have been established to make possible matching of bone marrow transplants between unrelated individuals. However, the polymorphism of HLA is so great that even with bone marrow registries of more than 100,000 potential donors, the chances of finding a match for any given recipient are still less than 50%. Clearly, it would be extremely difficult to find an exact match for all HLA antigens among potential cadaver organ donors.

Fortunately, in the case of bone marrow transplants and also kidney transplants, it is sometimes possible to find HLA identical donors among siblings of the potential recipient. This possibility arises because all of the HLA loci are inherited in a linked fashion on a single chromosome. Thus, every sibling from the same parents has a 25% chance of being HLA identical to a given sibling recipient (i.e., receiving the same two HLA chromosomes from the parents) (Fig. 98–2). When kidney transplantation is performed between HLA identical siblings, the results are remarkably good. Many patients are returned to a normal life after a

short hospital stay and on minimal long-term immunosuppression. However, it is obvious that HLA identical transplants are possible only from organs or tissues that permit removal without undo damage to the donor. Thus, although matching provides a reasonable approach to avoiding the immune response to kidney and bone marrow transplants, MHC matching alone is an unsatisfactory approach for heart transplants, and a controversial approach to transplants of other organs such as lung and liver, for which partial removal entails substantial risk to the donor.

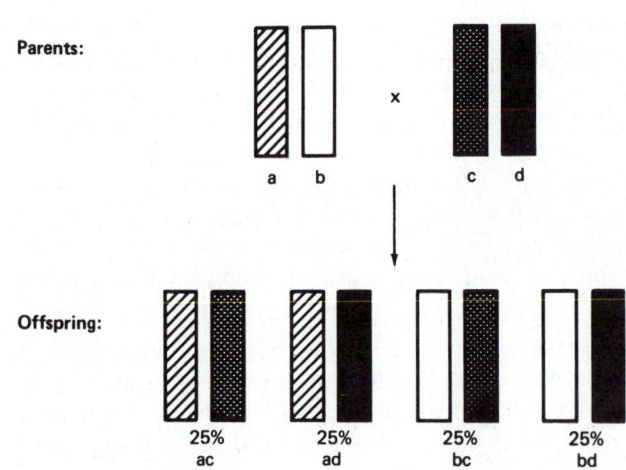

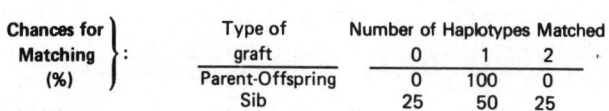

Figure 98–2. Segregation of HLA haplotypes in families. As illustrated, 25% of siblings are expected to share the same HLA genotype.

Antigen Presenting Cells

Foreign antigens of all sorts are presented to T lymphocytes on the surface of specialized, Class II-bearing cells termed antigen-presenting cell (APCs). Several types of cells have antigen-presenting capability, including dendritic cells, macrophages, and activated B cells.[10,11] The important role of APCs in graft rejection is illustrated best by the prolonged survival of some allografts when APCs in the donor organ have been eliminated.[12] APCs are unique, not only in their ability to present antigen, but in their ability to provide additional signals necessary for T cell activation. Together these additional components of T cell activation, are referred to as the *second signal* (occupancy of the T cell receptor being the first signal). The second signal is probably comprised of both the lymphokines secreted by APCs (i.e., interleukin-1 and interleukin-2), and the signals transmitted after binding of certain surface accessory and adhesion molecules, such as CD4 or CD8 with their determinants on Class II and Class I MHC molecules, respectively; LFA-1 with ICAM-1, -2, -3, CD2 (T11) with CD48 (LFA-3), and CD28 (CTLA-4) with B7.

An important aspect of the second signal is that in the absence of some or all of its components, T cells stimulated by foreign antigen may actually become inactivated.[13] This phenomenon, termed *anergy,* may explain the acceptance of APC-depleted grafts and the prolonged survival of subsequent grafts from the same organ donor that have not been APC-depleted.[14]

Alloreactivity

The immune response to an allograft differs from other immunological responses in two fundamental ways. First, allogeneic responses are much stronger than classic immune responses, and second, they can be stimulated by two different sets of APCs, one from the donor, expressing donor MHC antigens, and one from the recipient, expression recipient MHC antigens.

Most T cell-mediated immune responses in the body (e.g., against virally infected cells) occur when T cells recognize foreign antigens (e.g., viral proteins) that have been processed and presented by self-MHC molecules on the surface of the organism's own APCs.[15] In fact, the mechanism of this recognition has recently been elucidated by solving the structure of Class I[16] and Class II MHC molecules.[17] These molecules have a groove in their surface into which can fit a variety of peptides (Fig. 98–3). It turns out that APCs are able to acquire, process, and "present" (place in the groove of their MHC molecules) foreign peptide antigens, and in doing so, make them recognizable to T lymphocytes. This classic pathway of T cell activation, termed *self-restriction,* occurs, to some extent, in an immune response to an allograft (Fig. 98–4A). However, the extraordinary strength associated with an immune response to a

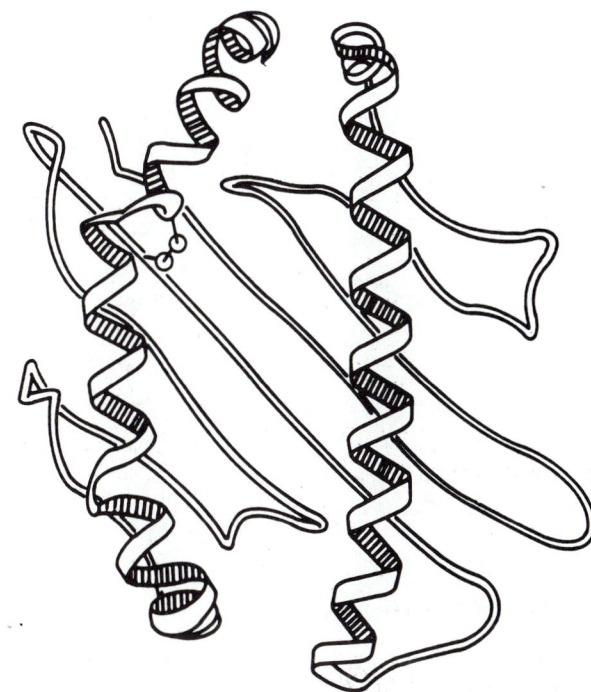

Figure 98–3. Structure of HLA-A2. A schematic representation of the outer surface of HLA-A2, which is contacted by the T cell receptor. The α-helices are represented by helical ribbons. The β-strands are shown as thin lines and form a eight-stranded β-pleated sheet on top of which lie the two α-helices. The antigen recognition site is defined by the deep groove running between the two long α-helices. *(Reprinted with permission from Nature,[16] copyright (1987) Macmillan Magazines Limited.)*

transplanted organ is due to a different mechanism. It involves T cells with the unique ability to respond to the foreign MHC molecules *directly,* without the usual requirement that peptides of the foreign MHC molecules be processed and presented by self-MHC antigens (Fig. 98–4B). This phenomenon, termed *alloreactivity,* is thought to be the predominant pathway in graft rejection.[14]

The simplest explanation for alloreactivity is that it results from the cross-reaction of T cells, normally specific for antigen and self-MHC (self-restricted), with allogeneic MHC molecules.[18] The peculiar strength of alloreactivity may be due, in part, to the fact that alloreactive T cells comprise sets of such cross-reactive cells and therefore outnumber T cells reactive with an exogenous protein (self-restrictive cells) by at least two orders of magnitude,[19] and that there is a greater density of allogeneic MHC determinants on the surface of APCs derived from any particular donor.[20]

T Helper Lymphocytes

The pivotal cells in rejection are T lymphocytes, in particular, T helper cells that predominantly express the CD4 molecular complex, or phenotypic marker, on their cell surface. CD4+ T helper cells recognize foreign Class II antigens, ei-

Allograft   Recipient

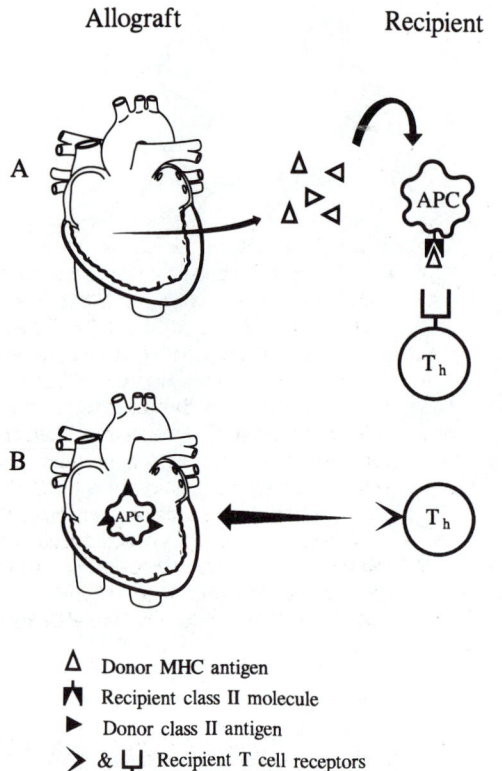

△   Donor MHC antigen
Ⱬ   Recipient class II molecule
▶   Donor class II antigen
⋟ & ⊔   Recipient T cell receptors

Figure 98–4. Direct and indirect routes of sensitization. Donor antigen shed from the graft can be taken up by recipient APCs to be processed and presented to recipient T cells. **A.** This is indirect sensitization via self-restricted T cells. Alternatively, alloantigens on donor APCs can directly activate host T cells. **B.** This is direct sensitization via alloreactive T cells. APC, antigen presenting cell; Th, helper T cell.

ther directly on donor-type APCs or on host-type APCs after they have been taken up, processed, and presented as peptides by recipient Class II molecules. As mentioned above, these two pathways of T cell activation are called allorestricted and self-restricted, respectively. In the jargon of transplant immunologists, these pathways are termed *direct* and *indirect sensitization.*

Once activated by foreign Class II antigens, CD4+ T cells produce an array of lymphokines in the graft that is essential for the growth and differentiation or activation of the other cells that mediate the effector phase of the rejection process. CD4+ T cells can be divided into Th1 and Th2 subpopulations according to the types of cytokines they produce.[21] The Th1 subpopulation secretes interleukin 2 (IL-2), interferon-γ (INF-γ), and tumor necrosis factor-β (TNF-β). IL-2 is required for the growth and differentiation of cytotoxic T lymphocytes (which usually express CD8), IFN-γ induces the expression of MHC Class II molecules within the graft, while the combination of IFN-γ and TNF-β stimulates macrophages to release prostaglandins and free oxygen or nitric oxide radicals. Therefore, Th1 cells are important in promoting specific cytotoxic, in addition to nonspecific inflammatory reactions.

In contrast, Th2 cells secrete Il-4, IL-5, and IL-10, which seem to augment B cell-mediated humoral responses, and also suppress Th1 cells. Thus, lymphokines secreted by one subpopulation can inhibit the lymphokines produced by the other.[22]

Effectors of Graft Rejection

Although virtually every known immunological effector mechanism has been shown to damage transplanted tissues, there is evidence that the three major components of graft rejection include (1) donor-specific T cytotoxic lymphocytes, (2) nonspecific inflammatory cells, and (3) antidonor antibodies (Fig. 98–5).

T cells, especially cytotoxic T cells, expressing the CD8 surface marker and recognizing Class I antigens, are thought to play the preeminent role in effecting graft rejection. Evidence for the importance of T cells in graft rejection comes from experimental studies demonstrating that athymic mice (with congenitally absent T cells) accept tissue grafts from other members of the same species and even from members of other species.[23] Furthermore, repopulation of these athymic mice with purified T cells reconstitutes their ability to reject grafts.[24] In humans, the efficacy of an immunosuppressive agent usually correlates with its ability to either eliminate T cells or block T cell responses which supports the central role of T cells in rejection.[4] The mechanism of CD8+ cytotoxic T cell activation is thought to involve the recognition of donor Class I antigen (first signal) in a setting of increased levels of IL-2 (second signal) secreted by activated CD4+ T helper cells. Although activated cytotoxic T cells have been assumed to cause graft destruction, how T cells actually destroy transplanted tissues in vivo is not clear. Recent evidence suggests a mechanism that involves direct physical contact and a process that resembles the cytologic changes of *apoptosis.*[25]

The contribution of other, nonspecific cellular mechanisms to the rejection of solid tissue is controversial. Natural killer (NK) cells and lymphokine-activated killer (LAK) cells have been defined in tumor allograft models and some xenograft models, but their relevance to the rejection of allogeneic organ transplants is not clear.[26] Activated macrophages, neutrophils, and mast cells, triggered by lymphokine release, may cause severe local inflammation resulting in nonspecific damage to bystander cells.

Although cell-mediated mechanisms predominate in the rejection of transplanted organs, either preformed or induced antibodies can contribute to the rejection process. Pre-existing blood group antibodies, anti-MHC antibodies, or natural antibodies that react with endothelial antigens of other species can cause almost immediate rejection of vascularized organ grafts. This type of rejection, called *hyperacute* rejection, results from the antibody-induced activation of several biological cascades, including the complement, coagulation, and kallikrein/bradykinin cascades. Together, these events lead to graft edema, hemorrhage,

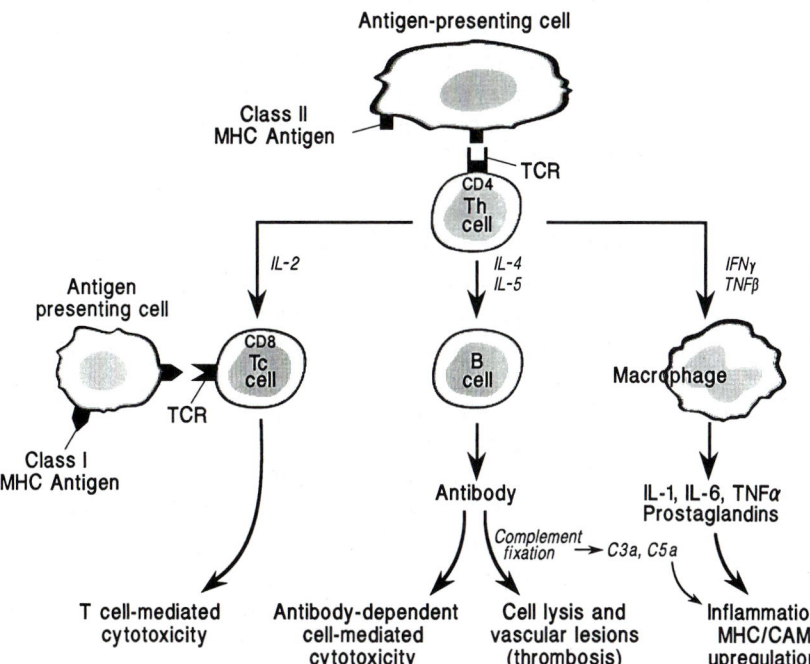

Antigen-presenting cell

Class II
MHC Antigen

TCR

CD4
Th
cell

IL-2

IL-4
IL-5

IFNγ
TNFβ

Antigen
presenting cell

CD8
Tc
cell

B
cell

Macrophage

TCR

Class I
MHC Antigen

Antibody

IL-1, IL-6, TNFα
Prostaglandins

Complement
fixation → C3a, C5a

T cell-mediated
cytotoxicity

Antibody-dependent
cell-mediated
cytotoxicity

Cell lysis and
vascular lesions
(thrombosis)

Inflammation,
MHC/CAM
upregulation

Figure 98–5. Pathway to acute cellular rejection. Foreign antigen is presented to the recipient's immune system via either the direct or indirect pathway. Activation of CD4+ T-helper cells leads to the production of lymphokines, which provide a second signal for CD8+ cytotoxic T cell activation, provide help for B cell-mediated antibody production, stimulate macrophages to secrete nonspecific mediators of inflammation, and up-regulate the expression of MHC antigens and endothelial cell adhesions molecules (CAM) on transplanted tissues. Activated cells migrate into the graft and cause specific cytotoxicity or inflammatory damage. *(Adapted from Hutchinson[26] by courtesy of Marcel Dekker, Inc.)*

and then vascular thrombosis destroying the graft within minutes or hours after transplantation. There is no known therapy for hyperacute rejection.

Rejection can also be mediated by either IgM or IgG antibodies formed in response to the donor graft. This has been termed *accelerated* rejection and on biopsy appears as predominant vascular destruction with a relative paucity of cellular infiltrate. Somewhat paradoxically, the injection of antidonor antibody into experimental recipients at about the time of transplantation can enhance the survival of the transplant and lead to long-term graft survival in some cases. This phenomenon is called *passive enhancement* and is, for the most part, restricted to rodent models of transplantation.

Leukocyte–Endothelial Interactions

The hallmark of cellular rejection is graft infiltration, which involves (1) the attachment of leukocytes to the vascular endothelium, (2) transmigration through the vessel wall, (3) migration within the graft, (4) selective retention of cells (activated) in the graft; and (5) local proliferation of cells.[26] Adherence of leukocytes to vascular endothelium is mediated by cell adhesion molecules (CAMs) of three general types including *selectins, integrins,* and *immunoglobulin superfamily-related* molecules. These act as receptors on leukocytes for ligands on vessel walls and in tissues.

Within minutes after stimulation, endothelial cells up-regulate P-selectin, then E-selectin, which make the endothelium more "sticky"—tethering flowing leukocytes to the vessel wall by loose adhesions and causing them to *roll* along the endothelium in the direction of blood flow. This *rolling effect* is mediated by selectins binding to carbohy-

drate moieties on leukocytes. Next, integrins such as LFA-1 and VLA-4 on the surface of lymphocytes and monocytes are activated to bind more strongly to their ligands—ICAM-1, -2, or -3 and VCAM-1 located on the endothelial surface. ICAM-1, -2, and -3 and VCAM-1 are members of immunoglobulin superfamily.

Thus, at sites of inflammation, the interaction of selectins with their ligands is responsible for the initial capture and subsequent rolling of leukocytes along the endothelium. These cells then become fixed and flattened to the vessel wall by integrin–immunoglobulin family interactions.[27] The molecular basis of diapedesis is unknown, although the ICAM-1–LFA-1 interaction appears to be critical. Leukocytes pass between the endothelium cell junctions where there is high density expression of cadherins and CD31 molecules. Leukocytes then penetrate the basement membrane to access tissues.[28]

PREVENTION OF ALLOGRAFT REJECTION

MHC-Matching

There are essentially three ways to overcome the immune response to a transplant: MHC-matching, nonspecific immunosuppression, and induction of tolerance.

It is standard medical practice for donor hearts and lungs to be allocated without consideration of the extent of HLA matching. The reasons for this include (1) time constraints, namely, the need to implant the donor organ within 6 hours of its procurement, (2) shortage of available organ donors, and (3) the continuing controversy over the significance of matching for the HLA complex in heart and/or lung transplant recipients. A number of studies have evaluated whether patient-graft survival, number of rejection episodes, time to onset of first rejection, histological rejection criteria, and death due to cardiac allograft vasculopathy correlated with the degree of donor–recipient HLA compatibility. Results have been mixed with some investigators reporting positive correlations,[29–32] while others were unable to demonstrate the significance of matching.[33,34] For instance, one of the largest single center study of 448 cardiac allograft recipients failed to show improved allograft survival with donor–recipient HLA matching.[33] However, the largest collaborative study to date in which 8331 patients were evaluated in 104 centers showed an impressive correlation between matching for HLA-A, -B, and -DR and graft survival at 3 years.[29] Matching for HLA-DR alone was associated with a beneficial effect, but not as marked as that of matching for all three HLA antigens.

Based on these findings, Opelz and Wujciak,[19] proposed that hearts be transplanted on the basis of prospective HLA matching, as is practiced in kidney transplantation. By HLA typing all potential recipients in a given region or country in advance, then combining waiting lists from neighboring geographic regions to create regional pools of 1000 patients, the authors predict that in under a 4-hour preservation limit, it would be possible to perform transplantations with no HLA-A, -B, or -DR mismatches or only one mismatch in 32% of patients, and in another 31% with only two mismatches. Based on their survival data, this would result in a 5% higher overall rate of transplant survival at 3 years.[29]

Would the expected outcome of prospective matching for cardiac transplantation—a 5% increase in 3-year graft survival—justify the effort and cost involved? Some argue that given the shortage of available hearts, the increased survival of HLA-matched hearts, and the risks of infection and lymphoproliferative diseases, a plan to initiate prospective HLA matching in cardiac transplantation be supported.[36] Others, however, make the point that minimizing ischemic time outweighs the advantages of matching.[33]

One would suspect that with improvements in cardiac allograft preservation[37] and HLA typing of peripheral blood from a potential donor before the heart is removed,[36] the percentage of HLA matched transplants could increase.

Immunosuppression

The second means for overcoming immune responses to a transplant involves administration of nonspecific immunosuppressive medications. This methodology has been responsible for the enormous success of the field of transplantation over the past three decades. In essence, nonspecific immunosuppression involves the administration of medications that depress all host immune responses. The amount of medications administered must be titrated such that the immune system is suppressed sufficiently not to reject the transplant, but not so extensively that the patient succumbs

to pathogens. Immunosuppressive agents such as prednisone, azathioprine, cyclosporin A, and, most recently, FK506 have all been chosen because of their relative selectivity for the kind of immunity involved in transplant rejection. Nevertheless, for all of these drugs, infections represent a major complication of therapy. In addition, immunosuppressive agents have tissue-specific toxicities and have been associated with increased incidence of malignancies in transplant recipients.

Immunosuppressive agents can be grouped into several broad categories by mechanism of action (Table 98–1). Drugs that block T cell activation do so by interfering with signal transduction pathways either early (cyclosporine, FK506) or late (rapamycin, leflunomide) in the cell cycle. Antimetabolites (azathioprine, mycophenolate) deplete nucleotides necessary for DNA synthesis. They inhibit lymphocyte proliferation in a semiselective manner because these cells, more than other cell types, depend on salvage pathways for nucleotide synthesis. Receptor antagonists are more specific in the cells they target. These drugs act by a variety of mechanisms and cause (1) lympholysis (immunotoxin conjugates), (2) inhibition of intercellular communication causing incomplete signaling (anti-ICAM, anti-LFA, anti-IL-1, and anti-IL-2), (3) induction of anergy by incomplete T cell stimulation (anti-CD4), and (4) inhibition of antigen presentation at the processing stage (deoxyspergualin) or at the presentation stage (soluble HLA antigen). Cytokine inhibitors target and potentially neutralize major inflammatory cytokines [IL-1, IL-6, tumor necrosis factor (TNF)]. Finally the inducers of suppression (SKF 105685, IL-2) are thought to expand natural suppressor activity.

It is beyond the scope of this chapter to review the immunology and pharmacology of all these drugs, however, some of the immunosuppressants currently in clinical use will be briefly reviewed along with potentially important experimental drugs. For a more in depth review the reader is referred to Thomson and Starzl[38] or Sollinger and Przepiorka.[39]

Cyclosporine (CyA) was originally discovered as an antifungal agent, but has had a profound impact on the field of transplantation. At present, the use of CyA, along with improvements in infection control, has increased the survival of cardiac allograft recipients to over 85% at 1 year.[40] FK506, discovered in 1984, is more potent than CyA and, though not similar structurally, has a similar spectrum of activity and mechanism of action. CyA and FK506 inhibit lymphocyte proliferation and lymphokine production by binding to intracellular receptors known as *immunophilins.* CyA specifically binds a subset of cytosolic immunophilins termed *cyclophilins* (CyPs), while FK506 binds to a subset termed *FK506 binding proteins* (FKBPs).[41] The complexes so formed (e.g., CyA/CyP or FK506/FKBP) work to inhibit *calcineurin,* an intracellular protein phosphatase that plays a crucial role in the induction of lymphokine genes, including the gene coding for IL-2.[42] With lymphokines such as IL-2 blocked, lymphocyte proliferation is suppressed.

TABLE 98–1. IMMUNOSUPPRESSIVE AGENTS

Therapeutic agent/strategy	Target	Major Toxicity	Status
Antimetabolites			
Cyclophosphamide	DNA alkylation	Marrow, GI	FDA-approved
Methotrexate	Dihydrofolate reductase	Marrow, mucosa	FDA-approved
Azathioprine	Purine biosynthesis	Marrow, GI, liver	FDA-approved
Mycophenolate mofetil	IMP dehydrogenase	GI	In clinical trials
Mizoribine (bredinin)	IMP dehydrogenase	GI, marrow	In clinical trials
Brequinar	Dihydroorate dehydrogenase	Marrow, mucosa	In clinical trials
T Cell Inhibitors			
Cyclosporine A	Calcineurin	Renal, CNS	FDA-approved
FK506 (Tacrolimus)	Calcinerurin	Renal, CNS	FDA-approved
SDZ IMM 125	SER/THR phosphatase	Renal, CNS	In clinical trails
Rapamycin	Unclear	Not reported	In clinical trials
Leflunomide (HWA 486)	Tyrosine kinase	Not reported	In clinical trials
Receptor Antagonists			
Antithymocyte globulin	Lymphocytes	Serum sickness	FDA-approved
Glucocorticoids	Steroid receptor family	GI, CNS, bone	FDA-approved
OKT3 (Muromonab-CD3)	CD3	Cytokine syndrome	FDA-approved
OKT4A	CD4	None	In clinical trails
H65-RTA	CD5	Capillary leak	In clinical trails
CTLA4-Ig	CD28	Not reported	In clinical trails
Anti-TAC	CD25 (IL-2R)	None	In clinical trails
DAB486-IL-2	CD25 (IL-2R)	Liver	In clinical trails
IL-1 receptor antagonist	IL-1 receptor	None	In clinical trails
Anti-LFA-1	LFA-1	None	In clinical trails
Anti-ICAM-1	ICAM-1	None	In clinical trails
15-Deoxyspergualin	Unknown	Marrow, GI	In clinical trials
Soluble HLA	TCR	Not reported	Preclinical
Cytokine Inhibitors			
Anti-IL-6	IL-6	Thrombocytopenia	In clinical trails
Anti-TNF	TNF	None	In clinical trials
Soluble IL-1 receptor	IL-1	None	In clinical trials
IK-10	Unknown	Not reported	Preclinical
Inducers of Suppression			
Aldesleukin (IL-2)	IL-2R	Capillary leak	Preclinical
SKF 105685	Unclear	Not reported	In clinical trials

Modified from Przepiorka D: Rational use of new immunosuppressive agents. In Przepiorka D, Sollinger H (eds): Recent Developments in Transplantation Medicine, volume I, New Immunosuppressive Drugs. Physicians & Scientists Publishing Co., Inc., Glenview, Illinois, 1995, pp 2–3, with permission.

Given their common mode of action, it is not surprising that CyA and FK506 have overlapping toxicities. Renal dysfunction and hypertension are their most frequent complications. Other side effects include neurological effects (headache, tremors, paresthesias, insomnia), gastrointestinal effects (nausea, vomiting, diarrhea), and diabetes.

OKT3 is a mouse monoclonal antibody directed against the human T cell receptor (CD3), which nonspecifically suppresses all T cell functions.[4] Although most frequently used to treat acute rejection episodes, OKT3 has also been shown to prevent rejection in prophylactic protocols. Following administration of OKT3, the number of peripheral lymphocytes drops dramatically, and T cells that reappear do not express CD3. The three problems associated with OKT3 therapy include (1) cytokine (TNF, INF-γ, IL-2) release causing fever, chills and pulmonary edema, (2) generation of antibodies against the murine antibody, which preclude repeated courses of OKT3, and (3) a dra-

matic increase in the incidence of lymphoproliferative disorders.[43]

Rapamycin is a structural homolog of FK506 that also binds FKBPs but does not inhibit calcineurin. Its mode of action is unclear. Rapamycin has exhibited impressive immunosuppressive activity in in vitro studies and rodent transplant models.[44] Of great interest is the fact that rapamycin prevented the development of cardiac allograft vasculopathy in rat allografts,[45] and thus may be effective in the prevention of chronic rejection.

15-Deoxyspergualin (DSG) is the derivative of the natural product spergualin, isolated from soil bacterium *Bacillus laterosporus*. Current data suggest that DSG acts by interfering with antigen presentation and T and B effector cell development by binding to the cytoplasmic protein Hsc70, a member of the heat shock protein family.[46] DSG is a potent suppressor of humoral responses; it is particularly effective in prolonging the survival of transplanted pancreatic islet cells, and, in comparison to other agents, it is remarkably effective in prolonging xenograft survival.[38] The major acute toxicity of DSG is myelosuppression.

Mycophenolate mofetil (RS-61443) is an exciting forerunner of the next generation of immunosuppressive agents. It is a fermentation product of several *Penicillium* species that acts as an antimetabolite, inhibiting inosine monophosphate dehydrogenase (IMPDH) and in doing so blocks the de novo pathway of purine synthesis. De novo purine synthesis is crucial for the proliferative responses of human T and B cells to antigens.[47] By inhibiting de novo purine metabolism in lymphocytes, both T and B cells are inhibited, leading to the depletion of immunocompetent cells.[48] Thus, mycophenolate mofetil should selectively inhibit lymphocyte proliferation with little effect on other major organs. Indeed, Phase I clinical trials have yielded encouraging results for the prevention and treatment of rejection with no concomitant nephrotoxicity, hepatotoxicity, or bone marrow suppression.[49]

Brequinar follows a similar immunosuppressive strategy as mycophenolate. It inhibits dihydroorotate dehydrogenase (DHO-DH) and thus blocks the de novo synthesis of pyrimidines. Stimulated T and B lymphocytes have limited pools of pyrimidines and are highly dependent on de novo pyrimidine synthesis for production of DNA and continued proliferation, more so than many other tissues. This differential sensitivity to brequinar allows low doses of the drug to be used for immunosuppression with correspondingly little toxicity.[50]

Preclinical experiments have demonstrated synergistic interactions between many of these drugs suggesting new and powerful combinations of immunosuppressive agents. Future clinical trials will likely include CyA supplemented by brequinar, rapamycin, and/or mycophenolate, to provide more effective suppression and at the same time a reduction in the side effects of any one drug alone.

Tolerance

The third method of preventing graft rejection and the major goal of modern transplantation immunology is the induction of transplantation tolerance. Transplantation tolerance refers to the elimination of the immune response to the antigens of the transplant while the immune response to all other antigens in the environment remains intact. Thus, although nonspecific immunosuppressive drugs eliminate immune cell populations with a broad range of reactivities, the induction of specific tolerance leads to loss or inactivation of only those immune cell populations with receptors specific for the antigens of the transplant. Such tolerance was demonstrated in the early 1950s by Billingham and colleagues,[1] who showed that injection of bone marrow across MHC barriers in neonatal mice was capable of producing animals that, in later life, remained specifically tolerant to tissue grafts from the bone marrow donor strain. Thus, an immature immune system such as that in a fetus or even a neonate is capable of being tricked by this procedure into considering the antigens of the donor as "self." However, to be of clinical use for transplants in adults, methods are needed to induce similar transplantation tolerance in animals whose immune system has already matured. This then is the goal of research in the field of specific transplantation tolerance.

Induction of tolerance in adult animals has been reported in many systems, but remains an elusive goal in clinical transplantation. There are three major ways in which a state of immunological tolerance to allogeneic transplants can be accomplished: (1) inactivation (but not elimination) of cells reactive to the foreign antigen (*anergy*); (2) elimination of cells reactive to the foreign antigens (*clonal deletion*); and (3) suppression of cells responsive to the foreign antigens by another, regulatory immunologic response (*suppression*).

Anergy refers to the presence of T cells that express the correct receptor for an antigen, but fail to respond when stimulated by the antigen. This unresponsive state is thought to be the result of T cells binding specific antigen but not receiving the appropriate "second signal" from antigen-presenting cells or helper T cells.[13] This concept follows from the basic two-signal model of lymphocyte activation suggested by Bretscher and Cohn; namely, that antigen–receptor occupancy alone leads to inactivation of the T cell, whereas this first signal in conjunction with a second costimulatory signal leads to activation.[51] The two-signal model of lymphocyte activation is supported by the fact that administration of IL-2 (a costimulatory signal) is able to reverse or prevent the induction of T cell anergy.[52] Evidence that T cell anergy, indeed, occurs is illustrated most clearly from work in which specific T cells from tolerant animals are shown to be unresponsive even to stimulation directly through their antigen receptor. In some models, anergy is associated with a down-regulation of cell surface proteins critical to T cell activation such as the T cell receptor (TCR) and/or accessory proteins like CD8.

Clonal deletion of T cells occurs predominantly in the thymus, where new T cells are formed, by a process known as *negative selection*. This process is involved during normal T cell differentiation as a means of avoiding self-reactive T cells that would otherwise cause autoimmunity. The induction of tolerance through establishment of chimerism (see below) depends predominantly on clonal deletion, and probably involves the presence of appropriate allogeneic bone marrow-derived cells in the thymus that participate (like their normal self counterparts) in negative selection of newly arising T cell clones.[60] Clonal deletion may also occur in the periphery, such as in the case of deletion of Vβ6+ cells in adult Mls-1[b] mice made tolerant to Mls-1[a]-expressing cells.[53] However, such clonal deletion would not be expected to eliminate new cells emerging from the thymus and, therefore, may not produce permanent tolerance.

Suppressor T cells have been invoked to explain why lymphoid cells isolated from recipients with long-term surviving allografts and adoptively transferred into syngeneic hosts can prolong the survival of a fresh graft from the same organ donor. For many years the hypothesis that suppressor cells controlled immune responses and were responsible for peripheral tolerance received wide acceptance.[54] However, many scientists have now abandoned this hypothesis, largely because it has not been possible to isolate and characterize the cells supposedly responsible for suppression. One possible explanation is that anergic T cells transfer tolerance to naive recipients by acting as incompetent competitors at sites of antigen presentation or by competing for cytokines, thereby preventing not only the initiation, but also the amplification of the rejection response.[55] Also, the microenvironment within the graft may be important for manifestations of suppressor cell function.[56] Another cell that may explain many suppressive phenomena is the *veto cell,* which is a cell defined by its ability to inhibit or eliminate the activity of T cells reactive with antigens on its surface. Such cells suppress, or "veto" the activity of the attacking cells, a function from which they derive their name.[57] Veto cells have been implicated in the mechanism of tolerance induction to Class I and Class II antigens expressed on donor lymphoid cells.

Finally, there is no reason to think that one mechanism alone must be responsible for graft acceptance in a given individual. Also, it should be remembered that these mechanisms for tolerance induction and maintenance have so far been demonstrated in experimental transplantation models in animals, and have yet to be extended to clinical transplantation.

Mixed Chimerism as an Approach to Transplantation Tolerance

It has been known for some time that adult mice can be made tolerant across MHC barriers by lethal irradiation and reconstitution with allogeneic bone marrow. However, there are two major problems with the use of bone marrow transplantation for induction of transplantation tolerance. If mature T cells are not removed from the donor bone marrow, the recipient that results often succumbs to the effects of *graft-versus-host disease.* If, on the other hand, mature T cells are removed from the bone marrow inoculum before transplantation, then chimerism and transplantation tolerance still occur, but the reconstituted recipient is relatively immunoincompetent. The reason for this relative immunoincompetence has been postulated to involve the failure of newly emerging T cells in an allogeneic host to develop appropriate MHC-restriction specificities for subsequent immune responses.[58] Thus, as illustrated in Figure 98–6A, when a lethally irradiated animal of strain A receives a T cell-depleted (TCD) bone marrow transplant from strain B, the new T cells that develop in the thymus are of strain B type. However, they are educated in the thymus by host type stromal cells of strain A, and therefore develop MHC-restriction specificities for MHC A plus anti-

genic peptide (i.e., A + X). However, when these cells reach the periphery, they encounter processed peptides of environmental antigens presented by antigen-presenting cells of strain B (i.e., B + X), because these cells are also replaced by the bone marrow transplant. This hypothesis to explain the relative immunoincompetence of allogeneic chimeras has been confirmed by the demonstration that new T cells arising in allogeneic chimeras are in fact immunocompetent if they are provided with appropriate presenting cells, such as those of an $(A \times B)F_1$.[59]

An alternative approach is to produce *mixed chimeras* in which a mixture of TCD host (A) and donor (B) bone marrow is used to reconstitute the irradiated strain A animal (Fig. 98–6B). The new T cells that develop therefore acquire restriction specificities for A + X. However, now there are appropriate strain A antigen-presenting cells in the periphery, leading to an appropriate immune response. In addition, cells (presumably of dendritic lineage) from strain B apparently enter the thymus, providing negative selection for cells alloreactive to strain B. Murine mixed chimeras prepared by this procedure show long-term specific tolerance to skin grafts from the donor strain while remaining capable of rejecting third-party skin grafts.[60]

The major problem with this procedure in terms of potential applicability to clinical transplantation is the requirement for lethal irradiation as a means of preparing the mixed chimeric recipient. Such irradiation is too toxic a procedure to be used as a preparative regimen for routine organ transplants. Thus, it was considered essential to develop less toxic preparative regimens for production of mixed chimeras if this phenomenon were to have further clinical applicability. Over the past several years, therefore, we have explored the use of anti-T cell monoclonal antibodies as a means of producing mixed chimeras without the need for lethal irradiation. We have demonstrated that treatment of recipient mice with monoclonal antibodies to the two mature T cells subsets, CD4 and CD8, followed by sublethal irradiation (300R) and a dose of irradiation to the thymus (700 R thymic irradiation) permits engraftment of a subsequent injection of allogeneic bone marrow, and the production of mixed chimerism.[61] Long-term mixed chimerism develops in all lymphohematopoietic compartments in such animals, and they are indistinguishable by two-color fluorescence-activated cell-sorting analysis from mixed chimeras prepared by lethal irradiation and reconstitution with mixtures of TCD syngeneic plus allogeneic bone marrow. Animals prepared by this nonmyeloablative preparative regimen show none of the premature graying shown after lethal irradiation, and they gain weight and remain healthy in a fashion similar to that of untreated cohorts. We therefore believe that this preparative regimen for production of mixed chimeras may have clinical applicability, and we are actively pursuing the extension of this procedure to nonhuman primates as a preclinical model (Kawai T, et al: *Transplantation,* in press).

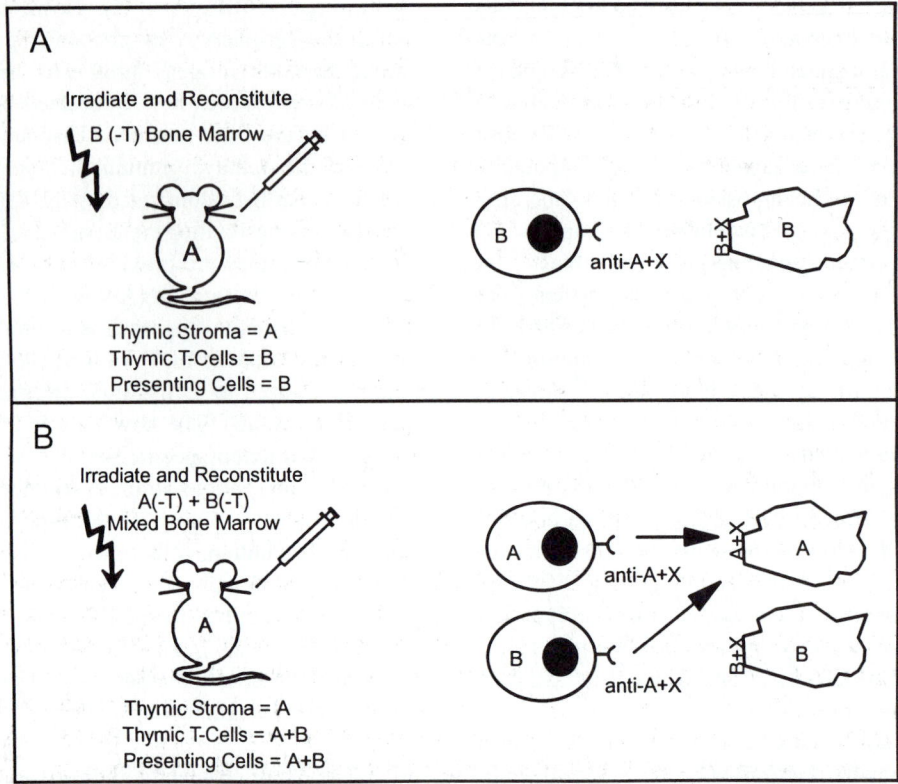

Figure 98–6. A. Fully allogeneic chimeras. Diagrammatic representation of the T cell interactions expected in fully allogeneic chimeras in comparison with those observed for syngeneically reconstituted or normal animals. T cells of MHC type B acquire MHC-restriction specificity for A + X in the host thymus, but find only B + X on presenting cells in the periphery. **B.** Mixed chimeras. Diagrammatic representation of the T cell interactions expected in mixed allogeneic chimeras in comparison with those observed for syngeneically reconstituted or normal animals. T cells of both MHC type A and B acquire MHC-restriction specificity for A + X in the host thymus, and find appropriate A + X presenting cells in the periphery.

CHRONIC REJECTION

The short-term results of heart transplantation have improved dramatically over the last 25 years with survival rates at 1 year increasing from 22% in 1969[62] to over 80% in 1993.[40] However, the progress made in the detection, prevention, and treatment of acute rejection has been overshadowed by the more difficult and perplexing problem of cardiac allograft vasculopathy (CAV) in long-term recipients. This disease is manifested by a diffuse and accelerated form of arteriosclerosis often involving entire lengths of coronary arteries. Autopsy findings reveal that virtually all transplant recipients who survive for more than a year demonstrate these intimal changes.[63] Intimal proliferation usually progresses rapidly to vessel occlusion and myocardial infarction. Indeed, cardiac allograft vasculopathy is now the leading cause of death or graft failure after the first posttransplant year.[64] The etiology and treatment of CAV remain elusive despite the recent burgeoning of interest in this area.

The dominant pathological finding in CAV is a diffuse, concentric intimal thickening and perivascular inflammation extending from large epicardial arteries into medium-sized arteries and arterioles. CAV differs from localized "naturally occurring" or nontransplant atherosclerosis in its generalized distribution throughout the coronary vasculature and its rapid progression. Despite these differences, there are significant morphologic and functional similarities between the vascular lesions of CAV and the lesions observed in nontransplant atherosclerosis. Indeed, there is mounting evidence that the complex events leading to CAV are very similar to those that occur in the pathogenesis of nontransplant atherosclerosis, the common denominator being the vessel wall's capacity to respond to injury.[65,66] It is well known that vessel wall injury activates endothelial and smooth muscle cells to produce multifunctional cytokines and growth factors that induce cell proliferation and migration, and that ultimately result in atherogenesis.[67] Perhaps the final pathway in the development of CAV is similar to, or the same as, that of nontransplant atherosclerosis. This is supported by reports demonstrating the presence of cytokines, growth factors, and endothelial receptors associated with nontransplant atherosclerosis in hearts exhibiting CAV.[68–70] In addition, histologic and immunocytochemical analyses of CAV suggest that, like nontransplant atherosclerosis, an inflammatory stage precedes the intimal and smooth muscle cell proliferation in the wall of the affected vessel.

Given the potentially critical role played by atherogenesis in the development of CAV, it is surprising that there is no clear cut correlation between known risk factors for atherosclerosis and CAV. For instance, the role of lipids in the initiation of the vessel wall damage of graft atherosclerosis is uncertain despite the known toxic effects of low-density lipoproteins and elevated cholesterol levels on vascular endothelium.[71] Recent reports failed to demonstrate any significant difference in lipid profiles among patients developing CAV and those who remained free of this complication.[72–74] Hypertension, smoking, diabetes, and a history of prior atherosclerosis in the transplant recipient have not correlated with an increased risk of CAV.[72,73,75] Thus, although the final molecular and cellular pathways of CAV and nontransplant atherosclerosis appear to have much in common, it is unclear what produces the initial endothelial damage that sets the biological machinery of atherogenesis in motion in an otherwise healthy, long-term allograft. Interestingly, only cytomegalovirus (CMV) infection has shown a strong association with either death or retransplantation from CAV.[76]

The fact that CAV is more widespread and rapidly progressive within the heart than conventional atherosclerosis, that it does not affect the native heart, and that vascular lesions develop much slower or not at all in syngeneic or isogeneic grafts suggests that immune mechanisms play an important role in the pathogenesis of CAV. Indeed, recent work by Russell et al[77] in the mouse heart transplant system strongly supports this idea. However, the immune mechanisms mediating this disease are not clear. Some groups have supported the predominance of antibodies specific for donor antigens,[78–80] while others have favored the predominance of cell-mediated immunity.[81,82] Of course, the possibility that both forms of immunity might participate in producing endothelial damage must also be acknowledged. What does seem to be clear is that the induction of CAV is not simply the result of the surgical transplant procedure itself.[83]

At present the only treatment for graft failure secondary to CAV is retransplantation, which carries with it survival rates that are a full 30% lower than first time operations. However, a variety of agents have shown some promise in small animal models. These include Amlodipine, a calcium antagonist, angiopeptin, a somatostatin analogue, Probucol, an antioxidant, and Iloprost, a prostacyclin analogue.

XENOTRANSPLANTATION

Clinical experience in xenotransplantation began in early 1960s when Reemtsma et al,[84] Starzl et al,[85] and Hitchcock et al[86] each performed primate-to-human kidney transplants. Surprisingly, one patient survived 9 months and died

of infection with a well-functioning transplant.[84] Twenty years later, in the cyclosporine era, one baboon-to-human heart transplant recipient died at postoperative day 20 from graft failure,[87] and more recently, two baboon-to-human liver transplant recipients died at days 28 and 70.[88]

Xenotransplants have been classified into two groups based on the phylogenetic distance between the species, speed of rejection, and levels of detectable preformed antibodies. Species that belong to disparate zoological classifications and reject organs in an hyperacute fashion are termed *discordant* (e.g., pig to human). Closely related species that reject transplants in a manner similar to an allograft are called *concordant* (e.g., baboon to human). For the purpose of clinical xenotransplantation, the most appropriate potential donor species remains controversial. Clearly, the most concordant donors would be nonhuman primates. However, there are serious problems in considering such animals as donors. The closest nonhuman primates phylogenetically would be chimpanzees, but these are far too rare to be considered seriously. The nonhuman primate species that has been most commonly suggested as a donor in terms of potential availability is the baboon. However, in addition to availability issues, the baboon is too small to be an appropriate donor for most organ transplants. The largest baboons weigh less than 40 kg, which would be inadequate as a heart donor for most adult human beings. In addition, questions about transmission of pathogenic viruses from nonhuman primates have been raised as a potential concern.[89]

There is a growing consensus that swine would make the optimal xenograft donor. Among the large number of similarities between swine and human beings with respect to parameters of importance to transplantation are

1. Size.
2. Digestive physiology.
3. Kidney structure and function.
4. Pulmonary vascular bed structure.
5. Coronary artery distribution.
6. Respiratory rate.
7. Cardiovascular anatomy and physiology.
8. Immunology mechanisms.[90]

In addition, swine have excellent breeding characteristics (large litter size, early sexual maturity, and frequent estrous cycles), lower risks of viral transmission, and pose fewer ethical concerns.

Over the past 20 years, this laboratory has developed miniature swine as a large animal model for studies of transplantation biology. Miniature swine were chosen both because of the similarities indicated above and because of their size and breeding characteristics. While domestic swine can attain weights in excess of 450 kg, fully adult miniature swine weigh 110 to 135 kg; a size much more similar to that of human beings. In terms of xenotransplantation, one can envision obtaining a xenograft organ of ap-

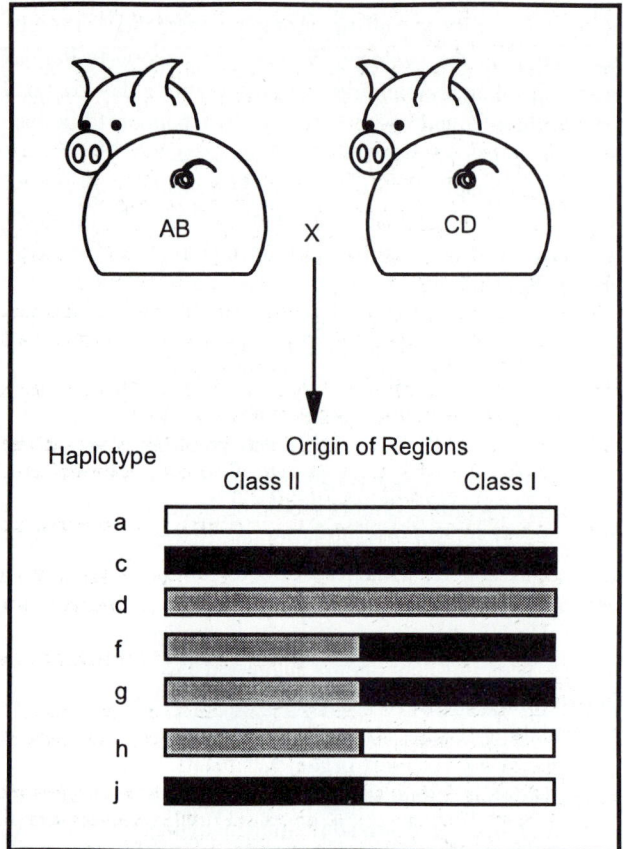

Figure 98–7. Origin of inbred miniature swine. Shown are the three inbred SLA haplotypes and four of the recombinant haplotypes that separate Class I from Class II antigens in this model.

propriate size for any potential human recipient, from a newborn baby to the largest adult.

As shown in Figure 98–7, three lines of miniature swine have been developed each homozygous for a different set of alleles at the MHC (termed SLA in swine). In addition, during subsequent breeding studies four intra-MHC recombinant haplotypes have been identified and bred to homozygosity, also illustrated in Figure 98–7. The availability of these recombinants makes miniature swine the only large animal model in which one can reproducibly study the effects of transplantation across selective MHC barriers. In addition, in inbreeding of these animals makes it possible to develop new treatment regimens that are directed toward induction of specific tolerance to a set of pig MHC genes, as opposed to the prospect of tailoring therapy for each particular donor to be used as the source of a xenograft.

Prevention of Xenograft Rejection

There are several unique problems in xenografting. First, there are widespread preformed or "natural" antibodies in humans that are reactive for antigens of other species. These natural antibodies, which recognize glycoproteins on the surface of endothelial cells, may be similar to blood group-specific antibodies and mediate hyperacute rejection. They currently preclude xenogeneic transplantation of most organs into humans. Second, cells and organs from one species may not be able to function in a xenogeneic environment. However, there are some examples of physiologic function across species barriers.[91] Third, the nature of cell-mediated xenograft rejection may be different from cell-mediated allogeneic rejection and thus require different forms of immunosuppression. Finally, there is the concern that pathogens introduced by organs from nonhuman donors may have unexpected sequelae.

Based on the findings discussed earlier, that mixed allogeneic chimerism can induce tolerance to fully MHC mismatched organs in mice,[92] and that this strategy is also effective in producing long-term survival of xenografts in concordant rat-to-mouse combinations,[60] mixed xenogeneic chimerism across a discordant barrier (pig-to-monkey) is being actively studied in this laboratory. The pig-to-monkey kidney model involves the use of nonlethal irradiation as a means of facilitating engraftment of xenogeneic bone marrow (Fig. 98–8). Natural antibodies are eliminated by absorption, the recipient's blood being perfused through the isolated donor's liver intraoperatively. Horse antihuman antithymocyte globulin and high dose CyA are added to deplete mature T cells in the host. Kidney transplantation is performed simultaneously with donor bone marrow infu-

Figure 98–8. Nonmyeloablative protocol for induction of tolerance in a discordant system. Absorption of the monkey's blood by passage through a pig liver has been found capable of avoiding hyperacute rejection. Long-term engraftment of pig bone marrow (BM) may lead to induction of long-term tolerance. ATG, antithymocyte globulin; mAbs, monoclonal antibodies; TI, thymic irradiation; Tx, transplantation; WBI, whole body irradiation.

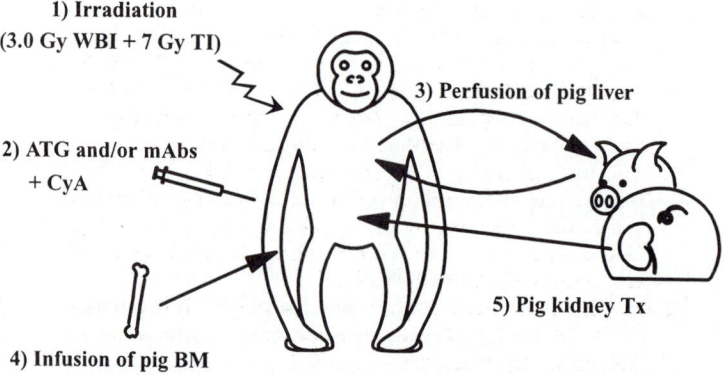

1) Irradiation
(3.0 Gy WBI + 7 Gy TI)

2) ATG and/or mAbs
+ CyA

3) Perfusion of pig liver

4) Infusion of pig BM

5) Pig kidney Tx

sion. Recently, pig-specific growth factors (stem cell factor and IL-3) have been added to enhance engraftment of pig stem cells. Using this approach, hyperacute rejection has been prevented, kidney survival of up to 15 days has been achieved, and evidence for at least transient xenogeneic chimerism in host bone marrow documented.

An alternative approach to the prevention of xenorejection is to manipulate the donor organ instead of manipulating the host's immune system. It is well recognized that the hyperacute rejection observed after discordant xenotransplantation involves the host's complement system, activated by natural antibodies. There exist, on the surface of endothelial cells, complement-inhibitory proteins that serve to prevent complement activation.[93] These proteins include decay accelerating factor (DAF) and membrane cofactor protein (MCP). One strategy is to exploit these proteins by creating transgenic swine whose tissues express human DAF. It is hoped that transplantation of a kidney or heart from a transgenic pig whose endothelium expresses DAF may be protected from complement-mediated hyperacute rejection.

Although the problems in xenotransplantation are daunting, the recent burgeoning interest in this field promises resolution of some important issues in the near future.

REFERENCES

1. Billingham RE, Brent L, Medawar PB: Actively acquired tolerance to foreign cells, twin diagnosis and the freemartin condition in cattle. *Nature* (London) **172**:603–606, 1953
2. Myburgh JA, Smit JA, Hill RR, Browde S: Transplantation tolerance in primates following total lymphoid irradiation and allogeneic bone marrow injection. *Transplantation* **29**:405–408, 1980
3. Najarian JS, Ferguson RM, Sutherland DER, et al: Fractionated total lymphoid irradiation as preparative immunosuppression in high risk renal transplantation: Clinical and immunological studies. *Ann Surg* **196**:442–451, 1982
4. Cosimi AB, Burton RC, Colvin RB et al: Treatment of acute renal allograft rejection with OKT3 monoclonal antibody. *Transplantation* **32**:535–539, 1981
5. Waldmann H: Manipulation of T-cell responses with monoclonal antibodies. *Annu Rev Immunol* **7**:407–425, 1989
6. Monaco AP, Wood ML, Russell PS: Studies on heterologous antilymphocyte serum in mice. *Ann NY Acad Sci* **129**:190–209, 1966
7. Cosimi AB, Wortis H, Delmonico F, Russell PS: Randomized clinical trial of antithymocyte globulin in cadaver renal allograft recipients. *Surgery* **80**:155–161, 1976
8. Chan GLC, Canafax DM, Johnson CA: The therapeutic use of azathioprine in renal transplantation. *Pharmacotherapy* **7**:165–177, 1987
9. Lagrange PH, Mackaness GB, Miller TE: Potentiation of T-cell-mediated immunity by selective suppression of antibody formation with cyclophosphamide. *J Exp Med* **139**:1529–1539, 1974
10. Steinman RM: Dendritic cells. *Transplantation* **31**:151–160, 1981
11. Glimcher LH, Kim KJ, Green I, Paul WE: Ia antigen-bearing B cell tumor lines can present protein antigen and alloantigen in a major histocompatibility complex-restricted fashion to antigen-reactive T cells. *J Exp Med* **155**:445–449, 1982
12. Lechler R, Batchelor J: Restoration of immunogenicity to passenger cell depleted kidney allografts by the addition of donor strain dendritic cells. *J Exp Med* **155**:31–41, 1982
13. Schwartz RH: A cell culture model for T lymphocyte clonal anergy. *Science* **248**:1349–1352, 1990
14. Auchincloss H Jr, Sachs DH: Transplantation and graft rejection. In Paul WE (ed): *Fundamental Immunol* 3rd ed. New York, Raven Press, 1993, pp 1099–1141
15. Zinkernagel RM, Doherty PC: Restriction of in vitro T cell-mediated cytotoxicity in lymphocytic choriomeningitis within a syngeneic or semiallogeneic system. *Nature* (*London*) **251**:547–548, 1974
16. Bjorkman PJ, Saper MA, Samraoui B, et al: Structure of the human class I histocompatibility antigen, HLA-A2. *Nature* (*London*) **329**:506–512, 1987
17. Jardetzky TS, Brown JH, Gorga JC, et al: Three-dimensional structure of a human class II histocompatibility molecule complexed with superantigen. *Nature* (*London*) **368**:711–718, 1994
18. Hunig T, Bevan MJ: Specificity of T-cell clones illustrates altered self hypothesis. *Nature* (*London*) **294**:460–462, 1981
19. Fischer-Lindahl K, Wilson DB: Histocompatibility antigen-activated cytotoxic T lymphocytes II. Estimates of frequency and specificity of precursors. *J Exp Med* **145**:508–522, 1977
20. Bevan MJ: High determinant density may explain the phenomenon of alloreactivity. *Immunol Today* **5**:128–130, 1984
21. Mosmann TR, Coffman RL: Two types of mouse helper T cell clones—Implications for immune regulation. *Immunol Today* **8**:223–228, 1986
22. Howard M, O'Garra RL: Biological properties of interleukin 10. *Immunol Today* **13**:198–200, 1992
23. Manning DD, Reed ND, Shaffer CF: Maintenance of skin xenografts of widely divergent phylogenetic origin on congenitally athymic (nude) mice. *J Exp Med* **138**:488–497, 1973
24. Rosenberg AS, Mizuochi T, Sharrow SO, Singer A: Phenotype specificity, and function of T cell subsets and T cell interactions involved in skin allograft rejection. *J Exp Med* **165**:1296–1310, 1987
25. Ando K, Guidotti LG, Wirth S, et al: Class I-restricted cytotoxic T lymphocytes are directly cytopathic for their target cell in vivo. *J Immunol* **152**:3245–3253, 1994
26. Hutchinson IV: Immunological mechanisms of long-term graft acceptance. In Paul LC, Solez K (eds): *Organ Transplantation: Long-Term Results*. New York, Marcel Dekker, 1992, pp 1–32
27. Springer TA: Traffic signals for lymphocyte recirculation and leukocyte emigration: The multistep paradigm. *Cell* **76**:301–314, 1994
28. Orosz CG: Lymphocyte-endothelial interactions and tolerance induction. *Clin Transplant* **8**:188–194, 1994
29. Opelz G, Wujciak MS: The influence of HLA compatibility on graft survival after heart transplantation. *N Eng J Med* **330**:816–819, 1994
30. DiSesa VJ, Kuo PC, Horvath KA, et al: HLA histocompatibility affects cardiac transplant rejection and may provide one basis for organ allocation. *Ann Thorac Surg* **49**:220–223, 1990
31. Zerbe TR, Arena VC, Kormos RL, et al: Histocompatibility and other risk factors for histological rejection of human cardiac allografts during the first three months following transplantation. *Transplantation* **52**:485–490, 1991
32. Cochrane A, Benson E, Williams T, et al: Effect of HLA-DR matching on rejection after cardiac transplantation. *Transplant Proc* **24**:169–170, 1992
33. Kerman RH, Kimball P, Scheinen S, et al: The relationship among donor-recipient HLA mismatches, rejection, and death from coronary artery disease in cardiac transplant recipients. *Transplantation* **57**:884–888, 1994
34. Kerman RH, Van Buren CT, Lewis RM: The impact of HLA A, B, and DR blood transfusions and immune responder status on cardiac allograft recipients treated with cyclosporine. *Transplantation* **45**:333–338, 1988
35. Opelz G, Henderson R: Incidence of non-Hodgkins lymphoma in kidney and heart transplant recipients. *Lancet* **342**:1514–1516, 1993
36. Morris PJ: HLA matching and cardiac transplantation. *N Eng J Med* **330**:857–858, 1994
37. Ferrera R, Marcsek P, Larèse A, et al: Simple storage or continuous

coronary perfusion for 24 hours heart preservation? *J Heart Lung Transplant* 12:463–469, 1993

38. Thomson AW, Starzl TE: New immunosuppressive drugs: Mechanistics insights and potential therapeutic advances. *Immunol Rev* 136:71–98, 1993

39. Sollinger H, Przepiorka D: *Recent Developments in Transplantation Medicine Volume I. New Immunosuppressive Drugs.* Glenview, IL, Physicians & Scientists Publishing, 1994

40. Kaye MP: The registry of the international society for heart and lung transplantation: Tenth official report-1993. *J Heart Lung Transplant* 12:541–548, 1993

41. Bierer BE, Somers PK, Wandless TJ, et al: Probing immunosuppressant action with a nonnatural immunophilin ligand. *Science* 250:556–559, 1990

42. O'Keefe S, Tamura J, Kincaid RL, et al: FK-506 and CsA-sensitive activation of the interleukin-2 promotor by calcineurin. *Nature (London)* 357:692–694, 1992

43. Swinnen LJ, Costanzo-Nordin MR, Fisher SG: Increased incidence of lymphoproliferative disorder after immunosuppression with monoclonal antibody OKT3 in cardiac transplant recipients. *N Eng J Med* 323:1723–1728, 1990

44. Morris RE: Rapamycin. In Sollinger H, Przepiorka D (eds): *Recent Developments in Transplantation Medicine Volume I. New Immunosuppressive Drugs.* Glenview, IL, Physicians and Scientists Publishing, 1994, pp 51–75

45. Gregory CR, Huie P, Billingham ME, Morris RE: Rapamycin inhibits arterial intimal thickening caused by both alloimmune and mechanical injury. *Transplantation* 55:1409–1418, 1993

46. Tepper M, Nadler S, Mazzuco C, et al: Mechanism of action of 15-deoxyspergualin, a novel immunosuppressive drug. *Ann NY Acad Sci* 685:122–135, 1993

47. Allison AC, Hovi T, Watts RWE, Webster ADB: Immunological observation in patients with Lesch-Nyhan syndrome and the role of de-novo purine synthesis in lymphocyte transformation. *Lancet* 2:1179–1183, 1927

48. Sollinger HW, Deierhoi MH, Belzer FO: RS-61443: A phase I clinical trial and pilot rescue study. *Transplantation* 53:428–432, 1992

49. Ensley RD, Bristow MR, Olsen SL, et al: The use of mycophenolate mofetil (RS-61443) in human heart transplant recipients. *Transplantation* 56:75–82, 1993

50. Cramer DV, Chapman FA, Jaffee BD: The effect of a new immunosuppressive drug, brequinar sodium, on heart, liver, and kidney allograft rejection in the rat. *Transplantation* 53:303–308, 1992

51. Bretscher P, Cohn M: A theory of self-nonself discrimination. *Science* 169:1042–1044, 1970

52. Essery G, Feldmann M, Lamb JR: Interleukin-2 can prevent and reverse antigen-induced unresponsiveness in cloned human T lymphocytes. *Immunology* 64:413–417, 1988

53. Webb MJ, Morris C, Sprent J: Extrathymic tolerance of mature T cells; clonal elimination as a consequence of immunity. *Cell* 63:1249–1258, 1990

54. Dorf ME, Benacerraf B: Suppressor cells and immunoregulation. *Annu Rev Immunol* 2:127–157, 1984

55. Qin S, Wise M, Cobbold SP, et al: Induction of tolerance in peripheral T cells with monoclonal antibodies. *Eur J Immunol* 20:2737–2745, 1990

56. Rosengard BR, Kortz EO, Guzzeta PC, et al: Transplantation in miniature swine: Analysis of graft infiltrating lymphocytes provides evidence for local suppression. *Human Immunol* 28:153–158, 1990

57. Rammensee HG: Veto function *in vitro* and *in vivo*. *Immunol Rev* 4:175–191, 1989

58. Zinkernagel RM, Althage A, Callahan G, Welsh RM Jr, On the immunocompetence of H-2 incompatible irradiation bone marrow chimeras. *J Immunol* 124:2356–2365, 1980

59. Singer A, Hathcock KS, Hodes RJ: Self-recognition in allogeneic radiation bone marrow chimeras. *J Exp Med* 153:1286–1301, 1981

60. Ilstad ST, Sachs DH: Reconstitution with syngeneic plus allogeneic or xenogeneic bone marrow leads to specific acceptance of allografts or xenografts. *Nature (London)* 307:168–170, 1984

61. Sharabi Y, Sachs DH: Engraftment of allogeneic bone marrow following administration of anti-T cell monoclonal antibodies and low-dose irradiation. *Transplant Proc* 21:233–235, 1989

62. Jamieson SW, Oyer PE, Baldwin JC, et al: Heart transplantation for end-stage ischemic heart disease: The Stanford experience. *Heart Transplant* 3:224–227, 1984

63. Uys CJ, Rose AG: Pathologic findings in long-term cardiac transplants. *Arch Pathol Med* 108:112–116, 1984

64. Billingham ME: Graft coronary disease: The lesions and the patients. *Transplantat Proc* 21:3665–3666, 1989

65. Hosenpud JD, Shipley GD, Wagner CR: Cardiac allograft vasculopathy: Current concepts, recent developments, and future directions. *J Heart Lung Transplant* 11:9–23, 1992

66. Häyry P, Paavonen T, Mennander A, et al: Pathophysiology of allograft arteriosclerosis. *Transplant Proc* 25:2070, 1992

67. Paul LC, Fellström B: Chronic vascular rejection of the heart and the kidney - have rational treatment options emerged? *Transplantation* 53:1169–1179, 1992

68. Adams DH, Russell ME, Hancock WW, et al: Chronic rejection in experimental cardiac transplantation: Studies in the Lewis-F344 Model. *Immunolog Rev* 134:5–19, 1993

69. Gordon D: Growth factors and cell proliferation in human transplant arteriosclerosis. *J Heart Lung Transplant* 11:7–13, 1992

70. Higgy NA, Davidoff AW, Grothman GT, et al: Expression of platelet-derived growth factor receptor in rat heart allografts. *J Heart Lung Transplant* 10:1012–1019, 1993

71. Pescovitz MD, Auchincloss H Jr, Thistlethwaite JR Jr, Sachs DH: Transplantation in miniature swine: Acceptance of class I antigen mismatched renal allografts. *Transplant Proc* 15:1124–1126, 1983

72. McDonald K, Rector TS, Braunlin EA, et al: Association of coronary artery disease in cardiac transplant recipients with cytomegalovirus infection. *Am J Cardiol* 64:359–362, 1989

73. Uretsky BF, Murali S, Reddy S, et al: Development of coronary artery disease in cardiac transplant patients receiving immunosuppressive therapy with cyclosporine and prednisone. *Circulation* 76:827–834, 1987

74. Butman SM: Hyperlipidemia after cardiac transplantation: Be aware and possibly wary of drug therapy for lowering of serum lipids. *Am Heart J* 121:1585–1590, 1991

75. Hess ML, Hastillo A, Mohanakumar, et al: Accelerated atherosclerosis in cardiac transplantation: Role of cytotoxic B-cell antibodies and hyperlipidemia. *Circulation* 68(suppl II), II-94–II-101, 1983

76. Grattan MT, Moeno-Cabral CE, Starnes VA, et al: Cytomegalovirus infection is associated with cardiac allograft rejection and atherosclerosis. *J Am Med Assoc* 261:3561–3566, 1989

77. Russell PS, Chase CM, Winn HJ, Colvin RB: Coronary atherosclerosis in transplanted mouse hearts. III. Effects of recipient treatment with a monoclonal antibody to interferon-gamma. *Transplantation* 57:1367–1371, 1994

78. Petrossian GA, Nichols AB, Marboe CC, et al: Relation between survival and development of coronary artery disease and anti-HLA antibodies after cardiac transplantation. *Circulation* 80:III-122–III-125, 1989

79. Rose EA, Peppino P, Barr ML, et al: Relation of HLA antibodies and graft atherosclerosis in human cardiac allograft recipients. *J Heart Lung Transplant* 11:S120–S123, 1992

80. Russell PS, Chase CM, Winn HJ, Colvin RB: Coronary atherosclerosis in transplanted mouse hearts. II. Importance of humoral immunity. *J Immunol* 152:5135–5141, 1994

81. Cramer DV, Chapman FA, Wu GD, et al: Cardiac transplantation in the rat: II. Alterations of the severity of donor graft arteriosclerosis by modulation of the host immune response. *Transplantation* 50:554–562, 1990

82. Libby P, Salomon RN, Payne DD, et al: Functions of vascular wall cells related to the development of transplantation-associated coronary arteriosclerosis. *Transplant Proc* **21:**3677–3684, 1989

83. Cramer DV, Qian S, Harnaha J, et al: Cardiac transplantation in the rat 1. The effect of histocompatibility differences on graft arteriosclerosis. *Transplantation* **47:**414–419, 1989

84. Reemtsma K, McCracken BH, Schlegal JU, Pearl M: Heterotransplantation of the kidney: Two clinical experiences. *Science* **143:**700–702, 1964

85. Starzl TE, Marchioro TL, Peters GN: Renal heterotransplantation from baboon to man: Experience with six cases. *Transplantation* **2:**752–776, 1964

86. Hitchcock CR, Kiser JC, Telander RL, Seljeskob EL: Baboon renal grafts. *J Am Med Assoc* **189:**934–936, 1964

87. Bailey LL, Nehlsen-Cannarella WSL: Observations on cardiac xenotransplantation. *Transplant Proc* **18:**88–92, 1986

88. Starzl TE, Fung J, Tzakis A, et al: Baboon to human liver transplantation. *Lancet* **341:**65–71, 1993

89. Kalter SS: The non-human primate as potential organ donor for man: Virological considerations. In Cooper DKC, Kemp E, Reemtsma K, White DJG (eds): *Xenotransplantation.* Heidelberg, Springer-Verlag, 1991 pp 457–479

90. Cooper DKC, Ye Y, Rolf LL, Zuhdi N: The pig as potential organ donor for man. In Cooper DKC, Kemp E, Reemtsma K, White DJG (eds): *Xenotransplantation.* Heidelberg, Springer-Verlag, pp 481–500

91. Auchincloss H Jr: Xenogeneic transplantation: A review. *Transplantation* **46:**1–20, 1988

92. Sharabi Y, Sachs DH: Mixed chimerism and permanent specific transplantation tolerance induced by non-lethal preparative regimen. *J Exp Med* **169:**493–503, 1989

93. Cary N, Moody J, Yannoutsos N, et al: Tissue expression of human decay accelerating factor, a regulator of complement activation expressed in mice: A potential approach to inhibition of hyperacute xenograft rejection. *Transplant Proc* **25:**400–401, 1993

99

Pharmacological Approach to the Management of the Cardiac Surgical Patient

Judith A. Mackall, Carol M. Buchter,
and Marc D. Thames

INTRODUCTION

Any physician involved in the postoperative management of the cardiac surgical patient recognizes that the initial week after surgery provides many challenges. Other chapters in this book address metabolic, renal, and respiratory challenges. This chapter focuses on cardiovascular issues that impact morbidity, mortality, cost of care, and length of hospitalization.

The two cardiovascular problems that continue to challenge us to the greatest degree are the management of cardiac arrhythmias and the management of low cardiac output states during the early hours and days after surgery. This chapter focuses on these two areas. The use of pharmacological agents and/or devices in their management is reviewed within the context of these clinical problems.

It is beyond the scope of this chapter to cover all pharmacologic agents that may be used in the postoperative cardiac surgery patient in general or even for these two selected areas in particular. It is our goal to develop a conceptual framework that includes an approach to the problems and to describe in some detail selected specific therapies that are used for their treatment. Thus, the major emphasis is on therapeutics rather than on pharmacology. Selected figures and tables have been included that we hope will prove useful to those involved in the care of the cardiac surgical patient.

THE PROBLEM OF LOW CARDIAC OUTPUT

Low cardiac output following cardiac surgery is a common problem that has a significant negative impact upon in-hospital morbidity and mortality.[1,2] The sections that follow will present a general overview of the problem of low cardiac output following bypass surgery including etiologic considerations and available diagnostic modalities. A discussion of the rationale for treatment with positive inotropes and vasodilators follows, including a review of the role of the adrenergic nervous system in regulation of cardiac performance. Similarities and differences in the treatment of acute versus chronic heart failure are highlighted. Lastly, consideration is given to specific modalities of treatment, focusing on the more commonly utilized inotropes and vasodilators.

The clinical recognition of inadequate cardiac output may predate cardiac surgery, developing acutely in the setting of myocardial infarction or acutely decompensated valvular heart disease. Alternatively, chronic congestive heart failure, due to one or more myocardial infarctions, ongoing myocardial ischemia, or on a valvular basis, may be present prior to cardiac surgery. Low cardiac output can be recognized in the operating room as failure to wean from cardiopulmonary bypass or may be recognized postoperatively in the surgical intensive care unit. It is important to be aware of the existence and duration of preoperative hemodynamic abnormalities as responses to pharmacologic therapy in the perioperative and postoperative period are modulated by individual patient characteristics, which are, in turn, influenced by preoperative hemodynamics.

Low cardiac output may be secondary to inadequate heart rate (either tachyarrhythmias or bradyarrhythmias), inadequate intravascular volume, interference with ventricular filling or emptying, inappropriately elevated afterload, or myocardial dysfunction. Decreased myocardial function occurring in the early postoperative period may be segmental, representing acute myocardial infarction, or global, representing diffuse myocardial damage. Despite improvements in surgical technique, methods of cardioplegia and intraoperative anesthesia and monitoring, acute myocardial dysfunction is a common problem early after coronary artery bypass surgery. In studies of patients with normal preoperative cardiac function undergoing uncomplicated coronary bypass surgery,[3] significant transient global biventricular dysfunction was seen in the vast majority of cases. This effect was maximal at 2 hours, improved at 8 to 10 hours, and had largely dissipated 24 to 48 hours postoperatively. This transient ventricular dysfunction occurred despite treatment with inotropes or pressors and was independent of preoperative medications, pump time, number of grafts placed, or postoperative core temperature. The mechanism of transient postoperative ventricular dysfunction is unknown but may represent reperfusion injury due to the generation of oxygen free radicals.[4] Even those patients who arrive in the surgical intensive care unit with preserved systolic function appear to have transient impairment of diastolic function.[5]

Several tools are available to ascertain the etiology of low cardiac output in the perioperative and immediate postoperative period. Direct visual inspection of the heart in the operating room can provide information regarding contractility, graft patency, and unsuspected valvular heart disease. Transesophageal echocardiography employed in the operating room is an important adjunct to visual inspection and is invaluable in assessing both stenotic and regurgitant valvular lesions. Mitral regurgitation often has an ischemic basis and may improve following revascularization, negating the need for valve repair or replacement.

Measurement of intravascular pressures and cardiac output via a Swan-Ganz thermodilution catheter is of critical importance in the management of postoperative patients. Previously unsuspected congenital or acquired intracardiac shunts can be evaluated by means of simultaneous oxygen saturations obtained from the proximal (central venous) and distal (pulmonary arterial) ports. Mixed venous oxygen saturation levels from the pulmonary artery can be monitored continuously as an aid on the ongoing evaluation of cardiac function. Mixed venous O_2 saturation falls as cardiac output declines and oxygen extraction increases.

The Frank–Starling curve describes the relationship between left ventricular end-diastolic volume and stroke volume or cardiac output (Fig. 99–1). The dysfunctional ventricle operates on the plateau portion of the Frank–Starling curve such that changes in end-diastolic volume produce little significant change in cardiac output. However, in cases of inadequate circulating blood volume, a significantly lowered end-diastolic volume will decrease cardiac output. The normal myocardial contractility curve is positioned upward and to the left of the curve of myocardial dysfunction. In both situations, excessive lowering of ventricular end-diastolic volume is to be avoided, as it can result in a progressive decrease in cardiac output.

The relationship between left ventricular end-diastolic volume and pressure is not linear, although pressure measurements are commonly utilized clinically as an estimation of volume status. As seen in Figure 99–2, at low ventricular volumes substantial changes in volume produce little change in pressure. At higher ventricular volumes, small changes produced exponentially greater increases in pressure. The property of ventricular compliance defines the position of the entire curve, with increased compliance shifting the curve to the right, allowing a greater end-diastolic volume at a lower pressure.

The treatment of low cardiac output in the perioperative period should initially be directed towards removing precipitating factors and correcting underlying mechanical abnormalities. The intra-aortic balloon pump can be an important temporizing measure that serves to lower systemic vascular resistance, increase coronary bloodflow, and increase cardiac output without increasing cardiac work. The mainstay of therapy for low cardiac output is pharmacologic and the discussion of these options is presented below.

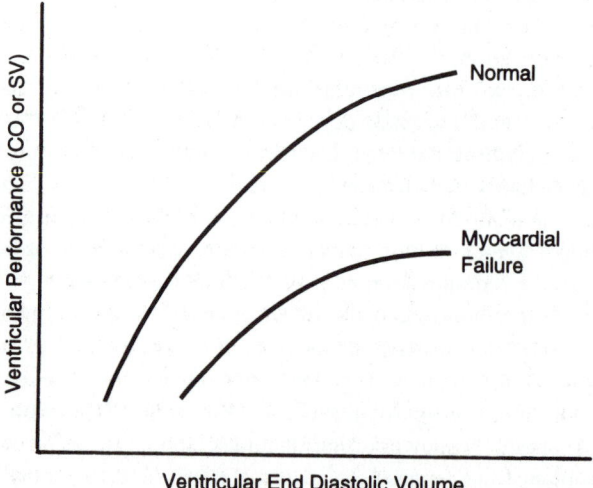

Figure 99–1. The relationship between ventricular end diastolic volume and ventricular performance as demonstrated by the Frank–Starling curve. As myocardial performance decreases, the curve shifts downward, to the right and flattens so that changes in end-diastolic volume cause proportionately smaller changes in performance.

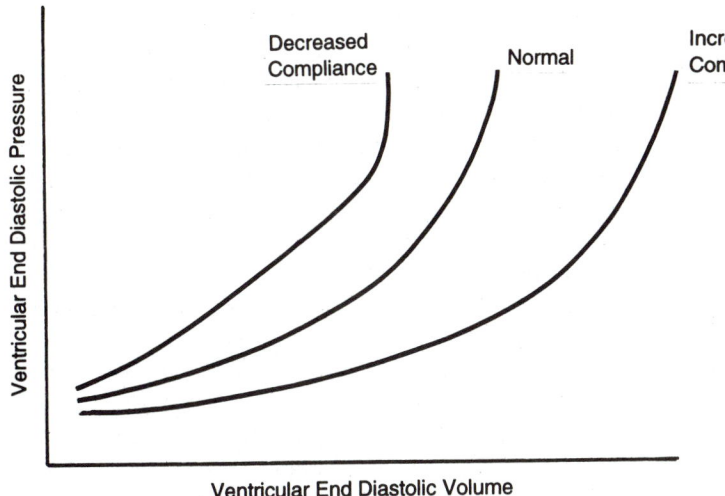

Figure 99–2. Relationship between ventricular end-diastolic volume and pressure. At low volumes, substantial changes in volume may occur with little effect upon pressure, whereas at higher volumes, small increments in volume produce substantial pressure changes. Ischemia and heart failure both lead to decreased compliance with proportionately greater pressure changes for any change in volume.

PHARMACOLOGICAL TREATMENT OF LOW CARDIAC OUTPUT

Positive inotropic agents can be subdivided into cardiac glycosides, directly acting catecholamines, β-adrenergic receptor agonists, and phosphodiesterase inhibitors. The direct acting agents include epinephrine, a naturally occurring circulating hormone, and norepinephrine, which is the neurotransmitter released from sympathetic nerves and is the biosynthetic precursor of epinephrine. Commonly used β-adrenergic receptor agonists include dopamine, the biologic precursor of norepinephrine, and dobutamine, a synthetic catecholamine structurally related to dopamine. Isoproterenol, as will be discussed below, rarely is utilized in the treatment of low cardiac output in the postoperative patient. Phosphodiesterase inhibitors such as amrinone and milrinone provide positive inotropic action by increasing the intracellular concentration of cyclic AMP via inhibition of its degradation. The cardiac glycosides such as digitalis, although of less inotropic potency than the above mentioned compounds, also play an important role in the treatment of postoperative low cardiac output syndrome in appropriately selected patients.

In addition to positive inotropic agents, vasodilators are of paramount importance in the treatment of low cardiac output. Vasodilators, which work by regulating tone of vascular smooth muscle cells, can be subdivided into venodilators, arteriolar dilators, and those with effects on both vascular segments. Vasodilators can be subdivided into three categories: (1) inhibitors of the renin–angiotensin–aldosterone system or angiotensin-converting enzyme (ACE) inhibitors, (2) direct smooth muscle relaxers such as nitroprusside or hydralazine, and (3) sympathetic nervous system blocking agents that act on α-adrenergic receptors such as phentolamine, prazosin, and trimethophan.

The efficacy of vasodilator therapy in the treatment of heart failure was first reported in 1971 when the α-adrenoreceptor antagonist phentolamine was reported to re-

sult in clinical improvement in patients with severe heart failure secondary to ischemic heart disease.[6] One year later, nitroprusside was shown to improve symptoms and hemodynamics in patients in cardiogenic shock following extensive myocardial infarction.[7] Since that time, innumerable reports have validated the efficacy of this treatment modality.[8–11]

The main goal of vasodilator therapy in low output syndromes is to counteract inappropriately vigorous and perhaps maladaptive compensatory vasoconstriction. Although vasoconstriction is partially adaptive in acute severe heart failure, serving to maintain adequate perfusion pressure and blood flow to vital organs, in chronic heart failure this increase in afterload can lead to further decrease in cardiac output. The greater the degree of myocardial dysfunction the more "afterload dependent" is the ventricle, such that small increases in systemic vascular resistance will lead to appreciable decreases in cardiac output. This relationship is illustrated in Figure 99–3, which compares patients with normal as opposed to depressed myocardial function. Increased systemic vascular resistance in normal ventricles leads to hypertension with no appreciable decreases in cardiac output, whereas increasing resistance to left ventricular ejection in dysfunctional ventricles leads to a significant decrease in cardiac output.

In the presence of adequate filling pressures, vasodilator therapy does not typically cause a significant decrease in systolic blood pressure. Although systemic vascular resistance decreases, cardiac output increases and the combination of these counterbalancing effects most commonly leads to stable blood pressure. If blood pressure decreases significantly with vasodilator therapy the possibility of inadequate filling pressure must be considered. Additionally, minimally impaired ventricular function, obstructive cardiac lesions such as aortic stenosis, mitral stenosis, or hypertrophic obstructive cardiomyopathy may cause a significant hypotensive response to vasodilator therapy. Severe cardiac dysfunction with lack of cardiac reserve may also present as

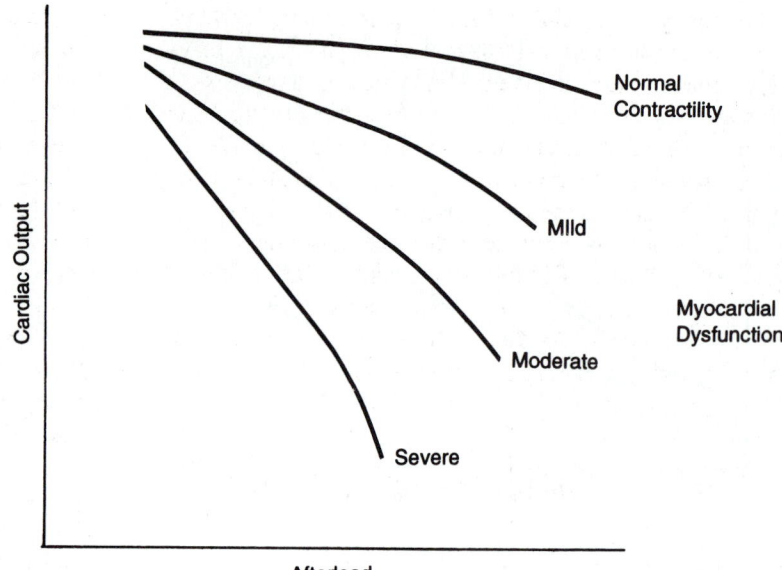

Figure 99–3. Relationship between ventricular performance (CO) and outflow resistance (afterload) in healthy and diseased hearts. A normal heart can maintain a constant output despite an increased resistance to outflow. Progressive degrees of systolic dysfunction are associated with progressively greater decreases in cardiac output as resistance increases.

vasodilator-induced hypotension as an end-stage ventricle cannot increase cardiac output despite manipulation of afterload.

Abundant evidence exists to support the efficacy of vasodilator therapy in improving hemodynamics and symptoms in patients with mild, moderate, and severe depression of myocardial function.[12,13] In addition, survival benefits are apparent in patients with chronic left ventricular dysfunction irrespective of the presence or absence of symptoms.[14–16] Thus, all patients with left ventricular dysfunction (generally defined as a left ventricular ejection fraction of less than 40%) should receive vasodilator therapy unless specific contraindications exist. Angiotensin-coverting enzyme inhibitors are preferred, although combination therapy with hydralazine and isosorbide dinitrate should be given to those patients unable to receive angiotensin converting enzyme inhibitor therapy.[8]

ADRENERGIC NERVOUS SYSTEM

The adrenergic nervous system is of crucial importance in the regulation of heart rate, intrinsic ventricular contractility, ventricular relaxation, and vascular tone, the latter controlling both preload and afterload. Thus, all major determinants of ventricular systolic performance are influenced by the sympathetic nervous system and are thus subject to pharmacologic manipulation. Adrenergic receptors, located at the cell surface in myocardial and vascular smooth muscle cells, are responsible for the transduction of signals from neurotransmitters and circulating hormones, either exogenous or endogenous, into altered cellular function. These receptors are present in three major subclasses; alpha (α), beta (β), and dopaminergic (DA) receptors. Each of

these classes is further subdivided into subtypes 1 and 2. α_1-receptors produce smooth muscle contraction. Although present predominantly on the surface of vascular smooth muscle cells, α_1-receptors are also present, albeit in lower concentrations, in myocardial cells where they produce a slow onset prolonged increase in inotropic state. α_2-receptors are presynaptic and inhibit norepinephrine release. β_1 receptors are located mainly in cardiac muscle and, when stimulated, produce increased inotropic activity, cardiac acceleration, and facilitation of A-V conduction. β_2-receptors are located primarily in vascular and bronchial smooth muscle where activation produces both bronchial and vascular smooth muscle cell relaxation. There are also β_2-receptors in the heart, compromising between 14 and 40% of ventricular β-receptors and 20 and 55% of atrial β-receptors.[17,18] DA_1 receptors are located on smooth muscle cells within the renal, splanchnic, coronary, and cerebral vascular beds. Activation of these receptors produces vasodilatation by increasing intracellular concentrations of cyclic AMP. Activation of DA_2-receptors promotes release of norepinephrine from sympathetic nerve endings and inhibits aldosterone synthesis and release from the adrenal cortex.

The responses to endogenous or exogenous catecholamines such as epinephrine, norepinephrine, and dopamine are dependent upon receptor density and responsiveness. This is a dynamic rather than a static condition, responding to levels of circulating hormones as well as prior agonist or antagonist therapy. In septic shock, α-receptor responsiveness is decreased and administration of potent sympathomimetics with vasoconstricting properties will not achieve the same increase in arterial perfusion pressure and vascular resistance seen in patients without sepsis.[19] In chronic heart failure β-receptor and stimulatory G protein densities are decreased in response to a chronic increase in locally released and circulating catecholamines.

Additionally the remaining β-receptors in chronic heart failure are desensitized and thus less responsive to catecholamine stimulation. Preoperative treatment with α- or β-receptor antagonists will increase receptor density. Thus appreciation of the likely concentration and responsiveness of adrenergic receptors will aid in the anticipation of responses to pharmacologic therapy.

The concept of receptor malleability raises the issue of continued efficacy versus tachyphylaxis with prolonged catecholamine usage. As will be discussed later, phosphodiesterase inhibitors do not act via cell surface receptors and thus may not lead to problems of tolerance.

THE USE OF POSITIVE INOTROPIC AGENTS

Epinephrine

Epinephrine is a circulating endogenous catecholamine released mainly from the adrenal medulla, whose effects are mediated mainly by β_1- and β_2-receptors and, to a lesser degree, by α-adrenoreceptors. Epinephrine acts as a circulating hormone and small changes in plasma concentration produce significant hemodynamic effects. At low doses (0.005 to 0.02 μg/kg per minute) β-receptor activation predominates with bronchial and vascular smooth muscle relaxation, tachycardia, and increased cardiac contractility leading to decreases in systemic and pulmonary vascular resistance with increases in stroke volume and cardiac output. At higher doses, α-mediated effects predominate with intense vasoconstriction. Epinephrine is a potent renal vasoconstrictor with doses as low as 0.03 μg/kg per minute decreasing renal bloodflow by as much as 10%. Additionally, epinephrine produces direct β-stimulation of the juxtaglomerular apparatus leading to renin release and secondary vasoconstriction via angiotensin II. These effects limit to a degree the clinical utility of epinephrine in treating low cardiac output.

Norepinephrine

Norepinephrine is the neurotransmitter of the sympathetic nervous system and the biosynthetic precursor of epinephrine. The endogenous compound is released from synaptic nerves and acts locally. As levels of sympathetic nerve activity increase norepinephrine "spills over" into the circulation where it also acts as a neurohormone. Plasma norepinephrine levels are directly correlated with sympathetic nerve activity in normal subjects as assessed by microneurographic techniques. However, the levels are affected by rates of release, reuptake, degradation at effector sites, and metabolic clearance, and these may be altered to varying degrees in patients subjected to cardiac surgery, especially those with heart failure.

Continuous intravenous infusions of norepinephrine act predominantly by binding to α-adrenergic receptors. The β_1-adrenergic receptors of the heart, and, to a very modest degree, β_2-adrenergic receptors of the bronchi and peripheral blood vessels are stimulated by norepinephrine, although the β effects of this neurohormone are less than those seen with either epinephrine or isoproterenol. At low doses β effects on the heart and α effects on the circulation are relatively balanced, but higher doses produce predominantly α stimulation leading to vasoconstriction and increased pulmonary and systemic vascular resistance. As with epinephrine, norepinephrine is a potent renal vasoconstrictor. Additionally, it acts to vasoconstrict the pulmonary circuit and must be used cautiously in patients with pulmonary hypertension. Its most common use is in septic shock unresponsive to volume or less potent inotropic and vasoconstricting agents. It is also used under conditions where combined α and β stimulation are desired. The usual maintenance dose for β effect is 2–4 μg/min, although doses of 8–12 μg/min are often needed for hypotensive patients.

Isoproterenol

Isoproterenol is a synthetic sympathomimetic structurally related to, but pharmacologically distinct from, epinephrine. It is a pure β-agonist that produces increased heart rate and contractility, decreased systemic and pulmonary vascular resistance, and bronchodilatation. It is rarely utilized for its inotropic properties since its profound chronotropic and vasodilator effects often lead to unacceptable degrees of tachycardia and hypotension.

Dopamine

Dopamine is an endogenous catecholamine that is the immediate precursor of norepinephrine. It has principally a direct stimulatory effect on the β_1-adregenic receptors but also appears to have an indirect effect of releasing norepinephrine from its storage sites. Dopamine also acts on specific DA receptors in the renal, mesenteric, coronary, and intracerebral vascular beds to cause vasodilatation, but has little or no effect on β_2-receptors. With the continuous intravenous infusion of 0.5–2 μg/kg per minute renal DA receptor activation predominates over other effects, resulting in increased renal blood flow and increased urine output. At intermediate dose ranges of 2–10 μg/kg per minute, β_1-receptors also are stimulated. At doses greater than 10 μg/kg per minute, α and β effects are seen with α effects dominating at doses greater than 20 μg/kg per minute.

Dopamine constricts pulmonary capacitance veins and may increase pulmonary capillary wedge pressure when used as monotherapy in treatment of low cardiac output. Dopamine's long-term usefulness in low output states is limited, since part of its action depends on the release of endogenous catecholamines that are reduced in chronic congestive heart failure.

When compared with other inotropes, dopamine, for the same increase in blood pressure, increases cardiac output and urine flow to a greater extent than does norepinephrine. It is not as potent a myocardial stimulant as is isoproterenol and produces less vasodilatation, but may be safer in patients who experience hypotension, tachycardia, or arrhythmias with the latter.

Dobutamine

Dobutamine is a synthetic sympathomimetic compound structurally related to dopamine developed as a result of a search for an agent with selective positive inotropic influence and little peripheral vascular effect. It is predominantly a β_1-receptor agonist with modest β_2 and α_1 effects leading to cardiac stimulation without significant change in vascular tone. Unlike dopamine, dobutamine exerts no influence on DA receptors and increases urinary output simply as a result of increased cardiac output. It does not rely upon release of endogenous catecholamines and thus may be more efficacious than dopamine in the treatment of chronic heart failure. Heart rate changes little at usual therapeutic doses and the tendency to provoke arrhythmias is less than is seen with dopamine. It generally is regarded as an inotropic agent superior to dopamine in the period immediately following coronary artery bypass surgery.[20,21]

The rate of infusion of dobutamine usually needed to increase cardiac output is 2–20 µg/kg per minute. At doses greater than 20 µg/kg per minute, tachycardia is more common, potentially exacerbating myocardial ischemia.

Amrinone

Amrinone is a bipyridine derivative that is chemically unrelated to the cardiac glycosides or catecholamine compounds. Its positive inotropic activity occurs via inhibition of phosphodiesterase, thereby enhancing intracellular concentrations of cyclic AMP. Amrinone has been classified by some as an "inodilator" due to its potent inotropic and vasodilating properties. Based on studies in isolated tissues, the vasodilating potency of this drug is 10 to 100 times greater than its inotropic action.[22] The actions of amrinone, and other phosphodiesterase inhibitors such as milrinone, do not depend upon direct activation of adrenergic receptors.

Single amrinone doses of 0.5–1.5 µg/kg administered over 2 to 3 min to patients with heart failure increase cardiac output within 5 min. Increases ranging from 28 to 61% have been reported. Preload and afterload reduction also occurs by relaxation of vascular smooth muscle with a resultant decrease in pulmonary capillary wedge pressure and systemic vascular resistance. Effects of a single bolus may persist for as long as 2 hours but longer benefit is maintained with continuous infusion, usually of 5–10 µg/kg per minute.[23] Combination therapy with epinephrine or norepinephrine has been of benefit in selected patients.[24,25] Ad-

ministered in this way amrinone augments cyclic-AMP levels above those that can be provoked by cathcholamines alone.

Thrombocytopenia occurs in 2–3% of patients receiving short-term amrinone therapy. This decrease in platelet count is dose dependent and usually occurs within 48–72 hours of initiation of therapy. For this reason, platelet counts should be measured frequently during amrinone therapy. Hepatotoxicity occurs in 0.2% of patients receiving this medication intravenously.

Digitalis

Digitalis is presently the only orally active positive inotrope available for treatment of low cardiac output. Its efficacy in the treatment of heart failure complicated by atrial fibrillation has been well known for decades, but only recently has its suitability for treatment of heart failure in patients with normal sinus rhythm been established.[26] Two recent placebo-controlled withdrawal trials[27,28] have demonstrated the utility of digoxin in controlling signs and symptoms of heart failure, maintaining exercise tolerance, and preventing clinical deterioration in chronic heart failure. The role of digoxin in prolonging survival in heart failure is not presently known but is the subject of a large ongoing multicenter trial.[29]

Digoxin exerts its positive inotropic action by inhibition of Na^+–K^+-activated ATPase, an enzyme required for active transport across myocardial cell membranes. The resultant increase in intracellular sodium concentration leads, via a separate exchange pump, to increased intracellular calcium concentration and thus to increased contractility. In addition to its positive inotropic activity, digoxin produces systemic vasodilatation in patients with low cardiac output,[30] although vasoconstriction is seen in patients with normal ventricular function. This vasodilator effect in heart failure is due to sympathoinhibition, perhaps as a result of its sensitizing effect on cardiac and arterial baroreceptors.[31] Digoxin also is used in the management of arrhythmias as discussed elsewhere in this chapter.

THE USE OF VASODILATORS

Nitroprusside

Sodium nitroprusside is a vasodilator structurally unrelated to other vasodilating agents. It is a balanced arteriolar and venous dilator that decreases preload (central venous pressure and capillary wedge pressure) and afterload (pulmonary and systemic vascular resistance) in the low cardiac output syndrome. Its action is mediated by nonenzymatic release of nitric oxide,[32] which acts directly on vascular smooth muscle without effects on vasomotor centers, sympathetic nerves, or adrenergic receptors. Nitroprusside has no effect on nonvascular smooth cells.

Although nitroprusside has no direct effect on the myocardium, it increases cardiac output in patients with depressed myocardial function by reducing afterload. It may be combined with relatively pure inotropes such as dobutamine to further augment cardiac performance in severe pump dysfunction.

Unlike nitroglycerin, which predominantly dilates the veins and the large epicardial coronary arteries while having a minimal effect on coronary resistance vessels less than 100 μm in diameter, nitroprusside produces intense vasodilatation of small resistance vessels. In the presence of coronary occlusive disease, this may serve to preferentially direct bloodflow away from ischemic areas causing the phenomenon of "coronary steal."[33] If clinically apparent myocardial ischemia is induced by nitroprusside, the infusion should be discontinued. This may be seen in patients such as those who are not completely revascularized at the time of coronary bypass surgery.

Nitroprusside infusion should be initiated at 0.25–0.3 μg/kg per minute and gradually titrated upward every few minutes until the desired hemodynamic response is obtained or a maximal dose of 10 μg/kg per minute is attained. Transient hypotension, promptly responding to discontinuation of the infusion, is the most commonly observed side effect of intravenous nitroprusside and frequently reflects inadequate intravascular volume. Thiocyanate or cyanide toxicity may be seen but rarely occurs with infusion rates less than 3 μg/kg per minute given for less than 72 hours. Thiocyanate toxicity is manifest by tinnitus, miosis, confusion, and hyperreflexia and is seen more commonly in patients with impaired renal function. Cyanide toxicity may manifest as venous hyperoxemia or lactic acidosis.

Nitroglycerin

Nitroglycerin is an organic nitrate whose principal pharmacologic effect is relaxation of vascular smooth muscle, resulting in generalized arterial and venous dilatation. The increased venous capacitance following nitroglycerin treatment results in venous pooling and decreased venous return to the heart. The effects of nitroglycerin on arteriolar resistance are not as great as is its action on the venous side. As a result of this combined action, preload and, to a lesser extent, afterload are reduced. Reduction in left ventricular end-diastolic pressure and volume results in reduction of ventricular size and wall tension. Nitroglycerin, in intravenous, oral, or topical forms, has been used to treat the elevated preload commonly seen in conjunction with the low cardiac output syndrome occurring following bypass surgery. In addition to its actions in the treatment of heart failure, nitroglycerin is commonly used to treat myocardial ischemia, including ischemia occurring after bypass surgery. In patients with coronary artery occlusive disease, nitroglycerin causes a beneficial redistribution of coronary bloodflow to the subendocardial regions of the heart. This redistribution of coronary bloodflow may occur due to pref-

erential dilation of the large conductance vessels rather than the arteriolar resistance vessels or to dilation of collateral vessels that may develop secondary to myocardial ischemia. In addition to vascular smooth muscle, the nitrates relax bronchial, biliary, gastrointestinal, ureteral, and uterine smooth muscle, irrespective of autonomic innervation.

Forty to 80% of intravenous nitroglycerin is absorbed by the polyvinylchloride (PVC) plastic of standard IV tubing. Special IV administration sets are available that are of non-PVC plastic and cause minimal drug absorption. Nitroglycerin should be administered intravenously through non-PVC tubing at an initial dosage of 5–10 μg/min with the dosage increased by 5–10 μg/min every 3–5 minutes until the desired response is obtained. Individual dosage requirements vary and, thus, titration is mandatory. For treatment of hypertensive emergencies, dosages as high as 100 μg/min may be required. Because of its modest arterial vasodilating effect, nitroglycerin is not ideal for control of arterial pressure in hypertensive patients; nitroprusside would be a better choice under these circumstances.

Common side effects of intravenous nitroglycerin include cutaneous flushing and pulsing headaches due to dilation of meningeal vessels. Postural hypotension may occur, occasionally leading to true syncope. Postural hypotension can be reversed with administration of intravenous fluids and placement of the patient in the Trendelenburg position.

Tolerance to organic nitrates is seen most commonly with high or sustained drug concentrations. This is seen with either intravenous, oral, or topical administration, but is rarely observed even with frequent administration of sublingual nitroglycerin. Tolerance does not develop to the same degree in all patients, and some evidence suggests that up to 50% of patients may receive benefit from continuous nitrate therapy. The majority of patients on chronic nitrate therapy should have a nitrate free interval of 8–10 hours incorporated into their treatment regimen to prevent tolerance. Unlike nitroprusside, intravenous nitroglycerine does not cause coronary "steal."

Angiotensin-Converting Enzyme Inhibitors

This class of medication produces a vasodilating effect by blocking the action of angiotensin-converting enzyme, necessary for the conversion of angiotensin-I to the potent vasoconstrictor angiotensin-II. Reduced production of angiotensin-II via competition with the physiologic substrate will lead to vasodilatation.

Enalaprilat is the active metabolite of the pro drug enalapril and is available in intravenous form for the postoperative patient. The affinity of enalaprilat for angiotensin-converting enzyme (ACE) is 200,000 times greater than that of angiotensin-1 and, in vitro on a molar basis, 300 to 1000 times that of oral enalapril. In vivo, however, the ACE-inhibitory effects of enalaprilat are similar to that of its pro drug due to extensive hepatic hydrolysis.

Intravenous ACE inhibition is indicated when a rapid

onset of action is desired and when, in the early postoperative period, oral medications cannot be administered. An initial dose of 1.25 mg, administered by slow infusion over a period of at least 5 minutes, will decrease systemic vascular resistance, lower blood pressure in hypertensive patients, and increase cardiac output in patients with impaired ventricular function.

The intravenous administration of enalaprilat may be repeated every 6 hours as the clinical situation warrants with occasional patients requiring intravenous doses as high as 5 mg. For patients receiving a diuretic, the recommended initial intravenous dose is 0.625 mg. This lower dose is used to avoid excessive hypotension. A blood pressure reduction is usually seen within 15 min. Although most of the effect is usually apparent within the first hour, the maximal hypotensive response may not occur for up to 4 hours after the initial dose.

When feasible, patients with low cardiac output syndrome as well as patients with asymptomatic left ventricular systolic dysfunction should be changed from intravenous to oral ACE inhibitor therapy. Many products are available for oral use and are shown in Table 99–1. Major side effects of ACE inhibition include progressive azotemia (most commonly seen in patients with bilateral renal artery stenosis or with vascular compromise to a solitary kidney), hyperkalemia, cough, headache, and rash.

Hydralazine

Hydralazine reduces peripheral resistance and blood pressure as a result of a direct relaxant effect on vascular smooth muscle; the effect on arterioles is greater than on veins. Reflex tachycardia may be seen in patients with normal cardiac function who are given hydralazine for control of hypertension. Additionally, sodium and water retention has been reported with hydralazine given as monotherapy for hypertension, partially secondary to activation of the renin–angiotensin–aldosterone system. However, these side effects are typically not seen in patients who receive hydralazine for low cardiac output syndrome.

Hydralazine may be given intravenously in the early postoperative period as needed to control hypertension or to treat elevated systemic vascular resistance in the face of low cardiac output. Initial intravenous doses of 10–20mg may be repeated as necessary, rarely as often as every 20–30 min in a hypertensive emergency. Oral doses of hydralazine typically range from 10 to 100 mg three times daily. As previously noted, hydralazine in combination with isosorbide dinitrate has been shown to improve symptoms and survival in patients with chronically reduced left ventricular systolic function. Its ability to improve hemodynamics and symptoms in patients with low cardiac output is superior to ACE inhibitors, although the impact on survival is somewhat less.[9] For this reason, hydralazine, in combination with isosorbide dinitrate, should generally be reserved for those patients with symptomatic reduction in left ventricular function who are not suitable candidates for ACE inhibitor therapy, or may be used in combination with ACE inhibition.

RECOMMENDATIONS FOR TREATMENT OF THE LOW CARDIAC OUTPUT SYNDROME

Treatment of low cardiac output in the early postoperative period must be based on the specific hemodynamic abnormalities present. Low cardiac output associated with low ventricular filling pressures should be treated with appropriate volume replacement. If low cardiac output persists despite adequate volume resuscitation, a positive inotrope should be administered. Epinephrine or norepinephrine are appropriate in the setting of concomitant hypotension, but their use is limited by potent renal and systemic arterial vasoconstricting properties. Dobutamine and amrinone will provide positive inotropic activity without vasoconstriction and are therefore preferable agents in patients with adequate blood pressure. Dopamine is useful in low doses to increase renal blood flow and at intermediate doses as an inotrope, but also produces undesirable vasoconstriction at high doses. Excessive tachycardia and precipitation of ventricular and supraventricular arrhythmias are most common with epinephrine and norepinephrine, less common with dopamine, and least often seen with dobutamine or amrinone.

Vasodilator therapy may be utilized in conjunction with inotropes, especially with agents such as epinephrine and norepinephrine that possess no vasodilatory action. Occasionally vasodilators are needed with dobutamine as well, but amrinone is a relatively potent vasodilator and rarely requires concomitant vasodilator therapy.

In the acute setting, nitroprusside is the vasodilator of choice because of its balanced effect (lowering both preload and afterload), its rapid onset of action, and the ease of titration. Intravenous enalaprilat is also an appropriate choice, although its considerably longer duration of action may present problems in the immediate postoperative period and can cause prolonged hypotension in patients with inadequate intravascular volume.

TABLE 99–1. ORALLY ACTIVE ACE INHIBITORS

Generic Name	Brand Name	Dose Range	Clearance
Benazepril	Lotensin	10–40 mg qd-bid	Renal, hepatic
Captopril	Capoten	6.25–100 mg tid	Renal
Enalapril	Vasotec	2.5–20 mg qd-bid	Renal
Fosinopril[a]	Monopril	10–40 mg qd	Renal, hepatic
Lisinopril	Zestril, Prinivil	5–20 mg qd	Renal
Ramipril[a]	Altace	2.5–20 mg qd	Renal
Quinapril	Accupril	5–20 mg bid	Renal

[a]Not FDA approved for treatment of heart failure.

If low cardiac output persists into the later recovery phase of cardiac surgery, long-term therapy should be initiated. Digitalis should be administered to all patients with symptomatic heart failure from systolic dysfunction and ACE inhibitors to all patients with a reduced LVEF regardless of the presence or absence of symptoms. If ACE inhibitors are not tolerated, combination therapy with hydralazine and isosorbide dinitrate should be initiated and titrated upwards as tolerated.

THE POSTOPERATIVE MANAGEMENT OF CARDIAC ARRHYTHMIAS

Cardiac arrhythmias occur frequently following cardiac surgery. The incidence has been reported to be 11 to 54% for supraventricular arrhythmias and 1.8 to 13% for ventricular arrhythmias.[34-36] Patients undergoing valvular surgery and correction of congenital cardiac anomalies tend to have a higher prevalence of atrial arrhythmias than do patients undergoing coronary artery bypass surgery.[37] Due to the high incidence of postoperative arrhythmias in all patients undergoing cardiac surgery, monitoring is recommended for the initial 3 days following surgery and longer if arrhythmias are present or antiarrhythmic therapy is being initiated.[38]

There are numerous factors that may contribute to the development of cardiac arrhythmias in the postoperative patient. These include electrolyte abnormalities such as hypokalemia or hypomagnesemia, myocardial ischemia or infarction, low cardiac output, hypotension or hypertension, respiratory difficulty with hypoxemia or respiratory alkalosis, anemia, pericarditis, an increased sympathetic drive and circulating catecholamines, and cardiotoxicity from ongoing pharmacologic therapy. Recognition and correction of these underlying abnormalities are essential for the prevention of malignant arrhythmias and for their successful treatment once present. By optimizing myocardial function and reversing myocardial ischemia, the conditions necessary for arrhythmogenesis, i.e., alterations in action potential propagation, heterogeneities of repolarization, and increased automaticity, can in most cases be reversed.

Diagnosis

The successful treatment of a cardiac arrhythmia depends on the accurate identification of the arrhythmia. Arrhythmias can be divided into bradyarrhythmias, those with rates less than 60 bpm, and tachyarrhythmias, those with rates greater than 100 bpm. They can also be classified by the origin of the rhythm as either supraventricular (originating above the bundle of His) or ventricular. Several modalities are available to aid in the diagnosis of the arrhythmia. These include the 12-lead electrocardiogram (ECG), the electrograms recorded from the atrial and ventricular epicardial wires, the response of the arrhythmia to overdrive

pacing, and the response of the arrhythmia to transient blockade of A-V node conduction. The 12-lead ECG and rhythm strip can be used to correctly diagnose a narrow complex tachycardia in up to 90% of the cases and wide complex tachycardias approximately 75% of the time.[39] The ability to accurately diagnose the arrhythmia is enhanced by the recording of atrial and ventricular electrograms.

Ventricular epicardial wires are routinely placed at the time of surgery to facilitate ventricular pacing postoperatively in cases of bradyarrhythmia such as complete heart block. The placement of atrial epicardial wires also should be routine because of their value in the diagnosis and treatment of atrial arrhythmias. Atrial electrograms can be recorded to clarify the underlying atrial activity, such as atrial flutter with 2:1 conduction, atrial tachycardia with 1:1 or 2:1 conduction and atrial fibrillation (Fig. 99–4). Ventricular tachycardia is diagnosed definitively when ventriculoatrial (V:A) dissociation can be demonstrated. The surface ECG P-wave may be hidden within the QRS complex or T-wave, thus making it difficult to demonstrate V:A dissociation. Recordings of atrial and ventricular electrograms can provide definitive proof of the ventricular origin of the arrhythmia or establish that there is normal and sequential A:V activation with aberrant ventricular conduction. Alternatively, ventricular tachycardia with retrograde V:A conduction may be demonstrated. Many of the postoperative tachyarrhythmias can be terminated or suppressed by pacing via the epicardial wires.[40-42] Overdrive pacing should be attempted only after verifying which wires are atrial and which are ventricular, so that inadvertent rapid ventricular pacing does not occur. A cardioverter-defibrillator should be present, especially when pace-terminating ventricular tachycardia as acceleration of the tachycardia to an unstable rate or degeneration of the rhythm to ventricular fibrillation can occur. Pacing thresholds via the epicardial wires may be as high as 15 to 20 mA postoperatively, due to depressed cardiac excitability and to the nature of the epicardial electrode.

Extra Beats

An isolated premature atrial contraction appears as a narrow QRS complex preceded by a P-wave, which may be hidden in the preceding T-wave. These are not ususally of hemodynamic significance and generally do not require treatment. Frequently they precede and initiate supraventricular arrhythmias. In this circumstance it is desirable to suppress the premature atrial contractions with digoxin, a β-blocker, or a type IA or type III antiarrhythmic drug.

Isolated premature ventricular contractions (PVCs), ventricular bigeminy, ventricular trigeminy, and couplets also are usually not hemodynamically significant and suppression of these rhythms with drug therapy is not indicated. Premature ventricular beats or an increase in the amount of ectopy can occur due to electrolyte abnormali-

LEAD II

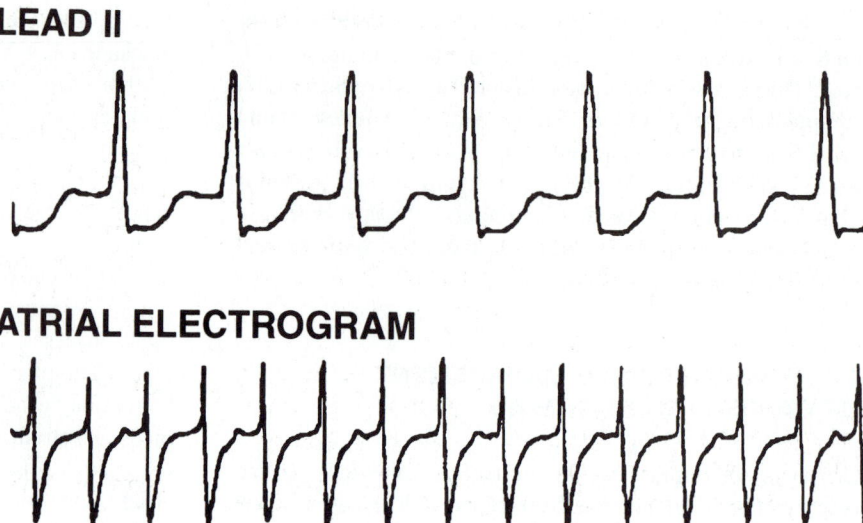

ATRIAL ELECTROGRAM

Figure 99–4. Surface ECG (lead II) recorded simultaneously with a bipolar atrial electrogram during an episode of atrial flutter. The atrial rate is 300 bpm and there is 2:1 A:V conduction.

ties, specifically potassium and magnesium. These abnormalities should be corrected to maintain a serum potassium level above 4.0 mEq/L and a magnesium level above 1.5 mEq/L. Both electrolytes can be repleted intravenously, with the replacement dose reduced in the presence of renal insufficiency. Severe bradycardia or antiarrhythmic therapy in the presence of hypokalemia or hypomagnesemia may predispose the patient to the development of torsades de pointes,[43] a form of polymorphic ventricular tachycardia that can occur in patients with a prolonged QT interval. Therapy for torsades de pointes is outlined in the section entitled Tachyarrhythmias. In the presence of normal electrolytes and in the absence of ongoing myocardial ischemia, isolated premature ventricular contractions generally do not require therapy. There is one exception regarding the treatment of PVCs that should be noted. Occasionally, patients with relatively slow sinus rates may develop ventricular bigeminy. This could result in a 50% reduction in the number of effective cardiac contractions and consequently a reduction in cardiac output and an increase in cardiac filling pressure. Treatment is directed at increasing the heart rate with either atrial pacing or A-V sequential pacing if heart block is present.

The presence of premature ventricular contractions is not associated with an increased incidence of ventricular fibrillation nor is the suppression of PVCs sufficient to prevent sudden cardiac death. This became evident during the cardiac arrhythmia suppression trial (CAST), which was undertaken to randomize postinfarction patients with PVCs to either suppressive therapy with an antiarrhythmic agent (flecainide, encainide, or moricizine) or placebo. The study was prematurely terminated due to a higher mortality in patients with suppressed PVCs who were treated with the antiarrhythmic agents.[44,45]

Bradyarrhythmias

Sinus bradycardia is defined as a sinus rate less then 60 beats per minute (bpm). In the immediate postoperative pe-

riod, where there is an increase in circulating catecholamines, a sinus rate less than 80 bpm is considered a relative bradycardia. The diagnosis is made from the surface ECG where there is a 1:1 relationship between the P-wave and the QRS complex and the axis of the P-wave is similar to the axis of the P-wave observed during sinus rhythm preoperatively. The atrial electrogram recording will exclude atrial begeminy with nonconducted premature atrial beats. Temporary atrial pacing or AV sequential pacing at 90 to 110 bpm should be considered for asymptomatic sinus bradycardia and relative sinus bradycardia in the early postoperative period. Patients with low cardiac output and bradycardia will frequently improve with temporary pacing. Atropine can be administered at 0.5 to 1.0 mg intravenously every 3 to 5 min up to a total of 3 mg until the sinus rate has increased or pacing has been initiated. Sinus bradycardia may be a manifestation of intrinsic sinus node dysfunction or myocardial ischemia.

Sinus node dysfunction or the sick sinus syndrome is characterized by inappropriate sinus bradycardia with a blunted response to atropine, and sinus pauses. In the postoperative patient this usually results from trauma to the sinus node, and, therefore, is often transient but may last for several days. Cardiac drugs that suppress sinus node function such as α-methyldopa and clonidine should be discontinued if possible. Long-term sinus node dysfunction is seen more frequently following orthotopic heart transplant[46] and corrective surgery for congenital heart disease.[47,48] The Mustard procedure, performed to correct transposition of the great vessels, is associated with a high risk of long-term sinus node dysfunction because the baffle is sutured in close proximity to the sinus node.[47] One recognized complication of ASD repair is sinus node dysfunction that can become manifest years after surgery.[48] Ten to 20% of children requiring pacemakers have sinus node dysfunction following ASD repair.[49] Sinus node dysfunction may have been present preoperatively, particularly in elderly patients subjected to coronary revascularization or valve replacement. This may contribute to the propensity for older patients to devleop either brady- or tachyarrhythmias postoperatively.

Atrial quiescence or standstill is a rhythm that, although rare, has been reported in patients following mitral or aortic valve surgery. In the postoperative period, the atria may become completely inexcitable and therefore cannot be paced. Fortunately this state is usually transient, lasting 24 to 36 hours, and when treatment is required, small doses of isoproterenol, administered at 1 μg/min, have been successful.[50] In some patients, ventricular pacing may be required to avoid inappropriate bradycardia.

Partial or complete A-V block may occur in the initial postoperative period and is most likely secondary to trauma and subsequent edema of the A-V node. This A-V nodal block resolves, although may require temporary pacing, in most patients undergoing coronary artery bypass grafting. Goldman et al. reviewed 5,942 patients undergoing cardiac surgery and found that 0.6% of patients undergoing coronary bypass grafting required permanent pacing, while patients undergoing valvular surgery had a 4.6% incidence of permanent A-V nodal block required pacing.[51] A:V sequential pacing is preferred over single chamber ventricular pacing due to the hemodynamic benefits of A:V synchrony.

Tachyarrhythmias

Patients exhibiting sustained tachycardia associated with hemodynamic compromise should be promptly electrically cardioverted after adequate anesthesia is administered. An attempt should be made to elucidate the mechanism of the tachycardia with a 12-lead ECG, a recording of the atrial and ventricular electrograms, and administration of adenosine if time permits. In the hemodynamically stable patient, it is important to accurately diagnose the arrhythmia prior to instituting either pharmacologic or electrical therapy, so that the appropriate treatment strategy can be initiated to terminate and avoid recurrences of the arrhythmia.

Narrow Complex Tachycardia

The algorithm in Figure 99–5 presents a step-by-step approach to the diagnosis of the narrow (QRS<0.15 sec) complex tachycardia. The initial step is the determination of whether the tachycardia has a regular or irregular R–R interval. Following this stratification an assessment of atrial activity is made by evaluation of the ECG, the atrial epicardial electrogram recordings and by unmasking atrial activ-

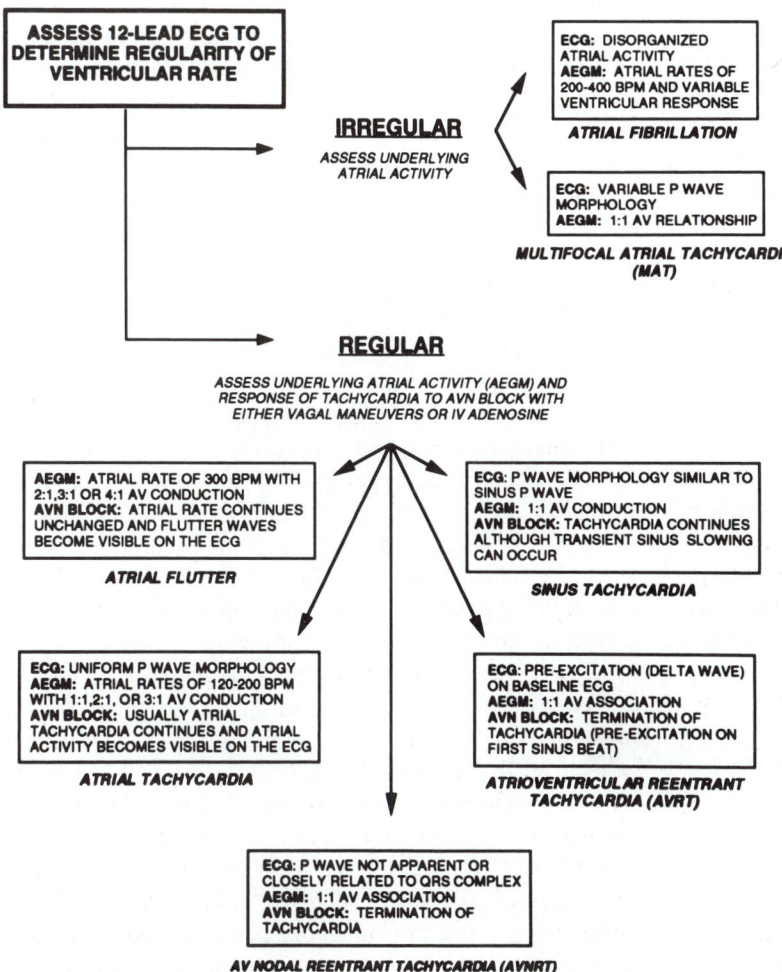

Figure 99–5. Algorithm for the diagnosis of the narrow complex tachycardia: AEGM, atrial electrogram.

ity during A-V nodal block. Finally, the response of the tachycardia to A-V nodal block is helpful to elucidate this underlying mechanism of the tachycardia. In the postoperative patient, the most common irregular tachyarrhythmias include multifocal atrial tachycardia (MAT) and atrial fibrillation. Characteristics of MAT include a differing P-wave morphology and a variable R–R interval on the surface ECG, as well as a 1:1 A-V relationship on the atrial electrogram recording. Finally, the development of A-V nodal block with either vagal maneuvers or administration of intravenous adenosine does not terminate this tachycardia. Therapy for MAT is primarily directed at correction of the underlying physiologic abnormalities (most commonly pulmonary insufficiency), although both β-blockers and calcium channel blockers have been used with success.[52] There is no indication for cardioversion.

Atrial fibrillation can be diagnosed from the 12-lead ECG by the presence of disorganized atrial activity and a variable ventricular response. The atrial electrogram clearly demonstrates rapid, irregular atrial activity at rates of 200 to 400 beats per minutes (Fig. 99–6). The response of the tachycardia to A-V nodal block is transient ventricular slowing with continued erratic atrial activity. Initial treatment is aimed at controlling the ventricular response, which can be done promptly either with intravenous diltiazem, verapamil, or a β-blocker. Intravenous administration allows closer titration of the desired ventricular response, which in patients with impaired cardiac function is a heart rate of 90 to 100 bpm. The use of intravenous β-blockers or calcium channel blockers is preferable to digoxin in the initial management of atrial fibrillation because of their more rapid onset of action. Several doses of digoxin over a 4- to

8-hour period may be required before significant therapeutic benefit is detected. In addition, the effect of digoxin on the A-V node is diminished in the presence of increased circulating catecholamines, and in the vagolytic state, which often is present postoperatively.

If digoxin therapy is instituted a loading regimen (usually 1 mg over 24 hours) should be employed. In the absence of such loading and administration of maintenance doses only, therapeutic digoxin levels will not be obtained for 5 to 7 days. Once the ventricular rate is controlled, a type 1A or type 3 agent can be used in an attempt to restore normal sinus rhythm (Table 99–2). Ideally, normal sinus rhythm should be restored within 48 hours to minimize the risk of a cardioembolic event. Elective cardioversion under anesthesia should be performed prior to discharge if medical cardioversion is unsuccessful. The continuation of an antiarrhythmic agent (in addition to anticoagulation) is recommended to maintain normal sinus rhythm and minimize the risk of thromboembolism during the initial 4 to 6 wk following surgery.

Atrial fibrillation can be difficult to recognize in the setting of complete heart block. In this case, the ventricular rate is governed by a regular junctional escape rhythm of 40 to 60 bpm (Fig. 99–6). Therapy includes temporary ventricular pacing to increase the ventricular rate and improve cardiac output as well as therapy to restore normal sinus rhythm as outlined above. Two important points should be kept in mind when digitalis glycosides are used in the treatment of atrial fibrillation for rate control. First, junctional rhythm or "regularization" of the R–R intervals in the presence of atrial fibrillation may indicate the presence of digitalis intoxication in patients treated with digoxin, ouabain,

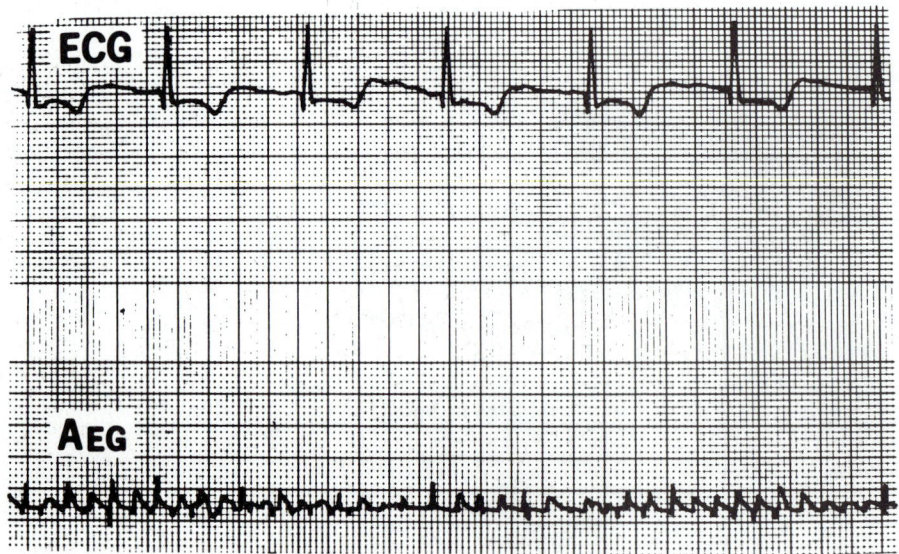

Figure 99–6. Surface ECG lead recorded simultaneously with a bipolar atrial electrogram (AEG). The atrial electrogram demonstrates disorganized atrial activity, while the surface ECG demonstrates a regular narrow QRS complex at 65 bpm. This is an example of atrial fibrillation with complete A-V block and a junctional rhythm. *(From Waldo AL, MacLean WAH: Diagnosis and Treatment of Cardiac Arrhythmias Following Open Heart Surgery. Futura Publishing Company, Mount Kisco, New York, 1980, p 73, with permission.)*

TABLE 99–2. ANTIARRHYTHMIC AGENTS[a]

Class	Drug	Indications	Dosage	Elimination Half-life	Adverse Effects
IA	Quinidine	AF, AFl, PACs, AT, AVRT, EP guided suppression of VT	Oral: gluconate 324–660 mg q8–12° sulfate 300–400 mg q6°	6–8 h	GI side effects—diarrhea Proarrhythmia—torsades de pointe
	Procainamide	As above	IV: 15 mg/kg at 20 mg/min (load) then 1–6 mg/min[b] (maintenance) Oral: 50/mg/kg/day[b] in 4 divided doses	2.5–4.7 h	Hematologic—marrow suppression, lupus-like illness Proarrhythmia Hypotension (with IV infusion)
	Disopyramide	As above	Oral: 150 mg q6° or 300 mg CR q12°	4–10 h	Anticholinergic effects—dry mouth, urinary retention Conduction disturbances Proarrhythmia
IB	Lidocaine	VT, PVCs in setting of ischemia	IV: 1 mg/kg bolus then 1–4 mg/min[b] (maintenance)	1.5–2 h	CNS—drowsiness, agitation, disorientation, tremulousness
IC	Flecainide	Atrial arrhythmias-AF, AFl, AT, AVRT, EP guided suppression of VT[c]	Oral: 50–150 mg q12°[b]	11–14 h	Proarrhythmia[c] CNS—dizziness, visual disturbances
II	Esmolol	Short-term rate control of AF, AFl, treatment of AVNRT, AVRT, MAT	IV: 500 µg/kg over 1 min (load) then 50 µg/kg per minute (maintenance)	2 min	Hypotension, CNS—dizziness, somnolence, headache, Bronchospasm at higher doses
	Metoprolol	Rate control of AF, AFl, treatment of AVNRT, MAT	Oral: 50–200 mg q12°	3–4 h	As above
	Atenolol	As above	Oral: 25–100 mg q day[b]	6–7 h	As above
	Propranolol	As above	IV: 0.5–3 mg repeat in 2–5 min then q 4° Oral 10–30 mg q6–8°	2 h (initial dose) 3.4–6 hrs	As above Bronchospasm due to β₂-antagonist activity
III	Sotalol	VT, atrial arrhythmias (not yet FDA approved)	Oral: 80–160 mg q12°[b]	12 h	Proarrhythmia—torsades de pointes, sinus bradycardia CHF CNS—dizziness, fatigue Bronchospasm
	Bretyllium	VT and VF refractory to other therapy (short-term therapy only)	IV: 5–10 mg/kg over 8–10 min	5–10 h	Significant hypotension
	Amiodarone	VT, VF	Oral: 800–1600 mg q day for 1–3 wk (load) 200–400 mg q day (maintenance)	9–44 days	Conduction disturbances—sinus bradycardia, heart block Abnormalities of thyroid function, liver function Pulmonary toxicity
		Atrial arrhythmias	Oral: 100–400 mg q day (maintenance)		
IV	Diltiazem	Rate control of AF, AFl, treatment of AVNRT, MAT	IV: 0.25 mg/kg over 2 min if no response in 15 min 0.35 mg/kg over 2 min then 5–15 mg/hr (maintenance) Oral: 30–120 mg tid, 120–300 mg CD q day	3.5–10 h	Hypotension Potentiation of sinus node dysfunction
	Verapamil	As above	IV: 5–10 mg may repeat in 15–30 min with 10 mg Oral: 60–120 mg q6–8° 120–240 mg SR q12–24°	2–8 h (IV) 4.5–12 h (oral)	Cardiac effects—congestive heart failure due to negative inotropic effect, hypotension GI effects—constipation

(continued)

TABLE 99–2. ANTIARRHYTHMIC AGENTS^a (Continued)

Class	Drug	Indications	Dosage	Elimination Half-life	Adverse Effects
other	Digoxin	Rate control of AF,AFl, treatment of AVNRT	IV/oral: 0.5 mg (initial) 0.25 mg q4–8° to total of 1.0 mg (load) 0.125–0.375 mg q day (maintenance)^b	30 min (IV) 34–44 h (oral)	Toxic side effects—nausea, accelerated junctional rhythm, high grade A-V block
	Adenosine	Termination of AVNRT,AVRT, occasionally MAT, and exercise-mediated VT	IV: 6 mg rapid bolus may repeat with 12 mg in 1 min and then 18 mg	0.6–1.5 sec	Dyspnea, chest pain, flushing Sinus tachycardia
	Magnesium	Torsades de pointes	IV: 1–2 g (load) 1–7.5 mg/min (maintenance)^b		Hypotension

^{a}AF, atrial fibrillation; AFl, atrial flutter; AT, atrial tachycardia; AVRT, atrioventricular reentry tachycardia; VT, ventricular tachycardia; AVNRT, atrioventricular nodal reentry tachycardia; MAT, multifocal atrial tachycardia; VF, ventricular tachycardia. The dosages and indications listed are based on current practice standards and therefore are subject to change in the future.
^{b}The dosage should be adjusted in the presence of renal insufficiency.
^{c}The Cardiac Arrhythmia Suppression Trial (CAST)[44] demonstrated an increase in mortality and cardiac arrest in patients receiving flecainide who had a history of myocardial infarction and decreased LV function, therefore Class IC agents are not recommended as first line therapy in this patient population.

or other cardiac glycosides. Administration of additional digoxin may lead to further acceleration of the A-V node resulting in nonparoxysmal junctional tachycardia. Continued digoxin administration under these circumstances is likely to provoke life-threatening ventricular arrhythmias. Second, when digitalis is used to induce A-V nodal block for rate control in the presence of hypokalemia, repletion of potassium may augment the effect of the glycoside, thereby increasing the degree of A-V node block that is present. This can result in profound junctional bradycardia, which requires ventricular pacing.

If the narrow complex tachycardia is regular, underlying atrial activity may not be readily apparent on the 12-lead ECG. The atrial electrogram recorded simultaneously with the surface ECG will demonstrate 1:1, 2:1, or even 3:1 A:V association. A tachycardia with an atrial rate of 300 bpm, which usually conducts 2:1 yielding a ventricular rate of 150 bpm, is atrial flutter (Fig. 99–4). Because the ventricular response is more difficult to control in atrial flutter than in atrial fibrillation, therapy is directed at termination of the atrial flutter. This includes overdrive atrial pacing to interrupt the atrial flutter circuit, administration of a type IA or type III agent, or rapid atrial pacing at 450 bpm to fibrillate the atria and allow better control of the ventricular rate. Alternatively, synchronized cardioversion (usually with 25–50 J) under anesthesia can be performed to restore normal sinus rhythm. Pharmacologic therapy is continued for maintenance of sinus rhythm during the initial 4 to 6 wk postoperatively. Cases of 2:1 or 3:1 A:V conduction with atrial rates of less than 300 bpm and 1:1 A-V node conduction with atrial rates of 120 to 200 bpm indicate atrial tachycardia. If there is uncertainty regarding the underlying atrial activity, intravenous adenosine can be administered and atrial activity on the surface ECG will be unmasked during the transient A-V node block (Fig. 99–7). Some types of

atrial tachycardia are successfully terminated with adenosine, vagal maneuvers, or overdrive atrial pacing;[53] however, cardioversion in addition to antiarrhythmic therapy is often necessary.

Termination of the tachycardia following A-V node block suggests that the A-V node is an integral part of the re-entrant circuit. Atrioventricular nodal reentrant tachycardia (AVNRT) occurs when dual A-V node pathways with

LEAD II

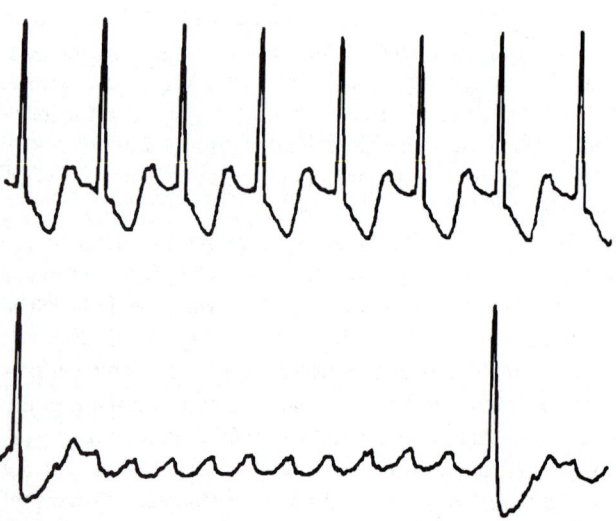

Figure 99–7. (Top) Surface ECG (lead II) demonstrates a narrow complex tachycardia with a ventricular rate of 150 bpm. **(Bottom)** Following the intravenous administration of adenosine (6 mg), transient A-V node block occurs and the underlying atrial flutter waves are easily visible.

differing refractory periods are present. The re-entrant circuit of AVNRT is initiated when antegrade conduction is blocked in one pathway but continues via the other pathway. During the antegrade conduction the blocked pathway recovers and is able to conduct retrograde. The re-entrant circuit continues within the A-V node and is terminated by maneuvers that cause A-V node block. The atrial electrogram demonstrates 1:1 A:V association with almost simultaneous A:V depolarization. Therapy includes long acting A-V nodal blocking agents such as digoxin, β-blockers, or calcium channel blockers. Since AVNRT as well as atrial tachycardias are frequently initiated by premature atrial beats, suppression of premature atrial beats may be indicated.

The presence of ventricular pre-excitation, seen as a delta wave on the surface ECG at baseline or following the administration of an A-V node blocking agent, indicates the presence of an accessory A-V connection. Atrioventricular re-entry tachycardia (AVRT) involves antegrade conduction via the A-V node and retrograde conduction via the accessory connection (narrow QRS complexes) or vice versa (wide QRS complexes). Therapy for this tachycardia is directed at altering the properties of the bypass tract to terminate the tachycardia and prevent its recurrence. The type 1A or 1C antiarrhythmic agents slow conduction in the accessory connection and are therefore effective in the treatment of tachycardias involving accessory connections. Patients with accessory connections should undergo electrophysiologic assessment to determine their risk for fatal arrhythmias and sudden cardiac death. Until the antegrade properties of the pathway are known, the administration of long acting A-V nodal blocking agents is contraindicated. If atrial fibrillation develops in the presence of A-V node block, conduction exclusively via the accessory pathway can occur with rates up to 300 bpm, precipitating ventricular fibrillation and hemodynamic collapse.[54] The use of adenosine (in contrast to longer acting agents such as verapamil) for these tachycardias is relatively safe because of its very short half-life (<10 seconds); however, it has been reported that adenosine as well as verapamil can precipitate atrial fibrillation following termination of the tachycardia.[54,55]

Finally, sinus tachycardia is frequently seen in the postoperative setting. The 12-lead ECG demonstrates a normal P-wave axis (inferior and leftward) and the atrial electrogram shows a 1:1 A:V relationship. While this is a regular narrow complex tachycardia, it demonstrates a progressive increase in heart rate and a gradual slowing as opposed to the sudden onset and termination seen in the re-entrant arrhythmias. A-V nodal blocking maneuvers will not terminate the tachycardia, although momentary slowing of the sinus rate may be observed with adenosine. Treatment of sinus tachycardia is directed at correcting the underlying abnormality including extreme pain, hypovolemia, hypotension, low cardiac output, myocardial ischemia, hypoxemia, and anemia.

Wide Complex Tachycardias

Diagnosing a wide complex tachycardia from the surface ECG is not always straightforward. All of the narrow complex tachycardias can present as wide complexes if aberrant ventricular conduction is present. In patients with coronary artery disease or a history of myocardial infarction, a wide complex tachycardia is ventricular tachycardia (VT) until proven otherwise.[56] As in all tachyarrhythmia management, if the patient is hemodynamically unstable, emergent synchronized cardioversion is indicated. If the patient is hemodynamically stable, or if there is the opportunity during preparation for cardioversion, a 12-lead ECG and atrial and ventricular epicardial electrograms should be obtained. Several authors have published ECG criteria to aid in the diagnosis of VT (Table 99–3).[57,58] As mentioned previously, the atrial electrogram can be diagnostic of ventricular tachycardia if A-V dissociation is clearly present. The absence of A-V dissociation does not exclude ventricular tachycardia as 1:1 retrograde V:A conduction can occur. Adenosine has been used to further differentiate VT from a supraventricular tachycardia.[39,59] Following the rapid intravenous injection of 6 to 12 mg of adenosine, transient A-V node block occurs. If there is termination of the tachycardia then the wide complex tachycardia is most likely a supraventricular arrhythmia, although there are certain types of ventricular tachycardia that are adenosine sensitive. Adenosine sensitive ventricular tachycardias are usually associated with a structurally normal heart or are exercise/catecholamine mediated. If the tachycardia continues uninterrupted then ventricular tachycardia is present. There is no role for verapamil in the diagnosis of a wide complex tachycardia. The peripheral vasodilation that occurs following verapamil administration has led to rapid cardiac decompensation and death in patients with ventricular tachycardia.[60]

Monomorphic ventricular tachycardia, either sustained or nonsustained, in the postoperative period requires prompt treatment. Lidocaine is usually the initial drug of choice. If lidocaine is unsuccessful, procainamide is the second line of therapy. Both drugs are associated with adverse side effects (Table 99–2) and the patient must be care-

---

TABLE 99–3. ECG CRITERIA THAT SUPPORT THE DIAGNOSIS OF VENTRICULAR TACHYCARDIA[57,58]

QRS complex width > 0.14 seconds

Left axis deviation

Configuration of QRS complex
  In RBBB: a mono- or biphasic complex in lead V_1
  In LBBB: a Q-wave in lead V_6
  Concordance in the precordial leads

A:V dissociation[a]

The absence of an RS complex in the precordial leads[a]

If the RS complex is present, an RS interval > 0.10 seconds[a]

[a]100% specific for ventricular tachycardia.

LEAD II

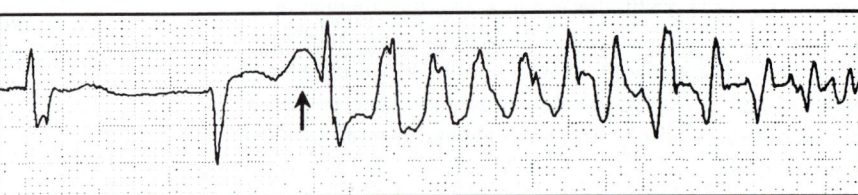

Figure 99–8. Surface ECG recorded from a patient receiving oral quinidine. Note the predominant U-wave (arrow) that is present following a pause, and the onset of torsades de pointes.

fully monitored during administration of these drugs. Patients with incessant ventricular tachycardia or polymorphic ventricular tachycardia should be carefully evaluated for myocardial ischemia secondary to incomplete revascularization or impending graft closure. Patients in the immediate postoperative period with refractory ventricular tachycardia and a low cardiac output may often be treated effectively with placement of an intra-aortic balloon pump. In some cases, monomorphic ventricular tachycardia can be pace terminated with overdrive ventricular pacing. Because of the possibility that overdrive pacing may result in acceleration of the tachycardia to a hemodynamically unstable ventricular tachycardia or ventricular fibrillation, equipment for emergency cardioversion and defibrillation should be present. Patients with recurrent ventricular tachycardia despite lidocaine or procainamide therapy may respond to amiodarone. Although the intravenous formulation of amiodarone is not widely available, oral loading regimens of 800 to 1600 mg/day for 1 to 2 wk have been used.[61] Suppression of recurrent ventricular tachycardia may take up to 1 week. Patients exhibiting sustained ventricular tachycardia in the postoperative period not associated with myocardial infarct or ischemia should undergo electrophysiologic study to guide pharmacologic therapy, to identify the need for implantation of a cardioverter-defibrillator, or to attempt radiofrequency ablation of the VT site.

Polymorphic ventricular tachycardia in the setting of a normal QT interval is often seen in association with myocardial ischemia. Lidocaine in addition to a β-blocker can be helpful in suppressing this ventricular tachycardia; however, treatment should be directed at reversing the underlying ischemia. Patients with prolonged QT interval from either ischemia or drug toxicity may develop a polymorphic ventricular tachycardia called torsades de pointes (Fig. 99–8). Because torsades de pointes frequently consists of recurrent and self-limiting episodes, treatment strategies are aimed at shortening the QT interval and preventing recurrence. Therapy for torsades de pointes includes temporary pacing, atrial if possible, to avoid pause-related initiation of ventricular tachycardia, and to shorten the QT interval; intravenous lidocaine, which shortens the QT interval; and intravenous magnesium, which is thought to have membrane stabilizing effects.[62] Drugs that further prolong the QT interval such as the type 1A or type 3 antiarrhythmics are contraindicated. Isoproterenol, although used to increase the heart rate and shorten the QT interval, is associated with

hypotension, and, therefore, epicardial atrial pacing to increase heart rate is preferable.

Ventricular fibrillation represents the electrical and mechanical disorganization of the ventricles. The atrial electrograms, however, may continue to demonstrate sinus rhythm. Ventricular fibrillation is incompatible with life and emergent nonsynchronized defibrillation at 360 J is indicated. For ventricular fibrillation that does not respond to three successive emergent defibrillation attempts, institution of pharmacotherapy including epinephrine, lidocaine, procainamide, and bretyllium may be required using the advanced cardiac life supprot (ACLS) protocols as described by the American Heart Association.[63]

REFERENCES

1. Kouchoukos NT, Oberman A, Kirklin JW, et al: Coronary artery bypass surgery: Analysis of factors affecting hospital mortality. *Circulation* **62** (suppl I):I–84–9, 1980

2. Davis KB: Operative mortality in the CASS registry. In Hammermeister KE (ed): *Coronary Bypass Surgery*. New York, Praeger, 1983, pp 93–128

3. Breisblatt WM, Stein KL, Wolfe CJ, et al: Acute myocardial dysfunction and recovery: A common occurrence after coronary bypass surgery. *J Am Coll Cardiol* **15**:1261–1269, 1990

4. Stewart JR, Blackwell WH, Crute SL, et al: Inhibition of surgically induced ischemia/reperfusion injury by oxygen free radical scavengers. *J Thorac Cardiovasc Surg* **86**:262–272, 1983

5. McKenney PA, Apstein CS, Mendes LA, et al: Increased left ventricular diastolic chamber stiffness immediately after coronary artery bypass surgery. *J Am Coll Cardiol* **24**:1189–1194, 1994

6. Majid PA, Sharma B, Taylor SH: Phentolamine for vasodilator treatment of severe heart-failure. *Lancet* **22**:719–726, 1971

7. Franciosa JA, Cuiha NH, Limas CJ, et al: Improved left ventricular function during nitroprusside infusion in acute myocardial infarction. *Lancet* **1**:650–654, 1972

8. Cohn JN, Franciosa JA, Francis GS, et al: Effect of short-term infusion of sodium nitroprusside on mortality rate in acute myocardial infarction complicated by left ventricular failure. *N Engl J Med* **306**:1129–1135, 1982

9. Cohn JN, et al: Effect of vasodilator therapy on mortality in chronic congestive heart failure: Results of a Veteran's Administration cooperative study. *N Engl J Med* **314**:1547–1552, 1986

10. Cohn JN, et al: A comparison of enalapril with hydralazine-isosorbide dinitrate in the treatment of chronic congestive heart failure. *N Engl J Med* **325**:303–310, 1991

11. The Consensus Trial Study Group: Effects of enalapril on mortality in severe congestive heart failure: Results of the Cooperative North Scandinavian Enalapril Survival Study. *N Engl J Med* **316**:1429–1435, 1987

12. Captopril-digoxin Multicenter Research Group: Comparative effects

of therapy with capropril and digoxin in patients with mild to moderate heart failure. *JAMA* **259**:539–544, 1988

13. Captopril Multicenter Research Group: A placebo-controlled trial of captopril in refractory chronic congestive heart failure. *J Am Coll Cardiol* **2**:755–763, 1983

14. The SOLVD Investigators: Effect of enalapril on survival in patients with reduced ejection fractions and congestive heart failure. *N Engl J Med* **325**:293–302, 1991

15. The SOLVD Investigators: Effect of enalapril on mortality and the development of heart failure in asymptomatic patients with reduced left ventricular ejection fractions. *N Engl J Med* **327**:685–691, 1992

16. Pfeffer MA, Braunwald E, Moye LA, et al: On Behalf of the SAVE Investigators: Effect of captopril on mortality in patients with left ventricular dysfunction after myocardial infarction. *N Engl J Med* **327**:669–677, 1992

17. Brodde O-E, Karad K, Zerkowski HR, et al: Coexistence of β_1-and β_2-adrenoreceptors in human right atrium. *Circ Res* **53**:752–758, 1983

18. Heitz A, Schwartz J, Velly J: β-Adrenoreceptors of the human myocardium: Determination of β_1- and β_2-subtypes by radioligand binding. *Br J Pharmacol* **80**:711–717, 1983

19. Sibbald WJ, Fox G, Martin C: Abnormalities of vascular reactivity in the sepsis syndrome. *Chest* **100** (suppl):155–159S, 1991

20. Fowler MB, Alderman EL, Oesterle SN, et al: Dobutamine and dopamine after cardiac surgery: Greater augmentation of myocardial blood flow with dobutamine. *Circulation* **70** (suppl I):I–103–11, 1984

21. Van Trigt P, Spray TL, Pasque MK, et al: The comparative effects of dopamine and dobutamine on ventricular mechanics after coronary artery bypass grafting: A pressure-dimension analysis. *Circulation* **70** (suppl I):I–112–117, 1984

22. Morgan JP, Gwathmey JK, DeFeo TT, Morgan KG: The effects of amrinone and related drugs on intracellular calcium in isolated mammalian cardiac and vascular smooth muscle. *Circulation* **73** (suppl III):III65–77, 1986

23. Ramsay JG, DeJesus JM, Wynands JE, et al: Amrinone before termination of cardiopulmonary bypass: Haemodynamic variables and oxygen utilization in the postbypass period. *Can J Anaesth* **39**:342–348, 1992

24. Royster RL, Butterworth JF, Prielipp RC, et al: Combined inotropic effects of amrinone and epinephrine after cardiopulmonary bypass in humans. *Anesth Analg* **77**:662–672, 1993

25. Hardy J-F, Searle N, Roy M, Perrault J: Amrinone, in combination with norepinephrine, is an effective first-line drug for difficult separation from cardiopulmonary bypass. *Can J Anaesth* **40**:495–501, 1993

26. Kelly RA, Smith TW: Digoxin in heart failure: Implications of recent trials. *J Am Coll Cardiol* **22** (suppl A):107–112A, 1993

27. Packer K, Gheorghiade M, Young JB, et al: Withdrawal of digoxin from patients with chronic heart failure treated with angiotensin-converting-enzyme inhibitors. *N Engl J Med* **329**:1–7, 1993

28. Uretsky BF, Young JB, Shahidi FE, et al: Randomized study assessing the effect of digoxin withdrawal in patients with mild to moderate chronic congestive heart failure: Results of the PROVED trial. *J Am Coll Cardiol* **22**:955–962, 1993

29. Yusuf S, Garg R, Held P, Gorlin R: Need for a large randomized trial to evaluate the effect of digitalis on morbidity in congestive heart failure. *Am J Cardiol* **69**:64–70G, 1992

30. Ferguson DW, Berg WJ, Sanders JS, et al: Sympathoinhibitory responses to digitalis glycosides in heart failure patients. *Circulation* **80**:65–77, 1989

31. Ferguson DW, Abboud FM, Mark AL: Selective impairment of baroreflex-mediated vasoconstrictor responses in patients with ventricular dysfunction. *Circulation* **69**:451–460, 1984

32. Harrison DG, Bates JN: The nitrovasodilators: New ideas about old drugs. *Circulation* **87**:1461–1467, 1993

33. Becker LC: Conditions for vasodilator-induced coronary steal in experimental myocardial ischemia. *Circulation* **57**:1103–1110, 1978

34. Chee TP, Prakash NS, Desser KB, Benchimol A: Postoperative supraventricular arrhythmias and the role of prophylactic digoxin in cardiac surgery. *Am Heart J* **104**:974–977, 1982

35. Johnson LW, Dickstein RA, Fruehan CT, et al: Prophylactic digitalization for coronary artery bypass surgery. *Circulation* **53**:819–822, 1976

36. Vecht RJ, Nicolaides EP, Ikweuke JK, et al: Incidence and prevention of supraventricular tachyarrhythmias after coronary bypass surgery. *Int J Cardiol* **13**:125–134, 1985

37. Smith R, Grossman W, Johnson L, et al: Arrhythmias following cardiac valve replacement. *Circulation* **45**:1018–1023, 1972

38. Atkins JM, Field JM, Francis CK, et al: Recommended guidelines for in-hospital cardiac monitoring of adults for detection of arrhythmia. *J Am Coll Cardiol* **18**:1431–1433, 1991

39. Rankin AC, Oldroyd KG, Chong E, et al: Value and limitations of adenosine in the diagnosis and treatment of narrow and broad complex tachycardias. *Br Heart J* **62**:195–203, 1989

40. Waldo AL, MacLean WAH, Karp RB et al: Continuous rapid atrial pacing to control recurrent or sustained supraventricular tachycardias following open heart surgery. *Circulation* **54**:245–250, 1976

41. Waldo AL, Wells JL, Cooper TB, MacLean WAH: Temporary cardiac pacing: applications and techniques in the treatment of cardiac arrhythmias. *Prog Cardiovasc Dis* **23**:451–474, 1981

42. Waldo AL, MacLean WAH, Cooper TB, et al: Use of temporarily placed epicardial atrial wire electrodes for the diagnosis and treament of cardiac arrhythmias following open-heart surgery. *J Thorac Cardiovasc Surg* **76**:500–505, 1978

43. Kay GN, Plumb VJ, Arciniegas JG, et al: Torsade de pointes: the long-short initiating sequence and other clinical features: observations in 32 patients. *J Am Coll Cardiol* **2**:806–817, 1983

44. Echt DS, Liebson PR, Mitchell LB, et al and CAST Investigators: Mortality and morbidity in patients receiving encainide, flecainide, or placebo. *N Engl J Med* **324**:781–788, 1991

45. The Cardiac Arrhythmia Suppression Trial II Investigators: Effect of the antiarrhythmic agent moricizine on survival after myocardial infarction. *N Engl J Med* **327**:227–233, 1992

46. Markewitz A, Schmoeckel M, Nollert G, et al: Long-term results of pacemaker therapy after orthotopic heart transplantation. *J Card Surg* **8**:411–416, 1993

47. Bink-Boelkens MTE, Velvis H, Homan van der Heide JJ, et al: Dysrhythmias after atrial surgery in children. *Am Heart J* **106**:125–130, 1983

48. Bink-Boelkens MTE, Meuzelaar KJ, Eygelaar A: Arrhythmias after repair of secundum atrial septal defect: The influence of surgical modification. *Am Heart J* **115**:629–633, 1988

49. Gillette PC, Shannon C, Garson S, et al: Pacemaker treatment of sick sinus syndrome in children. *J Am Coll Cardiol* **5**:1325–1329, 1983

50. Waldo AL, Vitikainen KJ, Kaiser GA, et al: Atrial standstill secondary to atrial inexcitability (atrial quiescence). *Circulation* **66**:690–697, 1972

51. Goldman BS, Hill TJ, Weisel RD, et al: Permanent cardiac pacing after open-heart surgery: acquired heart disease. *PACE* **7**:367–371, 1984

52. Kastor JA: Multifocal atrial tachycardia. *N Engl J Med* **322**:1713–1717, 1990

53. Chen SA, Chiang CE, Yang CJ, et al: Sustained atrial tachycardia in adult patients; electrophysiological characteristics, pharmacological response, possible mechanisms, and effects of radiofrequency ablation. *Circulation* **90**:1262–1278, 1994

54. Garratt C, Ward D, Camm AJ: Degeneration of junctional tachycardia to pre-excited atrial fibrillation after intravenous verapamil. *Lancet* **2**:219, 1989

55. McGovern B, Garan H, Ruskin JN: Precipitation of cardiac arrest by verapamil in patients with Wolff-Parkinson-White syndrome. *Ann Intern Med* **104**:791–794, 1986

56. Tchou P, Young P, Mahmud R, et al: Useful clinical criteria for the diagnosis of ventricular tachycardia. *Am J Med* **84**:53–56, 1988

57. Wellens HJJ, Bart FWHM, Lie KI: The Value of the Electrocardiogram in the differential diagnosis of a tachycardia with a widened QRS complex. *Am J Med* **64:**27–33, 1978

58. Brugada P, Brugada J, Mont L, et al: A new approach to the differential diagnosis of a regular tachycardia with a wide QRS complex. *Circulation* **83:**1649–1659, 1991

59. Griffith MJ, Ward DE, Linker NJ, Camm AJ: Adenosine in the diagnosis of broad complex tachycardia. *Lancet* **1:**672, 1988

60. Stewart RB, Bardy GH, Greene HL: Wide complex tachycardia: misdiagnosis and outcome after emergent therapy. *Ann Intern Med* **104:**766–771, 1986

61. Zipes DP, Prystowsky EN, Heger JJ: Amiodarone: electrophysiologic actions, pharmacokinetics and clinical effects. *J Am Coll Cardiol* **3:**1059–1071, 1984

62. Smith WM, Gallagher JJ: "Les Torasades de Pointes": an unusual ventricular arrhythmia. *Ann Intern Med* **93:**578–584, 1980

63. Emergency Cardiac Care Committee and Subcommittees, American Heart Association: Guidelines for resuscitation and emergency cardiac care. *JAMA* **268:**2171–2302, 1992

100

Anesthesia for Cardiac Surgery

Joseph P. Mathew and Paul G. Barash

The emergence of cardiac anesthesiology as a subspecialty has accompanied the advances in cardiac surgery. The relative youth of cardiac anesthesiology is reflected in the fact that it was only in 1946 that Harmel and Lamont[1] first described the anesthetic management and perioperative course of a hundred patients operated on by Blalock for treatment of congenital pulmonic stenosis. The safety of anesthetic techniques for cardiac surgery remained in question until 1969 when Lowenstein et al[2] demonstrated in a landmark study that large doses of intravenous morphine could be safely administered as an anesthetic in patients with minimal circulatory reserve. New developments in anesthetic agents used for cardiac surgery have also been accompanied by advances in intraoperative monitoring. The introduction of multiple lead electrocardiography,[3,4] pulmonary artery catheterization,[5] and transesophageal echocardiography[6] (TEE) have allowed complex surgical procedures to be safely undertaken in a population that can be best described as high-risk.

PREOPERATIVE EVALUATION

The preoperative evaluation of the patients undergoing cardiac surgery is directed at answering the question: *Is the patient in the optimum condition to withstand the stress of the perioperative period?* Implicit in this question is the ability to assess not only the patient's physiologic reserve but also to assess preoperative risk factors that contribute to both morbidity and mortality. Numerous studies have been performed in recent years in an attempt to define risk in cardiac surgery. The Montreal Heart Institute used factors known to be associated with greater operative morbidity and mortality to categorize patients into three risk groups.[7] Parsonnet et al[8] analyzed 17 variables and developed a scoring system that could prospectively predict operative morbidity and mortality. This early scoring system was limited by the fact

that some of the scoring factors were heavily influenced by the opinion of the evaluating physician. Recently, Higgins et al[9] developed a clinical severity score (Table 100–1) from a retrospective analysis of 5051 patients that was then found useful for preoperative estimates of morbidity and mortality (Figure 100–1).

The preoperative history should detail the status of the cardiovascular system at rest and when stressed by the patient's daily activity. Equally important is an assessment of pulmonary, renal, hematologic, and endocrine function. During the physical examination, specific attention is directed at the cardiopulmonary and neurologic systems to help further objectively evaluate physiologic reserve. The physical examination also provides information that is useful for intraoperative and postoperative management. The anatomy of the upper and lower respiratory tract is evaluated for any indication of difficulty in airway management and endotracheal intubation. Signs of cardiac decompensation such as jugular venous distension, rales, or an S_3 gallop may be detected. Potential sites of vascular cannulation are also evaluated preoperatively. Radial and ulnar pulses should be palpated as an aid in determining the site and ease of peripheral arterial cannulation. Since the internal or external jugular veins are commonly employed for central venous catheterization, the neck should be examined for anatomic deformity or carotid disease that may preclude the use of these routes (Fig. 100–2).

The medication history is extremely important to the conduct of a good anesthetic. A history of allergic reactions or adverse responses to anesthetic agents may be elicited. To preserve the balance between myocardial oxygen supply and demand, antianginal and antihypertensive medication should not be withdrawn prior to surgery.[10] Abrupt cessation of beta-blocker therapy can result in a hypersympathetic state with resultant rebound increases in ischemia.[11,12] Preoperative administration of Beta-blockers prevents most

TABLE 100–1. CLINICAL SEVERITY SCORING SYSTEM

Preoperative Factors	Score
Emergency case	6
Serum creatinine,	
$\geq$ 141 and $\leq$ 167 μmol/L	
($\geq$ 1.6 and $\leq$ 1.8 mg/dL)	1
$\geq$ 168 μmol/L ($\geq$ 1.9 mg/dL)	4
Severe left ventricular dysfunction	3
Reoperation	3
Operative mitral valve insufficiency	3
Age $\geq$65 and $\leq$74 years	1
Age $\geq$75 years	2
Prior vascular surgery	2
Chronic obstructive pulmonary disease	2
Anemia (hematocrit $\leq$0.34)	2
Operative aortic valve stenosis	1
Weight $\leq$65 kg	1
Diabetes, on oral or insulin therapy	1
Cerebrovascular disease	1

From Higgins TL, Estafanous F, Loop FD, et al: Stratification of mobidity and mortality outcome by preoperative risk factors in coronary artery bypass patients—a clinical severity score. JAMA 267:2344–2348, 1992, with permission. Copyright 1992, American Medical Association.

tachycardia-related ischemia and does not adversely affect intraoperative cardiovascular performance.[13,14] In contrast, chronic administration of calcium channel blockers alone does not appear to reduce perioperative myocardial ischemia.[10,13,15] Furthermore, concurrent Beta-blocker and

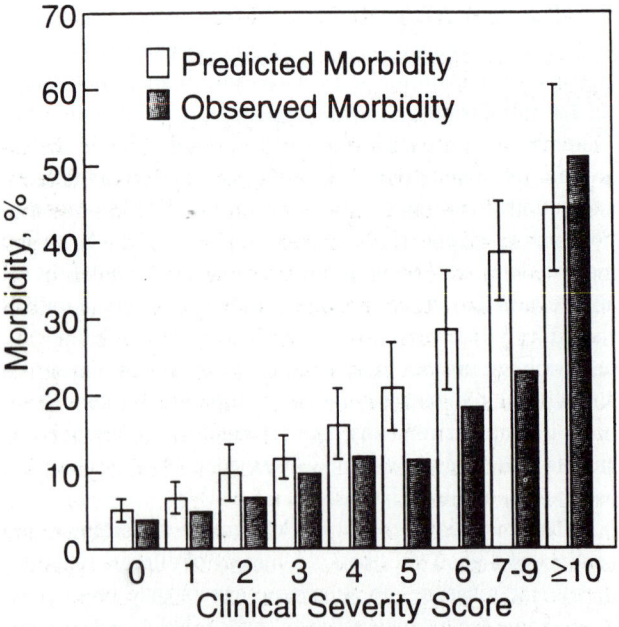

Figure 100–1. Predicted versus observed morbidity by severity score. *(From Higgins TL, Estafanous F, Loop FD, et al: Stratification of morbidity and mortality outcome by preoperative risk factors in coronary artery bypass patients—a clinical severity score. JAMA 267:2344–2348, Copyright 1992, American Medical Association, with permission.)*

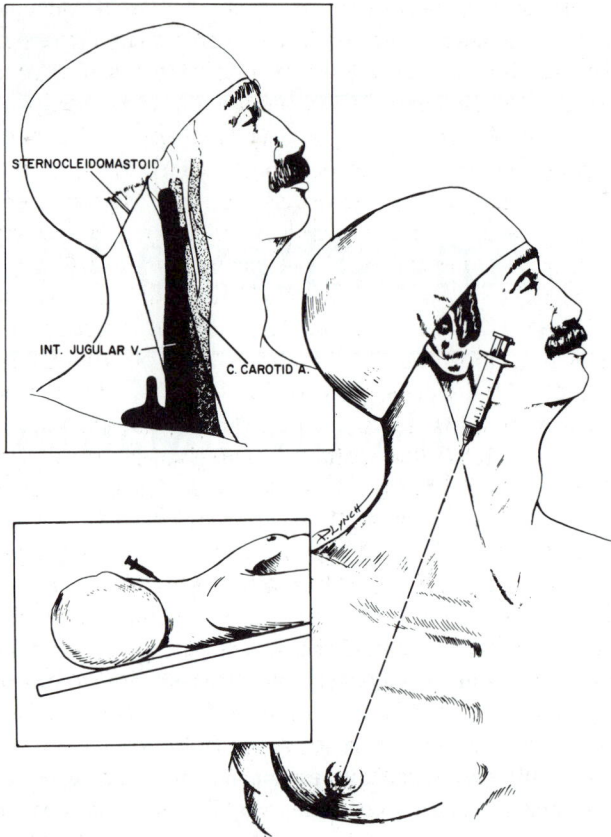

Figure 100–2. The anatomic landmark for right internal jugular vein catheterization is the midpoint of the medial border of the sternocleidomastoid muscle. The carotid artery is retracted medially and the needle aimed at the ipsilateral nipple (or middle of the breast) at a 30–45° angle to the skin. *(From Barash P, Dizon CT: An introducer for intraoperative percutaneous insertion of a Swan-Ganz catheter. Anesth Analg 56:444–445, 1977, with permission.)*

calcium channel blocker therapy may have an additive myocardial depressant and bradycardic effect. Such additive effects can precipitate hypotension and severe bradycardia during induction of anesthesia using opioids and muscle relaxants lacking vagolytic properties. Intravenous administration of diltiazem during anesthesia and surgery before cardiopulmonary bypass has also been reported to significantly decrease heart rate, mean arterial pressure, and cardiac index.[16] Nevertheless, calcium channel blockers are commonly continued in the perioperative period while the potential for side effects is accounted for in the anesthetic management plan.

Angiotensin-converting enzyme (ACE) inhibitors are increasingly being used to treat congestive heart failure as well as essential and renovascular hypertension. In addition to the regulation of extracellular fluid volume, the renin–angiotensin system maintains venous return and blood pressure during acute hemodynamic stresses.[17] Under general anesthesia, when blood pressure may frequently become angiotensin-dependent, ACE inhibition will lead to significant hypotension.[18] Case reports of low systemic vascular resistance, responsive only to an angiotensin II infusion, during and after hypothermic cardiopulmonary bypass in patients chronically treated with ACE inhibitors have been presented.[19] However, studies in both coronary artery bypass grafting and valvular surgery have not demonstrated significant deleterious hemodynamic events.[20,21]

Patients presenting for cardiac surgery have commonly undergone an extensive cardiac evaluation. The resting electrocardiogram provides information on dysrhythmias, conduction system disturbances, chamber hypertrophy or enlargement, and the location and severity of myocardial ischemia or infarction. Studies utilizing continuous ambulatory ECG monitoring (Holter) have recently established silent myocardial ischemia as a predictor of perioperative cardiac morbidity and mortality in patients undergoing peripheral vascular surgery.[22] Although Slogoff and Keats[23] were able to demonstrate that perioperative ECG detected ischemia did lead to myocardial infraction in CABG patients, Leung et al[6] have shown that ECG ischemia, in contrast to TEE ischemia, occurring in the prebypass, postbypass, or the first 4 hours in the intensive care unit was not predictive of adverse cardiac outcome in patients undergoing CABG surgery. Coronary angiography and ventriculography provide detailed information on the severity of disease and the extent of injury. Noninvasive tests of myocardial perfusion such as stress thallium testing or positron emission tomography may provide additional information on myocardial reserve and the functional significance of a coronary lesion.

Analysis of laboratory information completes the data base for preoperative evaluation. A reduced level of hemoglobin may significantly impair myocardial oxygen delivery. As previously described, preoperative anemia has been described as a risk factor for mortality following CABG surgery.[9] Diuretic therapy may be associated with hypokalemia reflecting large total body potassium deficits. While it has been traditionally taught that a surgical patient should have a serum potassium of ≥3.0 mmol/L before induction of anesthesia, recent studies have not demonstrated hypokalemia to be an independent risk factor for the development of ventricular dysrhythmias.[24,25] The decision to treat hypokalemia must be individualized and must account for the etiology and time course of the hypokalemia, use of medications such as digoxin, underlying cardiac function, ECG evidence of hypokalemia, and the urgency of the surgery.[26] Intraoperative hyperventilation and administration of calcium, sodium bicarbonate, glucose, and/or insulin may further alter the serum potasium level. Chronic hypokalemia frequently represents a large total body deficit (500–>1000 mEq in a 70 kg patient) that cannot be corrected by administering 20 mEq of potassium chloride the night prior to surgery. Furthermore, it must be noted that dangerous complications of repletion therapy occur in approximately 6% of patients. In one study, adverse effects of potassium were judged to have contributed to the death of seven patients.[27]

ANESTHETIC MANAGEMENT

Premedication

Patients with heart disease are aware of the severity of their disease and the risks and complications of the operation. These factors plus the need for preinduction monitoring (arterial and central venous cannulation) may lead to stress and anxiety in the patient. To blunt these adverse effects, good premedication is essential. We prefer a combination of morphine and scopalamine. Morphine is administered in doses of 0.05–0.1 mg/kg intramuscularly (IM) to those with diminished cardiac reserve, while 0.1–0.2 mg/kg is given to the more robust patient. Scopalamine (0.4 mg IM) not only supplies amnesia, but also enhances the central nervous system effect of morphine. A smaller dose of scopalamine (0.1–0.2 mg) is used in the elderly, since severe mental confusion resembling acute organic brain disease might be observed on the basis of scopalamine's autonomic effects. The desired effects of intramuscular morphine and scopalamine require at least 90 min to become apparent. Premedication with sedatives can affect blood gas tensions significantly.[28] To minimize the possibility of hypoxemia, especially in patients with ischemic heart disease, supplemental oxygen (via nasal prongs or face mask) should be administered at the time of premedication. In addition to sedatives, any drugs required for daily maintenance, such as insulin and corticosteroids, are administered at the time of premedication.

INTRAOPERATIVE MONITORING

Electrocardiography

The intraoperative electrocardiogram (ECG) aids in the diagnosis of arrhythmias, ischemia, and conduction defects. Limb lead II is most commonly monitored during anesthesia since its axis parallels the electrical axis of the heart and the P-wave is well seen, thus facilitating the diagnosis of arrhythmias. The recommendations for perioperative ECG monitoring of myocardial ischemia are, for the most part, based on results obtained from exercise treadmill studies. Kaplan and King, after reviewing results from exercise testing showing that 89% of the ST-segment information is found in lead V_5, presented three cases in which myocardial ischemia was diagnosed only in the V_5 lead.[3] London et al, in 1988, performed continuous 12-lead electrocardiography in 105 patients with known or suspected coronary artery disease undergoing noncardiac surgery under general anesthesia.[4] Sensitivity for detecting ECG ischemia using a single lead was greatest in lead V_5 (75%) followed by leads V_4 (61%), V_6 (37%), II (33%), and V_3 (24%). The standard clinical combination of leads II and V_5 was only 80% sensitive while combining leads V_4 and V_5 increased sensitivity to 90%. The greatest sensitivity (96%) was obtained by combining II, V$_4$, and V$_5$. Placement of a sternal retractor has been associated with a reduction in V$_5$ R-wave and S-wave amplitude and in absolute ST-segment deviation. Mark et al[29] have therefore proposed that inclusion of an R-wave gain factor may improve perioperative electrocardiographic monitoring.

Computer-assisted analysis has also been employed for the detection of myocardial ischemia and arrhythmias. For the ST-segments to be assessed, either a preset number of ECG complexes or a preset time period is required to develop a template to which all changes in the QRS complex are compared.[30] Since a number of complexes without artifact are required, intraoperative use of ST-segment trending is limited by the frequency of electrocautery use. Use of the ST-trend analyzer has been shown to improve the anesthesiologists' ability to detect ischemia intraoperatively.[31] Esophageal, intracardiac, and endotracheal electrocardiography has also been utilized but has not achieved wide clinical use. The esophageal ECG may be particularly helpful in diagnosing posterior ischemia because of its proximity to the posterior wall of the left ventricle.

In order to accurately diagnose ischemia, the ECG output must be calibrated such that a 1 mV deflection measures 10 mm on the strip chart recorder. Paper speed is set at 25 mm/s. The American Heart Association also recommends that ECG recordings be obtained at a bandwidth of 0.05–100 Hz. The high frequency limit ensures that the QRS morphology is accurately reproduced while the lower frequency limit is necessary for accurate reproduction of the ST-segment. Most ECG monitors do, however, employ filters in an attempt to reduce environmental artifacts. The high-frequency filters reduce artifacts due to 60 Hz electrical current and muscle movement, whereas the low-frequency filters produce a more stable baseline by decreasing respiratory and body motion artifacts. In the "monitor" mode of the ECG monitor, a low-frequency filter is used which can, in turn, distort the ST-segment. It is therefore imperative that all ST-segment information be analyzed in the "diagnostic" mode (lower filter limit = 0.05 Hz).

Pulmonary Artery Catheterization

Since its development more than two decades ago, the balloon-tipped pulmonary artery flotation (Swan-Ganz) catheter has become an important tool in assessing the hemodynamic function of the patient undergoing open heart surgery. Given that left ventricular end-diastolic pressure (LVEDP) measurements have traditionally been used to estimate preload, pulmonary capillary wedge pressures (PCWP) are a useful indirect measurement of LVEDP over a wide range of pressures (5–25 mm Hg). Exceptions to this include patients with mitral stenosis, left atrial myxoma, and elevated positive end-expiratory pressure (PEEP) wherein PCWP is greater than LVEDP and patients with a stiff (noncompliant) ventricle, LVEDP >25 mm Hg, or premature closure of the mitral valve (aortic insufficiency)

wherein PCWP is less than the LVEDP. To avoid frequent inflation of the pulmonary artery catheter (PAC) balloon, the pulmonary artery end-diastolic pressure (PAD) can be used as an estimate of PCWP. In a patient with normal pulmonary vascular resistance, the gradient between PAD and PCWP is 1–4 mm Hg. PAD may also be greater than PCWP in a patient with tachycardia as the diastolic filling time is decreased.

Pulmonary artery monitoring can lead to the early diagnosis of myocardial ischemia.[32] An acute decrease in left ventricular compliance is one of the first changes associated with myocardial ischemia. An increase in pulmonary artery diastolic or wedge pressures occurring in the absence of the administration of fluids or vasoactive drugs can then aid in the detection of myocardial ischemia. (Fig. 100–3) In addition, acute papillary muscle dysfunction secondary to ischemia may be detected by the appearance of "v"-waves in the pulmonary artery wedge tracing. Pichard et al[33] have shown however that patients can develop large "v"-waves simply by acutely increasing preload. Other studies have also shown that the majority of ischemia detected by ECG or wall motion abnormalities are not accompanied by significant changes in the pulmonary artery pressure or waveform.[34]

One modification of the standard PAC is the use of reflectance spectrophotometry and fiber optics to measure mixed venous oxygen saturation (SVO$_2$).[35] SVO$_2$ measurement is a representation of the balance between total body

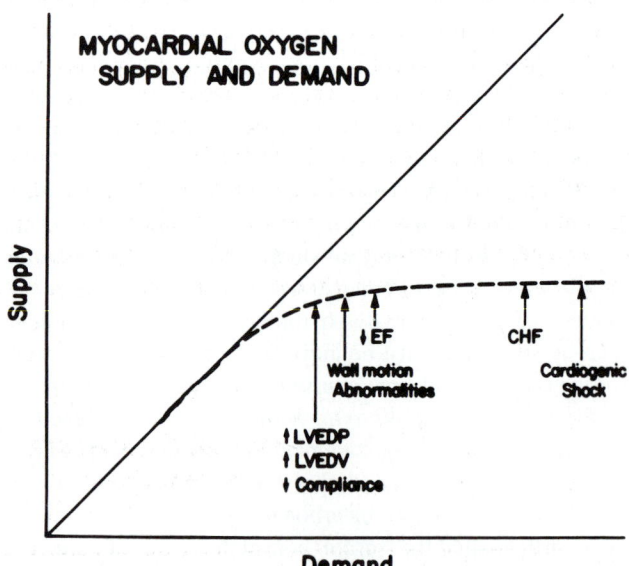

Figure 100–3. Hemodynamic consequences of myocardial ischemia. Ischemia occurs when demand exceeds supply. CHF, congestive heart failure; EF, ejection fraction; LVEDP, left ventricular end diastolic pressure; LVEDV, left ventricular end diastolic volume; ST, segment change. *(From Barash PG: Monitoring myocardial oxygen balance: Physiologic basis and clinical application. Am Soc Anesthesiol Ann Refresher Course Lect 13:21–32, 1985, with permission.)*

oxygen supply and demand. Since blood flow exhibits regional differences, a normal SVO₂ (75%) does not necessarily imply adequate perfusion in every organ system. In a study by Pearson et al,[36] SVO₂ monitoring in the intensive care unit produced a significant increase in cost from additional cardiac output and blood gas analysis without producing patient benefit. Furthermore, common errors in sampling occur with distal migration of the catheter or rapid aspiration such that blood is withdrawn from the pulmonary capillary system.

Incorporation of a thermistor into the PAC allows cardiac output measurements using the thermodilution method, a variant of the indicator dilution technique where "cold" is the trace indicator. Common errors in measurement result from the use of inaccurate injectate volumes and an inappropriate computation constant. Since the ability to measure cardiac output may be of greater value than measuring SVo₂, recent attention has been directed at providing a reliable continuous cardiac output monitor. "Stochastic,"[37] continuous arterial thermodeprivation,[38] and Doppler techniques have been utilized in developing a continuous cardiac output PAC. The higher cost of these newer catheters has prevented widespread use.

The capacity to pace the myocardium has been yet another modification to the standard PAC. Initially, a lumen placed 19 cm from the catheter tip allowed passage of a pacer wire for emergency right ventricular pacing. Subsequently a right atrial port was added to allow atrioventricular (A-V) sequential pacing. Successful atrial capture using this catheter occurred at a rate of 98% while the rate of ventricular capture was 100%.[39] A PAC with five pacing electrodes is also available.[40] This PAC is unique in its capacity to record an intracardiac ECG and, therefore, monitor electrical activity during cardioplegic arrest.[41]

The development of rapid response thermistors has facilitated the measurement of right ventricular ejection fraction (RVEF) and volumes. Radionuclear[42] and echocardiographic[43] studies have validated this technique; however, the accuracy of measurement in patients with tricuspid regurgitation or an irregular cardiac rhythm remains in ques-

tion. While providing useful information on right ventricular function, Hines and Barash[44] have, in particular, demonstrated the ability of the RVEF PAC to detect right ventricular ischemia in patients with right coronary artery disease.

There have been numerous reports of complications associated with the use of a PAC. These include arterial puncture, pneumothorax, air embolism, nerve injury, arrhythmias (especially the development of complete heart block in patients with preexistent left bundle branch block), intracardiac knotting, thrombosis, infection, pulmonary infarction, and pulmonary artery rupture. The most devastating of these complications is pulmonary artery perforation and subsequent hemorrhage. Advanced age, hypothermia, pulmonary hypertension, female gender, and deviations from standard insertion techniques have been associated with a greater risk of perforation. A common feature of perforation is the distal location of the PAC. "Overwedging" on the catheter waveform may help to identify a PAC that is in a distal location. (Fig. 100–4) The characteristic presentation of pulmonary artery perforation is the sudden appearance of hemoptysis. Usually this bleeding is related to balloon inflation or catheter manipulation including flushing the catheter in the wedge position. (Fig. 100–5) Management of perforation is supportive in nature. Anticoagulation should be reversed and massive blood and fluid replacement may be necessary. On occasion, operative intervention (wedge resection, pneumonectomy) may also be required. If the patient is anesthetized, a double lumen endotracheal tube may be used to protect the "good" lung. Alternatively, a standard endotracheal tube can be advanced into the left main stem bronchus since most PACs lie in the right lower lobe. Barash et al[45] in the early reports of perforation recommended that the PAC should be pulled back approximately 5–10 cm with the balloon deflated. Injecting contrast media into the distal port of the PAC would then permit localization of the rupture.

Variation does exist in the utilization of PACs in patients undergoing cardiac surgery.[46,47] Conservative clinicians argue that clinical experience, physical examination, preoperative cardiac catheterization data, and information

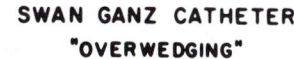

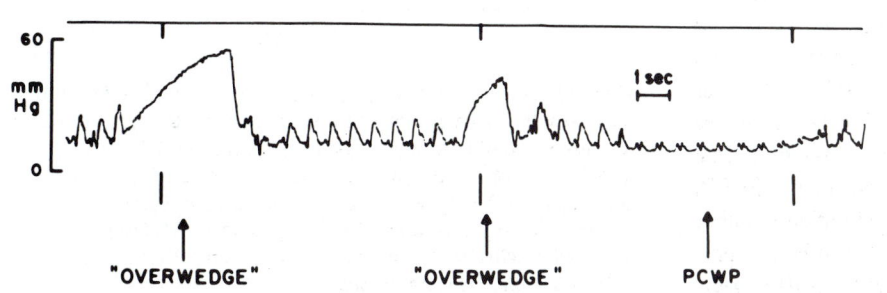

Figure 100–4. Intraoperative pulmonary artery pressure recording which demonstrates "overwedging" pattern observed with balloon inflation. This pattern results from the catheter tip impinging against the vessel wall or balloon herniation over the catheter tip. The pulmonary artery pressure catheter is withdrawn 3 cm and a normal transition pulmonary artery to pulmonary artery capillary wedge pressure is obtained. *(From Barash PG, Nardi D, Hammond G, et al: Catheter induced pulmonary artery perforation: Mechanisms, management, and modifications. J Thorac Cardiovasc Surg 82:5–12, 1981 with permission.)*

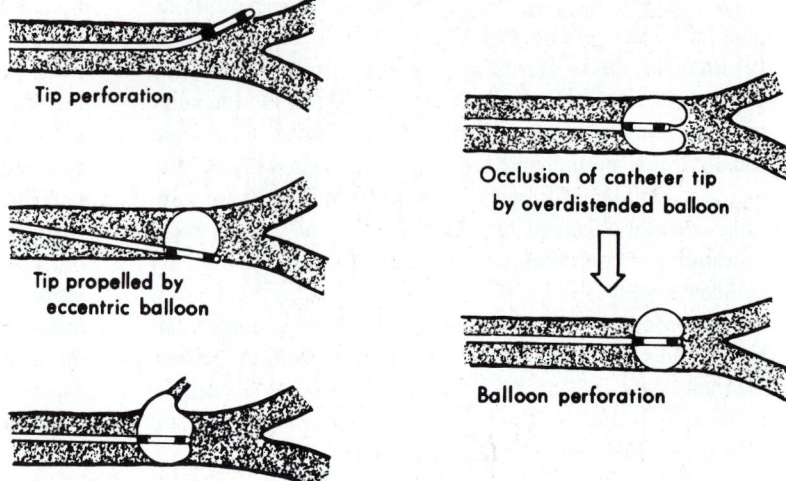

Figure 100–5. The various mechanisms involoved in pulmonary artery perforation. *(From Barash PG, Nardi D, Hammond G, et al: Catheter induced pulmonary artery perforation: Mechanisms, management, and modifications. J Thorac Cardiovasc Surg 82:5–12, 1981, with permission.)*

derived from invasive and noninvasive monitors are adequate to diagnose and treat hemodynamic abnormalities in the perioperative period, thereby making pulmonary artery catheterization unnecessary. However, "routine" clinical assessment has proven to be a poor predictor of a patient's hemodynamic status.[48] Attempts to determine if PAC use affects outcome in cardiac surgery patients have been mostly limited to uncontrolled observational studies.[49] Tuman et al[50] were unable to demonstrate a decrease in myocardial ischemia, infarction or mortality in 1094 patients receiving either a PAC or a central venous catheter. Unfortunately, assignment to either group was made at the discretion of the anesthesiologist assigned to the case thus preventing true randomization. The American Society of Anesthesiologists has recently published Practice Guidelines for Pulmonary Artery Catheterization after reviewing a total of 860 clinical trials, controlled observational studies, uncontrolled case reports, and individual reports.[51] While the data indicated a change in therapy as a result of PAC monitoring in 30–62% of all cases, these studies demonstrated no effect on mortality rates.

Transesophageal Echocardiography

Echocardiography has long been established as a diagnostic tool outside of the operating room. It has been only in the last decade that the use of transesophageal echocardiography (TEE) has expanded the ability of the anesthesiologist to evaluate cardiovascular performance, anatomy, and intravascular volume status. Technological advances such as biplane and multiplane imaging, Doppler, and color-flow mapping have made TEE ideally suited for perioperative hemodynamic monitoring. Although technological advances provide new and exiting applications for intraoperative TEE, proper use of this monitor requires not only an appreciation of the applications but also the limitations of TEE.

Central to the use of echocardiography as an ischemia

monitor has been the demonstration of its increased sensitivity in detecting reductions in coronary blood flow as compared with the ST segment changes seen with ECG.[52,53] The use of TEE as a monitor of ischemia is based on its ability to detect abnormalities in ventricular wall motion. Normal left ventricular (LV) wall motion is characterized by an inward movement of the endocardial surface and thickening of the LV wall, resulting in a net decrease in the size of the ventricular cavity. Historically, abnormal wall motion has been most frequently described qualitatively. Using this approach, decreased systolic wall thickening or inward endocardial movement is described as hypokinesia, while akinesia represents an absence of systolic wall thickening or inward endocardial motion. Dyskinesia is characterized by outward systolic endocardial motion that may be present with wall thinning rather than thickening. The validity of any intraoperative TEE evaluation depends on obtaining a consistent cross-sectional view. Clinically, the mid-papillary short-axis view (Fig. 100–6) is used to monitor for ischemia as it represents segments of myocardium supplied by all three major coronary arteries. These areas include the posterior and posteroseptal wall by the right coronary, the anterior and anteroseptal by the left anterior descending, and the lateral wall by the circumflex artery. The mid-papillary short-axis view has also become popular because changes in ventricular filling are more easily detected in this view than in a long-axis view.

Limitations to the use of TEE as a method of diagnosing myocardial ischemia arise because of variations in coronary artery distribution. Although the mid-papillary short-axis view is ideal for monitoring ischemia in areas supplied by major epicardial vessels, it may not reflect ischemia involving more peripheral and smaller coronary arterioles. As a result, basilar, apical, or right ventricular ischemia may go undiagnosed. In addition, operator inexperience, resulting in a poor quality image or "echo dropout" of segments, may lead to misinterpretation of a specific regional wall motion abnormality (RWMA). Errors may also result from at-

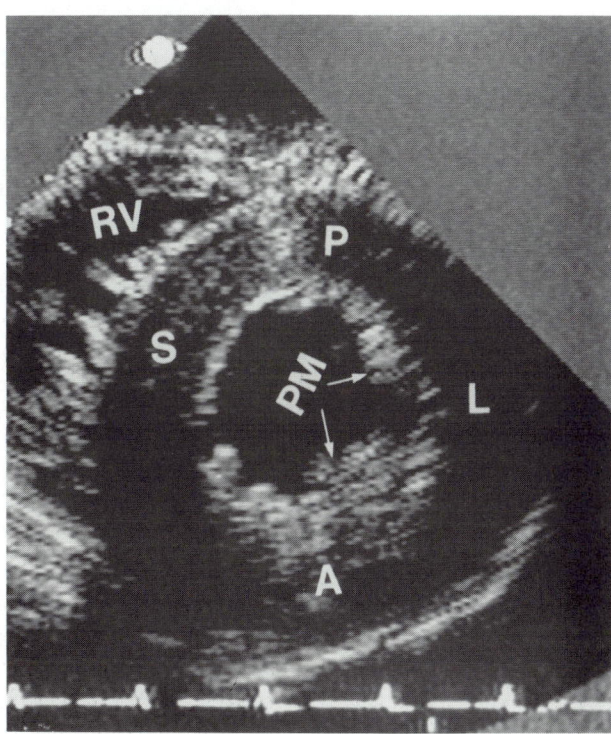

Figure 100–6. Mid-papillary short-axis view. S, septal wall; P, posterior wall; A, anterior wall; L, lateral wall; PM, papillary muscles; RV, right ventricle.

tempts to grade oblique views. A paced rhythm or the presence of a left bundle branch block may alter the timing of ventricular contraction, resulting in the impression of regional dysfunction. Finally, rotational changes in the position of the heart (particularly during the respiratory and cardiac cycle) may distort the TEE image. The difficulties associated with the specificity of TEE (when compared with ECG indices of ischemia) are best reflected in a study by London et al,[54] which describes the "natural history" of segmental wall motion abnormalities. In this study, the lack of concordance between ECG and TEE in monitoring for ischemic changes in patients undergoing noncardiac surgery was significant. Temporal overlap with these two monitoring modalities was present in only 5 of 19 patients. Similarly, Comunale et al[55] in 207 patients undergoing CABG surgery demonstrated temporal overlap in only 2 of 77 ischemic episodes.

The onset of a new, persistent, postcardiopulmonary bypass RWMA has been associated with adverse cardiac outcome. In a study of 50 patients undergoing CABG surgery, Leung et al[6] demonstrated that 6 of 18 patients with postbypass RWMA had adverse cardiac outcomes (2 deaths, 3 myocardial infarctions, and 1 ventricular failure). On the other hand none of the 32 patients without TEE ischemia experienced an adverse cardiac outcome. Similarly, Harris et al[56] in a series of 34 patients, reported the occurrence of myocardial infarction in 3 of 10 patients manifesting new RWMA in the postbypass period. When

an RWMA is accurately diagnosed, these studies suggest that the onset of persistent new RWMA increases the likelihood of a clinically meaningful adverse cardiac event.

In addition to ischemia detection, TEE has been useful in assessing LV preload. Typically, TEE uses the end-diastolic area as an approximation of LV volume. The accuracy of TEE in measuring LV volume is improved by increasing the number of cross-sectional images obtained.[57] Clinically, the transgastric short-axis view does not provide a good estimate of right ventricular volume and a reliance on this imaging plane alone in guiding volume replacement therapy can lead to right ventricular distention. Immediately following CABG surgery, the correlation between estimates of end-diastolic volume obtained from a single cross sectional short-axis TEE image and those obtained by scintigraphy is only fair ($r = 0.74$).[58] Nevertheless, when compared with more traditional hemodynamic parameters for measuring LV volume such as pulmonary artery diastolic pressures, central venous pressures, and heart rate changes, TEE appears to provide a more sensitive and reliable method for detecting intraoperative hypovolemia.[59]

The close anatomical relationship between the esophagus and the aorta allows for high-resolution images of the aortic intima. The potential for embolization from aortic atheromatous plaques during manipulation or cannulation before cardiopulmonary bypass has led to the use of TEE to define the nature and severity of aortic atherosclerotic disease. Marschall et al[60] recently demonstrated that plaques located in the aortic arch characterized by ≥5 mm thickness or a mobile component correlate significantly with the occurrence of postoperative stroke. Although the aortic arch and descending thoracic aorta are clearly imaged with TEE, imaging of the ascending aorta has been less successful. While studies indicate that palpation of the aorta clearly underestimates the presence and severity of atherosclerosis, especially when compared with ultrasonography,[61] epiaortic scanning is in fact better than TEE at assessing the ascending aorta.[62] Wareing et al[63] suggested that modification of cannulation and clamping techniques based on intraoperative epiaortic scanning may decrease the frequency of postoperative stroke.

Coagulation

The anesthesiologist can provide valuable help in assessing the state of anticoagulation during cardiopulmonary bypass (CPB) and in ensuring that adequate reversal of heparin with protamine has been accomplished following CPB. The activated coagulation time (ACT) is the hemostatic test most commonly used during cardiac surgery. The ease of performance of this test combined with its low cost and ready availability has led to the popularity of the automated form of ACT measurement. As with any single coagulation test, the ACT has limitations. Nevertheless, if used appropriately and interpreted correctly, the ACT can be tremendously beneficial during cardiac surgery.

Hattersley introduced the ACT into clinical medicine in 1966. The routine use of the ACT did not, however, gain wide acceptance until 10 years later when Bull et al[64-66] demonstrated wide variations in heparin sensitivity and half-life and therefore proposed a method for quantitative heparin administration and protamine reversal. In a control group the normal value for ACT is 107 ± 13 seconds. Heparin administration results in a linear prolongation of the ACT. The adequate level for ACT during bypass is greater than 400 seconds. During CPB, at ACT values below 400 seconds, abnormal levels of fibrin monomer appear and fibrin, platelet debris, and cells are deposited on the oxygenators.[67] Because aprotinin-mediated inhibition of the intrinsic pathway leads to elevation of the ACT, an ACT greater than 750 seconds has been recommended for those patients receiving aprotinin during CPB. At the end of CPB, the use of a heparin dose–response curve provides an easy means of determining the amount of "circulating" heparin. Bull's work demonstrated that administration of protamine 1.3 mg/1OO U of circulating heparin will result in return of the ACT to normal values in the vast majority of patients. Protamine administration has been associated with significant hemodynamic deterioration.[68] Various mechanisms have been suggested including myocardial depression, vasodilation, pulmonary vasoconstriction, and complement activation. Thus, protamine should be administered in a test dose, then by slow infusion in the smallest dose possible to achieve reversal of heparin.

Although the ACT is well suited to the measurement of anticoagulation during CPB, it must be remembered that the ACT is not a sensitive index of qualitative or quantitative platelet or procoagulant deficiency. The ACT measurement is also relatively insensitive to small concentrations of heparin. Low levels of plasma heparin can be measured using protamine titration methods. As samples of blood are added to tubes containing increasing concentrations of protamine, the time to clot formation decreases. Automated measurements of heparin levels such as the Hepcon (Hemotec Inc., Englewood, CO) are not measures of functional activity but of the absolute amount of circulating heparin. As such, these tests are primarily used following CPB to diagnose the presence of circulating heparin in the setting of continued bleeding despite protamine administration.

Recently, viscoelastic measures of coagulation have been evaluated as an indicator of post CPB coagulopathies.[69] Measurements from the thromboelastograph (TEG) trace (Fig 100–7) yield information on the abnormalities of clot formation and lysis. TEG has, however, not gained widespread use because of the nonspecificity of the findings. While some investigators have demonstrated its usefulness in differentiating hemorrhage due to a coagulopathy from that due to inadequate surgical hemostasis,[69] others have argued that the delay in obtaining results (>1 hour) prevents its use in guiding urgent therapeutic decisions.[70]

ANESTHESIA

Induction

The transition from the awake to the anesthetized state represents one of the most critical parts of the perioperative period. The goal of anesthetic induction is to maintain circulatory stability and the often tenuous balance between myocardial oxygen delivery and demand. Sodium pentothal is the most widely used induction agent in anesthesia. However, thiopental may cause significant hemodynamic alterations in patients with marginal cardiac reserve. In an extensive study of high-risk patients, Knapp and Dubow reported that 83% of patients receiving intravenous pentothal (2mg/kg) had a greater than 15% decrease in cardiac output associated with an average decrease in mean arterial blood pressure of 15 mm Hg.[71] Ketamine and etomidate, on the other hand, are intravenous agents that appear to preserve hemodynamic function during induction of anesthesia. Despite the occurrence of effects resembling sympathetic nervous system stimulation (hypertension, tachycardia) and emergence phenomena with administration of ketamine and the reports of adrenocortical inhibition induced by etomidate, these agents appear useful, particularly in the setting of hemodynamic instability (hypovolemia, cardiac tamponade).

Benzodiazepines such as diazepam are also associated with minimal circulatory changes. However diazepam can cause severe hypotension in an occasional patient. In addition, the ultimate elimination of diazepam can be prolonged

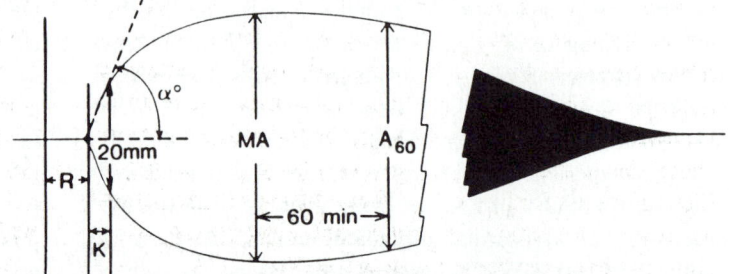

Figure 100–7. Schematic diagram of a normal thromboelastography tracing. *(From Spiess BD, Tuman KJ, McCarthy RJ, et al: Thromboelastography as an indicator of post-cardiopulmonary bypass caoagulopathies. Reprinted with permission from J Clin Monit 3:25–30, 1987.)*

(elimination half-life 46 hours). Midazolam is more potent than benzodiazepine and has a faster clearance rate but, like diazepam, can produce substantial decreases in systemic vascular resistance when given in combination with narcotics. Benzodiazepines also do not reliably attenuate the hemodynamic responses to endotracheal intubation.[72]

As an alternative, narcotic analgesics have been used for induction and maintenance of anesthesia.[73] In a classic study, Lowenstein et al[2] reported on the benefits of morphine "anesthesia" (0.5–3.0 mg/kg) in a group of patients undergoing valvular heart surgery. The reported advantages of morphine anesthesia include a lack of cardiac depression, modulation of the stress response, cardiovascular stability, decreased sensitization of the myocardium to arrhythmias, reversibility, and smooth transition to postoperative ventilatory support. However, certain pitfalls become evident. Rapid administration of high doses of morphine can result in life-threatening hypotension. Consequently, morphine should be administered slowly with the patient in the supine position. Histamine release and the associated decreases in systemic vascular resistance with the use of morphine requires that HI and H2 receptor antagonists be administered as part of the premedication. Hypovolemia must also be corrected prior to induction of anesthesia. Other disadvantages of morphine include the possibility of awareness and recall of intraoperative events and imperfect attenuation of the cardiovascular response to stress. As a result, other agents such as benzodiazepines are often added to supplement a morphine anesthetic. The interaction of these agents with morphine as previously described may be deleterious.

Although cardiovascular stability may be achieved during the initial part of the induction with either intravenous or inhalational agents (see below), the stress of laryngoscopy, endotracheal intubation, incision, or sternotomy may be deleterious to cardiac surgical patients. Using a diazepam, nitrous oxide, oxygen, and enflurane sequence, Giles et al[74] demonstrated a precipitous decline in the left ventricular ejection fraction during intubation from 49 to 32%. This decrease occurred within seconds of laryngoscopy despite the fact that laryngoscopy and intubation required less than 13 seconds. In a subsequent study, Barash et al[75] demonstrated that fentanyl, a synthetic narcotic (100 times as potent as morphine), could block this response. Due to the stabilizing effects on the circulation, high doses of fentanyl are now widely used in cardiac anesthesia. Sufentanil, 10 times more potent than fentanyl, was initially touted as a more complete anesthetic. Most studies, however, have demonstrated only the similarities between fentanyl and sufentanil. Like fentanyl, sufentanil demonstrates a ceiling effect such that breakthrough hypertension is common, especially in patients with normal left ventricular function. Studies examining the effects of narcotic choice on emergence and extubation have produced conflicting results. Sanford et al[76] found that sufentanil permitted earlier extubation, but Thompson et al[77] reported no clinical differences between the two drugs.

Maintenance

Following induction of anesthesia, supplementation is often required with either additional intravenous agents (narcotics, benzodiazepines, sedatives) as a bolus or infusion or with the use of potent inhalational anesthetics. Propofol, a new intravenous agent with sedative and hypnotic properties but lacking analgesic effects, has gained popularity in recent years primarily because of its short duration of action. Like thiopental, propofol produces ventilatory depression, peripheral vasodilatation, and decreases in cardiac output. The high clearance rate for propofol dictates that it be administered as a continuous infusion. In a prospective, randomized comparison of propofol and sufentanil administered with a computer-controlled infusion pump as a primary anesthetic for CABG surgery, propofol anesthesia was associated with a greater incidence of hypotension.[78] The severity of the hypotension was, however, similar in both groups. The occurrence of myocardial ischemia and infarction also did not differ between the sufentanil and propofol groups. The use of propofol intraoperatively as well as for sedation postoperatively in the ICU allows for early extubation of the cardiac surgical patient.[79,80] Early extubation in a suitable subgroup of cardiac surgical patients may, in turn, lead to decreased costs of hospitalization.

Initial studies on the use of nitrous oxide raised concerns over the occurrence of myocardial ischemia upon addition of nitrous oxide to a narcotic or inhalational anesthetic. More recent studies, however, indicate that if hemodynamics are controlled, then nitrous oxide does not worsen myocardial ischemia.[81] In patients undergoing CABG surgery, Slavik et al[82] were unable to demonstrate a relationship between the use of nitrous oxide and the onset of RWMAs. Nitrous oxide is contraindicated in the presence of a pneumothorax. Rapid diffusion of nitrous oxide into an air filled pneumothorax can increase the volume of a pneumothorax by 2-fold in 10 min. This problem may be observed following trauma (rib fractures), insertion of a subclavian catheter, or rupture of a pleural bleb.

Halothane and enflurane are halogenated inhalational anesthetics. Although these two agents are similar to each other in many respects, there are some notable differences. In a very small percentage of cases (1/10,000) severe and sometimes fatal hepatic dysfunction may follow halothane administration.[83] Enflurane administered in high concentrations can often produce an EEG pattern resembling seizure activity. This is easily reversed by decreasing the concentrations of enflurane and restoring the arterial carbon dioxide tension to normal. A small amount of enflurane is also metabolized to free fluoride ion. Prolonged exposure to enflurane can then result in a fluoride ion-related renal toxicity, particularly in those with preexisting renal disease.

Isoflurane is currently the most commonly used inhalational anesthetic. It suppresses ventricular dysrhythmias effectively and exhibits synergism with nondepolarizing neuromuscular blockers. Like enflurane and halothane, it is a potent myocardial depressant, but differs from both of the former agents in that it is a more potent peripheral vasodilator. Its vasodilating properties may be useful in unloading the diseased left ventricle. Controversy exists as to whether isoflurane causes "coronary steal." The debate was initiated by Reiz et al[84] when they reported coronary steal and myocardial ischemia in 10 of 21 patients with coronary artery disease undergoing vascular surgery under isoflurane anesthesia. Numerous publications[85–87] have since sought to develop an association between the use of isoflurane and the occurrence of ischemia and therefore steal phenomena. Of note, most of these studies were confounded by significant decreases in mean arterial pressure. Such decreases may by itself have been sufficient to produce ischemia. It is likely that the beneficial effects of isoflurane in decreasing myocardial oxygen demand are of greater importance than its effects on coronary tone. In a large trial of four different anesthetic regimens for patients undergoing CABG surgery, Slogoff and Keats[88] demonstrated no difference in the frequency of myocardial ischemia between isoflurane, enflurane, halothane, and sufentanil even in patients with steal prone anatomy.[89]

Desflurane is a newer inhalational agent with a low blood-gas solubility that allows a more rapid anesthetic induction and emergence. Its clinical properties are otherwise equivalent to isoflurane. Sevoflurane is an inhalational agent with greater potency than isoflurane but questions regarding its potential for neurotoxicity have delayed its availability.

Muscle relaxants are required during anesthesia to facilitate laryngoscopy, endotracheal intubation, and ventilation, and to prevent movement during the surgical procedure. Administration of muscle relaxants may be associated with significant cardiovascular effects. Historically, the nondepolarizing muscle relaxant d-tubocurarine was commonly employed. d-Tubocurarine (curare) causes hypotension on the basis of blockade of sympathetic autonomic ganglia and histamine release. These effects are magnified in the presence of inhalational anesthesia and hypovolemia. Pancuronium is five to six times more potent than curare and is associated with small increases in heart rate, blood pressure, and cardiac output. Pancuronium is predominantly excreted by the kidney. In contrast, vecuronium has no sympathomimetic effects but has been implicated in the generation of bradyarrhythmias when given with high doses of sufentanil.[90] Atracurium offers a unique pathway of elimination (Hoffman degradation) that makes it a useful drug in patients with renal failure. The histamine release and hypotension associated with atracurium have limited its widespread use during cardiac surgery. Doxacurium, pipecuronium, mivacurium, and rocuronium are newer neuromuscular blocking agents with varying durations of action that seem also to have no adverse hemodynamic side effects. The benefits of minimal side effects must be balanced against the increased cost of the newer agents.

Succinylcholine, a depolarizing muscle relaxant, produces small, if any, changes in hemodynamic performance. The bradycardia commonly observed in children following succinylcholine treatment is rarely seen in adults, unless multiple doses are administered. In trauma and burn patients, succinylcholine significantly increases serum potassium and can cause life-threatening cardiac arrhythmias. A similar hyperkalemic response is also reported in patients with neurologic disease (upper or lower motor neuron lesions), Succinylcholine is metabolized by the enzyme pseudocholinesterase. A genetically transmitted deficiency of this enzyme may prolong the action of succinylcholine to more than 8 hours (normal duration is 5 min).

Postoperative Pain Management

Postoperative analgesia, despite being extensively studied in the general surgical population, has received minimal study in the cardiac surgical patient. Since patients usually receive a high-dose opioid technique in the operating room, a PRN intravenous opioid dosing regimen is most commonly employed in the cardiothoracic intensive care unit. To facilitate extubation, such regimens may be supplemented with nonopioid analgesics.

Spinal and epidural analgesia may also be beneficial in the cardiac surgical patient. Despite concerns over the development of spinal hematomas during the placement of a spinal analgesic prior to systemic heparinization, studies indicate that if traumatic placement is avoided in a patient with adequate platelet counts (75,000–100,000), spinal and epidural analgesia can be a safe option for postoperative pain management.[91–93] Single-dose intrathecal morphine[94,95] or continuous epidural analgesia[96,97] use in cardiac surgery has been reported to produce good analgesic effects and associated decreases in stress hormone levels. Therapeutic options in the cardiac surgical patient are summarized in Table 100–2.

Emergence

Under certain circumstances (e.g., neurologic evaluation) one may want to reverse the effects of a narcotic anesthetic with naloxone (Narcan). Early reports indicated that naloxone possessed "pure" antagonist properties. The dangers of naloxone administration following a high-dose narcotic anesthetic are emphasized in a report by Flacke et al.[98] They observed acute left ventricular failure and pulmonary edema in a patient who underwent CABG surgery. It would be prudent to carefully titrate the dose of naloxone to patients with diminished cardiovascular reserve and perhaps to withhold its use entirely in the immediate postoperative period in patients who have undergone open heart surgery.

In summary, a well-planned and executed anesthetic starting with the preoperative evaluation and including pain management in the intensive care unit is one of the most important advances in the management of the cardiac surgi-

TABLE 100–2. ANALGESIC USE IN THE CARDIAC SURGICAL PATIENT

Postoperative Time Period	Analgesic	Route	Dosage
0–18 hours (intubated patient)	Morphine	IV	1–2 mg every 10–15 min until comfortable to maximum of 1 mg/kg, then maintain with 2–10 mg/h
	Fentanyl	IV	Continuous infusion 5–10 µg/kg per hour
	Sufentanil	IV	Continuous infusion 1 µg/kg per hour
	Morphine	Subarachnoid	0.5–1 mg given preoperatively
12–18 hours (period of weaning from mechanical ventilation)	Morphine (ms)/meperidine (mep)	IV	2–5 mg (ms) or 25–50 mg (mep) every 1 hour
	Ketorolac	IV	60 mg loading dose, then 30 mg every 6 hours (if creatine ≥ 2 use 30 loading 15 every 6 hours)
18 hours (postextubation period)	Morphine	IV-PCA	1 mg every 6 min PCA
	Ketorolac + morphine	IV	Morphine PCA as above to supplement IV ketorolac analgesia with 30 or 15 mg every 6 hours
	Ketorolac	IV	Continue 30 or 15 mg every 6 hours
	Meperidine	PO	50–100 mg every 2–3 hours
	Ketorolac + meperidine	IV/PO	IV ketorolac (30 or 15) with 50–100 mg meperidine PO every 2–3 hours PRN to supplement
	Morphine	Epidural	Thoracic (T) catheter: 60 µg/mL at 4–8 mL/h; Lumbar (L) catheter: 60 µg/mL at 10–14 mL/h
	Meperidine	Epidural	T catheter: 100 µg/mL at 4–8 mL/h; L catheter: 100 µg/mL at 10–14 mL/h
	Hydromorphone	Epidural	T catheter: 10 µg/mL at 4–8 mL/h; L catheter: 10 µg/mL at 10–14 mL/h

From Sevarino FB: Postoperative pain control in cardiac surgery. Sem Anesth 13:57–62, 1994, with permission.

cal patient. The ability to care for patients with impaired circulatory reserve has been enhanced by new technologies such as TEE. While newer drugs and monitoring modalities proliferate, the changing climate of medical economics will sustain efforts to provide cost-effective cardiac anesthetic care.

REFERENCES

1. Harmel MH, Lamont A: Anesthesia in the surgical treatment of congenital pulmonic stenosis. Anesthesiology 7:477–498, 1946
2. Lowenstein E, Hallowell P, Levine FH, et al: Cardiovascular responses to large doses of intravenous morphine in man. N Engl J Med 281:1389–1393, 1969
3. Kaplan JA, King SB: The precordial electrocardiographic lead (V5) in patients who have coronary artery disease. Anesthesiology 45:570–574, 1976
4. London MJ, Hollenberg M, Wong MG, et al: Intraoperative myocardial ischemia: Localization by continuous 12 lead electrocardiography. Anesthesiology 69:232–241, 1988
5. Swan HJC, Ganz W, Forrester J, et al: Catheterization of the heart in man with use of a flow-directed balloon-tipped catheter. N Engl J Med 283:447–451, 1970
6. Leung JM, O'Kelly B, Browser WS, et al: Prognostic importance of postbypass regional wall motion abnormalities in patients undergoing coronary artery bypass graft surgery. Anesthesiology 71:16–25, 1989
7. Paiement B, Pelletier C, Dyrda I, et al: A simple classification of the risk in cardiac surgery. Can Anaesth Soc J 30:61–68, 1983
8. Parsonnet V, Dean D, Bernstein AD: A method of uniform stratification of risk for evaluating the results of surgery in acquired adult heart disease. Circulation 79:(suppl I) 1-3–1-12, 1989
9. Higgins TL, Estafanous F, Loop FD, et al: Stratification of morbidity and mortality outcome by preoperative risk factors in coronary artery bypass patients—a clinical severity score JAMA 267:2344–2348, 1992
10. Knight AA, Hollenberg M, London MJ, et al: Perioperative myocardial ischemia: Importance of the preoperative ischemic pattern. Anesthesiology 68:681–688, 1988
11. Boudoulas H, Lewis RP, Kates RE, Dalamangas G: Hypersensitivity to adrenergic stimulation after propranolol withdrawal in normal subjects. Ann Intern Med 86:433–436, 1977
12. Rangno RE: Propranolol withdrawal: Practical considerations. Arch Intern Med 141:161–162, 1981
13. Slogoff S, Keats AS: Does chronic treatment with calcium entry blocking drugs reduce perioperative myocardial ischemia? Anesthisiology 68:676–680, 1988
14. Kopriva CJ, Brown ACD, Pappas G: Hemodynamics during general anesthisia in patients receiving propranolol. Anesthesiology 48:28–33, 1978
15. Chung F, Houston PL, Cheng DCH, et al: Calcium channel blockade does not offer adequate protection from perioperative myocardial ischemia. Anesthesioloqy 69:343–347, 1988
16. Colson P, Medioni P, Saussine M, et al: Hemodynamic effect of calcium channel blockade during anesthesia for coronary artery surgery. J Cardiothorac Vasc Anesth 6:424–428, 1992
17. Colson P: Angiotensin-converting enzyme inhibitors in cardiovascular anesthesia. J Cardiothorac Vasc Anesth 7:734–742, 1993
18. Coriat P, Richer C, Douraki T, et al: Influence of chronic angiotesin-converting enzyme inhibition on anesthetic induction. Anesthesioloqy 81:299–307, 1994
19. Thakur U, Geary V, Chalmers P, Sheikh F: Low systemic resistance during cardiac surgery: Case reports, brief review, and management with angiotensin II. J Cardiothorac Vasc Anesth 4:360–363, 1990
20. Colson P, Ribstein J, Mimran A, et al: Effect of angiotensin converting enzyme inihibition on blood pressure and renal function during open heart surgery. Anesthesiology 72:23–27, 1990
21. Taylor KM, Morton IJ, Brown JJ, et al: Hypertension and the renin-angiotensin system following open-heart surgery. J Thorac Cardiovasc Surg 74:840–845, 1977

22. Fleisher LA, Rosenbaum SH, Nelson AH, Barash PG: The predictive value of preoperative silent ischemia for postoperative ischemic cardiac events in vascular and nonvascular surgery patients. *Am Heart J* **122:**980–986, 1991

23. Slogoff S, Keats AS: Does perioperative myocardial ischemia lead to postoperative myocardial infarction? *Anesthesiology* **62:**107–114, 1985

24. Vitez TS, Soper LE, Wong KC, Soper P: Chronic hypokalemia and intraoperative dysrhythmias. *Anesthesiology* **63:**130–133, 1985

25. Hirsch IA, Tomlinson DL, Slogoff S, Keats AS: The overstated risk of preoperative hypokalemia. *Anesth Analg* **67:**131–136, 1988

26. Wong KC, Schafer PG, Schultz JR: Hypokalemia and anesthetic implications. *Anesth Analg* **77:**1238–1260, 1993

27. Lawson DH: Adverse reactions to potasium chloride. *Q J Med* **43:**433–440, 1974

28. Marjot R, Valentine SJ: Arterial oxygen saturation following premedication for cardiac surgery. *Br J Anaesth* **64:**737–740, 1990

29. Mark JB, Chien GL, Steinbrook RA, Fenton T: Electrocardiographic R-wave changes during cardiac surgery. *Anesth Analg* **74:**26–31, 1992

30. Muller JG, Barash PG: Automated ST-segment monitoring. *International Anesth Clinics* **31** (3):45–55, 1993

31. Kotrly KJ, Kotter GS, Mortara D, Kampine JP: Intraoperative detection of myocardial ischemia with an ST segment trend monitoring system. *Anesth Analg* **63:**343–345, 1984

32. Kaplan JA, Wells PH: Early diagnosis of myocardial ischemia using the pulmonary arterial catheter. *Anesth Analg* **60:**789–793, 1981

33. Pichard AD, Diaz R, Marchant E, Casanegra P: Large V waves in the pulmonary capillary wedge pressure tracing without mitral regurgitation: The influence of the pressure/volume relationship on the V wave size. *Clin Cardiol* **6:**534–541, 1983

34. Van Daele MERM, Sutherland GR, Mitchell MM, et al: Do changes in pulmonary capillary wedge pressure adequately reflect myocardial ischemia during anesthesia? A correlative preoperative hemodynamic, electrocardiographic, and transesophageal echocardiographic study. *Circulation* **81:**865–871, 1990

35. Hecker BR, Brown DL, Wilson D: A comparison of two pulmonary artery mixed venous oxygen saturation catheters during the changing conditions of cardiac surgery. *J Cardiothorac Anesth* **3:**269–275, 1989

36. Pearson KS, Gomez MN, Moyers JR, et al: A cost/benefit analysis of randomized invasive monitoring for patients undergoing cardiac surgery. *Anesth Analg* **69:**336–341, 1989

37. Yelderman M: Continuous measurement of cardiac output with the use of stochastic system identification techniques. *J Clin Monit* **6:**322–332, 1990

38. Beique F, Ramsay JG: The pulmonary artery catheter: A new look. *Sem Anesth* **13:**14–25, 1994

39. Trankina MF, White RD: Perioperative cardiac pacing using an atrioventricular pacing pulmonary artery catheter. *J Cardiothorac Anesth* **3:**154–162, 1989

40. Roth JV: Temporary transmyocardial pacing using epicardial pacing wires and pacing pulmonary artery catheters. *J Cardiothorac Vasc Aneth* **6:**663–667, 1992

41. Roth JV, Zaidman JR: Use of the pacing pulmonary arterial catheter to detect endocardial electrical activity during hypothermic cardioplegic arrest. *J Clin Monit* **4:**178–180, 1988

42. Kay HR, Afshari M, Barash P, et al: Measurement of ejection fraction by thermal dilution techniques. *J Surg Rev* **34:**337–346, 1983

43. Rafferty TD: Transesophageal two-dimensional echocardiography in the critically ill: Is the Swan-Ganz catheter redundant? *Yale J Biol Med* **64:**375–385, 1991

44. Hines R, Barash PG: Intraoperative right ventricular dysfunction detected with a right ventricular ejection fraction catheter. *J Clin Monit* **2:**206–208, 1986

45. Barash PG, Nardi D, Hammond G, et al: Catheter induced pulmonary artery perforation: Mechanisms, management, and modifications. *J Thorac Cardiovasc Surg* **82:**5–12, 1981

46. Weintraub AC, Barash PG: Pro: A pulmonary artery catheter is indicated in all patients undegoing coronary artery surgery. *J Cardiothorac Anesth* **1:**358–361, 1987

47. Bashein G, Ivey ID: Con: A pulmonary artery catheter is indicated in all patients undergoing coronary artery surgery. *J Cardiothorac Anesth* **1:**362–365, 1987

48. Kressin N, Laravuso RB: Hemodynamic measurements in patients for coronary artery surgery: Cath lab vs. operating room. *Anesthesiology* **59:**A6, 1983

49. Moore CH, Lombardo TR, Allums JA, Gordon FT: Left main coronary artery stenosis: Hemodynamic monitoring to reduce mortality. *Ann Thorac Surg* **26:**445–451, 1978

50. Tuman KJ, McCarthy RJ, Spiess BD, et al: Effect of pulmonary artery catheterization on outcome in patients undergoing coronary artery surgery. *Anesthesiology* **70:**199–206, 1989

51. Practice Guidelines for Pulmonary Artery Catheterization: A report by the American Society of Anesthesiologists task force on pulmonary artery catheterization. *Anesthesiology* **78:**380–394, 1993

52. Waters DD, DaLuz P, Wyatt HL, et al: Early changes in regional and global left ventricular function induced by graded reductions in regional coronary perfusion. *Am J Cardiol* **39:**537–543, 1977

53. Smith JS, Cahalan MK, Benefiel DJ, et al: Intraoperative detection of myocardial ischemia in high-risk patients: Electrocardiography versus two-dimensional transesophageal echocardiography. *Circulation* **72:**1015–1021, 1985

54. London MJ, Tubau JF, Wong MG, et al: The "natural history" of segmental wall motion abnormalities in patients undergoing noncardiac surgery. *Anesthesiology* **73:**644–655, 1990

55. Comunale ME, Body SC, Koch CG, et al: Concordance of TEE wall motion abnormalities and Holter ECG ST segment depression during CABG surgery. Presented at the Sixteenth Annual Meeting of the Society of Cardiovascular Anesthesiologists, Montreal, Canada, April 25, 1994

56. Harris SN, Gordon MA, Urban MK, et al: The pressure rate quotient is not an indicator of myocardial ischemia in humans—an echocardiographic evaluation. *Anesthesiology* **78:**242–250, 1993

57. Weiss JL, Eaton LW, Kallman CH, Maughan WL: Accuracy of volume determination by two-dimensional echocardiography: Defining requirements under controlled conditions in the ejecting canine left ventricle. *Cirulation* **67:**889–895, 1983

58. Urbanowicz JH, Shaaban JM, Cohen NH, et al: Comparison of transesophageal echocardiographic and scintigraphic estimates of left ventricular end-diastolic volume index and ejection fraction in patients following coronary artery bypass grafting. *Anesthesiology* **72:**607–612, 1990

59. Leung JM, Chan FW, Mangano DT: Transesophageal echocardiography: Prediction of intraoperative hypovolemia. *Anesth Analg* **70:**S236, 1990

60. Marschall K, Kanchuger M, Kessler K, et al: Superiority of transesophageal echocardiography in detecting aortic arch atheromatous disease: Identification of patients at increased risk of stroke during cardiac surgery. *J Cardiothorac Vasc Anesth* **8:**5–13, 1994

61. Davila-Roman V, Barzilai B, Wareing TH, et al: Intraoperative ultrasonographic evaluation of the ascending aorta in 100 consecutive patients undergoing cardiac surgery. *Circulation* **84:**III47–III53 (Suppl 3), 1991

62. Phillips KJ, Davila-Roman VG, Barzilai B, et al: Atherosclerosis of the ascending aorta: Intraoperative comparison of two ultrasound techniques to assess its severity. *J Am Coll Cardiol* **21:**342A, 1993

63. Wareing TH, Davila-Roman VG, Barzilai B, et al: Management of the severely atherosclerotic ascending aorta during cardiac operations: A strategy for detection and treatment. *J Thorac Cardiovasc Surg* **103:**453–462, 1992

64. Bull BS, Huse WM, Brauer FS, Korpman RA: Heparin therapy dur-

ing extracorporeal circulation. I. Problems inherent in existing heparin protocols. *J Thorac Cardiovasc Surg* **69**:674–684, 1975

65. Bull BS, Huse WM, Brauer FS, Korpman RA: Heparin therapy during extracorporeal circulation. II. The use of a dose-response curve to individualize heparin and protamine dosage. *J Thorac Cardiovasc Surg* **69**:685–689, 1975

66. Bull MH, Huse WM, Bull BS: Evaluation of tests used to monitor heparin therapy during extracorporeal circulation. *Anesthesiology* **43**:346–353, 1975

67. Young JA, Kisker CT, Doty DB: Adequate anticoagulation during cardiopulmonary bypass determined by activated clotting time and the appearance of fibrin monomer. *Ann Thorac Surg* **26**:231–240, 1978

68. Horrow JC: Protamine: A review of its toxicity. *Anesth Analg* **64**:348–361, 1985

69. Spiess BD, Tuman KJ, McCarthy RJ, et al: Thromboelastography as an indicator of postcardiopulmonary bypass caoagulopathies. *J Clin Monit* **3**:25–30, 1987

70. Van Riper DF, Horrow JC, Osborne D: Is the thromboelastograph a clinically useful predictor of blood loss after bypass? *Anaesthesiology* **73**:A1206, 1990

71. Knapp RB, Dubow H: Comparison of diazepam with thiopental as an induction agent in cardiopulmonary disease. *Anesth Analg* **49**:722–726, 1970

72. Kawar P, Carson IW, Clark RSJ, et al: Haemodynamic changes during induction of anesthesia with midazolam and diazepam (Valium) in patients undergoing coronary artery bypass surgery. *Anaesthesia* **40**:767–771, 1985

73. Barash P, Kopriva CJ: Narcotics and the circulation. In Kitahata LM, Collins JG (eds): *Narcotic Analgesics in Anesthesiology.* Baltimore, Williams & Wilkins, 1982, pp 91–132

74. Giles RW, Berger HJ, Barash PG, et al: Continuous monitoring of left ventricular performance with the computerized nuclear probe during laryngoscopy and intubation before coronary artery bypass surgery. *Am J Cardiol* **50**:735–741, 1982

75. Barash PG, Tarabadkar S, Giles R, et al: Preservation of global left ventricular function during intubation in patients with ishemic heart disease. *Anesthesiology* **55**:A6, 1981

76. Sanford TJ, Smith NT, Dec-Silver H, Harrison WK: A comparison of morphine, fentanyl, and sufentanil anesthesia for cardiac surgery: Induction, emergence, and extubation. *Anesth Analg* **65**:259–266, 1986

77. Thompson IR, Hudson RJ, Rosenbloom M, Meatherall RC: A randomized double-blind comparison of fentanyl and sufentanil anaesthesia for coronary artery surgery. *Can J Anaesth* **34**:227–232, 1987

78. Mora CT, Body S, Bellows W, et al: Propofol and hemodynamic stability: A comparison with sufentanil anesthesia in patients undergoing coronary revascularization. Presented at the Sixteenth Annual Meeting of the Society of Cardiovascular Anesthesiologists, Montreal, April, 1994

79. Karski JM, Teasdale SJ, Boylan J, et al: Propofol infusion for sedation after CABG: Hemodynamics and early extubation—preliminary results. *Can J Anaesth* **40**:A69, 1993

80. Roekaerts PMHJ, Huygen FJPM, De Lange S: Infusion of propofol versus midazolam for sedation in the intensive care unit following coronary artery surgery. *J Cardiothorac Vasc Anesth* **7**:142–147, 1993

81. Nathan HJ: Control of hemodynamics prevents worsening of myocardial ischemia when nitrous oxide is administered to isoflurane-anesthetized dogs. *Anesthesiology* **71**:686–694, 1989

82. Slavik JR, LaMantia KR, Kopriva CJ, et al: Does nitrous oxide cause regional wall motion abnormalities in patients with coronary artery disease? An evaluation with two-dimensional transesophageal echocardiography. *Anesth Analg* **67**:695–700, 1988

83. Ray DC, Drummond GB: Halothane hepatitis. *Br J Anaesth* **67**:84–99, 1991

84. Reiz S, Balfors E, Sorensen MB, et al: Isoflurane—a powerful coronary vasodilator in patients with coronary artery disease. *Anesthesiology* **59**:91–97, 1983

85. Reiz S, Ostman M: Regional coronary hemodynamics during isoflurane-nitrous oxide anesthesia in patients with ischemic heart disease. *Anesth Analg* **64**:570–576, 1985

86. Moffitt EA, Barker RA, Glenn JJ, et al: Myocardial metabolism and hemodynamic responses with isoflurane anesthesia for coronary arterial surgery. *Anesth Analg* **65**:53–61, 1986

87. Khambatta HJ, Sonntag H, Larsen R, et al: Global and regional myocardial blood flow and metabolism during equipotent halothane and isoflurane anesthesia in patients with coronary artery disease. *Anesth Analg* **67**:936–942, 1988

88. Slogoff S, Keats AS: Randomized trial of primary anesthetic agents on outcome of coronary artery bypass operations. *Anesthesiology* **70**:179–188, 1989

89. Slogoff S, Keats AS, Dear WE, et al: Steal-prone coronary anatomy and myocardial ischemia associated with four primary anesthetic agents in humans. *Anesth Analg* **72**:22–27, 1991

90. Starr NJ, Sethna DH, Estafanous FG: Bradycardia and asystole following the rapid administration of sufentanil and vecuronium. *Anesthesiology* **64**:521–523, 1986

91. Odoom JA, Sih IL: Epidural analgesia and anticoagulation therapy: Experience with one thousand cases of continuous epidurals. *Anesthesia* **38**:254–259, 1983

92. Rao TLK, El-Etr AA: Anticoagulation following placement of epidural and subarachnoid catheters: An evaluation of neurologic sequelae. *Anesthesiology* **55**:618–620, 1981

93. Owens EL, Kasten GW, Hessel EA: Spinal subarachnoid hematoma after lumbar puncture and heparinization: A case report, review of the literature, and discussion of anaesthetic implications. *Anesth Analg* **65**:1201–1207, 1986

94. Mathews ET, Abrams LD: Intrathecal morphine in open heart surgery (letter). *Lancet* **2**:543, 1980

95. Vanstrum GS, Bjornson KM, Ilko R: Postoperative effects of intrathecal morphine in coronary artery bypass surgery. *Anesth Analg* **67**:261–267, 1988

96. Robinson RJS, Brister S, Jones E, Quigley M: Epidural meperidine analgesia after cardiac surgery. *Can Anaesth Soc J* **33**:550–555, 1986

97. El-Baz N, Goldin M: Continuous epidural infusion of morphine for pain relief after cardiac operations. *J Thorac Cardiovasc Surg* **93**:878–883, 1987

98. Flacke JW, Flacke WE, Williams GD: Acute pulmonary edema following naloxone reversal of high-dose morphine anesthesia. *Anesthesiology* **47**:376–378, 1977

101

Cardiopulmonary Bypass for Open Heart Surgery

L. Henry Edmunds, Jr.

Simply stated, the heart–lung machine or cardiopulmonary bypass (CPB) is an apparatus that temporarily substitutes for the pumping and ventilatory functions of the natural heart and lungs. The apparatus permits open cardiac operations and modifications are used for temporary support of patients with reversible heart or lung disease.

HISTORICAL NOTE

After a long series of laboratory studies, Dr. John Gibbon of Philadelphia performed the first successful intracardiac operation with the aid of a heart–lung machine on May 6, 1953.[1] Unfortunately, Dr. Gibbon's achievement was followed by several unsuccessful efforts by both Dr. Gibbon and other surgical groups.[2,3] These failures cast doubt about the safety of extracorporeal circulation and prompted C. Walton Lillihei of Minneapolis in March 1954 to introduce a cross-circulation technique for oxygenation of venous blood during intracardiac operations. In this technique, an adult donor (usually a parent) served as the blood oxygenator. Dr. Lillihei and his group carried out 45 operations with cross-circulation,[3] and although no human oxygenators were lost, the procedure carried the possibility of a 200% mortality.

In March 1955, Dr. John Kirklin at the Mayo Clinic began the first successful series of intracardiac repairs using the heart–lung machine.[4] In that same month, Dr. Lillihei and his colleagues began to use other bypass methods including dog lung oxygenators, bubble oxygenators, and arterial blood reservoirs in low-risk patients. They continued to use the cross-circulation technique in higher-risk patients until July 1955, when a bubble oxygenator developed by

Drs. DeWall and Lillihei became the sole method of oxygenation for cardiopulmonary bypass at the University of Minnesota.[3] By the end of 1955, many surgical groups around the world began to perform intracardiac repairs with homemade heart–lung machines. Other techniques such as the atrial well, surface hypothermia, and in-flow occlusion were gradually abandoned, or used adjunctively, in favor of the versatility of the heart-lung machine.

THE HEART–LUNG MACHINE

The basic components of the heart–lung machine are one or more venous cannulas, a venous reservoir, oxygenator/heat exchanger, pump, arterial line filter, and arterial cannula. The machine is built from synthetic and nontoxic materials such as polycarbonate, polyvinylchloride, teflon, polyethylene, stainless steel, silicone rubber, and polyurethanes. Bloodflow paths are designed to minimize turbulence and stagnant areas and to minimize the volume of perfusate required for priming. The need to add perfusate and drugs, to salvage blood from the surgical field, obtain blood samples, and provide cardioplegic solutions requires multiple access ports. For most applications subsystems supplement the basic machine. A cardiotomy suction system aspirates blood from open cardiac chambers and the surgical field. This blood is filtered and debubbled, and added directly to the perfusate. Diluted field blood is retrieved by a separate "cell saver" system that filters and concentrates red cells before returning them to the perfusate. A cardioplegic delivery system consists of a separate pump, reservoir, and heat exchanger, and is designed to provide potassium-enriched blood or crystalloid solution directly into the coronary circulation. Current heart–lung machines and their subsystems have an open architecture with separated components connected by a maze of tubing. The open architecture permits the perfusionist to visually monitor the system and to correct problems, but exposes blood to large areas of synthetic materials, multiple air entry sites, and potential contamination.

Venous Cannulas

A venous cannula drains blood by gravity from the patient into the extracorporeal circuit or pump-oxygenator system. One or more venous cannulas are used depending on the type of cardiac surgical procedure, and, to some extent, the surgeon's preference. When one cannula is used, it is usually placed in the right atrium through the right atrial appendage. When two cannulas are used, the cannulas are passed through pursestring sutures in the right atrium into the superior and inferior vena cava. If there is an additional left superior vena cava and it drains into the coronary sinus, a third venous cannula can be inserted into the sinus from the right atrium. A single cannula or a "two-stage" cannula is used by many surgeons for operations involving the aortic valve, left ventricular outflow tract, ascending aorta, and coronary arterial bypass procedures. Two venous catheters with snares tightened around both cavas are necessary for work within the right atrium or right ventricle. In certain operations, either cava may be cannulated directly. Venous cannulas also can be inserted into either cava or the right atrium from the femoral, iliac, or jugular vein. Flow is limited if the cannula tip is greater than one-half the diameter of the great vein due to collapse of the vein around the cannula; therefore longer catheters that reach the right atrium and are inserted percutaneously or directly over a wire guide are preferred.[5] Peripheral cannulation is used for some reoperations, in occasional emergencies, and when long-term circulatory or respiratory support is needed.[5]

The size of the venous cannulas is determined by the number used, the size of the patient, and the anticipated flow rate.[6] During perfusion, central venous pressure must be kept below 15 mm Hg and negative pressure, which causes collapse of thin-walled great veins and obstucts flow, should not be allowed to develop.[5] In most extracorporeal perfusion systems, systemic venous blood drains by gravity into the venous reservoir. Thus, the venous reservoir is placed 25–30 inches below the plane of the systemic great veins.

Oxygenator

The oxygenator is where oxygen and carbon dioxide exchange takes place. There are two types of oxygenators, bubble and membrane. In bubble oxygenators, oxygen is directly infused into a column of systemic venous blood through a diffusion plate (sparger). The sparger produces thousands of small oxygen bubbles within blood. Gas exchange occurs across a thin film at the blood-gas interface around each bubble (Fig. 101–1A). Carbon dioxide diffuses into the bubble and oxygen diffuses outward into blood. Since oxygen diffuses slowly in plasma, many small bubbles improve oxygen exchange by effectively increasing the surface area of the gas–blood interface.[7] Carbon dioxide diffuses 25 times more rapidly than oxygen in plasma; its removal is facilitated by larger bubbles, which accommodate more CO_2 and are easier to remove from blood. Commercial oxygenator diffusion plates produce bubbles (approximately 36 μm) that efficiently remove carbon dioxide and fully saturate blood with oxygen. Carbon dioxide escapes into the gas phase when bubbles and blood are separated by defoaming surfactants, settling, and filtration in the arterial reservoir. Contemporary bubble oxygenators incorporate a reservoir and heat exchanger within the same unit and are placed upstream to the arterial pump.

Commercial bubble oxygenators are highly efficient and add 350 to 400 mL oxygen to blood and remove 300 to 330 mL CO_2 at flow rates from 1 to 7 L/min.[6,8] Priming volumes are less than 500 mL. Modern membrane oxygenators are equally efficient and add up to 470 mL of O_2 and remove up to 350 mL of CO_2 at 1 to 7 L/min flow.[6,8] Priming volumes range from 270 to 500 mL; pressure differences across the machines are approximately 12–15 mm Hg/L bloodflow. These specifications compare respectfully with the adult human lung at resting cardiac outputs. However, the human lung is capable of adding 2 L of O_2 and removing 1.6 L of CO_2 at flows up to 15 L/min with pressure differences across the lung of about 2 mm Hg/L.[9] The priming volume of the human lung is approximately 140 mL, but the surface area of the blood–gas interface is nearly 90 m². Surface areas of membrane oxygenators are around 2 m².

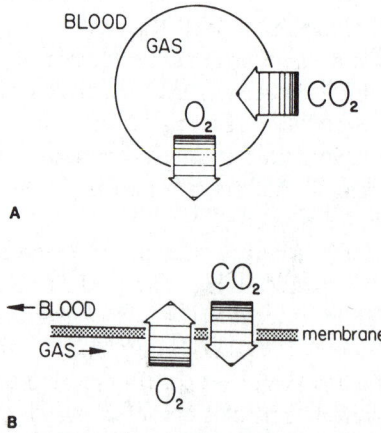

Figure 101–1. A. Oxygen diffuses out of the bubble into the blood and carbon dioxide diffuses from the blood into the bubble when a bubble-type oxygenator is used. **B.** Blood and gas are not in direct contact with a membrane oxygenator. Oxygen diffuses through a semipermeable membrane into the blood and carbon dioxide diffuses from the blood through the semipermeable membrane.

Gas does not come in direct contact with the blood in a membrane oxygenator. A silicone rubber membrane or a polypropylene microporous membrane separates blood and gas compartments. Oxygen diffuses into the blood driven by a high concentration gradient (approximately 640 mm Hg) (Fig. 101–1B). Because oxygen diffuses poorly in plasma, blood must be spread thinly over a relatively large surface area (2.0–5.4 M^2) to achieve complete saturation of hemoglobin. Areas of turbulence and secondary flows enhance the diffusion of oxygen within blood and therefore improve oxyhemoglobin saturation. Carbon dioxide diffuses outward across the membrane and is driven only by the carbon dioxide tension in systemic venous blood (35–50 mm Hg) and the rate carbon dioxide is washed out by gas flow. Oxygen content of the gas compartment is regulated by a blender that mixes oxygen and air to produce any desired oxygen concentration. The thin blood path and large blood–membrane surface area produce relatively high resistance to flow; therefore in most membrane oxygenator perfusion systems, the arterial pump is placed upstream to the oxygenator. A heat exchanger is integral to the unit. Current membrane oxygenators are disposable, single-use units (Fig. 101–2).

Two different designs to bring red cells near the membrane surface within the blood compartment are used. In the spiral coil oxygenator, which is largely used for prolonged perfusions for respiratory or circulatory support, an envelope of silicone rubber membrane is wound around a central spool. Oxygen enters the envelope and blood passes between the windings. The bloodflow path is irregular and produces secondary flows and turbulence. The other basic design is the hollow fiber membrane oxygenator that contains sheaves of hollow fibers (120–200) μm in diameter) connected to inlet and outlet manifolds within a chamber.[8] Usually oxygen is passed inside the fibers and blood passes between and over individual fibers (Fig. 101–2). Blood can also circulate through the fibers with gas outside; however, because of secondary flows and turbulence oxygenation is better with blood outside. Gas exchange efficiency is greatly increased by making fibers of microporous polypropylene. Plasma surface tension seals micropores to prevent gas emboli, but the holes greatly reduce the diffusion barrier to gas exchange.

Both membrane and bubble oxygenators activate blood elements and produce microemboli. However, because the blood contact surfaces of membrane oxygenators are constant, most of the blood injury occurs within the first few minutes before adsorbed proteins passivate the surface. In bubble oxygenators, blood trauma is progressive since each new bubble presents a new foreign surface to which blood elements react. Bubble oxygenators are very efficient gas exchangers; however, with development of microporous polypropylene membranes, membrane oxygenators are just as efficient and cause less blood trauma with perfusions that last more than 2 or 3 hours.[10–12]

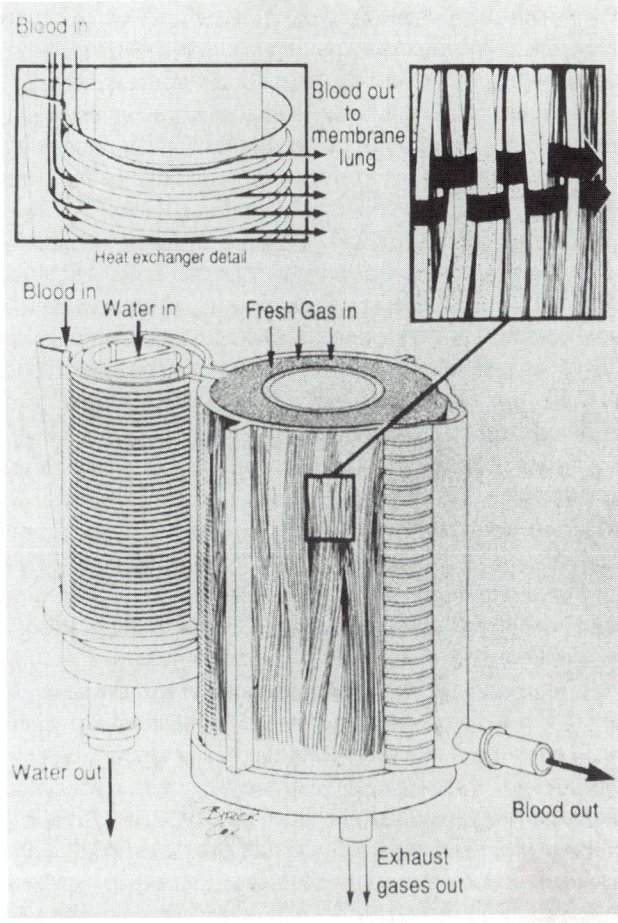

Figure 101–2. Diagram of a contemporary blood oxygenator–heat exchanger unit with a polycarbonate shell and microporous polypropylene hollow fibers. Venous blood enters the top of the heat exchanger, passes over water-filled coils, into the oxygenator and outside "woven" bundles of hollow fibers. Potting compound seals the oxygenator at either end. Oxygenated gas enters the cut ends of the hollow fibers from above and exits from below. *(From High KM, Snider MT, Basbein G: Principles of oxygenator function: Gas exchange, heat transfer, and blood-artificial surface interaction. In Gravlee GP, Davis RF, Utley JR (eds): Cardiopulmonary Bypass. Baltimore, Williams & Wilkins, 1993, p 40, reproduced with permission.)*

Heat Exchanger

Heat exchangers are necessary to control body temperature during cardiopulmonary bypass. Body temperatures are lowered during cardiopulmonary bypass for several reasons (see below). Water circulates within the heat exchanger between 1–2° and 42°C. Blood should not be heated above 42°C to avoid injury to blood proteins. Cooling usually occurs more rapidly than rewarming because greater temperature differences between blood leaving and entering the patient are more easily maintained. In adults, nasopharyngeal temperatures decrease at a rate of 0.7–1.5°C/min between 30° and 37°C and more slowly at lower temperatures.[10] During rewarming, temperature increases at the rate of

$0.2-0.5°C/min$. Caloric exchange is most rapid at the beginning of cooling or rewarming, but often temperature changes lag because of heat dissipation within the body.

Oxygen, carbon dioxide, and nitrogen are more soluble in cold blood. Therefore, perfusion of very cold blood into warm patients must be avoided so that microbubble formation does not occur within the patient. This danger develops if blood is too rapidly cooled during induction of hypothermia. Rapid warming of blood may produce microbubbles within the circuit, but these will dissolve after reaching the cold patient. The perfusionist should avoid temperature gradients of more than $12-14°C$ between patient and blood perfusate. Because of the importance of the brain, nasopharyngeal temperature (the probe is placed close to the base of the brain) is measured in addition to rectal or bladder temperature during hypothermic CPB.

Pumps

The two most commonly used blood pumps are the roller and the centrifugal. Valved pumps are rarely used for clinical CPB, but are often used in circulatory assist devices. The roller pump consists of two rollers, 180° apart, which rotate through a metal raceway that is an arc of approximately 200° (Fig. 101–3A). Polyvinyl, silicone rubber, or polyurethane tubing between $\frac{1}{4}$ and $\frac{5}{8}$ inches (i.d.) is placed between the rollers and raceway so that the rollers barely occlude the tubing at 180 mm Hg back-pressure. As one roller begins to compress the tubing, the opposite roller releases so that blood within the tubing is continuously propelled in one direction. Roller pumps are reliable, safe, comparatively inexpensive, and easy to operate, and maintain forward flow regardless of outflow line pressure. Pump output is proportional to the speed of rotation of the rollers and the diameter of the compressible tubing. In practice, rate of bloodflow is calculated or read from a chart that correlates roller speed, tubing diameter, and bloodflow. Roller pumps produce a sine wave pressure curve of low amplitude.

The centrifugal pump consists of a rapidly rotating impeller (either concentric cones or blades) within a blood compartment (Fig. 101–3-B). The impeller causes blood to rotate at high speed within the compartment, and the centrifugal force propels the blood forward when it reaches the pump outlet. The centrifugal pump is safe, reliable, disposable, and simple to operate; however flow varies as a function of outflow line pressure and must be monitored by an electromagnetic flowmeter. Centrifugal pumps have several advantages over the roller pump in that they do not produce high back-pressures when tubing is temporarily obstructed or kinked, do not produce spatulated emboli from compression of the tubing, and cannot pump large gas emboli. Centrifugal pumps produce continuous, nonpulsatile bloodflow.

A roller or centrifugal pump is used to pump oxygenated blood to the patient. A roller pump is used to produce negative pressures to operate the cardiotomy suction system or actively vent the left heart. A third pump, usually of the roller type, is used to deliver cardioplegic solution or to perfuse the coronary arteries directly during open operations involving the aortic root.

Filters

Blood filters are designed to trap particulate and gaseous emboli.[11] Arterial line filters are required for bubble oxygenator perfusion systems and are usually used with membrane oxygenator systems.[12] Currently most arterial line filters are screen (rather than mesh) filters made of nylon or polyester with pore sizes between 25 and 40 μm (Fig. 101–4). Surface areas vary between 650 and 800 cm^2. Flow rates up to 7 L/min produce pressure differences across the filter that are less than 30 mm Hg. Most filters require 200 mL of perfusate to prime. Other filters are included in cardiotomy suction systems and cell savers and are used temporarily during priming.

Arterial Cannulas

The arterial cannula is usually placed in the ascending aorta just proximal to the innominate artery, but can be placed in any major peripheral artery such as the axillary, iliac, or femoral. Femoral arterial cannulation is often used in patients with dissecting aortic aneurysms, in patients who require reoperation, and in emergencies when rapid cannulation of the femoral artery and vein is necessary to establish circulation with partial cardiopulmonary bypass. Percutaneous arterial (and venous) cannulas that are passed through a tiny skin incision into a peripheral artery over a guide wire are also available for special situations.

The size of the arterial cannula varies with the size of the patient and the anticipated bloodflow rate through the heart–lung machine. Internal diameters of commercially available arterial cannulas vary between 6 and 24 Fr. The pressure difference across the cannula is directly propor-

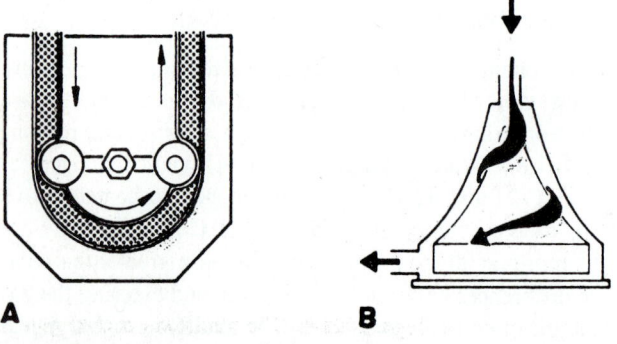

A　　　　　　**B**

Figure 101–3. **A.** With the roller pump, blood is propelled by rollers that compress the blood-filled plastic tubing. **B.** With the centrifugal pump, blood is propelled through the circuit by the centrifugal force of multiple, rapidly spinning impellers.

tional to bloodflow rate and inversely proportional to the internal diameter of the cannula.[13]

Cardiotomy Suction System

This system is necessary to return blood spilled in the operative field directly into the perfusion circuit. The system avoids potentially tremendous blood losses that might otherwise occur, but beyond filtering does not process blood. The cardiotomy suction system usually consists of two suckers, connecting tubing, one roller pump, and a combined blood filter and reservoir unit (Fig. 101–5). The suction system is a major cause of hemolysis because of the air–blood interface and the turbulence required to aspirate blood. Since debris may be aspirated from the field into the system, a filter in the cardiotomy suction system reservoir is mandatory.[11] The system also aspirates large volumes of air and is a major source of gaseous emboli if aspirated blood reaches the cardiotomy suction reservoir. The cardiotomy suction system is a major source of blood injury.

Left Ventricular Venting System

Decompression of the flaccid, noncontracting heart prevents ventricular distension and nonischemic myocardial creep.[14] Ventricular distention significantly reduces myocardial contractility and sometimes produces acute lung damage from increased pulmonary venous pressures. Left ventricular venting also facilitates exposure of the aortic

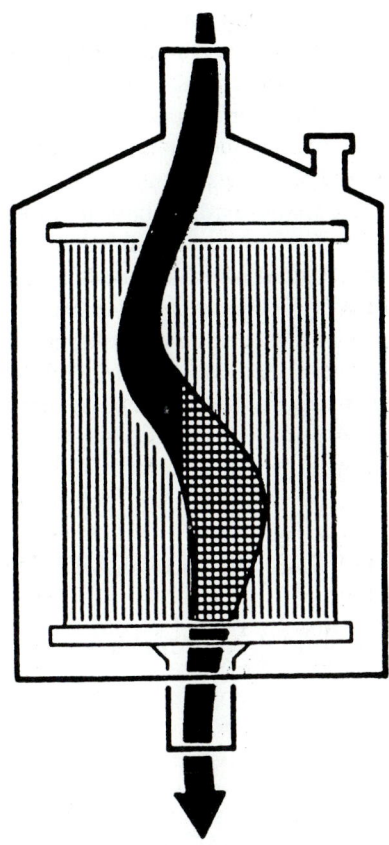

Figure 101–4. Arterial blood filters generally contain nylon screen of approximately 25–40 μm pore size and are designed to trap particulate matter and serve as a bubble trap.

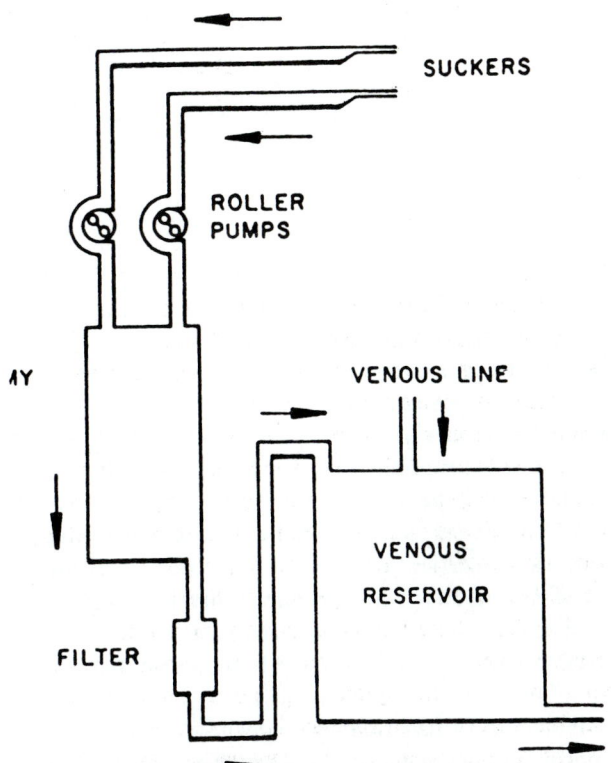

Figure 101–5. The cardiotomy sucker system usually consists of two suckers and roller pumps to create suction. In addition, there is a blood reservoir and blood filter. After the blood is filtered, it is returned to the venous reservoir of the heart–lung machine.

valve and root. Separate catheters are not usually necessary for venting the right ventricle; if the right atrium is closed, absence of caval snares ensures that right ventricular pressure will not exceed central venous pressure. The left ventricle may be vented directly through a catheter inserted into the left ventricular apex, left atrial appendage, or the junction of the right superior pulmonary vein and left atrium. The catheter tip is usually advanced across the mitral valve if the left atrial approach is used. The left ventricle may also be vented using a pulmonary arterial catheter. Pulmonary veins do not have valves; therefore, decompression of the pulmonary artery during CPB reduces all left-sided cardiac pressures and provides some protection against myocardial distention. Vented blood may be drained directly into the venous reservoir of the perfusion system by gravity. More commonly a roller pump is used to aspirate blood into the cardiotomy reservoir. One-way valves in the system prevent accidental air entry into the heart; however, after vent decompression, all air must be carefully removed from the heart before contractions begin.

Cell Saver

Only blood that is fully anticoagulated should pass through the heart–lung machine. Clotting within the perfusion circuit is a major disaster and results in abrupt termination of bypass with possible death of the patient. Large numbers of red cells may be lost if field blood diluted with topical cooling solutions and liquid blood, shed before the injection of heparin or after the injection of protamine, is not retrieved. For this reason, cell saver systems are used to conserve blood during open cardiac surgery. A cell saver system usually consists of one or two suckers powered by the wall vacuum system. As blood enters the sucker tip, heparin is immediately added; blood then passes through a 20-μm filter to a reservoir where the cells are washed and concentrated using a centrifuge.[15] Washed, concentrated red blood cells are placed in plastic bags to be reinfused as needed. Postoperatively blood collected from chest tubes may also be filtered and reinfused when collection systems that ensure sterility are used.

Perfusionist

Alert, attentive, well-trained perfusionists are required to assemble and operate the heart–lung machine. Current standards encourage assignment of two perfusionists to each case. Perfusionists are responsible for the safe, smooth, and continuous operation of the machine and operate under the direct control of the operating surgeon. Ideally the primary perfusionist is in constant contact with the operating surgeon; however many surgeons prefer to delegate this responsibility to the anesthesiologist. The perfusionist receives specific instructions regarding flow rates, temperature levels, and differential allocation of perfusate between patient and machine from the surgeon. The perfusionist is responsible for monitoring pressures within the system, maintenance of adequate oxygen and carbon dioxide transfer, and avoidance of air intake or obstructions to flow. During operation, the perfusionist is responsible through the operating surgeon for maintenance of adequate perfusion and metabolism of all of the patient's organs and tissues.

Schools for training cardiopulmonary perfusionists are accredited by the Council for Allied Health Education and Accreditation (CAHEA), which is the sole accrediting body recognized by the Department of Education of the United States government.[16] Courses of instruction include didactic material, hands-on training, and usually last 1–2 years. Matriculating students are examined by the American Board of Cardiovascular Perfusion and, if successful, receive a certificate.

CONDUCT OF CARDIOPULMONARY BYPASS

Assembly of Heart–Lung Machine

The heart–lung machine is partially assembled 30–60 min before bypass is scheduled to begin. Partial assembly of the various components of the system requires approximately 20 min for bubble oxygenator systems and 30 min for membrane oxygenator systems (Fig. 101–6). The various components are mounted on a roller pump chassis. Usually the venous, arterial, cardiotomy sucker, and cardioplegic delivery lines, which enter the operative field, are separately packaged, sterilized, and passed from the operative field to the perfusionist, or vice versa. The perfusionist connects these lines to the partially assembled machine. The system is primed with crystalloid and recirculated for several minutes through a sterile 0.5-μm filter to remove all air bubbles and particulate emboli from the system. During recirculation, the system is checked for leaks and problems and the performance of the monitoring devices is tested. The recirculation filter is discarded.

Priming

For adults, about 2 L of priming solution is required to prepare the extracorporeal perfusion circuit for bypass. The priming solution usually consists of balanced salt solution, sometimes with the addition of starch. Because of expense albumin and plasma are rarely used. Unless the adult patient is anemic, blood is generally not added to the system. Once CPB starts, the patient's hematocrit is kept in the range of 20–25%. Some surgeons accept lower hematocrits during perfusions at low temperatures.[17] If the hematocrit drops below a predetermined concentration, homologous blood or packed cells are added to the system. During perfusion, additional perfusate may be required to operate the system safely.

Infants and small children frequently require blood in the priming solution since the amount of perfusate to prime

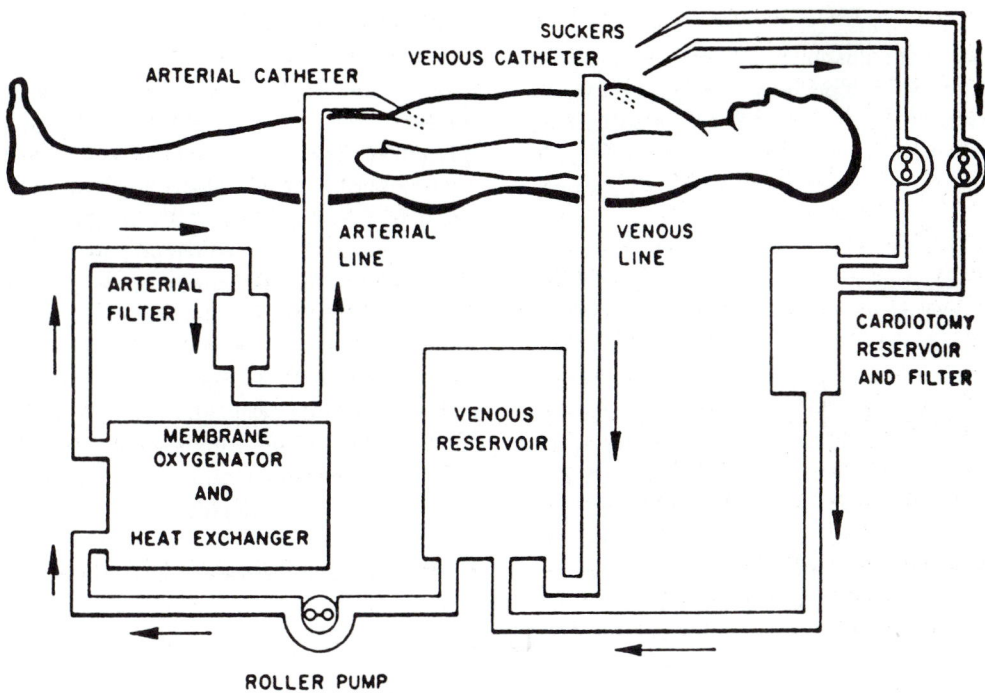

Figure 101–6. Diagram of a typical cardiopulmonary bypass setup with a membrane oxygenator.

the heart–lung machine is proportionately greater than that required for an adult. At least 800 mL of priming volume is required to prime the heart–lung machine for an infant. When the heart–lung machine is primed with bank blood, heparin must also be added. Calcium is then added to neutralize the citrate in donor blood. Bicarbonate is also added to bring the pH of the perfusate to 7.4.

Reducing hematocrit during cardiopulmonary bypass has a number of advantages. First, less blood is required for operation and the risk of serum hepatitis and viral borne pathogens is proportionately reduced. Second, trauma to blood cells and blood proteins is reduced since less blood is in the circuit. Less plasma hemoglobin is produced. Hemodilution also increases urine flow and clearance of sodium, potassium, and creatinine. The incidence of oliguria and acute tubular necrosis is less with hemodilution.[18] Since blood is less viscous, flow characteristics are improved through partially obstructed vessels and through smaller arterioles and capillaries, especially during hypothermia. Hemodilution, however, does reduce intravascular osmotic pressure and therefore increases interstitial edema. This disadvantage, however, does not offset the multiple advantages of hemodilution and blood conservation techniques.

Anticoagulation

CPB produces a powerful thrombotic stimulus and is not possible without heparin. However, heparin is not an ideal anticoagulant. Heparin acts near the end of the coagulation cascade and fails to suppress the series of enzymatic reactions that are amplified and accelerated at each step. These uninhibited reactions produce a number of powerful serine proteases during CPB even though clotting does not occur. Heparin prevents clotting by activating the natural plasma protein, antithrombin III (AT-III). AT-III is a large (62,000 D), abundant (290 µg/mL), plasma protease inhibitor of Factors IXa, Xa, and thrombin. AT-III primarily complexes with thrombin; inhibition of Factor Xa is partial and even less with Factor IXa. Heparin accelerates the action of AT-III approximately 1000-fold to achieve a second-order rate constant for thrombin of 3.7×10^7 M^{-1} s^{-1}.[19] Thus AT-III–heparin inhibits soluble thrombin very rapidly, but does not become part of the complex. After the reaction, heparin is released to catalyze another coupling and the AT-III–thrombin complex is excreted through liver and kidney.

Despite activated clotting times over 400 seconds thrombin is progressively formed during CPB in every patient.[20,21] CPB overwhelms the ability of AT-III–heparin to prevent thrombin production and circulation. Fl.2, a marker of the conversion of prothrombin to thrombin, and fibrinopeptide A (FPA), a fragment produced by conversion of fibrinogen to fibrin, increase progressively during CPB despite very rapid inhibition of thrombin and partial inhibition of Factor Xa.

Heparin has some additional drawbacks. Heparin preparations vary in anticoagulant effectiveness. Heparin also increases the sensitivity of platelets to various agonists[22] and slightly increases bleeding times.[23] AT-III–heparin does not inhibit thrombin bound to fibrin and cannot prevent thrombin activation of platelets and fibrinogen conversion within clots.[24] Heparin also contributes to the activation of neutrophils[25] and when complexed with protamine is a major stimulus to complement activation.[26] Heparin-induced thrombocytopenia is a serious postoperative problem for some patients (2–5%).[27] On rare occasions heparin-induced thrombosis is a catastrophic problem.[28] Thus heparin is not an ideal anticoagulant, but is the only one we have.

Sensitivity to heparin and metabolism of heparin vary among patients.[29] Hypothermia decreases the rate of heparin metabolism. Heparin monitoring is recommended during cardiopulmonary bypass to ensure that clotting does not occur. The activated clotting time is the most common and simplest method used to measure the degree of anticoagulation by heparin in the operating room, but is not as accurate as direct titration measurements using specially designed kits. Activated clotting times using celite tubes are affected by aprotinin, which artifactually delays clot formation and prolongs the time.[30] The activated clotting time is measured after the initial dose of heparin (usually 300 U/kg); CPB does not begin until the time is greater than 400 seconds.[31] Additional heparin is given if needed. Activated clotting time is rechecked every 30 min during bypass and supplemental heparin is added to maintain the activated clotting time over 400 seconds.

Protamine

After cardiopulmonary bypass has stopped, protamine (1 mg for each 100 U of heparin) is given to neutralize heparin. The heparin–protamine complex formed activates complement and in approximately 50% of patients causes transient hypotension and reduced cardiac output.[32] Activated complement causes vasodilation, cardiac dysfunction,[26] and an increase in capillary permeability, but also stimulates mast cells and basophils to release histamine.

In rare instances, protamine may cause anaphylactic reactions in certain diabetics or in patients with fish allergies. These patients often have pre-existing IgE or IgG antibodies to protamine.[33] In even rarer instances, administration of protamine causes synthesis and release of thromboxane A_2 from platelets.[34] This produces severe pulmonary vasoconstriction and may require reheparinization and restarting CPB.

Aside from protamine reactions, protamine may be cleared from the circulation faster than heparin is removed. Heparin is cleared from the circulation by the reticuloendothelial system, but rates of clearance vary widely between patients and are influenced by many other factors during CPB (e.g., hypothermia). Therefore after initial protamine, residual heparin ("heparin rebound") may continue to inhibit clot formation. In very high doses, protamine is a weak anticoagulant; however, this is not a clinical concern. If "heparin rebound" is suspected, additional protamine can be given safely without laboratory verification.

Patient Monitors

During intracardiac operations, a number of physiologic parameters are monitored. Electrocardiographic leads are placed before induction of anesthesia. Pads for external cardiac defibrillation are also placed over the back and left chest in selected patients. An arterial catheter is inserted, usually into the radial or femoral artery (or umbilical, temporal, or brachial in infants) to monitor arterial pressure continuously throughout the operation and the early postoperative period. A Swan-Ganz catheter is usually introduced into the jugular vein percutaneously before or after induction of anesthesia to monitor central venous, pulmonary arterial, and pulmonary capillary wedge pressures. Thermodilution cardiac outputs are often measured intermittently; catheters are also available to continuously measure pulmonary arterial oxygen saturation and cardiac output. The electrocardiogram is essential to monitor arrhythmias, ischemic changes, and loss of electrical activity with administration of cardioplegic solutions. Some anesthesiologists and surgeons also monitor the electroencephalogram in an effort to detect possible brain ischemia or injury during operation. Nasopharyngeal and rectal or bladder temperatures are routinely monitored; esophageal temperature is easily influenced by topical solutions in the field and proximity to the aorta. Nasopharyngeal temperature reflects the temperature of the base of the brain while rectal or bladder temperature reflects the mean temperature of the body mass. Urine output is continuously collected via a Foley catheter and periodically measured.

Perfusion flow rate and arterial and central venous pressures are measured continuously during cardiopulmonary bypass. In addition, pressure within the arterial perfusion line (upstream to the arterial line filter and arterial cannula) is monitored. If coronary arteries are directly perfused with cardioplegic solution, pressure in this perfusion line is monitored and maintained within prescribed ranges to avoid injury to coronary vessels. Temperatures of both inflow and outflow blood in the perfusion circuit and temperature of cardioplegic solutions are monitored routinely. Direct measurement of ventricular myocardial temperature during cardioplegic arrest is optional.

Arterial blood gases, hematocrit, and serum electrolytes including ionized calcium are periodically checked throughout the operative procedure, but, most importantly, immediately before stopping CPB. Digital pulse oximetry permits continuous observation of arterial oxygen saturation.

Optionally, an electronic level sensing device may be placed on the venous (or arterial) reservoir upstream to the pump to detect dangerously low levels of perfusate within the system. Some perfusionists also measure oxygen saturation in the arterial line. Use of an arterial line ultrasound bubble detector is another optional safety feature. These detectors can be connected to stop the arterial pump automatically, but the perfusionist must have the ability to override this feature.

Flow Rates and Pressures

Flow rates of 2.2 L/min per m^2 are adequate to meet metabolic requirements and to avoid metabolic acidosis during cardiopulmonary bypass in anesthetized adults at 37°C.[35] Oxygen consumption at normothermia is 80–125 cm^3/min per m^2 and is similar to that in the anesthetized adult not on bypass.[35,36] Hypothermia reduces metabolic requirements and therefore permits flow rates less than 2.2 L/m^2 per minute. Perfusate flow rates and oxygen-carrying capacity must always be adequate to meet the metabolic requirements of all tissues and organs, since oxygen is not stored in the body. Flow rates of 2.5 L/m^2 per minute are generally used at 37°C to perfuse the microcirculation and to add a margin of safety.

Blood pressure during normothermic cardiopulmonary bypass is generally kept in the range of 50–70 mm Hg (mean). Increased neurologic problems correlate with mean blood pressures less than 45 mm Hg.[37] With moderate hypothermia, blood pressures above 35 mm Hg are considered safe. During bypass, blood pressure is controlled by flow rate (which can be increased above 2.2 L/m^2 per minute) and by infusion of peripheral vasodilators (trimethaphan, nitroglycerin, nitroprusside) or vasoconstrictors (methoxamine, norepinephrine). Additional anesthesia or intravenous morphine also reduces blood pressure.

Temperature

Metabolic activity, and thus oxygen consumption, decreases with decreasing body temperature. Oxygen consumption decreases 50% for every 10°C decrease in body temperature.[35] There are several advantages of moderate hypothermia during cardiopulmonary bypass. Since the oxygen requirement is reduced, flow rates can be reduced without production of lactate or metabolic acidosis.[36] Below 28°C, flow rates of 1.6 L/m^2 per minute are safe for as long as 2 hours.[35] Reduced body temperature enhances the safe duration of cardiac ischemia after infusions of cold cardioplegia by reducing the temperature difference between the heart and body. Moderate hypothermia adds safety to the perfusion since more time is available for repairs if perfusion must be interrupted because of accidents in the surgical field or failure of the perfusion apparatus.

Various organs and tissues within the body cool and rewarm at different rates. In general, the rate of cooling or rewarming is proportional to the bloodflow per unit of tissue mass.[35,38] Thus, small organs with large proportionate bloodflows cool and rewarm rapidly (e.g., kidney, adrenal, heart); large tissue masses, such as skeletal muscle or fat, cool and rewarm slowly. Because of its sensitivity to ischemic injury, brain temperature, as estimated by nasopha-

ryngeal temperature, must be monitored closely. Brain bloodflow at 80–90 mL/100 g is intermediate between that of heart and nonworking skeletal muscle.[38]

Recent practice tends to carry out some relatively short operations at normothermia or only modest hypothermia (e.g., 32–34°C).[39] Improved cardioplegic techniques that provide continuous perfusion of the coronary vasculature at about 5°C or better maintain protective low cardiac temperatures underlie this option. Warmer perfusions obviate or attenuate rewarming and shorten the duration of CPB.

Deep Hypothermia and Circulatory Arrest

Nasopharyngeal temperatures below 20°C define clinical *deep* hypothermia. The techniques of deep hypothermia and low perfusion flow (0.5 L/m^2 per minute) or circulatory arrest are often useful when bloodflow to the brain must be interrupted (e.g., aneurysms involving the aortic arch or during repair of certain complex congenital heart lesions in infants). Cooling is usually achieved by perfusion in combination with a hypothermia blanket beneath the patient and ice packing around the head if the period of circulatory arrest is expected to exceed 20 min.[40] Both nasopharyngeal and rectal temperatures are monitored; occasionally esophageal temperature is also observed. Surface hypothermia without perfusion is no longer used because of the danger of arrhythmias at temperatures below 32°C and the threat of ventricular fibrillation at temperatures below 30°C. Infants cool and rewarm rapidly as compared to adults and caloric exchange is proportional to body mass, rate of perfusion flow, and temperature differences between perfusate and patient.[35] It is essential to cool long enough to reduce temperatures of the brain to desired levels; for adults at least 30 min of cooling before reducing or stopping flow is recommended.

Perfusion cooling requires special considerations. Cooling increases blood viscosity, but hemodilution reduces viscosity and facilitates uniform distribution of bloodflow even at low temperature.[38] Cooling also shifts the oxygen–hemoglobin saturation curve to the left causing hemoglobin to remain highly saturated (and not easily release oxygen) at low oxygen tensions. At very low temperatures cell metabolism depends primarily on dissolved oxygen, which is increased by cold. Below 18°C plasma oxygen tensions must decrease to very low pressures for hemoglobin to release bound oxygen. Lastly, hyperglycemia appears to be detrimental to the brain at low temperature and is associated with increased postoperative evidence of brain ischemia.[41]

Temperature also affects acid–base balance and management of both pH and CO_2 is of special concern during deep hypothermia.[42] If measurements of blood CO_2 below 37°C are corrected for temperature (pH-stat protocol), CO_2 must be added to blood to maintain pH at 7.4 at the low temperature. This protocol reduces cerebral autoregulation of bloodflow and produces an excess of hydrogen ions in the perfusate.[40] The alternative alpha-stat protocol does not correct blood measurements for temperature, produces a relative alkalosis, better maintains cerebral bloodflow autoregulation, and is easier. By not correcting for temperature the buffering capacity of an important blood buffer, the α-imidazole group of histidine is maximized.[40] Controversy rages over which protocol is associated with a greater number of postoperative neurologic problems.[40,43]

The safe duration of circulatory arrest below 20°C is not precisely known. The brain is susceptible to ischemic (metabolic) injury, emboli, and perhaps a poorly understood cold injury that occurs sporadically at temperatures below 12°C.[44] During cooling, temperature differences between patient and perfusate are limited to 10–14°C. Circulatory arrest is usually not initiated until the nasopharyngeal temperature is below 18°C; for longer anticipated periods of arrest, cooling is continued to 13–15°C.[40] At these temperatures circulation has been stopped for up to 2 hours without neurologic problems.[40,45] However, the incidence of stroke in adults and developmental abnormalities in infants correlates with longer arrest times.[40,43,45] Most surgeons try to avoid arrest times over 40 min. Other correlates with postoperative neurologic problems include history of cerebrovascular disease, age, and duration of CPB.

Retrograde cerebral perfusion[46–48] and "total body" retrograde perfusion[49] are adjunctive techniques to protect the brain during operations on the thoracic aorta. Both techniques are used with deep hypothermia. For retrograde cerebral perfusion the superior vena cava is perfused with cold blood at pressures around 25 mm Hg.[50] Blood exits the head via the carotid arteries and provision must be made to prevent back pressure if the aortic arch is not open. For total body retrograde perfusion separate caval catheters are perfused at a total flow of 300–500 mL/min at 13–15°C at pressures below 30 mm Hg.[49]

Cardioplegia

Various methods are employed to protect the myocardium during cardiac operations. Methods vary to some extent on the type of cardiac operation, and perhaps to a greater extent on the surgeon's preference. The most popular method of myocardial protection is cold cardioplegia in which cold blood or crystalloid (4–12°C) is infused antegrade through the aortic root or retrograde through the coronary sinus.[51] If the aortic root is opened, cardioplegia may be delivered directly into the coronary arteries by hand-held catheters. Retrograde cardioplegia uses a special catheter and low-pressure perfusion system to deliver the cardioplegic solution into the coronary sinus. The catheter is soft and has an end hole and a balloon to prevent backflow. Perfusion pressure in the delivery system is monitored and is kept below 40 mm Hg. The active ingredient is potassium, which causes the heart to arrest during diastole. The cold solution and arrest in diastole markedly decreases oxygen demand of the

heart. In addition, the pericardial well is filled with cold (4°C) saline to further cool the heart and surrounding structures. This method renders the heart flaccid and motionless and prevents ischemic damage. Return of electrical activity on the cardiogram or appearance of fibrillatory contractions indicates the need to repeat the infusion of cardioplegic solution. The reintroduction of cold potassium cardioplegic solution by Gay and Ebert in 1973 is an important reason for improved results of open cardiac operations.[52]

Cardioplegic solutions are given through a special perfusion system that uses a roller pump, reservoir, and heat exchanger. The solution is mixed in the reservoir by adding blood, crystalloid, potassium, and other additives to achieve the desired composition (see Chap. 102). Temperature, pressure, and flow rate of the perfusate are closely monitored. Many surgeons also monitor myocardial temperature with a thermistor inserted directly into the heart.

Blood Conservation

The cornerstone of any blood conservation program is meticulous surgical hemostasis; however, some additional techniques are useful. To reduce the risk of blood borne pathogens some patients are able to donate one or two units of their own blood before a scheduled operation. Autologous blood can also be protected from exposure to the heart–lung machine by removing one or two units of heparinized blood shortly before or at the time of starting CPB. This blood is reinfused after cardiopulmonary bypass ends. This blood is fresh and contains normal clotting factors and functioning platelets. Cell-saving devices scavenge shed, nonheparinized blood from the surgical field. A heparin-containing diluent must be added at the tip of the collection catheter to prevent clotting within the system. This blood is washed and centrifuged to prepare packed cells; no other blood constituents are saved by the method. Blood lost from chest tubes after operation may be reinfused directly after filtration[53] or as washed packed cells if the collection and processing are done aseptically. Filtered blood directly infused from chest tubes has few coagulation factors and has high concentrations of fibrinopeptide A.[54] Many open cardiac operations can be performed without the use of homologous blood and blood derivatives. Furthermore, many patients can tolerate postoperative anemias as low as 9 g of hemoglobin without difficulty and can replenish their own red cells within 1 mo if iron is added to their diet.

Dialysis and Ultrafiltration

Hemodialysis and/or ultrafiltration is easily accomplished during CPB.[55] The dialysis or filtration unit is connected to the arterial line of the perfusion system downstream to the pump. Processed blood is returned to the cardiotomy suction reservoir. The dialysate is pumped countercurrent through the unit by a separate pump and perfusion system or pulled through the filtration unit by vacuum. Additional heparin is not required.

Emergency Cardiopulmonary Bypass

In certain emergency situations, partial cardiopulmonary bypass can be rapidly started by cannulation of the femoral artery and vein. Percutaneous techniques using wire guided catheters can be used, but in emergencies usually the vessels are exposed by cutdowns. Heparin must be given (300 U/kg) before cannulas are inserted. Perfusion flow rates are generally limited by the volume of systemic venous blood returning to the heart–lung machine.[5] Preferably the right internal jugular vein can be cannulated and the tip of the cannula placed in the right atrium. Higher flows can be obtained if the cannula reaches the right atrium.[5]

If cardiac arrest or ventricular fibrillation occurs during early stages of operation, before the chest is opened, full bypass can be initiated by accelerating the operation, giving heparin and rapidly cannulating the aorta and right atrium. If pericardial and mediastinal adhesions preempt rapid cannulation, rapid insertion of groin cannulas permits partial bypass until central catheters can be placed. If massive bleeding occurs during the initial dissection, administration of heparin, cannulation of a femoral artery, and aspiration of shed blood by the cardiotomy suction permits partial perfusion until the site of hemorrhage is controlled.

PATHOLOGIC PHYSIOLOGY OF CARDIOPULMONARY BYPASS

Hemodynamics

During CPB blood is circulated without a pulse by a mechanical pump that is independent of physiologic controls. Intravascular pressures stray outside normal ranges. Plasma colloid osmotic pressure is reduced and capillary permeability increases. Many physiologic reflexes are set aside or modified by changes in temperature, acid–base balance, heart rate and volume, and changes in vasomotor tone caused by production and release of a host of vasoactive substances.

Clearly, nonpulsatile flow is abnormal; however, nonpulsatile extracorporeal perfusion is technically easier than pulsatile perfusion. Roller and centrifugal pumps deliver essentially nonpulsatile flow. Pulseless blood flow at 37°C does not alter the distribution of bloodflow from that during pulsatile extracorporeal perfusion,[56] and does not adversely affect calves perfused for 9–34 days.[57] However, various experimental studies suggest that at low bloodflow rates, pulsatile bloodflow improves tissue perfusion and capillary bloodflow over that produced by nonpulsatile flow.[58] Nevertheless no conclusive data indicate that nonpulsatile bloodflow is detrimental for short-term perfusions lasting several hours at recommended flow rates.[58,59]

Cardiopulmonary bypass increases blood flow to the stomach, intestines, and adrenal glands.[60] Pulsatility does not affect the distribution of bloodflow during extracorporeal circulation.[56] Deep perfusion hypothermia does not prevent the increase in stomach, intestinal, and adrenal bloodflow, but causes a decrease in brain and renal bloodflow.[38]

Cardiopulmonary bypass decreases systemic vascular resistance, but there is considerable variability between patients. Deep hypothermia reduces systemic vascular resistance.[61]

Activation of Blood Constituents

Blood mediates most of the morbidity caused by CPB because only blood touches the plastic and metal surfaces of the heart–lung machine. All other organs remain "in-situ." CPB causes massive fluid retention and intercompartmental fluid shifts,[62] multiple organ dysfunction,[63–65] showers of emboli,[66] and unique bleeding complications.[67] Blood elements are activated, plasma proteins are diluted and denatured and contaminants and foreign materials are introduced. A host of vasoactive substances[68] that affect capillary permeability[69] and vasomotor tone are generated. Temporary dysfunction of nearly every organ ensues. A massive defense reaction—aptly termed "the whole body inflammatory response"—is initiated.[70]

Adsorbed Plasma Proteins

When heparinized blood touches a nonendothelial cell surface, plasma proteins are instantly adsorbed onto the surface to produce a protein layer approximately 200 Å thick.[71] The chemical and physical characteristics of the surface influence the amounts and distribution of surface adsorbed proteins, but so far no physical or chemical attribute or attributes predict the molecular topography of the protein mosaic.[72,73] All nonendothelial cell surfaces produce a thrombotic stimulus, but the intensity of the stimulus varies between surfaces. Thromboresistant materials have relatively weaker thrombotic stimuli. Beyond the need for smoothness and chemical inertness, the physical and chemical characteristics of surfaces that reduce the thrombotic stimulus are not defined.

The amounts of adsorbed proteins are not proportional to bulk plasma concentrations. Hydrophobic surfaces adsorb more fibrinogen than hydrophilic materials.[73] Adsorbed fibrinogen, however, rapidly undergoes conformational changes and is partially displaced by an activated form of high-molecular-weight kininogen.[74] Other plasma proteins are also adsorbed. Albumin, Factor XII, prekallikrein, high-molecular-weight kininogen, von Willebrand factor, fibronectin, thrombospondin, hemoglobin, and immunoglobulins all adsorb onto the surface in various amounts that differ between surfaces.[75] A dynamic equilibrium between circulating and adsorbed surface proteins is quickly established for each synthetic material. Over time, adsorbed proteins desorb or are degraded and replaced by new proteins.[75]

Activation of Blood Elements

CPB activates at least five plasma protein systems and five "blood cells" during perfusion of heparinized blood. The vasoactive substances, enzymes, and microemboli produced by activation of these protein systems and cells mediate much of the morbidity associated with CPB.

Contact System

The contact system consists of four primary plasma proteins: Factors XII and XI, prekallikrein, and high-molecular-weight kininogen (HK).[76] When blood contacts a negatively charged surface, Factor XII cleaves into Factor XIIa and Factor XIIf. Prekallikrein and HK must be present. FXIIa cleaves prekallikrein to produce kallikrein. Kallikrein greatly accelerates cleavage of Factor XII in a feedback loop and thus amplifies activation of the contact system. Surface adsorbed proteins provide sufficient negative charges to activate Factor XII. The activated forms of Factor XII directly initiate activation of the intrinsic coagulation pathway, complement, and neutrophils.

Intrinsic Coagulation Pathway

In the presence of HK, Factor XIIa also activates Factor XI, the fourth protein of the contact system. Activation of Factor XI to Factor XIa initiates the intrinsic coagulation pathway that proceeds through Factor IX to activate Factor X. Factor Xa converts prothrombin to thrombin. Thrombin catalyzes the conversion of fibrinogen to fibrin. This pathway provides the major coagulation stimulus during all applications of extracorporeal perfusion technology.

Extrinsic Coagulation Pathway

Until recently the extrinsic coagulation pathway, which is the major pathway that provides hemostasis in wounds, was not considered important during CPB. Although there is overlap of the two pathways,[77] the intrinsic pathway is not particularly involved in wound hemostasis. Open heart operations, however, produce a sizable wound that produces tissue factor. There is evidence that tissue factor is also present in blood aspirated from the pericardial well during CPB.[78] Tissue factor is a integral membrane glycoprotein that is present and expressed on most nonvascular cells and is induced by various agonists in endothelial cells and monocytes. Tissue factor rapidly binds to Factors VII and VIIa to initiate the extrinsic pathway that proceeds to activate Factor X.[77] Factor X, produced by both the intrinsic and extrinsic coagulation pathways, is the gateway protein of the common coagulation pathway.

Complement

The fourth plasma protein system activated during extracorporeal perfusion is the complement system.[79] Like the co-agulation system, two separate pathways activate the gateway complement protein C3 to form C3a and C3b. Factor XIIa, produced by the contact system, activates C1 of the classical pathway. The alternative system, thought to be the principal complement activation pathway during CPB,[79] is activated by generation of C3b by the classical pathway or by hydrolysis of a third bond of C3[80] to produce C3bBb. C3bBb activates C5 to C5a and C5b. C5a directly activates neutrophils and C5b initiates formation of the membrane attack complex that is capable of producing cell lysis and death.

Complement is also activated by the classical pathway[25] which involves C1, C2, and C4 and in sequential steps forms C4b2a. This complex cleaves C3 to form C3a and C3b.[80] C4b2a, with the help of C3b, also activates C5 to form C5a and C5b. The classical pathway proceeds in sequential steps, but the alternative pathway contains a feedback loop that serves to amplify complement activation. Both the alternative and classical pathways are activated during CPB, but amplification of the alternative system predominates.

C3a and terminal complement proteins[79] increase progressively during CPB. Protamine also activates complement.[26] C3a and C5a, produced during CPB, and C4a, produced by the heparin–protamine complex, are anaphylatoxins that have vasoactive properties. C3a impairs cardiac function and C5a activates neutrophils. Complement activation during CPB is associated with significant morbidity.

Fibrinolysis

The fifth plasma protein system activated during CPB is the fibrinolytic system. During CPB, endothelial cells, stimulated by thrombin,[81] produce tissue plasminogen activator (t-PA),[82] which cleaves plasminogen to plasmin. t-PA primarily activates plasminogen adsorbed onto fibrin. Fibrinolysis, as demonstrated by detection of plasma D-dimer,[82] occurs during and after open heart surgery.

Platelets

Platelets are activated during CPB. The degree of activation and the effect of a decrease in platelet numbers and function on bleeding time and wound hemostasis appears to vary between perfusion systems and patients.[83,84]

Platelets are probably activated during CPB by thrombin, but this has not been proved. Once activated, platelets undergo shape change, aggregate, adhere to synthetic surfaces, and release granule contents and cause an increase in bleeding times.[83,84]

During CPB platelets adhere to binding sites located on surface-adsorbed fibrinogen[85] and form aggregates. Platelets also express GMP-140 receptors and form aggregates with circulating monocytes and, to a lesser extent, neutrophils.[86] Both surface adhesion of platelets and platelet aggregation primarily involve the GPIIb/IIIa receptor complex (fibrinogen receptor)[87] and do not involve the GPIb receptor. Platelet adhesion occurs almost instantly,[87] but the density of platelet accumulation varies with the chemical and physical attributes of the surface.[88] Rough surfaces accumulate more platelets than smooth surfaces. As perfusion continues, some adherent platelets detach, leaving behind fragments of platelet membrane.[85] Platelet membrane fragments also detach and circulate.[85,89] Platelet adhesion, platelet aggregation, and blood dilution are the major causes of thrombocytopenia during CPB.

A small percentage of platelets, both attached and circulating, release granule contents. Alpha granules contain several coagulation and chemotactic proteins and factors that increase capillary permeability and smooth muscle cell proliferation. Dense granules contain ADP and ATP, calcium, and serotonin. Lysosomes contain potent acid hydrolases and neutral proteases. Activated platelets also synthesize and release thromboxane A_2, a potent vasoconstrictor and powerful platelet agonist.[90] Thromboxane A_2 has a critical role in platelet hemostasis and a half-life in plasma of approximately 30 seconds. Release of thromboxane A_2 and granular contents contributes to the systemic inflammatory response.

At the end of CPB, the platelet population is a heterogeneous mixture that probably varies between patients and perfusion systems. Hemodilution, adhesion, aggregation, release, and destruction reduce platelet numbers by 30 to 50%.[83,84] Some platelets are intact and discoid and others show pseudopod formation.[84] Some larger platelets recently arrived from the bone marrow are present. Partially and completely degranulated platelets are also present, as are platelet membrane fragments and resealed platelets. The majority of the reduced numbers of platelets appear morphologically normal.[84]

The functional state of the circulating intact platelet during and early after CPB is reduced but it is not clear whether this functional defect is intrinsic or extrinsic to the platelet. Heparin increases bleeding times,[23] but bleeding times remain prolonged for several hours after protamine is given following CPB. Analysis of shed blood from bleeding time wounds shows reduced platelet sensitivity to agonists and reduced concentrations of plasma thromboxane B_2.[23] The relative contributions of extrinsic platelet inhibition and intrinsic change of the circulating platelets during CPB are under active investigation. The end result is an increase in bleeding times during and immediately after CPB.[67,83] Bleeding times usually return to the normal range within 4 to 12 hours.

Neutrophils

During CPB, leukocyte counts decrease in response to dilution and then increase moderately after operation. Only a few neutrophils attach to synthetic surfaces and platelets. Several agonists activate circulating neutrophils during CPB; C3a, C5a,[91] kallikrein, Factor XIIa, and, less strongly, neutrophil-activating peptide 2 (NAP-2) from platelets are all neutrophil agonists. The Mac-1 receptor, which is a cell adhesive protein, is also up-regulated during CPB.[92] Mac-1 (CD11b/18CR3) receptors also bind various

coagulation proteins and may have a role in thrombogenesis.[92]

During CPB, neutrophils release a variety of enzymes and cytotoxic substances including elastase, myeloperoxidase, several lysosomal enzymes, cytotoxic neutral proteases, and reactive chemicals that include hydroxyl radicals, hydrogen peroxide, and hypobromous and hypochlorous acids.[79,93–95] CPB induces activated neutrophils to accumulate in the lungs where they increase capillary permeability and interstitial edema.[63,96] Neutrophils mediate much of the inflammatory response associated with CPB.

Monocytes

Monocytes are also activated activated during CPB. Monocytes produce and release cytokines during and after extracorporeal perfusion. C3b may be a mechanism by which monocytes are activated. Interleukin-8 (IL-8) increases during CPB,[97] and IL-1, Il-2, IL-4, and IL-6 all increase after bypass.[97] Changes in plasma concentrations of tumor necrosis factor (TNF) are not conclusive. Monocytes also express tissue factor and up-regulate Mac-1 receptors during simulated extracorporeal perfusion of human blood.[98]

Endothelial Cells

Endothelial cells are the fourth "blood cell" activated by CPB. Endothelial cells over a surface area estimated to be between 1000 and 5000 m^2 in an adult.[99] Endothelial cells maintain the fluidity of blood, influence vascular tone, and maintain the integrity of the vascular system by active metabolic processes.[99] Endothelial cells produce prostacyclin, heparan sulfate, thrombomodulin, protease nexin 1, protein S, tissue factor pathway inhibitor, and tissue plasminogen activator (t-PA). Endothelial cells also produce vasoactive substances, such as nitrous oxide, PGI_2, endothelin-1,[68,100] and platelet-activating factor (PAF) and inactivate others, such as histamine, norepinephrine, and bradykinin.[99] During CPB, endothelial cells produce t-PA, probably in response to thrombin.[81] Plasminogen activator inhibitor increases only slightly.

Lymphocytes

CPB decreases the total number of lymphocytes and specific subsets of lymphocytes. CPB also inhibits certain T cell functions and the ability of monocytes to present antigen and to synthesize IL-1.[101] Responses to various agonists and mitogens are depressed.[102] Changes in lymphocytes, cytokines, complement proteins, and immunoglobulins and reduced white cell phagocytosis after CPB increase the susceptibility of postoperative patients to infection.

Consequences of Blood Activation during CPB

Bleeding

Nonsurgical bleeding complications associated with CPB are related to heparin, platelets, and fibrinolysis. Deficiency of soluble coagulation factors is a rare cause of bleeding during and after open heart surgery. Bleeding due to reduced plasma coagulation proteins is most likely seen in patients with congenital or acquired coagulation protein deficiencies, uremia, or severe cachexia, and in infants or children with deep cyanosis, polycythemia, and reduced plasma volumes.

Several CPB-related bleeding problems are related to heparin. These include AT-III deficiency, heparin-induced thrombocytopenia, and inadequate heparin neutralization.

Healthy newborns have about one-half adult concentrations of AT-III. Infants with liver disease, cachectic babies, and prematures have even less. If the standard dose of heparin (3 mg/kg) prior to CPB in a cachectic patient fails to increase the activated clotting to over 400 seconds, AT-III deficiency may be the cause. Fresh frozen plasma is all that is required.

Heparin-induced thrombocytopenia (HIT) occurs in 2–5% of the population.[27] In these patients, exposure to heparin, even in "heparin flushes," induces IgG antibodies against the Fc receptor of the platelet membrane.[103] Continued or subsequent exposure to heparin produces thrombocytopenia with platelet counts below 50,000, usually 5 to 10 days after the exposure. The major concern is bleeding; the condition should be distinguished from heparin-induced thrombocytopenia and thrombosis (HITT), which may or may not be related. Treatment of HIT requires stopping heparin and giving platelet transfusions to prevent internal bleeding.

The deficiency in platelet numbers and function after CPB is a major cause of postoperative bleeding. Thrombocytopenia is due to dilution, platelet adhesion to circuit surfaces, aggregation, and activation and removal of damaged platelets by the reticuloendothelial system. At the end of CPB, platelet counts are usually above 100,000 platelets/μL but are 30 to 50% lower than preoperative values.[82,83] Bleeding times are approximately double prebypass values. Over the next few hours, platelet counts do not change consistently, but bleeding times shorten progressively and return to normal within 4–12 hours; platelet counts reach the normal range in 3 to 7 days.

During CPB endothelial cells produce t-PA, which primarily converts fibrin-bound plasminogen to plasmin.[81] Although most plasmin is bound, production of D-dimer[81] indicates that plasmin also circulates. Lysis of bound fibrin tends to increase bleeding. The success of antifibrinolytic agents in reducing postoperative blood losses suggests that fibrinolysis contributes to bleeding. To be effective, antifibrinolytic agents must be given at the beginning of surgery to prevent binding of plasminogen to fibrin.[104]

Emboli and Thrombi

CPB produces a variety of large and small emboli that can be reduced but not totally prevented by filtration[11] (Table 101–1). A 40 μm (pore size) arterial line filter removes macroemboli; filters with smaller pore sizes increase the

TABLE 101–1. EMBOLI

Gas (nitrogen, oxygen)
Fibrin
Fat (free fat, denatured lipoproteins, chylomicrons)
Denatured protein
Platelet aggregates
Leukocyte aggregates
Red cell debris
Foreign material (calcium, tissue debris, fibrin, clot, fat, etc.)
Spallated material (primarily roller pumps)

pressure difference across the filter and interfere with pump flow. During CPB, arterioles, precapillaries, and capillaries are bombarded with microemboli, but cell death is diffusely distributed and involves relatively few cells in any one location. For the most part, microembolization during CPB is not detected, but can be documented.[105]

The majority of particulate emboli are aspirated by cardiotomy suckers and include fibrin, fat, calcium, cellular debris, talc, suture material, and other foreign materials.[11] In addition, aspiration of large quantities of air may result in production of nitrogen-containing microbubbles. Nitrogen is poorly soluble in plasma; therefore, these microbubbles are more dangerous than those of oxygen or carbon dioxide. All blood aspirated from the surgical field must be filtered and allowed to settle to enhance removal of microbubbles.

Blood activation and trauma produce fibrin emboli, macroaggregates of denatured proteins and lipoproteins, fat globules, and platelet and leukocyte aggregates[11,106] The amount is directly proportional to the duration of CPB.[20] Bubble oxygenators produce microbubbles of oxygen.[106] Foreign material also may enter the perfusion system. Homologous blood contains platelet and leukocyte aggregates, fibrin, lipid precipitates, and red cell debris and should be filtered before it is added to the perfusate.[11] Crystalloid solutions may contain inorganic debris, and dust may remain on the inside of commercially produced tubing. Roller pumps may cause spallation of bits of the compressed tubing.[11] Arterial line filters (20–40 m) remove most but not all emboli over 40 μm. Massive air embolism is a rare but catastrophic event.

Thrombosis during CPB can occur if the heparin dose is inadequate. There is no rationale for giving inadequate doses of heparin (activated clotting times < 400 seconds) to reduce bleeding. Such practice risks catastrophic thrombosis and is more likely to increase bleeding than to decrease it.

Heparin-induced thrombocytopenia and thrombosis (HITT) is a rare condition wherein arterial and/or venous thrombosis develops upon exposure to heparin. These patients usually have a history of a thrombotic event with exposure to heparin. When suspected, the diagnosis in the presence of heparin-induced platelet antibodies can be determined by measuring serotonin release or platelet aggregation when the patient's plasma is incubated with donor platelets.[28] Plasma from patients with HIT and HITT both contain heparin-induced antiplatelet antibodies, but it is unclear whether HITT is a severe manifestation of HIT. Patients with heparin-induced antibodies to platelets who require open heart surgery should receive full doses of heparin and one of several strategies to inhibit platelet activation during CPB.[28]

Vasoactive Substances and Endotoxin

CPB initiates a massive defense reaction that results in the production and release of a host of vasoactive hormones, autoacoids, and cytokines[68] (Table 101–2). Most of these potent substances do not normally circulate but act only on local, specific, cellular receptors. However, during CPB vasoactive chemicals circulate[68] and alter blood pressure and distribution, vascular permeability, fluid balance, and myocardial contractility. The massive production and release of vasoactive molecules during CPB mediate the whole body inflammatory response[70] and much of the morbidity associated with open heart surgery.

Endotoxins are structural fragments of bacteria that trigger the body's defense reaction. Lipopolysaccharides derived from the walls of Gram-negative bacteria are particularly powerful agonists. Endotoxins have been detected during CPB using the sensitive but nonspecific limulus amebocyte lysate test.[107] However, at present, the role of endotoxins in the defense reaction associated with CPB is not clearly defined.

Fluid Balance

CPB causes massive fluid retention and intercompartmental fluid shifts. Intermittent or sustained increases in systemic venous pressure raise capillary filtration pressure. Hemodilution dilutes plasma protein concentrations and decreases colloid osmotic pressure. Capillary permeability increases[69] due to circulating vasoactive substances[68] that contract endothelial cells and widen intercellular junctions. The coefficient for Starling's law of fluid exchange across capillaries increases,[69] enabling water, electrolytes, and small molecules to pour into the extracellular compartment. The inter-

TABLE 101–2. VASOACTIVE SUBSTANCES ALTERED DURING EXTRACORPOREAL PERFUSION

Hormones	Autacoids
Epinepherine, norepinepherine	Platelet-activating factor
Renin, angiotensin II	PGI_2, thromboxan A_2, PGE_2
Vasopressin, aldosterone	Endothelin-1, nitric oxide, serotonin, histamine
Atrial natriuretic factor	
Bradykinin	Leukotrienes LTB_4, LTC_4, LTD_4
Glucagon	Proteases
Thyroid: T_3, T_4	Free oxygen radicals
Complement: C3a, C4a, C5a	Lysosomal enzymes, interleukins 1, 2, 4, 6, 8
Electrolytes: Ca^{2+}, Mg^{2+}, K^+	

stitial compartment may increase 18 to 33%.[62] As compared to normothermic perfusions, hypothermia tends to reduce fluid accumulation. CPB does not alter intracellular fluid balance.

The increase in interstitial fluid is restrained by dilution of interstitial proteins and by increases in interstitial fluid pressure. Interstitial fluid pressure is influenced by the rapidity of lymph flow and by the compliance of the interstitial space,[108] which varies for different organs and tissues.

Organ Dysfunction

Heart

It is difficult to separate cardiac dysfunction due to CPB from that due to operative manipulations, the disease being treated, and the early consequences of surgery on ventricular mechanics and myocyte metabolism. However, CPB produces C3a, a negative inotrope,[109] and endothelin-1, which constricts coronary arteries. Intracardiac neutrophils release hydrogen peroxide[110] during and after aortic cross-clamping. Myocardial stunning is inevitable during aortic cross-clamping.[111] Both myocardial edema and distention of the flaccid cardioplegic heart[14] reduce contractility. When the heart contracts poorly, the high afterload produced by CPB during the weaning process increases wall stress and myocardial oxygen consumption.[112] The final performance of the heart depends upon many variables; the damage caused directly by CPB varies.

Lung

CPB temporarily impairs lung function. Activation of complement and neutrophils causes sequestration of neutrophils in the pulmonary microvasculature[113] and an increase in pulmonary capillary permeability. Pulmonary interstitial edema increases. Composition of alveolar surfactant changes[114] and becomes less effective in maintaining alveolar stability. Atelectasis develops and continues to be a problem during the first 48 hours after CPB ends. Functional residual volume and pulmonary compliance decrease.[115] The work of breathing increases. The physiologic shunt and alveolar arterial oxygen difference increase. In occasional patients blood extravasates into alveoli to produce the acute respiratory distress syndrome. Incisional pain, reduced compliance, increased atelectasis, increased work of breathing, increased shunting, and interstitial edema contribute to postoperative pulmonary dysfunction.

Central Nervous System

Cardiopulmonary bypass is associated with a significant incidence of stroke and other neurologic problems. The incidence of stroke ranges between 1 and 5%[116] and is higher in older patients, those with symptomatic carotid arterial disease[117] or with severe atherosclerotic disease of the ascending aorta.[118] The majority of strokes are embolic and related to cannulation, surgical manipulations, and CPB.[117]

Careful neuropsychologic tests demonstrate subtle neurologic injuries in up to 50% of patients.[65,119] In some patients deficits are temporary, but in as many as one-third of these patients, neuropsychologic deficits are still present at 1 year.[119] Microemboli are the most likely cause of these subtle deficits.

Deep hypothermia and circulatory arrest are associated with a significant number of postoperative neurologic injuries. The major causes of injury are ischemia and emboli, but excessive cooling below brain temperatures of 10°–12°C may also cause postoperative neurologic dysfunction.[40,45]

Kidney

Prolonged CPB, hemodilution, circulating hormones, low perfusion pressure, diuretics, hypothermia, microemboli, and hemolysis all affect renal function. Preoperative renal status and periods of low cardiac output after CPB are the most important predictors of postoperative renal insufficiency.[64] Reduced renal perfusion pressure stimulates renin release and angiotensin II production, which decreases renal blood flow. Increased aldosterone and vasopressin raise sodium and water resorption. When plasma binding proteins become saturated from excessive hemolysis, hemoglobin precipitates in renal tubules. Kidneys have high bloodflow and are bombarded with microemboli. Without hemodilution, renal blood and plasma flow, creatinine clearance, free water clearance, and urine volume decrease.[18]

Hemodilution attenuates most of the detrimental effects of CPB on renal function. Hemodilution improves outer cortical and total renal bloodflow, increases creatinine, electrolyte, and water clearances, and increases glomerular filtration and urine volume.[18] After CPB, renal function, which is so important for restoration of fluid balance, largely reflects preoperative renal function, postoperative cardiac output, any toxic drugs given, microemboli, and any ischemic injuries incurred during CPB.

Gastrointestinal Organs

The liver, pancreas, and intestinal tract are subjected to vasoactive substances and microemboli, but few clinical manifestations result. Some liver enzymes increase slightly early after CPB, and mild jaundice appears in 10 to 20% of patients.[120] The connection between CPB and occasional patients who develop severe jaundice and hepatic failure is unclear. Many patients develop a slight increase in blood amylase, but less than 1% of patients develop clinical pancreatitis.[121] Postoperative gastritis, ulcers, and occasional lower GI bleeding are not directly related to CPB. Rare patients may develop a vasculitis of mesenteric vessels that produces severe and often fatal intestinal ischemia postoperatively; this problem may be a late manifestation of a CPB injury.[122]

Other Complications of CPB

Massive Air Embolism

Massive air embolism occurs in 0.1–0.2% of perfused patients, and approximately half of these patients suffer permanent neurologic damage or death.[46,123] Large amounts of air can enter the perfusion system via many different portals. When recognized at operation retrograde cerebral perfusion with hypothermia and venting of the aortic arch may pre-empt permanent injury.[46] Prompt institution of hyperbaric compression also may alleviate some of the permanent sequelae of massive air embolism.

Arterial Catheters

Postoperative bleeding is the most common complication of aortic cannulation. Occasionally an atherosclerotic plaque may be dislodged during cannulation and become an embolus. Aortic dissection is a rare complication of aortic cannulation, but is more common after cannulation of the femoral artery.[124] Insertion of femoral or iliac catheters over guidewires reduces the possibility of dissection or rupture of the vessel. Femoral arterial cannulation may also produce postoperative ischemic complications of the ipsilateral leg and is associated with occasional groin wound infections.

Venous Cannulas

If air enters the venous cannula from a loose connection or from a leak around the cannula at its site of insertion during cardiopulmonary bypass, obstruction to venous return may occur from the air lock. Tubing kinks, forgotten clamps, and obstruction of the intake port of the cannula against the wall of the vein are other causes of obstruction to venous return during cardiopulmonary bypass. Tears in the thin-walled right atrium or cavae occasionally occur and sometimes are difficult to repair. Cannulas in the superior vena cava may partially obstruct venous return before and after bypass and decrease cardiac filling and output.

Pericardial Tamponade

This complication may occur with or without surgical closure of the pericardium. Accumulation of blood around atria and ventricles compromises ventricular filling and contractility and can occur even in the presence of patient mediastinal chest tubes. Reduced cardiac output, increased right atrial pressure (relative to left atrial pressure), blood pressure variation with respiration (pulsus paradoxicus), widening of the mediastinum, and a sudden decrease in mediastinal chest tube drainage raise the possibility of pericardial tamponade in the early postoperative period.

Postpericardiotomy Syndrome

This syndrome is characterized by one or more of the following signs or symptoms: malaise, fever, pericardial effusion, leukocytosis, pleuritic chest pain over the left chest, electrocardiographic abnormalities, and pericardial friction rub. This syndrome typically appears 0.5–2 wk after cardiac surgery, may last 3–5 wk, and is usually self-limited. Most patients respond to nonsteroidal anti-inflammatory compounds, but in more severe cases, steroids may be required. The etiology of the postpericardiotomy syndrome is not clear, but it has been associated with increased viral antibody titers in some patients, particularly children.[125]

CONTROL OF THE COMPLICATIONS OF CPB

The majority of complications of CPB are mediated by blood; it follows, therefore, that these complications can be prevented or attenuated by preventing blood activation and formation of vasoactive substances and microemboli. Two strategies have developed to accomplish this: discover or create surfaces that do not activate blood constituents or temporarily and selectively inhibit key blood elements during the period of CPB to prevent activation by surface contact.[126]

The endothelial cell is the only known nonthrombogenic surface and maintains the fluidity of blood by active metabolic processes. No other cell or surface is nonthrombogenic. Efforts to produce synthetic, nonthrombogenic surfaces for CPB have not succeeded, although a number of "thromboresistant" materials have been developed.[126] Beyond the need for smoothness, no general guidelines for thromboresistivity have been developed.

Heparin can be attached to certain plastic materials by ionic or covalent bonds. With ionic bonds heparin may leach into the circulation; covalent bonds prevent leaching. The commercially available Duraflo II heparin coating (Baxter Health Care Inc.) ionically binds standard heparin using a proprietary process that retards heparin leaching. The competing "Carmeda" (Medtronic Inc.) heparinized surface covalently binds partially degraded heparin attached to "spacer arms" that are about 100 Å long. Surface bound heparin reduces platelet adhesion.[127,128] Macroscopic clotting does not occur and plasma fibrinogen concentrations are not reduced when heparin-coated circuits are used without systemic heparin for up to 7 days in animal perfusions.[129] With full dose heparin, "Carmeda"-coated perfusion circuits reduce complement activation during clinical CPB for myocardial revascularization.[130]

"Carmeda" heparin-coated perfusion circuits have been used for treatment of trauma victims, certain operations on the descending thoracic aorta, postoperative circulatory assistance, and long-term perfusions for respiratory insufficiency.[131] More recently Duraflo II circuits have been used with one-half doses of systemic heparin for clinical myocardial revascularization operations.[132,133] In view of the fact that thrombin is formed during every operation with full doses of heparin, a risk of catastrophic clotting exists.[134] Reduced systemic heparin is not recommended until the ability of surface bound heparin has been shown to reduce concentrations of circulating thrombin.

An alternative strategy is to control activation of blood elements during CPB by selective inhibition of key blood elements. Several reversible platelet inhibitors are available to prevent platelet interaction with the CPB circuit during operations. Dipyridamole weakly inhibits platelet function and can partially preserve platelets during CPB[135]; however, it is not quickly reversible because of a long plasma half-life.[136] The prostaglandins are effective, quickly reversible platelet inhibitors, but are also powerful vasodilators and must be used with continuous infusion of a vasoconstrictor to maintain blood pressure.[137] The disintegrins are reversible, platelet fibrinogen receptor antagonists that inhibit the platelet GPIIb/IIIa receptor to prevent platelet adhesion and aggregation.[138] Temporary inhibition of platelet function by one or more of these drugs during the period of blood contact with the heart-lung machine may preserve platelet numbers and function for hemostasis postoperatively. This strategy is under active clinical investigation.

In 1989 Bidstrup and colleagues introduced aprotinin for cardiac surgery and demonstrated a 50% reduction in postoperative bleeding and a similar reduction in the need for blood and blood product transfusions.[139] They observed that the drug reduced postoperative bleeding times, but had no effect on platelet count.

Aprotinin is a natural serine protease inhibitor that strongly inhibits plasmin and weakly inhibits kallikrein.[140] Plasma concentrations of 4–10 KIU (Kallikrein inhibitory units) of aprotinin completely inhibit plasmin, but 250–400 KIU are required to completely inhibit kallikrein.[140] Clinical doses of aprotinin only partially inhibit kallikrein. Numerous studies have shown that aprotinin reduces fibrinolysis during and after CPB.[141,142] Despite low potency, the drug partially inhibits kallikrein-mediated activation of the intrinsic coagulation pathway, complement, and neutrophils[143] and thus attenuates the "whole body inflammatory response."

Nearly all of the enzymatic proteins of the coagulation and fibrinolytic systems are serine proteases. A large number of reversible and irreversible serine protease inhibitors are known and one or more of these or other inhibitors may prove more efficacious than heparin in controlling the activation of blood elements during CPB. These inhibitors of Factor XIIa, Factor XII fragments, Factor IXa, Factor Xa, kallikrein, Cls, t-PA, plasmin, thrombin, and neutrophil elastase have different rate and binding constants for each target protease. The most inviting targets for selective inhibition are Factors XIIa, kallikrein, and Factor Xa. Complete inhibition of these three serine proteases offers good prospects for attenuating activation of blood elements and the production of vasoactive substances and microemboli during CPB.

Temporary Left Ventricular Assistance

The most common indication for temporary left ventricular assistance is failure to wean from CPB after heart surgery.[144] Other indications include bridging to transplantation and treatment of cardiogenic shock after acute myocardial infarction or other causes of acute cardiac decompensation. The method complements and to some extent competes with long-term extracorporeal life support (ECLS) (formerly called ECMO for extracorporeal membrane oxygenation).

When a patient cannot be weaned from CPB, temporary left ventricular assistance is most easily implemented by inserting a wire wrapped catheter directly into the left atrium through either the left atrial appendage or the junction of the right superior pulmonary vein and left atrium. This catheter is connected to a centrifugal pump, which is connected to either the existing arterial cannula in the ascending aorta or to a new catheter inserted percutaneously or under direct vision into the femoral or iliac artery. The perfusion system consists of the two catheters, a centrifugal pump and a three-way stopcock for adding perfusate. The position of the left atrial catheter is critical for maintenance of flows of 2 to 4.5 L/min. Flows are sensitive to left atrial volume changes and blockage (by the atrial wall) of catheter inlet ports. Volume and flows are adjusted to maintain ejection by the native heart to prevent intracardiac clot formation. Activated clotting times are maintained between 140 and 180 seconds with an infusion of heparin.

ECLS is usually implemented by either percutaneous or direct insertion of a venous and an arterial catheter into the femoral vessels. The system includes a membrane oxygenator. Flow is best if the inlet ports of the venous catheter are in the right atrium.[5] ECLS is used after cardiotomy in patients with biventricular failure.[145]

Mechanical left ventricular assistance reduces left ventricular volumes of dilated, poorly contracting hearts at both end-diastole and at end-systole[146] (Fig. 101–7). In some instances, temporary left ventricular assistance actually improves myocardial contractility in postischemic hearts.[146] In effect, temporary left ventricular assistance "rests" the contracting, ejecting, injured heart and perhaps enhances the prospects for recovery. In contrast, ECLS increases left ventricular wall stress of poorly contracting hearts by increasing afterload[147] (Fig. 101–8). For this reason, ECLS is usually used with an intra-aortic balloon pump, which offsets the increase in afterload.[148]

Temporary left ventricular assistance can be used without thoracotomy. Two methods are available. One method uses a small impellor pump that resides in the descending thoracic aorta.[149] The pump is connected to a soft catheter that traverses the aortic valve and aspirates blood from the left ventricle. The pump is usually introduced into an iliac artery and rotated at approximately 30,000 rpm. Blood from the left ventricle is ejected from the back of the pump into the descending thoracic aorta. Alternatively, a catheter introduced into the jugular or femoral vein is passed across the interatrial septum into the left atrium

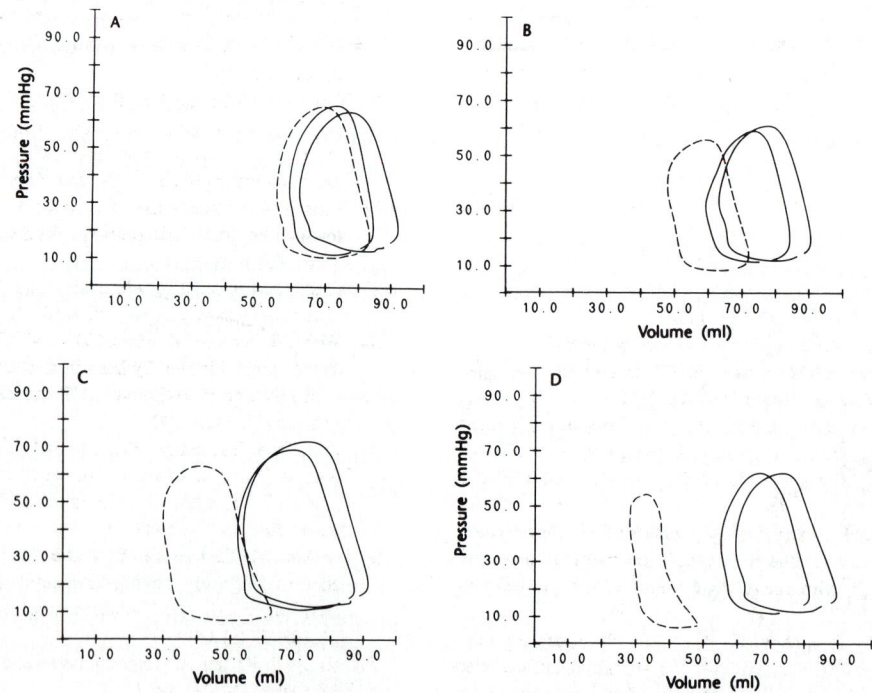

Figure 101–7. The effect of mechanical left ventricular assistance on cardiac pressure–volume loops after cardiac ischemia at flows of 20 (**A**), 40 (**B**), 60 (**C**), and 80 (**D**) mL/kg per minute in sheep. The solid lined loops represent pressure–volume loops immediately before and immediately after initiation of left ventricular assistance (dashed lined loop) at the flow indicated. Note that left ventricular assistance reduces both left ventricular end-systolic and end-diastolic volumes in the poorly contracting heart. (*Reprinted with permission from Ratcliffe et al.[146]*)

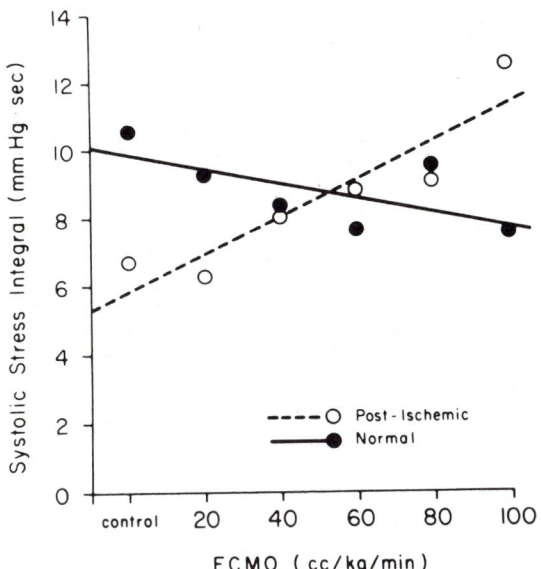

Figure 101–8. Integrated circumferential left ventricular systolic stress (SSI) in ejecting normal and poorly contracting, postischemic sheep hearts is plotted against increasing ECMO flows. Note that SSI decreases with increasing ECMO flow in the normal heart, but increases with increasing flow in the dilated, poorly contracting ischemic heart. *(Reprinted with permission from Bavaria et al.[147])*

using fluroscopy and/or echocardiography.[150] Left atrial blood is pumped using a centrifugal pump into an arterial catheter inserted into either a femoral or iliac artery. Heparin is required to prevent clotting with both methods.

Permanent mechanical circulatory assist devices, the intraaortic balloon pump, long-term ECLS, and the artificial heart are presented in Chapters 108 and 111.

REFERENCES

1. Gibbon JH Jr: Application of a mechanical heart and lung apparatus in cardiac surgery. *Minn Med* **37**:171, 1954
2. Gibbon JH Jr: Personal communication to F.B. Wagner, Jr., 1955
3. Lillehei CW: A personalized history of extracorporeal circulation. *Trans Am Soc Artif Intern Organs* **28**:5–16, 1982
4. Kirklin JW, DuShane JW, Patrick RT, et al: Intracardiac surgery with the aid of a mechanical pump-oxygenator system (Gibbon type): Report of eight cases. *Proc Staff Meet Mayo Clin* **30**:201, 1955
5. Wenger R, Bavaria JE, Ratcliffe MB, Edmunds LH Jr: Flow dynamics of peripheral venous catheters during extracorporeal membrane oxygenation (ECMO) with a centrifugal pump. *J Thorac Cardiovasc Surg* **96**:478–484, 1988
6. High KM, Snider MT, Bashein G: Principles of oxygenator function: Gas exchange, heat transfer, and blood-artificial surface interaction. In Gravlee GP, Davis RF, Utley JR (eds): *Cardiopulmonary Bypass.* Baltimore, Williams & Wilkins, 1993, pp 28–54
7. Hammond GL, Bowley WW: Bubble mechanics and oxygen transfer. *J Thorac Cardiovasc Surg* **71**:422–428, 1976
8. Pearson DT: Gas exchange; bubble and membrane oxygenators. *Sem Thor Cardiovas Surg* **2**:313–319, 1990
9. Weibel ER: Morphometrics of the lung. In *Handbook of Physiology,*

Section 3: *Respiration,* Vol 1. Washington, DC, American Physiologic Society, 1964 pp 285–308
10. May RD, Hackett JE, Crane TN, et al: A clinical evaluation of the Sci-Med Omnitherm and the Travenol normothermic miniprime heat exchangers. *Bull Texas Heart Inst* **6**:85, 1979
11. Edmunds LH Jr, Williams W: Microemboli and the use of filters during cardiopulmonary bypass. In Utley JR (ed): *Pathophysiology and Techniques of Cardiopulmonary Bypass,* Vol 2. Baltimore, Williams & Wilkins, 1983, pp 101–114
12. Dutton RC, Edmunds LH, Jr, Hutchinson JC, et al: Platelet aggregate emboli produced in patients during cardiopulmonary bypass with membrane and bubble oxygenators and blood filters. *J Thorac Cardiovasc Surg* **67**:258–265, 1974
13. Harshbarger HG, Kirklin JW, Donald DE: Studies in extracorporeal circulation: IV. Surgical techniques. *Surg Gyn Obstet* **106**:111, 1958
14. Downing SW, Savage EB, Streicher JS, et al: The stretched ventricle: Myocardial creep and contractile dysfunction after acute nonischemic ventricular distention. *J Thor Cardiovas Surg* **104**:996–1005, 1992
15. Ansell J, Parilla N, King M, et al: Survival of autotransfused red blood cells recovered from the surgical field during cardiovascular operations. *J Thorac Cardiovasc Surg* **84**:387–391, 1982
16. Anderson RP, Nolan SP, Edmunds LH Jr, et al: Cardiovascular perfusion: Evolution to allied health profession and status, 1986. *J Thorac Cardiovasc Surg* **92**:790–794, 1986
17. Housman L: Blood conservation during cardiopulmonary bypass. In Utley JR (ed): *Pathophysiology and Techniques of Cardiopulmonary Bypass,* Vol 2. Baltimore, Williams & Wilkins, 1983, pp 101–114
18. Utley JR: Renal function and fluid balance with cardiopulmonary bypass. In Gravlee GP, Davis RF, Utley JR (eds): *Cardiopulmonary Bypass.* Baltimore, Williams & Wilkins, 1993, pp 488–508
19. Olson ST, Bjork I: Predominant contribution of surface approximation to the mechanism of heparin acceleration of the antithrombin-thrombin reaction. *J Biol Chem* **266**:6353–6362, 1991
20. Brister SJ, Ofosu FA, Buchanan MR: Thrombin generation during cardiac surgery: Is heparin the ideal anticoagulant? *Thromb Haemost* **70**:259–262, 1993
21. Boisclair MD, Lane DA, Philippou H et al: Thrombin production, inactivation and expression during open heart surgery measured by assays for activation fragments including a new ELISA for prothrombin Fragment F1+2. *Thromb Haemost* **70**:253–258, 1993
22. Ellison N, Edmunds LH Jr, Colman RW: Platelet aggregation following heparin and protamine administration. *Anesthesiology* **48**:65–68, 1978
23. Kestin AS, Valeri CR, Khuri SF, et al: The platelet function defect of cardiopulmonary bypass. *Blood* **82**:107–117, 1993
24. Weitz JI, Hudoba M, Massel D, et al: Clot-bound thrombin is protected from inhibition by heparin-antithrombin III but is susceptible to inactivation by antithrombin III-independent inhibitors. *J Clin Invest* **86**:385–391, 1990
25. Wachfogel YT, Harpel PC, Edmunds LH Jr, Colman RW: Formation of Cls-Cl-inhibitor, kallikrien-Cl-inhibitor and plasmin-alpha 2-plasmin inhibitor complexes during cardiopulmonary bypass. *Blood* **73**:468–471, 1989
26. Kirklin JK, Chenoweth DE, Naftel DC, et al: Effects of protamine administration after cardiopulmonary bypass on complement, blood elements, and the hemodynamic state. *Ann Thorac Surg* **41**:193–199, 1986
27. King DJ, Kelton JG: Heparin-associated thrombocytopenia. *Ann Int Med* **100**:535–540, 1984
28. Kappa JR, Fisher CA, Bell P, et al: Intraoperative management of patients with heparin-induced thrombocytopenia. *Ann Thorac Surg* **49**:713–723, 1990
29. Bull BS, Korpman RA, Huse WM, et al: Heparin therapy during extracorporeal circulation: Problems inherent in existing heparin protocols. *J Thorac Cardiovasc Surg* **69**:674–684, 1975

30. Hunt BJ, Segal HC, Yacoub M: Guidelines for monitoring heparin by the activated clotting time when aprotinin is used during cardiopulmonary bypass. *J Thor Cardiovas Surg* **103**:211–212, 1992

31. Bull BS, Huse WM, Brauer FS, et al: Heparin therapy during extracorporeal circulation: The use of a drug response curve to individualize heparin and protamine dosage. *J Thorac Cardiovasc Surg* **69**:685, 1975

32. Shapira N, Schaff HV, Piehler JM, et al: Cardiovascular effects of protamine sulfate in man. *J Thor Cardiovasc Surg* **84**:505–514, 1982

33. Weiss ME, Nyhan D, Peng Z, et al: Association of protamine IgE and IgG antibodies with life-threatening reactions to intravenous protamine. *N Engl J Med* **320**:886–892, 1989

34. Lowenstein E, Johnston WE, Lappis DG, et al: Catastrophic pulmonary vasoconstriction associated with protamine reversal of heparin. *Anesthesiology* **59**:470–473, 1983

35. Davies LK: Hypothermia: Physiology and clinical use. In Gravlee GP, Davis RF, Utley JR (eds): *Cardiopulmonary Bypass*. Baltimore, Williams & Wilkins, 1993, pp 140–154

36. Hickey RF, Hoar PF: Whole-body oxygen consumption during low-flow hypothermic cardiopulmonary bypass. *J Thorac Cardiovasc Surg* **86**:903–906, 1983

37. Stockard JJ, Bickford RB, Schnauble JF: Pressure-dependent cerebral ischemia during cardiopulmonary bypass. *Neurology* **23**:521, 1973

38. Rudy LW Jr, Boucher JK, Edmunds LH Jr: The effect of deep hypothermia and circulatory arrest on the distribution of systemic blood flow in rhesus monkeys. *J Thorac Cardiovasc Surg* **64**:706–712, 1972

39. Christakis GT, Koch JP, Deemar KA, et al: A randomized study of the systemic effects of warm heart surgery. *Ann Thor Surg* **54**:449–459, 1992

40. Griepp RB, Ergin MA, Lansman SL, et al: The physiology of hypothermic arrest. *Sem Thorac Cardiovasc Surg* **3**:188–193, 1991

41. Ekroth R, Thompson RJ, Lincoln C, et al: Elective deep hypothermia with total circulatory arrest: Changes in plasma creatine kinase BB, blood glucose, and clinical variables. *J Thorac Cardiovasc Surg* **97**:30–35, 1989

42. Swan H: The importance of acid-base management for cardiac and cerebral preservation during open heart operations. *Surg Gynecol Obstet* **158**:391–414, 1984

43. Jonas RA, Bellinger DC, Rappapost LA, et al: Relation of pH strategy and developmental outcome after hypothermic circulatory arrest. *J Thorac Cardiovasc Surg* **106**:362–368, 1993

44. DeLeon S, Ilbawi M, Arcilla R, et al: Choreoathetosis after deep hypothermia without circulatory arrest. *Ann Thorac Surg* **50**:714–719, 1990

45. Svensson LG, Crawford ES, Hess KR, et al: Deep hypothermia with circulatory arrest. *J Thorac Cardiovasc Surg* **106**:19–31, 1993

46. Mills NL, Ochsner JL: Massive air embolism during cardiopulmonary bypass. *J Thorac Cardiovasc Surg* **80**:708–717, 1980

47. Lemole GM, Strong MD, Spagna PM, Karmilowicz P: Improved results for dissecting aneurysms. *J Thorac Cardiovasc Surg* **82**:249–255, 1982

48. Ueda Y, Miki S, Kusuhara K, et al: Surgical treatment of aneurysm of dissection involving the ascending aorta and aortic arch, utilizing circulatory arrest and retrograde cerebral perfusion. *J Cardiovasc Surg* **31**:553–558, 1990

49. Yasuura K, Okamoto H, Ogawa Y, et al: Resection of aortic aneurysms without aortic clamp technique with the aid of hypothermic total body retrograde perfusion. *J Thorac Cardiovasc Surg* **107**:1237–1243, 1994

50. Usui A, Hotta T, Hiroura M, et al: Retrograde cerebral perfusion through a superior vena caval cannula protects the brain. *Ann Thorac Surg* **53**:47–53, 1992

51. Guiraudon GM, Campbell CS, McLellan DG, et al: Retrograde coronary sinus versus aortic route perfusion with cold cardioplegia: randomized study of levels of cardiac enzymes in 40 patients. *Circulation* **74**(Suppl III): III105–III115, 1986

52. Gay WA Jr, Ebert PA: Functional, metabolic and morphological effects of potassium-induced cardioplegia. *Surgery* **54**:193, 1976

53. Schaff HV, Hauer JH, Bell WR, et al: Autotransfusion of shed mediastinal blood after cardiac surgery. *J Thorac Cardiovasc Surg* **75**:632–641, 1978

54. Hartz RS, Smith JA, Green D: Autotransfusion after cardiac operation. *J Thorac Cardiovasc Surg* **96**:178–182, 1988

55. Moore RA, Laub GW: Hemofiltration, dialysis, and blood salvage techniques during cardiopulmonary bypass. In Gravlee GP, Davis RF, Utley JR (eds): *Cardiopulmonary Bypass*. Baltimore, Williams & Wilkins, 1993, p 93–123

56. Boucher JK, Rudy LW, Edmonds LH Jr: Organ blood flow during pulsatile cardiopulmonary bypass. *J Appl Physiol* **36**:86–90, 1974

57. Golding LR, Jacob G, Groves LK, et al: Clinical results of mechanical support of the failing left ventricle. *J Thorac Cardiovasc Surg* **83**:597, 1982

58. Philbin DM: Pulsatile blood flow. In Gravlee GP, Davis RF, Utley JR (eds): *Cardiopulmonary Bypass*. Baltimore, Williams & Wilkins, 1993, pp 323–339

59. Edmunds LH Jr: Pulseless cardiopulmonary bypass. *J Thorac Cardiovasc Surg* **84**:800–804, 1982

60. Rudy LW Jr, Heymann MA, Edmunds LH Jr: Distribution of systemic blood flow during cardiopulmonary bypass. *J Appl Physiol* **34**:194–200, 1973

61. Kirklin JW, Barratt-Boyes BG: *Cardiac Surgery*. New York, Churchill Livingstone, 1993

62. Pacifico AD, Digerness S, Kirklin JW: Acute alterations of body composition after open intracardiac operations. *Circulation* **41**:331–341, 1970

63. Ratliff NB, Young WG Jr, Hackel D, et al: Pulmonary injury secondary to extracorporeal circulation; An ultrastructural study. *J Thorac Cardiovasc Surg* **65**:425–432, 1973

64. Abel RM, Buckley MJ, Austen WG, et al: Etiology, incidence and prognosis of renal failure following cardiac operations: Results of a prospective analysis of 500 consecutive patients. *J Thorac Cardiovasc Surg* **71**:32–43, 1976

65. Shaw PJ, Bates D, Aartidge NEF, et al: Neurologic and neuropsychological morbidity following major surgery: Comparison of coronary artery bypass and peripheral vascular surgery. *Stroke* **18**:700–707, 1987

66. Kurusz M, Butler BD: Embolic events and cardiopulmonary bypass. In Gravlee GP, Davis RF, Utley JR (eds): *Cardiopulmonary Bypass*. Baltimore, Williams & Wilkins, 1993, pp 267–290

67. Woodman RC, Harker LA: Bleeding complications associated with cardiopulmonary bypass. *Blood* **76**:1680–1697, 1990

68. Downing SW, Edmunds LH Jr: Release of vasoactive substances during cardiopulmonary bypass. *Ann Thorac Surg* **54**:1236–1243, 1992

69. Smith EEJ, Naftel DC, Blackstone EH, Kirklin JW: Microvascular permeability after cardiopulmonary bypass. *J Thorac Cardiovasc Surg* **94**:225–233, 1987

70. Blackstone EH, Kirklin JW, Stewart RW, Chenoweth DE: The damaging effects of cardiopulmonary bypass. In Wu KK, Roxy EC (eds): *Prostaglandins in Clinical Medicine: Cardiovascular and Thrombotic Disorders*. Chicago, Yearbook Medical Publishers, 1982, pp 355–369

71. Baier RE, Dutton RC: Initial events in interactions of blood with a foreign surface. *J Biomed Mater Res* **3**:191–206, 1969

72. Baier RE: The organization of blood components near interfaces. In Vroman L, Leonard EF (eds): *The Behavior of Blood and Its Components at Interfaces. Ann NY Acad Sci* **283**:17–36, 1977

73. Uniyal S, Brash JL: Patterns of adsorption of proteins from human plasma onto foreign surfaces. *Thromb Haemost* **47**:285–290, 1982

74. Brash JL, Scott CF, ten Hove P, et al: Mechanism of transient ad-

sorption of fibrinogen from plasma to solid surfaces: Role of the contact and fibrinolytic systems. *Blood* **71:**932–939, 1988

75. Ziats NP, Pankowsky DA, Tierney BP, et al: Adsorption of Hageman factor (factor XII) and other plasma proteins to biomedical polymers. *J Lab Clin Med* **116:**687–696, 1990

76. Colman RW: Surface-mediated defense reactions: The plasma contact activation system. *J Clin Invest* **73:**1249–1253, 1984

77. Edgington TS, Mackman N, Brand K, Ruf W: The structural biology of expression and function of tissue factor. *Thromb Haemost* **66:**67–79, 1991

78. Tabuchi N, de Haan J, Boonstra PW, van Overen W: Activation of fibrinolysis in the pericardial cavity during cardiopulmonary bypass. *J Thorac Cardiovasc Surg* **106:**828–833, 1993

79. Chenoweth DE, Cooper SW, Hugli TE, et al: Complement activation during cardiopulmonary bypass: Evidence for generation of C3a and C5a anaphylatoxins. *N Engl J Med* **304:**497–503, 1981

80. Sims PJ: Plasma proteins: Complement. In Hoffman R, Benz EJ, Jr, Shatteil SJ, et al: *Hematology.* New York, Churchill Livingstone, 1991, pp 1582–1591

81. Levin EG, Marzec U, Anderson J, Harker LA: Thrombin stimulates tissue plasminogen activator release from cultured human endothelial cells. *J Clin Invest* **74:**1988–1995, 1984

82. Gram J, Janetzko T, Jespersen J, Bruhn HD: Enhanced effective fibrinolysis following the neutralization of heparin in open heart surgery increases the risk of post-surgical bleeding. *Thromb Haemost* **63:**241–245, 1990

83. Edmunds LH Jr, Ellison N, Colman RW, et al: Platelet function during open heart surgery: Comparison of the membrane and bubble oxygenators. *J Thorac Cardiovasc Surg* **83:**805–812, 1982

84. Zilla P, Fasol R, Groscurth P, et al: Blood platelets in cardiopulmonary bypass operations. *J Thorac Cardiovasc Surg* **97:**379–388, 1989

85. Wenger RK, Lukasiewicz H, Mikuta BS, et al: Loss of platelet fibrinogen receptors during clinical cardiopulmonary bypass. *J Thorac Cardiovasc Surg* **97:**235–239, 1989

86. Rinder CS, Bonan JL, Rinder HM, et al: Cardiopulmonary bypass induces leukocyte-platelet adhesion. *Blood* **79:**1201–1205, 1992

87. Gluszko P, Rucinski B, Musial J, et al: Fibrinogen receptors in platelet adhesion to surfaces of extracorporeal circuit. *Am J Physiol* **252:**H615–621, 1987

88. Salzman EW, Lindon J, Brier D: Surface-induced platelet adhesion, aggregation and release. In Vroman L, Leonard E (eds): *The Behavior of Blood and Its Components in Interfaces. Ann NY Acad Sci.* 114–127, 1977

89. George JN, Pickett EB, Sauderman S, et al: Platelet surface glycoproteins: Studies on resting and activated platelets and platelet membrane microparticles in normal subjects, and observations in patients during adult respiratory distress syndrome and cardiac surgery. *J Clin Invest* **78:**340–348, 1986

90. Faymonville ME, Deby-Dupont G, Larbuisson R, et al: Prostaglandin E2, prostacyclin, and thromboxane changes during nonpulsatile cardiopulmonary bypass in humans. *J Thorac Cardiovasc Surg* **91:**858–866, 1986

91. Hammerschmidt DE, Stroncek DF, Bowers TK, et al: Complement activation and neutropenia during cardiopulmonary bypass. *J Thorac Cardiovasc Surg* **81:**370–377, 1981

92. Kappelmayer J, Bernabei A, Gikakis N, et al: Upregulation of Mac-1 surface expression on neutrophils during simulated extracorporeal circulation. *J Lab Clin Med* **121:**118–126, 1993

93. Wachtfogel YT, Kucich U, Greenplate J, et al: Human neutrophil degranulation during extracorporeal circulation. *Blood* **69:**324–330, 1987

94. Faymonville ME, Pincemail J, Duchateau MD, et al: Myeloperoxidase and elastase as markers of leukocyte activation during cardiopulmonary bypass in humans. *J Thorac Cardiovasc Surg* **103:**309–317, 1991

95. Craddock PR, Fehr J, Brigham KL, et al: Complement and leuko-

cyte-mediated pulmonary dysfunction in hemodialysis. *N Engl J Med* **296:**769–774, 1977

96. Finn A, Naik S, Klein N, et al: Interleukin-8 release and neutrophil degranulation after pediatric cardiopulmonary bypass. *J Thorac Cardiovasc Surg* **105:**234–241, 1993

97. Steinberg JB, Kapelanski DP, Olson JD, Weiler JM: Cytokine and complement levels in patients undergoing cardiopulmonary bypass. *J Thorac Cardiovasc Surg* **106:**1008–1016, 1993

98. Kappelmayer J, Bernabei A, Edmunds LH Jr, et al: Tissue factor is expressed on monocytes during simulated extracorporeal circulation. *Circ Res* **72:**1075–1081, 1993

99. Jaffe EA: Endothelial cell structure and function. In Hoffman R, Benz EJ Jr, Shatteil SJ, et al (eds): *Hematology.* New York, Churchill Livingstone, 1991, pp 1198–1213

100. Vane JR, Anggard EE, Botting RM: Regulatory functions of the vascular endothelium. *N Engl J Med* **323:**27–36, 1990

101. Markewitz A, Faist E, Lang S, et al: Successful restoration of cell-mediated immune respose after cardiopulmonary bypass by immunomodulation. *J Thorac Cardiovasc Surg* **105:**15–24, 1993

102. DePalma L, Yu M, McIntosh CL, et al: Changes in lymphocyte subpopulations as a result of cardiopulmonary bypass. *J Thorac Cardiovasc Surg* **101:**240–244, 1991

103. Kelton JG, Sheridan D, Santos A, et al: Heparin-induced thrombocytopenia: laboratory studies. *Blood* **72:**925–930, 1988

104. Horrow JC: Management of coagulopathy associated with cardiopulmonary bypass. In Gravlee GP, Davis RF, Utley JR (eds): *Cardiopulmonary Bypass.* Baltimore, Williams & Wilkins, 1993, pp 436–466

105. Blauth CI, Smith PL, Arnold JV, et al: Influence of oxygenator type on the prevalence and extent of microembolic retinal ischemia during cardiopulmonary bypass. *J Thorac Cardiovasc Surg* **99:**61–69, 1990

106. Clark RE, Magraf HW, Beauchamp RA: Fat and solid filtration in clinical perfusion. *Surgery* **77:**216–224, 1975

107. Nilsson L, Kulander L, Nystrom S-O, Eriksson O: Endotoxins in cardiopulmonary bypass. *J Thorac Cardiovasc Surg* **100:**777–780, 1990

108. Menninger FJ III, Rosenkranz ER, Utley JR, et al: Interstitial hydrostatic pressure in patients undergoing CABG and valve replacement. *J Thorac Cardiovasc Surg* **79:**181–187, 1980

109. Del Balza UH, Levi R, Polley MJ: Cardiac dysfunction caused by purified human C3a anaphylatoxin. *Proc Natl Acad Sci USA* **82:**886–890, 1985

110. Ko W, Hawes AS, Lazenby WD, et al: Myocardial reperfusion injury. *J Thorac Cardiovasc Surg* **102:**297–308, 1991

111. Bavaria JE, Furakawa S, Kreiner G, et al: Myocardial oxygen utilization after reversible global ischemia. *J Thorac Cardiovasc Surg* **100:**210–220, 1990

112. Bavaria JE, Ratcliffe MB, Gupta KB, et al: Changes in left ventricular systolic wall stress during biventricular circulatory assistance. *Ann Thorac Surg* **45:**526–532, 1988

113. Westby S: Complement and the damaging effects of cardiopulmonary bypass. *Thorax* **38:**321–325, 1983

114. McGowan FX, del Nido PJ, Kurland G, et al: Cardiopulmonary bypass significantly impairs surfactant activity in children. *J Thorac Cardiovasc Surg* **106:**968–977, 1993

115. Sladen RN, Berkowity DE: Cardiopulmonary bypass and the lung. In Gravlee GP, Davis RF, Utley JR (eds): *Cardiopulmonary Bypass.* Baltimore, Williams & Wilkins, 1993, pp 468–487

116. Tuman KJ, McCarthy RJ, Najafi H, Ivankovich AD: Differential effects of advanced age on neurologic and cardiac risks of coronary artery operations. *J Thorac Cardiovasc Surg* **104:**1510–1517, 1992

117. Clark RE, Davis DA, Lovell MR, et al: Microemboli during CABG. Genesis and effect on outcome. *J Thorac Cardiovas Surg* (in press)

118. Blauth CI, Cosgrove DM, Webb BW, et al: Atheroembolism from the ascending aorta. *J Thorac Cardiovasc Surg* **103:**1104–1112, 1992

119. Rogers AT, Newman SP, Stump DA, Prough DS: Neurologic effects of cardiopulmonary bypass. In Gravlee GP, Davis RF, Utley JR (eds): *Cardiopulmonary Bypass.* Baltimore, Williams & Wilkins, 1993, pp 542–576

120. Collins JD, Ferner R, Murray A, et al: Incidence and prognostic importance of jaundice after cardiopulmonary bypass surgery. *Lancet* 1:1119–1123, 1983

121. Fernandez-del Castillo C, Harringer W, Warshaw AL, et al: Risk factors for pancreatic cellular injury after cardiopulmonary bypass. *N Engl J Med* 325:382–387, 1991

122. Leitman IM, Paull DE, Barie PS, et al: Intra-abdominal complications of cardiopulmonary bypass operations. *Surg Gynecol Obstet* 165:251–254, 1987

123. Stoney WS, Alford WC, Burrus GR, et al: Air embolism and other accidents using pump oxygenators. *Ann Thorac Surg* 29:336, 1980

124. Salerno TA, Lince DP, White DN, et al: Arch versus femoral perfusion during cardiopulmonary bypass. *J Thorac Cardiovasc Surg* 76:681, 1978

125. Engle MA, Klein AA, Hepner S: The post-pericardiotomy and similar syndromes. *Cardiovasc Clin* 7:211, 1976

126. Edmunds LH Jr: The sangreal. *J Thorac Cardiovasc Surg* 90:1–6, 1985

127. Lindon JN, Salzman EW, Merrill EW, et al: Catalytic activity and platelet reactivity of heparin covalently bonded to surfaces. *J Lab Clin Med* 105:219–226, 1985

128. Stenach N, Korn RL, Fisher CA, et al: The effects of heparin bound surface modification (Carmeda Bioactive Surface) on human platelet alterations during simulated extracorporeal circulation. *J Am Soc Extracorpor Technol* 24:97–102, 1992

129. Mottaghy K, Oedekoven B, Poppel K, et al: Heparin free long-term extracorporeal circulation using bioactive surfaces. *Trans Am Soc Artif Intern Organs* 35:635–637, 1989

130. Videm V, Svennevig JL, Fosse E, et al: Reduced complement activation with heparin-coated oxygenator and tubings in coronary bypass operations. *J Thorac Cardiovasc Surg* 103:806–813, 1992

131. Anderson HL III, Delius RE, Sinard JM, et al: Early experience with adult extracorporeal membrane oxygenation in the modern era. *Ann Thorac Surg* 53:553–563, 1992

132. Borowiec J, Thelin S, Bagge L, et al: Decreased blood loss after cardiopulmonary bypass using heparin-coated circuit and 50% reduction of heparin dose. *Scand J Thorac Cardiovasc Surg* 26:177–185, 1992

133. von Segesser LK, Weiss BM, Garcia E, Turina MI: Risk and benefit of low systemic heparinization during open heart surgery. *Ann Thorac Surg* (in press)

134. Cheung AT, Levin SK, Weiss SJ, et al: Intracardiac thrombus: A risk of incomplete anticoagulation for cardiac operations. *Ann Thorac Surg,* (in press)

135. Teoh KH, Christakis GT, Weisel RD, et al: Dipyridamole preserved platelets and reduced blood loss after cardiopulmonary bypass. *J Thorac Cardiovasc Surg* 96:332–341, 1988

136. FitzGerald GA: Dipyridamole. *N Engl J Med* 316:1247–1257, 1987

137. Musial J, Niewiarowski S, Rucinski B, et al: Inhibition of platelet adhesion to surfaces of extracorporeal circuits by disintegrins. *Circulation* 82:261–273, 1990

138. Niewiarowski S, Edmunds LH Jr: Invited letter concerning: Fibrinogen receptor antagonists in cardiopulmonary bypass. *J Thorac Cardiovas Surg* 106:931–933, 1993

139. Bidstrup BP, Royston D, Sapsford RN, Taylor KM: Reduction in blood loss and blood use after cardiopulmonary bypass with high dose aprotinin (Trasylol). *J Thorac Cardiovasc Surg* 97:364–372, 1989

140. Gallimore MJ, Fuhrer G, Heller W, Hoffmeister HE: Augmentation of kallikrein and plasmin inhibition capacity by aprotinin using a new assay to monitor therapy. *Adv Exp Med Biol* 247B:55–60, 1989

141. Blauhut B, Klima U, Bettelheim P, et al: Comparison of the effects of aprotinin and tranexamic acid on blood loss and related variables following cardiopulmonary bypass. *J Thorac Cardiovasc Surg* 108:1083–1091, 1994

142. Lu H, Soria C, Commin P-L, et al: Hemostasis in patients undergoing extracorporeal circulation: The effect of aprotinIn (Trasylol). *Thromb Haemost* 66:633–637, 1991

143. Wachtfogel YT, Kucich U, Hack CE, et al: Aprotinin inhibits the contact, neutrophil, and platelet activation systems during simulated extracorporeal perfusion. *J Thorac Cardiovasc Surg* 106:1–10, 1993

144. Pae WE Jr, Miller CA, Matthews Y, Pierce WS: Ventricular assist devices for postcardiotomy cardiogenic shock. *J Thorac Cardiovasc Surg* 104:541–543, 1992

145. Magovern GJ Jr, Magovern JA, Benckart DH, et al: Extrascorporeal membrane oxygenation: Preliminary results in patients with postcardiotomy cardiogenic shock. *Ann Thorac Surg* 57:1462–1471, 1994

146. Ratcliffe MB, Bavaria JE, Wenger RK, et al: Left ventricular mechanics of ejecting, postischemic hearts during left ventricular circulatory assistance. *J Thorac Cardiovasc Surg* 101:245–255, 1991

147. Bavaria JE, Ratcliffe MB, Gupta KB, et al: Changes in left ventricular wall stress during biventricular circulatory assistance. *Ann Thorac Surg* 45:526–532, 1988

148. Bavaria JE, Furukawa S, Kreiner G, et al: Effect of circulatory assist devices on stunned myocardium. *Ann Thorac Surg* 49:123–128, 1990

149. Wampler RK, Frazier OH, Lansing AM, et al: Treatment of cardiogenic shock with the hemopump left ventricular assist device. *Ann Thorac Surg* 52:506–513, 1991

150. Edmunds LH Jr, Hermann HC, DiSesa VJ, et al: Left ventricular assist without thoracotomy: Clinical experience with the Dennis method. *Ann Thorac Surg* 57:880–885, 1994

102

Myocardial Protection Management During Adult Cardiac Operations

Gerald D. Buckberg and Bradley S. Allen

Perioperative myocardial damage remains the most common cause of morbidity and death following technically successful cardiac operations. Despite major advances in the surgical correction of acquired and congenital cardiac disease, as many as 90% of patients who do not survive the perioperative period show, at postmortem examination, varying combinations of gross, microscopic, or histochemical myocardial necrosis, which is most severe in the subendocardium of the left or right ventricle, depending on which chamber is affected by the basic cardiac lesion.[1-3] This necrosis occurs in the absence of coronary artery obstruction and may affect the entire ventricular shell in patients with valvular and congenital heart disease, as well as areas of myocardium supplied by patent grafts following myocardial revascularization. Patients suffering from intraoperative myocardial damage may require inotropic drugs or balloon counterpulsation support in the early perioperative hours, and may go on to develop late myocardial fibrosis despite a seemingly "uneventful" postoperative convalescence (Fig. 102–1).

This chapter details the recent progress in myocardial protection during cardiac operations that has allowed a significant reduction in perioperative injury. In our view, such damage is caused by an imbalance between myocardial energy supply and demand that reflects cumulative effects of unfavorable alterations in the supply–demand balance occurring before, during, and after extracorporeal circulation. Understandably, the major emphasis of the surgeon has been and will remain directed toward events occurring during extracorporeal circulation, especially during the necessary time that the heart must be arrested to provide a quiet, bloodless field during which the surgeon can work. It must be realized, however, that the avoidance of perioperative myocardial damage requires the coordinated efforts of the anesthesiologist and cardiologist who actively control hemodynamic events before and after extracorporeal circulation. The vital importance of this collaborative effort is emphasized by reports showing enzymatic signs of myocardial necrosis developing before extracorporeal circulation[4] as well as the knowledge gained from coronary care units showing that careful control of hemodynamic events after infarction can either decrease or increase its extent.

VULNERABILITY TO ISCHEMIC DAMAGE

Left ventricular subendocardial muscle is the most susceptible region of the left ventricle to ischemia[5] because it can receive its blood (oxygen) supply only during diastole; intramyocardial vessels are squeezed shut during systole. Conversely, the outer shell of the left ventricle and the normal right ventricle have lower compressive forces and can be perfused throughout the cardiac cycle. In normal hearts, coronary arteries can dilate and adjust flow (autoregulate) to meet oxygen needs; the reactive hyperemic response following transient coronary artery occlusion provides evidence of this vasodilator reserve capacity. When subendocardial vessels dilate maximally (in response to increased oxygen needs, reduced blood pressure, or lowered oxygen content), blood supply to subendocardial muscle becomes

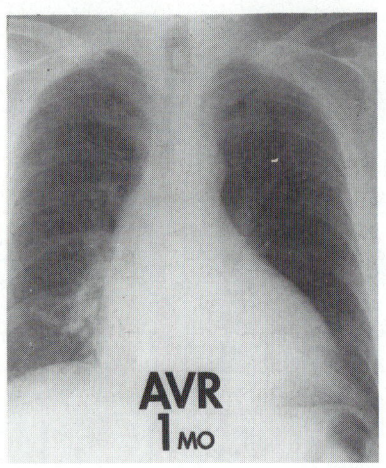
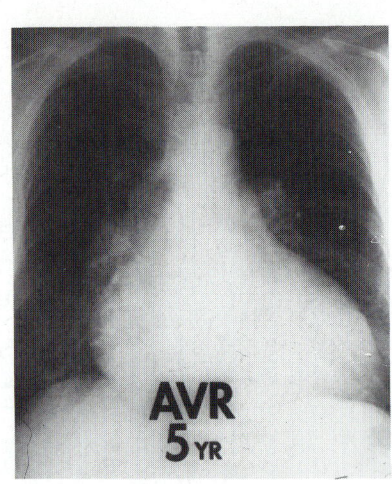

Figure 102–1. Postoperative x-rays films 1 mo and 5 years following technically successful aortic valve replacement (AVR), in a patient who developed late postoperative low output syndrome. Note the marked increase in cardiac silhouette at 5 years, despite a normally functioning mechanical prosthesis. The ejection fraction at time of this film was 0.19, where as it had been 0.50 preoperatively.

determined by the diastolic coronary driving pressure (aortic diastolic pressure) and the diastolic duration. We have shown previously[6] that the diastolic pressure–time index (DPTI = the area between aortic diastolic and left atrial or pulmonary artery wedge pressure curves in diastole) provides a reasonable bedside and catheterization laboratory estimate of potential subendocardial flow, and the product of DPTI × oxygen content predicts potential oxygen supply[7] (Fig. 102–2).

To assess the adequacy of bloodflow, however, we must know not only how much oxygen is supplied (blood flow × oxygen content), but how much is needed. The area beneath the left ventricular systolic pressure curve—the tension–time index (TTI)—is approximately proportionate to oxygen uptake.[8] This area underestimates oxygen demands by approximately 25–30% when inotropes are given.[9] The ratio DPTI/TTI allows a beat-to-beat guide to adequacy of subendocardial oxygenation (how well demands are met). Subendocardial ischemia occurs when this ratio is less than 0.80 when blood oxygen content is normal; a higher ratio is obviously needed with coronary disease because DPTI is lower beyond the stenotic lesion (Fig. 102–3) or during inotropic drug administration.[5,9] The usefulness of this index has been clinically confirmed,[10–13] and its limitations have been summarized.[5]

Subendocardial muscle is in greatest jeopardy in patients with ventricular hypertrophy or coronary artery disease, because both conditions cause resting vasodilatation and substantial reduction in the capacity of subendocardial vessels to dilate and regulate flow proportionate to changing oxygen needs. Myocardial ischemia can develop, therefore, because of minor imbalances of oxygen supply and

demand in these patients even before extracorporeal circulation is started.

CONSIDERATIONS BEFORE BYPASS

Subendocardial ischemia occurring before bypass is a particular concern because (1) it may go unrecognized except when severe, (2) it is added to the inevitable ischemia that occurs during bypass, and (3) it may contribute substantially to the subendocardial damage that impairs postoperative myocardial performance.

Hypotension should be avoided because subendocardial blood supply will fall and ischemia will occur in all hearts that have lost autoregulatory capacity. Ischemia may worsen, however, if appropriate decisions are not based on wedge pressure recordings. Myocardial depression by anesthetic drugs, for example, will reduce DPTI by lowering arterial blood pressure and raising left ventricular diastolic pressure. Treating this cause of hypotension with adrenergic drugs (e.g., Vasoxyl, Neosynephrine) may accentuate ischemia by increasing afterload, which raises left ventricular diastolic pressure further, while simultaneously augmenting left ventricular oxygen needs (TTI). A rise in arterial blood pressure may be transient and be followed by recurrent hypotension and the need to start extracorporeal circulation prematurely. Hypertension (e.g., insufficient anesthesia), however, may provide a false sense of security about the adequacy of subendocardial perfusion. High peripheral resistance (increased afterload) raises left ventricular oxygen requirements (TTI) markedly; left ventricular emptying becomes impaired, left ventricular diastolic pres-

Figure 102–2. Superimposed aortic and left ventricular pressure tracings (left) and left atrial pressure tracings (right) used to calculate the supply–demand (DTTI/TTI) ratio.

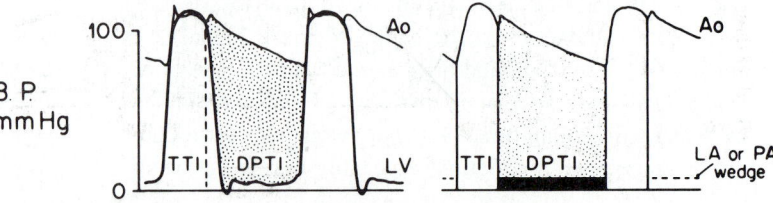

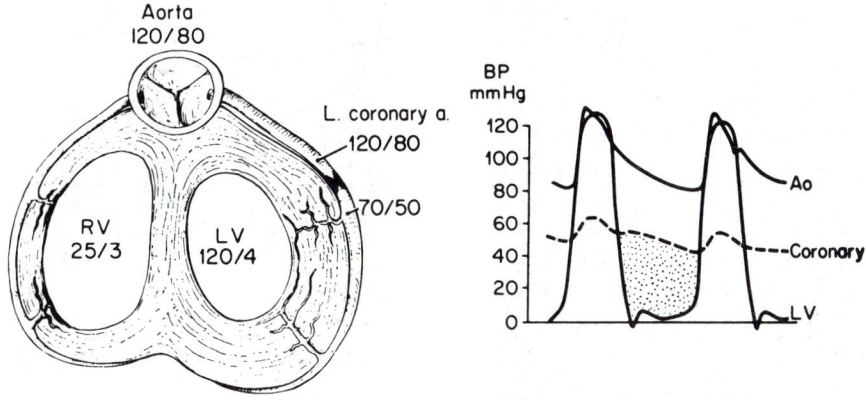

Figure 102–3. Coronary artery disease. Transmural ventricular section (left) with coronary stenosis. Note the pressure gradient beyond the stenosis. Right side indicates potential subendocardial blood flow (stippled area), beyond stenosis.

sure increases, DPTI falls, and subendocardial flow is impeded (Fig. 102–4). Pharmacologic vasodilators, such as nitroprusside or phentolamine, may cause a marked improvement in the myocardial supply–demand despite lowering diastolic blood pressure.[14] The effects of heart rate on various disease states must be taken into account so as to optimize heart rate before bypass. Tachycardia, for example, shortens the diastolic filling period of the coronary arteries and causes ischemia in patients who have coronary artery disease. Rapid heart rates should be avoided also in patients who have aortic stenosis because the diastolic interval is compromised even at slow heart rates, due to prolonged systolic ejection across the stenotic valve.[15] Conversely, very slow heart rates are deleterious to subendocardial perfusion in patients with aortic sufficiency because more time is available for regurgitation during bradycardia; DPTI is lowered markedly when aortic diastolic pressure falls and left ventricular diastolic pressure rises. Atrial pacing can improve the adequacy of subendocardial perfusion substantially in aortic insufficiency.[16] The use of balloon counterpulsation has been advocated[17] to optimize supply–demand balance before cardiopulmonary bypass. Although physiologically sound, this method is usually unnecessary if there is good monitoring and appropriate decision-making except in patients with unrelenting angina pectoris.

CONSIDERATIONS DURING BYPASS

Extracorporeal circulation was thought previously to cause subendocardial necrosis because of reports showing the severity of subendocardial damage to be proportionate to the duration of cardiopulmonary bypass. Prolonged extracorporeal circulation can theoretically impair the subendocardial microcirculation, because all pump oxygenator systems produce small particulate emboli, which go preferentially to the subendocardium.[18] Despite this potential problem, up to 3 hours of extracorporeal circulation with adequate coronary perfusion does not cause detrimental changes in coronary blood flow, its distribution, myocardial metabolism, or left ventricular performance[19] or ultrastructure.[20] Rather, it is the inadequate protection against supply–demand imbalances during cardiopulmonary bypass that is the major cause of subendocardial necrosis; more injury occurs when the imbalance is prolonged during lengthy operations. Almost all the determinants of subendocardial oxygen supply–demand, e.g., state of ventricular activity, temperature, blood oxygen content, coronary perfusion pressure, and flow, are controlled during cardiopulmonary bypass. As more is learned about how various interventions during extracorporeal circulation affect the supply–demand balance, the ways it has been disrupted unknowingly as in the past become more apparent.

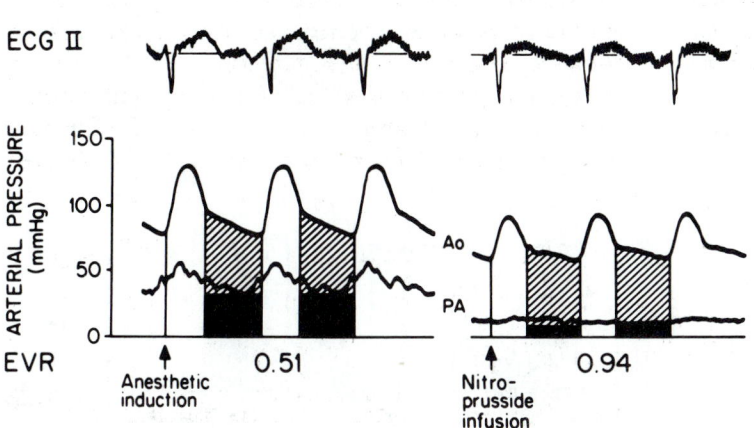

Figure 102–4. Effects of intraoperative afterload reduction on supply–demand balance. EVR is endocardial viability ratio, used synonymously with DPTI/TTI. Note the marked reduction in ratio (0.51) due to increased left ventricular end-diastolic pressure with anesthetic induction, and the marked improvement in ratio and electrocardiogram (lead following nitroprusside infusion despite lowering of arterial blood pressure).

TABLE 102–1. OPERATIVE TECHNIQUES

Hypothermia
Beating
Fibrillating
Arrest
Ischemic
Pharmacologic

Table 102–1 lists the techniques used intraoperatively to manage the heart during extracorporeal circulation. Until recently, hypothermia was used routinely to reduce metabolic demands and the surgeon has the option of either allowing the heart to beat, fibrillate, or be arrested. Figure 102–5 shows the effects of hypothermia in reducing metabolic requirements during each of these conditions while the heart is perfused continually with oxygenated blood.[21] Cardiac operations can be accomplished with greatest technical ease when the heart is arrested and bloodless. Arrest was achieved by shutting off coronary bloodflow by aortic clamping before the reintroduction of pharmacologic cardioplegia (to be discussed below). Ischemic arrest produces some cardiac injury despite hypothermic protection.

Many surgeons used the technique of ventricular fibrillation with continuous coronary perfusion in the past to (1) produce a quiet operative field and (2) be certain that the heart was not deprived of oxygen. They found, to their dismay, that hearts that were fibrillated during extracorporeal circulation frequently sustained some degree of ischemic subendocardial damage. The development of the microsphere method of bloodflow measurement enhanced our understanding of how subendocardial muscle can become damaged during open heart surgery.

In the normal left ventricle, the beating empty heart has a relatively low blood supply requirement. Conversely, when the normal heart fibrillates there is a marked increased blood supply to the inner shell of the left ventricle to provide oxygen for the high metabolic demands of normothermic ventricular fibrillation. However, it is not often that we operate on a normal left ventricle. We found that the hypertrophied beating empty left ventricle has a much higher oxygen or subendocardial flow need per gram than the normal left ventricle.[22] With fibrillation, hypertrophied ventricles failed to increase flow and this failure to augment flow in the face of a high energy requirement resulted in ischemia (Fig. 102–6).

The functional effects of electrical ventricular fibrillation are shown in Figure 102–7. Hearts that were fibrillated with constant application of an alternating current for 1 hour sustained the same degree of ischemic damage as hearts that were arrested ischemically with topical hypothermia for 60 min. As a consequence of these studies, we concluded that the use of either the electrical ventricular fibrillation or ischemic arrest with topical hypothermia alone provided a degree of subendocardial damage and subsequent functional depression that was unacceptable during clinical open-heart surgery.

CARDIOPLEGIA

Pharmacologic cardioplegia was not used widely in the United States until the past 25 years because of previous reports of left ventricular damage following cold hypertonic potassium citrate blood as introduced by Melrose et al in 1955.[23,24] Studies by Bretschneider et al[25] Kirsch et al[26] and Hearse et al[27] in Europe and by Gay and Ebert[28] provide a solid framework for the renewed interest in cardioplegia that has resulted in the intraoperative use of pharmacologic cardioplegic by most surgeons throughout the world. Tyers et al[29] showed that the problem with Melrose solution was inappropriate concentration of its constituents, rather than an inappropriate composition. Our studies fully support the original cardioplegic constituents of Melrose solution and we now use safe concentrations of alkaline, hypertonic, potassium citrate, and cold blood to stop the heart whenever we clamp the aorta during clinical surgery,[30] and the safety of this approach has been confirmed by others.[31–34]

Until recently, cold cardioplegic solutions have been used almost universally to prevent intraoperative myocardial ischemic damage during aortic clamping. This review shows that the inclusion of oxygen in the cardioplegic solution expands the therapeutic scope for clinical cardioplegia. It describes how these same solutions can be delivered warm to allow their use for *active resuscitation* before ischemia is imposed, and how to *avoid* and *reverse* ischemic and reperfusion damage before and after aortic unclamping.

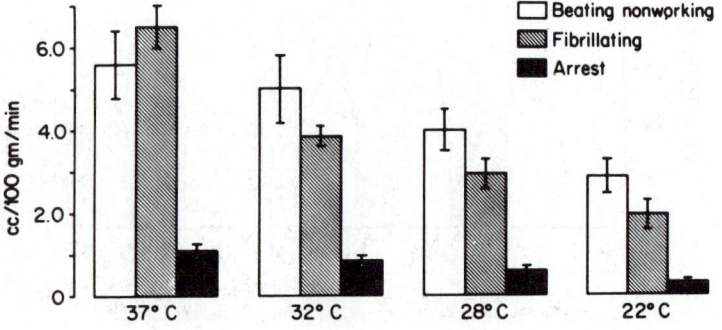

Figure 102–5. Left ventricular oxygen requirements during extracorporeal circulation in the continuously perfused heart. Note the high oxygen requirement of ventricular fibrillation, and the lowest oxygen requirement in the arrested heart at all myocardial temperatures.

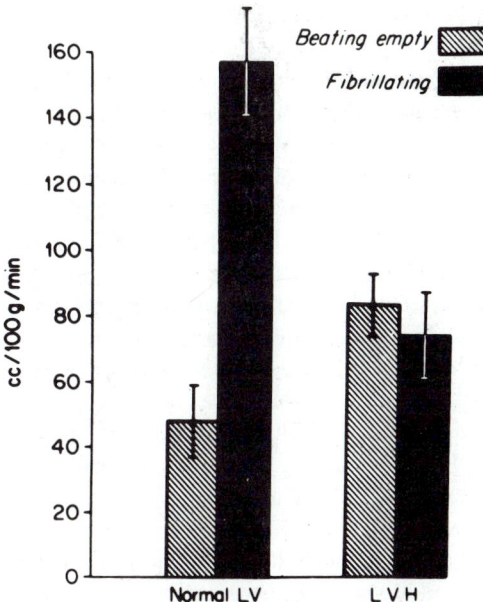

Figure 102–6. Myocardial oxygen uptake in beating empty and fibrillating normal and hypertrophied hearts. Note the marked increased subendocardial bloodflow during fibrillation in the normal left ventricle, and the failure to augment flow in hypertrophied ventricle that is allowed to fibrillate.

It reiterates briefly the principles that must underlie the composition of cardioplegic solutions and puts into perspective the commonality of apparently different pharmacologic approaches to myocardial protection.[35] It focuses primarily on the principles that form the basis for clinical strategies for cardioplegic delivery that can ensure that the selected cardioplegic solution can exert its desired effect and it describes how these can be implemented. Each proposed strategy can be used with oxygenated cardioplegic solutions (regardless of precise composition) and several are applicable to asanguineous cardioplegic solutions devoid of oxygen.

Table 102–2 lists the factors affecting the myocardial energy supply–demand balance during aortic clamping. The

two factors affecting supply include oxygenated blood coming from noncoronary collateral blood flow, and intrinsic or extrinsic substrate stores. All surgeons have noted noncoronary collateral flow during aortic clamping, as blood appears in the coronary ostia during aortic valve replacement or in the coronary arteriotomy site during coronary revascularization despite a flaccid aorta. The second determinant of supply is myocardial glycogen or exogenous glucose. Oxygenated hearts undergo aerobic metabolism, but the heart receiving little or no oxygen supply must undergo anaerobic metabolism to generate some energy to maintain cell membrane viability. Anaerobic glycolysis requires the presence of substrate (i.e., glucose of glycogen), and a metabolic environment (i.e., buffering) to allow anaerobic energy production. Myocardial oxygen demands are determined principally by electromechanical activity. The heart that is fibrillating or beating while ischemic has a much higher energy requirement than the heart that is arrested. The second determinant of demand is the wall tension within the myocardium, and the third is the myocardial temperature that governs metabolic rate directly.

CARDIOPLEGIC PREREQUISITES

Essential prerequisites for clinical use of cardioplegia include (1) use of a solution that has been shown to be safe through testing under experimental conditions, especially in models that simulate clinical circumstances, (2) assurance of distribution to all areas of the heart, (3) periodic replenishment to counteract noncoronary collateral washout, and (4) strategies for delivering and maintaining cardioplegia that can be adapted to various clinical conditions.

CARDIOPLEGIC COMPOSITION

The objectives of chemical cardioplegia are to stop the heart safely, create an environment for continued energy

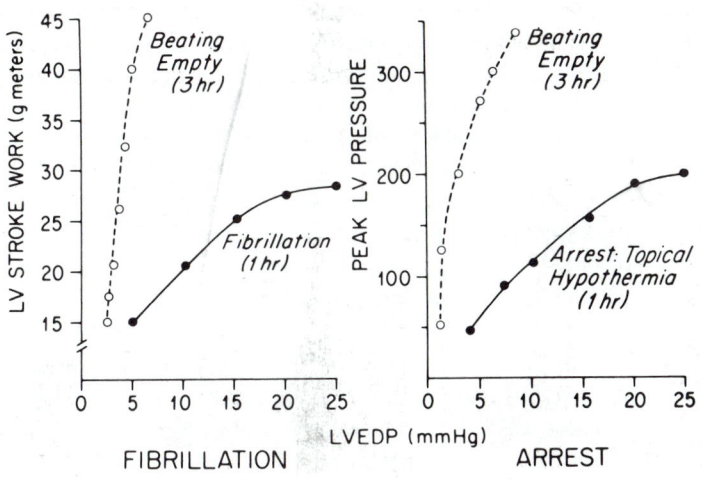

Figure 102–7. Left ventricular function curves following 3 hours of continuous coronary perfusion (beating empty heart) and after 1 hour of either ventricular fibrillation (left side) or ischemic arrest with topical hypothermia (right side). Note the comparable reduction in myocardial performance occurring with either ventricular fibrillation or topical hypothermic arrest.

TABLE 102–2. MYOCARDIAL SUPPLY–DEMAND BALANCE DURING AORTIC CROSS-CLAMPING

Supply	Demand
Noncoronary collaterals	Electromechanical activity
Intrinsic substrate stores (glycogen)	Wall tension
	Temperature (metabolic rate)

production, and counteract deleterious effects of ischemia. The principles that underlie the composition of any cardioplegic solution are enumerated in Table 102–3. Most clinically used solutions that embrace these principles likely confer comparably good myocardial protection during ischemia. First, immediate arrest should be produced to lower energy demands and avoid depletion by ischemic electromechanical work. This is especially true with nonoxygenated cardioplegic solutions. Conversely, high-energy stores may be enhanced when cardioplegia is induced with oxygenated solutions[36] and delay in asystole is less problematic. Studies[37] show substantial adenosine triphosphate (ATP) store reduction during the brief period of electromechanical activity preceding pharmacologic cardioplegia with asanguineous solutions. Arrest can be achieved either by use of potassium, magnesium, procaine, or perhaps some hypocalcemic solution. Second, myocardial temperature should be lowered to reduce metabolic rate if flow is to be interrupted. This can be achieved usually with perfusion hypothermia with a cold cardioplegic solution. Recurrence of electromechanical activity may, however, occur when the cardioplegic solution is washed away by noncoronary collateral flow, so that cardioplegic reinfusion at 4°–10°C are used and can be delivered safely with a blood vehicle.[38] Third, substrate (i.e., glucose or glycogen) should be provided for continued anaerobic or aerobic energy production (or both) during aortic clamping. The energy available during both induction of cardioplegia and with replenishments is far greater if oxygen (i.e., blood) is used in the cardioplegic vehicle, especially if the cardioplegic solution is enriched with precursors of Krebs cycle intermediates (i.e., glutamate or aspartate).[39] Fourth, there must be an appropriate pH to achieve a reasonable state of metabolism during hypothermia. Consequently, a buffer is necessary in all cardioplegic solutions. Tris(hydroxymethyl) aminoethane (THAM), bicarbonate, phosphate, or perhaps some other buffer may be used and reports confirm the benefits of opti-

TABLE 102–3. PHARMACOLOGIC CARDIOPLEGIA

Principle	Method
Immediate arrest	K^+, Mg^{2+}, procaine
Hypothermia	10°–20°C
Substrate	Oxygen, glucose, glutamate, aspartate
Appropriate pH (buffer)	THAM, bicarb, phosphate
Membrane stabilization	Ca^{2+} ($\geq$ 50 mM), ?steroids, ?procaine, Ca^{2+} antagonist, O^2 radical scavenger

mizing the small energy output of anaerobic glycolysis during ischemia by buffering the cardioplegic solution.[40] Fifth, there must be some degree of membrane stabilization in the form of exogenous additives or avoidance of intentional hypocalcemia; calcium-free cardioplegic solutions can damage the sarcolemmal membrane.[41] Calcium antagonists (i.e., verapamil, nifedipine, diltiazem, etc) that block calcium cellular entry may be important future cardioplegic additives.[42–44] Their routine incorporation in cardioplegic solutions must be delayed until more information is available about how to counteract their continuing action after extracorporeal circulation is discontinued and normal calcium homeostasis is needed. The role of steroids and procaine and how they affect membrane stabilization are uncertain, although many studies of these agents have been and will continue. Oxygen radical scavengers (i.e., superoxide dismutase,[45] catalase, allopurinol,[46] coenzyme Q_{10} [CoQ_{10}][47] or leukodepletion[48] may be useful potential cardioplegic additives to counteract the cytotoxic oxygen metabolites that can produce profound changes in membrane phospholipids during ischemia and reperfusion (see Chap. 97).[49] Sixth, ischemic damage produces myocardial edema, so that some attention must be directed to both the osmolarity and colloid osmotic pressure of the cardioplegic solution to avoid producing edema iatrogenically during cardioplegic infusions.[50]

BLOOD VERSUS ASANGUINEOUS CARDIOPLEGIA

The need to provide oxygen in the cardioplegic solution continues to be questioned despite experimental and clinical studies establishing the superiority of oxygenated cardioplegic solutions.[30–34] The vehicle for providing oxygen may be blood,[30] fluorocarbons,[51] stroma-free hemoglobin,[51] or oxygen dissolved in crystalloid.[52] We have selected blood as the cardioplegic vehicle, since this physiologic source of oxygen is available readily in the extracorporeal circuit, and its use limits hemodilution when large volumes of cardioplegia are needed.

An additional advantage of a blood cardioplegic vehicle is ensurance of the buffering capacity of blood proteins, especially histidine imidazole groups.[53] Furthermore, the rheologic benefits on the microvasculature afforded by erythrocytes enhance papillary muscle perfusion compared with oxygenated crystalloid cardioplegia and reduce coronary vascular resistance and edema formation.[52] The erythrocytes of blood cardioplegia also contain abundant endogenous oxygen free radical scavengers (i.e., superoxide dismutase, catalase, and glutathione),[54] which may reduce oxygen-mediated injury during reperfusion. Our experimental studies show that the salutary effects of controlled blood cardioplegic reperfusion are impaired markedly when endogenous red blood cell glutathione and catalase are blocked pharmacologically.[55]

Concern over use of cold blood cardioplegia stems from (1) producing possible unfavorable shifts in the oxyhemoglobin association curve with resultant impairment of oxygen unloading at the cellular level, (2) the theoretic potential of blood sludging if < 15°C temperatures are used, (3) potentially better distribution of asanguineous solutions beyond coronary stenoses, and (4) heretofore complex delivery systems with blood cardioplegia (the oxygen source).

We have addressed these concerns and found the following: First, O_2 uptake exceeds basal demands by as much as 10-fold during 4°C blood cardioplegic reinfusions during the period of prolonged aortic clamping[38] (Fig. 102–8). Second, intermittent infusions of 4°C blood cardioplegia at Hct 20–30% can be delivered safely for a period of up to 4 hours of aortic clamping so that a hypothermic blood cardioplegic perfusate can be used clinically without concern (Fig. 102–9).[56] Third, comparison of 250 mL/min infusions of asanguineous and blood 4°C cardioplegic solutions shows that the reduced viscosity of asanguineous cardioplegia results in a lower aortic pressure. The consequent higher aortic pressure with blood cardioplegia allows superior cardioplegic delivery beyond obstructed coronaries and better myocardial cooling (5°C) (Fig. 102–10). These findings suggest that the decreased viscosity of asanguineous cardioplegia causes diversion of cardioplegic solutions away from the obstructed vessels to the normal coronary bed.[57] Fourth, as shown in Figure 102–11, a disposable blood cardioplegic delivery system has been developed and used over the past several years to avoid the need for reservoirs, hand-mixing of solutions, and delay.[38] This system uses differential volumes of two tubing diameters to mix pump blood with cardioplegic solutions appropriately and instantaneously. Fifth cold noncardioplegic blood, after cardioplegic arrest, keeps the heart asystolic, ensures continued nourishment and hypothermia, and enhances right ventricular recovery when retroperfusion is used.[58]

The advantages of oxygenated cardioplegic solutions over oxygen-free solutions are obvious when attention is directed to the energy availability with these two vehicles. With asanguineous cardioplegia, myocardial viability must

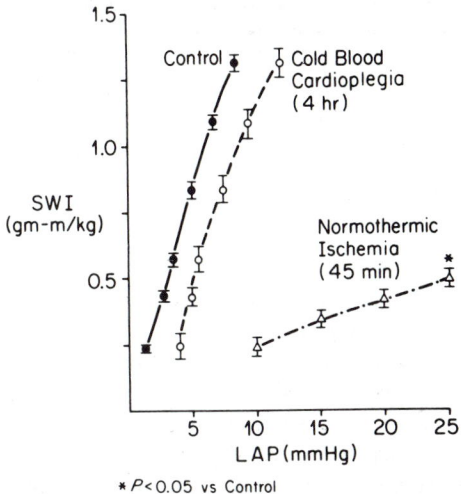

Figure 102–9. Postischemic myocardial performance during inscription of left ventricular function curves 30 min after unclamping the aorta. Note marked depression in function following 45 min of normothermic ischemia and normal function after 4 hours of multidose cold blood cardioplegia. LAP, left atrial pressure; SWI, stroke work index.

depend on the small amount of energy (2 mol of ATP/mol of glucose metabolized) produced by anaerobic metabolism. Bretschneider et al have emphasized the importance of maintaining aerobic metabolism (36 mol of ATP/mol of glucose metabolized) while the heart is stopped pharmacologically to avoid wasting energy stores uselessly by allowing the heart to do electromechanical work during asanguineous cardioplegic perfusion.[25] The use of blood as the vehicle for cardioplegic delivery (Table 102–4) has the ob-

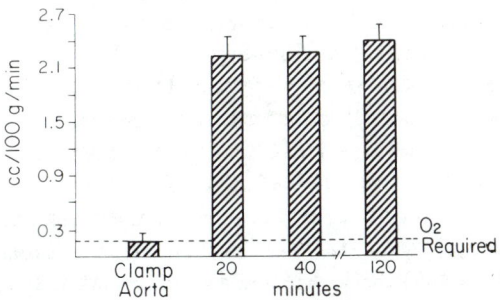

Figure 102–8. Myocardial oxygen uptake during 4°C blood cardioplegic infusions. Note very low myocardial oxygen demands (O_2 requirement), indicated by hatched line during cardioplegic induction (clamped aorta) and O_2 uptake 10 times in excess of basal demands with cardioplegic replenishment at 20 min intervals.

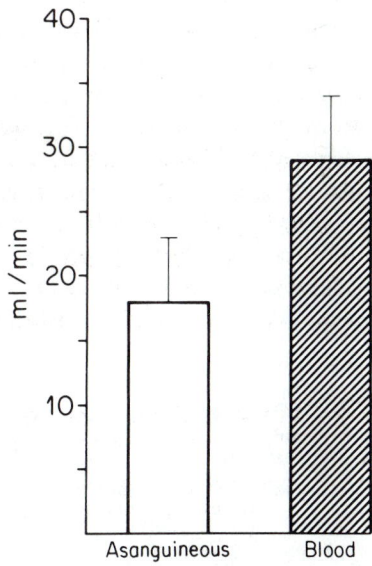

Figure 102–10. Cardioplegic flow beyond coronary stenosis when cardioplegic solution is given at 250 mL/min into aorta. Note the better flow beyond stenosis with blood than asanguineous cardioplegia.

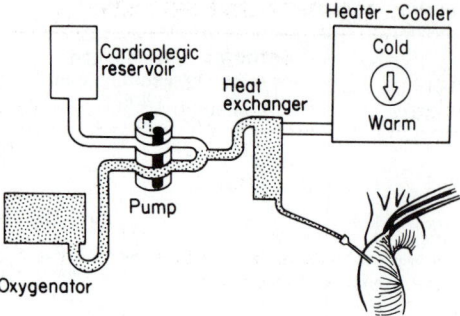

Figure 102–11. Cardioplegic delivery system for delivery of warm or cold blood cardioplegia.

TABLE 102–5. CARDIOPLEGIC SOLUTION[a]

Principle	Constituent	Final Concentration
Provide oxygen	Blood	Hct 20–30%
Maintain arrest	KCl	12–16 mg/L
Buffer acidosis	Tham	pH 7.5–7.6
Avoid edema	Glucose	> 400 mOsm
Restore substrate	Glucose	> 400 mg%
	Aspartate	13 mM
	Glutamate	13 mM
Limit calcium entry	CPD	500–600 µM Ca^{2+}
	Diltiazem	300 mg/kg body weight

[a]CPD, citrate phosphate dextrose; Hct, hematocrit.

vious advantages of (1) keeping the heart oxygenated while it is being arrested, (2) allowing reoxygenation when the cardioplegic solution is replenished, (3) avoiding reperfusion damage (to be discussed below), (4) minimizing hemodilution, and (5) having endogenous oxygen radical scavengers, buffers, and onconicity.

The critical importance of using an oxygenated cardioplegic solution was emphasized in a report[59] comparing asanguineous to oxygenated cardioplegia (blood and fluorocarbons) in hypertrophied hearts, whereby the experimental model simulates more closely the clinical conditions confronted when operations are performed in patients with advanced cardiac disease. Table 102–5 enumerates the principles that underlie a clinically tested blood cardioplegic solution that contains the blood constituents shown to provide for ideal reperfusion of ischemic myocardium.[60] Our standard cardioplegic solution contains 500–600 µmol/L, calcium without glutamate or aspartate, but the cardioplegic solution used for warm cardioplegic induction and warm reperfusion contains glutamate and aspartate and a lower ionic calcium (150–250 µmol/L) achieved by adding more citrate phosphate dextrose (CPD) (discussed later in this chapter). Diltiazem is used *only* in the regional reperfusate after revascularization for acute evolving myocardial infarction.[61,62] Figure 102–12 shows the protective effect of multidose blood vs. asanguineous cardioplegia using two solutions of comparable composition during 2 hours of aortic clamping in the experimental setting. The recovery of contractility is greater than normal with blood cardioplegia, reflecting perhaps the cardiac effects of the catecholamine

release occurring with extracorporeal circulation. Good recovery also occurs with asanguineous cardioplegia, but it is slightly less than complete. Figure 102–13 shows a similar early salutary effect in matched groups of 16 high-risk patients (i.e., extending MI, ejection fraction <0.30) where we compared the effects of blood cardioplegia to asanguineous cardioplegia with the same ingredients. Table 102–6 shows the pooled results and indicates that blood cardioplegia resulted in a lower incidence of postoperative ECG abnormalities and inotropic needs but did not avoid completely enzymatic evidence of myocardial damage (Table 102–7). No attempt was made to distribute either cardioplegia solution beyond stenoses in these patients. We continue to see the highest level of enzymes in patients who have coronary disease, hypertrophied left ventricles, or when these two lesions are combined. These data have led to the development of additional strategies to induce, distribute, maintain, and reperfuse with cardioplegic solutions that have increased

TABLE 102–4. BLOOD CARDIOPLEGIA ADVANTAGES

Oxygenation during arrest
Reoxygenation during replenishment
Limits reperfusion injury
Reduces hemodilution
Endogenous
  Oxygen radical scavengers
  Buffers
  Onconicity

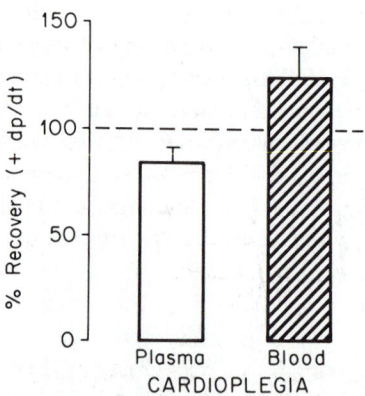

Figure 102–12. Myocardial performance (25 mL end-diastolic volume) after 2 hours of aortic clamping with either multidose asanguineous (plasma) or blood cardioplegia with comparable constituents. Note the slight depression in postischemic performance with asanguineous cardioplegia, and the better postischemic performance with blood cardioplegia. (The above normal contractility probably reflects the effects of catecholamines normally released during extracorporeal circulation on the well-protected myocardium.)

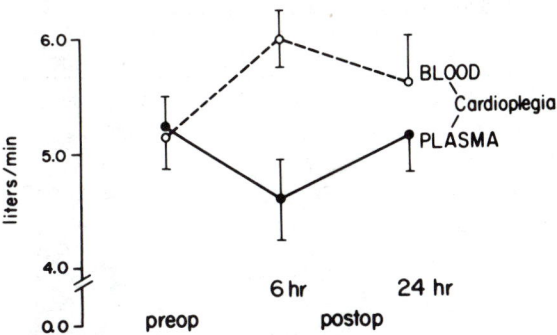

Figure 102–13. Postoperative cardiac output in patients undergoing comparable operations and receiving either blood or asanguineous (plasma) cardioplegia. Note the similarity in transitory increase in cardiac performance following blood cardioplegia and slight depression following asanguineous cardioplegia at 6 hours (see Fig. 102–15).

the safety of cardiac operations and expanded the uses of oxygenated cardioplegic solutions, and reduced perioperative morbidity and hospitalization in the increasing number of high-risk patients requiring cardiac surgery.

OPERATIVE STRATEGY

The strategies for clinical cardioplegia may be separated into the phases of (1) induction, (2) maintenance and distribution, and (3) reperfusion.

CARDIOPLEGIC INDUCTION

Cardioplegia may be given immediately after extracorporeal circulation has begun, provided the pulmonary artery is collapsed to attest to the adequacy of venous return. This avoids admixture of the cardioplegic solution with systemic blood that traverses the lung because it is not captured by the venous cannula. Starting the infusion shortly before aortic clamping ensures aortic valve competence. The volume, rate, and temperature of cardioplegic administration are determined by the mass and pathophysiologic status of the heart before arrest is initiated.

TABLE 102–6. RESULTS OF PHARMACOLOGIC CARDIOPLEGIA IN MATCHED GROUPS OF 16 HIGH-RISK PATIENTS

	Asanguineous (%)	Blood (%)
Infarcts	6	0
Abnormal ECG[a]	44	13
Circulatory support	12	0
Death	6	6

[a]ECG, electrocardiogram.

TABLE 102–7. POSTOPERATIVE ENZYMES[a]

Enzyme (at 18 hours)	Beating Empty or Intermittent Ischemia	Blood Cardioplegia
CPK	1251 ± 127	796 ± 43*
CPK-MB	20 ± 3	13 ± 1
SGOT	99 ± 18	59 ± 4

[a]CPK, creatine phosphokinase; CPK-MB, CPK-myocardial band; SGOT, serum glutamic-oxaloacetic transaminase.
*$p < 0.05$.

Cold Induction

Cardioplegic induction (Table 102–8) in operations on hearts with reasonably normal energy reserves is intended to (1) stop the heart promptly to lower oxygen demands, (2) produce hypothermia to reduce O_2 demands further, and (3) create an environment that allows continuous anaerobic energy production during intervals between cardioplegic replenishments to *prevent* ischemic damage. An initial cold (4°–8°C) solution containing a high concentration of the arresting agent (i.e., 20–25 mEq/L, KCl) will produce asystole promptly. Global arrest occurs usually within 30 seconds but may be delayed to 1–2 min in patients with coronary disease due to maldistribution of cardioplegia beyond stenotic or occluded arteries. Palpation of the aorta or measurement of infusion pressure will allow detection of aortic incompetence if it is caused inadvertently, but it is now routine to measure aortic pressure directly during antegrade cardioplegic administration.[63] Cardioplegic solutions stop the heart by depolarizing the cell membrane. The optimal concentration of cardioplegic agent (KCl) is that amount required to produce and maintain arrest. Higher cardioplegic potassium concentrations (15–30 mEq/L) are necessary to produce arrest than to maintain asystole, but raising $K^+ > 30$ mEq/L is unnecessary during cardioplegic induction and serves only to cause systemic hyperkalemia. Arrest occurs more quickly with crystalloid than with blood cardioplegia, since depolarization combines with anoxia and perfusion hypothermia to halt electromechanical activity. Cardioplegic K^+ can be reduced to 8–10 mEq/L during subsequent cold cardioplegic infusions (i.e., multidose cardioplegia; see Cardioplegic Maintenance below) since perfusion or topical hypothermia potentiates the effectiveness of any cardioplegic potassium concentration. Additionally, infusion of cold noncardioplegic blood retrograde will maintain arrest, and can be used during parts of the operation where visualization is not impeded such as performing

TABLE 102–8. BLOOD CARDIOPLEGIA INDUCTION

Cold
  Global hypothermia
  Prompt asystole
Warm
  "Active resuscitation"

(i.e., constructing) proximal anastomosis in the clamped vented aorta.[58] The initial cardioplegic flow rate differs with oxygenated and nonoxygenated cardioplegic solutions. Maintenance of the selected flow rate after arrest produces transmural cooling by delivering the total volume of cardioplegic solution. Global cardioplegia is usually induced with 4°–8°C blood cardioplegia at a flow rate of 250–350 mL/min depending on cardiac size, and the infusion continued for 3 min (750–1000 mL total dose in nonhypertrophied hearts). Greater volumes of cardioplegia (1000–1500 mL) are required when there is increased left ventricular mass.[64] There should be minimal concern over the duration of cardioplegic induction or rapidity of arrest with oxygenated cardioplegic solutions since the heart receives oxygen continually during the cardioplegic infusion. Conversely, delivery of asanguineous cardioplegic solutions at higher flow rates (400–500 mL/min) shortens the time to arrest and minimizes the duration of anoxic aortic clamping.

Failure to produce arrest within 1–2 min may be due to (1) incomplete aortic clamping, (2) aortic insufficiency produced by distortion of the noncoronary cusp by a large right atrial cannula, (3) incomplete decompression by the venous cannula resulting in admixture of venous blood returning to the left heart and diluting of the cardioplegic solution, and (4) inadvertent failure to add sufficient potassium to the cardioplegic solution. Palpation of the left ventricle during cardioplegic induction allows detection of left ventricular distention, which occurs if venous drainage is inadequate or aortic insufficiency has been produced. Corrective measures include readjusting the position of the venous cannula within the right atrium and/or moving it away from the coronary cusp. Discontinuation of the cardioplegic infusion and immediate ventricular venting are necessary if these maneuvers fail to produce decompression and primary cardioplegic reliance is placed upon retrograde delivery. Undue concern should not be directed toward reducing the temperature of the cardioplegic solution much below 10°C since minor differences in solution temperature (between 5° and 10°C) will not produce major differences in myocardial temperature or oxygen demands during the brief interval of cardioplegic infusion, especially after the heart is arrested. The oxygen requirements of the arrested heart at 20°C are extremely low at 0.3 mL/100 g per minute and are reduced only to 0.15 mL/100 per minute at 10°C.[21,25] Conversely, the oxygen requirements of the beating or fibrillating heart are 2–3 mL/100 g per minute at comparable temperatures.[21,31] Consequently, preoccupation with obtaining a predetermined level of myocardial cooling after arrest in areas supplied by occluded arteries or stenotic vessels will delay the operation unnecessarily. Deeper regional hypothermia can be achieved readily by distribution of cardioplegic solution through the grafts after they are constructed (see Cardioplegic Distribution, below) and by retrograde cardioplegic or noncardioplegic blood infusion when arterial conduits are used or when diffuse coronary disease is present.

Cardioplegic infusions may cause myocardial edema (especially if the myocardial cells are ischemic), if perfusion pressure is allowed to become excessive (> 80 mm Hg) since the myocardial contractile force and muscle tone that limit fluid flux mechanically are overcome by pharmacologic asystole, and hypothermia interferes with normal cell volume regulation by decreasing the effectiveness of the Na^+–K^+ pump. The extent of edema that can be produced during cardioplegic infusion is determined by the interaction of the Starling forces that govern fluid flux. These include the perfusion pressure as well as the oncotic and osmotic pressures of the solution, the electromechanical status of the myocardium, and the integrity of the capillary bed. We have, for example, caused temporary myocardial edema iatrogenically in a normal heart by inducing cold cardioplegia with a hypo-oncotic, hypo-osmotic crystalloid cardioplegic solution under experimental conditions.[50] Clinical cardioplegic perfusion pressures of 80–100 mm Hg are probably safe during cardioplegic induction since myocardial electromechanical activity persists during part of the infusion, the full extent of perfusion hypothermia is not instantaneous, and the integrity of the capillary bed has not yet been altered by ischemic damage. Conversely, keeping perfusion pressure at or below 50 mm Hg during reinfusions and reperfusion will limit edema when cardioplegic replenishments are delivered to myocardial regions containing capillary endothelial cells that may have been damaged because they did not receive adequate cardioplegic protection during previous infusions. Delivery of cardioplegia at predetermined pressure in coronary patients does not ensure even distribution beyond stenoses. Simultaneously, myocardium in regions supplied by unobstructed arteries may become edematous if the arrested heart is perfused at high perfusion pressures. The surgeon and perfusionist should always be aware of the actual or estimated perfusion pressure to avoid producing edema.

Pressure Monitoring During Infusions

Cardioplegic System Pressure

Pressure in the cardioplegic delivery system must be known to detect inadvertent occlusion (i.e., clamping or kinking) in the delivery line that might cause its disruption unless corrected. A pressure port is integrated into most commercial systems, and a high system pressure requires an immediate response to reduce or stop cardioplegic flow until the source of obstruction is identified and corrected. Before the availability of antegrade and retrograde cannulae with dual pressure lumina for direct pressure monitoring, intravascular pressures were estimated indirectly by observing the pressure recorded on the pressure port of the cardioplegic delivery system at the pump, and subtracting from it the known pressure drop in the delivery system. This required the perfusionist to intermittently calibrate the system (especially if different-sized cannulae were used), and made it necessary to calculate intravascular pressure with each change in cardioplegic flow rate.

Intravascular Pressure

Direct intravascular pressure measurement is the only reliable method for determining either aortic or coronary sinus pressure during cardioplegic delivery.[63] This conclusion was reached after intraoperative recording of mean pressure in the cardioplegic delivery system during simultaneous measurement of intravascular pressure in either the aorta or coronary sinus during cardioplegic infusions and comparing it to calculated pressure from the known pressure drop in the tubing system (containing either an antegrade or retrograde cannula) at flow rates ranging from 50 to 300 mL/min. Results comparing predicted versus measured vascular pressures for antegrade perfusion are shown in Figure 102–14 and led to the following conclusions:

1. Estimated pressure does not predict accurately the measured intravascular pressure during either antegrade or retrograde delivery, with differences ranging between +70 and 25 mm Hg, depending on flow rate.
2. The variability between predicted and measured intravascular pressure increases as either antegrade or retrograde cardioplegic flow rate is raised.
3. Predicted pressure tends to systematically underestimate the intravascular pressure, especially with retrograde delivery. This reduces the potential for excessive intravascular pressure, and limits the chance of coronary sinus or coronary artery barotrauma and edema. Simultaneously, the erroneous estimate of intravascular pressure may lead to systematic underperfusion with either antegrade or retrograde delivery.

We suspect the discrepancy between the predicted and measured intravascular pressure results from difference related to calibration with roller pumps; wide fluctuations in cardioplegic delivery system pressure develop when temperature and flow and viscosity are varied in systems containing rigid and compliant components, and preclude accurate measurement of pressure at the pump head. These fluctuations occur during calibration of the system while flow is delivered without an added vascular resistance component (i.e., into atmospheric pressure). They increase substantially when peripheral vascular resistance varies during cardioplegic administration (i.e., between doses in individual patients, and where vascular bed cross-sectional areas differ between patients). Direct intravascular measurement circumvents these sources of error and provides the surgeon with a more reliable pressure measurement.

Pressure Monitoring During Antegrade Infusions

The aorta is inspected and palpated to be sure the aortic valve is competent, and can be observed to billow as the root is filled by the cardioplegic infusion. Low aortic pressure (i.e., <50 mm Hg) occurs when there is (1) aortic insufficiency, (2) the vent port on the aortic cannula is not closed, or (3) the surgeon has not switched from retrograde delivery. Aortic insufficiency occurs sometimes from distortion of the noncoronary cusp by the two-stage cannula and can be relieved by retracting it downward and to the right. Compression of the RV outflow tract by a sponge stick will often push the septum onto the posterior LV wall and restore aortic pressure of more than 30 mm Hg at flow rates of more than 200 mL/min. If this cannot be achieved it implies that antegrade delivery is deficient, and primary reliance should be placed on retrograde perfusion. A less satisfactory alternative is opening the aorta to either provide direct coronary perfusion, or placing a temporary suture to coapt the aortic leaflets and closing the aorta and resuming antegrade flow. High aortic pressure (i.e., >100 mm Hg) occurs with extensive coronary disease and implies that the distribution of antegrade flow is unpredictable. Pressure monitoring during retrograde infusions will be discussed later (see Retrograde Delivery).

Warm Induction

Cardiac operations upon ischemic hearts (i.e., cardiogenic shock, extending myocardial infarction, hemodynamic in-

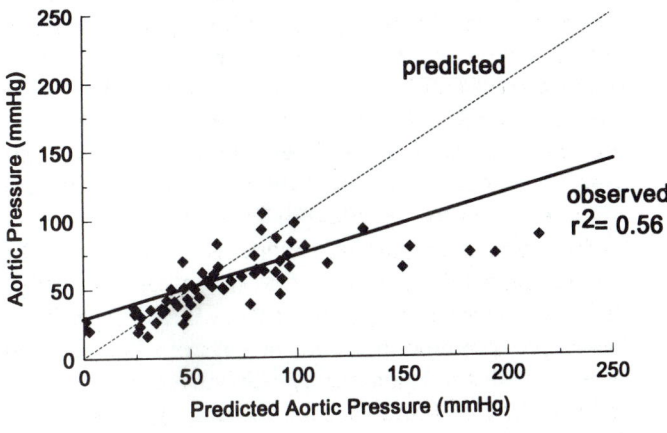

Figure 102–14. Predicted versus measured aortic pressure during antegrade cardioplegic infusion. (See text for description.)

stability before bypass) or in patients with advanced left or right ventricular hypertrophy or dysfunction pose more difficult problems in myocardial protection. Depletion of energy reserves and glycogen stores are common in such hearts; they (1) are less tolerant to ischemia during aortic clamping, (2) cannot sustain cell metabolism when blood supply is interrupted, and (3) use oxygen inefficiently during reperfusion.[65,66] Oxygenated cardioplegic solutions are particularly well suited for use in patients with energy-depleted hearts since they prevent further energy loss during induction, avoid reperfusion damage,[67] and improve metabolic recovery when administered warm.[68] The induction of blood cardioplegia in the energy-depleted heart is, in a sense, the first phase of reperfusion.

A brief (i.e., 5-min) infusion of warm oxygenated cardioplegic solution can be used as a form of *active resuscitation* in energy-depleted hearts[65] which must undergo prolonged (i.e., 2 hour) subsequent aortic clamping. Normothermia optimizes the rate of cellular repair, and enrichment of the oxygenated cardioplegic solution with amino acid precursors of Krebs cycle intermediates (aspartate and glutamate) improves oxygen utilization capacity. Substrate-enriched warm (37°C) blood cardioplegic induction results in myocardial oxygen uptake in energy-depleted hearts (subjected to 45 min of normothermic global ischemia), which exceeds basal requirements markedly (Fig. 102–15) and results in improved recovery despite 2 additional hours of aortic clamping with multidose blood cardioplegia (to simulate the time needed for operative repair)[69,70] (Fig. 102–16). The extra oxygen may be used to repair cell damage and to replace the energy stores (creatine phosphate) that can be used to sustain anaerobic metabolism during the

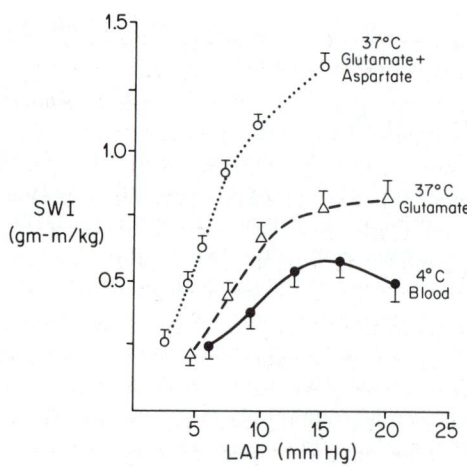

Figure 102–16. Left ventricular performance 30 min after blood reperfusion. Note normal ventricular performance after warm (37°C) induction of aspartate-enriched glutamate blood cardioplegia, moderate depression in ventricular performance after warm induction with glutamate blood cardioplegia, and severe depression in ventricular failure after cold (4°C) blood cardioplegia. LAP, left atrial pressure; SWI, stroke work index.

ischemic intervals until the next cardioplegic replenishment. Left ventricular venting during warm induction lowers wall tension maximally.[71]

In contrast to cold cardioplegic induction, the *duration* of cardioplegic delivery during normothermic induction is more important than the volume of cardioplegia given because the heart takes up oxygen over *time* and not by *dose*. Whereas the basal myocardial oxygen requirements of the healthy heart subjected to normothermic arrest are only 1 mL/100 g per minute or 5 mL/100 g during 5 min, the energy-depleted heart consumes approximately 25–30 mL O_2 over a 5-min induction interval under experimental conditions.[5,39] Administration of this same cardioplegic volume for 1 min would allow only 20% of the oxygen to be used compared to the 5-fold greater O_2 uptake, which can occur when the same volume of cardioplegia is given over 5 min.

The operation does not need to be prolonged during warm induction of oxygenated cardioplegia. Distal anastomoses into occluded left anterior descending or right coronary arteries can be constructed in coronary operations provided aortic insufficiency is not produced by distorting the heart. More immediate arrest during warm induction of blood cardioplegia occurs when the concentration of the cardioplegic agent is increased (i.e., to 25 mEq/L K+). Normothermia is assured by circulating warm water through the heat-exchanger used for cardioplegic mixing and delivery (Fig. 102–11). Warm cardioplegic induction *must* be followed by the administration of cold cardioplegia to provide perfusion hypothermia to *prevent* ischemic damage during the subsequent period of aortic clamping where intermittent ischemic intervals are imposed. The prolonged aortic clamping during cardioplegic induction (5 min of

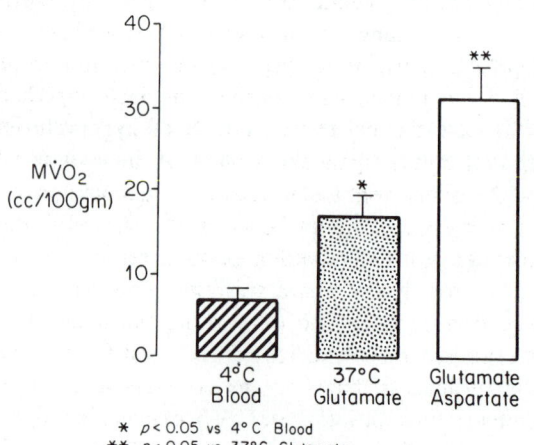

Figure 102–15. Oxygen consumption during induction of blood cardioplegia. Note twice as much oxygen consumed by hearts given warm (37°C) glutamate blood cardioplegia compared to cold (4°C) blood cardioplegia and > 3-fold increase in oxygen consumption by aspartate enrichment of warm glutamate blood cardioplegia. MVo₂, myocardial oxygen consumption.

warm and 3–5 min of cold blood cardioplegia) does not add ischemia when the cardioplegic ingredients are mixed with blood or some other form of oxygen (i.e., fluorocarbons, bubbled oxygen, or stroma-free hemoglobin).

A 5-min interval of warm blood cardioplegic induction has previously been used in hemodynamically unstable patients, particularly those in cardiogenic shock[72,73] (Fig. 102–17, see later discussion). It is now apparent that many hearts not exhibiting cardiogenic shock may also be energy depleted, as decreased levels of ATP are reported in hypertrophied hearts with pressure or volume overload and those with coronary artery disease.[74–76] In addition, the risk profile of patients requiring operation is increasing and recent studies[77] show that there is increased uptake of oxygen and glucose during warm substrate-enriched blood cardioplegic induction in noncardiogenic shock patients; this (1) is most pronounced in patients who were unstable preoperatively (CHF, left main disease, unstable angina, Fig. 102–18) or who are hypertensive with or without left ventricular hypertrophy, (2) persists throughout normothermic induction, and (3) correlates directly with the preoperative score described by Parsonnet[78] that predicts higher perioperative mortality. These observations have led to the use of warm blood cardioplegic induction in an increasing subset of patients. The infusion is restricted to 2–3 min in elective operations in patients who are not hypertensive, where the Parsonnet (severity) score is low, or where coronary artery disease is only moderate, as studies show that increased metabolic uptake normalizes after that time interval. Conversely, high metabolic uptake persists in high-risk patients (hypertension, urgent operation, high Parsonnet score, severe multivessel disease), and a 5-min warm induction interval is employed in them to attempt more thorough cellular repair before subsequent imposition of a period of ischemia to facilitate surgical precision. The normothermic infusion is delivered both antegrade and retrograde to ensure cardioplegic distribution as in cardiogenic shock patients (to be described subsequently).

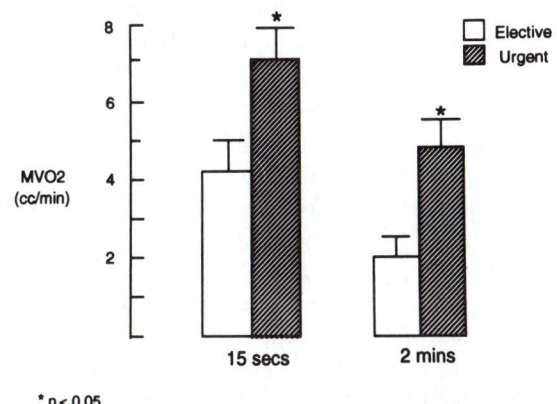

Figure 102–18. Myocardial oxygen (MVO$_2$) in 25 consecutive (hemodynamically stable) nonshock patients during warm blood cardioplegic induction. Note the increased oxygen consumption in patients undergoing urgent (*n* = 18 patients) vs. elective (*n* = 7 patients) operation both at 15 seconds and 2 min.

MAINTENANCE AND DISTRIBUTION OF CARDIOPLEGIA

Cardioplegic Maintenance

All hearts receive some noncoronary blood flow via pericardial connections. The volume of this flow is variable,[79] but is sufficient to wash away all cardioplegic solutions with the exception of those given to donor hearts excised for subsequent transplantation. Myocardial temperature increases after the cardioplegic solution is discontinued, as the heart is rewarmed by the noncoronary collateral blood-flow that has the same temperature as the systemic perfusate. Efforts at controlling noncoronary collateral flow by reducing either systemic flow rate or systemic perfusion pressure, or by using profound levels of systemic hypothermia (<25°C) must be tempered by the recognition of the possible hematologic consequences of deep hypothermia, and the potential deleterious effects of hypoperfusion of other vital organs (brain and kidney) at low systemic flow rates. Recurrent ventricular activity is uncommon if systemic temperature is kept between 32° and 34°C despite cardioplegic washout providing periodic reinfusions of cold blood cardioplegic or noncardioplegic blood are delivered (see section on Integrated Myocardial Management). The clinical presence of noncoronary collateral flow is evident by (1) refilling of blood in the coronary arteries during revascularization procedures, (2) back-bleeding from the coronary ostia during aortic valve replacement, and (3) recurrence of electromechanical activity after cardioplegic administration, especially during the systemic rewarming phase. Periodic replenishment of the cardioplegic solution at approximately 20-min intervals counteracts noncoronary collateral washout. Multidose cardioplegia is necessary even if electromechanical activity does not return since low-level electrical activity may precede recurrence of visi-

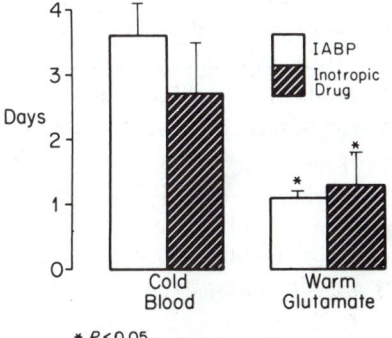

Figure 102–17. Days of postoperative hemodynamic support. Note the earlier discontinuation of intraortic balloon counterpulsation (IABP) and inotropic support in patients receiving warm glutamate cardioplegic induction (warm glutamate).

ble mechanical activity, and can lead to delayed recovery is cardioplegic replenishment is not provided.[80] Periodic replenishment (1) maintains arrest, (2) restores desired levels of hypothermia, (3) buffers acidosis, (4) washes acid metabolites away that inhibit continued anaerobiosis, (5) replenishes high-energy phosphates if the cardioplegic solution is oxygenated, (6) restores substrates depleted during ischemia,[81] and (7) counteracts edema with hyperosmolarity.

Cardioplegic replenishment with low-potassium (8–10 mg/L) solutions limits systemic hyperkalemia and can be limited further by delivering continuous noncardioplegic cold blood during portions of the procedure where perfusion does not compromise visualization (i.e., placing sutures from the valve annulus to the valve sewing ring or closing the aorta or atrium; see Integrated Myocardial Management). Replenishment of oxygenated cardioplegic solutions at 200–250 mL/min over 2 min ensures a gentle perfusion pressure to avoid edema, and allows enough time for the heart to use the delivered oxygen. Myocardial oxygen uptake may exceed basal demands by as much as 10-fold during each 2-min replenishment.[38] Asanguineous cardioplegic solutions without oxygen should be reinfused after similar intervals, but anoxic solutions should be given as a fixed volume and as rapidly as possible to limit the duration of anoxia, provided perfusion pressure does not exceed 50 mm Hg. Limiting perfusion pressure to reduce potential edema formation in newly revascularized myocardium also minimizes mechanical damage to the vein graft. High perfusion pressure during cardioplegic reinfusions should direct suspicion toward the possibility of (1) obstruction of the infusion cannula or (2) kinking or twisting of one of the grafts. Inspection and/or palpation of the aorta during reinfusions allows detection of aortic insufficiency that will interfere with cardioplegic delivery. The most frequent causes of aortic incompetence in the absence of aortic valvular disease are distortion of the aortic valve by (1) a large right atrial cannula against the noncoronary sinus, (2) the retractor or sutures during mitral valve replacement, or (3) failure to remove retrocardiac pads used to improve exposure during valve replacement and/or coronary revascularization.

Cardioplegic Distribution

Coronary Operations

Ensuring adequate cardioplegic solution distribution is especially important in patients with coronary disease where maldistribution of flow is the reason for operation. Our studies show that it is safer to clamp the aorta for up to 4 hours with good cardioplegic distribution than for as little as 30 min when the same cold cardioplegic solution is given without attempts to deliver it beyond coronary stenoses.[82–84] (Fig. 102–19). Homogeneous hypothermia is not a necessary immediate goal provided the heart remains arrested. The myocardial oxygen requirements of asystole are

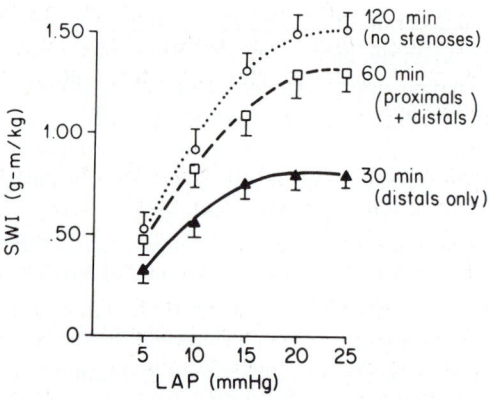

Figure 102–19. Left ventricular performance after blood cardioplegic infusion in dogs with no stenosis, and where attempts were made to distribute the cardioplegic solution beyond stenosis. Note the partial recovery following 30 min of aortic clamping when no attempt was made to distribute the cardioplegic solution, and the normal performance following 120 min of aortic clamping when cardioplegic distribution was unimpeded.

so low at 22°C (0.3 mL/100 g per minute) that they cannot be reduced substantially by reducing temperature further. Prompt fall in myocardial temperature will be achieved by perfusion of cardioplegia through the grafts after distal anastomoses are constructed, or by retrograde delivery. Determination of the order of grafts by review of the preoperative arteriogram allows planning for cardioplegic delivery regionally beyond stenosis if only antegrade methods are used. Myocardium supplied by totally occluded vessels is cooled more slowly than muscle supplied by stenotic or open arteries when cardioplegia is given only through the proximal aorta.[85] Optimal distribution may be achieved if totally occluded vessels with large coronary flow distribution are grafted first, followed by grafting of vessels with significant stenoses, and finally by grafting into areas with the least stenoses or regions receiving the smallest coronary flow distribution. The only exception to this suggested order of grafting is in patients with cardiogenic shock secondary to extending myocardial infarction (> 24 hours after coronary occlusion) and this will be discussed separately.

Possible strategies to ensure cardioplegic distribution include (1) constructing proximal grafts before aortic clamping, (2) constructing all anastomoses during a single period of aortic clamping, (3) perfusing cardioplegic solution through the grafts after each distal anastomosis is completed, and (4) delivering retrograde cardioplegia through either the right atrium or coronary sinus. Special techniques for graft perfusion into areas of recent myocardial infarction (i.e., naturally occurring occlusion or angioplasty occlusion) will be discussed in Reperfusion, below.

Proximal Grafts First. This method ensures that distribution of cardioplegia is determined by the resistance of the coronary vascular bed of the grafted vessel. The construction of proximal anastomoses on cardiopulmonary bypass avoids increasing left ventricular afterload unnecessarily and unknowingly. Precise estimation of graft length is essential as there is less margin for error than when distal anastomoses are made first.

All Anastomoses during Aortic Clamping. This method prolongs the duration of aortic clamping but ensures cardioplegic delivery provided each proximal anastomosis is accomplished immediately after each distal anastomosis. The obligatory prolongation of aortic clamping is counterbalanced by the improved cardioplegic distribution.[86] Prolongation of aortic clamping may be problematic if complete revascularization is not possible, as no protection can be offered to areas of contracting muscle that cannot be revascularized due to unsuitable distal vessels. Retrograde cardioplegic administration circumvents this problem by ensuring distribution to areas supplied by obstructed vessels,[87–89] and can be delivered during construction of proximal anastomoses to further limit the ischemic duration while the aorta is clamped. The construction of all anastomoses during a single period of aortic clamping also circumvents possible dislodgement of atheromatous intra-aortic debris during application of a tangential aortic clamp.

Perfusion Through Grafts. This method does not prolong aortic clamping and allows somewhat easier estimation of graft length, especially with sequential grafts. Care must be taken to avoid kinking during reinfusions. Each cardioplegic reinfusion should be delivered through *all* completed grafts. This can be accomplished with a cardioplegic delivery system that ensures equal resistance through the cannulae delivering cardioplegic solution to the aorta and grafted arteries. Use of a manifold with multiple sidearms allows the same system to deliver warm noncardioplegic blood to the distal myocardium while proximal anastomoses are constructed after aortic unclamping (see Reperfusion below). Recent studies indicate, however, that the incidence of cerebral atheroemboli is increased[90] when tangential clamps are applied to the aorta, so that it is currently recommended to do all anastomoses with a single period of aortic clamping. The use of continuous retrograde blood cardioplegic or noncardioplegic blood perfusion to the vented aorta will limit ischemia despite the prolongation of the duration of aortic clamping. Clinical adoption of retrograde techniques has been slow, despite abundant experimental and clinical data attesting to their usefulness.

Retrograde Cardioplegia. This method has several theoretical advantages, which include (1) distribution of cardioplegia in diffuse coronary disease, especially when all areas cannot be revascularized, (2) avoidance of the need for direct coronary cannulation and possible late ostial stenoses in patients undergoing aortic valve replacement, (3) exclusion of the need for aortotomy and cannulation of the coronary ostia in patients with minimal aortic regurgitation who do not require aortic valve replacement, and (4) ability to give cardioplegia during mitral valve operations without removing the valve retractor.[88]

The need for both routes of cardioplegic delivery in coronary operations is emphasized by experimental and clinical data[87–89, 91] documenting poor cardioplegic distribution to jeopardized myocardium with antegrade infusions under conditions of experimentally simulated coronary stenosis,[87,89] and redistribution of cardioplegic flow away from vulnerable subendocardial muscle. In addition, the inability of cold antegrade cardioplegia to protect ischemic myocardium has been confirmed by others.[92,93] Conversely, retrograde cardioplegia is directed preferentially toward subendocardial muscle despite occlusion of the arterial vessel supplying the jeopardized region. The right ventricle is not protected consistently by retrograde cardioplegia, as right ventricular cooling and postbypass functional recovery are somewhat variable in experimental studies of isolated cold retrograde cardioplegia. These experimental findings have recently been confirmed clinically[94] by contrast echocardiography that demonstrated poor right ventricular myocardial perfusion with retrograde delivery (Fig. 102–20). Preliminary clinical observations suggest also that antegrade and retrograde cardioplegia supply different vascular beds, as glucose and O_2 uptake increase, and lactate washout occurs when switching from antegrade to retrograde cardioplegia, or from retrograde to antegrade cardioplegia (Fig. 102–21A,B,C).[63]

Retrograde cardioplegia may become particularly useful in coronary patients who receive internal mammary or gastroepiploic artery grafts since antegrade cardioplegia cannot presently be delivered through the proximally intact arteries. The development of transatrial methods of coronary sinus cannulation[88] has overcome the need for double venous isolation and cannulation, control of the pulmonary artery, and decompression of the aorta. However, primary reliance on retroperfusion alone requires a greater volume of cardioplegia and longer intervals before arrest is produced because 30% of retroperfusion is non-nutritive, and nutritive right ventricular retroperfusion is only 20% of that to the left ventricle.[95] They also require a greater volume of cardioplegia and longer interval before arrest is produced, and may be less consistent than antegrade techniques.

The delay in arrest with retrograde cardioplegia can be offset by combining an initial antegrade cardioplegic infusion to provide for rapid asystole with subsequent retrograde cardioplegia to ensure cardioplegic distribution. The method of alternating between the antegrade and retrograde techniques in coronary patients enhances the cardioprotective benefit of each method as reported recently.[96] These data reinforce the conclusion that adding retrograde cardioplegic techniques increases the armamentarium of ways to ensure cardioplegic distribution.

Infusion of the cardioplegic solution through the right atrium with isolation of the right heart[97] cools the right ventricle directly by intracavitary hypothermia as well as by retrograde perfusion through thebesian veins. Failure to

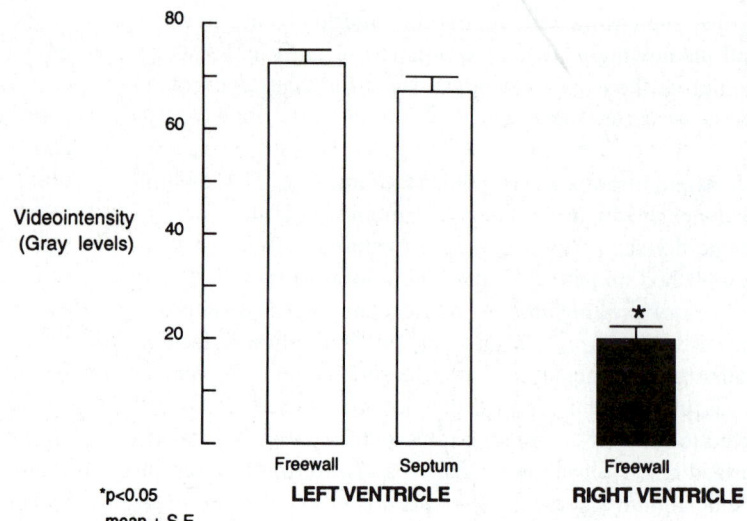

Figure 102–20. Myocardial perfusion assessed by contrast echocardiography of the right and left ventricular (freewall and septum) during retrograde cardioplegic delivery in 12 patients. Note the decreased right ventricular perfusion compared to the septum and left ventricular freewall.

maintain right ventricular distention occurs when the cavae or pulmonary artery are not occluded completely, or if there is an atrial septal defect. Direct coronary sinus cannulation as described by Menache requires right atriotomy and direct coronary sinus cannulation.[98] Coronary sinus cardioplegia alone is effective during aortic replacement but may not protect the right ventricle because of problems of distribution.[97] Additional efforts at right ventricular protection by topical hypothermia may be needed when this technique is used in patients with right ventricular hypertrophy or failure.

Antegrade/Retrograde Cardioplegia. Recently developed simplified clinical techniques of retrograde cardioplegia de-

livery, employing a self-inflating/deflating low-pressure balloon on a retrograde cannula, avoids the need for right heart isolation by allowing transatrial coronary sinus cannulation through a small puncture of the right atrium (Fig. 102–22). This method has allowed retrograde cardioplegia to be used without making cumbersome changes in the conduct of the operation and allows the superior cardioplegic distribution to compliment the advantages achieved via antegrade delivery.[63,88,91] *We now routinely use both antegrade and retrograde cardioplegia in all patients undergoing aortic coronary bypass grafting, and valve replacement or repair.* The blood cardioplegic volume is usually delivered equally via antegrade and retrograde routes during all phases of cardioplegic administration (i.e., warm induction,

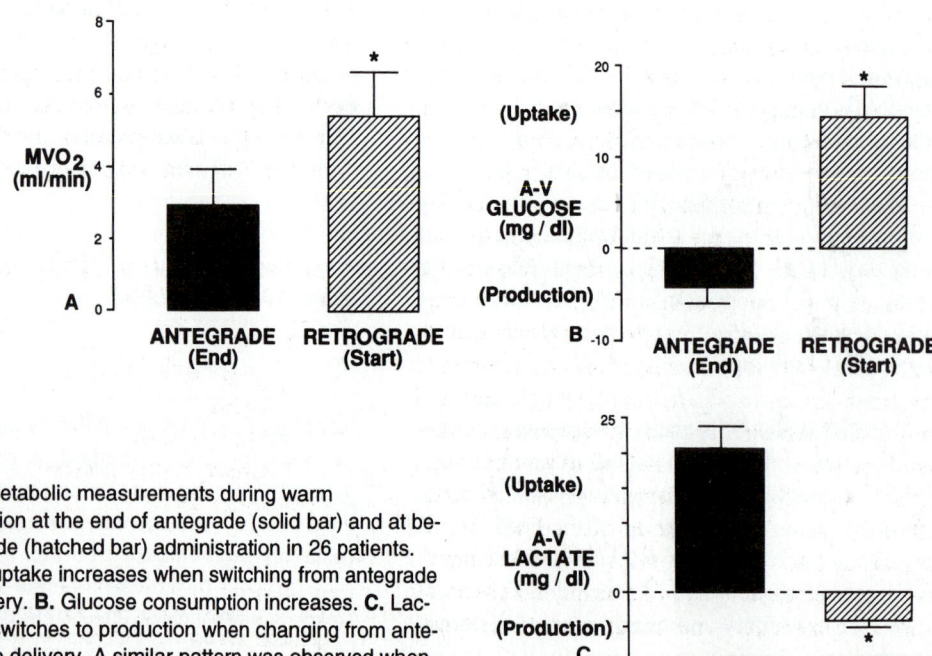

Figure 102–21. Metabolic measurements during warm cardioplegic induction at the end of antegrade (solid bar) and at beginning of retrograde (hatched bar) administration in 26 patients. **A.** Myocardial O_2 uptake increases when switching from antegrade to retrograde delivery. **B.** Glucose consumption increases. **C.** Lactate consumption switches to production when changing from antegrade to retrograde delivery. A similar pattern was observed when switching from retrograde to antegrade delivery in separate studies.

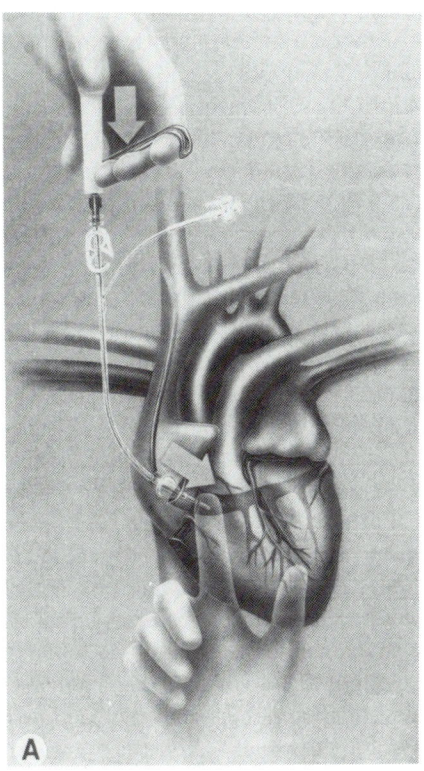
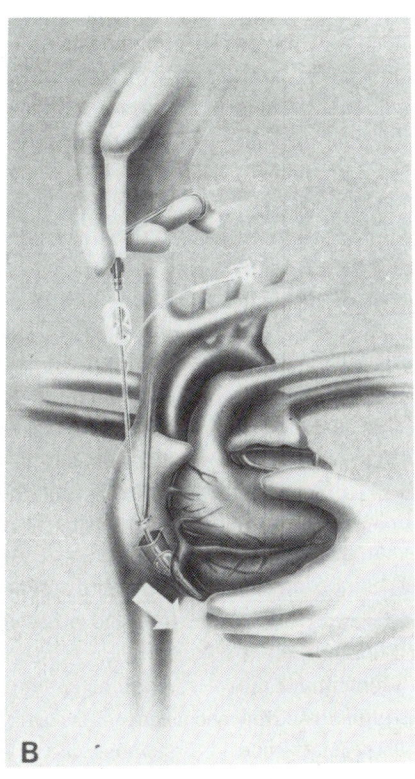

Figure 102–22. Coronary sinus cannulation can be carried out percutaneously using a self-inflating retrograde cardioplegic cannula without the need for bicaval cannulation. This can be done either off bypass (**A**) or on partial bypass (**B**) when coronary sinus visualization is necessary.

multidose cold blood cardioplegic replenishments, and warm reperfusion) and several reports confirm the benefits of the combined approach, compared to antegrade cardioplegia alone.[63,88]

Transatrial insertion of the retrograde cannula into the coronary sinus has been successful in 98–99% of patients, and can be accomplished before starting bypass in more than 90% of instances. Partial bypass to facilitate exposure of the coronary sinus surface has been needed in the others to aid in cannula placement. Right atriotomy is rarely needed (<2%) to remove a septum or cribriform sheet of tissue covering the coronary sinus and permit direct visual coronary sinus cannulation. Coronary sinus injury is rare and occurs only if forceful efforts are made to position the cannula or if infusion is continued with pressures exceeding 50 mm Hg.[63] Compression of the IVC–RA junction to raise coronary sinus pressure (> 25 mm Hg) is sometimes needed if the cannula retracts, but remains within the coronary sinus. Introducing the cannula through the low RA wall to minimize intra-atrial redundancy, advancing the cannula to the coronary sinus-left atrial junction, and using a textured balloon limit dislodgement. Transiently stopping cardioplegic infusion between the antegrade and retrograde dose, and raising the flow to 200–250 mL/min over 5–10 seconds limits recoil of the cannula from the coronary sinus. Encircling sutures around the coronary sinus to avoid cannula displacement has been described, but is rarely necessary as application of these maneuvers has made cannula dislodgement rare.

Overall mortality in a recent series was 2.8% (Table

102–9) and the majority of patients were in the high risk category. This combined antegrade/retrograde approach has expanded the safety of using IMA and other arterial grafts in high risk patients who otherwise would have received vein grafts because of previous inability to provide reliable cardioplegic distribution to the jeopardized muscle supplied by the left anterior descending coronary artery. Preliminary data in a subset of coronary operations show that deeper hypothermia of the anterolateral ventricle and septum (11° vs. 15°C, $p < 0.05$ range 9°–13°C vs. 12°–22°C) was achieved when the 4°–8°C blood cardioplegic infusions were given both antegrade and retrograde, versus only antegrade. Not infrequently, atheromatous debris is flushed retrograde from the distal cut orifices of previously placed vein grafts

TABLE 102–9. ANTEGRADE/RETROGRADE BLOOD CARDIOPLEGIA[a]

CABG	261
Shock or EF <0.2 or AMI	49
Reops	48
AVR and/or MVR	103
Dissecting aortic aneurysm	3
Pediatric CHD	123
	490 patients
Mortality	2.8%

[a]Types of operation where combined antegrade/retrograde blood cardioplegia was used. CABG, coronary artery bypass grafting; AVR, aortic valve replacement; MVR, mitral valve replacement; CHD, congenital heart disease.

so that retrograde perfusion likely reduces the damage produced by atheromatous embolization during dissection in coronary reoperations. It also provides a treatment option in the event of inadvertent coronary air embolism, together with the other advantages enumerated in Table 102–10. Experimental and clinical studies show that cardioprotective strategies are superior when perfusion is via both arterial (antegrade) and coronary sinus (retrograde) routes of delivery.[63,88,99] Retrograde perfusion techniques are used because antegrade cardioplegia is unable to deliver flow to vascular beds receiving arterial grafts and such conduits are used with increasing frequency in high risk patients. Antegrade techniques are advantageous because they produced more prompt arrest and overcome the deficient delivery to the right ventricle by retrograde coronary sinus perfusion.[87,100,101]

Currently, most surgeons alternate between arterial (antegrade) and coronary sinus retroperfusion because of concern over possible myocardial edema and hemorrhage if venous pressure exceeds 50 mm Hg. Venous hypertension during retroperfusion is less likely in the heart than in other organs, because most coronary venous drainage is via thebesian channels and enters the right atrium and right ventricle directly.[102–104] This unique coronary venous drainage pattern makes understandable the report showing that intermittent, and prolonged coronary sinus occlusion during antegrade cardioplegia enhances its distribution to jeopardized muscle and improves its protective property.[102,103] The distribution of retrograde and antegrade cardioplegic flow is also different within the left ventricle itself, and these two routes of delivery compliment each other providing more homogenous perfusion.[63,105]

Simultaneous Antegrade/Retrograde Perfusion. Based upon the aforementioned information, we reasoned that *simultaneous* antegrade and retrograde perfusion might combine the benefits of both routes of delivery and provide a further refinement to current myocardial protective strategies. Recent studies (1) confirm experimentally the safety of simultaneous arterial and coronary sinus perfusion[58] and (2) report initial clinical application of this combined strategy in 155 consecutive high-risk patients. Cardioplegic induction was warm in patients in cardiogenic shock and cold in most others, and all anastamoses were constructed during

a single interval of aortic clamping. Distal anastomoses were accomplished with cold intermittent ischemia followed by simultaneous coronary sinus and arterial perfusion via the vein graft. These sequential distal-proximal anastomosis are performed using an adapter whereby the long saphenous graft segment is attached to the arm of the retrograde line and multiple connections or tubing are avoided (Fig. 102–23).

Simultaneous arterial/coronary sinus perfusion provides several technical advantages, including retrograde flushing of the aorta followed by antegrade deairing before securing the suture line on distal grafts. The tendency to pursestring the anastomosis is reduced by securing the suture line with a distended perfused graft; the full graft expedites detection of kinking and leaks at the suture line or along the conduit. Appropriate graft length can be estimated without the need to fill the graft with syringes and saline and the aortic anastomosis site can be selected with a simultaneous distended graft and aorta. This avoids aortic distortion and possible dislodgement of atheroma during tangen-

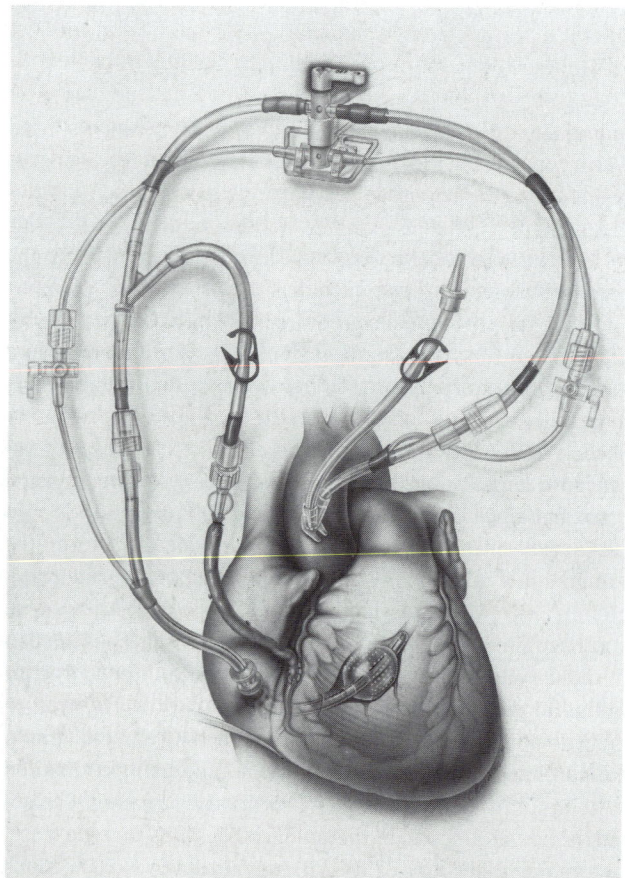

Figure 102–23. Clinical method of simultaneously delivering antegrade/retrograde cardioplegia to ensure protection to jeopardize myocardium. Note that this system allows for antegrade or retrograde delivery separately or simultaneous coronary graft and retrograde delivery. Also pressure monitoring is easily accomplished (see text for description).

TABLE 102–10. ADVANTAGES OF COMBINED ANTEGRADE/RETROGRADE CARDIOPLEGIC TECHNIQUES[a]

Prompt arrest

Ensure distribution (IMA, AI)

Limit CP volume

Uninterrupted valve procedures

Avoid ostial cannulation

Flush coronary debris/air

[a]IMA, internal mammary artery; AI, aortic insufficiency; CP, cardioplegia.

tial clamping. Finally, the continuity of the operation is not interrupted to deliver cardioplegia and cold ischemia permits a dry bloodless surgical field when technical precision is essential during construction of distal anastomosis (see Integrated Myocardial Management). Clinical results in this group of patients were essentially similar with simultaneous antegrade/coronary sinus perfusion to previous results, so that the principle of simultaneous perfusion does not appear to be detrimental and yet provides many technical advantages (Table 102–11). These data overcome perceived concerns that myocardial damage may ensue from simultaneous arterial and coronary sinus perfusion, and suggest that this technique may add to the armamentarium of the cardioprotective strategies currently available.

Integrated Myocardial Protection. Confusion about cardioplegic delivery continues, predominantly due to the surgical predilection for assuming adversarial predictions (i.e., warm versus cold blood cardioplegia, antegrade vs. retrograde, intermittent vs. continuous). All of these aforementioned individual modalities have been combined recently into a comprehensive cardioplegic strategy termed "integrated myocardial management." This approach provides a flexible and simple method to take maximal advantage of each aforementioned cardioprotective method (see Table 102–12). It evolved from concepts tested in our laboratory and incorporates the strategies of warm/cold blood cardioplegia, antegrade/retrograde delivery, continuous/intermittent infusion, and noncardioplegic blood/blood cardioplegia infusions during a single period of aortic cross clamping (a tangential aortic clamp is not used).

The method is based on the following principles: (1) surgical precision is optimized by a dry bloodless field so that *cold* intermittent arrest is used to avoid ischemic damage (no perfusion during distal anastomosis or when visualization is needed), (2) ischemia is unnecessary when visualization is not problematic (i.e., during construction of proximal anastomosis, placing sutures in valve annulas or valve sewing ring) so that *continuous* blood or blood cardioplegia is infused retrograde during this time, (3) continuous blood perfusion of the cold arrested heart does not require cardioplegia to maintain arrest,[106] thereby limiting hemodilution and hyperkalemia, (4) the continuity of the

TABLE 102–11. POSTOPERATIVE RESULTS AFTER SIMULTANEOUS ARTERIAL AND CORONARY SINUS PERFUSION

	Patients (n = 155)	%
Mechanical circulatory support (IABP)	18[a]	12
days postop	(1.2 ± 0.2)	
Perioperative myocardial infarction	3	2
Death	6	4

[a]Sixteen of 18 in preoperative cardiogenic shock

TABLE 102–12. INTEGRATED MYOCARDIAL MANAGEMENT

Warm/cold blood cardioplegia
Antegrade/retrograde delivery
Intermittent/continuous perfusion
Blood/blood cardioplegia
Limits cardioplegia overdose and hemodilution
Avoids tangential aortic clamping

operation should not be interrupted to deliver perfusion (blood or cardioplegia) while the aorta is clamped; the only exception is during cardioplegic induction when cardiac manipulation may make the aortic valve incompetent, and (5) the aorta is clamped as soon as satisfactory extracorporeal circulation is established (collapsed pulmonary artery) and cardiopulmonary bypass is discontinued within 5 min of aortic unclamping, as the last portion of each procedure is performed with continuous warm cardioplegic or blood perfusion.

The following description defines how this technique is used in a typical coronary artery operation. Similar methods are applied to valve operations where cardioplegic (or noncardioplegic) flow is interrupted only when visualization is needed (e.g., valve excision, placing sutures in annulas, and securing prosthesis sutures) and given continuously when visualization is nonproblematic (e.g., placing sutures from annulus to valve ring, closing atrium or aorta). Cardioplegic induction is either warm or cold (see Cardioplegic Induction) and the infusion is administered antegrade and retrograde in relatively equal proportions. This is the only time that the operation is interrupted to deliver cardioplegic flow. Systemic temperature is reduced to ~ 34°C to provide a margin of safety if a perfusion accident occurs. Cardioplegic flow is stopped after cold induction so that distal anastomoses can be constructed in a dry operative field required for surgical precision while hypothermia limits the rate of development of ischemic damage. A brief (1 min) cold blood cardioplegic infusion is delivered retrograde after completion of the distal anastomosis and followed by *continuous* retrograde cold *noncardioplegic* blood perfusion as the proximal anastomosis is constructed with the aorta vented. Conversion from cold blood cardioplegia to cold noncardioplegia blood maintains arrest, hypothermia, and cardiac nourishment to both the left and right ventricles,[106] while reducing cardioplegia dose and hemodilution. The safety of continuous cold noncardioplegic blood perfusion suggests that cold perfusion of the heart can be used to avoid ischemia during aspects of the operation when the aorta is clamped and visualization is not impeded by continuous coronary perfusion.[106] A brief antegrade cardioplegic infusion is delivered at the conclusion of each proximal anastomosis while the suture line is secured and the graft tip is fashioned for the next anastomosis. This antegrade infusion ensures cardioplegic distribution to the right ventricle, which may be perfused inadequately by retrograde delivery,[87,100,101] and keeps the heart arrested during the next ischemic interval.

The sequence is repeated for each distal and proximal anastomosis and the internal mammary anastomosis is performed during rewarming of the patient and cardioplegic solutions. The warm blood cardioplegic reperfusate is delivered first antegrade and then retrograde while the last proximal anastomosis is constructed. This is followed immediately thereafter by retrograde perfusion of warm non-cardioplegic blood to wash out the cardioplegic solution, and allow the heart to begin beating as the proximal anastomosis is completed. This method usually allows discontinuation of bypass within 5 min of removing the aortic clamp as continuous cardioplegic and noncardioplegic blood perfusion reduces ischemic time despite performance of all anastomoses during a single interval of aortic clamping.

Recent reports[90] confirm the concept that myocardial damage is related more to the method of myocardial protection than the duration of aortic cross-clamping and show also that the incidence of cerebral complications is reduced by avoiding the use of tangential aortic clamps. This probably reduces potential dislodgement of intra-aortic atheromatous debris.[107] Ischemic duration is also shortened during valve procedures since cold continuous blood or blood cardioplegia can be infused during much of the procedure, and interrupted only when visualization is desired. Table 102–13 shows results of the integrated myocardial management method in a consecutive series of adult patients undergoing revascularization and/or valve operations.[108]

Proponents of different techniques of intraoperative myocardial protection have traditionally, and for uncertain reasons, taken adversarial positions (i.e., warm vs. cold blood cardioplegia, antegrade versus retrograde and intermittent vs. continuous delivery, blood vs. blood cardioplegic perfusion). The fundamental issue is the development of a thoughtful strategy for cardioplegic distribution, and this can be achieved by combining the benefits of both

TABLE 102–13. INTEGRATED MYOCARDIAL PROTECTION[a]

Procedure	Patients	
CABG		979
Urgent, emergent	174	
Reoperation	143	
NYHA IV	356	
AVR/MVR		393
Reoperation	48	
NYHA IV	96	
Valve and CABG		102
Reoperation	9	
NYHA IV	31	
Total		1496
Mortality		1.6%

[a]CABG, coronary artery bypass grafting; AVR, aortic valve replacement/repair; MVR, mitral valve replacement/repair; NYHA IV, New York Heart Association Class IV.

antegrade and retrograde cardioplegic techniques. We suspect that application of this combined strategy will allow more critically ill patients to undergo safe internal mammary artery grafting and to experience the same complete immediate recovery of regional and global function shown in patients who receive vein grafts.

Myocardial Protection During Coronary Reoperations.
The increasing frequency of coronary reoperations requires special attention toward developing operative strategies that are flexible and provide protection against potential intraoperative damage that would not occur during primary coronary revascularization procedures. Intraoperative myocardial injury can occur sometimes before aortic clamping if vein grafts are compressed during dissection of the heart in preparation for cannulation or exposure of arteries for subsequent grafting since they frequently contain atheromatous debris that can embolize when compressed. This problem can be circumvented in several ways: First, the prebypass dissection is confined to exposing the aorta and right atrium to minimize graft compression, and the remainder of the dissection carried out after extracorporeal circulation is begun and the heart is decompressed and arrested with cardioplegic solution. Second transection of functioning grafts and construction of new anastomoses will avoid graft embolization and increase graft longevity. Third, retrograde cardioplegia is particularly well suited for flushing out atheromatous debris, as we have observed particulate matter become dislodged from grafts (presumably from coronary vessels) when retrograde doses are given, while inspecting the effluent from transected grafts. In some instances, the predominance of coronary bloodflow is provided by functioning grafts so that their presence ensures cardioplegic distribution during antegrade induction and multidose maintenance especially if retrograde is not used. The heart is particularly vulnerable to damage if they are occluded by the tangential clamp if proximal anastomoses are constructed during rewarming so that construction of all proximal and distal anastomoses during a single interval of aortic clamping is recommended in all reoperations where patent graft are present (as described in Cardioplegic Distribution, above).

The induction and maintenance of cardioplegic arrest are problematic in patients with functioning mammary grafts (or prior Vineburg operations), since these conduits carry noncardioplegic blood and delay arrest and/or cause early return of electromechanical activity. This potential problem can be circumvented by dissection of the mammary pedicle and temporary occlusion of the graft during aortic clamping. Retrograde cardioplegia is particularly useful when a functioning mammary graft supplies a substantial muscle mass. An alternate strategy in patients with functioning internal mammary artery (IMA) grafts is that of intermittent aortic clamping for each distal anastomosis with use of either ischemic arrest or, preferably, a dose of antegrade cardioplegia to protect areas supplied by patent coronary arteries. Under these circumstances, the proximal anastomoses are constructed while the aorta is clamped tangentially, and the temporary occluder is removed from the IMA pedicle to provide intermittent reperfusion after each interval of aortic clamping.

Aortic Valve Replacement. Preoperative coronary angiography is helpful to determine (1) if there are coronary arterial stenoses that require bypass grafting, (2) length of the left main coronary artery (i.e., separate cannulation of the left anterior descending and left circumflex may be necessary if the left main coronary artery is short or if branching occurs at the ostia), and (3) the distribution of the right coronary artery (i.e., if it is dominant and supplies the inferior left ventricular wall). Performance of distal grafts first and distribution of cardioplegia through *both* the newly constructed grafts and the coronary ostia will optimize the strategy for myocardial protection during combined aortic valve replacement in coronary revascularization if primary reliance is placed upon antegrade perfusion.

The underlying valvular lesion (i.e., stenosis or insufficiency) is the principal determinant of how cardioplegia is induced. The total volume of cardioplegia used during induction must be increased (i.e., to ~1500 mL) to provide satisfactory cooling of the increased left ventricular muscle mass caused by hypertrophy. Arrest can be achieved without opening the aorta in patients with aortic stenosis, but aortotomy and direct cannulation of the coronary ostia are required in patients with aortic insufficiency unless retrograde cardioplegia is used. Alternation of infusions through the left and right coronary cannula ensures distribution into the vascular bed supplied by each vessel if antegrade methods are used exclusively. Conversely, retrograde cardioplegia may negate the need for ostial cannulation and allow the operation to be accomplished without interruptions, since infusions can be delivered while the operation proceeds. Intermittent reinfusions are given every 20–30 min unless a very brief procedure is anticipated and cold noncardioplegic blood is given when visualization is not compromised (i.e., sutures from valve annulus to valve, closure of aorta; see Integrated Myocardial Management). Direct infusion into the right coronary artery is important if (1) there is right ventricular hypertrophy or pulmonary hypertension or (2) the right coronary artery supplies substantial branches to the diaphragmatic surface of the left ventricle. Exposure of the right coronary ostium is facilitated by eversion of the aortic lip and counterpressure on the right ventricular outflow tract as described recently.[109] To avoid prolonging the operation unnecessarily, attempts to cannulate the right coronary artery should be abandoned if there is failure after a reasonable effort. This limitation of right coronary cardioplegic delivery can be counterbalanced by provision and maintenance of topical hypothermia, use of *cold* retrograde infusion to provide conductance cooling of the right ventricle despite a limited nutritive flow, and delivery of a more prolonged warm cardioplegic reperfusate after aortic unclamping (see section of Reperfusion).

REPERFUSION

Reperfusion injury is defined as the functional, metabolic, and structural alterations caused by restoring bloodflow after a period of temporary ischemia (i.e., aortic clamping).[70] The potential for this damage exists during all cardiac operations because the aorta must be clamped to produce a quiet bloodless field. Reperfusion damage is characterized by (1) intracellular calcium accumulation,[110] (2) explosive cell swelling with reduction of postischemic blood flow and reduced ventricular compliance,[110,111] and (3) inability to effectively utilize delivered oxygen, even when coronary flow and oxygen content are ample.[60,112] Our studies show that the fate of myocardium jeopardized by global and regional ischemia is determined more by the careful control of the conditions of reperfusion and composition of the reperfusate than by the duration of ischemia itself.[113] *The cardiac surgeon is in the unique position to counteract the potential of reperfusion damage since the conditions of reperfusion and the composition of the reperfusate are under the surgeon's immediate control.*

Postischemic reperfusion damage after global ischemia can be *avoided* or minimized by substituting a brief (i.e., 3 to 5 min) warm (37°C) blood cardioplegic infusion during the initial phase of reoxygenation for the normal blood reperfusion that would be provided by aortic unclamping[60] (Fig. 102–24). The principles (Table 102–14) that are addressed during controlled reperfusion include (1) reoxygenation with blood to start aerobic metabolism for energy production to repair cellular injury, (2) delivery of the reperfusion over *time* rather than by *dose* to maximize O_2, utilization,[114] lowering energy demands by maintaining temporary cardioplegia to allow the limited O_2 ability to be channeled toward reparative processes,[115] (4) replenishing

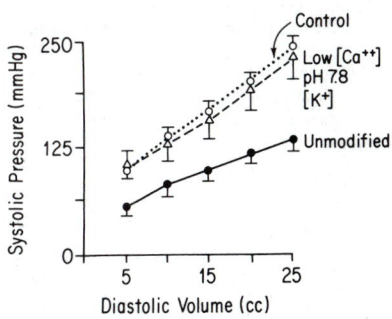

Figure 102–24. Left ventricular performance 30 min after 1 hour of topical hypothermic ischemic arrest. Note the normal postischemic performance when a blood cardioplegic reperfusate containing low calcium, high pH, was given just prior to removal of the aortic clamp, and the depressed myocardial performance when the reperfusate was unmodified.

TABLE 102–14. WARM CARDIOPLEGIC REPERFUSION

Principle	Method
Provide O_2	Blood
Optimize metabolism	Normothermia
Duration	5–10 min
Maintain asystole	KCl
Replenish substrate	Glutamate/aspartate
Reverse acidosis	Buffer
Limit Ca^{2+}	CPD[a]
Counteract edema	Hyperosmolarity
	Gentle pressure

[a]CPD, citrate phosphate dextrose.

substrate (i.e., glutamate), which allows optimal aerobic energy production to occur,[69] (5) making the reperfusate pH alkalotic to counteract tissue acidosis and optimize enzymatic and metabolic function during recovery,[116] (6) temporarily reducing ionic calcium available to enter the cell (i.e., chelation with citrate phosphate dextrose),[61] (7) inducing hyperosmolarity and decreasing perfusion pressure (i.e., 50 mm Hg to reduce and minimize reperfusion edema),[117,118] and (8) warming the reperfusate to 37°C to optimize the rate of metabolic recovery.[70,119] Hypothermic reperfusion is not used because it retards metabolic rate and slows repair.[120,121]

The metabolic and functional values of using a warm blood cardioplegic reperfusate strategy in elective coronary operations are well documented[122] and a warm blood reperfusate is delivered before aortic unclamping in *all* operations. The studies of Kirklin[123] provide added evidence that controlled warm blood cardioplegia reperfusion is a powerful tool to reduce the detrimental effects of prolonged aortic clamping (Fig. 102–25). The capacity to avoid or minimize reperfusion damage by reperfusion cardioplegia makes this technique a valuable adjunct to the cardiac surgeon's armamentarium, especially if cardioplegic distribution has been problematic, or if aortic clamping has been prolonged. Reperfusion cardioplegia may be used as the primary form of cardiac protection (to avoid reperfusion injury) if homogeneous cardioplegic delivery is questionable through a large right coronary artery or if early branching of left main artery requires selective cannulation of anterior descending and circumflex branches during aortic valve replacement. Starting systemic and cardioplegic rewarming about 5 min before unclamping the aorta ensures normothermia in the 8–10 mEq/L K^+ oxygenated blood cardioplegic reperfusate, which is the same level of hyperkalemia used during multidose cold cardioplegia. Delivery of this reperfusate at 150 mL/min for 3–5 min avoids high reperfusion pressure (i.e., 50 mm Hg). Longer infusions (i.e., 5–15 min) may be useful if there has been poor cardioplegic distribution during the preceding aortic clamping interval (i.e., through large right coronary artery that was not perfused during aortic valve replacement or if the last distal coronary anastomoses was made into a vessel with a large myocardial flow distribution).

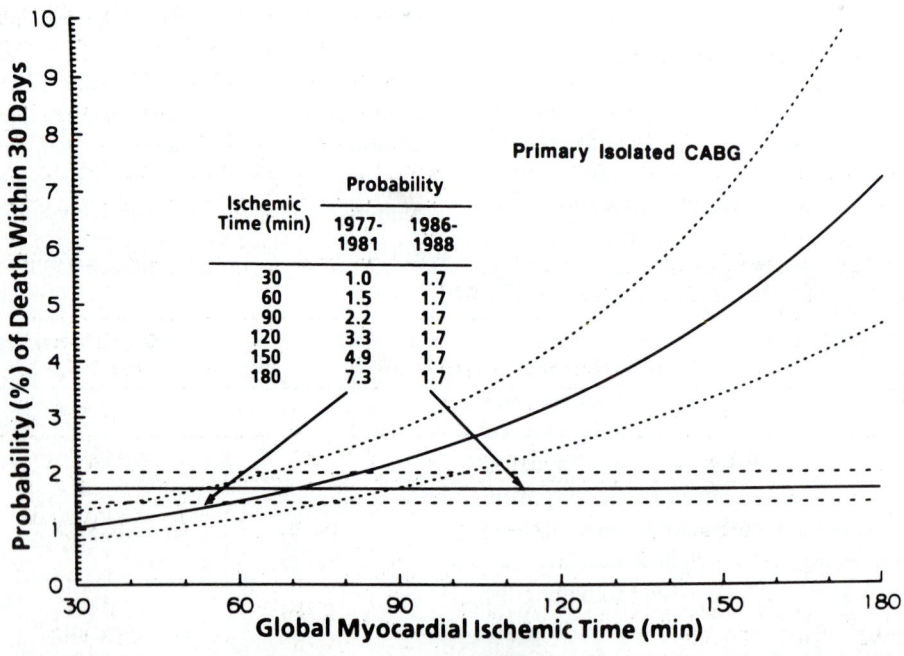

Figure 102–25. Relation between global myocardial ischemic time (in minutes) and the probability of death within 30 days of the operation. The two depictions are normograms of multivariate equations describing experiences with isolated primary coronary artery bypass grafting during 1977 to 1981 ($n = 3872$) and during 1986 to 1992 ($n = 2351$). In both eras, cold cardioplegia was used, but in the latter era controlled aortic root warm blood cardioplegia reperfusion was given in patients with long global myocardial ischemic times. The solid lines depict the continuous estimate of probability and the dash lines are 70% confidence intervals around the estimate: Note the decreased probability of death within 30 days in those patients who underwent warm reperfusion.

Reperfusion cardioplegia must be delivered into *all* grafts *and* into the aorta in coronary patients and its distribution is augmented when it is also given retrograde via the coronary sinus. The warm cardioplegic reperfusate may be used also to evacuate air from the aorta through the suture line during aortic valve replacement. Recurrence of cardiac electromechanical activity during reperfusion cardioplegia is rare despite the low potassium concentration. The warm reperfusate is discontinued and the aortic clamp removed if electromechanical activity recurs (i.e., beating or fibrillating) while it is being infused in routine operations. Conversely, a more hyperkalemic (20 mEq/L K^+) warm reperfusate is substituted if cardioplegic delivery was considered inadequate during operative repair as the period of warm arrested reperfusion is considered *critical* to compensate for the potentially inadequate myocardial protection. Electromechanical activity resumes usually 1–2 min after aortic unclamping unless there is systemic hyperkalemia. Failure to recover contractility requires temporary ventricular pacing to avoid the myocardial edema that may follow prolonged perfusion of the flaccid heart. Palpation of the left ventricle detects distention so that a vent can be inserted if necessary. Recurrent asystole after placing the tangential clamp in coronary operations suggests that coronary flow has been interrupted by the clamp. Routine palpation of the proximal aorta below the clamp allows estimation of the adequacy of coronary perfusion pressure and provides grounds for reapplication of the tangential clamp if the proximal aorta is flaccid.

Reperfusion After Acute Myocardial Infarction

Precise control of the conditions of reperfusion and composition of the reperfusate is especially important in patients undergoing revascularization for acute evolving myocardial infarction.[113] The principles of reperfusate composition discussed previously for use after global ischemia are applicable directly to reperfusion after regional ischemia and the same reperfusate may be used. Delivery of the warm reperfusate selectively into the ischemic region after removing the aortic clamp following completion of all distal anastomoses concentrates the reperfusate in the area most vulnerable to reperfusion damage. The duration of regional 37°C cardioplegic reperfusion (i.e., through the graft) is prolonged to 20 min because experimental studies show that postischemic O_2 uptake does not return to baseline levels until this interval has elapsed.[114] Shorter regional reperfusion intervals limit muscle salvage and hampers recovery. Other proximal anastomoses can be constructed during this prolonged segmental cardioplegic reperfusion and this is the only time that a tangential clamp is used during coronary operations. Keeping reperfusion pressure at or below 50 mm Hg limits edema and avoids disruption of microvasculature,[124,125] while decompression by venting ensures low energy demands in the reperfused segment.[71] Restriction of flow to a maximum of 50 mL/min simplifies the procedure, but low reperfusion pressure (i.e., < 50 mm Hg) may not revascularize subendocardial muscle optimally. Conversely, salvage of overlying midmyocardium and epicardial muscle may convert the potential transmural necrosis to a subendocardial infarction.

Initial application of the aforementioned technique has resulted in early recovery of regional contractility in a preliminary series of 16 patients revascularized after an average of 10 hours of acute coronary occlusion.[113] Subsequently, a multicenter analysis[62] of the treatment of acute coronary occlusion documented the superiority of surgically controlled reperfusion over medically uncontrolled reperfusion using percutaneous transluminal coronary angioplasty (PTCA) by showing that it accomplishes more completely the primary goals of revascularization, restoring segmental contractility and lowering mortality (Table 102–15, Fig. 102–26). This surgical experience[62] in 156 pa-

TABLE 102–15. RESULTS OF MEDICALLY UNCONTROLLED REPERFUSION BY PTCA VS. CONTROLLED SURGICAL REPERFUSION BY CABG AFTER ACUTE CORONARY OCCLUSION[a]

Reperfusion	PTCA (Uncontrolled) ($n = 1203$)			CABG (Controlled) ($n = 156$)	p value
Ischemic time[b] (hours)	3.9			6.3	< 0.05
	Patients	**Range**	**%**	**Patients %**	
Mortality					
Overall	105/1203	(7.2–11%)	(8.7%)	6/156 (3.9%)	< 0.05
High risk					
Subgroups[c]					
LAD occlusion	39/331	(10–12%)	(11%)	9/95 (5%)	NS
3 vessel disease	25/158	(15–20%)	(17%)	0/66 (0%)	< 0.05
Age > 70 years	21/109	(17–25%)	(19%)	1/22 (5%)	NS
Failure to reperfuse	26/82	(15–50%)	(32%)	0/0 (0%)	< 0.05
Preop shock	49/114	(41–57%)	(43%)	6/66 (9%)	< 0.05

[a]PTCA, percutaneous transluminal coronary angioplasty; CABG, coronary artery bypass grafting; *n*, number of patients.
[b]Time from chest pain to reperfusion (PTCA) or bypass (CABG).
[c]Each of the 5 reports did not include *all* subgroups.

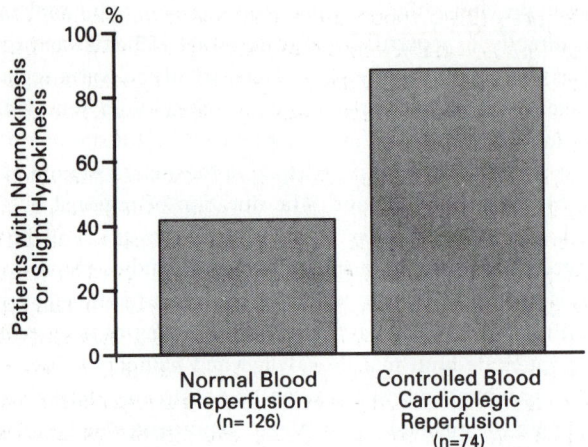

Figure 102–26. Results after emergency coronary artery bypass grafting in patients with acute coronary occlusion. The ordinate shows the percentage of patients having either normo-or slight hypokinesis in the previously ischemic area after normal blood reperfusion or regional controlled blood cardioplegic reperfusion, 7 to 14 days postoperatively. Significantly more patients show substantial recovery of regional wall motion after controlled regional reperfusion than after normal blood reperfusion. *p < 0.05.

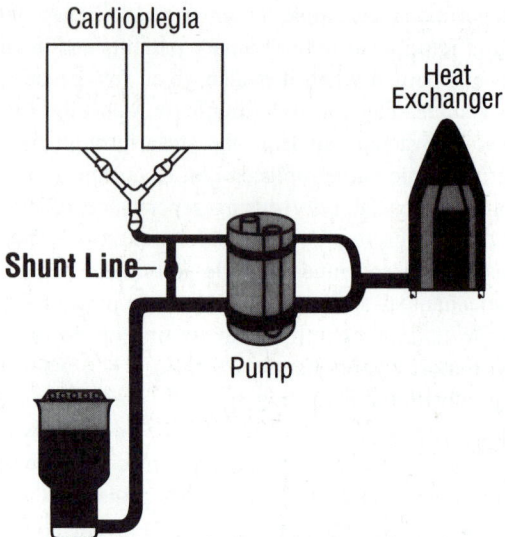

Figure 102–27. Schematic representation of cardioplegic delivery system containing a shunt line allowing alternation between blood cardioplegia and blood, a bifurcation line allowing alternation between high and low potassium solution, and an infusion for bolus injections or infusions of more concentrated cardioplegic constituents.

tients from six centers confirmed our preliminary findings of the benefits of the controlled reperfusion strategy[113,126] and is contrasted to the results in 5 major series of 1203 patients treated medically by PTCA.[127–131] The improved outcome, including substantial recovery of regional contractile function in 87% of patients, occurred despite longer ischemic time (6.3 vs. 3.9 hours) and where a larger proportion of surgical patients fell into the high-risk categories of LAD occlusion, 3-vessel disease, age >70 years, and cardiogenic shock, as defined in reports of medical revascularization with uncontrolled reperfusion.[127–140] The absence of a prospective randomized trial and failure to include the results of uncontrolled reperfusion from the participation centers are obvious limitations of this study design, but we do not believe that failure to provide this information nullifies the implications of this data.

Warm Noncardioplegic Flow Through Distal Grafts

Adequate reperfusion beyond coronary stenoses cannot occur when proximal anastomoses are constructed after aortic unclamping. Distal graft reperfusion with normal blood (1) hastens cardiac rewarming, (2) washes out residual cardioplegic solution, (3) ensures adequate reperfusion pressure beyond residual stenoses, and (4) facilitates estimation of graft length. Normal blood reperfusion can be provided by either removing the cardioplegic tube from the roller head used to deliver blood cardioplegia, interposing a shunt line in the system (Fig. 102–27), or via a side branch from the arterial line. The same vein introducer cannulae placed

into the proximal ends of the vein grafts for multidose cardioplegia can be used to deliver *both* the warm cardioplegic reperfusate and warm noncardioplegic blood as experimental and clinical studies show that lactate washout persists until the coronary obstruction is bypassed by connecting all the grafts to the aorta.[84,86]

Reversal of the order of proximal grafting from that used for cardioplegic delivery (i.e., connecting the most important graft to the aorta last) is recommended if proximal anastomoses are constructed *after* all distal anastomoses are complete and a tangential clamp is used, and optimizes an extended interval of normal blood reperfusion to the largest revascularized region.

Cardiogenic Shock Secondary to Extending Infarction

These aforementioned principles of myocardial protection were applied to a recent series of patients with cardiogenic shock secondary to left ventricular power failure, where medical mortality exceeds 75%[141,142] and surgical mortality is 30–60%.[142,143] Surgical mortality was reduced to approximately 7%[73] (Fig. 102–28) by (1) warm induction of blood cardioplegia to repair cellular processes and replenish energy stores before clamping,[72] (2) multidose cardioplegia to minimize energy loss during aortic clamping,[144] (3) glutamate and aspartate enrichment of blood cardioplegic solutions to replenish substrate utilized during ischemia,[39] (4) ensuring adequate distribution of cardioplegic solutions through the bypassed grafts and by retrograde perfusion to protect regions beyond stenosis,[84] (5) grafting viable areas

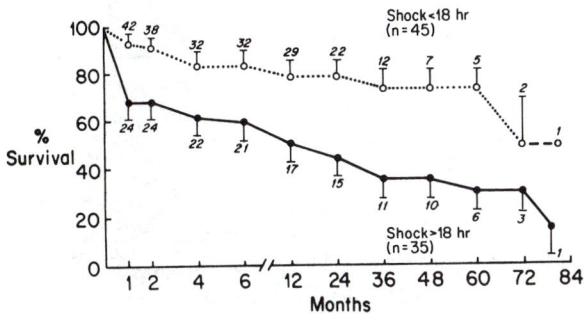

Figure 102–28. Coronary artery bypass grafting after cardiogenic shock: influence of time of operation after cardiogenic shock (n = 80, deaths = 35). p, Wilcoxin, mean ± standard error; italics indicate patients alive and well.

first to offer maximum protection of the portions of myocardium responsible for supporting the circulation, (6) warm reperfusion of blood cardioplegia to lessen reperfusion damage,[60] (7) ensuring adequate blood perfusion of grafted regions while proximal anastomoses are being constructed, and (8) early operation to prevent development of preoperative organ failure or progressive loss of ischemic remote myocardium. We ascribe the gratifying clinical results to careful application of *all* aspects of operative strategy (Table 102–16) that is based on our interpretation of the pathophysiology of cardiogenic shock with special reference to the remote myocardium.

Cardiogenic shock after acute myocardial infarction usually develops 24–72 hours after acute coronary occlusion even though acutely ischemic muscle stops contracting immediately, is maximally dysfunctional initially, and never contributes to cardiac output before operation.[145–150] Ischemic muscle remains viable for a variable period of time[145] and is a source of chest pain, but there is no evidence that infarct extension worsens infarcting muscle function. Maintenance of systemic output is dependent, therefore, on the ability of adjacent remote myocardium to develop and sustain compensatory hypercontractility. We observed experimentally that LV power failure after an otherwise nonlethal anterior (LAD) infarction (i.e., < 30% LV muscle mass) is caused principally by a progressive decline in remote muscle function when there is associated circumflex stenosis.[146,151,152] Remote muscle contractility becomes impaired if its volume is diminished by previous infarction or if it is ischemic. Consequently, delayed cardio-

TABLE 102–16. OPERATIVE STRATEGY— CARDIOGENIC SHOCK

Warm blood cardioplegic induction
Substrate enrichment (glutamate, aspartate)
Graft viable areas first
Multidose cold blood cardioplegia
Ensure distribution through grafts and retroperfusion
Warm blood cardioplegic reperfusate

genic shock (24–72 hours after acute myocardial infarction) occurs because viable muscle in the distribution of stenotic arteries fails to maintain the compensatory hypercontractility that is responsible for ensuring adequate cardiac output.[153]

The operative strategy is designed to ensure maximum myocardial protection and immediate optimal function of viable functioning muscle. Therefore, grafts are placed first into contracting muscle, especially into arteries with large flow distributions.[72] Vessels supplying regions with smaller functioning muscle mass are grafted next. The last graft(s) is placed into the infarcted region. For example, if cardiogenic shock evolves gradually after a large anterolateral infarction, the right coronary artery and circumflex arteries are grafted before the left anterior descending and diagonal vessels. Distribution of cold cardioplegia through all grafts into newly revascularized segments is accomplished after each anastomosis is completed to maximize perfusion of these regions. It is unlikely that one isolated aspect of our approach ensures success, just as no single component of the blood cardioplegic solution (i.e., temperature, hypocalcemia, buffering, substrate, hyperosmolarity, etc.) guarantees perfect protection.

Conventional treatment of cardiogenic shock includes maximum pharmacologic and mechanical support, with coronary artery bypass grafting only in intra-aortic balloon and inotropic drug-dependent patients or in those whose condition improves sufficiently to allow semielective revascularization. This concept of "stabilization to buy time" is not borne out by the results. Early operation (< 18 hours) has resulted in 93% early survival (Fig. 102–28) as it was undertaken before preoperative organ failure supervened. Conversely, delay of operation (> 18 hours) prolonged the need for inotropic support, caused more leg complications from the intraaortic balloon, allowed organ failure to develop, prolonged hospitalization, and increased early and late mortality rates. We suspect that progressive remote muscle necrosis occurred while the myocardium remained ischemic during prolonged circulatory support and resulted in impaired subsequent functional recovery.

Topical Hypothermia

Topical cooling is a useful adjunct when problems in cardioplegic distributions are anticipated (i.e., during aortic valve replacement when the right coronary artery cannot be perfused, especially if there is right ventricular hypertrophy, or in coronary patients with diffuse coronary disease or occluded right coronary arteries where right ventricular protection is not possible). Topical hypothermia is most helpful during valve replacement where there is ventricular hypertrophy, as cold solution can also be introduced directly into the ventricular cavity to achieve the endocardial cooling, which is more difficult from the myocardial surface.

Topical cooling retards the recurrence of electromechanical activity by keeping myocardial temperature low and counteracts the effects of coronary collateral washout of the cardioplegic solution. Surface cooling may not be essential with multidose cardioplegia and retroperfusion, since the oxygen requirements of the arrested heart below 20°C are extremely low. The value of topical hypothermia is limited most in coronary patients because (1) the heart must be removed from the pericardial well for all but very proximal left anterior descending and right coronary anastomoses, and (2) injury to the phrenic nerve (especially with ice slush) may cause otherwise avoidable respiratory complications.[154,155] A recent review of 150 consecutive coronary patients undergoing coronary artery bypass grafting with multidose cold blood cardioplegic and warm reperfusion shows that topical cooling, especially with ice slush, is associated with a higher incidence of phrenic nerve palsy, pleural effusion, and atelectasis without improving outcome as assessed by postoperative hemodynamics, ECG changes, postoperative enzymes, inotropic requirements, or deaths.[156] The comparable results in patients who did not receive topical cooling lead to the conclusion that surface hypothermia is unnecessary during coronary operations when complete revascularization is possible, even if cardiogenic shock is present.

Secondary Cardioplegia

Inadequate myocardial protection becomes apparent only when extracorporeal circulation is discontinued and cardiac performance is depressed. Temporary resumption of extracorporeal circulation results often in some hemodynamic improvement, but this may not be complete and requires further measures. Improvements are ascribed to lowering oxygen demands by "resting the heart" and simultaneously enhancing oxygen delivery by maintaining a perfusion pressure > 60–70 mm Hg. Delivery of abundant oxygen does not, however, ensure that the cell can use its oxygen efficiently enough to repair ischemic or reperfusion damage,[66–68] or reconstitute depressed energy stores. Further recovery and *reversal of damage* is possible if the heart is rearrested by providing a brief (5–10 min) continuous 37°C blood cardioplegic solution during the time frame allocated for prolonging extracorporeal circulation, especially when the cardioplegic solution is enriched with precursors of Krebs cycle intermediates (i.e., glutamate and aspartate).[36,68]

These observations infer limitation of the postischemic heart's capacity to utilize oxygen is related in part to myocardial loss of these key Krebs cycle intermediates, these can be replenished by enriching the warm cardioplegic induction and reperfusate solutions with exogenous glutamate and aspartate. Experimental studies show that use of a normothermic (37°C) blood cardioplegic solution to rearrest the heart frequently restores oxidative metabolism toward normal and results in near complete functional recovery (Fig. 102–29). We have termed this *secondary blood cardioplegia* and suspect that this intervention channels postis-

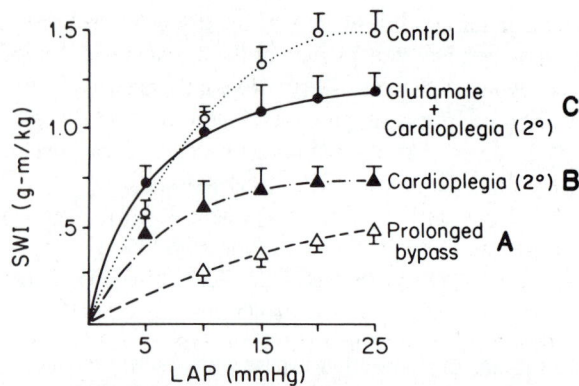

Figure 102–29. Left ventricular performance following 45 min of normothermic ischemic arrest when (**A**) bypass was prolonged without producing secondary cardioplegia, (**B**) secondary cardioplegia was administered for 5 min, and (**C**) glutamate was added to secondary cardioplegic solution. Note the near normal recovery with substrate enhancement of secondary cardioplegic solution with glutamate.

chemic oxygen uptake toward reparative processes rather than wasting the aerobic energy production on needless electromechanical work. In addition, a brief (i.e., 2 min) infusion of secondary cardioplegia restores syncronymous contraction when troublesome atrium or ventricular arrhythmias are refractory to conventional countershock and pharmacologic agents.[157] It is anticipated that it should be possible to develop cardioplegic solutions and reperfusates with the ions, substrates, and possible cofactors that will avoid or reverse completely ischemic and reperfusion damage. As more is learned about the characteristics of reperfusion injury this extended use of blood cardioplegia indicates that the surgeon may now play an active role in reversing myocardial injury due to the present limitations of cardioplegic techniques.

Intractable ventricular fibrillation (sometimes progressing to asystole) occasionally develops after an otherwise successful cardiac operation either in the operating room or in the intensive care unit. This results in severe energy depletion, since the diastolic pressure generated during CPR will not adequately perfuse the subendocardium.[158,159] Temporary cardiopulmonary bypass (which can be instituted percutaneously or directly) ensures more adequate peripheral perfusion, and facilitates defibrillation, but the beating heart requires substantial amounts of oxygen[21,22,160] and the damaged myocardial cells have a reduced capacity to take up oxygen.[67,68] Under these circumstances, decompression of the heart by venting and reclamping the aorta to deliver a prolonged (i.e., 20 min) infusion of amino acid-enriched cardioplegic solution may augment repair of ischemically damaged muscle. Application of secondary blood cardioplegia is based on the study of prolonged regional ischemia, where contractility and mitochondrial energy-generating capacity could be restored after 6 hours of LAD occlusion,[126] and resuscitation and salvage of hearts with 2 hours of intractable ventricular fibrillation under conditions of simulated multivessel disease were achieved.[151] Maintenance of the arrested state on total vented bypass to lower oxygen demands maximally (to 1 cm^3/100 g per minute) while the cardioplegic dose is given over 20 min to take maximum advantage of the fact that oxygen is consumed over time rather than by dose.

We have applied this concept successfully in patients who developed intractable ventricular fibrillation perioperatively after an otherwise successful surgical repair. Careful attention is directed toward maintaining adequate cerebral perfusion pressure during CPR, especially during transit to the operating room for placement on total vented bypass and prolonged secondary cardioplegic infusion for myocardial resuscitation. The clinical availability of percutaneous technology may allow prompt initiation of cardiopulmonary bypass to support the systemic circulation and facilitate defibrillation during transfer to the operating room for secondary cardioplegic administration. Total vented bypass is begun as quickly as possible, and aspartate/glutamate blood cardioplegia (37°C at 150 mL/min) is delivered antegrade for 20 min immediately after aortic clamping. The heart is kept in the beating empty state for 30 min after removing the aortic clamp and extracorporeal is then discontinued gradually. We achieved complete hemodynamic recovery in 13 patients, and survival of 11 of 14 patients who underwent secondary cardioplegia to treat intractable perioperative ventricular fibrillation.[161] Complete revascularization and/or otherwise patent coronary vessels is a prerequisite for success of this salvage application of secondary blood cardioplegia.[162] This aggressive approach may offer a more optimistic outcome for patients who would otherwise succumb after a seemingly successful operation.

Warm Blood Cardioplegia Without Hypothermia

Bigelow, in 1950 at the University of Toronto, introduced hypothermia as an important component of myocardial protection that slows cardiac metabolism while limiting ischemic injury during the periods of aortic cross-clamping needed to optimize operative conditions to provide a quiet bloodless field, and Shumway and Lower, in 1959, reinforced this cardioprotective strategy.[163] These observations led to the surgical axiom that "all is well if the heart is made as cold as possible" and that there is a "battle against the clock" when the aorta is clamped. Recent data on the cardioprotective benefits of warm blood cardioplegia suggest that these axioms are outdated, and that intraoperative damage is related more to "how the heart is protected" rather than "how long the aorta is cross-clamped."

Hypothermia may also impose certain adverse consequences, including shifting the oxygen–hemoglobin dissociation curve leftward, retarding Na$^+$–K$^+$-ATPase to promote edema, reducing membrane stability, increasing blood viscosity, and activating platelets, leukocytes, and complement.[164,165] These concerns led the surgical team at the University of Toronto (where hypothermia was introduced)

to suggest warm blood cardioplegia without hypothermia as a cardioprotective strategy, where the patient and the heart are maintained at 37°C and the cardioplegic flow is delivered continually when feasible. This concept is based on the fact that electromechanical arrest substantially decreases myocardial oxygen requirements to low levels (from 10 to 1 mL/100 g per minute) with little further reduction in O$_2$ demands accomplished by adding profound hypothermia. Therefore, they propose that myocardial oxygen demands can be met with continuous warm cardioplegia as long as the heart is kept arrested.[164,166] This occurs only if there is *homogeneous and adequate* distribution of cardioplegic solutions and this has yet to be proven.

There is no current experimental infrastructure for the clinical application of this attractive hypothesis, although preliminary results in patients are encouraging.[164,165,167] The continuous warm cardioplegic approach is in contrast to early attempts of 37°C continuous coronary perfusion with normal blood where the energy requirements remain high when the heart was either kept beating or fibrillated. An added potential advantage of this method is that ischemia is avoided if 37°C blood cardioplegic flow is continuous and postischemic reperfusion injury cannot occur by maintaining the heart in a constant aerobic state. Finally, systemic normothermia may limit the possible detrimental effects of hypothermic cardiopulmonary bypass on coagulation and other organ systems.

Efforts to avoid intentional ischemia by continuous coronary perfusion are not new, but it has remained impossible to provide homogeneous flow distribution in the past by continuous perfusion techniques. Every prior attempt has been accompanied by creation of "unintentional ischemia" because of the artificial conditions imposed by the various intraoperative methods, such as ventricular fibrillation that directs blood away from subendocardial muscle, especially in hypertrophied hearts.[21,159] These lessons of the past concerning "unintentional ischemia" have relevance today with the use of warm continuous retrograde blood cardioplegia. Coronary sinus retroperfusion results in systematic underperfusion of the right ventricle, which receives less than 20% of flow delivered to the left ventricle. Furthermore, in homogeneous left ventricular perfusion is more pronounced with retrograde vs. antegrade cardioplegia. The potential for impaired right ventricular performance may be accentuated with right ventricular hypertrophy. The nonhomogeneous distribution of nutritive left ventricular retrograde flow makes inhomogeneous perfusion more likely also in hypertrophied hearts, in which optimum flow rates are not yet established. Consequently, inadequate continuous warm blood cardioplegic infusion might cause the same on "unintentional ischemia" as occurred with ventricular defibrillation of ischemia without cardioplegia, but continuous perfusion.

Reports of superior clinical results using continuous warm antegrade or retrograde blood cardioplegia are made by comparison of retrospective analysis. The retrograde technique offers possible advantages in (1) patients with coronary disease where coronary stenosis might limit antegrade distribution and (2) valve operations where mitral valve retractors can make the aortic valve incompetent and to exclude the need for direct coronary perfusion catheters in aortic operations, since these may lead to late ostial injury. Although these early results were encouraging, they were not superior to results using techniques with an extensive experimental infrastructure in which warm and cold antegrade and retrograde methods are applied as described previously in this chapter. Subsequent experimental data now show some unforeseen problems of the warm continuous cardioplegic technique and many questions have arisen and remain unanswered (see below). Experimental studies show the superiority of intermittent cold antegrade and antegrade/retrograde blood cardioplegic techniques over continuous warm antegrade or retrograde cardioplegia, especially in protecting areas of jeopardized myocardium.[92,93] Intermittent interruption of continuous warm antegrade or retrograde cardioplegia as must be done clinically to optimize visualization during construction of distal anastomoses is particularly deleterious in vulnerable regions, whereas intermittent cold antegrade/retrograde cardioplegia provides superior results under these circumstances.[168] Recent studies (Fig. 102–30) show that right ventricular protection is enhanced when retroperfusion after arrest is with cold noncardioplegic blood, rather than warm blood cardioplegia. These observations suggest hypothermic lowering of metabolic demands compensates for reduced RV blood supply during continuous retroperfusion. It seems that both warm and cold cardioplegic techniques as well as antegrade and retrograde methods of delivering may be useful and complimentary rather than adversarial techniques in the cardiac surgeons armamentarium, especially when cardioprotective strategies are formulated to reduce and avoid damage to vascular beds in jeopardized myocardium.

Additional missing data on the role of warm heart surgical techniques include (1) what flow rates are needed to adequately supply the arrested heart, and will continuous infusion ensure all areas receive sufficient flow to meet metabolic needs (for example, the normal right ventricle, or when right or left ventricular hypertrophy is present), (2) how long can the blood flow be interrupted safely before ischemic changes take place, and how can these changes be overcome with resumption of cardioplegic flow, (3) what is the ideal cardioplegic composition (i.e., is it different from the composition used for intermittent cold blood cardioplegia), (4) does warm heart surgery, with the patient at 37°C, lead to increased bleeding due to the inherently higher flow rates that must maintained, (5) will cerebral complications increase if nonpulsatile flows with inherently lower perfusion pressure are used, and (6) will more fatal "perfusion accidents" occur due to the limited time (3–4 min) available to the perfusionists to stop extracorporeal circulation and correct the problem before cerebral damage occurs.

Finally, experimental and clinical studies have demonstrated that the normal and ischemically damaged heart can be protected safely for 2–4 hours of aortic clamping with intermittent cold blood cardioplegia especially if bracketed with an interval of warm induction and reperfusion to "resuscitate" the heart and "limited reperfusion injury" (see earlier sections on Blood Cardioplegia and Warm Induction). These intermittent cardioplegic techniques provide the ideal technical conditions of a bloodless field needed for surgical precision, while simultaneously ensuring metabolic correction of the consequences of ischemia, which are minimized by hypothermic protection. Consequently, abandonment of cold cardioplegic techniques in favor of the warm approach is not recommended until a sufficient infrastructure of data is accumulated to answer the aforementioned questions. Postoperative univentricular or biventricular failure or death after continuous warm retrograde blood cardioplegia reflects a problem that hypothermia and antegrade cardioplegia might avoid, and that is caused directly by an inflexible approach based on the misconception that "all is well if the heart is perfused continually." We suspect that warm blood cardioplegic techniques will become adjunctive to hypothermic techniques, rather than a replacement for them.

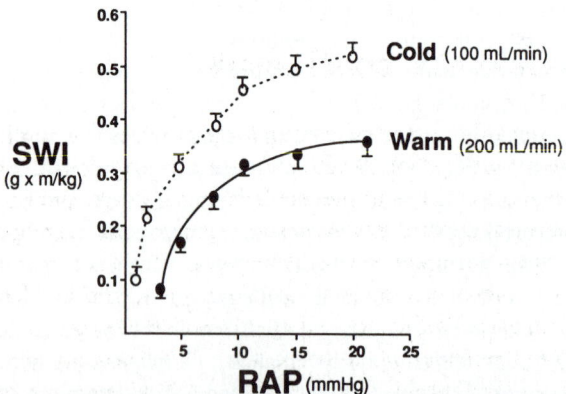

Figure 102–30. Right ventricular performance after 30 min of continuous retrograde perfusion via the coronary sinus. Note in the cold group, arrest was achieved by a 1-min infusion of antegrade 4°C blood cardioplegia (30 mEq/L), and noncardioplegia blood was delivered at 100 mL/min thereafter; in the warm group, arrest was achieved by a 1-min infusion of warm blood cardioplegia (30 mEq/L KCl), and maintained by retroperfusion of 10 mEq/L KCl blood cardioplegia for 30 min; superior recovery after cold retroperfusion despite 50% reduction of flow rate and no added KCl.

Warm Blood Cardioplegia: Starting Points, End Points, and Median Lethal Dose (LD₅₀)

Cardioplegic research has not, in general, followed established procedures for drug testing. The LD_{50} concept is used routinely in pharmacologic studies whereby the starting point is an intervention in a model that kills 50% of live organisms; its effectiveness or end point is compared with this starting point. Consequently, an intervention is (1) ineffective if it does not change the starting point, (2) toxic if less than 50% viability results, and (3) defined as effective by how much more than 50% viability it produces. The starting point of most studies of myocardial protection is the normal heart, so that the LD_{50} approach has no relevance to them, inasmuch as any intervention that fails to maintain biochemical and mechanical integrity must be considered ineffective. Consequently, the normal heart model is useful only to test the safety of interventions such as multidose cold blood cardioplegia that allows normal biochemical and mechanical function to recover completely after 4 hours of aortic clamping; the starting point is the same as the end point.

Cardiac surgeons rarely get the chance to operate on normal hearts, so our clinical starting point conforms more closely to the LD_{50} model in pharmacologic studies. Experimental study of the energy- and substrate-depleted heart model has been useful to develop strategies intended to metabolically resuscitate the heart, because cold cardioplegia confers no metabolic benefit other than offsetting further damage. The concepts of warm induction and reperfusion of blood cardioplegia developed from such models, whereby extensive testing of various cardioplegic modifications resulted in a regimen that restored function to ischemically damaged hearts, with the rationale for individual factors described previously. *Normothermia is only one element in this regimen and is included to optimize the rate of metabolic recovery, which is retarded by hypothermia.*

The objective of adding normothermic blood cardioplegia is to use a cardioprotective strategy in the impaired myocardium that acts in concert with mechanical repair to restore near normal biochemical and mechanical function (that is, a normal starting point). Conversely, cold cardioplegic techniques alone can *only* prevent further damage so that total reliance is placed on the mechanical benefits of operative correction to improve cardiac performance. For example, the operative mortality rate for the surgical treatment of cardiogenic shock is approximately 50% with conventional hypothermic cardioprotective techniques because left ventricular power failure progress unabatedly despite revascularization.[142,143] In contrast, use of warm blood cardioplegic induction and reperfusion lessens the duration of postoperative circulatory support and improves mortality.[73]

Intermittent Warm Blood Cardioplegia

Intermittent warm blood cardioplegia may theoretically prove beneficial *without* hypothermic supplementation if the formulations result in metabolic resuscitation and limitation of reperfusion damage, as documented previously when normothermic methods were used as an adjunct to intermittent cold ischemia in energy-depleted hearts.[82] Confirmation of this application of intermittent warm ischemia requires testing in globally ischemic hearts that would otherwise develop biochemical or mechanical dysfunction if no intervention was undertaken (for example, aortic un-

clamping without cardioplegia). The importance of this type of analysis is drawn from our previous studies showing cold intermittent blood cardioplegia that fully protected normal heart muscle for 4 hours, but failed to amplify function in the stressed myocardium.[39] Postmyocardial dysfunction imposed after 45 min of normothermic ischemia after 2 hours of aortic clamping (i.e., to simulate the time needed for operative repair) was comparable to that when the aorta was unclamped immediately. *The "end-point equalled the starting point."*

The strategic goal is to make the "end-point" *exceed* the "starting point" so that the intermittent warm cardioplegia would be considered ineffective if an "end-point" equalled a "starting point" of deranged metabolism and function as observed following simple aortic unclamping after a period of unprotected ischemia. Use of a normal heart to demonstrate that intermittent warm blood cardioplegia restores normal metabolic and contractile function may lead to the misleading conclusion that intermittent warm ischemia is safe in jeopardized muscle. For example, our previous studies showing the limitations of intermittent cold blood cardioplegia as the sole cardioprotective strategy in the stressed myocardium[39] paved the way for use of warm blood cardioplegic induction and reperfusion.

Hopefully, subsequent studies in damaged hearts will be undertaken, since the results may be of fundamental importance in planning cardioprotective strategies devoid of the recognized capacity of hypothermia to delay the rate of development of cell damage. Relatively homogeneous flow distribution via antegrade and retrograde delivery would probably be needed for intermitent normothermic cardioplegia to be effective. Additionally, metabolic interventions that precondition the heart[169] must be evaluated in the aforementioned way to justify their use in allowing exclusion of hypothermic techniques.

CARDIOPLEGIC CONCLUSIONS

The versatility of blood cardioplegia provides the cardiac surgeon with a tool to actively treat the jeopardized myocardium as well as to prevent ischemic damage, provided attention is directed toward ensuring adequate delivering of the cardioplegic solutions. No exogenous blood is needed to deliver blood cardioplegia, as a readily available blood source exists within the extracorporeal circuit during all cardiac operations when the patient's blood volume mixes with the clear priming fluid. The expense of depriving the patient of the potential benefits of blood cardioplegia includes increased perioperative mortality, prolonged intensive care unit stays, and development of late cardiac fibrosis owing to necrosis caused by less adequate protection, and far outweighs the monetary cost of its use.

The aforementioned benefits of enhanced oxygen-carrying capacity, active resuscitation, avoidance of reperfusion damage, limitation of hemodilution, provision of on-

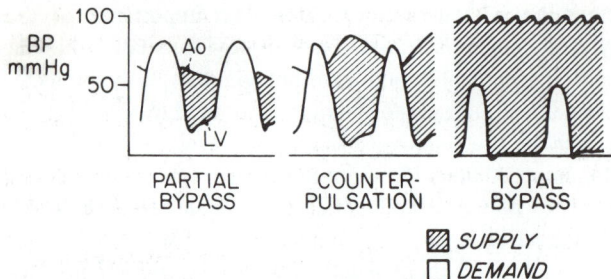

Figure 102–31. Subendocardial supply/demand balance (DPTI/TTI) in postischemic hearts receiving partial bypass, intraortic balloon counterpulsation, and total bypass. Note that the best supply–demand balance is achieved when total bypass is prolonged.

conicity, buffering, rheologic effects, and endogenous oxygen free radical scavengers enumerate only the known benefits of using blood as the vehicle for delivering oxygenated cardioplegia. We are confident that further studies will reveal other naturally occurring blood components (i.e., enzymes, cofactors, substrates, electrolytes) that are important and would otherwise need to be added to any artificially constructed solution.

CONSIDERATIONS AFTER BYPASS

Impaired myocardial performance immediately after bypass should lead to the suspicion that a technical or metabolic problem is present if myocardial protection has been adequate. Immediate resumption of total extracorporeal circulation will lower myocardial oxygen requirements (see previous discussion). Simultaneously, subendocardial oxygen supply (i.e., perfusion and O_2 content) can be raised by increasing aortic blood pressure and red cell mass, especially if extreme hemodilution has been used. Inotropic drugs

should be avoided during prolonged total bypass because they raise oxygen demands unnecessarily when no external cardiac work is needed.[170]

The effectiveness of cardiopulmonary bypass in reversing ischemic damage and relieving the heart of work is achieved only when the left ventricle is vented completely.[171] Conversely, partial bypass (diverting 50–90% of venous return) lowers left ventricular oxygen needs only slightly because ventricular wall tension remains high. Secondary cardioplegia should be used if ventricular performance remains depressed. Intra-aortic balloon counterpulsation is more sound physiologically than administering inotropic drugs that increase oxygen needs. Balloon deflation reduces afterload and lowers oxygen demands while inflation simultaneously augments supply. Figure 102–31 shows the hemodynamic improvement afforded by balloon counterpulsation on the supply–demand balance. Balloon counterpulsation has been found most effective when the supply–demand balance remains impaired (DPTI:TTI < 0.8) after discontinuation of total bypass. Clinical reports[10,12,13] suggest survival in patients who require balloon counterpulsation only when they could maintain a satisfactory supply and demand balance (DPTI/DTI > 0.8) without mechanical support. Intra-aortic balloon counterpulsation has certainly extended our ability to salvage patients who otherwise might die from severe subendocardial necrosis.

Failure of these interventions should lead to the use of left or right heart assist devices that can support the circulation for several days until ischemic and reperfusion damage has a chance for recovery. Postoperative follow-up studies[172] show return of reasonably intact left ventricular function in survivors of left ventricular assist devices. Unfortunately, survival is only ~ 25% but may be improved by earlier mechanical support when conventional methods fail, since it is likely that a substantial amount of dysfunctional heart muscle is "stunned" rather than necrotic.

Figure 102–32. Pre- and postoperative x-ray films of patients undergoing aortic valve replacement (AVR), mitral valve replacement (MVR), and tricuspid angioplasty (TA). Note that the enlarged heart preoperatively has assumed normal contour 1 mo postoperatively, suggesting that the improved mechanical performance was associated with good myocardial protection. These films should be compared with those in Figure 102–1, where myocardial protection was inadequate.

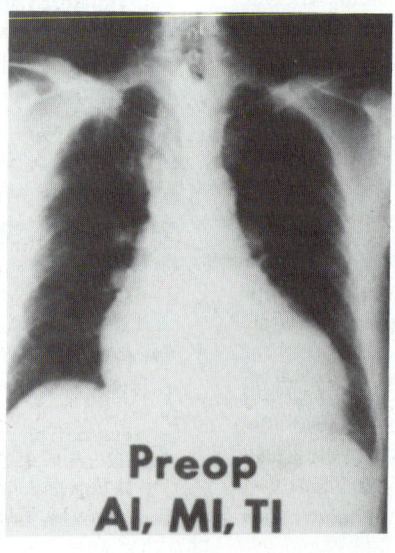

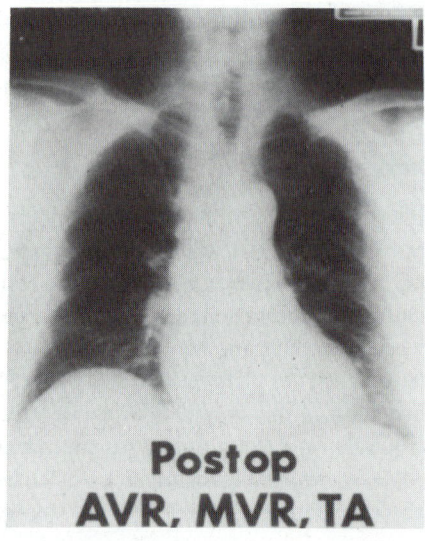

Significant advances have been made in protecting the heart against perioperative myocardial damage. The role of cardioplegic myocardial protection has expanded to allow cardioplegic solutions to be used for *active resuscitation*, to *prevent* ischemic injury, to *avoid* reperfusion damage, and to *reverse* ischemic and reperfusion damage. The persistent evidence of some enzymatic signs of myocardial necrosis in patients who do not need postoperative circulatory assistance suggests a more subtle form of intraoperative damage may still be occurring. It is to be hoped that we can avoid intraoperative myocardial damage completely as we learn more about the pathophysiology of ischemic and reperfusion injury, and that we can develop strategies for delivering and maintaining properly designed cardioplegic solutions to all myocardial segments (Fig. 102–32). The long-term effects of the more subtle forms of the cardiac damage that still exist will not be known until we develop both the impetus and simplified methodology for routine study of ventricular performance months and years after operation. We suspect strongly that we will find that delayed myocardial fibrosis, when present, reflects the healed results of perioperative myocardial injury (Fig. 102–31). The incidence of this injury has been reduced significantly in recent years, but we do not believe that the role of surgery in the natural history of congenital and acquired heart disease will be established until it is avoided completely.

REFERENCES

1. Buckberg GD: Left ventricular subendocardial necrosis. *Ann Thorac Surg* **24**:379–393, 1977
2. Najafi H, Henson D, Dye WS: Left ventricular hemorrhagic necrosis. *Ann Thorac Surg* **7**:550, 1969
3. Taber RE, Norales AR, Fine G: Myocardial necrosis and the postoperative low cardiac output syndrome. *Ann Thorac Surg* **4**:12, 1967
4. Isom OW, Spencer FC, Feigenbaum H: Prebypass myocardial damage in patients undergoing coronary revascularization; an unrecognized vulnerable period. *Circulation* **51/52**:II–119, 1975
5. Hoffman JIE, Buckberg GD: Transmural variation in myocardial perfusion. In Yu PN, Goodwin JF (eds): *Progress in Cardiology,* Philadelphia, Lea & Febiger, 1976
6. Buckberg GD, Fixler DE, Archie JP: Experimental subendocardial ischemia in dogs with normal coronary arteries. *Circ Res* **30**:67–81, 1972
7. Brazier J, Cooper N, Buckberg GD: The adequacy of subendocardial oxygen delivery: The interaction of determinants of flow, arterial oxygen content and myocardial oxygen need. *Circulation* **49**:968–977, 1974
8. Sarnoff SJ, Braunwald E, Welch GD: Hemodynamic determinants of oxygen consumption of the heart with special reference to the tension time index. *Am J Physiol* **192**:148, 1958
9. Buckberg GD, Ross G: The effects of isoprenaline on coronary blood flow, its distribution and myocardial performance. *Cardiovasc Res* **7**:429–437, 1973
10. Bregman D, Parodi EN, Edie RN: Intraoperative unidirectional intraaortic balloon pumping in the management of left ventricula power failure. *J Thorac Cardiovasc Surg* **70**:1010–1023, 1975
11. Buckberg GD, Towers B, Paglia D: Subendocardial ischemia after cardiopulmonary bypass. *J Thorac Cardiovasc Surg* **64**:669–684, 1972
12. Goldman BS, Gunstensen J, Gilbert BW: Increasing operability and survival with intraaortic balloon pump assist. *Can J Surg* **19**:69, 1976
13. Phillips PA, Marty AT, Miyamoto AM: A clinical method for detecting subendocardial ischemia after cardiopulmonary bypass. *J Thorac Cardiovasc Surg* **69**:30–39, 1975
14. Hoar PF, Hickey RF, Ullyot DJ: Systemic hypertension following myocardial revascularization. *J Thorac Cardiovasc Surg* **71**:859–864, 1976
15. Brazier JR, Buckberg GD: Effects of tachycardia on the adequacy of subendocardial oxygen delivery in aortic stenosis. *Am Heart J* **90**:222–230, 1975
16. Buckberg GD, Fixler DE, Archie JP: Variable effects of heart rate on phasic and regional left ventricular muscle blood flow in anesthetized dogs. *Cardiovasc Res* **9**:1–11, 1975
17. McEnany MT, Kay HR, Buckley JM: Clinical experience with intraaortic balloon pump support in 728 patients. *Cardiovasc Surg* **58**:124, 1978
18. Utley J, Carlson EL, Hofman JIE: Total and regional myocardial blood flow measurement with 25u, 9u, and filtered 1-10u diameter microspheres and antipyrine. *Circ Res* **34**:391, 1974
19. Follette DM, Steed DL, Foglia RP, Buckberg GD: Advantages of intermittent blood cardioplegia over intermittent ischemia during prolonged hypothermic aortic clamping. *Cardiovasc Surg* **58**:1–200, 1978
20. Stemmer EA, McCart P, Stanton WWJ: Functional and structural alterations in the myocardium during aortic cross clamping. *J Thorac Cardiovasc Surg* **66**:754–770, 1973
21. Buckberg GD, Brazier JR, Nelson RL, et al: Studies of the effects of hypothermia on regional myocardial blood flow and metabolism during cardiopulmonary bypass. I. The adequately perfused beating, fibrillating and arrested heart. *J Thorac Cardiovasc Surg* **78**:87–94, 1977
22. Hottenrott CE, Towers B, Kurkji HJ, et al: The hazard of ventricular fibrillation in hypertrophied ventricles during cardiopulmonary bypass. *J Thorac Cardiovasc Surg* **66**:742–753, 1973
23. Melrose DG, Dreyer B, Bentall HH: Elective cardiac arrest. *Lancet* **2**:21, 1955
24. Waldhausen JA, Braunwald NS, Bloodwell RD: Left ventricular function following elective cardiac arrest. *J Thorac Cardiovasc Surg* **39**:813, 1960
25. Bretschneider HJ, Hubner G, Knoll D: Myocardial resistance and tolerance to ischemia: Physiological and biochemical basis. *J Cardiovasc Surg* **16**:241, 1975
26. Kirsch U, Rodewald G, Kalmar P: Induced ischemic arrest. *J Thorac Cardiovasc Surg* **63**:121, 1972
27. Hearse DJ, Stewart DA, Braimbridge MV: Cellular protection during myocardial ischemia. *Circulation* **54**:193, 1976
28. Gay WAJ, Ebert PA: Functional, metabolic, and morphologic effects of potassium-induced cardioplegia. *Surgery* **74**:284, 1973
29. Tyers GFO, Todd GJ, Niebauer IM: The mechanism of myocardial damage following potassium citrate (Melrose) cardioplegia. *Surgery* **78**:45, 1975
30. Follette DM, Mulder DG, Maloney JVJ, Buckberg GD: Advantages of blood cardioplegia over continuous coronary perfusion and intermittent ischemia. *J Thorac Cardiovasc Surg* **76**:604–619, 1978
31. Roberts AJ, Moran JM, Sanders JH: Clinical evaluation of the relative effectiveness of multidose crystalloid and cold blood potassium cardioplegia in coronary artery bypass graft surgery. *Ann Thorac Surg* **33**:421–433, 1982
32. Cunningham JN, Catinella FP, Spencer FC: Blood cardioplegia—experience with prolonged cross-clamping. In Engleman RM, Levitsky S (eds): *A Textbook of Clinical Cardioplegia.* Mt. Kisco, NY, Futura, 1982, pp 242–264
33. Fabiani JN, Perier P, Chelly J: Blood versus crystalloid cardioplegia. In Engelman RM, Levitsky S (eds): *A Textbook of Clinical Cardioplegia.* Mt. Kisco, NY, Futura, 1982, pp 285–295

34. Catinella FP, Cunningham JN, Adams PX: Myocardial protection with cold blood potassium cardioplegia during prolonged aortic cross-clamping. *Ann Thorac Surg* **33**:228–233, 1982

35. Buckberg GD: A proposed "solution" to the cardioplegic controversy. *J Thorac Cardiovasc Surg* **77**:803–815, 1979

36. Catinella FP, Cunningham JNJ, Spencer FC: Myocardial protection during prolonged aortic cross-clamping. *J Thorac Cardiovasc Surg* **88**:422–423, 1984

37. Peyton RB, Van Tright P, Pellam GL: Improved tolerance to ischemia in hypertrophied myocardium by preischemic enhancement of adenosine triphosphate. *J Thorac Cardiovasc Surg* **84**:11–15, 1982

38. Buckberg GD, Dyson CW, Emerson RC: Techniques for administering clinical cardioplegia: Blood cardioplegia. In Levitsky S, Engelman RM (eds): *A Textbook of Clinical Cardioplegia*. Mt. Kisco, NY, Futura, 1982

39. Rosenkranz ER, Okamoto F, Buckberg GD, et al: Safety of prolonged aortic clamping with blood cardioplegia. III. Aspartate enrichment of glutamate-blood cardioplegia in energy-depleted hearts after ischemic and reperfusion injury. *J Thorac Cardiovasc Surg* **91**:428–435, 1986

40. Vander Woude JC, Christlieb IY, Sicard GA: Imidazole-buffered cardioplegic solution: Improved myocardial preservation during global ischemia. *J Thorac Cardiovasc Surg* **90**:225–234, 1985

41. Langer GA: Control of calcium movement in the myocardium. *Eur Heart J* **4**:5–11, 1983

42. Yamamoto F, Manning AS, Braimbridge MV: Cardioplegia and slow calcium channel blockers. Studies with verapamil. *J Thorac Cardiovasc Surg* **86**:252–261, 1983

43. Clark RE, Christlieb IY, Henry PD, et al: Nifedipine. A myocardial protective agent. *Am J Cardiol* **44**:825–831, 1979

44. Standeven JW, Jellinek M, Menz LJ, et al: Cold blood potassium diltiazem cardioplegia. *J Thorac Cardiovasc Surg* **87**:201–212, 1984

45. Steward JR, Blackwell WH, Crute SL: Inhibition of surgically induced ischemia/reperfusion injury by oxygen free radical scavengers. *J Thorac Cardiovasc Surg* **86**:262–272, 1983

46. Coghlan JG, Flitter WD, Clutton SM, et al: Allopurinol pretreatment improves postoperative recovery and reduces lipid peroxidation in patients undergoing coronary artery bypass grafting. *J Thorac Cardiovasc Surg* **107**:248–256, 1994

47. Okamoto F, Allen BS, Buckberg GD, et al: Studies of controlled reperfusion after ischemia: Reperfusate composition: X. Supplemental role of intravenous and intracoronary CoQ10 in avoiding reperfusion damage. *J Thorac Cardiovasc Surg* **92**:573–582, 1986

48. Pearl JM, Drinkwater DC, Laks H, et al: Leukocyte-depleted reperfusion of transplanted human hearts prevents ultrastructural evidence of reperfusion injury. *J Surg Res* **52**:298–308, 1992

49. McCord JM: Oxygen-derived free radicals in postischemic tissue injury. *N Engl J Med* **312**:159–163, 1985

50. Foglia RP, Steed DL, Follette DM, Buckberg GD: Iatrogenic myocardial edema with potassium cardioplegia. *J Thorac Cardiovasc Surg* **78**:217–222, 1979

51. Elert O, Ottermann U: Cardioplegic hemoglobin perfusion for human myocardium. In Anonymous (ed): *Myocardial Protection for Cardiovascular Surgery*. Köln, Pharmazeutische Verlagsgesellschaft, 1979, pp 134–143

52. Bodenhamer RM, DeBoer LV, Geffin GA: Enhanced myocardial protection during ischemic arrest. Oxygenation of a cyrstalloid cardioplegic solution. *J Thorac Cardiovasc Surg* **85**:769–780, 1983

53. Reeves RB: What are normal acid-base conditions in man when body temperature changes? In Rahn H, Prakash O (eds): *Acid-Base Regulation and Body Temperature*. Boston, Martinus Nijhoff, 1985, pp 13–32

54. Van Asbeck B, Hoidal J, Vercellotti GM, et al: Protection against lethal hyperoxia by tracheal insufflation of erythrocytes: Role of red cell glutathione. *Science* **227**:756–758, 1985

55. Julia PL, Buckberg GD, Acar C, et al: Studies of controlled reperfu-

sion after ischemia. Reperfusate composition. XXI. Superiority of blood cardioplegia over crystalloid cardioplegia in limiting reperfusion damage: Importance of endogenous oxygen free-radical scavengers in red blood cells. *J Thorac Cardiovasc Surg* **101**:303–313, 1991

56. Cauvin C, Loutzenhiser R, Hwang O, Van Breemen C: Alpha1-adrenoreceptors induce Ca influx and intracellular Ca release in isolated rabbit aorta. *Eur J Pharmacol* **84**:233–235, 1982

57. Robertson JM, Buckberg GD, Vinten-Johansen J: Comparison of distribution beyond coronary stenoses of blood and asanguineous cardioplegic solutions. *J Thorac Cardiovasc Surg* **86**:80–86, 1983

58. Ihnken K, Morita K, Buckberg GD, et al: The safety of simultaneous arterial and coronary sinus perfusion: Experimental background and initial clinical results. *J Card Surg* **9**:15–25, 1994

59. Novick RJ, Stefaniszyn HJ, Michel RP: Protection of the hypertrophied pig myocardium. A comparison of crystalloid, blood, and Fluosol-DA cardioplegia during prolonged aortic clamping. *J Thorac Cardiovasc Surg* **89**:547–566, 1985

60. Follette DM, Fey K, Buckberg GD, et al: Reducing postischemic damage by temporary modification of reperfusate calcium, potassium, pH, and osmolarity. *J Thorac Cardiovasc Surg* **82**:221–238, 1981

61. Allen BS, Okamoto F, Buckberg GD, et al: Studies of controlled reperfusion after ischemia: Reperfusate composition: IX. Benefits of marked hypocalcemia and diltiazem of regional recovery. *J Thorac Cardiovasc Surg* **92**:564–572, 1986

62. Allen BS, Buckberg GD, Fontan F, et al: Superiority of controlled surgical reperfusion vs. PTCA in acute coronary occlusion. *J Thorac Cardiovasc Surg* **105**:864–884, 1993

63. Buckberg GD, Beyersdorf F, Kato NS: Technical considerations and logic of antegrade and retrograde blood cardioplegic delivery. *Sem Thorac Cardiovasc Surg* **5**:125–133, 1993

64. Matsuda H, Maeda S, Hirose H: Optimum dose of cold potassium cardioplegia for patients with chronic aortic valve disease: Determination by left ventricular mass. *Ann Thorac Surg* **41**:22–26, 1986

65. Rosenkranz ER, Vinten-Johansen J, Buckberg GD, et al: Benefits of normothermic induction of cardioplegia in energy-depleted hearts, with maintenance of arrest by multidose cold blood cardioplegic infusions. *J Thorac Cardiovasc Surg* **84**:667–676, 1982

66. Kane JJ, Murphy ML, Bissett JK, et al: Mitochondria function, oxygen extraction, epicardial S-T segment changes and tritiated digoxin distribution after reperfusion of ischemic myocardium. *Am J Cardiol* **36**:218–224, 1975

67. Lazar HL, Buckberg GD, Manganaro AJ: Reversal of ischemic damage with amino acid substrate enhancement during reperfusion. *Surgery* **88**:702–709, 1980

68. Lazar HL, Buckberg GD, Manganaro AM, Becker H: Myocardial energy replenishment and reversal of ischemic damage by substrate enhancement of secondary blood cardioplegia with amino acids during reperfusion. *J Thorac Cardiovasc Surg* **80**:350–359, 1980

69. Rosenkranz ER, Okamoto F, Buckberg GD: The safety of prolonged aortic clamping with blood cardioplegia. II. Glutamate enrichment in energy-depleted hearts. *J Thorac Cardiovasc Surg* **88**:401–410, 1984

70. Rosenkranz ER, Buckberg GD: Myocardial protection during surgical coronary reperfusion. *J Am Coll Cardiol* **1**:1235–1246, 1983

71. Allen BS, Okamoto F, Buckberg GD, et al: Studies of controlled reperfusion after ischemia: Reperfusate conditions: XIII. Critical importance of total ventricular decompression during regional reperfusion. *J Thorac Cardiovasc Surg* **92**:605–612, 1986

72. Rosenkranz ER, Buckberg GD, Mulder DG, Laks H: Warm induction of cardioplegia with glutamate-enriched blood in coronary patients with cardiogenic shock who are dependent on inotropic drugs and intraaortic balloon support: Initial experience and operative strategy. *J Thorac Cardiovasc Surg* **86**:507–518, 1983

73. Allen BS, Rosenkranz ER, Buckberg GD, et al: Studies on prolonged regional ischemia. VI. Myocardial infarction with LV power

failure: A medical/surgical emergency requiring urgent revascularization with maximal protection of remote muscle. *J Thorac Cardiovasc Surg* **98**:691–703, 1989

74. Jones R, Peyton R, Sabine R: Transmural gradient in high-energy phosphate content in patients with coronary artery disease. **32**:546–553, 1981

75. Sink JD, Pellom GL, Currie WD: Response of hypertrophied myocardium to ischemia. *J Thorac Cardiovasc Surg* **81**:865–872, 1981

76. Peyton RB, Jones RB, Attarian D: Depressed high-energy phosphate content in hypertrophied ventricles of animal and man. **196**:278–284, 1982

77. Hanafy HM, Allen BS, Wiewall JM, Hartz RS: Warm cardioplegic induction: An underused modality. *Ann Thorac Surg* **58**:1589–1594, 1994

78. Serizawa T, Vogel WM, Apstein CS, Grossman W: Comparison of acute alterations in left ventricular relaxation and diastolic chamber stiffness induced by hypoxia and ischemia. *J Clin Invest* **68**:91–102, 1981

79. Brazier J, Hottenrott C, Buckberg GD: Noncoronary collateral myocardial blood flow. *Ann Thorac Surg* **19**:425–435, 1975

80. Ferguson TB, Smith PK, Buhrman WC: Studies on the physiology of the conduction system during hyperkalemic, hypothermic cardioplegic arrest. *Surg Forum* **34**:302–304, 1983

81. Penhkurinen KJ, Takala TES, Nuutinen EM: Tricarboxylic acid cycle metabolites during ischemia in isolated perfused rat heart. *Am J Physiol* **244**:H281–H288, 1983

82. Robertson JM, Vinten-Johansen J, Buckberg GD, et al: Safety of prolonged aortic clamping with blood cardioplegia: I. Glutamate enrichment in normal hearts. *J Thorac Cardiovasc Surg* **88**:395–401, 1984

83. Hilton CJ, Teubl W, Acker M, McEnany MT: Inadequate cardioplegic protection with obstructed coronary arteries. *Ann Thorac Surg* **28**:323, 1979

84. Becker H, Vinten-Johansen J, Buckberg GD: Critical importance of ensuring cardioplegic delivery with coronary stenoses. *J Thorac Cardiovasc Surg* **81**:507–515, 1981

85. Landymore RW, Tice D, Trehan N: Importance of topical hypothermia to ensure uniform myocardial cooling during coronary artery bypass. *J Thorac Cardiovasc Surg* **82**:832–836, 1981

86. Weisel RD, Hoy FBY, Baird RJ: Improved myocardial protection during a prolonged cross-clamp period. *Ann Thorac Surg* **36**:664, 1983

87. Partington MT, Acar C, Buckberg GD, et al: Studies of retrograde cardioplegia. I. Capillary blood flow distribution to myocardium supplied by open and occluded arteries. *J Thorac Cardiovasc Surg* **97**:605–612, 1989

88. Buckberg GD: Antegrade/retrograde blood cardioplegia to ensure cardioplegic distribution: Operative techniques and objectives. *J Card Surg* **4**:216–238, 1989

89. Partington MT, Acar C, Buckberg GD, Julia PL: Studies of retrograde cardioplegia. II. Advantages of antegrade/retrograde cardioplegia to optimize distribution in jeopardized myocardium. *J Thorac Cardiovasc Surg* **97**:613–622, 1989

90. Loop FD, Higgins TL, Panda R, et al: Myocardial protection during cardiac operations. *J Thorac Cardiovasc Surg* **104**:608–618, 1992

91. Buckberg GD: Recent advances in myocardial protection using retrograde blood cardioplegia. *Eur Heart J* **10**/Supple H:43–48, 1989

92. Matsuura H, Lazar HL, Yang X, et al: Warm vs. cold blood cardioplegia: Is there a difference? *Surg Forum* **42**:231–232, 1991

93. Diehl JT, Pontoriero M, Connolly R, et al: Alternative methods of retrograde cardioplegia delivery: Effects on preservation of the Ischemic left ventricle after acute coronary artery occlusion and reperfusion. *AATS* 60–61, 1992 (abstract)

94. Allen BS, Hartz RS, Wiewall J, et al: Retrograde cardioplegia does not adequately perfuse the right ventricle. *J Thoracic Cardiovasc Surg* **109**:1116–1126, 1995

95. Gates RN, Laks H, Drinkwater DCJ, et al: Gross and microvascular distribution of retrograde cardioplegia in explanted human hearts. **56**:410–417, 1993

96. Diehl JT, Eichhorn EJ, Konstam MA: Efficacy of retrograde coronary sinus cardioplegia in patients undergoing myocardial revascularization: A prospective randomized trial. *Ann Thorac Surg* **45**:595–602, 1988

97. Fabiani JM, Carpentier AF: Comparative evaluation of retrograde cardioplegia through the coronary sinus and the right atrium. *Circulation* **68**:III–251, 1983

98. Menasche P, Kural S, Fauchet M: Retrograde coronary sinus perfusion: A safe alternative for ensuring cardioplegic delivery in aortic valve surgery. *Ann Thorac Surg* **34**:647–658, 1982

99. Bhayana JN, Kalmbach T, Booth FVMcL, et al: Combined antegrade/retrograde cardioplegia for myocardial protection: A clinical trial. *J Thorac Cardiovasc Surg* **98**:956–960, 1989

100. Shiki K, Masuda M, Yonenaga K, et al: Myocardial distribution of retrograde flow through the coronary sinus of the excised normal canine heart. *Ann Thorac Surg* **41**:265–271, 1986

101. Stirling MC, McClanahan TB, Schott RJ, et al: Distribution of cardioplegic solution infused antegradely and retrogradely in normal canine hearts. *J Thorac Cardiovasc Surg* **98**:1066–1076, 1989

102. Sun RC, Raza ST, Tam SKC, et al: Effects of antegrade cardioplegic infusion with simultaneously controlled coronary sinus occlusion on preservation of regionally ischemic myocardium after acute coronary artery occlusion and reperfusion. *J Thorac Cardiovasc Surg* **96**:626–633, 1988

103. Mohl W: The relevance of coronary sinus interventions in cardiac surgery. *Thorac Cardiovasc Surgeon* **39**:245–250, 1991

104. Haan C, Lazar HL, Bernard S, et al: Superiority of retrograde cardioplegia after acute coronary occlusion. *Ann Thorac Surg* **51**:408–412, 1991

105. Aldea GS, Hou D, Fonger JD, Shemin RJ: Inhomogeneous and complimentary delivery of antegrade and retrograde cardioplegia in the absence of coronary artery obstruction. *J Thorac Cardiovasc Surg* 1993 (in press)

106. Ihnken K, Morita K, Buckberg GD: New approaches to blood cardioplegic delivery to reduce hemodilution and cardioplegic overdose. *J Card Surg* **9**:26–36, 1994

107. Wareing TH, Davila-Roman VG, Daily BB, et al: Strategy for the reduction of stroke incidence in cardiac surgical patients. *Ann Thorac Surg* **55**:1400–1408, 1993

108. Bomfim V, Kayser L, Bendz R: Myocardial protection during aortic valve replacement. Cardiac metabolism and enzyme release following continuous blood cardioplegia. *Scand J Thorac Cardiovasc Surg* **15**:141–147, 1981

109. Sud A: Identification of right coronary ostium. Correspondence to the Editor. *Ann Thorac Surg* **40**:97, 1985

110. Jennings RB, Ganote CE: Structural changes in myocardium during acute ischemia. *Circ Res* **35**:III–156–III–172, 1974

111. Kloner RA, Ellis SG, Lange R, Braunwald E: Studies of experimental coronary artery reperfusion. Effects on infarct size, myocardial function, biochemistry, ultrastructure and microvascular damage. *Circulation* **68**:I–8–I–15, 1983

112. Wood JA, Hanley HG, Entman JL: Biochemical and morphological correlates of acute experimental myocardial ischemia in the dog. IV. Early mechanisms during very early ischemia. *Circ Res* **44**:52–62, 1979

113. Allen BS, Buckberg GD, Schwaiger M, et al: Studies of controlled reperfusion after ischemia: XVI. Early recovery of regional wall motion in patients following surgical revascularization after eight hours of acute coronary occlusion. *J Thorac Cardiovasc Surg* **92**:636–648, 1986

114. Allen BS, Okamoto F, Buckberg GD, et al: Studies of controlled reperfusion after ischemia: Reperfusate conditions: XII. Considerations of reperfusate "duration" vs "dose" on regional functional, biochemical, and histochemical recovery. *J Thorac Cardiovasc Surg* **92**:594–604, 1986

115. Follette DM, Steed DL, Foglia RP: Reduction on postischemic myocardial damage by maintaining arrest during initial reperfusion. *Surg Forum* **28**:281–283, 1977

116. Follette D, Fey K, Livesay J, et al: Studies on myocardial reperfusion injury. I. Favorable modification by adjusting reperfusate pH. *Surgery* **82**:149–155, 1977

117. Foglia RP, Buckberg GD, Lazar HL: The effectiveness of mannitol after ischemic myocardial edema. *Surg Forum* **30**:320–323, 1980

118. Engelman RM, Spencer FC, Gouge TH: Effect of normothermic anoxic arrest on coronary blood flow distribution of pigs. *Surg Forum* **25**:176–179, 1974

119. Menasche P, Grousset C, de Boccard G: Protective effect of an asanguineous reperfusion solution on myocardial performance following cardioplegic arrest. *Ann Thorac Surg* **37**:222–228, 1984

120. Lazar HL, Buckberg GD, Manganaro A, et al: Limitations imposed by hypothermia during recovery from ischemia. *Surg Forum* **XXXI**:312–315, 1980

121. Metzdorff MT, Grunkemeier GL, Starr A: Effect of initial reperfusion temperature on myocardial preservation. *J Thorac Cardiovasc Surg* **91**:545–550, 1986

122. Teoh KH, Christakis GT, Weisel RD, et al: Accelerated myocardial metabolic recovery with terminal warm blood cardioplegia. *J Thorac Cardiovasc Surg* **91**:888–895, 1986

123. Kirklin JW: The science of cardiac surgery. *Eur J Cardiothorac Surg* **4**:63–71, 1990

124. Okamoto F, Allen BS, Buckberg GD, et al: Studies of controlled reperfusion after ischemia. Reperfusate conditions: XIV. Importance of ensuring gentle vs sudden reperfusion during relief of coronary occlusion. *J Thorac Cardiovasc Surg* **92**:613–620, 1986

125. Jennings RB, Reimer KA: Factors involved in salvaging ischemic myocardium: Effect of reperfusion of arterial blood. *Circulation* **68**:I25–I36, 1983

126. Allen BS, Okamoto F, Buckberg GD, et al: Studies of controlled reperfusion after ischemia. XV. Immediate functional recovery after 6 hours of regional ischemia by careful control of conditions of reperfusion and composition of reperfusate. *J Thorac Cardiovasc Surg* **92**:621–635, 1986

127. Stack RS, Califf RM, Hinohara T, et al: Survival and cardiac event rates in the first year after emergency coronary angioplasty for acute myocardial infarction. *J Am Coll Cardiol* **11**:1141–1149, 1988

128. Miller PF, Brodie BR, Weintraub RA, et al: Emergency coronary angioplasty for acute myocardial infarction. *Arch Intern Med* **147**:1565–1570, 1987

129. Rothbaum DA, Linnemeier TJ, Landin RJ, et al: Emergency percutaneous transluminal coronary angioplasty in acute myocardial infarction: A 3 year experience. *J Am Coll Cardiol* **10**:264–272, 1987

130. Erbel R, Pop T, Henrichs KJ, et al: Percutaneous transluminal coronary angioplasty after thrombolytic therapy: A prospective controlled randomized trial. *J Am Coll Cardiol* **8**:485–495, 1986

131. O'Keefe JHJ, Rutherford BD, McConahay DR, et al: Early and late results of coronary angioplasty without antecedent thrombolytic therapy for acute myocardial infarction. *Am J Cardiol* **64**:1221–1230, 1989

132. Wilcox RG, Olsson CG, Skene AM, et al: Trial of tissue plasminogen activator for mortality reduction in acute myocardial infarction. Anglo-Scandinavian study of early thrombolysis (ASSET). *Lancet* **II**:525–530, 1988

133. GISSI: Effectiveness of intravenous thrombolytic treatment in acute myocardial infarction. *Lancet* **I**:397–402, 1986

134. GISSI-2: A factorial randomised trial of alteplase versus streptokinase and heparin versus no heparin among 12,490 patients with acute myocardial infarction. *Lancet* **336**:65–71, 1990

135. ISIS-2: Randomised trial of intravenous streptokinase, oral aspirin, both, or neither among 17,187 cases of suspected acute myocardial infarction: ISIS-2. *Lancet* 349–360, 1988

136. Rogers WJ: Update on recent clinical trials of thrombolytic therapy in myocardial infarction. *J Invasive Cardiol* **3**:11A–19A, 1991

137. The ISAM Study Group: A prospective trial of intravenous streptokinase in acute myocardial infarction (I.S.A.M.). *N Engl J Med* **314**:1465–1471, 1986

138. AIMS Trial Study Group: Effect of intravenous apsac on mortality after acute myocardial infarction: Preliminary report of a placebo-controlled clinical trial. *Lancet* **I**:545–549, 1988

139. Ohman EM, Califf RM: Thrombolytic therapy: Overview of clinical trials. *Coronary Artery Dis* **1**:23–33, 1990

140. Topol EJ, Califf RM, George BS, et al: A randomized trial of immediate versus delayed elective angioplasty after intravenous tissue plasminogen activator in acute myocardial infarction. *N Engl J Med* **317**:581–588, 1987

141. Page DL, Caulfifeld JB, Kastor JA, et al: Myocardial changes associated with cardiogenic shock. *N Engl J Med* **285**:133–137, 1971

142. Johnson SA, Scalon RJ, Loeb HS: Treatment of cardiogenic shock in myocardial infarction by intraaortic balloon counterpulsation and surgery. *Am J Med* **62**:687–692, 1977

143. Mundth ED, Buckley JM, Daggett WF: Surgery for complications of acute myocardial infarction. *Circulation* **45**:1279–1291, 1972

144. Nelson R, Fey K, Follette DM: The critical importance of intermittent infusion of cardioplegic solution during aortic cross-clamping. *Surg Forum* **26**:241–243, 1976

145. Beyersdorf F, Allen BS, Buckberg GD, et al: Studies on prolonged acute regional ischemia: I. Evidence for preserved cellular viability after 6 hours of coronary occlusion. *J Thorac Cardiovasc Surg* **98**:112–126, 1989

146. Beyersdorf F, Acar C, Buckberg GD, et al: Studies on prolonged regional ischemia. III: Early natural history of simulated single and multi-vessel disease with emphasis on remote myocardium. *J Thorac Cardiovasc Surg* **98**:368–380, 1989

147. Beyersdorf F, Okamoto F, Buckberg GD, et al: Studies on prolonged regional ischemia. II. Implications of progression from dyskinesis to akinesis in the ischemic segment. *J Thorac Cardiovasc Surg* **98**:224–233, 1989

148. Banka VS, Helfant RH: Temporal sequence of dynamic contractile characteristics in ischemic and non-ischemic myocardium after acute coronary ligation. *Am J Cardiol* **34**:158–162, 1974

149. Kloner RA, Przyklenk K, Lange R, Ellis S: Reperfusion pathophysiology. In Roberts AJ (ed): *Myocardial Protection in Cardiac Surgery.* New York, Marcel Dekker, 1987, pp 29–52

150. Kerber RE, Marcus ML, Ehrhardt J, et al: Correlation between echocardiographically demonstrated segmental dyskinesis and regional myocardial perfusion. *Circulation* **520**:1097, 1992

151. Beyersdorf F, Acar C, Buckberg GD, et al: Studies on prolonged regional ischemia. IV. Aggressive surgical treatment for intractable ventricular fibrillation after acute myocardial infarction. *J Thorac Cardiovasc Surg* **98**:557–566, 1989

152. Beyersdorf F, Acar C, Buckberg GD, et al: Studies on prolonged regional ischemia. V. Metabolic support of remote myocardium during LV power failure. *J Thorac Cardiovasc Surg* **98**:567–579, 1989

153. Widimsky P, Gregor P, Cervenka V: Diffuse left ventricular hypokinesis in cardiogenic shock; its cause or consequence? *Gor Vasa* **26**:27–31, 1984

154. Benjamin JJ, Cascade PN, Rubenfire M, et al: Left lower lobe atelectasis and consolidation following cardiac surgery: The effect of topical cooling on the phrenic nerve. *Radiology* **142**:11–14, 1982

155. Buga GM, Griscavage JM, Rogers NE, Ignarro LJ: Negative feedback of endothelial cell function by nitric oxide. *Circ Res* **73**:808–812, 1993

156. Allen BS, Buckberg GD, Rosenkranz ER, et al: Topical cardiac hypothermia in patients with coronary disease: An unnecessary adjunct to cardioplegic protection and cause of pulmonary morbidity. *J Thorac Cardiovasc Surg* **104**:626–631, 1992

157. Robicsek F: Biochemical termination of sustained fibrillation occurring after artificially induced ischemic arrest. *J Thorac Cardiovasc Surg* **87**:143–145, 1984

158. Hottenrott C, Maloney JVJ, Buckberg GD: Studies of the effects of

ventricular fibrillation on the adequacy of regional myocardial flow. III. Mechanism of ischemia. *J Thorac Cardiovasc Surg* **68**:634–645, 1974

159. Buckberg GD, Hottenrott CE: Ventricular fibrillation: Its effect on myocardial flow, distribution and performance. *Ann Thorac Surg* **20**:76–85, 1975

160. Allen BS, Rosenkranz ER, Buckberg GD, et al: Studies of controlled reperfusion after ischemia: VII. The high oxygen requirements of dyskinetic cardiac muscle. *J Thorac Cardiovasc Surg* **92**:543–552, 1986

161. Beyersdorf F, Kirsh MM, Buckberg GD, Allen BS: Warm glutamate/aspartate-enriched blood cardioplegic solution for perioperative sudden death. *J Thorac Cardiovasc Surg* **104**:1141–1147, 1992

162. Mooney MR, Arom KV, Joyce LD: Emergency cardiopulmonary bypass support in patients with cardiac arrest. *J Thorac Cardiovasc Surg* **101**:450–454, 1991

163. Shumway NE, Lower RR: Hypothermia for extended periods of anoxic arrest. *Surg Forum* **10**:563, 1959

164. Lichtenstein SV, Ashe KA, el Dalati H, et al: Warm heart surgery. *J Thorac Cardiovasc Surg* **101**:269–274, 1991

165. Salerno TA, Houck JP, Barrozo CAM, et al: Retrograde continuous warm blood cardioplegia: A new concept in myocardial protection. *Ann Thorac Surg* **51**:245–247, 1991

166. Lichtenstein SV, Salerno TA, Slutsky AS: Warm continuous cardioplegia is preferable to intermittent hypothermic cardioplegia for myocardial protection during cardiopulmonary bypass: Pro and con. *J Cardiothorac Anesth* **4**:279–281, 1990

167. Lichtenstein SV, Abel JG, Panos A, et al: Warm heart surgery: Experience with long cross-clamp times. *Ann Thorac Surg* **52**:1009–1013, 1991

168. Matsuura H, Lazar HL, Yang XM, et al: Detrimental effects of interrupting warm blood cardioplegia during coronary revascularization. *AATS* 62–63, 1992 (abstract)

169. Schott RJ, Rohmann S, Braun ER: Ischemic preconditioning reduces infarct size in swine myocardium. *Circ Res* **66**:1133–1142, 1990

170. Lazar H, Foglia R, Manganaro AJ: Detrimental effects of premature use of inotropic drugs to discontinue cardiopulmonary bypass. *J Thorac Cardiovasc Surg* **82**:18–25, 1981

171. Pennock JL, Pierce WS, Waldhausen JA: Quantitative evaluation of left ventricular bypass in reducing myocardial ischemia. *Surgery* **79**:523, 1976

172. Pennington DG, Bernhard WF, Golding LR: Ventricular assist device salvage of cardiotomy patients long-term follow-up. *Circulation* **70**:I1–I72, 1984

Cardiac Catheterization in the Evaluation of Heart Disease

Michael S. Remetz and John Hennecken

Heart catheterization and angiography give critical diagnostic and anatomic information in the vast majority of patients being considered for cardiac surgery. It is therefore mandatory that the cardiac surgeon be able to understand information obtained from cardiac pressure recordings and angiographic studies. By understanding the nature of catheterization techniques and the risks involved in their application, the surgeon, in consultation with the cardiologist, can provide pivotal information regarding the appropriate therapy for an individual patient. This chapter focuses on basic interpretation of catheterization and angiographic data used in the evaluation of patients being considered for cardiac surgical procedures.

INDICATIONS FOR CARDIAC CATHETERIZATION

The indications for cardiac catheterization have changed since interventional technology has become available. The individual practice philosophy of physicians has a major impact on the use of cardiac catheterization, however, a variety of relatively well-accepted indications have evolved.

In the assessment of coronary artery disease the indications for cardiac catheterization can be divided into therapeutic and diagnostic categories. The diagnostic indications include the assessment of the patient with atypical chest pain and an indeterminate or positive exercise treadmill test. Angiography can also definitely evaluate atherosclerotic disease in the asymptomatic patient with significant cardiac risk factors and a markedly abnormal resting electrocardiogram. In these patients coronary angiography provides confirmatory information regarding the presence and severity of significant coronary atherosclerosis.

The therapeutic indications for cardiac catheterization are manifold and include incapacitating angina pectoris, un-

stable angina, or postinfarction angina. Patients with a strongly positive exercise treadmill test,[1,2] increased lung uptake on exercise thallium scintigraphy,[3,4] resting ST segment depression,[5] or acute pulmonary edema induced by ischemia[6,7] have a high prevalence of severe three vessel or left main coronary artery disease. Because these patients have an increased likelihood of morbid cardiac events, coronary arteriography is generally performed to assess the utility of aggressive treatment with coronary artery bypass grafting or angioplasty. Patients in the postinfarction period who have evidence of mechanical complications such as acute mitral regurgitation, ventricular septal perforation, pseudoaneurysm formation, or aneurysm formation with intractable congestive heart failure are candidates for cardiac catheterization to evaluate the functional abnormality in preparation for corrective surgical procedures.

Patients with significant symptomatic valvular heart disease who are candidates for surgical correction are studied with right and left heart catheterization. In these patients catheterization confirms the presence and severity of the valvular abnormality and also provides information regarding associated problems such as significant coronary artery disease that may require concomitant bypass grafting during surgical correction. Patients with critical aortic or mitral stenosis who are not surgical candidates are now being considered for therapeutic cardiac catheterization to perform palliative procedures such as percutaneous catheter balloon valvuloplasty.

TECHNIQUES OF CARDIAC CATHETERIZATION

Sones originally described cardiac catheterization using a brachial approach for vascular access.[8] Brachial access can be achieved percutaneously or by local arterial cut down allowing catheter insertion, measurements of intravascular pressure, and angiography. The percutaneous femoral approach has gained widespread use because of its ease and expediency. Development of ingenious preshaped catheters by Judkins and others has facilitated the straightforward, rapid, and safe application of this percutaneous femoral approach. However, femoral access may not be possible in patients with severe peripheral vascular disease, prior aortic or femoral vascular surgery, or abdominal aortic aneurysms. In these patients the brachial approach may be required.

The percutaneous approach involves needle insertion into the lumen of either the femoral or brachial artery. When free back flow is established a guide wire is inserted through the needle and passed into the arterial lumen. An 8 Fr sheath is inserted over the guide wire and arterial pressure is documented by connecting the sidearm of the sheath to an available pressure transducer. If a brachial cut down is required it is generally performed at a site 2 cm above the antecubital fossa. The brachial artery lies within a vascular sheath running below the insertion of the biceps aponeurosis of the biceps tendon. This sheath contains the basilic vein and is in close proximity to the median nerve. After careful dissection, ligatures are placed around the brachial artery and a small arteriotomy is performed to allow catheter insertion. Venous catheterization can be performed using similar maneuvers with the basilic vein.

INTERPRETATION OF CARDIAC ANGIOGRAPHY

Left Ventriculography

In most patients left ventriculography is performed as the first angiographic procedure. Following insertion of a ventriculographic catheter into the left ventricle, chamber pressures are recorded. Angiography is generally performed in the 30° right anterior oblique (RAO) projection. This projection visualizes the left ventricle perpendicular to its long axis so that the ventricular contour is seen in profile. The principle areas of importance visualized in this projection are the anterobasal, anterior, apical, inferior, and posterobasal segments of the left ventricle (Fig. 103–1). The septum and lateral wall are not seen in the RAO projection. These areas are visualized in the orthogonal 60° left anterior oblique (LAO) view (Fig. 103–2).

Left ventriculography allows assessment of global and regional contractile performance of the heart (Fig. 103–3). The severity of contractile dysfunction assists in defining the prognosis of patients with myocardial disease. Patients with depressed ventricular function are at higher risk for cardiac surgery than patients with preserved function.[9] In addition, anatomic abnormalities that can be corrected by surgery such as mitral regurgitation, ventricular septal defect, ventricular aneurysm, and ventricular pseudoaneurysm can be identified.

Coronary Angiography

Identification of Significant Coronary Artery Disease

Coronary angiography has become the gold standard in the identification and assessment of anatomic severity of coronary artery atherosclerotic lesions. Angiographic atherosclerotic stenoses are generally expressed as a percent reduction of the lesion lumen diameter compared to an area of adjacent normal vessel. The percentage of stenosis is generally estimated subjectively by an experienced angiographer. Quantitative techniques where the lumen diameter is measured by calipers can also be used to assess lesion severity. Generally the angiographic assessment of arterial stenoses can be divided into three major categories. The first group includes vessels with less than 50% luminal diameter narrowing. These lesions are generally considered not to be hemodynamically significant. The second group consists of lesions with 50–70% decrease in lumen diameter and the third group includes those with a greater than 70% decrease. Experimental studies demonstrate that a 75% reduction in the lumen cross-sectional area of large arteries is required to decrease flow reserve during exercise.[10] In practice, a reduction in the diameter of coronary arteries by 50% or more is generally considered significant since it represents a 75% reduction in cross-sectional area. A 75% decrease in luminal diameter results in 95% reduction in cross-sectional area. Long lesions or multiple sequential short segments of narrowing may worsen flow further and cause greater ischemia when compared to vessels with discrete single stenoses of similar severity.

There are a variety of potential sources of error in the assessment of coronary stenoses. Errors in coronary stenosis estimation may be based on vessel foreshortening, vessel overlap, eccentric lesions visualized in only one projection, lesions not well seen due to their proximal location, and long segments with uniform involvement. A major difficulty also lies in comparison of the coronary segment of interest to the presumed normal adjacent segment. Since atherosclerosis is a diffuse process, an adjacent segment interpreted as angiographically normal may actually be involved in the disease process.[11] Overestimation of the stenosis may be related to superimposed coronary spasm, myocardial bridging, and failure to fill some vessels because of selective engagement of the coronary and contrast streaming and layering effects. Technical errors such as slow contrast injection, poor filling, poor processing, and failure to recognize anatomic variations may also make a significant contribution to a lack of precision. A very important aspect in the angiographic assessment of coronary stenoses relates to visual interpretation. Several studies have shown significant inter- and intraobserver variability in the assessment of the degree of stenosis. In a study by Zir et al, in only 65% of cases did all four angiographic observers agree that a significant stenosis was present in the proximal or mid-left anterior descending coronary artery.[12]

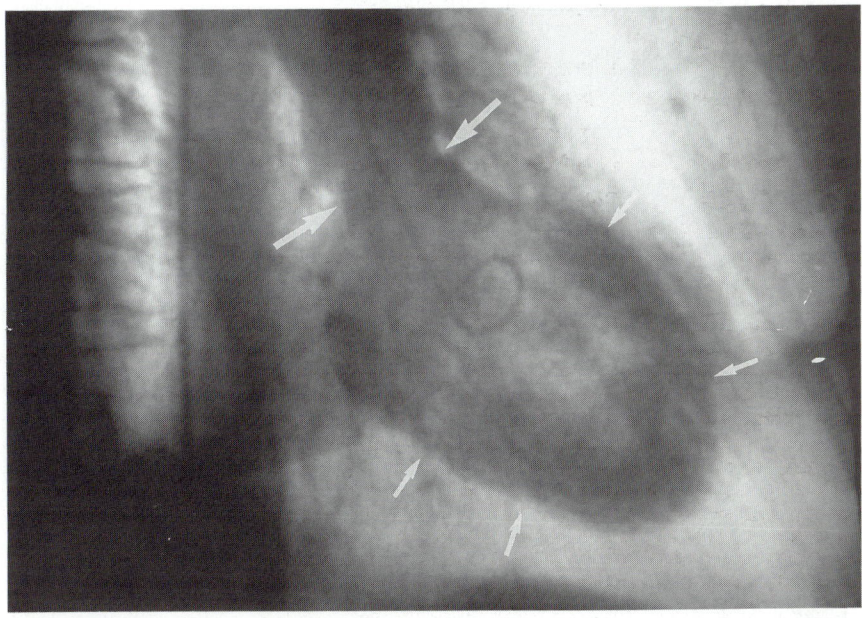

A

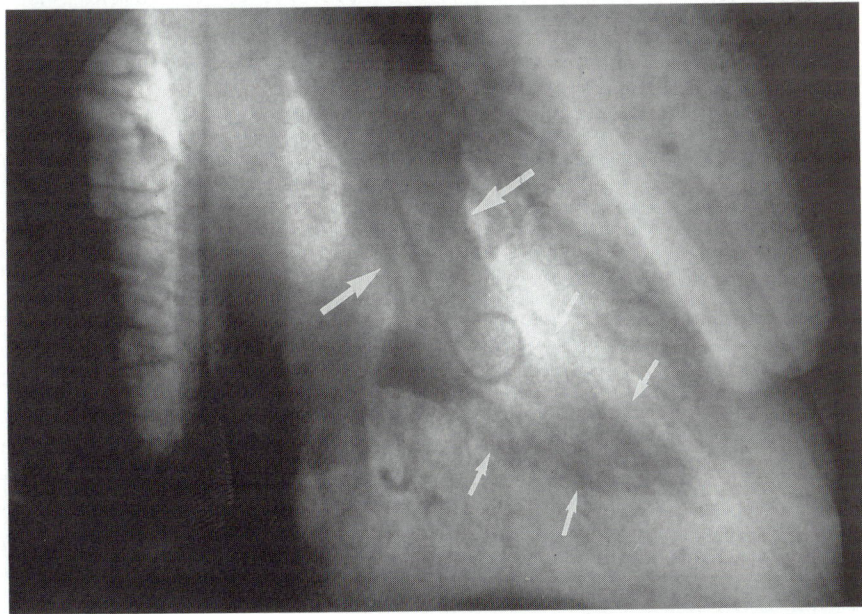

B

Figure 103–1. Thirty degree right anterior oblique (RAO) projection of a normal left ventriculogram at end-diastole (**A**) and end-systole (**B**). A pigtail angiographic catheter can be seen within the left ventricular chamber cavity. The large arrows show the plane of the aortic valve. The smaller arrows demarcate the five muscle segments visualized in this projection. Progressing from the top clockwise are the anterobasal, antero-lateral, apical, inferior, and posterobasal segments. Comparison of the diastolic and systolic frames reveals that all five segments move normally.

Another source of potential error is represented by the physical limitations of the method as evidenced by progressive increase in error as normal vessel size diminishes.

Right Coronary Artery Angiography

The right coronary artery, which runs in the right atrioventricular (A-V) groove, is angiographically well demonstrated in the standard left (LAO) and right (RAO) anterior oblique projections. Each of these projections avoids overlap with the spine and visualizes unique segments of the right coronary and its branches. In the LAO projection, the right coronary artery appears as a semicircle with its con-

vexity directed to the right side of the patient (Fig. 103–4). The course in either the anterior or posterior direction is foreshortened in this view. In the RAO view the plane of the A-V groove is projected tangentially. This makes the right coronary appear to course more or less straight downward with side branches arising either posterior to the right atrium or anterior to the wall of the right ventricle (Fig. 103–5). Identification of the U turn of the right coronary artery at the crux represents a landmark indicating the plane of the interventricular septum. At the crux the A-V nodal artery can be seen coursing superiorly in the LAO projection.

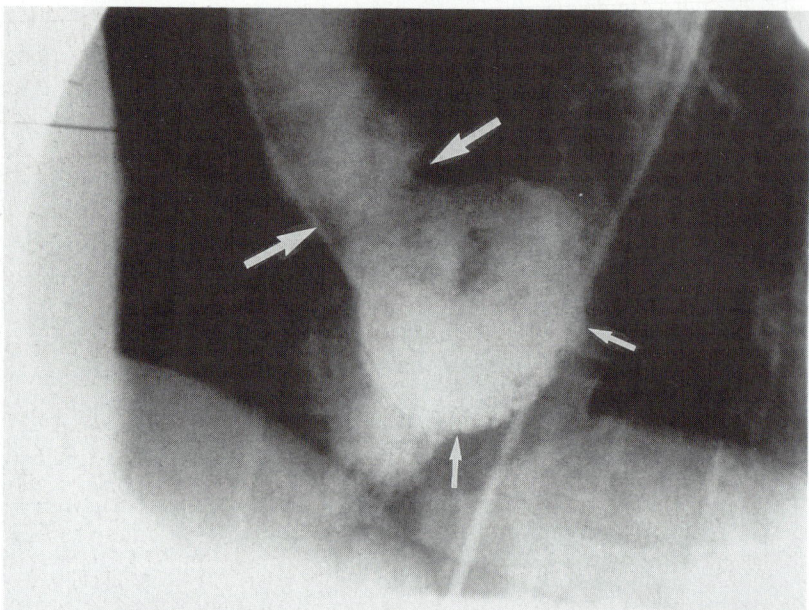

A

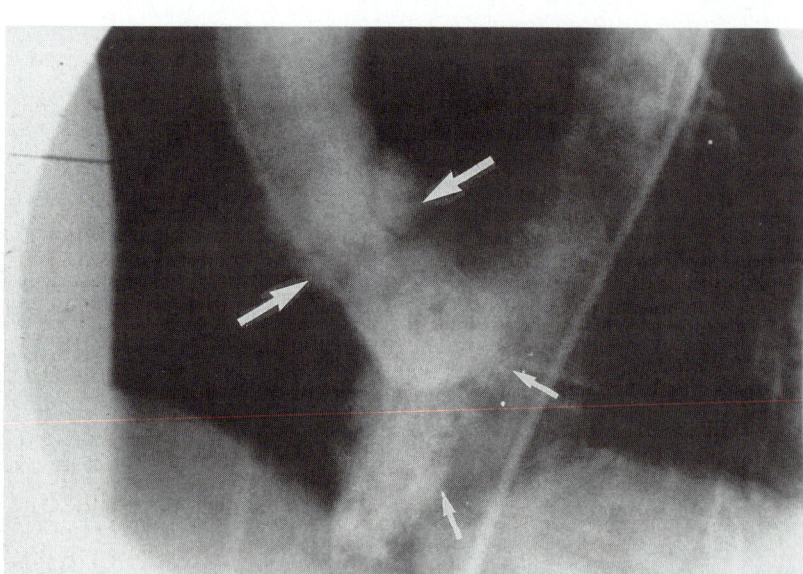

Figure 103–2. Sixty degree left anterior oblique (LAO) projection of an abnormal left ventriculogram at end-diastole (**A**) and end-systole (**B**). Large arrows show the plane of the aortic valve. The smaller arrows demarcate the three segments visualized in this projection. Progressing from the right clockwise are the lateral, inferoapical, and septal segments. Comparison of the diastolic and systolic frames shows that the apical septum is akinetic. The patient had suffered an anteroseptal myocardial infarction.

B

Other views may be required in some cases to view specific regions of this vessel (Figs. 103–6, 103–7, 103–8, and 103–9). Cranial angulation may be required in the LAO projection to show the crux and bifurcation of the right coronary artery into the PDA and posterolateral branches. This region can additionally be seen in a cranial RAO projection. The proximal segment of the right coronary artery can be more readily identified in a cranial posteroanterior (PA) projection. This may be particularly helpful in patients with a pronounced "shepherd's crook" type configuration to the proximal right coronary artery.

Left Coronary Artery Angiography

Multiple views are required for appropriate identification and assessment of the major branches of the left coronary artery. In our laboratory a shallow RAO projection is initially performed to assess the left main coronary artery (Fig. 103–10). Frequently this will also be helpful in the assessment of the mid and distal left anterior descending coronary artery (LAD). The LAD is generally assessed in a variety of views. A cranially angulated LAO projection separates the circumflex and LAD origins in most cases and, because of this, provides good visualization of the proximal LAD (Fig.

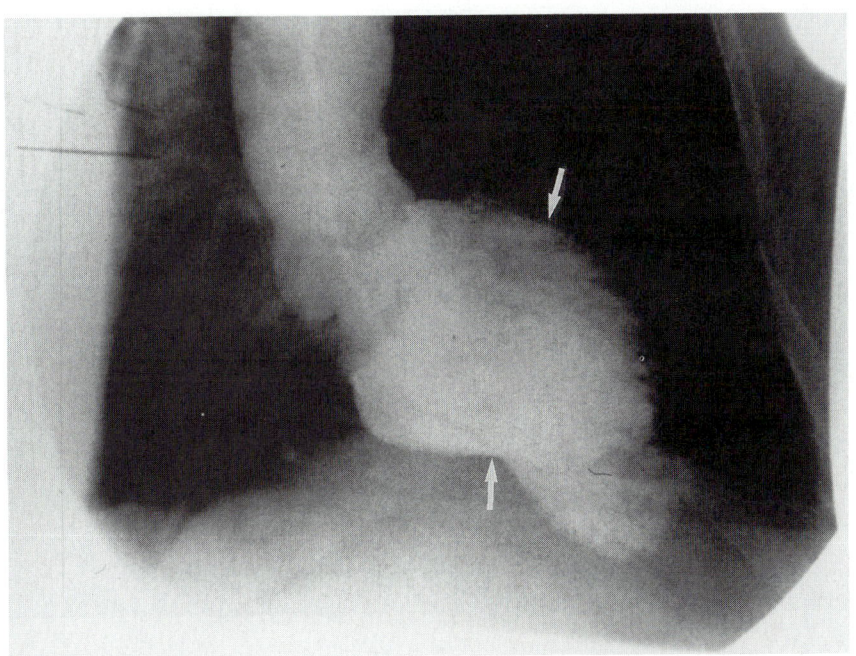

A

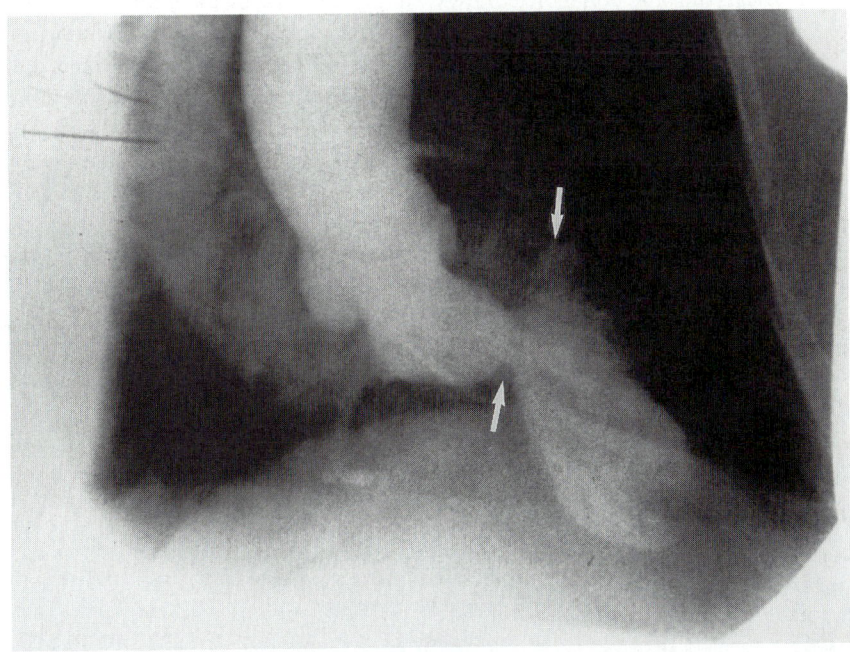

B

Figure 103–3. RAO ventriculogram of the same patient shown in Figure 103–2. The patient has suffered a large anteroseptal myocardial infarction. Comparison of the diastolic (**A**) and systolic (**B**) frames shows an extensive wall motion abnormality (indicated by arrows) involving the anterolateral, apical, and inferoapical segments. The anterobasal and posterobasal segments contract normally. The deformity of the diastolic apical contour would allow angiographic diagnosis of a left ventricular aneurysm.

103–11). It additionally demonstrates the mid and distal LAD as well as some of the major diagonal branches. In many cases this view is also helpful in the assessment of the left main coronary artery. The proximal portions of the LAD can also be assessed with a cranially angulated RAO or PA projection (Fig. 103–12). This view also allows assessment of the origin of major diagonal branches as well as the septal perforators. The cranial PA additionally offers adequate visualization of the mid and distal LAD. One further view that is used for assessment of both the left main coronary artery as well as visualization of the bifurcation of

the circumflex and LAD is a caudal LAO projection (Fig. 103–13). This view, however, is not particularly helpful in assessing the mid and distal vasculature.

The circumflex system can be visualized in the RAO projection, which outlines the A-V groove portion of the circumflex and obtuse marginal branches. This view, however, does not allow definitive assessment of the proximal portions of the circumflex. Other angulations that are helpful in the assessment of the proximal segments of this system are a caudally angulated RAO (Fig. 103–14) projection and a caudally directed PA projection (Fig. 103–15). In each of these

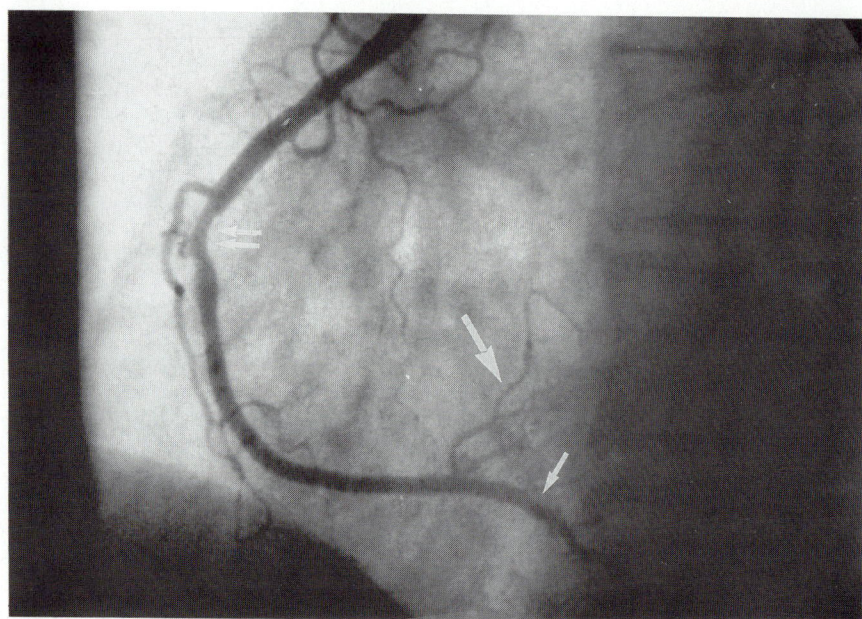

Figure 103–4. LAO projection of a right coronary artery. The crux and atrioventricular nodal artery (large arrow) can be seen at the origin of the posterior descending artery (small arrow). There is a 50% lesion in the mid-right coronary artery (double arrow). No posterolateral branches are seen identifying the system as codominant.

views the origin of marginal branches and the left posterior descending artery (PDA) when present can be well visualized.

CARDIAC CATHETERIZATION IN THE ASSESSMENT OF VALVULAR HEART DISEASE

Mitral Stenosis

Pathophysiology of Mitral Stenosis

The normal area of the adult mitral valve is 4–6 cm². When this area is significantly reduced by pathophysiologic processes, the signs and symptoms of mitral stenosis result.

Rheumatic mitral valve disease is overwhelmingly the most common etiology causing narrowing of the valve orifice. Very rarely mitral stenosis can be congenital or result from some other process such as the carcinoid syndrome. Left atrial myxoma can simulate mitral stenosis if the tumor mass obstructs the mitral orifice during diastole.

Mitral stenosis resulting from acute rheumatic fever is a chronic process. Over the course of years the mitral orifice is narrowed progressively by commissure fusion and chordal thickening. When the valve area is reduced to less than 2 cm² a pressure gradient between the left atrium and left ventricle is required to maintain diastolic mitral inflow at a rate great enough to sustain cardiac output. It has been demonstrated that flow is proportional to the square of the

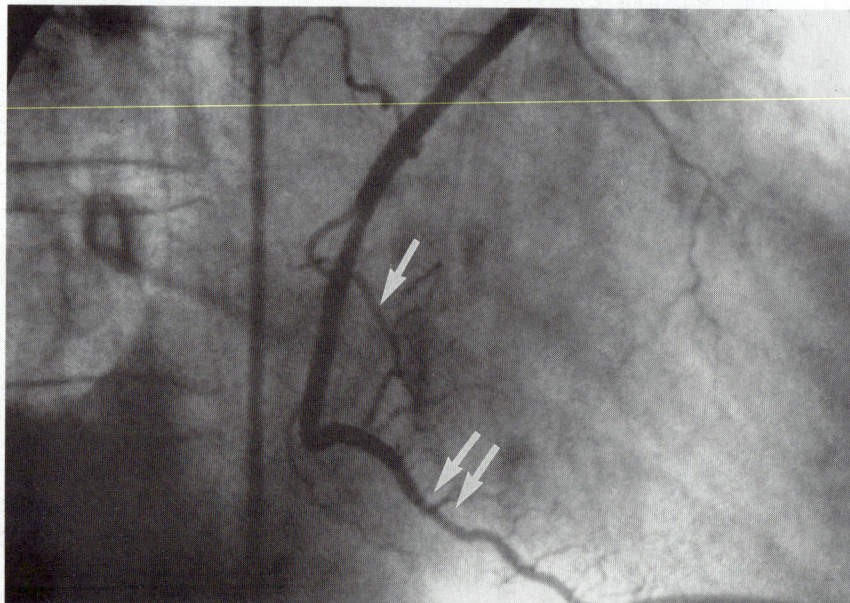

Figure 103–5. RAO projection of the right coronary artery from the patient in Figure 103–4. A large right ventricular marginal branch (single arrow) arises at the location of the high grade lesion. The posterior descending (double arrows) is seen coursing towards the apex along the inferior interventricular septum.

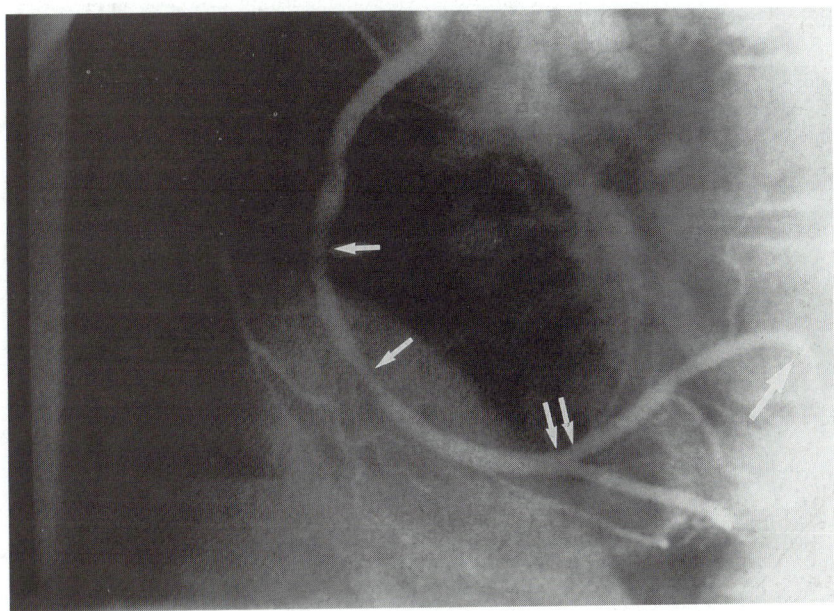

Figure 103–6. LAO projection of a dominant right coronary artery. The right coronary extends past the crux (double arrows) in the atrioventricular groove and gives off a large posterolateral left ventricular branch (large arrow) after the take-off of the posterior descending. Sequential 50% lesions are seen in the mid right coronary (small arrows).

pressure gradient across a fixed area orifice. Therefore, initially patients can maintain adequate resting cardiac output. However, with exercise the pressure gradient increases causing high left atrial pressure, high pulmonary capillary pressure, and symptoms of pulmonary congestion. It can be seen that with an increase in cardiac output during exercise a doubling of resting mitral flow will be associated with a 4-fold increase in mitral pressure gradient. As mitral area is further reduced to less than 1 cm^2 the clinical picture of severe mitral stenosis results. At this point there is a significant mitral pressure gradient at rest and cardiac output is reduced. Chronic increases in pulmonary capillary pressure cause reflex elevation of pulmonary artery and right ven-

tricular pressures. Pulmonary arterial resistance becomes elevated and this, in association with increased pulmonary lymphatic flow and decreased pulmonary capillary permeability, can limit pulmonary congestion. These compensatory mechanisms allow the patient with severe mitral stenosis to tolerate high pulmonary wedge pressures (greater than 25–30 mm Hg) without developing severe symptoms or pulmonary edema. Eventually, however, cardiac output is further reduced by the high pulmonary arterial and mitral valve resistance to forward flow. Both right and left heart failure result and the patient eventually succumbs to complications of low cardiac output and congestive heart failure. It is of note that the left ventricle in pure

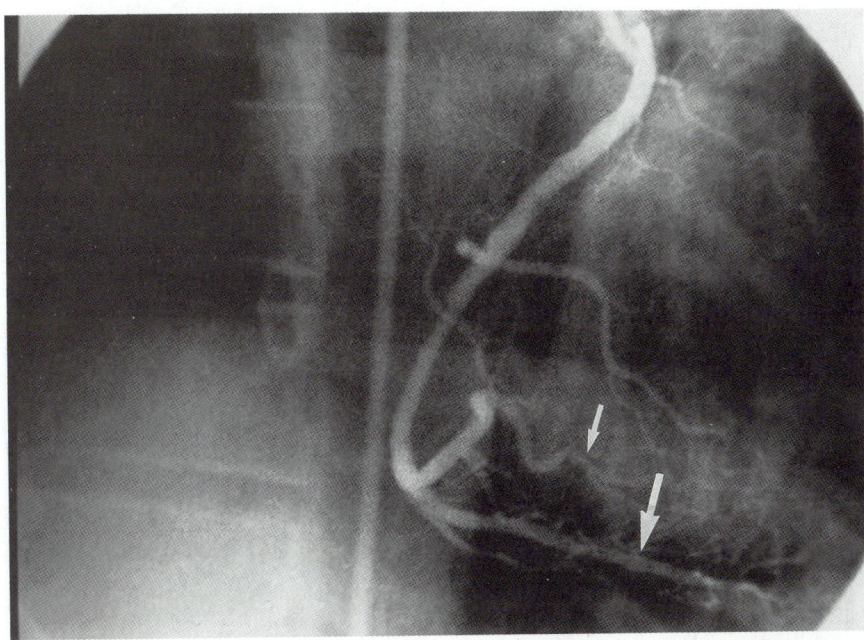

Figure 103–7. RAO projection of the right coronary from the patient in Figure 103–6. The courses of the posterior descending (large arrow) and posterolateral (small arrow) are both identified.

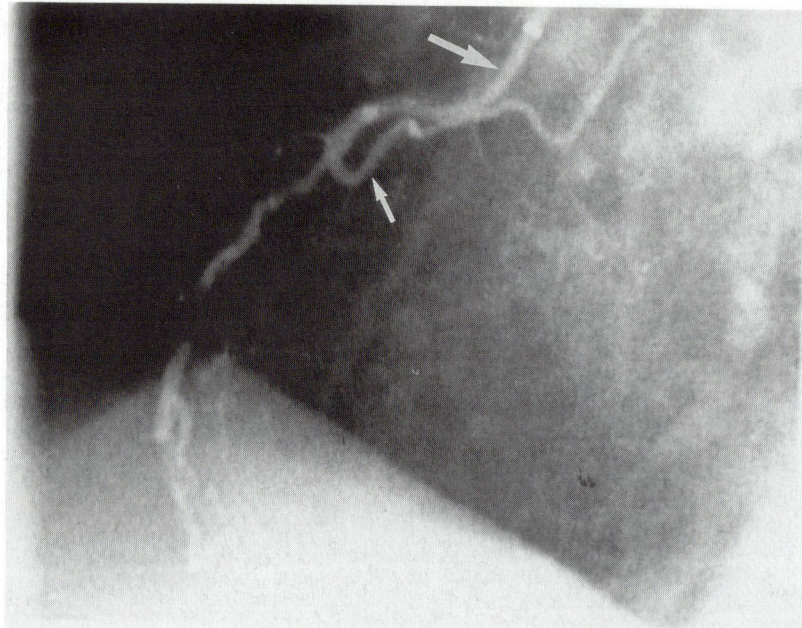

Figure 103–8. LAO projection of a nondominant right coronary artery. An angiographic catheter is seen engaged in the small right ostia (large arrow). A large atrial branch can be seen arising proximally (small arrow). The nondominant right artery does not reach the crux and does not supply the posterior descending.

mitral stenosis is not exposed to either a high pressure load as in aortic stenosis or an increased volume load as in mitral regurgitation. Because of this the left ventricle is protected from the damage that can result from these overload states and indices of ventricular function are usually well preserved even in patients with end-stage mitral stenosis.

Cardiac Catheterization in Mitral Stenosis

This procedure is performed to confirm the diagnosis, determine the stenosis severity, and evaluate the presence of associated disease that may impact on surgery. The diagno-

sis of mitral stenosis is confirmed by demonstrating a reduced mitral valve area. Gorlin has developed an equation that relates mitral or aortic valve flow and pressure gradient to valve area.[13,14]

The Gorlin formula is as follows:

$$\text{valve area} = \frac{\text{valve flow}}{(C) \times (44.3) \times \sqrt{(\text{pressure gradient})}}$$

The C represents an empiric constant that varies with the anatomic nature of the valve area to be calculated. For aortic valve area calculations $C = 1$, while in mitral valve cal-

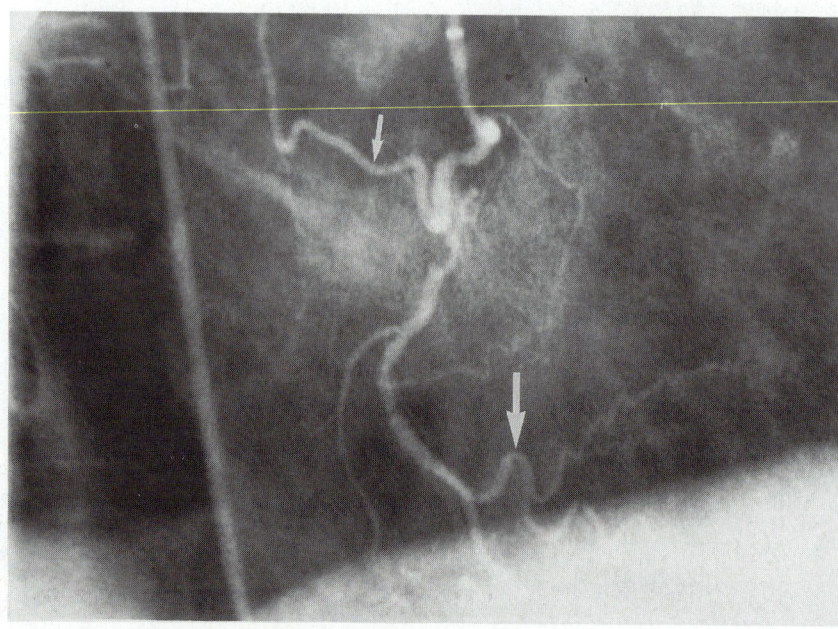

Figure 103–9. RAO projection of the nondominant right coronary from the same patient in Figure 103–8. The atrial branch (small arrow) can be seen coursing posteriorly and a right ventricular branch (large arrow) can be seen coursing anteriorly over the right ventricular surface.

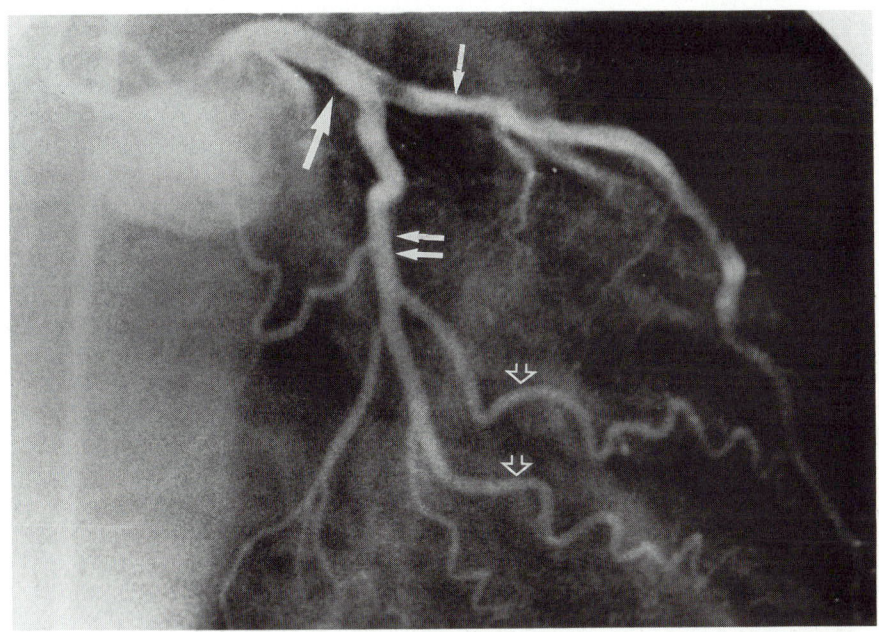

Figure 103–10. Shallow RAO projection of the left coronary artery. An angiographic left catheter can be seen in the left cusp engaged in the ostia of the left main coronary artery (large arrow). The left main gives rise to the left anterior descending artery (LAD, small arrow), and atrioventricular (A-V) groove circumflex artery (double arrows). The A-V groove circumflex gives off two large marginal branches (transparent arrows) that supply the lateral wall of the left ventricle.

culations $C = 0.85$. The pressure gradient across the mitral valve can be measured directly during catheterization by simultaneously recording pulmonary capillary wedge and left ventricular pressure. The mean pressure gradient in millimeters of mercury during diastole can be calculated. Mitral valve flow is determined simultaneously by measuring forward cardiac output and diastolic filing period. Forward cardiac output is measured using standard thermodilution, indicator dilution, or Fick techniques. Flow across the mitral valve can occur only during the time when the valve is open. This time during the cardiac cycle when mitral flow occurs is called the diastolic filling period. It can be calculated by multiplying heart rate by average diastolic time per cycle. The average diastolic time per cycle is determined from the left ventricular and pulmonary wedge pressure tracings. Total mitral valve flow (in milliliters per second) equals cardiac output (in milliliters per minute) divided by diastolic filling period (in seconds per minute). The patient in Figure 103–16 can be used as an example of valve area calculation.

This patient had the following data recorded:

cardiac output	= 5400 mL/min
diastolic time per cycle	= 0.37 s/beat
heart rate	= 84 beat/min
mean diastolic pressure gradient	= 12 mm Hg

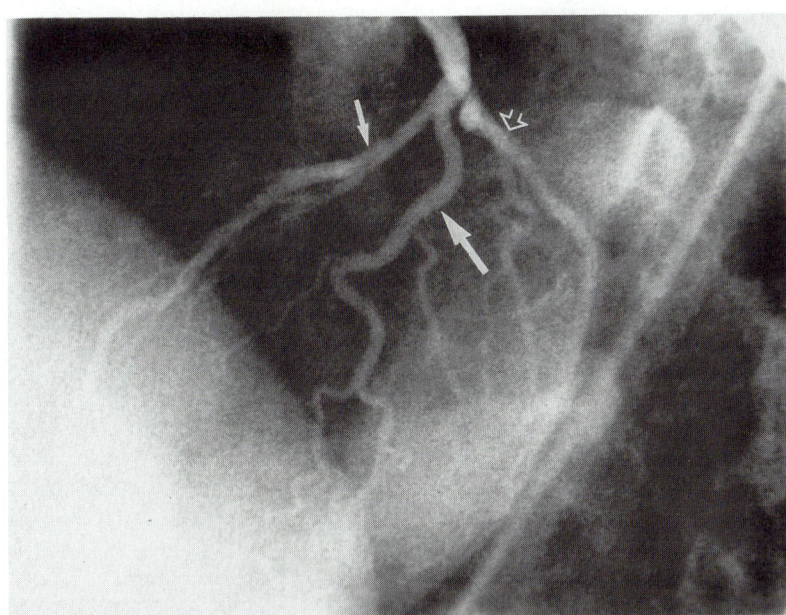

Figure 103–11. Cranially angulated LAO projection of the left coronary artery. The course of the LAD (small arrow) is well seen in this projection along with a large diagonal (large arrow) arising proximally from the LAD. The proximal A-V groove circumflex (transparent arrow) is also visualized.

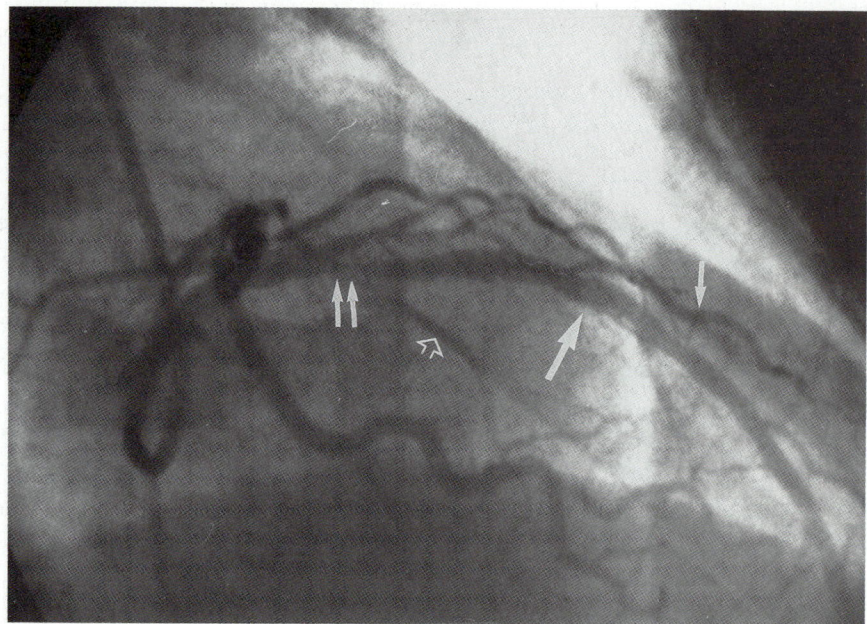

Figure 103–12. Cranially angulated PA projection of the left coronary artery. The entire course of the LAD can be visualized (large arrow). This projection allows visualization of both diagonal (small arrow) and septal (transparent arrow) branches as they arise from the LAD. A high grade lesion can be seen in the proximal LAD (double arrow).

The following parameters were then calculated:

$$\text{diastolic filling period} = \text{heart rate} \times \text{diastolic time per cycle}$$
$$= 84 \text{ beat/min} \times 0.37 \text{ s/beat}$$
$$= 31 \text{ s/min}$$
$$\text{mitral valve flow} = \text{cardiac output/diastolic filling period}$$
$$= 5400 \text{ mL/min per } 31 \text{ s/min}$$
$$= 174 \text{ mL/s}$$

mitral valve area

$$= \frac{\text{mitral valve flow}}{(0.85) \times (44.3) \times \sqrt{(\text{mean diastolic gradient})}}$$
$$= \frac{174 \text{ mL/s}}{(0.85) \times (44.3) \times \sqrt{12}}$$
$$= 1.3 \text{ cm}^2$$

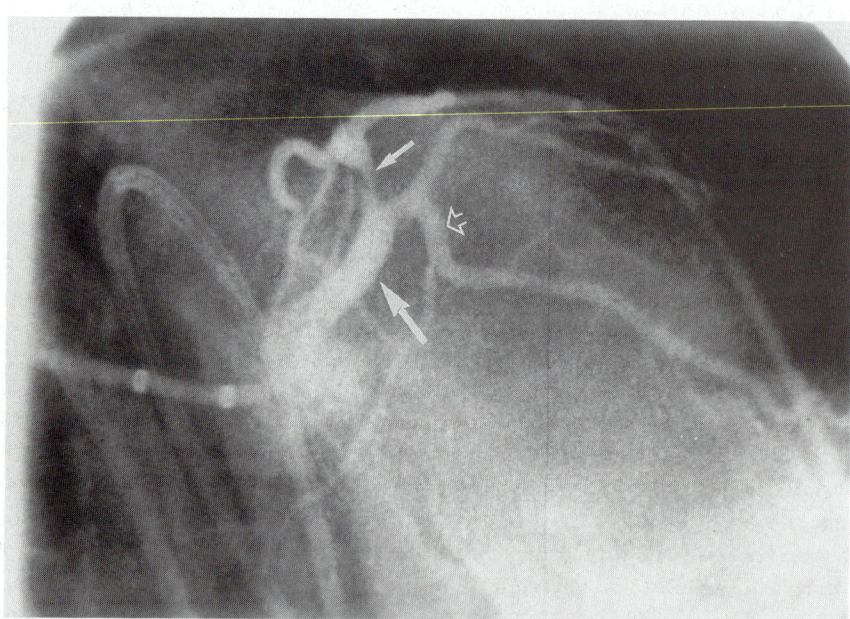

Figure 103–13. Caudally angulated LAO projection of the left coronary artery. This view allows visualization of the left main (large arrow), proximal LAD (small arrow), and proximal A-V circumflex (transparent arrow). There is a complex lesion in the proximal LAD at the arrow tip.

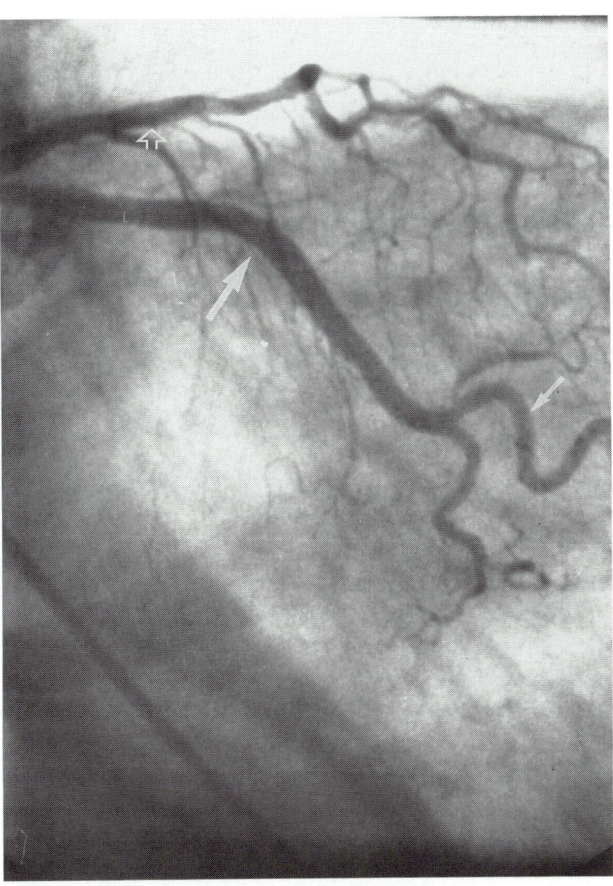

Figure 103–14. Caudally angulated RAO projection of the left coronary artery. This view is good for visualization of the A-V circumflex (large arrow) and circumflex marginal branch (small arrow). The course of the LAD (transparent arrow) is also seen, however it is frequently overlapped by diagonal branches.

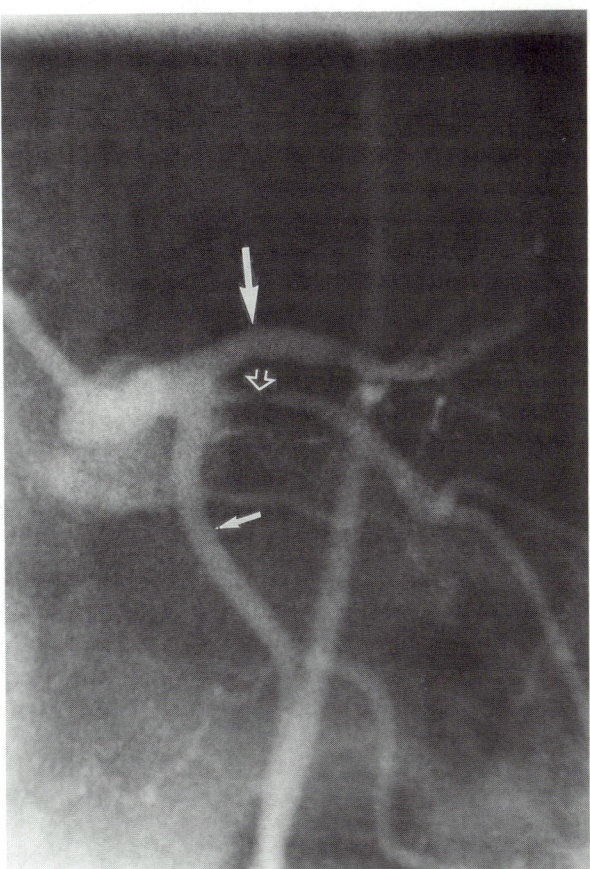

Figure 103–15. Caudally angulated PA projection of the left coronary artery. This view results in adequate visualization of the left main, proximal A-V circumflex (small arrow), and proximal LAD (large arrow). A ramus intermedius with a high grade lesion (transparent arrow) is seen arising between the A-V circumflex and the LAD.

It can be seen that with a calculated mitral valve area of 1.3 cm^2 this patient had moderately severe mitral stenosis. The Gorlin formula used in this manner is useful in categorizing patients with mitral stenosis.

Methodological errors leading to inaccurate valve area calculations are worth noting. It is important that measurements of pressure gradient and cardiac output be performed simultaneously. Pressure transducers must be accurately calibrated and referenced to zero. Occasionally, proper wedge position is not obtained and a gradient is recorded between a damped pulmonary artery tracing and left ventricular pressure. This will tend to overestimate the true gradient. A proper wedge can be confirmed by noting a high (>95%) hemoglobin percent saturation of blood obtained from the catheter tip while in the wedge position. This will contrast the lower (<85%) hemoglobin saturations obtained in the pulmonary artery. There is a time delay of pressure transmission from the left atrium through the pulmonary veins to the capillary wedge position. For this reason the wedge pressure is delayed in time compared to the left ventricular pressure. Proper realignment of these pressures using the A- or V-wave is necessary for accurate gradient

calculation. It is important to note that the cardiac output measured by thermodilution or Fick techniques measures only forward flow. If significant mitral regurgitation is present, which is frequently the case in rheumatic mitral valve disease, the actual diastolic flow across the valve is composed of both regurgitant and forward cardiac output. Substituting forward cardiac output, which is lower than true diastolic flow, therefore causes an underestimation of true mitral valve area. If significant mitral regurgitation is present, the calculated mitral valve area using only a measurement of forward cardiac output is thus said to be a "minimal valve area" estimate. Occasionally the resting mitral gradient is less than 4–6 mm Hg. If valve area is calculated with a small gradient, substantial error can result. Under these circumstances the patient should be exercised in the catheterization laboratory during the recording of cardiac output and pressure data. With the subsequent rise in cardiac output the gradient increases and allows a more accurate assessment of valve area.

Evaluation of right ventricular function and pulmonary vascular resistance aids in assessing the severity of mitral stenosis. With progressive narrowing of the valve there are

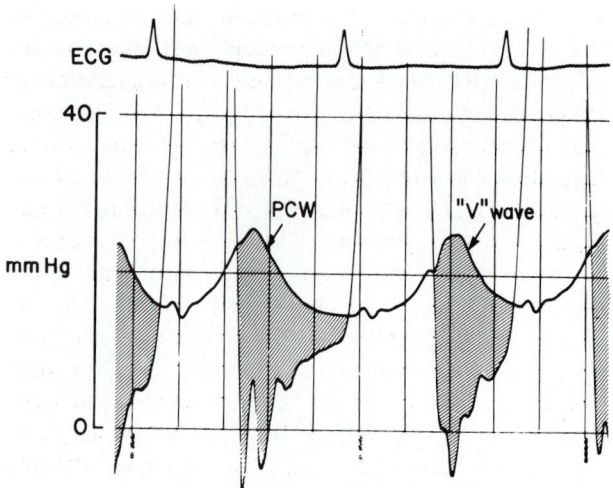

Figure 103–16. Simultaneous left ventricular (LV) and pulmonary capillary wedge (PCW) tracings from a patient with moderate mitral stenosis and 2 plus mitral regurgitation secondary to rheumatic heart disease. The patient is in atrial fibrillation. Note the large diastolic gradient between wedge and left ventricle (shaded area), the prominent V-waves in the wedge tracing (due to moderate mitral insufficiency), and the elevated mean-wedge pressure.

reactive increases in pulmonary vascular resistance due to chronically elevated left heart filling pressures. In late stages pulmonary artery pressure and vascular resistance can be greatly elevated and sometimes approach values seen in the systemic circulation. In this setting the right ventricle becomes overloaded and right atrial pressure becomes elevated. With progressive dilatation of the right ventricle and tricuspid annulus, functional tricuspid regurgitation can result causing large V-waves in the right atrial pressure tracing. Fortunately these changes respond well to relief of mitral stenosis and with valve replacement pulmonary pressure, pulmonary resistance, right heart failure, and tricuspid regurgitation usually show substantial improvement.[15–18] Tricuspid stenosis, a distinctly rare entity, can sometimes be associated with rheumatic mitral stenosis and careful evaluation of pressures while pulling the catheter back from the right ventricle to the right atrium should be performed to search for a tricuspid valve gradient.

Other conditions associated with mitral stenosis should be evaluated by cardiac catheterization. Mitral regurgitation is frequently associated with mitral stenosis and evaluation with left ventriculography to assess for mitral incompetence is indicated. If there is a history of chest pain or if the patient is older than 30 years, significant coronary artery disease should be ruled out by coronary angiography.

Factors that may influence operative approach are frequently evident from catheterization data. The presence of significant leaflet calcification seen on fluoroscopy or ventriculography generally precludes both open and closed mitral commissurotomy. Significant atrial thrombus or mitral regurgitation contraindicates closed mitral commissurotomy.

Aortic Stenosis

Obstruction to left ventricular outflow can be subdivided into three categories. Obstruction is most commonly localized at the aortic valve level. However, obstruction may also occur at the supravalvular level as a discrete aortic narrowing or may be subvalvular secondary to a stenotic membrane or hypertrophic obstructive cardiomyopathy. Isolated valvular aortic stenosis without accompanying mitral valve disease is more common in men and rarely occurs on a rheumatic basis. It is usually either congenital or degenerative in origin. The most common congenital malformation underlying aortic stenosis is a bicuspid aortic valve. Congenitally bicuspid valves may be stenotic from commissural fusion at birth. More commonly, bicuspid valves undergo progressive narrowing due to the abnormal turbulent flow that results in leaflet traumatization, fibrosis, increased rigidity, and calcification. Acquired aortic stenosis is most commonly due to rheumatic heart disease. Valvular lesions resulting from this systemic disease include adhesion and fusion of the commissures and cusps, along with vascularization of the leaflets and valve ring. This leads to retraction and stiffening of the free borders of the cusps and the formation of calcific nodules on both surfaces of the valve. Due to the cusps' immobility and valve fixation in the open position, rheumatic aortic stenosis is also frequently accompanied by aortic regurgitation. Other causes of acquired aortic stenosis include degenerative or senile calcific aortic stenosis and atherosclerotic aortic valvular stenosis. Atherosclerotic aortic stenosis is most frequently observed in patients with severe hypercholesterolemia and is frequently seen in children which homozygous type II hyperlipoproteinemia. Other rare causes of acquired aortic stenosis include rheumatoid arthritis and ochronosis.[19,20]

Pathophysiology of Aortic Stenosis
When outflow tract obstruction occurs the ventricle must generate much higher systolic pressures to maintain stroke volume and cardiac output. As the aortic valve area is reduced, a systolic pressure gradient develops between the left ventricle and the central aorta. The left ventricle generally responds to abrupt production of left ventricular outflow obstruction and pressure overload by dilatation and reduction in stroke volume. With long-standing obstruction compensatory mechanisms are called into play to maintain cardiac output. Stroke volume is generally maintained by an increase in left ventricular mass. There is a large increase in myocardial wall thickness and relatively less increase in chamber volume. This pattern of increasing muscle mass is termed *concentric left ventricular hypertrophy* and is characteristic of ventricular pressure overload states such as outflow tract obstruction and systemic hypertension. The increase in ventricular wall thickness in combination with minimal chamber dilatation allows the ventricle to sustain large increases in chamber pressure while maintaining relatively normal left ventricular wall stress. Because of com-

pensatory concentric hypertrophy, cardiac output, left ventricular end-diastolic volume, and left ventricular wall stress remain normal early in the course of aortic stenosis. As the valvular stenosis worsens there is a progressive increase in end-diastolic volume and left ventricular wall stress. Late in the course of aortic stenosis the ventricle decompensates and as wall stress further increases ejection fraction falls. If outflow obstruction is corrected, ejection fraction improves as the after load on the left ventricle is reduced; however, pressure overload can also cause some degree of muscle damage, which further depresses ventricular performance. Eventually both lowered contractility and increased afterload are operative when ejection fraction is depressed due to long-standing aortic stenosis.[19–21]

Cardiac Catheterization in Aortic Stenosis

The purpose of cardiac catheterization in aortic stenosis is to assess the area of the aortic valve. This is performed in a manner similar to that utilized in mitral stenosis (see discussion of calculating mitral valve area in Pathophysiology of Mitral Stenosis). Left ventricular and aortic pressure are recorded simultaneously and the mean transvalvular aortic valve pressure gradient is determined (Fig. 103–17). Access to left ventricular pressure can be achieved using several different catheter techniques. Although sometimes technically difficult and time consuming the reduced aortic orifice can be crossed in a retrograde fashion from the central aorta. The ventricle can also be entered by puncturing the interatrial septum using the transseptal technique and advancing a catheter into the left ventricle via the left atrium. Although there is risk of coronary laceration, bleeding, and tamponade, direct transthoracic left ventricular apical puncture can be used to obtain pressure recordings if entry into the ventricle is impossible using other techniques. Patients with prosthetic valves in the aortic position are best approached using the transseptal technique to prevent catheter-induced aortic insufficiency or catheter entrapment in the mechanical valve apparatus.

Aortic valve area is calculated using the Gorlin for-

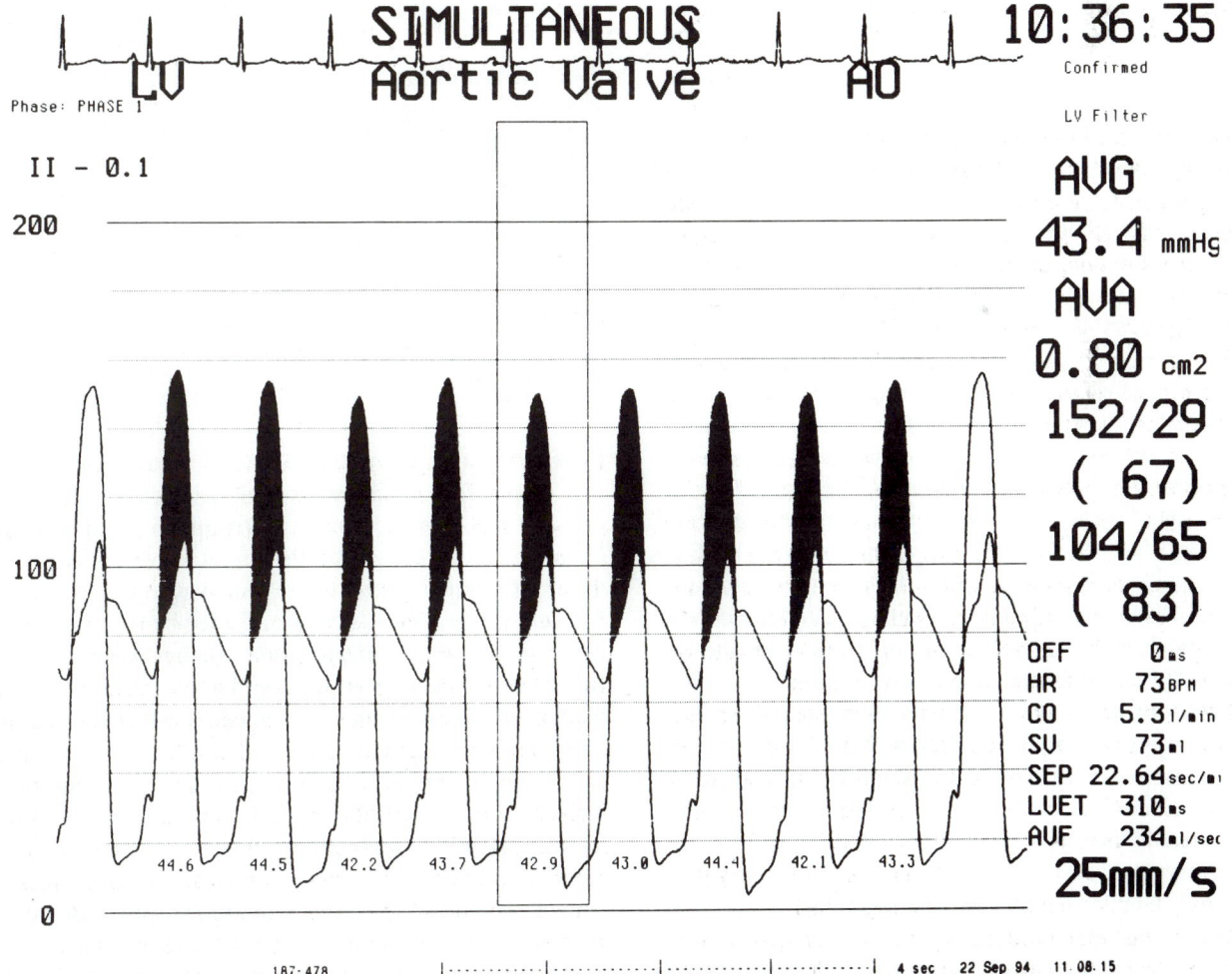

Figure 103–17. Simultaneous femoral artery and left ventricular pressures from a patient with severe aortic stenosis on a zero to 200 mm Hg scale. Note the large gradient between the left ventricle and femoral artery (shaded area). The peak-to-peak gradient is near 50 mm Hg. The average gradient is 43 mm Hg with a calculated aortic valve area of 0.80 cm². The left ventricular end-diastolic pressure (LVEDP) is markedly elevated at 30 mm Hg.

mula in a manner similar to that used in mitral stenosis.[22,23] Cardiac output, heart rate, systolic ejection period (SEP), and transvalvular aortic pressure gradient are all measured simultaneously. The systolic ejection period is the time interval in the cardiac cycle during which the aortic valve remains open and allows forward bloodflow. SEP is measured from the pressure recordings and is defined as the time interval during which left ventricular pressure is greater than aortic pressure. This parameter can be affected by a variety of factors including heart rate, afterload, and contractility. Aortic valve flow is then calculated by dividing cardiac output by the SEP. Aortic flow and mean pressure gradient are then entered into the Gorlin formula and the valve area determined. A peak systolic pressure gradient exceeding 50 mm Hg in the presence of a normal cardiac output or an effective aortic orifice less than 0.6 cm^2 (or an indexed measure less than 0.4 cm^2/m^2 of body surface area) is generally considered to represent critical left ventricular outflow obstruction.

Methodological errors can occur leading to miscalculation of valve area. As with mitral stenosis, it is important that cardiac output and pressure measurements are recorded simultaneously and that pressure transducers are properly balanced and standardized. Substituting peripheral arterial pressure for central aortic pressure can sometimes lead to error. Because of pressure waves reflected from the periphery, femoral or brachial artery systolic pressure can be significantly higher than central aortic pressure. This leads to underestimation of the aortic valve gradient and overestimation of the valve area.[24] To avoid this problem central aortic and peripheral pressures should be recorded simultaneously. If there is a significant discrepancy in systolic pressure then peripheral arterial pressure should probably not be used to calculate transvalvular gradient. In this case gradients should be calculated from either a "pull-back" pressure recording from the left ventricle to the central aorta, or from pressures recorded simultaneously from the ventricle and central aorta. With end-stage aortic stenosis ventricular function can be severely depressed and cardiac output can be critically reduced. Transvalvular pressure gradients recorded under these conditions can be less than 20–30 mm Hg even with critical aortic stenosis. During these low flow states small errors in gradient or cardiac output determination can lead to large errors in valve area calculation. It has been suggested that exercise or infusion of inotropic agents can increase valve flow and allow more reliable calculations, however, these maneuvers carry some risk in the patient with critical aortic stenosis and a severely reduced cardiac output.[25] If aortic regurgitation is present, the systolic flow across the valve is composed of both regurgitant and forward cardiac output. This increased flow tends to increase the measured gradient across the valve. Substituting forward cardiac output, which in the presence of aortic insufficiency is lower than true systolic flow, causes an underestimation of true valve area.

Evaluation of the coronary arteries is important in elderly patients with aortic stenosis because significant atherosclerotic obstruction is frequently found. Coronary arteriography is especially important when the patient is symptomatic with angina pectoris. Significant coronary obstruction may require concomitant bypass grafting when aortic valve replacement is performed. Evaluation of left ventricular function with ventriculography is generally of secondary importance in patients with aortic stenosis. Results of this test usually have little bearing on surgery for aortic stenosis, as with relief of outflow obstruction ventricular dysfunction usually improves. Similarly mild to moderate mitral regurgitation also improves after aortic valve replacement and if identified by ventriculography generally does not significantly influence surgical approach. Ventriculography is often omitted from the catheterization procedure because of the tenuous hemodynamic status of patients with aortic stenosis, the risk of hypotension secondary to contrast injection, and the reduced importance of diagnostic information obtained from the study.

Mitral Regurgitation

Pathophysiology of Mitral Regurgitation

Assessment of mitral regurgitation by catheterization techniques requires an understanding of the basic pathophysiologic and etiologic factors that are involved in producing the lesion. The mitral valve apparatus is composed of four major structures: the mitral annulus, mitral leaflets, chordae tendinae, and papillary muscles. Derangement of any one of these elements can cause the mitral valve to become incompetent. Mitral regurgitation can be classified according to different pathophysiologic processes which affect proper function of one or more of the structures comprising the valve. Ventricular and annular dilatation from any primary cardiomyopathy can cause secondary mitral regurgitation due to inability of the normal-sized leaflets to properly close in the enlarged annulus. Disruption of the chordae tendinae can be caused by the mitral valve prolapse syndrome, rheumatic fever, trauma, or bacterial endocarditis. The mitral valve leaflets can be affected by rheumatic fever and endocarditis. Papillary muscle dysfunction is primarily caused by ischemic heart disease, but can also result from infiltrative disorders of the heart such as sarcoidosis and amyloidosis.

Once the valve has become incompetent a portion of the ventricular stroke volume is ejected into the left atrium during systole. The regurgitant volume is again presented to the left ventricle during subsequent diastolic filling. This increase in volume of blood entering the left ventricle during each diastolic filling period causes a ventricle volume overload state. If the process causing valvular incompetence develops slowly over the course of months to years such as in rheumatic fever or mitral valve prolapse then significant compensatory mechanisms are called into play. To accommodate the increased volume, ventricular chamber size increases. Muscle sarcomeres will lengthen in series causing greatly increased end-diastolic volume, increased ventricular wall mass, and modestly increased wall thickness. This constellation of findings is termed *eccentric ventricular hypertrophy*. It is characteristic of volume overload states such as aortic and mitral regurgitation and is in contrast to the concentric hypertrophy seen in pressure overload states like aortic stenosis and systemic hypertension. Because of the increased sarcomere length, muscle fiber shortening is increased by the Frank–Starling mechanism. Initially, increased filling pressures are required to maintain the enlarged end-diastolic volume, however, with continued chronic volume overload left ventricular compliance increases significantly, resulting in lower ventricular filling pressure for a given diastolic volume.

Because a significant proportion of stroke volume is ejected into the low-pressure left atrium during systole, impedance to ventricular ejection or afterload is greatly reduced. Sarcomere shortening can occur against a low afterload early in systole even prior to opening of the aortic valve. This allows the ventricle to more efficiently expend energy in fiber shortening rather than in developing fiber tension and cavitary pressure. In addition, left ventricular wall tension decreases progressively as shortening occurs. Because of this low impedance to early systolic ejection, measures of ventricular function that are afterload dependent, such as ejection fraction, are usually well preserved. Ejection fraction is usually normal until very late in the course of chronic mitral regurgitation and when ejection fraction is moderately reduced severe depression of ventricular function is present.

Because of these adaptive processes that accompany chronic mitral regurgitation, patients can remain minimally symptomatic for many years. Eventually, however, the chronic volume overload damages the myocardium and the ability to maintain cardiac output is impaired. This damage causes further ventricular dilatation, worsening regurgitation, further increase in ventricular filling pressure, low cardiac output, pulmonary congestion, and eventually death. Unfortunately when the patient presents after the ventricle has been damaged by years of chronic volume overload the prognosis even with surgical valve replacement is poor. In fact, valve replacement at this stage removes the low impedance to ventricular ejection and can actually cause further functional and clinical deterioration.[26–28]

Cardiac Catheterization in Mitral Regurgitation

This procedure is performed to address several of the issues that impact on patient management. Foremost among these is confirmation of the diagnosis and assessment of hemodynamic severity. The presence and degree of regurgitation can be quantified by visual inspection of the contrast ventriculogram. This technique is performed by injecting radiopaque contrast medium into the ventricular cavity in the right anterior oblique projection. If mitral incompetence is present dye will reflux into the left atrium during systole.

The severity of regurgitation is graded from 1 to 4 plus. One plus is present when a small amount of dye enters the left atrium, does not fill the entire atrial cavity, and clears completely during subsequent beats. Two plus is defined by complete filling of the entire atrium, however the degree of opacification is less than that of the ventricle. Three plus fills the entire atrium and the opacification is equal to that of the ventricle. In 4 plus the entire atrium and pulmonary veins fill rapidly and are progressively opacified to a greater degree than the ventricle. Grades of 3 plus and 4 plus correlate with significant regurgitation.

Some pitfalls in the angiographic assessment of regurgitation are worth noting. Occasionally the angiographic catheter can become entrapped in the mitral apparatus, interfere with valve closure, and cause significant dye reflux. Premature ventricular contractions and ventricular tachycardia during contrast injection can also cause significant regurgitation. The size of the left atrium can also interfere with subjective assessment of reflux. A severely enlarged left atrium, which is sometimes present in chronic mitral regurgitation will not opacify to the same degree as a small atrium. This may cause some underestimation of the severity of mitral regurgitation in patients with large left atrial cavity size. Similarly if very small amounts of contrast are injected during ventriculography poor opacification of the left ventricle results. In this setting inaccurate assessment of mitral regurgitation is likely.

Quantification of regurgitation is made more objective by determination of regurgitant stroke volume and regurgitant fraction. Left ventricular volumes at end-diastole and end-systole can be calculated from the angiogram and stroke volume can then be determined. This volume represents the sum of forward cardiac output ejected into the aorta and regurgitant volume refluxing into the atrium. A total forward cardiac output can also be obtained by thermodilution or Fick techniques. Dividing forward output by heart rate yields forward stroke volume. *Regurgitant stroke volume* is the difference between total and forward stroke volume. *Regurgitant fraction* is the ratio of regurgitant stroke volume to total stroke volume and thus represents the percent of stroke volume ejected into the left atrium. A regurgitant fraction of greater than 60% characterizes severe mitral regurgitation. Generally regurgitant fraction correlates well with visual interpretation of regurgitation, however, its calculation depends on very accurate and relatively simultaneous assessment of stroke volume by two techniques. Compounding errors can result if all procedures are not performed meticulously.[29]

Hemodynamic Assessment of Mitral Regurgitation

Assessment of left ventricular filling pressures aids in determining the severity of mitral regurgitation. Severe, decompensated mitral regurgitation is characterized by elevated ventricular end-diastolic and mean pulmonary capillary wedge pressures. In addition, because of the large volume of blood ejected into the atrium during systole, the wedge pressure develops large V-waves, sometimes exceeding the mean wedge pressure by 3- to 3-fold. The large increase in diastolic flow across a normal-sized mitral valve sometimes produces a small diastolic gradient between the wedge and left ventricular pressures (Fig. 103–18). While this constellation characterizes severe regurgitation, it is of note that many patients with significant angiographic regurgitation can be compensated with normal mean wedge pressure and absent V-waves. In addition, very large V-waves can be seen in the absence of mitral regurgitation in patients with decompensated ischemic heart disease or other states characterized by poor left ventricular compliance[30,31] (Fig. 103–19).

Catheterization Data to Assess Prognosis in Mitral Regurgitation

Data from the catheterization are important in assessing prognosis post valve replacement. The most important factors for determining response to surgery relate directly to ventricular performance. As stated previously, when ejection fraction is even moderately depressed significant impairment of ventricular function is present. An ejection fraction of less than 40% predicts a generally poor clinical response to mitral valve replacement.[26–28] Ventricular volumes are also predictive of surgical outcome. A very dilated chamber indicates long-standing regurgitation with probable consequent damage from volume overload. End-systolic volume index has been shown to be an especially helpful indicator of clinical course post valve replacement. Patients with an end-systolic volume index of greater than 90 mL/m^2 are at high risk for postoperative mortality and persistent symptoms, while patients with an end-systolic volume index of less than 30 mL/m^2 fare much better.[32] Associated disease also impacts on prognosis. Patients with significant coronary stenoses are at higher operative risk than patients with normal coronary arteries. Patients with acute papillary muscle rupture or left ventricular aneurysm are at especially high risk.[33,34] Catheterization can be helpful in identifying patients with mitral regurgitation sec-

ondary to an underlying dilated cardiomyopathy. Secondary regurgitation is characterized by a depressed ejection fraction, dilated ventricular volumes, and less severe degrees of angiographic regurgitation. These patients respond poorly to mitral valve replacement.

Finally catheterization can provide information that is helpful in planning surgery. Mitral regurgitation caused by rheumatic fever, mitral valve prolapse, or ruptured chordae can frequently be repaired by valvuloplasty and annular placement of a Carpentier ring. Mitral regurgitation associated with significant annular calcification or transmural infarction, however, precludes valvuloplasty and would require insertion of a prosthetic valve.[35–37] Paravalvular abscess cavities or valvular vegetations associated with mitral regurgitation from bacterial endocarditis can sometimes be visualized during ventriculography. This would necessitate preparation for possible extensive surgical debridement. Significant coronary disease would require plans for concomitant bypass grafting while identification of a ventricular aneurysm may invoke contemplation of possible aneurysmectomy.

Aortic Regurgitation

Pathophysiology of Aortic Regurgitation

Aortic regurgitation, like mitral insufficiency, can be classified according to different pathophysiologic processes that affect proper function of the different structures comprising the aortic valve and its support apparatus. Dilatation of the aortic root from primary aortic disease can cause secondary aortic regurgitation due to inability of the leaflets to properly close in the dilated aortic root. Significant aortic root enlargement can occur in hypertensive heart disease, proximal aortic dissection, atherosclerotic aneurysm of the ascending aorta, syphilis, and connective tissue disorders such as Marfan's disease and rheumatoid arthritis. Incompetency of the aortic valve leaflets can be caused by bacterial endocarditis, rheumatic fever, trauma, and degenerative changes secondary to a congenital bicuspid valve.[19]

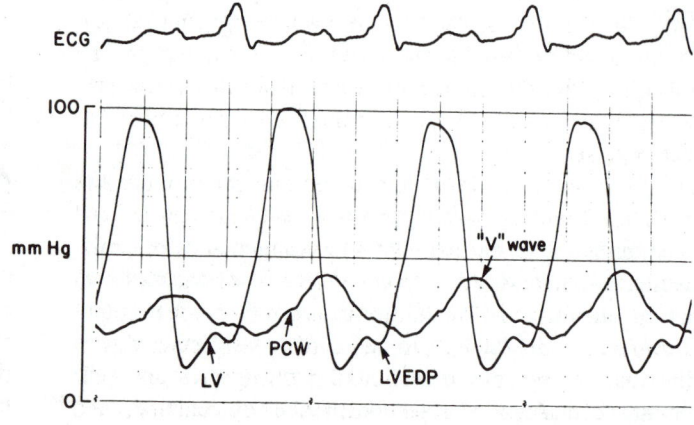

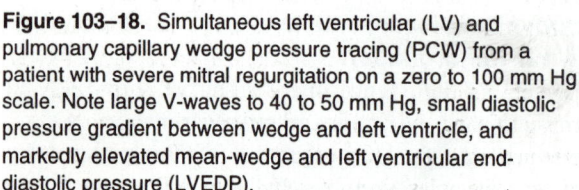

Figure 103–18. Simultaneous left ventricular (LV) and pulmonary capillary wedge pressure tracing (PCW) from a patient with severe mitral regurgitation on a zero to 100 mm Hg scale. Note large V-waves to 40 to 50 mm Hg, small diastolic pressure gradient between wedge and left ventricle, and markedly elevated mean-wedge and left ventricular end-diastolic pressure (LVEDP).

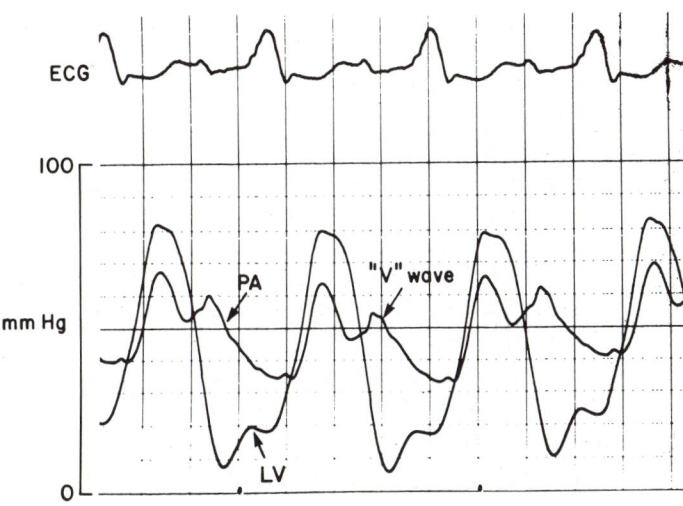

Figure 103–19. Simultaneous pulmonary artery (PA) and left ventricular (LV) pressures from the same patient as in Figure 103–18. Note large V-waves reflected into the pulmonary artery tracing.

Once the aortic valve becomes incompetent a portion of the ventricular stroke volume flows into the left ventricle during diastole. This increase in volume of blood entering the left ventricle during diastole causes a ventricular volume overload state very similar to that observed in mitral regurgitation. If the process causing valvular incompetence develops slowly over the course of months to years significant compensatory mechanisms similar to those seen in mitral regurgitation begin to develop. Eccentric hypertrophy occurs (see Mitral Regurgitation, above) with an increased end-diastolic volume, increased ventricular wall mass, and modestly increased wall thickness. Because of the increased sarcomere length, muscle fiber shortening is increased by the Frank–Starling mechanism. The regurgitant volume from the aorta initially causes an increase in left ventricular diastolic filling pressure, however, like mitral regurgitation, with continued chronic volume overload, left ventricular compliance increases significantly. This results in lower ventricular filling pressures for a given end-diastolic volume.

In severe aortic insufficiency, aortic pressure decreases rapidly during diastole because of rapid runoff into the left ventricle and periphery. Diastolic central aortic pressure is lowered and this in combination with the increased stroke volume causes a significant increase in pulse pressure. These changes cause the typical physical findings associated with aortic insufficiency such as a bounding arterial pulse, low diastolic blood pressure, a hyperdynamic precordium, and a leftward displacement of the point of maximal impulse.

Because of the adaptive changes that occur in chronic aortic insufficiency, the volume overload state can be well tolerated and patients can remain asymptomatic for years. Eventually, however, the chronic volume overload damages the myocardium and the ability to maintain cardiac output is impaired. This damage causes further ventricular dilatation, further increase in ventricular filling pressure, pulmonary congestion, further ventricular dysfunction, and

symptoms of low cardiac output. Like mitral regurgitation, if the patient presents after the ventricle has been damaged by chronic volume overload, the prognosis is worse with valve replacement. However, with improved techniques of myocardial protection during cardiopulmonary bypass, recent series have shown a 3-year survival of 85–90% even when valve replacement is performed in the presence of left ventricular dysfunction and significant chamber dilatation.[38]

Cardiac Catheterization in Aortic Regurgitation

Cardiac catheterization in aortic regurgitation is performed to document the presence and hemodynamic severity of the valvular insufficiency. The presence and degree of regurgitation can be quantified by subjective assessment of a contrast aortogram. This is performed by injecting contrast medium into the central aorta just above the plane of the aortic valve in the left anterior oblique projection. If aortic insufficiency is present, dye will reflux into the left ventricle during diastole. The severity of regurgitation is subjectively graded from 1 to 4 plus in a manner similar to that used in grading mitral insufficiency. One plus is present when a small amount of dye enters the ventricle, does not fill the entire cavity, and clears completely with each subsequent beat. Two plus is defined by complete filling of the entire ventricle, however, the degree of opacification is less than that of the aorta. In a rating of 3 plus, dye fills the entire ventricle and the opacification is equal to that of the aorta. In a rating of 4 plus aortic regurgitation, the entire ventricle fills rapidly and is progressively opacified to a greater extent than the aorta. Grades of 3 plus and 4 plus indicate the presence of severe aortic regurgitation.

Errors in the angiographic assessment of aortic insufficiency can occur. Occasionally the angiographic catheter can prevent proper closure of the aortic valve and falsely cause significant dye reflux. Similarly the angiographic catheter can enter the left ventricle during injection and interfere with the assessment of valvular insufficiency. If very small amounts of contrast are injected during aortography, poor opacification of the left ventricle results and this can result in inaccurate assessment of aortic regurgitation.[23]

Determination of regurgitant fraction (see above discussion) can be performed to assess aortic insufficiency in a manner similar to the calculations used in mitral regurgitation. Total ventricular stroke volume is calculated from the angiogram and compared to forward stroke volume determined from measurements of cardiac output. As in mitral insufficiency, regurgitant fraction correlates well with visual interpretation of angiographic regurgitation severity.[29]

Hemodynamic Assessment of Aortic Regurgitation

Measurement of left ventricular, pulmonary capillary wedge, and central aortic pressures aid in determining the severity of aortic regurgitation. In severe aortic insufficiency the diastolic regurgitant volume significantly elevates left ventricular end-diastolic and mean-wedge pressure. Because of the diastolic leak between the central aorta and left ventricle, diastolic aortic pressure falls off rapidly and tends to equilibrate with left ventricular end diastolic pressure. The aortic pressure trace shows a wide pulse pressure (at times greater than 100 mm Hg) with rapid systolic upstroke. In severe acute aortic insufficiency left ventricular pressure increases to high levels very early in diastole. Left ventricular diastolic pressure can elevate to levels above left atrial and pulmonary wedge pressures prior to the onset of mechanical systole. This can cause premature closure of the mitral valve. As in mitral regurgitation, the large increase in flow across a normal-sized aortic valve sometimes produces a small systolic gradient between the left ventricle and the aorta in the absence of significant aortic stenosis.[19,23]

Catheterization Data to Assess Prognosis in Aortic Regurgitation

Data from the catheterization are important in assessing prognosis after aortic valve replacement. As with mitral regurgitation, the most important factors for determining response to surgery relate directly to ventricular performance. Ventricular volumes are predictive of the development of postoperative congestive heart failure and death. A very dilated chamber indicates long-standing volume overload with probable ventricular muscle damage. End-systolic volume index can be used as an indicator of the clinical course post valve replacement. Patients with an end-systolic volume index of greater than 90 mL/m^2 are at high risk for postoperative mortality and persistent symptoms, while patients with an end-systolic volume index of less than 30 mL/m^2 fare much better.[32]

Catheterization can be helpful in providing information regarding the etiology of aortic regurgitation. Acute aortic dissection, aortic aneurysm, a bicuspid aortic valve, and paravalvular abscesses can be identified with aortogra-

phy. These coexistent processes are important to define prior to surgical repair.

CATHETERIZATION IN THE ASSESSMENT OF PERICARDIAL AND MYOCARDIAL DISEASE

Constrictive Pericarditis and Restrictive Cardiomyopathy

Constrictive pericarditis and restrictive cardiomyopathy are both disorders that affect diastolic filling of the heart. Because of this, the distinction of these two processes by clinical and hemodynamic criteria is frequently difficult. Unfortunately it is often critical to establish the diagnosis because constrictive pericarditis is surgically treatable with pericardial stripping, whereas restrictive cardiomyopathy is generally not a surgical condition. Constrictive pericarditis can be a sequela to pericardial inflammation. Any process that causes pericarditis can eventually result in constriction including tuberculosis, bacterial or viral pericarditis, idiopathic pericarditis, pericardial involvement from malignancy, chronic renal failure, connective tissue disease, or postradiation injury. Restrictive cardiomyopathy is a consequence of endomyocardial or intramyocardial infiltrative processes. Restriction results from hemochromatosis, amyloidosis, sarcoidosis, or endomyocardial fibrosis.

In both restriction and constriction the primary pathophysiologic process is interference with diastolic filling of the left and right ventricle. In constrictive pericarditis, impedance to filling is caused by the noncompliant, fibrous shell of pericardium surrounding the heart. In restriction the impedance to relaxation is a consequence of intramyocardial infiltration. This impairment of diastolic filling causes increased ventricular filling pressures for a given diastolic volume. End-diastolic volume is normal or small and cannot increase due to the constrictive or restrictive process. Myocardial reserve allows cardiac output to initially be maintained because of increased ventricular filling pressure, improved myocardial contractility, and increased heart rate. As the process worsens cardiac output and stroke volume fall and signs and symptoms of right and left sided congestive heart failure develop. Indices of systolic shortening such as ejection fraction are normal or even increased, however in some restrictive processes like amyloidosis and hemochromatosis muscular damage eventually occurs and late depression of ventricular function results.[39–41]

In constrictive pericarditis, because the entire heart is encased in a rigid shell in diastole, all chamber pressures are equal. This condition is seen in the catheterization laboratory as equal right and left ventricular diastolic pressures during simultaneous recording (Fig. 103–20). This equality of ventricular diastolic chamber pressures is a less consistent but frequently present finding in restrictive cardiomyopathy. In restriction, left ventricular diastolic pressure is sometimes higher than right ventricular pressure and can

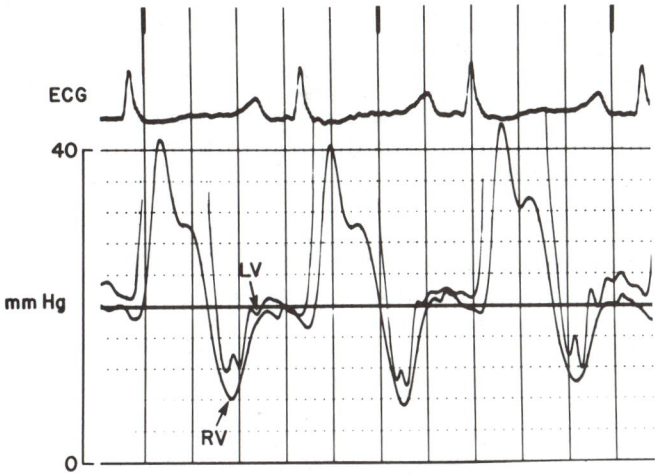

Figure 103–20. Pressure tracings recorded during catheterization of a patient with calcific pericardial constriction documented at pericardiectomy. Simultaneous recordings of left (LV) and right (RV) ventricular pressures are displayed on a zero to 40 mm Hg scale. Note equalization of diastolic pressures, diastolic dip and plateau (square root sign), and elevated right and left ventricular end-diastolic pressure of 20 mm Hg. Pressure remained equalized despite a 1000 mL fluid challenge, treatment with atropine, isometric exercise, and injection of contrast during ventriculography.

generally be dissociated by exercise or isoproterenol infusion. In both processes early diastolic filling is rapid and is abruptly halted shortly after the onset of diastole. The pressure correlate of this phenomenon is an early diastolic dip followed by an abrupt plateau in the right and left ventricular pressure tracings. This is descriptively termed the "square root sign." The right atrial pressure trace is characterized by an elevated mean pressure and a deep rapid Y descent. This rapid descent corresponds to the early diastolic dip in the right ventricular pressure curve (Fig. 103–21). Normally right atrial pressure falls with inspiration as intrathoracic pressure decreases. However, in constrictive pericarditis this negative pressure during inspiration is not transmitted to the right atrium and right ventricle because of the hard noncompliant pericardial shell. The right ventricle cannot dilate to accept the increased venous return during inspiration and consequently right atrial pressure rises. This paradoxical rise in central venous and right atrial pressure

during inspiration is termed *Kussmaul's sign*. It can be demonstrated during catheterization by recording right atrial pressure through several respiratory cycles.

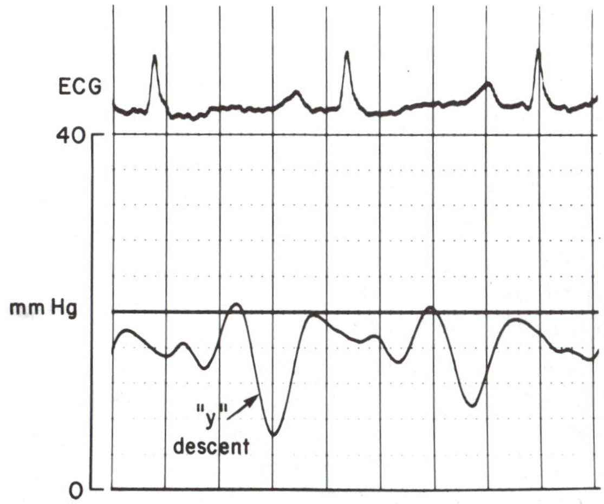

Right heart pressures can be used to help distinguish constrictive pericarditis from restrictive cardiomyopathy. Significant pulmonary hypertension is more common in restrictive cardiomyopathy. Similarly a diastolic plateau pressure less than one-third right ventricular systolic pressure suggests restriction while a plateau pressure greater than one-third right ventricular systolic pressure favors constriction.[42]

Frequently the distinction between constriction and restriction cannot be made from clinical or hemodynamic data. In this setting transvenous right ventricular biopsy can be used to search for histologic evidence of an infiltrative process that could cause restriction. In patients with constrictive/restrictive physiology by catheterization and right ventricular biopsy specimens that fail to show evidence of infiltration, a high incidence of occult constrictive pericarditis is demonstrated at subsequent exploratory thoracotomy.[43]

Endomyocardial Biopsy

With the increase in cardiac transplant operations myocardial biopsy techniques have also become more frequent. Pathologic review of samples of the right ventricular myocardium have become critical in assessing for the presence of cardiac transplant rejection. Microscopic analysis of myocardial tissue is also helpful in the diagnosis of inflammatory myocarditis,[44] hypertrophic and dilated cardiomyopathies, and infiltrative disorders such as sarcoidosis,[45] amyloidosis,[46] and hemochromatosis.[47] Myocardial biopsy is also useful in the evaluation of adriamycin cardiotoxicity[48] and in distinguishing restrictive myocardial infiltration from constrictive pericarditis (see above discussion in Catheterization in the Assessment of Pericardial and Myocardial Disease).[43]

The procedure is most commonly performed using the

Figure 103–21. Right atrial pressure recording from the same patient in Figure 103–20 on a scale of zero to 40 mm Hg. Note prominent Y descent and elevated mean right atrial pressure of 16 mm Hg.

Stanford Bioptome. This device consists of a flexible stainless-steel coil shaft fitted with two hemispherical cutting jaws that can be opened and closed via an attached handle similar to those used in transbronchial biopsy. The device is inserted through a 9 Fr sheath introduced percutaneously into the right internal jugular vein. The tip of the bioptome is advanced under fluoroscopic guidance into the right atrium, across the tricuspid valve, and into the right ventricle. The jaws are kept closed and positioned against the ventricular septum. The bioptome is then withdrawn to a point just off of the septal surface and the jaws are opened. The device is then advanced onto the septum, the jaws closed, and the bioptome is withdrawn. This procedure usually results in 1- to 2-mm diameter specimens of endocardium which are then fixed in formalin and processed for light microscopy. Several different types of bioptomes and positioning sheaths are now available that allow sampling from a femoral vein percutaneous approach and, if needed, biopsy of the left ventricle.[49]

When performed properly, right ventricular endomyocardial biopsy specimens can be obtained with a very low morbidity and mortality. Serial specimens can be obtained many times with no adverse effects. The overall mortality of the procedure is 0.05%. The major cause of morbidity and mortality is the risk of cardiac perforation, which occurs in 0.5% of cases.[50] Equipment and facilities necessary for pericardiocentesis must be readily available when endomyocardial biopsy is performed in the event that cardiac perforation and subsequent tamponade result as a complication of the procedure.

REFERENCES

1. Goldschlager N, Selzer A, Cohn K: Treadmill stress tests as indicators of presence and severity of coronary artery disease. *Ann Intern Med* **85:**277, 1976
2. Weiner DA, McCabe CH, Ryan TJ: Identification of patients with left main and three vessel coronary disease with clinical and exercise test variables. *Am J Cardiol* **46:**21, 1980
3. Kushner FG, Okada RD, Kirshenbaum HD, et al: Lung thallium-201 uptake after stress testing in patients with coronary artery disease. *Circulation* **63:**341, 1981
4. Boucher CA, Zir LM, Beller GA, et al: Increased lung uptake of thallium-201 during exercise myocardial imaging: Clinical, hemodynamic and angiographic implications in patients with coronary artery disease. *Am J Cardiol* **46:**189, 1980
5. Detre K, Peduzzi P, Murphy M, et al: Effect of bypass surgery on survival in patients with low and high-risk groups delineated by the use of simple clinical variables. *Circulation* **63**(1329), 1981
6. Clark LT, Garfein OB, Dwyer EM Jr: Acute pulmonary edema due to ischemic heart disease without accompanying myocardial infarction. *Am J Med* **75:**331, 1983
7. Dwyer ED, et al: Association between transient pulmonary congestion during acute myocardial infarction and high incidence of death in six months. *Am J Cardiol* **58:**900, 1986
8. Sones FM, Shirey EK, Prondfit WL, et al: Cine-coronary arteriography. *Circulation* **20:**773, 1959
9. Kennedy JW, Kaiser GC, Fisher LD, et al: Multivariate discriminant analysis of clinical and angiographic predictors of operative mortality from the Collaborative Study in Coronary Artery Surgery (CASS). *J Thorac Cardiovasc Surg* **80:**876, 1980
10. Gould KL, Lipscomb K, Hamilton GW: Physiologic basis for assessing critical coronary stenosis. *Am J Cardiol* **33:**87, 1974
11. Roberts WC: The coronary arteries and left ventricle in clinically isolated angina pectoris: A necropsy analysis. *Circulation* **54:**388, 1976
12. Zir LM, et al: Interobserver variability in coronary angiography. *Circulation* **54:**627, 1976
13. Cohen MV, Gorlin SG: Modified orifice equation for the calculation of mitral valve area. *Am Heart J* **84:**839, 1972
14. Gorlin R, Gorlin SG: Hydraulic formula for calculations of the area of the stenotic mitral valve, other cardiac valves, and central circulatory shunts. *Am Heart J* **41:**1, 1951
15. Walston A, Peter RH, Morris J, et al: Clinical implications of pulmonary hypertension in mitral stenosis. *Am J Cardiol* **32:**650, 1973
16. Jordan SC: Development of pulmonary hypertension in mitral stenosis. *Lancet* **2:**322, 1965
17. Braunwald E, Braunwald NS, Ross J, et al: Effects of mitral valve replacement on the pulmonary vascular dynamics of patients with pulmonary hypertension. *N Engl J Med* **273:**509, 1965
18. Zemer JC, Hancock EW: Regression of extreme pulmonary hypertension after mitral valve surgery. *Am J Cardiol* **30:**820, 1972
19. Braunwald E: Valvular heart disease. In Braunwald E (ed): *Heart Disease: A Textbook of Cardiovascular Medicine,* 4th ed. Philadelphia, W.B. Saunders, 1992, pp 1007–1077
20. Ross J, Braunwald E: The influence of corrective operations on the natural history of aortic stenosis. *Circulation* **37** (Suppl 5):61, 1968
21. Carabello BA, Green LH, Grossman W, et al: Hemodynamic determinants of prognosis of aortic valve replacement in critical aortic stenosis and advanced congestive heart failure. *Circulation* **62:**42, 1980
22. Carabello BA, Grossman W: Calculation of stenotic valve orifice area. In Grossman W (ed): *Cardiac Catheterization and Angiography,* 3rd ed. Philadelphia, Lea & Febiger, 1986, pp 143–154
23. Grossman W: Profiles in valvular heart disease. In Grossman W, Baim D (ed): *Cardiac Catheterization and Angiography,* 4th ed. Philadelphia, Lea & Febiger, 1991, pp 557–581
24. Folland ED, Parisi AF, Carbone C: Is peripheral arterial pressure a satisfactory substitute for ascending aortic pressure when measuring aortic valve gradients? *J Am Coll Cardiol* **4:**1207, 1984
25. Bache RJ, Wang Y, Jorgenson CP: Hemodynamic effects of exercise in isolated valvular aortic stenosis. *Circulation* **44:**1003, 1971
26. Philips HR, Levine FH, Carter JE, et al: Mitral valve replacement for isolated mitral regurgitation: Analysis of clinical course and late postoperative left ventricular ejection fraction. *Am J Cardiol* **48:**647, 1981
27. Dalby AJ, Firth BG, Forman R: Preoperative factors affecting the outcome of isolated mitral valve replacement: A 10 year review. *Am J Cardiol* **47:**826, 1981
28. Osbakken MD, Bove AA, Spann JF: Left ventricular regional wall motion and velocity of shortening in chronic mitral and aortic regurgitation. *Am J Cardiol* **47:**1055, 1981
29. Croft CH, Lipscomb K, Mathis K, et al: Limitations of quantitative angiographic grading in aortic or mitral regurgitation. *Am J Cardiol* **53:**1593, 1984
30. Pichard A, Kay R, Smith H, et al: Large V waves in the pulmonary wedge pressure tracing in the absence of mitral regurgitation. *Am J Cardiol* **50:**1044, 1982
31. Fuchs RM, Heuser RP, Yin Y, et al: Limitations of pulmonary wedge V waves in diagnosing mitral regurgitation. *Am J Cardiol* **49:**849, 1982
32. Borow KM, Green LH, Mann T, et al: End systolic volume as a predictor of postoperative left ventricular performance in volume overload from valvular regurgitation. *Am J Med* **68:**655, 1980
33. Gahl K, Sutton R, Pearson M, et al: Mitral regurgitation in coronary heart disease. *Br Heart J* **39:**13, 1977
34. Czer L, Gray RJ, DeRobertis M, et al: Mitral valve replacement: Im-

pact of coronary artery disease and determinants of prognosis after revascularization. *Circulation* **70**(Suppl 1):198, 1984

35. Carpentier A, Chauvaud S, Fabiani JN, et al: Reconstructive surgery of mitral valve incompetence. Ten-year appraisal. *J Thorac Cardiovasc Surg* **79**:338, 1980

36. Reed GE, Pooley RW, Moggio RA: Durability of measured mitral annuloplasty. *J Thorac Cardiovasc Surg* **79**:321, 1980

37. Lessana A, Ades F, Kara SM, et al: Mitral reconstructive operations. *J Thorac Cardiovasc Surg* **86**:553, 1983

38. Bonow RO, Rosing DR, Maron BJ, et al: Reversal of left ventricular dysfunction after aortic valve replacement for chronic aortic regurgitation: Influence of duration of preoperative left ventricular dysfunction. *Circulation* **70**:570, 1984

39. Gaasch WH, Peterson KL, Shabetai R: Left ventricular function in chronic constrictive pericarditis. *Am J Cardiol* **34**:107, 1974

40. Chew C, Ziady GM, Raphael MJ, et al: The functional defect in amyloid heart disease: The "stiff heart" syndrome. *Am J Cardiol* **36**:438, 1975

41. Cutler DJ, Isner JM, Bracey AW, et al: Hemochromatosis heart disease: An unemphasized cause of potentially reversible restrictive cardiomyopathy. *Am J Med* **69**:923, 1980

42. Shabatai R, Fowler NO, Guntheroth WG: The hemodynamics of cardiac tamponade and constrictive pericarditis. *Am J Cardiol* **26**:480, 1970

43. Parillo JE, Aretz HT, Palacios I, et al: The results of transvenous endomyocardial biopsy can frequently be used to diagnose myocardial diseases in patients with idiopathic heart failure. *Circulation* **69**:93, 1984

44. Fenoglio JJ, Ursell PC, Kellogg CF, et al: Diagnosis and classification of myocarditis by endomyocardial biopsy. *N Engl J Med* **308**:12, 1983

45. Lorell B, Alderman EL, Mason JW: Cardiac sarcoidosis: Diagnosis by transvenous endomyocardial biopsy and treatment with corticosteroids. *Am J Cardiol* **42**:143, 1978

46. Schroeder JS, Billingham ME, Rider AK: Cardiac amyloidosis: Diagnosis by transvenous endomyocardial biopsy. *Am J Med* **59**:269, 1975

47. Short EM, Winkle RA, Billingham ME: Myocardial involvement in idiopathic hemochromatosis: Morphologic and clinical improvement following venesection. *Am J Med* **70**:1275, 1981

48. Bristow MR, Mason JW, Billingham ME, et al: Doxorubicin cardiomyopathy: Evaluation by phonocardiography, endomyocardial biopsy, and cardiac catheterization. *Ann Intern Med* **88**:168, 1978

49. Fowles RE, Baim DS: Endomyocardial biopsy. In Grossman W (ed): *Cardiac Catheterization and Angiography,* 3rd ed. Philadelphia, Lea & Febiger, 1986, pp 359–381

50. Sekiguchi M, Take M: World survey of catheter biopsy of the heart. In Sekiguchi M, Olsen EGJ (ed): *Cardiomyopathy, Clinical, Pathological, and Theoretical Aspects.* Baltimore, University Park Press, 1980, pp 217–225

104

Echocardiography

John S. Child and Janine Krivokapich

INTRODUCTION

Echocardiographic imaging and hemodynamic evaluation of cardiovascular disease have revolutionized the diagnosis and management of heart disease and, at times, rendered cardiac catheterization unnecessary.[1] It is the goal of this chapter to introduce the cardiothoracic surgeon to the basics of normal echocardiographic anatomy, to the pathophysiologic processes that appropriately exploit the strengths of this technology, and to the issues that are specific to the practice of cardiothoracic surgery. The combination of high-quality transthoracic two-dimensional (2-D) and M-mode echocardiography in conjunction with color-flow imaging and pulsed- and continuous-wave spectral Doppler has made precise delineation of cardiac anatomy and function routinely available.[1-3] Transesophageal echocardiography (TEE) provides a complementary acoustic window to the heart and great vessels.[2-15] TEE is particularly effective at imaging the atria, atrial septum, pulmonary veins and branch arteries, atrioventricular valves, ventricular outflow tracts, and aorta.[2-15] Multiplane or biplane TEE imaging is essential for complete evaluation of the aorta, the right ventricular outflow tract, ventricular-to-arterial conduits, and other outflow tracts, and for more complete evaluation of ventricles and atrioventricular valves.[9-12] Intraoperative TEE allows excellent immediate evaluation of repairs of complex congenital cardiac malformations, the results of valvular repair, and evaluation of myocardial function.[11,12] Echocardiography has been utilized to guide pericardiocentesis, transseptal catheterization or atrial septostomy, percutaneous balloon valvotomy, and radiofrequency arrhythmia ablation.[13,14] Echocardiography, particularly TEE, is often required in the critical care units for clinical problem solving (Tables 104–1 and 104–2).[15]

NORMAL ANATOMY AND FUNCTION

Complete echocardiographic examination includes M-mode and 2-D echocardiographic imaging, and color-flow and spectral Doppler examination.[1-3] The M-mode echocardiogram, using 2-D echo to target specific portions of the heart, is useful for obtaining timing of events and chamber dimensions. The 2-D echocardiographic examination depicts cardiac anatomy in real-time motion, which permits direct evaluation of valve motion, muscle thickening, and ventricular function. At least five standard views of the heart are routinely recorded: left parasternal long axis and short axis views, and apical long axis, two chamber, and four chamber views are typically obtained (Fig. 104–1, see page 1713, and Figs. 104–2 and 104–3, see Color Plates following page 2072).[2,3] For a full introduction to the entire spectrum of normal anatomic imaging planes, the reader is referred to standard major current texts of echocardiography.[2,3] Two-dimensional examination allows a complete assessment of the wall motion and thickening characteristics of all of the ventricular walls from base to apex at rest and with exercise or pharmacologic stress and these segments can be related to expected coronary arterial distribution patterns (Fig. 104–1). The proximal anterior interventricular septum is visualized in the long axis view, along with the inferior lateral wall. The basal-mid inferior interventricular septum and mid-apical anterior interventricular septum, the lateral wall, and the right ventricular free wall are represented in the four-chamber view. The anterior wall and the inferior medial wall are seen on the two-chamber view. All of these walls are visible in the short axis view by sequentially sweeping the transducer from base to apex. Ejection fractions can be estimated visually or quantitated by on- or off-line computer algorithms.

TABLE 104–1. ECHO AND CLINICAL PROBLEM SOLVING IN CRITICAL CARE PATIENTS

Hypotension/low cardiac output
   Ventricular function
   Volume status/sepsis
   Tamponade
   Pulmonary embolism
   Aortic dissection
   Left ventricular outflow tract obstruction
   Complications of infective endocarditis
   Complications of myocardial infarction
Chest pain
   Aortic dissection
   Myocardial ischemia or infarction
   Pericarditis/effusion
   Pulmonary embolism
Cause of cardiac arrest
Sepsis/?endocarditis
Source of arterial embolus
Cyanosis
New murmur evaluation

Doppler echo uses ultrasound to reflect off moving red blood cells; the Doppler shift records the direction and velocity of bloodflow. Color flow Doppler is done in conjunction with 2-D echo imaging and entails conversion of the pulsed-wave Doppler signals into a mean velocity whereby specific velocities and direction are encoded into color images. Thus, intracardiac and vascular flow is imaged based on its velocity and directional characteristics and displayed in an "angiographic" format superimposed upon the anatomic and functional format of the 2-D echo image.[2,3]

Abnormal color-flow imaging patterns of valvular stenosis and regurgitation are easily recognizable (Figs. 104–2 and 104–3). It is important to recognize that trivial regurgitation of the mitral, tricuspid, and pulmonary valves is commonly present in healthy people. The degree of regurgitation is graded based on the dimensions of the regurgitant jet, including the size of the regurgitant jet at the regurgitant orifice, as well as the area of the jet relative to the distal chamber.[2,3,16] More sophisticated techniques (e.g., measuring regurgitant fractions) have been devised to quan-

TABLE 104–2. SPECIFIC ROLE OF TEE IN THE CRITICAL CARE PATIENT

Aortic dissection
Prosthetic valve dysfunction
Source of stroke or arterial embolus
Asymmetric tamponade postcardiac surgery
Patent foramen ovale/cyanosis
Complications of infective endocarditis
Positioning of intra-aortic balloon
Inability to obtain adequate transthoracic echo for
   important/appropriate question

titate regurgitation more precisely, but these techniques are not readily applicable and are not routinely used in most echocardiography laboratories. It is important to emphasize that the color-flow Doppler images of regurgitation do not represent volume, but velocity. Color-flow imaging of regurgitation echocardiographically is only semi-quantitative. Problems in accurately grading the degree of regurgitation arise because equal volumes of regurgitation may have different sizes on color-flow imaging depending on the velocity of the regurgitation. Higher velocity jets result in larger color-flow regurgitations despite equal volumes.[16]

Pulsed and continuous-wave Doppler are used to show direction and timing of blood flow and quantitate the velocities at particular locations within the heart (Figs. 104–4, 104–5, and 104–6). Flow going away from the transducer is usually displayed below the baseline and flow toward the transducer is usually displayed above the baseline. With pulsed-wave (PW) Doppler, a sample volume is placed anywhere within the heart where there is bloodflow, and the velocity and direction of flow at that spot is recorded (Fig. 104–4). The limitation of PW Doppler is that velocities ≥ 2 m/s cannot accurately be displayed.[14] Continuous-wave (CW) Doppler accurately measures high velocities but records all velocities along the "ice-pick" line of the Doppler beam. When a high velocity is recorded on CW Doppler, additional information regarding 2-D echo anatomy and PW mapping along the echo beam line is required to localize the source of the high velocity (Fig. 104–5). Normal velocity patterns have been described for the mitral and tricuspid inflow views, the right and left ventricular outflow tracts, the aorta and pulmonary artery, and the vena cavae and pulmonary veins.[2,3] For example, mitral inflow in normal sinus rhythm shows an early passive inflow velocity (the peak of which is called the "E" velocity) as the mitral valve opens and the atrium initially begins emptying into the left ventricle; with the onset of active atrial contraction, another velocity (the "A" velocity) is seen (Fig. 104–4). Pattern variations often indicate a specific pathology (e.g., mitral stenosis, diastolic dysfunction, and severe mitral regurgitation).[2,3] Velocities obtained across valves and septal defects represent pressure gradients; these gradients are calculated using the simplified Bernoulli equation (pressure gradient = 4 × maximum velocity^2) (Figs. 104–5 and 104–6).[14,15] An example of an important application is in the estimation of pulmonary artery systolic pressure using a tricuspid regurgitant jet (Fig. 104–6).[17] The systolic gradient across the tricuspid valve (tricuspid regurgitation) represents the pressure difference between the right ventricle and right atrium. The right atrial pressure can be estimated from the jugular venous pressure or assumed to be 10 mm Hg; the gradient across the tricuspid valve plus the right atrial pressure equals the right ventricular pressure. In the absence of right ventricular outflow obstruction, this measures the peak systolic pulmonary artery pressure.

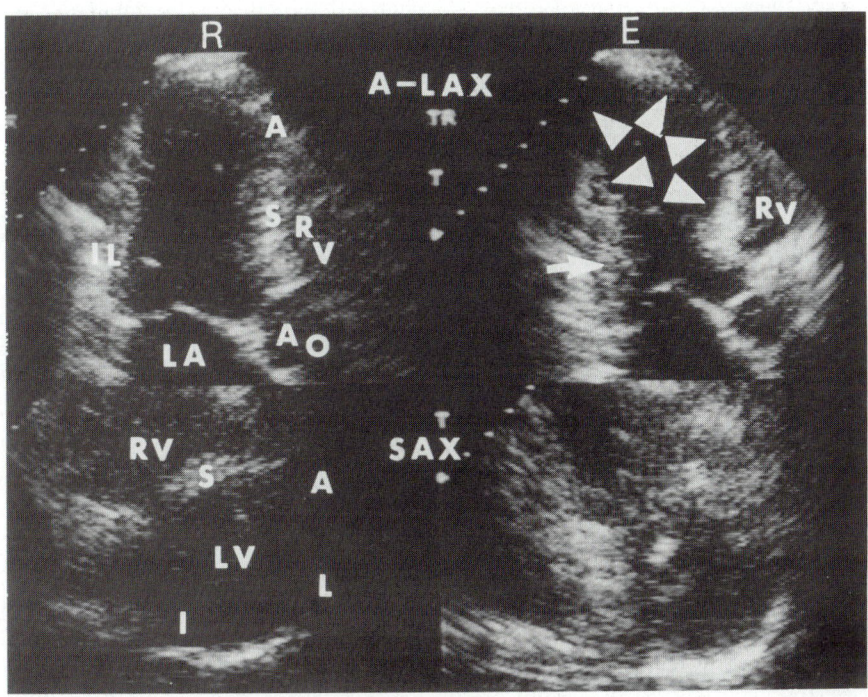

A

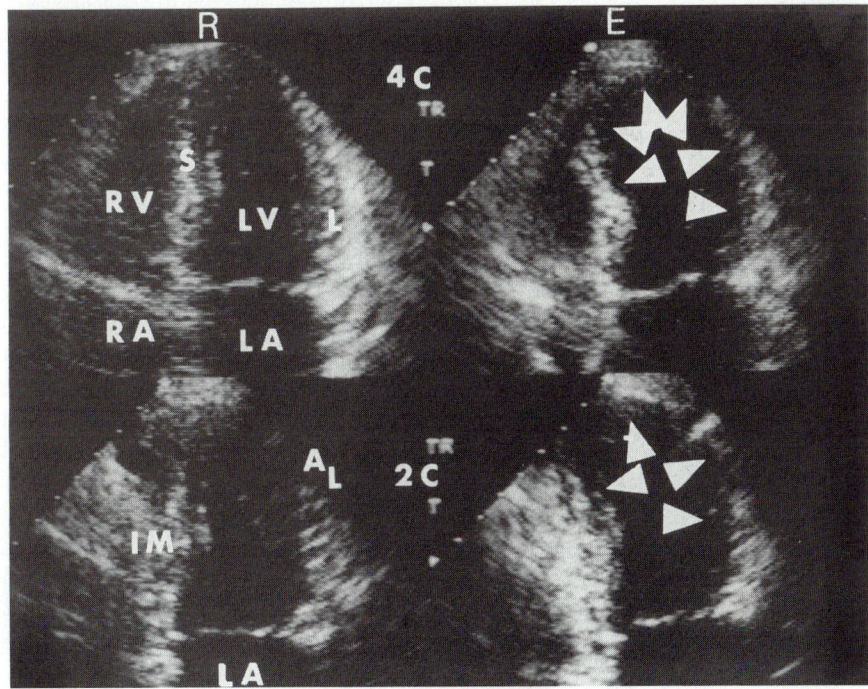

B

Figure 104–1. Quad-screen computer-captured display of treadmill stress echo showing rest (R, left hand panels) and exercise (E, right hand panels) images at end-systole to accentuate the stress-induced ischemia of the mid-apical anteroseptum and anterolateral and lateral wall, and inferoapex (white arrowheads) to the left anterior descending coronary artery disease. **A.** *Upper frames* are an apical long-axis view (A-LAX) with apex at the top showing the septum (S), anterior wall apex (A), and inferolateral wall (IL). The white arrow shows increased contractility of the base of the inferolateral wall with exercise. The *lower frames* show the parasternal short axis (SAX) at the basal ventricular level with septum (S), anterior wall (A), lateral wall (L), and inferior wall (I). AO, aorta; LA, left atrium; LV, left ventricle; RV, right ventricle. **B.** *Upper frames* are an apical four-chamber view (4C) with apex at the top, septum (S) and lateral wall (L). RA, right atrium; other abbreviations as above. The *lower panels* are the apical two-chamber (2C) view with left ventricular apex at the top with anterolateral wall (AL) and inferomedial wall (IM).

AORTIC DISEASE

Biplane/multiplane TEE and color-flow imaging performed by the experienced examiner provides high resolution imaging of all segments of the thoracic aorta. Bloodflow in the aorta and major branches can be well seen and aortic regurgitation is reliably detected and quantified. Standard transthoracic echocardiography, though excellent for detecting aortic regurgitation, aortic valve disease, the proximal portion of the ascending aorta, as well as portions of the transverse and descending aorta, is less reliable for complete thoracic aortic imaging than is TEE.[18]

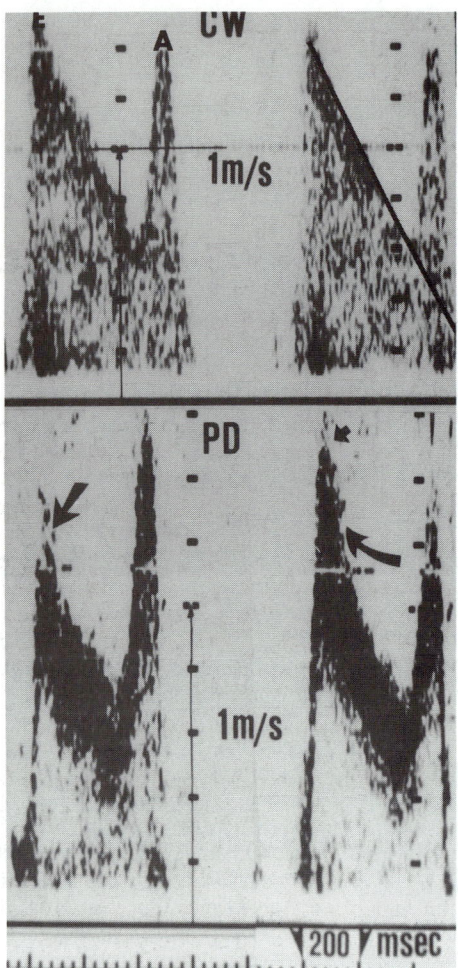

Figure 104–4. Mitral inflow profile in mitral stenosis. The *upper panel* shows the continuous-wave (CW) Doppler spectral profile of mitral stenosis; the early diastolic (E) velocity is increased (1.5 m/s) as is the late A velocity (1.4 m/s) because of an increased left atrial pressure as a result of the obstruction to left atrial emptying. The black line shows the slope of the falloff of the E velocity from which a pressure half-time can be measured. The *lower panel* shows the pulsed-wave Doppler (PD) recording of the same patient; the effect of having the sample volume at different positions in the mitral orifice (left = into annulus with lower E velocity, right = at tips of leaflets with higher E velocity) is shown emphasizing the need for recording the mitral velocities at the tips of the leaflets.

Aortic Aneurysms

Transthoracic echocardiography is relatively reliable at showing the proximal ascending aorta, annuloaortic ectasia, and aneurysms of the sinuses of Valsalva and evaluation of aortic regurgitation.[18,19] TEE is the procedure of choice for complete echocardiographic evaluation of the extent and location of true and false aneurysms. Intraoperative TEE imaging of the results of aneurysm surgery provides a baseline for follow-up. Early and late imaging of reparative techniques, i.e., Bentall procedure, is ideal with TEE including evaluation of the conduit, its connection to native aorta, the coronary artery anastomoses, and the prosthetic valve.[18,19]

Aortic Dissection

An intimal tear or intramural hematoma is the primary sign of "dissecting aortic hematoma" (Figs. 104–7 and 104–8). TEE is the most rapid, efficient, and accurate means of urgent early diagnosis and management in the hands of the experienced operator and has evolved as the first technique of choice in the urgent diagnosis of aortic dissection.[18–25] TEE can be performed at the patient bedside in the intensive care unit or emergency room without interference with the care of the critically ill patient. Biplane/multiplane TEE accurately confirms the presence, type, and extent of dissection, presence of true and false lumens, sites of entrance–exit points, and intimal tears. TEE is useful for finding other complications (pericardial and pleural effusion, involvement of branch vessels including coronary arteries, fistulae such as rupture into right heart) and can evaluate ventricular function and aortic regurgitation and can be readily utilized in the operating room.[18] TEE has equivalent sensitivity (97.7%) to magnetic resonance imaging (MRI) and computed tomography (CT); previously reported lower specificity (76.9%) was in those with single plane TEE only.[23] Biplane TEE was used by Ballal et al in 22 of 61 patients (36%) with proven dissections with a sensitivity = 97% and specificity = 100%.[24] They found that CT made a correct diagnosis in only 67% and misclassified the type of dissection in 33%. Of note, TEE correctly identified the involvement of the coronary arteries in 6 of 7 patients and the absence of involvement of the coronaries in 10 patients with aortic dissection. Technical artifacts that may mimic intimal flaps and methods to verify the presence of an intimal flap (flap seen in two orthogonal planes, characteristic flap motion, color-flow patterns in true and false lumen) must be familiar to the examiner to avoid false-positive diagnosis.[7,8,18] Skill must have been acquired in a variety of TEE expressions of the disease with emphasis on complete evaluation of the ascending aorta and transverse arch and the ability to recognize unusual variants [i.e., intramural hematoma (Fig. 104–8), penetrating aortic ulcer, and traumatic transection (Fig. 104–9)].[18,25]

Angiography, an imperfect "Gold-Standard," poses risks to those with renal dysfunction. Erbel et al, in a prospective study of 164 patients with suspected aortic dissection, found a sensitivity = 88% vs. 99% and specificity = 94% vs. 98% for angiography vs. TEE, respectively.[20] TEE plays an important role in subsequent follow-up of aortic dissections; routine follow-up angiographic study is cumbersome.[22] False-negative angiograms occur when the false lumen is thrombosed or faintly opacified, or, catheter tip placement is faulty and the false and true lumens are opacified simultaneously thereby obscuring the intimal flap. Intramural hematoma without an intimal flap can be missed by angiography.

CT is more sensitive and specific than angiography but also has limitations. Nienaber et al noted a sensitivity = 93.8% and specificity = 87.1% of CT for aortic dissection

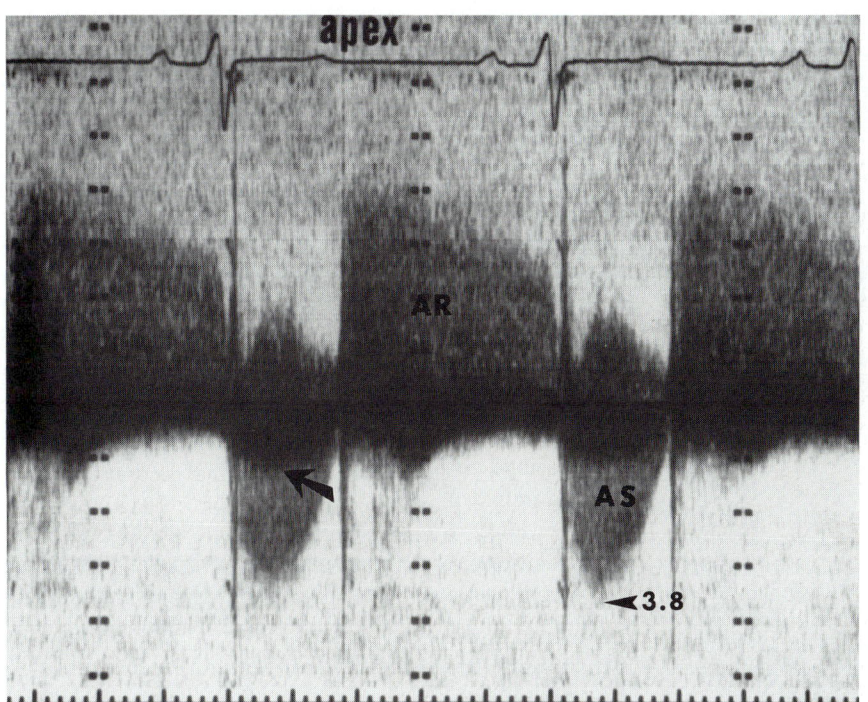

Figure 104–5. Continuous-wave Doppler recording of aortic stenosis (AS) and aortic regurgitation (AR) from the left ventricular apex. The AR enters the left ventricle in diastole toward the transducer, thus, AR is above the baseline. The AS exits the left ventricle into the aorta in systole and is shown as going away from the transducer below the baseline. The peak AS velocity = 3.8 m/s with a calculated peak instantaneous gradient = 58 mm Hg. Note that within the high velocity due to the AS is a darker superimposed profile (arrow) of the left ventricular outflow tract velocity reflecting the fact that the CW Doppler sees all velocities along its course in contrast to the local recording of velocities by pulsed-wave sample volumes.

but CT has the disadvantages of lack of mobility, inability to evaluate aortic regurgitation, use of nephrotoxic intravenous agents, inability to visualize branch vessel involvement, and, most importantly, low likelihood of detection of the intimal flap and entry site.[23]

MRI provides anatomic definition of the aorta that is uniformly equal or superior to other techniques and is noninvasive and does not require injection of nephrotoxic agents. Sensitivity and specificity are nearly 100%.[18,23] Nonetheless, it is time-consuming and requires on-site expensive equipment, and access to the patient can be difficult should there be clinical deterioration. MRI cannot be used in the patient with certain pacemakers or metallic prostheses.

Aortic Atheromata and Debris

Intraaortic debris, ranging from flat atheromatous plaques to protruding mobile thrombi on ulcerated plaques, is a potential cause of embolic disease. Epicardial echocardiography and biplane/multiplane TEE is useful in the operating room to identify significant ascending aortic atheromatous disease, which may have implications for the site of cross-clamping and cannula insertion.[26–28]

INTRACARDIAC TUMORS, MASSES, AND SOURCES OF EMBOLISM

Two-dimensional echocardiography is the technique of choice for detection, localization, and follow-up of intracardiac masses (tumors, thrombi, vegetations).[29–35] Standard

transthoracic 2-D echo does an excellent job in an echogenic patient of evaluating the ventricular apices, the tricuspid and pulmonic valves, and the inferior vena cava and hepatic veins because they are reasonably near the transducer; in addition, large atrial masses, e.g., atrial myxomas, are usually seen in echogenic patients (Figs. 104–10 and 104–11). TEE, with the position posterior to the heart and unimpeded by air, bone, or cartilege, provides a better acoustic window to evaluate the more posterior structures such as the atriums and their appendages, interatrial septum, superior vena cava, pulmonary artery branches and pulmonary veins, and the mitral and aortic valves, because these are in the near field (Figs. 104–12 and 104–13).[29,30] TEE can detect metastatic osteosarcoma or lung cancer growing through the pulmonary veins into the left atrium (Fig. 104–13) or small atrial myxomas not imaged from the chest surface. Tumors, thrombi, or central venous lines in the superior vena cava are best seen by TEE. Localized effusions adjacent to the atriums, common postcardiac surgery, are more reliably visualized by TEE.

TEE is an important modality in the search for the source of stroke or systemic arterial embolus.[31] The ascending and transverse aorta has been found to frequently be the site of atheromatous debris, which may be a source of embolism, and is well imaged using biplane or multiplane TEE.[32,33] Furthermore, sites in the heart commonly associated with thrombi, such as the left atrial appendage, are inadequately seen on standard 2-D echo. A patent foramen ovale, a potential site for paradoxical embolism, and the occasional culprit in significant postoperative hypoxemia, is readily identified with TEE and color-flow imaging combined with intravenous injection of agitated saline

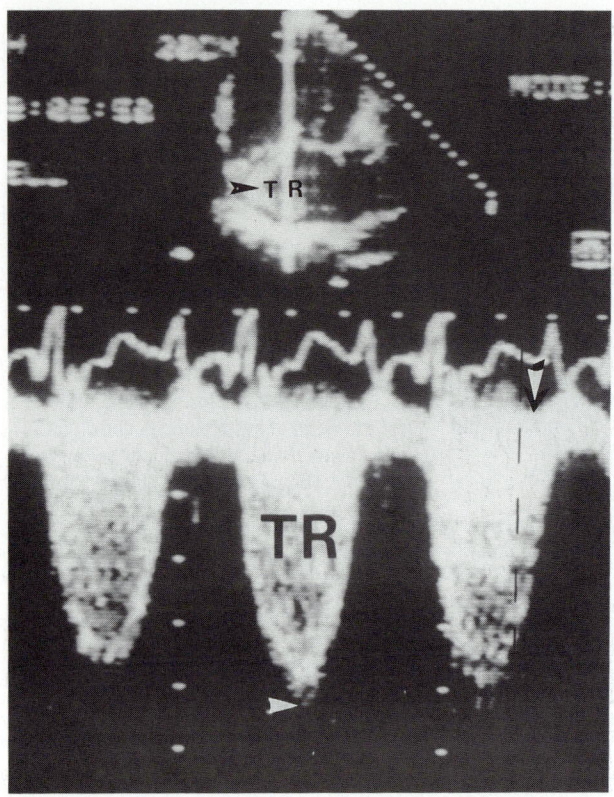

Figure 104–6. Tricuspid regurgitation (TR) and pulmonary hypertension. Continuous-wave Doppler recording with upper panel showing the beam aligned through a color flow image (shown in black and white) of TR; lower panel shows the TR velocity profile. The peak TR jet velocity = 4.3 m/s, consistent with a right ventricular to right atrial pressure gradient = 74 mm Hg. If the right atrial pressure = 10 mm Hg, the right ventricular systolic pressure and (in this patient with no right ventricular outflow tract obstruction) the pulmonary artery systolic pressure) = 84 mm Hg. The black dotted line shows that the TR velocity continues after the end of systole and, in fact, stops only after the onset of the P-wave (white arrowhead) reflecting diastolic TR due to a high right ventricular diastolic pressure.

(echocontrast). Vegetations and their complications are much more readily evaluated with TEE (discussed later).

ISCHEMIC HEART DISEASE

Acute and chronic myocardial ischemia is shown on 2-D echo as a decrease in segmental myocardial thickening (Fig. 104–1). The wall motion for each segment can be visually graded as having normal function, hypokinesis, akinesis, or dyskinesis. Unfortunately, a wall motion abnormality does not distinguish between infarcted and ischemic myocardium. Myocardium can be stunned, due to transient acute ischemia, or hibernating, due to chronic low flow, and exhibit wall motion abnormalities similar to infarcted myocardium. It can take days or weeks for previously stunned or hibernating myocardium to recover normal systolic func-

tion after normal perfusion is restored. A thinned and echodense segment makes a scar and infarction more likely; diffuse or global rather than segmental wall motion abnormalities can be due to nonischemic cardiomyopathy, hypertensive cardiovascular disease, end-stage valvular disease, or severe ischemic heart disease. Global left ventricular ejection fraction can be accurately estimated visually by experienced echocardiographers. Computer software is available to digitize images and quantitate the left ventricular ejection fraction, if required, using biplane apical views of the heart. TEE has also been used extensively to evaluate left and right ventricular function and volume status intraoperatively or in critically ill patients in whom transthoracic imaging is inadequate due to respirator interference, surgical dressings, and/or inability to properly position the patient.

Exercise electrocardiography had been traditionally used to detect stress-induced ischemia but the sensitivity and specificity for detecting ischemia average ≤70%. Imaging techniques, such as echocardiography or radionuclide angiography and flow imaging, significantly improve the detection of stress-induced ischemia.[36] The fact that myocardium reacts to ischemia with an immediate decrease in systolic contraction has been the basis of performing stress 2-D echocardiograms to detect ischemia. Images are obtained at rest, with or immediately after stress, and in the recovery period. Computer digital echocardiographic images are captured as a cine loop with each of four standard views of the heart at rest and with or immediately after stress displayed in a quad-frame format (four views at the same time with the rest and stress images for a particular view displayed side-by-side) (Fig. 104–1). Stress-induced ischemia is detected as a worsening of wall motion with the sensitivity and specificity of diagnosing coronary artery disease approximating 85%.[36–40]

Stress echocardiography can be performed with exercise or pharmacological stress. Most studies have utilized treadmill stress testing; motion artifact during exercise on the treadmill requires that imaging be performed immediately after treadmill exercise. Images must be obtained ≤2 min after completion of the exercise to ensure detection of transient wall motion abnormalities. Bicycle ergometry has also been used for stress echocardiography because imaging can be performed during the exercise with better sensitivity but lower specificity.

Pharmacological stress testing, recommended if the patient is unable to successfully complete an exercise test due to deconditioning, orthopedic problems, arthritis, peripheral vascular disease, recent surgery, or catheterization, is usually done with dobutamine, dipyridamole, or adenosine.[41–48] Dobutamine, usually given in progressive doses of 5 μg/kg starting with 5 μg/kg and increasing to a maximum of 40 μg/kg per minute, simulates exercise by increasing contractility and the heart rate.[41–44] Echocardiographic imaging with pharmacologic stress is easier than with exercise because there is no movement or respiratory-induced interference and allows imaging during the stress, unlike

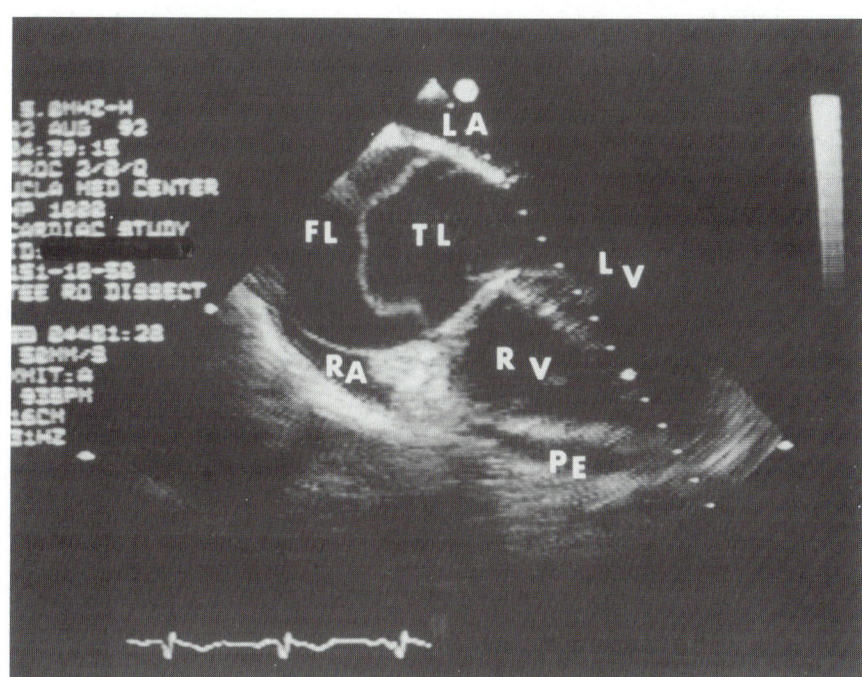

Figure 104–7. Transesophageal echo of ascending aortic dissection. The transverse plane shows a dilated ascending aorta that contains an intimal flap with a true lumen (TL) and a false lumen (FL). There was moderate aortic regurgitation (not shown) and a small pericardial effusion (PE) was developing because of leakage. LA, left atrium; LV, left ventricle; RA, right atrium; RV, right ventricle.

treadmill testing. Viability of myocardium can be assessed: improvement in a resting wall motion abnormality with low dose (5–10 μg/kg) dobutamine implies that viable myocardium (stunned or hibernating) is present, even if the wall motion decreases again with peak dobutamine dosing. Sensitivity and specificity are similar to exercise echocardiography.[41–45] Dipyridamole and adenosine are coronary vasodilators, which induce a flow imbalance and steal phenomenon in the presence of significant coronary artery

stenoses. They are most frequently employed with flow imaging using radionuclides, but have also been successfully used with echocardiography.[46–48]

Stress echocardiography has been demonstrated to be a useful tool to estimate prognosis of coronary artery disease.[49–51] Patients who develop new or worsened wall motion abnormalities on stress echocardiography have at least a 3-fold increased incidence of myocardial infarction, coronary artery bypass surgery, coronary angioplasty, and/

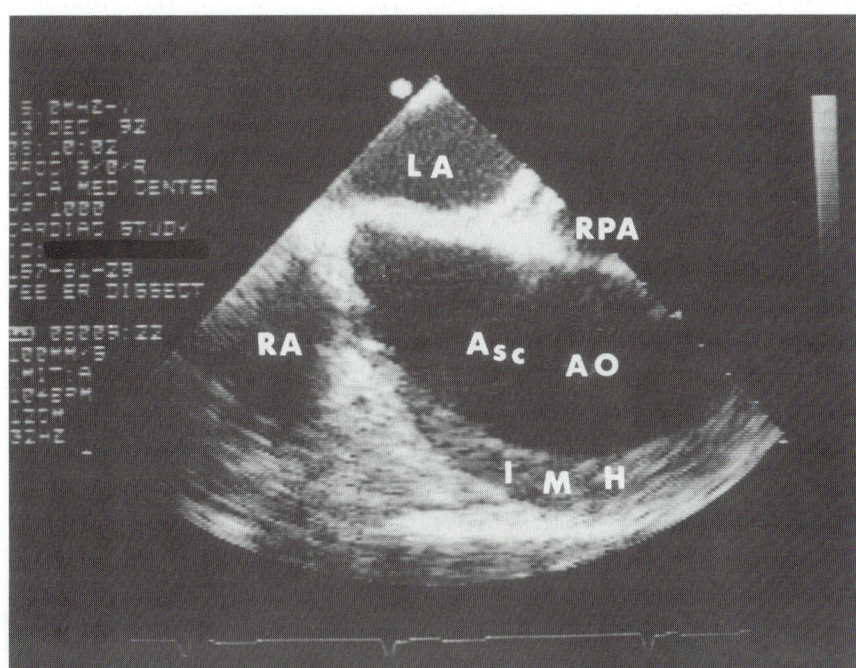

Figure 104–8. Transesophageal echo of intramural hematoma. A vertical plane of the ascending aorta (Asc AO) in an elderly lady with acute chest and back pain who later died (from aortic rupture) shows an acute intramural hematoma (IMH) (proven at necropsy). No intimal flap or false lumen is seen. LA, left atrium; RA, right atrium; RPA, right pulmonary artery.

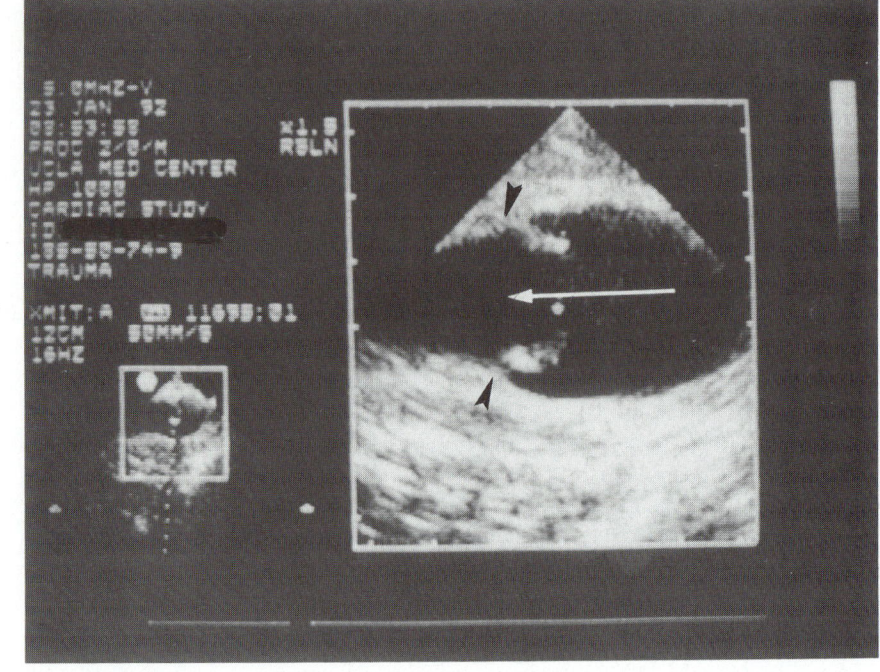

Figure 104–9. Traumatic descending aortic transection. Transesophageal echo of the descending aorta, performed emergently in the operating room of a trauma victim (with a widened mediastinum on chest x-ray) while he was undergoing emergency splenectomy. The descending aorta is shown in a longitudinal view with the proximal superior portion on the right shown just below the transition from the transverse aorta and the lower portion on the left. The direction of bloodflow is shown by the arrow. The transection flap can be seen with the aortic wall thickness below the flap (black arrowheads) seen to be thicker than the thinner proximal descending aortic wall above the flap, which was mainly adventitia.

or death than patients who do not develop new or worsened wall motion abnormalities.[49]

Echocardiography detects complications related to ischemic heart disease including pericardial effusion, aneurysm formation, thrombi (Fig. 104–10), intra- and extracardiac rupture (Fig. 104–14), and mitral regurgitation that is a result of "papillary muscle dysfunction." Echocardiography is the best technique available for detecting left ventricular thrombi (Fig. 104–10). Diastolic dysfunction, the earliest effect of ischemia, is evaluated by mitral and pulmonary venous flow profiles.[52–54] Life-threatening complications, i.e., ventricular septal rupture or papillary muscle rupture (Fig. 104–14), are detected with combined 2-D echo and color-flow imaging. Extracardiac rupture is usually detected as a pericardial effusion with evidence of tamponade or a false aneurysm.

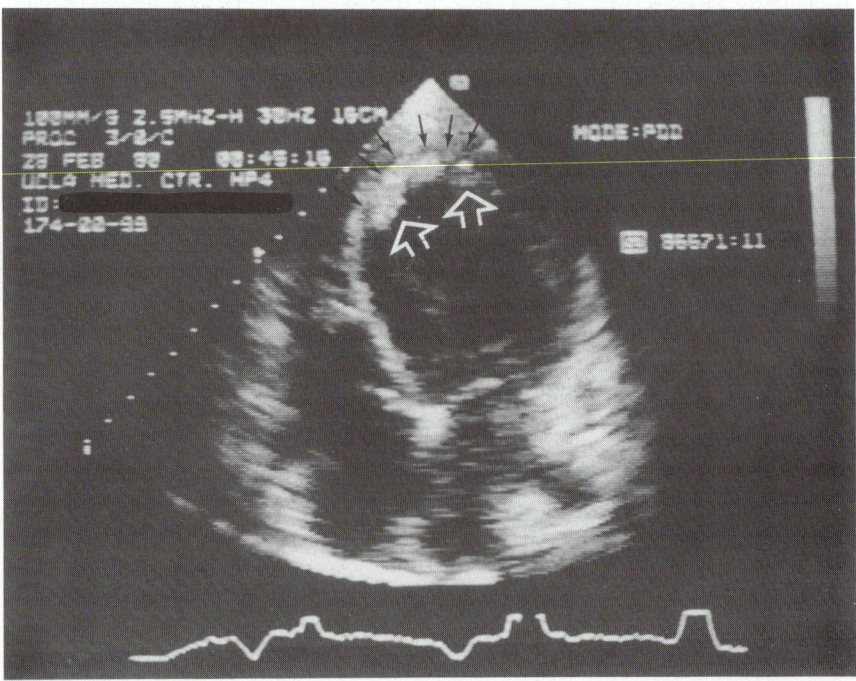

Figure 104–10. Left ventricular apical thrombi in a patient with dilated heart failure and multivessel coronary artery disease. The white arrows point to the lobulated apical thrombi. The black arrows show the inner margin of the endocardium.

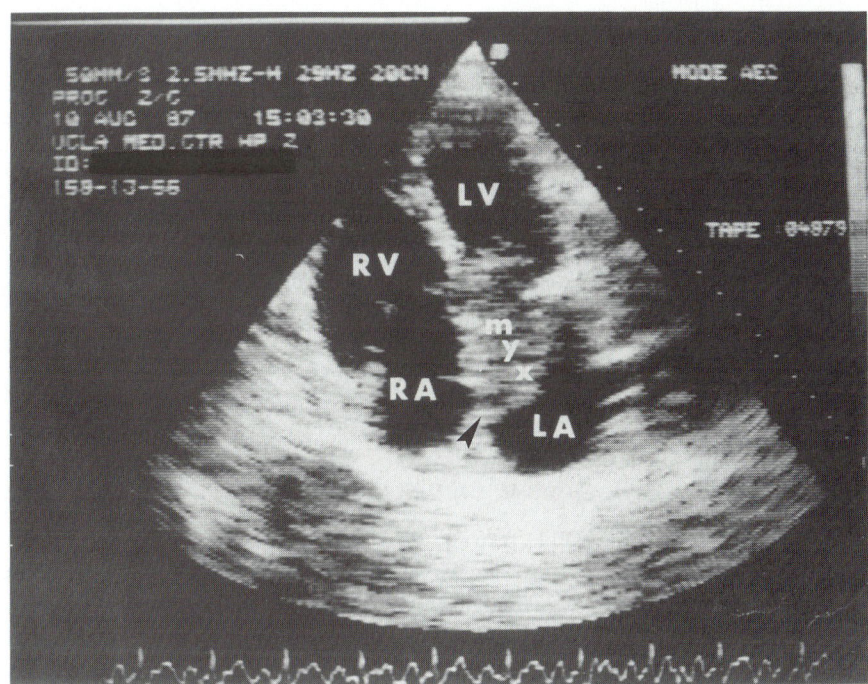

Figure 104–11. Left atrial myxoma (myx) seen attached to the interatrial septum (at black arrow) at the fossa ovalis and projecting through the mitral orifice in diastole in this four-chamber apical view. LA, left atrium; LV, left ventricle; RA, right atrium; RV, right ventricle.

CARDIOMYOPATHIES

Echocardiography and Doppler quantifies systolic and diastolic dysfunction, valvular regurgitation, and hemodynamic status and are invaluable in the diagnosis and follow-up of congestive heart failure because of one of the three main types of cardiomyopathic profiles (dilated, restrictive, hypertrophic).[55–61] The acute and chronic response to therapy can be evaluated and can provide important prognostic information, particularly important with advances in medical treatment and orthotopic cardiac transplantation.[58–60]

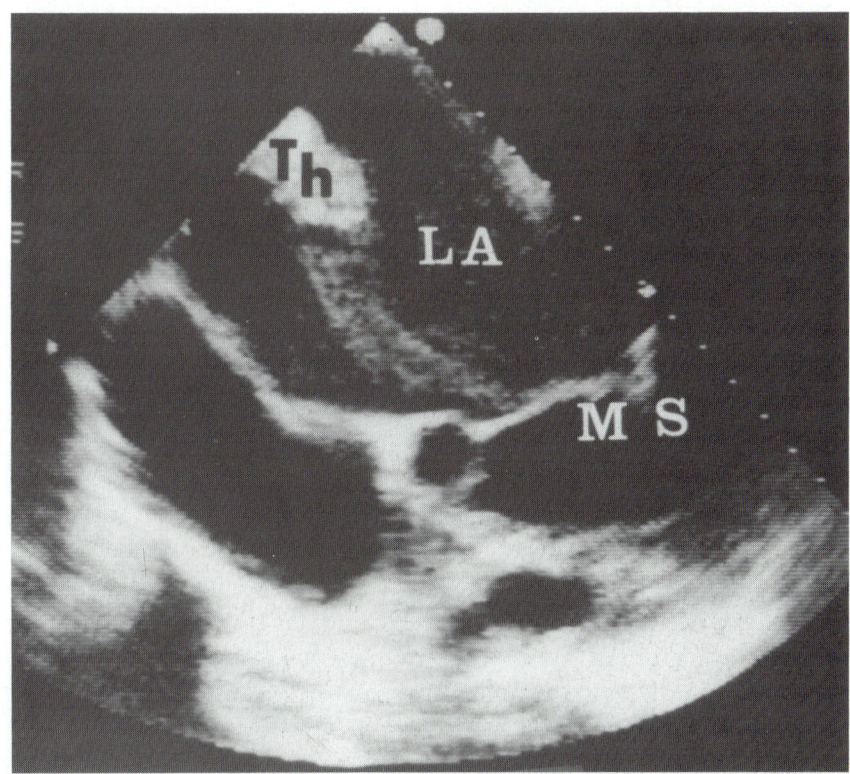

Figure 104–12. TEE of left atrial (LA) thrombus (Th) in mitral stenosis (MS). There is also a "smoking" appearance to the slow LA flow.

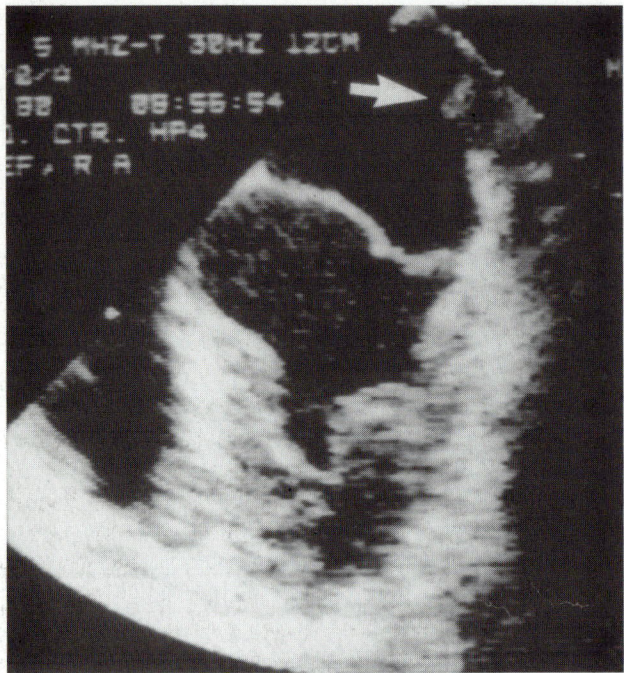

Figure 104–13. TEE of metastatic osteosarcoma into the left superior pulmonary vein (white arrow).

Dilated Cardiomyopathy

Dilated cardiomyopathy is characterized by dilated left and often right ventricular chambers, normal wall thickness, and reduced ejection fraction due to globally reduced myocar-

dial systolic thickening. Intracardiac thrombi may be seen at the apex (Fig. 104–10). "Idiopathic" versus ischemic etiologies may be indistinguishable, though ischemic cardiomyopathy may have detectable areas of thinned and scarred myocardium often with a greater severity of mitral regurgitation if the free wall base of a papillary muscle is infarcted. Ischemic cardiomyopathy more frequently has normal right ventricular function than the "idiopathic" type. Clinical deterioration may occur with less striking degrees of ventricular dilatation in the ischemic type. "Minimally" dilated cardiomyopathy forms a distinct entity with a poor prognosis and is recognized by poor systolic function with normal wall thickness and minimal, if any, ventricular dilatation.

Restrictive Cardiomyopathy

Idiopathic restrictive cardiomyopathy, a primary abnormality of diastolic dysfunction, has normal systolic function and wall thickness; ventricular volumes are often small to normal with biatrial enlargement.[56] Infiltrative myocardial diseases (e.g., amyloidosis), first detected as abnormalities of diastolic dysfunction and congestive heart failure when systolic function may be normal, cause increased wall thickness. Diastolic dysfunction, and ultimately systolic dysfunction, worsens as progressive infiltration occurs.[56,61]

Hypertrophic Cardiomyopathy

Hypertrophic cardiomyopathy, characterized by ventricular hypertrophy of unknown cause, may be nonobstructive or

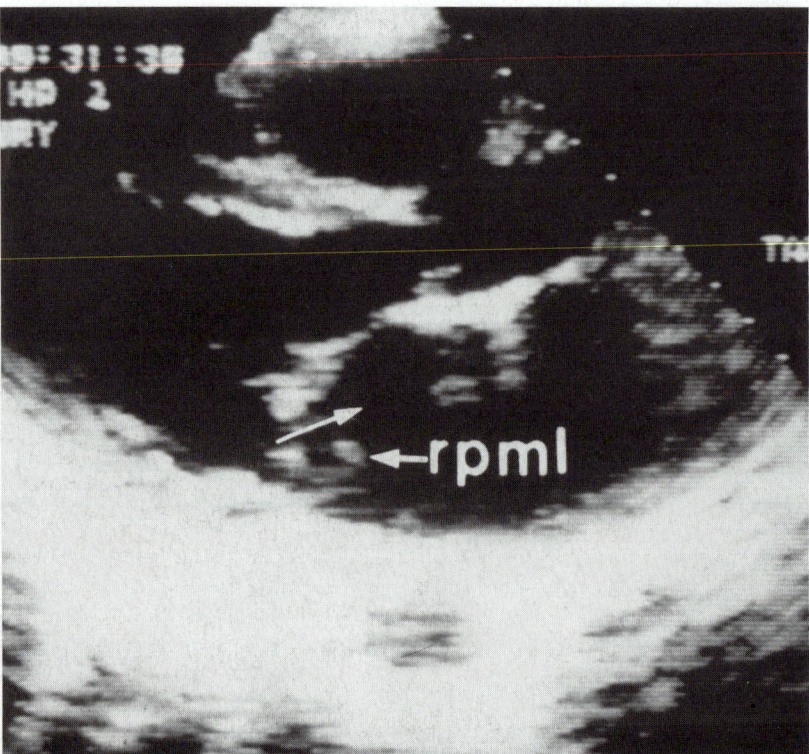

Figure 104–14. Ruptured papillary muscle (rpml) in acute inferior myocardial infarction resulted in systolic prolapse of that portion of the mitral apparatus into the left atrium on this parasternal long-axis view. There was severe mitral regurgitation through the area of malcoaptation (white arrow).

obstructive to ventricular outflow (Figs. 104–15 and 104–16).[55,57] Asymmetric septal hypertrophy is most common and concentric hypertrophy less common. Variations include focal apical or midseptal hypertrophy. Systolic anterior motion of the mitral valve coming into apposition with the ventricular septum and Doppler findings of an increased velocity across the left ventricular outflow tract reflects the pressure gradient in obstructive hypertrophic cardiomyopathy (Fig. 104–15). Dynamic obstruction may be present at rest or with provocation and has a characteristic continuous-wave Doppler late peaking profile in contrast to fixed left ventricular outflow tract obstruction (Fig. 104–16). Color-flow evidence of mitral regurgitation, almost invariable in the obstructive form, varies with the degree of obstruction and is a focus for infective endocarditis. Intraoperative transesophageal or epicardial echocardiography serves to evaluate the adequacy of septal myotomyectomy, search for an iatrogenic ventricular septal defect, and determine if significant residual mitral regurgitation exists.

Heart Transplantation

Follow-up for transplant rejection includes clinical, hemodynamic, endomyocardial biopsy, and echo-Doppler observations.[62] Echo-Doppler recordings are used to serially follow each individual as his own control. Markers for deterioration as a result of transplant rejection and accelerated coronary artery disease include increases in ventricular volumes, wall motion abnormalities, reduction in ejection frac-

tion, and development of a restrictive diastolic mitral inflow pattern due to high left atrial pressure.

PERICARDIAL DISEASES

Pericardial Effusion

2-D echocardiography detects the size, extent, and location of effusions, and permits the identification of loculated effusions (Fig. 104–17). The hemodynamic effects are dependent upon whether the intrapericardial pressure is increased and whether this increase interferes with diastolic filling of the heart. Tamponade is not "all-or-none," but a spectrum from minor to major interference of diastolic filling. Abnormal inspiratory increase in right ventricular size with compensatory decrease in left ventricular size reflects the reciprocal changes in ventricular filling due to tamponade. This is the pathophysiologic correlate of "pulsus paradoxicus." Late diastolic–early systolic inversion of the right atrial free wall (indentation, compression) lasting ≥one-third of the cardiac cycle, is a sensitive but nonspecific sign of tamponade; right ventricular early-diastolic indentation is less sensitive but more specific (Fig. 104–17).[63–67] Doppler echo records the reciprocal variation of right and left ventricular filling and ejection velocities caused by tamponade responsible for "pulsus paradoxicus."[67–69] The Doppler signs can be affected by positive-pressure respiratory breathing, loculated effusions with focal tamponade, abnormal left ventric-

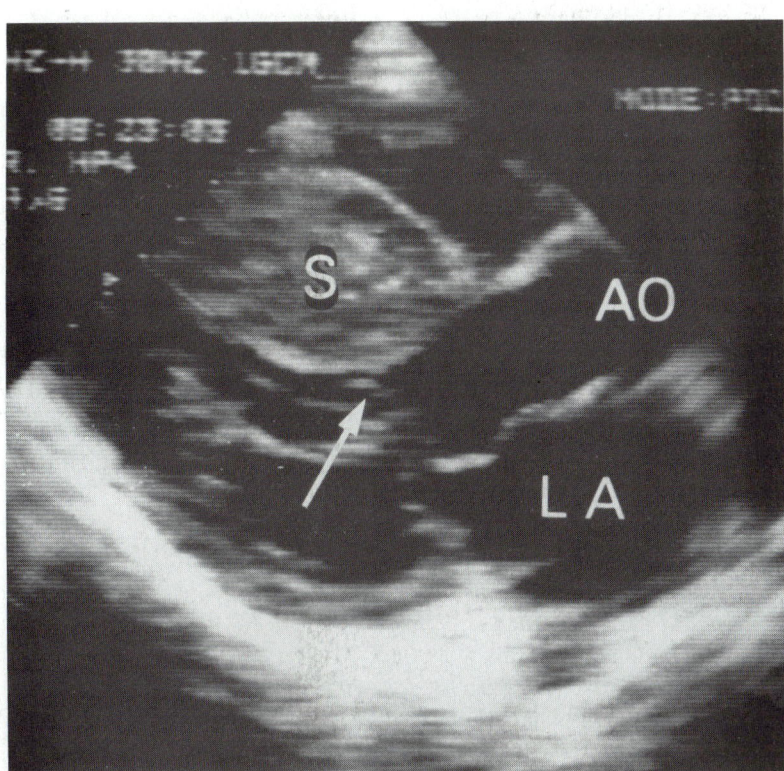

Figure 104–15. Hypertrophic obstructive cardiomyopathy. This parasternal long-axis view shows dynamic left ventricular outflow tract obstruction as a result of systolic anterior motion of the mitral valve (white arrow). The septum (S) is markedly thickened compared to the posterior left ventricular wall. AO, aorta; LA, left atrium.

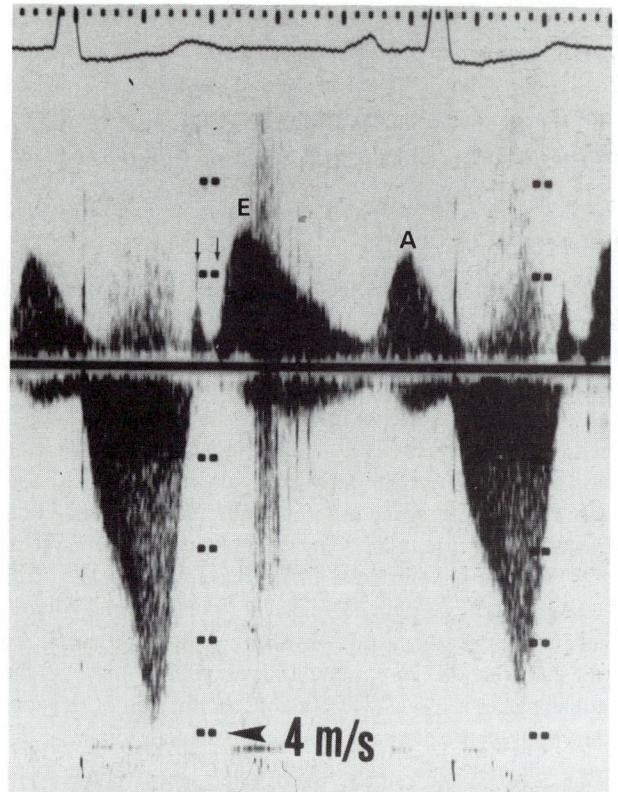

Figure 104–16. Continuous-wave Doppler recording through the left ventricular outflow tract in hypertrophic obstructive cardiomyopathy shows the typical late-peaking profile of dynamic left ventricular outflow tract obstruction. The maximum velocity = 4 m/s consistent with a peak instantaneous gradient = 64 mm Hg. Evidence of increased left atrial pressure is seen by the increased mitral E velocity (∿ 1.5 m/s) and A velocity (∿1.2 m/s). The deceleration time was 300 ms, which reflects abnormal left ventricular relaxation and diastolic dysfunction.

ular diastolic function, pulmonary hypertension, or a nonrestrictive atrial septal defect. The finding that is most likely to be associated with tamponade is a large pericardial effusion, and cardiac tamponade is first a clinical diagnosis.[70,71] 2-D echo assists in directing percutaneous pericardiocentesis.[72]

Constrictive Pericarditis

Detection of a thickened pericardium is unreliable by echocardiography. In constrictive pericarditis, an indirect sign may be abnormal septal motion with both an early and late ("atriosystolic") notch.[73] A dilated inferior vena cava is a nonspecific but useful sign of increased right atrial pressure secondary to constrictive physiology. A Doppler "restrictive physiology pattern" (i.e., elevated atrial pressure pattern) in conjunction with excessive respiratory variation of tricuspid and mitral inflow parameters similar to tamponade may be found.[74]

ACQUIRED VALVULAR HEART DISEASE

Aortic Stenosis

The anatomy of aortic valve is usually visible on a short axis view of the base of the heart. The most common abnormality of the aortic valve observed in adult patients is nonspecific degenerative thickening of a trileaflet aortic valve (Fig. 104–18). Commonly the degree of thickening precludes adequate assessment of the degree of restriction of leaflet motion and, therefore, Doppler pressure gradients are required to evaluate the degree of aortic stenosis (Fig.

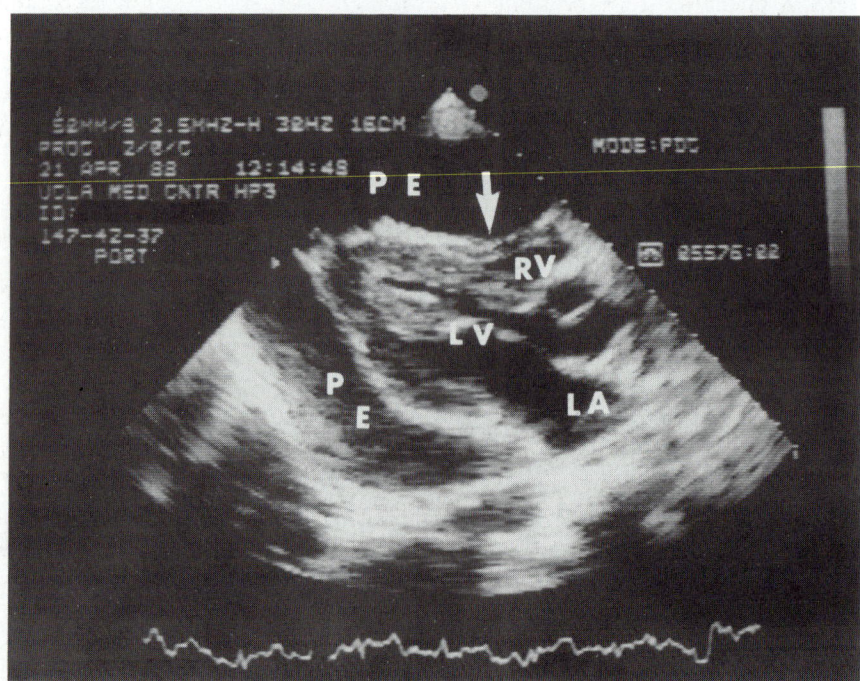

Figure 104–17. Pericardial effusion (PE) with tamponade. Parasternal long-axis view shows a large PE with diastolic compression (arrow) of the right ventricle (RV). LA, left atrium; LV, left ventricle.

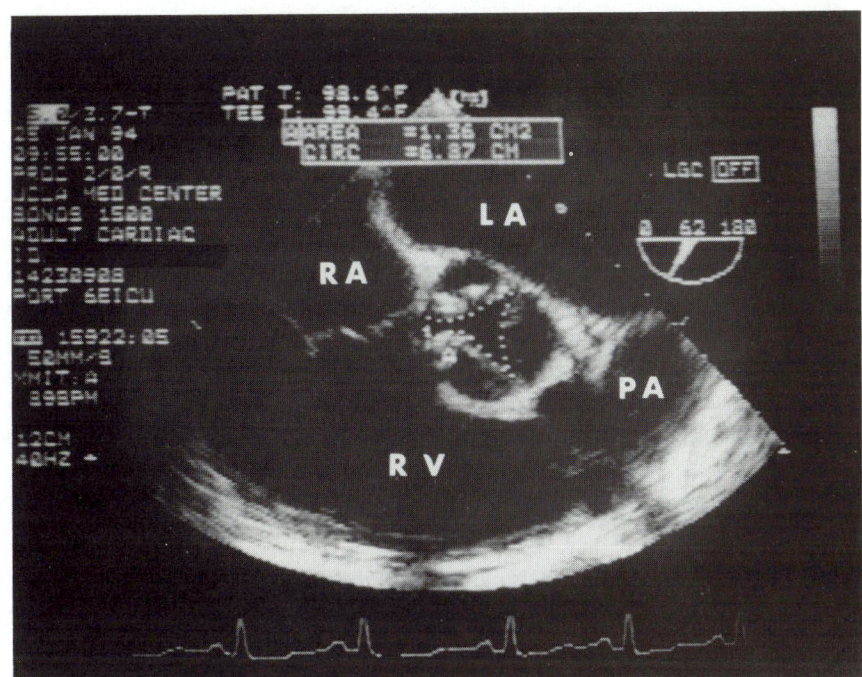

Figure 104–18. Aortic stenosis. The TEE planimetered valve area (outlined with dots) of the systolic orifice of this degenerative trileaflet valve was 1.36 cm^2, which correlated well with Doppler and catheter measurements.

104–5). Planimetered TEE aortic valve areas (Fig. 104–18) correlate well with catheterization and Doppler-derived measurements but will likely be applied only in those patients in whom transthoracic imaging is inadequate to accurately quantitate the aortic valve with Doppler echocardiography.[75]

Doppler echocardiography accurately quantitates the severity of valvular aortic stenosis and has eliminated the need for cardiac catheterization in many patients (Fig. 104–5).[76] Using the simplified Bernoulli equation, the instantaneous peak gradient can be estimated from the peak velocity obtained across the aortic valve. The gradient obtained is an instantaneous peak gradient and is higher than the peak–peak gradient from catheterization data. Aortic valve area calculations using Doppler echocardiography correlate well with Gorlin formula derived calculations.[76]

Echocardiography is useful in the postoperative period after aortic valve replacement to identify a subset of patients who develop hypotension as a result of development of an intraventricular gradient as a result of dynamic left ventricular contraction of a small hypertrophied ventricle.[77] These patients usually require volume and the discontinuation of inotropic agents.

Aortic Regurgitation

Aortic regurgitation is qualitatively graded as mild, moderate, or severe based on the size of the color-flow jet at aortic valve level (Fig. 104–3).[2,3] The area of the jet can directly be measured on the short axis view and compared with the aortic valve annular area. On long axis view, the diameter of the jet at valve level is compared with the diameter of the left ventricular outflow tract. A jet diameter which is >46%

of the left ventricular outflow tract diameter is consistent with moderately severe to severe regurgitation.[78,79]

The deceleration slope of the aortic regurgitant continuous-wave Doppler flow profile represents the decrease in pressure difference between the left ventricle and the aorta throughout diastole and reflects the severity of aortic regurgitation and/or left ventricular end-diastolic pressure.[80] Steep deceleration slopes or rapid pressure half-times (e.g., faster than 2 m/s^2 and less than 400 ms, respectively) are consistent with severe aortic regurgitation and/or an elevated left ventricular end-diastolic pressure. Calculation of aortic regurgitation orifice area using Doppler echocardiography and the continuity equation is feasible and offers the advantage of being load-independent.[81] Prolonged reversal of diastolic flow in the descending aorta is consistent with moderate or greater aortic regurgitation.[2,3]

Mitral Regurgitation

Mitral valve prolapse (MVP) is the most common etiology of severe mitral regurgitation requiring surgical intervention in the general population. Echocardiographic criteria for diagnosis of pathologic MVP includes moderate–severe superior systolic displacement of one or both of the mitral valve leaflets into the left atrium usually associated with some degree of mitral regurgitation (Fig. 104–2).[82] 2-D echocardiographic findings of true pathologic MVP include detection of evidence of myxomatous degeneration with redundant and elongated leaflets, often with a dilated mitral annulas, and of elongated or ruptured chordae tendineae. Left ventricular size and function are useful in evaluating the severity of the mitral regurgitation with mitral valve surgery often recommended based on clinical symptoms or when the end-systolic dimension exceeds 45 mm.[83]

TEE is useful in the preoperative evaluation of valve anatomy and function and to guide operative repair (Fig. 104–19, see Color Plates following page 2072).[84–87] Intimate knowledge by the surgeon and echocardiographer of the mitral apparatus components and mechanisms and etiologies of mitral regurgitation is required (Fig. 104–20, see Color Plates following page 2072). To successfully assist in the evaluation of the surgeon's repair the echocardiographer must be familiar with the various types of repair techniques and how to evaluate the amount of residual mitral regurgitation, and presence of iatrogenic stenosis or left ventricular outflow tract obstruction.

Mitral regurgitation is usually subjectively graded as mild, moderate, or severe based on the color-flow jet area into the left atrium (Fig. 104–2).[88] Estimation of regurgitation is less reliable when the jet is eccentric as opposed to central.[89,90] Because the area of the regurgitant jet alone can be unreliable as an indicator of the severity of mitral regurgitation, the experienced echocardiographer uses several additional findings including systolic reversals of pulmonary venous flow (Fig. 104–21).[92,93] TEE is more sensitive than transthoracic echocardiography in the detection and grading of severity of mitral regurgitation.[91,93–95]

Mitral Stenosis

Rheumatic mitral stenosis, detected as thickened mitral valve leaflets with abnormal tethering of the posterior leaflet to the anterior leaflet, may also have submitral valve apparatus thickening. The mitral valve area can be directly planimetered on the short-axis views and these measurements correlate well with Gorlin formula-derived calculations.[96,97] Mitral inflow Doppler velocity recordings measure the pressure half-time where mitral valve area (cm^2) = (220 ÷ pressure half-time), which correlates well with both planimetered mitral valve areas and Gorlin-derived calculations (Fig. 104–4).[96,97] Echocardiography helps to determine the suitability for balloon valvuloplasty based on the degree of leaflet thickening, submitral apparatus thickening, restriction of motion, and calcification.[2] TEE is used to exclude left atrial thrombi (Fig. 104–12) prior to attempting valvuloplasty and is used to guide positioning of the catheters and balloons.[97]

Right-Sided Valvular Regurgitations

Mild tricuspid and pulmonic regurgitation by color-flow imaging occurs in many normal patients.[2,3] The degree of regurgitation is graded from mild to severe depending on the width and extent of the regurgitant jet. Severe tricuspid regurgitation results in reversed hepatic vein systolic flow detected by Doppler imaging of the hepatic veins. The evaluation of pulmonary artery pressure from the peak tricuspid regurgitant velocity has been discussed; the peak velocity of pulmonary regurgitation can estimate pulmonary artery diastolic pressure. As with mitral valve disease, intraoperative TEE assists in determination of adequacy of tricuspid

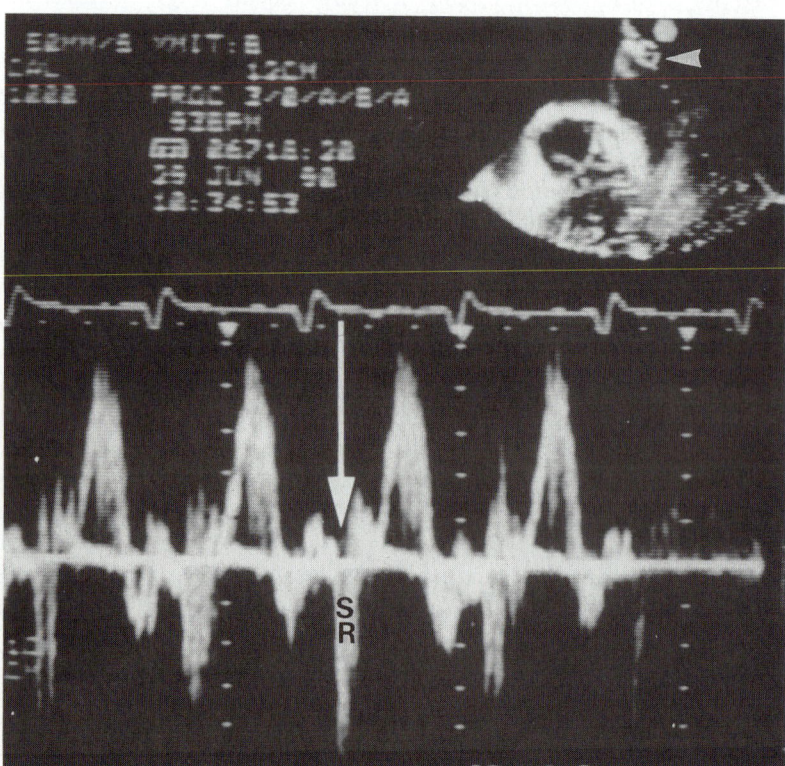

Figure 104–21. Severe mitral regurgitation. Systolic reversal of pulmonary venous flow. Upper panel shows a pulsed-wave Doppler sample volume in the left superior pulmonary vein (white arrowhead) on TEE. The lower panel shows the spectral Doppler recordings with systolic reversal (SR) (arrow shows timing with ECG) of pulmonary venous flow.

valve repair (Fig. 104–22, see Color Plates following page 2072).

Prosthetic Valves

Prosthetic valve function is evaluated by direct two-dimensional observation of leaflet, disc, or ball motion, by color-flow imaging to detect regurgitation, and by spectral Doppler imaging to evaluate prosthetic valve gradients and areas (Figs. 104–23 and 104–24, see Color Plates following page 2072). The echocardiographer must know the type and size of the prosthetic valve as each valve type and size has its own flow characteristics. Doppler echocardiographic examination prior to discharge establishes a normal baseline for the specific patient and valve type and size.[98] On occasion, Doppler-derived gradients significantly exceed catheterization-derived gradients; this has been described for the St. Jude valve, the Carbomedics valve, and the Duromedics valve.[99] The discrepancy results because the catheterization data are derived with placement of the pressure measuring catheter above the aortic valve and pressure recovery plays a role in the measured pressures, whereas Doppler measures gradients at the valve. The gradients associated with mechanical prosthetic valves are not homogeneously distributed across the valve.[100] TEE has greatly assisted in the functional evaluation of prosthetic valves that are not adequately visualized on transthoracic echocardiography for any reason (Fig. 104–23).[101–103] Thrombi, vegetations, and loose sutures can be distinguished from ring or leaflet-induced artifact. TEE is particularly useful in the

evaluation of mitral prostheses because it allows imaging of the left atrial side of the valve, which is poorly visualized by transthoracic echocardiography because of artifact as a result of the valve itself (Fig. 104–23).

Infective Endocarditis

Echocardiography is uniquely able to visualize valvular vegetations directly and quantify regurgitation, evaluate intracardiac hemodynamics, and measure affected chamber dimensions and ventricular function.[2,3] Vegetations (fuzzy, shaggy, irregularly shaped mobile masses attached to valvular tissue or endocardium that do not restrict valve motion) as small as 2 mm can be visualized. Nonspecific thickening, as often seen in degenerative valvular disease, can be difficult to distinguish from true vegetations. If the transthoracic echocardiogram is technically inadequate or if suspicious but nondiagnostic findings are present, TEE is indicated to further assess for the presence of vegetations with a greater than 90% sensitivity in detecting endocarditis (Figs. 104–25 and 104–26).[104–106,108]

Mitral valve vegetations may result in a higher incidence of emboli though studies conflict regarding the relationship of vegetation size and mobility to prognosis.[104–107] TEE is superior to transthoracic echocardiography in detecting abscesses and prosthetic valve vegetations.[108–110] Leaflet disruption (observed as torn or flail leaflets, ruptured chordae, and regurgitation), abscesses (e.g., in the annular rings of the aortic and mitral valves), and fistulae between cardiac chambers as a result of erosion through

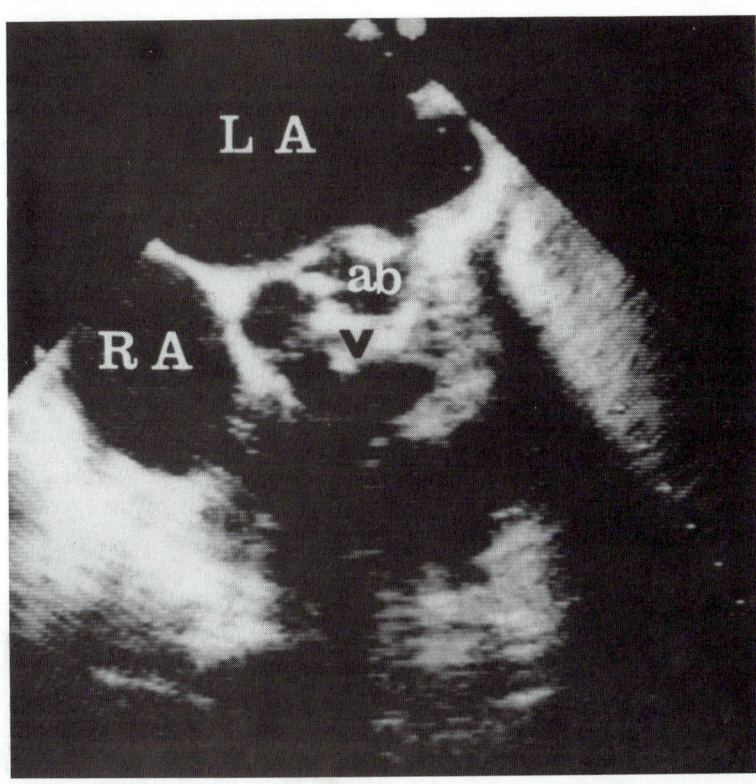

Figure 104–25. TEE in aortic valve endocarditis and ring abscess. The aortic valve vegetation (v) has extended into the annulus near the left coronary cusp and formed an abscess (ab). LA, left atrium; RA, right atrium.

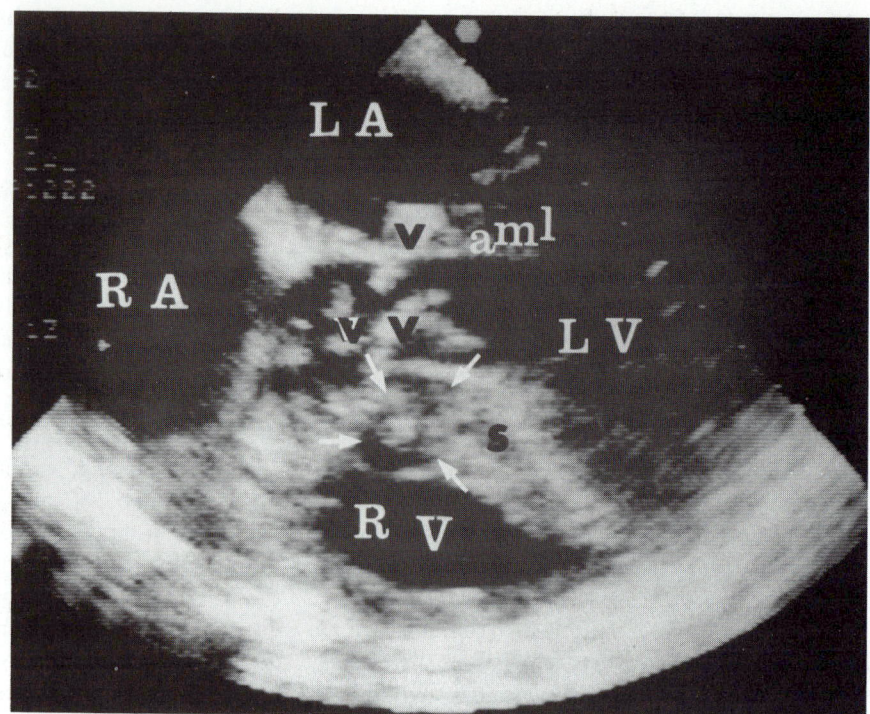

Figure 104–26. TEE in aortic valve endocarditis with septal abscess and invasion of aortic-mitral intervalvular fibrosa. The aortic valve vegetations (v) prolapse into the left ventricular outflow tract. A vegetation can be seen perforating the base of the anterior mitral leaflet (aml) where it attaches to the aortic annulus, i.e., the intervalvular fibrosa. An abscess is seen as an echolucent space involving the proximal ventricular septum (s) (white arrows). LA, left atrium; LV, left ventricle; RA, right atrium; RV, right ventricle.

chamber walls from direct extension of the infection have important surgical implications. Abscesses, most commonly seen at the aortic ring or with a prosthetic valve, more than double the risk of complications (Figs. 104–25 and 104–26). Aortic valve endocarditis can be associated with aneurysms formation at the level of the mitral–aortic intervalvular fibrosa with or without perforation or the mitral valve apparatus can be secondarily infected by an aortic regurgitant jet (Fig. 104–26).

A negative TEE for suspected endocarditis substantially reduces the likelihood of endocarditis, but does not explicitly rule it out.[111] If a patient continues to have unexplained bacteremia or is at high risk of endocarditis because of a prosthetic valve or other significant cardiac lesion, it is reasonable to repeat the TEE study as clinically indicated.

ECHOCARDIOGRAPHY IN THE CRITICAL CARE PATIENT

An important specific role for echocardiography, using the principles that have preceded this section, is in problem solving in the intensive care unit and the critically ill patient (Table 104–1).[15] Limited acoustic windows (due to bandages, wounds, or inability to properly position the patient) often preclude an adequate transthoracic echo and TEE is frequently needed for a complete evaluation (Table 104–2). Even when the transthoracic echocardiogram is technically good, some specific questions virtually require a transesophageal echocardiogram. Diagnosis of infective endocarditis and its complications were discussed earlier (Figs. 104–25, 104–26). Aortic dissection in the patient with chest

pain, aortic regurgitation, or hypotension must be promptly recognized using TEE (Fig. 104–7). Hypoxemia may be a result of pulmonary embolism, acute respiratory distress syndrome, pulmonary edema, etc., but can also be caused by elevated right atrial pressure and a patent foramen ovale that requires echocontrast to search for the right-to-left shunt at atrial level. Direct visualization of a patent foramen ovale often necessitates TEE. Search for an embolic source in general is more effective using TEE as is identification of thrombosis at the site of superior vena cava catheters or at anastomoses for lung or cardiac transplantation.

One of the most frequent reasons for requesting echocardiography in the critically ill patient is to search for the cause of hypotension, e.g., pericardial tamponade (Fig. 104–17), myocardial infarction or dysfunction, or pulmonary embolism. Hypovolemia or sepsis as a cause of hypotension may be suspected when the only finding is that the ventricles are small and contracting vigorously.

Another clinical problem is identification of the cause of chest pain, dyspnea, or pulmonary edema, e.g., pulmonary embolism, myocardial ischemia/infarction, or acute severe aortic or mitral regurgitation. Complications of myocardial infarction such as ventricular aneurysms or thrombi, intra- or extracardiac rupture, and mitral regurgitation as a result of "papillary muscle dysfunction" are well detected by echocardiography (Figs. 104–10 and 104–14).

Echocardiographic imaging can provide an adjunct to therapy. Transthoracic echocardiography can direct needle position for pericardiocentesis. TEE can evaluate the response to ventricular assist devices and can direct nonfluoroscopic positioning of an intraaortic counterpulsation balloon in the upper aorta below the left subclavian.

CONGENITAL HEART DISEASE

Simple lesions include isolated shunts and regions of obstruction or valvular regurgitation. Complex lesions are usually a combination of simple lesions, are usually cyanotic, and often have cardiac malpositions or transpositions.

Detection and Sizing of Shunts

Shunt location is usually readily anatomically identified by two-dimensional echocardiographic imaging if the shunt site is large and the acoustic window acceptable. Intravenous echo-contrast (e.g., agitated saline) reveals low-pressure right-to-left atrial shunts. Spectral and color-flow Doppler has proven indispensable in identifying the location and direction of shunts, particularly when small. Physiologic size of a shunt can qualitatively be inferred from the effects on the receiving chambers of the shunt.

Atrial Septal Defect

Atrial septal defect (ASD) type is defined by the location in the atrial septum (Figs. 104–27, see Color Plates following page 2072, and 104–28). Two-dimensional imaging reveals right ventricular dilatation and abnormal ventricular septal motion as a result of the volume overload. The sinus venosus ASD is the most difficult to image by transthoracic echo and TEE is usually required for this diagnosis in the adult (Fig. 104–28).[1,11,12] To determine the presence and degree of pulmonary hypertension, CW Doppler of the tricuspid regurgitant velocity is needed (Fig. 104–6).

Ventricular Septal Defect

Ventricular septal defect (VSD), classified by location, size, whether muscular or nonmuscular, and alignment (malalignment or alignment), is common as an isolated defect or as a component of a complex malformation. The most common location is in the perimembranous area; other sections of the ventricular septum include the inlet, trabeculated (muscular), and outflow (infundibular) regions. Malalignment defects occur with more complex anomalies including tetralogy of Fallot, double outlet ventricles, and truncus arteriosus. Infundibular defects (outlet, supracristal, subpulmonary) may be muscular or may be rimmed by a semilunar valve.

The functional disturbance of any VSD depends on the defect size and the level of pulmonary vascular resistance.[1] Defect size is best defined hemodynamically as nonrestrictive (left and right ventricular systolic pressures equalize) or restrictive (systolic gradient from left to right ventricle). The color-flow image can be used to align the continuous-wave Doppler beam with the vector of the VSD jet to provide the left-to-right ventricular gradient using the modified Bernoulli formula. Partial or complete spontaneous closure

is associated with septal aneurysm and/or overlying tricuspid tissue.

Ruptured Sinus of Valsalva Aneurysm

This is readily detectable by two-dimensional echo imaging with right and noncoronary cusps, the most frequently involved; color-flow imaging readily reveals the defect (Fig. 104–29, see Color Plates following page 2072).

Patent Ductus Arteriosus

Direct two-dimensional echo imaging of the patent ductus arteriosus (PDA) is done from high left parasternal and suprasternal notch windows to image the main pulmonary artery and bifurcation as well as the descending aorta and in conjunction with color-flow imaging shows continuous high velocity flow from the aorta, which emerges into the pulmonary trunk bifurcation.

Aorticopulmonary Window

Two-dimensional echo images may detect the defect but often have false dropout in this region. Color-flow imaging will show continuous flow from systole through diastole originating in the aorta and traversing the defect.

Coronary Artery Anomalies

These abnormalities are better detected by transesophageal than transthoracic echocardiography. Anomalous connections of the coronary arteries, such as anomalous origin of the left coronary artery from the pulmonary trunk, may cause shunting of blood from the coronary bed and may result in myocardial ischemia or infarction and a left-to-right shunt. Other coronary anomalies coronary arteriovenous fistulae isolated ostial malpositions (sometimes related to sudden death) and abnormal coronary connections and courses (transpositions, tetralogy of Fallot) and can have surgical significance.

OBSTRUCTIVE AND REGURGITANT LESIONS

Right Ventricular Inflow Lesions

Ebstein's anomaly, identified by apical two-dimensional echocardiography because of the abnormal apical displacement of the tricuspid leaflets, is used to evaluate the mobility of the anterior tricuspid leaflet and the function of the residual functioning right ventricle in anticipation of surgical repair.[1,113,114] Color-flow imaging semiquantitates the tricuspid regurgitant jet emerging from the apically displaced leaflets and can detect associated right-to-left shunting via an interatrial communication.

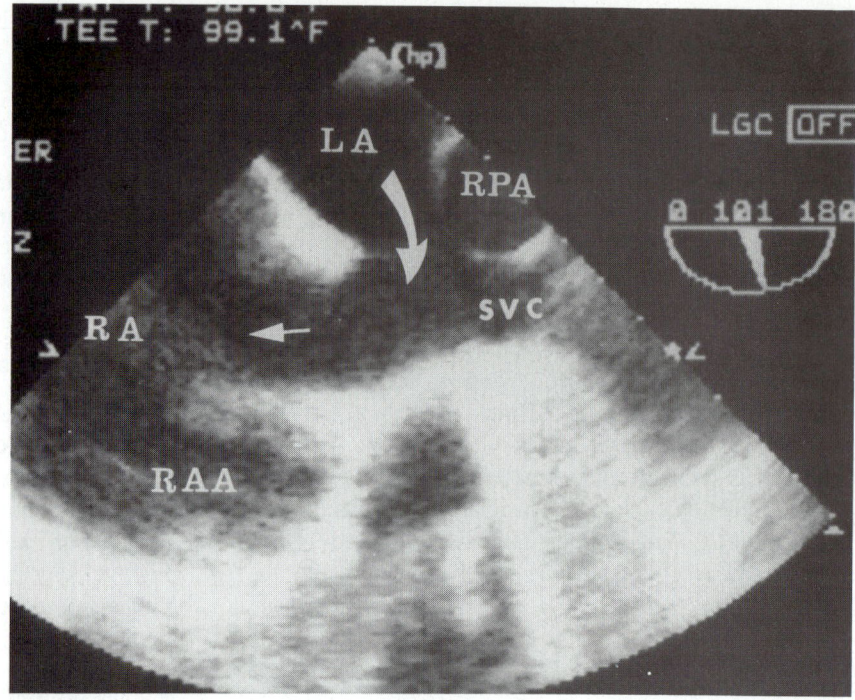

A

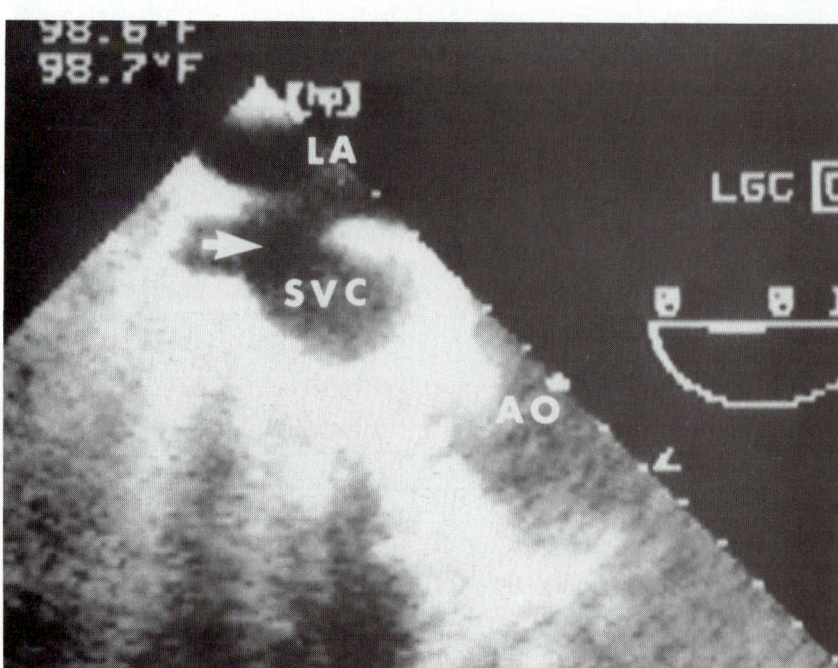

B

Figure 104–28. Sinus venosus atrial septal defect (ASD) and partial anomalous pulmonary venous connection (PAPVC). **A.** Vertical plane TEE view of the sinus venosus ASD (curved arrow) into the superior vena cava (SVC) from the left atrium (LA) before the SVC enters the right atrium (RA) (straight arrow). RAA, right atrial appendage; RPA right pulmonary artery. **B.** Transverse or horizontal plane TEE view of the SVC shows a PAPVC into the right side of the SVC. The sinus venosus ASD is seen at the 12 O'clock position of the SVC. AO, aorta.

Right Ventricular Outflow Obstruction

Isolated pulmonary valve stenosis is diagnosed by imaging a doming or thickened pulmonary valve with an increased velocity across the valve by Doppler.[1] Other sites of obstruction (subvalvar, supravalvar) are readily detected by combined two-dimensional echo and color-flow imaging and PW Doppler mapping and severity is best defined by CW Doppler.[1,112]

Left Ventricular Inflow Obstruction

Congenital obstruction to left ventricular inflow includes cor triatriatum, supravalvar mitral ring, double orifice mitral valve, and parachute mitral valve and is detected by combined echo and color-flow imaging. For pulmonary venous obstruction, best done with transesophageal echocardiography, careful attention must be directed to the entrance of the pulmonary veins as they enter the left atrium.[1,11,12]

Left Ventricular Outflow Obstruction

Left ventricular outflow obstruction may be valvar, sub-valvar (e.g., discrete membranous, muscular or tunnel) (Fig. 104–30), or supravalvar. Two-dimensional imaging reveals the anatomic deformity and ventricular dynamics whereas color-flow imaging shows the site of obstruction. CW Doppler is directed throughout the stenotic site from multiple windows to obtain the maximum velocity and the gradient determined. In the case of valvar aortic stenosis, the aortic valve area is derived from the continuity equation.

An unusual cause of "subaortic" outflow obstruction is a restrictive "VSD" at the bulboventricular foramen in some patients with single ventricle.[1,115] The bulboventricular foramen provides the connection from the main ventricular chamber to an outflow chamber, which gives rise to the aorta (thus, "subaortic stenosis"). Anatomic definition is readily achieved by combined two-dimensional and color-flow imaging with quantitation of the gradient by continuous-wave Doppler. Identification of this subgroup of patients with single ventricle is crucial prior to operative intervention because of their higher morbidity and mortality rate.

Aortic Coarctation

Coarctation of the aorta is often readily imaged on two-dimensional echocardiography in the young but is more difficult in the adult. Transesophageal echocardiography is virtually essential for complete echo evaluation.[11,12] With surface echo, from the suprasternal position, pulsed and continuous-wave Doppler can show obstruction even when the echo images are less than clear. The peak systolic velocity is useful in estimating the maximum gradient. Persistent diastolic high velocities signify diastolic obstruction, which confirms that the coarctation is hemodynamically important. The diameter of the color flow at the coarctation and the rate of narrowing of the zone of acceleration in the descending aorta proximal to the zone of obstruction are predictive of the angiographic severity.

CONOTRUNCAL AND COMPLEX MALFORMATIONS

Most of these malformations are cyanotic. They include a mix of septal defects, obstructive and regurgitant lesions, and malpositions of the cardiac chambers or arteries. Whether they reach adulthood unoperated depends upon the balance of pulmonary bloodflow. If excessive pulmonary flow exists, pulmonary hypertension usually develops. Pulmonary stenosis protects the pulmonary vasculature proportional to the degree of the stenosis; excessive stenosis results in pulmonary oligemia and increased right-to-left shunting with resulting excessive cyanosis and erythrocytosis. Examples include tetralogy of Fallot (the most severe form being pulmonary atresia with VSD and aorticopulmonary collaterals), transposition of the great arteries, trun-

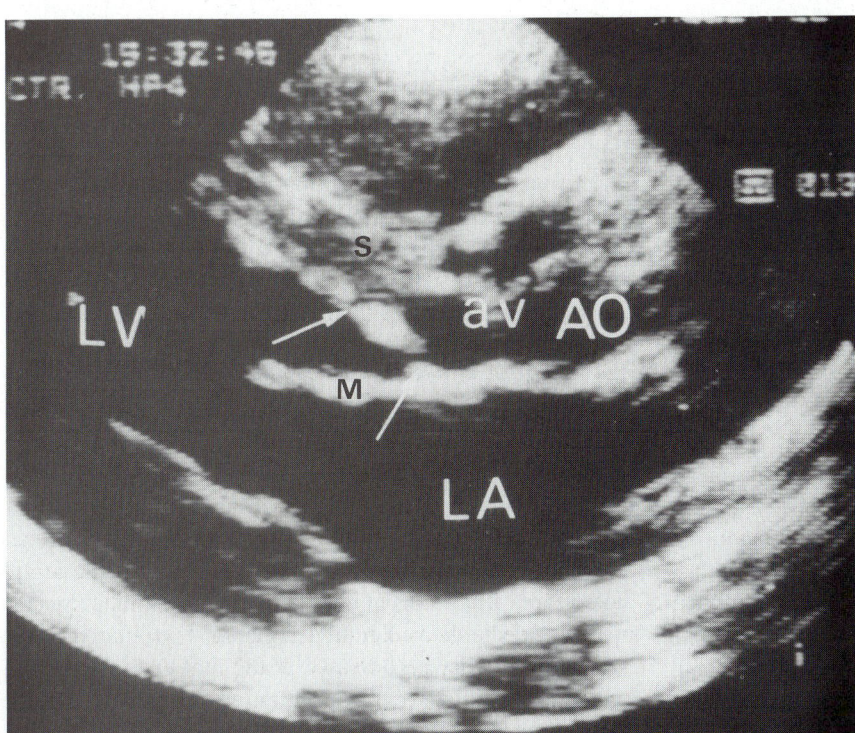

Figure 104–30. Discrete subaortic stenosis. Parasternal long-axis view shows a discrete fibrous obstruction (arrows) in the outflow tract of the left ventricle (LV) with attachments both to the ventricular septum (S) and base of the anterior mitral (M) leaflet. CW Doppler showed a 5 m/s velocity (100 mm Hg gradient) and the aortic valve (av) was mildly incompetent on color-flow imaging (not shown). AO, aorta.

cus arteriosus, univentricular hearts (tricuspid atresia, single ventricle), and total anomalous pulmonary venous connection.

The importance of integrating anatomic and hemodynamic information from all available imaging and flow data in these complex malformations is demonstrated by the tetralogy of Fallot (Fig. 104–31, see Color Plates following page 2072).[112] With coexistent right ventricular outflow obstruction and a nonrestrictive malaligned VSD, the greater the severity of the pulmonary stenosis the greater the right-to-left shunt, and, as such, the velocity across the pulmonary stenosis is lower than otherwise would be found for isolated right ventricular outflow obstruction of equivalent severity. A high-velocity tricuspid regurgitant jet will reflect a right ventricle ejecting simultaneously with the left ventricle at systemic pressure but given pulmonic stenosis should not be misinterpreted as demonstrating pulmonary hypertension.

"Double chambered right ventricle," an entity that may mimic but is separate from tetralogy of Fallot, must also be recognized.[1] This consists of a large perimembranous VSD with mid-right ventricular obstruction as a result of anomalous muscle bundles. These anomalous muscle bundles are hypertrophied and abnormally positioned (probably because of a malalignment between the trabecular and anteriorly displaced infundibular septum). They can be seen as echodense structures protruding at right angles to the infundibular septum and free wall, which divides the right ventricle into an upper chamber connected to the pulmonary artery and a lower chamber connecting with the VSD.

In transposition complexes, combined two-dimensional echocardiography and color-flow imaging not only allow easier definition of the course of each of the great arteries but also ease the task of assessing the common associated lesions. These include identification of the size and location of a VSD, presence and severity of pulmonic stenosis, detection of other shunts (ASD, PDA), and evaluation of the presence and severity of valvular regurgitation. Congenitally corrected transposition has a high incidence of an "Ebstein's-like" malformation of the left-sided atrioventricular valve (anatomically tricuspid) with consequent tricuspid regurgitation that may be mislabeled "mitral regurgitation."

In univentricular hearts, pulmonary artery pressure and bulboventricular foramen obstruction are two major determinants of the surgical outcome after Fontan repair. The function of the left or single ventricle, presence and amount of atrioventricular valve regurgitation, severity of pulmonary stenosis, and if present, size of any previous palliative aortopulmonary shunt help assess the likelihood of an increased mean pulmonary artery pressure.[1,115]

Anomalies of pulmonary venous connection are often difficult to assess using transthoracic two-dimensional echocardiography alone and suspicion of their presence dictates transesophageal examination if definition is clinically important preoperatively.[11,12]

POSTOPERATIVE CONGENITAL HEART DISEASE

Proper evaluation and care of postoperative congenital heart disease patients require knowledge of the type of operation, presence and extent of postoperative residua, sequelae, and complications. Intraoperative transesophageal and epicardial echocardiography are important adjuncts to direct surgical inspection when preoperative diagnostic studies are inconclusive or when the initial response to repair is unsatisfactory.[11,12]

Palliative Shunts

Palliative systemic arterial to pulmonary arterial shunts (Blalock–Taussig, Waterston, Pott's) are performed for malformations characterized by decreased pulmonary arterial flow, e.g., tetralogy of Fallot, more so in the past before intracardiac repairs were available. The shunts from the high pressure aorta to the low pressure pulmonary artery can be assessed for patency by the use of continuous-wave Doppler, which should reveal nonlaminar flow in both systole and diastole toward the pulmonary artery. The Waterston (ascending aorta–pulmonary artery) and Pott's (descending aorta–left pulmonary artery) are discrete side-to-side connections and can be assessed by continuous-wave Doppler. TEE effectively visualizes these shunts.[11,12]

Valvular Sequelae and Residua

Bicuspid aortic valves are frequent in patients with aortic coarctation and continue to pose risks of progressive stenosis, regurgitation, and endocarditis despite coarctation repair. Variations on a parachute mitral valve, also associated with coarctation and other stenoses in sequence on the left sided circulation, may be detected by searching for a decreased interpapillary muscle distance and Doppler evidence of inflow obstruction. Repair of an ostium primum atrial septal defect includes repair of the cleft mitral valve; residual mitral regurgitation may be noted. Furthermore, subaortic discrete stenosis may coexist and should be recognized. In the repair of tetralogy of Fallot, important valvar pulmonary regurgitation may be a sequel to a valvulotomy or transannular incision and patch performed to relieve valvar, subvalvar, or annular stenosis.[112] Isolated mild–moderate low-pressure pulmonic regurgitation is both common and well-tolerated. Severe pulmonic regurgitation may cause right ventricular failure and tricuspid regurgitation, particularly if there is any residual right ventricular outflow, pulmonary valve, or pulmonary artery (e.g., branch stenosis) obstruction.[112] Muscular ventricular septal defects may have been missed (or not sought preoperatively) and should be sought using color-flow imaging. Lesions associated with a dilated aortic root or trunk include tetralogy of Fallot, or transposition of the great arteries or single ventricle in association with pulmonic stenosis, and, of course, truncus arteriosus, commonly have aortic regurgitation that can become progressive.[1] Atrioventricular valve regurgitation is common preoperatively in Fontan candidates and may progress postoperatively. After either homograft aortic valve replacement or the Ross procedure (pulmonary autograft insertion into the aortic position, reimplantation of coronaries, tissue heterograft or homograft replacement of pulmonary valve) postoperative "neoaortic" regurgitation must be sought.[116] Evaluation of coronary anatomy pre- and postoperatively can in part be done by echocardiography.[117]

Intraventricular Surgery

In complex congenital malformations that are amenable to "biventricular repair," surgical interventions result in two well-formed functional ventricles with a subpulmonic ventricle and a subaortic ventricle that are able to provide a circulation in series without admixture of venous and systemic blood. A unifying theme includes patch closure of a ventricular septal defect and reconstitution of ventricular to pulmonary arterial bloodflow. Examples of anatomic substrates that are usually candidates for "biventricular repair" include conotruncal abnormalities such as tetralogy of Fallot (the most severe form being pulmonary atresia with ventricular septal defect and aortic-to-pulmonary arterial collaterals), transposition complexes of the great arteries, double outlet right or left ventricle, and truncus arteriosus.

In some anatomic substrates, e.g., double outlet right ventricle, the ventricular septal defect is baffled by an internal conduit to the aorta, which exits the right ventricle to allow left ventricular ejection of blood into the aorta. If pulmonic stenosis cannot be directly repaired for anatomic or conduction system reasons, a ventricular to pulmonary arterial conduit must be placed. Long-term survival depends upon a number of variables including age at operation, degree of relief of the loading conditions imposed upon the ventricular myocardium, myocardial protection during operation, electrophysiologic sequelae, and durability of prosthetic materials, especially valved or nonvalved conduits.

Intraatrial Surgery

Malformations where biventricular connections are not usually possible include functionally or anatomically univentricular hearts, complex straddling of atrioventricular valves, or criss-cross relationships whereby two functioning ventricles may not be effectively established. Many such patients may undergo one of the variations on Fontan connections or Glenn shunts, partially covered below, full details of which are found in a separate chapter.

Fontan Repair

The Fontan repair results in the complete or nearly complete (hemi-Fontan) separation of the pulmonary and systemic circulations in patients not eligible for biventricular

repair. The several variations are described elsewhere in this book. The most commonly encountered complications in the atrial portion of the Fontan circulation include cavo-atrial shunting, atrial septal shunting, thrombus, and right atrial to pulmonary artery obstruction. Surgical sequelae purposely left behind in high-risk patients include atrial fenestrations and adjustable ASDs. An important determinant of outcome is the function of the systemic ventricle and its atrioventricular valve, both of which are usually readily interrogated by transthoracic echo and Doppler. TEE is indicated for suspected complications or the Fontan atrial anatomy.[11,12]

With intraatrial switch surgical baffles (Mustard, Senning), mid-baffle obstruction and/or pulmonary or systemic venous obstruction may develop, which is reflected in a distinct high velocity turbulent flow pattern localized at the site of stenosis by color-flow imaging and pulsed Doppler.

Glenn Shunts

The classic Glenn shunt involves an end-to-side anastomosis of the right superior vena cava to the right pulmonary artery and ligation of the right pulmonary artery at its attachment to the main pulmonary trunk. Some with Glenn shunts develop arteriovenous fistulae in the right lung. Contrast echocardiography is a practical way to assess for these extracardiac right-to-left shunts in those with Glenn shunts and recurrence of cyanosis late postoperatively. These fistulae are amenable to catheter intervention and coil embolization.

REFERENCES

1. Child JS: Echo-Doppler and color-flow imaging in congenital heart disease. *Cardiol Clin* **8:**289–313, 1990
2. Weyman AE: *Principles and Practice of Echocardiography,* 2nd ed. Philadelphia, Lea & Febiger, 1994
3. Feigenbaum H: *Echocardiography,* 5th ed. Philadelphia, Lea & Febiger, 1994
4. Seward JB, Khanderia BK, Edwards WD, et al: Biplanar transesophageal echocardiography: Anatomic correlations, image orientation, and clinical applications. *Mayo Clin Proc* **65:**1193–1213, 1990
5. Nanda NC, Pinheiro L, Sanyal RS, Storey O: Transesophageal biplane echocardiographic imaging: Technique, planes, and clinical usefulness. *Echocardiography* **7:**771–788, 1990
6. Bansal RC, Shakudo M, Shah PM: Biplane transesophageal echocardiography: Technique, image orientation, and preliminary experience in 131 patients. *J Am Soc Echo Cardiogr* **3:**348–366, 1990
7. Seward JB, Khanderia BK, Oh JK, et al: Critical appraisal of transesophageal echocardiography: Limitations, pitfalls, and complications. *J Am Soc Echocardiogr* **5:**288–305, 1992
8. Blanchard DG, Dittrich HC, Mitchell M, McCann HA: Diagnostic pitfalls in transesophageal echocardiography. *J Am Soc Echocardiogr* **5:**525–540, 1992
9. Schneider AT, Hsu TL, Schwartz SL, Pandian NG: Single, biplane, multiplane and three-dimensional transesophageal echocardiography. Echocardiographic-anatomic correlations. *Cardiol Clin* **11:**361–387, 1993

10. Seward JB, Khanderia BK, Freeman WK, et al: Multiplane transesophageal echocardiography: Image orientation, examination technique, anatomic correlations, and clinical applications. *Mayo Clin Proc* **68:**523–551, 1993

11. Marelli AJ, Child JS, Perloff JK: Transesophageal echocardiography in congenital heart disease in the adult. *Cardiol Clin* **11:**505–520, 1993

12. Child JS, Marelli AJ: The application of transesophageal echocardiography in the adult with congenital heart disease. In Maurer G (ed): *Transesophageal Echocardiography.* New York, McGraw Hill, 1994, pp 159–188

13. Saxon LA, Stevenson WG, Fonarow GC, et al: Transesophageal echocardiography to guide catheter energy delivery and catheter position during radiofrequency catheter ablation of ventricular tachycardia. *Am J Cardiol* **72:**658–661, 1993

14. Lai WW, Al-Khatib Y, Klitzner TS, et al: Biplanar transesophageal echocardiographic direction of radiofrequency catheter ablation in children and adolescents. *Am J Cardiol* **71:**872–874, 1993

15. Foster E, Schiller NB: Transesophageal echocardiography in the critical care patient. *Cardiol Clin* **11:**489–503, 1993

16. Losordo DW, Pastore JO, Coletta D, et al: Limitations of color flow Doppler imaging in the quantification of valvular regurgitation: Velocity of regurgitant jet, rather than volume, determines size of color Doppler image. *Am Heart J* **126:**168–176, 1993

17. Schiller NB: Pulmonary artery pressure estimation by Doppler and two-dimensional echocardiography. *Cardiol Clin* **8:**277–287, 1990

18. Goldstein SA, Mintz GS, Lindsay J Jr: Aorta: Comprehensive evaluation by echocardiography and transesophageal echocardiography. *J Am Soc Echocardiogr* **6:**634–659, 1993

19. Aldrich HR, Labarre RL, Roman MJ, et al: Color flow and conventional echocardiography of the Marfan syndrome. *Echocardiography* **9:**627–636, 1992

20. Erbel R, Engberding R, Daniel W, et al: Echocardiography in diagnosis of aortic dissection. *Lancet* **1:**457–461, 1989

21. Simon P, Owen AN, Havel M, et al: Transesophageal echocardiography in the emergency surgical management of patients with aortic dissection. *J Thorac Cardiovasc Surg* **103:**1113–1118, 1992

22. Erbel R, Oelert H, Meyer J, et al for the European Cooperative Study Group on Echocardiography: Effect of medical and surgical therapy on aortic dissection evaluated by transesophageal echocardiography; implications for prognosis and therapy. *Circulation* **87:**1604–1615, 1993

23. Nienaber CA, von Kodolitsch Y, Nicolas V, et al: The diagnosis of thoracic aortic dissection by noninvasive imaging procedures. *N Engl J Med* **328:**1–9, 1993

24. Ballal RS, Nanda NC, Gatewood R, et al: Usefulness of transesophageal echocardiography in assessment of aortic dissection. *Circulation* **84:**1903–1914, 1991

25. Mohr-Kahaly S, Erbel R, Kearney P, et al: Aortic intramural hemorrhage visualized by transesophageal echocardiography: Findings and prognostic implications. *J Am Coll Cardiol* **23:**658–664, 1994

26. Marshall WG Jr, Barzilai B, Kouchoukas NT, Saffitz I: Intraoperative ultrasonic imaging of the ascending aorta. *Ann Thorac Surg* **48:**339–344, 1989

27. Sangwan S, Child JS, Laks H: Biplane transesophageal echocardiography (TEE) and intraoperative assessment of ascending aortic atheromatous plaque (abstr). *J Am Soc Echo* **6:**532, 1993

28. Katz ES, Tunick PA, Rusinek H, et al: Protruding aortic athroma predict stroke in elderly patients undergoing cardiopulmonary bypass: Experience with intra-operative transesophageal echocardiography. *J Am Coll Cardiol* **20:**70–77, 1992

29. Reeder GS, Khanderia BK, Seward JB, Tajik AJ: Transesophageal echocardiography and cardiac masses. *Mayo Clin Proc* **66:**1101–1109, 1991

30. Mugge A, Daniel WG, Haverich A, Lichtlen PR: Diagnosis of noninfective cardiac mass lesions by two-dimensional echocardiography. Comparison of transthoracic and transesophageal approaches. *Circulation* **83:**70–783, 1991

31. Hsu T-L, Hsiung M-C, Lin S-L, et al: The value of transesophageal echocardiography in the diagnosis of cardiac metastasis. *Echocardiography* **9:**1–7, 1992

32. Faletra F, Ravini M, Moreo A, et al: Transesophageal echocardiography in the evaluation of mediastinal masses. *J Am Soc Echocardiogr* **5:**178–186, 1992

33. Dressler FA, Labovitz AJ: Systemic arterial emboli and cardiac masses. Assessment with transesophageal echocardiography. *Cardiol Clin* **11:**447–460, 1993

34. DeRook FA, Commess KA, Albers GW, Popp RL: Transesophageal echocardiography in the evaluation of stroke. *Ann Intern Med* **117:**922–932, 1992

35. Pearson AC, Labovitz AJ, Tatineni S, Gomez CR: Superiority of transesophageal echocardiography in detecting cardiac source of embolism in patients with ischemia of uncertain etiology. *J Am Coll Cardiol* **17:**66–72, 1991

36. Armstrong WF, O'Donnell J, Dillon JC, et al: Complementary value of two-dimensional exercise echocardiography to routine treadmill exercise testing. *Ann Intern Med* **105:**829–835, 1986

37. Armstrong WF, O'Donnell J, Ryan T, Feigenbaum H: Effect of prior myocardial infarction and extent and location of coronary disease on accuracy of exercise echocardiography. *J Am Coll Cardiol* **10:**531–538, 1987

38. Ryan T, Vasey CG, Presti CF, et al: Exercise echocardiography: Detection of coronary artery disease in patients with normal left ventricular wall motion at rest. *J Am Coll Cardiol* **11:**993–999, 1988

39. Crouse LJ, Harbrecht JJ, Vacek JL, et al: Exercise echocardiography as a screening test for coronary artery disease and correlation with coronary arteriography. *Am J Cardiol* **67:**1213–1218, 1991

40. Marwick TH, Nemec JJ, Pashkow FJ, et al: Accuracy and limitations of exercise echocardiography in a routine clinical setting. *J Am Coll Cardiol* **19:**74–81, 1992

41. Cohen JL, Greene TO, Ottenweller J, et al: Dobutamine digital echocardiography for detecting coronary artery disease. *Am J Cardiol* **67:**1311–1318, 1991

42. Sawada SG, Segar DS, Ryan T, et al: Echocardiographic detection of coronary artery disease during dobutamine infusion. *Circulation* **83:**1605–1614, 1991

43. Segar DS, Brown SE, Sawada SG, et al: Dobutamine stress echocardiography: Correlation with coronary lesion as determined by quantitative angiography. *J Am Coll Cardiol* **19:**1197–1202, 1992

44. Marcovitz PA, Armstrong WF: Accuracy of dobutamine stress echocardiography in detecting coronary artery disease. *Am J Cardiol* **1269:**1269–1273, 1992

45. Marwick T, D'Hondt A, Baudhuin T, et al: Optimal use of dobutamine stress for the detection and evaluation of coronary artery disease: Combination with echocardiography or scintigraphy, or both? *J Am Coll Cardiol* **22:**159–167, 1993

46. Picano E, Lattanzi F: Dipyridamole echocardiography: A new diagnostic window on coronary artery disease. *Circulation* **83** suppl III:III 19–III 26, 1991

47. Picano E, Lattanzi F, Masini M, et al: High dose dipyridamole echocardiography test in effort angina pectoris. *J Am Coll Cardiol* **8:**848–854, 1986

48. Picano E, Masini M, Lattanzi F, et al: Role of dipyridamole-echocardiography test in electrocardiographically silet effort myocardial ischemia. *Am J Cardiol* **1986:**235–237, 1993

49. Krivokapich J, Child JS, Gerber RS, et al: Prognostic usefulness of positive or negative exercise stress echocardiography for predicting coronary events in ensuing twelve months. *Am J Cardiol* **71:**646–651, 1993

50. Ryan T, Armstrong WF, O'Donnell JA, Feigenbaum H: Risk stratification after acute myocardial infarction by means of exercise two dimensional echocardiography. *Am Heart J* **114:**1305–1316, 1987

51. Applegate RJ, Dell'Italia LJ, Crawford MH: Usefulness of two-

dimensional echocardiography during low-level exercise testing early after uncomplicated acute myocardial infarction. *Am J Cardiol* **60:**10–14, 1987

52. Nishimura RA, Abel MD, Hatle LK, et al: Assessment of diastolic function of the heart: Background and current application of Doppler echocardiography II. Clinical studies. *Mayo Clin Proc* **64:**181–204, 1989

53. Appleton CP, Galloway JM, Gonzalez MS, et al: Estimation of left ventricular filling pressures using two-dimensional and Doppler echocardiography in adult patients with cardiac disease. *J Am Coll Cardiol* **22:**1972–1982, 1993

54. Rossvoll O, Hatle LK: Pulmonary venous flow velocities recorded by transthoracic Doppler ultrasound: Relation to left ventricular diastolic pressures. *J Am Coll Cardiol* **21:**1687–1696, 1993

55. Shah PM, Child JS: Echocardiography of cardiac muscle disease. *In* Pohost GM, O'Rourke RA (eds): *Principles and Practice of Cardiovascular Imaging.* Boston, Little Brown, 1991, pp 599–626

56. Child JS, Perloff JK: The restrictive cardiomyopathies. *Cardiol Clin* **6:**289–316, 1988

57. Sasson Z, Rakowski H, Wigle ED, Popp R: Echocardiographic and Doppler studies in hypertrophic cardiomyopathy. *Cardiol Clin* **8:**217–232, 1990

58. Hamilton MA, Stevenson LW, Child JS, et al: Acute reduction of atrial afterload during vasodilator and diuretic therapy in advanced congestive heart failure. *Am J Cardiol* **65:**1209–1212, 1990

59. Pinamonti B, Di Lenarda A, Sinagra G, et al and the Heart Muscle Study Group: Restrictive left ventricular filling pattern in dilated cardiomyopathy assessed by Doppler echocardiography: Clinical, echocardiographic and hemodynamic correlations and prognostic implications. *J Am Coll Cardiol* **22:**808–815, 1993

60. Wong M, Johnson G, Shabetai R, et al for the V-HeFT Cooperative Studies Group: Echocardiographic variables as prognostic indicators and therapeutic monitors in chronic congestive heart failure. *Circulation* **87**[suppl VI]:VI65–VI70, 1993

61. Klein AL, Hatle LK, Burstow DJ, et al: Doppler characterization of left ventricular diastolic function in cardiac amyloidosis. *J Am Coll Cardiol* **13:**1017–1026, 1989

62. Hauptman PJ, Gass A, Goldman ME: The role of echocardiography in heart transplantation. *J Am Soc Echocardiogr* **6:**496–509, 1993

63. Kronzon I, Cohen ML, Winer HE: Diastolic atrial compression: A sensitive echocardiographic sign of cardiac tamponade. *J Am Coll Cardiol* **2:**770–775, 1983

64. Gillam LD, Guyer DE, Gibson TC, et al: Hydrodynamic compression of the right atrium: A new echocardiographic sign of cardiac tamponade. *Circulation* **68:**294–301, 1983

65. Schiller NB, Botvinick EH: Right ventricular compression as a sign of cardiac tamponade: an analysis of ventricular dimensions and their clinical implications. *Circulation* **56:**774, 1977

66. Singh S, Wann LS, Klopfenstein S, et al: Usefulness of right ventricular diastolic collapse in diagnosing cardiac tamponade and comparison to pulses paradoxus. *Am J Cardiol* **57:**652–656, 1986

67. Armstrong WF, Schilt BF, Helper DJ, et al: Diastolic collapse of the right ventricle with cardiac tamponade. An echocardiographic study. *Circulation* **55:**1491–1496, 1982

68. Appleton CP, Hatle LK, Popp RL: Cardiac tamponade and pericardial effusion: Respiratory variation in transvalvular flow velocities by Doppler echocardiography. *J Am Coll Cardiol* **11:**1020–1030, 1988

69. Schutzmann JJ, Obarski TP, Pearce GL, Klein A: Comparison of Doppler and two-dimensional echocardiography for assessment of pericardial effusion. *Am J Cardiol* **70:**1353–1357, 1992

70. Eisenberg MJ, Oken K, Guerrero S, et al: Prognostic value of echocardiography in hospitalized patients with pericardial effusion. *Am J Cardiol* **70:**934–939, 1992

71. Fowler NO: Cardiac tamponade; a clinical or an echocardiographic diagnosis? *Circulation* **87:**1738–1741, 1993

72. Kopecky SL, Callahan JA, Tajik AJ, Seward JB: Percutaneous peri-cardial catheter drainage: Report of 42 consecutive cases. *Am J Cardiol* **50:**633, 1986

73. Tei C, Child JS, Tanaka H, Shah PM: Atrial systolic notch on the interventricular septal echocardiogram: An echocardiographic sign of constrictive pericarditis. *J Am Coll Cardiol* **1:**907–912, 1983

74. Hatle LK, Appleton CP, Popp RL: Differentiation of constrictive pericarditis and restrictive cardiomyopathy by Doppler echocardiography. *Circulation* **79:**357–370, 1989

75. Hoffman R, Flachskampf FA, Hanrath P: Planimetry of orifice area in aortic stenosis using multiplane transesophageal echocardiography. *J Am Coll Cardiol* **22:**529–534, 1993

76. Judge KW, Otto CM: Doppler echocardiographic evaluation of aortic stenosis. *Cardiol Clin* **8:**203–216, 1990

77. Wiseth R, Skjaerpe T, Hatle L: Rapid systolic intraventricular velocities after valve replacement for aortic stenosis. *Am J Cardiol* **71:**944–948, 1993

78. Aurigemma G, Whitfield S, Sweeney A, et al: Color Doppler mapping of aortic regurgitation in aortic stenosis: Comparison with angiography. *Cardiology* **81:**251–257, 1992

79. Perry GJ, Helmcke MD, Nanda NC, et al: Evaluation of aortic insufficiency by Doppler color flow mapping. *J Am Coll Cardiol* **9:**952–959, 1987

80. Grayburn P, Handshow R, Smith M, et al: Quantitative assessment of the hemodynamic consequences of aortic regurgitation by means of continuous wave Doppler recordings. *J Am Coll Cardiol* **10:**135–141, 1987

81. Yeung AC, Plappert T, St John Sutton MG: Calculation of aortic regurgitation orifice area by Doppler echocardiography: An application of the continuity equation. *Br Heart J* **68:**236–240, 1992

82. Krivokapich J, Child JS, Dadourian BJ, Perloff JK: Reassessment of echocardiographic criteria for diagnosis of mitral valve prolapse. *Am J Cardiol* **61:**131–135, 1988

83. Crawford MH, Souchek J, Oprian CA, et al and Participants in the Veterans Administration Cooperative Study on Valvular Heart Disease: Determinants of survival and left ventricular performance following mitral valve replacement. *Circulation* **81:**1173–1181, 1990

84. De Simone R, Lange R, Saggan W, et al: Intraoperative transesophageal echocardiography for the evaluation of mitral, aortic and tricuspid valve repair: A tool to optimize surgical outcome. *Eur J Cardio-thorac Surg* **6:**665–673, 1992

85. Currie PJ, Stewart WJ: Intraoperative echocardiography in mitral valve repair for mitral regurgitation. *Am J Cardiac Imaging* **4:**192–206, 1990

86. Marwick TH, Stewart WJ, Currie PJ, Cosgrove DM: Mechanisms of failure of mitral valve repair: An echocardiographic study. *Am Heart J* **122:**149–156, 1991

87. Sheikh KH, Bengston JR, Rankin JS, et al: Intraoperative transesophageal Doppler color flow imaging used to guide patient selection and operative treatment of ischemic mitral regurgitation. *Circulation* **84:**594–604, 1991

88. Helmcke F, Nanda NC, Hsiung MC, et al: Color flow Doppler assessment of mitral regurgitation using orthogonal planes. *Circulation* **75:**175–183, 1987

89. Chen C, Thomas JD, Anconina J, et al: Impact of impinging wall jet on color Doppler quantification of mitral regurgitation. *Circulation* **84:**712–720, 1991

90. Enriquez-Sarano M, Tajik AJ, Bailey KR, Seward JB: Color flow imaging compared with quantitative Doppler assessment of severity of mitral regurgitation: Influence of eccentricity of jet and mechanism of regurgitation. *J Am Coll Cardiol* **21:**1211–1219, 1993

91. Schiller NB, Foster E, Redberg RF: Transesophageal echocardiography in the evaluation of mitral regurgitation. The twenty four signs of severe mitral regurgitation. *Cardiol Clin* **11:**399–408, 1993

92. Klein AL, Stewart WJ, Bartlett J, et al: Effects of mitral regurgitation on pulmonary venous flow and left atrial pressure: An intraoperative transesophageal echocardiographic study. *J Am Coll Cardiol* **20:**1345–1352, 1992

93. Kamp O, Dijkstra JW, Huitink H, et al: Transesophageal color flow Doppler mapping in the assessment of native mitral valvular regurgitation: Comparison with left ventricular angiography. *J Am Soc Echocardiogr* **4:**598–606, 1991

94. Smith MD, Harrison MR, Pinton R, et al: Regurgitant jet size by transesophageal compared with transthoracic Doppler color flow imaging. *Circulation* **83:**79–86, 1991

95. Mimo R, Sparacino L, Nicolosi GL, et al: Quantification of mitral regurgitation: Comparison between transthoracic and transesophageal color Doppler flow mapping. *Echocardiography* **8:**619–626, 1991

96. Hatle L: Doppler echocardiographic evaluation of mitral stenosis. *Clin Cardiol* **8:**233–247, 1990

97. Goldstein SA, Campbell AH: Evaluation and guidance of valvuloplasty by transesophageal echocardiography. *Clin Cardiol* **11:**409–425, 1993

98. Nihoyannopoulos P, Kambouroglou D, Athanassopoulos G, et al: Doppler haemodynamic profiles of clinically and echocardiographically normal mitral and aortic valve prostheses. *Eur Heart J* **13:**348–355, 1992

99. Baumgartner H, Khan S, Derobertis M, et al: Effect of prosthetic aortic valve design on the Doppler-catheter gradient correlation: An in vitro study of normal St. Jude, Medtronic-Hall, Starr-Edwards and Hancock valves. *J Am Coll Cardiol* **19:**324–332, 1992

100. Baumgartner H, Shima H, Kuhn P: Discrepancies between Doppler and catheter gradients across bileaflet aortic valve prostheses. *Am J Cardiol* **71:**1241–1243, 1993

101. Alton MD, Pasierski TJ, Orsinelli DA, et al: Comparison of transthoracic and transesophageal echocardiography in evaluation of 47 Starr-Edwards prosthetic valves. *J Am Coll Cardiol* **20:**1503–1511, 1992

102. Habib G, Cornen A, Mesana T, et al: Diagnosis of prosthetic heart valve thrombosis. The respective values of transthoracic and transoesophageal Doppler echocardiography. *Eur Heart J* **14:**447–455, 1993

103. Flachskampf FA, Lehmann C, Klues H, et al: Transesophageal echocardiography for prosthetic valve evaluation: Is it always necessary? *Echocardiography* **10:**303–310, 1993

104. Yvorchuk KJ, Chan KL: Application of transthoracic and transesophageal echocardiography in the diagnosis and management of infective endocarditis. *J Am Soc Echocardiogr* **14:**294–308, 1994

105. Rohmann S, Erbel R, Gorge G, et al: Clinical relevance of vegetation localization by transesophageal echocardiography in infective endocarditis. *Eur Heart J* **12:**446–452, 1992

106. Mugge A, Daniel WG, Frank G, Lichtlen PR: Echocardiography in infective endocarditis: Reassessment of prognostic implications of vegetation size determined by the transthoracic and the transesophageal approach. *J Am Coll Cardiol* **14:**631–638, 1989

107. Sanfilippo AJ, Picard MH, Newell JB, et al: Echocardiographic assessment of patients with infectious endocarditis: prediction of risk for complications. *J Am Coll Cardiol* **18:**1191–1199, 1991

108. Daniel WG, Mugge A, Grote J, et al: Comparison of transthoracic and transesophageal echocardiography for detection of abnormalities of prosthetic and bioprosthetic valves in the mitral and aortic positions. *Am J Cardiol* **71:**210–215, 1993

109. Rohmann S, Seifert T, Erbel R, et al: Identification of abscess formation in native-valve infective endocarditis using transesophageal echocardiography: Implications for surgical treatment. *Thorac Cardiovasc Surgeon* **39:**273–280, 1991

110. Karalis DG, Bansal RC, Hauck AJ, et al: Transesophageal echocardiographic recognition of subaortic complications in aortic valve endocarditis. *Circulation* **86:**353–362, 1992

111. Sochowski RA, Chan KL: Implication of negative results on a monoplane transesophageal echocardiographic study in patients with suspected infective endocarditis. *J Am Coll Cardiol* **21:**216–221, 1993

112. Child JS: Echocardiographic assessment of adults with tetralogy of Fallot. *Echocardiography* **10:**629–640, 1993

113. Seward JB: Ebstein's anomaly. Ultrasound imaging and hemodynamic evaluation. *Echocardiography* **10:**641–664, 1993

114. Calermajer DS, Bull C, Till JA, et al: Ebstein's anomaly: Presentation and outcome from fetus to adult. *J Am Coll Cardiol* **23:**170–176, 1994

115. Williams RG: Echocardiography in the management of single ventricle. Fetal to adult life. *Echocardiography* **10:**331–342, 1993

116. Kouchoukas NT, Davila-Roman VG, Spray TL, et al: Replacement of the aortic root with a pulmonary autograft in children and young adults with aortic-valve disease. *N Engl J Med* **330:**1–6, 1994

117. Sim EKW, Julsrud PR, Van Son JAM, et al: Preoperative diagnosis of coronary artery anatomy in dextrotransposition of the great arteries. *Mayo Clin Proc* **69:**28–32, 1994

Nuclear Imaging in the Assessment of Acquired Heart Disease

Bernard R. Chaitman and D. Douglas Miller

INTRODUCTION

The growth in the field of nuclear cardiac imaging in recent years has been sustained by changes in imaging technology, agents, clinical applications, and target populations. Initially, a major advantage of nuclear cardiac imaging procedures was their noninvasive nature, and their improved diagnostic accuracy over standard ECG stress testing alone. Increased access and clinical utility have fostered this growth, and have consolidated the diagnostic value of nuclear cardiac imaging, even as competitive cardiac stress testing modalities have become available. Both myocardial perfusion and cardiac functional information can be acquired under stress and rest conditions, providing unique physiologic information that cannot easily be obtained using other diagnostic techniques.

Pharmacologic stress agents can now be utilized as an alternative or adjunct to exercise testing in patients who are unable to exercise to a diagnostically useful workload. Whereas imaging techniques were once restricted to a few planar projections of the heart, myocardial tomography (using either gamma or positron emitting radionuclides) can now be used to improve spatial resolution and to better define the distribution of cardiac abnormalities. Tracer radionuclides are frequently used as biochemical probes of cardiac metabolism and as clinically important determinants of myocardial viability in patients under consideration for coronary revascularization. The capacity of accurately quantitate cardiac perfusion–function–metabolic parameters further enhances the diagnostic and prognostic capabilities

of nuclear cardiac imaging, thereby providing more clinically useful information on patients with known or suspected coronary artery disease, and a basis for appropriate referral for cardiac catheterization and surgery.

These factors have contributed to the establishment of nuclear cardiac imaging as an important noninvasive tool with the capacity to improve patient management before or after cardiovascular surgical procedures. This is particularly true of the complex and growing subset of patients with prior coronary revascularization, coexisting valvular heart disease and depressed left ventricular contractile function.

ASSESSMENT OF VENTRICULAR PERFORMANCE

First-Pass Radionuclide Angiography

This technique has been applied to assessing global and regional function of the right and left ventricles.[1] Left and right ventricular function can be assessed from a single study because there is temporal and anatomic separation of radioactivity within each chamber. In addition to calculating an ejection fraction, regional wall motion can be assessed and ventricular volumes determined. Technetium-99m (^{99m}Tc)-labeled (8–20 mCi/injection) radiopharmaceuticals usually are used for first-pass studies.

Critical to the first-pass technique is a compact intravenous radionuclide bolus and reliable high temporal frequency data acquisition. Injections usually are made into an antecubital basilic vein or external jugular vein.[1,2] Slow streaming or fragmentation of the bolus of radioactivity entering the central circulation will result in invalidation of data analysis.

Data are usually obtained using a multicrystal gamma camera on a high speed magnetic disc at framing rates of 10 to 50 ms. The temporal separation of the bolus of activity allows the analysis of right and left ventricular performance in the anterior and right anterior oblique positions, views that normally demonstrate anatomic overlap of both ventricles. Activity is analyzed in the ventricular region of interest while the bolus is passing through the background correction applied for scattered and overlying activity. Background correction is used in both right and left ventricular ejection fraction analysis. The various methods of analysis of left and right ventricular performance have been standardized and validated[1,3–6] (Fig. 105–1).

For the left ventricle, two to six beats at the peak of the background corrected-time activity curve are usually suitable for analysis. These individual beats are summed to form a single representative cardiac cycle. From the single representative cardiac cycle, the left ventricular ejection fraction is calculated as the difference between the background corrected end diastolic counts and end systolic counts divided by end diastolic counts. As assessment is limited to a few beats, arrhythmias or premature ventricular contractions can affect the accuracy of this technique.

Ejection fraction and assessment of regional wall motion abnormalities determined by the first-pass technique correlate well with that determined by contrast ventriculography.[3,4,7–9] The radionuclide technique has a low intrinsic inter- and intraobserver variability.[3,4,10] Other information

such as ejection rate, velocity of circumferential fiber shortening,[11] first third ejection,[12] and regional ejection fraction determination[8] also can be obtained from these studies.

Data of the summed representative cardiac cycle can be viewed as a temporal sequence of images, arranged as an endless loop movie display. These cine data, as well as static end diastolic and systolic images or perimeters, can be used for qualitative assessment of regional contraction.

Rapidly changing physiologic states can be readily studied because the actual data acquisition of a first pass study is 30 seconds or less. Individual ventricular chambers can be assessed without contamination of activity from the adjacent ventricle. The technique can be used for both supine and upright studies, which is advantageous since patients sometimes experience difficulty with supine exercise or are unable to exercise in the supine position.

Equilibrium Gated Blood Pool Imaging

The gated equilibrium study analyzes several hundred cardiac cycles, in contrast to the few cycles examined in first-pass studies. The radionuclide remains within the intravascular space during the study. The in vivo labeling of the patient's own red blood cells with 15 to 30 mCi of ^{99m}Tc sodium pertechnetate is employed in most laboratories.[13] Cardiac performance must be relatively stable and the patient must remain relatively still under the scintillation camera to reduce motion artifact during the 2 to 10 min data collection period.

Equilibrium studies are performed with a standard single-crystal gamma camera. The R-wave of the electrocardiogram is used as a physiologic triggering signal during

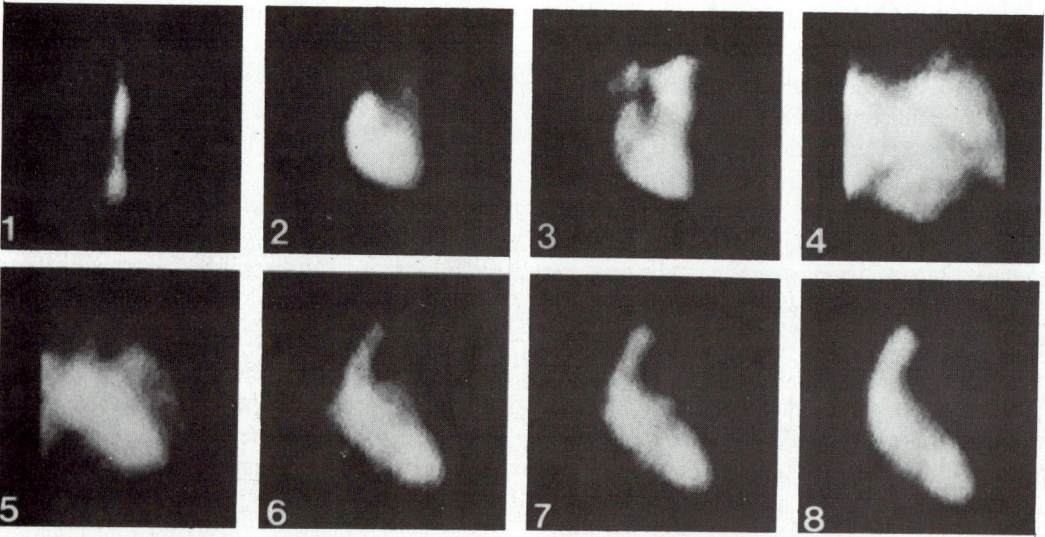

Figure 105–1. First-pass radionuclide cardioangiography showing sequential 1-s images obtained during passage of the bolus of radioactivity through the central circulation. The normal temporal and anatomic separation of radioactivity in the cardiac chambers is well seen. The right ventricle and pulmonary artery are seen in frame 3 and the left ventricle and ascending aorta are seen in frames 6–8. (From Berger HJ, Matthay RA, Pytlik LM, et al: First-pass radionuclide assessment of right and left ventricular performance in patients with cardiac and pulmonary disease. Semin Nucl Med 9:275,1979, with permission.)

data collection.[14-16] The R-R interval is divided into 16 to 28 equal time intervals. Data from each heart beat are collected during specific consecutive time intervals and sorted into the computer bin whose location is determined by the time elapsed from the R-wave signal. When the next R-wave signal is a single representative cycle made up of consecutive frames, each containing the sum of data from several hundred cardiac cycles (Fig. 105–2).

The left ventricular ejection fraction is based on computer analysis of a left ventricular time activity curve obtained from the left anterior oblique (LAO) view. Left ventricular ejection fraction measured using the equilibrium-gated blood pool technique correlates well with determinations made at the time of contrast ventricular angiography.[17,18] Poor ventricular separation or the presence of a large anterior aneurysm or a large left atrium can affect the left ventricular ejection fraction determinations. Although there is overlap of the left atrium and left ventricle in the LAO view, the contribution of the atrial activity usually is relatively small because of its distance from the detector and its relatively smaller size compared to the ventricle. In patients with large left atria secondary to mitral valve disease, the activity contribution increases and can falsely depress the left ventricular ejection fraction.

At least three views are obtained to assess wall motion,[19,20] the anterior, LAO 45°, and left lateral or left posterior oblique views. Additional views can be necessary in the presence of cardiac rotation or individual chamber enlargement. A qualitative assessment of regional wall motion is best evaluated on an endless loop radionuclide cineangiogram.[21] Developments in computer software have led to quantitative assessments of regional contraction patterns and the temporal sequence of contraction patterns.[22,23] A multigated technique also has been reported for measuring right ventricular ejection fraction, but is less reliable than the left ventricular study.[24]

Because radioactivity is proportion to blood volume, by comparing radioactivity from a blood sample to activity arising from the ventricle it should be possible to determine chamber volumes. After accounting for radiation attenuation by overlying structures, left ventricular volume can be estimated by the use of appropriate regression equations.[25] Additionally, the relative size and orientation of the great vessels can be appreciated.

The equilibrium blood pool technique has several advantages. Multiple studies in one or more views can be acquired after a single radionuclide injection. The equilibrium study allows a high count density in the ventricular region of interest, improving the statistical reliability of the technique. Because the radionuclide labeling is stable, sequential and multiple view data can be obtained in association with physiologic and pharmacologic interventions over several hours.

Analysis of ventricular function during exercise using the equilibrium technique is done most frequently in the supine or semierect position. This can present difficulty with reaching adequate work loads compared to the upright position. In addition, the patient has to remain in a steady state at maximum work load for at least 2 min during data collection. Excessive thoracic motion can produce significant artifact.

CLINICAL APPLICATION OF VENTRICULAR PERFORMANCE ANALYSIS

Resting Ventricular Performance

Global left ventricular ejection fraction and regional wall motion analysis are among the most important determinants of long-term prognosis in patients with ischemic heart disease. Analysis of resting right and left ventricular function by either technique is valuable in assessing the extent of myocardial dysfunction and designing and following pharmacologic or surgical therapy. Radionuclide studies also

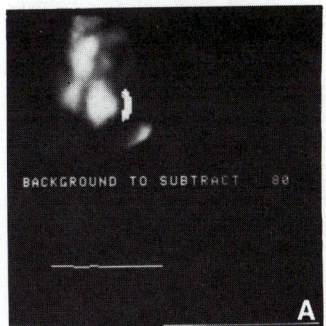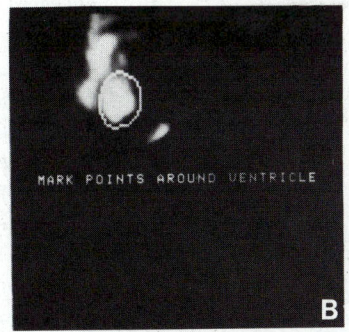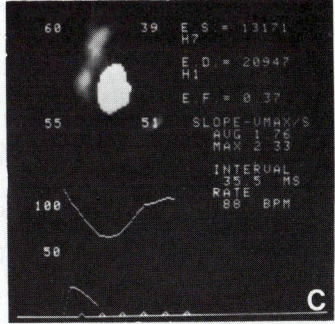

Figure 105–2. Images taken in the left anterior oblique showing the steps involved in processing a multigated equilibrium blood pool study. The image on the left (**A**) shows the region of background selected and flat time activity curve. The middle image (**B**) shows the left ventricular region of interest. The image on the right (**C**) shows the relative volume curve in the left ventricular region of interest and the ejection fraction (EF). These data are displayed step-by-step on the computer oscilloscope screen. *(From Berger HJ, Gottschalk A, Zaret BL: Radionuclide assessment of the left and right ventricular performance. Radiol Clin North Am 18:441, 1980, with permission.)*

are valuable in distinguishing cardiac from pulmonary causes of dyspnea in suspected or documented heart failure.

Studies during the acute stage of myocardial infarction have shown that anterior wall infarcts result in a greater depression of left ventricular function than inferior wall infarcts.[26] In contrast, inferior wall myocardial infarction frequently results in altered right ventricular function,[27,28] whereas this is uncommon in anterior wall myocardial infarction.[6,26] Risk stratification of patient subsets based on radionuclide parameters offers the opportunity to optimally select the high risk patients who might benefit from revascularization procedures.

Using a resting MUGA scan, the diagnosis of hypertrophic cardiomyopathy can be inferred from the relative thickness of the intraventricular septum.[29] A pericardial effusion or left atrial myxoma also can be suspected from the appearance of the cardiac image.[30] Application of the equilibrium technique to detection and measurement of aortic or mitral regurgitation has been described.[31] However, the right ventricular region of interest is often difficult to define, and there is a wide range of normal values, as well as potential difficulties in quantitating the tricuspid valve regurgitant fraction.[32]

Ventricular Performance During Exercise

Exercise ventricular function studies assessed with either the first-pass or equilibrium technique have diagnostic application in patients with known or suspected coronary artery disease.[2,21,33–34] The normal response to bicycle exercise is an absolute increase of at least 5% in ejection fraction of both right and left ventricles above resting values. This is associated with normal regional wall motion and little (<20%) increase in left ventricular end-diastolic volume.[2] In patients with coronary disease, the left ventricular ejection fraction generally decreases or does not augment appropriately with exercise and can be associated with abnormal segmental wall motion contraction and ventricular dilatation.[35] The presence of a new regional wall motion abnormality is a less sensitive but more specific finding for coronary disease than global left ventricular ejection fraction response. Abnormal responses are seen in 80–90% of patients with significant coronary artery disease. The ventricular response appears to be related to the degree of induced myocardial ischemia and adequacy of the stress.

Several studies indicate that exercise left ventricular function measurements improve the sensitivity for multivessel coronary disease over that of exercise perfusion imaging alone. In patients in whom a clinical suspicion of coronary artery disease remains after a normal or borderline perfusion imaging response, it can be worthwhile to perform a functional study. Normal responses using both exercise imaging studies are unlikely to occur in the presence of significant multivessel disease.[35–37] Abnormal exercise left ventricular function studies can occur in a variety of conditions, such as left ventricular hypertrophy, hypertension, aortic regurgitation, and prior myocarditis, and can give the false impression of coronary artery disease. In the postoperative coronary artery bypass patient in whom the question of adequate myocardial revascularization or recent graft closure arises, exercise perfusion imaging is the procedure of choice. Also, patients with baseline arrhythmia or exercise-induced arrhythmia in whom there could be sufficient artifact in the ventricular function analysis introduced by the arrhythmia should be studied by perfusion imaging.

Jones et al examined 496 patients who underwent rest and exercise radionuclide imaging and reported a sensitivity and specificity of 90% and 58% in 387 patients who had an optimal study using the first-pass technique.[38] Rozanski et al studied 77 angiography normal patients over a 4-year interval and noted a temporal decline in specificity because of a change in the population being tested and a preferential selection of patients with a positive test result for coronary angiography.[39] Thus, from a diagnostic standpoint, an abnormal global left ventricular ejection response to exercise has important limitations. Nevertheless, in clinical patient subsets with a high pretest risk or documented coronary artery disease, an abnormal response is a powerful prognostic indicator of long-term outcome in both acute and chronic ischemic heart disease.[40–44]

The exercise level achieved is important in assessing ventricular function. Ventricular function can be normal at submaximum myocardial oxygen consumption, whereas further increase of myocardial oxygen requirement can induce ventricular dysfunction in the presence of significant disease. Calcium-entry or β-blockade can blunt the normal heart rate response to exercise and result in a normal ventricular response to exercise in the presence of significant disease.[45] Achievement of maximum exercise levels improves the reliability of the procedure.

As with exercise ECG testing, several other means of stressing the ventricle have been evaluated using radionuclide techniques. These include atrial pacing, catecholamine infusions, isometric handgrip, and cold pressor tests.[46–49] The mechanisms of stress differ with each of these techniques, as do their sensitivities and specificities for the diagnosis of coronary artery disease.

Several studies have evaluated ventricular performance in patients with aortic regurgitation.[49,50] Abnormal exercise left ventricular responses have been demonstrated in asymptomatic as well as symptomatic patients who have normal ventricular function at rest. Preoperative abnormal exercise responses often revert to normal following aortic valve replacement.[51] However, the physiology of exercise performance in aortic regurgitation is complex.

MYOCARDIAL PERFUSION IMAGING

Thallium-201

Myocardial perfusion images provide information on relative regional myocardial perfusion and regional viability. Thallium(^{201}Tl) was introduced in 1975 for clinical imaging as a potassium analogue with physical properties more suitable for imaging than the prototype radionuclide, potassium-43.[52] It has a relatively low energy spectrum with a major 80 keV mercury x-ray photopeak and a physical half-life of 73 hours. Thallium-201 is a cyclotron-produced radionuclide.

The initial distribution of ^{201}Tl is determined primarily by regional myocardial perfusion.[53–55] Myocardial thallium (^{201}Tl) extraction is very efficient.[56] The peak myocardial concentration of ^{201}Tl is approximately 3–4% of the administered dose. Uptake is directly proportional to regional myocardial bloodflow within the normal range of blood flow. However, as with most perfusion radiotracers, extraction is less efficient at hyperemic blood flow rates.[53]

Following the initial high extraction of ^{201}Tl uptake, there is a continuous washout of cellular ^{201}Tl into the interstitial fluid space. In poorly perfused regions, ^{201}Tl accumulation is slow and washout is delayed. Thus, there is an efflux of ^{201}Tl from normally perfused regions and an in-

flux of ^{201}Tl to ischemic but viable myocardium. The process of gradual equilibration of myocardial ^{201}Tl concentrations is termed "redistribution."[55,57]

Usually 1.5–2.0 mCi of ^{201}Tl is injected for planar studies and 3.0–4.0 mCi for tomographic studies. Planar images should be obtained in multiple (3–4) views (Fig. 105–3).[58] When exercise images are obtained, the patient generally should exercise maximally to a symptom-limited end point. The radionuclide is injected at peak exercise, and the patient is exercised for a further 30–60 seconds. Because of the potential for rapid tracer clearance, ^{201}Tl imaging should commence within 5 min of administration of the radionuclide. Delayed ^{201}Tl images are obtained 3–4 hours following exercise to assess the presence of defect redistribution.[57] Various computer methods have been used to process image data involving quantification of regional ^{201}Tl uptake, various background correction methods, image enhancement, and color display.[59–74] Quantitation of planar ^{201}Tl images requires acquisition for a fixed time in

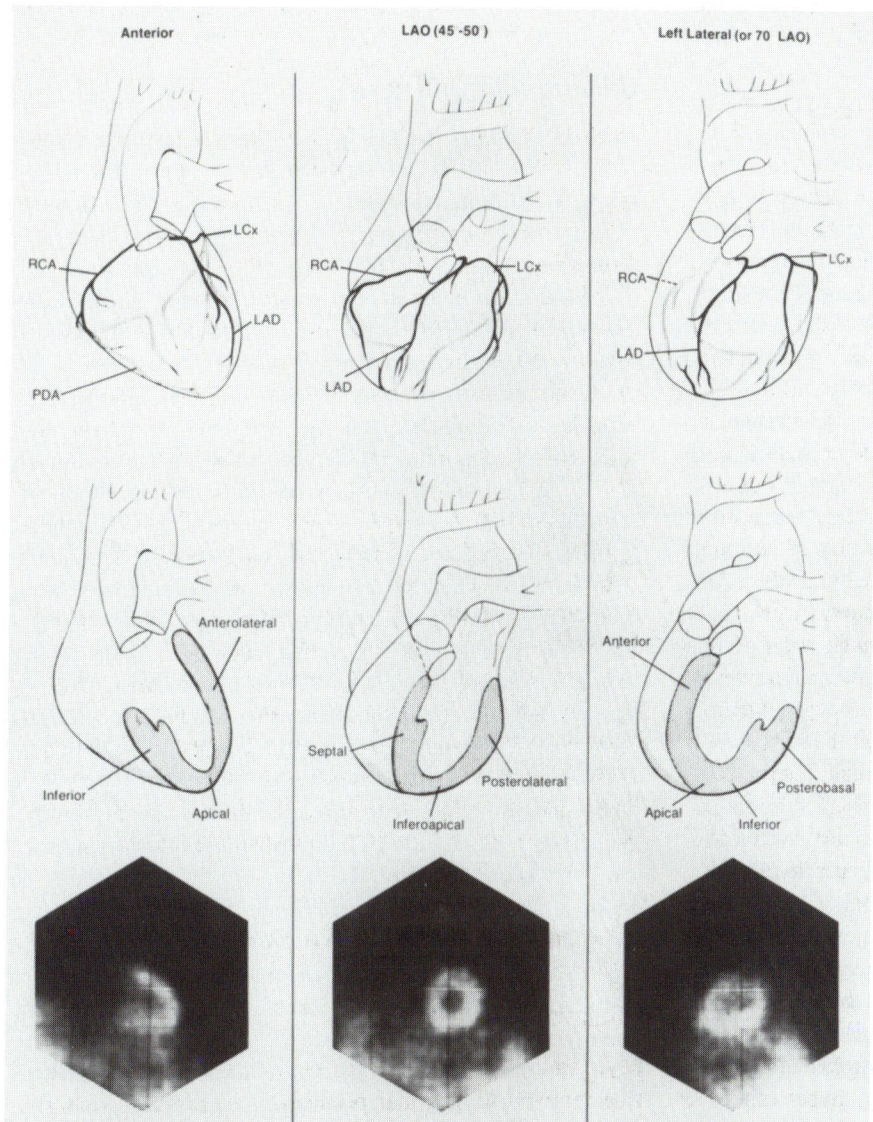

Figure 105–3. Three commonly used views for planar ^{201}Tl imaging are shown. The relationship of coronary artery distribution (upper panel) to left ventricular myocardial segments (middle panel) and normal thallium images (lower panel) is illustrated. *(Courtesy of DuPont Radiopharmaceutical Division.)*

each view (approximately 10 min), immediately post exercise and 2–4 hours later. Distribution and washout profiles are then generated and compared to lower limits of normal.[75]

A thorough familiarity with cardiac anatomy is essential for interpreting myocardial perfusion images and appreciating the range of normal variation and the causes of presumed false-positive defects.[75] Images normally demonstrate a homogeneous distribution of radioactivity in the left ventricular myocardium. Approximately 20% of normal subjects will have a small apical defect resulting from normal relative thinning of the myocardium at apex. Apparent fixed defects can be seen in patients with large breasts, thick chest walls, pacemakers, AICD devices, or overlying ECG electrodes. Diaphragmatic attenuation can result in a fixed inferior wall defect in the left lateral planar view when patients are imaged in the supine position. Small perfusion defects seen in only one view should be interpreted with caution, and perfusion defects should be confirmed in a second position.

Right ventricular uptake usually is not appreciated in normal resting images. In exercise studies, right ventricular uptake is seen because of increased right ventricular coronary bloodflow. Right ventricular uptake in resting images also can be seen in right ventricular hypertrophy, increased right ventricular afterload, or pulmonary hypertension.

Abnormal images at rest can be the result of acute transient myocardial ischemia or remote infarction. Abnormal rest images also have been seen in patients with unstable angina.[76,77] In patients with acute ischemic syndromes, the incidence of abnormal rest perfusion images is temporally related to the onset of chest pain. Reversible perfusion abnormality can be seen in instances of either spontaneous or ergonovine maleate-induced coronary artery spasm.[78]

In the absence of prior myocardial infarction, most patients with coronary artery disease will have normal resting ^{201}Tl images. During exercise, increased demand can exceed coronary vascular reserve in stenotic vessels, resulting in regional flow differences. These inequalities of regional bloodflow can be reflected in abnormal regional perfusion tracer uptake. Patients exercising only to modest workloads because of either fatigue or β-blockade therapy with a limited increase in heart rate and blood pressure have a higher incidence of false-negative images. Thus, as with exercise ventricular function studies, the patient must be maximally exercised for adequate ^{201}Tl exercise imaging.

Perfusion defects seen immediately after peak exercise will reflect relative hypoperfusion or prior myocardial infarction. Abnormal exercise images should be compared to either a redistribution[201]Tl image obtained 3–4 hours later or to a separate rest study. A reversible perfusion defect indicates relative hypoperfusion and transient ischemia during exercise. However, problems can occur in distinguishing between reversible and irreversible myocardial ischemia in patients with prior myocardial infarction.

Because differences in perfusion tracer uptake with exercise studies are related to relative rather than absolute regional perfusion, there need not be a close correlation between anatomic coronary artery lesions and regional perfusion defects. Frequently, patients with multivessel disease will show only a single exercise perfusion defect reflecting the most ischemic region. The functional significance of coronary narrowing and collateral blood supply also will influence the demonstrable perfusion patterns.

Increased pulmonary uptake has been observed in exercise images[79] and also in resting images obtained in patients with severe left ventricular failure. The increased pulmonary uptake indicates transient left ventricular failure during uptake and indicates transient left ventricular failure during exercise and presumably a slowed pulmonary transit. Increased thallium pulmonary uptake correlates with coronary disease extent and degree of exercise-induced left ventricular dysfunction, and has been shown to be a useful prognostic indicator of adverse coronary events in patients with obstructive coronary disease.[80] Transient ischemic dilation of the left ventricle on stress perfusion scintigraphy is another useful indicator of severe and extensive coronary disease.[81]

Pharmacologic Stress

In a number of patients, adequate exercise levels will not be achieved for orthopedic, neurologic, or other medical reasons. An alternative approach is to use a pharmacologic agent to increase coronary blood flow. Dipyridamole, a complex pyrimidine derivative, causes selective coronary hyperemia through an elevation of endogenous plasma adenosine levels.[82,83] The most commonly used protocol employs 0.14 mg/kg per minute administered over 4 min with the perfusion tracer infected 4 min after the termination of dipyridamole infusion.[84] Total coronary hyperemic blood flow in normal individuals increases approximately 2–5 times normal resting levels. A differential rate of myocardial radiotracer uptake occurs in vascular beds supplied by normal versus stenosed arteries which results in abnormal images. Quantitative analysis of thallium washout is variable.[85] In most consecutive series of patients undergoing IV dipyridamole stress imaging, chest pain, dipyridamole-induced ischemic ST segment depression, and noncardiac side effects such as headache, dizziness, or flushing occur in 25, 15, and 20% of patients, respectively.[86] In general, side effects can be reversed by theophylline and, when necessary, by sublingual nitroglycerin. Severe myocardial ischemic responses after IV dipyridamole infusion are rare, but have been described.[87] Xanthine derivatives need to be stopped prior to testing. However, patients with severe bronchospastic pulmonary disease should not undergo IV dipyridamole or adenosine stress imaging, nor should those who have shown myocardial ischemic instability within the previous 2 days of testing.

The use of intravenous dipyridamole or adenosine offers a suitable diagnostic and prognostic alternative as a noninvasive test to assess ischemic heart disease in patients unable to adequately exercise, and can identify preoperatively, patients at low and high risk of subsequent perioperative cardiac events.[88,89] Composite reported sensitivity and specificity from several series are 90 and 70%, respectively.

Tomographic Myocardial Perfusion Imaging

Myocardial tomography improves the accurate determination of the presence and extent of coronary artery disease by allowing detection of smaller perfusion defects. Tomographic approaches provide a mechanism for minimizing overlap of structures in the cardiac region (Fig. 105–4).

Single photon emission computed tomographic (SPECT) data are performed using a rotating single or multiheaded gamma camera system.[90] Images from this system can be reliably reoriented in multiple orthogonal planes, which permits examination of the myocardial perfusion image such that virtually all perfusion defects can be viewed transversely.[91] This standardized type of reorientation is also

very similar to the projections that are in other noninvasive cardiac imaging techniques such as two-dimensional echocardiography and magnetic resonance imaging.

Single photon emission tomography acquisition occurs as a large field of view gamma camera rotates around the thorax of the patient over a 180° or 360° angle. As the camera system rotates around the patient, most imaging systems make many individual discrete stops at three to six degree intervals during which time the count data are acquired. Depending on the number of tomographic camera heads (1–3), the overall collection time varies from 10 to 30 min with up to 10 million counts recorded within this imaging time. Whereas ^{201}Tl redistribution images are typically collected 3–4 hours later, a separate resting ^{99m}Tc sestamibi SPECT study must be acquired a few hours before or after, or on a separate day from the stress study. The data acquired at each angular position in the SPECT tomographic technique may then be reconstructed to provide tomographic images using several different types of mathematical algorithms.[92] The most common mathematical technique employed involves a filtered back-projection technique and is similar to

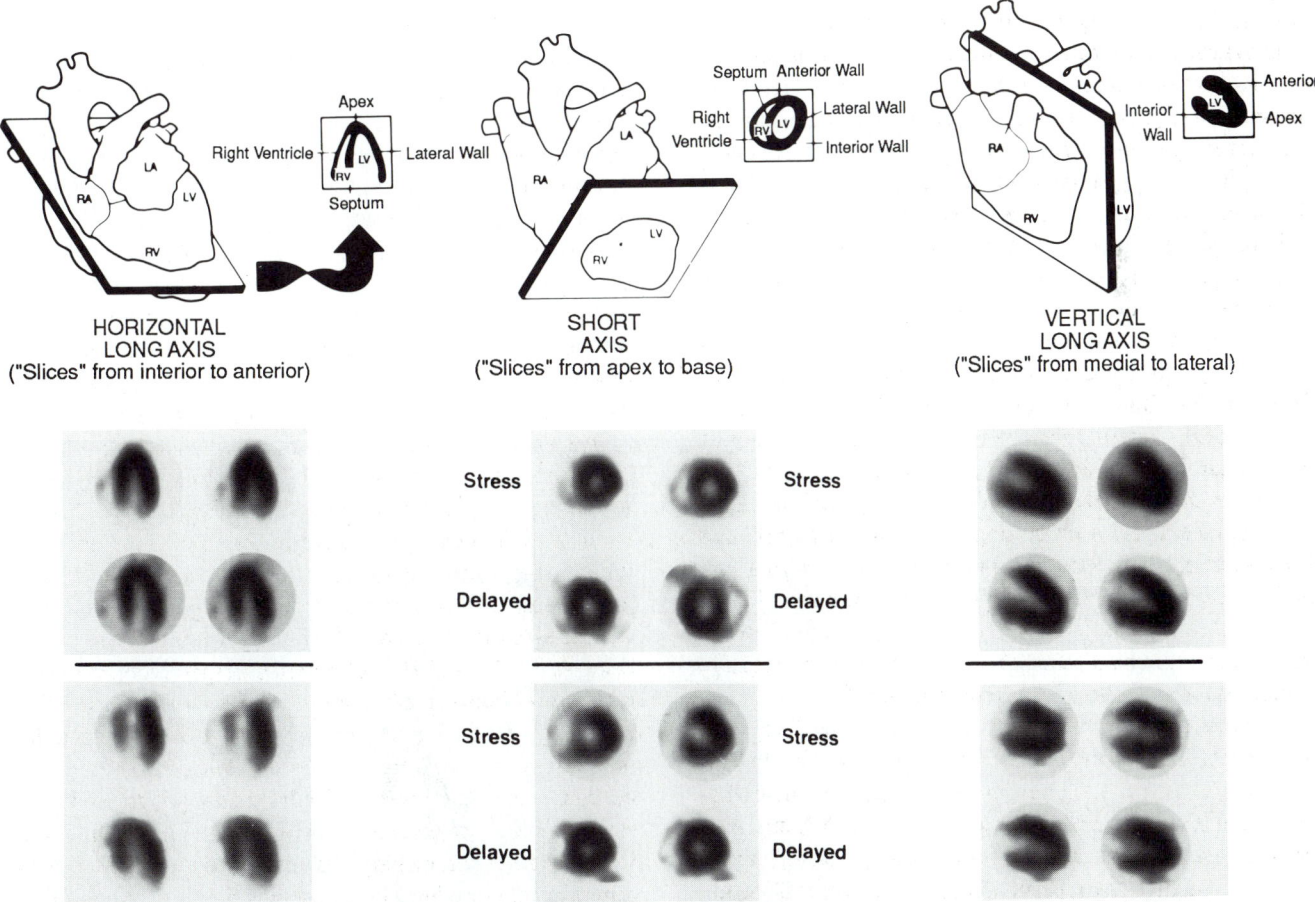

Figure 105–4. The three tomographic planes oriented to major cardiac axes are illustrated. The top panel of SPECT images shows a normal test; the bottom panel shows ischemia in the LAD distribution (see text). *(Courtesy of DuPont Medical Products and Dr. Ernest Garcia and E. Gordon DePuey of Emory University.)*

that employed in computerized axial tomography. The major advantage of SPECT imaging is that the three-dimensional imaging volume data can now be reoriented to form a series of tomographic planes oriented to the major cardiac axes (Fig. 105–5).

Quality control is a critical factor in tomographic imaging if artifacts, which may simulate myocardial abnormalities, are to be avoided. Quality control for tomographic imaging systems is much more rigorous than for planar imaging systems and must include assurance of detector uniformity, assurance of the completeness and adequacy of data collection, verification of the accuracy of the tomographic center of rotation, and testing the fidelity of the imaging characteristics of the system using appropriate phantoms.[93] Tomographic imaging will generate a relatively large number of slices for interpretation and review.

Image Quantitation

Quantitation of ^{201}Tl planar images has produced slight improvements in sensitivity and specificity, but the differences do not reach statistical significance.[94,95] A similar trend has been reported for SPECT myocardial imaging, however increased sensitivity with an accompanying loss in specificity can occur. SPECT myocardial perfusion imaging following exercise provides improved detection of individual coronary artery stenoses compared to qualitative planar imaging.[96] One inherent advantage of quantitative SPECT imaging is the improved reproducibility of lesion detection among different observers using quantitative tomographic analyses compared to simple visual assessment of tomographic polar coordinate images. These results do suggest an advantage with reduction of observer error as inexperienced observers using quantitative analyses can perform as well as experienced observers employing visual

analyses of SPECT myocardial perfusion images.[97] Another useful approach that has been employed to assist with this problem is a polar coordinate or "bulls eye" type of display.[98]

The profiles from the slice closest to the cardiac base are mapped onto the outer ring of the bullseye plot while data from each successive slice moving toward the ventricular apex are mapped into the next concentric ring moving to the center of the bullseye. Typical displays for the bullseye plot include color displays that show the uptake, redistribution, and washout of the tracer in regions that correspond to the distribution of the major coronary arteries. In addition, the distribution of activity can be compared to a reference normal population where regions with counts in the myocardium that fall more than two and a half standard deviations below the normal mean value are highlighted. In this fashion a severity map can be used to illustrate how far below the normal range each location in the myocardium falls.

Technetium-99m Radioisotopes

Technetium-99m-labeled perfusion tracers offer some advantages for myocardial perfusion imaging.[99] Technetium-99m has a 140 keV photon energy, which is optimal for gamma camera imaging and is more likely to produce high quality images than [201]Tl. The half-life of ^{99m}Tc and dosimetry make it possible to administer a 10–15 times higher dose of this radiopharmaceutical. This results in better images within a shorter time interval. Unlike ^{201}Tl, clinically significant redistribution of ^{99m}Tc agents such as sestamibi within the myocardium does not occur, necessitating both a stress and resting injection of this radiotracer. The timing of imaging after sestamibi administration is not as

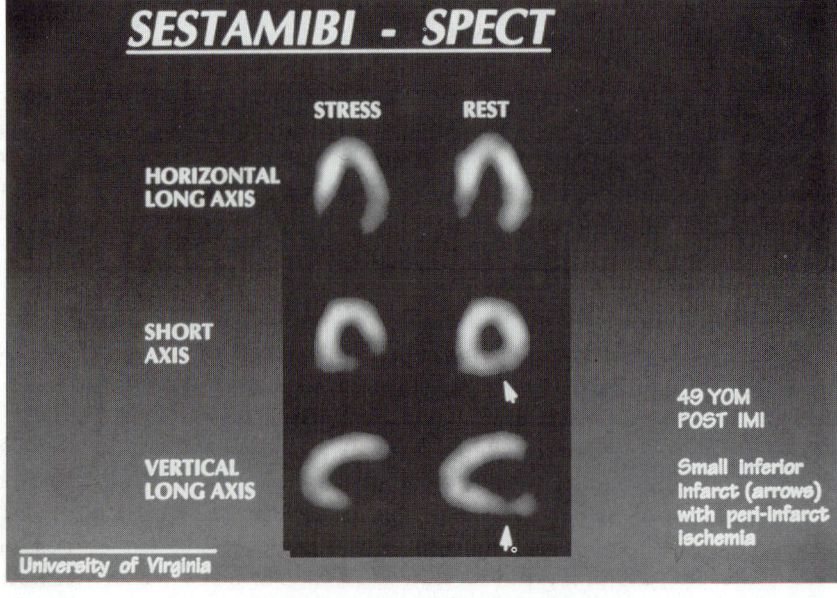

Figure 105–5. Representative tomographic slices in three orthogonal planes derived from a stress-rest ^{99m}Tc sestamibi myocardial perfusion study in a 49-year-old patient following inferior myocardial infarction. The stress images obtained in the short-axis and vertical long-axis views demonstrate a transmural defect in the inferolateral and posterior walls that is predominantly reversible in nature, as indicated by the increase in regional myocardial tracer uptake in these regions at rest (see arrows). This finding is compatible with a small inferior myocardial infarction with peri-infarction ischemia. There is no evidence of significant hypoperfusion of the left anterior descending coronary artery territory. This is a low-risk study for subsequent cardiac events.

critical as after injection of ^{201}Tl for detection of myocardial perfusion defects because of its prolonged myocardial retention. Myocardial images, which reflect regional myocardial bloodflow at the time of injection, can be acquired 2–3 hours after injection. Technetium-99m sestamibi is superior to ^{201}Tl for assessment of myocardium at risk in the setting of acute interventions such as thrombolytic therapy for acute myocardial infarction or coronary angioplasty. A report by Wackers et al in patients with significant coronary artery disease who had an abnormal stress planar ^{201}Tl image demonstrated that ^{201}Tl and sestamibi images correlated in 86% of patients who had either scar or ischemia on ^{201}Tl images, and that an exact concordance of segmental myocardial analysis was observed in 81% of segments.[100]

Technetium-99m sestamibi myocardial perfusion imaging has found numerous applications in the setting of coronary revascularization. In addition to its capacity to accurately detect, localize, and quantify the extent of myocardial hypoperfusion, this agent demonstrates a clinically useful capacity to predict myocardial viability, and recovery of function following coronary revascularization.[101] Whereas ^{201}Tl remains an excellent agent for myocardial viability detection, ^{99m}Tc sestamibi also serves as a marker of myocyte metabolism and nutritive perfusion.[102,103] The relative value of these agents in viability detection is being evaluated in a multicenter study of resting tomography with both agents prior to coronary revascularization, with postoperative recovery of left ventricular function as the "gold standard" of myocardial viability. In addition to its potential for viability determination, myocardial perfusion imaging with evidence of concomitantly increased sestamibi lung activity is a marker of multivessel coronary disease and extensive myocardial jeopardy, which portends a poor prognosis without coronary revascularization.[104] Technetium-99m perfusion agents may also offer some advantages in the diagnostic assessment of women with coronary disease, as compared to ^{201}Tl imaging in which significant attenuation artifacts may limit the diagnostic accuracy of perfusion studies.[105] It is anticipated that technetium-based perfusion agents will improve the diagnostic accuracy of myocardial imaging in the female population under evaluation for coronary revascularization.

Another significant advantage of ^{99m}Tc perfusion agents is the high count rates, which permit the performance of dual functional and perfusional imaging in the same study. A bolus injection of ^{99m}Tc sestamibi can be utilized to define the first-pass function of the left ventricle, and to quantitate regional wall motion and global left ventricular ejection fraction.[106] Tomographic wall motion and myocardial thickening can also be quantitated, and have demonstrated a good correlation with echocardiographic indices of ventricular function and ^{201}Tl indices of myocardial viability.[107] As such, the simultaneous assessment of myocardial perfusion and ventricular function during exercise with technetium sestamibi offers a significant advantage in the pre- and postoperative assessment of patients

with multivessel coronary disease, with the potential for demonstrating improvements in function and perfusion accrued by successful coronary revascularization.[108] Utilizing technetium agents, exercise radionuclide angiography can be combined with myocardial perfusion imaging to optimize the assessment of cardiac risk in patients with coronary artery disease.[109,110]

In summary, ^{99m}Tc sestamibi myocardial perfusion imaging can be applied for the evaluation of myocardial perfusion before and after coronary revascularization, and is a useful technique to document postrevascularization improvements in viability and cardiac function in patients with preoperative ventricular dyssynergy and global cardiac dysfunction.[111] As such, ^{99m}Tc perfusion agents are a reasonable alternative to ^{201}Tl perfusion imaging in the setting of coronary artery disease and surgical revascularization.

Diagnostic Considerations

The accuracy of any less than perfect noninvasive test in detecting coronary artery disease is dependent on test sensitivity and specificity, and pretest likelihood of disease in the population under study.[112] The sensitivity of a test for coronary artery disease can be said to define the percent of the population with coronary disease who have a positive test (true positive/true positive + false negative) and specificity to define the percent of the population without coronary artery disease who have a negative test (true negative/true negative + false positive). Once the sensitivity and specificity of the test are known, the predictive value of an abnormal or normal test result can be calculated over a wide range of clinical patient subsets using Bayesian theory.[113]

In general, the sensitivity and specificity of a test are not affected by the prevalence of coronary disease.[114] However, the sensitivity of most noninvasive tests for coronary artery disease is increased in patient populations with higher grade coronary lesions and in populations with more extensive coronary disease. Sensitivity is increased with maximal rather than submaximal exercise performed and may be decreased in patients with an extensive previous myocardial infarction. The sensitivity may be different when the test is performed in the supine versus upright position. The specificity of radionuclide diagnostic testing is decreased in patients who are hypoxic, severely anemic, or who are taking drugs known to alter exercise test performance.

Patients with severe left ventricular hypertrophy, and those with volume overload secondary to valvular heart disease will more likely have a "false-positive" response for coronary artery disease and decreased diagnostic specificity. The reported sensitivity and specificity of radionuclide tests may also vary because of interobserver variability in the interpretation of radionuclide data and angiographic coronary stenosis severity from within or different medical centers. Other factors that may impact on diagnostic test results at individual medical centers include age, gender, exercise end points, resting ejection fraction, and pharmacologic agents.

Optimal utilization of radionuclide tests for detection and severity of coronary disease take into consideration the pretest likelihood of coronary disease and are most useful in patients with an intermediate pretest risk of coronary disease. The pretest risk of coronary disease is enhanced in patients with multiple atherosclerotic risk factors. Tables of post-test risk after exercise perfusion imaging and computer programs that estimate post-test risk are available.[115]

Prognostic Considerations

[201]Tl stress scintigraphy is a powerful prognostic variable in determining future cardiac events in patients with suspected or proven ischemic heart disease. Wackers et al. studied a consecutive series of 344 patients referred with chest pain who underwent a planar ^{201}Tl stress scintigraphy.[116] Of 95 patients with a normal test, none died after an average follow-up of 22 mo and only two patients had a myocardial infarction. Similar data were reported by Pamelia et al in a consecutive series of 349 patients referred with chest pain, and by Wahl et al in a patient series of 455 patients referred for ^{201}Tl scintigraphy.[117,118] Several series report various myocardial hypoperfusion abnormalities associated with severe and extensive coronary disease and an adverse prognosis.[119–122] Silverman et al noted that prognosis following infarction could be related to presence and size of ^{201}Tl defects.[123]

Predischarge exercise ^{201}Tl scintigraphy after uncomplicated myocardial infarction is predictive of subsequent cardiac events. In a 140 patient series reported by Gibson et al 47 of the 50 patients who had a cardiac event were detected by ^{201}Tl scintigraphy.[124] The finding of more than one discrete vascular region, presence of delayed redistribution, or increased lung thallium uptake were more sensitive predictors of subsequent cardiac events than ST segment depression, angina, or extent of angiographic disease. In patients who cannot exercise or who perform inadequate levels of exercise, intravenous dipyridamole thallium scintigraphy is a useful prognostic test to risk stratify patients after an acute coronary event or who have chronic ischemic heart disease.[88,89,125] Several recent studies have demonstrated the prognostic value of dipyridamole and exercise ^{99m}Tc sestamibi perfusion imaging.[126,127]

Exercise radionuclide angiography is a powerful predictor of long-term outcome in patients with suspected or proven coronary artery disease. Of 79 patients followed for an average of 25 months after an abnormal exercise radionuclide angiogram in the absence of significant angiographic coronary artery disease, infarct-free survival at 4 years by life table analysis was 97%.[44] Of 386 consecutive medically treated symptomatic patients who underwent cardiac catheterization and exercise radionuclide angiography,[43] after an average follow-up of 4.5 years, univariate analysis revealed that the exercise ejection fraction was a variable most closely associated with future events. Multivariate analysis revealed that once the exercise ejection fraction was known, no other radionuclide or clinical variables contributed independent information about the likelihood of future events. In 117 patients with known coronary artery disease and mild symptoms with well-preserved left ventricular function, without left main coronary disease,[42] mortality during subsequent medical therapy was associated with three-vessel coronary disease and magnitude of ejection fraction response during exercise.

INFARCT AVID-IMAGING TECHNIQUES

Infarct avid-radionuclide-imaging agents accumulate in areas of acute myocardial necrosis resulting in a "hot spot," in contrast to ^{201}Tl perfusion images that outline region of necrosis as a cold spot. Of the currently available nuclear cardiology procedures, this is used least frequently (<1% of all nuclear cardiac imaging studies).

Technetium-99m stannous pyrophosphate, an agent used in bone imaging, can be used for infarct avid imaging.[128] Tissue uptake of pyrophosphate can be related in part to tissue calcium accumulation.[129,130] Regional accumulation of pyrophosphate also depends on adequate tissue delivery to necrotic tissue as well as the extent of the necrosis. Although a quantitative relationship between pyrophosphate uptake and calcium accumulation in zones of necrosis has not been demonstrated, there is a topographic relationship between areas of maximum pyrophosphate binding and maximum calcium accumulation in the periphery of an infarcted region. Thus, the actual intensity of ^{99m}Tc pyrophosphate binding in a myocardial region cannot be used to quantitate the degree of necrosis accurately. In addition, pyrophosphate binds to denatured protein or macromolecules that became available for chemical interaction only during myocardial necrosis.[131–133]

The optimum time for pyrophosphate myocardial infarct imaging is 2–3 days after the onset of necrosis. Imaging performed within 24 hours of infarction or later than 7–10 days after infarction is usually negative. However, in some patients in whom positive images were seen in the acute phase of myocardial infarction, there can be a persisting, less intense, diffuse uptake for several months after the acute event. Buja et al described an association between these persistently positive pyrophosphate images and ongoing myocytolytic degeneration.[134] Patients with presumed clinical diagnosis of unstable angina can have a positive scan in the absence of enzymatic or electrocardiographic changes of infarction.[135] Infarct avid-imaging was positive in approximately 93% of cases with acute infarction and negative in approximately 83% of cases in whom infarction was not present.[136] Others have reported low sensitivity, particularly in nontransmural infarction.[137]

Indium-111 (^{111}In)-antimyosin [Myoscint (antimyosin-Fab-DTPA-^{111}In)] imaging has a number of useful applications in the management of coronary artery disease. It is certainly of value in the diagnosis of myocardial infarction (MI), particularly in the presence of equivocal clinical, enzymatic, or ECG findings. For example, some patients admitted with suspected acute MI may hae ECG evidence of complete left bundle branch block. Also, if the acute event occurred 4 to 5 days prior to admission, serial determinations of creatine kinase may be nondiagnostic for acute necrosis. In such patients, ^{111}In-antimyosin imaging may be useful in confirming the diagnosis of recent myocardial necrosis. ^{111}In-antimyosin imaging can also detect subacute infarction that may be 7 to 10 days old. In addition, the use of [111] In-antimyosin imaging in the noninvasive estimation of infarct size may be helpful in risk stratification and prognostication.

The amount of residual viable myocardium, particularly after coronary reperfusion, may be evaluated as well with ^{111}In-antimyosin imaging. This application is most effective by a dual imaging approach with ^{201}Tl and ^{111}In-antimyosin. When correlated with wall motion, ^{111}In-antimyosin uptake may also be used to determine the degree of viability in an area of ischemic injury.

[111]In-antimyosin imaging is an effective diagnostic agent for a number of applications in the clinical management of MI. It has been used in the diagnosis of MI in patients with equivocal clinical, enzymatic, or electrocardiographic (ECG) findings. In addition, infarct-avid imaging with ^{111}In-antimyosin may be an excellent approach to noninvasive evaluation of infarct size. Because infarct size is a critical determinant of mortality risk after MI, ^{111}In-antimyosin imaging may prove to be useful in risk stratification and prognostication.[138–140]

Positron Emission Tomography

Positron emission tomography (PET) is imaging of positron emitting tracers: carbon-11, nitrogen-13, oxygen-15, and fluorine-18 are the most important of these very short lived "physiologic tracers." PET provides the ability to image and measure regional function and chemistry of tissues and organs.

Although a number of important areas of cardiac biochemistry and physiology can be measured with PET, including regional bloodflow,[141–143] myocardial substrate metabolism of fatty acid,[144,145] glucose[146,147] and protein metabolism,[148,149] one of the most important current PET applications is to distinguish ischemically compromised but viable myocardium from scar tissue. Assessment of viable myocardium has become important with the growth and development of new techniques for restoring blood flow as there is a need for accurate identification of ischemic but viable myocardium that will benefit from revascularization. PET assessment for coronary artery disease can be performed at rest or during drug stress with an identification of myocardial regions with reduced blood flow using N-13 ammonia. Alternatively, other positron emitting tracers that

are capable of measuring flow such as rubidium-82 can also be used.

The future of PET will depend largely on how well it competes with other less expensive and less complex modalities. The introduction of dedicated, simple minicyclotrons and methods for automated isotope production and radiochemistry has certainly assisted the successful introduction of PET as a routine clinical tool. PET offers unique ways of studying the neural control of the heart with tracers for evaluating neurotransmitters and the cardiac sympathetic and parasympathetic receptors. PET also offers the ability to directly measure the effects of drugs on the heart through the use of labeled drugs such as calcium antagonists, inotropic compounds, and β-blockers. Finally, the combined study of flow and fluorodeoxyglucose (FDG) uptake defines tissue viability more specifically than any other invasive or noninvasive technique currently available. This application alone favors an important future role for PET in the clinical management of coronary artery disease.

Assessment of Myocardial Viability

The increased availability of effective therapeutic interventions to promote the acute salvage of jeopardized myocardium following myocardial infarction, and the recognition of the salutory effects of coronary revascularization in patients with chronic ischemic left ventricular dysfunction, has driven the development of noninvasive diagnostic techniques for the detection of myocardial viability. These noninvasive techniques are probes for various components of the perfusion–metabolism–function coupling in the myocyte, which provide evidence as to the degree and distribution of residual nutritive blood flow, alternative metabolic activity, and recruitable ventricular function in severely ischemic myocardium. The predictive value of these diagnostic techniques for postrevascularization recovery of global and regional ventricular function is synergistic when more than one modality is utilized. Notwithstanding intraoperative myocardial injury, progressive and at times dramatic recovery of ventricular function frequently follows successful revascularization and bloodflow restoration to the viable tissue. This postrevascularization functional recovery remains the "gold-standard" against which tests designed to prospectively detect myocardial viability should be compared. The two syndromes of reversible ischemic left ventricular dysfunction are acute myocardial "stunning" and chronic myocardial "hibernation."[150,151]

The phenomenon of myocardial "stunning" was originally described in experimental studies of acute canine coronary occlusion and reperfusion.[152,153] Severe regional contractile dysfunction follows acute ischemic injury, which is associated with myocardial ATP depletion, reduced myocyte calcium responsiveness, and the potential for reversibility with sustained reperfusion. Unusual clinical examples of this syndrome include acute coronary spasm[154] and severe exercise-induced myocardial ischemia.[155] The use of acute interventional therapies for myocardial infarction has created a clinical subset of patients with the potential for myocardial "stunning" following coronary thrombolysis[156,157] and following acute coronary angioplasty.[158]

The "hibernation" syndrome of myocardial ischemic dysfunction as a result of sustained or repetitive episodes of hypoperfusion may represent an adaptive response to chronic hypoperfusion,[159,160] in which a concomitant protective decrease in ventricular function occurs in association with normal myocardial high energy phosphate content, and reduced myofilament calcium availability.[150,151] The dysfunctional state is frequently reversible upon coronary revascularization, or rarely with the use of aggressive anti-ischemic therapy. The observation that chronic ischemic left ventricular dysfunction (global or regional) could be reversed by coronary revascularization following bypass surgery[161,162] or angioplasty[163] underscores the clinical importance of this phenomenon.

Several clinical variables can effect the time course and degree of postischemic left ventricular recovery including the duration and severity of the ischemic insult, coexisting supply–demand imbalance due to multivessel disease, the mode of reperfusion, and the use of additional circulatory support.

In patients with unexplained congestive heart failure and a severely depressed left ventricular ejection fraction, without a prior history of angina or myocardial infarction, the question of whether the pathophysiology of heart failure is ischemic or idiopathic is clinically relevant, in that revascularization may offer significant functional benefits in the former subsets. Patients with known severe multivessel coronary artery disease and combined regional and global left ventricular dysfunction may require viability studies to determine whether "complete" revascularization by coronary bypass surgery or limited revascularization by angioplasty in selected viable zones is preferrable. Finally, the postinfarction patient with severe regional ventricular asynergy or aneurysm formation may have myocardial "stunning" that could functionally benefit from revascularization of the infarct-related coronary artery. Patients with these syndromes are selected for either percutaneous angioplasty or surgical revascularization to restore anatomy, overall left ventricular function, and the distribution and extent of ischemic but viable myocardium.

It is now possible to noninvasively prospectively detect viable tissue with a high positive predictive accuracy. The following techniques have been validated and are useful in this regard.

Thallium-201 Myocardial Perfusion Imaging

Thallium-201 has been widely utilized as a diagnostic imaging agent. Its initial myocardial extraction occurs in proportion to blood flow, but retention of ^{201}Tl ions is an active process requiring metabolic activity at the level of the sodium-potassium ATPase sarcolemmal complex. As such, ^{201}Tl is both a myocardial perfusion and viability

marker. Although limited "non-nutritive" passive uptake of ^{201}Tl may occur in infarcted myocardium, ^{201}Tl uptake is a good index of residual perfusion and myocyte metabolic activity.

The standard stress (exercise or drug) and 3–4 hour delay ^{201}Tl imaging protocol is suboptimal for viability detection, and is associated with a 40–50% false negative rate. Otherwise stated, 40–50% of 3–4 hour "fixed" nonreversible ^{201}Tl defects contain some residual viable myocardium. The use of delayed (8–24 hour) ^{201}Tl imaging further reduces the false negative rate to 15–25%[164,165] (Fig. 105–6). Reinjection of 1 mCi of ^{201}Tl on the same day as the stress-delay study, followed 3–4 hours later by repeat imaging, reduces the false-negative rate to 10–15%.[166] The combination of ^{201}Tl injection at rest (2–3 mCi) followed by 3–4 redistribution imaging reduces the false-negative rate to 5–10%.[167]

The general principle guiding this viability approach is that the availability of circulating ^{201}Tl to intact but is-

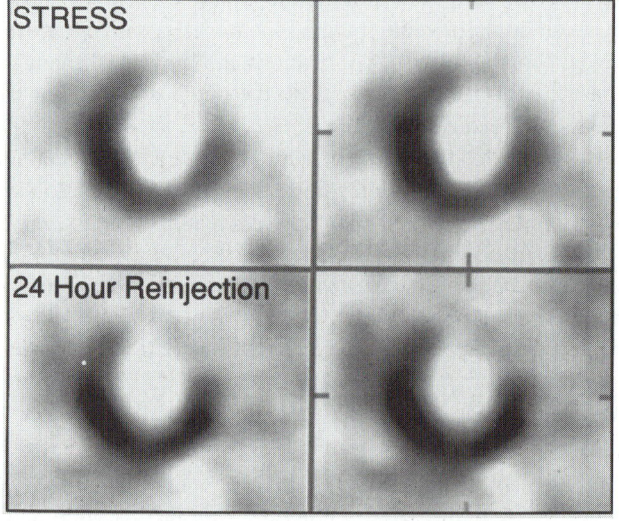

Figure 105–6. A dipyridamole stress thallium-201 tomographic study from a 54-year-old man with five previous myocardial infarctions who was admitted with unstable angina. The baseline ECG demonstrated lateral Q-waves, nonspecific ST-T-wave changes, and an intraventricular conduction delay. The patient was unable to perform exercise stress and underwent an IV dipyridamole stress study, which produced typical chest pain and accentuated the baseline ST-wave changes. An extensive anterior, lateral, and posterolateral perfusion defect was noted on the contiguous short-axis views (upper panels) through the mid-ventricle. No significant redistribution was observed on the 4-hour delay study. However, with thallium reinjection at 24 hours, repeat images demonstrated a decrease in left-ventricular chamber size and significant thallium redistribution in the posterolateral wall (lower panels). The patient underwent a high-risk angioplasty of the right coronary artery. He was subsequently stabilized with medical therapy and was discharged from the hospital without further complications. The 24-hour thallium reinjection study showed significantly viability in the previously hypokinetic posterolateral wall, which was amenable to coronary revascularization (PTCA), resulting in clinical improvement.

chemic myocyte membranes permits the gradual uptake and sustained retention of this potassium analog. The presence of any significant amount of residual ^{201}Tl activity at rest is generally a sign of viability, although the degree of radiotracer uptake is generally proportional to the degree of subsequent functional recovery. The severity (i.e., mild, moderate, or severe) of the myocardial ^{201}Tl defect is generally correlated with the likelihood of viability and subsequent functional recovery. On average, the presence of ^{201}Tl redistribution (with or without thallium-201 reinjection) is approximately 85–90% predictive of segmental ventricular functional recovery.[168,169] Even 75% of "fixed" 3–4 hour thallium-201 defect segments without akinesis recover ventricular function after revascularization.[170] The time course of post-revascularization ventricular function recovery and thallium-201 uptake may be significantly delayed (up to 6 months) following successful coronary bypass surgery[171] and angioplasty.[172]

Positron Emission Tomography

Positron emission tomographic (PET) correlations with the severity of 3–4 hour "fixed" ^{201}Tl defects have demonstrated that approximately 90, 60, and 30% of mild, moderate, and severe defects (respectively) have PET evidence of viability (i.e., FDG uptake), or exhibit further uptake of ^{201}Tl upon reinjection.[173–175] Of 24 hour "fixed" ^{201}Tl defects, approximately 80, 60, and 15% of mild, moderate, and severe defects show evidence of viability using FDG imaging of glycolytic metabolism.

Numerous studies have described the presence of relative increases in FDG activity (as compared to various perfusion markers) on PET studies of patients with subsequent postrevascularization ventricular function recovery (Fig. 105–7, see Color Plates following page 2072). This finding has been reported in patients undergoing coronary artery bypass graft surgery[176,177] and following percutaneous coronary angioplasty.[178] On average, 85–90% of segments with this FDG:flow "mismatch" pattern demonstrate improvements in segmental ventricular function following successful coronary revascularization. Although originally described in the setting of acute myocardial infarction,[179–181] this finding has been utilized as a method for distinguishing ischemic from nonischemic cardiomyopathy in patients with chronically depressed left ventricular dysfunction (i.e., hibernation).[182,183] Even irreversible (by reinjection) ^{201}Tl defects that are only mild-to-moderate in severity may contain viable myocardium, as evidenced by increased FDG uptake.[184]

Recent studies have pointed to the clinical benefits of viability screening for prediction of function recovery[185] and cardiac events[186] following revascularization. FDG:ammonia PET "mismatch" in heart failure patients (average EF = 25 ± 6%) was associated with 81% improvement in New York Heart Association Functional Class following revascularization.[185] Only 40% of patients with a "mismatch" pattern who are not revascularized improve in New York Heart Association Functional Class over 13.6 mo of

follow-up. Patients without the PET "mismatch" pattern do poorly, with functional class improvement in 27% of revascularized and 26% of nonrevascularized patients. An FDG:ammonia "mismatch" pattern, when revascularized is associated with an 88% cardiac event free survival over 1 year.[186] Patients with a similar imaging pattern who are not revascularized have a reduced 1 year cardiac event-free survival (50%). As such, it appears that these viability data have functional and prognostic importance.

Technetium-99m Sestamibi

The class of myocardial perfusion agents which are complexed with ^{99m}Tc to improve image resolution and myocardial activity has also been studied as potential markers of viability. Agents such as ^{99m}Tc sestamibi are known to have similar diagnostic and prognostic capabilities to ^{201}Tl. However, their uptake is not dependent on an intact sarcolemmal sodium potassium exchange pump. These agents are transported across membranes by facilitated transport, and are then complexed to the intracellular mitochondrial organelles. In vitro studies have demonstrated that intact mitochondrial metabolism is a prerequisite for sestamibi uptake.[187] The ^{99m}Tc sestamibi imaging approach has been useful in documenting the effects of acute reperfusion therapy for myocardial salvage.[188–190] Initial studies have demonstrated that regional myocardial ^{99m}Tc sestamibi activity >50% of that in normal zones is 90% predictive of nonakinetic and/or dyskinetic regional wall motion in the same zone.[111] Limited data exist on the positive predictive value of ^{99m}Tc sestamibi activity for recovery of ventricular function following revascularization.[101]

A reversible defect is 74% predictive of postrevascularization segmental recovery and a mild-to-moderate fixed defect is approximately 75% predictive.[191–193] As with ^{201}Tl, mild fixed defects are usually viable, whereas severe fixed defects are frequently nonviable. The moderate ^{99m}Tc sestamibi defect has an approximately 50% likelihood of being viable as compared to PET imaging, postrevascularization improvement in wall motion, or 24-hour ^{201}Tl redistribution. This has led some investigators to combine stress sestamibi imaging with rest ^{201}Tl reinjection, or to acquire ECG gated functional ^{99m}Tc sestamibi images to determine if regional wall motion and thickening are retained in defects of moderate severity.

Evaluation Following Coronary Artery Bypass Surgery

Given the premise that the most common causes of recurrent angina following bypass surgery are incomplete revascularization and bypass graft closure, selective coronary arteriography seems a logical "gold standard" for defining coronary anatomy as a prelude to repeat revascularization. However, confounding physiologic variables including coronary vasomotion, intermittent platelet-mediated thrombotic events, stenosis rheology, and competitive flow may complicate the coronary anatomic data and produce symptoms in the absence of progressive native circulation or bypass graft disease. Noninvasive testing may be applied to select high-risk patients who require coronary arteriography from the larger population with stable angina after bypass surgery. High-risk noninvasive markers, or a failure of medical therapy should be considered as appropriate indications for repeat angiography and revascularization as indicated by the coronary anatomy. Using this approach, the option of repeat revascularization will not be exercised prematurely. Noninvasive studies provide important information about the functional impact of bypass graft stenoses and assist in planning the type of repeat revascularization procedure.

Noninvasive Diagnostic Techniques for Detecting and Localizing Bypass Graft Stenoses

Although periodic noninvasive testing could theoretically be performed in low-risk patient subsets to detect disease progression and the development of recurrent myocardial ischemia, this approach would not be cost-effective. A more practical and common approach is to evaluate the functional capacity and inducibility of ischemia in the early postoperative setting as a baseline for subsequent evaluations to be performed if angina returns. The usual causes of myocardial ischemia at a 4- to 6-week postrevascularization study are incomplete revascularization or anastomotic closure. Patients with clearly abnormal postoperative studies are moderate-to-high-risk groups that may require more frequent follow-up. Serial studies in such patients may identify ischemic regions and permit subsequent identification of new ischemic zones as further native and graft atherosclerosis occurs.

Functional measurements of coronary flow using perfusion tracers may detect an unexpected suboptimal surgical result, even in those patients who receive grafts to each stenotic site.

It is important to reemphasize that graft flow and subsequent graft patency are determined primarily by the coronary flow reserve of the distal arterial beds beyond the anastomosis.[194] At 2.5 years postoperatively, 35% of vein grafts show important reductions in coronary flow (averaging 45%) as compared with early postoperative studies. This reduction in flow may result from morphological graft changes or from flow reserve abnormalities in the distal perfusion bed. Coronary flow reserve may improve but not return to normal following bypass surgery.[195–197] Thus, the postoperative myocardial perfusion and ventricular function result may not be entirely predicted by the anatomic site of graft placement or by preexisting coronary artery stenoses.

A comparison of precoronary and postcoronary bypass surgery treadmill testing usually demonstrates an improvement in functional capacity and reduced exercise-induced ischemia in the majority of patients tested. Preoperative exercise impairment in the heart rate response is improved

following bypass surgery, leading to an improved cardiac output and myocardial oxygen extraction, while reducing ischemic symptoms and ST segment depression.[198]

Exercise ECG and radionuclide imaging variables indicative of high-risk coronary artery disease have been derived from patients *without* previous coronary artery bypass surgery. The recurrence of high-risk markers following bypass surgery indicates continued or recurrent evidence of significant ischemia. Comparison with the immediate postoperative study may be valuable to determine whether a change has occurred. These findings are generally associated with significant angina pectoris; however, silent ischemia or anginal equivalents such as exertional dyspnea may be present. These findings objectify myocardial ischemia and reflect the extent of jeopardized and dysfunctional myocardium following bypass surgery in a manner that exercise ECG studies cannot.

Myocardial Perfusion Imaging

Myocardial perfusion imaging studies comparing the preoperative to postoperative states may be used to assess the adequacy of revascularization, and the postoperative study may be used as a baseline for subsequent studies that may be needed to evaluate recurrent symptoms. Perfusion imaging also may be useful in the frequent patients who demonstrate significant ST-T-wave changes due to drugs (e.g., digitalis) or conduction abnormalities (e.g., left bundle branch block) following bypass surgery.

In a 4-week preoperative and 8-week postoperative ^{201}Tl quantitative planar imaging study in 47 patients undergoing bypass surgery,[199] 93% of totally redistributing (i.e., ischemic) segments normalized postoperatively. Only 73% of myocardial segments with partial redistribution (i.e., severe ischemia and/or infarction) normalized postoperatively. A commensurate improvement in regional wall motion was usually noted in association with improved perfusion in these patients. The presence of persistent (i.e., 4 hour nonredistribution) ^{201}Tl defects postoperatively was associated with less frequent (45%) improvement to normal wall motion following bypass surgery. Only 14% of segments without postoperative improvement in perfusion demonstrated improved regional wall movement following revascularization. Thus, the density and reversibility of postoperative ^{201}Tl perfusion defects is significantly correlated with improvements in nutritive blood flow and regional wall motion postoperatively.

In another study of 23 patients with stable angina, resting left ventricular wall motion improved in 19 of 71 segments supplied by a patent bypass graft in association with improved ^{201}Tl perfusion.[200] Of 10 segments with abnormal regional wall motion postoperatively, 9 had an occluded graft or significantly stenotic graft and continued ^{201}Tl perfusion abnormalities postoperatively. Improvement in preoperative ^{201}Tl ischemia predicted graft patency with 90% accuracy.

Of 55 patients undergoing serial preoperative, 2-week,

and 1-year postoperative exercise ^{201}Tl imaging,[201] a sensitivity of 80%, a specificity of 88%, and a diagnostic accuracy of 86% were achieved for detecting or excluding graft occlusion. While graft lesions can be missed in the posterior circulation (right coronary artery, obtuse marginal circumflex arteries) and diagonal coronary arteries, 83% of the left anterior descending coronary artery (LAD) system lesions were successfully imaged. A high probability of graft occlusion exists in the presence of a new postoperative ^{201}Tl defect, particularly if work capacity is reduced and chest pain is present. The absence of new perfusion defects is 90% predictive of all grafts being patent, a frequent finding in patients with atypical chest pain or no symptoms.

Angina may be a useful guide to the timing of repeat exercise ^{201}Tl imaging in the postrevascularization setting.[201] In one study, 73% of patients with angina demonstrated an occluded graft, whereas only 27% of patients with atypical chest pain had graft occlusion at 1 year postoperatively. Eighty-three percent of patients with any type of chest pain (atypical or typical) and a new ^{201}Tl defect had occluded grafts, but only 5% of patients without new ^{201}Tl defects and without chest pain had an occluded graft.

In summary, postoperative myocardial perfusion imaging is useful to assess the functional status of bypass grafts.[202–207] The majority of preoperative ischemic perfusion defects are associated with some degree of preserved wall motion, and subsequent improvement in both perfusion and function can be expected postoperatively. By contrast, persistent or fixed defects without redistribution usually do not improve following revascularization, although 15–20% of mild persistent 4 hour poststress defects do improve. These zones may represent areas of severe ischemia perfused by high-grade stenoses, which require ^{201}Tl reinjection or delayed (24 hour) imaging to detect defect redistribution following ^{201}Tl stress testing.[208]

Thallium-201 redistribution during a symptom-limited stress test may precede the development of angina by several months. Exercise ^{201}Tl imaging may distinguish patients with atypical chest pain of noncardiac origin from those with significant myocardial ischemia. A normal maximal stress postbypass perfusion scan essentially excludes significant graft stenosis. Patients with patent bypass grafts should theoretically normalize previously abnormal regional ^{201}Tl distribution following surgery. Of patients with a normal exercise ^{201}Tl perfusion study following surgery, nearly 90% have patent bypass grafts. The causes for an abnormal postoperative ^{201}Tl scan with redistribution include graft occlusion or stenosis, incomplete revascularization, and progression of native coronary disease. The appearance of a new fixed defect (without ^{201}Tl redistribution) is frequently due to intraoperative myocardial infarction.

Assessment of Ventricular Function

During the interval between initial bypass surgery and reoperation, approximately one-third of patients suffer a decrease in left ventricular function in association with pro-

gressive age or coronary artery disease, and the onset of microvascular disease due to hypertension or diabetes mellitus.[209] Although regional wall motion analysis in a general chest pain population lacks specificity for detecting coronary stenoses as compared with ^{201}Tl perfusion imaging, the presence of a new exercise-induced transient regional wall motion abnormality in a zone perfused by a bypass graft frequently reflects graft stenosis or occlusion. Resting wall motion alone is not predictive of graft patency status. The presence of new exercise-induced global or regional ventricular dysfunction in a patient with recurrent angina following bypass surgery is strongly suggestive of myocardial ischemia. The higher sensitivity and specificity of perfusion imaging make it preferable to exercise radionuclide angiography in most patients.

Previous studies have demonstrated a variable effect of revascularization on resting left ventricular function, with improvement frequently observed in patients with preoperative unstable angina but little improvement noted in patients with stable angina. There may be no significant postoperative improvement in global left ventricular ejection fraction following limited revascularization (single- or double-vessel bypass). However, more complete revascularization usually improves both rest and exercise ejection fraction in addition to improving regional wall motion. Coronary bypass surgery also improves postoperative exercise performance, a parameter closely related to ventricular function. Following successful coronary bypass surgery, an abnormal ejection fraction response to exercise (any decrease or failure to rise 5%) is also often reversed.[210] This improvement in global function is frequently associated with the disappearance of exercise-related ischemia and exercise-induced regional wall motion abnormalities.

Rest and exercise first-pass radionuclide left ventriculography during supine bicycle exercise before and 3 mo after coronary bypass surgery in 20 patients with chronic stable angina demonstrated no improvement in rest ejection fraction, whereas exercise ejection fraction was significantly improved (53 ± 17 to 63 ± 17; $p < 0.01$) in association with a higher maximum work load and rate-pressure product.[211] Multiple gated (MUGA) ejection fractions during graded exercise also were significantly higher in the postoperative state (53 ± 17 to 63 ± 19; $p < 0.001$). This increase in exercise ejection fraction following bypass surgery was principally the result of decreased exercise end-systolic volumes. A subgroup of five patients with significantly decreased ejection fraction during postoperative exercise had one or more obstructed grafts.

Patients with more severe preoperative exercise-induced ischemia, for example, those with > 2 mm ST segment depression, often have the greatest postoperative improvement in ventricular function.[211]

Concomitant medication such as β-blockers or calcium antagonists may significantly diminish the ventricular response to exercise. Bypass alone is more likely to improve left ventricular performance than would cardiac medication by virtue of differences in the supply versus demand ratio provided by these two interventions. Only the improvement in bloodflow associated with coronary revascularization can reproducibly improve LV function in chronically ischemic (hibernating) myocardium. Perfusion defects noted in the immediate postoperative period may be associated with dysfunctional areas of myocardial stunning or hibernation, which can require up to 6 months to reverse.[212,213]

It is difficult to demonstrate a predictable relationship between exercise-induced changes in ejection fraction and patency of individual grafts. Multivessel disease, when present, may obscure the effects of individual occluded grafts. Also, overlap of perfusion zones and unexpected revascularization or distant zones by patent grafts complicates the assignment of regional wall motion abnormalities to a particular graft.

Positron Emission Tomography

Metabolic imaging using PET can distinguish hypoperfused but viable myocardium from infarcted tissue. The discordance between increased FDG and decreased nitrogen-13 ammonia uptake, which reflects a change to increased anaerobic glycolysis in the ischemic zone, can be used to predict recovery of function following myocardial stunning and revascularization procedures.[214] Of 22 patients who underwent a precoronary and postcoronary artery bypass PET study and MUGA radionuclide angiogram, 55 grafts (82%) were patent at 1 month postoperatively.[215] In this study, 62% (13 of 21) of the ischemic segments improved perfusion postoperatively, as compared with only 27% (8 of 30) of those classified as infarcted ($p < 0.05$). Nineteen of the 21 segments with improved perfusion had patent grafts. As measured by PET imaging, 46% of segments with patent grafts had increased perfusion, whereas regional wall motion improved in 61% of segments supplied by patent grafts. It is apparent that improved segmental FDG uptake following bypass surgery correlates well with graft patency and with improved wall motion.

Preoperative and postoperative metabolic PET imaging may be useful for noninvasively predicting and serially following the response to coronary revascularization. The relationship of metabolic activity to angina threshold and functional recovery is now being assessed.[216] The expense and technical complexity of PET imaging limit the widespread applicability of this technique. Less expensive and more widely applicable ^{201}Tl perfusion imaging, with reinjection to late (24 hour) studies to determine viability may provide a more practical, albeit less sensitive, alternative to PET imaging in this setting. Newer metabolic imaging techniques such as PET and single photon myocardial tomography with ^{123}I-labeled fatty acid analogs remain promising, but are clinically unproven as diagnostic tests for the evaluation of unselected patient populations presenting with recurrent angina following revascularization surgery.[217]

REFERENCES

1. Berger HJ, Matthay RA, Pytlik LM, et al: Firstpass radionuclide assessment of right and left ventricular performance in patients with cardiac and pulmonary disease. *Semin Nucl Med* **9**:275, 1979
2. Rerych SK, Scholz PM, Newman GE, et al: Cardiac function at rest and exercise in normals and patients with coronary disease: Evaluation by radionuclide angiography. *Ann Surg* **187**:449, 1978
3. Schelbert HR, Verba JW, Johnson AD, et al: Non-traumatic determination of left ventricular ejection fraction by radionuclide angiography. *Circulation* **51**:902, 1975
4. Marshall RC, Berger HJ, Costin JC, et al: Assessment of cardiac performance with quantitative radionuclide angiocardiography: Sequential left ventricular ejection fraction, normalized left ventricular ejection rate, and regional wall motion. *Circulation* **56**:320, 1977
5. Berger JH, Matthay RA, Loke J, et al: Assessment of cardiac performance with quantitative radionuclide angiocardiography: Right ventricular ejection fraction with reference to findings in chronic obstructive pulmonary disease. *Am J Cardiol* **41**:397, 1978
6. Tobinick E, Schelbert HR, Henning H, et al: Right ventricular ejection fraction in patients with acute anterior and inferior myocardial infarction assessed by radionuclide angiography. *Circulation* **57**:1073, 1978
7. Hecht HS, Mirell SG, Rolett EL, et al: Left ventricular ejection fraction and segmental wall motion by peripheral first-pass radionuclide angiography. *J Nucl Med* **19**:17, 1978
8. Bodenhiemer MM, Banka VS, Fooshee CM, et al: Quantitative radionuclide angiography in the right anterior oblique view: Comparison with contrast ventriculography. *Am J Cardiol* **41**:718, 1978
9. Jengo JA, Mena I, Blaufuss A, et al: Evaluation of left ventricular function (ejection fraction and segmental wall motion by single pass radioisotope angiography. *Circulation* **57**:326, 1978
10. Marshall RC, Berger HJ, Reduto LA, et al: Variability in sequential measures of left ventricular performance assessed with radionuclide angiocardiography. *Am J Cardiol* **41**:531, 1978
11. Steele P, LeFree M, Kirch D: Measurement of left ventricular mean circumferential fiber shortening velocity and systolic ejection rate by computerized radionuclide angiography. *Am J Cardiol* **37**:388, 1976
12. Slutsky R, Gordon D, Karliner J, et al: Assessment of early ventricular systole by first pass radionuclide angiography. *Am J Cardiol* **44**:459, 1979
13. Pavel DG, Zimmer AM, Paterson VN: In vivo labeling of red blood cells with ^{99m}Tc. A new approach to blood pool visualization. *J Nucl Med* **18**:305, 1977
14. Greene MV, Ostrow HG, Douglas MA, et al: High temporal resolution ECG-gated scintigraphic angiography. *J Nucl Med* **16**:95, 1975
15. Burow RD, Strauss HW, Singleton R, et al: Analysis of left ventricular function from multiple gated acquisition cardiac blood pool imaging. *Circulation* **56**:1024, 1977
16. Bacharach SL, Green MV, Borer JS, et al: A real time system for multi-image gated cardiac studies. *J Nucl Med* **18**:79, 1977
17. Wackers FJ, Berger HJ, Johnston DE, et al: Multiple gated cardiac blood pool imaging for left ventricular ejection fraction: Validation of the technique and assessment of variability. *Am J Cardiol* **43**:1159, 1979
18. Federman J, Brown ML, Tancredi RG, et al: Multiple gated acquisition cardiac blood pool imaging: Evaluation of left ventricular function correlated with contrast angiography. *Mayo Clin Proc* **53**:625, 1978
19. Freeman M, Berman D, Staniloff H, et al: A 70 degrees LAO view overcomes the inadequacies of standard views the scintigraphic assessment of inferior wall motion (Abstract). *Circulation* **60**(Suppl 2):136, 1979
20. Kelly MJ, Giles RW, Simon TS, et al: Multigated equilibrium radionuclide angiography: Improved detection of left ventricular wall motion abnormalities and aneurysms with the addition of the left lateral view. *Radiology* **139**:167, 1981

21. Borer JS, Bacharach SL, Green MV, et al: Realtime radionuclide cineangiography in the noninvasive evaluation of global and regional left ventricular function at rest and during exercise in patients with coronary artery disease. *N Engl J Med* **296**:839, 1977

22. Maddox DE, Wynne J, Vren R, et al: Regional ejection fraction: A quantitative index of left ventricular performance. *Circulation* **59**:984, 1979

23. Maddox DE, Hilman BL, Wynne J, et al: The ejection fraction images: A noninvasive index of regional left ventricular wall motion. *Am J Cardiol* **41**:1230, 1978

24. Maddahi J, Berman DS, Matsuoka DT, et al: A new technique for assessing right ventricular ejection fraction using multiple-gated equilibrium cardiac blood pool scintigraphy. Description, validation and findings in chronic coronary artery disease. *Circulation* **60**:581, 1979

25. Dehmer GJ, Lewis SE, Hillis LD, et al: Nongeometric determination of left ventricular volumes from equilibrium blood pool scan. *Am J Cardiol* **45**:293, 1980

26. Reduto LA, Berger HJ, Cohen LS, et al: Sequential radionuclide assessment of left and right ventricular performance after acute myocardial infarction. *Ann Intern Med* **39**:441, 1978

27. Rigo P, Murray M, Taylor DR, et al: Right ventricular dysfunction detected by gated scintigraphy in patients with acute inferior infarction. *Circulation* **52**:268, 1975

28. Sharpe DN, Botvinick EH, Shames D, et al: The noninvasive diagnosis of right ventricular infarction. *Circulation* **57**:483, 1978

29. Pohost GM, Vignola PA, McKusick KA, et al: Hypertrophic cardiomyopathy: Evaluation by gated cardiac blood pool scanning. *Circulation* **55**:92, 1977

30. Zaret BL, Hurley PJ, Pitt B: Noninvasive scintiphotographic diagnosis of left atrial myxoma. *J Nucl Med* **13**:81, 1972

31. Rigo P, Alderson PO, Robertson RM, et al: Measurement of aortic and mitral regurgitation by gated cardiac blood pool scans. *Circulation* **60**:306, 1979

32. Lam W, Pavel D, Byrom E, et al: Radionuclide regurgitant index: Value and limitations. *Am J Cardiol* **47**:292, 1981

33. Berger HJ, Reduto LA, Johnstone DE, et al: Global and regional left ventricular response to bicycle exercise in coronary artery disease: Assessment by quantitative radionuclide angiocardiography. *Am J Med* **66**:13, 1979

34. Jengo JA, Oren V, Conant R, et al: Effects of maximal exercise stress on left ventricular function in patients with coronary artery disease using first-pass radionuclide angiography. *Circulation* **59**:60, 1979

35. Caldwell JH, Hamilton GW, Sorensen SG, et al: The detection of coronary artery disease with radionuclide techniques: A comparison of rest exercise thallium imaging and ejection fraction response. *Circulation* **61**:610, 1980

36. Johnstone DE, Sands MJ, Berger HJ, et al: Comparison of exercise radionuclide angiocardiography and thallium-201 myocardial perfusion imaging in coronary artery disease. *Am J Cardiol* **45**:1113, 1980

37. Jengo JA, Greenman R, Brizendine M, et al: Detection of coronary artery disease: Comparison of exercise stress radionuclide angiocardiography and thallium stress perfusion scanning. *Am J Cardiol* **45**:535, 1980

38. Jones RH, McEwan P, Newman GE, et al: Accuracy of diagnosis of coronary artery disease by radionuclide measurement of left ventricular function during rest and exercise. *Circulation* **64**:586, 1981

39. Rozanski A, Diamond GA, Berman D, et al: The declining specificity of exercise radionuclide ventriculography. *N Engl J Med* **309**:518, 1983

40. Iskandrian A, Hakki AH, Goel I, et al: The use of rest and exercise radionuclide ventriculography in risk stratification in patients with suspected coronary artery disease. *Am Heart J* **110**:864–872, 1985

41. Iskandrian A, Hakki AH: Radionuclide evaluation of exercise left ventricular performance in patients with coronary artery disease. *Am Heart J* **110**:851–856, 1985

42. Bonow R, Kent K, Rosing D, et al: Exercise-induced ischemia in mildly symptomatic patients with coronary-artery disease and preserved left ventricular function. *N Engl J Med* **311**:1339–1345, 1984

43. Pryor DB, Harrell F, Lee K, et al: Prognostic indicators from radionuclide angiography in medically treated patients with coronary artery disease. *Am J Cardiol* **53**:18–22, 1984

44. Miller T, Taliercio C, Zinsmeister A, et al: Prognosis in patients with an abnormal exercise radionuclide angiogram in the absence of significant coronary artery disease. *J Am Coll Cardiol* **12**:637–641, 1988

45. Port S, Cobb FR, Jones RH: Effects of propranolol on left ventricular function in normal men. *Circulation* **61**:358, 1980

46. Bodenhiemer MM, Banka VS, Fooshee CM, et al: Detection of coronary heart disease using radionuclide-determined regional ejection fraction at rest during handgrip exercise: Correlation with coronary arteriography. *Circulation* **58**:640, 1978

47. Wainwright RJ, Brennand-Roper DA, Cueni T, et al: Cold pressor test in detection of coronary heart disease and cardiomyopathy using Technetium 99m gated blood pool imaging. *Lancet* **II**:320, 1979

48. Kurz RG, Brady TJ, Besozzi MD, et al: Cold pressor radionuclide ventriculography. *Clin Res* **28**:189A, 1980

49. Borer JS, Bacharach SL, Green MV, et al: Exercise-induced left ventricular dysfunction in symptomatic and asymptomatic patients with aortic regurgitation: Assessment by radionuclide cineangiography. *Am J Cardiol* **42**:351, 1982

50. Lewis SM, Riba AL, Berger HJ, et al: Radionuclide angiographic exercise left ventricular performance in chronic aortic regurgitation: Relationship to resting echographic ventricular dimensions and systolic wall stress index. *Am Heart J* **103**:498, 1982

51. Borer JS, Rosing DR, Kent KM, et al: Left ventricular function at rest and during exercise after aortic valve replacement in patients with aortic regurgitation. *Am J Cardiol* **44**:1297, 1979

52. Lebowitz E, Greene MW, Bradley-Moore P, et al: (201)Tl for medical use. *J Nucl Med* **14**:421, 1973

53. Strauss HW, Harrison K, Langan JK, et al: Thallium-201 for myocardial imaging. Relation of thallium-201 to regional myocardial perfusion. *Circulation* **51**:641, 1975

54. DiCola VS, Downing SE, Donabedian RK, et al: Pathophysiologic correlates of thallium-201 myocardial uptake in experimental infarction. *Cardiovasc Res* **11**:141, 1977

55. Pohost GM, Alpert NA, Ingwall JS, et al: Thallium redistribution: Mechanisms and clinical utility. *Semin Nucl Med* **10**:70, 1980

56. Welch HF, Strauss HW, Pitt B: Myocardial extraction fraction of thallium-201. *Circulation* **56**:188, 1977

57. Pohost GM, Zir LM, Moore RH, et al: Differentiation of transiently ischemic from infarcted myocardium by serial imaging after a single dose of thallium-201. *Circulation* **55**:294, 1977

58. Johnstone DE, Wackers FJ, Berger HJ, et al: Effect of patient positioning on left lateral thallium-201 myocardial images. *J Nucl Med* **20**:183, 1979

59. Goris ML, Daspit SG, McLaughlin P, et al: Interpolative background subtraction. *J Nucl Med* **17**:744, 1976

60. Narahara KA, Hamilton GW, Williams DL, et al: Myocardial imaging with thallium-201: An experimental model for analysis of the true myocardial and background image components. *J Nucl Med* **18**:781, 1977

61. Burow RD, Pond M, Schafer AW, et al: Circumferential profiles: A new method for computer analysis of thallium-201 myocardial perfusion images. *J Nucl Med* **20**:171, 1979

62. Garcia E, Maddahi J, Berman D, et al: Space/time quantitation of thallium-201 myocardial scintigraphy. *J Nucl Med* **22**:309–317, 1981

63. Areeda J, Train K, Garcia E, et al: Improved segment analysis of (abstr) thallium-201 myocardial scintigrams: Quantitative of distribution, washout, and redistribution. *J Nuc Med* **23**:18, 1982

64. Granato J, Watson D, Flanagan T, et al: Myocardial thallium-201 kinetics during coronary occlusion and reperfusion: Influence of

method of reflow and timing of thallium-201 administration. *Circulation* **73**:150–160, 1986

65. Kaul S, Chesler D, Newell J, et al: Regional variability in the myocardial clearance of thallium-201 and its importance in determining the presence or absence of coronary artery disease. *J Am Coll Cardiol* **8**:95–100, 1986

66. Watson DD, Norman C, Read E, et al: Spatial and temporal quantitation of plane thallium myocardial images. *J Nucl Med* **22**:577–584, 1981

67. Wackers F, Fetterman R, Mattera J, et al: Quantitative analysis of thallium-201 kinetics on initial and delayed resting scans: Patterns in normal volunteers. *J Am Coll Cardiol* **1**:1601, 1983

68. Clements J, Fetterman R, Wackers F: An improved thallium-201 stress circumferential profile for objective analysis of coronary artery disease. *Radiol Soc North Am* Scientific Program 1982. Chicago, Radiologic Society of North America, 1982, p 176

69. Heitzman M, Fetterman R, Mattera J, et al: Thallium-201 kinetics shortly after termination of exercise: Implications for quantitative analysis. *J Nucl Med* **24**:46, 1983

70. Wackers F, Fetterman R, Mattera J, et al: Optimal count rates for reliable assessment of thallium-201 myocardial washout. *J Nucl Med* **24**:28, 1983

71. Wackers F, Bales D, Fetterman R, et al: Nonuniform washout of thallium-201 (within normal range): Criterion for improved detection of single vessel coronary artery disease. *J Nucl Med* **24**:46, 1983

72. McCarthy DM, Makler PT: Potential limitations of quantitative thallium scanning. *Am J Cardiol* **55**:215, 1985

73. Berger BC, Watson DD, Taylor GJ, et al: Quantitative thallium-201 exercise scintigraphy for detection of coronary artery disease. *J Nucl Med* **22**:585, 1981

74. Gould KL: Quantitative imaging in nuclear cardiology. *Circulation* **66**:1141, 1982

75. Wackers FJ: Myocardial perfusion imaging. In Goctschalk A, Hoffer PB, Potchen EJ (eds): *Diagnostic Nuclear Medicine*. Baltimore, Williams & Wilkins, 1988, p 291

76. Wackers FJ, Busemann-Sokole E, Samson G, et al: Value and limitations of thallium-201 scintigraphy in the acute phase of myocardial infarction. *N Engl J Med* **295**:1, 1976

77. Wackers FJ, Lie KI, Liem KL, et al: Thallium-201 scintigraphy in unstable angina pectoris. *Circulation* **57**:738, 1978

78. Maseri A, Parodi O, Severi S, et al: Transient transmural reduction of myocardial blood flow, demonstrated by thallium-201 scintigraphy as a cause of variant angina. *Circulation* **54**:280, 1976

79. Kushner FG, Okada RD, Kirschenbaum HD, et al: Stress-induced pulmonary TI-201 uptake in patients with coronary artery disease (Abstract). *J Nucl Med* **20**:649, 1979

80. Liu P, Kiess M, Okada RD, et al: Increased thallium lung uptake after exercise in isolated left anterior descending coronary artery disease. *Am J Cardiol* **55**:1469, 1985

81. Canhasi B, Dae M, Botvinick E, et al: Interaction of "Supplementary" scintigraphic indicators of ischemia and stress electrocardiography in the diagnosis of multivessel coronary disease. *J Am Coll Cardiol* **6**:581, 1985

82. Gould KL: Noninvasive assessment of coronary stenosis by myocardial perfusion imaging during pharmacologic vasodilatation. I. Physiologic basis and experimental validation. *Am J Cardiol* **41**:267, 1978

83. Albro PC, Gould KL, Westcott RJ, et al: Noninvasive assessment of coronary stenosis by myocardial imaging during pharmacologic coronary vasodilatation. III. Clinical trial. *Am J Cardiol* **42**:751, 1978

84. Leppo JA: Dipyridamole-thallium imaging: The lazy man's stress test. *J Nucl Med* **30**:281, 1989

85. Francisco DA, Collins SM, Go RT, et al: Tomographic thallium-201 myocardial perfusion scintigrams after maximal coronary artery vasodilation with intravenous dipyridamole. Comparison of qualitative and quantitative approaches. *Circulation* **66**:370, 1982

86. Lam JY, Chaitman BR, Glaenzer M, et al: Safety and diagnostic accuracy of dipyridamole-thallium imaging in the elderly. *J Am Coll Cardiol* **11**:585, 1988

87. Lewen MK, Labovitz AJ, Kern MJ, et al: Prolonged myocardial ischemia after intravenous dipyridamole thallium imaging. *Chest* **92**:1102, 1987

88. Eagle KA, Singer DE, Brewster DC, et al: Dipyridamole thallium scanning in patients undergoing vascular surgery. Optimizing preoperative evaluation of cardiac risk. *JAMA* **257**:2185, 1987

89. Shaw L, Miller DD, Kong BA, et al: Determination of perioperative cardiac risk by adenosine thallium-201 myocardial imaging. *Am Heart J* **124**:861–869, 1992

90. Ritchie JL, Larsson S, Israelson A, et al: Single photon tomographic imaging of a standard heart phantom with 201-TI: A gamma camera based system. *Eur J Nucl Med* **7**:254, 1982

91. Borrello JA, Clinthorne NH, Rogers WI, et al: Oblique-angle tomography: A restructuring algorithm for transaxial tomographic data. *J Nucl Med* **22**:471, 1981

92. Budinger TF: Physical attributes of single-photon tomography. *J Nucl Med* **21**:579, 1980

93. Rogers WL, Clinthorne NH, Harkness BA, et al: Field-flood requirements for emission computed tomography with an anger camera. *J Nucl Med* **23**:162, 1982

94. Berger BC, Watson DD, Taylor GJ, et al: Quantitative thallium-201 exercise scintigraphy for detection of coronary artery disease. *J Nucl Med* **22**:585, 1981

95. Maddahi J, Garcia EV, Berman DS, et al: Improved noninvasive assessment of coronary artery disease by quantitative analysis of regional stress myocardial distribution and washout of thallium-201. *Circulation* **64**:924, 1981

96. Tamaki N, Yonekura Y, Mukai T, et al: Segmental analysis of stress thallium myocardial emission tomography for localization of coronary artery disease. *Eur J Nucl Med* **9**:99, 1984

97. DePasquale EE, Nody AC, DePuey EG, et al: Quantitative rotational thallium-201 tomography for identifying and localizing coronary artery disease. *Circulation* **77**:316, 1988

98. Jaszczak RJ, Greer K, Coleman RE: SPECT system misalignment: Comparison of phantom and patient images. In Essen PD (ed): *Emission Computed Tomography: Current Trends*. New York, Society of Nuclear Medicine, 1983, pp 57–70

99. Holman BL, Jones AG, Lister-James J, et al: A new Tc-99m-labeled myocardial imaging agent, hexakis (t-Butylisonitrile)-technetium(I) [Tc-99m TBI]: Initial experience in the human. *J Nucl Med* **25**:1350, 1984

100. Wackers FJ, Berman DS, Maddahi J, et al: Technetium-99m hexakis 2-methoxyisobutyl isonitrile: Human biodistribution, dosimetry, safety, and preliminary comparison to thallium-201 for myocardial perfusion imaging. *J Nucl Med* **30**:301, 1989

101. Udelson J, Coleman PS, Metherall J, et al: Predicting recovery of severe regional ventricular dysfunction: Comparison of resting scintigraphy with ^{201}Tl and ^{99m}Tc-sestamibi. *Circulation* **89**:2552, 1994

102. Marzullo P, Sambuceti G, Parodi O: The role of sestamibi scintigraphy in the radioisotopic assessment of myocardial viability. *J Nucl Med* **33**:1925–1930, 1992

103. Rocco TP, Dilsizian V, Strauss HW, Boucher CA: Technetium-99m isonitrile myocardial uptake at rest, II: Relation to clinical markers of potential viability. *J Am Coll Cardiol* **14**:1678–1684, 1989

104. Taillefer R, Costi P, Jarry M, et al: Increased ^{99m}Tc-sestamibi (MIBI) lung uptake in the diagnosis of coronary artery disease: Comparison between early (5 min) and delayed (60 min) post-stress MIBI and thallium (Tl) planar imaging (abstr). *J Nucl Med* **34**:121P, 1993

105. Shaw LJ, Miller DD, Romeis JC, et al: Gender differences in the noninvasive evaluation and management of patients with suspected coronary artery disease. *Ann Intern Med* **120**:559–566, 1994

106. DePuey EG, Nichols K, Dobrinsky C: Left ventricular ejection fraction assessed from gated technetium-99m-sestamibi SPECT. *J Nucl Med* **34**:1871–1876, 1993

107. Chua T, Kiat H, Germano G, et al: Gated technetium-99m sestamibi for simultaneous assessment of stress myocardial perfusion, postexercise regional ventricular function and myocardial viability. Correlation with echocardiography and rest thallium-201 scintigraphy. *J Am Coll Cardiol* **23**:1107–1114, 1994

108. Jones RH, Borges-Neto S, Potts JM: Simultaneous measurement of myocardial perfusion and ventricular function during exercise from a single injection of technetium-99m sestamibi in coronary artery disease. *Am J Cardiol* **66**:68E–71E, 1990

109. Jones RH, Johnson SH, Bigelow C, et al: Exercise radionuclide angiocardiography predicts cardiac death in patients with coronary artery disease. *Circulation* **84**:152–158, 1991

110. Stratmann HG, Williams GA, Wittry MD, et al: Exercise technetium-99m sestamibi tomography for cardiac risk stratification of patients with stable chest pain. *Circulation* **89**:615–622, 1994

111. Kam R, Chua T, Goh A, et al: Stress sestamibi myocardial perfusion SPECT before and after coronary angioplasty for the identification of viable, ischemic myocardium and post-angioplasty improvement. *Circulation* (Supp I):1–419, 1992

112. Epstein S: Implications of probability analysis on the strategy used for noninvasive detection of coronary artery disease: Role of single or combined use of exercise electrocardiographic testing, radionuclide cineangiography and myocardial perfusion imaging. *Am J Cardiol* **46**:491–500, 1980

113. Chaitman B, Bourassa M, Davis K, et al: Angiographic prevalence of high-risk coronary artery disease in patient subsets (CASS). *Circulation* **64**:360–367, 1981

114. Chaitman BR, Hanson JS: Comparative sensitivity and specificity of exercise electrocardiographic lead system. *Am J Cardiol* **47**:1335, 1981

115. Diamond GA, Staniloff HM, Forrester JS, et al: Computer-assisted diagnosis in the noninvasive evaluation of patients with suspected coronary artery disease. *J Am Coll Cardiol* **1**:444, 1983

116. Wackers F, Russo D, Russ D, et al: Prognostic significance of normal quantitative planar thallium-201 stress scintigraphy in patients with chest pain. *J Am Coll Cardiol* **6**:27–30, 1985

117. Pamella F, Gibson R, Watson D, et al: Prognosis with chest pain and normal thallium-201 exercise scintigrams. *Am J Cardiol* **55**:920–926, 1985

118. Wahl J, Hakki AH, Iskandrian A: Prognostic implications of normal exercise thallium-201 images. *Arch Intern Med* **145**:253–256, 1985

119. Brown K, Boucher C, Okada R, et al: Prognostic value of exercise thallium-201 imaging in patients presenting for evaluation of chest pain. *J Am Coll Cardiol* **4**:994–1001, 1983

120. Gewirtz H, Paladina W, Sullivan M, et al: Value and limitations of myocardial thallium washout rate in the noninvasive diagnosis of patients with triple-vessel coronary artery disease, *Am Heart J* **106**:681–686, 1983

121. Ladenheim M, Pollack B, Rozanski A, et al: Extent and severity of myocardial hypoperfusion as predictors of prognosis in patients with suspected coronary artery disease. *J Am Coll Cardiol* **7**:464–471, 1986

122. Weiss A, Berman D, Lew A, et al: Transient ischemic dilation of the left ventricle on stress thallium-201 scintigraphy: A marker of severe and extensive coronary artery disease. *J Am Coll Cardiol* **9**:752–759, 1987

123. Silverman KJ, Becker LC, Bulkely BH, et al: Value of early thallium-201 scintigraphy for predicting mortality in patients with acute myocardial infarction. *Circulation* **61**:996, 1980

124. Gibson RS, Watson DD, Craddock GB, et al: Prediction of cardiac events after uncomplicated myocardial infarction: A prospective study comparing predischarge exercise thallium-201 scintigraphy and coronary angiography. *Circulation* **68**:321, 1983

125. Younis LT, Byers S, Shaw L, et al: Prognostic value of intravenous dipyridamole thallium scintigraphy after an acute myocardial ischemic event. *Am J Cardiol* **64**:161–166, 1989

126. Miller DD, Tamesis BR, Wittry MD, et al: Dipyridamole technetium-99m sestamibi myocardial tomography as an independent predictor of cardiac event-free survival following acute ischemic events. *J Nucl Cardiol* **1**:72–82, 1994

127. Stratmann HG, Tamesis BR, Younis LT, et al: Prognostic value of dipyridamole technetium-99m sestamibi myocardial tomography in patients with stable chest pain who are unable to exercise. *Am J Cardiol* **73**:657–752, 1994

128. Parkey RW, Bonte FJ, Meyer SL, et al: A new method for radionuclide imaging of acute myocardial infarction in humans. *Circulation* **50**:540, 1974

129. Buja LM, Parkey RW, Dees JH, et al: Morphologic correlates of technetium-99m stannous pyrophosphate imaging of acute myocardial infarcts in dogs. *Circulation* **52**:596, 1975

130. Buja LM, Tofe AJ, Kulkarni PV, et al: Sites and mechanisms of localization of technetium-99m phosphorus radiopharmaceuticals in acute myocardial infarcts and other tissues. *J Clin Invest* **60**:724, 1977

131. Zaret BL, DiCola VC, Donabedian RK, et al: Dual radionuclide study of myocardial infarction: Relationships between myocardial uptake of potassium-43, technetium-99m stannous pyrophosphate, regional myocardial blood flow and creatine phosphokinase depletion. *Circulation* **53**:422, 1976

132. Dewanjee MK, Kahn PC: Mechanisms of localization of 99mTc-labeled pyrophosphate and tetracycline in infarcted myocardium. *J Nucl Med* **17**:639, 1976

133. Riba A, Downs J, Thakur ML, et al: Technetium-99m stannous pyrophosphate imaging of infective endocarditis. *Circulation* **58**:111, 1978

134. Buja LM, Poliner L, Parkey RW, et al: Clinicopathologic study of persistently positive technetium-99m stannous pyrophosphate myocardial scintigrams and myocytolytic degeneration after acute myocardial infarction. *Circulation* **56**:1016, 1977

135. Donsky MS, Curry GC, Parkey RW, et al: Unstable angina pectoris: Clinical angiographic and myocardial scintigraphic observations. *Br Heart J* **38**:257, 1976

136. Wynne J, Holman BL: Acute myocardial infarct scintigraphy with infarct-avid radiotracers. *Med Clin North Am* **64**:119, 1980

137. Walsh WF, Karunaratne HB, Resnekow L, et al: Assessment of diagnostic value of technetium 99m pyrophosphate myocardial scintigraphy in 80 patients with possible acute myocardial infarction. *Br Heart J* **39**:974, 1977

138. Khaw BA, Gold HK, Yasuda T, et al: Scintigraphic quantification of myocardial necrosis in patients after intravenous injection of myosin-specific antibody. *Circulation* **74**:501–508, 1986

139. Khaw BA, Strauss HW, Moore R, et al: Myocardial damage delineated by indium-111 antimyosin Fab and technetium-99m pyrophosphate. *J Nucl Med* **28**:76–82, 1987

140. Khaw BA, Yasuda T, Gold HK, et al: Acute myocardial infarct imaging with indium-111-labeled monoclonal antimyosin Fab. *J Nucl Med* **28**:1671–1678, 1987

141. Grover-McKay M, Huang SC, Hoffman EJ, et al: Noninvasive quantification of myocardial blood flow in dogs with rubidium-82 and PET (Abstract). *J Nucl Med* **27**:976, 1986

142. Schelbert HR, Phelps ME, Hoffman EJ, et al: Regional myocardial perfusion assessed with N-13 labeled ammonia and positron emission computerized axial tomography. *Am J Cardiol* **43**:209, 1979

143. Schelbert HR, Phelps ME, Huang SC, et al: N-13 ammonia as an indicator of myocardial blood flow. *Circulation* **63**:1259, 1981

144. Goldstein RA, Klein MS, Welch MJ, et al: External assessment of myocardial metabolism with C-11 palmitate in vivo. *J Nucl Med* **21**:342, 1980

145. Klein MS, Goldstein RA, Welch MJ, et al: External assessment of myocardial metabolism with C-11 palmitate in rabbit hearts. *Am J Physiol* **237**:H51, 1979

146. Krivokapich J, Huang SC, Phelps ME, et al: Estimation of rabbit myocardial metabolic rate for glucose using fluorodeoxyglucose. *Am J Physiol* **243**:H884, 1982

147. Ratib O, Phelps ME, Huang SS, et al: Positron tomography with deoxyglucose for estimating local myocardial glucose metabolism. *J Nucl Med* **23**:577, 1982

148. Krivokapich J, Barrio JR, Phelps ME, et al: Kinetic characterization of 13-NH$_3$ and 13-N-glutamine metabolism in rabbit heart. *Am J Physiol* **246**:H267, 1983

149. Baumgartner FJ, Barrio JR, Henze E, et al: 13-N-labeled L-amino acids for in vivo assessment of local myocardial metabolism. *J Med Chem* **24**:764, 1981

150. Ross J: Myocardial perfusion-contraction matching. Implications for coronary heart disease and hibernation. *Circulation* **83**:1076–1083, 1991

151. Marban E: Myocardial stunning and hibernation. The physiologic behind the collaquialisms. *Circulation* **83**:681–688, 1991

152. Braunwald E, Kloner RA: The stunned myocardium: Prolonged, postischemic ventricular dysfunction. *Circulation* **66**:1146–1149, 1982

153. Heyndrickx GR, Baig H, Nelkins P, et al: Depression of regional blood flow and wall thickening after brief coronary occlusions. *Am J Physiol* **234**:11653–11659, 1978

154. Scholl JM, Chaitman BR, David PR, et al: Exercise electrocardiography and myocardial scintigraphy in the serial evaluation of the results of percutaneous transluminal coronary angioplasty. *Circulation* **66**:380–390, 1982

155. Broderick T, Sawada S, Armstrong WF, et al: Improvement in rest and exercise-induced wall motion abnormalities after coronary angioplasty: An exercise echocardiographic study. *J Am Coll Cardiol* **15**:591–599, 1990

156. Rogers WJ, Hood WP Jr, Mantle JA, et al: Return of left ventricular function after reperfusion in patients with myocardial infarction: Importance of subtotal stenoses or intact collaterals. *Circulation* **69**:338–349, 1984

157. Touchstone DA, Beller GA, Nygaard TW, et al: Effects of successful intravenous reperfusion therapy on regional myocardial function and geometry in humans: A tomographic assessment using two-dimensional echocardiography. *J Am Coll Cardiol* **13**:1506, 1989

158. Renkin J, Wijns W, Ladha Z, Col J: Reversal of segmental hypokinesis by coronary angioplasty in patients with unstable angina, persistent T wave inversion and left anterior descending stenosis. *Circulation* **82**(3):913–921, 1990

159. Rahimtoola SH: A perspective on the three large multicenter randomized clinical trials of coronary bypass surgery for chronic stable angina. *Circulation* **72**(Suppl V):V123–V135, 1985

160. Rahimtoola SH, Griffith GC: The hibernating myocardium. *Am Heart J* **117**:211–221, 1989

161. Braunwald E, Rutherford JD: Reversible ischemic left ventricular dysfunction: Evidence for the "hibernating myocardium". *J Am Coll Cardiol* **8**:1467–1470, 1986

162. Bourassa MG, Lesperance J, Campeau L, Saltiel J: Fate of ventricular contraction following aortocoronary venous grafts. *Circulation* **46**:724–730, 1972

163. Van den Berg EK, Popma JJ, Dehmer GJ, et al: Reversible segmental left ventricular dysfunction after coronary angioplasty. *Circulation* **81**:1210–1216, 1990

164. Cloninger KG, DePuey EG, Garcia EV, et al: Incomplete redistribution in delayed thallium-201 single photon emission computer tomographic (SPECT) images: An overestimation of myocardial scarring. *J Am Coll Cardiol* **12**:955–963, 1988

165. Yang LD, Berman DS, Kiat H, et al: The frequency of late reversibility in SPECT thallium-201 stress redistribution studies. *J Am Coll Cardiol* **15**:334–340, 1990

166. Dilsizian V, Rocco TP, Freedman NMT, et al: Enhanced detection of ischemic but viable myocardium by the reinjection of thallium-201 after stress-redistribution imaging. *N Engl J Med* **323**:141–146, 1990

167. Dilsizian V, Smeltzer WR, Freedman NMT, et al: Thallium reinjection after stress redistribution imaging: Does 24 hour delayed imaging after reinjection enhance detection of viable myocardium? *Circulation* **83**:1247–1255, 1991

168. Rozanski A, Berman DS, Gray R, et al: Use of thallium-201 redistribution scintigraphy in the preoperative differentiation of reversible and non-reversible myocardial asynergy. *Circulation* **64**:936–940, 1981

169. Ohtani H, Tamaki N, Yonekura Y, et al: Value of thallium-201 reinjection after delayed SPECT imaging for predicting reversible ischemia after coronary artery bypass grafting. *Am J Cardiol* **66**:394–399, 1990

170. Liu P, Kiess MC, Okada RD, et al: The persistent defect on exercise thallium imaging and its fate after myocardial revascularization: Does it represent scar or ischemia? *Am Heart J* **110**:996–1001, 1985

171. Breisblatt WM: Reversibility of long-standing left ventricular aneurysm predicted by thallium-201 imaging. *J Am Coll Cardiol* **7**:1162–1166, 1986

172. Manyari DE, Knudston M, Kloiber R, Roth D: Segmental thallium-201 myocardial perfusion studies after successful percutaneous transluminal coronary artery angioplasty: Delayed resolution of exercise-induced scintigraphic abnormalities. *Circulation* **77**:86–95, 1988

173. Dilsizian V, Freedman NMT, Bacharach SL, et al: Regional thallium uptake in irreversible defects. Magnitude of change in thallium activity after reinjection distinguishes viable from nonviable myocardium. *Circulation* **86**:1125–1137, 1992

174. Bonow RO, Dilsizian V, Cuocolo A, Bacharach SL: Identification of viable myocardium in patients with chronic coronary artery disease and left ventricular dysfunction. *Circulation* **83**:26–37, 1991

175. Perrone-Filardi P, Bacharach SL, Dilsizian V, et al: Regional left ventricular wall thickening: Relation to regional uptake of fluorodeoxyglucose and Tl-201 in patients with chronic coronary artery disease and left ventricular dysfunction. *Circulation* **86**:1125–1137, 1992

176. Tillisch J, Brunken R, Marshall R, et al: Reversibility of cardiac wall-motion abnormalities predicted by positron tomography. *N Engl J Med* **314**:884–888, 1986

177. Tamaki N, Yonekura Y, Yamashita K, et al: Positron emission tomography using fluorine-18 deoxyglucose in evaluation of coronary artery bypass grafting. *Am J Cardiol* **64**:860–865, 1989

178. Nienaber CA, Brunken RC, Sherman CT, et al: Metabolic and function recovery of ischemic human myocardium after coronary angioplasty. *J Am Coll Cardiol* **18**:966–978, 1991

179. Marshall RC, Tillisch JH, Phelps ME, et al: Identification and differentiation of resting myocardial ischemia and infarction in man with positron-computed tomography, F-18 labeled fluorodeoxyglucose and N-13 ammonia. *Circulation* **67**:766–778, 1983

180. Schwaiger M, Brunken R, Grover-McKay, et al: Regional myocardial metabolism in patients with acute myocardial infarction assessed by positron emission tomography. *J Am Coll Cardiol* **8**:800–808, 1986

181. Brunken R, Schwaiger M, Grover-McKay M, et al: Positron emission tomography detects tissue metabolic activity in myocardial segments with persistent thallium defects. *J Am Coll Cardiol* **10**:557–567, 1987

182. Eisenberg JD, Sobel BE, Geltman EM: Differentiation of ischemia from nonischemic cardiomyopathy with positron emission tomography. *Am J Cardiol* **59**:1410–1414, 1987

183. Bonow RO, Dilsizian V, CuoColo A, Bacharach SL: Identification of viable myocardium in patients with chronic coronary artery disease and left ventricular dysfunction. Comparison of thallium scintigraphy with reinjection and PET imaging with F-18 fluorodeoxyglucose. *Circulation* **83**:26–37, 1991

184. Perrone-Filardi P, Bacharach SL, Dilsizian V, et al: Regional left ventricular wall thickening. Relation to regional uptake of 18-fluorodeoxyglucose and 201-Tl in patients with chronic coronary artery disease and left ventricular dysfunction. *Circulation* **86**:1125–1137, 1992

185. Sambuceti G, Giorgetti A, Marzullo P, et al: Residual coronary vasodilating capability despite reduction in resting myocardial blood flow in collateral dependent myocardium. *J Am Coll Cardiol* **21**:129A, 1993

186. Eitzman D, Al-Aouar Z, Kanter HL, et al: Clinical outcome of patients with advanced coronary artery disease after viability studies with positron emission tomography. *J Am Coll Cardiol* **20**:559–565, 1992

187. Beanlands RSB, Dawood F, Wen WH, et al: Are the kinetics of 99m-Technetium methoxyisobutyl isonitrile affected by cell metabolism and viability? *Circulation* **82**:1802–1814, 1990

188. Marzullo P, Sambuceti G, Parodi O: The role of sestamibi scintigraphy in the radioisotope assessment of myocardial viability. *J Nucl Med* **33**:1925–1930, 1992

189. Altehoefer C, Kaiser H-J, Dorr R, et al: Fluorine-18 deoxyglucose PET for assessment of viable myocardium in perfusion defects in Tc-99m-MIBI SPECT: A comparative study in patients with coronary artery disease. *Eur J Med* **19**:334–342, 1992

190. Sawada S, Beanlands R, Allman K, et al: Rest sestamibi detection of viable myocardium after infarction: Comparison with PET. *Circulation* **86**(Supp I):1–418, 1991

191. Wackers FJTH, Gibbons RJ, Verani MS, et al: Serial quantitative planar technetium-99m isonitrile imaging in acute myocardial infarction: Efficacy for noninvasive assessment of thrombolytic therapy. *J Am Coll Cardiol* **14**:861–873, 1989

192. St Gibson W, Christian TF, Pellikka PA, et al: Serial tomographic imaging with technetium-99m sestamibi for the assessment of infarct-related arterial patency following reperfusion therapy. *J Nucl Med* **33**:2080–2085, 1992

193. Rocco TP, Dilsizian V, Strauss HW, Boucher CA: Tc-99m isonitrile myocardial uptake at rest. II. Relation to clinical markers of potential viability. *J Am Coll Cardiol* **14**:1678–1684, 1989

194. Weisz D, Hamby RI, Aintalian A, et al: Late coronary bypass graft flow: Quantitative assessment by roentgendensitometry. *Ann Thorac Surg* **28**:429, 1979

195. Stinson EB, Olinger GN, Glancy DL: Anatomical and physiological determinants of blood flow through aortocoronary vein bypass grafts. *Surgery* **74**:390, 1973

196. Bittar N, Kroncke GM, Dacumos GC, et al: Vein graft flow and reactive hyperemia in the human heart. *J Thorac Cardiovasc Surg* **64**:855, 1972

197. Greenfield JC, Rembert JC, Young WG, et al: Studies of blood flow in aorta-to-coronary venous bypass grafts in man. *J Clin Invest* **51**:2724, 1972

198. Hossack KF, Bruce RA, Ivey TD, et al: Changes in cardiac functional capacity after coronary bypass surgery in relation to adequacy of revascularization. *J Am Coll Cardiol* **3**:47, 1984

199. Gibson RS, Watson DD, Taylor GJ, et al: Prospective assessment of regional myocardial perfusion before and after coronary revascularization surgery by quantitative thallium-201 scintigraphy. *J Am Coll Cardiol* **1**:804, 1983

200. Brundage BH, Bassie BM, Botvinick EH: Improved regional ventricular function after successful surgical revascularization. *J Am Coll Cardiol* **3**:902, 1984

201. Pfisterer M, Emmenegger H, Schmitt HE, et al: Accuracy of serial myocardial perfusion scintigraphy with thallium-201 for prediction of graft patency early and late after coronary artery bypass surgery. *Circulation* **66**:1017, 1982

202. Ritchie JL, Narahara KA, Trobaugh JB, et al: Thallium-201 myocardial imaging before and after coronary revascularization: Assessment of regional myocardial blood flow and graft patency. *Circulation* **56**:830, 1977

203. Verani MS, Marcus ML, Spoto G, et al: Thallium-201 myocardial perfusion scintigrams in the evaluation of aorto-coronary saphenous bypass surgery. *J Nucl Med* **19**:765, 1978

204. Greenberg GH, Hart R, Botvinick EH, et al: Thallium-201 myocardial perfusion scintigraphy to evaluate patients after coronary bypass surgery. *Am J Cardiol* **42**:167, 1978

205. Sbarbaro JA, Karunarantne H, Cantez S, et al: Thallium-201 imaging and assessment of aorto-coronary artery bypass graft patency. *Br Heart J* **42**:553, 1979

206. Robinson TS, Williams BT, Webb-Peploe MM, et al: Thallium-201 myocardial imaging and assessment of results of aorto-coronary bypass surgery. *Br Heart J* **42**:455, 1979

207. Hirzel HO, Nuesch K, Siale RG, et al: Thallium-201 exercise myocardial imaging to evaluate myocardial perfusion after coronary bypass surgery. *Br Heart J* **43**:426, 1980

208. Cloninger KG, DePuey EG, Carcia EV, et al: Incomplete redistribution in delayed thallium-201 single photon emission computed tomographic (SPECT) images: An overestimation of myocardial scanning. *J Am Coll Cardiol* **12**:955, 1988

209. Loop FD, Lytle BW, Gill CC, et al: Trends in selection and results of coronary artery reoperations. *Ann Thorac Surg* **36**:380, 1983

210. Kent KM, Borer JS, Green MV, et al: Effects of coronary-artery bypass on global and regional left ventricular function during exercise. *N Engl J Med* **298**:1434, 1978

211. Lim Ly, Kalff V, Kelly MJ, et al: Radionuclide angiographic assessment of global and sequential left ventricular function at rest and during exercise after coronary artery bypass surgery. *Circulation* **66**:972, 1982

212. Cohen M, Chamey R, Hershmann R, et al: Reversal of chronic ischemic myocardial dysfunction after transluminal coronary angioplasty. *J Am Coll Cardiol* **12**:1193, 1988

213. Manyari DE, Knudtson M, Kloiber R, et al: Sequential thallium-201 myocardial perfusion studies after successful percutaneous transluminal coronary artery angioplasty: Delay resolution of exercise-induced scintigraphic abnormalities. *Circulation* **77**:86, 1988

214. Brunken R, Schwaiger M, Grover-McKay M, et al: Positron emission tomography detects tissue metabolic activity in myocardial segments with persistent thallium perfusion defects. *J Am Coll Cardiol* **10**:557, 1987

215. Tamaki N, Yonekura Y, Yamashita K, et al: Positron emission tomography using fluorine-18 deoxyglucose in evaluation of coronary artery bypass grafting. *Am J Cardiol* **64**:860, 1989

216. Maddahi J, DiCarli M, Davidson M, et al: Prognostic significance of PET assessment of myocardial viability in patients with left ventricular dysfunction. *J Am Coll Cardiol* **19**(3):142A, 1992

217. Hansen CL: Preliminary report of an ongoing phase I/II dose range, safety and efficacy study of iodine-123-phenylpentadecanoic acid for the identification of viable myocardial. *J Nucl Med* **35**(No. 4 Suppl):38S–42S, 1994

Magnetic Resonance Imaging of Acquired Cardiovascular Disease

James M. Lieberman, Jeffrey L. Duerk,
and Lee P. Adler

There have been numerous technical advances in magnetic resonance imaging (MRI) since its introduction into clinical medicine in the early 1980s. MRI is now the preeminent imaging method in diseases of the nervous system. Although radiography remains the primary method of bone imaging, MRI, because of its excellent soft tissue contrast, is the method of choice for joint problems, tumor extent, and other soft tissue abnormalities. Even though early research showed both normal and abnormal anatomy with improved clarity, as compared to other noninvasive imaging modalities,[1-4] cardiac MRI has to date not enjoyed a similar degree of success. There are many reasons for this, but probably the most important is that the rapid and complex motion of the heart presents a considerable challenge for MRI. It is only recently that the problem of motion has been overcome with fast imaging sequences.

Nevertheless, there are established niches for MRI of acquired cardiovascular diseases. MRI has definite advantages over computed tomography (CT) and transesophageal ultrasound in the detection of aortic dissection.[5] MRI gives an excellent display of cardiac and pericardial neoplasms.[6]

In the future, there will probably be growth of the clinical applications of MRI in the cardiovascular system. The proximal coronary arteries have already been imaged. Pulmonary artery embolism has been detected. With the usage of three-dimensional imaging techniques, contrast material, and enhanced computer manipulation of the data, there is the potential for cardiac MRI to become an all purpose examination yielding both anatomic and functional data.[6]

BASIC MAGNETIC RESONANCE IMAGING

Magnetic resonance imaging works by virtue of various nuclei having a nucleus that has both a magnetic moment (like a compass needle) and angular momentum. Examples of biologically relevant nuclei that may be imaged include hydrogen-1, phosphorus-31, sodium-23, oxygen-17, and carbon-13. By far, hydrogen protons are the most abundant in the human body and are almost exclusively the nuclei imaged in conventional MRI.

When placed in a strong magnetic field, a small percentage of the proton nuclei eventually orient themselves in the same direction as the magnetic field. This development of magnetization along the direction of the main field over time is governed by a parameter called T1. Unfortunately, it is difficult to detect this development of magnetization because of its slow rate and its direction being parallel to the main field. However, because most tissues have different T1s, MRI pulse sequences often attempt to exploit these differences when generating contrast between tissues.

To detect the tissue magnetization, radio frequency (RF) pulse is applied: this addition of energy causes the magnetization to tip slightly and reorient itself (into what is known as the transverse plane) with respect to the main field. In this new orientation, the magnetization generates a time-dependent field of its own that can be detected with special antennas (often called "receiver coils"). The magnetization gradually disappears from this new orientation, governed by a parameter called T2, and returns to its alignment along the main field. As one might expect, different tissues have different T2's and many MRI pulse sequences attempt to generate contrast between tissues by exploiting T2 variations.

In summary, all MRI pulse sequences function by (1) allowing magnetization to develop as a function of T1, (2) applying RF pulses to reorient the tissue magnetization, (3) allowing the signal decay in the transverse plane by T2 processes (duration known as TE), (4) detecting the induced signals in receiver coils, and (5) allowing the magnetization some time to begin its return to its preferred alignment along the magnetic field direction (duration known as TR).

Unfortunately, this sequence of RF application and signal detection must be repeated a number of times (e.g., a few hundred) to generate enough "views" from which an image can be reconstructed. A useful analogy is that the MRI acquisition process is similar to taking a picture with a camera whose aperture is open for a long period of time. During the interval between "views" the heart beats, the patient breathes and swallows, and blood flows: these sources of patient motion can cause blurring and artifacts in the images similar to those one might expect with a conventional film camera using an extended aperture duration. Fortunately, a number of MRI pulse sequence methods have been developed to (1) combat the various types of patient motion that occur, (2) reduce the total acquisition time, and (3) generate contrast between tissues by virtue of their T1 and T2 differences. Some of these sequences and methods are described below.

MRI SEQUENCES AND METHODOLOGY

Methodology: Cardiac Gating

Prospective cardiac gating is a method of synchronizing the acquisition procedure to the ECG. Electrodes are placed on the patient's chest, the ECG is observed by electronic circuitry, and upon detection of the R-wave, the acquisition of each view is triggered. In this way, the heart appears to be "strobed," or imaged consistently at the same point in the cardiac cycle, thus eliminating apparent differences in the heart's position with each view. Retrospective gating is a method where MRI signal data and the ECG waveform are collected simultaneously. Following completion of MRI signal acquisition for all views, the MRI computer sorts the acquired data and selects only those views for reconstruction that were acquired at a consistent point in the ECG. The advantage of cardiac gating is the reduction of motion artifacts; the disadvantage is some loss of sequence flexibility (RF pulses applied each R-R interval), and long scan durations (hundreds of cardiac cycles).

Methodology: Gradient Moment Nulling

Motion of the heart and blood during each view causes these signals to disappear faster than if they were stationary

as a result of the nuclei interacting with the magnetic field gradients; the rate of signal loss is dependent on the speed with which the tissue is moving and the time duration of the waveforms. Gradient moment nulling implies that the gradient waveforms have been designed in such a way as to remove this source of signal loss, at the expense of slightly longer gradient durations. Motion artifacts can be reduced and signal from flowing blood can be returned to near its "full" intensity. However, additional methods for reducing motion artifacts are still required (e.g., gating).

Sequences: Gradient Echo

Gradient echo imaging pulse sequences are the simplest sequences used in cardiac imaging. They have a single RF pulse during each view (tip angle varies from a few degrees to upwards of 90°). The gradient waveform durations and TE are short, and hence their sensitivity to motion following the RF pulse is low. They can be combined with gradient moment nulling to further reduce sensitivity to motion, and they are (virtually) always used with some form of cardiac gating. They are most commonly associated with bright blood and cine type acquisitions (single spatial locations at multiple temporal points following the R-wave detection). Acquisition time is several hundred heart beats (e.g., 2–10 min).

Sequences: Spin Echo

Spin echo sequences utilize two RF pulses during the acquisition of each view: a 90° excitation pulse tips the magnetization, and a 180° refocusing pulse eliminates signal loss due to magnetic field inhomogeneities. They can be combined with gradient moment nulling and cardiac gating: they are most often associated with "black" blood imaging and hence evaluation of myocardium or examination of masses. Acquisition time is several hundred heart beats (e.g., 2–10 min).

Sequences: RARE, Turbo-Spin Echo, Fast Spin Echo

As mentioned earlier, many views must be acquired to have sufficient data for reconstruction of an image. Until recently, a single view was acquired following each RF excitation pulse. However, fast spin echo sequences apply multiple 180° pulses following the 90° pulse, and generate multiple views for a single excitation. The advantage is that the total imaging time is reduced (multiple views, rather than a single view, acquired following ECG detection of R-wave). These sequences can utilize gradient moment nulling and require some form of cardiac gating. Their use in cardiac MRI is new, yet it is presumed that they will fulfill a similar role to spin echo sequences, yet at the significantly reduced scan time. The disadvantage is some blurring as a result of signal decay during detection of the multiple views. Acquisition time is only a few heart beats (e.g., 10–60 seconds).

Sequences: Echo Planar Imaging

The fastest type of MRI pulse sequence is the echo planar sequence. Here, all of the views required for reconstruction are obtained following a single excitation pulse. However, nonstandard imaging hardware is required, and this hardware is expensive. The advantage, however, is that the acquisition duration is on the order of 50–100 ms for each image. MRI sequences can be designed to provide dark or bright blood, and the imaging time within the cardiac cycle can be controlled through gating circuitry. Because of the short imaging time, many types of motion artifact are reduced. However, images suffer from poor signal-to-noise ratios when compared to other sequences, and previously unappreciated types of motion artifact may result. For some conditions, the advantage of exceptionally fast imaging capability exceeds the loss of image quality associated with these sequences.

CLINICAL APPLICATIONS

Aortic Aneurysm/Dissection

MRI has distinct advantages in imaging diseases of the aorta. With the spin echo technique, there is inherent contrast between the flowing blood in the lumen, which lacks signal, and the wall of the vessel. Slow flowing blood, clot, and thrombus will elicit a signal (Fig. 106–1). Bright blood techniques using gradient echo imaging demonstrate luminal flow (Fig. 106–2), and may help to differentiate the true

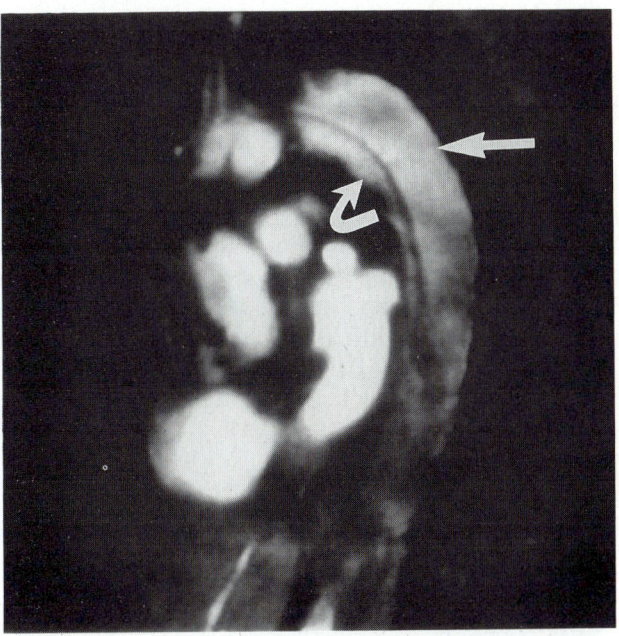

Figure 106–2. Aortic dissection, Type A (cine MRI; parasagittal). There is moving blood in both the true lumen (curved arrow) and false lumen (straight arrow).

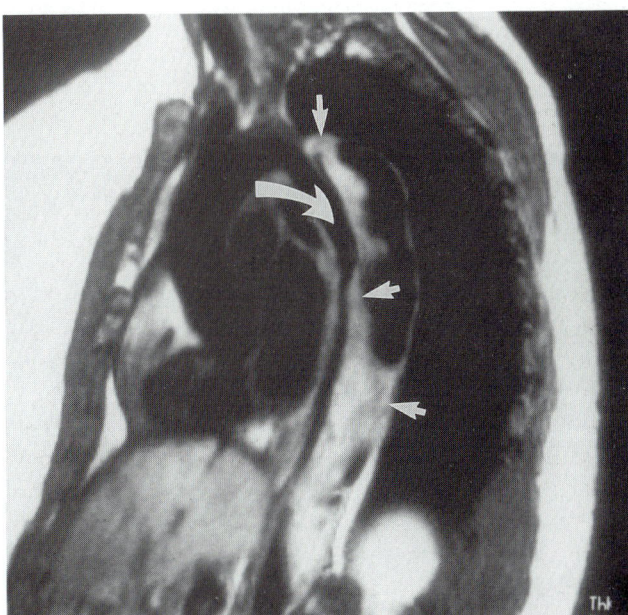

Figure 106–1. Aortic dissection (spin echo MRI; parasagittal). This is a Type B aortic dissection with high signal intensity in the false lumen indicating thrombus and/or slow flow (straight arrows). Curved arrow indicates the true lumen.

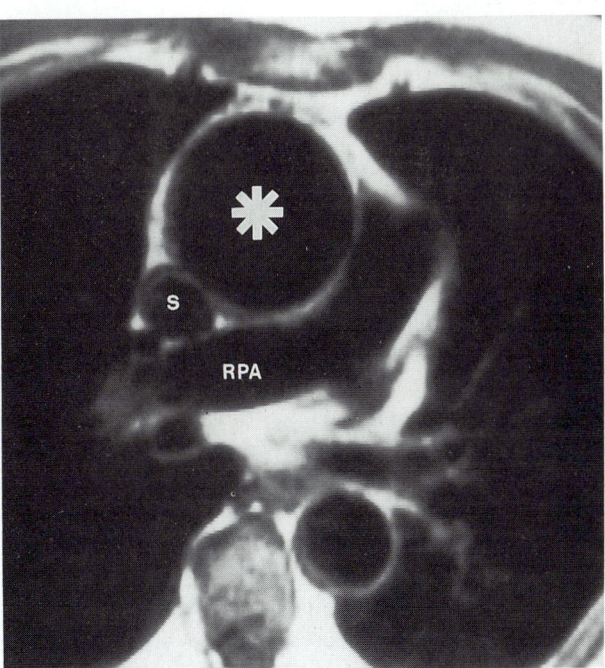

Figure 106–3. Ascending aortic aneurysm (spin echo MRI; transaxial). A large concentric aneurysmal dilatation of the ascending aorta (asterisk) is noted. Its intravascular space is filled with signal void of rapidly flowing blood; there is no evidence of dissection or thrombus. RPA, right pulmonary artery; S, superior vena cava. *(Reprinted from R. D. White, et al. Journal of Thoracic Imaging, Vol. 4, No. 2, pp. 34–50, with permission of Aspen Publishers, Inc., © April 1989.)*

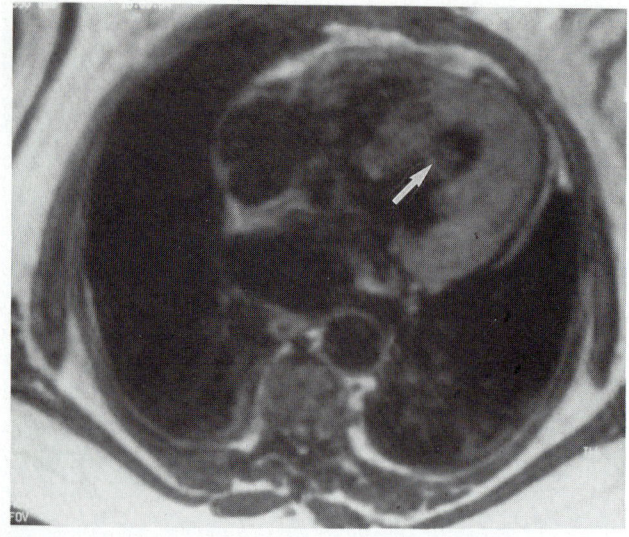

A

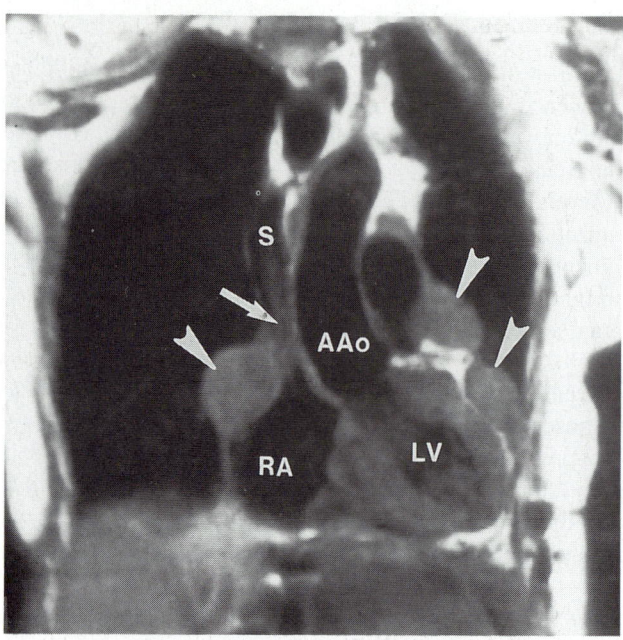

Figure 106–5. Metastatic adenocarcinoma to the pericardium (spin echo MRI; coronal). Three oval-shaped soft-tissue tumor masses (arrowheads) are identified on the percardium. The right-sided mass deviates the lower superior vena cava inward as it inserts into the deformed right atrium. Abnormal intravascular signal (arrow) within the superior vena cava above this level is consistent with slow blood flow as a result of obstruction. There is no evidence of direct invasion of the cardiovascular structures. AAo, ascending aorta; LV, left ventricle; RA, right atrium; S, superior vena cava.

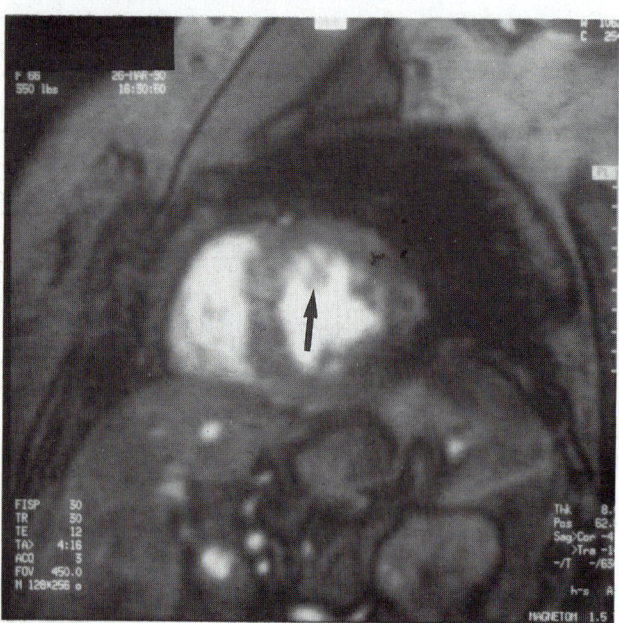

B

Figure 106–4. Left ventricular myxoma. **A.** Spin echo MRI, transaxial. **B.** Cine MRI, short-axis view. Arrow indicates myxoma.

from the false lumen. Competing modalities with MRI are angiography, CT, and transesophageal ultrasound. The advantages of MRI are that it is a noninvasive technique, contrast material is not required, imaging is not limited to the axial plane, both the ascending and descending portions of the aorta are completely evaluated, the wall and adjacent regions are imaged, and follow-up studies are easily obtained. The major disadvantage of MRI in the clinical situation is that this modality is not suitable for unstable patients. The accuracy of detection of an aortic dissection using MRI has

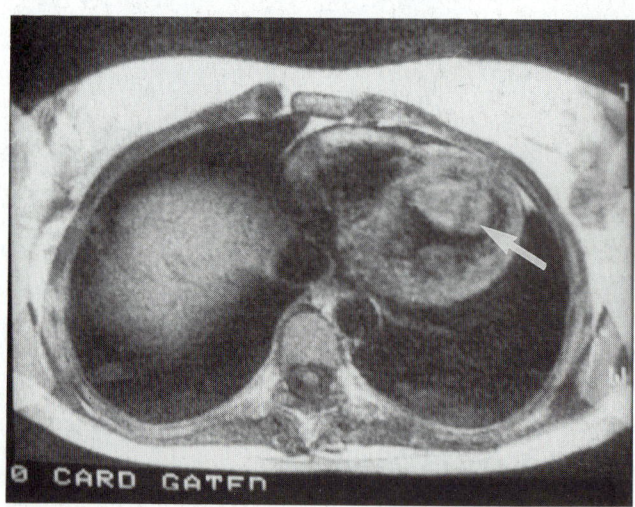

Figure 106–6. Acute thrombus (spin echo MRI; transaxial). Note that portions of the thrombus (arrow) have higher signal intensity than adjacent myocardium.

ranged from 83 to 100%.[7-10] As a multiplanar imaging modality, MRI is also useful in the evaluation of thoracic aortic aneurysms (Fig. 106–3).

CARDIAC AND PERICARDIAL MASSES

MRI is useful in the evaluation of neoplasms of the heart (Fig. 106–4) and pericardium (Fig. 106–5). These masses may be initially found with ultrasound or CT, and MRI will become a problem solver. For a cardiac mass, the differential diagnosis is usually between a neoplasm and thrombus. Many times this distinction can be made with use of the

cine gradient echo bright blood technique: tumors will usually have a medium signal intensity and thrombus will have a low signal intensity, although there can be overlap with acute thrombus (high signal intensity, Fig. 106–6), and atrial myxoma (some have low signal intensity).[6]

ISCHEMIC CORONARY ARTERY DISEASE

There has been considerable research effort invested into the MRI evaluation of ischemic coronary artery disease. MRI can display the proximal coronary arteries (Fig. 106–7), acute[11] and chronic myocardial infarctions (Fig.

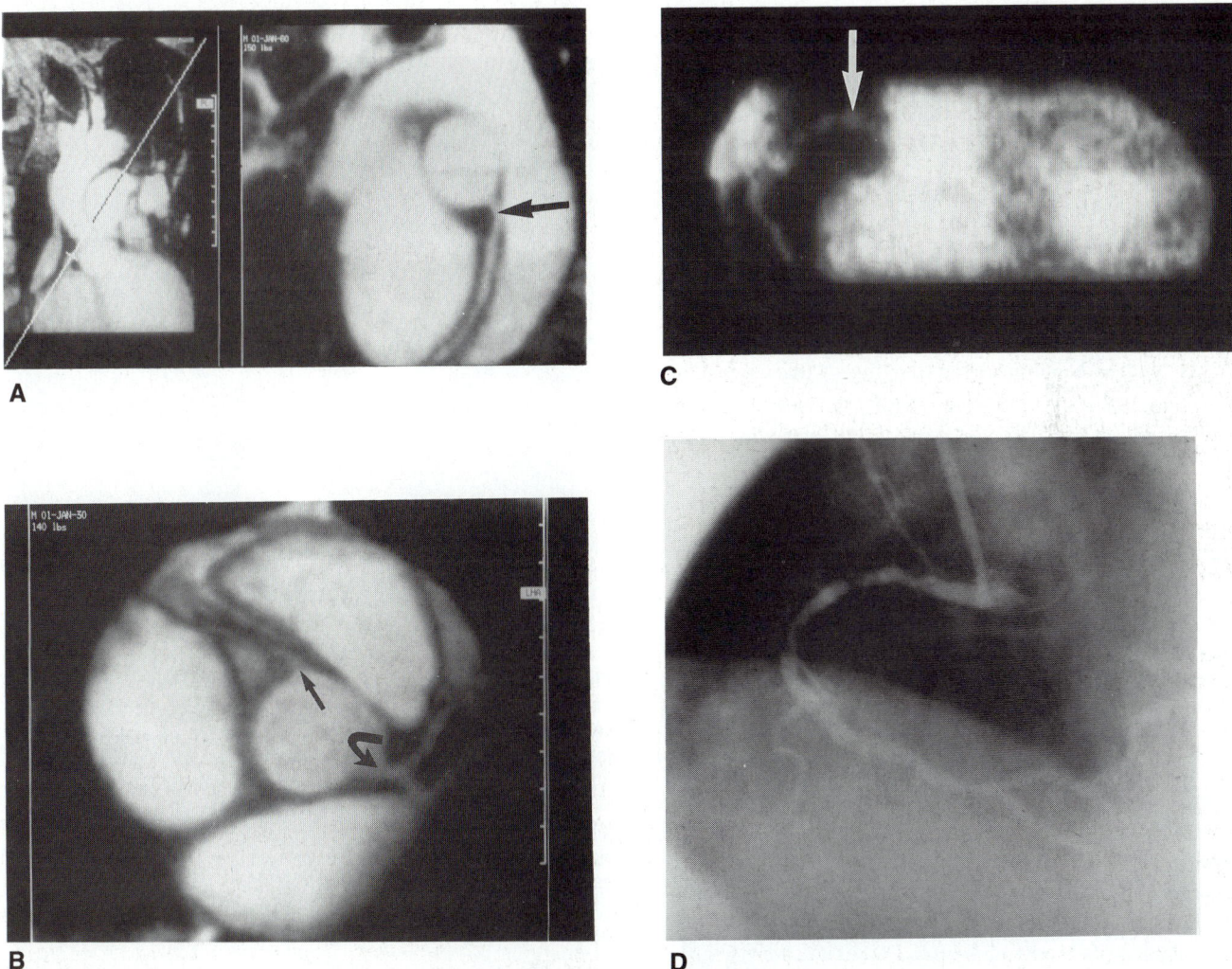

Figure 106–7. A. Coronary artery (cine MRI). Image on the left showing oblique plane of reconstruction that yields the image on the right of the right coronary artery (arrow). **B.** Origins of the coronary arteries (three-dimensional reconstructed image obtained from cine MRI). Straight arrow indicates right coronary artery; curved arrow indicates left coronary artery. **C.** Atherosclerotic right coronary artery (arrow). This image is a multiplanar reconstruction used with a cine MRI bright blood technique also with the subtraction of the adjacent fat. **D.** Right coronary artery arteriogram corresponding to **C.**

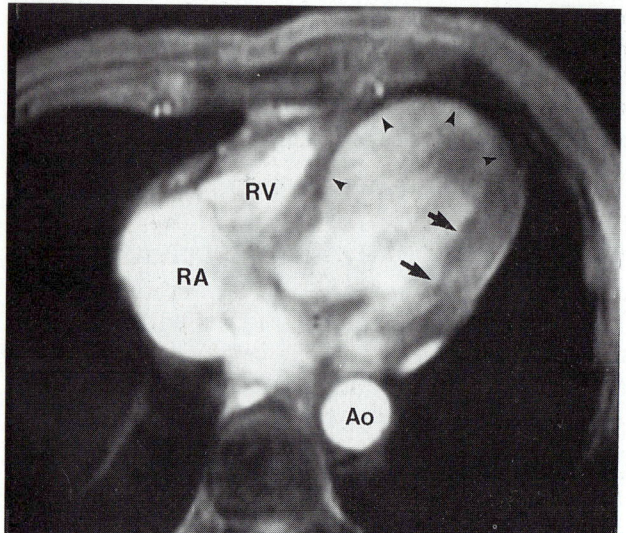

Figure 106–8. Anatomic and functional extent of MI (cine MRI; transaxial). A single systolic image clearly demonstrates the distribution of the MI. The area of thinning (arrowheads) involving the anterior and anteroseptal regions of the LV wall is clearly distinguishable from the normal thickened lateral LV wall (arrows). In fact, the MI region appears to be noncontractile and aneurysmal. Ao, ascending aorta; RA, right atrium; RV, right ventricle.

106–8), and coronary artery bypass grafts (Fig. 106–9). Wall motion can be evaluated using cine gradient echo techniques (Fig. 106–8). Despite these accomplishments, thallium myocardial nuclear medicine scans continue as the primary method of noninvasive imaging of this disease in the clinical realm. Noninvasive imaging of coronary artery bypass grafts is not part of current clinical practice; this

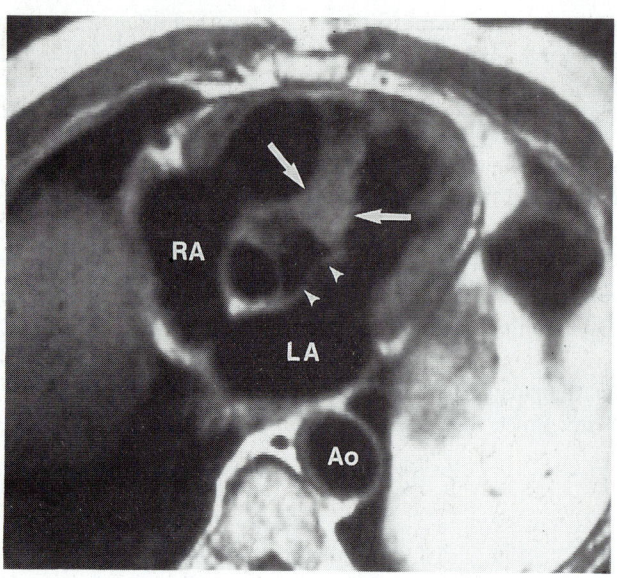

A

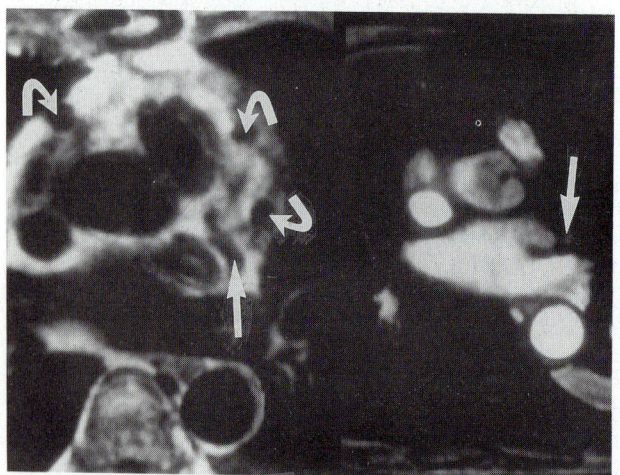

Figure 106–9. Coronary artery bypass graft (straight arrows). The left image is a spin echo transaxial image and the right is a transaxial cine MRI. The cine MRI confirms blood flow through the graft (straight arrow). Note, multiple artifacts from metal (curved arrows), which without the cine MRI could be confused with bypass grafts.

B

Figure 106–10. Anatomic and functional extent of hypertrophic CM (spin echo and cine MRI; transaxial). The static spin echo image (**A**) demonstrates asymmetric hypertrophy of the ventricular septum (straight arrows) in the LV outflow region. This area of thickening and the anterior leaflet of the mitral valve (arrowheads) causes relative narrowing of the LV outflow. On a corresponding systolic cine MRI image (**B**) the associated subaortic stenosis is manifested by signal void (curved arrow) located below the aortic valve. Ao, ascending aorta, LA, left atrium; RA, right atrium.

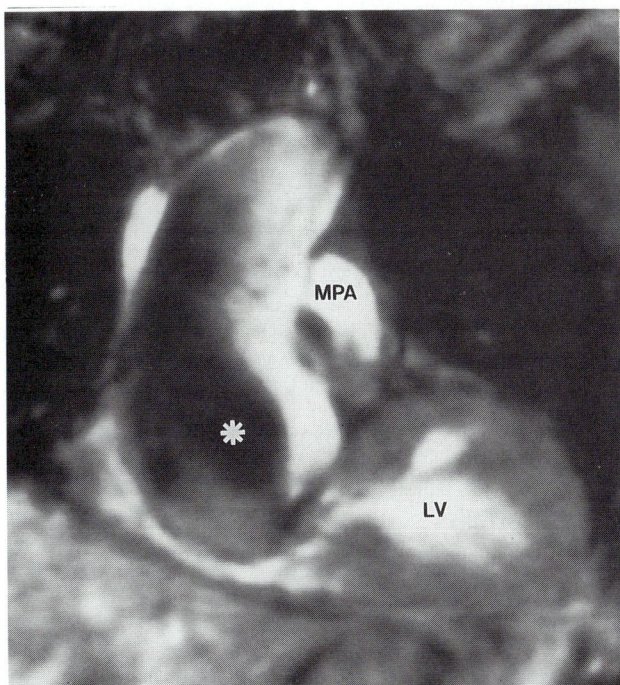

Figure 106–11. Aortic stenosis (cine MRI; coronal). The systolic cine image demonstrates a large stenosis "jet" (asterisk) extending from the aortic valve to the right wall of the proximal ascending aorta, which is dilated due to the poststenotic effect. LV, left ventricle, MPA, main pulmonary artery.

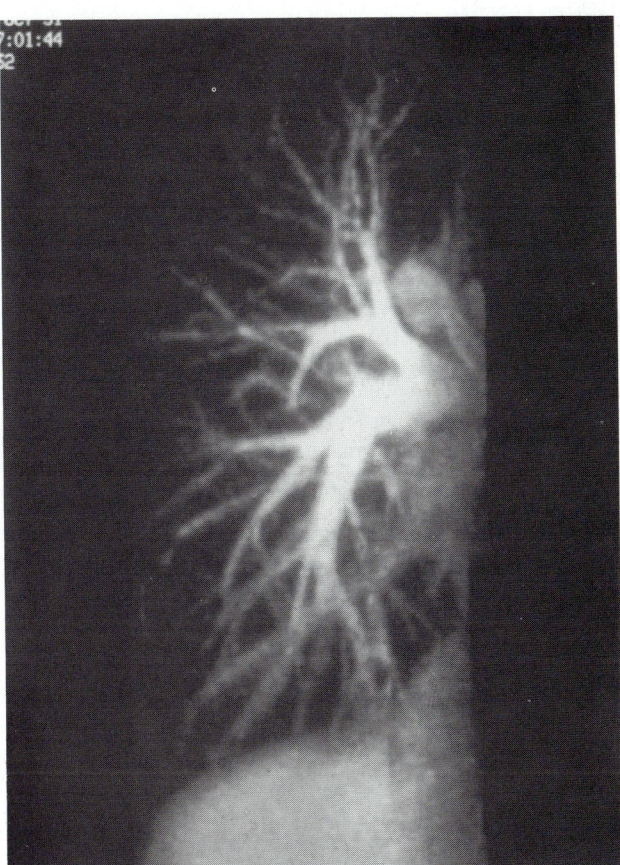

A

B

Figure 106–12. A. Three-dimensional bright blood reconstructed image of the pulmonary arteries in a normal volunteer. **B.** Saddle embolus in right pulmonary artery (spin echo MRI; transaxial). Note the high signal intensity of the embolism (arrow).

could become a role for either MRI or contrast-enhanced CT.

Recent research has been successful at imaging longer segments of the coronary arteries with MRI data obtained during a single breath-hold.[12] Perfusion of the myocardium after injection of gadopenetate dimeglumine, the MRI intravenous contrast agent, has been studied by Finelli and co-workers,[13] using rapid sequence imaging on a conventional MR scanner, and by Edelman and Li using echo-planar MRI.[14]

OTHER DISORDERS

MRI is capable of displaying the anatomic abnormality in the cardiomyopathies (Fig. 106–10), and both stenotic and regurgitant jets in the setting of valvular disease (Fig. 106–11). The ability to produce quantitative data in these entities enhances the value of MRI: ventricular function can be measured in the cardiomyopathies using cine MR,[15] and with velocity encoding the aortic valve pressure gradient is measured in patients with aortic stenosis.[16] The pulmonary arteries and pulmonary embolism (Fig. 106–12) have been demonstrated with MRI.[17,18] Although ventilation/perfusion lung scanning and angiography are still the primary methods for diagnosis of pulmonary embolism, there is potential for MRI in the future to replace these studies.

CONCLUSION

Although MRI to date has had only a limited role in the clinical evaluation of acquired cardiovascular diseases, the continuing technological development and the considerable research efforts by many groups suggest that there will be future growth in clinical applications.

ACKNOWLEDGMENT

The authors thank Richard D. White, M.D., for Figures 106–3, 106–5, 106–8, 106–10, and 106–11.

REFERENCES

1. Herfkens RJ, Higgins CB, Hricak H, et al: Nuclear magnetic resonance imaging of the cardiovascular system: Normal and pathologic findings. *Radiology* **147**:749&759, 1983
2. Lieberman JM, Alfidi RJ, Nelson AD, et al: Gated magnetic resonance imaging of the normal and diseased heart. *Radiology* **152**:465–470, 1984
3. Fletcher BD, Jacobstein JD, Nelson AD, et al: Gated magnetic resonance imaging of congenital cardiac malformations. *Radiology* **150**:137–140, 1984
4. Go RT, MacIntyre WJ, Yeung HN, et al: Volume and planar gated cardiac magnetic resonance imaging: A correlative study of normal anatomy with thallium-201 SPECT and cadaver sections. *Radiology* **150**:129–135, 1984
5. Webb WR, Sostman HD: MR imaging of thoracic disease: Clinical uses. *Radiology* **182**:621–630, 1992
6. Higgins CG, Caputo GR: Role of MR imaging in acquired and congenital cardiovascular disease. *AJR* **161**:13–22, 1993
7. Amparo EG, Higgins CB, Hricak H, Sollitto R: Aortic dissection: Magnetic resonance imaging. *Radiology* **155**:399–406, 1985
8. Geisinger MA, Risius B, O'Donnell JA, et al: Thoracic aortic dissections: Magnetic resonance imaging. *Radiology* **155**:407–412, 1985
9. Glazer HS, Gutierrez FR, Levitt RG, et al: The thoracic aorta studied by MR imaging. *Radiology* **157**:149–155, 1985
10. Petasnick JP: Radiologic evaluation of aortic dissection. *Radiology* **180**:297–305, 1991
11. Van Dijkman PRM, van der Wall EE, de Roos A, et al: Acute, subacute, and chronic myocardial infarction: Quantitative analysis of gadolinium-enhanced MR image. *Radiology* **180**:147–151, 1991
12. Edelman RR, Mannin WJ, Pearlman J, Li W: Human coronary arteries: Projection angiograms reconstructed from breath-hold two-dimensional MR images. *Radiology* **187**:719–722, 1993
13. Finelli DA, Adler LP, Paaschal CB, Haacke ME: Dynamic MR cardiac perfusion studies in patients with acquired heart diseases. Presented at the Radiologic Society of North America Annual Meeting, December, 1990
14. Edelman RR, Li W: Contrast-enhanced echo-planar MR imaging of myocardial perfusion: Preliminary study in humans. *Radiology* **190**:771–777, 1994
15. Semelka RC, Tomei E, Wagner S, et al: Interstudy reproducibility of dimensional and functional measurements between cine magnetic resonance studies in the morphologically abnormal left ventricle. *Am Heart J* **119**:1367–1373, 1990
16. Eichenberger AC, Jenni R, Von Schulthess GK: Aortic valve pressure gradients in patients with aortic valve stenosis: Quantification with velocity-encoded cine MR imaging. *AJR* **160**:971–977, 1993
17. Wielopolski PA, Haacke EM, Adler LP: Three-dimensional MR imaging of the pulmonary vasculature: Preliminary experience. *Radiology* **183**:465–472, 1992
18. Loubeyre P, Revel D, Douek P, et al: Dynamic contrast-enhanced MR angiography of pulmonary embolism: comparison with pulmonary angiography. *AJR* **162**:1035–1039, 1994

CHAPTER

107

Cardiopulmonary Resuscitation

William D. Spotnitz and Henry M. Spotnitz

The successful cardiothoracic surgeon must be capable of managing patients with life threatening pulmonary and cardiovascular compromise. Although advances in anesthetic management and postoperative care continue to improve survival and reduce complications after cardiothoracic surgery, understanding of cardiopulmonary resuscitation is an essential surgical skill. Immediate and appropriately aggressive interventions to restore effective gas exchange and circulation, as well as elimination of precipitating causes of cardiovascular decompensation, are often rewarded with successful resuscitation. This is particularly true in the postoperative cardiothoracic patient, for whom a wide armamentarium of interventions is available. The development of external defibrillation in 1956 and closed chest compression in 1960 was pivotal, but evolving technological and clinical improvements continue to enhance the success of resuscitation.

The need for cardiopulmonary resuscitation can occur in the cardiac catheterization laboratory, the operating room, the intensive care unit, standard patient rooms, or outside of the hospital. The focus of this chapter is on events occurring in the operating room or intensive care unit.

The proper conduct of cardiopulmonary resuscitation requires a working knowledge of hemodynamic management, treatment of arrhythmias, respiratory support, cardioversion and defibrillation, cardiac pacing, inotropic agents, mechanical circulatory support, and specific complications of cardiac and thoracic operations. Previously published resuscitation guides for management are a valuable adjunct to this summary.[1-4] This chapter reviews cardiopulmonary resuscitation from the viewpoint of the cardiothoracic surgeon and considers related controversies and new developments.

ASSESSMENT AND TREATMENT OF HEMODYNAMIC INSTABILITY

A variety of factors may cause hemodynamic instability after cardiothoracic surgery. The onset may be a sudden or gradual fall in blood pressure. Significant abnormalities in Swan-Ganz catheter readings, the electrocardiogram, or the O_2 saturation monitor may precede hemodynamic instability. Factors that may predispose to decompensation include hypovolemia, arrhythmias, acid–base imbalance, myocardial ischemia, hypoxia, electrolyte imbalance, and effects of drugs including sedatives, narcotics, β-blockers, calcium channel blockers, or angiotensin-converting enzyme inhibitors. Steps by the critical care team to evaluate the patient and intervene effectively in a brief period of time include:

1. *Evaluate Hemodynamics.* Spurious information about blood pressure can result from monitor malfunction. Confirm hypotension by palpation of the femoral pulse or by noninvasive cuff blood pressure determination. Arterial line patency and position should be quickly confirmed. The proper connection and function of electrocardiogram electrodes and O_2 saturation monitor should also be checked. A brief clinical assessment of body perfusion including mental status and periphial flow, as determined by capillary filling and skin warmth, can be rapidly performed. The evaluation should be completed within seconds, establishing whether intervention is warranted.

2. *Evaluate Arrhythmias.* Abnormalities should be quickly diagnosed via the electrocardiogram monitor and normal rhythm restored, if possible. Interventions include cardioversion, atrial, or ventricular pacing and pharmacologic manipulations.

3. *Confirm Ventilation.* Most hypotensive emergencies in the OR or ICU occur in patients on positive pressure ventilation. Confirm that ventilation is adequate during resuscitation, intubating the patient if necessary. If adequacy of mechanical ventilation is questioned, bag ventilation with 100% oxygen should be implemented.

4. *Correct Hypotension.* Treatment for mild to moderate hypotension includes intravenous fluids in the form of crystalloids, colloids, or blood and infusion of vasoactive agents. If severe hypotension occurs, Trendelenberg position raises filling pressures and boluses of calcium chloride or epinephrine can be used to increase myocardial contractility and, in the case of epinephrine, increase peripheral vasoconstriction. Calcium chloride is available in ampules containing 1 g in 10 mL of saline. One-half ampule (500 mg) to one ampule (1 g) can be used for moderate to severe hypotension via a central line. As will be discussed later, some data suggest that calcium chloride may be detrimental in a complete cardiac arrest. However, its use for hypotension in the postoperative cardiothoracic patient remains an option. Epinephrine, available in a 1:10,000 solution ampule containing 1 mg in 10 mL of saline, is also a valuable agent. Doses of epinephrine appropriate for hypotension vary from 0.1 to 0.3 mg. The entire ampule or 1 mg of epinephrine would be appropriate for treatment of a complete cardiac arrest. Higher doses of epinephrine in the range 5 mg should be considered only after a standard 1 mg dose has failed in an arrest setting. Epinephrine may contribute to ventricular tachycardia or fibrillation. Failure of these options may indicate the need for surgical intervention or implementation of mechanical circulatory assist in some cases.

Thus, a variety of options is available to treat mild, moderate, and severe hypotension. As the patient responds, a thorough search for the etiology of the hypotension to correct its cause should be expeditiously undertaken.

SUPPORT OF RESPIRATION AND CIRCULATION

Successful resuscitation requires artificial methods of maintaining adequate respiration and circulation. These efforts are necessary until the patient's cardiorespiratory system can resume these functions. Mechanical ventilation is instituted using an endotracheal tube and bag ventilation with 100% oxygen. This method of rapid gas exchange is used to correct hypoxia, hypercarbia, and acidosis. Circulatory support is provided by external cardiac compression. This is most effective with a board under the chest. Manual compression should be vigorous and can be monitored by an arterial line pressure trace if available. As will be discussed later in the chapter, new methods of cardiac compression are under evaluation. Circulatory support using external

compression may be inadequate early after median sternotomy, requiring rapid institution of open chest resuscitation using direct manual cardiac massage.

Effective respiratory and circulatory support are the mainstays of successful resuscitation. They are an absolute necessity and provide a period of time in which additional efforts at stabilizing and restoring the patient's intrinsic respiratory and cardiovascular system can be carried out.

MANAGEMENT OF ARRHYTHMIAS

Arrhythmias related to cardiac arrest include bradycardias and atrial or ventricular ectopy.

Bradycardias

The treatment of sinus bradycardia, nodal bradycardia, and asystole is similar and includes a series of increasingly aggressive interventions (Fig. 107–1).

1. Atropine is the first drug of choice. Atropine sulfate is a vagolytic drug that increases sinus node automaticity and arterial ventricular conduction through its parasympatholytic effects. Atropine is given in 0.4 to 0.5 mg/mL ampule boluses that can be repeated in 2–5 min intervals.

2. An infusion of isoproterenol or epinephrine can be used for treatment of bradycardia. The choice of agent depends on the desirability of vasodilation caused by

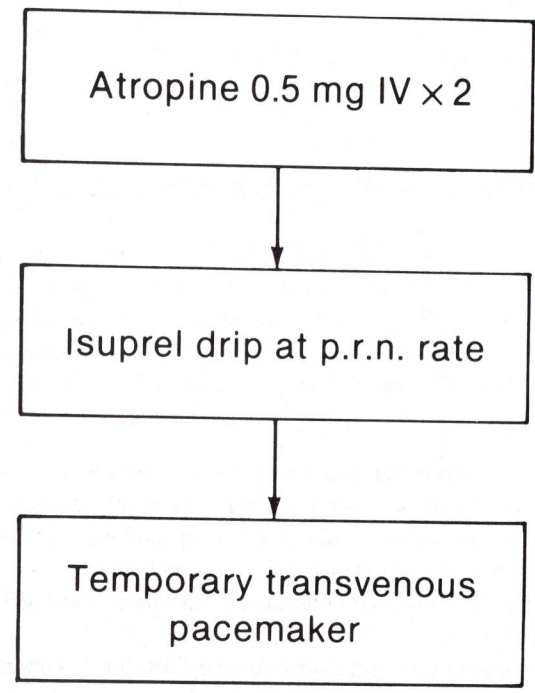

Figure 107–1. Stepwise management of urgent bradyarrhythmias.

isoproterenol and vasoconstriction caused by epinephrine. Thus, a hypertensive or normotensive patient under intensive care monitoring may be treated with isoproterenol, whereas a hypotensive patient should be treated with epinephrine. Isoproterenol is given by a drip (2 mg/500 mL) with rates between 30 and 120 mL/h. Epinephrine administration is also by drip (1 mg/500 mL) producing a concentration of 2 µg/mL, which can be infused at 2–10 µg/min.

3. If pharmacological support is ineffective, emergent temporary cardiac pacemaker support is required using a transcutaneous or transvenous approach. External pacemakers with adhesive cutaneous electrodes are often effective. However, dual chamber pacing is clearly preferable, if feasible, in patients with hemodynamic compromise.

Patients with denervated transplanted hearts will not respond to atropine. Bradycardia in these patients should be treated with isoproterenol, epinephrine, or cardiac pacing.

SUPRAVENTRICULAR TACHYCARDIAS

The onset of atrial flutter or fibrillation is detrimental to hemodynamics because of loss of the atrial contraction and shortening of diastolic filling time. Synchronized external cardioversion at 50–100 J should be employed immediately if hypotension is profound. Overdrive pacing of atrial flutter may be effective in atrial flutter, if the patient has atrial wires. Pharmacologic options include calcium channel blockers (verapamil, 5–10 mg), β-blockers, quinidine, and digoxin. Prophylactic use of these agents is desirable under appropriate circumstances. Their use can be detrimental in complex cases, which should be assessed on an individual basis.

PREMATURE VENTRICULAR CONTRACTIONS

Ventricular arrhythmias, particularly in the immediate postoperative patient, can often be traced to hypokalemia. Therefore a stat serum potassium should be measured and if <4 mEq/L a drip containing 50 mEq of potassium should be started immediately. If the potassium is >4 mEq/L, the following pharmacologic regime should be started:

1. Lidocaine is the drug of choice for ventricular ectopy. Initial dose is 1–1.5 mg/kg (given by intravenous push). A second dose of 0.5 mg/kg can be administered 5–10 min later if necessary. A lidocaine drip of 2–4 mg/min should be continued if lidocaine converted the arrhythmia.
2. Procainamide is the second line drug for treatment of ventricular arrhythmias. It is given as an infusion to provide 17 mg/kg at an infusion rate of 20–30 mg/min.

Procainamide should then be maintained as a continuous infusion of 1–4 mg/min. Procainamide administration can be associated with hypotension and widening of the QRS complex. Widening of the QRS complex reflects toxic levels of procainamide.

3. Bretylium can be used as a third agent for treatment of ventricular arrhythmias. A dose of 5 mg/kg should be administered as a continuous infusion over 8–10 min for ventricular premature contractions, as opposed to its use in ventricular fibrillation when it is administered as a bolus. If effective, a continuous infusion should be begun at 1–2 mg/min. Bretylium may cause hypotension as it is a significant vasodilator. Treatment consists of volume expansion, vasopressors, and inotropic support.

Ventricular Tachycardia

Ventricular tachycardia may be a stable rhythm with sufficient stroke volume to maintain cardiac output. When hemodynamics are stable, the treatment of choice is lidocaine with procainamide or bretylium as second and third line agents. If the patient is hemodynamically unstable with hypotension or other signs and symptoms of decreased cardiac output, immediate electrical cardioversion should be instituted.

Ventricular Fibrillation

Immediate defibrillation using electrical cardioversion is required for treatment of ventricular fibrillation. This rhythm does not provide adequate circulation for end-organ perfusion and thus requires emergency treatment. It has been previously noted that ventricular fibrillation may masquerade as ventricular standstill (asystole) and that evaluation of the rhythm in additional electrocardiogram leads should be performed prior to deciding against defibrillation.[5,6] Replacement of potassium and magnesium to prevent ventricular ectopy, as well as correction of other instigating factors such as myocardial ischemia, is required to prevent further recurrent arrhythmias.

DRUGS FOR RESUSCITATION

The following drugs are important components of a well supplied "code cart" and are available for immediate bolus intravenous infusion (Table 107–1).

Atropine

This drug provides the best initial treatment of bradycardia and has no significant negative effect during resuscitation. Dose is 0.4–0.5 mg.

TABLE 107–1. ESSENTIAL DRUGS IN CARDIAC ARREST

Drugs	Available Forms	Dose	Use(s)	Disadvantages
Sodium bicarbonate ($NaHCO_3$)	50 mL ampule (44 mEq/ampule)	1 mL/kg	Corrects acidosis	Considerable salt load
Atropine	0.4–0.5 mg/mL (vial) or 1 mg/10 mL (ampule)	0.4–0.5 mg; repeat × 1 p.r.n.	Corrects bradycardia	
Lidocaine	100 mg/10 mL (ampule)	1 mg/kg	Corrects ventricular ectopy	Seizures, myocardial depression
Calcium chloride ($CaCl_3$)	1 g/10 mL (ampule)	2.5–10 mL	Augments contractility	Ventricular irritability
Epinephrine	1:10,000 solution (ampule)	2.5–10 mL	Augments contractility; restores electrical activity in asystole; enhances defibrillation	Ventricular irritability
Norepinephrine	4 mg/4 mL (ampule)	Give by continuous infusion at 0.02–0.2 mg/kg per minute	Augments contractility; resores arteriolar tone and increases BP to improve coronary perfusion following restoration of cardiac rhythm	Renal vasoconstriction, increased afterload

Lidocaine

Lidocaine is the first line drug for treatment of ventricular arrhythmias. It can be used successfully to treat ventricular premature contractions and ventricular tachycardia, and to maintain a stable rhythm following electrical cardioversion for ventricular fibrillation. Initial therapeutic doses usually consist of a 100 mg bolus with continuous infusions varying from 1 to 4 mg/min. Lidocaine has mild negative inotropic effects and can cause central nervous system toxicity (disorientation, seizures).

Epinephrine

The beneficial effects of epinephrine during cardiopulmonary resuscitation are related to its α-adrenergic properties, which produce significant vasoconstriction, and its β-adrenergic effects, which augment myocardial contractility. Epinephrine can increase blood pressure, restore cardiac rhythm in asystole, and coarsen ventricular fibrillation, which may improve the likelihood of successful defibrillation. As outlined earlier, epinephrine can be given as a smaller bolus for hypotension and as a 1 mg bolus in the acute arrest setting. These boluses can be followed by a continuous infusion.

Negative effects of epinephrine include increased ventricular irritability, which can lead to ventricular fibrillation. Myocardial work is increased, which can cause or worsen subendocardial ischemia.

Calcium Chloride

This agent may be useful as treatment for hypotension. As discussed below, high levels of calcium may be injurious.

When hyperkalemia, hypocalcemia, or calcium channel blocker toxicity occur, treatment with calcium chloride is appropriate. Excessive use may increase ventricular irritability.

Sodium Bicarbonate

Mounting evidence suggests that sodium bicarbonate administration during cardiac arrest should be restricted to specific circumstances. Standard efforts such as intubation, mechanical ventilation, electrical defibrillation, cardiac compression, and epinephrine treatment should be used prior to consideration of bicarbonate. Rapid restoration of appropriate respiration and circulation is more important in control of acid–base balance during cardiac arrest than administration of exogenous buffer. However, preexisting metabolic acidosis, hyperkalemia, and phenobarbital overdose are appropriate circumstances for bicarbonate administration. Sodium bicarbonate comes in 50 mL ampules containing 44 mEq or approximately 1 mEq/mL. The initial dose of bicarbonate is 1 mEq/kg with 1/2 mEq/kg repeated every 10 min thereafter.

Proper acid–base management of patients during cardiac arrest can be enhanced by frequent blood gas determination with administration of bicarbonate guided by base deficit calculations. The efficacy of β-agonists is impaired by acidosis.

Negative effects of bicarbonate administration include shifting the oxyhemoglobin association curve to the left, thus inhibiting the release of oxygen, as well as hyperosmolarity, hypernatremia, and paradoxical acidosis as a result of carbon dioxide production. Further review of the controversial role of sodium bicarbonate is provided below.

Norepinephrine

Norepinephrine is a weak β-agonist and a potent α-agonist that can be used to restore blood pressure following cardiac arrest. However, clinical observation and experimental evidence indicates that norepinephrine is useful for its positive inotropic effects in the stunned heart. The vasoconstrictive effects of norepinephrine may be detrimental to the kidneys, but norepinephrine is less likely to cause ventricular arrhythmias than epinephrine. For this reason, it can be extremely valuable for short-term support in critically ill patients with hemodynamic compromise and ventricular arrhythmias.

OTHER AGENTS

Other agents that are valuable during a cardiac arrest or pre-arrest setting include administration of 100% oxygen via an endotracheal tube, which will correct hypoxemia and improve delivery of oxygen to end organs. Calcium channel blockers including verapamil and diltiazem, or adenosine, may be helpful in controlling paroxysmal supraventricular tachycardia. Diltiazem has also been recommended for coronary artery spasm. Magnesium can be used to correct hypomagnesemia and prevent ventricular fibrillation. Dopamine and dobutamine can be employed for inotropic support to maximize cardiac output, blood pressure, and end-organ perfusion. The hemodynamic effects of dopamine are dose dependent, and the effects of dobutamine are not always predictable in cardiac patients. Newer agents such as amrinone and milrinone may also be valuable.

UNUSUAL SITUATIONS AND PROBLEMS

Cardiac surgery results in situations in which expected effects of inotropic agents are altered. Unique problems apply to patients with intra-aortic balloon (IABP) or ventricular assistance devices (VAD), implanted pacemakers or defibrillators (ICD), epidural blocks, heart, lung, or heart–lung transplants, resected ventricular aneurysms, pulmonary hypertension after correction of mitral valve or congenital heart disease, negative inotropic agents (e. g., propranolol), incomplete myocardial revascularization, perioperative myocardial infarction, or myocardial stunning. These special clinical situations as well as the recent trend toward polypharmacy in which four or five vasoactive drips including antiarrhythmics, vasodilators, and inotropic agents are combined require special management that is best learned in a busy clinical center specializing in such care.

CARDIAC SURGERY

For management of low output states, four determinants of cardiac function should be optimized. These are preload, afterload, contractility, and heart rate.

Preload can be adjusted by volume expansion with crystalloid, colloid, or blood or by volume reduction by diuresis and venodilation with nitroglycerin. Physiologically, preload is the length of myocardial sarcomeres at end-diastole, which is most closely related to end-diastolic volume. Variation in end-diastolic volume cannot be conveniently measured clinically, the closest related measure being ventricular cross section by two-dimensional echocardiography. Clinical estimates of changes in preload are usually provided by (Swan-Ganz) ventricular filling pressures, estimated by capillary wedge pressure for the left ventricle and central venous pressure for the right side. However, these pressure measurements may be unreliable measures of preload if a change in ventricular compliance occurs. Common causes of changes in ventricular compliance are myocardial edema and cardiac tamponade (which reduce compliance of both ventricles), positive pressure ventilation (which reduces compliance of the left ventricle by shifting the interventricular septum to the left), and correction of congenital heart disease (which may increase compliance of the left ventricle by reducing right-sided filling pressures and shifting the septum to the right). In the presence of alterations in ventricular compliance, very high levels of filling pressure may be required to maintain adequate preload. Perhaps the best way to estimate optimum filling pressure in such situations is to monitor cardiac output, arterial blood pressure, and echocardiographic cross sections during adjustments in filling pressure. Such "Starling curves" are optimally determined in the operating room at the conclusion of cardiopulmonary bypass. The information obtained can then be used as a guide to management in the intensive care unit.

Afterload reduction can reduce the work of the heart and increase end-organ perfusion. Nitroprusside infusion is appropriate for this in the acute care setting. Nitroglycerine, amrinone, isoproterenol, dobutamine, and hydralazine also decrease afterload. The extent to which these agents are appropriate can be monitored by effects on end-organ function and cardiac output. In patients who may have critical stenoses of peripheral arteries, afterload reduction can result in diversion of flow from those arterial beds. One therapy that causes major reduction of afterload is intra-aortic balloon pumping.

Contractility can be maximized using inotropic agents that have been discussed above. A practical question is how much β-agonist can be safely administered to a given patient. As mentioned previously, the risks of β-agonists in the acute setting include increased myocardial irritability and provocation of myocardial ischemia, which could result in myocardial infarction. Practically speaking, an intrinsic heart rate of greater than 120 or the appearance of atrial and ventricular premature contractions and runs of atrial flutter or ventricular tachycardia is an indication that the level of inotropic agent being employed is becoming unsafe. Unfortunately, in critically ill patients it may not be possible to reduce the level of inotropic support without adding mechanical support. Patients with coronary artery disease on β-blocker therapy may be relatively refractory to therapy with β-agonists. Monitoring heart rate in these patients can be a useful guide to appropriate rate of infusion, and sensitivity to β-agonists is likely to change as the level of β-blockade subsides.

One strategy for managing low output states in patients after coronary artery bypass begins with dopamine in doses of less than 7.5 µg/kg per minute. If this is not sufficient, norepinephrine is added and titrated for desired effects on blood pressure and cardiac output. If norepinephrine, dopamine, and nitroglycerine do not stabilize the patient, then mechanical support is indicated. This strategy can be modified by addition or substitution of agents like dobutamine for dopamine, or epinephrine or amrinone for norepinephrine, if heart rate and ectopy levels allow. Nitroglycerine infusions should probably be maintained in any patient in whom myocardial revascularization is suspected to be incomplete.

In patients with valvular or congenital heart disease and no coronary disease, β-agonists may be emphasized because of their favorable effect on pulmonary hypertension and right ventricular function.

Heart rate as a determinant of cardiac output is particularly important in patients with fixed stroke volume as a result of ventricular dysfunction. Mean arterial pressure (but not peak systolic pressure) is directly related to cardiac output if resistance remains constant. In patients with permanent or temporary pacemakers, heart rate can be optimized by observing the effect of rate on mean arterial pressure. The lowest rate associated with a given level of performance is always preferable, particularly in relation to myocardial ischemia. The atrial kick should be preserved whenever possible in patients requiring inotropic support. In some patients with complete heart block, atrioventricular delay can have important effects on stroke volume. Impaired ventricles in such patients function better if intrinsic conduction is allowed to occur, even if very long atrioventricular delays are necessary for this. Fast heart rates adversely affect intra-aortic balloon pump function.

Another challenging problem is bleeding following cardiopulmonary bypass. This can be secondary to platelet dysfunction, fibrinolysis, or other clotting deficiencies, requiring appropriate replacement with blood, platelets, fresh frozen plasma, other blood products, or pharmacologic agents. Sudden cessation of bleeding may indicate obstruction of tubing by clot, and appropriate measures should be taken to exclude this possibility. Mediastinal re-exploration to rule out technical problems and to remove extensive clot prior to tamponade can be lifesaving and is now frequently performed within the intensive care unit. Pericardial tamponade, as a result of extensive clot formation from postoperative bleeding, is manifested by low cardiac output, equalization of right and left sided filling pressures, and decreased end-organ perfusion. If facilities for full re-explo-

ration of the median sternotomy incision are not readily available within the intensive care unit, re-exploration of the lower third of the incision may be important for relieving tamponade and improving cardiac output. (Fig. 107–2).

Myocardial ischemia may contribute to arrhythmias or low output states and should be ruled out, particularly in patients with known coronary artery disease. Electrocardiographic changes are not always dependable postoperatively, particularly in the presence of cardiac pacing, bundle branch block, or pericarditis. For this reason, two-dimensional echocardiography is an important adjunct for monitoring ventricular function in the postoperative period. Treatment of postoperative ischemia includes intravenous nitroglycerin, nifedipine for coronary spasm, reoperation for graft occlusion, and insertion of the intra-aortic balloon pump for low output states due to myocardial infarction or stunning.

Finally, failure of intrinsic or extrinsic pacemaking may occur requiring emergent intervention. Transcutaneous pacemaker units can be used with conversion to transvenous or epicardial pacing as required.

A review of autopsy findings in patients who died following cardiopulmonary resuscitation noted two diagnoses that were most frequently missed. Ninety percent of patients with ischemic bowel and 50% of patients with pulmonary emboli failed to be identified prior to death.[7] Ischemic bowel in this group of patients was associated with fever, leukocytosis, and, in the majority, with diarrhea. Surgical resection of involved bowel may be lifesaving in this setting, but a high index of suspicion is required for detection. Current treatment of pulmonary embolism is based on

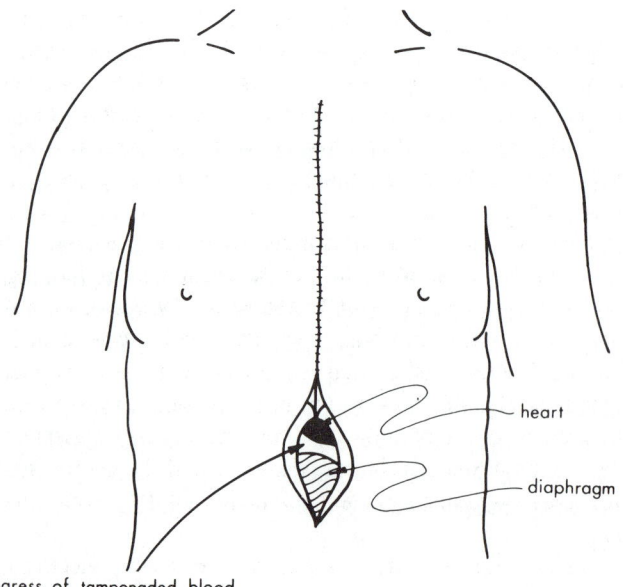

egress of tamponaded blood

Figure 107–2. Decompression of postoperative cardiac tamponade by opening the lower portion of the sternotomy incision and the linea alba.

thrombolytic therapy and anticoagulation, but cardiopulmonary bypass may be required for removal of clot in unstable patients. In rare cases, Trendelenberg surgical pulmonary embolectomy may still be performed.[8] Transvenous techniques for pulmonary embolectomy have also been successfully employed.

THORACIC SURGERY

Bleeding

Hemorrhage after pulmonary resection can occur from a major branch of the pulmonary artery or vein. Chest tubes will usually provide an adequate indication of the extent of bleeding, as will hemodynamic instability. Emergency re-exploration through the thoracotomy incision may be necessary to provide control of hemorrhage with manual compression followed by appropriate suturing.

Tension Pneumothorax

Despite the placement of chest tubes following pulmonary resection, tension pneumothorax can occur with life-threatening consequences. Chest tubes may be dysfunctional as a result of clotting, kinking, or occlusion by lung tissue. Tension pneumothorax may occur without lung resection in a patient who ruptures a previously existing bleb. Expeditious chest tube placement should not be delayed in patients on positive pressure ventilation.

Mediastinal Shift

An acute shift of the mediastinum following thoracic surgery may cause significant hemodynamic compromise. There may be severe restriction of venous return to the heart with resultant decreased cardiac output and hypotension. This clinical situation can occur during tension pneumothorax as noted above and can be treated with placement of an additional chest tube.

Position of the mediastinum following pneumonectomy surgery is an important consideration in performing the procedure. Again, significant hemodynamic compromise, arrhythmias, and pulmonary dysfunction can occur if the mediastinum is shifted significantly to either side. Specifically, a shift toward the operated side may enhance function of the remaining lung, but may cause significant obstruction of venous return. A shift toward the unoperated side may significantly reduce function of the remaining lung.

Thus, proper management of the pneumonectomy space is an important part of postpneumonectomy care. Diaphragmatic elevation, narrowing of intercostal spaces, and fluid accumulation tend to reduce the empty space on the operated side. However, the mediastinum may tend to shift

inappropriately for a variety of reasons. An overshift to the unoperated side may occur if fluid is secreted more rapidly than air is absorbed, or the opposite, a shift toward the operated side may occur if fluid secretion is slower than air absorption. Additional factors, such as positioning in the lateral decubitus position that tends to compress the down remaining lung, or loss of air through the incision postoperatively on the pneumonectomy side, may cause a shift of the mediastinum back toward the pneumonectomy side. The chest x-ray is the best means of evaluating the precise position of the mediastinum. A direct anterior–posterior or posterior–anterior film must be obtained without rotation to avoid an inaccurate assessment. Clinical observations that may be valuable include position of the trachea at the suprasternal notch and percussion of the cardiac apex location.

Interventions may be required to adjust the pressure in the postpneumonectomy space to achieve an adequate balance. Air can be added to the pneumonectomy space by needle injection if the mediastinum is shifted excessively far toward the operative side, or air can be removed from the pneumonectomy space if the mediastinum is shifted excessively far toward the unoperated side. In addition, a needle can be placed in the pneumonectomy space open to the atmosphere to allow for equilibration, which will usually achieve a balanced position of the mediastinum.

The above discussion relates to the acute management of the patient in the immediate postoperative period. A gradual long-term shift of the mediastinum toward the pneumonectomy space side may be advantageous by enhancing inflation of the remaining lung and is usually stable as a result of fibrosis.

Congestive Heart Failure

Many patients requiring pulmonary resection suffer from chronic forms of lung disease that may have significant effects on the pulmonary vasculature. Resection of lung tissue may raise pulmonary vascular resistance, which increases the work of the right heart and may predispose to right ventricular failure. This is particularly significant following pneumonectomy. Pneumonectomy may also precipitate an acute decompensation in patients predisposed to congestive heart failure. Mortality rates as high as 10% may be related to these issues.

The monitoring of cardiac performance following pneumonectomy may be problematic. A central venous line can provide an indication of right-sided heart pressures and incurs relatively little risk. A Swan-Ganz catheter, if placed preoperatively, must be positioned using fluoroscopy to avoid its placement on the operated side. Following pneumonectomy, insertion of a Swan-Ganz catheter can be associated with disruption of the pulmonary artery stump.

Thus, postoperative management of patients following major pulmonary resection requires consideration of right ventricular function as well as observation for development of pulmonary edema. Treatment of these conditions including inotropic support, positive end-expiratory pressure, tight fluid management, and treatment of other inciting causes can prevent cardiac decompensation.

Lobar Torsion

The remaining portions of the lung following pulmonary resection may twist on the mediastinal pedicle as mobilization of mediastinal and pleural attachments is used to facilitate resection. Thus, the remaining lung following lobectomy may become gangrenous if its blood supply is compromised due to torsion. The diagnosis can be entertained on the basis of opacification on chest x-ray in a lobar distribution following resection. The diagnosis may be confirmed by bronchoscopy, which will reveal a twisted lobar bronchus. Emergency resection of the involved lobe is the appropriate treatment.

Cardiac Herniation

Significant defects in the pericardium may be created when pneumonectomy is performed via an intrapericardial approach. A large defect may predispose the patient to cardiac herniation, which can be an immediately fatal event. Thus, the key to management of these patients is appropriate prevention of the herniation by closure of the defect at the time of surgery or leaving the pericardium widely and completely open. Although diagnosis may be reached on the basis of a chest x-ray, acute decompensation may be so rapid that immediate interventions are required. Thus, a significant index of suspicion for this complication is necessary.

ADVANCES AND DEBATES IN CARDIOPULMONARY RESUSCITATION

In this section, some of the more controversial as well as newer developments in cardiopulmonary resuscitation will be reviewed. Definitive judgments in these areas are not yet available. However, many of these concepts may prove valuable in patient management.

Physiologic Principles and Specific Methods

The mechanism of cardiopulmonary resuscitation (CPR) remains controversial.[16,17] Two explanations for the flow of blood from the chest to the body have been proposed. The traditional view is that bloodflow to the periphery occurs during external chest compression because the heart is directly compressed between the sternum and vertebral column. A newer theory suggests that changes in intrathoracic pressure created during CPR cause blood to flow from the chest to the periphery, with venous valves preventing simultaneous retrograde bloodflow. The original explanation is known as the "cardiac pump mechanism." The newer theory is known as the "thoracic pump mechanism." A large body of clinical and experimental evidence supports these theories (Fig. 107–3). Small animal data show much higher intravascular pressures than pleural pressures during CPR, supporting the cardiac pump mechanism.[18] However, clinical evidence of effective pulsatile arterial perfusion with coughing alone as a means of CPR supports the thoracic pump mechanism[19] (Fig. 107–4).

New approaches to CPR are based on these theories. The American Heart Association now favors high impulse CPR with chest compression 100 times per minute to improve end-organ perfusion.

Other methods under development include chest compression with a pneumatic vest, which has been shown to increase aortic and coronary perfusion pressure.[20] This method avoids loss of intrathoracic pressure by surrounding the entire chest with a simultaneously compressive vest. Interposed abdominal compression CPR has also been successful. The abdominal compressions may resemble an intraaortic balloon pump, enhancing coronary perfusion pressure, while compression of abdominal veins helps fill the heart.[21–23] Another new technique involves the use of active chest compression and decompression with a custom hand-held suction device (Fig. 107–5). This device produces chest compression in a standardized fashion and also provides for active chest decompression for improved effectiveness. Both significant hemodynamic and clinical benefits have recently been noted using this device.[24–26] Statistically significant improvements in 24 hour survival and neurologic outcome have also been demonstrated.[27]

Open chest massage as a means of performing more effective CPR has been demonstrated in animal models[28,29] with anecdotal reports of success compared to closed chest CPR in humans.[30,31] Therefore, if closed chest compression results in inadequate perfusion pressure as monitored by arterial line, open chest resuscitation should be considered. Balloon occlusion of the descending thoracic aorta during open chest massage in animal models has been demonstrated to improve coronary bloodflow.[32]

The use of a mechanical cardiopulmonary bypass circuit for assistance in resuscitation for hypothermic cardiac arrest following drowning or exposure has been documented.[33] The use of cardiopulmonary bypass for resuscitation following witnessed normothermic cardiac arrest has also been employed with percutaneous support via the femoral vessels.[34–37] The use of extracorporeal membrane oxygenation (ECMO) as means of CPR is under investigation and has been used successfully in the clinical arena.[38] The exact clinical role of the percutaneous technique has not yet been fully determined with costs and local vascular complications being significant limitations. Flows from 1.5 to 5.5 L/min have been achieved with this technique.

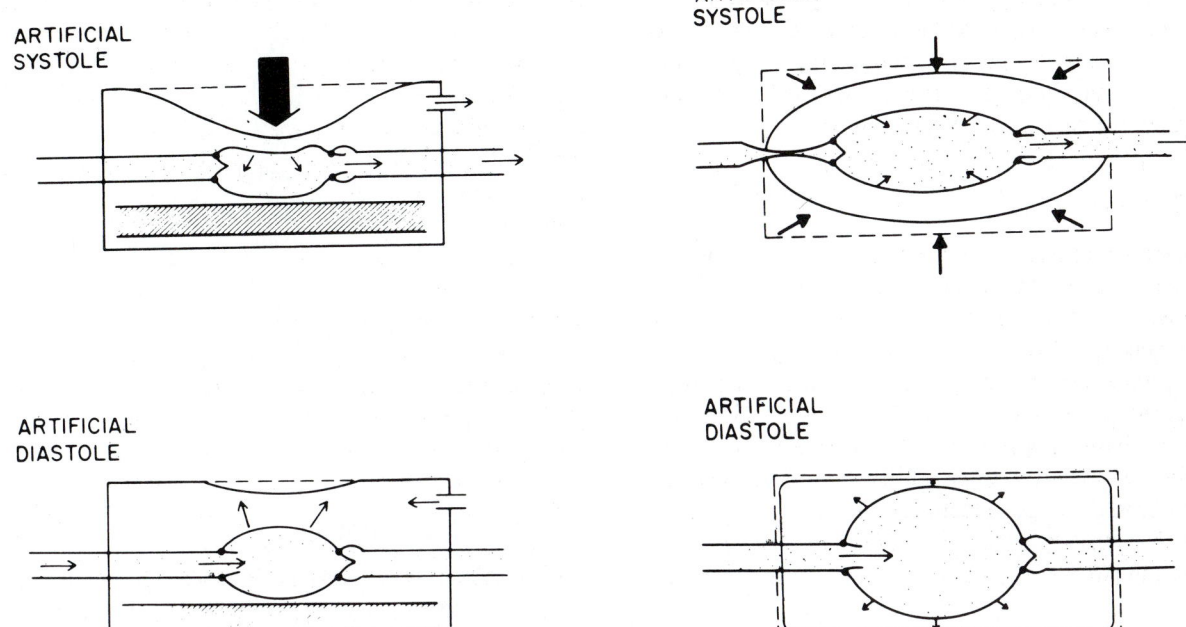

Figure 107–3. A. The cardiac pump mechanism. Central chest compression squeezes the heart against the spine. The cardiac valves work. Blood is forced out of the heart. Air is vented from the thorax via the tracheal (see opening at top right in schematic diagram). For simplicity, only one pumping chamber is shown. Between compressions, chest resiliency generates negative pressure and draws blood into the heart. **B.** The thoracic pump mechanism. Thoracic compression generates positive intrathoracic pressure, which is vented by arterial outflow to peripheral tissues. The cardiac valves are irrelevant. Between compressions, chest resiliency generates negative pressure and draws blood into the heart.

Pharmacologic Controversies

Sodium Bicarbonate

Mounting evidence now exists to suggest that routine administration of sodium bicarbonate at the time of initiation of CPR is no longer warranted. Attention to appropriate ventilation and circulation during resuscitation will lead to rapid correction of respiratory acidosis.[39] Administration of bicarbonate can lead to a variety of problems including excess salt loading, reduced coronary perfusion,[40] and paradoxical acidosis as a result of diffusion of carbon dioxide into myocardial and cerebral cells.[1] In fact, because of a paradoxical excess of pulmonary ventilation over perfusion during CPR, arterial carbon dioxide is low and pH is near normal whereas venous pH may be disproportionately low because of cellular acidosis. As satisfactory perfusion is re-

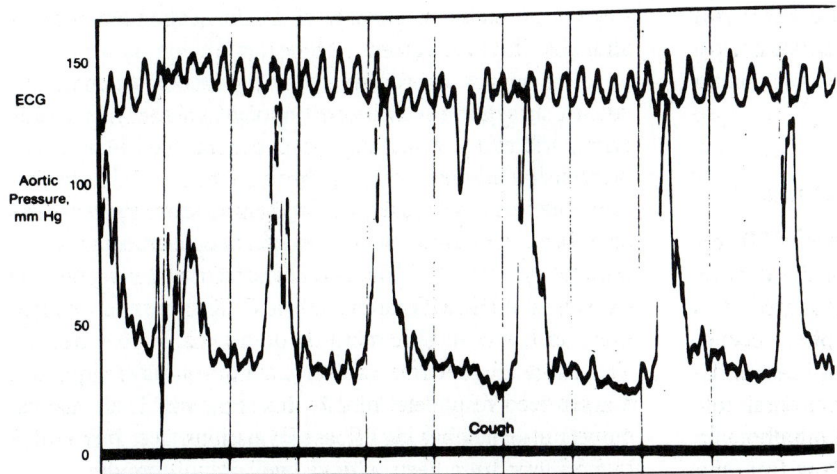

Figure 107–4. Cough-induced arterial pressure spikes during ventricular fibrillation.

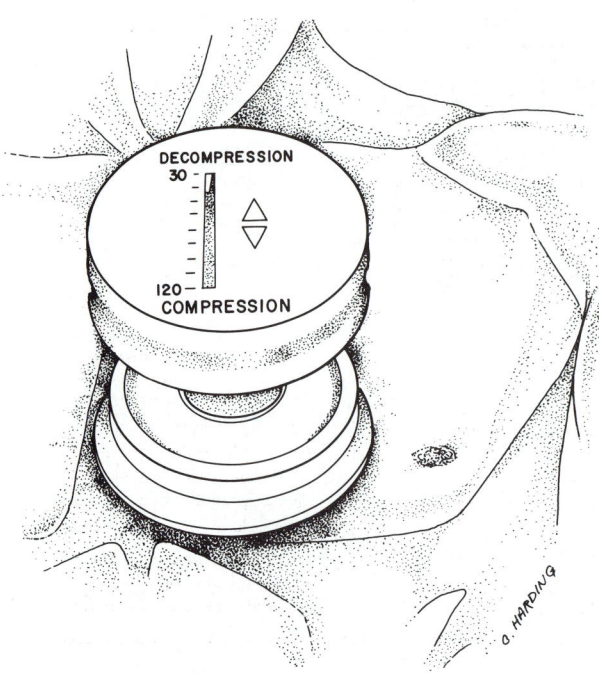

Figure 107–5. Mechanical device for use in active compression–decompression cardiopulmonary resuscitation.

stored, this arteriovenous pH difference normalizes. Therefore, the administration of bicarbonate would be best determined on the basis of mixed venous blood sampling.[41]

The correction of acidosis during CPR is best achieved by establishing early ventilation and tissue perfusion to allow for elimination of both respiratory and metabolic acidosis. The use of bicarbonate is indicated only to correct prearrest derangements of pH or in the case of prolonged CPR to correct persistent acid–base abnormalities as determined by mixed venous blood gas determinations.

Calcium

Present American Heart Association guidelines warn against routine use of calcium during CPR unless specific indications for its use exist, such as hyperkalemia and hypocalcemia (for example, following multiple blood transfusions), or following use of excessive calcium channel blockers. In fact, there may be significant deleterious effects of calcium chloride during CPR.[42–44] Although calcium can enhance normal myocardial cell function, in the presence of poor tissue perfusion related to cardiac arrest, administration of calcium can result in excessively high levels of intracellular calcium, which may have negative effects on cellular metabolism. In fact, the use of calcium channel blocking agents has been recently noted to enhance success of resuscitation in animal models of cardiac arrest.[45–47] Clinically, however, some cardiovascular and thoracic surgeons use calcium as an acute inotropic agent for treatment of hypotension as long as organ perfusion is judged to be satisfactory.

End-Tidal Carbon Dioxide Monitoring

End-tidal carbon dioxide ($ETCO_2$) monitoring can confirm proper placement of the endotracheal tube and monitor the success of end-organ perfusion. Using the assumption that the degree of carbon dioxide production and ventilation during CPR is relatively constant, the major determinant of $ETCO_2$ is cardiac output. During cardiac arrest, initial readings of $ETCO_2$ are low because of absence of flow. Successful restoration of end-organ washes out venous blood carrying carbon dioxide. When this blood returns to the lungs, $ETCO_2$ rises. Thus, $ETCO_2$ monitoring can measure the success of resuscitation efforts and has been noted to be 100% specific for successful endotracheal tube intubation[48–50] (Fig. 107–6).

Cerebral Resuscitation

The goal of CPR is the rapid restoration of ventilation and perfusion to maintain end organ viability. Investigations to maximize brain preservation during the period of cardiopulmonary resuscitation are in progress. The brain is extremely susceptible to injury during cardiac arrest. Within 15 seconds of arrest, unconsciousness develops as a result of cerebral hypoxia. Within 5 min, levels of stored glucose and adenosine triphosphate are exhausted. However, experimental work suggests that cerebral neurons can tolerate up to 20 min of normothermic ischemic anoxia. Thus, strategies to enhance revivability of brain neurons as well as cardiac myocytes are under investigation. A variety of explanations for the inability to rescue susceptible cells exist. These include perfusion failure, reperfusion injury (see Chap. 97), stasis of blood flow, and postarrest inflammatory processes.

The "no-reflow phenomenon" suggests that a combination of microcirculatory congestion caused by thrombosis, vasospasm, and vascular and cellular edema reduces capillary perfusion, thus perpetuating injury. In addition, even after reperfusion, a combination of oxygen free radicals and lysosomal enzyme release may continue to cause cascades of cellular necrosis. Also, the accumulation of additional noxious elements in the circulation as a result of renal or hepatic dysfunction may produce additional damage to susceptible neurons or myocytes. Finally, a significant postarrest inflammatory response may continue to have significant injurious effects throughout the body. In fact, improvements in survival in large animal models have been linked with improvements in reperfusion associated with open chest CPR, the early use of cardiopulmonary bypass, postresuscitation hypertension, calcium channel blocker treatment, and mild cerebral hypothermia.[51] Several other promising treatment modalities, however, have proved to have mixed results on further investigation. These include no improvements with the use of barbiturates, free radical scavengers, antiepileptic drugs, and amino steroids.

The use of 5% dextrose in water during CPR is contro-

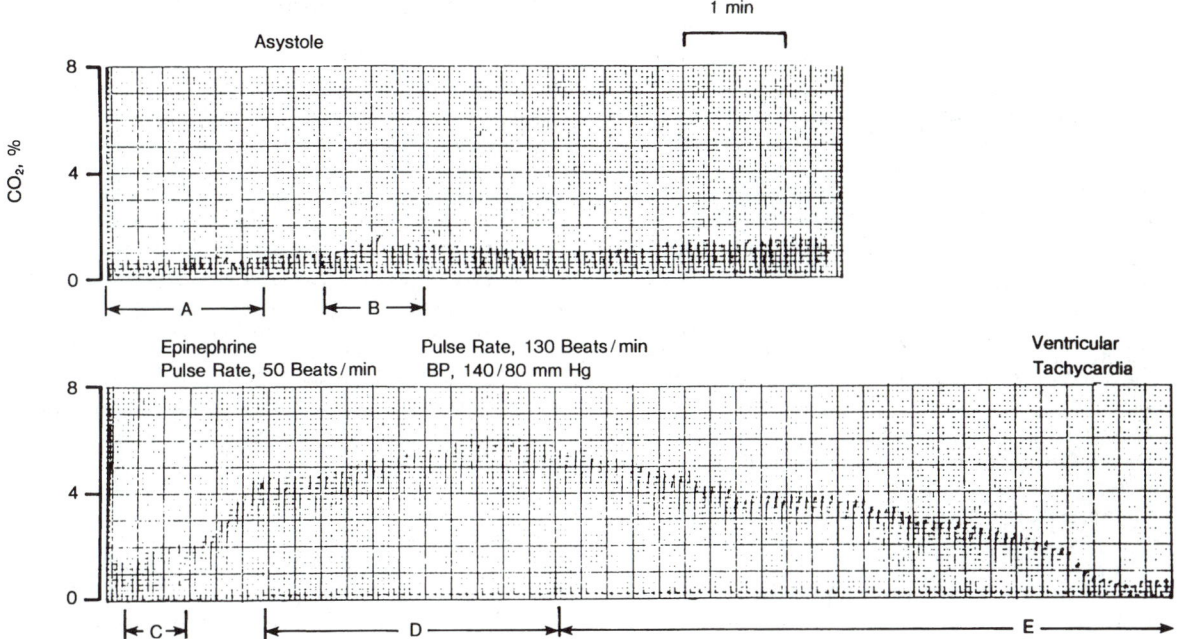

Figure 107–6. $ETCO_2$ as a monitor of resuscitation. **A.** Patient has arrived in emergency room. **B.** Medical and mechanical resuscitation has begun. **C.** Rise in $ETCO_2$ signals return of spontaneous activity (undetected clinically). **D.** Dramatic rise in $ETCO_2$ as hemodynamics improve. **E.** Fall in $ETCO_2$ as circulation deteriorates again.

versial as there are possible detrimental effects of high levels of glucose on neural cell function associated with ischemia. However, the data on this issue are not complete enough to allow conclusive recommendations.[52]

Although this field is progressing significantly, the latest American Heart Association guidelines suggest that no specific treatment is sufficiently proven to justify its routine use during CPR.[1]

SURVIVAL PREDICTIONS FOR CPR

A modern day review of CPR methods would not be appropriate without consideration of the efficacy of this technique and the factors influencing indications, ethics, and cost effectiveness of this modality. Recent data suggest that the length of CPR is related to the likelihood of success with duration of less than 30 min correlating with increased survival.[53] Also, data suggest that survival after CPR for those over 70 years of age is significantly decreased for in-hospital patients.[54,55] In addition, a recent study notes that physicians tend to overestimate the efficacy of CPR and overstate the value of this modality to patients and relatives.[56] These studies do not evaluate the role of CPR in postsurgical cardiothoracic patients. Thus, they do not provide specific conclusions applicable by specialty. However, outcomes research may be important in the future of our practice and should be considered during each of our interventions. One recent study attempted to use scoring systems to predict the survival of postcardiac arrest patients.[57] Such data, no doubt, will appear in our own future literature.

Fortunately, the unique position of the cardiothoracic surgeon with a vast armamentarium of clinical skills and technological support allows us a high success rate of CPR. Clearly, the goal of effective traditional CPR, which, at its best, restores only 30% of normal effective cardiac output,[30] is to resume effective respiration and circulation at the earliest possible time.

REFERENCES

1. Guidelines for cardiopulmonary resuscitation and emergency care. *JAMA* **268:**2171, 1992
2. Shoemaker WC, Ayres S, Grenvik A, et al: *Textbook of Critical Care,* 2nd ed. Philadelphia, W.B. Saunders, 1989
3. Schwartz GR, Cayten CG, Mangelsen MA, et al: *Principles and Practice of Emergency Medicine,* 3rd ed. Philadelphia, Lea & Febiger, 1992
4. Jaffe AS: *Textbook of Advanced Cardiac Life Support.* Dallas, American Heart Association, 1987
5. Ewy GA, Dahl CF, Zimmerman M, Otto C: Ventricular fibrillation masquerading as ventricular standstill. *Crit Care Med* **9:**392, 1981
6. McDonald JL: Course ventricular fibrillation presenting as asystole or very low amplitude ventricular fibrillation. *Crit Care Med* **10:**790, 1981
7. Bedell SE, Fulton EJ: Unexpected findings and complications at autopsy after cardiopulmonary resuscitation (CPR). *Arch Intern Med* **146:**1725, 1986
8. Weatherford SC, Lawrie GM: Trendelenberg pulmonary embolectomy for cardiac arrest secondary to massive pulmonary embolism. *Can J Surg* **29:**383, 1986
9. Young W, Perryman R: Complications of pneumonectomy. In Cordell A, Ellison R (eds): *Complications of Intrathoracic Surgery.* Boston, Little, Brown, 1979, pp 257–266
10. Kirsch M, Rotman H, Behrendt D, et al: Complications of pulmonary resection. *Ann Thorac Surg* **20:**216, 1975

11. Maier H: Pneumonectomy: Methods of improving morbidity and mortality rates. *Surg Clin North Am* **42:**1527, 1962

12. von Hippel A: *A Manual of Thoracic Surgery.* Springfield, Illinois, Charles C Thomas, 1978

13. Lanston H, Barker W: The adult thoracic surgical patient. In Neville W (ed): *Intensive Care of the Surgical Cardiopulmonary Patient.* Chicago, Year Book Medical, 1983, p 235

14. Gibbon J, Gibbon M, Kraul C: Experimental pulmonary edema following lobectomy and blood transfusion. *J Thorac Surg* **12:**60, 1942

15. Brooks J: Complications following pulmonary lobectomy. In Cardell A, Ellison R (eds): *Complications of Intrathoracic Surgery.* Boston, Little, Brown, 1979, pp 235–256

16. Babbs CF: New versus old theories of blood flow during CPR. *Crit Care Med* **8:**191, 1980

17. Chandra NC: Mechanisms of blood flow during CPR. *Ann Emerg Med* **22:**281, 1993

18. Maier GW, Tyson GS, Olsen CO, et al: The physiology of external cardiac massage: High impulse cardiopulmonary resuscitation. *Circulation* **70:**86, 1984

19. Criley JM, Blaufuss AH, Kissel GL: Cough-induced cardiac compression: Self-administered form of cardiopulmonary resuscitation. *JAMA* **236:**1246, 1976

20. Halperin HR, Tsitlik JE, Gelfand M, et al: A preliminary study of cardiopulmonary resuscitation by circumferential compression of the chest with use of a pneumatic vest. *N Engl J Med* **329:**762, 1993

21. Christienson JM, Hamilton DR, Scott-Douglas NW, et al: Abdominal compressions during CPR: Hemodynamic effects of altering time and force. *J Emerg Med* **10:**257, 1992

22. Sack JB, Kesselbrenner MB, Bregman D: Survival from in-hospital cardiac arrest with interposed abdominal counterpulsation during cardiopulmonary resuscitation. *JAMA* **267:**379, 1992

23. Babbs CF: Interposed abdominal compression-CPR: A case study in cardiac arrest research. *Ann Emerg Med* **22:**24, 1993

24. Cohen TJ, Tucker KJ, Lurie KG, et al: Active compression-decompression, a new method of cardiopulmonary resuscitation. *JAMA* **267:**2916, 1992

25. Tucker KJ, Redberg RF, Schiller NB, Cohen TJ: Active compression-decompression resuscitation: Analysis of transmitral flow and left ventricular volume by transesophageal echocardiography in humans. *J Am Coll Cardiol* **22:**1485, 1993

26. Lurie KG, Schultz JJ, Callaham ML, et al: Evaluation of active compression-decompression CPR in victims of out-of-hospital cardiac arrest. *JAMA* **271:**1405, 1994

27. Cohen TJ, Goldner BG, Maccaro PC, et al: A comparison of active compression-decompression cardiopulmonary resuscitation with standard cardiopulmonary resuscitation for cardiac arrests occurring in the hospital. *N Engl J Med* **329:**1918, 1993

28. Sanders AB, Kern KB, Ewy GA: Improved resuscitation from cardiac arrest with open-chest massage. *Ann Emerg Med* **13:**672, 1984

29. Bircher N, Safar P, Stewart R: A comparison of standard, "MAST"-augmented and open-chest CPR in dogs, a preliminary investigation. *Crit Care Med* **8:**147, 1980

30. Del Guericio LR, Feins NR, Cohn JD, et al: Comparison of blood flow during external and internal cardiac massage in man. *Circulation* **31** (Suppl I):171, 1965

31. Paradis NA, Martin GB, Rivers EP: Use of open-chest cardiopulmonary resuscitation after failure of standard closed-chest CPR: Illustrative cases. *Resuscitation* **24:**61, 1992

32. Spence PA, Lust RM, Chitwood WR Jr, et al: Transfemoral balloon aortic occlusion during open-cardiopulmonary resuscitation improves myocardial and cerebral blood flow. *J Surg Res* **49:**217, 1990

33. Lestou GV, Kopf GS, Elefteriades JA, et al: Is cardiopulmonary bypass effective for treatment of hypothermic arrest due to drowning or exposure? *Arch Surg* **127:**525, 1992

34. Phillips SJ, Ballentine B, Sinine D, et al: Percutaneous initiation of cardiopulmonary bypass. *Ann Thorac Surg* **36:**223, 1983

35. Moore CH, Rubin JM, Schnitzler RN, et al: Experience and directions using cardiopulmonary support in fifty-three consecutive cases. *ASAIO Transact* **37:**M340, 1991

36. Sugimoto JT, Baird E, Bruner C: Percutaneous cardiopulmonary support in cardiac arrest. *ASAIO Transact* **37:**M282, 1991

37. Rees MR, Brown T, Sivanthan UM, et al: Cardiac resuscitation with percutaneous cardiopulmonary support. *Lancet* **340:**513, 1992

38. Dembitsky, WP, Moreno-Cabral RJ, Adamson RM, Daily PO: Emergency resuscitation using portable extracorporeal membrane oxygenation. In Ott RA, Gutfinger DE, Jazzaniga AB, (eds): *Cardiac Surgery, State of the Art Reviews, Mechanical Cardiac Assist.* Philadelphia, Hanley & Belfus, 1993, pp 189–197

39. Von Planta M, Bar-Joseph G, Wilslund L, et al: Pathophysiologic and therapeutic implications of acid-base changes during CPR. *Ann Emerg Med* **22:**404, 1993

40. Kette F, Weil MH, Gazmuri RJ: Buffer solutions may compromise cardiac resuscitation by reducing coronary perfusion pressure. *JAMA* **266:**2121, 1991

41. Steedman DJ, Robertson CE: Acid base changes in arterial and central venous blood during cardiopulmonary resuscitation. *Arch Emerg Med* **9:**169, 1992

42. Stueven HA, Thompson BM, Aprahamian C, Darin JC: Use of calcium in prehospital cardiac arrest. *Ann Emerg Med* **136:**25, 1983

43. Stempien A, Katz AM, Messineo FC: Calcium and cardiac arrest. *Ann Intern Med* **105:**603, 1986

44. Hughes WG, Revdy JR: Should calcium be used in cardiac arrest? *Am J Med* **81:**285, 1986

45. Lindner KH, Prengel AW, Aknefeld FW, et al: Effects of diltiazem on oxygen delivery and consumption after asphyxial cardiac arrest and resuscitation. *Crit Care Med* **20:**650, 1992

46. Capparelli EV, Hanyok JJ, Dipersio DM, et al: Diltiazem improves resuscitation from experimental ventricular fibrillation in dogs. *Crit Care Med* **20:**1140, 1992

47. Schindler I, Weindlmayr-Goettel M, Susani M, et al: *Anesth Analg* **78:**87, 1994

48. Steedman DJ, Robertson CE: Measurement of end-tidal carbon dioxide concentration during cardiopulmonary resuscitation. *Arch Emerg Med* **7:**129, 1990

49. Varon AJ, Morrina J, Civetta JM: Clinical utility of a colorimetric end-tidal CO_2 detector in cardiopulmonary resuscitation and emergency intubation. *J Clin Monitoring* **7:**289, 1991

50. Ward KR, Menegazzi JJ, Zelenak RR, et al: A comparison of chest compressions between mechanical and manual CPR by monitoring end-tidal pCO_2 during human cardiac arrest. *Ann Emerg Med* **22:**669, 1993

51. Safar P: Cerebral resuscitation after cardiac arrest: Research initiatives and future directions. *Ann Emerg Med* **22:**324, 1993

52. Gonzalez ER: Pharmacologic controversies in CPR. *Ann Emerg Med* **22:**317, 1993

53. Rosenberg M, Wang C, Hoffman-Wilde S, Hickham D: Results of cardiopulmonary resuscitation, failure to predict survival in two community hospitals. *Arch Intern Med* **153:**1370, 1993

54. Bilsky GS, Banja JD: Outcomes following cardiopulmonary resuscitation in an acute rehabilitation hospital. *Am J Phys Med Rehab* **71:**232, 1992

55. Juchems R, Wahlig G, Frese W: Influence of age on the survival rate of out-of-hospital and in-hospital resuscitation. *Resuscitation* **26:**23, 1993

56. Miller DL, Gorbien MJ, Simbartl LA, Jahnigen DW: Factors influencing physicians in recommending in-hospital cardiopulmonary resuscitation. *Arch Intern Med* **153:**1999, 1993

57. Niskanen M, Kari A, Nikki P, et al: Acute physiology and chronic health evaluation (APACHE II) and glasgow coma scores as predictors of outcome after intensive care cardiac arrest. *Crit Care Med* **19:**1465, 1991

108

Postoperative Care of the Cardiovascular Surgical Patient

Jai H. Lee and Alexander S. Geha

Patients undergoing cardiac surgery have undergone an evolution in recent years. The clinical profile of these patients has changed to include increasing numbers of older, sicker, and more unstable patients.[1,2] These patients are at higher risk for increased morbidity and mortality, and demand greater scrutiny and intervention in the postoperative period by the surgeon. Although colleagues in critical care, anesthesiology, and medical subspecialties may provide valuable consultation during the postoperative period, it is the surgeon who has the knowledge, training, and personal commitment to the patient, and should therefore bear the primary responsibility for postoperative care.[3] This chapter focuses on the postoperative monitoring and management of these patients and particular emphasis will be placed on those with low cardiac output.

MONITORING SYSTEMS FOR POSTOPERATIVE CARDIAC PATIENTS

It has been recognized that the transfer of the patient from the operating room (OR) to the cardiac surgical intensive care unit (ICU) is associated with significant interruption in monitoring[4] and it is critical that the surgical and anesthesia teams adhere to a method to assure an orderly and safe transfer to the ICU. The transfer should be initiated only after the establishment of stable hemodynamics and respiratory function following chest closure. When the patient's condition remains unstable or becomes unstable following chest closure, invasive monitoring is continued in the OR

and appropriate measures are taken to stabilize the patient prior to transport.

Following transfer from the OR, careful monitoring of cardiopulmonary function is continued. Extensive monitoring of cardiac and pulmonary function allow measurement of the physiologic variables necessary to make sound clinical decisions. When the patient first arrives at the ICU, the arterial line is the first monitoring line connected to the bedside monitor. Arterial access allows systemic arterial blood pressure tracings to be continuously displayed graphically, as well as the ability to obtain arterial blood gases. Cuff blood pressures are often difficult to obtain in a cold patient and/or a patient with significant peripheral vasoconstriction. Although brachial and femoral sites are available, the radial artery is preferred due to its accessibility and good collateral circulation via the ulnar artery.[5] However, a pressure gradient may exist between central and radial arteries, related to hypovolemia, vasoconstriction, and central shunting,[6] in which case, femoral or brachial arterial catheters provide a more accurate estimation of central aortic pressure. The surface electrocardiogram (ECG) is recorded continuously to allow for rapid interpretation of arrhythmias, conductions defects, as well as ongoing ischemia. Lead V_5 has been shown to have the greatest sensitivity for detecting ECG ischemia.[7] In addition, pulse oximetry, which provides accurate and continuous determination of arterial oxygen saturation, is utilized. Finally, a Swan-Ganz pulmonary artery (PA) catheter, which is useful for measuring left-sided filling pressures, obtaining mixed venous oxygen saturation (SVO_2), and determining thermodilution cardiac outputs, is connected. Left artrial lines are utilized selectively in some patients with poor left ventricular function.

Since the adequacy of cardiovascular function is of chief concern in the postoperative period, the most important hemodynamic measurement in the early postoperative period is cardiac output. While objective data to support the use of PA catheters do not exist, routine measurements of cardiac output to permit effective therapy represents the normal standard of care in most centers performing cardiac surgery. Cardiac output measurements are based on the Fick principle and the Stewart–Hamilton principle as outlined below.

Special catheters and systems for continuous cardiac output and arterial blood gas tension measurements are now being evaluated. Where they will be helpful after cardiac operations has not been established.

The Fick Principle

Bloodflow through an organ can be determined if a substance is removed from or added to the blood during its flow through the organ. Applied to the lungs, the Fick principle is used to calculate the volume of blood required to transport the oxygen taken up from the alveoli per unit time. In the absence of intracardiac shunts, measurement of oxygen consumption and arterial and mixed venous oxygen contents would provide the necessary information to calculate cardiac output by the Fick method. Since measurement of oxygen consumption requires spirometric collection and analysis of exhaled air, the method becomes too cumbersome for bedside use. It is more commonly used in cardiac catherization laboratories.

Mixed venous oxygen levels, however, measure the relation of cardiac output to the function of other organs and systems and to the general metabolic activity. When mixed venous oxygen levels are normal, the relation between cardiac output and metabolic rate is normal unless there are nonperfused areas of the microcirculation in which an oxygen debt is developing. Samples of mixed venous blood (MVO_2) can be obtained through a catheter in the pulmonary artery. However, a new generation of PA catheters incorporates fiberoptic oximetry system in the catheter itself and allows continuous bedside monitoring of the MVO_2 saturation.[8] Although mixed venous oxygen saturation is normally about 75%, a level of 65% is adequate if most of the microcirculation is being perfused.

The Stewart–Hamilton Principle

The volume of fluid in a container can be calculated by adding a known quantity of indicator and measuring the concentration of the material after it has become evenly dispersed through the fluid. Stewart demonstrated that this method can also be applied to fluids in motion.[9,10] Hamilton and associates verified the usefulness of the method in

calculating the flow through glass models and in the circulation.[11,12] The introduction of a bedside thermodilution cardiac output computer, which uses a bolus of cold saline as the indicator, samples blood temperature distal to the site of injection, and computes output from the mean decrease in blood temperature and the transit time, has been a major advance in our clinical ability to measure cardiac output objectively. Injection is usually into the right atrium, and sampling is obtained from the pulmonary artery, using a flow-directed Swan-Ganz catheter.[13] It is assumed that right and left cardiac output values are the same. Modern thermodilution systems actually display the thermodilution curve, which is a graph of temperature over time (Fig. 108–1).[14]

In the postoperative surgical patient, a cardiac index of 3.0 L/min per m^2 usually indicates good cardiovascular function. Mild reduction in cardiac output is associated with an index ranging between 2.2 and 3.0 L/min per m^2, moderately severe reduction in cardiac output is reflected by an index between 1.5 and 2.2, and extremely severe depression of cardiac output is seen when the index is below 1.5; for postoperative cardiac patients, outputs in this range correlate with a high probability of cardiac death.[15]

GENERAL POSTOPERATIVE CARE

When the patient arrives in the ICU, the immediate goal after appropriate monitoring and infusion lines are connected is to establish mechanical ventilation and chest tube drainage. All patients arrive intubated, and are placed on a volume-cycled ventilator. The chest is auscultated with attention directed to heart sounds and examination of the lungs. Laboratory tests include complete blood count, elec-

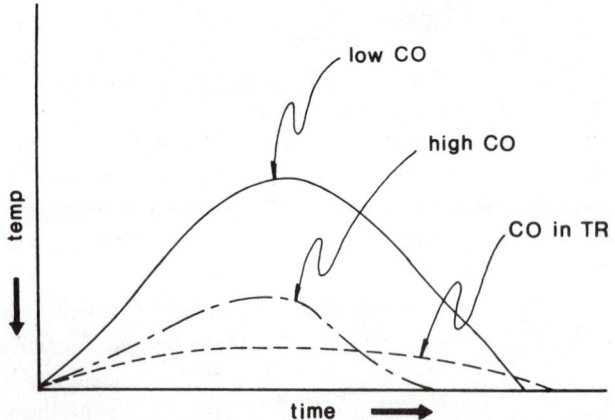

Figure 108–1. Thermodilution cardiac output (CO) curves (temperature versus time). The cardiac output is inversely proportional to the area under the curve (Stewart–Hamilton equation). Curves shown are normal CO, high CO, low CO, flat curve of tricuspid insufficiency (which underestimates actual CO). *(From Elefteriades et al.[14] reproduced with permission.)*

trolytes, prothrombin time (PT) and partial thromboplastin time (PTT), and cardiac isoenzymes, as well as a mixed venous gas from the distal PA catheter. A portable chest x-ray film is obtained and reviewed to confirm tube and line placements, the size of the mediastinal silhouette, and to rule out pneumothorax or atelectasis requiring therapy.

In the immediate postoperative period, patients are generally hypothermic and, consequently, peripherally vasoconstricted. Although these patients may be hypertensive, arterial blood pressure is an inaccurate guide to adequate hemodynamic performance due to the confounding influence of systemic vascular resistance (SVR). Hypothermia continues following termination from cardiopulmonary bypass (CPB) due to slower rewarming of the extremities, which eventually causes a drop in the core temperature, as equilibration with the periphery occurs. Hypothermia adversely affects hemodynamic performance by raising afterload and increasing myocardial oxygen consumption. Hypothermia also shifts the oxyhemoglobin dissociation curve to the left and the resulting increased affinity of hemoglobin for oxygen leads to less tissue oxygen delivery. During rewarming, shivering is common, which increases peripheral oxygen consumption. Some patients develop acute respiratory acidosis because carbon dioxide production increases with rewarming and patients on controlled ventilation are unable to increase spontaneous minute ventilation.[16]

The treatment of hypothermia includes careful ventilatory management, as well as control of shivering. In the ICU, warming is augmented by warming blankets, as well as radiant heat.[17] Demerol given in doses of 25–50 mg IV every 2 hours has been shown to control shivering.[18] If the balance between oxygen supply and demand is tenuous, shivering can be controlled with neuromuscular blocking agents such as pancuronium or vecuronium. In conjunction with rewarming, sodium nitroprusside is helpful by vasodilating arterial and venous smooth muscle and thus reducing SVR.

Close monitoring is required during the period of rewarming and vasodilation and adequate cardiac filling pressures should be maintained. The ideal filling pressure will depend on the state of myocardial contractility and compliance. Thus, observation of the response to fluid challenge is the most reliable method of assessing optimal filling pressures in each patient.

Volume expansion is begun with colloids, unless the hematocrit is less than 25%, in which case packed red blood cells should be used. Ringer's lactate and normal saline are poor volume expanders and generally not useful in the postoperative cardiac surgical patient who has typically sequestered 2–3 L of crystalloid prime. Hespan and 5% albumin have been shown to be equally efficacious as volume expanders in the setting of postoperative cardiac care.[19] They should be limited to 1500 mL to minimize their dilutional effect on clotting factors. During the re-

warming period, mean blood pressure may be low, compromising perfusion, despite adequate filling pressures and cardiac output. Vasopressor agents such as phenylephrine or norepinephrine are indicated to improve perfusion in such circumstance.

In the early postoperative phase, the phenomenon of acute hypertension resulting from arterial vasoconstriction has been reported in 30 to 80% of patients.[20–22] Although the precise mechanism is still unclear, elevated circulating catecholamines,[23,24] activation of the renin–angiotensin system during cardiopulmonary bypass,[25] surgical stimulation, and hypothermia all play a role. In addition to impairing optimal hemodynamics by increasing afterload, hypertension, if left untreated, can lead to hemorrhage, disruption of suture lines, cerebrovascular accidents, and myocardial ischemia. Thus prompt control of blood pressure is necessary.

Once it is ascertained that ventilation and sedation are adequate, vasodilator therapy is initiated for prompt control of hypertension. Nitroprusside and nitroglycerin are the agents most commonly used in the postoperative setting. Although other agents such as hydralazine, captopril, and esmolol are used, nitroprusside is preferred because of its rapid onset and short duration. However, the adverse effects of prolonged therapy or short-term dosage in excess of 10 μg/kg per minute include cyanide toxicity and elevated thiocyanate levels. Nitroglycerin can also be used, but it is primarily a venodilator, and thus less effective than nitroprusside as an arteriolar vasodilator. It, however, has the advantage of decreasing myocardial oxygen consumption and relieving myocardial ischemia by its vasodilatory effect on coronary arteries.[26]

Most patients are hypokalemic and hypomagnesemic in the immediate postoperative period due to hemodilution and the typical osmotic diuresis seen after CPB. Maintenance of adequate potassium levels is accomplished by administration of KCl through a central line at a rate of 10–20 mEq/h. KCl administration peripherally is not recommended due to potential thrombophlebitis and inflammation at the site of injection. Magnesium sulfate administration to raise the serum level to 2 mEq/L is beneficial in reducing the incidence of atrial and ventricular arrhythmias.[27,28]

There is a tendency for retention of sodium and water and most patients return from the operating room with an increase of between 2 and 5% total body weight. Full rewarming and cessation of the capillary leak syndrome, which occurs by 8 to 12 hours after an uneventful operation, are followed by a period of mobilization of interstitial fluid. Diuresis is initiated to excrete the excess salt and water and the body weight will decrease. This phase of mobilization of interstitial fluid and diuresis generally lasts 36 to 48 hours in a healthy patient with an uneventful perioperative course. However, the duration of this phase is prolonged and may be difficult in the unstable patient with severe myocardial dysfunction. This is anticipated if the surgical procedure has been difficult and complicated with prolonged ischemic and bypass times.

RESPIRATORY MANAGEMENT

It is routine practice to use a volume ventilator initially. The tidal volume is set at 10 to 12 mL/kg, and respiratory rate of 10 per minute, with an inspired oxygen percentage of 100%. Positive end-expiratory pressure of 5 cm is routinely added to prevent atelectasis, unless otherwise indicated. Arterial blood gases are monitored 15 min after arrival in the ICU and following any ventilatory adjustment, and the inspired oxygen is gradually lowered to less than 50%, as long as oxygenation is adequate. Intermittent mandatory ventilation is preferred since evidence suggests it is advantageous in the patient who is expected to awaken and be extubated early.[29]

Patients are weaned from the ventilator when they are hemodynamically stable, are warm, and have minimal mediastinal and pleural chest tube drainage. Additionally, they should be neurologically intact, and have no acid–base disturbances or electrolyte abnormalities (Table 108–1). In most centers, this generally occurs 16 to 18 hours postoperatively. During the weaning period, hemodynamics and vital signs are closely monitored. There are reports of cardiac decompensation occurring during transition from mechanical to spontaneous ventilation.[30,31] Extubation is suitable when the patient is able to tolerate spontaneous ventilation with assistance, and demonstrates a negative inspiratory force of greater then 25 cm H_2O (Table 108–2).

Early Extubation After Cardiac Surgery

In recent years, "early extubation" after cardiac surgery has become more prevalent. "Early extubation" has been defined as extubation within 8 hours postoperatively.[32] Although it may be technically feasible to extubate within the first hour, the advantages of waiting at least 4 hours postoperatively include adequate time for rewarming and adequate time for bleeding and hemodynamics to stabilize. Proponents of early extubation argue that spontaneous ventilation improves venous return, reduces right ventricular afterload, and augments left ventricular filling, thus improving cardiac output.[33] Furthermore, there is a possible reduction in pulmonary complications due to improved ciliary function

TABLE 108–1. WEANING CRITERIA

Awake, following commands
Adequate muscle strength
PaO_2 > 80 torr with FIO_2 < 50%
PEEP < 5 cm H_2O
pH > 7.32
$PaCO_2$ < 50 torr

TABLE 108–2. EXTUBATION CRITERIA

Tidal volume > 5 mL/kg
Vital capacity > 10 mL/kg
Negative inspiratory force > – 25 cm H_2O
Respiratory rate < 30
Satisfactory arterial blood gases

and earlier ability to cough, as well as earlier return to ambulation and oral intake. It is postulated that early extubation, by reducing cardiac and pulmonary morbidity, and by reducing the duration of ICU stay, ultimately leads to decreased cost.

The concept of early extubation after cardiac surgery has been described as early as 1977. Prakash et al[34] reported that 56 of 62 patients were successfully extubated within 3 hours following coronary bypass procedures. These patients needed fewer days of intensive care monitoring while having no increase in pulmonary morbidity. Since then, a number of studies have demonstrated the feasibility of early extubation after cardiac surgery in selected patients.[35–37] A randomized study reported by Quasha et al[35] demonstrated not only that early extubation was possible in the majority of cases, but was associated with less pulmonary morbidity than patients receiving routine extended ventilatory support.

However, the routine use of extended ventilatory support of cardiac surgical patients has been standard practice at most centers because of the unavailability of short-acting narcotics and sedatives, and the reported high incidence of postoperative ischemia, detected by clinical electrocardiography in up to 50% of the patients.[38] Thus it was firmly believed that adequate postoperative sedation and analgesia to prevent to keep stress under control were mandatory,[39,40] and the use of high-dose narcotics became popular. High-dose narcotics, however, result in a slow emergence from general anesthesia, and the need for prolonged postoperative ventilation. A balanced anesthetic technique, using short-acting narcotics (sufentanil), and short-acting hypnotics such as propofol, allows for acceptable hemodynamic stability and blunting of the stress response, in addition to earlier emergence from anesthesia.[41] A recent report suggests that earlier awakening with propofol had no effect on the incidence of ischemic events.[42]

Inherent in a successful program of early extubation after cardiac surgery is a coordinated effort among surgeons, anesthesiologists, ICU nurses, and respiratory therapists. Factors that must be considered include patient selection, changes in anesthetic techniques, changes in ventilator weaning, changes in postoperative sedation, and changes in nursing practices. Sedation and analgesia techniques in the ICU must allow for specific control of the level of sedation that avoids significant respiratory depression. Figure 108–2 outlines an algorithm used in our ICU for early extubation.

In terms of patient selection, although there are many preoperative factors that might be considered relative or ab-

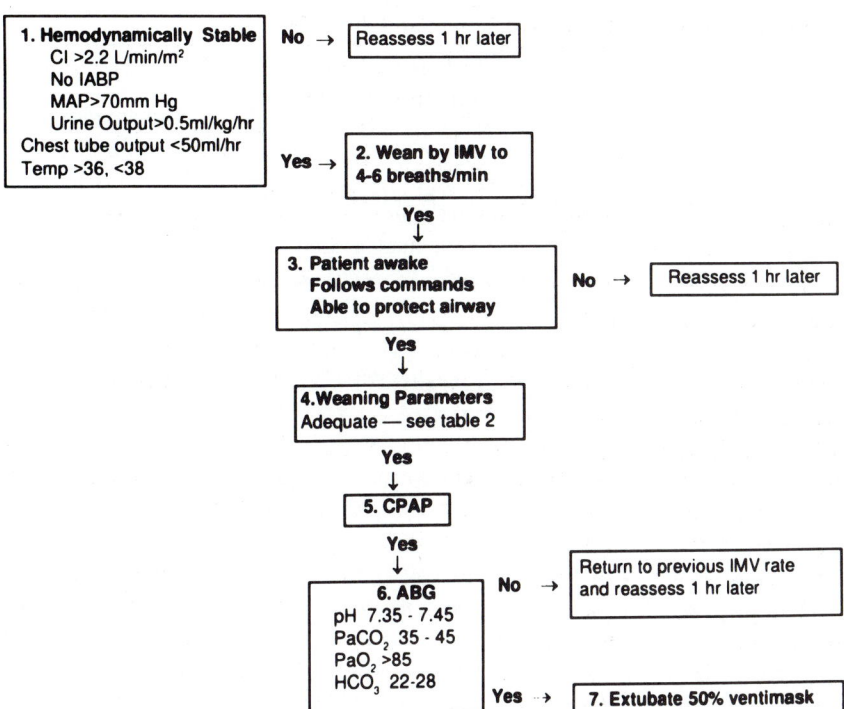

Figure 108–2. Early extubation algorithm at University Hospitals of Cleveland (assessment begins 4 hours postoperatively). Sections 1, 2, and 3 are assessed by the SICU nurses. Sections 4 through 7 are completed by Respiratory Therapy. The time and reasons for failure at any given step are recorded accordingly. At step 7, if the patient was found to be difficult to intubate, an anesthesiologist is consulted prior to extubation. CI, cardiac index; IABP, intra-aortic balloon pump; MAP, mean arterial pressure; IMV, intermittent mandatory ventilation; CPAP, continuous positive-airway pressure; ABG, arterial blood gas.

solute contraindications to early extubation, these factors may not necessarily correlate with the postoperative status of the patient. They may simply signify that the patient may have increased risk of not satisfying the postoperative criteria for extubation such as hemodynamic stability, mental alertness, and adequate pulmonary and renal function. Thus, each patient should be evaluated individually postoperatively, with the decision to extubate based on standard criteria for extubation. The absolute exclusion criteria for early extubation utilized in our ICU are listed in Table 108–3. The relative contraindications include prolonged CPB times (> 150 min), unstable arrhythmias, and inadequate urine output.

In summary, early extubation after cardiac surgery is possible, but its impact on outcome needs further evaluation. More research is also needed to clarify the issues of the impact of early extubation on stress response and myocardial ischemia. Nonetheless current concerns about health care costs and the need to minimize expensive resources such as ICU care will continue to drive the impetus for early extubation. In our ICU, length of stay after cardiac surgery is tracked in terms of hours, and patients who are extubated early stay in the ICU, on the average, 24 hours versus 48 hours for patients who undergo conventional recovery. However, in terms of cost containment, early extubation is a worthwhile effort only if it is accompanied by additional methods of reducing ICU stay, rehabilitation, and hospital stay.

Following extubation, continued attention is directed to maintenance of adequate oxygenation and mobilization of secretions. In this regard, adequate analgesia permitting effective cough is important. The effects of cardiac surgery on lung function and respiratory mechanics include reduction in functional residual capacity, atelectasis, and widened alveolar–arterial oxygen difference; thus the overall work of breathing is increased.[43] These effects are exaggerated in patients who have undergone internal mammary artery harvesting.[44–46] The oxygen is provided by face mask and incentive spirometry is begun to maintain functional residual capacity and prevent atelectasis.

Prolonged Ventilation

Most of the adverse consequences of cardiac surgery on pulmonary function have little consequence on the postoperative course of the majority of patients. Recent analysis of the Society of Thoracic Surgeons National Cardiac Surgery Database suggests that 2.5% of patients require prolonged ventilatory support (> 5 days) following isolated coronary

TABLE 108–3. ABSOLUTE EXCLUSION CRITERIA FOR EARLY EXTUBATION

Intraoperative complications
Inadequate rewarming
Significant mediastinal bleeding
Lack of return to consciousness
Unacceptable postoperative CXR
Unstable hemodynamics
   MAP < 80 mm Hg
   Mechanical assist devices
   Significant vasopressor/inotropic support

artery bypass surgery.[47] Factors that determine the need for prolonged ventilatory support include low cardiac output, preexisting pulmonary disease, and postperfusion adult respiratory distress syndrome. Increased technical sophistication of CPB has decreased the incidence of the latter from the postoperative course of a patient without preexisting pulmonary disease.

Management involves optimization of hemodynamic performance and nutritional status, as well as reduction of ventilatory demand. A more detailed discussion of prolonged ventilatory support can be found in Chapter 4. In unusual circumstances where intubation is expected for greater than 10 days, tracheostomy should be considered. Although tracheostomies tend to be deferred for 2–3 weeks postoperatively in cardiac patients due to the proximity of the median sternotomy incision and fear of increased risk of mediastinitis, early tracheostomy at about 10 days may reduce the incidence of laryngotracheal complications and shorten the duration of intubation.[48]

HEMODYNAMIC MANAGEMENT

A detailed review of the determinants of cardiac output and cardiovascular function is provided in Chapter 96. In brief, the clinical factors that influence cardiac output are heart rate and stroke volume (Fig. 108–3). Stroke volume is the end-diastolic volume of the ventricle minus the end-systolic volume. Diastolic filling is determined by effective filling pressure (preload) and resistance to distention offered by the ventricular wall. The degree of systolic ejection depends upon the degree of shortening that the ventricular myocardium can attain while working against the arterial resistance (afterload). The changes in contractile properties of the myocardium are included rather indiscriminately under the general term "contractility." Cardiac control clearly involves all five major factors:

1. Heart rate.
2. Ventricular filling or distending pressure (preload).
3. Ventricular distensibility.
4. Ventricular contractility.
5. Arterial resistance or impedance (afterload).

The major factors determining cardiac output are closely interrelated, and all these factors can be manipulated to optimize cardiac output. Although cardiac output is the most important hemodynamic variable, the essential primary goal of hemodynamic management is maintenance of oxygen transport adequate to meet tissue metabolic requirements.

CLINICAL MANIFESTATIONS AND DIAGNOSIS OF LOW CARDIAC OUTPUT

The cardiac output of normal subjects at rest averages 3.5 L/min per m^2 of body surface area, with a range between 2.5 and 4.4. Following major surgery, most patients require an increased cardiac output to meet the stress imposed by the operation and the accompanying elevation of oxygen consumption. In most postoperative situations, however, a cardiac index above 3.0 L/min per m^2 can be considered usual or adequate, with the exception of septic shock.

There is no single sign or symptom, nor a combination of signs or symptoms, that is absolutely pathognomonic of low cardiac output. Vigilance, however, is of utmost importance. Common clinical signs of low cardiac output include the appearance of anxiety, absent or weak peripheral pulses (dorsalis pedis, posterior tibial, and radial), cool and mottled skin of the extremities, blue fingernails and toenails, and moist skin. However, in the cardiac surgical patient, these clinical signs are unreliable due to the residual effects of anesthesia and systemic hypothermia. The arterial blood pressure is often low, and the pulse is thready and rapid. However, arterial pressure may be normal or elevated in a patient with low cardiac output. Oliguria (below 30 mL/h) is frequently an accompanying manifestation of inadequate cardiac output, but this sign is again not totally reliable, particularly in the presence of renal disease and/or administration of diuretics.

It is essential to obtain objective measurements of the level and adequacy of cardiac output in the postoperative

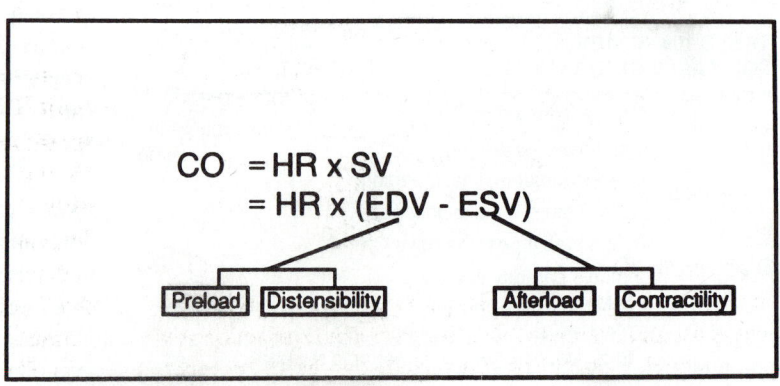

Figure 108–3. Determination of cardiac output (CO). HR, Heart rate; SV, stroke volume; EDV, end-diastolic volume; ESV, end-systolic volume.

cardiac surgical patient. Monitoring of left-sided pressures by either a left atrial line or a PA catheter is mandatory. The latter also allows measurement of thermodilution cardiac output.

TREATMENT OF POSTOPERATIVE LOW CARDIAC OUTPUT

The major factors determining cardiac output are usually intimately interrelated, and while it is extremely rare to find situations in postoperative patients where only one factor is deranged to the exclusion of the others, we will examine each of these factors separately from the point of view of evaluation and intervention.

It is also useful to identify the used and unused reserves of the cardiovascular system, to know its capability for increasing its performance when sudden new demands develop because of fever, atelectasis, increased work of breathing, arrhythmias, and the like. The components of cardiac output—rate, preload, distensibility, contractility, and afterload—define the reserves of the heart. Assessment of each of these determinants identifies which of the various components can be optimized to improve cardiac performance. Thus, when the cardiac rhythm is sinus, and the heart rate is increased, this reserve mechanism for increasing cardiac output is being employed. Systemic venous tone is a reserve mechanism and increases in it will result in increased preload, other things being equal. Systemic arteriolar resistance is a reserve mechanism also, and increases in it can maintain an arterial blood pressure adequate for perfusion of the brain, kidneys, and the heart when cardiac output is low. Peculiar properties of the hemoglobin molecule, as reflected in its oxygen dissociation curve, are an important reserve mechanism for oxygen transport when cardiac performance is poor.

Heart Rate

The optimal cardiac mechanism is sinus, and the optimal rate is proportional to the physiologic needs of the patient; deviations can affect cardiac output adversely. In the postoperative cardiac surgical patient, one may encounter a bradyarrhythmia, a slow heart rate, or, even more commonly, a tachyarrhythmia. Arrhythmias postoperatively result from electrolyte imbalance, particularly involving potassium metabolism, digitalis excess, hypothermia, myocardial ischemia, and the traumatic impact of the cardiac surgical procedure itself. Chapter 99 contains greater detail on the pharmacologic therapy of rhythm disturbances.

Bradyarrhythmias

The low heart rate of the postoperative cardiac surgical patient is usually associated with injury to the conduction system, although it may also reflect residual effects of preoper-

ative β-blockade. Knowledge of the anatomy of the conduction system, sufficient care during the cardiac procedure, as well as careful electrocardiographic monitoring during the procedure have markedly decreased problems. At the end of the procedure, temporary atrial and ventricular pacing wires should be placed in all patients with significant compromise of their cardiac function or arrhythmias, particularly those with a tendency toward development of heart block. The majority of patients who were taking β-blockers preoperatively will require pacing at a heart rate of 90–100 beats/min to achieve optimal hemodynamics. When the heart is in sinus rhythm, best control of rate is achieved by atrial pacing to maintain the atrial contribution to stroke volume. This atrial contribution can be quite sizable in a diseased heart and account for 20–25% of stroke volume. In cases of atrial fibrillation or atrioventricular (A-V) dissociation, ventricular pacing should be used to optimize the heart rate. Newer, sophisticated temporary pulse generators can provide DDD pacing, as well as a variety of other pacing modes.[49] The hemodynamics benefits of DDD pacing versus A-V sequential (DVI) pacing are derived from the ability to track the patient's intrinsic sinus rhythm, and, thus, the ventricular response is optimized by responding to changes in sinus rate mediated by metabolic demand.

Tachyarrhythmias

A recent large series documented the incidence of atrial tachyarrhythmias after isolated coronary bypass surgery to be over 30%, and as procedures increased in complexity, the incidence of atrial rhythm disturbances rose to as high as 90%.[50] Tachyarrhythmias, involving a heart rate above 120 beats/min, lead to hemodynamic impairment, particularly in an already compromised heart. Although an increase in the heart rate will increase cardiac output if the stroke volume remains constant, this does not occur above a rate of 120 beats/min. Stroke volume is compromised by decreased diastolic filling time, hence decreasing the effective preload. Myocardial contractility is diminished as a consequence of altered myocardial oxygen supply and demand. Because of the adverse hemodynamic consequences of tachyarrhythmias, control of the ventricular response is of primary importance.

Supraventricular Tachycardia. The majority of sustained supraventricular arrhythmias occurring after cardiac surgery will be atrial flutter or fibrillation. Less commonly, multifocal atrial tachycardia or atrioventricular nodal re-entrant tachycardia (AVNRT) can occur. Differentiation requires identification of atrial activity and determination of whether the rhythm is regular.[51] A regular rhythm is consistent with atrial flutter or AVNRT. An irregular rhythm is either atrial fibrillation or multifocal atrial tachycardia. Work by Waldo and colleagues [52] has demonstrated that an atrial electrocardiogram recorded from epicardial atrial wires is frequently helpful.

The most commonly identified risk factor associated

with the development of postoperative atrial arrhythmias has been increasing age.[50,53,54] Other factors include prolonged ischemic periods,[55,56] inadequate atrial and atrioventricular nodal hypothermia,[57] the presence of persistent atrial electrical activity during cardioplegic arrest,[58] as well as the consequences of the surgery itself, including pericardial inflammation, atrial distention, and hypoxemia.[59]

Although atrial fibrillation or flutter occurs most commonly on the second and third postoperative day, they can sometimes appear during the first 24 hours and usually require prompt therapy. In situations where the ventricular response is very rapid, immediate electrical cardioversion is required to prevent further hemodynamic compromise. The use of temporary epicardial atrial wires has proved useful in the therapy of atrial flutter.[60] Rapid overdrive atrial pacing at a rate approximately 125% of the atrial rate during flutter is done to capture the atrium. The pacer is then turned off abruptly and successul penetration of the flutter circuit will result in termination of the atrial flutter.

Pharmacologic agents that provide A-V nodal block and slow the ventricular rate such as digoxin, verapamil, and diltiazem provide the basis of therapy. Once the ventricular rate is controlled, addition of a Class I antiarrhythmic agent such as quinidine or procainamide is frequently necessary for conversion to sinus rhythm. Newer antiarrhythmic agents such as flecainide[61] or encainide or propafenone[62] can be used to prevent atrial flutter or fibrillation.

Ventricular Tachycardia. Although ventricular arrhythmias are frequently seen following cardiac surgery, the incidence has declined.[63] This decline is probably due to improvements in technical aspects of myocardial protection and cardiopulmonary bypass. Patients with an antecedent history of ventricular tachycardia are most at risk, and acute exacerbations can be precipitated by reversible factors such as electrolyte abnormalities, pharmacologic agents, hypotension, and hypoxia.

Ventricular ectopy occurring either early or late after surgery can be suppressed. However, the results of the Cardiac Arrhythmia Suppression Trial, which demonstrated that suppression of ventricular ectopy after myocardial infarction does not necessarily prolong survival,[64] have cast doubt on the impact of suppression on patient outcome. Nonetheless, it is prudent to assume that premature ventricular contractions (PVCs) that occur early postoperatively may reflect myocardial ischemia or herald a more serious arrhythmia and should be investigated. Frequent ectopy (greater than 6 times per minute) or complex ventricular ectopy requires treatment initially with either intravenous lidocaine or procainamide. In one study, intravenous tocainide suppressed postoperative ventricular ectopy better than lidocaine, with fewer side effects.[65] Intravenous amiodarone has also been used effectively in managing patients with intractable, sustained ventricular tachyarrhythmias that were resistant to other antiarrhythmic drugs.[66]

Ventricular arrhythmias that are sustained or compromise hemodynamics clearly require immediate electrical cardioversion or defibrillation. As soon as hemodynamic stability is established, underlying factors exacerbating the ventricular arrhythmias should be sought and corrected. Ventricular fibrillation is a rhythm that is always associated with profound circulatory collapse, and the protocol for cardiac arrest should be instituted immediately (see Chap. 107).

VENTRICULAR PRELOAD

An increase in filling pressure and ventricular diastolic volume (stretch) increases both stroke volume and ventricular contractility until stretch is excessive. This is described as the Frank–Starling effect on the ventricular function curve (Fig. 108–4). Thus, it is imperative that cardiac filling pressures be continuously monitored. Ideally, one would like to know the left ventricular end-diastolic pressure (LVEDP), which is the ultimate volume status criterion. In most patients with normal atrioventricular valves, end-diastolic pressure is similar to the mean pressure in the corresponding atrium. It must be realized however that right heart filling pressures, although more readily accessible, do not accurately reflect left heart pressure, especially in compromised hearts.[67]

Thus, after LVEDP, the mean left atrial pressure is the next most accurate index of volume status. The left heart filling pressure can be monitored by either a left atrial catheter brought out through the chest wall at the end of the operative procedure, or by a PA catheter. The PA catheter in its wedged position, closely approximates left atrial pressure. In patients with a normal heart rate and a normal pulmonary vascular bed, the pulmonary diastolic pressure closely approximates wedge pressure,[5] and inflation of the balloon is not essential. However, with tachycardia (heart rates above 120 beats/min), or pulmonary hypertension, the pulmonary artery diastolic pressure will exceed wedge pressure.[68]

In patients with heart disease and decreased myocardial contractility, increasing the filling pressure will increase cardiac output, although at a lower starting point and with smaller increments in output for each unit increase in filling pressure. Thus, the ventricular function curve of the diseased heart is lower than that of the normal heart (Fig. 108–4). For all states of contractility, there is a point on the plateau of the curves at which increased filling pressure will not increase cardiac output. This plateau is reached at lower levels of cardiac output and slightly higher levels of filling pressure in diseased hearts. Similarly, hypovolemia can set off a cycle of progressive fall in cardiac output, as demonstrated in Figure 108–4.

With measurements of ventricular filling pressure, hypovolemia should be quickly assessed, and the effect of fluid challenge evaluated, while increments in cardiac out-

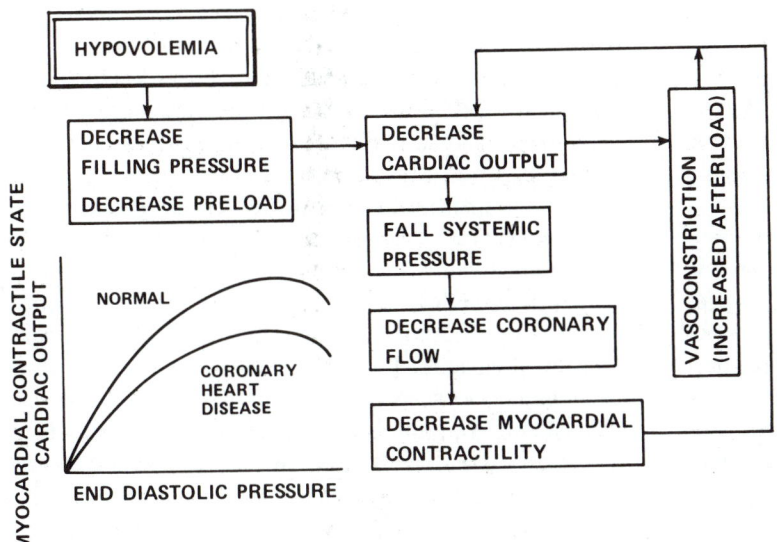

Figure 108–4. The indirective effects of hypovolemia in patients with decreased myocardial reserve due to heart disease. The Frank–Starling effect is shown in the left lower corner. In patients with heart disease, the increments in cardiac output are smaller for each increment in filling pressure. The boxes and arrows show how hypovolemia and decreased preload can set off a vicious cycle of progressive fall in cardiac output.

put are observed. In the normally convalescing patient, adequate preload may be all that is required for optimization of cardiac output. In situations of preexisting left ventricular dysfunction, or patients who experience transient global biventricular dysfunction in the early postoperative period, manipulation of preload often is not enough to achieve satisfactory cardiac output. Special catheters now assess right ventricular function with calculation of right ventricular ejection fraction and diastolic volume. This may be a good way to adjust preload as well.

VENTRICULAR DISTENSIBILITY

Alterations in ventricular distensibility and their effect on cardiac output are quite specific to the postoperative cardiac surgical patient. Myocardial ischemia may adversely affect distensibility, as may cardiopulmonary bypass itself with its activation of complement. Myocardial edema is also always present after cardiopulmonary bypass[69,70] and results in decreased compliance. Excessive clotted and unclotted blood in the confined mediastinal or pericardial space can also impinge on cardiac distensibility and lead to cardiac tamponade. This situation usually occurs when excessive postoperative bleeding has continued for a number of hours and may be associated with malfunctioning of the chest tubes without an excessive amount of measured blood loss.

Significant postoperative bleeding per se, even without cardiac tamponade, may lead to depression of myocardial contractility and reduction of cardiac output. This occurs through repeated dislocation of fluid compartments when excessive blood is lost and replaced with banked blood and other intravenous fluids as well as through metabolic and electrolyte aberrations that accompany excessive transfusions, in addition to the direct effects of hypovolemia when blood loss is underestimated. Patients who have no evi-

dence of coagulopathy, but continue to have excessive mediastinal drainage (in an adult, 150–200 mL/h for 4 hours without evidence of decreasing) should be re-explored. At the time of re-exploration, the blood in the mediastinum and pleura should be removed, and mechanical hemostasis carefully accomplished. If re-exploration is performed at a time when the patient is still in satisfactory hemodynamic condition, the procedure is well tolerated and usually results in control of the bleeding problem.

Cardiac Tamponade

To help avoid tamponade, most surgeons leave the pericardium widely open to ensure adequate drainage of the mediastinum and also place a tube in the most dependent part of the pericardial sac near the left ventricle. However, this does not preclude tamponade, which continues to be a complication of open heart surgery and should always be ruled out in the patient with low cardiac output, particularly during the early hours after operation. Late tamponade may also occur days or weeks postoperatively.[71]

Compression of the heart causes limitations of diastolic filling and decreases cardiac output by decreasing distensibility. Clinically, the blood pressure is usually somewhat low, and the pulse pressure is narrow. A precipitous fall in systolic pressure usually indicates severe tamponade and occurs rather late in the course of this hemodynamic abnormality. The filling pressure is elevated, unless the patient is grossly hypovolemic, and there may be significant paradoxical pulse. However, the diagnosis may be difficult to make because of low systemic blood pressure, and high right-sided pressure findings are also consistent with cardiac failure. In addition, the paradoxical pulse may be difficult to identify, or it may be difficult to ascertain the significance of the paradoxical pulse in a patient on a respirator. Although a portable chest x-ray or a bedside echocardiogram may be helpful in the diagnosis, this is primarily a clinical diagnosis. Once the diagnosis is established, expeditious re-exploration is undertaken. If the operating room is not immediately available, the lower end of the sternotomy incision can be opened in the ICU and blood evacuated from the substernal space. The hemodynamic response should be immediate.

Sudden massive bleeding with or without severe tamponade is a rare postoperative complication leading to low cardiac output. It may originate in the breakdown of a suture in one of the cardiac chambers or major vessels, or from a branch of a graft in cases of myocardial revascularization. Alertness to the situation and prompt, aggressive intervention can be lifesaving in these circumstances. Immediate exploration of the pericardial cavity in the intensive care unit to control bleeding and relieve the tamponade may avoid a fatal outcome. Therefore, a thoracotomy tray should always be immediately available in the ICU. This is the only postoperative complication after open heart surgery that can be significantly affected by bedside opening of the chest.[72,73]

MYOCARDIAL CONTRACTILITY AND AFTERLOAD

These two determinants of cardiac output are discussed together, since they are closely interrelated, and pharmacologic agents affecting one usually have a major effect on the other. The modern era of afterload reduction in the treatment of acute pump failure began in the late 1970s, after the initial investigations of Franciosa and associates[74] and Chatterjee and colleagues,[75,76] who demonstrated the salutory hemodynamic effects of phentolamine and, especially, nitroprusside in intractable pump failure due to acute myocardial infarction. The concept of using vasodilator drugs spread rapidly and has since been extended to the management of severe chronic heart failure of various etiologies.

The dynamics of the peripheral arterial and venous beds are closely linked with the state of left ventricular contractility. When the left ventricle is normal, reduction of aortic impedance in response to arterial vasodilation slightly augments stroke output, but a marked decrease in blood pressure also occurs in conjunction with reflex tachycardia.[77] Arterial resistance is increased in the presence of left ventricular dysfunction as a result of increased sympathetic tone[78,79] and, in contrast to the normal heart, cardiac output becomes very dependent on outflow resistance (afterload mismatch).[80] Thus, with impaired contractility, aortic impedance reduction affected by arteriodilation results in considerable increase in cardiac output, accompanied by little change in blood pressure and heart rate. Although systemic arterial pressure may be thought of as the hemodynamic connection between cardiac function and peripheral arterial dynamics and may reflect somewhat the afterload faced by the heart in ejecting blood, arterial pressure itself

is an unreliable measure of afterload or impedance. Similarly, the therapeutic effects of vasodilator drug therapy cannot be judged by arterial pressure alone. Ventricular afterload should be equated with aortic impedance, which, in turn, can be estimated clinically by systemic vascular resistance.

The influence of the systemic venous system on cardiac output bears a substantially different relation to ventricular contractility than does the peripheral arterial bed.[77] Thus, when the left ventricle is normal, the heart operates on the steep ascending limb on its Frank–Starling curve (outflow-preload relation) (Fig. 108–4). Hence, preload reduction in response to venodilation markedly decreases cardiac output. With impaired contractility, on the other hand, the Frank–Starling relation is depressed and flat, in contrast to the steep outflow-resistance curve. Thus, preload reduction affected by venodilation may not affect cardiac output in left ventricular dysfunction and as impedance reduction predominates over preload decline, cardiac output is increased.[78]

It is often necessary to use a combination of an inotropic agent and a vasodilator agent to achieve optimal increase in myocardial contractility and reduction in afterload. The concept of preload restoration has been demonstrated by Miller and colleagues, who showed that combined use of afterload reduction with nitroprusside and inotropic support with dopamine produced a greater increase in stroke index than either agent used alone.[81]

A rational approach to selection of inotropic agents in the management of low cardiac output is based on an understanding of the effect of various inotropic agents, vasodilators, and agents with combined properties on the heart and the peripheral circulation. The approach must be flexible and individualized and takes into account the observation that no specific agent or combination of agents is the most effective treatment in all cases of the low cardiac output syndrome. The proper choice of drug or drugs to be used requires a knowledge of both the hemodynamic disturbance and the specific pharmacology of the inotropic agent. Complete details of the pharmacokinetics of the various commonly used inotropic agents are given in Chapter 99. The most commonly used agents are described in the next sections.

Dopamine is a naturally occurring catecholamine that has β_1- and α_1-adrenergic and dopaminergic activities. At low doses (< 2 μg/kg per minute) the dopaminergic activity is maximal and results in increased renal, mesenteric, and coronary flow. Above 3 μg/kg per minute, dopamine induces β_1 cardiac receptors, leading to increased inotropic effects and impaired contractility. However, at doses above 7 μg/kg per minute, α-adrenergic effects predominate, and systemic vascular resistance, pulmonary vascular resistance, and blood pressure increase. Some of these effects may be secondary to release of endogenous norepinephrine. The end result of increased afterload is a detrimental increase in myocardial oxygen consumption. The chronotropic and arrhythmogenic effect increases, as the dose is increased.

Dobutamine is a positive inotrope that has a strong β_1 effect that enhances inotropy and a mild β_2 effect that reduces systemic vascular resistance. At commonly used doses from 5 to 20 µg/kg per minute, dobutamine increases coronary bloodflow[82] and reduces left ventricular wall stress by lowering preload and afterload.[83] Dobutamine appears to have less of a chronotropic effect than dopamine.[84]

Epinephrine is a naturally occurring catecholamine that possesses potent α- and β-adrenergic effects. At doses < 0.05 µg/kg per minute, epinephrine has a potent inotropic effect mediated through β_1 stimulation and minimal peripheral vasodilation due to the balance of β_2 and α_1 stimulation. At doses above 0.1 µg/kg per minute, α effects predominate and SVR is increased significantly, and this may have adverse effects on myocardial oxygen consumption.

Norepinephrine is a potent catecholamine that possesses both β_1- and α_1-adrenergic activity. The α_1 activity usually predominates as the dose increases and thus its inotropic effects are overshadowed by its peripheral vasoconstrictive effects. Although coronary bloodflow is maintained, the increased afterload increases myocardial oxygen demand and also reduces renal blood flow.

The phosphodiesterase (PDE)-inhibiting agents are either bypiridines (amrinone and milrinone) or imidazoles (enoximone). Amrinone, until 1992, was the only PDE inhibitor available for clinical use in this country. Although their mechanism of action is incompletely understood, they are not β-adrenergic agonists. These agents inhibit type III phosphodiesterase found predominantly in cardiac muscle.[85] This inhibition results in increased cellular cyclic adenosine monophosphate (cAMP), which enhances myocardial contractility by facilitating calcium utilization and mobility at the level of the sarcoplasmic reticulum and sarcolemma. Further, the PDE inhibitors also produce systemic and pulmonary vasodilation. These agents were initially used in a different population from postoperative cardiac patients: patients with congestive heart failure.[86,87] More recently, however, they have been successfully employed in weaning patients with low cardiac output from cardiopulmonary bypass.[88]

Because amrinone does not act via β_1 receptors, it appears to be synergistic with β_1 agents in augmenting inotropy.[89] Gage et al reported that when amrinone was used in combination with dobutamine, cardiac output was significantly increased compared to dobutamine therapy alone.[90] A distinct advantage of the PDE inhibitors is that the beneficial hemodynamic effects of increased cardiac output, decreased LVEDP and decreased SVR are accomplished without any significant increase in either heart rate or myocardial oxygen consumption.[91] PDE inhibitors have also been shown to decrease pulmonary vascular resistance,[92] and, thus, offer unique advantages over other inotropes in effectively managing right ventricular dysfunction as well as biventricular dysfunction.

Milrinone has a positive inotropic action approximately 12–15 times that of amrinone. In limited studies, it has demonstrated favorable short-term effects both in the management of congestive heart failure and ventricular dysfunction after CPB.[93–95] Enoximone is an imidazolam PDE inhibitor derivative that is currently undergoing trials in patients with congestive heart failure, those awaiting cardiac transplantation, and following CPB.

Although catecholamines are administered as a starting infusion, amrinone, milrinone, and enoximone must be administered initially as a loading dose to obtain therapeutic levels, followed by an infusion if levels are to be maintained in a therapeutic range.[96] Administering a loading dose alone will provide an initial therapeutic concentration for 30 to 60 min for most of the PDE inhibitors. If further therapeutic benefits are to be achieved, infusions must be begun at recommended doses. Table 108–4 lists the initial loading dose and concomitant infusion rates. Since all PDE inhibitors produce dose-dependent vasodilation, they should be given over 5 to 10 min to attenuate the associated vasodilation.

ASSISTED CIRCULATION

Should all the steps described to enhance cardiac output and decrease metabolic demands prove to be insufficient in restoring adequate cardiovascular function, the use of mechanical devices is indicated. The aim of improving circulatory failure, while allowing the heart to recover and cardiac function to return, is predicated upon the concept that the myocardium is capable of recovery with time.

The use of the intra-aortic balloon pump (IABP) for diastolic blood pressure and coronary blood flow augmentation has been one of the most successful techniques for managing such patients. The indications in the majority of cases are low cardiac output states as evidenced by the need for large doses of inotropes and failure to wean from cardiopulmonary bypass. Other situations where IABP has been of proven benefit are for perioperative ischemia and for mechanical complications of myocardial infarction such as ventricular septal defect and acute mitral regurgitation. In a recent review from Washington University, 10% of patients undergoing cardiac surgical procedures required an

TABLE 108–4. LOADING AND INFUSION DOSES FOR THE PHOSPHODIESTERASE INHIBITORS

Drug	Loading Dose	Infusion (µg/kg per minute)
Amrinone	1.5–2.0 mg/kg[a]	5–10
Enoximone	0.5–1.0 mg/kg	5–10
Milrinone	50 µg/kg	0.375–0.75

[a]Manufacturer's package insert recommends a loading dose of 0.75 mg/kg.
Data from Levy.[96]

IABP during their hospital course[97]; 52% were inserted in the operating room, 36% preoperatively, and the remainder postoperatively. This trend of increased IABP usage in the perioperative period has been documented by others.[98] Further details regarding IABP as well as other modalities of postcardiotomy support such as extracorporeal membrane oxygenation and ventricular assist devices are covered in Chapter 111.

SEQUELAE OF INADEQUATE CARDIOVASCULAR FUNCTION

A prolonged period of inadequate cardiovascular function will lead to multiple organ and system failure. In the early phases, the patient compensates by redistribution of flow away from cutaneous and splanchnic regions to preserve cerebral, coronary, and renal perfusion. With prolongation of low cardiac output state, renal perfusion suffers, and eventually coronary and cerebral perfusion will also manifest deleterious effects. Bowel ischemia, hepatic failure, and renal failure are common complications in patients with cardiovascular dysfunction who eventually recover sufficient cardiac function to survive the initial episode of severely decreased cardiac output. In 5924 cardiac operations at the St. Louis University Medical Center from 1985 to 1991, the incidence of multiple organ failure (MOF) was 2.16%.[99] Thus, MOF is not a frequent occurrence. However, the mortality in this group of patients was 78%. Low cardiac output was the most common contributing factor in most of these patients. Lung problems, central nervous system depression, sepsis, and the kidneys also initiated MOF in some patients. Postoperative renal failure, discussed below, is a relatively frequent occurrence in postoperative cardiac surgical patients with low cardiac output.

POSTOPERATIVE ACUTE RENAL FAILURE

Acute renal failure is defined as a relatively sudden cessation of renal function, leading to life-threatening changes in fluid–electrolyte and acid–base balances and the retention of dangerous drugs and toxic products. In the patient with low cardiac output postoperatively, prerenal factors usually account for the development of acute renal failure. The (potentially fatal) effects of prerenal failure are usually quickly reversible if treated effectively.[100] However, postoperative acute renal failure continues to carry a poor prognosis, and a survey of reports published during the last two decades indicates an overall mortality of approximately 50%.[101–104] Acute renal failure after cardiac surgery is also associated with a mortality rate approximating 50%.[105] Survival is limited not only by the severity of the renal failure itself, but also by the number of comorbid factors and the age of the patient. In comparison to younger patients, elderly patients have more comorbid diseases and are at greater risk of developing acute renal failure as a consequence of ischemic or nephrotoxic insult.

Specific preoperative and intraoperative circumstances influence the postoperative course. For example, with preoperative congestive heart failure, the renal blood flow is reduced and in patients with rheumatic valvular disease or cyanotic cardiovascular disease, the effective renal plasma flow is diminished even before cardiac failure takes place. Intraoperatively, although acute hemodilution that accompanies CPB increases total renal flow, the combination of systemic cooling and nonpulsatile flow diminishes outer cortical perfusion.[106]

MANAGEMENT OF POSTOPERATIVE ACUTE RENAL FAILURE

The most effective treatment is avoidance of renal failure. Thus, perioperative preparation in the high-risk patient includes adequate hydration to promote intravascular repletion and diuresis.[107] Patients undergoing cardiac catherization prior to operation should also be adequately hydrated, and if there is elevation of blood urea nitrogen (BUN) and creatinine levels, surgery should be delayed if possible. If this is not possible, intraoperative strategies include infusion of dopamine (3 µg/kg per minute) as well as mannitol and furosemide to initiate diuresis.

Aggressive therapy is indicated for patients who develop postoperative renal dysfunction or renal failure. The use of furosemide and mannitol in maintaining urine output to prevent oliguric renal failure from becoming anuric renal failure has been advocated by Kron et al.[108] Baek et al[103] and subsequently others[104,109] have shown that the mortality rate is substantially lower in patients who were nonoliguric. However, the large urine volume in nonoliguric renal failure tends to be fixed and relatively unresponsive to variations in fluid intake, making the patient subject to the dangers of volume overload and contraction unless the fixed urinary output is recognized. Certain drugs such as digitalis that depend upon the kidney for excretion will require alteration in dosage in nonoliguric renal failure, just as in the oliguric form. Nonetheless, a greater urine volume makes fluid and electrolyte management easier. Among patients with nonoliguric renal failure, only 50% require dialysis.[110]

Sodium is not given in the early phases of acute renal failure unless there is severe hyponatremia or continuing loss of sodium. In the recovery phase, with increasing urinary flow, sodium may have to be given, and perhaps potassium if losses are large. In the oliguric phase of renal failure, however, the major threat is hyperkalemia, which may develop rapidly, particularly in the postoperative patient with increased catabolism and acidemia, which is a potential cause of death. Serum potassium approaching 6 mEq/L is rapidly but transiently reduced by giving glucose and insulin or calcium salts intravenously. More permanent control is obtained by such ion-exchange resins as kayexalate given orally, by enema, or by dialysis.

Specific attention to nutrition and metabolic factors is important since the most important complications of acute renal failure are related to the accumulation of unexcreted waste products from catabolism of body proteins and dietary amino acids. BUN and creatinine levels may rise rapidly in the postoperative cardiac patient with acute renal failure, particularly in the presence of multisystem disease. The general principles of nutritional support include adequate calories in a minimal volume of water to avoid fluid overload and hyponatremia and adequate daily protein of approximately 1 g/kg per day to achieve neutral nitrogen balance. However, patients requiring dialysis should be given 1.5 g/kg per day due to increased protein requirements related to the loss of nutrients into the dialysate.

With these conservative measures, the patients may be supported until renal function returns. However, dialysis is often necessary. The indications for dialysis are presence of cardiovascular fluid overload, hyperkalemia, severe acidemia, uremia with altered mental state, usually with a BUN rising to > 120 mg/dL or rising at a rate > 20 mg/dL per day. In patients whose prospects are good, dialysis may be started before the state of low cardiac output causing acute renal failure is eliminated, to avoid additional consequences of renal insufficiency. When BUN and creatinine levels rise to 80–90 and 5–6 mg/dL, respectively, and serum potassium exceeds 6 mEq/L in spite of conservative therapy, including ion-exchange resins, dialysis is instituted.

The three methods of dialysis include hemodialysis, peritoneal dialysis, and continuous arteriovenous hemofiltration. Utilization of peritoneal dialysis is limited in the setting of acute renal failure,[107] but is useful in children, patients with vascular access problems, or hemodynamic instability.[108] Intermittent hemodialysis is effective in correcting volume overload, hyperkalemia, and acid–base imbalances. However, because large volume removal occurs in a limited period of time, its applicability is limited to patients who are hemodynamically stable.

Continuous arteriovenous hemofiltration (CAVH) is a newer method of dialysis and is the most effective method of controlling urea.[111] It is thus ideal for patients with high catabolic rates. The major advantage of CAVH is its continuity, which eliminates the fluctuations associated with intermittent forms of dialysis. Thus, the risk of hemodynamic instability is reduced. A systolic blood pressure of 80 mm Hg is sufficient for adequate filtration that is achieved through the natural flow of blood from artery to vein via the continuous circuit.

Despite increased sophistication in nutritional therapy and dialysis, a significant impact on the mortality of patients with acute renal failure has not been realized. This is undoubtedly due, in part, to the impact of comorbid diseases in an increasingly complex cohort of patients currently undergoing cardiac surgery.

REFERENCES

1. Jones EL, Weintraub WS, Craver JM, et al: Coronary bypass surgery: Is the operation different today? *J Thorac Cardiovasc Surg* **101**:108, 1991
2. Naunheim KS, Fiore AC, Wadley JJ, et al: The changing profile of the patient undergoing coronary artery bypass surgery. *J Am Coll Cardiol* **11**:494, 1988
3. Magovern GJ: The role of the thoracic surgeon in the intensive care unit. *Ann Thorac Surg* **38**:309, 1984
4. Barash PG, May M, Geha AS, et al: Patient transport following open heart surgery: A necessary evil? *Anesth Anal* **60**:238, 1981
5. Wiedermann HP, Matthay MA, Matthay RA: Cardiovascular-pulmonary monitoring in the intensive care unit (Part 1). *Chest* **85**:537, 1984
6. Mohr R, Lavee J, Goor DA: Inaccuracy of radial artery pressure measurement after cardiac operations. *J Thorac Cardiovasc Surg* **94**:286, 1987
7. London, MJ, Hollenberg M, Wong MG, et al: Intraoperative myocardial ischemia: Localization by continuous 12 lead electrocardiography. *Anesthesiology* **69**:232, 1988
8. Waller JL, Kaplan JA, Bauman DI, et al: Clinical evaluation of a new fiberoptic catheter during cardiac surgery. *Anesth Analg* **61**:676, 1982
9. Stewart GN: Researches on the circulation time and on the influences which affect it. *J Physiol* **22**:159, 1897.
10. Stewart GN: The output of the heart in dogs. *Am J Physiol* **57**:27, 1921
11. Hamilton WF, Remington JW: Comparison of the time concentration curves in arterial blood of diffusible and nondiffusible substances when injected at a constant rate and when injected simultaneously. *Am J Physiol* **84**:25, 1929
12. Kinsman JM, Moore JW, Hamilton WF: Studies on the circulation: Injection method: Physical and mathematical considerations. *Am J Physiol* **89**:321, 1929
13. Swan H, Ganz W, Forester JS, et al: Catherization of the heart in man with the use of a flow-directed balloon-tip catheter. *N Engl J Med* **238**:447, 1970
14. Elefteriades JA, Geha AS, Cohen LS: *House Officer Guide to ICU Care: Fundamentals of Management of the Heart and Lungs.* New York, Raven Press, 1994
15. Karp R, Kouchoukos N: Postoperative care of the cardiovascular surgical patient. In Baue AE, Geha AS, Hammond GL, et al (eds): *Thoracic and Cardiovascular Surgery,* 5th ed. Norwalk, CT, Appleton & Lange, 1991, pp 1535–1545
16. Hendren WG, Higgins TL: Immediate postoperative care of the cardiac surgical patient. *Sem Thorac Cardiovasc Surg* **3**:3, 1991
17. Sharkey A, Lipton JM, Murphy MT, et al: Inhibition of postanesthetic shivering with radiant heat. *Anesthesiology* **66**:249:1987
18. Guffin A, Girard D, Kaplan JA: Shivering following cardiac surgery: Hemodynamic changes and reversal. *J Cardiothorac Anesth* **1**:24, 1987
19. Kirklin JK, Lell WA, Kouchoukos NT: Hydroxyethyl starch versus albumin for colloid infusion following cardiopulmonary bypass in patients undergoing myocardial revascularization. *Ann Thorac Surg* **37**:40, 1984
20. Estafanous FG, Tarazi RC, Viljoen SF, et al: Systemic hypertension following myocardial revascularization. *Am Heart J* **85**:732, 1973
21. Viljoen SF, Estafanous FG, Tarazi RC: Acute hypertension immediately after coronary artery surgery. *J Thorac Cardiovasc Surg* **71**:548, 1976
22. Roberts AJ, Niarchos AP, Subramanian VA, et al: Systemic hypertension associated with coronary artery bypass surgery: Predisposing factors, hemodynamic characteristics, humoral profile, and treatment. *J Thorac Cardiovasc Surg* **74**:846, 1977
23. Kim YD, Jones M, Hanowell ST, et al: Changes in peripheral vascu-

lar and cardiac sympathetic activity before and after coronary artery bypass surgery: Interrelationships with hemodynamic alteration. *Am Heart J* **102**:972, 1981

24. Weinstein GS, Zabetakis PM, Clavel A, et al: The renin-angiotension system is not responsible for hypertension following coronary artery bypass grafting. *Ann Thorac Surg* **43**:74, 1987

25. Taylor KM, Morton IJ, Brown JJ, et al: Hypertension and the renin-angiotensin system following open-heart surgery. *J Thorac Cardiovasc Surg* **74**:840, 1977

26. Fremes SE, Weisel RD, Mickle DAG, et al: A comparison of nitroglycerin and nitroprusside. I. Treatment of postoperative hypertension. *Ann Thorac Surg* **39**:53, 1985

27. Fanning WJ, Thomas CS, Roach A, et al: Prophylaxis of atrial fibrillation with magnesium sulfate after coronary artery bypass grafting. *Ann Thorac Surg* **52**:529, 1991

28. England MR, Gordon G, Salem M, et al: Magnesium administration and dysrhythmias after cardiac surgery. A placebo-controlled, double-blind randomized trial. *JAMA* **268**:2395, 1992

29. Wolff G, Brunner JX, Ing DE, et al: Gas exchange during mechanical ventilation and spontaneous breathing: Intermittent mandatory ventilation after open heart surgery. *Chest* **90**:11, 1986

30. Lemaire F, Teboul J-L, Cinotti L, et al: Acute left ventricular dysfunction during unsuccessful weaning from mechanical ventilation. *Anesthesiology* **69**:171, 1988

31. Hurford WE, Lynch KE, Strauss W, et al: Myocardial perfusion as assessed by thallium-201 scintigraphy during the discontinuation of mechanical ventilation in ventilator-dependent patients. *Anesthesiology* **74**:1007, 1991

32. Higgins T: Pro: Early endotracheal extubation is preferable to late extubation in patients following coronary artery surgery. *J Cardiothorac Vasc Anesth* **6**:448, 1992

33. Gall SA, Olsen CO, Reves JG, et al: Beneficial effects of endotracheal extubation on ventilator performance. Implications for early extubation after cardiac operations. *J Thorac Cardiovasc Surg* **95**:819, 1988

34. Prakash O, Johnson B, Meij S, et al: Criteria for early extubation after intracardiac surgery in adults. *Anesth Analg* **48**:703, 1977

35. Quasha AL, Loeber N, Feeley TW, et al: Postoperative respiratory care: A controlled trial of early and late extubation following coronary artery bypass grafting. *Anesthesiology* **52**:135, 1980

36. Klineberg PL, Geer RI, Hirsh RA, et al: Early extubation after coronary artery bypass graft surgery. *Crit Care Med* **5**:272, 1977

37. Lichenthal PR, Wade LD, Niemyski PR, et al: Respiratory management after cardiac surgery with inhalation anesthesia. *Crit Care Med* **11**:603, 1983

38. Smith RC, Leung JM, Mangano DT, et al: Postoperative myocardial ischemia in patients undergoing coronary artery bypass graft surgery. *Anesthesiology* **74**:464, 1991

39. Siliciano D: Con: Early extubation is not preferable to late extubation in patients undergoing coronary artery surgery. *J Cardiothorac Vasc Anesth* **6**:494, 1992

40. Mangano DT, Siliciano D, Hollenberg M, et al: Postoperative myocardial ischemia: Effect on an intensive analgesic infusion. *Anesthesiology* **76**:342, 1992

41. Chong JL, Grebneik C, Sinclair M, et al: The effect of a cardiac surgical recovery area on the timing of extubation. *J Cardiothorac Vasc Anesth* **7**:137, 1993

42. Roekaerts P, Huygen F, DeLange S: Infusion of propofol versus midazolam for sedation in the ICU following coronary artery surgery. *J Cardiothorac Vasc Anesth* **7**:142, 1993

43. Matthay MA, Wiener-Kronish JP: Respiratory management after cardiac surgery. *Chest* **95**:424, 1989

44. Hurlbut D, Myers ML, Lefcoe M, et al: Pleuropulmonary morbidity: Internal thoracic artery versus saphenous vein graft. *Ann Thorac Surg* **50**:959, 1990

45. Shapira N, Zabatino SM, Ahmed S, et al: Determinants of pulmonary function in patients undergoing coronary bypass operations. *Ann Thorac Surg* **50**:268, 1990

46. Berrizbeitia LD, Tessler S, Jacobwitz IJ, et al: Effect of sternotomy and coronary bypass surgery on postoperative pulmonary mechanics. Comparison of internal mammary and saphenous vein bypass grafts. *Chest* **96**:873, 1989

47. Society of Thoracic Surgeons: *Data Analyses of the Society of Thoracic Surgeons National Cardiac Surgery Database: The Third Year—January 1994.* Minneapolis, MN, Summit Medical System, 1994

48. Rodriguez JL, Steinberg LM, Luchette FA, et al: Early tracheostomy for primary airway management in the surgical critical care setting. *Surgery* **108**:655, 1990

49. Ferguson TB Jr, Cox JL: Temporary external DDD pacing after cardiac operations. *Ann Thorac Surg* **51**:723, 1991

50. Creswell LL, Schuessler RB, Rosenbloom M, et al: Hazards of postoperative atrial bibrillation. *Ann Thorac Surg* **56**:539, 1993

51. Batsford WP: Arrhythmia complications following cardiac surgery. In Baue AE (ed): *Thoracic and Cardiovascular Surgery,* 5th ed. Norwalk CT, Appleton & Lange, 1991, pp 1837–1841

52. Waldo AL, MacLean WAH, Cooper TB, et al: Use of temporarily placed epicardial atrial wire electrodes for the diagnosis and treatment of cardiac arrhythmias following open-heart surgery. *J Thorac Cardiovasc Surg* **76**:500, 1978

53. Fuller JA, Adams GG, Burton B: Atrial fibrillation after coronary artery bypass grafting: Is it a disorder of the elderly? *J Thorac Cardiovasc Surg* **97**:821, 1989

54. Leitch JW, Thomson D, Baird DK, et al: The importance of age as a predictor of atrial fibrillation and flutter after coronary artery bypass grafting. *J Thorac Cardiovasc Surg* **100**:338, 1990

55. Caretta Q, Mercanti CA, Denardo D, et al: Ventricular conduction defects and atrial fibrillation after coronary artery bypass grafting. Multivariate analysis of preoperative, intraoperative and postoperative variables. *Eur Heart J* **12**:1107, 1991

56. Omerund OJM, McGregor CGA, Stone DL, et al: Arrhythmias after coronary bypass surgery. *Br Heart J* **51**:618, 1984

57. Smith PK, Buhrman WC, Levett JM, et al: Supraventricular conduction abnormalities following cardiac operations: A complication of inadequate atrial preservation. *J Thorac Cardiovasc Surg* **85**:105, 1983

58. Tchervenkov CI, Wynands JE, Symes JF, et al: Persistent atrial activity during cardioplegic arrest: A possible factor in the etiology of postoperative supraventricular tachyarrhythmias. *Ann Thorac Surg* **36**:437, 1983

59. Michelson EL, Morgonroth J, MacVaugh H: Postoperative arrhythmias after coronary artery and cardiac valvular surgery detected by long-term electrocardiographic monitoring. *Am Heart J* **97**:442, 1979

60. Waldo AL, MacLean WAH, Karp RB, et al: Entrainment and interruption of atrial flutter with atrial pacing. *Circulation* **56**:737, 1977

61. Wafa SS, Ward DE, Parker J, et al: Efficacy of flecainide acetate for atrial arrhythmias following coronary artery bypass grafting. *Am J Cardiol* **63**:1058, 1989

62. Blanconi L, Boccadamo R, Pappalardo A, et al: Effectiveness of intravenous propafenone for conversion of atrial fibrillation and flutter of recent origin. *Am J Cardiol* **64**:335, 1989

63. Abiden Z, Soares J, Phillips DF, et al: Ventricular tachyarrhythmias following surgery for myocardial revascularization. A follow-up study. *Chest* **72**:426, 1977

64. CAST Investigators: Preliminary report: Effect of Encainide and Flecainide on mortality in a randomized trial of arrhythmia suppression after myocardial infarction. *N Engl J Med* **321**:406, 1989

65. Morganroth J, Panidis IP, Harley S, et al: Efficacy and safety of intravenous tocainide compared with intravenous lidocaine for acute ventricular arrhythmias immediately after cardiac surgery. *Am J Cardiol* **54**:1253, 1984

66. Installe E, Schoevaerdts JC, Gadisseux PH, et al: Intravenous amio-

darone in the treatment of various arrhythmias following cardiac operations. *J Thorac Cardiovasc Surg* **81**:302, 1981

67. Forrester JS, Diamond G, McHugh TJ, et al: Filling pressures in the right and left sides of the heart in acute myocardial infarction. *N Engl J Med* **285**:190, 1971

68. O'Quin R, Marini JJ: Pulmonary artery occlusion pressure: Clinical physiology, measurement, and interpretation. *Am Rev Respir Dis* **128**:319, 1983

69. Utley JR, Michalsky GB, Bryant LR, et al: Determinants of myocardial water content during cardiopulmonary bypass. *J Thorac Cardiovasc Surg* **68**:8, 1974

70. Foglia RP, Steed DL, Follette DM, et al: Iatrogenic myocardial edema with potassium cardioplegia. *J Thorac Cardiovasc Surg* **78**:217, 1979

71. Borkon AM, Schaff HV, Gardner TJ, et al: Diagnosis and management of postoperative pericardial effusions and late cardiac tamponade following open-heart surgery. *Ann Thorac Surg* **31**:512, 1981

72. Fairman RM, Edmunds LH: Emergency thoracotomy in the surgical intensive unit after open cardiac operation. *Ann Thorac Surg* **32**:386, 1981

73. Kaiser GC, Naunheim KS, Fiore AC, et al: Reoperation in the intensive care unit. *Ann Thorac Surg* **49**:903, 1990

74. Franciosa JB, Guiha NM, Limas CJ, et al: Improved left ventricular function during nitroprusside infusion in acute myocardial infarction. *Lancet* **1**:650, 1972

75. Chatterjee K, Parmley WW, Ganz W, et al: Hemodynamic and metabolic responses to vasodilator therapy in acute myocardial infarction. *Circulation* **48**:1182, 1973

76. Chatterjee K, Parmley WW, Swan HJC, et al: Beneficial effects of vasodilator agents in severe mitral regurgitation due to dysfunction of subvalvular apparatus. *Circulation* **48**:684, 1973

77. Cohn JN, Franciosa J: Vasodilator therapy of cardiac failure, Part 1. *N Engl J Med* **297**:27, 1977

78. Krukenkamp IB, Silverman NA, Pridjian A, et al: Correlation between the linearized Frank-Starling relationship and myocardial energetics in the failing heart. *J Thorac Cardiovasc Surg* **93**:728, 1987

79. Zelis R, Brunner H, Zelis K, et al: Vascular sympathetic nerve function in congestive heart failure. *Am J Cardiol* **62**:63E, 1987

80. Ross J: Afterload mismatch and preload reserve: A conceptual framework for the analysis of ventricular function. *Prog Cardiovasc Dis* **18**:255, 1976

81. Miller DC, Stinson EB, Oyer PE, et al: Postoperative enhancement of left ventricular performance by combined inotropic-vasodilator therapy with preload control. *Surgery* **1980**:108, 1980

82. Fowler MB, Alderman EL, Oesterle SN: Dobutamine and dopamine after cardiac surgery: Greater augmentation of myocardial blood flow with dobutamine. *Circulation* **70** (Supp 1):105, 1984

83. Van Trigt P, Spray TL, Pasque MK, et al: The comparative effects of dopamine and dobutamine on ventricular mechanics after coronary artery bypass grafting: A pressure-dimension analysis. *Circulation* **70** (Supp 1):112, 1984

84. Benori JR, McCue JE, Alpert JS: Comparative vasoactive therapy for heart failure. *Am J Cardiol* **56**:19B, 1985

85. LeJemtel TH, Keunge E, Sonnenblick EH, et al: Amrinone: A new non-adrenergic cardiotonic agent effective in the treatment of intractable myocardial failure in man. *Circulation* **59**:1098, 1979

86. Benotti J, Grossman W, Braunwald E, et al: Hemodynamic assessment of amrinone: A new vasoactive agent. *N Engl J Med* **299**:1373, 1978

87. Benotti J, Grossman W, Braunwald E, et al: Effects of amrinone on hemodynamic and myocardial metabolism in patients with congestive heart failure from ischemic heart disease. *Circulation* **62**:28, 1980

88. Goenen M, Pedemonte O, Baele PH, et al: Amrinone in the manage-

89. Royster R, Butterworth J, Prielipp R, et al: Combined inotropic effects of amrinone and epinephrine after cardiopulmonary bypass in humans. *Anesth Analg* **77**:662, 1993

90. Gage J, Rutman H, Lucido D, et al: Additive effects of dobutamine and amrinone on myocardial contractility and ventricular performance in patients with severe heart failure. *Circulation* **74**:367, 1986

91. Hines R: Clinical applications of amrinone. *J Cardiothorac Anesth* **3**:24, 1989

92. Hess W, Arnold B, Viet S: The hemodynamic effects of amrinone in patients with mitral stenosis and pulmonary hypertension. *Eur Heart J* **7**:800, 1986

93. Feneck RO: The European Milrinone Multicentre Trial Group: Intravenous milrinone following cardiac surgery: I. Effects of bolus infusion followed by variable dose maintenance infusion. *J Cardiothorac Vasc Anesth* **6**:554, 1992

94. Feneck RO: The European Milrinone Multicentre Trial Group: Intravenous milrinone following cardiac surgery: II. Influence of baseline hemodynamics and patient factors on therapeutic response. *J Cardiothorac Vasc Anesth* **6**:563, 1992

95. Monrad ES, Baim DS, Smith HS, et al: Effects of milrinone on coronary hemodynamics and myocardial energetics in patients with congestive heart failure. *Circulation* **71**:972, 1985

96. Levy JH: Support of the perioperative failing heart with preexisting ventricular dysfunction: Currently available options. *J Cardiothorac Vasc Anesth* **7**:46, 1993

97. Creswell LL, Rosenbloom M, Cox JL, et al: Intraaortic balloon counterpulsation: Patterns of usage and outcome in cardiac surgery patients. *Ann Thorac Surg* **54**:11, 1992

98. Pennington DG, Swartz M, Codd JE, et al: Intraaortic balloon pumping in cardiac surgical patients: A nine-year experience. *Ann Thorac Surg* **36**:125, 1983

99. Baue AE: The role of the gut on the development of multiple organ dysfunction in cardiothoracic patients. *Ann Thorac Surg* **55**:822–829, 1993

100. Geha AS: Acute renal failure in cardiovascular and other surgical patients. *Surg Clin N Am* **60**:1151, 1980

101. Hall JW, Johnson WJ, Maher FT, et al: Immediate and long-term prognosis in acute renal failure. *Ann Intern Med* **73**:515, 1970

102. Merino GE, Buselmeier TJ, Kjellstrand CM: Postoperative chronic renal falire: A new syndrome? *Ann Surg* **182**:37, 1975

103. Baek SM, Makabali GG, Shoemaker WC: Clinical determinants of survival from postoperative renal failure. *Surgery* **140**:685, 1975

104. Rasmussen H, Ibels LS: Acute renal failure: Multivariate analysis of causes and risk factors. *Am J Med* **73**:211, 1982

105. Lange HW, Aeppli DM, Brown DC: Survival of patients with acute renal failure requiring dialysis after open heart surgery: Early prognostic indicators. *Am Heart J* **113**:1138, 1987

106. Utley JR, Rodd EP, Wachtell CC, et al: Effects of hypothermia, hemodilution and pump oxygenation on organ water content and blood flow. *Surg For* **27**:217, 1976

107. Paganini EP, Bosworth CR: Acute renal failure after open heart surgery: Newer concepts and current therapy. *Sem Thorac Cardiovasc Surg* **3**:63, 1991

108. Kron IL, Joob AW, Van Meeter C: Acute renal failure in the cardiovascular surgical patient. *Ann Thorac Surg* **39**:590, 1985

109. Bullock ML, Umen AJ, Finkelstein M, et al: The assessment of risk factors in 462 patients with acute renal failure. *Am J Kidney Dis* **5**:97, 1985

110. Schrier RW: Acute renal failure. *JAMA* **247**:2518, 1982

111. Stokke T, Kramu P, Schrader J, et al: Continuous arteriovenous hemofiltration. *Anesthesiology* **31**:579, 1982

Hemorrhagic and Thrombotic Complications of Cardiac Surgery

Michael Sobel and Cornelius M. Dyke

Cardiopulmonary bypass presents one of the greatest hemostatic challenges the cardiovascular surgeon will encounter. Profound anticoagulation with heparin is required to prevent pathologic clotting in response to the intense prothrombotic stimuli encountered in the extracorporeal circuits and oxygenator. At the conclusion of surgery, hemostatic mechanisms must be normalized very rapidly, to ensure safe and hemostatic closure of the chest. Success depends on a surgeon's ability to establish normal hemostatic mechanisms before surgery, to accurately control the effects of anticoagulants, and to diagnose and treat the hemostatic disorders that may arise during and after surgery. This chapter will review the fundamental effects of cardiopulmonary bypass on blood clotting mechanisms, and identify the clinical and pharmacologic factors influencing hemostasis. A framework of knowledge is provided for analyzing and treating hemorrhagic complications after open heart surgery. Finally, the indications and applications for chronic antithrombotic therapy are reviewed for arterial vascular grafts and heart valves.

A BRIEF HISTORY OF HEMOSTASIS AND CARDIAC SURGERY

The earliest animal experiments in extracorporeal oxygenation utilized cross-circulation of blood through the lungs of another animal. Gibbon's[1] first successful application of total cardiopulmonary bypass for open heart surgery in humans took place in 1953. In his screen oxygenator, the obligatory exposure to a large foreign surface and gas pro-

voked a myriad of changes in the blood that are still being investigated. The early disc, screen, and bubble oxygenators were traumatic to blood, and their use led to hemolysis, thrombocytopenia, and denaturation of plasma proteins. All patients suffered an incompletely understood bleeding diathesis after open-heart surgery; major hemorrhage was not uncommon, and the bleeding tendency often correlated poorly with the results of laboratory studies of hemostasis. Since those times, there has been significant progress in understanding the basic biology of vascular cells and blood proteins, and progress in the engineering and technical design of surfaces and devices that contact the blood.[2,3] New methods can now measure the responses of specific platelet receptors, the activities of individual fibrinolytic enzymes and inhibitors, and the interplay between plasma and cellular mediators of inflammation and coagulation can be assessed. But it is still clear that no single model can account for all cases of postbypass hemorrhage. These patients often develop a complex and heterogeneous hemostatic defect involving both platelet dysfunction and plasma coagulation, compounded by fibrinolysis and by the effects of heparin and protamine.

COMMON PREOPERATIVE HEMOSTATIC DISORDERS, THEIR DIAGNOSIS AND TREATMENT

The preoperative hemostatic assessment of a patient for cardiac surgery should raise three questions: (1) What, if any, are the pre-existing abnormalities? (2) What corrections need to be made? and (3) What special postoperative requirements for blood or blood products might be anticipated? A careful personal and family history and physical examination are the most important tools for detecting a bleeding diathesis. Laboratory assistance is required to rule out milder defects in plasma coagulation or thrombocytopenia, and to identify hemostatic disorders suspected from the history. Table 109–1 describes the basic tests that should be done preoperatively, along with common causes for abnormalities. Patients with pre-existing abnormalities of hemostasis will most often have either an inherited disorder of coagulation or an acquired platelet disorder stemming from their cardiac lesion or, more commonly, from drugs.

Hereditary Bleeding Disorders

Hereditary disorders of coagulation usually are caused by a deficiency of a single factor. The classic hemophilias A and B are due to deficits of Factors VIII and IX, respectively.[4] They are X-linked recessive disorders, and can exist in mild forms without manifestations of abnormal bleeding except after such major hemostatic challenges as surgery. Factor XI deficiency is usually a less severe disorder. In these syndromes, the activated partial thromboplastin time (aPTT) is prolonged, the prothrombin time (PT) usually normal, and platelet function and the bleeding time are normal. von Willebrand's Factor stabilizes Factor VIII, and is critical for normal platelet function. von Willebrand's disease is the most common inherited bleeding disorder, manifested by mucocutaneous bleeding and bruising, by a prolonged bleeding time, impaired platelet aggregation to ristocetin, and frequently a prolonged aPTT. Major surgery can be performed safely in patients with all of these disorders, provided that they are correctly identified in advance and that there is selective replacement of the necessary blood components. For hemophiliacs, individual factor assays can identify the specific deficiency. In the case of von Willebrand's disease, there are a number of variants that must be differentiated by specialized studies, to ensure the correct

therapy. Currently, Factor VIII concentrates are recommended for hemophilia A, and prothrombin complex or Factor IX concentrates for hemophilia B.[5,6] Treatment with fresh frozen plasma (or cryoprecipitate for Factor VIII or von Willebrand deficiency) is acceptable during emergency hemorrhage. For a more detailed discussion of the diagnosis and preoperative correction of these disorders, the reader is referred to several reviews.[7,8] Rarely, nonhemophiliacs may acquire autoantibodies to Factor VIII, presenting with a picture of "acquired hemophilia." Except for its association with pregnancy, this syndrome usually is a disease of the elderly with a systemic autoimmune disorder, malignancy, or infection.[9]

Acquired Bleeding Disorders

Platelet Dysfunction Caused by Abnormal Heart Valves or Assist Devices

As platelets flow turbulently past a diseased heart valve or intra-aortic balloon pump, the chronic activation and stimulation can consume platelets and impair the function of the remaining cells.[10] This dysfunction may be aggravated by the administration of platelet-inhibiting drugs. The bleeding time is an important preoperative screening test in this group of patients. If there is thrombocytopenia (less than 100,000 platelets/μl) due to consumption, platelet transfusions will only be transiently effective until the circulatory problem is corrected. Platelet transfusions are most effective after the conclusion of cardiopulmonary bypass, once the source of chronic platelet activation has been corrected.

Congenital Cyanotic Heart Disease

Children with congenital heart disease often have bleeding difficulties. Maurer et al[11] found impairment of platelet aggregation in 14% of children with acyanotic lesions and in 38% of those with cyanosis. The severity of thrombocytopenia, shortened platelet survival, and platelet dysfunction seems to be related to the degree of arterial hypoxemia

TABLE 109–1. ROUTINE HEMOSTATIC STUDIES FOR CARDIOPULMONARY BYPASS

Test	Evaluates	Normal Range	Common Causes for Abnormality
Platelet count	Platelet number	150,000–400,000 per mm³	Drugs Recent viral infection Primary hematologic disorders
Bleeding time	In vivo platelet function	4–8 min	Aspirin, indomethacin Valvular or cyanotic congenital heart disease Intra-aortic balloon pumping Uremia Thrombopathia

Prothrombin time	Factors X, VII, V, II (prothrombin), fibrinogen	No more than 3 seconds above control	Prolonged by
			  Warfarin
			  Hepatic dysfunction
			  Isolated factor deficiencies

Partial thromboplastin time	Factors VIII, IX, XI primarily; also X, II, V, fibrinogen	No more than 3–5 seconds above control	Prolonged by
			  Heparin
			  Factor deficiencies

and hemoconcentration.[12–14] With more profound hypoxemia, the hepatic synthesis of clotting factors may be depressed,[15] while the compensatory hemoconcentration leads to a relative plasma deficiency and impaired clot formation. Recent studies suggest that platelet receptors for von Willebrand factor may be diminished in cyanotic patients.[16] Preoperative phlebotomy and hemodilution to a hematocrit of 50 to 60% increase both platelet number and function and improve hemostasis in these children.[17] It is necessary to distinguish true abnormalities of coagulation from artifactual elevation of the prothrombin or partial thromboplastin times. When the patient is hemoconcentrated, the volume of anticoagulant in a blood sample should be reduced in proportion to the contraction of the plasma volume.

The Effects of Drugs

The most common cause for impaired hemostasis before cardiac surgery is drug ingestion. Table 109–2 details the effects of drugs frequently used by cardiac patients. It is rarely possible to withdraw all drugs that may affect hemostasis. Many of the medications have only mild, subclinical effects. Ongoing drug treatment up until the time of surgery may be essential, or surgery may be emergent. The following discussion focuses primarily on the challenging patient with a major drug-induced hemostatic defect who may be especially prone to bleeding.

Anticoagulants. When therapeutic anticoagulation cannot be suspended before surgery, several strategies using heparin or warfarin can be used. If the patient is on warfarin, it can be withheld for 1 to 2 days, while still preserving some modicum of residual anticoagulation.[18] During the operation, parenteral vitamin K and/or fresh frozen plasma can be given to correct the vitamin K deficiency-like state induced by warfarin. Heparin and protamine can then be administered during and after bypass, per routine. In emergencies, patients receiving intravenous heparin can be maintained on the infusion preoperatively. Heparin responses during bypass may be different in those receiving heparin preoperatively, so the effects of heparin and protamine administration should be monitored during surgery.

Drugs That Affect Platelets. An enormous number of drugs can impair platelet function.[19] Table 109–2 summarizes the major drug groups and their effects. If possible, aspirin should be discontinued 5–7 days preoperatively, because its use is associated with increased postoperative blood loss.[20] When the platelet count is normal, but impairment of function by aspirin is a concern, the bleeding time is helpful. If the bleeding time is prolonged by drug ingestion, 8 to 12 units of fresh platelets can usually correct the deficit, provided there is no active aspirin in the circulation. If the bleeding time is normal despite a history of aspirin ingestion, it is probably safe to proceed with operation, since the aspirin effect is then modest at most. The need for platelet transfusions postoperatively should be anticipated when the bleeding time is prolonged, especially when compounded by procedures prone to produce excessive destruction of platelets.

A number of cardiac drugs and antibiotics can cause thrombocytopenia. For idiosyncratic drug reactions (e.g., quinidine), discontinuation of the drug usually results in prompt recovery of the platelet count. A more dangerous type of immune-mediated platelet destruction can develop after exposure to heparin. Heparin-induced thrombocytopenia may affect up to 5% of patients who receive repeated exposures to heparin,[21] and is discussed later in this chapter.

Fibrinolytic Drugs. Tissue-type plasminogen activator (tPA), urokinase, and streptokinase all generate the endogenous fibrinolytic enzyme, plasmin.[18,22] Excessive fibrinolysis can reduce plasma fibrinogen to below safe levels (100 mg/dL), and the resulting fibrin(ogen) degradation products can interfere with platelet function and the coagulation cascade. This hemorrhagic state can be compounded by the coadministration of heparin. The effects of fibrinolytic

TABLE 109–2. ALTERATIONS OF HEMOSTASIS BY COMMON DRUGS

Drug	Mode of Action	Duration	Severity of Effect
Warfarin	Inhibits synthesis of Factors II, VII, IX, XI	5–7 days	Major
Heparin	Inhibition of clotting factor activation; immune thrombocytopenia	4–6 hr 2–4 days	Major variable
Aspirin	Block platelet secretion, aggregation	5–7 days	Major
Ticlopidine	Unknown	5–7 days	Major
Nonsteroidal anti-inflammatory drugs	Block platelet secretion, aggregation	1–2 days	Moderate
Dipyridamole	Inhibition of platelet aggregation	1–2 days	Mild
Dextran hydroxyethyl starch	Impair platelet adhesion, aggregation	3–5 days	Moderate
Ca^{2+} channel blockers	Inhibition of platelet aggregation (in large doses)	1 day	Mild
Vasodilators	Inhibition of platelet aggregation	Short	Mild
Quinidine	Immune thrombocytopenia	2–4 days	Variable
Various antibiotics	Inhibition of platelet aggregation	Few days	Variable

drugs are short lived. Systemic fibrinolytic activity, and its secondary effects will diminish within hours of stopping the drug. In severe hemorrhage, heparin should be stopped and cryoprecipitate administered if the plasma fibrinogen is low. Antagonists to heparin and fibrinolytic agents (protamine and ε-aminocaproic acid) can be given, but carry the risks of thrombosis.

Renal, Hepatic Failure, and Disseminated Intravenous Coagulation (DIC)

The bleeding tendency of uremia is primarily a defect in platelet function, due to the anemia of renal failure, and the accumulation of plasma factors not cleared by the kidney.[23,24] von Willebrand factor–platelet interactions and platelet metabolism are impaired.[25,26] Platelet transfusions are ineffective, because the problem is associated with the uremic plasma. Preoperatively, patients with renal failure should have their anemia corrected, and undergo thorough dialysis when indicated. Increasing the plasma levels of von Willebrand factor, by transfusion of cryoprecipitate or administration of desmopressin acetate (DDAVP, see below), can improve hemostasis in uremic patients.[27,28]

Major liver dysfunction presents a mixed picture of factor deficiency and DIC.[29] Synthesis of clotting factors is impaired (especially the vitamin K-dependent Factors II, VII, IX, and X). Fibrinogen and platelets may be low due to accelerated consumption, while there may be elevated products of fibrinolysis due to impaired clearance. If the PT is prolonged, parenteral vitamin K (10 mg) should be given preoperatively. If the PT does not normalize, or the aPTT or platelet count is abnormal, a more detailed hemostatic workup for DIC and pathologic fibrinolysis should be pursued. Preoperative infusions of fresh frozen plasma and platelets are indicated to restore the PT and platelet count to as normal as possible.

Bona fide DIC may develop in the patient with septic endocarditis, mediastinitis, or disseminated cancer. Elevated levels of fibrin degradation products, thrombocytopenia, and prolongation of both the PT and aPTT are typical. Treatment should be aimed at correcting the stimulus to clotting, if possible. Replacement therapy with fresh frozen plasma and platelets should be guided by laboratory values. Antithrombin III concentrates are now available, and may be useful.[30] Chronic or acute dissections or aneurysms of the aorta may induce a consumptive coagulopathy.[31,32]

EFFECTS OF CARDIOPULMONARY BYPASS ON HEMOSTASIS

Initial Events of Blood–Surface Interactions

The interactions of foreign surfaces and gases with the blood have been reviewed in detail elsewhere.[3,33–35] The adsorption of fibrinogen and other plasma proteins to the foreign surface is the initial event preceding the arrival of blood cells. Plasma coagulation may be induced by contact activation of Factor XII, and platelets adhere to the surface by a mechanism still not well characterized. They are stimulated to secrete the contents of their cytoplasmic granules, including platelet-specific proteins such as β-thromboglobulin and platelet Factor 4. There is also activation of prostaglandin synthetic pathways and generation of thromboxane A_2,[36] a potent vasoconstrictor. Subtle interactions between platelets and coagulation proteins result in the further stimulation and activation of both, to the extent permitted by the ever-present heparin.

Contact activation of the blood initiates the complement cascade and the kallikrein/kinin system.[37–39] This results in the activation of a broad range of proteases and inflammatory mediators. Various elements in the pump–oxygenator circuit contribute in different degrees to the stimulation and derangement of hemostatic processes. The reduced viscosity from hemodilution may actually reduce damage to the formed elements of the blood, decrease net blood loss, and improve capillary perfusion. Skillful engineering that ensures the streamlined flow of blood is extremely important in extracorporeal circuits. Stasis promotes the accumulation of activated procoagulant factors and platelet aggregates, as, for example, in the underperfused corners of an extracorporeal reservoir or in the headers of membrane oxygenators. Frothing, high shear rates, and turbulence in the pump and circuits are destructive of the formed elements of the blood, resulting in hemolysis and platelet activation. Membrane oxygenators offer a theoretical advantage by eliminating the direct blood–gas interface that occurs with a bubble oxygenator. Only when the total bypass time exceeds 2 to 3 hours does the constantly self-renewing air–blood interface in a bubble oxygenator become a major factor contributing to impaired hemostasis. Intracardiac suction devices are a major source of blood damage during open-heart surgery.[40] Blood recirculated from the operative field into the oxygenator is exposed to air and is often mixed with thromboplastic tissue juices, fat, and bone fragments from the sternotomy. Limitation of suction to the aspiration of pools of blood in the pericardium and chambers of the heart and the avoidance of frothing will reduce platelet destruction and the activation of coagulation.

Dynamics of Plasma Coagulation During Cardiopulmonary Bypass

Deficiencies of plasma coagulation proteins seldom contribute to the bleeding diathesis encountered after cardiopulmonary bypass. Detailed studies[41–43] have shown that (1) significant amounts of clotting proteins are not usually lost in the extracorporeal circuit, (2) although often diluted by the pump prime to concentrations of 50% of normal or less, clotting factor levels remain well above the minimum necessary for normal hemostasis, and (3) the occurrence of prolonged clotting times after operation correlates poorly with excessive postoperative bleeding. Perhaps the only exception to these generalizations is the profound hemodilution experienced by neonates during cardiopulmonary bypass—clotting factors can indeed be diluted below hemostatic levels.[44]

If adequate concentrations of clotting factors are usually present, what explains the derangements of clotting tests (and bleeding) in the early postoperative period? Excessive fibrinolysis may be one major factor. Activated plasmin degrades fibrinogen and fibrin. These fibrin(ogen) degradation products (FDP) act as anticoagulants by inhibiting platelet aggregations, and interfering with the coagulation cascade and fibrin polymerization. Even though absolute plasminogen concentrations are diluted during bypass, fibrinolytic activity increases. The concentrations of fibrin(ogen) degradation products (FDP) are often mildly elevated after open heart surgery (see Table 109–3); more sensitive biochemical markers for fibrinolysis confirm this.[45,46] This fibrinolysis is not associated with excessive bleeding in most cases, although recent trials using inhibitors of fibrinolysis suggest that suppression of fibrinolysis may reduce blood loss (see subsequent discussion of aprotinin). If there is inadequate anticoagulation during extracorporeal circulation, intravascular coagulation, and pathologic fibrinolysis may also occur.

Platelet Dynamics During Bypass

Abnormalities of platelet function remain a critical problem in cardiopulmonary bypass. Many aspects of the procedure adversely affect platelet function and number, most notably the extracorporeal circuits and oxygenator.[47–49] Hypothermia, heparin, and other drugs may also have an effect.

Platelet Number
During uneventful cardiopulmonary bypass, the platelet count usually falls to 40 to 50% of its baseline value within the first 10 to 15 min. This initial drop in platelet count is mainly attributable to dilution of the blood with the non-blood priming solution. The red cell mass and clotting factors are similarly diluted. The platelet count then stabilizes, pursuing a much slower decline or even a slight recovery toward the end of the bypass procedure. The count never falls to zero and rarely falls below 75,000/μL. Two contributory processes may be at work to produce these effects: the "passivation" of foreign surfaces after their initial exposure to blood, and reduced platelet adhesiveness, either because of loss of the more reactive members of the platelet population or development of a defect in all the platelets. The platelet count does not return to normal for 3 to 5 days after bypass, although the intraoperative hemodilution is corrected earlier. Temporary sequestration of platelets in the liver may play a role in this apparent loss of platelets.[50]

The formation of microemboli also contributes to the consumption of platelets. Postoperative dysfunction of the kidneys, lungs, and brain has been attributed to the embolic obstruction of the circulation in these organs by clumps of platelets, and to the vasoactive substances released by platelets. A micropore blood filter (25–40 μm) on the arterial side of the oxygenator is commonly used to reduce the microembolic complications of bypass, even though it may contribute somewhat to platelet depletion.

Platelet Function
Once platelets have been exposed to the extracorporeal circuit, their function is substantially altered. Plasma levels of thromboxane A_2 and platelet-specific proteins rise at the onset of bypass, indicating significant platelet activation. Platelet stores of ADP, ATP, and other procoagulant constituents are depleted.[10] The fate of platelet receptors during bypass remains controversial. Some studies suggest that receptors for von Willebrand factor (vWf) and fibrinogen are reduced in number and/or function.[39,51] In vitro tests of platelet aggregability show an impairment of function for 3 to 5 days postoperatively. The bleeding time is usually prolonged during bypass, but ordinarily returns more quickly

TABLE 109–3. EVALUATION OF EXCESSIVE BLEEDING AFTER CARDIOPULMONARY BYPASS

	PT	aPTT	Platelet Count	Thrombin Time	Thrombin Time Corrected by Protamine	FDP	Fibrinogen
Expected range after CBP	Less than 3 seconds prolonged	Less than 10 seconds prolonged	75,000–150,000/mm³	Up to 3 second > control	No change	< 12 μg/mL	> 150 mg/dL
Heparin excess	Normal or prolonged	Prolonged	Normal	Prolonged	Returns to normal	Normal	Normal
Platelet dysfunction	Normal	Normal	Normal	Normal	Normal	Normal	Normal
Pathologic fibrinolysis	Prolonged	Prolonged	0–75,000/mm³	Prolonged	Remains prolonged	Usually > 20 μg/mL	< 150 mg/dL
Massive transfusion	Normal or slightly higher	Normal or slightly higher	30,000–75,000/mm³	Normal	Normal	Normal	Normal

to the normal range than does in vitro platelet function. Clot retraction is the final phase of platelet hemostasis, in which platelet contractile proteins interact with the solid fibrin clot to stabilize and solidify it.[52] Clot retraction is impaired by heparin.[53] Greilich and colleagues have recently shown that reductions in clot retractile force in vitro correlate well with postbypass hemorrhage.[54] Heparin binds to vWf, and recent studies have shown that high concentrations of heparin will effectively block platelet–vWf binding.[55]

In addition to the effects of drugs, turbulence, and contact with foreign surfaces, several additional factors contribute to platelet dysfunction. Even moderate hypothermia significantly retards platelet function.[56] Platelets may be damaged or impaired by plasmin, other activated proteases, as well as their products of digestion.[39,57] Finally, activated platelets express a surface glycoprotein (GMP-140, or P-selectin) that adheres to neutrophils and monocytes. Increased numbers of platelet–monocyte aggregates can be observed during cardiopulmonary bypass,[16,58] and platelet activation may lead to neutrophil activation as well.

Many platelet-active agents have been studied in an effort to reduce thromboembolic events in the arterial circulation. Their administration during cardiopulmonary bypass, to block platelet consumption, has had mixed results. Platelet survival is often improved by paralyzing platelet reactivity during bypass, but the net effect of this may be unsatisfactory if one is left with a circulating population of functionless, drug-impaired platelets. Both dextran and aspirin have been associated with excessive hemorrhage after bypass, despite higher platelet counts. An ideal platelet survival agent would be one that protects platelets from the trauma and stimulation of bypass but whose effect is short-lived and reversible. Earlier attempts to achieve these effects with infusions of prostaglandins have not met with clinical success.

THE CONDUCT
OF CARDIOPULMONARY BYPASS

Heparin

The heparins are a heterogeneous family of sulfated glycosaminoglycans varying in size from 6000 to 20,000 D. Heparin accelerates by 2500-fold the neutralization of thrombin by antithrombin III (a natural inhibitor protein). The effect of heparin as an anticoagulant extends far beyond the simple neutralization of thrombin activity, and covers a large portion of the preceding coagulation cascade, including Factors IX, X, XI, and XII.[59,60] Heparin differs from most other drugs, because it is a polysaccharide, not a protein. In addition, heparin and heparin-like glycosaminoglycans are now known to have a range of other biologic activities, including activation of heparin Cofactor II (another natural anticoagulant),[61] inhibition of smooth muscle proliferation,[62] and cytoprotective effects.[63] The current focus will be on heparin's conventional anticoagulant effects.

During clotting, there is synergism between platelet activation and plasma coagulation. Activated platelets may vitiate some of the inhibitory effects of heparin by secreting platelet Factor 4, which is an antiheparin compound. Additionally, activated clotting factors, and particularly Factor V, can adsorb in high concentrations on the platelet surface, where they may be protected from inhibitors. The role of these subtle effects in the patient on bypass is unclear. Clinically, it is useful to know that thrombocytopenic patients show an increased sensitivity to heparin.

The source of the heparin (porcine gut mucosa or bovine lung) seems to make little practical difference in the coagulation effects that result.[64] Because heparin-associated thrombocytopenia is unlikely to develop after a single intraoperative exposure, heparin of either origin is acceptable for uncomplicated bypass. However, heparin-associated thrombocytopenia is reported more frequently after long-term administration of bovine lung heparin, so if the patient will require anticoagulation with heparin pre- or postoperatively, porcine mucosal heparin would be preferable.

There can be great variation in individual and institutional practice patterns for heparin dosing during open heart surgery. Some centers experienced in cardiac surgery use standard formulas for heparin and protamine dosage with apparent satisfaction, while others individualize and titrate dosages according to the activated clotting time (ACT). Regardless of the specific method, regular monitoring of heparin's anticoagulant effects is essential to ensure adequately intense anticoagulation during bypass, and adequate reversal with protamine. Typically, the ACT or an equivalent whole-blood clotting time is measured at least hourly, and enough heparin is given to maintain it at 400 to 600 seconds. Surprisingly, there is still no complete agreement regarding the optimal intensity of heparin anticoagulation. Using sensitive markers for activation of coagulation, such as fibrin monomer or fibrinopeptide A, investigators have suggested that sufficient heparin should be given to maintain the ACT above 350 to 400 seconds.[65,66]

There is growing evidence that heparin preparations differ, and that some may directly promote platelet clumping and enhance aggregation induced by other agents.[67] Despite these laboratory observations, studies have not demonstrated clinically significant in vivo activation of platelets after the intravenous injection of heparin,[68,69] except in the immune-mediated syndrome of heparin-induced thrombocytopenia (see below).

Protamine

Protamine is a small, highly positively charged protein derived from fish sperm.[70] It indiscriminately binds to heparin (and likely a host of other negatively charged endogenous molecules). A large excess of protamine can have an anticoagulant action, but this entity tends to be overrated as a factor in postbypass hemorrhage. More common are its other toxicities, including increased pulmonary vascular resistance, myocardial depression, and systemic vasodilation. While controversies remain about the role of complement activation by protamine,[71–73] the formation of protamine/heparin complexes can lead to the induction of systemic mediators of inflammation and anaphylaxis, producing granulocytopenia, pulmonary sequestration of leukocytes, and vasodilation. Rarely, a more severe allergic form of this reaction to protamine may occur, resulting in pulmonary edema, hypoxia, and systemic hypotension.[74] This most commonly occurs in diabetics already sensitized to protamine by NPH insulin.

In spite of its associated toxicities, protamine remains the sole effective antidote to heparin. The in vivo ratio of protamine to heparin for exact neutralization is about 1.0 mg of protamine per 100 units of heparin. Ideally, calculation of the protamine dose should be based on an estimate of the circulating heparin at the conclusion of bypass, using a ratio that will provide a slight excess of protamine.

Heparin "rebound" has long been observed by cardiac surgeons, but its pathogenesis has not been clearly understood. Typically, incoagulability of the blood (and prolonged clotting times) recurs hours after the initial protamine treatment had restored clotting times to normal. The problem is usually correctable by the administration of more protamine, suggesting that there was reappearance of heparin in the circulation. Recent work by Teoh and colleagues suggests a promising new theory for this phenomenon.[75] Some of the circulating heparin is inactive, bound to plasma proteins and inaccessible to neutralization by protamine. Once most of the anticoagulantly active heparin is cleared from the circulation as heparin/protamine complexes, a new equilibrium favors the release of the formerly inactive plasma protein-bound heparin. This leads to "rebound" anticoagulation. A second factor in this process may be the inadvertent administration of small quantities of heparin remaining in the washed autologous blood recycled from the operative field and extracorporeal reservoirs.

Perioperative Adjuncts to Hemostasis and Blood Conservation

Intraoperative Techniques

A number of topical hemostatic agents are available to the operating surgeon.[76] Bovine thrombin is both a potent platelet activator and also directly clots fibrinogen. Topical thrombin is especially useful in the heparinized patient. Oxidized cellulose induces contact activation of the plasma coagulation cascade and furnishes a physical surface on which fibrin can polymerize. Because of its acidic pH, it is not best employed in conjunction with topical thrombin, which depends on a neutral pH for optimal enzymatic activity. Instead, gelatin foam is a useful absorbent reservoir for

thrombin and native blood. Microcrystalline bovine collagen is commercially prepared in several physical forms. Collagen is primarily a platelet activator and adhesive, so it is helpful where platelet hemostasis is critical—at bleeding needle holes and suture lines.

Hemostatic glues have been developed from chemical or plasma protein sources.[77] Cyanoacrylate glues were pioneered by orthopedic surgeons, but can be effectively used to control difficult bleeding sites without recourse to human blood products. Fibrin glue eliminates reliance on the patient's own hemostatic competence. Typically, cryoprecipitate (a source of human fibrinogen) is mixed rapidly in situ with bovine thrombin to create an adhesive fibrin seal at the bleeding point(s).

Autotransfusion

Several techniques are available to conserve blood and reduce transfusion requirements during cardiopulmonary bypass. A frequent method of autotransfusion involves preoperative phlebotomy (either days or minutes before bypass is instituted) with reinfusion, after bypass, of this blood, which has never contacted the extracorporeal circuit. A rise in platelet count and improvement in platelet function have been observed after such reinfusion, and a reduction in postoperative blood loss has been demonstrated.[78] The same beneficial effects have been observed from the transfusion of autologous platelet rich plasma.[79,80]

While the patient is heparinized on bypass, shed blood is routinely scavenged from the operative field with special suction devices and recirculated into the oxygenator. If the blood has not been excessively activated by frothing and contact with tissue thromboplastins, the red cells, platelets, and clotting factors are all returned to the circuit.

After bypass, the blood remaining in the oxygenator reservoir can be rapidly washed to produce a suspension of viable red cells (absent platelets and clotting factors).[81,82] Postoperatively in the intensive care unit, many institutions routinely collect the shed mediastinal blood in special chest drainage units, which allow for the direct reinfusion after simple filtration. These postoperative techniques for autotransfusion have recently undergone a critical reappraisal by randomized trials. Several prospective studies have failed to show that postoperative autotransfusion of shed blood significantly reduces the transfusion of homologous banked blood.[83–85] Salvaged blood contains activated clotting factors, thromboplastins, and high levels of fibrin degradation products, even after washing.[86,87] Reinfusion of this activated blood may actually enhance fibrinolysis, and activation of complement and other inflammatory mediators. In large volumes (more than 800 mL), it may actually contribute to the postbypass bleeding diathesis.[84]

DDAVP

Desmopressin acetate (DDAVP) is an analog of vasopressin that transiently raises plasma levels of von Willebrand factor and Factor VIII through release from endogenous stores.

While initial trials of this drug in patients at high risk for hemorrhage showed significant reductions in blood loss,[88,89] the results were not confirmed by subsequent trials in broader, low-risk populations (and children).[90–92] As Salzman et al summarized the data,[93] DDAVP is probably beneficial only in those patients with significant impairment of von Willebrand factor-dependent hemostasis (either from reduced vWf levels, impaired platelet receptor function, or drug effects). Thus, the routine administration of DDAVP in low-risk patients is not indicated.

Aprotinin

Aprotinin (Trasylol, Miles Inc, Pharmaceutical Division) is currently approved by the FDA for prophylactic use to reduce perioperative bleeding and blood transfusion after cardiopulmonary bypass in patients undergoing repeat operations, in patients at high risk for bleeding, and in patients for whom transfusion is unavailable or unacceptable. Aprotinin is a naturally occurring protease inhibitor obtained from bovine lung tissue.[86] Even though precise mechanisms by which aprotinin reduces blood loss after cardiac surgery are not completely understood, the drug has clear effects. First, aprotinin is a potent inhibitor of kallikrein activity and thereby inhibits contact activation of the coagulation cascade. Second, aprotinin possesses antifibrinolytic activity as an inhibitor of the conversion of plasminogen to plasmin. Finally, a possibly secondary effect of aprotinin is its preservation of platelet adhesion and aggregation. Together, these actions of aprotinin seem to reduce the hemostatic defect associated with cardiopulmonary bypass.

Since the early observations of Royston et al,[94] numerous clinical trials of aprotinin in cardiac surgery have demonstrated reduced perioperative blood loss, reduced postoperative chest tube drainage, and reduced transfusion requirements.[95–97] Like the initial DDAVP trials, these have primarily focused on subgroups of patients recognized to be at higher risk for postoperative hemorrhage. Although both high- and low-dosage regimens have been studied, Wildevuur and colleagues have shown that aprotinin is especially effective in preventing the initial contact activation of blood and platelets upon first exposure to the extracorporeal circuit.[39]

Three main safety concerns have arisen with this new drug: anaphylaxis, renal impairment, and the induction of a prothrombotic state. Because aprotinin is a protein of animal origin, anaphylactic reactions can occur (incidence reported to be less than 0.5%). A test dose has been recommended to assess for allergic reaction. Additionally, re-exposure to aprotinin is not recommended. Although a recent study by Blauth et al demonstrated no nephrotoxicity associated with the use of aprotinin,[95] transient rises in serum creatinine have been reported. The dominant concern among cardiac surgeons is whether aprotinin initiates a prothrombotic state that would increase the incidence of graft occlusion or perioperative myocardial infarction. Cosgrove and colleagues found a higher (but not statistically significant) incidence of perioperative MI in the high-dose aprotinin group.[98] In contrast, Murkin et al found no differences in perioperative myocardial infarction, despite demonstrating efficacy in terms of reduced blood loss and transfusion requirements.[96] Their findings are supported by others, even when graft patency is studied with sensitive techniques.[97,99,100]

One explanation for the higher myocardial infarction rate found in the Cleveland Clinic study may be related to inadequate heparin anticoagulation. The ACT is the most common monitor of anticoagulation used in the operating room and is designed to test the intrinsic coagulation pathway, mimicking contact activation of the blood. Aprotinin markedly elevates the ACT (especially when measured by the Hemochron system, which uses celite as the activator). Therefore, a patient receiving aprotinin may have a seemingly therapeutic ACT, but actually be inadequately anticoagulated with heparin. During aprotinin treatment, if the ACT with celite activator is used to monitor heparin therapy, the therapeutic range should be revised upward (700–1000 seconds). Or, alternative clotting times that do not require celite activation can be used.

EVALUATION OF POSTOPERATIVE BLEEDING

Fewer than 3% of patients undergoing cardiac surgery now require early re-exploration, usually for hemorrhage or tamponade. Shorter operations, refined technology in the form of less traumatic extracorporeal circuits and oxygenators, more sophisticated pre- and postoperative hematologic management, and the use of autotransfusion have reduced the transfusion requirements of the uncomplicated cardiac surgical patient to 1 to 3 units of packed red blood cells.[101,102] Cardiopulmonary bypass can successfully be performed without any blood transfusion, albeit with a slightly increased mortality.[103] A transfusion requirement of 3 to 5 units or more might be anticipated with more complex cardiovascular surgery including valve replacement, endocardial resection, or redo procedures.[104]

How much bleeding is acceptable? The answer varies with different surgical teams and institutions. Many authors report the loss of from 800 to 1200 mL of blood from mediastinal drainage tubes in the first 24 hours following cardiac surgery. At our own institutions, loss of more than 100 mL/h for several hours in the immediate postoperative period is considered excessive.

Transfusion: Indications and Risks

An NIH consensus conference[105] has questioned the traditional wisdom of routine transfusion when the hemoglobin is less than 10 g/dL or when the hematocrit is less than 30%. Most cardiovascular surgeons still adhere to these guidelines when the patient is hemodynamically unstable, or if there is excessive postoperative bleeding. However, a hematocrit of 24% and a hemoglobin of 8 g/dL may be more reasonable indications for transfusion in the younger, stable patient. Newer critical care techniques for monitoring oxygen delivery (mixed venous pO_2, transcutaneous arterial O_2 saturation, etc.) now enable clinicians to more carefully and safely assess the adequacy of oxygen delivery.

The complications of excessive bleeding include transfusion transmitted infections. Despite the routine screening of donor blood for the hepatitis B antigen, post-transfusion hepatitis will develop in approximately 7% of transfusion recipients.[106-108] Hepatitis C makes up the majority of these cases, while hepatitis B is responsible for 10–15%. The source of donor blood is the most important risk factor for hepatitis.

Less than 2% of all cases of acquired immune deficiency syndrome (AIDS) have been contracted from blood transfusion, and these have been primarily infants or older patients with hereditary coagulation disorders.[109] Since screening of all donor blood for HTLV-III (HIV) antibody has begun, only 0.25% of the donor pool has been found positive for antibody.[109] This low incidence, combined with self-selection of donors and an effective screening test makes the risk of contracting AIDS extremely low for the average transfusion recipient. The Center for Disease Control has outlined the appropriate precautions for health care workers having contact with AIDS patients.[110,111]

Differential Diagnosis of Excessive Bleeding

Although surgically correctable causes for bleeding are frequently found at reoperation, the hemostatic defects in patients undergoing cardiac surgery play such an important role that it is often difficult to ascribe the bleeding either to a purely mechanical cause or to a hematologic problem. The experienced surgeon is often the first to notice abnormal hemostasis when there is excessive bleeding from arteriotomy closures, or prolonged bleeding from skin and subcutaneous tissues after heparin reversal. If clinical circumstances suggest a bleeding diathesis, blood samples should be sent immediately from the operating room for platelet count, PT, and activated partial thromboplastin times (aPTT) (Table 109–3).

Upon arrival in the intensive care unit, every cardiac patient should have a platelet count, PT, and PTT. The blood should be drawn by fresh venipuncture. For the stable patient, these tests are intended as screening tests to detect gross derangements in the intrinsic or extrinsic pathways of the coagulation cascade, or in the platelet count. Table 109–4 reviews the normal ranges and expected values for these tests after cardiopulmonary bypass. It is not uncommon to encounter mild elevations of the PT or aPTT immediately after bypass; yet the levels of individual clotting factors are usually more than adequate for normal hemostasis at this time. Without evidence of active hemorrhage, the patient who exhibits the mild abnormalities outlined in Table 109–4 deserves watchful waiting, since these abnormalities will usually resolve within 4 to 6 hours after bypass.

Significant prolongations of clotting times most commonly result from a circulating anticoagulant such as heparin or fibrin degradation products. Very rarely, there may be an actual deficiency of clotting factors resulting from their abnormal consumption during bypass or from a congenital coagulation deficiency not recognized preoperatively. If there are major abnormalities in the initial clotting studies, or if bleeding is excessive, further investigation and treatment are warranted (Table 109–3). This workup should evaluate (1) heparin excess, (2) the integrity of the coagulation cascade, and (3) platelets.

Excess Anticoagulants

The persistence or recrudescence of active heparin in the blood is the most likely cause for significant prolongations of the ACT or aPTT in the early postoperative period. Alternatively, high concentrations of FDP (from excessive fibrinolysis or autotransfusion) can act as anticoagulants. Administration of 25–50 mg of extra protamine over a period of several minutes is a simple clinical trial. The aPTT or ACT should promptly normalize if heparin is the cause. If time permits laboratory investigation, a thrombin time performed with and without protamine can identify the problem. Heparin greatly prolongs the thrombin time (FDP less so); the in vitro addition of a small amount of protamine will correct the heparin-prolonged thrombin time but

TABLE 109–4. ROUTINE HEMOSTATIC STUDIES AFTER CARDIOPULMONARY BYPASS

Test	Normal Range	Acceptable Range after Bypass	Common Causes for Major Abnormalities
Platelet count	150,000–400,000 per mm^3	75,000–150,000 per mm^3	Long pump run, excessive blood trauma Consumption by DIC Massive transfusion
Partial thromboplastin time	3–5 seconds above control	Less than 10 seconds above control	Heparin excess FDP from fibrinolysis/DIC Unrecognized preop factor deficiency
Prothrombin time	Less than 3 seconds above control	Less than 3 seconds above control	FDP from fibrinolysis/DIC Factor deficiency, warfarin

not that prolonged by FDP. Fresh-frozen plasma is *not effective* in reversing the effects of residual heparin.

Thrombocytopenia and Platelet Dysfunction

If there is thrombocytopenia (less than 75,000 platelets/µL) and bleeding, 8 to 12 units of fresh platelets should be transfused. Sometimes there is no abnormality of clotting tests and no thrombocytopenia, and yet the patient demonstrates a generalized hemorrhagic tendency. In such a case the problem is usually due to a major defect in platelet function, and may represent a valid indication for DDAVP infusion (0.3 µg/kg IV). The evaluation of platelet function after cardiopulmonary bypass is somewhat academic, since it is always impaired to some degree. The bleeding time may be unreliable due to peripheral vasoconstriction and poor perfusion. For the patient who is actively bleeding, platelets should be given even if the platelet count is not sufficiently low to meet standard indications for transfusion, since thrombopathy is always a contributory factor. On the other hand, *routine* use of prophylactic platelet transfusions is not indicated, for it does not reduce transfusion requirements.[112]

Pathologic Fibrinolysis

The consequences of excessive fibrinolysis can range from a mild anticoagulant-like effect (see above), to DIC with thrombocytopenia and hypofibrinogenemia. Inadequate suppression of clotting during extracorporeal circulation, sepsis, transfusion reactions, and large volumes of salvaged blood can all contribute to the laboratory profile described in Table 109–3. Intraoperatively, this syndrome can be recognized when blood clots at the operative field, but the clots quickly lyse. Postoperatively, severe pathologic fibrinolysis is manifest by a generalized bleeding tendency with derangement of all laboratory parameters. Here, therapy should not be delayed for the results of detailed laboratory diagnostics. The use of antifibrinolytic drugs[113] such as ε-aminocaproic acid or aprotinin should be considered, in addition to transfusions of fresh frozen plasma, platelets and red blood cells, to keep pace with consumptive and hemorrhagic loses. Cryoprecipitate contains supranormal concentrations of fibrinogen, von Willebrand factor, and Factor VIII. Its use is preferable over fresh frozen plasma only when there is severe hypofibrinogenemia (< 100 mg/dL) and bleeding.

The Effects of Massive Transfusion

Occasionally, the diagnosis of a bleeding problem may be complicated by attendant massive transfusion. Serious dilution of plasma proteins occurs after transfusion of 1 to 1-1/2 times the blood volume.[114] Since platelets survive poorly in banked blood, thrombocytopenia is the most frequent abnormality that occurs in this situation.[115] Factors V and VIII are also labile in stored blood, but deficiencies in these factors are less common due to their extravascular stores and synthesis. Typically, patients with this problem have

required long bypass runs, have received large volumes of homologous and salvaged autologous blood, and often had acquired clotting defects preoperatively. The course of their management should remain the same: (1) rule out heparin excess, (2) assess plasma coagulation and fibrinolysis, and (3) replace deficits in clotting factor platelets.

Hemodynamic stability and the rate of blood loss will dictate when and if the patient should be re-explored. If reoperation is indicated by the clinical status of the patient, waiting for the results of clotting studies should not delay the patient's return to the operating room, where the re-united team of surgeons and anesthesiologists can stabilize the patient, and correct both surgical and nonsurgical causes for hemorrhage.

SPECIAL HEMOSTATIC CHALLENGES

Jehovah's Witnesses

Personal or religious proscriptions against transfusion require the surgeon to integrate all of the known blood-conserving techniques. For elective surgery, the highest possible hemoglobin level should be sought with the use of hematinic vitamins, iron, and recombinant erythropoietin.[116] Detailed preoperative discussions with the patient should establish precisely what forms of autotransfusion are or are not acceptable. The Jehovah's Witnesses can provide useful reviews of the relevant clinical literature to assist the surgeon. One must remember that any drugs or fluids containing native human proteins (e.g., serum albumin) are usually forbidden. Lewis and colleagues have reported the largest experience, with a perioperative mortality rate of 7% in the recent era.[103] While self-evident, all of these factors contribute significantly to the success of open heart surgery without homologous transfusion: meticulous attention to hemostasis, use of prohemostatic drugs, maximal use of autotransfusion techniques when permitted, and limited postoperative blood sampling for laboratory tests.

The Patient at High Risk for Hemorrhage

Unlike the patient with a single identified bleeding risk, it is the complex patient with multiple hemorrhagic risk factors that poses the greatest challenge. The preoperative assessment of hemostasis is most important here, as it allows the surgeon to predict and correct the anticipated problems in a timely fashion. The severity and urgency of the cardiac derangement often contribute indirectly. The emergent cardiac patient may be receiving anticoagulants, fibrinolytics, and platelet inhibitors. Cardiac decompensation may be associated with hepatic or renal dysfunction, or the patient may be on a mechanical cardiac assist device. These latter patients enter surgery with significant platelet dysfunction, as well as the effects of drugs. Redo surgery and long pump runs are known to carry higher risks for postoperative hemorrhage. A successful hemostatic strategy should attempt to dissect the individual, predictable derangements and utilize treatments and corrective actions that are specific for each element of the bleeding diathesis. Once major hemorrhage and its attendant massive transfusion have complicated the picture, it is much harder to discern the specific causes for hemorrhage. It then becomes difficult to avoid a "shotgun" approach to the bleeding patient.

Heparin-Induced Thrombocytopenia

This syndrome is more commonly associated with thrombosis than hemorrhage. Its incidence is estimated at 5% of those receiving continuous heparin, but the frequency in cardiac patients is likely less.[117] Although it has been recently reviewed,[21] new reports have added to our understanding of its pathobiology.[118,119] It is now believed that the autoantibodies of this syndrome are directed against heparin-platelet factor four complexes. Platelet Factor four (PF4) is a native heparin-binding protein that is released from platelet granules upon activation. When a patient acquires antibodies to the heparin–PF4 complex, platelets become activated and aggregate in response to the circulating antigen–antibody complex. This is mediated by the Fc receptor of the platelet.

The typical cardiac patient may develop immune sensitization from exposures to heparin during cardiac catheterization, preoperative treatment of unstable angina, or previous cardiovascular surgery. Once established, the immune syndrome can be perpetuated by the small doses of heparin used to flush catheters, or heparin-coated catheters themselves.[120] The syndrome has also been recognized in neonates.[121] The hallmark of the clinical diagnosis is thrombocytopenia (< 100,000/μL) during heparin therapy that resolves within a few days of heparin withdrawal. Occasionally, there will be a dramatic drop in platelet count (> 50%), but not absolute thrombocytopenia. If heparin sensitization has been remote in time, the platelet count may be normal, although the patient still harbors active antibodies. Here, a high index of suspicion and review of old medical records are warranted. The diagnosis is confirmed by platelet aggregation testing. Newer methods based on the heparin–PF4 antigen may soon be developed.[122]

Continuation of heparin in a sensitized patient, or re-exposure at a later date may result in severe thrombocytopenia (5,000–30,000/μL) and pathologic venous and/or arterial thromboses. Olinger and colleagues[123] reported a useful strategy for such patients. If surgery was elective, operation was postponed, and in vitro sensitivity to heparin was monitored. The platelet aggregating factor tended to disappear with time, and when the patient no longer had a plasma factor that caused heparin-induced aggregation, open heart surgery could be performed with the usual doses of heparin. With this approach, exposure to heparin in any form must be scrupulously avoided in the pre- and postoperative periods to avoid recurrence of heparin–induced

thrombocytopenia. Aspirin and dextran can reduce heparin–mediated platelet aggregation,[124] and may be useful adjuncts to reduce the risks of this approach.

A number of strategies are available when vascular surgery cannot be postponed.[21] There is broad cross-reactivity among pharmaceutical heparins in sensitized patients, so substitution of beef heparin for porcine heparin is contraindicated. A number of sensitized patients have been successfully treated with low-molecular-weight heparins[125,126] as an alternative to standard heparin. But cross-sensitivity can occur.[127–129] One heparin-like drug has shown the lowest cross-reactivity of all, perhaps because it is not a true heparin: Org 10172 (Lomoparan, Organon Inc, West Orange, NJ) is made of a mixture of heparans and dermatans that have anticoagulant activity. This drug rarely induces aggregation in positive patient samples, and has been successfully used to anticoagulate patients with heparin-induced thrombocytopenia,[130,131] even those sensitive to other low-molecular-weight heparins.[128,132] Currently this drug is available in the United States for investigational and compassionate use.

If heparin-associated thrombocytopenia is suspected postoperatively, all heparin should be stopped, including the small doses used in intravenous infusion lines. Usually, the platelet count will recover promptly. If there are arterial thromboembolic complications, aspirin, dextran, or warfarin may be useful. If there has been venous thromboembolism, placement of a vena caval filter may be indicated during the interval until anticoagulation with warfarin can be instituted.

FUTURE TRENDS

Pharmacologic Control of Hemostasis

Important questions remain to be answered about the roles for prohemostatic drugs such as DDAVP and aprotinin: which patients should receive them, and what are the risks of pathologic thrombosis? A wealth of data now suggest that the routine administration of DDAVP to low-risk patients is not beneficial. We will have to await similar detailed studies of aprotinin to understand the optimal indications and dosages.

Novel Heparins and Other Anticoagulants

Low-molecular-weight heparins are increasingly popular as first line cardiovascular drugs in Europe, but have only now entered the United States market under limited indications for thromboprophylaxis. Depolymerization, and chemical modification have yielded a large number of heparin fractions and fragments with widely different characteristics regarding molecular weight, inhibition of thrombin and activated Factor X, and stimulation or inhibition of platelets.[133,134] Currently, low-molecular-weight heparins appear to offer few advantages for acute anticoagulation during cardiovascular surgery. Nevertheless, continuing research to develop heparin-based drugs with narrow and focused biologic activities holds the promise of truly unique drugs that may be beneficial in the pre- or postoperative period. Potentially useful heparin fractions would possess anticoagulant activity with fewer hemorrhagic side effects, would inhibit platelet–vessel interactions or restenosis with minimal anticoagulant activities.

Hirudin is the prototype of a new family of direct thrombin inhibitors. Native, recombinant or chemically derived, they all directly bind and neutralize circulating thrombin (see references 135,136 for recent reviews). At high doses, they can be used as anticoagulants like heparin, rendering the blood incoagulable. At lower doses they have been used as adjuncts to coronary angioplasty and thrombolysis, where thrombin–platelet interactions are thought to contribute to acute reclosure. Thrombin inhibitors prolong the aPTT in a dose-dependent manner. There are generally no antidotes, so the duration of effect depends on the half-life of the drug (minutes to hours, depending on dose).

Antiplatelet drugs are also under development in a similar strategy to interrupt the platelet-dominated thrombosis, which can complicate coronary angioplasty. Antibodies to the platelet integrin receptor for fibrinogen (glycoprotein IIb/IIIa), or synthetic peptides that mimic fibrinogen can be used to totally block platelet aggregation.[137,138] Like thrombin inhibitors, these platelet inhibitors have no antidotes and can induce a hemorrhagic diathesis at high doses. Clinical research trials are still exploring the optimal dose and indications.

Near-Patient Coagulation Testing

Portable, bedside coagulation testing devices are now available that can perform the equivalents of the PT, aPTT, and other tests within minutes.[139,140] They appear to be accurate. Access to immediate coagulation results may be very useful in the early postoperative management of patients. Early results suggest that these devices may be cost effective if they reduce unnecessary transfusions of blood products.[140]

THROMBOEMBOLIC COMPLICATIONS OF PROSTHETIC CARDIAC VALVES

Whenever a prosthetic or foreign surface is in contact with the blood, thrombosis and embolism are major hazards. In the eighteenth century, William Hewson[141] demonstrated the tendency of blood to clot when outside the normal lining of a blood vessel. In the nineteenth century Kirkes[142] observed that an abnormal endothelial surface could be the site for thrombosis and embolization. Ever since Hufnagel[143] first inserted a prosthetic valve in the descending aorta in 1951, the success of cardiac valve replacement has

been limited by the morbidity and mortality of consequent thromboembolism.

Prosthetic cardiac valves present a unique problem in the prevention of thrombosis.[144] Recirculating eddies and regions of relative stasis behind the sewing ring or the tilting disc are likely to develop a plasma coagulum, whereas the metal struts that project into the mainstream of blood-flow acquire predominantly platelet thrombi. Oral anticoagulation with vitamin K antagonists is partially successful in preventing thromboembolism, at the expense of an increased risk of hemorrhage. Tilting disc mechanical valves and biologic tissue valves have brought further improvements in hemodynamic performance, but have not totally eliminated thromboembolic complications.

The recommended optimal therapeutic range for oral anticoagulant therapy has recently been revised.[145] Thromboplastin reagents used to measure the prothrombin time differ in their sensitivity, so a new system for reporting the PT has been widely adopted. The international normalized ratio (INR) is a formula that takes into account the sensitivity of each individual laboratory's thromboplastin reagent.[145] Each reagent is assigned a sensitivity index (ISI). The PT is reported as an INR, ranging upward from 1.0 (normal). The INR is not simply a ratio of patient to control prothrombin times, so the value of the INR is not intuitively the same as the old PT ratios most clinicians recognize. New guidelines for the intensity of anticoagulation with warfarin have now been developed.[145] For example, for deep venous thrombosis, the recommended INR range is 2.0–3.0.[146]

Mechanical Valves

All patients with mechanical prosthetic heart valves should be treated indefinitely with warfarin.[147,148] The recommended INR is 2.5 to 3.5. With adequate anticoagulation, the incidence of thromboembolism ranges from 0.5 to 3 per 100 patient years.[148] Most reports find a higher incidence after mitral valve replacement (1–3 per 100 patient years) than after aortic valve replacement (0.5–2.0). Management of these patients without oral anticoagulation, the late discontinuation of anticoagulants, or substitution of antiplatelet agents all result in a prohibitively high incidence of thromboembolism.

The addition of a platelet-inhibiting drug to the oral anticoagulation regimen further reduces the incidence of thromboembolism from mechanical heart valves. Low-dose aspirin or dipyridamole combined with oral anticoagulants may offer additional protection from embolism.[148] However, there remains some controversy as to whether antiplatelet drugs add to the hemorrhagic risks of warfarin—they probably do so at higher doses,[147] but may not at lower doses. For the patient who suffers systemic embolism, the addition of aspirin 160 mg/day or dipyridamole 400 mg/day is recommended.

Bleeding complications from anticoagulation can be

anticipated at a rate of 0.7 to 6.3 per 100 patient years, depending on the intensity of therapy. Patients older than 70 years are at higher risk of bleeding (9 per 100 patient years). When full-dose warfarin cannot be given, a lower INR range of 2.0 to 3.0, combined with both dipyridamole 150 mg/day and aspirin 660 mg/day is a reasonable alternative.[148]

Bioprosthetic Valves

Biologic tissue valves produce the lowest incidence of thromboembolism of all valve replacements. Their nearly normal streamlined flow pattern, soft and pliable leaflets, and biologic (although still abnormal) surface all probably contribute to their freedom from thrombosis. The long-term incidence of thromboembolism from bioprosthetic valves is about 2% per patient year,[148] less in the aortic than the mitral position. In exchange for these advantages, they are less durable, and more prone to degeneration and mechanical failure.[149] In a recent review, Jamieson suggests that when structural, thromboembolic, and hemorrhagic complications are all considered, mechanical and bioprosthetic valves yield similar performances over a 10-year period.[149]

Embolism does occur even with bioprosthetic valves, more commonly in the first 6 to 12 weeks after operation. Currently, the use of oral anticoagulants at a lower intensity (INR 2.0–3.0) is recommended for the first three months, until there is coverage of the sewing rings and supports with endothelium and fibrous tissue. After warfarin has been discontinued, long-term aspirin therapy (325 mg/day) may provide additional protection and is recommended. Although relatively nonthrombogenic, tissue valves cannot yet be considered as durable as mechanical types. Especially in children and younger patients, there is a significant incidence of late degeneration and calcification of the leaflets.

Complicating Conditions

Several clinical factors will augment the risk of postoperative thromboembolism: the presence of atrial fibrillation, a dilated left atrium, or a preoperative history of embolism. These risk factors, even with a bioprosthetic valve, may tip the balance in favor of long-term oral anticoagulation.

In the pregnant woman with a prosthetic heart valve, treatment poses risks to mother and fetus.[150] Pregnant women appear to be at greater risk of thromboembolism, and pregnancy may accelerate calcification and failure of bioprostheses. Antiplatelet therapy may provide sufficient protection in women with tissue valves and without other risk factors.[151] Warfarin is teratogenic and may cause fetal hemorrhage because it crosses the placenta; therefore, warfarin is clearly contraindicated in the first and last trimesters, and its use in the middle trimester is still controversial.[152] Self-administration of subcutaneous heparin for

the duration of the pregnancy may be the safest alternative.[153] Heparin does not cross the placenta; its anticoagulant effect should be adjusted so that the mid-interval APTT is 1.5 to 2 times control. In pregnant patients with mechanical heart valves, heparin should be used in preference to warfarin during the first trimester and the last 2 weeks.[152] It is not known whether warfarin or subcutaneous heparin therapy is safer for the middle trimester.

Retrospective studies suggest that it is reasonably safe to briefly suspend long-term anticoagulation if surgery or other procedures are indicated.[148] Perhaps the best strategy is to simply lower the intensity of warfarin anticoagulation around the time of procedures that can be safely performed with a low level of anticoagulation (i.e., dental extractions). Alternatives include temporarily switching to platelet inhibitors alone, or hospitalizing the patient and using heparin anticoagulation pre- and postoperatively.

VASCULAR AND PROSTHETIC GRAFTS

Autogenous saphenous vein is currently the preferred substitute for peripheral arteries. Prosthetic grafts have generally been unsuccessful for small diameter vessels such as the coronary or tibial arteries, since they develop a lining of organized thrombus that impinges on the already narrow lumen of the prosthesis. The 1-year patency rate of coronary saphenous vein grafts ranges from 75 to 90%, with a much diminished attrition rate thereafter.[154] Aspirin combined with dipyridamole does improve coronary vein graft patency if dipyridamole is given preoperatively and the aspirin soon after surgery.[155,156] There is also evidence that aspirin alone is as effective.[157] The evidence supporting antiplatelet therapy in infrainguinal vascular bypasses is less conclusive. However, because this patient population is at higher risk for stroke and myocardial infarction, lifelong aspirin therapy is recommended.[158] Antiplatelet therapy may be effective in prolonging the patency of infrainguinal prosthetic grafts. A large multicenter trial of aspirin versus low intensity warfarin plus aspirin is currently under way. This Veterans Administration trial may help establish the optimal antithrombotic regimen for autogenous and prosthetic peripheral grafts.

In larger-caliber arteries, prosthetic grafts have been more successful, as their porosity permits the eventual ingrowth of well-vascularized fibrous tissue and endothelium from the ends of the graft and through its interstices. The long-term patency of such grafts in the aortoiliac position is excellent (greater than 85%) without antithrombotic therapy.[159] Lifelong aspirin therapy is indicated to prevent other arterial thrombotic complications. Frequent bending of the graft as it crosses a joint can result in cracking of the well-organized neointima, and can produce late thrombosis. Because of sluggish flow, prosthetic grafts in the venous system have not met with great success; there is no evidence from clinical studies that antithrombotic therapy improves their long-term results.

Mechanical seeding of small diameter prosthetic grafts with autogenous endothelial cells holds promise as a method to reduce their thrombogenicity.[160,161] Genetic engineering of the endothelial cells may make them more thromboresistant. Once a monolayer of cells has grown to cover the prosthesis these small grafts are more resistant to thrombosis.[162] However, during the first 4–6 weeks before complete endothelialization, they remain relatively thrombogenic. Substantial technical hurdles remain before this approach can be applied to small grafts in human beings.

REFERENCES

1. Gibbon JH Jr: The development of the heart lung apparatus. *Rev Surg* **27**:231, 1970
2. Woodman RC, Harker LA: Bleeding complications associated with cardiopulmonary bypass. *Blood* **76**:1680–1697, 1990
3. Edmunds LH JR: Blood-surface interactions during cardiopulmonary bypass. *J Card Surg* **8**:404–410, 1993
4. Gill FM: Congenital bleeding disorders: Hemophilia and von Willebrand's disease. *Med Clin North Am* **68**:601–615, 1984
5. Brown B, Steed DL, Webster MW, et al: General surgery in adult hemophiliacs. *Surgery* **99**:154–159, 1986
6. Nilsson IM, Hedner U, Ahlberg A, et al: Surgery of hemophiliacs—20 years' experience. *World J Surg* **1**:55–66, 1977
7. Montgomery RR, Coller BS: Von Willebrand Disease. In Colman RW, Hirsh J, Marder VJ, Salzman EW (eds): *Hemostasis and Thrombosis.* Philadelphia, J.B. Lippincott, 1994, pp 134–168
8. Brettler DB, Levine PH: Clinical manifestations and therapy of inherited coagulation factor deficiencies. In Colman RW, Hirsh J, Marder VJ, Salzman EW (eds): *Hemostasis and Thrombosis: Basic Principles and Clinical Practice.* Philadelphia, J. B. Lippincott, 1994, pp 169–183
9. Green D: Inhibitors of factor VIII in non-hemophiliacs. In Green D (ed): *Anticoagulants: Physiologic, Pathologic, and Pharmacologic.* Boca Raton, CRC Press, 1994, pp 97–12
10. Beurling Harbury C, Galvan CA: Acquired decrease in platelet secretory ADP associated with increased postoperative bleeding in post-CPB patients and in patients with severe valvular heart disease. *Blood* **52**:13, 1978
11. Maurer HM, McCue CM, Caul J, et al: Impairment in platelet aggregation in congenital heart disease. *Blood* **40**:207, 1972
12. Waldman JD, Czapek EE, Paul MH, et al: Shortened platelet survival in cyanotic heart disease. *J Pediatr* **87**:77, 1975
13. Ekert H, Gilchrist GS, Stanton R, et al: Hemostasis in cyanotic congenital heart disease. *J Pediatr* **76**:221, 1970
14. Ekert H, Sheers M: Preoperative and postoperative platelet function in cyanotic congenital heart disease. *J Thorac Cardiovasc Surg* **67**:184, 1974
15. Hennriksson P, Varendh G, Lundstrom NR: Haemostatic defects in cyanotic congenital heart disease. *Br Heart J* **41**:23, 1979
16. Rinder CS, Gaal D, Student LA, Smith BR: Platelet-leukocyte activation and modulation of adhesion receptors in pediatric patients with congenital heart disease undergoing cardiopulmonary bypass. *J Thorac Cardiovasc Surg* **107**:280–288, 1994
17. Jackson DP: Hemorrhage diathesis in patients with cyanotic congenital heart disease: Preoperative management. *Ann NY Acad Sci* **115**:235, 1964
18. Kessler CM: The pharmacology of aspirin, heparin, coumarin, and thrombolytic agents. Implications for therapeutic use in cardiopulmonary disease. *Chest* **99** Suppl.97S–112S, 1991
19. George JN, Shattil SJ: The clinical importance of acquired abnormalities of platelet function. *N Engl J Med* **324**:27–39, 1991
20. Torosian M, Michelson EL, Morganroth J, MacVaugh H: Aspirin and coumadin related bleeding after coronary artery bypass graft surgery. *Ann Intern Med* **89**:325–328, 1978
21. Sobel M: Heparin-induced thrombocytopenia. *Perspec Vasc Surg* **5**:1–30, 1992
22. Robbins KC: Fibrinolytic therapy: Biochemical mechanisms. *Semin Thromb Hemost* **17**:1–6, 1991
23. Remuzzi G: Bleeding in renal failure. *Lancet* **1**:1205–1208, 1988
24. Harker LA: Acquired disorders of platelet function. *Ann NY Acad Sci* **509**:188–204, 1987
25. Escolar G, Cases A, Bastida E, et al: Uremic platelets have a functional defect affecting the interaction of von Willebrand factor with glycoprotein IIb–IIIa. *Blood* **76**:1336–1340, 1990
26. Ware JA, Clark BA, Smith M, Salzman EW: Abnormalities of cytoplasmic Ca^{2+} in platelets from patients with uremia. *Blood* **73**:172–176, 1989
27. Zwaginga JJ, Ijsseldijk MJW, Beeser-Visser N, et al: High von Willebrand factor concentration compensates a relative adhesion defect in uremic blood. *Blood* **75**:1498–1508, 1990
28. Mannucci PM: Desmopressin: A nontransfusional hemostatic agent. *Annu Rev Med* **41**:55–64, 1990
29. Mammen EF: Coagulation abnormalities in liver disease. *Hematol Oncol Clin North Am* **6**:1247–1257, 1992
30. Fourrier F, Chopin C, Huart JJ, et al: Double-blind, placebo-controlled trial of antithrombin III concentrates in septic shock with disseminated intravascular coagulation. *Chest* **104**:882–888, 1993
31. ten Cate JW, Timmers H, Becker AE: Coagulopathy in ruptured or dissecting aortic aneurysms. *Am J Med* **59**:171–176, 1975
32. Fisher DF Jr, Yawn DH, Crawford ES: Preoperative disseminated intravascular coagulation associated with aortic aneurysms. A prospective study of 76 cases. *Arch Surg* **118**:1252–1255, 1983
33. Salzman EW, Merrill EW: Interaction of blood with artificial surfaces. In Colman RW, Hirsh J, Marder VJ, Salzman EW (eds): *Hemostasis and Thrombosis: Basic Principles and Clinical Practice.* Philadelphia, J.B. Lippincott Co, 1987, p 1335
34. Varco RL: Conference on mechanical surface and gas layer effects on moving blood. *Fed Proc* **30**:1485–ff, 1971
35. Leonard EF, Turitto VT, Vroman L: Blood in contact with natural and artificial surfaces. *Ann NY Acad Sci* **516**:1–688, 1987
36. Moncada S, Vane JR: Unstable metabolites of arachidonic acid and their role in haemostasis and thrombosis. *Br Med Bull* **34**:129, 1978
37. Moore FD, Warner KG, Assousa S, et al: The effects of complement activation during cardiopulmonary bypass: Attenuation by hypothermia, heparin, and hemodilution. *Ann Surg* **208**:95–103, 1988
38. Westaby S: Aprotinin in perspective. *Ann Thorac Surg* **55**:1033–1041, 1993
39. van Oeveren W, Harder MP, Roozendaal KJ, et al: Aprotinin protects platelets against the initial effect of cardiopulmonary bypass. *J Thorac Cardiovasc Surg* **99**:788–796, discus, 1990
40. Boonstra PW, VanImhoff CW, Eysman L, et al: Reduced platelet activation and improved hemostasis after controlled cardiotomy suction during clinical membrane oxygenator perfusions. *J Thorac Cardiovasc Surg* **89**:900, 1985
41. Mammen EF, Koets MH, Washington BC, et al: Hemostasis changes during cardiopulmonary bypass surgery. *Semin Thromb Hemostas* **11**:281–292, 1985
42. Bachmann F, McKenna R, Cole ER, et al: Hemostatic mechanism after open heart surgery. I. Studies on plasma coagulation factors and fibrinolysis in 512 patients after extracorporeal circulation. *J Thorac Cardiovasc Surg* **70**:76–85, 1975
43. Bick RL: Hemostasis defects associated with cardiac surgery, prosthetic devices, and other extracorporeal circuits. *Semin Thromb Hemostas* **11**:249–280, 1985
44. Kern FH, Morana NJ, Sears JJ, Hickey PR: Coagulation defects in

neonates during cardiopulmonary bypass. *Ann Thorac Surg* **54**:541–546, 1992

45. Kawasuji M, Ueyama K, Sakakibara N, et al: Effect of low-dose aprotinin on coagulation and fibrinolysis in cardiopulmonary bypass. *Ann Thorac Surg* **55**:1205–1209, 1993

46. Orchard MA, Goodchild CS, Prentice CRM, et al: Aprotinin reduces cardiopulmonary bypass-induced blood loss and inhibits fibrinolysis without influencing platelets. *Br J Haematol* **85**:533–541, 1993

47. Salzman EW: Blood platelets: Their behavior with respect to extracorporeal membrane oxygenation. In Zapol WM, Qvist J (eds): *Artificial Lungs for Acute Respiratory Failure*. Washington, Hemisphere, 1976, p 105

48. Mckenna R, Bachmann F, Whittaker B, et al: The hemostatic mechanism after open-heart surgery. II. Frequency of abnormal platelet functions during and after extracorporeal circulation. *J Thorac Cardiovasc Surg* **70**:298–308, 1975

49. Holloway DS, Summaria L, Sandesara J, et al: Decreased platelet number and function and increased fibrinolysis contribute to postoperative bleeding in cardiopulmonary bypass patients. *Thrombosis Haemos* **59**:62–67, 1988

50. Hope AF, Heyns AD, Lotter MG: Kinetics and sites of sequestration of indium III-labeled human platelets during cardiopulmonary bypas. *J Thorac Cardiovasc Surg* **81**:880–1081, 1981

51. Wenger RK, Lukasiewicz H, Mikuta BS, et al: Loss of platelet fibrinogen receptors during clinical cardiopulmonary bypass. *J Thorac Cardiovasc Surg* **97**:235–239, 1989

52. Bennett JS, Kolodziej MA: Disorders of platelet function. *Dis Mon* **38**:577–631, 1992

53. Carr MEJ, Park A, Zekert SL, et al: Anticoagulant and antiplatelet activities of heparin and low molecular weight derivatives. *Blood* **82**:603a, 1993

54. Greilich PE, Carr Jr, Carr SL, Chang AS: Preliminary investigation: Reductions in platelet force development by cardiopulmonary bypass are associated with hemorrhage. *Anesth Analg* (in press)

55. Sobel M, McNeill PM, Carlson P, et al: Heparin inhibition of von Willebrand factor in vitro and in vivo. *J Clin Invest* **87**:1787–1793, 1991

56. Kahn HA, Faust GR, Richard R, et al: Hypothermia and bleeding during abdominal aortic aneurysm repair. *Ann Vasc Surg* **8**:6–9, 1994

57. de Haan J, Schonberger J, Haan J, et al: Tissue-type plasminogen activator and fibrin monomers synergistically cause platelet dysfunction during retransfusion of shed blood after cardiopulmonary bypass. *J Thorac Cardiovasc Surg* **106**:1017–1023, 1993

58. Rinder CS, Bonan JL, Rinder HM, et al: Cardiopulmonary bypass induces leukocyte-platelet adhesion. *Blood* **79**:1201–1205, 1992

59. Rosenberg RD: The heparin-antithrombin system: A natural anticoagulant mechanism. In Colman RW, Hirsh J, Marder VJ, Salzman EW (eds): *Hemostasis and Thrombosis: Basic Principles and Clinical Practice*. Philadelphia, J.B. Lippincott, 1987, p 1373

60. Hirsh J, Fuster V: Guide to anticoagulant therapy part 1: Heparin. *Circulation* **89**:1449–1468, 1994

61. Pratt CW, Whinna HC, Meade JB, et al: Physicochemical aspects of heparin cofactor II. *Ann NY Acad Sci* **556**:104–115, 1989

62. Clowes AW, Reidy MA: Prevention of stenosis after vascular reconstruction: Pharmacologic control of intimal hyperplasia—a review. *J Vasc Surg* **13**:885–891, 1991

63. Sternbergh WC III, Makhoul RG, Adelman B: Heparin prevents postischemic endothelial cell dysfunction by a mechanism independent of its anticoagulant activity. *J Vasc Surg* **17**:318–327, 1993

64. Silverglade A: Biologic equivalence of beef lung and hog mucosal heparins. *Curr Ther Res* **18**:1, 1975

65. Young JA, Kisker CT, Doty DB: Adequate anticoagulation during cardiopulmonary bypass determined by activated clotting time and the appearance of fibrin monomer. *Ann Thorac Surg* **26**:231, 1978

66. Gravlee GP, Haddon WS, Rothberger HK, et al: Heparin dosing and monitoring for cardiopulmonary bypass: A comparison of techniques with measurement of subclinical plasma coagulation. *J Thorac Cardiovasc Surg* **99**:518–527, 1990

67. Salzman EW, Rosenberg RD, Smith MH, Lindon JN: Effect of heparin and heparin fractions on platelet aggregation. *J Clin Invest* **65**:64–73, 1980

68. Sobel M, Gervin CA, Qureshi GD, Greenfield LJ: Coagulation responses to heparin in the ischemic limb: Assessment of thrombin and platelet activation during vascular surgery. *Circulation* **76**(suppl III):8–13, 1987

69. Davies GC, Sobel M, Salzman EW: Elevated plasma fibrinopeptide A and thromboxane B2 levels during cardiopulmonary bypass. *Circulation* **61**:808–814, 1980

70. Hobbhahn J, Conzen PF, Habazettl H, et al: Heparin reversal by protamine in humans—Complement, prostaglandins, blood cells, and hemodynamics. *J Appl Physiol* **71**:1415–1421, 1991

71. Wakefield TW, Kirsh MM, Till GO, et al: Absence of complement-mediated events after protamine reversal of heparin anticoagulation. *J Surg Res* **51**:72–76, 1991

72. Cavarocchi NC, Schaff HV, Orszulak TA, et al: Evidence for complement activation by protamine-heparin interaction after cardiopulmonary bypass. *Surgery* **98**:525, 1985

73. Horrow JC: Protamine: A review of its toxicity. *Anesth Analg* **64**:348–361, 1985

74. Weiss ME, Nyhan D, Peng Z, et al: Association of protamine IgE and IgG antibodies with life-threatening reactions to intravenous protamine. *N Engl J Med* **320**:886–892, 1989

75. Teoh KHT, Young E, Bradley CA, Hirsh J: Heparin binding proteins. Contribution to heparin rebound after cardiopulmonary bypass. *Circulation* [2] **88**:II420–II425, 1993

76. Larson PO: Topical hemostatic agents for dermatologic surgery. *J Dermatol Surg Oncol* **14**:623–632, 1988

77. Lerner R, Binur NS: Current status of surgical adhesives. *J Surg Res* **48**:165–181, 1990

78. Wagstaffe JG, Clarke AD, Jackson PW: Reduction of blood loss by restoration of platelet levels using fresh autologous blood after cardiopulmonary bypass. *Thorax* **27**:410, 1972

79. Giordano GF, Rivers SL, Chung GKT, et al: Autologous platelet-rich plasma in cardiac surgery: Effect on intraoperative and postoperative transfusion requirements. *Ann Thor Surg* **46**:416–419, 1988

80. DelRossi AJ, Cernaianu AC, Vertrees RA, et al: Platelet-rich plasma reduces postoperative blood loss after cardiopulmonary bypass. *J Thorac Cardiovasc Surg* **100**:281–286, 1990

81. Keeling MM, Gray LA, Brink MA, et al: Intraoperative autotransfusion. Experience in 725 consecutive cases. *Ann Surg* **197**:536, 1983

82. Ansell J, Parilla N, King M, et al: Survival of autotransfused red blood cells recovered from the surgical field during cardiovascular operations. *J Thorac Cardiovasc Surg* **84**:387, 1982

83. Bouboulis N, Kardara M, Kessteven PJ, Jayakrishnan AG: Autotransfusion after coronary artery bypass surgery: Is there any benefit? *J Card Surg* **9**:314–321, 1994

84. Schonberger JP, vanOevern W, Bredee JD, et al: Systemic blood activation during and after autotransfusion. *Ann Thorac Surg* **57**:1256–1262, 1994

85. Axford TC, Dearani JA, Ragno G, et al: Safety and therapeutic effectiveness of reinfused shed blood after open heart surgery. *Ann Thorac Surg* **57**:615–622, 1994

86. Sieunarine K, Lawrence-Brown MMD, Brennan D, et al: The quality of blood used for transfusion. *J Cardiovasc Surg* **33**:98–105, 1992

87. Bull BS, Bull MH: The salvaged blood syndrome: A sequel to mechanochemical activation of platelets and leukocytes? *Blood Cells* **16**:5–20, discus, 1990

88. Salzman EW, Weinstein MJ, Weintraub RM, et al: Treatment with desmopressin acetate to reduce blood loss after cardiac surgery. A double-blind randomized trial. *N Engl J Med* **314**:142–146, 1986

89. Czer LSC, Bateman TM, Gray RJ, et al: Treatment of severe platelet dysfunction and hemorrhage after cardiopulmonary bypass: Reduc-

tion in blood product usage with desmopressin. *J AM Coll Cardiol* **9:**1139–1147, 1987

90. Seear MD, Wadsworth LD, Rogers PC, et al: The effect of desmopressin acetate (DDAVP) on postoperative blood loss after cardiac operations in children. *J Thorac Cardiovasc Surg* **98:**217–219, 1989

91. Andersson TLG, Solem JO, Tengborn L, Vinge E: Effects of desmopressin acetate on platelet aggregation, von Willebrand factor, and blood loss after cardiac surgery with extracorporeal circulation. *Circulation* **81:**872–878, 1990

92. Hackmann T, Gascoyne RD, Naiman SC, et al: A trial of desmopressin (1-desamino-8-D-arginine vasopressin) to reduce blood loss in uncomplicated cardiac surgery. *N Engl J Med* **321:**1437–1443, 1989

93. Salzman EW, Weinstein MJ, Reilly D, Ware JA: Adventures in hemostasis: Desmopressin in cardiac surgery. *Arch Surg* **128:**212–217, 1993

94. Royston D, Bidstrup BP, Taylor KM, Sapsford RN: Effect of aprotinin on need for blood transfusions after repeat open heart surgery. *Lancet* **2:**1289–1291, 1987

95. Blauth C, Gross C, Necek S, et al: Effects of high-dose aprotinin on blood loss, platelet function, fibrinolysis, complement, and renal function after cardiopulmonary bypass. *J Thorac Cardiovasc Surg* **101:**958–967, 1991

96. Murkin JM, Lux J, Shannon NA, et al: Aprotinin significantly decreases bleeding and transfusion requirements in patients receiving aspirin and undergoing cardiac operations. *J Thorac Cardiovasc Surg* **107:**554–561, 1994

97. Bidstrup BP, Underwood SR, Sapsford RN, Streets EM: Effect of aprotinin (Trasylol) on aortocoronary bypass graft patency. *J Thorac Cardiovasc Surg* **105:**147–152, 1993

98. Cosgrove DM 3d, Heric B, Lytle BW, et al: Aprotinin therapy for reoperative myocardial revascularization: A placebo-controlled study. *Ann Thorac Surg* **54:**1031–1036, discussion 1036–1038, 1992

99. Jegaden O, Vedrinne C, Rossi R: Aprotinin does not compromise arterial graft patency in coronary bypass operations. *J Thorac Cardiovasc Surg* **106:**180–181, 1993

100. Lemmer JH, Stanford W, Bonney SL, et al: Aprotinin for cardiopulmonary bypass operations: Efficacy, safety, and influence on early saphenous vein graft patency. *J Thorac Cardiovasc Surg* **104:**543–553, 1994

101. McCarthy PM, Popovsky MA, Schaff HV, et al: Effect of blood conservation efforts in cardiac operations at the Mayo Clinic. *Mayo Clin Proc* **63:**225–229, 1988

102. Love TR, Hendren WG, OKeefe DD, Daggett WM: Transfusion of predonated autologous blood in elective cardiac surgery. *Ann Thorac Surg* **43:**508–512, 1987

103. Lewis CTP, Murphy MC, Cooley DA: Risk factors for cardiac operations in adult Jehovah's Witnesses. *Ann Thorac Surg* **51:**448–450, 1991

104. Hardy JF, Perrault J, Tremblay N, et al: The stratification of cardiac surgical procedures according to use of blood products: A retrospective analysis of 1480 cases. *Can J Anaesth* **38:**511–517, 1991

105. NIH Consensus Development Conference Statement: Perioperative red cell transfusion. *NIH* **7:**1–19, 1988

106. Lawler J: The structural and functional properties of thrombospondin. *Blood* **67:**1197–1209, 1986

107. Leung LL, Nachmann RL, Harpel PC: Complex formation of platelet thrombospondin with histidine-rich glycoprotein. *J Clin Invest* **73:**5–12, 1984

108. Aach RD, Kahn RA: Post-transfusion hepatitis; current perspectives. *Ann Intern Med* **92:**539, 1980

109. Progress on AIDS. *FDA Drug Bulletin* **15:**1985

110. CDC: Acquired immune deficiency syndrome (AIDS): Precautions for clinical and laboratory staffs. *MMWR* **31:**577, 1982

111. CDC: Acquired immunodeficiency syndrome (AIDS): Precautions for healthcare workers and allied professionals. *MMWR* **32:**450, 1983

112. Simon TL, Akl BF, Murphy W: Controlled trial of routine administration of platelet concentrates in cardiopulmonary bypass surgery. *Ann Thorac Surg* **37:**359–364, 1984

113. Sherry S, Marder VJ: Therapy with antifibrinolytic agents. In Colman RW, Hirsh J, Marder VJ, Salzman EW (eds): *Hemostasis and Thrombosis.* Philadelphia, J.B. Lippincott, 1994, pp 335–352

114. Massive transfusion in surgery and trauma. Proceedings of annual scientific symposium of the American Red Cross DC, May 6–7, 1982. *Prog Clin Biol Res* **108:**1–319, 1982

115. Counts RB, Haisch C, Simon TL, et al: Hemostasis in massively transfused trauma patients. *Ann Surg* **190:**91–99, 1979

116. Gaudiani VA, Mason DW: Preoperative erythropoietin in Jehovah's Witnesses who require cardiac procedures. *Ann Thorac Surg* **51:**823–824, 1991

117. Walls JT, Curtis JJ, Silver D, et al: Heparin-induced thrombocytopenia in open heart surgical patients: Sequelae of late recognition. *Ann Thorac Surg* **53:**787–791, 1992

118. Greinacher A, Pötzsch B, Amiral J, et al: Heparin-associated thrombocytopenia: Isolation of the antibody and characterization of a multimolecular PF4-heparin complex as the major antigen. *Thromb Haemost* **71:**247–251, 1994

119. Visentin GP, Ford SE, Scott JP, Aster RH: Antibodies from patients with heparin-induced thrombocytopenia/thrombosis are specific for platelet factor 4 complexed with heparin or bound to endothelial cells. *J Clin Invest* **93:**81–88, 1994

120. Laster JL, Nichols WK, Silver D: Thrombocytopenia associated with heparin-coated catheters in patients with heparin-associated antiplatelet antibodies. *Arch Intern Med* **149:**2285–2287, 1989

121. Murdoch IA, Beattie RM, Silver DM: Heparin-induced thrombocytopenia in children. *Acta Paediatr* **82:**495–497, 1993

122. Greinacher A, Michels I, Kiefel V, Mueller-Eckhardt C: A rapid and sensitive test for diagnosing heparin-associated thrombocytopenia. *Thromb Haemost* **66:**734–736, 1991

123. Olinger GN, Hussey CV, Olive JA, Malik MI: Cardiopulmonary bypass for patients with previously documented heparin-induced platelet aggregation. *J Thorac Cardiovasc Surg* **87:**673–677, 1984

124. Sobel M, Adelman B, Greenfield LJ: Dextran 40 reduces heparin-mediated platelet aggregation. *J Surg Res* **40:**382–387, 1986

125. Roland JG, Masade E, Serrano M, et al: Thrombocytopenia under low molecular weight heparin with fraxiparin dependent anti-platelet antibodies. *Therapie* **46:**498, 1991

126. Robitaille D, Leclerc JR, Laberge R, et al: Cardiopulmonary bypass with a low-molecular-weight heparin fraction (enoxaparin) in a patient with a history of heparin-associated thrombocytopenia. *J Thorac Cardiovasc Surg* **103:**597–599, 1992

127. Blockmans D, Bounameaux H, Vermylen J, Verstraete M: Heparin-induced thrombocytopenia: Platelet aggregation studies in the presence of heparin fractions or semi-synthetic analogues of various molecular weights and anticoagulant activities. *Thromb Haemost* **55:**90–93, 1986

128. Greinacher A, Drost W, Michels I, et al: Heparin-associated thrombocytopenia: Successful therapy with the heparinoid Org 10172 in a patient showing cross-reaction to LMW heparins. *Ann Hematol* **64:**40–42, 1992

129. Gouault-Heilmann M, Huet Y, Adnot S, et al: Low molecular weight heparin fractions as an alternative therapy in heparin-induced thrombocytopenia. *Haemostasis* **17:**134–140, 1987

130. Ortel TL, Gockerman JP, Califf RM, et al: Parenteral anticoagulation with the heparinoid lomoparan (Org 10172) in patients with heparin induced thrombocytopenia and thrombosis. *Thromb Haemost* **67:**292–296, 1992

131. Rowlings PA, Evans S, Mansberg R, et al: The use of a low molecular weight heparinoid (Org 10172) for extracorporeal procedures in patients with heparin dependent thrombocytopenia and thrombosis. *Aust NZ J Med* **21:**52–54, 1991

132. Makhoul RG, Greenberg CS, McCann RL: Heparin-associated thrombocytopenia and thrombosis: A serious clinical problem and potential solution. *J Vasc Surg* **4:**522–528, 1986

133. Hirsh J, Levine MN: Low molecular weight heparin. *Blood* **79**:1–17, 1992

134. Hirsh J: Overview of low molecular weight heparins and heparinoids: Basic and clinical aspects. *Aust NZ J Med* **22**:487–495, 1992

135. Lefkovits J, Topol EJ: Direct thrombin inhibitors in cardiovascular medicine. *Circulation* **90**:1522–1536, 1994

136. Johnson PH: HIRUDIN: Clinical potential of a thrombin inhibitor. *Annu Rev Med* **45**:165–177, 1994

137. Use of a monoclonal antibody directed against the platelet glycoprotein IIb/IIIa receptor in high-risk coronary angioplasty. The EPIC Investigation. *N Engl J Med* **330**:956–961, 1994

138. Mousa SA, Bozarth JM, Forsythe MS, et al: Antiplatelet and antithrombotic efficacy of DMP 728, a novel platelet GPIIb/IIIa receptor antagonist. *Circulation* **89**:3–12, 1994

139. Despotis GJ, Santoro SA, Spitznagel E, et al: On-site prothrombin time, activated partial thromboplastin time, and platelet count. A comparison between whole blood and laboratory assays with coagulation factor analysis in patients presenting for cardiac surgery. *Anesthesiology* **80**:338–351, 1994

140. Despotis GJ, Santoro SA, Spitznagel E, et al: Prospective evaluation and clinical utility of on-site monitoring of coagulation in patients undergoing cardiac operation. *J Thorac Cardiovasc Surg* **107**:271–279, 1994

141. Gulliver G: *The Works of William Hewson, P.R.S.* London, The Sydenham Society, 1846

142. Major RH: *Classic Descriptions of Disease.* Baltimore, Charles C Thomas, 1939

143. Hufnagel CA: Aortic plastic valvular prosthesis. *Bull Georgetown Univ Med Ctr* **4**:28, 1951

144. Berger S, Salzman EW: Thromboembolic complications of prosthetic devices. In Spaet T (ed): *Progress in Hemostasis and Thrombosis.* New York, Grune & Stratton, 1974

145. Hirsh JW, Dalen JE, Deykin D, Poller L: Oral anticoagulants; mechanism of action, clinical effectiveness, and optimal therapeutic range. *Chest* **102**:312S–326S, 1992

146. Hyers TM, Hull RD, Weg JG: Antithrombotic therapy for venous thromboembolic disease. *Chest* **102**:408S–425S, 1992

147. Cannegieter SC, Rosendaal FR, Briet E: Thromboembolic and bleeding complications in patients with mechanical heart valve prostheses. *Circulation* **89**:635–641, 1994

148. Stein PD Jr, Alpert JS, Copeland J, et al: Antithrombotic therapy in patients with mechanical and biologic prosthetic heart valves. *Chest* **102**:445S–455S, 1992

149. Jamieson WR: Modern cardiac valve devices-bioprostheses and mechanical prostheses: State of the art. *J Card Surg* **8**:89–98, 1993

150. Ginsberg JS, Hirsh J: Use of antithrombotic agents during pregnancy. *Chest* **102**:385S–390S, 1992

151. Ionescu MI, Smith DR, Sasan SS, et al: Clinical durability of the pericardial xenograft valve: Ten years experience with mitral replacement. *Ann Thorac Surg* **34**:265, 1982

152. Salazar E, Zajarias A, Gutierrez N, et al: The problem of cardiac valve prostheses, anticoagulants and pregnancy. *Circulation* **70**:169, 1984

153. Hellgren M, Nygards EB: Long-term therapy with subcutaneous heparin during pregnancy. *Gynecol Obstet Invest* **13**:76, 1982

154. FitzGibbon GM, Leach AJ, Keon W, et al: Coronary bypass graft fate. Angiographic study of 1,179 vein grafts early, one year, five years after operation. *J Thorac Cardiovasc Surg* **71**:773, 1986

155. Chesebro JH, Fuster V, Eleveback LR, et al: Effect of dipyridamole and aspirin on late vein-graft patency after coronary bypass operations. *N Engl J Med* **310**:209, 1984

156. Rajah SM, Salter MCP, Donaldson DR, et al: Acetylsalicylic acid and dipyridamole improve the early patency of aorta-coronary bypass grafts. *J Thorac Cardiovasc Surg* **90**:373, 1985

157. Laupacis A, Albers G, Dunn MI, Feinberg WM: Antithrombotic therapy in atrial fibrillation. *Chest* **102**:426s, 1992

158. Clagett GP, Graor RA, Salzman EW: Antithrombotic therapy in peripheral arterial occlusive disease. *Chest* **102**:516s–528s, 1992

159. Ameli FM: Aortobifemoral bypass-an enduring operation. *Can J Surg* **35**:237–241, 1992

160. Bearn PE, McCollum CN, Marston A: Prosthetic graft seeding: Breathing new life into old grafts. *J R Coll Surg Edinb* **39**:1–5, 1994

161. Welch M, Durrans D, Carr HM, et al: Endothelial cell seeding: a review. *Ann Vasc Surg* **6**:473–484, 1992

162. Stanley JC, Burkel WE, Graham LM, Lindblad B: Endothelial cell seeding of synthetic vascular prostheses. *Acta Chir Scand* [Suppl] **529**:17–27, 1985

C H A P T E R
110

Pulmonary Embolism

Stuart W. Jamieson

Pulmonary embolism was first described by Laennec in 1819.[1] He related the condition to deep venous thrombosis, and Virchow later associated the three factors predisposing to venous thrombosis as stasis, hypercoagulability, and vessel wall injury.[2] Although a great deal of progress has been made in the understanding of the pathophysiology of deep venous thrombosis and subsequent embolism, this remains today a significant cause of morbidity and mortality. Dalen and Alpert,[3] in 1975, calculated that pulmonary embolism resulted in 630,000 symptomatic episodes in the United States yearly, making it at the time about half as common as acute myocardial infarction, and three times as common as cerebral vascular accidents. It was also estimated that acute pulmonary embolism was the cause of approximately 200,000 deaths a year (the sole contributing cause of death in 100,000 and the major contributing cause in another 100,000) and as such was the third most frequent cause of death. The incidence of pulmonary hypertension due to chronic pulmonary embolism is much more difficult to establish, since a majority of patients can give no history of a deep vein thrombosis or pulmonary embolism, and the clinical picture is nonspecific until right heart failure becomes evident. However, it is likely that this entity is very much more common than is usually appreciated.

Although pulmonary embolism can be caused by tumors, septic emboli, vegetations, and foreign bodies, the overwhelming occurrence is due to venous thromboembolism.

ACUTE PULMONARY THROMBOEMBOLIC DISEASE

The majority of pulmonary thromboembolic episodes are silent, and it is not until the amount of embolic material is substantial that the patient becomes symptomatic. After an acute, major thromboembolic episode, approximately 10–20% of patients die within 48 hours. Most of the remaining patients resolve the emboli substantially by a variety of mechanisms. It is in the subgroup of patients who have a sudden fatal outcome, therefore (approximately 100,000 annually) that invasive therapy for acute pulmonary embolism might be considered.

Although the role of surgical therapy for the sequelae of *chronic* pulmonary emboli with resultant pulmonary hypertension is now well established, the appropriate treatment for acute pulmonary embolism remains unclear. There are several reasons for this. Many patients die from massive pulmonary embolism in the terminal phases of another illness which would make aggressive therapy unwise. For patients in whom invasive therapy is potentially indicated, there is very substantial difficulty in defining which patients will be unable to themselves deal with an acute massive pulmonary embolism, in the limited amount of time that presents itself for both diagnosis and treatment before death occurs.

The hemodynamic response to a large, sudden pulmonary embolus relates to a variety of factors, but most notably the size of the embolus, the degree of obstruction that it produces in the pulmonary vascular bed, and the underlying function of the lung that remains perfused. The degree of vascular obstruction is obviously related to the number of segmental arteries that are occluded, but also to prior pulmonary vascular capacitance. Thus the hemodynamic consequences are also a reflection of factors such as the age of the patient and any possible previous embolic events. The pre-existing status of the right ventricle that governs the forward flow will also be significant, and will be affected by factors such as the degree of right ventricular hypertrophy and the presence of coronary artery disease.

In addition to the mechanical factor of pulmonary artery obstruction, there are reflex and hormonal factors that can also increase pulmonary vascular resistance. Serotonin and other vasoactive amines are released from platelets attached to the thrombi,[4] and thus some patients with a relatively small embolus may have a seemingly disproportionate response to the degree of pulmonary vascular obstruction.

It has been demonstrated that in those without pre-existing cardiac or pulmonary disease, an obstruction of less than 20% of the pulmonary vascular bed results in minimal hemodynamic consequences. It is only when the acute pulmonary obstruction exceeds 50 to 60% of the pulmonary vascular bed that cardiac and pulmonary compensatory mechanisms are overcome, and cardiac output begins to fall. Right ventricular failure occurs, and this is accompanied by systemic hypotension as the amount of blood reaching the left ventricle decreases. The dilated right ventricle causes a shift of the ventricular septum to the left, further compromising left ventricular filling. Although patients with *chronic* pulmonary artery obstruction can present with high pulmonary artery pressures that reflect the degree of obstruction, in acute pulmonary embolism the previously normal right ventricle cannot generate these pressures. Therefore, in acute massive pulmonary embolism pulmonary artery pressures may be normal, and a pulmonary artery mean pressure of 30 to 40 mm Hg represents severe pulmonary hypertension.

The characteristic ventilatory response to acute pulmonary thromboembolism is hyperventilation, leading to hypocarbia (usually a pCO_2 less than 30 mm Hg).[4,5] In addition, there is a regional loss of pulmonary surfactant, leading to alveolar collapse. Hypoxemia therefore also occurs, due to a combination of ventilation–perfusion imbalance, anatomic venoarterial shunting, and impaired oxygen diffusion as a result of interstitial pulmonary edema.[6] Reflex hypoxic vasoconstriction also occurs in underperfused areas of the lung.

The clinical picture of acute pulmonary embolization is variable and the signs and symptoms nonspecific. The commonest symptoms are dyspnea and pleuritic chest pain. Cyanosis is present in less than 20% of patients. Routine laboratory tests are often normal. The most common electrocardiographic abnormalities are tachycardia and nonspecific ST- and T-wave changes. The major value of the ECG is in excluding a myocardial infarction. Chest x-ray may show oligemia (Westermark's sign) or linear atelectasis (Fleischner lines), but again these are also nonspecific. The chest radiograph, as with the ECG, is of greatest help in excluding other intrathoracic pathology. Thus although the majority of screening laboratory tests are nonspecific for the diagnosis, thromboembolism is the most likely diagnosis in the hypoxemic, hypocarbic patient with tachycardia.

Currently, the most useful screening test for stable patients suspected of having pulmonary thromboembolism is a lung scan. In this examination radioisotope-tagged macroaggregates of albumin injected intravascularly are distributed to regions of normal small vessel bloodflow. However, the images can be affected by the lung volume, counting sensitivity, and resolution rates of the imaging equipment. Additionally, a number of pulmonary disorders other than pulmonary embolus can also alter pulmonary perfusion, for instance external pulmonary vascular compression, as in pneumothorax or pleural effusion; pulmonary venous hypertension, as with mitral valve disease or left ventricular failure; alveolar hypoxia (pneumonia, bronchial tumors or plugs); vascular bed compression or destruction by emphysema, tumors, abscess, or atelectasis; and increased alveolar compression from asthma or positive pressure ventilation.

To improve the diagnostic accuracy rate of about 60%[7] with perfusion lung scanning, a ventilation scan may be helpful, by excluding a ventilatory disorder. However, it cannot always be assumed that a normal ventilation scan with an abnormal perfusion scan means a pulmonary embolism, because ventilation can be altered by the bronchoconstriction that may follow thromboembolism, as well as the atelectasis and pulmonary infarction that may also occur. More importantly, the group of patients in whom the diagnosis is most difficult to make—those with chronic lung disease, will likely have regional alterations in ventilation and perfusion, thus making a ventilation scan unhelpful.

The definitive test for pulmonary embolism is therefore pulmonary arteriography. The diagnosis is established when there are filling defects or obstruction of larger branches, other signs are irregular filling defects or "streaming" of contrast material. A CT scan may also be diagnostic.

PROPHYLAXIS

Although prophylactic measures should be considered or used for all patients undergoing major surgery, certain patients fall into a potentially high-risk group. These include patients with previous embolism, malignancy, cardiac failure, prolonged immobility, obesity, or advanced age.[8]

Dextran has been demonstrated to decrease the incidence of venous thrombosis in patients undergoing general or orthopedic surgery. It is known to act as a volume expander and to decrease platelet adhesiveness, but the optimal dose and duration of this therapy remain undefined, as does its exact mechanism of action.

Multiple studies have now shown that low-dose heparin administered subcutaneously is effective in reducing the incidence of postoperative venous thrombosis and fatal pulmonary embolism after major surgery. Five thousand units of calcium heparin are administered subcutaneously 2 hours before surgery and every 8 hours thereafter until the patient is ambulatory. This reduction in thrombosis is not associated with an excessive risk of bleeding.[9]

Intermittent pneumatic compression devices for the legs have also proved to provide effective prophylaxis for patients undergoing major surgery. These devices eliminate concern over any hemorrhagic risk associated with low-dose heparin, and are available for the calf or the whole leg. They can provide a range of compression pressures, inflation and deflation duration, and sequential or nonsequential inflation, though a clear difference between these variations has not been demonstrated.

Though the risk of pulmonary embolism is probably lower for patients undergoing open heart surgery than for general or orthopedic surgery (probably related to intraoperative heparinization), it is probably prudent to treat all thoracic surgery cases with prophylactic heparin and/or lower limb compression devices perioperatively.

SUPPORTIVE AND THROMBOLYTIC THERAPY

The majority of patients who die of massive pulmonary embolism do so within 2 hours of the initial acute event, before the diagnosis can be firmly established, and obviously before effective therapy can be instituted. Once the diagnosis is made, treatment will either be medical (supportive and thrombolytic therapy) or surgical.

Oxygen should be administered to alleviate hypoxic pulmonary vasoconstriction, and it is likely that a severely affected patient will require intubation and ventilatory support. There is debate as to whether pulmonary artery catheters, though obviously helpful in management, should be used in this setting because of the risk of dislodging further thrombotic material. Inotropic and vasoconstrictive support may be used with caution. Patients should be heparinized to prevent further propagation of thrombus at its origin and also in the pulmonary artery. Heparin also acts to block the release of vasoactive and bronchoconstrictor substances at the site of an embolism.

The natural history of survivors of acute embolic events is survival through fragmentation and progressive lysis of embolic material. It would therefore seem logical that the use of agents that increase the rate of thrombolysis would be helpful. Although a definite improvement in survival has not yet been demonstrated with thrombolytic therapy, this probably reflects the difficulty of obtaining sufficient patients to provide a reasonable sample size. However, early hemodynamic benefits have been shown in individual patients, and there is growing evidence that thrombolytic therapy can rapidly improve hemodynamic abnormalities and may reverse the downward spiral of right ventricular function as assessed by echocardiography.[10,11]

Urokinase may be given with a loading dose of 4,400 unit/kg followed by 4,400 unit/kg per hour, or streptokinase may be used (250,000 unit loading dose followed by 100,000 units/h). Some trials have used recombinant tissue-type plasminogen activator (rt-PA) in the treatment of massive pulmonary embolism, though the optimal dose and duration of infusion have not been clearly established. Regimens have included 50 to 100 mg of rt-PA infused over a period of 2 to 6 hours.[12]

ACUTE PULMONARY EMBOLECTOMY

There is no indication for acute pulmonary embolectomy in a patient who is likely to survive, since with time the patient's own lytic mechanisms will resolve the emboli. The primary difficulty with the broad application of operative embolectomy is that it is almost impossible to determine which patients will die without intervention. Obviously, an embolectomy is most feasible (because of the time factor) and most successful in patients who ultimately may not require it, and this makes it difficult to establish the efficacy of the therapy. However, to delay emergency surgical intervention in a patient who otherwise will have a fatal outcome obviously will make this outcome certain. Patients referred for surgical therapy must therefore be in critical hemodynamic condition, and the diagnosis must be established with certainty. Unstable patients in whom thrombolytic therapy is absolutely contraindicated should also be considered for surgical intervention.

Acute pulmonary embolectomy was first described by Trendelenburg in 1908[13] using pulmonary artery and aortic occlusion, through a transthoracic approach. There were no surviving patients. Sharp performed the first successful open embolectomy, using cardiopulmonary bypass.[14]

Although this operation may still be performed with in-flow occlusion and normothermia, in centers with the appropriate facilities, cardiopulmonary bypass should be used. A median sternotomy is employed and the heart exposed. Tapes are placed around the superior and inferior vena cavae. After initiation of bypass a longitudinal incision is made in the main pulmonary artery trunk. The emboli are extracted using forceps, suction, and a balloon catheter. It may be necessary to briefly clamp the aorta for better exposure to the distal pulmonary vasculature. The aim of this operation is to remove most of the embolic material, and no attempt is made to perform an endarterectomy or to unnecessarily proceed distally into the segmental or subsegmental vessels. The balloon catheter may be passed blindly down the distal segmental branches. However, when using a balloon catheter, great caution must be exercised, since excessive inflation could traumatize or rupture the pulmonary vessels.

The mortality for acute pulmonary embolectomy has ranged from 10 to 80% in various reported series. The mortality in patients who have not suffered a cardiac arrest is considerably better than in those who have, though as mentioned above, this probably reflects a different subpopulation. Results reported by three separate groups[15–17] show a mortality rate of 10 to 20% in those who have not sustained a cardiac arrest, and over 60% in those who have.

CATHETER REMOVAL OF EMBOLI

The difficulty of establishing those patients in whom surgical therapy will be effective, and the time factor involved in stabilizing a patient to be brought to the operating room, means that a procedure in the catheterization laboratory after establishing the diagnosis might be particularly useful. Because simply relieving a proportion of pulmonary vascular obstruction is effective in the surgical setting, it has seemed reasonable to try and do this with a percutaneous catheter device. In 1971, Greenfield and co-workers reported the successful treatment of acute massive pulmonary embolism in two patients using an embolectomy catheter device.[18] In a later paper they reported significant clot extraction in 23 out of 26 patients with an in-hospital mortality rate of 27%.[19] More recently, Timsit and co-workers reported their results in eighteen patients.[20] Although hemodynamic data in the report are limited, thrombus extraction was successful in 11 patients (61%). Overall mortality was 28%, 11% in whom thrombus extraction was successful and 43% in those in whom it was not.

An alternative to catheter embolectomy is to attempt to fragment and distally disperse centrally occluding emboli using standard cardiac catheters. This has been tried both experimentally[21] and clinically,[22] with apparent success. However, again, it is difficult to compare the final outcome in all these cases with a group in whom continued conservative therapy had been applied.

CAVAL INTERRUPTION AND WARFARIN THERAPY

Regardless of whether an interventional approach has been used, when the patient is stable a vena caval filter should be placed if there are factors that might predispose to repetitive events or in the presence of chronic pulmonary embolism with pulmonary hypertension.

Although early techniques of vena caval interruption included surgical division or plication, transvenous filter placement is now preferred. A transvenous approach under local anesthesia was first proposed by Eichelter and Schenk,[23] who designed a catheter for temporary protection against embolism. This was then followed by permanent devices for caval narrowing such as the Pate clip,[24] total occlusion of the vena cava with a balloon,[25] or for more gradual occlusion with an umbrella device.[26]

The cone-shaped Greenfield filter[27] can be filled to 75% of its depth without impairment of bloodflow (Fig. 110–1), and long-term results with this filter show a patency rate of 97%, and a recurrent embolism rate of 5%. This is currently the device of choice.

Warfarin therapy is begun; the overlap of warfarin therapy with cessation of heparin should be at least 5 days. The recommendation for continuation of warfarin therapy is for 4 months, but this probably should be extended for patients with continuing predisposing factors, pulmonary hypertension, or a history of recurrent thromboembolism.

CHRONIC PULMONARY THROMBOEMBOLIC DISEASE

The true incidence of pulmonary hypertension due to chronic thromboembolic disease is difficult to determine. Of the over 600,000 cases of massive acute thromboembolism in the United States annually there are more than 500,000 survivors.[3,28,29] In addition, there are perhaps 3- to 4-fold more patients who have thromboembolic episodes that remain undiagnosed. Although the majority of these patients resolve their emboli substantially, if not completely, some patients fail to do so, and present with pro-

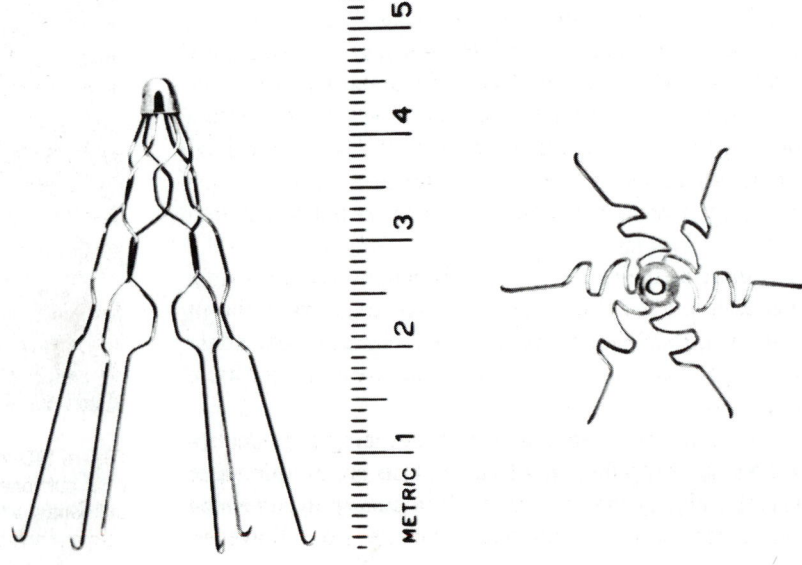

Figure 110–1. The Greenfield filter. It was designed to allow filling to 75% of its depth without interference with bloodflow. It can be inserted via either the jugular or femoral vein, and traps emboli 3 mm in diameter or larger, as seen in the axial view.

gressive pulmonary hypertension. Because of the difficulty in making the diagnosis, the absolute number of these patients is obscure, but probably is well in excess of 10,000 patients per year. Whether the failure to resolve embolic material is a result of abnormalities of clotting and lytic mechanisms, or repetitive emboli, or both, remains unclear. Studies of the pulmonary vascular endothelium in affected patients have failed to demonstrate abnormalities.

The prognosis for patients with chronic pulmonary hypertension due to thromboembolic disease is poor, and is proportional to the degree of hypertension. Riedel et al[30] followed 147 patients with serial right heart studies and pulmonary arteriograms, and found that those with mean pulmonary artery pressures over 30 mm Hg had a 30% 5-year survival rate; those with pressures over 50 mm Hg experienced a 10% survival at 5 years.

Medical therapy for this condition, using anticoagulants, vasodilators, or thrombolytic agents, does not affect the prognosis.[31,32] An important aspect of the pulmonary circulation, however, is that pulmonary embolization uncommonly results in tissue necrosis because of the bronchial circulation. Surgical endarterectomy thus will allow distal pulmonary tissue to be used once more in gas exchange.[33]

DIAGNOSTIC TESTS IN CHRONIC THROMBOEMBOLIC PULMONARY HYPERTENSION

The clinical presentation of chronic pulmonary embolism is often insidious. It is not until the late stages of the disease, and when over 50% of the pulmonary vasculature has been occluded, that the patient becomes symptomatic. Further, the two major symptoms, effort dyspnea and fatigue, are very nonspecific. Other symptoms that may occur, usually in the later stages of the disease, include exertional chest pain, cough, and hemoptysis.

Although it is estimated that at least 90% of thromboembolic material results from a deep venous thrombosis, less than half the patients with thromboembolic pulmonary hypertension can give a history of deep venous thrombosis or pulmonary embolism. The clinical history may therefore not be helpful, but predisposing causes for deep venous thrombosis should be sought, as should a history of leg swelling or anything to indicate episodes of pulmonary embolism.

Clinical examination is usually nonproductive if right heart failure has not occurred. One specific sign is that of flow murmurs,[33] heard especially over the back, due either to flow through stenotic pulmonary arteries, or aggressive bronchial flow.

Routine studies such as the chest radiograph, electrocardiogram, and pulmonary function tests are of little value in differentiating thromboembolic pulmonary hypertension from other forms of pulmonary hypertension. However,

these investigations often give the initial clues that pulmonary hypertension exists when the physical findings are less conclusive.

The radiographic signs of pulmonary hypertension on chest x-ray may be difficult to determine. Enlargement of the pulmonary artery and paucity of flow to the pulmonary vascular bed may indicate occlusion of major vessels. The typical appearance of an enlarged heart, enlarged main pulmonary artery shadow, and enlarged peripheral pulmonary arteries is shown in Figures 110–2 and 110–3. The lateral view shows the cardiac shadow close to the sternum as a result of right ventricular hypertrophy.

Echocardiography demonstrates enlarged right-sided heart chambers and varying degrees of tricuspid regurgitation. Standard two-dimensional echocardiography is also helpful in defining the presence and severity of pulmonary hypertension and excluding certain other causes such as Eisenmenger's syndrome. Continuous-wave Doppler of the tricuspid regurgitant jet is helpful in estimating the pulmonary artery systolic pressure.[34] Sometimes it is possible to visualize proximal, chronic, organized thrombus in the main pulmonary artery or main right and left pulmonary arteries with transthoracic echocardiography, but this technique lacks sensitivity and is inadequate for visualization of the lobar vessels, where the embolic material may be local-

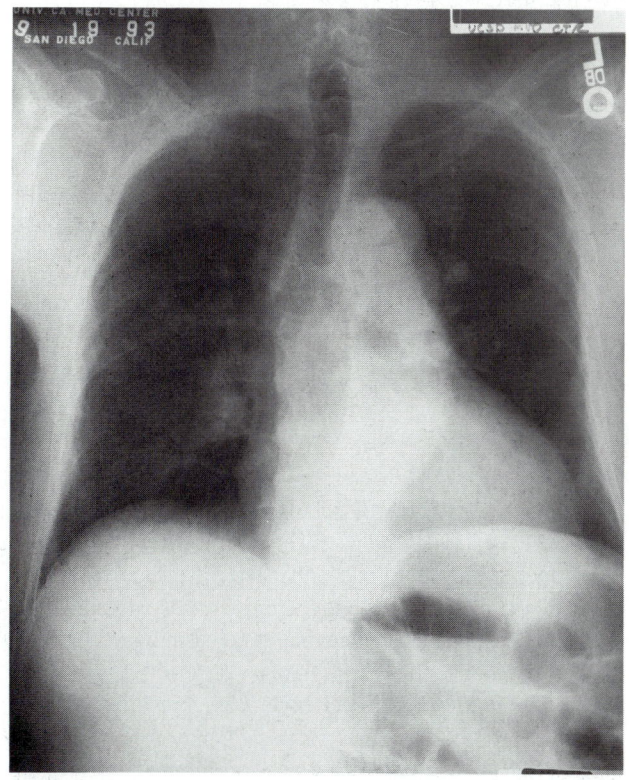

Figure 110–2. A typical x-ray in a patient with chronic thromboembolic pulmonary hypertension. PA view. Note the enlarged pulmonary artery shadow, some cardiomegaly, and enlarged hilar pulmonary artery shadows.

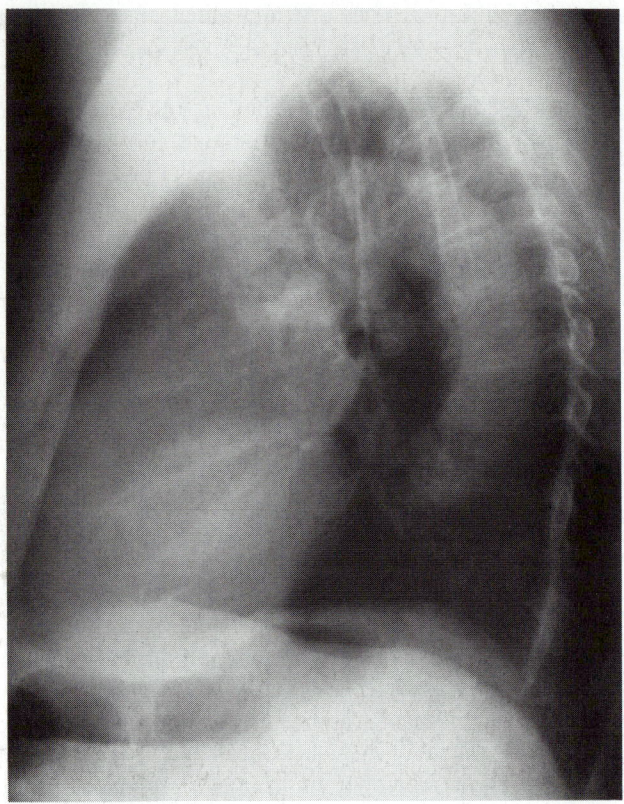

Figure 110–3. Same patient as in Figure 110–2. Chest x-ray—lateral view. Right ventricular enlargement with the anterior border of the heart close to the sternum.

ized. Transesophageal echocardiography has proven to be more promising, especially with newer multiplane probes that allow angulation of the imaging plane so that the origin of most of the lobar vessels can be identified. Early attempts are being carried out at visualizing the pulmonary arteries with transbronchial echocardiography.

A perfusion scan may be helpful. The major differential diagnosis is that of primary pulmonary hypertension, where the scan is usually normal, or has a patchy and mottled appearance, in contrast to the multiple punched-out lobar or segmental defects of chronic thromboembolic disease (Fig. 110–4). However, the perfusion scan tends to underestimate the degree of occlusion of the pulmonary vessels. A CT scan may be useful[35] and recent work has been performed using computer-enhanced images of CT scanning, both in the acute and chronic forms of this condition.[36] These images are capable of confirming occlusion in at least the main and lobar pulmonary arteries.

Once pulmonary hypertension as a result of chronic thromboembolic disease is suspected, the specific evaluation of the patient prior to planning surgical intervention hinges upon right heart catheterization and pulmonary angiography. Pulmonary angiography remains the "gold standard" for assessing the operative risk and surgical accessibility.[37] The classical signs of disease on pulmonary

angiography include an irregular lumen, indicating thrombus attached to the vessel wall, the appearances of bands or webs across the lumen of vessels, sometimes with poststenotic dilatation, and occlusion of branches with lack of filling out to the periphery, often with an abrupt termination of pulmonary vessels with a pouch-like appearance (Figs. 110–5 and 110–6).

Despite previous reports that pulmonary angiography is a high-risk procedure, we have found this not to be the case. Selective power injections of the right and left pulmonary trunks using nonionic contrast agents to prevent the cough response are well tolerated. In addition to pulmonary angiography, patients over 35 undergo coronary arteriography, and other cardiac investigation as necessary. If significant disease is found, additional cardiac surgery is performed at the time of pulmonary thromboendarterectomy.

In approximately 20% of cases, the differential diagnosis between primary pulmonary hypertension and distal and small vessel pulmonary thromboembolic disease remains unclear. In these patients pulmonary angioscopy has been found to be helpful.[38]

The pulmonary angioscope (Fig. 110–7) is a fiberoptic telescope that is advanced through central line access into the pulmonary artery. The tip contains a balloon that is then filled with saline and pushed against the vessel wall (Fig. 110–8). In this way a bloodless field can be obtained for visualization of the pulmonary artery wall.

The hallmark of pulmonary embolic disease by pulmonary angioscopy is the appearance of intimal thickening, with intimal irregularity including scarring and webs across small vessels. These webs are thought to be the residua of resolved occluding thrombi of small vessels, but are diagnostic of the presence of embolic disease. Occlusion of vessels or the presence of thrombotic material is diagnostic.

The thrombotic state of the patient is also evaluated. Abnormalities such as lupus anticoagulant, protein C deficiency, or antithrombin III deficiency are found in approximately 10% of patients. In addition, some patients with a paradoxical response to heparin have been identified. In such cases, special precautions must be taken during the perioperative period with the use of prostacyclin during cardiopulmonary bypass.

HISTORY OF SURGICAL THERAPY

Surgery for the chronic form of pulmonary embolism was first performed in 1951.[39] This was largely accidental, when a patient suspected of a pulmonary aneurysm was treated by pneumonectomy. Pulmonary thromboendarterectomy for pulmonary hypertension due to chronic pulmonary thromboembolism was suggested by Hollister and Cull[40] and the first planned pulmonary endarterectomy was performed in 1957.[41] The patient was operated upon using inflow occlusion and systemic hypothermia. The patient died, being unable to recover from cardiac arrest at the time of in-

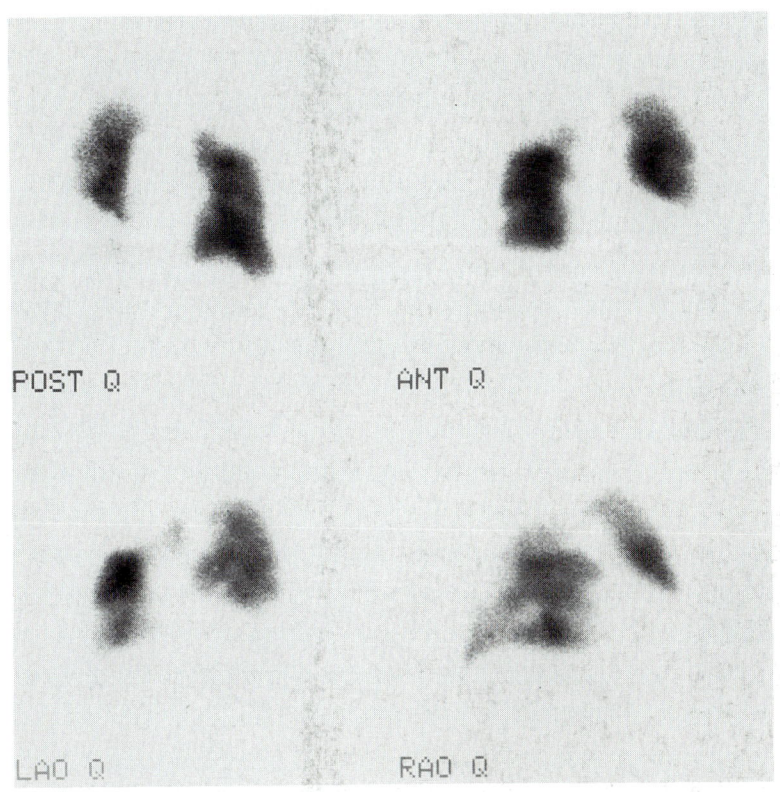

Figure 110–4. Perfusion scan—same patient. The typical punched-out defects due to lack of segmental pulmonary artery flow are shown.

flow occlusion. In 1958 Allison performed the first successful endarterectomy, again using inflow occlusion.[42] A right thoracotomy approach was used by Snyder et al[43] in 1963 in a 71-year-old man initially operated on for a suspected tumor. In the same year Houk and his associates[44] also reported a thromboendarterectomy through a thoracotomy approach, thus beginning the San Diego experience.

Cardiopulmonary bypass for this operation was used in 1964 by Castleman et al[45] and several other cases using either thoracotomy or median sternotomy with bypass were later reported over the next 20 years. In 1984 Chitwood et al[46] reviewed the world's literature and found 85 cases managed surgically, with a mortality of 22%.

Though there have been occasional other case reports, particularly from the groups at Duke University[46] and La Pitie Hospital in Paris,[47] the majority of the subsequent surgical experience in pulmonary thromboendarterectomy has been reported from the UCSD medical center.[48,49]

CURRENT STATUS OF PULMONARY THROMBOENDARTERECTOMY

Surgical therapy for pulmonary hypertension is possible whenever the etiology of the disease is thromboembolic. Over 500 operations for chronic pulmonary hypertension due to emboli have now been performed at the University of California San Diego (UCSD).

Specific preoperative evaluation of patients includes right heart catheterization and pulmonary angiography. Pulmonary artery pressures are confirmed, and the pulmonary artery anatomy examined, as outlined above. In cases where residual doubt exists, pulmonary angioscopy is then performed. Aside from the establishment of the diagnosis, the decision for operation will be made on the general condition of the patient, and the severity of symptoms. Patients accepted for surgery typically include those who have chronic thrombi judged to be surgically accessible, the absence of significant comorbid disease, and a pulmonary vascular resistance over 300 dyn/s per cm^{-5}.

None of these criteria is absolute. As the surgical experience has continued to grow, patients have been accepted for surgery with more distal thromboembolic disease, and with advanced (though presumed reversible) hepatic and renal dysfunction due to right-sided cardiac failure. Occasional patients have had a pulmonary vascular resistance below 300 dyn/s per cm^{-5}. These have been young patients with total unilateral pulmonary artery occlusion and unacceptable exertional dyspnea. The ages of the patients have ranged from 15 to 81 years.

An inferior vena cava filter is always placed prior to surgery unless an obvious upper extremity or cardiac (e.g., intraventricular pacing wire, ventriculoatrial shunt) source is present. In the latter case, removal of any foreign material is undertaken, with alternative sites used, as with replacement of intravascular pacing leads with epicardial electrodes. Patients are treated with warfarin until the time of surgery and this is continued lifelong after surgery.

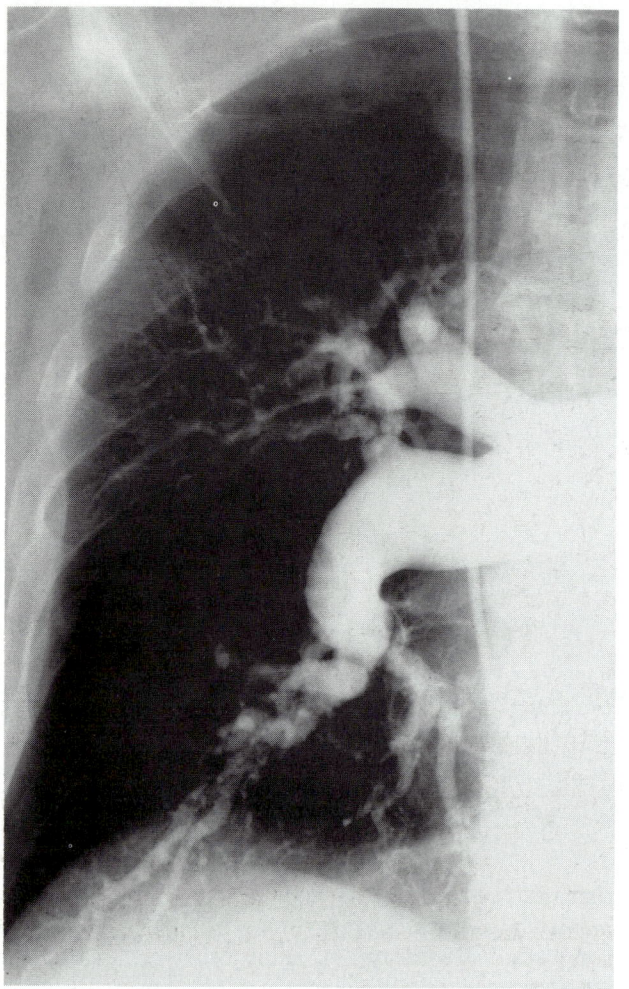

Figure 110–5. Typical right-sided angiogram—same patient. The middle and lower lobe arteries show a web, with some poststenotic dilatation. Some lateral branches are completely absent. There is distal disease in the right upper lobe (compare to specimen removed at surgery—Fig. 110–9).

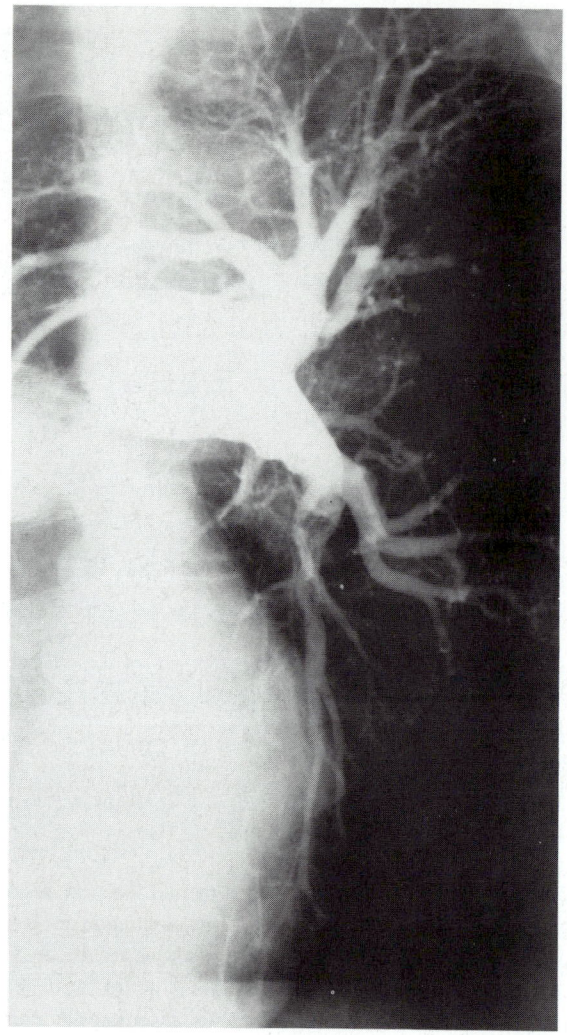

Figure 110–6. Typical left-sided angiogram—same patient. The left upper lobe shows predominantly good filling. The lower lobe artery shows an irregular lumen suggestive of clot. There is lack of filling with contrast to the periphery in the middle and lower lung fields (compare to specimen removed at surgery—Fig. 110–9).

The surgical procedure of pulmonary thromboendarterectomy has gradually evolved from a unilateral approach using a thoracotomy to a bilateral approach through a median sternotomy and using cardiopulmonary bypass. Other changes have been made to improve operative exposure and to minimize ischemic, bypass, and circulatory arrest times.

The operation of pulmonary thromboendarterectomy must be bilateral. This is an important concept, but one not always appreciated. Obviously, for pulmonary hypertension to be a major factor, both pulmonary arteries must be substantially involved, since a patient with a pneumonectomy is not necessarily pulmonary hypertensive. In chronic pulmonary embolism the right ventricle is hypertrophied, and pulmonary hypertension, even to suprasystemic levels, is

possible. A unilateral approach without bypass is therefore also more likely to result in an unstable intraoperative course, particularly after clamping one pulmonary artery.

The only reasonable approach to both pulmonary arteries is through a median sternotomy incision. Further, to define an adequate endarterectomy plane and to then follow the pulmonary endarterectomy specimen all the way out into the subsegmental vessels very good visibility is required, in a bloodless field. Therefore, cardiopulmonary bypass is required, with the institution of profound hypothermia and circulatory arrest.

The patient is prepared as for any open heart procedure, with arterial and pulmonary artery pressure, and EEG monitoring. However, a femoral artery line is also placed because the profound vasoconstriction that tends to occur

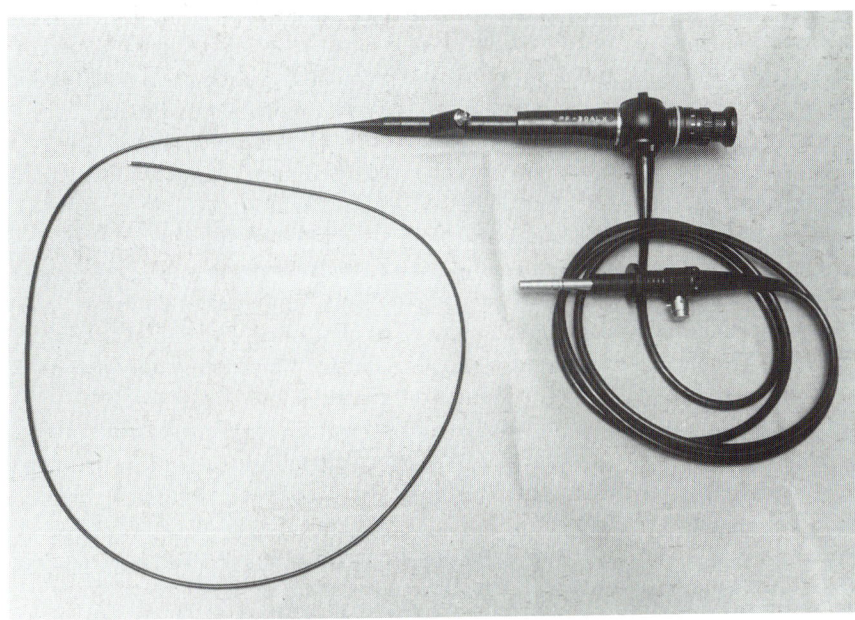

Figure 110–7. The pulmonary angioscope.

after hypothermic circulatory arrest makes readings from the radial artery catheter unreliable during the immediate postoperative course.

A median sternotomy incision is made and the sternum divided. Bypass is instituted with high ascending aortic cannulation and two caval cannulae. Standard flow for cardiopulmonary perfusion is used, and the patient cooled, maintaining a 10°C gradient between arterial blood and bladder or rectal temperature.[50]

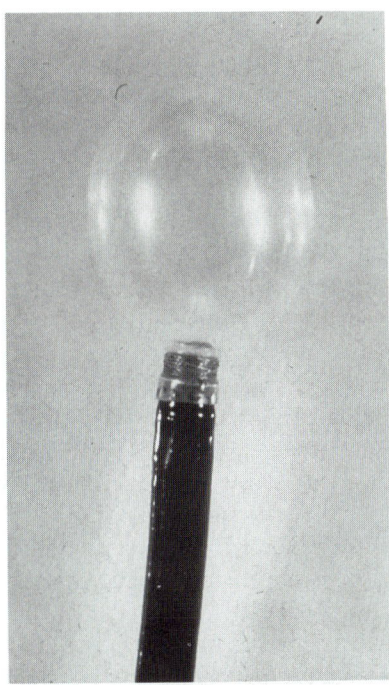

Figure 110–8. The balloon at the tip of the angioscope is filled with saline and pushed against the vessel wall.

The patient's head is packed in ice and the cooling blanket turned on. During perfusion the venous saturations increase; saturations of 80% at 25°C and 90% at 20°C are typical. Hemodilution is carried out to decrease the blood viscosity during hypothermia and to optimize capillary bloodflow; the hematocrit is maintained in the range of 18–25 during profound hypothermia. Phenytoin is administered IV during cooling at 15 mg/kg, to a maximum dose of 1 g.

A temporary pulmonary artery vent is inserted. As soon as the heart fibrillates, a further vent is placed in the left atrium through the right upper pulmonary vein. Exuberant bronchial arterial bloodflow is the rule with these patients. During the cooling period, preliminary dissection can be carried out, with full mobilization of the ascending aorta, and the superior vena cava. The superior vena cava is mobilized all the way to the innominate vein, and dissected free of the right pulmonary artery. The attachment of the right pulmonary artery to the left atrium is also divided. Most of this dissection is performed with electrocautery since with advanced right heart failure and hepatic congestion coagulation is usually abnormal. However, care must be taken to preserve the integrity of the right phrenic nerve lying lateral to the superior vena cava. All dissection of the pulmonary arteries occurs intrapericardially, and in the normal way neither pleural cavity is entered.

The right pulmonary artery is now exposed so that the take-off of upper and middle lobes can be seen. The upper pulmonary vein is usually not visualized, but reflected upward from the plane of the pulmonary artery wall. An incision is made in the right pulmonary artery from beneath the ascending aorta out under the superior vena cava and entering the lower lobe branch of the pulmonary artery just after the takeoff of the middle lobe. It is important that the incision stays in the center of the vessel. Only one incision is needed, and it is easier to endarterectomize the right upper lobe from a central incision than through a separate incision in the upper lobe artery. The distal limit of the lower lobe pulmonary artery incision is dictated by the accessibility required to repair this subsequently.

Any loose thrombus is now removed, and if the bronchial circulation is not excessive, the endarterectomy plane can be found. However, although a small amount of dissection can be carried out prior to the initiation of circulatory arrest, it is unwise to proceed unless perfect visibility is obtained. Surgical therapy for chronic thromboembolic pulmonary hypertension involves not only an embolectomy of chronic laminated thrombus where this is present, but a true endarterectomy of the pulmonary arterial bed. It is most important to recognize that first, embolectomy without endarterectomy is quite ineffective, and second, that in 90% of patients with chronic thromboembolic hypertension, direct examination of the pulmonary vascular bed at operation shows no obvious embolic material. Thus, to the inexperienced or cursory glance, the pulmonary vascular bed may appear normal.

When the patient's temperature reaches 20°C the aorta is cross-clamped and a single dose of cold cardioplegic solution administered. Additional myocardial protection is obtained by the use of a cooling jacket. The entire procedure is carried out with a single aortic cross-clamp period with no further administration of cardioplegic solution. After cross-clamping of the aorta thiopental is administered (500 mg to 1 g) until the EEG becomes isoelectric. When circulatory arrest is initiated, all monitoring lines to the patient are turned off, and the patient exsanguinated. The endarterectomy plane is then developed, and the endarterectomy specimen is progressively followed all the way to the subsegmental vessels. Each lobe is endarterectomized, and

then each segmental and subsegmental artery pursued distally. Although many of these vessels cannot be seen initially, progressive dissection and traction allow a complete endarterectomy of the entire pulmonary vascular bed (Figs. 110–9, 110–10, and 110–11). It is important that each subsegmental branch is followed and freed individually until it ends in a "tail."

Circulatory arrest periods are limited to 20 min, followed by, if necessary, a reperfusion period. Reperfusion is carried out at 18°C until the venous saturations reach 90%, or for a minimum of 10 min. However, with experience it is found that the entire unilateral endarterectomy can be performed within a 20-min circulatory arrest period.

When the endarterectomy on the right side has been completed, reperfusion is established, and the pulmonary arteriotomy repaired, using a running suture of polypropylene. Hemostasis of the suture line is absolutely necessary, as visualization of the distal incision can be obtained later only with the reinstitution of circulatory arrest.

Attention is now turned to the left side, and an incision made from the main pulmonary artery down, again intrapericardially, to the takeoff of the left upper lobe. Any loose thrombus is removed and an endarterectomy under profound hypothermia with circulatory arrest again carried out. The most difficult part of this operation on the left side is that of the left lower lobe, which proceeds posterior to the left bronchus, thus making visibility more difficult. Progressive traction and freeing of each segmental branch make this possible (Fig. 110–10).

After the completion of the endarterectomy, cardiopulmonary bypass is reinstituted and warming commenced. Methylprednisolone (500 mg) is administered IV, and during warming a 10°C temperature gradient is maintained between the perfusate and body temperature. If the systemic

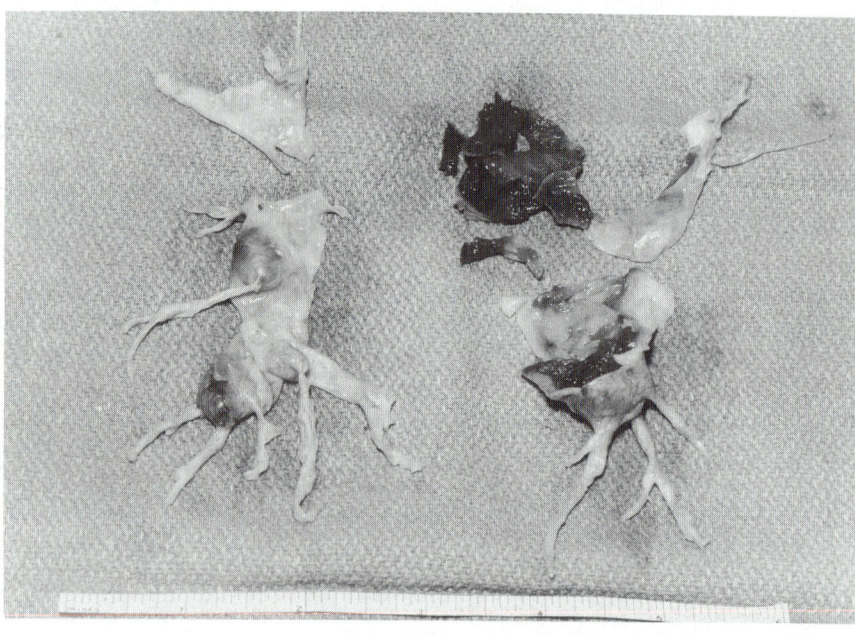

Figure 110–9. The specimen removed at surgery in the patient depicted in Figures 110–1 to 110–6.

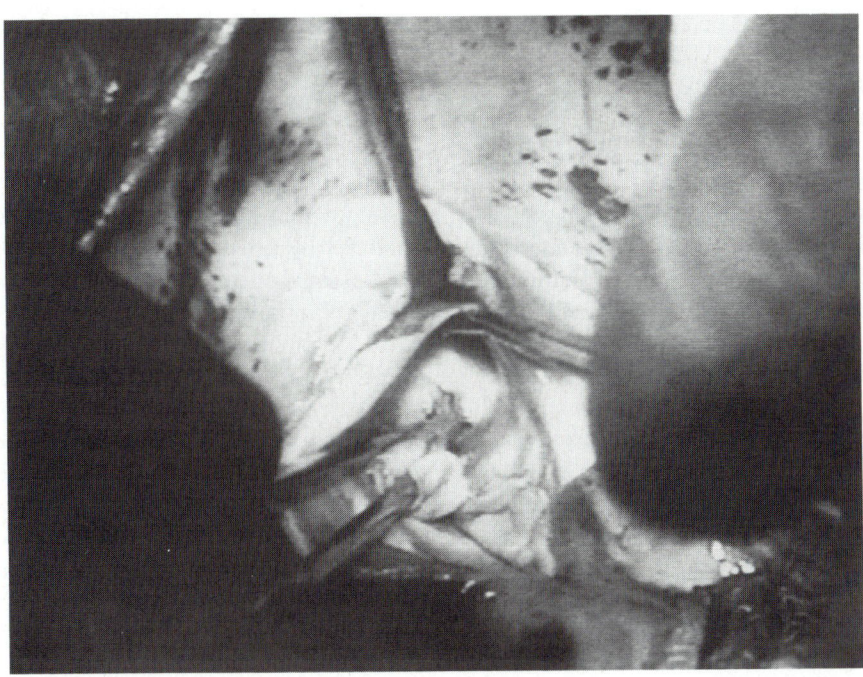

Figure 110–10. An operative view of the endarterectomy of the left lower lobe. Good visibility is obtained, even though the endarterectomy is now being carried out at the subsegmental level of the left lower lobe. Note the clear and bloodless field.

vascular resistance is high nitroprusside is administered to promote vasodilatation and warming. The rewarming period generally takes about 90 min, but varies according to the body mass of the patient.

The left pulmonary arteriotomy is repaired. The right atrium is then examined to remove any incidental thrombus and to close an atrial-septal defect or persistent foramen ovale if this is present. This is important since if pulmonary pressures do not immediately return to normal right-to-left shunting may contribute to postoperative hypoxemia. Although tricuspid valve regurgitation is invariable in these

patients, and is often severe, tricuspid valve repair is not performed. Right ventricular remodeling occurs within a few days[51] with return of tricuspid competence.

If other cardiac procedures are required, such as coronary artery or mitral or aortic valve surgery, these are conveniently performed during the systemic rewarming period.

Wound closure is routine, though both atrial and ventricular pacing wires are left in situ, and an additional posterior pericardial Jackson-Pratt drain left for 5–7 days because of the high incidence of late pericardial effusions in these patients.

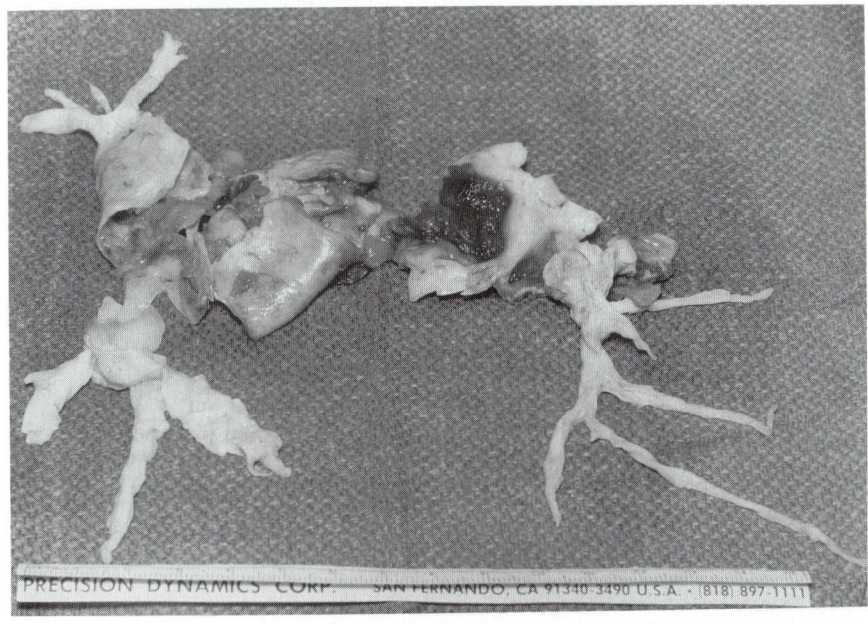

Figure 110–11. The specimen obtained from operation shown in Figure 110–10. Distal specimen on the left is 15 cm from the initial endarterectomy plane.

POSTOPERATIVE MANAGEMENT

As is the case with preoperative assessment, careful postoperative management is pivotal to a successful outcome. Although almost all patients have immediate resolution of high pulmonary artery pressures, some patients may have residual high resistance of the pulmonary vascular bed (usually patients with long-standing chronic thromboembolic disease), which resolves after about 24 hours. In addition, many patients develop some degree of reperfusion pulmonary edema. This is now seen in a distinct minority of patients, probably a result of the more complete and expeditious removal of the endarterectomy specimen that has come with a large experience over the last few years. Reperfusion edema is limited to the areas of the lung from which obstruction has been removed (Fig. 110–12).

Reperfusion pulmonary edema varies in severity from a mild form of edema seen commonly, to an acute and fatal complication seen in 1 or 2% of cases. However, some degree of postoperative hypoxemia is common from this complication. The areas of alveolar edema involve the segments of lung that are endarterectomized, and are now preferentially perfused. Blood is therefore diverted away from previously normal areas ("steal"), to those not contributing to oxygenation. In addition, the resulting hypoxemia results in pulmonary vasoconstriction, thus worsening the situation. Meticulous ventilatory management is thus required, together with very careful management of fluid balance. An aggressive diuresis should be instituted, and the hematocrit kept high to minimize an alveolar capillary leak. The patient's ventilatory status may be dramatically position-sensitive. Because this complication resolves with time, management hinges on adequate support until this occurs.

RESULTS

Over 500 patients have now been operated on for chronic thromboembolic pulmonary hypertension at the University of California Medical Center, the majority since 1990. The overall mortality (30 days or in-hospital if hospital course is prolonged) was 9% for the entire patient group. This encompasses a time span of 20 years, and during the early experience with this procedure mortality was related to many causes, including myocardial infarction, bilateral phrenic nerve paralysis, pulmonary hemorrhage, and sepsis. Of 196 patients operated on from July 1970 to December 1989, the mortality was 15%, with no appreciable change over the years. A change in the operative method, as described above, was instituted in 1990.[49] Since this time the mortality rate has been 5.7% in 315 patients, and 4% for the last 200 patients.

Residual causes of mortality are operation upon patients in whom thromboembolic disease was not the cause of the pulmonary hypertension, and the rare case of reperfusion pulmonary edema that progresses to a respiratory distress syndrome of long standing that is not reversible.

Long-term results show persistent hemodynamic and respiratory improvement.[52] The New York Heart Association (NYHA) functional classification improves markedly, with the majority of patients changing from NYHA III or IV to NYHA I functional status.

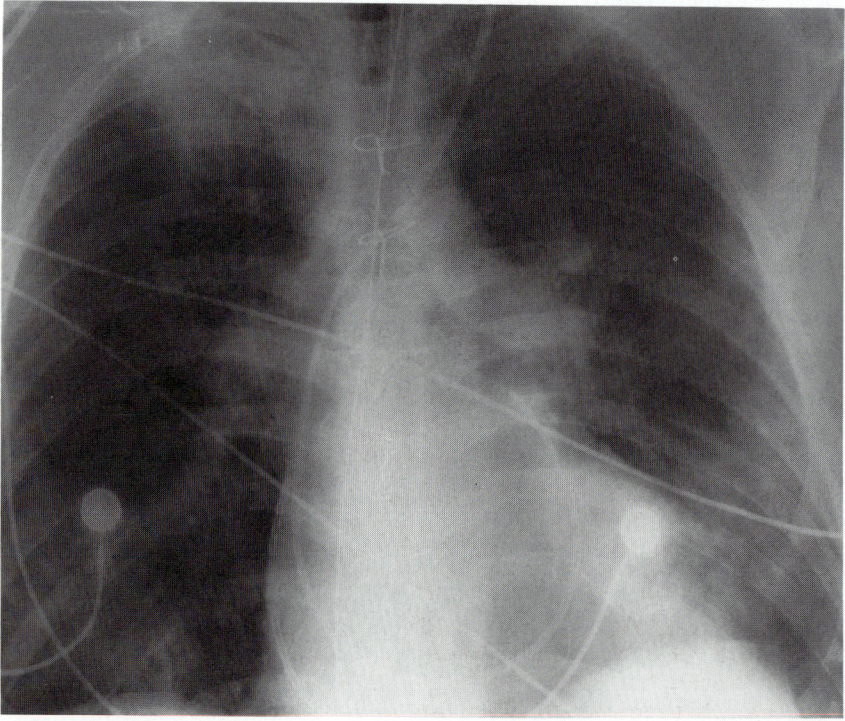

Figure 110–12. The postoperative chest x-ray in patient shown in Figures 110–10 and 110–11. Note reperfusion injury in areas supplied by right upper and lower, and left lower lobe arteries—those endarterectomized.

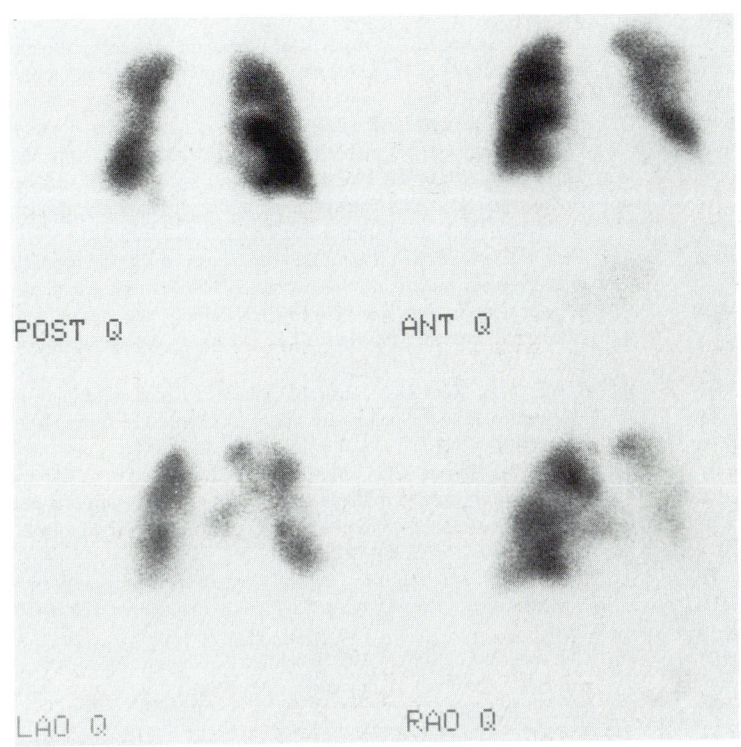

POST Q

ANT Q

LAO Q

RAO Q

Figure 110–13. The postoperative lung scan in the same patient. Compare to Figure 110–4. There is return of perfusion to most areas. Note some "steal" from the lingular area—the one area not endarterectomized.

It is increasingly apparent that pulmonary hypertension due to chronic pulmonary embolism is a condition that is underrecognized. Further, medical therapy is quite ineffective. Operation for the condition is technically demanding, and requires careful dissection of the pulmonary artery planes and the use of circulatory arrest. There is a distinct learning curve for the procedure. However, surgical therapy is curative, with currently excellent short- and long-term results.[52] Perhaps, with increased awareness of the efficacy of surgical treatment for this condition, more patients will be given the opportunity for relief from this disease.

REFERENCES

1. Laennec RTH: Traite de l'auscultation mediate et des maladies des poumons et du coeur. Paris, 1819. In Virchow R: Uber die Verstopfung der Lungenarterie. Reue Notizen auf Geb d Natur u Heilk. **37:**26, 1846

2. Virchow R: *Die Cellular Pathologie in Ihrer Begrundung auf Physiologische und Pathologische Gewebelehre.* Berlin, A. Hirschwald, 1858

3. Dalen JE, Alpert JS: Natural history of pulmonary embolism. *Prog Cardiovasc Dis* **17:**259–270, 1975

4. Gurewich V, Cohen ML, Thomas DP: Humoral factors in massive pulmonary embolism: An experimental study. *Am Heart J* **76:**784, 1968

5. Allgood RJ, Wolfe WG, Ebert PA, Sabiston DC: Effects of carbon dioxide on bronchoconstriction after pulmonary artery occlusion. *Am J Physiol* **214:**772, 1968

6. Moser KM: Pulmonary embolism. *Am Rev Respir Dis* **115:**829, 1977

7. Goodall RJR, Greenfield LJ: Clinical correlations in the diagnosis of pulmonary embolism. *Ann Surg* **191**(2):219, 1980

8. Greenfield LJ: Pulmonary embolism: Pathophysiology and treatment. In Baue AE, Geha AS, Hammond GL, et al (eds): *Glenn's Thoracic and Cardiovascular Surgery,* Vol II. Norwalk, CT, Appleton & Lange, 1991, pp 1561–1572

9. Collins R, et al: Reduction in fatal pulmonary embolism and venous thrombosis by perioperative administration of subcutaneous heparin. Overview of results of trials in general, orthopedic and urologic surgery. *N Engl J Med* **318:**1162–1173, 1988

10. Come PC, Ducksoo K, Parker JA, et al: Early reversal of right ventricular dysfunction in patients with acute pulmonary embolism after treatment with intravenous tissue plasminogen activator. *J Am Coll Cardiol* **10:**971–978, 1987

11. Goldhaber SZ, Haire WD, Feldstein ML, et al: Alteplase versus heparin in acute pulmonary embolism: Randomized trial assessing right-ventricular function and pulmonary perfusion. *Lancet* **341:**507–511, 1993

12. Goldhaber SZ: Evolving concepts in thrombolytic therapy for pulmonary embolism. *Chest* **101**(suppl):183–185, 1992

13. Trendelenburg F: Uber die operative behandlung der embolie der lungarterie. *Arch Klin Chir* **86:**686–700, 1908

14. Sharp EH: Pulmonary embolectomy: Successful removal of a massive pulmonary embolus with the support of cardiopulmonary bypass: A case report. *Ann Surg* **156:**1, 1962

15. Alpert JS, Smith RE, Ockene IS, et al: Treatment of massive pulmonary embolism: The role of pulmonary embolectomy. *Am Heart J* **89:**413–418, 1975

16. Miller GAH, Hall RJC, Paneth M: Pulmonary embolectomy, heparin and streptokinase; their place in the treatment of acute massive pulmonary embolism. *Am Heart J* **93:**568–574, 1977

17. Clarke DB: Pulmonary embolectomy re-evaluated. *Ann R Coll Surg Engl* **63:**18–24, 1981

18. Greenfield LJ, Bruce TA, Nichols NB: Transvenous pulmonary embolectomy by catheter device. *Ann Surg* **62**:890–897, 1971

19. Greenfield LJ, Langham MR: Surgical approaches to thromboembolism. *Br J Surg* **71**:968–970, 1984

20. Timset JF, Reynaud P, Meyer G, Sors H: Pulmonary embolectomy by catheter device in massive pulmonary embolism. *Chest* **100**:655–658, 1991

21. Stein PD, Sabbah HN, Basha MA, et al: Mechanical disruption of pulmonary emboli in dogs with a flexible rotating-tip catheter (Kensey Catheter). *Chest* **98**:994–998, 1990

22. Brady AJB, Crake T, Oakley CM: Percutaneous catheter fragmentation and distal dispersion of proximal pulmonary embolus. *Lancet* **338**:1186–1189, 1991

23. Eichelter P, Schenk WG: Prophylaxis of pulmonary embolism: A new experimental approach with initial results. *Arch Surg* **97**:348, 1968

24. Pate JW, Melvin D, Cheek RC: A new form of vena caval interruption. *Ann Surg* **169**:873, 1969

25. Hunter JA, Sessions R, Buenger R: Experimental balloon obstruction of the inferior vena cava. *Ann Surg* **171**:315, 1970

26. Mobin-Uddin K, McLean R, Bolooki H, Jude JR: Caval interruption for prevention of pulmonary embolism: Long-term results of a new method. *Arch Surg* **99**:711, 1969

27. Greenfield LJ, Zocco J, Wilk JD, et al: Clinical experience with the Kim-Ray Greenfield vena caval filter. *Ann Surg* **185**(6):692, 1977

28. Benotti JR, Ockene IS, Alpert JS, Dalen JE: The clinical profile of unresolved pulmonary embolism. *Chest* **84**:669–678, 1983

29. Moser KM, Auger WR, Fedullo PF: Chronic major-vessel Thromboembolic pulmonary hypertension. *Circulation* **81**:1735–1743, 1990

30. Riedel M, Stanek V, Widimsky J, Prerovsky I: Long term follow-up of patients with pulmonary embolism. Late prognosis and evolution of hemodynamic and respiratory data. *Chest* **81**:151–158, 1982

31. Dantzker DR, Bower JS: Partial reversibility of chronic pulmonary hypertension caused by pulmonary thromboembolic disease. *Am Rev Respir Dis* **124**:129–31, 1981

32. Dash H, Ballentine N, Zelis R: Vasodilators ineffective in secondary pulmonary hypertension. *N Engl J Med* **303**:1062–1063, 1980

33. Moser KM, Daily PO, Peterson KL, et al: Thromboendarterectomy for chronic, major vessel thromboembolic pulmonary hypertension in 42 patients: Immediate and long-term results. *Ann Intern Med* **107**:560–565, 1987

34. Chow L, Dittrich H, Hoit B, et al: Doppler assessment of changes in right heart hemodynamics following pulmonary thromboendarterectomy. *Am J Cardiol* **61**:1092–1097, 1988

35. Schwickert HC, Schweden F, Schild HH, et al: Pulmonary arteries and lung parenchyma in chronic pulmonary embolism: Preoperative and postoperative CT findings. *Radiology* **191**(2):351–357, 1994

36. Takamiya M, Kuribayashi S: *Personal Communication.* Osaka, National Cardiovascular Center, May 1994

37. Nicod P, Peterson K, Levine M, et al: Pulmonary angiography in severe chronic pulmonary hypertension. *Ann Intern Med* **107**:565–568, 1987

38. Shure D, Gregoratos G, Moser KM: Fiberoptic angioscopy: Role in the diagnosis of chronic pulmonary arterial obstruction. *Ann Int Med* **103**:844–850, 1985

39. Boucher H, Protar M, Bertein J: Aneurysme de la branche droite de l'artere pulmonaire par embol latent post-phlebitique. *J Franc Med Chir Thorac* **5**:421–427, 1951

40. Hollister LE, Cull VL: The syndrome of chronic thromboembolism of the major pulmonary arteries. *Am J Med* **21**:312–320, 1956

41. Hurwitt ES, Schein CJ, Rifkin H, Lebendiger A: A surgical approach to the problem of chronic pulmonary artery obstruction due to thrombosis or stenosis. *Ann Surg* **147**:157–165, 1958

42. Allison PR, Dunnill MS, Marshall R: Pulmonary embolism. *Thorax* **15**:273–283, 1960

43. Snyder WA, Kent DC, Baish BF: Successful endarterectomy of chronically occluded pulmonary artery. *J Thorac Cardiovasc Surg* **45**:482–489, 1963

44. Houk VN, Hugnagel CA, McClenathan JE, Moser KM: Chronic thrombosis obstruction of major pulmonary arteries. Report of a case successfully treated by thromboendarterectomy and review of the literature. *Am J Med* **35**:269–282, 1963

45. Castleman B, McNeely BU, Scannell G: Case records of the Massachusetts General Hospital. Case 32-1964. *N Engl J Med* **271**:40–50, 1964

46. Chitwood WR, Sabiston DC, Wechsler AS: Surgical treatment of chronic unresolved pulmonary embolism. *Clin Chest Med* **5**:507–536, 1984

47. Jault F, Cabrol C: Surgical treatment for chronic pulmonary thromboembolism. *Hertz* **14**:192–196, 1989

48. Daily PO, Dembitsky WP, Peterson KL, Moser KM: Modifications of techniques and early results of pulmonary thromboendarterectomy for chronic pulmonary embolism. *J Thorac Cardiovasc Surg* **93**:221–233, 1987

49. Jamieson SW, Auger WR, Fedullo PF, et al: Experience and results of 150 pulmonary thromboendarterectomy operations over a 29 month period. *J Thor Cardiovasc Surg* **106**:116–127, 1993

50. Winkler MH, Rohrer CH, Ratty SC, et al: Perfusion techniques of profound hypothermia and circulatory arrest for pulmonary thromboendarterectomy. *J Extracorporeal Technol* **22**:57–60, 1990

51. Dittrich HC, Nicod PH, Chow LC, et al: Early changes of right heart geometry after pulmonary thromboendarterectomy. *J Am Coll Cardiol* **11**:937–943, 1988

52. Moser KM, Auger WR, Fedullo PF, Jamieson SW: Chronic thromboembolic pulmonary hypertension—Clinical picture and surgical treatment. *Eur Respir J* **5**:334–342, 1992

111

Intra-aortic Balloon Counterpulsation, Ventricular Assist Pumping, and the Artificial Heart

Walter E. Pae, Jr., William S. Pierce, and John S. Sapirstein

INTRA-AORTIC BALLOON COUNTERPULSATION (IABC)

Historical Aspects

The concept of counterpulsation, which forms the basis for intra-aortic balloon pumping, was conceived by Harken[1] in 1958, and reported by Clauss et al[2] in 1961. Blood was removed from the body via one femoral artery during systole and rapidly reinfused during diastole through the other femoral artery, thereby producing diastolic augmentation. Unfortunately, practical considerations, as well as excessive hemolysis, were limiting factors with this technique. In 1962, Moulopoulos and co-workers[3] suggested that a balloon placed over a catheter located in the thoracic aorta could produce diastolic augmentation without the drawbacks of the external system. The balloon was inflated at the close of the aortic valve, producing diastolic augmentation, and deflated at the onset of systole, reducing ventricular afterload (Figs. 111–1 and 111–2). Kantrowitz et al[4] perfected the technique and reported the first successful clinical use in 1968. Since their report, numerous studies have indicated the importance of the timing of the IABC with cardiac contraction in order to maximally reduce afterload and to increase diastolic pressure, thereby increasing coronary bloodflow.[5–9]

The sophisticated hemodynamic monitoring of the early 1970s enabled widespread use of IABC, opening a new era in management of patients with severe left ventricular dysfunction. Following the introduction of percutaneous insertion techniques by Bregman and Casarella,[10] duplicated by Subramanian and associates[11] in 1978, the need for a surgical cutdown was reduced. Cardiologists mastered the IABC techniques, expanding the indications for use. Simultaneous biomedical engineering developments led to improved balloon catheters and sophisticated control consoles; accurate timing of inflation and deflation was simplied; cautery interferences were reduced; on-line hemodynamic monitoring and cardiac output calculations became available; and systems were scaled down for portable use. Thus, intra-aortic balloon counterpulsation has evolved into a safe, routine, and integral part of therapy for patients with severe cardiovascular disease complications.

Indications and Results

Indications for use of the intra-aortic balloon (IAB) and general incidence of use in the various subsets are illustrated in Figure 111–3. Current indications for the use of the IAB in various clinical situations are detailed with justification for use and presentation of results.

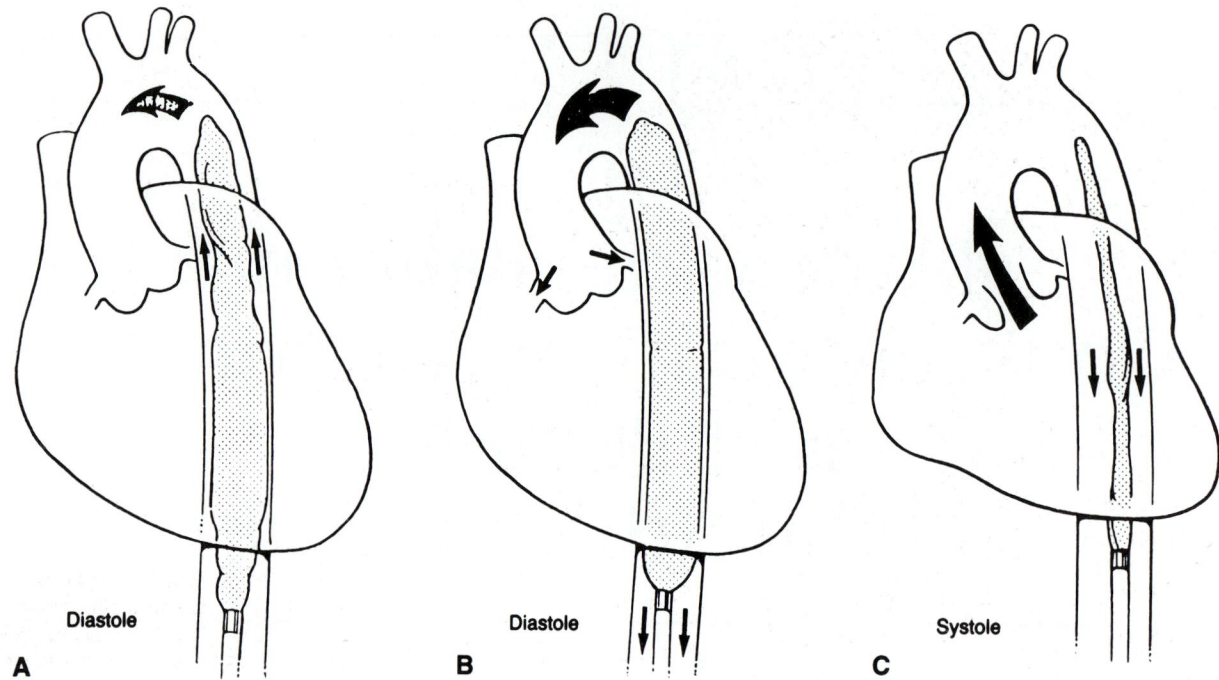

Figure 111–1. The intra-aortic balloon is a temporary left ventricular assist device utilizing the principle of counterpulsation. Counterpulsation refers to any system that raises aortic diastolic pressure and lowers left ventricular systolic pressure in synchrony. **A.** Rapid inflation of balloon in aortic arch during early diastole (just after aortic valve closure following patient's maximum ejection of ventricular volume). **B.** Aortic diastolic pressure is increased (diastolic augmentation by balloon inflation, which leads to increased coronary perfusion). A competent aortic valve is necessary to avoid regurgitation of blood. **C.** Deflation just prior to systolic ejection results in decreased intra-aortic pressure, which lowers resistance to flow (decreases afterload), thereby reducing myocardial oxygen consumption. *(From Crotta PR, Hollingsed MJ, Pierce WS, et al: Physician's Assistant 82:2(2):67–73, 1985. By permission of SCP Communications, Inc.)*

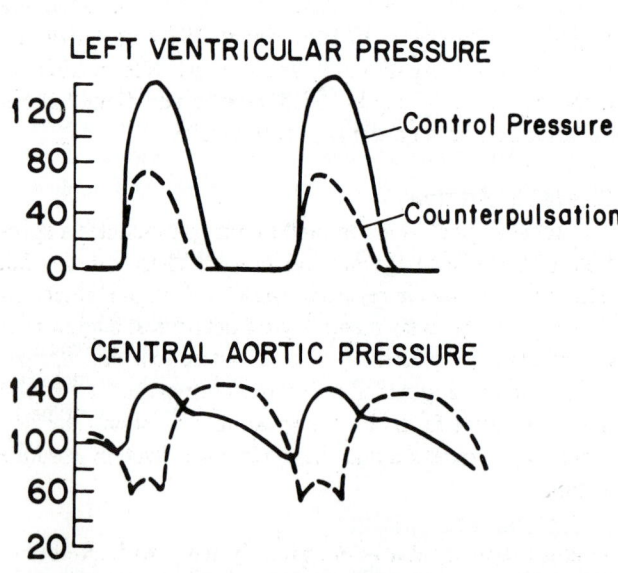

Figure 111–2. Effect of counterpulsation, left ventricular and aortic pressures. With counterpulsation, systolic pressure falls in both, while diastolic pressure increases in the aorta. *(From Sanders CA, Buckley MJ, Leinbach RC, et al: Circulation 45:1292, 1972. By permission of the American Heart Association.)*

Cardiogenic Shock

Cardiogenic shock following acute myocardial infarction is present in a patient when the mean arterial blood pressure is less than 60 mm Hg, or the peak systolic pressure is less than 90 mm Hg pulmonary capillary wedge pressure exceeds 18 mm Hg, cardiac index is less than 2.0 L/min per m², and urine output falls to less than 20–30 mL/h. Such patients have nearly 100% mortality if there is no response to medical therapy since the self-perpetuating effect of continuous decrease in perfusion in various organs, especially the myocardium, results in irretrievable damage.[12,13]

With invasive hemodynamic monitoring, appropriate medical therapy to correct hypovolemia, rhythm disturbances, and acidosis is begun, along with inotropic agents and/or vasodilators. A poor response to such interventions is an indication for IAB insertion and cardiac catheterization to delineate the coronary pathology. At least 75% of these patients will have hemodynamic improvement after balloon insertion with significant increases in mean and systolic blood pressure and cardiac index with decreased pulmonary capillary wedge pressure.[14,15] Unfortunately, this improvement has not led to increased survival with IABC alone.[16–18] At least 85% of patients who initially respond to the IAB remain device dependent, since the underlying coronary pathology has not been altered.[18,19,22,23]

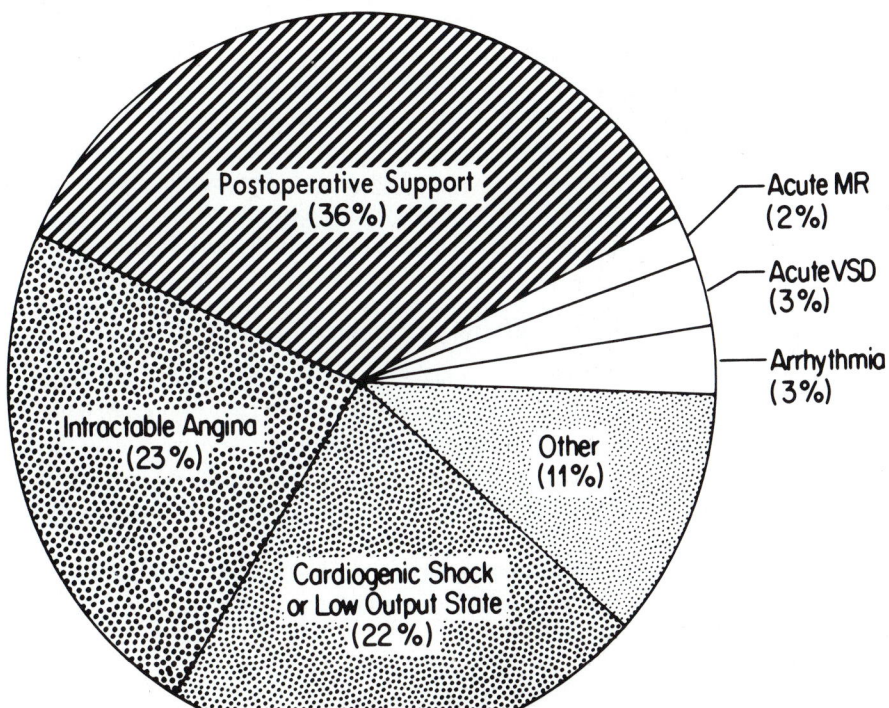

Figure 111–3. Relative frequency of major indications for insertion of the intra-aortic balloon. *(From Levine FH, Austen WG: Thoracic and Cardiovascular Surgery, 4th ed. 1983, Chap 79, pp 1155–1163. By permission of Appleton-Century-Crofts, Norwalk, CT.)*

These experiences have led investigators to combine IABC with revascularization at varying intervals after infarction and cardiogenic shock.[15,17,19–21,24–26] Early intervention is indicated in patients with operable coronary artery disease regardless of whether they are IAB dependent.[27] The operability rate has been reported as high as 75% and as low as 20%.[15,19–21,28] Patients who can be weaned from IAB support remain at high risk for subsequent problems and can benefit from myocardial revascularization before withdrawal of circulatory support. Thus the short- and long-term results of balloon-dependent patients rest on the coronary pathology and ventricular function. The best prognosis is in patients with no previous myocardial infarction, shock soon after infarction, short duration of shock with a good response to IABC, and reasonable ventricular function. Experience with this highly aggressive approach to cardiogenic shock indicates that those balloon-dependent patients who do not respond and those with inoperable coronary artery disease generally die in the hospital. In the patients with operable disease and prompt revascularization, early survival varies from 40 to 88%, with best results in patients operated on during the acute evolving infarct, less than 18 hours after the onset of shock, without a previous infarct or preoperative organ failure.[15,19,29–37] The mean 2-year survival rate has been reported at about 50%, and as high as 75% with no previous infarction.[29,36,37] It is not only reperfusion of the acutely ischemic area but also maximal protection of remote muscle that is responsible for the improvement in ventricular function which allows short- and long-term survival.[37,38] The impact of recent advances in interventional cardiology directed at re-establishing coronary flow and

salvaging jeopardized myocardium in acute myocardial infarction and cardiogenic shock remains to be defined. Thrombolysis appears less successful than angioplasty which, when successful, achieves short- and long-term results equal to those obtained with surgical revascularization, despite inattention to remote lesions.[18,39–48]

The risk of acute myocardial infarction with cardiogenic shock remains high, and optimal therapy has not been identified. Nevertheless, IABC is important in achieving hemodynamic stability to allow for cardiac catheterization, delineation of the pathology, and therapy. Reperfusion remains central to salvaging endangered myocardium, but optimal methods and timing are controversial.

Unstable Angina

"Unstable angina" is an umbrella term that includes a spectrum of acute ischemic pain syndromes. These patients fall into two categories in regard to IABC and surgical intervention: (1) patients with medically refractory rest angina with no evidence of recent myocardial infarction; and (2) patients with rest angina refractory to maximal medical efforts during recovery from acute myocardial infarction. The first group is preinfarction and the latter postinfarction unstable angina.

Preinfarction Unstable Angina. Patients with preinfarction unstable angina have a worse prognosis than patients with stable angina pectoris.[49–51] In the 1970s, the IAB was widely used and effective to reduce ischemia and abate symptoms in most patients with preinfarction angina. The counterpulsation mechanism decreased ventricular afterload, wall tension, and myocardial oxygen consumption while likely improving coronary bloodflow.[52] No controlled, prospective randomized trail of IAB counterpulsation in unstable angina pectoris was performed, but nonrandomized studies suggested benefit to IABC prior to myocardial revascularization.[53-55] With circulatory support during anesthetic induction and prior to cardiopulmonary bypass, ischemic injury during this critical period seemed to be lessened. In 130 patients with medically refractory unstable angina pectoris, Langou et al[56] reported 75 patients who received IABC prior to revascularization, with 55 control patients in whom the IAB could not be inserted or for whom the balloon was not available. Patients supported with the IAB had a 5.6% mortality and a 5.1% perioperative infarction rate, while bypassed "controls" had a 14.5% operative mortality and a 29% perioperative infarction rate. Weintraub et al[57] found similar results and encouraging late results. However, IABC is not without risk and cannot be used in all patients. With modern aggressive medical therapy, the majority of patients can be "cooled down."[58] Craver et al[59] and Pennington et al[60] indicate that extensive preoperative management that renders the patient nonischemic, coupled with judicious anesthetic techniques, obviates the need for and eliminates the morbidity and mortality of balloon insertion with equally favorable results. Thus, IABC should now be reserved for patients refractory to medical therapy or with hemodynamic instability prior to myocardial revascularization.

Postinfarction Unstable Angina. Unstable angina after an acute myocardial infarction suggests viable but threatened myocardium, and the syndrome is predictive of early reinfarction or death. Patients with ischemic chest pain at rest in the early postinfarction period have a particularly poor prognosis. Schuster and Bulckley found a 6-month mortality rate of 33% for patients with postinfarction rest pain and electrocardiographic (ECG) changes in the region of the infarct.[61] The 6-month mortality rate was 72% for patients with rest pain and ischemic changes electrocardiographically in areas distant from the acute infarct.[61] With this poor prognosis, aggressive medical and surgical management is justified. An IAB will usually stabilize the patient prior to catheterization and myocardial revascularization.[62] Bardet et al[62] found in 21 patients with postinfarction unstable angina that IABC eliminated further episodes of pain and ECG changes. Four patients were inoperable, three of whom had myocardial infarctions, and two died. Seventeen patients were operated on with one death, and 14 of the 17 patients were pain free 9-28 months following surgery. Nevertheless, IABC therapy has not been subjected to prospective randomized studies. Brundage et al,[63] Williams et al,[64] and Craver et al[59,65] do not support this view. In Craver et al's experience, ischemia can be controlled medically; catheterization and revascularization were performed in 58 patients with no early or late deaths, and a 3% perioperative infarction rate. Twenty percent of the patients re-

quired IABC postoperatively to achieve satisfactory hemodynamics. IAB insertion was avoided in the remaining three-quarters of patients, with equally favorable results. IAB support is indicated for hemodynamic compromise or for ischemic episodes that are prolonged or unresponsive to vigorous medical therapy prior to myocardial revascularization. Routine prophylactic balloon insertion is unnecessary, assuming judicious anesthetic and drug management.

Acute Ischemia Complicating PTCA

About 3-5% of patients undergoing percutaneous transluminal coronary angioplasty (PTCA) develop acute myocardial ischemia secondary to occlusion or dissection of the instrumented coronary vessels. Hemodynamic instability or ongoing ischemia is the rule, requiring urgent surgical revascularization. The IAB provides hemodynamic support of these patients during transport to the operating room, induction of anesthesia, and the prebypass part of the operation.

Mechanical Complications of Acute Myocardial Infarction

Ventricular Septal Defect
Septal rupture occurs through necrotic myocardial tissue, and usually occurs within 10-14 days after infarction[66] in 1-2% of patients.[67-70] Early mortality approaches 81% within a month; only 7% survive 1 year.[71,72] Unfortunately, vasoconstrictor therapy to support blood pressure increases left-to-right shunting, while afterload reduction to decrease shunting leads to a marked fall in systolic blood pressure and reduced coronary bloodflow. IABC decreases the left-to-right shunt without lowering mean aortic pressure while coronary perfusion is maintained or increased (Fig. 111-4).[73] IABC is intended to support the patient for catheterization and subsequent surgery, not to delay urgent definitive therapy.[74] Further hemodynamic deterioration usually occurs in a short time even with IABC.

With preoperative IABC and urgent operation there is an overall hospital mortality rate of 20-25%, with favorable long-term results in this group of patients.[75-77] Prolonged IAB support and deferred operation is reserved only for patients with a delay in diagnosis or multisystem failure, in whom the risk is a function of organs other than the heart.[74]

Mitral Regurgitation
After acute myocardial infarction, mitral valve dysfunction produces a variety of clinical syndromes. Most important is severe mitral insufficiency and cardiogenic shock due to simultaneous loss of myocardium and papillary muscle dysfunction or rupture. This catastrophic event usually occurs within a week of infarction, and 70% of patients die within 24 hours.[78,79] Mortality of acute postinfarction mitral re-

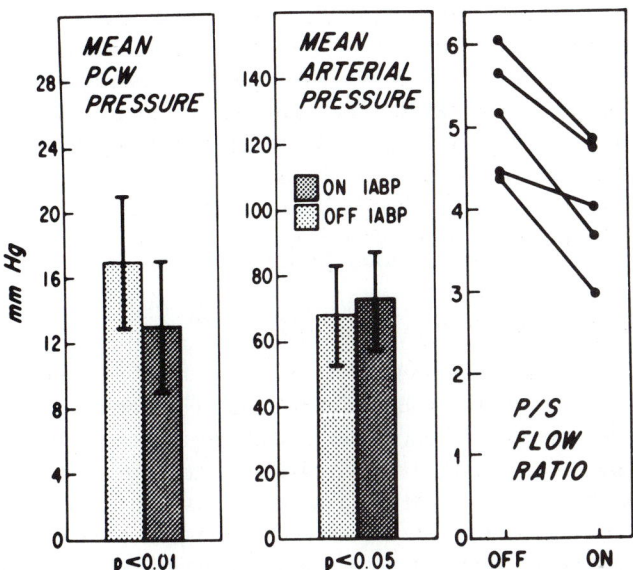

Figure 111–4. The hemodynamic response to IABC in patients with acute ventricular septal rupture. During IABC, the pulmonary wedge pressure falls, mean arterial pressure rises, and pulmonic/systemic flow ratio falls. *(From Gold, et al: Circulation 47:1191, 1973. By permission of the American Heart Association.)*

gurgitation and cardiogenic shock is 90%.[79–82] Nonetheless, this is a potentially correctable lesion because the amount of infarcted left ventricle cannot be quantitated before operation.[83] Therapy with inotropic drugs to restore contractility and cardiac output increases myocardial oxygen consumption and systemic vascular resistance, thereby aggravating mitral regurgitation and myocardial ischemia.[84] IABC, on the other hand, raises coronary perfusion pressure and reduces afterload, decreasing ischemic

dysfunction and mitral regurgitation (Fig. 111–5). This generally decreases pulmonary capillary wedge pressure and the V-wave amplitude, along with causing a rise in cardiac index.[84] After IAB insertion, emergency catheterization and mitral valve replacement with preservation of the subvalvular apparatus or repair and revascularization, when necessary, should be performed. Surgical mortality approaches 50% due to the extent of cardiac dysfunction.[82,83,85–87] Long-term results in general are not satisfactory and depend on residual ventricular contractility.[85,88] Mitral valve repair as opposed to replacement may improve results in this group.[89]

Ventricular Tachyarrhythmias

Persistent tachyarrhythmias are frequent with acute myocardial infarction. They can usually be suppressed by new drugs and overdrive pacing. The inability to control these malignant rhythms carries a poor prognosis. Ventricular tachyarrhythmias are generally due to ectopic impulses originating in ischemic areas surrounding an infarct zone. IABC may control tachyarrhythmias by increasing oxygenation in the ischemic zones.[90–94] Hanson et al[94] reported 86% improvement and 55% total resolution of postinfarction ventricular tachyarrhythmias in 22 patients using IABC. Most of these patients were balloon dependent and required operation; 12 of 22 (55%) survived. Increased survival occurs when ventricular tachyarrhythmias are related to ischemia and resolved with IABC; left ventricular functions preserved; and left ventricular aneurysm and only myocardial revascularization is required. Poor survival is associated with left ventricular aneurysm, poor left ventricular function, diffuse coronary artery disease, and poor control of ventricular tachyarrhythmias with the IAB. In the

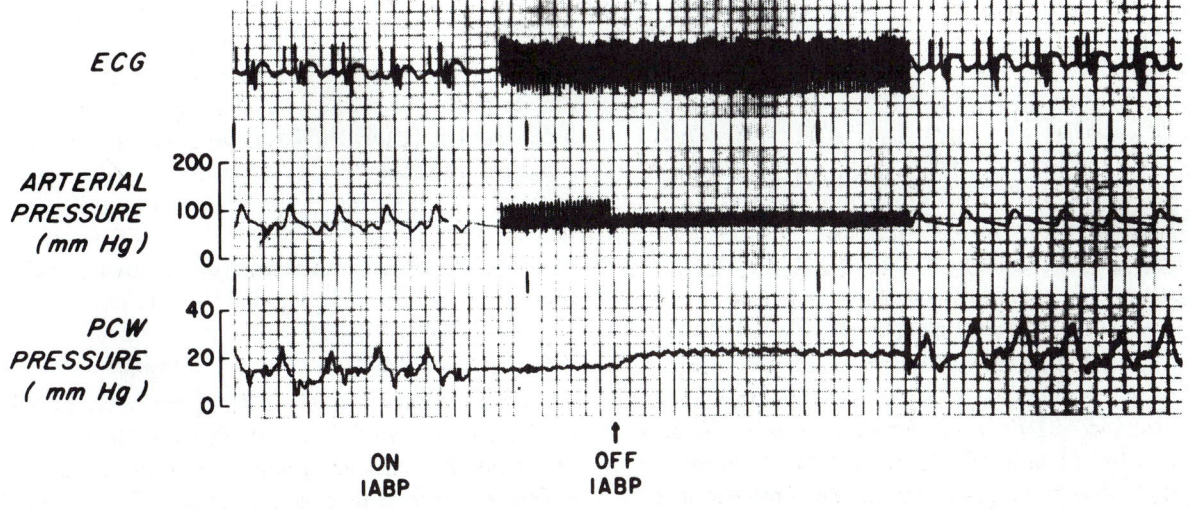

Figure 111–5. The effect of IABC on acute mitral regurgitation. When the balloon pump is turned off, the increase in systolic pressure is accompanied by a rise in pulmonary wedge pressure and an increase in the amplitude of systolic regurgitant V waves. *(From Gold, et al: Circulation 47:1191, 1973. By permission of the American Heart Association.)*

rare patient with ventricular irritability unresponsive to drug therapy and overdrive pacing after acute myocardial infarction, IAB insertion and catheterization are indicated. Electrophysiologic mapping followed by excision, exclusion, or catheter ablation of the arrhythmogenic focus should improve the prognosis for these patients.[95] The role of implantable automatic cardioverter-defibrillators with anti-tachycardia pacing capabilities is in evolution.

Postoperative Cardiac Dysfunction

Adults

IABC is generally the first method of circulatory support for patients who cannot maintain adequate hemodynamics despite medical therapy following a cardiac operation. This group represents 2–6% of all patients undergoing myocardial vascularization and/or valvular heart surgery.[96–98] Faulty myocardial preservation, intraoperative myocardial infarction, preoperative left ventricular dysfunction, prolonged cardiopulmonary bypass and ischemic times, and technical problems contribute to postoperative low-output syndrome.[98] The efficacy of IABC to reverse low-output syndrome has been established, with survival of approximately 30–60%.[36,60,98–101] Many contend that high mortalities in some series were due to delay in using IABC postoperatively.[100–103]

Late results in patients with preserved ventricular function receiving intraoperative IABC have been quite satisfactory and comparable to patients not requiring IAB assist.[100,101,103,104] Although stabilization of patients with poor left ventricular function preoperatively who receive additional intraoperative ischemic injury may be achieved, the long-term prognosis is poorer and related to baseline left ventricular dysfunction.[100,105,106]

It has been our policy to insert a percutaneous femoral arterial catheter in patients undergoing complex procedures with known cardiac dysfunction to facilitate IAB insertion, if necessary, after cardiopulmonary bypass. If a patient cannot maintain a peak systolic blood pressure above 90 mm Hg, pulmonary capillary wedge pressure below 18 mm Hg, and cardiac index above 1.8-2.0 L/min per m² despite volume loading, correction of acidosis, atrioventricular (A-V) sequential pacing, inotropic support, and afterload reduction, IABC is instituted.

Children

It is estimated that IABC is used in at least 75,000 adult patients annually, but there has been less experience in children following cardiac operations. A principal deterrent was the lack of balloon catheters small enough for children less than 5 years of age. The compliant aorta in young children may prohibit effective diastolic augmentation. Also synchronizing balloon action to higher heart rates is difficult. Limited success was achieved by Pollack et al,[107] with 6 of 14 patients being long-term survivors; survival did not

occur in patients less than 5 years of age. Veasy et al[108,109] miniaturized balloon catheters to fit the small child (about 80% of patients were less than 15 months of age), and short-term survival was seen in 50% of 18 patients. Long-term survival was 28%. The use of the IAB in children continues to be limited.

IAB in Staged Cardiac Transplantation

The IAB has been used successfully for partial cardiac assistance before transplantation. Reemstma et al[110] first reported patients who survived with such treatment. Recently, Hardesty et al[111] and O'Connell et al[112] reported results that compared favorably with those for patients who were not as ill and did not require aggressive hemodynamic support. IABC at present is indicated as a first-line measure in an otherwise suitable candidate for orthotopic heart transplantation who decompensates hemodynamically despite maximal medical therapy before a donor organ is available. We use the IAB for support lasting less than a week. If a donor organ is not obtained by then, a left ventricular assist pump is used.

Miscellaneous Indications

The IAB has been used in other problems of acute left ventricular dysfunction. Berger et al[113] reported the use of IABC in five patients with septic shock, two of whom survived. Since then, other attempts have been made, but the success rate has been small.[114]

There are many reports of IABC in high-risk cardiac patients undergoing general surgical procedures.[115–118] Most of these patients have (1) inoperable coronary disease or (2) develop acute ischemia or infarction before or after a general surgical procedure. If hemodynamic instability or ischemic symptoms persist, the IAB may be useful. Lastly, the IAB has been used during high-risk percutaneous transluminal coronary angioplasty.[119]

TECHNIQUES OF INSERTION AND REMOVAL

Femoral Arterial Route

The IAB is inserted most commonly through the common femoral artery. The side with the stronger pulse that is free of scarring and peripheral vascular disease should be chosen. The percutaneous route is our choice, unless the patient is obese or the artery cannot be cannulated after repeated attempts.

Using standard aseptic techniques, the femoral artery is cannulated with a 16-gauge needle approximately 3 cm below the inguinal crease, to remain above the profunda femoris artery and below the inguinal ligament (Fig. 111–6A). Entering the femoral artery below the inguinal

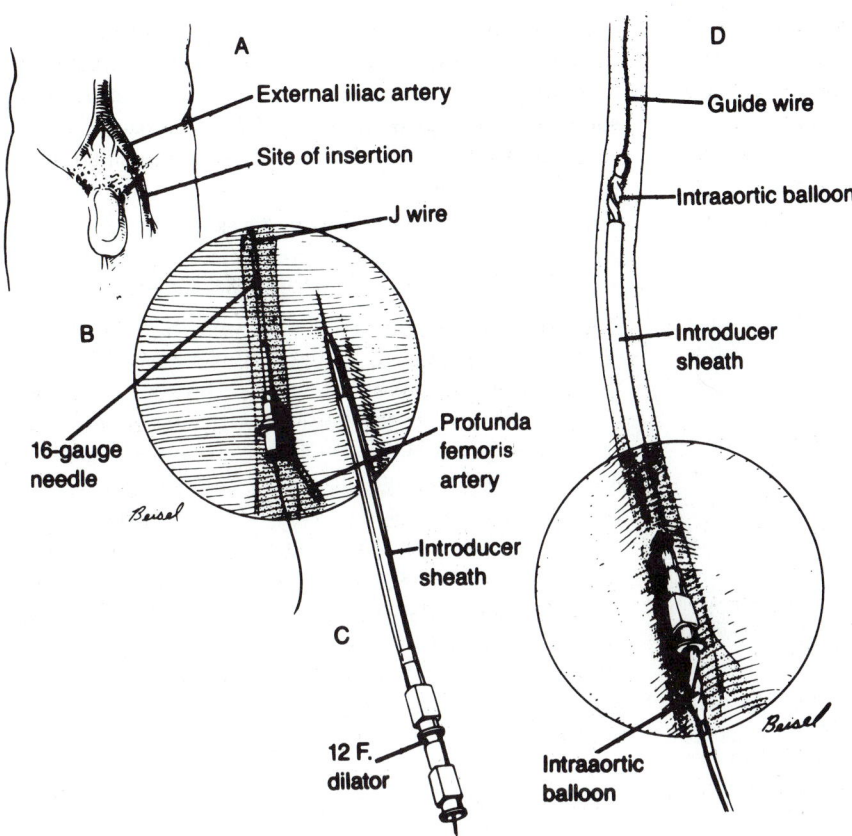

Figure 111–6. The technique for percutaneous IAB insertion. **A.** Site of insertion. **B.** Guidewire passed into external iliac artery. **C.** A dilator and introducer sheath slipped over guidewire. **D.** Balloon being inserted through introducer sheath and passed into abdominal aorta and into aortic arch. *(From Crotta PR, Hollingsed JJ, Pierce WS, et al: Physician's Assistant 85:2(2):67–73, 1985. By permission of SCP Communications, Inc.)*

ligament is important since manual hemostasis is difficult if the IAB has been inserted above the inguinal ligament. After suitable cannulation, a J-tipped guidewire is passed through the needle and into the abdominal aorta (Fig. 111–6B). A stab wound is made through the skin adjacent to the guidewire site, and the arteriotomy is sequentially dilated over the guidewire. The ideal anatomic location of the balloon is with the tip just distal to the left subclavian artery. This can be measured prior to insertion by externally positioning the balloon tip at the second intercostal space, and then placing a tie or the retainer provided by the manufacturer at the appropriate place on the catheter. The final dilator includes an introducer sheath (Fig. 111–6C). The dilator and guidewire are removed, the sheath is left in place, and arterial backflow is observed. The balloon is wrapped according to the manufacturer's instructions and inserted through the introducer sheath and positioned appropriately. If difficulty is encountered, a longer guidewire may be passed into the thoracic aorta, and the IAB inserted over it (Fig. 111–6D). The balloon is unwound and purged. Augmentation is begun and confirmed by the arterial waveform. Radiographic confirmation of proper balloon placement is required following insertion if fluoroscopic guidance was not employed. The largest balloon size possible should be used to provide for the greatest blood volume displacement. A 40-mL balloon is used in most adults. Recently, sheathless insertion to reduce the indwelling

catheter area and perhaps permit increased distal perfusion and fewer limb complications has been introduced.

Alternatively, the IAB may be inserted by direct exposure of the common femoral artery. A 5-cm segment of an 8- or 10-mm vascular graft is anastomosed to the common femoral artery at a 45° angle, and the balloon is inserted through this. It is held in place by multiple umbilical tapes passed about the vascular graft and tied tightly. Alternatively, the balloon is passed into the common femoral artery under direct vision through a purse-string suture held in place with a tourniquet. This allows rapid initiation of the IAB and easy removal at the bedside with local anesthesia.

With percutaneous removal, the balloon is deflated manually with a 50-mL syringe, and the catheter pulled back until the balloon engages the introducer sheath. The introducer sheath and balloon are pulled out together, and the artery allowed to bleed to pass any thrombus or debris. Direct pressure is applied a few centimeters above the skin insertion site with enough force to occlude the artery initially. The area is held for a minimum of 30 min, with enough pressure to avoid hemorrhage while allowing adequate distal perfusion of the extremity. The site is then inspected frequently for hematoma formation, and distal pulses are palpated or checked with a bedside Doppler unit to confirm distal perfusion. After the initial 30 min, a pressure dressing is placed along with sandbags to maintain pressure, but not occlusion. Sandbags are left in place for a minimum of 12 hours, and the patient is reminded not to flex the extremity.

Removal by operation is performed after high percutaneous insertion, in obese patients, in patients with limb ischemia after percutaneous insertion, or when the device has been inserted using a direct surgical approach. In the operating room, with local anesthesia, arterial control is achieved. The balloon is removed, and an appropriately sized Fogarty embolectomy catheter is passed down the femoral artery and its tributaries. The puncture site is then closed primarily or with a vein patch if necessary. After surgical insertion, the graft may simply be oversewn after removal of the balloon and appropriate embolectomy. If the purse-string technique was utilized, the wound is opened at the bedside under local anesthesia, the balloon removed, and the purse-string suture tied.

We use low-molecular-weight dextran (40,000 Da) at 10–20 mL/h not to exceed 10 ml/kg per 24 hours during IABC to decrease clot formation on the balloon in the postoperative patient. This is discontinued about 8 hours prior to anticipated balloon removal. If there are no contraindications to heparin, a continuous infusion to maintain the partial thromboplastin time at 1.5–2.0 times its normal value is administered at the onset of IAB pumping.

Balloon Catheter Insertion by the Ascending Aorta or Aortic Arch

These techniques are usually reserved for intra- or postoperative patients, when the femoral arteries are diseased or do not allow balloon passage for whatever reason. Numerous tech-

nical maneuvers have been used successfully to allow safe and easy insertion, as well as nonoperative removal.[119,120] A simple technique that does not require re-exploration for removal may be preferred (Fig. 111–7). A 10- to 12-mm aortotomy is made over a partial occlusion clamp and a long 10-mm, woven Dacron graft is beveled and sewn to the aortotomy. The IAB catheter is threaded distally through the graft while the partial occlusion clamp is removed. The graft may then be used to direct the catheter caudad or cephalad for exteriorization above or below the sternotomy incision. Ties are placed on the graft at a point close to the subcutaneous portion so that the extraction can be performed under local anesthesia. If a percutaneous balloon catheter type is used, the graft may be sewn to the aorta without an arteriotomy, introducing the balloon and sheath through a stab wound. The sheath is then withdrawn and externalized. In either case, a marker tie should be placed around the catheter to ensure proper position with the balloon tip lying at approximately the level of the diaphragm. Alternatively, insertion can be performed under a double tourniquet technique. A 2-0 polypropylene suture and an implantable grade silicone rubber tubing long enough to be brought out under the sternum and buried subcutaneously is used. When IABC is discontinued, the end of the tourniquet is exposed, momentarily loosened, the IAB catheter deflated and removed, the tourniquet retightened, and the skin closed.

Other Insertion Sites

In desperate situations, the intra-aortic balloon pump may be inserted via the iliac or axillary artery or abdominal aorta,

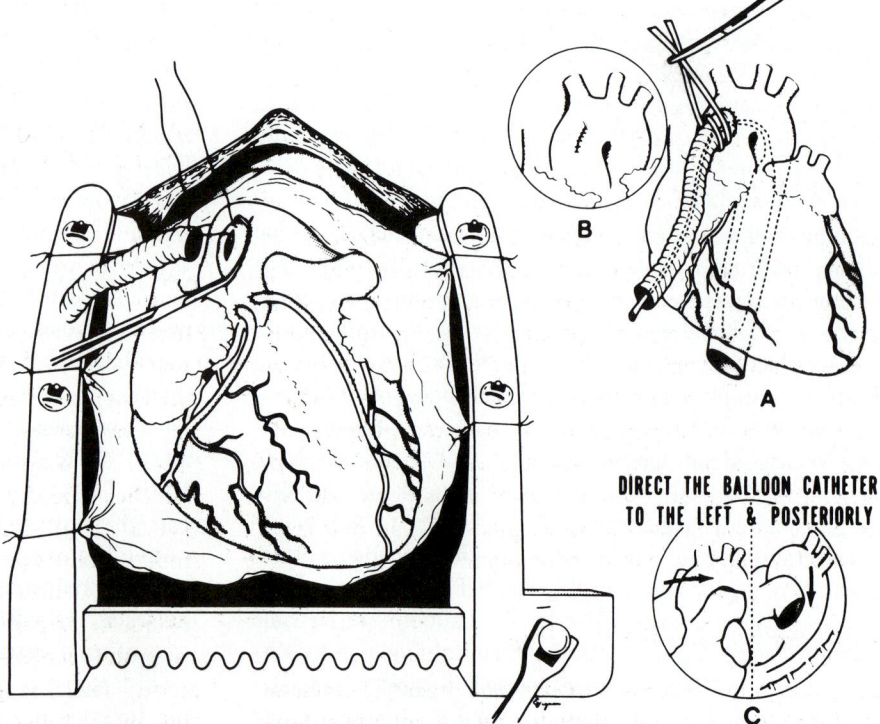

Figure 111–7. Technique for transthoracic IAB insertion. This drawing shows the ascending aorta and method of suturing a graft over the aorta. **A.** Position of the balloon catheter in the descending aorta and the graft on the ascending aorta. **B.** Insert shows closure of the graft over the aorta after removal of the balloon catheter. **C.** The correct direction that the balloon catheter should take and the method of guiding the catheter tip to the left and posteriorly is depicted. *(From Bolooki H: Clinical Applications of Intra-Aortic Balloon Pump, 2nd ed. 1984, Chap 9, pp 103–126. By permission of Futura Publishing Company, Inc.)*

but complications are more frequent and insertion techniques are more involved.[120] Insertion via the axillary route has been advocated to allow patient mobility when an IAB is a bridge to transplantation.[119,121]

Complications of Intra-aortic Balloon Counterpulsation

Complications of IABC result from insertion of the balloon, and are reported to range from 0 to 36%.[60,99,119,122–124] Injuries stem from intimal trauma to the vessel anywhere from the insertion site to the aortic arch. The status of the patient's native arteries, including size, presence of atherosclerotic occlusive disease, and tortuosity of vessels, is the ultimate determinant of balloon-related complications in an experienced operator's hands.

Difficulties With the Introduction

In 5–10% of patients, balloon catheter placement by the femoral approach is not possible.[36,119,125,126] Successful surgical catheter insertion is equal to or somewhat lower than that for percutaneous insertion techniques using a guidewire.[120] Problems with IAB catheter introduction may be decreased with the guidewire technique and percutaneous IABP insertion with a central lumen and fluoroscopic control.[127,128] Additionally, a long introduction sheath is frequently helpful.[120]

Vessel Perforation

Vessel perforation may occur in patients with severe aortoiliac disease, and it occurs more commonly in patients with cardiogenic shock.[129] Penetration through the superficial femoral artery frequently results in thrombosis and leg ischemia. High perforation may result in retroperitoneal hemorrhage and death.

Incorrect Position

This may cause inadequate counterpulsation, persistent or increased left ventricular failure, and inadequate peripheral circulation. Occlusion of the orifice of a large branch of the aorta (subclavian artery, renal artery, superior mesenteric artery) may result in distal ischemia.[60,130] Incorrect placement of the IAB across the aortic valve may also induce acute aortic insufficiency, resulting in increased heart failure.[130] These complications are avoided by careful preinsertion measurement of the length of the balloon catheter, use of fluoroscopic control when practical, and postinsertion confirmation by routine radiographic techniques.

Gas Escape/Catheter Fracture

Due to the safety features in modern equipment, if a balloon develops a gas leak, the volume of helium or carbon diox-

ide released is minute and generally nonfatal.[131] Appearance of blood within the balloon inflating chamber indicates balloon rupture and is usually associated with a difficult IAB insertion in which a sharp atherosclerotic plaque lacerates the balloon. Treatment is removal and reinsertion. Balloon catheter shaft fracture has also been reported with contact with cleaning agents, which can cause the polymer to stiffen and deteriorate.[132] Contact with such agents should be avoided, and the devices used only once.

Limb Ischemia

Leg ischemia is the most frequent complication of IABC, with an incidence of 5–19%.[60,99,119,129,133] It is related to cardiac output, vessel/catheter diameter, intimal injury, and thromboembolic phenomena.[129] Most cases are recognized as soon as insertion is completed by observing leg pallor and the absence of pulses. Low puncture of the femoral artery, with subsequent occlusion of the profunda femoris, may cause ischemia. In patients with a common femoral artery diameter only slightly larger than the balloon catheter, ischemia will almost certainly develop after balloon insertion. In a patient with an ischemic extremity, removal of the balloon is recommended, with possible thrombectomy and patch angioplasty, if the patient is not IAB dependent and limb ischemia persists. Investigators have recommended that femoral–femoral crossover grafts be used immediately when arterial occlusion occurs, thus avoiding premature balloon removal in the hemodynamically compromised patient.[134] Other surgeons recommend removal and replacement on the opposite side.[60] Nonetheless, persistence of leg ischemia after balloon catheter removal mandates emergency femoral exploration.

If limb ischemia develops because of peripheral thromboembolism to small arteries, restoration of circulation to the extremity may not be successful. Fasciotomy may be required in addition to reconstructive procedures.[135] In patients with vascular problems, the rate of amputation is quite low, in some series less than 1%.

Acute Aortic Dissection

Acute aortic dissection occurs in less than 5% of patients.[29,60,126,135] This figure may underestimate the true incidence since aortic dissection in autopsies on patients who died during balloon pumping is significantly higher than 5%.[122] Most dissections are unsuspected until autopsy, since the balloon may often function adequately while outside the vessel's true lumen.[36] Limb ischemia, back pain, flank pain, hematuria, and hypotension may be present. Diagnosis of a silent dissection may be made by the abnormal position of the balloon catheter in the thoracic aorta in relation to the vertebral column.[125,130] This complication is frequently fatal. Long-term survival after dissection of the aorta by the balloon catheter is infrequent.[126] Since the dissection is retrograde, removal of the catheter and antegrade flow may return the dissected intima to a normal position and remedy the problem.

Wound Problems

Local wound infection may occur when the balloon is inserted operatively using the graft technique. The graft stump, if left after balloon removal, may provide a nidus for infection necessitating removal and arterial repair with a vein patch. Postremoval hematoma may also provide a substrate for bacteria, requiring subsequent incision and drainage of the site and local wound care.

Septicemia can also develop in patients with prosthetic materials in place. Bacteria may spread from local wound sites via the bloodstream to seed areas of synthetic materials, such as heart valves. Discontinuation of pumping with catheter removal and appropriate antibiotic therapy guided by blood culture and sensitivity testing may be required. This complication has occurred more frequently in patients after percutaneous balloon catheter insertion.[126,130,133,135] These infectious complications are seen at a rate of 1–3%, and they warrant prophylactic use of antibiotics in all patients who receive the IAB.

The problems related to the lymphatic system respond to conservative treatment. Lymphedema can be treated with compression stockings and elevation of the affected extremity. Lymphocele may respond to repeated aspirations and compression.

Delayed Complications

Nearly 48% of patients who survive and who have had vascular complications of the IAB will have claudication.[99] This may develop due to partial obstruction of the femoral artery in which the balloon catheter was inserted, or it can be related to the insertion of the catheter, occurring as a result of extensive atherosclerosis at a level below or above the arterial puncture site.

Neuralgia, due to trauma during insertion of the catheter, usually dissipates in time.[136] Pseudoaneurysm of the femoral artery at the site of femoral artery puncture following percutaneous insertion may develop a few weeks or months after the procedure.[137] The diagnosis is made by development of a pulsatile mass at the skin puncture site. Treatment is by direct repair.

Summary

IABC is an effective means of supporting the circulation. Balloon support has proven to be an effective adjuvant in patients with circulatory instability, allowing time for subsequent diagnosis and selection of appropriate therapy.

Balloon support is not without complications. This risk must be weighed against possible benefits for any particular patient. Percutaneous insertion techniques have broadened

the cardiologist's scope of medical management of cardiogenic shock, and have facilitated the use of IAB in the cardiac catheterization laboratory and in the intensive care unit. The IAB has enabled cardiac surgeons to wean patients from cardiopulmonary bypass and allow the myocardium to rest following extensive surgery. With careful attention to insertion techniques and proper removal, complications can be minimized.

PULMONARY ARTERY BALLOON COUNTERPULSATION

Right ventricular failure is recognized as an important but infrequent cause of low cardiac output following cardiac operation in adult patients.[138,139] Isolated right ventricular failure following cardiac operations for acquired heart disease is less frequent than biventricular failure, but may be seen in acute inferior wall myocardial infarction.[140,141] To date, right ventricular failure following cardiac operations has been treated medically and with mechanical circulatory assistance. Although the IABC technique has had widespread application and acceptance for the failing left ventricle, applying this principle to the failing right ventricle has received much less attention.[142,143]

We define right ventricular failure on the basis of a central venous or right atrial pressure equal to or greater than 25 mm Hg, left atrial pressure less than 15 mm Hg, peak systolic pressure less than 90 mm Hg, and cardiac index less than 1.8 L/min per m^2 in the presence of tricuspid valve competence. The treatment of acute intraoperative right ventricular failure has consisted of volume loading to a central venous or right atrial pressure of 25 mm Hg, administration of inotropic agents (isoproterenol) to increase contractility of the right ventricle, and hyperventilation to lower the P_{CO_2} and thereby the pulmonary vascular resistance.[143] Infusion of prostaglandin E_1 into the right heart, coupled with norepinephrine infusion in the left atrium, has been reported with clinical successes.[144] Most recently, inhaled nitric oxide has been shown to be quite effective in the treatment of right ventricular failure after orthotopic heart transplantation,[145,146] and clinical trials are under way in other areas. If medical measures fail to improve hemodynamics, further circulatory support is indicated.

Experimental results of either intrapulmonary or extrapulmonary artery balloon counterpulsation indicate the ability to unload the failing right ventricle and maintain sufficient pulmonary bloodflow for adequate left-sided filling and output in moderate isolated right ventricular failure.[147–149] The successful use of the extrapulmonary artery counterpulsation for postcardiotomy cardiogenic shock in the face of IABC and maximal pharmacologic support has been described.[139,142,150] In these instances, pulmonary artery counterpulsation was provided by positioning a standard IAB within a side arm graft sutured to the main pulmonary artery. Intra-pulmonary artery counterpulsation is limited at the present time to animal experiments, since pulmonary artery balloons have not been made commercially available for patient use.[142,149] Experimental results indicate efficacy, and biomedical engineering improvements could lead to a device for percutaneous insertion.[151]

The role of pulmonary artery balloon counterpulsation in the treatment of right ventricular failure is undetermined. Indications for this type of support, balloon size and configuration, and technique of insertion are unanswered questions.

MECHANICAL VENTRICULAR ASSIST PUMPING

The counterpulsation mechanism of the IAB reduces left ventricular afterload and diminishes myocardial oxygen consumption. Still, to be beneficial, IABC requires a certain level of left ventricular function. Methods of circulatory assistance have been developed that take over a larger percentage of left ventricular work than is possible with the IABC techniques.[152–162] Ventricular bypass has evolved experimentally and clinically as a more aggressive form of circulatory support capable of maximal reduction of myocardial oxygen consumption while maintaining the systemic and/or pulmonary circulation.[97,152–163]

The relative safety and efficacy of temporary mechanical ventricular support for postcardiotomy cardiogenic shock have been demonstrated with different ventricular support systems. Ventricular recovery and hospital discharge occur in as many as 40–45% of those patients who otherwise would die.[164–167] Even more encouraging are reports that cardiac function and quality of life are excellent in long-term survivors.[168–172] Cardiac transplantation has become accepted therapy in certain patients with end-stage cardiomyopathy. However, the demand for donor organs greatly exceeds the supply. Since the prognosis for survival in these patients without transplantation is less than 1 year, timely availability of a suitable donor organ is of obvious importance. Transplantation and temporary ventricular support are complementary, since ventricular support is a safe method of maintaining systemic, and, at times, pulmonary, circulation in a patient whose hemodynamic condition deteriorates while awaiting transplantation.[173–176] Temporary ventricular support is appropriate in two groups of patients: (1) those with postcardiotomy cardiogenic shock where ventricular function is expected to recover, and (2) those requiring a bridge to transplantation, when no ventricular recovery is expected and the goal is hemodynamic support until a suitable donor organ is located. Patients in the former group may migrate into the latter group if ventricular function does not recover and the patient is otherwise a suitable candidate for cardiac transplantation. The role of temporary ventricular support in acute myocardial infarction and cardiogenic shock is yet to be defined. Protocols have

been suggested, but there is a dearth of clinical experience.[22,163,177,178] Temporary support under these conditions encompasses expectation of ventricular recovery, suitability for orthotopic transplantation, and hemodynamic stability to allow subsequent diagnostic and therapeutic maneuvers.

Mechanical circulatory support may play a role in end-stage cardiomyopathies as an alternative to transplantation.[157,176,179] Implantable long-term assist pumps capable of unloading the damaged ventricle and restoring cardiac output offer considerable promise in this large group of patients.[176,179,180]

Types of Ventricular Assist Pump Systems

Clinical experience has been obtained with ventricular support using four types of ventricular assist pump systems: (1) roller pumps, (2) centrifugal (vortex) pumps, (3) pneumatic pulsatile pumps, and (4) electric pulsatile pumps. Novel devices employing direct mechanical activation, Archimedes screw principles, or axial flow have had limited clinical applications and will not be discussed here.[176]

Roller Pumps
Roller pumps are available and familiar to all cardiac surgeons. They are inexpensive and many of the components are reusable. The systems typically consist of a 28- to 32-Fr venous cannula for inflow, a standard outflow arterial cannula, $\frac{3}{8} \times \frac{9}{16}$ inch silicone rubber medical grade pump tubing, and a portable roller pump (Sarns, Inc., Ann Arbor, MI).[169,171] Hemolysis as well as trauma to the formed blood elements may occur. When used for long-term support, tubing and position on the pump head must be changed on a relatively frequent basis to avoid tubing spatulation and fatigue. Since roller pumps are not pressure limited, care must be taken to ensure unobstructed inflow and outflow. If left atrial pressure or volume falls too low, air can be aspirated around the cannulation site to the inside of the heart. Likewise, should pump outflow obstruction occur, proximal hypertension and tubing connector rupture may occur. Accordingly, constant vigilance is necessary when employing such systems.[181]

Generally, the inflow cannulation is via the left atrial appendage with the tubing exiting the left chest tunneled parasternally by way of the second or third intercostal space (Figs. 111–8 and 111–9) or subxiphoid.[169,171] The outflow cannula is brought out through the sternotomy incision or tunneled subxiphoid.[169,171] Right heart bypass may be instituted alone or in combination with left heart bypass by inflow right atrial cannulation and outflow pulmonary artery cannulation. Pump removal requires repeat sternotomy.

Centrifugal (Vortex) Pumps
Currently, a number of centrifugal pumps are available. Principles of operation are similar, in that pressure is gener-

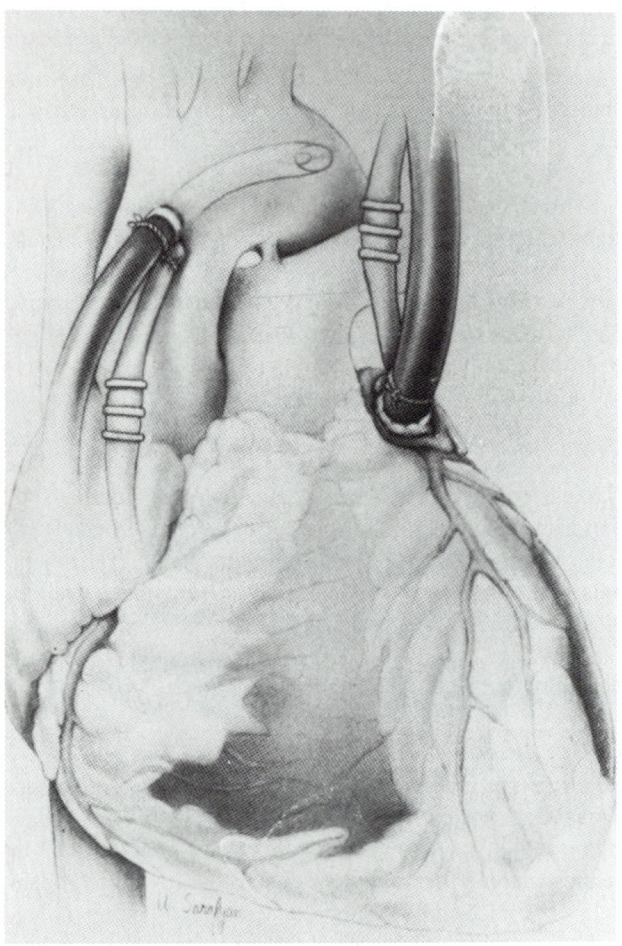

Figure 111–8. The intracardiac location of aortic and left atrial cannulas for roller pump support. Tips of arterial cannulas are inserted beyond the origin of the left subclavian artery. The left atrial cannula can also be inserted via the right superior pulmonary vein. *(From Rose DM, et al: World J Surg 9:11–17, 1985. By permission of Springer-Verlag, New York.)*

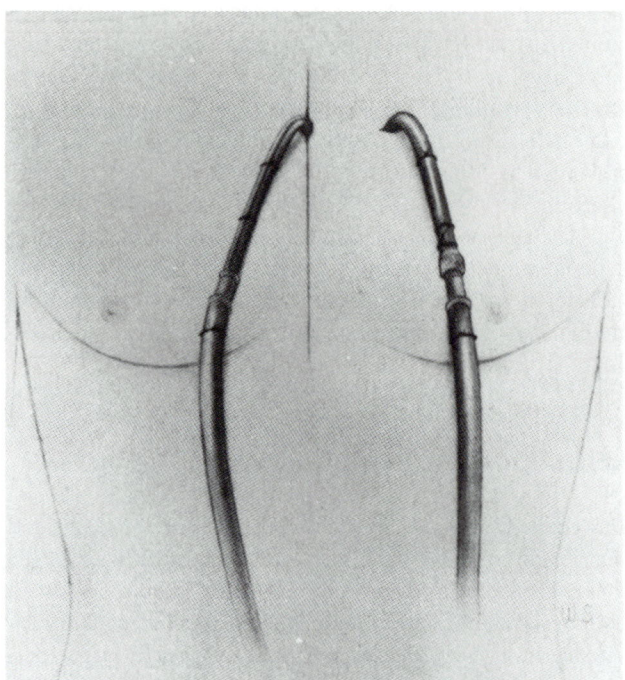

Figure 111–9. This drawing shows the location of cannulas as they exit from chest for roller pump support. Cannulas can exit through either the sternal incision or separate parasternal incisions. It is important to avoid kinking of cannulas. *(From Rose DM, et al: World J Surg 9:11–17, 1985. By permission of Springer-Verlag, New York.)*

ated by spinning the blood as a solid body vortex inside the rigid casing.[181] Theoretically, since the liquid rotates in nearly the same velocity of the impeller blades, there should be minimal frictional loss and heat generation. Kinetic energy imparted to this blood is recovered in the form of pressure at the exit diffuser. Replacement fluid enters through a central inlet.[182] The expense of these pumps is similar to the roller pump, although the reusable and disposable parts are more costly. Inflow and outflow cannulas and techniques of cannulation used with the system are similar to those used with roller pumps. Systemic anticoagulation is recommended since clot formation in the pump housing as well as systemic embolization has been reported.[183] Recently available, heparin-bonded circuits may offer the advantages of a decreased need for systemic anticoagulation. Varying degrees of hemolysis have also been reported.[183] However, tubing trauma is nonexistent, and these pumps are pressure-limited, lessening the chance of air embolus and connector rupture.[181] Left heart bypass, right heart by-

pass, or biventricular circulatory support is possible. Removal of the system requires repeat sternotomy.

Pneumatic Pulsatile Sac-Type Pumps

Pneumatic pulsatile ventricular assist devices, on the contrary, are more complex and costly. An Investigational Device Exemption is required for all, except the Abiomed BVS 5000 (Abiomed Cardiovascular Inc., Danvers, MA) and the HeartMate 1000 IP (Thermo Cardio Systems, Woburn, MA). Advantages, however, are significant in that the design may decrease the need for systemic anticoagulation, minimize blood trauma and potential thromboembolism, while allowing complete support of the systemic and/or pulmonary circulation with a pulsatile system.[140,166,183] The Pierce-Donachy ventricular assist device has been used clinically for nearly 20 years, and is the prototype of this class of device (Thoratec Laboratories Corp., Berkeley, CA).[97,140,164,168] The pump is a smooth, segmented polyurethane inner sac enclosed in a rigid polysulfone case (Fig. 111–10). Tilting disc inlet and outlet valves provide unidirectional flow. The device can be implanted as a right atrial-to-pulmonary artery right ventricular assist device, a left atrial-to-ascending aorta left ventricular assist device, or both pumps can be implanted for biventricular assistance. Blood is taken from the left atrial appendage using a curved 51-Fr, specially manufactured cannula, and returned to the ascending aorta through a com-

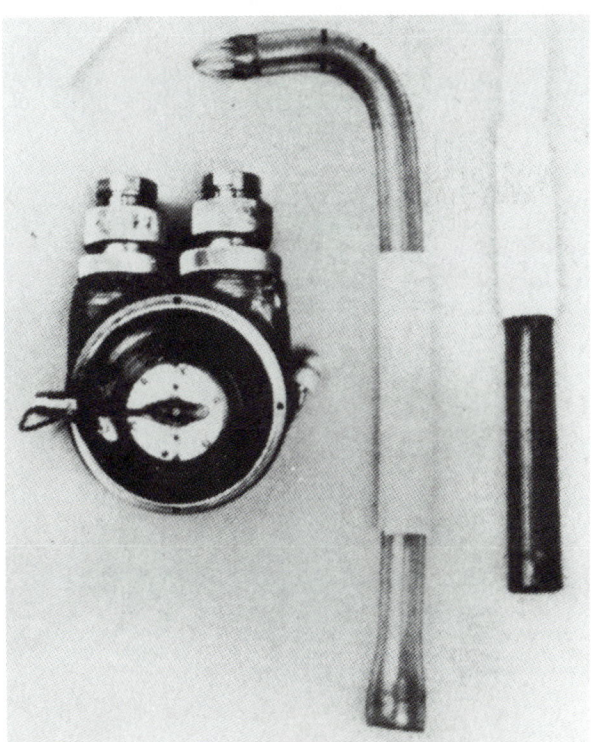

Figure 111–10. The ventricular assist device developed at The Pennsylvania State University. A highly smoothed, segmented polyurethane sac is enclosed within a rigid polysulfone housing. Tilting disc inlet and outlet valves provide unidirectional flow. The cannula in the middle is inserted into the respective atrium to provide pump inflow. The composite cannula to the far right is anastomosed to either the ascending aorta or the main pulmonary artery in an end-to-side fashion to provide pump outflow. Stroke volume is 65 mL.

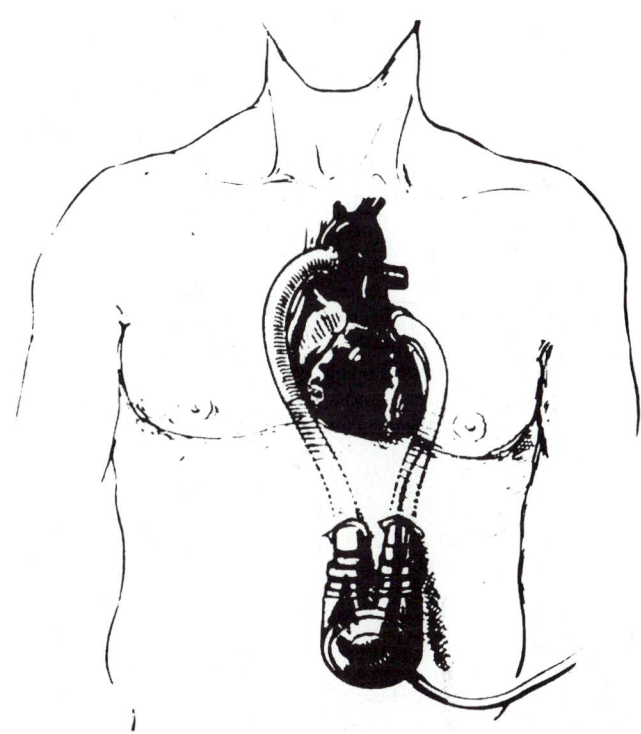

Figure 111–11. Left ventricular assistance with the pulsatile pump is achieved by withdrawing blood from the left atrium into the assist device and returning blood into the ascending aorta.

posite segmented polyurethane-woven 14-mm Dacron prosthesis treated with filler-free silicone rubber (Fig. 111–11). The two cannulas exit the chest below the costal margin, while the pump lies on the anterior abdominal wall. The pump is tethered to a control console by a 2-m-long vinyl tube. The pneumatic drive unit will function automatically in a full-to-empty mode, in a synchronous mode using an electrocardiographic signal, or in an asynchronous fixed rate mode. The stroke volume is approximately 65 mL, with a maximal blood-flow of 6.5 L/min. Pump removal requires re-entry through the sternotomy incision. The atrial cannula is removed as a previously placed purse-string suture is tied. The Dacron prosthesis is divided just above its anastomosis, and the stump oversewn. The device may also be utilized in a bridge-to-transplantation application where apical ventricular cannulation is preferred (see below).

The BVS 5000 Biventricular Support System recently received FDA approval.[184] The pump is a dual chamber device that incorporates an atrial as well as a ventricular chamber each composed of a smooth-surfaced 100-mL polyurethane bladder (Fig. 111–12). Polyurethane trileaflet inlet and outlet valves isolate the ventricular chamber. Atrial filling is passive throughout pump systole and dias-

tole, as no vacuum is employed. Inlet and outlet cannulation is similar to that described above. The device console operates asynchronously, relative to the native cardiac rhythm. The control system automatically adjusts duration of pump diastole and systole to compensate for changes in pre- and afterload, maintaining a constant 80 cm^3 stroke volume.

Unlike the other pneumatic devices, the HeartMate 1000 IP is implantable and has received exclusive use only in the bridge-to-transplantation application (Fig. 111–13).[185] The outer housing is titanium and the internal blood-contacting surface of the titanium shell is lined with sintered titanium microspheres. The polyurethane diaphragm is integrally textured and bonded to a rigid pusher plate. The textured surfaces are designed to promote the formation of a pseudointimal lining. The inflow and outflow conduits consist of Dacron grafts with 25 mm porcine xenografts at the inlet and outlet. Because of the design, full systemic anti-coagulation may not be necessary. In general, only anti-platelet agents are utilized. The pump lies pre- or intraperitoneally in the left upper quadrant with the driveline passing percutaneously through the lower abdominal wall. Inflow is by the left ventricular apex crossing the diaphragm to the pump. Outflow is by a conduit anastomosed to the ascending aorta. Programmed pulses of air drive the pusher plate to create a stroke volume of up to 83 mL. The pump can be run in a fixed-rate or a full-to-empty mode, with ejection each time the chamber is nearly full. A portable driver has been evaluated clinically for patient mobility.

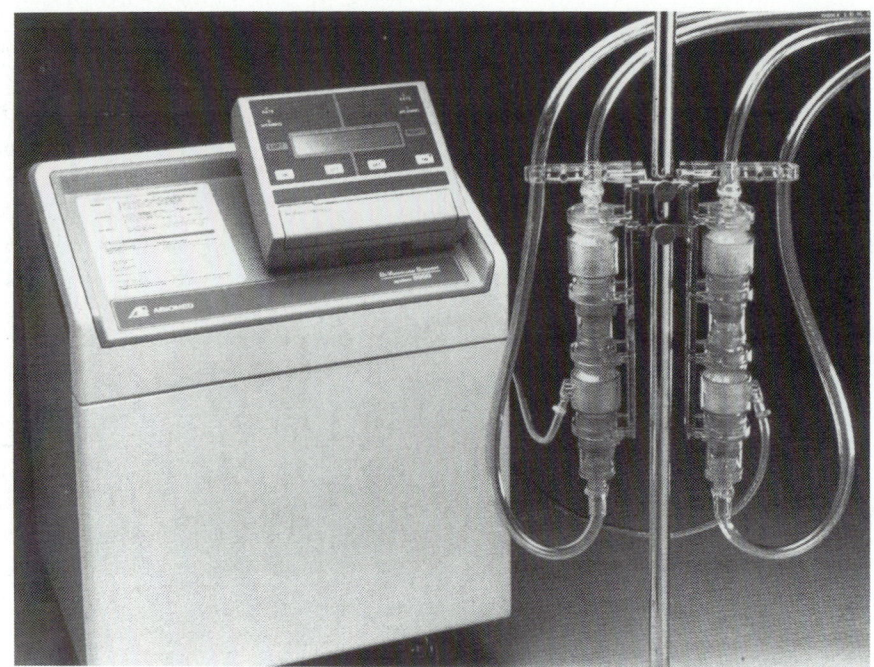

Figure 111–12. The BVS 5000 Biventricular Support System. The dual chamber device is passively filled and operates asynchronously relative to the native cardiac rhythm. The device is used for postcardiotomy cardiogenic shock.

Electric Pulsatile Pumps

Use has been limited to the bridge-to-transplantation experience and development for long-term support (see below).

Indications/Contraindications, Management, and Results of Temporary Ventricular Support

Postcardiotomy Cardiogenic Shock

Profound refractory heart failure is a significant cause of death in high-risk patients following corrective open heart procedures. Conventional medical therapy and IABC provide adequate circulatory support and survival in approximately one-half of the patients who cannot be weaned from cardiopulmonary bypass after a technically satisfactory cardiac operation.[36,99–101] When these measures fail, temporary ventricular support is necessary to maintain the systemic and/or pulmonary circulation and unload the depressed ventricles. In most series, the need for temporary ventricular support is 1% or less of adult patients undergoing cardiac operations in the modern era of myocardial protection with cold potassium cardioplegia.[165–167,177] Re-

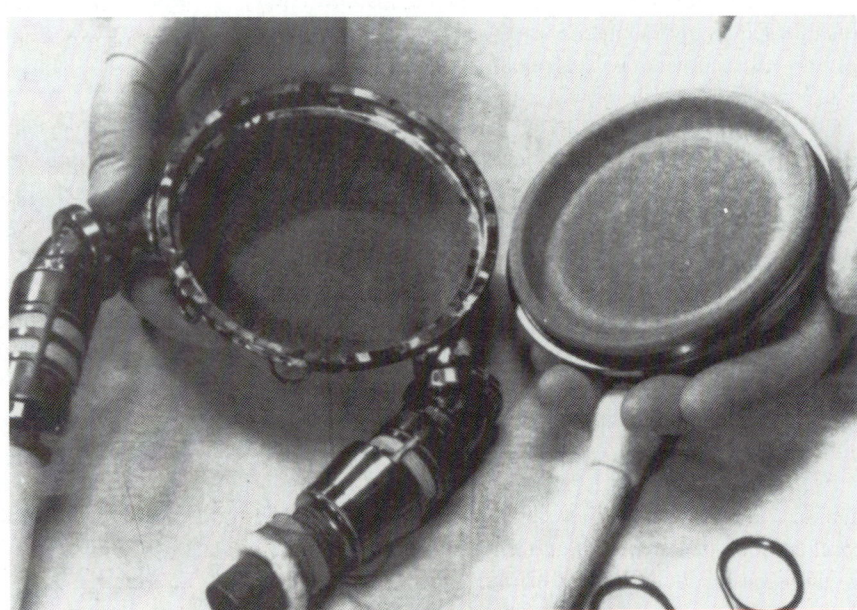

Figure 111–13. TCI HeartMate 1000 IP has a unique textured blood-containing surface and integral inlet and outlet xenograft valves.

gardless of the system used, the goal is to diminish myocardial oxygen consumption and work while allowing time for metabolic recovery of the "stunned myocardium."[152,154,155,158–162,186,187]

Indications for the Use of Ventricular Assist Devices

In high-risk patients, it is prudent to place a femoral arterial catheter prior to initiation of cardiopulmonary bypass to facilitate percutaneous insertion of the IAB. Following a technically satisfactory procedure, a patient who cannot be weaned is first treated by conventional medical therapy. Accurate monitoring of right and left atrial pressures, pulmonary artery and aortic pressures, and cardiac output is necessary to make intelligent and rational decisions in patient management. Patients with a cardiac index of less than 1.8 L/min per m^2, left atrial pressure above 18–25 mm Hg, right atrial pressure below 15 mm Hg, and an aortic pressure below 90 mm Hg peak systolic who are unable to be weaned from cardiopulmonary bypass using conventional therapy, including IAB, are candidates for left ventricular assistance. Right ventricular failure is manifested by a cardiac index of less than 1.8 L/min per m^2, peak systolic aortic pressure less than 90 mm Hg systolic, and left atrial pressure less than 15 mm Hg despite volume loading to a right atrial pressure of 25 mm Hg with a competent tricuspid valve. Right ventricular failure results in pulmonary bloodflow that is inadequate to provide sufficient preload to the left ventricle. This may occur as an isolated event, but also may not be apparent until left ventricular assistance is instituted. Medical treatment of right ventricular failure includes correction of acidosis, hypoxia, and hypercarbia as well as infusion of isoproterenol to lower the pulmonary vascular resistance and improve right ventricular contraction.[138,143,188] Infusion of prostaglandin E_1 and inhaled nitric oxide has recently been reported to be beneficial in these circumstances.[144–146] When these methods of supporting pulmonary circulation are unsuccessful, a right ventricular assist device is indicated. The role of intrapulmonary or extrapulmonary artery balloon counterpulsation in these circumstances remains to be defined.[139,142,147–150] In the future, this may be an intermediate support system much as the IAB is employed in left ventricular failure. Once refractory ventricular failure has been identified, delays in initiating support only prolong cardiopulmonary bypass and its associated complications.

Prior to institution of circulatory support, we have searched for a patent foramen ovale, present in approximately 25% of adult patients.[189] Closure is mandatory prior to circulatory support, particularly with right ventricular failure, to eliminate atrial right-to-left shunting and hypoxia. Also, we prefer left atrial cannulation for inflow to eliminate further myocardial damage, inflow cannula obstruction, and the possible long-term sequela of an intracardiac foreign body.[190] Proper cannula tip position is confirmed with transesophageal echocardiography. Although

theoretically left ventricular decompression by apical ventricular inflow may more effectively lower myocardial oxygen consumption and work, our clinical experience suggests that the risks of apical inflow cannulation outweigh the theoretic benefit when ventricular recovery might be expected. Lastly, systems that require vigorous anticoagulation with heparin are disadvantageous, as postoperative bleeding has been a significant problem in the majority of patients requiring mechanical circulatory support.[177,191,192] Hemodynamic parameters of right ventricular failure, inflow cannula obstruction, hypovolemia, and satisfactory ventricular support are illustrated in Table 111–1.

Contraindications to the Use of Ventricular Assist Devices

Implantation of an assist device should not be considered in a postcardiotomy patient who has had a technically imperfect procedure. This includes patients with residual hemodynamically significant lesions, such as paravalvular leak, a residual ventricular septal defect, or major segments of myocardium that are incompletely revascularized. A successful outcome is unlikely in a patient with well-documented preoperative organ dysfunction, such as renal failure, or an intercurrent condition, such as bacterial endocarditis. Advanced age is a relative contraindication, with most series reporting poor survival in patients over 70 years of age.[140,143,169,177]

Prolonged cardiopulmonary bypass prior to initiation of ventricular assistance sets the stage for significant problems. Elevated plasma hemoglobin levels and bleeding diatheses secondary to damaged blood components reduce survival with ventricular assistance, although they are not a definite contraindication.[177,193]

Postoperative Management and Weaning Procedures

There are numerous protocols for weaning a patient from circulatory support. Bernhard et al[143] recommend that weaning be attempted only when cardiovascular dynamics have improved sufficiently to maintain a cardiac index of

TABLE 111–1. HEMODYNAMIC STATUS FOLLOWING LEFT VENTRICULAR ASSIST PUMP INSERTION[a]

CVP (mm Hg)	LAP (mm Hg)	Systolic AoP (mm Hg)	CI (L/min per m^2)	Diagnosis
15–20	< 15	> 90	> 1.8	Satisfactory pumping
< 15	< 15	< 90	< 1.8	Hypovolemia
15–20	> 20	< 90	< 1.8	Inlet cannula obstruction
>20	< 15	< 90	< 1.8	Right ventricular failure

[a]CVP, central venous pressure; LAP, left atrial pressure; AoP, aortic pressure; CI, cardiac index.

greater than 2.0 L/min per m^2 with no concomitant rise in left atrial or pulmonary capillary wedge pressure, while the pump flow rate is reduced by 50%. Hemodynamics are checked at 15-min intervals, and, if unchanged after several hours, output is reduced by an additional 25%. If there is any indication of left ventricular failure, such as drop in cardiac index or systemic pressure or a rise in left atrial or pulmonary capillary wedge pressure, full support is reinstituted for an additional 8 to 12 hours.

Litwak and associates[170] use the percentage of left ventricular contribution to total systemic bloodflow as a guide to weaning. The percentage of the left ventricular contribution to flow was defined as total systemic bloodflow minus left heart assist device flow, divided by total systemic bloodflow, times 100, where the left heart assist device flow is the flow provided solely by the left heart assist device. Flow from the assist device is slowly decreased until the left ventricular contribution to total bloodflow is greater than 90% with a stable mean left atrial pressure less than 20 mm Hg. At this point, the device can be removed. Spencer and colleagues use a similar technique in discontinuing roller pump support, but state that a flow rate of 400–600 mL/min should be maintained for 6 to 12 hours prior to pump removal.[169]

We discontinue the pump daily for periods up to 60 seconds to permit sequential evaluation of ventricular function.[97,176,194] When the left ventricle can maintain a left atrial pressure less than 20 mm Hg, a systolic aortic pressure greater than 100 mm Hg, and a cardiac index of greater than 2.0 L/min per m^2 with the pump off for 60 seconds, pump output is progressively decreased at 6-hour intervals to permit the left ventricle to gradually assume complete circulatory support. Adequate left ventricular function may also be confirmed by transesophageal echocardiography under varied loading conditions.[195] Anticoagulation during weaning assessment differs according to device type and may require increases during low pump flow states.

Results/Complications
Roller Pumps. Left atrial-to-aortic temporary ventricular support has been employed with varying results by many investigators. Reports by Litwak et al[170] and Rose et al[169,171] are illustrative of exceptional results achieved. In the former report, 18 of 27 patients (67%) were weaned from the device, and half of these were discharged from the hospital, for an overall survival rate of 33%. Seven of nine patients discharged from the hospital are well, the longest survivor having been followed for 10 years. In the latter report, 21 of 46 patients (46%) were successfully weaned from the device, and 16 of those 21 patients (76%) were discharged from the hospital. Overall survival was 35%. Follow-up of 14 survivors from 6 to 54 months demonstrated that they had excellent cardiac function, with 13 being New York Heart Association (NYHA) functional class I or II, and one patient being NYHA functional class III.

Complications included severe coagulopathy, which caused death in nine patients, and neurologic injury, in two. The authors postulated that some patients did not survive, because of progressive right heart failure due to ischemia as a result of inadequate left heart bypass flows.[171] This limitation results from the cannula size. Advocates of the use of roller pumps cite their simplicity, availability, and low cost, while critics are concerned about thromboembolism, systemic anticoagulation, flow limitations, blood trauma, nonpulsatility, and constant attendance by trained personnel.

Centrifugal (Vortex) Pumps. Investigators who use modern vortex pumps cite their simplicity, availability, relative low cost, low amount of blood trauma, and perhaps little or no need to use systemic anticoagulants. Some authors suggest that the systems induce a state of controlled fibrinolysis that prevents thrombosis,[197] and covalently heparin-bonded circuits may reduce or eliminate the need for systemic anticoagulation.[196] Magovern et al[197] reported left atrial-to-aortic bypass in 21 patients, with 10 patients having been weaned (48%), and half of these (24%) being discharged from the hospital. All were alive 1 to 3 years following surgery.[197] Again, in the 11 patients who did not survive, the inability to maintain adequate flow with left ventricular assistance was associated with severe right ventricular failure. Recently, this group updated their experience in 77 patients.[196] Twenty-seven patients were long-term survivors with 16 of 17 being NYHA class I or II. Bleeding requiring transfusion and re-exploration was the primary complication in 83% of patients. Pennington et al[183] employed similar techniques and reported that bleeding was also the most frequent complication, requiring reoperation in 14 of 16 patients. Hemolysis was common and more than half of the patients had thrombi in the vortex pump system; one had a systemic embolus.[183] Because thrombi were visible, heparin therapy was recommended.

Pneumatic Pulsatile Ventricular Assist Devices. The advantages of pneumatic pulsatile ventricular assist devices are significant in that they reduce the need for systemic anticoagulation, minimize blood trauma and potential thromboembolism, and provide complete pulsatile support of the systemic and/or pulmonary circulations.[140,166,183] The Pennsylvania State and St. Louis University groups have employed these systems to treat postcardiotomy cardiogenic shock using atrial inflow cannulation and asynchronous pumping, and their experiences illustrate the results achieved. Pae et al reported on use of this system in patients who could not be weaned from cardiopulmonary bypass.[168] Thirteen of the 25 patients (52%) were weaned from ventricular support; the hospital discharge rate was 36%. In the nine long-term survivors followed-up to 60 months after hospital discharge, all but one were NYHA functional class I or II, and their cardiac status and quality of life were quite good.[168] Complications occurred in nearly half of these patients, including, most frequently, respiratory insufficiency. Bleeding that required reoperation occurred in one-third of the patients despite the fact that no anticoagulation was used. Hemolysis, infection, and thromboembolism were absent, as were neurologic events attributable to pumping. Pennington et al[165] reported similar experiences, with 17 patients having postcardiotomy cardiogenic shock who were treated over a 2-year period from February 1982 to March 1984. Overall survival and hospital discharge rates were 41%, while long-term survival and quality of life were reported as excellent.[165,172] The most common complication was bleeding; three of eight patients who were weaned required exploration for hemorrhage. Thromboembolism and hemolysis could not be attributed to the ventricular assist pumping, and neurologic events were absent.

Guyton et al,[184] in a prospective multicenter trial, evaluated the safety and efficacy of the BVS 5000 system in 55 patients with postcardiotomy cardiogenic shock. Only 31 patients met entry criteria, and 60% of these required biventricular support averaging 4.7 days. Seventeen of 31 were weaned from circulatory support (55%), and 9 of 31 (29%) were discharged, with 8 of 9 being long-term asymptomatic NYHA class I or II at 1-year follow-up. Seventy-six percent of patients had bleeding problems, with reoperation in two-thirds.

Summary of Results in Ventricular Assist Pumping for Postcardiotomy Cardiogenic Shock

The superiority of one support system over another can only be settled by careful controlled trials, but it seems that the available systems provide reasonable therapeutic options for patients who would otherwise die. In a recent analysis of data from a voluntary registry,[177] circulatory support was provided for approximately 4 days regardless of whether isolated left, right, or biventricular support was used. Patients supported with centrifugal devices were weaned on an average of 3 days, versus 6 days for those with pulsatile devices. In about 90% of surviving patients circulatory support was discontinued by 1 week postoperatively. Considering the original operations, the weaning status and hospital discharge rates were not different. Table 111–2 summarizes the results. A higher proportion of patients receiving univentricular support were weaned with a significant difference and trend toward overall diminished survival with biventricular support. When outcome was analyzed by pump design, twice as many patients were supported with the more readily available and less costly nonpulsatile centrifugal devices. Weaning and hospital discharge rates were not statistically different between the pulsatile and centrifugal devices. Although the overall hospital mortality rate was about 75%, in those patients discharged, 2-year actuarial survival averaged 82% and did not statistically differ by the type of support originally used. Most importantly, in those patients who survived to hospital discharge, 86% were NYHA functional class I or II.

TABLE 111–2. RESULTS OF VENTRICULAR ASSIST PUMPING IN POSTCARDIOTOMY CARDIOGENIC SHOCK[a]

Support	Number of Patients	Weaned	Discharged
LVAD	494	254 (51%)	137 (28%)
RVAD	121	47 (39%)	31 (26%)
BVAD	350	132 (38%)	69 (20%)
Total	965	433 (45%)	237 (25%)

[a]LVAD, left ventricular assist device; RVAD, right ventricular assist device; BVAD, biventricular assist device.

Complications during assist pumping were common, with multiple complications in individual patients. Univariate analysis indicated that bleeding, disseminated intravascular coagulation, renal and biventricular failure, cyanosis secondary to an unrecognized patent foramen ovale, inadequate cardiac output, and inlet cannula obstruction leading to low cardiac output were associated with the inability to wean a patient from mechanical support regardless of the type of support employed. Bleeding was more common with vortex pumps. In patients weaned from circulatory support, only renal failure, perioperative myocardial infarction, and infection had a significant negative impact on survival regardless of the type of support or the device. Biventricular failure nearly reached significance. Although there was no difference in the rates of weaning based on age, there was a significant decrease in hospital discharge in patients older than 70 years of age. A 13% salvage rate was recorded. Device dependency was seen only in 8% of unweanable patients, and three-quarters of those device-dependent individuals had no immediate contraindications to transplantation. Staged orthotopic heart transplantation was then carried out in 20 of the 32 patients, with 63% ultimately surviving after transplantation. These results were nearly equivalent to those seen in the standard bridge-to-transplantation application.

In conclusion, all the available devices provide reasonable and safe circulatory support with equivalent results for postcardiotomy cardiogenic shock. Myocardial recovery and acceptable short-term results can be expected in about 25% of patients who otherwise would have died. Complications during support are frequent, but those limiting patient survival are not exclusively device related. Some are technical errors in cannula positioning, unrecognized patent foramen ovule, or unrecognized or inadequately treated right ventricular failure. Many are patient-related, based on underlying disease, the surgeon's ability to correct myocardial pathology, the patient's physiologic reserve, and the duration of shock, as well as cardiopulmonary bypass time before the institution of circulatory support. Pump dependency is rare, but staged transplantation can be carried out with reasonable results in those patients without contraindications to transplantation. Caution is advised in instituting circulatory support in patients older than 70 years. Physiologic reserve is limited and the final outcome is less than desired. Future studies to define patient selection criteria, associated variables, and optimal timing for institution of circulatory support are indicated.

Circulatory Support in Conjunction With Cardiac Transplantation

Approximately one-fifth to one-third of all potential cardiac transplantation recipients die before a donor organ is located.[198] Cardiac complications including inadequate donor organ preservation, acute rejection, and right-sided failure account for a large percentage of early deaths after transplantation.[199]

Circulatory support with the IAB followed by cardiac transplantation was first reported by Reemstma et al.[110] Subsequently, Hardesty et al[111] reported that results compared favorably with those in patients who did not require aggressive hemodynamic support. A great deal of experience now demonstrates the ability of assist pumps to provide temporary circulatory support to patients who decompensate hemodynamically while awaiting a donor heart.[199] The systems designed and used for these bridging procedures minimize the likelihood of device-related complications (infection, bleeding, thromboembolism) that would lead to absolute contraindications to subsequent transplantation. In experienced hands, univentricular support with either paracorporeal pneumatic devices or internal pneumatic or electric devices has been adequate, despite the presence of varying degrees of biventricular failure.[201-203] Prospectively, the need for biventricular support is difficult to predict and the versatility of paracorporeal devices in this regard is an advantage.[173,204] Although more experience is necessary to define precise indications and contraindications, we feel that the simpler, pulsatile left ventricular assist device forms a third line of circulatory support for the patient with normal pulmonary vascular resistance who requires a bridging procedure. Left ventricular decompression and lowering of left atrial pressure has promoted satisfactory improvement of right heart function. In contrast to patients requiring mechanical circulatory support for postcardiotomy cardiogenic shock, we favor apical ventricular cannulation for inflow in bridging procedures. This eliminates atrial trauma and ventricular thrombosis, and it lowers left ventricular end-diastolic pressure and volume maximally. Internal placement of the Novacor left ventricular assist device (Novacor Division, Baxter Healthcare) and TCI HeartMate with small external devices/battery packs represents an important improvement in quality of life while awaiting transplantation.[205-207] Patients have left the hospital for extended times, which improves quality of life and potentially decreases costs.[207] It has been suggested that survival is improved in supported patients when compared with conventional Status I patients.[200]

No single institution has the number of cases needed to determine the survival rates of bridging procedures. Cumulative multicenter results can be tabulated in several years.

Five-hundred forty-four implants were reported in the voluntary combined registry,[199] with the age distribution for circulatory support in conjunction with heart transplantation paralleling that seen in those individuals undergoing isolated cardiac transplantation. The best results of patients receiving transplants and then being discharged were in the younger end of the age spectrum, with 80% receiving transplants and 81% of those surviving. The worst results, at the older end of the age spectrum, were 50% survival. Indications for mechanical circulatory support were hemodynamic deterioration before transplantation, in 436 patients, acute rejection in 40 patients, and postcardiotomy cardiogenic shock not considered related to acute rejection in 68 patients. In the 40 patients treated with circulatory support during rejection, only 23 (58%) underwent a second transplantation, and 8 of the 23 patients (35%) ultimately were discharged from the hospital. In the 68 patients suffering from post-transplantation cardiogenic shock not related to rejection but considered potentially reversible, the absolute salvage rate was about 19%; this was statistically equal to that seen in other types of procedures. The duration of circulatory support in these patients was quite variable, and it underscored the necessity that the devices used in conjunction with transplantation provide safe and reliable assistance over a wide range of times (range, 0 to 438 days). Shorter durations of circulatory support were not associated with a more favorable outcome. The overall results are illustrated in Table 111–3. Rates of transplantation were equal regardless of the type of support employed. Statistical analysis of survival indicated highly significant differences, with the best results obtained with univentricular support, then biventricular, and the least favorable with a total artificial heart. The rates of subsequent transplantation, as well as hospital discharge, were identical in patients who received either a pneumatic assist device, an electrically activated device, or a centrifugally driven left ventricular assist device. However, those patients receiving centrifugal devices did fare less well overall, and if the sample size was a bit larger, there would have been a statistical significance. The 30-day operative mortality with isolated orthotopic heart transplantation has remained at 10 to 12%. In those patients receiving transplants after circulatory support, the mean operative morality was about 18%. However, it was 9% for univentricular support, 18% for biventricular support, and 23% for total artificial hearts. The differences

TABLE 111–3. OVERALL RESULTS OF CIRCULATORY SUPPORT IN CONJUNCTION WITH TRANSPLANTATION

Type of Support	Number of Patients	Transplanted	Discharged
LVAD	122	87 (71%)	76 (87%)
BVAD	161	105 (65%)	73 (70%)
TAH	189	135 (71%)	67 (50%)
Total	476	328 (69%)	217 (66%)

LVAD, left ventricular assist device; BVAD, biventricular assist device; TAH, total artificial heart.

were highly significant between the ventricular assist devices and the total artificial heart. Kaplan–Meier survival estimates for all patients undergoing staged cardiac transplantation at 1 and 2 years after the procedures inclusive of the 30-day operative mortality were nearly 65%. This is in contrast to the nearly 90% actuarial survival in an isolated orthotopic cardiac transplant. When survival estimates were prepared for each type of mechanical support, the 1- and 2-year estimates for univentricular support were equivalent to isolated orthotopic cardiac transplantation, approximately 86 and 83%, respectively. Complications precluding transplantation after establishing circulatory support were numerous. Most of the patients suffered more than one complication. Stepwise logistic regression analysis indicated, in decreasing order of importance, that bleeding, neurologic events, and biventricular and renal failure had a significant negative effect on future transplantation. Univariate analysis indicated that bleeding, renal failure, persistent respiratory failure, infection, and rejection negatively affected hospital discharge. Multivariate analysis indicated that bleeding, infection, and renal failure were the most important predictors of hospital death. The causes of death after 30 days paralleled those of the general isolated cardiac transplantation population.

In conclusion, these results of bridging to transplantation are encouraging where support is instituted for hemodynamic instability and donor organ unavailability. Nearly three-quarters of the patients will undergo subsequent transplantation when the initial support is univentricular and with an electric or pulsatile pneumatic device. In patients who receive transplants, 30-day mortality and long-term survival are equivalent to those in patients having isolated orthotopic cardiac transplantation. Survival may exceed conventionally treated Status I patients. It would be advantageous to prospectively identify patients requiring only univentricular support. Information derived from staged cardiac transplantation will have an impact on future clinical trials of chronic, totally implanted devices.

The Future: Long-Term Mechanical Ventricular Assist Pump

In the early 1980s, the National Heart, Lung, and Blood Institute (NHLBI) released a request for a proposal entitled "Device Readiness Testing of an Implantable Ventricular Assist System." Proposals were prepared and funding made available. Clinical trials were slated for the late 1980s; unfortunately, these have been delayed. Nonetheless, a "permanent" implantable assist pump will offer an important mode of therapy for certain patients with end-stage congestive heart failure.

Several peer NHLBI committees have reviewed and confirmed the need for such pumps. Estimates have placed the number of patients who could benefit by such devices at more than 16,000–40,000 per year.[208] Most potential candidates have end-stage congestive heart failure as a result of

myocardial fibrosis following multiple myocardial infarctions. Corrective surgery is contraindicated because of inoperable coronary anatomy and poor left ventricular function. In some patients, no contraindications to cardiac transplantation exist, but in many, the procedure is not an option. In any case, recipient demand will continue to outstrip donor availability. Those patients who cannot be transplanted have a grim prognosis, and most expire within a year. Permanent ventricular assistance offers several advantages over a permanent total artificial heart (TAH). Extrapolation from currently available data suggests that many—perhaps most—candidates for a support device may not require replacement of both right and left ventricles. Furthermore, residual heart function could provide a "safety net" if a mechanical device were to fail. If univentricular support can suffice, implantation of a TAH would be inappropriate given the TAH's higher cost and operative risk, more complex control requirements, and greater psychological burden.

The design of long-term implantable assist pumps is not unlike pneumatically powered bladder pumps[163,179]; instead of a bulky external power unit, long-term pumps require an implantable energy converter. The converter actuates a pusher-plate that, in turn, compresses the blood-containing chamber. Two systems in particular hold promise for permanent, untethered left ventricular assist devices (LVADs). ThermoCardiosystems Inc.'s (TCI) Heart-Mate-1000 LVAD is an electromechanical device based upon the similar, pneumatically driven unit.[209] A diaphragm separates the pump's electric motor from its blood chamber. Compression of the diaphragm causes ejection of blood, and filling of the pump occurs passively. The LVAD is externally controlled; permanent percutaneous wires connect the pump to a wearable controller-battery pack. A permanent percutaneous vent permits the displacement of air from the pump as the LVAD diaphragm moves. This system is already being tested clinically under an IDE for bridging-to-transplantation, and work toward its permanent implantation continues.[207]

The implantable Novacor Left Ventricular Assist System consists of a polyurethane blood sac compressed by two opposing pusher-plates (Fig. 111–14). The pump is actuated by a pulsed-solenoid energy converter.[210] Bovine pericardial valves produce unidirectional bloodflow. Since 1984, the Novacor LVAD has supported bridge-to-transplantation patients in a clinical trial using an external controller/power console and percutaneous vent with excellent results.[205] Novacor has recently begun clinical testing of a wearable external controller/battery pack configuration to aid patient mobility.[211] Eventually, they hope to market a completely implanted device—including a transcutaneous energy transmission system (TETS) and intrathoracic compliance chamber—for permanent applications. Animal studies of this complete system have begun.[212]

Other investigators are also interested in pulsatile LVADs suitable for chronic use, although for the most part,

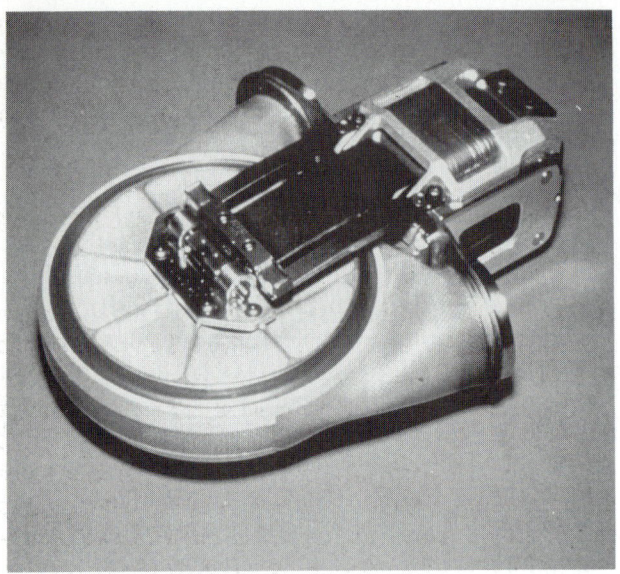

Figure 111–14. The implantable Novacor pump is actuated by a pulsed solenoid energy converter compressing the polyurethane blood sac by opposing pusher plates. Xenograft valves provide unidirectional flow.

they are now at the stage of early animal studies with partial systems.[213–215] For about 15 years, our group at The Pennsylvania State University has been developing a completely implanted LVAD for permanent use. Our goal was to avoid the need for any percutaneous lines or vents. We believe that the recipient should only be concerned with the rechargeable, extracorporeal battery pack. The 70 mL stroke volume LVAD shares much in common with our total artificial heart (see below). The pump uses the same roller screw mechanism, but only a single blood sac and pusher plate are present. An intrathoracic compliance chamber and implanted controller/back-up battery are included. The TETS is used to power the device as well as to modify the internal controller's algorithm if desired.[216] As in the TAH, telemetry is used with an implanted radio frequency transmitter. Figure 111–15 shows a representation of the implanted LVAD. Between March of 1988 and January of 1990, the system was tested with an external controller in nineteen Holstein calves. Our experience ranged from immediate mechanical failure to good pump performance for 235 days. After design and manufacturing modifications and refinement of the implanted control and

Figure 111–15. Artist's conception of The Pennsylvania State University totally implantable motor-driven apical left ventricular-to-aortic assist device for chronic use. Energy is supplied by a portable battery pack and transmitted across the skin via inductive coupling (transcutaneous energy transmission system, TETS). Implantable electronics for control, an emergency battery backup, and compliance chamber are necessary parts of the system. Air-volume regulation within the system is accomplished by a subcutaneously placed infusion port. The pump itself is positioned in the preperitoneal space in the left upper quadrant.

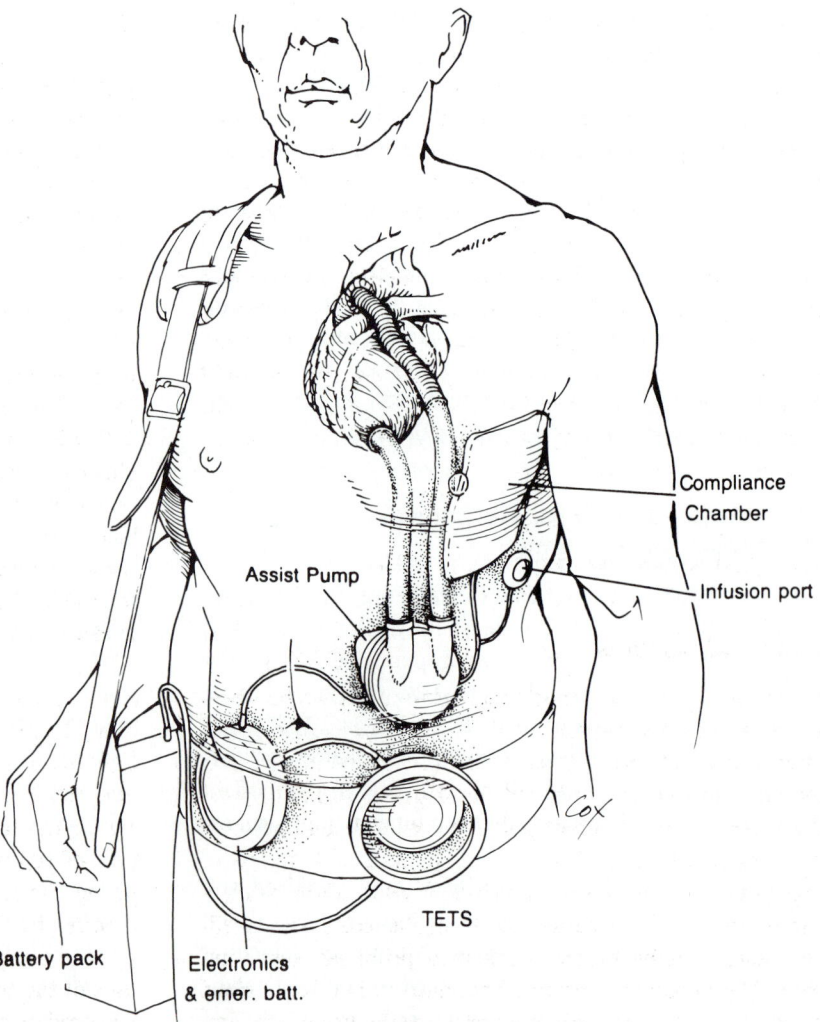

Compliance Chamber

Infusion port

Assist Pump

TETS

Battery pack

Electronics & emer. batt.

telemetry systems, in vivo testing of "wireless" LVADs commenced in November 1991 in the calf model. The implantation procedure, performed without cardiopulmonary bypass, positions all implanted components under abdominal fascial layers. The ventricular apex inlet cannula, descending aorta outlet graft, and compliance chamber are all passed into the chest through diaphragmatic tunnels. To date, in 20 calf implantations, one intraoperative pump failure occurred; the source of this malfunction was identified, and the same system has since been successfully placed within a second calf. Thirty-seven percent of the other 19 recipients lived and gained weight appropriately for more than 3 months, and one remains alive and healthy after surgery. Our longest surviving animal with the LVAD lived for more than 8 months; by the time of death, this calf's weight had doubled to 407 pounds. We expect to begin initial clinical study of this system within the next 5 years.

Nonpulsatile pumps are also attracting attention for permanent support given their small sizes and relative simplicity.[217–219] Such systems may ultimately serve as the mainstays of chronic ventricular support. However, developers must overcome the substantial hurdle of chronically maintaining these blood-contacting pumps' seals and bearings. The difficulty of this task suggests that clinical availability of permanently implanted, nonpulsatile LVADs will lag considerably behind the pulsatile systems.[219]

It is hard to argue against the need for cost-effective, reliable permanent circulatory support systems that offer reasonably normal lifestyles. The current environment of cost-consciousness will probably temper public enthusiasm for "high technology" interventions like mechanical circulatory support. In the end, our society will have to assign a concrete yet emotionally acceptable value to the extended life of a patient with end-stage heart failure. In the meantime, development of completely implantable systems moves ahead, but the issue of cost may prove to be the overriding determinant of how quickly the devices become available.

THE ARTIFICIAL HEART

Historical Aspects

Five years after the first successful clinical use of the heart-lung machine, Akutsu and Kolff[220] described canine experiments in which two compact blood pumps were placed in the chest to replace the heart of a dog. These initial prosthetic hearts were made of polyvinyl chloride and powered by an externally located compressed air source. A variety of ingenious artificial hearts, powered by solenoids[221] or electric motors,[222] were subsequently evaluated. These artificial hearts were bulky, and mechanical problems were common. The maximum period of animal survival was only 6 hours. Thereafter, investigators resumed studies of the sim-

pler, pneumatically powered hearts.[223] Calves were chosen for the animal studies because of their relatively large chest size, good tolerance to cardiopulmonary bypass, and docile nature, which facilitated long-term observation. By the late 1960s, several groups working with artificial hearts had survival in calves of 3 to 5 days.[224,225]

A major effort was made to improve the results of air-driven artificial hearts during the 1970s. Flexible blood-contacting membranes that had been fabricated of low-tensile-strength silicone rubber were refabricated in high-strength inert polyether polyurethane.[226] Pump design was improved to reflect a better understanding of the blood–material interface and bloodflow dynamics.[227] As a result of these improvements, device breakage and thromboembolic episodes became less common and animal survival times increased. Thus, by 1975, a calf survival of 100 days was reported following the implantation of an air-powered artificial heart[228]; this has now been extended to 353 days.

Disadvantages of an artificial heart powered by a large external air-pulse generator with percutaneous passage of large-diameter (12–14 mm) air tubes have been apparent since this type of heart was first employed. In the late 1960s and early 1970s, both the former National Heart and Lung Institute (now the NHLBI) and the former Atomic Energy Commission (AEC) supported efforts to develop a completely implantable, self-contained artificial heart using a plutonium-238 heat source to power a thermal engine of the Stirling or Rankine type.[229] The engine, in turn, actuated the two blood pumps. Considerable effort was expended in the design, fabrication, and bench testing of prototype systems.[230] However, long-term animal studies were not achieved. The National Heart and Lung Institute subsequently altered the direction of its efforts toward implantable left ventricular assist pumps, while the AEC discontinued its support. Kolff's laboratory[231] subsequently modified the blood pump to permit it to be powered by an electric motor. In 1978, they reported a 35-day survival of a calf with the implanted, motor-driven artificial heart.[232] However, the heart was large, mechanical failures were common, and no further work was done. Recently, motor hearts have been designed and fabricated with improvements in microelectronics and miniature brushless dc motors; animal survival with these motor hearts has been extended to 13 months.[233,234]

The first clinical use of a pneumatic artificial heart was reported by Colley and associates in 1969.[235] In this patient, the mechanical heart was used to support the circulation following an unsuccessful operation. A donor heart was obtained and implanted after 68 hours of mechanical circulatory support. Unfortunately, the patient subsequently died of sepsis. After a long hiatus, a successful use of the pneumatic artificial heart as a bridge for transplantation was reported by Copeland, who used a Jarvik-7 heart for 9 days prior to transplantation.[236] A number of similar successful uses of the bridge application of this pneumatic heart have occurred recently. An important step in the clinical application of the artificial heart occurred in 1982, when DeVries electively implanted a Jarvik-7 artificial heart in a patient with end-stage heart disease who was not a transplantation candidate.[237] Although the patient sustained a series of complications, he lived for 112 days with the mechanical heart, and served as the impetus for additional "permanent" artificial heart implants.

Current Status of the Artificial Heart

The ultimate goal of artificial heart research is to provide a readily available cardiac replacement for patients who have irreparable acute or chronic heart failure, much in the same way that the surgeon now has prosthetic valves and pacemakers. The recipient of an artificial heart should be able to lead as normal a life as possible. Certain concessions will have to be made in patients with artificial hearts, just as patients with prosthetic valves must take anticoagulants and patients with implanted pacemakers require periodic evaluations of the pacemaker.

In some ways, the heart is an ideal organ for prosthetic replacement. Each cardiac ventricle has a single, well-understood, mechanical function of providing an adequate flow of blood through the lungs or systemic circulation. Moreover, the function of the heart is now commonly and successfully supplanted temporarily during periods of open-heart surgery by the heart–lung machine, and on a more permanent basis by a donor heart, transplanted from another human.[238]

Has the availability of cardiac transplantation decreased or eliminated the need for an artificial heart? On the contrary, having the two therapeutic options will improve the treatment of end-stage heart disease. The availability of suitable donor hearts is, and promises to remain, a serious problem. The artificial heart may be used as a temporary device to support the patient's circulation for a period of days to months while a suitable donor heart is located. Rejection of the donor heart remains a second serious problem that generally limits the recipient's age to less than 60 years, and prevents the recipient from leading a normal life because of the need to take a variety of immunosuppressive drugs throughout the day. It is the age group between 60 and 70 years in which end-stage ischemic heart disease has its major impact, and in which the permanently implanted artificial heart would have its major therapeutic role.

The practical problems associated with the development of an ideal artificial heart center around our inability to match the high efficiency of the natural heart with prosthetic pumps. The adult human heart weighs 350 g and occupies a volume of approximately 500 mL. Yet this organ is capable of pumping well in excess of 10 L/min at a mean systemic arterial pressure of 80 mm Hg (left ventricle), and an equal flow rate at a mean pulmonary artery pressure of 20 mm Hg (right ventricle). Under these conditions, the left ventricle adds 2.5 W to the systemic arterial blood, while the right ventricle adds 1 W to the pulmonary arterial blood.

Mechanical pumps suitable for handling blood and having capacities similar to those of the right and left ventricles have overall efficiencies of less than 25%. Thus, a minimum of 14 W is required to power an artificial heart.

It would be desirable to power an artificial heart using an implantable power source such as an electrical storage battery as is used in a pacemaker, but the large power requirements of the artificial heart limit the available options. The power requirement of the artificial heart is over one million times that of an implantable pacemaker. With state-of-the-art technology, an implantable electrical storage battery of an acceptable size could provide the required power for only 8 hours.

At present, the only feasible, completely implantable artificial heart would use plutonium-238 as a radionuclide heat source for a Stirling- or Rankine-cycle thermal engine. A radionuclide-powered artificial heart system (Fig. 111–16A) requires neither an external apparatus nor wires or tubes through the skin. The major disadvantages are cost and safety. No active research is being done now on such a device, although compact, implantable thermal engines are being made for implantable left ventricular assist pumps.[239,240] Components of other types of artificial hearts may ultimately be applied to a radionuclide-powered unit.

Electrical energy can power a motor or solenoid to activate the two blood pumps of an artificial heart. Electrical energy can be transmitted across intact skin using inductive coupling (transformer) techniques (Fig. 111–16B). A raised secondary coil is placed under the skin of the abdomen, which serves to locate the external primary coil.[241] This system represents an attainable goal. A patient with this type of artificial heart would be mobile when using a portable battery pack, and when in the home or office, would use house current to energize the artificial heart and recharge the battery pack. A similar system uses electrical energy transmitted through the skin by a percutaneous wire (Fig. 111–16C). This also allows the patient to be mobile, but potential infection along the wire could result in fatal infection of the artificial heart components. Thus, the electrically powered hearts being evaluated represent satisfactory, but not ideal, artificial hearts. An electrical heart capable of satisfactorily maintaining the circulation in living systems remains a challenge of this decade.

The air-powered artificial heart (Fig. 111–16D) requires a bulky, externally located dual-air compressor. The air pulses are led into the thorax through separate tubes to energize each of the two pumps. While this system has the disadvantage of tethering the patient to a bulky power unit, and carries the risk of infection along the percutaneous tubes, its feasibility has been demonstrated both in animals and in humans. With this model, important problems relating to the long-term use of artificial hearts have been identified, and solutions to them are being discovered.

A typical, implantable air-powered artificial heart is shown in Figure 111–17. Separate right and left ventricles are employed. The blood chamber is alternately expanded

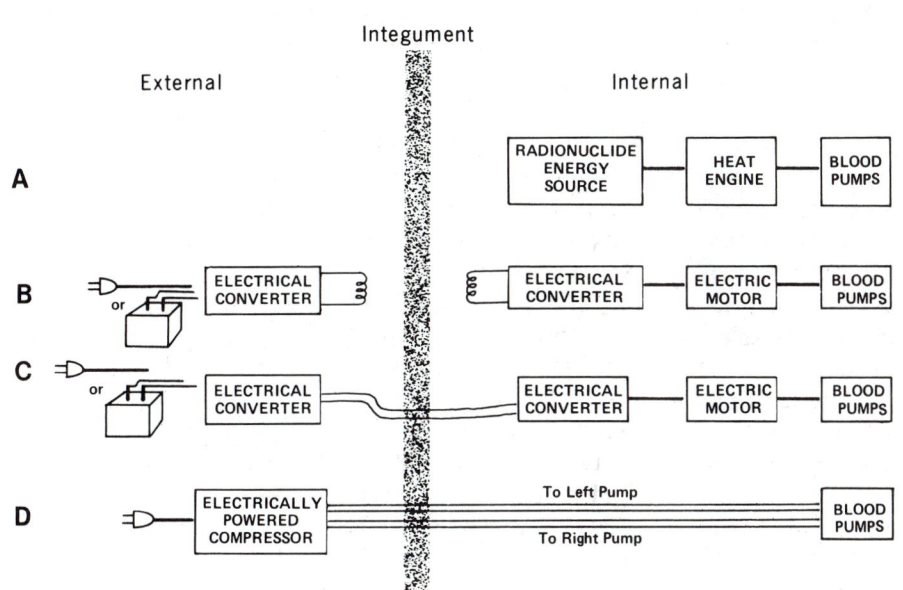

Figure 111–16. Four artificial heart systems are under consideration. **A.** The theoretically ideal system would use an implantable radionuclide power source to energize a thermal cycle engine, which, in turn, would actuate the blood pumps. **B.** Electrical energy can be transmitted across the skin using the principle of inductive coupling to power an electric motor artificial heart. As with **A,** no percutaneous wire or tube would be required. **C.** Electrical energy can be transmitted through the skin with tunneled, fabric-covered wires to power an artificial heart. The risk of infection at the skin puncture site would be small, but ever-present. In the systems shown in both **B** and **C,** the patient would be required to carry a battery pack or to be connected to an electrical outlet to ensure continuous heart function. **D.** To date, the only successful artificial heart system to function for months in patients has been powered by a rather bulky, pneumatic power unit located external to the body. Pneumatic power is transmitted through tubes to the blood pumps. This system lacks the portability inherent in the systems shown in **A, B,** or **C.**

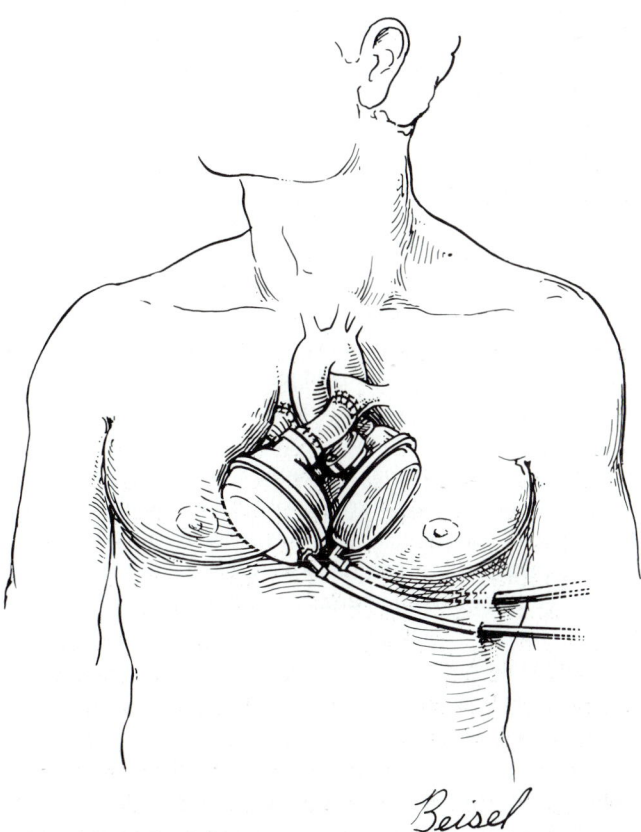

Figure 111–17. Pneumatic artificial hearts have been implanted in patients for temporary circulatory support, prior to cardiac transplantation, or for permanent circulatory support. The required percutaneous pneumatic power lines present a constant risk of infection.

and contracted by the motion of the air-driven diaphragm (Fig. 111–18). A one-way pumping action is imparted by the use of one-way inflow and outflow valves that are generally similar to those used for heart valve replacement. Highly smooth, seam-free blood-contacting surfaces are employed for the diaphragm and housing lining. These surfaces are generally fabricated of blood-compatible polyether polyurethene, which reduces the incidence of thromboembolic events and assures a long-functioning pump life. Each pump inlet port is encircled with a fabric sewing cuff for suture to the remnant of the biologic atria. Dacron fabric grafts at the outflow ports are designed for suture to the aorta and pulmonary artery.

A separate pneumatic power unit is employed to power each pump. The systolic pressure and diastolic or filling vacuum can be independently set for each ventricle, as are the systolic and diastolic times. It is now clear that the two ventricles can beat either synchronously or asynchronously at similar or dissimilar rates, with no pathophysiologic effect, provided the atrial pressures and cardiac index are maintained with a normal range. The pneumatic power units are highly reliable, and most have emergency power sources in the event that the electric power supply should fail. One obvious disadvantage of these power units has been their large size. A compact, portable, battery-powered pneumatic power unit has been evaluated in calf implants, and it has been used clinically to improve patient mobility.[242]

The air pulses in the pneumatically powered heart are supplied to the pumps through 10-mm-diameter tubing that is about 3-m long. These tubes are covered with velour fab-

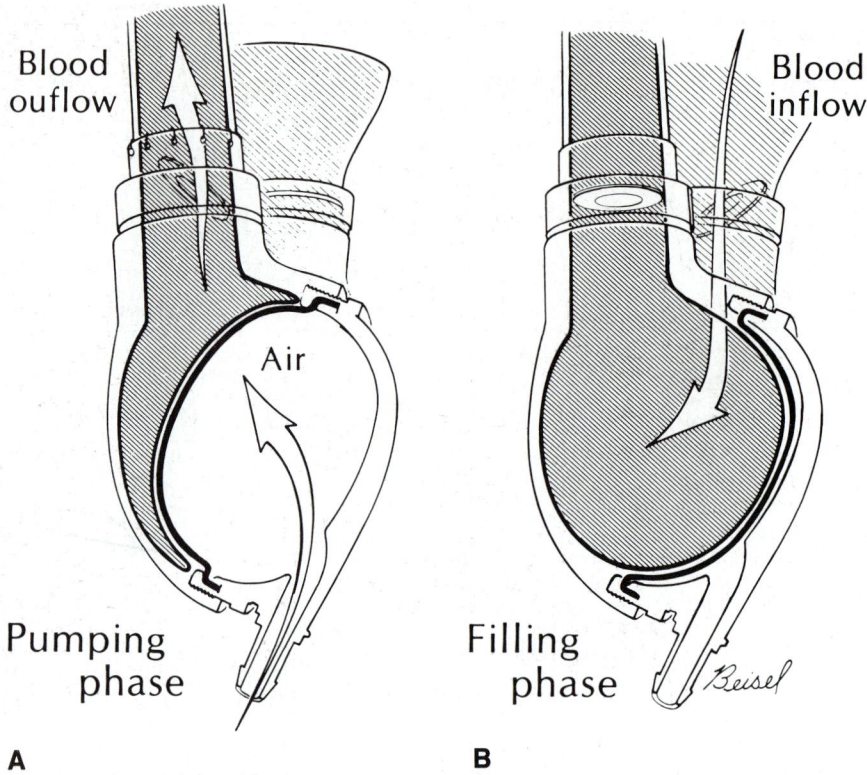

Blood ouflow

Blood inflow

Air

Pumping phase

Filling phase

Figure 111–18. A diagram indicating the function of an air-powered artificial heart. **A.** The end of pump ejection (systole). The air space is full and the outlet valve (shown open) will soon close. **B.** The end of pump filling (diastole). The inlet valve (shown open) will soon close (cross-hatched areas indicate blood-containing chambers). *(From Pierce WS: Trans Am Soc Artif Intern Organs 32:5, 1986 with permission.)*

A

B

ric in their transthoracic portion and are tunneled under the skin for a distance of at least 15 cm to permit a firm fixation to the transthoracic structures and to form a bacteria-proof seal.

Proper control of the output of the pumps is important to maintain the atrial pressures within the normal limits and to ensure an adequate cardiac index (generally > 100 mL/kg per minute). A limited degree of control can be achieved by operating the pumps in the fill-limited mode. In this mode, the time allotted for filling is inadequate to allow the ventricle to fill completely when the atrial pressure is within the normal range, while the systolic interval is sufficient to permit complete ventricular emptying. Any increase in atrial pressure will permit additional pump filling and thereby increase the pump output. This relationship between the atrial pressure and stroke volume affords a certain level of control and has been compared to the Frank–Starling mechanism of the normal ventricle.[243]

The automatic control system developed by Landis and associates[244] uses two negative-feedback servomechanisms. The left ventricular rate is adjusted to maintain the arterial pressure within a normal range. The right ventricular rate is adjusted to maintain a normal left atrial pressure. Moreover, the control system input signals are obtained indirectly, external to the patient, through pressures recorded in the left air line. This system has been used extensively in animals and has been shown to provide automatic increases in cardiac output in response to treadmill exercise. Clinical use, while limited, supports these findings.

An extensive series of animal implants with the pneumatic artificial heart has served as the foundation for clinical implants. The animal implants, in calves, sheep, or goats, are performed through a right fifth intercostal space thoracotomy. The operation proceeds similar to a cardiac transplantation, except that cuffs are sewn to the atria and great vessels, and the prosthetic ventricles are held in place with union nuts or snap fittings. The animals generally stand several hours after the operation. Blood element damage is within an acceptable range. Survival rates continue to improve and are generally limited to 4 to 8 months.[245–248] Causes of death include device breakage, infection, thromboemboli, blood sac calcification, and relative cardiac insufficiency due to rapid growth of young animals.

The excellent results and exponential growth of cardiac transplantation programs have served to highlight the need for a method of temporary circulation support.[238] Current estimates suggest that 20–30% of patients awaiting transplantation die prior to the availability of a donor heart.[249] Accordingly, a number of transplantation centers now have pneumatic artificial hearts available to serve as a bridge to cardiac transplantation.[250] Since 1980, approximately 250 patients have had the artificial heart implanted to provide circulatory support from a few hours to months, while a suitable donor heart was being identified.[251] The artificial heart offers excellent circulatory support provided the chest volume is ample for proper fit. In spite of the significant incidence of strokes, 70% of the recipients have undergone subsequent heart transplantation. Current needs

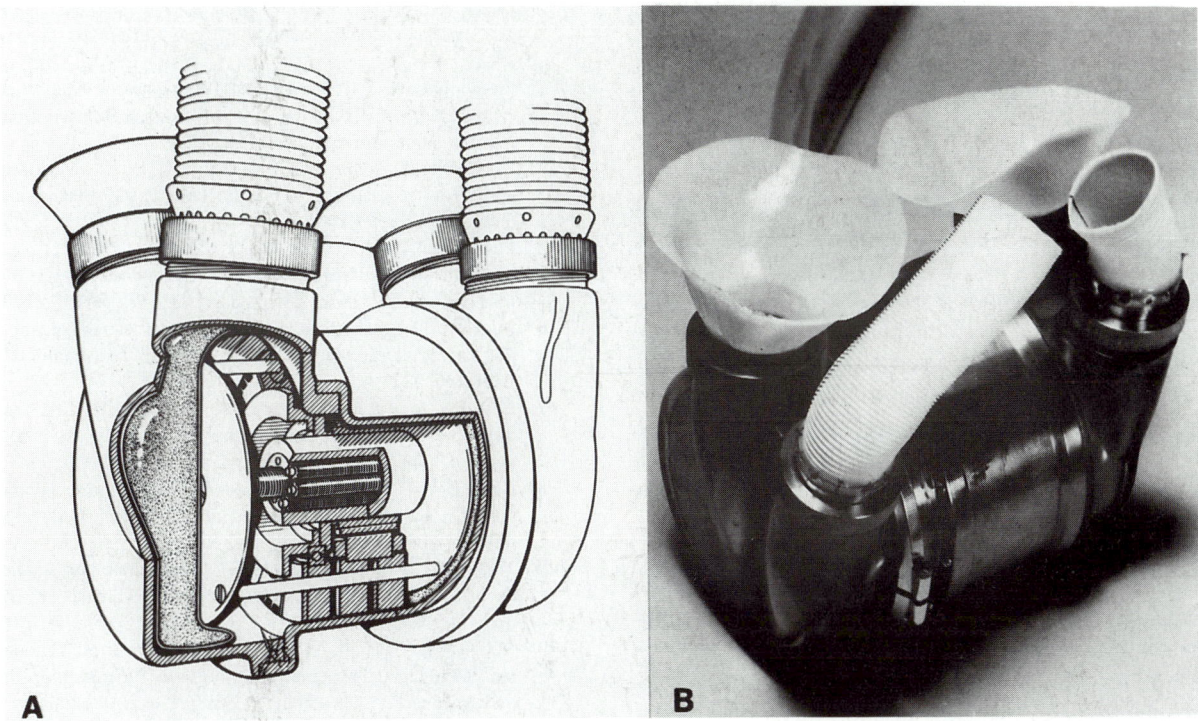

Figure 111–19. The electric motor artificial heart. **A.** This cutaway shows the roller screw motion translator surrounded by an electric motor. The pusher plate alternately compresses the two ventricles. **B.** Photograph of the electric motor heart showing the atrial and arterial sewing cuffs.

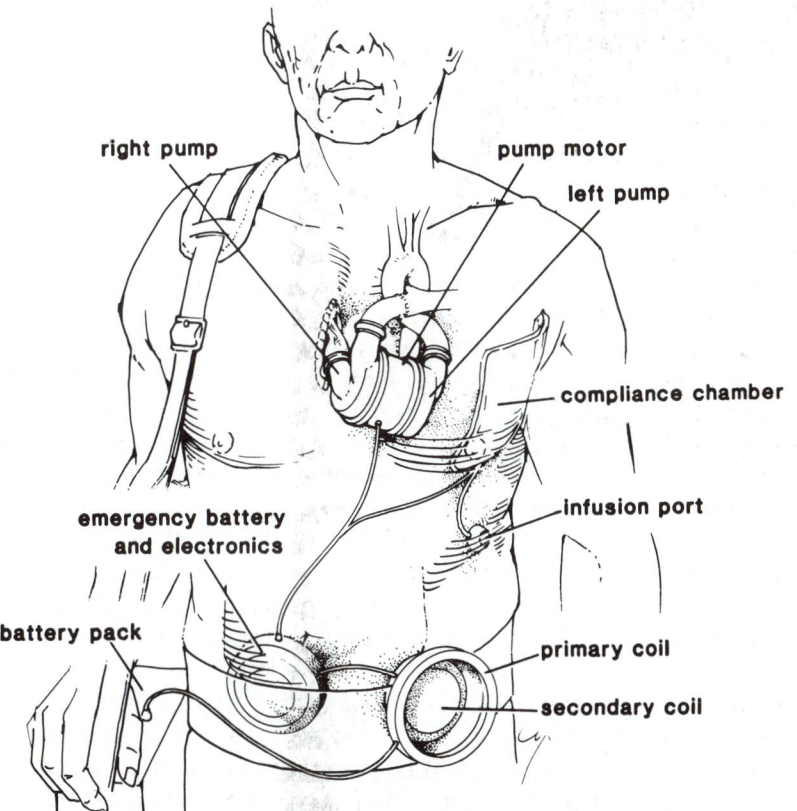

Figure 111–20. The electric motor heart as it will be used in clinical application. Electrical energy, from the battery pack, will be transmitted from the primary to the secondary coil by inductive coupling. The control electronics and emergency battery pack are implanted. An implanted compliance chamber with an infusion port is required to achieve differential pumping of the two ventricles.

center around a prosthetic heart having a smaller volume and improved design features, as well as effective antithrombotic regimens.[233]

The use of the pneumatic artificial heart as a permanent device in a small series of five patients who were not transplantation candidates has served to focus considerable attention not only on the effectiveness of the device in maintaining the circulation, but also on the problems associated with the risk of thromboemboli, long-term percutaneous tubes, and the bulky pneumatic power unit.[237] One patient has survived over 18 months. Considerable controversy exists as to the appropriateness of permanent clinical application of the current pneumatic devices and indeed on research in this field.[201,252] However, these initial results, when viewed in perspective with other advances in medicine, such as dialysis and open heart operations, are quite good and will clearly improve as refinement occurs.

An artificial heart powered by a small implantable motor (Fig. 111–16B and C) would eliminate the need for pneumatic lines across the chest wall and reduce the external apparatus to a compact, portable battery case. The unit being developed by Snyder and his associates uses a long-life, highly efficient, brushless dc motor and roller screw positioned between the right- and left-sac-type blood pumps (Fig. 111–19).[233] Pumping action is provided by pusher plates that alternately compress the two pumping sacs. The blood-pump design is similar to that in the air-powered artificial heart. The high-torque, low-speed motor rotates to and fro at six to twelve revolutions per second, and it has a long-functioning life. Pulse rates of 60 to 120 beats/min are attained. However, the system is large. Every effort is being made to conserve space and weight, while maintaining a maximum output of 8–10 L/min. Animal studies are now being performed; one animal has lived over 13 months with the motor heart. In the self-contained clinical system (Fig. 111–20), the blood pump and motor unit are positioned within the chest. An implanted battery will power the system for half-an-hour if the external battery pack is disconnected or disabled. Several other research groups are developing electric hearts.[253–255]

The development of a suitable artificial heart for clinical application is obviously in its infancy. Advances in material science and electronics that are made to solve industrial problems may have application to the artificial heart. There is a real need for research workers with expertise in many phases of engineering, technology, veterinary science, and medicine to pool their talents to bring the artificial heart to clinical use. Furthermore, the artificial heart promises to be the forerunner of a variety of artificial organs whose development will be based on the knowledge and experience gained with the artificial heart.

REFERENCES

1. Harken DE: Presented at the International College of Cardiology Meeting, Brussels, Belgium, 1958
2. Clauss RH, Birtwell WC, Albaertal G, et al: Assisted circulation. I. The arterial counterpulsator. J Thorac Cardiovasc Surg 41:447, 1961
3. Moulopoulos SD, Topaz S, Kolff WJ: Diastolic balloon pumping (with carbon dioxide) in the aorta: Mechanical assistance to the failing circulation. Am Heart J 63:669, 1962
4. Kantrowitz A, Tjonneland S, Krakauer JS, et al: Mechanical intra-aortic cardiac assistance in cardiogenic shock: Hemodynamic effects. Arch Surg 97:1000, 1968
5. Powell WJ, Daggett WM, Magro AE, et al: Effects of intra-aortic balloon counterpulsation on cardiac performance, oxygen consumption, and coronary blood flow in dogs. Circ Res 26:753, 1970
6. Buckley MJ, Leinbach RC, Kastor JA, et al: Hemodynamic evaluation of intra-aortic balloon pumping in man. Circulation 41(Suppl. II):II–130, 1970
7. Rose EA, Marrin CAS, Bregman D, Spotnitz HM: Left ventricular mechanics of counterpulsation and left heart bypass, individually and in combination. J Thorac Cardiovasc Surg 77:127, 1979
8. Baron DW, O'Rourke MD: Long-term results of arterial counterpulsation in acute severe cardiac failure complicating myocardial infarction. Br Heart J 38:285, 1976
9. Talpins NL, Kripke DC, Goetz RH: Counterpulsation and intra-aortic balloon pumping in cardiogenic shock: Circulatory dynamics. Arch Surg 97:991, 1968
10. Bregman D, Casarella WJ: Percutaneous intra-aortic balloon pumping: Initial clinical experiences. Ann Thorac Surg 29:153, 1980
11. Subramanian VA, Goldstein JE, Sos TA, et al: Preliminary clinical experience with percutaneous intra-aortic balloon pumping. Circulation 62(Suppl I):I–123, 1980
12. Scheidt S, Ascheim R, Killip T: Shock after acute myocardial infarction: A clinical and hemodynamic profile. Am J Cardiol 26:556, 1970
13. Page DL, Caulfield JB, Kastor JA, et al: Myocardial changes associated with cardiogenic shock. N Engl J Med 285:133, 1971
14. Levine FH, Austen WG: Intra-aortic balloon assistance. In Glenn W (ed): Thoracic and Cardiovascular Surgery. Norwalk, CT Appleton-Century-Crofts, 1983, p 1157
15. Dunkman WB, Leinbach RC, Buckley MJ, et al: Clinical and hemodynamic results of intra-aortic balloon pumping for cardiogenic shock. Circulation 46:465, 1972
16. Kantrowitz A, Tjonneland S, Freed PS, et al: Initial clinical experience with intra-aortic balloon pumping in cardiogenic shock. JAMA 203:113, 1968
17. Scheidt S, Wilner G, Mueller H, et al: Intra-aortic balloon counterpulsation with cardiogenic shock. N Engl J Med 288:979, 1973
18. Moosvi AR, Khaja F, Villaneuva L, et al: Early revascularization improves survival in cardiogenic shock complicating acute myocardial infarction. J Am Coll Cardiol 19:907, 1992
19. DeWood M, Notske R, Hensley G, et al: Intra-aortic balloon counterpulsation with and without reperfusion for myocardial infarction shock. Circulation 61:1105, 1980
20. Subramanian V, Roberts A, Zema M, et al: Cardiogenic shock following acute myocardial infarction: Late functional results after emergency cardiac surgery. NY State J Med 80(6):947, 1980
21. Resnekov L: Circulatory support and early cardiac surgery in the management of cardiogenic shock complicating myocardial infarction. Ann Clin Res 9:134, 1977
22. Pae WE Jr, Pierce WS: Temporary left ventricular assistance in acute myocardial infarction and cardiogenic shock: Rationale and criteria for utilization. Chest 79:692, 1981
23. Buckley MJ: Surgery for acute myocardial infarction: Evolution and current status. In Moran JM, Michaelis LL (eds): Surgery for Complications of Myocardial Infarction. New York, Grune & Stratton, 1980, p 247
24. Mundth ED: Mechanical and surgical interventions for the reduction of myocardial ischemia. Circulation 53(Suppl I)I:176, 1976
25. Willerson JT, Currey GC, Watson JT, et al: Intra-aortic balloon counterpulsation in patients in cardiogenic shock, medically refrac-

tory left ventricular failure and/or recurrent ventricular tachycardia. *Am J Med* **58**:183, 1975

26. Mundth ED, Yurchak PM, Buckley MJ, et al: Circulatory assistance and emergency direct coronary artery surgery for the treatment of cardiogenic shock complicating acute myocardial infarction. *N Engl J Med* **283**:1382, 1970

27. Leinbach RC, Dinsmore RE, Mundth ED, et al: Selective coronary and left ventricular cineangiography during intra-aortic balloon pumping for cardiogenic shock. *Circulation* **45**:845, 1972

28. Jackson G, Cullum P, Pastellopoulos A, et al: Intra-aortic balloon assistance in cardiogenic shock after myocardial infarction or cardiac surgery. *Br Heart J* **39**:598, 1977

29. Pierri MK, Zema M, Kligfield P, et al: Exercise tolerance in late survivors of balloon pumping and surgery for cardiogenic shock. *Circulation* **62**(Suppl I):I–138, 1980

30. Laks H, Rosenkranz E, Buckberg GD: Surgical treatment of cardiogenic shock after myocardial infarction. *Circulation* **74**(Suppl III):III–11, 1986

31. Guyton RA, Arcidi JM, Langford DA, et al: Emergency coronary bypass for cardiogenic shock. *Circulation* **76**(Suppl V):V–22, 1987

32. Phillips SJ, Zeff RH, Skinner JR, et al: Reperfusion protocol and results in 738 patients with evolving myocardial infarction. *Ann Thorac Surg* **41**:119, 1986

33. Miller MG, Weintraub RM, Hedley-Whyte J, et al: Surgery for cardiogenic shock. *Lancet* **2**:1342, 1974

34. Johnson SA, Scanlon PJ, Loeb HS, et al: Treatment of cardiogenic shock in myocardial infarction by intra-aortic balloon counterpulsation and surgery. *Am J Med* **62**:687, 1977

35. Bolooki H: Emergency cardiac procedures in patients in cardiogenic shock due to complications of coronary artery disease. *Circulation* **79**(Suppl I):I–137, 1989

36. McEnany MT, Kay HR, Buckley MJ, et al: Clinical experience with intra-aortic balloon pump support in 728 patients. *Circulation* **58**(Suppl I):I–124, 1978

37. Allen BS, Rosenkranz E, Buckberg GD, et al: Studies on prolonged acute regional ischemia VI. Myocardial infarction with left ventricular power failure: A medical/surgical emergency requiring urgent revascularization with maximal protection of remote muscle. *J Thorac Cardiovasc Surg* **98**:691, 1989

38. Braunwald E: The aggressive treatment of acute myocardial infarction. *Circulation* **71**:1087, 1985

39. Heuser RR, Maddoux GL, Goss JE, et al: Coronary angioplasty in the treatment of cardiogenic shock: The therapy of choice. *J Am Coll Cardiol* **7**:219A, 1986

40. Rothbaum DA, Linnemeier TJ, Noble RJ: Emergency percutaneous transluminal coronary angioplasty in acute myocardial infarction. *J Am Coll Cardiol* **7**:149A, 1986

41. Shani J, Rivera M, Greengart A, et al: Percutaneous transluminal coronary angioplasty in cardiogenic shock. *J Am Coll Cardiol* **7**:149A, 1986

42. Gruppo Italiano per lo Studio della Streptochinasi nell'Infarto Miocardico (GISSI): Effectiveness of intravenous thrombolytic treatment in acute myocardial infarction. *Lancet* **1**:397, 1986

43. Wilcox RG, von der Lippe G, Olsen CG, et al: Trial of tissue plasminogen activator for mortality reduction in acute myocardial infarction: The Anglo-Scandinavian Study of Early Thrombolysis (ASSET). *Lancet* **2**:525, 1988

44. AIMS Trial Study Group: Effect of intravenous APSAC on mortality after acute myocardial infarction: Preliminary report of placebo-controlled clinical trail. *Lancet* **2**:545, 1988

45. ISIS-2 Collaborative Group: Randomized trial of intravenous streptokinase, oral aspirin, both, or neither among 17,187 cases of suspected myocardial infarction. *Lancet* **2**:349, 1988

46. Lee L, Bates ER, Piti B, et al: Percutaneous transluminal coronary angioplasty improves survival in acute myocardial infarction complicated by cardiogenic shock. *Circulation* **78**:1345, 1988

47. Kaplan AJ, Bengston JR, Aronson LG, et al: Reperfusion improves survival in patients with cardiogenic shock after acute myocardial infarction (Abstract). *J Am Coll Cardiol* **15**:155A, 1990

48. Hibbard MD, Holmes DR, Gersh BJ, Reeder GS: Coronary angioplasty for acute myocardial infarction complicated by cardiogenic shock (Abstract). *Circulation* **82**(Suppl III):III–511, 1990

49. Fulton M, Lutz W, Donald KW, et al: Natural history of unstable angina. *Lancet* **1**:860, 1974

50. Gazes PC, Mobley EM Jr, Farais HM Jr, et al: Preinfarction (unstable) angina - A prospective study. Ten-year follow-up. Prognostic significance of electrocardiographic changes. *Circulation* **48**:331, 1973

51. Fischl SJ, Herman MJ, Gorlin R: The intermediate coronary syndrome. Clinical, angiographic, and therapeutic aspects. *N Engl J Med* **288**:1193, 1973

52. Baughman KL: Intra-aortic balloon pumping. In Plotnick GD (ed): *Unstable Angina: A Clinical Approach.* New York, Futura, 1985, p 327

53. Harris PL, Woollard K, Bartoli A, et al: The management of impending myocardial infarction using coronary bypass grafting and an intra-aortic balloon pump. *J Cardiovasc Surg* **21**:405, 1980

54. Levine FH, Gold HK, Leinbach RC, et al: Management of acute myocardial ischemia with intra-aortic balloon pumping and coronary bypass surgery. *Circulation* **58**(Suppl I):I–69, 1978

55. Gold HK, Leinbach RC, Buckley MJ, et al: Refractory angina pectoris: Follow-up after intra-aortic balloon pumping and surgery. *Circulation* **54**(Suppl III):III–41, 1976

56. Langou RA, Geha AS, Hammond GL, et al: Surgical approach for patients with unstable angina pectoris: Role of the response to initial medical therapy and intra-aortic balloon pumping in perioperative complications after aorto-coronary bypass graft. *Am J Cardiol* **42**:629, 1978

57. Weintraub RM, Aroesty JM, Paulin S, et al: Medically refractory unstable angina pectoris: Long-term follow-up of patients undergoing intra-aortic balloon pumping and operation. *Am J Cardiol* **45**:877, 1979

58. Plotnick GD: The role of coronary artery bypass graft surgery in unstable angina. In Plotnick DG (ed): *Unstable Angina: A Clinical Approach.* New York, Futura, 1985, p 49

59. Craver JM, Kaplan JA, Jones EL, et al: What role should the intra-aortic balloon have in cardiac surgery? *Ann Surg* **189**:769, 1979

60. Pennington DC, Swartz M, Codd JE, et al: Intra-aortic balloon pumping in cardiac surgical patients: A nine-year experience. *Ann Thorac Surg* **36**:125, 1983

61. Schuster EH, Bulkley BH: Early postinfarction angina. *N Engl J Med* **305**:1101, 1981

62. Bardet J, Rigaud M, Kahn JC, et al: Treatment of postmyocardial infarction angina by intra-aortic balloon pumping and emergency revascularization. *J Thorac Cardiovasc Surg* **74**:299, 1977

63. Brundage BH, Ullyot DJ, Winokur S, et al: The role of aortic balloon pumping in postinfarction angina. *Circulation* **62**(Suppl I):I–119, 1980

64. Williams DB, Ivey TD, Bailey WW, et al: Postinfarction angina: Results of early revascularization. *J Am Coll Cardiol* **2**:859, 1983

65. Jones EL, Douglas JS Jr, Craver JM, et al: Results of coronary revascularization in patients with recent myocardial infarction. *J Thorac Cardiovasc Surg* **76**:545, 1978

66. Mallory GK, White PD, Salcedo-Salgar J: The speed of healing of myocardial infarction. *Am Heart J* **18**:647, 1939

67. Lee W, Cardon L, Slodi S: Perforation of the interventricular septum. *Arch Intern Med* **109**:135, 1962

68. Kitamura S, Mendez A, Kay J: Ventricular septal defect following myocardial infarction. *J Thorac Cardiovasc Surg* **61**:186, 1971

69. Hutchins G: Rupture of the interventricular septum complicating myocardial infarction: Pathologic analysis of ten patients with clinically diagnosed perforations. *Am Heart J* **97**:165, 1979

70. Diaz-Rivera RS, Miller AJ: Rupture of the heart following acute myocardial infarction. *Am Heart J* **35**:126, 1948

71. Oyamada A, Queen FB: Spontaneous rupture of the interventricular septum following acute myocardial infarction with some clinico-pathologic observations on survival in five cases. Presented at the

First Pan-Pacific Pathology Congress, Tripler, U.S. Army Hospital, Honolulu, Hawaii, October 12, 1961

72. Sanders RJ, Kern WH, Blount SG: Perforation of the interventricular septum complicating myocardial infarction. *Am Heart J* **51**:736, 1956

73. Gold HK, Leinbach RC, Sanders CA, et al: Intra-aortic balloon pumping for ventricular septal defect on mitral regurgitation complicating acute myocardial infarction. *Circulation* **47**:1191, 1973

74. Heitmiller R, Jacobs ML, Dagget WM: Surgical management of postinfarction ventricular septal rupture. *Ann Thorac Surg* **41**:683, 1986

75. Daggett WM, Buckley WJ, Akins CW, et al: Improved results of surgical management of postinfarction ventricular septal rupture. *Ann Surg* **196**:269, 1982

76. Gaudiani VA, Miller DC, Stinson EB, et al: Postinfarction ventricular septal defect: An argument for early operation. *Surgery* **89**:48, 1981

77. Komeda M, Fremes SE, David TE: Surgical repair of postinfarction ventricular septal defect. *Circulation* **82**(Suppl IV):IV–243, 1990

78. Sander RJ, Neuberger KT, Ravin A: Rupture of papillary muscle. Occurrence of rupture of the posterior muscle and posterior myocardial infarction. *Chest* **31**:316, 1957

79. Wei JY, Hutchins GM, Bulkley BM: Papillary muscle rupture and fatal acute myocardial infarction. *Ann Intern Med* **90**:149, 1979

80. DePasquale NP, Burch GE: Papillary muscle dysfunction in coronary (ischemic) heart disease. *Annu Rev Med* **22**:327, 1971

81. DeBusk RF, Harrison DC: The clinical spectrum of papillary-muscle disease. *N Engl J Med* **281**:1458, 1969

82. Morrow AG, Cohen LS, Roberts WC, et al: Several mitral regurgitation following acute myocardial infarction and rupture of papillary muscle. *Circulation* **37**(Suppl. II):II–124, 1968

83. Tepe NA, Edmunds LH Jr: Operation for acute postinfarction mitral insufficiency and cardiogenic shock. *J Thorac Cardiovasc Surg* **89**:525, 1985

84. Mueller H, Aynes SM, Gianelli S Jr, et al: Cardiac performance and metabolism in shock due to acute myocardial infarction in man: Response to catecholamines and mechanical cardiac assist. *Trans NY Acad Sci* **34**:309, 1972

85. Radford MJ, Johnson RA, Buckley MJ, et al: Survival following mitral valve replacement for mitral regurgitation due to coronary artery disease. *Circulation* **60**(Suppl II):II–39, 1979

86. Magovern JA, Pennock JL, Campbell DB, et al: Risks of mitral valve replacement and mitral valve replacement with coronary artery bypass. *Ann Thorac Surg* **39**:346, 1985

87. DiSesa VJ, Cohn LH, Collins JJ Jr, et al: Determinants of operative survival following combined mitral valve replacement and coronary revascularization. *Ann Thorac Surg* **4**:482, 1982

88. Kay PH, Nunley DL, Grunkemeier G, et al: Late results of combined mitral valve replacement and coronary bypass surgery. *J Am Coll Cardiol* **5**:29, 1985

89. Connolly MW, Gelbfish JS, Jacobwitz IJ, et al: Surgical results for mitral regurgitation from coronary artery disease. *J Thorac Cardiovasc Surg* **91**:379, 1986

90. Williams DO, Scherlag BJ, Hope RR, et al: The pathophysiology of malignant ventricular arrhythmias during acute myocardial ischemia. *Circulation* **50**:1163, 1974

91. Mundth ED: Mechanical and surgical intervention for the reduction of myocardial ischemia. *Circulation* **53**(Suppl I):I–176, 1976

92. Ecker RR, Mullins CB, Grammer JC, et al: Control of intractable ventricular tachycardia by coronary revascularization. *Circulation* **44**:666, 1971

93. Cox JL: Anatomic-electrophysiologic basis for the surgical treatment of refractory ischemic ventricular tachycardia. *Am Surg* **198**:119, 1983

94. Hanson EC, Levine FH, Kay HR, et al: Control of postinfarction ventricular irritability with the intra-aortic balloon pump. *Circulation* **62**(Suppl I):I–130, 1980

95. Cox JL: The status of surgery for cardiac arrhythmias. *Circulation* **71**:413, 1985

96. Norman JC, Colley DA, Igo SR, et al: Prognostic indices for survival during postcardiotomy intra-aortic balloon pumping. *J Thorac Cardiovasc Surg* **74**:709, 1977

97. Myers JL, Parr GVS, Pae WE Jr, et al: The role of the ventricular assist pump for postcardiotomy cardiogenic shock: A four-and-one-half year experience. *Artificial Organs* **5**(Suppl):244, 1981

98. Bolooki H: Balloon pumping in cardiac surgery. In Bolooki H (ed): *Clinical Application of Intra-Aortic Balloon Pump*. New York, Futura, 1984, p 373

99. Sanfelippo PM, Baker NH, Ewy GH, et al: Experience with intra-aortic balloon counterpulsation. *Ann Thorac Surg* **41**:36, 1986

100. Creswell LL, Rosenbloom M, Cox JL, et al: Intra-aortic balloon counterpulsation: Patterns of usage and outcome in cardiac surgery patients. *Ann Thorac Surg* **54**:11, 1992

101. Naunheim KS, Swartz MT, Pennington DG, et al: Intra-aortic balloon pumping in patients requiring cardiac operations. *J Thorac Cardiovasc Surg* **104**:1654, 1992

102. Balooki H, Williams W, Thurer RJ, et al: Clinical and hemodynamic criteria for use of intra-aortic balloon pump in patients requiring cardiac surgery. *J Thorac Cardiovasc Surg* **72**:756, 1976

103. Golding LR, Loop FD, Peter M, et al: Late survival following use of intra-aortic balloon pump in revascularization operations. *Ann Thorac Surg* **30**:48, 1980

104. Davies R, Laks H, Berger H, et al: Follow-up radionuclide assessment of left ventricular function and perfusion in patients requiring intra-aortic balloon pump to wean from cardiopulmonary bypass. *Am J Cardiol* **45**:488, 1980

105. Buckley MJ, Craver JM, Gold HK, et al: Intra-aortic balloon assist for cardiogenic shock after cardiopulmonary bypass. *Circulation* **48**(Suppl III):III–90, 1983

106. Scanlon PJ, O'Connell J, Johnson SA, et al: Balloon counterpulsation following surgery for ischemic heart disease. *Circulation* **54**(Suppl III):III–90, 1976

107. Pollack JC, Charlton MD, Williams WG, et al: Intra-aortic balloon pumping in children. *Ann Thorac Surg* **29**:522, 1980

108. Veasy LG, Blaylock RC, Orth JL, et al: Intra-aortic balloon pumping in infants and children. *Circulation* **68**:1095, 1983

109. Veasy LG, Webster HF, McGough EC: Intra-aortic balloon pumping: Adaptation for pediatric use. *Crit Care Clin* **2**:237, 1986

110. Reemstma K, Drusin R, Edie R, et al: Cardiac transplantation for patients requiring mechanical circulatory support. *J Engl J Med* **298**:670, 1978

111. Hardesty RL, Griffith BP, Trento A, et al: Mortally ill patients and excellent survival following cardiac transplantation. *Ann Thorac Surg* **41**:126, 1986

112. O'Connell JB, Renlund DG, Robinson JA, et al: Effect of preoperative hemodynamic support on survival after cardiac transplantation. *Circulation* **78**(Suppl III):III–78, 1988

113. Berger RL, Saini VK, Long W, et al: The use of diastolic augmentation with the intra-aortic balloon in human septic shock with associated coronary artery disease. *Surgery* **79**:601, 1973

114. Mercer D, Doris P, Salerno TA: Intra-aortic balloon counterpulsation in septic shock. *Can J Surg* **24**(6):643, 1981

115. Bonchek LF, Olinger GN: Intra-aortic balloon counterpulsation for cardiac support during non-cardiac operations. *J Thorac Cardiovasc Surg* **78**:147, 1979

116. Foster ED, Olsson CA, Rutenberg AM, et al: Mechanical circulatory assistance with intra-aortic counterpulsation for major abdominal surgery. *Ann Surg* **183**:73, 1976

117. Grotyz RL, Yeston NS: Intra-aortic balloon counterpulsation in high-risk cardiac patients undergoing non-cardiac surgery. *Surgery* **106**(1):1, 1989

118. Georgen RF, Dietrick JA, Pifarre R, et al: Placement of intra-aortic balloon pump allows definitive biliary surgery in patients with severe cardiac disease. *Surgery* **106**:808, 1989

119. Kantrowitz A, Cardona RR, Av J, et al: Intra-aortic balloon pumping in congestive heart failure. In Hosenpud JD, Greenburg BH (ed): *Congestive Heart Failure: Pathophysiology, Diagnosis, and Comprehensive Approach to Management.* New York, Springer-Verlag, 1994

120. Balooki H: Methods of insertion of intra-aortic balloon catheter. In Bolooki H (ed): *Clinical Application of Intra-Aortic Balloon Pump.* New York, Futura, 1984, p 103

121. McBride LR, Miller LW, Naunheim KS, et al: Axillary artery insertion of an intra-aortic balloon pump. *Ann Thorac Surg* **48:**874, 1989

122. Isner JM, Cohen SR, Virmani R, et al: Complications of the intra-aortic balloon counterpulsation device: Clinical and morphologic observations in 45 necropsy patients. *Am J Cardiol* **45:**260, 1978

123. Gunstensen J, Goldman BS, Scully HE, et al: Evolving indications for preoperative intra-aortic balloon pump assistance. *Ann Thorac Surg* **22:**535, 1976

124. Cooper GN, Singh AK, Christian FC, et al: Preoperative intra-aortic balloon support in surgery for left main coronary stenosis. *Ann Surg* **185:**242, 1977

125. Bahn CH, Vitikainen KJ, Anderson CL, et al: Vascular evaluation for balloon pumping. *Ann Thorac Surg* **27:**475, 1979

126. Beckman DB, Geha AS, Hammond GL, et al: Results and complications of intra-aortic balloon counterpulsation. *Ann Thorac Surg* **24:**550, 1977

127. Vignola PA, Swaye PS, Gosselin AJ: Guidelines for effective and safe percutaneous intra-aortic balloon pump insertion and removal. *Am J Cardiol* **48:**660, 1981

128. Bregman D: Percutaneous intra-aortic balloon pumping. A time for reflection. *Chest* **82:**397, 1982

129. McCabe JC, Abel RM, Subramanian VA, et al: Complications of intra-aortic balloon insertion and counterpulsation. *Circulation* **57:**769, 1978

130. Harvey JC, Goldstein JE, McCabe JC, et al: Complications of percutaneous intra-aortic balloon pumping. *Circulation* **64**(Suppl II)II:114, 1981

131. Kunkler A, King H: Comparison of air, oxygen, and carbon dioxide embolization. *Ann Surg* **149:**95, 1959

132. Karayannacos PE, Shapiro IL, Kakos GS, et al: Counterpulsation catheter fracture: An unexpected hazard. *Ann Thorac Surg* **23:**276, 1977

133. Hauser AM, Gordon S, Gangadharan V, et al: Percutaneous intra-aortic balloon counterpulsation. Clinical effectiveness and hazards. *Chest* **82:**442, 1982

134. Alpert J, Bhaktan EK, Gielchinsky I, et al: Vascular complications of intra-aortic balloon pumping. *Arch Surg* **111:**1190, 1976

135. Martin RS, Moncure AC, Buckley MJ, et al: Complications of percutaneous intra-aortic balloon insertion. *J Thorac Cardiovasc Surg* **85:**186, 1983

136. Wolff GA, Kamadu RO, Collins JA, et al: Prolonged use of intra-aortic phase-shift balloon pumping in cardiogenic shock. *Chest* **62:**646, 1972

137. Cleveland RJ: IAB graft complications. *Ann Thorac Surg* **23:**389, 1977

138. Parr GVS, Pierce WS, Rosenberg G, et al: Right ventricular failure after repair of left ventricular aneurysm. *J Thorac Cardiovasc Surg* **80:**79, 1980

139. Miller DC, Moreno-Cabral RJ, Stinson EB, et al: Pulmonary artery balloon counterpulsation for acute right ventricular failure. *J Thorac Cardiovasc Surg* **80:**760, 1980

140. Pierce WS, Parr GVS, Myers JL, et al: Ventricular-assist pumping in patients with cardiogenic shock after cardiac operations. *N Engl J Med* **305:**1606, 1981

141. Cohn JN: Right ventricular infarction revisited. *Am J Cardiol* **43:**666, 1979

142. Speace PA, Weisel RD, Easdown J, et al: Pulmonary artery balloon counterpulsation in the management of right heart failure during left heart bypass. *J Thorac Cardiovasc Surg* **89:**264, 1985

143. Bernhard WF, Berger RL, Stetz JP, et al: Temporary left ventricular bypass. Factors affecting patient survival. *Circulation* **60**(Suppl II):II-131, 1979

144. D'Ambra MN, LaRara PJ, Philbin DM, et al: Prostaglandin E₁: A new therapy for refractory right heart failure and pulmonary hypertension after mitral valve replacement. *J Thorac Cardiovasc Surg* **89:**567, 1985

145. Dreyfus G, Guillemain R, Dubois C, et al: Right ventricular failure after heart transplantation: Treatment with nitric oxide. *J Heart Lung Transplant* **13**(Suppl II)II:552, 1994

146. Rich GF, Murphy GD Jr, Roos CM, Johns RA: Inhaled nitric oxide. Selective pulmonary vasodilation in cardiac surgical patients. *Anesthesiology* **78**(6):1028, 1993

147. Spence PA, Weisel RD, Easdown J, et al: Pulmonary artery balloon counterpulsation in the management of right heart failure during left heart bypass. *J Thorac Cardiovasc Surg* **89:**264, 1984

148. Opravil M, Gorman AJ, Krejcie TC, et al: Pulmonary artery balloon counterpulsation for right ventricular failure: I. Experimental results. *Ann Thorac Surg* **38:**242, 1984

149. Spence PA, Weisel RD, Easdown J, et al: The hemodynamic effects and mechanism of action of pulmonary artery balloon counterpulsation in the treatment of right ventricular failure during left heart bypass. *Ann Thorac Surg* **39:**329, 1984

150. Symbas PN, McKeown PP, Santora AH, et al: Pulmonary artery balloon counterpulsation for treatment of intraoperative right ventricular failure. *Ann Thorac Surg* **39:**437, 1985

151. Moran JM, Opravil M, Gorman AJ, et al: Pulmonary artery balloon counterpulsation for right ventricular failure. II. Clinical experience. *Ann Thorac Surg* **38:**254, 1984

152. Dennis C, Hall DP, Moreno JR, Senning A: Reduction of the oxygen utilization of the heart by left heart bypass. *Circ Res* **101:**298, 1962

153. Levine ID, Manoko PR, Bernstein EF: Comparison of intra-aortic balloon pumping and left ventricular decompression on myocardial ischemic injury after experimental coronary artery occlusion. *Surg Forum* **22:**149, 1971

154. Pennock JL, Pierce WS, Prophet GA, et al: Myocardial oxygen utilization during left heart bypass: Effects of varying percentage of bypass flow rate. *Arch Surg* **109:**635, 1974

155. Pennock JL, Pierce WS, Waldhausen JA: Quantitative evaluation of left ventricular bypass in reducing myocardial ischemia. *Surgery* **79:**523, 1976

156. Pierce WS, Aaronson AE, Prophet GA, et al: Hemodynamic and metabolic studies during two types of left ventricular bypass. *Surg Forum* **23:**1976, 1972

157. Pierce WS, Donachy JH, Landis DL, et al: Prolonged mechanical support of the left ventricle. *Circulation* **58**(Suppl I):I-133, 1978

158. Pennock JL, Pae WE Jr, Pierce WS, et al: Reduction of myocardial infarct size: Comparison between left atrial and left ventricular bypass. *Circulation* **59:**275, 1979

159. Davis PK, Pae WE Jr, Miller CA, et al: Myocardial oxygen consumption (MVO₂): Comparison between left atrial pulsatile synchronous and asynchronous bypass. *Trans Am Soc Artif Intern Organs* **35:**461, 1989

160. Davis PK, Pae WE Jr, Miller CA, et al: Reduction of myocardial oxygen consumption during left atrial-to-aortic bypass: Is pulsatility and synchronization important? *Surg Forum* **XL:**206, 1989

161. Quinn RD, Pae WE Jr, Pierce WS: Myocardial oxygen delivery and consumption during mechanical circulatory support. *Surg Forum* **43:**238, 1992

162. Kawaguchi O, Sapristein JS, Daily WB, et al: Left ventricular mechanics during synchronous left atrial-to-aortic bypass. *J Thorac Cardiovasc Surg* **107:**1503–1511, 1994

163. Pae WE Jr, Pierce WS: Mechanical left ventricular assistance: Current devices, future prospects. In Moran JM, Michaelis LL, (eds): *Surgery for the Complications of Myocardial Infarction.* New York, Grune & Stratton, 1980

164. Gaines WE, Pierce WS, Donachy JH, et al: The Pennsylvania State

University paracorporeal ventricular assist pump: Optimal methods of use. *World J Surg* 9:47, 1985

165. Pennington DG, Samuels LD, Williams G, et al: Experience with the Pierce-Donachy ventricular assist device in postcardiotomy patients with cardiogenic shock. *World J Surg* 9:37, 1985

166. Pennock JL, Pierce WS, Wisman CB, et al: Survival and complications following ventricular assist pumping for cardiogenic shock. *Ann Surg* 198:469, 1983

167. Pae WE Jr, Gaines WE, Pierce WS, Waldhausen JA: Mechanical circulatory assistance for postoperative cardiogenic shock. *Surg Rounds* July:49–63, 1985

168. Pae WE Jr, Pierce WS, Pennock JL, et al: Long-term results of ventricular assist pumping in postcardiotomy cardiogenic shock. *J Thorac Cardiovasc Surg* 93:434, 1987

169. Rose DM, Colvin SB, Culliford AT, et al: Long-term survival with partial left heart bypass following perioperative myocardial infarction and shock. *J Thorac Cardiovasc Surg* 83:483, 1982

170. Litwak RS, Koffsky RM, Jurado RA, et al: A decade of experience with a left heart assist device in patients undergoing open intracardiac operation. *World J Surg* 9:18, 1985

171. Rose DM, Laschinger J, Grossi E, et al: Experimental and clinical results with a simplified left heart assist device for treatment of profound left ventricular dysfunction. *World J Surg* 9:11, 1985

172. Pennington DG, Bernhard WF, Golding LR, et al: Long-term follow-up of postcardiotomy patients with profound cardiogenic shock treated with ventricular assist devices. *Circulation* 72(Suppl II):II–216, 1985

173. Pennock JL, Pierce WS, Campbell DB, et al: Mechanical support of the circulation followed by cardiac transplantation. *J Thorac Cardiovasc Surg* 96:994, 1986

174. Hill JD, Farrar DJ, Hershon JJ, et al: Use of a prosthetic ventricle as a bridge to cardiac transplantation for postinfarction cardiogenic shock. *N Engl J Med* 314:626, 1986

175. Pennock JL, Wisman CB, Pierce WS: Mechanical support of the circulation prior to transplantation. *Heart Transplant* I:299, 1982

176. Quinn RD, Pierce WS, Pae WE Jr: Ventricular assistance and replacement. In Hosenpud JD, Greenberg BH (eds): *Congestive Heart Failure: Pathophysiology, Diagnosis, and Comprehensive Approach to Management.* New York, Springer-Verlag, 1994

177. Pae WE Jr, Miller CA, Pierce WS: Ventricular assist device for postcardiotomy cardiogenic shock: A combined registry experience. *J Thorac Cardiovasc Surg* 104:541, 1992

178. Moritz A, Wolner E: Circulatory support with shock due to acute myocardial infarction. *Ann Thorac Surg* 55:238, 1993

179. Pierce WS: The implantable ventricular assist pump. *J Thorac Cardiovasc Surg* 87:811, 1984

180. Sapirstein JS, Pae WE Jr, Rosenberg G, Pierce WS: The development of permanent circulatory support systems. *Sem Thorac Cardiovasc Surg,* 6(3):188–194, 1994

181. Dembitsky W, Raney AA, Daily PO: Temporary extracorporeal postoperative circulatory support using the roller pump or rotor impeller pump. In Utley JR (ed): *Perioperative Cardiac Dysfunction,* Vol III. Baltimore, Williams & Wilkins, 1985, p 63

182. Bernstein EF, Dorman FD, Blackshear PL Jr, et al: An efficient, compact blood pump for assisted circulation. *Cardiovasc Surg* 63:865, 1972

183. Pennington DG, Merjavy JP, Codd JE, et al: Temporary mechanical support of patients with profound ventricular failure. In Unger F (ed): *Assist Circulation II.* New York, Springer-Verlag, 1984, p 85

184. Guyton RA, Schonberger JPAM, Everts PAM, et al: Postcardiotomy shock: Clinical evaluation of the BVS 5000 biventricular support system. *Ann Thorac Surg* 56:346, 1993

185. Frazier OH, Rose EA, Macmanus Q, et al: Multicenter clinical evaluation of the HeartMate 1000 IP left ventricular assist device. *Ann Thorac Surg* 53:1080, 1992

186. Braunwald E, Kloner RA: The stunned myocardium—Prolonged, post-ischemic ventricular dysfunction. *Circulation* 66:1146, 1982

187. Schoen FJ, LaFarge CG, Bernhard WF: Pathology and pathophysiology of temporary cardiac assist. *ASAIO J* 8:174, 1985

188. O'Neill MJ Jr, Pierce WS, Wisman CB, et al: Successful management of right ventricular failure with the ventricular assist pump following aortic valve replacement and coronary bypass grafting. *J Thorac Cardiovasc Surg* 87:106, 1984

189. Magovern JA, Pae WE Jr, Richenbacher WE, et al: The importance of a patent foramen ovale in left ventricular assist pumping. *Trans Am Soc Artif Intern Organs* 32:449, 1986

190. Pierce WS: Clinical left ventricular bypass: Problems of pump inflow obstruction and right ventricular failure. *ASAIO J* 2:1, 1979

191. Pae WE Jr, Rosenberg G, Donachy JH, et al: Mechanical circulatory assistance for postoperative cardiogenic shock: A three year experience. *Trans Am Soc Artif Intern Organs* 26:256, 1980

192. Copeland JG: Circulatory Support Panel II: Anticoagulation. *Ann Thorac Surg* 55:213, 1993

193. Pierce WS: Chairman, panel conference: Cardiac support. *Trans Am Soc Artif Intern Organs* 26:625, 1980

194. Aufiero TX, Pae WE Jr: Extracorporeal pneumatic ventricular assistance for postcardiotomy cardiogenic shock. *Card Surg State-of-the-Art Reviews.* 7:277, 1993

195. Barzilai B, Davila-Roman VG, Eaton MH, et al: Transesophageal echocardiography predicts successful withdrawal of ventricular assist devices. *J Thorac Cardiovasc Surg* 104(5):1410, 1992

196. Magovern GJ Jr: The biopump and postoperative circulatory support. *Ann Thorac Surg* 55:245, 1993

197. Magovern GJ, Park SB, Maher TD: Use of a centrifugal pump without anticoagulants for postoperative left ventricular assist. *World J Surg* 9:25, 1985

198. Copeland JG, Emery RW, Levinson MM, et al: The role of mechanical support and transplantation in treatment of patients with end-stage cardiomyopathy. *Circulation* 72(Suppl II):II–7, 1985

199. Pae WE Jr: Ventricular assist devices and total artificial hearts: A combined registry experience. *Ann Thorac Surg* 55:295, 1993

200. Reedy JE, Pennington DG, Miller LW, et al; Status I heart transplant patients: Conventional versus ventricular assist device support. *J Heart Lung Transplant* 11:246, 1992

201. Kormos RL, Borovetz HS, Gasior T, et al: Experience with univentricular support in mortally ill cardiac transplant candidates. *Ann Thorac Surg* 49:261, 1990

202. Kormos RI, Gasior T, Antaki J, et al: Evaluation of right ventricular function during clinical left ventricular assistance. *ASAIO Trans* 35:547, 1989

203. Pae WE Jr, Wisman CB, Pierce WS, et al: Staged cardiac transplantation: Total artificial heart or ventricular assist pump? *Circulation* 78(Suppl) Part II, (5):66, 1988

204. Farrar DS, Hill JD: Univentricular and biventricular Thoratec VAD support as a bridge-to-transplantation. *Ann Thorac Surg* 55:276, 1993

205. McCarthy PM, Portner PM, Tobler HG, et al: Clinical experience with the Norvacor ventricular assist system. Bridge-to-transplantation and the transition to permanent application. *J Thorac Cardiovasc Surg* 102:578, 1991

206. Portner PM, Oyer PE, Pennington DG, et al: Implantable electrical left ventricular assist system: Bridge-to-transplantation and the future. *Ann Thorac Surg* 47(1):142, 1989

207. Frazier OH: Chronic left ventricular support with a vented electric assist device. *Ann Thorac Surg* 55(1):273, 1993

208. O'Connell JB, Gunnar RM, Evans RW, et al: Twenty-fourth Bethesda conference: Organization of heart transplantation in the US. *J Am Coll Cardiol* 22:8, 1993

209. Jeevanandam V, Rose EA: TCI HeartMate left ventricular assist system: Results with bridge-to-transplant and chronic support. In Ott RA, Gutfinger DE, Gazzaniga AB (eds): *Cardiac Surgery: State-of-the-Art Reviews,* Vol 7. Philadelphia, Hanley & Belfus, 1993, pp 335–352

210. Jassawalla JS, Daniel MA, Chen H, et al: *In vitro* and *in vivo* testing

of a totally implantable left ventricular assist system. *Trans Am Soc Artif Intern Organs* **34**:470, 1988

211. Miller P, Billich J, LaForge D, et al: Development of a wearable controller for the Novacor LVAS. *Ann Biomed Eng* **21**:18, 1993 (Abstr Suppl)

212. Ramasamy N, Chen H, Miller PJ, et al: Chronic ovine evaluation of a totally implantable electric left ventricular assist system. *Trans Am Soc Artif Intern Organs* **35**:402, 1989

213. Diegel PD, Mussivand T, Holfert JW, et al: Electrohydraulic ventricular assist device development. *ASAIO J* **38**:M306, 1992

214. Sasaki T, Takatani S, Shiono M, et al: A biolized, compact, low noise, high performance implantable electromechanical ventricular assist system. *Trans Am Soc Artif Intern Organs* **37**:M249, 1991

215. Nakatani T, Anai H, Goto M, et al: An abdominally placed, implantable left ventricular assist system for long-term use. *ASAIO J* **38**:M631, 1992

216. Weiss WJ, Rosenberg G, Snyder AJ, et al: A completely implanted left ventricular assist device: Chronic *in vivo* testing. *ASAIO J* **39**:M427, 1993

217. Yamazaki K, Umezu M, Koyanagi H, et al: A miniature intraventricular axial flow blood pump that is introduced through the left ventricular apex. *ASAIO J* **38**:M679, 1992

218. Damm G, Mizuguchi K, Bozeman R, et al: *In vitro* performance of the Baylor/NASA axial flow pump. *Artif Organs* **17**:609, 1993

219. Butler KC, Maher TR, Borovetz HS, et al: Development of an axial flow blood pump LVAS. *ASAIO J* **38**:M296, 1992

220. Akutsu T, Kolff WJ: Permanent substitutes for valves and hearts. *Trans Am Soc Artif Intern Organs* **4**:230, 1958

221. Kolff WJ, Akutsu T, Dreyer B, et al: Artificial heart inside the chest and the use of polyurethane for making valves and aortas. *Trans Am Soc Artif Intern Organs* **7**:298, 1959

222. Akutsu T, Houston CS, Kolff WJ: Artificial hearts inside the chest, using small electro-motors. *Trans Am Soc Artif Intern Organs* **6**:299, 1960

223. Nosé Y, Topaz S, SenGupta A, et al: Artificial hearts inside the pericardial sac in calves. *Trans Am Soc Artif Intern Organs* **11**:255, 1965

224. Klain M, Mrava GL, Tajima K, et al: Can we achieve over 100 hours' survival with a total mechanical heart? *Trans Am Soc Artif Intern Organs* **17**:437, 1971

225. Ross NJ Jr, Akers WW, O'Bannon W, et al: Problems encountered during the development and implantation of the Baylor-Rice orthotopic cardiac prosthesis. *Trans Am Soc Artif Intern Organs* **18**:168, 1972

226. Boretos JW, Pierce WS: Segmented polyurethane: A new elastomer for biomedical application. *Science* **158**:1481, 1967

227. Dutton RC, Baier RE, Dedrick RL, et al: Initial thrombus formation on foreign surfaces. *Trans Am Soc Artif Intern Organs* **14**:57, 1968

228. Kolff WJ, Lawson J: Status of the artificial heart and cardiac assist devices in the United States. *Trans Am Soc Artif Intern Organs* **21**:620, 1975

229. Harmison LT: Totally implantable nuclear heart assist and artificial heart. National Heart and Lung Institute, National Institutes of Health, February 1972

230. Cole DW, Holman WS, Mott WE: Status of the USAEC's nuclear-powered artificial heart. *Trans AM Soc Artif Intern Organs* **19**:537, 1973

231. Smith L, Backman K, Sandquist G, et al: Development on the implantation of a total nuclear-powered artificial heart system. *Trans Am Soc Artif Intern Organs* **20**:732, 1974

232. Jarvik RK, Smith LM, Lawson JH, et al: Comparison of pneumatic and electrically powered total artificial heart *in vivo*. *Trans Am Soc Artif Intern Organs* **24**:593, 1978

233. Snyder AJ, Rosenberg G, Reibson J, et al: An electrically powered total artificial heart. Over one year survival in the calf. *ASAIO J* **38**(3):M707, 1992

234. Pierce WS, Rosenberg G, Snyder AJ, et al: An electric artificial heart for clinical use. *Ann Surg* **212**(3):105, 1990

235. Colley DA, Kiotta D, Hallman GL, et al: First human implantation of cardiac prosthesis for staged total replacement of the heart. *Trans Am Soc Artif Intern Organs* **15**:252, 1969

236. Levinson MM, Smith RG, Cork RC, et al: Thromboembolic complications of the Jarvik-7 total artificial heart: Case report. *Artif Organs* **10**:236, 1986

237. DeVries WC, Anderson JL, Joce LD, et al: Clinical use of the total artificial heart. *N Engl J Med* **310**:273, 1984

238. Pennock JL, Oyer PE, Reitz BA, et al: Cardiac transplantation in perspective for the future. Survival, complications, rehabilitation, and cost. *J Thorac Cardiovasc Surg* **83**:168, 1982

239. Balubaugh AL, Butler KG, Schnieder JA, et al: Thermally and electrically powered left ventricular assist devices. *Prog Artif Organs* **1**:91, 1983

240. White MA: Implantable energy source for artificial hearts. In *Artificial Heart: Proceedings of the First International Symposium on Current Problems for Further Development of the Artificial Heart and Assist Devices, Tokyo, Japan*. Berlin, Springer-Verlag, 1985, p 33

241. Sherman C, Daly BDT, Clay W, et al: *In vivo* evaluation of a transcutaneous energy transmission system. *Trans Am Soc Artif Intern Organs* **30**:143, 1984

242. Heimes HP, Klasen F: Completely integrated wearable TAH-drive unit. *Int J Artif Organs* **5**:157, 1982

243. Kwan-Gett CS, Wu Y, Collan R, et al: Total replacement artificial heart and driving system with interhent regulation of cardiac output. *Trans Am Soc Artif Intern Organs* **15**:245, 1969

244. Landis DL, Pierce WS, Rosenberg G, et al: Long-term *in vivo* automatic electronic control for the artificial heart. *Trans Am Soc Artif Intern Organs* **23**:519, 1977

245. Hughes SD, Butler MD, Holmberg DL, et al: Comparative hematological data from animals implanted with a total artificial heart containing different valves. *Trans Am Soc Artif Intern Organs* **31**:224, 1985

246. Bucherl ES: The artificial heart research program in Berlin, German. *Heart Transplant* **4**:510, 1985

247. Takatani S, Harasaki H, Koike S, et al: Optimum control mode for a total artificial heart. *Trans Am Soc Artif Intern Organs* **28**:148, 1982

248. Pae WE, Rosenberg G, Donachy JH, et al: A solution to inlet pannus formation in the pneumatic artificial heart. *Trans Am Soc Artif Intern Organs* **31**:12, 1985

249. Copeland JG: Heart transplantation, The Tucson Perspective. *Heart Transplant* **4**:499, 1985

250. Kawaguchi AT, Cabrol C, Pavie A, et al: Survival prediction in staged heart transplantation using Jarvik-7 artificial heart. *Circulation* **86**:II-311, 1992

251. Oaks TE, Pae WE Jr, Miller CW, Pierce WS: Combined registry for the clinical use of mechanical ventricular assist pumps and the total artificial heart in conjunction with heart transplantation: Fifth official report—1990. *J Heart Lung Transplant* **10**(5): Part I, 621, 1991

252. Preston TA: Who benefits from the artificial heart? *Hastings Cent Rep* **15**(1):5, 1985

253. Himley SC, Butler KC, Massiello A, et al: Development of the E4T electrohydraulic total artificial heart. *ASAIO Trans* **36**:M234, 1990

254. Orime Y, Takatani S, Shiono M, et al: Versatile one-piece total artificial heart for bridge-to-transplantation or permanent heart replacement. *Artif Organs* **16**:607, 1992

255. Rowles Jr, Kanwilkar PS, Diegel PD, et al: Development of a totally implantable artificial heart. *ASAIO J* **38**:M713, 1992

CHAPTER

112

Preservation of Intrathoracic Organs for Transplantation

John C. Baldwin

Since the first human (xenograft) cardiac transplant operation was performed by Hardy et al in 1964, and during the development of cardiac allografting by Shumway and his group at Stanford, one of the most critical and often poorly understood aspects of thoracic transplantation has been the procurement and preservation of donor organs.[1–3] When the numerical, political, and logistical difficulties of allograft organ procurement are obviated by successful strategies for xenografting, the fundamental technical and physiological aspects of organ procurement will remain critical to success. Investigation continues in this area in parallel with basic immunological work. A common reason for failure of cardiac, pulmonary, and cardiopulmonary transplant is poor graft function, usually related to lack of understanding of the details and nuances of organ procurement. In this chapter, I examine three major areas: the cardiac donor, the lung donor, and the heart–lung donor, concluding with comments on current investigative work and implications for future clinical practice.

CARDIAC GRAFT PROCUREMENT

Criteria for selection of suitable donors for cardiac transplantation have been established over the past 25 years, but they are in a continual state of evolution. Suitable grafts are obtained from donors who are brain dead, with no history of prior cardiac disease, or prolonged cardiopulmonary resuscitation, with normal electrocardiograms and echocardiograms, no chest trauma to result in cardiac contusion or other injury, and no excessive (greater than 5 µg/kg per minute of dopamine) pressor requirements (Table 112–1). At a recent Bethesda Conference sponsored by the Ameri-

can College of Cardiology, accepted criteria for donor selection were summarized, and are listed in Table 112–1.[4] Relative contraindications are described in Table 112–2.[5]

However, an "ideal" donor is a rare phenomenon. In nearly every case, some compromises must be made based upon clinical judgment. The exigencies of clinical cardiac transplantation require that the surgeon be able to "match" donor and recipient beyond simple blood group and cross-match criteria. Some recipients have medical problems that make it important to have a graft with vigorous cardiac function to maximize end-organ perfusion. Recipients with high pulmonary vascular resistance generally fare better with a graft from a donor of greater body weight and should never receive a heart from a donor with difficulties with right ventricular function or high filling pressures. In desperately ill recipients in whom it is imperative to remove mechanical support, donor criteria may have to be liberalized, although improved mechanical devices and better understanding of their proper use have made these situations rare. Finding a suitable donor for the recipient with high circulating levels of antibodies can be vexing and can frustrate expeditious organ procurement with delays from cross-matching. Occasionally, clinical circumstances require transplantation with a positive cross-match, and our Yale group has an innovative strategy of plasmapheresis and extracorporeal UV blood irradiation.[6]

Currently acceptable allograft donors are available to transplant approximately 5% of the total number of people dying of heart failure and treatable by transplant in this country every year. Therefore, while we work toward xeno-transplantation, we must expand the donor pool. There is some potential for improvement with public and physician education, but this has already been accomplished in large

TABLE 112–1. CLINICAL DEFINITION FOR LOSS OF ENTIRE BRAIN FUNCTION

1. Loss of cortical function
   a. Pressence of deep coma
   b. Lack of spontaneous motor activity (spinal reflexes may be present even with complete brain death)
   c. Absence of response to deep painful stimuli
2. Loss of brain stem activity
   a. Absence of respiratory effort (apnea) (Apnea is demonstrated by preoxygenating the patient with 100% fractional inspiratory oxygen for 10 min before disconnecting the ventilator. After the ventilator is disconnected, oxygen is provided by tracheal cannula at 8 L/min. The patient is observed for 5 to 10 min to allow carbon dioxide to accumulate and stimulate respiratory. If there are no respiratory efforts an arterial blood gas measurement is obtained and the ventilator is reconnected. If the arterial partial pressure of carbon dioxide is > 60 mm Hg, the test is considered to be valid and apnea to be present.)
   b. Lack of pupillary or corneal reflexes (Pupillary constriction in response to a bright light is best demonstrated in a darkened room. The cornea is tested by touching with a cotton swab. Absence of pupillary change in response to light or blinking in response to corneal touch indicates brain stem inactivity.)
   c. Lack of gag or cough reflex, even with tracheal suctioning
   d. Lack of oculocephalic or "doll's eye reflex" ("Doll's eye" test is performed by turning the head from side to side with the head tilted forward 30°. If the eyes passively follow the rotating head without a lag, the oculocephalic reflex is considered absent.)
   e. Lack of oculovestibular ("caloric") response (Instillation of 10 mL of ice water into the external ear canal should cause deviation of the eyes from the stimulated side. Absent eye movement response indicates lack of oculovestibular reponse.)

Irreversibility of loss of brain function requires that
1. Brain death has a defined etiology and there is no likelihood of recovery.
2. The patient is normothermic, defined as a core temperature > 32.5°C.
3. Pharmocologic agents capable of central nervous system depression, neuromuscular blockade, or disassociative coma are absent or below therapeutic levels.
4. These criteria for loss of brain function persist for a 12- to 24-hour observation period. A shorter observation period (6 hours) can be used if irreversibility can be confirmed by other means, such as demonstration of lack of cerebral bloodflow.

From Baldwin JC, et al: Task force 2, Reprinted with permission from the American College of Cardiology (Journal of the American College of Cardiology, July 1993, vol. 22)

TABLE 112–2. CONTRAINDICATIONS FOR CARDIAC DONORS

Absolute
1. HIV positivity (? except in cases of HIV-positive recipients)
2. Death from carbon monoxide poisoning, with blood carboxyhemoglobin level > 20%
3. Intractable ventricular arrhythmia
4. Inadequate oxygenation, with arterial saturation < 80% on ventilatory support
5. Documented previous myocardial infarction
6. Clinically significant structural heart disease, intracardiac tumor or severe global hypokinesis with ejection fracture < 10% as determined by echocardiogram
7. Severe occlusive coronary artery disease on arteriography

Relative
1. Hepatitis B surface antigen positivity (? except in cases of surface antigen positive recipients)
2. Bacterial sepsis
3. Hepatitis C positivity
4. History of metastatic cancer
5. Extensive chest wall trauma with evidence of cardiac contusion by ECG or echocardiography
6. Prolonged hypotension defined as a systolic blood pressure < 60 mm Hg for > 6 hours
7. Recurrent supraventricular arrhythmia
8. Prolonged need for inotropic support defined as a dopamine dosage > 20 μg/kg per minute for > 24 hours or comparable dosage of other β-agonist or epinephrine, norepinephrine, or dobutamine for the same period
9. Prolonged resuscitation time after cardiopulmonary arrest, defined as attempted cardiopulmonary resuscitation for > 30 min performed within 24 hours of organ harvest or multiple episodes of attempted cardiopulmonary resuscitation
10. Severe left ventricular hypertrophy on electrocardiogram or echocardiogram
11. Echocardiogram revealing moderate hypokinesia, which is typically segmental in brain injury, with shortening fraction 10 to 25%
12. Noncritical coronary disease on arteriogram
13. History of carbon monoxide inhalation with blood carboxyhemoglobin < 20%
14. History of intravenous drug abuse

From Baldwin JC, et al: Task force 2, Reprinted with permission from the American College of Cardiology (Journal of the American College of Cardiology, July 1993, vol. 22)

part. "Required request" laws exist in most states. In parts of Europe, "presumed consent" laws have been effective, but this approach may not be socially and politically feasible in this country. Thus, extending donor criteria must be considered, and proposals for such changes have been made.[4] While individual judgments to use "high-risk" donors are frequently being made, it will be in the best interest of the field (and certainly of individual programs responsible for their outcomes) to establish prospective studies with carefully defined criteria to analyze outcomes with the use of "high-risk" donor hearts.

Management of the potential cardiac donor requires attention to adequate red cell mass, correction of electrolyte imbalances, maintenance of physiologic blood gasses, treatment of diabetes insipidus with intravenous pitressin, and volume replacement. Rapid infusion of 1–2 L of crystalloid will often abruptly lower pressor requirements, but decisions regarding fluid administration must be tempered by consideration of the need to avoid excessive fluids when lungs are to be procured and by concern to avoid right ventricular distension. In most cases of multiple organ procurement there will be conflicts among the various organ teams, having to do with timing, fluid management, and other issues. Those concerned with extrathoracic organ procurement will favor larger volumes of fluids than those concerned with the heart and the lungs. The surgeon managing the cardiac donor should be judicious in the administration of volume, to reduce pressor requirements to an acceptable range. This can ordinarily be accomplished by treatment of diabetes mellitus with pitressin, a single fluid bolus, and replacement of hourly urine output with crystalloid. When lung donation is contemplated, fluid administration must be kept to an absolute minimum. General considerations in the management of the cardiac donor are outlined in Table 112–3.

The notion that technical features of the donor and recipient operations in cardiac transplantation are straightforward and even insignificant is common among inexperienced surgeons and leads to many of the failures. Thirty years ago, Lower and Shumway recognized the critical importance of donor procurement and preservation to the success of cardiac transplantation.[2] They recognized the two fundamental approaches—normothermic, perfused "maintenance" and hypothermic metabolic inhibition, instinctively favoring the latter with its greater simplicity. Their pioneering report of canine experiments in which hearts were statically cooled in saline at 2–4°C suggested that, with this method, 6–7 hours was the "maximum duration of anoxia" from which the normal heart can recover completely.[2] The basic Shumway system of topical hypothermia remains an effective and widely used method of cardiac preservation.

Other approaches, such as total body cooling, were applied in the early days of cardiac transplantation, but these were largely unsuccessful, while the simplicity of static hypothermia was compelling.[7] Angell, from the Stanford group, reported in 1969 that the viability of transplanted hearts could be predicted by knowing the storage temperatures and the length of the ischemic period, generating what he called "viability curves."[8] This work led to the first successful distant procurement of a cardiac graft by the same group.[7]

The concept of continuous perfusion or "autoperfusion" has never been completely abandoned. Robicsek was an early proponent of such methods, and Cooper reported successful orthotopic heart transplantation in baboons after 24 hours of perfusion.[9–11] However, the logistical complexity prevented these methods from gaining clinical acceptance. Also, perfusion techniques have the problem of free radical generation.[12] Free radicals are generated by reperfusion and reoxygenation after ischemia. "Free radical scavengers" have not consistently been of benefit in graft preservation.[13–15]

With the "cardioplegia era" in the 1970s, a standard method for heart allograft preservation evolved, with single-dose cardioplegia and static hypothermia. A variety of cardioplegia solutions, used in general cardiac surgery,

have been successfully employed. Recently, promising results were reported with the University of Wisconsin solution, but conflicting results concern the effect of relatively high potassium concentrations on coronary artery (and pulmonary artery) resistance during procurement.[16–22] Many other pharmacologic approaches to improve preservation are being considered.[23–25] Most exciting are those related to supplementation of the nitric oxide/cGMP pathway.[26]

Present methods for cardiac graft procurement are an assimilation of experience over the last 25 years in heart transplantation. The donor operation represents the last and best opportunity to assess the adequacy of the graft. After median sternotomy and incision and suspension of the pericardium, the heart is carefully inspected for evidence of unrecognized trauma, occult atherosclerosis, valvular disease, congenital anomaly, or abnormal contractility (Fig. 112–1).

The sequence of steps for successful excision of the heart are listed in Table 112–4. The aorta is encircled with an umbilical tape, and the venae cavae are also encircled, placing a heavy silk tie around the superior cava and an umbilical tape around the inferior cava. The patient is heparinized with 30,000 units of heparin administered into the right atrium. When communication with the other procurement teams indicates that the time for excision of the graft has arrived, a cardioplegic needle is inserted into the ascending aorta and connected to a 1-L bag of crystalloid cardioplegia at 4°C and pressurized to 150 mm Hg.

TABLE 112–3. GENERAL CONSIDERATIONS IN CARDIAC DONOR MANAGEMENT

Establishment and pronouncement of brain death by independent experts prior to involvement of transplant team

Adequate volume resuscitation with crystalloid to restore normal CVP

Aggressive treatment of diabetes insipidus with parenteral pitressin

Correction of electrolyte imbalances

Maximal weaning of inotropic support

Broad-spectrum prophylactic antibiotic coverage

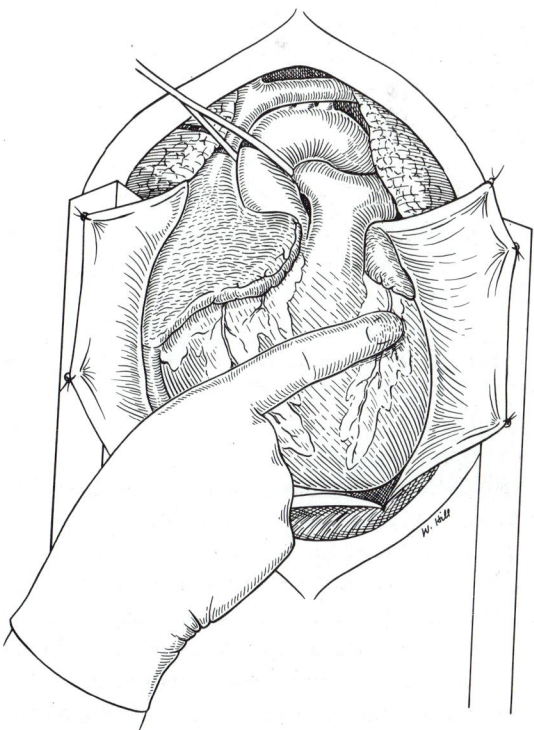

Figure 112–1. The first step in procurement is carefully to assess the heart for evidence of contusion, coronary atherosclerosis, congenital defects, thrills, and bruits. *(From Shumway N, Shumway S: Thoracic Transplantation. Reprinted by permission of Blackwell Scientific Publications, Inc., Cambridge, MA.)*

TABLE 112–4. STEPS IN HEART GRAFT PROCUREMENT

1. Donor assessment (ICU)
2. Sterile prep and median sternotomy
3. Examination of heart for trauma, atherosclerosis, valvular disease, congenital defects
4. Encircle aorta and venae cavae
5. Heparin 30,000 IU
6. Ligate SVC and clamp IVC
7. Clamp aorta
8. Start cardioplegia (pressurized to 150 mm Hg with pressure bag)
9. Incise right superior pulmonary vein and inferior vena cava
10. Apply topical saline (4°C)
11. Excise heart, dividing cavae, aorta, pulmonary veins, and pulmonary artery
12. Bag in saline, excluding air
13. Transport in ice

Excision of the heart takes precedence over other organs because of the greater sensitivity of the graft to hypotension and/or ischemia. When the other teams are ready to begin, the cardiac surgeon ligates the superior vena cava with a heavy silk tie. Next, anterior traction is placed on the inferior vena cava, and a straight, long vascular clamp ("spoon" Potts) is placed across the inferior vena cava at the level of the diaphragm. After inflow occlusion has been achieved, the surgeon waits for at least four full cardiac cycles, so that the heart is fully emptied. After thorough emptying of the heart, the aortic clamp is applied and antegrade crystalloid cardioplegia is given via the ascending aortic line placed as noted above. A single dose of cardioplegia (10 mL/kg) is sufficient.

The heart is excised, with transection of the superior vena cava and the inferior vena cava (above the Potts clamp). The aorta is transected proximal to the clamp, near the takeoff of the innominate artery. Pulling the apex of the heart up, the pulmonary veins are divided on the pericardium, and the pulmonary artery is divided last, as distally as possible, near its bifurcation. The donor surgeon must be aware of anatomic details affecting the performance of the recipient operation, such as congenital anomalies or previously observed tissue deficiencies in redo cases. Not uncommonly, it may be necessary to take greater lengths of either the pulmonary artery or the aorta.

The heart is placed in a plastic bag filled with normal saline at 4°C. The bag is tied shut, excluding all air from the bag. The first sterile bag is then placed in a second sterile plastic bag, and this bag is filled with enough saline to cover the first bag, and the air is again excluded. These are placed in a third bag, which is then placed in crushed ice for transport. Most centers use a simple drinks cooler type of container for transport. The container is opened in the recipient operating room, and the outer bag is cut open by the circulating assistant, allowing the operating surgeon to remove the inner sterile bag. This simple method with single-

dose cardioplegia and static hypothermia allows for up to six hours of safe preservation and is the standard method worldwide. The major pitfalls in this method, which are frequently encountered, are distension and inadequate cooling, as outlined in Table 112–5. Distension is the most common error, and its sequelae (particularly right ventricular dysfunction) are often impossible to overcome.

Cardiac graft preservation is an active area of investigation that relates to basic investigations of xenografting, the ultimate goal of "shelf availability" of organs. Some of the most interesting work relates to methods for "supercooling" the heart. Very low (subzero) temperatures are reached with major reduction in metabolism and expected improvement in ischemic graft preservation.[27,28] A critical feature is "intracellular antifreeze" solutions, which are hyperosmolar and contain supplementary quantities of high-energy phosphate compounds. Hyperosmolarity is achieved with glucose, ethylene glycol, and other solutions, and this results in retardation of intracellular crystal formation and resultant sudden entry of water into the cell and across the cell membrane in response to the increase in intracellular solute concentration. Use of these solutions has allowed extended (greater than 12 hour) storage of rat hearts at −9°C, with recovery of electrocardiographic and contractile function.[29] These methods contain considerable promise for preservation of all tissues for transplant.

Various substrates and additives for cardioplegia continue to be studied, and much of this work is directed toward transplantation.[30,31] Interest in the so-called "non-heart-beating" donor has been high in Japan, where there are continuing difficulties with acceptance of the concept of brain death. This approach involves waiting for the heart to stop beating in the terminally ill patient and immediately heparinizing, with some technique for immediate topical and/or systemic (via groin cannulation) cooling, and it has shown some prospects for success in kidney transplantation.[32] Clinical cardiac applications remain on the horizon.

It is well known that brain death and its endocrine ramifications have significant end-organ effects, including very noteworthy negative effects on myocardial contractility.[33] Clinically, the time of onset of these problems is highly variable, and the mechanisms of its occurrence are poorly understood. Unfortunately, there has been a tendency to approach this problem in a highly empirical way, with administration of thyroid hormone to donors. Heretofore, this has been done without any statistical control or valid study design, and the results have therefore been indiscernible. However, this problem is now being ap-

TABLE 112–5. PITFALLS IN HEART GRAFT PROCUREMENT

1. Failure to monitor heart closely during multiorgan dissection
2. Failure to heparinize
3. Allowance of right- or left-sided distension
4. Inadequate attention to cooling and storage for transport

proached mechanistically, and studies of basic mechanisms, which will lead to controlled clinical investigations of hormonal therapy, are being published.[34,35] Any inclusion of thyroid or other hormonal therapy in a routine clinical protocol should await the outcomes of prospective studies.

HEART–LUNG GRAFT PROCUREMENT

The need to replace the heart and lungs as a bloc has been evident for many years, because of frequent combined heart and lung failure, the incidence of end-stage lung disease resulting in heart failure, and, most important, the frequency of severe pulmonary hypertension with heart failure. Orthotopic heart transplant is not possible in this case because of inability of the normal donor right ventricle to pump against this high resistance. Despite realistic technical approaches to the recipient operation for heart and lung replacement, early attempts at this operation were uniformly unsuccessful, and even after the first successful operation at Stanford in 1981, survival remained problematic, because of the problem of lung preservation.[36] Unlike the heart, which is a solid organ and can be effectively cooled and preserved by static hypothermia, the lungs are "self-insulated" by the vast number of air pockets within them, and they are notoriously sensitive to ischemia. Early experience with heart–lung and lung transplantation revealed a high incidence of death due to "lung failure," and in fact, poor preservation. Recent experiences with isolated lung transplant reveal a high incidence of "early rejection," which was in reality poor preservation occurring well before rejection would be seen. This so-called "reimplantation response" was often not fatal in the single lung transplant patients because of the "life boat" role of the remaining (often diseased) lung, which allowed the patient to survive during the interval of ischemic graft dysfunction.

There have been two approaches to the problem of lung preservation—normothermic, "physiologic" perfusion and hypothermic metabolic inhibition.[37] Effort directed toward the perfusion approach has had some clinical success.[38] However, the complexity of these methods led to technical failures. Cooperation with other organ procurement teams and the frequency of distant procurements were incompatible with the complex technology required.

Metabolic inhibition through cooling is well established and would be simpler than preserving the "physiologic milieu." However, topical cooling of the lungs has been shown, through many laboratory and clinical failures, to be inadequate for cooling the lungs. Early successes with lung preservation involved pulmonary artery perfusion with "pulmonoplegia" solutions borrowed from other areas in organ preservation, but these operations were done with on-site donors, because of the inability of this approach to give safe longer-term preservation. Thus, donor and recipient were placed in adjoining operating rooms, and the heart–lung graft was hastily removed when the recipient organs

had been excised. The heart–lung bloc was then immediately implanted. Clearly, if heart–lung transplantation is to gain wider application and if lung transplantation is to be feasible, safe long-term preservation and distant procurement of the lungs are required.

Simple flush perfusion cooling of the lungs is ineffective because of the pulmonary artery baroreflex phenomenon described by Hyman and others.[38,39] Distension of the main pulmonary artery, by mechanical means or by increased flow as occurs in left-to-right shunts in congenital heart disease, results in a reflex, distal constriction of the pulmonary arterial bed. With positive pressure perfusion of the pulmonary artery, this reflex reduces the completeness and uniformity of distribution of the cooling solution. The solution to this clinical problem resulted from basic investigations of the mechanisms that control pulmonary vascular resistance and means to pharmacologically interrupt the pulmonary baroreflex.[41,42] Our early experimental work showed that prostaglandin E_1 was effective in blocking the pulmonary vasoconstrictive response to distension, and we therefore transferred this knowledge to the flush perfusion technique for lung cooling.[43] The method was effective in primate models, with marked extension of safe lung preservation time (to at least 6 hours) and significantly better oxygenation than with simple perfusion. The lung preservation technique using pretreatment with prostaglandin E_1 and extended (4 minute) flush perfusion cooling with modified Euro-Collins solution was introduced into the clinical program at Stanford where the first successful distant procurement and extended preservation of pulmonary tissue was accomplished in 1986.[44] A young woman with primary pulmonary hypertension and right ventricular failure established the clinical efficacy of this method of lung preservation. The technique is now universally used with minor variations.

The lung preservation method must be fully integrated into the donor operation, which is more complex in heart–lung procurement than in heart procurement. Donor criteria for a heart–lung graft include all those for a cardiac donor and several pulmonary criteria, listed in Table 112–6. In general, lung donors should be identified within 5 to 7 days after brain death, because the lungs develop atelectasis and infection, as well as the long-recognized and poorly understood problem of neurogenic pulmonary edema. The sputum should be carefully examined in the bacteriology laboratory and should not contain heavy amounts of organisms or polymorphonuclear leukocytes, nor should there be fungus on the KOH stain.[45] The pO_2 should be greater than 100 mm Hg on 40% inspired oxygen. We have observed

TABLE 112–6. CRITERIA FOR LUNG DONOR

Normal chest radiograph

Arterial pO_2 > 100 mg Hg on 40% FIO_2

Absence of fungus or gross purulence in tracheal aspirate

that the lungs of brain dead patients are susceptible to injury by high oxygen concentrations. Thus, the concept of "oxygen challenge," which has no physiologic rationale, may be injurious and should be abandoned in evaluation of heart–lung and lung donors. Potential lung donors should be maintained on 40% inspired oxygen with 5 cm positive end-expiratory pressure, and the pO_2 should remain stable at a level greater than 100. If the pO_2 begins to drop, this is usually an inexorable process. Rarely can a donor be salvaged with aggressive pulmonary toilet and therapeutic bronchoscopy. The lung fields should be clear radiographically in a suitable heart–lung donor.

Ventilation is maintained both in transport and in the operating room with an inspired oxygenation concentration not to exceed 40% and with 5 cm of positive end-expiratory pressure. It is important to explain this to the anesthesiologist prior to transport. The donor operation for heart–lung, double-lung, and single-lung transplantation is performed in exactly the same way up through the point of removing the heart–lung graft from the chest. After the sternum is divided, the heart is inspected, as is done in the donor operation for heart transplantation described previously (Fig. 112–1). The aorta is dissected out and encircled with an umbilical tape, as are the superior and inferior venae cavae. The pleural spaces are opened, and the lungs are inspected. Attention is given to avoid trauma to the lungs. Grasping the lungs with instruments and excessive compression are forbidden; the lungs should be touched as little as possible. Intrathoracic adhesions are taken down with electrocautery before the donor is heparinized. The anterior pericardium is

then excised posteriorly back to a point near the pulmonary hilum, meaning that the phrenic nerves will be excised at this point. Complete pericardial excision will make implantation of the graft easier, and will improve static cooling of the lungs (Fig. 112–2). The trachea is dissected incising the posterior pericardium between the aorta and the superior vena cava by retracting the superior vena cava to the right and the aorta to the left, to permit circumferential dissection of the trachea as high as possible (Fig. 112–3). This is important, since the security of the tracheal anastomosis in a heart–lung operation depends critically on coronary–tracheal collaterals that come from the tissue around the distal trachea and carina.[46] This tissue around the airway is equally important when the graft is to be used in a double-lung or isolated lung transplant. Once this portion of the dissection has been completed, and the trachea is encircled proximally with an umbilical tape, the surgeon is ready to harvest the heart–lung bloc in cooperation with the other organ procurement teams.

Fifteen minutes prior to clamping the aorta, a prostaglandin (PG) E_1 infusion is started via central venous catheter at an initial rate of 15 ng/kg per minute. The rate of infusion is gradually increased every 2–3 min and may reach 100 ng/kg per minute as long as the mean arterial pressure is not allowed to fall below 55 mm Hg. Heparin (30,000 units in the adult) is given into the right atrium where this is acceptable to the other organ procurement teams. During the PGE_1 infusion, the cardioplegia catheter should be connected to the ascending aorta and attached to a 1-L bag of crystalloid cardioplegia solution at 4°C. A 14-

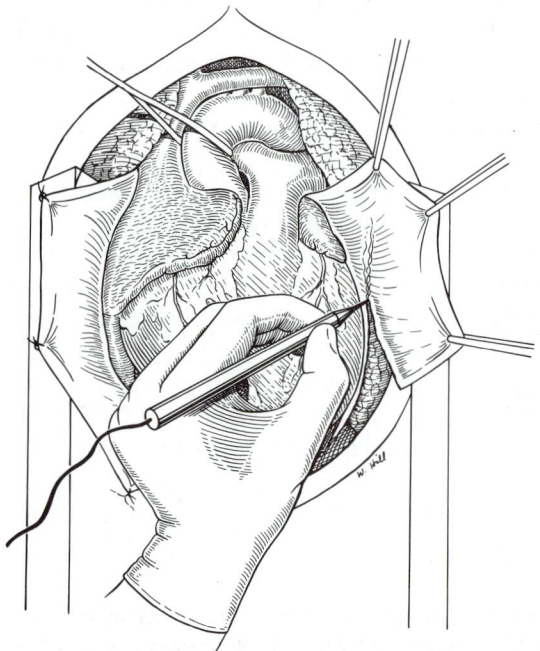

Figure 112–2. During procurement of the heart–lung block, the pericardium should be resected to facilitate removal of the block and improve static cooling of the lungs. *(From Shumway N, Shumway S: Thoracic Transplantation. Reprinted by permission of Blackwell Scientific Publications, Inc., Cambridge, MA.)*

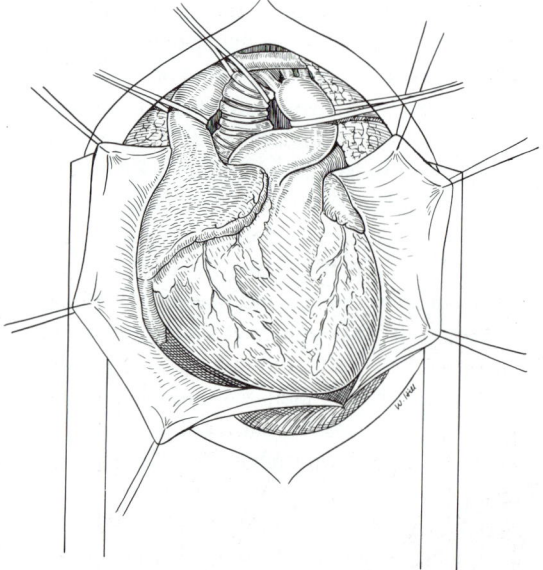

Figure 112–3. Exposure to the trachea is provided by retracting the superior vena cava to the right, the aorta to the left, incising the posterior pericardium, identifying the trachea by palpating the tracheal rings, and then encircling the trachea with umbilical tape. *(From Baldwin JC: Technique of combined heart–lung transplantation. J Cardiac Surg 7:1–11, 1992.)*

gauge pulmonary artery vent catheter is placed in the main pulmonary artery via a vertical stab wound made with a number 11 blade. This catheter is connected to the tubing from the rollerhead pump used to deliver the "pulmonoplegia" solution (Fig. 112–4). When the other surgical teams are ready for aortic clamping, the venae cavae are ligated, and the heart is allowed to beat through six cycles to empty. Then, the aorta is clamped, and the cardioplegia and pulmonoplegia infusions are begun. The pressure bag for the cardioplegia should be maintained at 150 mm Hg by the anesthesiologist, as the pressure will drop as the infusion proceeds. The pulmonary cooling solution is given by a technician using a simple single rollerhead pump at a rate of 15 mL/kg per minute for 4 min, delivering a total dose of 60 mL/kg. Higher doses should be avoided, as they are associated with increased lung water postoperatively. Immediately after clamping the aorta and beginning the two infusions, the inferior vena cava should be deeply incised, and the tip of the left atrial appendage should be amputated. A principal cause of graft failure is momentary distension of either the left or the right side of the heart. Amputation of the left atrial appendage is particularly important because of the large volume of cooling solution passing through the lungs. After these two critical maneuvers and the possibility of distension is obviated, cold (4°C) topical solution (Physiosol, Abbott Laboratories) is poured over the heart and lungs. Wet "lap pads" gently laid over the lungs anteriorly will keep them down in the cooling solution. Ventilation should be continued with 40% inspired oxygen and half-normal tidal volumes. The rate-limiting feature in this part of the operation is the infusion of the pulmonoplegia solution over 4 min. The aorta can be transected after the cardioplegia solution is in and while the pulmonoplegia infusion continues. This saves a step later and completely eliminates the possibility of left-sided distension. The prostaglandin E$_1$ is continued until the graft is excised.

When the infusions of cooling solutions have been completed, the lungs are briefly deflated. It is important, especially for the relatively inexperienced operator, to move at a deliberate pace during the remainder of the dissection and excision of the graft, as there is a significant risk of injury to the graft if one proceeds too hastily and/or without excellent exposure. Most surgeons will have had little experience with the anatomical approaches seen in the remainder of this operation. With the lungs deflated, the cavae are transected. The left hand of the operator is then placed on the diaphragmatic surface of the heart, and the dissection is carried down onto the esophagus. By dissecting in a cephalad direction on the esophagus, the surgeon avoids injury to the heart, the pulmonary vessels (most frequently injured), the lungs, and trachea. The pulmonary hilae are dissected well laterally, and the dissection directly on the esophagus is carried up to where the umbilical tape surrounds the trachea. With the lungs still deflated, a TA 55 stapler with 4.8-mm staples is placed across the trachea as high as possible in the area of the umbilical tape, and the tape is removed. The lungs are inflated to a normal tidal volume, with no visible atelectasis, and the stapler is then closed on the trachea. The trachea is divided proximal to the staple line. It is crucial for the lungs to remain inflated during transport (Fig. 112–5). The graft can then be withdrawn from the chest. The heart–lung graft is placed in a plastic container of appropriate size, which is filled with cold (4°C) physiologic solution (Physiosol, Abbott Laboratories). It is very important that the lungs are covered with wet "lap tapes," so that the lungs do not float up against the container and lose the full effect of the cooling solution. The container is completely filled with the cold solution, so that air does not surround any part of the graft. The plastic container is then placed in a sterile plastic bag filled with cold solution. This is then placed in a large ice-filled container for transport. This method, when correctly executed in a properly se-

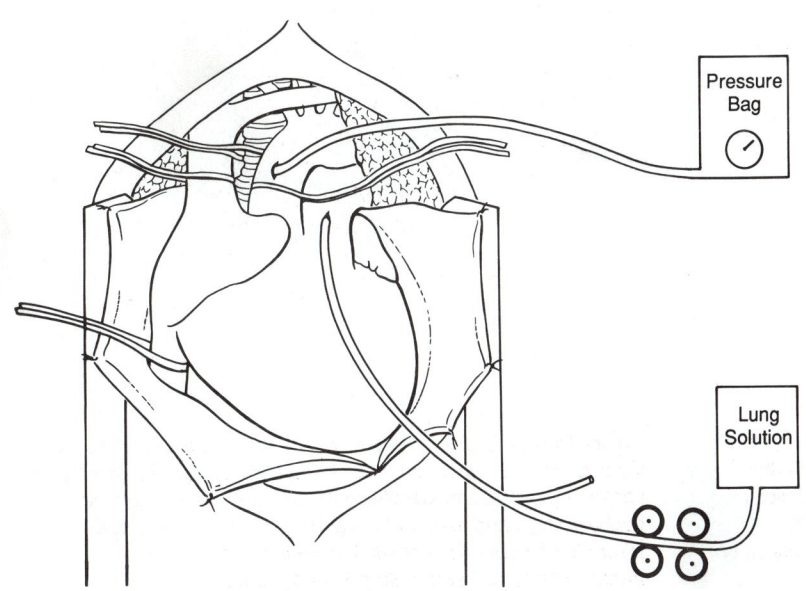

Figure 112–4. Schematic representation showing simultaneous delivery of cardioplegic and pulmonoplegic solutions. The cardioplegia is administered through a pressure bag while the pulmonoplegia is administered by roller pump. *(From Baldwin JC: Technique of combined heart–lung transplantation. J Cardiac Surg 7:1–11, 1992.)*

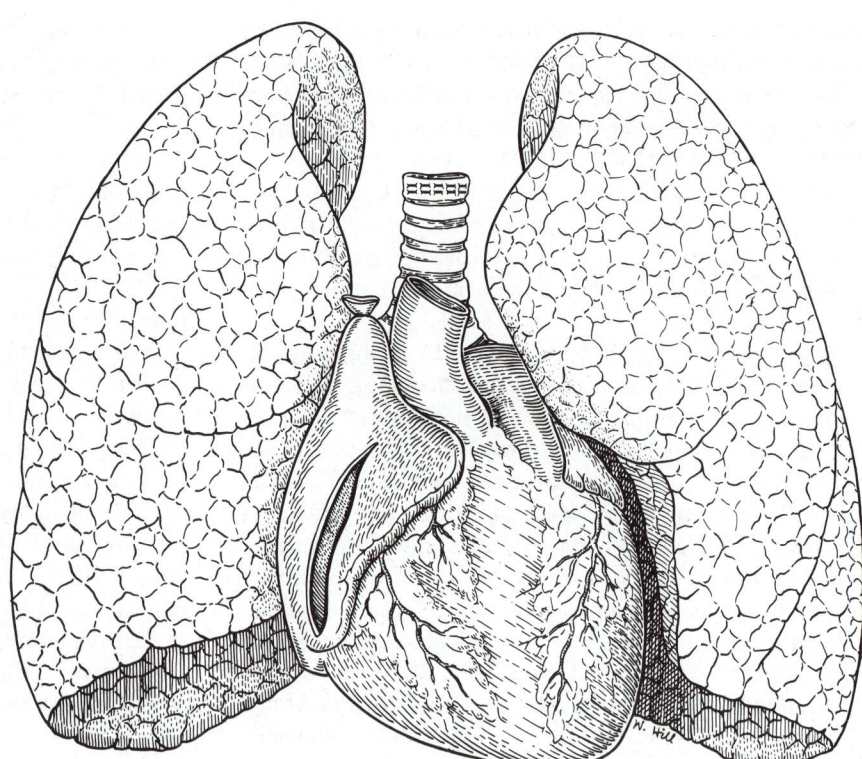

Figure 112–5. The heart–lung block is transported with the trachea stapled and the lungs inflated. *(From Shumway N, Shumway S: Thoracic Transplantation. Reprinted by permission of Blackwell Scientific Publications, Inc., Cambridge, MA.)*

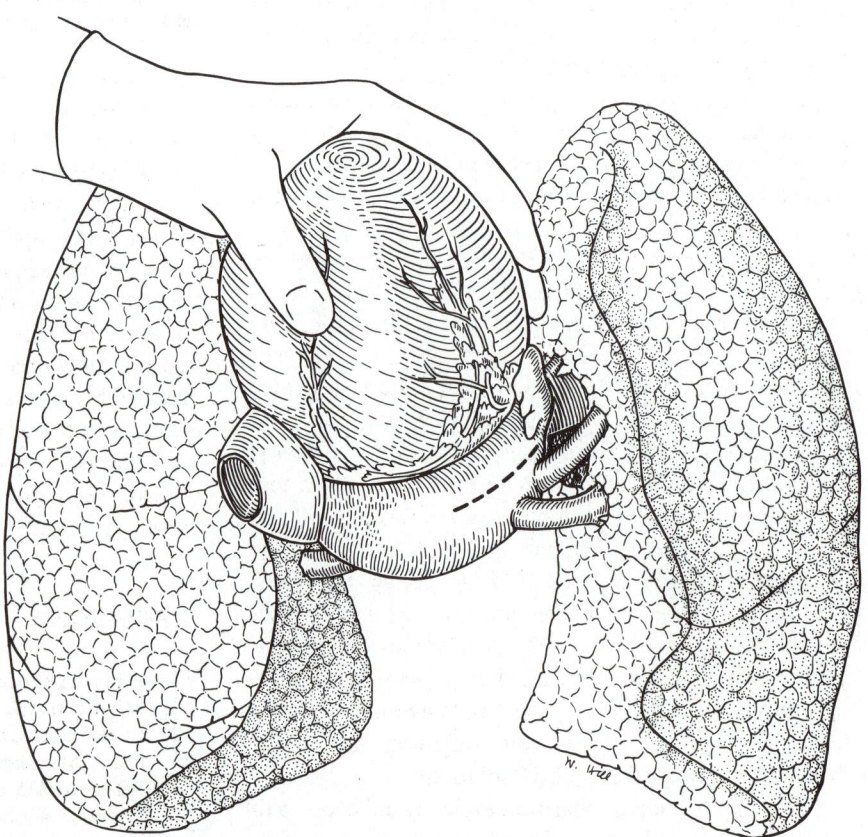

Figure 112–6. When separating the heart and lungs for separate harvesting teams, the division is best done with the resected heart–lung block on the back table. Both heart and lung procuring teams can then easily visualize, and agree upon, the line of division. The division should occur midway between the pulmonary veins and the left atrial ventricular junction. *(From Shumway N, Shumway S: Thoracic Transplantation. Reprinted by permission of Blackwell Scientific Publications, Inc., Cambridge, MA.)*

lected donor, is safe and effective for ischemic times up to 6 hours. It will result in pO$_2$s greater than 100 on 40% inspired oxygen and 3–5 cm positive end-expiratory pressure and in satisfactory cardiac function, usually with isoproterenol alone, to keep the heart rate at approximately 150 beats/min.

LUNG GRAFT PROCUREMENT

The method described above is a safe and effective way to procure heart–lung, heart, and lung grafts. In most instances, the intent will be to provide well-functioning grafts for three different patients—one for orthotopic heart transplantation, and two for single-lung transplantation. The division of the graft should be performed after the en bloc excision described above. Division of the grafts after en bloc excision allows for a more precise dissection and should be performed on the back table in the operating room where the donor operation has been performed. The surgeons on the lung and heart teams should collaborate in this crucial dissection.

First, the heart is excised from the lungs. The pulmonary artery is divided just proximal to its bifurcation. Maximum length of both pulmonary arteries is preserved. The left atrium is divided with great attention to detail. By dividing the left atrium exactly at the half-way point between the pulmonary veins and the left atrium, an intact full perimeter cuff can be preserved for both lung transplants and an adequate single perimeter cuff of left atrium is left on the heart, for performance of the heart transplant, as first described by Cass and Lord Brock.[47]

The traditional technique in orthotopic transplantation of interconnecting the transected orifices of the pulmonary veins to form a single left atrial perimeter is eliminated. One must be careful, in the recipient heart operation, to take small bites on the abbreviated left atrial perimeter (Fig. 112–6).

The heart is removed from the field and stored for transport in the manner described previously. The surgeon is then left with the pulmonary artery at its bifurcation and the posterior portion of the left atrium, with its four pulmonary veins (Fig. 112–7). The pulmonary artery is divided directly vertically at its bifurcation, preserving both pulmonary arteries. Next, the left atrium is divided vertically, retaining the two pulmonary veins on each side with an adequate perimeter of left atrial/pulmonary venous cuff for each of the single-lung transplants. At this juncture the lungs are still inflated. Dissection of the airway down onto and around the carina should preserve as much peribronchial tissue as possible. Both mainstem bronchi are encircled and stapled before they are divided, so that the lungs remain inflated for transport. The two lungs are stored as described for the heart–lung graft, weighing them down with wet gauze pads in the storage solution.

Using this method of pharmacologically enhanced pulmonary artery vasodilatation, flush perfusion cooling, sim-

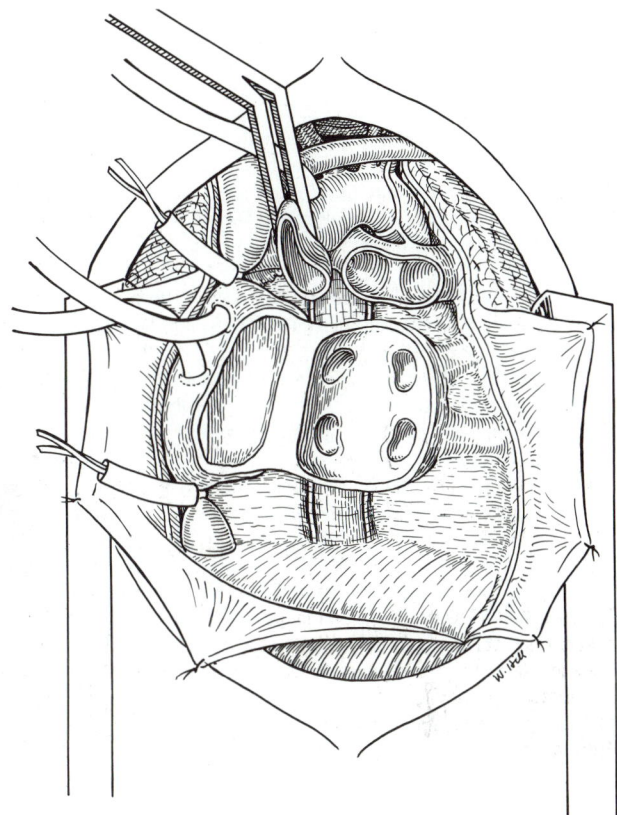

Figure 112–7. Diagram shows ideal appearance, after the heart has been removed, of the remaining pulmonary artery and left atrial cuffs on the lung block. The lungs can then be used separately for transplantation. *(From Baldwin JC: Technique of combined heart–lung transplantation. J Cardiac Surg 7:1–11, 1992.)*

ple crystalloid cardioplegia, and en bloc excision of the heart and lungs, safe procurement of tissue for heart, heart–lung, double-lung, and single-lung transplantation can be reliably achieved, with ischemic times up to 6 hours.

Methods for "supercooling" both the heart and lungs suggest the possibility of quantitatively greater reductions in metabolic activity. These techniques will afford the possibility of much longer transport and storage times for allografts and, most probably, indefinite storage times for xenografts. Other long-term possibilities for increasing the availability of lung donors include expansion of donor criteria, mechanically based changes in preservation solutions, and the use of non-heart-beating donors.[48–53] All of these approaches require laboratory study and careful prospective study in their clinical implementation.

REFERENCES

1. Hardy JD, Chavez CM, Karnes FD, et al: Heart transplant in man. *JAMA* **188:**1132, 1964
2. Lower RR, Stofer RC, Hurley EJ, et al: Successful homotransplantation of the canine heart after anoxic preservation for seven hours. *Am J Surg* **104:**302, 1962
3. Shumway NE, Lower RR, Stofer RC: Selective hypothermia of the heart in anoxic cardiac arrest. *Surg Gynecol Obstet* **108:**750–754, 1959

4. Baldwin JC, et al: Task Force 2. *Am Coll Cardiol* **22**(1):1–64, 1993

5. Baldwin JC: Cardiac transplantation. In Baue AE, Geha AS, Hammond GL, Laks H (eds): *Glenn's Thoracic and Cardiovascular Surgery*—Fifth Edition. Norwalk, CT, Appleton & Lange, 1991

6. Franco KL, Edelson RL, Snyder E, et al: Successful heart transplant with a positive T Cell crossmatch (by photochemotherapy and plasmapheresis). *J Thorac Cardiovasc Surg* (in press)

7. Watson DC, Dong E Jr, Shumway NE: Distant heart procurement for transplantation. *Surgery* **86**:56, 1979

8. Angell WW, Rikkers L, Dong E, Shumway NE: Organ viability with hypothermia. *J Thorac Cardiovasc Surg* **58**:619, 1969

9. Robicsek F, Tam W, Daughterty HK: Survival of heart grafts. *Arch Surg* **99**:750–752, 1969

10. Cooper DKC, Wicomb WN, Rose AG, Barnard CN: Orthotopic allotransplantation and autotransplantation of the baboon heart following 24-hr storage by a portable hypothermic perfusion system. *Cryobiology* **20**(4):385, 1983

11. Li G, Sullivan JA, Hall RI: Functional recovery in rabbit heart after preservation with a blood cardioplegic solution and perfusion. *Heart-Lung Transplant* **12**(2):263–270, 1993

12. Miller LW, Jellinek M, Codd JE, Kolata RJ: Improved myocardial preservation by control of the oxidation-reduction potential. *Heart Transplant* **IV**:319, 1985

13. Bando K, Teramoto S, Tago M, et al: Oxygenative perflurocarbon, recombinant human superoxide dismutase, and catalase ameliorate free radical induced myocardial injury during heart preservation and transplantation. *J Thorac Surg* **96**:930, 1988

14. Manasche P, Grousset C, Mouas C, Piwnica A: A promising approach for improving the recovery of heart transplants. *J Thorac Surg* **100**:13–21, 1990

15. Keith F: Oxygen free radicals in cardiac transplantation. *J Card Surg* **8**(2 suppl):245–248, 1993

16. Wiklund L, Svensson G, Nilsson F, et al: Six hour preservation of the isolated working rat heart improved with University of Wisconsin solution. *J Thorac Cardiovasc Surg* **27**(1):15–20, 1993

17. Karck M, Vivi A, Tassini M, et al: The effectiveness of University of Wisconsin solution on prolonged myocardial protection as assessed by phosphorus 31-nuclear magnetic resonance spectroscopy and functional recovery. *J Thorac Cardiovasc Surg* **104**(5):1356–1364, 1992

18. Lasley RD, Mentzer RM: The role of adenosine in extended myocardial preservation with the University of Wisconsin solution. *J Thorac Cardiovasc Surg* **107**(5):1356–1363, 1994

19. Human PA, Holl J, Vosloo S, et al: Extended cardiopulmonary preservation: University of Wisconsin solution versus Bretschneider's cardioplegic solution. *Ann Thorac Surg* **55**(5):1123–1130, 1993

20. Menasche P, Pradier F, Grousset C, et al: Improved recovery of heart transplants with a specific kit of preservation solutions. *J Thorac Cardiovasc Surg* **105**(2):353–363, 1993

21. Demertzis S, Wippermann J, Schaper J, et al: University of Wisconsin versus St. Thomas' Hospital solution for human donor heart preservation. *Ann Thorac Surg* **55**(5):1131–1137, 1993

22. Stringham JC, Paulsen KL, Southard JH, et al: Prolonging myocardial preservation with a modified University of Wisconsin solution containing 2,3-butanedione monoxime and calcium. *J Thorac Cardiovasc Surg* **107**(3):764–775, 1994

23. Kojima S, Wu ST, Wikman-Coffelt J, Parmley WW: Eighteen hour preservation of rat hearts with hexanol and pyruvate cardioplegia. *J Am Coll Cardiol* **21**(5):1238–1244, 1993

24. Hendry PJ, Labow RS, Keon WJ: A comparison of intracellular solutions for donor heart preservation. *J Thorac Cardiovasc Surg* **105**(4):667–673, 1993

25. Hisatomi K, Isomura T, Yomoda M, Ohishi K: The effect of the addition of albumin to cardioplegic and preservation solutions on the isolated rat heart. *J Heart-Lung Transplant* **12**(3):470–475, 1993

26. Pinsky DJ, Oz MC, Koga S, et al: Cardiac preservation is enhanced in a heterotopic rat transplant model by supplementing the nitric oxide pathway. *J Clin Invest* **93**(5):2291–2297, 1994

27. Storey KB, Storey JM: Frozen and alive. *Sci Am* **263**:92–97, 1990

28. Letsou GV, Braxton J, Liu, et al: Low temperature preservation at −4°C is safe and effective for rat cardiac transplantation after 12 hours. *FASEB J* **8**(5):A591, 1994

29. Braxton JH, Letsou GV, Schwann TA, et al: Effect of supercooling solutions on electromechanical activity. *Transplant Proc* **26**(4):2428–2430, 1994

30. Lopukhin SY, Southard JH, Belzer FO: University of Wisconsin solution containing 2,3-butanedione-monoxime extends myocardium preservation time. *Transplant Proc* **25**(6):3017–3018, 1993

31. Kawamura A, Meguro J, Takahashi M, et al: Artificial conditioner for stored organs. *Int J Artif Organs* **17**(1):53–60, 1994

32. Booster MH, Wijnen RM, Vroemen JP, et al: In situ preservation of kidneys from non-heart-beating donors—A proposal for a standardized protocol. *Transplantation* **56**(3):613–617, 1993

33. Galinanes M, Hearse DJ: Brain death-induced impairment of cardiac contractile performance can be reversed by explanation and may not preclude the use of hearts for transplantation. *Circ Res* **71**(5):1213–1219, 1992

34. Galinanes M, Smolenski RT, Haddock PS, Hearse DJ: Early effects of hypothyroidism on the contractile function of the rat heart and its tolerance to hypothermic ischemia. *J Thorac Cardiovasc Surg* **107**(3):829–837, 1994

35. Galinanes M, Smolenski RT, Hearse DJ: Brain death-induced cardiac contractile dysfunction and long-term cardiac preservation. Rat heart studies of the effects of hypophysectomy. *Circulation* **88**(5 Pt 2):II270–280, 1993

36. Feeley TW, Mihm FG, Downing P, et al: The effect of hypothermic preservation of the heart and lungs on cardiorespiratory function following canine heart-lung transplantation. *Ann Thorac Surg* **39**(6):558–562, 1985

37. Haverich A, Scott WC, Jamieson SW: Twenty years of lung preservation—A review. *Heart Transplant* **IV**:234–240, 1985

38. Ladowski JS, Kapelanski DP, Teodori MF, et al: Use of autoperfusion for distant procurement of heart lung allografts. *Heart Transplant* **IV**:300–333, 1985

39. Hyman AL: Pulmonary vasoconstriction due to non-occlusive distension of large pulmonary arteries in the dog. *Circ Res* **23**:401–413, 1968

40. Laks M, Juratsch CE, Garner D, et al: Chronic pulmonary artery (MPA) in the conscious dog. *Circulation* **7**(suppl IV):114, 1973

41. DeCampli WM, Baldwin JC, Hagbert RC, et al: Adrenergic characteristics of the pulmonary artery "baroreflex." *J Appl Cardiol* **5**:339–347, 1990

42. Starkey TD, Saskakibara N, Hagberg RC, et al: Successful six-hour cardiopulmonary preservation with simple hypothermic crystalloid flush. *Heart Transplant* **5**(4):291–297, 1986

43. Harjula A, Baldwin JC, Shumway NE: Donor deep hypothermia or donor pretreatment with prostaglandin E1 and single pulmonary artery flush for heart-lung graft preservation: An experimental primate study. *Ann Thorac Surg* **46**:553–555, 1988

44. Baldwin JC, Frist WH, Starkey TD, et al: Distant graft procurement for combined heart and lung transplantation using pulmonary artery flush and simple topical hypothermia for graft preservation. *Ann Thorac Surg* **43**:670, 1987

45. Harjula A, Baldwin JC, Stinson EB, et al: Recipient selection for heart-lung transplantation. *Scand J Thorac Cardiovasc Surg* **22**:193–196, 1988

46. Baldwin John C: Technique of combined heart-lung transplantation. *J Card Surg* **7**:1–11, 1992

47. Cass MH, Brock R: Heart excision and replacement. *Guy's Hosp Report* **108**:285, 1959

48. Higgins RS, Letsou GV, Sanchez JA, et al: Improved ultrastructural lung preservation with prostaglandin E1 as donor pretreatment in a

primate model of heart-lung transplantation. *J Thorac Cardiovasc Surg* **105**(6):967–971, 1993

49. Lin PJ, Hsieh MJ, Cheng KS, et al: University of Wisconsin solution extends lung preservation after prostaglandin E1 infusion. *Chest* **105**(1):225–261, 1994

50. Sundaresan S, Lima O, Date H, et al: Lung preservation with low-potassium dextran flush in a primate bilateral transplant model. *Ann Thorac Surg* **56**(5):1129–1135, 1993

51. Ulicny KS, Egan TM, Lambert CJ, et al: Cadaver lung donors: effect of preharvest ventilation on graft function. *Ann Thorac Surg* **55**(5):1185–1191, 1993

52. Sundaresan S, Trachiotis GD, Aoe M, et al: Donor lung procurement: Assessment and operative technique. *Ann Thorac Surg* **56**(6):1409–1413, 1993

53. Jenkinson SG, Levine SM: Lung transplantation. *Disease-A-Month* **40**(1):1–38, 1994

C H A P T E R

113

Cardiac Transplantation

Bartley P. Griffith and Mitchell J. Magee

HISTORY OF CARDIAC TRANSPLANTATION

The first experimental orthotopic cardiac transplant was described by Goldberg et al at the University of Maryland in 1958.[1] "The chief innovation," as the authors described, was to "circumvent the anastomosis of the several pulmonary veins" by utilizing a left atrial cuff anastomosis. The superior and inferior vena cavae were reconnected utilizing methylmethacrylate tubes, and aortic and pulmonary continuity was re-established utilizing suture techniques. The first description of the now standard anastomoses of the left and right atrial cuffs was by Cass and Brock from Guy's Hospital in London in 1959.[2] The experiment was, unfortunately, a technical failure due to bleeding from suture lines. In 1960, Lower and Shumway published the landmark paper on orthotopic cardiac transplantation in which methods of operative technique, graft preservation, and recipient support and protection are described in detail.[3] In continuing studies, Lower et al used echocardiograms as indicators of rejection and administered intermittent doses of azathioprine and methylprednisolone to achieve a survival of 250 days in an adult dog.[4] These experiments provided the foundation for the first successful clinical orthotopic cardiac transplant. Christiaan Bernard, who had visited centers in the United States experimenting in transplantation, returned to Groote Schuur Hospital in Capetown, South Africa, and on December 3, 1976, performed the surgery on a 54-year-old man dying of end-stage ischemic heart disease. He described the procedure as a culmination of "steady progress . . . made by immunologists, biochemists, surgeons, and specialists . . . of medical science all over the world during the past decades." In spite of his recipient's death from *Pseudomonas* pneumonia after 18 days, enthusiasm resulted in over 100 transplants being performed in 17 countries during the following year. Because survival was only 29 days in these early cases, all in-

stitutions, except Stanford University, the Medical College of Virginia, and Groote Schuur Hospital, abandoned the procedure. These tenacious groups, led primarily by Stanford, systematically and steadily improved the clinical results over the next decade, increasing the 1-year survival from 22% in 1968 to 65% in 1978. The introduction of cyclosporine and its early availability to our group in Pittsburgh ushered in a new era in immunosuppressive therapy, and resulted in the development of cardiac transplant activity at our center. Improved outcome with cyclosporine soon resulted in a burgeoning from 8 centers in the United States in 1981 to 156 in 1991. The widespread distribution of organs in the United States has resulted in low volume centers and has restricted clinical and laboratory experimentation. The continued evolution of cardiac transplantation as a solution to end-stage heart disease lies in the development of more specific immunosuppression, a better understanding of graft atherosclerosis, and perhaps, most importantly, strategies to deal with the shortage of donor organs, including regionalization of the procedure and continued work on artificial organs and xenotransplantation.

GUIDELINES FOR SELECTION OF POTENTIAL RECIPIENTS

Indications for cardiac transplantation have been based largely on subjective clinical observations.[5] Patients who have reached an "end-stage" of heart disease are so labeled based on perceived functional limitations and their physician's knowledge of therapeutic options. A failure to respond to maximal therapy is similarly subjective due to varying definitions of "maximal therapy." The primary underlying diseases leading to end-stage heart disease in adults are idiopathic dilated cardiomyopathy and ischemic cardiomyopathy.[6] Less common causes include end-stage

1869

valvular heart disease, congenital heart disease, nonresectable cardiac tumors, hypertrophic cardiomyopathy, angina or life-threatening dysrhythmias refractory to medical and surgical therapy, active myocarditis, sarcoidosis, and amyloidosis. Potential recipients with these latter three less common conditions should be selected with caution. Progression of systemic amyloidosis or sarcoidosis may limit long-term survival following successful transplantation, and a higher mortality and rate of rejection have been observed in patients transplanted with active acute myocarditis.[7,8]

A potential cardiac transplant recipient pool of greater than 16,000 annually (based on reported cause of death) can be generated if those up to age 55 years are considered, and the pool increases to greater than 40,000 when those up to age 65 are included.[9] For the latter it is likely that anticipated success with permanent left ventricular assist devices will provide another solution. It has been estimated that more than 900 candidates died waiting in 1993 and that between 75 and 85% of the listed candidates are not hospitalized. With an unchanging donor supply, it becomes apparent that more specific objective selection criteria that are intracenter consistent be established and applied to this increasingly large recipient pool to better utilize limited donor organs. The criteria for selection of recipients should identify those patients who are most likely to have sudden death or progressing heart failure. The New York Heart Association (NYHA) Class IV has traditionally been used to identify potential recipients, but in reality many patients are Class III. Based on a predicted 1-year survival of less than 50% in patients with NYHA Class IV symptoms of congestive heart failure and systolic dysfunction and from 40 to 70% in patients in NYHA Class III, life expectancy can be improved following cardiac transplantation.[10–15] Inclusion of patients in these classes, however, remains largely subjective and often does not take into consideration intensity or adequacy of medical therapy, including identification and treatment of potentially reversible factors contributing to decompensation.

Recent attempts to identify determinants of survival and provide guidelines for selection of candidates have met with limited success and should continue to be studied and refined. Patients with ejection fraction less than 20% are at a higher risk than patients with ejection fraction of 20% or greater.[16,17] Peak oxygen consumption measured during maximal exercise testing can provide an objective assessment of functional capacity and an indirect assessment of cardiovascular reserve in patients with heart failure and has been used as a tool in a prospective study to optimally time cardiac transplantation. Those patients with peak Vo_2 of less than or equal to 10 cc/kg per minute had the worse prognosis while those with Vo_2 greater than 14 cc/kg per minute had a 1-year survival rate 94%, allowing cardiac transplantation to be safely deferred in the absence of other clinical risk factors.[18] This index of prognosis is limited, as are other similar indices, by a variety of factors including

age, gender, conditioning status, muscle mass, angina, and perhaps, most importantly, the adequacy of therapy prior to evaluation. Additional conditions, which have been used by some programs as exclusion criteria due to notably less favorable outcomes after transplantation, should be given appropriate consideration. These include active myocarditis, active substance abuse, cerebral or peripheral vascular disease of significance that would limit rehabilitation, diabetes associated with severe secondary end-organ disease, and psychological factors, including a history of noncompliance or endogenous depression. Although it has been shown that older patients receive the same short-term benefits as their younger cohorts, transplantation of older recipients remains an ethical dilemma given the current short supply of donor hearts.[19] Recent pulmonary infarction is a relative contraindication to transplantation due to an observed increased incidence of post-transplant infection.[20] Current, absolute contraindications to transplantation include only uncontrolled infection or malignancy and severely elevated pulmonary vascular resistance in the potential orthotopic cardiac transplant recipient.[21] Most centers exclude patients with a pulmonary vascular resistance of more than 6–8 Wood units (mm Hg/L per minute) due to a higher observed incidence of right heart failure in the immediate postoperative period in these patients. Similarly an elevated transpulmonary gradient (mean pulmonary artery pressure minus pulmonary artery wedge pressure) greater than 15 mm Hg may also predict an increased incidence of right ventricular failure following transplantation.[22–26] It is important to determine whether the measured increased pulmonary vascular resistance is fixed or can be modulated by vasodilators such as oxygen, nitroprusside, or prostaglandin E_1.[27,28] Patients excluded from consideration for orthotopic cardiac transplantation should be periodically re-evaluated, following chronic administration of inotropic or vasodilator therapy as these patients occasionally will reduce their pulmonary vascular resistance over time to an acceptable level.

Patients referred to a cardiac transplantation center for consideration as a potential recipient undergo a battery of studies designed to aid the selection committee (Table 113–1). These studies should identify criteria for inclusion and exclusion, including predictors of outcome, as well as identify preoperative conditions that may affect postoperative management (Table 113–2). Examples of the former would include irreversible marked severe liver, kidney, or chronic lung disease, while examples of the latter would include hyperlipidemia, cholelithiasis, and diverticulitis. With an increasing interest in curbing health care costs, it will be important to better identify those studies that are truly predictive and essential to adequate evaluation. It should be emphasized that the evaluation process, like the patient, is a dynamic one and dependent on medical therapy and reversible factors. Periodic reassessment of patients will occasionally identify those who should not remain listed for transplantation. Although the actuarial survival in a stable group of outpatients awaiting transplantation is approxi-

TABLE 113–1. EVALUATION FOR CARDIAC TRANSPLANTATION

General data
  Comprehensive history and physical examination
  Blood chemistry determinations, including renal and liver function panels
  Complete blood count, differential, platelet count, prothrombin time, partial thromboplastin time, fibrinogen
  Urinalysis
  Stool for guaiac examination ×3
  24-hour collection of urine for creatinine clearance, total protein
  Mammography and Papanicolaou smear for women
  Dental examination
  Psychosocial consultation
  Pulmonary function testing
  Lung ventilation-perfusion scanning

Basic cardiovascular data
  Electrocardiogram
  Chest x-ray film
  Exercise test with oxygen consumption (peak Vo_2)
  Left or right cardiac catheterization
  Radionuclide ventriculogram
  Echocardiogram
  Myocardial biopsy when appropriate for myocarditis, amyloid, others

Basic immunologic data
  Blood type and antibody screen
  Human leukocyte antigen (HLA) typing
  Panel of reactive antibodies screen

Basic infectious disease background data
  Serology for
    Hepatitis HBsAg.HbsAb.HBcAb.C
    Herpes group virus
    Human immunodeficiency virus
    Cytomegalovirus IgM and IgG antibody
    Toxoplasmosis
    Varicella and rubella titers
    EB viral capsid IgG, IgM antibodies
    Lime titers when appropriate
    Histoplasmosis and coccidioidomycosis complement fixing antibodies
  Urine for viral cultures (cytomegalovirus, adenovirus)
  Throat swab for viral cultures (cytomegalovirus, adenovirus, herpes simplex virus)
  Skin testing for purified protein derivative with control, mumps, dermatophytid, histoplasmosis, and coccidioidomycosis

Data from ACC Bethesda Conference, November 1992.

TABLE 113–2. LIKELY EXCLUSION CRITERIA FOR CARDIAC TRANSPLANTATION

Coexistent systemic illness with poor prognosis
Irreversible pulmonary parenchymal disease
Irreversible renal dysfunction with serum creatinine >2 mg/dL or creatinine clearance <50 mL/min
Irreversible hepatic dysfunction
Severe peripheral and cerebrovascular obstructive disease
Insulin-dependent diabetes with end-organ damage
Active infection
Coexisting neoplasm
Pulmonary hypertension with irreversibly high pulmonary vascular resistance (pulmonary vascular resistance >6 Wood units or 3.0 Wood units after treatment with vasodilators)
Acute pulmonary embolism
Active diverticulitis
Active peptic ulcer disease
Myocardial infiltrative disease
Severe obesity
Severe osteoporosis
Psychosocial instability or substance abuse

Data from ACC Bethesda Conference, November 1992.

on blood type, body size, and, more importantly, length of recipient waiting time and severity of illness, which is classified as either Status I or Status II (Table 113–3). It is apparent with this simplified system that none of the more objective determinants of successful outcome is currently being used in donor allocation. This system encourages early listing of patients to accrue waiting-list time, leading to a longer list and longer waiting times. This rationale has also resulted in a reluctance of clinicians to remove patients from the list who have shown significant clinical improvement due to no provision for relisting these patients should the need arise, without jeopardizing their precious accrued waiting time. A lack of consistent criteria for patient eligibility among centers can result in patients selecting a center that is more sympathetic to their individual needs and, con-

TABLE 113–3. RECIPIENT STATUS CRITERIA OF THE UNITED NETWORK FOR ORGAN SHARING

Patients who require cardiac and/or pulmonary assistance with one or more of the following devices:
    Total artificial heart
  Left and/or right ventricular assist systems
  Intra-aortic balloon pump
  Ventilator
Patients meeting both of the following criteria:
  Patient in an intensive care unit and
  Patient requires inotropic agents to maintain adequate cardiac output
Patients less than 6 mo old
Status II

UNOS Executive Order, June 24, 1992.

mately 67% at 1 year, those who survive 6 months have an 83% chance of surviving the next year, suggesting that these patients should probably not remain on the recipient list.[29] Likewise, patients initially considered *not* to be candidates for transplantation may later be deemed appropriate. The importance of re-evaluating these patients was shown in a 1987 study in which 40% of such patients died within the year after their assessment at a transplant center.[30]

Once the patient is accepted for cardiac transplantation by an approved center, that patient is listed according to the guidelines of the United Network for Organ Sharing (UNOS). Distribution of donor organs by UNOS is based

versely, transplant centers may, through more strict criteria for selection of recipients, improve their statistics by not utilizing donor organs in critically ill patients who need them the most. The international registry demonstrates an operative mortality rate of 14% for critically ill patients compared with 6% for those in stable condition. While post-transplant survival is improved by transplanting the healthier patients, overall survival of recipients favors transplantation of the critically ill patient who is more likely to die awaiting transplantation.[5,31]

Patients considered for retransplantation should meet the same criteria as those considered for primary transplants, although the actuarial survival in patients with retransplants is lower.[32] Additional ethical, social, and financial concerns are raised when consideration is given to allocating a donor heart to a prior transplant recipient.

CARDIAC DONOR: SELECTION AND MANAGEMENT

Cardiac transplantation in the United States is currently limited primarily by donor availability.[33] While conservative estimates based on the cause of death listed on death certificates indicate that approximately 5200 donor hearts could be available each year, the number of cardiac transplants has reached a plateau of approximately 3000 per year.[34,35] Only 10 to 20% of brain dead patients with suitable hearts actually become heart donors.[36] The currently limited donor pool may be increased through public education and liberalization of organ donor criteria.

After establishing brain death according to individual state law and obtaining appropriate consent for organ donation, potential cardiac donors are screened initially by the local organ procurement agency. Pertinent information including body size, blood type, serologic and other laboratory data, and information related to cause of death and clinical course is relayed to cardiac surgeons or cardiologists responsible for determining the suitability of the donor for a given recipient matched by UNOS criteria. Most programs will accept hepatitis C seropositive recipients and seropositive donors accepted for selected recipients, although no prospective trials have reported the advisability of this practice.[37] Significant thoracic trauma that may have occurred around the time of brain death should be identified, and the level of inotropic support required to maintain stability should be determined. Pertinent past medical history, including cardiovascular risk factors or prescription/ use of illicit drugs that may affect cardiac function, should be obtained. An electrocardiogram, chest radiograph, arterial blood gas, and echocardiogram are routinely obtained, and on occasion a cardiac catheterization may be warranted. While efforts to increase the donor pool through liberalization of inclusion criteria have broadened the definition of a suitable cardiac donor, some absolute contraindications remain (Table 113–4). Relative contraindications to the use of

TABLE 113–4. ABSOLUTE CONTRAINDICATIONS TO THE USE OF A CARDIAC DONOR

Positive serology for HIV

Death from carbon monoxide poisoning with a blood carboxyhemo-globin level greater than 20%

Intractable ventricular dysrhythmias

Inadequate oxygenation with arterial saturation less than 80% on ventilatory support

Documented prior myocardial infarction

Clinically significant structural heart disease, including the presence of intracardiac tumor

Severe global hypokinesis with an ejection fraction estimated at less than 10% via echocardiography

Severe occlusive coronary artery disease on arteriography

a cardiac donor may vary from one transplant center to another. Even within a specific institution, the relative contraindications to cardiac donation may vary depending on the individual needs of the matched recipient. Acceptable donor body weight has traditionally been between 80 and 120% of the potential recipient's body weight, although the presence of moderate pulmonary hypertension may encourage the acceptance of a larger donor heart. Recent reports have shown no difference in survival or post-transplant hemodynamics in Status II recipients of undersized hearts, therefore these limits should not be considered absolute.[38,39] Previous age limits of 45 and 50 years for male and female donors, respectively, have been liberalized to include older donors at many transplant centers. A multicenter analysis of 911 patients identified older donor age as a risk factor for death after cardiac transplantation when donor age was analyzed as a continuous variable.[40] The appropriate use of an older donor heart for an older recipient is still debated. Liberal use of transesophageal echocardiography in the evaluation of potential heart donors with hemodynamic instability and increasing vasopressor requirements may improve selection of questionable cardiac donors.[41]

Function and survival are significantly impacted by ischemic times greater than 4 to 5 hours according to a 1992 multi-institutional study identifying pretransplant risk factors for death after cardiac transplantation.[40] Improved methods of organ preservation may allow extension of ischemic times.

Potential organ donors are best managed in the intensive care unit with hemodynamic stability as a priority. In an effort to minimize cerebral edema, potential donors are often relatively hypovolemic, which can be exacerbated by blood loss secondary to trauma, brain death-associated loss of vasomotor tone, or diabetes insipidus due to pituitary dysfunction. Central diabetes insipidus occurs in 38 to 87% of brain dead patients and may result in a massive diuresis.[42] Fluid replacement of 100–150 mL/h in excess of hourly urine output may be required to maintain a CVP of 8–12 cm^3/H_2O and thereby avoid hypotension (systolic blood pressure > 100). Low dose vasopressin infusions may be used to reduce urine output.[21] Hypotension with adequate filling pressures should be treated with low dose inotropic support (dopamine < 10 µg/kg per minute).

Thyroid dysfunction may occur with brain death and may be associated with clinically significant cardiac dysfunction believed due to decreased circulating levels of tri-iodothyronine (T_3). The utility and efficacy of T_3 infusions in such patients are currently under investigation and should not be routinely used at this time.[43–45]

DONOR CARDIECTOMY

Most cardiac donors are multiorgan donors, and the most challenging part of the donor cardiectomy can be retrieving a well-preserved, anatomically suitable organ without interfering with the other organ procurement surgeons' similar goals. The final decision regarding organ suitability is made by the procurement surgeon and is determined after careful visualization and palpation of the heart. It is important to exclude any significant hemodynamic deterioration that may have occurred since the initial offer of the donor and to ensure that the anesthetist maintains a proper balance between volume resuscitation and inotropic support throughout the donor operation. Volume overload of the right ventricle can sometimes result in an irretrievable state of failure. This can be determined by directly visualizing the heart, measuring the CVP, and observing the response to diuretics. The heart is palpated for the presence of coronary artery disease or a thrill suggestive of valvular disease or patent foramen ovale (PFO). The superior and inferior vena cavae, aorta, and pulmonary artery are dissected and the heparin is administered (Fig. 113–1). The technique of donor cardiectomy will vary a bit depending on the anticipated implant technique and whether or not the lungs are being simultaneously procured for transplant in another recipient. If the lungs are being used, Sondergaard's groove should be developed much as one might do for a left atrial incision. Ensure that the anesthetist removes any central venous catheter traversing the superior vena cava (SVC). The SVC is stapled closed, and the left superior pulmonary vein is divided followed immediately by incision of the inferior vena cava (IVC) to vent the left and right hearts, respectively. The left atrial appendage is cut instead of the pulmonary vein if the lungs are being procured. The aorta is *then* clamped distally at the takeoff of the innominate artery, and standard cold crystalloid cardioplegia is administered by a pressure bag into the aortic root (Fig. 113–2). Alternatively, the aorta may be stapled to allow for infusion of subsequent doses of cardioplegia prior to or during the implant procedure. A clear effluent, visualized from the left heart vent site, in addition to arrest of the heart ensures adequate delivery of cardioplegia. If the lungs are being used, incisions are made in the left atrium several centimeters anteriorly to the orifices of the pulmonary vein, nearing Sondergaard's

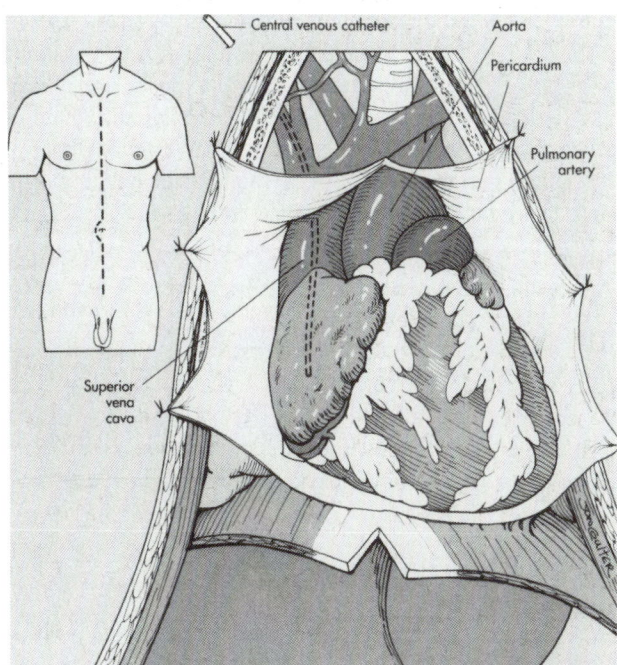

Figure 113–1. After extended sternotomy heart and associated great vessels are exposed.

groove on the right and the left atrial appendage on the left side. These incisions are then individually extended posteriorly, visualizing the pulmonary veins from inside the left atrium, to resect two atrial cuffs. If the lungs are not suitable for donation, the pulmonary veins may simply be cut individually and the entire left atrium removed. The SVC is

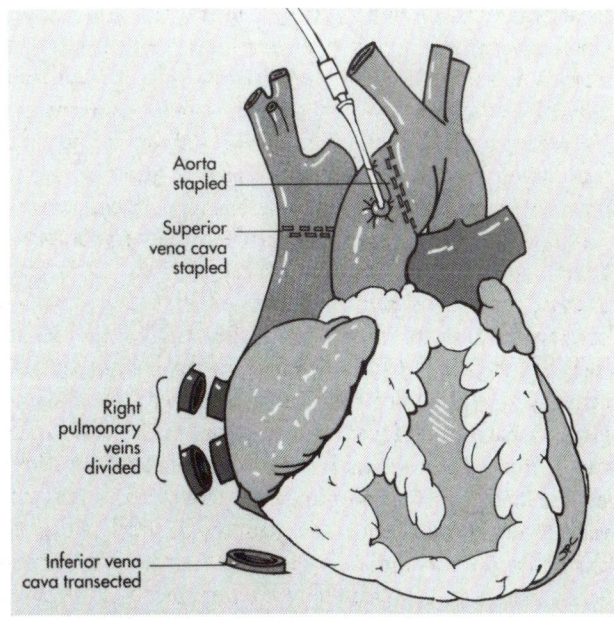

Figure 113–2. Donor cardiectomy begins with staple closures of SVC, transection of IVC, and, after decompression of LV, closure of aorta with induction of cardioplegia.

divided taking the staple line with the heart followed by the completion of the IVC incision. Caval length is a consideration only when individual caval anastomoses are planned for the recipient. Be cautious, however, of the "helpful" liver procurement team retracting the liver caudally in an attempt to maximize their SVC length as the opening of the coronary sinus can be jeopardized when the IVC is divided posteriorly. The heart may then be lifted anteriorly and toward the donor's right shoulder by the surgeon's left hand while the tissue around the transverse sinus is divided (Fig. 113–3). Division of the aorta and the main pulmonary artery distally completes the donor cardiectomy. The heart is then placed in a closed container of cold cardioplegia solution that is stored in an ice chest for transport to the recipient.

RECIPIENT OPERATION

The recipient operation begins with ensuring adequate venous access and placement of monitoring lines prior to induction of anesthesia. The pulmonary artery catheter is placed high in the superior vena cava where it will not interfere with the recipient cardiectomy. Immunosuppression is begun in the immediate preoperative period and continued in the operating room as outlined in the next section. Induction of anesthesia is withheld until confirmation is received from the donor surgeon of an acceptable donor heart. The transesophageal echocardiography probe is placed prior to draping and is most helpful when weaning from cardiopulmonary bypass to ensure adequate removal of air, volume

loading, and assessment of wall motion contractility and geometry. A standard sterile preparation and draping include both groins. Previous cardiac surgical procedures necessitate familiarity with the details of the procedure and exposure of the groin vessels for cannulation. Occasionally patients are placed on cardiopulmonary bypass prior to repeat sternotomy based on radiographic information, details of the previous operation, or hemodynamic instability on induction of anesthesia. Under most circumstances the arterial cannula is placed distally in the ascending aorta, and bicaval cannulation is accomplished via posterolateral right atrial purse strings or direct caval cannulation. The vena cavae are snared to complete the bypass and the recipient cardiectomy is begun when the donor heart arrives.

The aorta is cross-clamped close to the arterial cannula and the cardiectomy begins by opening the right atrium along the atrioventricular (A-V) groove anteriorly. The incision is extended inferoposteriorly to the opening of the coronary sinus, and superiorly, posterior to the right atrial appendage (Fig. 113–4). The aorta and main pulmonary artery are divided at the valve commissures, and an incision is made in the roof of the left atrium between the aorta and the SVC. The atrial incisions are connected and the left

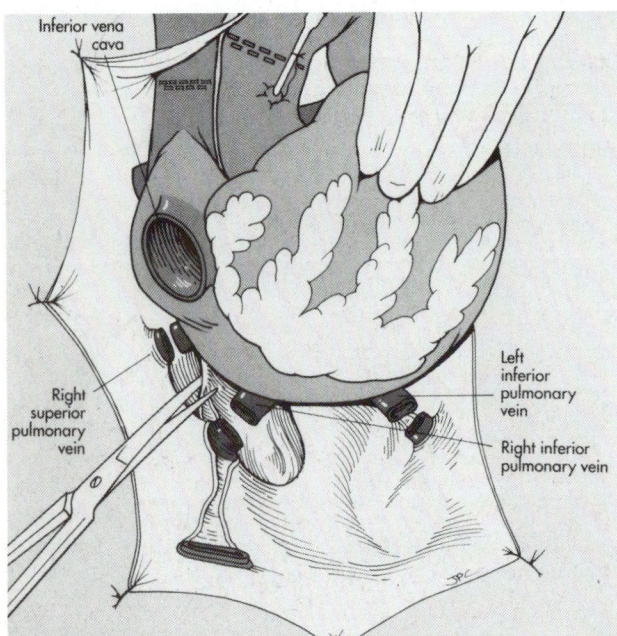

Figure 113–3. Donor cardiectomy requires separation of transverse sinus.

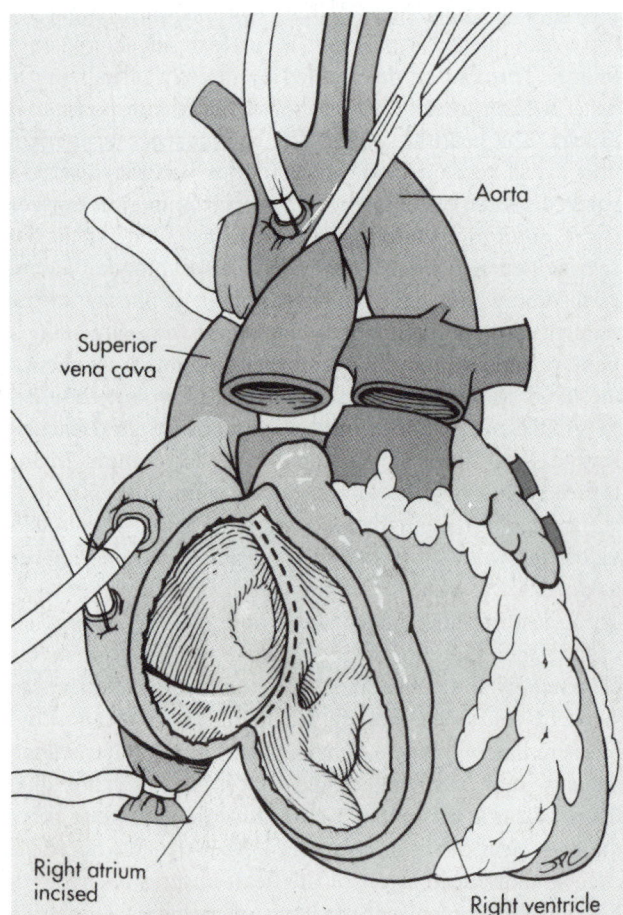

Figure 113–4. Recipient cardiectomy continues with right atriotomy.

atrial incision is then extended to the left toward the base of the left atrial appendage, which is removed (Fig. 113–5). The incision is then extended along the A-V groove just posterior to the coronary sinus to complete the cardiectomy (Fig. 113–6).

The donor heart is prepared by incising the right atrium from the opening of the IVC to the base of the right atrial appendage and closing any PFO present. The left atrial cuff is fashioned by incising through the pulmonary veins and then tailoring a rim of left atrial tissue at the level of the base of the appendage. A 54 inch, 3-0 double-armed polypropylene suture is passed through the recipient's left atrium where the appendage had been excised and then through the base of the donor left atrial appendage (Fig. 113–7). The donor heart is then lowered into the pericardium and cooled with ice slush or saline. Half of the continuous suture is run inferiorly from inside, ensuring proper alignment of the donor and recipient IVC as the interatrial septum is approached (Fig. 113–8). The other half of the suture is run along the roof of the left atrium superi-

orly to the right and down the interatrial septum to completion. A left ventricular vent is placed via the recipient's right superior pulmonary vein and positioned from the left atrium across the mitral valve under direct vision prior to completion of the left atrial anastomosis. The right atrial suture line is begun inferiorly near the septum at the IVC and

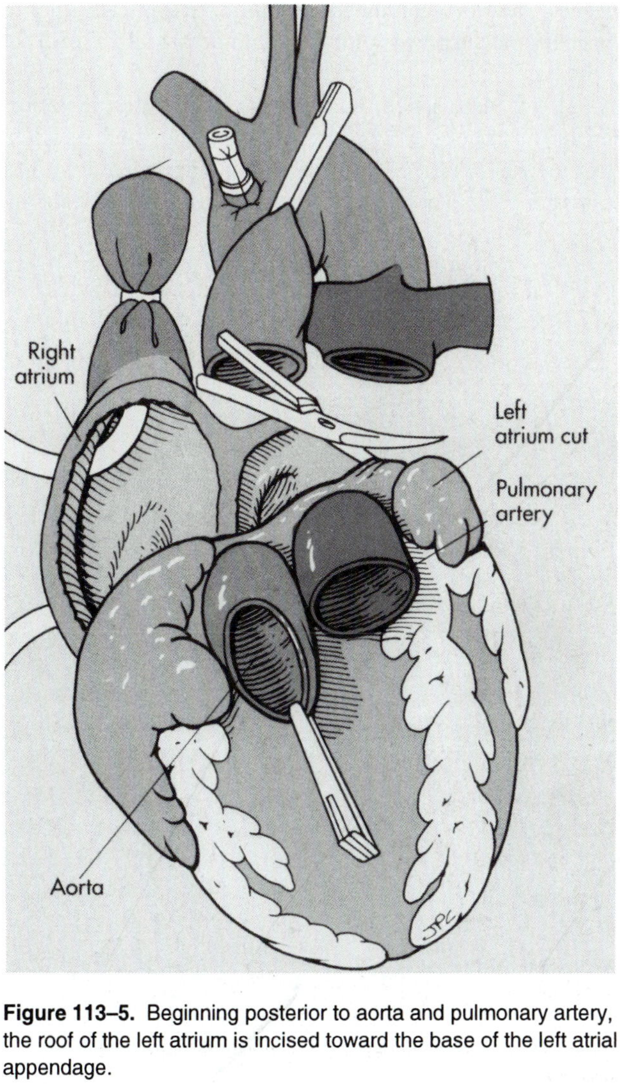

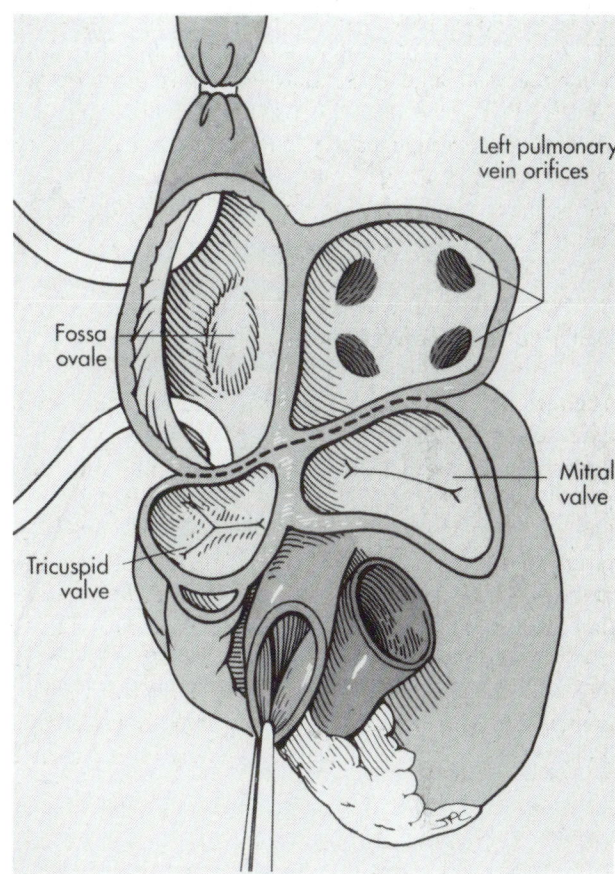

Figure 113–6. Recipient heart is removed with final incision excising the ventricles from the atriums. The coronary sinus generally remains on the ventricular side.

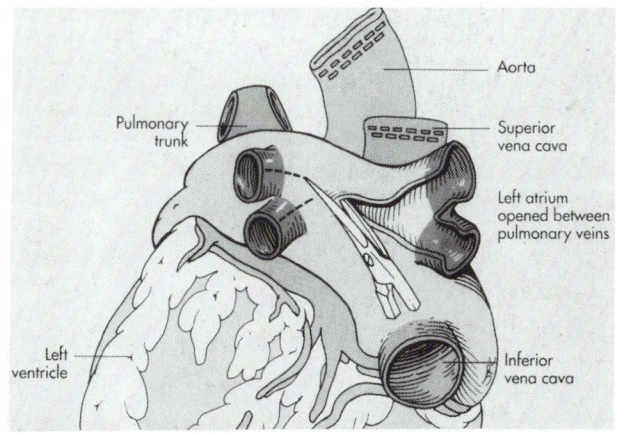

Figure 113–7. Donor pulmonary veins are connected to fashion the left atrial cuff.

Figure 113–5. Beginning posterior to aorta and pulmonary artery, the roof of the left atrium is incised toward the base of the left atrial appendage.

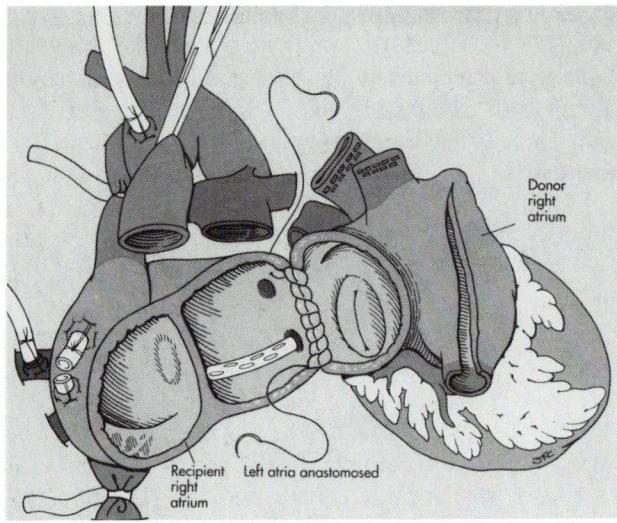

Figure 113–8. Left atrial anastomosis began at the base of the left atrial appendage of the donor and continued inferolaterally.

run up the interatrial septum to the base of the right atrial appendage. The other half of the same double-armed, 3-0 polypropylene suture is continued from below to meet at the appendage (Fig. 113–9).

The pulmonary artery and aorta are trimmed to eliminate any kinking due to redundancy (the tendency is to make these too long). The donor aorta may be cut at an angle to accommodate the often larger recipient aorta. The

pulmonary artery anastomosis is followed by the aortic anastomosis using a double-armed, simple vertical mattress stitch of 4-0 polypropylene suture. Each is begun posteriorly from inside and completed outside anteriorly where any discrepancy in size may be made up safely as any leak from the posterior suture line is troublesome (Fig. 113–10). The vent is temporarily clamped to allow the heart to fill with blood and displace air as the aortic suture line is completed. Deairing maneuvers are done prior to release of the aortic cross-clamp, which is done with the patient in the Trendelenburg position and with an active aortic root vent. Transesophageal echocardiography is used to ensure adequate removal of air from the left side of the heart as ventilation is resumed, and to assist with adequate preloads for the left ventricle as cardiopulmonary bypass is discontinued. Chronotropic support is always provided and inotropic support is occasionally needed. We have preferred dopamine for chronotropic and inotropic support with the addition of epinephrine when required. Atrial and ventricular temporary pacing wires are placed, and the right supraphrenic pericardium is resected to reduce postoperative pericardial effusions. While ventilatory support may be weaned and discontinued without reason for delay, chronotropic support should be continued at a low level for 48 hours.

Atrial size, shape, and orientation may be distorted, and asynchronous contraction of the donor and recipient atria may be observed following orthotopic cardiac transplantation.[46,47] These may contribute to A-V valvular in-

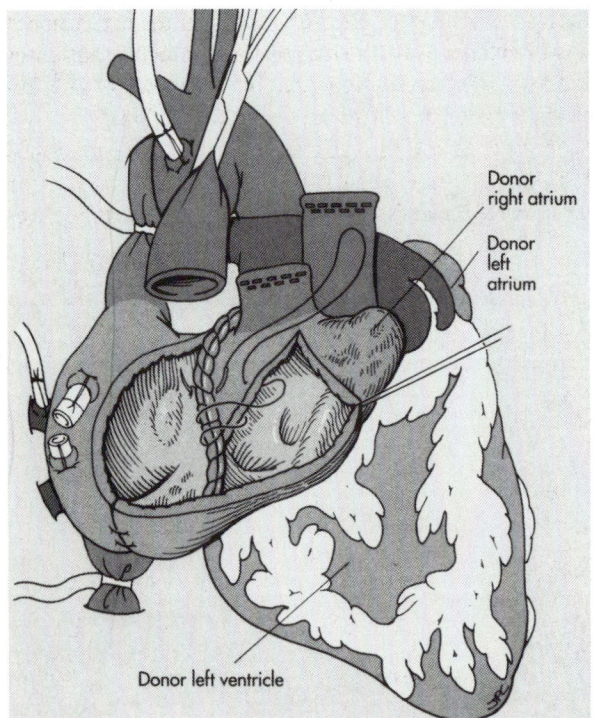

Figure 113–9. Closure of right atrial portion along the interatrial septum.

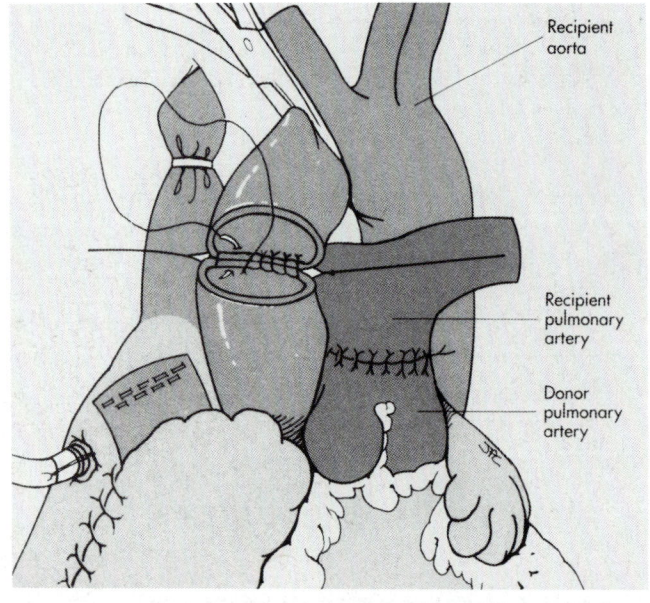

Figure 113–10. Anastomosis of the great vessels by continuous suture.

sufficiency. Alternative techniques of orthotopic cardiac transplantation have been recently described in an attempt to maintain more normal atrial geometry and to minimize conduction disturbances.[48–50] Individual caval anastomoses are performed and may include a modification in the left atrial anastomosis, requiring a bridge of tissue to be retained posteriorly between the right and left pulmonary vein orifices. The left atrial modification is difficult or impossible when donor lungs are procured. Less tricuspid and mitral valvular insufficiency and decreased permanent pacing requirements have been observed in patients in whom these techniques have been utilized.[49,50] Further investigation is needed to determine the clinical significance of these observations and any proven advantage these techniques may offer.

HETEROTOPIC CARDIAC TRANSPLANTATION

After median sternotomy and institution of cardiopulmonary bypass, an incision is made into the recipient's left atrium along the superior and inferior extent of the interstitial groove.[51,52] This incision is similar to that for the common approach to the mitral valve. The heart of the donor is placed in the right chest, anterior to the deflated lung and along the right side of the recipient's heart. The two left atriotomies are juxtaposed, and a continuous suture line of 4-0 polypropylene is carefully completed, beginning with the posterior lip (Fig. 113–11). Because this suture line will be inaccessible later, it is doubly sewn. A 5-cm right lateral atriotomy is made in the host, beginning 2 to 3 cm above the atriosuperior caval junction and extending 3 cm onto the right atrium (Fig. 113–12). A continuous anastomosis begins at the midpoint of the posterior lip of the incision in the recipient's atrium, which is sutured to the most caudal point of the opening in the atrium of the donor.

The open-ended aorta of the donor is sutured to the right side of the host's ascending aorta. The aorta of the

donor is usually trimmed just proximal to its innominate artery. If the aorta is too long, the heart of the donor will fall deeply into the right chest and onto the lung, and if the aorta is divided too short, the right atrial anastomosis will be distorted. A 22-mm Dacron graft is used to connect the end of the main pulmonary artery of the donor to an opening made in the anterior main pulmonary artery of the host (Fig. 113–13). A conduit is required because there is inadequate length of the donor's main pulmonary artery to reach without causing undesirable tension and kinking of the anastomosis. If desired, the intrapericardial portion of the donor's right pulmonary artery or a free graft of the donor's aorta can be used to avoid prosthetic material.

As with recipients of orthotopic hearts, these patients commonly require inotropic drugs, and isoproterenol is an excellent choice because it has the additional benefit of providing vasodilatation of the pulmonary arteries. Flexible bronchoscopy has been useful for the removal of airway secretions, which are often associated with compressive atelectasis of the right lower and middle lobes. Dominance of the host right and donor left ventricle is readily apparent by review of the electrocardiogram and traces of synchronous pulmonary and systemic arterial pressures.

POSTTRANSPLANT CONCERNS

Rejection and Immunosuppression

Infection and rejection contribute significantly to posttransplant morbidity and mortality. Currently available methods of immunosuppression require a delicate balance between excessive immunosuppression which predisposes the patient to infectious complications, and inadequate immunosuppression predisposing to acute rejection.

Three classic forms of rejection have been described and are characterized by their time of occurrence in relation to the transplant and the associated cellular mechanism. Re-

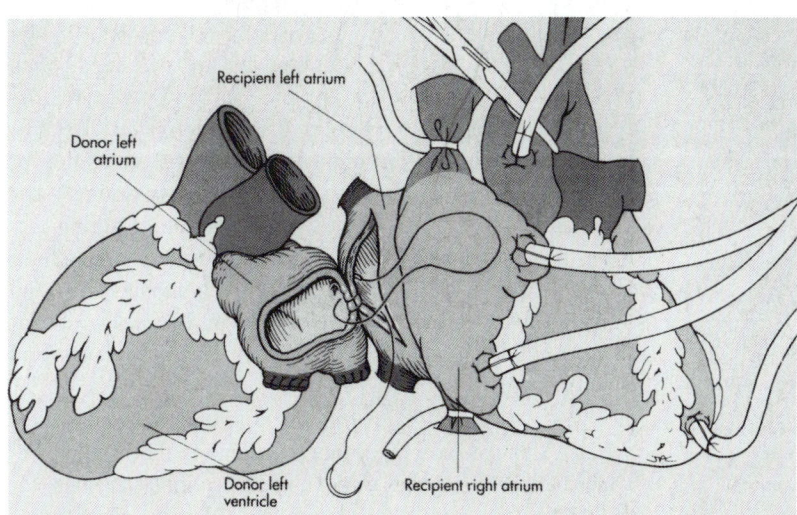

Figure 113–11. Positioning of the donor heart and left atrial anastomosis.

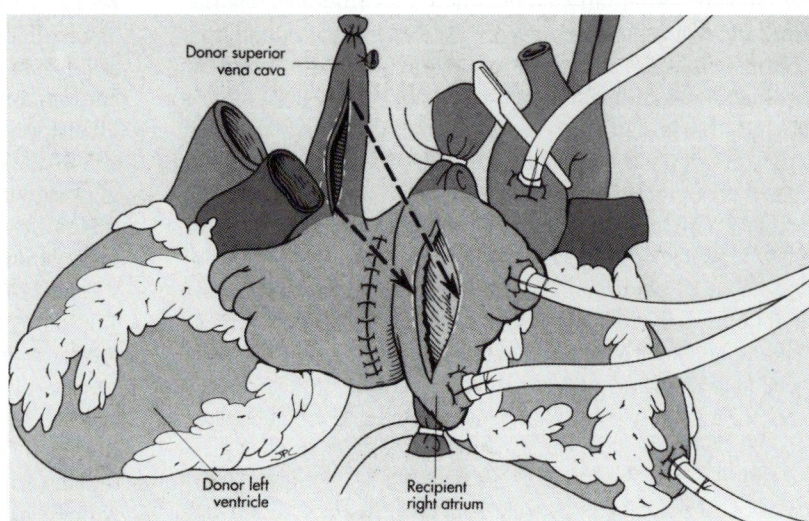

Figure 113–12. Right atrial superiocanal connection in heterotopic transplant.

jection that occurs within minutes to hours after transplantation is termed hyperacute rejection and is thought to be mediated by preformed antibody. The antibody is likely directed against antigens present on vascular endothelium, which may be tissue dependent. This type of rejection reaction is less commonly seen in the modern era of effective preoperative cross-matching.

Acute rejection typically occurs within the first weeks to months following transplantation and is the most common type of rejection treated by clinicians. Acute cellular rejection is T-lymphocyte mediated and involves a complex interaction between major histocompatibility (MHC) Class I and Class II antigens, antigen-presenting cells, and activated T-lymphocytes. T-lymphocytes may be divided into subpopulations based on cell surface antigenic determinants, i.e., CD-4[+] or CD-8[+] T cells. It has been suggested

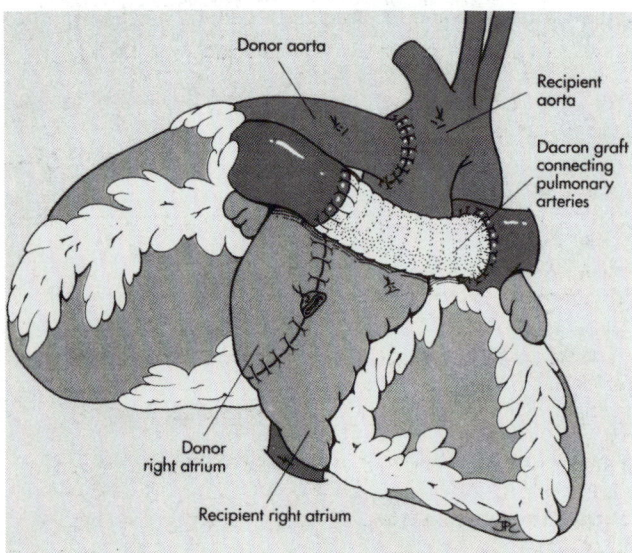

Figure 113–13. Completed heterotopic transplant.

that these antigenic determinants define a functional subset with the CD-4[+] subpopulation representing the "helper/inducer" group and the CD-8[+] population representing the "cytotoxic/suppressor" functional subset.[53,54] These functional subclassifications are not absolute, however, and it is probably more useful to define these subsets as being MHC antigen class-restricted.

Class I MHC antigens are present on all nucleated cells including antigen-presenting cells, while Class II MHC antigens are distributed primarily on antigen presenting cells, i.e., macrophages, dendritic cells, and B-lymphocytes. Various cytokines induce the expression of MHC Class II antigens on the cell surface of some lymphocytes and vascular endothelium.[55,56] CD-4[+] lymphocytes recognize foreign antigen when it is presented on the surface of antigen-presenting cells along with Class II MHC antigens. CD-8[+] T-lymphocytes, on the other hand, recognize foreign antigen when it is presented by antigen-presenting cells on their cell surface along with Class I MHC antigens.[57] These correlations are not perfect but tend to hold true much better than the functional (helper, cytotoxic, etc.) subdivisions mentioned previously.

CD-4[+] and CD-8[+] lymphocytes are activated when presented with a foreign antigen, initiating a cytokine-mediated chain of events involving activated T cells, macrophages, and B-lymphocytes. While the activation of specific subpopulations of T-lymphocytes is antigen-specific, and is MHC-antigen class restricted, the resulting cascade that occurs due to the release of important cytokines such as interleukin-2 (IL-2) is relatively nonspecific and may involve the recruitment of T-cytotoxic cells, T-suppressor cells, natural killer (NK) cells, B-lymphocytes, and macrophages.[58]

Currently available immunosuppressive agents intervene in this cascade of events to attenuate the immune response at various stages of development. This is the basis of multidrug therapy. Cyclosporine and the more recently introduced drug tacrolimus work early in the rejection cascade by restricting T-cell proliferation through limitation of calcium-dependent cytokine gene transcription factors, including IL-2, IL-3, and interferon-γ.[59] The major advance in organ transplantation in the last 15 years has been significantly related to the use of cyclosporine-based immunosuppression. Azathioprine works nonspecifically, by virtue of its antimetabolite effects, to inhibit lymphocyte proliferation. Corticosteroids act at various levels by negatively affecting the release of interleukin-1 and interleukin-6 from macrophages and thereby indirectly affecting the release of IL-2. Higher doses induce a nonspecific anti-inflammatory affect. Both rabbit antihuman thymocyte globulin (RATG) and OKT3 (a mouse monoclonal antibody to T-3) represent specific antisera to cell surface antigens present on human T-lymphocytes. Interaction of this antisera with the target antigen results in diminution of the specific effector cell from the rejection reaction cascade. Because the target of these antisera is a relatively undifferentiated human T cell, the effects again are nonspecific.

Rejection occurring over prolonged periods or later in the post-transplant course is often unresponsive to increased immunosuppression and is termed chronic rejection. Antibody production is thought to be responsible for many cases of chronic rejection, although this has been difficult to prove in the chronically immunosuppressed patient and may be confounded by graft antibody absorption. Cardiac allograft arteriosclerosis probably represents a chronic rejection process, although there is much unknown about the mechanisms and treatment of this process accounting for significant morbidity and mortality.

While various regimens have been successfully used (Table 113–5), the immunosuppression protocol currently used at the University of Pittsburgh includes oral azathioprine, 4 mg/kg preoperatively, and 1000 mg of methylprednisolone given intravenously at the time of reperfusion of the allograft in the operating room. Methylprednisolone is continued in the postoperative period at a dose of 125 mg IV every 8 hours for three doses followed by the administration of oral prednisone 20 mg/day. Azathioprine is continued on the first postoperative day at 2 mg/kg per day, either oral or IV, depending on the resumption of gastrointestinal function. Either cyclosporine or tacrolimus is added as a continuous intravenous infusion at a dose of 0.1 or 0.0015 mg/kg per hour, respectively. This is usually begun 6–12 hours postoperatively and is adjusted according to urine output and renal function. Cyclosporine and tacrolimus are switched to the equivalent oral doses when GI function has resumed and an effort is made to maintain a tacrolimus level of between 10 and 20 ng/mL (whole blood IMX) or a cyclosporine whole blood TDX level of 1000 ng/mL. Side effects of the various immunosuppressive

TABLE 113–5. COMMONLY EMPLOYED IMMUNOSUPPRESSIVE STRATEGIES

Drug	Dose	Comment
Preoperative		
Azathioprine	4.0 mg/kg IV	
Cyclosporine	5.0–10.0 mg po	Deleted in many centers due to acute nephrotoxicity
Intraoperative		
Methylprednisolone	500 mg	With reperfusion of the heart
Postoperative		
Azathioprine	2.0 mg/kg per day	Dose adjusted to keep WBC >5000
Cyclosporine	2.5–5.0 mg/kg per day po	Begun when pt is stable with diuresis (24–36 hours postop); adjust to
OR	0.1 mg/kg per hour IV	500–700 mg/mL whole blood RIA
Tacrolimus	0.075–0.15 mg/kg per day	As above; adjust to 15–20 mg/mL whole blood IMX
	0.0015 mg/kg per hour IV	
Methylprednisolone	125 mg q.8h × 3	
Prednisone	0.3–0.15 mg/kg per day	Wean over 3–6 mo
Rejection		
Methylprednisolone	1 g IV × 3 days	Mild or mod rejection
Antithymocyte globulin[a]	2.5 mg/kg × 5–7 days	Severe or recurrent rejection (For in-hospital preparation; dose varies per potency)
Orthoclone OKT3 and	5 mg IV qd × 14 days	Severe or recurrent rejection
Prednisone	1 mg/kg per day taper after 10 days	Steroid augmentation after OKT3 completed
Maintenance		
Cyclosporine	2.5–5.0 mg/kg per day	Dose adjustment based on individual history of rejection and drug toxicity
OR		
Tacrolimus	0.1–0.2 mg/kg per day	Dose adjustment based on individual history of rejection and drug toxicity
Prednisone	2.5–5.0 mg/kg per day	Dose adjustment based on individual history of rejection and drug toxicity
Azathioprine	1.0–2.0 mg/kg per day	Dose adjustment based on individual history of rejection and drug toxicity

[a]ATGAM, Upjohn.

drugs are related to their mechanism of action with the antimetabolite effects of azathioprine noted predominantly in bone marrow suppression, myelocyte suppression, dose-related leukopenia, thrombocytopenia, and GI disturbances. Since the inhibition of calcine urinphosphatase is the common biological action of both cyclosporine and tacrolimus, it is not surprising they share other toxicities. Both cause nephrotoxicity and this appears to be in part related to dose with significant nephrotoxicity observed with cyclosporine levels exceeding 1000 ng/dL (whole blood RIA) and tacrolimus above 20 ng/mL (IMX).[60] The problems of hypertension have not been as pronounced with tacrolimus when compared to cyclosporine, and the facial brutalization with hirsutism and gingival hyperplasia has not been seen with tacrolimus. Complications and side effects of steroid therapy affect multiple organ systems and include hypertension, diabetes, cushingoid features, poor wound healing, and aseptic bone necrosis. Lympholytic therapy with agents such as RATG or OKT3 has not been validated, and we have abandoned its routine use. We now only use RATG as induction therapy in patients with renal dysfunction who cannot tolerate cyclosporine or tacrolimus intravenously in the early postoperative period. Lympholytic agents are also used in steroid-resistant, persistent episodes of acute rejection. The incidence of acute rejection was recently analyzed in a multi-institutional study from 25 institutions involving 911 patients undergoing cardiac transplantation between January 1990 and July 1991. A varied analysis showed that the use of induction therapy was associated with a greater cumulative rejection frequency. Induction therapy did not delay the onset of first rejection nor did it reduce the cumulative number of episodes of rejection.[61]

Early recognition and treatment of acute cellular rejection were made possible by the introduction of transvenous myocardial biopsy by Caves et al in 1972.[62] Utilizing local anesthesia and fluoroscopic guidance, biopsy forceps are introduced through a sheath placed percutaneously into the internal jugular vein. Three to five specimens are taken from the septum of the right ventricle. Other less invasive methods of detecting rejection have not proven effective. Myocardia biopsies are performed weekly for the first 4 weeks following transplantation, with decreasing frequency over the first year or when clinical circumstances warrant, and then annually thereafter. Biopsy specimens are subjected to a standardized grading system established in 1990 by Billingham et al and published in the *Journal of Heart and Lung Transplantation*.[63]

We recently completed our analysis of tacrolimus as the major immunosuppressant after cardiac transplant. We first reported our experience with tacrolimus in adult cardiac recipients in 1991.[64] This and subsequent use after cardiac transplantation in our institution was not controlled prospectively against cyclosporine-based immunotherapy.[65] The adults received moderate doses of tacrolimus (0.15 mg/kg bid), prednisone (0.15 mg/kg), and azathioprine. Steroids were weaned relative to rejection whenever possi-

ble. A 93%, 1-year survival was achieved in this initial group in spite of the inclusion of a significant number of high-risk recipients. Freedom at 3 months from grade ≥3a was 41%, and the linearized rate was 0.95 per patient. At 1 year, 30% were not receiving steroids, and those who did averaged 8.5 mg/kg per day. Compared to our most contemporary cyclosporine-based protocols that included induction of therapy with the cytolytic monoclonal antibody OKT3, plus maintenance with prednisone and azathioprine, survival and freedom from rejection were similar, but only 28% of the tacrolimus versus 48% of the cyclosporine had repeat episodes of rejection. Left ventricular ejection fraction in this group of 70 patients averaged 66% and ranged between 48 and 75% at 1 year, and of the 35 who had annual coronary arteriography, 4 or 11% had evidence of mild coronary arteriopathy. The importance of this finding moderates initial concerns about the possibility of drug-associated vasculitis, previously seen in some animal species. Based on our continued experience with tacrolimus, it would appear the incidence of graft vascular disease is similar with both therapies. Side effects were not major problems and included hypertension in 54%, new onset diabetes in 18%, hyperkalemia in 10%, neuromuscular abnormalities including seizure, tremors, or hallucinations in 10%. Currently we are following 81 consecutive patients treated with FK506 (tacrolimus) (unpublished). This group has achieved an actual survival of 79% at 2.9±1.3 years of follow-up. Compared to cyclosporine plus cytolytic induction therapy, the FK group has had a higher incidence of grade > 2 rejection (57 vs 40%, $p = 0.07$). In contrast there appears to be less endocardial fibrosis and Quilty lesions (55 vs 89%, $p < 0.01$) in 12-month biopsies, suggesting a better long-term outlook for FK patients.

We have been fortunate to evaluate the usefulness of tacrolimus as a rescue from persistent cardiac rejection (≥3a) in an additional 26 recipients who have averaged 435 days of cyclosporine-based and augmented steroid plus cytolytic therapy.[65] All have been successfully treated. In 20, tacrolimus alone was successful within 2 weeks; two patients required additional methylprednisolone, and one required additional OKT3 and methylprednisolone. The average dose of prednisone was reduced in this group from 20 to 12.5 mg/day. Over the period of treatment, creatinine rose insignificantly from 1.5 to 2.0 mg%. Because of additive toxicities cyclosporine was discontinued for 2 to 3 days prior to tacrolimus that was slowly increased to 0.15 bid with a serum trough of 1.0 to 2.0 mg/mL (TDX). Serum creatinine was carefully followed during the conversion and thereafter. In view of the heavy immunosuppressants received by these patients, it is not surprising that four had major infections (disseminated tuberculosis 1, nocardiosis 1, mucormycosis 1, and aspergillosis, 1). Additionally four developed post-transplant lymphoproliferative disease. Six of the 26 have died between 4 months and 4 years of the switch to tacrolimus (PTLD 3, suicide 1, osteosarcoma 1, glioblastoma multiform 1). Since all patients stabilized their biopsies and none died with acute or chronic failure, we conclude that tacrolimus is an effective agent for refractory rejection and likely should be used earlier prior to heavy doses of adjunct immunosuppressive therapy.

Acute rejection is treated with IV methylprednisolone, 1000 mg/day for 3 days. Recurrent, recalcitrant, or severe rejection is treated with RATG or OKT3 as mentioned previously. Use of these lympholytic agents may be associated with the development of hives, fever, chills, local erythema, induration and pain, and other characteristics of anaphylaxis or a serum sickness-like reaction. Patients are pretreated with corticosteroids, antihistamines, and antipyretic agents to counteract these side effects. Because OKT3 and RATG are antibodies produced in mice and rabbits, respectively, patients generally respond in time to antibody production to the antigenic determinants of the foreign antibody that may preclude repeated use. The use of these agents has also been associated with an increased incidence of post-transplant lymphoproliferative disease.[66,67] OKT3 administration may also result in the development of pulmonary edema and bronchospasm.

Future developments in achieving symbiosis between the cardiac transplant recipient and their allograft will likely involve a state of antigen-specific immunosuppression whereby the immune response to donor alloantigens is suppressed without affecting the host response to other antigens. Alternatively, the development of tolerance to the transplanted organ either by clonal deletion or induction of an antigen-specific suppressor cell, or creation of mixed donor recipient bone marrow chimeras, thereby inducing tolerance to self and the donor organ, represents attractive possibilities under current investigation.

Coronary Graft Vasculopathy

Although short-term rates of survival have improved following cardiac transplantation due to better selection of candidates and detection, prevention, and treatment of acute rejection, allograft vasculopathy limits the long-term outlook and now is the major cause of death after 1 year.[68]

Findings at autopsy suggest virtually all recipients who survive more than 1 year demonstrate intimal changes[69] that usually progress to cause diffuse entire segment narrowing and ischemic injury. While initiating events likely differ, it is most likely that the arterial response leading to allograft vasculopathy is similar to those that occur in focal nonallograft atherosclerosis. The endothelial response to injury hypothesis likely forms the common bond.[70,71] Stimulated endothelial and smooth muscle cells produce cytokines and growth factors causing cell proliferation and smooth muscle and macrophage migration to the intima, resulting in concentric lipid-laden calcium-poor plaque.[72] Histologic and immunocytochemical analyses of allograft vessels have documented an inflammatory stage that precedes the intimal and smooth muscle cell proliferation in the vessel walls.[73] Finally, reduced vasodilatation after acetylcholine administration in cardiac allografts suggests impairment of endothelial-derived relaxation factor.[74] Identification of the cause of injury has been difficult as hypertension, smoking, diabetes, and a prior history of atherosclerosis in transplant recipients have not correlated with an increased risk.[75–77] It is reasonable to suggest that immune mechanisms are an important pathogenesis because the vasculopathy is selective for only the allograft that it affects diffusely.[78] While it appears that the induction of cardiac allograft vasculopathy is not simply a result of the surgical procedure, the alloimmune effector that causes endothelial injury is unknown.[79] Attempts to correlate rejection with coronary disease have resulted in inconsistent results.[80–82] Clinical studies that have attempted to relate histocompatibility to graft atherosclerosis have been confused primarily because of the inclusion of small numbers over short periods and various immunosuppressive regimens.[83,84] Both cell-mediated and antibody-mediated effector arms have been thought to be primary[85–88] in rodent studies. These studies also suggest that Class II MHC antigen expression is associated with the vascular lesion.[89]

Classically the standard for diagnosing graft atherosclerosis has been the annual coronary arteriogram. Because cardiac allografts are functionally denervated, ischemia is not reliably heralded by angina. Standard coronary arteriography is also limited because diffuse narrowing of small and large arteries. Recently intracoronary ultrasound has been proposed as a more sensitive tool.[90,91] Unfortunately nuclear scans, including thallium, have been relatively nonspecific again due to the diffuse nature of the disease.

Without a better understanding of the cause of injury, treatment will be suboptimal. Currently it is best addressed by retransplantation although this is associated with a 30% or greater lower rate of survival than primary transplantation.[92] Occasionally when the disease is associated with focal lesions, angioplasty can be performed but this therapy is far from definitive. Medical therapies, including exercise, cholesterol-lowering agents, antiplatelet and anticoagulant drugs, fish oil, and calcium blockers, have not been shown to alter the course of disease.[93–95]

Posttransplant Infection/Other

Early experience with cardiac transplantation and suppression of the normal immune response showed infection to be a frequent complication as 58% of patient deaths were from infection.[96–98] Fortunately there has been a reduced incidence of death and infection, choice of antibiotics, and greater clinical experience, and perhaps, most importantly, the introduction of cyclosporine. Infection has continued to be a major problem in our patients; it was thought to be the primary cause of death in 22% of them.[99]

Infections are most common early after transplantation, falling off after the first year to approximately one severe infection for every four patient years. The Registry of the International Society for Heart and Lung Transplantation has reported that the rate of early death from infection is 16%, the third most common cause of death after cardiac complications (40%) and rejection (19%). Infection, however, was the most significant factor in late deaths, accounting for 39% of them. Bacterial infections are the most common followed by viruses, fungi, and protozoans, which cause 35% of the severe infections. Severe viral infections were generally seen between 1 and 6 months postoperatively. Severe fungal infections were most common in the first 2 months; protozoal infections first appeared more than a month after transplantation and peaked in the third to sixth months. Cytomegalovirus, herpes virus, or bacterial infection is equally likely in the first 6 weeks, but late infection 2 or more years postoperatively is 10–20 times more likely to have a bacterial etiology.

Pneumonia, the most common infection, should be evaluated with sputum Gram's stain and culture at the time of the initial workup. If sputum is not available or if opportunistic pathogens are suspected, bronchoscopy and bronchoalveolar lavage will help to make a specific diagnosis. Open lung biopsy is being used less frequently because of improved clinical diagnosis and the increasing success of bronchoalveolar lavage.

Cytomegalovirus (CMV) can be cultured from 85 to 90% of cardiac recipients. But 18% of patients are symptomatic with fever and fatigue associated with atypical lymphocytosis, neutropenia, thrombocytopenia, and mild elevation of liver function tests, and about one-quarter of the symptomatic patients will also develop invasive gastrointestinal or pulmonary disease. Reactivation of CMV disease may minimally disturb the patient, but more severe illness occurs in those patients who are seronegative for CMV prior to transplantation and acquire the new infection from the donor organ or transfusion of blood products. In seronegative patients the illness is severe enough to justify transfusion of only seronegative blood products. Ganciclovir is the treatment of choice; recent studies have included the use of this agent (5 mg/kg bid) prophylactically for 2 weeks postoperatively, followed by oral acyclovir (600 mg bid) for 3 to 6 months.[100,101]

Herpes simplex and herpes zoster frequently cause minor but troublesome mucocutaneous infections. About half of the recipients will shed herpes simplex virus and half of these will have infection, most often oral ulcerations, usually in the first 3 weeks after transplantation. Genital herpes occurs, but less frequently, and is generally treated with oral acyclovir for 1 week.

The increased risk of developing a posttransplant lymphoproliferative disorder seems to be related to Epstein–Barr virus infection. Treatment of this lymphoproliferative disease with either radiation or chemotherapy has not been fruitful in our experience, and greater benefit has come from reduction of immunosuppression.[102,103] We currently also administer interferon-γ and pooled donor γ-globulin with high titers of anti-EBV antibodies.

Candidiasis is the most common severe fungal infection after transplantation and was seen in eight of 199 patients. Six of the eight patients had disseminated disease; all six were in the intensive care unit, were receiving broad spectrum antibiotics, and had other major infections. Illness in four of these six patients occurred more than 2 years after transplantation and was associated with renal, hepatic, or cardiac failure. Candidiasis also has caused esophagitis in one patient and was associated with staphylococcal mediastinitis in another. Candidiasis will continue to be a problem, but hopefully until it is easily diagnosed, less toxic antifungal agents like itraconazol will be helpful.

Aspergillosis was a major cause of death in the early experience and continues to be significant, affecting 4% of the patients reported by Dummer. Only one of the five patients survived treatment with amphotericin B. Cryptococcal infection must be considered, especially in patients who are debilitated at the time of transplantation. Fungal infections have been limited to these few organisms in our experience, but other species must be considered in particular geographic locations.

Pneumocystis carinii pneumonia (PCP) occurs in 3–15% of immunosuppressed transplant patients if they are not given prophylactic oral trimethoprim–sulfamethoxazole (TMP–SMX).[99] Patients typically have a fever, dry cough, and dyspnea for a few days or weeks associated with a diffuse infiltrate on chest x-ray. Diagnosis is confirmed by methenamine silver stains of fluid from a bronchoalveolar lavage. PCP may be slow to respond to therapy, and clinical and radiographic stability may not occur for at least a week. It has been suggested that a rapid reduction in immunosuppression may exacerbate the inflammatory process in the lung.[104] PCP can be effectively eliminated as a potential problem by the use of prophylactic low-dose trimethoprim–sulfamethoxazole (one single strength tablet once daily); in the case of allergic patients, monthly inhalation pentamidine (300 mg) is effective.

Renal Failure

Nephrotoxicity, which was noted when cyclosporine was first used for renal transplantation, continues to be the most important side effect of cyclosporine.[105,106] Early toxicity was seen in 58% of our first 43 patients treated with cyclosporine,[107] and 20% of them required temporary dialysis. While multiple factors are likely responsible, it is believed that nephrotoxicity is due to cyclosporine-induced vasoconstriction of the afferent arterioles and to a lesser extent from direct tubular cell injury.[108–110] To some extent, toxicity is dose related[111] and has plateaued as multidrug regimens have evolved with lower doses of cyclosporine. Oliguria occurs in the early form of renal failure; the BUN rises out of proportion to the serum creatinine, but both peak at 4 to 5 days. Volume depletion is associated with worse azotemia, and mortally ill transplant candidates who are being supported with inotropes and intra-aortic balloon counterpulsation are at greatest risk. Renal function rapidly improves after reduction in the dosage of cyclosporine.

Late nephrotoxicity is characterized by a slow rise in serum creatinine. In our experience, 45% of patients receiving cyclosporine had a serum creatinine greater than 1.7 mg/dL at 1 year, and all patients had a creatinine above 1.7 mg/dL at 4 years.[112] The reduction of doses of cyclosporine even late in the course of nephrotoxicity leads to some improvement in renal function, although the pathologic ranges are not completely reversible.[112] There are no known treatments that reliably prevent renal injury, but prostaglandin E_1 analogue has reduced the development in renal transplant recipients.[113]

Other Complications Associated With Immunosuppression

Hirsutism, tremor, and gingival hyperplasia are common sequelae to long-term use of cyclosporine but are less of a problem with tacrolimus. Hirsutism is handled with depilatories. Gingival hyperplasia usually is controlled with dental hygiene, but may require gingivectomy.[114] Tremor is usually mild with both agents and is well tolerated and may be controlled with small doses of propranolol.

Gout may be a troublesome complication during the follow-up period. Hyperuricemia is a common complication of cyclosporine therapy and is caused by decreased renal urate clearance. This is aggravated by the use of diuretics given to control hypertension.[115] Symptomatic relief can be obtained with anti-inflammatory agents. Allopurinol potentiates the bone marrow toxicity of azathioprine.

High cholesterol and low-density lipoprotein levels have been found as early as 3 months after transplantation and appear to be related to the cumulative doses of cyclosporine and steroids, of which the latter is a more important determinant.[116,117] Eight percent of 366 cardiac recipients who were not diabetic before transplantation have become diabetic, and most require insulin.[118] The influence of steroids on hyperglycemia is well known, but it appears that steroids unmask the tendency to become diabetic, rather than cause it. In the patients in our series who became diabetic following transplantation, there was no significant correlation with age, gender, race, HLA-type, steroid or cyclosporine dosage, or incidence of rejection. Coronary artery disease was demonstrated with similar frequency and severity, and infection and survival did not significantly differ from nondiabetic recipients.

Osteoporosis is another complication associated with corticosteroids and can result in fractures. Advanced age, postmenopausal status, and initial reduced bone density from inactivity increase the likelihood. It can be controlled with increased dietary intake of dairy products or with calcium and vitamin D supplementation.

Abdominal surgical complications occur with greater frequency after cardiac transplantation than after other types of cardiothoracic operations.[119,120] Opportunistic infections of the upper gastrointestinal tract and bleeding related to steroids lead to a more frequent need for upper gastrointestinal endoscopy.[121] Abdominal operations are tolerated, and a prompt and aggressive approach to abdominal complaints is appropriate for immunosuppressed patients.

SURVIVAL

As discussed in the brief historical review, cardiac transplantation burst into clinical medicine in 1978 and for only a few years enjoyed a near celebrity status before the harsh reckoning of dismal results eroded confidence in the procedure at most centers. Throughout the 1970s a core of determined surgeons worked to improve outcomes by perfecting techniques, postoperative schemes, and preoperative screening. However, between 1975 and 1981, the 36-month survival was just 40%, and were it not for the discovery of cyclosporine it is likely that further improvements would be quite marginal and delayed. Armed with cyclosporine the experienced Stanford center[122] and our own immature center at Pittsburgh were able to provide consistent survivals above 80% at 1 year and 70% at 3–5 years after transplantation.[123] In 1994 the Registry of the International Society for Heart and Lung Transplantation has reported on 26,704 heart transplant procedures.[124] The 1- and 12-year survivals were approximately 80 and 37%, respectively. 1- and 12-year survivals were approximately 80 and 37%, respectively. Significant risk factors ($p < 0.001$) from this large voluntary registry included previous transplantation (2.61 odds ratio), preoperative ventilator dependence (1.87 odds ratio), age < 5 years (3.75 odds ratio), and age > 60 years (1.42 odds ratio). While this report also indicated preoperative dependence on a ventricular assist device as a risk, the current bridge-to-transplant experience is associated with greater than 90% survival. Interestingly, donor-associated factors ($p < 0.001$) included age > 40 years (1.34), female sex (1.24 odds ratio), and ischemic time > 3.5 hours (1.27 odds ratio). While retransplantation represents only 2.3% of the cases, it is clear that those performed within 6 months fare worse than those after that period. Outcome in both groups of retransplants is inferior to primary transplantation, and given donor scarcity most question the advisability of repeat procedures.

The future of cardiac transplantation like that of other solid organ transplants will depend on further refinement in immunosuppression that will focus regulation specifically toward donor active endothelial receptors and responding host lymphocytes. Hopefully longer-term problems associated with allograft coronary disease will be mitigated by these or other improvements in regulating the host response. Progress with newer immunosuppressants is anticipated along with studies of bone marrow-induced tolerance and the development of transgenic animals proposed for xenografting. While much has been accomplished, it is likely that the future is equally promising.

REFERENCES

1. Goldberg M, Berman EF, Akman LC: Homologous transplantation of the canine heart. *J Int Coll Surg* **30:**575, 1958
2. Cass MH, Brock R: Heart excision and replacement. *Guys Hosp Rep* **108:**285, 1959
3. Lower RR, Shumway NE: Studies orthotopic homotransplantation of the canine heart. *Surg Forum* **11:**18, 1960
4. Lower RR, Dong E Jr, Shumway NE: Long-term survival of cardiac homografts. *Surgery* **58:**110, 1965
5. Mudge GH, Goldstein S, Addonizio LJ, et al: Task Force 3: Recipient Guideline/Prioritization. 24th Bethesda Conference on Cardiac Transplantation. *J Am Col Cardiol* **22:**1–21, 1993
6. Breen TJ, Keck B, Hosenpud JD, et al: Thoracic organ transplants in the United States from October 1987 through December 1991: A report from the UNOS Scientific Registry for Organ Transplant, United Network for Organ Sharing, Richmond, VA. In: Terasaki PI (ed): *Clinical Transplants 1992,* Los Angeles, CA, UCLA Tissue Typing Laboratory, 1992, pp 33–43
7. Hosenpud JD, Uretsky BF, Griffith BP, et al: Successful intermediate term outcome for patients with cardiac amyloidosis undergoing heart transplantation: Results of multi center survey. *J Heart Transplant* **9:**346–350, 1990
8. O'Connell JB, Deck GW, Goldenberg IF, et al: The results heart transplantation for active lymphocytic myocarditis. *J Heart Transplant* **9:**351–356, 1990
9. O'Connell JB, Gunnar RM, Evans RW, et al: Task force one: Organization of heart transplantation in the US. *J Am Coll Cardiol* **22:**8–14, 1993
10. The CONSENSUS Trial Study Group: Effects of enalapril on mortality in severe congestive heart failure. Results of the Cooperative North Scandinavian Enalapril Survival Study (CONSENSUS). *N Engl J Med* **316:**1429–1435, 1987
11. Wilson JR, Swartz JS, Sutton MS, et al: Prognosis in severe heart failure: Relation to hemodynamic measurements and ventricular ectopic activity. *J Am Coll Cardiol* **2:**403–410, 1983
12. Franciosa JA, Wilen M, Ziesche S, Cohn JN: Survival in men with severe chronic left ventricular failure due to either coronary heart disease or idiopathic dilated cardiac myopathy. *Am J Cardiol* **51:**831–836, 1983
13. Cohn JN, Levine TB, Olivari MT, et al: Plasma norepinephrine as a guide to prognosis in patients with chronic congestive heart failure. *N Engl J Med* **311:**819–823, 1984
14. Keogh AM, Freund J, Baron DW, Hickie JB: Timing of cardiac transplantation in idiopathic dilated cardiac myopathy. *Am J Cardiol* **61:**418–422, 1988
15. Creager MA, Faxon DP, Halperin JL, et al: Determinants of clinical response and survival in patients with congestive heart failure treated with Captopril. *Am Heart J* **104:**1147–1154, 1982
16. Keogh AM, Baron DW, Hickie JB: Prognostic guides in patients with idiopathic or ischemic dilated cardiomyopathy assessed for cardiac transplantation. *Am J Cardiol* **65:**903–908, 1990
17. DiBianco R, Shabetai R, Kostuk W, et al: A comparison of oral milrinone, digoxin, and their combination in the treatment of patients with chronic heart failure. *N Engl J Med* **320:**677–683, 1989
18. Mancini DM, Eisen H, Kussmaul W, et al: Value of peak exercise oxygen consumption for optimal timing of cardiac transplantation in ambulatory patients with heart failure. *Circulation* **83:**778–786, 1991
19. Olivari MT, Antolick A, Kaye MP, et al: Heart transplantation in elderly patients. *J Heart Transplant* **7:**258–264, 1988
20. Young JN, Yazbeck J, Esposito G, The influence of acute preoperative pulmonary infarction on the results of heart transplantation. *J Heart Transplant* **5:**20–22, 1986
21. O'Connell JB, Bourge RC, Costanzo-Nordin MR, et al: Cardiac transplantation: Recipient selection, donor procurement, and medical follow-up. *Circulation* **86:**1061–1079, 1992
22. Kormos RL, Thompson M, Hardesty RL, et al: Utility of perioperative right heart catheterization data as a predictor of survival after heart transplantation. *J Heart Transplant* **5:**391, 1986
23. Kirklin JK, Naftel DC, Kirklin JW, et al: Pulmonary vascular resistance and the risk of heart transplantation. *J Heart Transplant* **7:**331–336, 1988
24. Murali S, Uretsky BF, Reddy PS, et al: The use of transpulmonary pressure gradient in the selection of cardiac transplantation candidates, (Abstr). *J Am Coll Cardiol* **11:**45a, 1988
25. Erickson KW, Costanzo-Nordin MR, O'Sullivan EJ, et al: Influence of perioperative transpulmonary gradient on late mortality after orthotopic heart transplantation. *J Heart Transplant* **9:**526–537, 1990
26. Murali S, Kormos RL, Uretsky BF, et al: Preoperative pulmonary hypertension and mortality after cardiac transplantation, (Abstr). *J Heart Transplant* **9:**56, 1990
27. Costard-Jackle A, Fowler MB: Influence of preoperative pulmonary artery pressure on mortality after heart transplantation: Testing of potential reversibility of pulmonary hypertension with nitroprusside is useful in defining a high-risk group. *J Am Coll Cardiol* **19:**48–54, 1992
28. Murali S, Uretsky BR, Armitage JM, et al: Utility of prostaglandin E-1 in the pre-transplant evaluation of cardiac failure patients with significant pulmonary hypertension. *J Heart Lung Transplant* **11:**716–723, 1992
29. Stevenson LW, Hamilton MA, Tillisch JH, et al: Decreasing survival benefit from cardiac transplantation for out-patients as the waiting list lengthens. *J Am Coll Cardiol* **18:**919–925, 1991
30. Stevenson LW, Fowler MB, Schroeder JS, et al: Poor survival of patients with idiopathic cardiomyopathy considered too well for transplantation. *Am J Med* **83:**871–876, 1987
31. Stevenson LW, Warner SL, Hamilton MA, et al: Distribution of donor hearts to maximize transplant candidate survival. *Circulation* **84**(Suppl II):II–352, 1991
32. Karwande SV, Ensley RD, Renlund DG, et al: Cardiac retransplantation: A viable option? The Registry of the International Society for Heart and Lung Transplantation. *Ann Thorac Surg* **54:**840–844, 1992
33. Evans RW, Manninen DL, Garrison LP Jr, Maier AM: Donor availability as the primary determinate of the future of heart transplantation. *JAMA* **255:**1892–1898, 1986
34. Orians CE, Evans RW, Ascher NL: Evidence of organ specific availability for the United States. *Transplant Proc* **25:**1541–1542, 1993
35. Registry of the International Society for Heart and Lung Transplantation: Tenth official report. *J Heart Lung Transplant* **12:**541–548, 1993
36. Fragomeni LS, Rogers G, Kaye MP: Donor identification and organ procurement for cardiac transplantation. In Thompson MR (ed): *Cardiovascular Clinics: Cardiac Transplantation,* Vol. 20. Philadelphia, F.A. Davis, 1990
37. Milfred SK, Lake KD, Anderson DJ, et al: Practices of cardiothoracic transplant centers regarding hepatitis C—Seropositive candidates and donors. *Transplantation* **57:**568–572, 1994
38. Blackbourne LH, Tribble CG, Langenburg SE, et al: Successful use of undersized donors for orthotopic heart transplantation—with a caveat. *Ann Thorac Surg* **57:**1472–1475, 1994
39. Morley D, Boigon M, Fesniak H, et al: Post transplantation hemodynamics and exercise function are not affected by body-size matching of donor and recipient. *J Heart Lung Transplant* **12:**770–778, 1993
40. Bourge RC, Naftel DC, Costanzo-Nordin M, et al: Pre-transplant risk factors for death after cardiac transplantation: A multi institutional study. (Abstr). *J Heart Lung Transplant* **11:**191, 1992
41. Stoddard MF, Longaker RA: The role of transesophageal echocardiography in cardiac donor screening. *Am Heart J* **125:**1676–1681, 1993
42. Frist WH, Fanning WJ: Donor management and matching. *Cardiol Clin* **8:**55–71, 1990

43. Gifford RPM, Weaver AS, Burg JE, et al: Thyroid hormone levels in heart and kidney cadaver donors. *J Heart Transplant* 5:249, 1986

44. Novitsky D, Cooper DKC, Chaffin JS, et al: Improved cardiac allograft function following triiodothyronine therapy to both donor and recipient. *Transplantation* 49:311–316, 1990

45. Baldwin JC, Anderson JL, Boucek MM, et al: Task Force II: Donor guidelines. 24th Bethesda Conference: Cardiac transplantation. *J Am Coll Cardiol* 22:15, 1993

46. Angermann CE, Spes CH, Tammen A, et al: Anatomic characteristics and valvular function of the transplanted heart: Transthoracic versus transesophageal echocardiographic findings. *J Heart Transplant* 9:331–338, 1990

47. Stevenson LW, Dadourian BJ, Kobashigawa J, et al: Mitral regurgitation after cardiac transplantation. *Am J Cardiol* 60:119–122, 1987

48. Dreyfus G, Jebra V, Mihaileanu S, Carpentier AF: Total orthotopic heart transplantation: An alternative to the standard technique. *Ann Thorac Surg* 52:1181–1184, 1991

49. Sievers HH, Weyand M, Kraatz EG, Bernhard A: An alternative technique for orthotopic cardiac transplantation, with preservation of the normal anatomy of the right atrium. Department of Cardiovascular Surgery, University of Kiel, Germany. *Thorac Cardiovasc Surgeon* 39:70–72, 1991

50. Blanche C, Czer LS, Valenza M, Trento A: Alternative technique for orthotopic heart transplantation. *Ann Thorac Surg* 57:765–767, 1994

51. Griffith BP, Kormos RL, Hardesty RL: Heterotopic cardiac transplantation: Current status. *J Cardiac Surg* 2:283–289, 1987

52. Novitsky D, Cooper DKC, Barnard CN: The surgical technique of heterotopic heart transplantation. *Ann Thorac Surg* 36:476, 1983

53. Englemen EG, Benike CG: Antibodies to membrane structures that distinguish suppressor/cytotoxic and helper T lymphocyte subpopulations block the mixed leukocyte reaction in man. *J Exp Med* 154:193–198, 1981

54. Meur SC, Schlossman SF, Reinherz EL: Clonal analysis of human cytotoxic T lymphocytes: T4+ and T8+ effector T cells recognize products of different major histocompatibility complex regions. *Proc Natl Acad Sci USA* 79:4395–4399, 1982

55. Harris HW, Gill TJ III: Expression of class I transplantation antigens. *Transplantation* 42:109, 1986

56. Daar AS, Fuggle SV, Fabre JW, et al: The detailed description of MHC class II antigens in normal human organs. *Transplantation* 38:293, 1984

57. Swain SL: T cell subsets and the recognition of MHC class. *Immunol Rev* 74:129–141, 1983

58. Krensky AM, Weis A, Crabtree G, et al: T-lymphocyte antigen interactions in transplant rejection. *N Engl J Med* 322:510, 1990

59. Griffith BP, Bando K, Hardesty RL, et al: A prospective randomized trial of FK506 versus cyclosporine after human pulmonary transplantation. *Transplantation* 57:848–851, 1994

60. Griffith BP, Hardesty RL, Trento A, et al: Targeted blood levels of cyclosporin for cardiac transplantation. *J Thorac Cardiovasc Surg* 88:952, 1984

61. Kobashigawa JA, Kirklin JK, Naftel DC, et al: Pretransplantation risk factors for acute rejection after heart transplantation: A multi-institutional study. The Transplant Cardiologists Research Data Base Group. *J Heart Lung Transplant* 12:355–366, 1993

62. Caves PK, Stinson EB, Graham AF, et al: Percutaneous transvenous endomyocardial biopsy. *JAMA* 225:288, 1973

63. Billingham ME, Cary NRB, Hammond ME, et al: A working formulation for the standardization of nomenclature in the diagnosis of heart and lung rejection: Heart rejection study group. *J Heart Lung Transplant* 9:587, 1990

64. Armitage JM, Fricker FJ, del Nido P, et al: The clinical trial of FK506 as primary and rescue immunosuppression in pediatric cardiac transplantation. *Transplant Proc* 23:3058–3060, 1991

65. Armitage JM, Kormos RL, Fung J, Starzl TE: The clinical trial of FK506 as primary and rescue immunosuppression in adult cardiac transplantation. *Transplant Proc* 23:3054–3057, 1991

66. Swinnen LJ, O'Sullivan EJ, Johnson MR, et al: OKT3 therapy is associated with an increased incidence of lymphoproliferative disorder following cardiac transplantation. *N Engl J Med* 323:1723–1728, 1990

67. Brumbaugh J, Baldwin J, Stinson EB, et al: Quantitative analysis of immunosuppression in cyclosporine treated heart transplant patients with lymphoma. *Heart Transplant* 4:307–311, 1985

68. Billingham ME: Graft coronary disease: The lesions and the patients. *Transplant Proc* 21:3665–3666, 1989

69. Uys CJ, Rose AG: Pathologic findings in long-term cardiac transplants. *Arch Pathol Med* 108:112–116, 1984

70. Hosenpud JD, Shipley GD, Wagner CR: Cardiac allograft vasculopathy: Current concepts, recent developments, and future directions. *J Heart Lung Transplant* 11:9–23, 1992

71. Hayry P, Paavonen T, Mennander A, et al: Pathophysiology of allograft arteriosclerosis. *Transplant Proc* 25:2070, 1992

72. Paul LC, Fellstrom B: Chronic vascular rejection of the heart and kidney—have rational treatment options emerged? *Transplant* 53:1169–1179, 1992

73. Fellstrom B, Dimeny E, Larsson E, et al: Rapidly proliferating arteriopathy in cyclosporine-induced permanently surviving rat cardiac allografts simulating chronic vascular rejection. *Clin Exper Immunol* 80:288–297, 1990

74. Fish RD, Nabel EG, Selwyn AP, et al: Responses of coronary arteries of cardiac transplant patients to acetylcholine. *J Clin Invest* 81:21–31, 1988

75. Hess ML, Hastillo A, Mohanakumar T, et al: Accelerated atherosclerosis in cardiac transplantation: Role of cytotoxic B-cell antibodies and hyperlipidemia. *Circulation* 68:(vol. 3, part 2)94–101, 1983

76. Uretsky BF, Murali S, Reddy S, et al: Development of coronary artery disease in cardiac transplant patients receiving immunosuppressive therapy with cyclosporine and prednisone. *Circulation* 76:827–834, 1987

77. McDonald K, Rector TS, Braunlin Ea, et al: Association of coronary artery disease in cardiac transplant recipients with cytomegalovirus infection. *Am J Cardiol* 64:359–362, 1989

78. Cramer DV, Chapman FA, Wu GD, et al: Cardiac transplantation in the rat: II Alterations of the severity of donor graft arteriosclerosis by modulation of the host immune response. *Transplant* 50:554–562, 1990

79. Cramer DV, Qian S, Harnaha J, et al: Cardiac transplantation in the rat 1. The effect of histocompatibility differences on graft arteriosclerosis. *Transplant* 47:414–419, 1989

80. Uretsky BF, Murali S, Lee A, et al: Development of coronary atherosclerosis in the transplanted heart immunosuppressed with cyclosporine and prednisone (abstr). *J Am Coll Cardiol* 7(supp A):9A, 1986

81. Costanzo-Nordin MR: Cardiac allograft vasculopathy: Relationship with acute cellular rejection and histocompatibility. *J Heart Lung Transplant* 11:S90–103, 1992

82. Zerbe T, Uretsky B, Kormos R, et al: Graft atherosclerosis: Effects of cellular rejection and human lymphocyte antigen. *J Heart Lung Transplant* 11:S104–110, 1992

83. Watanaabe M, Suzuki T, Taniguchi M, Shinohara N: Monoclonal anti-Ia murine alloantibodies crossreactive with the Ia-homologues of other mammalian species including humans. *Transplant* 36:712–718, 1983

84. Costanzo-Nordin MR: Cardiac allograft vasculopathy: Relationship with acute cellular rejection and histocompatibility. *J Heart Lung Transplant* 11:S90–S103, 1992

85. Gravanis MB: Allograft heart accelerated atherosclerosis: Evidence for cell-mediated immunity in pathogenesis. *Modern Pathol* 2:495–505, 1989

86. Hruban RH, Beschomer WE, Baumgartner WA, Augustine SM: Accelerated arteriosclerosis in heart transplant recipients is associated with a T-lymphocyte-mediated endothelialitis. *Am J Pathol* 137:871–882, 1990

87. Bieber CP, Stinson EB, Shumway CP, et al: Cardiac transplantation in man. VII. Cardiac allograft pathology. *Circulation* **XLI**:753–772, 1970

88. Palmer DC, Tsai CC, Roodman ST, et al: Heart graft arteriosclerosis. *Transplant* **39**:385–388, 1985

89. Paigen B, Morrow A, Brandon C, et al: Variations in susceptibility to atherosclerosis among inbred strains of mice. *Atherosclerosis* **57**:65–73, 1985

90. Potkin BN, Bartorelli AL, Gessert JM, et al: Coronary artery imaging with intravascular high-frequency ultrasound. *Circulation* **81**:1575–1585, 1990

91. St Goar FG, Pinto FJ, Alderman EL, et al: Intracoronary ultrasound in cardiac transplant recipients: In-vivo evidence of "angiographically silent" intimal thickening. *Circulation* **85**:979–987, 1992

92. Hosenpud JD: Immune mechanisms of cardiac allograft vasculopathy: An update. *Transplant Immunol* **1**:237–249, 1993

93. deLorgeril M, Boissonnat P, Dureau G, et al: Low dose aspirin and accelerated coronary disease in heart transplant recipients. *J Heart Transplant* **9**:449–450, 1990

94. Sarris GE, Mitchell RS, Billingham ME, et al: Inhibition of accelerated cardiac allograft arteriosclerosis by fish oil. *J Thorac Cardiovasc Surg* **97**:841–855, 1989

95. Schroeder JS, Gao SZ, Alderman EA, et al: A preliminary study of diltiazem in the prevention of coronary artery disease in heart transplant recipients. *N Engl J Med* **328**:164–170, 1993

96. Remington JS, Gaines JD, Griepp RB, et al: Further experience with infection after cardiac transplantation. *Transplant Proc* **3**:699, 1972

97. Pennock JL, Oyer PE, Reitz BA, et al: Cardiac transplantation in perspective for the future. *J Thorac Cardiovasc Surg* **83**:168, 1982

98. Hofflin JM, Potasman I, Baldwin JC, et al: Infectious complications in heart transplant recipients receiving cyclosporine and corticosteroids. *Ann Intern Med* **106**:209, 1987

99. Dummer JS: Infectious complications of transplantation. In Thompson ME, Brest AN (eds): *Cardiac Transplantation*. Philadelphia, F.A. Davis, 1990, pp 163–178

100. Keay S, Petersen E, Icenogle T, et al: Gancyclovir treatment of serious cytomegalovirus infection in heart and heart-lung transplant recipients. *Rev Infect Dis* **10**(III):S563–572, 1988

101. Balfour HH, Chace BA, Stapleton JT, et al: A randomized placebo controlled trial of oral acyclovir for the prevention of cytomegalovirus disease in recipients of renal allografts. *N Engl J Med* **320**:1381–1387, 1989

102. Starzl TE, Nalesnik MA, Porter KA, et al: Reversibility of lymphomas and lymphoproliferative lesions developing under cyclosporine-steroid therapy. *Lancet* **1**:583–587, 1984

103. Nalesnik MA, Makowka L, Starzl TE: The diagnosis and treatment of posttransplant lymphoproliferative disorders. *Curr Probl Surg* **25**(6):367–472, 1988

104. Dummer SJ: Pneumocystis carinii infections in transplant recipients. *Semin Respir Infect* **5**:550–557, 1990

105. Myers BD, Ross J, Newton L, et al: Cyclosporine-associated chronic nephropathy. *N Engl J Med* **311**:699–705, 1984

106. Myers BD, Sibley R, Newton N, et al: The long-term course of CsA associated chronic nephropathy. *Kidney Int* **33**:590–600, 1988

107. Greenberg A, Egel JW, Thompson ME, et al: Early and late forms of cyclosporine nephrotoxicity: Studies in cardiac transplant recipients. *Am J Kidney Dis* **9**:12–22, 1987

108. Kahan BD: Cyclosporine. *N Engl J Med* **321**:1725–1738, 1989

109. Myers BD: Cyclosporine nephrotoxicity. *N Engl J Med* **30**:964–974, 1985

110. Mihatsch MJ, Thiel G, Ryffel B: Cyclosporine nephrotoxicity. *Adv Nephrol* **17**:303–320, 1988

111. Hamilton DV, Evans DB, Thiru S: Toxicity of cyclosporine A in organ grafting. In White DJB (ed): *Cyclosporine A. Proceedings of an International Conference on Cyclosporine A.* New York, Elsevier, 1982

112. Greenberg A: Renal failure in cardiac transplantation. In Thompson ME, Brest AN (eds): *Cardiac Transplantation.* Philadelphia, F.A. Davis, 1990, pp 189–198

113. Moran M, Mozes MF, Maddux MS, et al: Prevention of acute graft rejection by the prostaglandin E1 analogue misprostol in renal transplant recipients treated with cyclosporine and prednisone. *N Engl J Med* **322**:1183–1188, 1990

114. Wysocki GP, Gretzinger HA, Laupacis A, et al: Fibrous hyperplasia of the gingiva: A side effect of cyclosporine A therapy. *Oral Surg Oral Med Oral Pathol* **55**:274, 1983

115. Lin H-Y, Rocher LL, Mcquillan MA, et al: Cyclosporine-induced hyperuricemia and gout. *N Engl J Med* **321**:287–292, 1989

116. Becher DM, Chamberlain B, Swank R, et al: Relationship between corticosteroid exposure and plasma lipid levels in heart transplant recipients. *Am J Med* **85**:632–638, 1988

117. Ziady G, Ruffner R, Lee A, et al: Accelerated hyperlipidemia after heart transplant. Presented at the Pan American Congress of Diseases of the Chest, Puerto Rico, April 1990

118. Ladowski JS, Kormos RL, Uretsky BF, et al: Post-transplant diabetes in heart transplant recipients. *Heart Transplant* **8**(2):181–184, 1989

119. Steed DL, Brown B, Reilly JJ, et al: General surgical complications in heart and heart-lung transplantation. *Surgery* **28**:739, 1985

120. Parascandala SA, Wiseman CB, Burg JE, et al: Extracardiac surgical complications in heart transplant recipients. *Heart Transplant* **8**:400, 1989

121. Johnson R, Peitzman AB, Webster MW, et al: Upper gastrointestinal endoscopy after cardiac transplantation. *Surgery* **103**:300, 1988

122. Sarris GE, Moore KA, Schroeder JS, et al: Cardiac transplantation: The Stanford experience in the cyclosporine era. *J Thorac Cardiovasc Surg* **108**:240–252, 1994

123. Kormos RL, Armitage JM, Hardesty RL, et al: Cardiac transplantation at the University of Pittsburgh: 1980–1991. In Terasaki PI (ed): *Clinical Transplants,* Vol 9. Los Angeles, CA, UCLA Tissue Typing Laboratory, 1991, pp 87–95

124. Hosenpud JD, Novick RJ, Breen TJ, Daily OP: The Registry of the International Society for Heart and Lung Transplantation: Eleventh Official Report—1994. *J Heart Lung Transplant* **13**:561–570, 1994

C H A P T E R

114

Heart and Lung Transplantation

Jolene M. Kriett and Stuart W. Jamieson

The technique of combined heart–lung transplantation developed as a result of the growing experience and success of heart transplantation during the 1970s. Patients with pulmonary hypertension, including those with Eisenmenger's syndrome, of course, could not be helped by heart transplantation alone, and single lung transplantation, at that time, was associated with a high operative mortality.

Three heart–lung transplant procedures had been performed during the 1960s and 1970s by Cooley et al,[1] Lillehei,[2] and Barnard[3]; however, all three recipients died during the perioperative period, at 14 hours, 8 days, and 23 days, respectively. Experimental studies in primates with cyclosporine-based immunosuppression at Stanford University led to the first successful combined heart–lung transplant procedures in patients with pulmonary hypertension.[4–6] The early encouraging results with combined heart–lung transplantation with cyclosporine-based immunosuppression then led to a reintroduction of single lung transplantation in 1983[7] and the subsequent development of the double lung transplant technique in 1985.[8]

The application of clinical heart–lung transplantation gradually increased from five cases performed in 1981 at Stanford University, and the world experience through 1993 included over 1500 combined heart–lung transplant procedures from over 90 centers.[9] However, although the annual number of single and double lung transplantations continue to increase dramatically, the number of combined heart–lung transplant procedures has declined since 1989, as seen in Figure 114–1.

This shift away from heart–lung transplantation has been due to the expanded indications for and the success of single lung and double lung (using bilateral sequential single lung technique) transplantation as well as the limited availability of donor heart–lung blocks. In 1993 in the United States only 60 heart–lung transplant procedures were performed as compared to 665 single or double lung procedures.[10] Currently, heart–lung transplantation is primarily reserved for those patients with end-stage pulmonary vascular or parenchymal disease in conjunction with either significant irreversible cardiac dysfunction or complex cardiac defects not amenable to simultaneous surgical repair.

The selection of candidates for heart–lung transplantation, the donor and recipient surgical techniques, the management of recipients, and the current results are discussed below.

CANDIDATE SELECTION

The variety of cardiopulmonary diseases for which combined heart–lung transplantation has been used are shown in Table 114–1. However, recent experience has clearly demonstrated that single or double lung transplantation, rather than heart–lung transplantation, may be appropriate for the majority of these indications.

A thorough medical evaluation of each patient referred for consideration of lung transplantation is mandatory. Only those patients with severely restricted exercise tolerance and limited life expectancy in whom all other conventional medical or surgical therapies are either not effective or not applicable are appropriate candidates.

Factors that may compromise the patient's successful rehabilitation and survival after transplantation, e.g., active infection, malignancy, severe peripheral vascular or cerebrovascular disease, irreversible renal or hepatic disease, neurological impairment, major psychiatric disorder, or substance abuse history, must be carefully evaluated.

Many factors including patient age, previous thoracic surgical procedures, cardiac function and anatomy, and type of pulmonary disease influence the selection of a specific lung transplant procedure for each individual candidate. Our current approach to the selection of patients' for com-

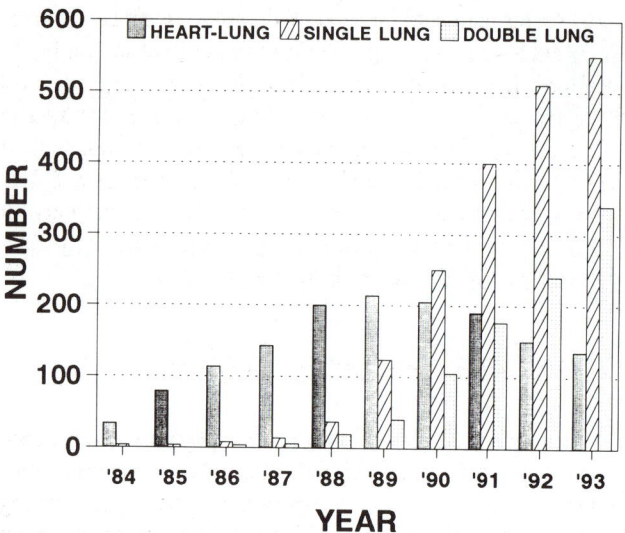

Figure 114–1. Number of lung transplant procedures by year 1984–1993. *(From the International Society for Heart and Lung Transplantation.)*

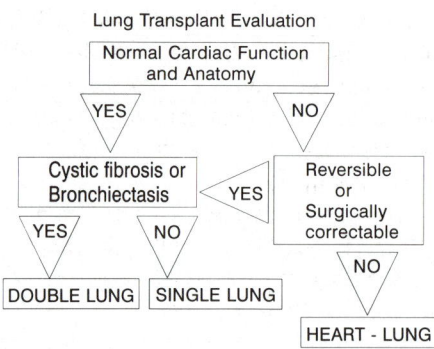

Figure 114–2. Selection of type of lung transplant procedure.

bined heart–lung, double lung, or single lung transplantation is shown in Figure 114–2.

In candidates with normal cardiac function, right ventricular dysfunction due to pulmonary hypertension, and congenital or acquired heart disease amenable to surgical correction, lung transplantation without the heart is preferable. The advantages of this approach include the avoidance of potential problems related to a cardiac allograft (such as accelerated atherosclerosis and cardiac denervation), the likelihood of a shorter waiting period prior to lung transplantation, and the most efficient use of the limited supply of donor lungs for the largest number of recipients.

The selection of single or double lung transplantation is then based on the type of pulmonary disease. While replacement of both lungs is required in patients with bilateral septic conditions such as cystic fibrosis and bronchiectasis, single lung transplantation has become the chosen procedure for all other patients. Right heart dysfunction rapidly reverses with normalization of pulmonary pressures, and single lung transplantation rather than heart–lung transplantation has been used in an increasing number of patients with primary and secondary pulmonary hypertension.[11–17] In patients with Eisenmenger's syndrome simultaneous repair of the congenital heart defect(s) in conjunction with single lung transplantation obviates the need for combined heart–lung replacement.[11–14,17]

There remains a small group of transplant candidates in whom heart–lung transplantation is the only possible option. This includes those patients with pulmonary vascular or parenchymal disease in conjunction with significant left ventricular dysfunction due to either congenital or acquired heart disease, and those patients with complex congenital heart defects that are not amenable to surgical correction.[17,18]

TABLE 114–1. PRIMARY DIAGNOSIS OF HEART–LUNG RECIPIENTS

Primary pulmonary hypertension
Eisenmenger's syndrome
Emphysema (includes α_1-antitrypsin deficiency)
Cystic fibrosis
Bronchiectasis
Idiopathic pulmonary fibrosis
Sarcoidosis
Connective tissue disease
Graft-versus-host disease
Bronchiolitis obliterans
Pulmonary hemosiderosis
Lymphangioleiomyomatosis
Acute respiratory distress syndrome
Bronchopulmonary dysplasia
Histiocytosis X
Pulmonary artery leiomyosarcoma

SELECTION CRITERIA AND MANAGEMENT OF HEART–LUNG DONORS

The possibility of heart and/or lung donation should be considered in all brain-dead individuals with well-maintained cardiopulmonary function. The early Stanford experience indicated that in less than 20% of heart donors were the lungs suitable for donation.[19] In 1993 in the United States the organ recovery rates in 4845 cadaveric donors were 95% for kidney, 77% for liver, 50% for heart, and only 16% for lung.[10]

The limited availability of suitable donor lungs has been related to the early onset of pneumonic changes and neurogenic pulmonary edema in ventilated brain-dead individuals, chest trauma, tracheobronchial aspiration, and advanced age. However, with careful donor management and selection the number of donor lungs can be significantly increased. In our experience the lung recovery rate has exceeded 30% for the past 2 years.

In donors with either unilateral abnormalities on chest radiography or unilateral chest trauma, the heart and contralateral lung may be suitable for donation. In donors who would meet criteria for bilateral lung donation the large number of heart transplant candidates further limits the number of heart–lung blocks.

Our criteria for acceptable heart–lung donors are shown in Table 114–2. For donors over the age of 40 years a coronary arteriogram is usually performed prior to procurement. Careful fluid management of potential lung donors is essential to prevent the development of pulmonary edema. Gentle tracheobronchial suctioning using sterile technique should be performed regularly, and specimens should be submitted for Gram stain, culture, and sensitivity. Prophylactic antibiotics (such as a second generation cephalosporine) to cover respiratory flora are used. Inotropic infusions may be added as needed to maintain hemodynamic stability and vasopressin may be required for the treatment of diabetes insipidus.

Matching of the donor and recipient for heart–lung or lung transplantation is primarily based on compatible blood type and size. Prospective cross-matching of donor lymphocytes against recipient serum is required only for those recipients who have tested positive against a random panel of lymphocytes.

In the past most lung transplant centers avoided cytomegaloviral CMV(+) donor to CMV(−) recipient mismatch because of the increased risk of a serious and potentially fatal CMV infection.[20–22] However, the availability of an effective and well-tolerated antiviral agent, gancyclovir, has significantly lessened the risks associated with CMV mismatch in lung recipients. With the addition of gancyclovir treatment during the early post-transplantation period CMV(+) donors may now be safely used for CMV(−) recipients.[22]

Size matching for heart–lung transplantation may be based on comparable donor and recipient height, chest radiograph measurements, or predicted total lung capacity. In recent years size matching criteria have been substantially liberalized. It is clear that small donor lungs will expand to fill the pleural space in a larger recipient, as demonstrated in Figure 114–3. We have noted no problems with residual air space, prolonged drainage of pleural effusion, or a difference in cardiac or pulmonary function in such patients. In contrast, however, difficulties may be encountered by placing larger lungs into smaller recipients.

HEART AND LUNG PROCUREMENT

In the early days of heart–lung transplantation, the donor was transported to the recipient hospital to allow organ procurement in an adjoining operating room thus limiting donor organ ischemic time. However, distant procurement is now the rule. Although several methods of lung preservation, including donor core cooling with cardiopulmonary bypass, have been used clinically, flush perfusion of the lungs with subsequent immersion of the partially inflated lungs into cold solution has proven simple and effective.[23–28]

We have been extremely satisfied with a simple flush lung perfusion using modified Euro-Collin's solution[29] for ischemic times extending to 8 hours. Other lung transplant centers have reported the use of a variety of perfusate solutions as well as addition of prostaglandin E_1[25] or prostacyclin.[26] Experimental work in our laboratory failed to demonstrate the beneficial effect of PGE_1 in "pulmonoplegia."[30] An increase in extravascular water has also been reported with prostacyclin.[27]

The operative technique for procurement of the heart–lung block may also be used if the heart and lungs are to be shared among two or three recipients. A median sternotomy incision is used. The pericardium is excised anteriorly and both pleural spaces opened. The trachea is mobilized between the aorta and superior vena cava, keeping dissection of the peritracheal tissue in the supracarinal region to a minimum. After all donor teams (heart–lung, liver, kidney, and pancreas) have completed their initial dissection the donor is systemically heparinized with 3–4 mg/kg heparin intravenously.

The superior vena cava and azygos vein are ligated and divided, carefully avoiding injury to the sinoatrial node at the superior vena caval–right atrial junction. The inferior vena cava is clamped. The ascending aorta is clamped and cardioplegic solution is infused into the aortic root. For lung preservation, cold flush solution (e.g., modified Euro-Collins 60 mL/kg) is infused via the main pulmonary artery. The tip of the left atrial appendage is amputated to prevent left heart distension. Even washout of the lungs can be seen as the color of the lungs changes to a homogeneous pale pink. During administration of the pulmonary flush solution, ventilation is continued using unwarmed room air. Topical cold saline solution is used for additional cooling.

TABLE 114–2. HEART–LUNG DONOR CRITERIA

Brain death declared; organ donation permit signed

Age < 60 years

Serology negative for hepatitis B and C, and HIV

History negative for significant cardiac or pulmonary disease, significant chest trauma, systemic or pulmonary infections

Hemodynamic stability: dopamine < 10 µg/kg per minute

Electrocardiogram negative for ischemia, infarction, arrhythmias, or conduction abnormalities

Echocardiogram negative for significant segmental or global wall motion abnormality or valve dysfunction

Chest radiograph negative for significant pulmonary vascular congestion, infiltrate or contusion

Normal gas exchange: PaO_2 > 100 mm Hg on 40% oxygen and PEEP of 5 cm H_2O; peak inspiratory pressure < 30 cm H_2O

Tracheal secretions: negative for large numbers of bacteria, fungi, or white cells

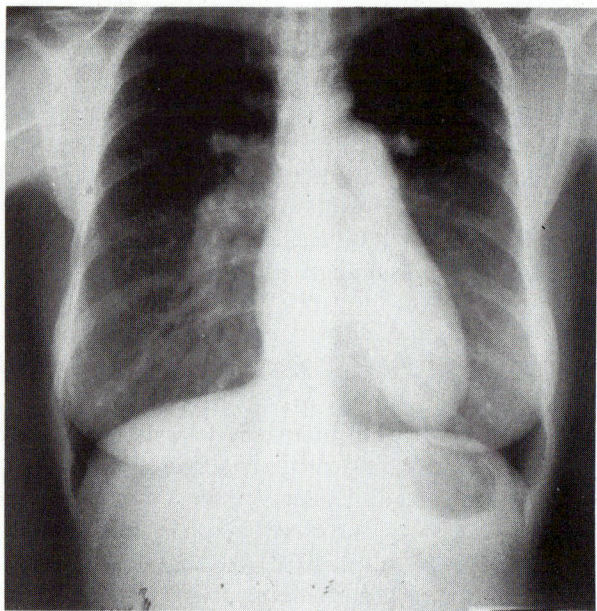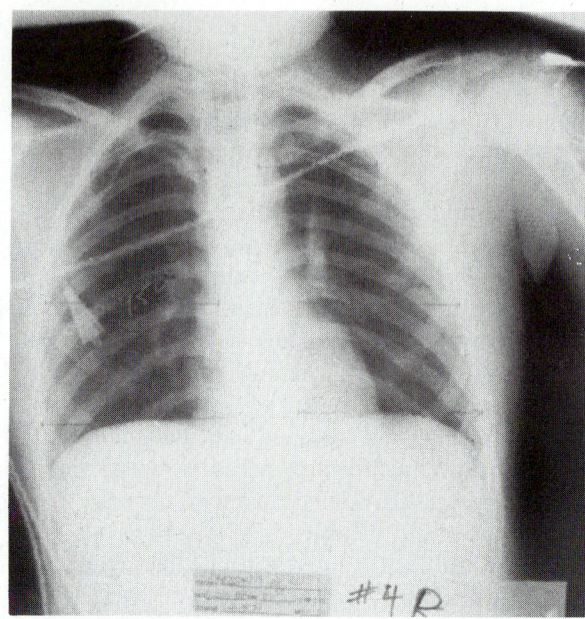

Figure 114–3. Preoperative recipient and donor chest radiographs for a heart–lung recipient with primary pulmonary hypertension (postoperative chest radiographs shown in Fig. 114–11).

The inferior vena cava is divided near the right atrial junction and the aorta is transected at the level of the innominate artery (if additional length is required the transverse arch and great vessels may be included). Following completion of lung flush perfusion the trachea is clamped or stapled approximately 5 cm above the carina and divided. The dissection in the posterior mediastinum is commenced from above downward, separating the posterior wall of the trachea from the esophagus. The combined heart–lung block is placed in cold solution in a storage container and packed in ice for transport to the recipient operating room.

RECIPIENT OPERATION FOR HEART–LUNG TRANSPLANTATION

The standard operative technique for heart–lung transplantation has remained essentially unchanged since the first cases at Stanford.[29] A modification was required for the "domino procedure," a technique that permitted use of the explanted heart from a heart–lung recipient as a donor heart for heart transplantation.[31,32] Separate caval anastomoses were required in order to preserve the sinus node of the explanted heart. Due to the success of double lung transplantation, domino transplantation is no longer used.

A median sternotomy has been the standard surgical approach for heart–lung transplantation. In patients who have had a prior thoracotomy we have found that a bilateral thoracosternotomy "clamshell" incision, as currently used for double lung transplantation, allows for better visualiza-

tion of posterior and apical pleural adhesions and mediastinal collaterals.

The major technical challenges of the heart–lung transplant procedure are removing the native heart and both lungs while preserving the vagus, phrenic, and recurrent laryngeal nerves and maintaining strict hemostasis. In recipients with diffuse vascularized pleural adhesions, large bronchial and mediastinal collaterals, or adhesions from prior thoracic surgical procedures careful dissection to assure adequate hemostasis is essential.

The pericardium is opened anteriorly and standard ascending aortic and bicaval cannulation for cardiopulmonary bypass is performed. The left and right pleural spaces are opened anteriorly. After institution of cardiopulmonary bypass with moderate hypothermia (28°C) the heart is excised as in orthotopic heart transplantation (Fig. 114–4). A pericardial incision is made posterior to the phrenic nerve and anterior to the hilum on each side, extending superiorly above the pulmonary artery and inferiorly to the diaphragm (Fig. 114–5).

The remaining posterior left atrium is divided vertically in the oblique sinus, allowing separation of the right and left pulmonary veins (Fig. 114–6). The left and right lungs are then removed separately. The pulmonary ligament is divided and the dissection of the hilar vessels is completed. A small cuff of pulmonary artery in the region of the ligamentum arteriosum is retained to prevent injury to the left recurrent laryngeal nerve.

With the lung retracted anteriorly the posterior pleura is divided taking care to preserve the vagus nerve and obtain hemostasis of mediastinal collaterals and bronchial ar-

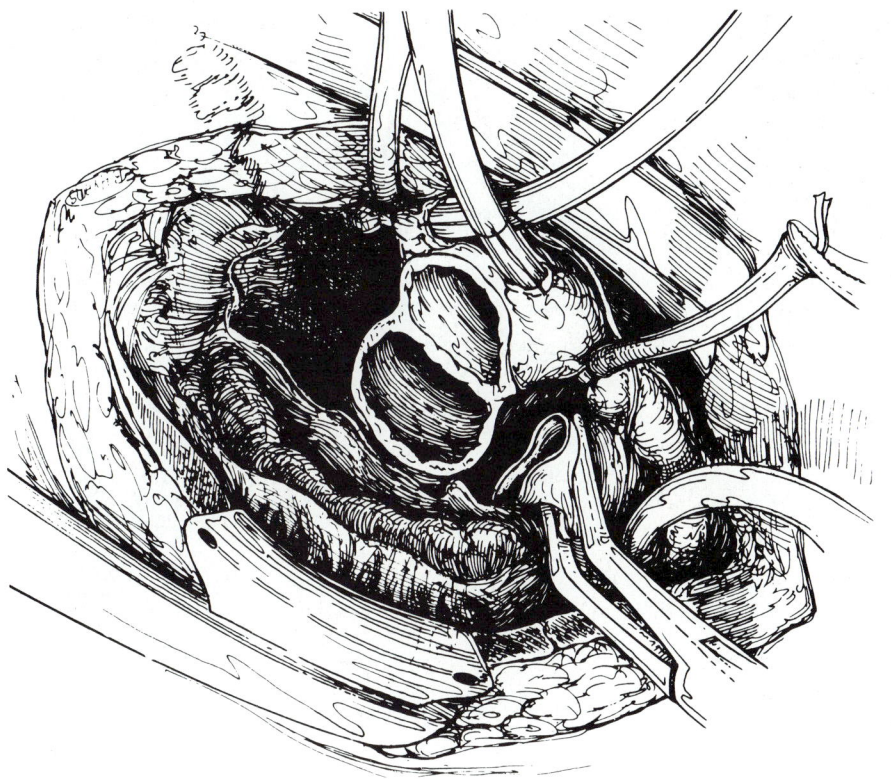

Figure 114–4. Excision of heart leaving right and left atria, ascending aorta, and pulmonary artery.

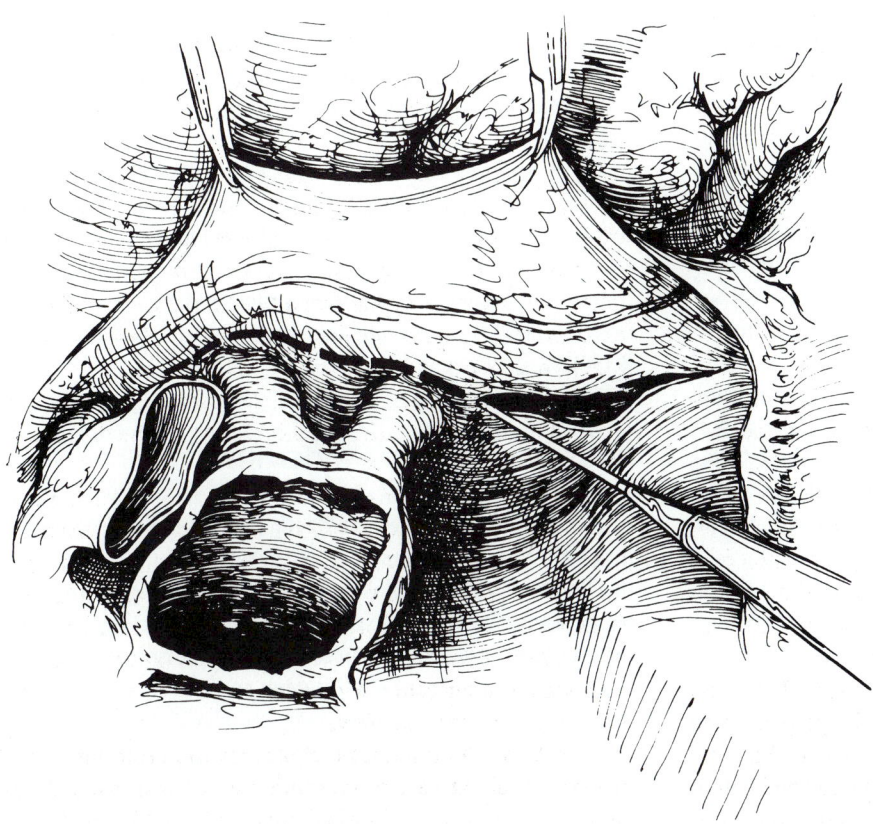

Figure 114–5. Pericardial pedicle created to preserve phrenic nerve.

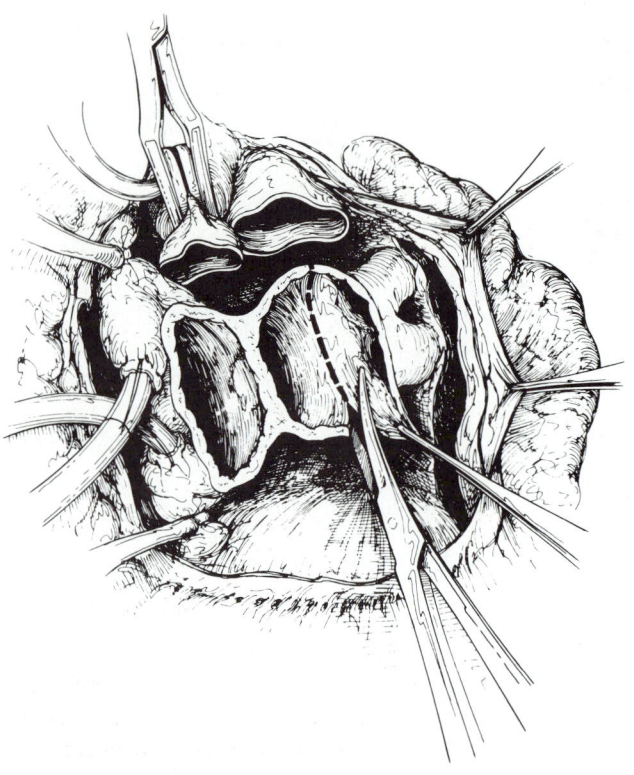

Figure 114–6. Division of left atrial remnant.

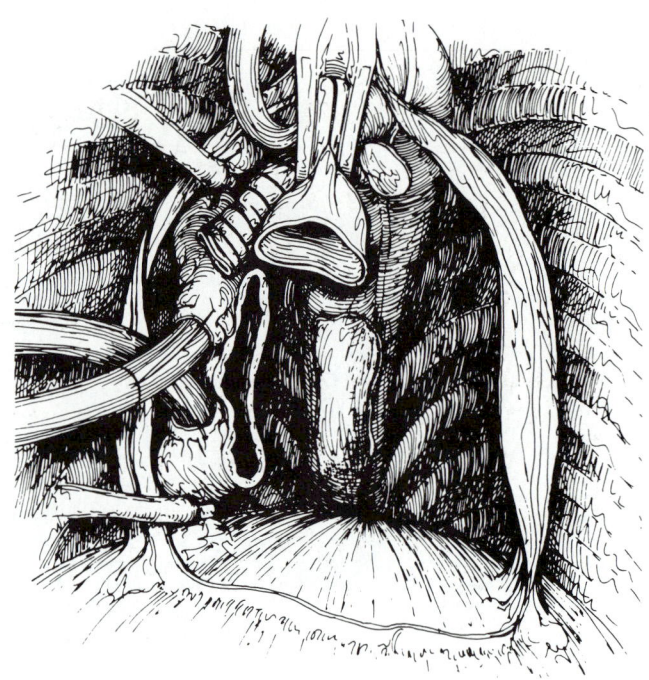

Figure 114–7. Completed explantation of heart and lungs.

teries. The bronchus is stapled and divided and the lung removed. Finally, the remaining right and left bronchial stumps are dissected free to the level of the carina.

Completion of the dissection leaves the distal trachea, ascending aorta, and right atrium as sites for subsequent anastomoses (Fig. 114–7). A patent foramen ovale must be closed since this portion of the atrial septum will form the posterior right atrial wall. During and following explantation of the heart and lungs, particular attention must be paid to meticulous hemostasis in the posterior mediastinum and at any sites of pleural adhesions. Bronchial arteries and mediastinal collaterals must be individually secured with hemoclips to prevent troublesome postoperative bleeding in relatively inaccessible areas.

The donor heart–lung block is then removed from cold storage. After specimens for culture are obtained, the donor trachea is divided one cartilaginous ring above the carina. The lungs are then placed into their respective pleural cavities posterior to the pericardial pedicles, passing the right lung behind the right atrium (Fig. 114–8).

The tracheal anastomosis is then carried out using running 3-0 polypropylene suture (Fig. 114–9). Any size disparity in donor/recipient tracheal diameter is compensated for in the membranous portion of the anastomosis. The atrial anastomosis is performed next. An incision in the donor right atrium is extended from the inferior vena cava toward the atrial appendage to accommodate the recipient right atrial cuff (Fig. 114–10).

Finally, the donor aorta is trimmed to a suitable length and anastomosed to the recipient aorta. Air is removed from the heart, the aortic cross-clamp is removed, and ventilation recommenced. The tip of the left atrial appendage, which had been incised during flushing of the donor lungs, is ligated. After completion of rewarming and return of adequate cardiac activity, cardiopulmonary bypass is discontinued.

An isoproterenol infusion may be used to maintain the heart rate at 100 to 120 beats per minute. The inspired oxygen concentration is gradually decreased to 0.40 as permitted by arterial saturations higher than 90%. Temporary ventricular pacing wires and bilateral pleural drainage tubes are inserted, satisfactory hemostasis is achieved, and the chest is closed.

POSTOPERATIVE MANAGEMENT

The early postoperative care of the heart–lung recipient differs little from that of any cardiac surgical patient except for the addition of immunosuppressive medications. Key aspects of the postoperative management of heart–lung recipients include aggressive diuresis, intensive respiratory physiotherapy, and diligent surveillance for infection and acute rejection. With careful fluid restriction and diuresis in the perioperative period lung function is usually excellent and extubation is generally possible within the first 24–28 hours.

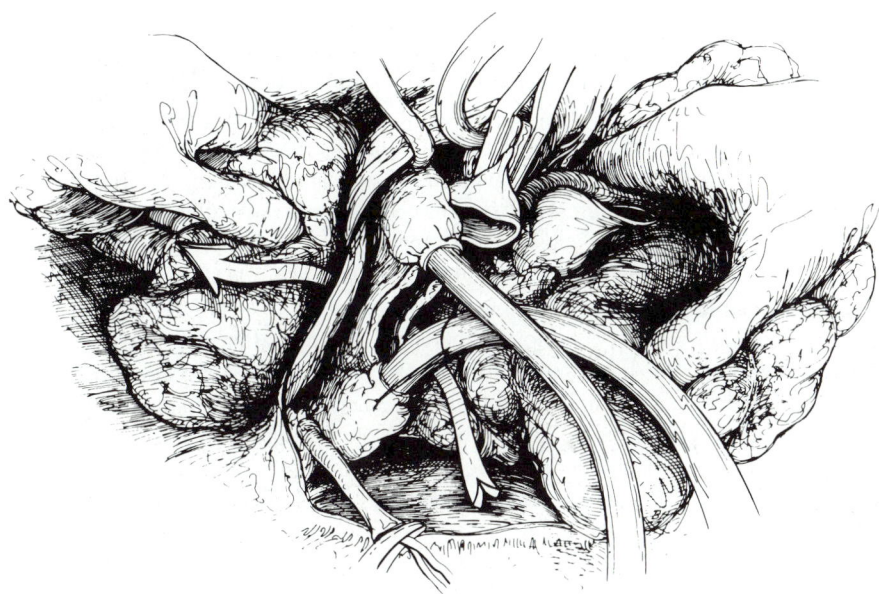

Figure 114–8. Placement of donor heart–lung block into chest.

In heart–lung recipients with evidence of preoperative renal impairment, cardiopulmonary bypass, fluid restriction, and cyclosporine nephrotoxicity may result in further renal dysfunction during the postoperative period. An infusion of low-dose dopamine (3 µg/kg per minute) may be helpful in ameliorating the nephrotoxic effects of cyclosporine.[33] Since fluid balance is critical continuous ultrafiltration may be useful in selected cases.

Emphasis is placed on early mobilization. Chest tubes are removed when chest drainage diminishes to less than 200 mL/day. Some patients may develop late pleural effusions that require drainage by thoracentesis. The potential risk for the development of bilateral pneumothoraces in heart–lung recipients has been reported[34] but these are rarely clinically significant.

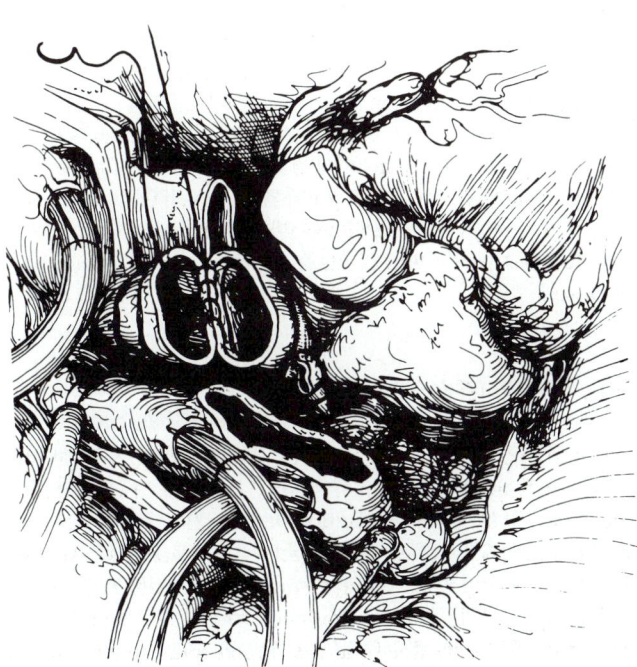

Figure 114–9. Tracheal anastomosis for heart–lung transplantation.

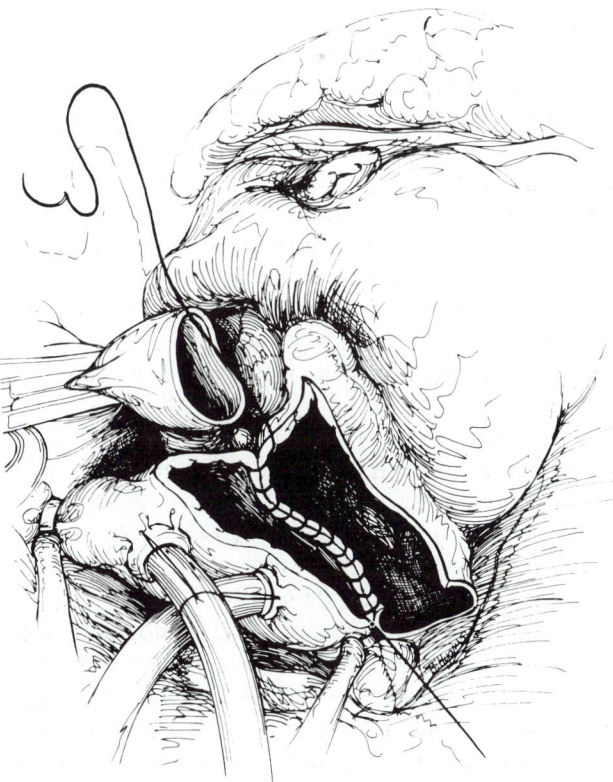

Figure 114–10. Right atrial anastomosis for heart–lung transplantation.

Most patients will be ready for hospital discharge within 2 to 3 weeks. With close follow-up in the outpatient clinic and participation in a pulmonary rehabilitation program, the majority of heart–lung recipients can expect to return to normal activity within 2 to 3 months.

IMMUNOSUPPRESSION

The immunosuppressive agents that are currently available and have been used in heart–lung and lung transplantation are shown in Table 114–3. Cyclosporine-based immunosuppression with induction cytolytic therapy (e.g., ATG, OKT3) was the most common regimen in lung transplantation during the past decade.[35–38] In our experience, a triple drug regimen (cyclosporine, azathioprine, and prednisone) without induction cytolytic therapy has shown a significant decrease in infection-related morbidity and mortality without any difference in the incidence of acute or chronic rejection.[39] This strategy also results in less cost and simplified patient care.

The majority of lung transplant programs have now discontinued the use of induction cytolytic therapy, reserving the antilymphocyte antibody preparations for the treatment of steroid-refractory acute rejection. Although there has been no experience to date in heart–lung recipients, a randomized trial of FK506 rather than cyclosporine in single and double lung recipients has been recently reported by the University of Pittsburgh group.[40]

COMPLICATIONS

Reimplantation Response

During the early experience in lung and heart–lung transplantation the development of progressive alveolar edema with deterioration in arterial saturation and decreased lung compliance within the immediate postoperative period was a common occurrence.[41–43] This entity (the "reimplantation response"), with characteristic radiographic and functional changes, has been attributed to interruption of lymphatic drainage, preservation injury, fluid overload, and neutrophil-mediated vascular injury with capillary leak.

The radiographic and functional changes associated with the reimplantation response follow a characteristic time course with initial appearance within the first 2 days, progression to a peak level 3 to 5 days after transplantation, and subsequent improvement both radiographically and clinically over several weeks. The rate of resolution can be highly variable.

Although aggressive diuresis after lung transplantation has significantly lessened the clinical significance of the reimplantation response, almost all recipients will show some evidence of the response during the early postoperative period, at least radiographically. If deterioration in lung function or new infiltrates develops more than 4 days after transplantation, another etiology, such as infection or acute rejection, must be considered. An example of the radiographic appearance of this entity is shown in Figure 114–11.

Tracheal Complications

Airway anastomotic complications were a significant factor in the initial failure of clinical lung transplantation. The lower incidence of tracheal anastomotic dehiscence following combined heart–lung transplantation was attributed to improved tissue healing with cyclosporine-based immunosuppression and the delayed initiation of steroid treatment. In addition, a collateral blood supply from the coronary circulation to the carina and distal trachea has been demonstrated angiographically.[44] Division of this collateral supply probably explains the significantly higher incidence of tracheal dehiscence following "en block" double lung transplantation as compared to the experience in heart–lung transplantation.[45,46]

In our experience, if disruption of the peritracheal tissues in both the donor heart–lung block and the recipient is minimized and the donor trachea is divided immediately above the carina, problems associated with healing of the tracheal anastomosis have not occurred.

Infection

The predominant cause of morbidity and mortality in heart–lung and lung transplant recipients has been infectious complications.[47–53] Although the types of infection have been similar to the experience in heart recipients, the incidence of serious infection, primarily viral and fungal infections, has been greater in lung recipients. The higher risk of infection and the predominance of pulmonary infection in lung recipients may be related to lung denervation, lymphatic obstruction, preservation injury, impairment of mucociliary function, and reduced local immunoglobulin production.

An increased incidence of infection has been associ-

TABLE 114–3. IMMUNOSUPPRESSIVE MEDICATIONS AND DOSAGES

	Range (mg/kg per day)	Adjustment
Prednisone	0.2–1	Tapered schedule
Cyclosporine	1–20	Based on CSA level
Azathioprine	0.5–2	Based on WBC count
FK506	0.15	Based on FK506 level
Antilymphocyte antibody preparations		
ATG	5–20	5–14 day course
OKT3	5–10	10–14 day course

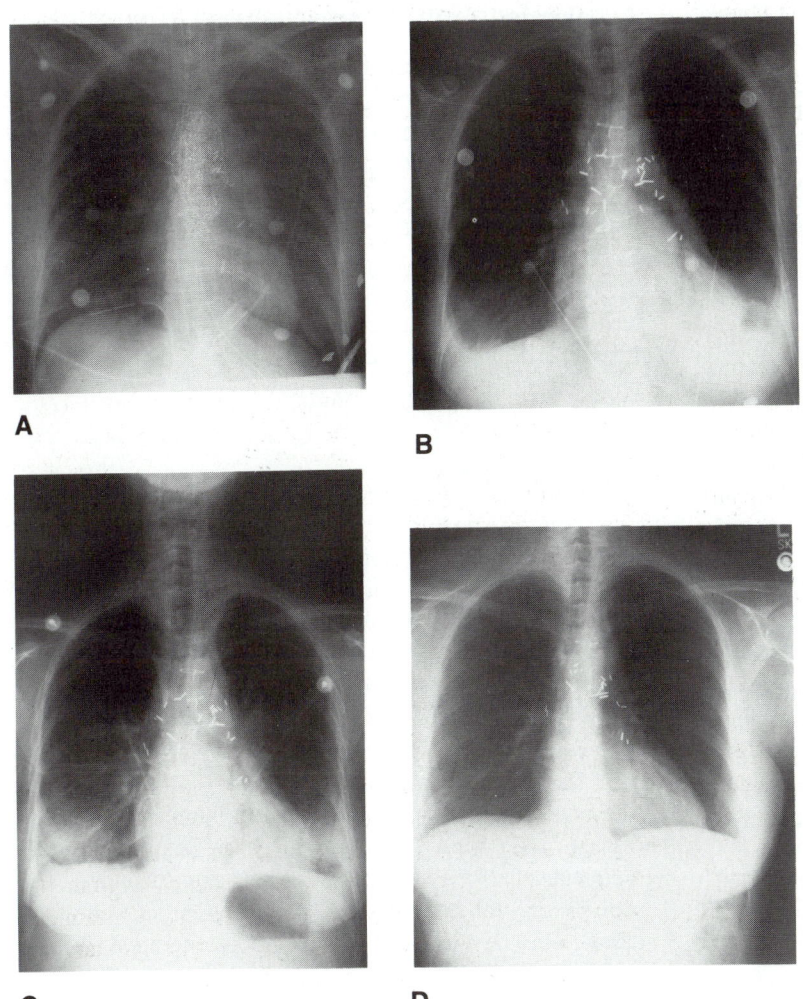

A

B

C

D

Figure 114–11. Reimplantation response and resolution of radiographic changes in a heart–lung recipient. **A.** Day 1. **B.** Day 5. **C.** Day 14. **D.** Three-month follow-up.

ated with the presence of large amounts of bacteria or fungi in the tracheobronchial secretions of the donor, CMV mismatch in CMV(−) recipients, the use of antilymphocyte antibody preparations, and augmented immunosuppression for the treatment of acute rejection episodes.[21,22,49,54,55] Mediastinitis and disruption of the aortic anastomosis related to donor-transmitted fungal infection have been reported.[55]

The use of triple drug immunosuppression, avoidance of induction cytolytic therapy, and CMV prophylaxis has significantly decreased the morbidity and mortality associated with infections after lung transplantation. The efficacy of trimethoprim–sulfamethoxazole prophylaxis for prevention of *Pneumocystis carinii* infection in lung recipients has also been demonstrated.[56]

Acute Rejection

The majority of heart–lung and lung recipients will experience one or more episodes of acute lung rejection with the highest incidence of rejection during the first 3 months after transplantation.[39,58,59] Fever, elevated white blood cell count with eosinophilia, acute deterioration in pulmonary

flow rates, oxygen desaturation, and progressive alveolar infiltrates with relative sparing of the upper lung fields are common signs of acute lung rejection.

A clinical diagnosis of acute lung rejection is often based on the exclusion of other etiologies, including infection, pulmonary edema, and the reimplantation response.[58] A decrease in pulmonary flow rates on home spirometry is a common early indication of acute lung rejection. Surveillance transbronchial biopsy[57,59–63] and bronchoalveolar lavage[64,65] for the early diagnosis of acute lung rejection has been advocated by some lung transplant centers.

The yield of positive biopsies in asymptomatic patients has been quite low. The selective use of bronchoscopic studies in heart–lung recipients with an acute deterioration in clinical status or spirometry may be useful in differentiating acute rejection from infection.[58,66] Rapid clearing of pulmonary infiltrates and associated clinical improvement is the rule following treatment of rejection with intravenous methylprednisolone.

The incidence of acute cardiac rejection in heart–lung recipients is much lower than in heart recipients.[53,67,68] In addition, because acute lung rejection is often asynchronous with cardiac rejection, surveillance endomyocardial biopsy has not proved useful in heart–lung recipients.[68–71] Signs of acute cardiac rejection include fever, elevation in white blood cell count, pericardial effusion, and atrial arrhythmias; however, many patients remain asymptomatic.

Obliterative Bronchiolitis

This entity remains the most serious impediment to successful long-term outcome following heart–lung and lung transplantation.[51–53,68,72–78] The etiology of obliterative bronchiolitis remains unclear, but is most likely related to chronic rejection.[73–76] Histologically, the acute phase of obliterative bronchiolitis is characterized by varying degrees of bronchiolar obstruction by plugs of granulation tissue (Masson bodies). In the chronic phase, although there may be only minimal inflammation, the bronchioles become partially or completely occluded by fibrosis.[72,76,79]

A diagnosis of obliterative bronchiolitis has been primarily based on progressive deterioration in pulmonary function studies rather than biopsy results.[76,80,81] A low sensitivity of transbronchial biopsy has been reported[81]; however, evidence of fibrosis or persistent peribronchial and perivascular infiltrates on biopsy may predict subsequent development of obliterative bronchiolitis.[62,63]

The chest radiographic picture of obliterative bronchiolitis progresses from lower-zone nodularity with peribronchial thickening to diffuse pulmonary infiltrates. High resolution chest computerized tomography may be useful in detecting early evidence of obliterative bronchiolitis.

On long-term follow-up of heart–lung transplant recipients up to 50% of patients develop obliterative bronchiolitis.[68,75] Factors associated with an increased risk for obliterative bronchiolitis have included CMV infection and more than three episodes of early acute lung rejection.[62,82] A higher incidence of obliterative bronchiolitis has also been reported in children.[78] A lower incidence of obliterative bronchiolitis has been reported with the use of triple drug immunosuppression and with early diagnosis and treatment of acute rejection episodes.[36,82]

Although early reports indicated that augmented immunosuppression may transiently slow progression of obliterative bronchiolitis,[83,84] no therapy has been effective in reversing the process or preventing continued deterioration in function. The rate of progression may be variable; however, an unrelenting downhill course toward retransplantation or death appears inevitable.

To date, the collective experience with heart–lung retransplantation has not been encouraging, with significant operative mortality (over 40%) and poor long-term survival (less than 40% at 1 year).[51,85] Although single lung retransplantation rather than heart–lung replacement may be utilized in most cases, a substantial improvement in the results with retransplantation has not been evident.[86]

Accelerated Graft Atherosclerosis

As is the case with heart transplant recipients, the development of accelerated graft atherosclerosis, characterized by diffuse concentric narrowing of both large and small coronary arteries, may occur in heart–lung recipients. This entity is probably related to chronic rejection with antibody-mediated injury of the coronary vascular endothelium. However, paralleling the lower risk for acute rejection of the heart, the incidence of accelerated graft atherosclerosis has also been much lower in heart–lung recipients.[53,68,75] Less than 5% of late deaths in heart–lung recipients have been related to graft coronary artery disease.

Other Complications

The common side effects of the current immunosuppressive agents include hypertension, renal dysfunction, diabetes, and osteoporosis. The majority of patients maintained on steroids and cyclosporine will require treatment for systemic hypertension. The chronic effects of cyclosporine on renal function have not been progressive or clinically significant. The degree of renal dysfunction in patients receiving FK506 appears similar to that with cyclosporine.

As is the experience with other types of solid organ transplantation, an increased risk of lymphoproliferative disease has been reported in heart–lung and lung recipients.[75,77,87] Evidence of primary or secondary Epstein–Barr viral infection has been present in almost all cases. The development of lymphoproliferative disease within the first year after lung transplantation rather than later has been associated with lower mortality due to the lymphoma (36 versus 70%), a greater probability of response to a reduction in immunosuppression (89 versus 0%), and a lower incidence of disseminated disease (23 versus 86%).[87]

CURRENT RESULTS

Operative Mortality

Based on data from the Registry of the International Society for Heart and Lung Transplantation (ISHLT) the early mortality for lung transplantation has remained higher than for heart transplantation. The worldwide experience since 1989 indicates an operative mortality (death within 30 days) of approximately 15–20% for heart–lung transplantation.[9,77] The results in heart–lung transplantation have been similar to the worldwide results with single and double lung transplantation.

Technical complications, including primary graft failure, cardiac complications (such as arrhythmias and myocardial infarction), and intraoperative hemorrhage have accounted for over 50% of early deaths following lung transplantation.[77] Factors that have been associated with an increased risk of early death following heart–lung transplantation have included advanced age (older than 40 years), history of prior cardiothoracic surgery, pre-existing hepatic dysfunction, primary pulmonary hypertension as the indication for transplantation, and preoperative ventilator dependence.[9,51,88,89]

Function

Pulmonary function studies in heart–lung transplant recipients without obliterative bronchiolitis have demonstrated normal lung volumes and flows.[53,75,90–93] During the early post-transplant period a reduction in lung volumes and compliance related to the sternotomy and reimplantation response is evident. Over the next 3 to 6 months progressive improvement toward normal lung function occurs.

The majority of heart–lung recipients are able to return to normal activity. Exercise studies have demonstrated normal gas exchange and ventilation during exercise.[91,93] As with the experience in heart transplantation, no clinically significant effects related to cardiac denervation have been apparent in the heart–lung recipients.

Long-Term Survival

The early collective experience in heart–lung transplantation (1981–1985) indicated 1 and 2 year actuarial survival rates of 52 and 44%, respectively.[94] The more recent ISHLT Registry data for heart lung transplantation (1988–1993) indicated a slight improvement in survival (60% at 1 year, 52% at 2 years).[9] The most common causes of late death following heart–lung transplantation have included infection, obliterative bronchiolitis, and lymphoproliferative disease.

THE FUTURE OF HEART–LUNG TRANSPLANTATION

Much progress has been made in thoracic transplantation during the past decade. Excellent results in heart–lung and lung transplantation have been achieved in a wide variety of patients with end-stage cardiopulmonary disease. Future developments in immunosuppression will possibly solve the problem of obliterative bronchiolitis while further decreasing the risk of infectious complications.

With three lung transplant options now available, the selection of a specific lung transplant procedure may be based on the candidate's cardiac function and pulmonary disease. The experience in single and double lung transplantation during the past 5 years indicates that heart–lung transplantation may be reserved for the small group of lung transplant candidates in whom replacement of both the heart and lungs remains the only option. This approach allows maximum utilization of the limited supply of donor hearts and lungs without compromising either functional results or patient survival.

REFERENCES

1. Cooley DA, Bloodwell RD, Hallman GL, et al: Organ transplantation for advanced cardiopulmonary disease. *Ann Thorac Surg* **8**:30–46, 1969

2. Lillehei CW, in discussion, Wildevuur CRH, Benfield JR: A review of 23 human lung transplants by 20 surgeons. *Ann Thorac Surg* **9**:489–515, 1970

3. Losman JG, Campbell CD, Replogle RL, et al: Joint transplantation of the heart and lungs. Past experience and present potentials. *J Cardiovasc Surg* **23**:440–52, 1982

4. Reitz BA, Burton NA, Jamieson SW, et al: Heart and lung transplantation. Autotransplantation and allotransplantation in primates with extended survival. *J Thorac Cardiovasc Surg* **80**:360–372, 1980

5. Reitz BA, Wallwork J, Hunt SA, et al: Heart-lung transplantation: Successful therapy for patients with pulmonary vascular disease. *N Engl J Med* **306**:557–564, 1982

6. Jamieson SW, Baldwin JC, Reitz BA, et al: Combined heart and lung transplantation. *Lancet* **1**:1130–1132, 1983

7. Toronto Lung Transplant Group: Unilateral lung transplantation for pulmonary fibrosis. *N Engl J Med* **314**:1140–1145, 1986

8. Patterson GA, Cooper JD, Dark JH, et al: Experimental and clinical double lung transplantation. *J Thorac Cardiovasc Surg* **95**:70–74, 1988

9. Hosenpud JD, Novick RJ, Breen TJ, Dailey OP: The Registry of the International Society for Heart and Lung Transplantation: Eleventh official report—1994. *J Heart Lung Transplant* **13**:561–570, 1994

10. *1994 Annual Report of the U.S. Scientific Registry for Transplant Recipients and the Organ Procurement and Transplantation Network—Transplant data: 1988–1993.* UNOS, Richmond, VA, and the Division of Organ Transplantation, Bureau of Health Resources Development, Health Resources and Services Administration, U.S. Department of Health and Human Services, Bethesda, MD

11. Fremes SE, Patterson GA, Williams WG, et al: Single lung transplantation and closure of patent ductus arteriosus for Eisenmenger's syndrome. Toronto Lung Transplant Group. *J Thorac Cardiovasc Surg* **100**:1–5, 1990

12. McCarthy PM, Rosenkranz ER, White RD, et al: Single-lung transplantation with atrial septal defect repair for Eisenmenger's syndrome. *Ann Thorac Surg* **52**:300–303, 1991

13. Pasque MK, Kaiser LR, Dresler CM, et al: Single lung transplantation for pulmonary hypertension. *J Thorac Cardiovasc Surg* **103**:475–481, 1992

14. Spray GL, Mallory GB, Canter CE, et al: Pediatric lung transplantation for pulmonary hypertension and congenital heart disease. *Ann Thorac Surg* **54**:216–225, 1992

15. Kriett JM, Smith CM, Hayden AM, et al: Lung transplantation without the use of antilymphocyte antibody preparations. *J Heart Lung Transplant* **12**:915–922, 1993

16. Chapelier A, Bauhe T, Macchiarini P, et al: Comparative outcomes of heart-lung and lung transplantation for pulmonary hypertension. *J Thorac Cardiovasc Surg* **106**:299–307, 1993

17. Lupinetti FM, Bolling F, Bove EL, et al: Selective lung or heart-lung transplantation for pulmonary hypertension associated with congenital cardiac anomalies. *Ann Thorac Surg* **54**:1545–1548, 1994

18. Kriett JM, Jamieson SW, Transplantation for congenital heart disease with special observations on pulmonary atresia and ventricular septal defect. *Prog Pediatr Cardiol* **1**:62–66, 1992

19. Harjula A, Baldwin JC, Starnes VA, et al: Proper donor selection for heart-lung transplantation. The Stanford experience. *J Thorac Cardiovasc Surg* **94**:874–880, 1987

20. Hutter JA, Scott J, Wreghitt T, et al: The importance of cytomegalovirus in heart-lung transplant recipients. *Chest* **95**:627–631, 1989

21. Smyth RL, Scott JP, Borysiewicz LK, et al: Cytomegalovirus infection in heart-lung transplant recipients: Risk factors, clinical associations, and response to treatment. *J Infect Dis* **164**:1045–1050, 1991

22. Novick RJ, Menkis AH, McKenzie FN, et al: Should heart-lung transplant donors and recipients be matched according to cytomegalovirus serologic status? *J Heart Transplant* **9**:699–706, 1990

23. Haverich A, Scott WC, Jamieson SW: Twenty years of lung preservation-a review. *J Heart Transplant* **4**:234–240, 1985

24. Wallwork J, Jones K, Cavarocchi N, et al: Distant procurement of organs for clinical heart-lung transplantation using a single-flush technique. *Transplantation* **44**:654–658, 1987

25. Harjula AL, Baldwin JC, Stinson EB, et al: Clinical heart-lung preservation with prostaglandin E-1. *Transplant Proc* **19**:4101–4102, 1987

26. Jurmann MJ, Dammenhayn L, Schafer HJ, et al: Prostacyclin as an additive to single crystalloid flush: Improved pulmonary preservation in heart-lung transplantation. *Transplant Proc* **19**:4103–4104, 1987

27. Fraser CD, Tamara F, Kontos GJ, et al: Evaluation of current organ preservation methods for heart-lung transplantation. *Transplant Proc* **20**:987–990, 1988

28. Kirk AJ, Colquhoun IW, Dark JH: Lung preservation: A review of current practice and future directions. *Ann Thorac Surg* **56**:90–100, 1993

29. Jamieson SW, Stinson EB, Oyer PE, et al: Operative technique for heart-lung transplantation. *J Thorac Cardiovasc Surg* **87**:930–935, 1984

30. Bonser RS, Fragomeni LS, Jamieson SW, et al: Effects of prostaglandin E1 in twelve hour lung preservation. *J Heart Transplant* **10**:310–315, 1991

31. Yacoub MH, Banner NR, Khagani A, et al: Heart-lung transplantation for cystic fibrosis and subsequent domino heart transplantation. *J Heart Transplant* **9**:459–466, 1990

32. Baumgartner WA, Traill TA, Cameron DE, et al: Unique aspects of heart and lung transplantation exhibited in the 'domino-donor' operation. *JAMA* **261**:3121–3125, 1989

33. Conte G, Sabbatini P, Napodano L, et al: Dopamine counteracts the acute renal effects of cyclosporine in normal subjects. *Transplant Proc* **20**(Suppl 3):563–567, 1988

34. Paranjpe DV, Wittich GR, Hamid LW, Bergin CJ: Frequency and management of pneumothoraces in heart-lung transplant recipients. *Radiology* **190**:255–256, 1994

35. Leval MR, Smyth R, Whitehead B, et al: Heart and lung transplantation for terminal cystic fibrosis. *J Thorac Cardiovasc Surg* **101**:633–642, 1991

36. McCarthy PM, Starnes VA, Theodore J: Improved survival after heart–lung transplantation. *J Thorac Cardiovasc Surg* **99**:54–59, 1990

37. Reichart B, Vosloo S, Holl J: Surgical management of heart-lung transplantation. *Ann Thorac Surg* **49**:333–340, 1990

38. Griffith BP, Hardesty RL, Armitage JM, et al: Acute rejection of lung allografts with various immunosuppressive protocols. *Ann Thorac Surg* **54**:846–851, 1992

39. Kriett JM, Smith CM, Hayden AM, et al: Lung transplantation without the use of antilymphocyte antibody preparations. *J Heart Lung Transplant* **12**:915–922, 1993

40. Griffith BP, Bando K, Hardesty RL, et al: A prospective randomized trial of FK506 versus cyclosporine after human pulmonary transplantation. *Transplantation* **57**:848–851, 1994

41. Siegelman SS, Sinha SB, Veith FJ: Pulmonary reimplantation response. *Ann Surg* **177**:30–36, 1973

42. Chiles C, Guthaner DF, Jamieson SW, et al: Heart-lung transplantation: The postoperative chest radiograph. *Radiology* **154**:299–304, 1985

43. Harjula AL, Baldwin JC, Silverman NE, et al: Implantation response following clinical heart-lung transplantation. *J Cardiovasc Surg* **31**:1–6, 1990

44. Jamieson SW, Stinson EB, Oyer PE, et al: Heart-lung transplantation for irreversible pulmonary hypertension. *Ann Thorac Surg* **38**:554–562, 1984

45. Patterson GA, Todd TR, Cooper JD, et al: Airway complications after double lung transplantation. *J Thorac Cardiovasc Surg* **99**:14–20, 1990

46. Colquhoun IW, Gascoigne AD, Au J, et al: Airway complications after pulmonary transplantation. *Ann Thorac Surg* **57**:141–145, 1994

47. Brooks RG, Hofflin JM, Jamieson SW, et al: Infectious complications in heart-lung transplant recipients. *Am J Med* **79**:412–422, 1985

48. Dummer JS, Montero CG, Griffith BP, et al: Infections in heart-lung transplant recipients. *Transplantation* **41**:727–729, 1986

49. Dummer JS, White LT, Ho M, et al: Morbidity of cytomegalovirus infection in recipients of heart and heart-lung transplantation who received cyclosporine. *J Infect Dis* **152**:1182–1191, 1985

50. Kriett JM, Kaye MP: The Registry of the International Society for Heart and Lung Transplantation: Eighth official report—1991. *J Heart Lung Transplant* **9**:323–330, 1991

51. Kriett JM, Jamieson SW: Risk assessment and prognosis in heart and heart-lung transplantation. In Kapoor AS, Singh BN (eds): *Prognosis and Risk Assessment in Cardiovascular Disease.* New York, Churchill-Livingstone, 1993, pp 521–537

52. Madden B, Radley-Smith R, Hodson M, et al: Medium-term results of heart and lung transplantation. *J Heart Lung Transplant* **11**:S241–243, 1992

53. Sarris GE, Smith JA, Shumway NE, et al: Long term results of combined heart/lung transplantation: The Stanford experience. *J Heart Lung Transplant* **13**:940–949, 1994

54. Wreghitt TG, Hakim M, Gray JJ, et al: Cytomegalovirus infections in heart and heart and lung transplant recipients. *J Clin Pathol* **41**:660–667, 1988

55. Dowling RD, Baladi N, Zenati M: Disruption of the aortic anastomosis in heart-lung transplant recipients. *Am J Med* **19**:118–122, 1990

56. Kramer MR, Stohr C, Lewiston NJ, et al: Trimethoprim-sulfamethoxazole prophylaxis for Pneumocystis carinii infections in heart-lung and lung transplantation—how effective and for how long? *Transplantation* **53**:586–589, 1989

57. Hutter JA, Stewart S, Higenbottam T, et al: Histologic changes in heart-lung transplant recipients during rejection episodes and at routine biopsy. *J Heart Transplant* **7**:440–444, 1988

58. Paradis IL, Duncan SR, Dauber JH, et al: Distinguishing between infection, rejection, and the adult respiratory distress syndrome after human lung transplantation. *J Heart Lung Transplant* **4**:S232–236, 1992

59. Starnes VA, Theodore J, Oyer P, et al: Evaluation of heart-lung transplant recipients with prospective, serial transbronchial biopsies and pulmonary function studies. *J Thorac Cardiovasc Surg* **98**:683–690, 1989

60. Stewart S, Higenbottam T, Hutter JA, et al: Histopathology of transbronchial biopsies in heart-lung transplantation. *Transplant Proc* **20**:764–766, 1988

61. Higgenbottam T, Stewart S, Penketh A, Wallwork J: Transbronchial lung biopsy for the diagnosis of rejection in heart-lung transplant patients. *Transplantation* **46**:532–539, 1988

62. Yousem SA, Dauber JA, Keenan R, et al: Does histologic acute rejection in lung allografts predict the development of bronchiolitis obliterans? *Transplantation* **52**:306–309, 1991

63. Clelland C, Higenbottam T, Otulana B, et al: Histologic prognostic indicators for the lung allografts of heart-lung transplants. *J Heart Transplant* **9**:177–185, 1990

64. Zeevi A, Rabinowich H, Paradis I, et al: Lymphocyte activation in bronchioalveolar lavages from heart-lung transplantation recipients. *Transplant Proc* **20**:189–192, 1988

65. Prior C, Klima G, Gattringer C, et al: Cell profiles in serial bronchoalveolar lavage after human heart-lung transplantation. *Acta Cytol* **36**:19–25, 1992

66. Otulana BA, Higenbottam T, Scott J, et al: Lung function associated with histologically diagnosed acute lung rejection and pulmonary infection in heart-lung transplant patients. *Am Rev Respir Dis* **142**:329–332, 1990

67. Baldwin JC, Oyer PE, Stinson EB, et al: Comparison of cardiac rejection in heart and heart-lung transplantation. *J Heart Transplant* **6**:352–356, 1987

68. Glanville AR, Baldwin JC, Hunt SA, Theodore J: Long-term cardiopulmonary function after human heart-lung transplantation. *Aust NZ J Med* **20**:208–214, 1990

69. McGregor CG, Baldwin JC, Jamieson SW, et al: Isolated pulmonary rejection after combined heart-lung transplantation. *J Thorac Cardiovasc Surg* **90**:623–626, 1985

70. Griffith BP, Hardesty RL, Trento A, et al: Asynchronous rejection of heart and lungs following cardiopulmonary transplantation. *Ann Thorac Surg* **40**:488–493, 1985

71. Glanville AR, Imoto E, Billingham ME, et al: The role of right ventricular endomyocardial biopsy in the long-term management of heart-lung transplant recipients. *J Heart Transplant* **6**:357–361, 1987

72. Burke CM, Theodore J, Dawkins KD, et al: Postoperative obliterative bronchiolitis and other late sequelae in human heart-lung transplantation. *Chest* **86**:824–829, 1984

73. Griffith BP, Paradis IL, Zeevi A, et al: Immunologically mediated disease of the airway after pulmonary transplantation. *Ann Surg* **208**:371–378, 1989

74. Burke CM, Glanville AR, Theodore J, et al: Lung immunogenicity, rejection, and obliterative bronchiolitis. *Chest* **92**:547–549, 1987

75. Madden BP, Hodson ME, Tsang V, et al: Intermediate-term results of heart–lung transplantation for cystic fibrosis. *Lancet* **339**:1583–1587, 1992

76. Scott JP, Higenbottam TW, Clelland C, et al: Natural history of chronic rejection in heart-lung transplant recipients. *J Heart Transplant* **9**:510–515, 1990

77. Kriett JM, Kaye MP: The Registry of the International Society for Heart and Lung Transplantation: Eighth official report—1991. *J Heart Lung Transplant* **10**:491–498, 1991

78. Whitehead B, Rees P, Sorenson K, et al: Incidence of obliterative bronchiolitis after heart-lung transplantation in children. *J Heart Lung Transplant* **12**:903–908, 1993

79. Yousem SA, Burke CM, Billingham ME: Pathologic pulmonary alterations in long-term human heart–lung transplantation. *Human Pathol* **16**:911–923, 1985

80. Burke CM, Morris AJR, Dawkins KD, et al: Late airflow obstruction in heart-lung transplant recipients. *J Heart Transplant* **4**:437–439,1985

81. Kramer MR, Stoehr C, Whang JL, et al: The diagnosis of obliterative bronchiolitis after heart-lung and lung transplantation: Low yield of transbronchial lung biopsy. *J Heart Lung Transplant* **12**:675–681, 1993

82. Scott JP, Higgenbottam TW, Sharples L, et al: Risk factors for obliterative bronchiolitis in heart-lung transplant recipients. *Transplantation* **51**:813–817, 1991

83. Allen MD, Burke CM, McGregor CGA, et al: Steroid-responsive bronchiolitis after human heart-lung transplantation. *J Thorac Cardiovasc Surg* **92**:449, 1986

84. Glanville AR, Baldwin JC, Burke CM, et al: Obliterative bronchiolitis after heart-lung transplantation: Apparent arrest by augmented immunosuppression. *Ann Interm Med* **107**:300–304, 1987

85. Adams DH, Cochrane AD, Khaghani A, et al: Retransplantation in heart-lung recipients with obliterative bronchiolitis. *J Thorac Cardiovasc Surg* **107**:450–459, 1994

86. Novick RJ, Andreassian B, Shafers HJ, et al: Pulmonary retransplantation for obliterative bronchiolitis. Intermediate-term results of a North American-European series. *J Thorac Cardiovasc Surg* **107**:755–763, 1994

87. Armitage JM, Kormos RL, Stuart RS, et al: Posttransplant lymphoproliferative disease in thoracic organ transplant patients: ten years of cyclosporine-based immunosuppression. *J Heart Lung Transplant* **10**:877–886, 1991

88. Kramer MR, Harshall SE, Tiroke A, et al: Clinical significance of hyperbilirubinemia in patients with pulmonary hypertension undergoing heart-lung transplantation. *J Heart Lung Transplant* **10**:317–321, 1991

89. Kaye MP: The Registry of the International Society for Heart and Lung Transplantation: Tenth official report—1993. *J Heart Lung Transplant* **12**:541–548, 1993

90. Theodore J, Jamieson SW, Burke CM, et al: Physiologic aspects of human heart-lung transplantation: Pulmonary function status of the post-transplanted lung. *Chest* **86**:349–357, 1984

91. Theodore J, Morris AJ, Burke CM, et al: Cardiopulmonary function following human heart–lung transplantation. *Chest* **92**:433–439, 1987

92. Williams TJ, Grossman RF, Maurer JR: Long-term functional follow-up of lung transplant recipients. *Clin Chest Med* **11**:347–358, 1990

93. Levy RD, Ernst P, Levine SM, et al: Exercise performance after lung transplantation. *J Heart Lung Transplant* **12**:27–33, 1993

94. Fragomeni LS, Kaye MD: The Registry of the International Society for Heart Transplantation: Fifth official report—1988. *J Heart Transplant* **7**:298–303, 1988

115

Cardiomyoplasty

James A. Magovern and Brian L. Cmolik

Great advances have been made in the past three decades in surgical treatment of diseased cardiac valves and coronary arteries, but management of the diseased myocardium continues to be problematic. Congestive heart failure (CHF) affects two million patients and causes 400,000 deaths per year in the United States.[1,2] Survival for patients with CHF continues to be poor. Mortality for patients with CHF, felt to be "too well" for heart transplantation, has been as high as 50% at 12 mo.[3] The addition of angiotensin-converting enzyme inhibitors to medical management with digoxin and diuretics has been a major advance for patients with CHF, but the mortality for patients with class IV heart failure is still greater than 45% after 1 year.[4] Cardiac transplantation is effective therapy for this disease, but is limited to less than 2500 operations per year due to a scarcity of donor organs. Implantable ventricular assist devices hold promise for the future, but clinical application will be hampered by high expense and regulatory delays.

The concept of using skeletal muscle power to augment ventricular function was considered several decades ago, but was abandoned because of the fatigability of skeletal muscle.[5,6] Renewed interest in this approach was generated by basic research in muscle physiology, which demonstrated that skeletal muscle could be made fatigue-resistant by chronic electrical stimulation.[7–9] The possibility of an autologous cardiac assist system that does not require immunosuppression or a mechanical blood pump is an attractive concept that has generated considerable recent attention.

Various approaches for using skeletal muscle for cardiac assistance have been proposed including (1) cardiomyoplasty, (2) skeletal muscle ventricles, and (3) diastolic aortic compression. Most of these concepts have been limited to the research laboratory, except cardiomyoplasty, which has also been applied clinically. This chapter will review the physiology of chronic skeletal muscle stimulation, sum-

marize recent clinical and experimental results with cardiomyopasty, and briefly outline the progress that has been made with other approaches, such as skeletal muscle ventricles and diastolic aortic compression.

SKELETAL MUSCLE TRANSFORMATION

Skeletal muscle contraction can generate a power output of approximately 6 mW/g of tissue, but under usual circumstances the power production drops rapidly due to muscle fatigue.[10] The fatigability of skeletal muscle is not an immutable property, but rather an adaptation to the fact that skeletal muscle contraction is needed only intermittently and usually at less than peak capacity. Skeletal muscle is a highly adaptable tissue and has a tremendous capacity to transform in response to physical demands. The hypertrophic physique of a body builder and the endurance capacity of the marathon runner are examples of the plasticity of skeletal muscle.

Skeletal muscle is composed of two primary fiber types.[11] Type II fibers are adapted for short periods of intense activity and are fatigue-prone, since they rely on glycolysis for metabolism. These fibers are also termed fast-twitch fibers because they contract and relax rapidly. Type I fibers are adapted for tasks that require prolonged muscle activity, usually at low levels of intensity. They are less powerful than type II fibers but are fatigue-resistant, since they obtain energy from oxidative metabolism. Type I fibers are also referred to as slow-twitch fibers because their rate of contraction and relaxation is slower than that of type II fibers. Muscles that are used intermittently, such as the latissimus dorsi, are primarily composed of type II fibers, whereas muscles that are used continuously for posture, such as the erector spinae, are composed primarily of type I fibers. Several intermediate fiber types having some properties of both type I and II fibers are also present in most muscles.

It was first demonstrated in the 1960s that muscle composed of fast-twitch, type II fibers could be transformed to slow-twitch, type I fibers. The initial experiments utilized cross-innervation studies in which the nerves to predominantly fast- and slow-twitch muscles were exchanged so that the nerve innervating a slow muscle was switched to a fast muscle.[8] Over time the type II fibers transformed into type I fibers. Salmons and Sreter demonstrated that this same phenomenon occurred if muscle was electrically stimulated at 10 Hz, which is a pattern that mimics the neural activity of a nerve innervating a slow muscle.[8] This work showed that muscle transformation was a response to the pattern of stimulation and not a function of the nerve innervating the muscle. These and other experiments gave rise to the basic science field of skeletal muscle transformation, which examines the process by which muscle adapts to chronic electrical stimulation. The studies reviewed in the next section have been done primarily in the tibialis anterior and extensor digitorum longus muscle of the rabbit. These are fast-twitch muscles that can be completely transformed to slow-twitch muscles in response to continuous electrical stimulation at 10 Hz.[12]

Metabolic Adaptation

As a result of chronic electrical stimulation, fast-twitch type II fibers change from glycolytic to oxidative metabolism.[9,13] Increases in the enzymes of aerobic oxidative metabolism and decreases in the enzymes of glycolysis and glycogenolysis are evident after a few weeks of stimulation. In addition, bloodflow to the stimulated muscle increases due to vasodilatation and an increase in capillary density.[14,15] Other changes include an increase in mitochondrial density and a decrease in myofibril size.[16–18]

Calcium Metabolism

Muscle contraction is ultimately controlled by calcium flux. Chronic low-frequency stimulation induces major changes in calcium metabolism in fast-twitch muscle. Early changes include structural alterations in the profile of the T-tubules, reductions in the calcium uptake capacity of the sarcoplasmic reticulum, and decreases in parvalbumin, a cytosolic calcium-binding protein.[19–21] Coincident with these changes is a decrease in the activity of the calcium-ATPase.[22] After several months of low-frequency stimulation, the calcium metabolism and sarcoplasmic reticulum of fast-twitch muscle become similar to that of slow-twitch muscle.

Fiber-Type Transformation

Chronic low-frequency stimulation eventually results in complete transformation of skeletal muscles to type I fibers, but the process involves a number of intermediate steps de-

fined by expression of different myosin heavy chain isoforms. The fiber type changes appear to occur in the following order: type IIB–type IID–type IIA–type IIC–type IC–type I.[12] Type I fiber expresses the slow myosin heavy chain isoform characteristic of a slow-twitch fiber. Stimulation also results in expression of slow isoforms of the thin, filament, regulatory proteins of tropomyosin and troponin.[23–25] Fiber-type transformations, which are not evident until after weeks or months of stimulation, are a late consequence of stimulation. There is a controversy about whether individual fibers actually transform or whether the observed transformation process results from replacement of senescent type II fibers with type I fibers derived from muscle satellite cells. Current evidence favors the replacement theory. Thus, muscle transformation is probably achieved by regeneration of new fibers rather than from modification of existing fibers.[12]

Latissimus Dorsi Stimulation

The latissimus dorsi is composed predominantly of type II fibers. Continuous electrical stimulation at 2 Hz or intermittent burst stimulation at 30 Hz results in transformation of the muscle to type I fibers in dogs, sheep, and goats.[11,26,27] This transformation not only results in fatigue resistance, but also some loss of muscle strength. A recent study has quantified the power generated by an unconditioned latissimus dorsi when the vascular supply of the muscle was not disturbed and when the muscle was allowed to contract in a linear fashion. Under these circumstances the latissimus dorsi generated 1.15 W or approximately 6 mW/g of tissue, which is comparable or slightly higher than the power generated by cardiac muscle.[10] There is a large body of basic science literature indicating that chronic electrical stimulation will reduce the power output of a skeletal muscle by as much as 50%.[28] By extrapolating experimental animal data to the human situation, it has been estimated that a human latissimus dorsi could produce between 50 and 75% of the power output of the left ventricle, which would be enough to provide significant circulatory support.

Very little work has been done to define the optimal stimulation pattern of skeletal muscle for cardiac assistance. Current protocols are designed to achieve full transformation of the muscle from type II to type I fibers, and not necessarily to optimize power production. Recent work has shown that dynamic training of the skeletal muscle, which allows the muscle to shorten rather than contracting isometrically, results in a fatigue-resistant muscle with no reduction in power production.[29] Fibrosis of the latissimus dorsi has been demonstrated after chronic burst stimulation in both animal and human studies of cardiomyoplasty.[30,31] The muscle damage is due primarily to muscle ischemia caused by mobilization of the muscle in a single stage without a vascular delay period, which results in vascular compromise in the distal 30% of the latissimus dorsi.[32] Continuous burst stimulation of the muscle without allowing rest periods is also a likely cause of muscle damage in the long term, especially in a muscle that is perfused solely by the thoracodorsal bundle. Additional research is needed to develop a muscle stimulation protocol that provides the optimal combination of fatigue resistance, muscle power, and muscle viability.

CARDIOMYOPLASTY: MECHANISM OF ACTION

Effects on Left Ventricular Systolic Function

The original intent of cardiomyoplasty was to augment left ventricular systolic function from compression of the heart by contraction of the latissimus dorsi.[27,33] In this conception, the procedure should increase stroke volume, ejection fraction, and cardiac output without increasing cardiac preload (Fig. 115–1). This hypothesis has been tested by several investigators in experimental animals. Lee et al studied the effects of cardiomyoplasty in animals with CHF induced by rapid ventricular pacing.[34] Cardiomyoplasty increased cardiac output and augmented shortening of the major and minor axis of the left ventricle, while decreasing left ventricular end-diastolic pressure. Cheng et al studied the effects of cardiomyoplasty in animals with adriamycin-induced heart failure and demonstrated an increase in regional function, global ejection fraction, and peak left ventricular filling rate, despite small decreases in the left ventricular end-diastolic pressure.[35] Millner et al demonstrated that dynamic cardiomyoplasty improved cardiac

performance in sheep with ischemic heart failure when the animals were given a large fluid challenge.[36] Park et al studied the effects of right latissimus dorsi cardiomyoplasty on left ventricular function and showed that the procedure improved left ventricular systolic function, as measured by an increase in preload recruitable stroke work.[37] Cho et al demonstrated that cardiomyoplasty improved left ventricular contractility, but did not improve cardiac output because the procedure also reduced left ventricular volume.[38]

The phase I study of cardiomyoplasty failed to show a consistent objective change in cardiac function in patients undergoing the operation.[39] However, this was an early feasibility study in which the endpoints for measuring cardiac function were not uniform from center-to-center. Recently, the results of the phase II study have shown a modest but consistent increase in stroke volume, left ventricular stroke work index, and left ventricular ejection fraction in patients at 6 and 12 mo after operation.[40] These findings are important in that they confirm the original hypothesis that cardiomyoplasty can improve systolic cardiac function.

Effects on Left Ventricular Volume

Another important aspect of cardiomyoplasty is its effect on left ventricular volume. Experimental publications have shown that cardiomyoplasty limits the left ventricular dilatation that occurs with heart failure induced by rapid ventricular pacing or multiple coronary ligations.[41,42] The stimulated latissimus dorsi muscle appears to provide a girdling effect on the left ventricle, which ameliorates the progressive remodeling and dilatation of the left ventricle that usually occurs with a failing heart. This probably results from a reduction of left ventricular wall stress.

Stabilization or reduction in left ventricular volume has also been consistently noted in clinical applications of the procedure. The natural history of CHF results in progressive left ventricular dilatation, even when cardiac filling pressures remain stable. Cardiomyoplasty appears to arrest this process as reported by both Carpentier and Magovern in long-term follow-up with patients undergoing cardiomyoplasty.[43,44] An example of this is shown in Figure 115–2. Kass et al have done pressure–volume analysis of ventricular function in patients before and after cardiomyoplasty. Striking reductions of left ventricular volume have been shown in several patients in the first 6–12 mo after operation.[45] This process has been termed reversed remodeling and is probably the primary long-term benefit of cardiomyoplasty. The changes in left ventricular systolic function after clinical cardiomyoplasty are small. In contrast, however, cardiomyoplasty is the first intervention that has consistently shown interruption in the progressive increase in left ventricular size that is typical in patients with CHF.

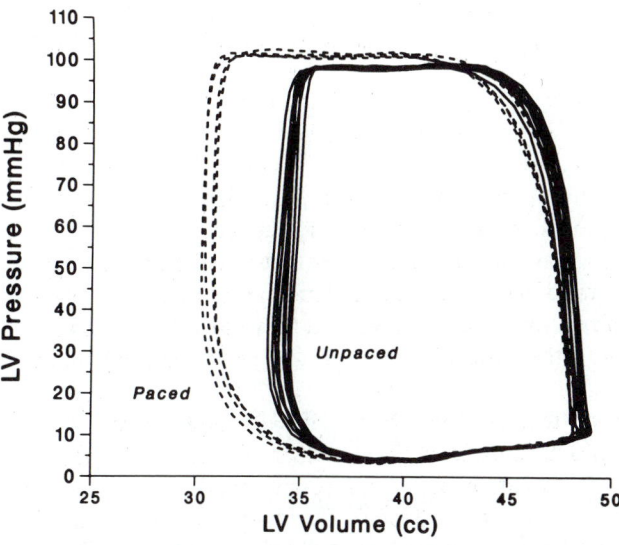

Figure 115–1. Pressure-volume loops obtained and without stimulation of a latissimus dorsi cardiomyoplasty. The area inscribed by the loops represents stroke work. Dynamic cardiomyoplasty increases ejection and stroke work without changing preload. *(From Park et al: Right latissimus dorsi cardiomyoplasty augments left ventricular systolic performance. Ann Thorac Surg 56:1295, 1993, reprinted with permission from the Society of Thoracic Surgeons.)*

Effects on Diastolic Function

The observation that cardiomyoplasty can reduce left ventricular size raises concerns that the procedure may impair

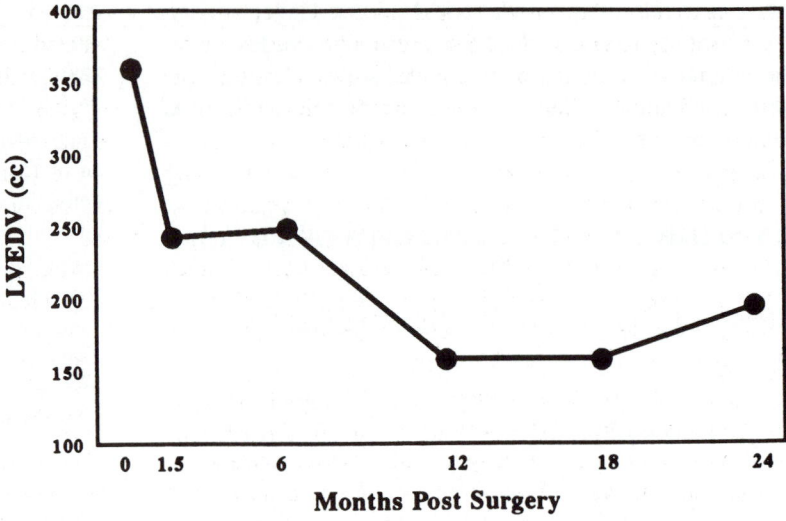

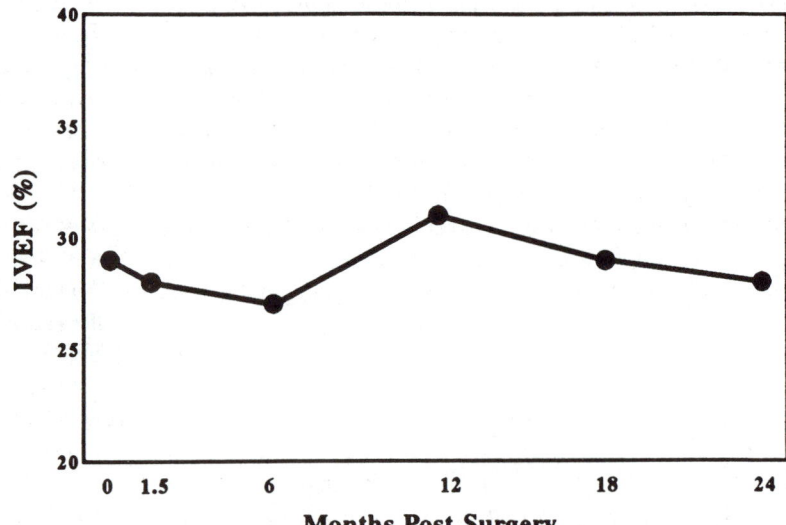

Figure 115–2. The graphs show measurements of left ventricular ejection fraction (LVEF) and left ventricular end diastolic volume (LVEDV) over time in a patient after cardiomyoplasty. Of note is the maintenance of LVEF with a marked reduction in LVEDV.

diastolic function. The experimental literature is divided on this question. In an acute experiment using animals with normal heart function, Corin et al showed that cardiomyoplasty can impair diastolic relaxation and increase left ventricular passive stiffness.[46] These observations are in contrast to work published by others.[47] The discrepancy may reflect slight differences in operative technique. It is certainly possible to disrupt diastolic function if the ventricles are wrapped tightly with the latissimus dorsi,[48] but this is not an inevitable consequence of the operation. In fact, it has been shown that cardiomyoplasty improves diastolic function in animals with adriamycin-induced cardiomyopathy.[35] The effects of cardiomyoplasty on diastolic function have been difficult to study in the clinical setting because all of the patients have abnormal diastolic function and some degree of mitral regurgitation prior to surgery. No obvious deterioration in diastolic function has been noted in any of the clinical studies, and patients do not develop con-

strictive pericarditis after the procedure. However, valid concerns remain about the long-term effects of cardiomyoplasty on diastolic filling and relaxation, especially during exercise when the heart rate increases. This issue will require further scrutiny in future studies of cardiomyoplasty.

TECHNICAL ASPECTS OF CARDIOMYOPLASTY

Mobilization of the Latissimus Dorsi

The latissimus dorsi is mobilized through a longitudinal flank incision extending from the axilla to just above the iliac crest. Skin flaps are developed to expose the underlying muscle. The latissimus dorsi is then lifted from the chest wall, starting with the anterior edge of the muscle and progressing posteriorly. Multiple chest wall perforating vessels supply the distal two-thirds of the latissimus dorsi and must be divided. The posterior and inferior attachments of the muscle are divided. Next, the thoracodorsal neurovascular bundle is identified and followed into the axilla. The fastest method for finding the thoracodorsal bundle is to find its branch to the serratus anterior, which runs in a superior to inferior direction and is easily found on the anterior surface of the serratus anterior (Fig 115–3). The other major branch of the thoracodorsal bundle is the circumflex scapular, which arises proximal to the serratus anterior branch and runs posteriorly toward the scapula. Both of these branches should be divided to provide greater mobility of the pedicle.

The next step is to implant the stimulating electrodes. In the experimental laboratory, nerve stimulating leads are used, but in the clinical setting intramuscular leads have been used in all cases. Two intramuscular wires are weaved into the axillary region of the latissimus dorsi, the first one adjacent to the branches of the thoracodorsal nerve and the second one 6 cm more distally. Transillumination of the muscle can help identify and avoid injury to the major neurovascular branches. Transposition of the latissimus dorsi into the thorax is done through the bed of the partially resected second or third rib. A 5-cm portion of the anterolateral rib is removed. Nonabsorbable sutures are then placed through the pleura, periosteum, and intercostal muscle and held with rubber-shod clamps. The muscle is then moved into the thorax. Next, the humeral tendon of the latissimus

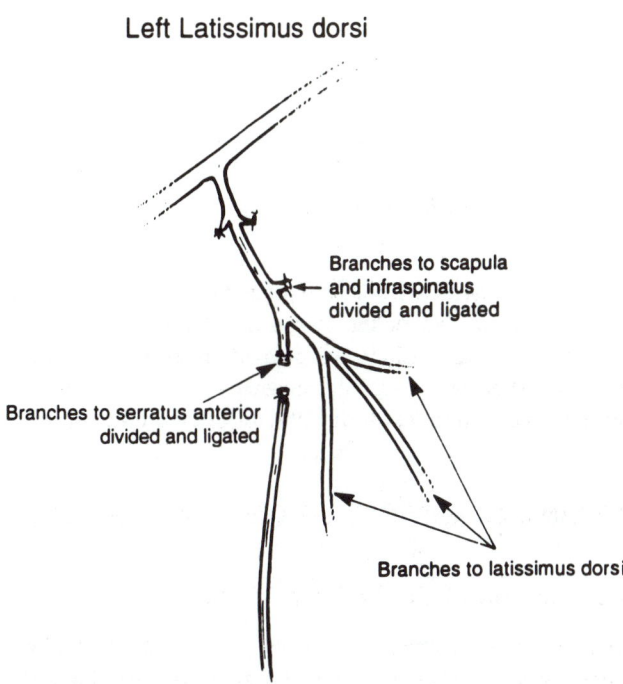

Left Latissimus dorsi

Branches to scapula and infraspinatus divided and ligated

Branches to serratus anterior divided and ligated

Branches to latissimus dorsi

Figure 115–3. The drawing shows the surgical anatomy of the thoracodorsal neurovascular bundle. The serratus anterior branch can always be traced back to identify the main bundle. Both the serratus anterior and the circumflex scapular branches should be divided to increase the mobility of the thoracodorsal pedicle.

dorsi is divided, and the previously placed sutures are passed through the tendon, which secures the muscle to the chest wall. Care must be taken to avoid twisting or tension on the vascular pedicle. The flank incision is then closed in layers over two closed suction drains. Serous fluid always collects under the skin flaps and failure to drain this space invariably leads to seroma formation. The cardiomyoplasty procedure is usually done through a midline sternotomy incision. Therefore, the patient is repositioned from the lateral to the supine position after mobilization of the muscle flap.

Operative Technique for Left Latissimus Dorsi Cardiomyoplasty

The technique for cardiomyoplasty is not difficult, but it can be confusing because there are several possible orientations for the muscle to be wrapped around the heart. The first decision is whether to start the wrap posteriorly or anteriorly. The next decision is whether to have the subcutaneous or the chest wall surface of the latissimus dorsi against the heart. Most surgeons have used the posterior wrap for cases of cardiomyopathy and have reserved the anterior to posterior wrap to repair the left ventricle after left ventricular aneurysm resection. The remainder of the operative description will concentrate on the posterior wrap. The most commonly employed technique places the anterior edge of the latissimus dorsi along the posterior atrioventricular groove, which requires that the subcutaneous surface of the muscle be against the heart. The challenging aspect of the procedure, especially in patients with dilated cardiomyopathy, is getting the muscle into place without disturbing ventricular function or causing arrhythmias.

Several key technical points are worth noting (Fig. 115–4). First, it is best to open the pericardium approximately 1 cm medial to the left phrenic nerve and create a broad-based pedicle of pericardium with its base on the right side. This improves exposure of the left ventricle and allows the substernal aspect of the muscle to be covered with pericardium, which prevents postoperative adhesions between the latissimus dorsi and the sternum. Second, sutures to secure the muscle flap on the heart should be placed into the pericardium rather than into the myocardium, since troublesome bleeding can occur posteriorly where it is difficult to repair if myocardial sutures tear through the tissue. Lastly, the heart should be lifted as little as possible when positioning the muscle. It is best to slide the latissimus dorsi behind the heart rather than lift the heart to directly suture the muscle in place. The distance that the flap must cover posteriorly extends from the left atrial appendage to the inferior vena cava. This distance can be measured with an umbilical tape before positioning the muscle. Pledgetted sutures of 2-0 polyester are placed into the anterior edge of muscle at a distance from each other as measured with the umbilical tape. The patient is then placed in steep Trendelenburg position with the table tilted toward the patient's right side. The apex of the left ventricle is then tilted

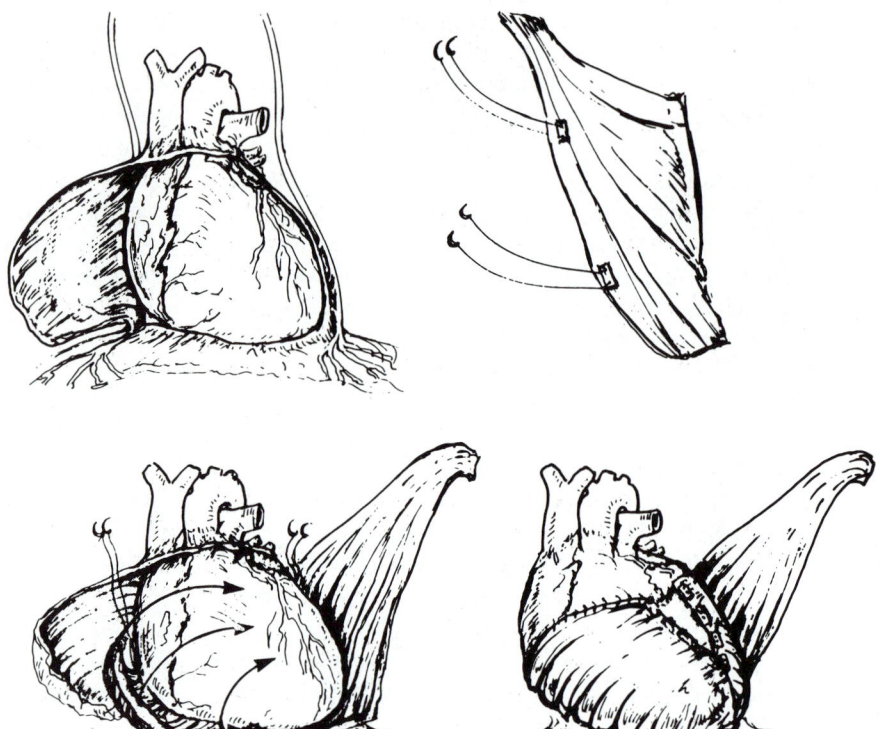

Figure 115–4. The drawing illustrates several important technical details of left cardiomyoplasty. The pericardium is opened close to the left phrenic nerve, which creates a flap of pericardium based on the right side. Sutures are inserted into the anterior edge of the latissimus dorsi. These sutures are used to slide the muscle behind the heart, and then to secure the muscle to the pericardium. The wrap is completed anteriorly, but often the outflow tract of the right ventricle is not covered.

slightly upward, and the latissimus dorsi flap is slipped around the ventricle with the aid of the previously placed sutures on the muscle. These sutures are then secured to the pericardium just below the origin of the left pulmonary artery, and just anterior and medial to the inferior vena cava. An epicardial sensing lead is then attached to the right ventricle for sensing the QRS complex. An R-wave of at least 5 mV amplitude and a slew rate of at least 0.5 V/sec are required for reliable operation of the cardiomyostimulator.

The remainder of the muscle is then folded around the heart and sutured to itself anteriorly, starting near the apex and proceeding cephalad. Often it is not possible to cover all of the right ventricle, especially the outflow portion. Carpentier and Chachques recommended bridging this area with pericardium, but we have generally not done this because of concern about constricting the outflow tract of the right ventricle. The muscle-stimulating leads and the sensing leads are then retrieved and tunneled into a subcutaneous pocket on the abdominal wall. The cardiomyostimulator is implanted in the subcutaneous pocket after the sternum is closed in the usual fashion.

Right Latissimus Dorsi Cardiomyoplasty

The right latissimus dorsi can also be used for cardiomyoplasty. This procedure was first done in the experimental laboratory as part of a bilateral latissimus dorsi cardiomyoplasty.[49] Subsequent experimental studies demonstrated that the procedure could augment left ventricular function

in animals.[37,50] The operation has also been done in a series of 16 patients.[51,52]

The technical details of right latissimus dorsi cardiomyoplasty are similar in most respects to those using the left muscle (Fig. 115–5). Mobilization of the right latissimus dorsi is done in the same fashion as the left, and the muscle wrap is done through a midline sternotomy incision. The anterior orientation is always used, because the right atrium and inferior vena cava are compressed if the muscle is positioned posteriorly. The pericardium is opened to the right of the midline and a pericardial flap is made that is based on the left side of the pericardium. The right latissimus dorsi cardiomyoplasty does not circumferentially encircle the heart, but rather comes across both ventricles and attaches to the posterior pericardium, creating a muscular sling around the heart. The costal surface of the muscle contacts the epicardium and the scapulospinal portion of the muscle covers the diaphragmatic surface of the heart. The same technique of using an umbilical tape to measure the distance of the posterior atrioventricular groove is used. To facilitate positioning of the flap with minimal heart retraction, we attach straps of autologous pericardium measuring 1 cm wide by 8 cm in length to the distal (iliac) edge of the muscle. One strap is placed on the most anterior edge of the flap, and the second one is placed at a distance from the first one as measured with the umbilical tape (Fig. 115–5). The patient is then placed in Trendelenburg position with the operating table turned toward the surgeon. The heart is gently lifted up and the muscle is passed around the apex and positioned posteriorly. A kidney pedicle clamp is then

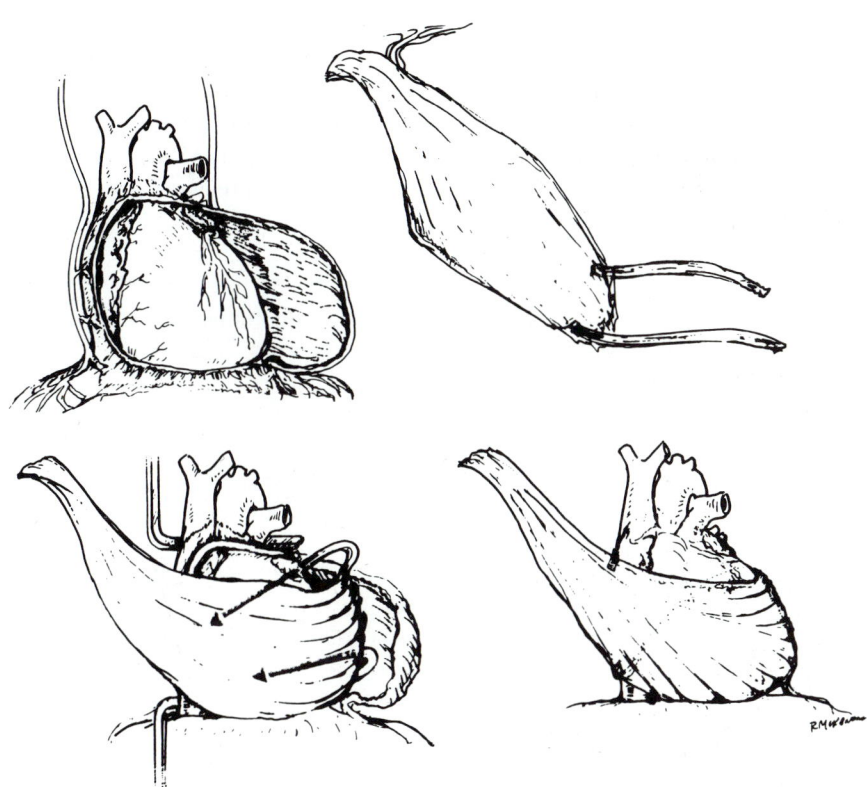

Figure 115–5. The drawing illustrates the important aspects of right latissimus dorsi cardiomyoplasty. The pericardium is opened close to the right phrenic nerve, which creates a pericardial flap based on the left side. Pericardial straps are sutured to the distal aspect of the muscle. The pericardial straps are grasped through the transverse sinus and behind the inferior vena cava to pull the latissimus dorsi into place.

passed through the transverse sinus and then behind the inferior vena cava to grasp the pericardial straps and pull the flap into place. The muscle is then secured to the pericardium between the left atrial appendage and left pulmonary artery on the left side and just anterior and medial to the inferior vena cava on the right side. The right latissimus dorsi has been long enough to reach the posterior atrioventricular groove, except when the cardiomegaly is extreme, as defined by a ventricular end-diastolic volume greater than 400 mL.

CLINICAL RESULTS WITH CARDIOMYOPLASTY

The first clinical cardiomyoplasty was done by Dr. Alain Carpentier in 1985 in a patient with a cardiac tumor that involved the majority of the left ventricle.[53] The tumor was resected and the left latissimus dorsi muscle was used to reconstruct the ventricular cavity. Within months of this procedure, Dr. George Magovern used the left latissimus dorsi to repair a left ventricular aneurysm.[33] Encouraged by a successful outcome in these initial cases, surgeons next attempted the procedure to improve cardiac function in patients with CHF secondary to cardiomyopathy. This technique used the latissimus dorsi to encircle or reinforce the ventricles, rather than to replace destroyed myocardium and therefore was potentially applicable to many more patients because of the high incidence of CHF. To date, the opera-

tion has been used to treat CHF in several hundred patients in Europe, North America, and South America. Objective data are available on the results of two prospective studies of cardiomyoplasty conducted from 1988 to 1991 and from 1991 to 1993. These two studies have been termed Phase I and Phase II, respectively.[39,40]

Phase I

Between January 1985 and August 1991, 118 patients underwent cardiomyoplasty in fourteen centers in Europe, South America, and North America. The major objectives of the study were to document the feasibility, safety, and reproducibility of the procedure in multiple centers, and to evaluate the performance and safety of the Medtronic Cardiomyoplasty System. Additional objectives were to determine patient selection criteria, document long-term muscle contraction, and determine the effects of the procedure on cardiac function.

Patient Population

There were 112 patients in the entire group who had predominant left ventricular failure: 62 (55.4%) had ischemic cardiomyopathy, 41 (36.6%) had idiopathic cardiomyopathy, 7 (6.3%) had Chagas disease, and 2 (1.7%) were for other unspecified reasons. Thirty-six percent (40/112) were in New York Heart Association (NYHA) functional class IV. Sixty-three percent (70/112) were class III, and two patients were in class II.

Operative Procedure

All but one of the operations used the left latissimus dorsi muscle. Approximately 90% of the procedures were done through a median sternotomy. The remainder used a left thoracotomy. The most common procedure was a posterior to anterior wrap using the technique originally described by Carpentier and Chachques.[27] A small number (< 10%) of patients had an anterior to posterior wrap as described by Magovern et al.[54] Isolated cardiomyoplasty was done in 77% (86/112) and cardiomyoplasty was combined with other procedures in 23% (26/112), including coronary artery bypass 13% (14/112), left ventricular aneurysm or tumor resection 12% (13/112), and valve replacement 3% (3/112). Four patients had more than one concomitant operation.

Survival

The operative mortality was 21% (24/112) and was higher for class IV patients than class III patients (38 vs 12%). Five patients subsequently had cardiac transplantation and were therefore withdrawn from the study. Long-term survival was related to preoperative functional class. The 18-mo probability of survival using Kaplan–Meier life table analysis was 75% for class III patients and 42% for class IV patients. Most of the late deaths were secondary to cardiac failure or ventricular arrhythmias.

Clinical Status of Survivors

Functional improvement occurred in 81% of survivors. The average improvement was 1.6 NYHA classes. Both class III and class IV patients improved to a similar degree. No consistent improvement in left ventricular function was noted as measured with radionuclide scanning or echocardiography. As cardiac catheterization was not part of the protocol, hemodynamic data were not available for analysis.

Phase II

Between May 1991 and September 1993, 68 patients had cardiomyoplasty at eight centers, including five in the United States, two in Canada, and one in Brazil. This group of patients constitute the Phase II study, in which data were collected to determine the effects of cardiomyoplasty on hemodynamics, exercise capacity, quality of life, ventricular function, and survival.

The selection criteria were broadly defined. Patients were required to have CHF (despite optimal medical therapy), a left ventricular ejection fraction (LVEF) of <40%, and a left ventricular end-diastolic pressure or pulmonary capillary wedge pressure of >15 mm Hg. All candidates were required to have the following preoperative testing: (1) right and left heart catheterization, (2) multigated acquisition cardiac scan (MUGA) and echocardiogram, (3) an exercise test with calculation of O_2 consumption, (4) chest x-ray, electrocardiogram, and 24-hour holter, (5) determina-

tion of NYHA functional classification, and (6) estimation of quality of life by a questionnaire.

The major exclusion criteria were (1) age > 80 or < 18; (2) creatinine clearance < 30 mL/min; (3) hepatic cirrhosis, chronic hepatitis, or hepatic tumor; (4) pulmonary dysfunction with a vital capacity < 55% of predicted; and (5) significant multiorgan dysfunction or cardiac cachexia. Patients who had or needed an automatic, implantable, cardioverter defibrillator (AICD) or valvular heart surgery were excluded, as were those who could not be weaned from intravenous inotropic drugs.

Patient follow-up visits were required at 6 wk and then every 6 mo. End-points for evaluating efficacy of the procedure were (1) right heart catheterization; (2) MUGA scan; (3) exercise testing; (4) chest x-ray, electrocardiogram, and holter monitor; and (5) evaluation of function class and quality of life.

Patient Population

There were 68 patients in the study group, of whom 78% were male and 22% female. Mean age was 57 ± 10 years. Cardiomyopathy was classified as idiopathic in 69% and ischemic in 31%. Preoperative NYHA functional class status was class III for 93%, class II for 5%, and class IV for 2%.

Operative Procedure

Cardiomyoplasty was done as the sole procedure in 88% and the procedure was combined with another procedure in 12% of the cases. Concomitant operations included coronary artery bypass or mitral valve surgery. The left latissimus dorsi was used in 52 patients and the right latissimus dorsi was used in 16 patients. Median sternotomy was the predominant approach, but in three cases the operation was done through a left thoracotomy incision. Cardiopulmonary bypass was used in all of the cases in which a concomitant procedure was done, but was avoided in the others if possible.

Survival

The operative mortality was 12%. Survival at 6 and 12 mo after operation was 75 ± 5% and 68 ± 6%, respectively. All deaths were cardiac in nature, with sudden death accounting for the majority and progressive heart failure causing the remainder. The survival rate after cardiomyoplasty did not differ from that of a reference group of patients with a similar degree of heart failure who were followed prospectively.

Clinical Status

Functional improvement occurred in the majority of the survivors. The average NYHA classes before and after surgery were 3 ± 0.04 and 1.8 ± 0.1, respectively. This improvement was also confirmed by a quality-of-life assessment, which was made before surgery and repeated at 6-mo intervals afterward. The assessment consisted of a questionnaire completed by the patient and family members, which yielded information on activities of daily living, social activities, quality of social interactions, and mental health. Significant increases in activities of daily living and social activities were found at 12 mo after operation for patients who had cardiomyoplasty. No improvement in maximum exercise capacity was seen, despite the evidence of improved functional capacity. Prior to cardiomyoplasty, the mean peak oxygen consumption for the group was approximately 15 mL O_2/kg per minute and this was not significantly different at 6 or 12 mo after operation. In addition, no changes in anaerobic threshold or total exercise time were detectable at 12 mo after operation (Table 115–1).

At first this discrepancy between functional capacity and maximum exercise capacity seems paradoxical. How can the patient be able to do more, but have no changes in exercise capacity? Two factors should be considered. First, maximum exercise capacity is measured in the laboratory and consists of very intense activity over a short period of time, usually less than 10 min. This type of activity is never performed by patients with CHF, except when they are evaluated in the laboratory. Submaximal exercise testing more closely approximates the activities of daily living. Second, the stimulation that was used in these patients has a fixed duration of 185 or 220 ms for muscle activation, regardless of the heart rate. Therefore, at heart rates greater than 120/min, which is the norm for peak exercise testing, performance of the patient may be limited by inadequate time for the latissimus dorsi muscle to fully relax between contractions. The next generation of cardiomyostimulators will avoid this potential problem by having a rate adaptation feature, which will reduce the duration of muscle stimulation as the heart rate increases.

Effects on Ventricular Function and Hemodynamics

Data obtained from MUGA scans showed modest but statistically significant improvement in cardiac function after surgery. Preoperative and 6-mo postoperative studies ($n =$ 33) showed increased LVEF (23.9 ± 7 vs 26.5 ± 11%), stroke volume (52.7 ± 16 vs 59.8 ± 20 mL/beat), and LV stroke work index (26.9 ± 10 vs 31.2 ± 12 g/m^2 per beat). No significant changes were found in cardiac index, pulmonary capillary wedge pressure, or heart rate. In fact, at 12 mo after operation there was a small increase in right atrial pressure and pulmonary artery mean pressure (Table 115–2).

Summary of Phase II Trial

The results of the recent experience with cardiomyoplasty provide cause for both optimism and pessimism about the

future of the procedure as therapy for cardiomyopathy. On the positive side, the procedure has now been shown to have measurable, beneficial effects on cardiac function. Improvements in LVEF, SV, and LVSWI are modest in magnitude, but are in direct contrast to the natural history of congestive heart failure, where progressive deterioration is the norm. The improved functional capacity has been noted many times before, but now has been confirmed by the quality-of-life assessment. From the patient's perspective, the improved functional capacity is the most important aspect of the operation and accounts for the enthusiastic comments that most patients have about the operation.

On the negative side, the failure to improve exercise capacity is disappointing. However, as noted before, maximum exercise testing is probably not a good measure of efficacy in this group of patients. Future studies will include measures of submaximal exercise capacity, such as a 6-min walk, which more closely reflects activities of daily living. The most disappointing aspect of the Phase II trial was the 1-year survival of only 68%, which is no better than the natural history of the disease without surgical intervention. It seems unlikely that the operation will become widespread until the survival rate is comparable to that after heart transplantation. Sudden death is the major problem in the first year after cardiomyoplasty, rather than CHF. A combination of an AICD with cardiomyoplasty is a logical potential solution to this problem, but this concept will need to be further evaluated before it can be recommended.

Future Studies

The next step in the development of cardiomyoplasty in the United States will be a multi-institutional, randomized, prospective study of medical therapy versus cardiomyoplasty. The study design calls for 300 patients to be randomized between these two options. End points for measuring efficacy will be survival, improved clinical status, submaximal exercise tolerance, and a need for subsequent hospitalizations for CHF. Due to the large number of patients, this trial will take several years to complete.

The Medtronic Corporation was recently granted approval to market the cardiomyostimulator in Europe; therefore, cardiomyoplasty is likely to develop more rapidly in Europe than in the United States. Surgeons in nonindustrialized countries have been doing cardiomyoplasty using commercially available dual-chambered pacemakers. The atrial channel senses a QRS and the ventricular channel stimulates the latissimus dorsi muscle with a single-spiked elec-

TABLE 115–1. MAXIMAL EXERCISE CAPACITY BEFORE AND AFTER CARDIOMYOPLASTY

	Preoperative ($n = 33$)	6 mo ($n = 33$)	Preoperative ($n = 20$)	12 mo ($n = 20$)
Peak Vo$_2$/kg (mL/min per kg)	14.99 ± 4.27	14.94 ± 4.52	15.69 ± 4.09	15.56 ± 5.66
Anaerobic threshold (mL)	904.63 ± 281.95	951.27 ± 380.72	902.88 ± 270.16	920.41 ± 372.38
Total exercise time (min)	6.79 ± 3.21	7.70 ± 3.25	7.12 ± 2.72	7.87 ± 3.58

TABLE 115–2. HEMODYNAMIC DATA BEFORE AND AFTER CARDIOMYOPLASTY

	Preoperative (*n* = 33)	6 mo (*n* = 33)	Preoperative (*n* = 20)	12 mo (*n* = 20)
Pulmonary capillary wedge pressure (mm Hg)	17.67 ± 10.15	17.20 ± 8.80	17.00 ± 7.65	18.89 ± 7.19
Left ventricular stroke work index (g/m per beat)	26.95 ± 10.39*	31.26 ± 12.15*	25.85 ± 8.74*	33.71 ± 13.47*
Right atrial pressure (mm Hg)	6.58 ± 3.39	7.74 ± 4.97	6.26 ± 2.73*	9.42 ± 3.89*
Cardiac index (L/min per m^2)	2.25 ± 0.58	2.34 ± 0.55	2.22 ± 0.65	2.47 ± 0.77
Stroke volume (mL/beat)	52.76 ± 16.35*	59.88 ± 20.24*	50.76 ± 13.81*	65.57 ± 19.54*
Mean pulmonary artery pressure (mm Hg)	25.84 ± 9.05	26.58 ± 10.05	25.89 ± 7.75*	29.05 ± 8.48*

*$p < 0.05$.

trical stimulus. This approach suffers from a lack of a burst stimulus to the skeletal muscle, but still may prove effective by limiting left ventricular dilatation and reducing left ventricular wall stress. Further information on the results of this approach will be forthcoming in the next several years.

OTHER APPLICATIONS OF SKELETAL MUSCLE CIRCULATORY SUPPORT

Diastolic Counterpulsation

Diastolic counterpulsation using paced diaphragm muscle was the first published use of skeletal muscle for circulatory support.[5] The problem of muscle fatigue and the lack of an implantable burst stimulator limited further work in this area for the next 20 years. Diastolic counterpulsation using paced-conditioned latissimus dorsi muscle has been the subject of multiple recent experimental publications.

Carpentier and Chachques developed an operation that has been termed aortomyoplasty, in which the ascending aorta is enlarged with a patch of pericardium and then encircled with the right latissimus dorsi muscle.[55] Contraction of the latissimus dorsi during diastole compresses the ascending aorta and causes augmentation of diastolic blood pressure. The enlargement of the ascending aorta increases the volume of blood that can be displaced by the muscle contraction, but creates an ascending aneurysm that increases the complexity of the procedure and raises concerns about the long-term safety of the operation. Studies in experimental animals show that the ascending aortomyoplasty can augment diastolic blood pressure and improve cardiac output in animals with heart failure.[56]

Most other researchers have used the descending aorta as the site for diastolic counterpulsation. Hymes et al and Hines et al confirmed that augmentation of diastolic blood pressure was possible using the latissimus dorsi.[57,58] Chiu et al used transformed skeletal muscle to compress an extra-aortic balloon, which then caused diastolic augmentation.[59] Pattison et al encircled the descending aorta with the left latissimus dorsi and demonstrated diastolic augmentation for up to 28 days after operation.[60] Lazzara et al developed a procedure in which a 4-cm-wide strip of the left latissimus

dorsi is used to encircle the distal transverse aortic arch and proximal descending aorta in an overlapping "barber-pole" fashion.[61] Diastolic aortic compression using this procedure has been compared to counterpulsation using an intra-aortic balloon pump in a series of acute and chronic experiments.[61–63] Diastolic aortic compression in animals with heart failure has been shown to increase diastolic blood pressure, reduce left ventricular end-diastolic pressure, and reduce left ventricular peak pressure by an amount equivalent to that achieved with an IABP.[63] Recent work has shown that the procedure can improve left ventricular regional function in an area of myocardial ischemia induced by occlusion of the LAD (Fig. 115–6).[64] Clinical application of the procedure will await further studies of the long-term effect of the operation on the aorta itself and its effects on the natural history of chronic congestive heart failure.

Skeletal Muscle Ventricles

The skeletal muscle ventricle (SMV) is another application of skeletal muscle power for circulatory support.[65] In this application the latissimus dorsi is fashioned into a neoventricle by wrapping it around a cylindrical plastic mandrel, allowing a 3-wk resting period, and then conditioning the muscle with a 2-Hz continuous stimulation for 6 wk. The mandrel is then removed and the SMV connected to the circulation. This requires the attachment of two valved conduits to the SMV, one for inflow and one for outflow.[66] Several configurations for SMVs have been tested, which means that an SMV can be used for right heart bypass, diastolic counterpulsation, or systolic left ventricular work.[67–70] The most efficient arrangement has been the LV apex to aorta, which has been able to pump approximately 50% of the systemic bloodflow over periods of weeks to months.[70]

There are several inherent problems with this approach to circulatory support.[71] The use of a blood-pumping chamber and prosthetic valves introduces the problem of thromboembolism and necessitates long-term anticoagulation. Another problem is the low compliance of the muscle pumping chamber. Over time the SMV becomes stiff and requires high filling pressures for optimal performance, which is necessary to provide adequate circulatory support and to prevent thromboembolism. This situation has limited

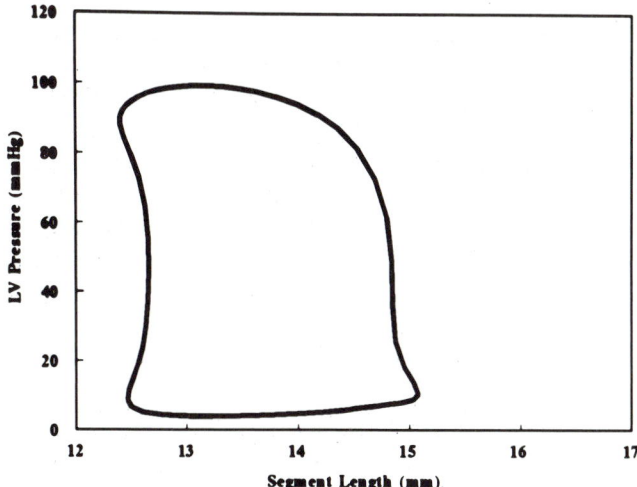

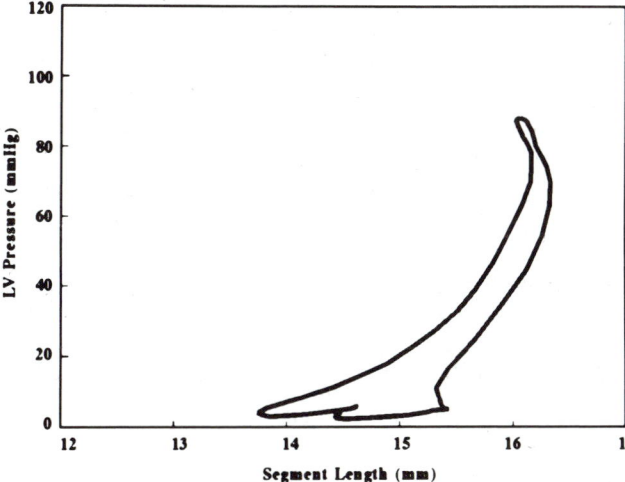

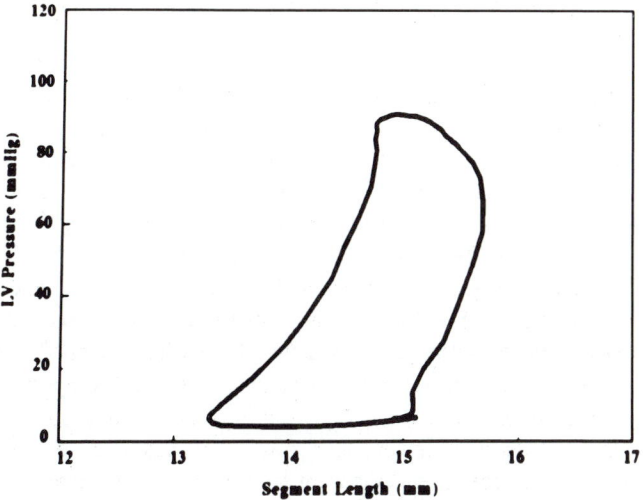

Figure 115–6. Three pressure–segment length loops are shown. The area inscribed by the loops is an estimate of regional stroke work. The top figure shows a normal loop, the middle figure shows the result of LAD ligation, and the bottom loop shows the effect of diastolic aortic compression after LAD ligation. Counterpulsation with the latissimus dorsi reduces paradoxical bulging of the ischemic myocardium during systolic and improves regional stroke work.

the usefulness of the left atrial to aortic configurarion, which is the most appealing approach from a practical viewpoint. Another problem with SMVs has been the structural integrity over time. Because the SMV operates at high filling pressures, generates systolic blood pressure, and cannot be allowed to rest, there have been problems with rupture of the ventricle, especially where the valved conduits are attached to the muscle ventricle.

None of these problems is insurmountable and active research continues in this area. The concept of a completely implantable, autogenous blood pump is a very attractive one. The capacity of an SMV to transfer systolic cardiac work from the left ventricle to the skeletal muscle is the chief advantage of this approach. Clinical application is the ultimate goal of the research and may be a feasible option within 5 years.

SUMMARY

Appreciation of the process of skeletal muscle transformation and advances in skeletal muscle training protocols have shown that contraction of the latissimus dorsi can provide sufficient power to assist the left ventricle. The major challenge now is to define and perfect the best method for harnessing and applying this power for circulatory support. To date, cardiomyoplasty has been the clinical method applied. The advantages of cardiomyoplasty over other types of circulatory support with skeletal muscle are (1) there is no added risk of thromboembolism since blood contact with artificial surfaces is avoided; (2) the technical aspects of the procedure have been defined and are easily learned; and (3) the procedure uses autogenous tissue and requires minimal implanted hardware. The clinical results of cardiomyoplasty have been inconsistent, which is not surprising for an operation in its early stage of development. The major problem with cardiomyoplasty from a fundamental perspective is that the procedure is an inefficient method for utilizing skeletal muscle power. The wrap configuration limits the power capacity of the latissimus dorsi, which is designed for linear shortening and not squeezing. Perhaps this is why the chronic effects of the operation of left ventricular function have been modest. However, the girdling effects of cardiomyoplasty on left ventricular volume have been striking and may form the rationale for more widespread application of the procedure for treatment of CHF.

Other forms of circulatory support using skeletal muscle are still in the experimental stage. Considerable work remains to be done before an SMV is ready for clinical application. Chronic diastolic counterpulsation using skeletal muscle is a less ambitious approach than others, but is more feasible from a technical perspective. Clinical trials of this procedure are planned pending additional chronic studies in animals.

REFERENCES

1. Parmley W: Pathophysiology and current therapy of congestive heart failure. *J Am Coll Cardiol* **13**:771–785, 1989
2. Smith WM: Epidemiology of congestive heart failure. *J Am Coll Cardiol* **55**(suppl):3A–8A, 1985
3. Stephenson LW, Fowler MB, Schroeder JS, et al: Patients denied cardiac transplantation for non-medical criteria: A control group. *J Am Coll Cardiol* **7**:9A, 1986
4. The CONSENSUS Trial Study Group: Effects of enalapril on mortality in severe congestive heart failure. *N Engl J Med* **316**:429–435, 1987
5. Kantrowitz A, McKennon WMP: The experimental use of the diaphragm as an auxiliary myocardium. *Surg Forum* **9**:266–268, 1959
6. Spotnitz HM, Merker C, Malin JR: Applied physiology of the canine rectus abdomenus. *Trans Am Soc Artif Int Organs* **20**:747–756, 1974
7. Buller AJ, Eccles JC, Eccles RM: Interaction between motor-neurons and muscles in respect of the characteristic speeds of their responses. *J Physiol* **150**:417, 1960
8. Salmons S, Sreter FA: Significance of impulse activity in the transformation of skeletal muscle type. *Nature* (*London*) **263**:30, 1976
9. Pette D, Smith ME, Staudte HW, et al: Effects of long-term electrical stimulation on some contractile and metabolic characteristics of fast rabbit muscles. *Pflügers Arch* **338**:257–272, 1973
10. Trumble DR, Magovern JA: Ergometric studies of untrained skeletal muscle demonstrate feasibility of muscle-powered cardiac assistance. *J Appl Physiol* **77**:2036–2041, 1994
11. Mannion JD, Bitto T, Hammond RL, et al: Histochemical and fatigue characteristics of conditioned canine latissimus dorsi muscle. *Circ Res* **58**:298–304, 1986
12. Pette D, Vrbová G: Adaptation of mammalian skeletal muscle fibers to chronic electrical stimulation. *Rev Physiol Biochem Pharmacol* **120**:115–202, 1992
13. Pette D, Staudte HW, Vrbová G: Physiological and biochemical changes induced by long-term stimulation of fast muscle. *Naturwissenschaften* **59**:469–470, 1972
14. Hilton SM, Jeffries MG, Vrbová G: Functional specialization of the vascular bed of the soleus muscle. *J Physiol (London)* **206**:543–562, 1970
15. Hudlická O, Brown M, Cotter M, et al: The effect of long-term stimulation of fast muscles on their blood flow, metabolism and ability to withstand fatigue. *Pflügers Arch* **369**:141–149, 1977
16. Brown MD, Cotter MA, Hudlická O, Vrbová G: The effects of different patterns of muscle activity on capillary density, mechanical properties and structure of slow and fast rabbit muscles. *Pflügers Arch* **361**:241–250, 1976
17. Reichmann H, Hoppeler H, Mathieu-Costello O, et al: Biochemical and ultrastructural changes of skeletal muscle mitochondria after chronic electrical stimulation in rabbits. *Pflügers Arch* **404**:1–9, 1985
18. Reichmann H, Wasl R, Simoneau J-A, Pette D: Enzyme activities of fatty acid oxidation and the respiratory chain in chronically stimulated fast-twitch muscle of the rabbit. *Pflügers Arch* **418**:572–574, 1991
19. Eisenberg BR, Salmons S: The reorganization of subcellular structure in muscle undergoing fast-to-slow type transformation. A stereological study. *Cell Tissue Res* **220**:449–471, 1981
20. Ramirez BU, Pette D: Effects of long-term electrical stimulation on sarcoplasmic reticulum of fast rabbit muscle. *FEBS Lett* **49**:188–190, 1974
21. Klug G, Wiehrer W, Reichmann H, et al: Relationships between early alterations in parvalbumin, sarcoplasmic reticulum and metabolic enzymes in chronically stimulated fast twitch muscle. *Pflügers Arch* **399**:280–284, 1983
22. Leberer E, Pette D: Immunochemical quantitation of sarcoplasmic reticulum Ca-ATPase, of calsequestrin and of parvalbumin in rabbit skeletal muscles of defined fiber composition. *Eur J Biochem* **156**:489–496, 1986
23. Schachat FH, Williams RS, Schnurr CA: Coordinate changes in fast thin filament and Z-line protein expression in the early response to chronic stimulation. *J Biol Chem* **263**:13975–13978, 1988
24. Härtner K-T, Pette D: Effects of chronic low-frequency stimulation on troponin I and troponin C isoforms in rabbit fast-twitch muscle. *Eur J Biochem* **188**:261–267, 1990
25. Roy RK, Mabuchi K, Sarkar S, et al: Changes in tropomyosin subunit pattern in chronic electrically stimulated rabbit fast muscles. *Biochem Biophys Res Commun* **89**:181–187, 1979
26. Kao RL, Trumble DR, Magovern JA, et al: Fatigue resistant muscle with preserved force and mass for cardiac assist. *J Cardiac Surg* **6**:210–217, 1991
27. Chachques JC, Grandjean PA, Schwartz K, et al: Effect of latissimus dorsi dynamic cardiomyoplasty on ventricular function. *Circulation* **78**:III206–216,1988
28. Ferguson AS, Stone HE, Roessmann U, et al: Muscle plasticity: Comparison of 30-Hz burst with 10-Hz continuous stimulation. *J Appl Physiol* **66**:1143–1151, 1989
29. Guldner NW, Eichstaedt HC, Klapproth P, et al: Dynamic training of skeletal muscle ventricles. A method to increase muscular power for cardiac assistance. *Circulation* **89**:1032–1040,1994
30. Lucas C, Van der Veen FH, Cheriex EC, et al: Long-term follow-up (12 to 35 weeks) after dynamic cardiomyoplasty. *J Am Coll Cardiol* **22**:758–767, 1993
31. Kalil R, Bocchi EA, Weiss R, et al: MRI evaluation of chronic morphologic changes in the latissimus dorsi cardiomyoplasty. *Circulation* **88**:A2889, 1993
32. Tobin G, Gu J-M, Tobin A-E, et al: Latissimus dorsi flap loss in cardiomyoplasty: Anatomic basis and prevention by delay. World Symposium on Cardiomyoplasty, Biomechanical Assist and Artificial Heart, Paris, France, May 24–26, 1993
33. Magovern GJ, Park SB, Magovern GJ Jr, et al: Latissimus dorsi as a functioning synchronously paced muscle component in the repair of a left ventricular aneurysm. *Ann Thorac Surg* **41**:116, 1986
34. Lee KF, Dignan RJ, Parmar JM, et al: Effects of dynamic cardiomyoplasty on left ventricular performance and myocardial mechanics in dilated cardiomyopathy. *J Thorac Cardiovasc Surg* **102**:124–31, 1991
35. Cheng W, Justicz AG, Soberman MS, et al: Effects of dynamic cardiomyoplasty on indices of left ventricular systolic and diastolic function in a canine model of chronic heart failure. *J Thorac Cardiovasc Surg* **103**:1207–1213, 1992
36. Millner RWJ, Burrows M, Pearson I, Pepper JR: Dynamic cardiomyoplasty in chronic left ventricular failure: An experimental model *Ann Thorac Surg* **55**:493–501, 1993
37. Park SE, Cmolik BL, Lazzara RR, et al: Right latissimus dorsi cardiomyoplasty augments left ventricular systolic performance. *Ann Thorac Surg* **56**:1290–1295, 1993
38. Cho PW, Levin HR, Curtis WE, et al: Pressure-volume analysis of changes in cardiac function in chronic cardiomyoplasty. *Ann Thorac Surg* **56**:38–45, 1993
39. Grandjean PA, Austin L, Chan S, et al: Dynamic cardiomyoplasty: Clinical follow-up results. *J Cardiac Surg* **6**:80–88, 1991
40. Furnary AP, Moreira LFP, Jessup M, et al: Dynamic cardiomyoplasty improves systolic ventricular function. Presented at the American Heart Association Meeting, Dallas, Texas, November 14–17, 1994
41. Capouya ER, Gerber RS, Drinkwater DC Jr, et al: Girdling effect of nonstimulated cardiomyoplasty on left ventricular function. *Ann Thorac Surg* **56**:867–871, 1993
42. Nakajima H, Niinami H, Hooper TL et al: Cardiomyoplasty: Probable mechanism of effectiveness using the pressure-volume relationship. *Ann Thorac Surg* **57**:407–415, 1994
43. Carpentier A, Chachques JC, Grandjean PA, et al: Dynamic cardiomyoplasty: A seven year clinical experience. *J Thorac Cardiovasc Surg* **106**:42–52, 1993
44. Magovern JA, Magovern GJ Sr, Maher TD Jr, et al: Operation for congestive heart failure: Transplantation, coronary artery bypass, and cardiomyoplasty. *Ann Thorac Surg* **56**:418–425, 1993

45. Kass DA, levin H, Cho P, et al: Mechanisms of ventricular improvement after cardiomyoplasty: Longitudinal report of a case studied by pressure-volume analysis. World Symposium on Cardiomyoplasty, Biomechanical Assist and Artificial Heart, Paris, France, May 24–26, 1993

46. Corin WJ, George DT, Sink JD, Santamore WP: Dynamic cardiomyoplasty acutely impairs left ventricular diastolic function. *J Thorac Cardiovasc Surg* **104**:1662–1671, 1992

47. Lazzara RR, Park SE, Cmolik BL, et al: Static left latissimus dorsi cardiomyoplasty: Effect on left ventricular function. *J Heart Lung Transplant* **12**:1024–1028, 1993

48. Cheng W, Avila RA, David BS, et al: Dynamic cardiomyoplasty: Left ventricular diastolic compliance at different skeletal muscle tensions. *Am Surgeon* **60**:128–131, 1994

49. Magovern JA, Furnary AP, Christlieb IY: Bilateral latissimus dorsi cardiomyoplasty. *Ann Thorac Surg* **52**:1259–1265, 1991

50. Furnary AP, Magovern JA, Christlieb IY, Trumble DR: Improved ventricular augmentation with right latissimus dorsi cardiomyoplasty. *Surg Forum* **42**:307–309, 1991

51. Magovern JA, Furnary AP, Christlieb IY, et al: Right latissimus dorsi cardiomyoplasty for left ventricular function. *Ann Thorac Surg* **53**:1120–1122, 1992

52. Magovern JA, Park SE, Cmolik BL, et al: Early effects of right latissimus dorsi cardiomyoplasty on left ventricular function. *Circulation* **88**:298–303, 1993

53. Carpentier A, Chachques J-C: Myocardial substitution with a stimulated skeletal muscle: First successful case. *Lancet* **1**:1267, 1985

54. Magovern GJ, Heckler FR, Park SB, et al: Paced latissimus dorsi used for dynamic cardiomyoplasty of ventricular aneurysms. *Ann Thorac Surg* **44**:379–388, 1987

55. Chachques JC, Grandjean PA, Cabrear-Fischer E, et al: Dynamic aortomyoplasty to assist left ventricular failure. *Ann Thorac Surg* **49**:225–230, 1990

56. Chachques JC, Haab F, Cron C, et al: Long-term effects of dynamic aortomyoplasty. *Ann Thorac Surg* **58**:128–134, 1994

57. Hymes W, Hines GL, Lenonick D, et al: Extra-aortic counterpulsation with a latissimus dorsi flap: Hemodynamic effects in a heart failure model. *J Cardiac Surg* **6**:184–189, 1991

58. Hines GL, Mishriki Y, Williams L, et al: Physiologic and pathologic evaluation of chronic extra-aortic counterpulsation with latissimus dorsi flap. *J Cardiovasc Surg* **32**:485–490, 1991

59. Chiu RCJ, Garret LW, Dewar LD, et al: Implantable extra-aortic balloon assist powered by transformed fatigue-resistant skeletal muscle. *J Thorac Cardiovasc Surg* **94**:694–701, 1987

60. Pattison CW, Cummings DVE, Williamson A, et al: Aortic counterpulsation for up to 28 days with autologous latissimus dorsi in sheep. *J Thorac Cardiovasc Surg* **102**:766–773, 1991

61. Lazzara RR, Trumble DR, Magovern JA: Autogenous cardiac assist with chronic descending thoracic aortomyoplasty. *Ann Thorac Surg* **57**:1540–1544, 1994

62. Lazzara RR, Park SE, Cmolik BL, et al: Static left latissimus dorsi cardiomyoplasty: Effect on left ventricular function. *J Heart Lung Transplant* **12**:1024–1028,1 993

63. Lazzara RR, Trumble DR, Magovern JA: Dynamic descending thoracic aortomyoplasty: Comparison with intraaortic balloon pump in a model of heart failure. *Ann Thorac Surg* **58**:366–371, 1994

64. Cardone J, Yoon P, Magovern JA: The effect of diastolic aortic compression on regional left ventricular function during coronary occlusion. Presented at the Circulatory Support Meeting of the Society of Thoracic Surgeons, Pittsburgh, PA, October 30, 1994

65. Acker MA, Hammond RL, Mannion JD, et al: An autologous biologic pump motor. *J Thorac Cardiovasc Surg* **94**:733–746, 1986

66. Acker MA, Anderson WA, Hammond RL, et al: Skeletal muscle ventricles in circulation: One to eleven weeks experience. *J Thorac Cardiovasc Surg* **94**:163–174, 1987

67. Bridges CR Jr, Hammond RL, DiMeo F, Stephenson LW: Functional right heart replacement with a skeletal muscle ventricle. *Circulation* **80**(Suppl III):183–191, 1989

68. Hooper TL, Hammond RL, Niimanni H, et al: Aortic counterpulsation with a valved skeletal muscle ventricle: Short term studies of coronary flow and left ventricular function. *BAM* **2**:159–168, 1992

69. Hooper TJ, Niimanni H, Hammond RL, et al: Skeletal muscle ventricles as left atrial-aortic pumps: Short-term studies. *Ann Thorac Surg* **54**:316–322, 1992

70. Lu H, Thomas GA, Hammond RL: Intrathoracic and extra thoracic skeletal muscle ventricles in circulation: Left ventricular apex-to-aorta configuration. *J Card Surg* **9**:332–342, 1994

71. Isoda S, Nakajima H, Hammond RL, et al: Skeletal muscle ventricle: 1993 update. *BAM* **3**:271–280, 1993

CHAPTER

116

Surgery for Bacterial Endocarditis

Robert W.M. Frater

Endocarditis can be defined as an infection that starts on the inner walls of the cardiac chambers and aortic root. It began to be recognized as a specific disease during the middle of the last century. Bacterial infection as the root cause, the relation of valvular disease as a predisposing factor, valvular incompetence as one lethal consequence, and embolism as another were brilliantly brought together by William Osler in the Goulstonian lectures delivered to the Royal College of Physicians of London in March 1885. The title of Osler's lectures was Malignant Endocarditis.[1] For the next 60 years the disease was indeed malignant. It took two main forms: subacute endocarditis with infection on valves or other cardiac structures damaged by disease; and acute endocarditis, in which normal valves became infected during the course of septicemia. The difference between the two forms was largely in the rate of progression to death. With the dawn of the antibiotic era after World War II the disease could finally be treated.[2,3] Success was limited to cases treated before hemodynamically significant valvular damage or the lethal consequences of embolism had occurred, and some cases remained in which the antibiotics for one reason or another failed to sterilize the infected tissue. For these cases it would be another 15 years before cardiac surgery would provide effective treatment. The role of the surgeon in the treatment of endocarditis had, however, been presaged in the preantibiotic era when Tubbs and Tourof cured cases of *Hemophilus* and *Streptococcus viridans* endocarditis associated with patent ductus arteriosus by ligation of the ductus.[4,5] The first case of active endocarditis undergoing a deliberate valve replacement was one of aortic endocarditis confined to the cusps reported in 1965 by Wallace et al. The essential contribution of this operation was the demonstration that, with the aid of antibiotics, a synthetic foreign body could be successfully implanted in the presence of bloodstream infection.[6]

PATHOGENESIS

There are five components determining the pathogenesis of bacterial endocarditis:

1. *Bacteremia.* Any infection can potentially cause bacteremia. Oral, urethral, and anal infections specifically are associated with bacteremias.[7,8] The relationship between benign and malignant colon disease and *Streptococcus bovis* endocarditis is well established.[8] Esophageal dilatation produces bacteremia, but esophagoscopy and echocardiography do not.[9] While dental manipulation provokes bacteremia, there are other more common dental causes of endocarditis. Guntheroth has shown that bacterial endocarditis follows a visit to the dentist in only 3.6% of cases (including those in which no bacterial prophylaxis was used). Dental extractions cause bacteremia lasting less than 15 min in 40% of patients. However, simple mastication produced transient bacteremia in 38% and brushing teeth or oral irrigation in 25% of subjects. Even more striking was the spontaneous occurrence of bacteremia without any specific activity in 11% of patients with acute dental disease waiting to be seen.[10] These data indicate that "physiological bacteremia" related to mastication[11] is a more important source of infection in cases of bacterial endocarditis.

Guntheroth also reports that in a 1-mo period with a diseased tooth leading to dental extraction on the last day of the month the accumulated hours of exposure to "physiologic" bacteremia is 900 times greater than that due to the extraction. Therefore dental hygiene is far more important than antibiotics in the prophylaxis of bacterial endocarditis.

All patients with intravascular lines are at risk for bacteremia as are patients who inject materials into their veins.

2. *Infected Endothelium.* Valves and other cardiac tissues with damaged endothelium are vulnerable to infection

1915

during bacteremia. Oka et al[12] created arteriovenous shunts in animals and showed a tendency for injected bacteria to infect an area of damaged endothelium on the venous wall by the jet of blood from the fistula. Rheumatic valves, regurgitant values, degenerative valves, and pulmonary artery adjacent to a patent ductus arteriosus, the right ventricular wall adjacent to a ventricular septal defect, and the bulging ventricular septum against which the anterior mitral leaflet makes contact during systolic anterior motion in IHSS (see Chapter 120) all have in common the presence of endothelium injured either by a primary disease or physical forces. Artificial heart valves present a variety of materials such as sewing rings of both mechanical and bioprosthetic valves and tanned xenograft tissue of biological valve cusps that are susceptible to infection.

3. *Hemodynamics.* Turbulence occurs at the areas of maximal narrowing in the circulation. Turbulence leads to high shear stresses, which, in contact with tissue, cause activation of "tissue factor," which in turn cause activation of platelets, important in the formation of vegetations. Beyond the high velocity turbulent area are areas of low velocity and low shear stresses; it is here that vegetations form and take root.[13,14] Classic experiments by Rodbard[15] using a Venturi tube of agar showed that bacterial colonies were localized just beyond the downstream orifice of the narrow part of the tube corresponding with the localization of vegetations on the atrial side of the incompetent mitral valve or on the ventricular side of an incompetent aortic valve. Bioprosthetic valves for the same reason develop vegetations on the downstream side of the cusps. In mechanical valves the change from high to low shear stresses occurs at the ring, and this is where vegetations are found in late cases of endocarditis, after satisfactory initial healing. Free floating, ultrasmooth occluders do not provide the opportunity for activation of tissue factors or a surface to which vegetations can adhere.

4. *The Nature of Infecting Bacteria.* The frequency of infection by various organisms is not directly related to the frequency of their occurrence in the bloodstream. For example, bacteremias due to *Escherichia coli* are common, while endocarditis due to this organism is relatively uncommon. *E. coli* are poorly invasive and a poor stimulus for platelet aggregation. Staphylococci, however, are a potent stimulus for platelet aggregation and are aggressively invasive: clumps of staphylococci within aggregations of platelets are thus more likely to adhere to areas of denuded endocardium. The properties of different organisms and their occurrence in the bloodstream determine their tendency to cause endocarditis.[14]

5. *Host Defenses.* Immune-compromised patients commonly have an indwelling access line or arteriovenous connection through which frequent injections are made. The combination of potential contamination and reduced resistance makes them continually at risk for endocarditis, as exemplified by renal dialysis patients. Also, patients who have undergone cardiopulmonary bypass have a temporar-

ily suppressed immune system.[15] Defenses against valvular infection also differ between the left and right side of the heart. Experimental and clinical evidence shows that antibiotic treatment is more effective on right-sided infections than left. The density of the bacterial inoculum, the extent of extravalvular infection, the frequency of intravegetation bacterial resistance, and lack of antimicrobial penetrance are all more marked on the left side. Some of these differences may be due to the differences in oxygenation between the left and right sides.[16]

PATHOLOGY

The initial stage of valvular infection is the surface vegetation, composed of platelets, fibrin, and microorganisms. Organisms multiply within the vegetations and are, to some extent, protected by this location from the defense mechanisms of the host and the action of antibiotics. They then migrate into the bloodstream producing repetitive bacteremias and may invade and destroy adjacent valves. Vegetations grow at variable rates and to variable sizes. They are initially soft and friable and often break away to produce the emboli characteristic of the clinical manifestations of endocarditis. Clinical manifestations may also be due to deposition of immune complex components and allergic vasculitis involving small arteries.[17] Fungal vegetations are particularly likely to grow to large sizes. As vegetations mature they become firmer and ultimately can become organized and calcified.

The larger the vegetation, the more likely is embolism, valve destruction, and failure of antibiotic cure. Penetration of antibiotics into the core of vegetations is inversely related to size. Continued bacterial activity gives more chance of digestion of the underlying valve tissue.

Vegetative material attached to underlying or earlier vegetative material is less secure than that attached directly to cusp tissue, and hence more likely to embolize. Vegetations of more than 1 cm in diameter are significantly more often associated with the indicators of failed treatment.[18,19] Conversely, the absence of echocardiographically detectable vegetations is accompanied by significantly less risk of embolism, congestive heart failure, need for surgery, and death.[20] Occasionally very large vegetations may block a valve.[21] Embolic vegetations may occlude a coronary artery, resulting in infarction.

The initial infection is on the surface of the valve. Depending on the invasiveness of the infecting organism and the duration of untreated infection, the underlying tissue may be variably involved. Once invasion takes place tissue damage is inevitable and so also is the potential for rupture of cusps or chordae.

When infection occurs at the annulus of natural valves and on the sewing ring of artificial valves, it can produce destruction of the adjacent cardiac skeleton. This may occur anywhere in the aortic root. The commissure between the left and the right coronary cusps is a common site for ex-travalvular extension and may cause compression of the left main coronary artery. Infection at the commissure between the right and noncoronary cusps and the membranous sep-tum can lead to a left bundle branch block, ventricular sep-tal defect, and secondary tricuspid infection.[22] Infection of the mitral annulus is almost entirely confined to the mural portion. At the medial side, the conducting system can be af-fected as an abscess burrows into the His bundle or its blood supply. Perivalvular extension is rarer around the tricuspid and pulmonic annulae. Perivalvular extensions, when acute, can contain gross pus even though open to the bloodstream.

Aortic valve endocarditis in IHSS may extend into the hypertrophied septum where it makes contact with the mitral valve.[23] A punched-out hole in the anterior leaflet of the mitral valve may result where the jet of aortic insufficiency is striking it.

COMPLICATIONS

Emboli

Emboli may be infected and produce ischemia, abscesses, and mycotic aneurysms. Renal infarcts may present as hy-persensitivity vasculitis.[24] Central nervous system compli-cations may be the result of diffuse arteritis producing widespread petechiae, sterile emboli producing white in-farcts, septic emboli producing erosive arteritis and cerebral hemorrhage, or, less often, a mycotic aneurysm with de-layed effects.[25,26]

Central Nervous System Complications and Cardiopulmonary Bypass

A common fear is that a hemorrhagic infarct will be aggra-vated by heparinization on bypass. Other mechanisms for deterioration of central nervous system function include (1) increased cerebrospinal fluid production associated with midbrain emboli (Fig. 116–1) and (2) raised central venous pressure from a blocked superior vena caval cannula, which, for example, will have more serious consequences if the brain is recovering from recent injury.

Cardiac Failure

Congestive failure is dependent upon the valve involved, the degree of valvular insufficiency, and compensation of the ventricle. Acute severe aortic insufficiency is less well tolerated by an uncompensated left ventricle than acute se-vere mitral insufficiency.

Indications for Surgery

When medical management has failed or is likely to fail, surgery is indicated. There is some difference between fail-ure or likelihood of failure in the treatment of natural valve and artificial valve infections.

NATURAL VALVES

Indications for Surgery With Left-Sided Endocarditis

1. *Congestive cardiac failure related to valve disrup-tion* is an unequivocal indication. If acute cardiac failure de-velops in the course of antibiotic treatment surgery should be performed as soon as possible. If the organism is antibi-otic sensitive, subsequent cultures may be negative after 2 or 3 days: there is thus no reason to wait a prescribed num-ber of weeks for antibiotic therapy before surgery in pa-tients who have developed congestive failure.

2. *Development of severe valvular insufficiency with-*

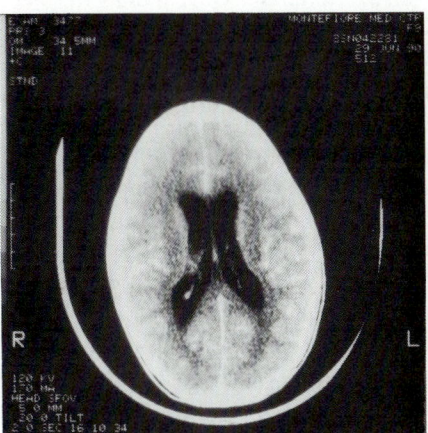 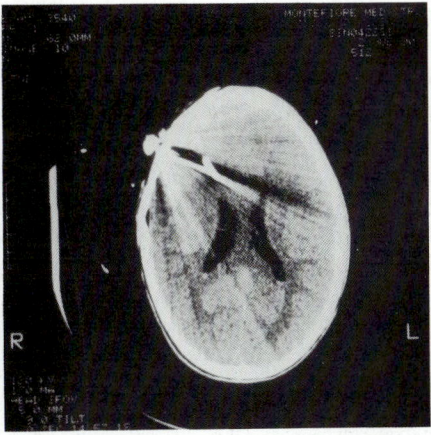 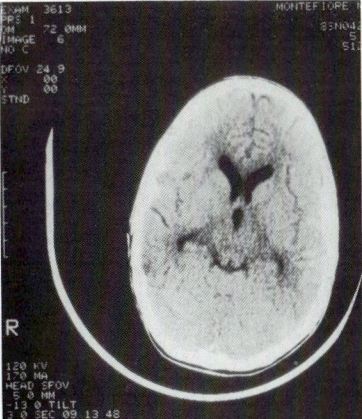

Figure 116–1. CT brain scans of a 5-year-old child with endocarditis. While on antibiotic therapy for endocarditis the patient became comatose due to a midbrain embolism producing acute hydrocephalus (left). Drainage of the cerebral ventricles relieved the coma (mid-dle). During cardiopulmonary bypass drainage increased dramatically. Postoperatively the tube was removed and the child made an ex-cellent recovery, the cerebral ventricle returning to normal (right).

out severe congestive failure is usually a compelling indication for surgery. Grade IV insufficiency, particularly of the aortic valve, presages the development of failure in a majority of cases so that delay is not recommended. In severe aortic insufficiency, an S3 gallop, mitral valve flutter, or premature closure and pulmonary congestion constitute clear indications for urgent surgery. The urgency is not quite so great with severe mitral insufficiency, but pulmonary edema usually occurs rapidly and therefore delay is not recommended.

3. *Extra valve extension* is an unequivocal indication of antibiotic failure and the potential for fatal complications. Perivalvular abscesses can heal and stabilize so that they present as nonexpanding smooth-walled cavities in the atrioventricular or ventriculoaortic annuli, but this outcome cannot be predicted in the active phase so that echocardiographic demonstration of a perivalvular abscess must be followed by urgent surgery.

4. *Multiple emboli* are usually an indication for surgery when endocarditis effects the *left-sided valves.* However, identification of multiple emboli is not always straightforward. Many of the clinical manifestations of endocarditis, such as Osler's nodes, retinal hemorrhage, and hematuria, may be caused by emboli. In the absence of significant valvular insufficiency, a small embolus causing, for example, a fingertip infarct, in the presence of Osler's nodes and microhematuria, does not necessarily indicate the need for urgent surgery. Autopsies may show infarctions that were never clinically manifest during life. Mycotic aneurysms may rupture or otherwise declare themselves weeks after the end of therapy without ever having presented earlier as emboli. Frontal lobe emboli are most often silent and a CT scan of the brain taken after an apparently single cerebral embolus may show several infarcts of various ages. The classical use of the term "Multiple" emboli therefore presumes that more than one embolus is a warning sign that further emboli may occur and produce cumulative critical damage, and acknowledges that many patients with one clinically detectable embolus never have another during a successful course of treatment.

Modern echocardiography allows a more rational approach to embolism as a surgical indication. All emboli are vegetations shed by the infected valve. If embolism occurs, the presence or absence of vegetations must be determined by transthoracic echocardiography and, if a clear answer is not obtained, should be followed by transesophageal echocardiography. In the absence of visible vegetations a single embolus does not constitute an indication for surgery. With an echocardiographically detectable vegetation, surgery is appropriately advised, since the patient has a type of vegetation that has already embolized and therefore is prone to further embolization.

The larger and more mobile the vegetation, the stronger the indication to proceed with surgery. The occurrence of multiple emboli remains an indication, although

the presence or absence of vegetations should help make the decision.

The type of organism is important: the frequency of embolic events is greater with infections caused by fastidious, slow-growing Gram-negative bacilli such as *Hemophilus parainfluenzae,* nutritionally variant *Streptococcus viridans,* and fungi that have a tendency to form large mobile vegetations.

Emboli from right-sided valves are a less pressing indication for surgery. Surgery is indicated if emboli produce multiple lung abscesses. Multiple bland infarcts are a more common consequence of tricuspid or pulmonic vegetations than abscesses and, by themselves, are not an indication for surgery.

5. *Persistent infection* may be defined as the persistence, despite proper antibiotic therapy, of positive blood cultures or systemic signs of infection in the form of leucocytosis, fever, and a raised sedimentation rate, usually combined with symptoms of "toxicity" such as tiredness, lassitude, and weakness. "Proper antibiotic therapy" is pivotal to this definition. The organism and its sensitivity to antibiotics must be known. The dosage schedule must be appropriate to achieve persistently high blood levels to achieve a cure.[27] There must be proof in the form of multiple measurements of blood levels that the goal is being achieved. If these criteria are met and infection continues it is appropriate to operate, even in the absence of other indications. Fever may, of course, be related to the antibiotics used; it is reasonable to assume this when it is the *only* manifestation of "persistent infection." Therefore, antibiotics should be stopped for 2 days and the patient recultured.

6. Infection by *resistant organisms* is an important indication for surgery. This situation takes two forms: (1) the organism may have been tested and found to be a strain resistant to all available antibiotics; or (2) the organism may be known from experience to respond poorly to antibiotic therapy. An obvious example is a blood culture positive for fungal species. Other poorly responsive organisms are *Herellia,* and Gram-negative organisms such as *Pseudomonas* and *Serratia. Staphylococcus aureus* is generally regarded as an organism that virtually always requires surgery for cure.

7. In various forms, echocardiographically defined *vegetations* are a relative indication for surgery. *Size* is the major determinant of this indication. Vegetations larger than 1 cm in two-dimensional size are more likely to be associated with embolism, valve disruption, and tearing of valve tissues during treatment.[18,19] However, these complications do not always occur with 1-cm vegetations. For example, in a new case with a *Streptococcus* infection that is sensitive to penicillin, and a valve that is intact and competent, but has a 1-cm vegetation, it is reasonable to continue antibiotic treatment. If the initial response shows an immediate fall in temperature and resolution of toxicity the importance of the 1-cm vegetation lessens. If infection persists

for more than a few days, a single embolus occurs, or the valve becomes insufficient, surgery is indicated. The larger the vegetation, the stronger is its relative importance. Mobile vegetations carry a special implication: they are always attached to a torn piece of cusp or broken chorda. Such vegetations do not always produce emboli: they may become organized, quite firm, and no longer likely to break away. Nor are they necessarily associated with significant incompetence: the torn cusp may be hemodynamically small or the broken chorda single. They are never attached by a stalk of pure vegetation, mobility always indicates some valve damage and therefore increases the importance of this as a relative indication for operation.

Rarely a large vegetation may block the mitral valve.[21] This is more likely to happen with fungal infections (Fig. 116–2). Conversely, cases without visible vegetations seldom need surgery.[20]

8. The indications for surgery are not always clear-cut. Good clinical judgment, even in the modern era of ever more precise and sophisticated diagnostic techniques, still requires the making of hard decisions on soft data. In cases of bacterial endocarditis this is common: when surgery is unequivocally indicated, the results are strikingly better than the results of medical treatment. It follows that when the indications are less certain, a wrong decision against surgery may carry more serious consequences for the patient than a wrong decision for surgery. The development of perivalvular extension, during a prolonged attempt at avoiding surgery, should be regarded as a mark of bad decision making: the surgery will be less beneficial to the patient and its risk will be increased. The development of a permanent crippling cerebral deficit or a central retinal occlusion must

be similarly regarded. Therefore, several "soft" indications for surgery are better taken as an indication than not. For example, the presence of a 1-cm vegetation, a persistent low-grade fever, and a white cell count of 13,000, and one transient cerebral ischemic episode after 8 days of antibiotics should constitute an indication for surgery.

Indications for Surgery With Right-Sided Endocarditis

The indications differ with right-sided disease partly because antibiotic therapy is more effective on the right[16] and, when it fails, the consequences of valve disruption and emboli are less. Patients can tolerate right heart failure in the resting state and the pulmonary vascular bed can absorb many emboli without critical long-term consequences. The indications then become modified in the following way:

1. *Heart failure* in the form of hepatomegaly, ascites, and peripheral edema is an indication for elective rather than emergency surgery. Any complication of right heart failure such as hepatic dysfunction is an indication for surgery.

2. *Gross valvular insufficiency* is similarly not an urgent indication. In the case of the pulmonary valve, gross insufficiency is well tolerated in the presence of normal right ventricular pressures and even with raised pressures, serious consequences may not occur for years. Although it is commonly believed that the same applies to gross tricuspid insufficiency,[28] this is in fact not so: even in the presence of normal right ventricular pressures patients have raised resting systemic venous pressure, an abnormal exercise tolerance, and a need for continued medical therapy.[29]

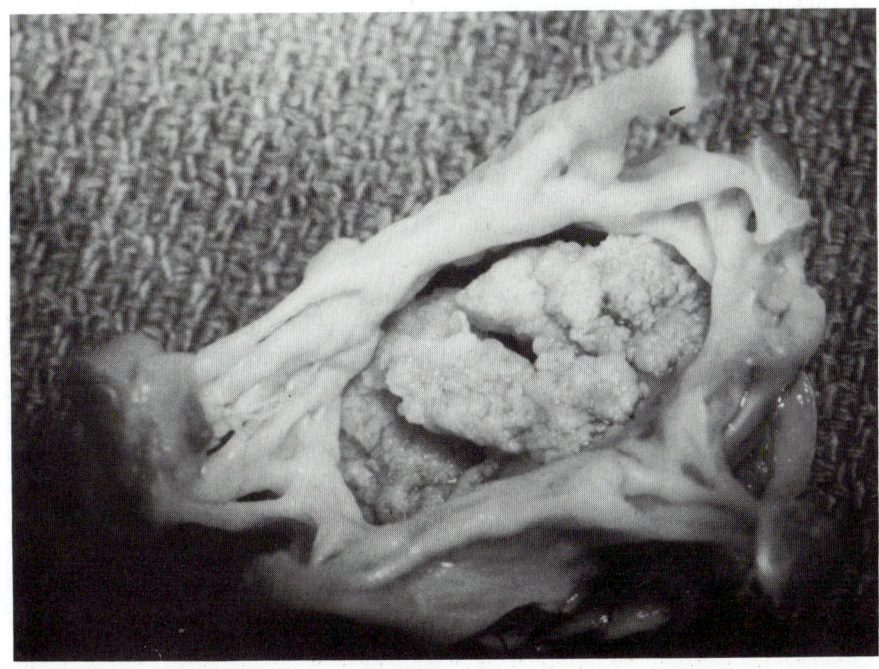

Figure 116–2. Fungal vegetation obstructing the mitral valve.

3. *Extravalvular extension* is an indication for surgery but rarely occurs.

4. *Multiple emboli* may produce multiple pulmonary abscesses. If these respond rapidly to antibiotic treatment they may be followed. When they lead to persistent fever, pyopneumothorax, or severe hemoptysis, surgery is indicated.

5. *Persistent infection, i.e., failure of antibiotic therapy,* is a prime indication for surgery of tricuspid endocarditis. In our experience most cases respond to antibiotic therapy. Only 25% of our cases required surgery and all were for failure of antibiotic therapy as judged by continued sepsis, or positive blood cultures.[19,22]

6. *Large and mobile vegetations* are associated with a greater chance of embolism, valve disruption, and antibiotic failure. In our experience with staphylococcal tricuspid endocarditis medical failures occurred only when there were vegetations larger than 1 cm in diameter. Nevertheless, the majority of cases presenting with vegetations of this size were successfully treated by antibiotic therapy.[19,22,29]

Indications for Surgery With Infection of Artificial Valves

Much of the published literature on infection of artificial valves describes extremely high mortality from both medical and surgical treatment. In one collective review the overall mortality for nonsurgical treatment was 65% and for surgical 46%.[30] Much of this literature also describes artificial valves that have dehisced or have extensive perivalvular infection. A distinction is also consistently made between infection occurring early (i.e., within 2 mo of valve replacement), and late, with nonsurgical mortality in this group being 81% while the surgical mortality was 63%. The early postoperative cases have a higher incidence of perivalvular extension. There is also a relationship between a long preoperative history and the presence of perivalvular infection. Finally, when infection occurs in the presence of foreign material, it is more difficult to cure with antibiotics. Indications include the following:

1. *Congestive cardiac failure* secondary to artificial valve dehiscence perivalvular leak, or high output failure secondary to sepsis.

2. *Multiple emboli* with abscess formation.

3. *Persistent infection* as demonstrated by a persistent low-grade fever and white count elevation after 6 wk of antibiotic therapy with or without positive blood cultures. The significance of bacteremia in the presence of an artificial heart valve was studied in 171 patients. During an observation period of 1 year 43% of the patients developed endocarditis, 56 at the time of the original bacteremia and 18 later. Indwelling intravascular lines accounted for 33% of the bacteremias, and skin infections and wounds for 28%.[31]

4. *Vegetations* are not particularly useful as an indication for surgery: whether transthoracic or transesophageal echocardiography is being used, vegetations are often poorly visible because of shielding or scattering of echo by the valve structures. When in the first week after valve surgery a positive blood culture has been obtained during a febrile episode in a patient with no other evidence of valve infection the presence of a vegetation confirms the diagnosis.[32]

In summary, valve infection occurring in the first 2 mo after valve replacement will virtually always require surgery. There is no virtue in an attempted cure by prolonged antibiotic therapy. The only exception is when infection is feared because of an isolated incidental positive blood culture with no known cause, without other evidence pointing to valve infection. The assumption is a bacteremia (possibly from manipulation of an intravascular line) that did not seed the valve. We prefer 2 to 3 wk of intravenous antibiotics and then observation for evidence of endocarditis over the next few weeks.

In late-occurring infection, mechanical valves, because of the sewing ring location of the infection, present significant dangers of early spread to the perivalvular tissues. There are cases that are successfully sterilized, but the emphasis must be on performing surgery early rather than late and on very careful post-treatment surveillance and strict criteria of successful treatment. Bioprosthetic valves, on the other hand, with vegetations usually located on the downstream side of the cusps rather than the sewing ring, may actually be cured by antibiotics if the treatment is started early enough. Bacteriologic cure may leave the valve with insufficiency due to cusp damage or with a tendency to premature calcification. In our experience this does not produce surgical mortality much different from that of endocarditis of natural valves, whereas late surgery for failed treatment of a mechanical valve infection certainly carries a higher morality than that for elective replacement. Endocarditis of homografts and from the early evidence, perhaps stentless xenografts, may be less common than infection of other devices.[33] In the absence of, or the presence of less, inorganic material the response of these devices seems closer to that of the natural valve. The indications for surgery are the same.

The late bacteriologically cured patient is treated as are other cases of valvular disease. The indications are the same as for valvular disease in general. They are commonly able to be repaired, and this will influence the willingness to perform early surgery in a young patient. Repair commonly demands the use of materials or tissue to replace or augment tissues previously destroyed by the infection.

HIV positive patients, because of the potentially long time before the transition to AIDS, have the same indication for surgery as HIV negative patients. However, our experience and that of others indicates that the patients with active sepsis at the time of surgery have a tendency for the infection to persist despite appropriate surgery.[34] The prognosis is therefore worse, but the indication for surgery is not changed. When the patient develops the criteria for the diagnosis of AIDS, it has been our policy to refuse surgery on the grounds that the results of surgery are too poor to justify operation. Patients with AIDS can survive the operation, but all die within months from progression of the disease.

Intravenous drug abuse is not a definite contraindication to surgery.[35] Enough addicts survive 10 years after surgery that contaminated intravenous injection, as the cause of the endocarditis, is not a reason to avoid operation. Addicts who survive 10 years after their initial operation are a heterogeneous group: some have given up intravenous drug abuse, with or without the use of an oral narcotic substitute such as methadone; some have continued to use intravenous drugs intermittently or continuously but seem to have learned to avoid bacterial contamination or drug overdoses. Since others die from continued use of drugs the question is whether those patients can be identified in advance. An indication of certain failure is the patient who takes intravenous drugs while on antibiotic therapy in the hospital. When there is no history of gainful employment there is little chance of success. When family and friends are involved and united in their desire to see the patient change there is a good chance of success. The patient who states unequivocally that he or she will not give up intravenous drug use presents a difficult problem: should they be required to sign up with a clean needle program as a condition of being accepted for surgery? There is no easy answer to these questions, which clearly extend beyond the scope of surgery to a combination of character analysis of individuals and general societal issues. The surgeons' prime duty is to the patient. There is an additional duty to the other patients needing attention and decisions can legitimately be made, when indications are equal, to take first the patients with the best chance of long-term success.

Preoperative Investigation

The preoperative investigation of patients with endocarditis is no different from that of other cardiac patients. The pathology needs to be precisely defined and it is valuable to quantitate the cardiac physiologic disorder. Since the advent of two-dimensional echocardiography it has rarely been necessary to use any other tool to define the pathology and measure the valvular regurgitation and ventricular function. For the last 15 years the only indication for coronary angiography in our practice has been the suspicion or fear of coronary disease, especially in the patient older than 50 years. The development of this policy was predicated by access to high-quality echocardiography and the incidence of diffuse cerebral embolism during cardiac catheterization in patients with aortic endocarditis.

The other necessary investigations are directed to the known complications of endocarditis: hematologic disorders and particularly platelet dysfunction, renal dysfunction, cerebral embolism, distal septic foci, and hepatic dysfunction, especially in addicts with hepatitis but also related to high right-sided pressures and sepsis.

Timing of the Operation

When a major indication for surgery exists the only justification for delay is the presence of a general condition that will make the mortality of the operation excessive unless corrected.

Acute central nervous system damage may be a reason for postponing surgery.[36] Patients with endocarditis who are in coma at the time of cardiopulmonary bypass generally do not recover neurologically. Evidence by CT scan or MRI that there is a hemorrhagic infarct presents a serious risk of aggravation by anticoagulation. The usual time recommended for healing of a hemorrhagic infarct is 10 days. The timing of surgery is dependent on daily evaluation of both neurologic and cardiac status. The determination of the cerebral pathology by CT or MRI is a very important aid in this decision.

Renal failure due to glomerulonephritis should be followed through the acute phase. Prerenal failure, on the other hand, is a reason to operate early to correct the causative hemodynamic abnormality. Whatever the cause, the ability to use a hemoconcentrator, venovenous hemodialysis, or peritoneal dialysis makes postponement unnecessary when the cardiac indication is severe.

Thrombocytopenia due to sepsis will improve as the infection comes under control, and is a reason for postponement if possible. Thrombocytopenia due to antiplatelet antibodies will not quickly improve and must be treated acutely with immune globulin and platelet transfusions prior to surgery.

Pericarditis is not a reason to delay surgery. Even when the fluid is cloudy, it is virtually always sterile, and does not influence the outcome of surgery.

Pneumonia should be treated but must not delay essential surgery.

THE OPERATION

Preparation

CNS injury can usually be helped when the cerebral ventricles are dilated following a midbrain embolus. A ventricular catheter allows increased cerebrospinal fluid production that occurs during extracorporeal circulation to drain off rather than produce a rise in intracranial pressure (Fig. 116–1). Rarely subarachnoid hemorrhage occurs as a result of rupture of a mycotic aneurysm of the circle of Willis. Surgical obliteration of the ruptured aneurysm must be achieved before proceeding to cardiac surgery.

Sites of extracardiac infection are sometimes present at the time of cardiac surgery. It is generally not necessary to treat these before the cardiac operation. Hepatic and even splenic abscesses can commonly be handled by percutaneous tube drainage. Splenectomy may be needed for the occasional large splenic abscess. Infected renal emboli generally need no treatment beyond antibiotics.

Dental consultation should always be obtained before surgery. If a source of infection is identified, the source should be eliminated preoperatively. This commonly requires extraction and drainage of abscess cavities.

Choice of Operation

The choice of operation is governed by the degree and acuity of the pathology as well as other issues such as age, the presence of other diseases, and the reliability and social circumstances of the patient.

Repair is a reasonable, perhaps even prefer e, option for mitral, tricuspid, and less often aortic en rditis in which the infection has been controlled. Whe antibiotic course has been completed the decision is dent on the proportion of functional to destroyed tissu ccess is more likely if the functional tissue is normal, i. f the endocarditis occurred on a normal valve. Ge rally the amount of damaged valve must be less than 50% of the total if there is to be much hope of success. Examples that have, in our experience, made repair quite feasible are perforations of the anterior leaflet of the mitral valve associated with aortic endocarditis, ruptured anterior leaflet main chordae, destruction of the base of the lateral half of the posterior leaflet and adjacent left atrial wall with atrioventricular separation, perforations of the aortic valve, and destruction of the anterior leaflet of the tricuspid valve. In each case there is a necessity to substitute new material for that which has been destroyed. For these purposes we use tanned xenograft pericardium or briefly tanned autogenous pericardium and Gore-Tex sutures. Currently available tanned xenograft pericardium will thicken and become stiff but so long as the remaining natural tissue is supple the repaired valve will remain functional. Briefly tanned autogenous pericardium promises to change less with time. The tanning should be no longer than 10 min: if tanned longer it will behave like tanned xenograft pericardium. New treatments of xenograft tissue will result in tissues that stay pliable and acquire endothelium.[37] Gore-Tex sutures are excellent substitutes for destroyed chordae, essentially providing the host with the opportunity to grow a new chorda complete with fibrous tissue and intima.[38] Partial homograft replacements have been used successfully for repair of partial destruction of both atrioventricular and semilunar valves.[39]

Depending on the pathology the question arises whether one should repair a valve if there has been only a few days of antibiotic therapy and proof of sterility is not known. The limiting factor is the quality of tissue that must hold sutures to make the repair possible. It must be possible to excise back to tissue that is obviously not inflamed and, by implication, weakened by the infectious process. This does not imply that there can be no organisms in the area of repair. Since endocarditis without vegetations can generally heal with antibiotic therapy so can repaired valves.[40] We have had no recurrent infections in patients treated by valve repair in the active stage of the infection (Figs. 116–3, 116–4, 116–5, and 116–6).

Valve excision has been advocated for tricuspid endocarditis in intravenous drug addicts.[28] The reasons given for choosing this treatment are: (1) that it is possible to survive without the tricuspid valve in the absence of pulmonary hypertension; (2) prevention of recurrent potential infection produced by a foreign body in an infected area, and (3) avoidance of infection of the prosthesis if the addict resumes his or her previous habit. One-third of these patients require subsequent tricuspid valve replacement.

The prime determinant of long-term prognosis in addicts is their ability to stop injecting contaminated material into their bloodstreams. It is likely that the success described by Dr. Arbulu is related to his exceptional success at following his patients and keeping them from returning to their former habits, rather than the absence of a tricuspid valve.[41] It must be emphasized that the surgeon's task in dealing with addicts is not confined to operating but carries with it a serious obligation to get the patient into a rehabilitation program and encourage him or her to stay in it. Dr. Arbulu achieves this by following his patients personally and indefinitely. The indefinite follow-up accepts that years of freedom from intravenous drug abuse do not guarantee no return to the practice. Thus a delayed replacement of the tricuspid valve is no guarantee that the device will not be subject to bacterial contamination during its life. Our approach to these patients is to oblige them to enter a rehabilitation program and replace their tricuspid valves: if they stay off drugs they will do well without need for heart failure therapy or a second tricuspid valve insertion; if they do not their prognosis is inevitably poor.

The Choice of Device

The choice between *mechanical, bioprosthetic,* and *biologic* devices may be made according to the usual criteria, which involve age, the presence of renal disease or hyperparathyroidism, risk of bleeding on anticoagulants, ability of the patient to take anticoagulants reliably, and, of course, the patient's preference. There is, however, strong opinion that a homograft valve or even a pulmonary autograft is less likely to be followed by recurrent infection than either a stent-mounted xenograft or a mechanical valve.[42–45] It has also been suggested that there is an advantage of a xenograft over a mechanical valve, although this has been challenged.[46,47] The reason recurrent infection does not always occur is that the infection is often confined to the cusp tissue, all of which is removed. The valvular foreign body is then sewn to uninfected tissue. It is in the bloodstream in direct contact with endogenous cellular and humoral defenses as well as exogenous antibiotics; this is very different from the situation in which a foreign implant is surrounded by soft tissues or bone. When there is perivalvular

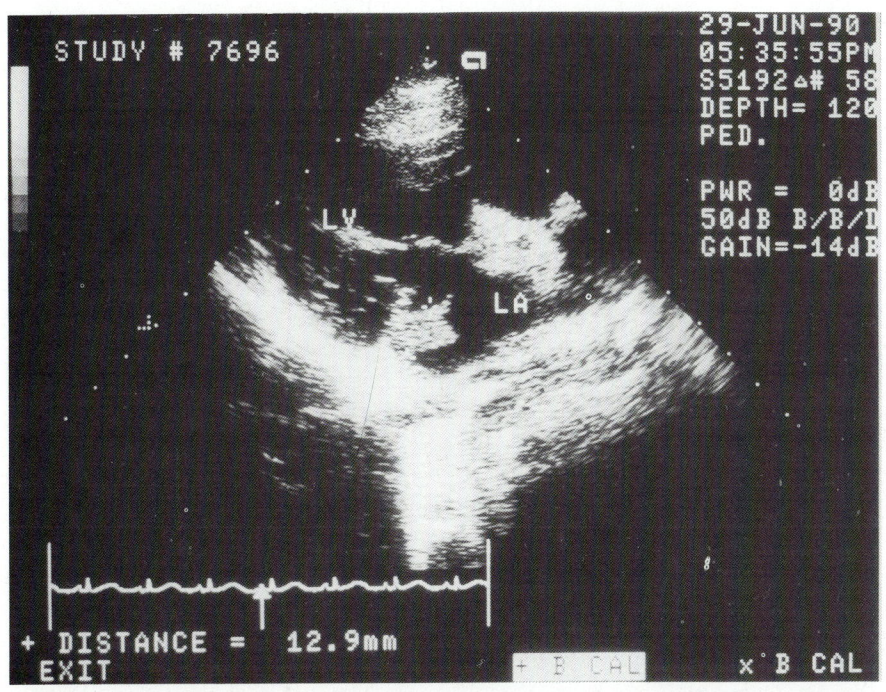

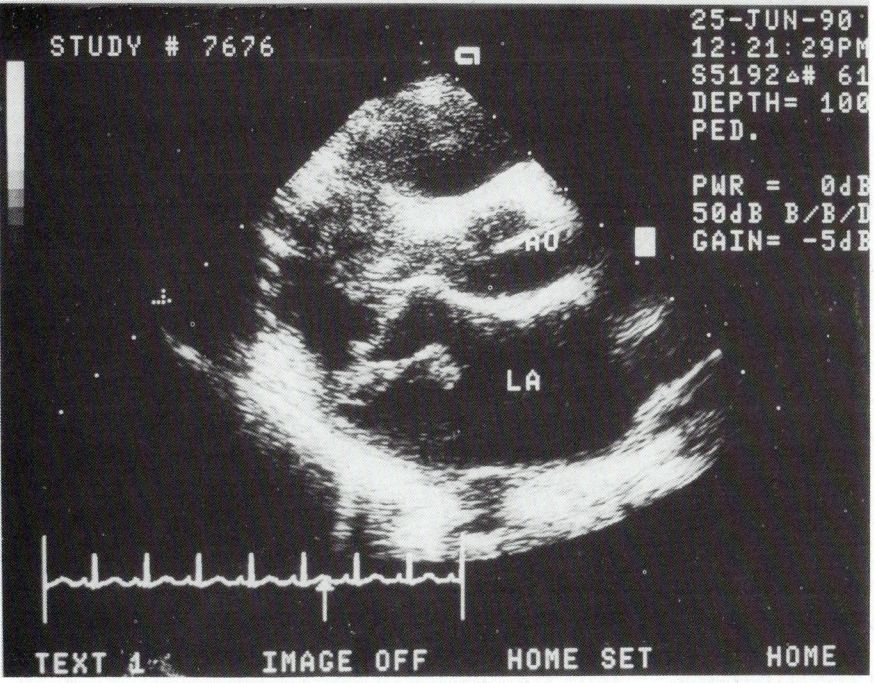

Figure 116–3. Preoperative echocardiogram of a 5-year-old child with endocarditis. Top: in diastole a large vegetation is seen to involve the mitral posterior cusp, the ventricle, and the atrium. Bottom: in systole the vegetation is elongated and a jet of insufficiency passes through it from ventricle to atrium.

extension the situation is changed: infected material left behind may be trapped between the annulus and the foreign materials of the sewing ring in a closed space and the classic predisposition of the foreign body to interfere with the control of bacterial infection is present. It should not then matter whether there is a mechanical occluder or a xenograft aortic valve inside the synthetic ring. It may, however, matter that the material in contact with the infected tissues is biological rather than synthetic, i.e., that the valve is a homograft rather than the synthetic fabric of a

stent-mounted valve. Users of homograft aortic valves uniformly report that the incidence of recurrent infection in the aortic position is less if a homograft is used. It remains to be seen whether the relatively thin layer of synthetic cloth that is present around the aortic remnant of some of the stentless aortic valves undergoing clinical trials will influence the rate of recurrent infection.

With perivalvular infection of the aortic valve resulting in aortoventricular discontinuity, an aortic valve-containing conduit may be needed.

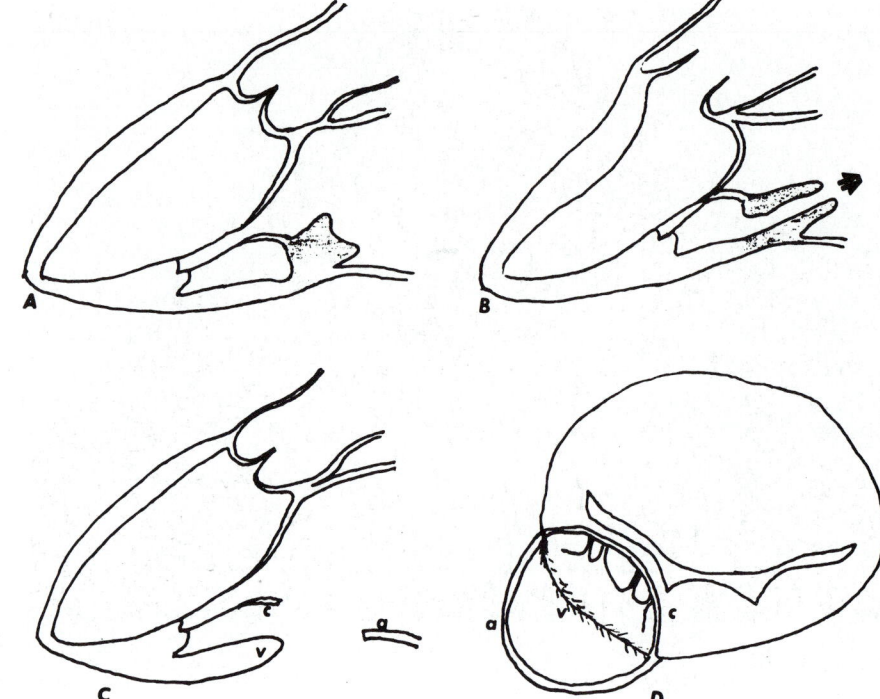

Figure 116–4. Drawings of the pathology shown in Figure 116–3 and the operation used to correct it. **A.** Long-axis view of the infected area (diastole). **B.** Same view in systole showing the vegetation elongated with a jet of insufficiency passing through it. **C.** Parts of the posterior cusp, left atrium, and the ventricular annulus have been excised to remove all infected tissue. **D.** Surgeon's transatrial view of the area of excision. a, atrium; c, cusp; v, ventricle.

Operative Technique

The operative techniques for valve replacement in endocarditis are similar to those used in noninfective cases.

The exposure often requires a more extensive cardiotomy since the critical hemodynamic disorder may have been only recently acquired and the size of the chamber through which access is obtained may be small. In acute mitral endocarditis, for example, the left atrium is still

nearly normal sized. The vertical transseptal incision provides excellent exposure in this situation. The incision starts at the foramen ovale and continues to the right of the coronary sinus (thereby avoiding the conducting tissue) to midway between the superior vena cava and the aorta. Damage to the sinoatrial (SA) node on the vena caval side and the risk of leaving too little atrium on the aortic side for safe closure, especially in view of the proximity of the left main and circumflex coronary arteries, are avoided. The artery to

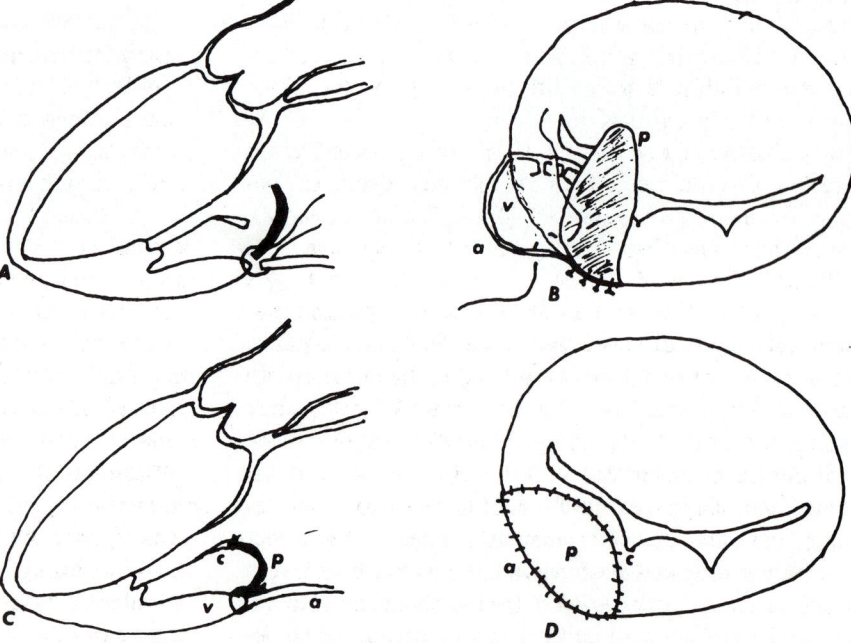

Figure 116–5. A,B. Long-axis and surgeon's view of the repair in progress: the atrium, ventricle, and a piece of tanned xenograft pericardium are being joined by multiple interrupted sutures. **C,D.** Same views of the completed repair: the pericardial patch, already attached to the atrium and ventricle, has been sutured to the remnant of the posterior cusp by multiple interrupted sutures. The result was eradication of the infection and a competent valve. The patient has remained infection free with a competent valve for 4 years. See Figure 116–6.

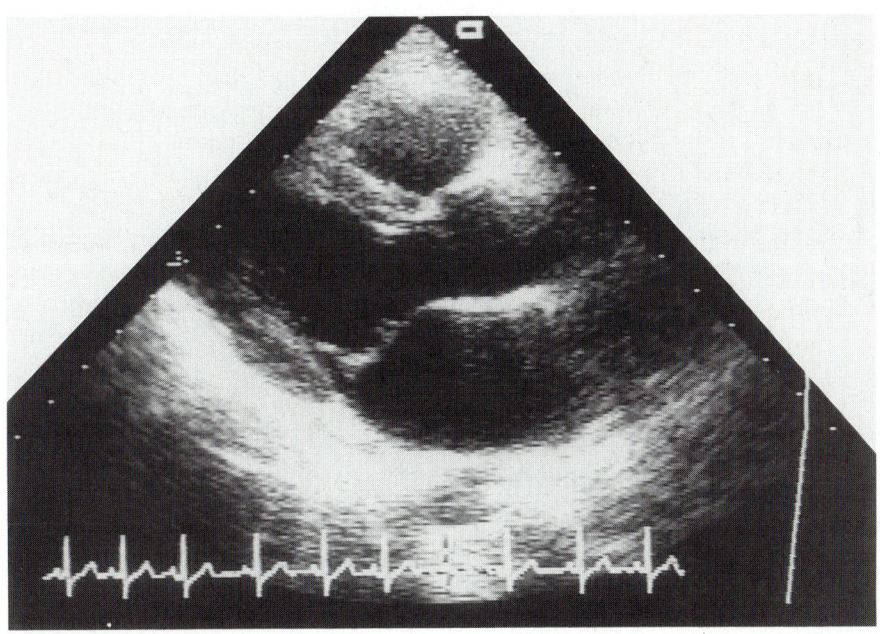

Figure 116–6. Long-axis echo of the patient 4 years after the repair.

the SA node is often cut in the right or left atrial wall at the upper end of this incision, but there appears to be no serious consequence. With both the DuBost transseptal incision, which avoids the dome completely, and the vertical transseptal incisions there is commonly a temporary nodal rhythm in the early postoperative period that usually reverts to the original rhythm. If there is any difficulty in closing the incision, a patch of tanned pericardium can be used. If the interatrial groove approach is used, it may require an extension behind the inferior vena cava.[48]

For the aortic valve the aortotomy can be carried down to the valve. Again, tanned xenograft pericardium is an excellent material for the commonly needed patch closure of the aortotomy. The valves to be operated on must be defined. With modern echocardiography this can usually be determined preoperatively. In at least the last 15 years, it has been possible to decide in advance of surgery which valves need to be exposed.

All infected tissues must be removed if possible. There should be no visible vegetations or fibrinous debris left before insertion of the new device. Tissue that is soft and inflamed should also be excised, although it may have been sterilized.

Extravalvular extensions are not always detected preoperatively. Consequently a deliberate effort must be made to find perivalvular extensions by wiping the annulus with gauze and by probing the circumference. A hockey stick probe is useful for this purpose. Common locations in the aorta area are at the left end of the left coronary cusp, and at the junction of the right and noncoronary cusps in the region of the membranous septum. Abscesses or disconnections may be proximal to, through, or distal to the aortoventricular junction. In the region of the membranous septum it must be determined whether there is a ventricular septal de-

fect. The mitral valve anterior leaflet must be inspected for vegetations or a hole at the site of impaction of the regurgitant jet. In the presence of obstructive cardiomyopathy, vegetations are looked for on the septum at the area of systolic contact of the anterior mitral leaflet. Extension to other chambers or large extracardiac false aneurysms are less likely in the mitral region.

Extracardiac extensions normally requires repair before valve insertion. Attempts to bring the edges of a defect together directly are often unsuccessful even if sutures are buttressed on one side and passed through the valve sewing ring on the other. The common consequence is a recurrence of an aueurysm or defect with or without a perivalvular leak. A tension-free closure of the margins of the defect is achieved by using a patch. We routinely use tanned xenograft pericardium for this purpose (Fig. 116–7 and 116–8). The material is strong and pliable and the host invariably heals to it. That it is a biological material may be an advantage. Residual aldehydes present in the tissue may inhibit recurrent infection.

Although contrary to surgical principles, closing an abscess does not usually cause problems. We have never seen a contained abscess develop behind a patch and have only once seen a false aneurysm develop in the aortic root as a result of suture line dehiscence between one edge of the aorta and a pericardial patch that had been used to repair an infected mycotic aneurysm. This was subsequently repaired with xenograft pericardium. We have not used autogenous pericardium for this purpose because it is also sometimes inflamed and because the thickness and strength of unselected pericardium is variable. Cloth patches should not be used for closing endocarditis-related defects to limit contact of infected tissue and synthetic material. Fortunately, in most cases the infection has not reached the annulus at the time of surgery and, after careful preparation, the valve is sewn to clean tissue. When the infection has reached the wall, it is then important to interpose biological tissue between the host and the synthetic material of the implant.[43,49,50] When there has been such destruction of the aortoventricular ring that an aortoventricular separation is imminent, some surgeons advocate excision of all infected tissue and then use of an aortic homograft conduit to bridge the defect. The published results, however, do not indicate a marked superiority of one technique over another[43,45,49,50] (Figs. 116–6, 116–7, and 116–8).

Sutures should be bolstered routinely whenever mechanical or stented xenograft valves are used since the tissues of the annulus are often weak and edematous. In aortic endocarditis it is often useful to pass the sutures from outside the aorta from a point just lateral to the left coronary orifice to the commissure between noncoronary and right coronary cusps passing under the right coronary orifice. Then proceed around the inferomedial portion of the aorta, between the aorta and superior vena cava to the left main coronary orifice. This technique can be performed with individually bolstered sutures or sutures passed through felt strips or xenograft pericardium. However, we have observed individually bolstered sutures originally placed outside the aorta erode through the wall over a 2- to 3-mo period in the absence of recurrent infection. This has not happened so far when the strip technique is used.

Perioperative Care

During surgery we favor a high flow (3.0 L/min per m^2) normothermic bypass with (in patients without renal failure) continuous retrograde normothermic blood cardioplegia with 1 min interruptions as needed for exposure. Since many patients with endocarditis have impaired platelet function the avoidance of hypothermia may be useful. A hemofilter to remove fluid in patients with severe heart failure or renal insufficiency is extremely valuable. Inotropes are

used routinely to aid in weaning from extracorporeal circulation. Atrial or atrioventricular pacing is used as needed and temporary leads are always placed since infective pathology may impair the conducting system. If renal function has deteriorated a catheter for peritoneal dialysis can be placed at the end of the operation. Dialysis may be started immediately in extreme cases.

Severe hemoptysis from lung abscesses may occur during surgery for tricuspid endocarditis. This can be managed by remaining on bypass and performing bronchoscopic irrigation and aspiration until the bleeding has slowed to manageable levels.

Postoperative Care

If failure to stop infection was the indication for surgery than a full course of antibiotics is clearly indicated postoperatively. Otherwise the decision to discontinue antibiotics is determined by the pathology at surgery. If cultures of the valve or surrounding tissues are positive, antibiotics should be continued for 6 wk. Even if cultures are negative, periannular involvement is also an indication for 6 wk of antibiotics. Healed chronic abscesses, with an established "neointima," are not an indication for long-term antibiotics. Histological demonstration of bacteria in the specimens may not indicate active infection but are probably more safely considered as such. If cultures and histology are negative and there was no perivalvular extension then there is no need for more than completion of the original course of antibiotics. Repeat blood cultures, of course, should be taken 3 to 4 days following the end of treatment. Peritoneal dialysis or venovenous hemodialysis is continued until renal function returns.

During the period of postoperative antibiotic therapy, the care of residual extracardiac infections and dental problems is completed. For addicts this period is very important for the establishment of a rehabilitation program, involving

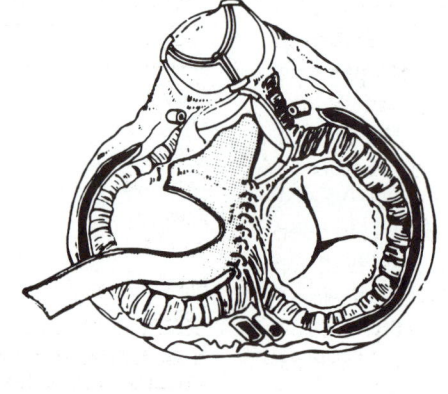

Figure 116–7. Pericardial patch used to reconstruct the mitral annulus and the intervalvar trigone and make possible the insertion of mitral and aortic replacement valves. *(From David et al: Circulation 76 (III): 102–107, 1987 by permission of the American Heart Association.)*

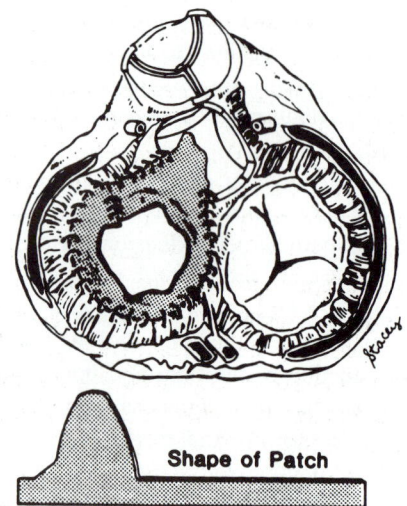

Shape of Patch

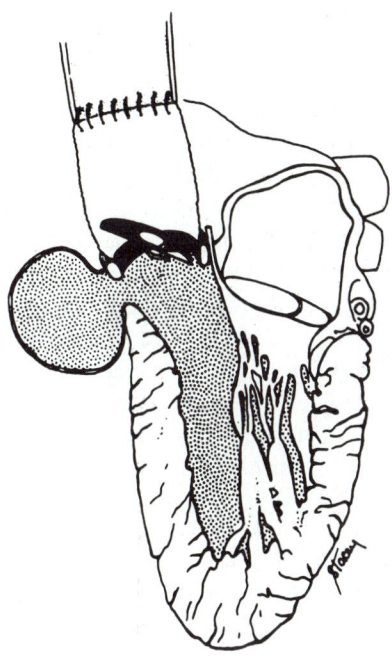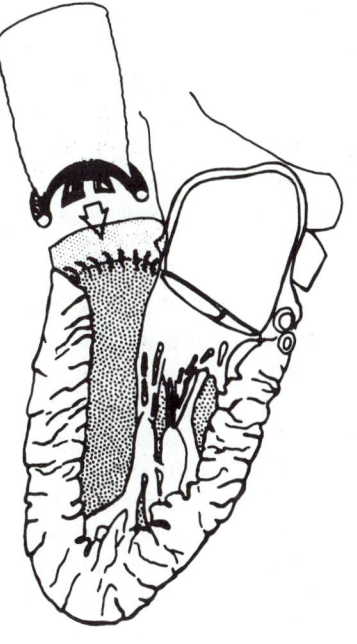

Figure 116–8. Aortoventricular separation with a mycotic aneurysm after conduit ascending aorta replacement. Pericardial reconstruction of the annulus with attachment of new conduit to the pericardium. *(From David et al: Circulation 76(III):102–107, 1987, by permission of the American Heart Association.)*

family, friends, religious support, and the appropriate agencies.

Results of Treatment for Endocarditis

The results of treatment for endocarditis need to be considered under specific headings:

1. Medical treatment for native valve endocarditis.
2. Surgical treatment for cases of failed medical treatment.
3. Medical treatment for infection of artificial valves: pure biological, stentless xenografts, stented xenografts, and mechanical.
4. Surgical treatment for infection of artificial valves.

1. For native valve endocarditis the published mortality for antibiotic therapy has for many years been approximately 30%. Deaths occur as a result of uncontrolled infection, unmanageable cardiac failure, and fatal embolism. When medical and surgical treatments are compared for cases in which the potential for these complications have developed the surgical results are better.[51,52] The risk factors for mortality are the infecting organism, the presence of cardiac failure, the persistence of sepsis, the occurrence of a major septic embolus, the presence of extravalvular extension, the presence of acute renal failure, and the size of vegetations. The medical mortality in the presence of these risk factors is >60%. On the other hand, the mortality with susceptible and favorable infecting organisms and no risk factors is <10%.

2. Surgical mortality. There are three issues to consider in evaluating the results of surgery: hospital mortality,

early recurrent endocarditis, and perivalvular leak, in the absence of recurrent infection.

Hospital mortality ranges between ░ d 20%. Statistically significant risk factors for mort; ░ re perivalvular infection, staphylococcal infection, ar ░ l and multiorgan failure.[53,54] The author's personal ░ ience with 107 primary cases is summarized in Table ░ . This series includes 56 addicts. In the early experien ░ double valve endocarditis presented technical problems that an understanding of the need to close abscess cavities with tension-free patches helped to solve. Other causes of mortality in primary infections were (1) surgery performed in patients with dense coma following preoperative neurological injury, (2) preoperative cardiogenic shock with uncorrectable severe acidosis and hepatorenal failure, and (3) technical problems

TABLE 116–1. ACTIVE NATIVE VALVE ENDOCARDITIS: 1968–1994[a]

Valves	Number	Hospital Mortality
Aortic	40	2
Mitral	25	1
Tricuspid	15	0
Pulmonic	1	0
Aor/mit	19	4
Aor/tri[b]	4	0
Mit/tri	3	0
Totals	107	7

[a]Perivalvular abscesses in a further 15 patients. Sixty-five patients were intravenous drug addicts. Three HIV+ hospital survivors not listed as hospital mortalities died 1–3 mo after discharge with recurrent sepsis without being offered further surgery.
[b]Ventricular septal defects in three.

with a small left atrium opened through the atrioventricular groove leading to bleeding and subsequent multiorgan failure. In the last 50 cases the only hospital mortality has been in an HIV positive patient with uncontrolled infection at the time of surgery. It should be noted, however, that 3 HIV positive patients who left the hospital alive died 1–3 mo after discharge with recurrent sepsis and without further surgery.

Recurrent endocarditis, due to the original organism that becomes apparent during the first two postoperative months, is traditionally attributed to persistence of the original infection. It is nevertheless clear that some recurrent infections occurring later than 2 mo after the initial operation can be attributed to an indolent persistence of the original infection. Therefore, it is more realistic to measure the time from the cessation of the antibiotic treatment. Unfortunately the definitions in the literature are variable. In our practice we presume an infection to be persistent rather than new if (1) the same organism is cultured, (2) the infection is in the annulus of the replacement device, (3) the original source of bacteria has been eliminated at the time of valve surgery or shortly thereafter, (4) the patient has not used intravenous drugs since surgery, and (5) the infection is manifest or seriously suspected within 2 mo of the cessation of antibiotic treatment. Results in the literature do not conform to this definition, although it has been recognized that operatively acquired infection may become manifest much longer than 2 mo following surgery.[55,56] Considering the conventional definition, the incidence of original infection persistence ranges from <5 to 20%. The data from the units where homografts are used appear to show that the use of aortic homografts rather than mechanical or stent-mounted xenografts is associated with a lower incidence of persistent infection. While there are conflicting opinions there is probably no difference in the risk of persistent infection for mechanical or stent-mounted xenografts.[54,55] In the author's experience, using the alternative definition given above, the incidence of persistent infection in nonaddicts is <2%. In the past 10 years the only important risk factor has been uncontrolled infection in HIV positive patients.

Perivalvular leaks occur more frequently in valve replacements for endocarditis even in the absence of recurrent or persistent infection.

Modern echocardiography can detect leaks with great sensitivity, but only hemodynamically significant leaks require reoperation. For the mitral valve this is best determined by transesophageal echocardiography. Cardiac catheterization with hemodynamic measurements may sometimes be needed for decision-making. In the literature significant perivalvular leaks occur in 3 to 7% of cases. In our experience the need for reoperation for perivalvular leaks in the absence of persistent infection in HIV negative patients has been 2%.

3. Medical treatment for infected artificial valves can be successful but the mortality is ≈70%.[57] The presence of valvular incompetence or perivalvular leaks severely diminishes the chance of medical cure.[55] Early postoperative endocarditis also responds poorly to medical treatment.[30] The ideal case for medical treatment would be a late infection by a *Streptococcus* on a biological valve with no more than a very small vegetation, no leak, and no perivalvular involvement. At this stage there are no data to determine whether the stentless valves will be more successfully treated medically than mechanical or stent-mounted valves.

4. Surgical treatment of prosthetic endocarditis once carried mortalities of 50 to 70%.[30] More recently mortalities of 0 to 22% have been reported.[54,58,59] Risk factors for failure are perivalvular extension, early postoperative onset, and delay in surgery. These three factors are all interrelated. The infecting organism is also significant, with staphylococcal, Gram-negative, and particularly fungal infections making surgical cure difficult but not impossible. The evidence shows that surgery should be performed early and should not be dependent upon an arbitrary period of antibiotic administration. With infection due to these organisms there should be no delay. If perivalvular extension becomes evident during a period of antibiotic treatment the case has been mismanaged. The hospital mortality in the author's series has been 2 of 23 cases (Table 116–2). Both deaths occurred in nonaddicts: one a patient with a mitral ball valve in whom treatment had been continued for 1 mo with staphylococcal infection and who was presented for surgery with a pH of 7, a potassium of 7, and renal failure; and the other a patient with a very indolent, late-occurring aortic valve infection with aortoventricular separation in which homograft root replacement together with pericardial reinforcement was unsuccessful. However, the long-term survivors include two nonaddicts with fungal endocarditis (one aortic and one mitral) and other cases with aortoventricular disruption and ventricular septal defect requiring extensive xenograft pericardial patch reconstruction. Only 2 of our nonaddict cases were early onset, giving an incidence of 0.26% of postvalve replacement intraoperative valve infections. An incidence this low has been achieved by others,[55,58] with the authors attributing their success to careful management of antibiotic prophylaxis. The principle of having cidal antibiotic levels before, during, and for at least 24 hours following valve replacement is well established. Selection of antibiotics according to the prevalence and sensitivity of the local flora is also important; and finally strict standards of management of all intravascular lines must be in operation in the operating room and the intensive care unit. We require a dental consult in every case of valve

TABLE 116–2. PROSTHETIC VALVE ENDOCARDITIS: 1970–1994[a]

	Number	Hospital Mortality
Addicts	13	0
Nonaddicts	10	2

[a]Two nonaddict survivors and one addict survivor had fungal infections.

surgery and in some of our patients with grossly neglected oral hygiene, emergency dental procedures have been performed. This practice avoids bacteremias during the early postoperative period before host coverage of the device has occurred and may have helped achieve low rates of perioperative infection.

SUMMARY

1. When infection of heart valves is confined to the cusps or leaflets, surgical treatment with complete replacement or repair is very satisfactory. When infection involves the annulus, the surgeon is obliged to break an important principle and implant foreign material in an infected location: the results are invariably less satisfactory.
2. Surgery for valvular endocarditis is indicated for failure of medical (i.e., antibiotic therapy).
3. Congestive cardiac failure, multiple emboli or a single major embolus, and persistence of infection are absolute marks of failed antibiotic therapy. Evidence of extravalvular extension of infection should be added to this classic triad.
4. The high probability of failure is an important extra indication: large vegetations, severe valve destruction and insufficiency even in the absence of cardiac failure, and infection by aggressive or resistant organism (e.g., staphylococci and fungi).
5. Extravalvular extension provides the most serious technical problems for the surgeon and the aim of timing should be to bring the patient to surgery before this happens.
6. In general the earlier the patient comes to surgery the better the results.
7. The indications for rereplacement of an artificial valve are the same but stronger: it is even more important to avoid delay in coming to surgery.
8. If there is an indication for surgery and antibiotics have been started there is no gain in waiting.
9. Cerebral hemorrhage and neurologic lesions producing coma are contraindications, but recovering neurologic injury and renal and hepatic complications are not.
10. At surgery remove all infected tissue and patch all defects that are left after this has been done: biologic tissue is best used for patching.
11. There is strong advocacy for the use of homografts or autografts for extensive aortic root infections, but when aggressive debridement is combined with patching, the results of surgery for even extensive disease are also good.

REFERENCES

1. Osler W: The Gulstonian lectures on malignant endocarditis. *Br Med J* **1**:467–470, 522–526, 577–579, 1889

2. Loewe L, Rosenblatt P, Green HJ: Combined penicillin and heparin therapy of subacute bacterial endocarditis: Report of seven consecutively successfully treated patients. *JAMA* **124**:144–149, 1944
3. Christie RV: Penicillin in subacute bacterial endocarditis. *Br Med J* **1**:1–13, 1948
4. Tubbs OS, Keele KD: Combined ligation of ductus arteriosus and sulphapyridine therapy in case of influenzal endocarditis. *St Bart's Hosp War Bull* **1**:175, 1940
5. Tourof ASW: Rationale of operative treatment of subacute bacterial endarteritis superimposed on patent ductus arteriosus. *Am Heart J* **23**:847–856, 1942
6. Wallace AG, Young WG, Osterhout S: Treatment of acute bacterial endocarditis by valve excision and replacement. *Circulation* **31**:450–453, 1965
7. Okell C, Elliot SD: Bacteremia and oral sepsis with special reference to the aetiology of subacute endocarditis. *Lancet* **2**:869–872, 1935
8. Bayliss R, Clarke C, Oakley CM, et al: The bowel, the genitourinary tract, and infective endocarditis. *Br Heart J* **52**:339–345, 1984
9. Hansen CP, Westh H, Brok KE, et al: Bacteremia following orotracheal intubation and oesophageal balloon dilatation. *Thorax* **44**:684–685, 1989
10. Guntheroth WG: How important are dental procedures as a cause of infective endocarditis? *Am J Cardiol* **54**:747–801, 1984
11. Lewis T, Grant RT: Observations relating to subacute infective endocarditis. *Heart* **10**:21–77, 1923
12. Oka M, Shirota A, Angrist A: Experimental endocarditis: Endocrine factors in valve lesions on AV shunt rats. *Arch Pathol* **82**:85–92, 1966
13. Rodbard S: Blood velocity and endocarditis. *Circulation* **27**:18–28, 1963
14. Clawson CC, White JG: Platelet interaction with bacteria. I Reaction phases and effects of inhibitors. *Am J Pathol* **65**:367–397, 1971
15. Utley JR: The effect of cardiopulmonary bypass on the immune system susceptibility to infection. In Gabbay S, Boncheck LI, Bortolotti U (eds): *Infective Endocarditis of Heart Valves.* Austin, Silent Partners, 1991, pp 29–44.
16. Bayer AS, Norman DC: Valve site specific pathogenetic differences between right-sided and left-sided bacterial endocarditis. *Chest* **98**:200–205, 1990
17. Gutman RA, Striker GE, Gilliland BC: The immune complex glomerulonephritis of bacterial endocarditis. *Medicine* **51**:1–25, 1972
18. Strom J, Becker RM, Davis R, Frater RWM: Echocardiographic and surgical correlations in bacterial endocarditis. *Circulation* **62**:164–167, 1980
19. Robbins MJ, Frater RWM, Soeiro R, Strom J: Influence of vegetation size on the clinical outcome of right sided infective endocarditis. *Am J Med* **80**:165–172, 1986
20. Buda AJ, Zotz RJ, Lemire MS: Prognostic significance of vegetations detected by two dimensional echocardiography in infective endocarditis. *Am Heart J* **112**:1291–1296, 1986
21. Ghosh PK, Miller HI, Vidne BA: Mitral obstruction in bacterial endocarditis. *Br Heart J* **53**:341–344, 1985
22. Frater RWM: Surgical management of endocarditis in addicts including long term results. *J Card Surg* **5**:63–67, 1990
23. LeJemtel TH, Factor SM, Koenigsberg M, et al: Mural vegetations at the site of endocardial trauma in infective endocarditis complicating idiopathic hypertrophic subaortic stenosis. *Am J Cardiol* **44**:569–574, 1979
24. Weinstein L, Schlesinger JJ: Pathoanatomic, pathophysiologic and clinical correlations in endocarditis. *N Engl J Med* **291**:1122–1126, 1974
25. Hart RG, Kagan-Hallet K, Joerns SE: Mechanisms of intracranial hemorrhage in infective endocarditis. *Stroke* **38**:1048–1056, 1987
26. Salgado AV, Furlan AJ, Keys TF: Mycotic aneurysms, subarachnoid hemorrhage and indications for cerebral angiography in infective endocarditis. *Stroke* **18**:1057–1060, 1987
27. Levison ME: Pharmadonymic considerations in the medical treat-

ment of bacterial endocarditis. In Gabbay S, Boncheck LL, Bortolotti U (eds): *Infective Endocarditis of Heart Valves.* Austin, Silent Partners, 1991, pp 53–63

28. Arbulu A, Holmes RJ, Asfaw I: Surgical treatment of intractable right sided infective endocarditis in drug addicts. *J Heart Valve Dis* **2:**129–137, 1993

29. Stern H, Sisto D, Strom J, Frater RWM: Immediate tricuspid valve replacement for endocarditis. *J Thorac Cardiovasc Surg* **91:**163–166, 1986

30. Wilcox BR: The role of surgery in the management of infective endocarditis. In Roberts AJ (ed): *Difficult Problems in Adult Cardiac Surgery.* St. Louis, Year Book, 1985, pp 199–218

31. Fang G, Keys TF, Gentry LO, et al: *Ann Intern Med* **119:**560–567, 1993

32. Iung B, Cornier B, Dadez E, et al: *J Heart Valve Dis* **2:**259–266, 1993

33. Kirklin JK, Pacifico AD, Kirklin JW: Surgical treatment of prosthetic valve endocarditis with homograft aortic valve replacement. *J Cardiac Surg* **4:**340–347, 1989

34. Frater RWM, Sisto D, Condit D: Cardiac surgery in human immunodeficiency virus (HIV) carriers. *Eur J Cardiothorac Surg* **3:**146–150, 1989

35. Frater RWM, Sisto D: Surgery for endocarditis in drug addicts: Is it worthwhile? In Gabbay S, Boncheck LI, Bortolotti U. (eds): *Infective Endocarditis of Heart Valves.* Austin, Silent Partners, 1991, 117–124

36. Ting W, Silverman NA, Levitsky S: Right and left side endocarditis. Cerebral emboli. In Gabbay S, Boncheck LI, Bortolotti U (eds): *Infective Endocarditis of Heart Valves.* Austin, Silent Partners, 1991, pp 3–15

37. Liao KJ, Frater RWM, Seifter E: Unpublished observations.

38. Frater RWM, Vetter HO, Zussa C, Dahm M: Chordal replacement in mitral valve repair. *Circulation* **82**(suppl IV):125–130, 1990

39. Dossche K, Vanerman H, Wellens F: Partial mitral valve replacement with a mitral homograft in subacute endocarditis. 1994

40. Gammage MD, Littler WA, Abrams LI: Conservative surgery of the mitral valve in bacterial endocarditis. *Thorax* **39:**868–871, 1984

41. Frater RWM: Tricuspid valvulectomy. *J Heart Valve Dis* **2:**138–139, 1993

42. Donaldson RM, Ross DN: Homograft aortic root replacement for complicated prosthetic valve endocarditis. *Circulation* **70**(suppl I):178–181, 1984

43. Kirklin JK, Kirklin JW, Pacifico AD: Aortic valve endocarditis with aortic root abscess cavity; surgical treatment with aortic valve homograft. *Ann Thorac Surg* **45:**674–677, 1988

44. Oswalt J: Management of aortic infective endocarditis by autograft valve replacement. *J Heart Valve Dis* **3:**377–387, 1994

45. Petterson G: The Ross operation in the treatment of native and prosthetic aortic valve endocarditis. *J Heart Valve Dis* **3:**371–376, 1994

46. Ivert TSA, Desmukis WE, Cobbs CG, et al: Prosthetic valve endocarditis. *Circulation* **69:**223–232, 1984

47. Reul GJ, Sweeney MS: Bioprosthetic versus mechanical valve replacement in patients with infective endocarditis. *J Cardiac Surg* **4:**348–351, 1989

48. Becker RM, Frishman W, Frater RWM: Surgery for mitral valve endocarditis. *Chest* **75:**314–319, 1979

49. David TE: Surgery for active endocarditis with perivalvular abscess. In Gabbay S, Boncheck LI, Bortolotti U (eds): *Infective Endocarditis of Heart Valves.* Silent Partners, 1991, pp 181–194

50. Yankah C, Hetzer R: Valve selection and choice in surgery of endocarditis. *J Card Surg* **4:**324–330, 1989

51. Croft CH, Woodward W, Elliott A, et al: Analysis of surgical versus medical therapy in active complicated native valve endocarditis. *Am J Cardiol* **51:**1650–1655, 1983

52. Horstkotte D, Schulte HD, Bircks W: Factors influencing prognosis and indications for surgical intervention in acute native valve endocarditis. In Hostkott D, Bodnar E (eds): *Infective Endocarditis.* London, ICR Publishers, 1991, pp 171–197

53. Miller DC: Determinants of outcome in surgically treated patients with native valve endocarditis. *J Card Surg* **4:**331–339, 1989

54. Larbalestier RI, Kinchla NM, Aranki SF, et al: Acute bacterial endocarditis. Optimising surgical results. *Circulation* **86,** II:68–74, 1992

55. Santinga JT, Kirswh M, Fekety R: Factors affecting survival. *Chest* **84:**471–475, 1984

56. Kuyvenhoven JP, vanRijk-Zwikker GL, Hermans J, et al: Prosthetic valve endocarditis: analysis of risk factors for mortality. *Eur J Cardiothorac Surg* **8:**420–424, 1994

57. Petheram IS, Boyce JMH: Prosthetic valve endocarditis: A review of 24 cases. *Thorax* **32:478–485, 1977**

58. Antunes MJ, Sanchez MF, Fernandes LE: Antibiotic prophylaxis and prosthetic valve endocarditis. *J Heart Valve Dis* **1:**201–205, 1992

59. Schulz R, Werner GS, Kreuzer H: Clinical outcome in prosthetic valve endocarditis as compared with native valve endocarditis in the era of transesophageal echocardiography. *J Am Coll Cardiol* 1994 Abstract 366A

CHAPTER

117

Acquired Disease
of the Tricuspid Valve

George C. Kaiser and Andrew C. Fiore

ACQUIRED TRICUSPID VALVE DISEASE

Acquired tricuspid valve disease is uncommon. The most frequent etiology of either stenosis or insufficiency is chronic rheumatic heart disease. Organic tricuspid involvement was observed postmortem in 46% of 144 cases of chronic rheumatic heart disease, but tricuspid stenosis was found in only three patients.[1] It almost always occurs in conjunction with mitral or aortic involvement or both.[1,2] Tricuspid insufficiency in patients with left-sided rheumatic heart disease and without involvement of the tricuspid valve by the rheumatic process has been felt to be functional. The left-sided valvular pathologic changes cause pulmonary arterial hypertension and eventual dilatation of the right ventricle and the tricuspid valve annulus resulting in functional tricuspid valve insufficiency. Whether the lesion is due to rheumatic fever or another cause and whether it is organic or functional, it is the degree of hemodynamic impairment that dictates the need for operative management.

TRICUSPID STENOSIS

Acquired tricuspid stenosis, while usually of rheumatic origin, may occur in carcinoid syndrome, fibroelastosis, endomyocardial fibrosis, and lupus erythematosus. A right atrial myxoma should be considered in the differential diagnosis.[3] As an isolated lesion, it occurs so rarely that observed cases have been published as case reports.[4] Clinically, it has been recognized in 3% of patients with mitral stenosis.[3,5]

The major deformity is fusion of the commissures,

which may be difficult to identify. The cusps are thickened but pliable. The valve orifice is generally oval and insufficient as well as stenotic. There is usually less fusion of the subvalvular apparatus than is seen in mitral valve disease. Unlike mitral valve disease, calcification is uncommon.[1,6]

Tricuspid stenosis has the same predilection for women in their fourth and fifth decades as does mitral valve disease. The most commonly observed symptoms are excessive fatigue, dyspnea, and peripheral edema.[3,5,6] Peripheral edema is almost uniformly present in patients with atrial fibrillation and rarely or only intermittently observed in patients in normal sinus rhythm.[5–7] With normal sinus rhythm, there is a pronounced A wave in the jugular venous pulse, often noticed by the patient as a flicking pulse.[3,5,7] Liver enlargement and ascites are uncommon in patients with tricuspid stenosis until late in the course and are usually associated with atrial fibrillation and tricuspid insufficiency.[6]

A well-localized diastolic murmur increasing in intensity with inspiration and decreasing in intensity with expiration is usually heard best along the left sternal border in the third, fourth, or fifth intercostal space. A systolic murmur is usually heard in patients with atrial fibrillation, but only rarely in patients with normal sinus rhythm.[7] If the stenosis is severe, inspiration may diminish the systolic murmur by reducing right ventricular systolic pressure.[7] A tricuspid valve opening snap may be difficult to separate from that of the mitral valve.[7] The presence of atrial fibrillation, increased venous pressure, and a diastolic murmur in the classic location should strongly suggest the possibility of significant tricuspid stenosis.

There are no specific diagnostic features of the electrocardiogram of patients with tricuspid stenosis. Approximately one-half of these patients have atrial fibrillation. Those with normal sinus rhythm have tall, peaked P-waves diagnostic of right atrial hypertension, hypertrophy, and dilatation, which may be encountered with disease processes other than tricuspid stenosis.[3,5–7]

The radiographic findings usually considered pathognomonic of tricuspid stenosis are right atrial enlargement, relative or absolute lack of pulmonary artery enlargement, and relatively clear lung fields.[3,5–7] Calcification of the tricuspid valve is rare.[3,6–8] The largest right atriums are seen in patients with tricuspid stenosis and insufficiency combined, atrial fibrillation, and a mean right atrial pressure greater than 12 mm Hg.[6,7]

The essential hemodynamic features of tricuspid stenosis are a tricuspid valve diastolic gradient greater than 5 mm Hg, an elevated right atrial pressure, and a reduced cardiac output. The diastolic gradient should be measured with simultaneous right atrial and right ventricular pressure measurements. The clinical and hemodynamic findings may be obscured by atrial fibrillation.[8] Reduction in valve orifice to less than 1.5 cm^2 usually results in significant hemodynamic changes and symptoms.[9] While the right atrial pressure is not related to the valve orifice size, the cardiac index has been shown to be highly correlative.[3,5,7–9]

Evaluation of the tricuspid valve by noninvasive techniques has been correlated with hemodynamic and operative assessment.[10–13] M-mode and two-dimensional echocardiography have demonstrated leaflet thickening, reduced

diastolic excursion, and doming of the valve to be diagnostic of tricuspid stenosis[11,12] (Fig. 117–1A). Doppler echocardiography is reliable in evaluating tricuspid valve lesions even in the presence of atrial fibrillation or congestive heart failure and is independent of right ventricular pressure.[10] The primary findings of tricuspid stenosis by Doppler echocardiography are an increased duration of diastolic analog wave and broadening of the corresponding time interval histogram[10] (Fig. 117–1B).

TRICUSPID INSUFFICIENCY

Isolated tricuspid insufficiency is rare.[14–17] Organic tricuspid regurgitation is usually due to trauma, endocarditis, carcinoid heart disease, or rheumatic heart disease.[1,2,18–26] In the majority of patients, tricuspid regurgitation has been felt to be functional rather than organic.[14–17]

Traumatic tricuspid insufficiency, reported infrequently, usually results from a blunt chest injury. There are two types of valve injury seen: (1) papillary muscle rupture or (2) chordae tendineae or valve laceration. Patients with papillary muscle rupture either die before diagnosis and treatment or require early operation. In those with chordae tendineae rupture, late operative repair has usually been undertaken, with good results.[19,20] Timing of the operation depends on the signs and symptoms. Some patients have been treated nonoperatively for many years.[21–23] Rarely,

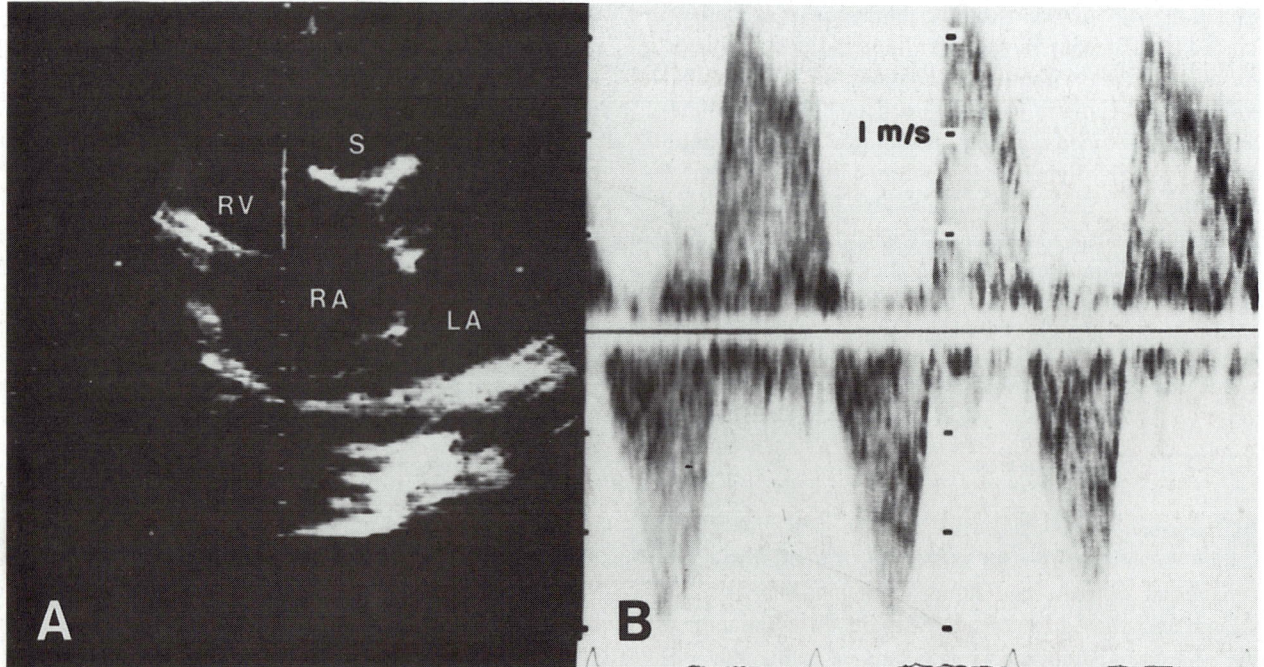

Figure 117–1. A. Two dimension short axis view of the tricuspid valve in a patient with tricuspid stenosis. The enlarged right atrium and thickened, domed septal leaflet (S) are shown. LA, left atrium; RA, right atrium; RV, right ventricle. **B.** The pulsed Doppler signal (white line) is placed across the valve annulus. The spectrum demonstrates an increase in peak diastolic velocity of 1.7 m/s with a prolonged pressure half-time consistent with tricuspid stenosis.

injury of the chordae tendineae may result from a cardiac catheter.[25] Tricuspid insufficiency following cardiac transplantation has been observed with increasing frequency. It has been felt to be due to chordal injury occurring during multiple right ventricular biopsies required as part of post-transplant follow-up.[25a,25b]

Destruction of valve tissue due to endocarditis, with resultant tricuspid insufficiency, has been recognized more frequently as drug abuse has increased. It is more completely discussed in Chapter 116.

In carcinoid heart disease, fibrous plaques are deposited on the endocardium of the valvular cusps and cardiac chambers. This fibrous tissue is usually deposited on the ventricular aspect of the tricuspid leaflets, frequently securing them rigidly to the adjacent ventricular wall. In spite of the stenosis resulting from this fibrosis, the tricuspid valve is fixed in the open position, producing predominantly tricuspid insufficiency. Valve replacement has been accomplished in some of these patients with symptomatic improvement.[26,27]

The most frequent cause of tricuspid insufficiency is rheumatic heart disease.[14–17] In patients with chronic rheumatic disease, organic tricuspid involvement has been observed in almost one-half of those who eventually came to autopsy.[1] The tricuspid valve has been felt by some to be especially vulnerable to incompetence under hemodynamic stress from left-sided lesions, thereby producing functional regurgitation.[16,28,29] In patients with mitral valve disease functional tricuspid regurgitation is more frequent than organic tricuspid regurgitation.[30] Functional tricuspid regurgitation has been observed in 62% of patients with pure mitral regurgitation.[30]

As with mitral stenosis, two-thirds of the patients with tricuspid insufficiency are female, with an average age of 40 years.[14,15,17] Dyspnea is common but its severity is frequently less than would be expected from the mitral stenosis alone.[14,15,17] Orthopnea, usually present, may be mild or absent.[15,17] Several authors have commented on this discrepancy between the symptoms and the severity of the valvular lesion.[14,15,17] They postulated that patients who have mitral stenosis and tricuspid regurgitation combined are less symptomatic because the tricuspid insufficiency acts as a decompressive mechanism. Under these circumstances, the right ventricle is working harder, but effective pulmonary flow is less.[16,17]

Distension of neck veins is common (50–90%), with venous pulsation occurring in up to three-fourths of these patients.[14,15,17] Hepatomegaly is present in 90% of the patients, but systolic pulsation is variable, usually paralleling the incidence of peripheral venous pulsation.[14,15,17] Venous and hepatic pulsation, dependent on the degree of fluid retention and congestion in patients with uncompensated right heart failure, frequently disappears with treatment.

A systolic parasternal murmur heard maximally in the right or left fourth or fifth intercostal spaces may be audible in less than 20% of patients with tricuspid regurgitation.[14,15,17] Increase in the intensity of the murmur with deep inspiration was pointed out by Carvallo in 1946.[17] The intensity of the murmur varies not only between patients but in the same patient. This may be further confounded by murmurs of associated left-sided lesions.

The majority of patients with tricuspid insufficiency have atrial fibrillation.[14,15,17,29] Some have felt that the occurrence of atrial fibrillation may actually contribute to the production of tricuspid insufficiency.[14] Regardless, it is rare to see patients with significant tricuspid insufficiency in normal sinus rhythm. In those occasional patients with normal sinus rhythm, the P-wave may demonstrate evidence of right atrial enlargement.[17]

Radiologically, right atrial enlargement is observed in 85% of the patients with tricuspid insufficiency.[15] Cardiomegaly is frequent but is dependent largely on the associated valvular defects. Pulmonary artery enlargement, less than expected from left-sided lesions, should make one suspect tricuspid insufficiency.[17]

Hemodynamic confirmation of significant tricuspid insufficiency may be difficult. The right atrial mean and pulmonary artery systolic pressures are elevated with a high right atrial V-wave. Hemodynamic factors relating to right ventricular dilatation correlate positively with the degree of tricuspid regurgitation.[29] The greater these levels, the more likely tricuspid insufficiency is present and the more frequent are the classic signs and symptoms.[14,15,29] Cardiac output at rest decreases as the severity of tricuspid regurgitation increases and is further adversely affected by exercise.[15,29] Right ventriculography performed with a catheter inserted through an arm vein may result in tricuspid regurgitation caused by the catheter, confusing the issue. Catheter insertion from the leg may reduce this possibility.[31]

Noninvasive techniques have added to the precision of tricuspid regurgitation assessment.[10,32–37] If the tricuspid valve can be examined easily by noninvasive techniques right ventricular enlargement is usually present.[36] Using contrast M-mode or two-dimensional echocardiography, microcavitation reflux patterns passing posteriorly through the tricuspid valve or into the inferior vena cava or hepatic veins during 80% or more of systole are considered specific for pathologic tricuspid regurgitation.[32–34,37] These patterns occurring at other times during the cardiac cycle are not pathognomonic of significant tricuspid regurgitation. Tricuspid regurgitation determined by Doppler echocardiography has been shown to correlate well with that demonstrated by contrast echocardiography and right ventriculography.[35,37] Early systolic backward flow, normally associated with tricuspid valve closure, should not exceed the first half of systole.[35,37] The Doppler signal of significant tricuspid regurgitation is a wide-band velocity spectrum parallel to the atrial septum extending from the tricuspid valve into the right atrium and lasting for at least 80% of systole[35,37] (Fig. 117–2B).

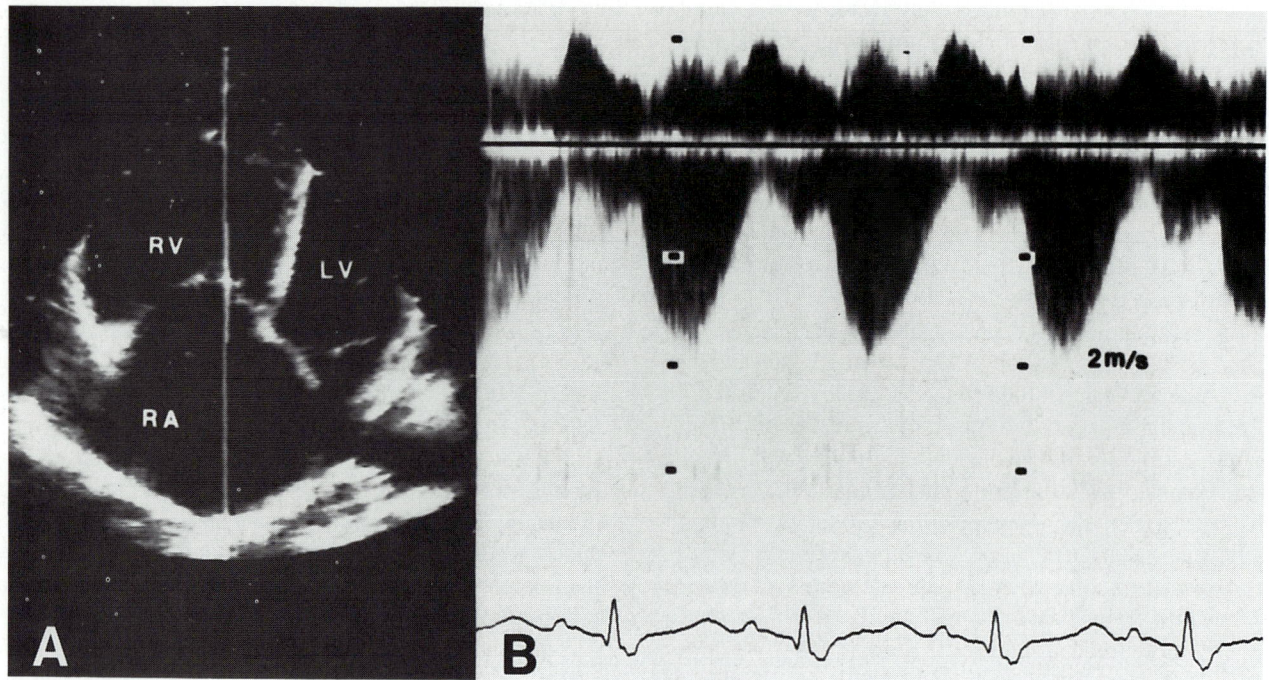

Figure 117–2. A. Two-dimensional apical four-chambered view of the tricuspid valve in a patient with tricuspid insufficiency. Enlarged right atrium and right ventricle are demonstrated. **B.** The pulsed Doppler signal (white line) is placed across the valve annulus. The spectrum demonstrates normal diastolic flow of 1.0 m/s and a holosystolic negative jet velocity of 1.7 m/s consistent with tricuspid regurgitation.

TRICUSPID VALVE COMMISSUROTOMY

To perform tricuspid valve plastic procedures properly, it is important to understand tricuspid valve anatomy and pathology. The essential features of tricuspid valve anatomy are shown in Figure 117–3.

In functional tricuspid regurgitation, dilatation of the annulus occurs chiefly in the right ventricular free wall. Carpentier et al indicated that the posterior leaflet increased 80% in length and the anterior leaflet 40% during its development while the septal leaflet attachment remained relatively unchanged.[38] Annular enlargement affects the commissures variably. The posteroseptal and anteroposterior commissure are enlarged 30% while the anteroseptal commissure increases minimally.[38] The relative stability of the septal leaflet size enables it to be used as an index to the size of a reconstructed valve.[31,38,39]

Tricuspid stenosis is almost always accompanied by some degree of regurgitation. Frequently, the leaflets remain thin and pliable, and the chordae tendineae are minimally involved. Lesser degrees of stenosis may be handled by commissurotomy. Commissurotomy is usually carried out at the anteroseptal and posteroseptal commissures[40,41] (Fig. 117–4). Incision of the anteroposterior commissure is avoided as this may result in tricuspid insufficiency.[40,41] Another method of commissurotomy incises the anteroseptal commissure and the posterior cusp.[38] Both commissur-

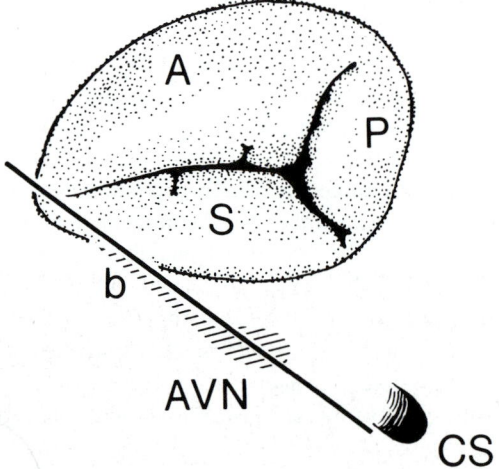

Figure 117–3. The most narrow portion of the egg-shaped tricuspid valve annulus is the anteroseptal commissure. The quadrangular anterior leaflet (A) is the largest, the triangular posterior leaflet (P) is the smallest. The septal leaflet (S) is semicircular. The anterior and septal leaflets may be notched, the posterior scalloped. The commissures, named for the abutting leaflets, are anteroseptal, anteroposterior, and posteroseptal. The bundle of His (b) courses along a line from the coronary sinus (CS) to the anteroseptal commissure, passing beneath the base of the septal leaflet just posterior to the anteroseptal commissure. The atrioventricular node (AVN) lies between this area and the coronary sinus.

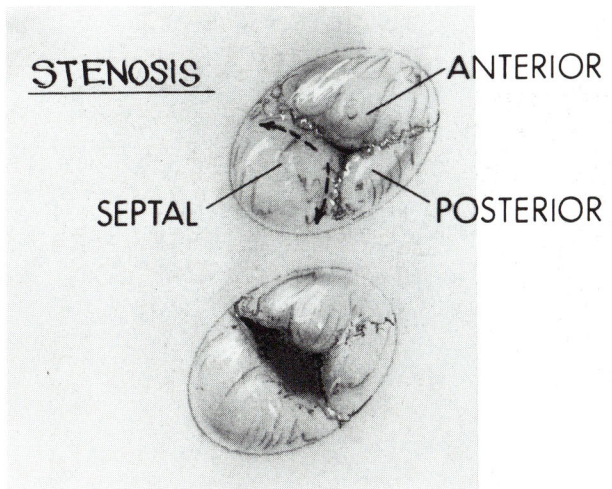

Figure 117–4. Tricuspid commissurotomy. The incision is made between the anterior and septal leaflets and between the posterior and septal leaflets. Fusion between the anterior and posterior and septal leaflets. Fusion between the anterior and posterior leaflets is not disturbed *(Reproduced with the kind permission of J. H. Kay, M.D., 1974.)*

otomy techniques produce a bicuspid valve. Annuloplasty is employed to correct any concurrent regurgitation.[31,38,40]

TRICUSPID ANNULOPLASTY

The three general techniques of tricuspid annuloplasty used to correct tricuspid regurgitation are (1) annular plication, (2) annular ring insertion, and (3) semicircular annuloplasty.

Annular Plication

Tricuspid annuloplasty by annular plication has been championed in the United States by Kay and Reed and their asso-

ciates[40,42–45] (Fig. 117–5). This technique, converting the tricuspid valve into a bicuspid valve by excluding the posterior leaflet, is accomplished by plication of the annulus over the posterior leaflet. Sutures in this area avoid the conduction system. The reported clinical results have been good and appear to have been maintained. One theoretical disadvantage of this technique is that it does not deal with the remainder of the tricuspid annulus in the right ventricular free wall. Annular plication is especially effective, however, in patients in whom there is loss of posterior leaflet substance.

Minale et al have modified the technique of annular plication by separating the anterior and posterior leaflets and the anteroposterior commissure from the annulus. After one half of the isolated annulus is plicated, the cut edges of the leaflets are sutured to the shortened annulus. This reduces the annulus circumference selectively without reducing the actual area of the leaflets, and allows improved coaptation of the three leaflets.[46]

Ring Annuloplasty

Disappointed with the results of annular plication and basing their technique on the pathologic anatomic studies of Deloche, Carpentier et al devised the ring annuloplasty.[47] They believed this technique distributed the tension over the entire annulus, while allowing maximal correction in the areas of greatest dilatation, i.e., over the insertion of the anterior and posterior cusps and their commissures (Fig. 117–6). Carpentier subsequently modified the original ring, making it flexible and creating an opening at the area of the anteroseptal commissure. He felt that these changes would improve the hemodynamic results by reducing the mechanical stress on the sutures and would reduce the incidence of conduction system injury by eliminating the ring and sutures in the area of the bundle of His.[48,49] Others have de-

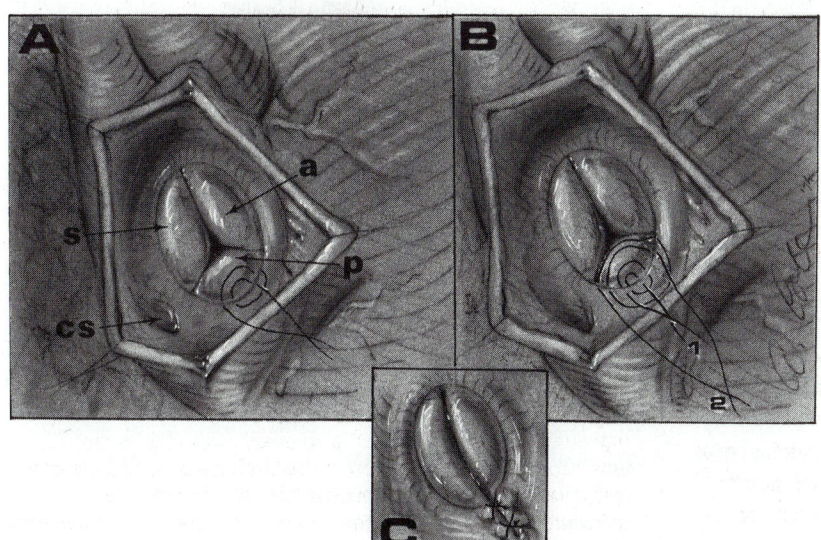

Figure 117–5. Method of repairing tricuspid insufficiency by plicating the annulus of the posterior leaflet with figure-of-eight sutures. (a) anterior leaflet; (cs) coronary sinus; (p) posterior leaflet; (s) septal leaflet. *(From Kay JH, Mendez AM, Zubiate P: A further look at tricuspid annuloplasty. Ann Thorac Surg 22:498, 1976, with permission of Little Brown & Co.)*

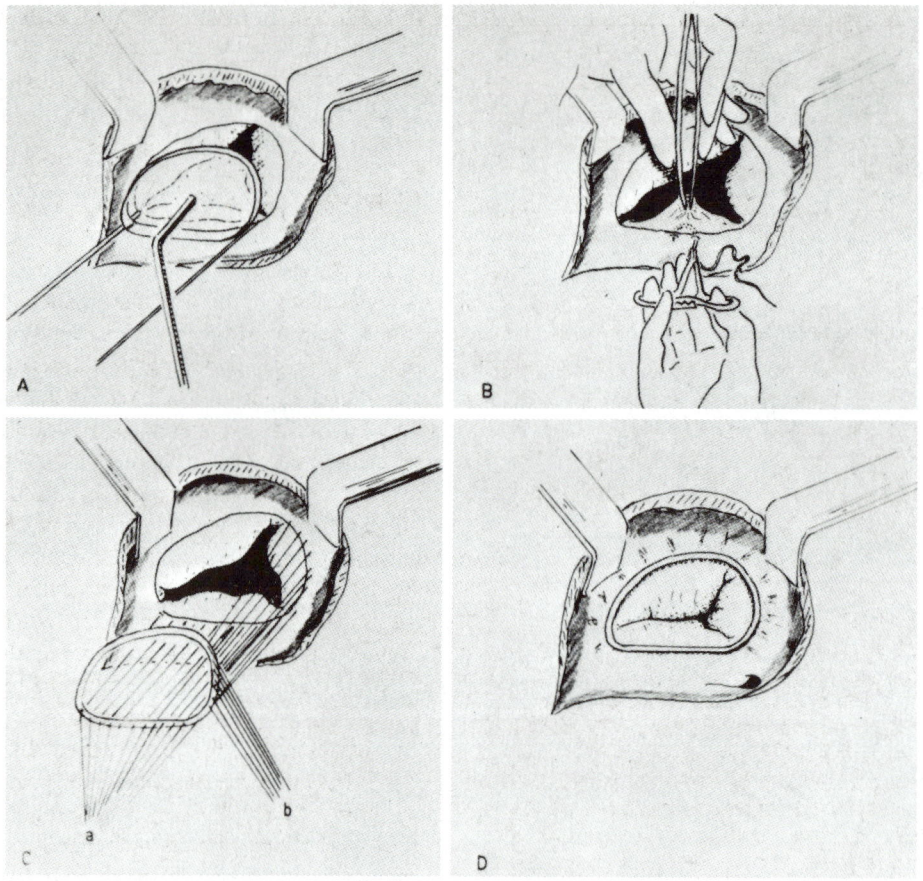

Figure 117–6. Technique of tricuspid ring valvuloplasty. **A.** Size of appropriate prosthetic ring is chosen according to measurement of base of septal cusp. **B.** The leaflet tissue is pulled perpendicular to the atrial wall to make the annulus more obvious. By directing the needle through the annulus toward the ventricular cavity, then back through it toward the atrium, injury to either the leaflet or the bundle of His is avoided. **C.** The sutures corresponding to the base of the septal cusp (a) are passed through the corresponding segment of the prosthetic ring with the same intervals between them. These intervals are reduced for the sutures arising from the posterior and anterior cusps and commissures (b). **D.** Result of the correction shows normal configuration and normal orifice area of the tricuspid valve. *(From Carpentier A, Deloche A, Hanania G, et al: Surgical management of acquired tricuspid valve disease. J Thorac Cardiovasc Surg 67:53, 1974.)*

vised similar flexible rings for atrioventricular valve competence.[50,51]

Semicircular Annuloplasty

Semicircular suture annuloplasty was developed independently by Cabrol in Paris and DeVega in Madrid to simplify the procedure, reduce the amount of intracardiac prosthetic material, maintain annular flexibility, and reduce the potential for conduction system injury.[52,53] It has since been modified by others.[54–56]

Frater's modification of semicircular annuloplasty, controlled tricuspid annuloplasty, allows further adjustment of the plication after the heart is closed and cardiopulmonary bypass is discontinued[54,55] (Fig. 117–7). The hemodynamic results are assessed by palpation, valvular gradient, and cardiac output determinations, or contrast echocardiography.[54–56] Digital examination off bypass usually will confirm the presence or absence of tricuspid regur-

gitation, but will not quantify it.[30] Intraoperative transesophageal Doppler echocardiography generally is used to semiquantify tricuspid regurgitation before and after repair.[57,58]

While tricuspid valve plastic procedures have been associated with encouraging clinical results, the variety of currently employed procedures suggests a lack of uniform success. Postoperative hemodynamic evaluation has confirmed this lack of complete physiologic correction, with persistent residual diastolic gradients in 40–50% of the patients and residual tricuspid insufficiency in 30–40% following valvuloplasty.[59,60] In general, those observed residual derangements have been mild.[59,60] These postoperative hemodynamic observations imply that annuloplasty by current techniques requires careful balancing of persistent residual tricuspid regurgitation against the potential production of tricuspid stenosis by narrowing the annulus too greatly. Ring annuloplasty preserves annular geometry more precisely than the semicircular technique. Follow-up

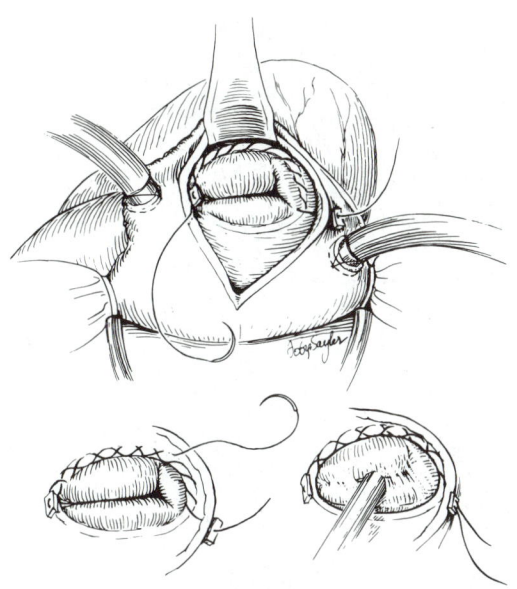

Figure 117–7. Technique of tricuspid semicircular valvuloplasty. A pledgeted 2-0 monofilament polypropylene suture is begun as a mattress suture at the anteroseptal commissure. One strand is sutured over and over the tricuspid annulus in the right ventricular free wall to the posteroseptal commissure and brought through the right atrial wall. The other strand is sutured crisscrossing the previous suture passing through the right atrial wall at the same level. After both sutures are brought through another pledget, they are tightened, judging the orifice size under direct vision with an appropriately sized tricuspid valve obturator. The suture is clamped atraumatially, the atrium is closed, and bypass discontinued. Assessment of the effectiveness of the annuloplasty can then be carried out and further adjustments made. The suture is then tied.

of patients 64 mo after semicircular annuloplasty revealed recurrence of significant tricuspid regurgitation in one-third to one-half of the patients while this occurred in 10% of those treated with ring annuloplasty for a similar period.[61] Others have reported a 5% incidence of severe tricuspid regurgitation requiring valve replacement of 85 mo following semicircular annuloplasty.[62] In spite of these observations, even severe forms of valvular stenosis and regurgitation have frequently responded well clinically to commissurotomy and annuloplasty and with clinically inconsequential residual hemodynamic abnormalities.[61–63]

Another significant factor in the success of tricuspid valvular plastic procedures is the completeness of correction of the associated left-sided lesions, with resolution of the attendant pulmonary hypertension and increased pulmonary vascular resistance.[60,61,61a] Residual tricuspid regurgitation is four times more likely to persist if pulmonary peripheral vascular resistance remains elevated than if it regresses.[60] If the degree of tricuspid regurgitation is moderate, semicircular annuloplasty will suffice. In patients with severe tricuspid regurgitation, particularly in the presence of pulmonary hypertension or increased pulmonary vascular resistance, ring annuloplasty should be employed to provide a fixed permanent annulus for the entire valve circum-

ference.[61b] It is generally conceded that tricuspid valvuloplasty, if feasible, is preferable to valve replacement.[47–56,60–64]

TRICUSPID VALVE REPLACEMENT

For severely deformed tricuspid valves, excision and replacement are required. If the decision is made to excise the tricuspid valve, a rim of cusp should be left. This is most important at the septal cusp to reduce possible conduction system injury. In some instances the valve may be left in place (Fig. 117–8). Interrupted buttressed horizontal mattress sutures are placed through the annulus. They should be superficial and through only the leaflet in the area of the bundle of His. If the sutures are placed in a beating heart, conduction disturbances may be detected, and the offending suture can be removed and repositioned. Since most of these patients have associated left-sided valvular lesions usually repaired with hypothermic cardioplegic arrest, myocardial perfusion should be resumed following their repair to facilitate resumption of spontaneous cardiac rhythm. Frequently, however, the preoperative rhythm has been atrial fibrillation. At operation, there may be a slow ventricular response or nodal rhythm, making conduction changes caused by suture placement difficult to detect. As in semicircular annuloplasty, another potential area of injury to other cardiac structures is at the anteroseptal commissure. Deep sutures in this area may injure the aortic root.

Patients undergoing tricuspid valve replacement should have permanent epicardial electrodes placed at that time. Provision should be made for control of the heart rate in the immediate postoperative period. Bradyarrhythmias becoming symptomatic in the late postoperative course may require permanent pacing at that time.[69] Depending on the type of tricuspid valvular procedure, it may be inadvisable or impossible to use a permanent transvenous pacemaker electrode. While the incidence of permanent postoperative complete heart block has ranged from 2 to 7% following tricuspid valve replacement, it has been reported as high as 45%.[65–70]

Initial enthusiastic reports of tricuspid valve replacement have been confirmed by many.[71,72] Operative mortality has varied between 7 and 40%. Five-year survival has been 55 to 80% with 10-year and 15-year survivals of 36 to 50% and 31 to 37%, respectively.[65,66,68–70,73–77b] Both operative and late survival are influenced negatively by impaired myocardial function.[65–67,69,70,73,74,76,77a,77b] The operative mortality of patients with New York Heart Association (NYHA) class IV is at least twice as high as, and the 5-year survival less than one-half of, that of patients in the NYHA class III.[65,67,69,74]

Mechanical valves inserted in the tricuspid position are associated with a significant rate of valve thrombosis. Right ventricular configuration has been felt to be detrimental to

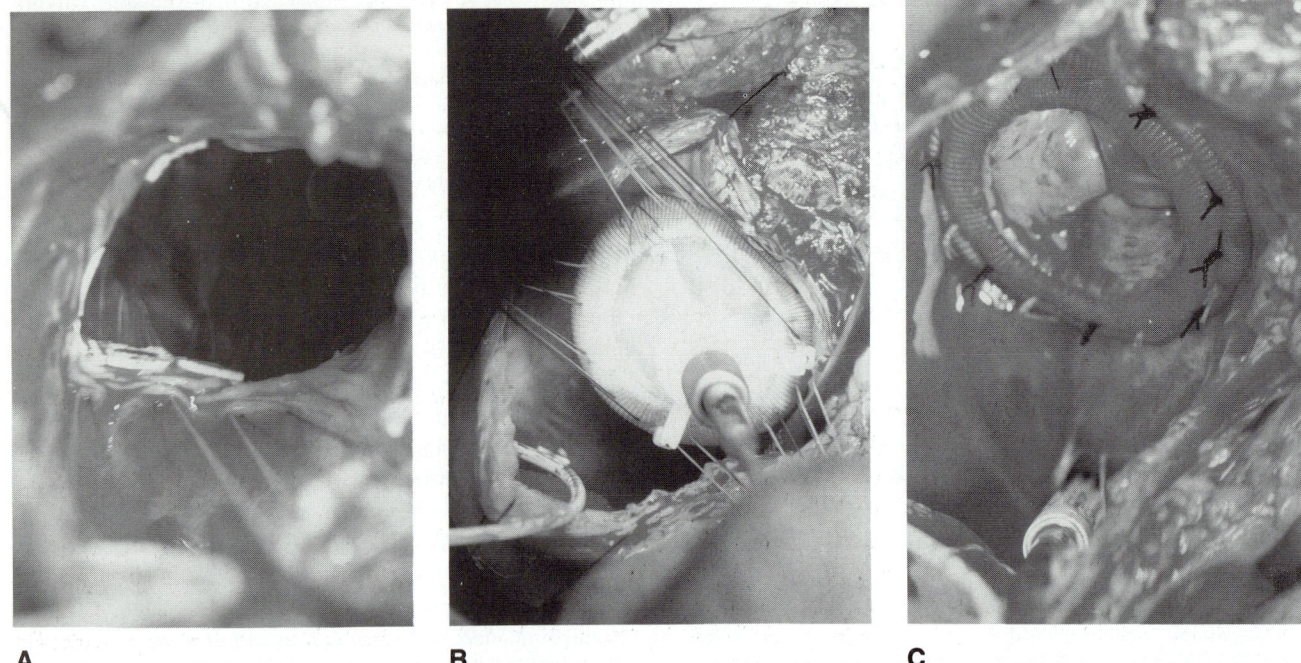

Figure 117–8. Technique of bioprosthetic tricuspid valve replacement. **A.** Interrupted mattress sutures buttressed with Dacron felt pledgets are passed through the annulus from the ventricular to the atrial side. As is shown, leaflet tissue is preserved for suture placement especially in the septal area to reduce possible conduction system injury. **B.** The interrupted sutures are placed through the prosthetic sewing ring. **C.** The valve is lowered in place and the sutures tied and cut. The Swan-Ganz catheter that had been placed preoperatively and withdrawn before valve replacement (lower left corner of illustration) may then be reinserted through the prosthetic valve under direct vision. A pulmonary artery monitoring catheter must not cross a mechanical valve.

ideal functioning of a ball valve prosthesis. However, poppet entrapment has been reported as a cause of malfunction in both ball and disc valves.[74,79] The bileaflet prosthesis because of its low profile and hemodynamics has been felt to offer an advantage in the tricuspid position.[77,78]

Thrombosis of mechanical prosthetic valves in the tricuspid position has varied between 4 and 30%.[66–69,73,74,76] Disc valves are five times more likely to thrombose than are ball valves.[68] While the chance of valve thrombosis is uniformly distributed over the life of the valve, disc valve thrombosis more often occurs early while ball valve thrombosis occurs late and may be secondary to pannus formation.[68,76] Bileaflet prostheses have the lowest thrombosis rate of the mechanical prostheses.[76,77] In contrast to mitral valve prosthetic thrombosis, the onset of tricuspid valve thrombosis may be insidious.[68] Reoperation has been associated with a low mortality.[68] Thrombolysis of thrombosed valves has been reported with all types of mechanical valves in the tricuspid position.[68,77,80–83] All mechanical valves require continual anticoagulation with Coumadin.

Bioprostheses have been shown to have low thrombogenicity in the atrioventricular position and are the valve of choice for tricuspid replacement.[68–70,76–77b,84,85] Rapid calcification of bioprostheses in younger patients may require a mechanical prosthesis for this group.[86,87] However, calcification of a tricuspid bioprosthetic replacement in children may not be as common as has been observed in

those inserted in the aortic or mitral position.[88,89] Less degenerative changes have been reported on late follow-up of bioprostheses implanted in the tricuspid position when compared to those simultaneously implanted in the mitral position.[77b,90] Of the mechanical prostheses, bileaflet valves have been shown to have the least thrombogenicity and should be the valve of choice if a bioprosthesis is not selected.[76,77] In patients who are or will require chronic anticoagulation, and in whom tricuspid valve replacement is contemplated, a bileaflet prosthesis should be considered.

Surgical treatment of tricuspid valvular lesions is not standardized. The surgeon should have at his command the various techniques of valvuloplasty and valve replacement. In planning and executing operative repair, one should understand the underlying anatomic and physiologic derangements not only of the tricuspid valve but also of the associated lesions. Based upon this information, one may then select the appropriate operative techniques to achieve the best possible correction.

If the tricuspid valve is stenotic and unable to be restored to a functional state, it should be replaced. The decision regarding whether any procedure should be performed in the presence of tricuspid insufficiency is much more difficult, and will depend upon the degree of regurgitation. In the presence of severe tricuspid regurgitation if there is loss of leaflet substance such that repair is impossible, valve replacement is necessary.

The most difficult decisions surround management of the insufficient valve usually secondary to left-sided valvular disease. In these instances of functional tricuspid insufficiency, the decision whether to perform a procedure or not will be determined by many factors. Preoperatively, if clinically severe tricuspid regurgitation as indicated by peripheral edema, venous distension, and/or hepatomegaly was present, repair will be required. However, the clinical signs of severe tricuspid insufficiency may not be present, depending upon the diuretic management of the patient. In these circumstances, and in the presence of severe tricuspid regurgitation as determined by Doppler echocardiography, ring annuloplasty should be performed.[61b]

If the degree of tricuspid regurgitation as determined by Doppler echocardiography is only moderate, semicircular annuloplasty should be employed. A modified semicircular annuloplasty with absorbable suture, the "vanishing annuloplasty" of Duran, may be appropriate.[61a] The major reason for performing annuloplasty in this group of patients is to assist their recovery during the operative and early postoperative periods until the long-term effects of the left-sided valve management have had time to reduce pulmonary vascular resistance and pulmonary artery pressure.[61b]

Generally nothing needs to be done for patients with minimal tricuspid regurgitation. These palliative procedures, properly applied, have achieved rewarding clinical results.

REFERENCES

1. Chopra P, Tandon HD: Pathology of chronic rheumatic heart disease with particular reference to tricuspid valve involvement. *Acta Cardiol* **32**:423, 1977
2. Clawson BJ: Rheumatic heart disease—an analysis of 796 cases. *Am Heart J* **20**:454, 1940
3. Kitchin A, Turner R: Diagnosis and treatment of tricuspid stenosis. *Br Heart J* **26**:354, 1964
4. Morgan JR, Forker AD, Coates JR, et al: Isolated tricuspid stenosis. *Circulation* **44**:728, 1971
5. Gibson R, Wood P: The diagnosis of tricuspid stenosis. *Br Heart J* **17**:552, 1955
6. Killip T III, Lukas DS: Tricuspid stenosis—clinical features in twelve cases. *Am J Med* **24**:836, 1958
7. El-Sherif N: Rheumatic tricuspid stenosis—a haemodynamic correlation. *Br Heart J* **33**:16, 1971
8. Sanders CA, Harthorne JW, DeSanctis RW, et al: Tricuspid stenosis—a difficult diagnosis in the presence of atrial fibrillation. *Circulation* **33**:26, 1966
9. Killip T III, Lukas DS: Tricuspid stenosis—physiological criteria for diagnosis and hemodynamic abnormalities. *Circulation* **16**:3, 1957
10. Veyrat C, Kalmanson D, Farjon M, et al: Noninvasive diagnosis and assessment of tricuspid regurgitation and stenosis using one and two dimensional echopulsed Doppler. *Br Heart J* **47**:596, 1982
11. Shimada R, Takeshita A, Nakamura M, et al: Diagnosis of tricuspid stenosis by M-Mode and two-dimension echocardiography. *Am J Cardiol* **53**:164, 1984
12. Guyer DE, Gillam LD, Foale RA, et al: Comparison of the echocardiographic and hemodynamic diagnosis of rheumatic tricuspid stenosis. *J Am Coll Cardiol* **3**:1135, 1984
13. Perez JE, Ludbrook PA, Ahumada GG: Usefulness of Doppler echocardiography in detecting tricuspid valve stenosis. *Am J Cardiol* **55**:601, 1985
14. Muller O, Shillingford J: Tricuspid incompetence. *Br Heart J* **16**:195, 1954
15. Sepulveda G, Lukas DS: The diagnosis of tricuspid insufficiency—clinical features in 60 cases with associated mitral valve disease. *Circulation* **11**:552, 1955
16. McMichael J, Shillingford JP: The role of valvular incompetence in heart failure. *Br Med J* **1**:537, 1957
17. Salazar E, Levine HD: Rheumatic tricuspid regurgitation. *Am J Med* **33**:111, 1962
18. Glancy DL, Marcus FI, Cuadra M, et al: Isolated organic tricuspid valvular regurgitation. *Am J Med* **46**:989, 1969
19. Brandenburg RO, McGoon DC, Campeau L, et al: Traumatic rupture of the chordae tendineae of the tricuspid valve. *Am J Cardiol* **18**:911, 1966
20. Katz NM, Pallas RS: Traumatic rupture of the tricuspid valve: Repair by chordal replacements and annuloplasty. *J Thorac Cardiovasc Surg* **91**:310, 1986
21. Morgan JR, Forker AD: Isolated tricuspid insufficiency. *Circulation* **43**:559, 1971
22. Marvin RF, Schrank JP, Nolan SP: Traumatic tricuspid insufficiency. *Am J Cardiol* **32**:723, 1973
23. Cahill NS, Beller BM, Linhart JW, et al: Isolated traumatic tricuspid regurgitation. Prolonged survival without operative intervention. *Chest* **61**:689, 1972
24. Sbar S, Diacoff G, Nightingale D, et al: Chronic tricuspid insufficiency. *South Med J* **66**:917, 1973
25. Smith WR, Glauser FL, Jemison P: Ruptured chordae of the tricuspid valve—the consequence of flow-directed Swan-Ganz catheterization. *Chest* **70**:790, 1976
25a. Votapka TV, Appleton RS, Pennington DG: Tricuspid valve replacement after orthotopic heart transplantation. *Ann Thorac Surg* **57**:752–754, 1994
25b. Huddleston CB, Rosenbloom M, Goldstein JA, Pasque MK: Biopsy-induced tricuspid regurgitation after cardiac transplantation. *Ann Thorac Surg* **57**:832–837, 1994
26. Roberts WC, Sjoerdsma A: The cardiac disease associated with the carcinoid syndrome (carcinoid heart disease). *Am J Med* **36**:5, 1964
27. Honey M, Paneth M: Carcinoid heart disease: Successful tricuspid valve replacement. *Thorax* **30**:464, 1975
28. Silver MD, Lam JHC, Ranganathan N, et al: Morphology of the human tricuspid valve. *Circulation* **43**:333, 1971
29. Hansing CE, Rowe GG: Tricuspid insufficiency—a study of hemodynamics and pathogenesis. *Circulation* **45**:793, 1972
30. Cohen SR, Sell JE, McIntosh CI, et al: Tricuspid regurgitation in patients with acquired, chronic, pure mitral regurgitation. I. Prevalence, diagnosis and comparison of preoperative clinical hemodynamic features in patients with and without tricuspid regurgitation. *J Thorac Cardiovasc Surg* **94**:481, 1987
31. Grondin P, Meere C, Limet R, et al: Carpentier's annulus and De-Vega's annuloplasty. *J Thorac Cardiovasc Surg* **70**:852, 1975
32. Lieppe W, Behar VS, Scallion R, et al: Detection of tricuspid regurgitation with two-dimensional echocardiography and peripheral vein injections. *Circulation* **57**:128, 1978
33. Chen CC, Morganroth J, Mardelli TJ, et al: Tricuspid regurgitation in tricuspid valve prolapse valve demonstrated with contrast cross-sectional echocardiography. *Am J Cardiol* **46**:983, 1980
34. Tei C, Shah PM, Ormiston JA: Assessment of tricuspid regurgitation by directional analysis of right atrial systolic linear reflux echoes with contrast M-mode echocardiography. *Am Heart J* **103**:1025, 1982
35. Miyatake K, Okamoto M, Kinoshita N, et al: Evaluation of tricuspid regurgitation by pulsed Doppler and two-dimensional echocardiography. *Circulation* **66**:777, 1982
36. DePace NL, Ross J, Iskandrian AS, et al: Tricuspid regurgitation:

Noninvasive techniques for determining causes and severity. *J Am Coll Cardiol* **3**:1540, 1984

37. Curtius JM, Thyssen M, Breuer HWM, et al: Doppler versus contrast echocardiography for diagnosis of tricuspid regurgitation. *Am J Cardiol* **56**:333, 1985

38. Carpentier A, Deloche A, Hanania G, et al: Surgical management of acquired tricuspid valve disease. *J Thorac Cardiovasc Surg* **67**:53, 1974

39. Grondin P, Lepage G, Castonguay Y, et al: The tricuspid valve: A surgical challenge. *J Thorac Cardiovasc Surg* **53**:7, 1967

40. Zubiate P, Kay JH: Tricuspid stenosis—Surgical treatment. *Circulation* **29**(Suppl 1):95, 1964

41. Kay JH: Personal communication, 1974

42. Kay JH, Mendez AM, Zubiate P: A further look at tricuspid annuloplasty. *Ann Thorac Surg* **22**:498, 1976

43. Boyd AD, Engelman RM, Isom OW, et al: Tricuspid annuloplasty—five and one-half years' experience with 78 patients. *J Thorac Cardiovasc Surg* **68**:344, 1974

44. Reed GE, Cortes LE: Measured tricuspid annuloplasty: A rapid and reproducible technique. *Ann Thorac Surg* **21**:168, 1976

45. Reed GE, Boyd AD, Spencer FC, et al: Operative management of tricuspid regurgitation. *Circulation* **54**(Supple 3):96, 1976

46. Minale C, Lambertz H, Messmer BJ: New developments for reconstruction of the tricuspid valve. *J Thorac Cardiovasc Surg* **94**:626, 1987

47. Carpentier A, Deloche A, Dauptain J, et al: A new reconstructive operation for correction of mitral and tricuspid insufficiency. *J Thorac Cardiovasc Surg* **61**:1, 1971

48. Carpentier A: In discussion of Grondin P, Meere C, Limet R, et al: Carpentier's annulus and DeVega's annuloplasty. *J Thorac Cardiovasc Surg* **70**:852, 1975 (ref. 24)

49. Carpentier A: In discussion of Breyer RH, McClenathan JH, Michaelis LL, et al: Tricuspid regurgitation—a comparison of nonoperative management, tricuspid annuloplasty, and tricuspid valve replacement. *J Thorac Cardiovasc Surg* **72**:867, 1976 (ref. 59)

50. Duran CG, Ubago JLM: Clinical and hemodynamic performance of a totally flexible prosthetic ring for atrioventricular valve reconstruction. *Ann Thorac Surg* **22**:458, 1976

51. Hecart J, Blaise C, Bex JP, et al: Technique for tricuspid annuloplasty with a flexible linear reducer. *J Thorac Cardiovasc Surg* **79**:689, 1980

52. Grondin P: In discussion of Breyer RH, McClenathan JH, Michaelis LL, et al: Tricuspid regurgitation—a comparison of nonoperative management, tricuspid annuloplasty, and tricuspid valve replacement. *J Thorac Cardiovasc Surg* **72**:867, 1976 (ref. 59)

53. DeVega NG: In discussion of Breyer RH, McClenathan JH, Michaelis LL, et al: Tricuspid regurgitation—a comparison of nonoperative management, tricuspid annuloplasty and tricuspid valve replacement. *J Thorac Cardiovasc Surg* **72**:867, 1976 (ref. 59)

54. Frater RWM: Technique of management in tricuspid disease. Syllabus of the 14th Postgraduate Program of the Society of Thoracic Surgeons. Atlanta, Georgia, The Society of Thoracic Surgeons, January 20, 1980, pp 37–41

55. Frater RWM, Becker RM, Strom J: Controlled tricuspid annuloplasty (CTA) for gross tricuspid insufficiency (GTI). *Circulation* **62**(Suppl 3):155, 1980

56. Meyer J, Bircks W: Predictable correction of tricuspid insufficiency by semicircular annuloplasty. *Ann Thorac Surg* **23**:574, 1977

57. Goldman ME, Guarino T, Fuster V, et al: The necessity for tricuspid valve repair can be determined intraoperatively by two-dimensional echocardiograpy. *J Thorac Cardiovasc Surg* **94**:542, 1987

58. Czer L, Maurer G, Khan S, et al: Reparative surgery for tricuspid regurgitation: Operative and follow-up evaluation by Doppler color flow mapping. *J Am Coll Cardiol* **11**(2):3A, 1988

59. Haerten K, Seipel L, Loogen F, et al: Hemodynamic studies after De-Vega's tricuspid annuloplasty. *Circulation* **58**(Suppl 1):28, 1978

60. Duran CMG, Pomar PL, Colman S, et al: Is tricuspid valve repair necessary? *J Thorac Cardiovasc Surg* **80**:849, 1980

61. Rivera R, Duran E, Ajuria M: Carpentier's flexible ring versus De-Vega's annuloplasty. *J Thorac Cardiovasc Surg* **89**:196, 1985

61a. Duran CMG: Tricuspid valve surgery revisited. *J Card Surg* **9**[Suppl]242–247, 1994

61b. Cohn LH: Tricuspid regurgitation secondary to mitral valve disease: When and how to repair. *J Card Surg* **9**[Suppl]:237–241, 1994

62. Chidambaram M, Abdulali SA, Baliga BA, et al: Long-term results of DeVega tricuspid annuloplasty. *Ann Thorac Surg* **43**:185, 1987

63. Mullany CJ, Gersh BJ, Orszulak TA, et al: Repair of tricuspid valve insufficiency in patients undergoing double (aortic and mitral) valve replacement. *J Thorac Cardiovasc Surg* **94**:740, 1987

64. Prabhakar G, Kumar N, Gometza B, et al: Surgery for organic rheumatic disease of the tricuspid valve. *J Heart Valve Dis* **2**:561–566, 1993

65. Kouchoukos NT, Stephenson LW: Indications for and results of tricuspid valve replacement. *Adv Cardiol* **17**:199, 1976

66. Stephenson LW, Kouchoukos NT, Kirklin JW: Triple-valve replacement; An analysis of eight years' experience. *Ann Thorac Surg* **23**:327, 1977

67. Peterffy A, Henze A, Jonasson R, et al: Clinical evaluation of the Bjork-Shiley tilting disc valve in the tricuspid position. *Scand J Thorac Cardiovasc Surg* **12**:179, 1978

68. Thorburn CW, Morgan JJ, Shanahan MX, et al: Long-term results of tricuspid valve replacement and the problem of prosthetic valve thrombosis. *Am J Cardiol* **51**:1128, 1983

69. Gersh BJ, Schaff HV, Vatterott PJ, et al: Results of triple valve replacement in 91 patients; perioperative mortality and long-term follow-up. *Circulation* **72**(1):130, 1985

70. Cohen SR, Sell JE, McIntosh Cl, et al: Tricuspid regurgitation in patients with acquired, chronic, pure mitral regurgitation: II. Nonoperative management, tricuspid valve annuloplasty, and tricuspid valve replacement. *J Thorac Cardiovasc Surg* **94**:488, 1987

71. Starr A, Herr R, Wood J: Tricuspid replacement for acquired valve disease. *Surg Gynecol Obstet* **122**:1295, 1966

72. Pluth JR, Ellis FH Jr: Tricuspid insufficiency in patients undergoing mitral valve replacement. *J Thorac Cardiovasc Surg* **58**:484, 1969

73. Sanfelippo PM, Giuliani ER, Danielson GK, et al: Tricuspid valve prosthetic replacement—early and late results with the Starr-Edwards prosthesis. *J Thorac Cardiovasc Surg* **71**:441, 1976

74. Jugdutt BI, Fraser RS, Lee SJK, et al: Long-term survival after tricuspid valve replacement—results with seven different prostheses. *J Thorac Cardiovasc Surg* **74**:20, 1977

75. Macmanus Q, Grunkemeier G, Starr A: Late results of triple valve replacement: A 14-year review. *Ann Thorac Surg* **25**:402, 1978

76. Wellens F, Leclerc JL, Deuvaert F, et al: *Tricuspid Valve Replacement—a Comparative Experience With Different Valve Substitutes.* Boston, Martinus Nijhoff, 1985, pp 91–97

77. Singh AK, Feng WC, Sanofsky SJ: Long-term results of St. Jude medical valve in the tricuspid position. *Ann Thorac Surg* **54**:538–540, 1992

77a. Scully HE, Armstrong S: Tricuspid valve replacement: Fifteen years of experience with mechanical and bioprostheses. *J Thorac Cardiovasc Surg* **109**:1035–1041, 1995

77b. Glower DD, White WD, Smith R, et al: In-hospital and long-term outcome after porcine tricuspid valve replacement. *J Thorac Cardiovasc Surg* **109**:877–884, 1995

78. Singh AK, Christian FD, Williams DO, et al: Follow-up assessment of St. Jude medical prosthetic valve in the tricuspid position: Clinical and hemodynamic results. *Ann Thorac Surg* **37**:324, 1984

79. Suwansirikul S, Glassman E, Raia F, et al: Late thrombosis of Starr-Edwards tricuspid ball valve prosthesis. *Am J Cardiol* **34**:737, 1974

80. Luluaga IT, Carrera D, D'Oliveira J, et al: Successful thrombolytic therapy after acute tricuspid-valve obstruction. *Lancet* **708**:1067–1068, 1971

81. Joyce LD, Boucek M, McGeough EC: Urokinase therapy for thrombosis of tricuspid prosthetic valve. *J Thorac Cardiovasc Surg* **85**:935, 1983

82. Boskovic D, Elezovic I, Boskovic D, et al: Late thrombosis of the Bjork-Shiley tilting disc valve in the tricuspid position: Thrombolytic treatment with streptokinase. *J Thorac Cardiovasc Surg* **91:**1, 1986

83. Kurzrok S, Singh AK, Most AS, et al; Thrombolytic therapy for prosthetic cardiac valve thrombosis. *J Am Coll Cardiol* **9:**592, 1987

84. McIntosh CL, Michaelis LL, Morrow AG, et al: Atrioventricular valve replacement with the Hancock porcine xenograft: A five year clinical experience. *Surgery* **78:**768, 1975

85. Breyer RH, McClenathan JH, Michaelis LL, et al: Tricuspid regurgitation—a comparison of nonoperative management, tricuspid annuloplasty and tricuspid valve replacement. *J Thorac Cardiovasc Surg* **72:**867, 1976

86. Geha As, Laks H, Stansel HC, et al: Late failure of porcine valve heterografts in children. *J Thorac Cardiovasc Surg* **78:**351, 1979

87. Ishihara T, Ferrans VJ, Jones M, et al: Calcific deposits developing in a bovine pericardial bioprosthetic valve three days after implantation. *Circulation* **63:**718, 1981

88. Dunn JM: Porcine valve durability in children. *Ann Thorac Surg* **32:**357, 1981

89. Pasque M, Williams WG, Coles JG, et al: Tricuspid valve replacement in children. *Ann Thorac Surg* **44:**164, 1987

90. Cohen SR, Silver MA, McIntosh CL, et al: Comparison of late (62 to 140 months) degenerative changes in simultaneously implanted and explanted porcine (Hancock) bioprostheses in the tricuspid and mitral valve positions in six patients. *Am J Cardiol* **53:**1599, 1984

C H A P T E R

118

Acquired Disease of the Mitral Valve

Julie A. Swain

STRUCTURE AND PATHOLOGY

To understand the pathological processes involving disease of the mitral valve, it is necessary to understand the anatomic components and relations of the mitral valve. In the past, valve replacement was the predominant operation involving the mitral valve. Since valve repair techniques have become advanced, it is critical to understand the anatomy to plan the appropriate corrective operation.

The mitral valve is composed of five separate components: the valvular leaflets, the annulus, the chordae tendinea, the papillary muscles, and the left ventricular wall. Abnormalities in one or several of these structural components lead to mitral valve dysfunction. Numerous operative procedures have been developed to address pathology in these components. The following sections will discuss the pathologic processes involving the mitral valve and the structural abnormalities associated with these processes. Chapter 119 will address the surgical techniques of mitral valve repair.

Ischemic Mitral Valve Disease

Myocardial ischemia from coronary artery disease affects mitral valve function in many ways. The integrity of the mitral valve apparatus, especially the papillary muscles and the attached left ventricular wall, is acutely affected by ischemia. Ischemia leads to loss of contractility and the resultant dyskinesis or akinesis of the left ventricular wall seriously affects mitral valve competence by distorting the normal dynamic papillary muscle interaction.

As viable myocardial structures containing functioning muscle, the papillary muscles are sensitive to ischemia be-

cause of their relative endartery vascularization. The anterior papillary muscle blood supply is most commonly from the left anterior descending coronary artery, but also may be from either a diagonal, a proximal marginal, or a ramus intermedius arterial branch. The posterior papillary muscle is supplied from the posterior circulation either by way of the right coronary artery or the distal circumflex artery. Myocardial infarction or ischemia in any of these distributions may lead to abnormalities of the papillary muscle–left ventricular wall complex. This is commonly referred to as papillary muscle dysfunction. Neither papillary muscle infarction nor left ventricular dilatation alone is sufficient to produce mitral regurgitation, but the combination of the two is necessary.[1] Necrosis of the papillary muscles can result in papillary muscle rupture either at the basilar attachment to the left ventricular wall (which is usually fatal) or at the chordal attachment on the tip of the muscle. Papillary muscle rupture typically leads to acute cardiac decompensation. Left ventricular aneurysm formation secondary to infarction may lead to mitral regurgitation and papillary muscle dysfunction because of the anatomic displacement of the muscles relative to one another and relative to the annulus.[2]

The chordae tendinea are not affected by ischemia since they are avascular structures. However, the connections of the chordae with the papillary muscle may be affected by infarction and necrosis. Likewise, the leaflets are avascular. However, leaflet coaptation is determined by annular size and motion. It is now accepted that the annulus undergoes shape change during the cardiac cycle. Left ventricular ischemia leading to cardiac chamber enlargement will cause annular dilatation and abnormal annular motion with subsequent lack of coaptation of the leaflet edges, leading to mitral regurgitation.

From the above description of the effects of ischemia on mitral valve function, it is apparent that there are multiple approaches to the correction of ischemic mitral regurgitation, depending on the level of involvement. One of the difficulties in management of mitral regurgitation is the determination of the need for mitral valve repair or replacement in myocardial ischemia. Up to 20% of patients undergoing surgery for coronary artery disease have some mitral regurgitation.[3] The amount of regurgitation is inversely proportional to myocardial function as manifest by the ejection fraction. Often, with correction of underlying myocardial ischemia, there is improvement of ejection fraction and a subsequent decrease in mitral regurgitation. Clinical judgment as to when to combine coronary bypass with a mitral valve procedure is important in patients with intermediate degrees of regurgitation secondary to ischemia.[4,5]

Rheumatic Disease

The inflammatory process invoked by rheumatic fever results in endocarditis and myocarditis with the mitral leaflets being the most common structures affected. The onset of mitral stenosis occurs at some time distant from the acute rheumatic fever episode. This may vary from 2 to 10 or more years after the acute process, being more fulminant in tropical climates. Controversy exists as to whether the rheumatic inflammatory process continues chronically, resulting in progressive destruction of the valvular tissue, or whether the initial insult is responsible for producing damage, leading to turbulence, which then chronically damages the valve.[6]

Rheumatic mitral valve disease can be manifest as either mitral stenosis, mitral insufficiency, or the more common mixed lesion found in older adults. Two primary processes occur at the mitral leaflets with the rheumatic involvement. There is generalized leaflet thickening, which may progress to calcification and retraction leading to the combination of stenosis and regurgitation. This thickening and calcification of the leaflets can progress in severe cases to periannular calcification and limitation of normal annular motion. The inflammation of the leaflets may result in fusion of the coapting edges, most commonly involving the commissural regions. This fusion may progress to the point where a "fish mouth" appearance occurs producing a central orifice.

Although the rheumatic process begins in the leaflets, the chordae tendinea are commonly involved. Involvement takes the form of chordal thickening, shortening, and fusion. This is most common in the commissural areas and progresses with more severe disease to the central chordae.

The rheumatic process can elicit an intense inflammation that affects papillary muscle length and function. In addition, myocarditis caused by rheumatic fever may affect the left ventricular wall and the attached valvular apparatus.

Myxomatous Degeneration

Myxomatous degeneration affects primarily the chordae tendinea and leaflets in older patients. The chordae elongate and may eventually rupture leading to acute worsening of the mitral regurgitation. The mitral leaflets thicken and become redundant with billowing into the left atrium. Degeneration and abnormal collagen synthesis occur in the central zona fibrosa area of the cusps near the chordal insertions.[7] This myxomatous degeneration with prolapse is a common cause for mitral valve operation.[8]

Endocarditis

Leaflet tissue is most commonly affected by endocarditis, resulting in vegetations and subsequent destruction of the leaflet or thickening and healing around chronic perforations. With progression of endocarditis, the annulus can be involved resulting in annular or periannular abscesses. Leaflet detachment from the annulus with massive regurgitation may ensue. Destruction of the edges of the leaflets may result in chordal detachment. Likewise, involvement of chordae or papillary muscles with endocarditis may result in rupture and leaflet prolapse. Infection in the body of the papillary muscle and of the left ventricular wall is rare. Annular involvement is important in that the mitral and aortic annulae share a common area. Annular involvement of one of the valves can progress to destruction of the annulus of the other valve and subsequent bivalvular regurgitation.

Other Diseases

There are other diseases that are unique to the mitral apparatus. Idiopathic calcification of the mitral annulus, particularly in the posterior area extending into the left atrium, is encountered more frequently in elderly women.[9] This calcification can lead to loss of the normal shape change of the mitral annulus during left ventricular contraction with subsequent mitral valve dysfunction. Calcification extending into the leaflets leads to fixation of the leaflets and prevention of normal motion.

Systemic diseases, such as Marfan's and Ehlers–Danlos syndromes, may lead to annular dilatation and chordal elongation. Other systemic diseases, such as polyarteritis, sarcoidosis, hypereosinophilia,[10] and amyloidosis can involve the papillary muscle–chordal system.

Hypertrophic cardiomyopathy commonly is associated with mitral regurgitation. Several mechanisms may be operative such as distortion of the anterior leaflet from contact with the septum during systolic anterior motion of the leaflet. Dilation of the left ventricle and of the annulus secondary to hypertrophic cardiomyopathy may also be responsible for the finding of mitral regurgitation. Thinning and redundancy of the leaflets can be corrected coincidentally by combining septal myotomy with anterior leaflet plication.[11]

Symptoms

Mitral Stenosis

Mitral stenosis is caused almost exclusively by rheumatic fever. The acute illness is followed one to two decades later by hemodynamic evidence of stenosis, which is usually asymptomatic until the stenosis becomes more severe. There is often a very slow onset of symptoms such that the patients deny a history of these symptoms. Their true debilitation only becomes clear after operative relief of the mitral stenosis. This onset can be over years, and generally starts with the limitation of exercise tolerance. This progresses to true dyspnea, which is due both to decreased cardiac output and to decreased lung compliance and vital capacity. In chronic mitral stenosis, any maneuver that increases the cardiac output will bring on symptoms of dyspnea. Orthopnea and paroxysmal nocturnal dyspnea follow. Pulmonary edema is a late symptom except in occasional patients who have a relatively acute onset of mitral stenosis and who present initially with pulmonary edema. This most commonly occurs when mitral stenosis appears during the third trimester of pregnancy.

Hemoptysis is another common symptom of severe mitral stenosis. Hemoptysis may present as profuse hemorrhage that is usually self-limiting; it may be manifest as pulmonary edema with bloody sputum or with bloody sputum secondary to bronchitis. Bronchitis is a common symptom because of the edema of the mucosa secondary to the pulmonary hypertension. End-stage mitral stenosis may be accompanied by pulmonary infarction.

The onset of atrial fibrillation often acutely worsens the symptoms of mitral stenosis due to a decrease in cardiac output because of decreased preload. Thromboembolism may be present in up to one-fifth of patients with atrial fibrillation and can be seen in patients with mitral stenosis without a history of atrial fibrillation. The incidence of thromboembolism correlates with the size of the left atrial appendage and the decrease in cardiac output. Embolism secondary to endocarditic vegetations must be considered.

The time of onset and the magnitude of pulmonary hypertension are variable in mitral disease. Pulmonary hypertension may be due to reflex constriction secondary to left atrial stretch, to increased lung water, or to increased left atrial pressure. Pulmonary hypertension usually decreases or disappears after valve correction.[12] Endstage pulmonary hypertension may be due to changes of arterial obliterans and may be irreversible. Mitral stenosis with severe pulmonary hypertension leads to right ventricular failure, which is manifest by peripheral edema, hepatomegaly, and ascites, and may be associated with tricuspid regurgitation. Chest pain is seen in a small portion of these patients and is

of unexplained etiology. It may be due to coexistent coronary disease or to right ventricular ischemia secondary to the pulmonary hypertension.

With the disturbance of flow patterns across the mitral valve, and subsequent turbulence, endocarditis may occur. Patients should have prophylactic antibiotic coverage before dental, urologic, or gastrointestinal procedures. The appearance of endocarditis and septic emboli is a relative indication for operation.

Mitral Regurgitation

The symptoms of mitral regurgitation depend on the acuteness of onset. In acute mitral regurgitation (such as occurs with chordal rupture, leaflet destruction secondary to endocarditis, or an infarcted and ruptured papillary muscle head), pulmonary edema and right heart failure secondary to acute pulmonary hypertension predominate. In these cases, the left atrial compliance and size are normal.

In contrast, patients with chronic mitral regurgitation have slow onset of symptoms over many years. Patients with mild mitral regurgitation may remain asymptomatic. Symptoms do not usually appear until left ventricular failure occurs, then dyspnea predominates secondary to the low cardiac output or decreased lung compliance with pulmonary congestion and hypertension. Dyspnea is often more prominent in mitral regurgitation than in stenosis. Common symptoms include chronic weakness and chronic fatigue, which is insidious in onset. The occurrence of atrial fibrillation in these patients is better tolerated than in mitral stenosis patients. Hemoptysis and pulmonary embolism are rare in patients with mitral insufficiency.

PHYSICAL EXAMINATION

Mitral Stenosis

The physical examination of patients with mitral stenosis reveals a normal-sized ventricle. The oscillatory findings are pathognomonic and include a loud first heart sound, a diastolic murmur, and, in some patients, an opening snap. The diastolic murmur is a low-pitched rumble that is heard best in the apex. While the loudness of the murmur is not proportional to the degree of mitral stenosis, the length of the murmur does correlate with severity. In severe cases of mitral stenosis with low cardiac output, the murmur may be extremely difficult to detect. The opening snap is characteristic of mitral stenosis when the leaflets are mobile. When the leaflets are rigid and calcified, there is no opening snap. This is an extremely important finding for predicting whether mitral valve repair will be possible. Peripheral vascular constriction is seen with severe mitral stenosis and low cardiac output. In patients who have suffered systemic embolism, the signs may be apparent by fundic examination and with examination of the peripheral arterial tree. Likewise, the signs of right ventricular failure, which include a right ventricular heave, tricuspid regurgitation, hepatomegaly, and ascites may be present.

Mitral Regurgitation

Moderate-to-severe mitral regurgitation leading to left ventricular enlargement will be evident on physical examination as an apical pulse that is displaced laterally. A precordial lift may be present and is secondary to left atrial or right ventricular enlargement. The auscultatory findings consist of a high-pitched apical systolic murmur that radiates to the axilla. In conditions affecting the posterior leaflet only, the murmur may radiate parasternally. However, in the case of prosthetic mitral regurgitation, the murmur may radiate in any direction depending on the location of the jet. There is little correlation between the loudness of the murmur and the severity of the mitral regurgitation. Systolic murmurs that occur late in systole are generally indicative of mild regurgitation, while holosystolic murmurs indicate more severe regurgitation. A diastolic rumble and a prominent S3 may be present because of rapid ventricular filling and increased flow velocity across the mitral valve. In ischemic regurgitation, the murmur may only transiently appear during papillary muscle dysfunction. Careful auscultation may reveal a transient regurgitation murmur in patients with episodes of chest pain or acute ischemic EKG changes. Severe mitral regurgitation will result in the predominance of symptoms of cardiac failure and low cardiac output. Findings of right ventricular failure, as in mitral stenosis, may occur in advanced disease.

Laboratory Examinations

Blood analysis may help to diagnose the etiology of acquired mitral disease. Blood cultures for endocarditis and tests for acute rheumatic fever are indicated when a clinical suspicion is present. The findings of an elevated erythrocyte sedimentation rate in left atrial myxoma mimicking stenosis may be present.

The electrocardiogram is diagnostic of left atrial enlargement with P-wave abnormalities in the majority of patients with mitral stenosis. Also, atrial fibrillation may be the first finding of mitral disease. Left and right ventricular hypertrophy is found in advanced mitral disease. Acute myocardial ischemia, especially in the posterolateral region, leads one to suspect ischemic mitral regurgitation. X-ray findings of left and right ventricular hypertrophy are present in severe mitral regurgitation, often accompanied by left atrial enlargement. Pulmonary hypertension leads to a prominence of the pulmonary vessels. Interstitial edema indicates severe mitral obstruction and progresses to pulmonary edema. Lateral chest x-ray may also show calcification of the posterior mitral annulus.

The echocardiogram, either transthoracic or transesophageal, remains the mainstay of mitral valvular pathology diagnosis. The M-mode echocardiogram demonstrates mitral leaflet thickening and abnormal excursion. Analysis of the specific abnormalities of valve motion may help the surgeon to plan operative repair. However, two-dimensional echocardiography is necessary to estimate the degree of mitral regurgitation or stenosis. Doppler echocardiography is used to estimate the velocity of flow across the mitral orifice and to give an estimate of the transvalvular gradient. The excellent visualization of all areas of the left atrium by transesophageal echocardiography allows a sensitive method for detection of atrial thrombi and valvular vegetations. Unsuspected aortic and tricuspid pathology may be demonstrated.

Cardiac catheterization is commonly performed prior to operative intervention for mitral valve disease in the United States. In the middle-aged/elderly population, coronary anatomy must be elucidated to determine the presence of silent coronary artery disease. Hemodynamic evaluation by right and left heart catheterization forms the basis for determination of the severity of the mitral pathology. The use of the modified Gorlin equation to calculate mitral valvular area in mitral stenosis is particularly helpful.[13] Systolic, diastolic, and ejection phase indices aid in determining the severity of disease.

Nuclear perfusion scintigraphy indicates the extent and location of myocardial ischemia and provides a physiologic correlation with anatomic evidence of coronary artery stenoses.

INDICATIONS FOR OPERATION

Mitral Stenosis

The natural history of mitral stenosis in the current era is difficult to determine because of the effectiveness of surgical therapy. Previous studies have shown that the onset of symptomatic mitral stenosis occurs approximately 10 years after acute rheumatic fever.[14] Over the next 5 to 10 years, the patients generally progress from class II to class IV symptoms.[15] The decrease in functional ability occurs in an exponential manner. It is generally agreed that asymptomatic patients should not undergo an operative procedure. Depending upon the patient's age (young) and coexisting medical conditions (few), patients with mild symptoms should be considered as candidates for operation. Elderly patients with coexisting diseases may tolerate mild-to-moderate mitral stenosis for long periods.

The hemodynamic definition of mitral stenosis is made at the time of left and right heart catheterization. The normal mitral valve orifice is 4 to 6 cm^2. Mild mitral stenosis occurs when the orifice is reduced to 2 cm^2; less than 1.0 cm^2 is severe stenosis. The symptoms and valvular gradient are affected by maneuvers that increase either bloodflow velocity across the mitral valve, as with tachycardia, or decrease cardiac filling, as with tachycardia or atrial fibrillation.

Certain indications for operation are generally agreed upon (Table 118–1). The appearance of atrial fibrillation usually heralds worsening symptoms because of the effect on left ventricular filling, and is a relative indication. Early correction of mitral stenosis may prevent atrophy of the atrial architecture that leads to irreversible atrial fibrillation.[16] The appearance of systemic embolism from the valve is an indication for operation. The incidence of embolism is increased fourfold in patients with atrial fibrillation.[17] Severe mitral disease with pulmonary hypertension, right heart failure, and hemoptysis are indications for operation. Patients with endocarditis accompanied by septic emboli, uncontrolled sepsis, or hemodynamic compromise are operative candidates. Early operation should be considered in patients with nonstreptococcal infections.[18]

Current noninvasive techniques of evaluation, especially echocardiography, allow a reasonable prediction of whether valve repair, rather than replacement, is possible. In patients who are candidates for a conservative operation, treatment may be considered earlier in the course of the disease.

A special situation occurs in young women who desire to become pregnant. It is expected that the increase in cardiac output will have a worsening effect on mitral stenosis symptoms. In this instance, mildly symptomatic patients with mild-to-moderate stenosis may be candidates for treatment (operative or percutaneous catheter-based) because of the predicted decline in functional status in the third trimester.

Mitral Regurgitation

The decision to recommend operation for patients with mitral regurgitation is more complex than for patients with mitral stenosis because of the variable etiology of regurgitation. In cases of endocarditis and acute ischemic mitral regurgitation, the indications for operation are relatively straightforward. However, with chronic mitral regurgitation secondary to rheumatic fever or myxoid degeneration, the course of myocardial involvement and the development of symptoms occur over a longer period. Patients often become symptomatic only after left ventricular function has been damaged irreversibly, at which time the results of surgery are not as favorable as in those patients with normal left ventricles. The evaluation of left ventricular function is different because most indices vary with preload and afterload. Ejection fraction is a poor way to evaluate function because it may be preserved even after irreversible left ventricular failure occurs because of the high volume of low-resistance regurgitant flow.

The pathophysiological effects of mitral regurgitation are dependent on the relative amount of left ventricular ejection into the aorta compared to regurgitation into the left atrium. These relative volumes depend on the three dynamic parameters of aortic pressure, left atrial pressure, and regurgitant orifice size. Maneuvers that increase aortic afterload also increase regurgitant volume. Likewise, afterload reduction can have dramatic effects on diminishing the regurgitant volume. Increases in preload may distort the mitral valve architecture by increasing left ventricular volume and regurgitant orifice size and lead to increased regurgitant fraction.

In chronic regurgitation, left ventricular forward output is preserved for a variable period by changes in left ventricular tension and fiber shortening resulting in normal cardiac output and ejection fraction. As mitral regurgitation progresses, left ventricular end-diastolic volume and left ventricular mass are increased, but the ejection fraction and velocity of circumferential fiber shortening (the ejection phase indices) may be near normal, even with irreversible left ventricular functional impairment. This is accompanied by ultrastructural evidence of increased myocyte length and decreased myofibril content.[19]

By the time the ejection fraction falls moderately (about 40%), left ventricular function may be severely impaired. Depressed cardiac output marks severe left ventricular dysfunction. Patients in whom irreversible ventricular changes have occurred generally have less improvement after mitral valve surgery because of the abolishment of the "pop-off" valve effect of the regurgitant leak and the subsequent increase in ventricular afterload and further decrease in ejection fraction and cardiac output.

It is important to assess the status of the left ventricle for prognostic reasons and to determine the optimal time for operation. For many years, attempts to find noninvasive parameters for following patients with mitral regurgitation and determining the optimal time for operation have been sought. Measurement of end-systolic volume or diameter recently have been found to be the most useful indices for evaluation of left ventricular function. The value of these parameters is confirmed by determining left ventricular function after mitral repair or replacement. In patients with end-systolic volume less than 30 mL/m², or end-systolic di-

TABLE 118–1. RELATIVE INDICATIONS FOR OPERATION

Mitral Stenosis and Regurgitation
Symptomatic to NYHA class II or greater
Systemic emboli
Hemoptysis
Pulmonary hypertension
Right heart failure
Endocarditis
Atrial fibrillation (?)
Mitral Stenosis
MV orifice area < 2 cm²
Mitral Regurgitation
Left ventricular dysfunction
Decreased ejection fraction
End-systolic LV diameter > 40–50 mm
End-systolic LV volume > 30–40 mm

ameter less than 40 mm, left ventricular function is normal postoperatively. In patients who have a preoperative elevation of end-systolic volume greater than 90 mL/m^2, or end-systolic diameter greater than 50 mm, left ventricular function is irreversibly impaired and surgical mortality is higher.[20,21] Still, without the operation, these patients have an even worse prognosis.

In patients who are minimally symptomatic (class II), but who have objective evidence of left ventricular dysfunction, operation is indicated unless contraindicated by other medical factors. Decision making in minimally symptomatic mitral regurgitation is difficult. Because mitral valve repair is less likely than in patients with mitral stenosis, there is more reticence to refer the minimally symptomatic patient. Class I and class II patients with normal ventricular function are better treated medically. Patients with class III and class IV disease are candidates for surgery unless other medical contraindications are present. Patients with continued infection from endocarditis or systemic embolization are also operative candidates. Generally, patients with acute onset of mitral regurgitation, secondary to chordal rupture or endocarditic involvement of the leaflets, should be considered for operation. The endstage symptoms of renal failure, low cardiac output, pulmonary edema, and paroxysmal nocturnal dyspnea, are indications for operation.

OPERATION

General Considerations

The surgical correction of mitral valve disease involves three general classes of techniques: repair, replacement, and transcatheter intervention. Valve repair is covered in Chapter 119.

Patient characteristics, demographic data, and preoperative evaluation, especially echocardiography, allow the surgeon to judge which operative technique to use. However, examination of the valve at the time of operation is necessary to make a final determination on whether replacement or repair is indicated. Patient-specific considerations, such as the ability to take anticoagulants and the reliability of long-term follow-up, will affect choice. In patients who require long-term anticoagulation because of chronic atrial fibrillation, giant left atrium, or the presence of other prosthetic valves, valve replacement may be the operation of choice. Valve replacement generally requires less ischemic time than valve repair. In patients who cannot afford to have a failure of repair, such as those in cardiogenic shock or with other hemodynamic instabilities, valve replacement is the operation of choice.

Transcatheter techniques will not be dealt with in this chapter. There is a place for this technique in a minority of patients with mitral stenosis who have optimum valvular characteristics. The current data indicate that balloon valvu-

loplasty by the percutaneous technique is equivalent in the short-run to closed mitral commissurotomy.[22,23] The majority of patients require either open repair or replacement.

Monitoring

The ability to monitor the patient during surgery and determine the adequacy of the operative procedure, especially valve repair, is important. Transesophageal and direct epicardial echocardiography allow intraoperative evaluation of valve motion and valvular or prosthetic valvular insufficiency. Echocardiography allows for the detection of thrombi or other solid particulate matter and is important in the determination of adequacy of deairing after open heart procedures.

Choice of Incision and Cannulation

Several chest incisions are used for exposure of the mitral valve (Table 118–2). Although the most common incision is a median sternotomy, isolated mitral valve replacement can be accomplished with excellent exposure and a more cosmetic result with a thoracotomy. The right thoracotomy approach may be particularly useful when the patient has had a previous median sternotomy and/or coronary bypass grafts with veins or mammary arteries. Either ascending aortic or femoral arterial cannulation is used with bicaval venous cannulation. Air evacuation is somewhat more difficult. Left thoracotomy also provides excellent exposure through the left atrium. Venous cannulation of the right ventricular outflow tract and femoral arterial cannulation are required. Thoracotomy may also be chosen when the patient has had chest wall abnormalities produced by trauma, radiation therapy, or skin or chest wall infections.

Cannulation for cardiopulmonary bypass is by any of the standard techniques. Mitral valve exposure may be improved with dual caval cannulation, but for the majority of the patients single cannulation is acceptable. Myocardial protection with retrograde cardioplegia is particularly advantageous because the replacement operation can be con-

TABLE 118–2. SURGICAL APPROACH TO THE MITRAL VALVE

Skin Incision
Median sternotomy
Right thoracotomy
Left thoracotomy
Atrial Incision
Right lateral
Superior
Trans-right atrial, septal
Superior-septal
Left lateral (with left thoracotomy)

tinued without interruption. When antegrade cardioplegia is used, retraction for exposure of the mitral valve annulus may produce aortic insufficiency and result in inadequate delivery in the antegrade direction to the coronary bed unless the mitral valve retractors are repositioned.

Left Atrial Incision

The approach to the mitral valve is through one of several different cardiac incisions (Table 118–2). The choice of incision is varied because of differences in atrial anatomy and body habitus of the patient. The standard approach is through an incision parallel to the intra-atrial groove into the lateral left atrium carried posterior to the superior and inferior vena cavae. Dissection of the intra-atrial groove is favored by some to increase exposure.[24] The superior septal approach by an incision in the roof of the left atrium between the aorta and superior vena cava also gives excellent exposure, and may be extended to include a septal incision for greater exposure (Fig. 118–1).[25,26] When concomitant procedures on the tricuspid valve or right atrium are needed, or when scarring or calcification at the site of previous left atrial incisions makes the standard approach difficult, a transseptal approach through the right atrium provides excellent exposure in addition to limiting the external cardiac incisions to a single incision in the low-pressure right atrium. The long-term effects on cardiac conduction through the atrium with the transseptal approach have not been completely determined.[25] It is essential that the surgeon be familiar with all of these techniques to deal with unexpected anatomic abnormalities.

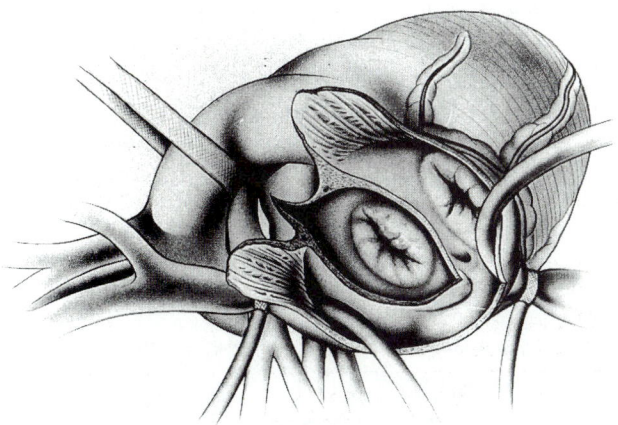

Figure 118–1. The superior septal approach to the mitral valve: The left atrium is opened beginning at the junction of the septal and right atrial incision and is extended across the left atrial dome toward the base of the left atrial appendage. A margin of atrial tissue must remain on the side of the atrioventricular groove to allow closure. The divided ends of the sinus node artery are illustrated in the muscle of the superior septum. *(From Smith CR: J Thorac Cardiovasc Surg 103:623–628, 1992.)*

Chordal Preservation

A controversial question in mitral valve replacement is how to deal with the native mitral valve. In the majority of cases of active endocarditis with infected tissue, complete excision of the valve is necessary. Resection is sometimes indicated in rheumatic mitral stenosis when severe leaflet calcification and thickening, and calcification and fusion of the subvalvular apparatus are present. It has long been known that too aggressive resection of the subvalvular apparatus, especially the posterior papillary muscle, can lead to atrioventricular groove dehiscence and myocardial rupture.

There is now a body of laboratory and clinical evidence showing the importance of the contribution of the intact mitral valve apparatus to myocardial shape and function.[27–33] Excision of the leaflets and chordae leads to disruption of the normal "suspender" function of the intact annuloventricular apparatus. Investigations have shown increased resting and exercise ejection fractions when valve replacement is accomplished with preservation of continuity of the leaflets, chordae, and papillary muscles.[34] A decrease in end-systolic circumferential left ventricular wall stress and increased contractility index and fractional shortening have been found with preservation of the valvular apparatus. The posterior leaflet seems particularly important. Significant differences in both global cardiac and myocyte function between mitral replacement with and without preservation of the subvalvular apparatus are well established.[20,28,35–38] A clinical study comparing mitral valve replacement with preservation of the subvalvular apparatus with mitral valve repair shows no differences in short- or long-term function between the two groups.[39] Reconstruction of papillary-annular integrity during prosthetic valve rereplacement has been advocated.[40,41]

The technical aspects of native valvular tissue preservation with mitral valve replacement are shown in Figures 118–2 and 118–3. With the exception of a very small number of patients with extreme calcification of the leaflets and the subvalvular apparatus, these leaflet preservation techniques can be used in nearly all patients. The posterior leaflet is the easiest to leave intact and contributes importantly to the suspensory function. The controversy about leaving the anterior leaflet intact centers on whether left ventricular outflow tract obstruction is produced.[42] This has not been reported in the larger series. Interference with mechanical valve function can occur if attention is not paid to subvalvular obstructions. With careful handling of the native valve leaflets, prosthetic leaflet obstruction can be avoided in both monoleaflet and bileaflet valves.[34]

Several techniques can be used to preserve the mitral apparatus. In the majority of patients, simply passing the valve suture through the free margin of the leaflet after it has been passed through the annulus will result in "tucking" the leaflet under the annulus. The suture is then passed through the prosthetic ring and the valve seated. Prior to plication, commissurotomy, chordal separation, and/or

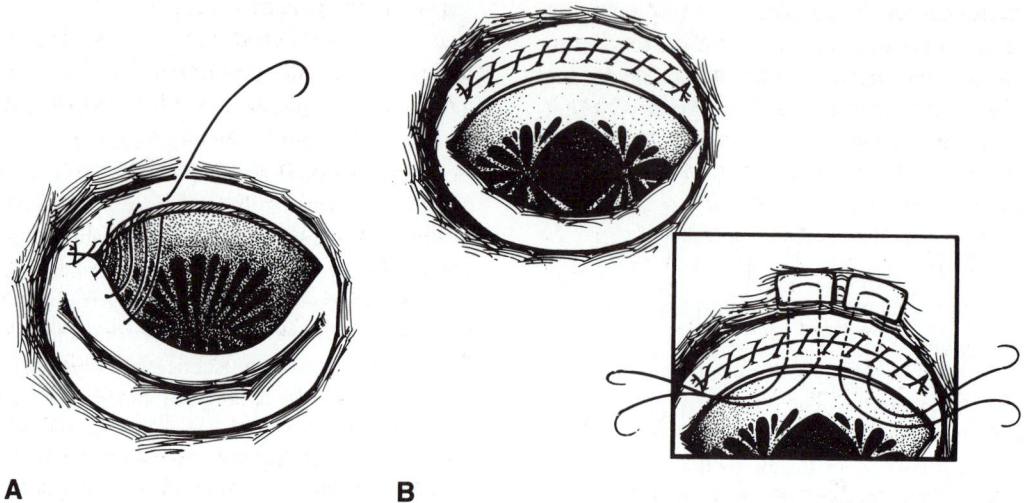

A   B

Figure 118–2. **A.** Preservation of the native mitral valve. The anterior leaflet of the mitral valve is stretched posteriorly and an ellipsoid incision is made 3 mm from the reflection from the atrium and close to the attachments of the anterior marginal chordae. The defect in the anterior leaflet is closed with a running 4-0 polypropylene suture placed parallel to the annulus. **B.** With the chordae and papillary muscles now attached to the rim of the anterior leaflet and retracted away from the subvalvular area, the valve sutures can be placed as is the custom of the surgeon. *(Reprinted with permission from the Society of Thoracic Surgeons (Rose EA, et al: The Annals of Thoracic Surgery 1994, 57:768–769).)*

valve calcium debridement may need to be performed for stenotic valves.[34] Other techniques have been developed to facilitate the subvalvular positioning of the leaflets. An incision can be made parallel to the annulus in either leaflet to excise the body of the leaflet to remove redundant leaflet tissue and preserve the chordal attachments (Fig. 118–2). The central portion of the anterior leaflet can be incised to

the annulus between the chordal attachments and each side of the leaflet suspended laterally (Fig. 118–3).[43,44]

Atrioventricular Groove Disruption

If it is chosen to excise the native leaflets and chordae, excision must be accomplished carefully to avoid damage to the

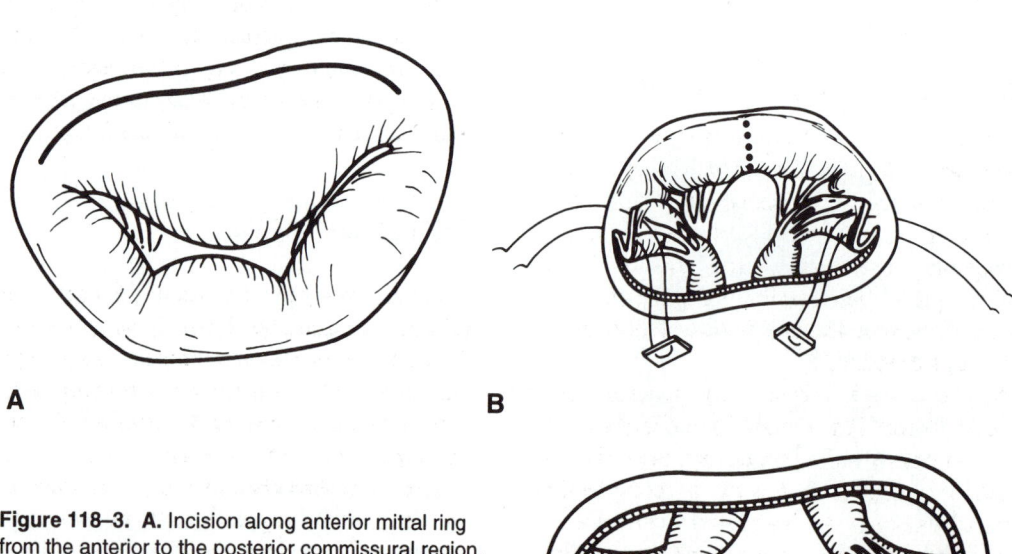

A   B

Figure 118–3. **A.** Incision along anterior mitral ring from the anterior to the posterior commissural region. **B.** The separated anterior and posterior segments are shifted and reaffixed to the mitral ring near the anterior and posterior commissures, respectively. **C.** Stitches for reaffixation are tied. The midportion of the posterior leaflet is incised from the edge to the base. *(Reprinted with permission from the Society of Thoracic Surgery (Miki S, et al: The Annals of Thoracic Surgery 1988, 45:28–34).)*

C

annulus and atrioventricular continuity. Atrioventricular groove disruption generally is a fatal complication. Resection of the papillary muscles has been implicated in this complication. Retention of the posterior leaflet and subvalvular apparatus has decreased the occurrence. Repair of atrioventricular groove disruption necessitates reinstituting cardioplegic arrest, removing the prosthetic valve, and reconstituting atrioventricular integrity with pledgeted sutures, followed by reinserting the valve. The mortality is high.

Valve Dysfunction

When using bioprosthetic valves, care must be taken that the valve sutures do not loop around the struts when the valve is seated, a cause of valve dysfunction and failure. With mechanical valves, careful attention must be paid to removing or displacing subvalvular tissue that could interfere with leaflet motion. The free ends of the sutures must be short and placed properly to avoid being caught in the closing prosthetic valve leaflets.

Intracardiac Deairing

The detection and removal of intracardiac air at the conclusion of the procedure are important. Cardiac venting may be by way of the left atrium, left ventricle, and/or ascending aorta. Aspiration of the cardiac chambers, inversion of the left atrial appendage, and tilting of the table from side to side with inflation of the lungs to dislodge any pulmonary vein bubbles are maneuvers that are used. Transesophageal echocardiography has improved the ability to detect gross intracardiac bubbles.

Left Atrial Calcification and Giant Left Atrium

A particularly difficult technical problem is encountered when the annulus and left atrial wall in the posterior area are calcified. Wide sutures in the annulus may compromise the circumflex coronary artery and/or lead to atrioventricular groove disruption. Superficial sutures may be inadequate and result in paravalvular leaks. Insertion of a left atrial baffle as an anchor for the prosthetic valve is an excellent solution to this problem.[45]

Longstanding end-stage mitral incompetence occasionally produces a "giant" left atrium. The enlargement of the left atrium can impinge on adjacent structures such as the bronchus and esophagus and result in compression symptoms. Stasis leads to an increased incidence of thrombi. For these reasons, left atrial tailoring procedures have been advocated by some.[46] Since this is a relatively uncommon condition, the efficacy of these tailoring procedures is not proven by controlled studies.

Associated Operations

The other cardiac operations most commonly performed with mitral valve replacement are coronary bypass and tricuspid valve repair/replacement. When mitral valve replacement is combined with coronary bypass, the vein bypasses are generally performed first. This allows for the delivery of cardioplegia past obstructions. Lifting the heart out of the pericardial cradle to approach the posterior vessels may result in myocardial rupture or atrioventricular groove dehiscence when a rigid prosthetic valve is in place and should be avoided. Therefore, the coronary bypasses are performed prior to mitral valve replacement. When porcine valves are used, it is advisable to size the mitral valve orifice so that the porcine valve can be washed while the coronary bypasses are being performed.

When tricuspid valve procedures are indicated at the time of mitral replacement, one may choose to expose the mitral valve through the intra-atrial septum. The tricuspid valve procedure is performed after the cardiotomy for the mitral valve is closed, the heart has been deaired, and the aortic cross-clamp has been removed. The patient is rewarmed and reperfused while the tricuspid procedure is accomplished in the beating heart, thus limiting cardiac ischemic time and allowing for the detection.

There is no longer controversy regarding whether coronary bypass operation should be combined with mitral operations when there is an indication for both.[47] Unbypassed significant coronary artery disease is an incremental risk factor for mitral valve replacement.

When aortic valve replacement is combined with mitral valve replacement, care must be taken in leaflet excision in the intra-annular region between the two valves to avoid damaging the aortic annulus. In cases where endocarditis has eroded the aortic annulus or the mitral annulus in this area, insertion of bridging prosthetic material may be necessary to reconstruct the annulus before valve replacement. Occasionally it may be necessary to suture the prosthetic ring of the aortic valve to the prosthetic ring of the mitral valve to reconstruct annular integrity.

CHOICE OF VALVE

There are two general types of prosthetic valves, mechanical and bioprosthetic. There is no general consensus as to the best type of valve for most patients requiring valve replacement and it is a matter of surgeon and patient preference. One must consider the risk/benefit ratio between the two types (Fig. 118–4). Bioprosthetic valves have a lower incidence of thromboembolism and valve thrombosis and do not generally require long-term anticoagulation, with its attendant bleeding possibilities. The trade-off is decreased durability, which averages in the 10 to 15 year range. Mechanical valves are extremely durable with valve life reported to exceed 20 years in some patients. However, all mechanical prostheses require systemic anticoagulation. Both bleeding and thromboembolic complications are higher in patients who have mechanical valves implanted.

There are a few patient groups in which the choice of valve prosthesis is clear. Mechanical valves are usually in-

MECHANICAL VALVE ADVANTAGE

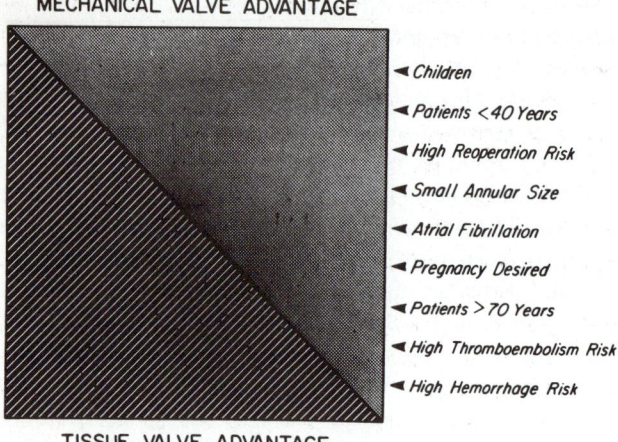

◄ *Children*

◄ *Patients <40 Years*

◄ *High Reoperation Risk*

◄ *Small Annular Size*

◄ *Atrial Fibrillation*

◄ *Pregnancy Desired*

◄ *Patients >70 Years*

◄ *High Thromboembolism Risk*

◄ *High Hemorrhage Risk*

TISSUE VALVE ADVANTAGE

Figure 118–4. Factors in the selection of mechanical and tissue valves. *(Reprinted with permission from the Society of Thoracic Surgeons (Akins CW: The Annals of Thoracic Surgery 1991, 52:161–172).)*

dicated in young patients (under age 30) because of the high rate of degeneration of bioprosthetic valves in the young. In patients who need chronic anticoagulation for chronic atrial fibrillation or other vascular problems, mechanical valves are indicated.[48] In patients with small left ventricular cavities, a low-profile mechanical valve should be used to prevent left ventricular outflow tract obstruction or myocardial impingement.

Bioprosthetic valves are indicated in patients who cannot take anticoagulation because of inherent bleeding disorders, coexisting diseases that predispose to bleeding such as gastrointestinal disorders, aneurysms, and arteriovenous malformations, or those who have high risk occupations or lifestyles. The need for close follow-up of the anticoagulation status after mechanical valve implantation makes socioeconomic considerations important in the choice of valve. The patient must be reliable and intelligent enough to be able and willing to participate in close monitoring of anticoagulation.

Porcine valves may be chosen in young female patients who wish to become pregnant. The teratogenic effects of Dicumarol as well as the risk of thrombosis when the patient cannot be anticoagulated at the time of birth make the risk of a mechanical valve substantial. However, in young patients, the accelerated degeneration does not make bioprosthetic valves an optimum choice.

The hemodynamic performance of mechanical and bioprosthetic valves is equivalent except in patients with small (less than approximately 27 mm) annuli. The effective orifice area of low profile mechanical valves in this situation is larger.

Bioprosthetic Valves

There are three types of bioprosthetic valves. The glutaraldehyde-preserved porcine tissue valves mounted on a stent are the most commonly used. The first glutaraldehyde-

preserved stented porcine valves were developed by Hancock at the Edwards laboratories in 1971. Several changes in preparation techniques, including low-pressure fixation, have served to increase the durability of these valves. Bovine pericardial valves were introduced in the 1980s, but were found to degenerate quickly.[49] The first attempts at valve replacement with bioprosthetic valves were with cadaver aortic homografts. These showed early degeneration and their use was abandoned. Other types of preserved homografts are currently being developed, but have not yet undergone widespread tests.[50]

Structural deterioration of the valves takes two forms. Mitral stenosis secondary to calcification occurs, especially in the young patient, those with chronic renal failure, and other patients with high calcium turnover. Mitral insufficiency from cuspal tearing and detachment is the second mode of dysfunction.[51] Advances in preservation, including low-pressure fixation and antimineralization pharmacological treatment, may improve long-term results.

The natural history of bioprosthetic valve degeneration and secondary stenosis or regurgitation is far different from that in natural valves. When bioprosthetic stenosis or insufficiency is detected, consideration of elective replacement, even before symptoms occur, should be made. Catastrophic cuspal rupture and embolism have been reported and the physiologic deterioration of the patients make valve rereplacement a higher risk procedure.

There is no consensus as to the anticoagulation regimen for patients with bioprosthetic valves. Some recommend that patients undergo 3 months of anticoagulation until the endocardial surfaces have repaired, since the incidence of embolism is increased in the early postoperative period. Although patients with bioprosthetic valves who are anticoagulated have a lower incidence of thromboembolism, most patients do not undergo long-term anticoagulation (although in one large series, 50% of the patients were on warfarin).[52] Most patients with chronic atrial fibrillation and bioprosthetic valves should undergo chronic anticoagulation therapy. All patients with a mechanical prosthetic valve, in combination with the bioprosthetic valve, need anticoagulation.

Mechanical Valves

There are three types of mechanical valves: caged-ball, tilting disc, and bileaflet. The Starr–Edwards caged-ball mechanical valve has been in use longer than any other type of mechanical valve. Model 6120, first implanted in 1965, consists of a silastic ball, bare metal struts, and a cloth-covered teflon sewing ring. The long-term durability of this valve has been proven and it has been found to be extremely reliable. There have been many modifications of the Starr–Edwards valve that have not survived the test of time, some having extremely high failure rates secondary to ball or cloth-covered strut wear. The incidence of thromboembolism is higher with this type valve compared to the bileaflet valves.[53] Caged-ball valves have a relatively high profile and are contraindicated in people with small left ventricles. The effective orifice area in the smaller sizes is less than with other mechanical valves.

The tilting disc valves, which are currently (June 1994) available in the United States, are the Medtronic-Hall and Omniscience valves. The Bjork–Shiley valve is no longer available. Tilting disc valves are low in profile and may be used with small ventricles. The effective orifice size is larger than that available with caged-ball valves in the smaller sizes and hemodynamic performance is better. Catastrophic valve thrombosis has been reported with disc valves, even in patients on excellent anticoagulation. Meticulous surgical technique must be employed in implanting these valves because of the possibility of subvalvular interference from retained chordae or leaflets. Suturing and knot tying must be precise to avoid wedging the sutures between the ring and the disc, resulting in failure to open and sudden death. These valves generally have a low failure rate, with the notable exception of the modification of the withdrawn Bjork–Shiley convexoconcave valve that resulted in a high incidence of structural failure.[54]

The bileaflet valves, as represented currently by the St. Jude and Carbomedics valves, are the most commonly implanted mechanical valves in the United States. The early postoperative hemodynamic and clinical performance is no different from the tilting disc valves.[55] Again, attention to surgical technique is important so that valve leaflet motion is not interfered with by subvalvular tissue and that the sutures in the sewing ring do not impinge upon the orifice. The incidence of valve thrombosis is low.

All patients with mechanical valves in the mitral position should be anticoagulated.[56] Previously it was recommended to adjust the INR (International Normalized Ratio) to 4.0, which roughly corresponds to a prothrombin time of twice control. The relatively high incidence of bleeding complications with this regimen, coupled with the decreased thrombogenic characteristics of the bileaflet valves, led to recommendations to decrease the anticoagulation level for valve replacements.[57] Currently, anticoagulation to an INR of 2.5 to 3.0 is used in many centers.[58,59] Lower levels of anticoagulation to a prothrombin time of 1.3 to 1.5 times control have been recommended for the St. Jude valve.[60] The advent of the INR for the monitoring of anticoagulation will help standardized anticoagulation regimens and allow for correlation of thromboembolic and bleeding rates with anticoagulation levels among reports from various institutions. Research is continuing on new methods of anticoagulation that may be extremely useful to patients with prosthetic valves.

RESULTS

Hospital Mortality

Mitral valve replacement carries a higher average mortality in all patient groups than aortic valve replacement. Im-

provement in preoperative preparation of the patient and intraoperative myocardial protection as well as advances in postoperative care have served to lower this mortality over the past two decades. Changing patient demographics, especially the increased incidence of mitral valve replacement in the face of coronary artery disease and ischemia and the inclusion of elderly patients once thought not to be operative candidates, serve to increase overall mortality. There are many excellent series of mitral valve replacement reports from the 1970s and early 1980s that are of historical interest. However, because of the above-mentioned changes in techniques and patient population, current data must be used for realistic decision making and counseling of patients and referring physicians. The Society of Thoracic Surgeons National Cardiac Surgery Database is the largest database of cardiac surgical procedures in the United States.[61] This database contains data from 345,000 cardiac procedures including 9,000 mitral valve replacements. Currently there are approximately 1300 surgeons at 650 institutions reporting data. This represents more than half of all institutions at which cardiac surgery is performed. These data represent the most complete data currently available to evaluate the risk of mitral valve replacement. The remainder of the data in this section on acute hospital mortality and morbidity will reflect the STS Database experience.

Univariate analysis of the Database with the 1991 to 1993 experience (3625 patients) reveals multiple risk factors as shown in Table 118–3. The operative mortality in mitral valve replacement for emergency, elective, and reoperations is shown in Figure 118–5. The ratio of first-time operation to reoperation has held constant at about 2 to 1. The operative mortality for males undergoing a first-time, elective operation is 2.5% and for females is 3.9%. Female mortality in all subgroups of mitral replacement is higher. The adverse affect of advancing age on mortality is shown in Figure 118–6. Whereas the operative mortality is 1.2% in patients under age 50 years, it is over 6% in those over 70 years. Hospital mortality most often is due to low cardiac output and multiorgan failure in the majority of patients.

TABLE 118–3. PREOPERATIVE UNIVARIATE RISK FACTORS FOR MORTALITY AFTER MITRAL VALVE REPLACEMENT (STS NATIONAL CARDIAC SURGERY DATABASE)

Factor	Mortality (%)
Unstable angina	11.56
Prior MI (< 21 days)	21.43
Prior MI (>21 days)	11.95
Cardiomegaly	3.28
Diabetes	8.54
Hypertension	6.52
Renal failure	14.48
COPD	8.80
Prior CAB OP	11.17
Prior other cardiac OP	11.27
Inotropes preop	15.54
NYHA class IV	10.00
Emergency operation	14.66

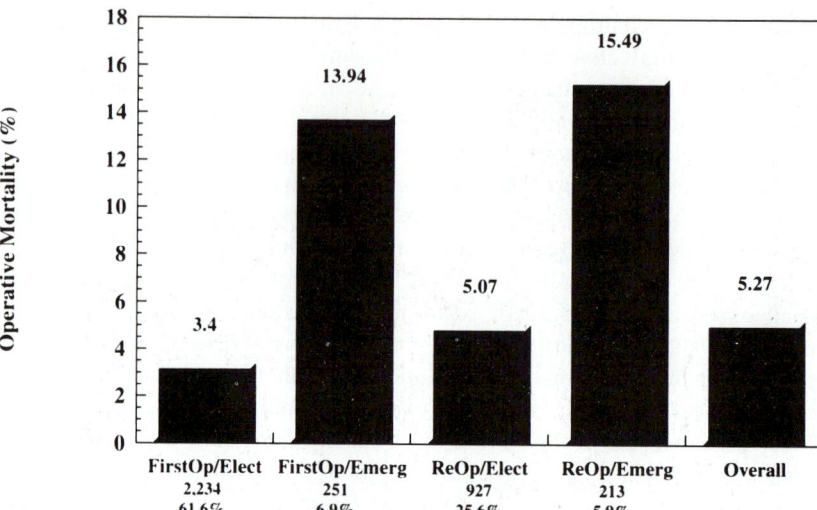

Figure 118–5. Operative mortality by status/incidence for mitral valve replacement, 1991–1993 (*n* = 3625). *(From STS Database.[61])*

Mitral valve replacement in combination with coronary bypass leads to increased operative risk (Fig. 118–7). The effect of gender is even more pronounced in patients undergoing a first elective mitral valve replacement and coronary bypass, with men having a mortality of 6.1% and 12.2% in women. Likewise, the effect of age is important. Patients under 50 years of age undergoing first-time, elective coronary bypass and mitral valve replacement have a mortality of 3.8%, while those over 65 years have a mortality of over 10% (Fig. 118–8).

Morbidity related to first mitral valve replacement includes a 6% incidence of early reoperation for bleeding or cardiac causes, a 4% incidence of stroke, a 3% incidence of renal failure, and a 6% need for mechanical ventilation over 5 days. In patients undergoing coronary bypass and first-time mitral valve replacement, the bleeding or cardiac reoperation rate was 10%, the stroke rate was 6%, and

the renal failure rate was 10%. Thirteen percent of the patients required mechanical ventilation for greater than 5 days.

Operative results depend on the patients' preoperative status and the presence of coexisting diseases. Patients who require reoperations and those who have coexisting coronary artery disease are at higher risk. The other factor not analyzed in these data is the effect of mitral valve pathology on outcome. Previous studies have shown that patients with ischemic mitral regurgitation and mitral regurgitation secondary to endocarditis are in the highest risk group, whereas those undergoing replacement for rheumatic mitral stenosis have the most favorable outcomes.[5,18,47] As mentioned previously, left ventricular end-systolic diameter is the most sensitive indicator of irreversible myocardial damage from mitral regurgitation and is a predictor of mortality.[62,63]

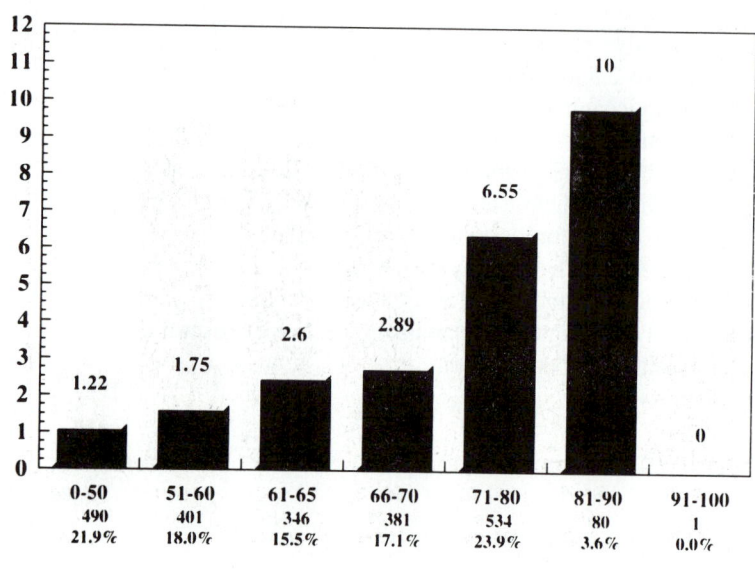

Figure 118–6. Effect of age on mitral valve operative mortality, 1991–1993 (*n* = 2233). *(From STS Database.[61])*

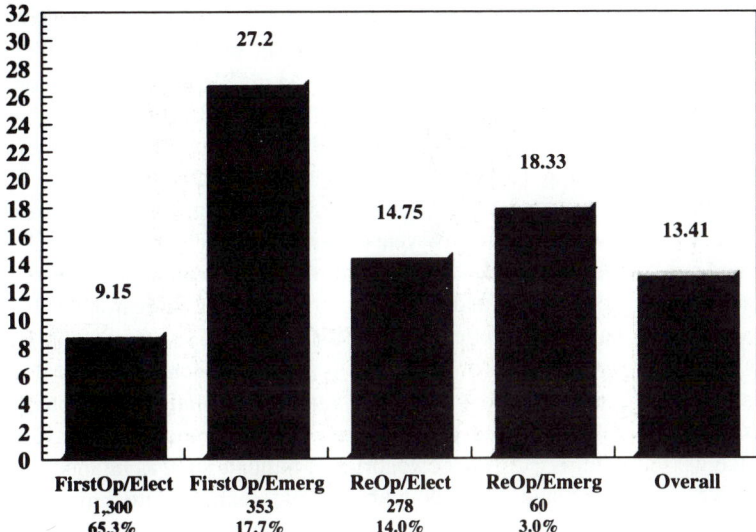

Figure 118–7. Operative mortality for combined coronary bypass and mitral valve replacement, 1991–1993 (*n* = 1991). *(From STS Database.[61])*

Late Results

Late results of mitral valve replacement depend on both patient-related factors and valve-related complications. The two most important patient factors are the postoperative left ventricular function and the age of the patient at the time of operation. Patients with impaired left ventricular function have decreased long-time survival. Other factors leading to late mortality include the presence of coronary artery disease, other associated valve disease and pathology, pulmonary hypertension, right ventricular failure, renal failure, thromboembolism, and cerebral vascular disease. Valve-related factors include bioprosthetic valve degeneration, mechanical valve dysfunction or thrombosis, thromboembolism and bleeding disorders, paravalvular leakage, hemolysis, and prosthetic valve endocarditis. Because of the changes in available valve types, bioprosthetic valve processing, and the introduction of new valves, it is important to consider new data. For this reason, most of the studies presented in this section have been published in the past decade. An excellent review of long-term results of specific prostheses and studies comparing different valve types was recently published by Akins.[64] There have been variations in the definitions of valve and patient-related mortality and morbidity, making comparison of previous studies difficult. In 1988, a joint committee from the Society of Thoracic Surgeons and the American Association for Thoracic Surgery made recommendations for valve reporting.[65] These have been utilized recently by most large series and form a standard method of valve reporting which allows for comparison of results among studies.

Overall Survival and Function

Actuarial 5-year survival after mitral valve replacement in recent series is approximately 80%, with 10-year survival between 50 and 87%.[49,66–74] In patients with poor left ven-

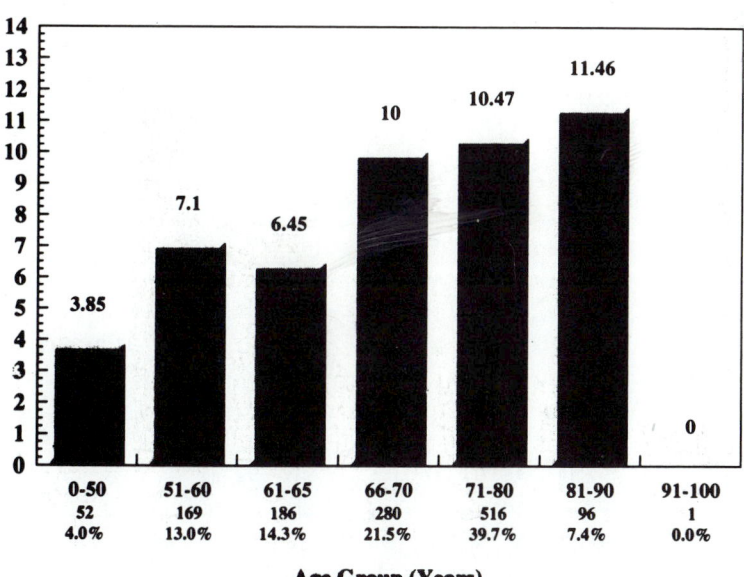

Figure 118–8. Effect of age on mortality after combined coronary bypass and mitral valve replacement, 1991–1993 (*n* = 1300). *(From STS Database.[61])*

tricular function preoperatively, the 7-year survival in one series is reported to be 17%.[72] In the future, more accurate assessment of left ventricular function using end-systolic diameter and volume should allow more precise estimation of long-term mortality.

Patients who have ischemic mitral regurgitation have a worse long-term prognosis. Patients who undergo combined mitral valve replacement and coronary revascularization can be divided into two groups with differing prognoses. Those who undergo mitral valve replacement for nonischemic mitral regurgitation and coincidental coronary bypass have better survival than those who undergo combined mitral valve replacement and coronary bypass because of ischemia.[47] The long-term survival of these patients is related to the severity of the left ventricular dysfunction.[3,5,75] A recent large series of patients undergoing combined coronary artery bypass and mitral valve replacement shows an actuarial 5-year survival of 66% and 10-year survival of 31%. Late risk factors include inhospital ventricular arrhythmias and left ventricular dysfunction. Patients who underwent bioprosthetic valve replacement who were not anticoagulated with warfarin had better event-free survival than either those with mechanical valves or those with bioprosthetic valves and long-term anticoagulation.[75] Other factors such as the degree of mitral regurgitation, the presence of congestive heart failure, acute presentation, and advanced age were also risk factors.[3]

Bioprosthetic Valve Failure

A major risk failure in the insertion of bioprosthetic valves is structural valve deterioration (SVD). Advances in the preparation of porcine valves, including low-pressure fixation and antimineralization regimes, are relatively recent. Data on short- and medium-term (10 to 15 years) durability

indicate that these valves have a low incidence of SVD. An excellent review of the long-term results of bioprosthetic valves has been compiled by Akins.[64] The two most commonly used glutaraldehyde-treated, porcine, stented valves (Hancock and Carpentier–Edwards) show no difference in SVD at 10 years.[70] Freedom from SVD at 10 years is between 60 and 78%.[52,70,76] However, SVD increases markedly after 14 years where the freedom from SVD is less than 45%. The freedom from reoperation at 14 years is between 27 and 43% (Fig. 118–9).[52,77] Pericardial valves have a freedom from SVD of only 44% at 10 years.[78] The age at valve implantation is the only factor that has been found to affect structural valve deterioration, the younger the age of the patient, the higher their incidence of valve failure.[52] Special categories of patients such as infants, children, and patients with chronic renal failure have been found in the past to have a high incidence of SVD and very few of these valves are implanted in these patient groups.

There have been many attempts to detect SVD in its early course, because leaflet detachment can result in catastrophic heart failure with a high operative mortality. Echocardiographic evaluation of bioprosthetic valve function has shown peak mitral flow velocity, mean mitral valve gradient, and left ventricular isovolumic relaxation time to correlate with valve failure.[79]

The position of the bioprosthetic valve influences SVD. Valves in the mitral position degenerate faster than those in the aortic position.[52]

Thromboembolism and Bleeding

Patient-related risk factors are the major cause of thromboembolism in the postoperative period. Atrial fibrillation, left atrial enlargement, and left ventricular dysfunction increase the risk of thromboembolism and are valve indepen-

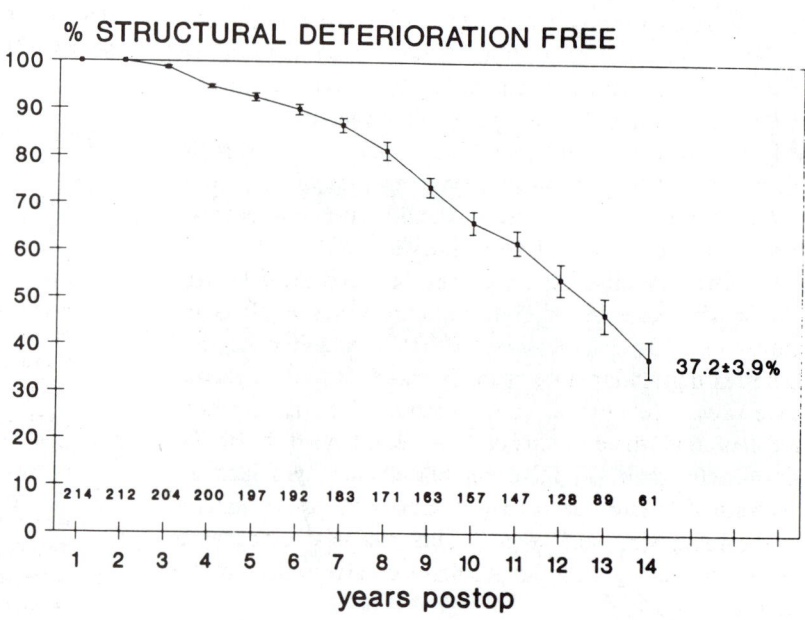

Figure 118–9. Actuarial freedom from structural valve deterioration of a series of aortic and mitral porcine valves (Hancock I). *(From Bernal JM, et al: Valve-related complications with the Hancock I porcine bioprosthesis. J Thorac Cardiovasc Surg 101:871–880, 1991.)*

dent. The attendant risk of anticoagulant-related hemorrhage is present both in patients with mechanical valves and those with bioprosthetic valves who undergo chronic anticoagulation. The main advantage of bioprosthetic valves is freedom from the need for long-term anticoagulation, but between 20 and 60% of patients in large series undergoing bioprosthetic valve implantation are anticoagulated long term.[48,52,80]

The percentage of patients free from thromboembolism at 10 years is similar whether mechanical or bioprosthetic valves are implanted. This rate varies between 77 and 87%[48,49,52,66,68,73,74,77,81,82] with a linearized rate of 1.6 to 2.9% per patient year. The only currently used mechanical valve that shows a higher incidence of thromboembolism is the Starr–Edwards valve. Only 55% of these patients have been found to be free of thromboembolism at 10 years,[53] for a rate of 3.1%.[71]

Anticoagulant-related hemorrhage (ACH) and thromboembolism are related. Because ACH is the most common cause of long-term morbidity, attempts have been made to decrease the level of anticoagulation. Bleeding is most commonly found in the central nervous system and gastrointestinal and urinary systems and is proportional to the prothrombin time. The incidence of anticoagulant-related hemorrhage is between 0.18 and 2.2 per patient year[23,66–69,73,74] and is similar when mechanical bioprosthetic valves are compared. Some studies have found ACH to increase with patient age[52] while others have not.[70]

Mechanical Valve Thrombosis and Structural Failure

Tilting disc valves are the most susceptible to valve thrombosis. Valve thrombosis usually presents as catastrophic valve failure and has a high mortality. The onset of thrombosis is often associated with suboptimal anticoagulation either because of the patient's inability to monitor coagulation or because anticoagulation is stopped for other medical reasons. The diagnosis is commonly made on clinical presentation, dynamic fluoroscopy of valve leaflet motion, and echocardiography. The Bjork–Shiley valve has a thrombosis rate of 0.28% per patient year in a series of 280 mitral valves studied over 10 years.[82] St. Jude valves have a valve thrombosis rate between 0.09 and 0.3%.[67–69]

Structural valve failure is rare in mechanical valves. No failures were found in three large series of St. Jude valves in a 10-year follow-up.[66,68,69] A notable exception has been high failure rate of the Bjork–Shiley convexoconcave valve. The decision to recommend elective rereplacement of this valve is difficult. A recent analysis of the risk/benefit ratio of valve rereplacement[54] provides an analysis of failure rates of Bjork–Shiley valves depending on position, size, and model. This analysis serves as a model for dealing with the problem of valve failure in the future.

Paravalvular Leak

Paravalvular leak is dependent on both patient risk factors and technical problems. The presence of active native valve endocarditis, especially that eroding the annulus, is a risk factor for paravalvular leak. Patients with annular and atrial wall calcifications also have a higher incidence of paravalvular leak because of the inability to seat the prosthetic valve. The incidence of paravalvular leak in a large series of St. Jude valves has been linearized to 0.3% per patient year.[73]

Prosthetic valve hemolysis is most often related to paravalvular leaks. However, certain valves have a higher basal state of hemolysis. One-third of patients with Bjork–Shiley valves have been shown to have mild chronic hemolysis.[83] Bileaflet valves have been found to be relatively free of chronic hemolysis.

Prosthetic Valve Endocarditis

The most important risk factor for prosthetic valve endocarditis is the presence of native endocarditis leading to valve replacement. In several series of porcine and mechanical valve replacements, the rate of endocarditis was between 0.06 and 0.4%.[66,67,69] In one series of patients who developed early prosthetic valve endocarditis, the mortality was 75% while those developing late endocarditis had a 25% mortality.[84] Other series show a 10% rate of endocarditis at 10 to 15 years.[52,70]

Indications for valve rereplacement with prosthetic valve endocarditis include septic emboli, persistent sepsis, and hemodynamic instability manifested by congestive heart failure. Large vegetations on echocardiography may also be an indication for valve replacement. Certain high-risk destructive organisms such as *Staphylococcus aureus*, Gram-negative organisms, and *Candida albicans* or other fungal disease should lead to early consideration of valve rereplacement. Early endocarditis often is accompanied by paraprosthetic valve leakage.

REFERENCES

1. Llaneras MR, Nance ML, Streicher JT, et al: Pathogenesis of ischemic mitral insuffiency. *J Thorac Cardiovasc Surg* **105**:439–443, 1993
2. Burch GE, Giles TD: Angle of traction of the papillary muscles in normal and dilated hearts. A theoretical analysis of its importance in mitral valve dynamics. *Am Heart J* **84**:141–144, 1972
3. Hickey MS, Smith LR, Muhlbaier LH, et al: Current prognosis of ischemic mitral regurgitation. Implications for future management. *Circulation* **78**(3 Pt 2):I51–I59, 1988
4. Dion R: Ischemic mitral regurgitation: When and how should it be corrected? *J Heart Valve Dis* **2**:536–543, 1993
5. Replogle RL, Campbell CD: Surgery for mitral regurgitation associated with ischemic heart disease. Results and strategies. *Circulation* **79**(6 Pt 2):I122–I125, 1989
6. Selzer A, Cohn KE: Natural history of mitral stenosis: A review. *Circulation* **45**:878–890, 1972

7. Henney AM, Parker DJ, Davies MJ: Collagen bio-synthesis in normal and abnormal human heart valves. *Cardiovasc Res* **2**:624–630, 1982

8. Roberts WC: Morphologic features of the normal and abnormal mitral valve. *Am J Cardiol* **51**:1005–1028, 1983

9. Korn D, DeSanctis RW, Sell S: Massive calcification of the mitral annulus. *N Engl J Med* **267**:900–902, 1962

10. Harley JB, McIntosh CL, Kirklin JJ, et al: Atrioventricular valve replacement in the idiopathic hypereosinophilic syndrome. *Am J Med* **73**:77–81, 1982

11. McIntosh CL, Maron BJ, Cannon RO, Klues HG: Initial results of combined anterior mitral leaflet plication and ventricular septal myotomy-myectomy for relief of left ventricular outflow tract obstruction in patients with hypertrophic cardiomyopathy. *Circulation* **86**:1160–1167, 1992

12. Kaul TK, Bain WH, Jones JV, et al: Escarous A: Mitral valve replacement in the presence of severe pulmonary hypertension. *Thorax* **31**:332–337, 1976

13. Cohen MV, Gorlin R: Modified orifice equation for the calculation of mitral valve area. *Am Heart J* **84**:839–840, 1972

14. Gorlin R: Natural history, medical therapy and indications for surgery in mitral valve disease. In Ionescu MI, Cohn LH (eds): *Mitral Valve Disease.* London, Butterworths, 1985, pp 105–123

15. Rapaport E: Natural history of aortic and mitral valve disease. *Am J Cardiol* **35**:221–227, 1975

16. Noble RJ, Fisch C: Factors in the genesis of atrial fibrillation in rheumatic valvular disease. *Cardiovascular Clinics* **5**:97–114, 1973

17. Coulshed N, Epstein EJ, McKendrick CS, et al: Systemic embolism in mitral valve disease. *Br Heart J* **32**:26–34, 1974

18. Larbalestier RI, Kinchla NM, Aranki SF, et al: Acute bacterial endocarditis. Optimizing surgical results. *Circulation* **86**(5 suppl): II68–II74, 1992

19. Spinale FG, Ishihra K, Zile M, et al: Structural basis for changes in left ventricular function and geometry because of chronic mitral regurgitation and after correction of volume overload. *J Thorac Cardiovasc Surg* **106**:1147–1157, 1993

20. Wisenbaugh T, Skudicky D, Sareli P: Prediction of outcome after valve replacement for rheumatic mitral regurgitation in the era of chordal preservation. *Circulation* **89**:191–197, 1994

21. Borow KM, Green LH, Mann T, et al: End-systolic volume as a predictor of postoperative left ventricular performance in volume overload from valvular regurgitation. *Am J Med* **68**:655–663, 1980

22. Cohen JM, Glower DD, Harrison JK, et al: Comparison of balloon valvuloplasty with operative treatment for mitral stenosis. *Ann Thorac Surg* **56**:1254–1262, 1993

23. Nobuyoshi M, Hamasaki N, Kimura T, et al: Indications, complications, and short-term clinical outcome of percutaneous transvenous mitral commissurotomy. *Circulation* **80**:782–792, 1989

24. Larbalestier RI, Chard RB, Cohn LH: Optimal approach to the mitral valve: Dissection of the interatrial groove. *Ann Thorac Surg* **54**:1186–1188, 1992

25. Smith CR: Efficacy and safety of the superior-septal approach to the mitral valve. *Ann Thorac Surg* **55**:1357–1358, 1993

26. Saksena DS, Tucker BL, Lindesmith GG, et al: The superior approach to the mitral valve. *Ann Thorac Surg* **12**:146–152, 1971

27. Shintani H, Glantz SA: Effect of disrupting the mitral apparatus on left ventricular function in dogs. *Circulation* **87**:2001–2015, 1993

28. Ishihara K, Zile MR, Kanazawa S, Tsutsui H: Left ventricular mechanics and myocyte function after correction of experimental chronic mitral regurgitation by combined mitral valve replacement and preservation of the native mitral valve apparatus. *Circulation* **86**(5 suppl):II16–II25, 1992

29. Yun KL, Rayhill SC, Niczyporuk MA, Fann JI: Mitral valve replacement in dilated canine hearts with chronic mitral regurgitation. Importance of the mitral subvalvular apparatus. *Circulation* **84**(5 suppl):III112–III124, 1991

30. Yun KL, Fann JI, Rayhill SC, et al: Importance of the mitral sub-

valvular apparatus for left ventricular segmental systolic mechanics. *Circulation* **82**(5 suppl):IV89–IV104, 1990

31. Salter DR, Pellom GL, Murphy CE, et al: Papillary-annular continuity and left ventricular systolic function after mitral valve replacement. *Circulation* **74**(3 Pt 2):I121–I129, 1986

32. Hansen DE, Cahill PD, Derby GC, Miller DC: Relative contributions of the anterior and posterior mitral chordae tendineae to canine global left ventricular systolic function. *J Thorac Cardiovasc Surg* **93**:45–55, 1987

33. Lillehei CW, Levy MJ, Bonnabeau RC Jr: Mitral valve replacement with preservation of papillary muscles and chordae tendineae. *J Thorac Cardiovasc Surg* **47**:532–543, 1964

34. Hennein H, Swain JA, McIntosh CL, et al: Comparative clinical assessment of mitral valve replacement with and without chordal preservation. *J Thorac Cardiovasc Surg* **99**:828–837, 1990

35. Vucinic M: Suspension of the papillary muscles during valve replacement for mitral stenosis. *J Heart Valve Dis* **2**:311–313, 1993

36. Horskotte D, Schulte HD, Bircks W, Strauer BE: The effect of chordal preservation on late outcome after mitral valve replacement: A randomized study. *J Heart Valve Dis* **2**:150–158, 1993

37. Rozich JD, Carabello BA, Usher BA, Kratz JM: Mitral valve replacement with and without chordal preservation in patients with chronic mitral regurgitation. Mechanisms for differences in postoperative ejection performance. *Circulation* **86**:1718–1726, 1992

38. David TE, Ho WC: The effect of preservation of chordae tendineae on mitral valve replacement for postinfarction mitral regurgitation. *Circulation* Sep:(3 Pt 2): I116–I120, 1986

39. Okita Y, Miki S, Ueda Y, Tahata T: Comparative evaluation of left ventricular performance after mitral valve repair or valve replacement with or without chordal preservation. *J Heart Valve Dis* **2**:159–166, 1993

40. Olinger GN: Rereplacement of the mitral valve with represervation of the subvalvular apparatus. *Ann Thorac Surg* **54**:189–190, 1992

41. Bonchek LI: "Chordal" preservation during mitral valve rereplacement. *Ann Thorac Surg* **55**:198, 1993

42. Come PC, Riley MF, Weintraub RM, et al: Dynamic left ventricular outflow tract obstruction when the anterior leaflet is retained at prosthetic mitral valve replacement. *Ann Thorac Surg* **43**:561–563, 1987

43. Rose EA, Oz MC: Preservation of anterior leaflet chordae tendinae during mitral valve replacement. *Ann Thorac Surg* **57**:768–769, 1994

44. Miki S, Kusuhara K, Ueda Y, et al: Mitral valve replacement with preservation of chordae tendineae and papillary muscles. *Ann Thorac Surg* **45**:28–34, 1988

45. Mills NL, McIntosh CL, Mills LJ: Techniques for management of the calcified mitral annulus. *J Card Surg* **1**:347–355, 1986

46. Kawazoe K, Beppu S, Takahara Y, et al: Surgical treatment of giant left atrium combined with mitral valvular disease. *J Thorac Cardiovasc Surg* **85**:885–892, 1983

47. Karp RB, Mills N, Edmunds LH JR: Coronary artery bypass grafting in the presence of valvular disease. *Circulation* **79**(6 Pt 1):I182–I184, 1989

48. Louagie YA, Jamart J, Eucher P, et al: Mitral valve Carpentier-Edwards bioprosthetic replacement, thromboembolism, and anticoagulants. *Ann Thorac Surg* **56**:931–937, 1993

49. Pelletier LC, Carrier M, Leclerc Y, et al: Porcine versus pericardial bioprostheses: A comparison of late results in 1,593 patients. *Ann Thorac Surg* **47**:352–361, 1989

50. Vrandecic M, Gontijo BF, Fantini FA, et al: Anatomically complete heterograft mitral valve substitute: Surgical technique and immediate results. *J Heart Valve Dis* **1**:254–259, 1992

51. Magilligan DJ Jr, Lewis JW, Tilley B, et al: The porcine bioprosthetic valve. Twelve years later. *J Thorac Cardiovasc Surg* **89**:499–507, 1985

52. Burdon TA, Miller DC, Oyer PE, et al: Durability of porcine valves at fifteen years in a representative North American population. *J Thorac Cardiovasc Surg* **103**:238–252, 1992

53. Miller DC, Oyer PE, Stinson EB, et al: Ten-to-fifteen year reassess-

ment of the performance characteristics of the Starr-Edwards Model 6120 mitral valve prosthesis. *J Thorac Cardiovasc Surg* **85:**1, 1983

54. Marrin CAS, Birkmeyer JD, O'Connor G: The Bjork-Shiley dilemma. *Ann Thorac Surg* **55:**1361–1364, 1993

55. Fiore AC, Naunheim KS, D'Orazio S, et al: Mitral valve replacement: randomized trial of St. Jude and Medtronic-Hall prostheses. *Ann Thorac Surg* **54:**68–73, 1992

56. Edmunds LH: Thrombotic and bleeding complications of prosthetic heart valves. *Ann Thorac Surg* **44:**430–445, 1987

57. Horstkotte D, Bergemann R, Althaus U, et al: German experience with low intensity anticoagulation (GELIA): Protocol of a multi-center randomized, prospective study with the St. Jude Medical valve. *J Heart Valve Dis* **2:**411–419, 1993

58. Gohlke-Barwolf C, et al: Guidelines for prevention of thromboembolic events in valvular heart disease. *J Heart Valve Dis* **2:**398–410, 1993

59. Butchart EG, Lewis PA, Bethel JA, Breckenridge IM: Adjusting anticoagulation to prosthesis thrombogenicity and patient risk factors. *Circulation* **84**(5 suppl):III61–III69, 1991

60. Kopf GS, Hammond GL, Geha AS, et al: Longterm performance of the St. Jude Medical valve: Low incidence of thromboembolism and hemorrhagic complications with modest doses of warfarin. *Circulation* **76**(3 Pt 2):III132–III136, 1987

61. Society of Thoracic Surgeons: *Data Analyses of the Society of Thoracic Surgeons National Cardiac Surgery Database: The Third Year—January 1994.* Minneapolis, MN, Summit Medical Systems, 1994

62. Reed D, Abbott RD, Smucker ML, Kaul S: Prediction of outcome after mitral valve replacement in patients with symptomatic chronic mitral regurgitation. The importance of left atrial size. *Circulation* **84:**23–34, 1991

63. Carabello BA, Williams H, Gash AK, et al: Hemodynamic predictors of outcome in patients undergoing valve replacement. *Circulation* **74:**1309–1316, 1986

64. Akins CW: Selection of cardiac valvular prostheses. *Ann Thorac Surg* **55:**801–802, 1993

65. Edmunds LH, Clark RE, Cohn LH, et al: Guidelines for reporting morbidity and mortality after cardiac valvular operation. *Ann Thorac Surg* **46:**257–259, 1988

66. Kratz JM, Crawford FA Jr, Sade RM, et al: St Jude prosthesis for aortic and mitral valve replacement: A ten-year experience. *Ann Thorac Surg* **56:**462–468, 1993

67. Nakano K, Koyanagi H, Hashimoto A, et al: Twelve years' experience with the St. Jude Medical valve prosthesis. *Ann Thorac Surg* **57:**697–703, 1994

68. Arom KV, Nicoloff DM, Kersten TE, et al: Ten years' experience with the St. Jude Medical valve prosthesis. *Ann Thorac Surg* **47:**831–837, 1989

69. Czer LSC, Chaux A, Matloff JM, et al: Ten-year experience with the St. Jude Medical Valve for primary valve replacement. *J Thorac Cardiovasc Surg* **100:**44–55, 1990

70. Sarris GE, Robbins RC, Miller DC, et al: Randomized, prospective assessment of bioprosthetic valve durability. Hancock versus Carpentier-Edwards valves. *Circulation* **88**(5 Pt 2):II55–II64, 1993

71. Schoevaerdts JC, Buche M, el Gariani A, et al: Twenty years' experience with the model 6120 Starr-Edwards valve in the mitral position. *J Thorac Cardiovasc Surg* **94:**375–382, 1987

72. Davis EA, Gardner TJ, Gillinov AM, et al: Valvular disease in the elderly: Influence on surgical results. *Ann Thorac Surg* **55:**333–338, 1993

73. Smith JA, Westlake GW, Mullerworth MH, et al: Excellent long-term results of cardiac valve replacement with the St Jude Medical valve prosthesis. *Circulation* **88**(5 Pt 2):II49–II54, 1993

74. Nitter-Hauge S, Abdelnoor M: Ten-year experience with the Medtronic Hall valvular prosthesis. A study of 1,104 patients. *Circulation* **80**(3 Pt 1):I43–I48, 1989

75. Lytle BW, Cosgrove DM, Gill CC, et al: Mitral valve replacement combined with myocardial revascularization: Early and late results for 300 patients, 1970 to 1983. *Circulation* **71:**1179–1190, 1985

76. Jones EL, Weintraub WS, Craver JM, et al: Ten-year experience with the porcine bioprosthetic valve: Interrelationship of valve survival and patient survival in 1,050 valve replacements. *Ann Thorac Surg* **49:**370–384, 1990

77. Bernal JM, Rabusu JM, Cagigas JC, et al: Valve-related complications with the Hancock I porcine bioprosthesis: A twelve-to-fourteen-year follow-up study. *J Thorac Cardiovasc Surg* **101:**871–880, 1991

78. Masters RG, Pipe AL, Bedard JP, et al: Long-term clinical results with the Ionescu-Shiley pericardial xenograft. *J Thorac Cardiovasc Surg* **101:**81–89, 1991

79. Nellessen U, Masuyama T, Appleton CP, et al: Mitral prosthesis malfunction. Comparative Doppler echocardiographic studies of mitral prostheses before and after replacement. *Circulation* **79:**330–336, 1989

80. Edmunds LH: Thromboembolic complications of current cardiac valvular prostheses. *Ann Thorac Surg* **34:**96–106, 1982

81. Akins CW, Carroll DL, Buckley MJ, et al: Late results with Carpentier-Edwards porcine bioprosthesis. *Circulation* **82**(5 suppl):IV65–IV74, 1990

82. Orszulak TA, Schaff HV, DeSmet JM, et al: Late results of valve replacement with the Bjork-Shiley valve (1973 to 1982). *J Thorac Cardiovasc Surg* **105:**302–312, 1993

83. Ahmad R, Manohitharajah SM, Deverall PB, Watson DA: Chronic hemolysis following mitral valve replacement. *J Thorac Cardiovasc Surg* **71:**212–219, 1976

84. Sett SS, Hudon MPJ, Jamieson WRE, Chow AW: Prosthetic valve endocarditis. *J Thorac Cardiovasc Surg* **105:**428–434, 1993

119

Surgical Anatomy
of Cardiac Valves and Techniques
# of Valve Reconstruction

Lawrence R. McBride and Alain Carpentier

Since the first prosthetic mitral valve implantation on September 21, 1960, by Albert Starr,[1] numerous valve substitutes have been proposed. None of them has yet been able to avoid totally the complications linked to the prosthesis itself, such as thromboembolism, valve dysfunction, infection, anticoagulation, hemolysis, and bleeding.

These persistent drawbacks explain and justify the efforts made to develop a reliable system of valve repair, and there is today no doubt that the mortality and morbidity associated with valvuloplasty are lower than after valve replacement. The key question is to determine whether reparative surgery is possible in each individual. The answer to the question presupposes a perfect knowledge of the anatomy and the pathology of cardiac valves.

MITRAL VALVE

The mitral apparatus is a complex, finely coordinated mechanism that requires for its normal performance the functional integrity of anatomic elements working in delicate harmony. These elements are the mitral leaflets, the annulus, the chordae tendinae, and the papillary muscles.[1a]

The interactions between the mitral valve and the left ventricle are complex and are not yet entirely understood. Experimental and hemodynamic studies, however, have demonstrated that the mitral valve plays an important role in left ventricular geometry and function.[2-4] This role is also indirectly documented by clinical studies.[5-7]

The Mitral Veil

The mitral valve forms a continuous veil attached to the circumference of the mitral annulus.

The free edge of this veil hangs into the left ventricle and is split by indentations, none of which reach the mitral ring. Two of the indentations are constant and well delineated: the anterolateral and the posteromedial commissures. They permit division of the mitral veil into the aortic (anterior) and mural (posterior) leaflets (Fig. 119–1).[8]

The Commissural Area

The commissures can be identified by the tips of the corresponding papillary muscles[8,9] and by the commissural chordae.[10] The commissural chordae arise from the tip of the papillary muscle as a single stem that branches radially in a fanlike fashion to insert into the free margin of the commissural regions.[11]

The Mitral Valve

The leaflets are covered with endocardium. They present on their atrial side a distinct ridge that follows the rim of the leaflets at a certain distance from the free edge. The ridge defines the line of leaflet closure and separates the leaflets into two zones (Fig. 119–2):

1. A rough zone distal to the ridge, which is the "closure area" and represents the surface of coaptation

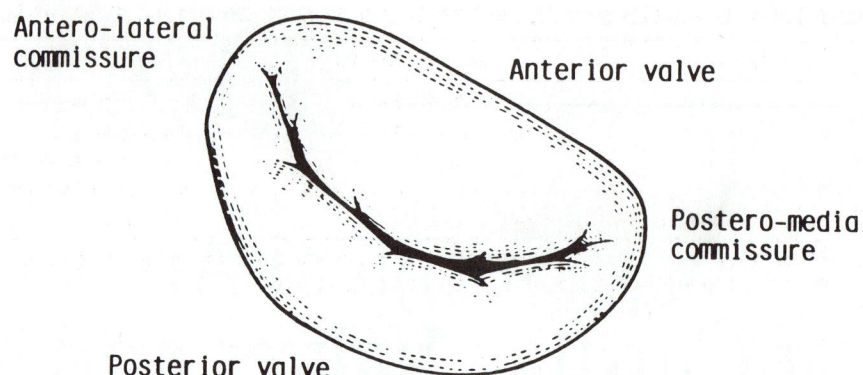

Figure 119–1. Mitral valve (atrial view). *(From Acar C, Deloche A: Anatomic et physiologie des valves mitrales et tricuspides. In Acar J (ed): Cardiopathies valvulaires acquises. Paris, Flammarian Médecine-Sciences, 1985, p. 3.)*

2. A proximal zone, membranous and clear on transillumination

The Anterior Mitral Leaflet

The anterior mitral leaflet is a semicircular or triangular structure. Its dimensions are specified in Table 119–1.[12] The rough zone receives the insertion of chordae tendinae on its ventricular surface. The anterior leaflet has a common attachment to the cardiac skeleton with the left coronary cusp and half of the noncoronary cusp of the aortic valve. There is a direct continuity between the anterior leaflet of the mitral valve and the aortic wall. The gap between the aortic valve and the mitral valve is filled with an intervalvular septum where the fibrous mitral annulus is absent (Fig. 119–3).[13,14] Thus the anterior mitral valve forms an important boundary dividing the inflow and the outflow tracts of the left ventricle.[15–17]

The Posterior Mitral Valve

The posterior mitral valve is quadrangular. It comprises all leaflet tissue posterior to the two commissural areas. Defined this way, the posterior valve has a wider attachment to the annulus than does the anterior leaflet.[18]

The margin of the mural leaflet has two indentations, giving rise to a scalloped appearance. A middle scallop, a posteromedial scallop, and an anterolateral scallop may be identified.[18] There are typical fan-shaped chordae tendinae that insert into and define the clefts between the individual scallops of the posterior leaflet. The dimensions of the posterior leaflets are shown in Table 119–1.[12]

Three zones can be identified on the leaflet surface: a rough zone forming the distal portion of the leaflet, a clear zone proximal to this, and a basal zone.[18] The rough zone, similar to that of the anterior leaflet, has chordal insertions on its ventricular surface. As in the anterior leaflet, this zone is broadest at the lowermost portion of the scallop, tapering toward the clefts between the scallops. The basal zone between the clear zone and the annulus receives the insertion of basal chordae tendinae that originate directly from trabeculum carnae of the left ventricular wall. This zone is most obvious on the middle scallop, because the majority of the basal chordae tend to insert in this region.

The Mitral Annulus

The mitral annulus is a zone of junction that serves as the attachment of the muscular fibers of the atrium and the ventricle and as the attachment of the mitral valve. Annular tissue is pliable, permitting sphincteric contraction during left atrial and left ventricular systole. The mitral annulus is attached to the two fibrous trigones. The right fibrous trigone forms a dense junction between the mitral, tricuspid, and aortic annuli (noncoronary cusp) and the membranous septum. The left fibrous trigone, situated more anteriorly and to the left, lies between the aortic (left cusp) and mitral annuli. Between these two trigones, the mitral valve is in continuity with the aortic wall and the fibrous mitral annulus does not exist in this region. The posterior portion of the annulus, to which the posterior leaflet is attached, has a variable thickness.

These anatomic data support the observation that during mitral valve insufficiency, the dilatation of the annulus occurs at its posterior level.[19]

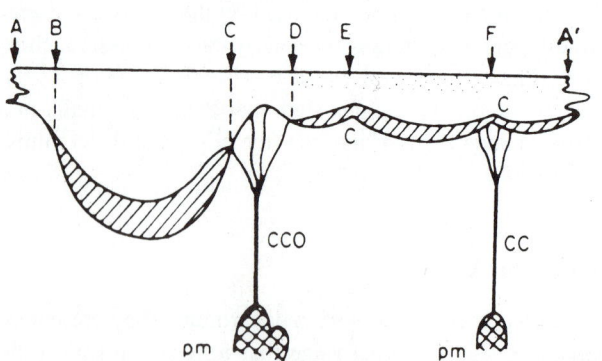

Figure 119–2. Mitral valve. AB, anterolateral commissure; BC, anterior valve, C, cleft; CC, cleft chordae; CCO, commissural chordae; CD, posteromedial commissure; DE, posteromedial scallop; EF, middle scallop; FA, anterolateral scallop; pm, papillary muscle. *(From Lam JH, Ranganathan N, Wigle ED, et al: Morphology of the human mitral valve: I. Chordae tendinae: A new classification. Circulation 41:449, 1970.)*

TABLE 119–1. DIMENSIONS OF THE ANTERIOR AND POSTERIOR LEAFLETS OF THE MITRAL VALVE

	Anterior Leaflet	Posterior Leaflet	
Insertion	32 ± 1.3 mm	55 ± 2.2 mm	
Height	23 ± 0.9 mm	Middle scallop	14 ± 0.9 mm
		Posteromedial scallop	9 ± 1 mm
		Anteromedial scallop	10 ± 2 mm
Rough zone	14 ± 1.1 mm	Middle scallop	8 ± 0.9 mm

Carpentier A, et al: Pathology of the mitral valve: Introduction to plastic and reconstructive valve surgery. In Kalmanson D (ed): The Mitral Valve, a Pluridisciplinary Approach. Acton, England, Publishing Science Group, 1976, with permission.

It has been shown that the mitral annulus decreases its diameter during each systolic contraction and as a consequence has a sphincterlike function, which reduces its area by approximately 26% during systole.[20]

This change in size and shape is thought to be secondary to the relaxation and contraction of the basoconstrictor muscles (bulbospiral and sinospiral bundles).[21]

Chordae Tendinae of the Mitral Valve

The chordae tendinae are fibrous strings that originate from tiny nipples on the apical portion of the two left ventricular papillary muscles or directly from the ventricular wall.

The majority of chordae branch either soon after their origin or just before their insertion into the leaflet.[11]

Commissural Chordae. The commissural chordae arise as a main stem that branches radially as do the struts of a fan to insert into the free margin of the commissural regions. Some of the fibers from these chordae continue within the leaflet toward its base. There are two commissural chordae, one at the anterolateral commissure and the other at the posteromedial commissure.

The extent of a commissural area is defined by the lateral spread of the attachment of the branches of a commissural chorda. The branches of the posteromedial chordae

are longer, thicker, and have a wider spread than those of the anterolateral commissural chordae. The average length of the commissural chordae is noted in Table 119–2.[12]

Chordae Tendinae of the Anterior Leaflet. The chordae of the anterior leaflet insert exclusively into the distal part of the leaflet, which is the rough zone.

Typically each chorda of the rough zone splits into three cords soon after its origin from the papillary muscle.

1. One branch inserts into the free margin of the leaflet.
2. One branch inserts beyond the free margin at the line of closure.
3. An intermediate cord is inserted between the other two branches.

Occasionally, each of the three cords branches further, giving rise to secondary branches that insert in the same area as the parent cord.

There are different types of chordae (Fig. 119–4) to the anterior leaflet.

The "Main" Chordae. Among the anterior leaflet rough-zone chordae, two are by far the thickest and largest; these are the "main chordae tendinae." They often originate from the tip of either the anterolateral or the posteromedial papil-

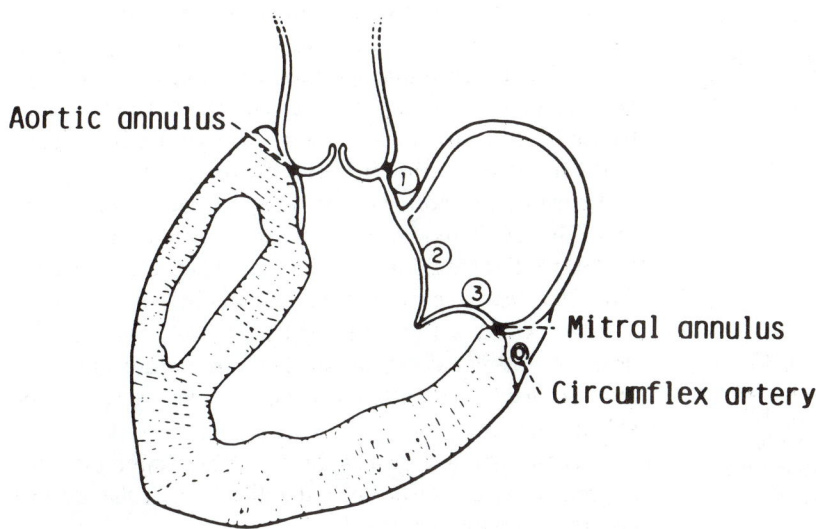

Figure 119–3. Oblique section of the heart. 1, intervalvular septum; 2, anterior valve; 3, posterior valve. *(From Acar C, Deloche A: Anatomie et physiologie des valves mitrales et tricuspides. In Acar J (ed): Cardiopathics valvulaires acquises. Paris, Flammarion Médecines-Sciences, 1985.)*

TABLE 119–2. AVERAGE LENGTH OF THE COMMISSURAL CHORDAE

Anterolateral commissural chordae	13 ± 0.2 mm
Posterolateral commissural chordae	15 ± 0.05 mm

Carpentier A, et al: Pathology of the mitral valve: Introduction to plastic and reconstructive valve surgery. In Kalmanson (ed): The Mitral Valve, a Pluridisciplinary Approach. Acton, England, Publishing Service Group, 1976.

lary muscle, and are inserted on the ventricular aspect of the rough zone near the closure line (between the four and five o'clock positions on the posteromedial side and between the seven and eight o'clock positions on the anterolateral side). Main chordae are present in more than 90% of the cases.

The Paramedial Chordae. These are thin chordae of the marginal type that insert near the middle of the free edge.

The Paracommissural Chordae. These are thin chordae of the marginal type that insert between the main chordae and the commissural chordae.

The mean length of the chordae of the anterior leaflet is shown in Table 119–3.[12]

Chordae Tendinae of the Posterior Leaflet. Three distinct types of chordae insert into the posterior leaflet (Fig. 119–5). Their mean length is shown in Table 119–3.[12]

The Basal Chordae. These are unique to the posterior leaflet. They arise as single strands directly from the left ventricular wall or from small trabeculum carnae to insert into the ventricular surface of the leaflet near the annulus.

The Rough-Zone Chordae Tendinae. These have a morphology similar to that of the rough-zone chordae tendinae

to the anterior leaflet, but are usually shorter and thinner. It should be noted that the posterior leaflet does not have "main" chordae among the rough-zone chordae.

The "Cleft" Chordae. These insert into the indentations of the posterior leaflet. Each gives rise to tiny radial branches similar to the struts of a fan. They insert into the free margin of the cleft or indentation. The main stem of a cleft chorda runs deep beneath the free margin of the cleft to insert into the adjacent rough zone on either side of the cleft.

The Number and Distribution of Chordae Tendinae. The chordae passing to the anterolateral commissure and the adjoining halves of the anterior and posterior leaflet arise from the anterolateral papillary muscle. The chordae passing to the posteromedial commissure and the adjoining halves of the anterior and posterior leaflet originate from the posterior papillary muscle.

The number and distribution of chordae tendinae are noted in Table 119–4.[12]

Left Ventricular Papillary Muscles

There are two groups of papillary muscles in the left ventricle: the anterolateral and the posteromedial. Each group supplies chordae tendinae to half of both leaflets. They are connected respectively to the anterior and posterior walls of the left ventricle.

Each papillary muscle group may have one or two distinct "bellies." Occasionally the posteromedial group has more than two bellies, while the anterolateral group often has only one belly. The tips of the papillary muscles usually point to the respective commissures. The left ventricular papillary muscle seems to have at least three recognizable morphologic types, depending on the attachment to the subjacent ventricular wall and the relative length of the body of

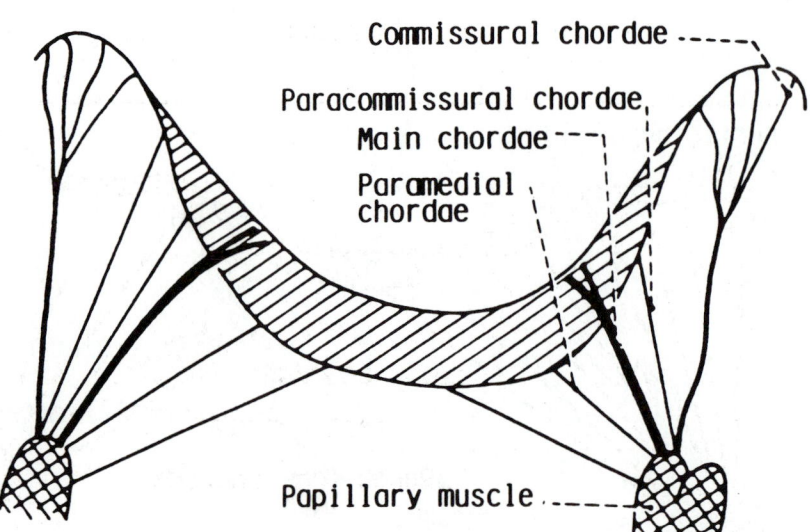

Figure 119–4. Chordae of the anterior valve. *(From Acar C, Deloche A: Anatomie et physiologie des valves mitrales et tricuspides. In Acar J (ed): Cardiopathics valvulaires acquises. Paris, Flammarion Médecines-Sciences, 1985.)*

TABLE 119–3. MEAN LENGTH OF THE CHORDAE OF THE ANTERIOR AND THE POSTERIOR LEAFLET OF THE MITRAL VALVE

Anterior Leaflet		Posterior Leaflet	
Anterolateral main cord	19 ± 0.4 mm	Marginal cord	14 ± 2.9 mm
Posteromedial main cord	17 ± 0.2 mm	Basal cord	8 ± 1.7 mm
Paracommissural cord	15 ± 0.5 mm	"Cleft" cord	13 ± 3.7 mm

Carpentier A, et al: Pathology of the mitral valve: Introduction to plastic and reconstructive valve surgery. In Kalmanson (ed): The Mitral Valve, a Pluridisciplinary Approach. Acton, England, Publishing Service Group, 1976.

the papillary muscle that protrudes freely into the ventricular cavity[22]:

1. Completely tethered papillary muscle fully adherent to the subjacent ventricular myocardium and protruding very little onto the left ventricular cavity with few trabecular attachments
2. Free and fingerlike papillary muscle with one third or more protruding freely into the ventricular cavity with few or no trabecular attachments
3. Intermediate-type with part of the body free but also with considerable trabecular attachments and tethering

Arterial Supply of the Mitral Valve

Mitral Leaflets
The arterial supply of the mitral valve is not well known. The arteries that vascularize the anterior leaflet are branches of Kugel's artery running at the base of the interatrial septum. Kugel's artery is a branch of either the first segment of the right coronary artery or of the proximal circumflex artery.

Papillary Muscles
The anterolateral papillary muscle receives branches from the anterior descending coronary artery and either from its diagonal branches or from the marginal branches of the left circumflex artery.[23–25] The posteromedial papillary muscle receives a variable supply from the left circumflex artery and branches of the right coronary artery. The epicardial branches of the coronary arteries course from the base to the apex of the heart, yielding penetrating intramyocardial branches.

The arterial vasculature of the papillary muscle seems to be related to its gross morphology.

The fingerlike papillary muscle usually receives a large central artery at its base; this artery arises from one of the epicardial arteries in that region. This central artery is often long and terminal and might measure as much as 900 μm at its entry into the papillary muscle. It enters the muscle mass toward the apex, dividing to form a network of anastomoses. After the fourth or the fifth division, it supplies almost the entire papillary muscle. Such free, fingerlike, papillary muscle bellies show few or no anastomotic connections with the extra-papillary endocardial plexus.

The tethered variety of papillary muscle often has a segmental distribution of the long penetrating intramyocardial vessels. The branches of these vessels not only connect with one another, but also have connections with the extra-papillary subendocardial plexus.

In the intermediate type of papillary muscle, a mixed arrangement is evident. When thick trabecular attachments

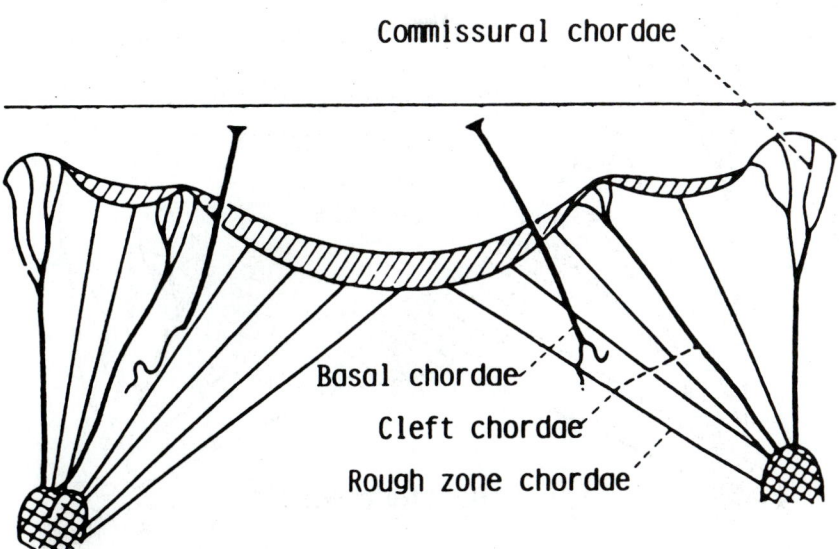

Figure 119–5. Chordae of the posterior leaflet. *(From Acar C, Deloche A: Anatomie et physiologie des valves mitrales et tricuspides. In Acar J (ed): Cardiopathics valvulaires acquises. Paris, Flammarion Médecines-Sciences, 1985.)*

TABLE 119–4. NUMBER AND DISTRIBUTION OF CHORDAE TENDINAE OF THE MITRAL VALVE

9 chordae insert into the anterior leaflet
  2 main chordae
  7 paramedial and paracommissural chordae
14 chordae insert into the posterior leaflet
  2 cleft chordae
  10 rough-zone chordae tendinae
  2 basal chordae
  2 commissural chordae

Carpentier A, et al: Pathology of the mitral valve: Introduction to plastic and reconstructive valve surgery. In Kalmanson (ed): The Mitral Valve, a Pluridisciplinary Approach. Acton, England, Publishing Service Group, 1976.

TABLE 119–5. TYPES OF VALVE PATHOLOGY

Type I: Normal leaflet motion
  Annular dilatation
  Leaflet perforation
Type II: Leaflet prolapse
  Chordal rupture
  Chordal elongation
  Papillary muscle rupture
  Papillary muscle elongation
Type III: Restricted leaflet motion
  a. Restricted opening: Commissural fusion, leaflet and chordal thickening
  b. Restricted closure: Excess tension on chordae during systole

are noted, one can often demonstrate penetrating intramyocardial vessels coursing through them as well.

This variation of the arterial vasculature significantly affects occlusive coronary disease in terms of resulting histopathologic damage to the papillary muscles. Occlusion of a large central artery would be expected to severely damage an entire papillary muscle. Tethering and trabecular attachments tend to preserve the integrity of the papillary muscle through the anastomotic plexus.

Closure of the Normal Mitral Valve

It is of interest to observe that the valvular surface area far exceeds the mitral orifice area. The relationship between the two areas is close to 2:1 in many cases[26] and there is always an excess of valvular tissue in relation to the area of the orifice. The difference becomes even greater in systole because of the sphincterlike action of the annulus that further reduces the area of the orifice.

The closure of the normal mitral orifice is a process involving three phases. (1) At first the leaflets meet edge to edge. (2) The leaflets then bulge upward, ballooning into the atrial cavity under the contraction of the myocardial fibers. (3) In the last phase, the surface of coaptation between the two leaflets becomes more and more extensive so that during systole the leaflets are disposed against each other in almost a vertical position.

MITRAL VALVE REPAIR

The Functional Approach

The lesions that may affect the mitral apparatus are manifold and complex, the problem being further complicated by the fact that several lesions usually affect the same valve. However, valvular reconstruction might be considered with the aim of restoring the function rather than the anatomy of the mitral apparatus.[12] Thus leaflet function may present only two anomalies: the opening and the closing of the leaflet is either increased or restricted.

The first functional anomaly, called *leaflet prolapse,* is present whenever the free edge of the leaflet overrides the plane of the annulus during systole. This condition can be assessed prior to the operation by echocardiography and during the operation under direct vision.

The second functional anomaly, *restricted leaflet motion,* is present when the leaflet does not open fully during diastole. Hence, whatever the complexity of the lesions, a leaflet presents either with a normal motion (type I), with an excessive motion or prolapse (type II), or with a restricted leaflet motion (type III) (Fig. 119–6). The functional status of each leaflet of a given valve must be assessed and defined according to this "functional approach."[27]

The lesions that can produce these dysfunctions can

Figure 119–6. Carpentier's functional classification. Drawings represent a mitral valve apparatus with the mural leaflet (left), the anterior leaflet (right), two papillary muscles, and the chordae tendinae. Dotted lines represent the course of the leaflet between the opening and the closing position. *(Modified from Carpentier A: Cardiac valve surgery. The "French correction." J Thorac Cardiovasc Surg 86:323–327, 1983.)*

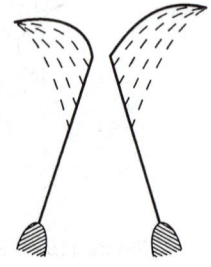
TYPE I
NORMAL LEAFLET MOTION

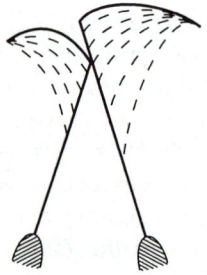
TYPE II
LEAFLET PROLAPSE

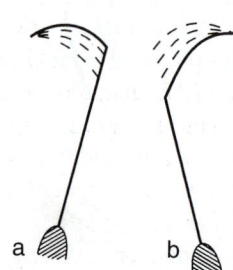
TYPE III
RESTRICTED LEAFLET MOTION

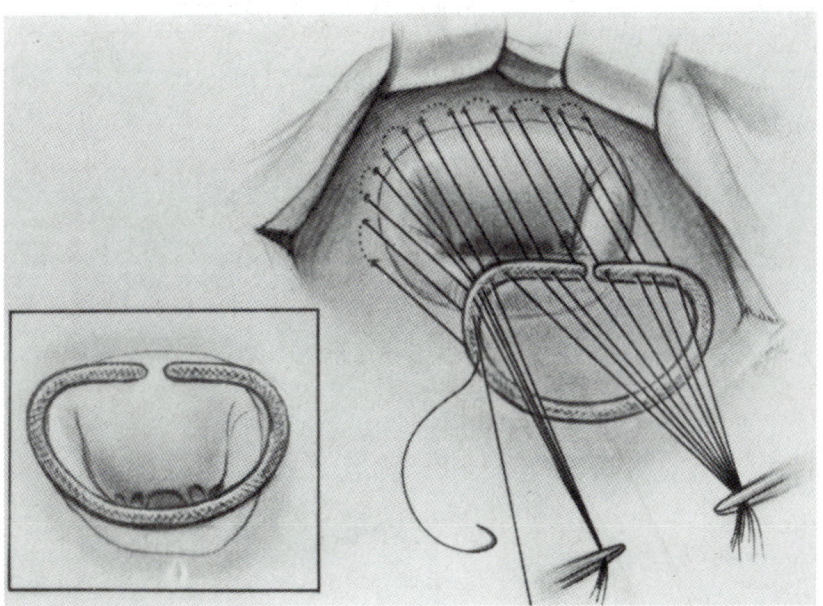

Figure 119–7. Annular remodeling using prosthetic ring. *(From Carpentier A: Cardiac valve surgery. The "French correction." J Thorac Cardiovasc Surg 86:323–327, 1983.)*

easily be recognized. For the mitral valve, for instance, the correspondence between the "functional type" and the causing lesions is presented in Table 119–5.

The Basis for Functional Repair

With the functional approach, the goal of valve repair may be simply defined as either limiting or increasing the leaflet motion in addition to remodeling the annulus by a prosthetic ring to obtain an optimal opening of the valve and a good surface of coaptation. This aim can be achieved by using a system of various techniques that are selected according to the valvular dysfunction and by analyzing the lesions prior to or during the operation. Preoperative and intraoperative echocardiography are useful in evaluating the pathology of the mitral valve as well as the feasibility of surgical repair.[28,29]

Valve Analysis

Valve analysis is the first and most critical step of mitral valve repair and as much time as necessary must be spent understanding the functional anomaly of the diseased valve that is being examined.

The atrium is first examined to determine if a jet lesion is present, which would indicate a prolapse of the opposing leaflet. The annulus is evaluated for annular distention.

The leaflet tissue is then examined to assess leaflet pliability and to check leaflet restricted motion or prolapse. Precise measurement of leaflet prolapse may be obtained by the "reference point" method.[27] Exerting traction with a nerve hook on different points of the free edge of the leaflets makes it possible to find a nonprolapsed area, usually on the posterior leaflet near the anterior commissure.

With this as a reference point, it is possible to measure the degree of prolapse of other areas.

Techniques of Repair

Prosthetic Ring Annuloplasty

Prosthetic ring annuloplasty is one of the major steps of valve reconstruction and is mandatory in most cases of mitral valve insufficiency.

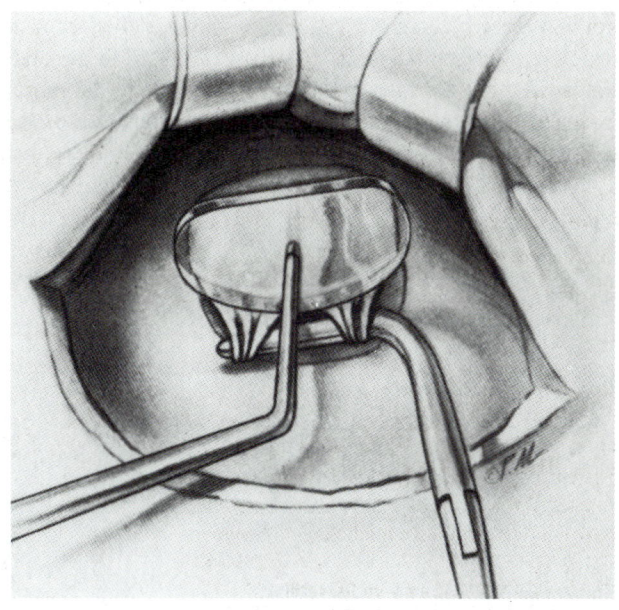

Figure 119–8. Ring selection. *(From Carpentier A: Cardiac valve surgery. The "French correction." J Thorac Cardiovasc Surg 86:323–327, 1983.)*

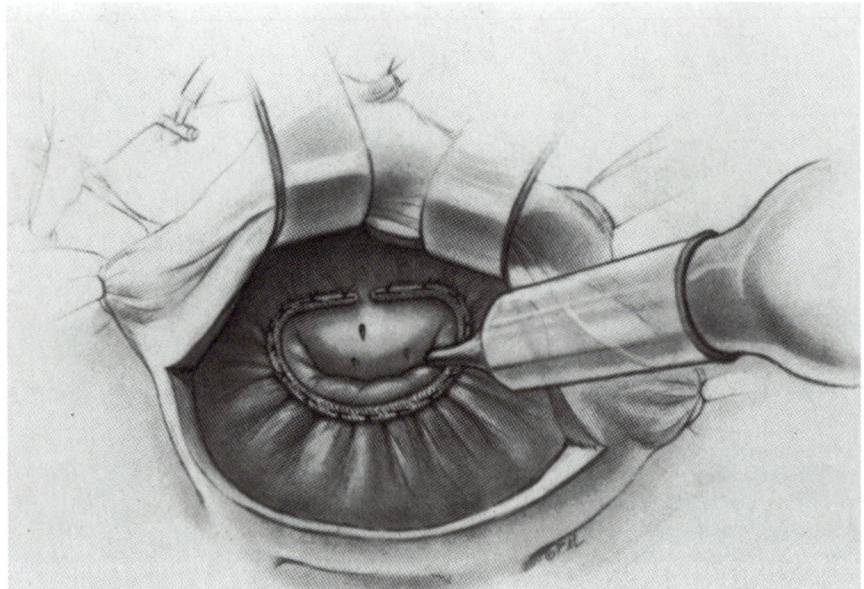

Figure 119–9. The result of testing. *(From Carpentier A: Cardiac valve surgery. The "French correction." J Thorac Cardiovasc Surg 86:323–327, 1983.)*

The basic principle of the ring annuloplasty is not only to reduce the size of the dilatated annulus, but also to restore the shape of the orifice. In fact, the dilatation of the annulus mainly affects the mural leaflet and the commissures leading to a gross deformation of the annulus with its anteroposterior diameter becoming greater than its transverse diameter (Fig. 119–7).[30]

Proper ring selection is based on measuring the surface area of the anterior leaflet with sized obturators (Fig. 119–8). The technique of ring implantation has been described previously.[27]

The repair is assessed by injecting saline into the left ventricle through the mitral valve. The adequacy of the repair is assessed by considering the functional rather than the anatomic aspect of the result. A repair is judged to be satisfactory if the line of leaflet closure is parallel to the mural part of the ring, since this indicates good apposition of the leaflets and a good surface of coaptation. A closure line that is not parallel to the posterior curve of the ring indicates a poor result, even in the absence of any leakage, since it indicates a poor coaptation of the leaflets (Fig. 119–9).

Repair of Mural Leaflet Prolapse

Prolapse of the posterior leaflet, caused by ruptured or elongated chordae, is treated by quadrangular resection of the prolapsed portion. The gap of the posterior leaflet is corrected either by annular plication (Fig. 119–10) or by a sliding plasty of the posterior leaflet (Fig. 119–11) and a subsequent suture of the edges of the leaflets. In about five percent of the patients, the mural leaflet will have excess tissue, which can result in systolic anterior motion of the leaflets and obstruction of the left ventricular outflow tract. In this situation, the quadrangular resection of the posterior scallop is completed by two triangular resections at the base of the posterior leaflet remnants, thereby reducing the height of the posterior leaflet and eliminating systolic anterior motion[31] (Fig. 119–12). A prosthetic ring annuloplasty is then used to reinforce the repair.

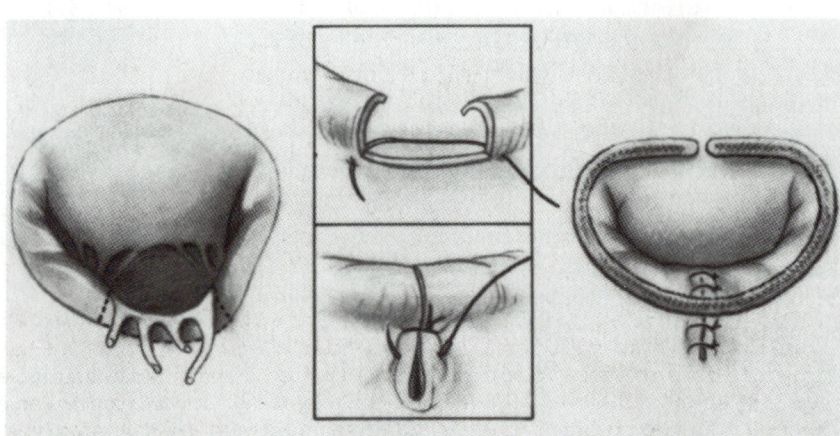

Figure 119–10. Repair of mural leaflet prolapse. Annulus plication. *(From Carpentier A: Cardiac valve surgery. The "French correction." J Thorac Cardiovasc Surg 86:323–327, 1983.)*

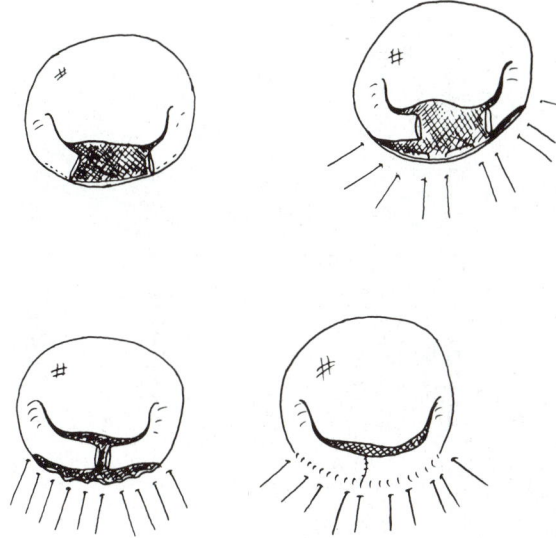

Figure 119–11. Repair of mural leaflet prolapse. Sliding technique. *(From Carpentier A: Cardiac valve surgery, The "French correction." J Thorac Cardiovasc Surg 86:323–327, 1983.)*

Repair of Anterior Leaflet Prolapse

Repair of prolapse of the anterior leaflet requires different techniques of repair depending on the nature of the lesions.

Chordal Rupture of the Anterior Leaflet

Leaflet Fixation on Secondary Chordae. The free edge of the prolapsed leaflet is sutured to adjacent secondary chordae close to the prolapsed area (Fig. 119–13).

Chordal Transposition. Strong chordae of the posterior leaflet, located opposite the prolapsed part of the anterior leaflet, are detached from the posterior leaflet and reattached to the free edge of the anterior leaflet. The gap in the mural leaflet is then treated either by a triangular or a quadrangular resection (Fig. 119–14). Secondary cords from the anterior leaflet can be used as well and can be transposed to the free margin of the leaflet.

Chordal Replacement. When chordal transposition is not feasible because of extensive scarring or degeneration of

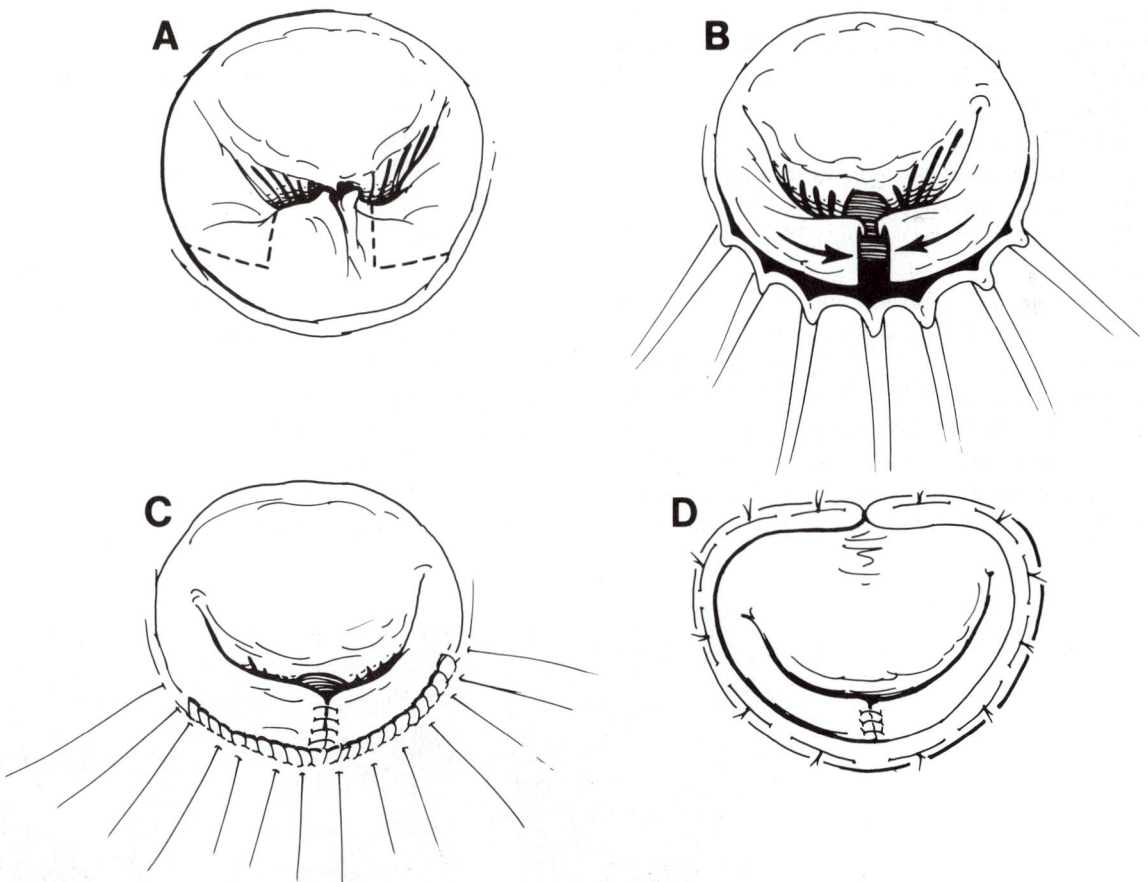

Figure 119–12. Technique for preventing systolic anterior motion: The sliding leaflet technique. **A.** In case of excess tissue of the mural leaflet, the quadrangular resection is completed by two triangular resections of the posterior leaflet remnants to correct excess tissue. **B.** Remnants are translated medially to close the gap. **C** and **D,** Repair is completed and the ring is inserted to reinforce the repair. *(Adapted from Jebara V, Mihaileanu S, Acar C, et al: Left ventricular outflow tract obstruction after mitral valve repair. Circulation 88:II–30, 1993. Reproduced with permission. Circulation. Copyright 1993 American Heart Association.)*

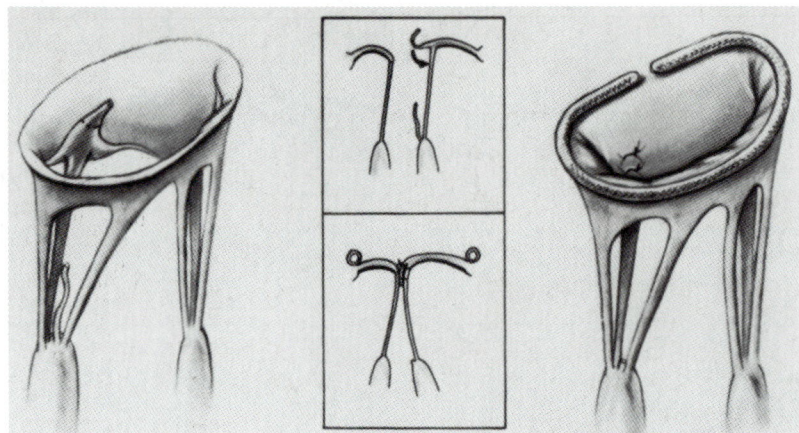

Figure 119–13. Repair of anterior leaflet prolapse by leaflet fixation on a secondary chordae. *(From Carpentier A: Cardiac valve surgery. The "French correction." J Thorac Cardiovasc Surg 86:323–327, 1983.)*

the posterior leaflet chordae, the anterior leaflet can be anchored by using polytetrafluoroethylene sutures as neochordae (Figure 119–15).[32]

Chordal Elongation of the Anterior Leaflet. Chordal elongation can be corrected by a shortening plasty of the chordae, which consists of invaginating the excess length of the chordae into a trench created in the papillary muscle (Fig. 119–16).

Papillary Muscle Elongation
Sliding Plasty of the Papillary Muscle. The portion of the papillary muscle to which the prolapsed area is attached is split longitudinally and resutured at a lower level (Fig. 119–17).

The Cuneiform Resection. A large papillary muscle with moderate prolapse (2–6 mm) can be shortened by a

cuneiform resection of its tip. The height of this resection is equal to the degree of shortening. The horizontal trench is then closed with separate sutures (Fig. 119–18).

The "Concertina" Technique. A thinner papillary muscle with moderate elongation can be treated by numerous superficial vertical sutures (Fig. 119–19), which can shorten 3–5 mm.

Repair of Restricted Leaflet Motion
Restricted leaflet motion results from commissural fusion, chordal fusion, chordal shortening, or chordal hypertrophy. Resection of secondary chordae (those attached to the ventricular surface of the leaflets) results in improved mobility of the leaflet tissue. Fused marginal chordae attached to the free edge of the leaflets are treated by triangular resection, called *fenestration*. These techniques are not difficult, but are somewhat tedious and time-consuming. It may be nec-

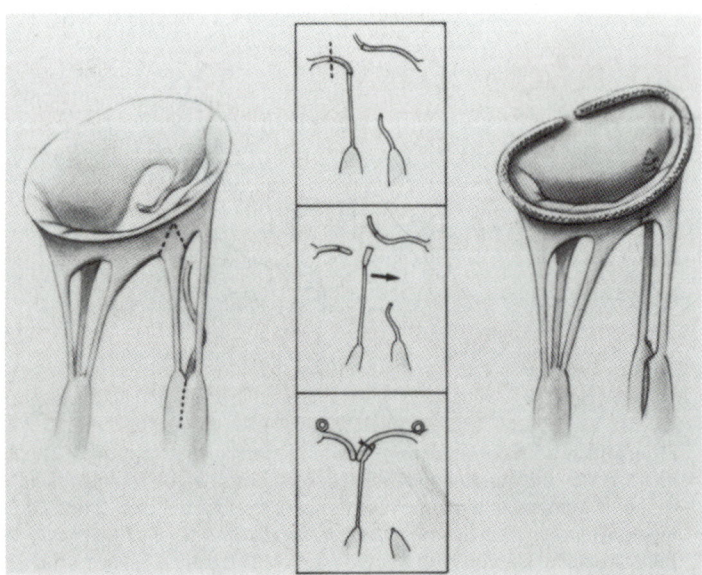

Figure 119–14. Repair of anterior leaflet prolapse by chordal transposition. *(From Carpentier A: Cardiac valve surgery. The "French correction." J Thorac Cardiovasc Surg 86:323–327, 1983.)*

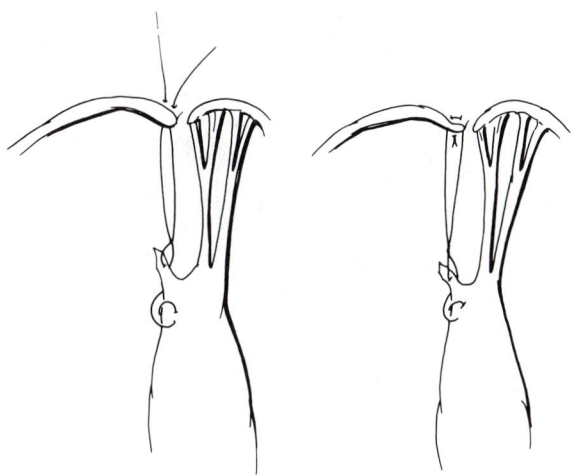

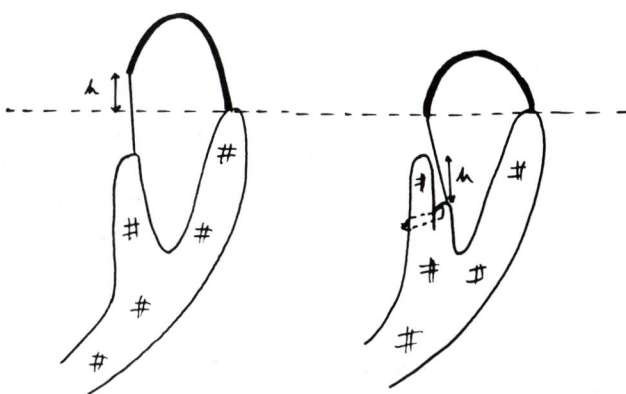

Figure 119–17. Repair of prolapse of the anterior leaflet by sliding plasty of the papillary muscle.

Figure 119–15. Replacement of a primary chorda with PTFE suture. *(From David TL, Bos J, Rakowski H: Mitral valve repair by replacement of chordae tendineae with polytetrafluoroethylene sutures. J Thorac Cardiovasc Surg 101:495, 1991.)*

essary to spend 15–20 min to mobilize the leaflet tissue adequately (Fig. 119–20). Although calcification of the mitral apparatus complicates valvuloplasty, it does not necessarily preclude it. If the mobility of the leaflets and annulus can be restored by decalcification and debridement, the valve can be repaired successfully utilizing standard valvuloplasty techniques.[33]

Intraoperative Assessment of Valve Repair

While the left atrium is open, the repair is assessed by injecting saline into the left ventricle through the mitral valve. The adequacy of the repair is assessed by considering the functional rather than the anatomic aspect of the result. A repair is judged to be satisfactory if the line of leaflet clo-

sure is parallel to the mural part of the ring, since this indicates good apposition of the leaflets and a good surface of coaptation. A closure line that is not parallel to the posterior curve of the ring indicates a poor result, even in the absence of any leakage, since it indicates a poor coaptation of the leaflets (Fig. 119–9).

After the patient has been weaned from cardiopulmonary bypass, a more physiologic assessment can be made with transesophageal or epicardial echocardiography. An echo-perfect result, although desirable, is not always attainable.[34] No or trivial residual insufficiency is seen in most instances. A residual regurgitation of 2 to 3+ may be seen immediately after discontinuing cardiopulmonary bypass. It is critical to analyze the cause of this insufficiency before deciding to replace the valve since most of them are functional and disappear some time after bypass. They may be due to temporary ventricular dysfunction, temporary ventricular dilatation, or temporary systolic anterior motion of the leaflets whenever the ventricle is too empty and hy-

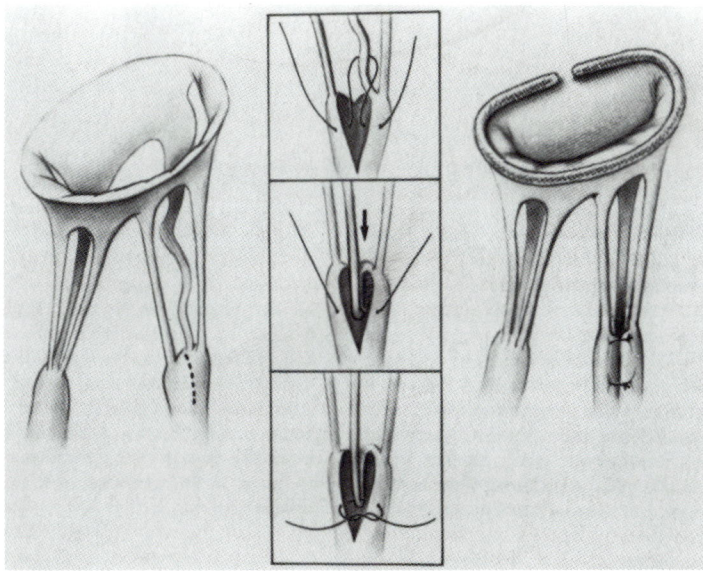

Figure 119–16. Repair of anterior leaflet prolapse by a shortening plasty of the chordae. *(From Carpentier A: Cardiac valve surgery. The "French correction." J Thorac Cardiovasc Surg 86:323–327, 1983.)*

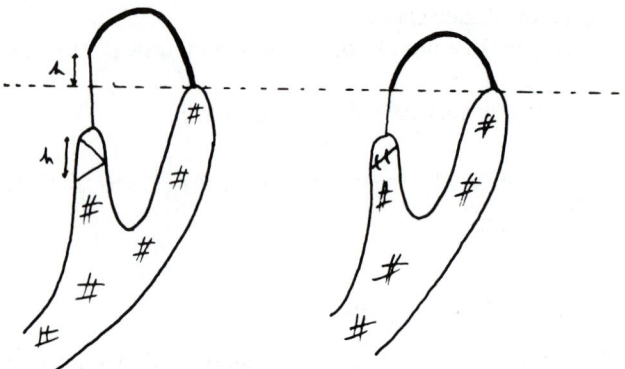

Figure 119–18. Repair of anterior leaflet prolapse by cuneiform resection of the papillary muscle.

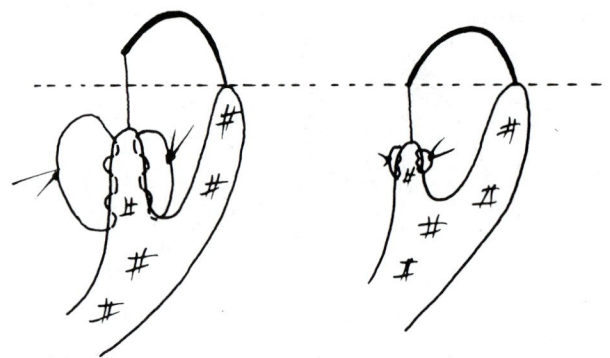

Figure 119–19. Repair of anterior leaflet prolapse by concertina technique.

perkinetic. Cardiac assistance, proper adjustment of filling pressures, and cautious use of inotropic agents usually restore normal ventricular function with no residual mitral regurgitation. A persistent 2–3+ mitral regurgitation or persistent systolic anterior motion of the leaflets with a transvalvar gradient above 40 mmHg after these precautions have been taken may require replacement of the valve.

Utilizing this approach, mitral valve replacement has been necessary in only 2% of our patients over the past three years.

THE TRICUSPID VALVE

Four anatomic elements constitute the tricuspid valve: the tricuspid veil, the tricuspid annulus, the chordae tendinae, and the papillary muscles.

The Tricuspid Veil

When viewed from its atrial aspect, the tricuspid valve orifice is roughly triangular with anterior, posterior, and septal sides (Fig. 119–21).

The leaflets of the tricuspid valve fall into the right ventricle like a curtain. Many indentations of variable length are observed in their free edge. Some of these have fan-shaped chordae inserting into them and may be distinguished as commissures[35,36] (Fig. 119–22).

The Commissures

The Anteroseptal Commissure
The basal attachment of the tricuspid valve reaches its highest level at the membranous interventricular septum, where the anterior and septal walls of the right ventricle join. At this point, a deep indentation is seen in

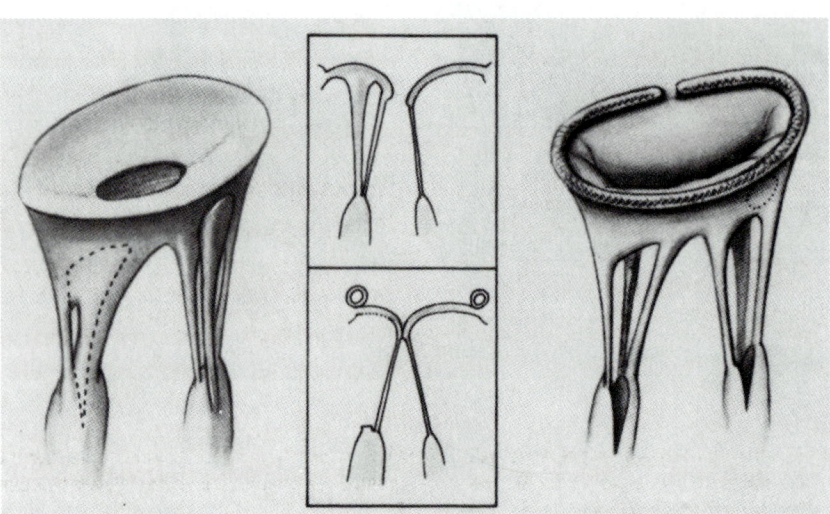

Figure 119–20. Repair of type III mitral valve incompetence. *(From Carpentier A: Cardiac valve surgery. The "French correction." J Thorac Cardiovasc Surg 86:323–327, 1983.)*

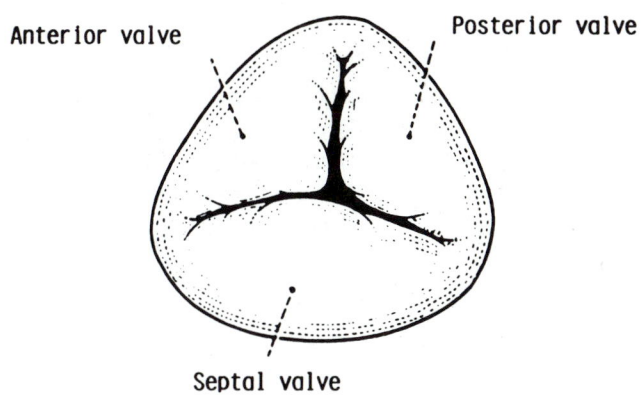

Figure 119–21. Tricuspid valve—atrial view. *(From Acar C, Deloche A: Anatomie et physiologie des valves mitrales et tricuspides. In Acar J (ed): Cardiopathics valvulaires acquises. Paris, Flammarion Médecines-Sciences, 1985.)*

the leaflet tissue; rarely is this indentation absent. This area is easily identified and marks the commissure between the anterior and septal leaflets. At this site there is a fan-shaped short corda which has ribbonlike branches. It arises either directly from the septal band of the crista supraventricularis or from a small papillary muscle on that band.[36]

The Anteroposterior Commissure

The anteroposterior commissure forms a deep indentation in the leaflet tissue between the anterior and posterior leaflets. Usually this commissure is well delineated by a fan-shaped chorda and is located roughly at the acute margin of the right ventricle. The anterior papillary muscle, which is usually the largest and has the moderator band attached to it, usually points toward this commissure.

The Posteroseptal Commissure

The posteroseptal commissure, which is a deep indentation in the leaflet tissue at the junction of the posterior and septal walls of the right ventricule, has three landmarks:

1. A fan-shaped chorda
2. A papillary muscle on the posterior wall of the ventricle
3. A fold in the tissue of the septal leaflet

The posteroseptal commissure has the widest spread of the three landmarks.

Tricuspid Valve Leaflets

The distal zone of the tricuspid leaflet is rough and thick on palpation. The area is neither as rough nor as thick as that on the mitral valve leaflet, and the zone does not extend into the commissural areas.

The basal zone of the tricuspid leaflet extends 2–3 mm into the leaflet from the annulus. As in the mitral valve, basal chordae insert into the ventricular aspect of the leaflet in this area.

Unlike the clear zones of the mitral valve, those of the tricuspid valve receive some chordal insertions on their ventricular aspect. The measurements of the basal attachment of the tricuspid valve is shown in Table 119–6.[37]

The Anterior Leaflet

The anterior leaflet is the largest of the three leaflets. Usually it is semicircular, but it may be quadrangular. On its free edge, close to the anteroseptal commissure, a notch can be observed. Sometimes it is large enough to suggest a commissure; however, the chordae that insert into the notch arise from the septal band of the crista supraventricularis and are almost invariably rough-zone chordae.

The Posterior Leaflet

The posterior leaflet lies between the anteroposterior and the posteroseptal commissures. The leaflet has several indentations in its free edge that give it a scalloped appearance.

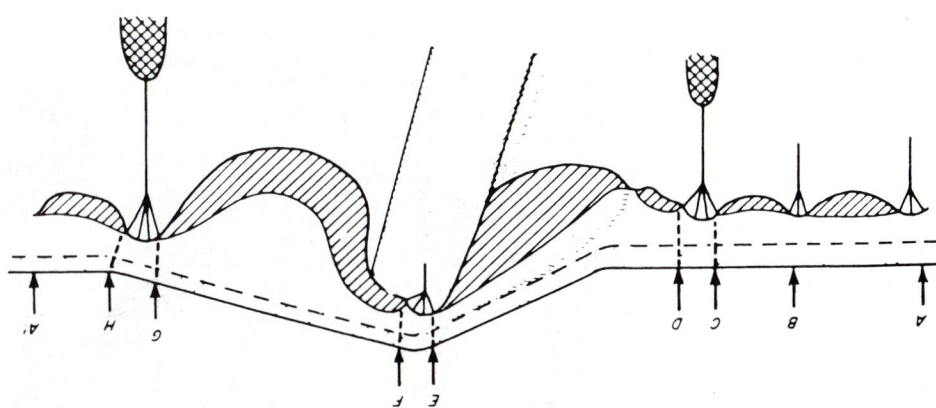

Figure 119–22. Tricuspid valve. AB, BC, HA, posterior valve; CD, posteroseptal commissure; DE, septal valve; EF, anteroseptal commissure; FG, anterior valve; GH, anteroposterior commissure. *(From Silver MD, Lam JHC, Ranganathan N, et al: Morphology of the human tricuspid valve. Circulation 43:333, 1971.)*

TABLE 119–6. MEASUREMENTS OF THE BASAL ATTACHMENT OF THE LEAFLETS OF THE TRICUSPID VALVE

Septal leaflet	35.9 ± 0.60 mm
Anterior leaflet	38.7 ± 0.47 mm
Posterior leaflet	37.8 ± 1.22 mm

The Septal Leaflet

The septal leaflet lies between the posteroseptal and anteroseptal commissures. Part of its basal attachment is to the posterior wall of the right ventricle but most is to the septal wall. Near the midpoint of the leaflet are its attachment angles. The angle marks the transition from the posterior wall to the septal wall of the ventricle. As a result of this angle, the septal leaflet appears to have a fold in its substance.

The Tricuspid Annulus

The tricuspid annulus is located at the junction between the right atrium and the ventricle. The tricuspid annulus is attached only to the right fibrous trigone where the septal leaflet and the anteroseptal commissure insert. Elsewhere the connective tissue in a leaflet joins the subendocardial tissue, and the anterior and posterior leaflets insert directly into the myocardium.[38] It is at this specific site that a dilatation of the annulus occurs in the "functional" tricuspid insufficiency.[37,39]

The Chordae Tendinae

Like the mitral valve, the tricuspid valve has fan-shaped chordae, rough zone chordae, and basal chordae. However, in the tricuspid valve two additional types of chordae are found: free-edge chordae and deep chordae.

- The *free edge chordae* are single, threadlike, often long chordae originating from the apex of a papillary muscle and inserting into a leaflet's free edge.
- The *deep chordae* are long chordae. They pass deep to a leaflet's free margin to insert on its ventricular surface, either in the upper part of the rough zone or in the clear zone. They may branch into two or three cords just before insertion. Often the cordlike branches have a triangular fold of membranous tissue passing between them and the leaflet tissue just before their insertion.

Number of Chordae Tendinae Attached to the Tricuspid Valve

On average, 25 chordae insert into the tricuspid valve. Of these, seven pass to the anterior leaflet, six to the posterior leaflet, nine to the septal leaflet, and three insert into the commissural areas.[36]

The Papillary Muscles

Three groups of papillary muscles are associated with the tricuspid valve.

- The *anterior papillary muscle* is attached to the anterior wall of the right ventricle. It is the largest. Its chordae tendinae are connected mainly to the anterior leaflet and few of them are connected to the posterior leaflet.
- The *posterior papillary muscle* is not always single, but sometimes consists of two or three muscular columns attached to the posterior wall of the right ventricle. Its chordae tendinae are connected to the posterior leaflet and few of them to the septal leaflet.
- The *chordae tendinae of the septal leaflet* spring directly from the ventricular septum or from small eminences on it.

TRICUSPID VALVE REPAIR

The same basic principles of repair that have been described for the mitral valve apply to the tricuspid valve.

Valve Analysis

Tricuspid valve incompetence, recognized prior to operation either clinically, by hemodynamic investigation, or by echocardiography, is analyzed by direct vision. Digital palpation has proved unreliable and has led to false-negative conclusions under the operative conditions.

The atrium is opened by a semicircular incision around the inferior vena caval cannula to avoid the intraparietal atrioventricular pathways of conduction. Leaflet tissue is analyzed for organic lesions, usually leaflet thickening and commissural fusion, rarely leaflet prolapse or leaflet tear or perforation.

The annulus is measured with obturators to assess with precision the degree of distension or deformation. Indications for valve repair are based on the following criteria: (1) annular size greater than the no. 34 obturator in women and the no. 36 in men; (2) organic lesions with or without annular dilatation.

Techniques of Repair

Remodeling of the Annulus

Anatomic studies[38] have shown that dilatation of the annulus affects the various parts of the annulus in an irregular manner: (in decreasing order of magnitude) the posteroseptal commissure, the anteroposterior commissure, the posterior leaflet, the anterior leaflet, and to a lesser degree the anteroseptal commissure and the septal leaflet (Fig. 119–23).

The annulus is not only dilated, but is also deformed, with the anteroposterior diameter being greater than the transverse diameter, contrary to the normal situation. Reducing the orifice size without restoring the shape of the orifice results in a 15% stenosis to achieve valve competence. This has been confirmed by hemodynamic studies.[40]

Dilatation and deformation of the tricuspid annulus can appropriately be corrected by suitably shaped and sized

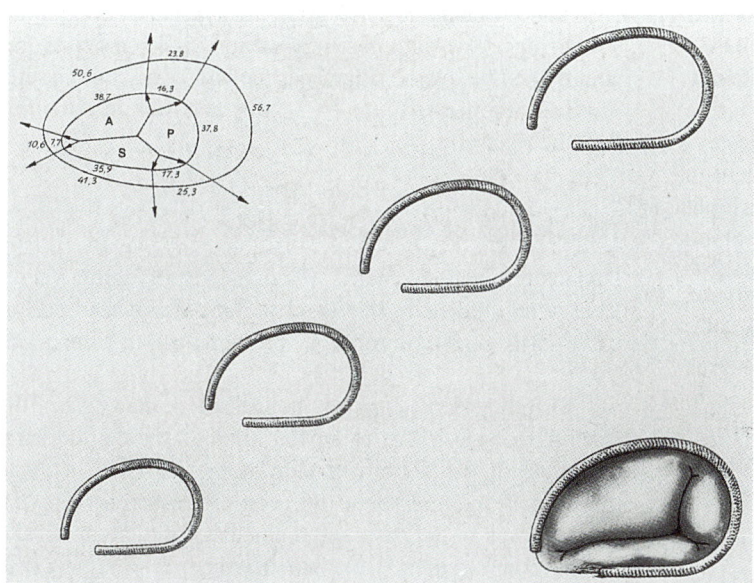

Figure 119–23. Tricuspid prosthetic ring annuloplasty. Upper left: anatomic study. Central numbers indicate normal dimensions in millimeters; peripheral numbers indicate dimensions of the distended annulus.

prosthetic rings. These rings are flexible, so that stress on the multiple points of fixation is reduced and they are open in the area of the bundle of His to avoid the risk of atrioventricular block (Fig. 119–24).

Repair of Organic Lesions

Commissural fusion is treated by a triple commissurotomy and subsequent remodeling of the annulus or bicuspidization whenever the posterior leaflet is retracted (Fig. 119–25). It may be necessary to resect some secondary chordae to mobilize the leaflet.

A prolapse of the leaflet can be corrected with the same techniques as those used for the mitral valve.

AORTIC VALVE

Anatomy of the Aortic Valve

The aortic valve is normally tricuspid and is composed of three basic components: a fibrous skeleton, three sinuses of Valsalva, and three thin and delicate cusps.

The Aortic Leaflets

The semilunar cusps are inserted along their scalloped outer edge within the connective tissue of the aortic annulus. The cusps meet at three commissures, which lie equally spaced

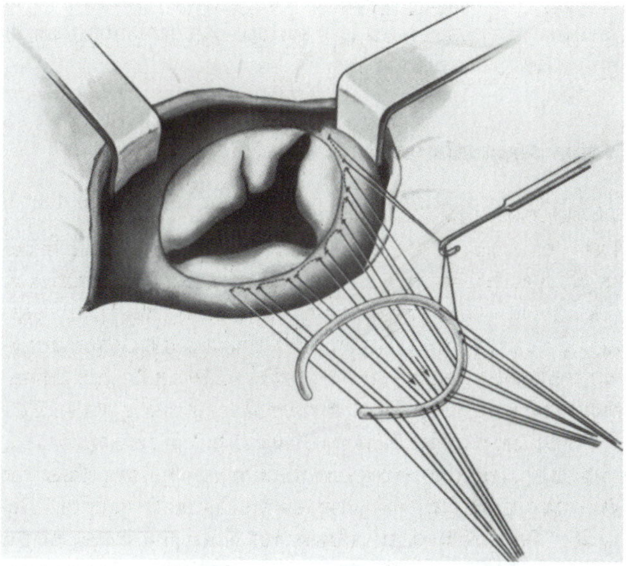

Figure 119–24. Suturing of the prosthetic ring using mattress sutures. (From Carpentier A: Cardiac valve surgery. The "French correction." J Thorac Cardiovasc Surg 86:323–327, 1983.)

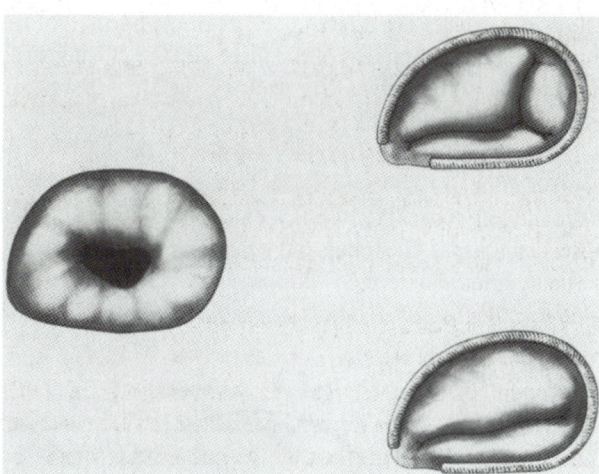

Figure 119–25. Repair of restricted leaflet motion of the tricuspid valve by triple commissurotomy and annular remodeling or bicuspidization whenever the posterior leaflet is retracted. (From Carpentier A: Cardiac valve surgery. The "French correction." J Thorac Cardiovasc Surg 86:323–327, 1983.)

on the supra-aortic ridge, to which they are firmly attached at identical levels.

The free edge of each cusp is of tougher consistency than the remainder of the cusp. At the midpoint of each free edge is a fibrous nodulus Aranti from which two ridges extend downward. These ridges mark the closure line on each cusp where it abuts on to its neighbor in the closed position. The portion of the valve below this line separates the blood in the aorta from the left ventricular cavity when the valve is closed. The portion of the valve above this line is known as the *lunula* and overlaps the neighboring cusp and serves as a supporting strut or cable. These portions form the area of coaptation during valve closure. The lunulae are occasionally fenestrated near the commissures (Fig. 119–26).

It should be noted that for a given aortic valve the cusps are often of different sizes.[41]

The Fibrous Skeleton

The base of the aortic valve is a circumferential region at the proximal attachment of the aortic leaflets. It has been described as a fibrous structure or annulus, which suggests a rigid and nonexpansile structure with no changes during the cardiac cycle.[42–44]

Others[45] have shown that the base of the aortic valve is capable of cyclic dimensional changes because it is partly composed of ventricular myocardium. At this level, two of the three trigonal regions forming the fibrous skeleton of the aortic valve consist almost entirely of obliquely or circularly oriented myocardium. Dense collagenous tissue present in these zones is limited to a thin intimal layer of tissue. Only the trigonal region between the posterior and right sinuses, which serves as the origin of the mitral valve leaflet, is composed of dense collagenous tissue.

The Sinuses of Valsalva

The aortic sinuses are dilated pockets of the aortic root that form the outer component of the three cuplike closing structures of the aortic valve. The walls of the sinuses are considerably thinner than the wall of the aorta proper.[46]

The origin of the coronary arteries is the basis of the nomenclature for the sinuses and cusps. The ostia of the right and left coronary arteries identify the right and left sinuses and cusps. The sinus and cusp without an associated coronary artery are termed "noncoronary."

The coronary arteries arise always below the supra-aortic ridge. The right coronary ostium (3–4 mm) rises frequently just below the ridge near the left–right commissure. The left coronary ostium (4–5 mm) is lower in the sinus than the right one.

The Design of the Aortic Valve

Dimensions and geometric relationships of aortic valves have been studied by different authors using methods of valve casts under physiologic pressures or in vivo models.[47–49]

Different parameters can be measured: the angle of the free edge of the leaflet to a plane through the commissure, the angle of the bottom surface of the leaflet to a plane through the commissures, the vertical distance from the commissures to the base, the diameter of the circle formed by the commissures (Dc), and the diameter of the circle formed by the base of the valve (Db). The proportion between these two diameters has a fundamental functional importance. If the ratio Dc/Db is 0.9 the valve is competent; if, on the other hand, this ratio is higher than 1, the valve is incompetent. There is a striking similarity in the basic design of all aortic valves and differences in valve design parameters are small.

AORTIC VALVE RECONSTRUCTION

Repair of the aortic valve follows the basic principles of valve reconstruction. The goal of the repair is to obtain a valve with the free edge of the three cusps at the same level and with a good surface of coaptation; however, the closing mechanism of the aortic valve is more precise than that of the mitral or tricuspid valves. This is partly because of the fact that the cusps have less surface of coaptation than the mitral and tricuspid leaflets.

Valve Analysis

The valve is analyzed in a systematic manner. Annular dilatation is demonstrated by a lack of apposition of otherwise pliable leaflets. Leaflet prolapse is recognized by evaluating the degree of elongation of the free edge of one or

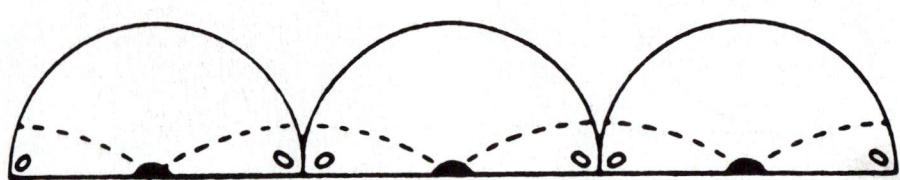

Figure 119–26. Aortic valve (view en face).

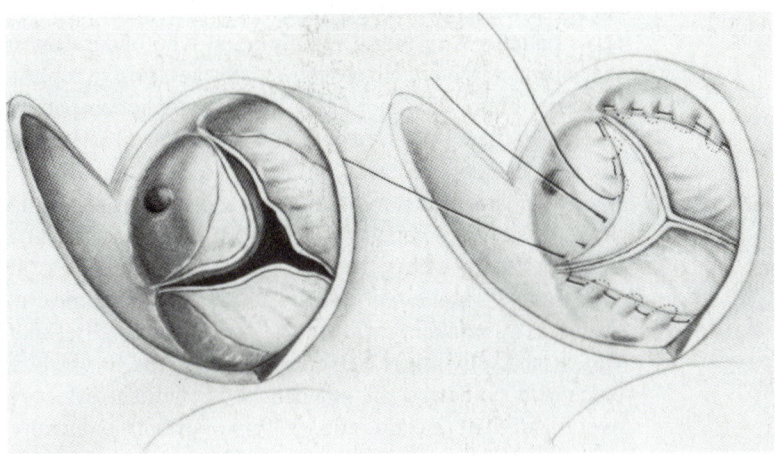

Figure 119–27. Repair of aortic annular dilatation by circular suture. *(From Carpentier A: Cardiac valve surgery. The "French correction." J Thorac Cardiovasc Surg 86:323–327, 1983.)*

several cusps below the plane of the annulus. Restricted leaflet motion is assessed by mobilizing the leaflets.

Valve Repair

Repair of Annular Dilatation

Annular dilatation is repaired by means of a circular suture. A circular suture is possible because of the circular configuration of the orifice as opposed to that of the mitral or tricuspid orifices. The circular suture is a continuous vertical mattress 2–0 Tevdek suture that is passed through the annulus successively downward from the aorta toward the ventricle and upward from the ventricle to the annulus twice the whole circumference[27] (Fig. 119–27). Annular dilatation can also be repaired by commissural annuloplasty. The aortic wall is plicated at each commissure with a pledgeted

vertically placed "U" stitch. This results in a reduced aortic circumference[50] (Figure 119–28). This technique, although appealing because of its simplicity, has been associated in our hands with less satisfactory long-term results than the circular annuloplasty.

Repair of Leaflet Prolapse

Leaflet prolapse is repaired by a triangular resection of the middle part of the distended cusp so as to restore normal length to the free edge.[27] The extent of this resection is calculated by measuring the free edge of the adjacent cusps (Fig. 119–29). Leaflet resuspension is another technique that can be utilized to correct prolapse of one or more cusps. After joining the three nodules of Aranti with a temporary suture, the free edge of the prolapsing cusp is plicated with a pledgeted suture and is anchored to the aortic wall[50] (Fig. 119–30).

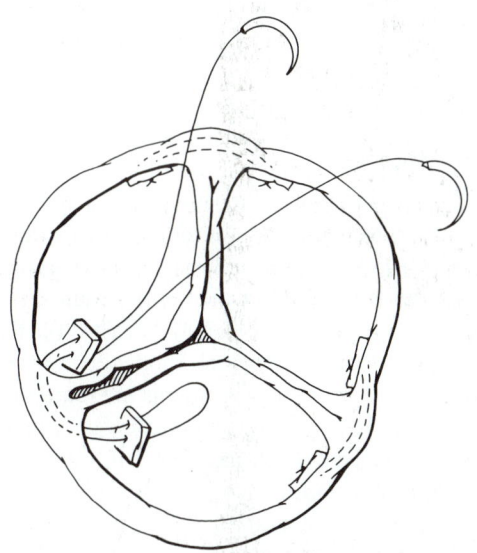

Figure 119–28. Commissural Annuloplasty. *(From Duran C: Present status of reconstructive surgery for aortic valve disease. J Card Surg 8:443, 1993.)*

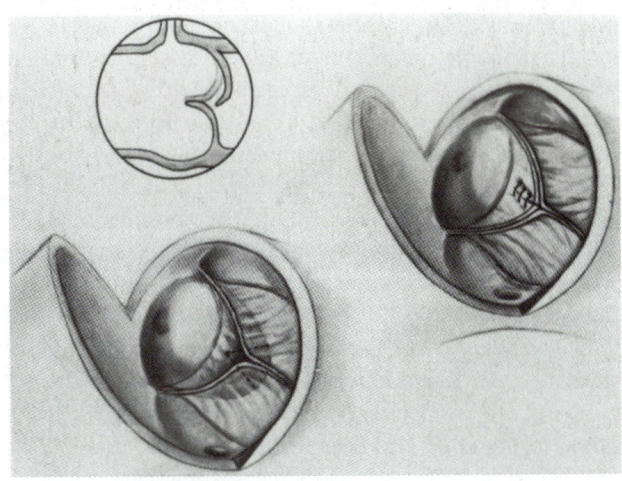

Figure 119–29. Aortic cusp prolapse treated by triangular resection. *(From Carpentier A: Cardiac valve surgery. The "French correction." J Thorac Cardiovasc Surg 86:323–327, 1983.)*

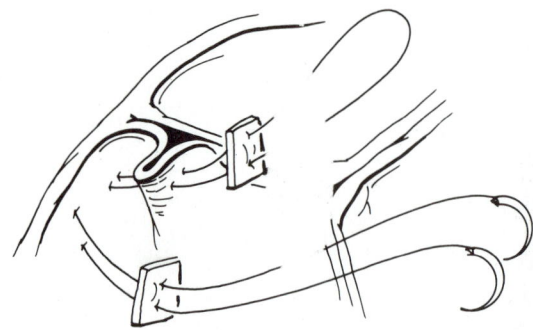

Figure 119–30. Free edge suspension. *(From Duran C: Present status of reconstructive surgery for aortic valve disease. J Card Surg 8:443, 1993.)*

Repair of Restricted Leaflet Motion

Restricted leaflet motion is corrected by commissurotomy and cusp shaving to thin out the leaflet tissue (Fig. 119–31).

RESULTS OF VALVE REPAIR

Mitral Valve Repair

We have studied consecutively 206 patients having undergone prosthetic ring mitral valve repair between 1972 and 1979 at our institution.[51] One hundred and ninety-five patients (94.5%) survived the operation. The age of the patients ranged from 18 to 79 years (mean 48.7 years). Mitral valve incompetence was secondary to degenerative valvular disease in 113 cases (58%), rheumatic disease in 74 cases (38%), and ischemia and other miscellaneous causes in 8 cases (4%). One hundred and eighty-eight patients were in New York Heart Association (NYHA) Class III and IV preoperatively and 94 (48%) had atrial fibrillation. Thirty-five patients (18%) had type I mitral valve incompetence, 147 (75%) type II, and 13 (7%) type III.

The techniques included prosthetic ring annuloplasty (185 patients), partial leaflet mobilization (10 patients), and papillary muscle reimplantation (2 patients). The survival was 72.4% at 15 years, with a valve-related survival of 82.8%. At 15 years, freedom from thromboembolism was 93.9%, freedom from endocarditis was 96.6%, and freedom from anticoagulant hemorrhage was 95.6%. At 15 years, 87.3% of patients were free from reoperation. It should be noted that the actuarial rate of freedom from reoperation was higher in the degenerative group (92.7%) than in the rheumatic group (76.12%). Among the 157 survivors, 117 (74%) were in NYHA Class I and II and 105 (66%) were in sinus rhythm. Echocardiography-Doppler studies showed normal contractility in 134 patients (84.5%) and absence of mitral regurgitation in 112 patients (71%), trivial mitral regurgitation in 27 patients (17%), and significant mitral regurgitation in 4 patients (2.5%). As more clinical data becomes available, mitral valve repair, when technically feasible, is emerging as the procedure of choice for mitral

regurgitation. Akins et al.[52] reported a series of 263 consecutive patients with mitral regurgitation who underwent either mitral valve reconstruction or prosthetic valve replacement between 1985 and 1992. The reconstruction patients had a significantly lower operative mortality (3% vs. 12% for replacement patients [$p < 0.01$]). In addition, freedom from all valve related morbidity and mortality was 85% for the reconstruction patients and 73% for the replacement patients ($p = 0.03$) during the followup period.

Similar results were found at the Mayo Clinic in a group of 409 patients with mitral regurgitation. By multivariate analysis, mitral valve repair compared to valve replacement conferred an independent beneficial effect on overall survival (hazard ratio, 0.39; $p = 0.00001$), operative mortality (odds ratio, 0.27; $p = 0.026$), and late survival (hazard ratio 0.44; $p = 0.001$).[53]

Tricuspid Valve Repair

Of 1345 tricuspid valve repairs performed in association with mitral valve repair (331) or with mitral or aortic valve replacement, 1210 were performed with prosthetic ring annuloplasty and 135 by the semicircular suture technique (De Vega) for comparative evaluation. The incidence of reoperation was 0.6% in the prosthetic ring annuloplasty group and 6.4% in the semicircular annuloplasty group. For further evaluation, 30 patients (15 with functional and 15 with organic disease) treated by prosthetic ring annuloplasty were subjected to follow-up catheterization, angiograms, dye dilution curves, and intracardiac phonocardiograms. A good result with no significant valve stenosis was observed in all patients but one, who had severe organic tricuspid disease.

Aortic Valve Repair

From January 1971 to December 1982, 95 patients with aortic valve incompetence were treated by reconstruction of the aortic valve. Fifteen patients had isolated aortic valve disease, and 50 had associated mitral valve insufficiency treated by either mitral valve repair (39 patients) or bioprosthetic valve replacement (11 patients). Thirty patients had triple valve reconstruction or aortic and tricuspid valve reconstruction associated with mitral valve replacement. Hospital mortality was 3.3% for the entire group. Reoperation was necessary eight times (13%) because of significant residual regurgitation. Residual moderate aortic insufficiency persisted in 15% of the patients not requiring reoperation. There were no thromboembolic complications. Duran[50] reported a similar incidence of significant aortic regurgitation after aortic valvuloplasty. In a series of 202 patients who underwent aortic valve repair, 17 patients (8.7%) developed severe aortic regurgitation requiring reoperation.

From these results we conclude that it is too early to recommend these techniques of aortic valve repair in the

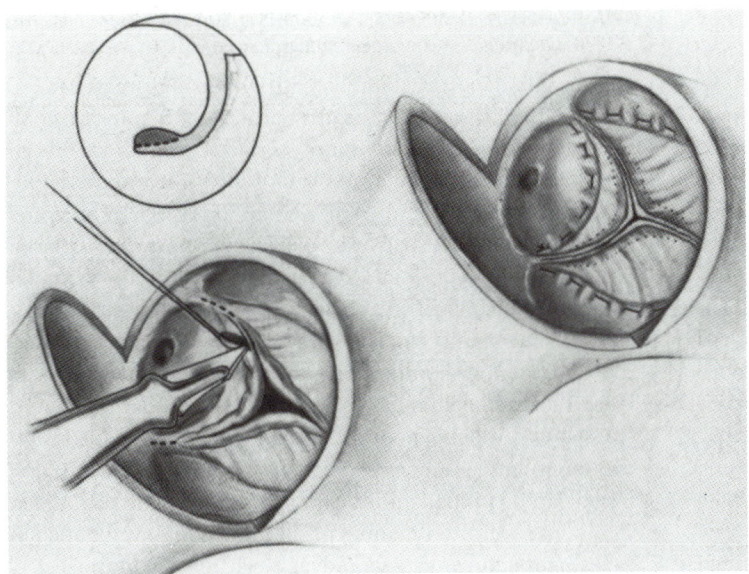

Figure 119–31. Restricted cusp motion treated by cusp shaving.

adult. However, they are a valuable alternative to valve replacement in children.

Twenty years after the introduction of the techniques of valve repair, good predictability and stability of the results have been demonstrated, particularly for the mitral and the tricuspid valves. When compared to other alternatives, whether they be mechanical valve replacement or bioprosthetic valve replacement, the advantages of reconstructive surgery (i.e., lower mortality, lower morbidity, and improved quality of life) are now well established. The arguments frequently advanced in opposition to this surgery (i.e., complexity of the lesions, difficulty of techniques, different patient population, and the evolving process of the diseases) are no longer valid. The complexity of the lesions can be minimized by the functional approach. The difficulty of the techniques can be overcome by adequate training so that when faced with a diseased valve the surgeon should always consider valve repair before proceeding to valve replacement.

REFERENCES

1. Starr A, Edwards ML: Mitral replacement: Clinical experience with a ball-valve prosthesis. *Ann Surg* **54:**726, 1961
1a. Perloff JK, Roberts WC: The mitral apparatus. *Circulation* **46:**227, 1972
2. Hansen DE, Cahill PD, Decampli WM, et al: Valvular-ventricular interaction: Interaction of the mitral apparatus in canine left ventricular systolic performance. *Circulation* **73:**1310, 1986
3. Sarris GE, Cahill POD, Hansen DE, et al: Restoration of left ventricular systolic performance after reattachment of the mitral chordae tendinae. The importance of valvular-ventricular interaction. *J Thorac Cardiovasc Surg* **95:**969, 1988
4. David TE, Burns RJ, Bacchus CM, et al: Mitral valve replacement for mitral regurgitation with and without preservation of chordae tendinae. *J Thorac Cardiovasc Surg* **88:**718, 1984
5. Perier P, Deloche A, Chauvaud S, et al: Comparative evaluation of mitral valve repair and replacement with Starr, Björk, and porcine valve prostheses. *Circulation* **70:**I 187, 1984
6. Sand ME, Naftel DC, Blackstone EH, et al: A comparison of repair and replacement for mitral valve incompetence. *J Thorac Cardiovasc Surg* **94:**208, 1987
7. Galloway AC, Colvin SB, Baumann FG, et al: A comparison of mitral valve reconstruction with mitral valve replacement: Intermediate-term results. *Ann Thorac Surg* **47:**655, 1989
8. Rusted IE, Schiefley CH, Edwards JR: Studies of the mitral valve: I. Anatomic features of the normal mitral valve and associated structures. *Circulation* **6:**825, 1952
9. Rusted IE, Schiefley CH, Edwards JE: Guides to the commissures in operations upon the mitral valve. *Pros Staff Meet Mayo Clin* **26:**297, 1951
10. Ranganathan N, Silver MD: The mitral valve in man. A review of anatomy and its clinical significance. *Anat Clin* **2:**361, 1980
11. Lam JH, Ranganathan N, Wigle ED, et al: Morphology of the human mitral valve: I. Chordae tendinae: A new classification. *Circulation* **41:**449, 1970
12. Carpentier A, Guerinon J, Deloche A, et al: Pathology of the mitral valve: Introduction to plastic and reconstructive valve surgery. In Kalmanson D (ed): The Mitral Valve, A Pluridisciplinary Approach. Acton, England, Publishing Science Group, 1976, p 65
13. Walmsley R, Watson H: *Clinical Anatomy of the Heart*. Edinburgh, Churchill Livingstone, 1978
14. Zimmerman J, Bailey CP: The surgical significance of the heart. *J Thorac Cardiovasc Surg* **44:**701, 1962
15. Gross L, Kugel MA: Topographic anatomy and histology of the valves in the human heart. *Am J Pathol* **7:**445, 1931
16. Zimmerman J: The functional and surgical anatomy of the heart. *Ann R Coll Surg* **39:**348, 1966
17. Walmsley R, Watson H: The out-flow tract of the left ventricle. *Br Heart J* **28:**435, 1966
18. Ranganathan N, Lam JH, Wigle ED, et al: Morphology of the human mitral valve. II. The valve leaflets. *Circulation* **41:**459, 1970
19. Carpentier A, Deloche A, Dauptain J, et al: A new reconstructive operation for correction of mitral valve insufficiency. *J Thorac Cardiovasc Surg* **61:**1, 1970
20. Ormiston JA, Shah PM, Tei C, et al: Size and motion of the mitral annulus in man: a two-dimensional echocardiographic method and findings in normal subjects. *Circulation* **64:**113, 1981

21. Sonnenblick EH, Napolitano LM, Dagett WR: An intrinsic neuromuscular basis for mitral valve motion in the dog. *Circulation* **21**:9, 1969

22. Ranganathan N, Burch GE: Gross morphology and arterial supply of the papillary muscles of the left ventricle of man. *Am Heart J* **77**:506, 1969

23. Estes EH, Dalton FM, Entman ML, et al: The anatomy and blood supply of the papillary muscles of the left ventricle. *Am Heart J* **71**:356, 1966

24. James TN: Anatomy of the coronary arteries in health and disease. *Circulation* **32**:1020, 1965

25. Fulton WFM: The Coronary Arteries: Arteriography, Microanatomy and Pathogenesis of Obliterative Coronary Artery Disease. Springfield, Illinois, Charles C Thomas, 1965

26. Chiechi M, Less WM, Thompson R: Functional anatomy of the normal mitral valve. *J Thorac Cardiovasc Surg* **32**:378, 1956

27. Carpentier A: Cardiac valve surgery: The French correction. *J Thorac Cardiovasc Surg* **86**:323, 1983

28. Skeikh K, De Brujin N, Rankin JS, et al: The utility of transesophageal echocardiography and doppler color flow imaging in patients undergoing cardiac valve surgery. *J Am Coll Cardiol* **15**:363, 1990

29. Stewart WJ, Currie PJ, Salcedol E, et al: Intraoperative doppler color flow mapping for decision-making in valve repair for mitral regurgitation: technique and results in 100 patients. *Circulation* **81**:556, 1990

30. Carpentier A: Plastic and reconstructive mitral valve surgery. In Kalmanson D (ed): The Mitral Valve, a Pluridisciplinary Approach. Acton, England, Publishing Science Group, 1976, p 527

31. Jebara VA, Mihaileanu S, Acar C, et al: Left ventricular outflow tract obstruction after mitral valve repair. *Circulation* **88**:II–30, 1993

32. David TL, Bos J, Rakowski H: Mitral valve repair by replacement of chordae tendineae with polytetrafluoroethylene sutures. J Thorac Cardiovasc Surg **101**:495, 1991

33. Grossi EA, Galloway AC, Steinberg BM, et al: Severe calcification does not affect long-term outcome of mitral valve repair. *Ann Thorac Surg* **58**:685, 1994

34. Fix J, Isada L, Cosgrove D, et al: Do patients with less than 'echoperfect' results from mitral valve repair by intraoperative echocardiography have a different outcome? *Circulation* **88**:II–39, 1993

35. Ranganathan N, Lam JHC, Wigle ED, et al: Morphology of the human tricuspid valve II. The valve leaflet. *Circulation* **41**:459, 1970

36. Silver MD, Lam JHC, Ranganathan N, et al: Morphology of the human tricuspid valve. *Circulation* **43**:333, 1971

37. Deloche A, Guerinon J, Fabiani JN, et al: Etudes anatomique des valvulopathies rhumatismales tricuspidiennes. *Ann Chir Thorac Cardiovasc* **12**:343, 1973

38. Tei C, Pilgrim JP, Shah PM, et al: The tricuspid valve annulus: Study of size and motion in normal subjects and in patients with tricuspid regurgitation. *Circulation* **66**:665, 1982

39. Carpentier A, Deloche A, Dauptain J, et al: A new reconstructive operation for correction of mitral and tricuspid insufficiency. *J Thorac Cardiovasc Surg* **61**:1, 1971

40. Haerten K, Seipel L, Loogen F, et al: Hemodynamic studies after De Vega tricuspid annuloplasty. *Circulation* **58**:I–28, 1978

41. Silver MA, Roberts WC: Detailed anatomy of the normally functioning aortic valve in hearts of normal and increased weight. *Am J Cardiol* **55**:454, 1985

42. Zimmerman J: The functional and surgical anatomy of the aortic valve. *Cardiac Surg* **5**:862, 1969

43. Swanson WM, Clark RE: Dimensions and geometric relationships of the human aortic valve as a function of pressure. *Circ Res* **35**:871, 1974

44. Mercer JL: Movement of the aortic annulus. *Br J Radiol* **42**:623, 1969

45. Thubrikar M, Nolan SP, Boscher LP, et al: The cyclic changes and structures of the base of the aortic valve. *Am Heart J* **99**:217, 1980

46. Reid K: The anatomy of the sinus of Valsalva. *Thorax* **25**:79, 1970

47. Mercer JL, Benedicty M, Bahnson HT: The geometry and construction of the aortic leaflet. *J Thorac Cardiovasc Surg* **65**:511, 1973

48. Carpentier A: Traitement des lésions valvulaires aortiques par des greffes heteroplastiques. Paris, *Thèse Med*, 1966

49. Thubrikar M, Piepgrass WC, Whaner TW, et al: The design of the normal aortic valve. *Am J Physiol* **241**:H795, 1981

50. Duran CM: Present status of reconstruction surgery for aortic valve disease. *J Card Surg* **8**:443, 1993

51. Deloche A, Jebara VA, Relland JYM, et al: Valve repair with Carpentier techniques—the second decade. *J Thorac Cardiovasc Surg* **99**:990, 1990

52. Akins CW, Hilgenberg AD, Buckley MJ, et al: Mitral valve reconstruction versus replacement for degenerative or ischemic mitral regurgitation. *Ann Thorac Surg* **58**:668, 1994

53. Enriquez-Sarano M, Schaff HV, Orszulak TA, et al: Valve repair improves the outcome of surgery for mitral regurgitation: a multivariate analysis. *Circulation* **91**:1022, 1995

120

Aortic Valve Disease and Hypertrophic Cardiomyopathies

Graeme L. Hammond and George V. Letsou

Aortic valve surgery continues to be the quest for an optimal valve prosthesis, along with renewed interest in aortic homografts and aortic repair techniques. The mainstay of our current treatment of aortic valve disease remains surgical. Building upon the remarkable contributions of surgeons such as Hufnagel, Gibbon, Harken, McGoon, Lillehei, Starr, and others in the late 1950s and early 1960s, the contemporary surgeon, armed with improved methods of myocardial protection, and better anesthesic and postoperative support, can operate with low mortality on a wide range of patients with aortic valve disease.

Acquired disease of the aortic valve may be divided into two categories: aortic stenosis (AS) and aortic regurgitation (AR).

AORTIC STENOSIS

Etiology

Obstruction of the left ventricular (LV) outflow tract may be subvalvular, valvular, or supravalvular. In the adult population, the majority of patients have obstruction at the level of the aortic valve. Valvular AS may be classified according to etiology: rheumatic versus nonrheumatic.[1,2]

Rheumatic aortic stenosis develops as a consequence of the pancarditis of acute rheumatic fever. A rheumatic etiology can be invoked in 30 to 40% of surgically excised aortic valves. The valve cusps become edematous and thickened and can be seen microscopically to contain an in-

flammatory cellular infiltrate. Vegetations consisting primarily of adherent platelet thrombi appear along the margins of closure and, following the acute phase, become organized. The cusps become deformed with progressive fibrosis and varying degrees of commissural fusion. Classically all three cusps are involved resulting in a small triangular opening. Rheumatic aortic valve stenosis is nearly always associated with an anatomically abnormal mitral valve which may be of varying clinical significance.[3]

Nonrheumatic AS falls into two categories: congenital and degenerative. The congenital variety of AS is the most common, and accounts for two-thirds of the nonrheumatic patients.[1] The bicuspid configuration is most often seen, having an incidence in the general population of 0.9 to 2.0%[4] and a frequency of 54% of all patients with valvular aortic stenosis >15 years.[1] The congenitally bicuspid valve may have normal function throughout life, may develop progressive calcification and stenosis, or may develop regurgitation with or without infection.[4] The mechanism for this variation in the natural history is not clear. Aortic stenosis may also result from a unicuspid valve, which may be stenotic from birth but may not come to clinical significance until adulthood.[5]

Aortic valvular stenosis of the degenerative type, also known as senile, idiopathic calcific, and atherosclerotic, includes older patients with extensive calcification of a tricuspid valve, without fusion of the commissures. This process of calcification may also involve the anterior leaflet of the mitral valve, or mitral annulus as well as the coronary arteries.[6,7]

Pathophysiology

Regardless of the specific etiology, the common endpoint in aortic stenosis is usually a heavily calcified valve with diminished valve area and a large transvalvular gradient which is required to maintain adequate flow. A degree of regurgitation is often present.

The normal aortic valve area is 2.5 to 3.5 cm^2.[8] At valve areas < 1.0 cm^2 many patients will become symptomatic and areas < 0.7 cm^2 represent critical stenosis. The heart adapts to this outflow obstruction or increased afterload by developing concentric hypertrophy. The wall thickness increases and the left ventricular mass increases two to three times, but the chamber size remains relatively constant.[9] Clinically, there is commonly a long latent period in which the left ventricle can meet the demands of the increased pressure and maintain adequate cardiac output with progressive hypertrophy. The gradient across the valve is a function of the aortic valve area and gradients of 90 to 180 mm Hg may be present in severe stenosis.[8]

Along with LV hypertrophy there is often an increase in diastolic stiffness, which may result from an increase in chamber wall thickness or from morphologic changes within the myocardium. As the compliance of the ventricle decreases, higher filling pressures, or preload, reflected in a higher left ventricular end-diastolic pressures, may be required to maintain adequate systolic ejection, especially in response to exercise. To maintain this preload, the left atrium undergoes hypertrophy resulting in a prominent "a"-wave on the atrial pressure curve. Eventually, the ventricle is unable to compensate and becomes dilated. This results in decreased cardiac output, elevated pulmonary pressures, and signs of congestive heart failure.

Hypertrophy of the left ventricle secondary to AS also plays a role in the important phenomenon of myocardial ischemia, usually effort related, in the presence of normal coronary arteries. Myocardial oxygen demand is increased proportionately to the increase in left ventricular mass and increase in systolic pressure. Myocardial oxygen supply is diminished in the subendocardium during diastole by the increased end-diastolic pressure and in systole by compression of the coronary microvasculature by the hypertrophied ventricle. This mismatch of supply and demand may result in angina or an anginal equivalent.[8]

The inability of the heart to increase cardiac output in response to exercise by the fixed obstruction at the level of the aortic valve may lead to cerebral hypoperfusion and syncope. This mechanism is often invoked in the patient with AS; however, care must be taken to exclude the numerous other causes of syncope in this population, namely, dysrhythmias and conduction abnormalities as well as cerebrovascular events.

Clinical Picture

Physical examination is remarkable for a loud harsh crescendo–descrescendo systolic aortic murmur that trans- mits to the neck. A faint diastolic blowing murmur may indicate associated aortic regurgitation. The second heart sound is usually closely split, but may be paradoxical; as the valve becomes less mobile the aortic closure sound becomes diminished.[10] With left atrial hypertrophy and forceful atrial contraction, an S4 is commonly heard and may be appreciated as a prominent presystolic impulse at the apex of the heart. The carotid pulse has a diminished upstroke and may have a palpable thrill.

The electrocardiogram typically demonstrates left ventricular hypertrophy and often left atrial enlargement. With calcification involving the bundle of His in its course along the junction of the muscular and membranous septum, complete heart block, bundle branch block, or intraventricular conduction delays may be present.[11]

The chest radiographs demonstrate relatively normal heart size with left ventricular prominence. End-stage hearts may show gross cardiomegaly as they dilate and fail. Calcification may be seen in the area of the aortic valve and poststenotic dilatation of the ascending aorta may be present.

Patients with AS may remain asymptomatic for many years; however, as the valve area decreases they typically present with all or part of the triad of congestive heart failure, angina, and syncope. After the appearance of symptoms the clinical course becomes malignant. Aortic stenosis is the most common fatal valvular lesion.[12] Sudden death may occur in up to 20% of patients and although often heralded by the onset of symptoms, it is a risk in any patient with aortic stenosis. Prior to the era of surgical replacement, Bergeron reported in 1954 that up to 30% of patients developed angina, 20% syncope, and 50% died within 2 years of the onset of symptoms.[13] In a postmortem analysis of patients dying from aortic stenosis, Ross and Braunwald showed that the average survival time after the onset of symptoms was 2 years for congestive heart failure, 3 years for syncope, and 5 years for angina (Fig. 120–1).[14] With the advent of current techniques of aortic valve replacement, these statistics have improved dramatically.

Patients with evidence of aortic stenosis on physical examination, with or without symptoms, should undergo investigation. Noninvasive evaluation should include ECG, chest x-ray film, and echocardiography. M-mode and two-dimensional (2-D) echocardiography can give useful information regarding the configuration and motion of the leaflets, but can be misleading in assessing the severity of the stenosis.[15] Doppler ultrasound can be useful in quantifying the pressure gradient across the valve, which has been found to correlate well with peak gradients obtained at cardiac catheterization.[16]

Following the noninvasive evaluation, any patient in whom the severity of the stenosis is uncertain, or in whom additional infarction is required, should undergo cardiac catheterization.[17] Simultaneous determination of pressure and flow (cardiac output) across the valve should be obtained via right and left heart catheterization. This data can

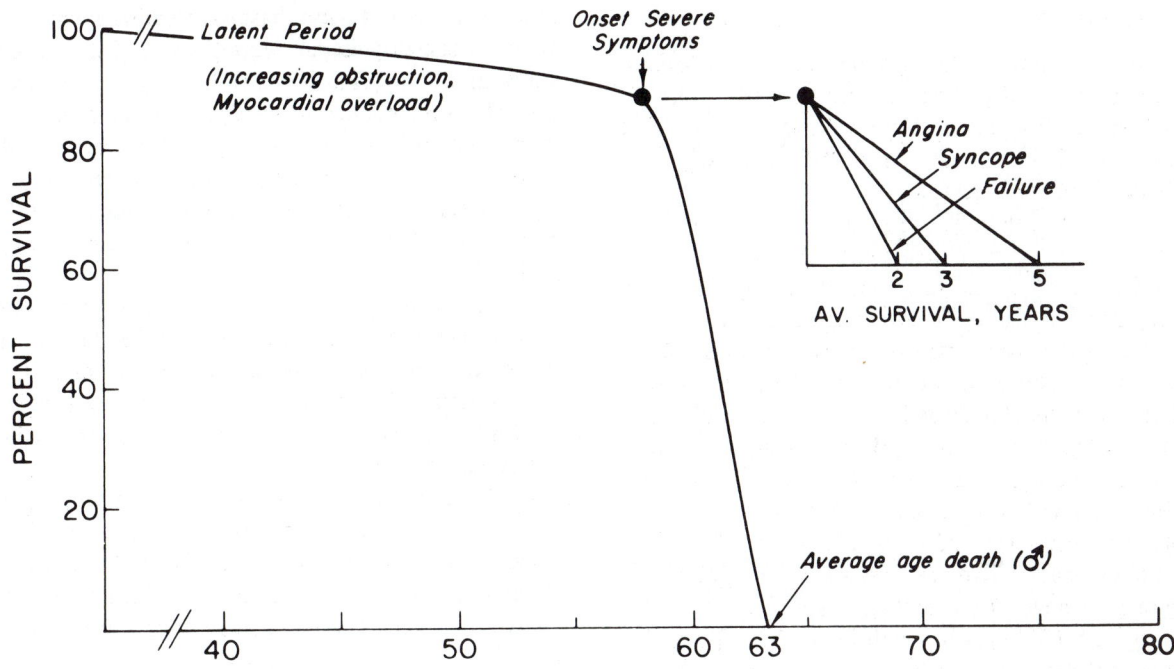

Figure 120–1. Average course of valvular aortic stenosis in adults. Data assembled from postmortem studies. *(From Ross J Jr, Braunwald E: Circulation 37(Suppl V):61, 1968.)*

then be used to calculate valve area according to the Gorlin formula,[18] which, in the simplified version, is expressed as

$$\text{valve area} = \text{cardiac output}/\sqrt{\text{gradient}}$$

Contrast angiography should generally be performed to assess the mitral valve, regional wall motion disturbances, and left ventricular function. However, care must be taken to weigh the risk of the contrast load in patients with left ventricular failure and high pulmonary capillary wedge pressures. Aortography may demonstrate the presence of aortic regurgitation or help to delineate supravalvular and subvalvular obstruction if these lesions are suspected.

Coronary arteriography is recommended in all patients and is mandatory in patients with symptoms of angina to assess the possible need for combined valve replacement and myocardial revascularization. Coronary anomalies of surgical significance can be identified and potential difficulties with cardioplegia administration through the coronary ostia assessed.

Indications for Surgery

The indications for aortic valve replacement in AS include (1) patients with aortic stenosis and symptoms of syncope, angina, or congestive heart failure and (2) asymptomatic patients with severe AS as documented by an aortic valve area $< 0.7 \text{ cm}^2$.

Obviously, there is an intermediate range of patients with moderately severe AS (valve area = 0.8 to 1.0 cm^2) and questionable symptoms in which recommendations must be individualized.

AORTIC REGURGITATION

Etiology

The most common cause of aortic regurgitation (AR) is rheumatic fever, accounting for up to one-half of patients requiring valve replacement.[19] Aortic regurgitation following acute rheumatic fever results from fibrous thickening and subsequent retraction of one or more cusps causing abnormal coaptation. Commissural fusion is minimal in pure AR but is a significant feature of aortic regurgitation when seen in combination with aortic stenosis.[2]

Unlike aortic stenosis, nonrheumatic causes of AR are numerous and involve both the valve per se and the aorta. Infective endocarditis is second to rheumatic fever as the most common cause of AR leading to valve replacement and is the most common cause of fatal isolated AR.[2] The mechanism of action varies from destruction or perforation of the valve cusps to abnormal coaptation secondary to vegetations. Endocarditis may affect either congenitally bicuspid or normal tricuspid valves. Bicuspid valves without endocarditis may produce AR, which is usually mild to moderate in severity, but may lead to valve replacement. Congenital ventricular septal defect may also produce AR when associated with prolapse of the valve cusps, particularly the right coronary cusp.

Aortic regurgitation is the most common valvular lesion in blunt chest trauma and may represent cuspal avulsion or laceration of the wall of the aorta.[20] Traumatic AR usually results in wide open regurgitation with rapid deterioration.

Other valvular causes of aortic regurgitation include myxomatous degeneration, rheumatoid arthritis, and systemic lupus arythematosis.[21]

Significant AR may result from disease of the ascending aorta in the presence of a histologically normal valve. Though in the past syphilis was a major cause of aortic regurgitation, it is uncommon today. Cardiovascular involvement represents a tertiary manifestation of the disease and usually does not appear until 15 to 20 years after contracting the infection. Dilatation of the aortic root, including the aortic annulus and ascending aorta, results from destruction of the elastic tissue and smooth muscle of the aortic media. The commissures are widened and the valve cusps no longer meet, giving rise to central regurgitation during diastole. The free margins of the cusps roll down and become fibrotic and thickened probably in response to the turbulent flow, further contributing to the regurgitation.

Marfan's syndrome is a hereditary disorder (single autosomal dominant; rarely, recessive) characterized by a basic defect in the formation of elastic fibers. Involvement of the aorta results in thinning and dilatation of the aortic wall due to a deficiency of elastic fibers in the media known as cystic medial necrosis.[22] Aneurysmal dilatation of the ascending aorta, including dilatation of the sinuses of Valsalva and the aortic annulus, "annuloaortic ectasia," produces AR as the cusps are unable to coapt. The aortic valve is usually normal. Acute AR can be seen in Marfan's syndrome in the event of acute aortic dissection.

Dilatation of the ascending aorta can also lead to aortic regurgitation in Ehler–Danlos syndrome and osteogenesis imperfecta as well as in a less well-defined group (idiopathic aortic root dilatation) in which no evidence of Marfan's or other systemic disease is present.

Acute aortic dissection may result in acute AR leading to sudden and severe congestive heart failure. Typically, retrograde dissection from a tear 2 to 3 cm above the valve produces detachment of the valve cusps.

Anklosing spondylitis may produce AR by a combination of aortic wall and aortic valve involvement. The valve cusps become thickened and fibrotic which may, in a small group of patients, lead to AR.[23]

Pathophysiology

The severity of acute regurgitation is a function of the size of the regurgitant orifice, the duration of diastole, and the difference in diastolic pressure between the aorta and the left ventricle. The physiologic response depends largely on the rate at which the regurgitation develops. The size of the regurgitant orifice producing significant AR may range from 0.5 cm^2 to as large as 1.0 cm^2.[24] Large volumes, up to 60 to 70% of the amount ejected, may regurgitate during diastole.[9]

The left ventricle must then increase its stroke volume to include the normal forward flow plus the volume regurgitated. This large increase in stroke volume during systole results in the typical hemodynamic profile of elevated systolic pressure, while the regurgitation results in lowered aortic diastolic pressure, i.e., widened pulse pressure.

In the chronic setting the left ventricle undergoes marked eccentric hypertrophy and dilatation. Eccentric hypertrophy refers to the relationship between increased wall thickness proportionate to increased ventricular diameter; the net result is a normal ratio between wall thickness and chamber radius. Eccentric hypertrophy should be distinguished from the concentric hypertrophy of aortic stenosis in which there is an increase in wall thickness without a corresponding increase in chamber radius. In AR this compensatory increase in end-diastolic volume allows the left ventricle to maximize ejection of the combined left atrial inflow and the volume regurgitated. In essence, both preload and afterload are elevated. Patients with severe AR undergo left ventricular hypertrophy initially, which is followed by the gradual onset of ventricular dilatation. Determining the point in the process at which to perform aortic valve replacement is the key issue in aortic insufficiency.

The left ventricle may be able to compensate in this manner for years, however, eventually the ejection fraction and cardiac output will fall and the patient will develop signs and symptoms of congestive heart failure. Patients may also present with angina in the face of normal coronary arteries, presumably secondary to decreased coronary perfusion during diastole and elevated oxygen demands of the hypertrophied ventricle.

The physiologic response to acute AR, most commonly caused by infective endocarditis and aortic dissection, usually varies considerably from that of chronic aortic regurgitation.[25] In the acute setting, the left ventricle does not have time to hypertrophy or to compensate with significant increases in stroke volume. The primary mechanism in maintaining cardiac output is tachycardia. Left ventricular end-diastolic pressure (LVEDP) rises dramatically as the ventricle fills with aortic root blood under arterial pressure. The rapid rise in LVEDP has a short-term protective effect by (1) equalizing the aortic diastolic pressure, which acts to limit the amount of diastolic regurgitation, (2) enhancing contraction as a function of increased sarcomere stretch, and (3) causing premature closure of the mitral valve (left ventricular diastolic pressure > left atrial pressure), which prevents transmission of the increased ventricular diastolic back into the pulmonary circulation and therefore delays the development of pulmonary edema. Ultimately, however, the rise in the mean left ventricular diastolic pressure produces left ventricular failure.[26] Although the time to onset of pulmonary edema may be variable, patients with acute severe AR usually require immediate aortic valve replacement as a lifesaving measure.

Natural History

Mild AR causes no symptoms. Patients with moderate to severe AR may remain asymptomatic for many years.

Those with hemodynamically significant AR in the adolescent period commonly remain asymptomatic until the fourth decade.[27] Early symptoms of exertional dyspnea may herald left ventricular dysfunction, however, the development of frank congestive heart failure often takes several more years. Angina pectoris, similar to that of coronary artery disease, is a common complaint in advanced AR. In contrast to the rapid downward trend in AS, in aortic insufficiency there is a 50% chance of death within 10 years of the onset of symptoms (Fig. 120–2).[28]

Physical examination in mild AR reveals a short high-pitched blowing diastolic murmur, while in severe cases a louder decrescendo blow can be heard along the left sternal border. When the regurgitant diastolic jet through the aortic valve hits the anterior leaflet of the mitral valve, it tends to close it, causing the classic Austin Flint murmur heard at the apex.[29] The first heart sound is frequently normal. The second sound may have a diminished aortic component. The presence of a third heart sound may be the first clinical indication of deteriorating ventricular function and at this point, aortic valve replacement should be considered.

The blood pressure reflects the widened pulse pressure and, in severe regurgitation, the so-called Korotkoff sounds may be present all the way to zero.[10] A fascinating constellation of signs related to the widened pulse pressure of severe AR may include (1) Corrigan's or water-hammer pulse, (2) de Musset's sign—bobbing of the head, (3) Quincke's pulse—pulsating nail beds, (4) Duroziez's sign—systolic and diastolic murmurs heard over the femoral arteries, and (5) Traube's sign—pistol shot sounds heard over the large arteries.

In acute AR, a high-pitched decrescendo murmur can be heard. A musical quality to the murmur may indicate torn or prolapsed aortic cusps. The second sound may be paradoxically split. An S3 and S4 are characteristically present. An Austin Flint murmur is often heard. The classic peripheral signs of chronic AR are minimal if not absent. In fact, while the patient may be in extremis, the diagnosis of acute aortic insufficiency on the basis of physical examination may be quite difficult.

In chronic AR the electrocardiogram demonstrates left ventricular hypertrophy. The chest x-ray shows enlargement of the left ventricle downward and to the left. Left atrial enlargement and dilatation of the aortic root may also be seen.

In acute AR, the ECG characteristically features sinus tachycardia. Nonspecific ST-T wave changes may be present, however, signs of LV hypertrophy secondary to acute aortic regurgitation may not become manifest for several days or weeks. The chest film will show normal or slightly increased heart size and may reveal signs of pulmonary edema depending on the severity of the regurgitation.

M-mode and 2-D echocardiography show only indirect evidence of AR and cannot directly quantitate the degree or regurgitation. Color-flow and Doppler echocardiography can document the presence of regurgitation and directly establish the diagnosis; however, at present they cannot accurately quantitate the degree. All of the echo modalities are

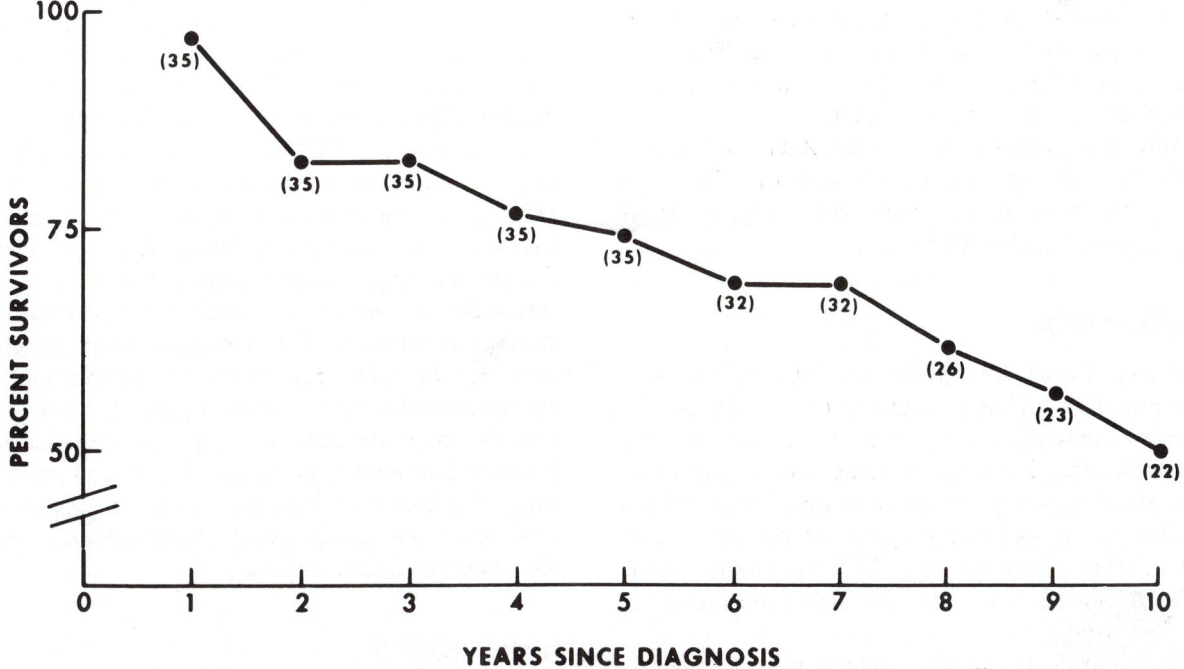

Figure 120–2. Percent survival of patients with aortic insufficiency treated medically. *(From Rapaport E: Natural history of aortic and mitral valve disease. Am J Cardiol 35:221, 1975.)*

helpful in documenting the amount of dilatation and hypertrophy of the ventricle and may delineate the etiology of the regurgitation, e.g., bicuspid valve, dilated aortic root, or a large vegetation or flail leaflet indicative of endocarditis.

The best method of demonstrating the dynamics of the regurgitation and estimating the severity is aortography. A scale of 1+ to 4+ is used:

- 1+: Mild regurgitation with contrast entering but not filling the left ventricle and clearing with each beat.
- 2+: Moderate regurgitation with faint filling of the entire chamber.
- 3+: Moderately severe regurgitation—the left ventricle is well opacified and equal in density with the ascending aorta.
- 4+: Severe regurgitation with complete opacification of the left ventricle (more dense than the aorta) with the first beat.

In addition to aortography, complete right and left heart catheterization should be performed to include determination of filling pressure and cardiac output. Coronary angiography should be performed, especially in the face of angina or a suspected ischemic component to the congestive heart failure and when replacement of the ascending aorta is being considered.

Indications for Surgery

The symptomatic patient with AR should undergo valve surgery. Improvement in symptoms and survival can be anticipated.[30] Depressed LV function is not a contraindication in this group.[31]

The surgical dilemma of chronic AR is the timing of operation in the asymptomatic patient with suspected severe AR based on clinical examination and noninvasive evaluation. At the extreme ends, operating too early exposes the patient to the operative mortality, and long-term morbidity and complications inherent in prosthetic valves; operating too late risks potentially irreversible LV damage. Asymptomatic patients with clinical AR should be divided into two groups, depending on whether there is normal or abnormal LV function.[32] This assessment can be made initially with noninvasive techniques including radionuclide studies and echocardiography. Asymptomatic patients with normal ventricular function should be treated medically until such time as early symptoms or noninvasive evidence of deteriorating LV function develop.[33]

These patients are generally followed at yearly intervals, and more frequently if there is evidence of borderline deterioration in LV function. In a series from the National Institutes of Health (NIH), Bonow et al concluded that if the end-systolic dimension is greater than 55 mm on repeated echo studies, and if the left ventricular fractional shortening, measured by echo, and ejection fraction measured by radionuclide ventriculography, demonstrate systolic dysfunction at rest, the patient should undergo cardiac

catheterization. If the catheterization confirms the presence of severe AR and LV dysfunction, the patient should undergo surgery. A majority of patients in this category, if treated medically, develop symptoms and require surgery within 3 years.[33] Consideration for surgery should be given early to prevent progressive LV dysfunction, rather than necessarily waiting for symptoms to develop in the face of documented LV deterioration.[32]

Patients with severe acute AR and congestive heart failure should be operated on as soon as possible. This includes patients with Marfan's syndrome and acute aortic dissection, as well as a subset of patients with native valve endocarditis who present with severe congestive heart failure.[34] Depending upon the virulence of the causative organism, patients with controlled symptoms and mild-to-moderate regurgitation may begin a 6-week course of antibiotics. A low threshold for surgical intervention should be maintained, however, should symptoms of congestive heart failure progress, or embolization occur. The development of heart block indicates possible abscess formation involving the atrioventricular (A-V) node and ventricular septum, which mandates surgical drainage and valve replacement.

Technical Considerations

With the rare but ever-present possibility of contamination of bank blood by HIV or hepatitis viruses a national trend to use less blood for major surgery has been operative for at least 10 years. At Yale, for example, the average blood usage in 1990 for aortic valve surgery was four units per case while in 1994 it was two units per case. This trend has been aided by the routine use of the Cell Saver for returning operative field, reservoir and oxygenator blood, and by removing a unit of fresh heparinized blood through the aortic cannula prior to cardiopulmonary bypass to be used after heparinization has been reversed. Blood usage will undoubtedly decline further. In a report of 79 patients with aortic valve disease who donated blood for their own use prior to surgery, 68% avoided any, homologous blood donor exposure during their subsequent hospitalization for aortic valve replacement. In contrast, the control group had a 31% change of avoiding homologous blood exposure.[35]

The median sternotomy is always the incision used for replacing the aortic valve or any combination of valves in which the aortic valve is included (Fig. 120–3). When only the aortic valve is being replaced, a single atrial cannula suffices. If the mitral valve is also being replaced, double atrial cannulas are usually safer, as, occasionally, the right atrium is inadvertently entered while opening the left atrium through the intra-atrial groove or by vigorous retraction. In cases of aortoatrial fistulae or suspected annular abscess, double cannulation of the cavae should be performed. Exposure of the valve is facilitated by venting the left ventricle. We prefer placing the vent through the right superior pulmonary vein. The vent can subsequently be used for air evacuation before coming off bypass. Aortic root cannulation

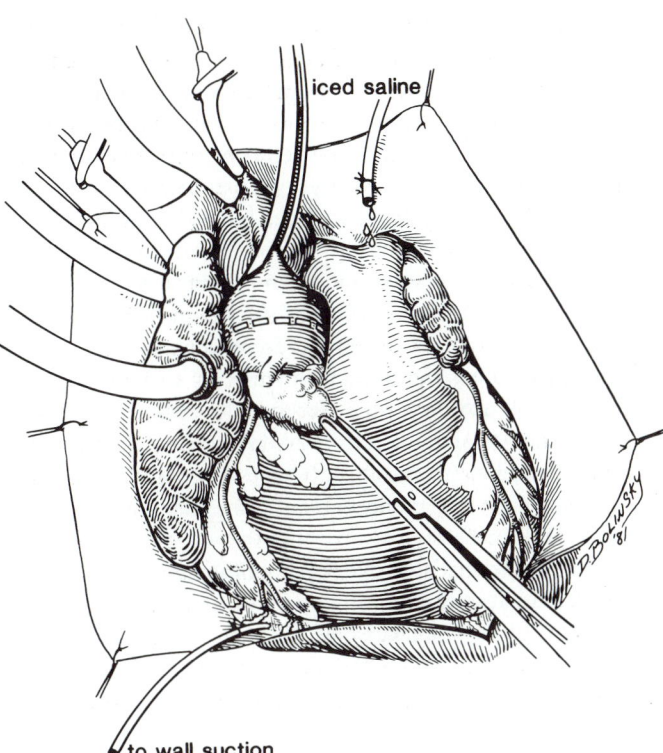

Figure 120–3. Exposure of heart for aortic valve replacement, showing placement of iced saline administration and withdrawal lines and site of aortotomy.

is standard and reduces the incidence of acute aortic dissections occasionally produced by femoral artery cannulation. In the repair of aortic dissection with AR, and in selected reoperations, femoral artery cannulation is employed. In patients with aortic insufficiency, one must be ready to immediately cross-clamp the aorta when going on cardiopulmonary bypass, as the sudden inrush of cold priming solution from the pump may cause ventricular fibrillation and distension of the left ventricle. Myocardial protection should include systemic cooling, cardioplegia, and topical hypothermia. After the patient is cooled to 28°C, the aorta is cross-clamped and in aortic stenosis, the first dose of cardioplegia (10 mL/kg) is given into the aortic root. In AR, depending upon the severity, the first dose of cardioplegia can either be given into the root while the aortic valve is manually closed by external pressure on the root of the aorta or directly into the coronary ostia. The aorta is opened through a transverse incision approximately 1 to 1.5 cm above the right coronary artery. The transverse incision runs parallel to the aortic stress lines. This tends to keep the incision closed after unclamping, as opposed to the vertical incision, which tends to open when the aorta is unclamped. After the aorta is opened, when necessary in AR, the initial dose of cardioplegia is infused directly into the coronary ostia. Cardioplegia is repeated every 20 to 30 min with 250 mL of solution.

There is usually no problem with resection of the purely fibrotic valve. The problems arise with heavy calcification of the valve and associated distortion of annular geometry (Fig. 120–4). The potential problems and pitfalls one must keep in mind during aortic valve replacement are

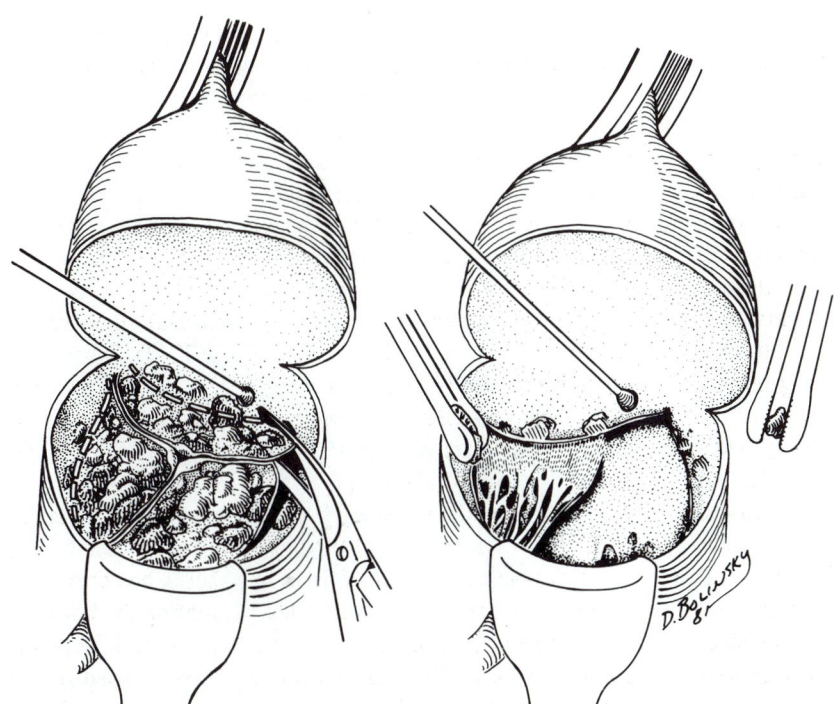

Figure 120–4. Removal of valve and decalcification of annulus. If excessive calcium is left behind, perivalvular leak may result.

(1) inadequate decalcification resulting in perivalvular leaks, (2) too vigorous decalcification resulting in perforations of the aorta of left ventricle and interruption of conduction pathways (Fig. 120–5), (3) detachment of the anterior leaflet of the mitral valve when removing the noncoronary leaflet of the aortic valve (Fig. 120–6), (4) heart block from sutures placed in or around the His bundle, (5) coronary occlusion by the prosthetic valve sewing ring placed at or above the coronary ostia (Fig. 120–7), and (6) detached calcium lodging in the left coronary artery or left ventricle, with subsequent embolization.

After resecting enough valve to permit visualization of the left ventricular chamber, it is good practice to place a sponge in this cavity to enmesh any calcium that may fragment from the annulus during decalcification. A culture stick placed in the left coronary orifice prevents embolization of calcium into this vessel, and the retractor providing exposure of the valve usually blocks the right coronary orifice (Fig. 120–8).

Suture technique using interrupted Teflon-backed mattress sutures of No. 0 Tycron is well suited for valve replacements. This technique has reduced our perivalvular leak rate to less than 1%. Approximately 12 mattress sutures are usually sufficient for providing secure anchorage of the valve (Fig. 120–9). The sutures should be placed through the junction of the leaflet to the aortic wall, i.e., the annulus (Fig. 120–10). There is usually a discrete color change between valvular and aortic wall tissue at this juncture that facilitates identification of the annulus and placement of sutures. Deeper bites can be taken in the area of attachment of the anterior leaflet of the mitral valve, provided the sutures go through mitral valve tissue and not through the aortic wall. In cases of acute annular abscesses from endocarditis, firm anchorage occasionally may be obtained only by placing sutures from outside the aorta. The bundle of His can usually be located by identifying the membranous septum in the area just below the cupola formed by the commissure of the noncoronary and right coronary leaflets. If the sutures are placed in or near the membranous septum but not the muscular septum, heart block can be avoided. The aorta is then closed with two layers of running 4-0 Prolene sutures, with the first layer mattressed and the second layer over and over. This provides a dry closure that rarely requires additional suturing for leaks. After the aorta has been unclamped, air evacuation procedures are immediately carried out while the heart is still fibrillating. These consist of (1) placing the patient in the Trendelenburg position before unclamping the aorta, allowing air to collect in the proximal ascending aorta rather than the carotid arteries; (2) puncturing the anterior surface of the ascending aorta with a No. 20 needle; (3) turning off the ventricular (LV) drain, disconnecting the pump tubing from the drain cannula, squeezing the heart, and inverting the left atrial appendage while the anesthetist is overinflating the patient's lung: this is carried out until blood freely egresses from the LV cannula; (4) tilting the heart out of the pericardial cavity, and venting the apex with a No. 18 needle while squeezing the heart and inflating the lungs; and (5) defibrillating the heart and, with the apex still everted, allowing the beating heart to pump air out through the apical venting needle. Venting through the aortic root needle continues until the patient is off bypass.

The choice of valve prosthesis is discussed in Chapter 122.

RESULTS

Operative mortality for isolated aortic valve replacement is less than 5%. Factors that have been implicated in contributing to mortality include age, preoperative functional classes New York Heart Association (NYHA) III–IV,

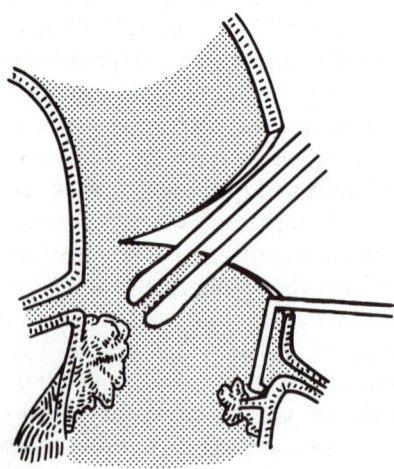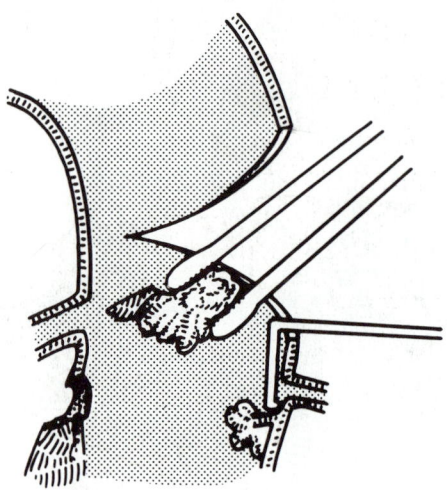

Figure 120–5. Complication from decalcification. Decalcification of aortic annulus must be conducted carefully, since vigorous decalcification can result in perforation.

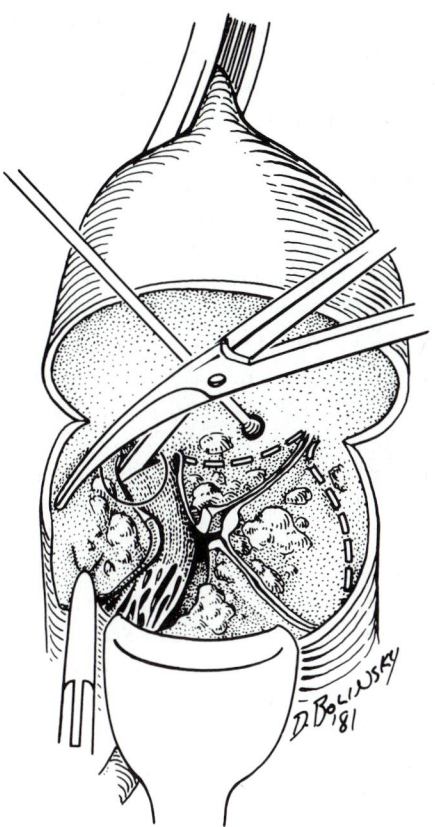

Figure 120–6. Distortion of valve annulus with loss of landmarks by heavy calcification can result in accidental detachment of anterior leaflet of mitral valve when removing noncoronary leaflet.

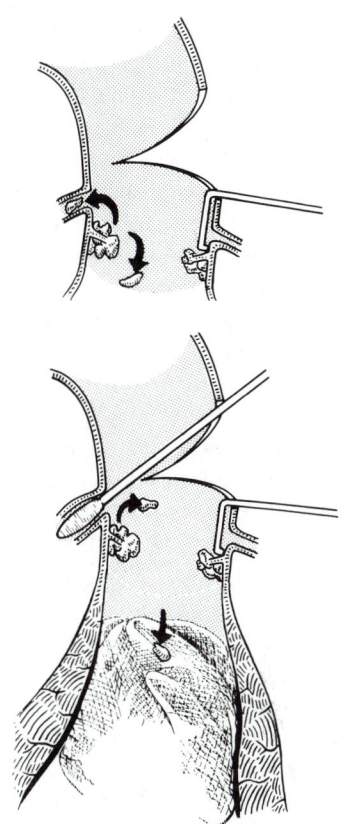

Figure 120–8. Further complications from decalcification. Calcium can lodge in coronary ostia or ventricular chamber, with subsequent embolization. This can be prevented by placing a culture stick (or coronary perfusion cannula) in left coronary orifice and sponge in left ventricle during decalcification. Retractor covers right coronary orifice.

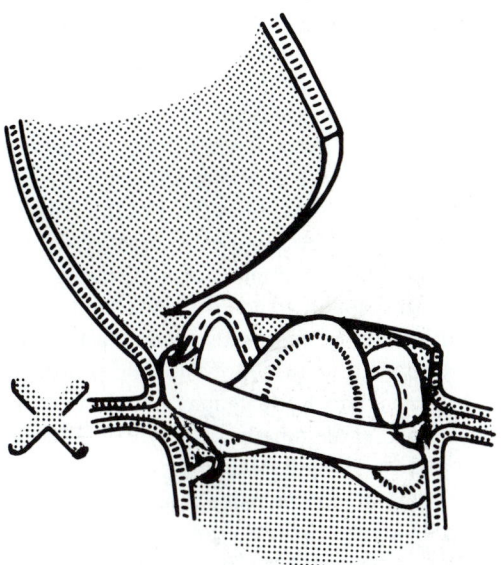

Figure 120–7. Occlusion of coronary ostia can result when attempting to implant an oversized valve or by not observing relationship of sewing ring to coronary ostia when tying sutures.

impaired LV function, and coexisting coronary artery disease. Consistently low mortality has been achieved by recognition of coronary disease and revascularization when indicated, improvements in myocardial protection, and earlier identification of LV deterioration using noninvasive testing.[36–39] The probability of long-term survival is approximately 80 to 90% at 5 years.[40] Patients with aortic stenosis generally have a better prognosis than those with aortic insufficiency, particularly in the face of reduced ventricular function. In a series of patients with aortic regurgitation, Bonow reported a mean 5-year survival of 63% for patients with depressed ejection fraction versus 96% for patients with normal ejection fraction.[41] Therefore, with a diagnosis of aortic insufficiency, it is imperative to operate upon the patient before ventricular function deteriorates.

With the advent of porcine and other tissue valves with their high rate of structural degeneration and the low but ever present incidence of endocarditis, perivalvular leak, valve thrombosis, and thromboembolism, common to all valves, the possibility of valve rereplacement must be considered when discussing with the patient the indications for initial valve replacement. There is an 8 to 17% chance of the need for future rereplacement[42,43] and the risk of

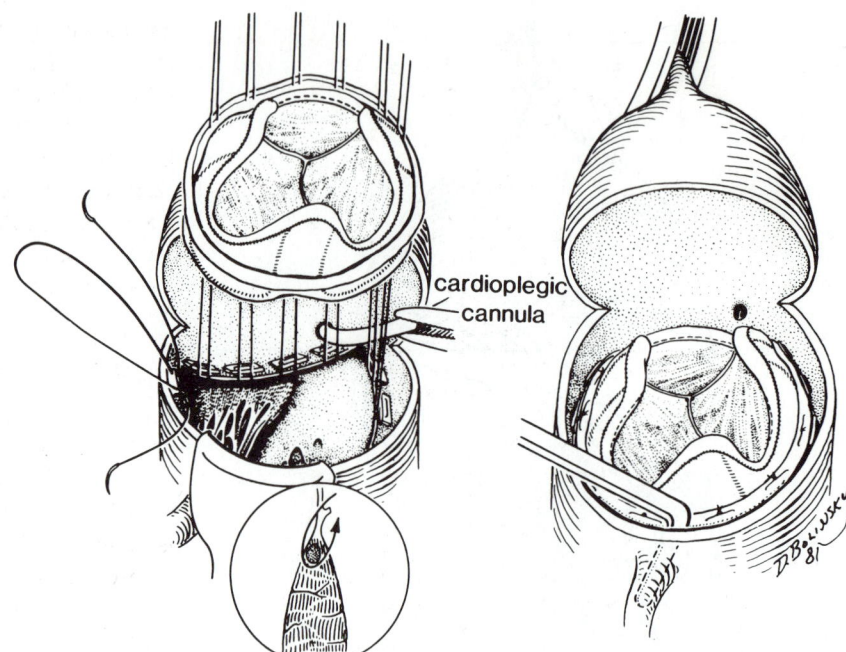

Figure 120–9. Insertion of Teflon-backed mattress sutures in annulus. Inset. Location of His bundle in upper part of muscular septum. Deep sutures placed in this area can interrupt the atrioventricular conduction pathway. Sutures should be placed no deeper than the membranous septum. After sutures have been tied, seating of sewing ring below right coronary orifice is checked with right angle clamp. Left coronary orifice can be visualized.

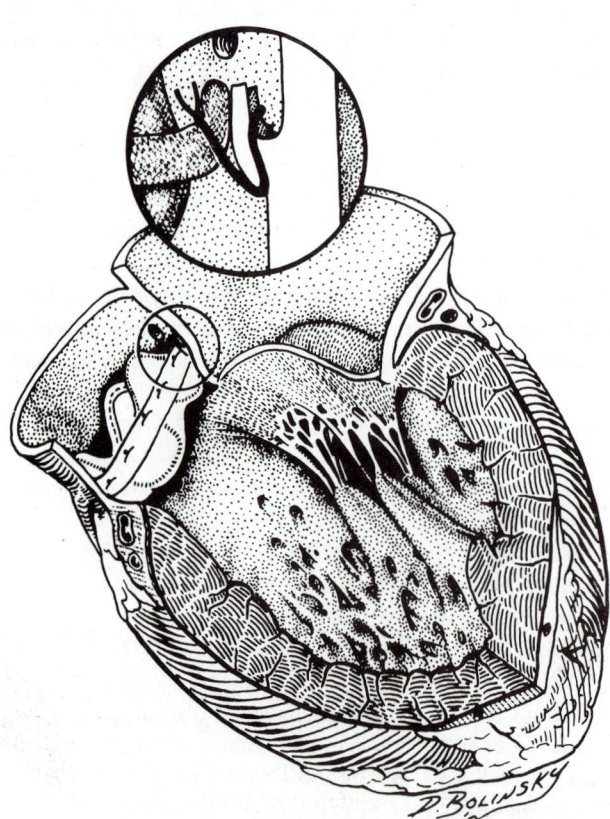

Figure 120–10. Valve in place, showing anchorage with Teflon-backed mattress sutures.

rereplacement is approximately twice the risk of the first operation. That is, the risk for rereplacement is approximately 10%.[43]

It is not for this chapter to address the impact of an aging population on the health care delivery system in the United States. Nevertheless, it should be pointed out that for patients with AS or AR and satisfactory ventricular contractions in the 77- to 83-year-old age range the operative mortality is 5% or less.[44,45]

The Small Aortic Annulus

Occasionally, the surgeon is faced with the dilemma of the small aortic annulus in which placement of a prosthetic device in the usual fashion will leave the patient with an unacceptable postoperative gradient. Porcine valves less than 21 mm should be avoided. In occasional patients, pericardial xenograft valves at the 19-mm size can be used. Of the mechanical valves, the St. Jude valve has the greatest effective orifice to annular ratio in the 19-mm size.[46] Ideally the need for an alternative technique of valve replacement due to a small aortic annulus should be made preoperatively. This would include patients with a hypoplastic aortic root, extensive subaortic stenosis, or a stenotic prosthetic valve already in place. Other patients may not be identified until the valve is sized at the time of surgery. It is unusual not to be able to place a 19-mm valve, although it may occasionally be necessary to seat the valve at an angle to the plain of the annulus. In other words, the sutures are placed in the annulus in the usual way but the valve is lowered into place so that the sewing ring is below the right and left coronary arteries but angled into the noncoronary sinus. The left and right coronary annular sutures are tied first thereby abutting

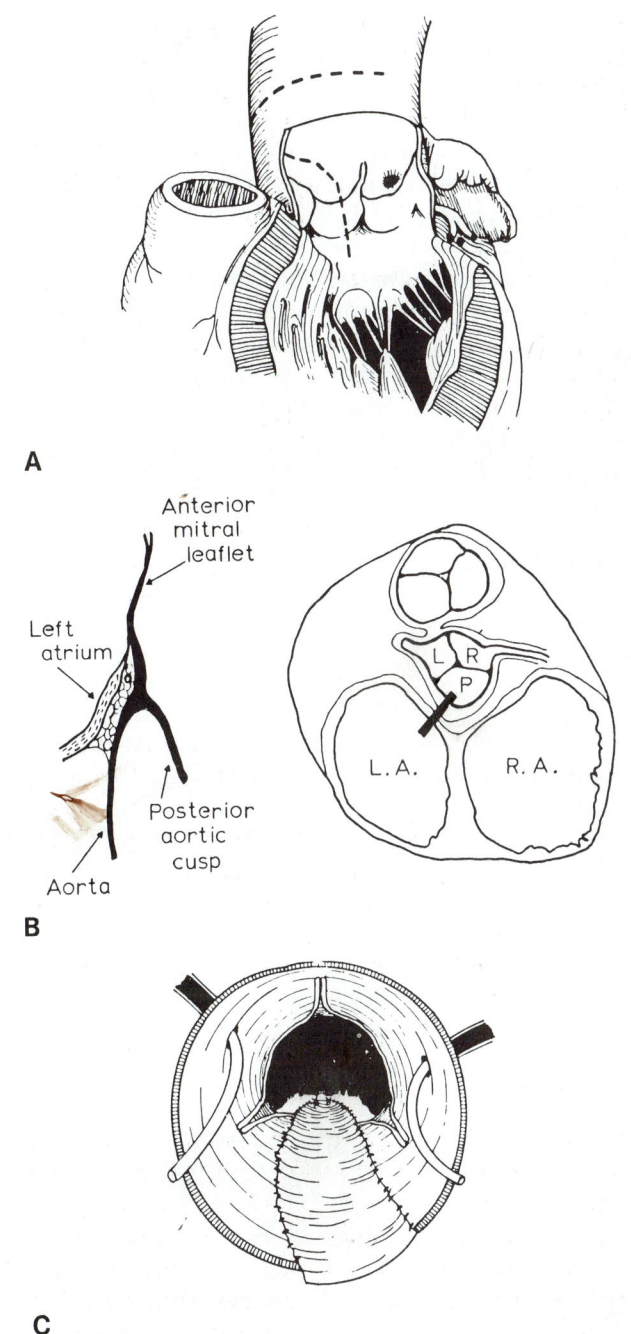

A

Anterior
mitral
leaflet

Left
atrium

Posterior
aortic
cusp

Aorta

B

L R
P

L.A.   R.A.

C

the sewing ring to the annulus below the coronary ostia. The noncoronary sutures are tied last, which then allows the valve to ride above the annulus in this portion of the aorta.

Annulus enlargement procedures should be reserved for those rare cases that will not accept a 19-mm valve. Techniques for dealing with the small aortic annulus include annular enlargement, either from an anterior or posterior approach, and ectopic placement of the valve as an apical aortic conduit.

Annular Enlargement

In many instances, enlarging the annulus 2 to 3 mm will be sufficient. This can be accomplished with little increase in morbidity with a posterior annular split through the midportion of the noncoronary cusp.[47,48] After initial sizing of the valve reveals that the natural annulus is too small, the aortotomy is extended through the annulus in the midportion of the noncoronary cusp, until an acceptable diameter valve sizer can be passed (Fig. 120–11). The split is patched with a broad-based Dacron patch through which the valve sutures in this area are passed. The remainder of the patch is incorporated in the aortotomy closure, which serves to widen the supravalvular region as well.[49]

When it is apparent that a more generous enlargement is needed, a more extensive posterior split can be made at the commissure between the left and the noncoronary cusp and carried down into the mitral apparatus as described by Manouguian and Seybold-Epting.[50] The incision is extended through the annulus and the intervalvular trigon into the center of the anterior leaflet of the mitral valve. Care must be taken to make the incision precisely in the midportion of the leaflet and to leave the free edge intact. The left atrium, which is entered at its attachment with the aortic root, can be opened further to facilitate exposure. A diamond-shaped Dacron patch can then be used to reconstruct the V-shaped defect in the anterior mitral leaflet. A larger valve can then be seated using the Dacron patch as part of the annulus. The superior portion of the patch is then incor-

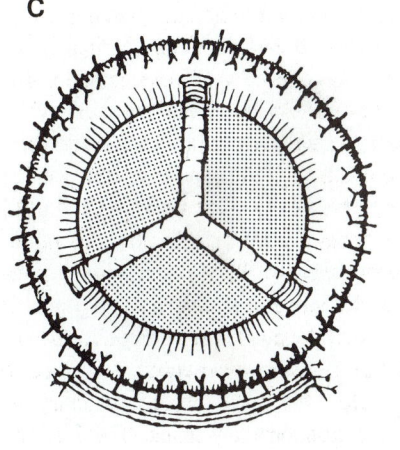

D

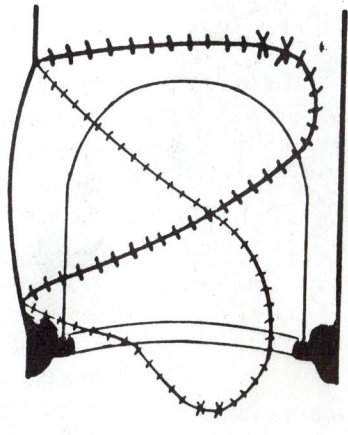

E

Figure 120–11. A. The incision. **B.** Anatomical section of aortic root through posterior sinus of Valsalva and origins of aortic and mitral valves (from above and as the surgeon approaches it). **C.** The patch in position. **D.** The valve firmly tied down. The arc attached to the patch is posterior. **E.** The lie of the patch is shown by the suture lines behind and in front. The valve attachment to the aortic ring and the cage within the aorta are sketched in.

porated into the aortotomy closure. The roof of the left atrium can then be closed with mattress sutures secured to the Dacron patch and sewing ring of the new valve (Fig. 120–12). Neither the conduction system nor the coronary arteries should be at risk with this maneuver. Concerns about mitral regurgitation secondary to distortion of the anterior leaflet have not proven to be significant. Using this technique, the annular circumference can be enlarged from 10 to 25 mm.

A mean 8.5 year follow-up of 15 patients undergoing annular enlargement by the Manouguian procedure was published in 1992.[51] The actuarial survival at 10 years was 62% and seven reoperative procedures were performed. These data indicate that the morbidity and mortality of enlargement procedures are not insignificant and should not be performed unless it is absolutely certain that the aorta will not accepts a 19-mm valve.

Enlargement of the aortic annulus from the anterior

approach, the Konno–Raastan procedure, involves a more complex reconstruction of the aortic outflow tract, the ventricular septum, and the right ventricular outflow tract.[52,53] A vertical anterior aortotomy is made and extended inferiorly through the annulus 4 to 5 mm to the left of the ostium of the right coronary artery, and then down into the interventricular septum. The pulmonary outflow tract is similarly opened along the same line of orientation, connecting with the aortotomy. The annulus, septal defect, and aortotomy can then be reconstructed with a diamond-shaped Dacron patch (Fig. 120–13) to which the prosthetic valve can be fixed. The right ventricular outflow tract in enlarged with a second patch. This technique can effect up to a 50% increase in the diameter of the annulus; however, it clearly represents a more formidable surgical challenge and is associated with a higher morbidity and mortality than the posterior annular approach. It is particularly useful in children with hypoplastic aortic roots, or in patients in whom previ-

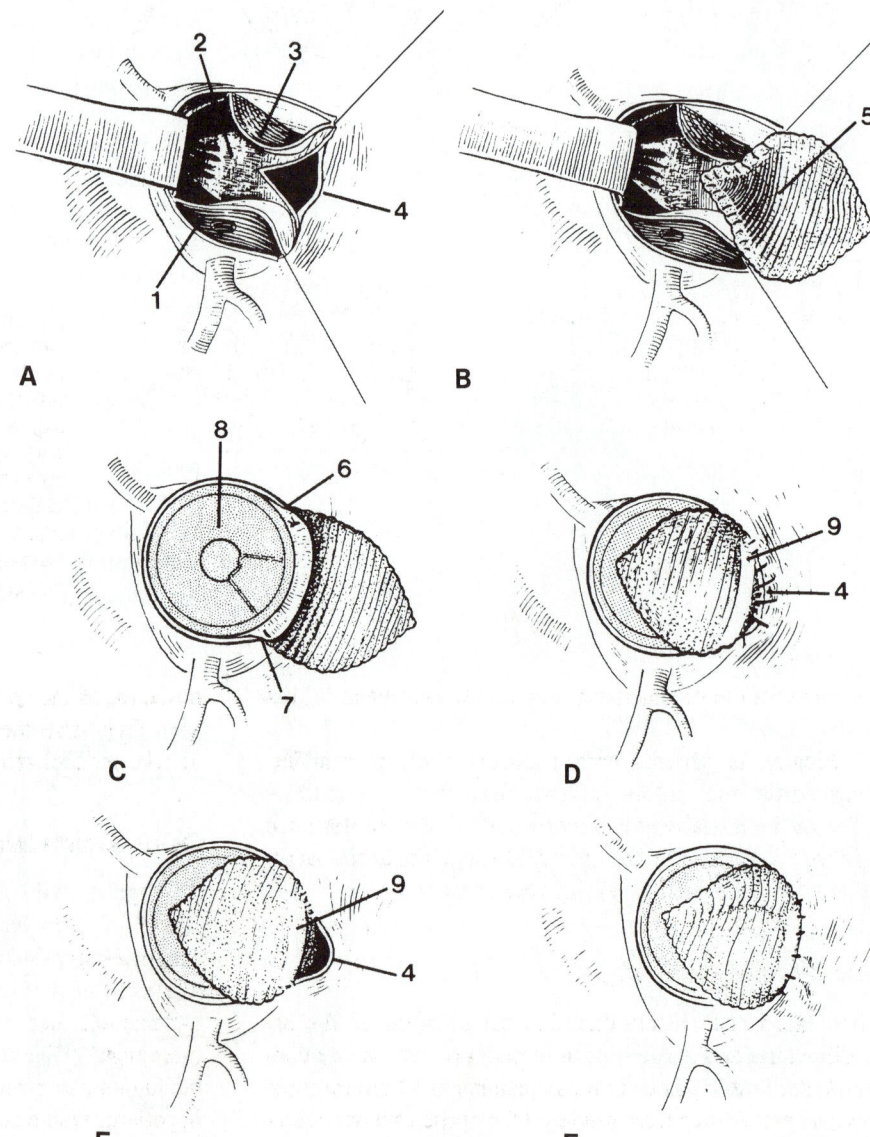

Figure 120–12. Operative technique. 1, Left semilunar cusp. 2, Anterior mitral leaflet. 3, Noncoronary semilunar cups. 4, Left atrial wall. 5, Patch. 6–7, Enlargement of the aortic valve ring. 8, Aortic valve prosthesis. 9, Sewing ring of the prosthesis. **A.** Aortotomy incision is carried down into the aortic leaflet of the mitral valve and free wall of the left atrium. **B.** Cleft in the aortic leaflet of the mitral valve is reconstructed with patch. **C.** Valve is sewn to aortic annulus and Dacron patch in area of noncoronary sinus. **D, E, F.** Free wall of left atrium is approximated to patch and sewing ring of valve.

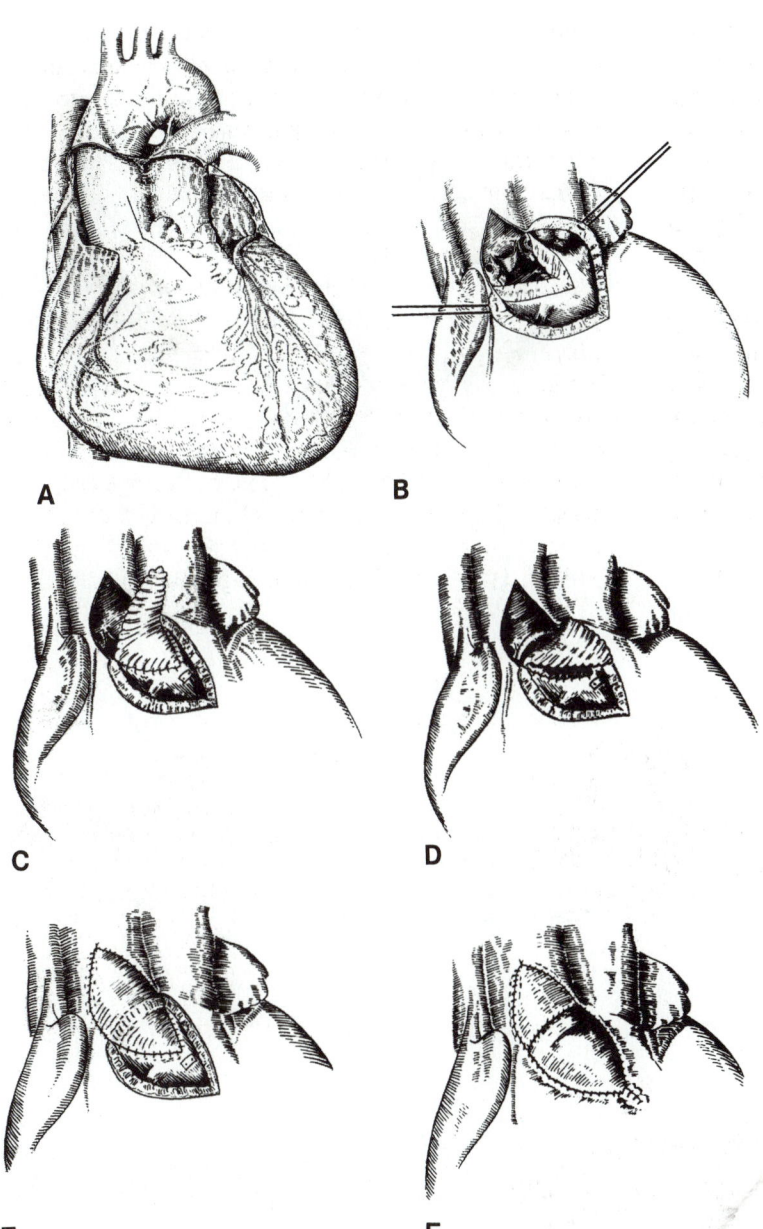

Figure 120–13. Operative technique of aorto-ventriculoplasty. **A.** Direction of incision on the aorta and right ventricular outflow tract. **B.** Opening of the aorta, right ventricle and interventricular septum. **C.** Widening of the subaortic area and the aortic ring by patching of the septal incision. **D.** Excision and replacement of the aortic valve. **E.** Closure of the aortic incision by the remainder of the same patch. **F.** Closure of the right ventricular outflow tract incision by a second Dacron patch which is sutured to the inner patch over the aorta.

ous conservative enlargement procedures have been unsuccessful.

Finally, in patients with a narrow aortic root undergoing aortic and mitral valve replacement, the anterior leaflet of the mitral valve, if not calcified, can be detached from its chordae, reflected upward through the aortic annulus and used as a patch to enlarge the aorta.[54]

Apical-Aortic Conduit

When faced with insurmountable calcification of the ascending aorta and aortic root or in patients with severe congenital aortic stenosis or in those patients in whom multiple previous procedures have rendered the aortic root and annulus unapproachable, a valved conduit can be placed from the apex of the left ventricle to the abdominal aorta.[55,56] This technique creates a double-outlet left ventricle and thereby reduces the LV outflow tract obstruction.

Other Alternatives

Homografts will be discussed in Chapter 121, but techniques of aortic valvuloplasty may also be considered in special circumstances. Mechanical debridement and decalcification of the valve leaflets have been used in selected patients not considered to be good candidates for valve replacement.[57] The technique may be of particular benefit in the higher risk group of patients with small aortic roots and in patients with a contraindication to anticoagulation.[58]

The St. Louis University group[59] reported ultrasonic

aortic decalcification procedures on 22 elderly patients. They were able to reduce the peak aortic gradient from 74 ± 34 mm Hg preoperatively to 20 ± 13 mm Hg postoperatively. However, there were two operative deaths and three late deaths and when aortic insufficiency was present, it was exacerbated by the procedure. Nevertheless, as experience in this area grows, the procedure may gain more generalized acceptance.

Aortic valve sparing operations for aortic insufficiency secondary to annuloaortic ectasia may also hold promise. In this operation the ectatic aorta is resected, the valve is left in place along with immediately adjacent scalloped aortic tissue and buttons of aorta with the coronary orifices. The valve is then sewn inside the Dacron graft, rather than to it, thereby releasing all subsequent pressure on the preserved aortic tissue. The coronary arteries are then reimplanted into the prosthetic graft (see Fig. 120–14, 120–15, 120–16, and 120–17). There have been two series[60,61] reporting the use of this procedure, or a modification of it, in a total of 20 patients with one death and two patients requiring subsequent aortic valve replacement for aortic insufficiency.

Percutaneous balloon valvuloplasty in aortic stenosis may be considered in patients with severe AS who are not candidates for surgery[62] or as a temporizing procedure to stabilize a patient for subsequent aortic valve replacement. The procedure, however, is still considered experimental and has not gained wide acceptance.

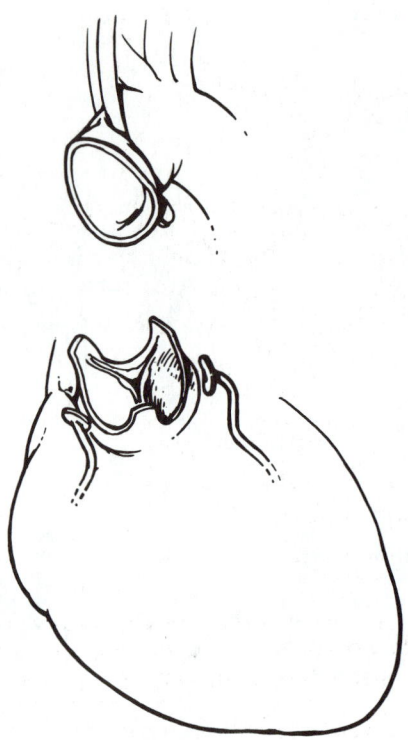

Figure 120–15. The aortic valve and a small portion of arterial wall are left attached to the left ventricular outflow tract. *(From David TE, Feindel CM: An aortic valve-sparing operation for patients with aortic incompetence and aneurysm of the ascending aorta. J Thorac Cardiovasc Surg 103:619, 1992.)*

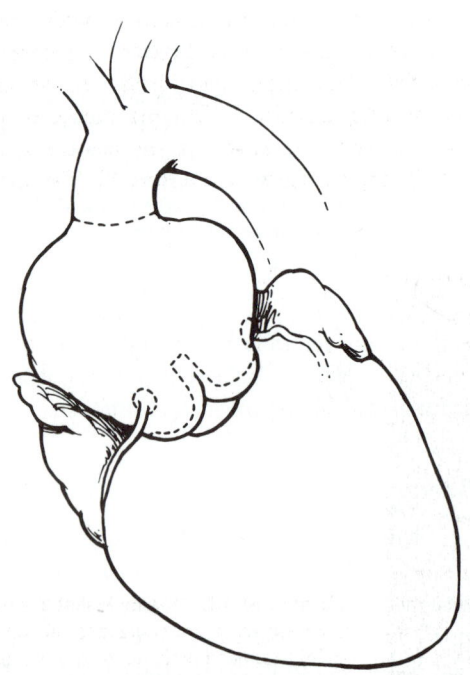

Figure 120–14. The dotted lines indicate the resection levels of the arterial wall. *(From David TE, Feindel CM: An aortic valve-sparing operation for patients with aortic incompetence and aneurysm of the ascending aorta. J Thorac Cardiovasc Surg 103:619, 1992.)*

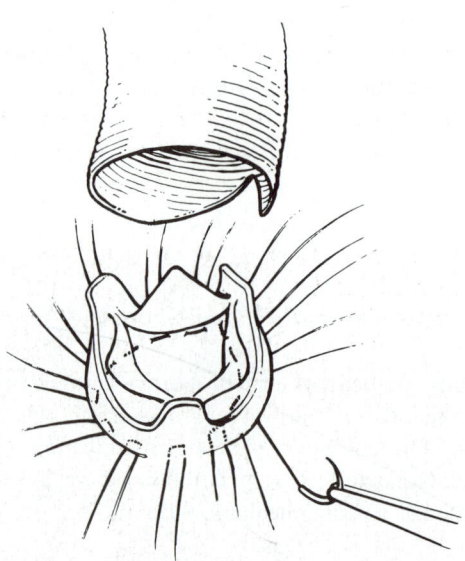

Figure 120–16. Multiple horizontal mattress sutures are passed from inside to outside the left ventricular outflow tract, immediately below the aortic valve on the left side and through a single horizontal plane on the right side. *(From David TE, Feindel CM: An aortic valve-sparing operation for patients with aortic incompetence and aneurysm of the ascending aorta. J Thorac Cardiovasc Surg 103:619, 1992.)*

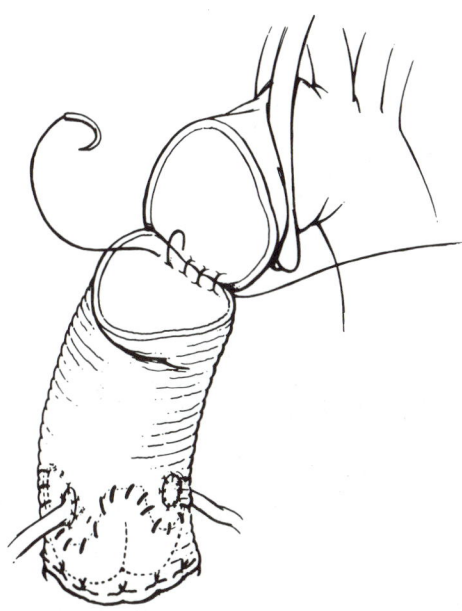

Figure 120–17. The aortic valve is reimplanted into the Dacron graft. It is secured at two levels: below the leaflets by the horizontal mattress sutures and above the leaflets by suturing the remnants of arterial wall to the Dacron graft. The coronary arteries are also reimplanted. *(From David TE, Feindel CM: An aortic valve-sparing operation for patients with aortic incompetence and aneurysm of the ascending aorta. J Thorac Cardiovasc Surg 103:620, 1992.)*

IDIOPATHIC HYPERTROPHIC SUBAORTIC STENOSIS

Idiopathic hypertrophic subaortic stenosis (IHSS) is a part of the spectrum of hypertrophic cardiomyopathies that includes idiopathic concentric hypertrophy. However, concentric hypertrophy is not a surgical disease and will not be considered in this chapter. IHSS is a primary disease of the myocardium in which anatomic and functional obstruction of the left ventricular outflow tract contributes to a clinical picture similar to that of aortic stenosis. IHSS has been demonstrated in a number of patients to be familial with an autosomal-dominant pattern, while in others no genetic link is evident.[63,64] Noninvasive screening of other family members with echocardiography is recommended.

The gross anatomic features usually include asymmetric left ventricular hypertrophy with marked thickening in the mid- and upper parts of the ventricular septum, however, variations in the pattern can be seen such as concentric, apical, or free-wall hypertrophy. The left atrium is usually dilated, the left ventricular cavity is small and nondilated, and the mitral valve is often abnormal. The upper septum may have a characteristic plaque representing fibroelastosis resulting from contact with the anterior leaflet of the mitral valve during systole.[65] As shown in Figure 120–18, the anterior leaflet of the mitral valve also may show an area of abrasion resulting from abutment against the septum. Histologically, the affected myocardium is characterized by a bizarre, whorling configuration of hypertrophied myofibrils and interstitial connective tissue best described as myocardial disarray.[66,67] The intramural coronary arteries may be thickened and show a decrease in luminal diameter.

Pathophysiology

Abnormal cardiac dynamics in IHSS center around the complex triad of a decrease in ventricular compliance in diastole, a hypercontractile left ventricle in systole, and the presence of an intraventricular outflow gradient. The decrease in diastolic compliance is associated with a prolongation of isovolemic relaxation in diastole, an increased reliance on atrial contraction, and decreased ventricular filling. The resulting abnormal diastolic pressure–volume curve shows the rate of rise in ventricular pressure to be disproportionately high relative to volume.[68] The diastolic

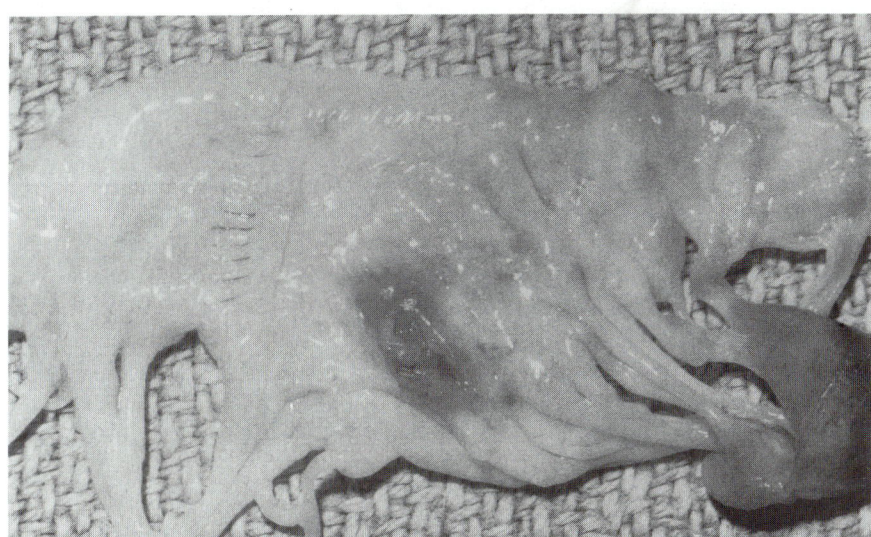

Figure 120–18. Anterior leaflet of a mitral valve removed from a patient with severe IHSS. Abrasion of the surface of the valve resulted from abutment against the hypertroph. *(From Cooley DA: Surgical techniques for hypertrophic left ventricular obstructive myopathy including mitral valve plication. J Card Surg 6:32, 1991.)*

dysfunction may result in a reduction in coronary blood flow, which may be partly responsible for producing angina.[69] During systole the ventricle ejects at an increased rate and often has an increased ejection fraction. The small ventricular chamber, already compromised in its ability to achieve maximal end-diastolic volume, is rapidly evacuated with near-apposition of the chamber walls.

Both the mechanism and the significance of the outflow gradient in IHSS are now well understood.[70] Unlike AS in which the gradient is at the level of the valve, in IHSS a gradient can be demonstrated between the left ventricular cavity and the left ventricular outflow tract (subaortic or intraventricular).[71] The outflow tract gradient in IHSS can be very fickle. It is not present in all patients, and in any given individual the gradient may be difficult to reproduce, depending on multiple factors. Decreasing preload, decreasing afterload, or increasing contractility will increase the gradient. This can be demonstrated in the cardiac catheterization laboratory with a Valsalva maneuver, the use of amyl nitrate or isoproteronol, or following a premature ventricular beat. The mechanism of actual obstruction to the outflow gradient appears to be a spectrum in which both bulging of the enlarged septum and systolic anterior motion of the mitral valve contribute.[72]

To date, the most lucid analysis and description of the pathophysiology of IHSS has been made by the cardiology and cardiovascular surgery divisions at the University of Toronto.[70] These observations were made by transesophageal Doppler echocardiography of IHSS patients and normal controls. The anterior mitral leaflet was approximately 1 cm longer and the posterior leaflet 0.5 mm longer in the IHSS patients. The coaptation point in the IHSS patients was approximately 1 cm from the anterior leaflet tip but only 3 mm from the tip in normal controls. Therefore, approximately 7 mm of extra anterior leaflet is free to abut against the hypertrophied septum during systole. Systolic anterior motion starts during early systole with the distal third to half of the anterior mitral leaflet angling sharply anteriorly and superiorly resulting in leaflet-septal contact and incomplete mitral leaflet coaptation in mid-systole. This causes the formation of a funnel composed of the distal parts of both leaflets that allows a jet of posteriorly directed mitral regurgitation to occur. As described by the Toronto group the sequence of events in systole is eject–obstruct–leak.

Clinical Picture

Although symptoms may develop at any age, patients commonly present in the second or third decade of life. The male/female ratio is approximately 2:1. The majority of patients who become symptomatic will have dyspnea and angina. A smaller number have syncope or presyncope. As in aortic stenosis with ventricular hypertrophy, angina may result from a combination of increased oxygen demand secondary to increased muscle mass or increased workload and decreased supply possibly secondary to decreased coronary flow, abnormal intramyocardial vessels, and compression of the intramyocardial vasculature during systole.[73] The cause of syncope is unknown but in most instances probably represents either an atrial or ventricular arrhythmia.[74] Certainly the greatest fear in IHSS is sudden death, which may be the initial presentation of the condition, and accounts for over 50% of all the deaths in this population.[75] The annual mortality from sudden death has been reported as 2 to 3% with young males with familial disease at highest risk.[76,77] As in syncope the etiology of the sudden death episodes is most likely an arrhythmia. The induction of both ventricular and supraventricular tachyarrhythmias has been reported during electrophysiologic studies in a number of survivors of sudden death or in patients with syncope.[78]

The usual physical findings in IHSS include a normal S1, a physiologically split S2, and an S4 and occasionally an S3 gallop. The S4 of atrial contraction may be palpable as a bifid apical impulse. A nonradiating systolic crescendo–decrescendo murmur is usually heard along the left sternal border. While there is little direct correlation between the quality of the murmur and the magnitude of the gradient, various maneuvers at the bedside will alter the murmur just as they will alter the gradient when applied in the cardiac catheterization laboratory. Decreasing preload with a Valsalva, or by standing up will increase the murmur while increasing filling by squatting will decrease the murmur. These maneuvers are particularly helpful in differentiating IHSS from aortic stenosis. A systolic thrill may also be palpable. A fascinating finding is the bifid carotid pulse (pulsus bisiferiens), which, as opposed to the slow upstroke of AS, has a rapid upstroke, a midsystolic drop, and finally a slower rise at the end of systole.

Both the chest x-ray and ECG usually show left ventricular hypertrophy. Holter monitor recordings frequently show premature ventricular contraction (PVCs), and may demonstrate either nonsustained ventricular or supraventricular tachycardias.[79]

Management

The goals of any therapy in IHSS are relief of symptoms and prevention of sudden death. Symptomatic improvement can be achieved medically in the majority of patients. Unfortunately there is no conclusive evidence that either medicine or surgery significantly impacts on the incidence of sudden death. Management of asymptomatic patients is controversial. Drug therapy may be indicated in a selected population of asymptomatic high-risk younger patients with either a family history of sudden death, marked hypertrophy of the ventricle or marked obstruction.[80] Endocarditis prophylaxis is routinely indicated because of an increased risk of bacterial endocarditis.

Symptomatic patients are treated primarily with β-blockers, calcium channel blockers, and disopyramide in high doses. β-blockers such as Inderal act to decrease myocardial oxygen demand by decreasing heart rate and contractility, especially in the face of sympathetic stimulation, and thereby decrease outflow obstruction.[81] Verapamil, the most extensively studied of the calcium channel blockers, has been shown to improve symptoms even in patients who have failed β-blockade. Verapamil appears to act by decreasing contractility, decreasing heart rate, and increasing diastolic relaxation, thereby improving diastolic filling.[82,83] Ventricular and supraventricular arrhythmias are prevented or controlled with disopyramide.[84]

Indications for Surgery

As in most other acquired cardiac surgical diseases the decision to operate is based on failure of medical management. This is true of IHSS and all patients, before being considered for myomectomy or mitral valve replacement, should have failed treatment with β-blockers, verapamil, and disopyramide. DDD pacing is also being used experimentally. The surgical management of IHSS has been the subject of significant and at times bitter controversy. The primary mode of treatment described by Morrow et al at the NIH has been relief of obstruction by left ventricular myotomy and myomectomy. An alternative approach popularized by Cooley is relief of obstruction by eliminating systolic anterior motion of the native mitral valve by replacing it with a low profile prosthetic valve.[85] The obstructive lesions that provide the rationale for both operations is represented in the schematic diagram in Figure 120–19.

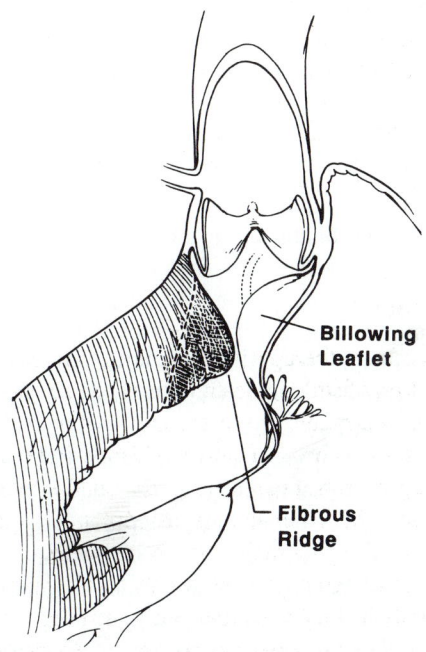

Figure 120–19. Schematic diagram showing mechanism of left ventricular outflow tract obstruction in IHSS. *(From Cooley DA: Surgical techniques for hypertrophic left ventricular obstructive myopathy including mitral valve plication. J Card Surg 6:30, 1991.)*

McIntosh et al at the NIH have reported their experience, which reinforces the idea that both myomectomy and mitral valve replacement may have specific roles in the treatment of IHSS and that proper patient selection is essential.[86,87] Indications for surgical intervention outlined by McIntosh include

1. patients in New York Heart Association (NYHA) class III or IV who have failed medical management and have resting and provocable gradients. The emphasis should remain on the degree of symptoms.
2. patients who have survived sudden death episodes and have significant (>50 mm Hg) resting or provocable gradients.

Judgment must be exercised in considering patients without a resting gradient and in those with chronic atrial fibrillation or unreconstructible coronary artery disease. Contraindications to surgery include primary patients previously known to have normal ventricular function who now have evidence of significant left ventricular dysfunction with reduced ejection fraction and only a mild gradient.[87] In most centers, left ventricular myotomy and myomectomy remains the procedure of choice for IHSS. A further contraindication is the presence of concentric hypertrophy.

McIntosh has attempted to resolve a portion of the controversy by suggesting specific guidelines for selecting patients for mitral valve replacement over LV myotomy and myomectomy.[86] These include

1. intraventricular septum dimension < 18 mm in the area of resection.
2. atypical septal morphology in which the hypertrophied region lies outside of the field of the standard myotomy and myomectomy.
3. persistent symptoms and obstruction following an adequate myomectomy.
4. patients with IHSS and severe mitral regurgitation secondary to organic mitral disease.

Pulmonary hypertension and mitral regurgitation in the absence of the above criteria are not an indication for mitral valve replacement and these patients should be treated with myomectomy alone.[88] Essential to these criteria is the use of both preoperative echocardiography and intraoperative echocardiography to clearly visualize septal anatomy in the area to be resected.

The theoretical rationale behind DDD pacemaker insertion is to address two fundamental properties of IHSS. Since diastolic dysfunction and abnormalities of relaxation cause a low volume, rapid rise in ventricular pressure during early systole a cracking of the whip effect is produced on the abnormally lengthened anterior leaflet of the mitral valve that contributes to systolic anterior motion. The effect of pacing is to prolong the rate of ventricular relaxation.[89] The second mechanism is to induce paradoxical movement of the ventricular septum by initiating contraction at the apex of the right ventricle and right side of the septum before septal contraction is initiated uniformly through the His bundle.[90] Excitation initiated through this pathway causes the septum to move away from the left ventricular wall during systole, thereby increasing left ventricular outflow tract dimensions, which reduces left ventricular outflow tract velocities and hence Venturi forces pulling the anterior leaflet of the mitral valve toward the ventricular septum.

Technique

The technique of left ventricular myotomy and myomectomy was pioneered by Morrow at the NIH.[91,92] Our current technique includes median sternotomy, standard aortic cannulation, and a double caval cannulation through the right atrium. Left ventricular venting is accomplished through the right superior pulmonary vein. Myocardial protection is provided with systemic cooling to 28°C, topical cooling, and crystalloid cardioplegia given initially into the aortic root, followed by direct coronary infusion at 20-min intervals. When performing the resection of interventricular septum several pitfalls must be kept in mind at all times to prevent technical errors; (1) the aortic valve, particularly the right coronary leaflet, can be damaged by excessive retraction or by the scalpel blade during myomectomy; (2) the mitral valve and chordae tendinae can be damaged if not retracted; (3) the A-V node and the membranous portion of the septum can be injured if the resection is started too far to the right, under the commissure between the right and the noncoronary cusps; and (4) a ventricular septal defect (VSD) can be created if too much septum is resected or if the area of septal hypertrophy is misjudged.

The aorta is opened through a transverse incision approximately 1 cm above the right coronary artery. The aortic valve is inspected. The extent of septal hypertrophy, previously visualized via echocardiography, is further examined by bimanual palpation with the left index finger inserted through the aortic annulus into the left ventricle and the left thumb or right index finger over the exterior surface of the heart in the area of the left anterior descending coronary artery. The right coronary cusp is retracted anteriorly and slightly to the patient's left, and at the same time a sponge stick is used to apply counterpressure on the anterior surface of the heart (Fig. 120–20B). This allows visualization of the septum. In some patients the characteristic plaque identifying maximal contact between the bulging septum and the anterior leaflet of the mitral valve can be clearly seen. This plaque when present, or the portion of septum identified by echocardiography as the maximum point of contact in patients without plaque, should be the area of maximal resection.

A specially designed lighted ribbon retractor, if available, or standard ribbon retractor is inserted through the annulus taking care to retract but not damage the mitral valve. The first incision is then made into the septum just to the right of the center of the right coronary cusp, using an an-

gled No. 10 blade (Fig. 120–20C,D). Alternatively, the CO_2 laser has been used for resection.[93] The incision is started 5 to 10 mm below the aortic annulus and extends 4 cm toward the apex. A second parallel myotomy is then made 10 to 12 mm to the left of the first, under the commissure between the right and the left coronary cusps (Fig. 120–20E). The final transverse myotomy is then made connecting the two linear myotomies and the portion of septum is removed. Care must be taken to stay in the same plane and at the same depth to avoid making the distal portion of the resection too shallow. Ideally, half of the thickness of the septum at the point of maximal contact is resected (Fig. 120–20F,G,H). Additional trimming of the septum can be individualized depending on the particular configuration of the septal hypertrophy. The LV cavity is then copiously irrigated and the aortotomy closed. The presence of aortic regurgitation secondary to injury to the aortic valve can be assessed by the amount of LV vent flow. Intraoperative echo should be used to assess the myomectomy and if additional resection appears needed or if it appears that mitral valve replacement will be necessary to obviate the outflow obstruction, it can be performed.[94] Loosening of the caval slings and decreasing venous return to the pump will fill the right ventricle with blood and allow identification of an iatrogenic VSD, which, if detected, must be repaired. Patients with a history of sudden death, or with EPS-documented severe ventricular arrhythmias, should be considered for placement of patches for use with an AICD. Most patients will have left-bundle branch block following the resection. In the unusual event of complete heart block, a permanent pacemaker should be inserted.

Mitral valve replacement when indicated is performed in the usual fashion. Our current choice of valve is the St. Jude, and in patients with contraindications to anticoagulation, the Carpentier–Edwards low-pressure fixation valve.

Results

Since no patient should be operated upon, or treated with DDD pacing, who has not failed medical management, there is no point in comparing medical or surgical figures. Also, the diagnosis is not always clear. For example, cavity obliteration identified as IHSS may be due to concentric hypertrophy, a condition that generally leads to death or poor results no matter how treated. Complicating the issue, there is a full spectrum of gradations between IHSS and concentric hypertrophy. This needs to be remembered when making the decision to operate and when reviewing the results of both medical and surgical management. When the diagnosis is in question, hemodynamic, angiographic, and echocardiographic evaluation is essential.

The earliest large series of patients with IHSS undergoing surgery remains at the NIH. In Morrow's series of patients (1960–1982) undergoing left ventricular myomectomy, operative mortality was 8% and symptomatic improvement was achieved in 82% of patients at 5 years. In a

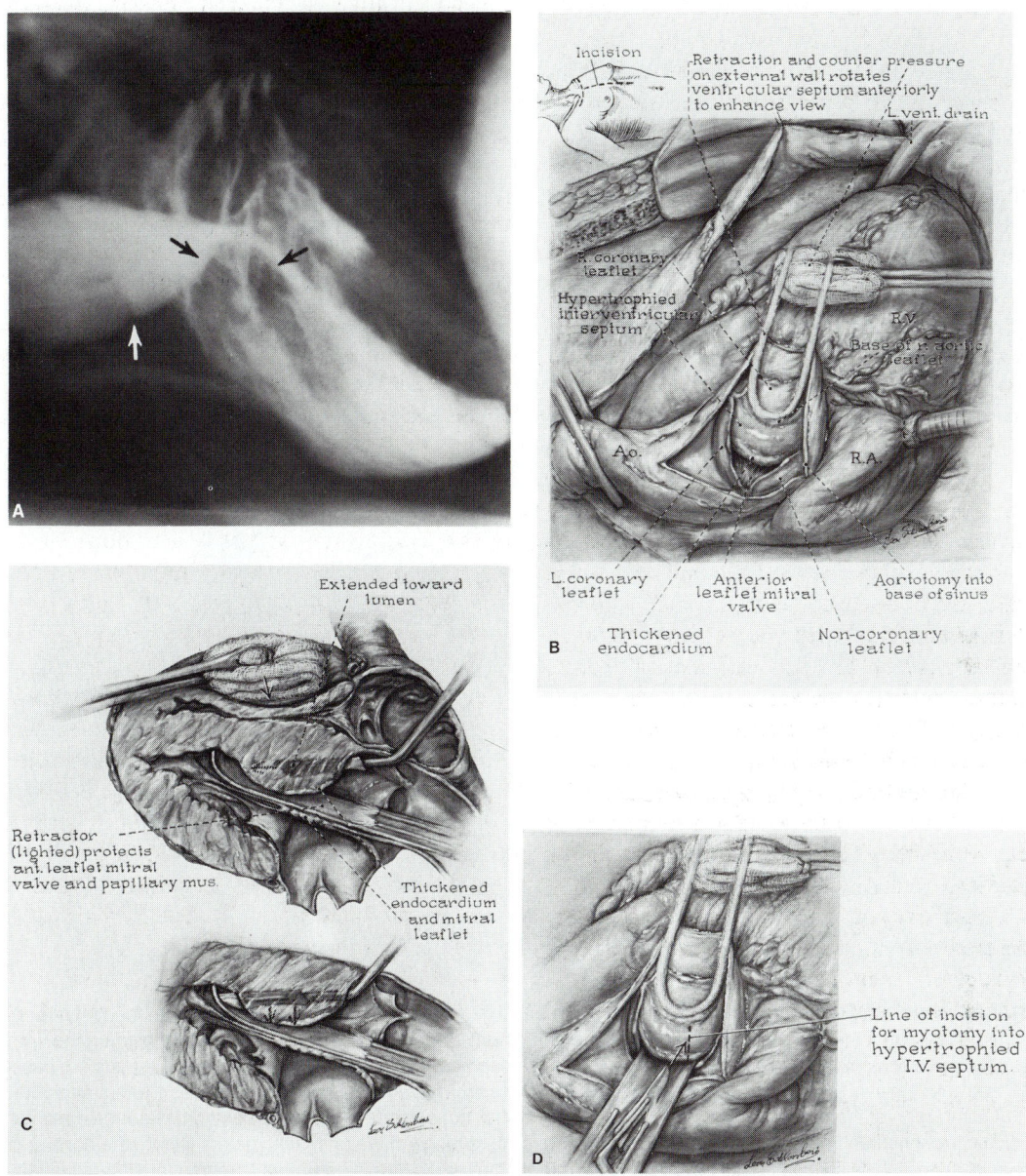

Figure 120–20. **A.** A left ventriculogram obtained in a patient with asymmetrical septal hypertrophy producing left ventricular outflow-tract obstruction. The narrow outflow tract of the left ventricle, resulting from the near coaptation of the asymmetrically hypertrophied septum and the anterior leaflet of the mitral valve, is apparent. Black arrows mark the hypertrophied septal mass. A white arrow marks a normal aortic valve. **B.** Operative exposure of the interventricular septum in preparation for left ventriculomyotomy and myectomy. After median sternotomy, bypass is instituted, general body hypothermia induced (30°C), and the aorta is opened vertically. The bulging, hypertrophied septum is visible below the right coronary valve leaflet. A ridge of thickened white endocardium is always evident on the most prominent part of the septum, the site at which it is opposed by the anterior mitral leaflet during systole. Exposure in the flaccid heart is facilitated by (1) traction on the right coronary leaflet by the cloth-covered retractor, and (2) counterpressure on the exterior wall of the left ventricle. **C.** A lighted ribbon retractor is passed through the annulus to the apex; it protects the mitral valve and papillary muscles. The first myotomy is made with an angled knife just to the right of the center of the right coronary leaflet. The blade is inserted into the septum in the long axis of the ventricle for a distance of at least 4 cm, and its tip can be felt to contact the retractor. The knife is withdrawn as its edge incises the septum with a sawing motion directed toward the ventricular lumen and the retractor. **D.** Site of first myotomy incision: 2 to 3 mm to the right (clockwise) of the center of the right coronary leaflet. *(Continued.)*

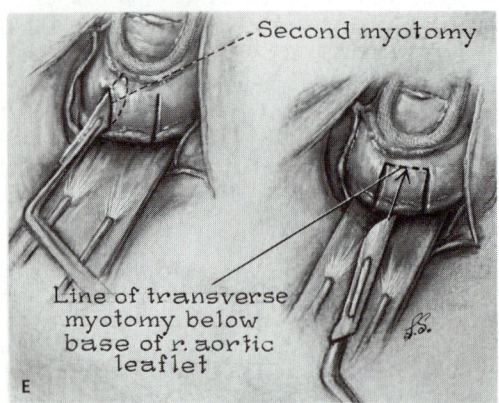

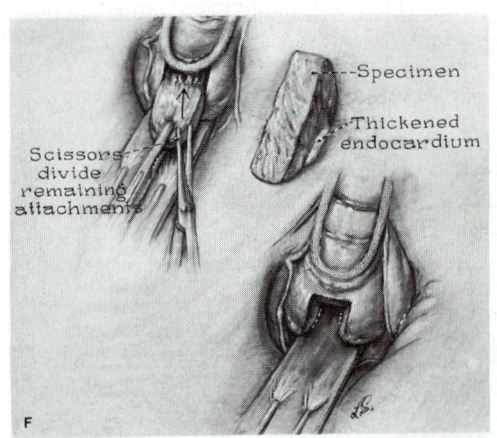

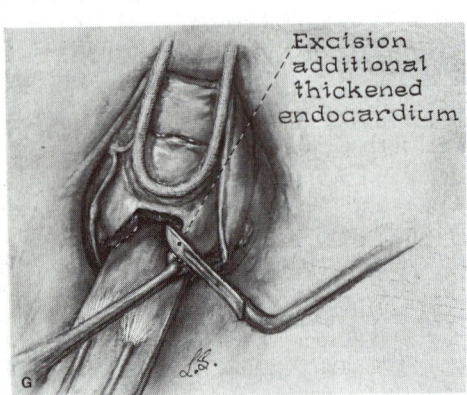

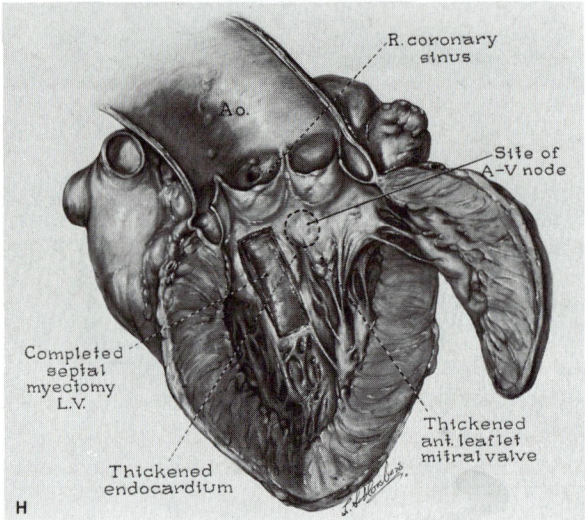

Figure 120–20. *(Continued.)* **E.** A second vertical myotomy is made 10 to 12 mm to the left of and parallel to the first one. A transverse incison is then made, connecting the vertical ones at the base of the right coronary leaflet. With this knife, angled on the flat, the bar of muscle between the vertical myotomies is largely detached from the septum. **F.** The tip of the cloth-covered retractor is passed into the left ventricle, and any remaining attachments of the muscle bar to the septum are divided under direct vision with a straight Potts scissors. After completion of the resection, a rectangular channel 1 × 1.5 cm extends from the valve ring toward the apex for about 4.5 cm. **G.** Additional thickened and scarred endocardium is trimmed from the edge of the channel created. Before the aorta is closed, the left ventricle is lavaged with saline solution to remove any particulate matter. **H.** Semidiagrammatic representation of the left ventricle after completion of the septal resection. The relations of the channel to the valve leaflets and to the adjacent membranous septum (and conduction tissue) are shown. The apical end of the floor of the channel blends smoothly onto the wall of the distal left ventricle. *(Parts B–H from Morrow AG: Hypertrophic subaortic stenosis operative methods utilized to relieve left ventricular outflow obstruction. J Thorac Cardiovasc Surg 76:423–430, 1978.)*

series of patients undergoing LV myotomy and myomectomy from 1982 to 1987, McIntosh reports an operative mortality of 2.7% and symptomatic improvement in approximately 80%.[87] McIntosh has reported the recent experience from the NIH in which patients underwent mitral valve replacement according to the criteria listed previously. The 30-day mortality after mitral valve replacement was 8.6% with symptomatic improvement in 83% of patients at a mean follow up of 24 months.[86] Neither operation appears to eliminate the risk of sudden death.

With the many deficiencies inherent in clinical studies and recognizing that patients managed surgically generally reflect those refractory to medical management, the mortal-

ity per year of patients with IHSS receiving no treatment, medical treatment, or surgical treatment is amazingly similar. In a review of the literature Seiler et al[95] reported that 255 patients receiving no treatment followed for an average of 5.8 years had an average yearly mortality of 4.7%, 869 patients receiving various forms of medical treatment for an average of 5.2 years had an average yearly mortality of 2.8%, and 764 surgical patients with an average yearly follow up of 26.6 years had an average yearly mortality of 2.5%. The message from Seiler's study is that patients with IHSS should receive medical treatment and that those failing medical management have an equal chance of survival with surgical management.

It is too soon to make any judgment about DDD pacing on yearly mortality. However, an interesting finding in DDD pacing is that the left ventricular outflow tract gradient is reduced by about 50%[90] and when the pacemaker is turned off, the reduction in gradient is maintained, at least for a while. The reasons for this are speculative, but may be due to ventricular remodeling.[96] Nevertheless, DDD pacing is still an experimental procedure and cannot be recommended for routine use in patients who are symptomatic despite medical management.[97] For the present, DDD pacing as a treatment for IHSS should remain in academic centers following NIH protocols.

REFERENCES

1. Roberts WC: Valvular, subvalvular and supravalvular aortic stenosis. Morphologic features. *Cardiovasc Clin* **5**(1):97, 1973
2. Waller BF: Rheumatic and non-rheumatic conditions producing valvular heart disease. *Cardiovasc Clin* **16**(2):17, 1986
3. Roberts WC, Virmani R: Aschoff bodies at necropsy in valvular heart disease. Evidence from an analysis of 543 patients over 14 years of age that rheumatic disease at least anatomically is a disease of the mitral valve. *Circulation* **57**:803, 1978
4. Roberts WC: The congenitally bicuspid aortic valve. A study of 85 autopsy patients. *Am J Cardiol* **26**:72, 1970
5. Falcone MW, Roberts WC, Morrow AG, et al: Congenital aortic stenosis resulting from a unicommissural valve. *Circulation* **44**:272, 1971
6. Roberts WC, Perloff JD, Constantino T: Severe valvular aortic stenosis in patients over 65 years of age. *Am J Cardiol* **27**:497, 1971
7. Sells S, Scully RE: Aging changes in the aortic and mitral valves. *Am J Pathol* **46**:345, 1965
8. Cohn PF: *Clinical Cardiovascular Physiology*. Philadelphia, PA, W.B. Saunders, 1985
9. Reichek N, Devereux RB: Reliable estimation of peak left ventricular systolic pressure by M-mode echocardiographic-detemined end diastolic relative wall thickness: Identification of severe valvular aortic stenosis in adult patients. *Am Heart J* **103**:202, 1982
10. Stapleton JF: The natural history of chronic valvular disease. *Cardiovasc Clin V* **16**(2):105, 1986
11. Punidis IP, Segal BL: Aortic valve disease in the elderly. *Cardiovasc Clin* **16**(2):289, 1986
12. Roberts WC: Morphologic features of the normal and abnormal mitral valve. *Am J Cardiol* **51**:1005, 1983
13. Bergeron J, Abelmann W, Vasquez-Milan H, Ellis L: Aortic stenosis-clinical manifestations and course of the disease. *Arch Intern Med* **94**:911, 1954
14. Ross J Jr, Braunwald E: Aortic stenosis. *Circulation* **37** Suppl **V**:61, 1968
15. Langou RA: Diagnostic procedures in acquired heart disease. In Glenn WWL, Baue AE, Geha AS, et al (eds): *Thoracic and Cardiovascular Surgery*. Norwalk, CT, Appleton-Century-Crofts, 1983, p 992
16. Stamm RB, Martin RP: Quantification of pressure gradients across stenotic valves by Doppler ultrasound. *J Am Coll Cardiol* **2**:707, 1983
17. Rahmintoola SH: The need for cardiac catheterization is not disproven. *Ann Intern Med* **97**:433, 1982
18. Gorlin R, Gorlin SG: Hydraulic formula for calculation of area of stenotic mitral valve, other cardiac valves, and central circulatory shunts. *Am Heart J* **41**:1, 1951
19. Roberts WC, Morrow AG, McIntosh CL, et al: Congenitally bicuspid aortic valve causing severe, pure aortic regurgitation without superimposed infective endocarditis. *Am J Cardiol* **47**(2):206–209, 1981
20. Parmley LF, Manion WC, Mattingly TW: Non-penetrating traumatic injury of the heart. *Circulation* **18**:371, 1958
21. Roberts WC, Dangel JC, Buckley BH: Non-rheumatic valvular cardiac disease: A clinicopathologic survey of 27 different conditions causing valvular dysfunction. *Cardiovasc Clin* **5**(2):334, 1973
22. Roberts WC, Honing HS: The spectrum of cardiovascular disease in the Marfan syndrome-A clinicopathologic study of 18 necropsy patients and comparison to 151 previously reported patients. *Am Heart J* **104**:115, 1982
23. Bulkley BH, Roberts WC: Anklylosing spondylitis and aortic regurgitation. Description of the characteristic cardiovascular lesion from study of 8 necropsy patients. *Circulation* **48**:1014, 1973
24. Rees JR, Epstein EJ, Criley JM, Ross RS: Hemodynamic effects of severe aortic regurgitation. *Br Heart J* **26**:412, 1964
25. Mann T, McLaurin L, Grossman W, et al: Assessing the hemodynamic severity of acute aortic regurgitation due to injective endocarditis. *N Engl J Med* **293**:108, 1975
26. Dervan J, Goldberg S: Acute aortic regurgitation. Pathophysiology and management. In Frankel WS, Brest AN (eds): *Valvular Heart Disease: Comprehensive Evaluation and Mangement, Cardiovascular Clinics*, Vol. 16, No. 2. Philadelphia, F.A. Davis, 1986
27. Segal J, Harvey WP, Hufnagel C: A clinical study of one hundred cases of severe aortic insufficiency. *Am J Med* **21**:200, 1956
28. Rapaport E: Natural history of aortic and mitral valve disease. *Am J Cardiol* **35**:221, 1975
29. Fortuin NJ, Craige E: On the mechanism of the Austin Flint murmur. *Circulation* **45**:558, 1972
30. Copeland JG, Griepp RB, Stinson EB, et al: Long term follow up after isolated aortic valve replacement. *J Thorac Cardiovasc Surg* **74**:875–889, 1977
31. Fioretti P, Roelandt J, Bos RJ, et al: Electrocardiography in chronic aortic insufficiency: Is replacement too late when left ventricular end systolic dimension reaches 55 mm? *Circulation* **67**:216–221, 1983
32. Gaasch WH: Aortic valve disease: Timing of valve replacement surgery. In Starek PJK (ed): *Heart Valve Replacement and Reconstruction*. St. Louis, Year Book Medical, 1987
33. Bonow RO, Rosing DR, Kent KM, Epstein SE: Timing of operation for chronic aortic regurgitation. *Am J Cardiol* **50**:325–336, 1982
34. Richardson JV, Karp RB, Kirklin JW, et al: Treatment of infective endocarditis: A 10 year comparative analysis. *Circulation* **58**:589, 1978
35. Dzik WH, Fleisher AG, Ciavarella D, et al: Safety and efficacy of autologous blood donation before elective aortic valve operation. *Ann Thorac Surg* **54**:1177–1181, 1992
36. Rahimtoola SH: Valvular heart disease: A perspective. *J Am Coll Cardiol* **1**:199–215, 1983
37. Christakis GT, Weisel RD, Fremes SE, et al: Can the results of contemporary aortic valve replacement be improved? *J Thorac Cardiovasc Surg* **92**:37–46, 1986
38. Bessone LN, Pupello DF, Hiro SP, et al: Surgical management of aortic valve disease in the elderly: A longitudinal analysis. *Ann Thorac Surg* **46**:264–269, 1988
39. Sethi GK: Should aortic valve replacement be performed in elderly patients? Editorial. *Ann Thorac Surg* **46**:262–263, 1988
40. Cohn LH: The long term results of aortic valve replacement. *Chest* **85**:387–396, 1984
41. Bonow RO, Picone AL, McIntosh CL, et al: Survival and functional results after valve replacement for aortic regurgitation from 1976 to 1983: Impact of preoperative left ventricular function. *Circulation* **72**:1244–1256, 1985
42. Hammond GL, Geha AS, Kopf GS, Hashim SW: Biological versus mechanical valves. *J Thorac Cardiovasc Surg* **93**:182–198, 1987
43. Cohn LH, Aranki SF, Rizzo RJ, et al: Decrease in operative risk of reoperative valve surgery. *Ann Thorac Surg* **56**:15–21, 1993
44. Elayda MAA, Hall RJ, Reul RM, et al: Aortic valve replacement in

patients 80 years and older. Operative risks and long-term results. *Circulation* **88**:II11–II16, 1993

45. Aranki SF, Rizzo RJ, Couper GS, et al: Aortic valve replacement in the elderly. Effect of gender and coronary artery disease on operative mortality. *Circulation* **88**:II17–II23, 1993

46. Morgan RJ, Davis JT, Fraker TD: Current status of valve prosthesis. *Surg Clin N Am* **65**(3):699, 1985

47. Blank RH, Pupello DF, Besson LN, et al: Method of managing the small aortic annulus during valve replacement. *Ann Thorac Surg* **22**:356–361, 1976

48. Nicks R, Cartmill T, Bernstein L: Hypoplasia of the aortic root. The problem of aortic valve replacement. *Thorax* **25**:339–346, 1970

49. Pupello DF, Bank RH: Valve replacement in the small aortic annulus in difficult problems. In Roberts AJ (ed): *Adult Cardiac Surgery*. St. Louis, Year Book Medical, 1985

50. Manouguian S, Seybold-Epting W: Patch enlargement of the aortic valve by extending the aortic incision into the anterior mitral leaflet: New operative technique. *J Thorac Cardiovasc Surg* **78**:402–412, 1979

51. Kawachi Y, Tominaga R, Tokunaga K: Eleven-year follow-up study of aortic or aortic-mitral anulus-enlarging procedure by Manouguian's technique. *J Thorac Cardiovasc Surg* **104**:1259–1263, 1992

52. Konno S, Imai Y, Nakajima M, et al: A new method for prosthetic valve replacement in congenital aortic stenosis associated with hypoplasia of the aortic valve ring. *Bull Heart Inst Jpn* **15**:1–17, 1974

53. Raasten H, Koncz J: Aortoventriculoplatsy. A new technique for treatment of left ventricular outflow obstruction. *J Thorac Cardiovasc Surg* **71**:920, 1976

54. Yener A, Ozdemir A, Sinav A, et al: New technique to enlarge the aortic annulus. *Ann Thorac Surg* **55**:1260–1261, 1993

55. Cooley DA, Norman JC, Reul GJ, et al: Surgical treatment of left ventricular outflow tract obstruction with apico-aortic valved conduit. *Surgery* **80**(6):674–680, 1976

56. Norman JC, Nihill MR, Cooley DA: Valved apico-aortic composite conduits for left ventricula outflow obstructions. *Am J Cardiol* **45**:1265–1271, 1980

57. King RM, Pluth JR, Giuliani ER, Piehler JM: Mechanical decalcification of the aortic valve. *Ann Thorac Surg* **42**:269–272, 1986

58. Mindich BP, Guarino T, Goldman ME: Aortic valvuloplasty for acquired aortic stenosis. *Circulation* **7**(Suppl 1):130–135, 1986

59. McBride LR, Naunheim KS, Fiore AC, et al: Aortic valve decalcification. *J Thorac Cardiovasc Surg* **100**:36–43, 1990

60. David TE, Feindel CM: An aortic valve-sparing operation for patients with aortic incompetence and aneurysm of the ascending aorta. *J Thorac Cardiovasc Surg* **103**:617–622, 1992

61. Sarsam MA, Yacoub M: Remodeling of the aortic valve anulus. *J Thorac Cardiovasc Surg* **105**:435–438, 1993

62. McKay RG, Safian RD, Lock JE, et al: Balloon dilatation of calcified aortic stenosis in elderly patients: Post-mortem, intraoperative, and percutaneous valvuloplasty studies. *Circulation* **74**:119–125, 1986

63. Clark CE, Henry WL, Epstein SE: Familial prevalence and genetic transmission of idiopathic hypertrophic subaortic stenosis. *N Engl J Med* **289**:709–714, 1973

64. Maron BJ, Mulvihill JJ: The genetics of hypertrophic cardiomyopathy. *Ann Intern Med* **105**:610–613, 1986

65. Roberts WC: Valvular, subvalvular, and supravalvular aortic stenosis: Morphologic features. *Cardiovasc Clin* **5**(1):97–126, 1973

66. Olsen EGJ: The pathology of cardiomyopathies: A critical analysis. *Am Heart J* **98**:385–392, 1979

67. Teare D: Asymmetrical hypertrophy of the heart in young adults. *Br Heart J* **20**:1–8, 1958

68. Hanrath P, Mathey DG, Siegert R, Bleifeld W: Left ventricular relaxation and filling pattern in different forms of left ventricular hypertrophy: An echocardiographic study. *Am J Cardiol* **45**:15–23, 1980

69. St John Sutton MG, Tajik AJ, Gibson DG, et al: Echocardiographic assessment of left ventricula filling and septal and posterior wall dy-

namics in idiopathic hypertrophic subaortic stenosis. *Circulation* **57**:512–520, 1978

70. Grigg LE, Wigle ED, Williams WG, et al: Transesophageal doppler echocardiography in obstructive hypertrophic cardiomyopathy: Clarification of pathophysiology and importance in intraoperative decision making. *J Am Coll Cardiol* **20**:42–52, 1992

71. Ross J Jr, Braunwald E, Gaul JH, et al: The mechanism of the intraventricular pressure gradient in idiopathic hypertrophic subaortic stenosis. *Circulation* **34**:558–578, 1966

72. Shah PM, Gramiak R, Adelman AG, Wigle ED: Role of echocardiography in diagnostic and hemodynamic assessment of hypertrophic subaortic stenosis. *Circulation* **44**:891–898, 1971

73. Pichard AD, Meller J, Teichholz LE, et al: Septal perforator compression in idiopathic hypertrophic subaortic stenosis. *Am J Cardiol* **40**:310–314, 1977

74. McKenna WJ, England D, Doi YL, et al: Arrhythmia in hypertrophic cardiomyopathy. I. Influence on prognosis. *Br Heart J* **46**:168–172, 1981

75. Maron BJ, Epstein SE: Clinical course of patients with hypertrophic cardiomyopathy. *Cardiovasc Clin* **10**(1):253–265, 1979

76. Maron BJ, Savage DD, Wolfson JK, Epstein SE: Prognostic significance of 24 hour ambulatory electrocardiographic monitoring in patients with hypertrophic cardiomyopathy: A prospective study. *Am J Cardiol* **48**:252–257, 1981

77. Hardarson T, DelaCalzada CS, Curiel R, Goodwin JF: Prognosis and mortality of hypertrophic obstructive cardiomyopathy. *Lancet* **2**:1462–1467, 1973

78. Kowley PR, Eisenberg R, Engel TR: Sustained arrhythmias in hypertrophic obstructive cardiomyopathy. *N Engl J Med* **310**:1566–1569, 1984

79. McKenna WJ, Chetty S, Oakley CM, Goodwin JF: Arrhythmia in hypertrophic cardiomyopathy: Exercise and 48 hour ambulatory electrocardiographic assessment with and without beta adrenergic blocking therapy. *Am J Cardiol* **5**:1–5, 1980

80. Maron BJ, Bonow RO, Cannon RO, et al: Hypertrophic cardiomyopathy. Interrelations of clinical manifestations, pathophysiology, and therapy (part 2). *N Engl J Med* **316**:844–852, 1987

81. Frank MJ, Abdulla AM, Canedo MI, Saylors RE: Long-term medical management of hypertrophic obstructive cardiomyopathy. *Am J Cardiol* **42**:993–1001, 1978

82. Rosing DR, Idanpaan-Heikkila U, Maron BJ, et al: Use of calcium channel blocking drugs in hypertrophic cardiomyopathy. *Am J Cardiol* **55**Suppl:185B–195B, 1985

83. Wigle ED: Impaired left ventricular relaxation in hypertrophic cardiomyopathy. Relation to extent of hypertrophy. *J Am Coll Cardiol* **15**:814–815, 1990

84. Wigle ED, Sasson Z, Henderson MA, et al: Hypertrophic cardiomyopathy. The importance of the size and the extent of hypertrophy. A review. *Prog Cardiovasc Dis* **28**:1–83, 1985

85. Cooley DA, Wukasch DC, Leachman RD: Mitral valve replacement for idiopathic hypertrophic subaortic stenosis: Results in 27 patients. *J Cardiovasc Surg* **17**:380–387, 1976

86. McIntosh CL, Greenburg GH, Maron BJ, et al: Clinical and hemodynamic results after mitral valve replacement in patients with obstructive hypertrophic cardiomyopathy. *Ann Thorac Surg* **47**:236–246, 1989

87. McIntosh CL: Idiopathic hypertrophic subaortic stenosis. In Grillo HC, Austen WG, Wilkins EW, et al (eds): *Current Therapy in Cardiothoracic Surgery*. Philadelphia, Toronto, B.C. Decker, 1989

88. Stone CD, Hennein HA, McIntosh CL, et al: The results of operation in patients with hypertrophic cardiomyopathy and pulmonary hypertension. *J Thorac Cardiovasc Surg* **100**:343–352, 1990

89. Zile MR, Blaustein AS, Shimizu G: Right ventricular pacing reduces the rate of left ventricular relaxation and filling. *J Am Coll Cardiol* **10**:702–709, 1987

90. Fananapazir L, Cannon RO, Tripodi D, Panza JA: Impact of dual-chamber permanent pacing in patients with obstructive hypertrophic

cardiomyopathy with symptoms refractory to verapamil and β-adrenergic blocker therapy. *Circulation* **85:**2149–2161, 1992

91. Morrow AG, Reitz BA, Epstein SE, et al: Operative treatment in hypertrophic subaortic stenosis: Techniques, and the results of pre and postoperative assessment in 83 patients. *Circulation* **52:**88–102, 1975

92. Morrow AG: Hypertrophic subaortic stenosis. Operative methods utilized to relieve left ventricular outflow obstruction. *J Thorac Cardiovasc Surg* **76:**423–430, 1978

93. Dowling RD, Landreneau RJ, Gasior TA, et al: Septal myectomy with a carbon dioxide laser for hypertrophic cardiomyopathy. *Ann Thorac Surg* **55:**1558–1560, 1993

94. Marwick TH, Stewart WJ, Lever HM, et al: Benefits of intraoperative echocardiography in the surgical management of hypertrophic cardiomyopathy. *J Am Coll Cardiol* **20:**1066–1072, 1992

95. Seiler C, Hess O, Schoenbeck M, et al: Long-term follow-up of medical versus surgical therapy for hypertrophic cardiomyopathy: A retrospective study. *J Am Coll Cardiol* **17:**634–642, 1991

96. McAreavey D, Fananapazir L: Altered cardiac hemodynamic and electrical state in normal sinus rhythm after chronic dual-chamber pacing for relief of left ventricular outflow obstruction in hypertrophic cardiomyopathy. *Am J Cardiol* **70:**651–656, 1992

97. Cannon RO, Tripodi D, Dilsizian V, et al: Results of permanent dual-chamber pacing in symptomatic nonobstructive hypertrophic cardiomyopathy. *Am J Cardiol* **73:**571–576, 1994

121

Homografts and Autografts

Mark F. O'Brien

HOMOGRAFTS AND AUTOGRAFTS

The "ideal" replacement valve, that is, one with perfect hemodynamics, devoid of early and late morbid events, readily available, and usable by all surgeons for all patients with any type of valve disease, does not exist and probably is unattainable. Nevertheless such a valve would offer a curative procedure if an operation was performed before severe cardiopulmonary disease had eventuated. Throughout our quest for this "ideal valve," the homograft or allograft, and more recently the pulmonary autograft, have always been appealing because human valve tissue is used to replace a human diseased valve. Over the last three decades, the continuing evolution of tissue preservation has produced improvements in valve durability. In addition, implantation techniques for allograft and autograft valves, both in acquired valve disease and congenital heart disease, have improved markedly. Consequently, with some confidence, it can be stated that the aortic allograft presents a very appealing device for the treatment of all pathological lesions of the aortic valve and root. A pulmonary autograft progresses one step further for selected patients. As the trend over the years has been one of improving quality and clinical performance, today's surgeon can be optimistic that further refinements are being evaluated. Continuing research and analysis obviously must continue.

This chapter focuses on some historical landmarks of the use of the allograft valve with emphasis on the importance of different preparations and storage techniques and their influence on the long-term durability. A standard protocol of procurement and preservation is outlined with either early implantation of a "fresh" valve or use of an early cryopreserved allograft valve. The evolution of the various implantation techniques, ranging from subcoronary to root replacement for allograft aortic or pulmonary autograft valves, is detailed step by step. The use of allografts as

valve conduits for right ventricular problems is left to other authors in this book. The importance of viability and the consequent host immunological response of allograft valve transfer together with the controversy of the need and value of immunosuppression are addressed. The pathological changes and the biomechanical analyses of explanted tissues are highlighted to determine predictors of long-term durability. In this chapter, reference is also made to specific technical concerns of reoperation, implantation techniques for endocarditis, and the small aortic root. The possibilities of using allograft atrioventricular valve tissue for mitral and tricuspid valve surgery are reviewed.

The autologous pulmonary valve and the newer autologous pericardial stented valve with their specific indications, technical aspects of retrieval and implantation, historical and current clinical results are more briefly detailed. They are superimposed on the allograft experience. The future place of both valves, the expectations of clinical results, and the apparent avenues for future research are expressed.

Finally, some aspects of tissue donation and a global viewpoint are put forward in reference to the influence of race, creed, law, and custom.

Terminology

The *homograft* valve is a graft from a donor of the same species. *Xenograft* is the converse term, namely a graft derived from a different species. An *allograft* is one from a donor of the same species but which is not genetically identical to the graft recipient. Its opposite term is an *autograft,* which is a graft from "self" tissue. All allografts are therefore homografts, but the allograft recipient recognizes genetic dissimilarity. However, identical twins are considered as genetically identical, being from the same germ line. A tissue graft from one twin to the other would not be an allograft but is described by the complimentary term *isograft* (Fig. 121–1). Such identical twins, although their germ line genetic information is identical, do have a different immune system repertoire as this is developed through somatic mutation. This does not influence the isograft as there is no host B and T cell response to grafted tissue from one twin to the other. Practically, the two terms, homograft and allograft, are currently used interchangeably. Historically, homograft was the term used three decades ago and is still currently the favored terminology in European and Asian countries, whereas the term allograft is predominantly used on the North American continent and is more frequently used in the current medical literature. The term allograft is favored by immunologists and transplant specialists.

In summary, the allograft is a more modern currently used term and as it does recognize the genetic differences and therefore the inherent immunological expression from the recipient, this terminology is adopted in this chapter.

The autograft may refer to a pulmonary valve taken from and implanted into the same patient in another location, such as the aortic root, or it may be an autograft pericardial valve implanted into any location in the heart. Both autografts are discussed in this chapter.

Historical Background

One of the earliest experimental animal studies was reported in 1952 by Lam et al[1] who implanted an allograft aortic valve into the descending aorta of the dog. This followed, within 3 years, with the clinical implantation of the allograft aortic valve into the human descending aorta by Murray[2] and Beall et al.[3] Eight years later, the technique for subcoronary implantation of allograft using a single suture method was reported by Duran and Gunning.[4] During the same year in 1962, the first subcoronary implant (with a freeze-dried aortic valve) in a human being was performed by Ross of London[5] and shortly after by Barratt-Boyes of New Zealand, who commenced with an initial series of fresh allograft valves.[6]

Because valves were procured in a totally unsterile manner, many methods were introduced to sterilize and store the aortic valve. These methods ranged from formaldehyde,[7] chlorhexidine, propiolactone, ethylene oxide, gamma irradiation, and storage using a carbon dioxide freezer at −70°C. These valves were all nonviable with a denatured protein matrix. The late postimplant morphologic picture remained one of acellularity with amorphous collagen and degenerating elastin. Such chemically sterilized allograft valves had an unacceptable incidence of late cusp rupture leading to discontinuance of their use by many surgeons throughout the world. Some fortunately persisted with the allograft valve, switching to antibiotic sterilization with storage at 4°C refrigeration.[8,9] There was still considerable variation of sterilization techniques with the antibiotic type and strength ranging from excessively high to pharmacological doses and exposure times from 24 hours to several weeks. Improvement occurred in valve durability using these techniques with an obvious reduction in late cusp rupture.[8,9] Nevertheless, the high dose antibiotics and prolonged exposure were damaging to leaflet tissue. In 1975, after a 5-year laboratory study[10] on the most appropriate method of preserving viability by cryopreservation, O'Brien and colleagues at The Prince Charles Hospital (TPCH) Brisbane commenced the clinical implantation of allografts from their cryopreservation valve bank. These valves were collected soon after donor death and were sterilized by short-term exposure to low-dose antibiotics, the details of which are described. Angell working in parallel and with some collaboration also established a cryopreservation heart valve bank.[11]

Preparation and Cryopreservation Protocol

Some 25 years ago in 1969, the aortic allograft valve for aortic valve replacement (AVR) was first used at TPCH. The early valves were sterilized in low-dose antibiotics for 24 hours and stored in nutrient medium at 4°C. Subsequently from mid-1975 all valves have been cryopreserved immediately after sterilization. The purpose of this method of storage was to retain the viability of the fibroblasts within the leaflets, with the aim of markedly enhancing subsequent valve durability.[12,13] Valves could be stored indefinitely.

At TPCH, the procurement, sterilization, and preservation have been implemented according to a *rigid* protocol with little variation from this methodology at any particular time over the past 19 years. Possible deviations from the protocol, for example valves that could have been obtained outside the 24-hour time limits of donor death to collection, have not been accepted. Hence the clinical long-term results with the maintenance of a relatively uniform "product"[14] using such a protocol have been more meaningful and reliable.

Procurement from the autopsy donor has always been within 24 hours of donor death (mean 15 hours). Donors must be less than 55 years of age and have no evidence of systemic infection or malignant neoplasia (excluding primary cerebral tumor). A donor blood sample is checked for blood group, human immune deficiency virus, hepatitis,

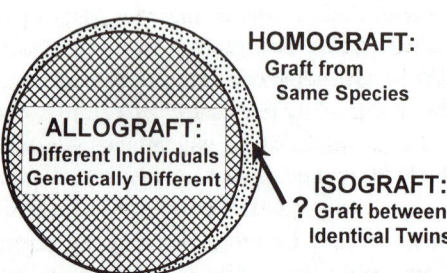

Figure 121–1. Diagramatic relationship of the terms "allograft," "isograft," and "homograft."

syphilitic, cytomegalovirus, and serology. From the beginning in 1969, accurate records at TPCH have been kept in relationship to all donor characteristics, including life style, age, sex, blood group, cause of death, and time of death to collection and to cryopreservation. Confidentiality of records is maintained. The precise valve characteristics of measurement, quality, and sterility at all stages of the preservation are recorded.

The heart, including the pulmonary bifurcation and aortic arch, is either removed under the usual sterile operating room conditions for organ donors or removed as aseptically as possible in the autopsy room. The ventricular mass is transected, leaving the base of the heart attached to the great arteries. The tissue is then placed in nutrient medium (Medium 199—cell culture medium, Commonwealth Serum Laboratories, Melbourne, Australia) containing antibiotics and brought immediately to TPCH. When procurement has occurred in a remote center, the heart is packed in ice and rapidly transported. The aortic and pulmonary valves are then separated and trimmed of excess tissue. The sizing of valves is carried out by aortic pressure distension to 80 mm Hg. An annular measurement of the valve from the ventricular aspect is made *without* passing any cone or instrument through the valve. Following dissection, each valve is rinsed in 100 mL of sterile M199 (without antibiotics) to remove any blood. The pulmonary valve is used for right-sided reconstruction of congenital lesions or for pulmonary valve replacement during the pulmonary autograft operation (Ross Procedure).

The leaflet of the tricuspid valve is cut into three pieces. One piece is placed in a bottle of M199 with antibiotics, and viability of the allograft valves is inferred from the subsequent demonstration of a positive cell culture from this tissue. One other piece of tricuspid valve is cryopreserved with the aortic and pulmonary valves each.

Valve sterilization is by incubation at 37°C for 6 hours in nutrient medium containing penicillin 30 μg/mL (50 IU/mL) and streptomycin 50 μg/mL. Prior to 1988 amphotericin B 10 μg/mL was added, but because of its deleterious effects on living cells its use was discontinued.[15] A warm incubation was used to obtain maximum antibacterial effectiveness with the low-dose antibiotic. The antibiotic concentrations used at TPCH are very low, unlike all other antibiotic protocols. This has been possible first because the valves are taken "sterile" in a clean room as the first autopsy procedure on the donor and second because the valve is collected as soon as possible after death, thereby minimizing postmortem contamination. Any delay with collection has been due to the time in waiting for next of kin permission. While many newer antibiotics have been available throughout the 25 years of this program, other than the omission of amphotericin B, no change from the original use of penicillin and streptomycin has been made. Because no antifungal agent is used, the presence of any fungus, although infrequent, generally leads to discard of the valve. At TPCH a 5-year analysis of the effectiveness of this antibiotic regime[16] has shown excellent tissue sterilization. Very few valves are contaminated and need to be discarded. For any one valve during the many steps of collection, trimming, incubation, pre- and post-thawing phases, some 12 samples are taken for bacteriologic analysis.

After incubation, the valves are cryopreserved in a manner identical to valves obtained from an organ donor. Valves obtained in an operating room from multiorgan donors are incubated because of the small incidence of contamination as the abdominal cavity is opened and the liver is taken simultaneously. Those valves from cardiac transplant recipients are cyropreserved immediately after trimming in 90 mL of cold M199 without antibiotics plus 10 mL dimethyl sulfoxide (DMSO) as the cryoprotectant. This 10% DMSO solution is placed in a Fenwal bag (Baxter Healthcare Corp., Deerfield, Illinois), along with the aortic valve and a piece of the tricuspid valve. The solution in the bag is kept at approximately 4°C because DMSO is toxic to cells at temperatures above 10°C. The top of the bag is enclosed in a piece of nylon foil and heat sealed, the foil maintaining sterility of the bag. This bag is placed in another plastic bag and heat sealed. All of these steps are repeated for the pulmonary valve. Identification tags are attached to both aortic and pulmonary valve bags. The bags are placed in a controlled rate freezer, cooled at the rate of −1°C/min to −40°C and transferred to the vapor phase large liquid nitrogen tank where the liquid temperature is −196°C and the vapor approximately −170°C. The freezing solution (M199 and DMSO) and a specimen of tissue trimmings are sent for microbiologic culture. Valves are not used if any microbiologic cultures consistently demonstrate the presence of organisms, or if cells cannot be cultured from the leaflet of the tricuspid valve. Valves are released for clinical use after the completion of serologic, microbiologic, and mycologic tests at 3 wk.

On the day after collection, the autopsy diagnosis of death is verified. This is a double check to ensure that the recipient had no communicable disease that may not have been initially identified.

Valve Thawing

If the supply is satisfactory, two or three valves of varying sizes are transported to the operating room in portable liquid nitrogen dewar. The selected valve is removed from its outer bag and, while still in its inner bag with a piece of tricuspid valve leaflet, is thawed rapidly in a sterile saline bath at 40°C. After approximately 5–10 min, the tissues are removed from this bag and rinsed stepwise for 2 min each in each of four bowls: The first contains 500 mL of M199 with 5% DMSO, the second contains M199 with 2.5% DMSO, and the last two each contain M199 without DMSO at 4°C. At the time of valve thawing, the corresponding piece of tricuspid valve leaflet is also thawed and viability is assessed by cell culture, which gives a qualitative index of leaflet viability after cryopreservation and thawing.

This thawing process takes almost 15–20 min from the time of selection of the valve to the time that the valve is available at the operating table for final examination and trimming. If the required size of the allograft is known, as is the situation when a root replacement is to be performed (size matching less critical), the valve can be thawed much earlier and be available for trimming prior to instituting cardiopulmonary bypass. This also permits time for thorough inspection of the allograft.

General Comments on the TPCH and Other Protocols. All valves are retrieved only after consent has been obtained, either from the donor, who has previously indicated on his or her driver's license a willingness to donate, or from the next of kin. The next of kin are contacted where possible not only to comply with the present legal guidelines but also to enhance the education of organ and tissue donation.

The whole protocol of valve collection and preservation does center around maximizing viability with low-dose antibiotic sterilization and avoidance of instrumental damage and abrasion of leaflet tissue during handling. A well-trained, dedicated, small group of scientists/technicians is responsible for valve collection, preservation, tissue culturing, and data collection. Some of these scientists are also responsible for detailed follow-up surveillance. The surgeon, although overseeing the valve bank, needs only notify the valve size required and when it becomes available, the operation can be scheduled. Urgent requirements are prioritized and met from the valve bank. There is always a short supply of grafts but at TPCH some 90 aortic valve implants and 40 to 50 pulmonary and other implants for right-sided lesions are performed annually.

The key aspects of TPCH protocol have been

1. Early "sterile" valve collection (which is at aortic cross-clamp from multiorgan donors or the transplant recipient patient, and at a mean of 15 hours after death from autopsy donors).
2. Short time exposure (6 hours) to the low-dose antibiotics penicillin and streptomycin for the autopsy and multiorgan donor valves. The valves from the heart of the transplant recipient are washed with nutrient medium containing antibiotics but not incubated.
3. Early cryopreservation [within 1 to 2 hours from collection from the transplant patient, 8–12 hours with valves from the multiorgan donor, and 22 hours (mean) from death for autopsy donors].

In the maintenance of the valve bank, it is important that the valves are neither moved around excessively in the cryopreservation tank, nor taken out and returned to the tank too often. Excessive rapid temperature changes may be deleterious to the valve and may contribute to the cracking of the aortic wall, especially in larger valves from older donors.

The protocol of valve preparation may be very different from one center or tissue bank to another. For example, in some centers delayed collection has caused valve sterilization not to commence for 48 hours. Antibiotic regimes have included cefoxitin, lincomycin, polymyxin B, vancomycin, ampicillin.[17] In addition, cryopreservation has not been commenced for 3 to 7 days after collection. It is maintained by the author that these variabilities may be critical to the durability of allograft tissue. Consequently, the clinical results may vary so much that they are not typical of the true best performance of an allograft valve. There are, therefore, many types of aortic allografts.[14] Age of donor[9] and recipient (younger less satisfactory), the valve warm ischemic time (death to collection), death to cryopreservation, type, strength, and duration of exposure to antibiotics are but a few factors that may influence the fate of the allograft valve. The most important determinants of long-term valve function are the preservation of the fibrous matrix, the viability of leaflet fibroblasts, and the techniques of implantation.

Viability Studies

At TPCH, tritiated proline (L-[5-^{3}H]proline) uptake autoradiography has been conducted as a quantitative analysis of viability of the leaflet fibroblast. Segments of valve leaflets from hearts of both multiorgan donors and from autopsy sources have been used. Viability of valves, processed with the current clinical protocol of preservation, has been compared with that of valves undergoing variations of exposure and type of antibiotic, before and after cryopreservation and after thawing with and without dilutions of the cryoprotectant DMSO. Leaflet segments prior to treatment acted as controls.

The ratio of living cells in leaflet segments from multiorgan donors (warm ischemic time < 1 hour) was over 90% with antibiotic exposure of 60 min prior to cryopreservation. Once cryopreservation was introduced the percentage of living cells dropped to 58% (+63% of the control). Leaflet segments analyzed from valves from autopsy sources showed the effects of longer warm ischemic times (mean 15 hours). The ratio of living cells in valve segments processed with the present clinical protocol was initially 58%. Viability did not decrease following 6 hours incubation at 37°C with penicillin and streptomycin. Following cryopreservation viability decreased to 43% (54% of the controls).

These studies have shown some loss of viability due to the effect of warm ischemia and of cryopreservation and thawing. The antibiotics penicillin and streptomycin at the concentrations used were not injurious to cell viability. This quantitative analysis proved that patients receiving allograft aortic valves at TPCH since 1975 had received "viable cryopreserved" valves.

The comparative clinical study of valve durability of "nonviable" allografts (1969–1975) and "viable cryopreserved" allografts (1975–1994) demonstrated the superiority of the viable tissue.[12,18] In addition, the results of these tritiated proline uptake studies have been confirmed by reports of electron microscopy studies of leaflet viability in relationship to warm ischemic times.[19,20] They demonstrated that significant rapid loss of viability of fibroblasts occurred after 12 hours of warm ischemia. Nevertheless, in spite of this work on viability and the obvious enhanced clinical results, the specific importance of leaflet viability and its effect of durability are still unanswered.

By preserving cell viability, the noncellular matrix of valve leaflets should be maximally protected as well. Understanding the nature and varying degrees of the host reaction and the remodelling of implanted allograft valves still remains the challenge. Until these are ascertained more fully, the importance of cellular viability as opposed to or together with the quality of the valve matrix is still to be determined.

The Aortic Root and Implantation Techniques

The aortic allograft valve has been implanted in three ways:

1. Complete root replacement with coronary artery implantation. The length of the ascending aorta is variable and no native aorta is wrapped over the graft (Fig. 121–2A).
2. An intraluminal tube or cylinder that necessitates side-to-side coronary artery reimplantation. The native aorta must be closed over the cylinder (Fig. 121–2B).
3. Subcoronary implantation using a scalloped valve. There are a number of variations of this method (Fig. 121–2C).

These techniques are described in some detail after the basic concept of the aortic root is outlined.

The Concept of the Aortic Root (Normal and Abnormal)

The aortic valve and root is a three-dimensional structure and viewed as a cylinder it has breadth and length (Fig. 121–3), the aortic valve leaflets being at its base and the commissural posts being a part of its side wall. The transverse and longitudinal axes are descriptive parts of this cylinder, which may be quite asymmetric when the valve annulus and sinotubular (transcommissural) diameters are neither equal nor parallel. Nevertheless even in such situations of asymmetry, the tube-like or cylinder-like appearance is the most important concept to visualize. In some congenital bicuspid valve roots, the "cylinder" is grossly distorted.

In addition, implanting a normal symmetric allograft aortic valve into an asymmetric aortic root may not be easy for several reasons:

1. The extent of the asymmetry of the host may not be fully appreciated particularly in the nondistended open root at operation.
2. The likelihood of distorting the allograft is high and the

subsequent degree of leaflet coaptation and valve competence is less assured.
3. Once the allograft is trimmed for subcoronary implantation, it becomes far more difficult to conceptualize this floppy piece of tissue as a three-dimensional structure or cylinder.

Workshops focusing on implantation techniques have been conducted in several countries over the last decade. Several implantation techniques are available but the decision as to which one to use can be confusing. Should the valve be rotated and inverted, should the noncoronary sinus wall be retained, and should the valve be implanted as a scalloped graft in the subcoronary position with continuous or interrupted sutures, as an intra-aortic cylinder or as a full root replacement? Both the latter two techniques entail coronary artery reimplantation. Many surgeons are unwilling to embark on an allograft program because of these complexities. The obvious learning curve has been aggravated further by the variety of published techniques,[21–23] making the judgment of which method to use and on which occasion difficult to make.

With the advent of intraoperative and early postoperative color Doppler echocardiography, sensitive as it is, it has been possible to see minor degrees of valve incompetence, not clinically detectable, which reflect failure to maintain the perfect geometry of the symmetrical allograft valve. In the author's experience, only the allograft implanted as a root replacement consistently produces the best results of valve competence as ascertained by echo Doppler. The important principle and objective is to preserve the symmetry of the allograft, basically disregarding the asymmetry of the host valve and aortic root. *The allograft should not be made to fit the host.* With this principle, distortion of the graft is minimized and possibly in most situations even abolished. In addition, the size of graft to host is far less critical and on most occasions the graft can be thawed prior to bypass, avoiding some 15 min delay. The only remaining problem is perhaps that of the coronary artery reimplantation. Some judgment is required in siting the coronary arteries for implantation. It is possible to produce some leaflet distortion with the coronary reimplantation. This is generally of a minor degree.

The Measurements of the Host Root

Pathological lesions of the aortic root present variable architecture ranging from perfect symmetry to gross asymmetry and disorganization, as in some cases of staphylococcal aortic root infection. For the purposes of deciding the appropriate surgical procedure, it is convenient to categorize the aortic root and annulus on the basis of two measurements, the valve annulus diameter (VAD) and the sinotubular or transcommissural diameter (STD). In the normal aortic root, the STD is usually 2 to 3 mm larger than the VAD. These measurements and the overall configuration of the root can be calculated preoperatively from the cineaor-

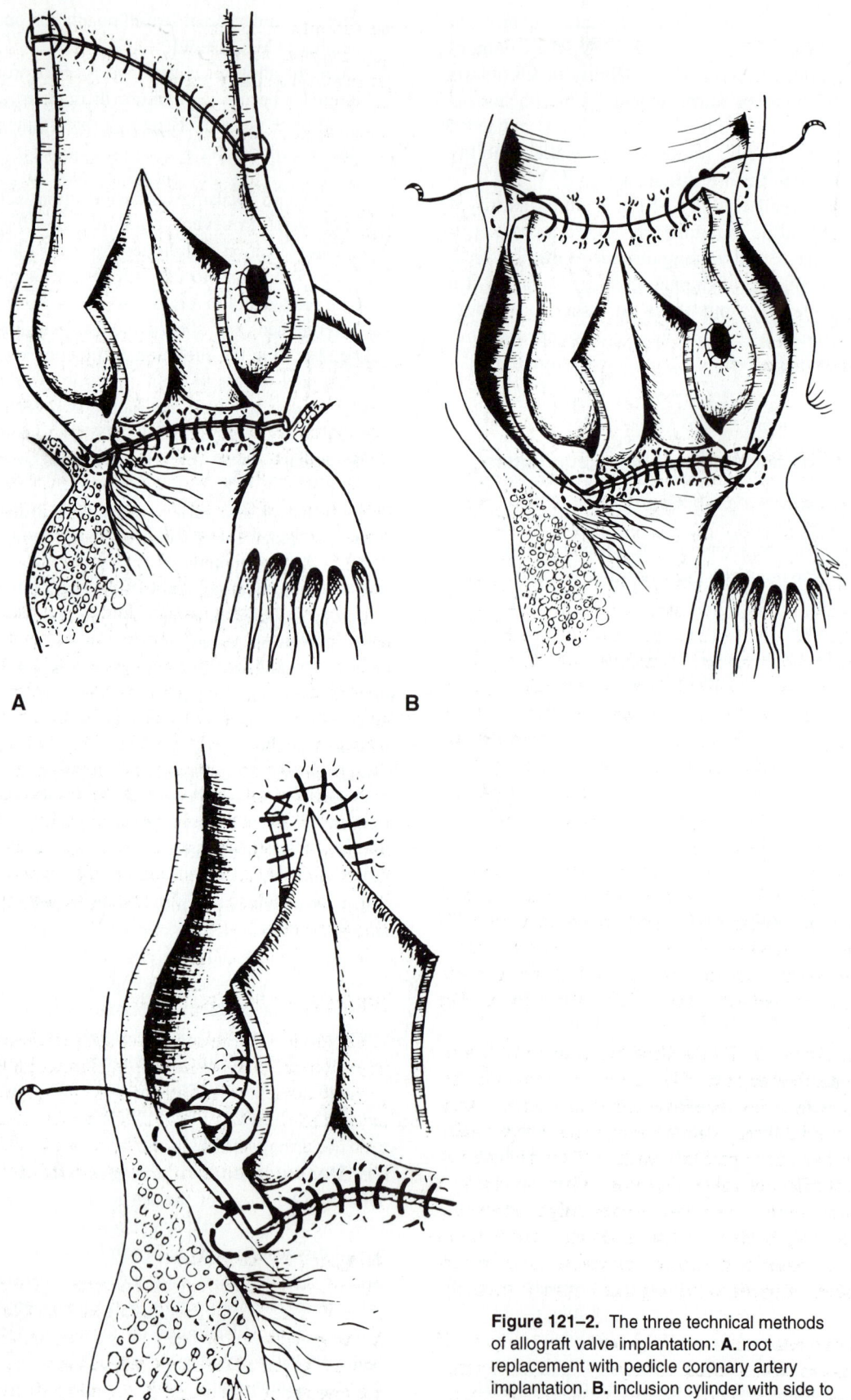

A

B

C

Figure 121–2. The three technical methods of allograft valve implantation: **A.** root replacement with pedicle coronary artery implantation. **B.** inclusion cylinder with side to side anastomoses, **C.** subcoronary, scalloped.

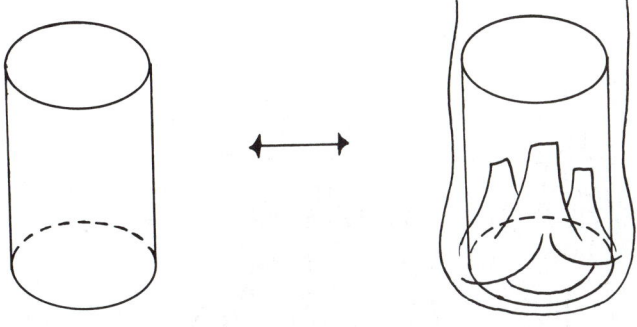

Figure 121–3. Conceptualization of the aortic root—annulus and its diameter, leaflets, sinuses, and commissures, and sinotubular diameter—as parts of a cylinder.

togram if a measuring grid is incorporated into the film[23] (Fig. 121–4A). The width of the contrast in the immediate subvalvar region on a left ventricular injection or reflux of contrast from an aortic root injection in the presence of aortic regurgitation can provide a reasonably accurate measurement of the VAD (Fig. 121–4B). Echocardiography is often used to estimate these diameters. Experience at TPCH has shown that the VAD estimations, especially with a calcific immobile valve, may be less accurate with either technique of measurement. Nevertheless the purpose of these calculations is to give the surgeon an appreciation of the aortic root asymmetry and to select a range of appropriate sized valves than can be brought to the operating room.

Lack of aortic root symmetry with a substantial discrepancy between the VAD and STD is often seen in aortic root pathology. The STD is greater than the VAD in poststenotic dilatation and in aneurysmal aortic root disease (Fig. 121–5A). Occasionally, removal of a stenotic bicuspid aortic valve results in the VAD being greater than the STD (Fig. 121–5B). In situations in which the noncoronary sinus alone is aneurysmal, or at least considerably larger than the other two sinuses, the VAD and STD may not be parallel (Fig. 121–5C).

In most instances of a calcified bicuspid aortic valve, there is an anteroposterior slit-like orifice and heavily calcified leaflets with a left lateral rudimentary raphe. After valve excision, the three sinuses surprisingly are generally virtually equal and little problem exists with the insertion of a symmetrical trileaflet valve. However, when the bicuspid valve has a transverse orifice, two sinuses only exist and the coronary ostia may be directly 180° opposite. This requires special care to ensure that none of the commissural pillars of the trileaflet allograft valve impinges upon a coronary ostium.

The above estimations are a guide to the surgeon. If the valve bank is well stocked, a range of sizes of allograft valves can be brought to the operating room. An experienced surgeon may find measuring of little help, but for the surgeon who is learning to use the allograft, this process of measuring helps in the understanding of the aortic root and

the varieties of anatomic configurations. For the subcoronary implant, the VAD must be accurately determined and preferably physically measured at operation before selecting and thawing the valve. The consequent delay is not particularly appreciated by surgeons. However, with the root replacement, the host–allograft size matching is less critical. Consequently, providing an echo measurement has been previously obtained, the valve can be thawed immediately after the pericardium is opened and the ascending aorta and root externally visualized.

The Training of a Surgeon in Allograft Valve Implantation Techniques

The techniques can be straightforward and easily learned by cardiac surgeons who perform many more technically demanding procedures than any of these. Nevertheless, the use of stentless tissue valves does require more spatial judgment, akin to that required in reparative procedures in congenital cardiac surgery. *The initial steps to learn these valve implantation techniques should be practiced on animal hearts.* Unfortunately, this sometimes requires more discipline than the surgeon is prepared to exercise. The implantation of small pig aortic valves into larger pig hearts is an ideal way to familiarize the surgeon with the techniques and the handling of valve tissue to avoid leaflet damage. The author believes no surgeon should insert a stentless valve in a human without such practice (Fig. 121–6). The author personally did this animal valve practice in the mid-1960s with stentless xenografts and allografts and periodically has returned to this at demonstration workshops. The cold storage room at TPCH has a readily available supply of animal hearts and dissected porcine aortic valves as cylinders. These are available for the annual workshop on implantation techniques.

Aortic Root Replacement

A full aortic root replacement with pedicle coronary artery implantation is the technique preferred by the author for primary aortic valve pathology or for primary ascending aortic wall pathology (Marfan's syndrome, annuloaortic ectasia requiring valve replacement as well.) *This technique is therefore used for all replacements and is now described in detail.*

Allograft Preparation

After thawing, the allograft is trimmed. The proximal muscle cuff is left 3 to 4 mm thick and 3 to 4 mm long below the hinge point of the belly of the leaflets. Excess tissue is excised but the adventitia is left on the aorta, which itself is not resected at this stage. If the allograft can be prepared early and its suitability checked, then the subsequent operative steps of preparing the native root with the coronary artery pedicles can proceed uninterrupted.

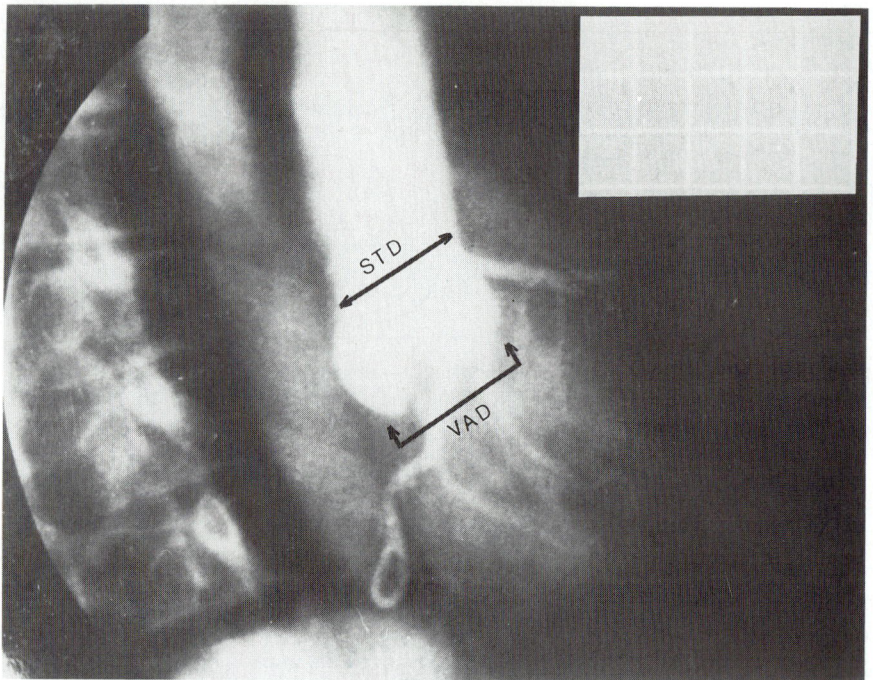

A

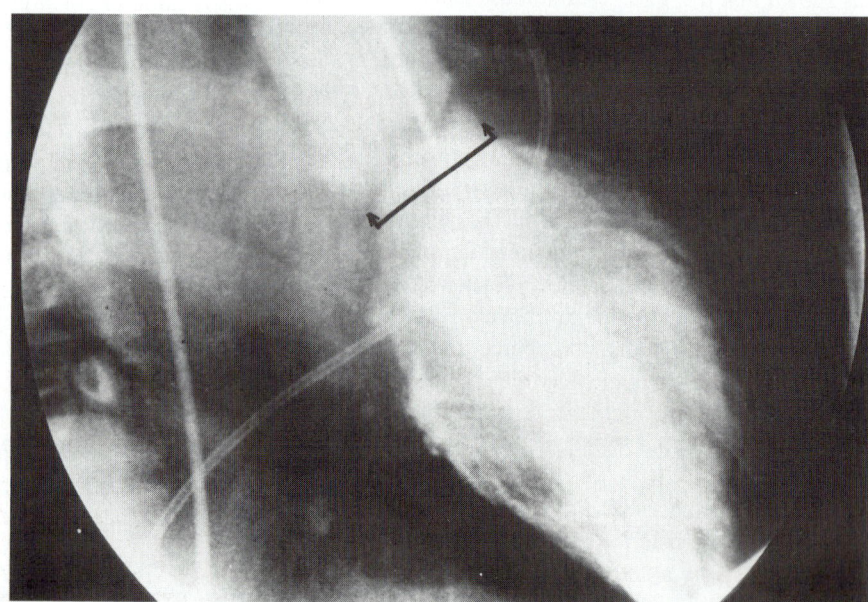

B

Figure 121–4. A. Cineaortogram demonstrating the VAD and STD. A 1.0-cm grid has been incorporated in the film. **B.** Left ventriculogram demonstrating the immediate subaortic valve dimension, which approximates the VAD. *(From O'Brien MF, McGiffin DC, Stafford EG: Allograft aortic valve implantation: Techniques for all types of aortic valve and root pathology. Ann Thorac Surg 48:600, 1989, with permission.)*

Aortic Root Exposure

After establishing cardiopulmonary bypass using the standard technique of mild hypothermia and myocardial protection with antegrade and retrograde cardioplegia, the native aorta is transected just above the sinotubular junction, approximately 1 cm distal to the right coronary ostium. A right angle extension is then made into the noncoronary sinus (Fig. 121–7A). Stay sutures are then placed to splay open the root. The distal ascending aorta is retracted away.

The exposure is uniformly excellent irrespective of the size of the aortic root.

Coronary Artery Pedicles

Leaving at least 5 mm of aortic cuff around the coronary ostia, both pedicles are fashioned with scissors. Care is taken with the right coronary artery always to include the conus branch, which often has a separate orifice. The coronary arteries are mobilized by dissecting outside the aorta

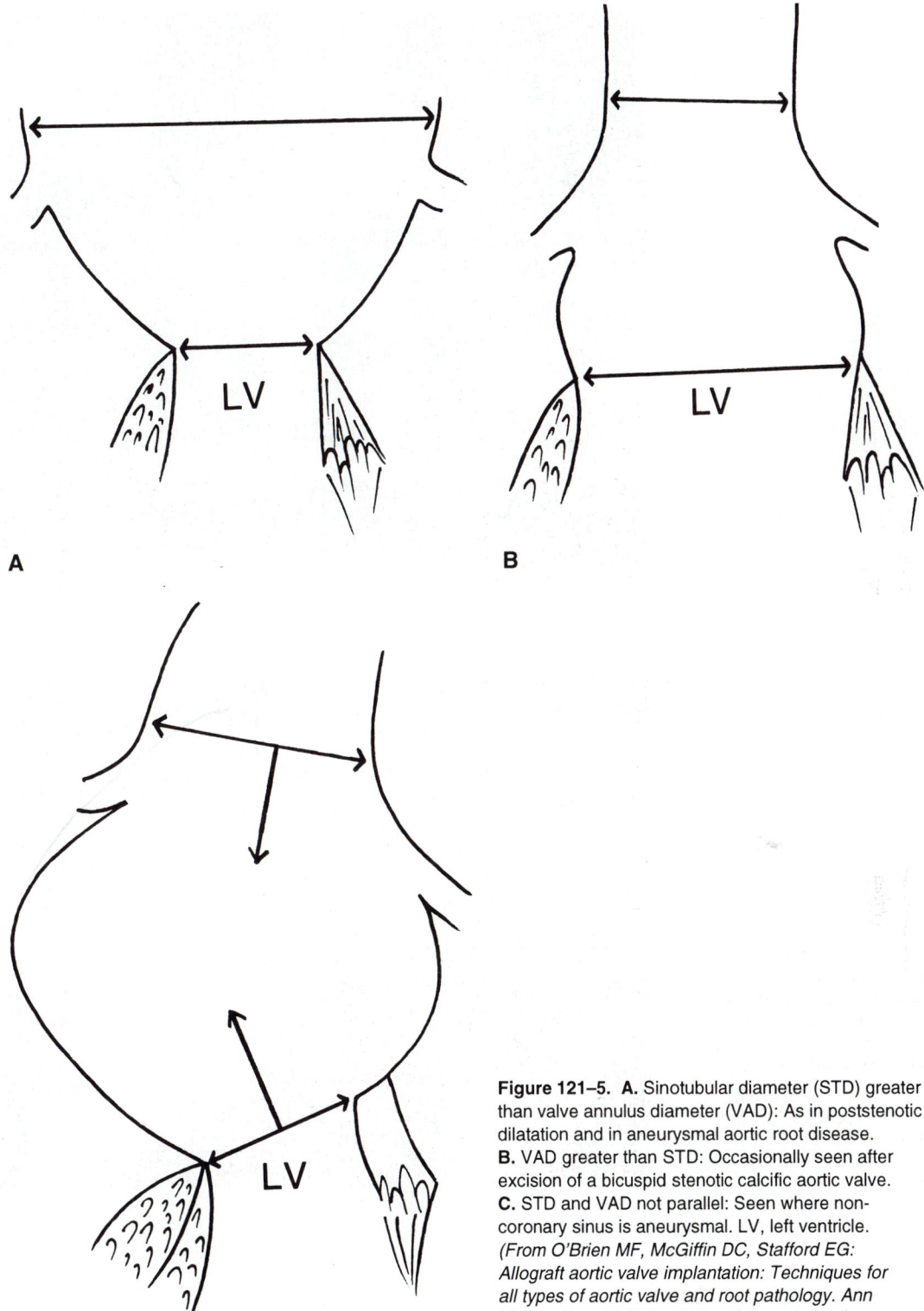

Figure 121–5. A. Sinotubular diameter (STD) greater than valve annulus diameter (VAD): As in poststenotic dilatation and in aneurysmal aortic root disease. **B.** VAD greater than STD: Occasionally seen after excision of a bicuspid stenotic calcific aortic valve. **C.** STD and VAD not parallel: Seen where non-coronary sinus is aneurysmal. LV, left ventricle. *(From O'Brien MF, McGiffin DC, Stafford EG: Allograft aortic valve implantation: Techniques for all types of aortic valve and root pathology. Ann Thorac Surg 48:600, 1989, with permission.)*

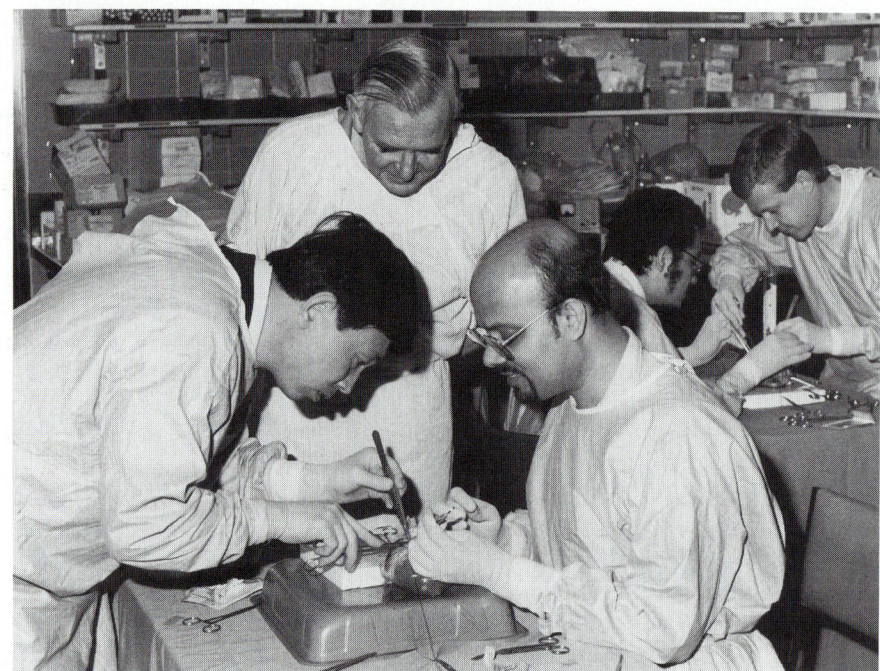

Figure 121–6. A group of young trainee cardiac surgeons from China, India, Saudi Arabia, and Australia practicing implantation techniques (stentless xenograft, pulmonary autograft retrieval, allograft aortic root) at The Prince Charles Hospital in 1992.

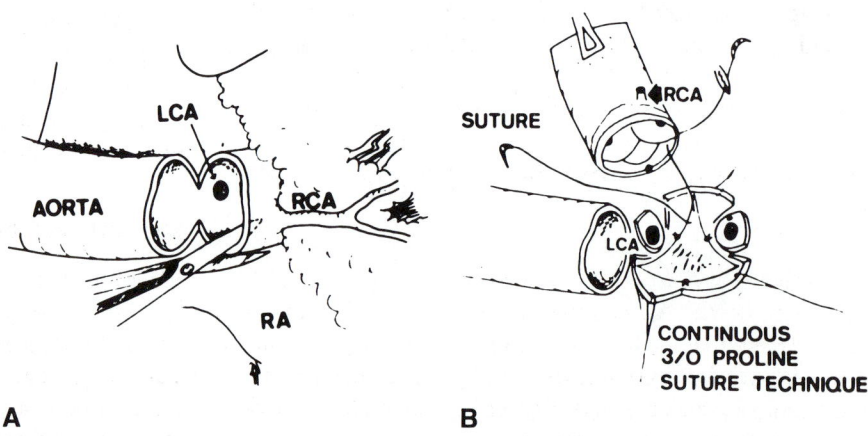

A   B

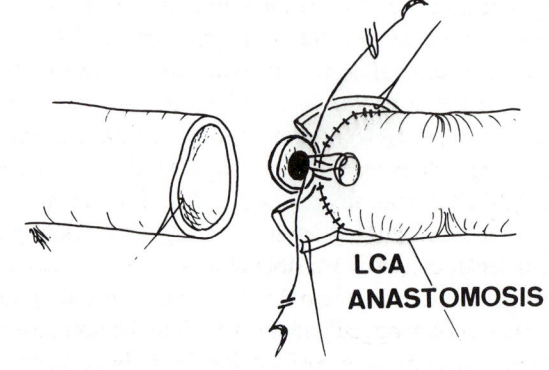

Figure 121–7. A. Aortic incision for root replacement: Transection with T incision into noncoronary sinus. **B.** Transection and coronary pedicles complete. Three equidistant markers in host annulus (fine black silk sutures) and in proximal allograft rim (pencil markers). Continuous 3-0 Prolene suture commences below left lateral commissure. **C.** Left coronary artery pedicle anastomosis with continuous 5-0 Prolene suture. *(From O'Brien MF: Allograft aortic valve replacement. In Trehan N, Kumar A (eds): New Developments in Cardiology and Cardiac Surgery. New Delhi, India, Escorts Heart Institute and Research Center, 1994, pp 313–326, with permission.)*

C

close to its wall. The pedicles should be freed and not tethered by surrounding connective tissue.

Alignment

The allograft is implanted in the anatomic position. To ensure correct alignment of graft and host at annular level, 5-0 black silk marker sutures are placed in the host annulus, first under the left coronary ostium and then at 120° on either side. These points will correspond to the nadir of each cusp of the allograft, which are marked with a surgical pencil (Fig. 121–7B).

Proximal Suture Line

A continuous 3-0 Prolene suture (No. 8936 on a small taper cut V5 half-circle needle) is used. Suturing commences at the left lateral side passing the needle through the allograft from outside to inside at the base of its commissure between the right and left leaflets (Fig. 121–7B). The needle is then passed through the corresponding point of the host annulus. The first few sutures anticlockwise around the posterior annulus are backhand while the rest are forehand. Good bites of both host and allograft tissue are taken approximately 2 to 3 mm apart. This posterior suture is continued around to the anterior position of the noncoronary annulus, the markers (black silk and pencil marks) serving as appropriate matching points. The other arm of the continuous suture is then used to secure the allograft anteriorly from left to right. Sutures through the host annulus follow an imaginary horizontal line passing across the base of each commissure, rising anteriorly to avoid the conducting bundle. The small half-circle needle is ideal to negotiate any slightly difficult access. A constant tension on the suture by the assistant is vital to ensure hemostasis as parts of this suture line are unapproachable once the implantation is complete.

Coronary Pedicle Anastomoses

Occasionally the host coronary buttons or pedicles do not align ideally with the allograft coronary ostia. If such is the case a new 6- to 7-mm hole is made by aortic punch proximal to and occasionally separate from the allograft coronary ostium which may have to be separately closed with a 6-0 double layer continuous Prolene suture. The coronary anastomoses are carried out with continuous 5-0 Prolene. This suture, with smaller needle holes, is more hemostatic than a 4-0 suture. A simple forehand technique again is used for both the left and right anastomoses, running anticlockwise for the lower half and clockwise for the upper half (121–7C). Suture spacing of 2 to 3 mm is critical.

If a satisfactory length of allograft ascending aorta is available, then it is possible at this stage to insert a cardioplegic infusion line into the distal end of the allograft aorta. This can be snugged and infusion into the aorta used to distend it. The precise position for the right coronary anastomosis can be determined. Cardioplegic infusion via the left coronary is achieved by this technique and the anastomosis can be checked at the same time.

Distal Aortic Anastomosis

The allograft is cut to length and tailored to the diameter of the host aorta. Some redundancy in length of aorta is maintained in order to avoid tension and stitch hole bleeding. A forehand technique is again used with 5-0 Prolene commencing on the left through the distal host aorta proceeding anticlockwise posteriorly.

An open appositional technique is used without aortic wrapping. Hemostasis has not been a problem, with only one re-exploration for bleeding in the early postoperative period in over 200 patients undergoing allograft root replacement. This has been accomplished without the use of felt or fibrin glue. In addition, with three deaths in this total consecutive series of allograft aortic root replacements the 30 day mortality has been only 1.5% at The Prince Charles Hospital.

A concern raised by some surgeons is the potential problem of reoperation, as the patient's aortic root is often replaced for valve pathology alone. The argument against this concern is a personal experience with four reoperations. In all cases the allograft did not pose a problem. In two patients a mechanical valve was implanted within the allograft aorta at annular level. And in another two, repeat root replacement with a second allograft was performed. Extensive calcification of the allograft has not been a problem.

The use of the allograft as a root replacement increases the applicability of the valve for the treatment of all pathologies of valve and root. The best valve function from the outset appears to be obtained with this approach. By inference, the long-term durability may further enhance the reasonably good results already attainable with the aortic allograft.

Implantation as Intraluminal Tube or Cylinder

Many of the advantages of the total root replacement over the subcoronary implantation are maintained with the use of the intra-aortic cylinder implantation technique (Fig. 121–8). The native aortic root is preserved—considered by some to be important and advantageous. Coronary anastomoses are still required. The main disadvantage is that the allograft can still be "compressed," as it does not have complete freedom to take its own position. In addition, the position of the side to side coronary anastomosis is far more critical and leaflet deformity in the form of prolapse is still possible, particularly if the allograft coronary ostium is made to oppose the native ostium instead of making a new more proximal hole in the allograft sinus (Fig. 121–9). Nevertheless for those surgeons hesitant to sacrifice the native root or not familiar with root replacement, the cylinder technique has some appeal particularly for a 28- to 30-mm aortic VAD. An annulus of this dimension is seen in the patient with symmetrical trileaflet rheumatic valve incompetence in whom there is leaflet retraction and annular dilata-

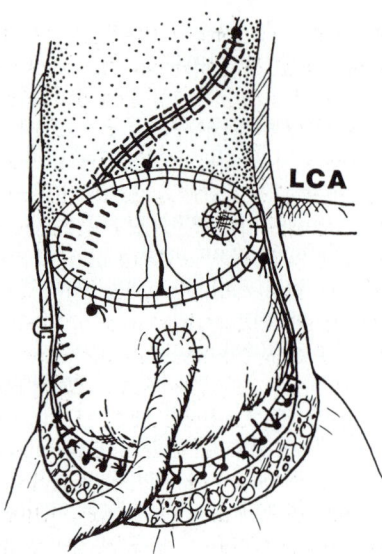

Figure 121–8. Allograft intra-aortic cylinder with side to side coronary artery anastomoses.

tion. Some men with congenital calcific valve stenosis have an annulus larger than 30 mm with associated poststenotic aortic dilatation. The allograft implanted as a scalloped subcoronary valve into an orifice of these sizes often becomes centrally incompetent. For the annulus over 29–30 mm, the preferable options are root replacement or cylinder implantation rather than tailoring the host–aortic annulus and root. By using the allograft valve intact with its aortic sinuses as a short cylindrical tube, in most cases competence can be obtained. An allograft with an internal diameter of 26 mm can be used for a host annulus of 28 to 30 mm.

The allograft is trimmed leaving a 3 to 4 mm cuff

below the leaflets, and superiorly the aortic wall is transected approximately 5 mm above the top of the allograft commissures. The exposure is generally excellent through an oblique or vertical aortotomy incision. The allograft is not rotated and no inversion is performed. The proximal continuous 3-0 or 4-0 Prolene suture line is carried out exactly as for aortic root replacement (Fig. 121–7B). Some surgeons prefer interrupted Prolene sutures (Fig. 121–8). The sinus walls around or more proximal to the coronary ostia of the graft are excised to create appropriate holes. The coronary anastomoses are performed in the same manner as for aortic root replacement except that they are side to side aortic approximations.

Suturing with 5-0 Prolene in a continuous forehand technique taking good close bites of both host and graft tissue is a safe and effective method. Because of the frequent presence of an accessory conus artery arising adjacent to the right coronary artery ostium, this anastomosis may have to be wide transversely to incorporate this vessel. For the distal suture line, three simple 4-0 Prolene sutures approximate the top of the allograft commissure against the host aorta around the sinotubular ridge. These sutures are tied making allowance for the aortotomy, which can be partly closed first. Almost full-thickness bites of the host aortic wall are taken. Should a suture be full thickness, there is generally no major problem with hemostasis later. To minimize or obliterate the space between the cylinder and host aorta, it is wise to appose the two sinus walls in the noncoronary position, either by inserting two mattress sutures or by tacking the host wall to the allograft as the aortotomy incision is closed (Fig. 121–8). The native aorta is not easy to close over the allograft, which may well indicate that this technique does compress the cylinder. To circumvent this

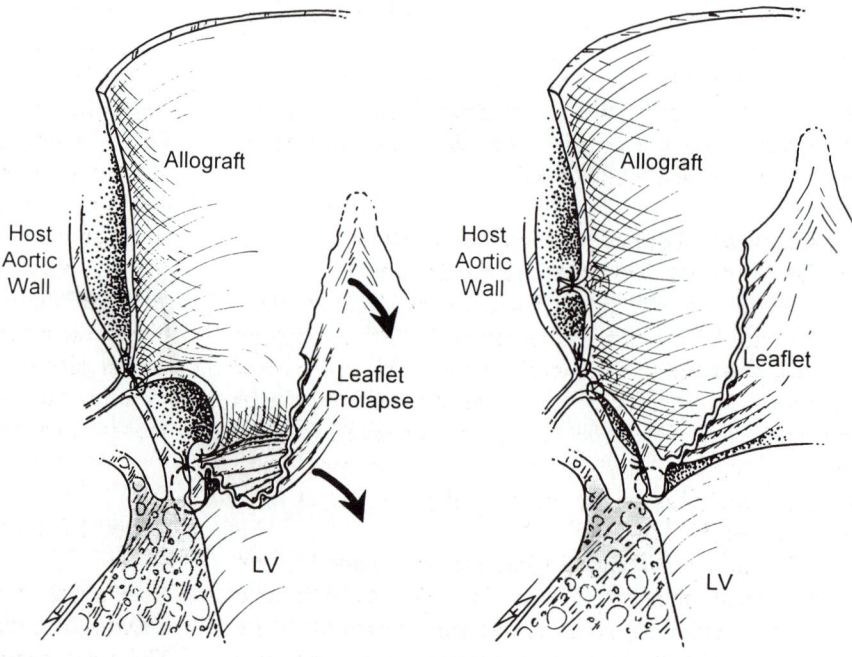

Figure 121–9. A. If coronary ostia are made to approximate one another and are too high, the leaflet may be deformed and may prolapse. **B.** A new more proximal hole in the allograft sinus for the coronary anastomosis prevents the prolapse.

A   B

problem, the surgeon can close the deficiency in the aortotomy above the cylinder with a pericardial patch.

The cylinder allograft is advantageous in providing valve competence for a large host annulus, which is a contraindication to the use of freehand subcoronary implantation techniques.

Subcoronary Implantation

Although since mid-1992 the author no longer uses the subcoronary implantation technique, it is still employed by many and therefore is described.

Valve Trimming

After thawing, the muscle beneath the base of the valve is carefully trimmed down to a thickness of 3 mm. Where a small allograft (18 mm or less in internal diameter) is being used, the muscle should be thinned more than for a larger valve to avoid obstruction by tissue bulk in a small valve orifice. Either at this stage or later, the valve pillars supporting the commissures are fashioned by excising the intervening aortic wall in a "U" shape. This leaves a rim of aorta that is approximately 3 mm wide around the base of each leaflet (Fig. 121–10A). Many surgeons leave the noncoronary sinus aortic wall intact. In addition, variations in this technique include rotating the valve 120° to have the muscle posteriorly and inverting the valve in order to have a clear view (Fig. 121–10B–G). Legitimate arguments against these preferences include the following: Inversion and eversion potentially change the structural support of the leaflet attachment and alter the spatial and precise match of the annular measurements of allograft and host. Rotation changes the normal natural outflow relationship, i.e., the right coronary leaflet is anterior. The author believes that the allograft should be implanted in its natural position and relationship. The published reports of a technique by Barratt-Boyes[22] and by the author[23] are considered now by the latter as inferior methods. Nevertheless, as some surgeons still practise the subcoronary, inversion–eversion rotation technique, it is described in detail.

Subcoronary Technique of Implantation (Valve Annulus Diameter 22 to 29 mm)

The valve is turned inside out and inverted, and the three double-armed 3-0 braided polyester or 3-0 Prolene sutures are then passed in turn through the allograft at the base of each cusp. The equidistant placement of these three sutures in both the host annulus and the graft is considered a most important technical step. The symmetrical insertion of the valve is dependent on the accuracy of placement of these three sutures (Fig. 121–10B).

The allograft is lowered into the left ventricular outflow tract and each suture is tied (Fig. 121–10C). The proximal suture line is begun using one arm of each of the sutures (Fig. 121–10D) in a continuous over and over technique. The important feature of this suture line is that it does not follow the scallops of the host annulus but proceeds in a horizontal line beneath the commissures. The only exception to this is in the region of the membranous septum anteriorly, where the suture line should be through or just below the annulus to avoid injury to the conduction system, which is very close by when the membranous septum is small. The allograft valve is everted back into normal orientation by drawing the pillars up into the aortic root and then placing a stay suture at the top of each pillar (Fig. 121–10E). The distal suture line is performed using three similar sutures. Taking the knots of the previous three sutures of the proximal suture line as the guide, each suture is placed exactly cephalad to this knot.

Therefore, if the first three equidistant sutures of the horizontal layer are correct, then these last three sutures of the distal suture line will also be correct. After tying these three sutures, the distal line is then begun at the noncoronary sinus. One arm of the suture proceeds with an over and over technique along the posterior half of this sinus up to the top of the pillar. The limb of the left coronary suture is then taken along the right side of this sinus to the top of the same posterior pillar. The two sutures at the top are then brought through the pillar, through the host aortic wall and tied outside the aorta without Dacron felt. The other two pillars are sutured in a similar manner (Fig. 121–10F–H). It is very important that each pillar is fixed to the host aortic wall about 1 cm above the top of the host commissural leaflets. This is more likely to ensure leaflet coaptation. In some instances, if one arm of the suture is completed to the top of a pillar, the visualization of the corresponding arm may be more difficult. Therefore it is sometimes easier to suture half-way up on one side and then go to the adjacent suture to complete this to the top of the same pillar. The tops of the pillars 1 cm above the host commissure need to be correctly sited in both the vertical and horizontal planes, particularly the two pillars on each side of the aortotomy incision. The distance between these pillars should be a little greater than the distance between the other pillars to allow for the aortotomy closure. Otherwise a pericardial patch must be incorporated into the aortotomy closure to separate the pillars. On most occasions at least two of the residual host commissures serve as vertical markers over which the allograft pillars can be sutured. If the STD is greater than the VAD, the excess is often corrected by a generous closure of the aortic incision. If it is too small by some 3 to 4 mm in diameter, then a pericardial patch is indicated; it should be inserted before the distal suture line of the allograft is begun and before the allograft pillars are sited.

Special Situations

Small Aortic Root (Valve Annulus Diameter Less Than 21 mm)

This small annulus is seen more frequently in women and children with congenital valve stenosis. The valve is

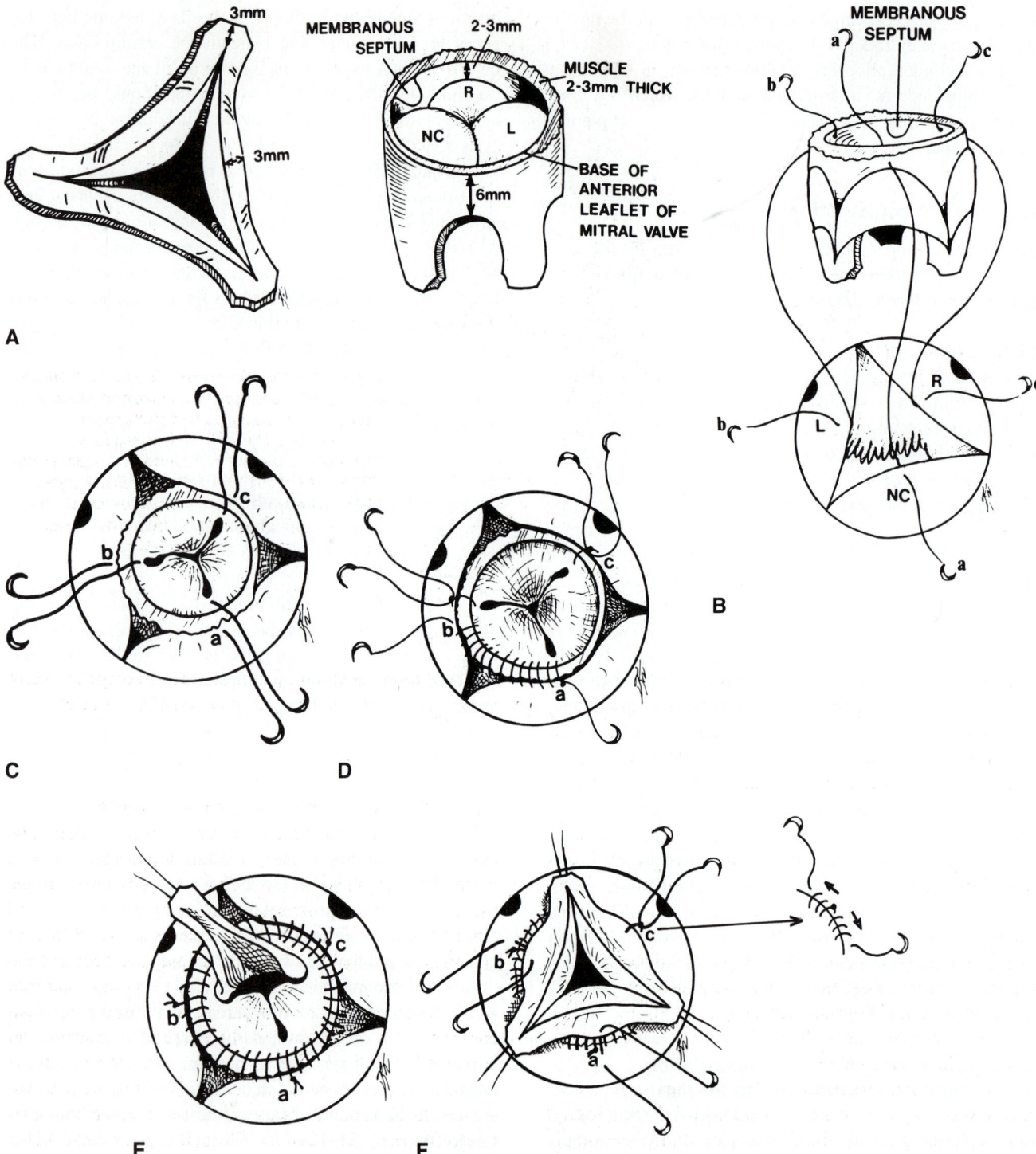

Figure 121–10. A. Appearances and dimensions of the allograft after trimming. **B.** The valve is turned inside out and then inverted. Three sutures (a,b,c) are placed for the proximal suture line. **C.** The valve is lowered into the left ventricular outflow tract. **D.** The proximal suture line is commenced. **E.** The commissures or pillars are brought up into the aortic root. Stay sutures are attached to the adventitia of each pillar. **F.** Sutures for the distal suture line are placed. *(Continued.)*

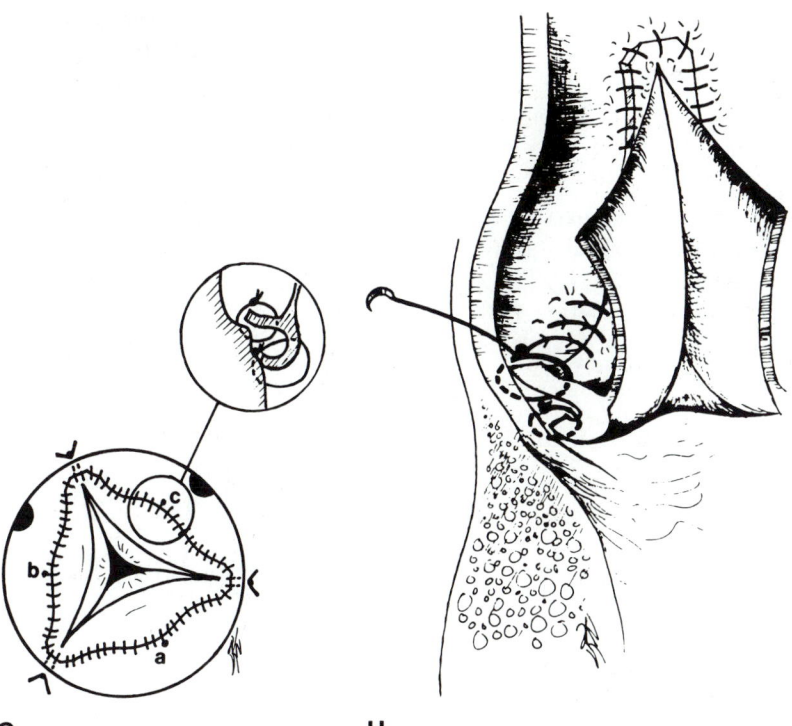

G   **H**

Figure 121–10. *(Continued.)* **G.** The distal suture line is performed, beginning at the noncoronary sinus. **H.** The subcoronary implantation is complete. Inversion-eversion technique is illustrated. L, left; NC, noncoronary; R, right. *(From O'Brien MF, McGiffin DC, Stafford EG: Allograft aortic valve implantation: Techniques for all types of aortic valve and root pathology. Ann Thorac Surg 48:600, 1989, with permission.)*

trileaflet in the elderly as a degenerative lesion, or bicuspid or rarely unicuspid. A previous valvotomy has often been performed. The small root is seen in tunnel aortic stenosis with marked obstruction of the left ventricular outflow tract. This may require aortic root replacement[24] or aortoventriculoplasty[25] techniques combined with aortic valve replacement.

A small annulus of 19 mm diameter in an *active* patient whose body surface area is greater than 1.5 m^2 is enlarged by a pericardial or Dacron gusset.[26,27] A 7-mm-wide patch (after suturing) enlarges the VAD from 19 to 21 mm, enabling an allograft valve of 19 mm internal diameter to be inserted. In smaller patients annular enlargement may not be necessary as an allograft with an internal diameter of 16 mm can be inserted into a 19-mm host root without a clinically significant gradient.[28]

The technical modifications for allograft implantation into the small aortic root are to avoid inverting the allograft while performing the proximal suture line and to use simple interrupted 4-0 Prolene sutures. Without inversion of the valve, excessive allograft tissue bulk in the left ventricular outflow tract is avoided (Fig. 121–11). Likewise, continuous suturing is not feasible in the small root as the valve needs to be held out of the aortic root to provide exposure. Although rotating the valve 120° to the left is not essential, it does bring the allograft muscle bulk posteriorly with less turbulence possibly than if it were left in the natural anterior position. The distal continuous suture line is the same as described for the subcoronary technique. The selected allograft with an internal diameter 2 mm less than the annular

diameter of the host should still produce a competent valve in this small root (see later for selection of valve size).

Large Asymmetrical Noncoronary Sinus

When the noncoronary leaflet is larger than the other two leaflets, its coronary sinus is often aneurysmal or vice versa. This anatomical anomaly presents difficulty with the usual implantation technique. The allograft commissural posts should not be aligned with the nonequidistant host commissures, otherwise leaflet prolapse and poor coaptation would occur and the incidence of valve incompetence would be unacceptable. This can be minimised if the noncoronary sinus aortic wall of the allograft is retained and implanted. The distal suture line of the noncoronary sinus is horizontally placed around the host sinotubular ridge as advocated by Ross and associates[29] for the implantation of all allografts (Fig. 121–12). The allograft is not rotated and is best not inverted for the first proximal horizontal suture layer. The excess host aneurysmal sinus wall can be excised, or incorporated into a generous aortotomy closure, which is commenced before the distal allograft wall is sutured into place. If the space between the two walls is excessive, it may be wise to insert one or two through and through mattress sutures to minimize this space or as previously to include the allograft sinus in the aortotomy closure. Retaining the allograft sinus wall reduces the chance of malalignment of the three valve pillars and is more likely to provide a competent valve.

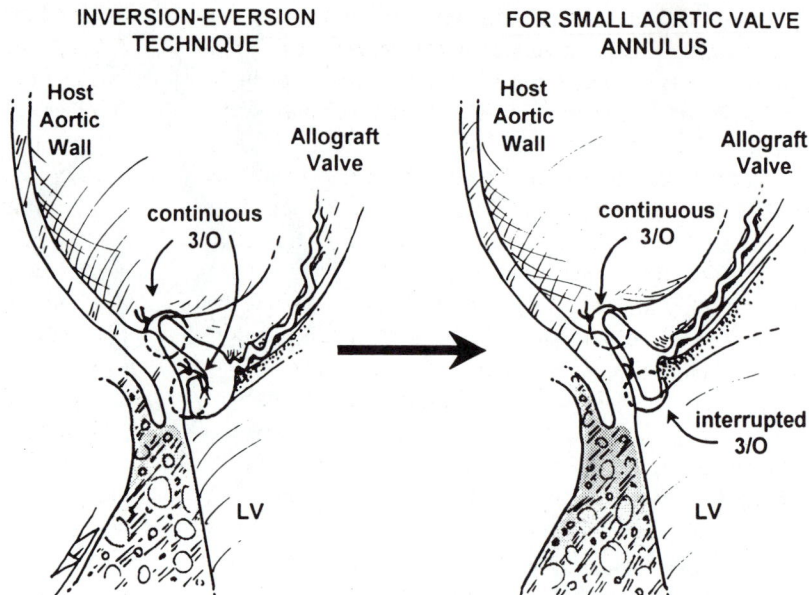

INVERSION-EVERSION TECHNIQUE

FOR SMALL AORTIC VALVE ANNULUS

Figure 121–11. With the small aortic valve annulus, avoidance of the inversion technique minimizes the amount of allograft tissue within the annulus.

Aortic Root Infection and Implantation Techniques

If endocarditis is confined to the native valve leaflets, some surgeons use the allograft as a subcoronary implant or as an intraluminal cylinder depending upon the root measurements. With annular or subannular abscesses into the mitral

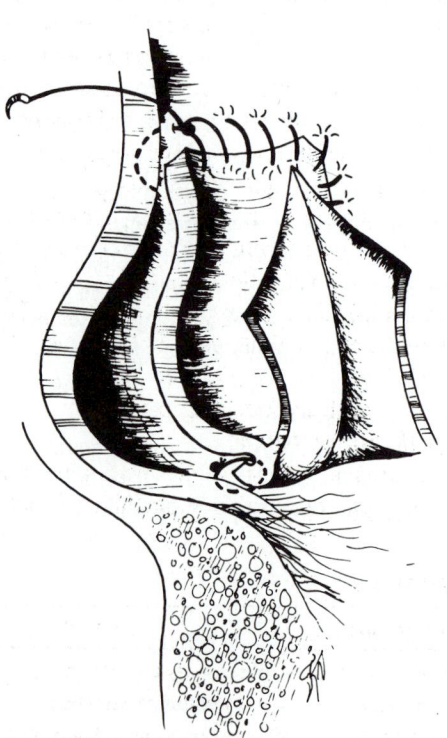

Figure 121–12. Retention of the noncoronary sinus wall of the allograft when the host noncoronary sinus is aneurysmal. *(From O'Brien MF, McGiffin DC, Stafford EG: Allograft aortic valve implantation: Techniques for all types of aortic valve and root pathology. Ann Thorac Surg 48:600, 1989, with permission.)*

valve annulus or into the ventricular muscle, the aortic root may be extensively destroyed even to the degree of left ventriculoaortic discontinuity. *The important principle is to exclude abscess cavities from the circulation.* Closing an abscess cavity with attempts to reapproximate the discontinuity or cover it with pericardium may leave a blood-filled space and an ideal culture medium. Ross and associates[30,31] have demonstrated the efficacy of total root replacement, excluding the abscess cavities from the circulation. Nevertheless, in less extensively destroyed roots, Kirklin and colleagues[32] have sutured the proximal rim and distal sinus wall of the scalloped subcoronary allograft to the edges of the cavities, obliterating or roofing over the abscess with allograft tissue. In this small experience, the allograft has remained competent. However, if the cavity is an active infective pocket, the chances of obtaining a good result may be marred with persistent infection. In general, for the treatment of aortic valve endocarditis, the author sees an even stronger indication for the use of the root replacement technique.

Selecting the Appropriate Allograft Size

Mistakes have been made in the past by selecting too small an allograft. Although the combined thickness of opposite sides of the base of the allograft valve (muscle on one side, mitral valve leaflet remnant on the other—Fig. 121–10A) is approximately 3 to 4 mm, much of this tissue especially the muscle is absorbed after implantation. Consequently the amount of leaflet coaptation changes. If too small a valve is inserted, subsequent incompetence is likely to occur. In the past,[23] we recommended that the internal diameter of the selected allograft be 3 to 4 mm less than the measured host valve annulus diameter. As leaflet distortion is more likely with subcoronary artery techniques, coupled with this muscle absorption, this undersizing error increased the incidence of mild postoperative incompetence. It is now recommended that, for *subcoronary implantation* except in the small aortic root (see previously), the internal diameter of the allograft should be the same as that of the host annulus.

For both the *cylinder* and *root replacement* techniques, a longer proximal allograft tissue cuff can be left, the diameter of which is larger than the actual valve annulus diameter. Therefore differences of as much as 3 to 5 mm between host and allograft annuli have been acceptable. If a long proximal cuff is left and the valve is not sutured well down virtually below the host annulus, the coronary artery ostia rarely match. New holes in the allograft sinus are necessary and these may finish up being very close to the leaflet attachment. So, if more than one allograft is available for selection, it is preferable to use that valve that approximates the host size. For *root replacement* with coronary artery pedicles or buttons for anastomoses, size matching is less critical. For example, the author has inserted a 25- to 26-mm allograft valve with a good proximal cuff, into a patient, very anxious to have an allograft valve, with a host annulus of 35 mm. The valve has remained competent long-term.

Summary of Technical Methods

It is of some importance for the surgeon to be familiar with the *range of options* of techniques, even though many of these are considered by the author as obsolete. These options have been previously summarized[23] in relationship to the host–graft annulus diameters, inversion, rotation, continuous or interrupted proximal suture line, and overall method, and are summarized in Table 121–1.

The reader is reminded that Table 121–1 epitomizes the complexity of techniques. It reinforces the author's argument that these variations are too difficult for the surgeon who is fully aware that a quick St Jude mechanical valve implant guarantees a high survival with minimal potential technical risks.[33] What gives best results for the individual patient must always "call the tune."

The author has, therefore, long since dispensed with these options and replaced everything with the one standard total root replacement irrespective of whatever variations (anatomic and pathologic) are present in the aortic root.

Is Root Replacement Too Radical?

When primary aortic wall disease in association with valve dysfunction is present, root replacement is essential. However, for primary valve disease, the standard technique of implantation of any device has generally been, for the last three decades, into the subcoronary position. In all situations, is complete root replacement with an allograft unnecessary and too radical? In spite of the many advantages already outlined, the theoretical problems relate to "dismantling" the root, the extent of aortic calcification at reoperation, and the type of surgery required at rereplacement if such becomes necessary.

Five of the 193 patients in the TPCH series (November 1985 to October 1994) have required repeat AVR. Two patients with endocarditis had a repeat allograft aortic root replacement without problem. Two patients with dysfunction due to structural degeneration at 2.7 and 7.5 years had implanted at reoperation a St Jude mechanical valve implanted within the allograft aortic wall at reoperation. The remaining patient with leaflet prolapse of uncertain cause at 6 mo postimplant also had a St Jude valve inserted within the allograft aorta. No undue operative problems were encountered due to the patient's aortic root having been "sacrificed" at the first operation and all patients had uncomplicated recoveries.

Yacoub,[34] with a longer clinical experience of root replacement since 1976, performed 15 reoperations in 14 patients at a mean of 109 mo (range 19 to 204). They were for degeneration (*n* = 9) and endocarditis (*n* = 6). Linear eggshell calcification was common but never involved the host coronary artery "buttons." In six patients a mechanical valve was inserted within the allograft and four patients had a subcoronary allograft. A second root replacement with repeat coronary artery reimplantation was carried out for five patients. There was no 30 day mortality nor any reoperation for hemorrhage. These results led Yacoub and colleagues to state that "reoperations following aortic root replacement can be accomplished by using one of several options without an increased risk of either early or late death."[34]

Comparison of Surgical Techniques of Allograft Implantation

With the continuing debate on the most appropriate technique for allograft aortic valve implantation[35] and with the

---

TABLE 121–1. ALLOGRAFT AORTIC VALVE REPLACEMENT: TECHNICAL VARIATIONS

Host Annulus Diameter	Inversion	120° Rotation	Proximal Suture Line	Method
1. Small ≤ 21 mm	No	Yes	Interrupted Proline 3-0 or 4-0	*Subcoronary* implantation
2. Normal size 22–29 mm	Yes/No	Yes/No	Interrupted or continuous	*Subcoronary* implantation
3. Asymmetrical, large noncoronary sinus	Yes/No	No	Interrupted or continuous	*Subcoronary* implantation, retention of noncoronary sinus wall of allograft
4. Moderately large annulus ≥ 30 mm	No	No	Continuous	*Intraluminal cylinder* (side to side coronary anastomoses)
5. Annuloaortic ectasia ascending aortic aneurysm	No	No	Continuous	*Root replacement* with coronary pedicle implantation

author's recommendation that all allografts should be implanted as root replacements, it is relevant to compare techniques under 10 headings (Table 121–2). The *subcoronary implantation* produces a valve with a risk of distortion and incompetence, with reasonable difficulty in implantation but with minimal actual and potential risks of technical complications (excluding malalignment). The *intraluminal cylinder* scores better on most points compared to the subcoronary implantation. *Root replacement* scores well in most aspects. Potential, but not actual in most clinical series, is the risk of operative hemorrhage. Rereplacement still has all options open, but excessive calcification of the allograft wall, in particular, may necessitate repeat root replacement. Rereplacement with a mechanical prosthesis within the allograft aorta has been a satisfactory and proven option.

THE CLINICAL PERFORMANCES OF ALLOGRAFT AORTIC VALVE SURGERY

The aim of surgery is to select the optimal timing in recommending to our patient an operation of low mortality and morbidity using an implant device that carries long-term the lowest incidence of morbid complications for that particular individual in his or her particular environment.

A complex interaction takes place between the severity of the aortic valve disease of the particular sick patient, who probably has associated or other system pathologies, the technical expertise of the whole hospital team, and the particular attributes of the implant tissue with one valve type being subtly different from that of another valve of the same type (see later in Comparisons: The Problems).

Brisbane Experience (The Prince Charles Hospital—1969 to January 1994)

Allograft aortic valve replacement has been performed on 804 patients.[18,36,37] From December 1969 to May 1975, 124 patients received a nonviable valve sterilized by incubation with low dose antibiotics (see protocol previously) and stored for weeks by refrigeration at 4°C (nonviable allograft, NVA). From June 1975 to January 1994, 680 patients received a viable cryopreserved allograft (VCA). Of this latter group, 146 have received a total aortic root replacement.

The patient characteristics of the two groups (NVA and VCA) were similar in age at operation (median ages 50.5 and 54 years). The age range of patients was 13 to 72 and 3 to 80 years with males predominating at 67 and 61.6%, respectively. The follow-up of this analysis had a closing date at 1 July 1994 for the inclusion of events and was 98.3% complete. Several patients in Pacific Islands were difficult to contact. The 30 day mortality was $8.9 \pm 5\%$ (95% confidence limits, CL) for NVA patients and $2.8 \pm 1\%$ (95% CL) for VCA patients. The actuarial patient survival (Fig. 121–13) at 15 years was $56 \pm 5\%$ (NVA) and $62 \pm 5\%$ (VCA). As with all published series [38] with a wide age range of patients, this drop in survival is primarily due to nonvalve cardiac and noncardiac reasons.

Thromboembolism

The freedom from thromboembolism was high for isolated AVR ± CABG and all allografts having associated mitral valve surgery (Fig 121–14). This is typical of the allograft and without the need for anticoagulants, this freedom from such a morbid event is very appealing. While the allograft

TABLE 121–2. AORTIC ROOT REPLACEMENT COMPARISON OF TECHNIQUES

	Subcoronary Implantation	Intra-aortic Cylinder	Root Replacement
Risk of allograft distortion	Moderately high	Minimal	Almost nil; allograft geometry maintained
Immediate competence	Less likely	Moderate guarantee	High guarantee
Surgical difficulty 0–4 grades, 4 = most difficult	3–4	3	2–3
Operative hemorrhage	Very low	Very low	Potentially high (not in this study and 34 others)
Compression of allograft	Nil	Moderate risk (if blood flow between the layers)	Nil
False aneurysm	Nil	Low risk	Low risk
Coronary artery problems	Virtually nil	Low risk (coronary artery distortion if blood flow between layers)	Low risk of malalignment
Fate of host root	Root preserved	Root preserved	Root "sacrificed"
Reoperation procedure with second allograft	Repeat AVR with all three options still available	Difficult allograft removal, repeat cylinder difficult, root replacement still possible	Requires second root replacement (other options possible)
Possibility of mechanical valve	Yes—no problem	Yes—may be possible within allograft cylinder	Yes—no problem unless aorta excessively calcified

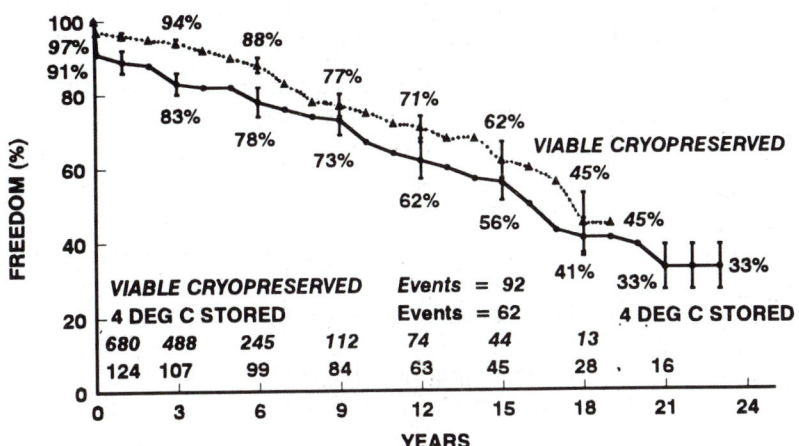

Figure 121–13. The actuarial percent survival after allograft aortic valve replacement using the 4°C stored valve (n = 124, deaths = 62) and the cryopreserved valve (n = 680, deaths = 92). Hospital mortality is included in all actuarial analyses. For this and subsequent figures, the patient numbers at risk in each series are expressed at 3 year intervals. The percent freedom and the standard error (±1) are indicated.

is considered not to have thromboembolic events in the absence of endocarditis, cardiovascular patients do have a baseline level of such events. It is presumed that intracardiac chambers or atheromatous aortacarotids can be the foci of thromboembolism in this patient series.

Endocarditis

Nine and 14 patients in the NVA and VCA groups, respectively, developed endocarditis following implantation. The actuarial freedom from endocarditis at 15 years was 91 ± 3% and 94 ± 2%, respectively for the two series (Fig. 121–15). Table 121–3 expresses the number of patients who died, underwent reoperation, or were cured medically. Eight of the 23 patients having endocarditis were cured medically.

Studies at TPCH confirm those of others[39,40] showing that the instantaneous risk of the development of early or late postoperative infection of the allograft aortic valve is low and constant. This risk compares favorably with that of infection of mechanical and bioprosthetic valves with their higher early phase of risk declining to emerge with a low

and constant risk. In addition, specifically in the treatment of active aortic valve endocarditis, the persistence of infection or late recurrence risk was similarly low for the allograft in the TPCH analysis[41] compared to the risk with mechanical and xenograft valves (Fig. 121–16). This was confirmed by Haydock and colleagues.[42]

Reoperation

Reoperation was performed for significant allograft valve dysfunction due to valve leaflet degeneration, endocarditis, or technical reasons (including valve repair in four patients). Table 121–4 summarized the operative indications. The actuarial freedom from reoperation for these causes at 15 years for NVA valves was 58 ± 6% and for VCA valves 78 ± 4% (Fig. 121–17). The differences between the two series became apparent at 12 years. There was 1 patient and 17 patients in the two groups, respectively, who had subsequent cardiac operations for other reasons such as CABG or mitral valve surgery. They are not included in this analysis as the allograft was left untouched.

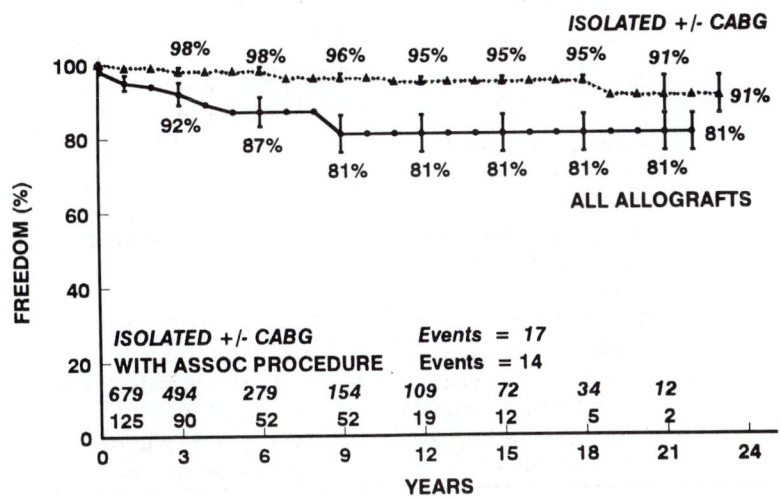

Figure 121–14. The actuarial percent freedom from thromboembolism for patients having AVR ± coronary artery bypass grafts (17 events) and AVR ± associated procedures (mitral valve surgery etc) (14 events). The presentation is as in Figure 121–13.

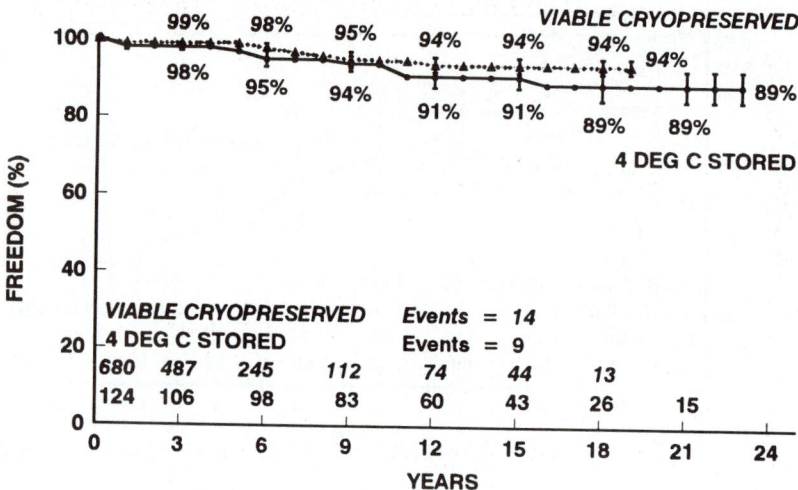

Figure 121–15. The actuarial percent freedom from allograft valve endocarditis for the NVA valves (9 events) and for the VCA valves (14 events). The presentation is as in Figure 121–13.

Structural Deterioration

The incidence of reoperation alone is an underestimation of the prevalence of structural deterioration (SD). An analysis was therefore made of the SD detected at reoperation, on clinical assessment of the presence of moderate or severe aortic valve incompetence or at death with a dysfunctional valve. Table 121–5 categorizes the patient numbers in each group. At 15 years, the actuarial freedom from SD was $45 \pm 6\%$ for NVA valves and $80 \pm 5\%$ for VCA valves (p value for the difference is zero) (Fig. 121–18). A reasonable extrapolation of the VCA curve suggests a freedom from SD of 70 to 75% at 20 years.

Clinical Analysis of Allograft Root Replacement

An additional clinical analysis of root replacement has been made with the aim of subsequently comparing this subset to the subcoronary implant series. From November 1985 to October 1994, 192 patients have received an allograft aortic root replacement (AARR) with 3 postoperative deaths (30 day mortality 1.5%). A more detailed study of the first 146 patients to January 1994 has been made.[43] The follow-up was 100% complete. Valve dysfunction (91 patients), primary aortic wall disease (45 patients), and a combination of both (10 patients) were the indications for AARR. Four late deaths gave an 8 year actuarial survival of 85 ± 8 (95% confidence limits). Important morbid events have included en-

docarditis (two events), thromboembolism (four events), and structural deterioration (two events). Comparing the subcoronary implanted cryopreserved valves, the AARR at 8 years is showing no statistical difference in patient survival, freedom from reoperation (all causes), and freedom from structural deterioration. As the major problems of durability become apparent during the second decade of follow-up, one would not expect the AARR series to show any difference at this stage. The freedom from both minor and major degrees of incompetence with the AARR and the reduction in reoperation due to technically induced valve incompetence constitute the major superior difference in the root compared with the nonroot groups at this stage.

Comparison of Clinical Results: The Problems

Mechanical valve models are "stable products" and the performance of such a model can be validly compared from one unit to another. However, a clinical comparative analysis of the aortic allograft valve is virtually impossible to make because of the large number of variables.[14] These factors include donor characteristics, procurement, sterilization, preservation, and storage protocols, the *uniform adherence* to these protocols, the implantation techniques, and the overall experience of the surgical team.

The surgeon must realize that the allograft is not a "uniform product." The donor age influences the extensibil-

TABLE 121–3. ALLOGRAFT AORTIC VALVE ENDOCARDITIS

Group	n	Incidence		Cured Medically	Totally
		Death	Reoperation		
NVA (4°C stored)	124	3[a]	3[a]	4	9 (7.3%)
VCA (cryopreserved)	680	3[b]	8[b]	4	14 (2.0%)

[a]One patient in both groups.
[b]One patient in both groups.

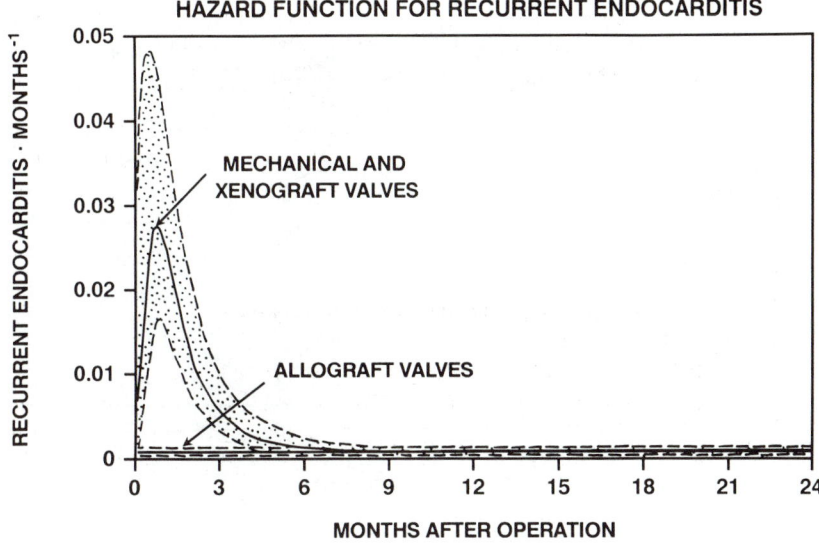

HAZARD FUNCTION FOR RECURRENT ENDOCARDITIS

Figure 121–16. Instantaneous risk or hazard function for recurrent endocarditis for mechanical, xenograft, and allograft valves with 70% confidence limits (dotted lines). *(From McGiffin DC, Galbraith AJ, McLachlan GJ, et al: Aortic valve infection: Risk factors for death and recurrent endocarditis following aortic valve replacement. J Thorac Cardiovasc Surg 104:511, 1992, with permission.)*

ity of leaflet tissue.[44] The warm ischemic time (death to collection) and the many factors of the preservation protocol influence qualitatively the leaflet viability and the integrity of noncellular fibrin and nonfibrin matrix.[14,19,45] For instance, in the TPCH series, an autopsy derived valve has a mean death to cryopreservation time of 22 hours, multiorgan valve (8 to 12 hours), and valve from a transplant patient (1 to 2 hours). Many valves in other institutions and tissue banks are not cryopreserved for days after collection. Homovital valves (supposedly used without antibiotic sterilization within 24 hours of collection) are often not implanted for 36 to 72 hours. Most valves are given 48 hours of antibiotic sterilization. In the TPCH experience, the antibiotic exposure period never exceeded 24 hours and since 1988 has been 6 hours. From the author's experience in reviewing the protocols from tissue banks and hospital valve banks, there is a vast range of every variable such that comparison of the clinical results even from within the one institution using the same valve bank is difficult. The TPCH protocol is the most rigid and yet the author believes that grouping all TPCH cryopreserved valves together still sees a heterogeneous group. Multivariable analyses of factors within the one institution are necessary. For this reason, the TPCH group have always compared its results of the antibi-

otic sterilized 4°C stored series with its cryopreserved series (the viability of which has always been qualitatively tested).

A multivariable analysis helps in predicting important factors such as age of donor, recipient, and ABO matching,[36] but the finer points of valve characteristics are often not known in many institutions. This creates difficulties when one is deciphering the factors controlling 15 and 20 year freedoms from structural deterioration. Lastly, the designation of a valve as being "cryopreserved" is often accepted as a valve that is "viable." This is obviously not correct. In essence, no two "cryopreserved" valves are the same and they may not behave the same. Therefore the clinical results of cryopreserved valves from one institution can hardly be compared in a meaningful statistical manner to those of another institution. The methodology requires detailed description in any report.[14]

Clinical Results from Other Units

Bodnar, Ross, and colleagues[46,47] analyzed 619 allograft valves implanted from June 1964 to December 1988. The antibiotic-sterilized nutrient medium-stored valves behaved no better than the freeze-dried irradiated valves. The 10-year freedom from primary tissue failure [defined as death

TABLE 121–4. ALLOGRAFT AORTIC VALVE REOPERATION

Operative Indication	NVA 4°C Stored Group		VCA Cryopreserved Group	
	n = 40	% of 40	n = 43	% of 43
Deterioration (70% confidence limits)	35	88 (74–96)	15	35 (21–53)
Endocarditis (70% confidence limits)	3	8 (2–21)	9	21 (38–11)
Technical (70% confidence limits)	2	5 (1–17)	19	44 (28–62)

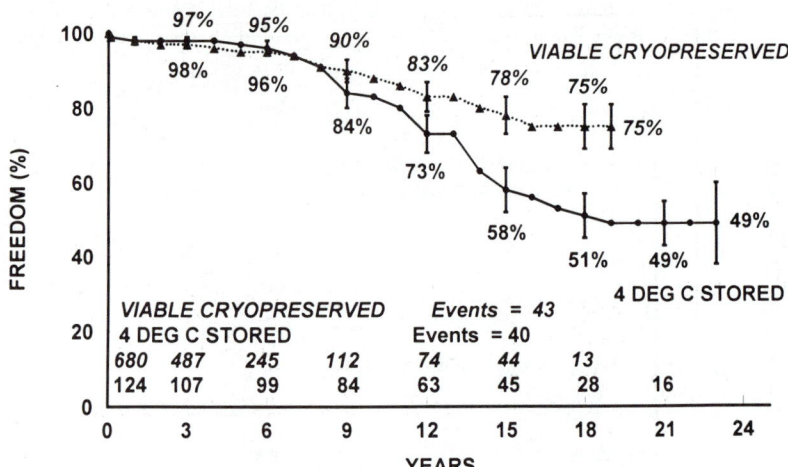

Figure 121–17. The actuarial percent freedom from reoperation for *all causes* (degeneration, endocarditis, and technical) for NVA group (events = 40) and for VCA (events = 43). The presentation is as in Figure 121–13.

due to structural deterioration (SD) or reoperation for SD] was 59 ± 5% and 50 ± 7% (NS), respectively. This 1989 analysis was described as follows: "Aortic homografts have proven themselves as an excellent choice for aortic or pulmonary valve replacement."[46] However, in this decade of the 1990s, it is hoped that the 10-year freedom from intrinsic failure would be a far higher percentage, otherwise the use of such a valve should be discontinued. Homografts are not "an excellent choice" unless clinical results are obtained that are much better than those described above.

Barratt-Boyes et al[48] analyzed the long-term results of the antibiotic sterilized aortic valves. A series of 252 aortic allografts were followed for a mean of 10.8 years. Freedom from significant incompetence due to "valve wear" was 95% at 5 years, 78% at 10 years, and 42% at 14 years. If the poor risk patients are excluded, i.e. donor age ≥ 55 years, recipient age < 15 years and aortic root diameter over 30 mean, the freedom from significant incompetence due to valve wear is 98% at 5 years, 94% at 9 years, and 56% at 13 years. Not stated, however, in this publication, is the important fact that beginning at 10 years is a rapid decline, the actuarial freedom being at this time approximately 83%. *Within 4 years* there is a fall from 94 to 56% (i.e., 38%) in the freedom from significant incompetence.

These results were similar to the published data from Khaghani, Yacoub and colleagues,[49] SD being defined as degeneration of the valve at death, reoperation, or in patients with severe incompetence. This definition is the same as that of TPCH. Freedom from valve failure (SD) at 10

years was 77% and 48% at 15 years. These several results, coupled with the initial TPCH antibiotic 4°C series (NVA group), highlighted the *one significant feature,* namely, that the antibiotic-stored valve gave acceptable results for approximately 8 to 9 years and then the valve failure rate increased markedly. In the subsequent 6 years to the 15-year follow-up point the percentage freedom from SD fell approximately 40%, expecting to reach the 15% freedom from SD at 20 years. These are inferior results and, in the opinion of the author, they do not justify the continuing use of this type of homograft (TPCH group discontinued its use in 1975).

A comparative study of allografts, xenografts, and mechanical valves from TPCH indicates that the St Jude mechanical disc valve gives far superior results compared to those of the antibiotic-sterilized 4°C stored allograft in terms of freedom from all death and morbid events.

Yacoub and co-workers[50] analyzed a specific group of 270 patients who received allografts taken sterile and kept at 4°C in tissue culture medium for a mean of 3.9 days before insertion. These "unprocessed aortic valve homografts" gave the probability of freedom from valve failure due to any cause at 97.8 and 91.2% at 5 and 10 years. These results of "homovital" valves and near homovital valves (implanted beyond 24 hours) must be considered as very satisfactory at 10 years with no evidence of accelerated rejection. The 15 year results of this series will be crucial in providing important data for our understanding of the performance from "early" valve implantation of a noncryopreserved valve. They can then be compared to the TPCH experience with early valve cryopreservation.

An important contribution came from Alabama in 1993. Kirklin et al[51] analyzed their 10-year results of cryopreserved aortic allografts in 178 patients. This study is essentially the only intermediate-term analysis that commences to match the TPCH long-term experience. Although there are differences in valve source (all from multiorgan donors), tissue preservation (different antibiotics, longer duration of exposure, and longer time interval before cryo-

TABLE 121–5. STRUCTURAL DETERIORATION FOR ALLOGRAFT AORTIC VALVES

	NVA (n = 54)	VCA (n = 21)
Clinical valve dysfunction	4	5
Reoperation for SD	35	15
Death with valve SD	15	1

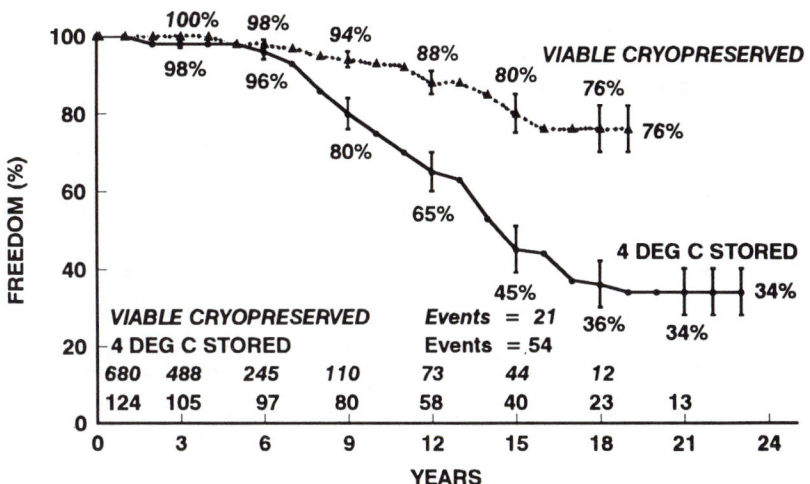

Figure 121–18. The actuarial percent freedom from structural deterioration for NVA valves (events = 54) and for VCA valves (events = 21). The *p* value for the difference is close to zero. The presentation is as in Figure 121–13.

preservation), the study is very relevant to the total knowledge of the fate and function of the allograft valve. The median age of the patient cohort was 46 years (range 9 months to 80 years). The overall survival at 8 years was 85% and for those patients who had isolated aortic valve replacement the survival was 94% at 8 years. Freedom from explantation was 95% at 8 years and from presumed leaflet failure (including also patients with Grade 3/4 aortic insufficiency) was 85% at 8 years. By multivariable analysis, younger patient age was the only risk factor identified for leaflet failure. In patients aged 20 to 50 years, the 8-year freedom from presumed leaflet failure was approximately 75% after 8 years. It would appear that these 8 to 10 year results are marginally inferior to those of Yacoub using the "unprocessed aortic valve homografts."

The author believes that there are many deficiencies in our knowledge and many challenging improvements yet to institute. But, at the present time, the only allograft for aortic valve replacement that should be used is the homovital valve (inserted within 24 hours of collection from beating

heart donors) or the cryopreserved valve that has been sterilized and preserved preferably well within 24 hours of donor death. Although these are personal views, they are derived from the above data and appear justified. It does suggest that many of the valves in use today would not fall within these recommendations. This rigid protocol of early use or early cryopreservation may perhaps explain why the TPCH results are far superior to those of other workers.

Comparative Analysis of Reoperation with Other Tissue Valves

A separate comparative analysis of the TPCH allografts and xenografts depicts the probability of a patient having a second operation for any reason at some stage in the lifetime before death (Fig. 121–19). The cryopreserved allografts are superior to xenografts up until the approximate age of 60 years at the time of the first operation. For young patients, the probabilities are much higher and different. For example, a 20-year-old patient receiving a TPCH *cryopre-*

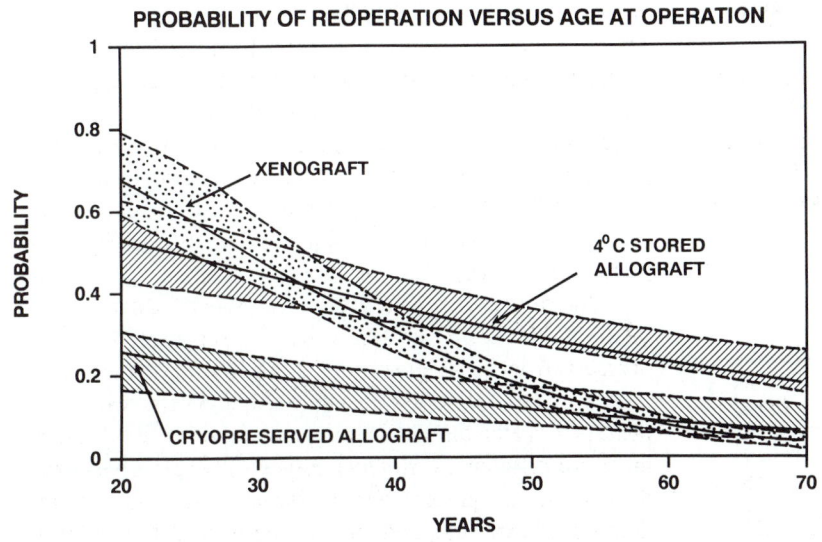

Figure 121–19. Nomogram of the probability of rereplacement before death for any reason for patients with xenograft valves, 4°C stored (NVA) and cryopreserved allograft (VCA) valves, as a function of increasing age at initial valve replacement. The solid lines are the parametric estimates with the 70% confidence limits indicated by the dotted lines. (*From McGiffin DC, Galbraith A, McLachlan GJ, et al: An analysis of aortic valve re-replacement following biological valve failure. J Thorac Cardiovasc Surg, in press.*)

served allograft has approximately a 25% probability of requiring a rereplacement at some time during the remainder of that patient's life. With a *TPCH 4°C stored allograft* in a 20-year-old patient the probability is 53% and for xenografts it is almost a 70% probability. Therefore beyond 60 years of age at first operation, there appears to be no difference in the probability of reoperation prior to death in patients receiving xenograft valves compared to those with cryopreserved allograft valves. This useful informative age-related rereplacement nomogram emanates from an analysis of the TPCH results by McGiffin and colleagues.[52] This analysis accepted death as a "competing risk" and in this statistical domain the unconditional probability (actual risk) of valve rereplacement before death has been depicted using a mixture model approach described by McLachlan and colleagues.[53] It crystallizes the information required as we fully inform our patients of the probabilities of future events. It also highlights in a clear form, first the limitations of valves such as the 4°C stored and xenografts for the young and middle aged patients and second that allografts function better in the middle age patient than they do in the young child or young adult. Lastly, the need for improved devices and further research is evident.

PATHOLOGIC ANALYSIS

The Immunologic Response to the Allograft Valve

At The Prince Charles Hospital, in conjunction with the Brisbane Princess Alexandra Hospital Department of Immunology, experimental[54] and preliminary human studies have shown cellular and humoral immune responses are evoked following the implantation of viable allograft aortic valves. Sera taken at 10, 30, 90, and 180 days and at 1 year after operation from allograft valve recipients have been tested against the cryopreserved splenic cells of the donor to ascertain the presence and degree of an immune response. Flow cytometry studies, which measure IgG antibody against surface antigens on B and T lymphocytes,

show increased binding of IgG. The degree of binding of the patient's sera was always greater to donor B and T cells (from the spleen) compared with third party control cells (Fig. 121–20). It was interesting that the immune response was never detected at day 10 but was uniformly present at 30 and 90 days. Even at 12 mos, recipients have shown persisting antidonor antibodies. These studies demonstrated that an immune response against the allograft valve does occur.

Other workers[55] have demonstrated the presence of endothelial cells and their consequent expression of MHC Class I and II molecules on the surfaces of optimally preserved cryopreserved allograft valves explanted up to 3 years. Allografts stored in antibiotic/nutrient media failed to show endothelia cell viability or Class I antigens.[56] The antigenic presence and antibody response has been described by others both experimentally and clinically.[57–60] Accepting that allografts are antigenic and evoke an antibody reaction, this immune response can be determined and quantified. However, laboratory analysis is time consuming and expensive and demands the availability of donor lymphocytes.

The translation of these findings to the clinical picture in relationship to valve durability is difficult. Clinically ABO match or mismatch has failed to influence long-term valve durability.[36] Pathologically, is the loss of cellularity in the matrix of an implanted allograft due to an immunological response? Is the patchy thickening (occasionally extreme) due to donor–host reactivity of an immunological type? The author believes the answer to both of these questions is yes. Such thickening, although sometimes ultimately deleterious, may minimize the risks of leaflet rupture or perforation and therefore extend durability. However, in children and especially young babies[61] the excessive calcification and fibrotic degenerative stenosis are almost certainly immunologic in origin and are unfavorable sequelae. The need for immunosuppression is evident. However, as the present evidence of durability of the allografts is reasonably good, a patient would need to have the guarantee that immunosuppressive therapy would have to be at a risk lower than that of anticoagulant hemor-

Figure 121–20. Flow cytometry cross-match measures the antibodies from human recipient's serum as IgG binding to the surface antigens on B and T lymphocytes collected and cryopreserved from the donor's spleen at the original organ retrieval. The vertical axis is a logarithmic scale representing the degree of IgG binding, the numbers expressing the mean intensity as a channel number on the flow cytometric photoreceptors. Binding, not detectable at 10 days, increased from 30 to 90 days after allograft implantation.

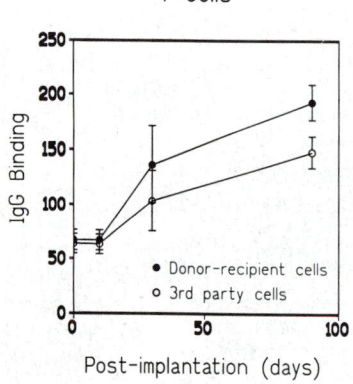

T cells

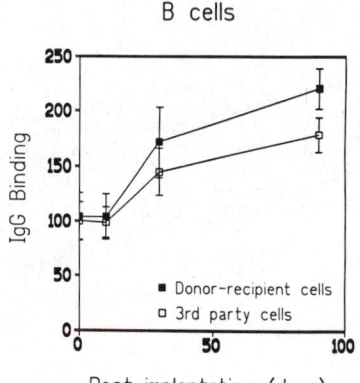

B cells

rhage/thromboembolic events. Otherwise a mechanical valve would be preferable to receiving an allograft valve and immunosuppression. Looking at Figure 121–19 it would appear that *once safer immunosuppressives become available,* children and young adults may warrant such medication. Even if a pulmonary autograft valve (see later) is implanted for AVR, immunosuppression may be indicated for the young patient to safeguard the long-term function of the pulmonary valve allograft in the right ventricular outflow tract.

Histopathologic Appearances

Many publications have focused on the pathologic features of the allograft valve. Differences of opinion, involving interpretation[62–66] of specific findings, suggest that, at least, over the months to early years, the appearance of the implanted allograft reflects its preimplant preservation characteristics, which differ widely with respect to viability and matrix integrity. Ultimately, a basic pattern of features becomes apparent. The hallmark paper in 1969 by Kosek and colleagues[67] still stands today as an excellent summary of the pathologic events of the implanted allograft and is added to more recently by contributions from Schoen.[45,68]

The *"dead"* valve (irradiated, chemically denatured, freeze-dried) used in the 1960s remained acellular, calcified, and ruptured or perforated. Its durability was poor. The *"nonviable" antibiotic 4°C stored* value remained acellular (Fig. 121–21) except for a host surface fibrosis and pseudo-endothelial–fibrin layer encroaching over the base of the allograft aortic wall and leaflet. Host tissue (endothelial cells or fibroblasts) does not grow into or over the leaflet. Very rarely, as occasionally occurs with a stented xenograft, an excessive proliferative tongue of host fibrosis

extends on to the body of the leaflet. This has been misinterpreted as recellularization. The elastic and collagen fibers or matrix remain surprisingly intact although some homogeneous amorphous appearance is evident. Surface thrombosis is macroscopically nonexistent but fibrin deposition and the occasional surface hemorrhage are microscopically apparent. Thin areas of the leaflet develop and are the site of rupture or perforation, the incidence of which is less than the freeze-dried valve but still substantial enough to produce the classical structural deterioration after the eighth to ninth year.

The *viable cryopreserved valves* in the TPCH series have shown a range of features. The occasional valve (explanted from the younger patient) has shown features of calcific fibrotic stenosis of the leaflet. This, having occurred within several years of initial implantation, is considered an immunological host response. The features are rare but are in keeping with those of others.[61] The majority of valves show in a vague chronological order the slow disappearance of donor cellular elements in the leaflets to the point where small islands only of persisting fibroblasts remain (Fig. 121–22). Essentially the valve becomes close to being virtually acellular. The tissue is more likely to be slightly thicker, although this is far from uniform. It is considered to indicate that a minor host/donor reaction may have led to some leaflet thickening. In this respect the reaction may be advantageous for the frequent cusp perforation of the nonviable valve is less frequently seen in valves that have been cryopreserved very early after donor death. Nevertheless, appearances from one leaflet to another can vary within the same valve.[66] In most implanted allografts, the surface endothelium and convoluted collagen bundle appearance is lost.[69] Fibrin deposition smooths out the surface and probably leads to the loss of extensibility and elasticity.[70,71]

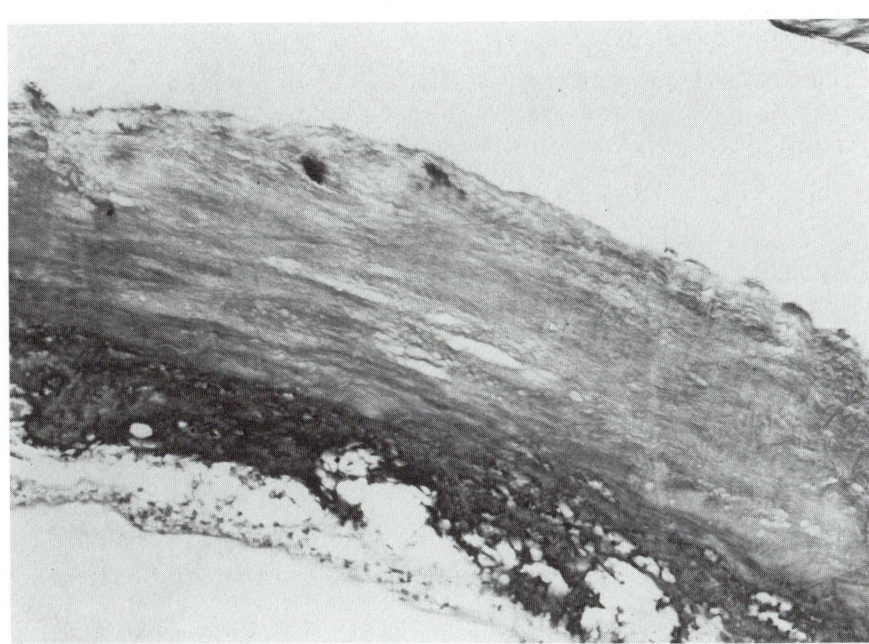

Figure 121–21. Typical acellular appearance of the explanted nonviable valve.

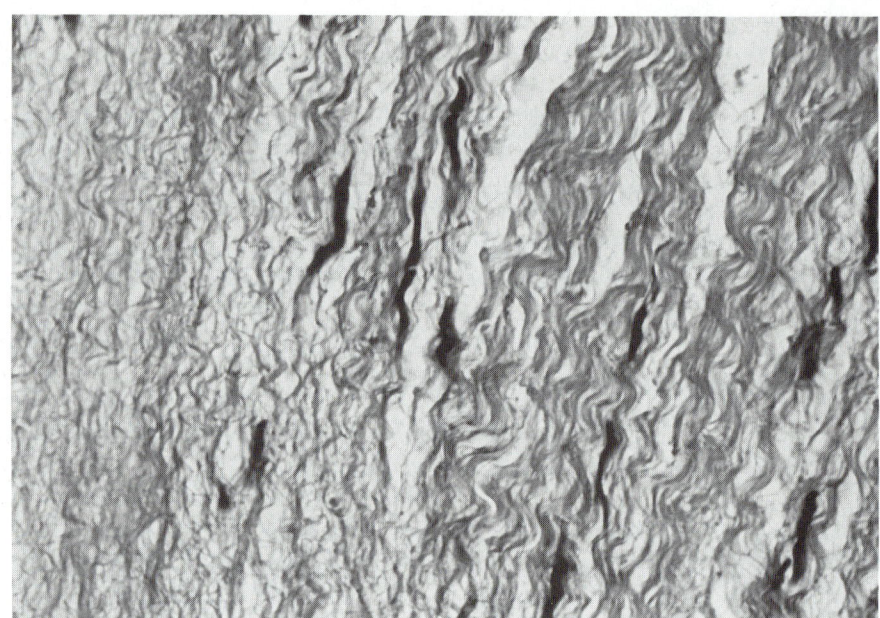

Figure 121–22. Histological appearance of a viable cryopreserved valve explanted at 22 mo: The occasional fibroblast is evident. The cell population has decreased markedly. Hematoxylin–eosin, × 400.

Very rarely, cellularity can be marked and even near normal[18,66] (Fig. 121–23). Such valves probably inhabit a favorable environment with the patient maintaining an immune tolerance to the living foreign tissue. Tissue culture of explanted leaflets are performed at The Prince Charles Hospital on every occasion. It is generally possible to grow some cells, presumably even from leaflets that have small remaining cellular islands in a predominantly acellular tissue. On three occasions, where there has been a host–donor sex mismatch, these cultured cells have verified the cell origin to be *donor* on chromosomal analysis. In 25 years of allograft experience, the TPCH group have not seen any evidence of host ingrowth into leaflet tissue except 2 to 3 mm basally. Recellularization does not occur. This may be a significant finding for some current and future proposed valve research that is directed to methods to encourage and stimulate host ingrowth into implanted tissues. However, in a simplistic description "remodeling," on the whole, is scarring. The author considers such research unlikely to be successful in vivo. In addition, leaflet tissue must remain mobile and flexible and therefore the patient reaction needs to be minimal.

All methods of allograft valve preservation, including cryopreservation, result in pathological features that are

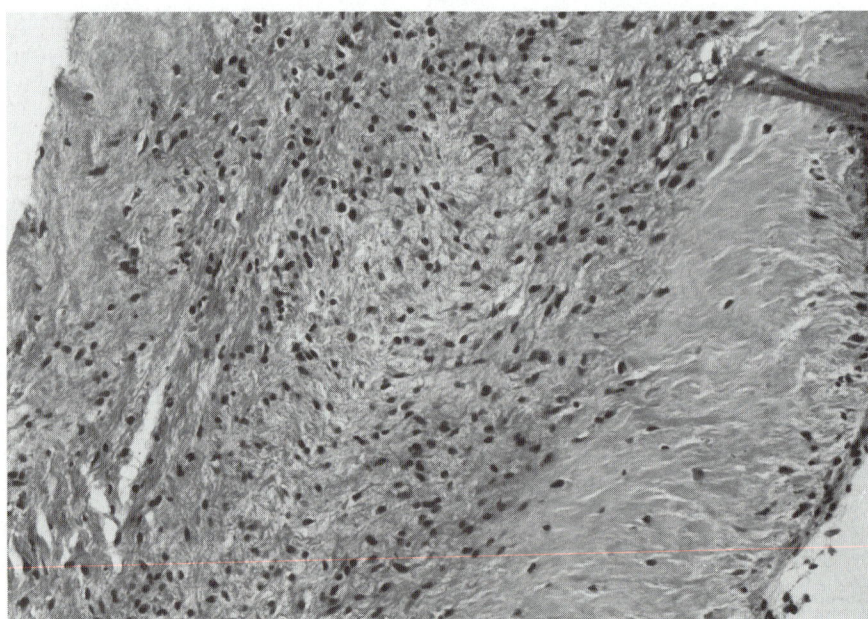

Figure 121–23. Histological appearance of a viable cryopreserved valve at 9.5 years. Viable fibroblasts are evident. This is a rare appearance. Hematoxylin–eosin, × 100.

very different from the normal valve, the autograft pulmonary valve in the subcoronary position (see later) and the aortic valve of the transplant heart (Fig. 121–24). These three valves demonstrate dense cellularity, normal collagen and elastin, and preserved sternal architecture. In these valves the convoluted collagen bundles that are responsible for the preservation of normal extensibility in both radial and circumferential direction are preserved.

The maintenance of normal valve structure is the primary goal in preserving normal valve function. To achieve this an allograft valve probably must be implanted within hours of retrieval and immunosuppression needs to be given. The logistics of performing this, except for the occasional individual patient, may be too great. The most appropriate type, strength, and duration of immunosuppression is also unknown. In the TPCH study of the immune response, further research is planned to continue with a group of immunosuppressed patients to compare any changing patterns of antibody production. The possible reappearance of antibodies after cessation of immunosuppression must also be assessed.

The Future of the Allograft Aortic Valve

The allograft aortic valve, now in its fourth decade of clinical implantation, has almost reached its zenith. The "viable cryopreserved" allograft used as a root replacement does produce excellent immediate and intermediate results and probably gives good long-term function. Perhaps only the "ultrafresh," homovital allograft, retrieved from a beating heart donor at cross-clamp and implanted without cryopreservation well within 24 hours, may be superior. Improvements are needed to modify the unfavorable immunologic response in infants, children, and some young adults.

Much information is required as to appropriate type, concentration, and especially duration of immunosuppression for the group. The influence of such therapy on valve durability is awaited and certainly these data will take more than a decade to collate. The TPCH studies on the quantification of recipient antibody levels will certainly provide an excellent model to determine the effects of immunosuppression on these levels during and after therapy. In the meanwhile aortic allografts will continue to be used according to their supply by those few surgical centers where surgeons have been exposed in their training to allograft valve use and who have seen and understood the advantages that this valve can offer over other devices for particular patients in specific circumstances (young females, endocarditis). Those patients unsuitable for anticoagulants and who live in remote areas benefit from the choice of an allograft.

ALLOGRAFTS FOR MITRAL AND TRICUSPID VALVE SURGERY

Frame mounted aortic allografts were used in the late 1960s and early 1970s with unfavorable results in both aortic and mitral positions. Surprising durability in the tricuspid valve position has been observed such that it may be one of the best devices for tricuspid valve replacement. The device has to be made on site by the surgical team using a specially purchased unmounted xenograft type prosthesis. This constitutes its major disadvantage.

There has been recent renewed interest and early small clinical experience with *unstented mitral valve allografts* (leaflet, chordae, and papillary muscle stump) in the tricuspid and mitral location.

Pomar et al[72] implanted a cryopreserved human mitral

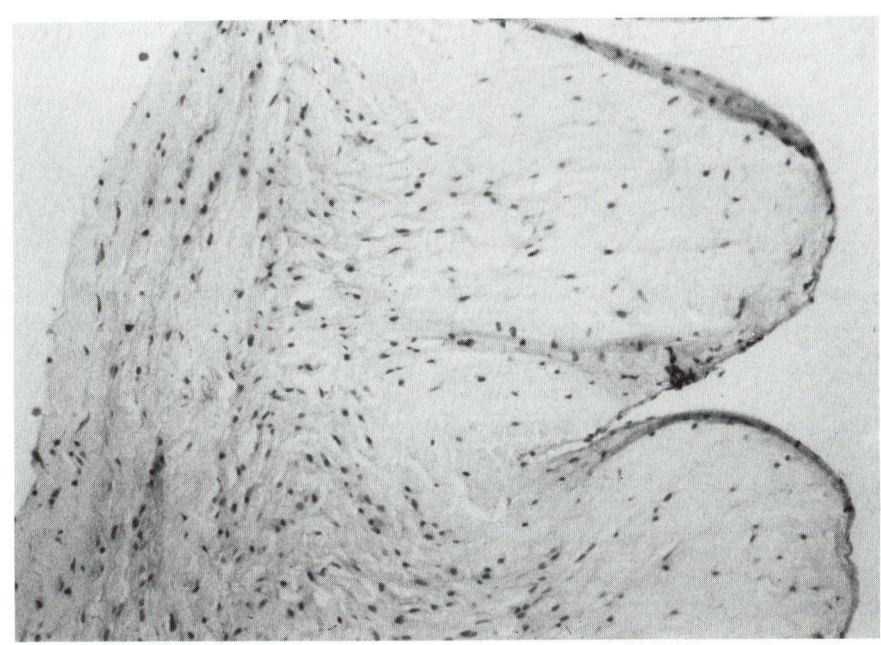

Figure 121–24. Histological appearance of the aortic valve of a transplant heart at 3.5 years from a previously immunosuppressed patient. Note normal cellularity and tissue convolutions. Hematoxylin–eosin, × 120.

valve complex into the tricuspid position in three patients with tricuspid valve endocarditis, two of whom also had blood cultures growing candida yeast. All three were HIV positive and actively using heroin. The papillary muscles and the annulus were supported with pericardium pledgetted sutures and pericardial strips respectively. All three survived and have been followed up for 20 mo. Echocardiography has shown trivial central incompetence in two patients and moderate regurgitation in the third patient.

Acar and associates[73,74] reported the use of partial and total replacement of the mitral valve with a cryopreserved mitral allograft in over 30 patients, many of whom had acute mitral valve endocarditis. In one patient with recurrent endocarditis *both* mitral and tricuspid valves were replaced with mitral allografts. Prosthetic ring annuloplasty was used for both annuli, which seems inappropriate in the setting of endocarditis when the primary objective was to use allograft tissue with its potential resistance to early recurrent infection. At four months postoperatively in this individual, the graft in the mitral location was competent on echocardiography while in the tricuspid there was a "minimal residual leak." A further case report by Kumar and Trehan[75] from India described the use of a fresh antibiotic preserved mitral homograft for a young 25 year old with calcific rheumatic mitral valve restenosis. No annuloplasty was performed, but all suture lines were generously supported by glutaraldehyde tanned autogenous pericardium. Experimental data from 1964 revealed uniform early successful results in the experimental animal.[76–78] The problems were primarily related to the suturing at the annulus rather than to papillary muscle fixation.

These recent successful clinical experiences are small and are specifically applied to patients with endocarditis. The feasibility is proven, but long-term results are unknown and awaited. It is highly likely that such allograft use for atrioventricular valve replacement will be small and performed with enthusiasm by only a few surgeons. Except in the treatment of endocarditis, it is difficult to envisage a widespread application when both bioprostheses and mechanical valves continue to improve an already established performance.

THE PULMONARY VALVE AUTOGRAFT

The pulmonary valve autograft procedure for aortic valve replacement (Fig. 121–25A–B) entails

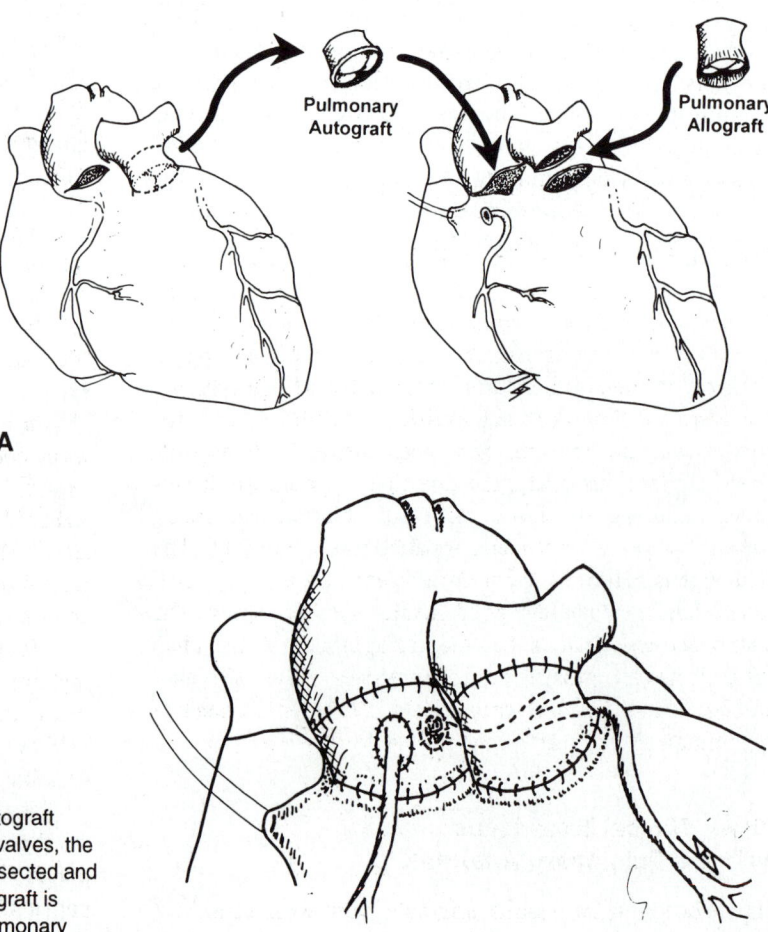

Figure 121–25. Schematic depiction of the pulmonary autograft operation. **A.** After inspection of the pulmonary and aortic valves, the pulmonary valve cylinder is excised. The aortic root is transected and the coronary artery buttons fashioned. The pulmonary allograft is implanted as a right ventricular outflow conduit. **B.** The pulmonary autograft and allograft implanted.

1. Excision of the pulmonary valve as a small cylinder with its main pulmonary artery.
2. Implantation of the valve into the aorta as an intraluminal cylinder or as a free standing total root replacement and coronary artery pedicle anastomoses.
3. Reconstruction of the right ventricular outflow tract with a pulmonary allograft valved conduit.

In 1960, Lower, from Stanford University, transplanted the autologous pulmonary valve into the canine descending thoracic aorta[79] and in another experimental series replaced the canine mitral valve with a pulmonary valve autograft.[80] Pillsbury and Shumway, also from Stanford, in 1966 experimentally replaced the aortic valve with a pulmonary autograft.[81] This was the first publication of this concept. One year later in 1967, Ross performed the pulmonary autograft replacement of the aortic valve in humans.[82] This has now become known as the "Ross Procedure." He persisted with this operation with only a few supporters, basically because the concept of converting single valve disease into a double valve operation was not easy to accept, recommend, or perform. These hurdles have now been overcome. The work of Ross et al[83–87] has only more recently been duplicated by Elkins, Stelzer, and colleagues[88,89] from Oklahoma, commencing a careful well documented clinical series in 1986. Consequently interest has been renewed. Now a worldwide pulmonary autograft registry of the Ross Procedure exists with well over 1000 procedures at the end of 1994.[90]

THE ADVANTAGES OF THE PULMONARY AUTOGRAFT

The autograft shares all the attributes of the allograft valve. It is noiseless, nonthrombogenic with no anticoagulant therapy required, has the good hemodynamics of a normal aortic valve, and a resistance to early endocarditis. Storage, sterilization, and preservation techniques are unnecessary and therefore tissue damage avoided. In addition, with the growth potential that has now been proven,[91–93] and the near excellent durability, the question is posed to all surgeons replacing the aortic valves of children and young adults: "Why am I not using a pulmonary autograft?" The challenge is before us, for many surgeons have as yet small series, but are obtaining good results with low risks. The pulmonary autograft is our closest approach to the ideal valve. It has the prospects of a permanent valve. The only problem, small that it appears, is the future replacement of the pulmonary allograft on the right side.[94]

Ross' Clinical Experience with the Pulmonary Autograft

The only long-term results originate from Ross et al.[86,87] An analysis of 339 implants from 1967 with the longest fol-

low-up of 24 years revealed an overall hospital mortality of 7.4% (25 patients). Since 1976, there has been one death with the current operative mortality being below 1% in this series. With late deaths (38 patients) the actuarial survival was 80% at 20 years. It is to be remembered that the majority of these patients were young (median age 29.3 years) and therefore survival expected to be high in comparison with results with other devices in older patients.

The commonest causes of in-hospital mortality were arrhythmias and hemorrhage, the former being due, in the early experiences, to operative injury to the first septal branch of the left anterior descending coronary artery (see later).

Eighty-five percent of the survivors have not required reoperation, which is the key point to analyze in this series over a 24-year span. Of the 33 patients requiring reoperation, nine have been for endocarditis and 19 for technical malinsertions during the early learning phase. There was no incidence of leaflet *"calcification, tears or thinning."*[87] In addition, 70% of patients were free from any event including reoperation, endocarditis, degeneration of the replacement valve, and death. Consequently, there are three salient features to analyze. First, the likelihood of malinsertion is being reduced in this modern era with the preferred technique of cylinder and root replacement of the autograft.[95] Second, there appeared a higher incidence of endocarditis in the early years of the Ross experience, which has not occurred with other workers over these last nine years. Third, the absence of leaflet degeneration explains the excellent valve durability of the pulmonary autograft—*this being the hallmark of the living autologous tissue of valvular origin.* The freedom from reoperation of the pulmonary autograft was 85% at 20 years.

Progressive regurgitation has not occurred, unlike the fate of the allograft aortic valve. In its natural state, the pulmonary valve dilates in response to pulmonary hypertension because it has a total circumferential base of right ventricle muscle. Once implanted into the aortic annulus it is prevented from dilating. The leaflets themselves have been shown to withstand immediate systolic pressures and biomechanical stress testing has verified more than adequate tensile strength.[96] Complications and reoperation on the right-sided conduit are reported as small in the Ross series.[85] The 20-year actuarial freedom from right-sided valve related death was 97%; freedom from valve failure or reoperation was 81% at 20 years.

Histologic examination of explanted pulmonary valves highlights the full complement of living cells with no evidence of calcification (Fig. 121–26A,B). Degeneration is unlikely and if turbulence is minimal, the valve may only be subject to the normal process of aging.

In the Ross series of 1988 with 249 patients, the actuarial patient survival including operative deaths was reported as 57.3 ± 9.6% at 19 yeas.[85] The 1991 report of 339 patients showed a patient survival of 80%[87] at 20 years. In the early Ross series the actuarial freedom from reoperation

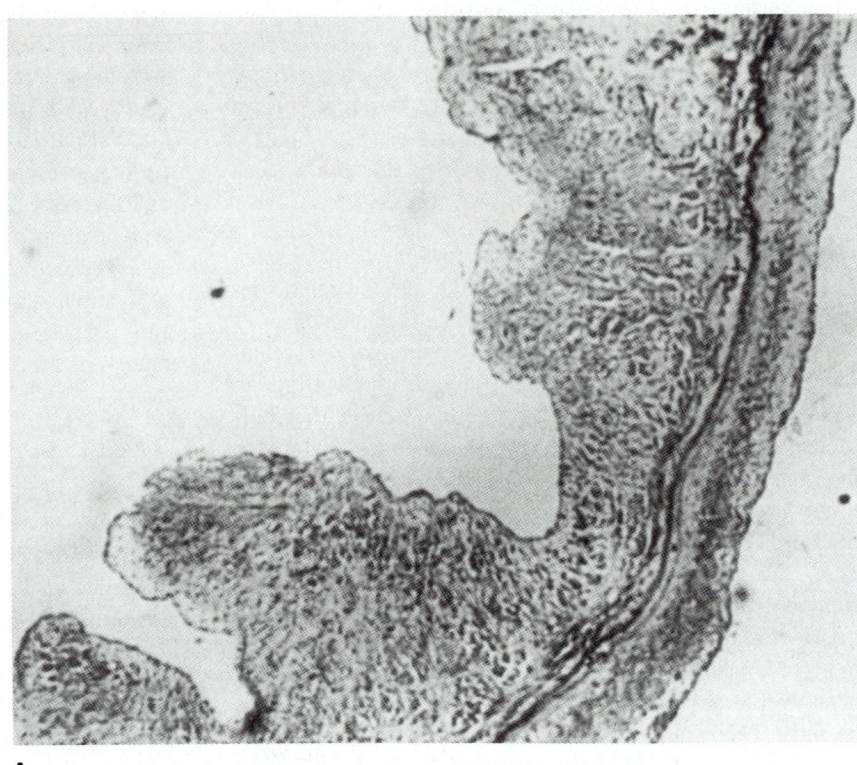

A

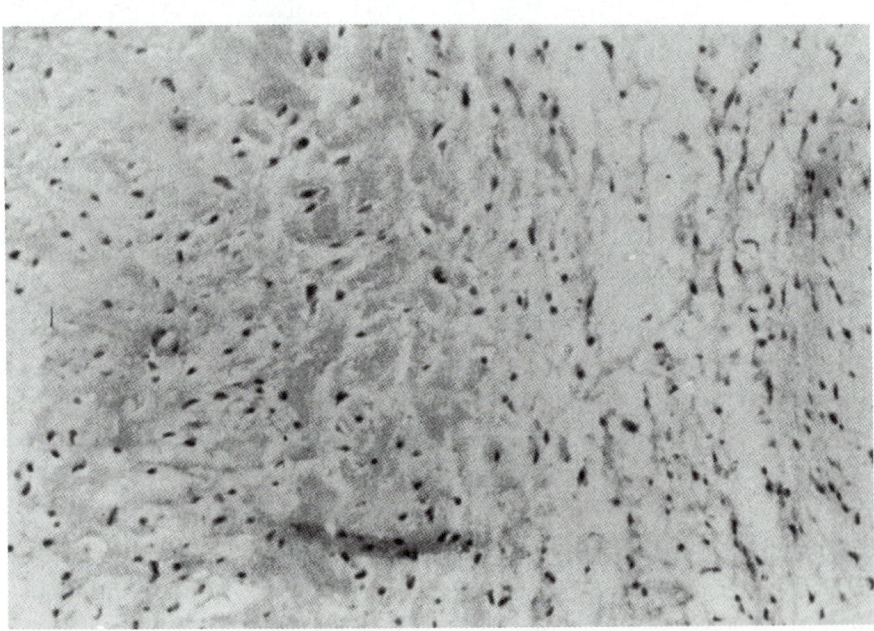

Figure 121–26. A. Histology of explanted pulmonary autograft valve at 13 mo showing retained structure and normal convolutions. **B.** Histology of explanted pulmonary autograft at 10 years showing normal cellularity. *(From Ross DN: Pulmonary valve autotransplantation (The Ross Operation). J Cardiac Surg. 3:313, 1988, with permission.)*

B

(presumably for all causes) was $40.5 \pm 11.9\%$ at 19 years.[84] Technical failures were said to be responsible for 24 of 36 reoperations, most of which were subcoronary implants. One would anticipate that in this modern era of surgery, root and cylinder implantations will produce improved results with the autograft. What appears already most important and relevant are first the strikingly normal histological appearances of explanted valves and second the awaited results of other workers with this procedure.

Recent Experience of Other Workers

Elkins[97] in a series of 56 patients followed for up to 6.3 years (mean 2.3 years) had to reoperate on one pulmonary autograft patient at 14 mo postoperatively for progressive aortic regurgitation due to dilatation of the aortic annulus and sinotubular ridge. Failure of the pulmonary autograft has been due more often to bacterial endocarditis or technical errors at the time of operation producing inadequate leaflet coaptation with resultant immediate and progressive regurgitation.

The actuarial freedom from reoperation of either the pulmonary autograft or the allograft in the right ventricular outflow tract was 92 ± 4% at 7 years in a series of 86 children (0.9 to 21 years) personally operated on by Elkins et al.[93] In this series patients receiving the autograft as an intraluminal or inclusion cylinder had the highest freedom from reoperation on the autograft (100%); the results with the scalloped subcoronary or intra-aortic implant were 90 ± 7% and with the root replacement 96 ± 4%. Yet in comparing the three techniques of implantation on echocardiographic assessment, at least 13 children had Grade 2+ insufficiency.[93] The incidence was dependent on the technique, the subcoronary implant having the highest incidence of incompetence and the intraluminal tube or cylinder the lowest.

Kouchoukos et al[98] reported results with the pulmonary autograft in 33 patients as a root replacement. With nil operative and late mortality and a follow-up to 48 mo (mean 21 mo) there were no episodes of endocarditis, thromboembolism, or autograft reoperation. Importantly, echocardiography demonstrated no progressive dilatation of the autograft. With color-flow Doppler imaging, 22 patients had trivial or no regurgitation and 9 patients had mild regurgitation of the autograft. No patient had moderate or severe regurgitation. One patient required reoperation for stenosis of the pulmonary allograft on the right side. Seven other patients had gradients across the allograft (mean 26 ± 14 mm Hg; range 12 to 45 mm Hg).

Gonzalez-Lavin et al[99] reported a small series of 12 patients operated on between 1969 and 1971. With a mean follow-up of 12.4 years, there was no incidence of pulmonary autograft degeneration. The TPCH group have performed 15 autograft procedures without early or late mortality. One patient has Grade 2 autograft valve incompetence and another young patient has developed a moderate gradient across the pulmonary allograft, considered probably to be of immunologic cause rather than technical.

PULMONARY AUTOGRAFT AORTIC VALVE REPLACEMENT

Technique

Selection and Sizing of the Autografts

The autograft is difficult to size and perioperative echocardiography is somewhat inaccurate. Likewise, intraoperative obturator measurement is not reliable with the relaxed heart. Estimating the probable size of the pulmonary root and that of the aorta by eye appears just as feasible and no more inaccurate. Ross speaks of the "forgiving" nature of the autograft in that the size matching has a wide range for acceptable error. Nevertheless, care needs to be exercised when the aortic annulus is large, i.e., 29 mm and greater. The autograft is probably contraindicated in these circumstances. As a general rule the autograft should be no smaller than 2 to 3 mm than the aortic annulus. As with the allograft, intraluminal cylinder implantation or root replacement decreases the possible errors from size mismatching.

Retrieval

The retrieval of the pulmonary valve and artery probably presents the major hurdle for the surgeon. The knowledge of the possible position of the septal branch or branches of the anterior descending coronary artery is essential[100] (Fig. 121–27). Once the decision has been made to perform the Ross Procedure, the midpoint of the main pulmonary artery is marked by pencil or diathermy prior to instituting cardiopulmonary bypass. The aortic valve is examined through a transverse aortotomy. This valve is excised and the aortic annulus measured. The pulmonary artery is then dissected from the aorta, transected at the mark, and the leaflets examined. The proximal pulmonary artery is swung forward and dissected posteriorly from all surrounding tissue down to a point where right ventricular muscle just becomes visible. As seen from within the pulmonary artery, the right ventricular outflow tract anteriorly is transversely incised about one centimeter below the pulmonary leaflets. The right ventricle is then circumferentially incised to the left and to the right ensuring a good 7 to 8 mm cuff of right ven-

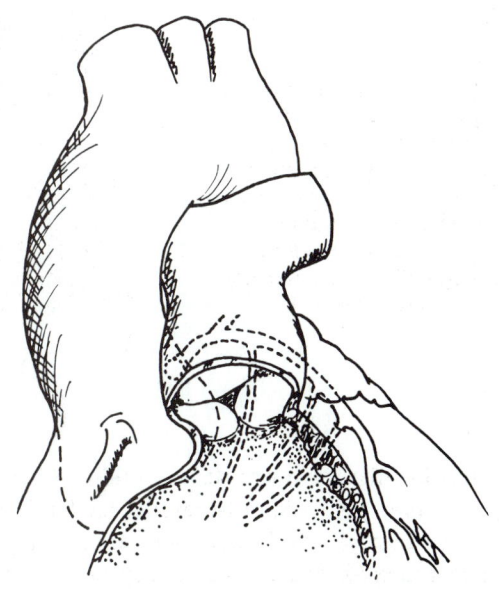

Figure 121–27. The first septal artery may vary in its origin and may have several branches, but is almost always in close posterior proximity to the pulmonary valve.

tricular muscle. Posteriorly, care around the septal artery is required. While anteriorly and laterally a right angle cut in the muscle is made, posteriorly, this cut is tangential or oblique, the scissors being angled almost parallel with the posterior right ventricular outflow tract (Fig. 121–28). As a result, the posterior muscle is bevelled, the cut edge being almost 1 cm broad, and consequently the posterior muscular rim of the autograft is thinner. Knowing that the septal artery rests just deep to the surface of this cut edge, in the reconstruction of the right side, the pulmonary allograft is later sutured to the most proximal or right ventricular edge of this muscular cut, exteriorizing the rest of the bevelled muscle outside the allograft conduit. The pulmonary valve is trimmed up evenly around its proximal rim ready for implantation. All adventitia is left intact and the valve immersed in autologous heparinized blood.

The author considers it important to practice pulmonary autograft excision with animal hearts, examining the proximity to the septal artery on each occasion. Probably the commonest error is the excision through the right ventricular muscle being made too close to the leaflet attachment.

Implantation Techniques

The options of a subcoronary scalloped valve, an inclusion cylinder, or a free standing root replacement are similar to those for the aortic allograft.[95,101] A description of the technical aspects is therefore unnecessary except to state that the fresh pulmonary valve tissue is strong and very easy to work with, unlike the friable muscle of the aortic allograft. The author prefers to complete the autograft root implantation prior to the right-sided reconstruction. This allows reperfusion of the myocardium enabling a good inspection of the posterior right ventricular muscle to identify any sep-

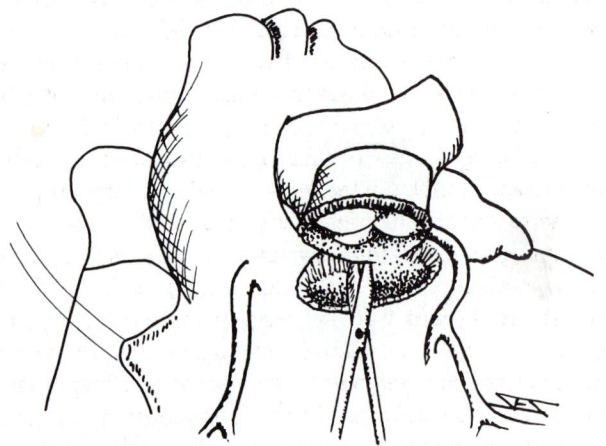

Figure 121–28. Excision of the pulmonary autograft in the vicinity of the septal artery. The scissors are virtually parallel with the posterior right ventricular wall. The cut is tangential or bevelled.

tal artery bleeding. The continuous 5-0 Prolene suture used for the distal pulmonary allograft artery anastomosis should be interrupted or locked in two to three places to minimize risk of purse-stringing. The pulmonary allograft, in size similar to the aortic annulus, is implanted without rotation. The pulmonary valve has one cusp posteriorly and a cusp on each side with an anterior commissure. The order of suturing appears unimportant and is purely dependent on the surgeon's preference. The potential risk of bleeding is high, but in all series hemorrhage has been infrequent and transfusion uncommon.[98]

Immediate postbypass assessment by transesophageal color Doppler provides an excellent teaching medium for the surgeon. The reasons for any minor leaflet prolapse or regurgitation can best be understood if the analysis is made during the operation rather than several days later prior to patient discharge.

Elkins has preferred not to use a pulmonary autograft in the presence of annuloaortic ectasia or if the aortic valve annulus is greater than 27 mm. He prefers to use a root replacement in patients who have a small aortic annulus (<20 mm), a dysplastic annulus, combined valve and subvalvular stenosis, distortion of a coronary sinus, or when coronary arteries are located directly opposite each other (180°C apposed).[101]

The Growth of the Pulmonary Valve in Children

Evidence has accumulated to prove that the pulmonary valve grows with the child. Growth can be inferred if cell viability is demonstrated, autograft enlargement occurs proportional to somatic growth, and if function remains normal. The cells of the living valve leaflets metabolize, replenish the matrix, and respond to growth factors. The lack of progression of incompetence is indicative of nondiseased leaflet tissue. Gerosa et al[91] and Elkins et al[93,102] in clinical series have demonstrated this potential to grow in proportion to the somatic growth of the child. The aortic annulus and sinotubular diameters were compared with normal valves predicted by body surface area. In the intra-aortic cylinder implants, the early and late postoperative annulus diameters were in the normal range and increased proportionally to somatic growth. In the root replacements, the annulus increased in diameter and became dilated. The sinotubular junction also increased from its small size early to normal range. The absence of valve failure, i.e., continuing durability, was considered confirmatory evidence of growth.

Kouchoukos et al,[98] however, found no change in diameters of the autograft in 16 patients followed for 19 to 24 mos. Most of these patients were adults and all autografts were implanted as root replacements. Sievers et al[103] also reported no increase in autograft root diameter in 7 patients up to 21 mo after surgery.

The Justification of the Pulmonary Autograft

Many arguments opposing the use of the autograft have been raised.

1. The operation converts single valve disease to a double valve replacement.
2. Even accepting the permanency of the pulmonary autograft, at the end of the operation there remains a potential for single valve disease, i.e., the pulmonary allograft.
3. The data on the likelihood of RV rereplacement may be underestimated.

At best, Ross reports 81% freedom from right-sided rereplacement at 20 years. The younger the patient the lower this figure will be. In young patients hoping for 40 or more years of life after operation, it is highly likely that far more than half will require a second or third operation in their lifetime.

Elkins[97] believes that "the use of the pulmonary autograft has decreased the number of cardiac procedures that an individual child may require, since there is no need to perform palliative procedures to avoid the insertion of a mechanical prosthesis, with its constant risk of thromboembolism and the difficulties associated with anticoagulation." In addition, "normalization of ventricular function by one postoperative year, enlargement of the autograft proportional to somatic growth and a low risk of valve-related complications suggest that pulmonary autograft replacement of the aortic valve is the ideal valve replacement for the potential parent."[104]

Kouchoukos et al[98] maintains that the pulmonary autograft may be the best available substitute for the diseased aortic valve in children and younger adults. Elkins[97] has extended this recommendation to include all patients with aortic valve disease and a life expectancy of more than 20 years.

In conclusion, if we can provide our patient with a "near normal" aortic valve substitute essentially for the life span of that patient, we have achieved a major therapeutic goal in spite of the rereplacement of the right-sided valve. The author adds a cautionary note that the incidence of autograft insufficiency of the Grade 2+ degree appears to be 10 to 20%. This needs careful long-term evaluation for possibly we may not as yet have a perfect valve. As with the allograft, the implantation technique of the pulmonary autograft is a critical determinant of the long-term function.

The Autologous Pericardial Valve

Autologous tissue (pericardium, fascia lata) of nonvalvar origin has been used for total valve replacement, cusp extension, and leaflet patches for many years. These tissues have behaved in one of two ways depending on their viability or chemical denaturation at the time of implantation.

Fresh living tissue, such as fascia lata, was never de-signed to be a moving valve leaflet and in its new locus is deprived of its nutritional vascular pathways and replaced with nutrients by diffusion. The tissue thickens and shrinks, fibroses, and hyalinizes, may calcify, and may rupture from its stent at points of greatest flexion. Lincoln et al[105] and Silver et al[106] confirmed these findings in studies of explanted fascia lata valves. These lessons were learned in the early 1970s.[107]

The behavior of pericardial tissue appears very different if it is autologous *and* preserved for a short time in glutaraldehyde. No longer is the tissue viable, no longer does it require a new blood supply, and no longer will host–graft remodeling lead to thickening, retraction or leaflet fibrosis.

The experimental work by Love and associates,[108,109] of California, examining the fate of the autologous pericardial constructed valve as an aortic valve implant in juvenile sheep, showed that it was resistant to calcification up to 5 mo after implantation in the mitral position, in marked contrast to the calcified xenograft and allograft tissue mounted in the same stent assembly.

These studies suggest very cogently that autologous glutaraldehyde- (10 min fixation) preserved tissue is resistant to calcification whereas, in the experimental animal, *non*autologous glutaraldehyde-preserved tissue (i.e., xenograft) does calcify. Because this autologous tissue is non-valvar it must be rendered nonviable otherwise it would remodel, fibrose, and shrink. Glutaraldehyde, as of 1994, appears adequate to achieve this tissue "inertness." Love and associates following this meaningful experimental work are now clinically trialing a stented autologous short-time glutaraldehyde-fixed pericardial valve, which is rapidly constructed prior to cardiopulmonary bypass.[110,111] The engineering construction of the valve is simple and quick. Pericardium after 10 min in 0.6% buffered glutaraldehyde is cut to measurement and clamped between two mating stents without the need for suturing.

Several European cardiac surgical centers have implanted the valve into 164 patients from September 1992.[112] The age range has been 2 wk to 86 years (mean 66 years) and the aortic implants have ranged in size from 19 to 25 mm. The valve function appears satisfactory at this early follow-up. The longer term results are awaited.

Further applications of this autologous preserved pericardium are possible. In the Ross Procedure it appears possible to reconstruct the right ventricular outflow tract with an autologous pericardial constructed valve and conduit with or without a stent. Prabhakar, Duran, and co-workers have shown the feasibility in an experimental study.[113] The operation would then be totally autologous. It would avoid the immunological response to the pulmonary allograft and may reduce the incidence of right-sided reoperations. Love is also examining the possibilities of right-sided reconstruction.[112]

An alternative interpretation to the absence of calcification in the autologous rapid fixed glutaraldehyde pericardial valve is offered by Liao, Frater, and co-workers.[114] They considered that the short-term fixation and not the "autologous" nature of the tissue is the important issue. Using the rat subcutaneous models, the calcium content of autologous and xenogenic pericardium 1 cm^2 pieces, either fresh or glutaraldehyde fixed for 15, 60, and 120 min was quantitatively measured after 45 days implantation. Frater showed the calcium content was solely glutaraldehyde time-dependent. The short fixation tissue had the least calcium. Once treated with glutaraldehyde, autologous tissues behaved biologically like glutaraldehyde treated xenogenic tissue. Nevertheless the use of tissue following short-time fixation has to be balanced by the risk of reduced tissue strength.

The removal of cells from leaflets fixed in glutaraldehyde has also been shown experimentally to minimize or prevent calcification.[115] If this facet, rather than the autologous nature or the short-time fixation, is the key, then maybe the "surface glazing" of short duration glutaraldehyde-fixed autologous pericardial valves fails to fix the cells within the substance of the leaflet, which subsequently autolyze or dissolve away. Such a sequence would leave the valve acellular and supposedly unlikely to calcify. It is worthy of comment to recall that in the 1960s xenografts preserved in formaldehyde failed to adequately and "permanently" fix stromal cells. Explants were acellular and characteristically devoid of calcification.[116]

The Choice of Valve

There is no one valve that is universally indicated or suitable for all patients. Age, sex, geographic location and abode, the pathological valve disease and associated conditions, the likelihood of adequate maintenance of long-term anticoagulant therapy, coupled with the patient's preference and the surgeon's experience are strong determinants in choosing the best valve for any particular patient. The patient–valve selection criteria for aortic valve replacement by the author at The Prince Charles Hospital are summarized in Table 121–6.

TABLE 121–6. PATIENT–VALVE SELECTION CRITERIA

Age of Patient	First Choice	Second Choice
Children and young adults < 40 years	Pulmonary autograft (Ross procedure)	Aortic allograft
Adults up to 65–70 years (approx)	Aortic allograft	St Jude valve
Adults > 65 years	Stentless xenograft—Cryolife–O'Brien model 300 or for large orifice > 29 mm the Stented xenograft (X-cell St Jude Medical)	St Jude valve

In clinical practice, for most reoperations a St Jude valve has been used, although a number of patients, having had an allograft tissue valve at the first operation, request a similar type of valve because of the good life style and the desire to continue avoiding anticoagulation. For the small aortic root, any of the above valves are suitable and ideal. The more specific added indications for the allograft aortic valve, such as endocarditis as mentioned previously, are adhered to and may therefore modify the choices for any individual patient. The pulmonary valve autograft is still in its "infancy" and will undoubtedly receive close scrutiny and reporting by those few committed to the procedure.

ALLOGRAFT TISSUE DONATION CREED AND CUSTOM

Most medical and paramedical practitioners and recipient patients of tissue and organ transplantation see donation as "the gift of life." Yet, the demand far surpasses the supply. Organ procurement groups within hospital and in central city areas have to constantly educate and publicize in spite of the well-known patient success stories that transplantation has provided.

Organ donation permission on drivers' licenses, laws allowing retrieval of tissue unless specifically denied (some European countries), and the establishment of in-hospital organ donor coordinators (Spain) have been of major benefit. Yet, family members of recently deceased, as a whole, are sometimes reluctant to give permission for tissue retrieval. Compassion, ongoing support, and follow-up information to donor relatives of the successful transplantation are quality duties required of organ procurement teams and tissue bank personnel.

Surrounding all these aspects are the innate beliefs and customs of a people. Table 121–7 summarizes briefly the acceptance of limitations of many religious groups to tissue donation and transplantation. It is evident that a large proportion of the world's population encompasses the religions of Buddhism, Hinduism, Islam, and Shintoism. As a broad statement across these groups, there are some religious limitations and customs that limit or restrict the pathways of organ and tissue donation. The clinical experience with both organ and tissue transplantation is interestingly limited in these predominantly Asian countries.

THE FUTURE: A PERSONAL, GLOBAL VIEWPOINT

The past 10 years have seen clearer pictures of both the advantages and limitations of most valves. Many publications have outlined these features. The ease of insertion, satisfactory hemodynamics, and durability of the *mechanical* valve, particularly the double disc, are evident. But thromboembolism and anticoagulant complications still occur. Al-

TABLE 121–7. RELIGIOUS GROUP ACCEPTANCE

	Religion
Donation and transplant acceptable and encouraged	Anglican, Baha'i (sect within Buddhism), Baptist, Greek Orthodox, Liberal Judaism, Parsi (Indian), Quakers (Religious Society of Friends), Roman Catholic, Salvation Army, Unitarian Universalist, Uniting Church
Special limitation	Islam (organs to be transplanted immediately not stored in tissue banks) Orthodox Judaism (donation acceptable only from living donors)
Individual choice or conscience	Buddhism, Christian Scientists, Jehovah's Witness, Maori, Mormons, Pacific Islanders, Seventh Day Adventists
Custom	Hindu (custom dictates burial as a whole—donation unlikely)
Generally opposed	Gypsy, Shinto (transplantation acceptable to some)

though they have been lessened, the problem of microembolism to myocardium and brain, mostly undetectable and certainly not quantifiable, may always exist. The *xenograft,* while enjoying the short- and intermediate-term advantages of tissue valves, has shown too high an age-related structural deterioration and reoperation factor. It is highly likely that the *unstented* xenograft may extend its durability.

Much of the data on valve performance and durability have been generated from Western countries and it is not immediately transferable to the needs of developing countries. In the West, the accent is toward using the mechanical prosthesis for the young and middle-aged and the xenograft valve for the elderly. The actual watershed cross-over of age has institutional variation. Only in a small number of cardiac units, unfortunately, is there a strong accent on using tissue valves such as autografts and allografts for young and middle-aged patients. After a slow rate of change, one is now seeing an increasing number of units offering the whole range of tissue and mechanical valves.

In developing countries the needs are different. The valve population age is much younger. For instance, Carlos Duran and colleagues[117] from Saudi Arabia report in their 1052 patients that the mean age was 32 years with a median of 30 years, two-thirds of the patient group having had rheumatic valve disease and over one-third of the total group having multivalvar pathology. The xenograft is used frequently, particularly in young females, to avoid anticoagulants. The different cultural, social, economic, and pathologic characteristics of the patients modify the surgical judgements in favor of

- Repair if possible.
- Avoidance of anticoagulants as almost half of the patients are female with a median age of 30 years.

- Delaying operation for as long as possible and replacing the valve only if absolutely necessary.

Different again is the problem in India and in China where the cost of reoperation has seen almost the virtual discontinuance of the use of bioprostheses in many surgical centers. So the mechanical valve is preferred. Patients must accept the burden of anticoagulation. Yet the control of anticoagulation of patients from near and remote villages is far from ideal. The morbidity and mortality from anticoagulation and thromboembolism are not low. As patients fail to attend for follow-up at their surgical centers, their absence is not always recognized and thromboembolic complications and reoperation are not an apparent problem. Consequently the surgeon may be unaware that the long-term results are unsatisfactory. Therefore in many developing countries, for the present, the reoperation factor, its costs, and its risks are determinants dictating the valve choice at the initial operation. Nevertheless, in countries and in areas within countries where anticoagulant control is not ideal, the choice of a xenograft over a mechanical valve for the first operation would probably lead to more patients surviving for more decades, providing reoperation, when valve deterioration has occurred, is appropriately timed and performed with the low risk that should be attainable in this era. The unnecessary delaying of an operation until the patient status has deteriorated excessively and the consequent high operative mortality are both avoidable and unacceptable. Lastly, the cost of reoperation in some countries needs specific strategies such as cost factoring into the initial procedure.

Surgeons have failed, in many instances, to address the issues of all parties concerned. It is highly likely that more patients would survive longer with an allograft or xenograft at first and second operation than similar patients having a mechanical valve at a single once-only operation with the subsequent morbidity and mortality of thromboembolism and anticoagulation therapy at varying levels of control.

Newer nonaldehyde and anticalcification methods of xenograft preservation, the use of unstented xenografts, the possible extension of durability by newer mounting techniques for heterologous pericardial valves and autologous pericardial valves deserve an optimistic but watchful eye.

The pulmonary valve autograft is the "gold standard" for the young patient. The aortic allograft valve will not attain the durability of the aortic valve of the transplant heart (immunosuppressed patient) but will be a good second best. Unfortunately, because of supply problems, too few recipients will receive one. Adequate supply is not an insurmountable problem but its solution should probably be the major target for the future.

REFERENCES

1. Lam CR, Aram HH, Munnell ER: An experimental study of aortic valve homografts. *Surg Gynecol Obstet* **94:**129, 1952

2. Murray G: Homologous aortic-valve-segment transplants as surgical treatment for aortic and mitral insufficiency. *Angiology* **7:**466, 1956

3. Beall AC, Morris GC, Cooley DA, et al: Homotransplantation of the aortic valve. *J Thorac Cardiovasc Surg* **42:**497, 1961

4. Duran CG, Gunning AJ: A method for placing a total homologous aortic valve in the subcoronary position. *Lancet* **2:**488, 1962

5. Ross DN: Homograft replacement of the aortic valve. *Lancet* **2:**487, 1962

6. Barratt-Boyes BG: Homograft aortic valve replacement in aortic incompetence and stenosis. *Thorax* **19:**131, 1964

7. Paneth M, O'Brien MF: Transplantation of human homograft aortic valve. *Thorax* **21:**115, 1966

8. Barratt-Boyes BG, Roche AHG, Whitlock RML: Six year review of the results of freehand aortic valve replacement using an antibiotic sterilized homograft valve. *Circulation* **55:**353, 1977

9. Khanna SK, Ross JK, Monro JL: Homograft aortic valve replacement: Seven years' experience with antibiotic-treated valves. *Thorax* **36:**330, 1981

10. Watts LK, Duffy P, Field RB, et al: Establishment of a viable homograft cardiac valve bank: A rapid method of determining homograft viability. *Ann Thorac Surg* **21:**230, 1976

11. Angell JD, Christopher BS, Hawtrey O, Angell WM: A fresh viable human heart valve bank: Sterilization, sterility testing and cryogenic preservation. *Transplant Proc, Suppl 1* **8:**139, 1976

12. McGiffin DC, O'Brien MF, Stafford EG, et al: Long-term results of the viable cryopreserved allograft aortic valve: Continuing evidence for superior valve durability. *J Cardiac Surg Suppl* **3:**289, 1988

13. O'Brien MF, Johnston N, Stafford G, et al: A study of the cells in the explanted viable cryopreserved allograft valve. *J Cardiac Surg Suppl* **3:**279, 1988

14. Grunkemeier GL, Bodnar E: Comparison of structural valve failure among different "models" of homograft valves. *J Heart Valve Dis* **3:**556, 1994

15. O'Brien MF, Stafford EG, Gardner MAH, et al: The cryopreserved viable allograft aortic valves. In Yankah AC, Hetzer R, Miller DC, et al (eds): *Cardiac Valve Allografts 1962–1987*. Damstadt, West Germany, Steinkopff Verlag, 1988

16. Gall K, Smith S, Willmette C, et al: Allograft heart valve sterilization: A six year in depth analysis of a twenty-five year experience with low dose antibiotics. *J Thorac Cardiovasc Surg* 1995 (in press)

17. Kirklin JK, Barratt-Boyes BG: Aortic valve disease: In Kirklin JW, Barratt-Boyes BG (eds): *Cardiac Surgery*. New York, Churchill Livingstone, 1993, p 561

18. O'Brien MF, McGiffin DC, Stafford EG, et al: Allograft aortic valve replacement: Long-term comparative clinical analysis of the viable cryopreserved and antibiotic 4°C stored valves. *J Cardiac Surg Suppl 4* **6:**534, 1991

19. Crescenzo DG, Hilbert SL, Barrick MK, et al: Donor heart valves: Electron microscopic and morphometric assessment of cellular injury induced by warm ischemia. *J Thorac Cardiovasc Surg* **103:**253, 1992

20. Wiwaya K, Kitamura S, Kawachi K, Sakaguchi H: Effect of warm ischemia to cell viability of allograft valves. *VI Int Symp Cardiac Bioprostheses* 144, 1994 (abstr)

21. Ross D: Technique of aortic valve replacement with a homograft: Orthotopic replacement. *Ann Thorac Surg* **52:**154, 1991

22. Barratt-Boyes BG: A method for preparing and inserting a homograft aortic valve. *Br J Surg* **52:**847,1965

23. O'Brien MF, McGiffin DC, Stafford EG: Allograft aortic valve implantation: Techniques for all types of aortic valve and root pathology. *Ann Thorac Surg* **48:**600, 1989

24. Sommerville J, Ross D: Homograft replacement of aortic root with reimplantation of coronary arteries. Results after one to five years. *Br Heart J* **47:**473, 1982

25. McKowen RL, Campbell DN, Woelfel FG, et al: Extended aortic root replacement with aortic allografts. *J Thorac Cardiovasc Surg* **93:**366, 1987

26. Piehler JM, Danielson GK, Pluth JR, et al: Enlargement of the aortic root or annulus with autogenous pericardial patch during aortic valve replacement. Long-term follow-up. *J Thorac Cardiovasc Surg* **86:**350, 1983

27. Manouguian S, Seybold-Epting W: Patch enlargement of the aortic valve ring by extending the aortic incision into the anterior mitral leaflet. New operative technique. *J Thorac Cardiovasc Surg* **78:**402, 1979

28. Kirklin JW, Barratt-Boyes BG: Acquired valvular heart disease. In Kirklin JW, Barratt-Boyes BG (eds): *Cardiac Surgery*. New York, John Wiley, 1986, p 416

29. Ross DN, Martelli V, Wain WH: Allograft and autograft valves used for aortic valve replacement. In Ionescu MI (ed): *Tissue Heart Valves*. London, Butterworth, 1979, pp 127–172

30. Donaldson RM, Ross DM: Homograft aortic root replacement for complicated prosthetic valve endocarditis. *Circulation Suppl I* **70:**178, 1984

31. Lau JKH, Robles A, Cherian A, Ross DN: Surgical treatment of prosthetic endocarditis. Aortic root replacement using a homograft. *J Thorac Cardiovasc Surg* **87:**712, 1984

32. Kirklin JK, Kirklin JW, Pacifico AD: Aortic valve endocarditis with aortic root abscess cavity: Surgical treatment with aortic valve homograft. *Ann Thorac Surg* **45:**674, 1988

33. Ibrahim M, O'Kane H, Cleland J, et al: The St Jude Medical Prosthesis: A thirteen-year experience. *J Thorac Cardiovasc Surg* **108:**221, 1994

34. Sundt TM, Rasmi N, Wong K, et al: Aortic valve reoperation following homograft root replacement: Surgical options and results. *VI Int Symp Cardiac Bioprostheses* 41, 1994 (abstr)

35. Jones EL: Aortic valve replacement in the young. *J Card Surg Suppl* **9:**188, 1994

36. O'Brien MF, Stafford EG, Gardner MAH, et al: A comparison of aortic valve replacement with viable cryopreserved and fresh allograft valves, with a note on chromosomal studies. *J Thorac Cardiovasc Surg* **94:**812, 1987

37. O'Brien MF, Strafford EG, Gardner RH, et al: Allograft aortic valve replacement: Long-term follow-up. *Ann Thorac Surg* 1995 (in press)

38. Mitchell RS, Miller DC, Stinson EB, et al: Significant patient-related determinants of prosthetic valve performance. *J Thorac Cardiovasc Surg* **91:**807, 1986

39. Kirklin JW, Barratt-Boyes BG: Acquired valvular heart disease. In Kirklin JW, Barratt-Boyes BG (eds): *Cardiac Surgery*. New York, John Wiley, 1986, p 412

40. Kirklin JK, Barratt-Boyes BG: Acquired valvular heart disease. In Kirklin JW, Barratt-Boyes BG (eds): *Cardiac Surgery*. New York, Churchill Livingstone, 1993, p 546

41. McGiffin DC, Galbraith AJ, McLachlan GJ, et al: Aortic valve infection: Risk factors for death and recurrent endocarditis after aortic valve replacement. *J Thorac Cardiovasc Surg* **104:**511, 1992

42. Haydock D, Barratt-Boyes B, Macedo T, et al: Aortic valve replacement for active infectious endocarditis in 108 patients: A comparison of freehand allograft valves with mechanical prostheses and bioprostheses. *J Thorac Cardiovasc Surg* **103:**130, 1992

43. O'Brien MF, Finney RS, Stafford EG, et al: Root replacement for all allograft aortic valves: Preferred technique or too radical? *Ann Thorac Surg* (in press)

44. Christie GW, Barratt-Boyes BG: The effect of donor age on the mechanical properties of cryopreserved aortic allograft leaflets. *VI Int Symp Cardiac Bioprostheses* 44, 1994 (abstr)

45. Schoen FJ, Mitchell RN, Jonas RA: Structure-function correlations in explanted cryopreserved human valvular allografts: Collagen preservation without cellular viability. *IV Int Symp Cardiac Bioprostheses* 147, 1994 (abstr)

46. Bodnar E, Parker R, Davies I, et al: Non-viable aortic homografts. In Bodnar E, (ed): *Surgery for Heart Valve Disease*. London, ICR Publishers, 1990, pp 494–500

47. Bodnar E, Ross DN: Valvular homografts. In Bodnar E, Frater REW

(eds): *Replacement Cardiac Valves.* New York, Pergamon, 1991, pp 287–306

48. Barratt-Boyes BG, Roche AHG, Subramanyan R, et al: Long-term follow-up of patients with the antibiotic-sterilized aortic homograft valve inserted freehand in the aortic position. *Circulation* **75:**768, 1987

49. Khaghani A, Dhalla N, Penta A, et al: Patient status 10 years or more after aortic valve replacement using antibiotic sterilized homografts. In Bodnar E, Yacoub M (eds): *Biologic and Bioprosthetic Valves.* New York, Yorke Medical Books, 1986, pp 38–46

50. Yacoub M, Rasmi N, Sundt T, et al: Long term performance of the "unprocessed" aortic valve homograft. *VI Int Symp Cardiac Bioprostheses* 40, 1994 (abstr)

51. Kirklin JK, Smith D, Novick W, et al: Long-term function of cryopreserved aortic homografts. *J Thorac Cardiovasc Surg* **106:**154, 1993

52. McGiffin DC, Galbraith A, O'Brien MF, et al: An analysis of aortic valve re-replacement following biological valve failure. *J Thorac Cardiovasc Surg* (in press)

53. McLachlan GJ, McGiffin DC, Galbraith AJ, Adams P: Modeling via finite mixture of time to reoperation following aortic valve replacement. Research Report No 11, Brisbane, Centre of Statistics, The University of Queensland, 1994

54. Zhao XM, Green M, Frazer IH, et al: Donor-specific immune response after aortic valve allografting in the rat. *Ann Thorac Surg* **57:**1158, 1994

55. Lang SJ, Giordano MS, Cardon-Cardo C, et al: Biochemical and cellular characterization of cardiac valve tissue after cryopreservation or antibiotic preservation. *J Thorac Cardiovasc Surg* **108:**63, 1994

56. el-Khatib H, Lupinetti F: Antigenicity of fresh and cryopreserved rat valve allografts. *Transplantation* **49:**765, 1990

57. Fischlein T, Schultz A, Haushofer M, et al: Immunologic reaction and cellular viability of cryopreserved homografts. *VI Int Symp Cardiac Bioprostheses* 151, 1994 (abstr)

58. Yacoub M, Suitters A, Khaghani M, Rose M: Localization of major histocompatibility complex (HLA, ABC and DR) antigens in aortic homografts. In Bodnar E, Yacoub M (eds): *Biologic and Bioprosthetic Valves.* New York, Yorke Medical Books, 1986, pp 65–72

59. Yankah AC, Dreyer W, Wottge HU, et al: Kinetics of endothelial cells of preserved aortic valve allografts used for heterotopic transplantation in inbred rat strains. In Bodnar E, Yacoub M (eds): *Biologic and Bioprosthetic Valves.* New York, Yorke Medical Books, 1986, pp 73–87

60. Yankah AC, Wottge HU, Muller-Ruchholtz W: Prognostic importance of viability and a study of a second set allograft valve. An experimental study. *J Cardiac Surg* **3:**263, 1988

61. Clarke DR, Campbell DN, Hayward AR, Bishop DA: Degeneration of aortic valve allografts in young recipients. *J Thorac Cardiovasc Surg* **105:**934, 1993

62. Livi U, Addulla AK, Parker R, et al: Viability and morphology of aortic and pulmonary homografts: A comparative study. *J Thorac Cardiovasc Surg* **93:**755, 1987

63. Gavin JB, Monro JL, Wall FM, et al: Fine structural changes in the fibroblasts of canine heart valves prepared for grafting. *Thorax* **28:**748, 1973

64. Armiger LC, Gavin JB, Barratt-Boyes BG: Histological assessment of orthotopic aortic valve leaflet allografts: Its role in selecting graft pre-treatment. *Pathology* **15:**67, 1983

65. Armiger LC, Thomson RW, Strickett MG, et al: Morphology of heart valves preserved by liquid nitrogen freezing. *Thorax* **40:**778, 1985

66. O'Brien MF, Johnston N, Stafford EG, et al: A study of the cells in the explanted viable cryopreserved allograft valve. *J Card Surg* **3:**279, 1988

67. Kosek JC, Iben AB, Shumway NE, et al: Morphology of fresh heart valve homografts. *Surgery* **66:**269, 1969

68. Schoen FJ: Pathology of bioprostheses and other tissue heart valve replacements. In Silver MD (ed): *Cardiovascular Pathology,* 2nd ed. New York, Churchill Livingstone, 1991, pp 1547–1605

69. Lupinetti FM, Tsai TT, Kneebone JM, Bove EL: Effect of cryopreservation on the presence of endothelial cells on human valve allografts. *J Thorac Cardiovasc Surg* **106:**912, 1993

70. Christie GW, Barratt-Boyes BG: Identification of a failure mode of the antibiotic sterilized aortic allograft after 10 years: Implications for their long-term survival. *J Card Surg* **6:**462, 1991

71. Christie GW, Barratt-Boyes BG: The Biaxial mechanical properties of leaflets from explanted aortic allograft heart valves. *VI Int Symp Cardiac Bioprostheses* 209, 1994 (abstr)

72. Pomar JL, Mestres CA, Pae JC, Miro JM: Management of persistent tricuspid endocarditis with transplantation of cryopreserved mitral homografts. *J Thorac Cardiovasc Surg* **107:**1460, 1994

73. Acar C, Iung B, Cormier B, et al: Double mitral homograft for recurrent bacterial endocarditis of the mitral and tricuspid valves. *J Heart Valve Dis* **3:**470, 1994

74. Acar C, Deloche A, Farge A, et al: Partial and total replacement of the mitral valve using a cryopreserved mitral homograft. *Eur Heart J Suppl* **15:**230, 1994 (abstr)

75. Kumar AS, Trehan H: Homograft mitral valve replacement—a case report. *J Heart Valve Dis* **3:**473, 1994

76. Berghuis J, Rastelli CG, Van Vliet PD, et al: Homotransplantation of the canine mitral valve. *Circulation* (Suppl I) **29:**47, 1964

77. O'Brien MF, Gerbode F: Homotransplantation of the mitral valve: Preliminary experimental report and review of the literature. *Aust NZ J Surg* **34:**81, 1964

78. Rastelli GC, Berghuis J, Swan HJC: Evaluation of function of mitral valve after homotransplantation in the dog. *J Thorac Cardiovasc Surg* **49:**459, 1965

79. Lower RR, Stofer RC, Shumway NE: Autotransplantation of the pulmonary valve into the aorta. *J Thorac Cardiovasc Surg* **39:**680, 1960

80. Lower RR, Stofer RC, Shumway NE: Total excision of the mitral valve and replacement with the autologous pulmonic valve. *J Thorac Cardiovasc Surg* **42:**696, 1961

81. Pillsbury C, Shumway NE: Replacement of the aortic valve with the autologous pulmonic valve. *Surg Forum* **17:**176, 1966

82. Ross DN: Replacement of aortic and mitral valves with a pulmonary autograft. *Lancet* **2:**956, 1967

83. Somerville J, Saravalli O, Ross DN, et al: Long-term results of pulmonary autograft for aortic valve replacement. *Br Heart J* **42:**533, 1979

84. Matsuki O, Okita Y, Almeida RS, et al: Two decades' experience with aortic valve replacement with pulmonary autograft. *J Thorac Cardiovasc Surg* **95:**705, 1988

85. Ross D: Pulmonary valve autotransplantation (The Ross Operation). *J Card Surg* Suppl **3:**313, 1988

86. Ross D: Replacement of the aortic valve with a pulmonary autograft: The "switch" operation. *Ann Thorac Surg* **52:**1346, 1991

87. Ross D, Jackson M, Davies J: Pulmonary autograft aortic valve replacement: Long-term results. *J Card Surg* **6** (Suppl):529, 1991

88. Stelzer P, Elkins RC: Pulmonary autograft: An American experience. *J Cardiac Surg* **2:**429, 1987

89. Stelzer P, Jones DJ, Elkins RC: Aortic root replacement with pulmonary autograft. *Circulation* (Suppl 3) **80:**209, 1989

90. Oury JH, Angell WW, Eddy AC, Cleveland JC: Pulmonary autograft—past, present and future. *J Heart Valve Dis* **2:**365, 1993

91. Gerosa G, McKay R, Ross DN: Replacement of the aortic valve or root with a pulmonary autograft in children. *Ann Thorac Surg* **51:**424, 1991

92. Walls JT, McDaniel WC, Pope ER, et al: Letter to the Editor: Documented growth of autogenous pulmonary valve translocated to the aortic valve position. *J Thorac Cardiovasc Surg* **107:**1530, 1994

93. Elkins RC, Knott-Craig CJ, Ward KE, et al: Pulmonary autograft in children: Realized growth potential. *Ann Thorac Surg* **57:**1387, 1994 (Discussion, p 1393)

94. Livi U, Kay P, Ross D: The pulmonary homograft: An improved conduit for RVOT reconstruction. *Circulation* (Suppl II) **74**:250, 1986

95. O'Brien MF: Editorial: Aortic valve implantation techniques—should they be any different for the pulmonary autograft and the aortic homograft? *J Heart Valve Dis* **2**:385, 1993

96. Gorcynski A, Trenkner M, Anisimowicz L, et al: Biomechanics of the pulmonary autograft valve in the aortic position. *Thorax* **37**:535, 1982

97. Elkins RC: Editorial: Pulmonary autograft—the optimal substitute for the aortic valve? *N Engl J Med* **330**:59, 1994

98. Kouchoukos NT, Davila-Roman VG, Spray TL, et al: Replacement of the aortic root with a pulmonary autograft in children and young adults with aortic-valve disease. *N Engl J Med* **330**:1, 1994

99. Gonzalez-Lavin L, Robles A, Graf D: Morbidity following the Ross operation. *J Card Surg* **3**:305, 1988

100. Geens M, Gonzalez-Lavin L, Dawbarn C, et al: The surgical anatomy of the pulmonary artery root in relation to the pulmonary valve autograft and surgery of the right ventricular outflow tract. *J Thorac Cardiovasc Surg* **62**:262, 1971

101. Elkins RC, Santangelo KL, Stelzer P, et al: Pulmonary autograft replacement of the aortic valve: An evolution of technique. *J Card Surg* **7**:108, 1992

102. Elkins RC, Santangelo KL, Randolph JD, et al: Pulmonary autograft replacement in children: The ideal solution? *Ann Surg* **216**:363, 1992 (Discussion, p 370)

103. Sievers HH, Leyh R, Loose R, et al: Time course of dimension and function of the autologous pulmonary root in the aortic position. *J Thorac Cardiovasc Surg* **105**:775, 1993

104. Elkins RC, Knott-Craig CJ, Razook JD, et al: Pulmonary autograft replacement of the aortic valve in the potential parent. *J Card Surg*, Suppl 2 **9**:198, 1994

105. Lincoln JCR, Riley DA, ReVignas A, et al: Viability of autologous fascia lata in heart valve replacement. *Thorax* **26**:277, 1971

106. Silver MD, Hudson REB, Trimble AS: Morphologic observations on heart valve prostheses made of fascia lata. *J Thorac Cardiovasc Surg* **70**:360, 1975

107. Cooper E: Aortic and mitral valve replacement with autologous fascia lata valves. *Med J Aust, Spec Suppl* **2**:47, 1972

108. Love JW: *Autologous Tissue Heart Valves.* Austin, TX, RG Landes Co, 1993, pp 92–110

109. Love JW, Schoen FJ, Breznock EM, et al: Experimental evaluation of an autologous tissue heart valve. *J Heart Valve Dis* **1**:232, 1992

110. Love JW, Calvin JH, Phelan RF, Love CS: Rapid intraoperative fabrication of an autogenous tissue heart valve: A new technique. In Bodnar E, Yacoub M (eds): *Proceedings of the Third International Symposium on Cardiac Bioprostheses.* New York, Yorke Medical Books, 1986, pp 691–698

111. Love CS, Love JW: The autogenous tissue heart valve: Current status. *J Cardiac Surg* **6**:499, 1991

112. Love JW: Personal communication (1994)

113. Prabhakar G, Kumar M, Kumar N, et al: Autologous pericardial valved right ventricular outflow tract conduit: An experimental study. *VI Int Symp Cardiac Bioprostheses* 163, 1994 (abstr)

114. Liao K, Frater RWM, LaPietra A, et al: Time dependent effect of glutaraldehyde on the tendency to calcify of both autograft and xenograft implants. *VI Int Symp Cardiac Bioprostheses* 168, 1994 (abstr)

115. Jaffe NR, Hancock W: Absence of intrinsic dystrophic mineralization in cell extracted porcine heart valve bioprosthesis: In vivo studies. *New Dimensions in Prosthetic Heart Valves Symposium,* Whistler, British Columbia, p 11, July 1994 (abstr)

116. Stephens BJ, O'Brien MF: Pathology of xenografts in aortic valve replacement. *Pathology* **4**:167, 1972

117. Gometza B, Kumar N, Prabhakar G, et al: The challenge of valve surgery in a developing population. *J Heart Valve Dis* **2**:194, 1993

122

Selection and Complications of Cardiac Valvular Prostheses

Lawrence H. Cohn and Wayne Lipson

Since the first successful human valve implantation by Starr and Edwards[1] and Harken et al,[2] many advances in the design, material selection, and manufacturing have been made. Despite these advances none of the currently available prosthetic or bioprosthetic heart valves approaches the normal human valve in either hemodynamic function or long-term freedom from valve-related complications. Mechanical prosthetic valves offer acceptable hemodynamics and long-term durability, however, they are thrombogenic and thus require anticoagulation, which is associated with the risk of anticoagulant-related hemorrhage. Bioprosthetic valves do not require anticoagulation, since they are less thrombogenic, however, their long-term durability is limited by structural degeneration, which is markedly accelerated in younger patients.

This chapter will outline the characteristics of available FDA-approved prosthetic and bioprosthetic valves and will include hemodynamics, thromboembolism and anticoagulant hemorrhage, structural and nonstructural degeneration and failure, periprosthetic leak, and risk of endocarditis. These characteristics will be examined to appropriately match valve characteristics to specific patient requirements.

MECHANICAL VALVES

There are three types of commercially available mechanical valves: caged ball, tilting disc, and bileaflet (Fig. 122–1). Typically, mechanical valves are chosen for younger patients (less than 70 years of age) without history of bleeding problems. Since anticoagulation is required, the patient's social and geographic situation must allow for adequate follow-up. Low profile mechanical valves are preferable in pa-

tients with a narrow aortic root or a small left ventricle; bileaflet valves appear to be more suited for patients with a small annulus. Late survival in patients with currently available mechanical valves is shown in Table 122–1.[3–15] Most studies indicate that over half the late deaths are related to valve complications and other deaths are related to nonvalvular cardiac complications such as progressive heart failure and coronary disease-related infarction and/or arrhythmia.

Hemodynamics

When evaluating prosthetic valve hemodynamics, certain design characteristics should be considered. First, the valve should function free of mechanical failure for the life span of the patient. Second, the valve should not increase the work of the heart. Third, the valve should not cause cellular damage to blood components or stimulate the coagulation cascade. Each valve type may be compared with the respective design characteristics to determine which would be best suited to the particular patient in terms of the above qualities as well as pressure differential across the valve and effective valve orifices.

Heart valve prostheses consist of an orifice, through which blood flows and an occluder mechanism, which opens and closes the occluder. The occluder mechanisms in prosthetic valves are manufactured biomaterials. In a bioprosthesis, either porcine or bovine pericardial, the occluder is the natural biologic leaflet made from animal tissue.

For mechanical valves, the occluder is a ball, a disc, or two hemispherical leaflets. The disc valve, more commonly referred to as a tilting disc valve, and the bileaflet valve are considered to be low profile. The caged ball valve, in con-

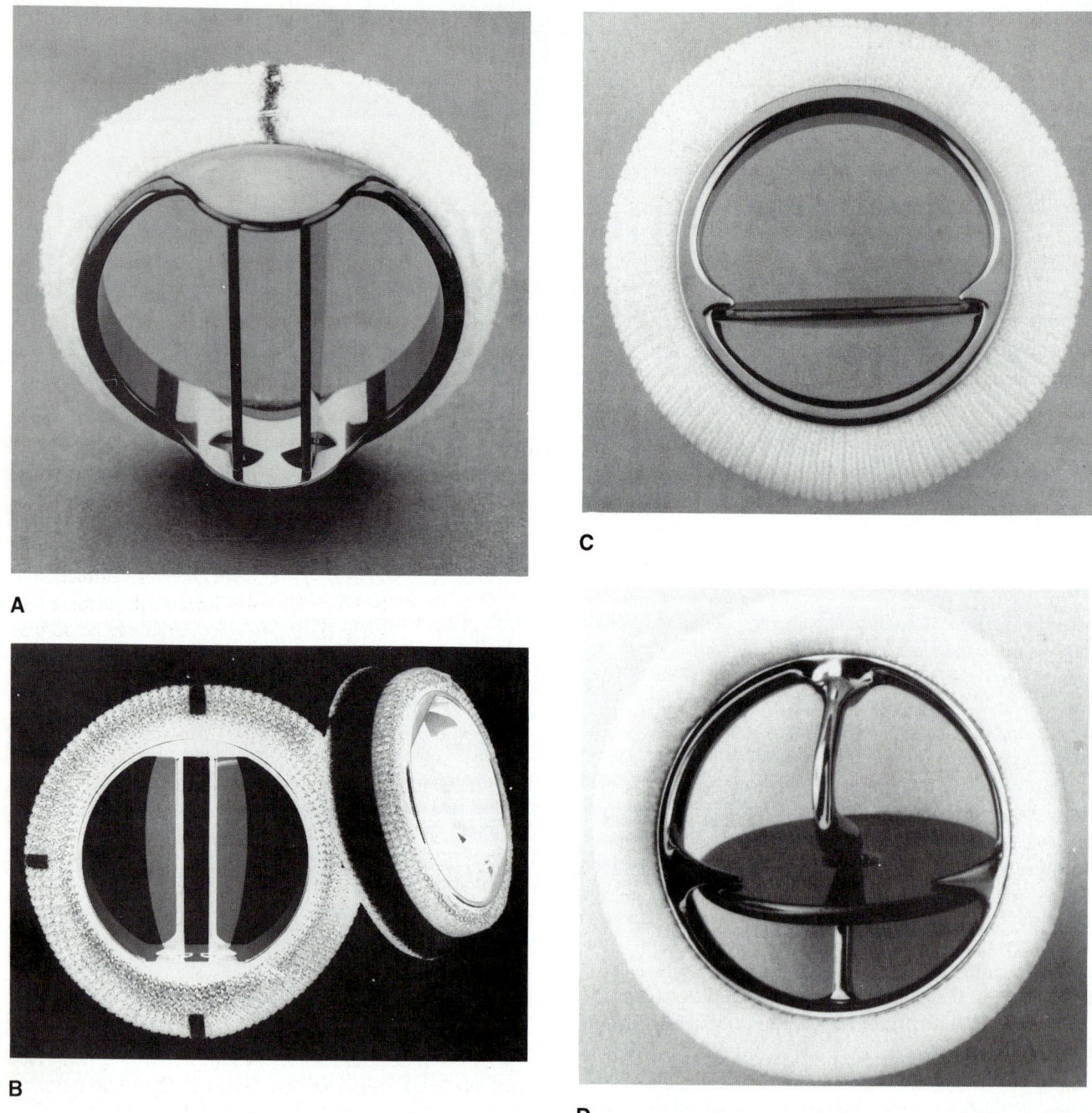

Figure 122–1. Commercially available mechanical valves. **A.** St. Jude Medical (bileaflet). *(Courtesy of St. Jude Medical.)* **B.** CarboMedics (bileaflet). *(Courtesy of CarboMedics.)* **C.** Omniscience (tilting disc). *(Courtesy of Omniscience.)* **D.** Medtronic Hall (tilting). *(Courtesy of Medtronic.) (Continued.)*

trast, has a high profile. The profile, that is the size, shape, degree of opening or opening angle, weight of the occluder and the dimensional relationship between the external valve, tissue annulus diameter, and internal orifice, all contribute to the degree of stenosis caused by the prosthesis. The volume of regurgitation, called leakage regurgitation, that occurs as the valve is closing is dependent on the size

of the gap between the occluder and internal valve housing. This amount of regurgitation allows backwashing while the valve is closing, which facilitates flushing of microemboli from the prosthesis. Regurgitation must be differentiated from periprosthetic leak, which occurs around the valve due to inadequate seal between the sewing ring and host tissue. Finally, all mechanical valves give rise to some slight de-

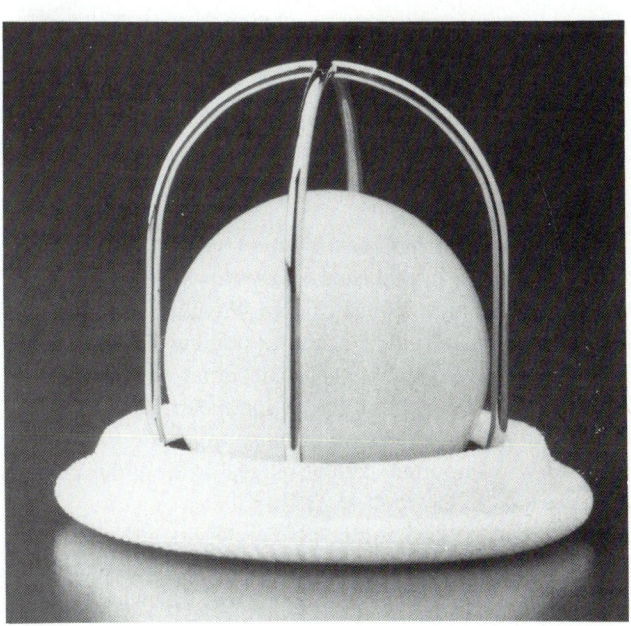

E

Figure 122–1. *(Continued.)* Commercially available mechanical valves. **E.** Starr–Edwards 6120 (caged ball).

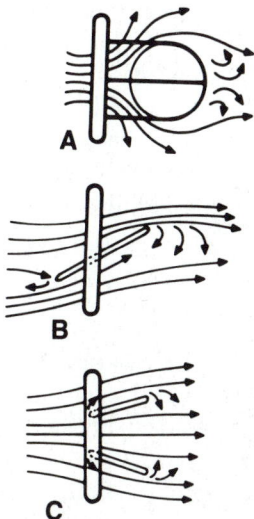

Figure 122–2. Flow patterns for different forms of prosthetic valves. **A.** Caged-ball valve. **B.** Tilting disc valve. **C.** Bileaflet valve.

gree of subclinical hemolysis as a result of flow abnormalities particular to each valve design.[16–20]

The Starr–Edwards caged ball valve prosthesis consists of a ball, usually silicone, entrapped in a cage. The ball sits directly on the orifice ring. This minimizes leakage through the closed valve. Due to the central obstruction of the ball, flow through the open orifice creates an annular area available for flow resulting in turbulent flow (Fig. 122–2a).[21] However, flow downstream becomes evenly distributed.[17] The disadvantages of this high profile valve are encountered in relation to the position of the valve. In the mitral position the ventricular outflow tract may be partially occluded. Also the cage may contact the ventricular wall during contraction. In the aortic position, size difference may lead to partial obstruction caused by the ball itself.[17–19,21]

The tilting disc prostheses (Medtronic Hall and Omni-

science) have significantly lesser degrees of obstruction to bloodflow. Most tilting disc valve have peak pressure values of 6 to 7 mm Hg (peak pressure values can be defined as the systolic pressure differences calculated from the left ventricle and the aorta). The specific opening angle is important in the disc valve because increased pressure differences can be attributed to a small opening angle of 60° or less that results in higher flow deflections.[20] However, the regurgitation volume is dependent on this opening angle. Therefore, a larger opening angle results in a longer time for disc closure, which ultimately leads to a higher value of regurgitation.[20] This increased regurgitation may be clinically significant in the setting of low cardiac output. As stated previously, regurgitation may reduce thrombus formation by virtue of the circular gap (found in most valves) between the occluder and the valve ring, which enhances backwash. However, flow through these narrow gaps may lead to increased shear stress resulting in hemolysis. Some tilting valve designs have a circular ceiling ring integrated into the inner valve ring that decreases flow through these gaps, thereby resulting in a decreased hemolysis.

Orientation of the valve, especially in the aortic position, may significantly affect hemodynamics. When blood flows through the valve, the disc is free to rotate, which divides the valve into a major or minor orifice (Fig. 122–2b). Approximately 70% of the blood flows through the major orifice. If the major orifice is directed toward the lesser curvature of the aorta, flow is not uniform and stasis may occur along the greater curvature.[17,22]

The bileaflet prostheses (St. Jude Medical and Carbo-Medics) have the lowest peak pressures due in large part to the wide opening angle. The wide opening angle, thin leaflets, and large cross section of the valve may result in minimal disturbance to flow when the valve is open. The valve can be divided into one minor and two major orifices

TABLE 122–1. LATE SURVIVAL FOLLOWING MECHANICAL VALVE REPLACEMENT[a]

Time	Implant Site	Type of Prosthesis		
		Caged Ball (%)	Tilting Disc (%)	Bileaflet (%)
5 years	AVR	78–82	92–96	76–92
	MVR	75–79	82–87	59–90
10 years	AVR	57–63	89–91	69–90
	MVR	54–60	78–82	48–84

[a]Pooled from analysis of several reports.[3–15]

(Fig. 122–2c). The wide opening angle does, however, result in larger regurgitant fractions. Leakage regurgitation in the bileaflet valves is increased due in part to the additional central gap between the leaflets.[23,24] Bileaflet valves, in general, have somewhat decreased values of hemolysis when compared to other valves except in the instance of periprosthetic leakage resulting in very high hemolysis.[25]

Thromboembolism

Thromboembolism is defined as any valve thrombosis or embolus exclusive of infection. Valve thrombosis can be obstructive or nonobstructive. Obstructive thrombosis can be defined as an accumulation of thrombus on the valve with potentially catastrophic hemodynamic or embolic consequences. This category includes all peripheral emboli and nonhemorrhagic strokes as well as transient ischemic attacks, reversible ischemic neurologic deficit, or major cerebral vascular accident. Nonobstructive valve thrombosis is usually a noncatastrophic event.[26,27] When selecting a valve, it should be understood that the thrombogenicity of prosthetic valves depends on valve design, surface area and texture, hemodynamic profile, turbulence, and stagnant areas.[28] Lack of endothelialization is also thought to contribute to a device's thrombotic potential. The incidence of thromboembolism for each type of mechanical valve is listed in Table 122–2.[3–15,28–32]

Thromboembolism and anticoagulant hemorrhage represent the most frequently cited complications (75%) in prosthetic valves. Most studies have noted that the highest risk for thromboembolism occurs in the first 14 mo after valve replacement and that the rate appears to drop to a steady level (approximately 0.5% per patient year).[28] The majority of thromboembolism has occurred in patients whose anticoagulation therapy was disrupted or discontinued, or in patients exhibiting an inadequate prothrombin time prior to the event. Therapeutic prothrombin times are defined as a prothrombin ratio of 1.5 to 1 or an INR of 2.5 or greater.[33,34] All patients with mechanical heart valves should be treated with anticoagulation therapy. To obtain an adequate INR, warfarin therapy should be instituted shortly after the operative procedure. Patients at high risk, that is, previously implanted heart valves, prior embolic complications, or with atrial fibrillation, may benefit not only from warafin but platelet inhibitors such as aspirin or dipyridamole.[33,35]

Patients with prosthetic valves in the aortic position are less prone to thromboembolic events because the majority of patients are in sinus rhythm. Prosthetic valves in the mitral position result in a higher number of thromboembolic events secondary to chronic atrial fibrillation (AF) and enlarged left atrium and/or intraventricular thrombus. AF is a common arrythmia in most prosthetic valve series and is a very important patient-related factor in thromboembolism.[36]

Patients with multiple valve replacement have demonstrated in some series a higher thromboembolic rate, possibly because of the increased debility of the patients undergoing this type of surgery. These patients typically have a low cardiac output and a high incidence of chronic atrial fibrillation. Other series, however, have demonstrated that results are better than either single valve alone, possibly because of the complete hemodynamic improvement resulting from double valve operation.[37–40] Although replacement of the severely diseased mitral valve decreases left atrial pressure, the affective valve orifice of any mitral prosthetic valve is relatively restricted compared to that of the natural valve. Intraventricular stasis can also occur with advanced left ventricular dysfunction resulting in the transmission of elevated left ventricular diastolic pressures to the left atrium. This may cause atrial mechanical dysfunction and stasis, which may result in thrombus formation.[36] Mechanical prostheses usually form thrombus in typical locations: above the struts, below the sewing rings, and at functional or engineered hinge points. These characteristics, along with the lack of endothelium, may give rise to the unique flow patterns that induce thrombus on the valve.[41–43] When anticoagulation is not appropriate, small bits of thrombotic material that form begin to organize and eventually lead to

TABLE 122–2. COMPARISON OF VALVE-RELATED MORBIDITY[a]

| Event | Implant Site | Events per Patient Year | | | | |
		Starr–Edwards	St. Jude Medical	Medtronic Hall	Omniscience	CarboMedics
Thromboembolism	AVR	1.4–3.3	0.7–2.8	0.8–4.7	0–2.9	0.5–0.87
	MVR	1.5–5.7	0.4–4.0	0.5–4.2	1.0–2.3	0.5–4.27
Anticoagulant-related hemorrhage	AVR	0.8–3.1	0.2–7.9	0.7–2.6	0–1.6	1.55–1.58
	MVR	1.0–3.7	0.3–2.9	0.5–4.8	0.6–2.7	1.56–1.70
Endocarditis	AVR	0.4–1.1	0.1–2.1	0–1.2	0.2–1.3	0.4–0.6
	MVR	0.3–0.8	0.1–2.2	0–1.7	0.5–0.8	0.35
Periprosthetic leak	AVR		0–3.4	0–0.4	0–1.8	0.78–1.21
	MVR		0.7–2.2	0.3–0.6	0–1.6	

[a]Pooled from analysis of several reports.[3–15, 28–32]

thrombosis and a low output syndrome due to the valve inlet or outlet obstruction. Thrombosis of a prosthetic valve can be a catastrophic event. This usually results from patients on long-term oral anticoagulation in whom such therapy is stopped in preparation for a minor surgical procedure or a major operation. Traditionally, therapy for thrombosed heart valves has been surgical. The diagnosis of the thrombosed prosthetic heart valve prompts emergency surgery to remove the clot and usually to rereplace the patient's valve. Due to the inability to remove all the prosthetic thrombotic material that is present in varying degrees of age, meticulous aspiration and removal are required. The thrombus may be organized to the point that it has become quite fibrotic. If the thrombus is on the underside of the ventricular aspect of some valves, it is impossible to remove all the clot unless the valve is completely excised. Recently, the use of thrombolytic agents such as streptokinase, urokinase, and tissue plasminogen activator (t-PA) has been employed to reduce and relieve thrombotic obstruction and allow nonoperative treatment of acute thrombosis of prosthetic valves.[44–47] Thrombolysis should be used only in patients with reasonable hemodynamics; patients in the low output syndrome should be operated on emergently.

Hemorrhage

This complication is defined as any episode of internal or external bleeding that causes death, stroke, or operation or requires transfusion.[26,27] Hemorrhage in this setting is restricted to patients who are receiving anticoagulants and/or antiplatelet drugs. The incidence of hemorrhage for each type of mechanical valve is found in Table 122–2.[3–15,28–32] The incidence of hemorrhage is approximately the same for valves placed in either aortic or mitral valve position. The risk of anticoagulated related bleeding is known to be closely associated with high anticoagulation levels (INR greater than 4.5).[48] This is evidenced by patients who have had a previous embolic history and have thus been treated with higher levels of anticoagulants. However, recent studies indicate that high (INR greater than 4.5) levels of anticoagulation confer no advantages over moderate anticoagulation (INR approximately 2.5) in terms of minimizing embolic risk. Maintaining INR levels at 2.5 to 3.5 will reduce hemorrhagic complications and should provide adequate thromboembolic prevention. At these levels the incidence of anticoagulated related death is approximately 0.2% per patient year.[49–51] In a patient with intractable bleeding following placement of mechanical valve, the use of a bioprosthesis should be considered despite the rate of mortality associated with re-operation.[52]

Endocarditis

Any infection involving a prosthetic valve is considered to be prosthetic valve endocarditis (PVE). This diagnosis is based on clinical criteria including an appropriate combination of positive blood cultures, fever, new, or altered cardiac murmurs, splenomegaly, and systemic emboli.[26] Morbidity associated with PVE includes severe systemic sepsis, valve thrombosis, septic emboli, and severe periprosthetic leak.[3–15,28–32] Although occurring at a relatively low rate (Table 122–2) PVE is associated with a high mortality ranging from 23 to 69%.[53,54] PVE occurs most frequently in the first several months postoperatively due to preoperative and intraoperative contamination and early postoperative surgical infection from line sepsis and other nosocomial infections. The incidence of PVE then diminishes to about 0.17% per patient year. Late infections are likely to be caused by bacteremia associated with surgical and dental procedures or other noncardiac infectious sources.[55] The most common morphologic feature of PVE is the occurrence of infection at the tissue-prosthesis site of attachment (sewing ring) resulting in a valve ring abscess.[56] This tends to burrow outward into the annulus. The burrowing nature of this infection makes antibiotic therapy ineffective in most cases, thus requiring early and aggressive surgical intervention.[57]

Periprosthestic Leakage

Periprosthetic leakage is leakage of blood around the valve due to an inadequate seal between the sewing ring and the host tissue. The incidence of periprosthetic leakage for each mechanical valve is found in Table 122–2.[3–15,28–32] Etiologies that predispose to periprosthetic leakage include (1) annular calcification, (2) infection, (3) annuloprosthetic mismatch, (4) excessive tension on sutures or annulus or both, (5) specific technique of suture placement and insufficient number of sutures, and (6) inadequate fibrous ingrowth or abnormal annulus tissue.[58,59]

Endocarditis, one of the most frequent causes of leakage, should be suspected in patients who have repeated leaks. Also, leaks that occur in the late postoperative period should be considered to be from an infectious cause.

Annular calcification makes placement of the valve into the annulus more difficult. Debridement may remove the calcium but may also leave a friable, thin, tissue annulus that may not effectively hold any suture. Both circumstances may lead to the development of a periprosthetic leak.[59]

Valvular mismatch usually occurs when a prosthetic valve is too large for the annulus. This is a result of improper valve seating with one portion of the sewing ring remaining above the annulus. Mismatch can also occur when the prosthetic valve is too small for the annulus. This may result in sutures pulling the annulus tissue towards the sewing ring. This is totally dependent on the strength of the sutures and tissues. Any tear in the tissue caused by the suture can lead to a leak.[58–60]

Suture placement may also lead to periprosthetic leak. Some studies have suggested that a continuous suture method is associated with a high rate of leakage in aortic or mitral valve replacement, whereas others have concluded that a continuous suture technique and the individual pledgetted mattress suture technique prevent postoperative periprosthetic leakage. Findings also noted that well-placed, pledget-reinforced sutures, rather than multiple deep interrupted sutures, prevent postoperative leak.[58,61]

Fibrous ingrowth occurs at the sewing ring where tissue from myocardium or the aortic wall grows into and over fabric covering the rough surface with partial anchoring of the valve. Clinical evidence has demonstrated that fibrous ingrowth alone may be inadequate to secure the valve sewing ring completely. Morphologic studies revealed that much of this strength between the tissue and valve bond is provided by sutures.[62,63]

Structural Valve Degeneration

Structural failure due to intrinsic mechanisms (that is related to valve design and/or material selection and properties) is an extremely rare occurrence in presently available mechanical valves. Most reported failures are due to leaflet fracture with one report attributing failure to cracks in the pivot guards.[64–66] Structural failure that occurs in the intraoperative or early postoperative period may result from mishandling during the surgical procedure. Sharp instruments can cause a deep scratch in the leaflet or disc resulting in early fracture once valve function begins. Failure in the late postoperative period may be due in part to a fatigue mechanism where a subcritical deep scratch, material defect, or inconspicuous microfracture progresses slowly under physiologic stresses until fracture occurs.[67]

Nonstructural Valve Dysfunction

Nonstructural dysfunction is defined as any abnormality resulting in stenosis or regurgitation at the valve that is not intrinsic to the valve itself. Sterile or infected thrombus and pannus formation can lead to interference with the occluder mechanism. Pannus formation occurs more commonly in the mitral position at approximately 0.3% per patient year.[10] This pannus formation as well as overgrowth of other fibrous tissue can result in obstruction of the inflow orifice preventing full opening and/or closure of the occluder. Retained strands of chordal tissue and unraveled or excessively long sutures can become trapped between a disc edge and the valve ring. This may result in the failure of the occluder mechanism causing the occluder to be jammed in the closed position.[69,70] Interference with the free movement of the occluder may also occur from impingement of the ventricular myocardium, intraventricular septum, or from intimal debris. Some studies have attributed this to improper sizing of the prosthesis. Annular calcific nodules have also been shown to prevent full opening and closure of the occluder as evidenced by calcified internal plaque that came into contact with the occluder mechanism.[70] Finally, valve orientation may affect the occluder

mechanism (specifically tilting disc valves where the occluder slips beyond the axis of bloodflow).[72]

BIOPROSTHETIC CARDIAC VALVES

This category of valves include prostheses that are made from biological tissue. This includes homografts, glutaraldehyde-preserved porcine valve, and bovine pericardial protheses. Because of the lower incidence of thrombosis and a virtual lack of indications for anticoagulation, tissue valves are ideal for patients at risk for hemorrhage, those who cannot receive adequate anticoagulation follow-up, or those who want to have children. Late survival of bioprosthetic valves is shown in Table 122–3.[73–81] As with mechanical valves, most late deaths result primarily from myocardial factors contributing to left ventricular failure, acute myocardial infarction and arrhythmias. Currently available bioprotheses are illustrated in Figure 122–3.

Glutaraldehyde-Preserved Porcine Valves

Porcine valves are stent-mounted heterografts. The occluding mechanism consists of porcine leaflets mounted on a cloth-covered flexible wire or plastic frame called a stent. The frame is designed to give the prosthesis the minimal profile height. The leaflets are treated with glutaraldehyde at low pressure to maintain leaflet structure and pliability.[16,17]

Hemodynamics

Porcine valves open into an irregular cone shape that allows for central unimpeded flow (Fig. 122–4a). Flow disturbances may occur from projection of the stent posts into the flow field and by buckling of leaflet free edges producing an irregular outflow orifice. Leakage through the closed valve is minimal as the leaflets are forced tightly under back pressure.[16] There are extensive data on the hemodynamics of porcine bioprotheses.[82–88] In the aortic position, the small sizes (19 and 21 mm) of prostheses have been found to be relatively stenotic. In the larger sizes, flow characteristics are improved over the mechanical valves and

TABLE 122–3. LATE SURVIVAL FOLLOWING BIOPROSTHETIC VALVE REPLACEMENT[a]

Time (years)	Implant Site	Porcine (%)	Bovine[b] Pericardial (%)
5	AVR	78–84	84–89
	MVR	76–80	
10	AVR	51–59	79–86
	MVR	40–49	

[a]Pooled from analysis of several reports.[73–81]
[b]Data for aortic valve replacement only.

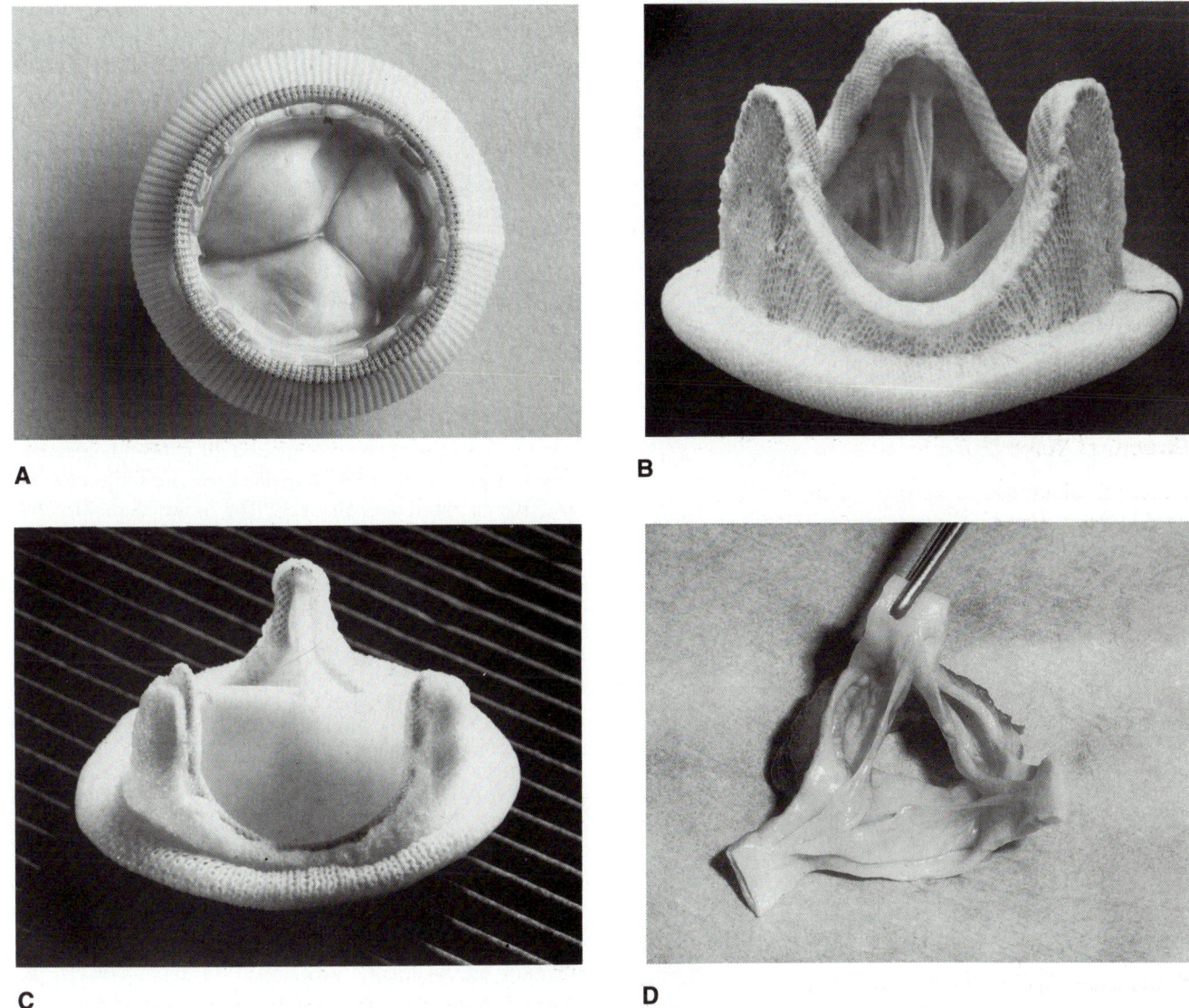

Figure 122–3. **A.** Hancock MO (porcine) **B.** Carpentier–Edwards (porcine) **C.** Carpentier–Edwards pericardial (bovine) **D.** Cryolife homograft. *(Courtesy of CryoLife Cardiovascular.)*

there is less shear stress to blood elements.[82] A supraannular bioprosthesis was developed to allow for supraannular placement of the prosthesis in the aortic position. This maximized the effective orifice of the bioprostheses and minimized turbulent carried by the seating of the valve into the annulus. The inner support is flared between the commissures to accommodate the much wider opening characteristic of the low-pressure fixed leaflets, thus minimizing the risk of abrasion of the leaflets against the stent.[81,83–85] The supraannular bioprosthesis demonstrates a hemodynamic improvement over the standard porcine valves at 19 to 23 mm. The newer generation bioprostheses have been constructed for supraanular implantation. In these prostheses the orifice can be of the same diameter as the patient's valve annulus if the supra-aortic space can accommodate the prosthesis.[85] Since the orifice is central, porcine valves do not require orientation in any special direction, although prevention of impingement of the left ventricular outflow track or on aortic wall closure by the high profile stents should be taken into account. Hemodynamic performance in the mitral position has been demonstrated to be satisfactory under both rest and exercise conditions.[86]

Thromboembolism

The incidence of thromboembolism is low in porcine bioprostheses. As noted in Table 122–4, the incidence was as high as 2.8% per patient year in the aortic position and 5.8% per patient year in the mitral position. The usual incidence ranges from 0.7 to 1.2% per patient year for the aortic prosthesis and is approximately 1.7% per patient year in the mitral position.[78–81] The incidence of thromboembolism in

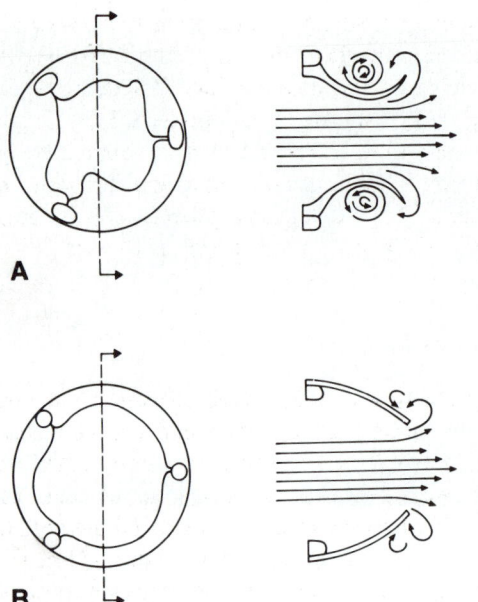

Figure 122–4. Flow patterns for bioprosthetic valves. **A.** Porcine bioprosthesis. **B.** Pericardial bioprosthesis.

the mitral position is higher than that for the aortic position. This may be related to pre-existing atrial dysfunction and chronic atrial fibrillation. It is therefore recommended that patients with atrial fibrillation and low cardiac output who have porcine valves in the mitral position be anticoagulated after valve implantation. An INR of 2.0 to 3.0 has been determined to be adequate.[50] Anticoagulation therapy in patients with porcine valves in the aortic position who have good cardiac function and are in sinus rhythm is unnecessary. Thrombosis of porcine valves is a rare event in the mitral and aortic position and usually occurs as a result of low cardiac output.

TABLE 122–4. COMPARISON OF VALVE-RELATED MORBIDITY FOR PORCINE BIOPROSTHETIC VALVES[a]

Event	Implant Site	Events per Patient Year	
		Medtronic Hancock	*Carpentier– Edwards*
Thromboembolism	AVR	0.7–0.97	1.0–1.2
	MVR	1.7–1.93	1.4–1.7
Anticoagulant- related bleeding	AVR	0.3–0.8	0.3–0.7
	MVR	0.6–1.2	1.2–2.1
Endocarditis	AVR	0.6–0.9	0.2–0.9
	MVR	0.2–0.5	0.5–1.0
Structural valve deterioration	AVR	0.4–1.11	0.4–1.0
	MVR	1.1–1.93	1.1–2.6
Periprosthetic leak	AVR	N/A[b]	0–0.3
	MVR		0.1–0.2

[a]Pooled from analysis of several reports.[73–81]
[b]N/A, not available.

Hemorrhage

The incidence of anticoagulant-related hemorrhage for each porcine valve is found in Table 122–4.[73–81] The lack of need for long term anticoagulation therapy is the major advantage of porcine valves over prosthetic valves. As noted, rates are higher in the mitral position due primarily to the fact that anticoagulation therapy is used to treat chronic atrial fibrillation, which is found in a significant number of patients with mitral valve disease. Lately, patients in chronic atrial fibrillation are generally given a prosthetic because of the necessity of anticoagulants for patients in atrial fibrillation.

Structural Valve Dysfunction

Despite the advantages of decreased thromboembolism and hemorrhage, porcine bioprosthetic valves are subject to progressive degenerative changes. The finite durability has been a major impediment to the long-term success of most biologic valve prostheses. The overall incidence of structural deterioration is found in Table 122–4.[73–81] The reasons for valve failure are twofold: first, calcification in valves causes stiffening or tearing and second, collagen degeneration-associated cuspal defect. Regurgitation through tears forming secondary to calcific nodules is the most frequent failure mode; pure stenosis due to calcific cuspal isolated stiffening and noncalcific tears or perforation are less frequent.[89–91] Noncalcific tears, revealed by scanning electron microscopy as fraying and disruption of collagen fibers, usually reflect direct mechanical damage to collagen.[92,93] Deterioration is time dependent, which accounts for the accelerated rate of valve failure beginning 8 to 10 years after operation.[89] Moreover, valve failure and calcification are markedly accelerated in bioprostheses implanted in children, adolescents, and young adults.[94,95] Although structural deterioration usually leads to gradual and progressive dysfunction thereby allowing elective reoperation, precipitous deterioration can occasionally occur requiring emergent reoperation. Studies have demonstrated that tissue degeneration was responsible for approximately two-thirds of all porcine prosthetic reoperations.[79]

Mitral valve prostheses have a higher failure rate than that of aortic valve prostheses. Mechanisms suggested include the increased compressive stresses seen by the mitral valve compared to that seen by the aortic valve prostheses during closure. Also, the rate of closure is expected to be greater with the mitral valve compared to that of the aortic valve. Lastly, atrial fibrillation can be implicated.[97]

Endocarditis

Prosthetic valve endocarditis (PVE) is not a common problem with porcine prostheses and the incidence is similar to that of prosthetic valves. The overall incidence of PVE is found in Table 122–4. The incidence by position is similar.

PVE in the porcine valve, like that of the mechanical valve, can be localized to the sewing ring and is complicated by ring abscess and its sequelae. Infections may also involve cuspal tissue, which can be treated successfully with antibiotic therapy alone, without surgery.[98] In isolated cuspal infection, valve incompetence may result in cuspal tearing, perforation, or destruction. Bacteria within cuspal vegetations can undergo extensive calcification.[93,97]

Periprosthetic Leak

The etiology of periprosthestic leak is similar to that found in mechanical valves. Overall incidence is found in Table 122–4.

PERICARDIAL VALVES

The pericardial valve uses bovine pericardium as a material to fabricate a trileaflet valve that is cut, fitted, and sewn onto a stent. Hemodynamically, pericardial valves provide the best solution to flow problems. The design of the valve makes maximum use of the available flow area, which results in minimal resistance to flow.[17] As illustrated in Figure 122–4b, the cone shape of the open valve and circular oriface minimize flow disturbance. Previous studies indicated poor durability of pericardial valves, namely the Ionescu-Shiley, was caused by leaflet tearing. This led to significant changes in design, including mounting of the pericardium completely within the stent.[99] This resulted in less abrasion to the leaflets with the hope of increasing long-term durability.[100] Valve-related complications are found in Table 122–5.[101,102] These are similar to that demonstrated by porcine prosthetic valves. With new design changes intermediate results appear to be markedly improved. Further long term follow-up is necessary.

HOMOGRAFT VALVE PROSTHESES

The use of homograft valves for aortic valve replacement was accomplished by Ross[103] and by Barratt-Boyes[104] in the early 1960s. However, problems in obtaining fresh valves, sterilization, storage, and technically demanding surgical expertise delayed widespread acceptance of the homograft. Early methods of sterilization and preservation resulted in structural deterioration.[105] Recent reports confirming cell viability in cryopreserved homografts and demonstration of long-term clinical durability have renewed interest in the use of homographs for aortic valve replacement.[106–109] Long-term patient survival has ranged from 85 to 94% at 7.5 years to 71% at 14 years.[107–109]

Durability

Homografts were initially preserved fresh in antibiotic solution with sterilization by irradiation and chemical means that did not provide acceptable long-term durability.[110–112] Failure was attributed to cusp rupture and calcification.[105,113] Freedom from valve tissue failure with this type of preservation at 14 years was noted to be 51%.[109] Pathology of explanted valve found homographs to be acellular when preserved in this manner. Homograft durability has improved substantially with cryopreservation. Using the method of 24-hour storage in antibiotic solution followed by cryopreservation, freedom from structural deterioration as found in Table 122–6 ranges from 95 to 98% at 10 years and decreases to 85% at 14 years.[107,109] It has been suggested that cryopreservation retains the viability of fibroblasts within the leaflets. This maintains the capacity of the homograft to regenerate, to replace dead or damaged cells, and to repair itself. The ability of the homograft to regenerate would then result in an improved structural integrity and increase long term durability.[109,114] A potential disadvantage of the viable homograft is the possibility of a greater immunologic response. One study suggested that cryopreserved homografts result in the loss of endothelial cells just leaving fiberblasts intact. Loss of endothelium may diminish this immunologic stimulus.[115]

Thromboembolism

The incidence of thromboembolism has been extremely low in adults and children. Freedom from thromboembolism found in Table 122–6 has ranged from 95 to 97% at 10 years and 94% at 14 years.[107,109] Freedom from thromboembolism was 100% at 7.5 years in children.[108] The low

TABLE 122–5. VALVE-RELATED MORBIDITY IN CARPENTIER–EDWARDS BOVINE PERICARDIAL BIOPROSTHESES[a]

Event	% per Patient Year
Thromboembolism	1.45
Anticoagulant-related hemorrhage	0.2
Endocarditis	0.9
Structural valve deterioration	0.1

[a]Pooled from analysis of two reports.[101,102]

TABLE 122–6. CYROPRESERVED HOMOGRAFT VALVE; PERCENT FREEDOM FROM EVENTS[a]

Event	At 10 Years (%)	At 14 Years (%)
Structural deterioration	95–98	85
Thromboembolism	95–97	94
Endocarditis	92–94	94

[a]Analysis pooled from several reports.[105–114]

incidence of thromboembolism noted was achieved without the need for anticoagulant therapy.

Loss of endothelium from cryopreservation techniques may result in a higher incidence of thromboembolism, however, studies of explanted valves were not covered by endothelium, suggesting that endothelium may not be an important factor in preventing thrombogenicity in homografts.[114,115]

Endocarditis

The incidence of endocarditis has also been low. Freedom from endocarditis as shown in Table 122–6 has ranged from 92 to 94% at 10 years to 94% at 14 years.[107,109] Studies have found *Staphylococcus aureus* to be one of the major organisms responsible for endocarditis in homografts.[108] In one study, all cases of endocarditis were treated successfully using IV antibiotics.[107] Homografts have not been associated with early postoperative endocarditis as demonstrated by mechanical and bioprosthetic valves.[114] However, endocarditis is an indication for homograft removal and reoperation when failure of IV antibiotics occurs. Implantation of homografts has been performed using a variety of surgical techniques. Implantation is technically more demanding, with little or no margin for technical error. The incidence of early aortic homograft valve incompetence is considered to be primarily technical in origin. Appropriate sizing, valve placement, and technical modifications have decreased valve incompetence.[107,109,116] The applicability of homografts has been limited to the aortic and pulmonary valves, however, recent work using homografts in the mitral position and in congenital heart lesions has been successful.[117–120] Availability of homografts has improved with the commercialization of cryopreserved homografts, however, the need for intact hearts for transplantation may limit its use.

VALVE SELECTION

The decision about which type of valve to use should be based on patient parameters such as age, risk of reoperation, underlying medical and surgical problems, and the risk of hemorrhage or thromboembolism. Figure 122–5 suggests a selection method for valves according to patient-related variables.[29]

Bioprosthetic valves should be used primarily in an elderly age group as the incidence of structural valve degeneration is reduced in this patient group. Lack of anticoagulation is also a distinct advantage in the elderly age group because they will have more concomitant medical and surgical problems. However, in any patient, regardless of age, in whom long-term anticoagulation is relatively or absolutely contraindicated, it is preferential to use a biologic valve. An example of this is a woman in the childbearing years who requires valve surgery. Such a patient

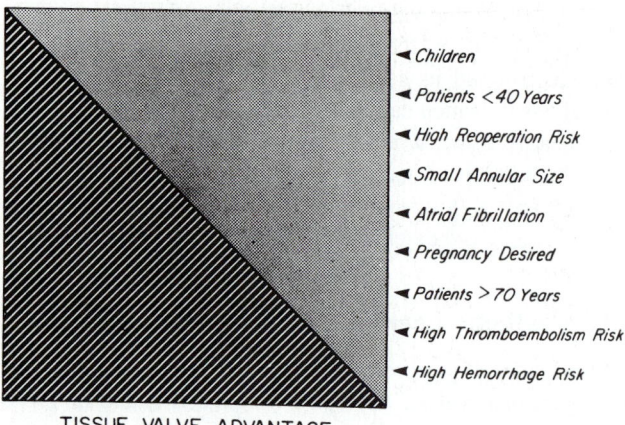

Children
Patients < 40 Years
High Reoperation Risk
Small Annular Size
Atrial Fibrillation
Pregnancy Desired
Patients > 70 Years
High Thromboembolism Risk
High Hemorrhage Risk

TISSUE VALVE ADVANTAGE

Figure 122–5. Relative advantage of mechanical valves or tissue valves according to patient-related variables.

would be a perfect candidate for a biologic valve since anticoagulation with warfarin is contraindicated. Mechanical bioprosthesis have an advantage in children, young adults, and patients who have a high risk at reoperation. A patient with a small annulus should also preferentially receive a mechanical prostheses or, if available and suitable, a homograft valve.

Reoperation for a failed valve has a mortality of 5 to 20%, with mortality statistics becoming increasingly worse with each subsequent reoperation.[121–123] Reoperation mortality is dependent on age, function of the heart, whether the procedure is elective or emergent, and whether the prosthesis is infected.[123]

In conclusion, improved survival and better quality of life will improve with better matching of valve characteristics to patient parameters. With continuing design, material, and manufacturing innovations, patients will benefit from better functional results and an increased long-term survival.

REFERENCES

1. Starr A, Edwards ML: Mitral replacement: Clinical experience with a ball valve prosthesis. *Ann Surg* **154:**726, 1961
2. Harken DE, Soroff HS, Taylor WJ, et al: Partial and complete prostheses in aortic insufficiency. *J Thorac Cardiovasc Surg* **40:**744, 1960
3. deLuca L, Vitale N, et al: Midterm follow-up after heart valve replacement with Carbo Medics bileaflet prostheses. *J Thorac Cardiovasc Surg* **106:**1158, 1993
4. O'Kane H, Cleland B, Gladstone D, et al: The St. Jude prosthesis. A thirteen year experience. *J Thorac Cardiovasc Surg* **108:**221, 1994
5. Hayashi J, Oguma F, Tsuchida S, et al: Review of ten years' use of the St. Jude Medical prosthetic valve replacement and post operative management at Nigata University Hospital. *Acta Med Biol* **41:**81, 1993
6. Fiore AC, Nauheim KS, D'Orazio S, et al: Mitral valve replacement: Radomized trial of St Jude and Medtronic Hall prostheses. *Ann Thorac Surg* **54:**68, 1992
7. Czer LSC, Chaux A, Matloff J, et al: Ten year experience with the

St. Jude Medical valve for primary valve replacement. *J Thorac Cardiovasc Surg* **100:**44, 1990

8. Arom KV, Nicoloff DM, Kersten TE, et al: Ten years' experience with the St. Jude Medical valve prosthesis. *Ann Thorac Surg* **47:**831, 1989

9. Akalin H, Corapcioglu ET, Ozyurdu U, et al: Clinical evaluation of Ominiscience cardiac valve prosthesis. *J Thorac Cardiovasc Surg* **103:**259, 1992

10. Damle A, Coles J, Teijeira J, et al: A six year study of the Omniscience valve in five Canadian centers. *Ann Thorac Surg* **43:**513, 1987

11. Akins CW, Buckley MJ, Daggert WM, et al: Ten year follow-up of the Starr-Edwards prosthesis. In Rabago G, Cooley DA (eds): *Heart Valve Replacement and Future Trends in Cardiac Surgery*. New York, Futura, 1987, p 137

12. Miller DC, Oyer PE, Mitchell RS, et al: Performance characteristics of the Starr-Edwards model 1260 aortic valve prosthesis beyond ten years. *J Thorac Cardiovasc Surg* **88:**193, 1984

13. Miller DC, Oyer PE, Mitchell RS, et al: Ten to fifteen year reassessment of the performance characteristics of the Starr-Edwards 6120 mitral valve prosthesis. *J Thorac Cardiovasc Surg* **85:**1, 1983

14. Keenan RS, Armitage JM, Trento A, et al: Clinical experience with the Medtronic-aortic valve prosthesis. *Ann Thorac Surg* **50:**748, 1990

15. Antunes MJ, Wessels A, Sadowski RG, et al: Medtronic valve replacement in a third world population group. A review of the performance of 1,000 prosthesis. *J Thorac Cardiovasc Surg* **95:**980, 1988

16. Grunkemeir GL, Starr A, Rahimtoola SH: Prosthetic heart valve performance: Long term follow-up. *Curr Probl Cardiol* **17:**335, 1992

17. Black MM, Cochrame T, Lawford PV, et al: Design and flow characteristics. In Bodner E, Frater R (eds): *Replacement Cardiac Valves*. New York, McGraw-Hill, 1992, p 1

18. Hammond GL, Laks H, Gieha AS: Development of aortic valve prostheses. *Conn Med* **44:**348, 1980

19. Gabbay S, Kresh JV: Bioengineering of mechanical and biological heart valve substitutes. In Morse D, Steiner RM, Fernandez J (eds): *Guide to Prosthetic Cardiac Valves*. New York, Springer-Verlag, 1985, p 9

20. Knott E, Rene H, Krock M, et al: In vitro comparison of aortic heart valve prosthesis: Part one: Mechanical valves. *J Thorac Cardiovasc Surg* **96:**959, 1988

21. Cobanoglu A, Grunkemein EL, Arm GM, et al: Mitral replacement: Clinical experience with the ball valve prosthesis. *Ann Surg* **202:**376, 1988

22. Chandran KB, Khalighi B, Chen CJ, et al: Effect of valve orientation on flow development post aortic valve prosthesis in a model human aorta. *J Thorac Cardiovasc Surg* **94:**20, 1987

23. Johnston RT, Weerasena NA, Butterfield R, et al: Carbomedics and St. Jude medical bileaflet valves: An "invito" and "invivo" comparison. *Eur J Cardiothorac Surg* **6:**267, 1992

24. Ihlea H, Molstad P, Simonson S, et al: Hemodynamic evaluation of the Carbomedics prosthetic heart valve in the aortic position: Comparison of non-invasive and invasive techniques. *Am Heart J* **123:**151, 1992

25. Okita Y, Mik S, Kusuhora, et al: Intractable hemolysis caused by peri-valvular leakage following mitral valve replacement with St. Jude medical prosthesis. *Ann Thorac Surg* **46:**89, 1988

26. Edmunds LH, Clark RE, Cohn LH, et al: Guidelines for reporting morbidity and mortality after cardiac valvular operations. *J Thorac Cardiovasc Surg* **96:**351, 1988

27. Bodnar E, Butchant EG, Bamford J, et al: Proposal for reporting thrombosis, embolism and bleeding after heart valve replacement. *J Heart Valve Dis* **3:**120, 1994

28. Edmunds LH: Thrombotic and bleeding complications of prosthetic heart valves. *Ann Thorac Surg* **44:**430, 1987

29. Akins CW: Mechanical cardiac valvular prostheses. *Ann Thorac Surg* **52:**161, 1993

30. Peter M, Weiss P, Jenzer HR, et al: The omnicarbon tilting-disc heart valve prosthesis. *J Thorac Cardiovasc Surg* **106:**599, 1993

31. Dewall R, Pelletier U, Panebianco A, et al: Five-year experience with the omniscience cardiac valve. *Ann Thorac Surg* **38:**3, 1984

32. Copeland JG, Sethi GK, et al: Four-year experience with the Carbomedics valve: The North American experience. *Ann Thorac Surg* **58:**630, 1994

33. Ad Hoc Committee of the working group on valvular heart disease, ELS, Gohlke-Barwolfe, et al: Guidelines for prevention of thromboembolic events on valvular heart valve disease. *J Heart Valve Dis* **2:**389, 1993

34. Issues and answers: *International Normalized Ratio*. Dupont Pharma, Wilmington, DE, 1993

35. Israel DH, Shanna SK, Foster V: Anti-thrombotic therapy in prosthetic heart valve replacement. *Am Heart* **127:**400, 1994

36. Butchart C: Thrombosis, embolism and bleeding. In Bodnar E, Frater R (eds): *Replacement Cardiac Valves*. New York, McGraw-Hill, 1992, p 77

37. Cohn LH: Thromboembolism in different anatomical positions. In Rabago G, Cooley DA (eds): *Heart Valve Replacement and Future Trends in Cardiac Surgery*. New York, Futura, 1987, p 259

38. Cohn LH, Alfred EN, DiSesa V, et al: Early and late risk of aortic valve replacement. *J Thorac Cardiovasc Surg* **88:**695, 1984

39. Oyer PE, Stinson EB, Miller DC, et al: Thromboembolic risk and durability of the Hancock bioprosthetic cardiac valve. *Eur Heart J* (Suppl D):81, 1984

40. Brais MP, Bedard JP, Goldstein W, et al: Mitral valve replacement with Hancock porcine valve prostheses: Up to 7-year follow-up. *Can J Surg* **28:**119, 1985

41. McKay C: Prosthetic heart valve thrombosis: "What can be done with regard to treatment?" *Circulation* **87:**294, 1993

42. Zelen L, Klatt EC: Cardiac valve prostheses at autopsy. *Arch Pathol Lab Med* **114:**933, 1990

43. Westaby S, Karp RB, Blackstone EH, et al: Adult human valve dimensions and their surgical significance. *Am J Cardiol* **53:**552, 1984

44. Mortinelli J, Jimenez A, RaSago G, et al: Mechanical cardiac valve thrombosis: Is thrombectomy justified? *Circulation* **84:**70, 1991

45. Silber A, Khan SS, Matloff JM, et al: The St Jude valve. Thrombolysis as the first line of therapy for cardiac valve thrombosis. *Circulation* **87:**30, 1993

46. Ledain LD, Ohayon JP, Colle JP, et al: Acute thrombotic obstruction with disc valve prostheses: Diagnostic considerations and fibrinolytic treatment. *J Am Coll Cardiol* **7:**743, 1986

47. Roudant R, Labbe T, Lorient-Randaut, et al: Mechanical cardiac valve thrombosis. Is fibrinolysis justified? *Circulation* **86** (Suppl II), II–8, 1991

48. Saour JN, Sieck JO, Mamo LAR, et al: Trial of different intensities of anticoagulation in patients with prosthetic heart valves. *N Engl J Med* **322:**428, 1990

49. Butchart EB, Lewis PA, Gunkemeinar GL, et al: Low risk of thrombosis and serious embolic events despite low intensity anticoagulation. Experience with 1004 Medtronic valves. *Circulation* **78** (Suppl):I–66, 1988

50. Stein PD, Alpent JS, Copeland J, et al: Anti-thrombotic therapy in patients with mechanical and biological prosthetic heart valves. *Chest* **192** (Suppl):445S, 1992

51. Butchant EG, Lewis PA, Bethel JA, et al: Adjusting anticoagulation to prosthesis thrombogenicity and patient risk factors: Recommendations for the Medtronic Hall valve. *Circulation* **84** (Suppl III) III–61, 1988

52. Reitz BA, Stinson EB, Griepp RB, et al: Tissue valve replacement of prosthetic heart valves for thrombo-embolism. *Am J Cardiol* **44:**512, 1980

53. Scott WC, Miller SC, Haverich A, et al: Determinants of operative mortality for patients undergoing aortic valve replacement. *J Thorac Cardiovasc Surg* **89:**400, 1985

54. Wilson WR, Danielson GK, Givliani ER, et al: Prosthetic valve endocarditis. *Mayo Clin Proc* **57:**155, 1982

55. Rutledge R, Kim J, Appelbaum RE: Actuarial analysis of the risk of prosthetic valve endocarditis in 1,598 patients with mechanical and bioprosthetic valves. *Arch Surg* **120**:469, 1985

56. Arnett EN, Roberts WC: Prosthetic valve endocarditis. Clinicopathological analysis of 22 necropsy patients with comparison of observations in 73 necropsy patients with active ineffective endocarditis involving natural left-sided cardiac valves. *Am J Cardiol* **38**:281, 1976

57. Sett SS, Hudson MP, Jamieson WR, et al: Prosthetic valve endocarditis. *J Thorac Cardiovasc Surg* **105**:429, 1993

58. Ozszulak TA, Schaff HV, Danielson GK, et al: Results of reoperation for peri-prosthetic leakage. *Ann Thorac Surg* **35**:584, 1983

59. Figuera D, Montero CG: Techniques in mitral valve implantation. In Rabago G, Cooley D (eds): *Heart Valve Replacement and Future Trends in Cardiac Surgery.* New York, Futura, 1987, p 55

60. Dhasmana JP, Blackstone EH, Kirklin JW, et al: Factors associated with peri-prosthetic leakage following primary mitral valve replacement: With special consideration of the suture technique. *Ann Thorac Surg* **35**:170, 1983

61. Beddermann C, Borst HG: Comparison of two suture techniques and materials: Relationship to perivascular leaks after cardiac valve replacement. *Cardiovasc Dis (Bull Tex Heart Inst)* **5**:354, 1978

62. Schoen FJ, Levy RJ, Piehler HR: Pathologic consideration in replacement cardiac valves. *Cardiovasc Pathol* **1**:29, 1992

63. Roberts WC, Bulkley BH, Morrow AG: Pathologic anatomy of cardiac valve replacement: A study of 224 necropsy patients. *Prog Cardiovasc Dis* **15**:539, 1973

64. Orsinelli DA, Becker RC, Guenoud AF, et al: Mechanical failure of a St Jude medical prosthesis. *An J Cardiol* **67**:906, 1991

65. Burckhardt D, Striebel D, Vogt S, et al: Heart valve replacement with St Jude medical valve prosthesis: Long-term experience in 743 patients in Switzerland. *Circulation* **78** (Suppl I): I–18, 1988

66. Odell TA, Durandt J, Sharma DM, et al: Spontaneous embolization of a St Jude prosthetic mitral valve leaflet. *Ann Thorac Surg* **39**:569, 1985

67. Teijeira FJ, Mikhail M: Cardiac valve replacement with mechanical prosthesis: Current status and trends. In Hwang NHC (ed): *Advances in Cardiovascular Engineering.* New York, Plenum Press, 1992, p 197

68. Jorvinen A, Virtanen K, Peltola K, et al: Postoperative disc entrapment following cardiac valve replacement. A report of ten cases. *J Thorac Cardiovasc Surg* **32**:152, 1984

69. Moke CK, Cheung DLC, Chin CSW, et al: An unusual lethal complication of preservation of chordae tendineae in mitral valve replacement. *J Thorac Cardiovasc Surg* **95**:534, 1988

70. Pai GP, Ellison RG, Rubin JW, et al: Disc immobilization of Bjork-Shiley and Medtronic Hall valves during and immediately after valve replacement. *Ann Thorac Surg* **44**:73, 1987

71. Roberts WC, Sullivan MF: Clinical and necropsy observations early after simultaneous replacement of the mitral and aortic valves. *Am J Cardiol* **58**:1067, 1987

72. Antunes MJ, Colsen PR, Kinsley RH: Intermittent aortic regurgitation following aortic valve replacement with the Hall-Kaster prosthesis. *J Thorac Cardiovasc Surg* **84**:751, 1982

73. Bortolotti U, Milano A, Mazzaro E, et al: Hancock II Porcine bioprosthesis: Excellent durability at intermediate-term follow-up. *J Am Coll Cardiol* **24**:676, 1994

74. Kawachi Y, Tanaka J, Tominaga R, et al: More than ten years' follow-up of the Hancock porcine bioprosthesis in Japan. *J Thorac Cardiovasc Surg* **104**:5, 1992

75. Cohn LH, Couper GS, Aranki SF, et al: The long term follow-up of the Hancock modified orifice porcine bioprosthetic valve. *J Cardiac Surg* **6**:557, 1991

76. Cohn LH, Collins JJ, DiSesa V, et al: Fifteen-year experience with 1,678 Hancock porcine bioprosthetic heart valve replacements. *Ann Surg* **210**:435, 1989

77. Burdon TA, Miller DG, Oyer PE, et al: Durability of porcine valves at fifteen years in a representative North American patient population. *J Thorac Cardiovasc Surg* **103**:738, 1992

78. Al-Khaja N, Rashid M, El-Gatit A, et al: The influence of age on the durability of Carpentier-Edwards biological valves. *Eur J Cardiothorac Surg* **5**:635, 1991

79. Akins CW, Carroll DC, Buckley JM, et al: Late results with Carpentier-Edwards porcine bioprosthesis. *Circulation* **82** (Suppl IV): IV–65, 1990

80. Jamieson WR, Allen P, Miyagishima RT, et al: The Carpentier-Edwards standard porcine bioprosthesis. *J Thorac Cardiovasc Surg* **99**:543, 1990

81. Jamieson WR, Munroai D, Miyagishimu RT, et al: The Carpentier-Edwards supra-annular porcine bioprosthesis. *J Thorac Cardiovasc Surg* **96**:652, 1988

82. Yoganatham AP, Chaux A, Gray R, et al: Bileaflet tilting disc and porcine aortic valves substitutes: In vitro hydrodynamic characteristics. *J Am Coll Cardiol* **3**:313, 1984

83. Carpenter A, Dubost C, Lane E, et al: Continuing improvements: Valvular bio-prostheses. *J Thorac Cardiovasc Surg* **83**:27, 1982

84. Jamieson WRE, Gullucci V, Thiene AW, et al: Porcine valves. In Bodnar E, Traten R (eds): *Replacement Cardiac Valves.* New York, McGraw-Hill, 1992, p 229

85. Jamieson WRE, Gerein AN, Ricci DR, et al: Carpentier-Edwards supraannular porcine bioprosthesis: A new generation tissue (clinical and hemodynamic assessment). In Bodnar E, Yacoub M (eds): *Biologic and Bioprosthetic Valve: Proceedings of the Third International Symposium.* New York, Yorke Medical Books, 1986, p 141

86. Jaffe WM, Coverdale A, Roche AHG, et al: Rest and exercise hemodynamics of 20 to 23 mm allograft, Medtronic intact (porcine) and St. Jude medical valves in the aortic position. *J Thorac Cardiovasc Surg* **100**:167, 1990

87. Baumgartner H, Khan S, DeRobertis M, et al: Effect of prosthetic aortic valve design on the Doppler catheter gradient A correlation: An "in vitro" study of normal St. Jude, Medtronic Hall, Starr-Edwards and Hancock valves. *J Am Coll Cardiol* **19**:324, 1992

88. Khan SS, Mitchell RS, Derby GL, et al: Differences in Hancock and Carpentier-Edwards porcine xenograft aortic valve hemodynamics. *Circulation* **82** (Suppl IV):IV–177, 1990

89. Schoen FJ, Levy RJ: Bioprosthetic heart valve failure: Pathology and pathogenesis. *Cardiol Clin* **2**:717, 1984

90. Schoen FJ: Cardiac valve prosthesis: Pathological and bioengineering considerations. *J Cardiac Surg* **2**:65, 1987

91. Ishihara T, Ferrones VJ, Boyce SW, et al: Structure and classification of Luspol tears and perforations in porcine bioprosthetic cardiac valves implanted in patients. *Am J Cardiol* **48**:665, 1981

92. Schoen FJ, Kujovich JL, Levy RJ, et al: Bioprosthetic valve failure. *Cardiovasc Clin* **8**:289, 1988

93. Ferrons VJ, Tomita Y, Hilbent SL, et al: Pathology of bioprosthetic cardiac valves. *Human Pathol* **18**:586, 1987

94. Jamieson WRE, Rosau LTJ, Munro AI, et al: Primary tissue failure (structural valve deterioration) by age groups. *Ann Thorac Surg* **46**:216, 1988

95. Miller DC, Stinson EB, Oyer PE, et al: The durability of porcine xenograft valves and conduits in children. *Circulation* **66** (Suppl I):I–72, 1982

96. Sanders JP, Levy RJ, Freed MD, et al: Use of porcine xenografts in children and adolescents. *Am J Cardiol* **46**:429, 1980

97. Shoen FJ, Collins JJ, Cohn LH, et al: Long-term failure rates and morphologic correlations in porcine bioprosthetic heart valves. *Am J Cardiol* **51**:957, 1983

98. Baumgartner WA, Miller DC, Reitz BA, et al: Surgical treatment of prosthetic valvular endocarditis. *Ann Thorac Surg* **35**:87, 1987

99. Duran CG: The pericardial heart valve: An open question. In Bodnar E, Frater R (eds): *Replacement Cardiac Valves.* New York, McGraw-Hill, 1992, p 277

100. Relland J, Perier P, Leconte B: The third generation Carpentier-Edwards bio-prothesis: Family results. *J Am Coll Cardiol* **6**:1149, 1985

101. Pelletier LL, Leclerc Y, Bonon R, et al: The Carpentier-Edwards bovine pericardial prosthesis. Clinical experience with 301 valve replacements. In Bodnar E (ed): *Surgery for Heart Valve Disease.* London, ICR, 1990, p 691

102. Aupant M, Neville X, Dreyfus Y, et al: The Carpentier-Edwards pericardial aortic valve: Intermediate results in 420 patients. *Eur J Cardiothorac Surg* **8:**277, 1994

103. Ross DW: Homograft replacement of the aortic valve. *Lancet* **2:**487, 1962

104. Barratt-Boyes BG: Homograft aortic valve replacement in aortic incompetence and stenosis. *Thorax* **19:**131, 1964

105. Angell WW, Iben AB, Shumway NE: Fresh aortic homografts for multiple valve replacements. *Arch Surg* **97:**826, 1968

106. Brockbank KGM, Bank HL: Measurement of post cryopreservation viability. *J Cardiac Surg* **2** (Suppl):145, 1987

107. Kirklin JK, Smith D, Novick WS, et al: Long term function of Cryopreserved aortic homografts: A ten year study. *J Thorac Cardiovasc Surg* **106:**154, 1993

108. Doby DB, Guido M, Wang N-D, et al: Replacement of aortic valve with Cryopreserved aortic allograft. *Ann Thorac Surg* **56:**228, 1993

109. O'Brien MF, McGiffin DC, Stafford EG, et al: Allograft aortic valve replacement: Long term clinical analysis of viable Cryopreserved and antibiotic 4-degree-C stored valves. *J Cardiac Surg* **6** (Suppl):543, 1991

110. Borratt-Boyes BG, Roche AHG, Subranenyan R, et al: Long-term follow-up of patients with the antibiotic sterilized aortic homograft valve inserted free hand in the aortic position. *Circulation* **75:**768, 1987

111. Barratt-Boyes BG: A method for preparing and inserting a homograft aortic valve. *Br J Surg* **52:**847, 1965

112. Pacifico AD, Kurp RB, Kirklin JW: Homografts for replacement of the aortic valve. *Circulation* **45,46** (Suppl):36, 1992

113. Mitsuki O, Robles A, Gibbs S, et al: Long term performance of 555 aortic homografts in the aortic position. *Ann Thorac Surg* **46:**187, 1988

114. O'Brien MF, Stafford EG, Gardner MAH, et al: A comparison of aortic valve replacement with cryopreserved and fresh allograft valve with a note on chromosomal studies. *J Thorac Cardiovasc Surg* **94:**812, 1987

115. Lupinetti FM, Tsai TT, Kreobone JM: Endothelial cell replication in an "in vivo" model of aortic allografts. *Ann Thorac Surg* **56:**237, 1993

116. Moreno-Cabral LE, Miller DC, Shumway NE: A simple technique for AVR using free hand allografts. *J Cardiac Surg* **3:**69, 1989

117. Albert JD, Bishop DA, Fullerton DA, et al: Conduit reconstruction of the right ventricular outflow tract: Lessons learned in a 12-year experience. *J Thorac Cardiovasc Surg* **106:**228, 1993

118. Mestres CA, Ginel A, Cartona R, et al: Cryopreserved homografts in aortic and mitral prosthetic endocarditis. *J Heart Valve Dis* **2:**679, 1993

119. Michler RE, Chen JM, Quaegebeur J: Novel technique for extending the use of allografts in cardiac operations. *Ann Thorac Surg* **57:**83, 1994

120. Milsom FP, Doty SB: Aortic valve replacement and mitral valve replacement with allograft. *J Cardiac Surg* **8:**350, 1993

121. Hammermeister KE, Sethi G, Henderson WG, et al: A comparison of outcomes in men 11 years after heart-valve replacement with a mechanical valve or bioprosthesis. *N Engl J Med* **328:**1290, 1993

122. Jones EL, Weintraub WS, Craver JM, et al: Ten-year experience with porcine bioprosthetic valve: Interrelationship of valve survival and patient survival in 1,050 valve replacements. *Ann Thorac Surg* **49:**370, 1990

123. Cohn LH, Aranki SF, Rizzo RJ, et al: Decrease in operative risk of reoperative valve surgery. *Ann Thorac Surg* **56:**15, 1993

Surgical Anatomy
of the Coronary Arteries

Claude M. Grondin

The anatomy of the coronary arteries is fascinating and most varied. Nowhere, except perhaps in the brain, does the organ function depend so much—literally from one moment to the other—on the integrity and constancy of the blood supply. Yet, until recently, the coronary anatomy was of interest only to anatomopathologists. Raymond Vieussens first described the coronary anatomy in 1706.[1] The clinical account of angina pectoris by Heberden[2] followed nearly a century later and the correlation with occlusive coronary artery disease was established by Parry and Jenner[3] some 200 years after the description by the French anatomist.

With the advent of open heart surgery, the interest rose but again the information was gathered by a minority of individuals who during the correction of tetralogy of Fallot or the repair of a ventricular septal defect would observe a single coronary artery or an aberrant left anterior descending branch. Angiograms in those days served to delineate cardiac chambers, sites of cardiac shunts, or the position of the great vessels. Selective coronary arteriography by Mason Sones was a decade away.[4] In fact, in the early years of indirect myocardial revascularization, indications and results of the operation, by necessity, relied solely on symptoms. With the development of selective coronary angiography in the mid-1960s, Sones not only legitimized internal mammary artery implantation but also opened the modern era of treatment of myocardial ischemia, which now ranges from thrombolysis[5] to percutaneous angioplasty[6] and direct surgical repair of complex coronary arterial disease.[7] None of today's sophisticated techniques would be possible without selective coronary angiography, a procedure that now appears pedestrian as more than one million are performed annually in the United States.[8]

Following the angiographic breakthrough, interest and knowledge grew rapidly as did the number of anatomical classifications and nomenclatures. No one description is complete or entirely satisfactory, however. The classification most commonly used today is the one proposed by the National Heart, Lung, and Blood Institute for the Coronary Artery Surgery Study (CASS).[9] In general, the classifications follow three lines: the number of arteries, the site of origin, and the course of the vessels and their branches. Surprisingly, even the number of coronary arteries is the focus of occasional debate. Clinicians speak of triple vessel disease while conceding that there are but the left (LCA) and the right (RCA) coronary arteries. In fact, the number of coronary arteries arising from the aortic sinuses may vary with age as postmortem studies have shown that the incidence with which the conus artery arises from the aorta rather than from the main RCA increases with age.[10] Be that as it may, for practical purposes, two coronary arteries are recognized, the RCA and the LCA.

The RCA perfuses the right ventricle, the LCA, the anterolateral portion of the left ventricle. The posterior part of the left ventricle and the posterior third of the left ventricular (LV) septum may be perfused by either the RCA or the LCA depending on the dominance of either vessel. The posterior papillary muscle depends for its supply on the RCA and the circumflex (Cx) artery; the anterior depends on the left anterior descending artery (LAD) and its branches.

Seventy-five percent of patients have a dominant RCA (Figs. 123–1 and 123–2). By convention, this indicates that the RCA not only supplies the posterior septum, but also gives off at least one branch beyond the posterior descending artery (PDA). In a balanced circulation, only the PDA originates from the RCA, the remainder of the circulation to the posterior left ventricle is assumed by the circumflex

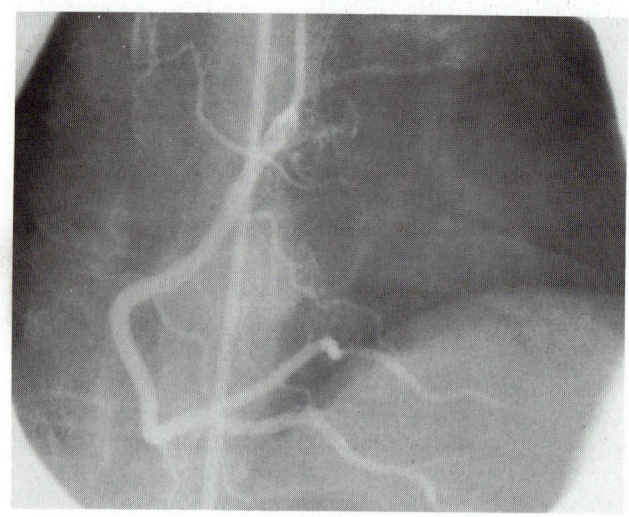

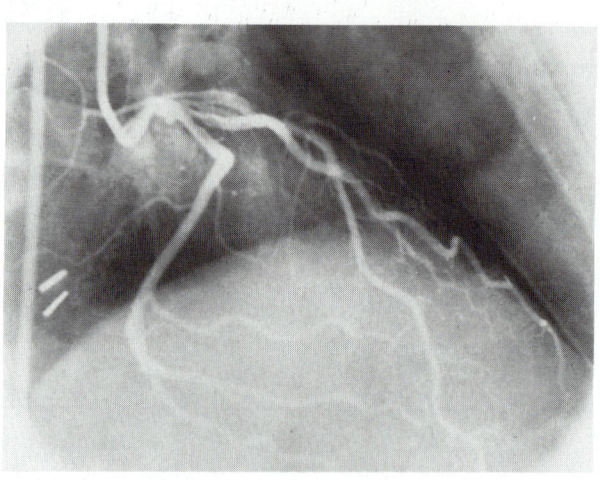

A

B

Figure 123–1. **A.** Dominant RCA anteroposterior view. Note first two branches taking off in opposite directions, the SA node upward and to the left, the conus branch downward and to the right, followed by two anterior ventricular branches parallel to the conus branch. The RCA takes on a C configuration in this view; from the lower limb of the C are the posterior descending and posterolateral branches. The segment between these two is the crux segment or the artery to the crux. **B.** Dominant LCA, anteroposterior view. Note that Cx in this view stays in the A-V groove creating a 90° angle with its first portion. In a nondominant circumflex, the distal segment leaves the A-V groove early and the angle opens up to 130° or so. There often is in dominant Cx a large gap—as in this instance—between the distal branches (the posterolateral and the PDA) and the first marginal branch.

artery. When, on the other hand, the PDA arises from the Cx, the LCA is said to be dominant (Fig. 123–3). Approximately 10% of patients have a balanced circulation; 15% have a dominant LCA. The incidence of dominant LCA doubles in cases of congenital aortic stenosis suggesting a developmental complex.[11]

THE RIGHT CORONARY ARTERY

The RCA arises from the right (anterior) sinus and the LCA from the left (posterolateral) sinus. Both orifices are located in the middle of their respective sinus at a point level with the free edge of the leaflet. At times, the orifice is close to a commissure. The RCA originating closer to the anterior commissure constitutes a point of surgical interest in procedures designed to enlarge the aortic valve annulus (such as the Konno operation[12]) where a vertical incision across the aortic annulus must be made to the left of that orifice. Also of interest is the fact that the coronary ostia may be located above the sinuses in the tubular portion of the aorta in 30% of cases for the LCA and 8% for the RCA.[13] Origin of a coronary artery from the posterior (noncoronary) sinus is almost unheard of in humans.[14] Conversely, origin of the

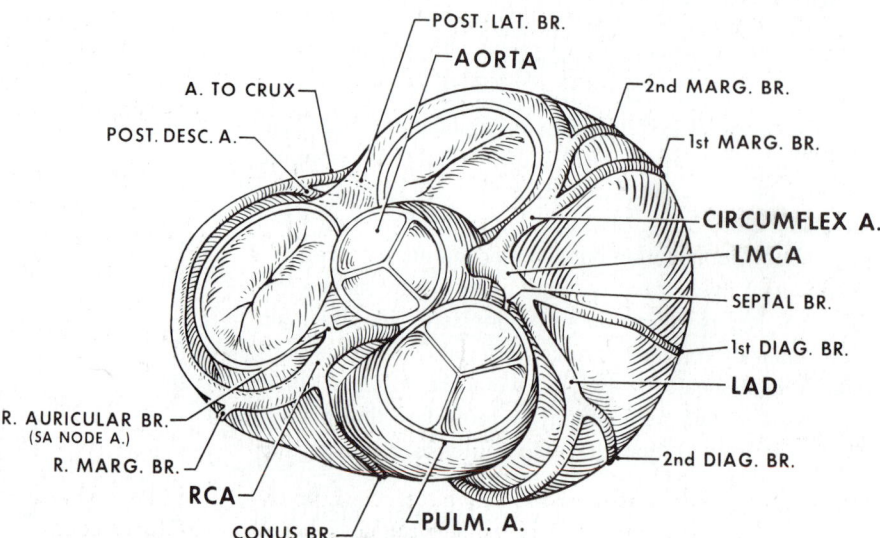

Figure 123–2. Drawing depicting overhead view of both coronary arteries in a dominant right system. Note various branches of the right, LAD, and circumflex arteries.

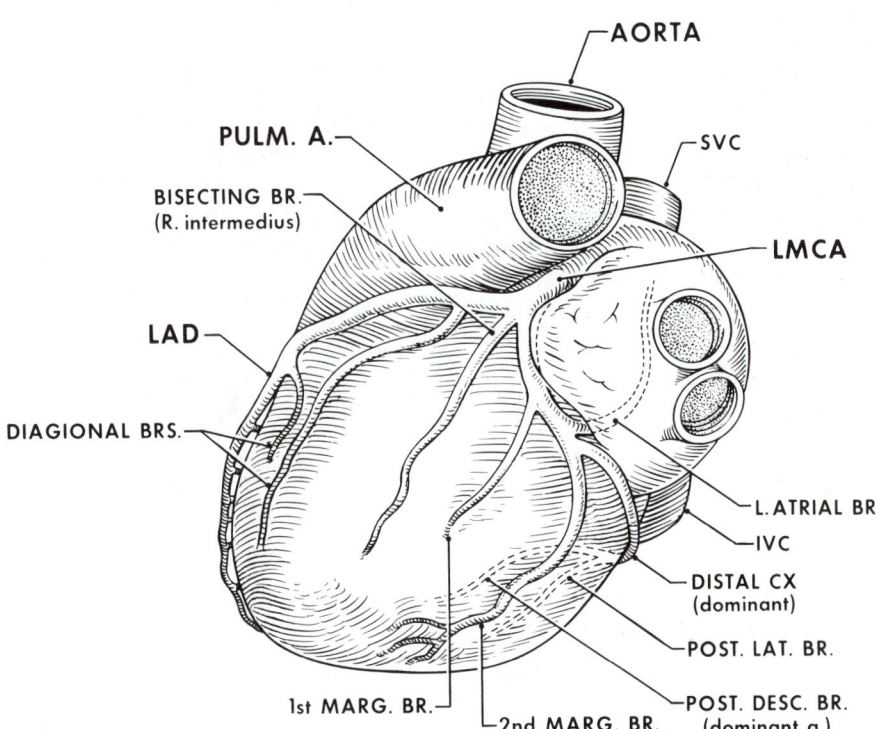

Figure 123–3. Drawing of lateral view of left coronary artery in a dominant Cx including bisecting branch (ramus intermedius), marginal branches, left posterolateral, and posterior descending branches.

conus artery from the right sinus is not rare, and origin of both coronaries (a true anomaly) from the right sinus is much more frequent than from the left sinus[13] (Fig. 123–4). The left anterior descending (LAD) (branch of the LCA) may originate anomalously from either the RCA or the right sinus and like the conus branch artery cross anteriorly below the pulmonary valve enroute to the interventricular septum (Fig. 123–4D).

The most frequent anomaly remains that of the origin of the Cx from the right sinus or more commonly from the RCA (Fig. 123–4C). The Cx will then course behind the aorta and, typically, will be underdeveloped, i.e., will taper off in the hight lateral myocardium (see also Fig. 123–6A). In the adult with atherosclerosis, the segment of Cx behind the aorta may display severe narrowing often over a long segment and the territory involved may be so small that bypass grafting is not warranted. In other instances, it may be large enough and require grafting behind the aorta, on the right side.[15] In cases of aberrant Cx, the LAD and the RCA usually cover a larger area and have several high diagonal branches or posterolateral branches.

Beyond its takeoff at a right angle from the aorta, the RCA turns right and downward and gives off two branches that head in opposite directions. The first one—the conus branch—heads anteriorly toward the conus or that part of the right ventricle located immediately below the pulmonary valve, the other—the sinus node artery—goes up and posteriorly on its way of the medial aspect of the superior vena cava–right atrium junction (Fig. 123–1). The conus branch, as indicated earlier, may have a separate aortic orifice (30%) and often acts as a major collateral branch

in cases of occlusion of the LAD. This source of collateral may not be apparent (because the tip of the catheter lies beyond the origin of the conus branch) or may not be demonstrated at angiography, but should be suspected whenever the LAD fails to opacity distal to an obstruction in the presence of a normal contraction of the anterior portion of the left ventricle.

The next branches—the anterior ventricular arteries—vary in number and are usually small, except the most distal one called the marginal branch, which courses along the right border of the heart. Like the conus branch, it serves as a collateral to the LAD and also to the distal RCA and the PDA, the next division branch of the right coronary artery. The inferior border of the RV is usually devoid of branches. In 30% of cases, however, the PDA originates early and courses diagonally across the inferior RV en route to the septum. This particularity allows the right internal mammary artery (IMA) to reach the PDA with greater ease when grafting of the latter is necessary. The PDA does not follow the septum with enough regularity to be called the posterior interventricular branch. In only 25% of cases does the PDA reach the apex and in another 25%, it reaches only the midpoint between the apex and the base.[16] The PDA serves as a major collateral source to the LAD either via the apex or through septal branches. The true septal branches originate from the LAD and supply most of the septum. The septal branches from the PDA, when present, are usually small, multiple, and have a short course into the septum.

Beyond the PDA is the crux. The latter designates an ill-defined area where all four chambers are in apposition. Often a collateral branch from the RCA (right atrial branch)

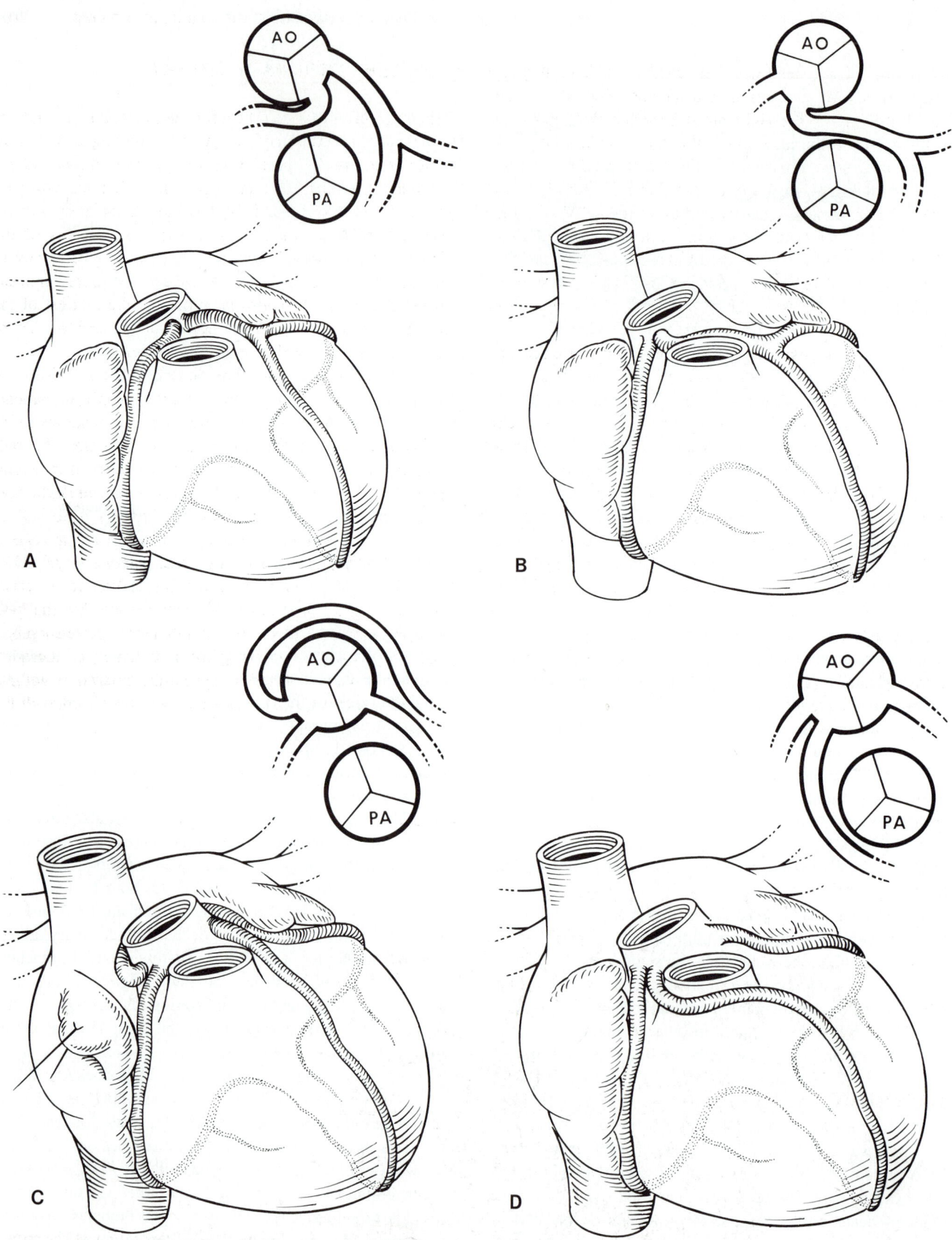

Figure 123–4.A–D. Drawing depicting most common anomalies in origin of coronary arteries. **A** and **B** show the origin of both arteries from either the right or the left sinus. Note the possibility of compression of either vessel between aorta and pulmonary artery. **C** shows aberrant origin of the circumflex from the right sinus or more frequently from the early portion of the RCA. **D** shows the less common origin of the left anterior descending artery from the right sinus or the right coronary artery. Like a conus branch, the LAD courses anterior to the pulmonary artery (see also Fig. 123–6B).

or at times from the LCA (left atrial branch or Kugel's artery, which by extension now designates a collateral from either the left or the right atrial branches[16,17]) joins the main RCA via the atrioventricular (A-V) node artery and creates an *arterial* cross (crux) with the main RCA horizontally and the PDA vertically (Fig. 123–5). The artery to the crux (the anatomical crux) according to the CASS classification is the "horizontal" segment located between the PDA and the first posterolateral branch of the RCA. Beyond that segment are one or several branches named LV branches of the RCA or right posterolateral branches (RPL). When the RCA is truly dominant or in cases of aberrant Cx, these posterolateral branches are responsible for the arterial supply of a large portion of the posterior LV. They often need separate grafting during revascularization and may be bypassed either singly or in a sequential manner with the PDA or the proximal RCA. When only the posterolateral branches need grafting, the vein segment may be routed behind the inferior vena cava and course to the right of the right atrium toward the ascending aorta.

Rarely, the PDA may have an intramyocardial course. Even the RCA may course in the wall of the right atrium instead of in the A-V groove. Ultimately, it surfaces before the crux or in the upper part of the A-V groove.[18] Different techniques have been described to reach the RCA in these circumstances when proximal grafting of this vessel is necessary,[19] a most unusual situation since the distal PDA may usually be used for grafting.

THE LEFT CORONARY ARTERY

The LCA takes off from the left posterolateral sinus and immediately dips inferiorly and laterally, creating a crest or incisura that may be more evident at postmortem than at angiography. A short left main portion [left main coronary artery (LMCA)] of the LCA has been associated with increased incidence of atherosclerosis.[20] Anomalies of the left coronary artery are more frequent, of greater consequences than those of the RCA and deserve more emphasis here. The incidence varies according to the interest of the reports, whether surgical[21] or purely anatomic[22] (see Chapter 94 on anomalies of the coronary vessels).

The LCA may arise from the right sinus of Valsalva or from the right coronary artery in about 0.05% of patients (Fig. 123–4A, B).[21] In most instances of anomalous LCA, the vessel courses anterior to the aorta behind the pulmonary artery. Rarely, it runs behind the aorta as an anomalous Cx arising from the RCA. Cases of sudden death have been described in young adults who displayed no atherosclerosis at postmortem examination and have an anomalous LMCA coursing behind the pulmonary artery.[21] Most of these sudden deaths occurred in relation to exercise, which suggests a mechanical compression by the pulmonary artery in patients with pulmonary hypertension or a kink of the LMCA resulting from stretching of the aorta during exercise.[23] Anterior myocardial infarction without coronary atherosclerosis has also been associated with the

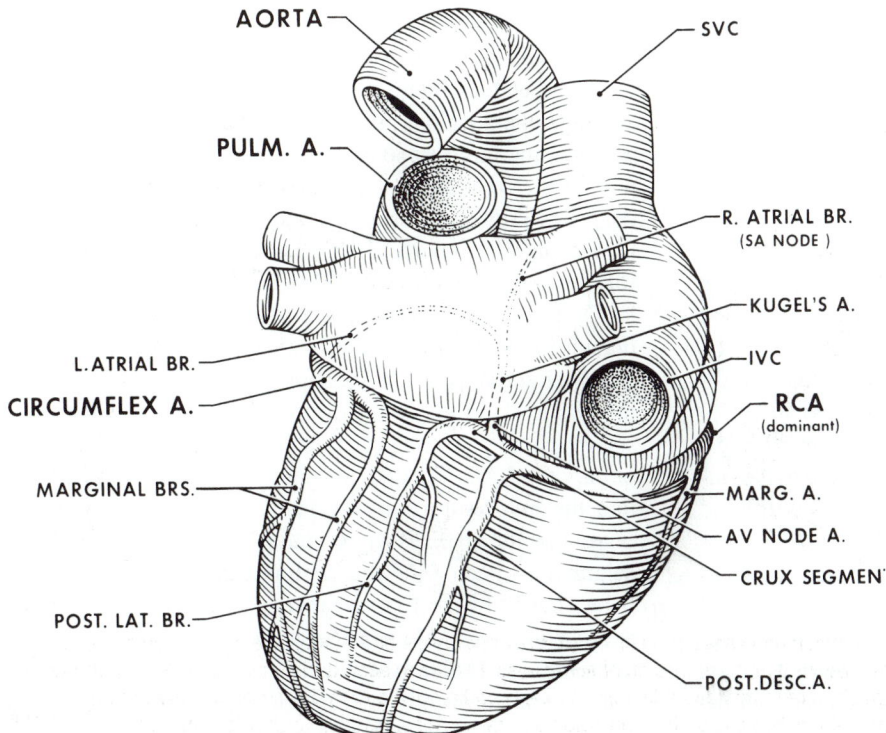

Figure 123–5. Drawing of posterior aspect of heart in dominant RCA showing A-V node artery that, when joined by either the left or right atrial branch, forms Kugel's anastomatic collateral artery in cases of obstruction of the RCA.

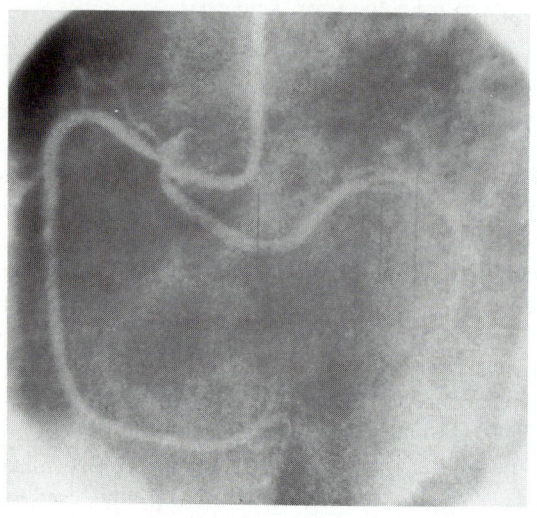 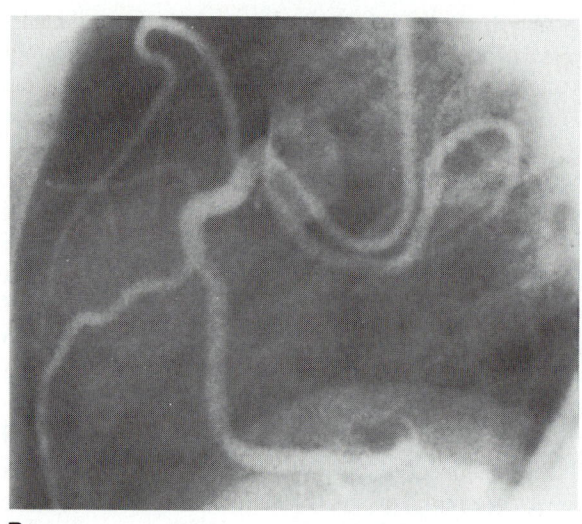

A **B**

Figure 123–6. A. Aberrant circumflex from RCA, lateral view. Note long course behind the aorta and termination height on the lateral LV by small "insignificant" branch. **B.** Single coronary artery, lateral view. In this case, as in **A**, the Cx is aberrant and courses (here along catheter) behind the aorta. The LAD originates anteriorly like a conus branch across from the origin of the aberrant Cx branch.

LMCA coursing behind the aorta.[24] More rarely, the LMCA may course anterior to the pulmonary artery or the LAD may arise separately from the right sinus or the RCA and also course anterior to the pulmonary artery (Figs. 123–4D and 123–6B).[24] The first septal branch may also arise separately from the right sinus or the RCA.[23] Rare instances of origin of the PDA from the LAD have also been described.[25]

The LMCA divides into the LAD and the circumflex branch 2 to 20 mm from the aortic orifice.[14] In 10 to 15% of patients, a branch often equal in size to the LAD and the Cx bisects those two structures. This branch is neither a marginal nor a diagonal branch and, appropriately, is called a bisecting branch (or ramus intermedius). The nomenclature for the branches of the Cx has varied over the years. Formerly, these branches were called the lateral and posterolateral branches depending on their position, but since considerable overlap existed, the simpler terms used by the CASS group of first, second, third marginal branches, and so on, have gained acceptance. The Cx may remain in the A-V groove (it does so when dominant) or may course diagonally across the posterolateral LV giving off marginal branches (often only one major one), which themselves divide in two (usually) or three branches. In the latter instance, the A-V groove segment of the Cx is minuscule and does not participate to vascularization of the LV but becomes more or less a left atrial branch. In the case of a dominant Cx, the distal branches are called the posterolateral branches and the very last is called the PDA. Not infrequently the marginal branches are intramyocardial except for their initial 1 or 2 cm. They may be seen through the muscle layer like fish frozen in ice and may be dissected out of their tunnel or approached proximally in their epicardial

portion for bypass grafting. The dominant Cx is often made of multiple small branches hanging down from the A-V groove portion. These branches are often small and barely adequate for grafting; this type of dominant Cx is a handicap to grafting if not a disease in itself.

The LAD offers more constancy of size and course than the Cx. Its first branch is often a small conus branch that, when linked with the right side counterpart, forms the ring of Vieussens.[1] The next branch of the LAD is usually the septal branch. The term "septal perforator" is a misnomer since all coronary branches ultimately "perforate" to reach the endocardium. The septal branch is rarely unique although the first one is logically—like the first diagonal branch—the largest one. It is easily identified at angiography on the right anterior oblique (RAO) projection as taking off at a right angle and posteriorly from the LAD and on the left anterior oblique (LAO) as the "only" vessel [except for tiny right ventricular (RV) branches] medial to the LAD. Often its orifice lies opposite the first diagonal branch forming a trifurcation with the LAD and anchoring the latter at that position. Perhaps as a result of this anchoring, this very point is a site of predilection for atherosclerosis, which may involve all three members of the trifurcation or only the LAD. Beyond this point, the LAD often plunges into the myocardium to resurface 3 or 4 cm below or at times near the apex. Most exceptionally, the LAD is several centimeters deep into the septum and cannot really be fished out.[14] In the first instance, grafting is fashioned by approaching the LAD near the apex and freeing the artery of its muscle bridge under cardiac arrest. The artery may also be grafted distally as it resurfaces or, more frequently, through one of the communicating diagonal branches.

The LAD gives off three to six septal branches and

several smaller and inconsistent branches to the right ventricle medially. At times the LAD is bifid with one of the limbs giving off the diagonal branches and the other the septal. Usually one LAD is small and the other is long. When the one giving off the septal branches is the longer one, it is usually intramyocardial and resurfaces near the apex.[26] Occasionally, the first septal branch originates from the first diagonal branch and not from the LAD.

In 80% of cases, the LAD goes around the apex and supplies a portion of the posterior septum. In half of those cases, the LAD will go up more than 2 cm toward the base of the posterior left ventricle.[16] Frequently the LAD terminates like an anchor; one branch curling up toward the lateral wall and the other toward the posterior interventricular septum. Atherosclerotic narrowing is commonly seen on the LAD at the point of bifurcation near the apex.

CORONARY VENOUS CIRCULATION

In humans, the coronary venous return is through multiple routes. The coronary venous circulation is composed of a large network at the postcapillary level that communicates with itself and (for the most part) with the right sided chambers. It is estimated that 75% of the venous return is through the coronary sinus whose orifice lies at the posterior septal base of the right atrium above the tricuspid valve, medial and above the entrance of the inferior vena cava. Several coronary veins whose distribution follows the general pattern of the arteries empty into the coronary sinus, which courses transversely at the base of the LV in the atrioventricular groove.[27] Embryologically, the sinus develops alongside the left superior vena cava with which it communicates and this communication disappears when the left SVC regresses.[28] Some drainage does occur through the lymphatic system—perhaps 5%—and the remaining 20% of the venous return is through the Thebesian veins, which empty into all four cardiac chambers—although most do so on the right side.

During mechanical occlusion of the orifice of coronary sinus, the secondary system is capable of assuming all venous returns without engorgement (partial ligation of the coronary sinuses was at one time used to promote better distribution of the coronary arterial flow,[29] a procedure later found to have little effect on either circulation). Atresia of the coronary sinus orifice in the right atrium is associated with a persistent left superior vena cava and does not have hemodynamic consequences, although it is accompanied by other congenital cardiac malformations in 50% of cases.[30]

With the recent use of retrograde coronary sinus perfusion during aortic clamping, interest in the anatomy of the coronary sinus has been rekindled. No longer an anatomopathologic curiosity,[28] variations and anomalies of the coronary sinus, although innocuous as some may be in the normal setting, have come to have an influence on surgical

techniques. Inadequate protection using retrograde coronary perfusion has been blamed on anatomical variants (probably rare), on improper positioning of the catheter (e.g., beyond a major cardiac vein), as well as on the presence of one-way valves that, akin to those present in the saphenous vein, could prevent blood from flowing in a direction opposite (i.e., retrograde) the normal pathway. These valves do exist, not in the coronary sinus proper, but at the entrance of the major coronary veins into the sinus. Recent studies have suggested that venous valves may impede retrograde flow (especially if the perfusion pressure is kept low and, therefore, incapable of overcoming the valves).[31] Coronary venous valves vary from species to species and, in humans, may be less functional in the adult heart.[32] Inadequate protection using retrograde cardioplegia may also occur in the beating heart, i.e., when retrograde perfusion is used to initiate arrest, as retrograde flow is impeded by the systolic squeeze.

INTERCORONARY ANASTOMOSES

A large network of anastomoses between coronary arteries has been demonstrated in man both at autopsy and at angiography.[33] They occur both in health and in disease but, understandably, have been the subject of greater scrutiny in pathologic states. There are natural connections such as Vieussens's ring, the atrial branches, Kugel's artery (Fig. 123–7A), the septal arteries, and so on. Others develop probably as a result of occlusion such as those between the LAD and the diagonal artery, and between the marginal and diagonal branches. The possibility exists, however, that these collateral branches are there, but become angiographically apparent only when proper conditions arise. At postmortem, their sizes have been shown to be related to the presence of disease. In cases of complete occlusion, collaterals with a diameter of 20 to 200 μm may increase by 10- to 20-fold.[34] Typically, a well-developed collateral is tortuous; since it develops between fixed points, it has to buckle. The most frequently observed collaterals at autopsy are between the RCA and the LAD.[35] The most common source of collateral flow, on the other hand, appears to be from the LAD.

Contrary to the macroscopic finding, the RCA is the most common source of collaterals at angiography and probably the most frequent recipient, while the Cx is the least frequent recipient.[36] The LAD may be the least frequent source, in total contradiction to what is usually found at autopsy.[35]

In occlusion of the RCA, the suppliers other than the parent vessel are the septal branches of the LAD, the periapical connection between the LAD and PDA, and the periapical connection between the latter and the Cx marginal branches. In occlusion of the LAD, the most frequent collateral is from the acute marginal branch of the RCA and connections between the septal branches of the LAD. The

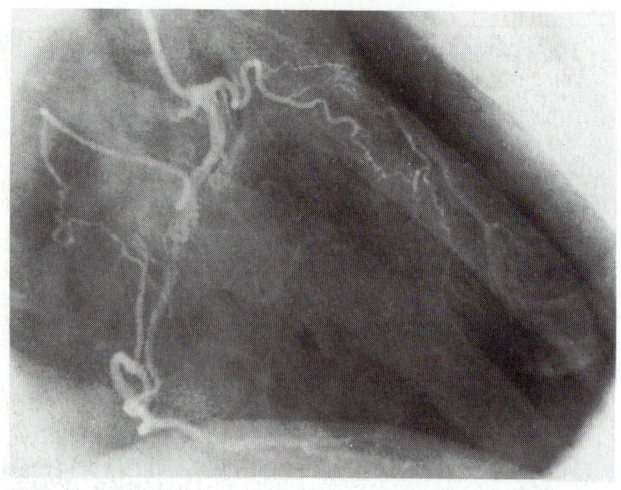

A

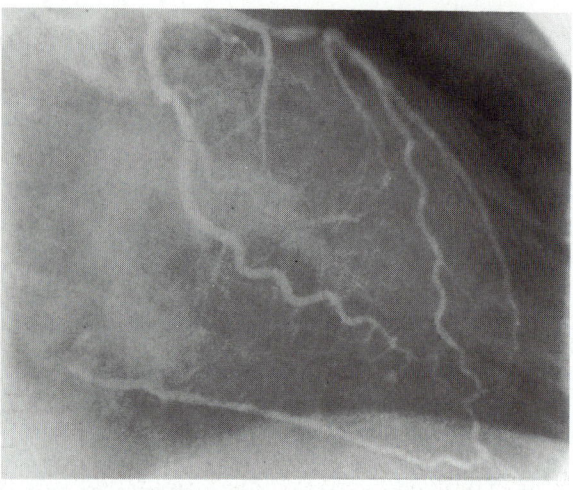

B

Figure 123–7. A. Right anterior oblique view of RCA showing occlusion of midportion with collateral circulation from the right atrial branch (in horizontal left direction on this view) down the A-V node branch (Kugel's anastomosis, here in a vertical direction) to the distal RCA. Note also collateralization to the LAD via the conus branch, going horizontally in this picture from left to right. **B.** Right anterior oblique view of LCA showing tight narrowing of LAD and direct collateralization of PDA around the apex by the LAD. Despite appearance, narrowing is likely not greater than 80% in diameter (see text), otherwise flow would not be seen this early (same as in Cx) in LAD and up posterior descending branch.

conus branch, although ideal, is not as frequent a supplier as anticipated. The Cx appears to suffer from a lack of good collateral vessels. The left atrial branch, the diagonal branches of the LAD, and the distal RCA are the more frequent sources for the Cx.[37]

Collaterals regress angiographically when the conditions provoking their development no longer prevail. Following reduction or correction of a proximal stenosis by dilatation or bypass grafting, collaterals literally disappear and, on the other hand, reappear almost instantaneously when either dilatation or grafting fails.[38,39]

At angiography, collaterals increase with the severity of the disease and the number of vessels involved.[36,40] Usually all totally occluded arteries are collateralized,[38] while those with narrowing of less than 70% rarely show collateralization.[41] When no collaterals are demonstrated at angiography, the severity of stenosis or the adequacy of the examination should be questioned. In the latter case, either the late phase of the injection was cut off or "traveling" of the camera was improper. Failure to inject the artery selectively or to catheterize the conus branch, for instance, may have occurred. More often than not, however, overestimation of the degree of stenosis is responsible. Although pathologic studies have showed the lesions to be worse at autopsy than at angiography,[42] visual assessment when compared to computer analysis, as a rule, tends to overestimate the severity of stenosis.[43] There is probably no such thing as a 95%, or worse a 99% diameter stenosis (Fig. 123–7B) since in surface area this is equivalent to a 99.999 occlusion through which dye could not be seen to flow and opacify the distal artery. An 80% reduction in diameter corresponds to a 96% reduction in area. Such a stenosis is in-

compatible with viable myocardium distally unless adequate collateral circulation exists.[44]

QUANTITATIVE CORONARY ARTERIOGRAPHY (QCA)

Because of enormous variations in the visual estimation of coronary artery stenosis—both inter- and intraobserver variations—it has become difficult to reproduce measurements and compare results between centers or interventions.[45] Therapeutic decisions are taken for both medical and surgical treatment of coronary artery disease which, at best, rest on debatable interpretation of what remains the gold standard in diagnostic tools. During the past decade, computer analysis of coronary arteriograms—quantitative coronary arteriography (QCA)—has come to the rescue.[46] It is generally agreed that visual assessment tends to overestimate the severity of tight lesions and underestimate the severity of mild lesions. It has facetiously been stated that the efficacy of a therapeutic agent capable of reducing by one-third postangioplasty restenoses would not be recognized by current angiographic reading techniques.[45]

Systems for computer analysis are now available worldwide and within the present decade will be required by all agencies for the study of therapeutic interventions in coronary artery disease be they mechanical (bypass, angioplasty) or pharmacologic (lipid lowering agents). In essence these QCA systems, through image enhancement, videodensity assessment, can measure with precision the edge of the lumen, the degree of narrowing, and the size of the "normal" lumen (Fig. 123–8A, B). These calculations still

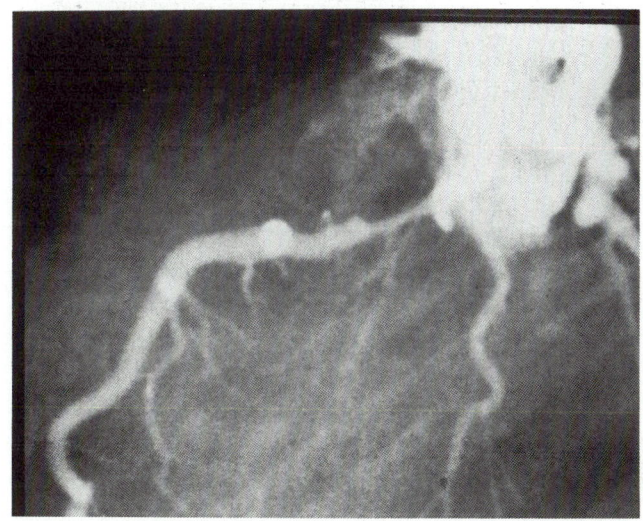

A

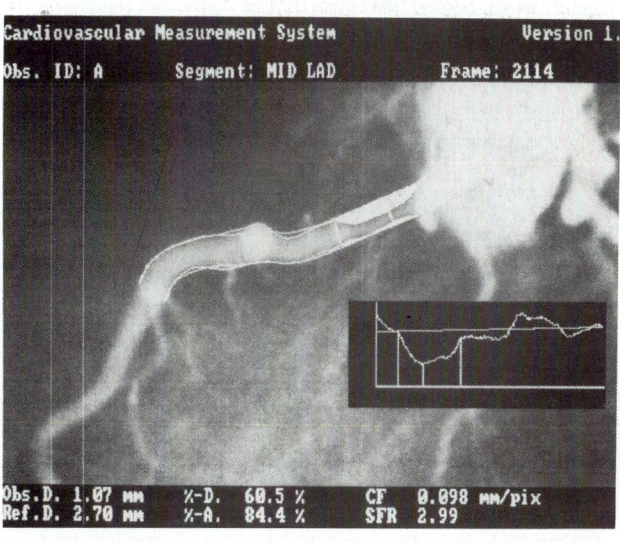

B

Figure 123–8. A. Cineangiogram showing long narrowing of mid-LAD stenosis beyond a diagonal branch. Note variable size of LAD with a small localized dilatation beyond lesion. **B.** Quantitative analysis of the same lesion using optimal frame. The computer, through measurement of videodensity, traces the edge of the lumen at the site of narrowing as well as proximal and distal to it. In the window are depicted the variations of the diameter as well as the average diameter (semihorizontal line slashed across the peaks and valleys) of the segment of artery analyzed. Below the line are the stenotic points and above the site of dilatation. Vertical lines represent points of measurement of the lumen diameter. The diameter (D) is expressed in millimeters and in percentage of reduction, e.g., diameter of obstruction = 1.07 mm, reference diameter (mean diameter of segment analyzed) = 2.70 mm. The percentage (%D) of stenosis is 60.5%, the percentage of surface area reduction (%A) is 84.4%. By measuring pixel sizes (CF=0.098 mm/pix), the computer arrives at the theoretical flow reduction (S FR) at the site of stenosis (<3.0 = significant). Visual estimation of the degree of narrowing might arrive at a higher percentage than the QCA analysis. Reproducibility of the visual technique is low and that of the QCA is high (see text).

depend[47] on the choice of frames by a physician and, most importantly, on optimal arteriographic equipment, the latter, regrettably, not a universal property. Although the severity of a lesion, contrary to expected logic, does not predict clinical outcome[48] (but does help predict angiographic changes[49]), precise knowledge of the extent and severity of coronary artery disease is paramount to the decision process. Whereas visual interpretation is reproducible to about 30%, quantitative coronary arteriography interpretation reaches 85%.[47] QCA has made enormous progress in the past 5 years and has become a most valuable tool.

SUMMARY

In depth knowledge of the coronary arterial anatomy has become a necessity for radiologists, cardiologists, surgeons, as well as for the anatomopathologist. In recent years, nomenclatures have become standardized and simplified. Variations in the anatomy of coronary arteries are not uncommon. In the adult, the most common include aberrant Cx (from the RCA) and origin of the LCA from the right sinus. In the infant, origin of the LCA from the PA and AV fistulae (usually RCA to RV) are the most common. Intramyocardial course of the LAD or of any branch of the Cx—not a true anomaly—is probably the most frequent

"bête noire" of the coronary surgeon. With the advent of retrograde cardioplegia, interest in the coronary venous circulation has risen. Anomalies of the coronary venous network are rare and of occasional significance to adult cardiac surgery.

Proper interpretation of the coronary arteriogram by the cardiac surgeon and last minute review of the location and severity of coronary stenoses are paramount and part of good clinical judgment. Current reading techniques remain less than ideal. Computer analyses—although time consuming—can help the decision process and soon will be part of the armamentarium.

REFERENCES

1. Vieussens R: *Nouvelles découvertes sur le coeur*. Paris, 1706
2. Heberden W: Some account of a disorder of the breast. *Med Trans R Col Phys* **II:**59, 1786
3. Herrick JB: *A Short History of Cardiology*. Springfield, IL, Charles C Thomas, 1942
4. Sones FM Jr, Shirey EK: Cine coronary arteriography. *Mod Concepts Cardiovasc Dis* **31:**7–35, 1962
5. Kennedy JW, Ritchie JL, David KB, et al: Western Washington randomized trial of intracoronary streptokinase in acute myocardial infarction. *N Engl J Med* **309:**1477, 1983
6. Gruentzig AR: Transluminal dilatation of coronary artery stenosis. *Lancet* **1:**263, 1986

7. Kirklin JW, Akins CW, Blackstone EI, et al: Guidelines and indications for coronary artery bypass graft surgery, A report of the ACC/AHA Task force. *J Am Coll Cardiol* **17**:543–589, 1991

8. National Center for Health Statistics: Health, United States, 1992. Hyattsville, MD, Public Health Service, 1993

9. Principal investigators of CASS and their associates: The national Heart, Lung and Blood Institute Coronary Artery Surgery Study (CASS). *Circulation* **63** (Suppl I):1, 1981

10. Edwards BS, Edwards WD, Edwards JE: Aortic origin of conus coronary artery. Evidence of postnatal coronary development. *Br Heart J* **45**:55, 1981

11. Hutchins GM, Nazarin IH, Bulkley BH: Association of left dominant coronary arterial systems with congenital bicuspid aortic valve. *Am J Cardiol* **42**:51, 1978

12. Konno S, Imai Y, Iida Y, et al: A new method for prosthetic valve replacement in congenital aortic stenosis associated with hypoplasia of the aortic ring. *J Thorac Cardiovasc Surg* **70**:909, 1975

13. Vlodaver Z, Neufeld HN, Edwards JE: *Coronary Arterial Variations in the Normal Heart and in Congenital Heart Disease.* New York, Academic Press, 1975

14. McAlpine WA: *Heart and Coronary Arteries. An Anatomical Atlas.* Berlin, Springer-Verlag, 1975

15. Killen DA, Wathanacharden S: Proximal bypass to anomalous circumflex artery. *J Thorac Cardiovasc Surg* **107**:447–449, 1994

16. James TN: *Anatomy of the Coronary Arteries.* New York, Hoeber Medical Division, 1961

17. Kugel MA: Anatomical studies on the coronary arteries and their branches. I. arteria anastomotica auricularis magna. *Am Heart J* **3**:260, 1927

18. Hutchinson MC: A study of the atrial arteries in man. *J Anat* **125**:39, 1978

19. Oschsner JL, Mills NL: Surgical management of diseased intracavitary coronary arteries. *Ann Thorac Surg* **38**:356, 1984

20. Saltissi S, Webb-Reploe MM, Coltart DJ: Effect of variation in coronary artery anatomy on distribution of stenotic lesions. *Br Heart J* **42**:186, 1979

21. Fernandes ED, Kadivar H, Hallman GL, et al: Congenital malformations of the coronary arteries. *Ann Thorac Surg* **54**:732–740, 1992

22. Levin DC, Fellows KE, Abramns HL: Hemodynamically significant primary anomalies of coronary arteries. Angiographic aspects. *Circulation* **58**:25–34, 1978

23. Kimbiris D, Iskandrian AS, Segal BL, et al: Anomalous aortic origin of the coronary arteries. *Circulation* **58**:606, 1978

24. Chaitman BR, Lesperance J, Saltiel J, et al: Clinical, angiographic and hemodynamic findings in patients with anomalous origin of the coronary arteries. *Circulation* **53**:122, 1976

25. Clark VL, Brymer JF, Lakier JB: Posterior descending artery origin from the left anterior descending: An unusual coronary artery variant. *Cathet Cardiovasc Diagn* **11**:167, 1985

26. Spindola-Franco H, Grose R, Solomon N: Dual left anterior descending coronary artery: Angiographic description of important variants and surgical implications. *Am Heart J* **105**:445, 1983

27. Netter FH: *Atlas of Human Anatomy.* Ciba-Geigy, Summit, NJ, 1989

28. Mantini E, Grondin CM, Lillehei CW, Edwards JE: Congenital anomalies involving the coronary sinus. *Circulation* **33**:317–327, 1966

29. Beck CS, Leighninger OS: Operations for coronary artery disease. *Ann Surg* **141**:24–37, 1955

30. Gerlis LM, Gibbs JL, Williams GS: Coronary sinus orifice and persistent left superior vena cava. *Bri Heart J* **26**:648–653, 1984

31. Pan-Chih, Huang AH, Dorsey LMA, Guyton RA: Hemodynamic significance of the coronary vein valves. *Ann Thor Surg* **57**:424–430, 1994

32. Mohl W: Invited commentary on reference 31. *Ann Thor Surg* **57**:430–431, 1994

33. Cohen MV: *Coronary Collaterals. Clinical and Experimental Observations.* Mount Kisco, Futura Publishing, 1985

34. Fulton WFM: The dynamic factor in enlargement of coronary arterial anastomoses, and paradoximal changes in the subendocardial plexus. *Br Heart J* **26**:39, 1984

35. Robbina SL, Solomon M, Bennett A: Demonstration of intercoronary anastomosis in human hearts with a low viscosity perfusion mass. *Circulation* **33**:733, 1966

36. Hambry RI, Aintablia A, Schwartz A: Reappraisal of the functional significance of the coronary collateral circulation. *Am J Cardiol* **38**:305, 1976

37. Gensini GG, daCosta BCB: The coronary collateral circulation in living man. *Am J Cardiol* **24**:393, 1969

38. Bourassa MG, Solignac A, Goulet C, et al: Regression and appearance of coronary collaterals in humans during life. *Circulation* **50**(Suppl II):127, 1974

39. Gruntzig A, Pyle R, Goebel N, et al: The fate of collaterals after PTCA. *Circulation* **62**(SupplIII):161, 1980

40. Sheldon WC: On the significance of coronary collaterals. *Am J Cardiol* **24**:303, 1969

41. Nieminen MS, Valle M, Lassila E: Global and regional left ventricular contractility and coronary collaterals in stable ischemic heart disease. *Clin Cardiol* **3**:163, 1980

42. Grondin CM, Dyrda F, Pasternac A, et al: Discrepancies between cineangiographic and postmortem findings in patients with coronary artery disease and recent myocardial revascularization. *Circulation* **49**:703, 1974

43. Serruys RW, Reiber JHC, Wijns W, et al: Assessment of percutaneous transluminal coronary angiography: Diameter versus densitometric area measurements. *Am J Cardiol* **54**:482, 1984

44. McMahon M, Brown BG, Cukingman R, et al: Quantitative coronary angiography: Measurements of the "critical" stenosis in patients with unstable angina and single-vessel disease without collaterals. *Circulation* **60**(1):106, 1979

45. Ross AM: Interpretation of Coronary angiograms. *J Am Coll Cardiol* **16**:114, 1993

46. Reiber JHC, Serruys PW, Kooijman CJ, et al: Assessment of short medium and long term variations in arterial dimensions from computer-assisted quantisation of coronary cineangiograms. *Circulation* **71**:280–288, 1985

47. Vogel RA: Quantitative coronary arteriography: Uses and misuses. *Am Coll Cardiol-Current Review* **3**:53–54, 1994

48. Waters D, Craven TE, Lesperance J: Prognostic significance of progression of coronary atherosclerosis. *Circulation* **87**:1067–1075, 1993

49. Parisi AF, Fulland ED, Hartigan P: The VA Acme investigations. A comparision of angioplasty with medical therapy in the treatment of single vessel coronary artery disease. *N Engl J Med* **326**:10–16, 1992

C H A P T E R

124

Indications for Nonsurgical Coronary Revascularization

Spencer B. King, III

INTRODUCTION

Coronary angioplasty, developed by Andreas Gruentzig in 1977, has had a dramatic effect on the treatment of obstructive coronary artery disease.[1] The number of angioplasty procedures has increased so that by 1993 over 350,000 procedures were performed in the United States alone.[2] Although somewhat competitive with bypass surgery, this activity has not resulted in a decrease in the number of bypass operations, so the total number of myocardial revascularization procedures and the cost of this activity have increased greatly over the past 10 years. Currently, angioplasty is being used as an alternative both to bypass surgery and to medical therapy in patients with stable angina pectoris, unstable angina pectoris, and acute myocardial infarction. Before exploring the current recommended indications for balloon angioplasty, it is important to understand some of the background data that have led to these recommendations.

BACKGROUND

Balloon Angioplasty

Balloon angioplasty was originally conceived as a therapy for single obstructive lesions in patients with angina pectoris refractory to medical therapy as an alternative to bypass surgery. The patients originally selected by Gruentzig were those with significant symptoms and documented ischemia on exercise stress testing who had a single culprit lesion that was felt to be responsible for the ischemic syndrome. These patients were chosen for two reasons: First, they had anatomic problems that could be addressed by bal-

loon angioplasty and second, they had such clear documentation of the source of ischemia that the results of the angioplasty procedure could be easily measured by relief of the symptoms and by objective exercise testing.

ACUTE RESULTS AND COMPLICATIONS

Long-Term Follow-up

The original series treated by Gruentzig has been followed completely at 10 years.[3,4] Of 169 patients treated, 133 were successfully dilated. Relief of angina and objective measures of improved exercise performance were evident early. The 10-year completed follow-up showed that the patients with involvement of only one coronary artery had a 95% survival whereas the smaller group of patients with more than one vessel involved had an 81% 10-year survival. Coronary bypass surgery was ultimately performed in 23% of the patients by 10 years. After Gruentzig joined our group at Emory University, we collected another series of patients treated in the year 1981.[5] Those patients also have been followed completely at 10 years. There were 427 patients treated; the average age was 54, 77% were males, 88% had single-vessel disease, and 12% multivessel disease. A single site was dilated in 94% of the patients. There was no in-hospital mortality and 91% of the patients remained alive at 10 years. Additional angioplasty was required in 30% and bypass surgery was required in 23% over the 10-year follow-up period. Freedom from death, MI, or bypass surgery was 55% at the 10-year mark. These patients are typical of the single-vessel patients undergoing angioplasty. Even though the angioplasty equipment has undergone dramatic improvement, it is unlikely that the successfully treated patients will have a course very different from those patients treated in 1981.

Multivessel disease patients began to undergo angioplasty in increasing numbers in the mid-1980s.[6] Reports from Hartzler suggested that initial angioplasty results in selected patients were comparable to those found with single-vessel disease, however, long-term survival has not been as good.[7] In 1985 the NHLBI collaborated with 16 centers in setting up a registry of patients undergoing angioplasty. That registry was composed of approximately 50% single-vessel disease patients and 50% patients with multivessel disease. Since this was a multicenter registry, it may be more representative of the long-term outcome of patients selected for angioplasty. The single vessel patients in that registry had a 5-year survival of 93% and the multivessel patients 87%.[8]

There has also been significant experience with angioplasty in patients who have undergone previous bypass surgery. Douglas reported a series of patients who had prior bypass surgery and received angioplasty in the 1980s.[9] The initial success rate in dilating vein grafts was 94%. It was apparent that the long-term success depended largely on the location of the vein graft lesions. Those lesions located at the distal anastamotic site showed a very good long-term patency with an overall restenosis rate of 24%. However, the vein grafts diseased in the mid-portion and the proximal anastamosis with the aorta had a much higher incidence of restenosis. Some other studies have shown lower restenosis rates, but the follow-up period has been shorter and from the Douglas paper it is clear that the attrition of vein grafts is a continuum rather than a healing process that is time limited within the first 6 months. There is continuing attrition of patent grafts after 2 years. We also observed that older vein grafts have a much higher restenosis rate than vein grafts dilated within the first 1 to 2 years. When vein graft occlusion has occurred, dilatation of the native coronary artery feeding the same zone is often the preferred approach.

Angioplasty in the setting of acute myocardial infarction has been used in several situations. First, it was used following myocardial infarction to treat residual stenoses in the setting of recurrent ischemia. In addition, angioplasty has been used as a primary therapy for acute myocardial infarction as a substitute for thrombolytic therapy.[10] The TIMI II trial showed that angioplasty performed very early following thrombolysis was not associated with additional benefit.[11] Finally, elective angioplasty following thrombolysis has been used in the days to weeks following the infarction often preceded by an exercise stress test. There are few data to prove that this practice has improved overall mortality and morbidity. Recently primary angioplasty for interruption of acute myocardial infarction has been advocated. The Primary Angioplasty in Myocardial Infarction (PAMI) trial[10] demonstrated that primary angioplasty could be performed in high volume centers with angioplasty facil-

ities available 24 hours a day with a high level of success. The overall mortality rates with primary angioplasty were somewhat lower than those found with thrombolysis in this study. There was a particular high-risk subgroup composed of patients with anterior myocardial infarction and older patients who benefitted the most. Overall mortality in patients with anterior infarctions was 1.4% with PTCA compared to 11.9% with thrombolysis. Mortality in patients over 65 was 5.7% with angioplasty compared to 15% with thrombolytic therapy. Patients in the lower risk subgroups, namely those that were younger and with inferior infarctions, did not show additional benefit for primary angioplasty compared to thrombolysis.

NEW DEVICES

Examination of the pathology following balloon angioplasty, both early and late, has encouraged the development of the new technologies to open obstructed coronary arteries. Each of the new devices opens arteries by different mechanisms and each alters the pathology of the arterial obstruction in a somewhat different way.

Directional atherectomy removes strips of atherosclerotic plaque by means of a cylindrical cutting piston that entraps the material into a nose cone from which it can be removed along with the catheter.[12,13] Rotary ablation atherectomy removes tissue by the action of a high-speed rotating burr covered with diamond microchips.[14,15] This abrading activity removes tissue and causes smaller microparticles to embolize distally passing through the arteriolar and capillary circulation to be removed by the reticuloendothelial system. The transluminal extraction atherectomy catheter (TEC) operates by rotation of a conical cutting head on the distal end of the catheter that minces portions of the plaque and aspirates it through the catheter by suction.[16]

Several forms of laser energy have been used, however, in recent years excimer laser has been the most widely accepted.[17–19] This energy source is delivered via a fiberoptic bundle in a catheter configuration directly at the atherosclerotic plaque. By contacting the plaque and activating the laser, the tissue is removed by a combination of photoablation and mechanical disruption. The effects on the arterial wall are different from those of earlier argon lasers in that very little heat damage occurs, however, there is a shock wave and gaseous expansion within the artery and some particles are liberated.

Endovascular stent devices have been made primarily of stainless steel and come in various configurations ranging from an interdigitating mesh to wire coils of various configurations and a slotted cylindrical tube that is expanded by a balloon. All these devices act to exert radial force on the artery and to maintain that force once the delivery system has been removed. These retained stents have the ability to resist elastic recoil and to create a smoother lumen by sealing cracks and flaps. A major disadvantage is that they are metallic foreign bodies within the lumen of the vessel and have a thrombogenic potential. Several evaluations have been performed on these devices to judge their superiority compared to standard balloon angioplasty.

The directional atherectomy catheter has been compared to balloon angioplasty in the recently published CAVEAT and C-CAT trials.[20,21] Although the artery was opened more completely by the directional atherectomy device, at the end of 6 months the repeat angiograms showed that there was very little difference in the final residual lumen diameter or the restenosis rate defined as 50% occlusion. There was one subset in the CAVEAT trial that did show a reduction in restenosis, that being the proximal portion of the anterior descending coronary artery not involving the origin of that vessel. The Canadian trial, C-CAT, however, failed to show proximal anterior descending artery restenosis improvement with the atherectomy device. Further trials are being planned to investigate whether a more complete opening of the artery with the atherectomy catheter would result in an improved restenosis rate. To accomplish that, centers committed to vigorous atherectomy aimed at achieving almost zero residual stenosis will compare their results to randomly treated patients who undergo balloon angioplasty. Results of this trial are expected in 1996.

No major trials have been carried out testing the excimer laser, the rotablator, or the TEC extraction atherectomy device. Various registries, including industry-sponsored registries, have recorded the results of these devices, however. An NHLBI-sponsored registry of these new devices, called NACI (new approaches to coronary intervention), has collected cases from 37 participating sites.[22] Interdevice comparison is difficult because the devices were selected for specific applications. The rotablator and the excimer laser devices have been used largely in longer lesions with the rotablator being concentrated on calcific and hard fibrotic lesions while the excimer laser has been used predominantly in long lesions and ostial lesions. Examination of the 1 year event rates in 330 rotablator patients and over 750 excimer laser patients shows 1 year mortality rates that do not seem very different from that expected with balloon angioplasty. The TEC atherectomy device has been used primarily in thrombotic vein grafts[23] and in other vessels with a high thrombus burden or very bulky irregular plaque. The 1-year mortality and complication rates with the TEC device are somewhat higher than a broad population of angioplasty patients, but this may be related to the type cases that were selected for its use.[22,23] None of these three devices has laid claim to reduction in restenosis rates compared to balloon angioplasty.

Finally, the endovascular stents have been used for two indications. First in patients who have acute closure or severe dissection following balloon angioplasty.[24–26] Most of these patients formerly would have gone for bypass surgery and, therefore, the stenting is used either as a bridge

to bypass surgery or as a substitute for bypass surgery. The other use for stents is in attempting to reduce the restenosis rate. Two recent studies have examined this possibility. They are the Benestent trial in Europe[27] and the STRESS trial in the United States.[28] Each trial randomized over 1000 patients and the primary endpoint was similar, namely the diameter of the lesion at its narrowest point measured angiographically on the 6-mo follow-up angiogram. The two trials were consistent in showing a significantly larger lumen at follow-up in the stent group. This increased luminal size was apparently achieved through maximizing lumen size at the time of the initial angioplasty. In the STRESS trial, the average lumen postprocedure diameter and follow-up diameter in the balloon group were 1.99 and 1.56 mm, whereas they were 2.49 and 1.74 mm in the stent group. Translating this information into the familiar dichotomous definition of 50% stenosis at follow-up, the balloon angioplasty group had a restenosis rate of 42.1% compared to 31.6% in the stent group. Similar findings were reported in the Benestent study. These improved restenosis rates did influence the need for repeat intervention on the target vessel. That requirement for repeat intervention in the STRESS trial was 15% in the balloon group and 10% in the stent group resulting in a 5 percentage point improvement in target vessel revascularization in the stented group. Similar findings were obtained in the Benestent trial with a 7.5 percentage point difference favoring stents. This improvement in need for additional procedures, however, was obtained at a cost. There were more bleeding complications in the stent patients in both studies due to the use of vigorous anticoagulation regimes and there was a significantly longer hospital stay averaging over 5 days in the stent group.

Although new devices have been important in dealing with specific lesion types, they have not replaced balloon angioplasty. A survey of four large interventional cardiology programs in 1992 revealed that 80% of patients treated received balloon angioplasty only. On a national level this exclusive use of balloon angioplasty probably occurred in close to 90% of patients treated in 1992 and 1993. It is therefore concluded that angioplasty can be thought of as a procedure performed with various tools heavily dominated by balloon angioplasty with other devices being used for specific type lesions largely to improve the initial result without dramatically impacting the long-term restenosis rate. There will undoubtably be a shift toward more stent usage if the bleeding complications can be solved.

ANGIOPLASTY VS. CORONARY BYPASS SURGERY

Although many observational studies of angioplasty have been carried out over the past 15 years, it was not until the latter part of the 1980s that organized randomized trials were begun. The first of these trials is also the only single center trial, the Emory Angioplasty Surgery Trial (EAST).

This trial, sponsored by the NHLBI, was quickly followed by the larger multicenter trial, the Bypass Angioplasty Revascularization Investigation (BARI). In Europe three trials have been performed—the RITA trial in the United Kingdom,[29] the CABRI trial on the European continent, and the GABI trial in Germany.[30] Entry criteria for the RITA trial included patients with single and multivessel disease with approximately 50% of the patients having only one vessel involved. The RITA trial included only patients who could undergo attempted revascularization to every lesion with either surgery or angioplasty. The other trials were largely strategy trials comparing patients who could be selected either for angioplasty or surgery allowing the angioplasty procedure and the surgery to be performed at the discretion of the operator without any requirement for attempting to open all lesions.

The first trial to be completed is the EAST trial[31] and the results of that trial will be discussed in further detail. There were 392 patients randomized and 450 additional eligible patients who were not randomized either because of physician or patient preference. Sixty percent of the patients who were eligible had double-vessel disease and 40% had triple-vessel disease. There were no differences in baseline variables between the randomized cohorts. The average age was 62 years, ejection fraction was 62%, 40% had triple-vessel disease and 60% double-vessel disease, the proximal anterior descending artery was involved in 72%, and there were 3.4 lesions per patient. Those patients with left main disease, old total occlusions, and severe left ventricular dysfunction were excluded from the trial. The surgery and the angioplasty patients exhibited similar in-hospital mortality (1% in each group). At the end of 3 years the mortality was also the same, 6.3% in the surgery group and 7.1% in the angioplasty group. The predefined primary endpoint was a composite of death, myocardial infarction, and a large amount of ischemia demonstrated on stress thallium scanning at the end of the trial. There was no difference between the two groups in the occurrence of the primary endpoint. The major differences seen in the trial are related to the number of repeat procedures. Freedom from subsequent bypass surgery occurred in 79% of the angioplasty patients and 99% of the surgery patients. Freedom from repeat angioplasty occurred in 60% of the angioplasty patients and 88% of the surgery patients. Despite the increased use of repeat procedures in the angioplasty group, the surgery patients remained more completely revascularized at the end of the 3 years. One measure of symptomatic improvement, the occurrence of class II, III, or IV angina, occurred in 12% of the surgery group and 20% of the angioplasty group. The conclusions from this trial are that angioplasty can be chosen in patients with this form of multivessel coronary artery disease suitable for either angioplasty or surgery without jeopardizing safety; however, additional repeat procedures are frequently required in the angioplasty group.

The other trials have reported interim results that are not dramatically dissimilar from the results shown in EAST. The need for bypass surgery in the angioplasty group at 1 year was 20% in the European CABRI trial and 21% in the German GABI trial. The largest trial, the BARI (Bypass vs. Angioplasty Revascularization Investigation), will be reporting average 5-year follow-up information in 1995. BARI is a 16-center NHLBI-sponsored trial following over 1800 patients with very similar baseline features to EAST. Both trials have been funded by NHLBI for an additional 5 years clinical follow-up.

Although randomized trials are essential to understand the true value of angioplasty compared to bypass surgery, much can be learned from observational studies of patients who have undergone these procedures. An obvious shortcoming of this approach is the fact that all patients are selected for their assigned therapies and therefore the treatment groups cannot be identified. A recent study from the Duke database[32] suggested that based on their experience with patients undergoing surgery, angioplasty, or medical therapy, predictions could be made. For patients with single-vessel disease either medical therapy or angioplasty had essentially comparable results with angioplasty-treated patients exhibiting reduction in angina. Those patients with simpler forms of two vessel disease were improved by both angioplasty and surgery compared to medical therapy with little to choose between angioplasty and surgery. For those patients with more complex two-vessel disease and patients with three-vessel disease, both angioplasty and surgery performed better than medical therapy with surgery outperforming angioplasty. It will be interesting to see whether the randomized trials or the meta-analysis of multiple trials will support this observational information.

INDICATIONS

Recently the American Heart Association and the American College of Cardiology Task Force on New Technology Assessment have published an updated revision of the guidelines for indications for percutaneous transluminal coronary angioplasty.[33] For the reasons enumerated above, all techniques for angioplasty including the new devices are included together in these recommendations.

Several considerations should be made prior to selecting angioplasty: Will angioplasty have a reasonable chance of addressing the problem at hand, if successful? Is the chance of angioplasty success with the available devices and experience high? What is the risk of acute closure of the artery or arteries treated? What is the risk of serious complications including death or myocardial infarction should the vessel close? What is the chance of long-term success with the procedure or with additional procedures? Finally, what results would be expected from alternative therapies such as bypass surgery or medical therapy?

The indications are divided for single-vessel disease patients who are asymptomatic or mildly symptomatic, single-vessel disease patients who are significantly symptomatic, multivessel disease patients who are asymptomatic or mildly symptomatic, and multivessel disease patients who are significantly symptomatic. In addition, guidelines for patients undergoing angioplasty in the setting of acute myocardial infarction are given and recommendations for training in angioplasty, maintenance of competence, and need for surgical back-up are also discussed.

Angioplasty indications are divided into three classes. Class I: Conditions for which there is general agreement that coronary angioplasty is justified. A Class I indication does not mean that angioplasty is the only acceptable therapy. Class II: Conditions for which there is a divergence of opinion with respect to the justification for coronary angioplasty in terms of value and appropriateness. Class III: Condition for which there is general agreement that angioplasty is ordinarily not indicated.

The indications are divided for significantly symptomatic vs. asymptomatic or mildly symptomatic patients. In brief, the Class I and II indications for symptomatic patients include those shown to have lesions amenable to angioplasty plus ischemia on therapy, angina unresponsive to therapy, or patients intolerant of therapy side effects who have a high to moderate chance of angioplasty success with a low to moderate risk of mortality or morbidity.

Asymptomatic patients or those with mild or easily controlled symptoms should show more severe ischemia on laboratory testing, or be rescued from cardiac arrest, or be in need of high-risk noncardiac surgery. They should have a high likelihood of successful angioplasty with a low risk of morality and morbidity.

Recommendations for PTCA in the setting of myocardial infarction are also enumerated. Class I and II indications in the setting of acute myocardial infarction are AMI with a duration less than 6 hours, persisting or recurrent pain within 12 hours of MI, cardiogenic shock or continued ischemia following thrombolysis. Angioplasty following the acute phase of myocardial infarction can be indicated for recurrent pain, recurrent ischemia on laboratory testing, recurrent or refractory VT or for severe lesions in arteries serving viable myocardium. Elective angioplasty immediately following thrombolysis is not recommended because of adverse results of this strategy shown in previous trials. The full document should be read to understand the recommendations put forward in the guidelines.

The Committee preparing the guidelines re-emphasized the requirement for a surgical program in the institution where angioplasty is performed. This was in recognition of the important role of backup surgery when angioplasty fails or complications occur as well as providing on-site consultation about high-risk cases in which heightened surgical backup support is warranted. Although the type of backup will vary with the experience of the institution, the number of operating rooms, and the acuity of the cases, the availability of surgery is considered essential. Cardiac surgery in the institution is also important in that it

provides the opportunity for patients to access the broad range of revascularization procedures. The choice of procedures is not limited by availability.

Recently, guidelines for management of unstable angina have been developed under a grant from the Agency for Health Care Policy and Research (AHCPR).[34] These guidelines provide multiple pathways for management of patients with unstable angina ranging from "watchful waiting" with delayed exercise tests in patients deemed to be at "low risk" to an invasive strategy for physicians more comfortable with early angiographic risk stratification in unstable angina patients. This document is available by calling AHCPR Clearinghouse at 800-358-9295.

SUMMARY

The greatest role for angioplasty remains the first role, that is in those significantly symptomatic patients with single-vessel disease or single lesions producing the ischemia that can be effectively dilated thereby alleviating the symptoms. Angioplasty in such a setting may be done as an alternative to bypass surgery since it is associated with less costs and morbidity or as an alternative to medical therapy because it is more completely effective. Such patients must expect a certain incidence of recurrence ranging from 25 to 50% depending on the size of the vessel, the location and severity of the lesion, the device used, and many other factors. Fortunately recurrence is rarely associated with myocardial infarction and can be treated with repeat angioplasty.

Multivessel angioplasty is more problematic because of a higher initial risk and a greater chance of restenosis. Nonetheless, many multivessel cases are adequately managed with angioplasty and the randomized trials are now helping to evaluate the relative value of angioplasty and surgery for these patients. Although there are exceptions, current practice favors surgery in patients with diffuse three-vessel disease, especially those with chronic total occlusions.

Previously operated patients comprise an increasing proportion of angioplasty procedures. The patients treated most successfully are those with vein grafts of recent vintage with distal anastamotic lesions and patients with dilatable native arteries. Ostial lesions and old vein graft disease remain problematic and it is hoped that new technologies, especially stents, may help palliate these patients more effectively. Angioplasty as a primary therapy for acute infarction has been shown to be a viable technique when applied in experienced centers. It seems most valuable in high-risk MI patients.

In the future, nonsurgical revascularization will continue to evolve as will other forms of less invasive surgery. The next major impact on surgery volume will occur when restenosis is brought into better control. Because of the diffuse nature of the disease in many patients, angioplasty cannot replace bypass surgery in the foreseeable future. However, improved understanding of long-term outcomes will lead to better selection of these two complementary revascularization therapies.

REFERENCES

1. Gruentzig AR: Transluminal dilatation of coronary artery stenosis (letter). *Lancet* **2:**263, 1978
2. Feinleib M, Halvik RJ, Gillum RF, et al: Coronary heart disease and related procedures: National hospital discharge survey data. *Circulation* **79:**13–18, 1989
3. Gruentzig AR, King SB, Schlumpf M, Siegenthaler W: Long term follow-up after percutaneous transluminal coronary angioplasty: The early Zurich experience. *N Engl J Med* **316:**1127–1132, 1987
4. King SB, Schlumpf M: Ten year completed follow-up after percutaneous transluminal coronary angioplasty: The early Zurich experience. *J Am Coll Cardiol* **22:**353–360, 1993
5. Talley JD, Hurst JW, King SB, et al: Clinical outcome 5 years after attempted percutaneous transluminal coronary angioplasty in 427 patients. *Circulation* **77:**820–829, 1988
6. Cowley MJ, Vetrovec GW, DiSciasio G, et al: Coronary angioplasty of multiple vessels: Short term outcome and long-term results. *Circulation* **72:**1314–1320, 1985
7. O'Keefe JH Jr, Rutherford BD, McConahay DR, et al: Multivessel coronary angioplasty from 1980–1989: Procedural results and long-term outcome. *J Am Coll Cardiol* **16:**1079–1102, 1990
8. Detre K, Holubkov R, Kelsey S, et al: Percutaneous transluminal coronary angioplasty in 1985–1986 and 1977–1981. *N Engl J Med* **318:**265–270, 1988
9. Douglas JS Jr: Percutaneous interventional in patients with prior coronary bypass surgery. In: Topol EJ (ed): *Textbook of Interventional Cardiology*. Philadelphia, W.B. Saunders, 1990
10. Grines CL, Browne KF, Marco J, et al: A comparison of immediate angioplasty with thrombolytic therapy for acute myocardial infarction. *N Engl J Med* **328:**673–679, 1993
11. Timi Study Group: Comparison of invasive and conservative strategies after treatment with intravenous tissue plasminogen activator in acute myocardial infarction. Results of the Thrombolysis in Myocardial Infarction (TIMI) Phase II Trial. *N Engl J Med* **320:**618–627, 1989
12. Ellis SG, DeCesare NB, Pinkerton CA, et al: Relation of stenosis morphology and clinical presentation to the procedural results of directional coronary atherectomy. *Circulation* **84:**644–653, 1991
13. Hinohara T, Rowe M, Robertson GC, et al: Effect of lesion characteristics on outcome of directional coronary atherectomy. *J Am Coll Cardiol* **17:**1112–1120, 1991
14. Bertrand ME, Lablanche JM, Fourrier JL, et al: Percutaneous coronary rotary ablation. *Herz* **15:**285–291, 1990
15. Ellis SG, Popma JJ, Buchbinder M, et al: Relation of clinical presentation, stenosis morphology, and operator technique to the procedural results of rotational atherectomy and rotational atherectomy-facilitated angioplasty. *Circulation* **89:**882–892, 1994
16. Sketch MH Jr, Phillips HR, Lee M, et al: Coronary transluminal extraction endatherectomy. *J Intervent Cardiol* **3:**23–28, 1991
17. Forrester JS, Litvack F, Grundfest WS: Laser angioplasty in cardiovascular disease. *Am J Cardiol* **57:**990–992, 1986
18. Litvack F, Margolis J, Cummins F, et al and the ELCA investigators: Excimer Laser Coronary (ELCA) Registry: Report of the first consecutive 2080 patients. *J Am Coll Cardiol* **19:**276A, 1992
19. Safian RD, Freed M, O'Neill WW, et al: Are residual stenoses ater excimer laser angioplasty and coronary atherectomy due to inefficient or small devices? Comparison with balloon angioplasty. *J Am Coll Cardiol* **22:**1628–1634, 1993
20. Topol EJ, Leya F, Pinkerton CA, et al: A comparison of directional atherectomy with coronary angioplasty in patients with coronary artery disease. *N Engl J Med* **329:**221–227, 1993
21. Adelman AG, Cohen EA, Kimball BP, et al: A comparison of directional atherectomy with balloon angioplasty for lesions of the left anterior descending coronary artery. *N Engl J Med* **329:**228–233, 1993
22. Baim DS, Kent KM, King SB, et al: Evaluating new devices. Acute (in-hospital) results from the new approaches to coronary interventional registry. *Circulation* **89:**471–481, 1993
23. Safian RD, Grines CL, O'Neill WW, et al: Clinical and angiographic results of transluminal extraction coronary atherectomy in saphenous vein bypass grafts. *Circulation* **89:**303–312, 1994
24. Roubin GS, King SB III, Douglas JS Jr, et al: Intracoronary stenting during percutaneous transluminal coronary angioplasty. *Circulation* **81**(Suppl IV):IV92–IV100, 1990
25. Hearn JA, King SB III, Douglas JS Jr, et al: Clinical and angiographic outcomes after coronary artery stenting for acute or threatened closure after percutaneous transluminal coronary angioplasty. Initial results with a balloon-expandable, stainless steel design. *Circulation* **88**(part 1):2086–2096, 1993
26. Sigwart U, Urban P, Golf S, et al: Emergency stenting for acute occlusion after coronary balloon angioplasty. *Circulation* **78:**1121–1127, 1988
27. Serruys PW, de Jaegere P, Kiemeneij F, et al for the Benestent study group: A comparison of balloon-expandable stent implantation with balloon angioplasty in patients with coronary artery disease. *N Engl J Med* **331:**489–495, 1994
28. Fischman DL, Leon MB, Baim D, et al: A randomized comparison of coronary stent placement and balloon angioplasty in the treatment of coronary artery disease. *N Engl J Med* **331:**496–501, 1994
29. Henderson RA for the RITA trial participants: Coronary angioplasty versus coronary artery bypass surgery: The randomized intervention treatment of angina (RITA) trial. *Lancet* **341:**573–580, 1993
30. Hamm CW, Reimers J, Ischinger T, et al for the G.A.B.I. study group: A randomized study of coronary angioplasty compared with bypass surgery in patients with symptomatic multivessel coronary disease. *N Engl J Med* **331:**1037–1043, 1994
31. King SB III, Lembo NJ, Weintraub WS, et al for the EAST investigators. The Emory angioplasty vs. surgery trial (EAST): A randomized trial comparing coronary angioplasty to coronary bypass surgery. *N Engl J Med* **331:**1044–1050, 1994
32. Mark DB, Nelson CL, Califf RM, et al: Continuing evolution of therapy for coronary artery disease. *Circulation* **89:**2015–2025, 1994
33. Ryan TJ, Bauman WB, Kennedy WJ, et al: Guidelines for percutaneous transluminal coronary angioplasty. A report of the American Heart Association/American College of Cardiology Task Force on Assessment of Diagnostic and Therapeutic Cardiovascular Procedures (Committee on Percutaneous Transluminal Coronary Angioplasty). *Circulation* **88:**2987–3007, 1993
34. Unstable Angina: Diagnosis and Management. Clinical Practice Guideline. Number 10. U.S. Department of Health and Human Services. AHCPR Publication No. 94-0602, March 1994

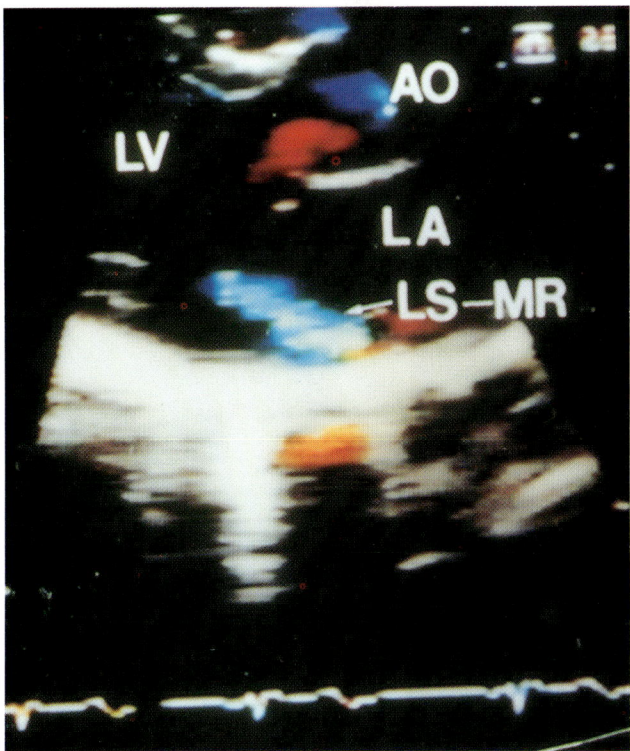

Figure 104–2. Parasternal long-axis view of mild late-systolic mitral regurgitation (LS-MR) due to mitral valve prolapse. The MR is seen as a light blue oval jet during systole entering the left atrium (LA) through the mitral valve. AO, aorta; LV, left ventricle.

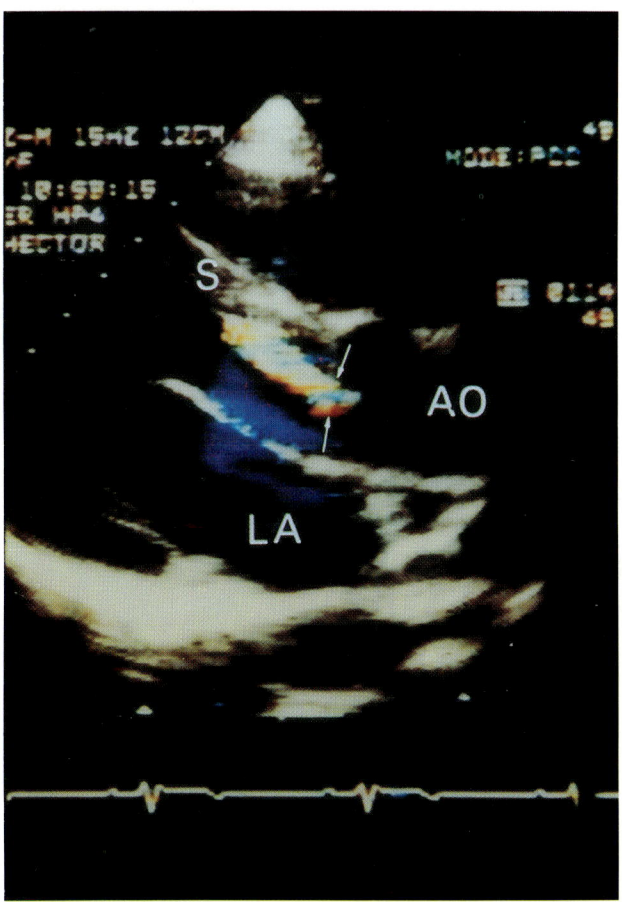

Figure 104–3. Moderate aortic regurgitation is seen as a bright yellow jet entering the left ventricular outflow tract in diastole through the closed aortic valve (white arrows show width of regurgitant orifice outlined by the color flow jet). AO, aorta; LA, left atrium; S, proximal anterior ventricular septum.

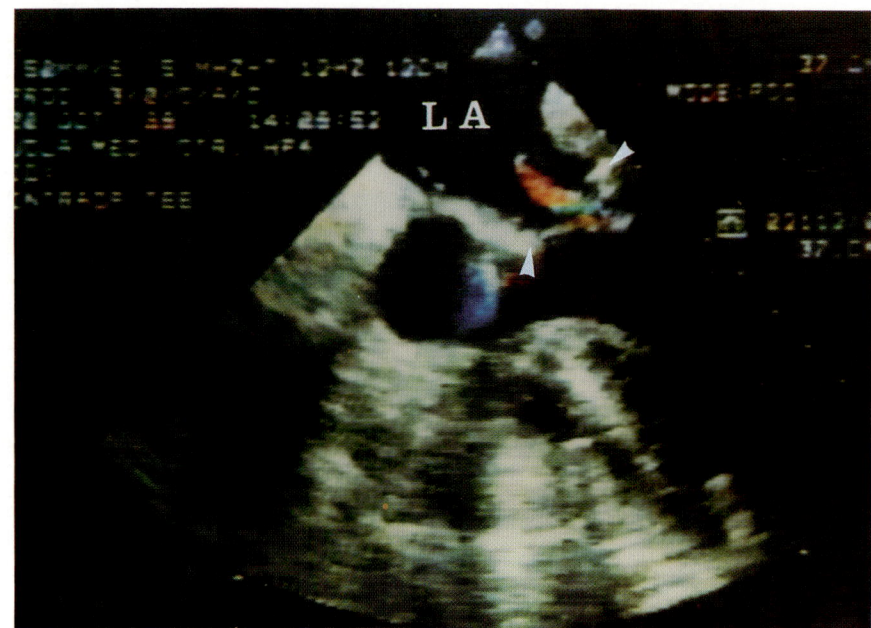

Figure 104–19. Mitral valve repair. Intraoperative TEE results of mitral valve repair with annuloplasty (arrowheads) and resection of flail portion of the posterior leaflet; there is trivial residual mitral regurgitation. LA, left atrium.

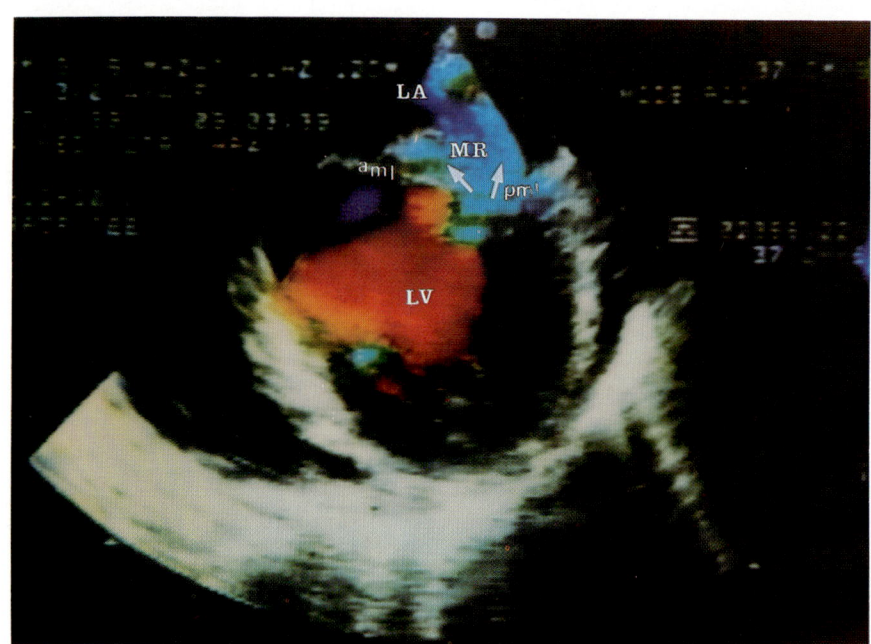

Figure 104–20. TEE in mitral regurgitation (MR). Severe MR in a patient with mitral valve prolapse with elongated anterior mitral leaflet (aml) and hooded posterior mitral leaflet (pml) and dilated mitral annular dimensions (annular size measured 4.3 cm with upper limit of normal = 3.5 cm). LA, left atrium; LV, left ventricle.

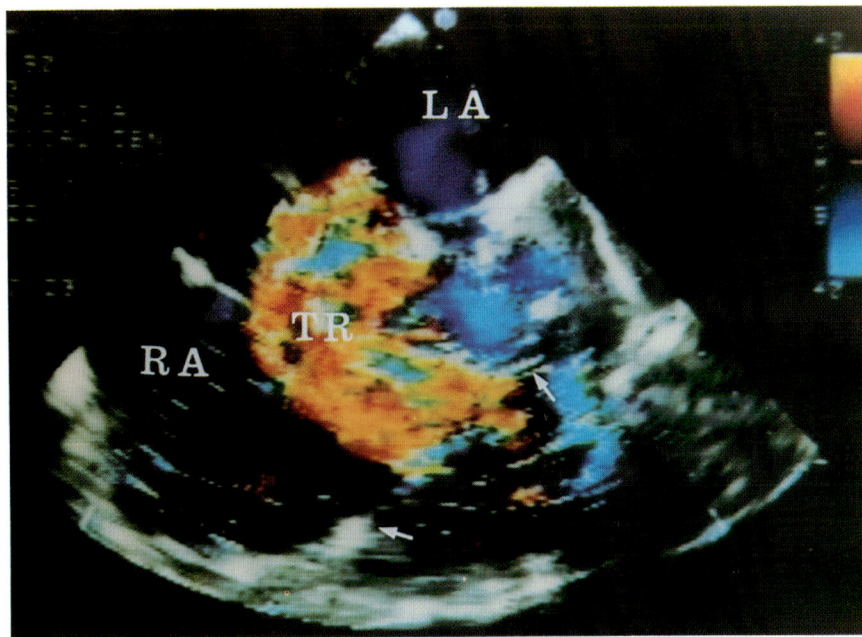

A

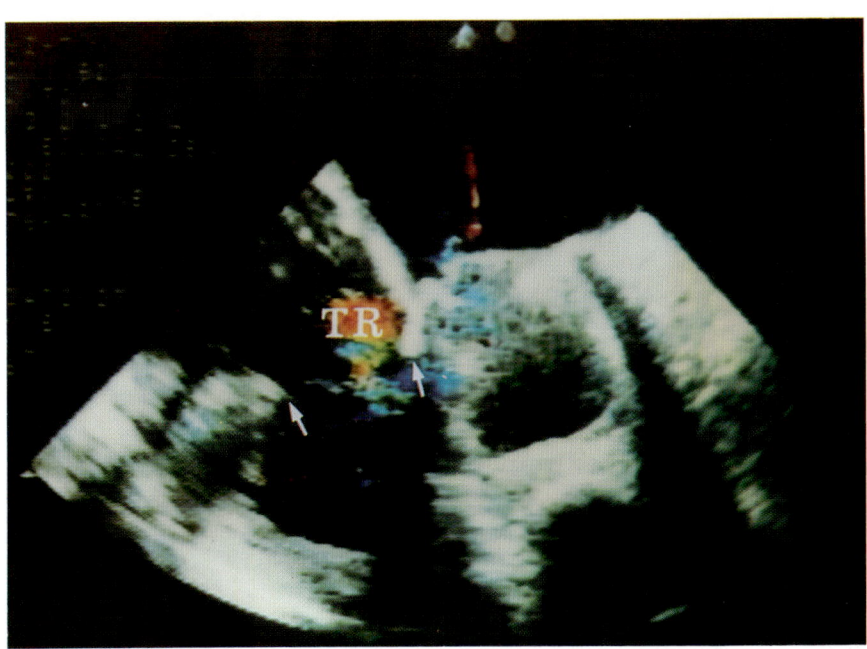

B

Figure 104–22. Tricuspid valve repair. Intraoperative TEE evaluation before and after tricuspid valve repair for functional tricuspid regurgitation (TR). **A.** Prerepair, the tricuspid annulus is dilated (arrows) with severe TR by color-flow imaging into a dilated right atrium (RA). LA, left atrium. **B.** After repair, the annuloplasty (arrows) shows the smaller annulus with trivial TR by color flow imaging.

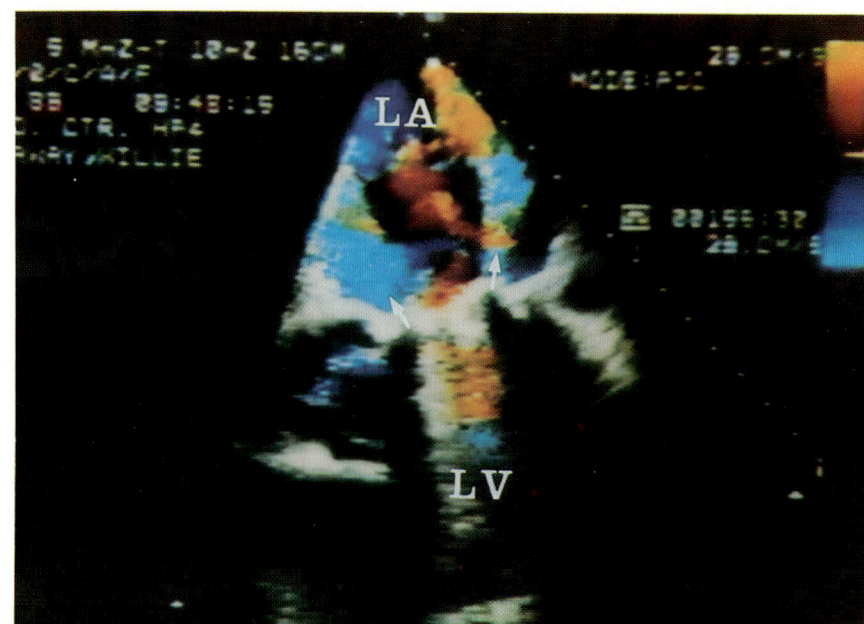

Figure 104–23. TEE of severe paraprosthetic mitral regurgitation (arrows) around a St. Jude's mitral valve prosthesis. LA, left atrium; LV, left ventricle.

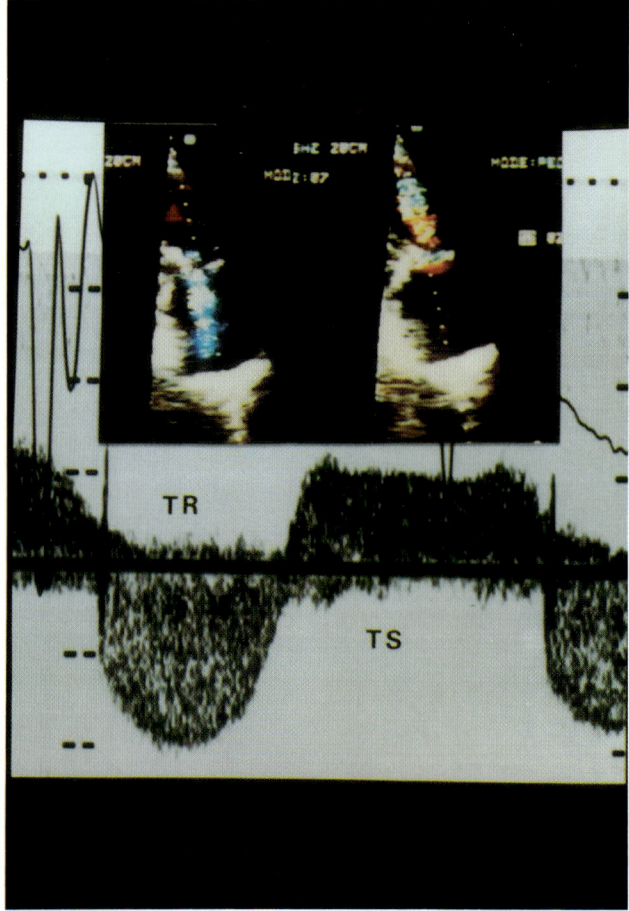

Figure 104–24. Transthoracic echo of degenerated bioprosthetic tricuspid valve. Color-flow imaging (upper panel) shows moderate tricuspid regurgitation (TR) with (lower panel) a low peak systolic velocity (2 m/s) and tricuspid stenosis (TS) by both color-flow and spectral Doppler.

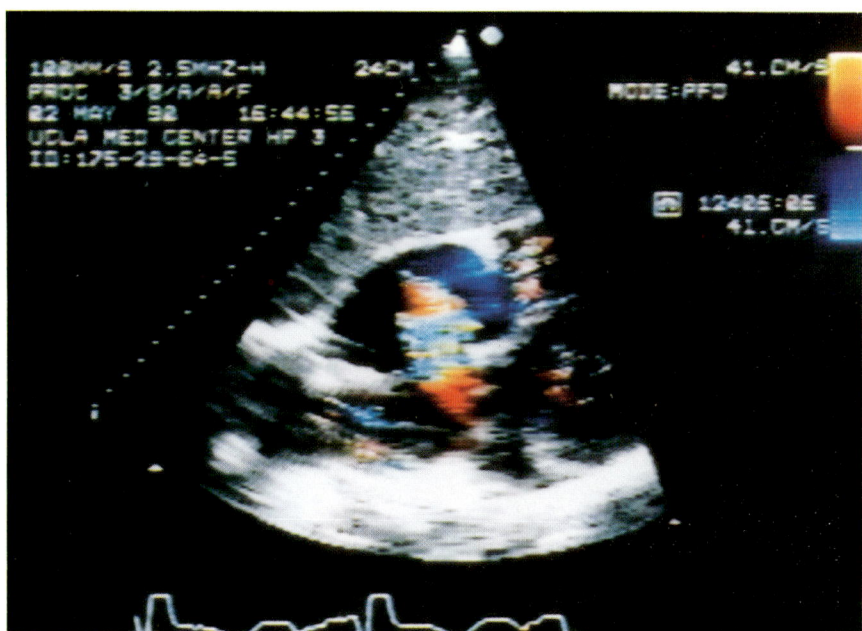

Figure 104–27. Secundum atrial septal defect. Subcostal 2-D echo shows the defect with a large left to right shunt (black arrow) by color-flow imaging.

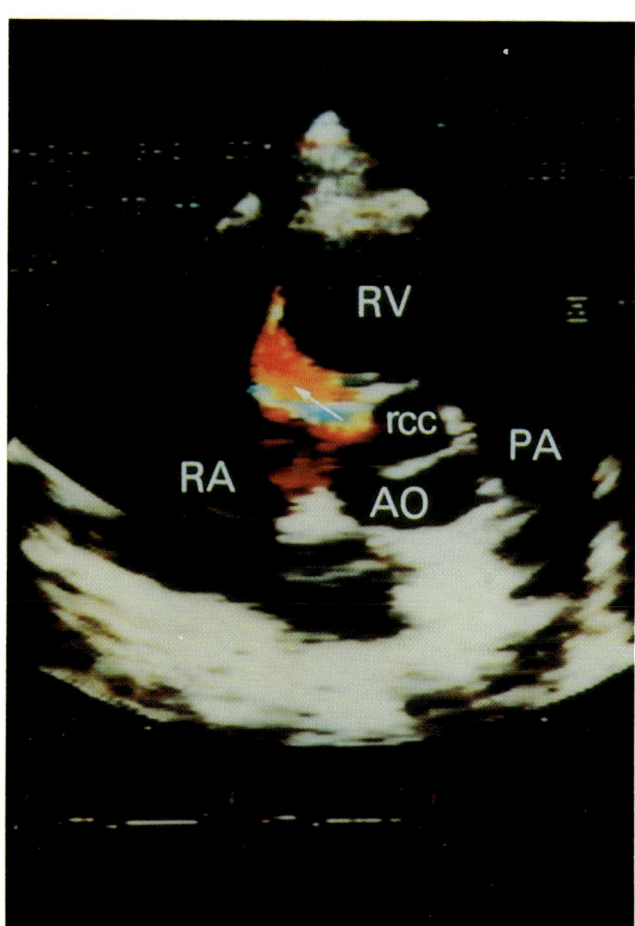

Figure 104–29. Ruptured sinus of Valsalva. This parasternal short axis shows a ruptured sinus of Valsalva (arrow shows direction of continuous flow) from the right coronary cusp (rcc) into the inflow tract of the right ventricle (RV). AO, aorta; PA, pulmonary artery; RA, right atrium.

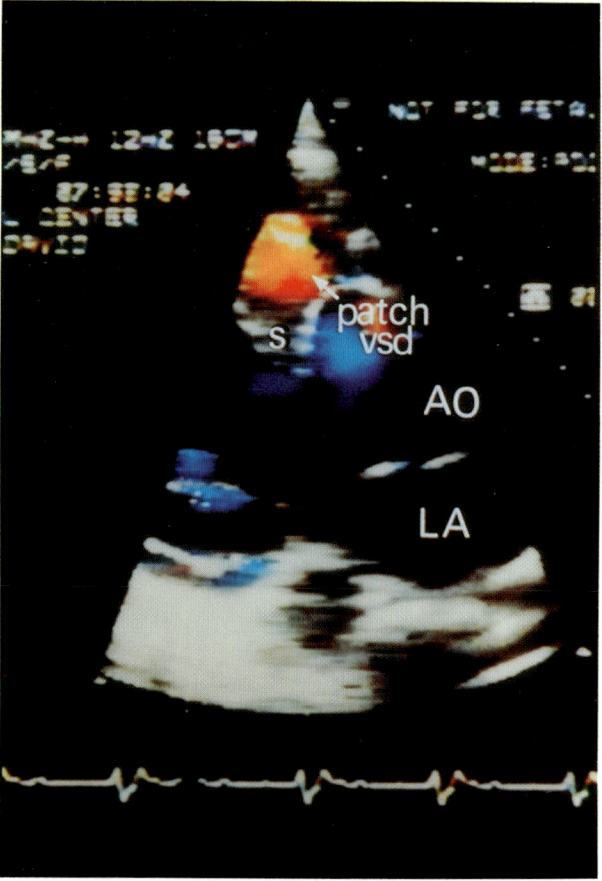

Figure 104–31. Tetralogy of Fallot with patch ventricular septal defect (VSD). This parasternal long axis shows a small residual patch VSD (arrow) after repair of tetralogy of Fallot. AO, aorta; LA, left atrium; S, ventricular septum.

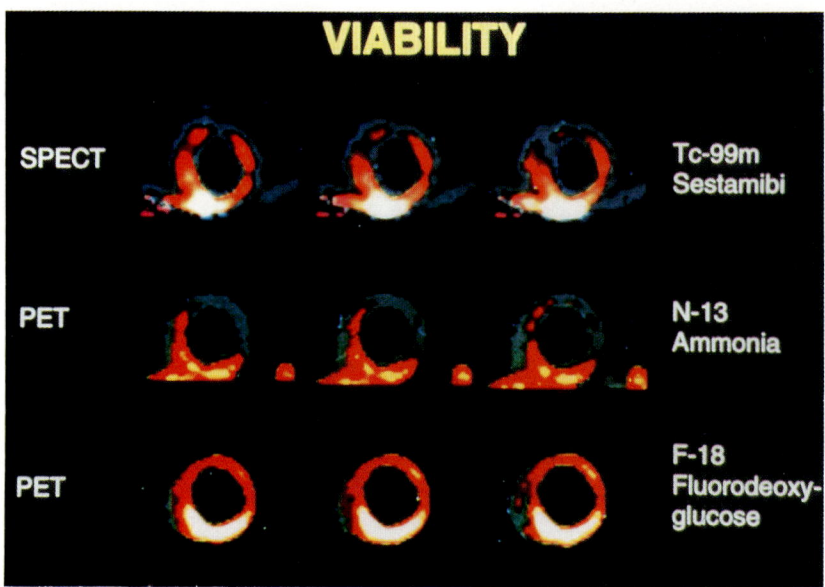

Figure 105–7. This case presents a 57-year-old man with a 5-year history of progressive dyspnea and a previous diagnosis of heart failure. The patient was referred for heart transplant evaluation with a presumed diagnosis of idiopathic cardiomyopathy. At the time of presentation, he was in the New York Heart Association functional class 4, and was dyspneic at rest. Cardiac catheterization showed left ventricular ejection fraction=20% with multiple and severe regional wall motion abnormalities. Although the patient had no history of chest pain or prior infarction, there was 90% stenosis in the left main coronary artery, 100% stenosis in the proximal left circumflex artery, and moderate disease in the right coronary artery. Based on the coronary anatomy and the patient's symptoms, bypass would improve survival and symptoms only if the dysfunctional tissue was viable. Because catheterization does not provide viability information, a series of nuclear imaging studies were performed to evaluate viability: SPECT perfusion imaging using technetium-99m sestamibi, PET perfusion imaging using nitrogen-13 ammonia, and PET metabolic imaging using fluorine-18 fluorodeoxyglucose (FDG). The figure presents contiguous short-axis views for the technetium-99m sestamibi SPECT study (top row), the PET nitrogen-13 ammonia perfusion study (middle row), and the PET fluorine-18 FDT metabolism study (bottom row). The heart was shown to be markedly dilated using all three techniques. The extensive nitrogen-13 ammonia perfusion defect was not matched with a defect in fluorine-18 fluorodeoxyglucose metabolism (perfusion metabolism "mismatch"), suggesting residual glucose metabolism, which has been shown to be a viability marker. Based on preliminary studies, however, the significant residual technetium-99m sestamibi uptake would be interpreted as indicating myocardial viability. The patient was judged to not be a transplant candidate. The patient underwent bypass, with grafts placed into the left anterior descending and posterior descending coronary arteries. A leaking mitral valve that led to moderately severe mitral regurgitation was also repaired. The echo ejection fraction improved modestly up to 30%. The patient improved from the New York Heart Association functional class 4 to class 2 after surgery.

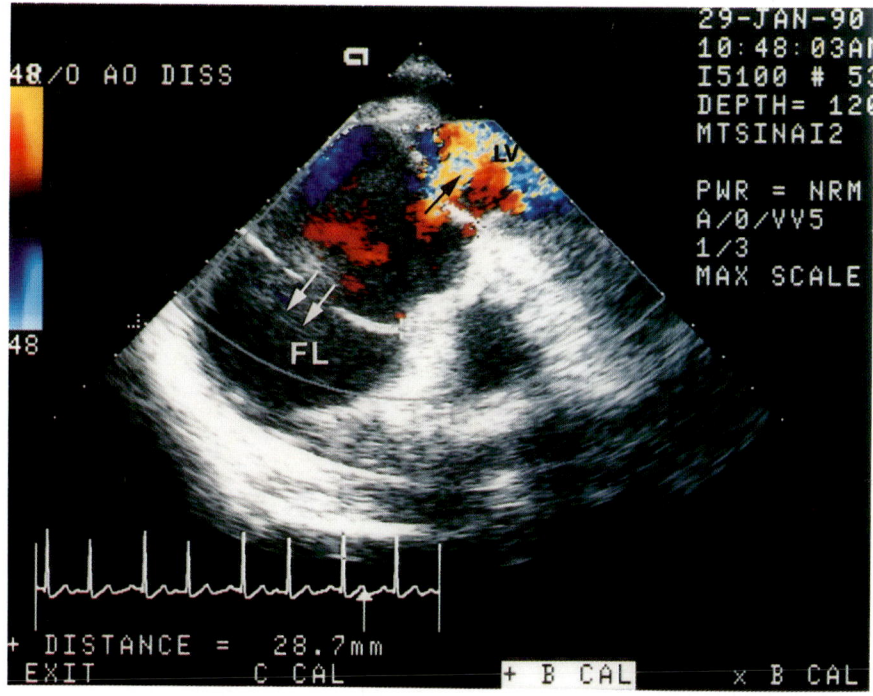

A

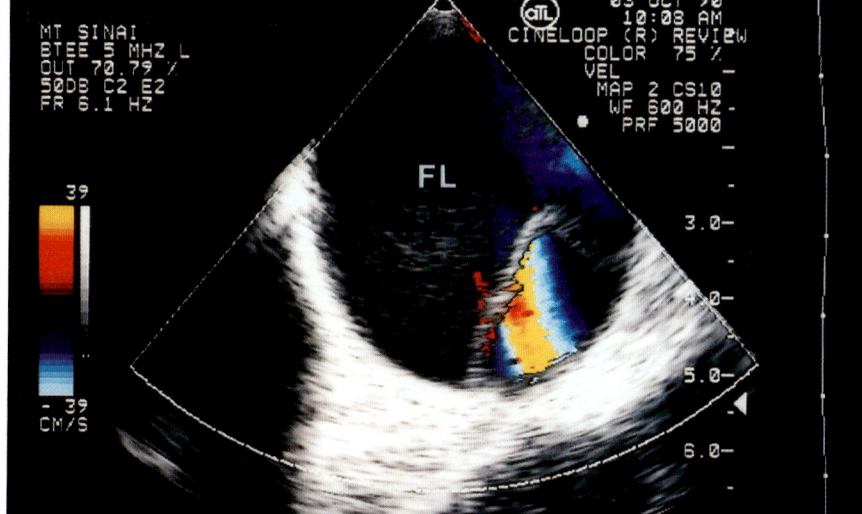

B

Figure 138–3. A. TEE showing the primary tear in the ascending aorta. The true and false lumens are clear with the arrows pointing through the tear a few centimeters above the aortic valve. Color Doppler also shows moderate degree of aortic regurgitation. **B.** Color Doppler demonstration of secondary tear in the descending aorta. Notice the enlarged false lumen and compressed true lumen. FL, false lumen. *(From Goldman ME: Clinical Atlas of Transesophageal Echocardiography. Mount Kisco, NY, Futura, 1993, with permission.)*

Surgical Indications for Coronary Revascularization

Kenneth L. Franco and Graeme L. Hammond

Coronary artery bypass surgery was introduced 25 years ago and has proved to be a viable and durable operation with approximately 1 in every 1000 persons in the United States receiving this operation today.[1]

The potential objectives of coronary artery bypass surgery are to relieve ischemia and the symptoms of angina, prolong survival, prevent myocardial infarction, preserve left ventricular (LV) function, and improve exercise tolerance. Several studies have examined the relationship between the extent of coronary artery disease, the relief of angina, and improvement in survival, to determine the relative benefits of medical, percutaneous therapeutic, or surgical management. Results of these studies are used to determine which patients are appropriate candidates for bypass surgery. There are several factors that must be evaluated in patients being considered for any form of management. These include the degree of symptoms and the presence of associated medical problems, a determination of the physiologic significance of coronary disease (evidence of reversible ischemia), documentation of the angiographic abnormalities of the coronary arteries, and an assessment of left ventricular function. The patient can then be categorized into one of several subsets to which the results of clinical trials can be applied.

The majority of patients with coronary artery disease come to medical attention because of angina. It should be determined whether the patient has stable or unstable angina, two conditions that have a different prognosis with medical treatment. Chronic stable angina refers to a pain pattern that has been stable for 4 to 6 wk without significant change. Most patients have typical symptoms of exertional substernal chest pain or other anginal equivalents including shortness of breath or fatigue. The severity of symptoms

should be classified into the Canadian Cardiovascular Society categories I–IV.[2] Class I angina occurs only with strenuous or prolonged exertion at work or recreation and does not occur with ordinary physical activity. Class II angina occurs with rapid walking on level ground or climbing stairs. Walking at a normal pace for less than two blocks on level ground or climbing one flight of stairs does not cause angina, except when walking occurs during the first few hours after awakening, after meals, under emotional stress, in the wind, or in cold weather. Class II angina implies slight limitation of ordinary activity. Class III angina occurs when walking less than two blocks on level ground, at a normal pace, under normal conditions, or when climbing one flight of stairs. This implies marked limitation of ordinary physical activity. Class IV angina occurs with even mild activity and may occur at rest, but must be brief, i.e., less than 15 min. If the angina is of longer duration, it is called unstable angina. This implies the inability to carry out even mild physical activity. Unstable angina refers to a variety of clinical conditions of varying significance.[3] It has been defined as the new onset of severe angina within the past 2 mo, acceleration of a previously stable pattern, or angina occurring at rest. For patients with rest angina, it is important to note whether it is occurring in the early postinfarction period (within 2 weeks of an MI), within the last 48 hours, and whether angina is associated with ECG changes.[4] In any event, unstable angina is taken as clear evidence of important reversible myocardial ischemia.

Documentation of myocardial ischemia includes radionuclide exercise testing. Stratification to the various therapeutic modes depends upon reversible or irreversible defects in one or more areas of myocardium, increased lung uptake (reflecting pulmonary edema), exercise induced reduction in ejection fraction greater than or equal to 10%, and the development of segmental wall motion abnormalities.[5]

In acute myocardial infarction, the newly occluded vessel often does not have a pre-existing stenotic lesion, which is consistent with the idea that the myocardium supplied by the diseased vessel is usually devoid of important collateral vessels. Current available information suggests that rupture of an unstable atheromatous plaque is the genesis of the acute reduction in luminal diameter often accompanied by thrombosis and platelet aggregation.[6] The greater the number of myocardial infarctions suffered by a patient, the greater the likelihood that he or she will have subsequent infarcts. This may indicate that some patients generate more unstable plaques than others.

Coronary arteriography is indicated for patients who have angina or anginal variants, a positive stress test, and those with previous documented myocardial infarction. The number of major vessels involved, the location of the stenosis, and the status of the distal vessels must be assessed. A stenosis is important when it produces a 70% or greater reduction in the luminal diameter of the vessel. An exception is the left main coronary artery in which a greater than 50% reduction in luminal diameter is important. Functional status of the left ventricle can be determined by ventriculography, echocardiography, or radionuclide ventriculography. Ejection fraction greater than 50% is normal and an ejection fraction less than 35% reflects moderate to severe LV dysfunction.

Major randomized trials of medical vs. surgical management of coronary artery disease were initiated in the early 1970s to determine whether there was any survival advantage to bypass surgery in patients with stable angina. These studies demonstrated that surgery provided superior relief of angina and improvement in functional capacity, a reduction in the incidence of fatal myocardial infarction, but no difference in the incidence of late nonfatal myocardial infarction.[7] It was shown that patients with left main disease or three-vessel disease with moderate left ventricular dysfunction also had survival advantage with surgery. The advantage diminished with time due to vein graft occlusion. Application of these studies to patients undergoing coronary artery bypass grafting today requires an understanding of the limitations and exclusion criteria of each study and appreciation of the changes in medical and surgical practice that have occurred during the past 25 years. Randomized studies correlated survival with the severity of angina, the extent of coronary disease as documented by coronary arteriography, and the level of ventricular function. There have been three major studies: the VA study, the European Cooperative Surgical Study (ECSS), and the Coronary Artery Surgery Study (CASS). Only one of three trials used ischemia as a basis of entry into the study and none of them stressed the relationship between the extent of ischemia, or myocardium in jeopardy, and survival. In fact, many patients did not have evidence of inducible ischemia

by stress testing. Patients with moderate to severe ventricular dysfunction were not included in two studies and application of the results of these trials to women and patients over age 65 is limited because so few patients in these categories were included. Since these studies were performed, numerous changes have occurred in the conduct of the surgical operation, patient monitoring, and postoperative care. They include (1) the studies were performed before the widespread use of β-blockers and (2) cardioplegia, (3) many patients managed with single- or two-vessel disease are now treated by percutaneous transluminal coronary angioplasty (PTCA), (4) the internal mammary artery was not used in any study, (5) transesophageal echocardiography is now used intraoperatively to detect ischemic regional wall motion abnormalities, and (6) antiplatelet therapy has improved the patency of vein grafts.

The VA study began its pilot phase in 1970.[8] The randomized trial involved 686 patients recruited over a 3-year period from January 1972 through December 1974. Thirteen centers participated in the study. The angiographic criteria for inclusion in the VA study were (1) at least a 50% narrowing in one or more coronary arteries, and (2) graftable distal vessels and acceptable ventricular function as measured by a number of criteria. Of the 686 patients in the study, there were 90 with left main coronary artery disease. The overall operative mortality at 30 days for all patients was 5.6%. The incidence of perioperative myocardial infarction calculated on the basis of the development of new Q-waves was 9.9%. Vein graft angiography was performed in 79% of surgical patients between 10 and 15 mo after surgery. Of 503 grafts placed, 357 (70%) were patent at 1 year and 87% of patients had at least one patent graft.

At 36 mo, there was no significant overall difference in mortality between patients treated medically or surgically. The overall survival in the medical cohort was 87% and that in the surgical cohort 88%. Although the overall mortality was equivalent in the medical and surgically treated patients, the one subgroup that benefitted from operation was patients with left main coronary artery stenosis. At 4 years, 93% of the surgically treated patients were alive while only 58% of the medically treated patients were alive. The 7-year survival rates for all patients were 70% with medical treatment and 77% with surgery. At 11 years, the rates were 57 and 58%, respectively.[9] Certain small subsets of patients in the VA trial, such as that group with three-vessel disease and impaired left ventricular function, continued to show benefit from surgical therapy at 11 years, but beyond 7 years, the survival benefit gradually diminished. The surgical cohort with normal left ventricular function, single- or double-vessel disease, and minimal initial symptoms showed, if anything, a survival disadvantage at 11 years when compared with the medical cohort.

The ECSS trial included 768 men under the age of 65 with angina pectoris of 3 mo, obstructions in at least two major coronary arteries of greater than 50%, and a left ventricular ejection fraction above 50%.[10] Survival was significantly better for the total group of patients randomized to surgery than for the total group randomized to medical therapy. Survival rate at 16 mo was 93.5% for the surgical group and 84.1% for the medical group. A significant improvement in survival was found in the surgical subgroup of patients with left main coronary disease and in patients with triple-vessel disease. No significant difference in survival was found in patients with two-vessel disease. The exception to this statement was a subgroup of patients for whom a proximal left anterior descending stenosis was one of the two vessels involved. The ECSS, therefore, reported that the symptomatic patient with stable angina benefitted from surgery if left main coronary artery disease or triple- or double-vessel disease that included a proximal left anterior descending stenosis was present.

The CASS study consists of a Registry containing data on 24,959 patients at 15 participating centers.[11] The registry is made up of consecutive patients undergoing angiography because of the suspicion of coronary artery disease. From this number, many patients were excluded from randomization for a variety of reasons such as prior coronary bypass surgery, unstable or progressive angina, angina more severe than Canadian Class II, congestive heart failure, or a coexisting illness that would increase the likelihood of death within 5 years. These exclusions left 2099 patients eligible for randomization to the CASS protocol. Of these 780 patients agreed to be assigned randomly to either medical or surgical treatment. After randomization, the 780 trial participants were stratified into three groups. In Group A, 514 patients had angina and ejection fraction greater than 50%, Group B, 106 patients had angina and an ejection fraction between 35 and 50%, and Group C, 160 patients were free of angina after myocardial infarction. Medically and surgically treated groups were similar in terms of age, sex, work status, severity of angina, history of myocardial infarction, hypertension, congestive heart failure, or use of medications. Twenty-seven percent of the patients had single-vessel disease, 40% double-vessel disease, and 33% triple-vessel disease. The remaining 1219 patients eligible for randomization declined to be randomized because they or their physicians wanted specific medical or surgical therapy or were uneasy with the decisions being made by the computer. This group of patients was also followed and is called randomizable, but not randomized patients. Of these randomizable patients, 57% chose medical therapy and 43% elected to undergo bypass surgery.

It should be emphasized that the CASS protocol was specifically directed toward patients with less severe angina (Canadian Class I or II) or those who were asymptomatic after a documented myocardial infarction. At the inception of the study, it was already clear that bypass grafting was an effective therapy for patients with symptomatic angina in Canadian Class III or IV. The primary question asked by CASS was which form of therapy, medical or surgical, was the most appropriate initial therapy for mildly symptomatic patients. Therefore, it was not a trial of medical therapy vs.

surgical therapy. It was a trial that evaluated the most appropriate initial therapy for minimally symptomatic patients. A secondary aim was to determine if coronary artery bypass grafting reduced the rate of subsequent myocardial infarction.

Randomization took place between August 1975 and May 1979. Intensive follow-up was continued through April 1983. Of 390 patients assigned to receive medical therapy, 23.5% (4.7% per year) crossed over and had bypass surgery in the first 5 years because of progression of symptoms. Patients with triple-vessel disease were heavily represented in the crossover group. In the patients randomly assigned to surgery, operative mortality defined as death occurring within 30 days of surgery was 1.4%. Perioperative myocardial infarction occurred in 6.4% of patients assigned to surgical therapy. In the patients assigned to the surgical group, there were 954 distal anastomosis constructed or an average of 2.7 per patient. Graft patency was assessed in 129 patients within 60 days of surgery. Ninety percent of the grafts were open, 97% of patients had at least one open graft, and in 81% of patients, all grafts were patent.

At 5 years, the average annual mortality in patients assigned to surgical treatment was 1.1%. The annual mortality in those receiving medical therapy was 1.6%. These differences are not statistically significant. At 5 years, 92% of medical and 95% surgical patients were alive. At the time of initial data reporting (5 years) life table analyses showed no significant differences in survival between any subgroup. The annual mortality rates in medically treated patients with single-, double-, and triple-vessel disease were 1.4, 1.2, and 2.1%, respectively. In patients assigned to medical treatment who have moderately impaired ventricular function (ejection fractions less than 50%) the annual mortality rate was 3.3%. Mortality rates in surgical patients with single-, double-, and triple-vessel disease were 0.7, 1, and 1.5%, respectively. In the surgically assigned patients with ejection fractions less than 50%, there was an annual mortality rate of 1.7%.

Although there was a trend toward increased survival in the surgical subgroup with ejection fractions between 35 and 50%, this did not reach a statistical significance until the seventh year follow-up report.[12] There were 160 patients with ejection fractions above 34%, but below 50% at baseline examination. Eighty-two patients were randomized to medical therapy and 78 to surgery. In seven years, 84% of the patients in the surgical group were alive as compared with 70% of the medical group. Nearly half of the patients with impaired ventricular function had triple-vessel disease at entry. At 7 years, observed survival in this group was 88 and 65% for those assigned to the surgical and medical treatment, respectively. Survival of patients with single-vessel or double-vessel disease was similar in the two groups. Therefore, one of the conclusions of CASS is that patients with mild angina, triple-vessel disease, and an ejection fraction higher than 34%, but lower than 50% had an improved 7-year survival with elective bypass surgery.

The question of whether coronary artery bypass surgery can prevent myocardial infarction is also often raised. In CASS, there was no difference in infarction rate between the medical and surgical cohorts.[13] The likelihood of nonfatal Q-wave myocardial infarction was 11 and 14%, respectively, in the medical and surgical cohorts. The 5-year probability for remaining alive and free of infarction was 82% in the patients assigned to medical therapy and 83% in the patients assigned to surgery. There were no statistically significant differences in the survival rate or in the myocardial infarction rate between subgroups of patients randomly assigned to medical or surgical therapy when they were analyzed according to the initial group assignment, number of diseased vessels, or ejection fraction. Surgery did decrease the incidence of fatal infarction and sudden death.

In summary, these three excellent clinical trials illustrate different aspects of the surgical approach of the patient with stable angina pectoris. It is quite clear from the VA trial that patients with a greater than 75% stenosis of the left main coronary artery have a better outlook after coronary artery bypass surgery. ECSS pointed out that severity of symptoms correlated with a more favorable prognosis if surgery was performed. In the CASS study, patients who were less symptomatic showed a benefit from surgery only if left ventricular function was compromised.

At present, the major indications for coronary artery bypass grafting are summarized in Table 125–1.

INDICATIONS FOR SURGERY

With the advent of percutaneous approaches for relieving coronary obstruction, there are numerous gray zones and controversial areas regarding who should undergo surgery vs. those who should undergo balloon angioplasty or relief by other catheter-introduced devices. Indications for percutaneous approaches are changing rapidly as experience is gained and new devices are approved by the FDA. Accordingly, the indications for surgery discussed below must be considered in light of advances in catheter techniques that are discussed in Chapter 124.

TABLE 125–1. INDICATIONS FOR CORONARY ARTERY BYPASS GRAFTING

1. Failure of medical therapy
2. Unstable angina
3. Left main CAD
4. Symptomatic three vessel CAD with depressed LV function
5. Postinfarction angina
6. Acute myocardial infarction with cardiogenic shock
7. Failed PTCA
8. Reoperation for recurrent symptoms
9. Congenital anomalies of coronary arteries (see Chapter 94)
10. Kawasaki's disease (see Chapter 94)

Failure of Medical Therapy

When a patient develops severe disabling angina or is unable to tolerate medical therapy, surgery may be beneficial for the relief of symptoms. There have been no randomized trials of medical vs. surgical therapy comparing survival or the incidence of infarction for patients with Class III–IV symptoms, but conclusions can be drawn from large nonrandomized studies. The most important of these is the CASS registry that followed over 4000 patients with Class III–IV angina treated medically or surgically. It showed that surgery improved 5-year survival for all patients with CLASS III–IV angina and three-vessel disease regardless of ventricular function, 87 vs. 65% at 5 years.[14] The benefit was greatest for patients with poor ventricular function. For patients with proximal stenosis of one or two vessels, surgery improved survival only in the presence of moderate to severe left ventricular dysfunction.[15] The CASS registry also showed that surgery lowered the relative risk of development of a subsequent infarction by one-half in patients with three-vessel disease and CLASS III–IV symptoms. This was significant for patients with impaired left ventricular function, but a trend was also noted for patients with normal left ventricular function.[16]

Unstable Angina

The features of unstable angina include angina at rest with episodes lasting longer than a few minutes, incomplete or no relief with nitrates, and an unstable electrocardiogram with no new Q-waves. Several randomized studies were conducted in the 1970s to determine the relative merits of medical and surgical management in the prevention of infarction and death in patients with unstable angina. These studies demonstrated that surgery produced superior long-term relief of symptoms, but not long-term survival.[17] It was demonstrated that urgent surgery could improve the results in patients with ischemia refractory to medical therapy, especially when there was evidence of ventricular dysfunction and left main or three vessel disease. Careful follow-up of medically treated patients was advised because these studies reported that 35% of patients crossed over to surgical therapy within $2\frac{1}{2}$ years of randomization due to recurrent symptoms.[18]

At the present time, it is recommended that patients presenting with unstable angina be stabilized medically, including a regimen of nitrates, β-blockers, calcium channel blockers, and heparin. If the patient is already on such a program and develops unstable angina, elective cardiac angiography is undertaken after the unstable angina episode has subsided, usually following treatment with intravenous nitroglycerin. If unstable angina does not abate in patients who have received an adequate antianginal regimen including intravenous nitroglycerine and intra-aortic balloon pump, then emergency coronary angiography should be performed. Patients will require balloon angioplasty or aortocoronary bypass grafting as soon as possible if their symptoms are not controllable by medical therapy. In a review of 14 major series published between 1978 and 1988 of patients undergoing bypass surgery for unstable angina, operative mortality averaged 3.7% with a perioperative infarction rate of 10%.[19] These rates are approximately two to three times higher than those seen in patients with stable angina. Excellent long-term results were noted with 80% of patients surviving 10 years and 80% free of significant angina. The annual rate of nonfatal infarction was about 3 to 4%. A VA randomized study initiated in 1982 of medical vs. surgical therapy of patients with various forms of unstable angina demonstrated improved survival with surgery for all patients with three-vessel disease with progressively increasing benefit for those with depressed left ventricular ejection fraction. No difference was demonstrated in the 5-year incidence of nonfatal myocardial infarction.[20]

Left Main Coronary Artery Disease

The significance of left main stenosis lies in the potential damage to a large area of myocardium should an occlusion occur. The overall annual mortality of medically treated patients with left main coronary artery disease is about 10 to 15%.[21] The VA, ECSS, and the CASS registry data have demonstrated that surgery improved survival from 60 to 90% at 4 years in patients with left main stenosis exceeding 50%. This benefit was realized in symptomatic and asymptomatic patients and was independent of ventricular function.[22] However, the greatest benefit was realized in patients with impaired ventricular function, stenoses greater than 75%, and the presence of high-grade right coronary artery disease.[23]

Three-Vessel Coronary Artery Disease and Depressed Left Ventricular Function

The VA and CASS randomized studies demonstrated that surgery improved survival in patients with three-vessel coronary artery disease and impaired left ventricular function.[24] CASS registry data have also shown that a positive stress test was predictive of improved surgical survival in these patients.[25] The CASS randomized study showed that the percentage of patients with three-vessel disease and abnormal LV function who were alive and free from infarction was greater in those who had undergone surgery.[26] In addition, the CASS registry showed that surgery lowered the risk of developing a subsequent fatal or nonfatal infarction in these patients.[27]

Postinfarction Angina

The prognosis following a myocardial infarction is determined by the presence of ischemia in remaining viable muscle, the extent of left ventricular dysfunction, and the development of ventricular arrhythmias. If the patient is sta-

ble, a submaximal stress test should be performed prior to hospital discharge for risk stratification. One year mortality of patients with a positive stress test was 27% compared to 2.1% if the test was normal. Therefore, early coronary angiography is indicated in patients with a positive stress test to identify those who might benefit from PTCA or bypass surgery.[28] Because of the high incidence of recurrent ischemic events following a non-Q-wave infarction, coronary angiography is usually recommended often without stress testing. Approximately 40 to 50% of patients with non-Q-wave infarction and 15% of patients with Q-wave infarction will develop early postinfarction angina either with or without ECG changes.[29] Coronary artery bypass surgery is indicated for most patients with multivessel disease and can be performed with an operative mortality of approximately 5%. Although the timing of surgery after infarction does not appear to be an independent risk factor for nonemergent surgery, the operative mortality is significantly increased when a patient requires emergent surgery within 24 hours of infarction. Generally, when a patient develops postinfarction angina, surgery should not be delayed in an attempt to decrease operative morality because reinfarction or death may occur in the interim. The perioperative infarction rate in patients with unstable postinfarction angina is between 5 and 10%. The relief of angina and long-term survival following surgery are similar to those achieved for stable and unstable angina.

Acute Myocardial Infarction With Cardiogenic Shock

The syndrome of acute myocardial infarction with cardiogenic shock carries a mortality in excess of 80%. Attempts at reperfusion for cardiogenic shock are based on the principle that survival is dependent on the salvage of areas of reversible ischemia in the peri-infarct zone or in the areas of hypercontractile muscles subtended by stenotic vessels at a distance from the infarct zone. Although coronary bypass surgery has been helpful in isolated cases, the mortality in this syndrome is still overwhelming, even in patients brought to operation. Leinbach reported the results of bypass surgery in a series of cardiogenic shock patients treated initially with an aortic balloon pump.[30] Sixty-eight patients were balloon dependent. Sixteen of them were treated medically and all of them died. Forty-two balloon-dependent patients underwent coronary arteriography. Twenty-two patients were considered inoperable and all of them died. Of the 30 patients considered to be operable, six did not have an operation and they all died. Twenty-four patients underwent coronary artery bypass grafting associated with infarctectomy and repair of mechanical defects when indicated. There were nine survivors (37%). This experience suggests that in the occasional patient with balloon-dependent cardiogenic shock, bypass surgery may be lifesaving. If a mechanical defect such as an acquired ventricular septal defect, mitral regurgitation, or a left ventricular aneurysm is also present, repair of the mechanical defect plus bypass surgery may carry an even greater likelihood of patient survival. It would seem reasonable to treat a patient with cardiogenic shock with optimal fluids using Swan–Ganz monitoring. A certain number of such patients, particularly those with right ventricular infarction, respond to optimal fluid management and reverse their shock state. In those with clear-cut left ventricular failure, an intra-aortic balloon pump will usually temporarily reverse many of the hemodynamic abnormalities. The decision must then be made whether to study the patient angiographically to determine the coronary anatomy and diagnose any mechanical problems that may contribute to the shock state. Since the mortality in balloon-dependent patients approaches 100%, operation may be offered to appropriate patients. Recently, successful reperfusion with thrombolytic therapy or PTCA of the culprit vessel within 4 hours of occlusion has resulted in survival of up to 70% of patients with cardiogenic shock, in contrast to a 20% survival when reperfusion cannot be accomplished successfully.[31] In addition, Buckberg and associates have achieved a 70% survival rate (as late as 12 to 18 hours after infarction) with an operative strategy that includes active resuscitation of the ischemic zone using warm induction and terminal warm blood cardioplegia enriched with substrates to aid in the salvage of reversibly damaged myocardium.[32]

Failed PTCA

Since its initial use in the late 1970s, the success for PTCA has improved with advances in angioplasty catheters and refinement of selection criteria. Currently about 90% of lesions can be dilated successfully with a mortality rate of <1%. Myocardial infarction is noted in about 3% of patients and commonly results from dissection within the vessel wall complicated by vessel occlusion from thrombus formation.[33] When PTCA fails and results in vessel closure, the patient usually develops angina, ischemic ECG changes, or hemodynamic instability resulting in cardiogenic shock or cardiac arrest. The current incidence of emergency surgery for failed PTCA is 3 to 4% and carries a 30 to 40% incidence of Q-wave infarction and an overall mortality of 5 to 6%.[34] Improved techniques of myocardial protection during the operative procedure in combination with complete revascularization have improved the surgical results in this challenging group of patients.

Reoperations for Recurrent Symptoms

Coronary artery bypass surgery should be considered a palliative operation because of the progressive nature of the atherosclerotic process. Although the use of postoperative aspirin minimizes the risk of early graft closure and may decrease the extent of intimal hyperplasia, progressive atherosclerosis leads to stenosis or occlusion of 50% of vein grafts by 10 years.[35] Coronary bypass grafting accelerates

the progression of proximal bypass disease, such that occlusion of native vessels is a very common finding of late postoperative coronary arteriograms. Even if grafts remain patent, recurrent ischemia may result from progressive disease in previously nonbypassed vessels and from distal disease beyond patent grafts. Factors associated with decreased reoperation survival include failure to use the internal mammary artery, younger age, incomplete revascularization, and continued smoking.[36] Coronary reoperation should be restricted to patients with refractory angina symptoms because the operative mortality and long-term results are not as good as those with primary revascularization. Mortality rate for reoperation is generally two to three times higher due primarily to technical factors and less satisfactory revascularization. Long-term survival following reoperation is slightly inferior to that following primary revascularization with 80% 5-year and 65% 10-year survival rates in contrast to 90 and 75%, respectively, for primary operations.[37]

Due to advances in surgical techniques, myocardial preservation, and postoperative care, many patients, including the elderly, are undergoing coronary artery bypass grafting with good results. Quoted mortality rates at many major medical centers across the country include 1% for stable angina, 3% for unstable angina, 5% for postinfarction angina or failed PTCA, and 30% for cardiogenic shock. The Cleveland Clinic has developed a clinical severity scoring system (Table 125–2) based on preoperative factors to assess an individual patient's operative mortality.[38] Scoring systems such as this can help individual hospitals and practicing surgeons predict postoperative mortality. Bypass surgery has clearly improved the quality of life of many pa-

TABLE 125–2. THE CLEVELAND CLINIC—CLINICAL SEVERITY SCORING SYSTEM[a]

Preoperative Factors	Score
Emergency case	6
Serum creatinine (mg/dL)	
≥ 1.6 and ≤ 1.8	1
≥ 1.9	4
Severe LVD	3
Reoperation	3
Operative mitral valve insufficiency	3
Age ≥ 65 and ≤ 74 years	1
Age ≥ 75 years	2
Prior vascular surgery	2
Chronic obstructive pulmonary disease	2
Anemia (hematocrit ≤ 34%)	2
Operative aortic valve stenosis	1
Weight (<65 kg)	1
Diabetes (oral or insulin therapy)	1
Cerebrovascular disease	1

[a]A total score above 6 is associated with a mortality of 10%. Scores above 10 have a mortality near 30%.
Reproduced from Higgins TL et al: JAMA 267:2346, 1992, copyright 1992, American Medical Association, with permission.

tients with coronary artery disease. As the indications for coronary artery bypass grafting become more refined, we would expect continued improvement in terms of operative results, and with the use of the internal mammary artery as the conduit of choice fewer reoperations will be needed in the future. The role of PTCA will require close scrutiny as was done with bypass surgery in the past. Coronary artery bypass grafting remains a valid operation for the treatment of coronary artery disease.

REFERENCES

1. Lytle BW, Cosgrove DM: Coronary artery bypass surgery. *Curr Probl Surg* **29:**743, 1992
2. Campean L: Grading of angina pectoris. *Circulation* **54:**522, 1976
3. Kirklin JW, Akins CW, Blackstone EH, et al: Guidelines and indications for coronary artery bypass graft surgery. *J Am Coll Cardiol* **17:**543, 1991
4. Braunwald E: Unstable angina. *Circulation* **80:**410, 1989
5. Ross J, Brandenburg RO, Dinsmore RE, et al: Guidelines for coronary angiography. A report of the ACC/AHA Task Force of Assessment of Diagnostic and Therapeutic Cardiovascular Procedures. *J Am Coll Cardiol* **10:**935, 1987
6. Trip MD, Cats VM, Vrecken J: Platelet hyperreactivity and prognosis in survivors of myocardial infarction. *N Engl J Med* **322:**1549, 1990
7. Kaiser GC: CABG-Lessons for randomized trials. *Ann Thorac Surg* **42:**3, 1986
8. Murphy ML, Hultgren HN, Detre K, et al: Treatment of chronic stable angina: A preliminary report of survival data of the randomized Veterans Administration Cooperative Study. *N Engl J Med* **297:**621, 1977
9. The Veterans Administration Coronary Artery Bypass Surgery Cooperative Study Group, 1984: Eleven year survival in the Veterans Administration Randomized Trial of Coronary Bypass Surgery for stable angina. *N Engl J Med* **311:**133–139, 1984
10. European Coronary Surgery Study Group: Long-term results of prospective randomized study of coronary artery bypass surgery in stable angina pectoris. *Lancet* **2:**1173–1180, 1982
11. CASS Principal Investigators and their Associates: Coronary artery surgery study (CASS): A randomized trial of coronary artery bypass surgery. Survival data. *Circulation* **68:**939–950, 1983
12. Passamani E, Davis KB, Gillespie MJ, et al: A randomized trial of coronary artery bypass surgery. Survival of patients with a low ejection fraction. *N Engl J Med* **312:**1665–1671, 1985
13. CASS Principal Investigators and their Associates: Myocardial infarction and mortality in the coronary artery surgery study (CASS) randomized trial. *N Engl J Med* **310:**750–758, 1984
14. Myers WO, Schaff HV, Gersh BJ, et al: Improved survival of surgically treated patients with triple vessel coronary artery disease and severe angina pectoris. A report from the Coronary Artery Surgery Study (CASS) registry. *J Thorac Cardiovasc Surg* **97:**487, 1989
15. Mock MB, Fisher LD, Holmes DR Jr, et al: Comparison of effects of medical and surgical therapy on survival in severe angina pectoris and two-vessel coronary artery disease with and without left ventricular dysfunction: A Coronary Artery Surgery Study registry study. *Am J Cardiol* **61:**1198, 1988
16. Myers WO, Schaff HV, Fisher LD, et al: Time to first new myocardial infarction in patients with severe angina and three-vessel disease comparing medical and early surgical therapy: A CASS registry study of survival. *J Thorac Cardiovasc Surg* **95:**382, 1988
17. Unstable angina pectoris: National Cooperative study group to compare surgical and medical therapy. II. In-hospital experience and initial follow-up results in patients with one, two and three vessel disease. *Am J Cardiol* **42:**839–848, 1978
18. Goldman BS, Weisel RD: Surgical reperfusion of acute myocardial ischemia: A clinical review. *J Cardiac Surg* **1:**167, 1986
19. Kaiser GC, Schaff HV, Killip T: Myocardial revascularization for unstable angina pectoris. *Circulation* **79**(Suppl I):60, 1989
20. Parisi AF, Khuri S, Deupree RH, et al: Medical compared with surgical management of unstable angina. 5-year mortality and morbidity in the Veterans Administration study. *Circulation* **80:**1176, 1989
21. Chaitman BP, Fisher LD, Bourassa MG, et al: Effect of coronary bypass surgery on survival patterns in subsets of patients with left main coronary artery disease. Report of the Collaborative Study in Coronary Artery Surgery (CASS). *Am J Cardiol* **48:**765, 1981
22. Taylor HA, Deumite NJ, Chaitman BR, et al: Asymptomatic left main coronary artery disease in the Coronary Artery Surgery Study (CASS) registry. *Circulation* **79:**1171, 1989
23. Takaro T, Pifarre R, Fish R: Left main coronary artery disease. *Prog Cardiovasc Dis* **28:**229, 1985
24. Gersh BJ, Califf RM, Loop FD, et al: Coronary bypass surgery in chronic stable angina. *Circulation* **79**(Suppl I):46, 1989
25. Weiner DA, Ryan TJ, McCabe CH, et al: The role of exercise testing in identifying patients with improved survival after coronary artery bypass surgery. *J Am Coll Cardiol* **8:**741, 1986
26. Alderman EL, Bourassa MG, Cohen LS, et al: Ten year follow-up of survival and myocardial infarction in the randomized Coronary Artery Surgery. *Circulation* **8:**1629, 1990
27. Myers WO, Gersh BJ, Fisher LD, et al: Time to first new myocardial infarction in patients with mild angina and three-vessel disease comparing medicine and early surgery: A CASS registry study of survival. *Ann Thorac Surg* **43:**599, 1987
28. Gibson RS: Management of acute non-Q-wave myocardial infarction: Role of prophylactic pharmacotherapy and indications for predischarge coronary arteriography. *Clin Cardiol* **12:**26, 1989
29. Gibson RS, Young PM, Boden WE, et al: Prognostic significance and beneficial effect of diltiazem on the incidence of early recurrent ischemia after non-Q-wave myocardial infarction: Results from the multicenter diltiazem reinfarction study. *Am J Cardiol* **60:**203, 1987
30. Leinbach RC, Gold HK, Dinsmore RE, et al: The role of angiography in cardiogenic shock. *Circulation* **48**(Suppl 3):95–98, 1973
31. Lee L, Erbel R, Brown TM, et al: Multicenter registry of angioplasty therapy of cardiogenic shock: Initial and long-term survival. *J Am Coll Cardiol* **17:**599, 1991
32. Laks H, Rosenkranz E, Buckberg GD: Surgical treatment of cardiogenic shock after myocardial infarction. *Circulation* **74**(Suppl III):11, 1986
33. King SB III, Talley JD: Coronary arteriography and percutaneous transluminal coronary angioplasty. Changing patterns of use and results. *Circulation* **79**(Suppl I):19, 1989
34. Talley JD, Jones EL, Weintraub WS, King SB III: Coronary artery bypass surgery after failed elective percutaneous transluminal coronary angioplasty. A status report. *Circulation* **79**(Suppl I):126, 1989
35. Bourassa MG, Enjalbert M, Campeau L, Lesperance J: Progression of atherosclerosis in coronary arteries and bypass grafts: Ten years later. *Am J Cardiol* **53:**102, 1984
36. Cosgrove DM, Loop FD, Lytle BW, et al: Predictors of reoperation after myocardial revascularization. *J Thorac Cardiovasc Surg* **92:**811, 1986
37. Salomon NW, Page US, Bigelow JC, et al: Reoperative coronary surgery. Comparative analysis of 6591 patients undergoing primary bypass and 508 patients undergoing reoperative coronary artery bypass. *J Thorac Cardiovasc Surg* **100:**250, 1990
38. Higgins TL, Estafanous FG, Loop FD, et al: Stratification of morbidity and mortality outcome by pre-operative risk factors in coronary artery bypass patients. *JAMA* **267:**2344, 1992

Coronary Artery Operations and Reoperations

Techniques and Conduits

Brian L. Cmolik and Alexander S. Geha

Techniques of coronary artery bypass surgery have evolved over the past 35 years in response to the changing technical problems presented to the surgeon, as well as the changing patient base. Constant refinements of technique are required in order to minimize morbidity and mortality risks for the patient.

An excellent working knowledge of coronary anatomy and its variations, and the relationship of this anatomy to the angiographic findings for a particular patient are crucial to the successful performance of any coronary revascularization. Various cardioplegic techniques have allowed at least 2 hours of safe myocardial protection. The addition of microsurgical instrumentation, headlight illumination, loupe magnification, and complete myocardial revascularization has contributed to decreased risk during coronary artery bypass, even in patients with acute, unstable angina or left main coronary artery stenosis. However, more recently there has been a rise in the overall mortality of coronary artery bypass grafting, and this may well continue. (Table 126–1)

CORONARY ARTERY REVASCULARIZATION: PRIMARY OPERATION

Because of the attention paid by many surgeons to the preparation of vein grafts, cannulation is often delegated to less experienced members of the operating team. Proper cannulation techniques will influence the quality of a smooth "pump run" and ultimate outcome. After median sternotomy and division of the mediastinal fat in the midline, a pericardial well is created. Inspection of appropriate available targets is accomplished, and an assessment of the quality of the ascending aorta for cannulation is made. The internal mammary artery is then taken down, if it is intended to be used as a bypass conduit. Heparin in adequate doses is then delivered to the central circulation. The adequacy of heparinization is monitored by measurement of the activated clotting time.

Prior to cannulation, digital palpation of the ascending aorta is mandatory to determine whether this vessel is affected by atherosclerotic disease and calcified plaques. Transesophageal echocardiography may be used as a tool to guide the site for cannulation. Areas of periaortic fat and adventitial inflammation or adhesions are suggestive of friable, intimal disease. These areas should be avoided in the cannulation process, and also in the placement of the proximal anastomoses. When the site for cannulation is selected, two concentric 2-0 polypropylene sutures are placed, the inner suture tagged with a small curved hemostat and the outer suture tagged with a straight hemostat. A small aortotomy is made and a high-flow aortic cannula is inserted, with the bevelled position downward. The cannula is placed in such a fashion as to direct the flow away from the head vessels selectively, so that any debris that is showered during cannulation will be directed beyond the arch vessels and into the descending thoracic aorta. The right atrial appendage is then encircled, snared, and opened, and the trabeculations are divided. A two-staged venous cannula is placed and then secured. Positioning of the venous cannula

TABLE 126–1. REASONS FOR RECENT HIGHER MORTALITY FOR CORONARY ARTERY BYPASS GRAFT

1. Poor left ventricular function
2. Increased number of reoperations
3. Older patient population
4. More women in coronary artery bypass grafting population
5. Complexities of new drug interactions with use with cardiopulmonary bypass
6. Poor nutritional status
7. Patients referred later due to early management of PTCA

should be confirmed by palpation with the tip of the cannula in the inferior vena cava and not obstructing the hepatic veins. A small catheter is then placed in the ascending aorta for the delivery of cardioplegia and for aortic root venting. A pursestring suture is then placed in the distal third of the right atrium for the placement of a retrograde cannula, which is positioned in the coronary sinus after the patient is placed on bypass. Cardiopulmonary bypass is begun at the request of the operating surgeon. Both the surgeon and the perfusionist must ensure there are no remaining clamps on any of the inflow or outflow lines prior to the initiation of cardiopulmonary bypass.

Various choices for venting the heart are available to the surgeon. The use of a bifurcated needle in the ascending aorta provides for delivery of antegrade cardioplegia and subsequently for venting of left ventricle via the ascending aorta. This technique provides for adequate ventricular decompression and also for adequate coronary visualization when doses of cold retrograde cardioplegia are used for myocardial protection. The use of a left superior pulmonary vein vent to decompress the left ventricle is reserved for cases of redo coronary bypass surgery, in instances where aortic insufficiency is encountered, and in patients with extremely poor left ventricular function. Pulmonary artery venting is also an option that can provide right ventricular decompression, as well as adequate coronary visualization.

EXPOSURE OF DISTAL CORONARY ARTERIES

Exposure of the distal coronary artery targets that are to be grafted may be difficult. This is especially true in instances of left ventricular hypertrophy, large transverse globular hearts, arteries within the myocardium, bypasses to certain areas of the circumflex system, and reoperations. Exposure of the left anterior descending and diagonal branches on the anterior surface may be facilitated by the use of either epicardial traction sutures of 2-0 silk, or a special spring-supported epicardial retractor used after a laparotomy pad has been placed under the heart. When using a self-retaining, spring-loaded retractor, one must avoid spreading the epicardium too much, as this distorts the arteriotomy. When the coronary arteries are located intramyocardially or even in an intracavitary position, the vessel can be identified by

tracing a branch back to the parent vessel. Other techniques, such as opening of a distal branch with retrograde advancement of a small probe and the use of a sterile Doppler ultrasound device, have been reported.[1,2] To expose the ramus intermedius and circumflex branches, the heart can be rotated toward the right, thereby allowing excellent exposure. The table can also be tilted slightly to the right for added visualization. Various sling type nets have been reported to aid exposure. Opening of the right hemithorax with rotation of the heart into the right pleural cavity has also been reported. Exposure of the main circumflex or distal right coronary artery is difficult, especially when the arteries are covered by the great cardiac vein or coronary sinus. Traction sutures in the epicardium and division of small venous branches facilitate such exposure, as can a rubberized traction loop placed around the coronary artery. Bypass to the main circumflex or circumflex marginal artery as an isolated graft may be performed by way of a left thoracotomy, and the proximal anastomosis can be made to the left subclavian artery or descending thoracic aorta.[3] Exposure of the distal right coronary artery may be facilitated with traction sutures. Cephalad traction on the acute margin, or apex of the heart exposes the posterior descending coronary artery. Previous pericarditis or adhesions from prior operation may make it extremely difficult to locate coronary arteries after the heart is exposed. This is especially true when the arteries are buried in fat or covered by myocardial bridges. Because of this, it is absolutely imperative that one be familiar with the preoperative angiograms. This includes identification and location of the veins on the late filling phase of the angiogram (Fig. 126–1). These veins are almost invariably located on the surface of the heart and can be helpful in identifying the proper coronary artery to be bypassed.[4]

CONSIDERATIONS FOR VASCULAR ANASTOMOSIS

The optimal environment for the construction of a vascular anastomosis is a motionless, dry field. This can be attained by total cardiopulmonary bypass and cardioplegia techniques to arrest the heart. Although it is possible to graft certain vessels without cardiopulmonary bypass, the indications for such an approach are rare.[5,6] A patient with marginal pulmonary function in whom even minimal lung water from cardiopulmonary bypass would be detrimental and in whom the coronary artery, such as a left anterior descending or proximal right coronary artery, could be easily exposed, may benefit from not using extracorporeal circulation. An additional indication may be a patient with marginal renal function who is not presently on dialysis.

Venting of the left ventricle is not universally used during coronary artery bypass surgery.[6,7] Gentle massage of the heart while the pump is temporarily shut off with ventilation of the lungs empties the cardiac chambers just

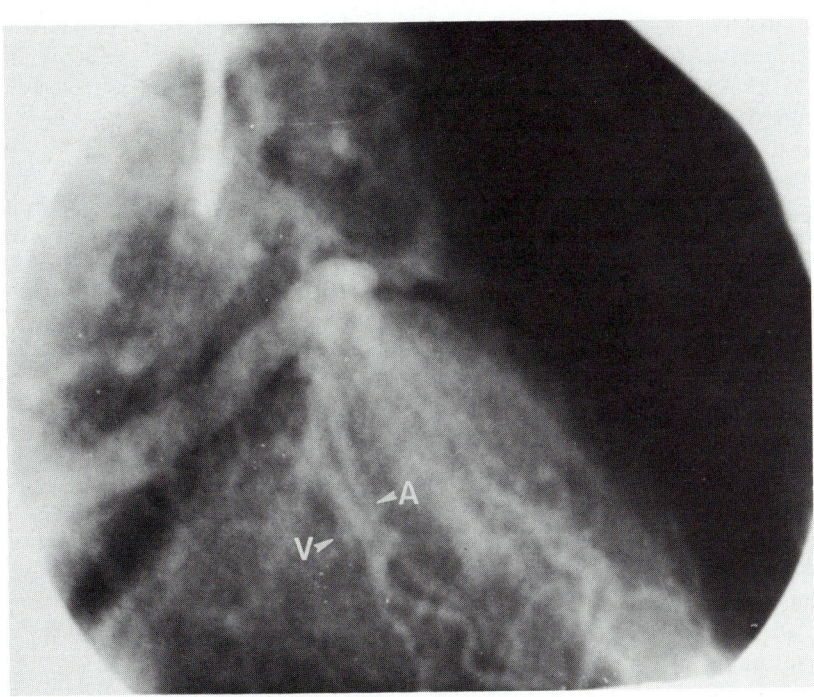

Figure 126–1. Follow-up on cineangiogram to the venous phase enables one to identify coronary veins and their anatomic relation to coronary arteries. During operation, even with severe adhesions, coronary veins can be readily identified and serve as landmarks when one is locating the artery to be bypassed.

before the aorta is crossclamped. A small negative fluid gradient in relation to the patient is maintained while the patient is on cardiopulmonary bypass. This avoids left ventricular distention but allows a more even distribution of cardioplegic solution and avoids air in the cardiac chambers.

Handling of the Ascending Aorta

As previously mentioned, the ascending aorta should be routinely palpated to determine the location of areas of atherosclerosis that would be unsuitable for cannulation, application of clamps, or the placement of grafts.[8–12] Moreover, areas in which the adventitia is inflamed or densely adherent to the aortic media should be avoided, as this indicates the presence of intimal atherosclerotic disease. Increasing experience with ascending aortic disease has allowed modification of surgical techniques to circumvent this potentially disastrous situation. Alternatives include interposition of a segment of Dacron graft for placement of the saphenous bypass, selection of a suitable site on the subclavian, innominate, or carotid arteries for proximal anastomosis, or avoidance of the ascending aorta completely. In this circumstance cannulation of the inferior aspect of the distal transverse arch is effected with pledgeted polypropylene sutures and positioning of the cannula into the descending aorta to avoid embolization into the arch vessels. If this is not possible, the femoral or right axillary artery may be cannulated; however, these can be associated with embolic strokes as well. One or both internal mammary arteries and even a right gastroepiploic artery graft can be used to avoid manipulation of the aorta. In the presence of significant aor-

tic disease, myocardial protection can be achieved with cold fibrillatory arrest. If additional vein grafts are necessary, the proximal anastomoses can be placed onto the pedicled internal mammary artery.[13]

Distal Anastomoses

One may use any of a number of techniques to obtain a dry operative field while performing a distal anastomosis. Aspiration of the ascending aorta has been reported.[14] However, this can introduce air into the aortic root either from around the needle or in a retrograde fashion from the open coronary artery. Soft bulldog clamps may be applied to the proximal coronary artery with a generous amount of tissue being included in the clamp to avoid damage to the coronary artery. Occluders in the shape of a T, or Parsonnet probes may be introduced into the opened artery. The use of small tubes as plastic shunts has been reported when techniques that do not use cross-clamping and cardioplegia are preferred. An incomplete wire-ring hand-held with pressure around the coronary artery has been used with success. Slow, continued irrigation of the vein graft with clear solution is helpful when minimal amounts of back-bleeding are encountered.

Before beginning the distal anastomosis, the sequence and location of grafting should be planned out. Once cardiopulmonary bypass is instituted, the vessels to be grafted are dissected out and the appropriate spot is chosen for the anastomosis. Matching the diameter of the vein to the diameter of the coronary artery is important to effect a perfect anastomosis. Large veins anastomosed to small coronary arteries produce turbulent flow, with the risk of graft closure or buildup of graft disease. The sequence of grafting is also important. As more grafts are applied, further manipulation of the heart increases the risk of tearing a previous anastomosis. Generally, the vein graft anastomoses are performed first, followed by internal mammary grafts. If the right gastroepiploic artery is to be used as a graft, this is done last.

The surgeon begins a distal anastomosis by performing an arteriotomy with an appropriate knife, taking care to open the middle of the coronary artery. The arteriotomy is then increased to a minimum of $1\frac{1}{2}$ times the diameter of the graft with Dietrich scissors. Reverse angle scissors are useful for opening circumflex marginal branches. The internal diameter of the coronary artery is calibrated and the size recorded. The graft should be cut at an angle of 45° or less to achieve a desired angle of takeoff of the anastomosis, and a matching length for the coronary artery (Fig. 126–2). A continuous suture of 7-0 polypropylene is begun on the side of the graft opposite the surgeon and continued to construct the heel of the anastomosis before parachuting the graft onto the coronary artery. Any larger suture is more rigid and has less tendency to align properly. Bites of approximately 1 mm are taken. This is continued around the toe, with use of even smaller bites to avoid constriction of the distal end of the anastomosis. The same needle is used to construct the complete anastomosis on the contralateral side, and the anastomosis is terminated at the midpoint of the arteriotomy (Fig. 126–3). A flush of clear, balanced electrolyte solution through the needle during the performance of the distal anastomosis may help to keep the anastomotic area free of blood. Anastomotic patency is checked

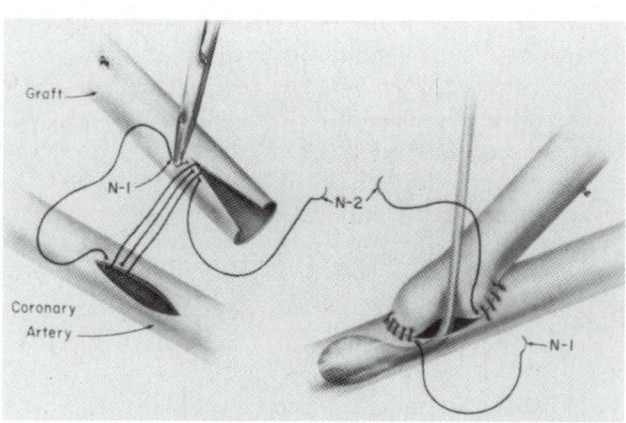

Figure 126–3. End-to-side anastomosis constructed with one continuous suture of polypropylene, using the same needle (N-1) to go around the entire anastomosis while the two vessels are held apart; the suture is tightened and the anastomosis is probed just before its completion. *(From Geha AS, Kron RJ, McCormick JR, Baue AE: Selection of coronary bypass: anastomosis, physiologic and angiographic considerations of vein and mammary grafts. J Thorac Cardiovasc Surg 70:414–433, 1975, with permission of the publisher.)*

in both directions prior to lightly tying final stitches to avoid pursestringing. Cardioplegia solution with a high concentration of potassium should be flushed from the vein graft and not allowed to "stagnate" in the graft during the performance of other anastomoses (Fig. 126–4).

An interrupted suture technique is preferred by some groups. The sutures are laid in place circumferentially

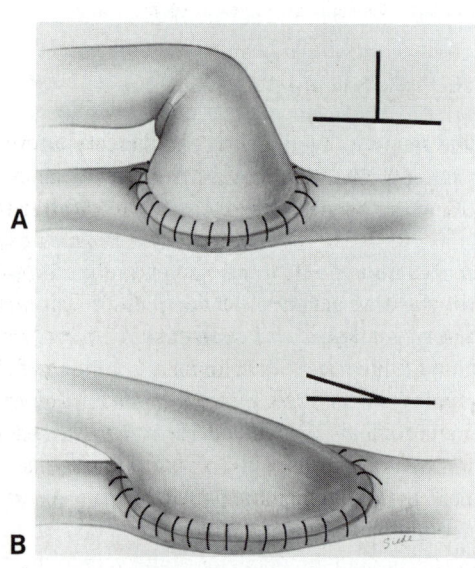

Figure 126–2. A. A minimal-angle cut on the transected graft results in kinking after takeoff from the saphenous coronary anastomosis. **B.** A more acute angle results in smooth takeoff of the vein graft and less disturbance of laminar flow.

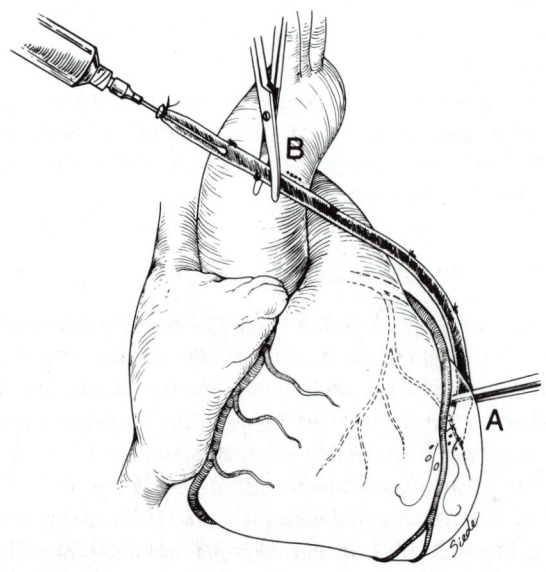

Figure 126–4. A. Flush of the vein graft during anastomosis and as the final sutures are tied provides a clear field, clears potential debris, and eliminates prolonged contact of high-potassium cardioplegia solution with the vein intimal wall. **B.** Gentle dilation of the saphenous graft before proximal anastomosis allows graft length to be measured precisely without tension or twist.

around the whole of the anastomosis, and the graft is brought down after all sutures are in place. This can be accomplished rapidly by a two-team surgical effort in which one surgeon puts one end of the double-ended suture in the vein graft while the other puts the opposite end of the suture in the coronary artery.[15] A monofilament suture with little or no tissue drag is essential in both techniques. A good endothelium-to-endothelium approximation is the objective of every anastomosis, and care should be taken to avoid any inclusion of adventitia or debris in the suture line. Alternatively, continuous anastomoses to very small coronary arteries may be augmented by interrupted sutures at the toe end of the anastomosis to avoid constriction.

In rare instances, it may be helpful to construct the toe of the distal coronary-saphenous anastomosis before constructing the heel. This technique is useful when bypassing the right coronary artery at the takeoff of the posterior descending artery. A Parsonnet probe may be placed in the distal coronary artery to serve as a guide. Before the last sutures are tied, the probe is removed, and distal patency is thereby ensured.

Suturing calcified coronary arteries is sometimes necessary and may be technically challenging. It can be achieved by piercing the calcified area with a cutting-edge needle against a buttress of peanut sponge. The needle is then removed, and suturing is continued with polypropylene (Fig. 126–5).

Occasionally, there will be an anastomosis in which side branches are present or a "bad" area of the coronary artery is found after the arteriotomy is made. Extending the arteriotomy in such a fashion to locate this "bad" area or side branch in the middle of the anastomosis avoids luminal compromise.

After the completion of the distal coronary anastomosis, the conduit should be flushed with a solution with a pH of 7.4. The anastomosis should be flushed prior to tieing to remove any remaining air in the conduit. After flushing, the distal anastomosis is tied, the graft is measured, and then cut to the appropriate length.

Sequential Anastomoses

Sequential side-to-side anastomoses connecting longitudinal incisions in the grafts to the coronary arteries as a graft crosses over stenotic vessels are popular because of decreased operating time and the possibility of increased patency resulting from increased total distal outflow.[16–19] When the arteries are lined up perpendicular to the graft, longitudinal incisions are made in each vessel. The midpoint of the vein graft is sutured to the apex of the arteriotomy, a "diamond anastomosis" thus being formed, which holds the anastomosis open. A continuous or interrupted technique may be used. The coronary arteriotomy should be at least the internal diameter of the coronary artery itself and never more than one-third of the diameter of the saphenous vein graft to avoid a depression in the vein graft.

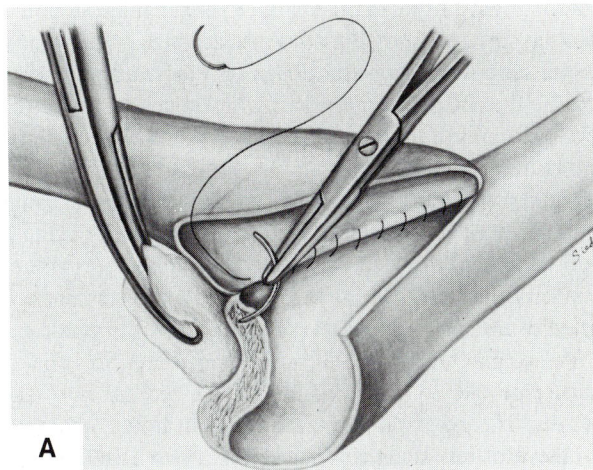

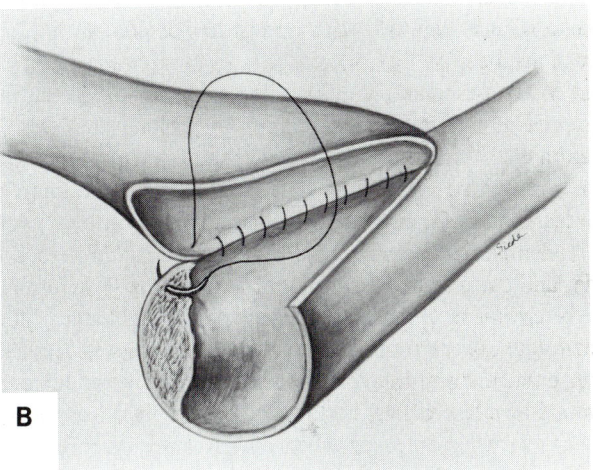

Figure 126–5. A. Calcified coronary wall may be pierced with a cutting-tip needle against a "peanut sponge." **B.** Suturing is continued with a BV-1 needle on Prolene suture.

Internal Mammary Artery Anastomosis

The anastomosis between the internal mammary artery and coronary artery is constructed in essentially the same way as for saphenous grafts. The excess mammary artery is trimmed off before the distal end of the anastomosis is reached. In this case, 7-0 or 8-0 polypropylene may be used, and the adjacent pedicle is tacked to the epicardium to avoid torsion or damage to the anastomosis by inadvertent traction on the graft after the anastomosis is completed. The internal mammary artery anastomosis is performed as the final distal anastomosis to avoid subsequent manipulation of the heart and traction on the graft. This reduces the chance of damage to the mammary vessel.

Proximal Anastomosis

The circumference of the proximal vein graft is enlarged with a Pott's scissors so that it is 20% longer than that of the circular opening of the aortotomy. 5-0 polypropylene suture is used for the construction of proximal anastomosis when the saphenous vein graft is of usual size (4 to 5 mm). The anastomosis is constructed along the same principles used for the distal anastomosis. A "lozenge" technique is used employing a total of 8 bites to construct a geometrically uniform circular anastomosis. To obtain adequate visualization, the vein graft can be suspended either by using the suture to hold the graft onto the pericardium, or using a hemostat to hold the graft onto a towel or laparotomy pad at the side of the field. During the construction of the anastomosis the mouth of the vessel is held apart by the gentle insertion of fine forceps into the vein. The vein graft is parachuted into place after completion of the heel of the anastomosis, and the suture is continued around the vein until the anastomosis is completed. An atraumatic clamp is placed distally on the vein graft and the partial occlusion clamp is removed allowing the vein to fill antegradely. The anastomosis is then tied. The vein is then deaired with a 27-gauge needle.

When saphenous grafts are inserted near the left atrial appendage and atrioventricular groove along the obtuse margin of the heart, they have a tendency to kink if brought anteriorly to the aorta. This is especially true when there is a large, anteriorly located, bulbous pulmonary artery. Even with reoperation, such grafts can be brought through the transverse sinus and the proximal anastomosis performed on the right side of the ascending aorta. The right side of the aorta offers more room for proximal anastomoses. This is helpful when multiple grafts must be anastomosed to a small, short ascending aorta. Grafts brought through the transverse sinus are used when bypasses are performed to the ramus intermedius, laterally located diagonal branches from the left anterior descending coronary artery, and proximal marginal branches from the circumflex coronary artery. Grafts to the inferior ventricular branches of the distal right coronary artery system may be brought under the inferior vena cava, again for a more comfortable lie and to prevent kinking (Fig. 126–6).

CONDUITS FOR BYPASS GRAFTING

Saphenous Vein Grafts

The greater saphenous vein remains the most commonly used conduit for coronary bypass surgery. Harvest and preparation of the saphenous vein are important parts of coronary bypass surgery.[20–22] Atraumatic technique while dissecting the saphenous vein cannot be overemphasized. Scanning and electron microscopy have shown that saphenous veins may have intimal disruption immediately after removal, before any attempts at dilatation. If one chooses to use multiple skin incisions, care should be taken to avoid excess traction on the saphenous vein grafts while bringing the graft through the skin tunnels. The single incision technique may avoid the use of excess traction on the saphenous

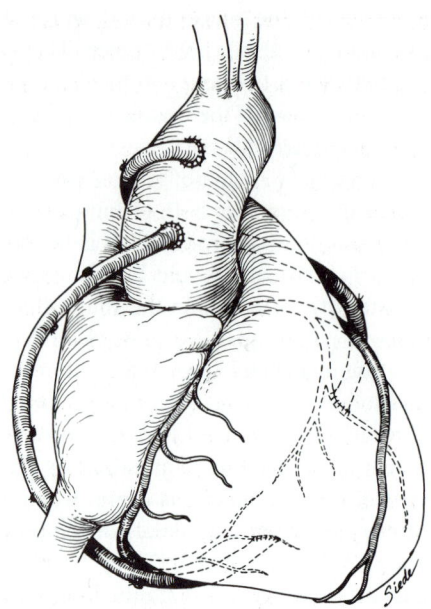

Figure 126–6. Grafts to the ramus marginalis, proximal diagonal, and proximal marginal branches may kink if brought through over a bulbous pulmonary artery. However, when brought through the transverse sinus, a comfortable lie is achieved. Grafts to distal right coronary branches also take a straight, kinkfree pathway when placed posterior to the inferior vena cava.

vein during harvesting and preparation (Fig. 126–7). Manipulation or direct grasping of the vein should be avoided while dissecting the vein sharply from its bed. The vein may be manipulated by gently grasping the adventitial portion of the vein and moving it from side to side. Side branches should be divided well away from the body of the vein using ties or clips. During the dissection, if one is unsure of the presence of side branches from the vein, tissue

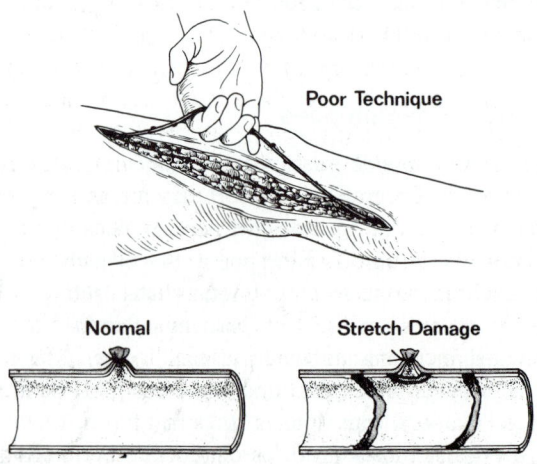

Figure 126–7. A carefully performed technique to avoid stretch damage during harvest of the saphenous vein is imperative. A "no-touch" technique, in which only the adventitia of the graft is held, is preferable.

should be divided well away from the vein to allow the side branches to be tied or clipped later. In the lower portion of the leg, the saphenous nerve runs in close continuity proximity to the vein. Care should be taken to preserve the saphenous nerve to avoid numbness and hyperesthesia in the lower extremities postoperatively. Once the vein is completely freed from the areolar tissues, it is divided both proximally and distally and prepared using 4-0 silk ties or stainless-steel clips. During preparation, a balanced electrolyte solution (pH 7.4) is used to flush any clot or platelet deposits from the vein. Some advocate the use of heparinized blood during preparation.[23] Areas of the vein that have extravasation from avulsed branches, bulbousness, or varicosities should be discarded, if this is possible. A small amount of pressure is used to sequentially inject the vein and make sure that it is free of any spasm. Care should be taken to avoid undue dilatation, which would result in intimal disruption. Using a sterile marking pen, one side of the vein should be marked along its entire length to avoid twisting during the construction of the anastomoses and allow proper orientation of the grafts.

In patients with visible varicosities of the lower extremities, previous vein stripping or harvesting, noninvasive vein mapping may be very useful to evaluate the presence of usable veins in either the greater or lesser saphenous systems. When leg veins are unobtainable, arm veins may be a rare source of conduit, but they have a significantly decreased patency and tend to become dilated with time.[24] Due to the availability of other arterial conduits, such as the internal mammary artery, the right gastroepiploic artery, the inferior epigastric artery, the need for arm veins and cryopreserved banked veins has decreased.

In most series, the 1-year patency rate for aortocoronary veins grafts is between 80 and 90%.[24–26] Modifications in technique and increased operative experience have been shown to have a role in early graft patency.[27–30] Important factors in determining long-term patency include preservation of the vein endothelium during procurement, techniques used in vein preparation, relationship of the coronary vein to coronary artery diameter, and recipient arterial run-off in the coronary artery grafted. Vein grafts to the anterior descending coronary artery show consistently higher patency than those to the right or circumflex coronary systems. The use of sequential vein grafting techniques may theoretically improve patency rates by providing better distal run-off. Early patency of sequential vein grafts has been shown to be as good as that of grafts with a single distal anastomosis.[31–33] Concerns regarding sequential vein grafts are that they are technically more difficult to construct and measure, and that proximal graft occlusion might jeopardize a large myocardial territory.

Long-term follow-up of patients who have undergone coronary bypass grafting has shown that the limitation of saphenous vein grafts is late degeneration. Although diffuse intimal thickening is found in most grafts, late occlusion of saphenous vein grafts is related to the development of graft atherosclerosis.[34] The etiology of vein graft atherosclerosis may be related to intimal injury at the time of preparation or exposure to systemic arterial pressure. It differs from arterial atheromatous disease in that it has no fibrous cap over the atheromatous process, tends to be concentric rather than eccentric, and shows a variable but often dense subintimal inflammatory reaction. Vein graft atherosclerosis may progress faster than native vessel atherosclerosis.[35]

Long-term patency of saphenous vein grafts has been investigated by angiography after bypass surgery. In one study, vein graft atherosclerosis was found in 17% of grafts at the 5 to 7 year postoperative mark, and in 49% of grafts studied 10 to 12 years postoperatively.[36] In another study, angiograms were performed at 1 and 5 years postoperatively. The 1-year patency was noted to be 82%, and the 5-year patency was only 45%.[36] Multivariant analysis in the second study identified increasing postoperative interval, interim myocardial infarction, angina, diabetes, hypercholesterolemia, and hypertriglyceridemia as factors associated with late occlusion of vein grafts patent at the time of the earlier study. Both studies concluded that 50% of the aortocoronary grafts had closed at the 10-year postoperative mark. Furthermore, of those that remained open, about half showed wall alterations consistent with graft atherosclerosis.

Internal Mammary Artery Grafts

The internal mammary artery was described as a conduit for bypass grafting in the 1960s.[37,38] This graft is appealing because of its documented long-term patency. The late patency rate is reported to be 90% or greater.[39] Barner and associates reported significantly better patency for internal mammary artery grafts than for saphenous vein grafts at varying postoperative intervals: 95.7 versus 93.4% at 1 year, 87.9 versus 74.0% at 5 years, and 83.0 versus 41.0% at 10 years, respectively.[40]

In addition to patency advantages, the internal mammary graft appears to confer a survival benefit when compared to those patients who have had saphenous vein grafting to the anterior descending coronary artery. The 10-year actuarial survival was significantly better for patients with internal mammary grafts, regardless of the extent of disease, preoperative ventricular function or gender, when compared to those patients without an internal mammary artery graft.[39] The risk of subsequent myocardial infarction after bypass grafting also seems to be decreased; in the same study, the vein-graft-only group had 1.4 times the risk of late myocardial infarction, 1.25 times the risk of hospitalization for cardiac events, and 2.0 times the risk of cardiac reoperation when compared to those patients that had the use of the internal mammary artery as bypass conduit. Geha also found significantly better survival and freedom from cardiac events for patients who had received one or more internal mammary artery grafts compared with those who had received vein grafts only.[41]

The reason for the superior performance of the internal mammary artery is not completely understood. The internal mammary artery seems to be free of the progressive intimal thickening noted in coronary arteries with advancing age.[42,43] In addition, the preserved vasa vasora of the arterial graft may be a factor that contributes to its increased patency rate. Prostacyclin production from the internal mammary artery endothelium, when compared to that of harvested saphenous vein, may well be a biochemical basis for the improved patency rate.[44]

The right and left internal mammary arteries can be used to revascularize a large territory of myocardium. The anterior two-thirds of the septum and the anterior lateral and proximal halves of the inferior wall of the left ventricle are all able to be easily reached with the use of this conduit.[41,45]

Harvesting of the internal mammary is aided by the use of various specialized retractors. After the pericardium is opened and the left anterior descending coronary artery is inspected and assessed for grafting, a chest wall retractor is placed and the undersurface of the thoracic cage is visualized. The pleural space is entered and the mammary artery is exposed from the first rib to the xyphoid process. The artery is palpated along its course and two parallel incisions are made with the electrocautery device, each one to 1.5 cm away from the artery. Using the spatula of the cautery device as a dissecting tool, the tissues holding the mammary to the chest wall are freed. Branches from the mammary are found at each intercostal space. Each branch is clipped next to the mammary artery and the distal portion of the branch is electrocauterized using a low level of coagulating energy. The electrocautery device should be used with caution above the level of the first rib on the left, and near the entrance of the superior vena cava to the pericardium on the right, to avoid injury to the phrenic nerves. After the dissection of the mammary artery is completed, the graft should be wrapped in a papaverine-soaked sponge to eliminate any component of spasm. Once the patient is heparinized, the distal end of the mammary artery is divided and spatulated with fine scissors in preparation for anastomosis.

ALTERNATE CONDUITS

Gastroepiploic Artery

The use of the gastroepiploic artery as a conduit for coronary bypass grafting was initially described in 1987.[46,47] The artery is harvested by extending the median sternotomy incision toward the umbilicus, and harvesting the artery from its course along the greater curvature of the stomach. It is of technical importance to avoid twisting the artery, thus compromising its flow. Some authors have suggested marking the course of the artery with fine ties to prevent the possibility of twisting the conduit. The grafting of targets in the right coronary and circumflex coronary distributions re-quires that the graft be routed in a retrogastric fashion. If the target is in the distribution of the left anterior descending coronary artery, routing the graft in an antegastric fashion is recommended. Short-term studies of graft patency show good results with rates in the 90 to 100% patency range.[48-50] Long-term studies of the patency of the gastroepiploic artery are not yet available.

Inferior Epigastric Artery

The inferior epigastric artery has also been used as an arterial conduit for coronary artery bypass grafting.[51,52] The artery is exposed by performing a paramedian incision and retracting the rectus muscle. The artery itself is harvested as a free graft. Lengths of conduit between 10 and 15 cm can be obtained by dissecting the artery from its origin from the external iliac artery. Long-term patency rates of the inferior epigastric artery are not available at this time, although short-term studies of the graft show encouraging (98%) patency rates.[53]

Radial Artery

The use of the radial artery for an alternative arterial bypass conduit was initially reported by Carpentier in 1973.[54] He has recently revisited the use of this alternate arterial conduit as an option for coronary bypass grafting. The initial experience with the radial artery graft was disappointing because high occlusion rates were reported.[55,56]

Modifications in both the harvest technique and the pharmacologic treatment of the radial artery graft have improved its immediate patency rate. The use of intraoperative and postoperative calcium channel blockers, as well as harvesting the artery as a pedicle graft including the vein, and not skeletonizing the artery, may improve its long-term patency.

Cryopreserved Homograft Veins

Cryopreserved homograft veins matched by blood type to the patient are now available. The patency rates for the cryopreserved veins remain marginal and are reported to be under 50% at 7 mo.[57] Because of the low patency rate, this form of conduit should be used only when no other conduit is available.

CORONARY ENDARTERECTOMY

Coronary endarterectomy without the use of extracorporeal circulation represented the initial attempts at coronary revascularization.[58,59] Because of the technical limitations resulting from the lack of cardiopulmonary bypass or adequate preoperative evaluation of the location and distribution of the coronary artery disease, the early results were disappointing.[60-62] The advent of extracorporeal circulation and its combination with coronary artery bypass grafting were two factors that enabled adequate results with coronary endarterectomy to be accomplished.

The indications for coronary endarterectomy include patients with severe diffuse coronary disease whose distal coronary target is unsuitable for bypass. The most frequent indication for coronary endarterectomy is in those vessels that are completely occluded. The large right coronary artery that is completely occluded but supplies viable myocardium is a candidate for coronary endarterectomy. While an endarterectomy of an occluded left anterior descending coronary artery can be undertaken, the combination of endarterectomy of the LAD with bypass grafting carries a significantly higher operative risk.

Contraindications to coronary endarterectomy include aneurysmal coronary arteries, vessels of less than 2 mm in diameter, small nondominant vessels, and vessels supplying nonviable myocardium.

The technique for right coronary endarterectomy in-

volves an arteriotomy at the crux of the right coronary and encircling the plaque at the level of the crux. Using special endarterectomy tools, a dissection plane is developed between the plaque and the media of the coronary artery. The tools are used to dissect both the posterior descending branch and the left ventricular branch, and gentle traction is applied to the distal plaque while countertraction is applied to the adventitia of the coronary artery. In this way, the plaque is everted and peeled away from the arterial wall. The eversion endarterectomy is completed distally, and a similar technique is used for the proximal vessel. At the site of the arteriotomy, the vessel is bypassed using the saphenous vein (Fig. 126–8).

The technique for endarterectomy of the left anterior descending coronary artery differs from right coronary endarterectomy in that a long arteriotomy, anywhere between 6 and 8 cm long, is employed to expose the diseased vessel and the septal perforators. The endarterectomy is carried out and involves each separate septal perforator. The plaque

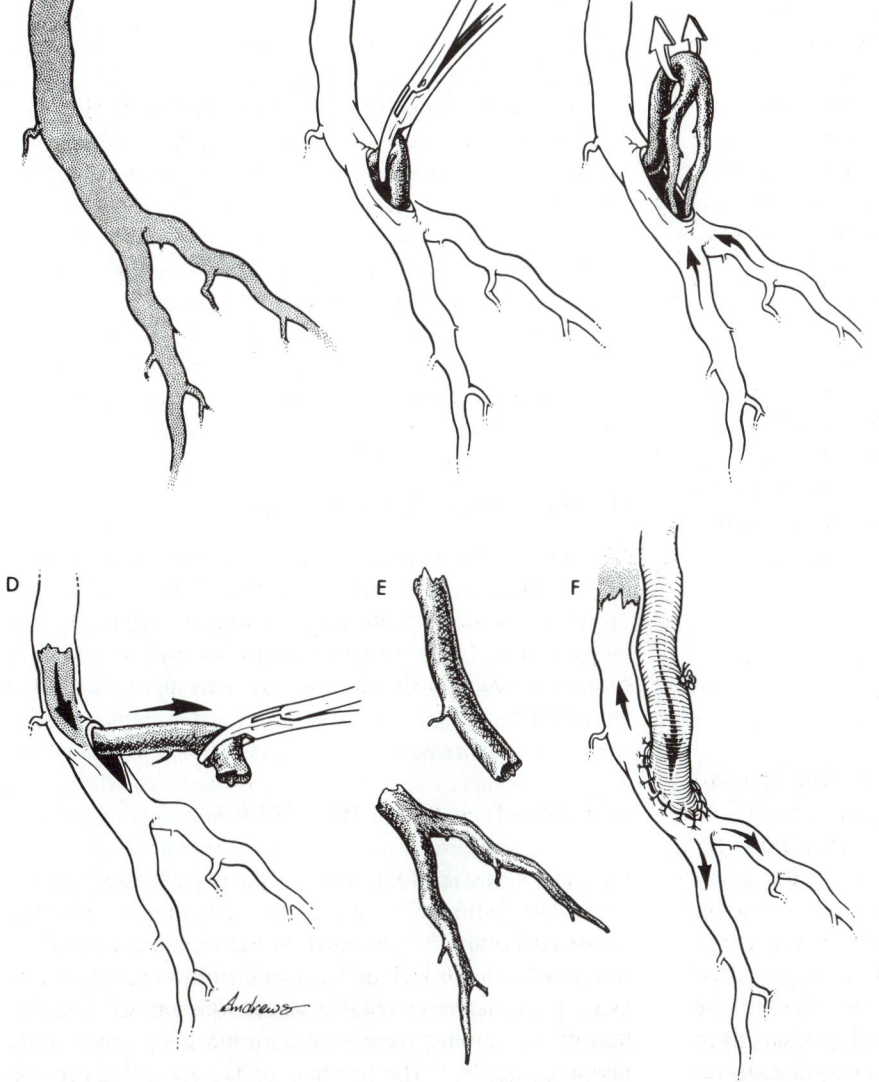

Figure 126–8. Technique for right coronary endarterectomy. **A.** An occluded right coronary artery is considered for endarterectomy. **B.** The incision is made just above the crux and the core brought out through the incision. Gentle traction is exerted on the distal portion while the artery is peeled back. **C,D.** A complete endarterectomy results when all the distal branches are free of plaquing. The distal vessels should be cleared individually. The proximal portion is then removed by gentle traction until it breaks free from the proximal area. It is not important to obtain a clearly feathered proximal portion. **E.** The specimen is considered satisfactory when the distal specimen and small branches have feathered ends. **F.** A vein graft is then placed to the arteriotomy to assure flow in both directions. *(Reprinted with permission from Cooley DA: Techniques in Cardiac Surgery, 2nd ed. Philadelphia, Saunders, 1984.)*

is elevated in a similar fashion to the right coronary artery, and traction and countertraction are used to deliver the plaque from the septal perforators. In contrast to right coronary endarterectomy, eversion endarterectomy of the proximal segment is not performed on the left anterior descending coronary artery. Endarterectomy of the left anterior descending involves a sharp dissection of the plaque proximally, and tacking of the wall of the plaque to the native coronary artery. In this manner, blood supplied by the bypass graft cannot dissect between the layers of the proximal left anterior descending coronary artery. The long arteriotomy is closed using a saphenous vein bypass graft as an onlay patch (Fig. 126–9).

Complications that are seen following endarterectomy include myocardial infarction, which can be secondary to dissection by blood within the wall of the endarterectomized vessel thus occluding the residual lumen, thrombosis of the vessel, or obstruction of branches that could not be endarterectomized. Perforation of the coronary may also occur, either from improper dissection of the plaque or improper traction on the plaque.

The patency rates for arteries that require endarterectomy, as opposed to those that do not require endarterectomy, are lower for the endarterectomized vessels. The patency rates at 1 year for endarterectomized right coronary arteries range from 73 to 86%, and for the left coronary artery, from 62 to 86%. Endarterectomized circumflex coronary artery patency rates are approximately 75%.[63] Antiplatelet therapy is used to improve graft patency following routine bypass grafting. The extension of antiplatelet therapy to those patients requiring coronary endarterectomy for revascularization is both sensible and practical, and may improve both early and long term graft patency.

CORONARY REOPERATIONS

Coronary reoperations may represent up to 15% of total revascularizations performed today. Important aspects of the evaluation of a patient for repeat coronary operation include the presence of conduit, the quality of targets both at the initial operation and at proposed reoperation, and the presence of reversible myocardial ischemia. Contraindications for reoperative coronary artery bypass grafting include previous irradiation of the anterior mediastinum, a previous Beck operation, and lack of a conduit.

The risk of coronary revascularization is higher than for first operations. The risk of death is three to four times that of the initial operation, the risk of stroke over two times that of the initial operation, and the risk of perioperative myocardial infarction can be as high as eight times that of the primary operation. Patients and their families must be made aware of the increased morbidity and mortality associated with coronary reoperation.

The reasons for repeat coronary revascularization have changed over time. Initially, progression of native coronary artery atherosclerosis was the primary reason for requiring redo coronary artery bypass grafting. In recent years, the patient profile has changed such that a majority of patients now require bypass grafting to be performed for progression of disease in vein graft conduits. Failure of vein graft conduits may occur from subintimal hyperplasia, the use of a suboptimal conduit, or venous valve disease.

Once the patient has been found to be a candidate for reoperative bypass grafting, a thorough review of the previous procedure's operative note should be undertaken.

The conduct of the operation begins with the approach to sternotomy. The pump should be ready and the perfusionist should be present in the room at the time of sternotomy. We recommend that the lines be cut and on the field, ready for cannulation of either the ascending aorta or the femoral artery in an emergency. Both femoral arteries should be prepared so that rapid exposure can be accomplished in the event that inadvertent entry into either a major vessel or cardiac chamber occurs during sternotomy. Preoperative review of both the lateral chest x-ray and the cineangiograms for location and course of existing bypass grafts in relation to the proposed sternotomy incision is mandatory. Although some surgeons use the standard sternal saw for repeat sternotomy, we recommend the use of the oscillating saw in these operations.

Once repeat sternotomy is successfully performed, the electrocautery device is used to divide the tissues on the undersurface of the sternum (Fig. 126–9). Dissection of the heart should be undertaken with the initial goal of safe and expeditious cannulation of the patient as a primary concern. Exposure of the right atrium and the ascending aorta for cannulation is the primary task after sternotomy. We employ a no-touch technique in regards to the previous existing saphenous vein bypass grafts. If a mammary artery is present, this is dissected and isolated in one segment, so that the artery can be clamped and cardioplegia can be delivered. Once adequate atrium and aorta are exposed for cannulation, the internal mammary is dissected, if it has not been previously used as bypass conduit. The remainder of the dissection takes place while the heart is decompressed on cardiopulmonary bypass.

Both antegrade and retrograde cardioplegia are routinely used for myocardial protection and, in addition, a left ventricular vent is placed to facilitate decompression of the left ventricle. Again, a no-touch technique is employed with regards to the diseased bypass grafts. After cannulation, the aorta is clamped, cardioplegia is delivered, and dissection of the heart is completed. If the distal targets are small and the vein graft disease does not extend to the distal portion of the graft, the hood of the vein graft may be used as a target for bypass grafting. The old vein grafts are ligated after the completion of the distal anastomosis to ensure that no atherosclerotic debris is ejected through the old vein graft. Once the distal anastomoses are completed, the operation is conducted in a similar fashion as during primary myocardial revascularization.

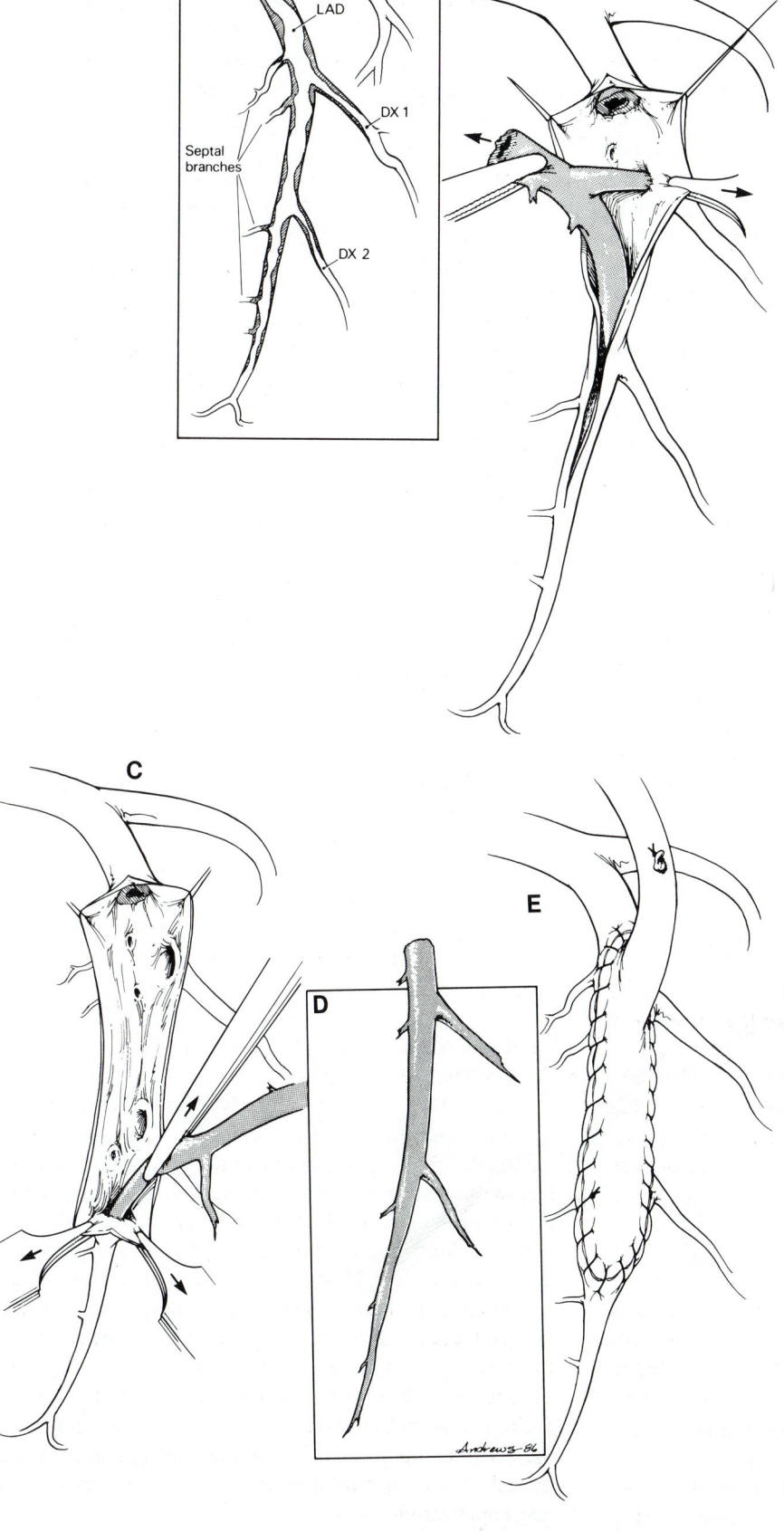

Figure 126–9. Technique for endarterectomy of the left anterior descending coronary artery. **A.** Diffuse coronary atherosclerosis is found obstructing all major tributaries and precluding effective bypass. **B.** A lengthy incision is made in the midportion of the artery to allow plaque removal under direct vision. The proximal plaque is sharply divided. Gentle traction is applied to the core with countertraction of the arterial wall, extracting the plaque from each major tributary. **C.** The distal plaque is removed by gentle traction on the core with countertraction, peeling away the arterial wall. **D.** The specimen is examined to insure complete extraction of plaque from each tributary. **E.** The artery is reconstructed with a long anastomosis using an onlay saphenous vein graft.

CALCIFIED ASCENDING AORTA

The calcified or porcelain ascending aorta should be suspected on the preoperative chest roentgenogram or when examining the cineangiograms prior to revascularization. The calcified aorta presents a unique challenge to the cardiovascular surgeon in terms of both cannulation and placement of proximal anastomoses. Cannulation techniques for approaching the calcified ascending aorta include cannulation of the axillary artery, cannulation of the femoral arteries, and cannulation of the under surface of the aortic arch. Conduct of the operation involves the use of a left ventricular vent via the superior pulmonary vein, and hypothermic fibrillatory arrest for the construction of distal anastomoses. Proximal anastomoses can be constructed using the internal mammary artery as a site for the proximal vein graft anastomosis, or possibly the innominate artery, which may have been spared from the atherosclerotic disease. It is of paramount importance to avoid cross-clamping the aorta to avoid the complications of stroke in these patients.

REFERENCES

1. Robinson G, Brodman R: Letter to the editor. *Ann Thorac Surg* **31**(4):396, 1981
2. Robinson G: Location of the proximal left anterior descending coronary artery. *Ann Thorac Surg* **15**:299–300, 1973
3. Ungerlider RM, Mills NL, Wechsler AS: Left thoracotomy for reoperative coronary artery bypass procedures. *Ann Thorac Surg* **40**(1):11–15, 1985
4. Ochsner JL, Mills NL: *Coronary Artery Surgery.* Philadelphia, Lea & Febiger, 1978, p 48
5. Ankeney JL: Editorial: To use or not to use the pump oxygenator in coronary bypass operation! *Ann Thorac Surg* **19**(1):108–109, 1975
6. Atkins CW, Austen WG: Revascularization of the myocardium. *Curr Probl Surg* **18**(1):44, 1981
7. Alinger GN, Bonchek LI: Ventricular venting during coronary revascularization: Assessment of benefit by intraoperative ventricular function curves. *Ann Thorac Surg* **26**:525–534, 1978
8. Miller DW Jr, Hessel EA II, Winterscheid LC, et al: Current practice of coronary bypass surgery: Results of a national survey. *J Thorac Cardiovasc Surg* **73**(1):75–83, 1977
9. Lam R, Robinson MJ, Morales AR, et al: Aortic dissection complicating aortocoronary saphenous vein bypass. *Am J Clin Pathol* **68**(6):729–735, 1977
10. Boruchow IB, Lyengar R, Lude JR, et al: Injury to ascending aorta by partial-occlusion clamp during aortocoronary bypass. *J Thorac Cardiovasc Surg* **73**(2):303, 1977
11. Michelson WJ, Cravley IS, Logue RB, et al: Aortic root dissection complicating coronary bypass surgery. *Am J Cardiol* **41**(1):103–107, 1978
12. Kimbiris D, Dreifus LS, Adam A, et al: Dissection and rupture of the ascending aorta: Unusual complications of aortocoronary bypass surgery. *Chest* **68**(3):303–316, 1975
13. Mills NL, Everson CT, Rigby CS, et al: Atherosclerosis of the ascending aorta and coronary artery bypass: Pathology, clinic correlates and operative management. Presented at annual meeting of the American Association of Thoracic Surgery, Boston, MA, May 1989
14. Harlan BJ, Kygen ER, Reul GJ Jr, Cooley DA: Needle suction of the aorta for left heart decompression during aortic crossclamping. *Ann Thorac Surg* **23**(3):259–260, 1977

15. Stiles AT: Technique of saphenous vein aorto-coronary bypass grafting. *J Thorac Cardiovasc Surg* **78**(2):305–308, 1979
16. Sewell WH, Sewell KV: Technique for the coronary snake graft operations. *Ann Thorac Surg* **22**(1):58–65, 1976
17. Cleveland JC, Lebenson IM, Twobey RJ, et al: Further evaluation of the circular sequential vein graft technique of coronary artery bypass. *Ann Thorac Surg* **30**:336, 1980
18. Ochsner JL, Mills NL: *Coronary Artery Surgery.* Philadelphia, Lea & Febiger, 1978, p 203
19. Sewell WH: Should we do Y and sequential grafts for coronary bypass? *Ann Thorac Surg* **27**(5):397–398, 1976
20. Boerboom LE, Bonchek LI, Kissebah AH, et al: Effect of surgical trauma on tissue lipids: Primate vein grafts in relation to plasma lipids. *Circulation* **62**(2)(Suppl I):142–147, 1980
21. Roth JA, Cukingnan RA, Brown Ba, et al: Factors influencing patency of saphenous vein grafts. *Ann Thorac Surg* **28**(2):176–183, 1979
22. Bonchek LI: Prevention of endothelial damage during preparation of saphenous veins for bypass grafting. *J Thorac Cardiovasc Surg* **79**(6):911–915, 1980
23. Guidry SR, Jones M, Takuhiro I, et al: Optimal preparation techniques for human saphenous vein grafts. *Surgery* **88**:785–794, 1980
24. Stoney WS, Alford WC, Burrus GR, et al: The fate of arm veins used for aorta-coronary bypass grafts. *J Thorac Cardiovasc Surg* **88**(4):522–526, 1984
25. Kouchoukos NT, Karp RB, Oberman A, et al: Long-term patency of saphenous veins for coronary bypass grafting. *Circulation* **58**(Suppl I):96, 1978
26. Lytle BW, Loop FD, Cosgrove DM, et al: Long-term (5 to 12 years) serial studies of internal mammary artery and saphenous vein coronary bypass grafts. *J Thorac Cardiovasc Surg* **89**:248, 1985
27. Loop FD, Cosgrove DM, Lytle BW, et al: An 11 year evolution of coronary arterial surgery (1967–1978). *Ann Surg* **190**:444, 1979
28. Campeau L, Lesperance J, Corbara F, et al: Aortocoronary saphenous vein bypass graft changes 5 to 7 years after surgery. *Circulation* **58**(Suppl I):179, 1978
29. Campeau L, Crochet D, Lesperance J, et al: Postoperative changes in aortocoronary saphenous vein grafts revisited: Angiographic studies at two weeks and at one year in two series of consecutive patients. *Circulation* **52**:369, 1975
30. Bourassa MG, Campeau L, Lesperance J, Grondin CM: Changes in grafts and in coronary arteries after saphenous vein aortocoronary bypass surgery. In Hammermeister KE (ed): *Coronary Bypass Surgery. The Late Results.* New York, Praeger, 1983
31. Grondin CM, Vouhe P, Bourassa MG, et al: Optimal patency rates obtained in coronary artery grafting with circular vein grafts. *J Thorac Cardiovasc Surg* **75**:161, 1978
32. Sewell WH: Should we do Y- and sequential grafts for coronary bypass? *Ann Thorac Surg* **27**:397, 1979
33. Yeh TJ, Heidary D, Shelton L: Y-grafts and sequential grafts in coronary bypass surgery: A critical evaluation of patency rates. *Ann Thorac Surg* **27**:409, 1979
34. Smith SH, Geer JC: Morphology of saphenous vein-coronary artery bypass grafts: 7-116 months post-operative. *Arch Pathol Lab Med* **107**:13, 1983
35. Grondin CM: Graft disease in patients with coronary bypass grafting. *J Thorac Cardiovasc Surg* **92**:323, 1986
36. Campeau L, Enjalbert M, Lesperance J, et al: Atherosclerosis and late closure of aortocoronary saphenous vein grafts: Sequential and angiographic studies at 2 weeks, 1 year, 5–7 years, and at 10–12 years after surgery. *Circulation* **68**(Suppl II):1, 1983
37. Kolessov VI: Mammary artery-coronary artery anastomosis as method of treatment for angina pectoris. *J Thorac Cardiovasc Surg* **54**:535–544, 1967
38. Green GE, Stertzer SH, Reppert EH: Coronary arterial bypass grafts. *Ann Thorac Surg* **5**:443–450, 1968
39. Loop FD, Lytle BW, Cosgrove DM, et al: Influence of the internal

mammary artery graft on 10-year survival and other cardiac events. *N Engl J Med* **314**:1–6, 1986

40. Barner HB, Standeven JW, Reese J: Twelve year experience with internal mammary artery for coronary artery bypass. *J Thorac Cardiovasc Surg* **90**:688–675, 1985

41. Geha AS, Hammond GL, Stephan RN et al: Late results of revascularization with crossed double internal mammary versus saphenous vein bypass grafts. *Surgery* **102**:667–673, 1987

42. Sims FH: A comparison of coronary and internal mammary arteries and implications of the results in the etiology of arteriosclerosis. *Am Heart J* **106**:560, 1983

43. Barbour DJ, Roberts WC: Additional evidence for relative resistance to atherosclerosis of the internal mammary artery compared to saphenous vein when used to increase myocardial blood supply. *Am J Cardiol* **56**:488, 1985

44. Chaikhouni A, Crawford FA, Kochel PJ, et al: Human internal mammary artery produces more prostacyclin than saphenous vein. *J Thorac Cardiovasc Surg* **92**:88–91, 1986

45. Tector AJ, Schmahl TM, Canino VR: Expanding the use of the internal mammary artery to improve graft patency in coronary artery bypass grafting. *J Thorac Cardiovasc Surg* **91**:9–16, 1986

46. Pym J, Brown PM, Charrette EJP, et al: Gastroepiploic-coronary anastomosis: A viable alternative bypass graft. *J Thorac Cardiovasc Surg* **94**:256, 1987

47. Suma H, Fukumoto H, Takeuchi A: Coronary artery bypass grafting by utilizing in situ right gastroepiploic artery: Basic study and clinical application. *Ann Thorac Surg* **44**:394, 1987

48. Lytle BW, Cosgrove DM, Ratliff NB, Loop FD: Coronary artery bypass grafting with the right gastroepiploic artery. *J Thorac Cardiovasc Surg* **97**:826, 1989

49. Isshiki T, Yamaguchi T, Nakamura M, et al: Post-operative angiographic evaluation of gastroepiploic artery grafts: Technical considerations and short-term patency. *Cathet Cardiovasc Diagn* **21**:233, 1990

50. Suma H, Wanibuchi Y, Terada Y, et al: The right gastroepiploic artery graft. Clinical and angiographic midterm results in 200 patients. *J Thorac Cardiovasc Surg* **105**:615–623, 1993

51. Milgalter E, Pearl J, Laks H, et al: The inferior epigastric arteries as coronary bypass conduits: Size, preoperative duplex scan assessment of suitability, and early clinical experience. *J Thorac Cardiovasc Surg* **103**:463, 1992

52. Mills NL, Everson CT: Technique for use of the inferior epigastric artery as a coronary bypass graft. *Ann Thorac Surg* **51**:208, 1991

53. Buche M, Schoevaerdts J, Louagie Y, et al: Use of the inferior epigastric artery for coronary bypass. *J Thorac Cardiovasc Surg* **103**:665, 1992

54. Carpentier A, Guermonprez JL, Deloche A, et al: The aorta-to-coronary radial artery bypass graft. *Ann Thorac Surg* **16**:111, 1973

55. Curtis JJ, Stoney WS, Alford WC Jr, et al: Intimal hyperplasia: A cause of radial artery aortocoronary bypass graft failure. *Ann Thorac Surg* **20**:268,1975

56. Fisk RL, Brooks CH, Callaghan JC, Dvorkin J: Experience with the radial artery graft for coronary artery bypass. *Ann Thorac Surg* **21**:513, 1976

57. Laub GW, Muralidharan S, Clancy R, et al: Cryopreserved allograft veins as alternative coronary artery bypass conduits: Early phase results. *Ann Thorac Surg* **54**:826, 1992

58. Bailey CP, May A, Lewman WM: Survival with coronary endarterectomy in man. *JAMA* **164**:641–646, 1957

59. Longmire WP, Cannon JA, Kattus AA: Direct-vision coronary endarterectomy for angina pectoris. *N Engl J Med* **259**:993–999, 1958

60. Ellis PR, Cooley DA: The patch technique as an adjunct to coronary endarterectomy. *J Thorac Cardiovasc Surg* **42**(2):236–243, 1961

61. Effler DB, Groves KL, Sones FM, Shirey EK: Endarterectomy in the treatment of coronary artery disease. *J Thorac Cardiovasc Surg* **47**:98–108, 1964

62. Dilley RB, Cannon JA, Kattus AA, et al: The treatment of coronary occlusive disease by endarterectomy. *J Thorac Cardiovasc Surg* **50**:511–526, 1965

63. Qureshi SA, Halim MA, Pillai R, et al: Endarterectomy of the left coronary system. Analysis of a 10 year experience. *J Thorac Cardiovasc Surg* **89**:852–859, 1985

C H A P T E R

127

Combined Coronary and Carotid Artery Disease

Ellis L. Jones and George T. Hodakowski

Atherosclerotic cerebrovascular disease in its many presentations continues to be a major health problem throughout the world.[1] Due to the diffuse nature of atherosclerosis, the coexistence of cerebrovascular and coronary artery disease in some patients is to be expected. The surgical management of this subset of patients has remained controversial; however, experience gained with patients having coronary artery bypass (CAB) and concomitant asymptomatic carotid artery disease has increased our understanding of this condition. The routine use of intraoperative echocardiography has implicated the ascending aorta and transverse arch as major sources of atherosclerotic cerebral emboli in some patients suffering a perioperative stroke following CAB.

Although the association between coronary and carotid artery disease is well documented, the true incidence is unknown due to the many asymptomatic individuals. Nonetheless, in patients undergoing myocardial revascularization, the incidence of hemodynamically significant carotid artery stenosis (>70% diameter narrowing) has been reported to be between 2.8 to 11.8%, depending on the screening methods used.[2–4] Despite advances in surgical technique, the overall incidence of stroke following coronary artery bypass continues to be a source of great morbidity occurring with an overall incidence of 1 to 3%, but is significantly higher in patients greater than 70 years of age.[5–8]

There is a constant stroke risk in patients with combined disease, with significant, but nonoperated carotid artery stenoses. The stroke rate in these patients during the first 4 years after CAB is approximately 4% per year.[3] The presence of significant carotid stenosis in coronary artery bypass patients increases the risk of either transient is-

chemic attack (TIA) or stroke from 1.9 to 9.2%.[9] Interestingly, patients with coronary artery and coexistent carotid disease have three times the incidence of left main coronary obstruction when compared to patients without associated carotid artery disease.[10] Whether carotid disease is the major culprit of perioperative stroke after CAB, or merely represents one manifestation of generalized atherosclerosis, has not been determined.

Approximately one-half of patients with extracranial cerebrovascular disease manifest signs and symptoms of coronary artery disease.[11] Myocardial infarction is the most common cause of early and late death following carotid endarterectomy.[4,12–14] Fatal myocardial infarction following carotid endarterectomy has been reported to occur with a frequency of 3 to 5%, but the true incidence depends on the clinical state of the patient.[15–17] In patients with no history of coronary artery disease this incidence is as low as 1%, but increases to 7% in patients with a history of coronary artery disease and even to 17% in patients with unstable angina pectoris.[11,18] As many as 50 to 70% of late deaths following carotid endarterectomy are attributable to myocardial infarction.[19–21]

EVALUATION OF THE PATIENT WITH COMBINED DISEASE

The preoperative evaluation of a patient for CAB requires a thorough history (from both patient and family members) and physical examination, with particular emphasis not only on the heart and lungs but also the vascular system. A comprehensive history will frequently elicit symptoms of extracranial cerebrovascular disease, such as prior stroke,

TIA, amaurosis fugax, or a previous history of carotid endarterectomy (CEA). The physical examination should include auscultation of the carotid arteries, with notation of the extension of the bruit into diastole, evaluation of peripheral pulses, and a basic screening neurologic examination. Patients with symptomatic cerebrovascular disease, a history of previous carotid endarterectomy or stroke, and those asymptomatic patients with a highly suspicious carotid bruit should undergo noninvasive studies of the carotid arteries by duplex scanning. In most institutions, a positive duplex scan will be an indication for a cerebral arteriogram to further delineate the atherosclerotic lesion prior to planning the operative strategy.

Nonetheless, the presence of a carotid bruit alone is not diagnostic of a significant carotid stenosis. Asymptomatic cervical bruits are said to be present in 4.4% of the population older than 45 years of age without a previous history of stroke, TIA, or overt heart disease.[13] Historically carotid bruits have been identified in approximately 7% of patients undergoing CAB.[10] Yet, no direct correlation has been identified between a carotid bruit, the severity of carotid disease, and the incidence of perioperative stroke.[13,22] Their presence, however, dictates further diagnostic studies to precisely define the underlying pathology. In one prospective study, Barnes reported that cervical bruits were associated with significant carotid stenoses in only 38% of patients. Conversely, of carotid arteries with significant stenosis only one-third will have an associated bruit.[23] For *asymptomatic* patients with a cervical bruit, a significant carotid artery stenosis is present in approximately one-third of patients with approximately 5% having internal carotid artery occlusion.[24] In data extracted from The North American Symptomatic Carotid Endarterectomy Trial (NASCET), a multicenter randomized controlled trial of CEA in symptomatic patients, a focal ipsilateral carotid bruit had a sensitivity of 63% and a specificity of 61% for high grade stenoses (70 to 90% diameter stenosis). Furthermore, the frequency of carotid bruits concomitantly increased with the degree of stenosis, but peaked at the 70 to 89% stenosis range, with a subsequent decline in the frequency of bruits with stenoses greater than 90% diameter reduction.[25]

The NASCET study and the European Carotid Surgery Trial (ECST), a multicenter randomized trial of carotid endarterectomies in patients with prior nondisabling ischemic strokes, have important implications for patients with combined coronary and carotid disease. These studies have reported the beneficial effect of carotid endarterectomy in reducing the risk of subsequent stroke and early death in symptomatic patients with high grade stenosis (70 to 99% diameter) of the internal carotid artery. The NASCET results revealed a cumulative ipsilateral stroke free rate at 2 years of 91% in the surgical group versus 74% in the medical group ($p < 0.001$).[26] Similarly, in the ECST study the cumulative risk of ipsilateral stroke at 3 years following the perioperative period was 2.8% in the surgical group versus

16.8% in the medically treated group ($p < 0.0001$), a sixfold reduction in stroke risk.[27] Thus, patients presenting for CAB who are experiencing *symptoms* of documented extracranial cerebrovascular disease should undergo a carotid endarterectomy, either as a staged procedure (prior to CAB) or simultaneously with the CAB procedure. However, the exact etiology of cerebral symptoms in patients with combined disease is uncertain. Spontaneous embolization of atherosclerotic material from the ascending or transverse arch of the aorta, or a fibrillating left atrium, may result in a stroke or TIA, indistinguishable from that of carotid disease.

ETIOLOGY OF CEREBRAL INJURY DURING CORONARY BYPASS SURGERY

Strokes have become a major source of morbidity following CAB, however, the exact etiology of the neurologic event is usually unknown. Possible mechanisms of perioperative stroke include a reduction in cerebral blood flow through a stenotic extracranial or intracranial vessel, embolization of atherosclerotic debris from an ulcerated carotid artery plaque or aorta, and embolization of postinfarction left ventricular mural thrombus or an atrial thrombus. Embolization of air, inadequately evacuated from the heart or aorta, is another cause of neurologic injury following CAB.

It is possible that cardiopulmonary bypass alters cerebral arterial autoregulation such that cerebral blood flow becomes proportional to cerebral perfusion pressure.[28] This may be particularly true in patients with diffuse intracerebral vascular disease. Consequently, a decrease in arterial perfusion pressure results in a parallel decline in blood flow to the brain. Cerebral blood flow may be further impaired by a reduction in perfusion pressure distal to a carotid artery stenosis, especially when the vessel diameter is reduced greater than 70%.[29,30] In this case, the collateral circulation to the internal carotid artery functions as a compensatory source of cerebral blood flow. This important collateral system includes (1) the circle of Willis, which joins the carotid and basilar systems, (2) anastomotic channels between the internal and external carotid arteries, such as the meningeal, ophthalmic, and caroticotympanic arteries, and (3) anastomoses between the external carotid artery and the subclavian and vertebral arteries.[31] A poorly developed collateral system increases the risk of stroke in patients with severe atherosclerosis of the internal carotid arteries. Though hypothermia during surgery decreases the metabolic demand of the brain, episodes of normothermic hypotension, both during and after bypass, may expose the relatively hypoperfused brain to ischemic insult. Thus, maintenance of perfusion pressure at a level >70 mm Hg may counteract the decrease in cerebral blood flow associated with stenotic lesions.

The significance of embolism of atherosclerotic debris in the etiology of strokes during CAB has been previously reported.[32] These findings have been recently confirmed by others.[33-36] A review of 100 autopsied hearts in patients with clinically significant atherosclerosis revealed that 40 patients had atherosclerotic plaques within the ascending aorta. Most of the plaques were located anteriorly, posteriorly, and on the right side (greater curvature) of the ascending aorta.[37] In an autopsy series of 500 patients with cerebrovascular or neurologic disease, ulcerated plaques of the ascending aorta or aortic arch were identified in 26% of patients with cerebrovascular disease, but only 5% of patients with other neurologic diseases.[34] Patients with severe atherosclerosis of the ascending aorta were reported to have a 2.4 times an increased risk for stroke.[38] In addition, the presence of atherosclerotic disease in the ascending aorta or arch has been shown to be strongly correlated with increasing age.[8,38] Approximately 33% of patients over 80 years exhibited moderate to severe atherosclerosis of the ascending aorta.[33] Though atheromatous debris originating in the ascending aorta most frequently embolize to the brain, other sites include the spleen, kidney, pancreas, and gastrointestinal tract in decreasing order of frequency.[39]

Three pathologically distinct patterns of atherosclerosis within the ascending aorta have been described[35]: Type I—extensive, circumferential medial calcification of the ascending aorta producing a "porcelain aorta"; Type II—ragged, friable, ulcerated intraluminal disease; and Type III—liquid, toothpaste-like cholesterol debris, which oozes from within the aorta during aortotomy. Type III atherosclerosis is the most difficult to identify prior to aortotomy, but is frequently found to coexist with abdominal aneurysms. Atherosclerosis of the ascending aorta is suggested by the adherence of the adventitia to the ascending aorta, which is pale and leathery in appearance, or the lack of bleeding when the aorta is opened with the scalpel.

Direct palpation of the ascending aorta significantly underestimates the presence and severity of atherosclerosis.[8] Preoperative chest radiographs also lack sensitivity in quantifying atherosclerosis of the ascending aorta.[40] However, intraoperative ultrasonographic scanning of the ascending aorta appears to be a sensitive technique for identifying specific atheromatous plaques within the ascending aorta (Fig. 127–1).[36,40,41] Yet, despite this sensitivity, ulcer craters filled with loose atherosclerotic material may appear as a smooth image. Intraoperative ultrasonography involves filling the pericardial cradle with normal saline and placing a 5- to 10-MHz ultrasonic transducer within a sterile plastic sheath containing conducting gel. The probe is guided from the aortic valve superiorly to the aortic arch, obtaining multiple images in both the transverse and longitudinal planes. Areas of atherosclerosis are noted and optimally protected from further manipulation. The ultrasonographic findings may require modification of the standard operative technique to include alterations of cannulation sites within the ascending aorta, femoral artery cannulation, retrograde delivery of cardioplegia, use of hypothermic fibrillatory arrest, adjustments in the position of the aortic clamp and proximal vein grafts, and replacement of the ascending aortic root when large segments of the aorta are involved. Kouchoukos reports a reduction in the incidence of stroke in older patients undergoing cardiac surgery with the aggressive treatment of carotid occlusive disease combined with meticulous attention to the presence of moderate or severe ascending aortic atherosclerosis. Using this protocol, perioperative stroke occurred in only 1% of 500 patients undergoing complex cardiac surgical procedures (89% CAB).[42]

Left ventricular mural thrombi are most frequently discovered in patients with a large prior myocardial infarction.

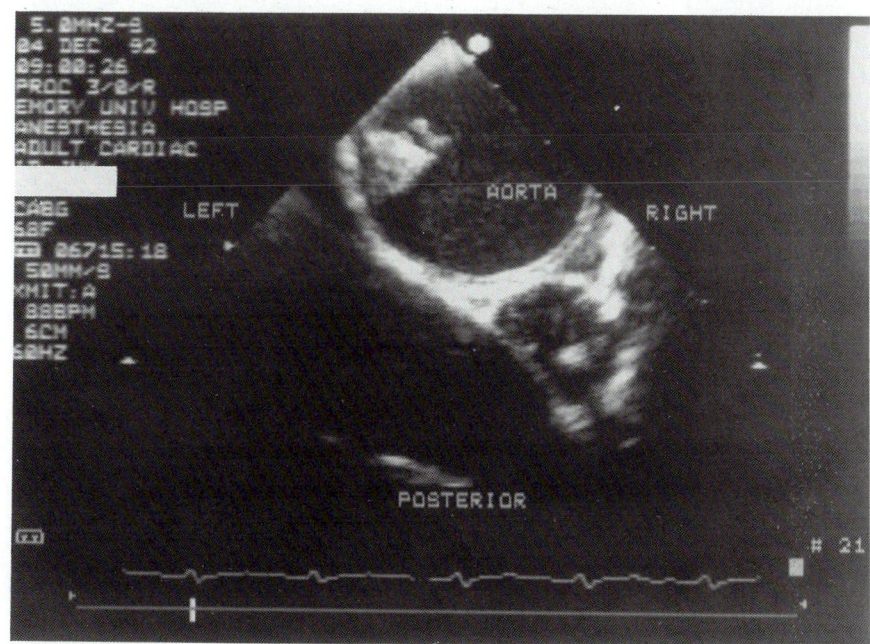

Figure 127–1. Friable, intraluminal atherosclerosis. Cross-clamp, cardioplegia cannula, and proximal vein grafts placed at atherosclerotic free sites documented by intraoperative ultrasonography. Aortotomy performed to extract intraluminal atherosclerotic mass.

It has been noted that the incidence of stroke in patients with preoperative angiographic evidence of left ventricular thrombus was 9% versus 2% in patients without angiographically identifiable thrombi. Intraoperative cardiac manipulation may dislodge mural thrombi resulting in an embolic infarct.[32]

Embolization of air intraoperatively is also a potential cause of cerebral vascular accidents. Air embolization may occur with residual bubbles infused through the arterial inflow line, inadequate deairing of the aorta following removal of the side-biting exclusion clamp for proximal vein anastomoses, venting of the left ventricle, or following combined valve and coronary operations. Classic risk factors previously associated with an increased postoperative stroke rate are advanced age,[6,34,38] severe left ventricular dysfunction,[43] long standing diabetes mellitus,[8] protracted cardiopulmonary bypass time, severe perioperative hypotension,[38] history of previous stroke,[32,44] and bilateral carotid disease.[9,10,15]

OPERATIVE STRATEGY FOR PATIENTS WITH COMBINED DISEASE

In patients with combined coronary and symptomatic carotid disease, the sequence of operative procedures is determined by the most unstable system, either neurologic or cardiac. The surgical approach in patients with significant *asymptomatic* carotid stenosis is more controversial. Several authors have proposed the nonoperative management of significant asymptomatic carotid stenosis in patients undergoing myocardial revascularization with no significant increase in the incidence of stroke.[9,45–49] Yet, other authors maintain that carotid endarterectomy should be performed in patients with significant asymptomatic carotid stenosis to minimize the risk of late neurologic events.[4,12,50–53]

Of the various surgical options available for patients with combined coronary and carotid artery disease, the one favored here is a staged operation performed to treat significant carotid obstructions first if the patient's cardiac status is stable. The CEA can be safely performed on a neurologically unstable patient utilizing local anesthetic, followed by CAB several days later. This same sequence of procedures can be performed on those patients with significant asymptomatic carotid stenoses. The advantages of a staged operation are the total operative time under general anesthesia is reduced, there is a decreased risk of hematoma formation in the neck, the distinct physiological requirements of each operation can be optimized, and a postoperative neurologic deficit may be localized to either the CEA or CAB, with possible subsequent intervention.

CEA and CAB operations may be performed as a combined procedure under the same general anesthetic, with the carotid portion of the operation performed immediately prior to placing the patient on cardiopulmonary bypass. This should be considered whenever the patient presents with cerebrovascular symptoms associated with cardiac instability, diffuse multivessel disease, or a critical left main coronary obstruction. In addition, patients with unstable

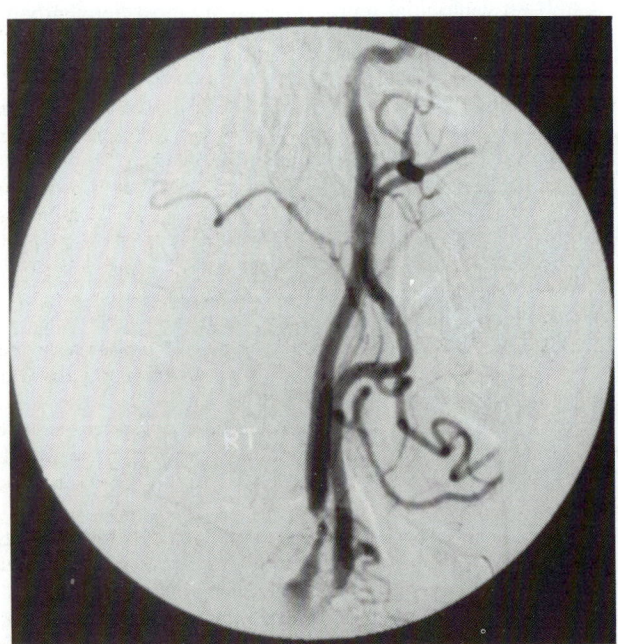 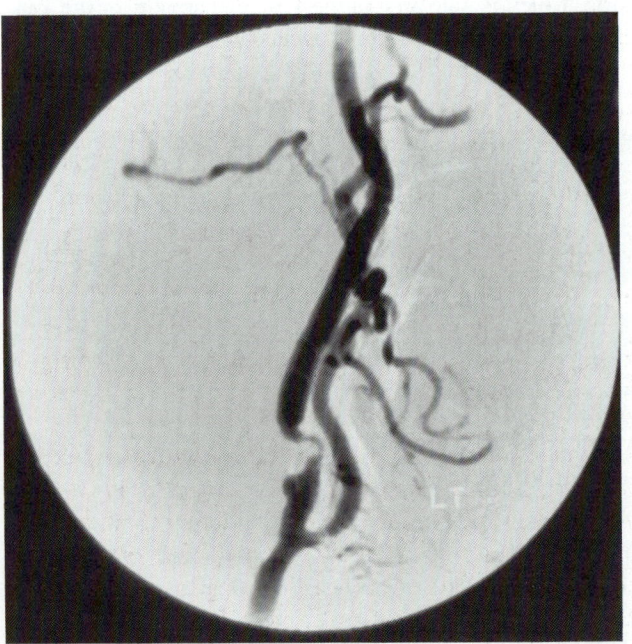

A   **B**

Figure 127–2. A. Right common carotid injection. **B.** Left common carotid injection. Severe bilateral carotid disease (>90% stenosis). An indication for combined CEA and CAB.

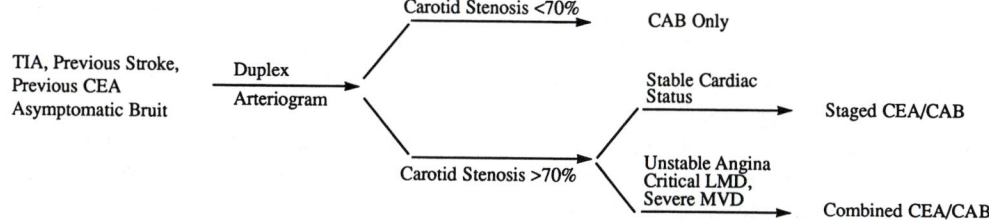

Figure 127–3. Algorithm for combined carotid and coronary disease. Carotid duplex is screening test prior to cerebral arteriogram. CAB, coronary artery bypass; CEA, carotid endarterectomy; LMD, left main disease; MVD, multivessel disease.

angina or advanced coronary disease and severe bilateral carotid disease, should undergo a combined procedure (Fig. 127–2). The first CEA is performed on the carotid artery with the greater stenosis or the one that supplies the dominant hemisphere, followed by CAB. A few days later, the second CEA is undertaken.

The combined approach of carotid endarterectomy and myocardial revascularization was first reported by Bernhard and colleagues in 1972.[54] This procedure was proposed in response to those patients who, having undergone a recent carotid endarterectomy, developed unstable angina or an acute myocardial infarction in the early postoperative period, or those patients with known significant carotid disease who developed a perioperative or late stroke following CAB. These results have since been corroborated by several other authors.[10,55,56] However, with close hospital supervision, it is rare for a patient with combined disease, who has just undergone a CEA, to decompensate before urgent or emergent CAB can be safely performed.

During combined CEA–CAB operations, the carotid endarterectomy is performed while the saphenous vein is harvested from the leg; but in unstable patients or those with severe left main coronary stenosis, the median sternotomy is completed in the event that rapid cannulation is necessary for hemodynamic instability. Some surgeons have advocated institution of cardiopulmonary bypass, with the accompanying hypothermia and hemodilution, adding a protective effect during the carotid endarterectomy.[57,58] The use of a internal carotid artery shunt, EEG monitoring, and vein or Gortex patch angioplasty of the carotid artery is left to the discretion of the individual surgeons. To minimize bleeding complications, the cervical incision is reapproximated following closure of the sternotomy. An algorithm for patients with combined carotid and coronary disease is presented in Figure 127–3.

Patients with significant coexistent carotid and coronary artery disease represent a higher risk population than those patients with isolated carotid or coronary atherosclerosis. These patients have an increased incidence of left main coronary artery disease,[10,59] hypertension,[43] diabetes,[43] history of smoking,[43] impaired left ventricular function,[60] multivessel coronary disease,[60] and female gender.[60] The pathogenesis of atherosclerosis requires a high index of suspicion for combined coronary and carotid artery disease. Selecting the appropriate operative strategy will

help minimize postoperative morbidity and mortality. A staged operation may be safely performed in which the most symptomatic subsystem is the first to be corrected; nonetheless, in those patients with both neurologic and cardiac instability, a combined CEA–CAB can be undertaken with equally satisfactory results.

REFERENCES

1. Hoyert DL, Hudson BL: Advance report of final mortality statistics, 1991. *National Center for Health Statistics. Monthly Vital Statistics Report* **42**(2):1–61, 1993
2. Faggioli GL, Curl GR, Ricotta JJ: The role of carotid screening before coronary artery bypass. *J Vasc Surg* **12**:724–731, 1990
3. Barnes RW, Nix ML, Sansonetti D, et al: Late outcome of untreated asymptomatic carotid disease following cardiovascular operations. *J Vasc Surg* **2**:843–849, 1985
4. Hertzer NR, Loop FD, Beven EG, et al: Surgical staging for simultaneous coronary and carotid disease: A study including prospective randomization. *J Vasc Surg* **9**:455–463, 1989
5. Loop FD, Lyte BW, Cosgrove DM, et al: Coronary artery bypass graft surgery in the elderly: Indications and outcome. *Cleve Clin J Med* **55**:23–34, 1988
6. Gardner TJ, Horneffer PJ, Manolio TA, et al: Major stroke after coronary artery bypass surgery: Changing magnitude of the problem. *J Vasc Surg* **3**:684–694, 1986
7. Reed GL, Singer DE, Picard EH, DeSanctis RW: Stroke following coronary artery bypass surgery: A case control estimate of the risk from carotid bruits. *N Engl J Med* **319**:1246–1250, 1988
8. Davila-Roman VG, Barzilai B, Wareing TH, et al: Intraoperative ultrasonographic evaluation of the ascending aorta in 100 consecutive patients undergoing cardiac surgery. *Circulation* **84**:III 47–53, 1991
9. Brener BJ, Brief DK, Alpert J, et al: The risk of stroke in patients with asymptomatic carotid stenosis undergoing cardiac surgery: A follow up study. *J Vasc Surg* **5**:269–279, 1987
10. Mehigan JT, Buch WS, Pipkin RD, Fogarty TJ: A planned approach to coexistent cerebrovascular disease in coronary artery bypass candidates. *Arch Surg* **112**:1403–1409, 1977
11. Ennix CL Jr, Lawrie GM, Morris GC Jr, et al: Improved results of carotid endarterectomy in patients with symptomatic coronary disease: An analysis of 1,546 consecutive carotid operations. *Stroke* **10**:122–125, 1979
12. Thompson JE, Patman RD, Talkington CM: Asymptomatic carotid bruit: Long term outcome of patients having endarterectomy compared with unoperated controls. *Ann Surg* **188**:308–316, 1978
13. Heyman A, Wilkinson WE, Heyden S, et al: Risk of stroke in asymptomatic persons with cervical bruits: A population study in Evans County, Georgia. *N Engl J Med* **302**:838–841, 1980
14. Mattos MA, Hodgson KJ, Londrey GL, et al: Carotid endarterectomy: Operative risks, recurrent stenosis, and long term stroke rates in a modern series. *J Cardiovasc Surg* **33**:387–400, 1992

15. Hertzer NR, Loop FD, Taylor PC, Beven EG: Staged and combined surgical approach to simultaneous carotid and coronary vascular disease. *Surgery* **84:**803–811, 1978

16. Okies JE, MacManus Q, Starr A: Myocardial revascularization and carotid endarterectomy: A combined approach. *Ann Thor Surg* **23:**560–563, 1977

17. Thompson JE, Austin DJ, Patman RD: Carotid endarterectomy for cerebrovascular insufficiency: Long term results in 592 patients followed up to thirteen years. *Ann Surg* **172:**663–679, 1970

18. Sundt TM, Sandok BA, Whisnant JP: Carotid endarterectomy: Complications and preoperative assessment of risk. *Mayo Clin Proc* **50:**301–306, 1975

19. Hertzer NR, Lees DC: Fatal myocardial infarction following carotid endarterectomy: Three hundred thirty-five patients followed 6–11 years after operation. *Ann Surg* **194:**212–218, 1981

20. Thompson JE, Talkington CM: Carotid endarterectomy. *Ann Surg* **184:**1–15, 1976

21. Nunn DB: Carotid endarterectomy: An analysis of 234 operative cases. *Ann Surg* **182:**733–738, 1975

22. Hart RG, Easton JD: Management of cervical bruits and carotid stenosis in preoperative patients. *Stroke* **14:**290–297, 1983

23. Barnes RW, Marszalek PB: Asymptomatic carotid disease in the cardiovascular surgical patient: Is prophylactic endarterectomy necessary? *Stroke* **12:**497–500, 1981

24. Roederer GO, Langlois YE, Jager KA, et al: The natural history of carotid arterial disease in asymptomatic patients with cervical bruits. *Stroke* **15:**605–613, 1984

25. Sauve JS, Thorpe KE, Sackett DL, et al: Can bruits distinguish high-grade from moderate symptomatic carotid stenosis? *Ann Intern Med* **120:**633–637, 1994

26. North American Symptomatic Carotid Endarterectomy Trial Collaborators (NASCET): Beneficial effect of carotid endarterectomy in symptomatic patients with high-grade carotid stenosis. *N Engl J Med* **325:**445–453, 1991

27. European Carotid Surgery Trialists' Collaborative Group: MRC European Carotid Surgery Trail: Interim results for symptomatic patients with severe (70–99%) or mild (0–29%) carotid stenosis. *Lancet* **337:**1235–1243, 1991

28. Lundar T, Lindegaard KF, Froysaker T, et al: Dissociation between cerebral autoregulation and carbon dioxide reactivity during nonpulsatile cardiopulmonary bypass. *Ann Thorac Surg* **40:**582–587, 1985

29. Archie JP Jr, Feldtman RW: Critical stenosis of the internal carotid artery. *Surgery* **89:**67–72, 1981

30. DeWeese JA, May AG, Lipchik EO, Rob CG: Anatomic and hemodynamic correlations in carotid artery stenosis. *Stroke* **1:**149–157, 1970

31. Lazorthes G, Gouaze A, Salamon G: *Vascularisation et circulation de l'encephale*, Vols I, II. Paris, Masson Editeur, 1978

32. Jones EL, Craver JM, Michalik RA, et al: Combined carotid and coronary operations: When are they necessary? *J Thorac Cardiovasc Surg* **87:**7–16, 1984

33. Wareing TH, Davila-Roman VG, Daily BB, et al: Strategy for the reduction of stroke incidence in cardiac surgical patients. *Ann Thorac Surg* **55:**1400–1408, 1993

34. Amarenco P, Duyckaerts C, Tzourid C, et al: The prevalence of ulcerated plaques in the aortic arch in patients with stroke. *N Engl J Med* **326:**221–225, 1992

35. Mills NL, Everson CT: Atherosclerosis of the ascending aorta and coronary artery bypass: Pathology, clinical correlates and operative management. *J Thorac Cardiovasc Surg* **102:**546–553, 1991

36. Ohteki H, Tsuyoshi I, Natsuaki M, et al: Intraoperative ultrasonic imaging of the ascending aorta in ischemic heart disease. *Ann Thorac Surg* **50:**539–542, 1990

37. Tobler HG, Edwards JE: Frequency and location of atherosclerotic plaques in the ascending aorta. *J Thorac Cardiovasc Surg* **96:**304–306, 1988

38. Gardner TJ, Horneffer PJ, Manolio TA, et al: Stroke following coronary artery bypass grafting: A ten-year study. *Ann Thorac Surg* **40:**574–81, 1985

39. Blauth CI, Cosgrove DM, Webb BW, et al: Atheroembolism from the ascending aorta. *J Thorac Cardiovasc Surg* **103:**1104–1112, 1992

40. Marshall WG Jr, Barzilai B, Kouchoukos NT: Intraoperative ultrasonic imaging of the ascending aorta. *Ann Thorac Surg* **48:**339–344, 1989

41. Barzilai B, Saffitz JE, Miller JG, Sobel BE: Quantitative ultrasonic characterization of the nature of atherosclerotic plaques in human aorta. *Circ Res* **60:**459–463, 1987

42. Wareing TH, Davila-Roman VG, Barzilai B, et al: Management of the severely atherosclerotic ascending aorta during cardiac operations: A strategy for detection and treatment. *J Thorac Cardiovasc Surg* **103:**453–462, 1992

43. Vermeulen FEE, Hamerlijnck RPHM, DeFaux JJAM, Ernest SMPG: Synchronous operation for ischemic cardiac and cerebrovascular disease: Early results and long term follow-up. *Ann Thorac Surg* **53:**381–390, 1992

44. Rizzo RJ, Whittemore AD, Couper GS, et al: Combined carotid and coronary revascularization: The preferred approach to the severe vasculopath. *Ann Thorac Surg* **54:**1099–1109, 1992

45. Gerraty RP, Gates PC, Doyle JC: Carotid stenosis and perioperative stroke risk in symptomatic and asymptomatic patients undergoing vascular or coronary surgery. *Stroke* **24:**1115–1118, 1993

46. Barnes RW: Asymptomatic carotid disease in patients undergoing major cardiovascular operations: Can prophylactic endarterectomy be justified? *Ann Thorac Surg* **42:**S36–40, 1986(Suppl)

47. Ivey TD, Strandness DE Jr, Williams DB, et al: Management of patients with carotid bruit undergoing cardiopulmonary bypass. *J Thorac Cardiovasc Surg* **87:**183–189, 1984

48. Breslau PJ, Fell G, Ivey TD, et al: Carotid arterial disease in patients undergoing coronary artery bypass operations. *J Thorac Cardiovasc Surg* **82:**765–767, 1981

49. Turnipseed WD, Berkoff HA, Belzer RO: Postoperative stroke in cardiac and peripheral vascular disease. *Ann Surg* **192:**365–368, 1980

50. Anderson RJ, Hobson RW, Padberg FT, et al: Carotid endarterectomy for asymptomatic carotid stenosis: A ten year experience with 120 procedures in a fellowship training program. *Ann Vasc Surg* **5:**111–115, 1991

51. Moneta GL, Taylor DC, Nicholls SC, et al: Operative versus nonoperative management of asymptomatic high-grade internal carotid artery stenosis: Improved results with endarterectomy. *Stroke* **18:**1005–1010, 1987

52. Hertzer NR, Flanagan RA Jr, O'Hara PJ, Beven EG: Surgical versus nonoperative treatment of symptomatic carotid stenosis: 211 patients documented by intravenous angiography. *Ann Surg* **204:**154–162, 1986

53. Moore DJ, Miles RD, Gooley NA, Summer DS: Noninvasive assessment of stroke risk in asymptomatic and nonhemispheric patients with suspected carotid disease: Five-year follow-up of 294 unoperated and 81 operated patients. *Ann Surg* **202:**491–504, 1985

54. Bernhard VM, Johnson WD, Peterson JJ: Carotid artery stenosis: Association with surgery for coronary artery disease. *Arch Surg* **105:**837–840, 1972

55. Morris GC, Ennix CL, Lawrie GM, et al: Management of coexistent carotid and coronary artery occlusive atherosclerosis. *Cleve Clin Q* **45:**125–127, 1978

56. Urschel HC, Razzuk MA, Gardner MA: Management of concomitant occlusive disease of the carotid and coronary arteries. *J Thorac Cardiovasc Surg* **72:**829–834, 1976

57. Minami K, Sagoo KS, Breymann T, et al: Operative strategy in combined coronary and carotid artery disease. *J Thorac Cardiovasc Surg* **95:**303–309, 1988

58. Kouchoukos NT, Daily BB, Wareing TH, Murphy SF: Hypothermic circulatory arrest for cerebral protection during combined carotid and

cardiac surgery in patients with bilateral carotid artery disease. *Ann Surg* **219:**699–706, 1994

59. Schwartz RL, Garrett JR, Karp RB, Kouchoukos NT: Simultaneous myocardial revascularization and carotid endarterectomy. *Circulation* **66**(Pt 2):I97–101, 1982

60. Hertzer NR, Loop FD, Taylor PC, Beven EG: Combined myocardial revascularization and carotid endarterectomy: Operative and late results in 331 patients. *J Thorac Cardiovasc Surg* **85:**577–589, 1983

128

Cardiogenic Shock Secondary to Myocardial Infarction

K. Francis Lee and Andrew S. Wechsler

INTRODUCTION

Since the introduction of coronary intensive care units over 30 years ago,[1,2] efforts to reduce ischemia in acute myocardial infarction have led to improved survival and quality of life for most patients. However, a subset of patients still develops profound cardiac failure and face a grim prognosis. The incidence of cardiogenic shock complicating acute myocardial infarction (AMI) ranges from 5 to 15% in most studies,[3–8] and the rate has not varied significantly over the past two decades.[9] A multivariate analysis from the Multicenter Investigation of Limitation of Infarct Size (MILIS) study has shown that independent predictors for developing cardiogenic shock are old age (>65 years), low left ventricular ejection fraction at admission (<35%), large infarct size as determined by serial isoenzyme levels (peak CPK-MB >160 IU/L), history of diabetes mellitus, and previous myocardial infarction.[7] The incidence of cardiogenic shock in AMI is much greater among patients with a previous history of heart failure. Prior history of stroke and peripheral vascular disease have also been reported as independent predictors of developing cardiogenic shock.[8]

Whereas the overall mortality from AMI has decreased from 30 to 40% to 5 to 10% in the last three decades, the in-hospital mortality from cardiogenic shock with conservative medical management has remained fairly high, ranging from 80 to 100%.[3–6] The risk of mortality increases 15-fold when a patient in acute myocardial infarction develops cardiogenic shock,[7] and, in fact, cardiogenic shock is the leading cause of in-hospital death in acute myocardial infarction. The average time from admission to the development of cardiogenic shock is 3 to 4 days, although one-third to one-half of the patients develop the syndrome within the first 24 hours.[7,8] The cause may be a single, large myocardial infarction leading to immediate shock, or repetitive episodes of ischemia deteriorating to a low-output state. The latter form may be due to multivessel coronary artery disease including the left anterior descending coronary artery.[4,10,11]

Although precise mechanisms for development of cardiogenic shock may still be elusive, there is growing evidence that favorable clinical outcome may be contingent upon patency of the infarct-related coronary artery. A retrospective analysis from Duke University reported an in-hospital mortality rate of only 53% among patients in cardiogenic shock.[12] With an aggressive reperfusion strategy consisting of pharmacologic thrombolysis, angioplasty, and coronary bypass surgery, the authors discovered that the mortality rates among patients with patent vs. closed infarct-related arteries were 33 vs. 75%, respectively.[12] Others have reported mortality rates as low as 27 and 41% using thrombolytic therapy and angioplasty in such patients.[13,14] Some postulate that early intervention focusing on patent infarct-related vessels may reduce the incidence of cardiogenic shock with AMI.[15]

The prognosis for patients in cardiogenic shock is mostly dependent upon the extent of left ventricular injury and dysfunction.[7,12] The cornerstone of management is myocardial protection and early reperfusion of the ischemic zone. The coming decade will see growth of clinical investigation in this area. Both cardiac surgeons and interventional cardiologists will have a number of therapeutic modalities at their disposal. Success will depend upon the pathophysiology, patient selection, and rationale behind each therapeutic modality. This chapter focuses on cardiogenic shock secondary to primary pump failure following myocardial infarction. Cardiogenic shock with mechanical complications—mitral regurgitation, ventricular septal defect, left ventricular aneurysm, free wall rupture and pseudoaneurysm—are reviewed elsewhere (see Chapters 118, 129, and 130).

PATHOPHYSIOLOGY

The definition of cardiogenic shock has not changed much from Killip and Kimball's original classification of patients in extreme heart failure.[3] According to the Myocardial Infarction Research Units of the National Heart and Lung Institute,[16] the cardinal manifestations of cardiogenic shock, or Killip Class IV acute heart failure, are (1) hypotension, i.e., systolic blood pressure of less than 90 mm Hg or 30 mm Hg below the previous basal level, and (2) evidence of reduced bloodflow as shown by all three signs—oliguria (urine output <20 mL/h), impaired mental function, and peripheral vasoconstriction associated with cold, clammy skin.[3,16-18] The hemodynamic measurements by Swan–Ganz monitoring typically reveal a low cardiac index (<1.8–2.0 L/min per m²), elevated left ventricular filling pressure (mean pulmonary capillary wedge pressure >18 mm Hg), increased systemic vascular resistance (>30 Wood units), and tachycardia.[16]

Traditional teaching has been that cardiogenic shock occurs when greater than 40% of the left ventricle is infarcted. A postmortem analysis reported that left ventricular damage was 51% (range 35 to 68%) among patients who died in cardiogenic shock, compared to only 23% (range 14 to 31%) among those who died due to other complications of acute myocardial infarction.[19] In another report, all 20 patients who died in cardiogenic shock—and only one of 14 without shock—had greater than 40% left ventricular infarction.[20] These clinicopathologic results appeared to correlate with the laboratory data. In hemodynamic studies of rats 3 weeks after left coronary artery occlusion, animals with greater than 46% left ventricular infarctions developed congestive heart failure, whereas those with 4 to 30% infarctions showed no discernible hemodynamic impairment.[21] These data have been widely embraced on conceptual grounds that small infarcts may lead to compensatory mechanisms, e.g., increased sympathoadrenal activity, increased left ventricular end-diastolic volume, and hyperfunctioning of the noninfarcted, normally perfused remote myocardial segments,[22] that may allow the injured heart to produce adequate output and avoid end-organ failure.

Infarcted and ischemic myocardial segments have been noted to stretch and lengthen in the immediate postinfarction phase, producing what has been called "infarct expansion."[23,24] This contributes to left ventricular enlargement, remodeling of left ventricular geometry, and increased wall stress.[23] Larger infarcts, however, may lead to failure of the above mechanisms. With a 40% infarct, for example, afterload mismatch develops in which compliance

of the left ventricular cavity and contractility decrease acutely to such an extent that cardiac output is not adequate, especially when catecholamine-induced vasoconstriction and increased systemic vascular resistance are present.[16,22,25,26] Acute end-organ hypoperfusion then leads to cardiogenic shock.

Cardiogenic shock may develop with infarct sizes less than 40% of the left ventricle.[27-29] In a postmortem, quantitative analysis of 20 patients with cardiogenic shock, infarcted left ventricular mass ranged from 24 to 72%, and 7 of 20 patients showed infarct sizes less than 40%.[28] Others have shown that 50% of patients who died with cardiogenic shock had an average infarct size of 19% only in the subendocardium.[27] These findings may be explained by the fact that hypofunction of the left ventricle may be due to large areas of ischemic, noncontractile but viable myocardium, which do not stain necrotic in the postmortem studies. An area of infarcted myocardium typically is surrounded by a concentric ring or "ischemic border zone," which shows profound systolic and diastolic dysfunction that may recover in time with reperfusion.[22] An acute occlusion of one coronary artery could lead to a large ischemic area of myocardium supplied by another coronary artery if the latter were significantly stenotic and dependent on collateral bloodflow from the first coronary artery. So-called ischemia at a distance (or ischemia of the remote myocardium) was involved in 40% of deaths from acute myocardial infarction according to one retrospective study.[30] While the postmortem study showed small infarct sizes, perfusion of significant areas of myocardium was angiographically demonstrated to be dependent upon the collateral bloodflow from the infarct-related coronary artery.

Mechanisms such as ischemic border zone and ischemia of the remote myocardium lead to the strategy of myocardial salvage for cardiogenic shock. The initial infarction may be small but hypocontractility of the ischemic zone may lead to a low-output state, hypotension, low coronary perfusion, increased preload and afterload, and, ultimately, unfavorable imbalance of myocardial oxygen supply and demand. The nonviable area may increase in size with further hypofunction of the left ventricle producing a vicious cycle of myocardial ischemia, infarct extension, and deterioration.[23] Attempts at improving hemodynamics and decreasing myocardial oxygen debt may only temporize this vicious cycle. Thus an ischemic insult causing cardiogenic shock usually is not reversed with conservative management alone. The prognosis of cardiogenic shock is not altered by pharmacologic treatment and an intraaortic balloon pump.

Rescue of myocardium at risk requires timely reperfusion of the ischemic zone. Experimental data have shown a "wavefront phenomenon" of myocardial cell death with increasing duration of coronary occlusion.[31] This begins in the subendocardial myocardium and progresses toward the subepicardial myocardium in a concentric, outward fashion. In dogs, transmural necrosis was 38% after 40 min of coronary occlusion, 57% after 3 hours, 71% after 6 hours, and 85% after 24 hours.[31] This suggests the presence of a subepicardial zone of ischemic but viable myocardium that may be rescued by angioplasty or surgery, preferably within less than 6 hours from the onset of ischemia.[31] Thus an early reperfusion strategy might be lifesaving for patients developing cardiogenic shock within a few hours after a myocardial infarction. For patients with multivessel disease who develop late cardiogenic shock due to stuttering myocardial necrosis, the optimal timing of intervention is less clear. Because the risk of infarct extension is higher among patients with recurrent ischemic pain, aggressive attempts to revascularize ischemic myocardium at any point during the hospital course may be important.[33,34]

MANAGEMENT OF CARDIOGENIC SHOCK

General Consideration

All patients in cardiogenic shock require invasive hemodynamic monitoring because estimates of changes in volume status and cardiac output can be erroneous up to 30% of the time.[35] Knowledge of hemodynamic subsets is critical in titrating inotropic agents, initiating an intraaortic balloon pump, and predicting mortality.[36,37] Monitoring should include a flow-directed Swan-Ganz pulmonary artery catheter, a pulse oximeter, an arterial line, EKG leads, and a urinary catheter.[18] Relative hypovolemia is present in as many as 20% of patients in cardiogenic shock,[38] and fluid should be administered to raise pulmonary capillary wedge pressure. Graded fluid boluses during measurement of Frank–Starling curves of preload vs. cardiac output will indicate optimal filling pressure.[38] Heart block and arrhythmias require treatment because they can cause up to 40% of postinfarction deaths.[2] Arterial hypoxemia complicated by systemic hypotension or acidosis may limit cardiac function. Endotracheal intubation should not be delayed in patients whose mental status is deteriorating, or with moderate to severe hypoxemia, acid–base disturbances, or other signs of end-organ hypoperfusion. Lastly, patients in cardiogenic shock are frequently apprehensive, frightened, and in considerable pain; comfort measures, pain medication, and verbal reassurance are important.[38]

Pharmacologic Therapy

The goal of pharmacotherapy is to optimize myocardial oxygen consumption and supply. Vasodilators should be used to decrease systemic vascular resistance when blood pressure permits. Arterial hypotension from relative hypovolemia jeopardizes coronary perfusion; therefore, intravenous fluid should be administered to ensure adequate intravascular volume and left ventricular preload prior to vasodilator therapy. *Nitroglycerin* causes relaxation of vascular smooth muscle, resulting in generalized vasodilation

greater on venous capacitance vessels than on arteriolar resistance vessels. The drug also causes dilation of collateral coronary vessels and beneficial redistribution of bloodflow to ischemic myocardium. Its efficacy in the treatment of angina pectoris is well established. Although nitroglycerin can be used at high doses to achieve systemic vasodilation, *nitroprusside* is more often used to lower arteriolar resistance. By lowering the afterload in heart failure, nitroprusside increases the stroke volume and cardiac index while decreasing myocardial oxygen consumption. Cyanogen (cyanide radical) and thiocyanate toxicities are rare side-effects of nitroprusside manifested by an elevated cyanogen level, metabolic acidosis, or marked clinical deterioration. The drug is stopped and nitrites given to form methemoglobin, an important step in the breakdown of cyanogen.[39]

Inotropic agents are commonly used to increase myocardial contractility, stroke work, and arterial blood pressure. There has been debate as to whether these effects may increase myocardial oxygen consumption with ischemia. However, an inotropic agent such as epinephrine decreases myocardial oxygen consumption in the failing heart. It may favorably alter ventricular dimensions in the dilated, failing heart, restoring the normal ellipsoidal configuration and lowering systolic wall stress.[40,41] Left ventricular wall stress is the primary determinant of myocardial oxygen consumption in an epinephrine-treated heart rather than stroke work or cardiac output.[40] *Dopamine* is an immediate precursor of norepinephrine, and its benefit in cardiogenic shock is derived from its direct effect on the β_1-adrenergic receptors in moderate dose of 3 to 10 μg/kg per minute. It increases cardiac output, blood pressure, and urine output. In high dose, >10 μg/kg per minute, it also has α-adrenergic effects, while in low dose of 0.5 to 3 μg/kg per minute, it acts on specific dopaminergic receptors in the renal, mesenteric, coronary, and intracerebral circulation to cause vasodilation. The net hemodynamic effects of moderate-dose dopamine make the drug particularly useful in patients with mild hypotension, low cardiac output, and refractory oliguria. Ectopic heartbeats and conduction abnormalities are important side effects of the drug. *Dobutamine* is a selective agonist on the β-adrenergic receptors, stimulating adenyl cyclase activity and increasing intramyocardial cyclic adenosine monophosphate (cAMP) level. Augmentation of contractility and lowering of peripheral resistance make it the preferred inotrope for cardiogenic shock with acute myocardial infarction. Although dobutamine may cause a slight increase in myocardial oxygen consumption, it increases cardiac output without increasing infarct size or causing malignant cardiac arrhythmias.[38]

A new class of cardiotonic drugs is specific phosphodiesterase inhibitors (*amrinone, milrinone, enoximone,* and *pimobendan*). By blocking the breakdown of cAMP, they may enhance the effects of dobutamine.[42] Their positive inotropic action is also associated with increased cAMP levels in vascular smooth muscle, causing vasodilatory effects on the peripheral circulation. Both amrinone and milrinone are helpful for congestive heart failure.[39,42] Their role in cardiogenic shock continues to evolve. *Norepinephrine* and *epinephrine* are classic catecholamines that effect both the α- and the β-adrenergic receptors. They are reserved for patients with severe cardiogenic shock refractory to other inotropes. Their use should suggest the need for intraaortic balloon counterpulsation.

Intraaortic Balloon Counterpulsation (IABC)

IABC can rapidly stabilize patients whose cardiogenic shock is refractory to initial measures. IABC is instituted usually within 9 to 24 hours following the onset of shock symptoms,[43–45] with maximal benefit generally derived within 24 to 48 hours of circulatory support.[43,44,46] Cardiac output typically increases by 10 to 20%, mean arterial blood pressure is raised by 10 to 20%, heart rate shows a mild slowing, and pulmonary capillary wedge pressure decreases by 20 to 30%.[43–46] Improved end-organ perfusion is manifested by increased urine output and mixed venous oxygen saturation. These hemodynamic changes are due to reduced afterload during systole and augmented coronary perfusion during diastole. IABC is particularly helpful for cardiogenic shock with mechanical complications, e.g., mitral regurgitation and ventricular septal defect.

The efficacy of IABC in cardiogenic shock is well documented. However, in-hospital mortality on IABC alone remains high and many patients cannot be weaned successfully. IABC and pharmacotherapy can optimize clinical variables and restore a favorable balance between myocardial oxygen supply and demand; they cannot reestablish blood flow through the infarct-related coronary artery or salvage areas of ischemic but viable myocardium. Thus, long-term survival among cardiogenic shock patients is less on IABC alone, vis-à-vis that of patients on IABC with revascularization of the infarct-related artery.[43,45] In 40 patients treated only with an IABC, long-term survival was 47.3% but 71.4% survived who also had emergent surgical revascularization in addition to the IABC.[45] In-hospital deaths were 25 and 71% in patients who were revascularized within 16 hours or beyond 16 hours. An early IABC and revascularization have shown favorable results in patients with complicated acute myocardial infarction.[47,48] Thus an IABC alone cannot reverse cardiogenic shock, and the major determinant of survival is in supplying blood to the ischemic, but viable, myocardium.

Thrombolytic Therapy

In an uncomplicated acute myocardial infarction, early thrombolysis reduces infarct size, preserves left ventricular function, and increases survival.[49] Data are lacking, however, to show that thrombolytic therapy improves outcome of patients in cardiogenic shock. Only a few of the 92 thrombolytic therapy trials reported as of January 1994 have adequate data on efficacy in patients in cardiogenic shock.[50] In a study in Italy, in-hospital mortality rates in Killip Class IV patients with streptokinase vs. placebo treatments were 69.9 and 70.1%, respectively.[51] An earlier clinical trial in 1971 also showed that streptokinase therapy did not improve mortality, and data from the International Study on Infarct Size (ISSI) in 1990 showed no difference in outcome between streptokinase and recombinant tissue plasminogen activator in cardiogenic shock patients.[52,53]

It has been postulated that cardiogenic shock has physiologic and metabolic features that limit the efficacy of thrombolytic agents. Effective thrombolytic therapy appears to require adequate cardiac output.[54] In a low-flow state, decreased transport and slowed delivery of fibrinolytic agents to an occlusive thrombus may diminish the thrombolytic potential. Also, in a relatively hypoperfused, acidotic state, alterations in blood pH may adversely affect the conversion of plasminogen to plasmin, impairing both physiologic thromboresistance and thrombolytic efficacy.[55] Improved survival from thrombolytic therapy depends upon early and sustained patency of the infarct-related coronary artery. Hypotension and vasoconstriction in cardiogenic shock may compromise open but stenotic vessels.

These theories have been supported in part by a report in which thrombolytic reperfusion by streptokinase was less likely for patients in cardiogenic shock than for those not in shock, 43 vs. 71%, respectively.[56] When thrombolysis was successful and patency of the artery was maintained, benefit was demonstrated. In 44% of shock patients with successful thrombolytic reperfusion, the mortality rate was only 42%. In the patients with unsuccessful thrombolytic therapy, however, the mortality rate was 84%.[56] Thus current thrombolytic therapy has limited efficacy in patients with cardiogenic shock. However, when lysis is successful, outcome is improved due to patency of the infarct-related artery.

Coronary Angioplasty

There is growing evidence of the efficacy of percutaneous transluminal coronary angioplasty (PTCA) for cardiogenic shock.[57–67] The success rate of reperfusion ranges from 54 to 100% (average, 75%).[66] Mortality rates for successful versus failed angioplasty were 17 to 39% vs. 71 to 93%, respectively.[57–62] These data are impressive, but all of the studies were retrospective analyses, and pertinent questions are unanswered. The number of patients per study is typically small, ranging from 7 to 69 patients,[57–66] they lack control groups, and their objectives were to compare outcomes of patients retrospectively identified as angioplasty failures or successes. Characteristics inherently different between the two groups may influence outcome and lead to an overestimate of true efficacy. For example, in a multicenter registry analysis, the preprocedural cardiac indices of failed vs. successful angioplasty patients were 1.8 ± 0.5 vs. 2.2 ± 0.6 L/min per m^2, respectively.[61] The difference was reported as statistically insignificant, but the small size of the unmatched groups, 20 vs. 49 patients, raises the question of a Type II statistical error.

Inclusion and exclusion criteria also have not been well documented, and indications for angioplasty are largely undefined. The high success rate of reperfusion is based on patients with favorable coronary anatomy as determined by the angiographer. Data on patients in cardiogenic shock not eligible for angioplasty but amenable to surgical bypass are usually absent. In one study, patients on whom angioplasty was not attempted had a 30-day survival rate of 14%, which was higher than patients with failed angioplasty, 7%.[62] The lower survival of failed angioplasty patients compared to those excluded from angioplasty may be due to complications of the procedure.

Major complications from angioplasty include stroke (0.5%), bleeding (2.8%), and early reocclusion of the infarct vessel with or without acute cardiopulmonary collapse (13%).[63] Technical complications such as acute occlusion, dissection, or perforation of a coronary vessel occur in about 5%.[69] Eccentric, nondiscrete, and >90% stenotic coronary lesions have a greater chance of failing angioplasty and requiring emergent coronary bypass.[70,71] Risks of a contrast medium load on marginally perfused kidneys should also be considered. Without detailed knowledge of why angioplasty was performed on some patients but not others, risk–benefit data are difficult to interpret. The additive risk of performing the procedure in cardiogenic shock is unknown.

Patients in some of the studies had rescue angioplasty after failed thrombolytic therapy rather than angioplasty as primary therapy. Thrombolytic therapy may complicate angioplasty by increasing hemorrhage at the site of vascular access, at remote sites (brain or intestinal tract) or at a traumatized coronary placque or ulcer.[63] Patients in cardiogenic shock after failed thrombolysis have a lower patency with angioplasty than those who undergo primary angioplasty.[65] Since over half of patients with acute myocardial infarction are not candidates for thrombolysis, direct angioplasty may be more applicable than previously thought.[72]

Direct angioplasty may be particularly helpful in patients with prior bypass surgery. Occlusion of a bypass graft is involved in 76% of acute myocardial infarctions in patients after bypass surgery.[63,68] The morbidity and mortality of re-do bypass surgery in acute cardiogenic shock may be prohibitive. O'Keefe et al reported that angioplasty can successfully recanalize acutely occluded vein grafts in 86% of cases.[63] In comparison, thrombolytic therapy produced successful reperfusion of an occluded graft in only 25%.

The long-term reocclusion rate of percutaneously dilated coronary arteries in cardiogenic shock is not known. In three retrospective studies, survival after hospital discharge ranged from 80 to 92% with mean follow-up of 12 to 32 months.[60,61,69] Hibbard et al reported that 80% of late deaths occurred in patients with three-vessel disease and low ejection fractions. They suggest that consideration be given to surgical revascularization before discharge.[60] Lee et al reported that two-thirds of patients who died despite successful angioplasty had multivessel disease.[61] If these patients were inadequately revascularized, they could have done better with surgical bypass. Mean follow-up of 1 to 3 years is hardly adequate and the 5- and 10-year reocclusion rate is unknown. The role of follow-up catheterization and bypass surgery with a myocardial infarction and cardiogenic shock must also be determined.

SURGICAL REVASCULARIZATION

Preoperative Considerations

The indication for operation in patients with cardiogenic shock is the presence of bypassable arteries with significant proximal stenosis leading to the area of ischemia.[73] Surgery is indicated especially with multivessel disease. Between 80 and 90% of deaths after angioplasty for cardiogenic shock occur in patients with multivessel disease.[60,61] Angioplasty for cardiogenic shock is associated with 31% mortality with single vessel disease, whereas multivessel disease increases mortality twofold.[61] The high failure rate of angioplasty and attendant mortality of cardiogenic shock with multivessel coronary disease indicate treatment by operation. This approach was evident in a retrospective multicenter study, in which patients with three-vessel disease had twice the likelihood of being treated by surgery than those with single-vessel coronary disease.[74] Surgical patients underwent an average of 2.3 bypass grafts per procedure, but angioplasty tended to involve only the infarct-related coronary vessel.[74] A bypass should provide more complete revascularization than angioplasty. In the NHLBI PTCA registry, angioplasty failure requiring emergent surgery was correlated with eccentric coronary lesions.[71] Thus adverse appearances of coronary lesions should influence the decision for surgery. Relative benefits of operation versus angioplasty in cardiogenic shock are not known, calling for prospective randomized trials.[75]

Cardiogenic shock after PTCA failure requires surgical intervention. Indications for emergency operation after PTCA include coronary dissection or occlusion, coronary spasm, prolonged angina, and myocardial infarction.[71] Class IV angina, three-vessel disease, urgent angioplasty, and failed LAD dilatation are risk factors for cardiogenic shock or cardiac arrest after PTCA.[76] In retrospective clinical series, approximately 3 to 5% of all patients undergoing PTCA developed complications and required emergent surgery.[70,76–79] About 25% of these patients arrived in the operating room in either cardiogenic shock or cardiopulmonary arrest.[73,76,77] Most patients were already on IABC and inotropic support. If available, circulatory assist devices were utilized on the way to the operating room: hemopump, percutaneous cardiopulmonary bypass, or percutaneous left heart bypass.[62,80] These patients were gravely ill because emergency surgery following failed angioplasty had a mortality rate of about 10% (range 2.6 to 19%). Most deaths occurred in patients with preoperative cardiogenic shock.[70,76–79] Survival depended upon prompt reversal of myocardial ischemia and salvage from myocardial infarction. In keeping with this, the time from onset of ischemia during angioplasty to bypass was an independent predictor of perioperative myocardial necrosis.[79]

In AMI with shock, the strategy to delay surgery to "stabilize the patient" is not warranted, and earliest possible reperfusion is crucial to increasing survival. In acute myocardial ischemia after failed angioplasty, operation is typically performed within 140 to 180 min.[70,73,77,81] Klepzig and associates reported that the duration of postangioplasty ischemic time correlated with the surgical outcome. The ischemic times of survivors with no or small perioperative infarct, and survivors and nonsurvivors of large perioperative infarct were 179 ± 80, 231 ± 87, and 273 ± 161 min, respectively.[79] Early surgery (<3 hours) in acute myocardial infarction was associated with smaller thallium defects and higher ejection fraction of the involved segments than controls in postoperative period.[81] The late surgical group (>3 hours) showed irreversible mitochondrial damage and cell membrane rupture of the ischemic myocardium, compared to a reversible histologic picture in the early surgical group.

In uncomplicated AMI, six hours from the onset of symptoms to surgical revascularization has been considered the time beyond which there is little reduction in the size of myocardial necrosis.[82,83] Surgery performed within 6 hours of the onset of symptoms was associated with increased preservation of left ventricular function and long-term survival.[82–87] In AMI and cardiogenic shock, however, infarct extension into the ischemic border zone and collateral-dependent ischemic area appears to continue for a considerably longer period, and operation well beyond 6 hours has been beneficial. Emergency bypass in cardiogenic shock after almost 7 hours of ischemic time resulted in a low mortality rate of 12%.[73] Both Dewood and co-workers and Allen and associates reported that surgical reperfusion of shock patients with less than 16 to 18 hours ischemic time decreased mortality three- to fivefold.[45,88] Moosvi et al showed that mean ischemic time of survivors of cardiogenic shock was 12.4 ± 15 hours. That of nonsurvivors was 58.5 ± 93 hours.[89] Laks et al reported that 92% of the patients with left ventricular power failure showed reversal of the shock syndrome following surgical revascularization at an average of 4.3 ± 1.0 days after the AMI.[90] Hines and Mohtashemi found that 71% of patients who failed to wean from IABC left the hospital after bypass grafting 8 to 21 days after balloon insertion.[91]

The time to operation and salvage of ischemic but live myocardium, restoring its contractile function, is critical. Diagnostic techniques most commonly used to assess myocardial viability are thallium-201 (^{201}Tl) scintigraphy, positron emission tomography (PET), technetium-99m (^{99m}Tc) sestamibi imaging, and dobutamine echocardiography.[92,93] On stress-^{201}Tl scintigraphy, viable myocardium

is suggested when a region is asynergic with normal thallium uptake, or when a defect in thallium uptake shows redistribution. In resting ^{201}Tl scintigraphy, regional thallium uptake in the infarct zone may correlate with the extent of the viable myocardium. Asyngergic regions with normal thallium uptake suggest postoperative improvement in ejection fraction after operation.[93]

The PET scan is considered by many as the gold standard. Myocardial viability is suggested when perfusion defects show uptake of metabolic tracers such as [1-^{11}C] palmitate for fatty acid metabolism and [^{18}F]fluorodeoxyglucose for glucose utilization.[94] Predictive value of PET scans using [^{18}F]fluorodeoxyglucose has been reported to be between 75 and 85%, and the specificity of the technique has been reported to be as high as 92%.[92,94,95] The PET scan has been helpful in predicting which ischemic patients with severe left ventricular dysfunction may improve cardiac function following operation.[92] ^{201}Tl scintigraphy with reinjection technique and PET scan have been comparable in identifying viable myocardium in patients with left ventricular dysfunction from ischemic cause.[96] Dobutamine-echocardiography is a promising tool more applicable to the bedside of a critically ill patient. Increase of regional wall-thickening in response to dobutamine supposedly detects the presence of viable myocardium in both acute and chronic ischemic myocardial dysfunction.[97] Dobutamine-echocardiography has been compared favorably in preliminary studies with those of resting ^{201}Tl SPECT scintigraphy and PET scan.[97]

These diagnostic techniques may assume a greater role in management of AMI with cardiogenic shock, because in patients surgical or angioplastic revascularization is not cost-effective. Dobutamine-echocardiography may be modified for acute clinical situations. Assessment of salvageable myocardium would separate patients whose severe left ventricular dysfunction would improve with revascularization from those patients whose cardiac impairment has become fixed, or irreversible, despite any reperfusion strategy. This is particularly important in the setting of hibernating myocardium following acute myocardial infarction. Ventricular function may be depressed with stenotic coronary vessels because diminished coronary blood flow may maintain basal cell function and viability, but insufficient to support normal contractile function. Hibernation has been proposed as an adaptive mechanism for ischemic myocardium to maintain viability in an oxygen-debt environment. This may partly explain the chronic low-output state for patients who do not recover fully from cardiogenic shock. Support for this notion comes from reports in which coronary bypass grafting improved left ventricular regional wall-motion abnormalities long after the initial myocardial infarction and the onset of severe cardiac dysfunction occurred.[91,98] When cardiogenic shock follows a large myocardial infarction, careful assessment of myocardial viability is crucial because of the relative importance of the still viable muscle mass. Preservation of every myocardial fibril should contribute directly to long-term survival. On the other hand, in some patients in clinical shock, the risk of perioperative mortality and the absence of viable myocardium in the area of the stenotic coronary vessels should discourage heroic surgical efforts. Using magnetic resonance spectroscopy, we have demonstrated that differentiation among normal, ischemic but viable, and infarcted myocardium is possible in the controlled laboratory setting.[99] Whether the same accuracy can be achieved clinically remains an active area of research.

Perioperative Considerations

Surgical treatment of ischemic cardiogenic shock requires rapid revascularization. Coordination of the catheterization laboratory, operating room, and blood bank should minimize wasted time and efforts. IABC is preferable to the overusage of inotropic and vasoconstrictive drugs to achieve hemodynamic stability. Antegrade bloodflow can be provided with variable success by placing a "bailout catheter" with multiple proximal and distal sideholes across a stenotic coronary artery.[80] Intraoperatively, these catheters can deliver cardioplegia to the ischemic myocardium. When a coronary artery is completely occluded and does not allow the passage of a catheter, alternative techniques include synchronized retrograde perfusion and pressure-controlled intermittent coronary sinus occlusion. These methods increase bloodflow to the jeopardized myocardium via the coronary sinus, and, in recent years, have gained renewed interest and utilization.[80]

With cardiovascular collapse, percutaneous bypass can provide circulatory support on the way to the operating room. Cannulating the femoral artery and vein for inflow and outflow, one can achieve flow rates of 3.5 to 5.0 L/min[80] and support patients in cardiac arrest. This technique has had acceptable clinical results when the arrest occurs in the catherization laboratory and percutaneous bypass is achieved within 20 min.[80] The Nimbus hemopump withdraws blood from the left ventricle and pumps nonpulsatile blood to the descending aorta. Flow rates of up to 3.5 L/min can be achieved with this technique. Time should not be wasted attempting to institute these devices. Expeditious transport to the operating room is critical.

In the operating room, cardiopulmonary bypass should be established as quickly as possible, and saphenous veins should be harvested with equal speed. Some authors report that use of the internal mammary artery (IMA) is safe in the absence of hemodynamic compromise.[80,100] However, in the presence of shock, most surgeons would use only veins, saving time by not taking down the IMA and avoiding IMA vasoconstriction with the use of vasopressors postoperatively. Once on bypass, the heart is examined to discern the infarcted area from the still viable myocardium, and correlated with the coronary angiogram. When the aortic cross clamp is applied and cardioplegia is delivered, careful attention should be paid to optimal myocardial protection. Ef-

fective local and systemic cooling should be achieved. Ventricular distension must be avoided and flaccidity of a well-protected myocardium should be maintained. Coronary sinus retrograde cardioplegia is widely used with acute coronary occlusion to protect myocardium unreachable by the antegrade route.

As a general rule, the order of bypass grafting should follow the coronary vessels corresponding to the largest area of viable but threatened myocardium. The first vein graft should be placed on the coronary vessel involved in acute ischemia, and cardioplegia should be infused through the vein afterward to protect the myocardium from further ischemia. Using a multiple-line delivery catheter, cardioplegia should be infused through the vein graft after each distal anastomosis. This is not possible when an IMA is used, another reason why IMAs are not commonly utilized with cardiogenic shock. After the aortic cross-clamp is removed, the proximal anastomoses may be performed using a side-biting aortic clamp to shorten global ischemic time. If the coronary disease is particularly severe, e.g., left main artery stenosis with right coronary artery occlusion, the proximal anastomoses can be done during the same aortic cross-clamp.[73] After revascularization, reperfusion on cardiopulmonary bypass should be provided for as long as necessary for recovery of the ventricular function.

To date, there is no prospective randomized study demonstrating the best form of myocardial protection in cardiogenic shock. A range of techniques include hypothermic fibrillatory arrest,[101,102] oxygenated crystalloid cardioplegia,[73,101] blood cardioplegia,[103,104] and substrate-enriched blood cardioplegia with controlled reperfusion.[101,103] Some have reported an overwhelming advantage of using blood over crystalloid cardioplegia in cardiogenic shock patients,[101] whereas others have reported excellent clinical results with crystalloid cardioplegia alone.[73] A few important concepts in myocardial protection are worth considering. Survival in cardiogenic shock directly correlates with the capacity of reperfused, viable myocardium to compensate for infarcted myocardium. Thus it is important to protect the muscle mass in the ischemic border zone and in the collateral-dependent, remote ischemic zone during surgery.

The ischemic myocardium has depleted energy reserves and glycogen storage, and is less tolerant to ischemia during aortic cross clamping.[105] Rosenkranz and associates report an advantage of using a brief period of warm induction of substrate-enriched oxygenated blood cardioplegia with cardiogenic shock.[104] This theoretically resuscitates ischemic myocardium, so it can better tolerate aortic cross-clamping. Normothermia facilitates return of basal cell function and metabolism. Various substrates restore energy stores. Glutamate can be deaminated to α-ketoglutarate and replenish the Krebs cycle intermediates used for ATP production.[105] Glutamate also has an important role in the malate–aspartate shuttle for mitochondrial oxidation and ATP production. Aspartate is transaminated to glutamate and oxylacetate. The oxylacetate enters the Krebs cycle and facilitates anaerobic ATP production via glycolysis.[105] These substrates with warm induction-blood cardioplegia resulted in superior postoperative left ventricular performance and survival.[104]

Allen et al stressed the importance of controlling the conditions of reperfusion and the composition of the reperfusate to minimize reperfusion injury.[74] Reperfusion injury is characterized by intracellular calcium accumulation, cell swelling, ventricular stiffening, and inefficient oxygen utilization.[106] The consequence of reperfusion injury is myocardial stunning. The purpose of controlled reperfusion is to (1) provide oxygenated blood to begin aerobic metabolism; (2) lower energy demands by maintaining asystole with potassium chloride; (3) restore aerobic substrates with glutamate and aspartate; (4) reverse tissue acidosis with buffered solution; (5) minimize the intracellular calcium exposure by adding citrate phosphate dextrose, a calcium-chelating agent; and (6) reduce tissue edema with a hyperosmolar solution perfused at low pressure.[106] After completing distal anastomoses, warm blood cardioplegia enriched with metabolic substrates and the above protective components is infused for 2 min into the aortic root and all grafts. This is followed by unclamping of the aorta and further infusion of the warm blood cardioplegia into the appropriate vein grafts for 18 min while proximal anastomoses are performed.[107] The heart is allowed to recover in an empty, beating state on bypass for 30 min or more, as aerobic metabolism gradually supports return of regional contractile function. Using warm induction and controlled reperfusion Allen et al demonstrated that the period of irreversible ischemic damage can be extended significantly. The method of reperfusion may be more important than the speed with which coronary occlusions are bypassed.[74]

Results

Controlled reperfusion in patients with cardiogenic shock yielded a mortality of 3%, in contrast to 17% with "uncontrolled" brief global reperfusion.[74] These results were superior to the 43% mortality of cardiogenic shock patients after angioplasty. Allen et al ascribed these differences to making the myocardium more tolerant of ischemia and protection from reperfusion injury, which preserves contractility of remote myocardium and better compensates the work of nonfunctioning myocardium.[74] In 87% of the patients, regional wall motion abnormalities improved from akinesia/dyskinesia to mild/moderate hypokinesia following 6.3 hours of ischemia. This functional improvement was seen immediately following reperfusion of previously ischemic areas.[74,101,103] Patients receiving standard reperfusion had continued depression of function in the ischemic areas. It is difficult to assess whether hypocontractility of a reperfused segment is due to ischemic necrosis or "myocardial stunning." Ventricular dysfunction due to stunned myocardium

is almost as undesirable as the nonfunctioning infarcted myocardium in the immediate postoperative period. Buckberg's proposition that controlled reperfusion increases immediate postoperative regional function is a critical notion.[107] Even after an average of 45 hours of shock, left ventricular power failure was reversed by surgery in 93% of patients, and perioperative survival was 83%.[88] This supports the claim that warm induction can resuscitate ischemic myocardium and controlled reperfusion helps minimize reperfusion injury. However, there has not been a prospective controlled, randomized study to test this hypothesis. Most of the data are retrospective, reported by a few select centers, and not accepted by everyone.

Perioperative mortality (<30 days) ranges from 12 to 60[74,88–90,108] and this may, in part, reflect the change in death rate from the 1970s to 1980s. Frequent causes of early mortality are multiorgan system failure, pump failure, and cardiac arrhythmia.[74,88,90,108] Postoperative multiorgan system failure is frequently a continuation of the preoperative state. Thus patients with severe organ system failure preoperatively may not survive. The longer the operation is delayed from the onset of shock, the more likely is preoperative organ failure. Organ failure for more than 18 hours preoperatively is likely to be irreversible, and has been proposed as a relative contraindication to surgery.[90] Perioperative morbidity occurs in 47% of patients, and the causes include reexploration for bleeding, sepsis, wound infection, and respiratory failure.[90] Late mortality has been reported to range between 0 and 33% at a mean follow-up of 10 to 36 mo.[74,88,90] The cause of late death is usually progressive congestive heart failure, presumably due to inadequate normal myocardium to meet the physiologic demand. Nonsurvivors have a greater incidence of perioperative infarction and postoperative regional wall motion abnormalities.[90] Survivors of cardiogenic shock with extensive functional abnormalities are at increased risk of late death. They should receive aggressive medical treatment and be considered for cardiac transplantation if appropriate (see Chapter 113). The quality of life for long-term survivors of cardiogenic shock has been reported as satisfactory.[109] In a small series with a mean follow-up of 22 mo, 46% of patients resumed preoperative work activity, and the rest either retired or are permanently disabled. On average, their exercise capacity on a Bruce protocol equalled that of patients with uncomplicated myocardial infarction. This suggests that with aggressive surgical revascularization, survivors of cardiogenic shock may enjoy an acceptable lifestyle.

SUMMARY

Cardiogenic shock is the leading cause of death in acute myocardial infarction. Its incidence is only 5 to 15%, however, it has an 80 to 100% mortality when treated conservatively. Cardiogenic shock develops when the infarct size is >40% of the myocardium, or when the noninfarcted myocardium cannot compensate for a smaller infarction. The cornerstone of treatment is to perfuse the viable myocardium in the ischemic border zone or remote ischemic areas dependent upon collateral flow from the occluded artery. Pharmacologic therapy, intraaortic balloon counterpulsation, and thrombolytic therapy have not been effective in improving survival in cardiogenic shock. Percutaneous coronary angioplasty and surgical bypass have been shown to be efficacious, but lack of prospective randomized clinical trials makes interpretation difficult. Multivessel coronary disease and eccentric coronary lesions should be treated by operation. Preoperative assessment of myocardial viability should be helpful. Rapid revascularization and optimal myocardial protection are crucial to salvage the ischemic but viable myocardium. Survival with aggressive management ranges between 50 and 90%. Long-term quality of life is possible for a patient in cardiogenic shock, provided physicians understand the pathophysiology of acute infarct extension and the strategy of revascularization and myocardial salvage.

REFERENCES

1. Brown KW, Macmillan RL, Forbath N, et al: An intensive care center for acute myocardial infarction. *Lancet* **2**:349–352, 1963
2. Lee TH, Goldman L: The coronary care unit turns 25: Historical trends and future directions. *Ann Intern Med* **108**:887–894, 1988
3. Killip T IIId, Kimball JT: Treatment of myocardial infarction in a coronary care unit: A two year experience with 250 patients. *Am J Cardiol* **20**:457–464, 1967
4. Alpert JS, Becker RC: Mechanisms and management of cardiogenic shock. *Crit Care Clin* **9**(2):205–218, 1993
5. Swan HJC, Forrester JS, Danzig R, Allen HN: Power failure in acute myocardial infarction. *Prog Cardiovasc Dis* **12**:568–600, 1970
6. Rackley CE, Russell RO Jr, Mantle JA, Rogers WJ: Cardiogenic shock. *Cardiovasc Clin* **11**:15–24, 1981
7. Hands ME, Rutherford JD, Muller JE, et al: The In-hospital development of cardiogenic shock after myocardial infarction: Incidence, predictors of occurrence, outcome and prognostic factors. *J Am Coll Cardiol* **14**:40–46, 1989
8. Leor J, Goldbourt U, Reicher-Reiss H, et al: Cardiogenic shock complicating acute myocardial infarction in patients without heart failure on admission: Incidence, risk factors, and outcome. *Am J Med* **94**:265–273, 1993
9. Goldberg RJ, Gore JM, Alpert JS, et al: Cardiogenic shock after acute myocardial infarction: Incidence and mortality from a community-wide perspective, 1975 to 1988. *N Engl J Med* **325**:1117–1122, 1991
10. Gutovitz AL, Sobel BE, Roberts R: Progressive nature of myocardial injury in selected patients with cardiogenic shock. *Am J Cardiol* **41**:469–475, 1978
11. Wackers FJ, Lie KI, Becker AE: Coronary artery disease in patients dying from cardiogenic shock or congestive heart failure in the setting of acute myocardial infarction. *Br Heart J* **38**:906–910, 1976
12. Bengston JR, Kaplan AJ, Pieper KS, et al: Prognosis in cardiogenic shock after acute myocardial infarction in the interventional era. *J Am Coll Cardiol* **20**:1482–1489, 1992
13. Stack RS, O'Connor CM, Mark DB, et al: Coronary perfusion during acute myocardial infarction with a combined therapy of coronary angioplasty and high-dose intravenous streptokinase. *Circulation* **77**:151–161, 1988
14. O'Neill W, Erbel R, Laufer N, et al: Coronary angioplasty therapy of cardiogenic shock complicating acute myocardial infarction (abstr). *Circulation* **72**(Suppl III):III–309, 1985
15. Killip T: Cardiogenic shock complicating myocardial infarction. (Editorial) *J Am Coll Cardiol* **14**:47–48, 1989
16. Swan HJC, Forrester JS, Diamond G, et al: Hemodynamic spectrum of myocardial infarction and cardiogenic shock: A conceptual model. *Circulation* **45**:1097–1110, 1972
17. Lavie CJ, Gersh BJ: Mechanical and electrical complications of acute myocardial infarction. *Mayo Clin Proc* **65**:709–730, 1990
18. Gay WA Jr: Cardiogenic shock secondary to myocardial infarction. In Baue AE, Geha AS, Hammond GL, et al (eds): *Glenn's Thoracic and Cardiovascular Surgery, Fifth Edition,* Vol. II. Norwalk, CT, Appleton & Lange, 1991, pp 1809–1816
19. Alonso DR, Scheidt S, Post M, Killip T: Pathophysiology of cardiogenic shock: Quantification of myocardial necrosis, clinical, pathologic and electrocardiographic correlations. *Circulation* **48**:588–596, 1973
20. Page DL, Caulfield JB, Kastor JA, et al: Myocardial changes associated with cardiogenic shock. *N Engl J Med* **285**:133–137, 1971
21. Pfeffer MA, Pfeffer JM, Fishbein MC, et al: Myocardial infarct size and ventricular function in rats. *Circ Res* **44**:503–512, 1979
22. Cercek B, Shah PK: Complicated acute myocardial infarction: Heart failure, shock, mechanical complications. *Cardiol Clin* **9**:570, 1991
23. Chatterjee K: Complications of acute myocardial infarction. *Curr Probl Cardiol* 5–79, 1993
24. Erlebacher JA, Weiss JL, Weisfeldt M, et al: Early dilation of the infarcted segment in acute transmural myocardial infarction: Role of infarct expansion in acute left ventricular enlargement. *J Am Coll Cardiol* **4**:201–208, 1984
25. Herman MV, Heinle RA, Klein MD, et al: Localized disorders in myocardial contraction. *N Engl J Med* **227**:222, 1967
26. Klein M, Herman M, Gorlin R: A hemodynamic study of left ventricular aneurysm. *Circulation* **35**:614, 1967
27. Grande P, Christiansen C, Hansen BF: Myocardial infarct size and cardiogenic shock. *Eur Heart J* **4**:289–294, 1983
28. Harnarayan C, Bennett MA, Pentecost BL, Brewer DB: Quantitative study of infarcted myocardium in cardiogenic shock. *Br Heart J* **32**:728–732, 1970
29. Wackers FJ, Lie KI, Becker AE, et al: Coronary artery disease in patients dying from cardiogenic shock or congestive heart failure in the setting of acute myocardial infarction. *Br Heart J* **38**:906–910, 1976
30. Schuster EH, Bulkley BH: Ischemia at a distance after acute myocardial infarction: A cause of early postinfarction angina. *Circulation* **62**:509–515, 1980
31. Reimer KA, Lowe JE, Rasmussen MM, Jennings RB: The wavefront phenomenon of ischemic cell death: 1. Myocardial infarct size vs. duration of coronary occlusion in dogs. *Circulation* **56**:576–594, 1977
32. McKay RG, Pfeffer MA, Pasternak RC, et al: Left ventricular remodelling following myocardial infarction: A corollary to infarct expansion. *Circulation* **74**:693–702, 1986
33. Marmor A, Sobel B, Roberts R: Factors presaging early recurrent myocardial extension. *Am J Cardiol* **48**:603, 1981
34. Muller JE, Rude RE, Braunwald E, et al: Myocardial infarct extension: Occurrence, outcome, and risk factors in the Multicenter Investigation of Limitation of infarct size. *Ann Intern Med* **108**:1–6, 1988
35. Alpert JS, Becker RC: Mechanisms and management of cardiogenic shock. *Crit Care Clin* **9**:205–219, 1993
36. Forrester JS, Diamond G, Chatterjee K, et al: medical therapy of acute myocardial infarction by application of hemodynamic subsets (first of two parts). *N Engl J Med* **295**:1356–1362, 1976
37. Forrester JS, Diamond G, Chatterjee K, et al: Medical therapy of

acute myocardial infarction by application of hemodynamic subsets (second of two parts). *N Engl J Med* **295:**1404–1413, 1976

38. Alpert JS, Becker RC: Pathophysiology, diagnosis, and management of cardiogenic shock. In Schlant RC, Alexander RW (eds): *The Heart, Arteries and Veins,* Vol. 1. New York, McGraw-Hill, 1994, pp 907–927

39. McEvoy GK (ed): *AHFS Drug Information 1994.* Bethesda, MD, American Society of Hospital Pharmacists, 1994, pp 1163–1166

40. Dyke CM, Lee KF, Parmar J, et al: Inotropic stimulation and oxygen consumption in a canine model of dilated cardiomyopathy. *Ann Thorac Surg* **52:**750–758, 1991

41. Borrow KM, Lang RM, Neumann A, et al: Physiologic mechanisms governing hemodynamic responses to positive inotropic therapy in patients with dilated cardiomyopathy. *Circulation* **77:**625–637, 1988

42. Gage J, Rutman H, Lucido D, LeJemtel TH: Additive effects of dobutamine and amrinone on myocardial contractility and ventricular performance in patients with severe heart failure. *Circulation* **74:**367–373, 1986

43. Dunkan WB, Leinbach RC, Buckley MJ, et al: Clinical and hemodynamic results of intraaortic balloon pumping and surgery for cardiogenic shock. *Circulation* **56:**465–477, 1972

44. Bardet J, Masquet C, Kahn JC, et al: Clinical and hemodynamic results of intraaortic balloon counterpulsation and surgery for cardiogenic shock. *Am Heart J* **93:**280–288, 1977

45. DeWood MA, Notske RN, Hensley GR, et al: Intraaortic balloon counterpulsation with and without reperfusion for myocardial infarction shock. *Circulation* **61:**1105–1112, 1980

46. Ehrich DA, Biddle TL, Kronenberg MW, Yu PN: The hemodynamic response to intraaortic balloon counterpulsation in patients with cardiogenic shock complicating acute myocardial infarction. *Am Heart J* **93:**274–279, 1977

47. Leinbach RC, Gold HK, Harper RW, et al: Early intraaortic balloon pumping for anterior myocardial infarction without shock. *Circulation* **58:**204, 1978

48. Levine H, Gold HK, Leinbach RC, et al: Safe early revascularization for continuing ischemia after acute myocardial infarction. *Circulation* **60**(suppl I):1–5, 1979

49. Schlant RC, Alexander RW: Part VII. Coronary heart disease. In Schlant RC, Alexander RW (eds): *The Heart, Arteries and Veins,* Vol. 1. New York, McGraw-Hill, 1994, pp 1124–1180

50. Col NF, Gurwitz JH, Alpert JS, Goldberg RJ: Frequency of inclusion of patients with cardiogenic shock in trials of thrombolytic therapy. *Am J Cardiol* **73:**149–157, 1994

51. Gruppo Italiano per lo Studio della Streptochianasi nell'Infarto Miocardioco (GISSI): Effectiveness of intravenous thrombolytic treatment in acute myocardial infarction. *Lancet* **1:**397–401, 1986

52. Dioguardi N, Lotto A, Levi GF, et al: Controlled trial of streptokinase and heparin in acute myocardial infarction. *Lancet* **2:**891–895, 1971

53. International Study Group: In-hospital mortality and clinical course of 20,891 patients with suspected acute myocardial infarction randomized between alteplase and streptokinase with or without heparin. *Lancet* **336:**71–75, 1990

54. Collins R: Optimizing thrombolytic therapy of acute myocardial infarction: Age is not a contraindication. *Circulation* **84**(suppl):II-230, 1991

55. Becker RC: Hemodynamic, mechanical, and metabolic determinants of thrombolytic efficacy: A theoretic framework for assessing the limitations of thrombolysis in patients with cardiogenic shock. *Am Heart J* **125:**919–929, 1993

56. Kennedy JW, Gensini GG, Timmis GC, Maynard CM: Acute myocardial infarction treated with intracoronary streptokinase: A report of the Society for Cardiac Angiography. *Am J Cardiol* **55:**871–877, 1985

57. Lee L, Bates ER, Pitt B, et al: Percutaneous transluminal coronary angioplasty improves survival in acute myocardial infarction complicated by cardiogenic shock. *Circulation* **78:**1345–1351, 1988

58. Disler L, Haitas B, Benjamin J, et al: Cardiogenic shock in evolving myocardial infarction: Treatment by angioplasty and streptokinase. *Heart Lung* **16:**649–652, 1987

59. Heuser RR, Maddoux GL, Goss JE, et al: Coronary angioplasty in the treatment of cardiogenic shock: The therapy of choice (abstr). *J Am Coll Cardiol* **7:**219A, 1986

60. Hibbard MD, Holmes DR, Bailey KR, et al: Percutaneous transluminal coronary angioplasty in patients with cardiogenic shock. *J Am Coll Cardiol* **19:**639–646, 1992

61. Lee L, Erbel R, Brown TM, et al: Multicenter registry of angioplasty therapy of cardiogenic shock: Initial and long-term survival. *J Am Coll Cardiol* **17:**599–603, 1991

62. Gacioch GM, Ellis SG, Lee L, et al: Cardiogenic shock complicating acute myocardial infarction: The use of coronary angioplasty and the integration of the new support devices into patient management. *J Am Coll Cardiol* **19:**647–653, 1992

63. O'Keefe JH, Bailey WL, Rutherford BD, Hartzler GO: Primary angioplasty for acute myocardial infarction in 1000 consecutive patients: Results in an unselected population and high-risk subgroups. *Am J Cardiol* **72:**107G–115G, 1993

64. Ghitis A, Flaker GC, Meinhardt S, et al: Early angioplasty in patients with acute myocardial infarction complicated by hypotension. *Am Heart J* **122:**380–384, 1991

65. Klein LW: Optimal therapy for cardiogenic shock: The emerging role of coronary angioplasty (editorial). *J Am Coll Cardiol* **19:**654–656, 1992

66. Bates ER, Topol EJ: Limitations of thrombolytic therapy for acute myocardial infarction complicated by congestive heart failure and cardiogenic shock. *J Am Coll Cardiol* **18:**1077–1084, 1991

67. Verna E, Repetto S, Boscarini M, et al: Emergency coronary angioplasty in patients with severe left ventricular dysfunction or cardiogenic shock after acute myocardial infarction. *Eur Heart J* **10:**958–966, 1989

68. Grines CL, Booth DC, Nissen SE, et al: Mechanism of acute myocardial infarction in patients with prior coronary artery bypass grafting and therapeutic implications. *Am J Cardiol* **65:**1292–1296, 1990

69. Stack RS, Califf RM, Hinohara R, et al: Survival and cardiac event rates in the first year after emergency coronary angioplasty for acute myocardial infarction. *J Am Coll Cardiol* **11:**1141–1149, 1988

70. Lazar H: Emergency coronary artery bypass graft surgery after failed percutaneous transluminal coronary angioplasty. In Lazar H (ed): *Current Therapy for Acute Coronary Ischemia.* Mount Kisko, NY, Futura, 1993, pp 149–168

71. Cowley MJ, Dorros G, Kelsey SF, et al: Emergency coronary bypass surgery after coronary angioplasty: The National Heart, Lung, and Blood Institute's percutaneous transluminal coronary angioplasty registry experience. *Am J Cardiol* **53:**22C–26C, 1984

72. Berman JN, Faxon DP: The current role of percutaneous transluminal coronary angioplasty for acute coronary ischemic syndromes. In Lazar H (ed): *Current Therapy for Acute Coronary Ischemia.* Mount Kisko, NY, Futura, 1993, pp 85–110

73. Guyton RA, Arcidi JM, Langford MD, et al: Emergency coronary bypass for cardiogenic shock. *Circulation* **76**(suppl V):V22–V27, 1987

74. Allen BS, Buckberg GD, Fontan FM, et al: Superiority of controlled surgical reperfusion versus percutaneous transluminal coronary angioplasty in acute coronary occlusion. *J Thorac Cardiovasc Surg* **105:**864–884, 1993

75. O'Neill WW: Angioplasty therapy of cardiogenic shock: Are randomized trials necessary? *J Am Coll Cardiol* **19:**915–917, 1992

76. Bredee JJ, Bavinck JH, Berreklouw E, et al: Acute myocardial ischemia and cardiogenic shock after percutaneous transluminal coronary angioplasty; risk factors for and results of emergency coronary bypass. *Eur Heart J* **10**(suppl H):104–111, 1989

77. Buffet P, Danchin N, Villemot JP, et al: Early and long-term outcome after emergency coronary artery bypass surgery after failed coronary angioplasty. *Circulation* **84**(suppl III):III254–259, 1991

78. Tebbe U, Ruschewski W, Knake W, et al: Will emergency coronary bypass grafting after failed elective percutaneous transluminal coronary angioplasty prevent myocardial infarction? *Thorac Cardiovasc Surg* 37:308–312, 1989

79. Klepzig H, Kober G, Satter P, Kaltenbach M: Analysis of 100 emergency aortocoronary bypass operations after percutaneous transluminal coronary angioplasty: Which patients are at risk for large infarctions? *Eur Heart J* 12:946–951, 1991

80. Lazar H: Methods of reducing myocardial necrosis after failed percutaneous transluminal coronary angioplasty in patients undergoing emergent coronary artery bypass surgery. In Lazar H (ed): *Current Therapy for Acute Coronary Ischemia.* Mount Kisko, NY, Futura, 1993, pp 167–186

81. Sergeant P, Flameng W, Vanhaecke J, Suy R: Time constraints in the emergency coronary bypass surgery for acute evolving myocardial infarction. *J Cardiovasc Surg* 28:68–74, 1987

82. DeWood MA, Spores J, Berg R, et al: Acute myocardial infarction: A decade of experience with surgical reperfusion in 701 patients. *Circulation* 68(suppl II):II8–16, 1983

83. Cohen LH: Surgical treatment of acute myocardial infarction. *Cardiology* 76:167–172, 1989

84. Berg R Jr, Selinger S, Leonard JJ, et al: Immediate coronary artery bypass for acute evolving myocardial infarction. *J Thorac Cardiovasc Surg* 81:493–497, 1981

85. Flameng W, Sergeant P, Vanhaecke J, Suy R: Emergency coronary bypass grafting for evolving myocardial infarction: Effects on infarct size and left ventricular function. *J Thorac Cardiovasc Surg* 94:124–131, 1987

86. Koshal A, Beanlands DS, Davies RA, et al: Urgent surgical reperfusion in acute evolving myocardial infarction: A randomized controlled study. *Circulation* 78(suppl I):I171–178, 1988

87. Selinger SL, Berg R, Leonard JJ, et al: Surgical intervention in acute myocardial infarction. *Texas Heart Inst J* 11:44–51, 1984

88. Allen BS, Rosenkranz E, Buckberg GD, et al: Studies on prolonged acute regional ischemia. VI. Myocardial infarction with left ventricular power failure: A medical/surgical emergency requiring urgent revascularization with maximal protection of remote muscle. *J Thorac Cardiovasc Surg* 98:691–703, 1989

89. Moosvi AR, Khaja F, Villanueva L, et al: Early revascularization improves survival in cardiogenic shock complicating acute myocardial infarction. *J Am Coll Cardiol* 19:907–914, 1992

90. Laks H, Rosenkranz E, Buckberg GD: Surgical treatment of cardiogenic shock after myocardial infarction. *Circulation* 74(suppl III):III11–16, 1986

91. Hines GL, Mohtashemi M: Delayed operative intervention in cardiogenic shock after myocardial infarction. *Ann Thorac Surg* 33:132–138, 1980

92. Ragosta M, Beller GA: The noninvasive assessment of myocardial viability. *Clin Cardiol* 16:531–538, 1993

93. Beller GA: New directions in myocardial perfusion imaging. *Clin Cardiol* 16:86–94, 1993

94. Bergmann SR: Use and limitations of metabolic tracers labeled with positron-emitting radionuclides in the identification of viable myocardium. *J Nucl Med* 35(suppl):15S–22S, 1994

95. Tillisch J, Brunken R, Marshall R, et al: Reversibility of cardiac wall-motion abnormalities predicted by positron tomography. *N Engl J Med* 314:884–888, 1986

96. Bonow RO, Dilsizian V, Cuocolo A, Bacharach SL: Identification of viable myocardium in patients with chronic coronary artery disease and left ventricular dysfunction: Comparison of thallium scintigraphy with reinjection and PET imaging with ^{18}F-fluorodeoxyglucose. *Circulation* 83:26–37, 1991

97. Smart SC: The clinical utility of echocardiography in the assessment of myocardial viability. *J Nucl Med* 35(suppl):49S–58S, 1994

98. Brill DA, Deckelbaum LI, Remetz MS, et al: Recovery of severe ischemic ventricular dysfunction after coronary artery bypass grafting. *Am J Cardiol* 61:650–651, 1988

99. Rehr BR, Fuhs BE, Lee KF, et al: Differentiation of reperfused-viable (stunned) from reperfused-infarcted myocardium at 1 to 3 days postreperfusion by in vivo phosphorus-31 nuclear magnetic spectroscopy. *Am Heart J* 122:1571–1582, 1991

100. Ferguson TB, Muhlbaier LH, Salai DL, Wechsler AS: Coronary bypass grafting after failed elective and failed emergent percutaneous angioplasty. *J Thorac Cardiovasc Surg* 95:761–772, 1988

101. Beyersdorf F, Mitrev A, Sarai K, et al: Changing pattern of patients undergoing emergency surgical revascularization for acute coronary occlusion: Importance of myocardial protection techniques. *J Thorac Cardiovasc Surg* 106:137–148, 1988

102. Akins CW: Early and late results following emergency isolated myocardial revascularization during hypothermic fibrillatory arrest. *Ann Thorac Surg* 43:131–137, 1987

103. Beyersdorf F, Sarai K, Maul FD, et al: Immediate functional benefits after controlled reperfusion during surgical revascularization for acute coronary occlusion. *J Thorac Cardiovasc Surg* 102:856–866, 1991

104. Rosenkranz ER, Buckberg GD, Laks H, Mulder DG: Warm induction of cardioplegia with glutamate-enriched blood in coronary patients with cardiogenic shock who are dependent on inotropic drugs and intraaortic balloon support: Initial experience and operative strategy. *J Thorac Cardiovasc Surg* 86:507–518, 1983

105. Rosenkranz ER, Okamoto F, Buckberg GD, et al: Safety of prolonged aortic clamping with blood cardioplegia: III. Aspartate enrichment of glutamate-blood cardioplegia in energy-depleted hearts after ischemic and reperfusion injury. *J Thorac Cardiovasc Surg* 91:428–435, 1986

106. Buckley GD: Myocardial protection during adult cardiac operations. In Baue AE, Geha AS, Hammond GL, et al (eds): *Glenn's Thoracic and Cardiovascular Surgery, Fifth Edition,* Vol II. Norwalk, CT, Appleton & Lange, 1991, pp 1417–1441

107. Beyersdorf F, Buckberg G: Principles of myocardial protection during acute coronary ischemia and reperfusion. In Lazar H (ed): *Current Therapy for Acute Coronary Ischemia.* Mount Kisko, NY, Futura, 1993, pp 111–148

108. Miller MG, Weintraub RM, Hedley-Whyte J, Restall DS: Surgery for cardiogenic shock. *Lancet* 1342–1345, 1974

109. Subramanian VA, Roberts AJ, Zema MJ, et al: Cardiogenic shock following acute myocardial infarction: Late functional results after emergency cardiac surgery. *NY State J Med* 947–952, 1980

Postinfarction Ventricular Septal Rupture

Joren C. Madsen and Willard M. Daggett, Jr.

INTRODUCTION

Evolution of surgical techniques for repair of postinfarction ventricular septal rupture initially involved differentiation of these lesions from prior experience with surgical approaches to congenital ventricular septal defects, which were, for the most part, not applicable. Understanding the significance of differing anatomical locations of postinfarction ventricular septal defects led to innovations in terms of the location of the cardiotomy and the type of repair necessary to achieve a successful result in any given patient. In addition, the gradual appreciation of different clinical courses pursued by patients after postinfarction ventricular septal rupture both in terms of location of the defect and the degree of right ventricular functional impairment has led to increased urgency relative to the timing of surgical repair. The incorporation of specific anatomical concepts of surgical repair and better understanding of the time course of physiological deterioration of patients can ultimately lead to an integrated approach aimed toward improved salvage of patients suffering this catastrophic complication of acute myocardial infarction.[1]

HISTORY

In 1845 Latham[2] described a postinfarction ventricular septal rupture at autopsy, but it was not until 1923 that Brunn[3] made the first diagnosis antemortem. Sager[4] in 1934 added the eighteenth case to the world literature and established specific clinical criteria for diagnosis, stressing the association of postinfarction septal rupture with coronary artery disease. The treatment of this entity was medical and strictly palliative until 1956 when Cooley et al[5] performed the first successful surgical repair in a patient 9 wk after the diagnosis of septal rupture. These first patients who underwent similar repairs in the early 1960s usually presented with congestive heart failure, having survived for more than a month after acute septal perforation.[6–9] The success of operation in these patients and the precipitous, acute course of other patients with this complication[10] gave rise to the belief that operative repair should be limited to patients surviving for 1 mo or longer.[6,11] This, purportedly, allowed for scarring at the edges of the defect which was thought to be crucial to the secure and long-lasting closure of the septal rupture.[7,12] In the late 1960s, more rapid recognition of septal rupture following infarction led to the recommendation that operation be attempted earlier in patients who were hemodynamically deteriorating.[13,14] The use of improved prosthetic materials accompanied the successful surgical repair of defects from 1 to 11 days old, as reported by Allen and Woodwark[14] in 1966, Heimbecker et al[15] in 1968, and Iben et al[16] in 1969. Notable among these was Heimbecker and associates' superb early study of infarctectomy and clinical application to patients with postinfarction ventricular septal defects. The surgical management of these patients was further refined by the inclusion of infarctectomy[15,17] and aneurysmectomy[18,19] and the development of techniques to repair perforations in different areas of the septum.[20,21] Over the last 15 years, it has become increasingly clear that in the majority of cases postinfarction ventricular septal rupture constitutes a surgical emergency. More recently, improved surgical techniques, newer prosthetic materials, enhanced myocardial protection, and improved perioperative mechanical and pharmacological support have led to more favorable results in the surgical management of patients with postinfarction septal rupture.[22-29]

INCIDENCE AND PATHOGENESIS

Whereas autopsy studies reveal an 11% incidence of myocardial free wall rupture following acute infarction,[30] septal perforation is found much less frequently, with an incidence of 1 to 2%.[30-32] It occurs in men more often than women (3 to 2), but more women experience rupture than what would be expected from the incidence of coronary artery disease in women.[10] The age of patients with this complication ranges from 44 to 81 years, with a mean of 62.5 years. There is some evidence that the average age is increasing.[28,29,32,33] The vast majority of patients who experience ventricular septal rupture do so after their initial infarction.[32,33] The overall incidence of postinfarction ventricular septal rupture may have decreased slightly during the past decade as a result of aggressive pharmological therapy in patients with evolving myocardial infarction and the prompt control of hypertension in these patients.[33] Angiographic evaluation of these patients indicates that septal rupture is usually associated with complete occlusion, rather than severe stenosis of a coronary artery.[34] In addition, on average, they have less extensive coronary artery disease, as well as less developed septal collaterals than do other patients with coronary artery disease.[35] The lack of collateral flow noted acutely may be secondary to anatomical configuration, edema, or associated arterial disease. Hill and associates,[27] in reviewing 19 cases of postinfarction ventricular septal rupture, found single-vessel disease in 64%, double-vessel disease in 7%, and triple-vessel disease in 29%. The defect is most commonly located in the anterioapical septum as the result of an anterior infarction (over 60%), while in 20 to 40% of patients the rupture occurs in the posterior septum following an inferior infarction.[36] Thus, epidemiologically, septal perforations occur most frequently in 65-year-old men with single-vessel coronary disease and poor collateral flow who present with their first anterior infarction.

The infarct associated with septal rupture is transmural and generally quite extensive, involving a mean 26% of the left ventricular wall in hearts with septal rupture, compared with only 15% in other acute infarctions.[32] There are two types of rupture: simple, consisting of a direct through and through defect usually located anteriorly; and complex, consisting of a serpiginous dissection tract remote from the primary septal defect which is usually located inferiorly.[37] Multiple defects, which may develop within several days of each other, occur in 5 to 11% of cases. Since a successful surgical outcome is related to adequacy of closure of septal defects, multiple defects must be sought preoperatively if possible, and certainly at the time of operative repair. The rupture itself occurs through a zone of necrotic myocardial

tissue generally within 2 wk after myocardial infarction. The average time from infarction to rupture has been reported to be between 2.6 and 8 days.[32,38,39] These observations correlate well with the pathologic findings of Mallory and co-workers,[40] which demonstrate that four to 21 days following a myocardial infarction, necrotic tissue is most abundant and ingrowth of blood vessels and connective tissue is only beginning.

Of the small number of patients who survive the early period of ventricular septal rupture, 35 to 68% go on to develop ventricular aneurysms.[27,38] This compares with a 12% incidence of aneurysm formation in patients suffering an infarction but no septal rupture,[41] and probably relates to the transmural nature of the infarction associated with septal rupture. Postinfarction septal rupture, especially in the posterior septum, may be accompanied by mitral valve regurgitation due to papillary muscle infarction or dysfunction. In approximately one-third of cases of septal rupture, there is a degree of mitral insufficiency, usually functional in nature secondary to left ventricular dysfunction with mitral annular dilation, which usually resolves with repair of the defect.

Although sample sizes were small, reviews by both Oyamada and Queen[42] and Sanders et al[10] revealed that nearly 25% of patients with infarction and septal rupture died within the first 24 hours, 65% within 2 wk, and of the unoperated patients with postinfarction septal rupture, only 7% lived longer than 1 year. The dreadful natural history of patients with postinfarction ventricular septal rupture is a consequence of the sudden increase in hemodynamic load imposed upon a heart already compromised by acute infarction, and possibly by a ventricular aneurysm, mitral valve dysfunction, or a combination of these problems. Ultimately, persistence of a low cardiac output state results in peripheral organ failure. Despite the many advances in the nonoperative treatment of congestive heart failure and cardiogenic shock, including the intra-aortic balloon pump and a multitude of new inotropic agents and vasodilators, these methods have not and will not supplant the need for operative intervention for these critically ill patients.

DIAGNOSIS

The typical presentation of a ventricular septal rupture is that of a patient who has suffered an acute myocardial infarction and who, after convalescing for a few days, develops a new systolic murmur, recurrent chest pain, and an abrupt deterioration in hemodynamics. The development of a loud systolic murmur, usually within the first week following an acute myocardial infarction, is the most consistent physical finding of postinfarction ventricular septal rupture (present in over 90% of cases). The murmur is usually harsh, pansystolic, and best auscultated at the left lower sternal border. Depending on the location of the septal defect, the murmur may radiate to the left axilla, thereby mimicking mitral regurgitation.[39] Up to half of these patients experience postinfarction chest pain in association with the appearance of the murmur.[32] Coincident with the onset of the murmur, there is usually an abrupt decline in the patient's clinical course with congestive failure and often cardiogenic shock. The findings of cardiac failure that occur acutely in these patients are primarily the result of right-sided heart failure, with pulmonary edema being less prominent than that occurring in patients with acute mitral regurgitation due to ruptured papillary muscle.[43]

The electrocardiographic findings in patients with acute septal rupture relate to the changes associated with antecedent anterior, inferior, posterior, or septal infarction. The localization of infarction by ECG correlates highly with the location of the associated septal perforation. In our review[33] of 55 patients with postinfarction septal rupture, the location of the defect corresponded to the territory of transmural infarction as determined by ECG in all but three patients. Up to one-third of patients develop some degree of atrioventricular conduction block (usually transient) that may precede rupture,[44] but there is no pathognomonic prognostic indicator of impending perforation. The chest radiograph usually shows increased pulmonary vascularity consistent with pulmonary venous hypertension.

It is important to realize that the sudden appearance of a systolic murmur and hemodynamic deterioration following infarction may also result from acute mitral regurgitation due to ruptured papillary muscle. Distinguishing these two lesions clinically is difficult but a number of points may help. First, the systolic murmur associated with a septal rupture is more prominent at the left sternal border, whereas the murmur resulting from a ruptured papillary muscle is best heard at the apex. Second, the murmur associated with septal perforation is loud and associated with a thrill (in over 50% of patients), whereas the murmur of acute mitral regurgitation is softer and is not associated with a thrill.[10] Third, septal rupture is often associated with anterior infarctions and conduction abnormalities, whereas papillary muscle rupture is commonly associated with an inferior infarction and no conduction defects.[45] Finally, it should be noted that septal rupture and papillary muscle rupture may coexist following infarction.[46,47]

Until recently, the mainstay of differentiating septal rupture from mitral valve dysfunction has been right heart catheterization using the Swan–Ganz catheter.[48] With septal rupture, there is an oxygen saturation step-up between the right atrium and pulmonary artery. Step-up in oxygen saturation greater than 9% between the right atrium and pulmonary artery confirms the presence of a shunt.[49] The pulmonary-to-systemic flow ratios, Q_p/Q_s, obtained from oxygen saturation samples, range from 1.4:1 to greater than 8:1 and roughly correlate with the size of the defect.[50] In contrast, with acute mitral regurgitation secondary to papillary muscle rupture there are classic giant V-waves on the

pulmonary artery wedge pressure trace. It should be noted, however, that up to one-third of patients with septal ruptures also have mild mitral regurgitation secondary to left ventricular dysfunction.[51]

Recent advances in transthoracic and transesophageal echocardiography, especially the advent of color-flow Doppler mapping, have revolutionized the diagnosis of both the presence and site of septal rupture.[52,53] Smyllie et al[53] reported a 100% specificity and 100% sensitivity when color-flow Doppler mapping was used to differentiate ventricular septal rupture from acute severe mitral regurgitation following acute myocardial infarction. It also correctly demonstrated the site of septal rupture in 41 of 42 patients. Widespread use of this technology has, for the most part, replaced thermodilution catheter insertion, which in outlying hospitals, where patients are often seen first, may be time-consuming, difficult to accomplish, and occasionally harmful to the patient. Indeed, the trend toward early surgical referral and prompt operative repair is at least partially explained by the more widespread use of color Doppler echocardiography for diagnosis in peripheral centers.[29]

The necessity of preoperative left heart catheterization with coronary angiography has been a matter of debate. On one hand, left heart catheterization provides important information concerning associated coronary artery disease, left ventricular wall motion, and specifics of valvular dysfunction, which are all important in planning operative correction of postinfarction septal rupture. In most series[54–56] over 60% of patients with septal rupture have significant involvement of at least one vessel other than the one supplying the infarcted area. We recently reported that bypassing associated coronary artery disease significantly increased long-term survival when compared with patients with unbypassed coronary artery disease.[57] As will be discussed later, we and others[54] prefer to have a left heart catheterization with coronary angiography and left ventriculography before proceeding to the operating room. However, there are significant disadvantages in performing left heart catheterization with coronary angiography. It is time consuming and can contribute to both the mortality and morbidity of these already compromised patients.[29] Thus, some centers do not carry out preoperative left heart catheterization.[24,59] Others use it selectively, avoiding invasive studies in patients with septal rupture caused by anterior wall infarction, which is associated with a much lower incidence of multiple-vessel disease than septal defects resulting from posterior infarctions.[29] Our studies indicate that while both patients with anterior septal rupture and patients with posterior septal rupture gain a longevity advantage by carrying out complementary bypasses at the time of septal rupture repair, this improved long-term survival is greatest in the patients with anterior septal rupture.[57] Because hospital survival is not adversely influenced by complementary coronary bypass grafting, but long-term survival is significantly enhanced, we confidently advocate coronary arteriography prior to surgery and grafting of major stenotic vessels in all of these patients.

PREOPERATIVE THERAPY

As the natural course of the disease in unoperated patients is so dismal, the diagnosis of postinfarction ventricular septal rupture can be regarded as its own indication for operation.[31] Preoperative management is directed toward stabilization of the hemodynamic condition so that peripheral organ perfusion can be best maintained while any further diagnostic studies are obtained and while deciding on the optimal time for surgical intervention. Although the early clinical course of patients with postinfarction ventricular septal rupture can be quite variable, 50 to 60% present with severe congestive heart failure and a low cardiac output state requiring intensive therapy.[23]

The goals of preoperative management are to (1) reduce the systemic vascular resistance and, thus, the left-to-right shunt, (2) maintain cardiac output and arterial pressure to ensure peripheral organ perfusion, and (3) maintain or improve coronary artery bloodflow. This is best accomplished by the intraaortic balloon pump (IABP). Counterpulsation reduces left ventricular afterload, thus increasing cardiac output and decreasing the left-to-right shunt, as reported by Gold and associates in 1973.[60] In addition, IABP support is associated with decreased myocardial oxygen consumption, as well as improved myocardial and peripheral organ perfusion. Although counterpulsation produces an overall improvement in the patient's condition, a complete correction of the hemodynamic picture cannot be obtained.[61] Peak improvement occurs within 24 hours and no further benefit has been observed with prolonged balloon pumping.[55]

Pharmacologic therapy with inotropic agents and diuretics should be instituted promptly. The addition of vasodilators (i.e., sodium nitroprusside or intravenous nitroglycerine) makes good theoretical sense—decreasing the left-to-right shunting associated with the mechanical defect, and, thus, increasing cardiac output. However, this is often associated with a marked fall in mean arterial blood pressure and reduced coronary perfusion, both poorly tolerated in these critically ill patients. In fact, vasoconstrictors may be necessary to maintain blood pressure pending placement of an intraaortic balloon pump or surgical repair. It must be stressed that pharmacologic therapy is intended primarily to support the patient in preparation for operation and should not in anyway delay urgent operation in the critically ill patient. We now admit patients with postinfarction septal rupture directly to the surgical intensive care unit rather than to the coronary care or medical intensive care unit.

Other techniques that have been tried in an effort to improve the hemodynamics of patients with intraventricular septal rupture include venoarterial extracaporeal membrane oxygenation (ECMO)[25] and inflation of a balloon in the right ventricular outflow track to decrease the left-to-right shunt.[62] Neither has been proven reliable in clinical application.

TIMING OF OPERATION

It has become clear that the early practice of waiting for several weeks after ventricular septal rupture before proceeding with surgery only selects out the small minority of patients in whom the hemodynamic insult is less severe and is better tolerated.[20,26,63] It has also become clear that to manage most patients supportively in hopes of deferring operation is to deprive the great majority of those with postinfarction ventricular septal rupture of the benefits of definitive surgery before irreversible damage due to peripheral organ ischemia has occurred.[31,54]

While we,[22] as well as others[64] have advocated early surgery since the middle of the 1970s, some continue to prefer to defer operation in patients who are easily supported and exhibit no further hemodynamic deterioration.[65] Persistence of congestive heart failure or marginal stabilization with rising blood urea nitrogen (BUN) and borderline urine output necessitate aggressive therapy and prompt operation. The routine use of IABP, whenever technically feasible, frequently results in *transient* reversal of the hemodynamic deterioration. This period of stability often makes it possible to complete left-heart catheterization before proceeding to operation but should not significantly delay definitive surgical treatment. Patients with septal rupture rarely die of cardiac failure per se, but rather of end-organ failure as a consequence of shock. Shortening the duration of shock by operating early is the only therapeutic solution for this group of patients and can yield dramatic results.[33,57] As long as one adheres to a policy of proceeding with surgery before the point of irreversible end-organ failure due to prolonged shock, no patient need be considered "too sick" for emergency operation.

Radford and associates[66] reviewed 41 consecutive patients with postinfarction ventricular septal rupture at the Massachusetts General Hospital between 1971 and 1975 and found the presence or absence of cardiogenic shock to be the most important determinant of operative mortality. Thereafter, we have employed intra-aortic balloon pumping and immediate operative repair in all patients with cardiogenic shock. In 1982, we again reviewed our experience[33] and compared the results achieved before 1975 with those achieved after 1975 with a program of early surgery for all unstable patients. Overall, hospital survival was 59% for the group before 1975 and 75% for the group after 1975. Significantly, the difference in hospital survival was most dramatic for patients in cardiogenic shock preoperatively; 27% before 1975 vs. 67% after 1975. Most other groups have reported success with early operative repair, and emphasize the importance of early operation before the development of multisystem failure.[64,67–69]

Overall, these results suggest the following approach to the surgical management of patients with postinfarction ventricular septal rupture. Those patients in cardiogenic shock represent a true surgical emergency requiring immediate operative repair. As deaths in these patients result from multisystem failure secondary to end-organ hypoperfusion, delay in operative repair represents a "failed strategy." Those few patients who are completely stable, with no clinical deterioration, and who require no hemodynamic support, can undergo operative repair when convenient during that hospitalization. The large group of patients who are in an intermediate position between those with shock and those in stable condition should be operated on early (usually within 12 to 24 hours) after appropriate preoperative evaluation. Since the group of patients in stable condition constitutes 5% or less of the total population of patients with postinfarction ventricular septal rupture, the overwhelming majority of patients require prompt surgical treatment.

Rarely, because of delayed referral, a patient will be seen for surgical therapy who is already in a state of multisystem failure or has developed septic complications. Such a patient is unlikely to survive an emergency operation, and thus may benefit from prolonged IABP support before an attempted operative repair. We have found it necessary to treat a rare patient (2 of 92) in this fashion. Baillot and colleagues[70] have reported individual successes with such an approach, which we consider the exception rather than the rule.

OPERATIVE TECHNIQUE

The first repair by Cooley et al[5] of an acquired ventricular septal defect was accomplished using an approach through the right ventricle with incision of the right ventricular outflow tract. This approach, which was adapted from surgical techniques for closure of congenital ventricular septal defects, proved to be disadvantageous for many reasons. Exposure of the defect was frequently less than optimal, particularly for defects located in the apical septum. It involved unnecessary injury to normal right ventricular muscle and interruption of collaterals from the right coronary artery. Finally, it failed to eliminate the paradoxical bulging segment of infarcted left ventricular wall. Subsequently, Heimbecker et al[15] introduced, and others adopted,[71,72] a left-sided approach (left ventriculotomy) with incision through the area of infarction. Such an approach frequently incorporates infarctectomy and aneurysmectomy, together with repair of septal rupture. Experience with a variety of techniques for closure of postinfarction ventricular septal rupture has led us to the evolution of the following eight principles: (1) expeditious establishment of total cardiopulmonary bypass with moderate hypothermia and meticulous attention to myocardial protection; (2) transinfarct approach to ventricular septal defect with the site of ventriculotomy determined by

the location of the transmural infarction; (3) thorough trimming of the left ventricular margins of the infarct back to viable muscle to prevent delayed rupture of the closure; (4) conservative trimming of the right ventricular muscle as required for complete visualization of the margins of the defect; (5) inspection of the left ventricular papillary muscles and concomitant replacement of the mitral valve only if there is frank papillary muscular rupture; (6) closure of the septal defect without tension, which in most instances will require the use of prosthetic material; (7) closure of the infarctectomy without tension with generous use of prosthetic material as indicated, and epicardial placement of the patch to the free wall to avoid strain on the friable endocardial tissue; (8) buttressing of the suture lines with pledgets or strips of Teflon felt or similar material to prevent sutures from cutting through friable muscle. Adherence to these principles in the closure of septal defects in different locations has led to the evolution of individualized approaches to apical, anterior, and inferoposterior septal defects.

Apical Septal Rupture

The technique of apical amputation was described by Daggett and associates in 1970.[71] Incision is made through the infarcted apex of the left ventricle. Excision of the necrotic myocardium results in amputation of the apical portion of the left ventricle and septum (Fig. 129–1). The remaining apical portions of the left and right ventricle free walls are then approximated to the apical septum. This is accomplished by means of a row of interrupted mattress su-

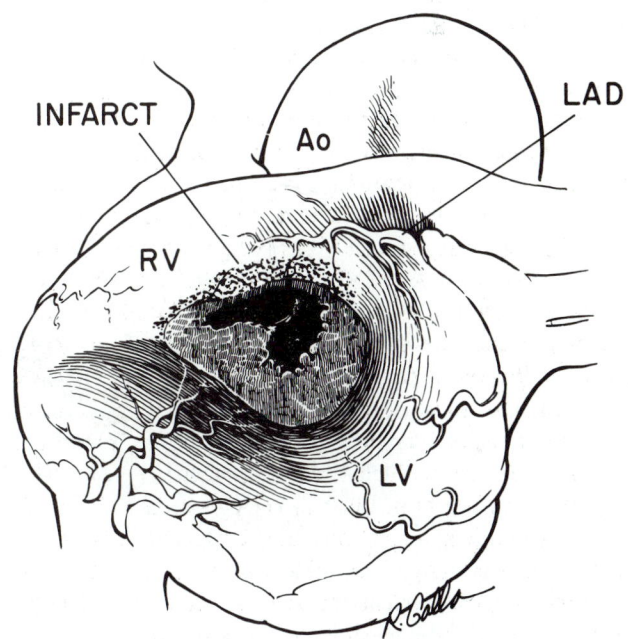

Figure 129–1. View of apical septal rupture, which is exposed by amputating apex of left and right ventricles. Ao, aorta; LAD, anterior descending branch of the left coronary artery; RV, right ventricle; LV, left ventricle.

tures that are passed sequentially through a buttressing strip of felt, the left ventricular wall, a second strip of felt, the interventricular septum, a third strip of felt, the right ventricular wall, and a fourth strip of felt (Fig. 129–2). After all sutures have been tied, the closure is reinforced with an additional over-and-over suture.

Anterior Septal Rupture

The approach to these defects is by a left ventricular transinfarct incision with infarctectomy (Fig. 129–3). Small defects beneath anterior infarcts can be closed by the technique of plication as suggested by Shumaker.[73] This involves approximation of the posterior rim of the anterior defect to the right ventricular free wall using mattress sutures over strips of felt. The transinfarct incision is then closed with a second row of mattress sutures buttressed with strips of felt (Fig. 129–4). An over-and-over running suture completes the ventriculotomy closure.

Most anterior defects require closure with a prosthetic patch (DeBakey Elastic Dacron fabric made by U.S.C.I., Division of C.R. Bard, Inc., Billerica, MA) (Fig. 129–5) to avoid tension that could lead to disruption of the repair. After debridement of necrotic septum and left ventricular muscle, a series of pledgeted interrupted mattress sutures are placed around the perimeter of the defect. Along the posterior aspect of the defect, sutures are passed through the septum from right side to left. Along the anterior edge of the defect, sutures are passed from the epicardial surface of the right ventricle to the endocardial surface. All sutures are then passed through the edge of a synthetic patch, which is seated on the left side of the septum. Each suture is then passed through an additional pledget and then all are tied. The edges of the ventriculotomy are then approximated by a two-layer closure consisting of interrupted mattress su-

tures passed through buttressing strips of Teflon felt, and a final over-and-over running suture.

Inferoposterior Septal Rupture

Closure of inferoposterior septal defects, which result from transmural infarction in the distribution of the posterior descending artery, has posed the greatest technical challenge.[21] Early attempts at primary closure of these defects by simple plication techniques similar to those used in the repair of anterior defects was frequently unsuccessful because of the sutures tearing out of soft, friable myocardium that had been closed under tension. This resulted in either reopening of the defect or catastrophic disruption of the infarctectomy closure. It was, in large part, the analysis of such early results that led to the evolution of the operative principles enumerated above.

Use of the following techniques have been associated with a greatly improved operative survival. After the establishment of bypass with bicaval cannulation, the left side of the heart is vented via the right superior pulmonary vein. The heart is retracted out of the pericardial well as for bypass to the posterior descending coronary artery. The margins of the defect may involve the inferior aspects of both ventricles, or of the left ventricle only (Fig. 129–6A). A transinfarct incision is made in the left ventricle, and the left ventricular portion of the infarct is excised (Fig. 129–6B), exposing the septal defect. The left ventricular papillary muscles are inspected. Only if there is frank papillary muscle rupture is mitral valve replacement performed (when it is indicated, we prefer to perform mitral valve replacement through a separate conventional left atrial incision, to avoid trauma to the friable ventricular muscle). After all infarcted left ventricular muscle has been excised, a less aggressive debridement of the right ventricle is ac-

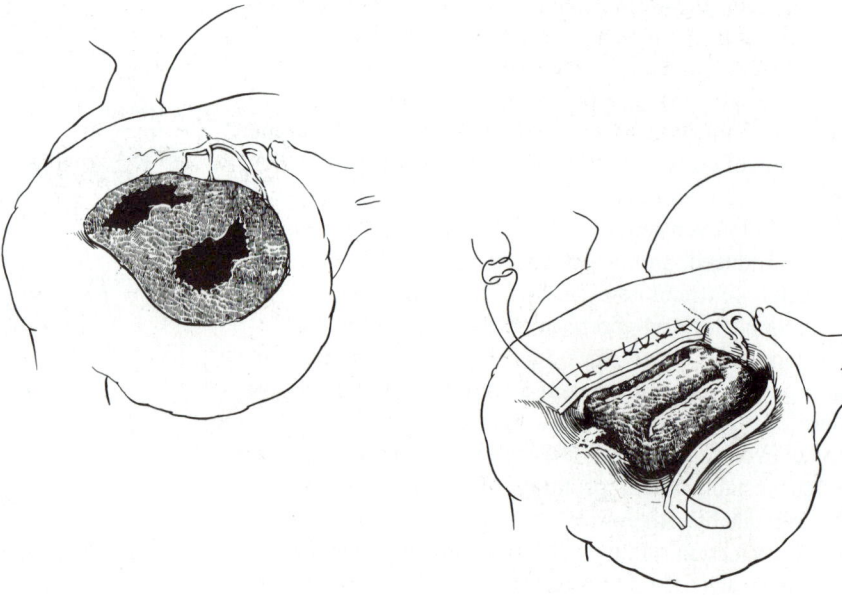

Figure 129–2. Left: Necrotic infarct and apical septum have been debrided back to healthy muscle. **Right:** Repair effected by approximation of left ventricle, apical septum, and right ventricle; interrupted mattress sutures of O Tevdek with buttressing strips of Teflon felt are used within the interior of the left and right ventricles as well as on the epicardial surface of each ventricle. All sutures are placed before any are tied. A second running suture (not shown) is used, as in left ventricular aneurysm repair, to ensure a secure hemostatic ventriculotomy closure.

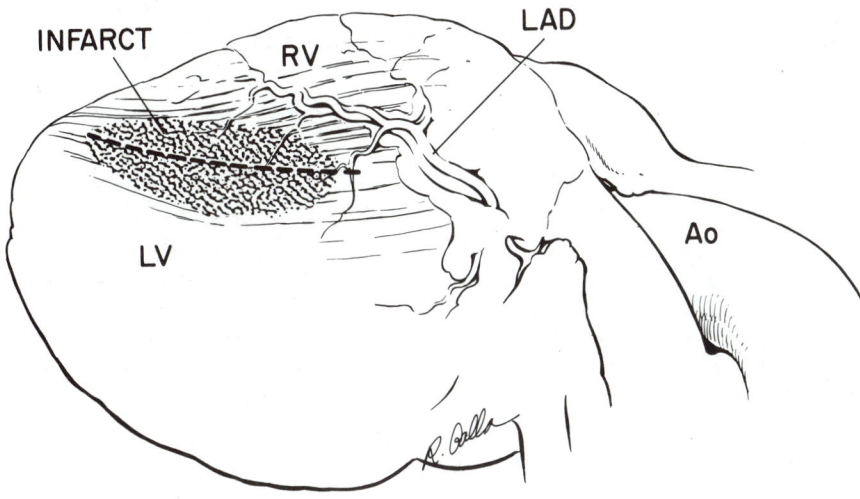

Figure 129–3. Transinfarct left ventricular incision to expose anterior septal rupture. Incision (dashed line) is made parallel to anterior descending branch of left coronary artery (LAD) through center of infarct (stippled area) in anterior left ventricle (LV). Ao, aorta; RV, right ventricle.

complished, with the goal of resecting only as much muscle as is necessary to afford complete visualization of the defect. With the technique described, delayed rupture of the right ventricle has not been a problem. If the posterior septum has cracked or split from the adjacent ventricular free wall without loss of a great deal of septal tissue, then the septal rim of the posterior defect may be approximated to the edge of the diaphragmatic right ventricular free wall using mattress sutures buttressed with strips of Teflon felt (Fig. 129–6C). Larger defects require patch closure. Pledgeted mattress sutures are placed from the right side of the septum and from the epicardial side of the right ventricular free wall (Fig. 129–6D). All sutures are passed through the

perimeter of the patch and then through additional pledgets, and are then tied (Fig. 129–6F). Thus, as in closure of large anterior defects, the patch is secured on the left ventricular side of the septum. Direct closure of the remaining infarctectomy is rarely possible because of tension required to pull together the edges of the gaping defect. A prosthetic patch is generally required. Originally we cut an oval patch from a Cooley low porosity woven Dacron tube graft (Meadox Medicals, Inc. Oakland, NJ). Currently we cut this patch from a Hemashield woven double velour Dacron collagen-impregnated graft (Meadox Medicals,Inc.). Pledgeted mattress sutures are passed out through the margin of the infarctectomy (Fig. 129–6G) and then through the patch

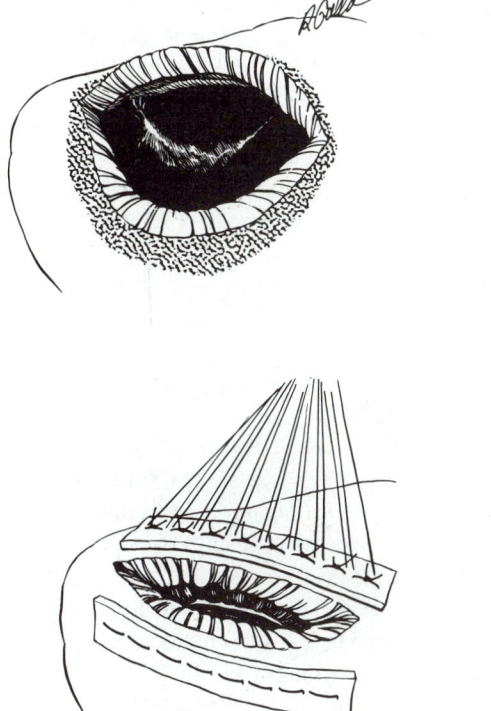

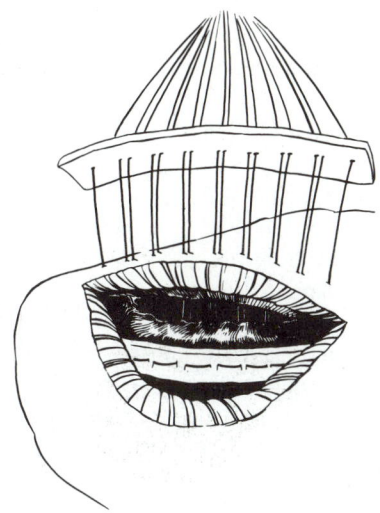

Figure 129–4. Repair of anterior septal rupture by plicating free anterior edge of septum to right ventricular free wall with interrupted O Tevdek mattress sutures buttressed with strips of Teflon felt. Orientation as in Figure 129–3. Left ventriculotomy (lower illustration) is closed as a separate suture line, again with interrupted mattress sutures buttressed with felt. A second running suture (not shown) is used to ensure a secure left ventriculotomy closure.

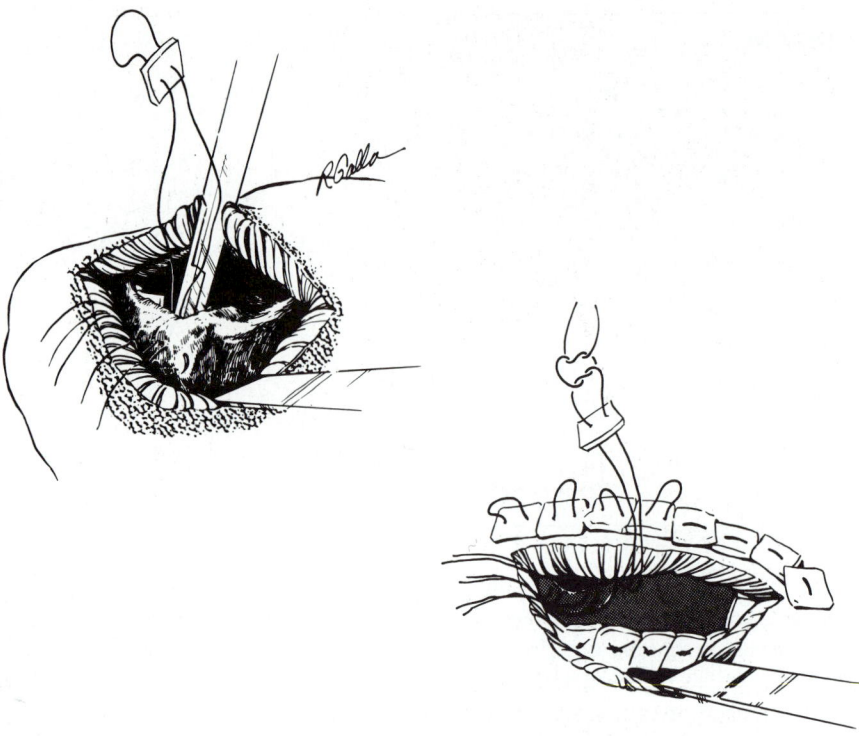

Figure 129–5. Larger anterior defects require a patch [DeBakey Dacron fabric (elastic) made by United States Catheter and Instrument Corporation, Billerica, MA], which is sewn to the left side of the ventricular septum with interrupted mattress sutures, each of which is buttressed with a pledget of Teflon felt on the right ventricular side of the septum and anteriorly on the epicardial surface of the right ventricular free wall. All sutures are placed before the patch is inserted. We use additional pledgets on the left ventricular side overlying the patch (lower right illustration) to cushion each suture as it is tied down to prevent cutting through the friable muscle.

(Fig. 129–6H), which is seated on the epicardial surface of the heart. After each suture is passed through an additional pledget, all sutures are tied (Fig. 129–6I). The cross-sectional view of the completed repair (Fig. 129–7) illustrates the restoration of relatively normal ventricular geometry, which is accomplished by the use of appropriately sized prosthetic patches.

Other Operative Techniques

Most of the other operative techniques that have resulted in successful management of postinfarction of ventricular septal rupture have adhered to the same general principles described above. An example is the method described in 1989 by da Silva and associates, whereby a nontransfixing running suture has been used to secure a large prosthetic patch to the left side of the ventricular septum with little or no resection of septum muscle.[74] This method, which has been used successfully in the management of anterior defects, is based upon transinfarct incision into the left ventricle, securing a patch to the left side of the septum, and closure of the infarctectomy with sutures buttressed with the prosthetic material.

In 1987 Rousou and associates reported successful cases of closure of an acquired posterior ventricular septal defect by means of a transatrial approach.[75] Such a technique does not, of course, involve infarctectomy, and thus cannot achieve the hemodynamic advantages of elimination of a paradoxically bulging segment of ventricular wall. Filgueira and colleagues have used the transatrial approach

for *delayed* repair of chronic acquired posterior septal defects.[76] We would concur with that group's cautionary statement that while this approach may be used selectively for the closure of chronic defects, it is unlikely to be an appropriate choice for the closure of acute defects except under rare circumstances.

In the early 1990s the technique of intracavitary placement of an endocardial patch supported by an epicardial patch was introduced by David,[69] and then by Cooley,[77] and Ross.[68] This so-called endocardial repair consists of exposing the septum through a left ventriculotomy in the infarcted wall in the now standard fashion. Then, a single patch of either Dacron fabric or glutaraldehyde-fixed bovine pericardium[77] is sutured to the healthy endocardium all around the infarct with a continuous polypropylene suture,[69] which may be reinforced with pledgeted mattress sutures.[68,77] This excludes the septal defect, the infarcted septum, and the infarcted free wall from the left ventricular chamber (Fig. 129–8A). The left ventriculotomy is closed either primarily (Fig. 129–8B) or it is reinforced with an epicardial patch (Fig. 129–8C). Thus, instead of closing the septal defect, it is simply *excluded* from the high pressure zone of the left ventricle. There are several theoretical advantages in this technique. It does not require resection of myocardium, which, if excessive, results in depression of ventricular function and if insufficient predisposes to recurrence of septal rupture. It also maintains ventricular geometry, which could enhance ventricular function; and it avoids tension on friable muscle, which may diminish postoperative bleeding. However, it is too early to tell if endocardial

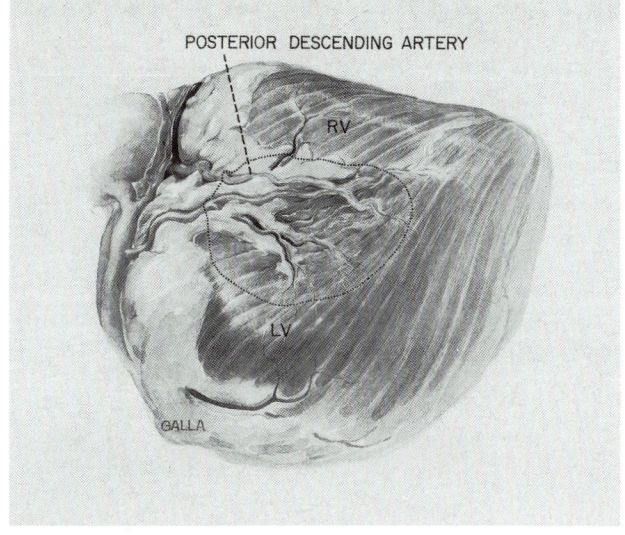

A

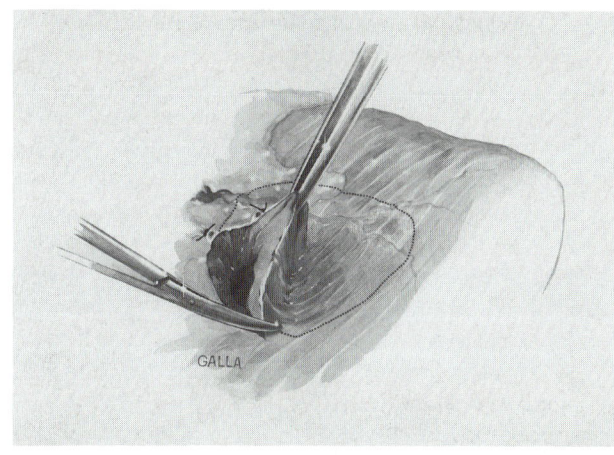

B

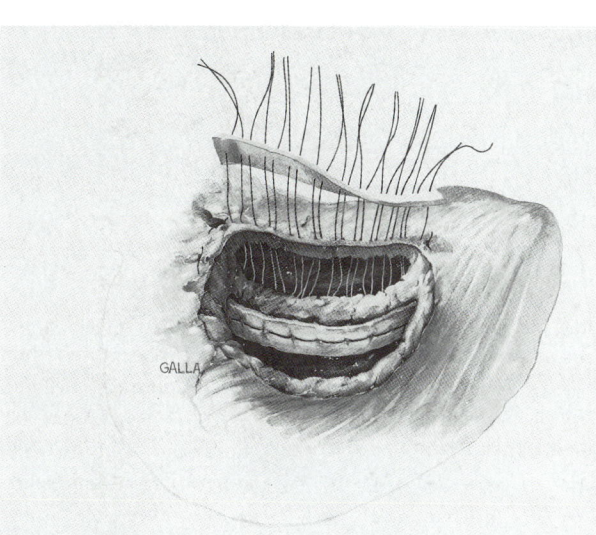

C

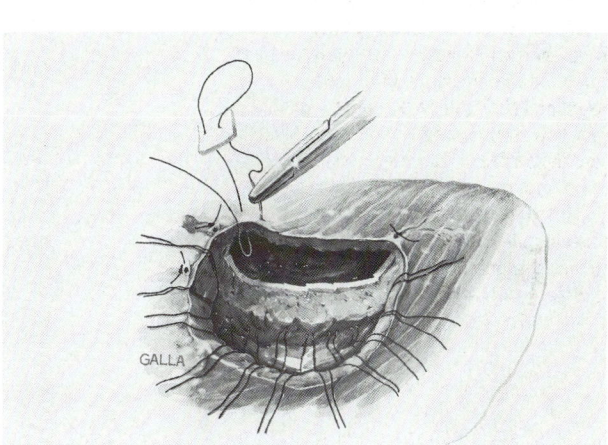

D

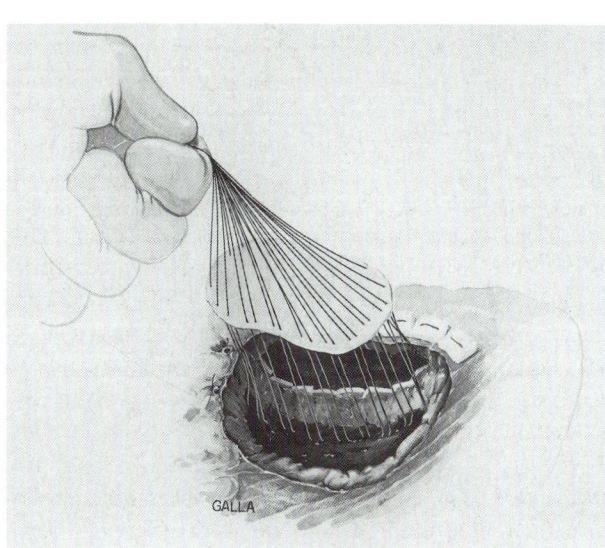

E

Figure 129–6. A. View of inferior infarct (circumscribed by dotted line) associated with posterior septal rupture. Apex of the heart is to the right. Exposure at operation is achieved by dislocating the heart up out of the pericardial sac and retracting the heart cephalad as in the performance of distal vein bypass and anastomosis to the posterior descending artery. RV, diaphragmatic surface of right ventricle; LV, posterior left ventricle. **B.** The inferoposterior infarct is excised to expose the posterior septal defect. Complete excision of the left ventricular portion of the infarct is important to prevent delayed rupture of the ventriculotomy repair. The free edge of the right ventricle is progressively shaved back to expose the margins of the defect clearly (see Fig. 129–6C). **C.** Repair of the posterior septal rupture by approximating the edge of the posterior septum to the free wall of the diaphragmatic right ventricle with felt-buttressed mattress sutures. The repair is possible when the septum has cracked or split off from the posterior ventricular wall without necrosis of a great deal of septal muscle. The surgeon can perform repair of posterior septal rupture to best advantage by standing at the left side of the supine patient. **D.** Repair of posterior septal rupture wherein there has been necrosis of a substantial portion of the posterior septum. Interrupted mattress sutures are placed circumferentially around the defect. These sutures are buttressed with felt pledgets on the right ventricular side of the septum and on the epicardial surface of the diaphragmatic right ventricle. **E.** All sutures are placed and then the patch (DeBakey elastic Dacron fabric) is slid into place on the left ventricular side of the septum. *(Continued.)*

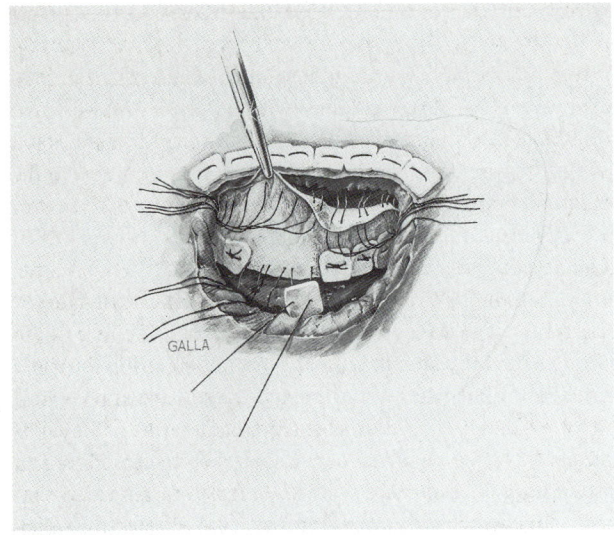

F

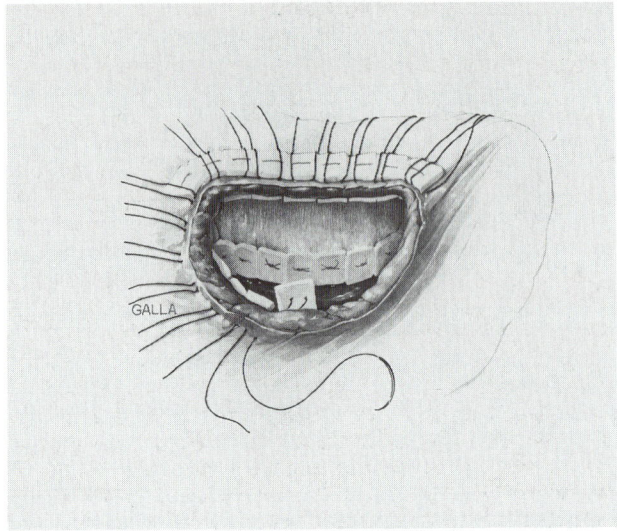

G

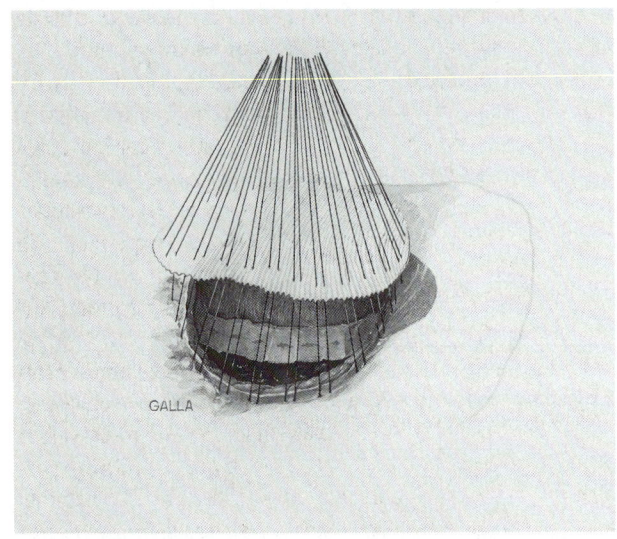

H

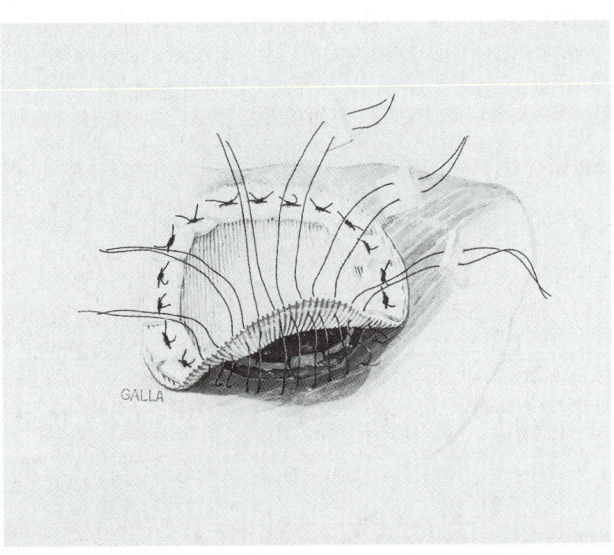

I

Figure 129–6. *(Continued.)* **F.** The patch sutures are tied down with an additional felt pledget placed on top of the patch (left ventricular side), as each suture is tied, to cushion the tie and prevent cutting through the friable muscle. The maneuvers illustrated in **G,H,** and **I** are viewed by the authors as essential to the success of early repair of the posterior septal rupture. **G.** The patch repair of the posterior septal defect has been completed. Remaining to be repaired is the posterior left ventricular free wall defect created by infarctectomy. Mattress sutures of 2-0 Tevdek are placed circumferentially around the margins of the posterior left ventricular free wall defect. Each suture is buttressed with a Teflon felt pledget on the endocardial side of the left ventricle. **H.** With all sutures in place, a circular patch, fashioned from a Cooley low-porosity woven Dacron tube graft (Meadox Medicals Inc., Oakland, NJ), is slid down onto the epicardial surface of the left ventricle. This onlay technique of patch placement prevents the cracking of friable left ventricular muscle that occurred with the eversion technique of patch insertion. **I.** An additional pledget of Teflon felt is placed under each suture (on top of the patch) as it is tied to cushion the tie and prevent cutting through the friable underlying muscle. *(From Daggett WM: J Thorac Cardiovasc Surg 84:306, 1982.)*

repair of postinfarction ventricular septal rupture will significantly affect short- and long-term outcome of this life-threatening condition. It appears particularly applicable to anterior defects.

Recently Tashiro et al[78] described an extended endocardial repair in which a saccular patch of glutaraldehyde-fixed equine pericardium was used to exclude an anterior

septal rupture. Usui et al[79] reported the successful repair of a posterior septal rupture using two sheets of equine pericardium to sandwich the infarcted myocardium including the septal defect and ventriculotomy.

Immediately postpump, patients should undergo transesophageal echocardiography to examine ventricular function and search for the presence of any residual shunt. Peri-

ANTERIOR

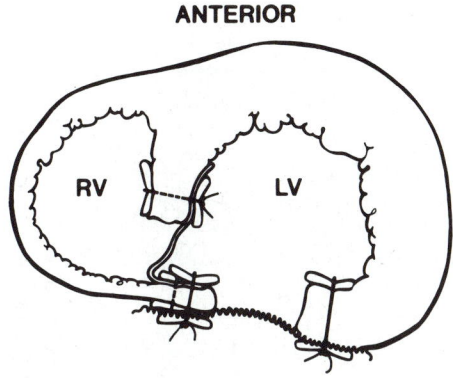

Figure 129–7. Cross-sectional view of the completed repair of posterior septal rupture with prosthetic patch placement of the posterior left ventricular free wall defect created by infarctectomy. RV, right ventricular cavity; LV, left ventricular cavity. *(From Daggett WM: J Thorac Cardiovasc Surg 84:306, 1982.)*

operative bleeding may be reduced by application of a fibrin sealant to the ventricular septum around the septal defect prior to formal repair.[80]

Percutaneous Closure

Successful transcatheter closure of congenital ventricular septal defects[81] and postinfarction ventricular septal rupture[82] has been reported using a double umbrella prosthesis. In one case, a balloon catheter was introduced percutaneously to abolish the shunt in a poor-risk patient with postinfarction septal rupture. Hemodynamic improvement was immediate and sustained, and 3 wk later the septal defect was closed operatively with a good result.[83]

Technical improvements in the experimental devices being tested to obliterate intracardiac shunts percutaneously may one day become an important tool in the treatment of postinfarction ventricular septal rupture, and currently are used successfully for recurrent or residual defects after primary surgical repairs (L. Cohn, personal communication).

CORONARY REVASCULARIZATION

There has been much controversy in the literature concerning the advantages and disadvantages of concurrent coronary artery grafting in patients undergoing emergent repair of postinfarction ventricular septal rupture.[24,28,57–59] Some have argued that the revascularization provides no benefit and subjects patients to preoperative left heart catheterization, a time-consuming and potentially dangerous diagnostic procedure.[24,59] Loisance et al[84] base their recent policy of not revascularizing patients with postinfarction septal ruptures on the fact that none of their 20 long-term survivors (five of whom were bypassed) had incapacitating angina or recurrent myocardial infarction. Piwnica and associates[58] reported a series of 28 survivors of early opera-

tive closure of postinfarction ventricular septal rupture, among whom only one had coronary artery grafting. Among the 24 patients for whom follow-up was complete, there were only 2 late deaths of cardiac origin. However, it is not clear from their report what the impact of associated coronary artery disease (revascularized or not) may have been on the course of the other 32 patients who did not survive operation.

Some groups use left heart catheterization and coronary bypassing selectively.[28,29] Davies and colleagues[28] found that of 60 long-term survivors (median 70 mo; range 1 to 174 mo) only five patients developed exertional angina during follow-up and none required revascularization. Their current policy is to avoid left heart catheterization on patients in whom an acquired septal defect is suspected to be a consequence of their first anterior infarction, provided that the patients have no history of angina or electrocardiographic evidence of previous infarction in another territory.[28] This approach is also based on the findings that multivessel disease is much less prevalent in those with an apical septal rupture as a result of anterior infarction.[29]

We[57] and others[23,63,68,69,85] have employed coronary revascularization with increasing frequency. Our policy is to place aortocoronary grafts to principal epicardial coronary arteries that have severe proximal stenoses. To investigate the early and late effects of coronary artery revascularization, we have recently reviewed our experience in patients undergoing repair of postinfarction septal rupture.[57] Between June 1968 and April 1991, 75 patients underwent coronary angiography and repair of postinfarction septal rupture. Thirty-three patients had two- or three-vessel proximal coronary artery disease and underwent complete revascularization, 19 patients also had two- or three-vessel coronary disease but did not have bypass grafting performed with the closure of the septal defect, and 23 patients had only single-vessel coronary artery disease that corresponded to the region of the infarct: they underwent ventricular septal defect repair only. Cumulative 30-day mortality was similar in all three groups (21 to 26%), however, patients undergoing revascularization demonstrated significantly improved *long-term survival* when compared with patients who were unbypassed despite each group having a similar extent of coronary artery disease and similar preoperative hemodynamics. With follow-up after 5 and 10 years, survival was 72.2 and 47.8%, respectively, in the bypassed group, 29.2 and 0%, respectively, in the unbypassed group, and 52.2 and 36.5%, respectively, in the cohort with single-vessel disease. Not only do these data support concomitant revascularization during the repair of postinfarction septal rupture, but they also support the use of coronary angiography preoperatively in all patients who have suffered this lesion.

It is interesting that in our series, patients with anterior septal defects benefited from bypassing associated coronary disease to a greater extent than did patients with posteriorly located septal defects. Specifically, in patients with an ante-

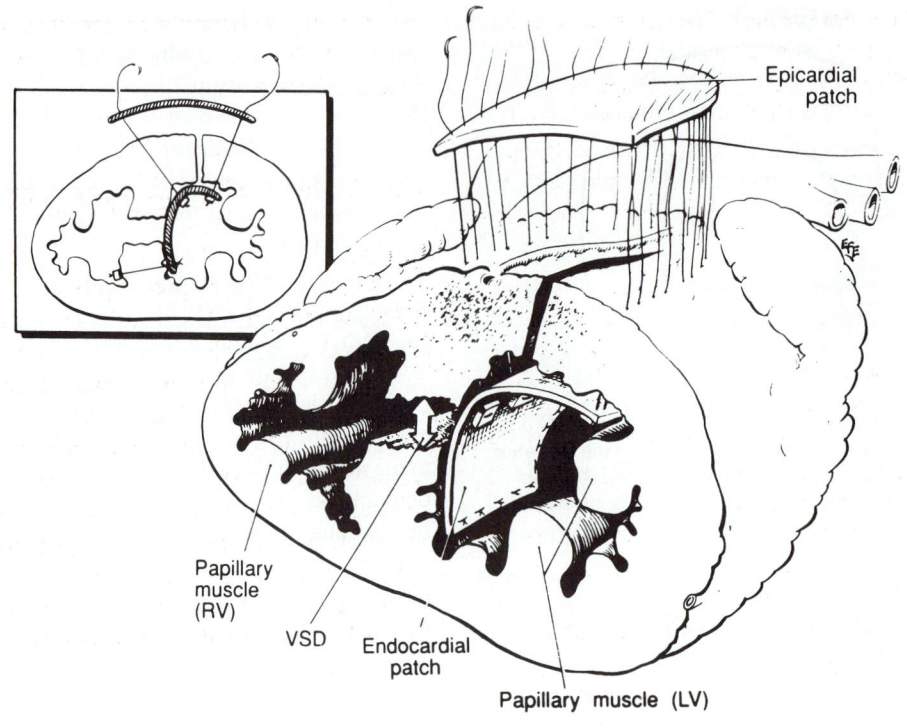

A

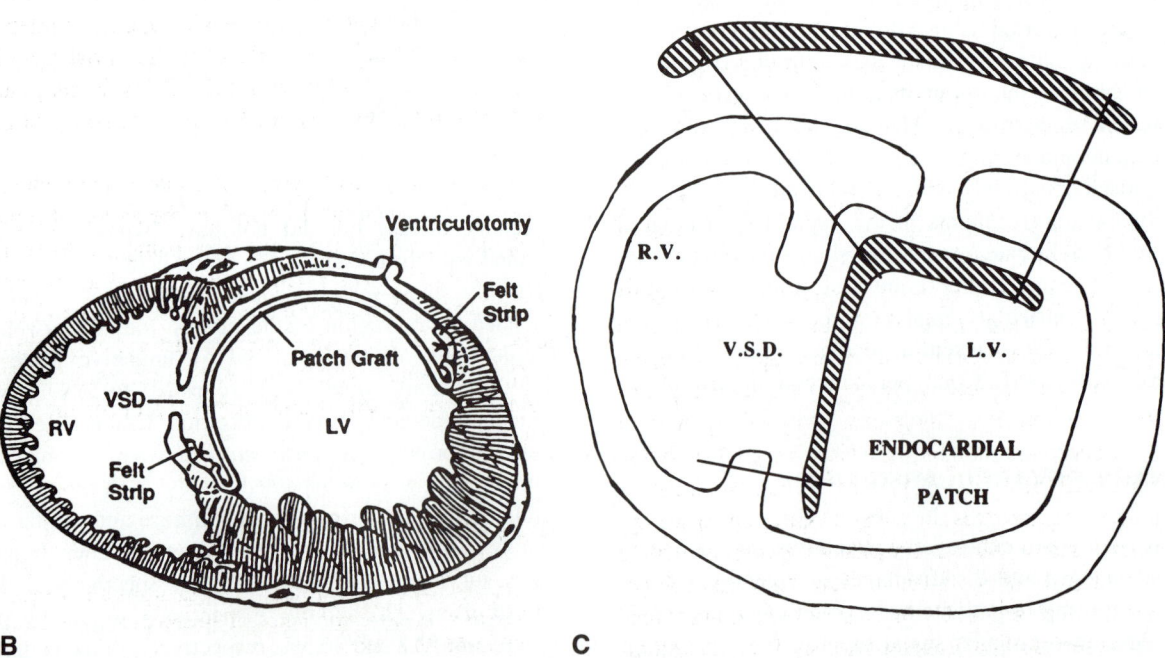

B   **C**

Figure 129–8. A. Endocardial repair of postinfarction ventricular septal rupture. The standard ventriculotomy is made in the infarcted area of left ventricular free wall. An interior patch of either Dacron(Meadox Medicals Inc., Oakland, NJ), polytetrafluoroethylene, or glutaraldehyde-fixed pericardium is fashioned to replace and/or cover the diseased areas (septal defect, septal infarction, free wall infarction). The internal patch is secured to normal endocardium with a continuous monofilament suture which may be reinforced for pledgeted mattress sutures. There is little, if any, resection of myocardium and no attempt is made to close the septal defect. **B.** The ventriculotomy, which is outside the pressure zone of the left ventricle, may be repaired with a continuous suture. **C.** Alternatively, the sutures can be passed through the ventricular free wall and through a tailored external patch of Teflon or pericardium. On transverse section, one can see that the endocardial patch is secured at three levels, above and below the septal rupture and beyond the ventriculotomy. *(From Alvarez JM, et al: J Card Surg 7:198, 1992, with permission.)*

riorly located septal perforation, only 16% of those with unbypassed coronary disease were alive after 5 years of follow-up, however, after revascularization of all epicardial disease, 92% were alive. This finding puts into question the policy of avoiding coronary angiograms in patients with apical septal rupture due to anterior myocardial infarction.[28]

SURVIVAL

Adhering to the policy of early operative intervention described above, we reported an overall hospital mortality of 25% in patients treated since 1975.[31] Mortality varied with anatomic location of the septal defect. Mortality was 34% for correction of posterior defects and 15% for closure of anterior defects. Skillington et al[29] reported an overall early mortality of 20.8% in 101 patients who underwent surgical correction of postinfarction ventricular septal defects between 1973 and 1988 (32.6 for posterior defects and 12.1% for anterior defects). However, their most recent experience with 36 patients (1987 to 1988) has seen early mortality decline to 11.1%.[29] Deville and colleagues[63] reported a similar improvement in mortality. Using their endocardial patch technique, Komeda et al[69] report an operative mortality of 10% in 31 patients operated on between 1980 and 1989.

Factors found to increase the risk of early death are (1) posterior infarctions, which are technically more difficult to repair and associated with right ventricular dysfunction,[20,56,57,86] (2) a short time interval between infarction and operation which selects for sicker patients,[22,25,87] and (3) the presence of cardiogenic shock.[23,25,63,69,88]

Long-term results have been favorable as regards to survival and functional rehabilitation. Sixty-four percent of our patients treated since 1975 are long-term survivors. In our series, 8 of the 19 long-term survivors were in New York Heart Association functional class I, and 10 were in New York Heart Association functional class II.[33] In a recent review, our data revealed that patients over the age of 70 could expect excellent long-term survival, with over 90% of these survivors remaining in New York Heart Association functional class I or II. Gaudiani and associates reported similar long-term results using an early operative approach. In their series, 88% of hospital survivors were alive at 5 years, with 74% of survivors in New York Heart Association functional class I and 21% of survivors in functional class II. In the series of patients reported by Piwnica and associates, there were 20 long-term survivors, of whom 8 were in New York Heart Association functional class I and 12 were in class II. Finally, in what is probably the largest follow-up study to date (60 long-term survivors), Davies et al[28] reported 5-, 10-, and 14-year survivals of 69, 50, and 37%. Eighty-two percent of patients were in New York Heart Association functional class I or II.

Thus, it is clearly the case that aggressive management of postinfarction ventricular septal rupture with a program of early surgical intervention can be anticipated to yield favorable long-term results in terms of both survival and functional palliation.

RECURRENT VENTRICULAR SEPTAL DEFECTS

Recurrent or residual septal defects have been diagnosed by Doppler color-flow mapping early or late postoperatively in 10 to 25% of patients.[29] They may be due to reopening of a closed defect, to the presence of an overlooked defect, or to the development of a new septal rupture during the early postoperative period. These recurrent defects should be closed when they cause symptoms or signs of heart failure. When they are small ($Q_p:Q_s < 2.0$) and either asymptomatic or controlled with minimal diuretic therapy, a conservative approach is reasonable and late spontaneous closure can occur.[29] Intervention in the catheterization laboratory with a clam-shell device may be useful in closing symptomatic residual or recurrent defects postoperatively.

SUMMARY

Postinfarction ventricular septal rupture constitutes a surgical emergency. The presence of cardiogenic shock is an indication for prompt surgical repair. Operative intervention should be accomplished early after the initial stabilization of patients who are not in shock. Delay in surgical treatment is appropriate only for the select minority of patients who are truly stable.

The principles of operative management include a left ventricular transinfarct approach to the region of septal rupture, and reconstructive techniques using prosthetic materials to restore cardiac geometry and avoid undo tension of the repair. Such a therapeutic approach results in dramatic alterations of the dismal natural history of postinfarction ventricular septal rupture with long-term results that are favorable with regard to both survival and functional palliation.

REFERENCES

1. Daggett WM: Postinfarction ventricular septal defect repair: Retrospective thoughts and historical perspectives. *Ann Thorac Surg* **50:**1006–1009, 1990

2. Latham PM: *Lectures on Subjects Connected with Clinical Medicine Comprising Diseases of the Heart.* 2nd edn. London, Longman Rees, 1845

3. Brunn F: Diagnostik der erworbenen ruptur der kammerscheidewand des herzens. *Wien Arch Inn Med* **6:**533–535, 1923

4. Sager R: Coronary thrombosis: Perforation of the infarcted interventricular septum. *Arch Intern Med* **53:**140–145, 1934

5. Cooley DA, Belmonte BA, Zeis LB, Schnur S: Surgical repair of ruptured interventricular septum following acute myocardial infarction. *Surgery* **41:**930–935, 1957

6. Effler DB, Tapia FA, McCormack LJ: Rupture of the ventricular my-

ocardium and perforation of the interventricular septum complicating acute myocardial infarction. *Circulation* 20:128–134, 1959

7. Dobell ARC, Scott HJ, Cronin RFP, Reid EAS: Surgical closure of interventricular septal perforation complicating myocardial infarction. *J Thorac Cardiovasc Surg* 43:802–809, 1962

8. Bressie JL, Snyder DD, Williams GR et al: Ruptured interventricular septum: Successful repair after myocardial infarction. *J Am Med Assoc* 182:1043–1050, 1962

9. Payne WS, Hunt JC, Kirklin JW: Surgical repair of ventricular septal defect due to myocardial infarction: Report of a case. *J Am Med Assoc* 183:603–607, 1963

10. Sanders RJ, Kern WH, Blount SG: Perforation of the interventricular septum complicating myocardial infarction. *Am Heart J* 51:736–742, 1956

11. Lee WY, Cardon L, Slodki SV: Perforation of infarcted interventricular septum. *Arch Intern Med* 109:135–140, 1962

12. Daicoff AR, Rhodes ML: Surgical repair of ventricular septal rupture and ventricular aneurysms. *J Am Med Assoc* 203:457–461, 1968

13. Barnard PM, Kennedy JH: Postinfarction ventricular septal defect. *Circulation* 32:76–83, 1965

14. Allen P, Woodwark G: Surgical management of postinfarction ventricular septal defects. *J Thorac Cardiovasc Surg* 51:346–353, 1966

15. Heimbecker RO, Lemire G, Chen C: Surgery for massive myocardial infarction. *Circulation* 11–3 (Suppl 2):37–44, 1968

16. Iben AB, Pupello DF, Stinson EB, Shumway NE: Surgical treatment of postinfarction ventricular septal defects. *Ann Thorac Surg* 8:252–260, 1969

17. Lojos TZ, Greene DG, Bunnell IL, et al: Surgery for acute myocardial infarction. *Ann Thorac Surg* 8:452–457, 1969

18. Stinson EB, Becker J, Shumway NE: Successful repair of postinfarction ventricular septal defect and biventricular aneurysm. *J Thorac Cardiovasc Surg* 58:20–28, 1969

19. Freeny PC, Schattenberg TT, Danielson GK, et al: Ventricular septal defect and ventricular aneurysm secondary to acute myocardial infarction. *Circulation* 43:360–364, 1971

20. Daggett WM, Guyton RA, Mundth ED, et al: Surgery for post-myocardial infarct ventricular septal defect. *Ann Surg* 186:260–271, 1977

21. Daggett WM, Mundth ED, Gold HK, et al: Early repair of ventricular septal defects complicating inferior myocardial infarction. *Circulation* 50 (Suppl 3):112–119, 1974

22. Daggett WM: Surgical management of ventricular septal defects complicating myocardial infarction. *World J Surg* 2:753–758, 1978

23. Gaudiani VA, Miller DC, Stinson EB, et al: Post-infarction ventricular septal defect: An argument for early operation. *Surgery* 89:48–55, 1981

24. Matsui K, Kay JH, Mendez M, et al: Ventricular septal rupture secondary to myocardial infarction: Clinical approach and surgical results. *J Am Med Assoc* 245:1537–1539, 1981

25. Loisance DY, Cachera JP, Poulain H, et al: Ventricular septal defect after acute myocardial infarction. *J Thorac Cardiovasc Surg* 80:61–67, 1980

26. Donahoo JS, Brawley RK, Taylor D, Gott VL: Factors influencing survival following postinfarction ventricular septal defects. *Ann Thorac Surg* 19:648–654, 1975

27. Hill JD, Lary D, Keith WJ, Gerbode F: Acquired ventricular septal defects: Evolution of an operation, surgical technique and results. *J Thorac Cardiovasc Surg* 70:440–446, 1975

28. Davies RH, Dawkins KD, Skillington PD, et al: Late functional results after surgical closure of acquired ventricular septal defect. *J Thorac Cardiovasc Surg* 106:592–598, 1992

29. Skillington PD, Davies RH, Luff AJ, et al: Surgical treatment for infarct-related ventricular septal defects. *J Thorac Cardiovasc Surg* 99:798–808, 1990

30. Lundberg S, Sodestrom J: Perforation of the interventricular septum in myocardial infarction: A study based on autopsy material. *Acta Med Scand* 172:413–420, 1962

31. Heitmiller R, Jacobs ML, Daggett WM: Surgical management of postinfarction ventricular septal rupture. *Ann Thorac Surg* 41:683–690, 1986

32. Hutchins GM: Rupture of the interventricular septum complicating myocardial infarction: Pathological analysis of 10 patients with clinically diagnosed perforation. *Am Heart J* 97:165–170, 1979

33. Daggett WM, Buckley MJ, Akins CW, et al: Improved results of surgical management of postinfarction ventricular septal rupture. *Ann Surg* 196:269–277, 1982

34. Skehan JD, Carey C, Norrell MS, et al: Patterns of coronary artery disease in post-infarction ventricular septal rupture. *Br Heart J* 62:268–276, 1989

35. Miller S, Dinsmore RE, Greene RE, Daggett WM: Coronary, ventricular, and pulmonary abnormalities associated with rupture of the interventricular septum complicating myocardial infarction. *Am J Radiol* 131:571–584, 1978

36. Swithingbank JM: Perforation of the interventricular septum in myocardial infarction. *Br Heart J* 21:562–567, 1959

37. Edwards BS, Edwards WD, Edwards JE: Ventricular septal rupture complicating acute myocardial infarction: Identification of simple and complex types in 53 autopsied hearts. *Am J Cardiol* 54:1201–1205, 1984

38. Kitamura S, Mendez A, Kay JH: Ventricular septal defect following myocardial infarction: Experience with surgical repair through a left ventriculotomy and review of the literature. *J Thorac Cardiovasc Surg* 61:186–192, 1971

39. Selzer A, Gerbode F, Keith WJ: Clinical, hemodynamic and surgical considerations of rupture of the ventricular septum after infarction. *Am Heart J* 78:598–604, 1969

40. Mallory GK, White PD, Salcedo-Salgar J: The speed of healing of myocardial infarction: A study of the pathologic anatomy in seventy cases. *Am Heart J* 18:647–659, 1939

41. Abrams D, Edilist A, Luria M, Miller A: Ventricular aneurysms. *Circulation* 27:164–170, 1963

42. Oyamada A, Queen FB: Spontaneous rupture of the interventricular septum following acute myocardial infarction with some clinico-pathologic observations on survival in five cases. Unpublished, 1961

43. Campion BL, Harrison CE, Guiliani ER, et al: Ventricular septal defect after myocardial infarction. *Ann Intern Med* 70:251–261, 1969

44. Vlodaver Z, Edwards JE: Rupture of ventricular septum or papillary muscle complicating myocardial infarction. *Circulation* 55:815–821, 1977

45. Honey M, Belcher JR, Hasa M, Gibbons JRP: Case reports: Successful early repair of acquired ventricular septal defect after myocardial infarction. *Br Heart J* 29:453–459, 1967

46. Rawlins MO, Mendel D, Braimbridge MV: Ventricuolar septal defect and mitral regurgitation secondary to myocardial infarction. *Br Heart J* 34:323–330, 1972

47. Taylor FH, Citron DS, Robicsek F, Sanger PW: Simultaneous repair of ventricular septal defect and left ventricular aneurysm following myocardial infarction. *Ann Thorac Surg* 1:72–80, 1965

48. Meister SG, Helfant RH: Rapid differentiation of ruptured interventricular septum from acute mitral insufficiency. *N Engl J Med* 287:1024–1026, 1972

49. Hillis LD, Firth BG, Winniford MD: Variability of right-sided cardiac oxygen saturations in adults with and without left-to-right intracardiac shunt. *Am J Cardiol* 58:129–132, 1986

50. Heikkilä J, Karesoja M: Ruptured interventricular septum complicating acute myocardial infarction. *Chest* 66:675–682, 1974

51. Buckley MJ, Mundth ED, Daggett WM, et al: Surgical therapy for early complications of myocardial infarction. *Surgery* 70:814–820, 1971

52. Harrison MR, MacPhail B, Gurley JC, et al: Usefulness of color Doppler flow imaging to distinguish ventricular septal defect from acute mitral regurgitation complicating acute myocardial infarction. *Am J Cardiol* 64:697–701, 1989

53. Smyllie JH, Sutherland GR, Geuskens R, et al: Doppler color flow

mapping in the diagnosis of ventricular septal rupture and acute mitral regurgitation after myocardial infarction. *J Am Coll Cardiol* **15:**1449–1455, 1990

54. Blanche C, Khan SS, Matloff JM, et al: Results of early repair of ventricular septal defect after an acute myocardial infarction. *J Thorac Cardiovasc Surg* **104:**961–965, 1992

55. Scanlon PJ, Monotoya A, Johnson SA: Urgent surgery for ventricular septal rupture complicating myocardial infarction. *Circulation* **72** (Suppl 2):185–190, 1985

56. Jones MT, Schofield PM, Dark JF: Surgical repair of acquired ventricular septal defect: Determinants of early and late outcome. *J Thorac Cardiovasc Surg* **93:**680–686, 1987

57. Muehrcke DD, Daggett WM, Buckley MJ, et al: Postinfarct ventricular septal defect repair: Effect of coronary artery bypass grafting. *Ann Thorac Surg* **54:**876–883, 1992

58. Piwnica A, Menasche P, Beaufils P, Julliard JM: Long-term results of emergency surgery for postinfarction ventricular septal defect. *Ann Thorac Surg* **44:**274–279, 1987

59. Kaplan MA, Harris CN, Kay JH, et al: Postinfarctional septal rupture: Clinical approach and surgical results. *Chest* **69:**734–738, 1976

60. Gold HK, Leinbach RC, Sanders CA, et al: Intra-aortic balloon pumping for ventricular septal defect or mitral regurgitation complicating acute myocardial infarction. *Circulation* **47:**1191–1196, 1973

61. Montoya A: Ventricular septal rupture secondary to acute myocardial infarction. In Pifarre R (ed): *Cardiac Surgery: Acute Myocardial Infarction and Its Complications.* Philadelphia, Hanley & Belfus, 1992, pp 159–167

62. Babb JD, Waldhausen JA, Zelis R: Balloon induced right ventricular outflow obstruction: A new approach to control of acute interventricular shunting after myocardial infarction in canines and swine. *Circ Res* **40:**372–376, 1977

63. Deville C, Fontan F, Chevalier JM, et al: Surgery of post-infarction ventricular defect: Risk factors for hospital death and long-term results. *Eur J Cardiothorac Surg* **5:**167–175, 1991

64. Kay HR: In discussion of Daggett WM: Surgical management of ventricular septal defects complicating myocardial infarction *World J Surg* **2:**753, 1978

65. Estrada-Quintero T, Uretsky BF, Murali S, Hardesty RL: Prolonged intraaortic balloon support for septal rupture after myocardial infarction. *Ann Thorac Surg* **53:**335–337, 1992

66. Radford MJ, Johnson RA, Daggett WM, et al: Ventricular septal defect following myocardial infarction: Factors affecting survival. *Clin Res* **26:**262A, 1978

67. Guiliani ER, Danielson GK, Pluth JR: Postinfarction ventricular septal rupture. *Circulation* **49:**455–460, 1974

68. Alvarez JM, Brady PW, Ross DE: Technical improvements in the repair of acute postinfarction ventricular septal rupture. *J Cardiac Surg* **7:**198–202, 1992

69. Komeda M, Fremes SE, David TE: Surgical repair of the postinfarction ventricular septal defect. *Circulation* **82**(Suppl 4):243–247, 1990

70. Baillot R, Pelletier C, Trivino-Marin J, Castonguay Y: Postinfarction ventricular septal defect: Delayed closure with prolonged mechanical circulatory support. *Ann Thorac Surg* **35:** 138–145, 1983

71. Daggett WM, Burwell LR, Lawson DW, Austen WG: Resection of acute ventricular aneurysm and ruptured interventricular septum after myocardial infarction. *N Engl J Med* **283:**1507–1514, 1970

72. David H, Hunter JA, Najafi H, et al: Left ventricular approach for the repair of ventricular septal performation and infarctectomy. *J Thorac Cardiovasc Surg* **63:**14–24, 1972

73. Shumaker H: Suggestions concerning operative management of postinfarction ventricular septal defect. *J Thorac Cardiovasc Surg* **64:**452–457, 1972

74. daSilva JP, Cascudo MM, Baumgratz JF, et al: Postinfarction ventricular septal defect: An efficacious technique for early surgical repair. *J Thorac Cardiovasc Surg* **97:**86–89, 1989

75. Rousou JA, Engelman RM, Breyer RH, et al: Transatrial repair of postinfarction posterior ventricular septal defect. *Ann Thorac Surg* **43:**665–661, 1987

76. Filgueira JL, Battistessa SA, Estable H, et al: Delayed repair of an acquired posterior septal defect through a right atrial approach. *Ann Thorac Surg* **42:**208–215, 1986

77. Cooley DA: Repair of postinfarction ventricular septal defect. *J Cardiac Surg* **9:**427–429, 1994

78. Tashiro T, Todo K, Haruta Y, et al: Extended endocardial repair of postinfarction ventricular septal rupture: New operative technique modification of the Komeda-David operation. *J Cardiac Surg* **9:**97–102, 1994

79. Usui A, Murase M, Maeda M, et al: Sandwich repair with two sheets of equine pericardial patch for acute posterior post-infarction ventricular septal defect. *Eur J Cardiothorac Surg* **7:**47–49, 1993

80. Seguin JR, Frapier JM, Colson P, Chaptal PA: Fibrin sealant for early repair of acquired ventricular septal defect. *J Thorac Cardiovasc Surg* **104:**748–751, 1992

81. Bridges ND, Perry SB, Keane JF, et al: Preoperative transcatheter closure of congenital muscular ventricular septal defects. *N Engl J Med* **324:**1312–1315, 1991

82. Lock JE, Block PC, McKay RG, et al: Transcatheter closure of ventricular septal defects. *Circulation* **78:**361–369, 1988

83. Hachida M, Nakano H, Hirai M, Shi CY: Percutaneous transaortic closure of postinfarction ventricular septal rupture. *Ann Thorac Surg* **51:**655–667, 1991

84. Loisance DP, Lordez JM, Deleuze PH, et al: Acute postinfarction septal rupture: Long-term results. *Ann Thorac Surg* **52:**474–478, 1991

85. Weintraub RM, Thurer RL, Wei J: Repair of postinfarction ventricular septal defect in the elderly: Early and long term results. *J Thorac Cardiovasc Surg* **85:**191–196, 1983

86. Moore CA, Nygaard TW, Kaiser DL, et al: Postinfarction ventricular septal rupture: The importance of location of infarction and right ventricular function in determining survival. *Circulation* **74:**45–55, 1987

87. Hill JD, Stiles QR: Acute ischemic ventricular septal defect. *Circulation* **79**(Suppl 1):112–114, 1989

88. Radford MJ, Johnson RA, Daggett WM, et al: Ventricular septal rupture: A review of clinical and physiological features and an analysis of survival. *Circulation* **64:**545–553, 1981

Surgical Treatment of Left Ventricular Aneurysm

Andrew C. Fiore and Adib D. Jatene

HISTORICAL PERSPECTIVE

Modern surgical treatment of left ventricular (LV) aneurysms was initiated in 1955 when Likoff and Bailey performed a closed resection of an LV aneurysm utilizing a special side-biting clamp introduced through a thoracotomy incision.[1] In 1958, Cooley and colleagues utilized extracorporeal circulation in the performance of an aneurysmectomy utilizing a buttressed linear suture technique that is still in wide use today.[2] In 1977, Daggett et al introduced the concept of substituting Dacron material for part of the ventricular wall. This was undertaken to avoid deformity of the ventricular cavity in patients undergoing inferior wall infarctectomy due to postinfarction ventricular septal defect.[3] Utilizing this concept, Jatene and colleagues* introduced the concept of a geometric reconstruction of the left ventricle with the use of a Dacron patch. In 1978, Cooley proposed this treatment for the infarcted septal wall.[4] In 1985, Jatene defined the aneurysmectomy, not as a resection, but as a reconstruction of the geometry of the ventricular cavity most commonly utilizing a Dacron patch.[5]

INCIDENCE AND NATURAL HISTORY

Aneurysmal dilatation of the left ventricle occurs in between 10 and 35% of the patients experiencing a transmural myocardial infarction. The reported incidence varies depending upon the definition of aneurysm utilized by the au-

thor. Different types of ventricular contractility alterations may result from myocardial infarction. The most frequent are akinesia (noncontractile area) and dyskinesia, defined as an area that does not contract but rather expands during systole. Although ischemic, traumatic, or congenital aneurysms of the right ventricle do occur, these are most uncommon.

Variable mortality rates are reported in clinical and necropsy series. Schlichter and colleagues reviewed 102 necropsy cases and observed that in 73%, the aneurysm had been present for less than 3 years and in 88%, less than 5 years.[6] Proudfit, in 1978, studied a group of 74 patients with angiographically proven ventricular aneurysms and found a mortality of 53% at 5 years and 88% at 10 years.[7] Bruschke and colleagues demonstrated different mortality rates in patients with LV aneurysms and concomitant one-, two-, or three-vessel coronary artery disease.[8] Both the survival rate and the quality of life can be significantly affected by the complications of LV aneurysm: cardiac insufficiency, arrhythmias, arterial embolization, and the occurrence of angina.

PATHOPHYSIOLOGY

Postinfarction aneurysm of the left ventricle is a consequence of the transmural fibrous scar that forms following ischemic myocardial damage. There are few or no residual muscle cells within the aneurysm wall. The "border zone" surrounding the frank scar consists of a partially damaged myocardium that functions suboptimally. These factors express themselves clinically in the complications common to ventricular aneurysm.

---

*Presented at the XXXIV Brazilian Congress of Cardiology: Belo Horizonte, Brazil, July, 1978.

LV Dysfunction

An LV aneurysm results in both diastolic and systolic ventricular dysfunction. During systole, the aneurysm scar fails to contract, which leads to a reduced ejection fraction and cardiac output. In diastole, the fibrotic aneurysm scar does not undergo normal distension as does the undamaged myocardium. This failure to distend results in elevated left ventricular end diastolic pressure (LVEDP). The combination of the elevated LVEDP and the systolic ventricular dysfunction can lead to congestive heart failure with an increased diameter of the left ventricular cavity. Increased ventricular cavity size results in increased tension of the ventricular wall according to Laplace's Law. This increased wall tension can result in higher oxygen consumption in the remaining normal myocardium and decreased oxygen supply during diastole, both of which can eventually lead to additional damage with clinical deterioration.

Mural Thrombus

Following infarction, the normally smooth endocardial surface is transformed into a damaged, inflamed surface that promotes platelet adherence and aggregation. Contractility changes in the myocardium as well as geometric changes in the left ventricular configuration may result in relative stasis of the blood. These two factors often lead to the development of a thrombus adherent to the rough endocardial surface. Although, in the majority of cases this progresses harmlessly toward thrombus organization, portions of the thrombus can break off and embolize into the systemic, mesenteric, or cerebral circulations, often resulting in dire clinical consequences. The incidence of this occurrence is exceedingly low.

Ventricular Arrhythmias

The "border zone" surrounding an aneurysmal scar is a mixture of fibrous tissue and viable myocardium. As such, the normal electrophysiologic pathways are significantly altered and the stage is set for re-entrant ventricular arrhythmias, which can be life-threatening at times. Patients with ventricular arrhythmias and coexisting ventricular aneurysms are candidates for mapping with excision of the re-entrant circuit at the time of ventricular aneurysm repair (see Chapter 131). Alternatively, Dor and co-workers advocated nonguided endocardiectomy with LVA reconstruction for patients with LVA and ischemic ventricular arrhythmias.[9]

Ventricular Rupture

Cardiac rupture usually occurs only during the acute phase of myocardial infarction. Ventricular rupture is, therefore, not a routine indication for surgery on a ventricular aneurysm, although it certainly can lead to a pseudo-aneurysm that requires treatment. Rupture of a mature ventricular aneurysm is a distinctly infrequent event.

Mitral Insufficiency

If the posterior papillary muscle is infarcted, the resulting left ventricular aneurysm can be associated with mitral insufficiency. This carries a significant increase in operative mortality. Rarely will concomitant coronary revascularization reverse mitral insufficiency in these patients. If the insufficiency is severe, valve repair or replacement may be accomplished through the ventriculotomy.

SYMPTOMS AND DIAGNOSIS

The most frequent clinical manifestation of LV aneurysms is congestive heart failure. Angina pectoris is also a frequent symptom, occurring in 44 to 98% of patients with LV aneurysm due in most cases to concomitant obstructive lesions in noninfarct-related arteries.[10,11] Significant ventricular arrhythmias appear less frequently, occurring in about 20% of large aneurysms and 3% of smaller aneurysms.

On physical examination, signs of congestive heart failure may be present. In cases of anterior wall aneurysms, diffuse apical systolic thrust and double impulse are frequently present. On auscultation, heart murmurs are seldom heard except when associated mitral regurgitation is present.

Persistent ST segment elevation and T-wave changes are electrocardiographic signs suggestive of ventricular aneurysm. Fluoroscopy and chest roentgenograms may demonstrate bulging of the heart contour. Echocardiography provides a noninvasive and precise evaluation of the ventricular shape and, to some extent, function. Two-dimensional echocardiography may allow identification of an aneurysm of the aneurysm sac and can often detect the presence of mural thrombosis on the endocardial surface. The recent availability of intraoperative transesophageal Doppler echocardiography may allow even more precise anatomic and functional evaluations to be made. The presence of mural thrombis and the degree of mitral insufficiency can be accurately determined. Global left ventricular function can be noninvasively evaluated using the gated blood pool scintigraphy. This scan is highly accurate for the identification of aneurysms in the anterior and apical area but somewhat less sensitive in the posterobasal area. Because it is a safe, accurate, and noninvasive technique for identifying ventricular aneurysms and evaluating function, it is useful as a screening test. However, because it does not delineate the coronary artery anatomy, it does not replace contrast ventriculography. Computed tomography scans and magnetic resonance imaging of the chest are useful only in delineating anatomy. Because of the sharp contrast between flowing blood and static tissues in an MRI scan, this modality is particularly well-suited to delineating the anatomy of an aneurysmal sac. However, it is an expensive and time consuming test to perform, which gives little or no information as to cardiac function or coronary anatomy and, therefore, has no real role in the diagnosis of left ventricular aneurysms.

Contrast ventriculography remains the single most useful test in the workup of left ventricular aneurysm. It defines the cardiac function and coronary anatomy. These are critical determinations to make, since it is on the basis of these findings that a surgeon must decide whether or not to operate and what procedure should be undertaken. If one looks only at the standard ventriculogram, it is possible to misinterpret how much muscle has been destroyed and replaced by fibrosis, especially if the aneurysm is a large one. It is very important that ventriculography be undertaken from several views lest superimposition of the fibrosis and normal muscle lead to an inaccurate assessment. If misinterpretation occurs, patients eligible for aneurysmectomy may be inappropriately rejected or referred for heart transplantation. The motion of the coronary arteries supplying myocardium outside the infarcted area is particularly important to determine. The shape and movement of these arteries during the cardiac cycle are different from those in the hypokinetic or the noninvolved area. It is possible to make a reasonable distinction between distention and muscular destruction by assessing the motion of these arteries. When one looks at late results following surgery, the amount of preserved muscle and the technique of reconstruction are the two main contributing factors to a beneficial outcome. Naturally, it is extremely important that the anatomy of coronary arteries and the sites of obstruction be identified so that concomitant revascularization can be undertaken at the time of aneurysmectomy.

Impairment of Nonaneurysmal Myocardium

Mills and his associates pointed out that the presence of a left ventricular aneurysm involving more than 25% of the LV surface, burdens nonaneurysmal myocardial fibers, and ultimately decreases the ejection fraction of the noninfarcted area of the heart.[12] This phenomenon of LV stress is similar to the problem of aortic valvular insufficiency, in which patients are seen to change from an acceptable ejection fraction with an acceptable operative mortality to an inordinately low ejection fraction with an almost prohibitive operative mortality within a time frame of as little as 1 year. Mills has emphasized that some authors have advised repair of LV aneurysms only if medical measures fail.[13] A more current understanding of the pathophysiology has led clinicians to advise repair before such irreversible changes secondary to progressive impairment of nonaneurysmal muscle by increased wall tension, if an acceptable mortality rate can be achieved by the surgical team.[14–16]

Contraindications for Operation

Small asymptomatic aneurysms in patients without elevation of left ventricular end diastolic pressure should be treated medically and followed with noninvasive techniques, unless tachyarrhythmias develop.

The majority of patients with symptomatic or asymptomatic moderate to large size aneurysms should be treated surgically, particularly if they have associated coronary artery disease. If these patients are managed medically, it is possible that over time the contractile ejection fraction can decrease, thus increasing the subsequent operative risk. As pointed out by Dor and his associates, patients can be treated surgically even if the ejection fraction is between 25 and 30%, provided the mean pulmonary artery pressure is less than 40 mm Hg and the cardiac index is greater than or equal to 2.1 L/min per m². However, in selected patients transplantation should be performed as a treatment of choice when the contractile ejection fraction is less than 25% and when there is right ventricular dysfunction, permanent mitral insufficiency, and poor target coronary arteries for bypass.[17]

SURGICAL TECHNIQUE

Aneurysmectomy, as classically described, is a resection of the fibrotic area leaving a 1 to 2 cm border of fibrous tissue. The closure of the ventricular chamber is then accomplished utilizing interrupted mattress sutures tied over Teflon felt strips. This simplistic approach may be acceptable for small aneurysms, but in large ones, it can lead to varying degrees of ventricular dysfunction. This may explain the high mortality rate reported in this subset of patients in whom heart failure and not angina is the indication for surgery.

In patients with large aneurysms, reconstruction of the ventricular cavity may be warranted. This is a complex task, because the left ventricle has a peculiar architecture with superficial and deep muscle bundles crossing in opposite directions. In some areas, there is a spiral architecture to the myocardium with bundles that span across the cavity, both in a superficial and deep layer. Many of these bundles originate in critical structures such as the papillary muscle. Overall, there is an elaborate architecture to the myocardial bundles that allows them to contract with maximum efficiency. The muscular complex originates in the fibrous skeleton of the heart and inserts in the mitral valve leaflets through the chordae tendineae. Obstruction of a coronary artery induces infarction with damage to myocardial bundles, which course in several directions. If, during the healing process, distention does not occur, the size of the cavity remains essentially unchanged and the spared muscle bundles maintain their normal direction (Fig. 130–1A,B). However, if the infarcted area comes distended, the cavity size

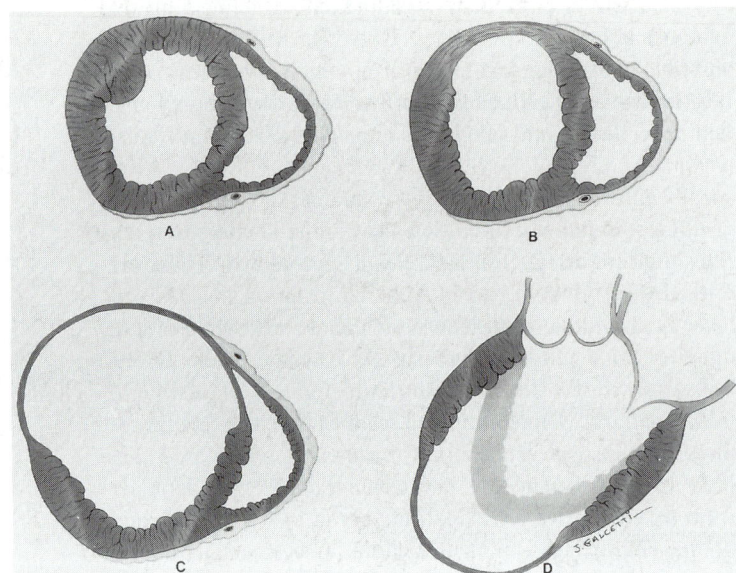

Figure 130–1. A,B. Postinfarction scarring without aneurysm formation, leaving normal muscle orientation intact. **C,D.** Postinfarction aneurysm formation with alteration of remaining normal muscle architecture.

increases and distortion of the normal bundles occurs in the transverse direction (Fig. 130–1C) as well as in the longitudinal direction (Fig. 130–1D). As seen in Figure 130–1A,B, it is clear that normal muscle contraction would produce reduction in the size of the myocardial cavity. However, in the distended ventricle (Fig. 130–1C,D), normal muscle contraction does not produce the same effect, since the distended area is unable to give the necessary support and, therefore, the efficiency of the contraction is decreased.

Because of this complex architecture, mere reapproximation of the fibrotic edges following aneurysmectomy may not result in adequate function due to alteration of the ventricular geometry. The direction of the normal muscle bundles distorted by the distended area must be returned as much as possible to their original position and orientation to induce a reduction of the ventricular diameter and shortening of ventricular cavity during systole. One needs to reshape the left ventricular cavity in such a way that it resembles an infarcted ventricle in which distention did not occur. In other words, the noninvolved muscle must be brought to its normal position leaving only an akinetic area the size of the original infarcted area before the occurrence of distention. Several fundamental steps should be observed in pursuing this goal: (1) determination of the limits of the aneurysm prior to opening the ventricular cavity; (2) careful removal of thrombi; (3) decision as to the extent of the area to be excised; (4) elimination of septal paradoxical motion; and (5) careful ventricular reconstruction utilizing a prosthetic patch if necessary. This latter step is easier if the operation is conducted on the beating heart.

The procedure is performed through midline sternotomy. Opening of the pericardium should be carried out carefully since firm adhesions may be present. The initial dissection exposes the right heart chambers, the aorta, the pulmonary artery, and the venae cavae to permit usual can-

nulation. Dissection of the aneurysm is more safely performed after cardiopulmonary bypass is established. This avoids undue manipulation of the heart, which might dislodge thrombi from the ventricular cavity or aggravate cardiac dysfunction during dissection of pericardial adhesions. In large aneurysms, this dissection may be difficult and produce increased postoperative bleeding if the pericardial adhesions are particularly firm. In this situation, it is wiser to open the aneurysm and leave a portion of the wall attached to the pericardium. To delineate the border of the LV aneurysm, suction is applied to the left ventricle after cross-clamping the aorta. This is achieved with a small bore cannula introduced in the ascending aorta or in the left ventricle via the right superior pulmonary vein. After careful evaluation, the aortic clamp is released, thus reestablishing the coronary circulation. Only after coronary perfusion is so established is the depressed, aneurysmal area incised.

A linear incision is made through the fibrotic area. The presence of thrombus in the aneurysm is common, especially in those aneurysms produced by obstruction in the left anterior descending artery. Removal of the thrombus must be complete, including the area of its attachment to the wall. This maneuver can be more easily accomplished if one utilizes a tangential scalpel dissection just between the aneurysmal fibrous tissue and the base of the thrombus. By this maneuver, the entire thrombus can be incised without breaking it and losing parts of it in the ventricular cavity. In many cases, the thrombus reaches the normal muscular area underneath the trabeculae, making its removal more difficult. During removal of the thrombus, the ventricular cavity is packed with gauze to avoid loose debris and subsequent embolization. Intermittent periods of aortic clamping sometimes make thrombus removal easier.

To decide what portion of ventricle should be resected, the ventricular wall is palpated circumferentially while the heart is beating. One of the fingers is kept on the epicardial surface and the other one inside the cavity. Myocardial thickening is felt with each contraction of the normal muscle *but not in the aneurysmal area.* With this maneuver, one can accurately identify all the area to be resected. On the other hand, if there is contraction in segments of the area corresponding to the obstructed artery, revascularization of this vessel is indicated. Thus, the extent of resection, determined after careful examination with the beating heart, may be quite different from the preoperative assessment.

When the intraventricular septum is involved by the aneurysm, it bulges into the right ventricle, a situation that is difficult to evaluate prior to opening the left ventricular cavity (Fig. 130–2A). This distortion must be corrected to avoid a residual paradoxical bulge that may detract from optimal results. Elimination of the fibrotic septal area can be accomplished either by plication or by suturing this area to a nondistensible patch of Dacron or glutaraldehyde-fixed bovine or autologous pericardium. Plication is performed with two or three horizontal mattress stitches of 00 braided

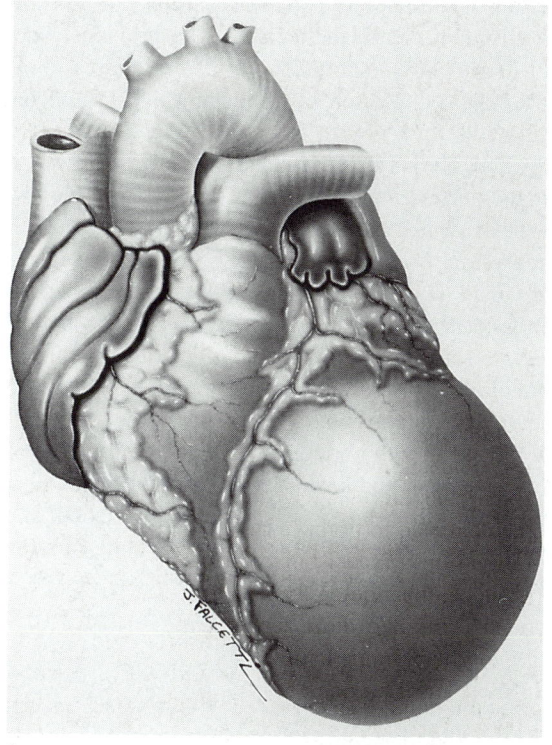

A

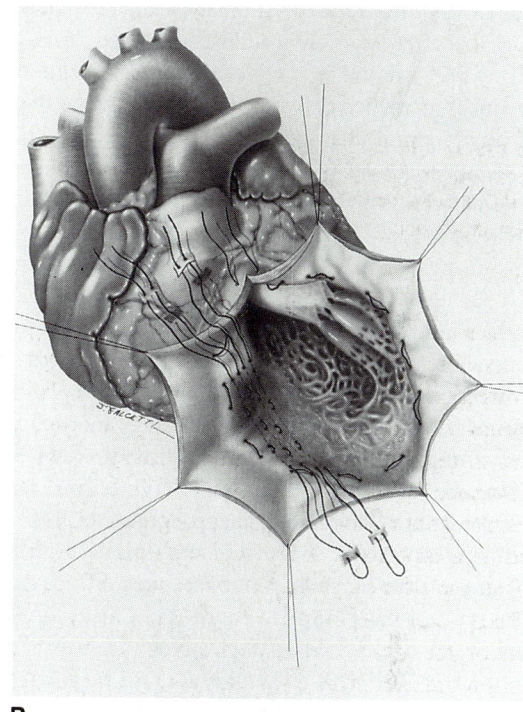

B

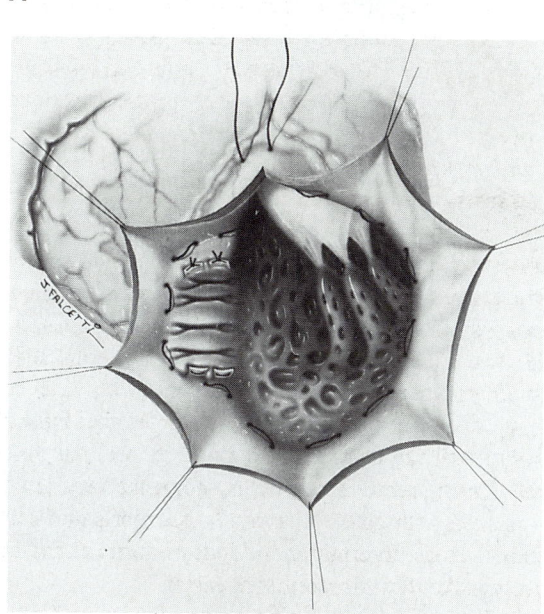

C

Figure 130–2. A. Anterior wall aneurysm prior to its opening. **B,C.** Septal aneurysm plication technique. Suture placement (**B**) and finished results (**C**).

suture anchored at both ends by Teflon felt pledgets. When these stitches are tied, the fibrous distended area is reduced and this eliminates the bulge into the right ventricle (Fig. 130–2B,C). A similar result can be obtained by suturing a nondistensible patch to the fibrous borders.[24] This technique is particularly useful because it distributes the tension of the suture line equally along the patch, which is important to prevent tearing when an irregular surface is present following removal of septal thrombi. This is common when the aneurysm is operated upon in its acute phase.

After determination of the extension of the aneurysm, removal of the thrombi and elimination of the septal dysfunction, the ventricular cavity must be closed. This is the most critical step in the procedure. Distention of the infarction produces an orifice between the aneurysm and the ventricular cavity larger than the original infarcted area. Figure 130–3 demonstrates how a relatively small aneurysm undergoing correction by simple linear suture can produce a deformity in the left ventricular cavity due to the long suture line changing the direction of normal muscle bundles. In such small aneurysms, this modest distortion can be compensated for with no major problem. However, when an aneurysm results from a more extensive muscle loss, distortion may produce significant dysfunction in the immediate postoperative period with a resultant high morbidity and mortality. An aneurysm resulting from distention of a larger infarcted area (Fig. 130–2) has a very large orifice, rendering a linear suture line entirely inappropriate. In this situation, it is best to reduce the aneurysmal orifice to the estimated size of the original infarcted area. This area is

deduced from evaluation of the ventriculogram and careful observation of the noninvolved arteries. This reduction of the orifice is accomplished by a pursestring suture placed exactly at the junction of the fiber scar and normal muscle (Figs. 130–2B,C and 130–4). If one is operating on a beating heart, this limit is easily detected by palpation (vide supra).

In the septal region, the pursestring suture is placed parallel to the anterior descending artery to avoid distortion of the right ventricle. When the ventricular cavity is reshaped by tightening the pursestring suture and tying it over Teflon or autologous pericardial strips, the fibrotic septal area is then clearly delineated. The previously described plication is now undertaken in this septal area to eliminate paradoxical distention by producing a firm noncontractile wall.

The size of the ventricular defect produced by tightening the pursestring should be as close as possible to the size of the original infarcted area. If it is small, the now reduced aneurysmal orifice may be closed by direct suture, taking care to avoid distortion. Two stitches at the superior and inferior corners should be placed in the junction between normal muscle and fibrotic scar. The intermediate sutures should leave a small margin of fibrous tissue so as to close the ventriculotomy without deforming the cavity. The closure is made with horizontal mattress sutures of braided 00 polypropylene tied over Teflon or autologous pericardial strips (Fig. 130–5A). After each stitch is tied, it is used again to close the borders tightly providing more efficient hemostasis (Fig. 130–5B).

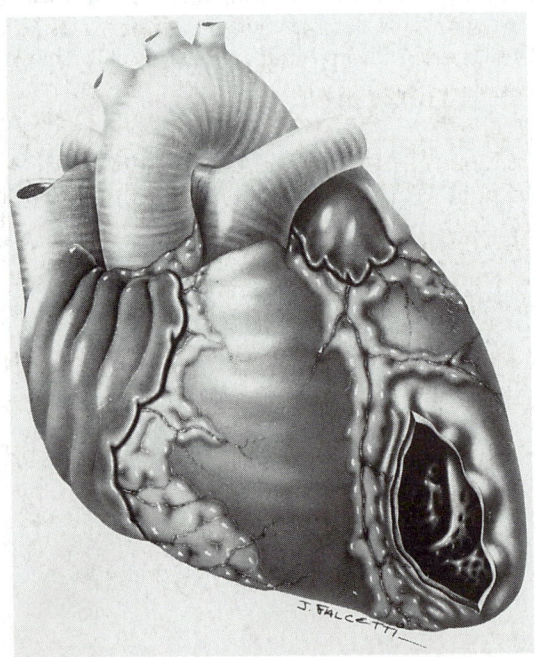

A

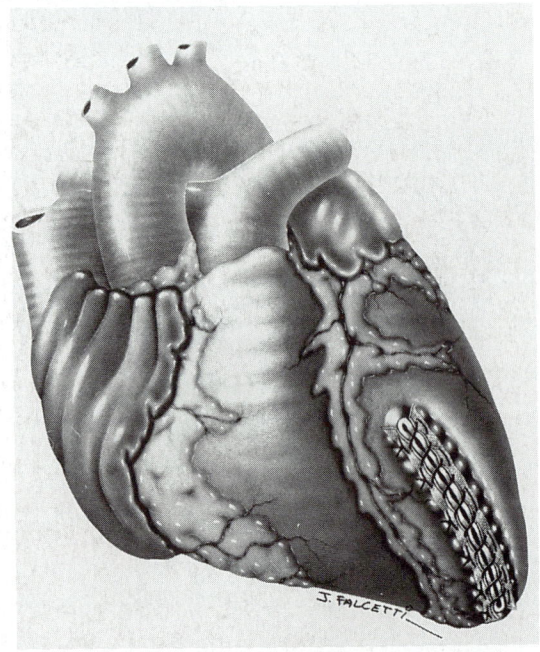

B

Figure 130–3. A,B. Linear repair of LV aneurysm with longitudinal distortion of normal muscle orientation.

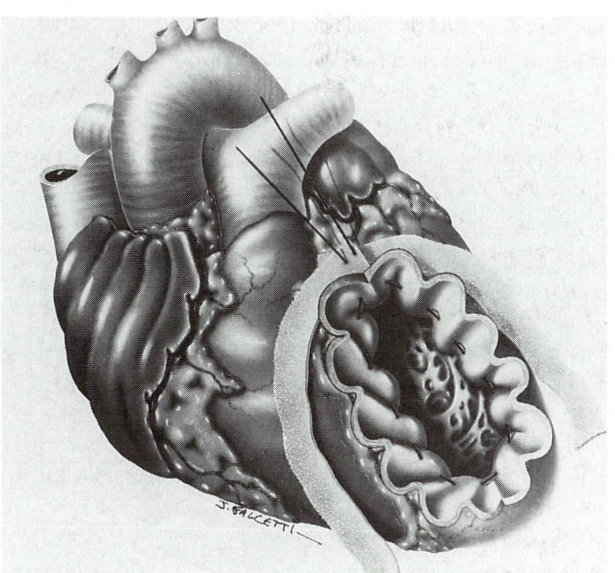

Figure 130–4. Pursestring suture placed at junction of scar and normal muscle and cinched so as to approximate original infarct size.

When direct suture of the defect would produce inordinate ventricular distortion, a Dacron patch is used. This was considered necessary in about 15% of our patients. A double layer #35 arterial woven Dacron prosthesis or a double layer glutaraldehyde-preserved bovine pericardium patch is sutured with horizontal mattress polypropylene sutures to the fibrous border of the aneurysm (Fig. 130–6A). The stitches are placed from inside through a Teflon felt strip into the double layer patch. The stitch is then continued through the fibrotic edge of the aneurysm and up through

the outer Teflon felt strip (Fig. 130–6B). After the sutures are tied, any excess patch is trimmed and each stitch is passed again through all layers. The stitches are tied individually (Fig. 130–6C).

This technique is particularly useful for aneurysms located in less favorable regions such as the inferior or lateral walls. In the acute phase when fibrosis is not well-established, the patch used to treat the septum can be sutured directly to the free borders of the aneurysm (Fig. 130–7).

A relatively common occurrence is the combination of an anteroseptal aneurysm and a distended previously infarcted area in the inferior wall. In this situation, it is possible to exclude the inferior distension by utilizing plication technique. This procedure is easily performed since the cavity is open and sutures can be placed from inside outward under the direct vision guided by palpation of the borders of the aneurysm and the beating heart. The same principles of reconstruction can be applied for a repeat procedure when the first operation has failed, leading to recurrence of symptoms.

In patients who require concomitant coronary artery bypass grafting, we have modified the above techniques. After opening the pericardium and placing the patient on hypothermic cardiopulmonary bypass, the heart is arrested with antegrade–retrograde blood cardioplegia. After lysing adhesions, opening and decompressing the left ventricle, as described above, any thrombus is carefully removed from the wall of the aneurysm. The coronary arteries are bypassed and subsequently the crossclamp is removed as the patient is brought to a normothermic core temperature. The aneurysm is then reconstructed with the heart beating and completely revascularized.

Alternatively, myocardial revascularization could be

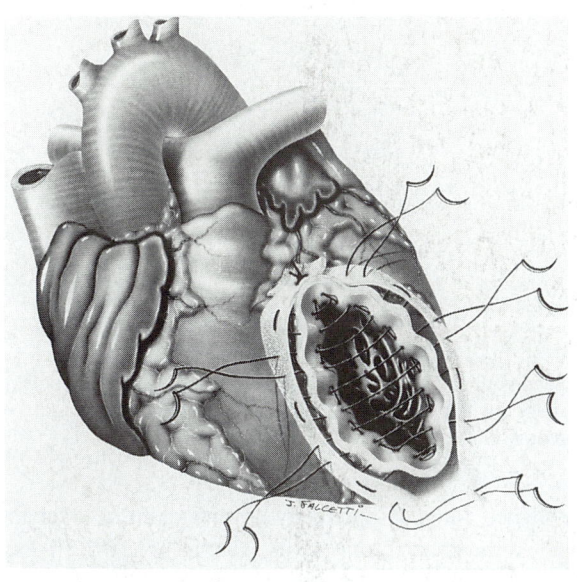

A

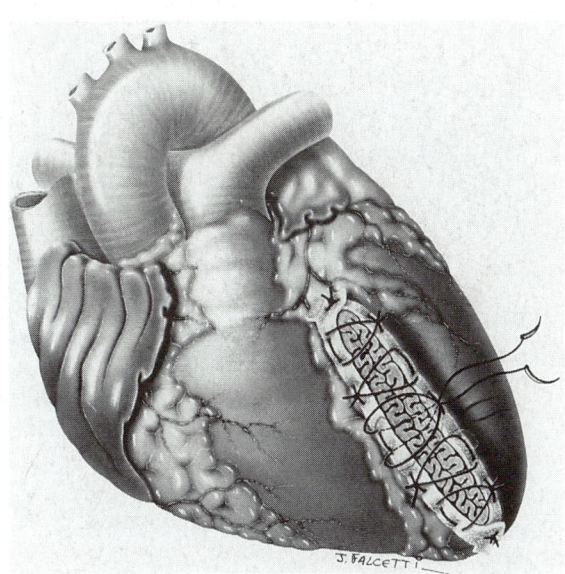

B

Figure 130–5. A. Closure of ventricular cavity, after pursestring reduction of orifice size, with individual sutures placed through Teflon felt strips. **B.** Completed closure after second placement of sutures through all layers.

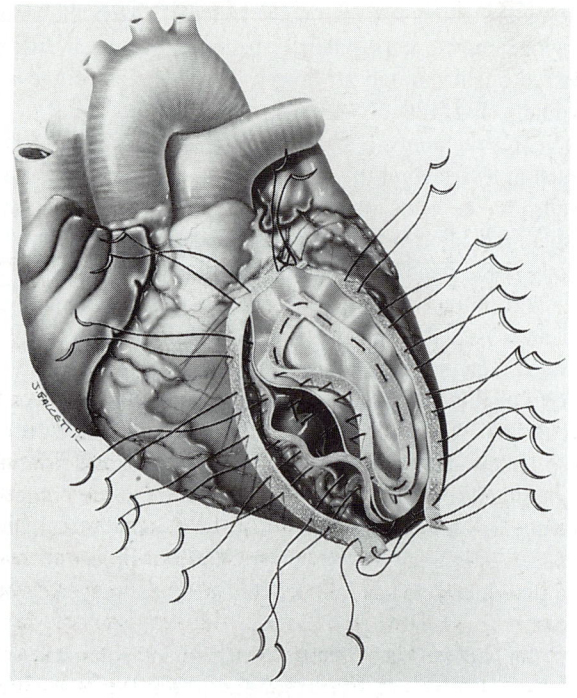

A

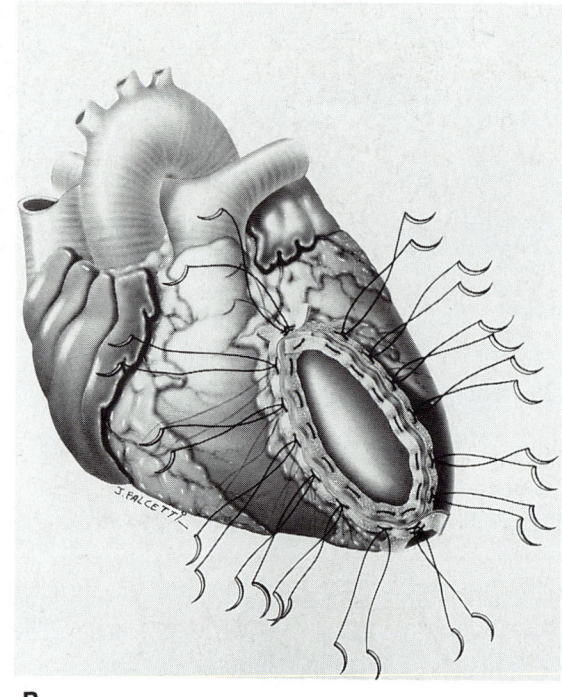

B

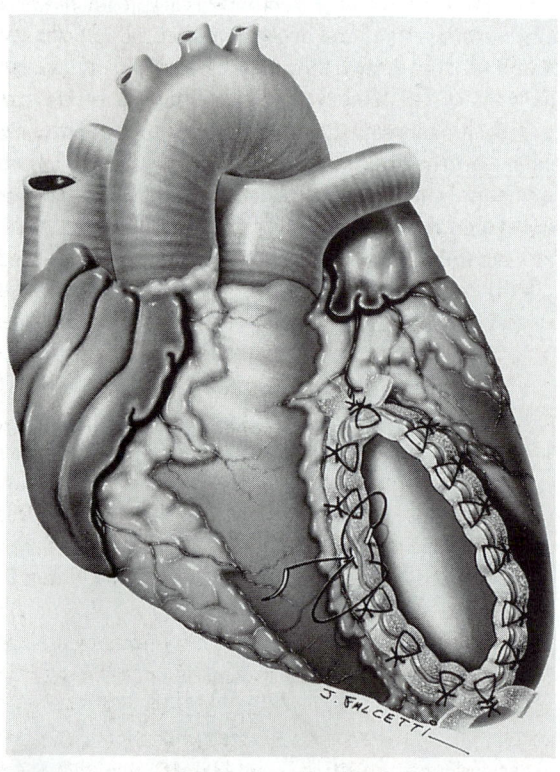

C

Figure 130–6. Reconstruction of ventricular cavity using a patch. **A.** Initial placement of sutures through inner felt strip, patch, aneurysm wall, and outer felt strip. **B.** Sutures tied and excess patch trimmed. **C.** Reinforcement of lines of closure.

performed using cold (25°C) fibrillatory arrest provided aortic insufficiency is not severe.[18]

The question of which material to use for left ventricular reconstruction still remains controversial. Different authors recommend their favorite implant material (e.g., scar tissue, Dacron, pericardium, and Teflon). There is no strik-

ing evidence for the superiority of one of these over the other.[19] At the present time we use Hemashield woven double velour patch material (Meadox Medical, Inc.). If the ventriculotomy requires additional external support for hemostatic closure, autologous pericardial strips are employed.[20]

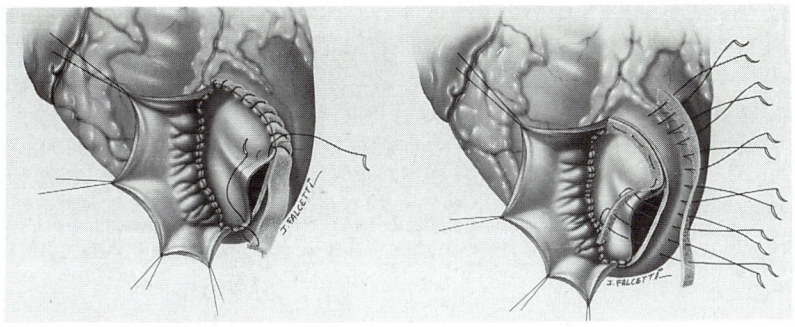

Figure 130–7. Septal patch anchored to the base of the septum and then sutured directly to the lateral fibrous border of the aneurysm.

RESULTS

Left ventricular aneurysm patients are not a homogeneous population. The size and clinical consequences of the aneurysm depend on the amount of myocardium destroyed, the degree of resultant ventricular distention, and the presence or absence of concomitant coronary artery obstruction. The reported operative mortality varies significantly from series to series and much of this difference can be explained by comparing these factors in the different patient populations. Operative mortality ranges from 4% in some series[21,22] up to 48 to 50% in others.[23,24] In those series with a 50% incidence of single vessel disease, the reported operative mortality ranges from 4 to 12%.[21,22] In other clinical series in which the incidence of single vessel disease is much lower (4 to 27%), the operative mortality can range up to 50%.[23–27] This partially explains the difference in mortality stressed by Cohen et al, who found operative risk varying from 4 to 50% and, as a result, concluded that ventricular aneurysmectomy is indicated only after maximal medical treatment has failed.[13] With the institution of more refined surgical techniques, the hospital mortality has been reduced and, more importantly, the functional status of hospital survivors is improving as documented in recent reports.[5,28] In our own early experience from 1962 to 1977, the hospital mortality among 214 patients was 11.6%, and the late mortality at 20 months was 12.6%. In our more recent series from 1977 to 1987 (1381 cases), hospital mortality was 5.8%, and late mortality was 4.5%. Only 25% of these patients overall had single vessel disease. Despite the greater complexity of the procedure, the present results of left ventricular reconstruction, with or without myocardial revascularization, are better than in the past. Although advances in myocardial protection have significantly contributed to this improvement, we feel that superior reconstructive techniques account for most of the improved outcomes.

The operative results after repair of left ventricular aneurysms by endoventricular patch plasty report low perioperative mortality ranging from 3.5 to 6.5%, compared with the reported figures of 2 to 23% after resection and linear closure.[29] The tendency toward increased survival seems to reflect the better functional results associated with patch reconstruction. In some patients, the inadequacy of the residual ventricular volume after linear resection of large aneurysms may account for the slightly higher mortality following convental repair.[30] Kesler and associates compared linear closure with circular techniques in a small patient population and reported no difference in clinical outcome or hemodynamics. The significantly lower number of patients requiring intra-aortic balloon pump support in the group with circular repair of the aneurysm might indicate improved hemodynamic performance after this procedure, but the sample size of this study limits its usefulness.[31]

Salate and associates demonstrated that restoration of left ventricle geometry is at least partly responsible for the improvement in functional outcome.[32] More recently Kowata and co-workers clearly demonstrated improvement in systolic and diastolic function after patch reconstruction of left ventricular aneurysms.[33] In their patients, the ejection fraction increased significantly from 0.28 to 0.39 at rest, and from 0.32 to 0.41 during exercise. In addition, the left ventricular end-diastolic pressure and left ventricular end-diastolic volume index were reduced significantly following circular geometric reconstruction. These results remain improved up to 16 to 24 months following operation. This elegant study demonstrates that patch reconstruction of the left ventricle resulted in the recovery of systolic and diastolic function soon after operation, which has persisted into the late postoperative period.

Another major advantage of circular reconstruction compared with linear closure is the potential to revascularize the left anterior descending coronary artery. This should be attempted if possible by an internal mammary artery graft irrespective of whether the vessel is small or fibrosed. After studying early and late determinants of survival following LV aneurysm repair, Rizzoli and associates in 1988 insisted on revascularization of the left anterior descending.[34] A report on LV aneurysms from the Montreal Heart Institute noted a favorable outcome influenced primarily by revascularization of residual territory of the LAD.[35] This has been confirmed in a recent report by Jindani and co-workers.[36] Mills and his associates have demonstrated a 5-year survival of 88% in patients undergoing ventricular aneurysm repair who had a concomitant internal mammary artery graft to the LAD.[12] The 5-year survival of patients having a saphenous vein graft to that vessel was 72%. When no graft was placed to the LAD system in the course of left ventricular aneurysmorrhaphy, the 5-year survival dropped to 65%. Therefore, our present philosophy incorporates complete revascularization including the left anterior descending whenever possible in patients requiring patch reconstruction of left ventricular aneurysm.

The statement that operation for ventricular aneurysm is indicated only when all medical measures fail must be reconsidered. Earlier operation can prevent the development of reversible damage to the remaining normal muscle, which results from the chronic overload imposed by the paradoxical movement of the aneurysmal wall.

REFERENCES

1. Likoff W, Bailey CP: Ventriculoplasty. Excision of myocardial aneurysm. *JAMA* **158**:915, 1955
2. Cooley DA, Collins HA, Morris GC Jr, Chapman DW: Ventricular aneurysm after myocardial infarction. Surgical excision with use of temporary cardiopulmonary bypass. *JAMA* **167**:557, 1958
3. Daggett WM, Guyton RA, Mundth AD, et al: Surgery for post-myocardial infarct ventricular septal defect. *Ann Surg* **186**:260, 1977
4. Cooley DA: Ventricular aneurysms and akinesis. *Cleve Clin Q* **45**:130, 1978
5. Jatene AD: Left ventricular aneurysmectomy. Resection or reconstruction. *J Thorac Cardiovasc Surg* **89**:331, 1985
6. Schlichter J, Hellerstein HK, Katz LN: Aneurysm of the heart. A correlation study of one hundred and two proved cases. *Medicine* **33**:43, 1954
7. Proudfit WL, Bruschke AVG, Sones FM Jr: Natural history of obstructive coronary artery disease. Ten years of 601 nonsurgical cases. *Prog Cardiovasc Dis* **21**:53, 1978
8. Bruschke AVG, Proudfit WL, Sones FM Jr: Progress study of 590 consecutive nonsurgical cases of coronary disease followed 5–9 years. II. Ventriculographic and other correlations. *Circulation* **47**:1154, 1973
9. Dor V, Subatier M, Montiglio F, et al: Results of nonguided subtotal endocardiectomy associated with left ventricular reconstruction in patients with ischemic ventricular arrhythmias. *J Thorac Cardiovasc Surg* **107**:1301–1308, 1994
10. Burton NA, Stinson EB, Oyer PE, Shumway N: Left ventricular aneurysm. Preoperative risk factors and long-term postoperative results. *J Thorac Cardiovasc Surg* **77**:65, 1979
11. Jones EL, Craver JM, Hurs JW, et al: Influence of left ventricular aneurysm on survival following the coronary bypass operation. *Ann Surg* **193**:733, 1981
12. Mills NL, Everson CT, Hockmuth DR: Technical advances in the treatment of left ventricular aneurysm. *Ann Thorac Surg* **55**:797–800, 1993
13. Cohen M, Packer M, Gorlin R: Indications for left ventricular aneurysmectomy. *Circulation* **67**:717, 1983
14. Froehlich RT, Falsetti HL, Doty DB, Marcus ML: Prospective study of surgery for left ventricular aneurysm. *Am J Cardiol* **45**:923, 1980
15. Dor V: Surgery for left ventricular aneurysm. *Curr Opin Cardiol* **5**:773, 1990
16. Komeda M, David TE, Malik A, et al: Operative risks and long-term results of operation for left ventricular aneurysm. *Ann Thorac Surg* **53**:22–29, 1992
17. Dor V, Sabatier M, Montiglio F: Clinical, hemodynamic and electrophysiologic results of 207 left ventricular patch reconstructions for infarction left ventricular aneurysm. Presented at the 72nd Annual Meeting of the American Association for Thoracic Surgery, Los Angeles, CA, April 26–29, 1992
18. Atkins CW: Resection of left ventricular aneurysm during hypothermic fibrallatory arrest without aortic occlusion. *J Thorac Cardiovasc Surg* **91**:610, 1986
19. Juidbashian JP, Follette DM, Contino JP, et al: Pericardial patch repair of left ventricular aneurysm. *Ann Thorac Surg* **55**:1022–1024, 1993
20. Fiore AC, McKeown PP, Misbach GA, et al: The use of autologous pericardium for ventricular aneurysm closure. *Ann Thorac Surg* **45**:570–571, 1988
21. Rogers WJ, Oberman A, Kouchoukos NT: Left ventricular aneurysmectomy in patients with single vs multivessel coronary artery disease. *Circulation* **58**:50, 1978
22. Cosgrove DM, Loop FD, Irarrazaval MJ, et al: Determinants of long-term survival after ventricular aneurysmectomy. *Ann Thorac Surg* **26**:357, 1978
23. Akins CW: Resection of the left ventricular aneurysm during hypothermic fibrillatory arrest without aortic occlusion. *J Thorac Cardiovasc Surg* **91**:610, 1986
24. Novick RJ, Stefaniszyn HJ, Morin JE, et al: Surgery for postinfarction left ventricular aneurysm. Prognosis and long-term follow-up. *Can J Surg* **27**:161, 1984
25. Olearchyk AS, Lemole GM, Spagna PM: Left ventricular aneurysm. Ten years' experience in surgical treatment of 244 cases. Improved clinical status, hemodynamics, and long-term longevity. *J Thorac Cardiovasc Surg* **88**:41, 1984
26. Barrett-Boyes BG, White HD, Agnew TM, et al: The results of surgical treatment of left ventricular aneurysms. An assessment of the risk factors affecting early and late mortality. *J Thorac Cardiovasc Surg* **87**:87, 1984
27. Skinner JR, Rasak C, Kongtahworn C, et al: Natural history of surgically treated ventricular aneurysm. *Ann Thorac Surg* **38**:42, 1984
28. Dor V, Saab M, Coste P, et al: Left ventricular aneurysm. A new surgical approach. *J Thorac Cardiovasc Surg* **37**:11, 1989
29. Di Donato M, Barletta G, Maioli M, et al: Early hemodynamic results of left ventricular reconstructive surgery for anterior wall left ventricular aneurysm. *Am J Cardiol* **60**:886–890, 1992
30. Cooper CS, Bunton RW, Birjinuik V, et al: Relative risk of left ventricular aneurysmectomy in patients with akinetic scars versus true dyskinetic aneurysms. *Circulation* **8**(suppl IV):248–256, 1990
31. Kesler KA, Fiore AC, Naunheim KS, et al: Anterior wall left ventricular aneurysm repair. *J Thorac Cardiovasc Surg* **103**:841–848, 1992
32. Salati M, DiBlasi P, Paje A, et al: Functional results of left ventricular reconstruction. *Ann Thorac Surg* **56**:316–322, 1993
33. Kawata T, Kitamura S, Kawachi K, et al: Systolic and diastolic function after patch reconstruction of left ventricular aneurysms. *Ann Thorac Surg* **59**:403–407, 1995
34. Rizzoli G, Bellotto F, Gallucci V, et al: Early and late determinants of survival after surgery of left ventricular aneurysm. *Eur J Cardiothorac Surg* **2**:265, 1988
35. Louagie Y, Alouini T, Lesperance J, Pelletier LC: Left ventricular aneurysm complicated by congestive heart failure; an analysis of long-term results and risk factors of surgical treatment. *J Cardiovasc Surg* **30**:648–655, 1989
36. Jindani A, Williams BT: Survival after left ventricular aneurysmectomy with or without coronary artery bypass graft. *Coron Artery Dis* **3**:739–744, 1992

CHAPTER

131

Surgery for Supraventricular Arrhythmias

T. Bruce Ferguson, Jr., and James L. Cox

INTRODUCTION

The therapy of supraventricular cardiac arrhythmias has undergone dramatic changes over the past several years.[1] For certain types of reentrant arrhythmias, surgical therapy has been supplanted by radiofrequency (RF) ablative therapy as the treatment of first choice. These include atrioventricular reentrant tachycardias due to the presence of accessory pathways in the Wolff-Parkinson–White syndrome, atrioventricular nodal tachycardias resulting from perinodal pathways, ectopic atrial tachycardias, and certain forms of simple Type I atrial flutter. Those patients who now come to surgery have failed RF ablation or have concomitant cardiac disease processes.

Finally, a new surgical cure for chronic paroxysmal or sustained atrial flutter/fibrillation has been demonstrated to be clinically efficacious over the past five years. This operation, termed the maze procedure, may well become the most frequently performed surgical procedure for cure of supraventricular arrhythmias over the next few years. The concept of a maze is used to produce multiple "blind alleys" off the main conduction route between the S-A node and the A-V node. Its role in the treatment of patients with combined valvar disease and atrial fibrillation is currently under active investigation throughout the world.

This chapter will discuss the basic principles involved in the surgical treatment of these various arrhythmias.

ACCESSORY ATRIOVENTRICULAR CONNECTIONS

Anatomy

For localization of accessory pathways responsible for reciprocating tachycardias seen in the Wolff–Parkinson–White (WPW) syndrome, the heart can be sectioned in the horizontal plane at the level of the atrioventricular (A-V) groove and divided into the left free wall, the right free wall, the posterior septal and the anterior septal spaces (Fig. 131–1). The posterior and anterior septal spaces are in fact epicardial spaces that abut onto the atrial septum posteriorly and anteriorly. The two fixed boundaries defining these spaces are the left and right fibrous trigones of the skeletal structure of the heart. Since the other boundaries are defined by adjacent anatomic landmarks, several additional subdivisions have been described to facilitate pathway localization, including the left and right paraseptal regions (Fig. 131–2). The subdivisions have been especially helpful in defining regions for RF ablation.

However, the fibrous skeleton of the heart is not entirely horizontal. The tricuspid anulus is more apical in position than is the mitral anulus; as a result the anterior part of the central fibrous body extends into the ventricles beneath the attachment of the tricuspid valve, and the interventricular component of the membranous septum between

2141

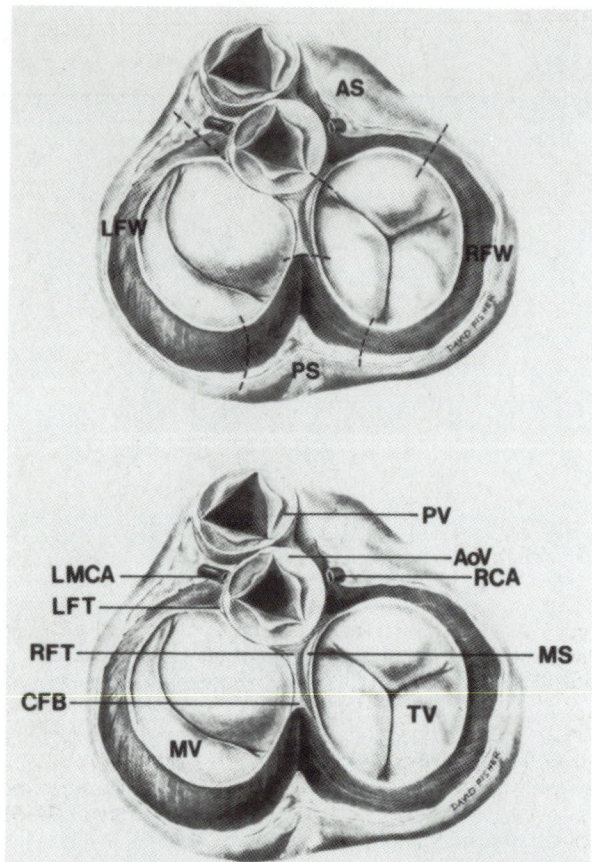

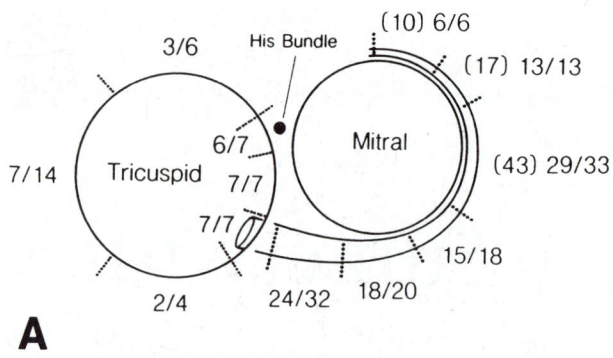

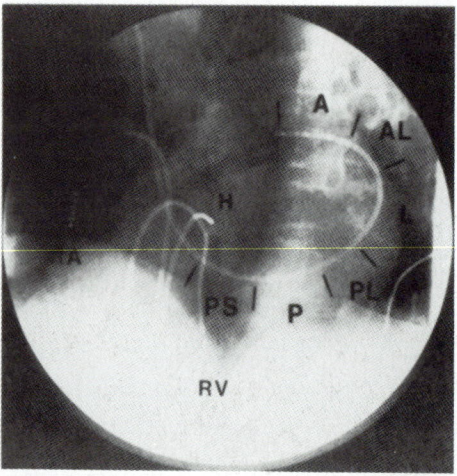

Figure 131–1. A superior view of the heart with the atria removed demonstrates the four anatomic areas in the horizontal plane where accessory connections can occur. These connections are not found between the left and right fibrous trigones along the area of contiguity between the mitral and aortic anuli. PV, Pulmonary valve; AoV, aortic valve; RCA, right coronary artery; MS, membranous system; LMCA, left main coronary artery; LFT, left fibrous trigone; RFT, right fibrous trigone; CFB, central fibrous body. *(From Lowe JE: Surgical treatment of the Wolff-Parkinson-White syndrome and other supraventricular tachyarrhythmias. J Cardiac Surg 1:117–130, 1986 with permission.)*

Figure 131–2. A. Schematic representation of the tricuspid and mitral anuli seen fluoroscopically in **B** in the left anterior oblique projection. The numerators in **A** represent the number of recorded pathway potentials, while the denominators represent the number of pathways located in these regions: A, left anterior; AL, left anterior lateral; L, left lateral; PL, left posteolateral; P, left posterior; PS, left posteroseptal or paraseptal. *(From Jackman W, et al: Catheter recordings of accessory atrioventricular pathway activation. In Zipes DL, Jalife J (eds): Cardiac Electrophysiology. Philadelphia, W.B. Saunders, 1991, pp 491–502, with permission; B is from Jackman W et al: Circulation 78:598–610, 1988.)*

the aortic outflow tract and the right atrium actually lies cephalad to the tricuspid anulus. For this reason RF ablation of right-sided pathways is feasible from the atrial septum above the tricuspid valve while ablation of left-sided pathways is performed from beneath the mitral valve anulus.[2]

The A-V groove between the left fibrous trigone and the right fibrous trigone (the anterior portion of the central fibrous body) does lie in the horizontal plane and represents the site of continuity between the anterior leaflet of the mitral valve and the aortic valve anulus (Fig. 131–3). This is the only area in the A-V groove where atrial muscle is not in juxtaposition to ventricular muscle, and for this reason accessory atrioventricular pathways are not found between the left and right fibrous trigones. In the vertical plane, the initial surgical experience suggested that these pathways can exist anywhere between the valve anuli and the epicardial surface of the heart (Fig. 131–4).[3] More recently, the

success of electrophysiologic identification of the accessory pathway potentials and the results with radiofrequency ablation suggest that the majority of accessory pathways are in fact juxta-anular,[4,5] at least on the left side. Right-sided pathways appear to be more variable in location, due in part to the infolding of the right atrial and ventricular tissue (Fig. 131–5). Posterior septal and anterior septal pathways are variable in location, as indicated by the multiple techniques that are necessary for successful ablation. Those pathways that are not able to be ablated by the RF technique are probably disparate in location from the true anulus.

Finally, when the horizontal and vertical planes are combined, it is clear that these accessory pathways can tangentially traverse this three-dimensional space.[6,7] This conceptualization has been confirmed by intraoperative map-

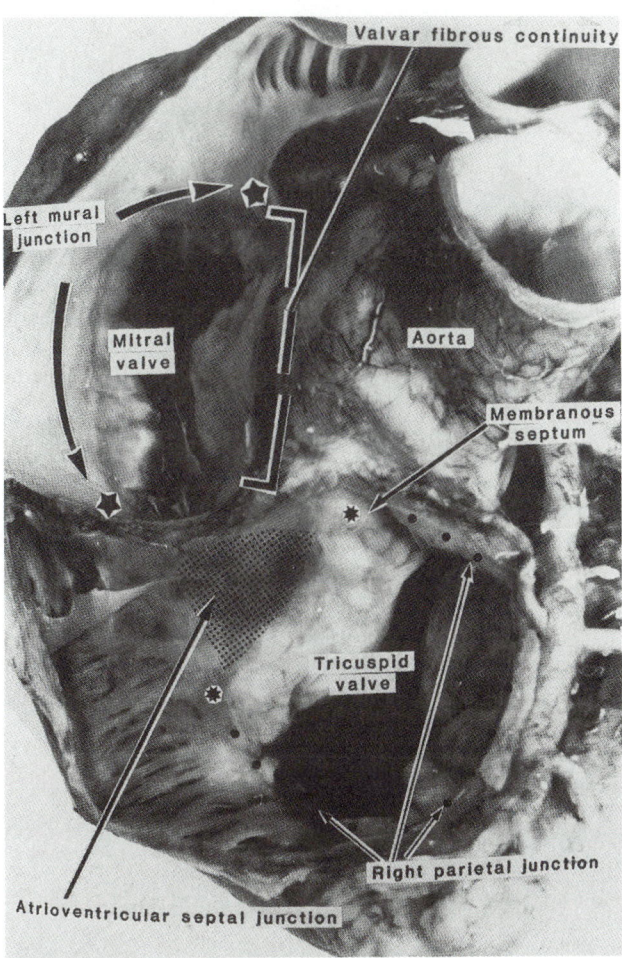

Figure 131–3. This dissection shows the overall structure of the atrioventricular junctions of the normal heart. Pathways may exist anywhere around the mitral or tricuspid anuli except along the mitral-aortic valvar fibrous continuity. *(From Anderson RH, Becker AE: Anatomy of the conduction tissues and accessory atrioventricular connections. In Zipes DL, Jalife J (eds): Cardiac Electrophysiology. Philadelphia, W.B. Saunders, 1991, pp 240–249, with permission.)*

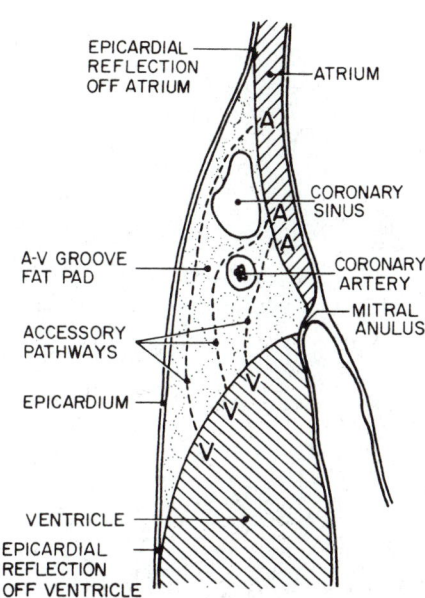

Figure 131–4. Cross-section of the left side of the heart in the vertical plane. Based on the surgical experience, pathways can be located at any depth between the valve anuli and epicardium. However, recent experience with radiofrequency ablation suggests that the majority of left sided-pathways are juxta-anular, while right-sided pathways tend to be more variable in depth. *(From Cox JL, Ferguson TB JR: Surgery for the Wolff-Parkinson-White syndrome: The endocardial approach. Sem Thorac Cardiovasc Surg 1:34–46, 1989, with permission.)*

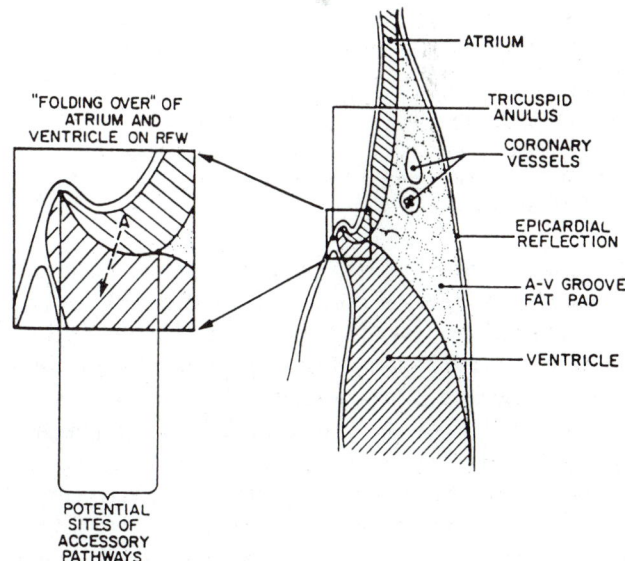

Figure 131–5. Folding over of the right atrium and right ventricle near the tricuspid anulus on the right free wall. Note that simple dissection of the A-V groove fat pad away from this folded-over tissue will not divide accessory pathways connecting the atrium and ventricle if they are near the tricuspid anulus. *(From Cox JL, Ferguson TB Jr: Surgery for the Wolff-Parkinson-White syndrome: The endocardial approach. Sem Thorac Cardiovasc Surg 1:34–46, with permission.)*

ping in preparation for surgery (Fig. 131–6) as well as by intracardiac mapping at the time of RF ablation (Fig. 131–7).

Surgical Treatment

Currently, candidates for surgical ablation of accessory pathways include patients with recurrent reciprocating tachycardia who are poorly controlled on medical therapy or have developed significant toxicity to an otherwise successful medical regimen and who (1) have failed attempted RF ablation or (2) have concomitant cardiac disease requiring surgical intervention.

Patients with symptomatic arrhythmias due to atrio-His, nodoventricular, and fasciculoventricular fibers should undergo surgery if they are resistant or intolerant to medical

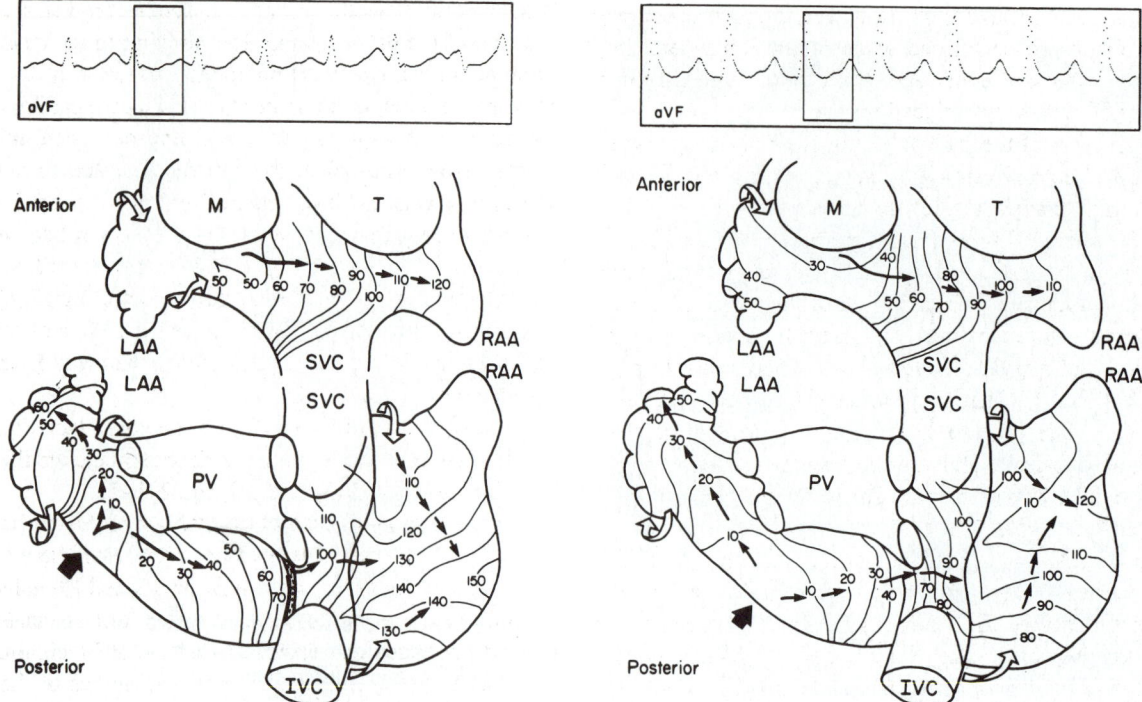

Figure 131–6. Atrial activation map during reciprocating tachycardias in two patients with the Wolff-Parkinson-White syndrome. The thick black arrow marks the site of atrial insertion of the accessory pathway on the posterior left atrium. **Left:** narrow, discrete area of initial atrial activation. **Right:** broad band of initial activation, encompassing several centimeters of atrial tissue. LAA, left atrial appendage; SVC, superior vena cava; IVC, inferior vena cava; RAA, right atrial appendage; PV, pulmonary veins; M, mitral valve; T, tricuspid valve. *(From Canavan TE, et al: Ann Thorac Surg 46:223–231, 1989, with permission.)*

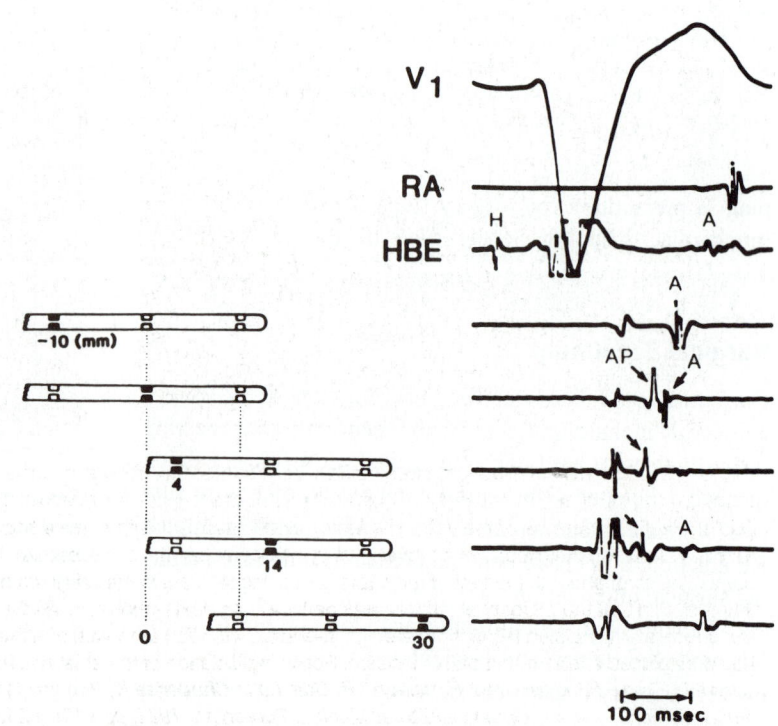

Figure 131–7. Composite of coronary sinus electrograms recorded during A-V reentrant tachycardia demonstrating a 14-mm lateral component in the course of the accessory pathway between ventricle and atrium. RA, right atrium; HBE, His bundle electrogram; V, ventricular potential; A, atrial potential; H, His potential; AP, accessory pathway potential; V_1, surface lead. *(From Jackman W: In Benditt DG, Benson DW, (eds): Cardiac Preexcitation Syndromes. Boston, Martinus Nijhoff, 1986, pp 413–434, with permission.)*

100 msec

therapy and fail RF ablation[8]; however, these procedures should probably be performed at an institution where the surgeon has extensive experience with these more complicated types of accessory connections.

The location of the pathway(s) is determined from the preoperative electrophysiologic data and from intraoperative epicardial mapping; the techniques for this are described elsewhere.[9] Intraoperative mapping is most commonly performed with a multipoint computerized mapping system. Activation sequence mapping of the ventricular and atrial sides of the atrioventricular groove determines the earliest site(s) of activation over the accessory atrioventricular connection.[1] In decreasing order of frequency, accessory pathways are located in the left free-wall, posterior septal, right free-wall, and anterior septal positions. Approximately 20% of patients in surgical series have multiple (two to four) pathways.[10]

Two surgical approaches have been developed to divide accessory A-V connections. The endocardial technique is designed to divide the ventricular end of the accessory pathway (analogous to the RF ablation techniques most commonly used)[1,10] and the epicardial technique is directed toward division of the atrial end of the pathway.[11,12]

Since 1981 we have used an endocardial technique and an anatomically based operation for division of all accessory pathways. The principles of this operative approach[3] are (1) accurate intraoperative localization of the pathway(s) to one of the four anatomic areas in the horizontal plane; (2) appreciation that the location of the pathway in the vertical plane may be variable; (3) appreciation that the endocardial dissection technique divides the ventricular insertion of the pathway and does nothing to the atrial insertion of the pathway; (4) complete dissection of the appropriate anatomic space(s) in every patient regardless of the location of the pathway within that space as determined by intraoperative mapping; (5) appreciation that certain pathways may exist as "broad bands" and that when the ventricular insertion site is located at the junction of two anatomic areas (e.g., left paraseptal region), complete dissection of both anatomic spaces should be performed; and (6) isolation of the atrial rim of tissue above the anulus of the valve is necessary to prevent a juxta-anular pathway from retrogradely activating the atrium.

The endocardial surgical dissection techniques for each of the four spaces in the horizontal plane are illustrated in Figs. 131–8, 131–9, 131–10, and 131–11.

The epicardial dissection techniques for pathways in these four locations have been described elsewhere.[11,12]

Surgical intervention following a failed RF ablation attempt does not seem to be more difficult or associated with increased morbidity, provided that the RF technique used places the ablation catheter below the anulus of the mitral valve and that excessive energies are not used on the right side of the heart. There does appear to be a direct correlation between the total amount of energy delivered to an area and the degree of endocardial and subendocardial scarring and fibrosis that occurs. Direct RF ablation of the left atrial side of the A-V groove has resulted in complete destruction of normal tissue planes and injury to circumflex coronary and coronary sinus vessels; excessive application of RF en-

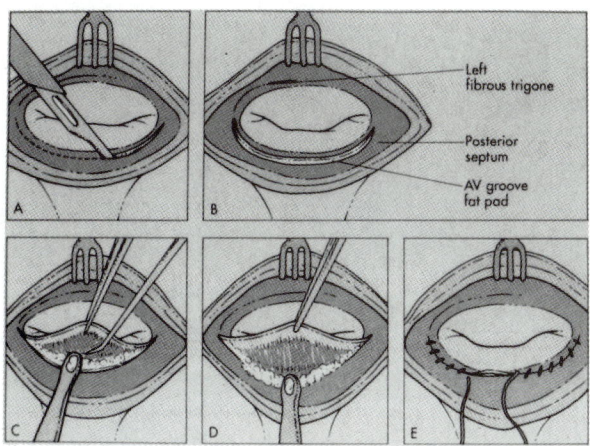
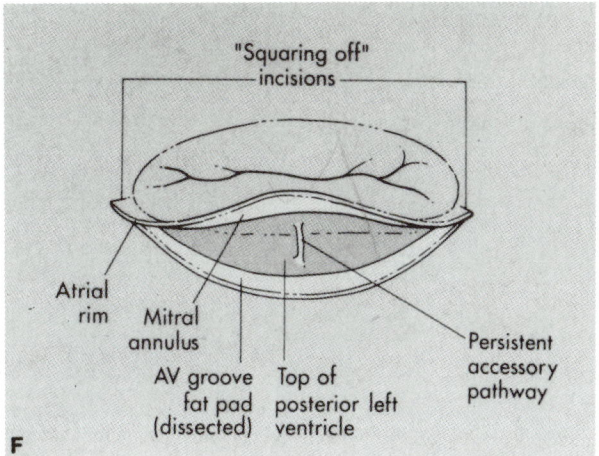

Figure 131–8. Left: Left free-wall endocardial dissection for the WPW syndrome. After exposure of the mitral valve through a left atriotomy, an incision 2 mm above the posterior anulus of the valve is made (**A**). This incision extends from the left fibrous trigone to the posteromedial comissure of the valve (**B**). Using blunt dissection with a nerve-hook the anulus is exposed and the posterior A-V groove fat pad containing the circumflex coronary artery and coronary sinus is separated from the top of the left ventricle (**C**). This dissection is completed throughout the extent of the supra-anular incision out to the reflection of the epicardium off the left ventricle (**D**). **Right:** Appreciation that the majority of left free wall pathways are juxta-anular resulted in addition of a "squaring-off" incision at either end of the supra-anular incision (**F**); this isolates juxta-anular activation to the rim of atrium above the anulus. Alternatively, a 3-mm cryolesion could be placed at either end of this incision. Following isolation of the atrial rim, the supra-anular incision is closed with a multifilament suture (**E, Top**). (*Modified from Ferguson TB, Cox JL: In Chatterjee K, Parmley WW (eds): Cardiology: An Illustrated Text/Reference. Philadelphia/New York, Lippincott/Gower Medical Publishing, 1991, pp 6185–6215, with permission.*)

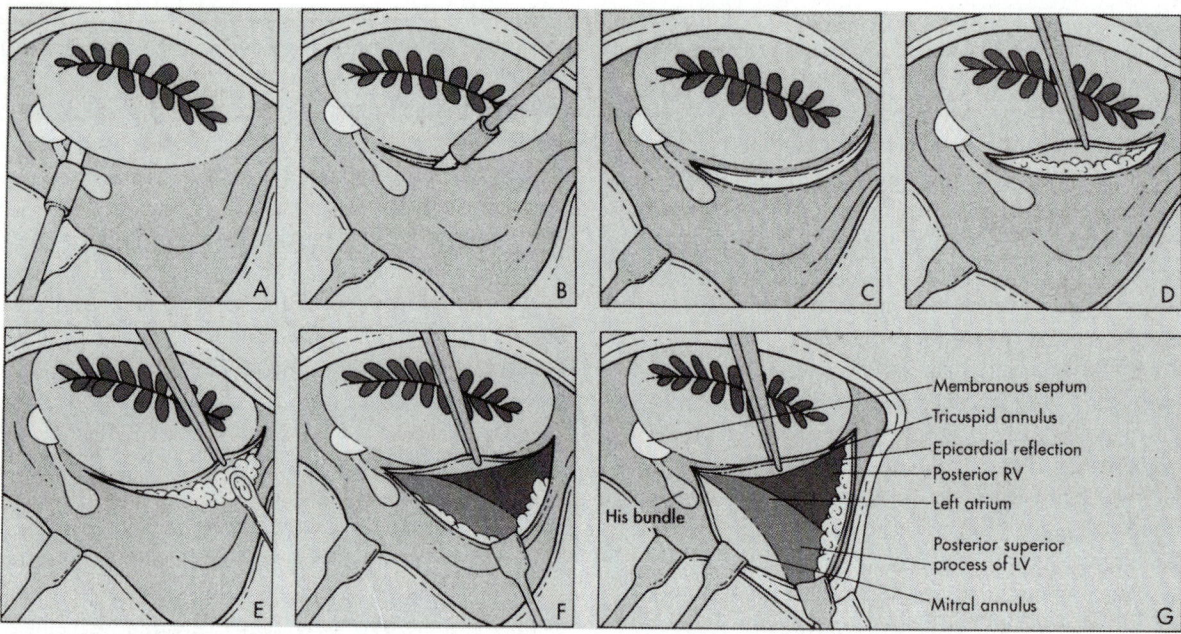

Figure 131–9. Endocardial dissection for surgical division of accessory pathways located in the posterior septal space. The right atrial septum is exposed in the standard fashion. Endocardial mapping, if necessary, is performed with a hand-held probe **A.** A supra-anular incision is made behind the A-V node-His bundle and extended out onto the right atrial free wall (**B,C**); this extension permits entry into the posterior septal space from behind (**D**). The fat pad is dissected off the top of the right ventricle and posterior septum, out to the epicardial reflection (**E**). The dissection is then carried medially using the mitral anulus as a guide to identify the junction of the mitral and tricuspid anuli, which is the posterior aspect of the central fibrous body (**F**); dissection onto the fibrous body will result in inadvertent heart block. The completed dissection is shown in **G**. *(From Ferguson TB, Cox JL: In Chatterjee K, Parmley WW (eds): Cardiology: An Illustrated Text/Reference. Philadelphia/New York, Lippincott/Gower Medical Publishing, 1991, pp 6185–6215, with permission.)*

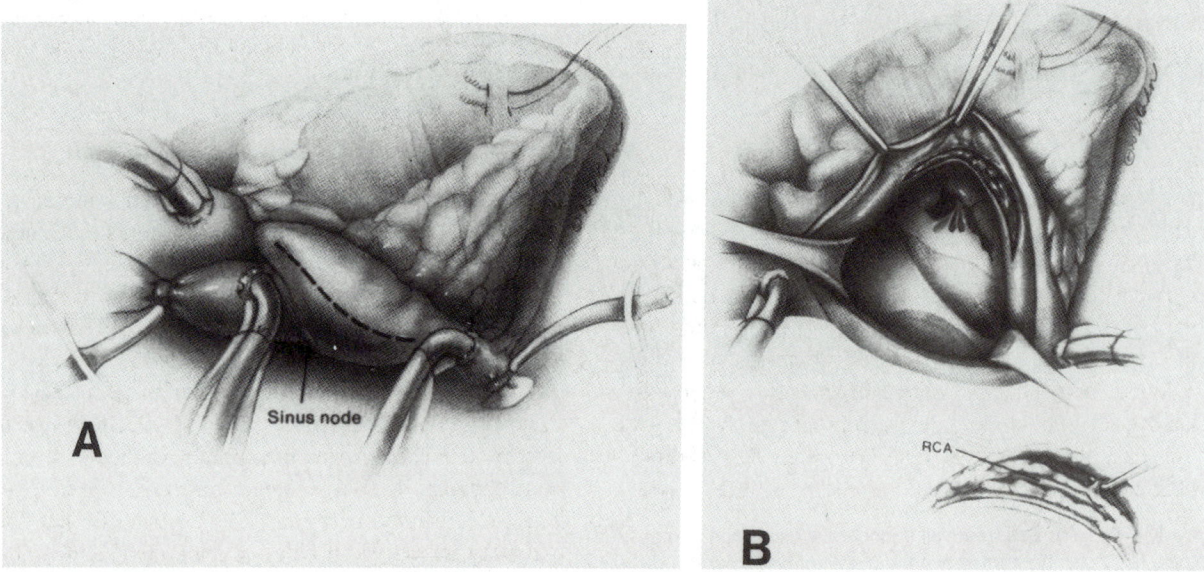

Figure 131–10. Right free-wall endocardial dissection for the WPW syndrome. **A.** The right atriotomy incision following bicaval cannulation and institution of cardiopulmonary bypass. This incision is made well away from the sinus node region. **B.** Exposure of the right atrium. A supra-anular incision is made 2 mm above the tricuspid anulus extending from the posterior septal-right free-wall junction to the pulmonary outflow tract anteriorly; the A-V groove fat pad over this entire space is dissected off the right ventricular free wall out to the epicardial reflection. The supra-anular incision is "squared-off" and closed. *(Modified from Hammon JW: In Cox JL (ed): Cardiac Arrhythmia Surgery. Cardiac Surgery, State of the Art Reviews, Vol. 4., Philadelphia, Hanley & Belfus, 1990, pp 279–286, with permission.)*

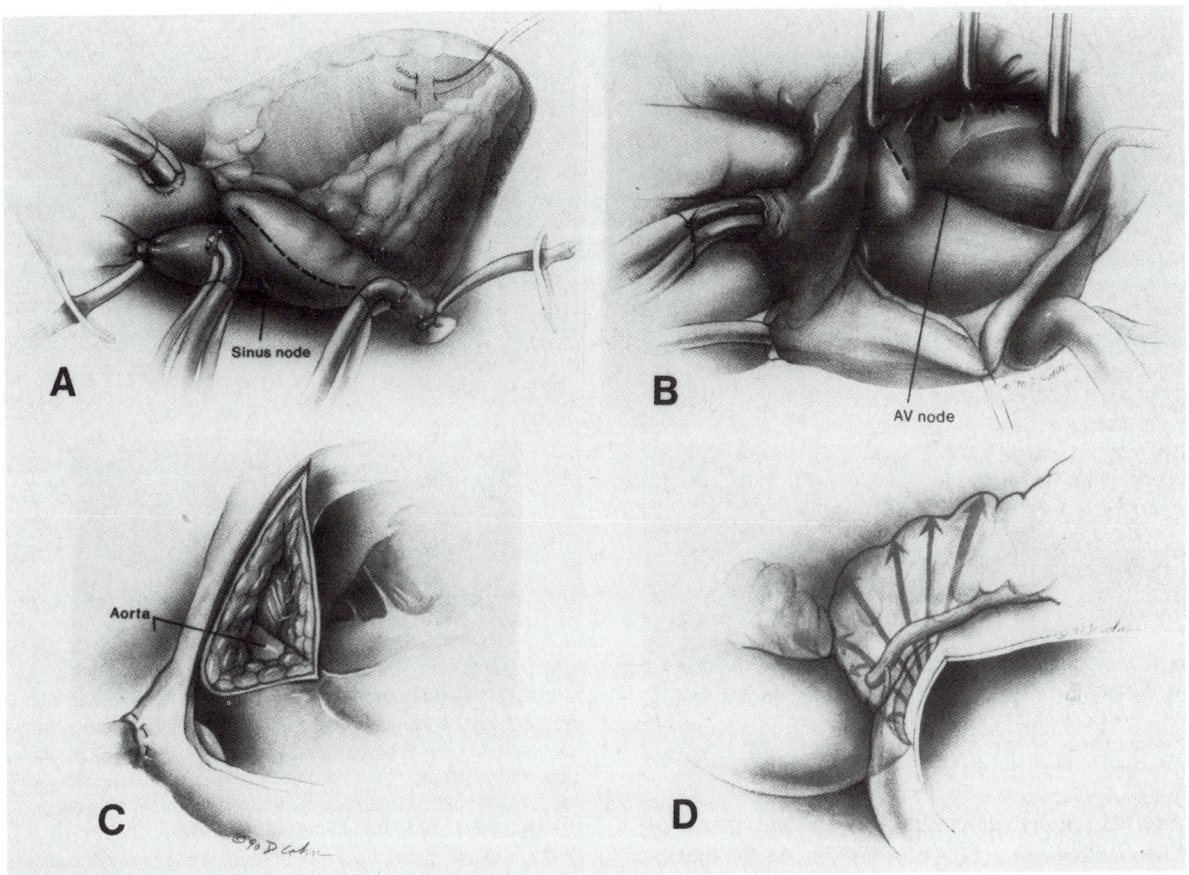

Figure 131–11. Endocardial anterior septal space dissection for the WPW syndrome. **A.** Exposure is obtained through the right atrium as for free-wall dissections. **B.** Initial supra-anular incision is made anterior to the membranous septum after endocardial mapping confirms the location of the pathway in the anterior septal space. **C.** Schematic conceptualization of the extent of the anterior septal dissection, which extends from the aorta medially to the right free-wall epicardium laterally, and out to the pulmonary outflow tract anteriorly. This dissection removes the fat pad containing the proximal right main coronary and its branches off the anterior intraventricular septum. **D.** Completed dissection. *(Modified from Hammon JW: In Cox JL (ed): Cardiac Arrhythmias Surgery. Cardiac Surgery, State of the Art Reviews, Vol. 4., Philadelphia, Hanley & Belfus, 1990, pp 279–286, with permission.)*

ergy to the right atrial septum has likewise resulted in obliteration of normal tissue planes. Placement of a recording catheter in the coronary artery for mapping purposes has been associated with early development of severe atherosclerotic coronary disease, and RF application in the coronary venous branches draining into the coronary sinus has been associated with perforation and tamponade. In this regard, patients with documented coronary sinus diverticuli associated with accessory pathways should probably undergo surgical ablation rather than attempted RF ablation[8] unless the electrophysiologist has extensive experience with these techniques.

Surgical Results

In over 300 patients operated upon for the WPW syndrome and/or other accessory pathways since 1981, the incidence of successful surgical correction of the WPW syndrome using the techniques described is 100% with the initial operation, with an operative mortality for elective, uncompli-

cated cases of 0.5%.[1,13] Approximately 20% of patients have had multiple pathways, 13% Ebstein's anomaly, 22% congenital heart disease other than Ebstein's, 35% other arrhythmias, 6% cardiomyopathy, and 6% coronary artery disease requiring concomitant revascularization. There have been no early or late recurrences following surgery using the endocardial technique described here.

When the recent surgical experience at Washington University with RFCA failures for tachycardias due to accessory connections was examined, two major points became apparent.[14] There were 15 patients referred to Washington University between 1990 and 1993 for surgery following unsuccessful ablation attempts (Table 131–1).[14] The first point was that the majority of RFCA failures were a result of anatomic abnormalities that were documented at surgery; these included Ebstein's anomaly, anomalous coronary sinus/aneurysm, persistent left superior vena cava, iatrogenic perforation of the right ventricle with pericarditis, or broad bundles of muscle (8 to 10 mm) adherent to the coronary sinus tissue that in fact was the accessory connec-

TABLE 131–1. SURGICAL INTERVENTION
FOLLOWING FAILED RFCA

	Number	%
Patients	15	
Mean age 33 years (7–72 years)		
12/15 (80%) with associated anomalies		
Anomalous coronary sinus anatomy	4	27
Ebstein's anomaly	3	20
Morbid obesity	2	13
Mitral insufficiency, coronary artery disease	1	7
Perforated right ventricle at EPS	1	7
Small heart due to age	1	7
10/15 (66%) had significant findings at surgical intervention		
Severe endocardial scarring due to RFCA	5	33
Large A-V muscle bundle	3	20
Severe pericarditis	1	7
Destruction of A-V groove and left atrial tissue	1	7

*From Ferguson TB Jr: The future of arrhythmia surgery. J Card
Electrophysiol 5:621–634, 1994.*

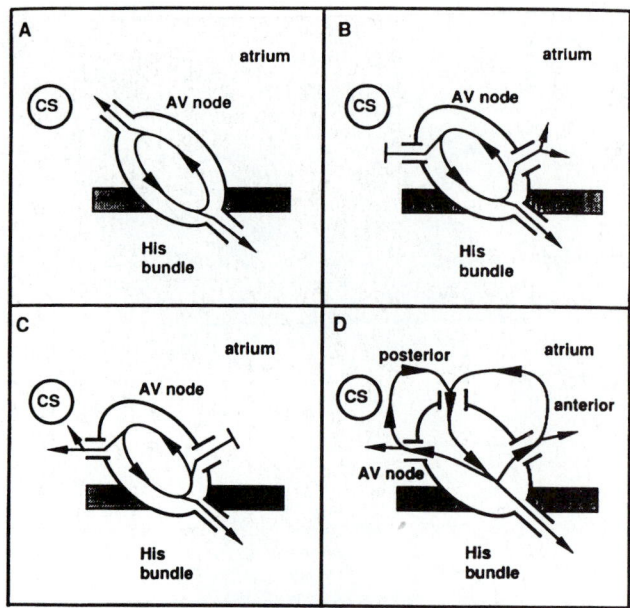

Figure 131–12. Possible mechanisms of atrioventricular (A-V)
junctional reentrant tachycardia. **A.** Commonly accepted
mechanism—intranodal reentry with a common pathway of nodal
tissue above and below reentrant circuit. **B.** Intranodal reentry without common pathway above site of reentry. Different sequences of
atrial activation may be a result of multiple atrial exits from A-V
node. In this case, atria are activated from anterior end of node.
C. Same as **B** but with atria activated from posterior end of node.
D. Reentry using perinodal atrium as part of circuit. Multiple atrial
exits form substrate for reentry. This model allows different
sequences of atrial activation, VA intervals, and tachycardia cycle
lengths and is compatible with selective surgical interruption of one
circuit or the other. Two tachycardia circuits are shown, one
anterior and one posterior. Multiple entry sites may be present, but
for the sake of clarity only one has been depicted. CS, coronary
sinus. *(From McGuire MA, et al: Circulation 83:1232–1246, 1991,
with permission.)*

tion. All of these anatomic variants would be expected to
complicate the anatomic localization of the accessory path-
way(s); similarly, knowledge of these anatomic variations
would be important at the time of surgical intervention. In
the remainder of cases, operator error was presumed to be
the cause of the failure, as manifest by a clinical history of
multiple applications of RFCA lesions but no visible lesions in the appropriate region at the time of surgery.

The second and most important point was that it was
possible to render a patient surgically incurable by inappropriately aggressive RFCA therapy. The result of this excessive application of RF energy is to obliterate the normal tissue planes that exist in the A-V groove of the heart, and in
the worst case to render the tissues so friable as to prohibit surgical correction altogether. In these circumstances, appropriate judgment should be used by the electrophysiologist in determining when maximal RFCA efficacy has been reached.

With this one exception, surgical results and morbidity
for WPW surgery in this circumstance were identical to
previous experience with this arrhythmia.

AV NODAL REENTRANT TACHYCARDIA

Anatomy

The electrophysiologic substrate for both the typical and
atypical forms of A-V nodal reentrant tachycardia is the
presence of "dual A-V conduction pathways," one fast and
one slow, through the A-V node or the perinodal tissues
(Fig. 131–12).[15] Histologic analysis of the A-V nodal and
perinodal tissue has not identified the anatomic correlate of
the electrophysiologic substrate for A-V nodal reentrant
tachycardia.[16] The recent experience with surgical[17] and
RF ablation[18] suggests that perinodal tissue is involved, ei-

ther tissue posterior to the compact node (most commonly)
or tissue anterior to the node.

Surgical anatomy of the right atrial septum is critically
important in the treatment of this arrhythmia (Fig. 131–13).
The A-V node and His bundle are contained in the Triangle
of Koch, bounded superiorly by the Tendon of Todaro, inferiorly by the tricuspid anulus, and posteriorly by the coronary sinus. The apex of the triangle is the atrial portion
of the membranous septum. The penetrating bundle passes
through the central fibrous body of the cardiac skeleton just
posterior to the membranous septum; the location of the His
bundle can be localized slightly more posterior within the
triangle. While the A-V node is always contained within the
Triangle, the exact position of the node within the Triangle
must be considered to be variable.

Surgical Treatment

Currently, the initial ablative treatment of choice is RF, and
surgical intervention is reserved for failed RF ablation or

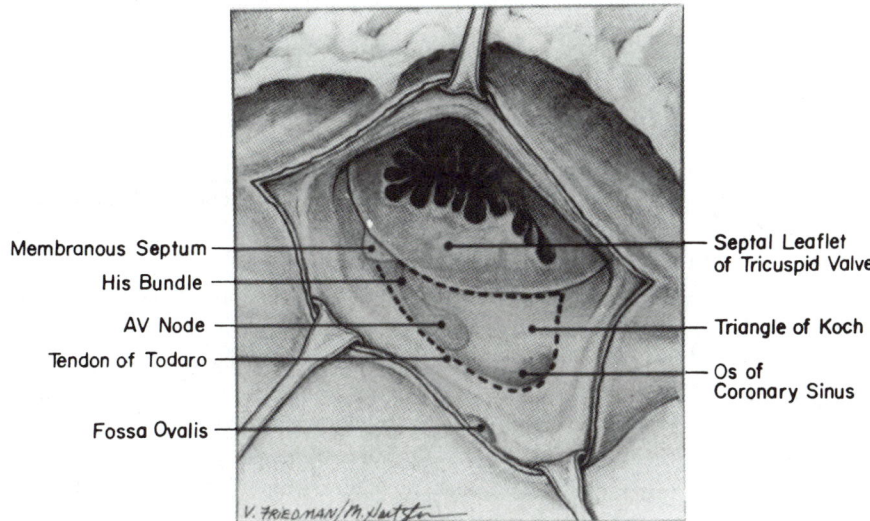

Membranous Septum —
His Bundle —
AV Node —
Tendon of Todaro —
Fossa Ovalis —

Septal Leaflet of Tricuspid Valve
Triangle of Koch
Os of Coronary Sinus

V. FRIEDMAN/M. Hartston

Figure 131–13. Surgical anatomy of the right atrial septum, including the triangle of Koch. *(From Cox JL, et al: Surgery for the Wolff-Parkinson-White syndrome. The endocardial approach. Sem Thorac Cardiovasc Surg 1:34–46, 1989, with permission.)*

when concomitant surgery is performed. However, since much of what was learned from the surgical dissection and cryoablation techniques provided the information necessary to permit successful RF ablation, a brief description of the surgical techniques is indicated.[1,17]

The exposure for the discrete cryosurgical procedure is the same as for a posterior septal pathway dissection. During application of the cryolesions the A-V conduction time is monitored on a beat-to-beat basis. A nitrous oxide cryoprobe with a 3-mm tip is used to place cryolesions along the borders of the Triangle of Koch, initially along the Tendon of Todaro, and then along the anulus of the tricuspid valve beginning just beneath the os of the coronary sinus (Fig. 131–14). When the cryolesion approaches the nodal tissue the A-V interval prolongs in a nearly linear fashion; impending complete heart block is heralded by a prolonga-

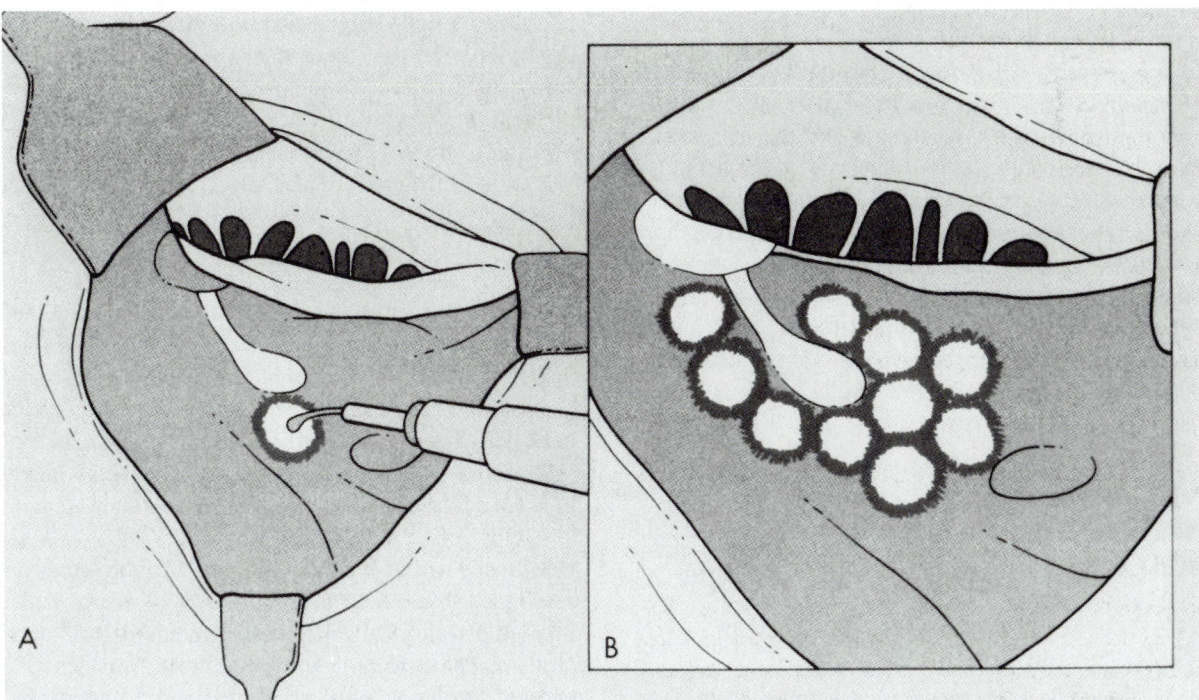

Figure 131–14. Discrete cryosurgical procedure for the treatment of A-V node reentry tachycardia. A 3-mm cryoprobe is used to place a series of cryolesions around the periphery of the A-V node (**B**), beginning at the os of the coronary sinus along the Tendon of Todaro (**A**). Thus the entire perinodal tissue is cryoablated without causing permanent damage to the A-V node proper or adversely affecting A-V node function. *(From Ferguson TB, Cox JL: In Chatterjee K, Parmley WW (eds): Cardiology: An Illustrated Text/Reference. Philadelphia/New York, Lippincott/Gower Medical Publishing, 1991, pp 6185–6215, with permission.)*

tion of the A-V interval by 200 to 300 ms. When block occurs cryothermia is terminated instantly and the A-V interval shortens back to baseline. Used in this way the cryoprobe acts as a "reversible knife." After outlining the borders of the Triangle, subsequent cryolesions are placed to "fill in" the Triangle of Koch as much as possible without causing block. Electrophysiologically, this procedure probably "silently" eliminates the slow pathway (regardless of whether it is anterior or posterior to the nodal tissue); the A-V prolongation and heart block are produced after elimination of the alternative pathway of conduction due to proximity of the cryolesion to the remaining pathway for A-V conduction. Patients with accessory A-V connections and A-V nodal reentrant tachycardia should have both entities treated at the time of the initial operation. Whether patients with WPW syndrome and dual A-V nodal conduction demonstrated on electrophysiologic evaluation should undergo both procedures has been a point of controversy in the past; there are no contraindications to treating both entities.[19] However, interruption of the accessory connection should be performed first so as to prevent inadvertent interruption of the A-V node-His bundle during the cryosurgical procedure while A-V conduction is maintained over the accessory pathway.

Patients with accessory nodoventricular connections and accessory atrio-His connections have been treated with this technique with excellent results.

Surgical Results and Complications

The discrete cryosurgical procedure has been performed on over 35 patients at our institution. In all cases postoperative electrophysiologic study has demonstrated the persistence of only a single A-V conduction pathway, and the reentrant tachycardia could not be induced. There have been no instances of permanent heart block, and no late recurrences.[3]

Two other surgical techniques have been developed for this arrhythmia, both involving surgical dissection either anterior or posterior to the A-V nodal tissue.[1,20,21] While effective, these techniques have been complicated by a small but finite incidence of permanent heart block, and a rather high late recurrence rate.

ECTOPIC OR AUTOMATIC ATRIAL TACHYCARDIAS

Anatomy

Ectopic or automatic atrial tachycardias can originate from foci occurring anywhere within the left or right atrial tissue or atrial septum.[22] However, these occur most commonly on the right side of the heart, can be incessant, and are often markedly refractory to medical therapy. In addition, there may be multiple foci present, some of which may be latent

and become manifest only at some interval following ablation of a different ectopic focus.

Surgical Treatment

Accurate preoperative localization is particularly important in patients with automatic atrial tachycardias if surgical ablation of the focus is contemplated,[3] for several reasons: (1) general anesthesia frequently suppresses the ectopic focus; (2) intraoperative mapping without sophisticated computerized multipoint systems can be prohibitively difficult and time-consuming; and (3) ectopic tachyarrhythmias are not inducible by standard programmed stimulation techniques. If the tachycardia focus can be localized, a variety of techniques have been advocated for surgical treatment including cryoablation, wide excision with pericardial patch repair, a combination of cryoablation and resection, or isolation.[3,22]

Foci on the left atrium have tended to be near the vein of Marshall and the left superior pulmonary vein; localized isolation procedures have met with limited success. In these instances, ectopic foci should be excluded from the remainder of the heart using the left atrial isolation procedure as described by Williams et al[23] (Fig. 131–15). Following the left atrial isolation procedure patients remain in normal sinus rhythm despite the presence of an incessant tachycardia confined to the left atrium. This therapy is preferable to the other therapeutic alternative, that of elective His bundle ablation and pacemaker insertion.

Right atrial tachycardias are usually confined to the body of the right atrium, and may be multifocal. If the arrhythmia circuit or focus cannot be localized at surgery, then a right atrial isolation procedure that isolates the body of the right atrium while leaving the atrial pacemaker complex in continuity with the atrial septum and ventricles should be performed (Fig.131–16).[24]

Surgical Results

If the ectopic focus can be adequately localized in the operation room, then the operative procedures for isolation and/or ablation of the arrhythmias should be uniformly successful.[3,22] Since 1982 the left atrial isolation procedure has been performed on six patients, and the right atrial isolation procedure has been performed on three patients; there have been no adverse sequelae from these operations to date.

Our recent (1988 to 1991) experience with ectopic atrial tachycardias includes 14 patients, 5 of whom initially responded to medical therapy, and 9 of whom underwent map-guided surgical ablation using computerized intraoperative mapping techniques.[25] Of these 9 patients, 3 had cryoablative procedures performed and 6 underwent some form of isolation procedure. Long-term follow-up of these 14 patients has resulted in tachycardia recurrence in 3 of 5 patients treated medically, with no recurrences in the surgically treated patients.

These excellent surgical results will have to be com-

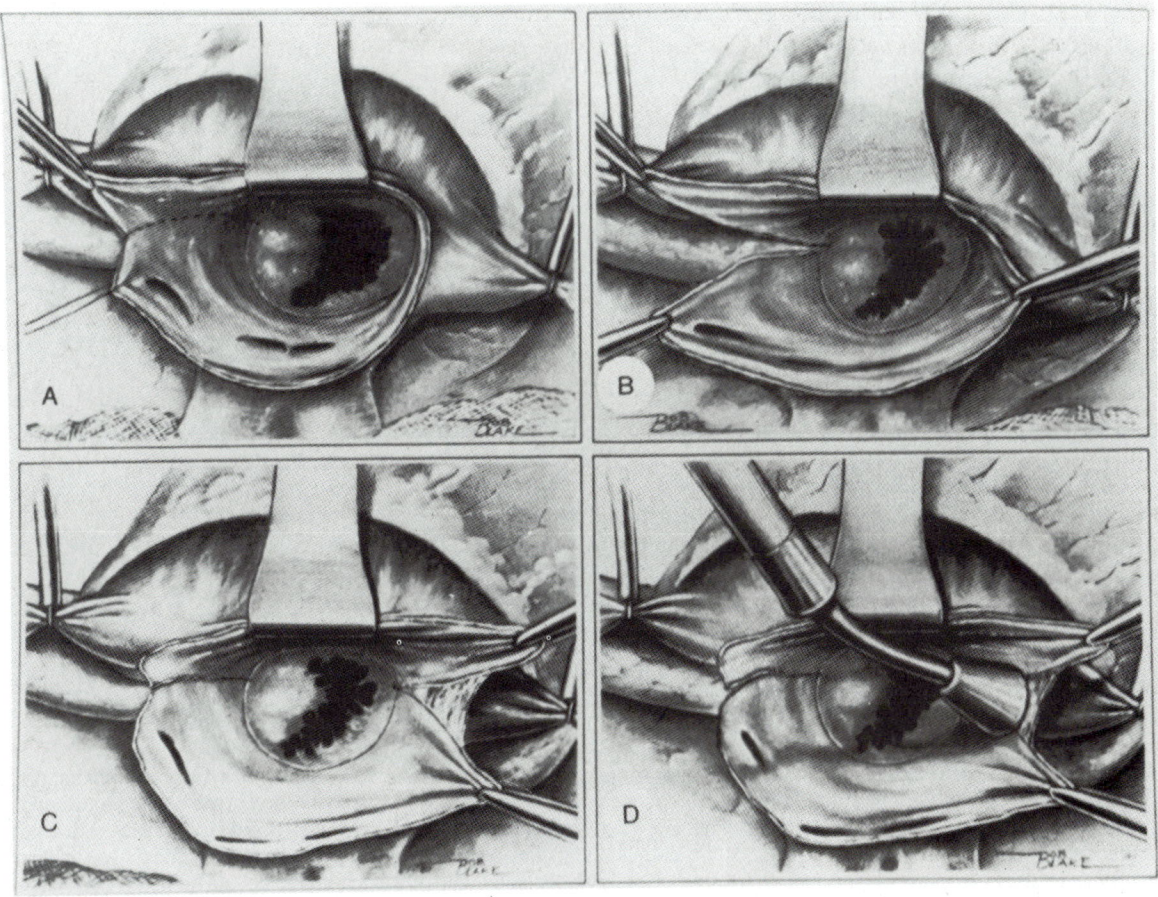

Figure 131–15. Left atrial isolation procedure. **A.** A standard left atriotomy incision is made, and then extended anteriorly (dashed line) across Bachmann's bundle to the level of the mitral anulus just to the left of the left fibrous trigone (**B**). The transmural atriotomy is then extended posteriorly (**C**) to the level of the coronary sinus. The remaining portion of the incision is made through the endocardium extending across the mitral anulus posteriorly. The coronary sinus and A-V groove fat pad are separated from the atrium using blunt dissection in similar fashion to endocardial dissections for left free-wall pathways and to the Maze procedure. To isolate the atrial fibers that are contained within the sinus, cryolesions are placed on the endocardial and epicardial aspects of the dissected coronary sinus at this point (**D**). The left atriotomy is closed with a continuous 4-0 nonabsorbable suture. *(From Ferguson TB, Cox JL: In Chatterjee K, Parmley WW (eds): Cardiology: An Illustrated Text/Reference. Philadelphia/New York, Lippincott/Gower Medical Publishing, 1991, pp 6185–6215, with permission.)*

pared to the results obtained with attempted RF ablation of these arrhythmias in experienced hands. This therapy appears promising based upon short-term results.

ATRIAL FLUTTER AND FIBRILLATION

The Electrophysiologic and Anatomic Aspects of Atrial Fibrillation

Moe and colleagues[26,27] using experimental models and computer simulations, hypothesized that atrial fibrillation was maintained by multiple independent wavelets activating the atria irregularly, very rapidly, and in random fashion. Allessie and colleagues[28] generally confirmed this hypothesis but estimated that an average of only four to six independent wandering wavelets must be present to maintain the fibrillatory process.[29] A recent study from this

group[30] has demonstrated regional entrainment of atrial fibrillatory wavelets, suggesting that stimulating a short excitable gap in the macroreentrant circuits could interfere with the fibrillatory process.

Documenting the correlation between this electrophysiologic concept and the complex anatomy of the atrium has been more difficult. In an isolated right atrial preparation, Schuessler et al[31] showed that at short refractory periods (< 95 ms), atrial reentrant circuits unassociated with anatomic obstacles can become stable and dominate activation. Moreover, the "three-dimensional" nature of these electrophysiologic circuits superimposed upon the thin, flat atrium has also been recently demonstrated by these investigators.[32] Waldo has recently demonstrated in the sterile pericarditis model[33] the conversion of flutter to fibrillation and vice versa; flutter in this model is dependent on the presence of a line of functional block in the right atrium, which upon shortening resulted in the subsequent develop-

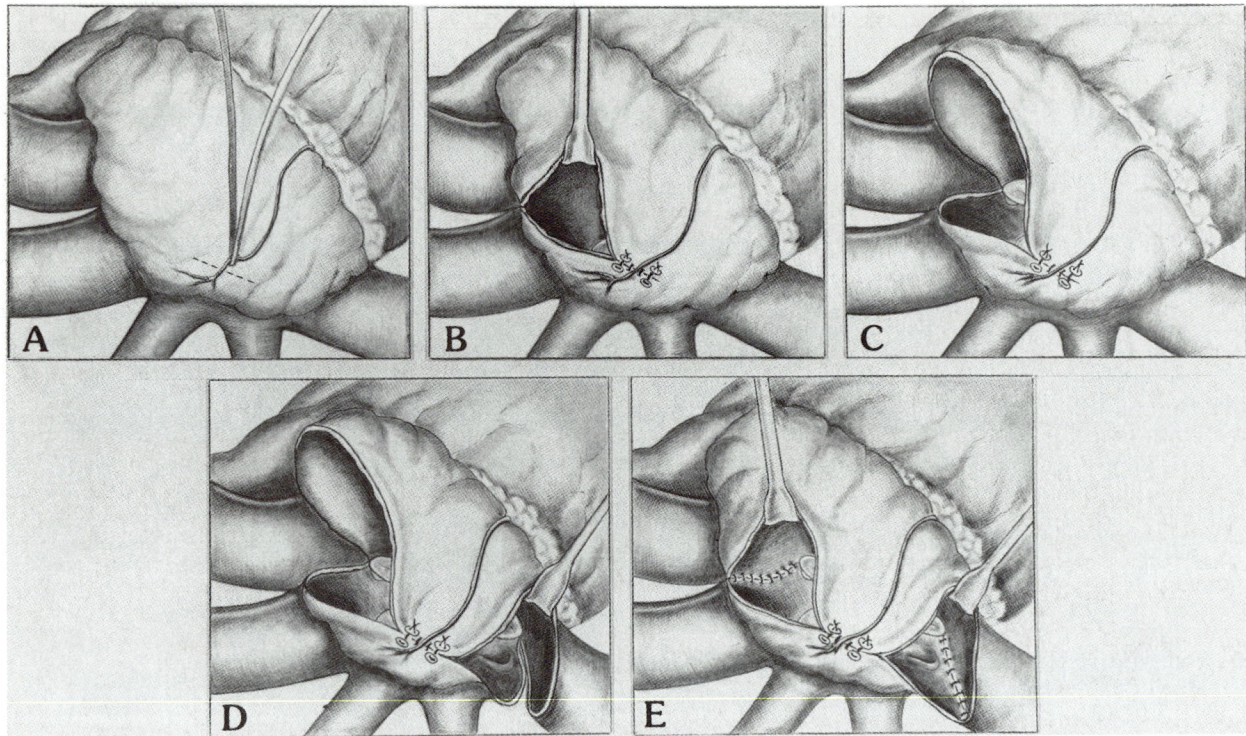

Figure 131–16. Right atrial isolation procedure: **A.** The sinus node artery is dissected and elevated off the atrial epicardium. An incision is made beneath this artery and then closed. **B.** This incision is carried anteriorly to the junction of the superior cava and the right atrial appendage, and then along the anterior limbus of the fossa ovalis to the anteromedial tricuspid valve anulus, just anterior to the membranous inter-atrial septum (**C**). Caudad extension of the atriotomy around the posterior right atrial-inferior caval junction to the posterolateral tricuspid valve anulus is performed. A cryolesion is placed at the end of this incision to ensure complete interruption of connecting atrial muscle fibers between the body of the right atrium and the remainder of the heart. **D,E.** The incision is closed with running nonabsorbable suture. *(From Ferguson TB, Cox JL: In Chatterjee K, Parmley WW (eds): Cardiology: An Illustrated Text/Reference. Philadelphia/New York, Lippincott/Gower Medical Publishing, 1991, pp 6185–6215, with permission.)*

ment of fibrillation. Other studies[34–36] have suggested that a critical mass of atrial tissue, again by definition primarily in a two-dimensional array, is necessary to maintain the fibrillatory process. It is still unclear whether it is the actual weight mass or simply the surface area of tissue that is necessary for sustained fibrillation to occur. Further complicating these issues are the effects of intra-atrial pressure[37,38] and volume[39–41] on the development, maintenance, and ablation of atrial fibrillation.

Several additional important electrophysiologic considerations have been demonstrated in the work of Boineau,[42] Cox,[43–45] and colleagues at Washington University in St. Louis. These studies have suggested that both experimental and clinical atrial flutter/fibrillation can be thought of as a continuum, extending from a single, macroreentrant circuit of right-sided atrial flutter at one end to multiple simultaneous macroreentrant circuits over the entire surface of the right and left atria. In addition, as reported by Ferguson et al,[46] these studies suggested that flutter was dependent upon anatomic obstacles on the right and left sides of the heart (e.g., the superior and inferior caval orifices, the annuli of the atrioventricular valves, and the pulmonary veins). Fibrillation, on the other hand, was

demonstrated to be independent of any anatomic obstacles for either initiation or maintenance, in contrast to all other types of supraventricular and ventricular arrhythmias previously evaluated. This "anatomic independence" allowed these circuits to be transient in both time and space on the surface of the atrium, again suggesting that considerations such as number of wavelets, surface area of tissue, and perhaps intra-atrial size, volume, or pressure are the most important factors to consider in the ablation of atrial fibrillation. At a minimum, these studies from Washington University suggested that any type of map-directed intervention to interrupt these circuits would be difficult.[45] This fact distinguished atrial fibrillation from all other types of supraventricular and ventricular arrhythmias that had been cured with map-directed surgical therapy prior to this time.

The Concept of a "Surgical Cure" of Atrial Fibrillation

The definition of "surgical cure" as applied to atrial fibrillation[46,47] includes (1) elimination of the clinical arrhythmia; (2) maintenance of sinoatrial nodal tissue as the driving impulse for the heart; (3)maintenance of intact atrioventricular conduction; and (4) restoration of atrial transport function. Ideally, if criteria 1 to 4 could be accomplished, then the risk of subsequent thromboembolic events related to the presence of atrial fibrillation could be reduced as well. The appropriateness of any intervention, then, needs to be judged against these five criteria; to the degree that one or more are not successfully achieved, the surgical therapy may be considered less than optimal.

In general, the greater the risk for morbidity and mortality associated with a procedure, the closer to a complete cure the procedure should come; this conceptualization was used in deriving these five criteria for a successful procedure for curing the arrhythmia of atrial fibrillation. None of the other surgical or nonsurgical treatments for atrial fibrillation treatment approaches this rigorous definition of cure, however. Recently, other investigators have argued that there are limits to this association between surgical risk and surgical cure as they pertain to combined procedures for atrial fibrillation and other associated cardiac diseases. For example, the electroanatomic circumstances in which the fibrillation occurs (e.g., idiopathic, associated with a congenital heart defect such as atrial septal defect, or associated with mitral valvar disease) may also need to be taken into account when examining the criteria for applicability and efficacy of procedures designed to surgically eliminate atrial fibrillation. Therefore, the surgical approaches discussed in this paper will be divided into those reported in patients with primarily idiopathic, nonrheumatic atrial fibrillation, and those reported in patients with atrial fibrillation in association with other significant structural cardiac disease as an indication for surgical intervention.

Procedures to Surgically Cure Idiopathic Atrial Fibrillation (Table 131–2)

The Maze Procedure

As reported by Cox et al,[47] this operation is the only surgical procedure described to date that has been demonstrated to cure patients of atrial fibrillation, that is, to meet the first four criteria described above. It is also the only procedure demonstrated to reduce (cf. eliminate) the critical number of reentrant circuits available to maintain the fibrillatory process (Fig. 131–17). The development of this operation and its validation both experimentally and clinically has been previously reported, as has the initial operative technique (Fig. 131–18)[48] as well as its subsequent modification (Fig. 131–19).[49]

The demographics of this selected population reveal that the majority of patients had drug-resistant, medically refractory symptomatic idiopathic (nonrheumatic) atrial fibrillation. The mean age of this surgical population is 56 ± 12 years. Approximately 28% of patients have undergone a concomitant procedure at the time of the maze procedure. The great majority of patients have had normal or near-normal ventricular function at the time of operation; thus far,

TABLE 131–2. SURGICAL RESULTS WITH THE MAZE PROCEDURE: WASHINGTON UNIVERSITY SCHOOL OF MEDICINE/BARNES HOSPITAL, ST. LOUIS, MO

	Number of Patients	%
1. Demographics		
9/87–8/93:	100 Consecutive	
72 males, 28 females		
Mean age 56 +/– 12 years		
(22–75 years)		
2. Duration of arrhythmia		
Paroxysmal fibrillation/flutter ($n=52$):		
8 years (0.5–30 years)		
Chronic fibrillation ($n=19$): 11 years		
(0.3–39 years)		
Paroxysmal fibrillation/flutter to		
chronic fibrillation ($n=29$): 13 years		
(0.5–45 years)		
3. Concomitant surgical procedures	28	
CABG	15	15
Valve repair	8	8
Other	6	6
4. Mid-term (>3 mo postoperative)		
results:	86	
Cure	85/86	99
Surgery alone	77/86	90
With drugs (late recurrence of flutter)	8/86	9
A-V synchrony restored	85/86	99
Without atrial pacing	52/86	61
With atrial pacing	33/86	38
Preserved atrial transport function	85/86	99
Surgical failure	1/86	1

From Ferguson TB Jr: The future of arrhythmia surgery. J Card Electrophysiol 5:621–634, 1994.

severe left ventricular dysfunction has been a relative contraindication to performance of this procedure at Washington University.

Approximately 40% of patients have required pacemaker implantation following the Maze procedure, for atrial chronotropic incompetence. Careful analysis of these patients,[50] however, has revealed that the overwhelming majority of these patients have evidence of underlying sick sinus syndrome as the etiology for the postoperative sinoatrial nodal dysfunction; effective AAIR pacing treats this problem, and in a small number of patients late recovery of adequate chronotropic competence of the sinus node has occurred.

Atrial transport function has been demonstrated in late follow-up by one of several techniques (dynamic magnetic resonance imaging scan, hemodynamic effect of atrial pacing versus ventricular pacing, transthoracic echocardiography) in 100% of the right atrium of patients, and in 81% of the left atrium of patients.

This clinical experience, therefore, with its excellent results, represents the current "state of the art" for surgical cure of idiopathic, nonrheumatic atrial fibrillation that is medically refractory.

SCHEMATIC ATRIAL ANATOMY

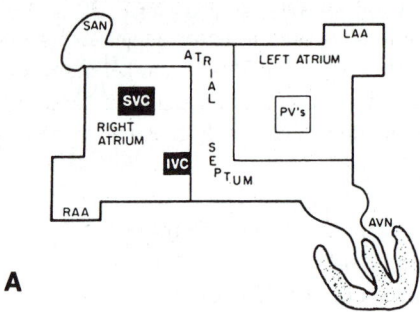

A

NORMAL ATRIAL ACTIVATION

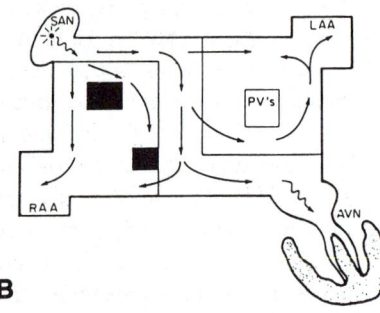

B

ATRIAL FIBRILLATION
(Multiple Macro-Reentrant Circuits)

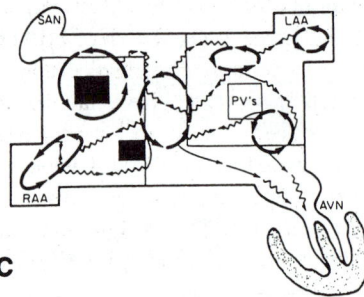

C

Figure 131–17. Schematic diagram of (**A**) normal atrial anatomy; (**B**) normal atrial activation; and (**C**) atrial fibrillation. The fixed obstacles on the right side of the heart are the superior vena cava (SVC) and inferior vena cava (IVC), while on the left side the fixed obstacle is the pulmonary veins (PV). Remaining structures include the right atrial (RAA) and left atrial(LAA) appendages, along with the atrial septum. In **B,** normal activation begins at the sinoatrial node (SAN) to depolarize the atrioventricular node (AVN). The multiple macroreentrant circuits responsible for clinical atrial fibrillation are shown in **C** superimposed on the schematic atrial anatomy. *(Modified from Cox JL, et al: J Cardiovasc Electrophysiol 2:541–561, 1991, with permission.)*

Additional results with the maze procedure have been recently acquired at the Cleveland Clinic, where a total of 14 patients were reported upon in full.[51] The surgical results were quite similar to the Washington University experience, in a similar patient population. They described two variations on the surgical technique; in the first, two patients had concomitant mitral valve repair for degenerative disease of the mitral apparatus, and the Maze procedure was completed in

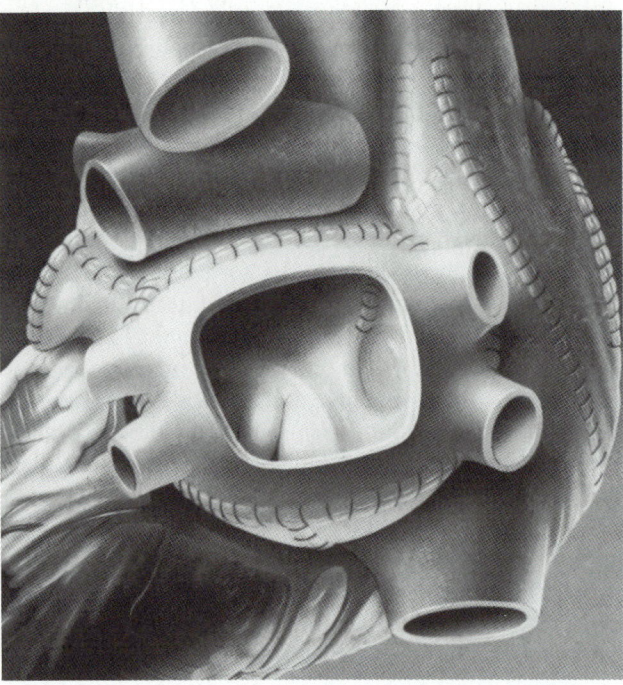

Figure 131–18. The completed Maze procedure (original) for cure of atrial fibrillation as viewed from the posterior aspect. *(From Ferguson TB Jr, Cox JL: Successful surgical treatment for atrial fibrillation. Primary Cardiol 18:15–25, 1992, with permission.)*

these patients only after successful repair was demonstrated intraoperatively, and in the second, three patients had what were judged to be markedly enlarged atria and resection of a portion of both left and right atrial tissue was performed as part of the procedure to reduce overall size postoperatively.

These surgical experiences have generated additional considerations regarding the electroanatomical origin of atrial flutter/fibrillation in these patients with primarily idiopathic disease[52]: (1) the local effective refractory periods (ERPs) of the left atrium appear to be shorter than those in the right atrium; (2) due to the longer ERPs (and therefore longer reentrant circuits) on the right side, atrial flutter is more likely to occur on the basis of reentry in the right atrium; (3) due to the shorter ERPs (and therefore shorter reentrant circuits) on the left side, atrial fibrillation is more likely to occur on the basis of reentry in the left atrium. To eliminate the recurrence of both flutter and fibrillation, a procedure involving both sides of the atrial tissue appears to be necessary in this setting.

Procedures to Surgically Cure Atrial Fibrillation in Association with Structural Diseases of the Heart

The Maze Procedure and Degenerative Mitral Valve Disease (Table 131–3)

As discussed by Cox,[52,53] there has been limited experience in combining the Maze procedure with other types of struc-

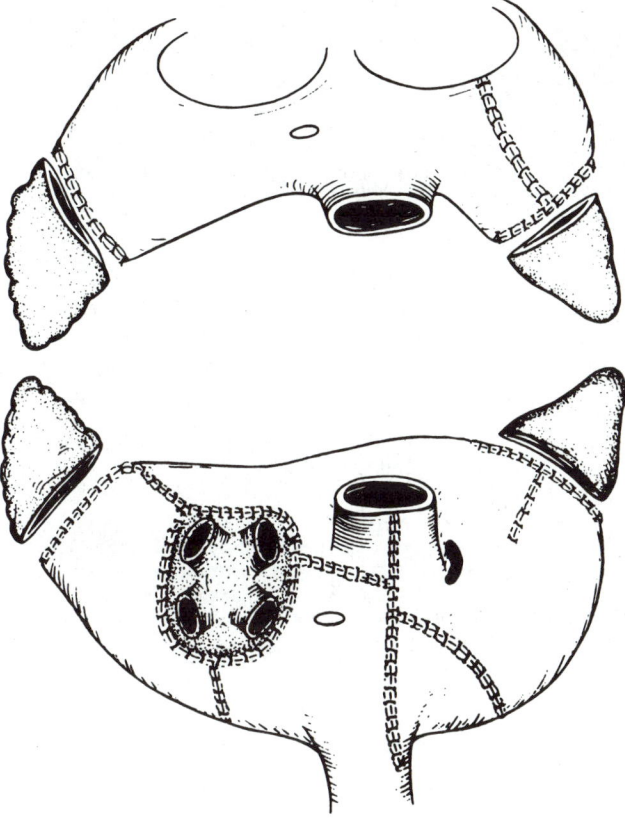

Figure 131–19. Current modification to the surgical technique for the Maze procedure. Note the difference in the right atrial incisions as well as the simplification in the incision across the top of the atrial septum. *(From Cox JL: Evolving applications of the Maze procedure for atrial fibrillation. Ann Thorac Surg 55:578–580,1993, with permission.)*

tural cardiac disease in this country. While the results from Washington University (six patients) and the Cleveland Clinic (two patients) in patients undergoing a combined procedure for atrial fibrillation and degenerative disease of the mitral apparatus are promising, this operation is a complex one that even under the best circumstances will be associated with a finite morbidity. As suggested by McCarthy et al,[51,54] patients with concomitant disease should ideally be less than 70 years of age, have normal ventricular function, have had embolic events related to long standing (greater than 1 year duration) fibrillation, be medically refractory and severely symptomatic, have a left atrial dimension greater than 60 mm, and have an easily reparable valve lesion.

These selection criteria were independently addressed by the Mayo Clinic group in reviewing their experience with mitral valve repair in 323 patients with preoperative atrial fibrillation between 1980 and 1991.[55] At late follow-up in this series, atrial fibrillation was present in 5% of patients with preoperative sinus rhythm, 80% of patients with preoperative chronic atrial fibrillation, and 0% of patients with preoperative recent onset atrial fibrillation. Prevalence

of late thromboembolic events was similar in patients with preoperative sinus rhythm as compared to preoperative atrial fibrillation, and survival between the two groups was not different. They suggested that a concomitant procedure for atrial fibrillation in this setting should have negligible morbidity and no adverse affect on operative mortality to be indicated.

Modifications to the Maze Procedure and Rheumatic Mitral Valve Disease (Table 131–3)

Around the world, where the incidence of rheumatic mitral disease remains high, a number of investigators have modified the maze procedure in its application to combined procedures. The majority of these appear to be in the setting of rheumatic mitral disease; presumably the motivation for the modifications is to simplify the overall operative procedure as a response to similar concerns as those expressed by the Mayo group. Others have suggested on the basis of preliminary mapping studies of human fibrillation in association with valvar heart disease that the fibrillatory mechanism in this setting may primarily involve the left side of the atria,[56,57] and, as a result, surgical procedures that address only the left atrium are all that are required in this setting.

Brodman et al[57] described a case where only the left-sided portion of the maze was performed in a patient undergoing mitral commissurotomy, to shorten operative time. Interestingly, atrial flutter but not atrial fibrillation was inducible at a late postoperative electrophysiologic evaluation in this asymptomatic patient, perhaps related to the ERP observations noted above. Hioki et al[58] reported a modification of the Maze procedure in a mitral valve replacement for mitral stenosis where the pulmonary veins were not encircled but were divided (left from right) instead; no recurrence of atrial fibrillation was reported in this one case.

The largest experience with combined antifibrillatory and valve procedures has been apparently accumulated in Japan, where the nationwide response to survey was reported at the recent meeting of the International Society of Cardio-thoracic Surgeons (Japan). From 30 institutions a total of 230 patients were reported; 196 patients underwent some form of combined mitral plus (modified) Maze procedure. Twenty-one patients had concomitant repair of an atrial septal defect, and only 3 of 230 had idiopathic atrial fibrillation.

The majority of these procedures were modifications of the Maze technique. Kawaguchi et al[59] reported on 51 patients undergoing a modified Maze procedure plus valvar surgery, and compared these results to historical disease- and procedure-matched controls without an antifibrillatory procedure. Morbidity and mortality were similar in both groups; recurrence rate for fibrillation in the surgical group was 8%, as compared to 90% in the non-AF group. Sueda et al[60] described a modified left-sided Maze technique that isolates the pulmonary veins, amputates the left atrial appendage, and uses cryolesions to regionally isolate a large

TABLE 131–3. SURGERY FOR ATRIAL FIBRILLATION[a]

Author	Oprn	Atrial Fibrillation Disease	Eliminates Reentrant Circuits	Decrease Fibrillatory Mass	Surgical Technique (Side)	Tech Diff	SR	Eliminates AF	Restores ATF	Number of Patients
Cox[53]	1	Idiopathic	Y	N	L, R	3+	Y(100%)	Y (99%)	Y (80%)	75
McCarthy et al[54]	1	Idiopathic	Y	N	L, R	3+	Y(100%)	Y (99%)	Y (80%)	14
DeFauw[71]	2	Idiopathic	N	Y	L, R	1+	Y	N	N	21
Brodman et al[57]	3	Rheumatic	Y	N	L	2+	Y	Y	Y	1
Hioki et al[58]	4	Rheumatic	Y	N	L, R	3+	Y	Y	Y	1
Kawaguchi et al[59]	5	Rheumatic	Y(?)	N(?)	L, R	2+	Y (92%)	Y (92%)	Y	51
Sueda et al[60]	6	Rheumatic	Y	Y	L	2+	Y(85%)	Y(85%)	Y(82%)	13
Shyu et al[61]	7	Rheumatic	N	Y	L, R	1+	Y(64%)	Y(64%)	Y(64%)	22
Itoh et al[62]	1	Rheumatic	Y	N	L, R	3+	Y(100%)	Y	Y	15
Graffigna et al[63]	8	Rheumatic	N	Y	L	1+	Y (70%)	N	N	100
Blitz et al[69]	1	HOCM	Y	N	L, R	3+	Y[b]	Y	Y	1
Bonchek et al [70]	1	ASD	Y	N	L, R	3+	Y	Y	Y	1

[a]Oprn, operation: 1 = Maze procedure; 2 = corridor procedure; 3 = left-sided maze procedure only; 4 = maze with modification to pulomonary vein isolation; 5 = unspecified modification to maze procedure; 6 = pulmonary vein isolation + areas of cryoablation; 7 = L and R compartmentalization procedure; 8 = left atrial isolation procedure. Idiopathic, primary atrial fibrillation in the absence of valvar disease in the majority of patients; rheumatic, almost all patients with underlying valvar disease and concomitant valve surgery; HOCM, hyperobstructive cardiomyopathy; ASD, atrial septal defect; L, left; R, right; Tech Diff, technical difficulty of antiarrhythmic portion of the operative procedure; SR, patients in sinus rhythm late postoperatively; AF, atrial fibrillation; ATF, late atrial transport function.
[b]Late atrial flutter, medically controlled.

portion of the posterolateral left atrial tissue. They have used this technique in 13 patients with mitral valve disease, demonstrating sinus rhythm and atrial transport in 11 of 13 patients at late follow-up; interestingly, all 11 patients had right atrial contraction by echocardiography, while 9 (82%) had left atrial contraction, similar to the experience accrued with the standard Maze technique. Shyu et al[61] recently reported 22 patients (16 with rheumatic heart disease) who underwent an atrial compartment procedure in combination with mitral valve surgery; this procedure was either a left atrial isolation procedure[23] or a biatrial isolation procedure.[24] Of 22 patients 14 were in sinus rhythm at 6-mo follow-up; all 14 (the majority with rheumatic disease) had evidence of both left and right atrial mechanical function at this time point, although in many patients it took between 2 and 6 mo for detectable function to return following surgery.

Itoh and colleagues[62] performed a combined Maze/valve procedure in 15 patients. Postoperative echocardiographic findings in this group demonstrated that in elderly patients (>60 years) with significant increases in left atrial volume (up to three times normal), effective left atrial systole despite sinus rhythm could not be demonstrated; in younger patients with smaller atria, contractions were readily apparent.

Graffigna et al[63] performed a left isolation procedure[23] in 100 patients with atrial fibrillation secondary to mitral valve disease undergoing operative intervention, with 70% of patients maintaining sinus rhythm at follow-up. Duration of fibrillation preoperatively longer than 6 mo was a risk factor for recurrence. It was not anticipated that the risk of thromboembolism was decreased by isolation of the left atrium, which could continue to fibrillate. Sinoatrial func-

tion was satisfactory in all patients who maintained persistence of sinus rhythm; during the same time interval in their institution, a nonrandomized group of patients with atrial fibrillation undergoing mitral procedures without the left atrial isolation had persistent fibrillation postoperatively in 80%.[63]

Thus, in the setting of concomitant mitral valve disease, particularly of rheumatic origin, there has been widespread consideration given to applying of the concept of a Maze-type procedure to reduce or eliminate concomitant atrial fibrillation. Most of these applications to date have utilized some modification of the Maze technique, in an attempt to simplify the overall operative procedure. At this point it is unclear if these (or any) modifications of the Maze technique can be as effective as the Maze procedure itself in the setting of concomitant valvar disease; alternatively, it is unclear whether it is justified to accept a slightly higher fibrillation recurrence rate in order to minimize overall operative mortality and morbidity in this setting of combined procedures for mitral valve disease. Cox[52,53,64] has effectively argued against such modifications, based upon the clinical experience to date.[49] Further complicating this dilemma, however, is the fact that a significant number of patients with rheumatic mitral disease have impaired ventricular function at the time of surgery; from a functional point of view it is precisely this group of patients in whom restoration of sinus rhythm and atrial transport would be expected to be of greatest benefit.[59,61,65]

Are there fundamental differences between fibrillation resulting from mitral valvar disease and fibrillation arising as the idiopathic form of the arrhythmia? Recent demographic,[34,35,39] echocardiographic,[37,38] and electrophysiologic[31–33] data are suggestive. If this could be demonstrated, then these differences might possibly permit an alteration in the surgical technique that does not significantly compromise the concept or the success rate of the procedure in this setting. Both volume overload and hypertrophy would be expected to play a role in the setting of valvar disease that might not be as prominent in idiopathic disease.

Overall, the results from these reported surgical experiences and experimental studies suggest that regional isolation of larger segments of left atrium (Sueda, Shyu), or the entire left atrium, (Graffigna) might be feasible in selected, higher risk patients. Data demonstrating improvement of transport function with these procedures are limited[59,66] at this time. The degree to which these modifications may decrease the success rate for curing atrial fibrillation must be weighed against the perceived increase in operative risk by performance of a "complete" Maze operation; to date, no modifications have been able to produce the efficaciousness in eliminating atrial fibrillation that the Maze procedure has achieved.

Finally, additional recent data suggest that sinus node automaticity[67] may play a role in the reinitiation of fibrillation in certain circumstances; this may be in contrast to the clinical association between sick sinus syndrome and atrial fibrillation, however.[68] Interestingly, approximately 30 to 35% of patients in the Washington University Maze group had evidence of sick sinus syndrome preoperatively in primarily idiopathic disease; does this suggest a higher degree of the contribution of right atrial electrophysiology to fibrillation in idiopathic patients as compared to earlier observations about the left atrial contribution in valvar patients?

The Maze Procedure in the Setting of Other Structural Diseases of the Heart (Table 131–3)

Blitz et al reported a successful case of the Maze procedure and a septal myectomy for hyperobstructive myopathy.[69] Postoperative atrial arrhythmias were effectively suppressed by atrial inhibited pacing. Bronchek et al[70] reported a patient with a secundum atrial septal defect and atrial fibrillation who underwent a successful combined procedure; several patients in the Washington University experience also had septal defects. This report raised the question of whether the Maze procedure should be performed *prophylactically* in adult patients undergoing ASD closure, since the incidence of subsequent development of atrial fibrillation was thought to be as high as 50%.[65,70] This would constitute the first application of a cardiac surgical procedure as a prophylactic as opposed to therapeutic procedure.

CONCLUSIONS

The surgical treatment of supraventricular arrhythmias other than atrial fibrillation is now reserved for complex cases following RF ablation failure or patients with combined cardiac disease.[71]

With respect to atrial fibrillation, the Maze procedure

has been demonstrated to cure the majority of patients with idiopathic, nonrheumatic atrial fibrillation who are refractory to medical therapy. Restoration of sinus rhythm (by atrial pacing in approximately 40%) has occurred in all patients and restoration of some degree of atrial transport function has been demonstrated in the majority of patients postoperatively, making this the procedure of choice in these patients.[71]

Combining the Maze procedure with mitral valve repair in patients with degenerative disease has demonstrated promising results thus far, provided that ventricular function is normal and that repair can be easily accomplished.

Worldwide in the setting of rheumatic mitral disease, some authors have tried to modify (e.g., simplify) the Maze procedure as part of a concomitant procedure in circumstances where the criteria outlined above for valve repair are not met. The long-term results of these modifications and their impact on the overall morbidity of these combined procedures remain to be determined.

Finally, the Maze procedure has been performed in conjunction with a number of other structural heart defects with success. Whether the success of the procedure in idiopathic atrial fibrillation warrants its performance as a prophylactic procedure remains to be determined.

REFERENCES

1. Ferguson TB Jr, Cox JL: Surgical treatment of cardiac arrhythmias. In Chatterjee K, Cheitlin MD, Karliner J, et al (eds): *Cardiology. An Illustrated Text/Reference.* Philadelphia, Lippincott/Gower, 1991, pp 6.185–6.214
2. Jackman WM, Kuck K-H, Friday KJ, Lazzara R: Catheter recordings of accessory atrioventricular pathway activation. In Zipes DP, Jalife J (eds): *Cardiac Electrophysiology.* Philadelphia, W.B. Saunders, 1990, pp 491–502
3. Ferguson TB Jr, Cox JL: Surgical therapy for patients with supraventricular tachycardia. In Scheinman MM (ed): *Cardiology Clinics.* Philadelphia, W.B. Saunders, 1990, pp 535–556
4. Jackman WM, Wang X, Friday KJ, et al: Catheter ablation of accessory atrioventricular pathways (Wolff-Parkinson-White syndrome) by radiofrequency current. *N Engl J Med* **324**:1605–1611, 1991
5. Calkins H, Sousa J, el-Atassi R, et al: Diagnosis and cure of the Wolff-Parkinson-White syndrome or paroxysmal supraventricular tachycardias during a single electrophysiologic test. *N Engl J Med* **324**:1612–1618, 1991
6. Canavan TE, Schuessler RB, Boineau JP, et al: Computerized global electrophysiological mapping of the atrium in patients with the Wolff-Parkinson-White syndrome. *Ann Thorac Surg* **46**:223–231, 1989
7. Jackman WM, Friday KJ, Yeung-Lai-Wah JAF, et al: New catheter technique for recording left free-wall accessory atrioventricular pathway activation: Identification of pathway fiber orientation. *Circulation* **78**:598–610, 1988
8. Ferguson TB Jr: The endocardial approach for posterior septal accessory pathways. In Cox JL (ed): *Cardiac Arrhythmia Surgery.* Philadelphia, Hanley & Belfus, 1990, pp 155–174
9. Cain ME, Lindsay BD: The preoperative electrophysiologic study. In Cox JL (ed): *Cardiac Surgery: State of the Art Reviews.* Philadelphia, Hanley & Belfus, 1990, pp 1–39
10. Cox JL, Ferguson TB Jr: Surgery for the Wolff-Parkinson-White syn-

drome: The endocardial approach. *Sem Thorac Cardiovasc Surg* **1:**34–46, 1989

11. Guiraudon GM, Klein GJ, Sharma AD, et al: Closed-heart technique for Wolff-Parkinson-White syndrome: Further experience and potential limitations. *Ann Thorac Surg* **42:**651, 1986

12. Guiraudon GM, Klein GJ, Sharma AD, et al: Surgery for the Wolff-Parkinson-White syndrome: The epicardial approach. *Sem Thorac Cardiovasc Surg* **1:**21–33, 1989

13. Ferguson TB JR, Cox JL: Complications related to the surgical treatment of supraventricular and ventricular cardiac arrhythmias. In Waldhausen JA, Orringer MB (eds): *Complications in cardiothoracic Surgery.* St. Louis, Mosby Year Book, 1990

14. Cox JL, Ferguson TB Jr., Lindsay BD, et al: Lessons learned from surgery from failed radiofrequency catheter ablation of accessory pathways. *J Am Coll Cardiol* 1993 (abstract)

15. Sung RJ, Huycke EC, Keung EC, et al: Atrioventricular node reentry: Evidence of reentry and functional properties of fast and slow pathways. In Zipes DP, Jalife J (eds): *Cardiac Electrophysiology.* Philadelphia, W.B. Saunders, 1990, pp 513–525

16. Holman WL, Hackel DB, Lease JG, et al: Cryosurgical ablation of atrioventricular nodal reentry: Histologic localization of the proximal common pathway. *Circulation* **77:**1356–1362, 1988

17. Cox JL, Ferguson TB Jr, Lindsay BD, Cain ME: Peri-nodal cryosurgery for AV nodal reentrant tachycardia in 23 patients. *J Thorac Cardiovasc Surg* **99:**440–450, 1990

18. Leon A, El-Atassi R, Borganelli M, et al: A prospective randomized comparison of anterior and posterior approaches for radiofrequency catheter modification of AV node reentry tachycardia. *J Am Coll Cardiol* **19:**145A, 1992 (abstract)

19. Cox JL, Ferguson TB Jr: Surgery for dual atrioventricular node physiology in the Wolff-Parkinson-White syndrome. *J Am Coll Cardiol* **17:**1568–1569, 1991

20. Guiraudon GM, Klein GJ, Sharma AD, et al: Skeletonization of the atrioventricular node for AV node reentrant tachycardia: Experience in 32 patients. *Ann Thorac Surg* **49:**565–573, 1990

21. McGuire MA, Lau K-C, Johnson DC, et al: Patients with two types of atrioventricular junctional (AV nodal) reentrant tachycardia: Evidence that a common pathway of nodal tissue is not present above the reentrant circuit. *Circulation* **83:**1232–1246, 1991

22. Lowe JE, Hendry PJ, Packer DL, Tang AS: Surgical management of chronic ectopic atrial tachycardia. *Sem Thorac Cardiovasc Surg* **1:**58–66, 1989

23. Williams JM, Ungerlieder GK, Lofland GK, et al: Left atrial isolation. New technique for the treatment of supraventricular arrhythmias. *J Thorac Cardiovasc Surg* **80:**373–380, 1980

24. Harada A, D'Agostino HJ, Boineau JP, Cox JL: Right atrial isolation procedure: A new surgical treatment of supraventricular tachycardia. II. Hemodynamic effects. *J Thorac Cardiovasc Surg* **95:**651–657, 1988

25. Prager NA, Cox JL, Lindsay BD, et al: Long-term effectiveness of medical and surgical treatment of automatic atrial tachycardia. *J Am Coll Cardiol* **22:**85–92, 1992

26. Moe GK, Abildskov JA: Atrial fibrillation as a self-sustaining arrhythmia independent of focal discharge. *Am Heart J* **58:**59–70, 1959

27. Moe GK, Rheinboldt WC, Abildskov JA: A computer model of atrial fibrillation. *Am Heart J* **67:**200–220, 1964

28. Allessie MA, Lammers WJEP, Bonke FIM, et al: Experimental evaluation of Moe's multiple wavelet hypothesis of atrial fibrillation. In Zipes DP, Jalife J (eds): *Cardiac Electrophysiology and Arrhythmias.* Orlando, FL, Grune & Stratton, 1985, pp 265–275

29. Allessie MA, Brugada J, Boersma L, et al: Mapping of atrial fibrillation in man. *New Trends Arrhyt* **6:**787–790, 1990

30. Kirchhof CJHJ, Chorro F, Scheffer GJ, et al: Regional entrainment of atrial fibrillation studied by high-resolution mapping in open-chested dogs. *Circulation* **88:**736–749, 1993

31. Schuessler RB, Grayson TM, Bromberg BI, et al: Cholinergically mediated tachyarrhythmias induced by a singe extra stimulus in the isolated canine right atrium. *Cir Res* **71:**1254–1267, 1992

32. Schuessler RB, Kawamoto T, Hand DE, et al: Simultaneous epicardial and endocardial activation sequence mapping in the isolated canine right atrium. *Circulation* **88:**250–263, 1993

33. Ortiz J, Niwano S, Abe H, et al: Mapping the conversion of atrial flutter to atrial fibrillation and atrial fibrillation to atrial flutter. *Circ Res* **74:**882–894, 1994

34. Petersen P, Kastrup J, Brinch K, et al: Relation between left atrial diameters and duration of atrial fibrillation. *Am J Cardiol* **60:**382–384, 1987

35. Sanfilippo AJ, Abascal VM, Sheenan M, et al: Atrial enlargement as a consequence of atrial fibrillation. *Circulation* **82:**792–797, 1990

36. York TC, Landa FJ: Minimal mass required for induction of a sustained arrhythmia in isolated atrial segments. *Am J Physiol* **202:**232–236, 1962

37. Barbier P, Alioto G, Buazzi MD: Left atrial and ventricular filling in hypertensive patients with paroxysmal atrial fibrillation. *J Am Coll Cardiol* **24:**165–170, 1994

38. Vulliemin P, Bufalo AD, Schlaepfer J, et al: Relation between cycle length, volume and pressure in Type I atrial flutter. *PACE* **17:**1391–1398, 1994

39. Gosselink ATM, Crijns HJGM, Hamer HPM, et al: Changes in left and right atrial size after cardioversion of atrial fibrillation: Role in mitral valve disease. *J Am Coll Cardiol* **22:**1666–1672, 1993

40. Vaziri SM, Larson MG, Benjamin EJ, et al: Echocardiographic predictors of nonrheumatic atrial fibrillation. *Circulation* **89:**724–730, 1994

41. Allessie MA, Rensma PL, Brugada J, et al: Pathophysiology of atrial fibrillation. In Zipes DP, Jalife J (eds): *Cardiac Electrophysiology: From Cell to Bedside.* Philadelphia, W.B. Saunders, 1990, pp 548–559

42. Boineau JP, Schuessler RB, Mooney CR, et al: Natural and evoked atrial flutter due to circus movement in dogs. Role of abnormal atrial pathways, slow conduction, nonuniform refractory period distribution and premature beats. *Am J Cardiol* **45:**1167–1181, 1980

43. Cox JL, Schuessler RB, Boineau JP: The surgical treatment of atrial fibrillation. I. Summary of the current concepts of the mechanisms of atrial flutter and atrial fibrillation. *J Thorac Cardiovasc Surg* **101:**402–405, 1991

44. Cox JL, Canavan TE, Schuessler RB, et al: The surgical treatment of atrial fibrillation. II. Intraoperative electrophysiologic mapping and description of the electrophysiologic basis of atrial flutter and atrial fibrillation. *J Thorac Cardiovasc Surg* **101:**406–426, 1991

45. Cox JL, Schuessler RB, D'Agostino JH, et al: The surgical treatment of atrial fibrillation. III. Development of a definitive surgical procedure. *J Thorac Cardiovasc Surg* **101:**569–583, 1991

46. Ferguson TB Jr, Schuessler RB, Hand DE, et al: Lessons learned from computerized mapping of the atrium: Surgery for atrial fibrillation and atrial flutter. *J Electrocardiol* **26:**210–219, 1993

47. Cox JL, Boineau JP, Schuessler RB, et al: A review of surgery for atrial fibrillation. *J Cardiac Electrophysiol* **2:**541–561, 1991

48. Cox JL: The surgical treatment of atrial fibrillation: IV. Surgical Technique. *J Thorac Cardiovasc Surg* **101:**584–592, 1991

49. Cox JL, Boineau JP, Schuessler RB, et al: Five year experience with the Maze procedure for atrial fibrillation. *Ann Thorac Surg* **56:**814–824, 1993

50. Ferguson TB Jr, Kater KM, Boineau JP, et al: The requirement for permanent pacemaker therapy following the Maze procedure for atrial fibrillation: Incidence and therapeutic indications. *PACE* **17:**862, 1994 (abstr)

51. McCarthy PM, Castle LW, Maloney JD, et al: Initial experience with the Maze procedure for atrial fibrillation. *J Thorac Cardiovasc Surg* **105:**1077–1087, 1993

52. Cox JL: Combined treatment of mitral stenosis and atrial fibrillation with valvuloplasty and a left atrial Maze procedure (reply). *J Thorac Cardiovasc Surg* **107:**622–624, 1994

53. Cox JL: Surgical treatment of atrial fibrillation (reply). *J Thorac Cardiovasc Surg* **104:**1492–1494, 1992

54. McCarthy PM, Cosgrove DM, Castle LW, et al: Combined treatment

of mitral regurgitation and atrial fibrillation with valvuloplasty and the Maze procedure. *Am J Cardiol* **71:**483–486, 1992

55. Chua YL, Schaff HV, Orszulak TA, et al: Outcome of mitral valve repair in patients with preoperative atrial fibrillation. Should the Maze procedure be combined with mitral valvuloplasty? *J Thorac Cardiovasc Surg* **107:**408–415, 1994

56. Harada A, Sasaki K, Fukushima T, et al: Atrial activation during chronic atrial fibrillation in patients with isolated mitral valve disease. *Ann Thorac Surg* (in press)

57. Brodman RF, Frame R, Fisher JD, et al: Combined treatment of mitral stenosis and atrial fibrillation with valvuloplasty and a left atrial Maze procedure (letter). *J Thorac Cardiovasc Surg* **107:**622, 1994

58. Hioki M, Ikeshita M, Iedokoro Y, et al: Successful combined operation for mitral stenosis and atrial fibrillation. *Ann Thorac Surg* **55:**776–778, 1993

59. Kawaguchi AT, Kosaki Y, Isobe F, et al: Risk and benefit of combined Maze procedure for atrial fibrillation associated with valvular heart diseases. *J Am Coll Cardiol* **February:** 459A, 1994 (abstr)

60. Sueda T, Shikata H, Orihashi K, et al: Modified left atrial isolation for chronic atrial fibrillation associated with mitral valve disease. *Ann Thorac Surg* (in press)

61. Shyu K, Cheng J, Chen J, et al: Recovery of atrial function after atrial compartment operation for chronic atrial fibrillation in mitral valve disease. *J Am Coll Cardiol* **24:**392–398, 1994

62. Itoh T, Okamoto H, Ogawa Y, et al: Left atrial function after the Cox/Maze operation in mitral valvular disease patients. *Jpn Heart J* 1994 (abstr)

63. Graffigna A, Pagani F, Minzioni G, et al: Left atrial isolation associated with mitral valve operations. *Ann Thorac Surg* **54:**1093–1098, 1992

64. Cox JL: Evolving applications of the Maze procedure for atrial fibrillation. *Ann Thorac Surg* **55:**578–580, 1993

65. Kono T, Sabbah HN, Rosman H, et al: Left atrial contribution to ventricular filling during the course of evolving heart failure. *Circulation* **86:**1317–1322, 1992

66. Manning WJ, Silverman DI, Katz SE, et al: Impaired left atrial mechanical function after cardioversion: Relation to the duration of atrial fibrillation. *J Am Coll Cardiol* **23:**1535–1540, 1994

67. Kirchhof CJHJ, Allessie MA: Sinus node automaticity during atrial fibrillation in isolated rabbit hearts. *Circulation* **86:**263–271, 1992

68. Page PL: Sinus node during atrial fibrillation. *Circulation* **86:**334–336, 1992

69. Blitz A, McLoughlin D, Gross J, et al: Combined Maze procedure and septal myectomy in a septuagenarian. *Ann Thorac Surg* **54:**364–365, 1992

70. Bonchek LI, Burlingame MW, Worley SJ, et al: Cox/Maze procedure for atrial septal defect with atrial fibrillation: Management strategies. *Ann Thorac Surg* **55:**607–610, 1993

71. Ferguson TB Jr: The future of arrhythmia surgery. *J Cardiovasc Electrophysiol* **5:**621–634, 1994

C H A P T E R
132

Surgery for Ventricular Tachyarrhythmias

Alexander S. Geha and Jai H. Lee

Up to the mid-1950s, patients who suffered sustained ventricular tachycardia or ventricular fibrillation in the hospital were not likely to survive. With the development of external defibrillators, the likelihood of successful resuscitation changed abruptly and dramatically. Most of these lethal arrhythmias, however, occur outside the hospital setting, and the outcome for victims of an out-of-hospital event depends on how quickly defibrillation can be achieved. Sudden cardiac death remains a major cause of morbidity and mortality in the United States.[1] It is estimated that 350,000 to 400,000 people die suddenly each year. In the majority, this sudden cardiac death is felt to be of arrhythmogenic origin (ventricular tachycardia or fibrillation).[2,3] However, the number of survivors of sudden cardiac death is increasing, probably as a result of increasing sophistication in prehospital and emergency medical care, and of the rising number of lay people trained in cardiopulmonary resuscitation. Furthermore, noninvasive and invasive techniques have been developed to predict those patients at greatest risk for sudden cardiac death *prior* to their first event.

Despite the introduction of many new antiarrhythmic drugs in the last 15 years, it is still possible to suppress arrhythmias by electrophysiologic criteria in only 50% of patients. In addition, all of the antiarrhythmic drugs currently available have significant cardiac and extracardiac toxicity.[4] Nonpharmacologic therapy for this refractory population is now well established and in widespread use. In the last two decades, the nonpharmacologic approach has undergone a dramatic change, from the development of surgical mapping and ablative techniques aimed at eliminating the arrhythmia to the introduction and refinement of implantable cardioverter defibrillators to detect and correct the arrhythmia when it occurs. This chapter aims at identifying the patient populations at greatest risk, reviewing the pathophysiology of "sudden cardiac death" and discussing the surgical (nonpharmacologic) options available and their rationale, and reviewing new and experimental techniques that may alter future therapy of these life-threatening arrhythmias.

Ventricular tachycardias (VT) encompass a spectrum of arrhythmias that range from nonsustained, asymptomatic VT to sustained arrhythmia, which can produce hemodynamic compromise and cardiac arrest. These tachycardias may be uniform in morphology or polymorphic.

PATIENT POPULATIONS AT RISK

Ventricular tachycardia most often occurs in the setting of some form of cardiac disease. The patient populations who will most likely sustain a left-threatening ventricular arrhythmia include (1) patients sustaining sudden cardiac death without prior identified cardiac disease, (2) patients with known ischemic heart disease (including a subpopulation of postmyocardial infarction patients), and (3) patients with structural heart defects with known arrhythmogenic potential (e.g., long QT syndrome and arrhythmogenic dysplasia).

Sudden cardiac death usually occurs without warning or symptoms, often during mild to moderate exercise.[5] Largely due to advances in prehospital and emergency care, more than 30% of these patients will survive and leave the hospital without major neurologic deficit.[2,3] These survivors, however have a 60% chance of recurrence during the first 2 years after hospitalization resulting in sudden death.[2,6] Overall sudden cardiac death survivors have an approximate 5-year survival rate of 50%, as compared to more than 80% for an age- and sex-matched similar population.[7] Frequently, the initial result of sudden death is not concurrent or associated with an acute transmural myocardial infarction (MI).[8] These non-MI patients (about 70% of all sudden death patients) are at even greater risk for recurrence,[8] and approximately two-thirds of them will have significant coronary artery disease when catheterized. Upon multivariant prospective analysis, significant proximal left anterior descending coronary artery stenosis and regional left ventricular dysfunction show up as strong predictors of recurrence of sudden death.[9] Additionally, retrospective review shows left ventricular failure (congestive heart failure) as another strong predictor of such recurrence.[10]

Patients with known ischemic heart disease are also at risk for sudden cardiac death, and ventricular tachycardia most often occurs in the setting of some form of cardiac disease. Although the overall incidence is low (approximately 3 to 4%),[11] high-risk subpopulations exist. Patients with ventricular tachyarrhythmias following myocardial infarction have early mortalities of 40 to 80%.[12] Especially vulnerable are those whose prior infarction is associated with aneurysm formation. These patients usually manifest sustained monomorphic VT.[13] In patients who have angiographically significant coronary lesions, bypass grafting is clearly superior to antianginal medical therapy in preventing subsequent cardiac death.[14,15] In the high-risk subpopulation with triple-vessel disease and congestive heart failure, 91% of surgically treated (coronary bypass grafting) vs. 69% of medically treated patients were free from sudden cardiac death during a 5-year follow-up.[11]

Patients with structural heart disease with known arrhythmigenic potential (long QT syndrome, arrhythmogenic right ventricular dysplasia),[16] with cardiomyopathy, valvular heart disease, as well as postoperative congenital heart patients [particularly tetralogy of Fallot, ventricular septal defect, complete atrioventricular (A-V) canal, and transposition of the great arteries], complete the list of patients at risk for sudden cardiac death/ventricular tachyarrhythmias.[13,17] In contrast to patients with uniform sustained VT primarily associated with coronary artery disease (in more than 90% of instances), patients presenting with nonsustained arrhythmias (uniform or polymorphic) and cardiac arrest are more heterogeneous groups. Occasionally, any of these forms of VT can occur in patients with normal hearts.[13]

PATHOPHYSIOLOGY

Classically, a wide QRS complex exceeding 0.14 seconds in duration (normal QRS < 80 ms) has been considered characteristic of ventricular tachycardia.[18] This rhythm, originating in the ventricle, will not travel along the major conduction pathways and therefore this conduction is

slower. Uniform VT has a single, stable QRS morphology. Polymorphic or multiform VT has a changing QRS morphology; for practical purposes, a tachycardia is considered polymorphic if it has no constant morphology for more than 5 complexes, has no clear isoelectric baseline, or has QRS complexes that are asynchronous in multiple simultaneously recorded leads.[13] Polymorphic VT frequently degenerates into ventricular fibrillation (VF). Rapid sustained uniform VT can also degenerate into VF, usually following a stage of polymorphic tachycardia. This is a fairly common mechanism of sudden cardiac death recorded by Holter monitor.[18,20] This observation suggests a link between uniform sustained VT and VF and provides a rationale for using suppression of induced VT as a goal for therapy in patients with cardiac arrest.

Tachycardia is considered sustained if it lasts at least 15 seconds, although some investigators use 30 seconds as the duration required for a "sustained VT."[13] Most tachycardias that last 15 seconds continue for 30 seconds. The significance of the requirement of a specified duration is related to the evolution of antitachycardia pacing or defibrillating devices in which a specific duration of a tachycardia will activate the device.

Potential mechanisms of VTs include re-entry, normal and abnormal automaticity, and triggered activity that is due to early or delayed after-depolarizations. Most of the recent knowledge of cellular mechanisms of arrhythmias is derived from isolated atrial, Purkinje, and ventricular muscle fibers exposed to a variety of conditions.[21–23] By comparing the mode of initiation of tachycardias and the influence of stimulation during tachycardias in vitro and in vivo experimental preparations to comparable situations in humans, and by extrapolating from activation mapping and other laboratory investigations in humans, the bulk of evidence suggests that re-entry is the mechanism of sustained uniform tachycardias associated with coronary artery disease.[30–32] Furthermore, nonsustained VT and VT producing cardiac arrest may have a similar mechanism because they have a qualitatively similar, although quantitatively less, substrate of abnormal conduction. The evidence supporting re-entry is based on the ability to reproducibly initiate and terminate the tachycardia by program stimulation, response of the tachycardia to stimulation, the effect of drugs on the tachycardia, and activation mapping demonstrating re-entrant excitation.[13]

The underlining mechanism for VF and for the entire spectrum of nonsustained and polymorphic ventricular arrhythmias in patients with cardiomyopathy, electrolyte imbalance, valvular disorders, and so on is not understood. However, the mechanism of sustained uniform VT, regardless of the underlying cardiac disorder, appears most consistent with re-entry (including patients with congenital heart disease, cardiomyopathy, and those with no organic heart disease), based on similar observations as those noted for uniform VT encountered in the setting of coronary artery disease.[13]

Action Potential

During electrical diastole the resting membrane potential is approximately −85 mV. When an electrical (most common), mechanical, or chemical signal reaches the cell, a current flows across the membrane, reducing the membrane potential (Fig. 132–1). If the stimulus is sufficient to raise the potential to a critical threshold, the membrane will depolarize (fire). At this point, current rushes across the cell membrane (Phase 0) and the membrane reverses polarity to +30 mV. Sinoatrial (S-A) node tissue, Purkinje fibers, and ventricular muscle then repolarize (Phase 1–3). Interestingly, as the heart rate increases (shorter cycle length), the action potential duration decreases, as if to quickly prepare itself for the next depolarization.

Automaticity

The resting membrane potential (Phase 4) of beating myocardial cells characteristically remains constant. Some specialized cells, however, automatically depolarize during diastole until they reach threshold and fire. This spark is propagated as an electrical excitatory wave across adjacent cells resulting in a synchronized beat. The capacity to produce impulses spontaneously is termed automaticity. Diastolic depolarization is clearly necessary for automaticity. Normally, this prerequisite is found only in specialized conduction systems such as the sinus node, internodal conduction pathways, A-V node, bundle branches, and peripheral Purkinje network. The rate of diastolic depolarization varies in automatic cells. This depolarization is typically most rapid in the sinus node, and therefore this node usually dominates the cardiac rhythm. The activity of this normal automatic mechanism, however, can be influenced by several factors, including alterations in automatic tone, is-

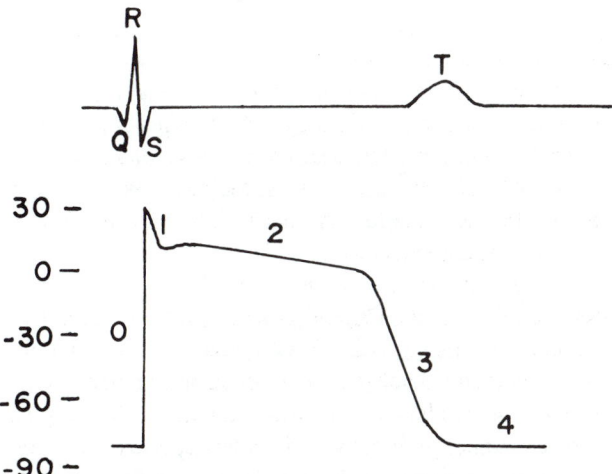

Figure 132–1. Diagrammatic representation of an action potential and a unipolar electrocardiogram. Note that the electrocardiographic R-wave and phase 0 are synchronous. Phase 3 repolarization and the T-wave also occur concurrently.

chemia, hypoxemia, electrolyte fluxes, and drugs. All these factors affect Phase 4 diastolic depolarization. Automatic tachyarrhythmias are common in the perioperative and peri-MI periods.[33,34] These tachyarrhythmias are associated with hypoxemia,[35] hypokalemia,[36] hypocalcemia,[37] and increased catecholamines whether endogenous or exogenous,[38,39] and drugs (typically digitalis).[40,41] These arrhythmias usually respond to lidocaine or procainamide, discontinuation of infused sympathomimetic amines, or β-blockade. Phase 4-dependent automatic tachyarrhythmias are not induced or terminated by electrophysiologic testing (programmed electrical stimulation); they are rarely approached surgically.[40]

Triggered automaticity is an abnormal rhythm that arises during the repolarization phase of a previous impulse rather than arising de novo.[41] It occurs when a spontaneous or paced stimulus is followed by late after-depolarizations that reach membrane threshold and excite the cell. As the spontaneous or paced rate increases, the amplitude of the after-potentials increases (thereby increasing the chance of an after-potential reaching threshold). Triggered automaticity cannot always be distinguished from re-entry. Triggered arrhythmias do, however, appear to be more sensitive to calcium channel-blocking agents than are re-entry-based tachyarrhythmias. While this triggered activity has been unquestionably shown to occur experimentally, its role in human ventricular arrhythmias remains unclear; its most likely clinical occurrence might be in patients with right ventricular outflow tract tachycardias.

Re-entrant Arrhythmias

Re-entry is a well proven mechanism for ventricular arrhythmias. For it to occur, two or more electrically heterogeneous pathways of varying conduction and refractoriness must have proximal and distal connections. Specifically, the two pathways are characterized by nonconduction (unidirectional block) and slow conduction. An impulse must travel in only one direction along one of these pathways (unidirectional block). If this impulse arises at the distal connection, it may return by the initially blocked pathway. If conduction of the impulse is sufficiently slow (slow conduction) to allow the initially blocked site to recover excitability, the impulse may re-enter the circuit (Fig. 132–2). The requirements for such a re-entrant mechanism are (1) unidirectional block, (2) slow conduction over an alternative route, (3) delayed excitation just distal to the blocked tissue, and (4) re-excitation of the proximal tissue upon return of the impulse.[42,43]

Pathophysiologic Substrate for Ventricular Tachyarrhythmias

Nonsustained VT, hemodynamically tolerated sustained monomorphic VT, and arrhythmias producing cardiac arrest have different anatomic and electrophysiologic substrates. The most common anatomic substrate for all these arrhyth-

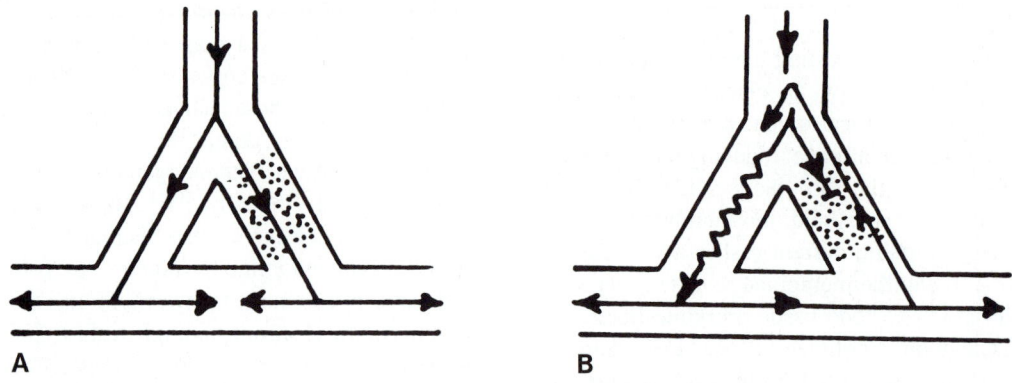

Figure 132–2. Schema for re-entry: An area of ventricle is depicted in each panel. **A.** The depolarization wave front proceeds down both limbs of the potential circuit, meets, and extinguishes at the bottom. **B.** The wave front proceeds, very slowly (sawtooth line) (slow conduction) down the left limb and is blocked (unidirectional block) in the right limb. If conduction is sufficiently slow down the left limb, the origin will have time to repolarize by the time the impulse returns retrograde up the right limb. In this instance, the returning impulse will re-excite the origin and re-enter the circuit.

mias is chronic coronary artery disease, usually associated with prior infarction. The vast majority of spontaneous, recurrent sustained ventricular tachycardias occurring in this setting are due to re-entrant mechanisms.[44] Ischemia alters both conduction and refractoriness.[44,45] The requirements for a re-entry arrhythmia appear to be met within ischemic myocardium.[46] The origin of these arrhythmias appears to involve peri-ischemic areas of abnormal but viable tissue.[44,45] This boundary between healthy, oxygenated myocardium and muscle that is either infarcted or reversibly or partially damaged may contain the electrophysiologic requirements for the initiation and perpetuation of arrhythmias (Fig. 132–3).[47–49] The delineation of the peri-ischemic area has been well documented[50,51] and it is here that conduction and refractoriness are altered.[52] Adjacent cells in a milieu of interdigitated normal, infarcted, and jeopardized but reversibly damaged myocardium have markedly different refractory periods;[53] a propagated impulse will be blocked in one direction but will propagate in another. In the chronic situation, cells that appear normal and well perfused, but that adjoin ischemic or infarcted tissue, may also behave abnormally, similarly satisfying the condition for re-entry.[54,55]

In experimental studies, the initiation of ventricular tachycardia was most likely to occur when an infarct was heterogeneous, namely consisting of normal myocardium interdigitating with ischemic/infarcted myocardium.[56–58] On the other hand, animals with homogeneous infarcts of comparable size were no more susceptible to the initiation of arrhythmia than were noninfarcted controls.[58,59] The presence of a heterogeneous infarction with multiple interfaces of surviving, but altered myocardium interdigitating with both normal and infarcted tissue apparently provides an adequate milieu for re-entry arrhythmias. Fenoglio et al encountered this heterogeneous pattern in endocardial resections from patients with ventricular tachycardia (Figs. 132–4 and 132–5).[60] Furthermore, thallium scintigraphic

scans in patients presenting with ventricular arrhythmias following myocardial infarction show partial redistribution (heterogeneous pattern) within the infarction zone, while non-arrhythmia-prone counterparts failed to demonstrate this heterogeneous pattern.[61]

Thus, the geometry of the ischemic area determines both the susceptibility and characteristics of a re-entrant ventricular arrhythmia. Notably, *heterogeneous* infarctions are more arrhythmogenic than dense homogeneous infarctions. Heterogeneous infarctions are capable of sustaining an impulse along a circuitous pathway and thereby when the conditions of re-entry are met, ventricular tachycardia ensues. Although sustained uniform monomorphic tachycardia may occur in the presence of either hypertropic or idiopathic dilated cardiomyopathy, or even in patients with normal hearts, it is uncommon in these settings. In these instances, the pathophysiologic basis for the arrhythmia is not understood.[13]

Regardless of the underlying cardiac pathophysiology, sustained uniform tachycardia can be studied electrophysiologically such that interpretation of the mechanism and development of therapy is possible.[13] Nonsustained VT is found in patients with a variety of disorders; thus, the pathophysiologic substrate for this arrhythmia is variable and the utility of program stimulation to study patients with cardiac arrest or nonsustained VT is not established.

Effect of Thrombolytic Therapy on the Arrhythmogenic Substrate

Thrombolytic therapy, which is currently widely used and administered immediately once the symptoms of infarction occur, has brought about a significant reduction in the numbers of the previously common large left ventricular infarcts, with or without aneurysmal formation. Initially, there was concern that such therapy would create an arrhythmogenic substrate.[62] This concern was based on the observations in canine experimental studies where the left

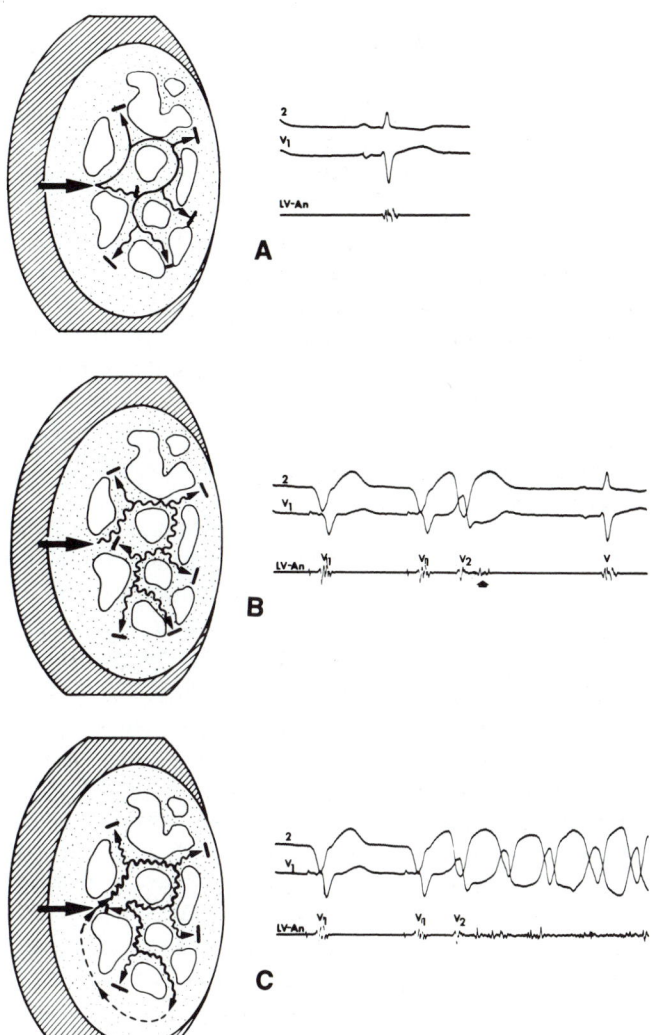

Figure 132–3. Schema of the mechanism of ventricular tachycardia associated with coronary artery disease. **Left:** A portion of the left ventricle is shown with normal muscle shown in oblique lines and ischemically damaged muscle in the stippled area. Islands of dead tissue are represented by the empty spaces enclosed with the ischemic area. An electrocardiogram and an electrogram from this area that represent the border of an infarct at the left ventricular aneurysm (LV-An) is shown alongside each of the panels. **A.** During sinus rhythm the cardiac impulse enters the ischemically injured area and conducts slowly but cannot exit since the surrounding area is refractory. The slow conduction is shown by a fractionated electrogram in the LV-An recording. **B.** During ventricular pacing (V_1) a premature ventricular stimulus (V_2) is delivered that results in marked slowing of impulse propagation through this damaged area. This is associated with more marked fractionation of the electrogram in the LV-An. **C.** A slightly more premature impulse is introduced during ventricular pacing and conduction of the impulse is slow enough to allow recovery of the surrounding tissue. Re-entry occurs resulting in ventricular tachycardia. Note that the fractionated electrogram in the LV-An extends through diastole, becoming continuous before and between complexes of the tachycardia.

anterior descending coronary artery was permanently occluded in one group and temporarily occluded for 2 hours in another group. In animals undergoing temporary occlusion, induced ventricular arrhythmia was more common. Histopathologic studies of all infarcts showed that permanent occlusion caused uniform necrosis but temporary occlusion resulted in areas of viable myocardium located within the necrotic region.[63] It was feared that these "salvaged" myocardial cells might not be electrically normal and could foster electrical instability of the heart.

However, clinical experience with reperfusion with thrombolytic agents has not led to a significant incidence of life-threatening ventricular arrhythmias in humans. Kersschot et al[64] reported on 62 patients who had sustained acute infarction and who were randomly assigned to either receive or not receive streptokinase therapy. Subsequent programmed stimulation was found to induce sustained ventricular arrhythmias less commonly in patients with early reperfusion brought about by the streptokinase treatment than in patients without reperfusion of the myocardium.

Our clinical experience and that of others[62] support this conclusion.

PROGRAMMED ELECTRICAL STIMULATION

Although mechanisms of arrhythmias had been clearly elucidated in animal models for many years, delineation of human arrhythmias was not feasible until 1967 when the technique of programmed electrical stimulation (EPS) was developed.[65] EPS techniques include rapid ventricular pacing and the introduction of progressively premature ventricular stimuli during sinus rhythm or ventricular pacing.[66] The premature ventricular depolarization is initially introduced in late diastole and then progressively earlier until no ventricular response is elicited (ventricular refractoriness) (Fig. 132–6). If this fails to induce ventricular tachycardia, double premature stimuli are introduced 50 to 100 ms following the effective ventricular refractory period. Essen-

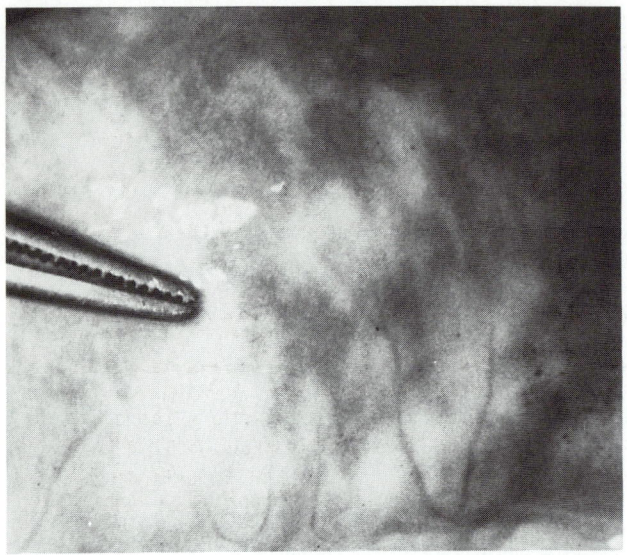

Figure 132–4. The inferior surface of a heart during a myocardial revascularization procedure. Note the heterogeneous (mottled) infarction. This corresponds to the infarction diagrammatically depicted in Figure 132–3.

tially, the heart is paced with a stimulus (S_1) at a fixed rate resulting in a fixed ventricular response. A premature stimulus (S_2) is then introduced in diastole, producing a paced premature ventricular response, and the coupling interval between S_1 and S_2 is decreased in 10-ms steps until no ventricular response is elicited (ventricular refractoriness). In this way, S_2 is scanned throughout "electrical diastole." When S_2 no longer initiates a ventricular response, an additional premature stimulus (S_3) is incorporated into the pac-

ing protocol and the S_2–S_3 interval is then decreased in 10-ms steps until ventricular refractoriness occurs (Fig. 132–6). Ultimately either a re-entrant arrhythmia or a refractoriness of both S_2 and S_3 occurs. Multiple right and left ventricular sites are studied. If single (S_2), double (S_3), and triple (S_4) extra stimuli failed to induce a tachycardia, "burst" pacing may be used. The number of extra stimuli used to induce a tachycardia is limited at two to three; arrhythmias induced with additional extra stimuli appear to be clinically nonrelevant.[67] Rapid atrial or ventricular pacing at a rate of 250 beats per minute may then be introduced for short "bursts." Once ventricular tachycardia is induced, programmed single, double, and triple extra stimuli are introduced in an attempt to terminate the arrhythmia. Induced ventricular tachycardia with hemodynamic instability may require cardioversion.

Induction of ventricular tachyarrhythmias by EPS is taken as evidence for re-entry as the mechanism for the arrhythmia.[47,68,69] The reasoning is as follows: during programmed stimulation, at a critical coupling interval, one pathway in the re-entrant circuit becomes blocked (unidirectional block) and the activation wave front proceeds exclusively along the other arm of the circuit slowly (slow conduction). Impulses may be conducted through diseased myocardium at markedly different rates. If a ventricular impulse were detoured and slowed through diseased muscle, it seems possible that the excitation wave front might wind its way back so slowly that the origin might have a chance to repolarize and become excitable again. The slowly returning impulse might then "re-enter" the diseased circuit, perpetuating the arrhythmia. It is clear that by EPS scanning of "electrical diastole," a premature stimulus at just the right

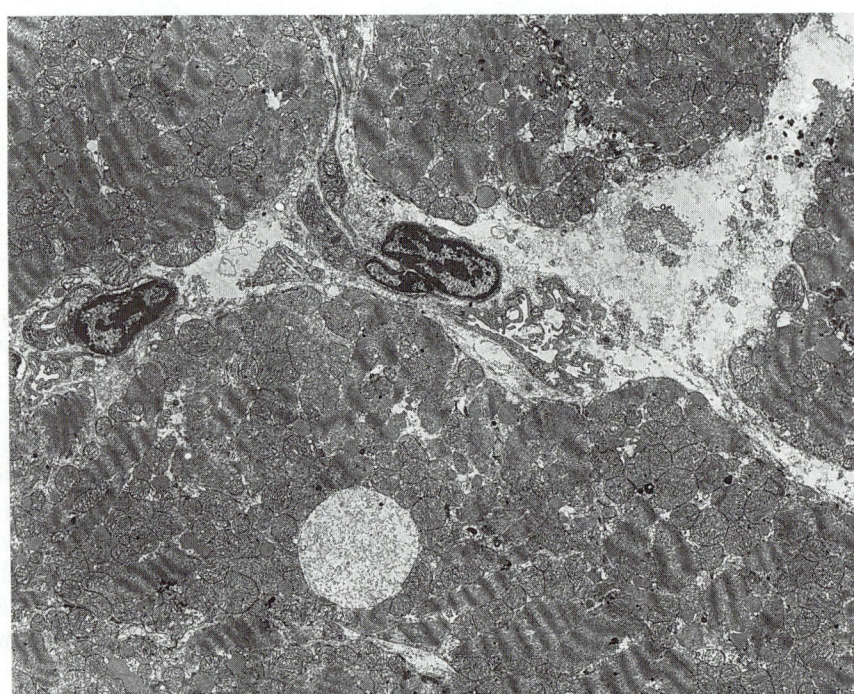

Figure 132–5. Electromicrograph of ventricular muscle cells at the area of the anoxic–perfusion border zone. Normal cellular structure is interspersed with damaged cellular elements (disrupted myofibrils, swollen mitochondria). Magnification ×7700.

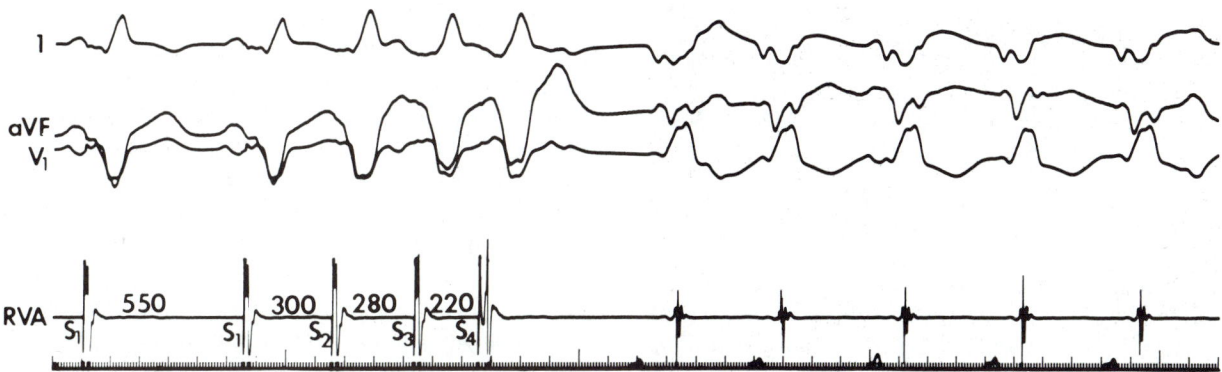

Figure 132–6. Induction of ventricular tachycardia with programmed electrical stimulation. The ventricle is captured with basic drive beats (S_1) and premature paced stimuli (S_2, S_3, S_4). 1, V, and aVF are electrocardiographic leads; RVA is the right ventricular apex-plunge electrode recording. Numbers indicate milliseconds between paced stimuli. In this record, three extrastimuli (S_2, S_3, S_4) have induced ventricular tachycardia.

critical time might establish a re-entrant rhythm in diseased myocardium.[13]

Slow response activity and the substrates for re-entry have been documented in human ventricular aneurysm tissue excised at operation (Fig. 132–5).[60–70] In contrast, timed premature stimuli cannot induce a tachyarrhythmia caused by automaticity because slow conduction and altered refractories are not prerequisites for automatic tachyarrhythmias. Thus, inducibility of a ventricular arrhythmia is accepted as evidence for a re-entrant mechanism. The success of direct surgical therapy of arrhythmias lies in the induction, localization, and physical disruption of these re-entrant pathways. Automatic arrhythmias, although arising from a theoretically resectable focus, usually cannot be induced and therefore are difficult to localize, precluding a direct surgical approach.

Evaluation of the Patient with Malignant Arrhythmia

The initial hospital evaluation of a patient admitted for control of lethal cardiac arrhythmias includes studies to (1) determine whether the mechanism of the arrhythmia is automatic or re-entrant, (2) identify the origin of the arrhythmia as supraventricular or ventricular, (3) identify the inducibility of the arrhythmia by programmed electrical stimulation, (4) assess the suppressibility of these induced arrhythmias with pharmacologic agents, and (5) localize the origin of the ventricular tachycardia by catheter mapping. Such an extensive work-up clearly should be carried out in patients who have survived an episode of sudden cardiac death, since they are at high risk for recurrence (60% recur within the first two years).[2,6] Patients with recurrent sustained ventricular tachycardia without sudden death, and those with known arrhythmogenic disease states should also be studied invasively to provide guidelines for treatment.[71] Efficacy of specific antiarrhythmic therapy can be predicted by EPS as opposed to Holter monitoring or other non-EPS methods.[72,73] The importance of specificity in antiarrhythmic

pharmacologic therapy cannot be overstated, as these drugs are not benign. They can have significant side-effects and can also be "proarrhythmic." As a matter of fact, the results of the Cardiac Arrhythmia Suppression Trial (commonly referred to as CAST) demonstrated a higher mortality with potent antiarrhythmia medications than with placebo drugs.[74]

The challenge remains in identifying those patients who are at risk for sudden cardiac death *prior* to their first event. A group from which most of these patients will arise are MI survivors as well as patients with chronic left ventricular failure and coronary artery disease. Yet even this group remains too large to screen by EPS, and the study would not be cost-effective. A noninvasive method to accurately identify those patients at greatest risk would allow for their selective study and treatment to prevent cardiac death. Though initially promising, computerized signal-averaging of the electrogram has not proven to be predictive.[13] Heart rate variability on ambulatory Holter monitoring is currently being investigated as a potential tool for noninvasive screening of patients at risk of sudden cardiac death.

In contrast with surgery for supraventricular arrhythmias where the mortality and morbidity are low,[75] direct surgical therapy of ventricular tachycardia is higher risk and less successful.[62] Patients have extensive coronary artery disease, poor ventricular function, LV aneurysms, multiple previous episodes of life-threatening arrhythmias, and high circulating concentrations of negatively inotropic antiarrhythmic agents.

SURGICAL THERAPY

Since the pathologic basis for most sustained ventricular tachycardias is the result of severe coronary artery occlusive disease, the earliest surgical interventions focused upon the restoration of coronary bloodflow. However, despite successful revascularization with aortocoronary bypass grafting and control of angina, simultaneous arrhythmia control was usually not achieved.[76,78] Myocardial revascularization has a very limited role because it has an effect only in those patients who have purely reversible ischemia as the cause of their arrhythmias.[78] Subsequent attempts at revascularization with concomitant resection of ventricular aneurysm also failed to prevent these arrhythmias. This so-called blind aneurysmectomy (nondirected, without electrophysiologic mapping) failed because the epicardial border of the aneurysm was often distant from the endocardial origin of the re-entrant focus.[80] The overall success rate of these indirect surgical techniques for the treatment of refractory ischemic VT is approximately 50%, and this figure is consistent regardless of the indirect procedure employed.[81,82] Because these indirect surgical approaches were associated with high surgical mortality rates, averaging 25%[81] and with a probability of cure that was little better than chance, interest turned toward more direct surgical approaches guided by preoperative and intraoperative electrophysiological studies.

Encircling Endocardial Ventriculotomy

The development of direct surgical approaches to ventricular arrhythmias began with the report in 1978 by Guiraudon and colleagues,[83,84] who introduced the encircling endocardial ventriculotomy. This was the first surgical technique developed on the basis of the knowledge of the mechanism of VT and its location. Cox and Boineau[85,86] had earlier demonstrated the presence of microentry circuits in the border zone of the region of myocardial infarction, giving origin to ischemic ventricular arrhythmias. These re-entrant circuits were located in the "twilight zone" of tissue between healthy and infarcted myocardium. It was thought that this border zone was always included in the visible area of endocardial fibrosis (Fig. 132–7). In the encircling endocardial ventriculotomy (EEV), an incision is made perpendicular to the endocardial surface and completely encircles the endocardial fibrosis. By creating a transmural fibrous scar barrier, the EEV isolates the arrhythmogenic substrate and re-entrant circuit from electrical continuity with the re-

mainder of the normal functioning myocardium. Intraoperative mapping was not performed in Guiraudon's series. Further studies designed to clarify the electrophysiological effects of this procedure demonstrated that although it may be capable of isolating ischemic ventricular arrhythmias to the encompassed myocardium, its mode of action usually is ablation of the electrophysiological substrate necessary for the genesis and perpetuation of these arrhythmias.[87]

The encircling endocardial ventriculotomy is performed on cardiopulmonary bypass, and involves entering the left ventricle through an area of infarction or aneurysm. The ventriculotomy is performed through a perpendicular ventricular incision, sparing only the epicardial surface and coronary vessels. When the septum is involved, the ventriculotomy is approximately 1 cm deep on the septal side, but not transmural. By sparing the overlying coronary vessels, it was believed that bloodflow to the encompassed myocardium might remain normal. However, the perpendicular ventricular incision profoundly decreases myocardial blood in the encircled tissue, especially the subendocardium.[88] This surgically induced regional ischemia, although effective from the viewpoint of ablating electrical activity in the encompassed myocardium, results in a concomitant hemodynamic impairment of an already compromised left ventricle.[89] Decreases in diastolic compliance and impairment of systolic excursion in the EEV-enclosed regions have been demonstrated. These sequelae of the EEV partly explained the observation that it is associated with a higher operative mortality rate in comparison to that observed following endocardial resection.[90,91] Therefore, although the historical importance of this procedure in initiating surgery directed toward eradication of VT is well established, its current applications are extremely limited.

Electrophysiologically Directed Endocardial Resection

Almost simultaneously, in 1979, Josephson et al[92] proposed a new surgical approach in which preoperative and intraoperative electrophysiological mapping was used to identify a

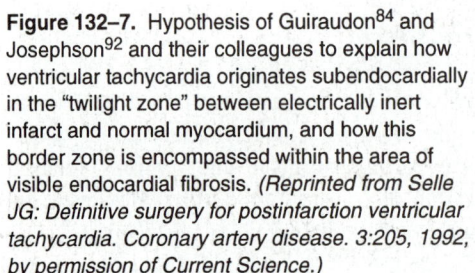

Figure 132–7. Hypothesis of Guiraudon[84] and Josephson[92] and their colleagues to explain how ventricular tachycardia originates subendocardially in the "twilight zone" between electrically inert infarct and normal myocardium, and how this border zone is encompassed within the area of visible endocardial fibrosis. *(Reprinted from Selle JG: Definitive surgery for postinfarction ventricular tachycardia. Coronary artery disease. 3:205, 1992, by permission of Current Science.)*

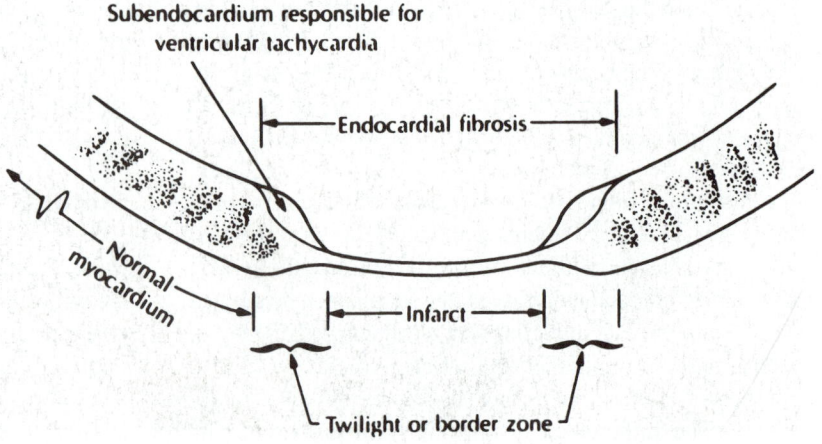

specific site of origin of the arrhythmia, and thus guide the surgeon toward resecting the arrhythmogenic region of the left ventricle.[93] Their findings agreed with those of Guiraudon as to location of this tissue, but they postulated it was subendocardial in origin (Fig. 132–7). This procedure is also performed on cardiopulmonary bypass following electrophysiological mapping to define the mechanism and identify the site of the arrhythmia. Aneurysmectomy is performed in the normothermic beating heart and, following operative mapping to confirm the endocardial origin of the arrhythmia (Fig. 132–8), core cooling of the patient to 30°C is established. Following cardioplegic arrest, a 5 to 25 cm^2 area of endocardium, to which the origin of the arrhythmia had been mapped, is elevated and excised (Fig. 132–9). Unlike the encircling endocardial ventriculotomy, ventricular function is generally well preserved with endocardial resection, accounting for a lower operative mortality.[94]

After the popular introduction of directed methods of treatment, a number of studies were mounted in an attempt to improve on these early ideas. Guiraudon et al modified their initial procedure by making cryolesions rather than sharp surgical incisions to isolate arrhythmogenic myocardium.[95] Mesnildrey et al used neodymium:yttrium–aluminum–garnet laser photocoagulation for this purpose instead.[96] EEV never gained wide popularity, particularly in the United States. Ostermeyer and co-workers[97] in Dusseldorf, however, studied this method extensively, recommending a partial endocardial ventriculotomy that encircled only those areas of myocardium identified by mapping to be arrhythmogenic.

Aggressive resection procedures were described by some. Moran et al[98] performed extensive subendocardial resections of all visible endocardial fibrosis, including sites distant from infarct or aneurysm. Papillary muscles were resected in five of their patients. Balooki and colleagues[99] recommended myocardial debulking and septal isolation along with coronary revascularization in patients when intraoperative mapping was not possible. Laser photocoagulation and cryoablation were used to neutralize arrhythmogenic myocardium, particularly in anatomic areas where resection would be difficult or hazardous, including the papillary muscles and interventricular septum.[100,101]

Kron et al[102] advocated a sequential approach in which myocardial cooling is not used, to preserve the inducibility of VT. Once induced, the VT is mapped and the area of responsible myocardium ablated until that form of VT disappears. Further attempts are made to induce additional forms of VT and, when successful, the process repeated. This method addresses the common situation in which more than one form of VT can exist. To avoid performing a ventriculotomy, Lawrie and colleagues approached the ventricular endocardium through the atrioventricular or aortic valves.[103] Downar and associates[104] have studied intracavitary balloon computer mapping and electric shock ablation of endocardial arrhythmogenic foci. All the results of these modifications appear to provide an efficacy similar to that of the standard endocardial resection, and it is clear that the operative mortality can be improved if diffusely poor left ventricular contractility is prevented.

Thus the decade of the 1980s witnessed the application of electrophysiological concepts to the surgical therapy of VT, along with the significant improvements in the surgical results both in terms of operative mortality and postopera-

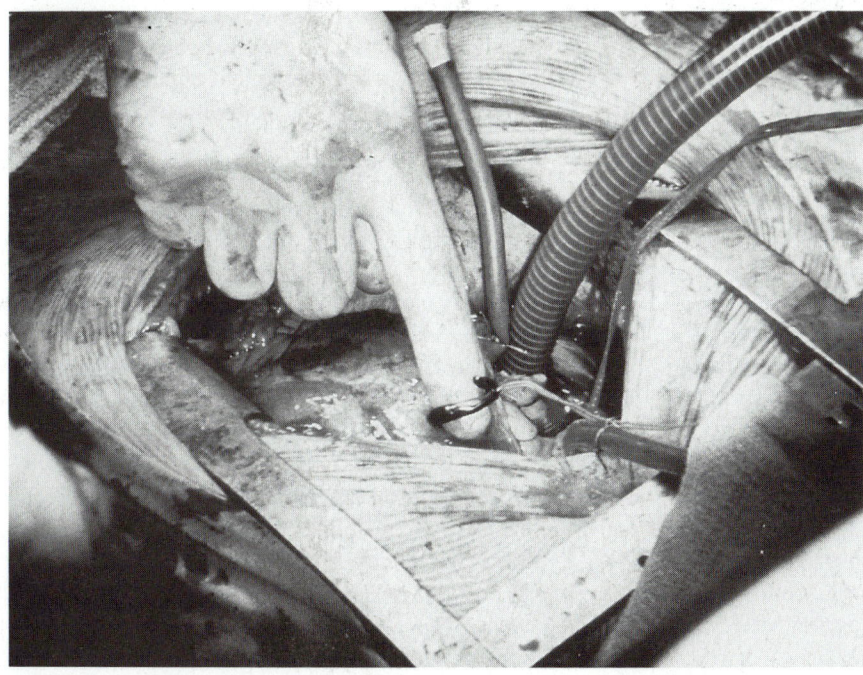

Figure 132–8. The earliest site of activation (tachycardia origin) is located by EPS-guided mapping. An epicardial map is recorded using a ring electrode on the index finger. The tachycardia is induced following initiation of normothermic cardiopulmonary bypass. Endocardial maps are obtained in a similar fashion through a left ventriculotomy (usually through a left ventricular aneurysm).

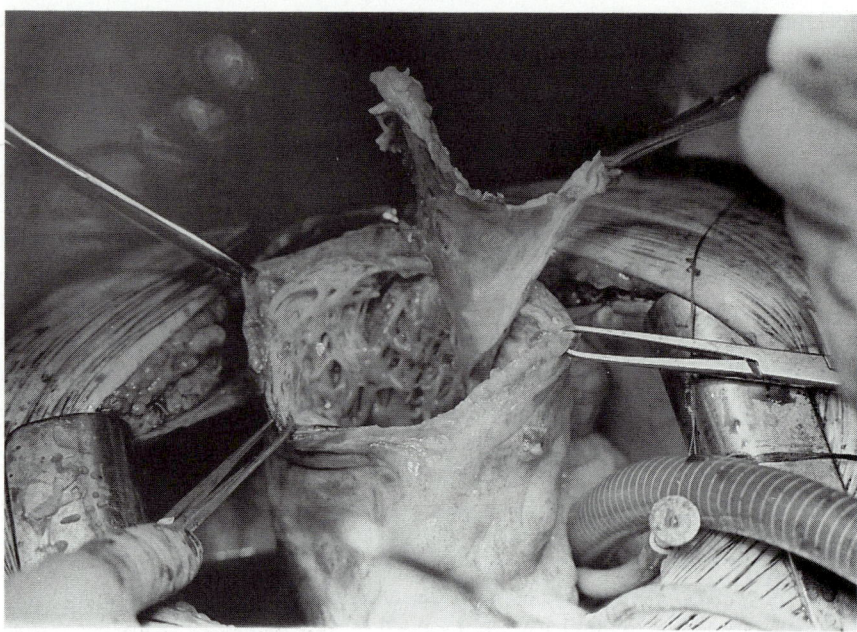

Figure 132–9. Endocardial resection. A standard left ventricular aneurysmectomy has been performed. Excision of the septal and lateral walls of the endocardium has been completed, but the base is still attached.

tive inducibility as compared to indirect approaches. However, a persistent concern with these direct approaches has been that they represent formidable operative procedures on a subset of patients who have compromised left ventricular function from previous infarctions. As compiled by Cox in a review of 16 published reports encompassing a total of 844 patients, there were 105 operative deaths yielding an operative mortality rate of 14.4%.[105] Although from a historical perspective these figures are good, the desire to reduce the mortality to an irreducible minimum encouraged the development of other modalities.

The Implantable Cardioverter Defibrillator

Internal cardioverter defibrillator (ICD) therapy has evolved from over a decade of development, pioneered by Michael Mirowski, through the first clinical implant in 1980[106] to a widely used modality for treatment of sustained VT or VF. The initial devices were able only to recognize ventricular fibrillation and deliver a high-energy shock. These have evolved to extremely sophisticated programmable devices.[107,108] Currently, all clinical available devices also recognize ventricular tachycardia. Many devices in clinical use or in development have tiered therapy, with antitachycardia pacing, cardioversion, defibrillation, and bradycardia pacing,[109,110] as well as memory to store electrograms or data regarding detected arrhythmias. The device was approved by the Food and Drug Administration for clinical use in the United States in 1986, and the early implants were restricted largely to patients with episodes of threatened sudden death due to sustained ventricular tachycardia and/or ventricular fibrillation, and who had failed antiarrhythmic therapy either clinically or by serial electrophysiologic testing. Historical control studies have demon-

strated the dismal outlook for such patients[111,112] with 1-year risk of sudden arrhythmic death being 26%, whereas actuarial 1-year freedom from sudden cardiac deaths for patients undergoing ICD implantation is reported to range from 98 to 99%.[83,94,113–115] Moreover, the operative mortality rates were consistently reported to be less than 3%. Thus the clinical efficacy of the ICD was established early, and the device proved to be a powerful deterrent to most episodes of life-threatening arrhythmias in these high-risk patients. Even in patients with severe LV dysfunction, the ICD has been shown to be very effective in preventing sudden death.[116,117] It is now a matter of record that the ICD can reliably terminate VT and/or VF, and it now dominates the clinical management of malignant ventricular arrhythmias. Indeed, some have suggested that the ICD should be considered the treatment of choice for virtually all patients who have been resuscitated from sudden cardiac death.[118]

The earlier models of the ICD required implantation with epicardial patches placed around the heart. However, the technology has evolved so much that currently this approach is extremely rare, and most ICDs have endocardial sensing electrodes and defibrillating coils, and occasionally may require the addition of a subcutaneous defibrillating patch (Fig. 132–10). Thus the method of implantation has become significantly simplified, and the magnitude of the procedure to implant the ICD has become much less extensive.[119–121]

Concepts of appropriate therapy for patients with sustained ventricular arrhythmias continue to evolve and questions have been raised as to which patients should have electrophysiologically directed procedures and which should have the ICD implanted.[122–124] There are considerations that favor one option over another for individual cases, beginning with the outcome expected from each therapeutic modality.

RESULTS OF NONPHARMACOLOGIC THERAPY

The most commonly used mapping-guided surgical technique is the subendocardial resection.[62] However, despite a number of studies which reported the results of electrophysiologically directed surgery, only a few series with more than 50 patients each and a follow-up of 5 years or more

have been published. We have recently reviewed six such series, including our own which includes patients treated at Yale-New Haven Hospital and University Hospitals of Cleveland between September 1984 and November 1991 with a follow-up ranging from 7 mo to 9 years.[124] Table 132–1 summarizes the characteristics of these six series of patients and the short- and long-term results obtained in each.

The basic operation of electrophysiologically directed subendocardial resection as originally described by the University of Pennsylvania group was used exclusively in the

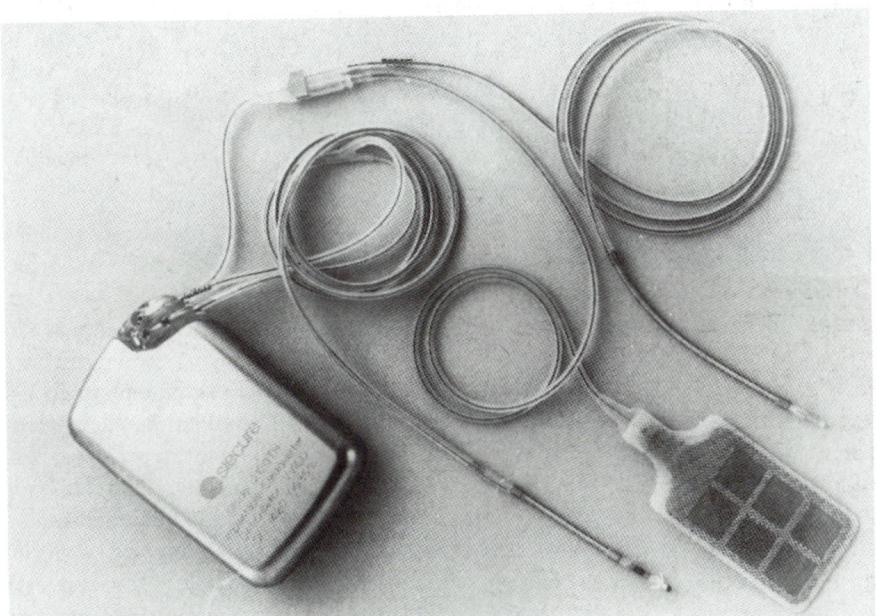

A

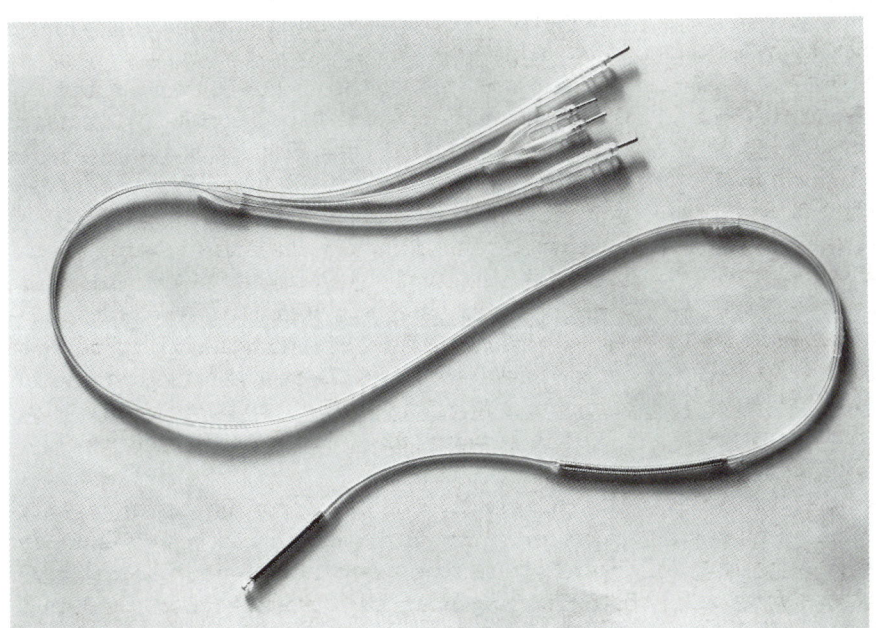

B

Figure 132–10. Implantable cardioverter defibrillator with tiered therapy including antitachycardia pacing and bradycardia pacing in addition to cardioversion and defibrillation. **A.** The device, the sensing and pacing electrode with the distal defibrillating coil (cathode), the subcutaneous patch (which is occasionally needed), and the superior vena cava-right atrial defibrillating coil (anode). **B.** ICD with tiered therapy capabilities. *(Continued.)*

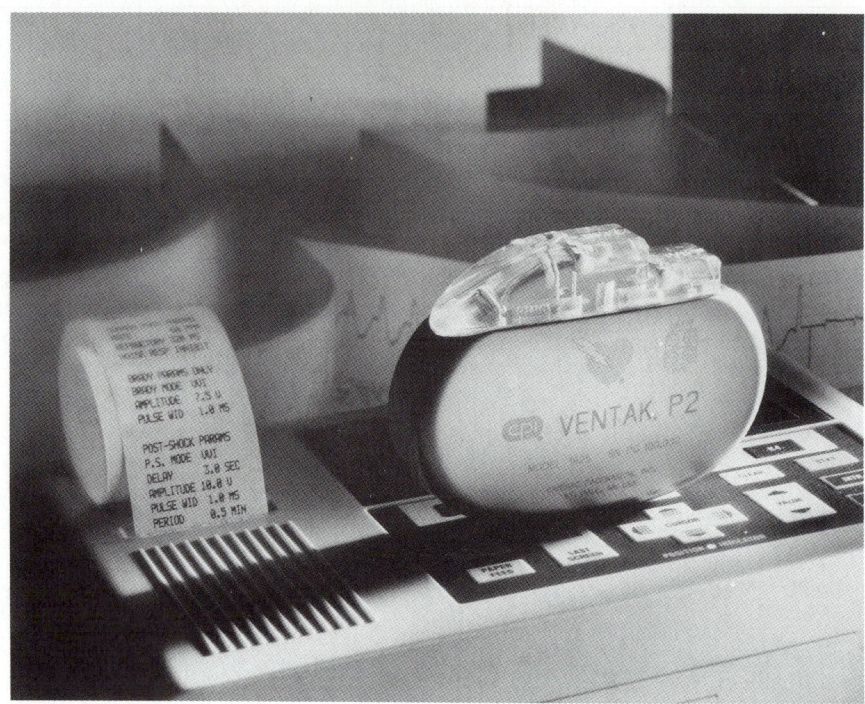

Figure 132–10. *(Continued.)* **C.** ICD with single lead sensing, pacing, and defibrillating electrode.

C

initial part of our experience.[82] We judiciously utilized preoperative placement of the intra-aortic balloon pump in higher risk patients to optimize perioperative hemodynamics. The resection was guided by epicardial and endocardial mapping using a single-handed roving electrode during induced ventricular tachycardia. In all but six patients, the resection was done under cold cardioplegic arrest. For arrhythmogenic foci arising from the posterior papillary muscle, resection of the papillary muscle with concomitant mitral valve replacement was done in four patients early in our experience; we replaced the mitral valve through the ventriculotomy. However, more recently we have tended to utilize cryoablation (−60°C for 2 min) as an adjunct to our endocardial resection over the ventricular septum and papillary muscle.

Seventeen percent (9/53) of patients undergoing endo-

cardial resection had inducible sustained monomorphic VT at postoperative electrophysiologic evaluation. We considered the test positive even if the rhythm induced was different from the clinical arrhythmia. Only 11% (6/53) of patients who survived endocardial resection required antiarrhythmic medications during the follow-up period.

Analysis of long-term results (Table 132–1) reveals 5-year survival rates that range from 33 to 70%. These results of the reported series listed in Table 132–1 include all operative deaths as well as all late cardiac and noncardiac deaths. The 5-year actuarial rates of our own patients are shown in Figure 132–11.

Technically, the definitive operation is a simple procedure. It continues, however, to be quite lengthy because of the time needed for induction, mapping, and ablation of the myocardium responsible for VT. Although it had been an-

TABLE 132–1. CHARACTERISTICS OF REPORTED SERIES OF ELECTROPHYSIOLOGICALLY DIRECTED SURGERY WITH LONG-TERM FOLLOW-UP

Series	Number of Patients	Operative Technique	Operative Mortality Rate %	Postoperative Reinducibility (%)	5-Year Survival (%)
Miller et al[125,126]	100	Localized SER	15	32	67
Swerdlow et al[127]	98	Multiple procedures	17	32	53
Ostermeyer et al[97]	93	EEV	5	19	70
McGiffin et al[128]	123	Multiple procedures	21	38	33
Cox[105]	65	EERP and cryosurgery	14	2	68
Geha et al[94]	58	SER and cryosurgery	9	17	70

SER, subendocardial resection (same as localized endocardial resection procedure); EEV, encircling endocardial ventriculotomy; EERP, extended endocardial resection procedure.

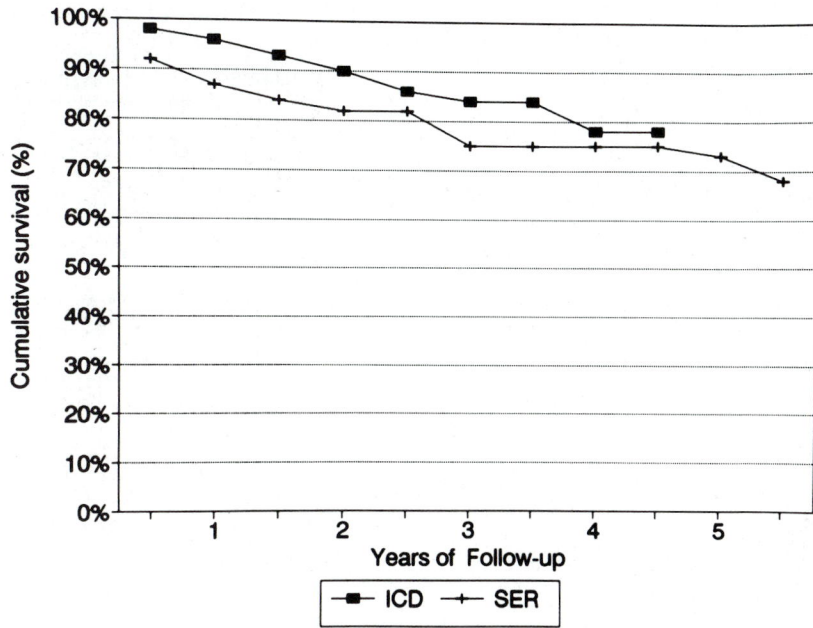

Figure 132–11. Actuarial survival following ICD implantation and subendocardial resection. Time 0 is the time of operation.

ticipated that the procedure would become more efficient with evolving experience, this did not prove to be the case. If anything, the operation appears to have become even longer because of a developing philosophy that the cure of VT depends on making sure that all potential forms of VT are discovered and treated.

To analyze the results of ICD implantation, we have used the database maintained by CPI (Cardiac Pacemakers, Inc., Minneapolis, MN), since CPI has had the longest experience with a FDA-approved ICD device and has had the widest worldwide distribution with an excellent record-keeping system. We also analyzed the results in our own group of patients treated with the ICD at Yale and Case Western Reserve Universities. As of June 1990, over 12,000 patients have had the ICD implanted. The patient characteristics from the CPI database as of February 1990 are listed together with our patient characteristics in Table 132–2. The operative mortality (defined as any death within 30 days of operation in our own series) was 1.5% (3/197), which is consistent with mortality data ranging from 1.2 to 4.4% reported in the literature.[113–115, 117,130] A variety of

complications related to the hardware have been reported to occur including infections, hematomas, sensing lead problems, constrictive pericarditis, patch migration, erosion of bypass grafts, and symptomatic shocks.[94] In our series, the morbidity related to the ICD consisted primarily of late infection, which was noted in eight (2%) of our patients. In four of them, this necessitated removal of the entire hardware system. In the other four, with *Staphylococcus epidermidis* infection of the ICD system, debridement of the infected subcutaneous abdominal pocket was carried out, and the ICD device was then soaked in broad spectrum antibiotics and replaced into the same pocket that was irrigated with an antibiotic solution over a period of 2 wk. After stopping the irrigation and establishing that the effluent was sterile over the ensuing 2 days, the irrigation system was removed, and the patients placed on chronic oral antibiotic therapy, usually with ciprofloxacin. These patients have remained asymptomatic on follow-up up to 48 mo. On the other hand, we have not seen in our patient population any of the other complications described above.

Table 132–3 lists the survival data in patients with im-

TABLE 132–2. ICD PATIENT CHARACTERISTICS

	CPI Database[129] (n = 9807)	Geha et al[94] (n = 197)
Male/female	80.7%/19.3%	76.1%/23.9%
Mean age (years)	60.9	62.2
Mean preop LVEF	33%	33.8%
Concomitant antiarrhythmic medications	55.1%	48.2%

TABLE 132–3. SURVIVAL DATA AFTER ICD IMPLANTATION (KAPLAN–MEIER)

	CPI Database[129] (n = 9807)		Geha et al[94] (n = 290[a])	
Freedom from	At 1 year	At 5 years	At 1 year	At 4 years
Sudden cardiac death	98%	95%	98%	96%
Death from all causes	92%	78%	90%	73%

[a]Includes 93 patients with concurrent CABG.

planted ICDs as reported to the CPI clinical database and in our patient population. The results of ICD therapy demonstrate a reduction of the sudden death rate to less than 2% per year, a figure far superior to that reported previously with antiarrhythmic therapy only—with its associated 1-year sudden death rate of 20 to 30% and a survival rate of 20 to 30% at 4 to 5 years.[111,112,131]

The foregoing discussion demonstrates that with either mode of therapy, the freedom from sudden death is similar and long-term survival is virtually identical with 5-year survival of approximately 70% (Fig. 132–11). It would thus appear that the important goal of improving patient selection to minimize the risk of sudden death has been accomplished in current surgical practice. However, the goal of further reducing this risk and providing a better overall quality of life for these patients requires ongoing evaluation for proper selection of the appropriate therapeutic modality in any given patient.[124]

STRATEGIES FOR THE CHOICE OF THERAPY

There are currently some ongoing studies randomizing patients between ICD treatment and amiodarone as first line therapy for malignant VT.[132,133] Other ongoing studies are testing the hypothesis that use of an ICD in patients at high risk for sudden death undergoing planned bypass surgery will decrease the mortality,[132] or evaluating the prophylactic use of ICD in those patients at high risk for sudden cardiac death.[134] However, there have been no randomized trials comparing electrophysiologically guided surgery to the ICD. It is safe to say that due to logistical and even ethical considerations, such trials will not occur. The evidence that comparable long-term results can be achieved with the two modes of therapy suggests that each modality acts as a crucial component in the overall contemporary therapy of ventricular arrhythmias.

In broad terms, a direct ablative surgical procedure provides an opportunity for cure rather than palliation of the problem with the additional benefit that patients are not committed to the continuous administration of potent antiarrhythmic medications. However, the reported high operative mortality rates as well as inadequate cure rates in some series have led to a preference for ICD implantation in some centers. The advantages are low operative mortality rates and efficacy in aborting sudden death.

In analyzing our patient database as listed in Table 132–4 for those who had only ICD implantation and those who had endocardial resection, we find that direct comparisons between these two groups of patients are not totally appropriate. The ICD cohort tended to be more heterogeneous, and includes all patients whose cardiac anatomy does not lend itself to endocardial resection such as those patients without discrete aneurysms or those patients with ventricular fibrillation as the preoperative rhythm.

The premise that patients with severely depressed left

TABLE 132–4. CLINICAL CHARACTERISTICS BY PROCEDURE

Variable	ICD Implantation	Subendocardial Resection
Number of patients	197	58
% male	76%	81%
Mean preoperative LVEF	33.8%	25.3%
Cardiac arrest	61%	7%
Electrophysiological morphology		
Noninducible	15%	0%
VT (monomorphic)	71%	100%
VT (polymorphic) or VF	14%	0%

ventricular function who are not candidates for extensive electrophysiologically directed surgery are mainly referred for ICD therapy may be accurate. The availability of the ICD has allowed the luxury of avoiding extensive operations on terminally ill patients with overwhelming comorbid factors and poor left ventricular ejection fraction (LVEF).

Analysis of our experience and that of others[94,131] indicates that LVEF is the most important determinant of both early and late mortality. Regardless of the surgical procedure used, pump failure was the major cause of early as well as late mortality. In our own experience, the group of patients who underwent endocardial resection had significantly more compromised left ventricular function in that their mean LVEF was 25 vs 34% for the ICD group. However, this depression of LVEF may be given more significance than it warrants, since most of the resection patients had discrete aneurysms that detract from the overall ejection fraction.

Our basic therapeutic strategy is based on the belief that endocardial resection is the therapy of choice if electrophysiological testing suggests that an arrhythmogenic focus can be ablated. We do not necessarily exclude patients simply on the basis of low LVEF. When assessing a patient for directed resection, we pay particular attention to the ventriculogram at the level of function of the remaining viable muscle outside the infarct zone from which the arrhythmia originates. If this muscle appears to have contractile properties, we would be inclined to proceed with resection, as opposed to a situation in which there are multiple areas of infarction giving rise to an overall picture of globally impaired contractility. Current sophisticated mapping techniques, improved surgical techniques, and postoperative care can result in excellent outcome with moderate operative risk and we would emphasize that, for carefully selected patients, endocardial resection remains a highly effective form of therapy.[124]

A single site of monomorphic VT, especially when associated with a discrete aneurysm, and particularly an anterior one is ideally suited for endocardial resection. All of our patients presenting for resection had inducible, sustained monomorphic or bimorphic tachycardia, while 30% of our patients who had the ICD implanted had either no inducible arrhythmias or multiple diffuse sites of polymorphic VT or VF.

Ventricular arrhythmias originating in the inferior wall of the left ventricle have been shown to have a failure rate of 41% following endocardial resection.[125] The inferior wall represents a difficult area for adequate endocardial resection because of the proximity of the mitral valve apparatus and the highly trabeculated nature of the endocardium. Endocardial resection can be extended to include a large area of resection with concomitant mitral valve replacement to totally eradicate an arrhythmogenic region. However, if such a preoperative anatomic substrate exists, ICD therapy should weigh heavily as a method of treatment. Electrophysiological characteristics such as polymorphic VT or VF as the arrhythmogenic substrate do not respond consistently to endocardial resection, and ICD implantation would be the preferred option.

A similar strategy would be utilized for patients with nonischemic VT, as endocardial resection is currently not applicable. Only 24% of the patients with nonischemic VT have inducibility following programmed electrical stimulation.[135] Because these arrhythmias are difficult to induce by standard measures, they are also difficult to localize precisely by standard cardiac mapping techniques. Therefore, the likelihood of a successful surgical cure is reduced, and endocardial resection is currently not applicable for such patients.

If, however, critical coronary artery stenoses are present, and there is no evidence of a scar on the ventriculogram, we believe that myocardial revascularization is frequently a necessary component of therapy. In such patients, we do coronary artery bypass grafting and a week later perform postoperative testing for inducibility. Although the importance of revascularization and its beneficial effect on malignant ventricular arrhythmias are well substantiated,[136,138] we have found that the ICD is a frequently required additional therapeutic adjunct in this group of patients.

There is a wide range in the frequency with which patients manifest their ventricular arrhythmias. A few have only a single event. However, in patients with incessant VT or frequent arrhythmic episodes, the ICD is not an option due to its finite generator capacity. In general, if the frequency of arrhythmic events is more than once every 2 wk despite concurrent antiarrhythmic medication, we would favor endocardial resection if at all possible.

It has become apparent that each therapeutic modality has its own unique advantages and disadvantages. Endocardial resection is curative in the majority of patients and prevents the recurrence of the arrhythmia. The patients enjoy a better life style because they require fewer drugs and have fewer arrhythmias. The ICD offers palliation in that its event-triggered action prevents sudden death. In our experience, about half of these patients require some form of an-

tiarrhythmic medication even with the ICD implanted, whereas only 11% of patients following endocardial resection required concomitant antiarrhythmic medications.

In addition, we noted that more than half (59%) of our patients experienced at least one device discharge during follow-up. These device discharges, if spurious, constitute a major source of morbidity. An inappropriate ICD discharge resulting in a random shock in a conscious patient is a frightening experience for that patient. Recent technological advances, such as antitachycardia pacing capabilities and improved sensing, have diminished the incidence of spurious ICD discharges. However, the prospect of being vulnerable to a discharge at any time can lead to fear, anxiety, and depression in some patients.

Although most patients do not lose consciousness before the device terminates an arrhythmia, the time from arrhythmia onset to its termination by the ICD is frequently in excess of 20 to 25 seconds. The patient may not be able to perform adequately, especially if he or she is carrying out a critical funcion. The bulk of cumulative clinical experience suggests that patients with ICD implantation have a restricted life style.[139] Theoretically, a patient should not drive an automobile. The ICD also may render him or her unemployable in certain occupations. The need for frequent follow-up visits and the cost of periodic generator replacement must also be considered. Nonetheless, continued improvements in technology and the development of devices that require less invasive procedures for implantation have rendered the ICD an even more flexible and powerful tool in the current management of medical refractory arrhythmias.

In conclusion, it is evident that in patients with previous sustained ventricular tachycardia or fibrillation, and in patients at high risk for these arrhythmias, management strategies continue to emerge based on the evolving knowledge of the risks and benefits of the available therapies. If a patient has no inducible arrhythmia at the initial drug-free study, or if spontaneous or induced arrhythmias are not suppressed with a limited number of drug trials, nonpharmacologic options should be considered. Mapping-guided subendocardial resection would be reasonable in a patient with a discrete aneurysm and preserved function of the nonaneurysmal portion of the ventricle. ICD therapy would provide optimal sudden death protection in those who have no inducible arrhythmia at baseline or who are still inducible on drugs. Each procedure has its unique advantages and disadvantages and because either operation may suffice for some patients, other factors such as the patient's acceptance and compliance may play a role. In others, both the ICD and endocardial resection may be required in combination to give the best and safest control of the arrhythmias. Thus the two modalities of therapy should be viewed as complementary rather than mutually exclusive. Continued examination of contemporary results to determine the criteria for appropriate application of each procedure and to evaluate the extent of their efficacy, including the quality of life after recovery from the procedure, the natural history of the dysfunctional ventricle that is not remodeled with an aneurysmectomy, the long-term survival and freedom from electrical events, and the cost of the therapy over the lifetime of the patient, will provide the information necessary to help the clinician make reliable recommendations concerning the proper surgical approach to the patient with malignant ventricular arrhythmias.

FUTURE TRENDS OF NONPHARMACOLOGIC MANAGEMENT OF ARRHYTHMIAS

Refinements in current techniques as well as ongoing clinical and basic research on arrhythmias will continue to impact significantly on this field. Some promising developments on the new horizon include the following:

Electrode catheter ablation involves localizing the site of the origin of the tachycardia and then delivering radiofrequency energy to modify the anatomic substrate. Although radiofrequency ablation has been extremely successful in managing patients with supraventricular arrhythmias from dual A-V node nodal pathways or bypass tracts,[75] the reported experience with ventricular tachycardia has been limited to small series of patients without long-term follow-up.[140] It may be curative in patients with sustained monomorphic VT, with highest efficacy rates reported in those with right ventricular outflow tract tachycardias.[108]

Percoronary techniques of arrhythmia ablation with intracoronary ethanol[141,142] have been tried in highly selected patients, based on stability of their tachycardia and suitability of their coronary anatomy. In one perspective randomized trial efficacy was achieved in one-third of patients.[142]

Implantable atrial defibrillators. Atrial fibrillation has been discussed in great detail in the previous chapter. Transvenous defibrillation of the atrium has been accomplished at a variety of centers worldwide. Using biphasic shocks delivered between the coronary sinus and the right atrium, atrial fibrillation has been successfully converted at low energies (1.7 ± 1.7 J) in over 80 patients. No ventricular tachyarrhythmias were noted during the shock deliveries. Complications that were noted included transient pauses, sinus bradycardia, and A-V block.[143] Implantable atrial defibrillators are currently being tested in animal modes. The implantable system used a three-lead atrial defibrillation configuration, including a spiral-shaped lead positioned in the coronary sinus, a standard screw-in atrial lead, and a bipolar pacing lead in the right ventricular apex for shock synchronization. Adult sheep were successfully defibrillated at low energy (< 2 J), and no ventricular arrhythmias were noted.[144] Much work remains to be done before human implantation of these devices can take place. The early results are promising; however, concerns regarding patient selection, induction of ventricular arrhythmias,

back-up pacing capabilities, and patient tolerance of these shocks remain to be addressed.

Further enhancement and refinement of signals are obtained from *surface electrograms* to allow construction of the activation sequence, and potentially identify patients whose arrhythmia arises from the subepicardial layer.[145] Such patients might benefit from myocardial revascularization combined with cryoablation of the subepicardial arrhythmic foci.

The outlook for patients with medically refractory malignant ventricular tachyarrhythmias has been tremendously improved and continues to be brightened by the sound pathophysiologic principles employed in developing surgical procedures and electrical approaches to the management of arrhythmias.

REFERENCES

1. Hinkle LE, Thaler HT: Clinical classification of cardiac deaths. *Circulation* **65**:457–464, 1982
2. Liberthson RR, Nagel EL, Hirschmann JC, et al: Pre-hospital ventricular defibrillation: Prognosis and follow-up course. *N Engl J Med* **291**:317–321, 1974
3. Cobb LA, Werner JA, Trobaugh GB: Sudden cardiac death. A decade's experience with out-of-hospital resuscitation. *Med Concepts Cardiovasc Dis* **49**:32–42, 1980
4. DiMarco JP: Nonpharmacological therapy of ventricular arrhythmias. *PACE* **13**:1527–1533, 1990
5. Josephson ME: *Clinical Cardiac Electrophysiology: Techniques and Interpretations.* Malvern, PA, Lea & Febiger, 1993
6. Myerburg RJ, Kessler KM, Estes D, et al: Long-term survival after prehospital cardiac arrest: Analysis of outcome during an 8-year study. *Circulation* **70**:538–546, 1984
7. Eisenberg MS, Hallstrom A, Bergner L: Long-term survival after out-of-hospital cardiac arrest. *N Engl J Med* **306**:1340–1343, 1982
8. Cobb LA, Baum RS, Alvarez H, et al: Resuscitation from out-of-hospital ventricular fibrillation: 4-year follow-up. *Circulation* **52** (Suppl 3):223–238, 1975
9. Vlay SC, Kallman CH, Weisfeldt JL, Reid, PR: Anatomic substrate and clinical outcome in survivors of sudden cardiac death: A multivariate analysis. *Cardiovasc Rev Rep* **7**:861–875, 1986
10. Swerdlow CD, Winkle RA, Mason JW: Determinants of survival in patients with ventricular tachyarrhythmias. *N Engl J Med* **308**:1436–1442, 1983
11. Holmes DR, Davis KB, Mock MB, et al: The effect of medical and surgical treatment on subsequent cardiac death in patients with coronary artery disease: A report from the Coronary Artery Surgery Study. *Circulation* **73**:1254–1264, 1986
12. Wellens HJJ, Bar FWHM, Vanagot EJDM, Brugada P: Medical treatment of ventricular tachycardia: Considerations in the selection patients for surgical treatment. *Am J Cardiol* **49**:186–193, 1983
13. Josephson ME: Recurrent ventricular tachycardia. In Josephson ME (ed): *Clinical Cardiac Electrophysiology: Techniques and Interpretations.* Malvern, PA, Lea & Febiger, 1993, pp 417–615
14. Hammermeister KE, DeRouen TA, Murray JA, Dodge HT: Effect of aortocoronary saphenous vein bypass grafting on death and sudden death: Comparison of nonrandomized, medically and surgically treated cohorts with comparable coronary disease and left ventricular function. *Am J Cardiol* **39**:925–934, 1977
15. Kaiser GA, Ghahramani A, Bolooki H, et al: Role of coronary artery surgery in patients surviving unexpected cardiac arrest. *Surgery* **78**:749–756, 1975

16. Schwartz PJ, Periti M, Malliani A: The long QT syndrome. *Am Heart J* **89:**378–390, 1975

17. Horowitz LN, Vetter VL, Harken AH, Josephson ME: Electrophysiologic characteristics of sustained ventricular tachycardia occurring after repair of tetralogy of fallot. *Am J Cardiol* **46:**446–452, 1980

18. Kastor JA, Horowitz LN, Harken AH, Josephson ME: Clinically electrophysiology of ventricular tachycardia. *N Engl J Med* **304:**1004–1020, 1981

19. Josephson ME, Horowitz LN, Spielman SR, Greenspan AM: Electrophysiologic and hemodynamic studies in patients resuscitated from cardiac arrest. *Am J Cardiol* **46:**948, 1980

20. Kempf FC, Josephson ME: Cardiac arrest recorded on ambulatory electrocardiograms. *Am J Cardiol* **53:**1577, 1984

21. Vassalo JA, Cassidy DM, Kindwall KE, et al: Nonuniform recovery of excitability in the left ventricle. *Circulation* **78:**1365, 1988

22. Johnson NJ, Rosen MR: The distinction between triggered activity and other cardia arrhythmias. In Brugada P, Wellens JHJ (eds): *Cardiac Arrhythmias: Where to Go from Here?* Mount Kisco, NY, Futura, 1987, p 129

23. Cranefield PF, Aronson RS: *Cardiac Arrhythmias: The Role of Triggered Activity and Other Mechanisms.* Mount Kisco, NY, Futura, 1988

24. Moak JP, Rosen MR: Induction and termination of triggered activity by pacing in isolated canine Purkinje fibers. *Circulation* **69:**149, 1984

25. Le Marec H, Dangman KH, Danilo P Jr, Rosen MR: An evaluation of automaticity and triggered activity in the canine heart one to four days after myocardial infarction. *Circulation* **71:**1224, 1985

26. Dangman KH, Danilo P Jr, Hordof AJ, et al: Electrophysiologic characteristics of human ventricular and Purkinje fibers. *Circulation* **65:**362, 1982

27. Johnson N, Danilo P Jr, Wit AL, Rosen MR: Characteristics of initiation and termination of catecholamine-induced triggered activity in atrial fibers of the coronary sinus. *Circulation* **74:**1168, 1986

28. Dangman KH, Hoffman BF: The effects of single premature stimuli on automatic and triggered rhythms in isolated canine Purkinje fibers. *Circulation* **71:**813, 1985

29. Damiano BP, Rosen MR: Effects of pacing on triggered activity induced by early after-depolarizations. *Circulation* **69:**1013, 1984

30. Josephson ME, Almendral JM, Buxton AE, et al: Mechanisms of ventricular tachycardia. *Circulation* **75(3):**41, 1987

31. Brugada P, Wellens HJJ: The role of triggered activity in clinical arrhythmias. In Rosenbaum MB, Elizari MV (eds): *Frontiers of Cardiac Electrophysiology.* Boston, Nijhoff, 1983

32. Josephson ME, Marchlinski FE, Cassidy DM, et al: Sustained ventricular tachycardia in coronary artery disease—Evidence for re-entrant mechanism. In Zipes DP, Jalife J, (eds): *Cardiac Electrophysiology and Arrhythmias.* Orlando, FL, Grune & Stratton, 1985, p 409

33. Spear JF, Michelson EL, Spielman SR, et al: The origin of ventricular arrhythmias 24 hours following experimental anterior septal coronary artery occlusion. *Circulation* **55:**844–852, 1977

34. Horowitz LN, Spear JF, Moore EN: Subendocardial origin of ventricular arrhythmias in 24 hour-old experimental myocardial infarction. *Circulation* **53:**56–63, 1995

35. Trautwein W: Membrane currents in cardiac muscle fibers. *Physiol Rev* **53:**793–835, 1973

36. Carmeliet EE: *Chloride and Potassium Permeability in Cardiac Purkinje Fibers.* Brussels, Bruxelles Presses Academiques Europeennes, 1961

37. Ferrier GR, Moe GK: Effect of calcium on acetylstrophanthidin-induced transient depolarization in canine Purkinje tissue. *Circ Res* **33:**508–515, 1973

38. Armour JA, Hageman GR, Randall WC: Arrhythmias induced by local cardiac nerve stimulation. *Am J Physiol* **223:**1068–1075, 1972

39. Tsien RW: Effects of epinephrine on the pacemaker potassium current of cardiac Purkinje fibers. *J Gen Physiol* **64:**293–319, 1974

40. Josephson ME, Spear JF, Harken AH, et al: Surgical excision of au-

41. Wit AL, Cranefield PF: Triggered activity in cardiac muscle fibers of the simian mitral valve. *Circ Res* **38:**85–98, 1976

42. Wellens HJJ: Observations on the pathophysiology of ventricular tachycardia in man. *Arch Intern Med* **135:**473–479, 1975

43. Wellens HJJ, Durken R, Lie KI: Observations on the mechanism of ventricular tachycardias in man. *Circulation* **54:**237–244, 1976

44. Scherlag BJ, El-Sherif N, Hope E, et al: Characterization and localization of ventricular arrhythmias resulting from myocardial ischemia and infarction. *Circ Res* **35:**372–383, 1974

45. Han J: Mechanisms of ventricular arrhythmias associated with myocardial infarction. *Am J Cardiol* **24:**800–813, 1969

46. El-Sherif N, Mehra R, Gough WB, Zeiler RH: Re-entrant ventricular arrhythmias in the late myocardial infarction period. Interruption of re-entrant circuits by cyrothermal techniques. *Circulation* **68:**644–656, 1983

47. Wellens HJJ: *Electrical Stimulation of the Heart in the Study and Treatment of Tachycardias.* Baltimore, University Park Press, 1971, pp 14–22

48. Boineau JP, Cox JL: Slow ventricular activation in acute myocardial infarction: A source of re-entrant premature ventricular contractions. *Circulation* **48:**702–713, 1973

49. Janse MJ, Van Capelle FJL, Morsink H, et al: Flow of "injury" current and patterns of excitation during early ventricular arrhythmias in acute regional myocardial ischemia in isolated porcine and canine hearts; evidence for two different arrhythmogenic mechanisms. *Circ Res* **47:**151–165, 1980

50. Simson MB, Harden W, Barlow CH, et al: Visualization of the distance between perfusion and anoxia along an ischemic border. *Circulation* **60:**1151–1155, 1979

51. Wetstein L, Nussbaum MS, Barlow CH, et al: Decrease in acute myocardial ischemia by hyaluronidase in isolated, perfused rabbit hearts. *J Surg Res* **30:**489–496, 1981

52. Gessman LJ, Agarual JB, Endo T, Helfant RH: Localization and mechanism of ventricular tachycardia by ice mapping one week after the onset of myocardial infarction in dogs. *Circulation* **68:**657–666, 1983

53. Pham TD, Fenoglio JJ, Harken AH, et al: Structural basis for recurrent sustained ventricular tachycardia. *Circulation* **64** (Suppl):87, 1981

54. Spear JF, Michelson EL, Moore EN: Cellular electrophysiologic characteristics of chronically infarcted myocardium in dogs susceptible to sustained ventricular tachyarrhythmias. *Circulation* **1:**1099–1110, 1983

55. El-Sherif N, Scherlag BJ, Lazzara R, et al: Re-entrant ventricular arrhythmias in the late myocardial period: I. Conduction characteristics in the infarction zone. *Circulation* **55:**686–702, 1977

56. Michelson EL, Spear JF, Moore NE: Elecrophysiologic and anatomic correlates of sustained ventricular tachyarrhythmias in a model of chronic myocardial infarction. *Am J Cardiol* **45:**583–590, 1980

57. Karagueuzian HS, Fenoglio JJ, Weis MB, et al: Protracted ventricular tachycardia induced by premature stimulation of the canine heart after coronary artery occlusion and reperfusion. *Circ Res* **44:**833–846, 1979

58. Grosso MA, Simson MB, Kobayashi K, et al: Myocardial ischemic pattern determines predisposition to ventricular arrhythmias. *Surg Forum* **34:**239–241, 1983

59. Wetstein L, Michelson EL, Simson MB, et al: Increased interphase between normoxic and ischemic tissue as the cause for re-entry ventricular tachyarrhythmias. *J Surg Res* **32:**526–534, 1982

60. Fenoglio JJ, Pham TD, Harken AH, et al: Recurrent sustained ventricular tachycardia: Structure and ultrastructure of subendocardial regions in which tachycardia originates. *Circulation* **68:**518–533, 1983

61. Huikuri HV, Korhonen UR, Linnaluofo MK, Takkunen JT: The re-

lationship of ventricular arrhythmias to the angiographically and scintigraphically estimated extent of ventricular damage late after myocardial infarction. *Clin Cardiol* **10**:175–179, 1987

62. Selle JG: Reflections on definitive surgical treatment of postinfarction ventricular tachycardia. *Ann Thorac Surg* **58**:1287–1290, 1994

63. Karagueuzian HS, Fenoglio JJ, Weiss MB, et al: Protracted ventricular tachycardia induced by premature stimulation of the canine heart after coronary artery occlusion and reperfusion. *Circ Res* **44**:833–846, 1979

64. Kersschot IE, Brugada P, Ramentol M, et al: Effects of early reperfusion in acute myocardial infarction on arrhythmias induced by programmed stimulation: A prospective, randomized study. *J Am Coll Cardiol* **7**:1234–1242, 1986

65. Durrer D, Roos JP: Epicardial excitation of the ventricles in a patient with WPW Syndrome. *Circulation* **35**:15–21, 1967

66. Josephson ME, Howowitz LN, Farshidi A, et al: Recurrent sustained ventricular tachycardia: Mechanisms. *Circulation* **57**:440–447, 1978

67. Wetstein L, Michelson EL, Simson MB, et al: Initiation of ventricular tachyarrhythmias with programmed stimulation: Sensitivity and specificity in an experimental canine model. *Surgery* **92**:206–211, 1982

68. Curry PVL: Fundamental of arrhythmias: Modern method of investigation. In Krickler DM, Goodwin JF (eds): *Cardiac Arrhythmias: The Modern Electrophysiological Approach.* London, W.B. Saunders, 1975, pp 65–76

69. Josephson ME, Horowitz LN, Farshidi A, et al: Sustained ventricular tachycardia: Evidence for protected localized reentry. *Am J Cardiol* **42**:416–424, 1978

70. Spear JF, Horowitz LN, Moore EN, Wyse DG: Verapamil sensitive slow response activity in infarcted human ventricular myocardium. *Circulation* **54** (Suppl II):75, 1976

71. Wilbur DJ, Garan H, Finkelstein D, et al: Out-of-hospital cardiac arrest. Use of electrophysiologic testing in the prediction of long-term outcome. *N Engl J Med* **318**:19–24, 1988

72. Mitchell LB, Duff HJ, Manyar DE, et al: A randomized clinical trial of the noninvasive approaches to drug therapy of ventricular tachycardia. *N Engl J Med* **317**:1681–1687, 1987

73. Kim SG, Seiden SW, Felder SD, et al: Is programmed stimulation of value in predicting the long-term success of anti-arrhythmic therapy for ventricular tachyarrhythmias? *N Engl J Med* **315**:356–362

74. CAST Investigators: Preliminary Report: Effect of Encainide and Flecainide on mortality in a randomized trial of arrhythmia suppression after myocardial infarction. *N Engl J Med* **321**:406–412, 1989

75. Geha AS, Biblo LA, Carlson MD, Waldo AL: Selective surgical approach for atrioventricular re-entrant tachycardia. *Ann Thorac Surg* **53**:200–206, 1992

76. Tilkian AG, Pfeifer JF, Barry WH, et al: The effect of coronary artery bypass surgery on exercise-induced ventricular arrhythmias. *Am Heart J* **92**:707–714, 1976

77. DeSoyza N, Murphy ML, Bissett JK, et al: Ventricular arrhythmia in chronic stable angina pectoris with surgical or medical treatment. *Ann Intern Med* **89**:10–14, 1979

78. Tabry IF, Geha AS, Hammond GL, et al: Effect of surgery on ventricular tachyarrhythmias associated with coronary arterial occlusive disease. *Circulation* **58** (Suppl 1):166–170, 1978

79. Manolis AS, Rastegar H, Estes NAM III: Effects of coronary artery bypass grafting on ventricular arrhythmias: Results with electrophysiologic testing and long-term follow-up. *PACE* **16**:984–999, 1993

80. Mason JW, Stinson EB, Winkle RA, et al: Relative efficacy of blind left ventricular aneurysm resection for the treatment of recurrent ventricular tachycardia. *Am J Cardiol* **49**:241–248, 1982

81. Boineau JP, Cox JL: Rationale for a direct surgical approach to control ventricular arrhythmias. *Am J Cardiol* **49**:381–396, 1982

82. Elefteriades JA, Biblo LA, Batsford WP, et al: Evolving patterns in

83. Guiraudon G, Fontaine G, Frank R: La ventriculotomie circulaire d'exclusion: Traitement chirurgical des tachycardias ventriculaires compliquant un infartus du myocarde. *Ach Mal Coeur* **71**:1255, 1978

84. Guiraudon G, Fontaine G, Frank R: Encircling endocardial ventriculotomy: A new technique for life-threatening ventricular tachycardias resistant to medical treatment following myocardial infarction. *Ann Thorac Surg* **26**:438–444, 1978

85. Cox JL, Daniel TM, Sabiston DC Jr, Boineau JP: Desynchronized activation in myocardial infarction: A reentry basis for ventricular arrhythmias (abstract). *Circulation* **39**(Suppl 3):63, 1969

86. Boineau JP, Cox JL: Slow ventricular activation in acute myocardial infarction. A source of re-entrant premature ventricular contractions. *Circulation* **48**:702–713, 1973

87. Ungerleider RM, Holman WL, Stanley TE III, et al: Encircling endocardial ventriculotomy (EEV) for refractory ischemic ventricular tachycardia. I. Electrophysiological effects. *J Thorac Cardiovasc Surg* **83**:840–849, 1982

88. Ungerleider RM, Holman WL, Stanley TE III, et al: Encircling endocardial ventriculotomy (EEV) for refractory ischemic ventricular tachycardia. II. Effects on regional myocardial blood flow. *J Thorac Cardiovasc Surg* **83**:850–856, 1982

89. Ungerleider RM, Holman WL, Calcagno D, et al: Encircling endocardial ventriculotomy (EEV) for refractory ischemic ventricular tachycardia. III. Effects on regional left ventricular function. *J Thorac Cardiovasc Surg* **83**:857–864, 1982

90. Cox JL, Gallagher JJ, Ungerleider RM: Encircling endocardial ventriculotomy (EEV) for refractory ischemic tachycardia. IV. Clinical indications, surgical technique, mechanism of action, and results. *J Thorac Cardiovasc Surg* **83**:865–872, 1982

91. Swerdlow CD, Mason JW, Stinson EB et al: Results of operations for ventricular tachycardia in 105 patients. *J Thorac Cardiovasc Surg* **92**:105–113, 1986

92. Josephson ME, Harken AH, Horowitz L: Endocardial excision. A new surgical technique for the treatment of recurrent ventricular tachycardia. *Circulation* **60**:1430–1439, 1979

93. Harken AH, Josephson ME, Horowitz LN: Surgical endocardial resection for the treatment of malignant ventricular tachycardia. *Ann Surg* **190**:456–460, 1979

94. Geha AS, Elefteriades JA, Hsu J, et al: Strategies in the surgical treatment of malignant ventricular arrhythmias. *Ann Surg* **216**:309–317, 1992

95. Guiraudon GM, Klein GJ, Jones DL, et al: Encircling endocardial cryoablation for ventricular arrhythmias after myocardial infarctions: further experience [abstract]. *Circulation* **72**(Suppl 3):222, 1985

96. Mesnildrey P, Laborde F, Piwnca A, et al: Encircling Thermo-exclusion by Nd: YAG laser without mapping: a new surgical technique for ischemic ventricular tachycardia [abstract] *Circulation* **72** (Suppl 3):389, 1985

97. Ostermeyer J, Borggrefe M, Breithardt G, et al: Direct operations for the management of life-threatening ischemic ventricular tachycardia. *J Thorac Cardiovasc Surg* **94**:848–865, 1987

98. Moran JM, Kehoe RF, Loeb JM, et al: Extended endocardial resection for the treatment of ventricular tachycardia and ventricular fibrillation. *Ann Thorac Surg* **34**:843–871, 1982

99. Bolooki H, Palatianos GM, Zaman L, et al: Surgical management of post-myocardial infarction ventricular tachyarrhythmia by myocardial debulking, septal isolation, and myocardial revascularization. *J Thorac Cardiovasc Surg* **92**:716–725, 1986

100. Selle JG, Svenson RH, Sealy WC, et al: Successful clinical laser ablation of ventricular tachycardia: A promising new therapeutic method. *Ann Thorac Surg* **42**:380–384, 1986

101. Guiraudon GM: Cryoablation, a versatile tool in arrhythmia surgery. *Ann Thorac Surg* **43**:129–130, 1987

102. Kron IL, Lerman BB, Nolan SP, et al: Sequential endocardial resection for the surgical treatment of refractory ventricular tachycardia. *J Thorac Cardiovasc Surg* **94**:843–871, 1987

103. Lawrie GM, Pacifico A, Kaushik RR: Transannular cryoablation of ventricular tachycardia. *J Thorac Cardiovasc Surg* **98**:1030–1036, 1989

104. Downar E, Mickleborough LL, Harris L, Parson I: Intraoperative electrical ablation of ventricular arrhythmias: A "closed heart" procedure. *Am J Coll Cardiol* **10**:1048–1056, 1987

105. Cox JL: Patient selection criteria and results of surgery for refractory ischemic ventricular tachycardia. *Circulation* **79** (Suppl 1):1163–1177, 1989

106. Mirowski M, Reid PR, Mower MM, et al: Termination of malignant ventricular arrhythmias with an automatic defibrillator in human beings. *N Engl J Med* **303**:322–324, 1980

107. DiMarco JP, Haines DE: Sudden cardiac death. *Curr Probl Cardiol* **18**:232, 1990

108. Estes NAM III: Strategies for management of malignant arrhythmias: Role of pharmacotherapy, surgery, ablation, and the implantable cardioverter defibrillator. In Estes NAM III, Manolis AS, Wang PJ (eds): *Implantable Cardioverter Defibrillators.* New York, Marcel Dekker, 1994, pp 229–255

109. Borggrefe M, Podczeck A, Ostermeyer J, et al: Long-term results of electrophysiologically-guided antitachycardia surgery in ventricular tachyarrhythmias: A collaborative report on 665 patients. In Griehardt G, Borggrefe M, Zipes DP (eds): *Nonpharmacological Therapy of Tachyarrhythmias.* Mt. Kisco, NY, Futura, 1987, pp 109–132

110. Thomas A, Moser S, Smutka ML, Wilson PA: Implantable defibrillation: Eight years of clinical experience. *PACE* **11**:1278–1286, 1988

111. Swerdlow CD, Winkle RA, Mason JW: Determinants of survival in patients with ventricular tachyarrhythmias. *N Engl J Med* **308**:1436–1442, 1983

112. Wilber JD, Garan H, Finkelstein D, et al: Out-of-hospital cardiac arrest: Use of electrophysiologic testing in the prediction of long-term outcome. *N Engl J Med* **318**:19–24, 1988

113. Gabry MD, Brodman R, Johnson D, et al: Automatic implantable cardioverter defribrillators: Patients survival, battery longevity and shock delivery analysis. *J Am Coll Cardiol* **9**:1349–1956, 1987

114. Winkle RA, Mead RH, Ruder MA, et al: Long-term outcome with the automatic implantable cardioverter defibrillator. *J Am Coll Cardiol* **16**:1353–1361, 1989

115. Kelly PA, Cannom DS, Garan H, et al: The automatic implantable cardioverter defibrillator efficacy, complications and survival in patients with malignant ventricular arrhythmias. *J Am Coll Cardiol* **11**:1278–1286, 1988

116. Axtell K, Tchou P, Akhtar M: Survival in patients with depressed left ventricular function treated by implantable cardioverter defibrillator. *PACE* **14**:291–296, 1991

117. Tchou PJ, Kadri N, Anderson J, et al: Automatic implantable cardioverter defibrillators and survival of patients with left ventricular dysfunction and malignant ventricular arrhythmias. *Ann Intern Med* **109**:529–534, 1988

118. Lehmann MH, Steinman RT, Schuger CD, Jackson K: The automatic implantable cardioverter defibrillator as antiarrhythmic treatment modality of choice for survivors of cardiac arrest unrelated to acute myocardial infarction (editorial). *Am J Cardiol* **62**:803–805, 1988

119. Spotnitz HM: *Research Frontiers in Implantable Defibrillator Surgery.* Austin, TX, R.G. Lanes, 1992

120. Markewitz A, Kaulbach H, Mattke S, et al: One-incision approach for insertion of implantable cardioverter defibrillators. *Ann Thorac Surg* **58**:1609–1613, 1994

121. Hammel D, Block M, Geiger A, et al: Single-incision implantation of cardioverter defibrillators using non-thoracotomy lead systems. *Ann Thorac Surg* **58**:1614–1616, 1994

122. Hargrove WC III, Josephson ME, Marchlinski FE, Miller JM: Surgical decisions in the management of sudden cardiac death and malignant ventricular arrhythmias. *J Thorac Cardiovasc Surg* **97**:923–928, 1989

123. Fogoros RN, Fiedler SB, Elson JJ: The automatic implantable cardioverter defibrillator in drug-refractory ventricular tachyarrhythmias. *Ann Intern Med* **107**:635–641, 1987

124. Geha AS, Lee JH: Selective strategies in the surgical management of malignant ventricular arrhythmias. In Spotnitz HM (ed): *Research Frontiers in Implantable Defibrillator Surgery.* Austin, TX, R.G. Landes, 1992

125. Miller JM, Kienzle MG, Harken AH, Josephson ME: Subendocardial resection for ventricular tachycardia: Predictors of surgical success. *Circulation* **70**:624–631, 1983

126. Miller JM, Marchlinski FE, Harken AH, et al: Subendocardial resection for sustained ventricular tachycardia in the early period after acute myocardial infarction. *Am J Cardiol* **55**:980–984, 1985

127. Swerdlow CD, Mason JW, Stinson EB, et al: Results of operations for ventricular tachycardia in 105 patients. *J Thorac Cardiovasc Surg* **92**:105–113, 1986

128. McGiffin DC, Kirklin JK, Plumb VJ, et al: Relief of life-threatening ventricular tachycardia and survival after direct operations. *Circulation* **76**:V93–103, 1987

129. Nisam S, Mower M, Mozer S: ICD clinical update: First decade, initial 10,000 patients. *PACE* **14**:255–262, 1991

130. Manolis AS, Tan-DeGuzman W, Lee MA, et al: Clinical experience in 77 patients with the automatic implantable cardioverter defibrillator. *Am Heart J* **118**:445–450, 1989

131. Roy D, Waxman HL, Kienzle MG, et al: Clinical characteristics and long-term follow-up in 119 survivors of out-of-hospital cardiac arrest: Relation to inducibility at electrophysiologic testing. *Am J Cardiol* **52**:969–974, 1989

132. Bigger JT: Future studies with the implantable cardioverter defibrillator. *PACE* **14**:883–889, 1991

133. Epstein AE: AVID necessity. *PACE* **16**:1773–1775, 1993

134. MADIT Executive Committee: Multicenter automatic defibrillator implantation trial (MADIT): Design and clinical protocol. *PACE* **14**:920 (Part II), 1992

135. Lemery R, Grugada P, Della Bella P, et al: Non-ischemic ventricular tachycardia: Clinical course and long-term follow-up in patients without clinically overt heart disease. *Circulation* **79**:990–999, 1989

136. Holmes DR, Davis KB, Mock MB, et al: The effect of medical and surgical treatment on subsequent sudden cardiac death in patients with coronary artery disease: A report from the Coronary Artery Surgery Study. *Circulation* **73**:1254–1263, 1986

137. Tresch DD, Wetherbee JN, Sierger R, et al: Long-term follow-up of survivors of prehospital sudden cardiac death treated with coronary artery bypass surgery. *Am Heart J* **110**:1139–1145, 1986

138. Garan H, Ruskin JN, DiMarco JP, et al: Electrophysiologic studies before and after myocardial revascularization in patients with life-threatening ventricular arrhythmias. *Am J Cardiol* **51**:519–524, 1983

139. Biblo LA, Carlson MD, Waldo AL: Follow-up of patients with implantable cardioverter defibrillator devices. In Estes NAM, Manolis AS, Wang PJ (eds): *Implantable Cardioverter Defibrillators.* New York, Marcel Dekker, 1994, pp 425–435

140. Oeff M, Langberg JJ, Chin M, et al: Ablation of ventricular tachycardia using multiple sequential transcatheter application of radiofrequency energy. *PACE* **15**:1167–1176, 1992

141. Brugada P, de Swart H, Smeets JL, et al: Transcoronary chemical ablation of ventricular tachycardia. *Circulation* **79**:475–482, 1989

142. Plumb V, Epstein AF, Kay NW: A prospective trial of intracoronary ETOH ablation for recurrent sustained ventricular tachycardia. *Circulation* 1989

143. Murgatroyd FD, Johnson EE, Cooper RA, et al: Safety of low en-

ergy transvenous atrial defibrillation—World experience. *Circulation* **90**:4 (Part II) p I–14, 1994

144. Ayers GM, Griffin JC, Kina MB, et al: An implantable atrial defibrillator: Initial animal experience with a novel device. *PACE* **17**:4 (Part II) p 769, 1994

145. Svenson RH, Littman L, Gallagher JJ, et al: Termination of ventricular tachycardia with epicardial laser photocoagulation: A clinical comparison with patients undergoing successful endocardial photocoagulation alone. *J Am Coll Cardiol* **15**:163–170, 1990

Pacemaker Therapy for Cardiac Arrhythmias

T. Bruce Ferguson, Jr.

INTRODUCTION

The implantable cardiac pacemaker was first developed in 1960 by Chardack and associates, using a single-chamber device that paced the ventricle asynchronously and was implanted through a left thoracotomy incision.[1] Additional milestones in bradypacing therapy are depicted in Table 133–1. Many individuals have made seminal contributions to this field over the ensuing 35 years.

At the present time, the developments in bradypacing have been shown to clearly prolong life and improve the quality of that life.[2–7] Technologic developments in pacing are proceeding at a remarkable rate, such that current devices are capable of more than 15 different pacing modes, pace both the atria and ventricles synchronously under a variety of conditions, and are less than one-tenth the size of the original devices. The rapid advances in microcomputer technology assure that these developments are certain to continue well into the next century.

This chapter will discuss the fundamental anatomic, electrophysiologic, and technical aspects of modern brady-pacing therapy, with emphasis on those aspects of therapy that pertain to the cardiothoracic surgeon with an interest in bradypacing therapy.

ANATOMIC PRINCIPLES

It is the goal in most instances of cardiac pacing to restore as closely as possible the normal electrophysiologic function of the conduction system. Where possible, this is done by taking advantage of anatomic relationships of the con-

duction tissue in the heart, and thus a working knowledge of normal anatomy is useful.[8]

Anatomy of the Mature Conduction System

The sinoatrial node is a spindle-shaped structure with the head extending toward the interatrial groove while the tail extends toward the orifice of the inferior vena cava (Fig. 133–1). Electrophysiologically, early investigators demonstrated the importance of pacemakers both above and below the sinus node in animal preparations. Sealy and Seaber[9] demonstrated persistence of atrial rhythm after isolation of the sinus node region, and Boineau et al[10] concluded that there is an extensive system of atrial pacemakers widely distributed in the right atrium and centered about the sulcus terminalis, extending inferiorly below the sinus node and anteriorly superiorly to the sinus node (Fig. 133–1). Additionally, lateral right atrial pacemakers, atrial septal pacemakers, and left atrial pacemakers in association with the inferior pulmonary veins have been demonstrated both experimentally and clinically.[11,12]

Controversy over the nature of internodal atrial myocardial tissue has been present since the early part of this century. It is generally agreed that there are preferential conduction, but not discrete anatomic, pathways for the spread of excitation from the sinus to the atrioventricular (A-V) node.[8,13] Well-oriented atrial muscle tracts made up of fibers running in parallel are found in the anterior limbus of the fossa ovalis, the crista terminalis, and its continuation into the sinus septum; activation of adjacent myocardium along these bands as broad wavefronts explains the preferential conduction known to occur in the atrium. The ulti-

TABLE 133–1. HISTORICAL DEVELOPMENTS IN CARDIAC PACING

Gerbezius	1719	Noted slow pulse among patients with apoplexy
Bichat	1791	Determined fundamentals of electrical cardiac stimulation
Walshe	1862	Proposed cardiac galvanic current
Gaskell	1883	Postulated the existence of a cardiac conduction system
Kent and His	1893	First described the cardiac conduction system
Tawara	1906	First described the atrioventricular (A-V) node
Kieth and Flack	1907	First described the sinoatrial (S-A) node
Gould	1929	Resuscitated a baby by direct electrical stimulation of the heart
Butterworth	1942	Described an experimental synchronous pacemaker
Bigelow, Callahan	1951	Developed a functional pacemaker
Zoll	1952	Restarted a human heart with electrical pacing
Hopps, Bigelow	1954	Described transvenous endocardial pacing in animals
Furman, Robinson	1958	Reported transvenous endocardial pacing
Elmquest, Senning	1959	Described rechargable implantable pacemaker system
Chardack	1960	Transistorized pacemaker implanted by thoracotomy
Parsonnet, Ekestrom	1962	Transvenous bipolar pacemaker insertion technique
Keleor	1964	Developed a synchronous atrioventricular pacemaker
Goetz	1966	Developed a demand pacemaker
Tarjan	1972	Developed external programmability
Camilli	1976	First rate-responsive pacing system (pH sensor)
Humen	1983	First activity rate-responsive pacing system
Multiple investigators	1985–on	Establishment of physiologic dual-chamber pacing

mate substrate for preferential conduction within these bands remains to be established.

There are no gross anatomic landmarks to indicate the locations of the A-V node and bundle of His.[14] These structures are contained within the triangle of Koch, which is bounded by the anulus of the tricuspid valve inferiorly, the Tendon of Todaro superiorly, and a line drawn between the coronary sinus and the tricuspid anulus posteriorly (Fig. 133–2). The apex of the triangle is the central fibrous body of the heart and the supra-anular portion of the membranous intraventricular septum. The node is usually far removed (anteriorly) from the coronary sinus; the transitional cell zones extend backward and superiorly from the compact node but are contained within the boundaries of the triangle.

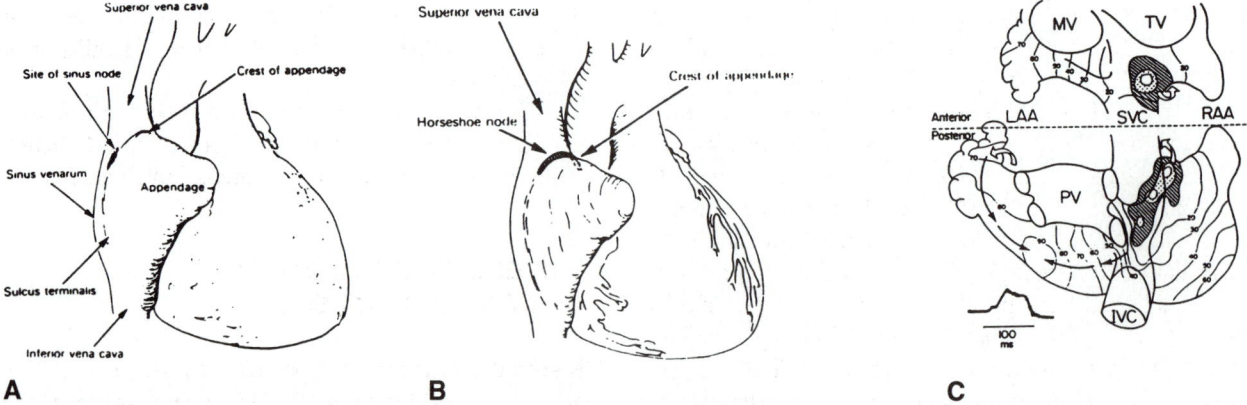

A   **B**   **C**

Figure 133–1. A. The usual depiction of the sinus node. *(From Davies MJ, Anderson RH, Becker AE: Embryology of the conduction tissues. In The Conduction System of the Heart. London, Butterworths, 1983, pp 81–94, with permission.)* **B.**The horseshoe disposition of the sinus node (10% of cases). *(From Anderson KR, Ho SY, Anderson RH: The location and vascular supply of the sinus node in the human heart. Br Heart J 41:28, 1979, with permission.)* **C.**The human atrial pacemaker complex. An epicardial activation map during normal sinus rhythm. The anterior atria are shown above as if unfolded along dotted line. The posterior atria are shown below. Note that there are four separate sites of impulse origin distributed over an area of approximately 6 cm extending from the anterior superior right atrium, inferiorly to the intercaval region. *(From Boineau JP, Schuessler RB: Reflections on the establishment of the electrophysiologic basis for cardiac arrhythmia surgery. In Cox JL (ed): Cardiac Arrhythmia Surgery, Vol. 4. Philadelphia, Hanley & Belfus, 1990, p 4, with permission.)*

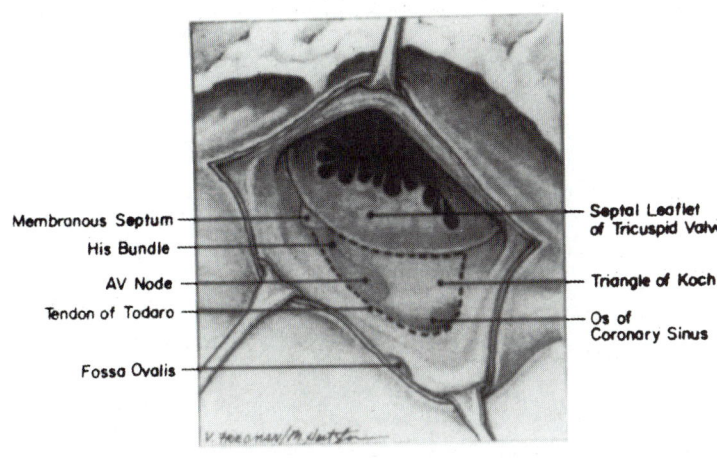

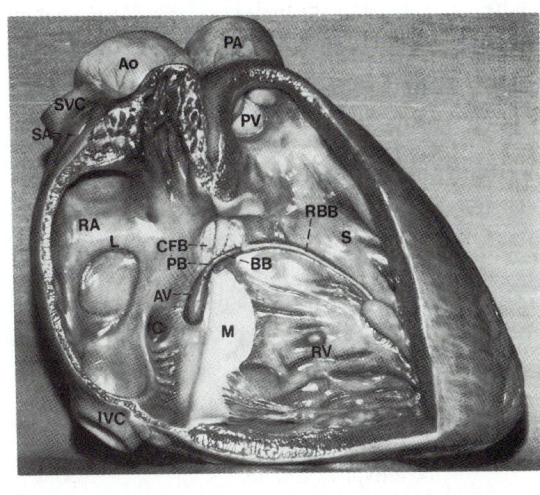

A   **B**

Figure 133–2. A. The right atrium viewed through a longitudinal right atriotomy. The patient's head is to the left and the feet are to the right. The boundaries of the triangle of Koch are the tendon of Todaro, the tricuspid valve annulus, and a line connecting the two at the level of the os of the coronary sinus. Within the triangle of Koch resides the A-V node and proximal portion of the His bundle, which enters the ventricular septum immediately posterior to the membranous portion of the interatrial septum. *(From Cox, et al: Surgery for the Wolff-Parkinson-White syndrome: The endocardial approach. Semi Thorac Cardiovasc Surg 1:34–46, 1989, with permission.)* **B.** Diagrammatic sketch of the right side of the heart, showing the conduction system. RA, right atrium; RV, right ventricle; L, limbus fossae ovalis; C, coronary sinus; SVC, superior vena cava; IVC, inferior vena cava; M, medial leaflet of the tricuspid valve; AV, A-V node; PB, bundle of His, penetration portion; BB, bundle of His, branching portion; RBB, right bundle branch; PA, pulmonary artery; Ao, aorta; SA, S-A node; PV, pulmonary valve; S, septal band; CBF, central fibrous body. *(From Bharati S, Lev M: The Cardiac Conduction System in Unexplained Sudden Death. Mount Kisco, NY, Futura, 1990, p 22A.)*

The compact A-V node becomes the penetrating bundle at the apex of the triangle and passes into the ventricular septum beneath the attachment of the tendon of Todaro to the central fibrous body, and just posterior to the membranous septum (Fig. 133–2). The nonbranching and branching bundles are sandwiched between the muscular ventricular septum and the membranous septum; branching of the bundle takes place on the muscular septum beneath the commissure between the right coronary and noncoronary cusps of the aortic valve.[15] Importantly, the compact node, penetrating bundle, and branching bundle form a continuous axis of cells that runs the length of the muscular ventricular septum; the atrial component lies above the anulus, the penetrating bundle passes through the anulus, and branching bundles lie beneath the anulus fibrosis of the heart. As explained below stimulation of and recording from areas within the right ventricular cavity result in different paced and sensed electrograms, in part depending on the proximity to the right ventricular bundle branch fibers. Finally, capture of the most caudad portion of the heart in the setting of an intact distal conduction system yields the most physiologic approximation of normal conduction for the patient, and, therefore, localization of the site of the conduction abnormality is important.

Additional Anatomic Considerations

Current endocardial pacemaker lead technology relies on certain anatomic features of the right atrium and ventricle for stable chronic positioning of the electrode tip. The atrial leads are designed for placement in the right atrial appendage, which has small trabeculae that engage and stabilize the acute placement of the electrode tip. Similarly, the apex of the right ventricle contains multiple trabeculations that function in a similar fashion. Other areas of the atrium (crista terminalis, fossa ovalis, right atrial free wall) and ventricle (high interventricular septum, pulmonary infundibulum) are devoid of trabeculations and in the absence of active-fixation mechanisms (see below) will not provide long-term electrode-myocardial interface stability in most circumstances.

The anatomic considerations that pertain to implantation of pacemaker systems are discussed in the section on Clinical Aspects of Cardiac Pacemaker Implantation.

THE ELECTROPHYSIOLOGY OF CARDIAC PACING

Myocardial cells can be depolarized by means of artificially applied electrical stimuli. This is a unique property of myocardial tissue, and forms the basis for bradypacing therapy. This section will discuss the pertinent electrophysiologic aspects of pacing.

Cardiac Impulse Initiation and Propagation

The cardiac membrane is a lipid bilayer containing ion channels through which the flow of ions is regulated.[16] In addition, biochemical pumps can distribute ions across the membrane using a process that requires energy in the form of ATP (see Chapter 97). The disparate distribution of ions against their gradient is responsible for the electronegative resting membrane potential seen in cardiac muscle, −90 mV in ventricular specialized conduction tissue, −70 to −80 mV in ventricular and atrial myocardial tissue, and −50 mV in the sinoatrial and atrioventricular nodal tissues.

The membrane potential is a function of the intracellular and extracellular K concentration, which is high intracellularly and low extracellularly. This potential, E, is described for a cell by the Nernst equation[17]:

$$E = RT/f \ln([K^+]_i/[K^+]_o) \qquad (1)$$

where R = the gas constant, T = the absolute temperature, and f = the Faraday constant. Below a $[K^+]_o$ of 5 mM, the linear relationship between $[K^+]_o$ and membrane potential is no longer linear and other intracellular and extracellular ions (e.g., Ca^{2+}, Na^+) play a role in determining the membrane potential.[16]

The transmembrane action potential is generated due to abrupt alterations in the ion fluxes across the membrane through the respective channels.[18] Channels have the characteristics of voltage sensitivity; for example, a depolarizing stimulus normally causes sodium channels to open and potassium channels to close. The extent to which a channel can move from one state to another is controlled by channel gates, known as activation and inactivation gates. The interaction of these gates is complex, and specific for a specific channel type. Ion specificity is in large part controlled by selectivity filters near the external surface of the gates. Finally, not all channels of the same type open and close with the same specificity.

In an idealized Purkinje fiber in the resting state at −90 mV, sodium and calcium channels tend to be closed. A small leak of K^+ ions through a small number of open potassium channels maintains electronegativity (Fig. 133–3). With delivery of a depolarizing stimulus (from the specialized conduction tissue or a pacemaker stimulus) the sodium channels will open and the potassium channels will close.[17–19] The influx of positively charged sodium ions along chemical and electrical gradients causes depolarization of the cell to +20 mV, and is phase 0 of the action potential (Fig. 133–4). This sodium influx secondarily causes calcium and potassium channels to open, resulting in an outward voltage and concentration-driven efflux of K^+ ions, and is phase 1 repolarization. An inward current carried by calcium as well as a persistent inward current carried by sodium is responsible for the plateau or phase 2 of the action potential. Increasing ionic flow out of the potassium channel, lesser inward flow through the calcium and sodium channels is responsible for the subsequent phase 3 repolarization, and repolarization is complete as a result of potassium leaving the cell. This sodium-dependent action potential is called the fast-response because of the rapid phase 0 depolarization and rapid propagation associated

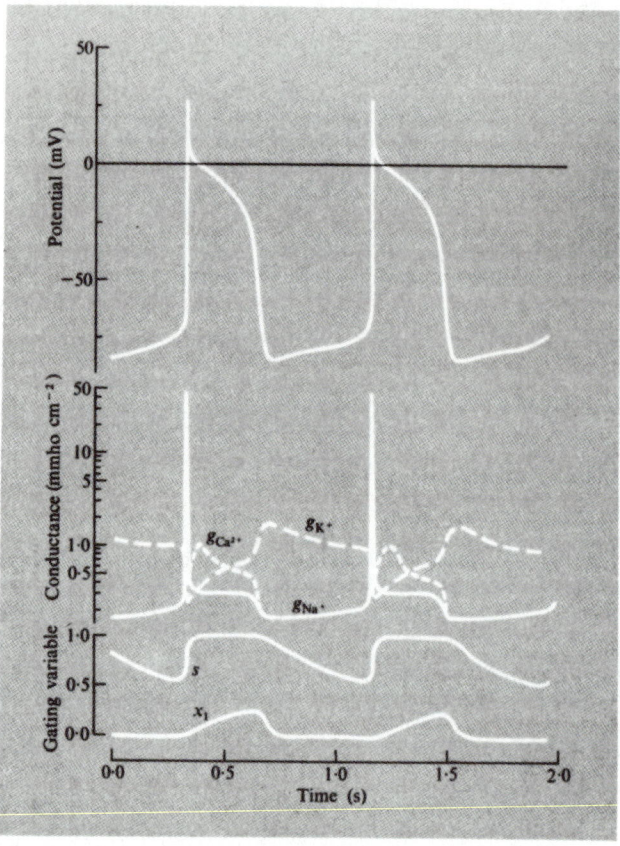

Figure 133–3. Diagram depicting the relationship between the cardiac action potential (top), conductance changes of the calcium (gCa^{2+}) and sodium (gNa^+) currents, and the potassium current (gK^+), controlled by the gating variables s and x1. *(From Noble D: Cardiac action potentials and pacemaker activity. In Linden RJ (ed): Recent Advances in Physiology. London, Churchill, pp 1–50.)*

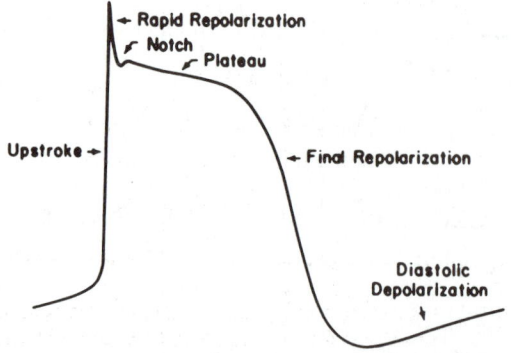

Figure 133–4. Protypical cardiac Purkinje fiber action potential. The upstroke is a rapid depolarization (phase 0) similar to that seen in nerve. After the overshoot, there is a rapid partial repolarization phase (phase 1), before the 200- to 400-ms plateau (phase 2). After repolarization (phase 3), there is slow depolarization that can lead to spontaneous firing (phase 4). *(From Fozzard HA, Arnsdorf MF: Cardiac electrophysiology. In Fozzard HA, Jennings RB, Haber E, et al (eds): The Heart and Cardiovascular System, 2nd ed. New York, Raven Press, 1991, pp 63–98, with permission.)*

with it; it is characteristic of normal cells of atrial and ventricular myocardium and specialized conduction tissue outside of the sinus and A-V nodal tissues.

A second type of action potential is characteristic of these two tissues, as well as cells on the atrial surfaces of the atrioventricular valves.[18,19] At the normal level of membrane potential of these cells, negative to −70 mV, the sodium channel is voltage-inactivated, and the calcium channel carries the inward current. An action potential is generated that has a slow rate of rise with slow propagation characteristics, and is called the slow response (Fig. 133–5). This slow response can be elicited from tissue normally capable of a fast response under pathophysiologic conditions.[20,21]

There are a number of factors involved in the cell-to-cell propagation of the cardiac impulse, without which cardiac pacing would not be feasible. A copper electrical wire, with insulation, coupled to a battery (electrical power source) and a variable resistor, provides the idealized ingredients for depolarization of the myocardium. The lipid bi-

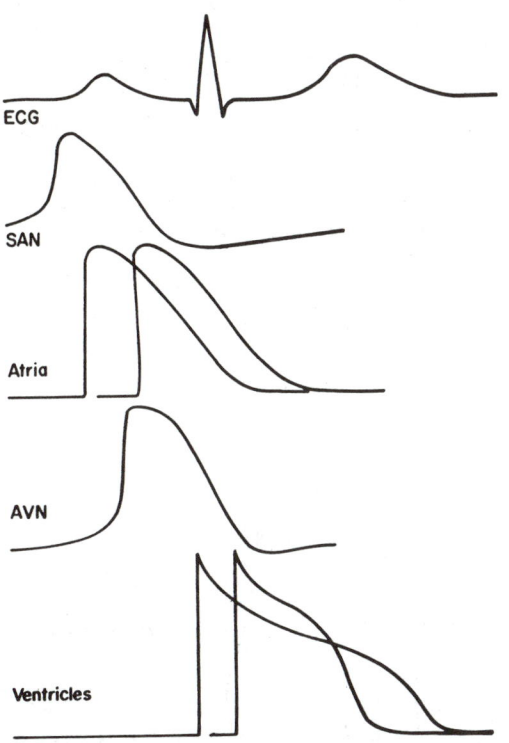

Figure 133–5. Examples of action potentials from various parts of the heart. The upper trace is a standard lead II electrogram (ECG) for time reference. The first action potential of the cardiac cycle is that of the sinoatrial node (SAN). The next action potentials are those of the atria, generating the P-wave of the ECG. Next is the atrioventricular node (AVN) action potential, followed by the ventricular conduction system (not shown, see Fig. 133–4). Finally, ventricular action potentials produce QRS on depolarization and T-wave on repolarization. Ventricular cells do not have uniform action potential durations. *(From Fozzard HA: Electrophysiologic basis of arrhythmias. In DasGupta DS (ed): Acute Cardiac Care. Chicago, Year Book, 1984.)*

layer provides excellent insulation, preventing dissipation of current between the highly conductive aqueous solutions within the cell and the extracellular space. A pathway of low resistance through which current can flow from cell to cell is provided by the nexal junctions, which are highly complicated structures at which cardiac cells are tightly apposed and which permit minute low-resistance pathways of communication.[22] The action potential generated by the first cell, if sufficient in amplitude, generates current flow between the first cell and a second cell sufficient to depolarize the second cell to threshold potential and generating an action potential in this second cell. The velocity of propagation also depends upon a number of factors.[23,24] Since the velocity of propagation increases with the square of the radius of the fiber, Purkinje fibers conduct more rapidly than myocardial cells. Propagation along fibers is much faster than across fibers, a principle termed anisotropy, and thus fiber orientation is important. Additional factors include the strength of the depolarizing stimulus (e.g., sodium-dependent or calcium-dependent), and the relationship of the membrane potential of a fiber to its threshold potential; the greater the disparity between these two potentials, the greater the displacement of membrane potential necessary to bring the fiber to threshold. Also, the coupling of cells is important; a stimulus of certain size may depolarize a cell tightly coupled to a small number of cells surrounding it but the current may be dissipated in a subthreshold manner if a large number of cells are coupled to the stimulated cell. Furthermore, a number of pathophysiologic factors[20] uncouple cells as a result of physical separation (e.g., tissue edema) or interposition of a poorly conducting medium (e.g., connective tissue). Overall, an organization of high and low resistance pathways is responsible for the organization of electrical activation of the heart in a repetitive fashion under normal circumstances.

Certain cells have a property termed "automaticity," the ability to generate an action potential de novo.[21,23] Normally these include the sinus node (which has the fastest intrinsic pacemaker rate), the pacemaker potential cells of the atrial, atrioventricular junctional, and ventricular specialized conduction tissues (Fig. 133–6). Under pathologic conditions, a number of other cells are capable of automaticity as well.

In the sinus node, a decay in outward current carried by potassium causes depolarization of the membrane and attainment of threshold on completion of full repolarization of the action potential and restoration of the transmembrane current to resting level. In the Purkinje fibers, there is an onset of inward sodium current through a channel designated i_f; this channel carries positive charge into the cell; if the charge accumulates faster than the membrane pump activity can remove it, then the cell will reach threshold potential. These two inward currents have different kinetics, which is in part responsible for the normal dominance of the sinus node in generating the depolarizing wavefront. Additionally, the principle of overdrive suppression[23] is im-

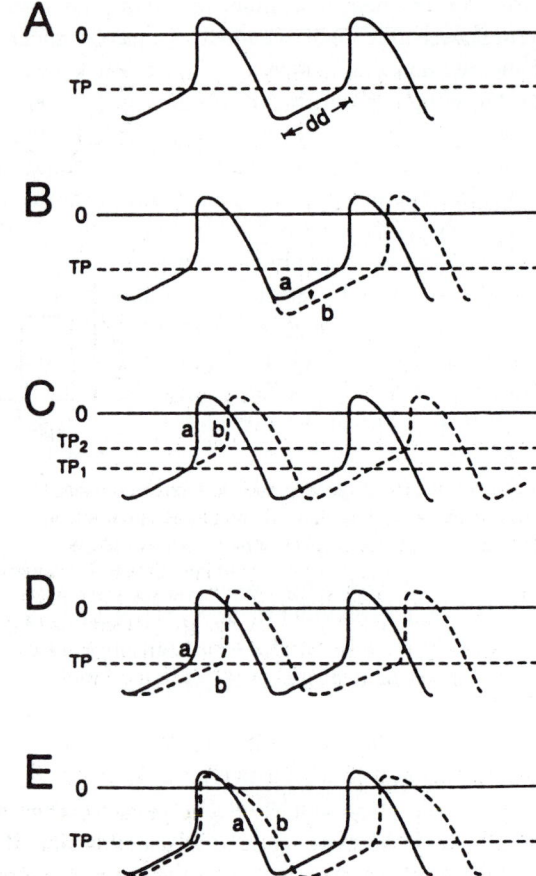

Figure 133–6. Diagrams of sinus node action potentials illustrating normal automaticity caused by spontaneous diastolic depolarization and the factors that change the rate of impulse initiation. **A.** A typical sinus node action potential with spontaneous diastolic depolarization, "dd." **B.** The change in rate that occurs when the maximum diastolic potential is shifted to a more negative level (from a to b). **C.** The change in rate caused by a change in threshold potential to a less negative level (from TP1 to TP2). **D.** The change in rate that occurs when the slope of phase 4 depolarization is decreased (from a to b). **E.** The change in rate that occurs when the action potential duration is increased (from a to b). *(Reproduced from Wit AL, Janse MJ: The Ventricular Arrhythmias of Ischemia and Infarction. Electrophysiologic Mechanisms. Mount Kisco, NY, Futura, 1993.)*

portant. This term refers to the stimulation of a pacemaker cell at a rate faster than its intrinsic rate, resulting in suppression of its pacemaker activity. In cells having low (less negative) potential and less sodium entry during phase 0 (such as the sinus node), there is a lower degree of overdrive suppression than occurs in the ventricle. Thus the sinus node is the primary pacemaker of the heart because of the relatively rapid rate of impulse initiation and its ability to overdrive suppress other cardiac pacemaker sites.

Cardiac Stimulation and Engineering Aspects of Output Circuits

In applying an external stimulating impulse to the my-ocardium, several conditions must be met to initiate my-

ocardial depolarization.[24] First, the myocardium must be excitable. Second, the stimulus current density (current per unit of cross-sectional area) must be sufficiently high, and of sufficient duration, to depolarize a large enough group of cells to initiate impulse propagation in the myocardium.

In cardiac pacing, a voltage is applied across two electrodes connected to the myocardium. These electrodes may be configured as a bipole, where the two electrodes are in close proximity to each other (typically 0.8 to 1.2 cm) and therefore both in proximity to the myocardium, or as a unipole, where one electrode is in contact with the myocardial tissue and the other is elsewhere in the body (typically an exposed portion of the generator).[25]

The interrelationship between current, voltage, and energy or charge required for reliable capture of the myocardium during electrical diastole with a stimulus of given duration is defined as the threshold of stimulation. This interrelationship is defined at first by Ohm's law:

$$V = I \times R \tag{2}$$

where V = voltage (in volts), I = current (in milliamperes), and R = resistance (in kiloohms). Energy is defined as

$$E = V \times I \times t \tag{3}$$

where E = energy (in microjules), V = voltage in (volts), I = current (in milliamperes), and t = time expressed as pulse width, PW (in milliseconds). A more useful expression of energy combines Eqs. (2) and (3):

$$E = (V)^2 \times PW/R \tag{4}$$

Energy (output) thus increases expotentially as a function of voltage, and linearly as a function of pulse width. Importantly, the behavior of each parameter (voltage, current, charge or energy) is dependent upon the duration of the stimulus (Fig. 133–7). These relationships can be simplified as the "strength–duration curve" representing the threshold of stimulation for cardiac muscle. The amplitude is expressed as voltage, or charge (the total quantity of current consumed during the time the stimulus is applied) or potential (work/unit charge to move an electron in an electric field from one point to another) as a function of pulse width. The *rheobase* is defined as the voltage at infinite pulse width; the *chronaxie* is the duration of a stimulus at the threshold of stimulation whose mean amplitude is twice the rheobase. All combinations of voltage and pulse width on or to the right of the potential line will effect capture of the myocardium; some combinations are more energy efficient than others, leading to important considerations regarding generator longevity.[26]

This relationship assumes that over the pulse-width interval the resistance remains constant. In fact, the resistance to flow of electrons (or impedance) rises with time over the duration of the pacemaker spike. The distal tip of a bipolar is negatively charged, while the proximal ring is positively charged. Polarization of the distal tip resists the flow of

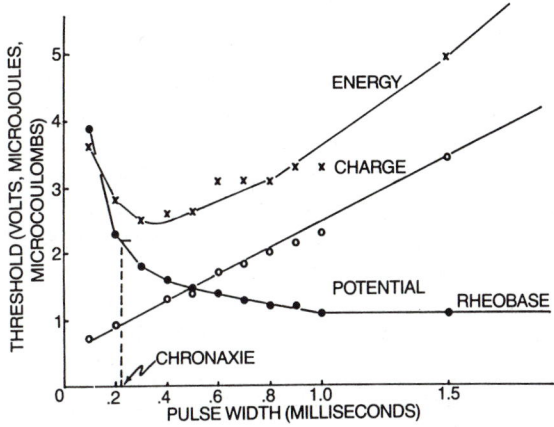

Figure 133–7. Strength–duration curve for cardiac pacing. Relationships between chronic ventricular (canine) constant-voltage threshold strength–duration curves expressed in terms of potential, charge, and energy for a tined unipolar lead with a 8-mm² ring tip. Thresholds were obtained with increasing stimuli. *(From Stokes K, Bornzin G: The electrode-biointerface: Stimulation. In Barold SS (ed): Modern Cardiac Pacing. Mount Kisco, NY, Futura, 1985, p 33, with permission.)*

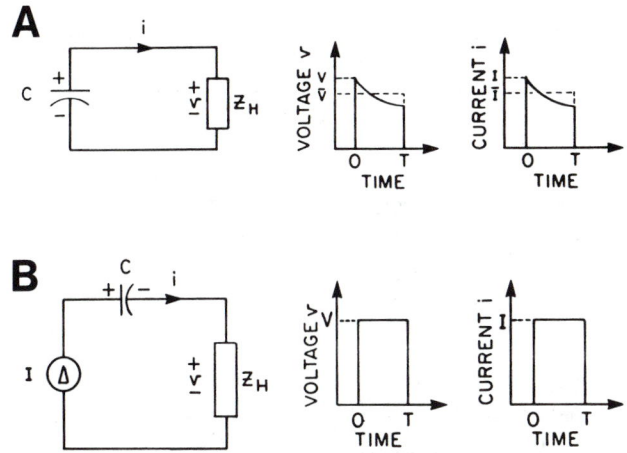

Figure 133–8. A. Voltage-source pacing. A charged capacitor (C) discharges through the heart. i, instantaneous current; v, instantaneous voltage; Io, initial current; Vo, initial voltage; I, mean current; V, mean voltage; Z_H, heart impedance; T, stimulus duration. **B.** Current-source pacing. A constant current (I) flows through the coupling capacitor (C) and the heart impedance (Z_H) producing a constant voltage (V) across the heart for the duration (T) of the stimulus. *(From Bernstein and Parsonnet,[24] with permission.)*

electricity through the electrode, and this polarization increases with the duration of current application.[25] This polarization effect is less with unipolar electrodes since the area of exposed metal surfaces (e.g., the generator can as compared with the proximal ring) is greater with unipolar systems; for this reason the impedance in unipolar systems is less than in bipolar ones.

The size of the distal electrode tip is inversely related to the concentration of the electrical charge, and therefore the amount of energy required to capture the myocardium. Unfortunately the surface area of the electrode tip is directly related to the ability to sense from the electrode, and these two considerations must be balanced in electrode tip designs.[26,27]

There are two basic types of pacing circuitry, voltage source and current source. In the former, the stimulus voltage and stimulus current decay during the stimulus as the charged capacitor discharges through the cardiac impedance (Fig. 133–8A). The peak voltage and current values are greater than the mean values of these parameters used in establishing a safety margin relative to the strength–duration curve. Voltage source pacemakers are sometimes referred to as constant voltage generators; this is a slight misnomer, since due to small capacitor size and varying impedance maintenance of an absolutely constant voltage during the pacemaker spike is not possible. Most permanent pacemaker systems are voltage source, sometimes called constant-voltage capacitor-coupled generators.[24]

Alternatively, current source pacing generates a current through the series combination of the coupling capacitor and the heart impedance (Fig. 133–8B); both stimulus voltage and stimulus current are constant for the duration of

the stimulus. The mean values of voltage and current are the same as the corresponding peak values; this simplifies relating measured amplitudes to the voltage or current threshold. Constant current pacing is used in temporary external pacemaker generators with replaceable battery supplies and where size is not a consideration.[25]

Sensing of Intramyocardial Electrical Activity

Strictly defined, sensing is the detection of real or apparent spontaneous cardiac depolarizations.[24] The majority of conventional sensing circuitry includes three or more components (Fig. 133–9): a sensing amplifier, which magnifies the voltage difference that appears across the two electrodes; a bandpass filter, to isolate the components of the amplified input signal that most clearly represents the cardiac depolarization; and a threshold comparator that performs the actual detection by comparing the instantaneous voltage at the filter output with a fixed reference voltage. A logic signal is produced whenever the filter output exceeds the reference voltage in amplitude, and this signal is used by the control circuitry of the pulse generator for resetting the pacemaker's escape timing or for other purposes.

To increase or decrease the sensitivity of a sensing circuit, the gain of the sensing amplifier is increased or decreased with the threshold detection voltage held constant.[24] The sensing threshold represents an approximation of the minimal rapid deflection amplitude that will be detected at a given sensitivity setting. To lower the sensing threshold, the amplifier gain is increased, and vice versa.

Factors that affect sensing include electrode size and

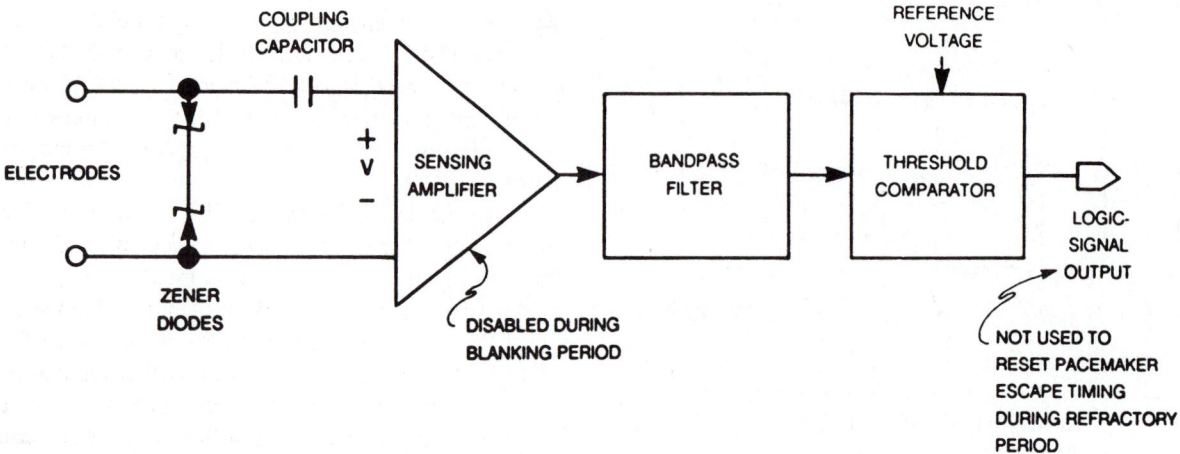

Figure 133–9. A block diagram of the basic elements of a conventional analog sensing circuit, showing Zener diodes (for protection against high applied voltages), the sensing amplifier, the bandpass filter, and the threshold comparator. The sensing amplifier is disabled during a blanking period, and the logic output is not used to reset pacemaker escape timing during a refractory period. *(From Bernstein and Parsonnet,[24] with permission.)*

the unipolar or bipolar electrode configuration of the system, as well as the position of the lead tip within the heart. Because of the distance between the two electrodes, unipolar sensing detects activity between the myocardial electrode and the generator, and is subject to considerable non-myocardial electrical noise such as myopotentials from the chest wall musculature or inappropriate sensing of pacemaker depolarization spikes from the second channel of a dual chamber pacing system, so-called "crosstalk." Bipolar leads sense activity between the two closely spaced electrodes, but bipolar sensing is more dependent upon electrode size and the vector of wavefront propagation than unipolar sensing. For example, if the wavefront is exactly parallel to the bipolar pair then the sensed signal will be extremely small (Fig. 133–10). Other factors affecting sensing include the setting of the bandpass filter of the pacemaker (Fig. 133–11). Both low-frequency (<40 Hz) and high-frequency (80 to 125 Hz) noise are filtered out of the amplified intrinsic deflection that is sensed.[26] Additionally, the positive and negative amplitudes and rate of change across the isoelectric line are instantaneously recorded in modern

sensing circuitry, yielding the *dV/dt* or slew rate of the electrogram. The slew rate can be used to differentiate between the initial rapid deflection of the electrogram and the later slow deflection of acute injury or repolarization; ideally, the amplitude recorded in millivolts of the intrinsic atrial or ventricular electrogram is the rapid deflection and excludes low-frequency (slow deflection) and high-frequency (myopotential) components. To further complicate the issue, most pacemaker systems have different bandpass filters for the atrial and ventricular channels (Fig. 133–11).[24, 26]

CURRENT PACEMAKER TECHNOLOGY

Permanent Pacemaker Leads

Endocardial pacing leads consist of wire insulated with a polyurethane or silicon external coating; there may be one (unipolar) or two (bipolar) wires in the lead body (Fig. 133–12A and B). The electrode is the uninsulated tip that

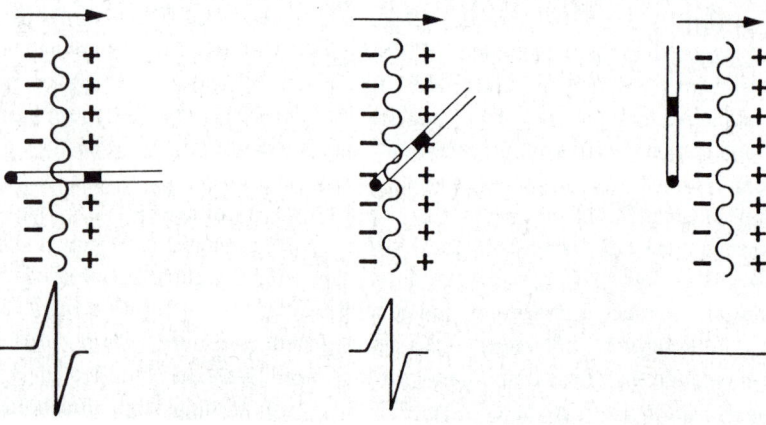

Figure 133–10. Bipolar sensing. The angle of the electrode relative to the depolarizing wave front affects both the amplitude and frequency of the detected signal. *(From Adams,[36] with permission.)*

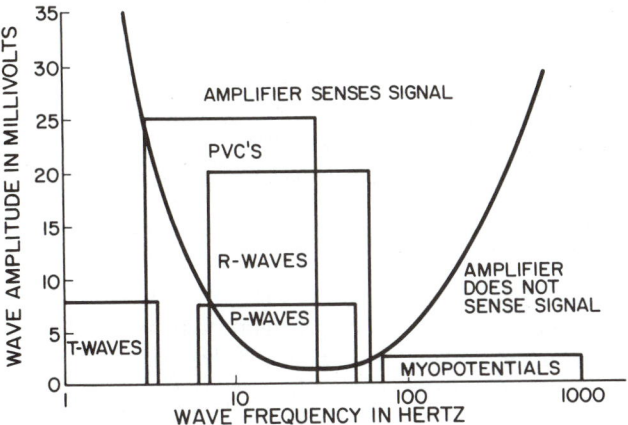

Figure 133–11. Typical pacemaker sensing parameters. Low-frequency signals (T-waves) and high-frequency signals (myopotentials) are excluded from sensing by frequency and wave amplitude parameters. Signals within the parabolic curve are sensed.

the most commonly used.[28–31] Steroid-eluting electrode tips have also been developed; the concept is that chronic leakage of a small amount of steroid at the tip over time will minimize the tissue reaction at the electrode–myocardial interface and result in lower chronic pacing thresholds.[31–34]

Attachment of the endocardial transvenous electrode lead tip to the myocardial tissue is accomplished either actively or passively; active-fixation leads have a tiny screw mechanism that is secured into the endocardial tissue (Fig. 133–12a–d). Passive-fixation lead tips consist of three or more tines of polyurethane or silicon that are designed to insinuate themselves into the trabeculations of the apical right ventricular endocardium or the atrial trabeculations in the atrial appendage. Chronic ventricular pacing thresholds tend to be lower with passive leads, particularly if a steroid-eluting lead is used,[27,35] but the lead dislodgement rate is somewhat higher; atrial lead stability is greater with active fixation leads. Sensing characteristics are similar between both active and passive leads.[36]

Epicardial electrodes (Fig. 133–12e) are screwed into the epicardium of the ventricle or hooked into the atrial myocardial tissue (Fig. 133–12f).[37,38] The electrode tip is usually the noninsulated distal portion of the screw or hook. They may be either unipolar (single electrode) or two may be placed adjacent to one another for a bipolar configuration. Epicardial electrodes must in general be placed at the time of cardiac surgery or through an anterior thoracotomy or subxiphoid approach. Ventricular epicardial electrodes

comes in contact with the myocardial tissue. As mentioned, the ability to capture the myocardial tissue and the ability to sense the patient's intrinsic electrical activity are affected by the size of the electrode tip; typical electrode surface areas for pacing are 8 to 10 mm, which provides a high enough current density for low chronic pacing thresholds. The exposed tip of the endocardial electrode is usually made of platinum, iridium, nickel alloys, or activated carbon.[27] Porous or solid platinum–iridium electrode tips are

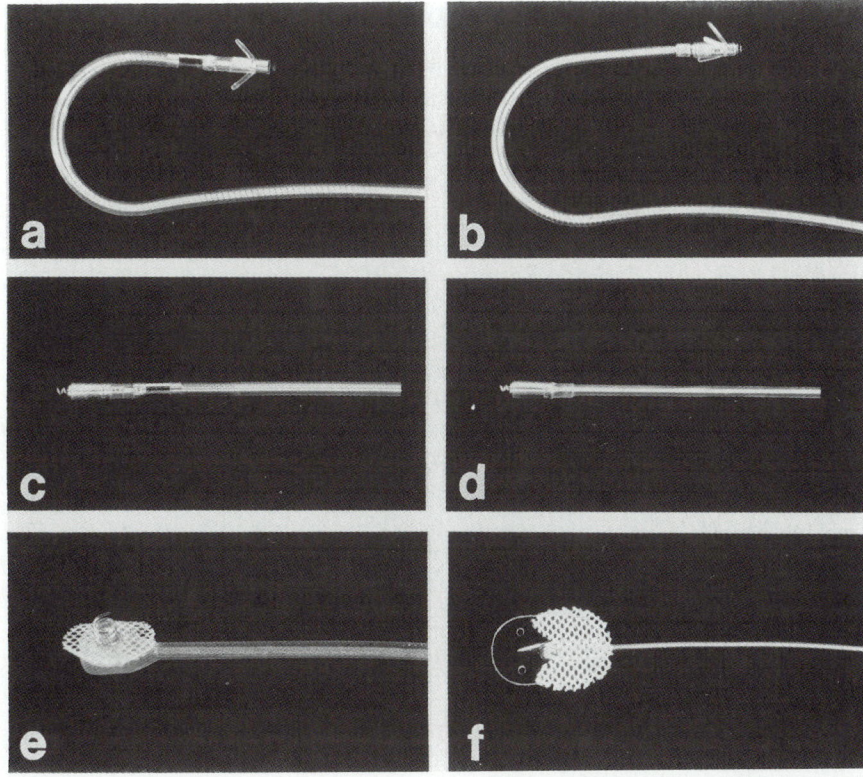

Figure 133–12. Examples of currently available endocardial and epicardial pacemaker leads. **a.** Unipolar endocardial passive fixation (tined) lead. **b.** Bipolar endocardial passive fixation (tined) lead. **c.** Unipolar endocardial active fixation lead. **d.** Bipolar endocardial active fixation lead. **e.** Unipolar epicardial screw-in lead. **f.** Unipolar epicardial fishhook lead.

are placed either on the diaphragmatic surface of the right ventricle or the left ventricular free-wall myocardium in an area of muscle devoid of epicardial fat; atrial electrodes should be placed on the free wall of the right atrium.[39] Epicardial electrodes historically have poorer performance characteristics long-term than endocardial electrodes; as such, endocardial electrode placement is preferred when possible.

The Pulse Generator

The modern pulse generator contains a power source, timing circuitry, sensing circuitry, and output circuitry for one or two channels connected to the electrodes, and a transceiver for telemetric communication with the programming device. All of the electrical components are now contained on a microchip, with programming and parameter setting changes performed by software alterations.

A large number of substrates have been used as power sources for implantable pacemakers, including early attempts at biologic and rechargeable chemical power sources.[40] Nuclear-powered pulse generators have excellent longevity but have not met widespread acceptance due to patient fear and regulatory considerations. Most commonly, chemical power sources consisting of a cathode, anode, and an electrolyte are used; a dry, crystalline electrolyte is present between the anode and cathode. Electric current is produced by ionization at the anode, with subsequent migration of the positively charged metallic ions through the electrolyte to the cathode. The electrons that remain at the anode can then flow through a connected conductive pathway to the cathode. The higher the resistance in the electrolyte conductor, the longer the life expectancy of the power cell. Most currently available generators contain a lithium–iodine power cell or a derivative.

The power source is a reservoir of charge, with a capacity (in ampere-hours) that passes charge through an electric circuit as current (charge per unit time).[24] The power source's ability to pump charge through an external load decreases over time, although all of the charge drawn from a power source as current returns to the source. With depletion, the voltage (electrical potential energy per unit charge) becomes progressively lower.

In the past, power sources have demonstrated considerable variation in life expectancy, both within a given type of power source and between different types of sources. With lithium–iodine sources, however, this has been less of a problem. Older generators also have widely variable indices of end of life (EOL) characteristics, making battery depletion difficult to detect in certain instances. In most current generators, however, battery voltage is monitored internally, and thus EOL parameters for that particular generator are detectable with telemetry and by transtelephonic monitoring.

Overall, battery longevity of currently available devices is determined by a number of factors; output voltage, resistance, pulse duration, number of electrodes, pacing rate (± activity pacing), percent of time the patient is paced, the adequacy of patient follow-up and programming, the characteristics of the electrode–myocardial interface, and specific considerations regarding safety margins for a patient.[41] Industry data on longevity of a device are therefore just estimates for an individual patient.[40]

As mentioned, modern pacemaker functions are integrated in circuitry embedded on microchips that function essentially as microcomputers. These systems contain central processing units, some memory capability, and the input–output circuits that perform all pacing, sensing, and timing functions. As with most small computers, re–programming can be done by software rather than hardware changes. The most dramatic advances in pacing technology that will occur over the next decade will be in the area of memory storage and on-line telemetry of electrophysiologic information.

These advances in microchip technology have permitted the interface of pacing with physiology over the past 8 years, leading to the development of rate-responsive "activity" pacemaker systems that provide "physiologic pacing."[42] Characteristics of these systems are discussed in greater detail below.

Finally, the size of bradypacing devices continues to decline. Most dual-chamber pacemakers weigh less than 30 g and are less than 4 mm thick, without a concomitant loss in the expected longevity of the device. The smallest single chamber device available is only slightly larger in diameter than a quarter.

CLINICAL CARDIAC PACING

Pacemaker Terminology and Principles of Timing Intervals

Standard nomenclature for describing the types of pacing modes available has been adopted, and is illustrated on Table 133–2.[43] The Inter-Society Commission for Heart Disease Resources (ICHD) code uses the letters A for atrium, V for ventricle, I for inhibit (inhibits pacemaker output), O for none (no output or no sensing or no response to sensing), T for triggered (triggers pacemaker output), and D for dual (atrium and ventricle, or triggered and inhibited).[44] In addition, R stands for rate-programmability. Other nomenclature for antitachyarrhythmia functions is shown on Table 133–2.

The position of the letter in the code refers to the following parameters: chamber paced, chamber sensed, response to sensing, programmability, and antitachyarrhythmia features. Currently, as many as 15 programmable pacing modes are available in state-of-the-art dual-chamber devices; however, a number of these (e.g., triggered pacing and completely asynchronous pacing) are used for diagnostic purposes only.

TABLE 133–2. THE NASPE/BPEG GENERIC (NBG) CODE

Position[a] and Category				
I **Chamber(s)** **Paced**	**II** **Chamber(s)** **Sensed**	**III** **Response to** **Sensing**	**IV** **Programmability, Rate** **Modulation**	**V** **Antitachyarrhythmia** **Function(s)**
O = None	O = None	O = None	O = None	O = None
A = Atrium	A = Atrium	T = Triggered	P = Simple Programmable	P = Pacing
V = Ventricle	V = Ventricle	I = Inhibited	M = Multiprogrammable	S = Shock
D = Dual (A+V)	D = Dual (A+V)	D = Dual (T+I)	C = Communicating	D = Dual (P+S)
			R = Rate Modulation	
Manufacturers' designation only	S = Single (A or V)	S = Single (A or V)		

[a]Positions I through III are used exclusively for antibradyarrhythmia function.
From Bernstein AD, Camm AJ, Fletcher RD, et al: The NASPE/BPEG generic pacemaker code for antibradyarrhythmia and adaptive-rate pacing and antitachyarrhythmia devices. PACE 10:794–799, 1987, with permission.

A complete discussion of timing intervals for cardiac pacing is beyond the scope of this chapter.[45] However, an understanding of the basic essentials is necessary for any of the pacing modes and especially for DDD pacemakers, which now represent the majority of implanted generators in most large centers.[46–48]

The term *blanking period* (Fig. 133–13A) refers to the turning off of the sensing amplifier itself to avoid its being driven into saturation by an anticipated high input voltage resulting from a stimulus delivered elsewhere in the heart (e.g., a ventricular pacing stimulus sensed by the atrial channel).[49,50] *Refractory periods* are time intervals incorporated in the timing cycles so that the device will not respond to a sensing system output by resetting the pace-

maker's escape timing during those portions of the cardiac cycle when one may safely anticipate that what is actually triggering the sensing circuit is an appropriate signal, such as T-waves following ventricular pacing stimulus being sensed as R-waves by the ventricular channel.

The *lower rate interval* (LRI) is the longest interval between consecutive ventricular paced events or from a sensed ventricular signal to a subsequent ventricular stimulus, in both cases without an intervening sensed P-wave. The *A-V interval* (AVI) is the programmed interval from the atrial stimulus to the ventricular stimulus (paced A-V), or from the sensed atrial depolarization to the ventricular stimulus (sensed A-V). The *atrial escape interval* (AEI) is the interval from a ventricular pacing stimulus or sensed

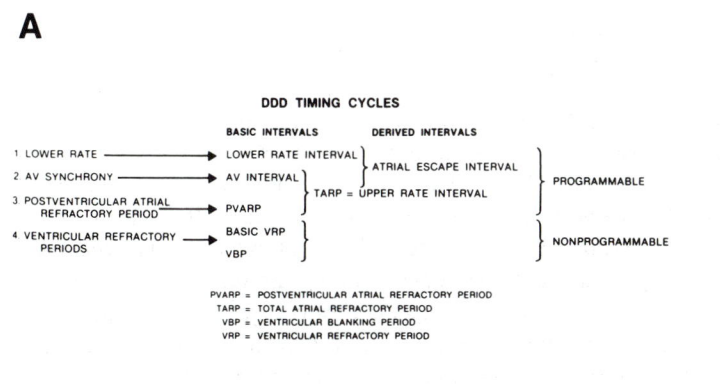

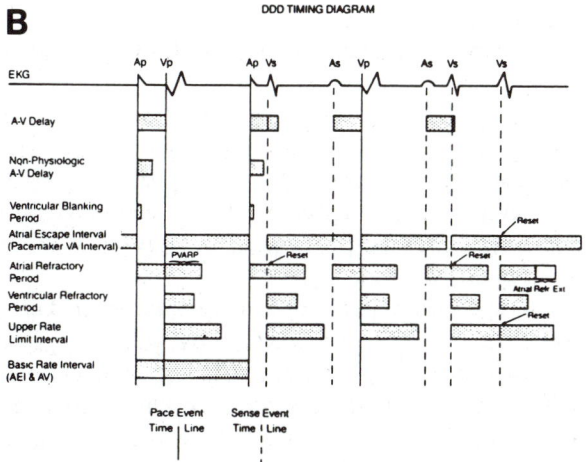

Figure 133–13. A. Basic and derived timing cycles of a simple DDD pulse generator. A simple DDD pulse generator requires three fundamental timing cycles (LRI, A-V, Interval, and PVARP), all of which must be programmable. The atrial escape (pacemaker VA) interval, the TARP, and the URI may be derived from these three basic intervals. As in a VVI pulse generator, the ventricular channel of a DDD pulse generator must generate a VRP. The VPB is necessary to prevent crosstalk; programmability of the VRP and VBP is not essential. *(From Barold et al,[50] with permission.)* **B.** Diagrammatic representation of the timing cycles of a DDD pulse generator. Ap, atrial paced event; As, atrial sensed event, Vp, ventricular paced event; Vs, ventricular sensed event; AEI, atrial escape (pacemaker VA) interval; PVARP, postventricular atrial refractory period; Atrial Refr Ext, arterial refractory period extension, which can be programmed to begin with the onset of a sensed PVC. *(From Barold et al,[49] with permission.)*

ventricular depolarization to the following atrial stimulus (AEI = LRI − AVI). The *ventricular refractory period* is the interval during which the lower rate interval cannot be reset (and reinitiated) by any signal whether or not it is actually recognized by the pulse generator. During this interval the ventricular sensing amplifier is completely (or partially, in certain devices) insensitive to incoming signals. The *post-ventricular atrial refractory period* (PVARP) is the pacemaker atrial refractory period occurring after the emission of a ventricular stimulus or a sensed ventricular event. This refractoriness prevents the atrial channel from sensing the ventricular pacing stimulus or the paced QRS complex. Similarly, the PVARP is programmed longer than the retrograde ventriculoatrial conduction time to prevent atrial sensing of ectopic premature or retrograde atrial depolarization. The *total atrial refractory period* (TARP) is the sum of the AVI and PVARP. The TARP starts with an atrial sensed or paced event, extends through the programmed AV delay, and continues through the PVARP, which is initiated by a ventricular sensed or paced event. The duration of the TARP always defined the shortest upper rate limit interval (or the fastest ventricular tracking rate). The upper rate limit interval can apply to either the atrial or ventricular channel of a dual chamber pacemaker, but is easiest to understand if applied to the ventricular channel. The URI is the shortest interval between two consecutive ventricular stimuli or from a sensed ventricular event to the subsequent ventricular stimulus while maintaining 1:1 A-V synchrony with sensed atrial events. These timing intervals are outlined in Figure 133–13B for the five possible combinations of atrial pacing/sensing shown.[49]

Timing cycles are more readily understood if their historical evolution is understood (Fig. 133–14). A simple VVI pacemaker consists of two timing cycles, the LRI and VRP. A simple DDD generator consists of four: LRI, AV, PVARP, and VRP (Fig. 133–18A). A complex DDD system consists of eight or nine cycles, each of which has been added for a particular feature (pacing or safety).[50]

Base (lower) rate behaviors of DDD, DVI, and DDI modes are similar but not identical, although they can appear similar on the surface ECG with stable A-V sequential pacing. In dual-chamber pacing systems, the VEI is divided into two sub-intervals; the atrial escape interval begins at a sensed or paced ventricular event to the ensuing atrial output pulse. This is followed by a second interval from the atrial output pulse to the ventricular output pulse, which is the atrioventricular interval. The sum of the AVI and AEI equals the VEI or basic pacing interval.[51]

Because of the absence of an atrial sensing circuit, two basic timing cycles are found in the DVI pacing mode, ventricular-based timing and atrial-based timing.[51] In ventricular-based timing, a sensed R-wave will always inhibit the ventricular output and reset the atrial escape interval. In an atrial-based timing system, a sensed R-wave will always inhibit the ventricular output pulse; its effect on the basic timing of the pulse generator will depend on where the R-wave was sensed within the sequence of events. If it is sensed within the AEI it resets the base rate, which is defined by the AA interval. If sensing occurs within the A-V interval, the ventricular output pulse is inhibited but the timing interval is not reset. In devices with atrial sensing capability (e.g., DDD), timing may be either atrial-based or ventricular-based; the majority are ventricular-based, however, where sensing a native P-wave terminates the AEI and initiates the A-V interval, but this then takes the system out of lower rate behavior. Finally, a newer mode of pacing is the DDI mode,[51, 52] where A-V sequential pacing is present with intact atrial sensing but without the ability to track the sensed P-wave. A sensed P-wave that occurs during the AEI will cause inhibition of the atrial output pulse but will not terminate the atrial escape interval timer (Fig. 133–15).

Upper rate behavior is one of the more complex fea-

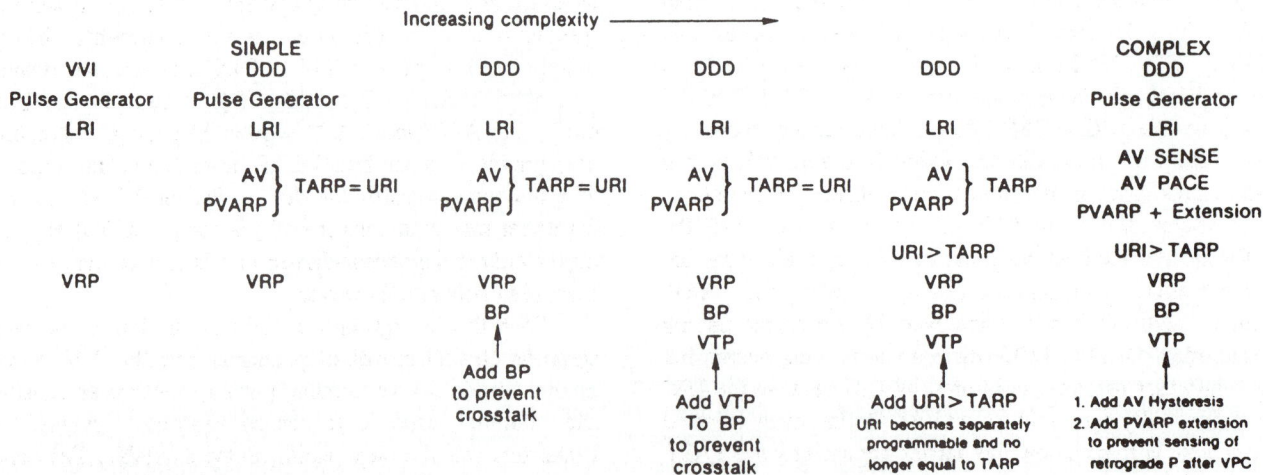

Figure 133–14. The progressive addition of new timing cycles to a simple DDD pacemaker (left) creates a more complex device. *(From Barold et al,[45] with permission.)*

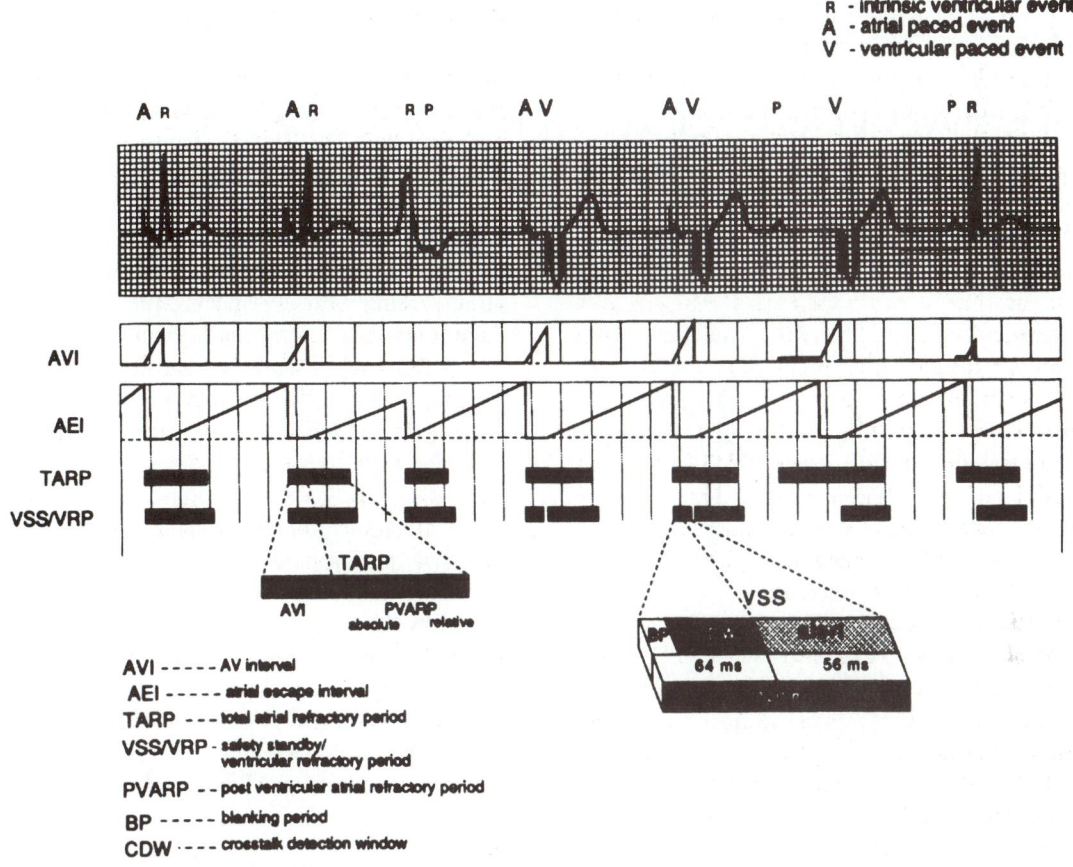

P - intrinsic atrial event
R - intrinsic ventricular event
A - atrial paced event
V - ventricular paced event

AVI ----- AV interval
AEI ----- atrial escape interval
TARP --- total atrial refractory period
VSS/VRP - safety standby/
          ventricular refractory period
PVARP -- post ventricular atrial refractory period
BP ----- blanking period
CDW ---- crosstalk detection window

Figure 133–15. Schematic diagram of the DDI mode including all the critical timing cycles. The timing intervals have been previously described. A sensed P-wave as shown on the next to last complex on this rhythm inhibits the atrial output but does not affect the atrial escape interval, which continues to time out. The sensed P-wave does, however, begin the atrial refractory period, which is primarily involved with sensing and not timing. *(From Floro et al,[53] with permission.)*

tures of dual-chamber pacing.[50,51,54] A pulse generator can track atrial activity at increasingly fast rates until the lower rate interval equals the upper rate interval. As mentioned, the upper rate behavior is governed by the TARP duration, and this limits the paced ventricular response to fast atrial rates because 1:1 tracking of atrial activity can occur only outside the TARP. In these devices, if the URI > TARP a pseudo-Wenckebach response occurs (Fig. 133–16); if the programmable URI = TARP then a fixed ratio of block occurs since the upper rate behavior is controlled by the TARP. This block is symptomatically abrupt but maintains A-V synchrony. If the P–P interval is shorter than the TARP the Wenckebach response cannot occur since the behavior in this circumstance is also governed by the TARP. Further "control" can be achieved by changing pacing modes, from DDD to DDI where atrial sensing occurs but the ventricular response is limited by LRI because the URI is automatically set equal to the LRI. Refinements to atrial rate control at rates below the barrier imposed by the TARP are features on multiprogrammable generators available today. Independent programming of the URI independently of the PVARP permits generators to respond in a pseudo-

Wenckebach fashion to fast atrial rates, which avoids the sudden occurrence of fixed-rate block.

Upper rate response (Fig. 133–17A) is further complicated by the addition of physiologic sensor-driven capability to the basic DDD timing cycles;[52–54] sensor-driven rate responsiveness is discussed more thoroughly below. Briefly, at the upper rate limit, a DDDR device may display several behaviors (Fig. 133–17B): pseudo-Wenckebach block, 2:1 A-V block, A-V sequential pacing, P-synchronous pacing, or a combination of these. The actual response depends upon the particular device. Pseudo-Wenckebach or 2:1 upper rate behavior (or both) is seen in a DDDR pacemaker only if the sensor-driven rate is slower than the patient's intrinsic rate, however.

With this background, a brief discussion of the most common clinical modes of pacing is possible. VVI terminology stands for ventricular pacing, ventricular sensing, and inhibited response to sensed ventricular events. For years, this was the only pacing mode available. The capability for ventricular sensing distinguishes it from VOO, or totally committed asynchronous ventricular pacing. VOO pacing runs the risk of ventricular arrhythmia induction by

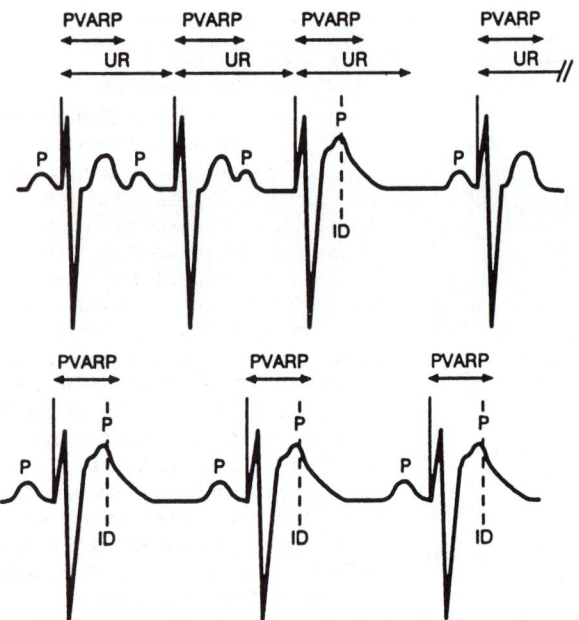

Figure 133–16. Upper panel: In the DDD pacing mode, the programmed UR interval cannot be violated regardless of the sinus rate. When a P-wave is sensed after the PVARP, the AVI is initiated. If, however, at the termination of the AVI delivering a ventricular pacing artifact would violate the UR interval, the ventricular pacing artifact cannot be delivered. The pacemaker waits until completion of the UR interval and then delivers the ventricular pacing artifact; this delay results in prolonged AVI, or pseudo-Wenckebach behavior. **Lower panel:** If the sinus rate becomes so rapid that every other P-wave occurs within the PVARP, effective 2:1 atrioventricular block occurs, that is, every other P-wave is followed by a ventricular pacing artifact. ID, intrinsic deflection. *(From Hayes,[54] with permission.)*

pacing on the T-wave of an intrinsic depolarization, and is currently used for diagnostic purposes only. The VVI pacing mode provides single chamber support, but does not restore A-V synchrony and patients are subject to the pacemaker syndrome, the signs and symptoms related to the adverse hemodynamic and electrophysiologic consequences of ventricular pacing,[55] which can in some patients be quite hemodynamically significant (Fig. 133–18). More recently it has become appreciated that "pacemaker syndrome" can occur with most pacing modes.[56,57] The AAI pacing mode is used infrequently in patients with intact A-V conduction for atrial chronotropic support. Controversy exists as to whether the majority of patients with sick sinus syndrome who are candidates for AAI pacing will eventually require ventricular support as well, and therefore should have a dual-chamber device implanted initially.[58,59] The available data demonstrate that AAI/AAIR pacing is superior to VVI pacing, and that the incidence of subsequent heart block in these patients is low.[59] The DVI pacing mode provides dual chamber support without the benefit of atrial sensing; for years, this was the only form of permanent dual-chamber pacing available; today it remains the commonest mode for temporary external pacing. Two types of DVI systems have

been developed, committed and non-committed; the committed systems deliver the ventricular pacing stimulus at the programmed A-V interval even in the presence of a ventricular sensed event during the A-V interval, which risks pacing during the vulnerable period of the QRST segment. The noncommitted DVI devices ventricular sensing during the A-V interval inhibits ventricular output, even if the sensed activity is inappropriate; this latter circumstance renders the patient at risk for atrial cross-talk and dropped ventricular paced beats. It remains unresolved whether the absence of atrial sensing with DVI pacing predisposes patients to induction of atrial arrhythmias, including atrial fibrillation.[60] The VDD pacing mode senses the atrium and paces the ventricle, and is quite effective in patients with normal sinus node function and various forms of heart block.

The DDD mode incorporates three simpler modes of pacing into the pacemaker logic, namely AAI, DVI, and VDD,[61] and therefore pulse generators limited only to these latter two pacing modes are no longer available. The mode of pacing for a single DDD pacemaker cycle may be determined by the way the cycle terminates in none, one, or two pacemaker stimuli (Fig. 133–19). This simplification is useful in analysis of DDD pacing electrograms and in conceptualizing the function of universal DDD pacemakers under circumstances or changing atrial activity (DVI, VDD) or ventricular activity (AAI, DVI, VDD).

Rate Responsiveness

Perhaps the most dramatic advance in cardiac pacing in the past 5 years has been the clinical implementation of rate responsiveness into all forms of single- and dual-chamber pacing. The goal of all sensor-driven rate adaptive pacing is to control heart rate changes as a function of level of activity, and to control heart rate as a function of time before, during, and after activity. As demonstrated in Figure 133–17, this physiologic sensor activity is superimposed over the basic elements of single- or dual-chamber pacing described above.[54]

The theoretical basis for rate-adaptive pacing derives from the fact that in the normal heart, the chronotropic responsiveness that accompanies physical exertion is the primary mechanism for increasing forward cardiac output.[62–64] The general consensus now is that similar improvement can be demonstrated in pacemaker patients.[65] Multiple studies have demonstrated both subjective and objective improvement with VVIR as compared to VVI pacing, independent of whether A-V synchrony was maintained;[62,63] other studies have demonstrated similar exercise responses (oxygen consumption with exercise) with VVIR as compared to DDD pacing, independent of the A-V interval.[5,7,67] The sustained benefit of DDDR as compared to VVIR pacing has been demonstrated by some investigators,[3] but these results require additional confirmation.[65]

The programmable parameters that affect heart rate

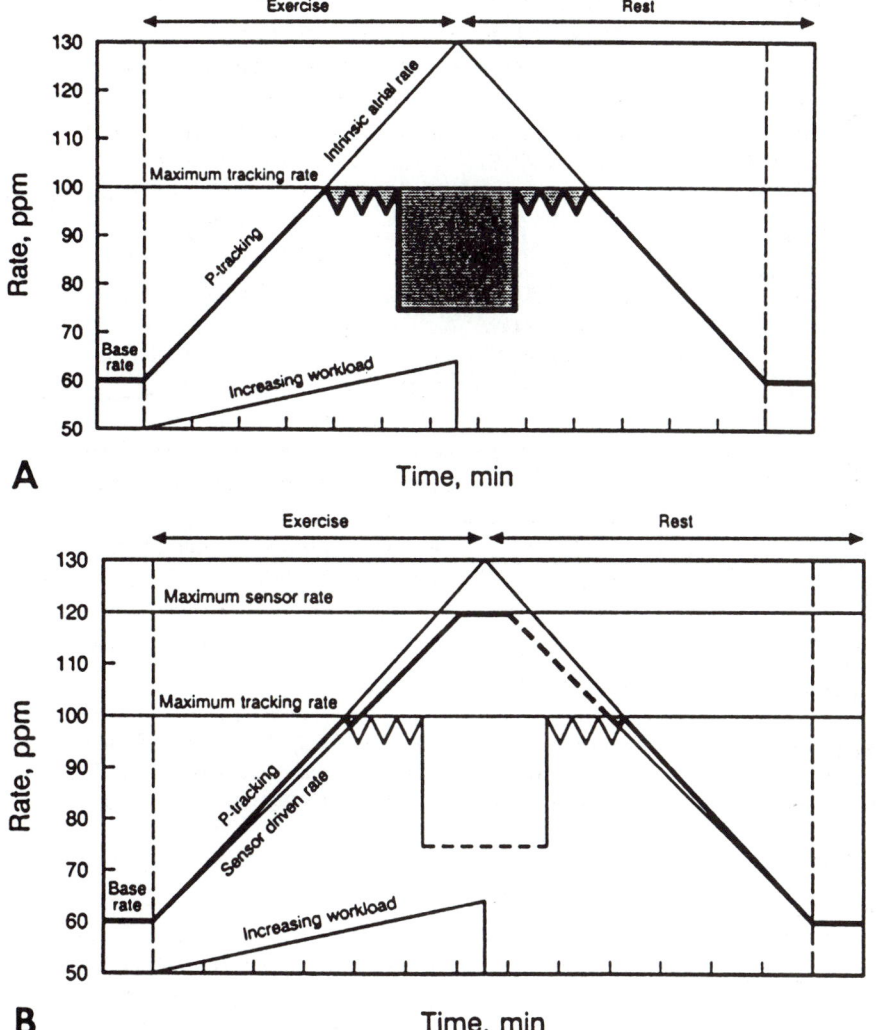

Figure 133–17. A. Diagram illustrating the rate response of a DDD pacemaker with Wenckebach-type block at the upper rate limit (100 ppm). The heavy black line represents the ventricular paced rate, assuming complete heart block. Note the varying RR intervals during Wenckebach-type block as the atrial rate exceeds the maximum tracking rate. (The shaded area is meant to represent potential paced ventricular rates that may occur during DDD upper rate behavior.) After termination of exercise, if the patient's atrial rate had increased to the point that the pacemaker was responding to every other P-wave, that is 2:1 block the paced ventricular rate will actually increase to the maximum tracking rate as the atrial rate slows and fewer P-waves fall within the PVARP. **B.** Diagram illustrating the rate response of the DDDR pacemaker and its behavior at both the maximum tracking and the maximum sensor rates. The heavy black line shows the ventricular paced rate, assuming complete heart block, as it progresses from the P-tracking mode to atrioventricular sequential pacing through a period of Wenckebach-type block. The rate may increase to the programmed maximum sensor rate. At termination of exercise, the ventricular paced rate gradually decreases to the base rate or lower rate limit unless activity resumes. Pseudo-Wenckebach activity can be minimized by optimal programming of the sensor rate response parameters. *(From Hayes,[54] with permission.)*

changes as a function of activity are the lower rate and the upper rate, the rate above which the clinician does not want the device to pace. All types of sensors have a programmable calibration factor, which determines the relative heart rate change for any given change in sensor output. For certain types of sensors, the rate response (slope of the rate vs. activity curve) and the activity (sensor) threshold (minimum level of activity required to engage the sensor) are also programmable. Acceleration and deceleration parameters that affect the heart rate as a function of time at the beginning of activity and after activity is completed have been incorporated into some circuits.[65] Finally, rate-adaptive A-V delay has been incorporated into the timing cycles of newer dual chamber rate-responsive devices.

Clinical studies have demonstrated an improved sense of well-being at rest[66] with a decrease in the tendency to develop congestive heart failure over time[67] with these devices. Preservation of an organized rhythm by atrial pacing in the setting of A-V synchrony is associated with a reduced risk of atrial fibrillation and its complications.[68] Compared to VVIR pacing, rate adaptive A-V sequential pacing with

presumably more optimal timing provided a small but consistent improvement of cardiac output during exertion.[69,70]

The current and investigational sensor technology is listed in Table 133–3. *Direct metabolic indicators* include central venous pH[71,72] and mixed venous oxygen saturation[73,74]; a fall in either of these parameters was concomitant with the onset of exercise and an indication for chronotropic responsiveness. Problems with sensor stability have occurred with both systems, but advances with the mixed venous system continue to be made and this may ultimately be demonstrated to be clinically beneficial.[75] *Indirect metabolic sensors* include respiration rate and minute ventilation. The relationship between respiratory frequency and heart rate is relatively linear over a broad range in most patients.[45] A low-amplitude high-frequency signal to measure transthoracic impedance is used to assess chest movement and thereby respiratory rate; this same technology has been incorporated to estimate minute ventilation (the product of respiratory rate and tidal volume), which closely reflects the metabolic demands of exercise, stress, and pyrexia.[76] A strong correlation was shown to exist between

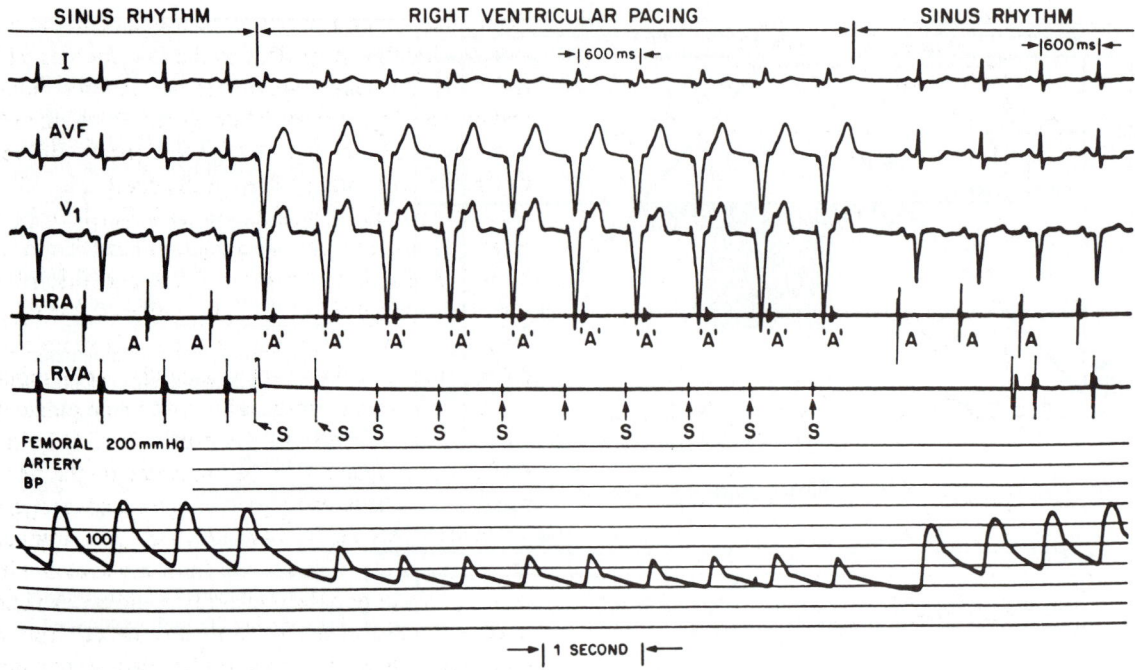

Figure 133–18. Hemodynamic consequences of ventricular pacing with retrograde atrial conduction in a patient with hypertensive heart disease and symptoms of the pacemaker syndrome. The patient is initially in sinus rhythm at 100 bpm. Ventricular pacing is initiated at an identical rate and is associated with retrograde atrial activation (A). Despite a constant identical ventricular rate, an abrupt and marked decline in systolic arterial pressure, from 145 to 85 mm Hg, is observed during ventricular pacing. Cessation of ventricular pacing is associated with gradual recovery of normal arterial pressure. HRA, high right atrium; RVA, right ventricular apex; A, antegrade atrial activation; S, pacing stimulus; BP, blood pressure. *(From Goldschlager N, Saksena S: Hemodynamics of cardiac pacing. In Saksena S, Goldschlager N (eds): Electrical Therapy for Cardiac Arrhythmias. Philadelphia, W. B. Saunders, 1990, pp 163–172, with permission.)*

transthoracic impedance and minute ventilation; with the development of an algorithm to link recorded intravascular electrical impedance from bipolar pacing leads and tidal volume, minute ventilation-based rate-adaptive pacing became clinically feasible.[77,78] The first generation of these devices had a slow pacing rate acceleration as well as a delayed onset of rate response; these problems have been addressed in the second generation of these devices, both by programmable parameters.[79] Other *indirect metabolic sensors* include mixed venous temperature.[80] Temperature changes of the blood pool result in alteration of thermistor impedance and signal the need for adjustment of pacing rate. However, as indicated on Table 133–3, a special endocardial pacing lead is needed and this has lessened enthusiasm for this approach. *Nonmetabolic physiologic indices* include QT interval detection,[81] evoked ventricular potential indicators,[82] systolic indices,[83] and pressure sensors to measure dP/dy[84]; of these, only stim-T (QT) detection has achieved widespread clinical use. The rest remain investigational or have been shown to be of no additional benefit above current sensor technology due to algorithm or lead considerations.

The most commonly utilized technology is a *direct estimation of physical activity,* either as a direct activity sensor or accelerometer.[85,86] Both use a piezoelectric crystal in the pacemaker to sense direct musculoskeletal activity from the chest wall.[86] The first configuration responds to vibra-

tory (pressure wave) activity, principally induced from the shock of footsteps hitting the ground; this approach forms the basis for the most clinically utilized rate-adaptive devices.[87–89] In the accelerometer approach, the small seismic mass responds to acceleration or deceleration caused by total body movement. Accelerotometer signals are centered in the low-frequency range at less than 4 Hz, while vibratory piezoelectric sensors are mainly in the range of 10 Hz.[86]

Rate-adaptive pacing has become a mainstay of current pacemaker technology and therapy. It requires careful implant follow-up and programming to optimize and individualize therapy for a particular patient. Active research into combining sensor technology into a multiple sensor system is ongoing, leading ultimately to the development of a truly "smart" pacemaker system capable of autoprogramming and self-adjustment to meet clinical demands.[90]

CLINICAL ASPECTS OF CARDIAC PACEMAKER IMPLANTATION

Indications for Cardiac Pacemaker Implantation

With the advent of this technology, the indications for cardiac pacing have grown from complete heart block, which was the first indication for pacing, to a large number of relatively complicated supraventricular and ventricular con-

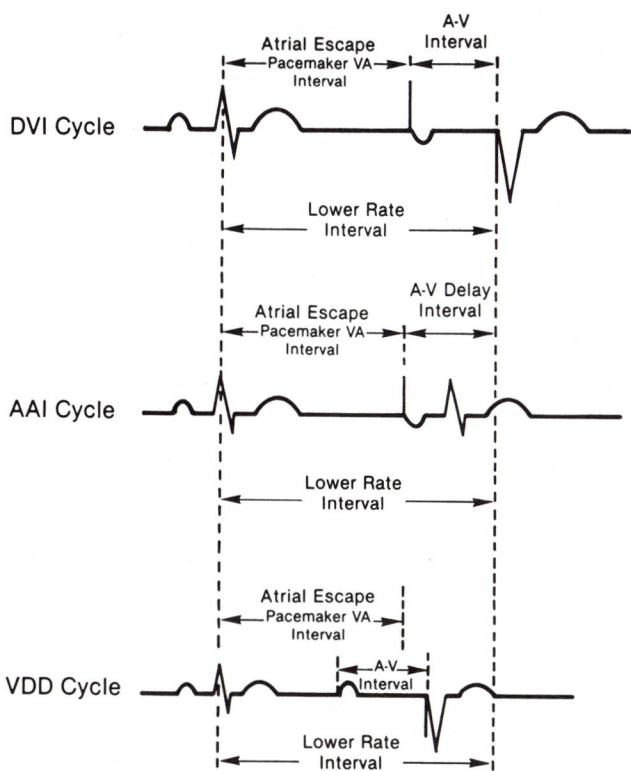

Figure 133–19. Behavior of a DDD pacemaker based on examination of a single cycle. Starting with either a paced or sensed ventricular event, DVI, AAI, or VDD may be seen. The mode described for a single pacemaker cycle is determined by the way the cycle terminates. *(From Barold et al,[45] with permission.)*

duction disturbances. In 1991, the ACC/AHA task force published the latest guidelines for implantation of cardiac pacemakers.[91] These guidelines are summarized in Table 133–4. These guidelines emphasize (1) their applicability to chronic, although sometimes intermittent, disorders of cardiac rhythm, and only after careful analysis of each patent and the patient's problem; and (2) the association of clinical symptoms with the arrhythmia (particularly bradycardia) for which the device is being implanted.

The final decision regarding pacemaker implantation should ideally be made in conjunction with the primary care provider, a cardiology and/or electrophysiology consultant, and the implanting physician.[48] The practice of self-referral in pacemaker therapy, like any other therapy for cardiovascular disease, should be heartily discouraged. Given the variability of certain of the underlying arrhythmias, and the multiprogrammability of the devices, the options for pacing in the present era are multiple and complex and require a great deal of expertise to maximally benefit the individual patient[92] (Fig. 133–20). The implanting physician is responsible for assuming a major role in this decision.

Implantation Techniques for Permanent Pacemaker Systems

The most common approach to permanent transvenous pacemaker implantation is subclavian cannulation tech-

nique, most often performed on the patient's nondominant side. Positioning the patient on the fluoroscopic table with a roll down the spine hyperflexes the anterior thoracic cage and makes venous cannulation easier. Anatomic considerations are important, since there are subtle differences between the right and left sides of the chest (Fig. 133–21). On the left, the vein is medial and superficial to the artery in most patients, and can be cannulated just lateral to the fibrous junction between the clavicle and first rib articulation. On the right side, the angle of entry of the right subclavian vein into the superior vena cava is more abrupt, and therefore cannulation of the subclavian vein slightly more laterally allows for additional room to manipulate the guide wire and introducers; this is particularly helpful when a dual chamber system is to be implanted on the right side. In patients who have had previous open heart surgery the innominate artery tends to be pulled caudad. Cannulation of the vein too far medially has been associated with an increased incidence of lead (electrode and/or insulation) fracture, especially when two leads are placed. This has been attributed to pressure on the lead by the fibrous junction of the clavicle and first rib articulation with chest wall and arm movement.[93]

The subclavian technique has been well-described. With high-fidelity ECG monitoring, the patient is positioned supine on the fluoroscopic operating table. The majority of implants can be performed under straight local xylocain anesthesia; a few patients will need light intravenous sedation as well. All patients should be covered with three doses of prophylactic perioperative intravenous antibiotics. After sterile preparation of the skin and creation of a sterile field (Fig. 133–22A), an incision is made on the anterior chest wall 1 to 1.5 cm below the middle third of the clavicle. This site permits access to both the subclavian and the cephalic vein through the same skin incision. A generator pocket is created, following the plane of the anterior pectoralis fascia. Electrocautery is used, which effectively prevents subsequent hemorrhage and hematoma formation, even in patients on anticoagulation. The patient is placed in steep Trendelenburg position and the subclavian vein is cannulated with an 18-gauge 4-cm needle (Fig. 133–22B). Nonpulsatile flow is confirmed and a flexible guidewire is advanced into the vein and into the superior vena cava, where the position is confirmed by fluoroscopy. If difficulty is encountered in cannulating the vein or passing the guidewire, injection of a small amount of dilute radiographic dye can be helpful in delineating the vascular anatomy.

The endocardial lead(s) are prepared for insertion by placing a gentle curve in the stylet of the ventricular lead and using a preformed J stylet in the atrial lead. A 10.0 or 10.5 F sheathed introducer is passed over the guidewire under fluoroscopic visualization and the lead is introduced through the vein. The guidewire is left in place as the sheath is withdrawn, and the second sheath is passed over the wire with introduction of the second lead (Fig. 133–22C). Alternatively, after placement of the first lead, the subclavian

TABLE 133–3.   MAJOR CLASSES OF SENSORS USED IN RATE-RESPONSIVE PACEMAKER TECHNOLOGY

Physiologic Methods	Physiologic Parameters	Manufacturer	Model
Generator-Based Sensor Mechanisms			
Impedance sensing	Respiratory rate	Biotec	Biorate
	Minute ventilation	Telectronics	Meta
	Stroke volume	CPI	Precept
	Preejection period		
	Right ventricular ejection time		
Ventricular-evoked response and output pulse parameter sensing	Evoked QT interval	Viatron	Quintex, TX Rhythmx
	Evoked R-wave area ("gradient") trailing edge of output pulse	Telectronics	Prism-CL
Activity sensing	Musculoskeletal vibration	Medtronic	Activitrax
			Legend
			Elite
			Thera DR
		Pacesetter	Synchrony I-III
			Solus I-II
	Accelerometer	CPI	Excel
		Intermedics	Relay
			Dash
Electrode-Based Sensor Mechanisms			
Physical parameters	Central venous temperature	Cook	Kelvin 500
		Intermedics	Nova MR
	dP/dt		
	Average atrial rate	Medtronic	Deltatrax
	Right atrial pressure	CPI	RS4
	Pulmonary artery pressure		
Chemical parameters	pH		
	Mixed venous oxygen satruation	Medtronic	
		Pacesetter	
	Catecholamine levels		

Adapted from Lau C-P: Clinical comparison of currently available sensor-based rate adaptive pacing systems. In Benditt BG (ed): Rate Adaptive Pacing. Boston, Blackwell Scientific Publications, 1993, p 201.

vein may be cannulated a second time, using the first lead as a marker; this can be helpful in thin or asthenic patients where the angle between the clavicle and first rib is small.

The ventricular lead is then passed under fluoroscopic visualization into the right atrium, across the tricuspid valve, into the right ventricle, and into the pulmonary outflow tract (Fig. 133–22D). From the right subclavian approach, the lead tip is allowed to curl in the right atrium and then flip across the tricuspid valve. The curved stylet is withdrawn and replaced with the straight stylet, which is carefully advanced out to the tip of the lead. The entire lead is gently withdrawn, permitting the tip to follow the course of the pulmonary outflow tract down into the ventricular chamber. When the tip flips into the distal right ventricular chamber the position is usually acceptable without further manipulation. If additional positioning is necessary over a small distance (0.5 cm), then the stylet should be withdrawn 2 to 3 cm before this is performed to prevent possible perforation of the free wall. Pacing and sensing parameters are obtained as outlined below, and if acceptable the lead is secured in place (Fig. 133–22E). This process may need to be repeated to adequately position the lead into the apex of the right ventricle and/or meet implant criteria.

The atrial lead is passed from the superior vena cava into the right atrium with the J stylet in place. In patients without previous open heart surgery this maneuver will usually locate the tip of the lead in the appendage (Fig. 133–22F). In patients without an appendage the lead tip will usually need to be manipulated and pace-mapping performed to locate an adequate site. Final positioning is checked by fluoroscopy, and these positions should correlate with the findings on a postoperative chest roentgenogram (Fig. 133–23A).

If subclavian access is difficult, the cephalic vein provides an alternate access route after dissection from within the deltopectoral groove (Fig. 133–21). Following distal ligation of the vein and placement of a proximal self-retaining (Pott's) ligature, the vein is opened. One lead may conveniently be passed into this vein and from there into the subclavian vein, but two leads are often too large. Additional options in this circumstance are to pass the guidewire into the opened cephalic vein, confirm its position in the subclavian vein, and pass the sheaths over this wire, or to use the first lead/wire to guide subsequent cannulation of the subclavian vein. In difficult access situations the external or internal jugular veins may be used, but these ap-

TABLE 133–4. SUMMARY OF IMPLANTATION GUIDELINES FOR PACEMAKER SYSTEMS*a*

1. AAI/AAIR mode
  A. Indications
    1. Symptomatic sinus node dysfunction with demonstrated adequate A-V conduction (AAI)
    2. Hemodynamic enhancement through rate adjustment in patients who have bradycardia and symptoms of impaired cardiac output, with demonstrated adequate A-V conduction (AAI)
    3. 1 and 2, above, in the presence of chronotropic incompetence and an anticipated high level of physical activity, normal A-V conduction, and little evidence for intrinsic or drug-induced A-V block (AAIR)
  B. Contraindications
    1. Preexisting A-V conduction delay or block, or if decremental conduction is demonstrated at slow paced rates by testing
    2. Inadequate atrial pacing/sensing thresholds
    3. Inexcitable atrial tissue

2. VVI/VVIR mode
  A. Indications
    1. Symptomatic bradyarrhythmia in the setting of no significant atrial hemodynamic contribution to cardiac output (e.g., chronic atrial fibrillation/SVT (VVI)
    2. No evidence of pacemaker syndrome (VVI)
    3. Symptomatic bradycardia where pacing simplicity is a prime concern (e.g., senility, terminal disease, etc.) (VVI)
    4. 1 and 2, above, with the presence of chronotropic incompetence and an anticipated high level of physical activity (VVIR)
  B. Contraindications
    1. Known pacemaker syndrome
    2. Retrograde VA conduction with angina pectoris or CHF
    3. CHF where atrial contribution to cardiac output is important

3. DDD/DDDR mode
  A. Indications
    1. Requirement for A-V synchrony over a wide range of rates (DDD)
    2. Complete heart block or sick sinus syndrome and stable atrial rates (DDD)
    3. When simultaneous control of atrial and ventricular rates can be demonstrated to inhibit tachyarrhythmias directly or by programming changes (DDD)
    4. 1–3, above, in patients with chronotropic incompetence and an anticipated moderate to high level of activity and in whom there is a stable atrial rhythm (DDDR)
  B. Contraindications
    1. Frequent or persistent supraventricular tachyarrhythmias, including atrial fibrillation and/or flutter
    2. Inadequate atrial pacing/sensing thresholds
    3. Severe ischemic heart disease where angina is precipitated by an increased rate

4. DDI/DDIR mode
  A. Indications
    1. Patients who require dual-chamber pacing and who have frequent, but not constant, supraventricular arrhythmias; atrial arrhythmias caused by competitive pacing are avoided because the atrial output is inhibited by an atrial or ventricular event (DDI)
    2. 1, above, in patients with chronotropic incompetence and an anticipated moderate to high level of activity and in whom dual-chamber pacing is needed (DDIR).
  B. Contraindication
    1. Same as for 3B, above

*a*The benefits of DDI/DDIR pacing can also be achieved by mode switching, a feature that automatically changes the mode of the pacemaker to a nonatrial tracking mode when an atrial tachycardia occurs, and back to an atrial tracking mode when the tachycardia ceases.

proaches require passage of the lead(s) either anterior to the clavicle with risk of subsequent lead fracture, or posterior to the clavicle with a risk of vascular trauma.

Epicardial Pacemaker Implantation

The subxiphoid or anterior thoracotomy approach is used for epicardial ventricular lead implantation in adults with difficult endocardial pacing problems and occasionally in children. Most commonly this is due to multiple endocardial lead failures, abnormalities of thoracic venous anatomy, the presence of congenital heart disease, the presence of a tricuspid valve prosthesis, or repeated development of exit block of endocardial leads. However, with the advances in technology even small infants who require pac-

ing for congenital conduction defects can usually undergo transvenous implantation of a device; the leads are positioned so as to permit growth of the child.[94,95] Furthermore, lead extraction techniques, discussed below, now permit removal of almost all types of endocardial leads in experienced hands.

The subxiphoid approach is the preferred epicardial route in patients who have not undergone previous cardiac surgery. Under local anesthesia, a subcostal incision is made below the xiphoid process and the midline of the abdomen identified (Fig. 133–24A). The xiphoid process is removed or retracted superiorly, exposing the fascial attachments of the rectus muscle sheaths to the anterior diaphragm. After dissecting the subcutaneous fat underneath the xiphoid the pericardial reflection off the diaphragm is

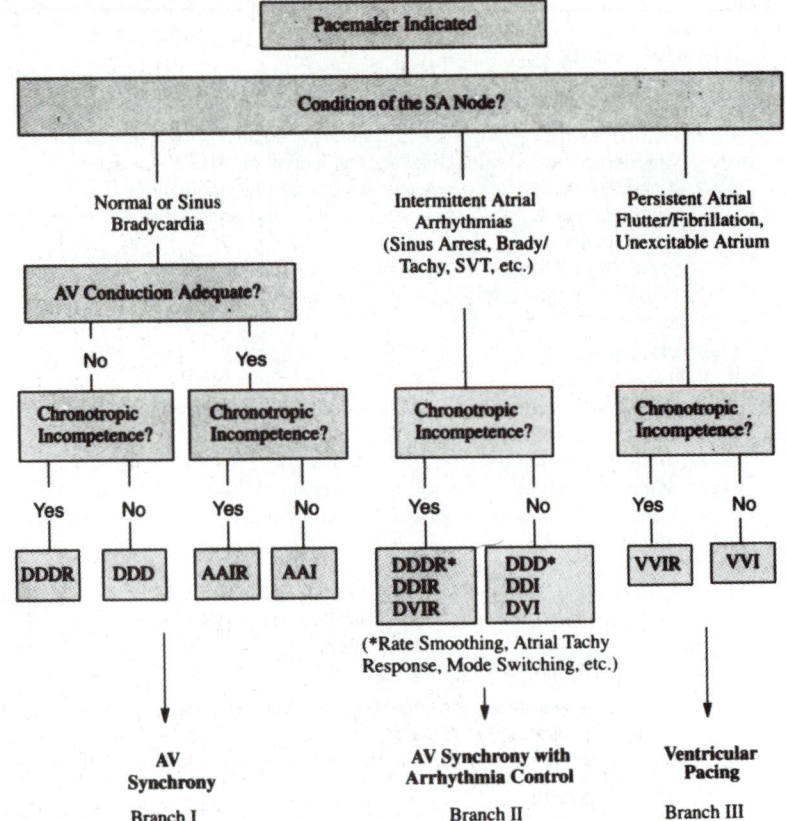

Figure 133–20. Algorithm for selection of the optimal pacing mode. The decision tree considers three basic points: (1) the status of the sinoatrial node; (2) the status of atrioventricular conduction; and (3) the presence of chronotropic incompetence. *(Modified from Bodenhamer RM, Grantham RN: Mode selection—the therapeutic challenge. In Adaptive Rate Pacing: Perspectives in Cardiac Rhythm Management. St. Paul, Cardiac Pacemakers, 1993, p 43.)*

exposed and incised (Fig. 133–24B and C). The epicardial screw-in electrodes are secured to the diaphragmatic surface of the heart to the right side of the interventricular septum, or onto the anterior right ventricular free wall (Fig. 133–24D). The pericardium is closed around the leads, and the generator is placed in the subcutaneous tissue or in extremely asthenic individuals below the left rectus muscle. Lead position is confirmed on the postoperative roentgenogram (Fig. 133–23B).

The anterior thoracotomy approach is useful for patients who have undergone previous cardiac surgery. Access is obtained through the fifth intercostal space anteriorly, allowing exposure of the anterolateral left ventricular free wall as the site for electrode placement. The lead(s) are tunneled into a generator pocket in the left upper abdominal quadrant subcutaneous tissue.

A major limitation of both of these approaches is the lack of access to the right atrium for dual-chamber lead placement. Epicardial pacing from the left atrial appendage can be accomplished through an anterior thoracotomy approach. Alternatively, a median sternotomy may be performed; however, the limitations in longevity of atrial epicardial leads make this approach less ideal than the endocardial approach, or placement of a rate-responsive VVIR device through the subxiphoid approach.

Electrophysiologic Testing of Acute Endocardial and Epicardial Pacemaker Leads

Optimal placement of endocardial leads is a combination of (1) acceptable electrophysiologic parameters, (2) visualization assessment on fluoroscopic exam, and (3) adequate securing of the lead. The electrophysiologic data obtained need to be interpreted in light of the acute and chronic natural history of the lead parameters, discussed earlier. The acute parameters measured for each lead at the time of implant include pacing threshold energy requirements, atrial and ventricular endocardial electrogram amplitudes, slew rates (if necessary), lead resistance, and the current at the threshold level for capture of the chamber being paced and at the voltage and pulsewidth parameters of the generator to be implanted (usually 4 to 5 V output at a pulsewidth of 0.4 to 0.5 ms). These recordings are made with a Pacing System Analyzer capable of independently altering each of these parameters that is directly connected to the lead being tested.

After lead placement, voltage parameters are measured by pacing at 0.5 ms and progressively lower voltages until capture is lost, as dictated by the strength–duration curve. Acute threshold measurements depend upon (1) the type of lead (active fixation or passive, steroid eluting, etc.), (2) the

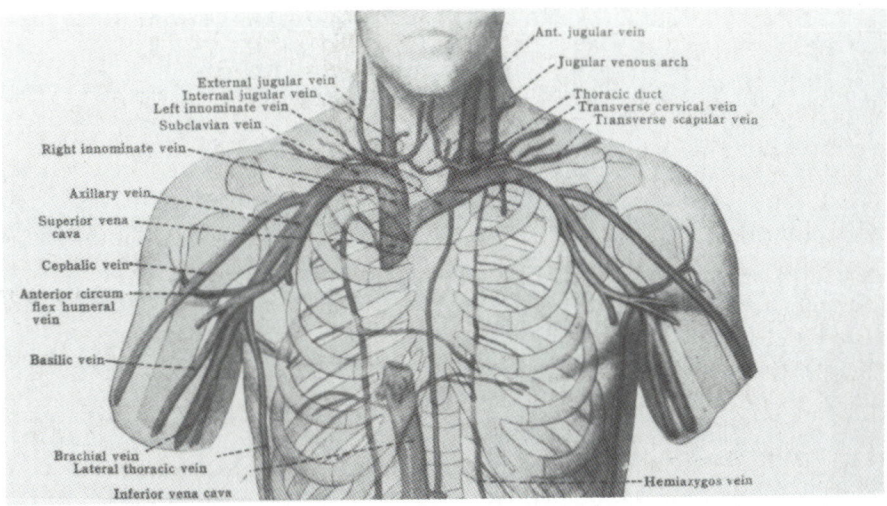

A

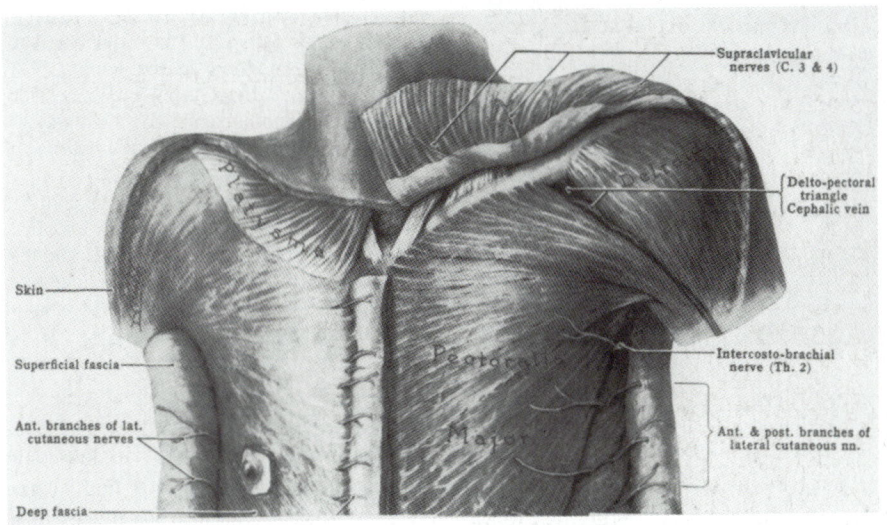

B

Figure 133–21. A. Anatomy of subclavian vein on left and right sides. *(From Schaeffer JP: Morris' Human Anatomy, 10th ed. Philadelphia, Blakiston, 1942, p 703.)* **B.** Position of the cephalic vein in the deltopectoral groove on the anterior chest wall. *(Modified from Grant JCB: Grant's Atlas of Anatomy, 6th ed. Baltimore, Williams & Wilkins, 1972, plate 13.1, with permission.)*

lead–tissue interface, (3) the location within the heart of the lead, and (4) with active fixation leads the duration of time following fixation that the recordings are made. This is because active fixation leads induce a current of injury in the surrounding myocardium with engagement of the fixation mechanism, which can take 5 to 10 min to dissipate the majority of this current. Low capture thresholds are necessary because as the lead–tissue interface matures over time there is an influx of inflammatory cells that produces an acute rise in pacing threshold over the first 2 to 3 wk postimplant that may be two or three times the voltage at implant. Over the next 2 to 3 wk, as the inflammatory response subsides and fibrotic scar tissue is formed around the tip of the lead, the thresholds become chronic and are elevated approximately twice over the implant data recordings on the average. Steroid-eluting leads with a small reservoir of corticosteroid at the tip, which is eluted over the first 6 mo, have been demonstrated to ameliorate this

initial acute rise in threshold, and have remained low chronically over time.[32] In general, active fixation leads tend to have higher chronic thresholds than tined passive fixation leads, but whether this translates into shortened battery longevity is difficult to demonstrate.

As indicated in Eq. (2), Ohm's law dictates that the resistance on the lead at 5 V (nominal generator output) is calculated by dividing the voltage output by the current at 5 V; with standard pacing leads, resistance should vary between 300 and 800 Ω. Low resistances can be caused by a number of factors, including electrode malposition within the ventricle or a parallel electrical pathway (e.g., current flowing through a stimulating and nonstimulating pathway, such as an insulation break). Resistances below 300 Ω cause higher currents and are unsatisfactory for pacing, because current is wasted and battery life is shortened; leaking current has been associated with exit block or muscle stimulation. High resistance (> 800 Ω) increases battery life for

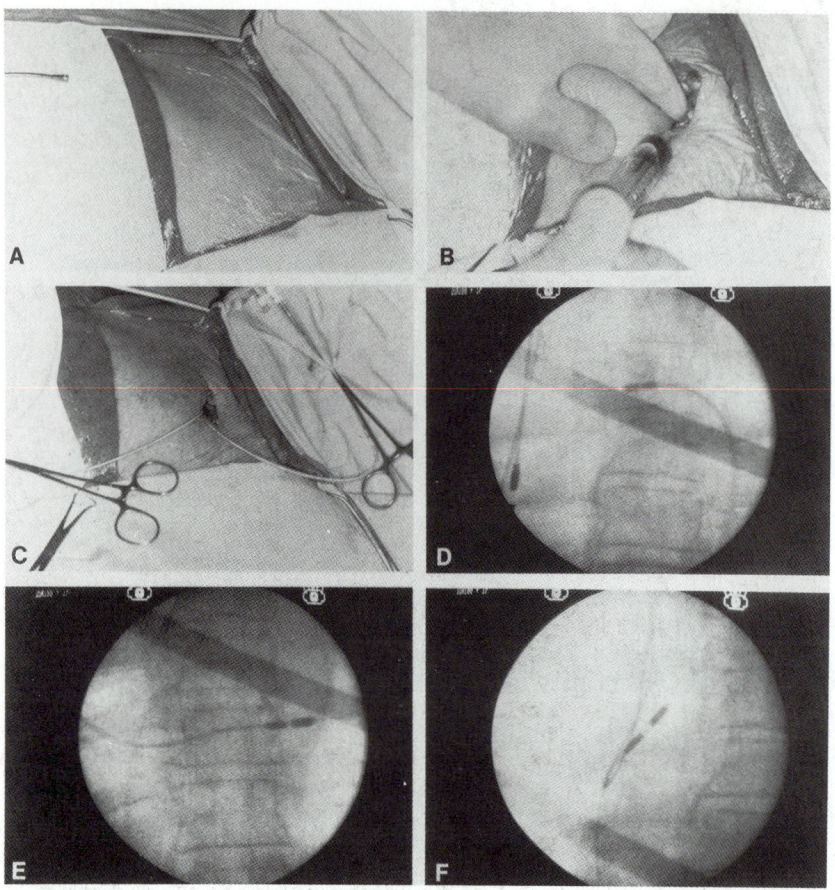

Figure 133–22. A. Sterile surgical preparation for a left-sided implant. **B.** After making the infraclavicular incision and creating the pacemaker pocket, the patient is placed in Trendelenburg position and the subclavian vein is cannulated. **C.** Both leads may be passed over a single guidewire, using a standard peel-away sheath technique. **D.** The ventricular lead tip is positioned into the pulmonary artery confluence with a curved stylet, and its position is confirmed by fluoroscopy. Note the atrial lead tip temporarily positioned in the right atrium (on the right of the screen). **E.** The ventricular stylet is exchanged for a straight stylet and the entire lead is withdrawn into the right ventricle; the lead tip is positioned into the apex of the right ventricular chamber under fluoroscopy. **F.** Fluoroscopic position of the atrial lead in the right atrium.

both constant current and constant voltage pacemakers but may decrease the current delivered to the heart to inadequate levels.

Along with pacing and system parameters, the filtered amplitude of the P- or R-wave is measured as depicted above. Both the amplitude (minivolts) and frequency (slew rate) of the waveform are measured by the Pacemaker System Analyzer. In general, acute bipolar electrograms greater than 6 mV for tined ventricular leads and 1.5 mV for tined atrial leads are acceptable acute parameters that will provide for adequate chronic sensing; slightly higher electrograms should be achieved for acutely placed active fixation leads. Acute ventricular slew rate parameters for bipolar leads should be 0.75 mV/s or higher while atrial slew rates should be 0.5 mV/s or greater.

Testing for diaphragmatic (ventricular lead) and phrenic (atrial lead) nerve pacing is performed by a 10-V PSA output with deep inspiration, exhalation, and coughing. The leads are secured proximally and connected to the generator, which has been programmed to specifications, including lower and upper rate, and pulse width, voltage, current, sensitivity, refractory period, and polarity for each channel as well as A-V interval(s).

As indicated by Eq. (4), the energy output of a genera-

tor can be calculated to determine the safety factor for acute pacing parameters. Most generators are nominally programmed to 4 or 5 V output and 0.4 or 0.5 ms pulsewidth. This results in a greater than four- to fivefold safety factor (defined as generator output divided by threshold at a given pulsewidth) for the acute implant if threshold criteria are met. The recommended chronic safety factor for energy is 3, while for voltage it is 1.75; these parameters can be achieved by testing threshold for both voltage and pulsewidth, then increasing pulsewidth by a factor of 3, or increasing the voltage by a factor of 2 at the same pulsewidth.

For epicardial leads, a similar sequence of measurements are made with the PSA prior to generator implantation. In general, the pacing threshold should be 0.5 V (bipolar) and the R-wave amplitude should be greater than 6 mV. The slew rate should be greater than 0.75 mV/s.

Follow-up of Pacemaker Patients

The majority of pacemaker implants done electively can be performed on an outpatient basis or 23-hour overnight observation. Three doses of perioperative intravenous antibi-

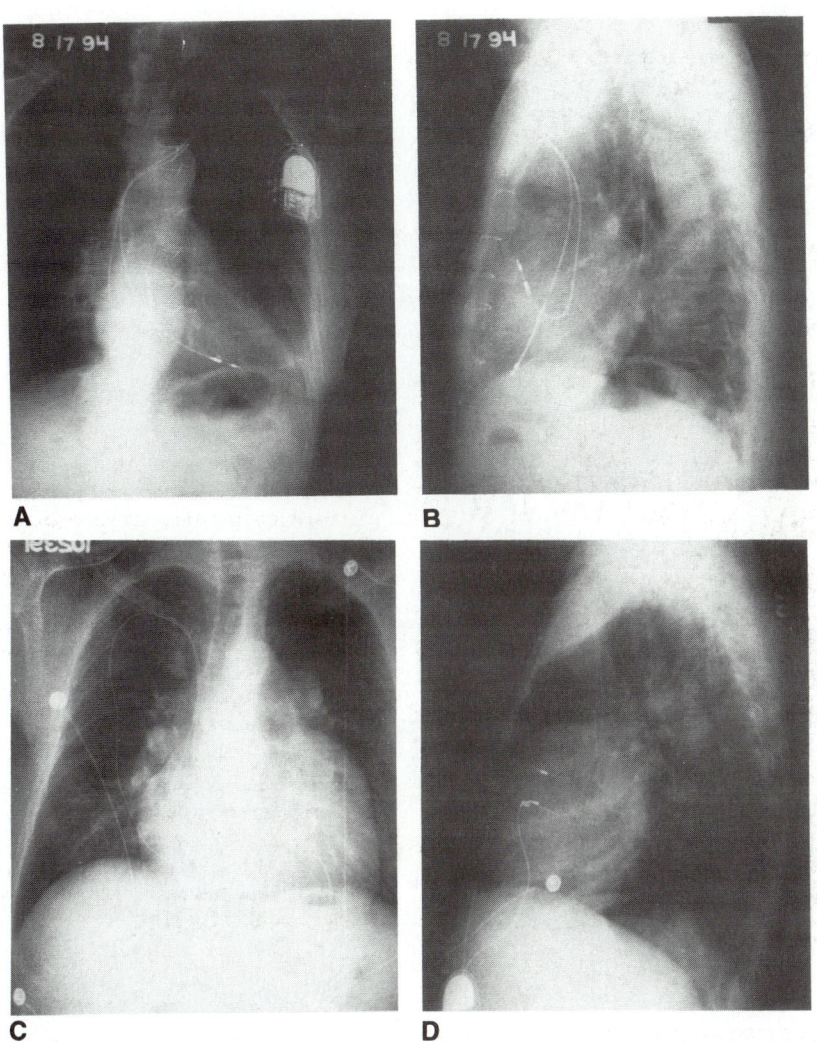

Figure 133–23. Posteroanterior (**A**) and lateral (**B**) chest roentgenogram of endocardial leads following coronary revascularization in a 78-year-old patient who required dual chamber pacing for intermittent atrial flutter. Posteroanterior (**C**) and lateral (**D**) chest roentgenogram of an epicardial ventricular lead combined with an endocardial atrial lead; both leads were tunneled into a generator pocket in the left upper quadrant of the abdomen.

otic coverage are provided according to the prevailing microbiology at the implantation institution. An absorbable subcuticular closure with Steri-Strips (3M Company, Minneapolis, MN) provides excellent cosmesis.

Given the complexity of the pacemaker technology, adequate follow-up of these patients is absolutely mandatory.[96] In general this has gone beyond the scope of many practitioners not actively involved in electrophysiologic cardiovascular disease. Postimplant, all patients undergo a complete pacemaker system evaluation; all devices are multiprogrammable, using a radiofrequency induction coil to communicate with the device. The sensing and pacing characteristics of the generator are fine-tuned to provide an adequate safety factor for pacing and sensing. In patients with rate responsiveness, the activity mode is activated and the parameters for this (slope, acceleration, deceleration, and upper rate) are set. Follow-up after discharge is usually by pacemaker telephone telemetry, where the basic characteristics of the pacemaker system can be determined over a special telephone connection. Occult problems with programming, generator end-of-life, or changes in the underlying rhythm can readily be detected with these simple yet effective devices. The complexity of the current pacemaker systems requires that most patients return to the pacemaker center for a complete evaluation once or twice a year.

Temporary External Cardiac Pacing

Most commonly, temporary cardiac pacing is used following all types of open heart surgery, both in adults and children. Temporary atrial and ventricular pacing wires are placed at the time of the operation and brought out through the skin; these wires are removed prior to discharge. Until recently, only single chamber (VVI or AAI) or atrially committed dual chamber (DVI) devices were available for temporary pacing in this setting. While helpful in restoring atrioventricular synchrony, the committed pacing of the atrium in the setting of the atrial ectopy that frequently occurs following open heart surgery undoubtedly resulted in "creation" of the substrate for atrial fibrillation/flutter. More recently, the dual-chamber pacing technology developed for permanently implantable devices has been applied to temporary pacing, with good results.[60] These new temporary pacemakers have an atrial sensing circuit, capable of detect-

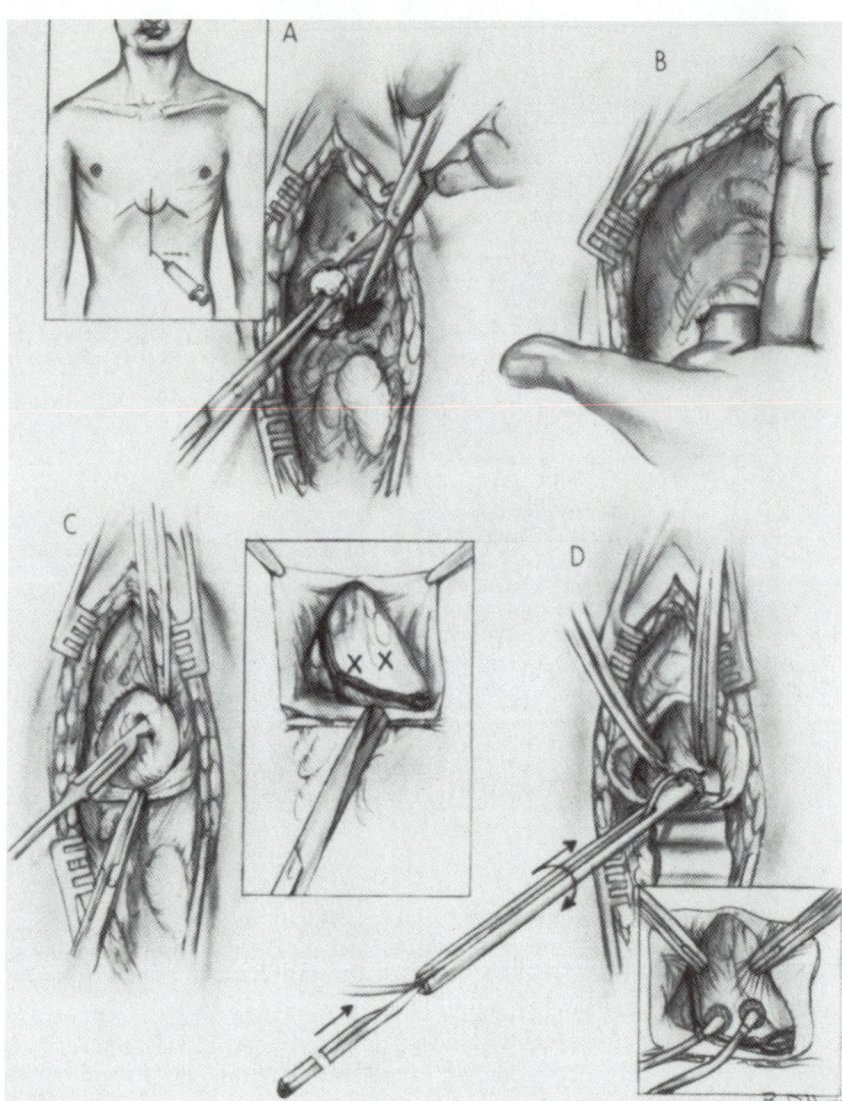

Figure 133–24. Subxiphoid approach.
A. Upper midline incision and excision of the xiphoid. **B.** Retrosternal space developed. **C.** Pericardium and (if necessary) diaphragm (inset) incised. **D.** Epicardial leads applied. *(From Stewart S: Placement of sutureless epicardial pacemaker lead by the subxiphoid approach. Ann Thorac Surg 18:310, 1974, with permission.)*

ing the patient's intrinsic atrial rhythm(s) and inhibiting the atrial output of the device when appropriate. Accurate placement of the atrial bipolar electrode pair is extremely important for atrial sensing function (Fig. 133–25A); the interelectrode distance and relationship of the electrode pair to the long axis of the atrial muscle fibers are also important.[60] Using this technique, adequate long-term (6 to 7 days) atrial sensing has been accomplished in the great majority of patients.

These external pacing devices are capable of providing effective AAI, VDD, or DVI pacing when programmed to the DDD mode (Fig. 133–25B). Their use may decrease the incidence of supraventricular arrhythmias in the postoperative period in many cardiac surgical patients.

Temporary endocardial pacing can also be accomplished by percutaneously placed pacing leads passed into the right ventricle under fluoroscopic guidance, or by passage of a Swan–Ganz catheter with pacing electrodes for the atrium and ventricle. Modifications of this approach in-

clude pacing guidewires that can be passed down a channel of a Swan catheter to selectively permit pacing. Percutaneous temporary atrial pacing wires are also available, but the stability of these in patients in the coronary care setting is less than ideal. Finally, electrodes may be passed down the esophagus to pace either the atrium or ventricle from behind in emergent situations. More recently the indications for esophageal pacing have broadened to less acute situations[97, 98] as well.

Each of these leads are connected to available temporary pacing devices, either single-channel (AAI, VVI) or dual-chamber (DVI, DDD) external pacemakers. In most instances of temporary pacing in this setting the output of the device (in milliamps, since these are constant-current devices) is set to maximum at a rate that provides optimal hemodynamic support.

External temporary pacing capability has recently become available with the Zoll external pacing system. Large cutaneous pads are placed anteriorly and posteriorly on the

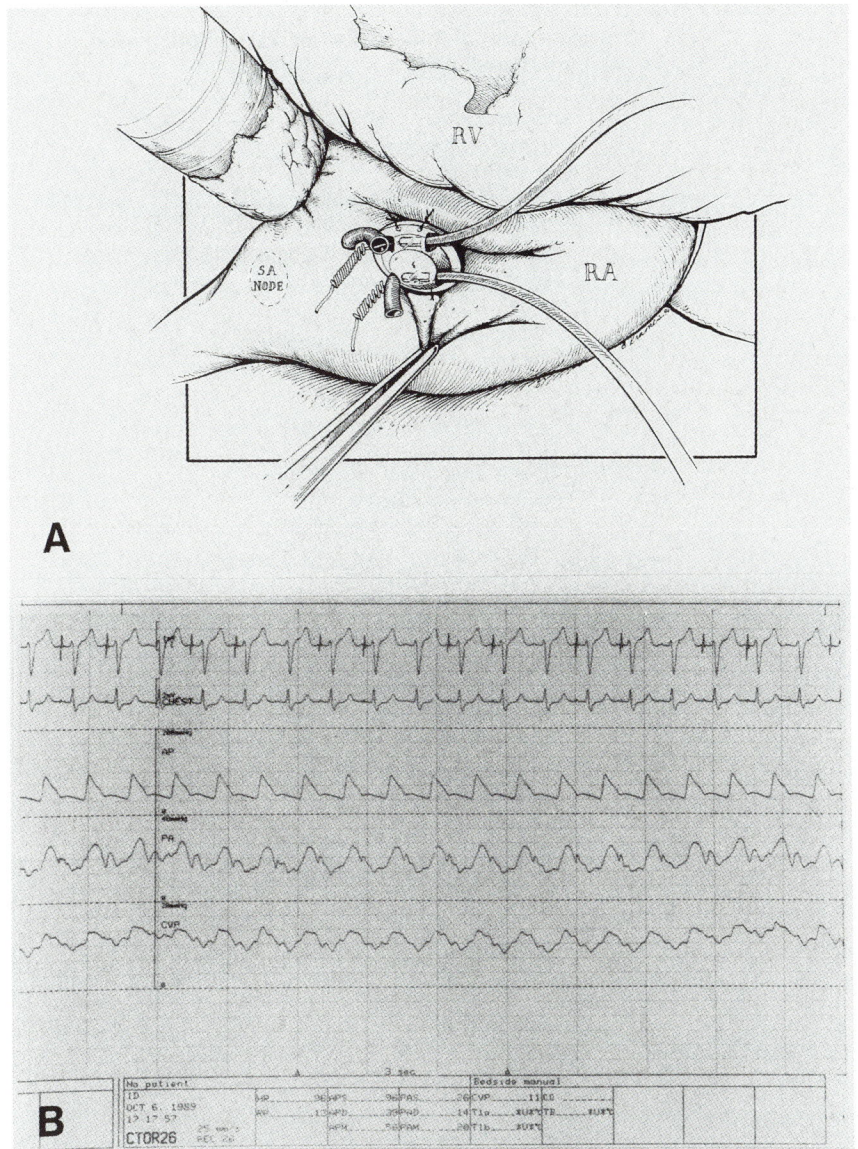

A

B

Figure 133–25. A. Schematic illustration of placement of temporary atrial bipolar wires for pacing and sensing following open heart surgery. Placement on the free wall of the right atrium, with the bipole perpendicular to the long axis of the atrial myocardial fibers at that site, provides the best sensing parameters for the leads. With this arrangement, no tissue necrosis from suturing the electrode directly to the epicardium can occur. **B.** External DDD pacing. Intraoperative electrophysiologic and hemodynamic data obtained after termination of cardiopulmonary bypass. Adequate atrial tracking of the patient's own sinus rhythm is illustrated. The pulse generator was programmed into the DDD mode with a lower rate approximately equal to the patient's own sinus rate. When the sinus rate drops below the lower rate of the pacemaker, the patient's atrium is paced; when the sinus rate speeds up and exceeds the programmed rate, adequate atrial and ventricular sensing are demonstrated and a normal sinus depolarization occurs. Atrioventricular conduction is intact throughout, and there are no hemodynamic alterations that result from the change to atrial sensing from atrial pacing. Ap, radial arterial pressure; CHEST, chest electrocardiographic lead; CVP, central venous pressure; PA, pulmonary artery pressure; II, surface electrocardiographic limb-lead II. *(From Ferguson and Cox,[60] with permission.)*

chest wall, and under emergent conditions transmediastinal external pacing can be accomplished in the majority of patients. Once the patient has been stabilized, temporary endocardial pacing leads can be placed for more reliable pacing.

COMPLICATION OF PACEMAKER SYSTEMS

The list of potential complications associated with cardiac pacing is rather long, but fortunately the incidence of individual complications is low (Table 133–5).

Complications Related to Implantation

The complications related to endocardial lead positioning include acute atrial or ventricular chamber perforation, car-

diac tamponade, or induction of complete heart block with asystolic arrest.[99,100] Any of these conditions may lead to death in inexperienced hands. Experience in manipulating leads and avoidance of excessive force during lead placement are necessary to avoid these complications. Acute lead dislodgment is also a relatively frequent complication of lead positioning. Positioning the lead too far out in the apex or placement through the endocardium can result in chest wall or diaphragmatic stimulation; performance of breathing and Valsalva maneuvers at the time of implant will detect most of these circumstances.

Complications related to venous access include pneumothorax, hemothorax, venous air embolism, arterial vascular injury, or brachial plexus injury. These complications are almost all related to subclavian vein cannulation, and occur much less commonly with the cephalic vein approach. However, with the prevalence of dual-chamber de-

TABLE 133–5. COMPLICATIONS OF PACEMAKER SYSTEMS AND IMPLANTATION

Complications of Pacemaker Systems	Complications of Pacemaker System Implantation

A. Pacemaker malfunction: sensing
  1. Skeletal myopotentials
   Pectoral
   Abdominal
   Diaphragmatic
  2. Cardiac events
   T-wave
   Atrial R-wave sensing
   Ventricular P-wave sensing
   Concealed extrastystoles
  3. Generator malfunction
   Programming error—high sensitivity or output
   Programming error—short refractory period
   Microchip malfunction
  4. Connector malfunction
   Loose set screw
   Current leak from header
  5. Lead malfunction
   Conductor fracture
   Insulation break
   Polarization potentials
  6. Environmental interference
   Electromagnetic
B. Pacemaker malfunction: pacing
  1. Lead position
   Displacement
   Microdislodgement (retraction)
   Perforation
   Poor placement at implantation
  2. Inadequate device output
   Power source failure (end of life)
   Programming error below safety factor
   Microchip component failure
  3. Increased pacing threshold
   Acute postimplant rise
   Late fibrotic exit block
   Myocardial infarction
   Metabolic, toxic or electrical influence
  4. High resistance in lead system
   Lead fracture
	A. Early Complications
	  1. Surgical
	   Pneumothorax
	   Arterial or venous vascular injury
	   Air embolism
	   Cardiac chamber perforation
	   Cardiac tamponade
	   Lead dislodgment due to inadequate fixation
	   Neural (brachial plexus) injury
	  2. Wound
	   Hematoma
	   Infection
	   Drainage
	B. Late complications
	  1. Surgical
	   Venous thrombosis
	   Pulmonary embolism
	   Constrictive pericarditis (following asymptomatic
	    perforation)
	   Pulmonary embolism
	   Tricuspid valvar insufficiency
	  2. Wound
	   Infection
	   Generator migration
	   Skin erosion
	   Device manipulation by patient (Twiddler's syndrome)
	C. Early or late electrophysiologic complications
	  1. Pacemaker syndrome
	   Ventricular
	   Atrial
	  2. Pacemaker mediated tachycardia

vices implanted, the subclavian approach is necessary and most efficient in most instances; these complications can be almost completely avoided in experienced operators' hands.

Complications related to the generator pocket include hematoma formation, generator migration, skin erosion, or skeletal muscle stimulation. Use of electrocautery for dissection of the pocket, securing of the generator on the pectoralis fascia, creation of a large enough pocket to prevent tension on the suture line, and use of bipolar pacing instead of unipolar pacing where possible will limit these complications.

Postsurgical Complications

Late lead perforation is rare, but can occur (Fig. 133–26). Late vascular access complications include subclavian vein

thrombosis and pulmonary embolus, with patients with right-sided heart failure at greatest risk. With current lead technology the incidence of tricuspid valvar abnormalities that are clinically symptomatic is rare. Twiddler's syndrome can occur in patients with Munchausen's syndrome (Fig. 133–27).

The majority of late complications relate to pacemaker system malfunction.[94,101,102] Loss of capture or sensing in a chronic lead suggests (1) a lead conductor fracture, (2) an insulation break, or (3) development of exit block (Fig. 133–28); these may be differentiated by lead impedance measurement in later model generators by telemetry; in general, insulation breaks are associated with low impedance measurements ($<250\ \Omega$), while conductor fractures are associated with high impedances ($<1000\ \Omega$). In exit block, the fibrosis around the electrode–myocardial interface becomes sufficient to inhibit conduction of the normal pace-

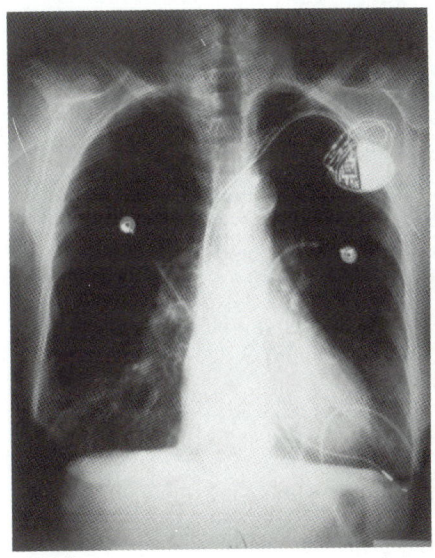

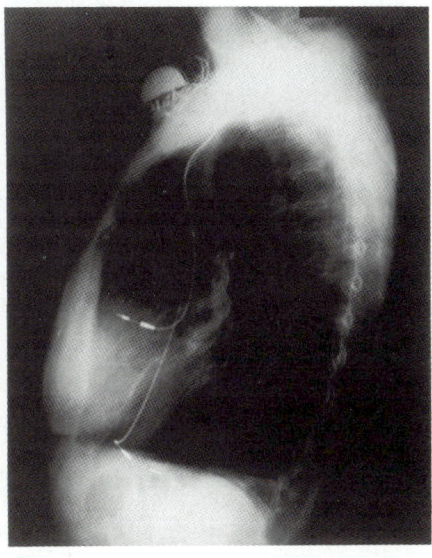

A   **B**

Figure 133–26. Posteroanterior (**A**) and lateral (**B**) chest roentgenogram of a patient transferred to Barnes Hospital with late right ventricular lead perforation; the patient had a sudden onset of excruciating left-sided chest pain due to chest wall stimulation by the pacing system.

maker depolarization impulse to the surrounding myocardium; the use of steroid-eluting leads has been shown to be useful in this situation,[32,103] which fortunately is unusual.

Pacemaker mediated tachycardia is a circumstance where a macroreentrant circuit is formed between the patient's conduction system and the implanted dual chamber pacemaker; the impulse is conducted to the ventricle with retrograde conduction to the atrium; this retrograde P-wave resets the upper rate timing cycle and starts a tachycardia at

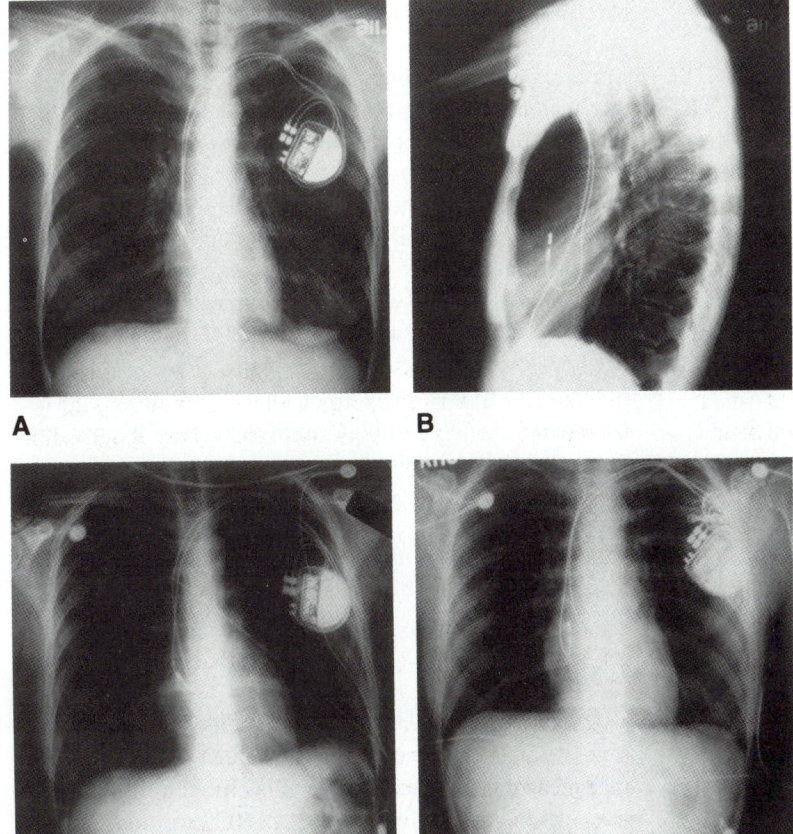

A   **B**

C   **D**

Figure 133–27. A,B. Posteroanterior (left) and lateral (right) chest roentgenograms of a patient with "Twiddler's syndrome." Films taken predischarge following DDDR implant in a young female with supraventricular tachyarrhythmias and intermittent block. **C.** Film taken 3 wk later when pacemaker malfunction was diagnosed with transtelephonic monitoring; the generator was reprogrammed at this time. **D.** Film taken 2 wk later upon representation with pacemaker system malfunction; note coiled leads in left upper chest.

Figure 133–28. Posteroanterior (**A**) and lateral (**B**) chest roentgenograms of a 51-year-old patient with uncorrected Tetralogy of Fallot, compensated Eisenmenger's syndrome, and chronic hypoxia who developed exit block almost exactly 6 mo following implant of ventricular leads into the common left ventricular chamber (same patient as in Fig. 133–22B). The exit block was due to the chronic hypoxemic effect on the lead–tissue interface. Use of steroid-eluting leads prolonged this interval from about 3 to 6 mo. Over a 3-year period, he had one subxiphoid, one anterior thoracotomy, and four endocardial ventricular lead placement procedures.

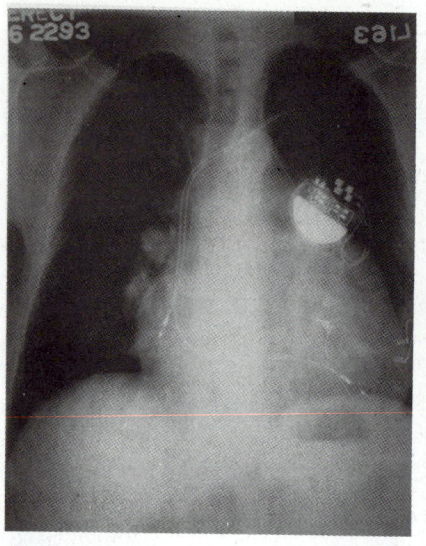 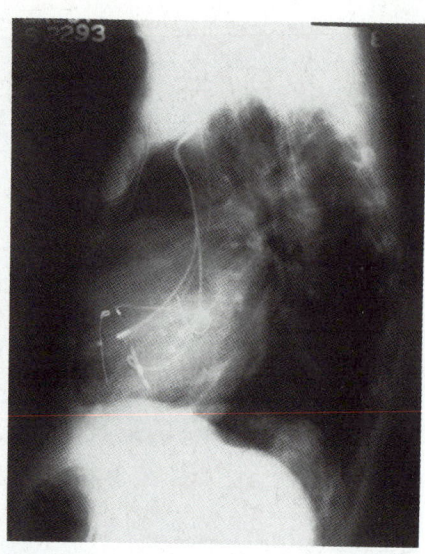

A   B

the upper rate limit of the device. The problem can be addressed by lengthening the atrial refractory period so that atrial sensing of the retrograde P-wave does not occur.

Other system malfunction complications include the development of myopotential inhibition, where the pacemaker senses skeletal muscle activity as cardiac electrical activity and is inhibited from firing, as well as a number of problems related to older model generators, including electromagnetic interference. All pacemaker systems are susceptible to radiation damage, and should be removed from the radiation port in that circumstance.

Infection and Lead Extraction

Infection of a pacemaker system[48,102–105] is a life-threatening complication that can occur at any time during the lifetime of the system. Acute infections are most often due to skin organisms in the perioperative period, while later infections can be caused by poor dentition or other organ system infections that seed the bloodstream. Once established, pacemaker system infections can rarely be cured without removal of the infected components.

Removal of the generator is straightforward, and should be performed after establishment of adequate levels of systemic antibiotic therapy. Endocardial lead removal[106,107] remains a technically complicated procedure that can result in a number of life-threatening complications including avulsion of right atrial or ventricular myocardial tissue, cardiac tamponade, avulsion of the tricuspid valve with acute valvar insufficiency, embolism of infected material to the pulmonary circulation, and hemothorax from laceration of the vasculature within the chest. In addition, approximately 25% of patients will require cardiopulmonary bypass for infected lead extraction following failure of other extraction efforts.

Active fixation leads, which have a constant diameter, are easier to remove than passive fixation leads. Even

chronic leads may be removed by passing a stylet down the lead and disengaging the active fixation mechanism; since this portion of the lead is often all than is imbedded in fibrous tissue, gentle traction under fluoroscopic visualization may permit lead removal. Excessive traction, however, will result in injury to the heart.

Passive fixation leads are best removed by extraction using a system of locking stylets and sheaths that permit placement of countertraction at the lead–myocardial interface to prevent avulsion of the myocardial tissue. The telescoping sheaths are advanced over the lead to disrupt the fibrous tissue surrounding the infected lead. If the lead has not been freed by the time the sheath has reached the tip of the lead, then the sheath is used to provide traction force at the electrode–myocardial interface, which ruptures the fibrous tissue and permits removal of the lead.

This commercially available system (Cook Pacemaker System, Inc.) requires considerable expertise but in experienced hands can be successful in a majority of cases.[108] A femoral venous approach can be used for removal of broken or free-floating fragments of leads. Failing these approaches, a thoracotomy or median sternotomy approach can be used, with or without cardiopulmonary bypass, to remove the infected material.

Once the infectious material has been removed and an appropriate duration of antibiotic therapy administered, the patient can undergo implantation of a new pacemaker system, usually on the contralateral chest wall.

CURRENT PRACTICE OF CARDIAC PACING

Pacing therapy has been targeted as a likely candidate for close scrutiny in the health care reform process because of issues of manpower, technology, and costs. By way of addressing these issues, the current status of cardiac pacing for bradyarrhythmias at Washington University was recently summarized.[48]

Over the past 3 years, in which over 200 new devices were implanted per year by a cardiothoracic surgeon working as a member of a combined medically and surgically staffed Pacemaker Service, the percent of dual chamber implants has been 70%. Complication rates have been extremely low (Table 133–6), and complete follow-up has been provided for all patients by telephone and office visits by the Pacemaker Service. Other institutions performing large volumes of pacing implantations have had similar experiences recently, particularly those in whom a defined Pacemaker Service has been established.[46,48,104,109]

The establishment of a pacemaker service consisting of input from cardiologists, surgeons, and electrophyisiologists (if available) has several advantages, as was demonstrated by this experience; it (1) eliminates the problems associated with self-referral and single-physician provider from diagnosis through therapy, (2) maximizes the effectiveness of the multispecialty involvement in pacing that exists at many institutions, and (3) provides for complete follow-up of this expensive technology, both in terms of patient welfare and in terms of issues of quality of care. Furthermore, this experience demonstrated that (1) active cardiothoracic surgical involvement in cardiac pacing can be an integral component in a "state-of-the-art" approach to pacing; (2) expertise in "state-of-the-art" pacing technology can be readily acquired by cardiothoracic surgeons interested in pacing, thus eliminating the need for an adjunctive nonsurgeon's presence at the implant; (3) surgical involvement in cardiac pacing contributes to minimization of implant-related complications and the expenses involved in

treating those complications; (4) additional training of cardiothoracic residents in cardiac pacing principles and techniques will be necessary above what has been done in the past to allow them to keep abreast of pacing technology and therapy; and (5) the advantages of surgical involvement in pacing that were paramount in the beginning of pacing (infection rates, complication rates, ability to handle the complications induced by a specific procedure) are still present and increasingly important.

As demonstrated in the latest NASPE Survey on Cardiac Pacing, the majority of pacemaker implantations in this country are done by individuals performing less than 12 implants per year.[46] Other studies have shown that complication rates for pacemaker implantation increase significantly in implanters performing less than 12 implants per year.[104] In the future, the financial impact of complications, as well as the medical impact, will need to be addressed in the discussion of quality of service and outcomes. To date, the American Board of Thoracic Surgery remains the only speciality board that requires exposure to pacemaker implantation. It is unlikely, however, that the present requirement provides adequate exposure to the more subtle aspects of dual-chamber, rate-responsive bradypacing without a concerted effort on the part of the resident and faculty.

An additional current issue in pacing is the need to justify additional technologic developments in this field. For example, developments such as the DDI and DDIR modes of pacing and mode switching have made dual-chamber pacing applicable to a larger number of patients, particularly those with paroxysmal or intermittent supraventricular arrhythmias. Considerable interest in pacing therapy for various cardiomyopathies[110,111] and in congestive failure[112] is developing, with promising early results. Demonstrating a clear beneficial effect of these therapies in a majority of patients, however, has been and will continue to be difficult.

TABLE 133–6. EXPERIENCE BETWEEN JULY 1989 AND DECEMBER 1992[a]

Total procedures	875	
Total new implants	709	(81.0% of total procedures)
Transvenous SC	308	(43.4% of new implants)
Transvenous DC	382	(53.9% of new implants)
Epicardial SC	11	(1.6% of new implants)
Epicardial DC	8	(1.1% of new implants)
Battery changes	79	(9.0% of total procedures)
Repositioned IH leads	36	(3.3% of endocardial leads placed)
Peri-oprepositionings	32	(3.0% of endocardial leads placed)
Outside repositionings	13	(26.5% of leads repositioned)
Lead changes	12	(1.1% of endocardial leads placed)
Infected IH explants	5	(0.6% of total procedures)
Infected outside explants	3	(37.5% of all infected explants)
Noninfected procedures	21	(2.4% of total procedures)

[a]SC, single chamber; DC, dual chamber; IH, in-hospital; peri-op, perioperative (30-day); outside, leads/systems implanted at outside hospital. *From Ferguson et al,[48] with permission.*

SUMMARY

Rapid advances in pacing technology will continue to impact on the quality of life of many patients with cardiovascular disease. A truly "smart" device that seemed fanciful 30 years ago now seems to be a virtual certainty early in the next century.

The surgical contributions and expertise of individuals trained in cardiothoracic surgery in these bradypacing developments are highly desirable to minimize morbidity to the greatest possible degree, optimize the outcome of the procedure for the individual patient, and conserve health care costs as much as is feasible. To maintain this cardiothoracic presence in cardiac pacing, acquisition of knowledge and expertise in the basic electrophysiology and technology of cardiac pacing, to go along with their surgical expertise, is necessary on the part of individuals with the interest and opportunity to do so.

REFERENCES

1. Chardack WM, Gage AA, Greatbatch W: A transistorized self contained implantable pacemaker for the long-term correction of heart block. *Surgery* **48:**643–649, 1960

2. Sulke N, Chambers J, Dritas A, Sowton E: A randomized double-blind crossover comparison of four rate responsive pacing modes. *J Am Coll Cardiol* **17:**696–706, 1991

3. Jutzy RV, Feenstra L, Florio J, Levine P: Evaluation of DDDR vs. VVIR pacing in patients with associated cardiac and pulmonary disease. *Eur J CPE* **2:**101–105, 1992

4. Sutton R, Bourgeois I: *The Foundations of Cardiac Pacing, Part I: An Illustrated Practical Guide to Basic Pacing.* Mount Kisco, NY: Futura, 1991, pp 319–324

5. Zanini R, Facchinetti AI, Gallo G, et al: Morbidity and mortality of patients with sinus node disease: Comparative effects of atrial and ventricular pacing. *PACE* **13:**2076–2079, 1990

6. Camm AJ, Katritsis D: Ventricular pacing for sick sinus syndrome-a risky business. *PACE* **13:**695–699, 1990

7. Rosenqvist M, Brandt J, Schuller HL: Long-term pacing in sinus node disease: Effects of stimulation mode on cardiovascular morbidity and mortality. *Am Heart J* **116:**16–22, 1988

8. Ferguson TB Jr: Anatomic and electrophysiologic principles in the surgical treatment of cardiac arrhythmias. In Cox JL (ed): *Cardiac Arrhythmia Surgery,* Vol 4. Philadelphia, Hanley & Belfus, 1990, pp 19–51

9. Sealy WC, Bache RJ, Seaber AV, Bhattacharga SK: The atrial pacemaking site after surgical exclusion of the sinoatrial node. *J Thorac Cardiovasc Surg* **65:**841–850, 1973

10. Boineau JP, Schuessler RB, Hackel DB, et al: Widespread distribution and rate differentiation of the atrial pacemaker complex. *Am J Physiol* **239** (Heart and Circulatory Physiol 8):J406–H415, 1980

11. Sealy WC, Seaber AV: Surgical isolation of the atrial septum from the atria: Identification of an atrial septal pacemaker. *J Thorac Cardiovasc Surg* **80:**742–749, 1980

12. Ferguson TB Jr, Schuessler RB, Hand DE, et al: Lessons learned from computerized mapping of the atrium. *J Electrocardiol* **26** (Suppl):210–219, 1993

13. Spach MS, Miller WT, Barr RC, Beselowitz DB: Electrophysiology of the internodal pathways: Determining the differences between anisotropic cardiac muscle and a specialized track system. In Little RC (ed): *Physiology of Atrial Pacemakers and Conductive Tissues.* Mt. Kisco, NY, Futura, 1980, pp 367–380

14. Davies MJ, Anderson RH, Becker AE: Anatomy of the conduction tissues. In *The Conduction System of the Heart.* London, Butterworths, 1983, pp 9–79

15. Anderson RH, Becker AH: *Cardiac Anatomy: An Integrated Text and Atlas.* London, Gower Medical, 1980, pp 6.15–6.29

16. Rosen MR: Mechanisms of cardiac impulse initiation and propagation. In Saksena S, Goldschlager N (eds): *Electrical Therapy for Cardiac Arrhythmias.* Philadelphia, W. B. Saunders, 1990, pp 3–8

17. Hille B: *Ionic Channels of Excitable Membranes.* Sunderland, MA, Sinauer Associates, 1984

18. Hondeghem L, Katzung B: Time and voltage dependent interactions of antiarrhythmic drugs with cardiac sodium channels. *Biochim Biophys Acta* **472:**373–398, 1977

19. Jack JJB, Noble D, Tsien RW: *Electric Current Flow in Excitable Cells.* Oxford, Clarendon, 1975

20. Rosen MR, Hoffman BF: Electrophysiologic determinants of normal cardiac rhythms and arrhythmias. In Rosen MR, Hoffman BF (eds): *Cardiac Therapy.* Boston, Martinus Nijhoff, 1983, pp 1–19

21. Giles W, van Ginneken A, Shibata EF: Ionic currents underlying cardiac pacemaker activity: A summary of voltage-clamp data from single cells. In Nathan RD (ed): *Cardiac Muscle: The Regulation of Excitation and Contraction.* Orlando, FL, Academic Press, 1986, pp 1–27

22. Katz AM: Membrane structure. In Fozzard HA, Jennings RB, Haber E, et al (eds): *The Heart and Cardiovascular System,* 2nd ed. New York, Raven Press, 1991, pp 51–62

23. Vassalle M: The relationship among cardiac pacemakers: Overdrive suppression. *Circ Res* **41:**269–277, 1977

24. Bernstein AD, Parsonnet V: Engineering aspects of pulse generators for cardiac pacing. In Saksena S, Goldschlager N (eds): *Electrical Therapy for Cardiac Arrhythmias.* W B Saunders, Philadelphia, 1990, pp 21–34

25. Moses HW, Taylor GJ, Schneider JA, Dove JT: *A Practical Guide to Cardiac Pacing,* 2nd ed. Boston, Little Brown, 1987, pp 43–58

26. Furman S: Rate-modulated pacing. *Circulation* **82:**1081–1094, 1990

27. Timmis GC: The electrobiology and engineering of pacemaker leads. In Saksena S, Goldschlager N (eds): *Electrical Therapy for Cardiac Arrhythmias.* Philadelphia, W. B. Saunders, 1990, pp 35–90

28. Bornzin GA, Stokes KB, Wiebush WA: A low threshold, low polarization platinized endocardial electrode. *PACE* **6:**A–70, 1983

29. Mujica J, Henry L, Attuel P, et al: Clinical experience with 910 carbon tip leads: Comparison with polished platinum leads. *PACE* **9:**1230–1238, 1986

30. Molajo AO, Bowes RJ, Fananapazir L, et al: Comparison of vitreous carbon and Elgiloy transvenous ventricular pacing leads. *PACE* **8:**261–265, 1985

31. Parsonnet V, Werres R: Clinical experience with a porous-tip steroid-loaded ventricular pacing electrode. *PACE* **6:**319, 1983

32. Crossley GH, Kay GN, Ferguson TB, et al: Treatment of patients with prior exit block using a novel steroid-eluting active fixation lead (abstr). *PACE* **17:**870, 1994

33. Timmis BC, Helland J, Westveer, DC, et al: The evolution of low threshold leads. *Clin Prog Pacing Electrophysiol* **1:**313–334, 1983

34. Tyers GFO, Brownlee RR, Hughes HC, et al: Myocardial stimulation impedance: The effects of electrode, physiological and stimulus variables. *Ann Thorac Surg* **27:**63–69, 1979

35. Fontaine G, Frank R, Aldakar M: The electrode-biointerface: Stimulation. In Barold SS, Mugica J (eds): *New Perspectives in Cardiac Pacing,* Mount Kisco, NY, Futura, 1988, pp 3–16

36. Adams T: The electrode-biointerface: Sensing. In Barold SS, Mugica J (eds): *New Perspectives in Cardiac Pacing.* Mount Kisco, NY, Futura, 1988, pp 17–25

37. Naclerio EA, Varriale P: The sutureless electrode for cardiac pacing: Problems, advantages and surgical technique. *PACE* **3:**232–235, 1980

38. Michalik RE, Williams WH, Zorn-Chelton S, et al: Experience with a new epimyocardial pacing lead in children. *PACE* **7:**831–838, 1984

39. Stokes K, Stephenson NL: The implantable cardiac pacing lead—just a simple wire? In Barold SS, Mujica J (eds): *The Third Decade of Cardiac Pacing: Advances in Technology and Clinical Applications.* Mount Kisco, NY, Futura, 1982, pp 365–416

40. Bilitch M, Hauser RG, Goldman BS, et al: Performance of implantable cardiac rhythm management devices. *PACE* **10:**389–398, 1987

41. Birnbaum M: *Pacing Reference Guide,* 5th ed. Medtronic, 1991

42. Benditt DG (ed): *Rate-Adaptive Pacing.* Boston, Blackwell Scientific, 1993

43. Bernstein AD, Camm AJ, Fletcher RD, et al: The NASPE/BPEG generic pacemaker code for antibradyarrhythmia and adaptive rate pacing and antitachycardia devices. *PACE* **10:**794, 1987

44. Parsonnet V, Furman S, Smyth NP: A revised code for pacemaker identification. *PACE* **4:**400, 1981

45. Barold SS, Falkoff MD, Ong LS, Heinle RA: Timing cycles of DDD pacemakers. In Barold SS, Mugica J (eds): *New Perspectives in Cardiac Pacing.* Mount Kisco, NY, Futura, 1988, pp 69–120

46. Bernstein AD, Parsonnet V: Survey of cardiac pacing in the United States in 1989. *Am J Cardiol* **69:**331–338, 1992

47. Clarke M, Sutton R, Ward D, et al: Recommendations for a pacemaker prescription for symptomatic bradycardia. Report of a work-

ing party of the British Pacing and Electrophysiology Group. *Br Heart J* **66:**185–191, 1991

48. Ferguson TB, Lindsay BD, Boineau JP: Should surgeons still be implanting pacemakers? *Ann Thorac Surg* **57:**588–597, 1994

49. Barold SS, Falkoff MD, Ong LS, Heinle RA: Function and electrocardiography of DDD pacemakers. In SS Barold (ed): *Modern Cardiac Pacing.* Mt. Kisco, NY, Futura, 1985, p 645

50. Barold SS, Falkoff MD, Ong LS, Heinle RA: Electrocardiography of contemporary DDD pacemakers. In Saksena S, Goldschlager N (eds): *Electrical Therapy for Cardiac Arrhythmias.* Philadelphia, W. B. Saunders, 1990, pp 225–264

51. Levine PA: Base rate behavior of dual chamber pacing systems. In Barold SS, Mujica J (eds): *New Perspectives in Cardiac Pacing,* Vol 3. Mount Kisco, NY, Futura, 1993, pp 215–232

52. Floro J, Castellanet M, Fiorio J, Messenger J: DDI: A new mode for cardiac pacing. *Clin Prog Pacing Electrophysiol* **2:**255–260, 1984

53. Hayes DL, Levine PA: Pacemaker timing cycles. In Ellenbogan KA (ed): *Cardiac Pacing.* Cambridge, MA, Blackwell Scientific, 1991, pp 263–308

54. Hayes DL: DDDR timing cycles: Upper rate behavior. In Barold SS, Mugica J (eds): *New Perspectives in Cardiac Pacing,* Vol 3. Mount Kisco, NY, Futura, 1993, pp 233–257

55. Ausubel K, Furman S: The pacemaker syndrome. *Ann Intern Med* **103:**402, 1985

56. Schuller H, Brandt J: The pacemaker syndrome: Old and new causes. *Clin Cardiol* **14:**336, 1991

57. Barold SS: The pacemaker syndrome during "physiologic" pacing. *Intell Rep Cardiac Pacing Electrophysiol* **11**(4):1–7, 1993

58. Barold SS, Falkoff MD, Ong LS, et al: Cardiac pacing in the nineties: Technologic, hemodynamic and electrophysiologic considerations in the selection of the optimal mode of pacing. In Rackley CE (ed): *Challenges in Cardiology.* Mount Kisco, NY, Futura, 1992, pp 30–42

59. Barold SS: Sick sinus syndrome: Is single chamber atrial pacing still a viable option? *Intell Rep Cardiac Pacing Electrophysiol* **12**(4): 1–3, 1994

60. Ferguson TB Jr, Cox JL: Temporary external DDD pacing after cardiac operations. *Ann Thorac Surg* **51:**723–732, 1991

61. Garson A Jr, Coyner T, Shannon CE, Gillette PC: A systematic approach to the fully automatic (DDD) pacemaker electrocardiogram. In Gillette PC, Griffin JC (eds): *Practical Cardiac Pacing.* Baltimore, Williams & Wilkins, 1986, p 181

62. Fananapazir L, Srinivas V, Bennett DH: Comparison of resting hemodynamic indices and exercise performance during atrial synchronized and asynchronous ventricular pacing. *PACE* **6:**202–209, 1983

63. Ausubel K, Steingart RM, Shimshi M, et al: Maintenance of exercise stroke volume during ventricular versus atrial synchronous pacing: Role of contractility. *Circulation* **72:**1037–1043, 1985

64. Mukharji J, Rehr RB, Hastillo A, et al: Comparison of atrial contribution to cardiac hemodynamics in patients with normal and severely compromised cardiac function. *Clin Cardiol* **13:**639–643, 1990

65. Benditt DG: Sensor-triggered rate-adaptive cardiac pacing: An overview. In Benditt DG (ed): *Rate-Adaptive Pacing.* Boston, Blackwell Scientific, 1993, pp 9–29

66. Jutzy R, Florio J, Isaeff D, et al: Comparative evaluation of rate modulated dual chamber and VVIR pacing. *PACE* **13:**1838–1846, 1990

67. Santini M, Alexidou G, Ansalone G, et al: Relation of prognosis in sick sinus syndrome to age, conduction defects and models of permanent cardiac pacing. *Am J Cardiol* **65:**729–735, 1990

68. Stangl K, Seitz K, Wirtzfeld A, et al: Differences between atrial single chamber pacing (AAI) and ventricular single chamber pacing (VVI) with respect to prognosis and antiarrhythmic effects in patients with sick sinus syndrome. *PACE* **13:**2080–2085, 1990

69. Janosik DL, Pearson AC, Buchingham TA, et al: The hemodynamic benefit of differential atrioventricular delay interval for sensed and

70. Higano ST, Hayes DL: Hemodynamic importance of atrioventricular synchrony during low levels of exercise. (abstr) *PACE* **13:**509, 1990

71. Camilli L, Alcidi L, Papeschi G: A new pacemaker autoregulating the rate of pacing in relation to metabolic needs. In Watanabe Y (ed): *Cardiac Pacing.* Amsterdam, Exerpta Medica, 1977, p 4149

72. Camilli L, Alcidi L, Paeschi G, et al: Preliminary experience with the pH-triggered pacemaker. *PACE* **1:**448–457, 1987

73. Stangl K, Wirtzfeld A, Gobl G, et al: Rate control with an external SO2 closed loop system. *PACE* **9:**992, 1986

74. Wirtzfeld A, Heinze R, Liess HD, et al: An active optical sensor for monitoring mixed venous oxygen saturation for an implantable rate regulating pacing system. *PACE* **6:**494, 1983

75. Faerestrand S, Ohm O-J: Mixed venous oxygen saturation for rate-adaptive pacing. In Benditt DG (ed): *Rate-Adaptive Pacing.* Boston, Blackwell Scientific, 1993, pp 335–348

76. Nappholz T, Lubin M, Maloney J, Simmons T: Measuring minute ventilation with a pacing catheter. *PACE* **8:**785, 1985 (abstr)

77. Mond H, Strathmore N, Kertes P, et al: Rate responsive pacing using a minute ventilation sensor. *PACE* **11:**1866–1874, 1988

78. Lau CP, Antoniou A, Ward DE, Camm AJ: Initial clinical experience with a minute ventilation sensing rate modulated pacemaker: Improvements in exercise capacity and symptomatology. *PACE* **11:**1815–1822, 1988

79. Mond HG: Minute ventilation based rate adaptive pacing. In Benditt DG (ed): *Rate-Adaptive Pacing.* Boston, Blackwell Scientific, 1993, pp 285–296

80. Sellers TD, Fearnot NE, Smith HJ, et al: Right ventricular blood temperature profiles for rate responsive pacing. *PACE* **10:**467–479, 1987

81. Mehta D, Lau CP, Ward DE, Camm AJ: Comparative evaluation of chronotropic responses of QT sensing and activity sensing rate responsive pacemakers. *PACE* **11:**1405–1412, 1988

82. Callaghan F, Wollmann W, Livingston A, et al: The ventricular depolarization gradient: Effects of exercise, pacing rate, epinephrine, and intrinsic heart rate control on the right ventricular evoked response. *PACE* **12:**1115–1130, 1989

83. McKay RG, Spears JR, Aroesty JM, et al: Instantaneous measurement of left and right ventricular stroke volume and pressure-volume relationships with an impedance catheter. *Circulation* **69:**703–710, 1984

84. Sutton R, Sharma A, Ingram A, et al: First derivative of right ventricular pressure as a sensor for an implantable rate responsive VVI pacemaker (abstr). *PACE* **11:**487, 1988

85. Benditt DG, Mianulli M, Fetter J, et al: Single chamber cardiac pacing with activity-initiated chronotropic response: Evaluation of cardiopulmonary exercise testing. *Circulation* **75:**184–191, 1987

86. Anderson KM: Activity-based rate adaptive pacing systems—Piezoceramic crystals, accelerometers. In Benditt DG (ed): *Rate-Adaptive Pacing.* Boston, Blackwell Scientific, 1993, pp 267–276

87. Smedgard P, Kristensson BE, Druse I, Ryden L: Rate responsive pacing by mean of activity sensing versus single rate ventricular pacing; a double blind crossover study. *PACE* **10:**902–915, 1987

88. Lau C-P, Butrous GS, Ward DE, Camm AJ: Comparison of exercise performance of six rate-adaptive right ventricular cardiac pacemakers. *Am J Cardiol* **63:**833–838, 1989

89. Linde-Edelstam C, Norlander R, Unden A-L, et al: Quality of life in patients treated with atrioventricular synchronous pacing compared to rate modulated ventricular pacing: A long term, double blind crossover study. *PACE* **15:**1467–1476, 1992

90. Mugica J, Barold SS, Ripart T: The smart pacemaker. In Barold SS, Mugica J (eds): *New Perspectives in Cardiac Pacing,* Vol. 2. Mount Kisco, NY, Futura, 545–577, 1991

91. Dreifus LS, Fisch C, Griffin JC, et al: Guidelines for implantation of cardiac pacemakers and antiarrhythmia devices. A report of the

American College of Cardiology/American Heart Association Task Force on Assessment of Diagnostic and Therapeutic Cardiovascular Procedures (Committee on Pacemaker Implantation). *J Am Coll Cardiol* **18:**1–13, 1991

92. Love CJ: Clinical followup of rate adaptive pacing systems. In Benditt DG (ed): *Rate-Adaptive Pacing.* Boston, Blackwell Scientific, 1993, pp 215–232

93. Magney JE, Flynn DM, Parsons JA, et al: Anatomical mechanisms explaining damage to pacemaker leads, defibrillator leads and failure of central venous catheters adjacent to the sternoclavicular joint. *PACE* **16:**445–457, 1993

94. Garson A, Kanter RJ: Rate-adaptive pacing in children: Requirements and clinical application. In Benditt DG (ed): *Rate-Adaptive Pacing.* Boston, Blackwell Scientific, pp 183–198, 1993

95. Walsh CA, McAlister HF, Andrews CA, et al: Pacemaker implantation in children: A 21 year experience. *PACE* **11:**1940–1944, 1988

96. Gertz E, Goldschlager N, Furman S: Principles of outpatient followup of the cardiac pacemaker patient. In Saksena S, Goldschlager N (eds): *Electrical Therapy for Cardiac Arrhythmias,* Philadelphia, W. B. Saunders, 1990, pp 191–205

97. Ferguson TB, Cox JL: Cardiac rhythm disturbances. In Barie PS, Shires GT (eds): *Surgical Intensive Care.* Boston, Little, Brown, 1993, pp 365–416

98. Greco EM, Manfredini R, Arlotti M, et al: Reliability of transient ventricular pacing triggered by atrial esophageal waves during acute myocardial infarction complicated by 3rd degree atrioventricular block (abstr). *PACE* **17:**802, 1994

99. Phibbs B, Marriott HJL: Complications of permanent transvenous pacing. *N Engl J Med* 312:1428–1432, 1985

100. Stoney WS, Addelstone RB, Alford WC Jr, et al: The incidence of venous thrombosis following long-term transvenous pacing. *Ann Thorac Surg* **22:**166–170, 1976

101. Tyers GFO: FDA Recalls: How do pacemaker manufacturers compare? *Ann Thorac Surg* **48:**390–396, 1989

102. Gross JN, Moser S, Benedek ZM, et al: DDD pacing mode survival in patients with a dual-chamber pacemaker. *J Am Coll Cardiol* **19:** 1536–1541, 1992

103. Dohrmann ML, Goldschlager NF: Myocardial stimulation threshold in patients with cardiac pacemakers: Effect of physiologic variables, pharmacologic agents and lead electrodes. *Cardiol Clin* **3:**527–537, 1985

104. Parsonnet V, Bernstein AD, Lindsay BD: Pacemaker implantation complications rates: An analysis of some contributing factors. *J Am Coll Cardiol* **13:**917–921, 1989

105. Brodman R, Frame F, Andrews C, Furman S: Removal of infected transvenous leads requiring cardiopulmonary bypass or inflow occlusion. *J Thorac Cardiovasc Surg* **103:**649–654, 1992

106. Byrd CL, Schwartz SJ, Hedin N. Cardiac pacing. Lead extraction: Indications and techniques. *Cardiol Clin* 735–748, 1992

107. Sellers TD, Smith HJ: Specialized pacing leads for rate adaptive cardiac pacing systems. In Benditt DG (ed): *Rate-Adaptive Pacing.* Boston, Blackwell Scientific, 1993, pp 111–124

108. Fearnot NE, Smith HJ, Goode LB, et al: Intravascular lead extraction using locking stylets, sheath and other techniques. *PACE* **13:**1971–1975, 1990

109. Furman S: Letter to the Editor. *Ann Thorac Surg* (in press)

110. Gross JN, Keltz TN, Cooper JA, et al: Profound "pacemaker syndrome" in hypertrophic cardiomyopathy. *Am J Cardiol* **70:**1507–1511, 1992

111. Hochleitner M, Hortnagl H, Fridich L, Gschnitzer F: Long-term efficacy of physiologic dual-chamber pacing in the treatment of end-stage idiopathic dilated cardiomyopathy. *Am J Cardiol* **70:**1320–1325, 1992

112. Linde C, Gadler F, Edner M, et al: Is DDD pacing with short AV delay a beneficial treatment in patients with severe heart failure? (abstr) *PACE* **17:**744, 1994

134

Blunt and Penetrating Trauma to the Great Vessels

Ralph L. Warren, Alan D. Hilgenberg, and Charles J. McCabe

Trauma has been referred to as "the neglected disease of modern society":[1] 140,000 to 160,000 lives are lost in the United States annually. Trauma is the leading cause of death in patients under 40 years of age and the third leading cause of death from all diseases overall; chest injuries are responsible for one quarter of these. The economic impact is staggering: the estimated direct and indirect costs of trauma care in the United States is on the order of $140 to 150 billion per year.

Deaths caused by trauma can be separated by timing into three groups, as described by Trunkey.[2,3] Immediate deaths—50% of the total—occur at the time of the accident, and result from lacerations of the brain, heart, major arteries, the high spinal cord, or obstruction of the airway. The next phase, accounting for approximately one-third of the total, is "the golden hour" (actually the first 1 to 6 hours after injury): death results from visceral hemorrhage resulting in subdural or epidural hematomas, hemoperitoneum, hemothorax, or external exsanguination. The final phase occurs at an average of 10 days to 2 wk after injury, at which time death results from sepsis and/or the multiorgan dysfunction syndrome.

There are two general mechanisms of injury. Penetrating injuries (knife and gunshot wounds) are more common in urban areas,[4–7] while blunt injuries, primarily secondary to motor vehicle accidents, are prominent in rural areas.[8] In both environments, illicit drugs and/or alcohol are commonly involved.[9–11] Firearm deaths are directly related to handgun availability in the United States (Table 134–1): there are an estimated 200,000,000 guns in America of which 60,000,000 are handguns, and an estimated 3,000,000 are military-type assault weapons. Since 1933, there have been over 500,000 deaths due to firearms in America; gunshot wounds are now the most common cause of death in Afro-American teenagers. Motor vehicles cause approximately 50,000 deaths per year and a significantly larger amount of morbidity.

EVALUATION OF THE INJURED PATIENT

All thoracic injuries should be considered "lethal" until proven otherwise. The initial approach to management should be one that creates order out of chaos, and provides for rapid treatment of the immediately life-threatening injuries that are discovered. The principles of Advanced Trauma Life Support should be followed.[12] The first priority is always to ensure a patent airway and adequate ventilation. External hemorrhage should be controlled by digital pressure, and the intravascular volume should be restored with appropriate intravenous fluids to restore perfusion. With massive hemorrhage, resuscitation may not be possible until the injury is surgically controlled. X-rays of the lateral cervical spine, chest, and pelvis in patients that have suffered blunt trauma are routine; additional diagnostic radiographs are often necessary. In patients who have suffered blunt chest trauma, a widened mediastinum is often the presenting abnormality on admission chest x-ray and implies great vessel injury. In patients with penetrating injuries, a massive hemothorax implies major vascular disruption.

Management of patients with chest trauma and multi-

TABLE 134–1. FIREARM DEATHS

In 1992, handguns killed
33 people in Great Britain
36 in Sweden
97 in Switzerland
60 in Japan
13 in Australia
128 in Canada
13,220 in the United States

From Handgun Control, Inc., 1225 Eye Street, N.W., Washington, D.C.

ple injuries is often difficult. The patient with a widened mediastinum often has a head injury, extremity fractures, and intra-abdominal injuries. High abdominal injuries and low thoracic penetrating wounds often cause injuries distant to the surface entrance site due to trajectory and the variable position of the diaphragm on inspiration and expiration. An impaled object must remain in place and be removed only when the viscera from which it is being removed can be repaired immediately upon its removal. Chest tubes should be used liberally. Blood should be drawn for type and cross-match, and blood for transfusion should be made rapidly available. The managing physician must establish priorities and ensure that the lethal potential of the thoracic injury remains in focus.

BLUNT INJURIES OF THE GREAT VESSELS

Traumatic Disruption of the Thoracic Aorta

The most common injury of the great vessels is disruption of the thoracic aorta secondary to blunt trauma: of the 50,000 traffic accident fatalities in the United States per year, approximately 15% (7500) are due to rupture of the thoracic aorta. Injuries to the aorta caused by blunt trauma consist of transverse, usually circumferential, tears of the intima and varying amounts of media and adventitia. If the full thickness of media and adventitia is torn, as is the case in 85% of those with the injury, immediate death due to exsanguination into the pleural cavity occurs. In the remaining 15%, at least the outer layers of the adventitia and mediastinal pleura are intact, and the patient can survive to reach a hospital. The tear is most often a well-localized lesion: actual dissection of the aortic wall rarely occurs in the absence of pre-existing degenerative changes (Fig. 134–3A).

The most common location for the tear to occur, accounting for 90 to 95% in surgical series, is at the aortic isthmus: the most proximal portion of the descending thoracic aorta just distal to the origin of the left subclavian artery. This part of the aorta is relatively fixed by the ligamentum arteriosum to the main pulmonary artery, while the aortic arch and more distal descending aorta are both more free to move during rapid decelerations (as with a motor vehicle crash or a fall from height) or accelerations (as when a

pedestrian is struck by a car). The second most common location, accounting for roughly 5% in surgical series (but 25% in autopsy series: this lesion is immediately fatal in 95% of victims), is in the ascending aorta a few centimeters above the aortic annulus (the same area that is the site of most intimal tears in cases of spontaneous aortic dissection). A few percent occur in the more distal thoracic aorta (and even fewer in the abdominal aorta), most often adjacent to a spinal fracture; a few percent occur at the origins of the great vessels, and up to 5% of patients have more than one tear.

Diagnosis

Making the diagnosis of traumatic aortic disruption requires a high index of suspicion: most patients have other more obvious injuries, there are no pathognomonic symptoms or signs, and, if treatment is not instituted expeditiously, the consequence is likely to be sudden death.

Patients at Risk. The vast majority of aortic tears occur secondary to high-speed (greater than 20 miles per hour) motor vehicle accidents. The incidence is higher in car occupants if they are driving, if they are unbelted,[13] and if they are ejected;[14] both head-on and side impact collisions can disrupt the aorta. Pedestrians struck by vehicles and patients who fall from height (the minimum height reported in the literature is 8 feet)[15] are the two other groups with a high likelihood of suffering a torn aorta. Victims of blunt trauma with a pelvic fracture have a several-fold higher chance of having an aortic disruption than those without.[16] Aortic tears occur in all age groups, though they are relatively rare in children.[17]

Findings. The *symptoms* of aortic tear are nonspecific and most often overshadowed by symptoms of associated injuries. Chest and/or upper back pain and dyspnea are the most frequent, but are usually attributable to overlying chest wall injury: up to 75% of patients have rib and/or sternal fractures. Symptoms suggestive of a mediastinal mass, e.g., stridor or wheezing, dysphagia, hoarseness, or superior vena cava obstruction, are present only rarely. Commonly associated injuries include extremity and/or pelvic fractures in two-thirds, serious head injuries in half, pulmonary and/or cardiac contusions in half, and intra-abdominal injuries in one-third. Of note, there are reports of patients with aortic disruption who are completely asymptomatic.[18]

Physical *findings* are likewise usually nonspecific: external evidence of chest wall injury is present in 70 to 90%. (Note that this means 10 to 30% of patients with aortic disruption do *not* have apparent chest injury; most of these are young patients with compliant, elastic chest walls.) Less than one-third of patients have unequal arm blood pressures and/or upper extremity hypertension with diminished femoral pulses and decreased lower extremity blood pressure—the so-called "pseudocoarctation" syndrome. Ten to 20% have a precordial systolic and/or interscapular murmur. Importantly, 2 to 5% will present with paraplegia, due either to concomitant direct cord trauma, or to spinal cord ischemia secondary to the aortic disruption. Moreover, since spinal cord ischemia is one of the most important complications of both the injury itself and of the operative repair, it is vital to fully document and carefully follow the neurologic status of the lower extremities.

The chest radiograph (*CXR*) (Fig. 134–1) is the single most helpful initial test: it shows evidence of mediastinal bleeding in 90 to 95% of all those with disrupted aorta. But it is quite nonspecific: 80% of mediastinal bleeding in victims of blunt trauma is caused by injuries other than aortic disruption. Moreover, up to 5% of patients with an aortic tear have a *normal* CXR.

The most common abnormality on CXR is widening of the mediastinum. There are, however, several complicating factors in the interpretation of mediastinal widening. First, as mentioned above, most mediastinal widening is caused by bleeding from small vessels rather than from the aorta or its large branches. Second, any CXR performed in an anteroposterior (AP) direction—as is done with most multiple trauma patients—will have an apparent widening of the mediastinum due to geometry alone; this effect is aggravated if the distance from x-ray tube to plate is less than the standard 6 feet (again as is the case with routine portable films). Third, the very definition of "widened" is problematic. Many authorities use a figure of 8 cm as the upper limit of normal for the width of the mediastinum at the level of the aortic knob; others use the ratio of the mediastinal width at this level to the width of the chest from in-side of rib to inside of rib at the same level, with any figure greater than 0.25 indicating abnormal widening.[19]

Several other chest radiographic signs of thoracic aortic injury have been described, and all should be consciously looked for, since they can be rather subtle. The most important are obscuration of the normally quite distinct "aortic knob" and/or obliteration of the window between the aortic knob and the left main pulmonary artery: these signs are present in 75 to 90% of patients. Rightward deviation of the trachea and/or a nasogastric tube in the esophagus is found in up to two-thirds, and depression of the left main bronchus to an angle of more than 140 degrees from the trachea is seen in up to half. Fluid in the left pleural cavity is visible in one-third to one-half; widening of the paratracheal or paraspinous stripes is found in one-third. A left "apical cap," which is a result of blood dissecting from the mediastinum up over the dome of the hemithorax, is found in one-half to two-thirds of patients.

Diagnostic Imaging. Once the presence of thoracic aortic disruption is suspected, the diagnosis must then be either established or completely ruled out. There are four imaging techniques currently available to do so: contrast angiography, computed tomography, transesophageal echocardiography, and magnetic resonance imaging.

Angiography is the "gold standard": it has high—nearly 100%—sensitivity and specificity, and it provides the surgeon with a complete "road map" of the aorta and its branches, as well as of the exact extent of the injury itself (Fig. 134–2). Despite the fact that aortography is usually performed via the femoral vessels and thus the catheters must traverse the site of the tear, there is a documented very low complication rate. The drawbacks of angiography are the need to use potentially nephrotoxic intravenous contrast, and the time it takes to assemble the vascular radiology team and perform the procedure.

The value of computed tomography (CT) of the chest is controversial, and is evolving with the increasing sophistication of CT scanners. Miller et al[20] in 1989 found that CT had a sensitivity of only 55% in diagnosing traumatic aortic tears. Since then, however, dynamic contrast-enhanced CT using newer, faster, and higher resolution machines has been demonstrated by many groups to be highly sensitive and quite useful, especially for excluding aortic disruption in patients in whom the suspicion of aortic tear is low. To maintain high sensitivity, however, the criteria outlined by Agee et al in 1992[21] used to properly interpret CT scans must be strictly adhered to (Table 134–2). Unless all five criteria for a negative scan are fulfilled, the study cannot reliably exclude aortic injury, and aortography is mandated. Moreover, the presence of any positive finding on CT necessitates aortography for confirmation and more detailed delineation.

Transesophageal echocardiography (TEE) has emerged since 1990 as an excellent tool for examining both the heart and the aorta after chest trauma.[22,23] TEE offers several ad-

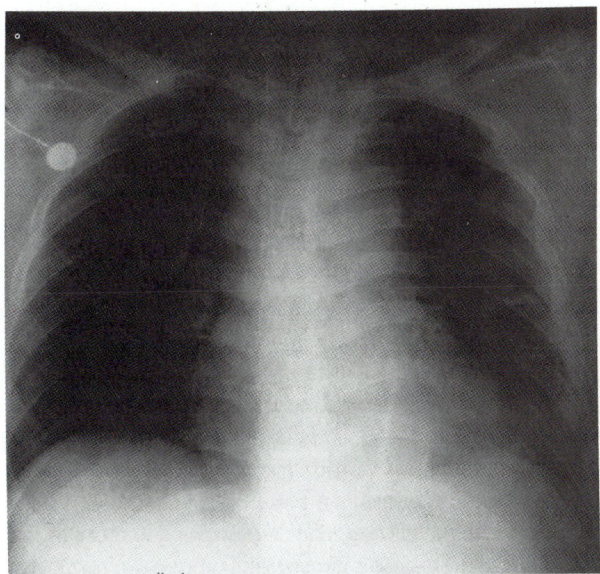

Figure 134–1. Upright anteroposterior (AP) chest radiograph of a 35-year-old male driver in a high-speed motor vehicle accident. There is widening of the mediastinum, obscuration of the aortic knob, and aortopulmonary window, deviation of the trachea, and nasogastric tube to the right, depression of the left mainstem bronchus, and widening of the upper left paraspinal stripe.

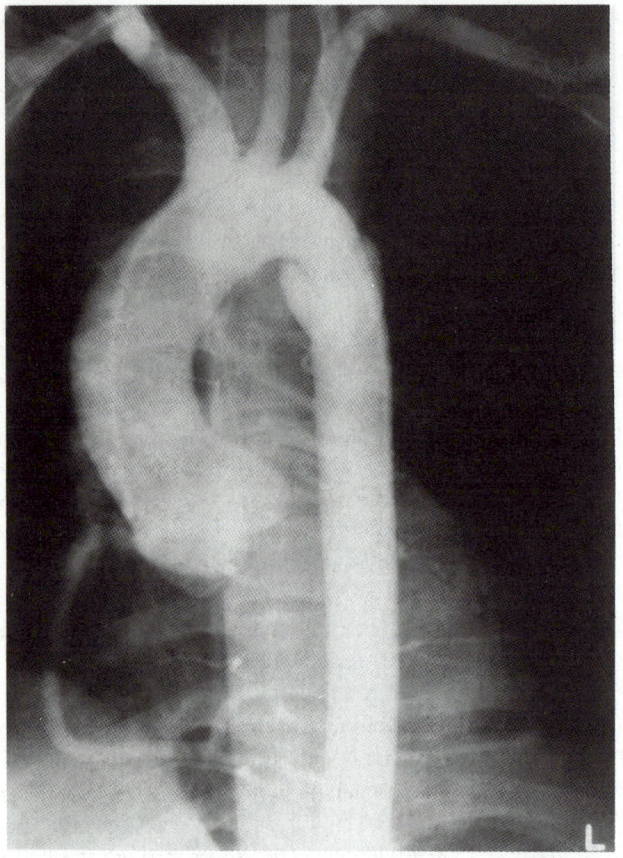

Figure 134–2. Aortogram of the same patient as in Figure 134–1, demonstrating the classic appearance of a disruption of the aorta in the aortic isthmus, with an intimal/medial "flap" and false aneurysm.

vantages over aortography. It is less invasive, and theoretically less dangerous, since the injured aorta is not directly instrumented; it is usually less time-consuming, and can be done in the emergency department or in the operating room even while other procedures are being performed; no nephrotoxins are required; and TEE can examine the heart for evidence of blunt cardiac injury as well as study the aorta. There are two significant problems with TEE. First is

TABLE 134–2. CRITERIA FOR CT SCANS IN PATIENTS WITH SUSPECTED AORTIC INJURY

Criteria for Reliably Negative CT Scans
    Good contrast enhancement of aorta
    No interfering artifacts
    A complete study
    Film read by an experienced CT radiologist
    Absence of "positive" criteria
Criteria for Positive CT Scans
    Mediastinal hematoma contiguous with the aorta
    False aneurysm
    Irregular aortic contour
    Divided aortic lumen
    Intimal flap

From Agee CK, et al: J Trauma 33:877, 1992.

its inability to always visualize the aortic arch and its main branches adequately. This can be a serious problem, since injuries to these vessels present as mediastinal widening on CXR, and thus a negative TEE may not reliably rule out significant thoracic vascular injury. Second, there are currently few operators available who have the considerable experience with traumatic aortic injuries required to perform a reliable exam.

Magnetic resonance imaging (MRI) has proved to be an excellent modality to visualize the thoracic aorta, especially for aneurysms and dissections. Its use in the evaluation of traumatic aortic injuries, however, is limited for two main reasons. First is its lack of ready availability to most trauma resuscitation areas in emergency situations. Second is the inability to closely monitor unstable or potentially unstable patients while they are in the scanner. At present, the role of MRI is limited to follow-up of postoperative patients and those stable patients with medically treated chronic lesions.

In summary, for patients in whom the suspicion of aortic injury is high, contrast aortography remains the diagnostic procedure of choice. As experience with TEE grows, it may come to supplant aortography; for now, its use is confined to centers where experienced echocardiographers and cardiac and trauma surgeons work together to further define its strengths and limitations. Dynamic contrast chest CT is best suited to exclude aortic injury in patients in whom the suspicion of aortic disruption is low; moreover, proper use of CT demands close adherence to strict guidelines concerning interpretation of findings.

Treatment

The treatment of choice in most cases of traumatic aortic disruption is urgent operative repair. However, (1) in the multiply injured patient, some injuries, such as expanding epidural hematoma or massive intraabdominal hemorrhage, must be treated *before* repair of the aorta can be done, (2) in the hemodynamically stable patient, *pharmacologic* intervention[24–27] should begin as soon as the diagnosis of aortic tear is suspected, and should continue until operative control of the aorta has been obtained, and (3) there are four groups of patients in whom pharmacologic treatment should be extended and aortic repair *delayed* for periods varying from days to months.

Initial Management. The initial approach to the patient with suspected thoracic aortic disruption is the same as for all seriously injured trauma patients, as outlined in the American College of Surgeons' Advanced Trauma Life Support guidelines. As soon as the diagnosis of aortic tear is suggested, usually by a combination of mechanism of injury, physical findings on the primary and secondary surveys, and CXR, pharmacologic treatment of hemodynamically stable patients is begun, while arrangements are made to perform one of the diagnostic tests discussed above.

Pharmacologic treatment is directed at minimizing the

stress on the injured aortic wall to forestall free rupture, and is the same as that used in the pharmacologic treatment of aortic dissection, first introduced by Wheat in 1965.[28] The aortic intraluminal pressure, and especially the rate of rise of the aortic pressure wave (*dP/dt*),[29] should be carefully controlled and, if not actually lowered to less than normal, at least prevented from increasing excessively. The *dP/dt* is best controlled by decreasing the force of left ventricular ejection with negative inotropic agents, and the mean aortic pressure is then controlled with systemic arterial vasodilators. Pure vasodilators, if used alone, increase rather than decrease the *dP/dt,* because they lower diastolic pressure more than systolic pressure; medical treatment should always begin with negative inotropic agents, adding vasodilators as needed.

With continuous heart rate and blood pressure monitoring, preferably via an indwelling right radial artery catheter, a negative inotropic agent such as propanolol or labetolol is administered intravenously. The goal is to lower the systolic blood pressure to 90 to 110 torr, and the mean pressure to 60 to 70 torr. β-Blockade is increased until this goal is reached, or until the heart rate is 55 to 60. If the heart rate gets to this level but the blood pressure remains higher than desired, nitroprusside is added; further β-blockade is unwise, as it will only predispose to unwanted conduction defects. Analgesics and sedatives are used cautiously but are important adjuncts for blood pressure control. In particular, topical and local anesthetics and systemic analgesics are vital prior to performing any painful procedure such as insertion of nasogastric or thoracostomy tubes. (Of note, it is safe to place NG and chest tubes, if indicated, as long as the chest tube is not inserted too far.) Strict control of blood pressure (*dP/dt*) is continued until operative repair of the aortic injury is accomplished.

Antihypertensive treatment is used only for hemodynamically stable patients. For unstable patients, expeditious evaluation and treatment of other injuries are essential. In general, aortic disruption does not cause hemodynamic lability: if free rupture occurs, exsanguination results and nothing short of operative control of the aorta will be able to restore the circulation. Hemodynamic instability in a patient with a torn aorta is caused by some other injury, most often hemorrhage—intra-abdominal, pelvic, etc. Treatment of these other injuries takes precedence over treatment, and even diagnosis, of the aortic tear. Thus, a patient with an abdominal paracentesis positive for gross blood, or with a cranial CT showing an epidural hematoma, should undergo laparotomy or craniotomy *prior* to aortography and subsequent aortic repair; a patient with ongoing bleeding into an unstable pelvic fracture should have an external fixator placed first. At all times during these diagnostic and therapeutic procedures, careful attention to blood pressure control should be continued.

There are four groups of patients in whom operative repair should be delayed while continuing strict antihypertensive treatment. First, patients with severe head injuries whose prognosis for neurologic survival is uncertain should not undergo aortic repair until they have made significant neurologic recovery. Clamping and unclamping the thoracic aorta even with the most careful anesthesia induces profound swings in cerebral perfusion pressure, which can only worsen cerebral perfusion abnormalities. Second, patients with established sepsis should undergo aortic repair only after their sepsis is adequately under control. For example, a patient in whom the diagnosis of aortic tear has been made several days after concomitant colon injury and who now has an intra-abdominal abscess, would be at high risk of infecting a new aortic intravascular graft. Likewise, a patient with extensive burns is at high risk for developing recurrent septicemia until all the burn wounds have been excised and grafted; such patients should undergo aortic grafting only after the likelihood of sepsis has been reduced. Finally, patients with severe right lung contusions may not be able to tolerate having their left lung collapsed for an operation on the descending aorta; aortic repair in these patients should be delayed until the right lung has recovered.

Operative Repair. Once the diagnosis of aortic disruption is made, the treatment of choice is operative repair. Tears of the descending aorta are approached through a standard posterolateral thoracotomy incision, entering the chest through the fourth intercostal space (or through the bed of the subperiosteally resected fifth rib in patients over 50 years of age) with or without aortic bypass, whereas tears of the ascending aorta are approached via median sternotomy using full femoral–femoral cardiopulmonary bypass. In all cases, an autotransfusion device should be used, and ample homologous blood should be in the operating room.

There are four general methods used to accomplish descending thoracic aortic repair, differing in respect to temporary bypass of the injured segment. These four methods represent different approaches to the avoidance of the dreaded main complication of thoracic aortic surgery: ischemic injury of the spinal cord, causing the anterior spinal syndrome with paralysis of the lower extremities. To date, *none* of these four methods has been definitively shown to be superior to the others.[30] First is the use of full cardiopulmonary bypass, femoral vein to femoral artery; the main drawback to this method is the requirement for complete heparin anticoagulation in a patient with multiple blunt injuries. Second is the use of partial bypass using the centrifugal Biomedicus® pump, for which heparinization is not required; the bypass can be from the left atrium or the left superior pulmonary vein, depending on the operator's preference, to the descending thoracic aorta distal to the tear or to the left femoral artery. Third is the use of partial bypass using a so-called "Gott" shunt (Fig. 134–3B): a plastic (tridodecylmethyl ammonium chloride, or TDMAC) tube to whose internal surface heparin has been bonded, inserted into the left ventricular apex or ascending aorta and into the distal descending aorta or femoral artery[31]; the main draw-

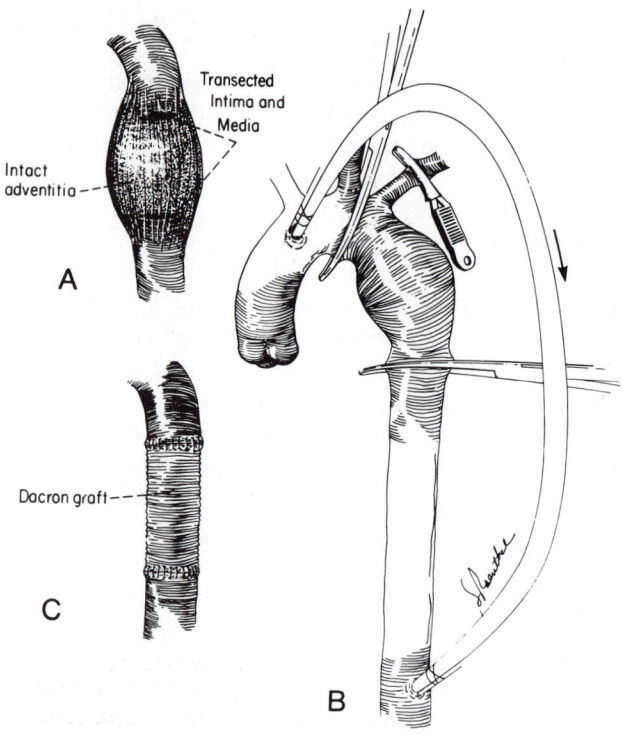

Figure 134–3. The "Gott" shunt. **A.** Acute traumatic false aneurysm of the descending thoracic aorta. The intima and media have been circumferentially disrupted, and the ends have retracted and are separated by several centimeters. The aortic adventitia remains intact to form the wall of the false aneurysm. **B.** With the aorta clamped on either side of the injured segment, bloodflow to the lower body is maintained via the heparin-coated shunt tubing. The proximal end of the shunt can be inserted into the proximal aorta or the left ventricular apex; the distal end can be inserted into the distal thoracic aorta or the left femoral artery. **C.** The completed repair, using a short segment of dacron graft. *(From Burke/ Boyd/McCabe: Trauma Management. St. Louis, Year Book Medical, 1988, p 165.)*

back of the Gott shunt is the inability to control the amount of bloodflow through the shunt. Fourth, the "clamp and sew" technique, where no bypass is used, and the cross-clamp time is kept to a minimum (preferably less than 30 min, though there are no data showing 30 min to be either the upper limit of safe or the lower limit of unsafe). Although none of these four approaches has been shown to be superior in preventing spinal cord ischemia, it *is* reasonable to assume that some form of bypass should be used if there is a concomitant blunt injury of the myocardium. Moreover, vasodilators must be used very carefully if at all during aortic cross-clamping, since they can further lessen distal aortic blood flow to the cord and to the kidneys.

Regardless of the type of bypass used, the disrupted descending aorta is approached through the left chest, with a double-lumen endotracheal tube or a bronchial blocker used to deflate the left lung. Before any manipulation of the injured area, proximal control and distal control of the aorta are obtained by placing circumferential umbilical tapes

using minimal dissection. Proximal control is most often obtainable between the origins of the left carotid and the left subclavian arteries; the proximal left subclavian is encircled and controlled separately (Fig. 134–3B). Care is taken when encircling the aortic arch to keep the plane of gentle sharp and blunt dissection close on the outer wall of the aorta, to avoid injury to the surrounding structures, including the pulmonary artery and the vagus and recurrent laryngeal nerves (Fig. 134–4). Distal control is obtained as close to the distalmost injured area as practical, to preserve flow to as many intercostals as possible. If a bypass is to be used, it is then inserted. The anesthesiologists should be given a five minute warning prior to aortic clamping, so that they can give intravenous mannitol, and be ready to start infusion of vasodilators (nitroprusside or nitroglycerin) as needed and/or monitor bypass blood flow. If a graft is to be used, the proper size is selected, in most cases a 16-, 18-, or 20-mm knitted (woven if the patient is heparinized) dacron tube, and the proximal suture of 3-0 or 4-0 prolene placed in the proximal end. When all is prepared, the bypass, if any, is opened, and the proximal and distal aortic and left subclavian clamps are placed, noting the time. The disrupted aortic segment is opened in the most injured area in a transverse direction, and the extent of injury assessed. Most often one finds that the intima and media have been completely transected, with a gap of several centimeters between the proximal and distal ends. Minimal debridement, just enough to remove debris from the lumen, is necessary. It is usually not necessary, and not desirable, to ligate any intercostal orifices: the distal clamp can often be repositioned closer to the injury if needed. The repair is carried out either by primary anastomosis using a single running 3-0 prolene suture, ensuring intima-to-intima coaptation, or more often by inserting a short (3 to 4 cm) graft (Fig. 134–3C), again using a single running 3-0 prolene for each anastomosis. The proximal anastomosis is tested prior to performing the distal anastomosis; the aorta is flushed of air and clot just before completing the distal anastomosis. The distal aortic and subclavian clamps are released first, then the proximal clamp is slowly opened (again after giving the anesthesia team a minute or two of advanced warning) little by little to prevent precipitous falls in blood pressure. Any leaks can be repaired with mattress sutures of 4-0 prolene with pledgets, partially occluding the aorta with a clamp or with fingers to decrease wall tension during placement and tying.

The operative mortality of patients undergoing repair of thoracic aortic disruption is mostly dependent on the patients' associated injuries. The most serious complication is paraplegia due to spinal cord ischemia, which occurs in 4 to 20%. To date, no one method of aortic bypass (or speed without bypass) has been definitively shown to be superior to the others in preventing cord ischemia; research on methods of spinal cord preservation during descending thoracic aortic surgery continues.

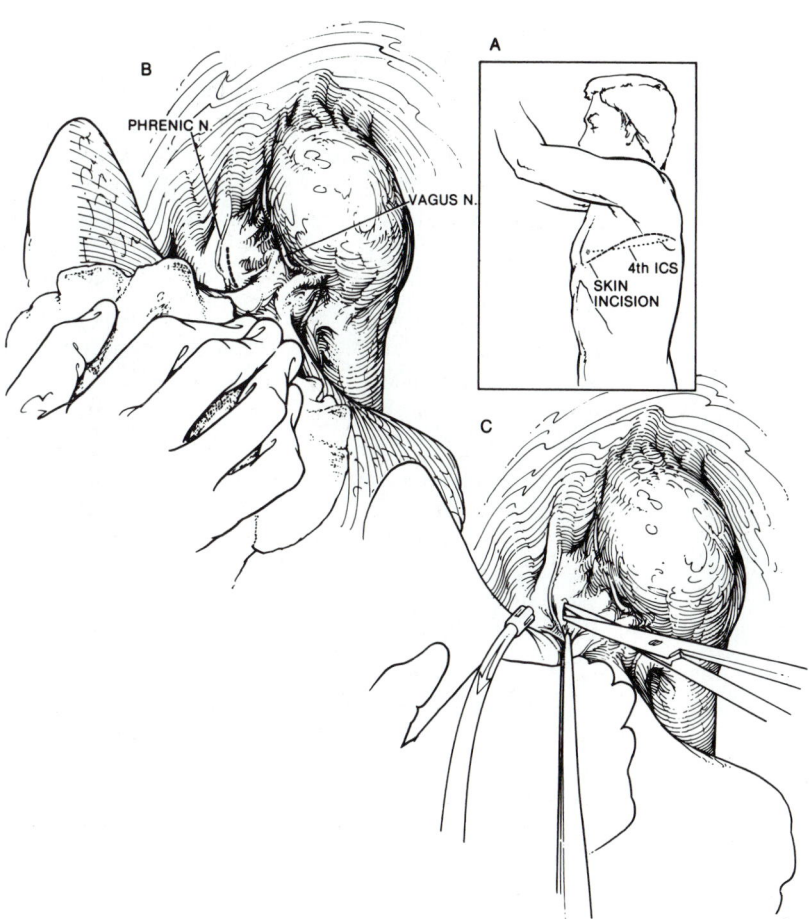

Figure 134–4. A. The descending aorta is approached via a left posterolateral thoracotomy through the fourth intercostal space. **B,C.** Careful dissection is used to obtain control of the proximal aorta between the left carotid and left subclavian arteries, just posterior to the phrenic nerve and anterior to the vagus and recurrent laryngeal nerves. *(From Cooley, Denton A: Surgical Treatment of Aortic Aneurysms. Philadelphia, Saunders, 1986, p 189.)*

Ascending Aortic Tears. The principles of treatment of tears of the ascending aorta are somewhat different from that of the much more common descending disruption. As with spontaneous dissections of the ascending aorta, surgery for this lesion must be emergent: there is no role for planned delay. Craniotomy and laparotomy for bleeding, if needed, must be performed simultaneously with the aortic repair. The operative approach is via median sternotomy, with full femoral–femoral cardiopulmonary bypass, ascending aortic clamping, and cardioplegia. The operative technique is essentially the same as for repair of an ascending aortic aneurysm, except that the sinuses of Valsalva, coronary arteries, and aortic valve are rarely involved, and length of graft needed will be less.

Blunt Injuries of the Great Vessels of the Arch

The same mechanism of injury that causes disruption of the thoracic aorta—rapid deceleration or acceleration—may cause disruption of the proximal portions of the arch vessels. The most commonly injured arch vessel is the innominate artery; blunt injuries of the left common carotid and left subclavian are quite rare. These injuries all present as upper mediastinal widening on CXR (Fig. 134–5A), usually

accompanied by an apical cap and deviation of the trachea. Diagnosis is made by angiography (Fig. 134–5B); TEE is often quite limited in visualizing the arch vessels. The principles of treatment are the same as for descending aortic disruption, with the same schemes for setting of injury priority, antihypertensive medical therapy, and planned delay if indicated.

Operative repair of the innominate artery is carried out via median sternotomy, with a right neck extension of the incision for control of the distal vessel. Aortic bypass is not required. If there is active bleeding, it is controlled with a side-biting clamp (e.g., Satinsky) placed tangentially on the aorta at the origin of the innominate (Fig. 134–6), and the proximal end of the vessel oversewn with 4-0 or 5-0 prolene. A 5- or 6-mm dacron graft is sewn onto the ascending aorta with running 5-0 prolene, again using a side-biting clamp, in side-to-end fashion. The other end of the graft is then anastomosed end-to-end or end-to-side to the distal innominate. If there is no active bleeding, the graft anastomoses are performed first to minimize cerebral ischemic time. Intraoperative EEG monitoring is used if possible, and a temporary intravascular shunt is employed if there are EEG changes with innominate occlusion.

The operative approach to the left carotid and left sub-

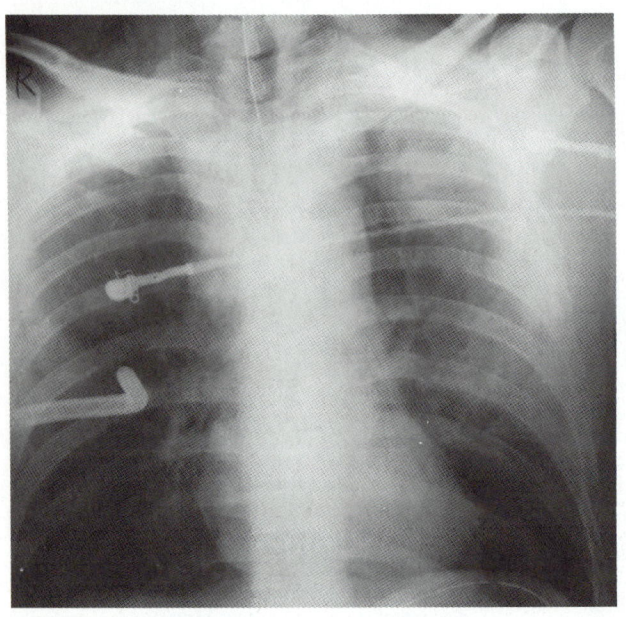

A

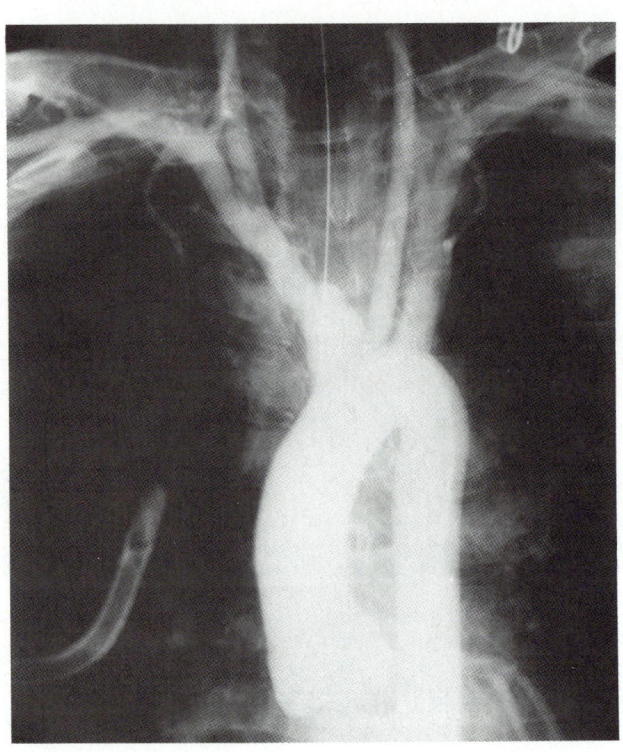

B

Figure 134–5. Chest x-ray (**A**) and aortogram (**B**) of a patient with disruption of the origin of the innominate artery. The chest x-ray shows widening of the mediastinum indistinguishable from that seen with rupture of the descending aorta.

clavian arteries is either through a high (third or fourth interspace) left thoracotomy, through a median sternotomy, or a combination of the two, depending on the patient's body habitus and the rapidity of exposure required. For unstable patients, a left anterior thoracotomy provides the most rapid access for proximal control; this incision is also required for patients with a large anteroposterior diameter of the thorax. A left neck incision, anterior to the sternocleidomastoid for the carotid or supraclavicular for the subclavian, is needed for distal control (Fig. 134–7). The proximal part of the injured vessel is oversewn, and a dacron graft from the ascending aorta side-to-end is then connected end-to-end to the distal vessel.

PENETRATING INJURIES OF THE GREAT VESSELS

The evaluation and treatment of penetrating injuries are, in general, conceptually more straightforward than that of blunt injuries: the structures at risk are those that are in proximity to the entry wound and the subsequent path of the blade or projectile (although it is an oft-repeated maxim that bullets do not always follow a straight line from point of entrance to point of exit or point of rest within the body). The clinical manifestations of the vascular injury depend somewhat on the wounding agent. Knife wounds cause he-

morrhage, false aneurysms, and occasionally arteriovenous fistulae. Projectiles—bullets and shrapnel—can cause hemorrhage, aneurysms, and arteriovenous fistulae by disrupting the full thickness of the vessel wall, or thrombosis by disrupting, by blast effect, only a partial thickness of the wall. Moreover, the greater degree of vessel damage caused by projectiles tends to cause unremitting bleeding, while knife wounds often stop bleeding spontaneously.[32–35] Hemorrhage from either type of agent can be external, internal, or both. External hemorrhage is immediately apparent, and is best temporarily controlled by direct pressure, if possible; however, with injury to the large thoracic vessels, emergent operative exposure of the proximal vessel will not infrequently be required to obtain adequate control. Internal hemorrhage can be into the pleural cavity, the pericardial space, the extrapericardial mediastinum, or the soft tissues of the chest wall and neck. Systemic arterial bleeding into the pleural space will *not* be tamponaded by the lung, even during positive pressure ventilation, whereas systemic venous and pulmonary arterial and venous bleeding can be. *Any* bleeding into the pericardium—arterial, venous, or capillary—can cause acute pericardial tamponade (as can arterial bleeding into the mediastinum next to but outside the pericardium). Arterial bleeding into the soft tissues will appear as an expanding, possibly pulsatile, hematoma; if close enough to the trachea, such bleeding can cause acute airway compromise.

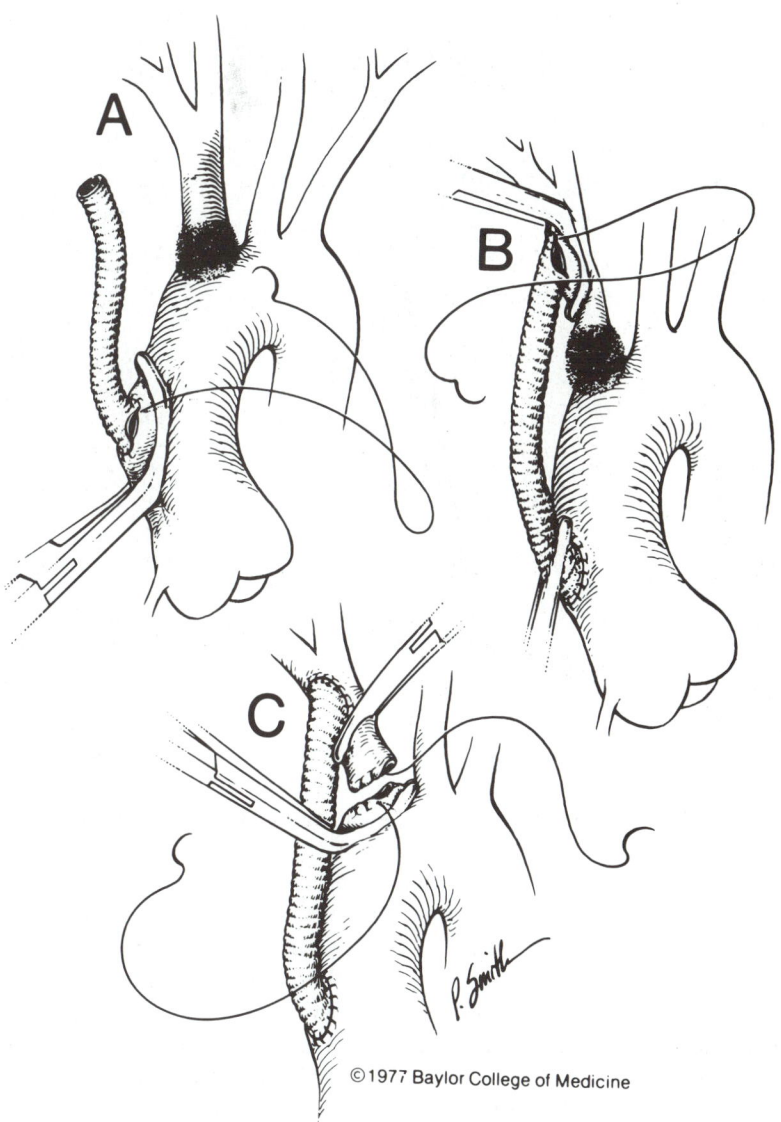

©1977 Baylor College of Medicine

Figure 134–6. Repair of innominate artery disruption. **A.** Anastomosis of the proximal graft to the ascending aorta. **B.** Anastomosis of the distal end of the graft to the innominate artery distal to the injury. **C.** Oversewing of the injured segment. *(From Flanigan D, Preston: Civilian Vascular Trauma. Philadelphia, Lea & Febiger, 1992, p 171.)*

Injuries to the Vessels of the Thoracic Outlet

While the aorta and proximal innominate artery are the great thoracic vessels most often injured by blunt trauma, penetrating injuries most frequently damage the other, less well-protected great vessels that traverse the thoracic outlet: the carotid and subclavian arteries and their branches, and the jugular, subclavian, and innominate veins and the superior vena cava. Injuries to the vessels of the thoracic outlet are relatively uncommon, but they are also highly lethal, with contemporary series still showing a mortality over 50%.[32–34] Among the reasons for such a high mortality are the high flow through the vessels, which causes rapid exsanguination when the vessels are injured; they supply blood to the head, thus injury to them often causes devastating neurologic insults; and finally, the thoracic outlet is a difficult area to access, both for diagnosis and for treatment.

The initial approach to the patient with a penetrating injury in the region of the thoracic outlet depends on the pa-

tient's hemodynamic status. After expeditiously securing the airway, assuring adequate ventilation, and obtaining large-bore intravenous access (the "A, B, Cs"), those patients in profound shock unresponsive to fluid administration should undergo emergency department (ED) thoracotomy via a left anterolateral incision. (Fig. 134–8) Entry into the chest is made through the fourth intercostal space, after positive pressure ventilation via an endotracheal tube has been instituted. The first priority is relief of pericardial tamponade: if the pericardium is full of blood, it is opened by an incision parallel and 2 cm anterior to the phrenic nerve. Bleeding from a hole in the ventricle is controlled with the index finger, and suture repair carried out with horizontal matress sutures of nonabsorbable material; a laceration of the ascending aorta or of the atria can be temporarily closed with a side-biting clamp. Bleeding from larger holes in the heart that cannot be controlled with the fingers or a clamp can sometimes be temporarily controlled by inserting a Foley catheter through the hole, inflating the balloon, and

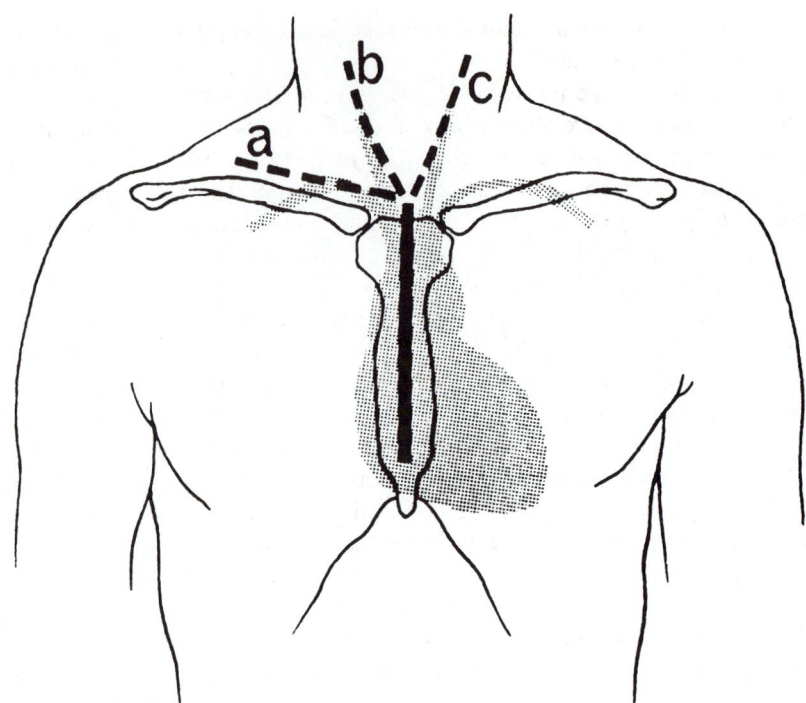

Figure 134–7. Extensions of the median sternotomy incision for exposure of the great vessels: **a,** the right subclavian artery; **b,** the right carotid; **c,** the left carotid. A supraclavicular mirror-image of **a** could be used for the left subclavian. *(From Hunt TK, et al: Vascular injuries of the base of the neck. Arch Surg 98:589, Copyright 1969, American Medical Association.)*

applying gentle traction. If there is no tamponade, the pericardium need not be opened. Whether or not the pericardium is opened, internal massage of the heart must be performed continuously, or intermittently while repairing the heart, so that some perfusion to the head and heart is maintained.

The next step is to clamp the descending aorta, to restore adequate blood pressure and flow to the head and heart. This is done primarily by feel, passing the left hand from the posterior part of the pleural space along the ribs, medially up to the vertebral column. The aorta is just anterior to the vertebrae and smaller than one expects it to be (since most victims are young and relatively free of degenerative changes, and since the systemic pressure is low). The mediastinal pleura is divided with the fingers or with the tips of the vascular clamp, which is then placed on the aorta at the most convenient location, usually at the level of

the fifth or sixth vertebral body. A tube in the esophagus aids in avoiding placing the clamp across that more muscular structure. Volume and cardiac resuscitation continues. Control is then obtained of any vessel or vessels that are bleeding, using fingers to start with, followed by clamps if possible. Extension of the incision across the sternum (clam shell) into the right chest allows access to the right side of the heart and ascending aorta.

If resuscitation is successful, the patient is taken to the operating room for definitive control of the injuries and formal chest closure. There, additional incisions for adequate exposure, including median sternotomy and neck extensions (Figs. 134–7 and 134–8), should be used as needed for repair of the arch and great vessels. The results of ED thoracotomy for penetrating injuries of the chest can be quite good, with up to 90% survival for stab wounds of the heart[35]; as long as there were measureable vital signs or

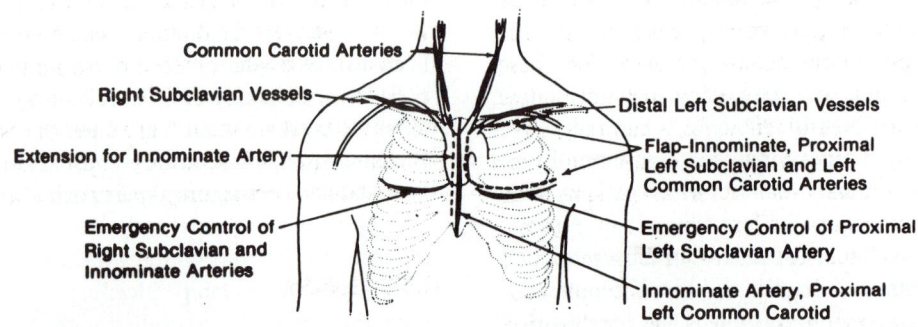

Figure 134–8. Incisions and extensions required for control and repair of major injury to common carotid, subclavian, and innominate arteries and their associated veins. *(From Flint LM, et al: Management of major vascular injuries in the base of the neck. Arch Surg 106:409, Copyright 1973, American Medical Association.)*

some signs of life within 5 min of arrival at the hospital, ED thoracotomy is justified.[36]

Patients who are unstable but who have a reasonable blood pressure—as are about one-third of all patients with great vessel injury—should be taken directly to the operating room for emergency thoracotomy. The incision of choice for most wounds of the great vessels is a median sternotomy, if time allows, with extensions into the neck or the supraclavicular areas as needed for distal control. (Figs. 134–7 and 134–8) The groins must be prepped and draped for access to both the saphenous veins for use as autogenous graft and the femoral vessels for possible cardiopulmonary bypass; intravenous access in both the upper and lower extremities is advisable, and the autotransfusion apparatus should be set up. As in all vascular surgery, the basic principles of first obtaining proximal and distal control, repair without narrowing the lumen, and anastomosis without tension must be followed. The great arteries should be repaired or bypassed if at all possible, since most often they have insufficient collateral flow: one-third of patients who undergo unilateral carotid ligation have serious neurologic damage. (Ligation of a vertebral artery, on the other hand, carries only a 3% risk of neurologic complication.) Synthetic dacron or Gortex grafts are preferable for bypassing the large arteries, while patches are more readily made from autogenous vein. The subclavian vessels are particularly fragile, and cannot be significantly mobilized; interposition grafts should be used in most instances. The great veins, with the exception of the superior vena cava itself, may in general be ligated without serious sequelae; if a patch graft is used, it should be autogenous vein.

Stable patients with penetrating wounds of the chest require careful and thorough evaluation in the emergency department: as stated by Debakey and associates in their 1970 report, "no matter how stable patients with such injuries may appear, they are in imminent danger of circulatory collapse from exsanguinating hemorrhage, which very likely will be irreversible if operative exposure has not already been obtained before it occurs."[37] Thoracostomy, using a 36 Fr or larger tube with an autotransfusion setup, should be performed in the mid-axillary line at nipple level if there is evidence of hemo- and/or pneumothorax on physical exam or chest x-ray. A blood pressure differential between the two arms suggests subclavian artery injury. A bruit or thrill suggests an arteriovenous fistula (but the absence of a bruit or thrill does not rule it out). The chest x-ray may show widening of the mediastinum, an apical cap, and/or hemothorax. Neurologic deficits can be caused by carotid injury or by direct spinal cord injury from gunshot wounds. However, nearly one-half of all patients with significant great vessel injury will not have any external findings. "Nonoperative" mediastinal exploration should be carried out, with contrast aortography, bronchoscopy, esophagoscopy, and gastrograffin swallow. (The combination of endoscopic and contrast radiologic examination of the esophagus approaches 100% sensitivity—better than the 80% of either one alone.) Angiography will be able to iden-

tify all injuries of the arteries that require operative intervention. It will not show venous injuries, but these do not need surgical repair unless they cause ongoing bleeding, manifest as hemodynamic compromise, continued chest tube drainage, and/or continued drop in hematocrit. Angiography may also be used to embolize small arterial bleeders, including the vertebral, internal mammary, and intercostal arteries. Angiographic placement of an intravascular balloon catheter to aid in proximal control of bleeding during subsequent operative repair has been reported.[38] The principles of operative management are delineated above. Repair of these injuries in stable patients should have little morbidity and mortality due to the vascular injury itself: these are principally determined by concomitant injuries.

For all patients, stable and unstable, it is important to have a high index of suspicion that other mediastinal structures may have been injured. Thus bronchoscopy and esophagoscopy should be carried out in all patients with wounds in proximity to these structures, and any injuries should be dealt with at the initial operation. The thoracic duct may be ligated with impunity. Somatic nerves (e.g., brachial plexus) and the recurrent laryngeal nerves should be identified and tagged with prolene sutures, and intraoperative consultation with a plastic/reconstructive specialist obtained, if the patient's stability allows.

Injury of the Vessels of the Pulmonary Hilum

Most injuries of the pulmonary hilum are caused by gunshot wounds. Shock, massive hemothorax, respiratory compromise, and hemoptysis are usually present. The optimum approach to the pulmonary hilum is via lateral thoracotomy in the fourth intercostal space on the side of injury. The pulmonary vessels, both arterial and venous, are very thin walled and fragile, making repair of injuries difficult at best. The entire hilum can be occluded manually or with a large vascular clamp. The exact extent of the injury is then determined, and the injured segments ligated; resection of the distal parenchyma is most often required.

Systemic air embolism, caused by air entering the damaged pulmonary veins, is the unique problem associated with injuries of the pulmonary hilum. Air embolism usually presents as sudden lateralized neurologic deficit and/or ventricular fibrillation, often beginning just after the institution of positive pressure ventilation. Immediate thoracotomy and clamping of the pulmonary hilum, with deairing of the heart via the LV apex and the ascending aorta via its topmost part, are necessary. Open chest resuscitation follows, and pneumonectomy will usually be required.

REFERENCES

1. *Accidental Death and Disability; The Neglected Disease of Modern Society.* Division of Medical Services, Washington, DC, The National Academy of Sciences, The National Research Council, 1965
2. Trunkey DD: Trauma. *Sci Am* **249**:28–35, 1983

3. Trunkey DD: The Presidential Address on the nature of things that go bang in the night. *Surgery* **92**:125–132, 1983

4. Tardiff K, Marzuk PM, Leon AC, et al: Homicide in New York City, cocaine use in firearms. *JAMA* **272**:43–46, 1994

5. Symbas PN, Kourias E, Tyras DH, et al: Penetrating wounds of great vessels. *Ann Surg* **179**:757–762, 1974

6. Schwab CW: Violence: America's uncivil war—Presidential Address, 6th Scientific Assembly of the Eastern Association for the Surgery of Trauma. *J Trauma* **35**:657–665, 1993

7. Mattox KL, Feliciano DV, Burch J, et al: Five thousand seven hundred and sixty cardiovascular injuries in 4,459 patients. *Ann Surg* **209**:698–707, 1989

8. Muellerman RL, Walker RA, Edney JA: Motor vehicle deaths: A rural epidemic. *J Trauma* **35**:717–719, 1993

9. Brewer RD, Morris PD, Cole TB, et al: The risk of dying in alcohol-related automobile crashes among habitual drunk drivers. *N Eng J Med* **331**:513–517, 1994

10. Brookoff D, Cook CS, Williams C: Testing reckless drivers for cocaine and marijuana. *N Eng J Med* **331**:518–522, 1994

11. Angell M, Kassirer JP: Alcohol and other drugs—toward a more rational and consistent policy. Editorial. *N Engl J Med* **331**:537–539, 1994

12. Advanced Trauma Life Support Program for Physicians, 1993 Committee on Trauma, American College of Surgeons

13. Arajarvi E, Santavirta S, Tolonen J: Aortic ruptures in seat belt wearers. *J Thorac Cardiovasc Surg* **98**:355–361, 1989

14. Greendyke RM: Traumatic rupture of the aorta—special reference to automobile accidents. *JAMA* **195**:527–530, 1966

15. Fabian T: Personal communication

16. Ochsner MG, Hoffman AP, DiPasquale D, et al: Associated aortic rupture-pelvic fracture: An alert for orthopedic and general surgeons. *J Trauma* **33**:429–434, 1992

17. Eddy AC, Rusch VW, Fligner CL, et al: The epidemiology of traumatic rupture of the thoracic aorta in children: A 13-year review. *J Trauma* **30**:989–991, 1990

18. Plume S, DeWeese JA: Traumatic rupture of the thoracic aorta. *Arch Surg* **114**:240–243, 1979

19. Seltzer SE, Orsi CD, Kirshner R, DeWeese JA: Traumatic aortic rupture: Plain radiographic findings. *AJR* **137**:1011–1014, 1983

20. Miller FB, Richardson D, Thomas HA, et al: Role of CT in diagnosis of major arterial injury after blunt thoracic trauma. *Surgery* **106**:596–603, 1989

21. Agee CK, Metzler MH, Churchill RJ, Mitchell FL: Computed tomographic evaluation to exclude traumatic aortic disruption. *J Trauma* **33**:876–881, 1992

22. Sparks MB, Burchard KW, Marrin CAS, et al: Transesophageal echocardiography. Preliminary results in patients with traumatic aortic rupture. *Arch Surg* **126**:711–714, 1991

23. Buckmaster MJ, Kearney PA, Johnson SB, et al: Further experience with transesophageal echocardiography in the evaluation of traumatic aortic injury, EAST abstract. *J Trauma* **35**: 983, 1994

24. Akins CW, Buckley MJ, Daggett WM, et al: Acute traumatic disruption of the thoracic aorta: A ten-year experience. *Ann Thorac Surg* **31**:305–309, 1981

25. Warren RL, Akins CW, Conn AKT, et al: Acute traumatic disruption of the thoracic aorta: Emergency department management. *Ann Emerg Med* **21**:391–396, 1992

26. Walker WA, Pate JW: Medical management of acute traumatic rupture of the aorta. *Ann Thorac Surg* **50**:965–967, 1990

27. Lee RB, Stahlamn GC, Sharp KW: Treatment priorities in patients with traumatic rupture of the thoracic aorta. *Am Surg* **58**:37–43, 1992

28. Wheat MW, Palmer RF, Bartley TD, et al: Treatment of dissecting aneurysms of the aorta without surgery. *J Thorac Cardiovasc Surg* **50**:364–373, 1965

29. Prokop EK, Palmer RF, Wheat MW: Hydrodynamic forces in dissecting aneurysms. *Circ Res* **27**:121–127, 1970

30. Hilgenberg AD, Logan DL, Akins CW, et al: *Ann Thorac Surg* **53**:233–239, 1992

31. Donahoo JS, Brawley RK, Gott VL: The heparin-coated vascular shunt for thoracic aortic and great vessel procedures: A ten-year experience. *Ann Thorac Surg* **23**:507–510, 1977

32. Buscaglia L, Walsh JC, Wilson JD, et al: Surgical management of subclavian artery injury. *Am J Surg* **54**:88–92, 1987

33. Ordog GJ, Wasserberger J, Balasubramanium S, et al: Asymptomatic stab wounds of the chest. *J Trauma* **36**:680–684, 1994

34. Bladergroen M, Brockman R, Luna G, et al: A twelve-year survey of cervicothoracic vascular injuries. *Am J Surg* **157**:483–486, 1989

35. Schwab CW, Adcock OT, Max MH: Emergency Department thoracotomy (EDT). A 26-month experience using an "agonal" protocol. *Am Surg* **52**:20–29, 1986

36. Lorenz HP, Steinmetz B, Liberman J, et al: Emergency thoracotomy: Survival correlates with physiologic status. *J Trauma* **32**:780–788, 1992

37. Bricker DL, Noon GP, Beall AC, et al: Vascular injuries of the thoracic outlet. *J Trauma* **10**:1–15, 1970

38. Scalea TM, Sclafani SJA: Angiographically placed balloons for arterial control: A description of a technique. *J Trauma* **31**:1671–1677, 1991

135

Aneurysms of the Ascending Aorta

Nicholas T. Kouchoukos

The first accurate description of an arterial aneurysm is attributed to Galen in the second century. In 1542, Fernelius recognized that aneurysms arose as a result of localized thinning of the arterial wall. Vesalius is credited with the first correct clinical diagnosis, which he made in 1557.[1]

Until the development of synthetic vascular grafts and prosthetic valves and the perfection of techniques for extracorporeal circulatory support, surgical treatment of ascending aortic aneurysms was limited to wrapping of the aorta or aneurysmorrhaphy.[2] In 1956, Cooley and DeBakey described a technique for supracoronary graft replacement of the ascending aorta with a synthetic graft.[3] In 1960, Mueller et al combined supracoronary graft replacement with bicuspidization of an incompetent aortic valve.[4] In 1963, Starr et al described supracoronary graft replacement and replacement of the aortic valve.[5] In 1964, Wheat et al described a technique of radical resection of the aortic wall, leaving small buttons of tissue adjacent to the coronary ostia, replacement of the aorta with a graft, and prosthetic replacement of the aortic valve.[6] In 1968, Bentall and de Bono described a technique for replacing the ascending aorta and aortic valve with a composite graft.[7] Modifications of the technique described by Bentall and de Bono, which involved direct attachment of the aortic tissue surrounding the coronary ostia to the aortic graft and wrapping of the aorta around the graft to minimize bleeding (inclusion-wrap), were subsequently introduced to reduce the frequency of false aneurysm formation, a complication of the inclusion-wrap method.[8–10]

PATHOLOGY AND NATURAL HISTORY

The majority of aneurysms of the ascending aorta are associated with cystic degenerative changes in the medial layer of the aorta (Fig. 135–1). These aneurysms are often associated with marked dilatation of the sinuses of Valsalva and the aortic annulus. This entity has been termed annuloaortic ectasia.[11] The aortic valve is usually normal on gross examination. Aortic valvular regurgitation, present in the majority of cases, results from dilatation of the aortic sinuses and aortic annulus, with resulting loss of coaptation of the aortic leaflets. Annuloaortic ectasia is frequently present in patients who manifest the clinical stigmata of the Marfan syndrome but may occur in the absence of these findings. Localized intimal tears confined to the ascending aorta are often present. Frank aortic dissections also occur. Other causes of ascending aortic aneurysms include arteriosclerosis, chronic aortic dissection, aortitis (giant cell, granulomatous, syphilitic), primary pyogenic infection (mycotic aneurysm), trauma, and false aneurysms that result from previous surgical procedures or infected vascular grafts.

The natural history of ascending aortic aneurysms is related to a number of factors, including the cause of the aneurysmal disease. For patients with cystic medial degeneration, follow-up of 257 patients with the Marfan syndrome by Murdoch et al[12] showed a 5-year survival of approximately 30%. Of 56 patients for whom the cause of death was known, 52 deaths were from cardiac causes and 39 of these were due to aortic dilatation and its complica-

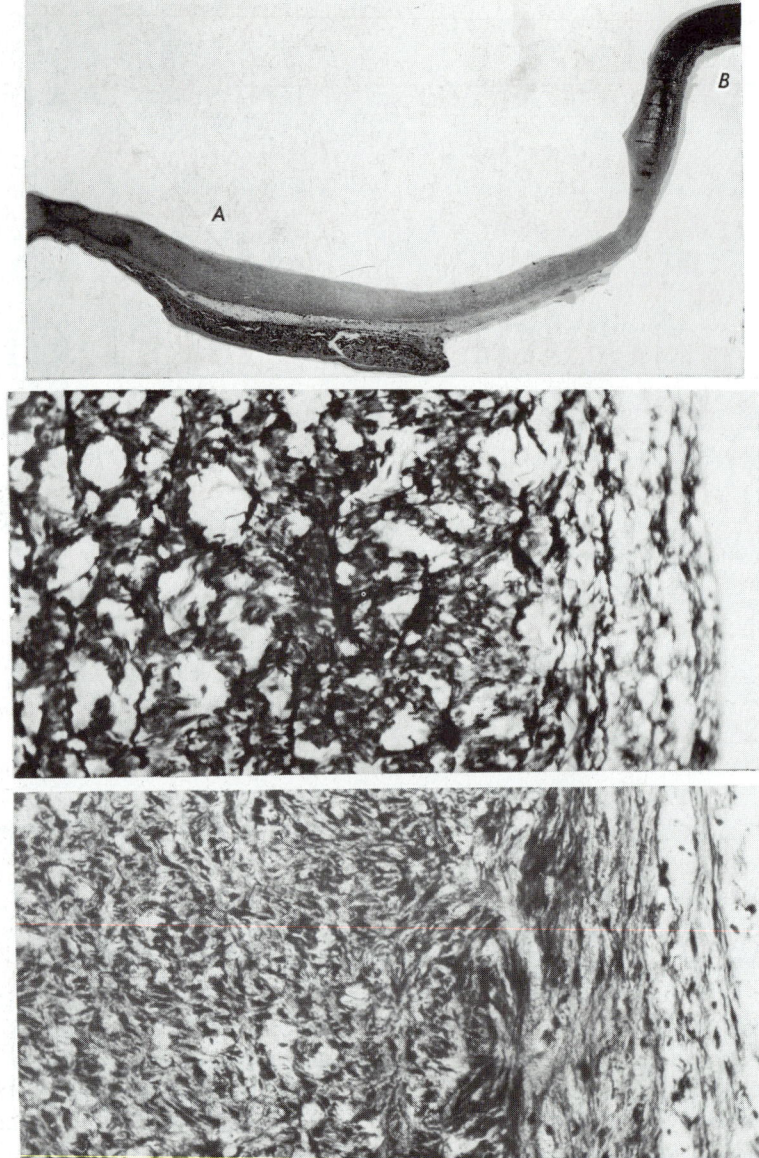

Figure 135–1. Ascending aortic aneurysm and aortic insufficiency associated with cystic medial degeneration. **Top.** Longitudinal section of ascending aorta carried upward from the aortic valve. Elastic-ven Gieson (Verhoeff) stain. **Center.** Enlargement at Level B of top panel. Abundant elastica. Small foci of cystic change occupied by basophilic ground substance. **Bottom.** Masson stain at level A of top panel. Abundant smooth muscle. Small foci of cystic change. Note absence of scarring.

tions. In an additional eight patients who died of congestive failure, aortic regurgitation probably was the underlying cause of the failure. For patients with arteriosclerotic aneurysms, rupture is the most common cause of death.[13–15] Approximately half of the deaths are the result of associated cardiovascular disease.

DIAGNOSIS

Many patients with ascending aortic aneurysms are asymptomatic at the time of presentation. When moderate or severe aortic regurgitation is present, peripheral signs (widened pulse pressure, bounding pulses) and an aortic diastolic murmur are generally present. The electrocardiogram (ECG) may show evidence of left ventricular hyper-

trophy (increased QRS voltage) and "strain" (ST depression and T-wave inversion). The chest roentgenogram often shows enlargement of the ascending aorta and left ventricle (Fig. 135–2A). The aortic enlargement may be confined to the retrosternal area, so that the aortic silhouette appears normal. The diagnosis is then established by aortography (Fig. 135–2B). With cystic medial degenerative disease, the aortic sinuses and ascending aorta are usually dilated, and the aorta tapers to a relatively normal size at the level of origin of the brachiocephalic vessels. The roentgenographic features of a syphilitic aneurysm of the ascending aorta are shown in Figure 135–2C,D. Aortography will also document the degree of cephalad displacement of the coronary ostia and the severity of the aortic valvular regurgitation. Computed tomography (CT), magnetic resonance imaging (MRI), and two-dimensional echocardiography are useful to

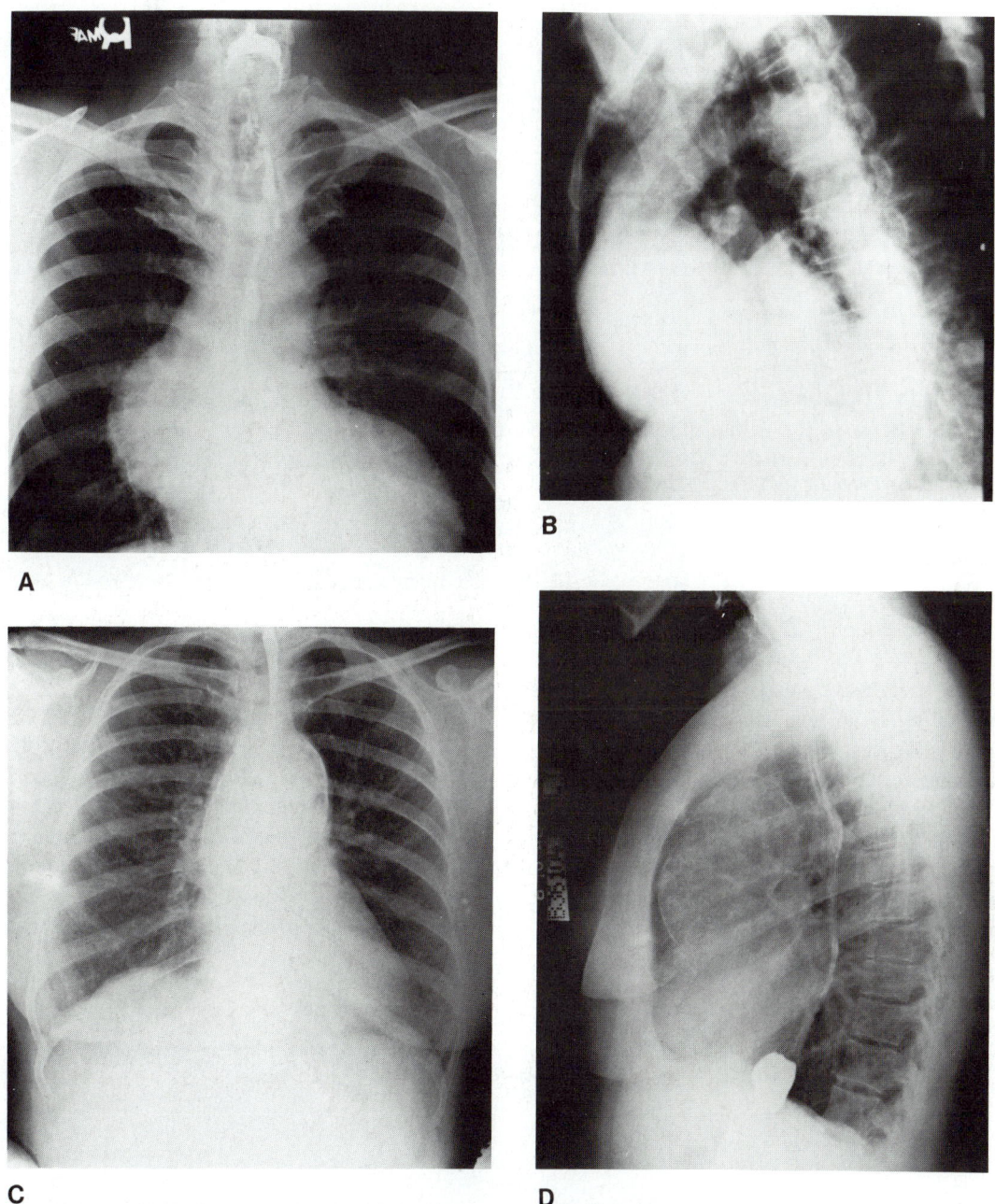

Figure 135–2. Aneurysm of ascending aorta. **A.** Cystic medial degeneration with associated aortic regurgitation. Plain roentgenogram demonstrates enlargement of the ascending aorta and left ventricle. **B.** Aortogram demonstrates symmetric dilatation of the aortic root with return to normal contour just proximal to the brachiocephalic vessels. **C,D.** Aneurysm in a 48-year-old woman with syphilis. Frontal and lateral roentgenograms demonstrate an aneurysm of the ascending aorta with extensive calcification.

document the size of the ascending aorta and for periodic evaluation of aneurysms that are not large enough to require resection (Figs. 135–3 and 135–4).

Coronary angiography is usually performed preoperatively in patients with aneurysms of the ascending aorta who are over the age of 40 years or who have a history of coronary artery disease. This study can be performed in conjunction with thoracic aortography to minimize the dose of intravenous contrast agents.

INDICATIONS FOR OPERATION

The majority of ascending aortic aneurysms are discovered in the course of evaluation of patients with symptoms and signs of aortic regurgitation. Progressive aortic valvular regurgitation is thus the most frequent indication for operation. Patients with symptoms attributable to the aneurysm should have urgent surgical treatment. Acute or chronic aortic dissection and rupture are other indications. Patients

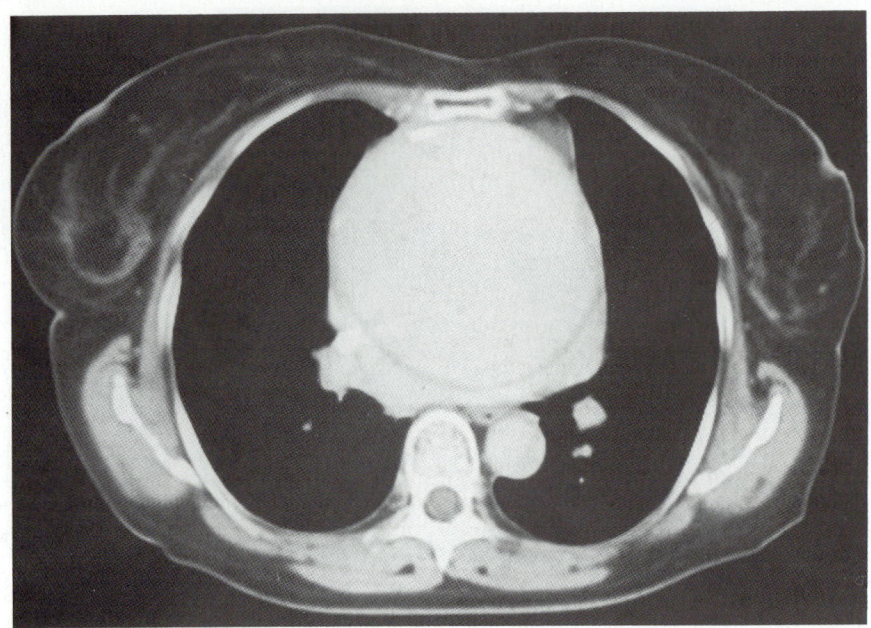

Figure 135–3. Computed tomogram with enhancement by intravenous injection of contrast medium of a patient with a degenerative aneurysm of the ascending aorta.

with evidence for progressive enlargement of the ascending aorta documented by serial roentgenograms, CT, MRI, or echocardiographic studies, even in the absence of symptoms or significant aortic valvular regurgitation, should be considered for operation to prevent dissection or rupture. Based on recent experience,[8,16,17] patients with the Marfan syndrome and ascending aortic aneurysms greater than 5 to 6 cm in diameter should have elective replacement of the ascending aorta and aortic valve.

OPERATIVE TECHNIQUES

Surgical treatment is directed at removal of the aneurysmal segment of the aorta and, when necessary, correction of the aortic valvular regurgitation. Venous access is obtained with a 14-gauge central and two large bore peripheral venous catheters. A 20-gauge cannula for monitoring of arterial pressure and blood gases is placed in a radial artery. Leads II and V5 of the electrocardiogram are continuously

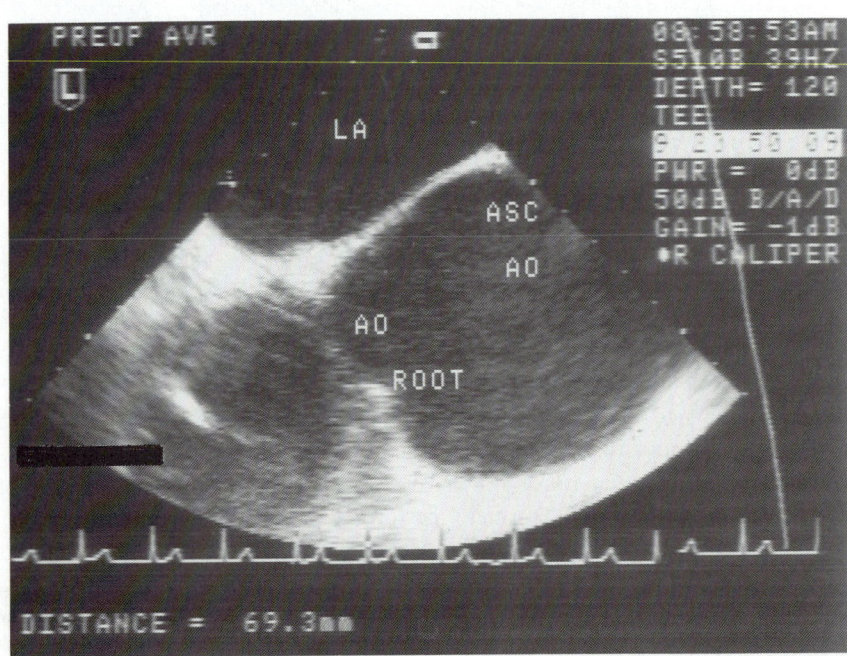

Figure 135–4. Two-dimensional, transesophageal echocardiogram of a patient with the Marfan syndrome and an aneurysm of the ascending aorta associated with dilatation of the aortic root (annuloaortic ectasia).

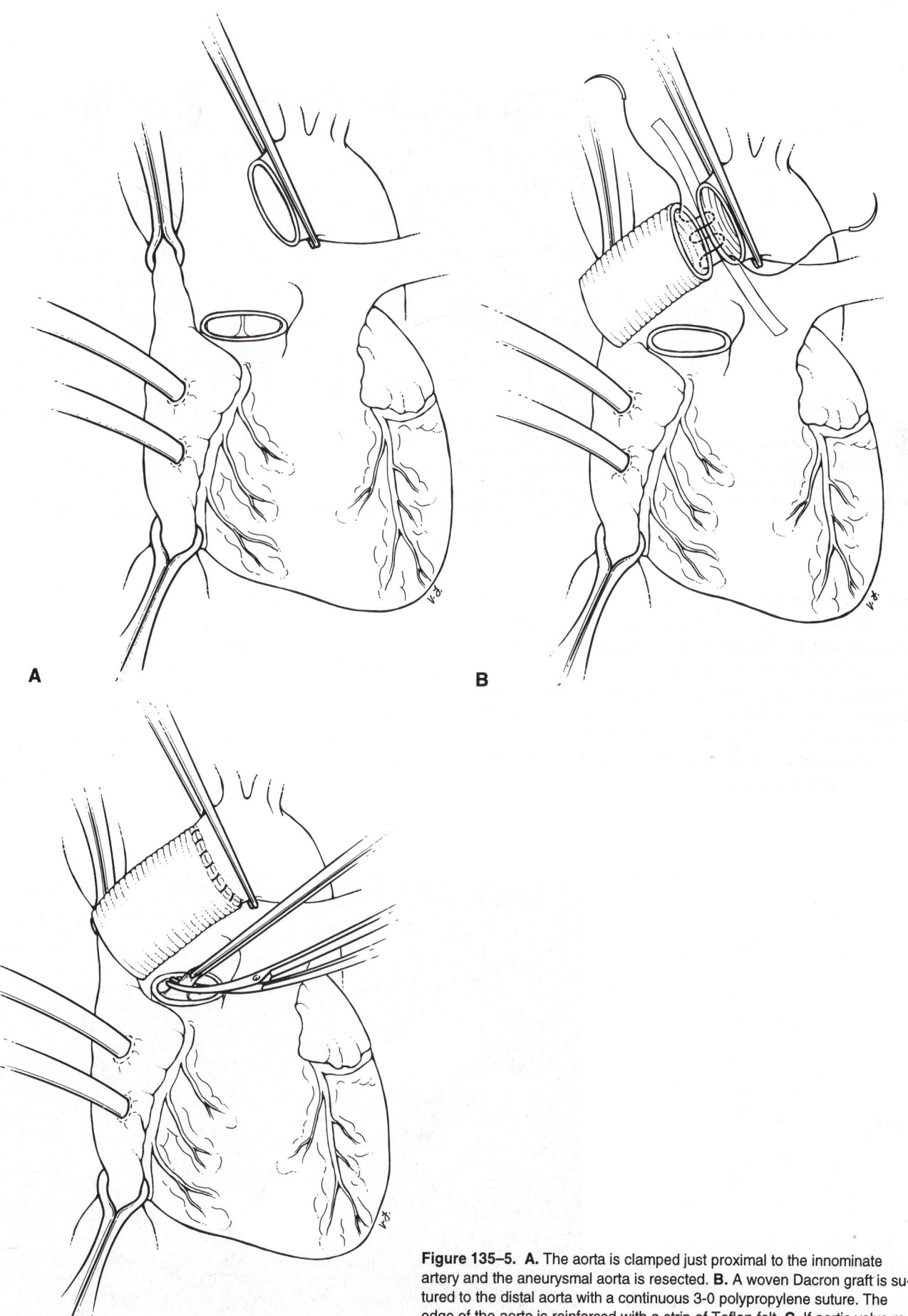

A

B

C

Figure 135–5. A. The aorta is clamped just proximal to the innominate artery and the aneurysmal aorta is resected. **B.** A woven Dacron graft is sutured to the distal aorta with a continuous 3-0 polypropylene suture. The edge of the aorta is reinforced with a strip of Teflon felt. **C.** If aortic valve replacement is indicated, the aortic valve is excised. *(Continued.)*

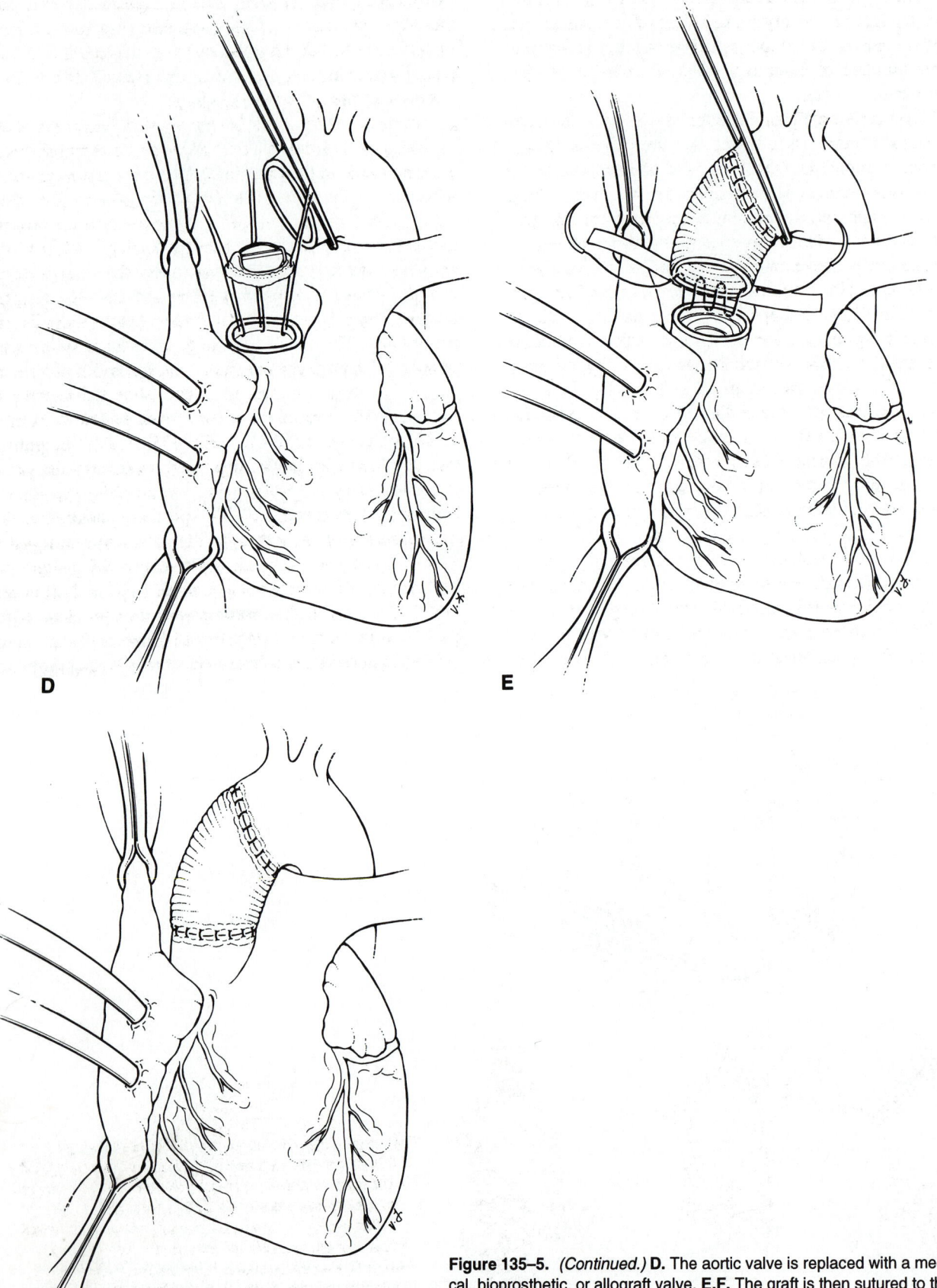

D

E

F

Figure 135–5. *(Continued.)* **D.** The aortic valve is replaced with a mechanical, bioprosthetic, or allograft valve. **E,F.** The graft is then sutured to the proximal aorta using 3-0 polypropylene suture and a strip of Teflon felt.

monitored. A pulmonary artery catheter is placed for monitoring of pulmonary artery pressure, mixed venous oxygen saturation, and cardiac output. Thermistor probes are placed for measurement of nasopharyngeal and rectal or bladder temperatures.

A median sternotomy incision is used, and the common femoral artery is exposed for cannulation. If the aneurysm is not large, the distal ascending aorta or the proximal aortic arch may be used for arterial return. A large single two-stage venous cannula or separate superior and inferior caval cannulas are inserted into the right atrium for venous return to the extracorporeal circuit. A vent is inserted into the left ventricle through the right superior pulmonary vein. Total cardiopulmonary bypass is established at an initial flow of 2.2 L/m^2 per minute using hemodilution (hematocrit 20 to 30%) and moderate systemic hypothermia (24° to 28°C). Lower temperatures and flows are often used for short intervals. The pericardial cavity is intermittently irrigated with 4°C Ringer's solution to cool the myocardium. If the aortic occlusion time is likely to exceed 1 hour, a cooling jacket is placed around the ventricles. A balloon-tipped cannula is placed through the right atrium and is passed into the coronary sinus. A cold (4°C) oxygenated blood cardioplegic solution containing 30 mEq/L of potassium chloride is infused through this cannula every 20 to 30 min during the period of aortic clamping at a flow rate of 250 mL/min for 3 to 4 min. If the aortic valve is competent, an initial dose of cardioplegic solution is in-

fused directly into the aortic root through a large-bore needle. The temperature of the myocardium is continuously monitored with a thermistor probe that is placed into the anterior ventricular septum and is maintained below 15°C during the period of aortic clamping.

A standard approach has involved replacement of the ascending aorta from the level of the aortic commissures to a site proximal to the origin of the innominate artery, and, if indicated, separate replacement of the aortic valve (Fig. 135–5). The aorta is clamped just proximal to the innominate artery and after infusion of cardioplegic solution, the aorta is completely transected just above the coronary ostia and just below the aortic clamp (Fig. 135–5A). A collagen- or gelatin-impregnated woven Dacron graft, which is impermeable to blood, is sutured to the distal aorta with a continuous 3-0 polypropylene suture incorporating a strip of Teflon felt (Fig. 135–5B). If aortic valve replacement is necessary, the diseased valve is removed and the valve substitute is inserted at this time (Fig. 135–5C,D). The graft is then cut to the appropriate length and is sutured to the proximal aorta using 3-0 polypropylene suture (Fig. 135–5E,F). If the right coronary ostium is displaced cephalad, it is detached from the aorta with a small rim of aortic wall and is sutured directly to the aortic graft using a 4-0 polypropylene suture and incorporating a small strip of Teflon felt (Fig. 135–6A,B). If this anastomosis cannot be done without excessive tension, a segment of 6 mm or 8 mm collagen-impregnated knitted Dacron graft is interposed between

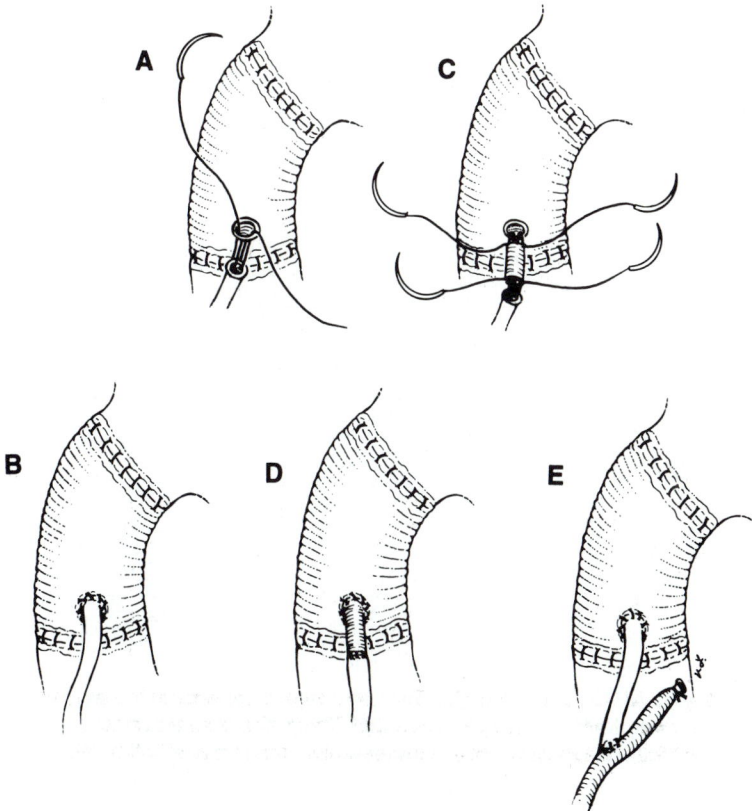

Figure 135–6. Attachment of the right coronary artery. **A,B.** If the right coronary artery is of sufficient length, it is mobilized and sutured to an opening in the Dacron graft with a 4-0 polypropylene suture incorporating a strip of Teflon felt. **C,D.** If the right coronary artery is not of sufficient length to reach the aortic graft, a segment of 8- or 10-mm collagen-impregnated Dacron graft is interposed between the aortic graft and the coronary artery. **E.** Alternatively, a segment of saphenous vein can be interposed between the aortic graft and the right coronary artery.

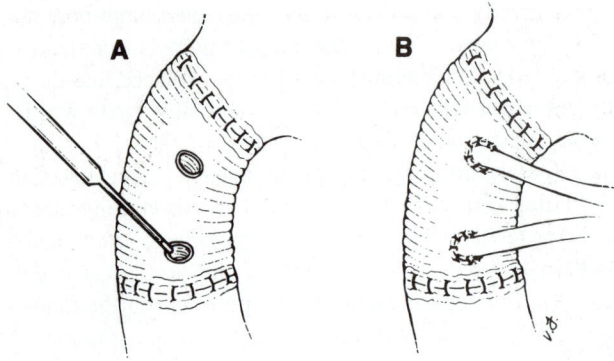

Figure 135–7. A,B. Saphenous vein bypass grafts to the coronary arteries are sutured to 5-mm openings in the aortic graft that are made with a cautery.

the right coronary artery and the aortic graft (Fig. 135–6C,D). Alternatively, a segment of saphenous vein can be inserted between the right coronary artery more distally and the aortic graft (Fig. 135–6E). If coronary artery disease is present that requires bypass grafting, the proximal ends of the vein grafts are sutured to circular openings in the aortic graft with 5-0 polypropylene suture (Fig. 135–7A,B).

This general technique does not eliminate the potential for subsequent dilatation and aneurysm formation of the sinuses of Valsalva that can occur in patients with cystic medial degenerative disease of the aorta, particularly those with the Marfan syndrome. This is a late complication, and

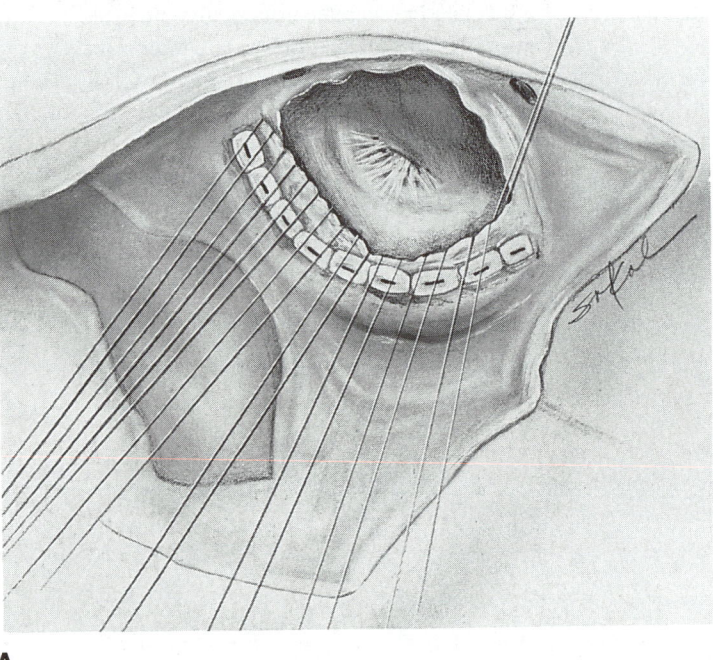

A

Figure 135–8. Replacement of the ascending aorta and aortic valve with a composite graft. **A.** Pledgeted double armed 2-0 suture are placed with the pledgets in the supraannular position and immediately adjoined to one another to ensure a water-tight closure. **B.** The sutures are placed in the upper half of the sewing ring of the valve prosthesis to permit seating of the valve deeply in the annulus. *(From Kouchoukos NT, Marshall WG Jr: J Card Surg 1:333, 1986, with permission.)*

B

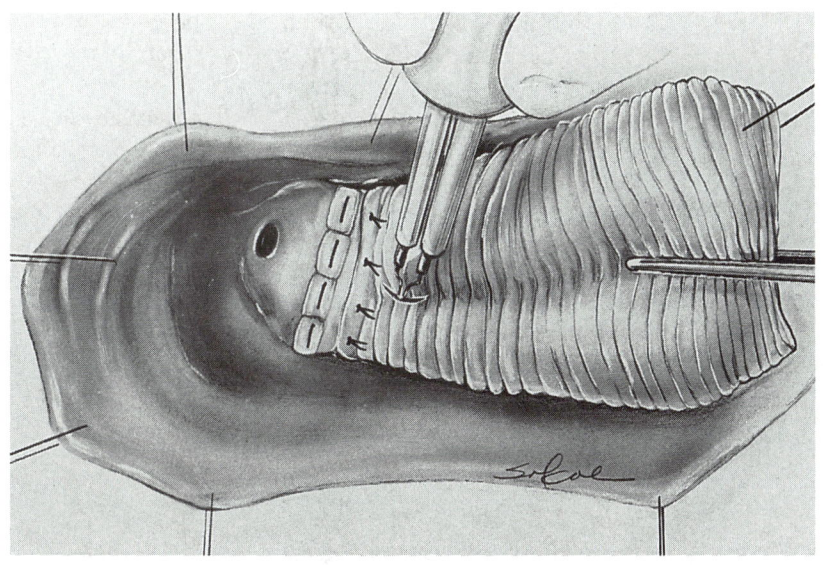

Figure 135–9. Button of graft opposite the coronary ostium is excised with a cautery.

is usually detected 5 to 7 years after the initial operation.[18–20] However, the technique has proved to be highly satisfactory for aneurysms that are not associated with cystic medial degenerative disease.

When the sinuses of Valsalva are enlarged, and the coronary ostia are displaced cephalad, the aortic valve, the aortic sinuses, and the ascending aorta are replaced with a composite graft that contains a mechanical valve prosthesis and a woven Dacron graft. Commercially prepared composite grafts in which the Dacron grafts are impregnated with collagen or gelatin to make them impermeable to blood are now available throughout the world, and preclotting of composite grafts by any of several other techniques is no longer necessary.

After the aorta is occluded and the cardioplegia solution has been administered, the aneurysm is opened and the aortic valve is excised. The sewing ring of the graft-valve prosthesis is then sutured to the aortic annulus with interrupted pledgeted mattress sutures of 2-0 braided polyester

that are placed immediately adjacent to one another to assure a watertight closure (Fig. 135–8A,B). Buttons of the Dacron aortic graft opposite the coronary ostia are excised with a wire cautery (Fig. 135–9). The aortic tissue surrounding the coronary ostia can be sutured to the openings in the graft with 4-0 polypropylene suture or, preferably, the coronary arteries are mobilized and excised from the aorta, maintaining a small rim of aortic tissue that is sutured to the graft with 4-0 or 5-0 polypropylene suture (Fig. 135–10A,B). A thin strip of Teflon felt is often incorporated into this suture line. The latter technique reduces the likelihood of development of false aneurysms at the sites of these anastomoses when compared to the inclusion technique.[8] The distal end of the composite graft is cut to the appropriate length and is sutured to the completely transected distal aorta with 3-0 polypropylene suture, incorporating a strip of Teflon felt (Fig. 135–11A,B). If there is marked displacement of the coronary ostia because of marked dilatation of the aortic sinuses or if there is consid-

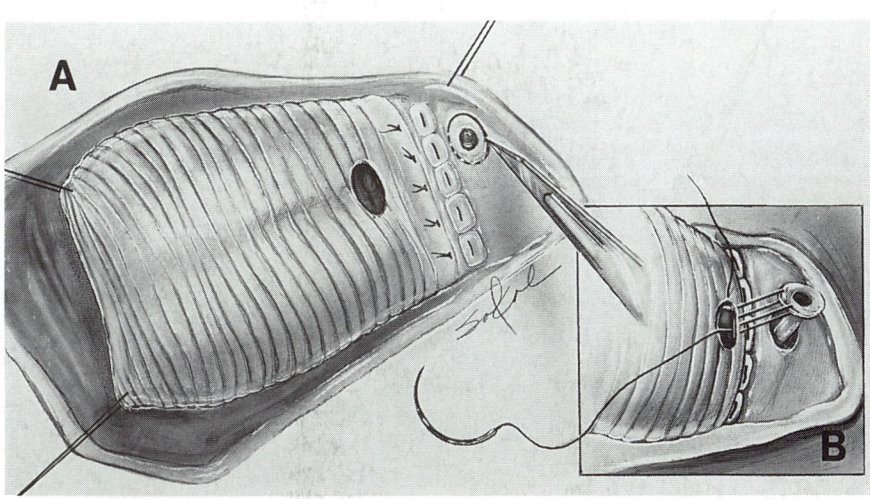

Figure 135–10. A. A full-thickness rim of aortic tissue is excised with the coronary artery. **B.** The coronary artery is mobilized and is anastomosed to the aortic graft with a 4-0 or 5-0 polypropylene suture.

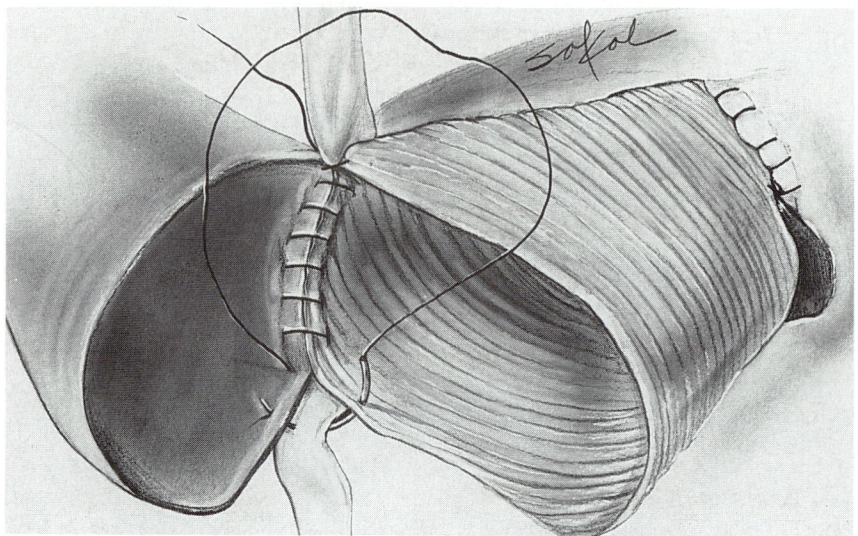

A

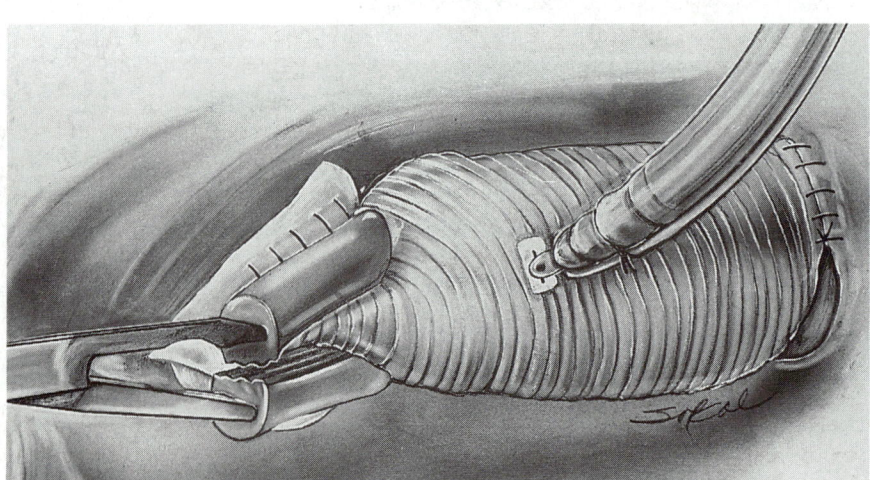

B

Figure 135–11. A,B. The distal aorta is completely transected and is sutured to the Dacron graft with a 3-0 polypropylene suture incorporating a strip of Teflon felt.

Figure 135–12. The aortic clamp is removed and is placed in a partially occlusive position. Air is aspirated from the graft with a 13-gauge needle.

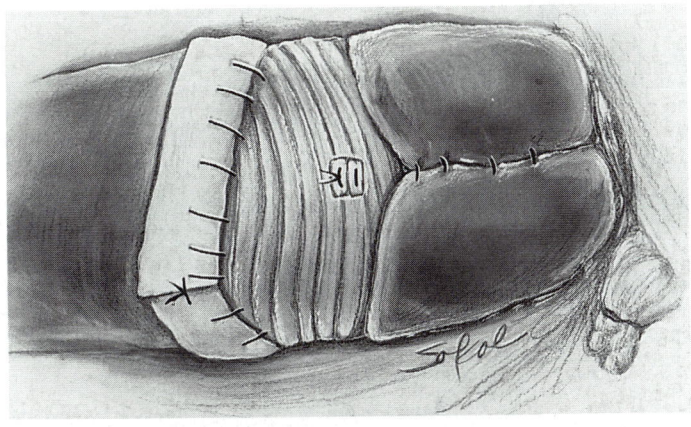

Figure 135–13. After decannulation, the aorta is wrapped loosely around the graft.

erable scarring around the aortic root which prohibits adequate mobilization of the coronary arteries, short segments of 6-, 8-, or 10-mm collagen-impregnated knitted Dacron grafts are sutured end-to-end to the aortic tissue surrounding the coronary ostia. These grafts are cut to the appropriate length and are sutured to openings in the aortic graft with 4-0 polypropylene suture.

The aortic clamp is then removed and replaced in a partially occlusive position downstream from a 13-gauge needle that is inserted into the graft through a small incision and is connected to continuous low suction for evacuation of air (Fig. 135–12). When rewarming is complete and strong cardiac contractions have resumed, air is evacuated from the left atrium and left ventricle, the left ventricular vent is removed, and cardiopulmonary bypass is discontinued. After decannulation, administration of protamine sulfate, and careful examination of all suture lines, the remaining aorta is loosely wrapped around the graft (Fig. 135–13). When a preclotted graft and the open technique for anastomosis are used, it is not necessary to wrap the aorta tightly around the graft or to attempt to cover the entire graft. With the use of blood conservation techniques that include preoperative blood donation, intraoperative use of a cell-saving device, and reinfusion of mediastinal drainage postoperatively, it is possible to perform many of these procedures without transfusion of homologous blood products.

Because of limited durability, particularly in younger patients, porcine or pericardial bioprostheses are not generally used in composite grafts for aortic root replacement unless there is a contraindication to use of warfarin, which is required for all grafts that contain a mechanical valve. Aortic allografts and pulmonary autografts can also be used to replace the aortic root.[8,21] They do not require anticoagulation with warfarin or the use of antiplatelet agents such as aspirin or dipyridamole.

For patients who develop aneurysms of the sinuses of Valsalva following graft replacement of the ascending aorta and require operation, the dilated noncoronary sinus is incised (Fig. 135–14A), and the operation is performed as described above except that the tube graft is sutured distally to the previously inserted graft (Fig. 135–14B).

Concomitant procedures may be necessary. These include mitral valve replacement or repair, particularly in patients with the Marfan syndrome, and coronary artery bypass grafting. Anastomosis of the internal mammary artery or saphenous veins to the coronary arteries and repair or re-

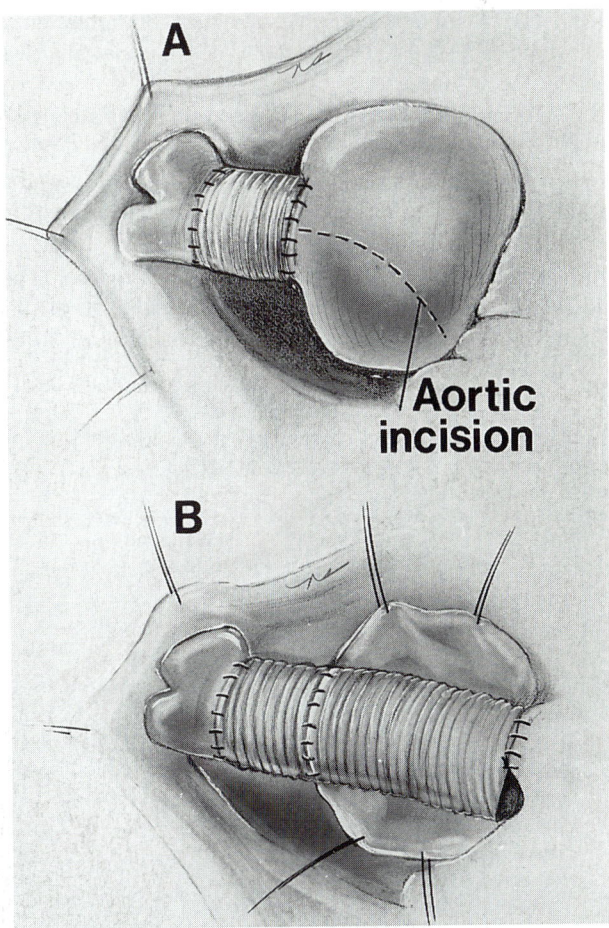

Figure 135–14. A. Line of incision for composite graft replacement of the aortic valve and sinuses of Valsalva following previous graft replacement of the ascending aorta. **B.** Composite graft is sutured distally to the previously inserted aortic graft. *(From Kouchoukos NT, Marshall WG Jr: J Card Surg 1:333, 1986, with permission.)*

placement of the mitral valve are performed during the single period of hypothermic ischemic arrest. Anastomosis of the vein grafts to the tube graft or to the aorta distal to the graft are performed after completion of the distal aortic anastomosis but before removal of the aortic clamp.

RESULTS OF OPERATION

The early (hospital) mortality rate in recently reported series containing heterogenous groups of patients has ranged from 5 to 14% and is importantly related to the year of operation, older age of the patient, the need for emergency operation, coexisting disease of the aortic arch or descending thoracic aorta, and duration of cardiopulmonary bypass.[8,22–25] In our own experience with 168 patients who underwent 172 aortic root replacements, hospital mortality was related to the etiology of the aortic disease (Table 135–1).[8] Using multivariate analysis, the duration of cardiopulmonary bypass was the only significant predictor of early death. For patients with cystic medial degenerative disease of the ascending aorta, even with associated chronic aortic dissection, or those in whom aortic root replacement was done as a secondary procedure, hospital mortality was under 3%.

The late survival following operation is approximately 65% at 5 years and 55% at 7 years.[8,22,23,25] In our series of 168 patients who were followed for up to 15 years, actuarial survival was 72% at 5 years and 48% at 12 years (Fig. 135–15). The survival rate at 12 years for the 81 patients with annuloaortic ectasia was higher than that for the 63 patients with aortic dissection (54 vs. 44%) although the difference was not statistically significant. Survival of 30 pa-

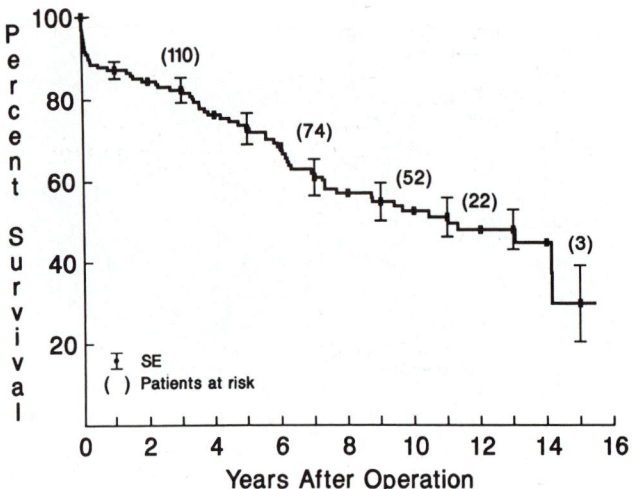

Figure 135–15. Actuarial survival rates for 168 patients undergoing replacement of the ascending aorta and aortic valve. The vertical bars enclose the standard error (5E). The numbers in parentheses indicate the number of patients traced at that time. *(Reproduced from Kouchoukos NT, Wareing TH, Murphy SF, Perrillo JB: Sixteen-year experience with aortic root replacement. Ann Surg 214:308, 1991, with permission.)*

tients with the Marfan syndrome was 44% at 12 years. Advanced age, presence of the Marfan syndrome, and increasing New York Heart Association functional class at the time of operation were significant independent predictors of late death.[8]

Reoperations on the ascending aorta and aortic valve for reasons other than postoperative hemorrhage have been necessary with all operative techniques.[8,18,25] With the composite graft technique, reoperations for pseudoaneurysm formation, prosthetic endocarditis, technical problems, thrombotic obstruction of the prosthetic valve, and other complications were required in 21 (14%) of 148 hospital survivors during a mean follow-up interval of 81 months.[8] By actuarial analysis, the probability of remaining free from reoperation on the ascending aorta or the aortic valve (exclusive of early reoperations for bleeding) following insertion of a prosthetic graft was significantly lower for patients in whom the open technique of anastomosis was performed than in patients in whom the inclusion-wrap technique was used (Fig. 135–16). Other important complications with all techniques include thromboembolic events, hemorrhage related to anticoagulant therapy, heart block, life-threatening arrhythmias, congestive failure, and myocardial infarction.[8,25]

Symptomatic improvement in the patients surviving operation has been excellent. Approximately 90% of patients are asymptomatic or mildly symptomatic (New York Heart Association Functional Class I or II).[8] Since the entire aorta can be affected by cystic medial degenerative disease, arteriosclerosis, or other conditions, aneurysms or dissection of the aortic arch, the descending thoracic aorta, and the abdominal aorta can develop after surgical treatment of

TABLE 135–1. HOSPITAL MORTALITY FOLLOWING REPLACEMENT OF THE ASCENDING AORTA AND AORTIC VALVE

Aortic Disease	Number of Patients	Hospital Deaths No.	Hospital Deaths %	CL[a]
Annuloaortic ectasia	93	2	2.2	0.6–3.8
Chronic dissection	47	1	2.1	0–4.3
Acute dissection	16	4	25.0	13.8–36.2
Other Syphilitic aortitis, endocarditis, post-stenotic dilatation, tunnel aorta stenosis, aortic valve disease, prosthetic valve malfunction	16	2	12.5	3.9–21.1
Total	172	9	5.2	3.4–7.0

[a]CL, 70% confidence limits.
Reproduced from Kouchoukos NT, Wareing TH, Murphy SF, Perrillo JB: Sixteen-year experience with aortic root replacement. Ann Surg 214:308, 1991, with permission.

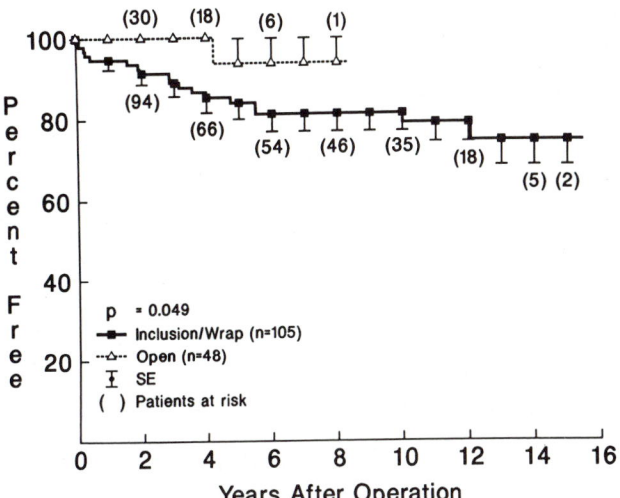

Figure 135–16. Actuarial freedom from reoperation on the ascending aorta or aortic valve (exclusive of early reoperations for hemorrhage) according to operative technique for the patients receiving prosthetic grafts. *(Reproduced from Kouchoukos NT, Wareing TH, Murphy SF, Perillo JB: Sixteen-year experience with aortic root replacement. Ann Surg 214:308, 1991, with permission.)*

the ascending aortic disease.[8,16,25] Close surveillance of these patients is essential since approximately one-third of the late deaths following operation on the ascending aorta are due to distal aortic disease.[25] This is especially important for patients with the Marfan syndrome.

Important technological advances such as the development of pliable woven arterial grafts that are impregnated with collagen or gelatin to render them impervious to blood, improved aortic valve substitutes, safer pump-oxygenator systems, superior methods of intraoperative myocardial protection, and improved diagnostic, anesthetic, and surgical techniques have contributed to the substantial reduction in hospital mortality and morbidity following operations on the ascending aorta in recent years, and will positively affect the long-term results. Early surgical intervention can now be considered in patients with cystic medial degenerative disease, particularly those with the Marfan syndrome, who have aneurysms of the aortic root or ascending aorta that are greater than 5 cm in diameter but are without symptoms, dissection, or substantial aortic regurgitation, to prevent the serious and often fatal complications of this disorder.

REFERENCES

1. Hirst AE Jr, Johns VJ, Kime SW Jr: Dissecting aneurysm of the aorta: A review of 505 cases. *Medicine* **37**:217, 1958
2. Bahnson NT: Definitive treatment of saccular aneurysms of the aorta with excision of sac and aortic suture. *Surg Gynecol Obstet* **96**:383, 1953
3. Cooley DA, DeBakey ME: Resection of entire ascending aorta in fusiform aneurysm using cardiac bypass. *JAMA* **162**:1158, 1956
4. Mueller WH, Dammann FJ, Warren WD: Surgical correction of cardiovascular deformities in Marfan's syndrome. *Ann Surg* **152**:506, 1960
5. Starr A, Edwards ML, McCord CW, et al: Aortic replacement. *Circulation* **27**:779, 1963
6. Wheat MW Jr, Wilson JR, Bartley TD: Successful replacement of the entire ascending aorta and aortic valve. *JAMA* **188**:717, 1964
7. Bentall H, deBono A: A technique for complete replacement of the ascending aorta. *Thorax* **23**:338, 1968
8. Kouchoukos NT, Wareing TH, Murphy SF, Perrillo JB: Sixteen-year experience with aortic root replacement. *Ann Surg* **214**:308, 1991
9. Cabrol C, Pavie A, Mesnildrey P, et al: Long-term results with total replacement of the ascending aorta and reimplantation of the coronary arteries. *J Thorac Cardiovasc Surg* **91**:17–25, 1986
10. Cabrol C, Pavie A, Ganjbakhch I, et al: Complete replacement of the ascending aorta with reimplantation of the coronary arteries. *J Thorac Cardiovasc Surg* **81**:309, 1981
11. Ellis PR, Cooley DA, DeBakey ME: Clinical considerations and surgical treatment of annuloaortic ectasia. *J Thorac Cardiovasc Surg* **42**:363, 1961
12. Murdoch JL, Walker BA, Halpern BL, et al: Life expectancy and causes of death in the Marfan syndrome. *N Engl J Med* **286**:804, 1972
13. Joyce JW, Fairbairn JF, Lomcaod OW, et al: Aneurysms of the thoracic aorta: A clinical study with special reference to prognosis. *Circulation* **29**:176, 1964
14. Pressler V, McNamara JJ: Thoracic aortic aneurysm: Natural history and treatment. *J Thorac Cardiovasc Surg* **79**:489, 1980
15. Bickerstaff LK, Pairolero PC, Hollier LH, et al: Thoracic aortic aneurysm: A population-based study. *Surgery* **92**:1103, 1982
16. Crawford ES: Marfan syndrome: Broad spectral surgical treatment of cardiovascular manifestations. *Ann Surg* **198**:487, 1983
17. Gott VL, Pyeritz RE, Magovern GJ Jr, et al: Surgical treatment of aneurysms of the ascending aorta in the Marfan syndrome. *N Engl J Med* **314**:1070, 1986
18. Symbas PN, Raizner AE, Tyras DH, et al: Aneurysms of all sinuses of Valsalva in patients with Marfan syndrome: An unusual late complication following replacement of aortic valve and ascending aorta for aortic regurgitation and fusiform aneurysm of ascending aorta. *Ann Surg* **174**:902, 1971
19. McCready RA, Pluth JR: Surgical treatment of ascending aortic aneurysms associated with aortic valve insufficiency. *Ann Thorac Surg* **28**:307, 1979
20. Kouchoukos NT, Karp RB, Blackstone EH, et al: Replacement of the ascending aorta and aortic valve with a composite graft: Results in 86 patients. *Ann Surg* **192**:403, 1980
21. Kouchoukos NT, Dávila-Román VG, Spray TL, et al: Replacement of the aortic root with a pulmonary autograft in children and young adults with aortic valve disease. *N Engl J Med* **330**:1, 1994
22. Galloway AC, Colvin SB, LaMendola CL, et al: Ten-year operative experience with 165 aneurysms of the ascending aorta and aortic arch. *Circulation* **80**(suppl I):I–249, 1980
23. Crawford ES, Svensson LG, Coselli JS, et al: Surgical treatment of aneurysm and/or dissection of the ascending aorta, transverse aortic arch, and ascending aorta and transverse aortic arch. *J Thorac Cardiovasc Surg* **98**:659, 1989
24. Lytle BW, Mahfood SS, Cosgrove DM, Loop FD: Replacement of the ascending aorta. *J Thorac Cardiovasc Surg* **99**:651, 1990
25. Lawrie GM, Earle N, DeBakey ME: Long-term fate of the aortic root and aortic valve after ascending aneurysm surgery. *Ann Surg* **217**:711, 1993

Aneurysms of the Transverse Aortic Arch

Joseph S. Coselli

The transverse aortic arch is the segment of aorta from which the brachiocephalic arteries arise. Aneurysmal involvement of this region is less common than other aortic sites and probably represents about 10% of all thoracic aortic aneurysms.[1] These are serious lesions that lead to death from complications in most cases. Aortic aneurysms here, as elsewhere, gradually enlarge and eventually rupture; however, the location, unlike aneurysms of other aortic segments, poses special problems that make treatment one of the more formidable undertakings in cardiovascular surgery. In addition to special reconstructive techniques to restore circulation to the head and upper extremities, the heart and brain must be protected during the operation. Nevertheless, safe, effective, and reproducible approaches to aneurysmal disease of the aortic arch have evolved.

HISTORY

Resection and replacement of transverse aortic arch aneurysms have clearly been a very special surgical challenge. In 1955 Cooley, Mahaffey, and DeBakey reported the unsuccessful resection of an aneurysm of the entire transverse aortic arch using a method of temporary shunting to the brachiocephalic vessels without cardiopulmonary bypass.[2] The technique employed mild, surface-induced hypothermia and temporary end-to-side bypass shunts made from polyvinyl sponge extending from the ascending aorta to the descending thoracic aorta with sidearms to both the innominate and the left common carotid arteries. On March 21, 1957, DeBakey et al first successfully replaced an aneurysm involving the ascending aorta and transverse aortic arch with an aortic homograft using total cardiopul-

monary bypass with separate innominate and left common carotid artery perfusion.[3] As experience with this technique increased, survival never exceeded 75%, with most deaths being due to cerebral complications, indicating that the methods employed were not reliably protective. Griepp and his associates in 1975 adopted total cardiopulmonary bypass, profound total body hypothermia (10° to 15°C, esophageal) and cerebral circulatory arrest for brain protection and to simplify aortic reconstruction.[4] Crawford and Saleh in 1980 advocated arch reconstruction using the graft inclusion technique and direct reattachment of the brachiocephalic arterial origins to openings made in the graft.[5] In 1981, Cooley and Livesay reported the adoption of circulatory arrest for routine use in patients with acute Type I aortic dissection describing the "open distal anastomosis technique" for ascending and transverse aortic arch resection.[6] Crawford and co-workers in 1993 reported an extensive experience with 656 patients using deep hypothermia and circulatory arrest for arch repair in which early mortality was 90% and the transient permanent stroke rate was only 7%.[7] Retrograde cerebral perfusion, with perfusion of oxygenated blood to the brain via the superior vena caval cannula during circulatory arrest for cerebral protection was revived in 1990 by Ueda and associates.[8] The "elephant trunk" technique was introduced by Borst et al in 1983 as an alternative for the treatment of patients with extensive aortic aneurysmal disease involving the arch and descending or thoracoabdominal aorta.[9] As a first stage, the arch is repaired by replacement with a Dacron graft, leaving a portion of the graft in the proximal descending thoracic aorta for a second stage. The latter provides for minimal dissection to achieve proximal aortic control at the second operation.

PATHOLOGICAL MANIFESTATIONS

The majority of aneurysmal lesions are due to medial degeneration and/or aortic dissection. Atherosclerosis is frequently a superimposed process. In all conditions, a weakness develops in the aortic wall leading to dilatation as a result of the relationships expressed in LaPlace's law as the wall stresses increase. The weakness secondary to degenerative disease results from a breakdown of elastin, collagen, and other structural elements within the aortic wall. Dissection results in a thinning of the outer wall of the false channel leading to progressive dilatation over time. Traumatic aortic transection produces a disruption of part or all of the aortic circumference. Aortitis, either granulomatous or secondary to syphilis, results in a destruction and weakening of the aortic media.

Aneurysms of the aortic arch are frequently associated with aneurysmal disease of the ascending aorta, aortic root, descending thoracic aorta, thoracoabdominal aorta, and abdominal aorta. In many cases the entire aorta may be involved. Associated diseases frequently include aortic valve pathology, coronary artery occlusive disease, and chronic obstructive pulmonary disease. The mean age of patients with aortic arch aneurysms in most series is approximately 66 years of age.

CLINICAL MANIFESTATIONS

With aortic aneurysmal enlargement, eventually there is compression or obstruction of adjacent mediastinal structures including the superior vena cava, innominate veins, pulmonary artery, trachea, bronchi, lung, and left recurrent laryngeal nerve. Symptoms include dyspnea, stridor, hoarseness, hemoptysis, cough, and chest pain. Many patients are entirely asymptomatic with the aneurysm discovered incidentally on chest x-ray or computed tomography scanning performed for unrelated problems. Physical findings may include distended veins of the upper body, cardiovascular murmurs, left vocal cord paralysis, abnormal pulsations of the upper anterior chest wall, signs of pleural fluid, and congestive heart failure. Erosion and fistula formation between the aneurysm and the great veins, pulmonary artery, right atrium, or right ventricle may occur producing the hemodynamic changes of a large arteriovenous fistula, which may result in sudden and fatal heart failure. Rupture generally occurs into the pericardium, bronchial airway, or pleural cavity causing death from tamponade in the former and exsanguination in the latter.

DIAGNOSIS

The aneurysm may first be discovered on routine chest x-ray. Ascending aortic aneurysms produce a convex shadow to the right of the cardiac silhouette while aneurysms of the transverse aortic arch present as an enlargement of the superior mediastinal silhouette or a left-sided shadow. Thoracic aortography remains an important diagnostic procedure. Digital techniques currently require minimal contrast exposure. Aortography allows for visualization of the entire aorta allowing for evaluation of the aortic valve and brachiocephalic vessels (Figs. 136–1 and 136–15). Anomalies of the branch vessels may be clearly delineated. Computed tomography scanning and magnetic resonant imaging are very useful methods for the evaluation of patients with thoracic aortic aneurysms and are particularly useful in the long-term follow-up of patients with aortic dissection (Figs. 136–2 and 136–3). Echocardiography (transthoracic and transesophageal) is valuable in assessing the extent of transverse aortic arch aneurysms and is additionally informative in establishing cardiac function and evaluating concomitant

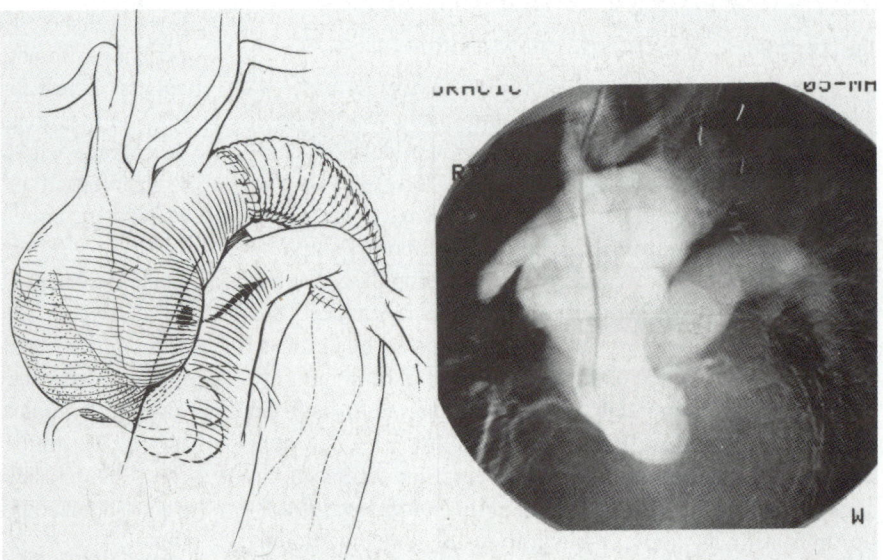

Figure 136–1. Illustration and aortogram demonstrating rupture into the main pulmonary artery.

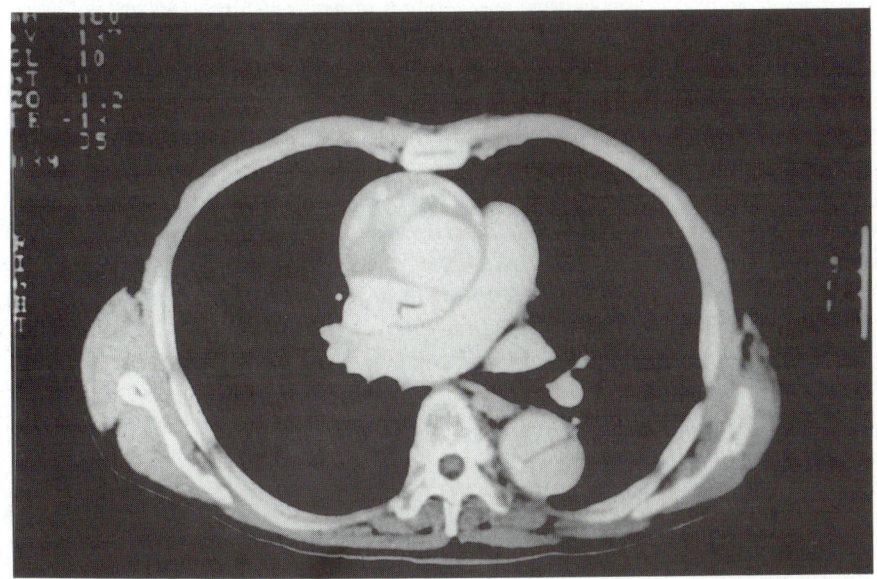

Figure 136–2. Computed tomography scan demonstrating chronic Type I aortic dissection involving the ascending aorta and descending thoracic aorta. In the ascending aorta the false lumen is anterior and partially clot-filled.

valvular abnormalities such as aortic valvular insufficiency. Cardiac catheterization is performed when necessary to evaluate coronary artery occlusive disease.

INDICATIONS FOR SURGERY

All patients with aneurysm of the transverse aortic arch who are symptomatic are treated with surgical intervention.

Patients who have fusiform medial degenerative type aneurysms are recommended for elective resection and replacement when the aortic diameter is 5 cm or greater. All patients with acute dissection involving the proximal aorta, including the arch, are operated upon emergently. Patients with chronic dissection are operated upon with the development of symptoms or when the combined diameter of the true and false lumens exceeds twice the normal size or approximately 4 to 5 cm. Patients with Marfan syndrome are

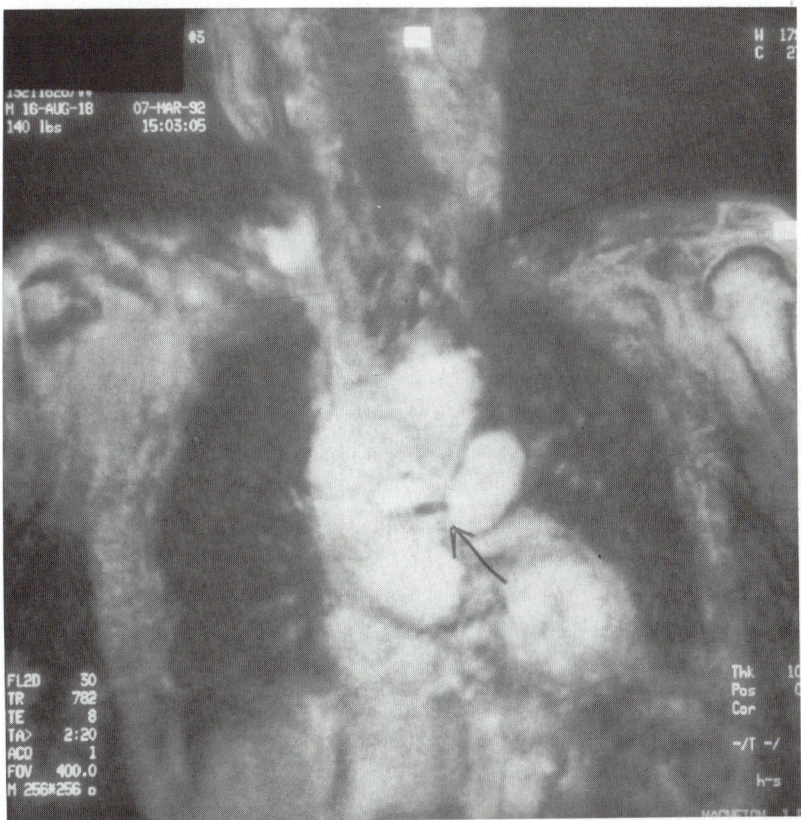

Figure 136–3. Magnetic resonance imaging scan of patient with ascending and transverse aortic arch aneurysm and dissection with rupture into the pulmonary artery.

treated somewhat more aggressively as are patients with concomitant aortic valvular insufficiency, stenosis, or coronary artery occlusive disease.[10] The natural history of saccular aneurysms of the transverse aortic arch is one of particularly unpredictable progressive enlargement and consequently saccular aneurysms 3 to 4 cm in size should be treated electively. Virtually all false aneurysms at the suture lines or cannulation sites of prior surgery should be treated prior to the development of symptoms.

SURGICAL TREATMENT

Treatment is by graft replacement and the approach depends upon the extent of involvement, including the need for cardiac and cerebral protection. Since Griepp and associates introduced profound hypothermia and circulatory arrest to support graft replacement in 1975, this technique has been the preferred method of cerebral protection.[4] This technique of excision and graft replacement with hypothermic circulatory arrest simplified operation and provided good brain protection, but was complicated by bleeding through the interstices of the graft due to coagulopathies that developed during the warm-up period. The problem of bleeding using this technique was significantly reduced in 1980 by Crawford's introduction of the graft inclusion technique of replacement and reattachment of the brachiocephalic vessels by suturing them directly to an opening made in the graft as successfully employed in the treatment of thoracoabdominal aortic aneurysms. In the performance

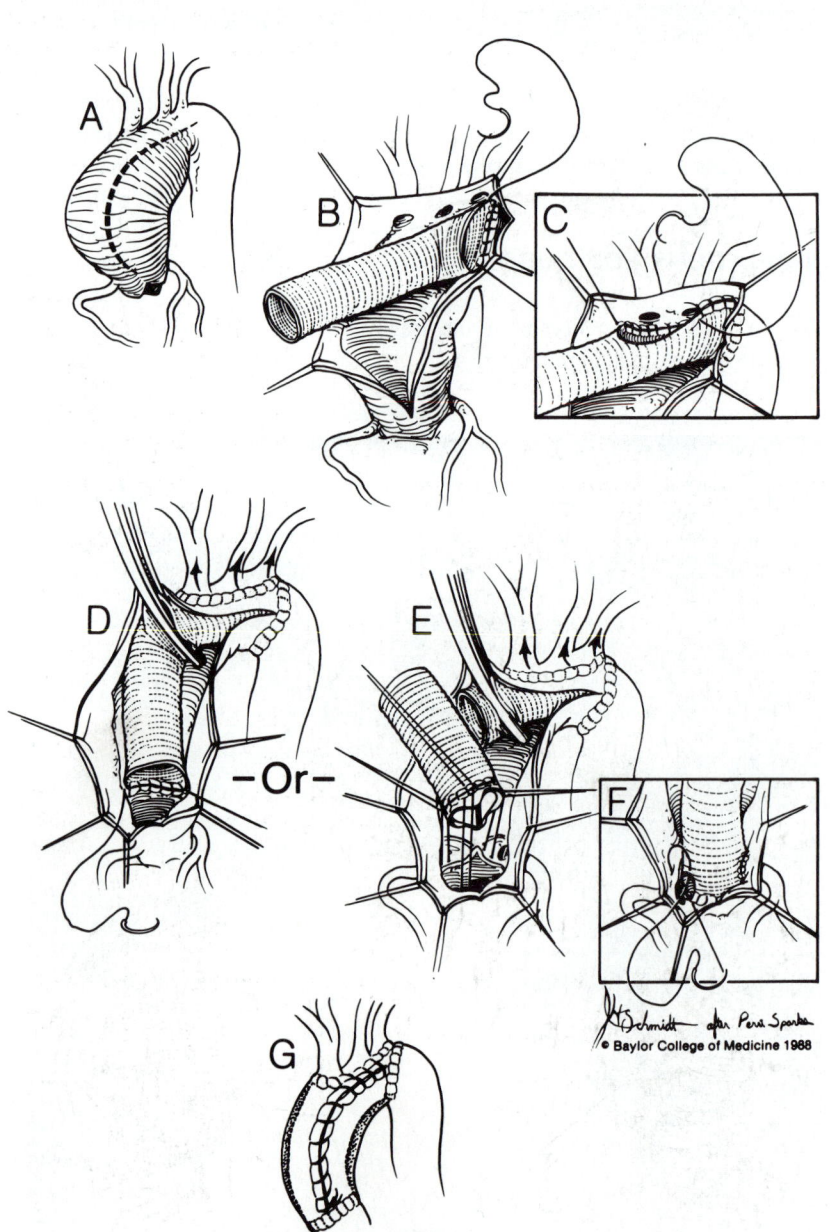

Figure 136–4. A–G. Drawing of operative technique for transverse aortic arch replacement and **D** supraannular proximal anastomosis or **E,F** composite valve graft replacement of the aortic root with direct reattachment of coronary artery origins.

of this operation, the aneurysm wall was sutured around the aortic graft to reduce bleeding that occurred through even preclotted grafts. Further improvements have been made in graft material with the use of presealed grafts employing albumin or collagen, as well as the pharmacological utilization of Amicar (aminocaproic acid) and aprotinin.

When the aortic root or sinuses are involved, the proximal aorta and aortic valve are replaced with a composite valve graft attaching the coronary arteries directly to openings made in the aortic graft (Fig. 136–4).[11] Associated coronary artery obstruction is treated by saphenous vein bypass grafting attached either to the side of the aortic graft or to uninvolved brachiocephalic vessels. In selected cases the right or left internal mammary arteries may be utilized for coronary artery grafting.

The insertion of a composite valve graft with direct reattachment of the coronary arteries was certainly an important step in the treatment of aortic aneurysmal disease extending into the aortic root. Disadvantages of this particu-

lar approach, however, have included suture line bleeding in locations difficult to control and late development of false aneurysms at the coronary artery reattachment sites secondary to tension. Modifications currently employed to prevent such problems have included the mobilization of the coronary arteries on buttons of aortic tissue that are attached to openings appropriately positioned in the aortic graft in a tension-free fashion allowing for improved access to control suture line bleeding (Fig. 136–5). In selected patients with extensive aortic aneurysmal disease of the aortic root and redo operations, the technique described by Cabrol is employed (Fig. 136–6). In this technique, a transversely positioned separate smaller Dacron tube graft is anastomosed end-to-end to the aorta surrounding the origins of each of the right and left coronary arteries and attached side-to-side to the aortic graft.

The technique diagrammed in Figure 136–7A–D is employed in patients in whom the aortic root is normal, but the ascending aorta is aneurysmally dilated with extension

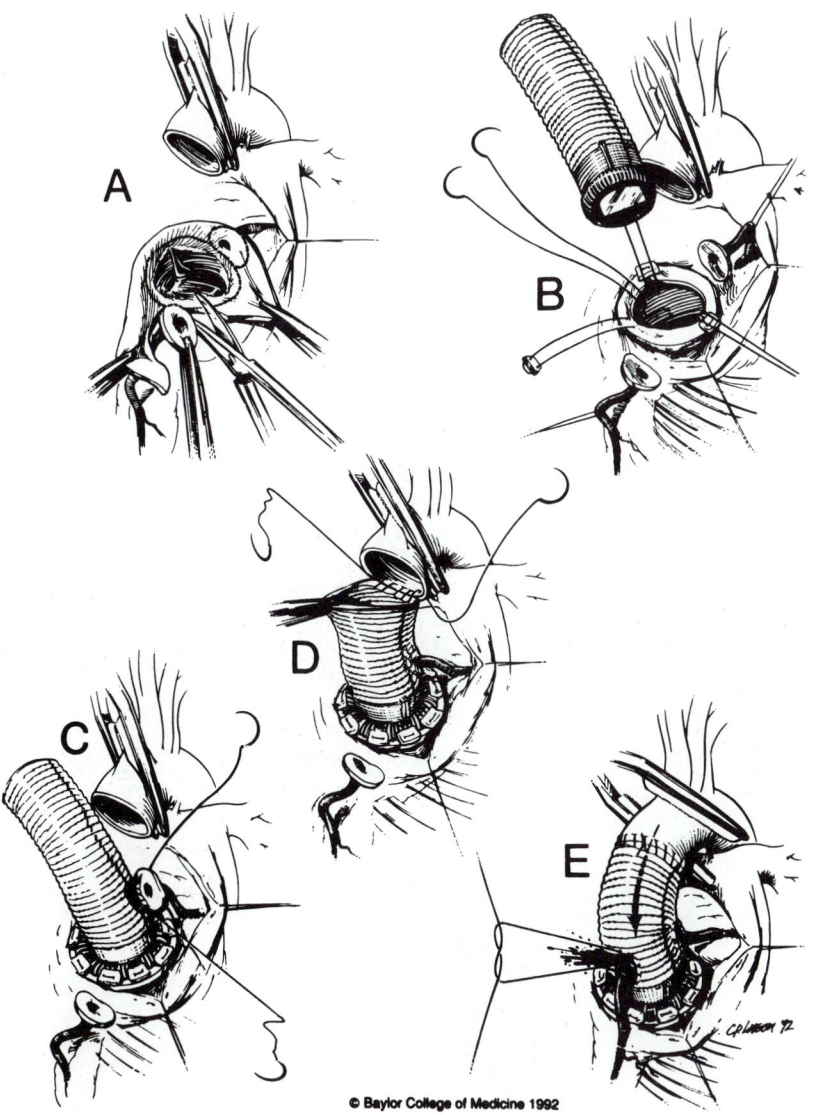

© Baylor College of Medicine 1992

Figure 136–5. A–E. Illustration of preferred operative technique for composite valve graft replacement of the aortic root with button reattachment of coronary arteries to composite valve graft without tension following complete resection of aortic root aneurysm.

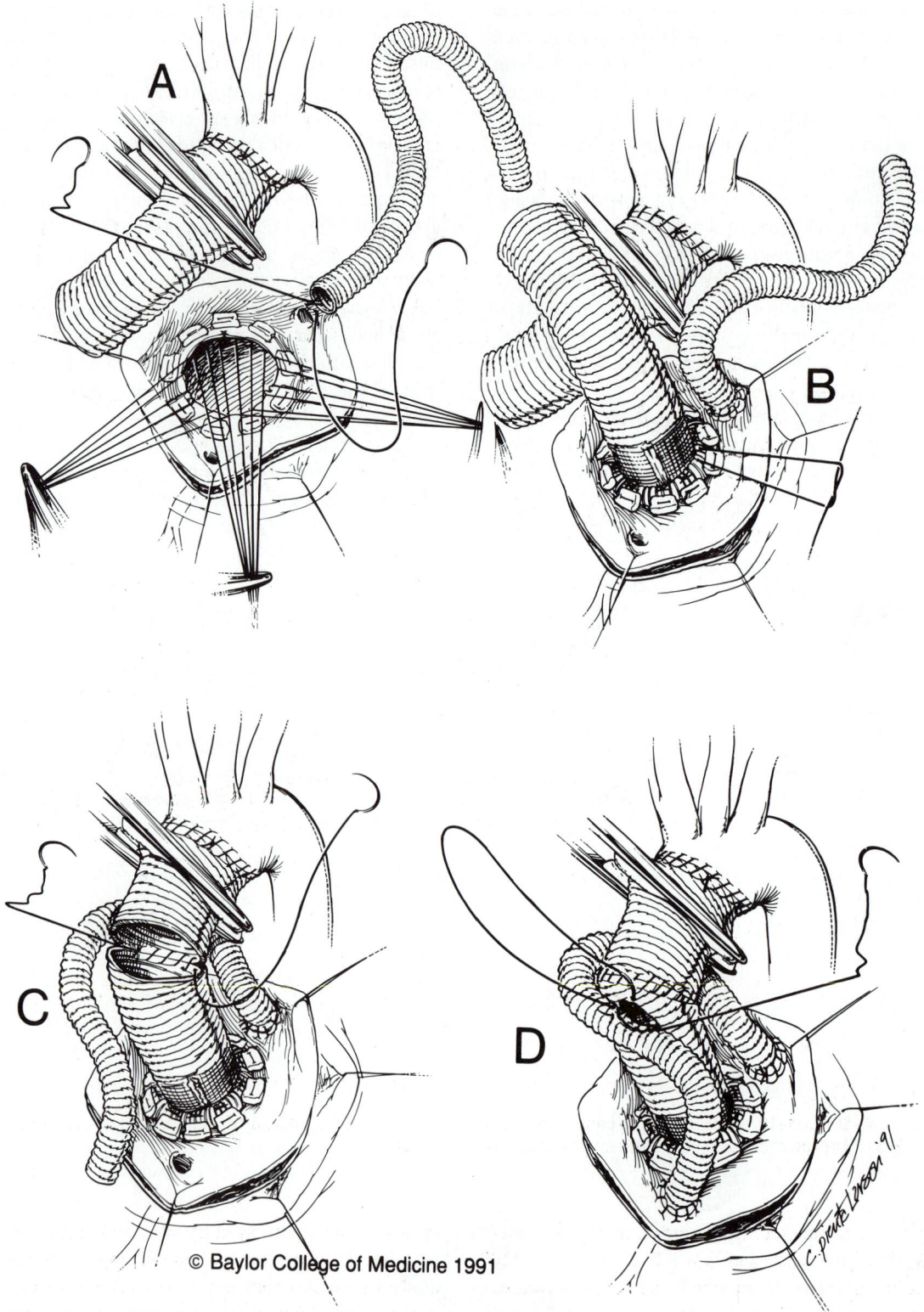

© Baylor College of Medicine 1991

c. preus Larson '91

Figure 136–6. A–D. Illustration of operative technique for partial arch replacement followed by composite valve graft replacement of the aortic root employing the Cabrol technique with a transversely placed graft to the coronary artery origins.

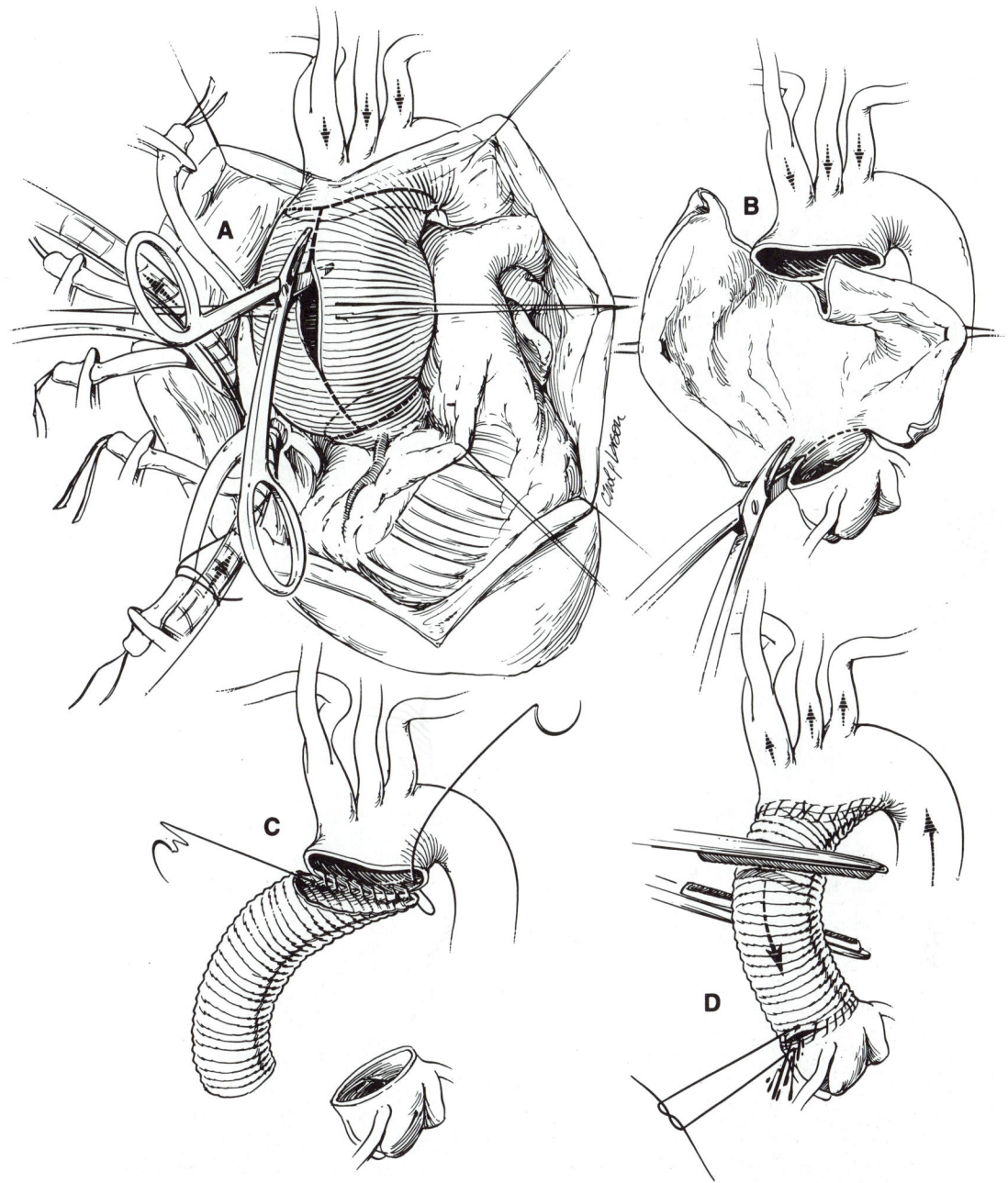

Figure 136–7. A–D. Illustration of operative technique for resection and replacement of ascending aortic and lesser curvature transverse aortic arch aneurysm using the bevel distal anastomosis approach.

into the transverse aortic arch, involving primarily its lesser curvature. Most of the lesser curvature is excised with the residual greater curvature from which the brachiocephalic arteries arise preserved for a bevelled end-to-end distal anastomosis.

Atriofemoral total cardiopulmonary bypass is utilized employing deep hypothermia and circulatory arrest for the arch portion of the reconstruction. Following completion of the distal anastomosis with the patient in the head-down position, the graft and aorta are flushed of blood and air, followed by clamping of the graft proximal to the distal anas-

tomosis. This is followed by proximal aortic root construction based upon extent of involvement. Options here include a supracoronary proximal anastomosis only, separate aortic valve replacement, or composite valve graft replacement of the entire aortic root. The technique diagrammed in Figure 136–8A–D is employed in cases where the entire transverse aortic arch is involved in the aneurysm except for the dome of the greater curvature from which the brachiocephalic vessels arise. An end-to-end anastomosis is first fashioned to the proximal descending thoracic aorta. This is followed by reattachment of the dome of the aorta

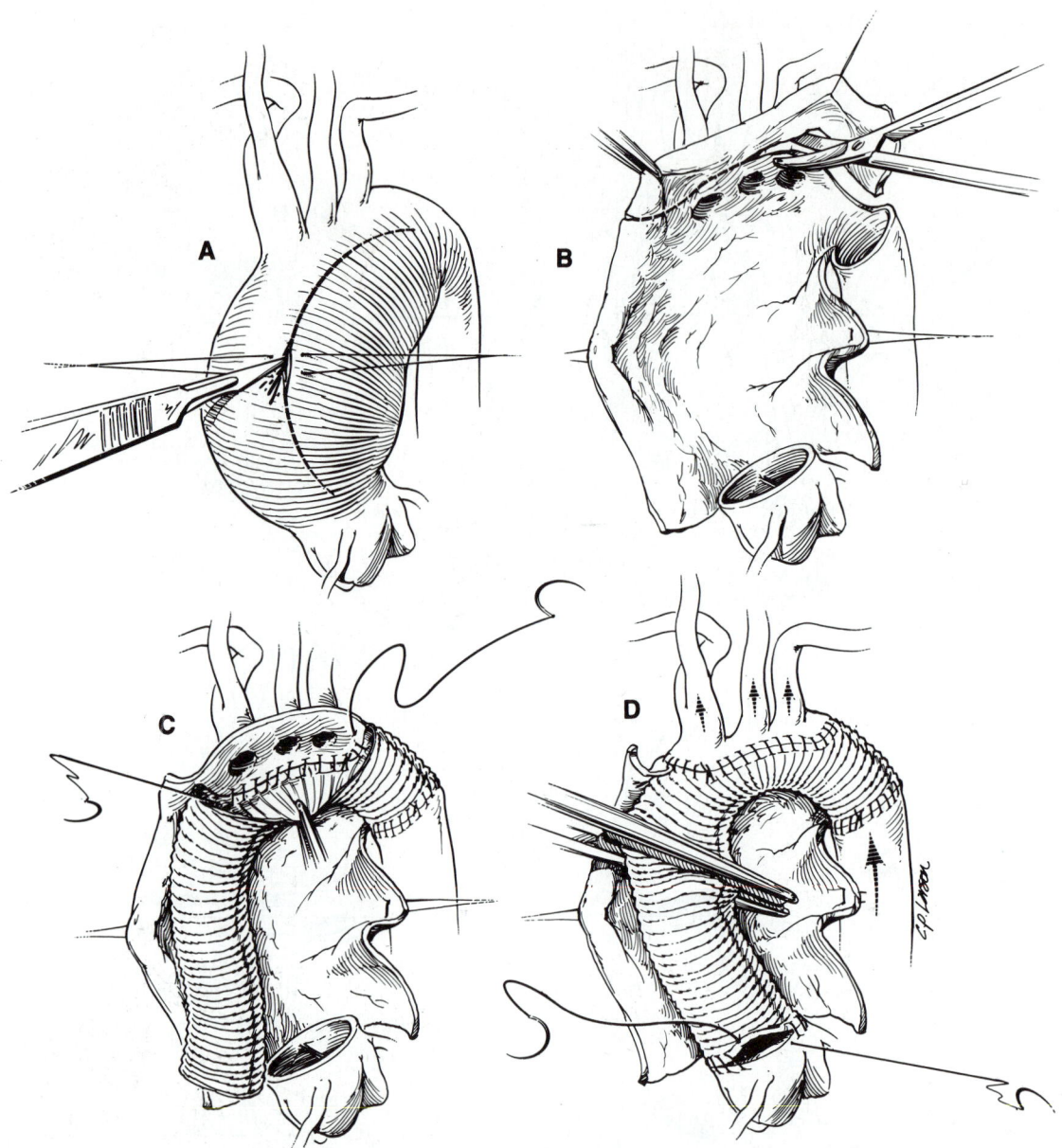

Figure 136–8. A–D. Illustration of operative technique for total transverse aortic arch replacement on a patient with fusiform aneurysm of ascending and transverse aortic arch showing reattachment of brachiocephalic vessels and supracoronary proximal anastomosis.

containing the brachiocephalic vessels to an opening in the aortic graft.

Patients with extensive aneurysmal disease involving the ascending, transverse arch, and descending or thoracoabdominal aorta are treated in a staged fashion with the ascending aorta and transverse aortic arch treated initially.[12,13] The aneurysm of the ascending aorta and arch is preferably replaced first through a midsternal incision to eliminate cardiac risks at the second operation and because recovery is usually more rapid from arch replacement than after distal operation; however, the more distal aneurysmal segment may be more symptomatic, larger, or even ruptured and require operation first. The technique used is similar to that described by Borst and referred to as the "ele-

phant trunk" technique.[14] The initial stage of the treatment of such a patient is illustrated in Figure 136–9A–F. Following opening of the ascending and transverse portion of the aortic aneurysm, an appropriately sized Dacron graft is folded upon itself and placed within the descending thoracic aorta. The graft is anastomosed to the proximal descending thoracic aorta. Following this, the graft is reverted back to its full length leaving a portion dangling within the proximal descending thoracic aorta for later use. The brachiocephalic vessels are reattached to an oval opening in the graft, following which proximal aortic reconstruction is carried out based upon extent of involvement. The advantages of this technique are related to the need for minimal dissection in the region of the distal transverse aortic arch at

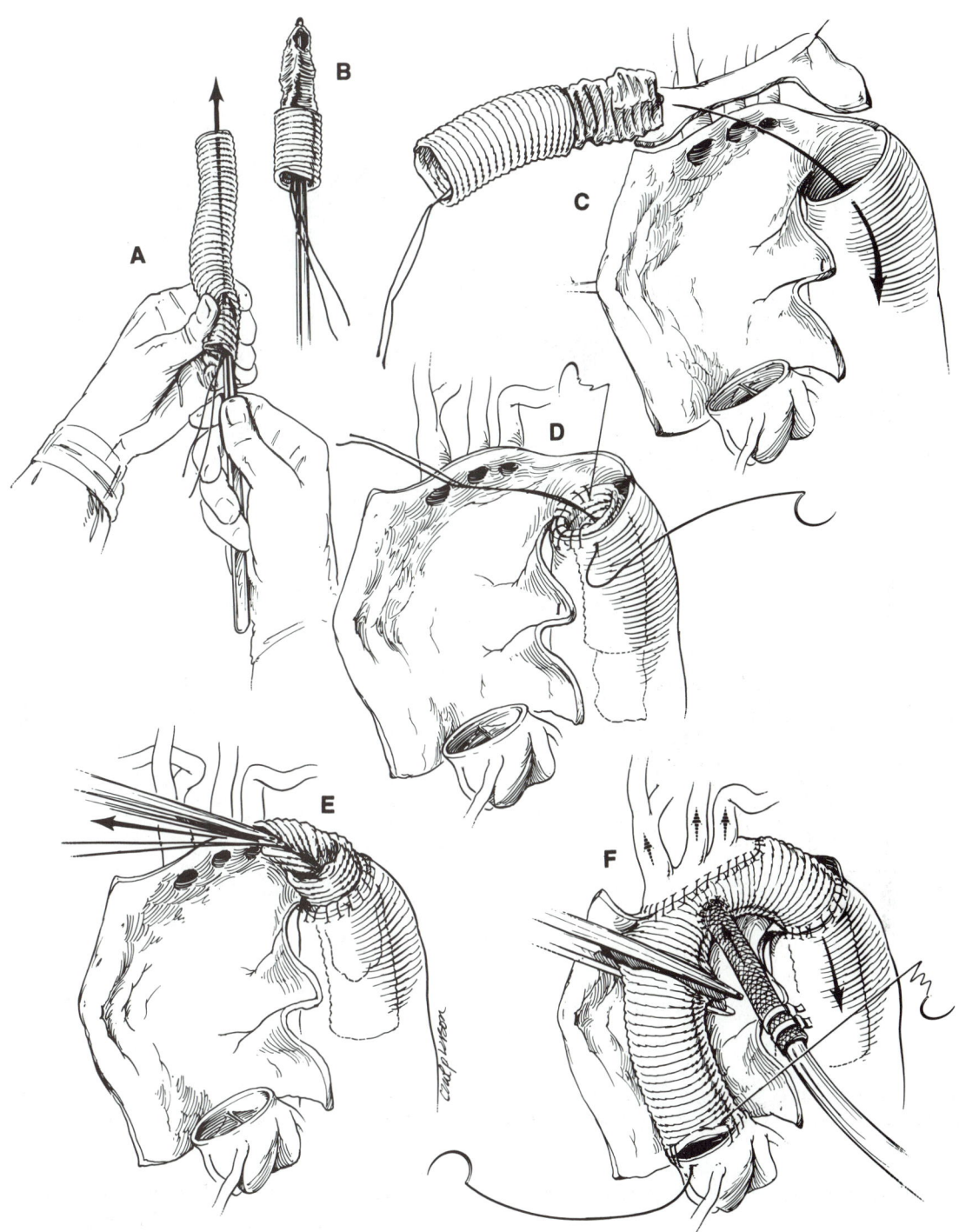

Figure 136–9. A–F. Illustration of operative technique for first stage of treatment of patient with mega aortic aneurysm showing the "elephant trunk" technique for replacement of the transverse aortic arch.

the second operation reducing risk of injury to the recurrent laryngeal nerve, esophagus, and pulmonary artery. The second stage of the treatment of such a patient is illustrated in Figure 136–10. Following opening the proximal descending thoracic aorta, the distal end of the graft is grasped and clamped, after which a thoracoabdominal reconstruction is carried out.

The approach to acute Type I aortic dissection is demonstrated in Figure 136–11A–E. All such patients are treated using deep hypothermia and circulatory arrest. An appropriately sized Dacron graft is anastomosed end-to-end to the transected aorta at the level of the proximal aortic arch. The false lumen is obliterated either in the suture line or with reinforcing Teflon felt strips placed internally and

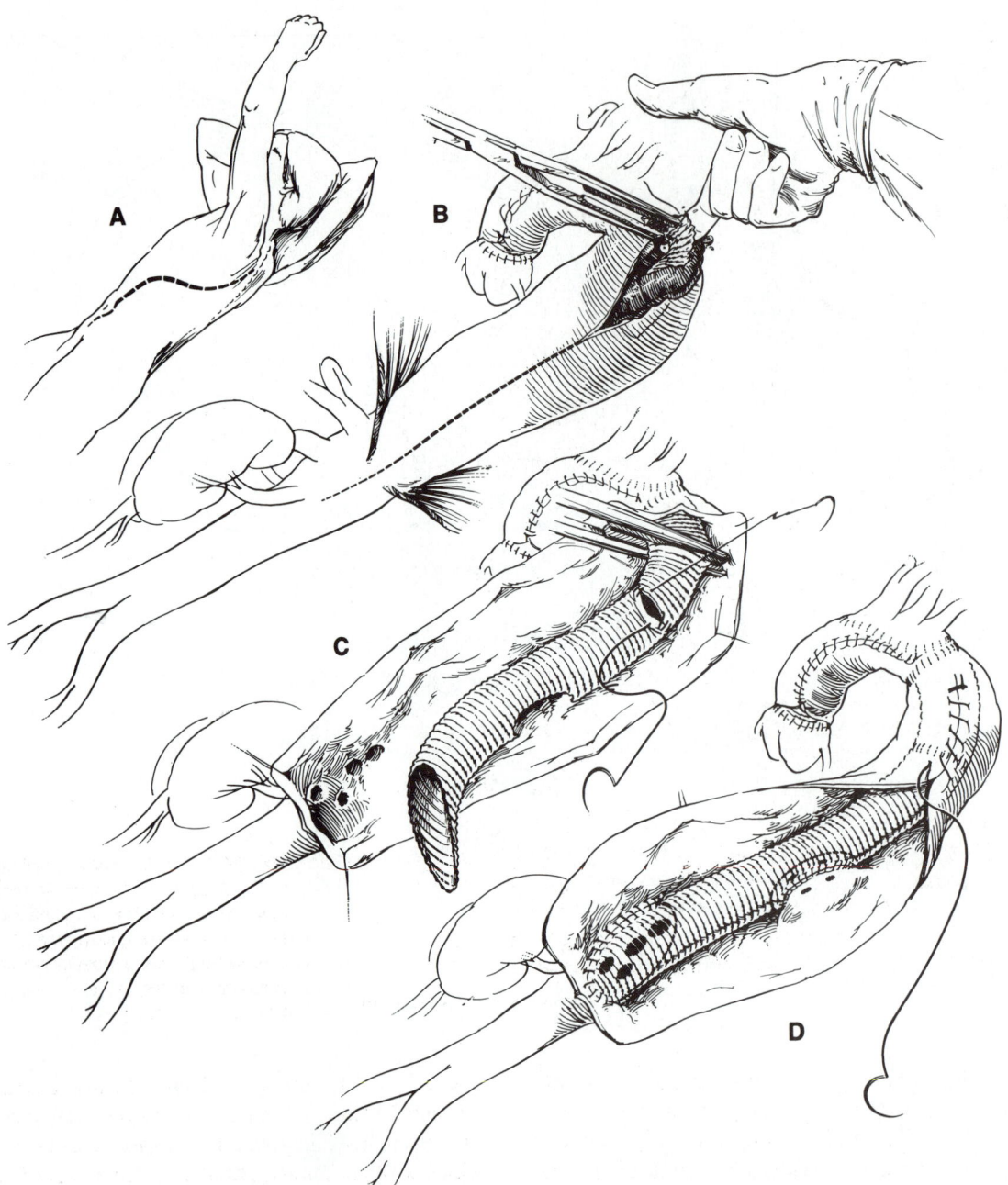

Figure 136–10. A–D. Illustration of operative approach for the second stage of treatment of patient with mega aorta with resection and replacement of thoracoabdominal aortic aneurysm following "elephant trunk" technique replacement of the transverse aortic arch.

externally. Fine suture, 5-0 or 4-0, is used. Following completion of the distal anastomosis, a clamp is applied to the aortic graft and rewarming is begun. A clamp is never applied to the aorta to prevent fracture of the friable internal layers. Additionally, the technique allows for visualization of the internal aspects of the arch should additional resection be required for tears within the transverse arch, and allows for maximal resection of the proximal aorta.[15]

The approach to chronic dissection of the transverse aortic arch is illustrated in Figure 136–12A–E. The concepts described earlier are employed; however, the wall between the true and the false lumen is excised throughout all of the transverse aortic arch and a wedge of aortic wall between the true and the false lumen is excised distally prior to distal anastomosis in the proximal descending aorta. The latter allows for perfusion beyond the distal anastomosis into both the true and the false lumen should a distal branch vessel such as the visceral, intercostal, renal, or iliac vessels be dependent upon flow through the false lumen. The remaining aspects of reconstruction are similar to those described previously.

The best approach to saccular aneurysms involving the lesser curvature of the transverse aortic arch and those in-

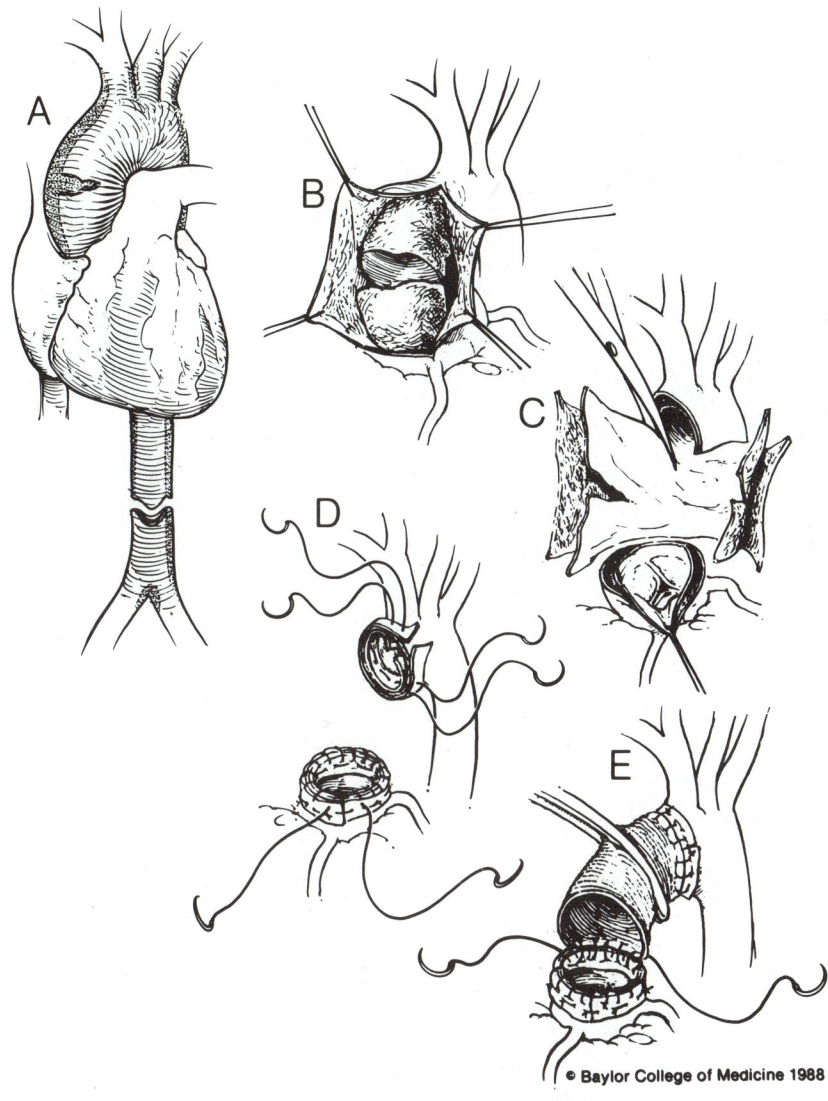

© Baylor College of Medicine 1988

Figure 136–11. A–E. Illustration of operative technique using open distal anastomosis approach with deep hypothermia and circulatory arrest for treatment of a patient with acute Type I aortic dissection with interposition tube graft replacement of ascending aorta and proximal transverse aortic arch.

volving the distal transverse aortic arch is frequently through a median sternotomy. Deep hypothermia and circulatory arrest are initiated, following which the saccular aneurysm is opened and a Dacron patch is applied to the defect in the aortic wall provided the defect encompasses only 50% or less of the circumference of the aorta (Fig. 136–13). In those in whom the opening is larger, tube graft insertion is employed. For those aneurysms that clearly involve the distal segment in the region of the origin of the left subclavian artery and/or left common carotid artery, a simple cross-clamp technique through a left thoracotomy may be employed. The aorta is clamped distal to the innominate artery along with separate clamps placed upon the left common carotid and left subclavian arteries.

HYPOTHERMIC TECHNIQUES

It has been our preference to employ total cardiopulmonary bypass in virtually all cases. Exposure is provided via an anterior midsternotomy incision. Bicaval cannulation for venous drainage to a membrane oxygenator with pump return is provided through femeral arterial cannulation. In patients with concomitant thoracoabdominal aortic aneurysm disease and severe atherosclerotic intimal involvement, antegrade perfusion with cannulation initially through the ascending aorta and later through direct cannulation of the aortic graft is utilized. Partial femoral vein to femoral artery bypass is employed in patients in whom posterolateral incisions are used and in patients with extremely large aneurysms in whom anterior incisions are required and with access to the right heart limited. Additionally, an occasional patient will have a large aneurysm eroding the posterior portion of the sternum. Frequently, this is a patient with a false aneurysm where a median sternotomy is unsafe prior to cardiopulmonary bypass, profound hypothermia, and circulatory arrest.[16]

Patients are systemically cooled until the EEG is isoelectric, usually around 18° to 20°C. Electroencephalographic monitoring is carried out using a standard 10-lead

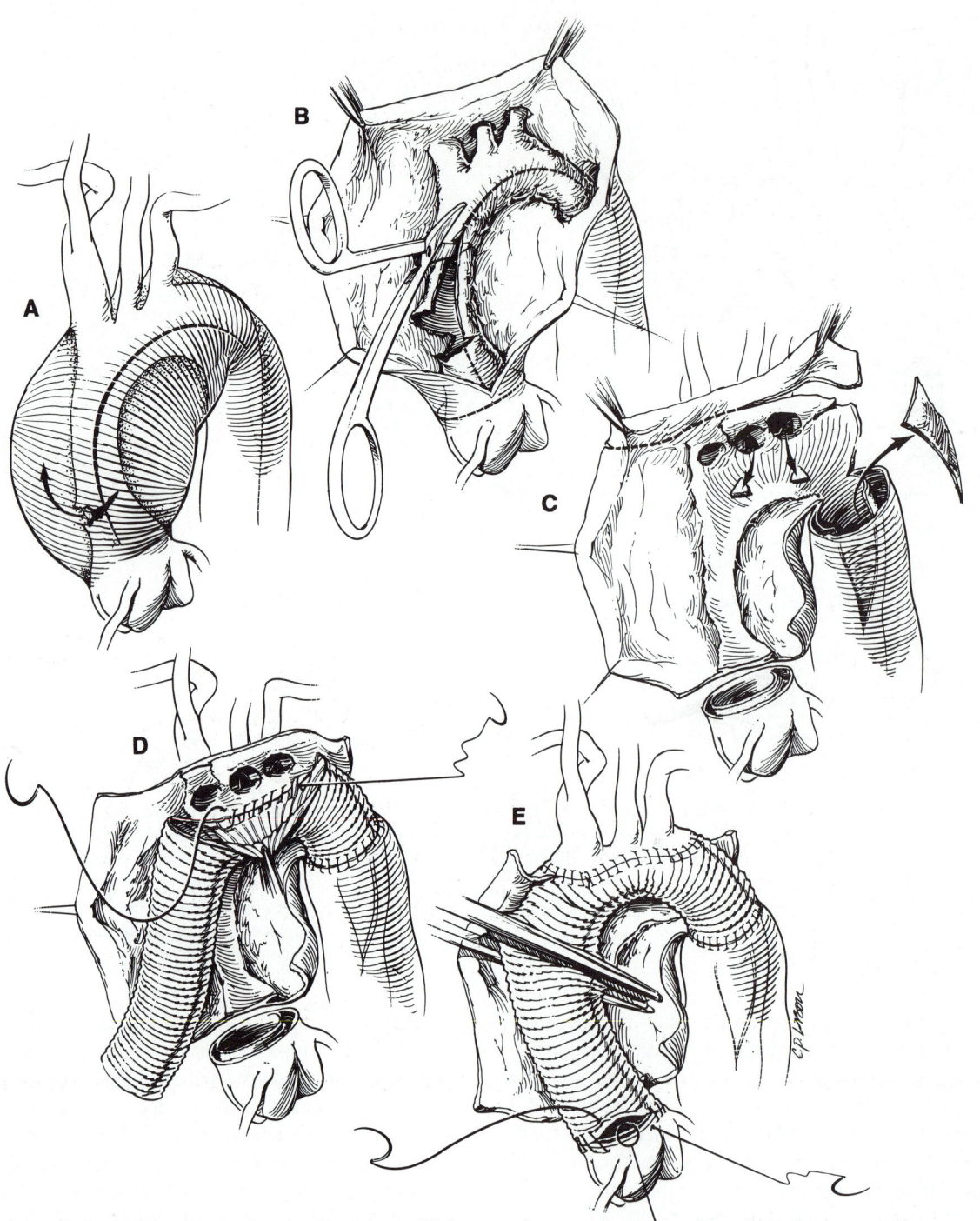

Figure 136–12. A–E. Illustration of operative technique for resection and replacement of ascending aortic and transverse aortic arch aneurysm in patient with chronic Type I aortic dissection.

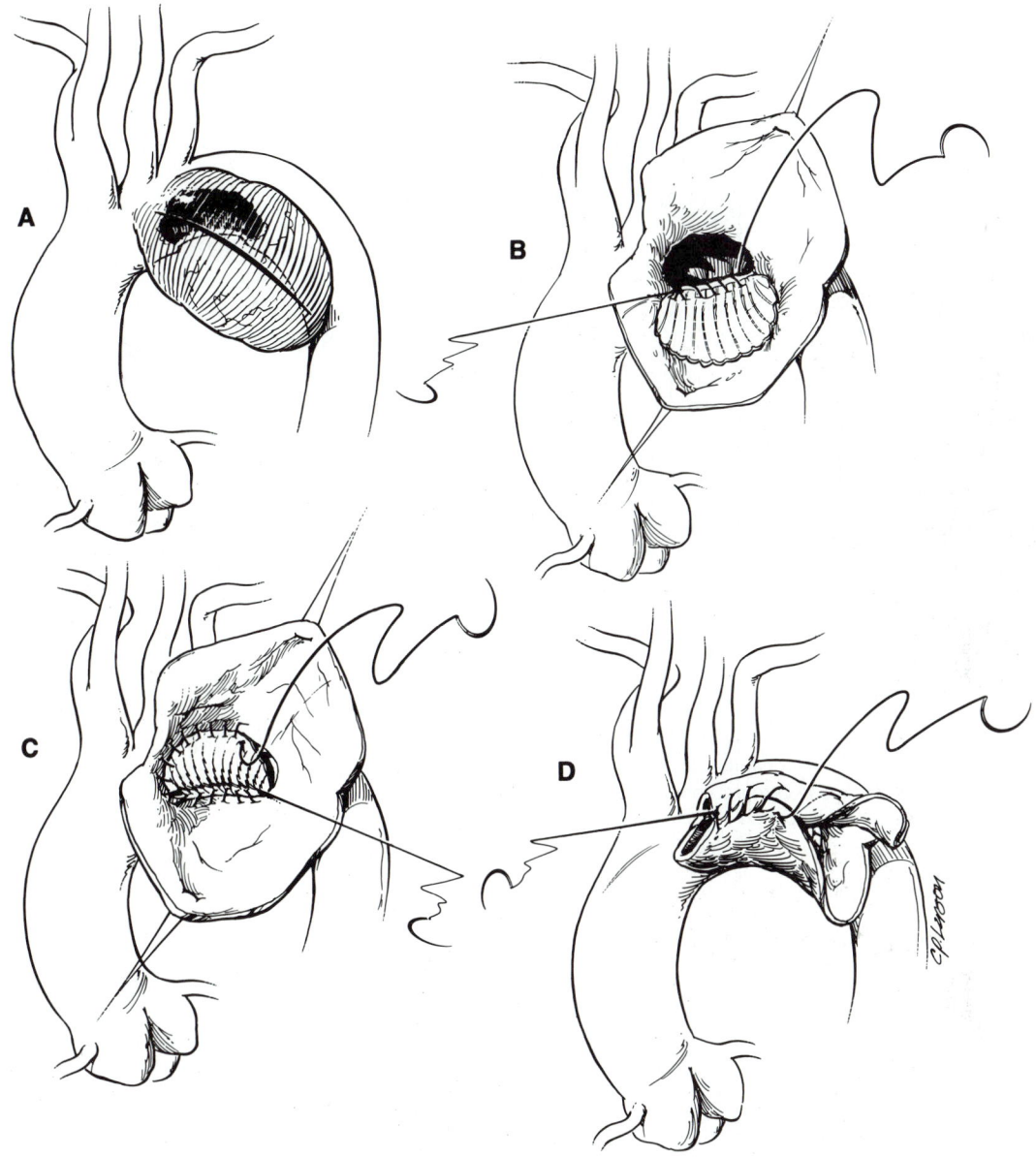

Figure 136–13. A–D. Illustration of operative technique for patch graft repair of saccular aneurysm involving the distal transverse aortic arch.

montage.[17] The period of cooling generally requires 20 to 25 min. Barbiturates and steroids are not routinely administered. Acid–base balance is maintained using the alphastat method of pH control. Five grams of aminocaproic acid (Amicar) or 1 g of transacemic acid (Cyclocapron) is administered at the initiation of cardiopulmonary bypass. Hemodilution to a hemoglobin of 6 to 7 mg/dL is employed until rewarming is initiated at which time hemoconcentration is begun. Specific dissection of the brachiocephalic vessels and clamping of such vessels is not employed. Aortic repair is carried out with the head in the extreme down position to allow for pooling of blood and to prevent air embolization. The arch segment is replaced first and this seg-

ment of the graft is filled with blood to remove air. The graft is then clamped adjacent to the brachiocephalic vessels with perfusion and rewarming begun and continued while the remaining proximal aortic segment is reconstructed. Rewarming is continued to a rectal temperature of 36° to 37°C. The period of circulatory arrest varies from 15 to 75 min, but generally averages 25 to 30 min.

More recently, retrograde cerebral perfusion has been applied for cerebral protection during the period of circulatory arrest. The circuitry for this technique is diagrammed in Figure 136–14.[18] A "Y" connection is placed on the arterial line and in the superior vena caval line to allow for connection and oxygenated perfusion via the superior vena

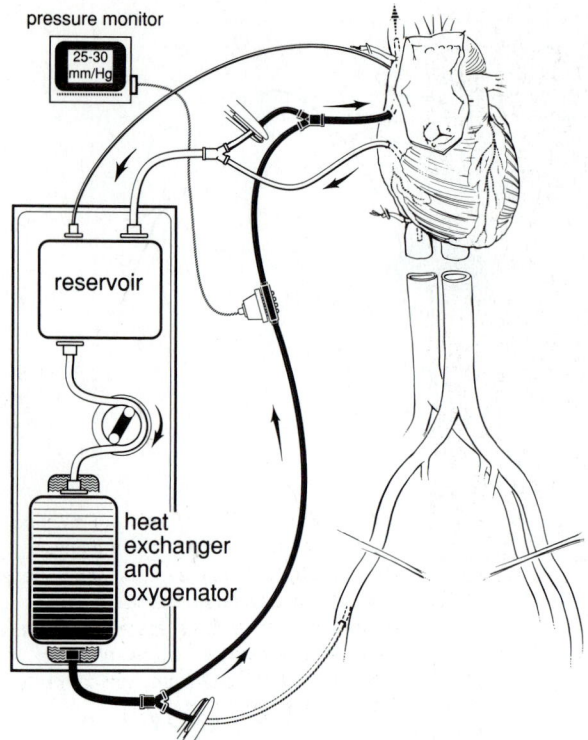

Figure 136–14. Illustration of circuitry for cardiopulmonary bypass with bicaval cannulation and retrograde cerebral perfusion via the superior vena caval cannula during the period of circulatory arrest.

cava during the arrest with flows maintained at no more than 500 mL/min. Proximal venous pressures are monitored and kept at 25 mm Hg or less to prevent cerebral edema.

RESULTS

These techniques of hypothermic circulatory arrest, as described, have provided an excellent method of cerebral protection for replacement of transverse aortic arch pathology. Crawford and his group reported upon an experience with deep hypothermia and circulatory arrest in 656 patients.[7] They found that the occurrence of stroke was observed to increase after 40 min of circulatory arrest and that the mortality rate increased significantly after 65 min of circulatory arrest.

During the period between January 1987 and December 1993 the author treated 227 patients for aortic disease involving the transverse aortic arch (Fig. 136–15).[19] Acute aortic dissection was present in 21%, chronic dissection in 30%, and nondissecting fusiform saccular aneurysm in 49%. The techniques described herein were employed in all cases including retrograde cerebral perfusion through the superior vena caval cannula in 111 patients. The in-hospital mortality was 6% and the long-term mortality was 9%. There were three patients, all with dissection, who suffered perioperative stroke. Currently, replacement of the trans-

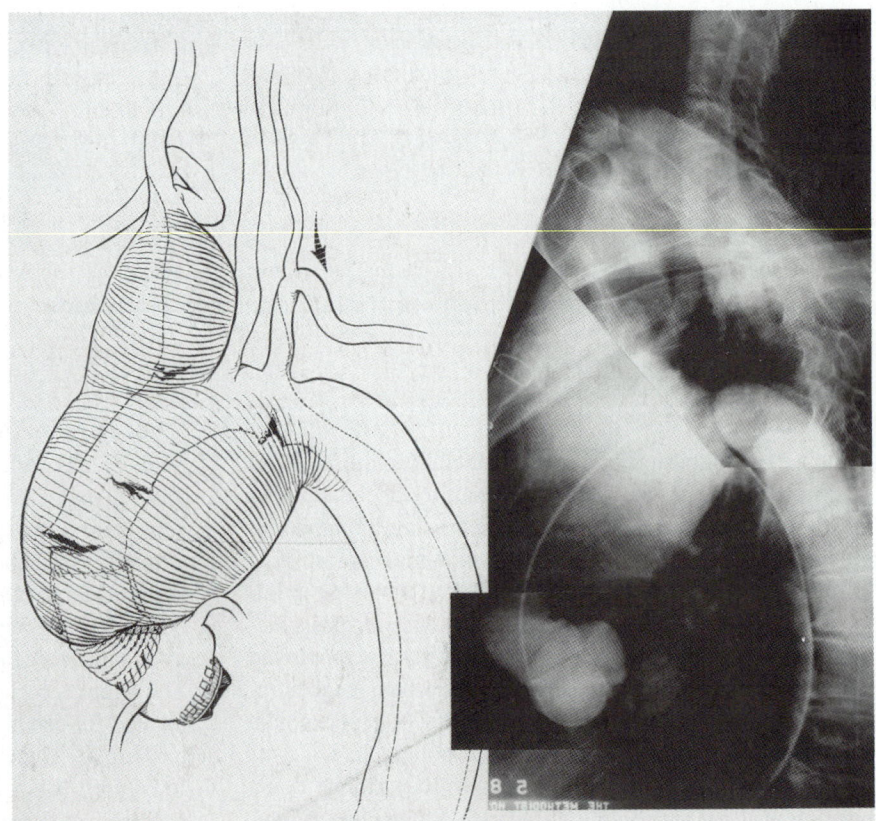

Figure 136–15. A. A preoperative drawing and arteriogram (composite photograph) of patient with aneurysm of the distal ascending aorta and transverse aortic arch and innominate artery secondary to aortic dissection following prior aortic valve and proximal ascending aortic graft replacement. *(Continued.)*

A

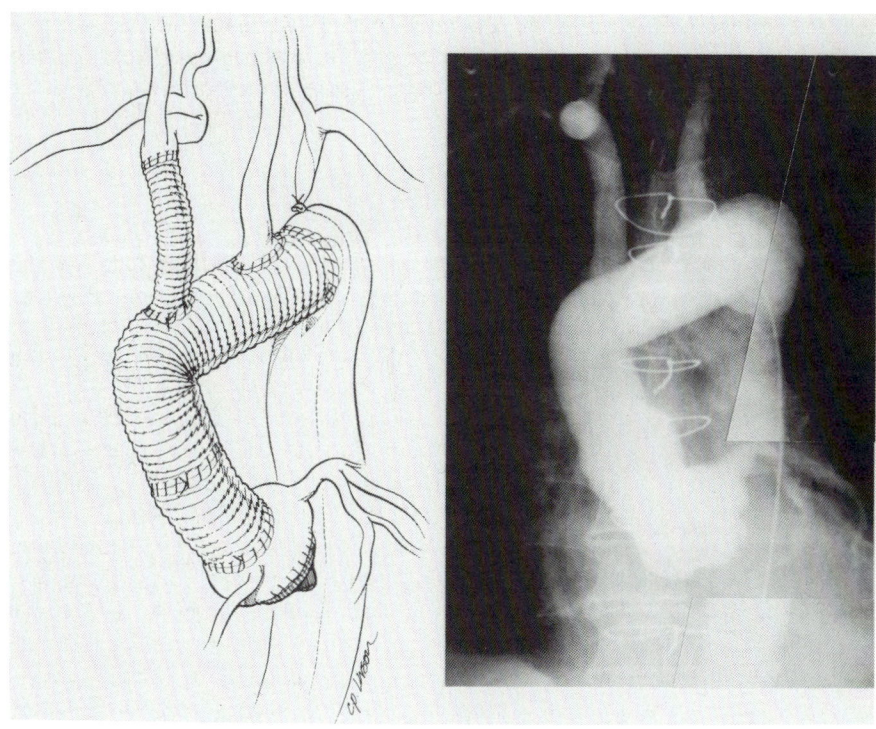

Figure 136–15. *(Continued.)* **B.** Postoperative drawing and arteriogram (composite photograph) following resection and replacement of distal ascending aorta and transverse aortic arch with separate graft replacement of the innominate artery and direct reattachment of the left common carotid to the transverse aortic arch graft.

B

verse aortic arch can be safely accomplished with very acceptably low morbidity and mortality.

REFERENCES

1. Bickerstaff LK, Pairolero PC, Hollier LH, et al: Thoracic aortic aneurysms: A population based study. *Surgery* **92:**1103, 1982
2. Cooley DA, Mahaffey DE, DeBakey ME: Total excision of the aortic arch for aneurysm. *Surg Gynecol Obstet* **101:**667, 1955
3. DeBakey ME, Cooley DA, Crawford ES, Morris GC Jr: Successful resection of fusiform aneurysm of aortic arch with replacement by homografts. *Surg Gynecol Obstet* **105:**656–664, 1957
4. Griepp RB, Stinson EB, Hollingsworth JF, Buehler D: Prosthetic replacement of the aortic arch. *J Thorac Cardiovasc Surg* **70:**1051–1063, 1975
5. Crawford ES, Saleh SA: Transverse aortic arch aneurysm: Improved results of treatment employing new modifications of aortic reconstruction and hypothermic cerebral circulatory arrest. *Ann Surg* **194:**180–188, 1981
6. Cooley DA, Livesay JJ: Technique of "open" distal anastomosis for ascending and transverse arch resection. *Bull Tex Heart Inst* **8:**421–466, 1981
7. Svensson LG, Crawford ES, Hess KR, et al: Deep hypothermia with circulatory arrest: Determinants of stroke and early mortality in 656 patients. *J Thorac Cardiovasc Surg* **106:**19–31, 1993
8. Ueda Y, Miki S, Kusuhara K, et al: Surgical treatment of aneurysm or dissection involving the ascending aorta and aortic arch, using circulatory arrest and retrograde cerebral perfusion. *J Cardiovasc Surg* **31:**553–558, 1990
9. Borst HG, Walterbusch G, Schaps D: Extensive aortic replacement using "elephant trunk" prosthesis. *J Thorac Cardiovasc Surg* **31:**37–40, 1983
10. Crawford ES, Coselli JS, Svensson LG, et al: Diffuse aneurysmal disease (chronic aortic dissection, Marfan, and mega aorta syndromes) and multiple aneurysm: Treatment by subtotal and total aortic replacement emphasizing the elephant trunk operation. *Ann Surg* **211:**521–537, 1990
11. Cabrol C, Pavie A, Gandjbakheh I, et al: Complete replacement of the ascending aorta with reimplantation of coronary arteries. New surgical approach. *J Thorac Cardiovasc Surg* **81:**309–315, 1981
12. Crawford ES, Stowe CL, Crawford JL, et al: Aortic arch aneurysm: A sentinel of extensive aortic disease requiring subtotal or total aortic replacement. *Ann Surg* **199:**742, 1984
13. Crawford ES, Coselli JS: Replacement of the aortic arch. *Semin Thorac Cardiovasc Surg* **3**(3):194–212, 1991
14. Lass J, Jurmann MJ, Heinemann M, Borst HG: Advances in aortic arch surgery. *Ann Thorac Surg* **53:**227–232, 1992
15. Crawford ES, Kirklin JW, Naftel DC, et al: Surgery for acute ascending aortic dissection: Should the arch be included? *J Thorac Cardiovasc Surg* **104**(1):46–59, 1992
16. Coselli JS, Crawford ES, Williams TW Jr, et al: Treatment of postoperative infection of ascending aorta and transverse aortic arch. *Ann Thorac Surg* **50:**868–881, 1990
17. Coselli JS, Crawford ES, Beall AC Jr, et al: Determination of brain temperatures for safe circulatory arrest during cardiovascular operation. *Ann Thorac Surg* **45:**638–642, 1988
18. Coselli JS: Retrograde cerebral perfusion via superior vena caval cannula for aortic arch aneurysm surgery. *Ann Thorac Surg* **57:**1668–1669, 1994
19. Coselli JS, Büket S, Djukanovic B: Aortic arch surgery: Current treatment and results. *Ann Thorac Surg* **59:**19–27, 1995

137

Descending Thoracic Aortic Aneurysms

James I. Fann and D. Craig Miller

HISTORY

Aortic aneurysm and its associated complications have been recognized since antiquity.[1-3] In the second century, Galen described a traumatic false aneurysm of an artery. Aetius reported a ruptured nontraumatic aneurysm four centuries later. Fernel discussed aortic and visceral artery aneurysms as early as 1542. In the late sixteenth century, Amboise Pare speculated on the various etiologies of aneurysm formation and noted the relationship to syphilis. In the early eighteenth century, Morgagni reported a ruptured ascending aortic aneurysm in a young woman with syphilis. In 1757 Hunter described a case of a thoracic aortic aneurysm that had eroded through the chest wall; he also defined true and false aneurysms. The principle of aneurysm ligation proximal to the dilatation was enunciated by Anel in 1710. Unsuccessful attempts at aortic aneurysm ligation were undertaken in the nineteenth century; other early therapeutic modalities included introduction of huge lengths of wire into the aneurysm sac, endoaneurysmorrhaphy, reinforcement with cellophane, and simple excision with oversewing of the aneurysmal neck. Experimentally, Hufnagel employed plastic prostheses to replace the thoracic aorta in 1947.[4] Surgical replacement of a descending aortic aneurysm using an aortic homograft was reported by Lam and Aram in 1951; postoperatively, the patient developed paraparesis and empyema and expired 3 mo later.[5] In 1953, Bahnson presented a limited series of successful thoracic aortic aneurysm repairs by lateral resection and aortorrhaphy.[3] In the same year, DeBakey and Cooley described the first successful replacement of a descending thoracic aortic aneurysm using a prosthetic graft.[6] Since these early publications, the risk of paraplegia has continued to be a vexing problem in the surgical management of this disease. This chapter focuses on the diagnosis and surgical treatment of descending thoracic aortic aneurysm. Because they are not true aneurysms, aortic dissections with aneurysmal dilatation will not be covered here because to be semantically correct they actually are "false aneurysms."

EPIDEMIOLOGY AND NATURAL HISTORY

The incidence of thoracic aortic aneurysms is estimated to be 5.9 cases per 100,000 person-years.[7] The mean age at diagnosis in those with aneurysms involving the descending thoracic aorta as a result of atherosclerosis is between 59 and 69 years.[8-12] Men predominate over women with a ratio of 2–4 to 1. Often, these patients have coexistent major medical problems, including hypertension in 59 to 63% of cases, coronary artery disease in 29%, chronic obstructive pulmonary disease in 29%, and congestive heart failure in 10%.[8,10,11,13] Additionally, peripheral vascular disease is common in this patient population, with abdominal aortic aneurysm occurring in 13 to 29% of cases, previous stroke in 6%, and peripheral arterial occlusive disease in 4%.[9-13]

The natural history of untreated thoracic aortic aneurysms is progressive expansion and rupture. In 1978, McNamara and Pressler reported the outcome of 22 patients with atherosclerotic descending thoracic aortic aneurysms who were not surgically treated.[13] Of these, 40% died from aneurysm rupture (all except one occurred in aneurysms larger than 10 cm in diameter), and 32% died from unrelated cardiovascular disease. Mean survival was less than 3 years. A recent increase in size preceded rupture in all patients in whom serial radiographic studies were available.[13]

In a subsequent update, rupture remained the cause of death in 44% of patients; 91% of ruptures occurred in the chronic phase of watchful observation, with 68% occurring more than 1 mo after the time of diagnosis.[9] The likelihood of death from rupture did not appear to be influenced by aneurysm location. In a group of 72 patients with thoracic aortic aneurysms, Bickerstaff et al from the Mayo Clinic reported a rupture rate of 74% in a population-based study; the aneurysm rupture was fatal in 94% of cases.[7] Importantly, the diagnosis was *not known* prior to rupture in 70%. For the remaining 30% of patients, the median interval between diagnosis and rupture was only 2 years. The actuarial 1- and 5-year survival estimates for patients with thoracic aortic aneurysms not surgically treated has been reported to be between 60 and 20%, respectively.[7,9]

PATHOGENESIS AND PATHOPHYSIOLOGY

The etiology of thoracic aortic aneurysm has changed dramatically since the early 1900s when more than 80% of the cases were secondary to syphilis, and atherosclerosis was infrequent.[1,2] The average interval from active syphilis to development of symptoms due to an aneurysm was 20 years.[2] In the modern antibiotic era, the incidence of syphilitic aneurysm has decreased to less than 5%; the majority of thoracic aortic aneurysms are the result of either medial degeneration or atherosclerosis.[8–10,14] Approximately 90% of cases of descending thoracic aortic aneurysms are atherosclerotic in origin, while medial degeneration is the most common etiology of ascending and arch aortic aneurysms. Less frequently, approximately 9% of patients present with mycotic or traumatic aneurysms. Other causes of descending thoracic aortic aneurysms include postoperative false aneurysms in approximately 1% of cases, the Marfan syndrome in 1%, and associated congenital anomalies of the aorta in about 0.6%. The majority of thoracic aortic aneurysms are chronic; however, some aneurysms, particularly those of infectious etiology, can present acutely.[14]

Because of LaPlace's law, aneurysm formation is a progressive and self-propagating phenomenon; as the aortic radius increases, wall tension becomes higher, leading to further aneurysm expansion and a higher likelihood of rupture. Aortic dilatation is associated with accentuated turbulent flow and deposition of laminated thrombus along the walls of the aneurysm; it should be emphasized that this clot formation confers no protection whatsoever against further expansion or rupture. The role of hypertension contributing to the development of aneurysmal dilatation is paramount. Although thoracic aortic aneurysm associated with the Marfan syndrome is more likely to rupture at a smaller absolute diameter, surgical intervention should be considered in any patient with a thoracic aortic aneurysm twice the diameter of the relatively normal sized contiguous aortic segment.

Thoracic aortic aneurysms are often classified according to location, etiology, and morphology. Aneurysms may involve the ascending thoracic aorta, the transverse arch, and/or the descending thoracic aorta.[7,9,14] Of all thoracic aortic aneurysms, the ascending aorta is affected in approximately 50% of cases, the aortic arch in 10%, and the descending aorta in 40%.[7] Descending thoracic aortic aneurysms, generally resulting from degenerative or atherosclerotic changes, usually begin just distal to the left subclavian artery. Morphologically, the fusiform configuration of descending thoracic aortic aneurysm is more common than is the localized (or saccular) type.[14]

DIAGNOSIS

At the time of diagnosis, often made after a routine chest radiograph or during evaluation for some other disorder, 21 to 50% of patients with descending thoracic aortic aneurysms are asymptomatic.[9–11,13] In the remainder, the only symptom occurring with any frequency is back or chest pain, generally localized to the area of the aneurysm. The pain may gradually increase in severity as the aneurysm enlarges, or it may be sudden with rapid expansion and impending rupture. Except for hypertension, physical examination often proves unrevealing. Nonetheless, symptoms and signs can result from compression or erosion of adjacent structures. Symptoms may include hoarseness from stretching or compression of the left recurrent laryngeal nerve (8.6%), tracheal deviation and respiratory symptoms resulting from local airway compression (8%), hemoptysis from bronchial or pulmonary parenchymal erosion, dysphagia (or even hematemesis) from esophageal compression (5%), hypotension and hemothorax from aneurysm rupture (3%), neurologic deficits from spinal cord ischemia (2.6%), and upper body venous distention from superior vena cava syndrome.[11,13,15]

Electrocardiography, generally obtained to rule out cardiac ischemia as the cause of the chest pain, may demonstrate left ventricular hypertrophy secondary to long-standing hypertension. A chest radiograph often reveals enlargement of the descending thoracic aorta.[11,13] Lateral or oblique views are essential to distinguish aneurysmal dilatation from marked aortic tortuosity. Calcification in the aneurysm wall is sometimes visualized. Occasionally, an aneurysm limited to the descending aorta may displace the arch to the right, giving the appearance of an arch aneurysm on plain chest radiograph. Mediastinal widening or the presence of a left pleural effusion suggests impending thoracic aortic aneurysm rupture.

Although atherosclerotic aneurysms occasionally can be difficult to distinguish from aortic dissection with aneurysmal dilatation using this modality, aortography is an important preoperative study to delineate the location and extent of the aneurysm, assess critical side branches, and aid in operative planning[11,13] (Fig. 137–1). Laminated intra-

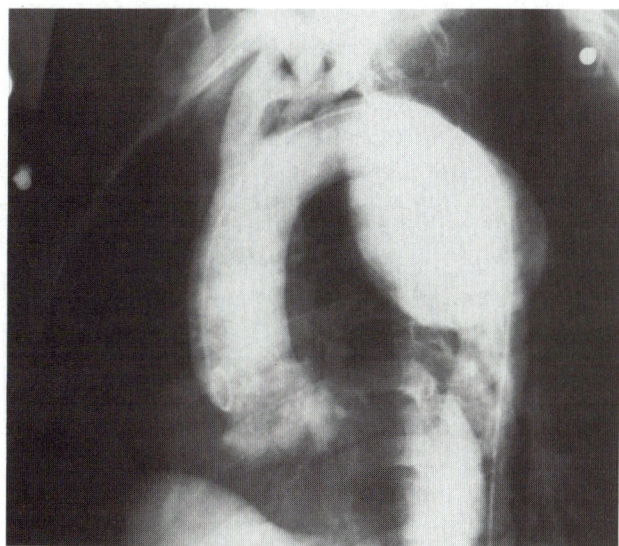

Figure 137–1. Oblique view of an aortogram of a patient with proximal descending thoracic aortic aneurysm.

luminal thrombus, however, leads to an underestimation of the actual aneurysm size. Digital subtraction angiography can also provide high quality images with the advantage of a lower contrast volume and radiation exposure. Coronary arteriography should be considered in older patients and those suspected on clinical grounds of having coronary artery disease. Additional diagnostic studies, such as com-

puted tomography (CT, axial or spiral) or magnetic resonance imaging (MRI), can document the pathoanatomic changes and morphology, assess involvement of surrounding structures, provide very accurate measurements of aneurysm size, and differentiate aortic aneurysm from dissection (Fig. 137–2). In general, CT or MRI scans are the preferred diagnostic tests, with aortography being reserved for those who are being considered for operation.

TREATMENT

The high risk of rupture of patients with untreated descending thoracic aortic aneurysms mandates surgical evaluation in essentially all cases, taking into account the patient's age and overall medical condition. The presence of coexistent cardiac or cerebrovascular disease remains an important factor in assessing the patient preoperatively. Our current recommendation for operation includes all symptomatic patients.[8,13] In those who are asymptomatic, aneurysm external diameter that is twice the size of a relatively normal contiguous segment of thoracic aorta or greater than 6 cm, or documented aneurysm enlargement should prompt consideration of operation. The purpose of operative treatment is to eliminate the diseased portion of the aorta; occasionally, operation is staged with initial attention directed toward the most diseased or most symptomatic segment. Smaller aneurysms can be followed with serial CT or MRI scans every 6 to 12 mo, proceeding with surgical interven-

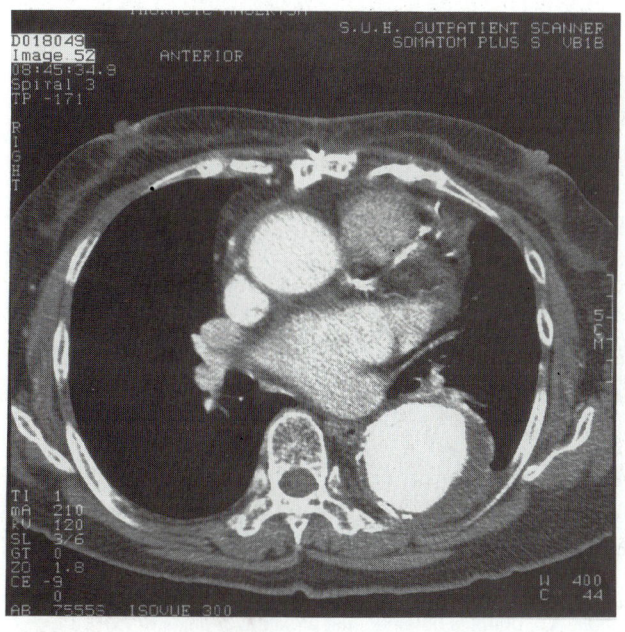

A

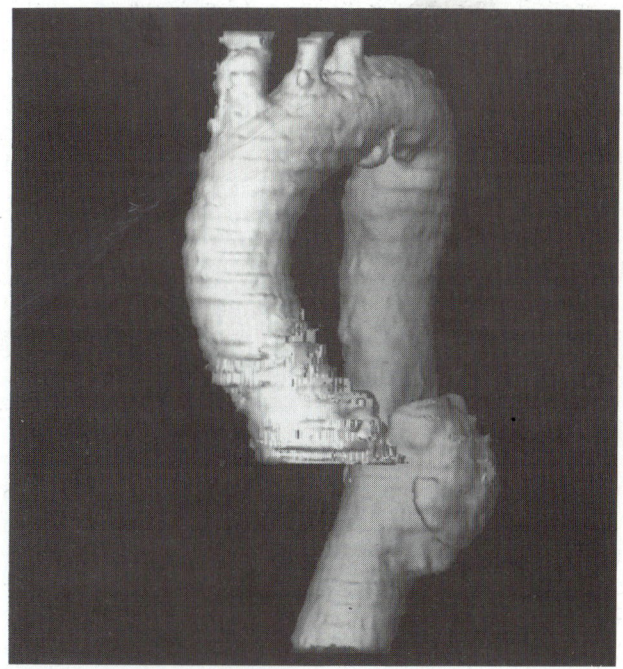

B

Figure 137–2. **A.** Computed tomography of a patient with descending thoracic aortic aneurysm. **B.** Spiral computed tomographic reconstruction of a patient with mid-descending thoracic aortic aneurysm.

tion if progressive expansion occurs. Medical therapy is integral to optimal management, primarily aimed at controlling associated diseases, such as hypertension and chronic obstructive pulmonary disease. In particular, patients with the Marfan syndrome or other inherited connective tissue disorders should have life-long β-blocker therapy.

Surgical Technique

The patient is positioned in the right lateral decubitus position for a left posterolateral thoracotomy[8,16] (Figs. 137–3 and 137–4). Selective endobronchial intubation greatly facilitates the procedure and lessens the risk of left lung injury. In our experience, partial cardiopulmonary bypass

(CPB, femoral artery and pulmonary artery or femoral vein cannulation) with systemic heparinization (300 U/kg) and an oxygenator has been used; alternatively, left atrial–femoral artery bypass using a Bio-Medicus centrifugal pump [with a reservoir and heat exchanger in the circuit and low dose (100 U/kg) heparinization] can be employed safely.

If partial CPB is used, the left common femoral artery is preferred for arterial cannulation; the main pulmonary artery is preferred for venous drainage. If a long venous cannula is planned for femoral–femoral bypass, it should be preferentially inserted in the right femoral vein because of the higher probability of passing the cannula into the right atrium. The aorta proximal and distal to the aneurysm is

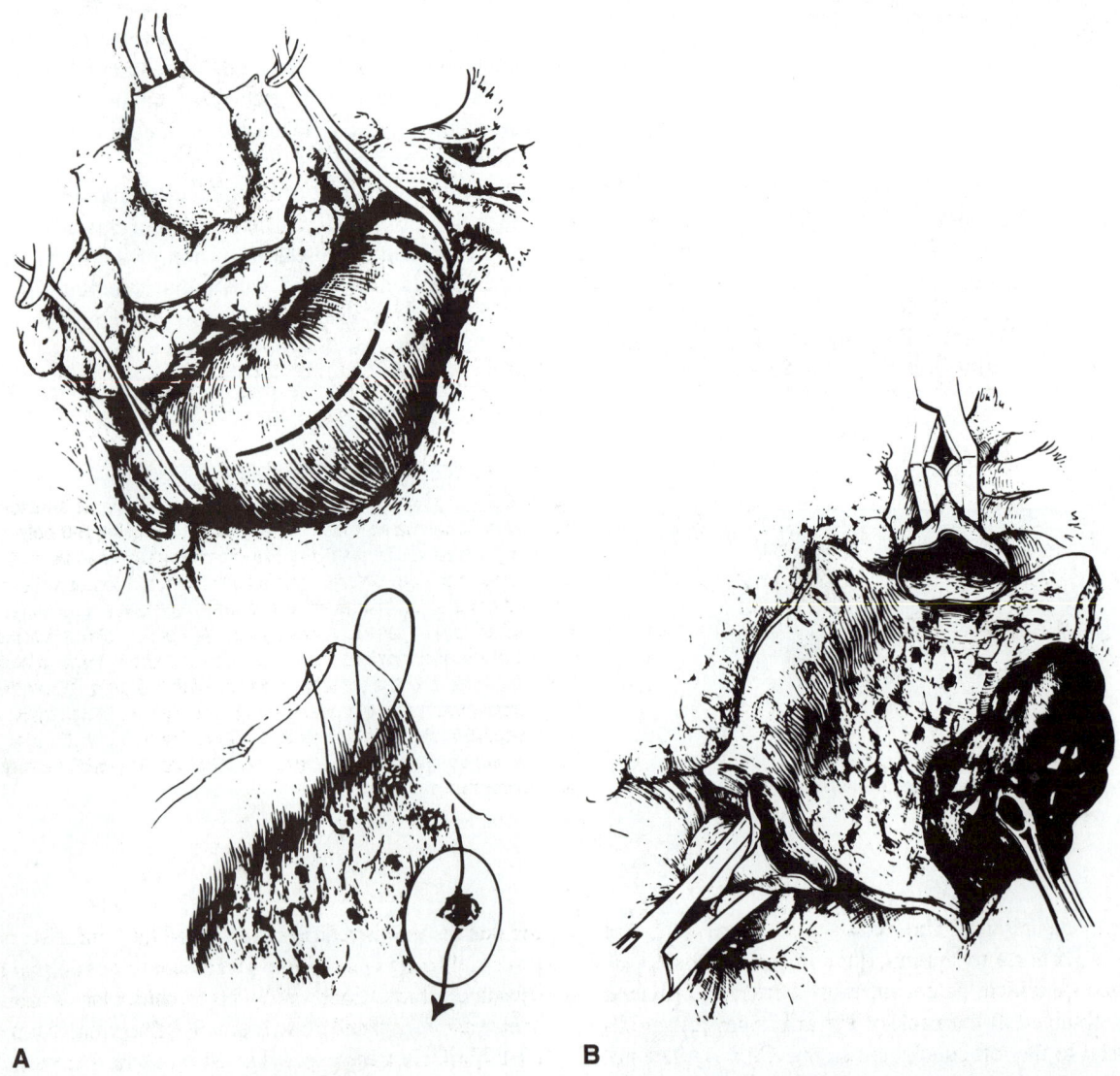

Figure 137–3. Surgical approach to descending thoracic aortic aneurysm repair. **A.** Control is obtained just proximal or distal to the left subclavian artery, depending on the extent of the aneurysm. Once the patient's hemodynamics are stable by pharmacologic and/or mechanical support, the distal descending thoracic aorta is cross-clamped, followed by cross-clamping the proximal aorta. **B.** The aneurysm is opened longitudinally, and the aortotomy is extended proximally and distally. The thrombus is evacuated and the intercostal vessels oversewn. Proximal and distal full-thickness aortic cuffs are dissected free. *(Continued.)*

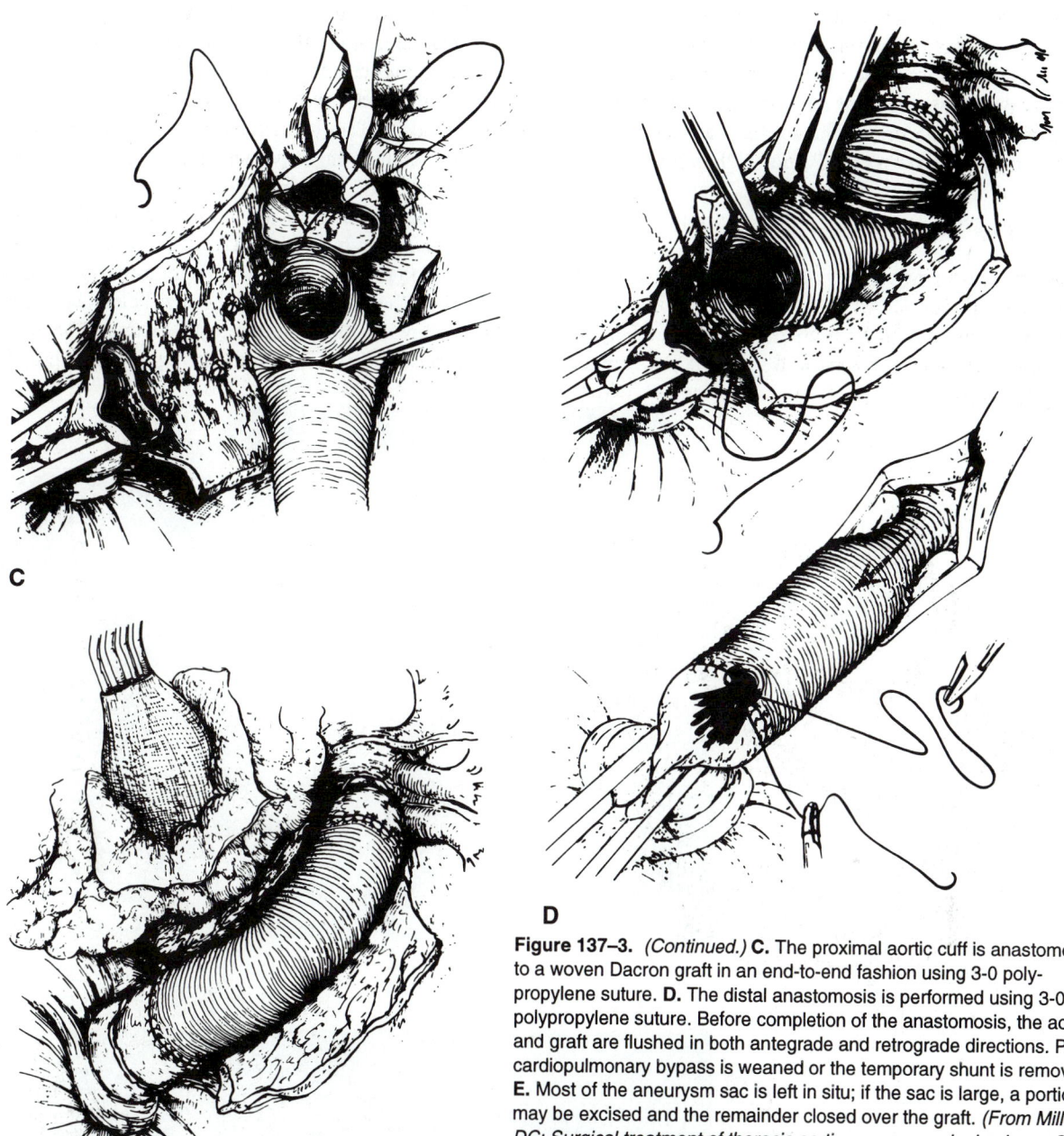

Figure 137–3. *(Continued.)* **C.** The proximal aortic cuff is anastomosed to a woven Dacron graft in an end-to-end fashion using 3-0 polypropylene suture. **D.** The distal anastomosis is performed using 3-0 polypropylene suture. Before completion of the anastomosis, the aorta and graft are flushed in both antegrade and retrograde directions. Partial cardiopulmonary bypass is weaned or the temporary shunt is removed. **E.** Most of the aneurysm sac is left in situ; if the sac is large, a portion may be excised and the remainder closed over the graft. *(From Miller DC: Surgical treatment of thoracic aortic aneurysms. In Jamieson SW, Shumway NE (eds): Rob and Smith's Operative Surgery: Cardiac Surgery, 4th ed. London, Butterworths, 1986, pp 519–525, reproduced with permission.)*

mobilized and encircled. The extent of resection is limited to the diseased aorta to minimize the chance of disruption or exclusion of critical patent intercostal arteries. Proximal control is obtained at the neck of the aneurysm just proximal or distal to the left subclavian artery. Care is taken not to injure the phrenic, vagus, and recurrent laryngeal nerves, the left lung, and the esophagus. If the aneurysm is densely adherent to a portion of the lung, only minimal dissection of the lung off the aneurysm is performed before the aorta is clamped and opened. Once CPB is instituted, adjustment in the rate of venous return and/or vasodilator infusion permits proximal aortic cross-clamp placement with minimal hemodynamic fluctuations and left ventricular strain. The aneurysm is opened longitudinally. Bleeding from intercostal branches are controlled with suture ligatures. When there is a large, patent left-sided intercostal artery in the region of T8–L1 that is not copiously back-bleeding, reimplantation of this vessel into the graft is performed. A woven, double velour Dacron graft impregnated with collagen (Hemashield Woven Double-Velour, Meadox Medical,

Oakland, NJ) is anastomosed end-to-end to the proximal and distal aortic cuffs in a full-thickness manner. Before completion of the distal anastomosis, the aorta and graft are flushed in both antegrade and retrograde directions, and air is removed from the graft. The residual aneurysm sac is closed loosely over the graft. Partial CPB is discontinued and the femoral artery and pulmonary artery (or femoral vein) are repaired.

"Elephant Trunk" Adjunctive Procedures

Developed in 1983 by Borst from Hannover, Germany, the elephant trunk technique has been used to facilitate replace-

ment of the descending thoracic aorta after initial total aortic arch replacement[17,18] or the supraceliac and distal descending thoracic aorta after graft replacement of the proximal descending thoracic aorta. This technique permits anastomosis of an interposition graft to the elephant trunk, thereby eliminating any need for proximal aortic surgical dissection and clamping (Fig. 137–5). For the first stage, our preferred variation of this technique is to initially invaginate the arch graft and direct the invaginated graft segments into the descending thoracic aorta for the distal arch (or "waist") anastomosis.[19] A suture is attached to the inner graft allowing this segment to be extracted once the distal arch anastomosis between the invaginating fold and the de-

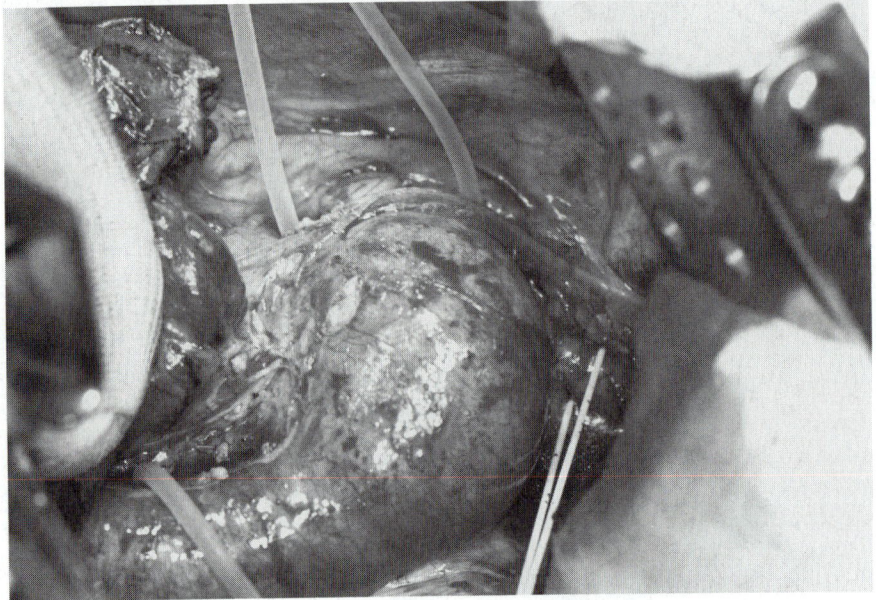

A

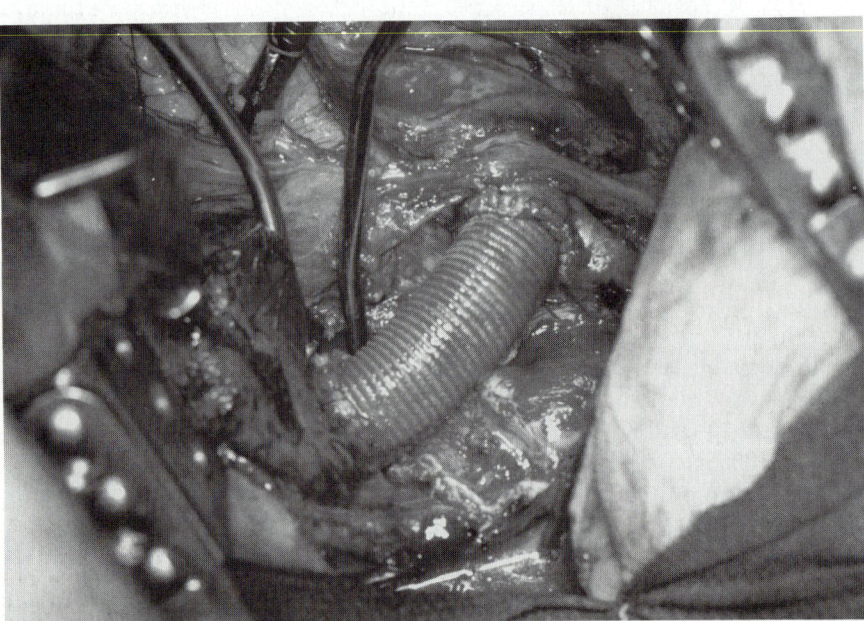

Figure 137–4. A. Intraoperative photograph of proximal descending thoracic aortic aneurysm. **B.** Replacement with woven Dacron graft. *(Continued.)*

B

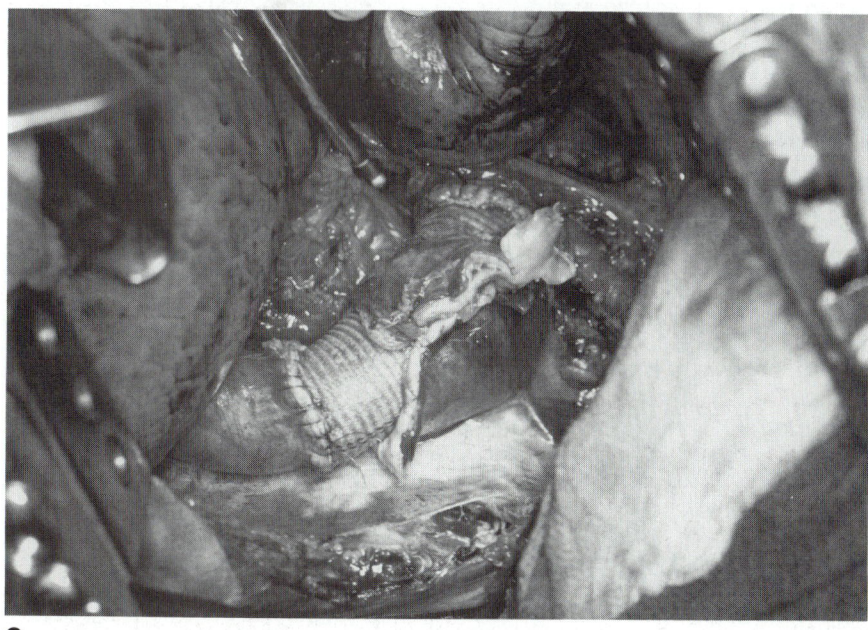

Figure 137–4. *(Continued.)* **C.** Closure of the aneurysm sac over the graft.

scending aorta is completed. Antegrade CPB perfusion is established by inserting the cannula into the arch graft after reimplantation of the great vessels to prevent possible kinking of the elephant trunk graft due to retrograde flow. The proximal aortic anastomosis is then performed. The length of the graft inserted into the descending aorta should not be excessively long (especially in cases of chronic aortic dissection). At the second stage for the replacement of the descending aorta in a patient who previously underwent aortic arch grafting with the elephant trunk technique, the proximal descending aorta need not be isolated. After exsanguinating the patient into the CPB reservoir and incising the aneurysm, the free end of the elephant trunk is identified and quickly clamped; the blood volume is then returned to the patient. The elephant trunk graft is anastomosed to another segment of graft or the distal aorta.

Results

Expected operative mortality risk for all patients (emergency or elective cases) undergoing resection of descending thoracic aortic aneurysms should be less than 20%, with an average operative mortality rate of 11%[8,10,11,12,14,20–30] (Table 137–1 to 137–4). The operative mortality rate for emergency procedures (16 to 67%) is up to sevenfold higher than that for elective procedures (5 to 12%)[8,12,14,21]

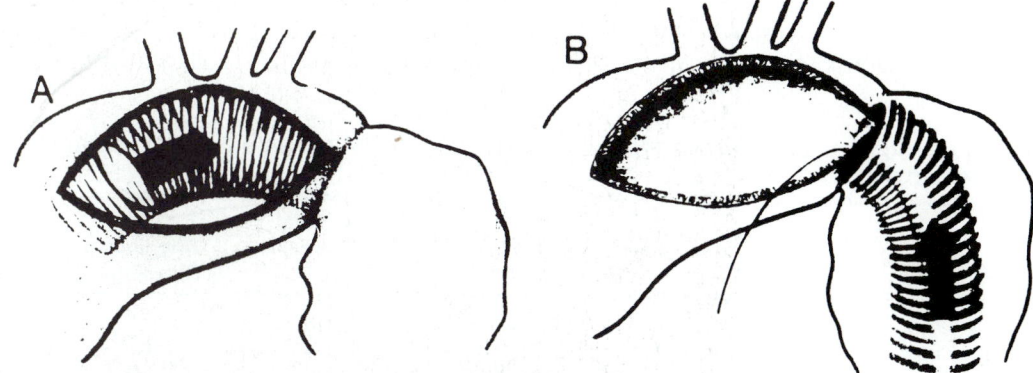

Figure 137–5. Two variations of the elephant trunk technique used in conjunction with total arch replacement. **A.** The trunk has been invaginated into the arch portion of the graft and will be pushed out distally after the distal arch anastomosis and before arch vessel reimplantation to the graft. **B.** The arch graft has been invaginated into the trunk. After performing the anastomosis between the origin of the descending aorta and the invaginating fold, the arch portion of the graft is pulled proximally using the stay suture. *(From Borst HG, Laas J: Surgical treatment of thoracic aortic aneurysms. In Karp RB, Laks H, Wechsler AS (eds): Advances in Cardiac Surgery, Vol. 4. St. Louis, Mosby Year Book, 1993, pp 47–87, reproduced with permission.)*

TABLE 137–1. EARLY OUTCOME OF DESCENDING THORACIC AORTIC ANEURYSM REPAIR USING NO DISTAL CIRCULATORY SUPPORT[a]

Author	Ref	Year	N	OM (%)	Emergency (%)	Paraplegia (%)	Severe Renal Dysfunction/Failure (%)	Significant Bleeding (%)	Pulmonary Insufficiency (%)
DeBakey	(11)	1978	117	9	NR	3	NR	NR	3
Najafi	(23)	1980	18	0	28	0	11	0	17
Crawford	(24)	1981	112	9	NR	1	3	NR	NR
Culliford	(22)	1983	11	18	NR	18	0	0	0
Carlson	(25)	1983	10	NR	NR	10	20	10	NR
Livesay	(12)	1985	263	11	8	7	5	6	NR
Hamerlijnck	(14)	1989	52	12	21	4	15	12	12
Cooley[b]	(26)	1992	31	13	NR	13	26	NR	NR
Cooley[c]	(26)	1992	24	17	NR	4	0	NR	NR
von Segesser	(27)	1993	42	19	NR	9	14	10	NR

[a]All series include a combined patient population of atherosclerotic aneurysms, aortic dissections, and post-traumatic aneurysms. OM, operative mortality; NR, not reported.
[b]Closed distal anastomosis.
[c]Open distal anastomosis.

(Table 137–4). Similarly, the risk of paraplegia and renal dysfunction is substantially higher for emergency cases compared to elective resections (Table 137–4).

The cause of death for patients undergoing descending thoracic aortic aneurysm graft replacement included preoperative aneurysm rupture, low cardiac output, renal failure, pulmonary insufficiency, myocardial infarction, postoperative hemorrhage, pulmonary embolism, and sepsis.[8,11,22] In the Stanford experience, emergency operation and congestive heart failure were independent risk factors portending a higher likelihood of operative death.[8] Patients with congestive heart failure had a 60% operative mortality risk compared to 14% for those without congestive heart failure.[8] Factors that did not correlate significantly with hospital mortality included age, hypertension, chronic lung disease, previous myocardial infarction, angina, etiology of aneurysm, and aneurysm location.[8]

In addition to emergency operation, Livesay et al found advanced age (older than 70 years) and atherosclerotic etiology to be significant risk factors for early mortal-

ity and morbidity.[12] Bleeding complications were more frequent in emergency operations, cases where the cross-clamp time exceeds 30 min, and in patients with more extensive aneurysms.[12] Operative risk appeared not to be influenced by the method of adjunctive distal perfusion (simple aortic cross-clamping, temporary shunt, or partial CPB), but was more influenced by patient-related and disease-related variables, such as the nature and extent of the aneurysm.[12]

In the Stanford experience, the actuarial survival estimates for discharged patients were 70 and 49% at 5 and 10 years, respectively[8] (Fig. 137–6). In other series, overall actuarial survival was 85% at 1 year, 79% at 5 years, 40% at 10 years, and 25% at 20 years depending on whether the aneurysm resection was performed electively.[10,11,14,29] Hypertension and preoperative congestive heart failure were independent predictors of late mortality in our experience.[8] Causes of late death included cardiovascular and cerebrovascular events in 41 to 59% of cases and ruptures of another aortic aneurysm in another 20 to 25% of cases.[8,11]

TABLE 137–2. EARLY OUTCOME OF DESCENDING THORACIC AORTIC ANEURYSM REPAIR USING A TEMPORARY PASSIVE SHUNT (E.G., GOTT TDMAC SHUNT)[a]

Author	Ref	Year	N	OM (%)	Emergency (%)	Paraplegia (%)	Severe Renal Dysfunction/Failure (%)	Significant Bleeding (%)	Pulmonary Insufficiency (%)
Lawrence	(28)	1977	23	13	NR	4	NR	4	NR
Hilgenberg	(29)	1981	12	8	42	0	NR	NR	NR
Culliford	(22)	1983	30	20	NR	0	0	0	7
Carlson	(25)	1983	56	NR	NR	2	4	6	NR
Livesay	(12)	1985	22	9	0	9	9	18	NR
Verdant	(21)	1992	267	15	4	0	0.4	4	6

[a]All series include a combined patient population of atherosclerotic aneurysms, aortic dissections, and post-traumatic aneurysms. OM, operative mortality; NR, not reported.

TABLE 137–3. EARLY OUTCOME OF DESCENDING THORACIC AORTIC ANEURYSM REPAIR USING ACTIVE PARTIAL CARDIOPULMONARY BYPASS[a]

Author	Ref	Year	N	OM (%)	Emergency (%)	Paraplegia (%)	Severe Renal Dysfunction/Failure (%)	Significant Bleeding (%)	Pulmonary Insufficiency (%)
Hilgenberg	(29)	1981	23	9	48	0	NR	NR	NR
Culliford	(22)	1983	7	0	NR	0	0	14	0
Carlson	(25)	1983	19	NR	NR	5	0	5	NR
Moreno-Cabral	(8)	1984	51	18	16	2	14	10	16
Livesay	(12)	1985	75	16	13	7	7	12	NR
Najafi	(30)	1993	37	3	8	0	0	5	8
von Segessor[b]	(27)	1993	49	10	NR	9	8	2	NR
Borst	(20)	1994	132	3	NR	2	2	NR	NR

[a]All series (except reference 8) include a combined patient population of atherosclerotic aneurysms, aortic dissections, and post-traumatic aneurysms except one; reference 8 includes only descending thoracic aortic aneurysms. Partial cardiopulmonary bypass is defined as pulmonary artery–femoral (or iliac), femoral–femoral, iliac–iliac, left atrial–femoral, or left atrial–aortic cardiopulmonary bypass. OM, operative mortality; NR, not reported.
[b]Heparin-coated circuit with low systemic heparin dose.

MAJOR SURGICAL COMPLICATIONS

Numerous methods have been attempted to minimize the deleterious effects of aortic cross-clamping during repair of descending thoracic aortic aneurysms. Notwithstanding improved surgical techniques, the major operative complications include paraplegia and renal insufficiency due to hypoperfusion of the anterior spinal cord tracts and kidneys and acute left ventricular strain due to proximal hypertension.[14,22,23] To improve patient outcome, proper emphasis has been placed on elective operation prior to rupture, preservation of spinal cord perfusion when feasible, expeditious operation, and prevention of hemorrhage and hypotension. Although distal circulatory support, including extracorporeal circulation or temporary extravascular shunting, is useful in providing cardiac decompression and reducing distal ischemic injury, it does not necessarily eliminate the risk of paraplegia or renal insufficiency.[12,23,31] The aneurysm may involve critical intercostal arteries, which are supplying the distal anterior spinal artery; therefore, no method of adjunctive perfusion can provide circulation during cross-clamping and graft placement. When these arteries cannot be successfully reimplanted within a short period of time, the period of ischemia may be minimized by sequential clamping (when it is feasible) and adjunctive distal CPB perfusion.[20]

Paraplegia

The incidence of paraplegia in patients undergoing descending thoracic aortic aneurysm repair ranges from zero to 18%, with an average rate of 4%[8,11,12,14,20–30] (Tables 137–1 to 137–3). Although attractive in theory, the use of distal circulatory support has not been demonstrated rigorously to reduce the risk of postoperative paraplegia.[12,23,31,36]

Anatomically, the blood supply to the spinal cord in humans is segmental and variable.[12,22,32] The majority of the 62 radicular arteries in the embryo regress to 6 to 8 arteries that supply the anterior spinal trunk and 10 to 23 arteries for the posterior spinal trunk in adults. The anterior spinal artery provides 75% of the perfusion to the spinal cord and is narrowest in its mid-dorsal region. The main arterial supply to the dorsal lumbosacral or lower spinal cord is derived from the artery described by Adamkiewicz, which usually arises from a left-sided intercostal or lumbar artery in 80% of individuals. In 85% of humans, it reaches

TABLE 137–4. COMPARISON OF OPERATIVE MORTALITY, PARAPLEGIA, AND RENAL FAILURE DEPENDING OF ELECTIVE VS EMERGENT PROCEDURES[a]

Author	Ref	Year	Operative Mortality Elective n	Elective (%)	Emergent n	Emergent (%)	Paraplegia Elective (%)	Paraplegia Emergent (%)	Renal Failure Elective (%)	Renal Failure Emergent (%)
Moreno-Cabral	(8)	1984	43	12	8	50	0	13	NR	NR
Livesay	(12)	1985	330	10	30	27	6	17	5	13
Hamerlijnck	(14)	1989	41	5	11	37	NR	NR	NR	NR
Verdant	(21)	1992	225	12	12	67	NR	NR	NR	NR

[a]All series (except reference 8) include a combined patient population of atherosclerotic aneurysms, aortic dissections, and post-traumatic aneurysms except one; reference 8 includes only descending thoracic aortic aneurysms. OM, operative mortality; NR, not reported.

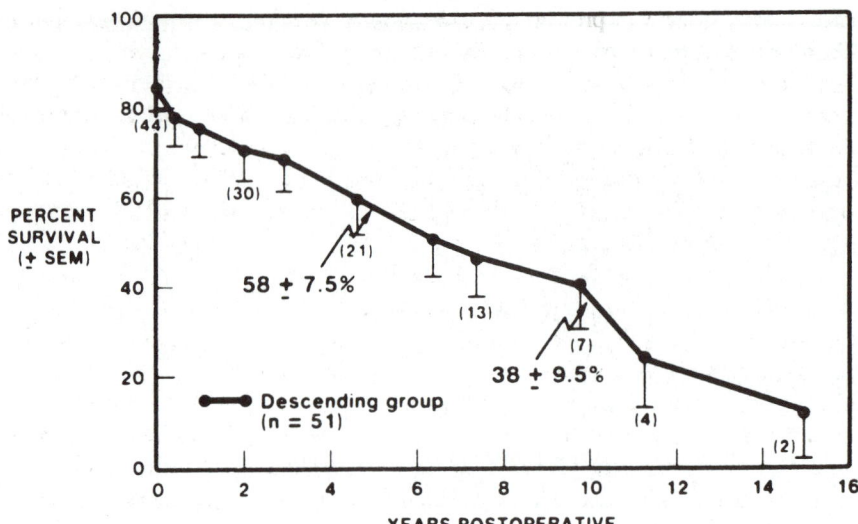

Figure 137–6. Actuarial survival for patients who underwent repair of descending thoracic aortic aneurysm. *(Modified from Moreno-Cabral CE, Miller DC, Mitchell RS, et al: Degenerative and atherosclerotic aneurysms of the thoracic aorta. J Thorac Cardiovasc Surg 88:1020–1032, 1984, reproduced with permission.)*

the cord accompanying a nerve root between T9 and L2 (75% are between T9 and T12 and 10% between L1 and L2). In the remaining 15% of individuals, it arises between T5 and T8. When the origin of the artery of Adamkiewicz is high (T5–T8), arterial perfusion to the distal anterior spinal artery is supplemented by a vessel that arises in the lower part of the lumbar region. If the artery of Adamkiewicz is compromised, blood supply to the dorsal lumbar region of the cord is derived from an anastomotic arch to the conus and the anterior and posterior lumbosacral radicular arteries.

Factors contributing to postoperative paraparesis or paraplegia include the degree of spinal cord ischemia during the aortic cross-clamp period (which is dependent on the extent of aneurysmal disease, available collateral channels, cross-clamp time, and possibly failure to maintain adequate distal CPB perfusion) and permanent exclusion of critical intercostal arteries during aortic graft replacement.[33–35] The influence of cross-clamp time on the risk of paraplegia in man remains controversial, but there appears to be a marked increase in the incidence of paraplegia when the aortic cross-clamp time exceeds 30 min without active distal CPB perfusion.[12,22,36,37] Reimplantation of the intercostal arteries around the level of the diaphragm, however, has not eliminated the risk of spinal cord injury; nonetheless, reimplantation of patent intercostal arteries between T8 and L1 should be considered in most distal descending aortic repairs. In chronic thoracic aortic aneurysms, the intercostal arteries are usually not patent within the diseased segment due to the laminated thrombus, and distal cord perfusion is already largely dependent on collateral channels. Thus, pre-existent collateral circulation may lessen the risk of paraplegia since arterial perfusion of the caudad spinal cord does not rely on intercostal arteries arising within the resected aneurysmal segment. In aneurysms limited to the proximal descending thoracic aorta, the risk of paraplegia as a result of oversewing intercostal arteries is negligible.[14]

In acute processes such as traumatic aortic disruption, however, spinal cord collateral arterial circulation may not be adequate; therefore, aortic cross-clamping and graft replacement can directly compromise spinal cord perfusion.

The concept of spinal cord perfusion pressure [perfusion pressure = mean distal aortic pressure – mean cerebral spinal fluid (CSF) pressure] is useful in understanding the pathophysiology of spinal cord ischemia.[12,31,34] Sustained hypotension in the lower body may lower spinal cord perfusion pressure during the aortic cross-clamp period and increase the risk of neurologic complications; a concomitant rise in CSF pressure may further impair spinal cord circulation. Without distal circulatory support, significant amounts of vasodilators are required during the aortic cross-clamping interval to control proximal blood pressure; however, this maneuver may actually decrease collateral bloodflow and thereby potentially harm the spinal cord. Pre-, post-, and intraoperative CSF drainage may confer some protection against spinal cord ischemia during descending thoracic aortic repair.[26,38,39] Experimentally, CSF pressure rises immediately after aortic cross-clamping and then subsequently declines, even though proximal systemic arterial pressure remains elevated. A reduction in CSF pressure by spinal fluid drainage via a lumbar subarachnoid drain can help maintain a sufficient perfusion gradient between the local spinal arterial and venous pressures and thus maintain some cord bloodflow.

Laschinger, Cunningham and others have suggested use of intraoperative measurement of somatosensory evoked potentials (SEP) to alert the surgeon to a problem with distal spinal cord perfusion.[34,35,40–42] Interruption of normal SEP signals is indicative of inadequate perfusion or exclusion of a critical spinal artery and corrective measures (e.g., increasing distal circulation using CPB or shunting, or intercostal artery reimplantation) can be attempted to try to reverse these changes. This strategy assumes that the spinal artery at risk can be identified correctly and revascularized successfully in time to prevent anterior spinal cord injury. Crawford et al, however, showed that measuring SEP was associated with a 13% false-negative rate and 67% false-positive rate and that this method has no significant impact on the prevention of neurologic deficits in the highest risk patients (e.g., Crawford extent II, chronic dissection etiology) undergoing repair of thoracoabdominal and descending thoracic aortic aneurysms.[43]

Although it is possible to demonstrate the anatomy of the anterior spinal cord arterial circulation using selective intercostal angiography, this procedure per se carries a small risk of neurologic deficits and paraplegia. Svensson et al have developed a technique of intraoperative localization of segmental spinal cord blood supply using a hydrogen-induced current impulse.[33] Experimentally, preservation of arteries thus localized substantially reduced the rate of paraplegia.[33] This technique has been used in patients to identify arteries at risk and guide expeditious reimplantation of such critical arteries; however, clinical experience is limited and these results should be considered preliminary.

Delayed paraparesis and paraplegia can occur 24 to 48 hours after resection of descending thoracic aortic aneurysms in patients who are initially neurologically intact postoperatively.[33,37] This phenomenon is probably the result of late thrombosis of arterial collaterals due to low flow states or compromise of marginal collateral circulation. Other possible etiologic factors include cord edema, reperfusion injury, and arterial spasm. Intensive postoperative monitoring is thus necessary to avoid hypotensive episodes, which can reduce collateral cord bloodflow especially when critical segmental arteries have been sacrificed. If a postoperative spinal cord deficit occurs, immediate treatment with CSF drainage and intravenous naloxone infusion should be initiated.[44]

Renal Insufficiency

The incidence of temporary renal failure in patients undergoing descending thoracic aortic aneurysm resection varies from zero to 26%, with a mean incidence of 5%[8,12,14,20–27,30](Tables 137–1 to 137–3).

Distal circulatory support probably reduces the risk of renal dysfunction, although this remains debated.[12,25,31,45] Laboratory studies in dogs have demonstrated that maintenance of a distal aortic pressure above 70 mm Hg and a bypass flow rate of at least 20 mL/kg per minute is necessary to preserve renal cortical bloodflow during aortic cross-clamping.[46] Conversely, others have shown postoperative impairment of renal function even if distal adjunctive CPB support was employed.[12,14,45] Experimentally, Roberts et al demonstrated a marked decrease in urine output, glomerular filtration rate, and renal plasma flow within 1 hour of aortic cross-clamping with or without distal perfusion adjuncts (bypass or shunt).[45] One hour after release of the aortic cross-clamp, renal function returned to approximately 90% of baseline levels in both groups.[45] Cartier et al showed that

postoperative renal function did not decline significantly when active circulatory support was used during aortic cross-clamping, but serum creatinine rose transiently in patients without circulatory support.[31]

Important clinical risk factors portending postoperative renal failure include advanced age, atherosclerotic etiology, emergency operation, and preoperative renal dysfunction.[12,47] Intraoperative hypotension may also be a possible risk factor for postoperative renal dysfunction, although this is controversial.[14,25] The duration of aortic cross-clamp time (range of 15 to 60 min) appears to have no demonstrable effect on the incidence of renal failure.[12] Although not conclusively proven, the use of partial CPB may be a prudent method to optimize renal perfusion during these procedures on the descending thoracic aorta, particularly in elderly patients with preexistent renal dysfunction.[25]

Left Ventricular Systolic Dysfunction

Aortic cross-clamping and the attendant proximal systemic hypertension can lead to left ventricular (LV) distension and/or failure, as reflected by decreased cardiac output and elevated LV filling pressure.[48,49] The increase in proximal systolic blood pressure is sustained with simple aortic cross-clamping and transient with temporary shunts, while there is no increase in systolic blood pressure using partial CPB.[31] Upon cross-clamp release, LV filling pressure decreases rapidly in patients without distal circulatory support.[31] Although the hemodynamic fluctuations associated with aortic cross-clamping can be mitigated by adjunctive CPB support, cardiac output and LV stroke work remain below baseline levels even with distal perfusion.[48] The LV dilatation during aortic cross-clamping is associated with a marked increase in LV wall stress, which may lead to compromised subendocardial myocardial perfusion. Decompression of the proximal aorta using distal CPB support may improve cardiac function by eliminating the augmented myocardial oxygen requirements and increasing subendocardial LV perfusion.[48] If Gott shunts are used, proximal aortic cannulation provides better LV decompression and maintains higher distal flow compared to ventricular cannulation in experimental models.[31]

Different Approaches to Distal Perfusion

Some surgeons have reported that descending thoracic aortic aneurysms can be replaced safely by simply cross-clamping the aorta without distal circulatory support, thereby expediting the operation and eliminating the potential complications of bypass and heparinization.[11,23,24,36] Adequate hemodynamic monitoring, blood pressure control using pharmacologic agents, and appropriate fluid management are critical. Clamping the left subclavian artery does not appear to increase the risk of paraplegia.[24]

In contrast to the conventional two-clamp technique

during thoracic aortic aneurysm repair, Cooley et al have utilized a method incorporating partial exsanguination and an "open" distal aortic anastomosis; they argue that maintaining distal aortic flow or pressure is unnecessary.[26,50] Short aortic clamp times have been the factor that consistently was related to lower mortality and morbidity rates in their experience; the average distal ischemic time was lower with an open distal anastomosis compared to a closed (or clamped) anastomosis (26 vs. 31 min, respectively). In Cooley's experience, renal insufficiency and spinal cord complications occurred slightly less frequently with the open technique. Favorable results with the use of an open distal anastomosis (which effectively lowers the abdominal aortic pressure to zero) underscores the poor correlation between distal aortic pressure and spinal cord bloodflow.[26,50]

Because of the complexities of extracorporeal circulation, the tridodecylmethylammonium chloride (TDMAC)-heparin bonded shunt developed by Gott has been employed as a means of temporary distal perfusion without requiring systemic heparinization.[12,21–23,51] In addition to descending thoracic aortic aneurysms, the Gott shunt has been used for traumatic injuries to the aorta and the great vessels, aortic coarctation, and stenotic and aneurysmal lesions of the great vessels. Inadequate distal perfusion can occur if shunts less than 9 mm in diameter are used.[12] The Gott shunt should be inserted in the ascending aorta if the aneurysm involves the transverse aortic arch. Advantages of shunts include avoiding systemic anticoagulation, lessening proximal hypertension during cross-clamping, and providing some degree of distal perfusion without an interposed extracorporeal CPB circuit.[12,51] Reported complications of temporary shunts include shunt dislodgement, bleeding from cannulation sites, and embolic stroke.[12]

Some surgeons have advocated the routine use of pulmonary artery–femoral or femoral–femoral partial CPB with an oxygenator for distal circulatory support.[8,30] The advantage of partial CPB includes ease in maintaining hemodynamic stability and adequate, controlled distal arterial perfusion thereby lessening systemic acidosis. In addition, partial CPB provides supplementary oxygenation, decreases reliance on vasoactive agents, facilitates rapid volume resuscitation after the reconstruction, and assists in patient rewarming.[30,31] Disadvantages include the extra time, added complexity, and need for systemic heparinization (300 U/kg). Reported complications of partial CPB include pulmonary problems, technical difficulty with the circuit and/or the pump, air embolism, and femoral arterial injury.[11] Systemic heparinization has not been linked to increased bleeding in some series, whereas it has in others.[12,30] The benefits of partial CPB in patients with chronic descending thoracic aneurysms have been debated extensively; however, in acute traumatic disruptions, provided there is no neurologic injury, it should be strongly considered to optimize distal spinal, visceral, and renal perfusion during the aortic repair.

Circulatory support with a centrifugal (Bio-Medicus,

Medtronic, Minneapolis, MN) pump may offer additional advantages compared to passive temporary shunts and partial CPB techniques.[27,31] Left atrial–femoral or left atrial–aortic bypass can be performed with newer heparin-coated circuits (Carmeda, Medtronic, Minneapolis, MN) with no or minimal systemic heparinization without major bleeding complications. Compared to patients supported with a Gott shunt, cardiac output decreases less, LV decompression is more reliable, and better control of distal aortic flow is obtained in those supported with left atrial–femoral bypass.[27,31]

Total cardiopulmonary bypass with profound hypothermia circulatory arrest (PHCA) has been used for spinal cord protection in patients at high risk of paraplegia (Crawford extent II thoracoabdominal aortic aneurysms due to chronic aortic dissection and certain extensive descending thoracic aortic aneurysms) with encouraging early results.[34,52] Nonetheless, paraparesis and paraplegia can occur despite PHCA protection of the spinal cord pointing to the cardinal importance of the vascular anatomy in the development of spinal cord ischemic injury. The mechanism by which hypothermia exerts a protective effect on spinal cord function is not well characterized; recent investigations have implicated the role of excitatory amino acids in the extracellular space in irreversible neuronal damage following central nervous system (CNS) ischemia.[53,54] Dextrophan, a noncompetitive N-methyl-D-aspartate (NMDA) receptor antagonist, has been shown to be protective against nervous system damage following focal ischemia, perhaps from decreasing the release of excitatory amino acids in the ischemic spinal cord.[53] Specifically, the brain regions most vulnerable to injury during prolonged PHCA have the highest density of glutamate receptors. Using dizocilpine, a selective NMDA-glutamate receptor antagonist, Redmond et al have shown the importance of glutamate excitotoxicity in the development of brain injury during PHCA.[54] Thus, selective glutamate receptor antagonists may be neuroprotective during prolonged periods of PHCA.[54]

General Recommendation

In a favorable situation, such as a proximal atherosclerotic descending thoracic aneurysm with thrombosed intercostal arteries, it is possible to insert an interposition graft in well under 30 min of aortic cross-clamping.[22,30] In these selected cases, simple aortic cross-clamping without distal circulatory perfusion may be sufficient with intensive hemodynamic monitoring and the use of vasoactive agents to avoid excessive proximal hypertension and left ventricular strain. On the other hand, descending thoracic aortic aneurysms are frequently extensive, not all intercostal arteries in the diseased segment are thrombosed, and the aortic cross-clamp time often exceeds 30 min. These patients are usually in their seventh or eighth decades of life and are likely to have some degree of coronary artery disease. Thus, in these more challenging patients, active distal circulatory support should be included in the operative plan. The choice between a passive bypass conduit (such as a Gott shunt) or partial CPB (LA–femoral or pulmonary artery–femoral perfusion) depends largely on the surgeon's familiarity with any given technique.

EARLY EXPERIENCE WITH ENDOVASCULAR STENT-GRAFTS

Endovascular catheter stent-graft techniques have been employed recently to treat patients with descending thoracic aortic pathology, including aneurysmal disease[55,56] (Fig. 137–7). The self-expanding stent-graft is composed of a stainless steel frame ("Z"-stents) covered by a commercially available woven Dacron graft (Cooley Verisoft, Meadox Medicals, Oakland, NJ) with the crimp ironed out. The

stent-graft is introduced through a 24 Fr sheath placed via a femoral or iliac arteriotomy or distal abdominal aortotomy (using a retroperitoneal approach).

The present Stanford University experience spans only 25 mo (July 1992 to August 1994) and includes over 30 patients with descending thoracic aortic pathology who have been treated with endovascular stent/graft methods. The majority had atherosclerotic or degenerative aneurysms, a few had acute or chronic aortic dissections, one had a chronic post-traumatic aneurysm, one had a postoperative false aneurysm (previous patch coarctation repair), and one had a recurrent aortobronchial fistula. The majority of patients were approached using a femoral arteriotomy (native femoral artery or old aortofemoral bypass graft), but several required an infrarenal abdominal aortotomy or attachment of a 10-mm side limb to an infrarenal aortic graft. CT and angiographic follow-up have been obtained in all patients.

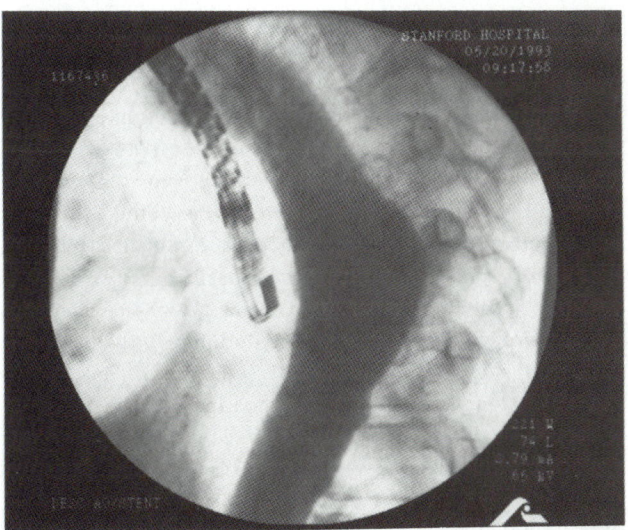

A

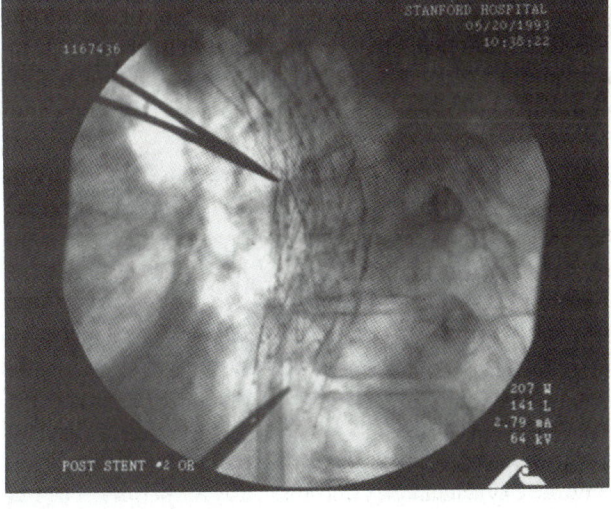

B

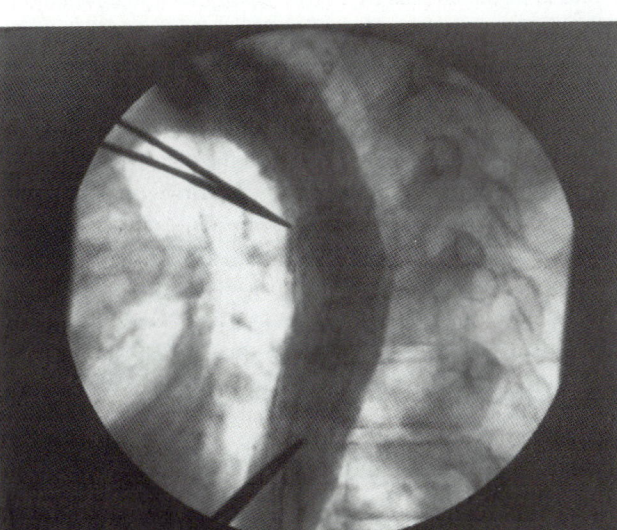

C

Figure 137–7. Fluoroscopic demonstration of deployment of stent-graft in the repair of descending thoracic aortic aneurysms. **A.** Intraoperative angiography is obtained outlining the aneurysm. **B.** The aneurysm is externally marked using hemostats. The stent-graft is positioned in the descending thoracic aorta via a femoral arteriotomy. **C.** Follow-up angiogram demonstrates full expansion of the stent-graft and exclusion of the aneurysm.

The mean follow-up period remains short (range 1 to 25 mo). Most patients had complete exclusion of the diseased native aortic segment following initial placement of the stent-graft, but some patients required a second endovascular stent-graft extension proximally or distally to complete stent-grafting of extensive aortic pathology. One patient had only partial thrombosis of the aneurysm after 9 mo of follow-up. There were three device misplacements: One patient with proximal descending thoracic aortic aneurysm near the origin of the left subclavian artery required a left subclavian–carotid transposition for left upper extremity ischemia 4 days after the initial stent-graft procedure. Two late hospital deaths occurred in elderly patients due to multisystem failure, which were not directly related to the endovascular stent-grafting. A major complication occurred in a 66-year-old woman who developed paraparesis, cardiogenic shock, and renal failure; a minor residual neurologic deficit remained after several months of follow-up. Minor complications included pleuritic chest pain and/or left pleural effusions. This preliminary experience suggests that stent-graft placement may offer a promising alternative treatment in highly selected patients, assuming that further follow-up confirms that this method is efficacious over the long-term.

SUMMARY

Thoracic aortic aneurysms are a relatively common disorder with an estimated incidence of 5.9 cases per 100,000 person-years. These patients are usually older and have other coexistent medical and cardiovascular illnesses. The natural history of untreated thoracic aortic aneurysms is progressive expansion and eventual aneurysm rupture. Mean survival of untreated patients is less than 3 years, with rupture being the cause of death in nearly one-half of cases. Of those who sustain aneurysm rupture, over 90% die. The majority of thoracic aortic aneurysms are chronic. Approximately 90% of cases of descending thoracic aortic aneurysms are atherosclerotic in origin. Less frequently, patients may have mycotic or traumatic aneurysms, postoperative false aneurysms, or associated heritable or congenital aortic anomalies. At the time of diagnosis, often by routine chest radiograph, up to 50% of patients are asymptomatic. If present, symptoms may include chest pain or be the result of compression or erosion of adjacent structures. Aortography is an important preoperative investigation to delineate the location and extent of the aneurysm, assess critical side branches, and aid in operative planning. Additional useful diagnostic studies, such as CT or MRI scans, document the pathoanatomic features of the aneurysm and provide an accurate and reproducible measurement of the aneurysm size. Surgical intervention should be considered in most cases, taking into account the patient's age and overall medical status. Current recommendations for operation include all symptomatic patients, individuals with an aneurysm diameter twice the size of a normal contiguous aortic segment or

greater than 6 cm, and those with documented aneurysm enlargement. Patients with smaller aneurysms can be followed with serial CT or MRI scans. The expected operative mortality risk for all patients undergoing resection of descending thoracic aortic aneurysms is around 11%. In the Stanford experience, the actuarial survival rates for discharged patients were 70 and 49% at 5 and 10 years, respectively. Major surgical complications include paraplegia and renal insufficiency and acute LV decompensation due to excessive proximal hypertension. To improve outcome, recent emphasis has properly been placed on elective operation prior to rupture, preservation of spinal cord perfusion, expeditious operation, and prevention of hemorrhage and hypotension. Although distal circulatory support, including partial CPB or shunts, is useful in providing proximal decompression and reducing distal ischemic injury, it does not necessarily eliminate the risk of paraplegia or renal failure. Approaches to descending thoracic aortic aneurysms include simple aortic cross-clamping without distal perfusion, passive shunting with a Gott shunt, pulmonary artery–femoral or femoral–femoral partial CPB, left atrial–femoral CPB with heparin-coated circuits and minimal heparinization, and total CPB with hypothermic circulatory arrest. Because of the challenging nature of these patients, active distal circulatory support should be included in the operative plan when feasible. Endovascular stent-graft techniques have been developed recently to treat patients with descending thoracic aortic aneurysms; the early Stanford experience suggests that stent-graft placement offers a promising therapeutic alternative in some highly selected patients.

ACUTE TRAUMATIC AORTIC DISRUPTION

Approximately one among every 6 to 10 fatal accident victims sustains rupture of the descending thoracic aorta.[57–59] Death is instantaneous in 80 to 90% of cases; the remaining 10 to 20% of victims survive temporarily because the rupture is contained by the aortic adventitia, the pleura, and the surrounding mediastinal tissue.[57,58,60,61] In a review by Parmley et al of 275 cases of traumatic aortic rupture due to nonpenetrating injury, 14% survived more than 30 min after the acute injury. Of these survivors, 21% died within 6 hours, 32% died by 24 hours, 61% by 8 days, and 84% within four mos.[60] In a recent analysis of aortic injury due to vehicular trauma, Williams et al noted that 94% of patients died within 1 hour of injury, and an additional 5% died between 1 and 24 hours later; thus, 99% of the victims died within the first 24 hours.[59] Aortic rupture generally results from abnormal stresses at points of aortic fixation caused by horizontal or vertical deceleration of different aortic segments. Sixty-five to 80% of all traumatic aortic tears occur at the aortic isthmus, the region of greatest stress.[57,59] The incidence of isthmus traumatic rupture is much more frequent in clinical series than that reported in autopsy series;[60,62] conversely, the incidence of multiple sites of aortic rupture is much higher in the autopsy series (8 to 13 vs. 1%) since these other rupture sites are almost universally fatal.[59,60,62] Other regions of aortic involvement include the ascending aorta or aortic arch (14%), the mid- and distal descending thoracic aorta (12%), and, rarely, the abdominal aorta (9%).[57,59,60] The mechanism of injury in mid-descending aortic ruptures usually involves direct aortic trauma, such as in spine injuries.[62]

Diagnosis of Acute Traumatic Aortic Tear

It is imperative that the diagnosis of acute traumatic aortic tear be established expeditiously and definitive surgical repair performed early. A high index of suspicion for thoracic aortic injury should be present in patients who sustain a high-speed deceleration injury, whether or not there is external evidence of blunt chest trauma.[57,58,60,62] In fact, up to one-half of patients have no evidence of external thoracic injury at the time of initial examination.[57] If a complaint is expressed (assuming the patient is conscious and oriented), the most common symptom is retrosternal or interscapular pain. Important clinical findings, although rarely present, include the acute onset of upper extremity hypertension associated with ongoing blood loss, difference in pulse amplitude between the upper and lower extremities, and the presence of a harsh systolic murmur over the precordium or the posterior triangle of ascultation.[57]

A chest radiograph may be normal or reveal only subtle findings (e.g., widened mediastinum, apical cap, depressed left mainstem bronchus, obscured aortic knob or aortopulmonary space, multiple rib fractures, tracheal deviation, or left pleural effusion) that require further investigation with transesophageal echocardiography (TEE), CT, or biplane aortography[57-60] (Fig. 137–8). The presence of a thoracic vertebral fracture should increase the suspicion for a possible descending thoracic aortic tear.[62] Of all aortograms obtained in patients with a suspected traumatic injury, only 10 to 20% are positive.[58] Characteristically, the aortogram demonstrates the presence of a pseudoaneurysm at or near the ligamentum arteriosum.[57] False-positive aortograms that lead to unnecessary surgery can occur in 1% of cases; the angiographic appearance of a ductus diverticulum or an ulcerated plaque may be misinterpreted as a traumatic pseudoaneurysm.[57,63]

CT, which has been advocated as a screening diagnostic modality, may not provide an adequate degree of sensitivity (i.e., excessive number of false negative examinations) or specificity. Nonetheless, CT has been utilized, especially when aortography is not immediately available (Fig. 137–9). An unsuspected mediastinal hematoma seen on a CT scan warrants aortography provided the patient is hemodynamically stable. Increasing experience with TEE in the assessment of thoracic aortic pathology suggests that this modality can provide a rapid bedside determination of

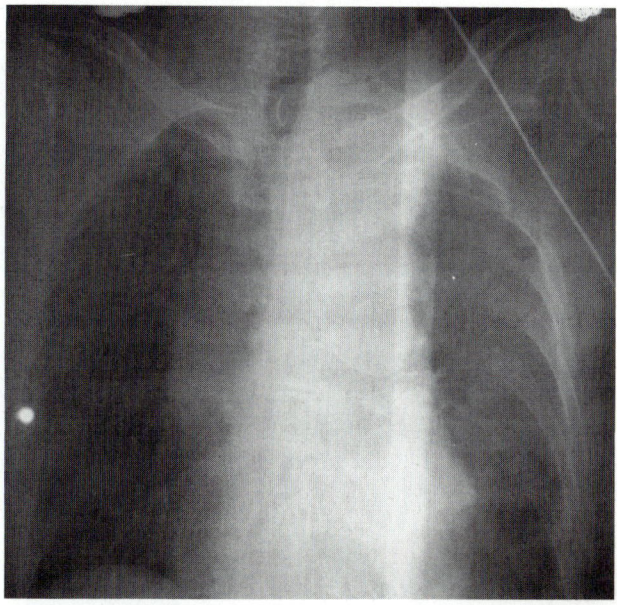

Figure 137–8. Chest radiograph of patient who suffered an acute traumatic aortic disruption at the aortic isthmus after a motor vehicle accident.

acute aortic injury anywhere (e.g., emergency room, ICU, or operating room) and thereby expedite therapy. In our opinion, TEE is the preferred diagnostic screening test of choice today because of its rapidity, ability to be performed anywhere in unstable patients, high sensitivity rates, and acceptable incidence of false-negative results.

Surgical Treatment of Acute Traumatic Aortic Tear

Because of the risk of rupture of the aortic false aneurysm, surgical intervention should be instituted as soon as the diagnosis is made unless other compelling life-threatening problems exist. Except for massive intracranial or intra-abdominal or pelvic injuries, traumatic aortic rupture has the highest therapeutic priority.[57,58] Most acute traumatic tears of the isthmus can be repaired with a short Dacron interposition graft approached through a posterolateral thoracotomy in the fourth interspace; however, those with limited tears not involving the entire thoracic aortic circumference and those with small false aneurysms may be amenable to primary aortic repair without graft interposition. In patients with ascending traumatic aortic ruptures, the approach is a median sternotomy with graft replacement of the ascending aorta or arch. In highly selected cases, such as in patients with severe concomitant injuries, elective delay of operation pending stabilization of the other injuries has been achieved with the utilization of β-blockade and antihypertensive therapy.[64–66]

The incidence of postoperative paraplegia is generally higher in patients with traumatic aortic rupture compared to

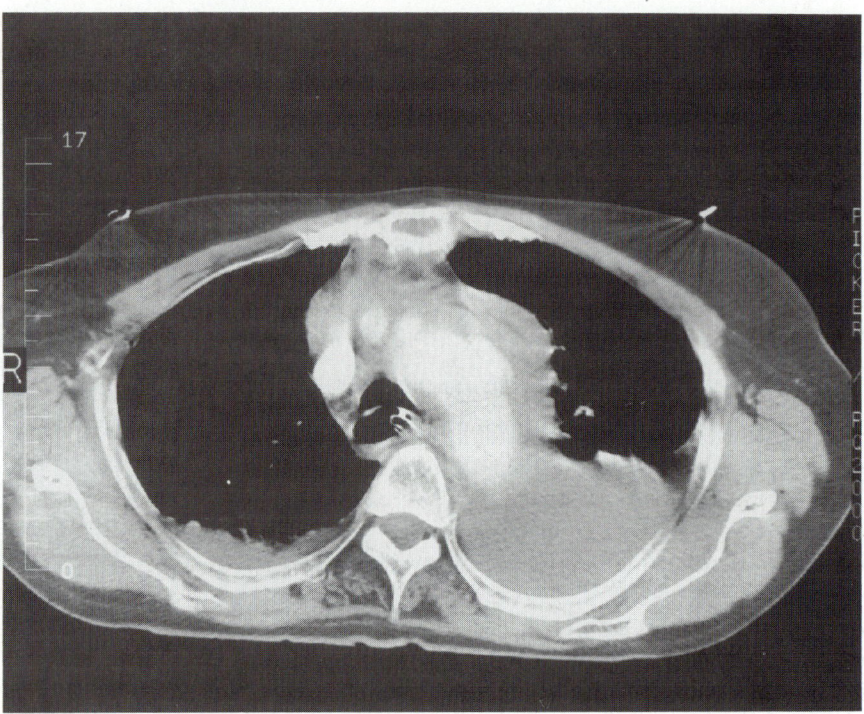

Figure 137–9. Computed tomography of patient with acute rupture of the aortic isthmus.

those with chronic thoracic aortic aneurysms, probably because of inadequate collateral circulation. Because it is impossible to predict preoperatively the length of aortic cross-clamp time necessary (with the average time frequently exceeding 30 min), the most prudent approach is to employ either conventional partial CPB with systemic heparinization or heparinless left atrial–femoral perfusion. Systemic heparinization, however, should not be used in patients with associated closed head or massive pelvic injuries, because of the risk of exacerbating the cerebral injury or inducing exsanguination from the pelvic injuries.

Surgical Results for Acute Traumatic Aortic Tear

The hospital mortality rate for patients with acute traumatic aortic rupture who undergo surgical intervention ranges from 14 to 32%.[57,58,61,64,67,68] Importantly, it should be emphasized that not infrequently patients exsanguinate while undergoing diagnostic tests or awaiting operation; indeed, an in-hospital rupture rate of 12% has been reported.[58,64,67] The operative mortality rate may possibly be higher with active distal CPB perfusion (18%) compared to active distal bypass without heparin (e.g., centrifugal pump and left atrial–femoral CPB) (10%).[68]

The incidence of spinal cord injury has not been shown conclusively to be lower if distal CPB techniques are employed. Merrill et al have reported two cases of paraparesis (for a rate of 5%), yet both patients were supported with a temporary shunt during the aortic repair.[58] On the other hand, Olivier et al noted a 20% rate of paraplegia in patients undergoing operation without any distal circulatory

adjuncts, compared to zero percent in those supported with left atrial–femoral CPB using a Bio-Medicus centrifugal pump.[61] A recent, illustrative meta-analysis of 1492 patients revealed a paraplegia rate of 10%.[68] The paraplegia rate was less with active distal perfusion (1.4 to 2.3%) compared with passive bypass (8.7 to 14.6%) and simple cross-clamping (19%).[68] Gott shunts inserted into the LV apex did not decrease the risk of paraplegia.[68]

The postoperative renal failure rate in this high-risk population with multiple injuries is 27%.[69] The development of renal failure did not correlate with patient age, injury severity score, initial blood pressure, interval between accident and thoracotomy, or total cross-clamp time.[67] The risk of renal failure correlated weakly with simple aortic cross-clamping (without using a shunt or bypass).

In conclusion, the diagnosis of acute traumatic aortic disruption should be suspected in patients who sustain a high-speed deceleration injury, even if external evidence of major chest trauma is absent or the chest radiograph is normal. If the integrity of the aorta is of concern, emergent investigation with TEE, CT, or biplane aortography is mandatory. Typically, the aortogram will demonstrate the presence of a pseudoaneurysm at or near the ligamentum arteriosum. Once the diagnosis is confirmed, definitive surgical repair should be promptly instituted; however, temporary medical stabilization may be considered in highly selected cases. With the exception of severe intracranial or intra-abdominal injury, traumatic aortic rupture has the highest therapeutic priority. Most patients can be treated using a short Dacron interposition graft or a primary aortic repair. The operative mortality rate and the risk of rupture while awaiting the correct diagnosis to be made remain substantial.

REFERENCES

1. Kampmeier RH: Saccular aneurysm of the thoracic aorta: A clinical study of 633 cases. *Ann Intern Med* **12**:624–651, 1938

2. Boyd LJ: A study of four thousand reported cases of aneurysm of the thoracic aorta. *Am J Med Sci* **168**:654–668, 1924

3. Bahnson HT: Definitive treatment of saccular aneurysms of the aorta with excision of sac and aortic suture. *Surg Gynecol Obstet* **96**:383, 1953

4. Hufnagel CA: Permanent intubation of the thoracic aorta. *Surgery* **54**:382, 1947

5. Lam CR, Aram HH: Resection of the descending thoracic aorta for aneurysm: A report of the use of a homograft in a case and an experimental study. *Ann Surg* **134**:743–752, 1951

6. DeBakey ME, Cooley DA: Successful resection of aneurysm of the thoracic aorta and replacement by graft. *JAMA* **152**:673, 1953

7. Bickerstaff LK, Pairolero PC, Hollier LH, et al: Thoracic aortic aneurysms: A population-based study. *Surgery* **92**:1103–1108, 1982

8. Moreno-Cabral CE, Miller DC, Mitchell RS, et al: Degenerative and atherosclerotic aneurysms of the thoracic aorta. *J Thorac Cardiovasc Surg* **88**:1020–1032, 1984

9. Pressler V, McNamara JJ: Thoracic aortic aneurysm: Natural history and treatment. *J Thorac Cardiovasc Surg* **79**:489–498, 1980

10. Pressler V, McNamara JJ: Aneurysm of the thoracic aorta. *J Thorac Cardiovasc Surg* **89**:50–54, 1985

11. DeBakey ME, McCollum CH, Graham JM: Surgical treatment of aneurysms of the descending thoracic aorta. *J Cardiovasc Surg* **19**:571–576, 1978

12. Livesay JJ, Cooley DA, Ventemiglia RA, et al: Surgical experience in descending thoracic aneurysmectomy with and without adjuncts to avoid ischemia. *Ann Thorac Surg* **39**:37–46, 1985

13. McNamara JJ, Pressler VM: Natural history of arteriosclerotic thoracic aortic aneurysms. *Ann Thorac Surg* **26**:468–473, 1978

14. Hamerlijnck RP, Rutsaert RR, DeGeest R, et al: Surgical correction of descending thoracic aortic aneurysms under simple aortic cross-clamping. *J Vasc Surg* **9**:568–573, 1989

15. Cooke JC, Cambria RP: Simultaneous tracheobronchial and esophageal obstruction caused by a descending thoracic aneurysm. *J Vasc Surg* **18**:90–94, 1993

16. Miller DC: Surgical treatment of thoracic aortic aneurysms. In Jamieson SW, Shumway NE (eds): *Rob and Smith's Operative Surgery: Cardiac Surgery*, 4th ed. London, Butterworths, 1986, pp 519–525

17. Borst HG, Frank G, Schaps D: Treatment of extensive aortic aneurysms by a new multiple-stage approach. *J Thorac Cardiovasc Surg* **95**:11–13, 1988

18. Borst HG, Laas J: Surgical treatment of thoracic aortic aneurysms. In Karp RB, Laks H, Wechsler AS (eds): *Advances in Cardiac Surgery*, Vol. 4. St. Louis, Mosby Year Book, 1993, pp 47–87

19. Crawford ES, Coselli JS, Svensson LG, et al: Diffuse aneurysmal disease (chronic aortic dissection, Marfan, and mega aorta syndromes) and multiple aneurysm. *Ann Surg* **211**:521–537, 1990

20. Borst HG, Jurmann M, Buhner B, Laas J: Risk of replacement of descending aorta with a standardized left heart bypass technique. *J Thorac Cardiovasc Surg* **107**:126–133, 1994

21. Verdant A: Descending thoracic aortic aneurysms: Surgical treatment with the Gott shunt. *Can J Surg* **35**:493–496, 1992

22. Culliford AT, Ayvaliotis B, Shemin R, et al: Aneurysms of the descending aorta. *J Thorac Cardiovasc Surg* **85**:98–104, 1983

23. Najafi H, Javid H, Hunter J, et al: Descending aortic aneurysmectomy without adjuncts to avoid ischemia. *Ann Thorac Surg* **30**:326–335, 1980

24. Crawford ES, Walker HSJ, Saleh SA, Normann NA: Graft replacement of aneurysm in descending thoracic aorta: Results without bypass or shunting. *Surgery* **89**:73–85, 1981

25. Carlson DE, Karp RB, Kouchoukos NT: Surgical treatment of aneurysms of the descending thoracic aorta: An analysis of 85 patients. *Ann Thorac Surg* **35**:58–69, 1983

26. Cooley DA, Baldwin RT: Technique of open distal anastomosis for repair of descending thoracic aortic aneurysms. *Ann Thorac Surg* **54**:932–936, 1992

27. von Segesser LK, Killer I, Jenni R, et al: Improved distal circulatory support for repair of descending thoracic aortic aneurysms. *Ann Thorac Surg* **56**:1373–1380, 1993

28. Lawrence GH, Hessel EA, Sauvage LR, Krause AH: Results of the use of the TDMAC-heparin shunt in the surgery of aneurysms of the descending thoracic aorta. *J Thorac Cardiovasc Surg* **73**:393–398, 1977

29. Hilgenberg AD, Rainer WG, Sadler TR: Aneurysm of the descending thoracic aorta. *J Thorac Cardiovasc Surg* **81**:818–824, 1981

30. Najafi H: 1993 Update: Descending aortic aneurysmectomy without adjuncts to avoid ischemia. *Ann Thorac Surg* **55**:1042–1045, 1993

31. Cartier R, Orszulak TA, Pairolero PC, Schaff HV: Circulatory support during crossclamping of the descending thoracic aorta. *J Thorac Cardiovasc Surg* **99**:1038–1047, 1990

32. Djindjian R: Summary of the anatomy of the blood supply to the spinal cord. In Djindjian R (ed): *Angiography of the Spinal Cord*, 1st ed. Paris, Masson, 1970, pp 2–26

33. Svensson LG, Patel V, Robinson MF, et al: Influence of preservation or perfusion of intraoperatively identified spinal cord blood supply on spinal motor evoked potentials and paraplegia after aortic surgery. *J Vasc Surg* **13**:355–365, 1991

34. Laschinger JC, Izumoto H, Kouchoukos NT: Evolving concepts in prevention of spinal cord injury during operations on the descending thoracic and thoracoabdominal aorta. *Ann Thorac Surg* **44**:667–674, 1987

35. Laschinger JC, Cunningham JN, Nathan IM, et al: Experimental and clinical assessment of the adequacy of partial bypass in maintenance of spinal cord blood flow during operations on the thoracic aorta. *Ann Thorac Surg* **36**:417–426, 1983

36. Crawford ES, Rubio PA: Reappraisal of adjuncts to avoid ischemia in the treatment of aneurysms of descending thoracic aorta. *J Thorac Cardiovasc Surg* **66**:693–704, 1973

37. Katz NM, Blackstone EH, Kirklin JW, Karp RB: Incremental risk factors for spinal cord injury following acute traumatic aortic transection. *J Thorac Cardiovasc Surg* **81**:669–674, 1981

38. Blaisdell FW, Cooley DA: The mechanism of paraplegia after temporary thoracic aortic occlusion and its relationship to spinal fluid pressure. *Surgery* **51**:351–355, 1962

39. Bower TC, Murray MJ, Gloviczki P, et al: Effects of thoracic aortic occlusion and cerebrospinal fluid drainage on regional spinal cord blood flow in dogs: Correlation with neurologic outcome. *J Vasc Surg* **9**:135–144, 1988

40. Cunningham JH, Laschinger JC, Merkin HA, et al: Measurement of spinal cord ischemia during operations upon the thoracic aorta. *Ann Surg* **196**:285–296, 1982

41. Laschinger JC, Cunningham JN, Catinella FP, et al: Detection and prevention of intraoperative spinal cord ischemia after cross-clamping of the thoracic aorta: Use of somatosensory evoked potentials. *Surgery* **92**:1109–1117, 1982

42. Coles JG, Wilson GJ, Sima AF, et al: Intraoperative detection of spinal cord ischemia using somatosensory cortical evoked potentials during thoracic aortic occlusion. *Ann Thorac Surg* **34**:299–306, 1982

43. Crawford ES, Mizrahi EM, Hess KR, et al: The impact of distal aortic perfusion and somatosensory evoked potential monitoring on prevention of paraplegia after aortic aneurysm operation. *J Thorac Cardiovasc Surg* **95**:357–367, 1988

44. Acher CW, Wynn MM, Hoch JR, et al: Combined use of cerebral spinal fluid drainage and naloxone reduces the risk of paraplegia in thoracoabdominal aneurysm repair. *J Vasc Surg* **19**:236–248, 1994

45. Roberts AJ, Nora JD, Hughes WA, et al: Cardiac and renal responses to cross-clamping of the descending thoracic aorta. *J Thorac Cardiovasc Surg* **86:**732–741, 1983

46. Connolly JE, Kountz SL, Boyd RJ: Left heart bypass: Experimental and clinical observations on its regulation with particular reference to maintenance of maximal renal blood flow. *J Thorac Cardiovasc Surg* **44:**577–588, 1962

47. Schepens MA, Defauw JJ, Hamerlijnck RP, Vermeulen FE: Risk assessment of acute renal failure after thoracoabdominal aortic aneurysm surgery. *Ann Surg* **219:**400–407, 1994

48. Kouchoukos NT, Lell WA, Karp RB, Samuelson PN: Hemodynamic effects of aortic clamping and decompression with a temporary shunt for resection of the descending aorta. *Surgery* **85:**25–30, 1979

49. Hug HR, Taber RE: Bypass flow requirements during thoracic aneurysmectomy with particular attention to the prevention of left heart failure. *J Thorac Cardiovasc Surg* **57:**203–213, 1969

50. Scheinin SA, Cooley DA: Graft replacement of the descending thoracic aorta: Results of "open" distal anastomosis. *Ann Thorac Surg* **58:**19–23, 1994

51. Donahoo JS, Brawley RK, Gott VL: The heparin-coated vascular shunt for thoracic aortic and great vessel procedures: A ten-year experience. *Ann Thorac Surg* **23:**507–513, 1977

52. Westaby S: Hypothermic thoracic and thoracoabdominal aneurysm operation: A central cannulation technique. *Ann Thorac Surg* **54:**253–258, 1992

53. Rokkas CK, Choi DW, Lobner DC, Kouchoukos NT: Hypothermia and dextrophan inhibit the release of excitory amino acids in spinal cord ischemia. Abstract presented at the Aortic Surgery Symposium IV, Mount Sinai Medical Center, New York, 1994, 68

54. Redmond JM, Gillinov AM, Zehr KJ, et al: Glutamate excitotoxicity: A mechanism of neurologic injury associated with hypothermic circulatory arrest. *J Thorac Cardiovasc Surg* **107:**776–787, 1994

55. Dake MD, Semba CP, Rubin GD, et al: Endovascular stent/graft treatment of thoracic aortic aneurysms. Abstract presented at the meeting of the Radiological Society of North America, December 1993

56. Moon MR, Dake MD, Walker PJ, et al: Endovascular stent-grafts for descending thoracic aortic pathology. Abstract presented at the Aortic Surgery Symposium IV, Mount Sinai Medical Center, New York, 1993, 74

57. Kirsch MM, Behrendt DM, Orringer MB, et al: The treatment of acute traumatic rupture of the aorta. *Ann Surg* **184:**308–316, 1976

58. Merrill WH, Lee RB, Hammon JW, et al: Surgical treatment of acute traumatic tear of the thoracic aorta. *Ann Surg* **207:**699–706, 1988

59. Williams JS, Graff JA, Uku JM, Steinig JP: Aortic injury in vehicular trauma. *Ann Thorac Surg* **57:**726–730, 1994

60. Parmley LF, Mattingly TW, Manion WC, Jahnke EJ: Nonpenetrating traumatic injury of the aorta. *Circulation* **17:**1086, 1958

61. Olivier HF, Maher TD, Liebler GA, et al: Use of the Biomedicus centrifugal pump in traumatic tears of the thoracic aorta. *Ann Thorac Surg* **38:**586–591, 1984

62. Rabinsky I, Sidhu GS, Wagner RB: Mid-descending aortic traumatic aneurysms. *Ann Thorac Surg* **50:**155–160, 1990

63. Morse SS, Glickman MG, Greenwood LH, et al: Traumatic aortic rupture: False-positive aortographic diagnosis due to atypical ductus diverticulum. *Am J Roentgen* **150:**793–796, 1988

64. Akins CW, Buckley MJ, Daggett W, et al: Acute traumatic disruption of the thoracic aorta: A ten-year experience. *Ann Thorac Surg* **31:**305–309, 1981

65. Walker WA, Pate JW: Medical management of acute traumatic rupture of the aorta. *Ann Thorac Surg* **50:**965–967, 1990

66. Pate JW: Is traumatic rupture of the aorta misunderstood? *Ann Thorac Surg* **57:**530–531, 1994

67. Shorr RM, Crittendon M, Indeck M, et al: Blunt thoracic trauma. *Ann Surg* **206:**200–205, 1987

68. von Oppell UO, Dunne T, DeGroot M, Zilla P: Spinal protection if no collaterals: Meta-analysis of mortality and paraplegia in acute traumatic aortic rupture. Abstract presented at the Aortic Surgery Symposium IV, Mount Sinai Medical Center, New York, 1994, 70

69. Sturm JT, Billiar TR, Luxenberg MG, Perry JF: Risk factors for the development of renal failure following the surgical treatment of aortic rupture. *Ann Thorac Surg* **43:**425–427, 1987

138

Dissections of the Aorta

M. Arisan Ergin and Randall B. Griepp

Acute dissection of the aorta is the most frequent catastrophic disease involving the aorta and remains the leading cause of death from aortic pathology.[1] Chronic aortic dissections account for a substantial proportion of aneurysms of the thoracic aorta. A thorough understanding of the pathology is important for rapid diagnosis and effective treatment of both. Advances in diagnostic techniques, operative and perioperative management, and long-term medical treatment have dramatically changed the outlook for patients with this otherwise lethal condition.

HISTORY

There are several early anatomical descriptions that closely resemble the dissection of the aorta, including Nicholls's famous autopsy report on King George II in 1776.[2] Most of these authors, however, failed to recognize this pathology as a separate entity. Even Laennec, while coining the popular misnomer "Aneurysme Dissequant" in 1826, believed that this represented an early stage of a common saccular aneurysm.[3] Maunoir is credited with the first clear description of a dissection and recognition of this as an entity.[2] Peacock published the first comprehensive review on the subject in 1843.[4] Until the middle of the twentieth century, dissections of the aorta remained in the pathologist's domain. Erdheim described the histologic changes in 1930 and introduced the descriptive term, "cystic medionecrosis."[5] A correct diagnosis prior to autopsy remained elusive for a long time. A correct antemortem diagnosis was made in only 6 of the 300 cases collected by Shennan in 1934.[2] The first radiologic confirmation of a clinical diagnosis was reported by Davy and Gates in 1922.[6] Paullin and James, in 1948, reported the use of contrast angiography for diagnosis.[7] The first attempt at surgical treatment was made by Gurin and associates in 1935; a fenestration in the iliac artery restored the circulation to the limb, but the patient

succumbed to renal failure.[8] Later, Abbott used cellophane wrapping to prevent rupture of the dissected aorta.[9] The first series of surgically treated patients with dissections were reported by DeBakey and associates in 1955.[10] The use of extracorporeal circulation during clamping of the descending aorta was introduced by Cooley and associates in 1957.[11] The DeBakey classification was described in 1965.[12] Intensive medical treatment was introduced by Wheat et al in 1965.[13] These developments in the late 1960s, combined with the advances in diagnostic, anesthetic, and surgical techniques, and the introduction of improved prosthetic grafts and new pharmacological agents, set the stage for the formulation of a rational treatment plan for acute dissections of the aorta.

DEFINITION

The dissection of the aorta is a catastrophic event that is characterized by the separation of the layers of the media by a column of circulating blood with variable proximal and distal extension throughout the entire length of the aorta. This acute event is not associated with the presence of an aneurysm. The widely used misnomer "dissecting aortic aneurysm" is inappropriate, and "acute dissection of the aorta" is a better term in describing the acute process.[14] In cases who survive the acute period, there is gradual aneurysmal dilatation of the false lumen, with or without re-entry tears, and double-lumen aorta. "Dissecting aortic aneurysm" is better reserved for the definition of these chronic dissections.

INCIDENCE

The incidence of acute aortic dissection is approximately 5.2 per million population per year, and is almost twice as frequent as ruptured abdominal aortic aneurysm.[1] It is found in 1 to 2.5% of coroner's autopsies.[15,16] It is seen in all age groups, although it is rare in the extremes of life. Seventy-five percent of the cases cluster between the fourth and the seventh decade, and the peak incidence is in the 50 to 69 year age group.[15] There is a 2 to 3:1 male-to-female ratio. It is rare among Orientals, and there is a slight apparent increase among individuals of African descent. This link probably reflects the racial predisposition to hypertension, rather than a racial predilection to dissection.[15]

ETIOLOGY

Although the etiology of aortic dissections is not well defined there are several predisposing conditions that show a significant association with dissection.

Hypertension

Of the various factors implicated in the etiology of acute dissections of the aorta, arterial hypertension remains the most consistent. The reported incidence of hypertension in acute dissections is about 75% (range 51 to 93%).[15,17,18] The presence of hypertension is more common among patients with Type B dissections (more than 75%).[18] There is evidence to indicate that hypertension accelerates the degenerative changes in the aging aorta, setting the stage for dissection.[19] Although there is no solid link between hypertension and the initiation of the dissecting process, hypertension is the major factor in promoting its progress.[13]

Heredity, Connective Tissue Disorders, and Marfan's Syndrome

The role of heredity in aortic dissections in the general population is poorly defined except for patients with connective tissue disorders like Ehler–Danlos and Marfan's syndromes. Familial occurrence of dissections[20] and familial annuloaortic ectasia in association with a mutation in the gene for type III procollagen have been reported.[21] Advances in molecular biology have provided important insight into the molecular basis of these disorders and their relation to the aortic involvement. The prime example of this is Marfan's syndrome. This autosomal dominant trait with variable penetration presents a clinical spectrum manifest at one extreme with a full blown constellation of abnormalities of the skin, the skeleton, the eyes, and the cardiovascular system (typical Marfan's syndrome) and at the other extreme with only the cardiovascular manifestations of the syndrome without the other anomalies (so-called "forme fruste" of the syndrome).[22,23] The phenotypic expression was recently linked causally to missense mutations of the large fibrillin gene (FBN1) on human chromosome 15.[24] This information may be important in genetic counseling of these individuals and cardiac follow-up of their families.[25] The most common cardiovascular manifestation of the syndrome or the "forme fruste" is pear-shaped aneurysms of the ascending aorta with or without aortic regurgitation. Aorta-related complications, especially acute dissections, are the leading cause of death in Marfan's syndrome.[26] Dilatation of the ascending aorta and a family history of acute dissection are associated with an increased risk of dissection in Marfan's syndrome.[27,28] Aortic dissections develop in 33% of patients with Marfan's syndrome.[29] The incidence of Marfan's in clinical series of acute dissections is 4 to 12%.[17,30]

Aortic Stenosis and Coarctation of the Aorta

Congenital aortic stenosis, bicuspid aortic valve, and coarctation of the aorta are associated with a higher incidence of dissections, especially in younger patients.[31,32] The risk of dissection in patients with bicuspid aortic valves is reported to be 9 times higher.[18] The overall incidence of bicuspid aortic valves among dissections is between 7 and 13%.[31,33] Dissections associated with bicuspid aortic valves frequently start in the ascending aorta.[31] Aortic valve replacement in patients with bicuspid valve carries a risk of perioperative dissection. Perioperative dissections occurred in 0.07% of 3785 patients undergoing aortic valve replacement.[34] Other forms of congenital heart disease may be seen with dissections as an incidental finding.

Iatrogenic Trauma and Dissections

There is a minute incidence of dissection during cardiac catheterization. These are usually self-limited localized dissections rarely requiring surgical treatment. Surgical trauma inducing dissections leads to more serious consequences. A 3% incidence of retrograde dissection of the aorta was reported for femoral cannulation for perfusion on cardiopulmonary bypass.[35] The other surgical causes of dissection are the cannulation of the ascending aorta,[36] cross-clamp injury,[37] and partial occluding clamp injury complicating coronary bypass grafting.[38] The overall incidence of operative dissections in close to 7000 cases over a 10-year period was reported to be 0.3%.[39] Significantly, a third of the operative mortality for coronary revascularization was due to this complication in one report.[40]

Pregnancy

Acute dissections in pregnancy are a result of the increased hemodynamic stresses of the pregnancy in predisposed individuals. About 50% of acute dissections in women younger than 40 years of age have occurred during pregnancy, mostly in patients with congenital malformation of the aorta or connective tissue disorders.[41]

Other Rare Associations

Localized dissections involving the descending aorta may be associated with an intimal disruption at the site of an atherosclerotic plaque.[42] Otherwise, atherosclerotic changes in the ascending aorta are quite rare in patients with ascending dissections. Dissections may also rarely be seen in patients with syphilitic aortitis, endocarditis, or mycotic infections of the aorta,[15] giant cell aortitis, polyarteritis nodosa, and systemic lupus,[43,44] in Cushing's syndrome or pheochromocytoma, and following thyroidectomy.[44] Other rare associations are familial hypercholesterolemia, cystinosis,[45] and Turner's syndrome with or without coarctation.[33,46]

ANATOMIC AND CLINICAL CLASSIFICATION

Clinically, dissections seen within the first 2 weeks following onset of symptoms are considered *acute* and beyond this period, *chronic*. The acute mortality in the critical first 2-wk period varies from 57 to 89%.[15,47,48] The attrition rate is slower in patients who survive this critical period.[47] There are major differences between acute and chronic dissections in pathology as well as physiologic derangement, response to treatment, surgical approach, and prognosis.

The original DeBakey anatomic classification of dissections[49] was subsequently simplified into three basic types.[12] DeBakey type 1 is a dissection starting in the ascending aorta and involving the entire length of the aorta, type 2 is limited to the ascending aorta, and type 3 starts distal to the left subclavian artery, but spares the ascending aorta and the arch. DeBakey type 2 dissection is frequently seen in chronic dissections with aneurysmal dilatation of the ascending aorta. The simpler Stanford classification was proposed as a logical guide for optimal treatment.[50] According to Stanford classification type A (proximal dissections) includes all dissections that involve the ascending aorta regardless of the site of the initial intimal tear and type B (distal dissections) includes dissections not involving the ascending aorta, dissection starting distally to the left subclavian artery, and extending along the aorta distal to this point (Fig. 138–1).[50] There are distinct clinical features and guidelines for treatment of these two types (Table 138–1). Recently other classifications have been proposed to include in the definition the site of the primary tear and the distal or proximal propagation of the dissecting process.[51,52]

PATHOLOGY AND PATHOGENESIS

Intimal Tear

The pathologic characteristic of acute dissection of the aorta is the progressive separation of the layers of the media by a column of blood. The communication between the "true

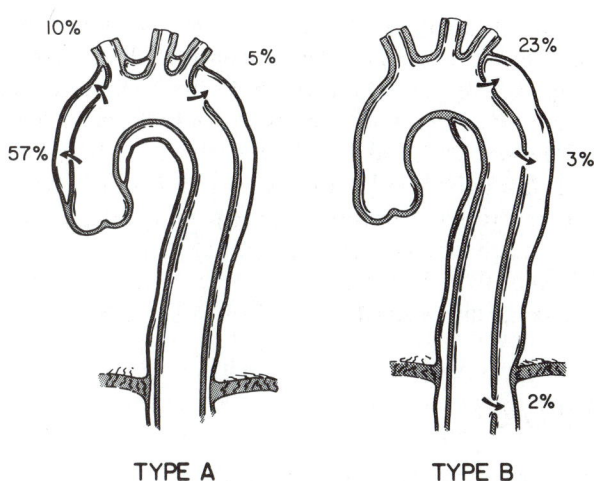

Figure 138–1. Classification of aortic dissections and distribution of the sites of the intimal tear.

lumen" of the aorta and the separated layer of the media, "the false lumen," is formed by the "primary or entry intimal tear." The intimal tear is a consistent feature of an acute dissection. Whether the occurrence of the intimal tear in all dissections is the primary event that leads to the separation of the layers or it is only secondary to the initial separation of the layers remains controversial. Only 2 to 4% of dissections present without an intimal tear, and most of these are confined to the descending aorta.[15] In the majority of dissections without an intimal tear the false lumen is totally thrombosed, so called "intramural hematoma of the aorta." With routine use of transesophageal echocardiography and CT scanning these cases are recognized more frequently. Whether this pathology in fact is a separate entity from dissections is not clear.[53–55] There is some evidence indicating that the intramural hematoma may represent the early stages of a typical dissection that culminates in the creation of an intimal tear with blood entering the false lumen previously occupied by the hematoma.[53,55] These observations may give credence to one of the oldest theories of pathogenesis, which suggests the rupture of vasovasorum and the result-

TABLE 138–1. CHARACTERISTICS OF TYPE A AND TYPE B DISSECTIONS

	Type A	Type B
Frequency	65–70%	30–35%
Male/female ratio	2:1	3:1
Average age	50–55	60–70
Associated hypertension	50%	80%
Hypertension on admission	+,–	++
Associated atherosclerosis	+,–	++
Aortic regurgitation	50%	10%
Intimal tear	Present	Absent in 5–10%
Acute mortality	57–90%	15–40%

ing hematoma in the media as the initiating event in the dissecting process. An intimal rupture then follows at points of fixation along the aorta where the hydraulic stress is more pronounced. These points, at the sinobulbar junction and the isthmus aortae, closely correlate with the observed distribution of the intimal tears. The majority of intimal tears are located within the first few centimeters of the ascending aorta, and the second most common site is the initial portion of the descending aorta. About 10 to 15% of the intimal tears are located in the arch of the aorta[15,17] (Fig. 138–1). An arch tear carries an especially grave prognosis and therefore has important surgical significance.[56–58] Very few primary tears are found beyond the thoracic aorta (2%).[15,59] The primary intimal tear usually is transverse in normal appearing intima, and rarely exceeds more than half the circumference of the aorta. In rare instances there is total disruption of intimal continuity with a circumferential intimal tear leading to "intimointimal intussusception." Recognition of this latter complex is important because of surgical implications.[60–63]

False Lumen

Once initiated the dissecting process progresses rapidly along the length of the aorta, usually in the outer third of the media. The dynamic forces that promote the progression of the dissection have been studied in detail.[13,64] Two major forces identified by Wheat and Palmer are directly related to the velocity of the ejection and to the rate of myocardial fiber shortening, *dp/dt*. Treatment aimed at reduction of these forces is the mainstay of intensive medical treatment of the dissections.[13,65]

The longitudinal dissection and the false lumen occupy the right anterior portion of the ascending aorta and the medial third or half of the ascending aorta remains mostly intact. In the arch the false lumen usually runs along the greater curvature and frequently extends into the innominate left carotid and the left subclavian arteries. In the descending aorta the false lumen follows the anterolateral wall of the aorta and the extension into the abdomen is also along the anterolateral walls; therefore the dissection frequently involves the left renal artery.[15]

The progress of the dissecting process in the false lumen has several important pathologic and clinical consequences. The dissection can interrupt the blood supply to the major branches of the aorta by extrinsic compression due to the false lumen or by actually shearing off the branches from the true lumen. Both mechanisms may lead to the so called "malperfusion syndrome" with distal organ or limb ischemia and associated functional consequences.[66–68] Proximal extension of the dissection toward the aortic root causes detachment of the aortic commissures, leading to prolapse of the leaflets and acute aortic insufficiency. Proximal dissection can also cause dissection of the coronary arteries, usually the right, leading to myocardial ischemia and infarction. The pressurized false

lumen tends to rupture readily into the pericardial or the pleural spaces, commonly in the area close to the primary intimal tear. Rupture into the pericardium is the most common cause of death in the first 2 weeks[15] (Table 138–2). The incidence of rupture into the pleural or the pericardial spaces through the thinner outer wall of the dissection is more common than the occurrence of a re-entry tear or internal rupture downstream back into the true lumen.[69] Re-entry tears frequently occur at sites of shorn side branches in the inner tube, especially along the intercostal arteries in the descending aorta. Creation of a re-entry tear, once thought to represent "an imperfect natural cure of the disease,"[4] forms the basis for the infrequently required surgical procedure of primary fenestration.[70]

The end-point of the dissecting process along the aorta is determined by scarring of the media, usually atherosclerotic in origin. A natural barrier such as coarctation or a repaired coarctation will also interrupt the dissection.[69] In patients who survive the acute episode, the false lumen either thromboses and goes on to healing or remains patent and continues to enlarge, forming an aneurysmal dilatation.[71–74] The presence of a re-entry tear prevents thrombosis of the false lumen. The persistence of the false lumen is a negative prognostic indicator associated with a higher incidence of aneurysmal dilatation in the chronic stage.[75,71] The interior of the false lumen contains fibrin and thrombus that later organize into fibrous tissue consisting mostly of collagen. In time, the wall of the false lumen may become much thicker than the true aortic wall, but will continue to dilate or rupture because of the structural weakness of the fibrous tissue.[69]

Histology

Since Erdheim's first description, "cystic medial necrosis" was believed to be the histologic sine qua non of dissection.[5] The degenerative changes that Erdheim described consist of fragmentation of elastic fibers, and loss of smooth muscle cells, with increase in the ground substance and collagen, which leads to structural weakening of the media. There are no cysts nor is necrosis present. Thus, like "dissecting aneurysm," "cystic medial necrosis" is a popular misnomer. "Medial degeneration" is a better descriptive term. Subsequent studies have proved some of these changes to be a common finding of the aging process, representing the spectrum of response to injury in the human

TABLE 138–2. PRIMARY TEAR AND SITE OF RUPTURE[a]

Location of the Tear	Site of Rupture
Ascending	intrapericardial 70%, left pleura 6%
Arch	intrapericardial 35%, left pleura 32%
Descending	intrapericardial 12%, left pleura 44%

[a]Hemopericardium cause of death in 70% of cases in the first 2 weeks.

aortic media.[76–79] The frequency of loss of muscle cells in the media of the aging aorta correlates well with the age-related peak incidence of dissection and the associated hypertension.[78] On the other hand pronounced "medial degeneration" with significant elastic tissue loss and accumulation of ground substance, more closely resembling Erdheim's original description, is frequently seen in younger patients with dissections or Marfan's' syndrome and related disorders with abnormal aortic histology.[18] These considerations suggest that there is no single histopathologic correlate of dissection, except in some younger patients and Marfan's syndrome. Rottino, justifiably, summed up these thoughts almost 60 years ago; "Dissection is essentially an accident in a fairly common process."[80]

CLINICAL PRESENTATION

Certain clinical features are common to all patients with aortic dissections. *Sudden or accelerated death* may be the presentation and the true diagnosis made only at autopsy. *Pain* is the most constant and dramatic symptom of aortic dissection. Unless the sensorium is clouded because of neurological impairment, pain is present and prominent in virtually all patients with dissection. The pain typically is described by the patient as "agonizing," "tearing," and "ripping," and is accompanied by the fear of imminent death. Pain is substernal in most patients with type A dissections, and is in the back in those with distal dissections. The pain of dissection reaches peak intensity instantly and remains constant in contrast to the sine-wave pain of the myocardial infarction. The pain does not radiate but may shift from the chest to the back and the epigastrium. Presence of a shifting pain may be a helpful hint in the differential diagnosis.[15] The pain is commonly associated by pallor, cold sweats, nausea, and vomiting, signs of intense neurohumoral response to the severity of the pain, in spite of an adequate and in most cases hypertensive arterial pressure.[15] Very rarely "painless" dissections may go unnoticed until their presentation with chronic aneurysmal dilatation of the ascending aorta as in some patients with Marfan's syndrome.

Syncope is the second most common presenting symptom of dissection. It is usually transient and related either to the intensity of the pain or to temporary ischemia of the central nervous system.[81]

Other neurologic manifestations such as temporary blindness, degrees of hemi-/paraparesis or plegia, and even deep coma, may be seen on presentation.[82]

Dyspnea and *hemoptysis* may be seen in acute dissections. They are more common in chronic dissections, representing manifestations of congestive heart failure due to aortic regurgitation or bronchial erosion due to an enlarging false lumen.[83]

Initial physical examination usually shows a distressed patient with a normal or high blood pressure, who otherwise may appear to be in shock. The blood pressure on admission is normal or high in over 80% of patients.[15] Occasional patients exhibit severe *hypertension,* which may be difficult to control. The severe hypertensive response in dissection is thought to be related to renal ischemia, destruction of the baroreceptor mechanism in the aortic arch, or, in rare cases, the presence of a "pseudocoarctation" due to extreme narrowing of the true lumen.[84,85] The presence of *hypotension,* on the other hand, is an ominous sign indicating either cardiac tamponade due to hemopericardium or hypovolemia due to rupture into the pleural cavity. Occasionally hypotension may be due to compromise of the coronary perfusion and resultant myocardial ischemia or infarction.

Differential or absent pulses accompanied by varying degrees of *limb ischemia* are among the best clinical signs of acute dissections, and are present in about 40% of the patients at admission.[67,83] Acute development of an *aortic regurgitation murmur* is a highly reliable sign of type A dissection and is present in about half the patients.[17,86] Depending on the severity of the aortic valve incompetence, *congestive heart failure* may be present during the acute phase. Other clinical findings include *distention of the neck veins* bilaterally in pericardial tamponade and compression of the superior vena cava or unilaterally due to occlusion of the innominate vein by the mediastinal hematoma,[15] pulsating neck masses due to extension of the dissection along the carotid arteries, and occasionally ecchymosis extending into the suprasternal area.[15]

A *pericardial friction rub* is present in about 5% of patients.[15] Paralytic *ileus* is common.[83] *Hematuria* and *oliguria* with flank pain accompany significant renal involvement. *Hematemesis* and *melena* are rare and when present indicate intestinal ischemia and a very poor prognosis.[15]

Five to 6% of patients present with frank *strokes* and other neurologic findings may be present in as many as 42% of patients.[82,87] The most common symptoms are syncope and altered states of consciousness without localizing signs.[15,81] Localized neurologic signs may be due to central infarction or peripheral neuropathy due to limb ischemia or nerve compression by the hematoma (Table 138–3).[15]

DIAGNOSIS

The clinical diagnosis of aortic dissection is dependent on a high index of suspicion. The diagnosis can be strongly suspected from the clinical presentation and findings in most patients. The sudden severe pain with typical progression in a hypertensive patient, especially in the presence of a new diastolic murmur and detection of a pulse differential, would make the diagnosis of acute dissection very likely.

Laboratory

The laboratory findings in acute dissections are nonspecific in nature and to a large extent should be used to rule out

TABLE 138–3. COMMON SYMPTOMS AND SIGNS OF ACUTE AORTIC DISSECTION

	Type A	Overall Frequency	Type B
Pain	Anterior substernal		Posterior, midscapular, abdominal
Syncope	+++		Rare
Dyspnea	+		–
Blood pressure	Elevated 50%, low 20%		Elevated 80%
Asymmetric pulses	Upper and lower extremity	30–50%	Lower extremity
Diastolic murmur	50%		10%
Pericardial effusion	+++		Rare
Pleural effusion	+,–		+++
Hemiparesis or plegia	+	5–6%	–
Paraparesis or plegia	+	2–6%	+
Renal, intestinal infarction	+	3–5%	+
Myocardial infarction	+	10%	Rare

other possible diagnoses. Common findings in aortic dissections are *hematuria* and *leukocytosis* with a left shift, which may sometimes be accompanied by a febrile reaction. Elevations of blood urea nitrogen (*BUN*) and *creatinine,* either due to hypertensive renal disease or as a result of hypoperfusion of both kidneys, may be present.[15] *Anemia* during the acute state is indicative of blood loss, usually into the left pleural space. Abnormalities seen in the serum chemistries are related to the severity of the accompanying organ dysfunction. SGOT commonly is normal and may serve as a useful guide in the differential diagnosis between myocardial infarction and dissection. *LDH elevations* are seen regularly, and reflect excess hemolysis of red cells within the false lumen.[15] High levels of amylase may occasionally be seen and they are usually associated with serious renal shutdown or ischemic bowel.[15] Subtle changes in the coagulation parameters, such as prolongation of the partial thromboplastin time (PTT), and increase in fibrin-split products may be present in acute dissections. This may be associated with a fall in the platelet count. Rarely, a full blown picture of disseminated intravascular coagulation is seen. The underlying mechanism of these changes is thought to be consumption of clotting factors in the dissecting hematoma.[88]

Electrocardiogram

The most common electrocardiographic finding is a sign of preexisting hypertension with *left ventricular hypertrophy* and left ventricular strain.[15,45] The major role of the electrocardiogram is in the differential diagnosis. Changes compatible with *myocardial infarction* are seen in 10 to 20% of patients with dissections.[15] Therefore the presence of a pattern suggestive of myocardial ischemia does not rule out the possibility of a dissection; however, absence of such changes favors the diagnosis of dissection. *Pericarditic changes* are seen in about 10% of the patients.[83] Occasional *heart block* may be seen with involvement of the interatrial and membranous septum by the dissecting hematoma.[89]

Diagnostic Imaging

The main points of interest for the surgeon are (1) presence of ascending aortic involvement, (2) location of the intimal tear, (3) the size of the aortic root and presence of aortic regurgitation, (4) state of perfusion to the major branches, (5) the extent and patency of the false lumen, (6) presence of a re-entry tear, (7) presence of pericardial effusion, and (7) state of the coronary circulation, especially in chronic dissections. Currently available and developing imaging techniques will in most cases answer all these questions adequately (Table 138–4).

Chest X-ray

The radiological findings seen on the plain films of the chest in acute dissections are all based on the distortion created by the false lumen and the leakage of blood into the pleural space. In over 80% of the patients widening of the mediastinum and obliteration or blurring of the aortic knob can be seen.[90,91] Intimal calcification separated more than 6 mm from the edge of the aortic contour is highly suggestive of dissection.[91] The other common and suggestive finding is the presence of a left pleural effusion.[90,91] These findings in the proper setting are valuable in leading to the correct diagnosis.

Transesophageal Echocardiography (TEE)

Transesophageal echocardiography (TEE) has become an indispensable tool for diagnosis, intraoperative management, and postoperative follow-up of dissections of the aorta.[71,92,93] Ready availability and ease of application at the bedside combined with a superior sensitivity and specificity (99 and 98%, respectively) have made the TEE the diagnostic modality of choice in acute dissection of the aorta.[94,95] With TEE accurate demonstration of important features of an acute dissection like the intimal flap and its extension, true and false lumens, primary and secondary in-

TABLE 138–4. DISSECTION OF THE AORTA: DIAGNOSTIC IMAGING MODALITIES AND INDICATIONS

	Accuracy (%)	Intimal Flap	Tear	Aortic Reg.	Other Cause	Logistics	Indication
TEE	98	++++	++++	++++	+	++++	Acute Dx
CT w contrast.	85	++	+	0	+++	++	Follow-up
Angiograp HY	95	+++	++	++++	++	+	Malperfusion
MRI	90	++	++	0	+++	0	Follow-up

Adapted from Fuster V et al: Sem Thorac Cardivasc Surg 3:219, 1991 with permission.

timal tears, presence of intramural hematoma, periadventitial leak, pericardial and pleural effusions, aortic regurgitation, size of the aortic root, coronary or brachiocephalic artery dissection is possible. The demonstration of a mobile "intimal flap" within the lumen of the aorta with flow seen by color Doppler imaging on either side of the flap, i.e., true and false lumens is specific (Fig. 138–2A,B). With the use of biplane probes primary tears can be demonstrated in nearly 90% of the cases[92] (Fig. 138–3A,B; see Color Plates following page 2072). The developing technology of intravascular ultrasonography has been applied to diagnosis of acute dissections, however, its utility as a routine diagnostic tool remains to be defined.[96] There are two potential problems associated with TEE. The procedure commonly induces a hypertensive response that may be dangerous in the presence of an acute dissection. Therefore use of adequate monitoring, sedation, and topical and when necessary general anesthesia is imperative. The principle technical limitation of the TEE is related to the blind window created by the air interface in the trachea interposed between the probe and the distal ascending aorta and the portions of the aortic arch. However, lack of preoperative information about this limited segment of the aorta should rarely influence any clinical decisions.

Computed Tomography and Magnetic Resonance Imaging

Using an intravenous infusion of contrast, CT can precisely demonstrate the extent of the dissection, the false lumen, the intimal flap, and the displacement of the true lumen.[97] With dynamic CT scanning, differential contrast flow in the true and false lumens, and further definition of the intimal flap is possible.[97,98] CT has also proved to be useful for noninvasive, postoperative follow-up of surgically treated patients.[73,74] Recent development of ultrafast CT, spiral CT technology, and associated three-dimensional CT angiography with powerful computer manipulation of the images has yielded definitions of aortic pathology of unsurpassed clarity.[99,100] This may prove to be the most accurate diagnostic tool in the near future (Figs. 138–4, 138–5, and 138–6A,B).

Magnetic resonance imaging (MRI) is valuable in evaluation of aortic pathology and allows a refined definition of the dissection.[101,102] The absence of contrast requirement for imaging is a distinct advantage of the MRI. However, the logistical problems involved in performing an adequate MRI examination in critically ill patients with acute dissection have limited the utility of this modality mostly to stable patients with chronic dissections and follow-up studies of treated patients[103–105] (Fig. 138–7A,B).

Aortography

Advances in the other noninvasive diagnostic modalities, i.e., TEE, CT, and MRI, have reduced angiography from the gold standard of diagnostic tests to a secondary role in acute dissections of the aorta.[95,106] However, angiography still remains superior in delineating the perfusion of various branches of the aorta and as such is indispensable in planning the operative strategy in chronic dissections.[100,107] The most specific angiographic sign of dissection of the aorta is the demonstration of two channels in the aorta.[75] Commonly because of flow differences in both lumens, differential opacification and washout of the dye in the lumen with the reduced flow can be seen (Fig. 138–8A,B). At times a single injection at a certain level in the aorta will not fill both lumens. The status of the main branches of the aorta is determined by the arrangement of the intimal flaps at the time of the injection. Determination of the perfusion characteristics of the major branches is much more crucial in chronic dissections where the false lumen has persisted and may be serving as the only source for visceral branches. False-negative aortograms commonly are seen in association with the intramural hematoma of the aorta (dissections without an intimal tear or thrombosed false lumen).[54,55] In these cases, TEE and CT scanning are more reliable by showing the intramural hematoma. The low diagnostic and therapeutic yield of coronary arteriography in acute dissections does not justify routine preoperative study of the coronary anatomy.[108] Recent development of catheter fenestration techniques has expanded the role of angiography from a diagnostic modality to one of therapeutic value in selected cases.[109–111]

TREATMENT

The treatment of acute dissections of the aorta has evolved with the improvement in diagnostic tools, operative techniques, and pharmacologic means. The impact of the changing technology on the outcome is reflected in results of both medical and surgical treatment of acute

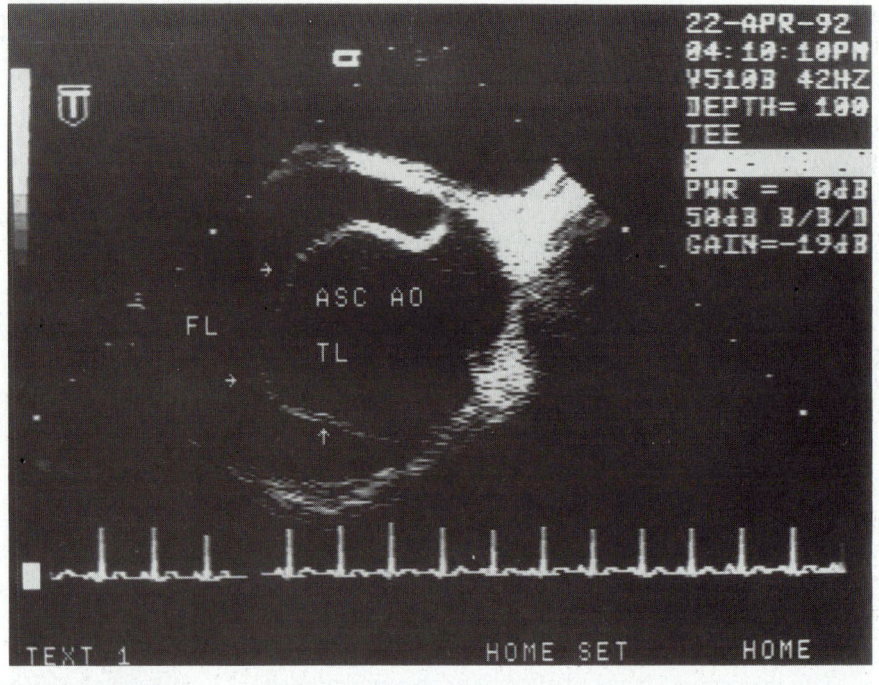

A

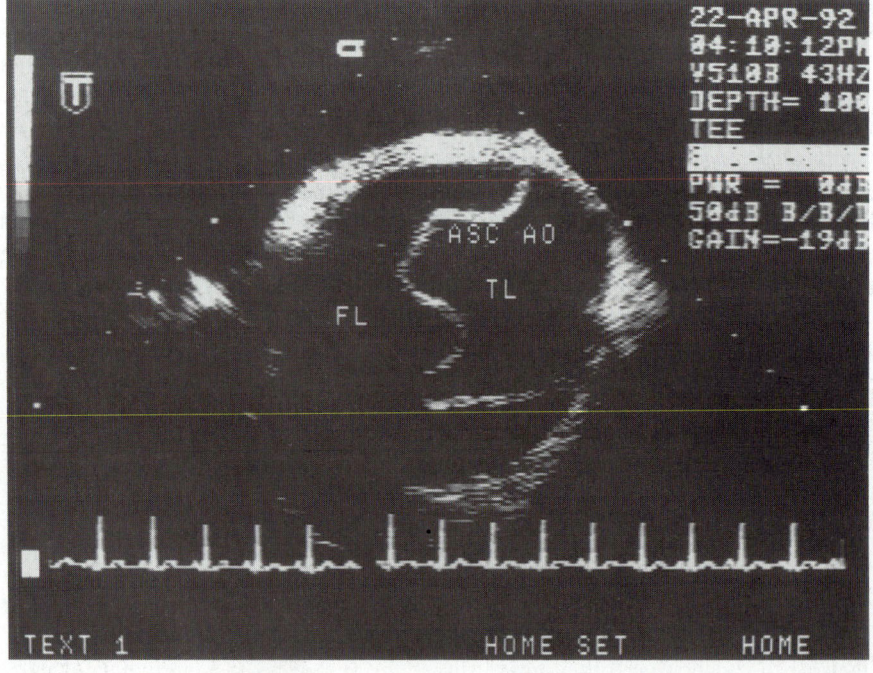

Figure 138–2. Intraoperative TEE in acute type A dissection demonstrating the oscillating intimal flap in the ascending aorta. **A.** In systole. **B.** In diastole. ASC AO, ascending aorta; FL, false lumen; TL, true lumen. *(Courtesy of Dr. S. Konstadt, Mount Sinai Medical Center Department of Anesthesiology, New York.)*

B

dissections.[112,113] The age-adjusted mortality rate from aortic dissection from 1968 to 1980 has declined more than 50% in the United States.[114] Improved medical treatment of acute type A dissection in the current era of rapid diagnosis, intensive monitoring, and modern pharmacology still carries a 57% mortality within the first 2 wk of the event.[47] Mortality of medically treated acute type B dissection has decreased in the last four decades from approximately 40% in 1960 to 10% most recently.[115] Surgical treatment of

acute type A dissection has shown significant improvement from an average of 25% mortality to less than 10% recently.[115,116] Current clinical management is dictated by this cumulative experience, with medical therapy employed for uncomplicated acute type B dissection and urgent surgery for all acute type A dissections and acute type B dissections with complications. Surgical indications in chronic dissections in general follow the same guidelines as in other aneurysms of the thoracic aorta.

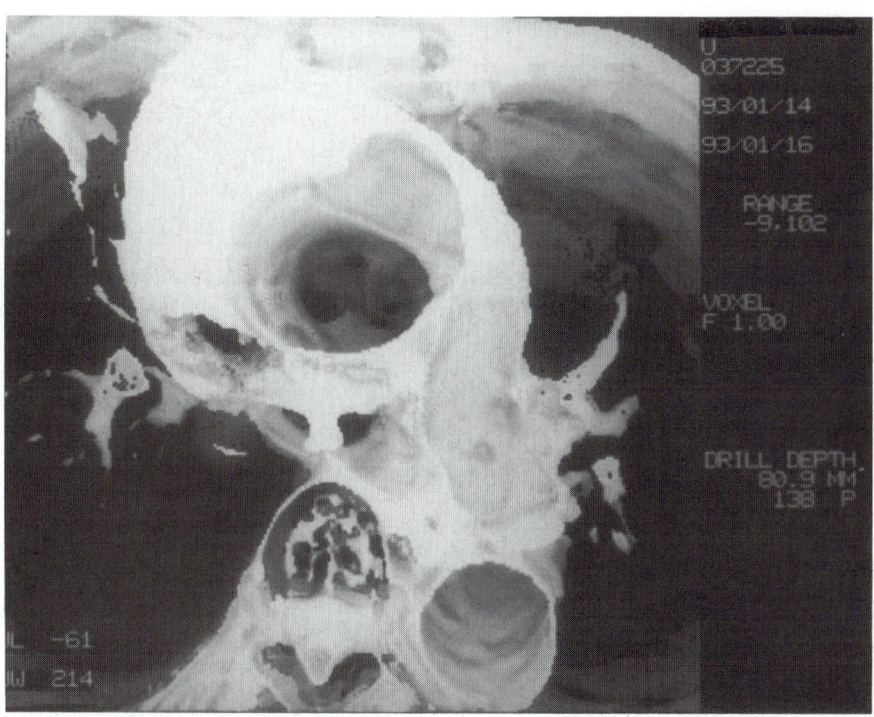

Figure 138–4. Three-dimensional spiral CT angiography (3D spiral CTA) in a patient with acute type A dissection. The false lumen confined to the ascending aorta is partially thrombosed. The intimal flap separating the two channels is clearly defined. *(Courtesy of Dr. H. Adachi, Omiya Medical Center, Jichi Medical School, Omiya, Japan.)*

ACUTE DISSECTIONS

Medical Treatment

The medical treatment is started upon clinical suspicion, and should be continued through all phases of the diagnostic work-up to confirm or rule out the diagnosis of acute dissection. The goal of medical therapy is to relieve the pain, control blood pressure, and arrest the dissecting process. Initially, the patient should be monitored in an intensive care unit with indwelling arterial, central venous or pulmonary artery catheters, and a urinary catheter, and evaluated continuously. Continued pain in spite of adequate pressure control or changes in the central nervous system and spinal cord function, peripheral pulses, aortic valve sounds, abdomen, and extremities indicate progression of

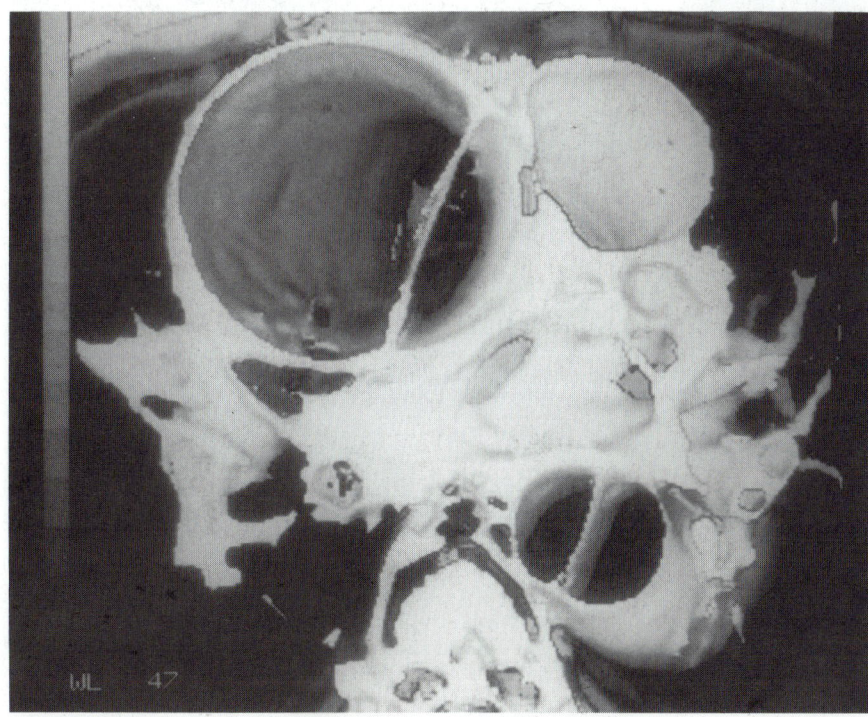

Figure 138–5. 3D spiral CTA in chronic type A dissection. The ascending aorta is dilated with a large false lumen. Intimal flap seen in both the ascending and descending aorta. *(Courtesy of Dr. H. Adachi, Omiya Medical Center, Jichi Medical School, Omiya, Japan.)*

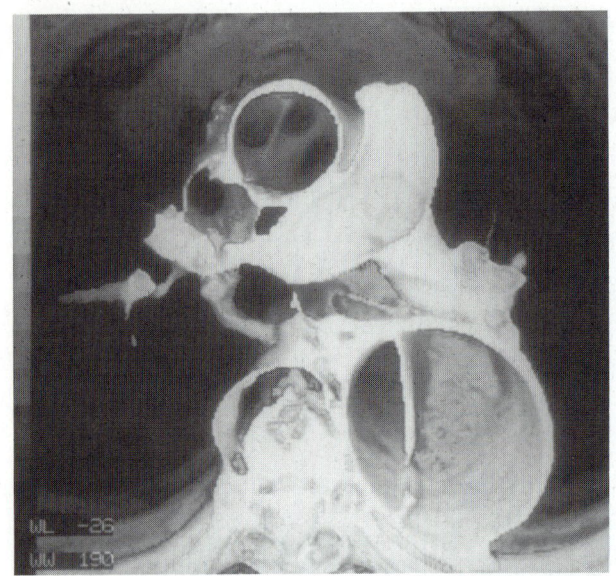

A

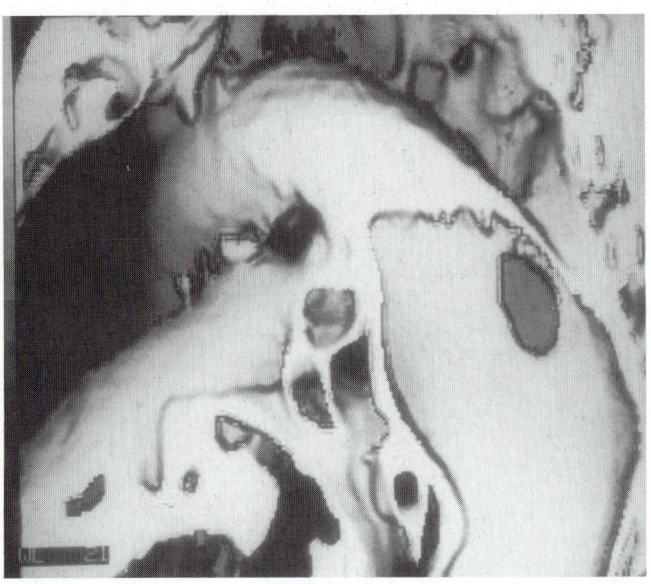

B

Figure 138–6. **A.** 3D Spiral CTA in chronic type B dissection. Enlarged descending aorta with a large false lumen and compressed true lumen, separated by the intimal flap. Notice the defect in the intimal flap at the site of the primary intimal tear. The ascending aorta is of normal size and is not involved. **B.** Longitudinal view of the same descending aorta demonstrating the shape and the size of the intimal tear later confirmed at surgery. *(Courtesy of Dr. H. Adachi, Omiya Medical Center, Jichi Medical School, Omiya, Japan.)*

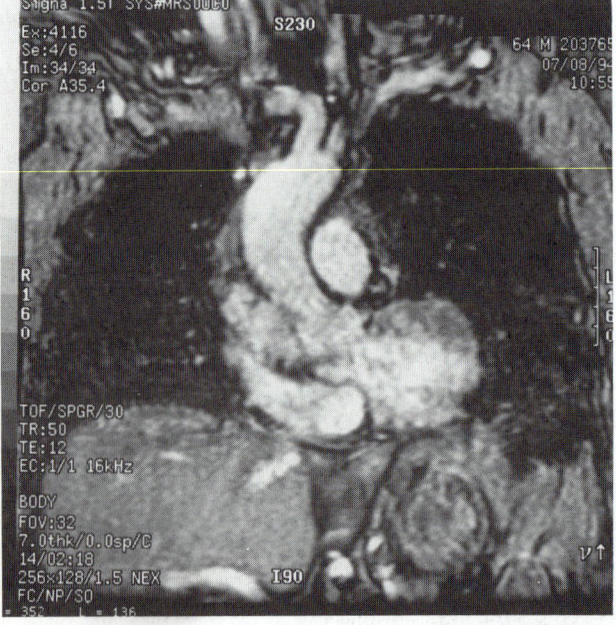

A

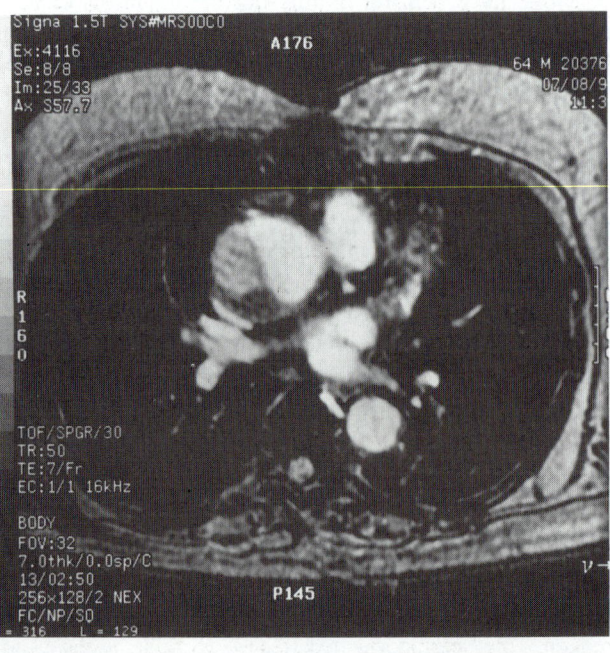

B

Figure 138–7. **A.** Sagittal magnetic resonance image (MRI) in a patient with chronic type A dissection 6 mo after coronary artery bypass grafting. Notice the false lumen extending towards the arch and the tear three centimeters above the aortic valve. **B.** Transverse cut proves that the dissection is limited to the dilated ascending aorta with the intimal flap clearly demarcating false lumen from the true lumen.

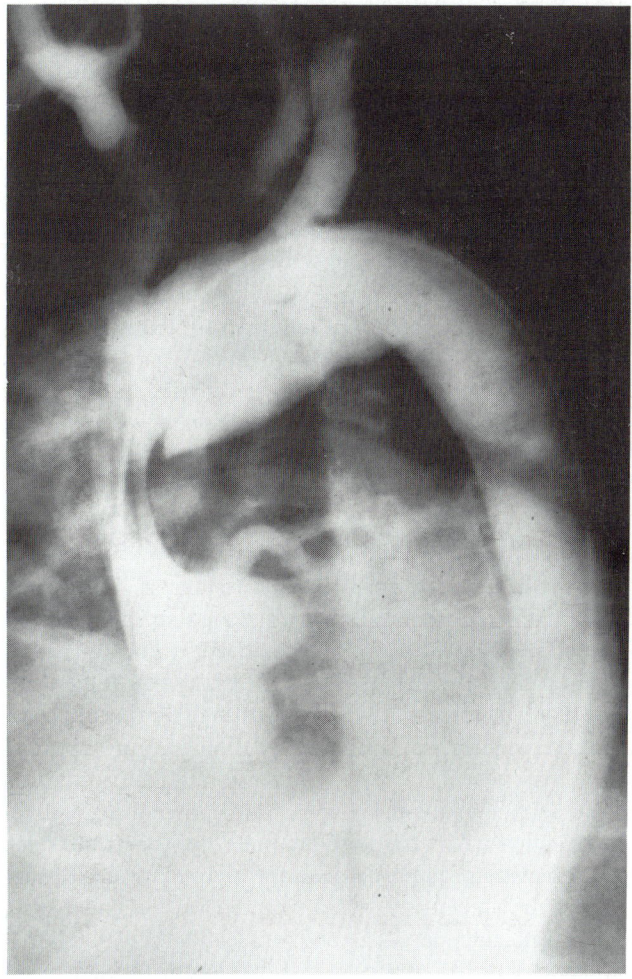
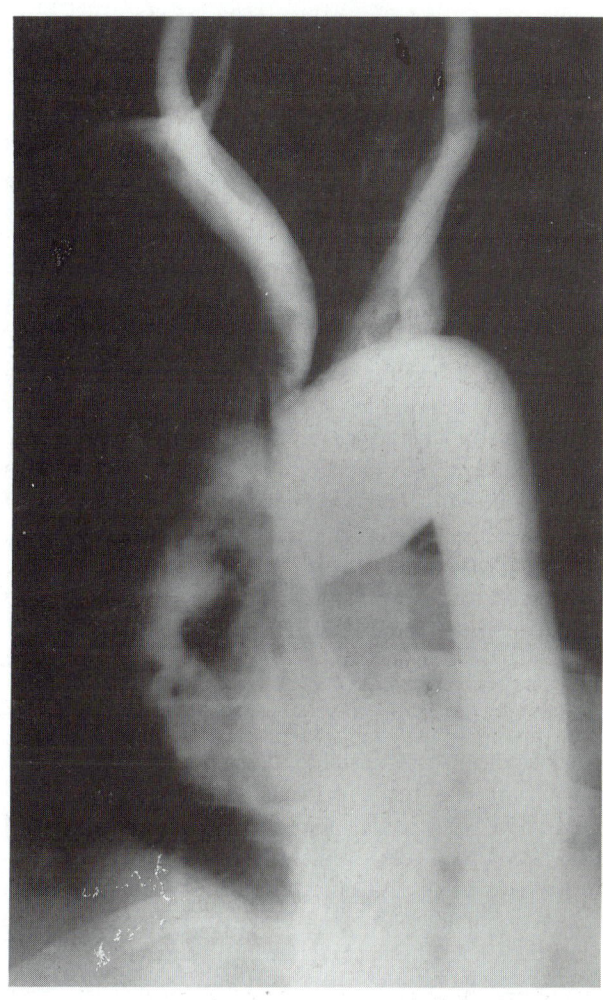

A   **B**

Figure 138–8. Aortography in acute Type A dissection. **A.** Injection into narrowed true lumen in the ascending aorta. Early filling of the false lumen in the arch indicates that the intimal tear is located in this region. **B.** Late filling of the false lumen in the ascending aorta with significant compression of the true lumen is apparent.

the dissection. Similarly, serial ECG, urinary output, and serum creatinine determinations may indicate new myocardial or renal compromise.

The principles of medical therapy for acute aortic dissections, developed by Wheat during the 1960s, are based on observations linking progression of experimental dissections to both mean arterial pressure and the rate of rise (*dp/dt*) of the arterial pulse.[13,65] "Anti-impulse" therapy, aimed at reducing mean arterial pressure and myocardial contractility, is initiated immediately via a central venous line. β-Blockade is achieved with propranolol (2 to 5 mg IV q4 to 6h) as tolerated. Labetalol, which combines selective α_1-adrenergic blockade with nonselective β-blockade, and reduces the peripheral resistance without significantly changing the heart rate or cardiac output, is reserved for patients who do not tolerate or respond to propranolol. Esmolol, a safe, intravenous, cardioselective β-blocking agent has also been used in the initial management of acute dissections. Its ultrashort half-life permits rapid achievement of stable blood levels and its effects are easily titratable (25

to 300 μg/kg per minute). Blood pressure reduction to a level compatible with adequate peripheral perfusion is accomplished by the use of unloading agents, primarily sodium nitroprusside (0.5 to 5.0 μg/kg per minute IV titrated to blood pressure). Since nitroprusside alone will increase the *dp/dt* it is started only following adequate β-blockade. Secondary choice for blood pressure control is trimethaphan (0.2 to 6.0 mg/min IV). One of the actions of trimethaphan is reduction of *dp/dt,* and it can be used without prior β-blockade. Trimethaphan may be the drug of choice in patients who cannot tolerate β-blockers.

SURGICAL TREATMENT

Indications and Rationale

Presence of acute type A dissection and failure of medical therapy in type B dissection—inability to control pain or hypertension or evidence of progressive dissection with

signs of impaired organ perfusion or impending rupture—
are indications for urgent surgical treatment.

Aortic rupture, the primary cause of early mortality,
most commonly occurs in the proximity of the primary intimal tear, the ascending aorta in acute type A dissection, and
the proximal descending aorta in acute type B dissection
(Table 138–2). The goals of current surgical therapy are to
prevent proximal and distal extension of the dissection, excise the intimal tear, and replace the portion of the aorta
most prone to rupture. In most cases, graft replacement of
the aortic segment containing the intimal tear, the ascending
aorta in type A and the initial portion of the descending
aorta in type B dissections, achieves these goals. Ideally, resection of the intimal tear and repair of the involved aortic
segment redirects flow back to the true lumen, and converts
the false lumen to a contained hematoma in the absence of
distal tears, allowing for complete healing of the dissection.
Clinical evidence suggests that the resection of the primary
tear including arch tears reduces the incidence of dissection
related long term complications.[112,117,118]

General Considerations

Inadequate hemostasis has been the most significant technical difficulty in surgery for acute dissection. Friable dissected aortic wall and hypothermic perfusion compound
routine hemostatic derangements arising from cardiopulmonary bypass and several techniques have evolved to address these problems. To improve hemostasis at the graft to
aorta suture lines, primary repair and inclusion techniques
have been used in the past. However, these repairs are associated with unacceptably high failure rates and are inferior
to total excision and replacement of the dissected aorta with
full thickness graft to aorta anastomosis.[119–126] Graft to
aorta suture lines may be secured with Teflon felt,[127] fibrin
glue,[128] gelatin resorcine formol biologic glue (GRF),[128–131]
or ringed intraluminal grafts.[132,133] Both the GRF and fibrin glues are used to seal the dissected layers at the suture
line and to strengthen the tissues for secure placement of
the sutures. The GRF glue has been widely used in Europe
and elsewhere with apparently good results and seems to

have helped in eliminating the difficulties associated with
friable dissected tissues in acute dissections.[130,131,134] It is
not approved for clinical use in the United States mainly because of concerns about the toxic effects, especially the car-
cinogenic potential of its formol component. Since the
major effect of the glue is related to its aldehyde components, 25% glutaraldehyde has been used as an alternative
to toughen the dissected tissues with good preliminary results.[135] In the past bleeding from graft interstices during
prolonged cardiopulmonary bypass had been a significant
problem requiring the use of low porosity grafts in spite of
their poor healing and handling qualities. This problem has
been totally eliminated by the development of pliable
double velour grafts, presealed with collagen impregna-
tion.[136–138]

Open Aortic Anastomosis and Arch Dissections

The routine use of open aortic anastomosis during hypothermic circulatory arrest for distal anastomosis and excision of the segment of aorta traumatized by the aortic cross
clamp has greatly helped in hemostasis at this suture line.
Inspection of the aortic arch has led to detection of unsuspected arch tears in many cases and effective elimination of
all primary tears.[56,139] Most intimal tears in the aortic arch
occur near the innominate artery orifice, permitting arch reconstruction with a single suture line (Fig. 138–9). In some
cases because of the location of the arch tear or the disruption of the arch it is necessary to replace the entire arch,
with reimplantation of the arch vessels.[56,139] Careful construction of the distal anastomosis has also reduced the incidence of postoperative false lumen patency related to suture
line leaks at this site.[74]

Type A Dissections

Type A dissections, approached via median sternotomy, are
repaired on right atrial–femoral bypass, using the strongest
pulsating femoral artery for cannulation.[140] If the artery is
dissected it is important to cannulate the true lumen to assure safe perfusion. As cardiopulmonary bypass is gradu-

Figure 138–9. Partial arch replacement and open aortic anastomosis for acute arch dissection. **A.** The primary tear frequently
is located in the initial segment of the arch in the majority of
arch dissections. **B.** Resection of the intimal tear can be
accomplished with partial resection of the arch and a single
suture line, during hypothermic circulatory arrest. The distal aortic cuff is prepared with reinforcing Teflon strips inside and
outside the aorta as dictated by the friability of the aortic wall.
Sandwiching the dissected layers between the felt strips effectively obliterates the false lumen at this site and allows for a
secure graft to aorta anastomosis. **C.** Completed partial arch replacement. The tear has been resected and all flow directed into
the true lumen.

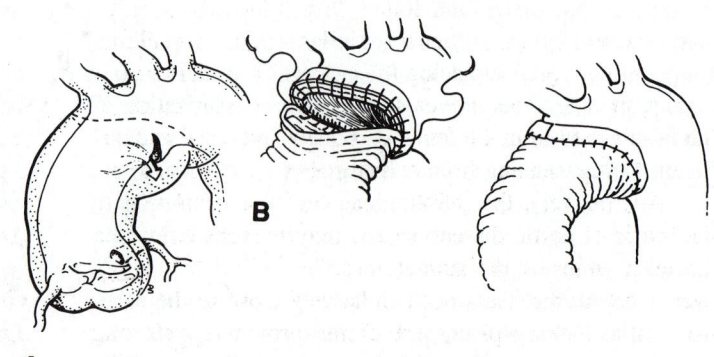

A   **C**

ally initiated the aorta is dissected from the pulmonary artery, unloaded by venous exsanguination to the pump oxygenator, and clamped at the base of the innominate artery. The initiation of the bypass represents the period of maximum risk of malperfusion as the circulation shifts from an antegrade direction to one of retrograde direction coming from the femoral artery. Continuous monitoring by TEE color Doppler of flow patterns in the descending aorta will give adequate forewarning of this complication and prevent the consequences of unrecognized malperfusion.[141] Systemic hypothermia (20°C) with hemodilution permits low flow (1000 to 1500 mL/min per m[2]), low-pressure (30 to 50 mm Hg), bypass, minimizing risk of aortic trauma during perfusion. The aorta is inspected via a longitudinal aortotomy to locate the intimal tear and the coronary ostia are perfused with cold cardioplegic solution as profound local hypothermia is induced for myocardial protection. The aortic valve is inspected; valvular competence, if compromised by commissural dissection, may be restored by resuspending the commissures.[142] The aorta is then transected immediately above the commissures and reinforced with Teflon felt strips, thereby obliterating the proximal false lumen and forming a sewing "cuff" for the proximal anastomosis (Fig. 138–10A–C). If tissues are friable a strip of autologous pericardium is used on the intimal side in addition to the Teflon strip on the adventitial side for effective bolstering of the proximal cuff. Alternative techniques use Teflon felt in between the dissected layers to occupy this space and to remodel the aortic root.[116,143] The GRF glue has been used for the same purpose and reportedly does eliminate the need for Teflon reinforcement of the aortic cuff.[134] The graft is anastomosed to the proximal "aortic cuff" with running 4-0 or 3-0 polypropylene suture, placing the graft inside the aorta effectively sandwiching the dissected layers between the graft and the outside Teflon felt. This results in a secure and hemostatic proximal suture line (Fig. 138–10D). During a period of hypothermic (16° to 18°C) circulatory arrest the aortic cross-clamp is removed and the distal aorta is trimmed at the base of the innominate artery to include the cross-clamp site and all proximal tears in the resected segment of the aorta. A reinforced distal "cuff" is prepared and the graft anastomosed in the same fashion, obliterating the distal false lumen. A 3-cm band of Teflon felt incorporated into the anastomosis to reinforce the suture line is also used to compress the distal false lumen (Fig. 138–10E–G). Cardiopulmonary bypass is then resumed through a cannula inserted into the graft replacing the ascending aorta in an antegrade manner. This prevents retrograde pressurization of the false lumen from the femoral cannula and distal malperfusion during weaning from extracorporeal perfusion.

Alternatively, the intraluminal graft has been used in the repair of aortic dissection and may prevent leaks into the false lumen at the suture lines.[74,132,133,144–146] However, most intimal tears occur relatively close to the coronary ostia, making placement of the proximal graft ring hazardous at this location. We have therefore reserved the

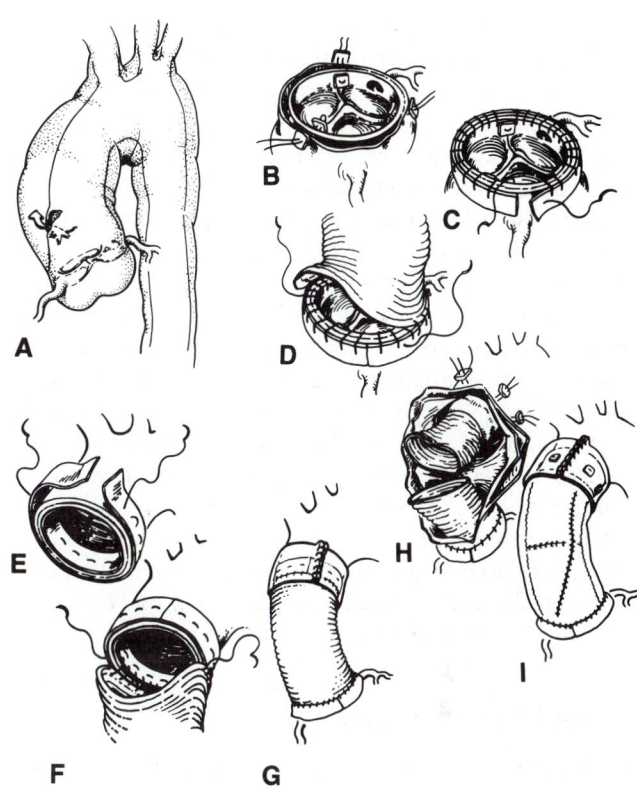

Figure 138–10. Steps and alternative methods in the surgical treatment of acute type A dissections. **A.** Pathology with the tear in the proximal portion of the ascending aorta. **B.** Resuspension of the aortic valve to restore competence. **C.** Preparation of the proximal cuff with reinforcing Teflon strip. **D.** Proximal anastomosis between the graft and the prepared cuff with running suture. **E.** The ascending aorta including the cross-clamp site has been totally resected, the inside of the arch is inspected, and the distal cuff is prepared again with reinforcing strips of Teflon felt. If tissues are friable a separate strip of felt is used on the intimal side of the cuff to bolster the dissected layers prior to the anastomosis of the graft. **F.** Graft is anastomosed to the cuff of aorta at the base of the innominate artery. The anastomosis completed carefully placing the graft inside the aorta. **G.** The distal anastomosis may further be wrapped with a wide strip of Teflon to compress the false lumen and take tension off the anastomosis. **H.** Alternatively the distal anastomosis may be performed with an intraluminal graft. The rigid ring is inserted into the aorta at the base of the innominate artery and tied in place. **I.** Graft-to-graft anastomosis completes the reconstruction. The remnant of the aorta may be wrapped around the graft. A separate wide strip of Teflon felt is used to wrap the aorta around the tied ring of the prosthesis to induce fibrosis and prevent migration or erosion of the ring.

intraluminal graft for the distal anastomosis, placing it at the base of the innominate artery during a brief period of circulatory arrest. In this fashion a relatively rapid, secure anastomosis is accomplished under direct vision. A simple graft-to-graft anastomosis connects the intraluminal prosthesis to a proximal graft implanted in the usual manner. We feel it is prudent to wrap the aorta overlying the intraluminal ring with Teflon felt to provide reinforcement and induce fibrosis[145] (Fig. 138–10H,I).

Preservation of the Aortic Valve and Composite Aortic Root Replacement

Preservation of the native valve is possible in 70 to 80% of patients with acute type A dissection.[125,134,147–149] The competence of the aortic valve can be restored with either simple resuspension of the commissures[142] and with Teflon remodeling of the root[143] or with the recently described valve preserving root replacement.[150] Preservation of the aortic valve in most series does not affect the immediate mortality or long-term survival. Postoperative freedom from valve replacement at 10 years varies between 80[147,148] and 90%.[123] However, preservation of the valve in a dilated root frequently leads to failure and is one of the leading causes of reoperation following type A dissection repair.[117]

Patients with dilated aortic roots, aortic annular ectasia, or Marfan's syndrome require composite root replacement rather than resuspension or repair of the aortic valve.[116,147,148,151] The long-term results of separate valve and graft replacement of the ascending aorta in patients with medial degenerative disease of the aorta including dissections are less than optimal.[152,153] Therefore, if the valve cannot be saved, a composite valved-graft should be implanted into the aortic root and the coronary ostia reanastomosed to the graft, the Bentall procedure[154,120] (Fig. 138–11A–D). Similarly if the root is dilated to more than 36 mm a composite replacement is indicated. The role of the valve preserving root replacement technique in routine treatment of such dilated aortic roots in the presence of acute dissection remains to be established.[150] The direct extension of the dissection into the ostia of the coronary arteries represents a technical challenge since repair of the root under these circumstances may be difficult. The most expeditious and safe solution to this problem is the composite replacement of the root and the aortic valve with the Cabrol modification of the Bentall procedure.[155,156] The dissected coronary ostia are isolated on buttons of aortic tissue which is reinforced with a collar of Teflon felt washer to buttress the dissection and coronary perfusion is reconstituted with a

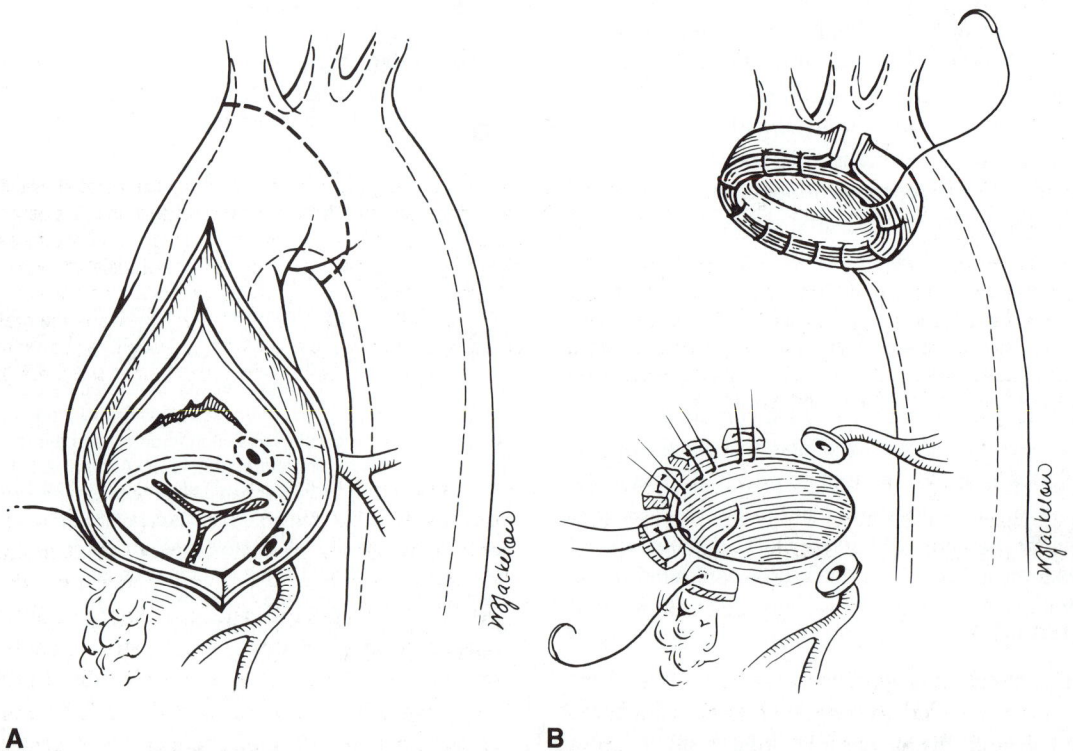

A   **B**

Figure 138–11. Modified Bentall procedure for composite replacement of the aortic valve and the ascending aorta in type A dissection with a dilated root and aortic regurgitation or Marfan's syndrome. **A.** The aorta is opened with a longitudinal aortotomy exposing the intimal flap separating false and true lumens of the dissection. The intimal tear is shown posteromedially close to the orifice of the left coronary artery. The dotted lines indicate the limits of the aortic resection at the proximal arch and the preparation of the coronary ostia on buttons of surrounding aortic tissue. **B.** Steps in the proximal and distal repairs following complete resection of the ascending aorta. Initially the aorta is completely transected across the area of the tear, the incompetent aortic valve excised, the coronary buttons dissected, and the aortic remnant is resected from the root. The mattress fixation sutures for the composite graft are placed from outside the perimeter of the root through the annulus, without any gaps between the pledgets. This technique yields a secure proximal repair with absolute hemostasis at the root. Following reimplantation of the coronary buttons the aortic cross-clamp is removed, the arch trimmed as indicated, and the distal aortic cuff is prepared as described in Figure 138–9. *(Continued.)*

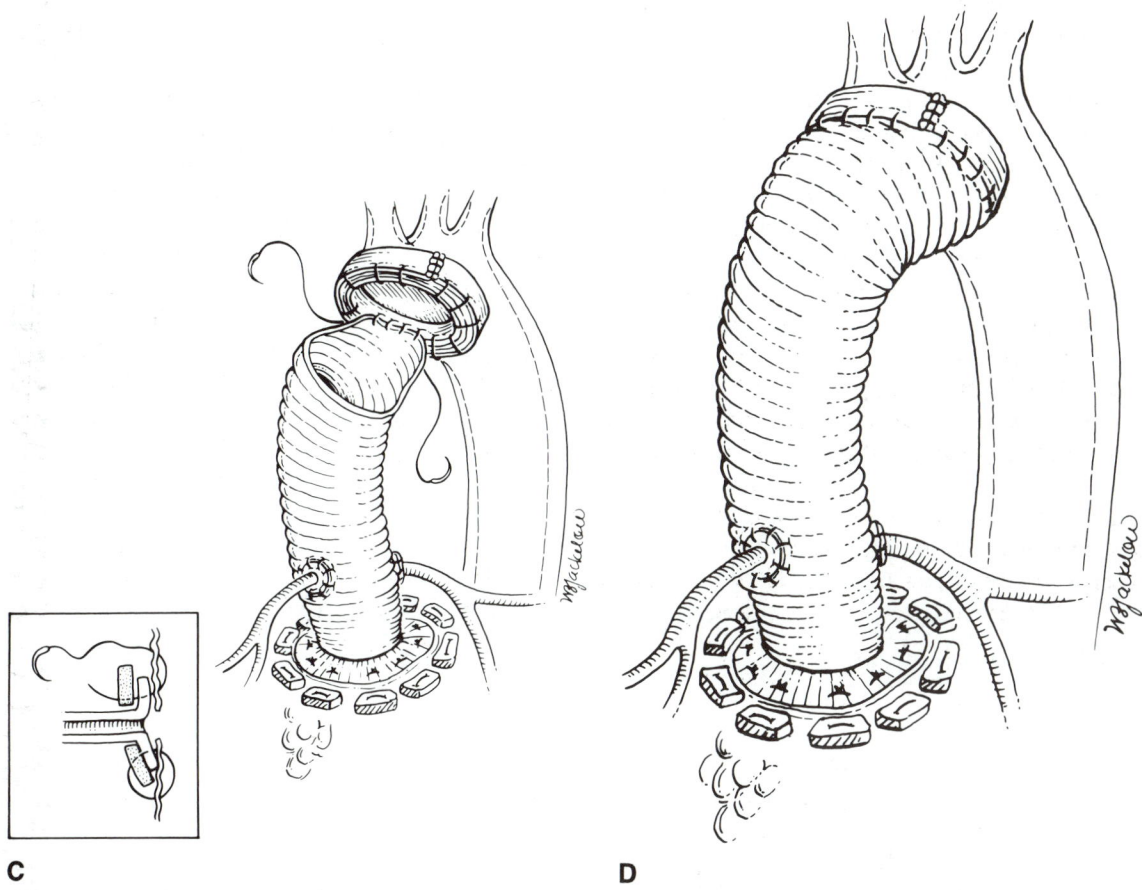

C   **D**

Figure 138–11. *(Continued.)* **C.** Completed proximal repair and anastomosis of the graft to the distal aortic cuff. Inset shows the details of the technique of coronary button anastomosis to the graft. The holes for coronary anastomoses are created with a hot ophthalmic cautery to prevent fraying at the edges of the graft fabric. These holes are made slightly larger than the native coronary orifices but considerably smaller than the diameter of the coronary button. A Teflon felt washer is incorporated into the anastomosis and the coronary button lies flat up against the graft material sandwiched between the felt and the graft (see inset). This method yields a leak proof suture line at these critical anastomoses. The distal anastomosis between the graft and the prepared aortic cuff shows the graft being placed into the cuff as the suture line progresses. **D.** Completed composite replacement of the aortic valve, ascending aorta, and the proximal arch. Notice the reinforcing Teflon felt strip at the distal anastomosis, which has been tightened to further compress the false lumen and take the tension off the anastomosis.

separate tube graft (Fig. 138–12). Alternative techniques have involved closure of the coronary ostia and saphenous vein bypass grafting with poor long-term results.[157]

Type B Dissections

Type B aortic dissection is approached via left lateral thoracotomy, the hips swiveled to permit femoral cannulation. With proximal and distal control, the aorta is cross-clamped, the segment containing the intimal tear and the dilated portion of the descending aorta resected, and a graft interposed, obliterating proximal and distal false lumens and redirecting flow to the true lumen. As in type A dissection, suture lines are reinforced with Teflon strips. The intraluminal graft may be used to perform the distal and, sometimes, if adequate true lumen exists between the tear and the left subclavian artery, the proximal anastomosis (Fig. 138–13A–G).

Provision of distal perfusion is important in most cases to provide a margin of safety since repair of the dissected aorta may require prolonged periods of clamping of the descending aorta associated with increasing risk of paraplegia.[158,112] Pump-oxygenator techniques of distal perfusion, heparin-bonded shunt,[159] and atriofemoral left heart bypass[160] have been used to provide distal perfusion with oxygenated blood and to unload the left ventricle during cross-clamping. We prefer a method of centrifugal pump perfusion from the left atrium or the left ventricle (LV) apex to the femoral artery with the added advantage of a means for rapid volume infusion requiring only low dose heparinization.[161] When the extension of the dissection retrogradely to the aortic arch makes the placement of the proximal clamp hazardous, hypothermic circulatory arrest can be utilized to replace the descending aorta containing the intimal tear and portions of the aortic arch or the distal ascending aorta as dictated by the local pathology.[162,163]

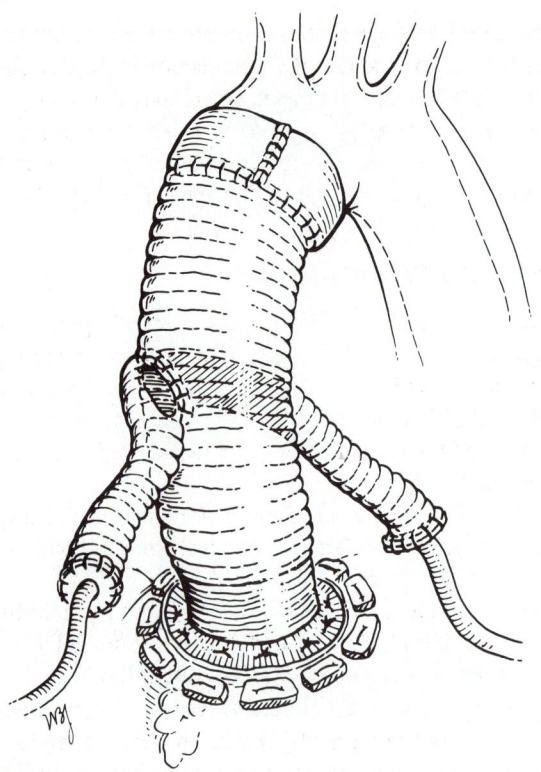

Figure 138–12. Cabrol modification of the Bentall procedure for composite replacement of the aortic root in acute type A dissection when the tear or the dissection extends into the coronary orifices. Coronary buttons are dissected reinforced with felt washers and anastomosed to a separate graft, which is connected to the composite graft. This technique allows tension free anastomosis of the dissected coronary ostia and easy access for hemostasis.

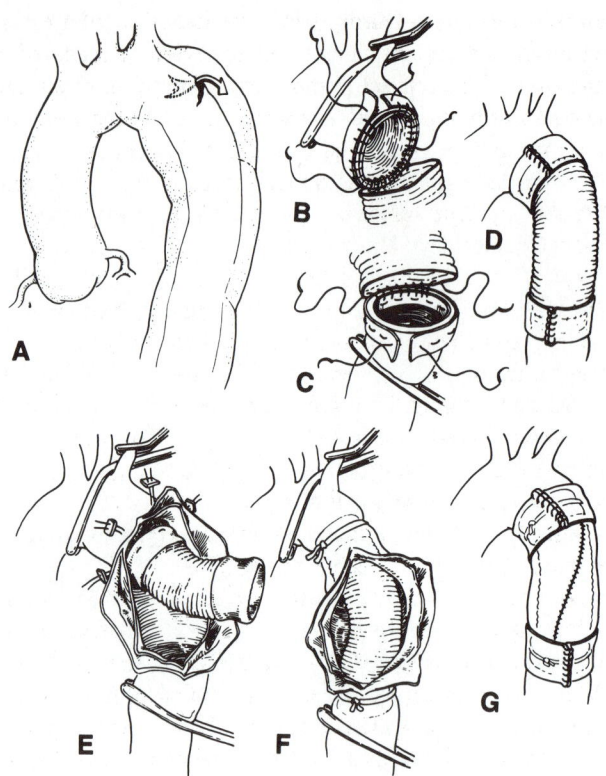

Figure 138–13. Surgical treatment of acute type B dissection. **A.** Pathology with the intimal tear in the initial segment of the descending aorta. **B,C.** Alternative techniques of preparing the proximal and distal cuffs, with single strip felt reinforcement on the outside (shown for proximal anastomosis) or double strip inside and outside felt reinforcement (shown for distal anastomosis) are used as dictated by the local conditions. **D.** Both anastomoses are wrapped with wide strips of Teflon felt for further hemostasis with compression of the false lumen. **E–G.** Use of the intraluminal graft for both anastomoses is possible only if the intimal tear is located away from the left subclavian artery to allow room for safe fixation of the proximal ring. If the intraluminal graft is used the aorta is closed around the graft and both ring ties reinforced with a collar of Teflon felt.

MANAGEMENT OF DISSECTION RELATED ACUTE COMPLICATIONS

Prevention and Treatment of Intraoperative Malperfusion Syndrome

After rupture of the aorta, malperfusion syndrome is the second leading cause of mortality due to acute dissection.[66] The incidence of major malperfusion in clinical series is as high as 33% with a resultant mortality ranging from 38 to 50%.[66,68,87,157] Malperfusion can occur either spontaneously as is the case in most patients presenting with cerebral symptoms and ischemic extremities or it may develop during the surgical treatment.

Intraoperative malperfusion, observed to occur in 13% of patients by TEE monitoring,[141] can be an insidious problem with catastrophic consequences. Monitoring of the right radial artery pressure during all phases of the operation will ensure that there is adequate perfusion of the innominate artery and will help prevent development of cerebral malperfusion.[66] Slow induction of the perfusion,

allowing the heart to eject initially, is a useful maneuver to prevent the sudden shift in the arrangement of the intimal flaps due to retrograde perfusion from the femoral cannula. Monitoring of flow patterns in the true and false channels with TEE or epiaortic echo Doppler[141] may give the earliest warning of intraoperative malperfusion. At the completion of the repair perfusion is restarted antegradely through the ascending graft into the true lumen and femoral retrograde perfusion is not used during the remainder of the operation.[74] This completely eliminates the possibility of retrograde pressurization of the false lumen from residual secondary tears, and prevents nonperfusion of the aortic root due to compression of the true lumen in the descending aorta or the arch.

Detection of intraoperative malperfusion requires immediate action to correct the situation and prevent major neurological injury. During a brief period of circulatory arrest a separate arterial cannula on a previously prepared Y extension of the arterial pump line is rapidly inserted into the completely transected ascending aorta and secured with an umbilical tape in an area that is later included in the resected aortic segment. It is important to place this soft cannula into the true lumen and advance it into the proximal descending aorta well beyond the arch vessels to prevent inadvertent selective cannulation of the arch branches. This maneuver can be accomplished in virtually every patient within a short period of time. It is also the only effective measure in the presence of a circumferential ascending aortic tear and intimointimal intussusception of the inner tube into the arch of the aorta.[62,63] Under circulatory arrest the prolapsing inner tube is pulled back into the ascending aorta and the cannula inserted into the true lumen and secured around the ascending aorta as described. Others have used cannulation of the ascending aorta through the left ventricular apex or excision of the membrane separating the two lumens in the arch to assure flow into the arch branches.[157] Both of these have disadvantages. Continued perfusion through the cannula in the left ventricle, especially in the presence of an incompetent aortic valve, is not practical. The forced fenestration in the arch may leave the arch supported only by the tenuous adventitial layer of the dissection and mandate an otherwise avoidable arch resection.

Fenestration and Treatment of Postoperative Malperfusion

In patients who present with malperfusion symptoms urgent proximal repair and direction of the flow into the true lumen are effective in preventing malperfusion in over 90% of the cases.[67] Treatment of persisting peripheral malperfusion is best tailored to the particular patient. In its simplest form lower limb ischemia can be treated with a crossover graft. More serious malperfusion like total obstruction of the bifurcation of the aorta, or visceral or renal ischemia has been effectively treated with abdominal aortic fenestration. Fenestration is done in the infrarenal aorta with isolation of the aorta from the renal arteries to the bifurcation between clamps. The aorta is opened longitudinally through its nondissected perimeter and the dissecting membrane is excised completely in the isolated segment of the aorta, with primary suture closure of the aortotomy.[157] Alternatively the aorta is completely transected close to the distal clamp, generous portion of the membrane up to the proximal clamp excised, and the aorta repaired with end-to-end anastomosis after obliteration of the distal false lumen with a separate suture. This method leaves part of the suture line vulnerable at the anastomosis made to the adventitial layer of the dissected aorta. In spite of this potential problem abdominal fenestration with this technique has had good long-term results.[68,70] Surgical fenestration in the abdomen is a simple and well-tolerated procedure and may be the procedure of choice in patients with type B dissections and malperfusion

of the distal aortic branches who are otherwise not candidates for proximal repair of the dissection in the descending aorta.[164] Radiological catheter techniques that create controlled re-entry tears in the abdominal aorta for reestablishment of flow to compressed branches of the aorta provide recent alternatives to surgical fenestration.[109,110,165]

Stroke and Paraplegia

Of patients with acute dissections 5 to 6% present with symptoms of stroke.[82,87] The incidence of neurological symptoms is as high as 42% when the tear is located in the aortic arch.[166] Most strokes occur with type A dissection and 85% of completed strokes are associated with carotid occlusion.[68]

Stroke in acute aortic dissection represents a therapeutic dilemma. The conversion of an ischemic cerebral infarct to a hemorrhagic one on cardiopulmonary bypass with catastrophic neurologic consequences is a real possibility.[82] Extra-anatomical bypass of the carotid arteries prior to primary repair of ascending aortic dissection has been used in the past.[68,167] However, current consensus favors direct repair of the ascending aorta, which in the majority of the cases results in total correction of the cerebral malperfusion with improvement in neurologic function.[82,157] Presentation with neurologic deficit in acute dissection is not a contraindication to surgery, although stroke by itself denotes a poor outcome and is a predictor of postoperative mortality.[67,168] Stroke-related mortality in the Stanford series of acute dissections was 14%, but neurologic recovery and satisfactory long-term outcomes were seen in 43%.[82]

The incidence of paraplegia in acute dissections ranges from 2 to 6%, and most paraplegias occur in acute type A dissection.[67] In patients presenting with paraplegia the possibility of neurologic recovery after surgery is slim. Nevertheless urgent operation is still indicated to prevent other lethal complications of the dissection.[67,68]

Pulse Deficits and Limb Ischemia

Pulse loss may occur in as many as 30 to 50% of patients with acute type A dissection. Local peripheral vascular operations are inappropriate since they will delay definitive treatment of the dissection and increase the acute mortality.[67] Persistent limb ischemia following aortic repair can currently be treated with catheter fenestration techniques and surgical fenestration or bypass grafting should rarely be necessary.[109–111]

Renal Failure

The dissection involves the renal arteries in 60% of patients. Clinically important renal dysfunction, however, occurs in only 5[68] to 8%,[67] but carries a high mortality (50%).[67] Prompt proximal repair of the dissection restores renal perfusion in the majority of the cases. Renal perfusion should be assessed postoperatively with renal perfusion scan to indicate further local treatment in the form of catheter fenestration[109,165] or abdominal aortic fenestration.[70] In most patients renal function recovers and the need for permanent dialysis is rare in the survivors.

Visceral Ischemia

Evidence of compromised visceral perfusion is seen in 3[87] to 5%[67] of patients, and is associated with a high mortality (43%).[67] In the absence of frank bowel necrosis urgent treatment should be directed to the proximal aorta. Awareness of the possibility of visceral ischemia and early diagnosis is the best prevention since once frank necrosis is established any strategy is doomed to failure. If there is doubt about the viability of abdominal contents after the proximal repair, further examination through a limited laparotomy should be carried out before leaving the operating room.[66,157] This may be aided by local Doppler examination of the visceral flow[141] in determining the need for further local treatment of visceral malperfusion with catheter or surgical fenestration or vascular bypass.[67,68,70,109]

Compression of the True Lumen and Pseudocoarctation

The compression of the true lumen in rare cases may lead to coarctation like obstruction of the descending aorta and significant pressure gradient across the narrowed segment of the aorta. This condition commonly occurs in the distal descending aorta and may lead to uncontrollable proximal hypertension. The treatment is by replacement of the involved segment of the aorta. Because of its general location in lower descending aorta the risk of postoperative paraplegia is increased. In high-risk patients with type B dissection an extra-anatomical bypass from the ascending aorta to the infrarenal aorta is an option.[66]

QUESTIONS AND CONTROVERSIES

Inclusion Technique, Total Aortic Replacement

Most experienced surgeons agree that best short- and long-term results are obtained with total excision of the dissected aorta at the site of the resection, with full thickness anastomosis of the graft to the distal aorta.[112,122,151,169] The graft inclusion techniques when used in acute dissections of the aorta are associated with high incidence of perigraft leakage and related findings of a poor repair.[121] In some series the inclusion technique was found to be an independent predictor of operative mortality.[170] Similarly the reoperation rate following the use of inclusion techniques is substantially higher (40% at 10 years)[123] when compared to series with total excision of the dissected ascending aorta (23% at 10 years).[118] Some have taken this observation one step further and suggested total replacement of the entire dissecting

process throughout the aorta as a curative treatment at the initial stage.[171] Although attractive in concept, the magnitude of the operation and associated risk as well as the long-term results (25% mortality, 19% reoperation rate) do not justify such an extensive undertaking during the acute stage.[171]

Arch Dissection

Presence of an arch tear decidedly portends a poor prognosis.[58,123] In spite of this the treatment of acute arch dissection (intimal tear in the aortic arch) remains controversial because of technical difficulties of direct arch replacement.[56,166,172–174] Clearly the old strategies of conservative treatment by withholding surgery in the presence of a primary tear in the aortic arch or wrapping the arch are ineffective and associated with high mortality. Similarly, operative therapy for acute type A dissection with limited resection of the ascending aorta, leaving intimal tears in the arch or proximal descending aorta leads to poor immediate and long-term results, with risk of continued dissection and rupture of the aorta.[17,118,117] Current experience indicates that the arch can be replaced with reasonable surgical risk in acute dissection, and therefore we would, as do others, resect the arch tears and replace the arch as indicated in all cases.[56,117,172,173,175]

Marfan's Syndrome

There is general agreement that patients with Marfan's syndrome, overt or forme fruste, with acute dissection of the aorta are best treated with root replacement.[117,124,148,151,176,177] Failure to do so invariably leads to long-term complications at the aortic root and is the leading cause of morbidity and even death in these patients.[117,124,151] The incidence of late reoperation (50%) is significantly higher in patients that did not receive a composite replacement at the initial operation.[124] The role of the valve preserving root replacement in Marfan's syndrome and acute dissection remains to be defined.[150]

Flow Reversal and Thromboexclusion

Flow reversal and thromboexclusion were proposed as a simpler alternative to resection and graft replacement for type B dissections by Carpentier et al.[178] It involves an extra-anatomical bypass graft from the ascending aorta to the infrarenal abdominal aorta and closure of the proximal descending aorta with a specially designed permanent clamp. The goal is to promote clotting of the descending aorta by reversing the direction of the flow and maintain perfusion of the lower most intercostal arteries to reduce the risk of paraplegia. However, there have been complications related to the use of the clamp. Visceral embolization with intestinal infarction and pancreatitis have occurred. In addition, paraplegia has not been an entirely avoidable problem.[164,179–181] We have reserved this approach only to poor risk patients with type B dissections, especially those with severe COPD, and used stapling of the descending aorta to avoid the problems associated with the permanent clamp.[182]

Coarctation and Type A Dissection

Acute dissection of the aorta in the presence of untreated coarctation presents a truly rare problem, since early detection and surgical correction of coarctation have virtually eliminated this interesting combination. There are only a few reported cases referring to this problem.[183–185] The main intraoperative concern revolves around provision of adequate proximal perfusion by retrograde femoral route through the coarctation. Monitoring of the arterial pressure in the right radial artery is imperative to ensure adequate proximal perfusion on cardiopulmonary bypass. Retrograde perfusion through the coarctation was possible in all reported cases.[184] Staged repair of the coarctation first followed by the repair of the ascending aorta can be used with chronic aneurysms.[185] However, acute dissection of the ascending aorta should be treated first to prevent rupture.[183,184] Either approach is a compromise leaving the patient at risk of rupture of the ascending aorta in the first instance or the stress of hypertension due to residual coarctation in the second. We would prefer a single stage complete repair through median sternotomy.

PREVENTION

Once the aorta is dissected, even after successful surgical treatment during the acute stage, the patient's life expectancy is drastically altered.[186] Therefore prevention of acute dissection of the aorta is of particular importance. Early detection and treatment of hypertension, Marfan's syndrome, and dilatation of the ascending aorta may help reduce the incidence of acute dissections of the aorta.

The increasing emphasis on the importance of treatment in hypertension may be largely responsible for the substantial reduction in mortality from dissections of the aorta since 1968.[18,114,186]

Marfan's Syndrome

Aortic dissection occurs in 33 to 44% of patients with Marfan's syndrome,[18,177] and portends a poor prognosis even after successful initial treatment.[118] Timely surgical treatment has made a substantial impact in the prognosis of patients with Marfan's syndrome.[29,176] Patients who had elective replacement of the ascending aorta prior to the occurrence of the dissection are less prone to aneurysmal disease of the remaining aorta[187] and the majority of patients requiring subsequent total replacement of the aorta have had prior dissections.[176,188] The incidence of life threatening events including acute dissection in Marfan's rises with increasing diameter of the ascending aorta.[189,190]

These considerations lead to compelling arguments in favor of preventive measures in Marfan's. Chronic β-blockade retards the dilatation of the aortic root;[191] close follow-up and more aggressive surgical treatment of asymptomatic aortic dilatation (5 cm, or twice the size of the normal aortic segment) should ideally reduce the incidence of acute dissection and the late sequelae in Marfan's.[112,187,192]

Dilated Aorta

Although aortic dissection can occur in a normal sized aorta, preexisting dilatation of the aorta is a common finding in patients with especially type A dissections.[193] In one study one-third of patients, with ascending aortic diameters between 4.0 and 5.4 cm, developed ascending aorta related complications including dissection (20%) during 6-year follow-up after aortic valve replacement for regurgitation.[194] A diameter of 6 cm in descending dissections is also associated with a 50% risk of rupture or reoperation.[123] The significant association of aortic dilatation with congenital bicuspid valves and the increased tendency to dissection are well documented.[18] In view of the low operative risk of elective replacement of the ascending aorta,[187,195,196] and the high mortality of dissections following cardiac surgery,[39] a more aggressive approach to the dilated ascending aorta in patients who require valve replacement or other cardiac operations is justified. We would recommend elective replacement of the ascending aorta in patients without associated cardiac disease at an ascending aortic diameter of 6 cm. In most of these patients a valve-preserving replacement of the ascending aorta and the root is possible. In younger patients with diseased or bicuspid valves the ascending aorta should be replaced at the time of the valve replacement if the diameter of the aorta is larger than 4.5 cm. In older patients a properly performed tailoring and external reinforcement of the ascending aorta may be a viable option, although this may not prevent dissection.[197]

POSTOPERATIVE FOLLOW-UP AND LATE COMPLICATIONS

The patient with repaired acute aortic dissection remains at risk for development of aorta-related complications.[87,118,198] Complications at the proximal repair usually are a result of surgical decisions or technique used for the reconstruction of the aortic root, like the use of the inclusion technique, primary repair of the dissected aorta, failure to replace the root in Marfan's or in the presence of a dilated aortic root, or use of an intraluminal graft in the proximal anastomosis.[117,123,124,169,198] Complications along the distal aorta are directly related to the patency of the distal false lumen and constitute the leading cause of long term attrition in these patients.[117,123,199] Reported rates of patency of the false lumen varies between 70 and 100% in the literature even with the use of GRF glue.[73,131,200–202] A patent distal false lumen correlates with aneurysmal dilatation of the distal aorta,[200] late reoperation,[199] and death due to rupture.[87] Reported late mortality due to aortic rupture varies from 9.4 to 29% and reoperation rate from 13 to 30% at 5 to 10 years.[87,118,171,199] Use of the techniques outlined above has reduced the incidence of patency of the false lumen to less than 50% with associated improvement in survival and incidence of late events during follow-up.[74]

The importance of strict blood pressure control and careful follow-up of all patients with dissections of the aorta cannot be overemphasized. Therefore, "anti-impulse" therapy is maintained indefinitely. The follow-up starts at the discharge of the patient when baseline postoperative angiographic, CT and MRI studies are obtained, and noninvasive follow-up is continued on a regular schedule. In patients with stable repairs or distal aortas these studies are repeated on a yearly basis, otherwise closer follow-up with more frequent surveillance is indicated to determine the optimal time for elective surgical treatment during the chronic stage.

Chronic Dissections

Indications

Surgery for chronic dissection is generally performed for distal aorta related symptoms (primarily pain and other symptoms of expansion), due to dilatation of the distal false lumen and late aneurysm formation or for problems at the aortic root and chronic aortic insufficiency. In asymptomatic patients the most important indication for operation is the size (5 cm) and the rate of expansion of the distal aorta. The size recommendation is based on the observation that 88% of ruptures in chronic dissections occurred with aortic diameters less than 10 cm and 23% with less than 6 cm.[112,169] Likewise the diameter of the dissected aorta greater than 5 cm was found to be the most important predictor of late death in a series of medically treated patients.[47] Other indications in chronic ascending aortic dissections are "persistent or new cardiac complications and complications of previous aortic or heart operations."[112,203] In some cases irregular expansion with bulges in areas of local weakening of the aneurysmal wall may indicate need for early surgery. In recommending elective operations on the descending aorta for asymptomatic patients other factors besides the size of the aorta like the patients age, associated pulmonary dysfunction, or other medical conditions, required extent of the resection and the risk of postoperative paraplegia have to be seriously considered.[112]

Surgical Treatment

Chronic dissections usually require extensive aortic resection and reconstruction. Chronic type A dissections in most cases require composite graft replacement of the aortic valve and root (Fig. 138–11). In some chronic type A dissections a valve preserving root replacement may be possible. Not infrequently the ascending arch and the descending portions of the aorta have to be replaced because of significant dilatation of these areas. This is usually done with the staged replacement technique, "Elephant trunk," originally described by Borst et al[204,188] (Fig. 138–14A–C).

In chronic type B dissections, it is necessary to replace the entire descending aorta in most patients and thoracoabdominal aorta in some. In chronic dissections, perfusion of vital structures may be dependent on the persistent false lumen, necessitating direction of the flow into both true and false channels. This is generally accomplished by creating a generous communication between true and false lumens (fenestration) and performing the distal anastomosis to the outer wall of the chronically dissected aorta (Fig. 138–14A–C). Tissue friability in chronic dissections is not problematic; however, operative morbidity is higher in direct proportion to the extent of aortic resection.

RESULTS

Hospital Mortality

Advances in diagnosis, intensive care, pharmacology, anesthesia, and surgery have improved surgical mortality for aortic dissection. There have been significant reductions in the operative mortality for repair of type A dissection, a trend reported by many centers. (Baylor series period before 1986 33% after 1986 5%,[112] Stanford series to 7%,[168,205] Hannover series from 20 to 10.5% after 1986 for arch replacement,[175] and in our experience from 24 to 5% since 1986.) In fact operation in the recent era emerges as the most important determinant of operative risk and late survival in several series.[112,116] This undoubtedly reflects the maturing surgical understanding of the pathology and effective eradication of causes of proximal failure. The intangible factors of institutional and surgeon experience may also play a role in these improvements.[123] In most series, besides the year of the operation, the determinants of operative risk are extent of resection,[112,118,123] associated medical disease, and postoperative cardiac renal and neurological complications.[112]

Survival following medical and surgical treatment in acute type B dissection differed only slightly.[112,206–208] This also has shown considerable improvement. Mortality with medical treatment decreased from 25 to 30% to 10 to 15% currently,[112,209] and with surgical treatment from 45 to 50%[112,186] to 6 to 16%.[87,112,168] However 15 to 20% of patients "successfully" treated with medical therapy require later surgery.[168,205] In view of these current surgical mortality figures, achieved in spite of the increased risk of operation for complicated type B dissection, arguments in favor of early surgery in selected patients may be justified.

Long Term Survival

Several groups have reported long-term follow-up of patients with aortic dissections. DeBakey et al described the

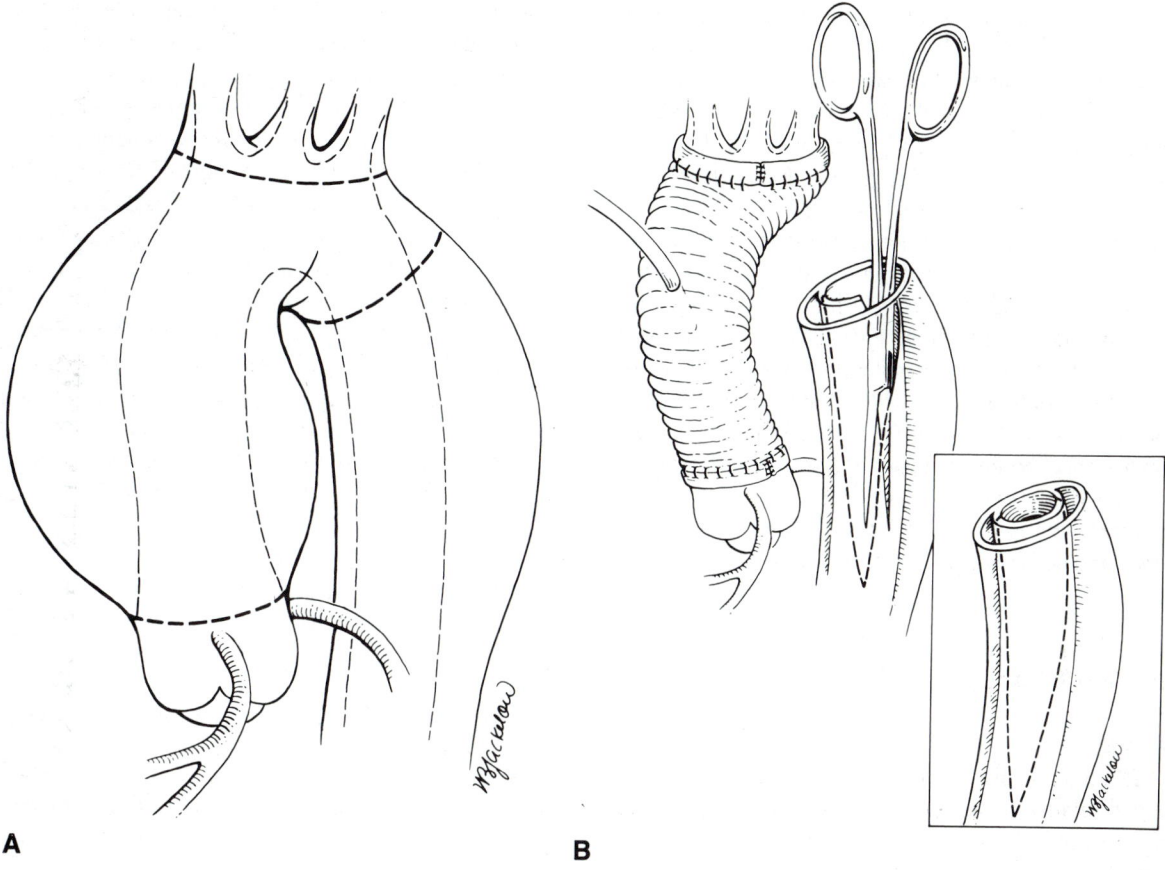

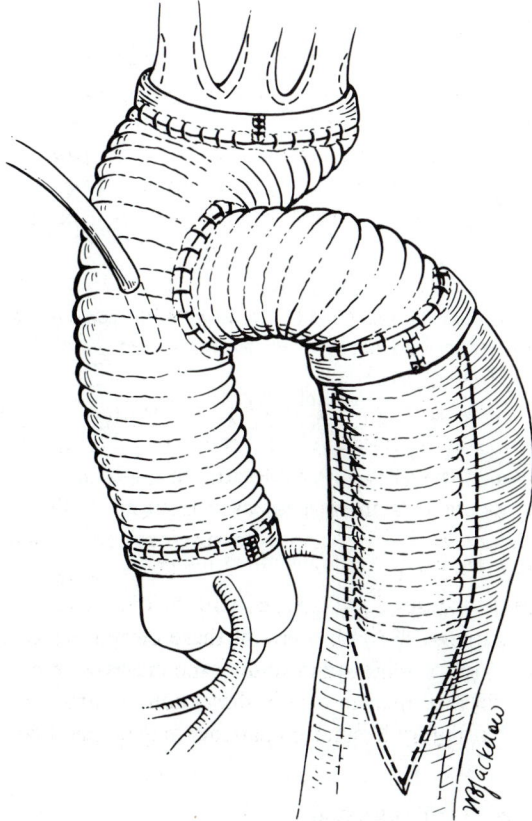

Figure 138–14. Chronic type A dissection with a competent aortic valve and dilatation of the ascending and descending aorta and the arch requiring replacement of these segments. Treatment with the modified "Elephant Trunk" method.[204]
A. Pathology showing the dilatation of the aorta; the dotted lines indicate the limits of the resection. **B.** Through median sternotomy the ascending aorta and the arch are replaced preserving the aortic valve. The arch anastomosis is made to the island of aortic tissue containing the origins of the brachiocephalic vessels during hypothermic circulatory arrest. At the completion of this anastomosis an arterial cannula is inserted into this graft and hypothermic antegrade cerebral perfusion started, while the distal body is not perfused during construction of the descending aortic anastomosis. This simple method of selective perfusion has helped reduce the prolonged circulatory arrest times necessary for these complex repairs. In the descending aorta the intimal flap is excised with long scissors, creating a generous communication between the false and true lumens. The inset shows the extent of the fenestration to assure perfusion of both lumens. **C.** A separate graft is then anastomosed to the narrowest segment of the proximal descending aorta allowing a length of the graft to hang down into the fenestrated area. The proximal end of this graft is connected to the ascending graft and antegrade perfusion and warming of the entire body carried out via the arterial cannula in the ascending aortic graft. In the second stage of the Elephant Trunk procedure through a left thoracotomy the descending aorta is opened, and the end of the graft in the descending aorta controlled and sutured to normal sized aorta distally.

20-year follow-up of 527 patients treated surgically, with overall survival at 5, 10, and 20 years of 57, 32, and 5%, respectively.[87] Significantly, subsequent development and rupture of an aneurysm resulted in 29.3% of late deaths, most commonly with distal aortic involvement in type A (30%) and type B (38%) dissections.[87] This indicates the important influence of the false lumen on survival. In our experience actuarial survival at 5 years following surgical treatment of type A dissection in discharged patients with a closed false lumen was 95% versus 76% with patent false lumen.[74] The Stanford group published actuarial survival data for 135 hospital survivors of surgical therapy, with follow-up extending to 15 years. Survival at 5 and 10 years was 82 and 64%, respectively, with a reoperation incidence of 13 and 23%, respectively. The overall rate of dissection-related death and reoperation was 5%/pt-y and 2%/pt-y, respectively.[118] In uncomplicated type B dissections the long-term results of medical and surgical treatment appear to be comparable (94, 87, and 32% survival at 1, 5, and 10 years, respectively, with medical and 90, 80, and 50% with surgical treatment).[113] However, 77% of all late deaths in these patients were due to residual aortic disease, cardiac causes, or sudden death, underscoring the extent to atherosclerotic involvement in this group.[113] These results can be improved upon only with scrupulous follow-up and timely intervention for developing aortic complications.

REFERENCES

1. Sorenson HR, Olsen H: Ruptured and dissecting aneurysms of the aorta: Incidence and prospects of surgery. *Acta Chir Scand* **128**:644, 1964

2. Shennan T: *Dissecting Aneurysms Special Report Medical Research Council Series No. 193.* London, His Majesty's Stationary Office, 1934

3. Laennec RTH: *Traite de L'Auscultation Mediate et des Maladies des Poumons et du Coeur,* 2nd ed, Vol. 2. Paris, Chaude, 1826, p 696, cited in ref 2

4. Leonard JC: Thomas Bevill Peacock and the early history of dissecting aneurysm. *Br Med J* **2**:260, 1979

5. Erdheim J: Medionecrosis aortae idiopathica cystica. *Virchows Arch Pathol Anat Physiol* **276**:187, 1930

6. Davy H, Gates M: Case of dissecting aneurysm of aorta. *Br Med J* **1**:471, 1922

7. Paullin JE, James DF: Dissecting aneurysm of aorta. *Postgrad Med* **4**:291, 1948

8. Gurin D, Bulmer JW, Derby R: Dissecting aneurysm of the aorta. Diagnosis and operative relief of acute arterial occlusion due to this cause. *NY State J Med* **35**:1200, 1935

9. Abbott OA: Clinical experiences with application of polythene cellophane upon aneurysms of thoracic vessels. *J Thorac Surg* **18**:435, 1949

10. DeBakey ME, Cooley DA, Creech O Jr: Surgical considerations of dissecting aneurysm of the aorta. *Ann Surg* **142**:586, 1955

11. Cooley DA, DeBakey ME, Morris GC Jr: Controlled extracorporeal circulation in surgical treatment of aortic aneurysm. *Ann Surg* **146**:473, 1957

12. DeBakey ME, Henly WS, Cooley DA, et al: Surgical management of dissecting aneurysms of the aorta. *J Thorac Cardiovasc Surg* **49**:130, 1965

13. Wheat MW, Palmer RF, Bartley TB, Seelman RC: Treatment of dissecting aneurysms of the aorta without surgery. *J Thorac Cardiovasc Surg* **50**:364, 1965

14. Burchell HB: Aortic dissection (dissecting hematoma; dissecting aneurysm of the aorta). *Circulation* **12**:1068, 1955

15. Hirst AE Jr, Johns VJ Jr, Kime SW: Dissecting aneurysm of the aorta: A review of 505 cases. *Medicine* **37**:217, 1958

16. Talbot S: Clinical features and prognosis of dissecting aneurysm and ruptured saccular aneurysms. *Chest* **66**:256, 1974

17. Miller DC, Stinson EB, Oyer PE, et al: Operative treatment of aortic dissections: Experience with 125 patients over a sixteen year period. *J Thorac Cardiovasc Surg* **78**:365, 1979

18. Larson EW, Edwards WD: Risk factors for aortic dissection: A necropsy study of 161 cases. *Am J Cardiol* **53**:849, 1984

19. Carlson RG, Lillehei CW, Edwards JE: Cystic medial necrosis of the ascending aorta in relation to age and hypertension. *Am J Cardiol* **25**:411, 1970

20. Nicod P, Bloor C, Godfrey M, et al: Familial aortic dissecting aneurysms. *J Am Coll Cardiol* **13**:811, 1989

21. Kontusaari S, Tromp G, Kuivaniemi H, et al: A mutation in the gene for type III procollagen (COL3AI) in a family with aortic aneurysms. *J Clin Invest* **86**:1465, 1990

22. Emanuel R, Ng RAL, Marcomichelakis J, et al: Forme frustes of Marfan's syndrome presenting with severe aortic regurgitation: Clinicogenetic study of 18 families. *Br Heart J* **39**:190, 1977

23. Hirst AE Jr, Gore I: Marfan's Syndrome: A review. *Prog Cardiovasc Dis* **16**:187, 1973

24. Kainulainen K, Pulkkinen L, Savolainen A, et al: Location on chromosome 15 of the gene defect causing Marfan syndrome. *N Engl J Med* **323**:935, 1990

25. Francke U, Furthmayr H: Genes and gene products involved in Marfan syndrome. *Sem Thorac Cardiovasc Surg* **5**:3, 1993

26. Murdoch JL, Walker BA, Halpern BL, et al: Life expectancy and causes of death in the Marfan syndrome. *N Engl J Med* **286**:804, 1972

27. Pyeritz RE: Predictors of the dissection of the ascending aorta in Marfan syndrome. *Circulation* **84**:351, 1991

28. Pyeritz RE: Marfan syndrome: Current and future clinical and genetic management of cardiovascular manifestations. *Sem Thorac Cardiovasc Surg* **5**:11, 1993

29. Marsalese DL, Moodie DS, Vacante M, et al: Marfan's syndrome: Natural history and long-term follow-up of cardiovascular involvement. *J Am Coll Cardiol* **14**:422, 1989

30. Seybold-Epting W, Meyer J, Hallman GL, Cooley DA: Surgical treatment of acute dissecting aneurysm of the ascending aorta. *J Cardiovasc Surg* **18**:43, 1977

31. Roberts CS, Roberts WC: Dissection of the aorta associated with congenital malformation of the aortic valve. *J Am Coll Cardiol* **17**:712, 1991

32. Heikkinen LO, Ala-Kulju KV, Salo JA: Dilatation of ascending aorta in patients with repaired coarctation. *Scand J Thorac Cardiovasc Surg* **25**:25, 1991

33. Edwards WD, Leaf DS, Edwards JE: Dissecting aortic aneurysm associated with congenital bicuspid aortic valve. *Circulation* **57**:1022, 1978

34. Muna WF, Spray TL, Morrow AG, Roberts WC: Aortic dissection after aortic valve replacement in patients with valvular aortic stenosis. *J Thorac Cardiovasc Surg* **74**:65, 1977

35. Kay JH, Dykstra PC, Tsuji HK: Retrograde ilioaortic dissection: A complication of common femoral artery perfusion during open heart surgery. *Am J Surg* **111**:464, 1966

36. Reinke RT, Harris RD, Klein AJ, Daily PO: Aortoiliac dissection due to aortic cannulation. *Ann Thorac Surg* **18**:295, 1974

37. Litchford B, Okies JE, Sugimura S, Starr A: Acute aortic dissection from cross-clamp injury. *J Thorac Cardiovasc Surg* **72**:709, 1976

38. Nicholson WJ, Crawley IS, Logue RB, et al: Aortic root dissection complicating coronary bypass surgery. *Am J Cardiol* **41**:103, 1978

39. Murphy DC, Carver JM, Jones EL: Recognition and management of ascending aortic dissection complicating cardiac surgical operations. *J Thorac Cardiovasc Surg* **85**:247, 1983

40. Jones EL, Craver JM, King SB, et al: Clinical anatomic and functional descriptors influencing morbidity, survival and adequacy or revascularization following coronary bypass. *Ann Surg* **192**:390, 1980

41. Kitchen DH: Dissecting aneurysm of the aorta in pregnancy. *J Obstet Gynecol Br Common* **81**:410, 1974

42. Cooke JP, Kazmier FJ, Orszulak TA: The penetrating aortic ulcer: Pathologic manifestations, diagnosis, and management. *Mayo Clin Proc* **63**:718, 1988

43. Walts AE, Dubois EL: Acute dissecting aneurysm of the aorta as the fatal event in systemic lupus erythematosus. *Am Heart J* **93**:378, 1977

44. Leonard JC, Hasleton PS: Dissecting aortic aneurysms: A clinicopathological study: I. Clinical and gross pathological findings. *Q J Med New Series* **XLVIII:** (No. 189):55, 1979

45. Strayer DS: Cystinosis and dissecting aortic aneurysm in a 7 year old boy. *Am J Dis Child* **133**:436, 1979

46. Lin AE, Lippe BM, Geffner ME, et al: Aortic dilation, dissection, and rupture in patients with Turner syndrome. *J Pediatr* **109**:820, 1986

47. Masuda Y, Yamada Z, Morooka N, et al: Prognosis of patients with medically treated aortic dissections. *Circulation* **84**:1117, 1991

48. Brindley P, Sternbridge VA: Aneurysms of the aorta, a clinicopathologic study of 369 necropsy cases. *Am J Pathol* **32**:67, 1956

49. DeBakey ME, Henly WS, Cooley DA, Crawford ES: Surgical treatment of dissecting aneurysm of the aorta. Analysis of seventy-two cases. *Circulation* **24**:290, 1961

50. Daily PO, Trueblood HW, Stinson EB, et al: Management of acute aortic dissections. *Ann Thorac Surg* **10**:237, 1970

51. Guilmet D, Bachet J, Goudot B, et al: Aortic dissection: Anatomic types and surgical approaches. *J Cardiovasc Surg Torino* **34**:23, 1993

52. Lansman SL, Ergin MA, Griepp RB: Treatment of acute aortic arch dissection [editorial]. *Ann Thorac Surg* **55**:816, 1993

53. Mohr-Kahaly S, Erbel R, Kearney P, et al: Aortic intramural hemorrhage visualized by transesophageal echocardiography: Findings and prognostic implications. *J Am Coll Cardiol* **23**:658, 1994

54. Lui RC, Menkis AH, McKenzie FN: Aortic dissection without intimal rupture: Diagnosis and management. *Ann Thorac Surg* **53**:886, 1992

55. Zotz RJ, Erbel R, Meyer J: Noncommunicating intramural hematoma: An indication of developing aortic dissection? *J Am Soc Echocardiogr* **4**:636, 1991

56. Ergin MA, O'Connor J, Guinto R, Griepp RB: Experience with profound hypothermia and circulatory arrest in the treatment of aneurysms of the aortic arch. Aortic Arch replacement for acute arch dissections. *J Thorac Cardiovasc Surg* **84**:649, 1982

57. Crawford ES, Kirklin JW, Naftel DC, et al: Surgery for acute dissection of ascending aorta. Should the arch be included? *J Thorac Cardiovasc Surg* **104**:46, 1992

58. Roberts CS, Roberts WC: Aortic dissection with the entrance tear in transverse aorta: Analysis of 12 autopsy patients. *Ann Thorac Surg* **50**:762, 1990

59. Roberts CS, Roberts WC: Aortic dissection with the entrance tear in abdominal aorta. *Am Heart J* **121**:1834, 1991

60. Liotta D, Hallman GL, Milam JD, Cooley DA: Surgical treatment of acute dissecting aneurysm of the ascending aorta. *Ann Thorac Surg* **12**:582, 1971

61. Symbas PN, Kelly TF, Vlasis SE, et al: Intimo-intimal intussusception and other unusual manifestations of aortic dissection. *J Thorac Cardiovasc Surg* **79**:926, 1980

62. Reitknecht FL, Bhayana JN, Lajos TZ: Circumferential intimal tear causing obstruction of the aortic arch: An unusual complication of aortic dissection. *Ann Thorac Surg* **46**:100, 1988

63. DeBakey ME, Lawrie G: Intimal intussusception: Unusual complication of dissecting aneurysm. *J Vasc Surg* **1**:566, 1984

64. Prokop EK, Palmer RF, Wheat MW: Hydrodynamic forces in dissecting aneurysm: In-vitro studies in a tygon model and in dog aortas. *Circ Res* **27**:121, 1970

65. Wheat MW Jr, Palmer RF: Dissecting aneurysms of the aorta: Present status of drug versus surgical therapy. *Prog Cardiovasc Dis* **11**:198–210, 1968

66. Laas J, Heinemann M, Schaefers HJ, et al: Management of thoracoabdominal malperfusion in aortic dissection. *Circulation* **84**:11120, 1991

67. Fann JI, Sarris GE, Mitchell RS, et al: Treatment of patients with aortic dissection presenting with peripheral vascular complications. *Ann Surg* **212**:705, 1990

68. Cambria RP, Brewster DC, Gertler J, et al: Vascular complications associated with spontaneous aortic dissection. *J Vasc Surg* **7**:199, 1988

69. Roberts WC: The aorta: Its acquired diseases and their consequences as viewed from a morphologic perspective. In Lindsay J Jr, Hurst JW (eds): *The Aorta*. New York, Grune & Stratton, 1979, p 51

70. Elefteriades JA, Hammond GL, Gusberg RJ, et al: Fenestration revisited. A safe and effective procedure for descending aortic dissection. *Arch Surg* **125**:786, 1990

71. Erbel R, Oelert H, Meyer J, et al: Effect of medical and surgical therapy on aortic dissection evaluated by transesophageal echocardiography. Implications for prognosis and therapy. The European Cooperative Study Group on Echocardiography [see comments]. *Circulation* **87**:1604, 1993

72. Roudaut RP, Marcaggi XL, Deville C, et al: Value of transesophageal echocardiography combined with computed tomography for assessing repaired type A aortic dissection. *Am J Cardiol* **70**:1468, 1992

73. Turley K, Ullyot DJ, Godwin JD, et al: Repair of dissection of the thoracic aorta. Evaluation of false lumen utilizing computed tomography. *J Thorac Cardiovasc Surg* **81**:61, 1981

74. Ergin MA, Phillips RA, Galla JD, et al: Significance of distal false lumen after Type A dissection repair. *Ann Thorac Surg* **57**:820, 1994

75. Dinsmore RE, Willerson JT, Buckley MJ: Dissecting aneurysm of the aorta. Aortographic features affecting prognosis. *Radiology* **105**:567, 1972

76. Schlatmann TJM, Becker AE: Histologic changes in the normal aging aorta: Implications for dissecting aortic aneurysm. *Am J Cardiol* **39**:13, 1977

77. Schlattmann TJM, Becker AE: Pathogenesis of dissecting aneurysm of aorta: Comparative histopathologic study of significance of medical changes. *Am J Cardiol* **39**:21, 1977

78. Hirst AE, Gore I: Is cystic medionecrosis the cause of dissecting aortic aneurysm. *Circulation* **53**:915, 1976

79. Stovin PGI: Editorial: Dissecting the dissecting aneurysm. *Thorax* **33**:273, 1978

80. Rottino A: Medial degeneration of the aorta. A study of two hundred and ten routine autopsy specimens by a serial block method. *Arch Pathol* **28**:377, 1939

81. Anagnostopoulos CE: *Acute Aortic Dissections*. Baltimore, University Park Press, 1975, p 70

82. Fann JI, Sarris GE, Miller DC, et al: Surgical management of acute aortic dissection complicated by stroke. *Circulation* **80**:1257,1989

83. Anagnostopoulos CE, Prabhakar MJS, Kittle CP: Aortic dissections and dissecting aneurysms. *Am J Cardiol* **30**:263, 1972

84. Rose EA, McNicholas KW, Bethea MC, et al: Renovascular hypertension following surgical repair of dissecting aneurysm of the thoracic aorta. *Surgery* **83**:235, 1978

85. Roan PG, Buja LM, Grammer JC: Ascending aortic obstruction produced by dissected intimal flap. *Br Heart J* **46**:452, 1981

86. d'Allarnes CL, Blondeau PH, Piwnica A, et al: Surgery for aortic dissection: 53 operated cases with 32 in the acute phase. *J Cardiovasc Surg* **18**:261, 1977

87. DeBakey ME, McCollum CH, Crawford ES, et al: Dissection and dissecting aneurysms of the aorta: Twenty year follow-up of five hundred twenty-seven patients treated surgically. *Surgery* **92**: 1118, 1982

88. Scott J, Humphreys DR: Dissecting aortic aneurysm and disseminated intravascular coagulation. *Br Med J* **1**:24, 1977

89. Yacoub MH, Schottenfeld M, Kittle CF: Hematoma of the interatrial septum with heart block secondary to dissecting aneurysm of the aorta: A clinicopathologic entity. *Circulation* **46**:537, 1972

90. Slater EE, DeSanctis RW: Clinical recognition of dissecting aortic aneurysm. *Am J Med* **60**:625, 1976

91. Itzchak Y, Rosenthal T, Adar R, et al: Dissecting aneurysm of thoracic aorta: Reappraisal of radiologic diagnosis. *Am J Roentgenol* **125**:559,1975

92. Adachi H, Omoto R, Kyo S, et al: Emergency surgical intervention of acute aortic dissection with the rapid diagnosis by transesophageal echocardiography. *Circulation* **84**:III14, 1991

93. Mohr Kahaly S, Erbel R, Rennollet H, et al: Ambulatory follow-up of aortic dissection by transesophageal two-dimensional and color-coded Doppler echocardiography. *Circulation* **80**:24, 1989

94. Erbel R, Engberding R, Daniel W, et al: Echocardiography in diagnosis of aortic dissection. *Lancet* **1**:457, 1989

95. Laas J, Schluter G, Daniel W, et al: Acute type-A dissection of the aorta: Which diagnostic modes remain for surgical indication? *Eur J Cardiothorac Surg* **1**:169, 1987

96. Weintraub AR, Schwartz SL, Pandian NG, et al: Evaluation of acute aortic dissection by intravascular ultrasonography. *N Engl J Med* **323**:1566, 1990

97. Godwin JD, Herfkens RL, Skiodebrand CG, et al: Evaluation of dissections and aneurysms of the thoracic aorta by conventional and dynamic CT scanning. *Radiology* **136**:125, 1980

98. Cigarroa JE, Isselbacher EM, De Sanctis RW, Eagle KA: Diagnostic imaging in the evaluation of suspected aortic dissection. Old standards and new directions. *N Engl J Med* **328**:35, 1993

99. Hamada S, Takamiya M, Kimura K, et al: Type A aortic dissection: Evaluation with ultrafast CT. *Radiology* **183**:155, 1992

100. Rubin GD, Dake MD, Napel SA, et al: Three-dimensional spiral CT angiography of the abdomen: Initial clinical experience. *Radiology* **186**:147, 1993

101. Geisinger MA, Risius B, O'Donnell JA, et al: Thoracic aortic dissections: Magnetic resonance imaging. *Radiology* **155**:407, 1985

102. Akins EA, Carmichael MJ, Hill JA, Mancuso AA: Preoperative evaluation of the thoracic aorta using MRI and angiography. *Ann Thorac Surg* **44**:499, 1987

103. Nienaber CA, Spielmann RP, von Kodolitsch Y, et al: Diagnosis of thoracic aortic dissection. Magnetic resonance imaging versus transesophageal echocardiography. *Circulation* **85**:434, 1992

104. Di Cesare E, Di Renzi P, Pavone P, et al: Postsurgical follow-up of aortic dissections by MRI. *Eur J Radiol* **13**:27, 1991

105. Mendelson DS, Apter S, Mitty HA, et al: Residual dissection of the thoracic aorta after repair: MRI-angiographic correlation. *Comput Med Imaging Graph* **15**:31, 1991

106. Goldman AP, Kotler MN, Scanlon MH, et al: Magnetic resonance imaging and two-dimensional echocardiography. Alternative approach to aortography in diagnosis of aortic dissecting aneurysm. *Am J Med* **80**:1225, 1986

107. Rackson ME, Lossef SV, Sos TA: Renal artery stenosis in patients with aortic dissection: Increased prevalence. *Radiology* **177**:555, 1990

108. Kern MJ, Serota H, Callicoat P, et al: Use of coronary arteriography in the preoperative management of patients undergoing urgent repair of the thoracic aorta. *Am Heart J* **119**:143, 1990

109. Saito S, Arai H, Kim K, et al: Percutaneous fenestration of dissecting intima with a transseptal needle. A new therapeutic technique for visceral ischemia complicating acute aortic dissection. *Cathet Cardiovasc Diagn* **26**:130, 1992

110. Faykus MH Jr, Hiette P, Koopot R: Percutaneous fenestration of a type I aortic dissection for relief of lower extremity ischemia. *Cardiovasc Intervent Radiol* **15**:183, 1992

111. Williams DM, Brothers TE, Messina LM: Relief of mesenteric ischemia in type III aortic dissection with percutaneous fenestration of the aortic septum. *Radiology* **174**:450, 1990

112. Svensson LG, Crawford ES, Hess KR, et al: Dissection of the aorta and dissecting aortic aneurysms. Improving early and long-term surgical results. *Circulation* **82**:IV24, 1990

113. Glower DD, Fann JI, Speier RH, et al: Comparison of medical and surgical therapy for uncomplicated descending aortic dissection. *Circulation* **82**:IV39, 1990

114. Lilienfeld DE, Gunderson PD, Sprafka JM, et al: Epidemiology of aortic aneurysms: I. Mortality trends in the United States, 1951 to 1981. *Arteriosclerosis* **7**:637, 1987

115. Nienaber CA, von Kodolitsch Y: Metaanalyse zur Prognose der thorakalen Aortendissektion: Letalitat im Wandel der letzten vier Jahrzehnte. *Herz* **17**:398, 1992

116. Miller DC: Surgical management of acute aortic dissection: New data. *Sem Thorac Cardiovasc Surg* **3**:225, 1991

117. Bachet JE, Termignon JL, Dreyfus G, et al: Aortic dissection: Prevalence, cause, and results of late reoperations. *J Thorac Cardiovasc Surg* **108**:199, 1994

118. Haverich A, Miller DC, Scott WC, et al:Acute and chronic aortic dissections—determinants of long-term outcome for operative survivors. *Circulation* **72**:II22, 1985

119. Galloway AC, Colvin SB, Grossi EA, et al: Surgical repair of type A aortic dissection by the circulatory arrest-graft inclusion technique in sixty-six patients. *J Thorac Cardiovasc Surg* **105**:781, 1993

120. Kouchoukos NT, Wareing TH, Murphy SF, Perrillo JB: Sixteen-year experience with aortic root replacement. Results of 172 operations. *Ann Surg* **214**:308, 1991

121. Rofsky NM, Weinreb JC, Grossi EA, et al: Aortic aneurysm and dissection: Normal MR imaging and CT findings after surgical repair with the continuous-suture graft-inclusion technique. *Radiology* **186**:195, 1993

122. Massimo CG, Presenti LF, Favi PP, et al: Excision of the aortic wall in the surgical treatment of acute type-A aortic dissection. *Ann Thorac Surg* **50**:274, 1990

123. Glower DD, Speier RH, White WD, et al: Management and long-term outcome of aortic dissection. *Ann Surg* **214**:31, 1991

124. Carrel T, Pasic M, Jenni R, et al: Reoperations after operation on the thoracic aorta: Etiology, surgical techniques, and prevention. *Ann Thorac Surg* **56**:259, 1993

125. Jex RK, Schaff HV, Piehler JM, et al: Repair of ascending aortic dissection. Influence of associated aortic valve insufficiency on early and late results. *J Thorac Cardiovasc Surg* **93**:375, 1987

126. Olinger GN, Schweiger JA, Galbraith TA: Primary repair of acute ascending aortic dissection. *Ann Thorac Surg* **44**:389, 1987

127. Hufnagel CA, Conrad PW: Intimo-intimal intussusception in dissecting aneurysms. *Am J Surg* **103**:727, 1962

128. Seguin JR, Frapier JM, Colson P, Chaptal PA: Fibrin sealant improves surgical results of type A acute aortic dissections. *Ann Thorac Surg* **52**:745, 1991

129. Guilmet D, Bachet J, Goudet B: Use of biological glue in acute aortic dissection: Preliminary results with a new surgical technique. *J Thorac Cardiovasc Surg* **77**:516, 1979

130. Laas J, Jurmann MJ, Heinemann M, Borst HG: Advances in aortic arch surgery. *Ann Thorac Surg* **53**:227, 1992

131. Bachet J, Goudot B, Teodori G, et al: Surgery of type A acute aortic dissection with Gelatine-Resorcine-Formol biological glue: A twelve-year experience. *J Cardiovasc Surg (Torino)* **31**:263, 1990

132. Dureau G, Villard J, George M, et al: New surgical technique for the operative management of acute dissections of the ascending aorta: Report of two cases. *J Thorac Cardiovasc Surg* **76**:385, 1978

133. Ablaza SG, Gosh SC, Grana VP: Use of a ringed intraluminal graft in the surgical treatment of dissecting aneurysms of the thoracic aorta: A new technique. *J Thorac Cardiovasc Surg* **76**:390, 1978

134. Weinschelbaum EE, Schamun C, Caramutti V, et al: Surgical treatment of acute type A dissecting aneurysm, with preservation of the native aortic valve and use of biologic glue. Follow-up to 6 years. *J Thorac Cardiovasc Surg* **103**:369, 1992

135. Vasseur B, Hammond GL: New technique for repair of ascending thoracic aortic dissections. *Ann Thorac Surg* **47**:318, 1989

136. Westaby S, Parry A, Giannopoulos N, Pillai R: Replacement of the thoracic aorta with collagen-impregnated woven Dacron grafts. Early results. *J Thorac Cardiovasc Surg* **106**:427, 1993

137. Hirt SW, Aoki M, Demertzis S, et al: Comparative in vivo study on the healing qualities of four different presealed vascular prostheses. *J Vasc Surg* **17**:538, 1993

138. Jonas RA, Schoen FJ, Levy RJ, Castaneda AR: Biological sealants and knitted Dacron: Porosity and histological comparisons of vascular graft materials with and without collagen and fibrin glue pretreatments. *Ann Thorac Surg* **41**:657, 1986

139. Cooley DA, Livesay JJ: Technique of "open" distal anastomosis for ascending and transverse arch resection. *Cardiovasc Dis Bull Texas Heart Inst* **8**:421, 1981

140. Pappas G, Starzl TE: Retrograde false channel perfusion: A complication of cardiopulmonary bypass during repair of dissecting aneurysms. *Ann Thorac Surg* **9**:263, 1970

141. Kyo S, Takamoto S, Omoto R, et al: Intraoperative echocardiography for diagnosis and treatment of aortic dissection. Utility of color flow mapping for surgical decision making in acute stage. *Herz* **17**:377, 1992

142. Najafi H, Dye WS, Javid H, et al: Acute aortic regurgitation secondary to aortic dissection: Surgical management without valve replacement. *Ann Thorac Surg* **14**:474, 1972

143. Collins JJ, Cohn LH: Reconstruction of the aortic valve: Correcting valve incompetence due to acute dissecting aneurysm. *Arch Surg* **106**:35, 1973

144. Lemole GM, Strong MD, Spagna PM, Karmilowicz NP: Improved results for dissecting aneurysms. Intraluminal sutureless prosthesis. *J Thorac Cardiovasc Surg* **83**:249, 1982

145. Lansman SL, Ergin MA, Galla JD, et al: Intraluminal graft repair of ascending, arch descending and thoracoabdominal aortic segments for dissecting and aneurysmal disease: Long-term follow-up. *Sem Thorac Cardiovasc Surg* **3**:180, 1991

146. Ergin MA, Galla JD, Lansman S, Griepp RB: Acute dissections of the aorta. Current surgical treatment. *Surg Clin North Am* **65**:721, 1985

147. Mazzucotelli JP, Deleuze PH, Baufreton C, et al: Preservation of the aortic valve in acute aortic dissection: Long-term echocardiographic assessment and clinical outcome. *Ann Thorac Surg* **55**:1513, 1993

148. Fann JI, Glower DD, Miller DC, et al: Preservation of aortic valve in type A aortic dissection complicated by aortic regurgitation. *J Thorac Cardiovasc Surg* **102**:62, 1991

149. Borst HG, Laas J, Frank G, Haverich A: Surgical decision making in acute aortic dissection type A. *Thorac Cardiovasc Surg* **35**(2):134, 1987

150. David TE, Feindel CM: An aortic valve-sparing operation for patients with aortic incompetence and aneurysm of the ascending aorta. *J Thorac Cardiovasc Surg* **103**:617, 1992

151. Crawford ES, Crawford JL, Safi HJ, Coselli JS: Redo operations for recurrent aneurysmal disease of the ascending aorta and transverse aortic arch. *Ann Thorac Surg* **40**:439, 1985

152. Karck M, Laas J, Heinemann M, Borst HG: Long-term follow-up after separate replacement of the aortic valve and ascending aorta. *Herz* **17**:394, 1992

153. Lawrie GM, Earle N, De Bakey ME: Long-term fate of the aortic root and aortic valve after ascending aneurysm surgery. *Ann Surg* **217**:711, 1993

154. Bentall H, Debono A: A technique for complete replacement of the ascending aorta. *Thorax* **23**:338, 1968

155. Cabrol C, Pavie A, Mesnildrey P, et al: Long-term results with total

156. Svensson LG, Crawford ES, Hess KR, et al: Composite valve graft replacement of the proximal aorta: Comparison of techniques in 348 patients. *Ann Thorac Surg* **54**:427, 1992

157. Borst HG, Laas J, Heinemann M: Type A aortic dissection: Diagnosis and management of malperfusion phenomena. *Sem Thorac Cardiovasc Surg* **3**:238, 1991

158. Katz NM, Blackstone EJ, Kirklin JW, et al: Incremental risk factors for spinal cord injury following operation for acute traumatic aortic transection. *J Thorac Cardiovasc Surg* **81**:669, 1981

159. Gott VL: Heparinized shunts for thoracic vascular operations (editorial). *Ann Thorac Surg* **14**:219, 1972

160. Oliver HF, Maher TD, Liebler GA, et al: Use of the Biomedicus Centrifugal pump in traumatic tears of the thoracic aorta. *Ann Thorac Surg* **38**:586, 1984

161. Ergin MA, Galla JD, Lansman SL, et al: Distal perfusion methods for surgery of the descending aorta. *Sem Thorac Cardiovasc Surg* **3**:293, 1991

162. Kouchoukos NT, Wareing TH, Izumoto H, et al: Elective hypothermic cardiopulmonary bypass and circulatory arrest for spinal cord protection during operations on the thoracoabdominal aorta. *J Thorac Cardiovasc Surg* **99**:659, 1990

163. Ergin MA, Galla JD, Lansman SL, et al: Hypothermic circulatory arrest in operations on the thoracic aorta: Determinants of operative mortality and neurologic outcome. *J Thorac Cardiovasc Surg* **107**:788, 1994

164. Elefteriades JA, Hartleroad J, Gusberg RJ, et al: Long-term experience with descending aortic dissection: The complication-specific approach. *Ann Thorac Surg* **53**:11, 1992

165. Williams DM, Andrews JC, Marx MV, Abrams GD: Creation of reentry tears in aortic dissection by means of percutaneous balloon fenestration: Gross anatomic and histologic considerations. *J Vasc Interv Radiol* **4**:75, 1993

166. Carrel T, Pasic M, Vogt P, et al: Retrograde ascending aortic dissection: A diagnostic and therapeutic challenge. *Eur J Cardiothorac Surg* **7**:146, 1993

167. Walterbusch G, Oelert H, Borst HG: Restoration of cerebral blood flow by extraanatomic bypass in acute aortic dissection. *J Thorac Cardiovasc Surg* **32**:381, 1984

168. Miller DC, Mitchell RS, Oyer PE, et al: Independent determinants of operative mortality for patients with aortic dissections. *Circulation* **70**:I153, 1984

169. Svensson LG, Crawford ES, Hess KR, et al: Dissection of the aorta and dissecting aortic aneurysms. Improving early and long-term surgical results. *Circulation* **82**:IV24, 1990

170. Ikonomidis JS, Weisel RD, Mouradian MS, et al: Thoracic aortic surgery. *Circulation* **84**:III1, 1991

171. Massimo CG, Presenti LF, Marranci P, et al: Extended and total aortic resection in the surgical treatment of acute type A aortic dissection: Experience with 54 patients. *Ann Thorac Surg* **46**:420, 1988

172. Bachet J, Teodori G, Goudot B, et al: Replacement of the transverse aortic arch during emergency operations for type A acute aortic dissection. Report of 26 cases. *J Thorac Cardiovasc Surg* **96**:878, 1988

173. Lansman SL, Raissi S, Ergin MA, Griepp RB: Urgent operation for acute transverse aortic arch dissection. *J Thorac Cardiovasc Surg* **97**:334, 1989

174. Yun KL, Glower DD, Miller DC, et al: Aortic dissection resulting from tear of transverse arch: Is concomitant arch repair warranted? *J Thorac Cardiovasc Surg* **102**:355, 1991

175. Heinemann M, Laas J, Jurmann M, et al: Surgery extended into the aortic arch in acute type A dissection. Indications, techniques, and results. *Circulation* **84**:III25, 1991

176. Svensson LG, Crawford ES, Coselli JS, et al: Impact of cardiovascular operation on survival in the Marfan patient. *Circulation* **80**:I233, 1989

177. Pasic M, von Segesser L, Carrel T, et al: Surgical treatment of car-

diovascular complications in Marfan syndrome: A 27-year experience. *Eur J Cardiothorac Surg* **6:**149, 1992

178. Carpentier AF, Deloche A, Fabiani JN, et al: New surgical approach to aortic dissection. Flow reversal and thromboexclusion. *J Thorac Cardiovasc Surg* **81:**659, 1981

179. Cabrol CE, Gandjbakhch I, Pavie A, et al: Surgical treatment of aortic dissection at La Pitie Hospital. *Sem Thorac Cardiovasc Surg* **3:**245, 1991

180. Morishita Y, Tabata F, Saigenji H, Taira A: Disseminated intravascular coagulopathy associated with thromboexclusion for dissecting aortic aneurysm. *J Cardiovasc Surg (Torino)* **27:**731, 1986

181. Carpentier A:Thromboexclusion: An alternative for type B dissection. *Sem Thorac Cardiovasc Surg* **3:**242, 1991

182. Ergin MA, O'Connor J, Blanche C, Griepp RB: Use of stapling instruments in surgery for aneurysms of the aorta. *Ann Thorac Surg* **36:**161, 1983

183. Lawson RA, Fenn A: Dissection of an aneurysmal ascending aorta in association with coarctation of the aorta. *Thorax* **34:**5, 1979

184. Hovaguimian H, Aru GM, Floten HS: Acute type I aortic dissection with coarctation of the aorta: Discussion of management and the report of a successful brain perfusion across an aortic coarctation [letter]. *J Thorac Cardiovasc Surg* **100:**152, 1990

185. Sampath R, O'Conner WN, Noonan JA, Todd EP: Management of ascending aortic aneurysm complicating coarctation of the aorta. *Ann Thorac Surg* **34:**125, 1982

186. Doroghazi RM, Slater EE, De Sanctis RW, et al: Long-term survival of patients with treated aortic dissection. *J Am Coll Cardiol* **3:**1026, 1984

187. Gott VL, Pyeritz RE, Cameron DE, et al: Composite graft repair of Marfan aneurysm of the ascending aorta: Results in 100 patients. *Ann Thorac Surg* **52:**38, 1991

188. Crawford ES, Coselli JS, Svensson LG, et al: Diffuse aneurysmal disease (chronic aortic dissection, Marfan, and mega aorta syndromes) and multiple aneurysm. Treatment by subtotal and total aortic replacement emphasizing the elephant trunk operation. *Ann Surg* **211:**521, 1990

189. Treasure T: Elective replacement of the aortic root in Marfan's syndrome [editorial]. *Br Heart J* **69:**101, 1993

190. el Habbal MH: Cardiovascular manifestations of Marfan's syndrome in the young. *Am Heart J* **123:**752, 1992

191. Shores J, Berger KR, Murphy EA, Pyeritz RE: Progression of aortic dilatation and the benefit of long-term B-adrenergic blockade in Marfan's syndrome. *N Engl J Med* **330:**1335, 1994

192. Fuster V, Ip JH: Medical aspects of acute aortic dissection. *Sem Thorac Cardiovasc Surg* **3:**219, 1991

193. Sutsch G, Jenni R, von Segesser L, Turina M: Predictability of aortic dissection as a function of aortic diameter. *Eur Heart J* **12:**1247, 1991

194. Michel PL, Acar J, Chomette G, Lung B: Degenerative aortic regurgitation. *Eur Heart J* **12:**875, 1991

195. Crawford ES, Svensson LG, Coselli JS, et al: Surgical treatment of aneurysm and/or dissection of the ascending aorta, transverse aortic arch, and ascending aorta and transverse aortic arch. Factors influencing survival in 717 patients. *J Thorac Cardiovasc Surg* **98:**659, 1989

196. Kouchoukos NT: Composite graft replacement of the ascending aorta and aortic valve with the inclusion-wrap and open techniques. *Sem Thorac Cardiovasc Surg* **3:**171, 1991

197. Carrel T, von Segesser L, Jenni R, et al: Dealing with dilated ascending aorta during aortic valve replacement: Advantages of conservative surgical approach. *Eur J Cardiothorac Surg* **5:**137, 1991

198. Svensson LG, Crawford ES: Aortic dissection and aortic aneurysm surgery: Clinical observations, experimental investigations, and statistical analyses. Part II. *Curr Probl Surg* **29:**913, 1992

199. Heinemann M, Laas J, Karck M, Borst HG: Thoracic aortic aneurysms after acute type A aortic dissection: Necessity for follow-up. *Ann Thorac Surg* **49:**580, 1990

200. Cachera JP, Vouhe PR, Loisance DY, et al: Surgical management of acute dissections involving the ascending aorta. Early and late results in 38 patients. *J Thorac Cardiovasc Surg* **82:**576, 1981

201. Yamaguchi T, Guthaner DF, Wexler L: Natural history of the false channel of type A aortic dissection after surgical repair: CT study. *Radiology* **170:**743, 1989

202. Gustavsson CG, Gustafson A, Albrechtsson U, et al: Diagnosis and management of acute aortic dissection, clinical and radiological follow-up. *Acta Med Scand* **223:**247, 1988

203. Crawford ES, Svensson LG, Coselli JS, et al: Aortic dissection and dissecting aortic aneurysms. *Ann Surg* **208:**254, 1988

204. Borst HG, Frank G, Schaps D: Treatment of extensive aortic aneurysms by a new multiple-stage approach. *J Thorac Cardiovasc Surg* **95:**11, 1988

205. Miller DC: Surgical management of aortic dissections: Indications, perioperative management and long-term results. In Doroghazi RM, Slater EF (eds): *Aortic Dissection.* New York, McGraw-Hill, 1983, p 193

206. Eagle KA, DeSanctis RW: Aortic dissection. *Curr Probl Cardiol* **14:**225, 1989

207. DeSanctis RW, Doroghazi RM, Austen GW, Buckley MD: Aortic dissection. *N Engl J Med* **317:**1060, 1987

208. Applebaum A, Karp RB, Kirklin JW: Ascending vs. descending aortic dissections. *Ann Surg* **183:**296, 1976

209. Tanaka K, Teruo T, Sasaki K, et al: Medical vs surgical treatment of acute aortic dissection in an intensive care unit. *Jpn Circ J* **55:**815, 1991

139

The Pericardium

Alden H. Harken, Alden W. Hall, and Graeme L. Hammond

HISTORICAL NOTE

Operations on the pericardium date back to Galen (A.D. 129–200), who described the treatment of two patients with apparent supperative pericarditis by surgical drainage.[1] Congenital absence of the pericardium was first described by Columbo in 1559 and then by Baille in 1793.[2] The original description of the paradoxical pulse with tamponade was by Adolph Kussmaul.[3] The modern treatment of pericardial disease, particularly constrictive pericarditis, is linked with the names of many surgical pioneers including Rehn, Sauerbruch, and Schmieden.[4] Weill, in 1895, first recognized that the rational treatment of constrictive pericarditis was within the possibilities of surgery. This was translated by Churchill in 1929 as follows: "After the adhesions have reached a fibrous stage, they act independently of their cause, and medical measures are illusory. No one has ventured to attempt a debridement on such a case, less perhaps from resignation than from the uncertainty of diagnosis. There would be good reason to make an attempt of this kind aimed at liberating a part of the heart, for example the apex and anterior surface. Surgery will one day deliver the heart from the shell that strangles it."[4] Delorme demonstrated the feasibility of a pericardiectomy by dissection of autopsy material.[5] In 1902 Brauer[6] introduced his operation of precardial thoracolysis, a much simpler and technically less hazardous operation. G. Rehn in 1920[7] and Volhard and Schmieden[8] in 1923 each reported a small series of cases. In the United States, the first completely successful recorded case was that of Churchill, performed in 1928.[4] The treatment of pericardial disease moved on rapidly after these important and significant events.

ANATOMY AND FUNCTION

The pericardium—like the pleura and peritoneum—consists of two mesothelial-lined tissue layers. The visceral pericardium is synonymous with the epicardium. Except in disease, the visceral pericardium has little clinical significance. The parietal pericardium is typically a thin, tough fibrous tissue layer separated from the epicardium by several milliliters of lubricating fluid. The heart moves freely in the pericardial space. The parietal pericardium attaches to the ascending aorta superiorly just below the innominate vein. It fixes across the superior vena cava (SVC) just above the sinoatrial node, then courses down over the right superior and inferior pulmonary veins to encircle the inferior vena cava (IVC). Thus, the surgeon should be able to pass a clamp completely around the IVC *inside* the pericardial space by cutting only a thin bit of coapted pericardial tissue posterior to the IVC. From the IVC, the pericardial attachment courses above the atrioventricular groove, attaching to the left atrium. This is important when explanting a diseased heart prior to cardiac transplantation. The surgeon can easily leave a 1-cm rim of left atrium (below the pericardial attachment) for anastomosis to the donor heart.

The parietal pericardium is sturdy, tough, and noncompliant. Thus, it capably secures the heart in the middle mediastinum. Should fluid accumulate in the pericardial space, however, it can push in against the compliant right atrium and right ventricle much more easily than it can push out against the stiff pericardium (Fig. 139–1A,B). This clinically important (and relatively common) postoperative cardiac surgical phenomenon is important to understand. A small elevation in pericardial fluid increases the intraperi-

2299

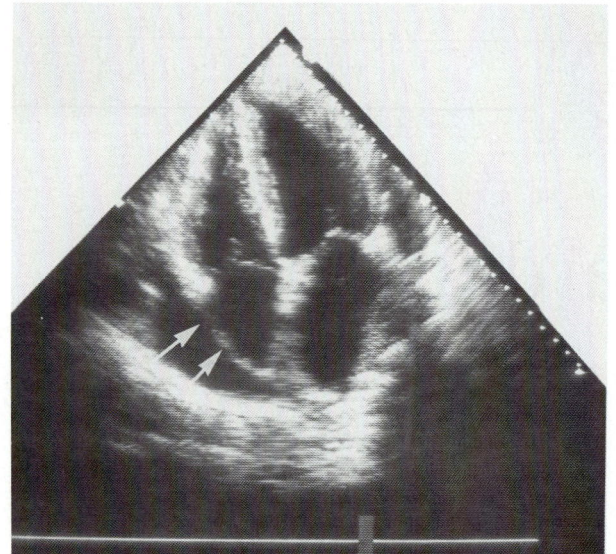

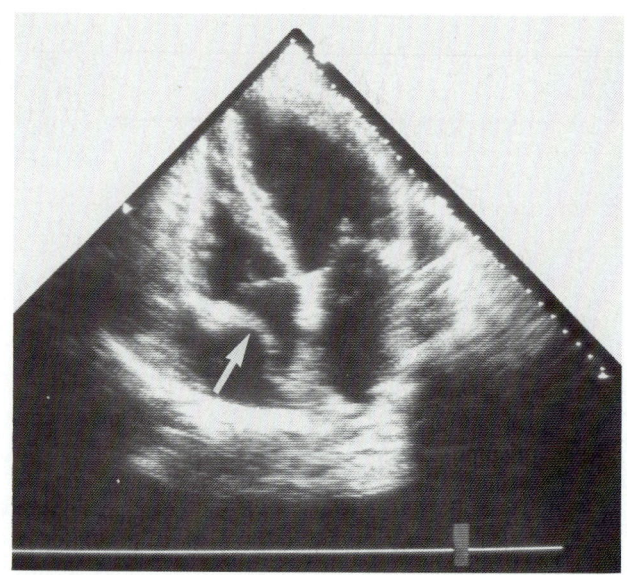

A   **B**

Figure 139–1. Transthoracic echocardiography provides an apical four-chamber view. **A.** Systolic frame depicting moderately large pericardial effusion. Arrows indicate right atrial wall during systole. **B.** Diastolic frame from the same patient as **A.** Arrow reveals right atrial collapse due to diastolic compression from pericardial fluid. Note that this is *early* "pericardial tamponade" in that there is minimal leftward shift of the interventricular septum. This patient was able to compensate completely and exhibited negligible hemodynamic compromise.

cardial pressure negligibly (Fig. 139–2). As soon as the elastic limit of the pericardium is exceeded, however, the pressure shoots up dramatically. A patient may, therefore, acutely accumulate a small amount of pericardial fluid with a big increase in pressure. Conversely, the slow development of a large chronic pericardial effusion may produce negligible hemodynamic consequences (Fig. 139–3). It is very important to recognize that pericardial fluid volume and pericardial pressure are *not linearly related*. For practical purposes, we will define a "pericardial effusion" as an abnormal accumulation of fluid with negligible hemodynamic sequelae. Similarly, "tamponade" requires clinical definition and is fluid (either a lot or a little) under suffi-

cient pressure to inflict hemodynamic consequences. Obviously, the spectrum between an effusion and tamponade is a continuum. But, a "pericardial effusion" is an anatomic diagnosis while "pericardial tamponade" is a physiologic one.

The dynamic orientation of parietal pericardial fibroelastic elements reduces friction and the serosal cell microvilli facilitate fluid and ion exchange.[9] Cardiopericardial lymphatics drain fluid from the subepicardium into mediastinal nodes and ultimately via the thoracic duct back into the venous system.[10] Pericarditis, resulting in fluid accumulation, typically results from inflammation of both the pericardium and the underlying myocardium. As the cardiopericardial lymphatics become progressively clogged with

Figure 139–2. In a healthy person (solid line) the pericardial space will accept 20 or 30 mL of fluid with a negligible increase in pericardial pressure. When the elastic limit of the pericardial space is reached however, small additional fluid volume raises the pressure dramatically. In a patient who has gradually developed a pericardial effusion (dashed line), the pericardial space may dilate substantially. Thus, the pericardium may contain a huge chronic effusion with minimal increase in pressure. A patient may acutely accumulate a small amount of fluid with a big increase in pressure. Conversely, the slow development of a chronic pericardial effusion may produce negligible hemodynamic consequences. It is very important to recognize that pericardial volume and pericardial pressure are *not linearly related*.

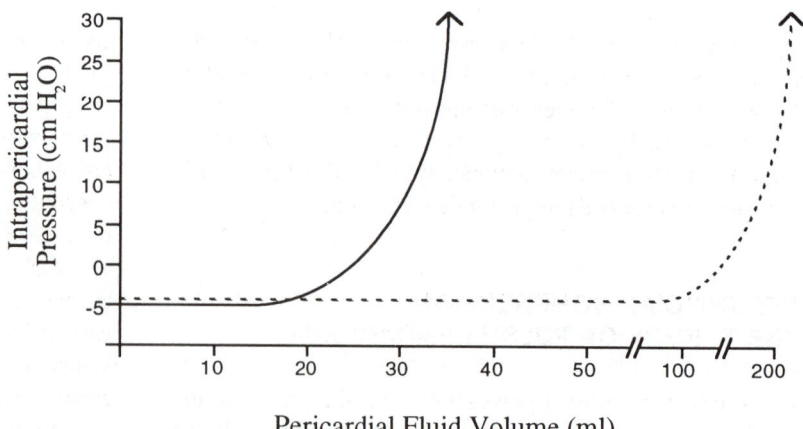

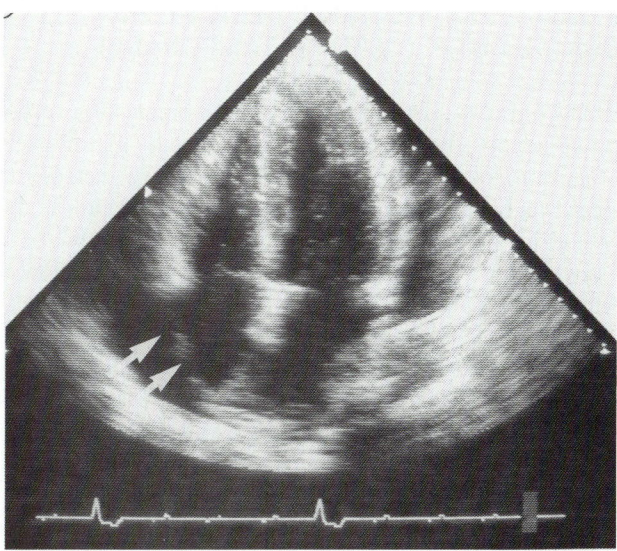

A

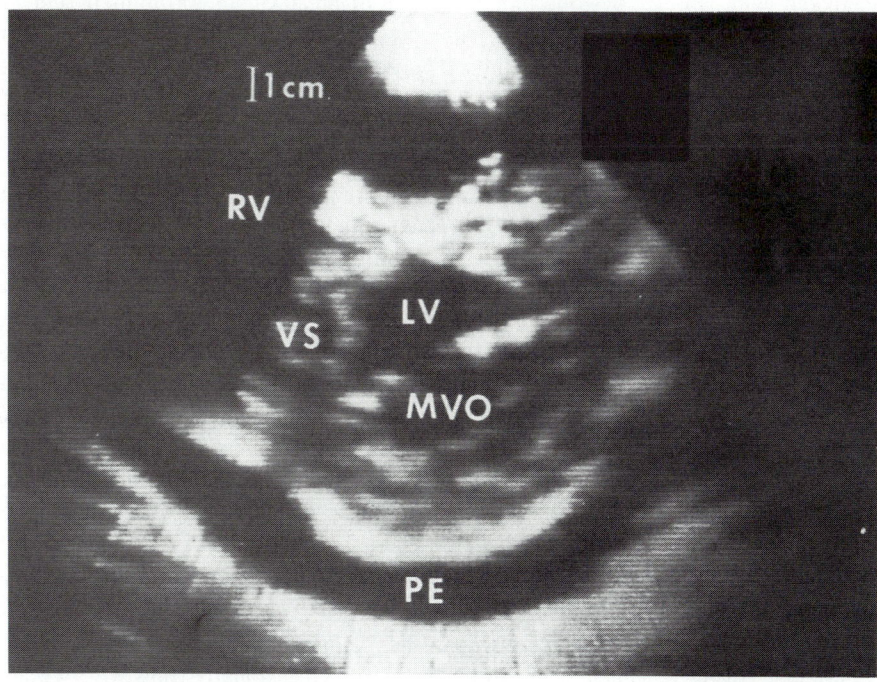

B

Figure 139–3. A. Transthoracic echocardiography provides the apical four-chamber view (same view but different patient as Fig. 139–1). Note the large pericardial effusion with *no* hemodynamic or echocardiographic evidence of pericardial tamponade. **B.** Two-dimensional ECHO. Short axis view of the heart at the level of the mitral valve orifice (MVO) along the right ventricular lumen (RV), the ventricular septum (VS), and the left ventricular lumen (LV). A posterior pericardial effusion (PE) can be easily seen. *(From Giuliani ER, et al: Two-dimensional echocardiography in acquired heart disease. Curr Probl Cardiol 5:25, 1981, with permission.)*

inflammatory debris — fluid accumulates. This characteristically concurrent myocardial inflammation explains the electrocardiographic features distinguishing pericarditis from ischemia/coronary artery spasm. The electrocardiogram (ECG) in acute pericarditis typically exhibits a tachycardia and only reciprocal ST segment depression in lead V1.[11]

PERICARDIAL COMPRESSION: THE THEORY OF PULSUS PARADOXUS

If you watch the arterial pressure tracing of a patient in the surgical intensive care unit you will note a fluctuation in the systolic pressure concurrent with respiration. Although this association has been noted for 100 years, its mechanistic etiology continues to foster delight within the physiologic community. The fashionable explanation of pulsus paradoxus is now both intuitively appealing and is sufficiently concordant with echocardiographic observations that explanation has clinical relevance.

Only two mechanisms seem to be involved: (1) under normal circumstances, pleural and pericardial pressures are essentially identical. Indeed, all intrathoracic organs are subject to comparable pressure changes associated with respiration/ventilation. Where veins and arteries enter or leave the thorax, however, breathing produces a pressure gradient. During spontaneous inspiration, negative pressure pulls venous flood into the chest augmenting right atrial and right ventricular filling. Equally important, however, negative intrathoracic pressure is transmitted to the distensible left ventricle, thus increasing the force the ventricle must exert (relative to the extrathoracic arteries) in order to maintain a stable systemic arterial pressure. This is like increasing the afterload. The left ventricle empties incompletely during spontaneous inhalation. Both systolic pressure and pulse pressure decrease.[12] (2) The left and right ventricles are separated by a pliable, mobile interventricular septum. Thus distention of the right ventricle displaces the septum leftward, compromising left ventricular diastolic filling. Decreased left ventricular filling translates into decreased stroke volume with resultant reduced systolic and pulse pressures. These two mechanisms should conspire to reduce blood pressure during negative pressure inhalation (breathing) and reciprocally augment blood pressure during positive pressure inhalation (ventilation). As a logical extrapolation, this phenomenon should be exacerbated with an increase in pericardial pressure (tamponade). It should also be possible to reproduce this process in animals and document it in patients.

LABORATORY CONFIRMATION OF PULSUS PARADOXUS

Rankin and colleagues[13] have provided elegant delineation of the physiology of paradoxical pulse and cardiac tamponade in conscious dogs. At peak inspiration, during tamponade, right ventricular filling increases while the interventricular septum shifts leftward and the septal arc decreases. In control animals, inspiration decreases left ventricular end-diastolic volume (LVEDV) by 10% while LVEDV decreased by almost one-third during tamponade. As predicted, decreased LVEDV was associated with both pulsus paradoxus and a decreased cardiac output. Several groups[14,15] have also produced acute tamponade in spontaneously breathing dogs. With inspiration, right ventricular filling occurred at the expense of left ventricular filling. Right ventricular dimensions increased, provoking a decrease in LVEDV. Mean pericardial pressure was increased from 1.2 to 10.5 mm Hg. This increased pericardial pressure decreased systolic blood pressure from 126 to 82 mm Hg, while pulsus paradoxus increased from a normal 4.3 to an abnormal 10.5 mm Hg.[14] For the purposes of clinical relevance, we want to emphasize that an effusion is pericardial fluid *without hemodynamic consequences* while tamponade exacerbates pulsus paradoxus, compromises left ventricular filling and decreases cardiac output. In surgical patients, this is a tremendously important distinction. Again, pericardial fluid volume *does not* relate to pericardial pressure in a linear fashion. Comprehension of this physiology should direct our diagnostic attention in a clinically practical fashion.

CLINICAL DIAGNOSIS OF PERICARDIAL COMPRESSION (CARDIAC TAMPONADE)

With clinically significant pericardial compression, echocardiography should be helpful. Indeed, transthoracic echocardiography does reveal an inspiratory increase in right ventricular diastolic diameter and a reciprocal decrease in left ventricular dimensions.[14] Similarly, peak early tricuspid flow velocity is increased and mitral flow is reduced.[16] A decrease in cardiac output triggers a formidable array of neuroendocrine compensatory systems. With a decrease in stroke volume, the early line of defense is a tachycardia. A more chronic decrease in cardiac output prompts a mineralocorticoid-mediated increase in intravascular blood volume that augments preload. Interestingly this entire compensatory spectrum has been delineated in a group of 56 medical patients.[17] With right ventricular dimensions increased and left ventricular dimensions decreased during inspiration, 36 of 56 patients maintained a systolic blood pressure of greater than 100 mm Hg and 27 of 56 had a pulse pressure of more than 40 mm Hg—for practical clinical purposes, these patients had an effusion *not* tamponade! Yet 52 of the 56 patients had an enlarged cardiac silhouette—again, pericardial fluid is *not* synonymous with hemodynamically significant tamponade. Forty-three of the 56 patients required a heart rate of more than 100 beats per minute to maintain adequate peripheral perfusion; but 13 of 56 did not. The spectrum is clear. When the patient has sufficient time to expand his intravascular volume and enlarge his pericardial space, a very large effusion produced little hemodynamic damage. When the elastic limits of the pericardial space are exceeded acutely, however, tamponade can snuff out forward flow with only subtle clinical clues.

CHRONIC FORMS OF PERICARDIAL COMPRESSION

For the surgeon, the diagnostic/therapeutic challenge is acute pericardial pressure. Occasionally, however, we are asked to see a patient with a more indolent, progressive form of pericardial compression. Both antibiotics (favorably) and innovative technologies (unfavorably) have changed the complexion of pericarditis during the recent decades.

Iatrogenic Pericarditis

As will soon be examined, dialysis, radiation, and drugs each affects the pericardium and the efflux of pericardial fluid. Procainamide (with or without drug induced lupus) and hydralazine can lead to pericarditis but do not commonly produce constriction. The mechanical irritation of cardiac surgical procedures inflicts an obligate pericardial irritation typically associated with mediastinal thrombus, which is surprisingly rarely associated with hemodynamically significant pericardial compression. With more patients now surviving massive myocardial infarction (the mortality of an acute myocardial infarction has halved in the past two decades), the associated myopericardial inflammation (Dressler's syndrome) does cause pericardial–epicardial fibrosis, which unusually results in hemodynamic compromise. Antibiotics and radiation have transformed the etiology, if not the frequency, of pericarditis.

TRADITIONAL DEFINITION OF CONSTRICTIVE PHYSIOLOGY

At cardiac catheterization, "constrictive physiology" has been defined by the following components:[18]

1. Equalization of the diastolic pressures of the ventricles within 5 mm Hg of each other.
2. Elevation of the mean atrial pressures to greater than 10 mm Hg.
3. A "dip-plateau" pattern (square root sign) of the ventricular filling pressure curves.
4. Prominant Y descent in the right atrial pressure tracing.
5. Right ventricular end-diastolic pressure more than one-third of the right ventricular systolic pressure.
6. Left ventricular ejection fraction greater than 40%.

DIFFERENTIATION OF RESTRICTIVE CARDIOMYOPATHY FROM PERICARDIAL CONSTRICTION

This distinction is critically important for the surgeon in both acute and chronic circumstances. A restrictive cardiomyopathy is intrinsic heart muscle disease. Stiff, fibrotic, inflamed heart muscle not only has not surgical therapy (short of transplantation), but these patients tolerate surgical stress very poorly.[18] Conversely, the only effective therapy for hemodynamically significant pericardial constriction is surgical excision. Endomyocardial biopsy may identify muscle disease and even suggest therapy, but when it exhibits myocyte hypertrophy or interstitial fibrosis, it does not exclude concurrent pericardial constriction.[19] Echocardiography can qualitatively distinguish normal from thickened pericardium. Much like the presence of pericardial fluid, however, the existence of a thick pericardium does not mandate hemodynamic significance.[18] Characteristic echocardiographic features of abnormal septal motion, flattening of left ventricular posterior wall diastolic motion, and left ventricular wall thickness have each been proposed as indicative of restrictive versus constrictive disease.[18,20] In *medical patients* this issue is typically easier because the disease is usually either myocardial or pericardial—but not both. With constriction, systolic function is preserved. Echocardiography reveals no impairment

of ventricular or atrial filling during *early* diastole (Fig. 139–3). The pericardial compression is ubiquitous, and mean atrial and ventricular end-diastolic pressures are, therefore, similar. Restrictive muscle disease, however, compromises both systolic and diastolic function. The ejection fraction may be reduced. The ventricular muscle is stiffer, and echocardiography can identify even early diastolic filling problems. Unlike the global pericardial compression of constrictive pericarditis, however, myocardial restrictive disease tends to be heterogeneous. Thus, although the end-diastolic pressures may be fortuitously comparable in restrictive disease, they should splay out at differing intravascular volumes (filling pressures). With the global cardiac compression associated with constrictive pericarditis, the end-diastolic pressures should track with each other in response to a volume challenge. Conversely, with infused fluid, the end-diastolic pressures should separate when restrictive disease predominates.

In *surgical patients* the issue is more complex because it is almost never isolated. The all-too-familiar scenario is the postoperative cardiac surgical patient whose mediastinal tubes are draining 100 mL/h. The blood pressure is 85/65 (reduced blood pressure and pulse pressure), heart rate is 125 beats per minute, pulmonary artery diastolic and right atrial mean pressures are both 20 mm Hg, the cardiac index is 1.8 L/min per m^2, and, with ventilation, the pulsus paradoxus is 20 mm Hg. This patient had an ejection fraction of 35% *prior to* cardiac surgery. We all already know (and our cardiology colleagues document by echocardiography) that this patient has some mediastinal thrombus. The critical question is: Can we help this patient by re-exploring him to evacuate the pericardial "compressive" clot? This frequent and important clinical problem has been exhaustively examined. In the vast majority of instances, it is probably fair to say that chest x-ray, echocardiography, computerized tomography, nuclear magnetic resonance, radionuclide angiography, and physical examination are all useless. This patient almost certainly has *both* restrictive and constrictive disease. You need to know the magnitude of the surgically correctable constrictive component. With a fluid challenge,[21] the contribution of the potentially correctable constriction can be assessed by the degree to which the end-diastolic pressures track with each other. With infused fluid, if the pressures splay out, your patient's problem is likely (and unfortunately) primary muscle disease. Conversely, if the right atrial mean and ventricular end-diastolic pressures respond similarly to infused volume, the patient may benefit by a return to the operating room.

BENIGN PERICARDIAL DISEASE

Congenital Pericardial Defects

Congenital defects of the pericardium are rare, with less than 200 cases reported in the world's literature.[22] The vast majority of pericardial defects occur on the left side and result from premature atrophy of the left common cardinal vein or Duct of Cuvier.[23] The left Duct of Cuvier should atrophy to form a portion of the left superior intercostal vein. The right Duct of Cuvier becomes the superior vena cava, ensuring closure of the right pleuropericardial membrane. Thus, pericardial defects are more common on the left. Unilateral complete absence of the pericardium may occur as frequently as one in 14,000 births, with a male predominance, but is rarely clinically significant.[22] In 30% of instances, congenital pericardial absence is associated with other congenital anomalies.[14] Resultant displacement of the heart into the pleural space has also been associated with incarceration[24] and surgically correctable tricuspid insufficiency.[23]

Total absence of the pericardium is rarely symptomatic, so treatment of a symptomatic partial defect may dictate pericardial resection.[22] Pericardial resection may be accomplished thoracoscopically, or the absent pericardium may be replaced with patch material at thoracotomy. Although the latter is more intuitively appealing, experience suggests that both therapies work.

Pericardial Cysts

Most pericardial cysts are initially appreciated on routine chest x-ray (Fig. 139–4). Although they have been associated with nonspecific chest pain, there is little evidence suggesting the pericardial cysts as the cause. The cysts contain clear, yellow fluid and uncommonly communicate with the pericardial space. The majority of these cysts are located at

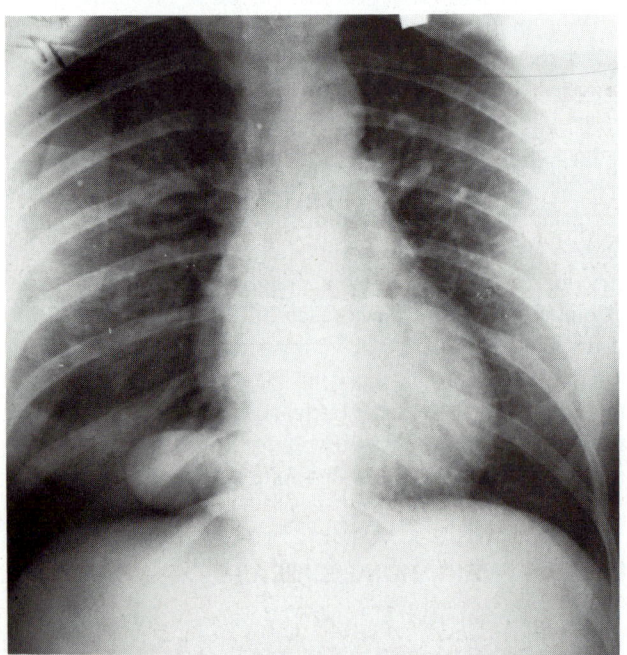

Figure 139–4. Chest x-ray. Pericardial cyst in a 39-year-old asymptomatic woman located in the right costophrenic angle.

the pericardiophrenic angle (right more common than left), but they can be located anywhere contiguous with the pericardium. If a pericardial cyst is asymptomatic and can be identified as a fluid-filled cyst by CT scan, it is safe to watch. In symptomatic patients or in patients in whom the cystic nature of the mass cannot be confirmed, surgical excision is warranted. Recently, thoracoscopic resection has been described.[25]

Infectious Pericardial Disease

Microorganisms may invade the pericardial space via spread from contiguous heart, lung, or diaphragm. A septicemia may seed the pericardial space, especially in immunosuppressed patients with concurrent burns or neoplastic disease.[26] Perhaps surprisingly, only one-third of patients with a purulent pericarditis exhibit tamponade physiology. This is a lethal disorder. Aggressive surgical drainage and treatment with a bactericidal antibiotic will avert significant mortality.[26] The organisms cultured from the pericardium include all of the usual suspects: *Staphylococcus, Pneumococcus, Haemophilus,* and fungi—depending primarily upon the immune status of the host. Although tuberculous pericarditis was formerly uncommon, it has experienced a resurgence (Fig. 139–5A,B). Like other pericardial infections, tuberculous pericarditis requires aggressive surgical drainage and antituberculous chemotherapy.[27] Fortunately triple drug therapy is typically very effective. Nine months of pharmacologic therapy is recommended, with at least 6 months of therapy following culture conversion. Quale and colleagues[28] advocate early surgical intervention for patients with tuberculous pericarditis. This group proposes a pericardial window for both diagnosis and therapy in patients with suspected tuberculous pericarditis. Further they propose a formal pericardiectomy for pericardial thickening, even in the absence of tamponade.

Postmyocardial Infarction Syndrome

The myopericardial inflammation associated with an acute myocardial infarction was first described by Dressler.[29] This pericardial inflammation, secondary either to cardiac muscle damage or postsurgical cardiotomy, can lead to pain, a friction rub, and electrocardiographic changes suggestive of ischemia. This process is important to the surgeon for two reasons: (1) When opening the pericardium in any patient who has had a myocardial infarction, the surgeon should anticipate potentially dense pericardial adhesions, and (2) when a patient is sufficiently fortunate to suffer a postinfarction cardiac rupture into a zone of dense pericardial adhesions, he may contain and eventually re-endothelialize this false aneurysm rather than experiencing the rapid demise associated with a free intrapericardiac rupture. Interestingly, pericardial mesothelial cells harbor plasminogen activating activity, which is rapidly depleted by inflammation.[30] Thus, all forms of pericarditis not only promote

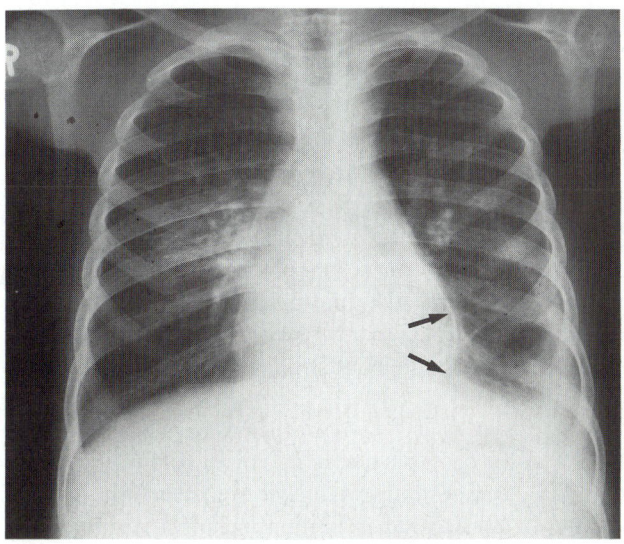

A

Figure 139–5. A. Antero-posterior chest x-ray of a 12-year-old girl with calcific tuberculous pericarditis. Arrows indicate calcified pericardium. **B.** Lateral chest x-ray of the patient with calcified tuberculous pericarditis. Also note the apparent absence (or minimal degree) of tuberculous pulmonary involvement.

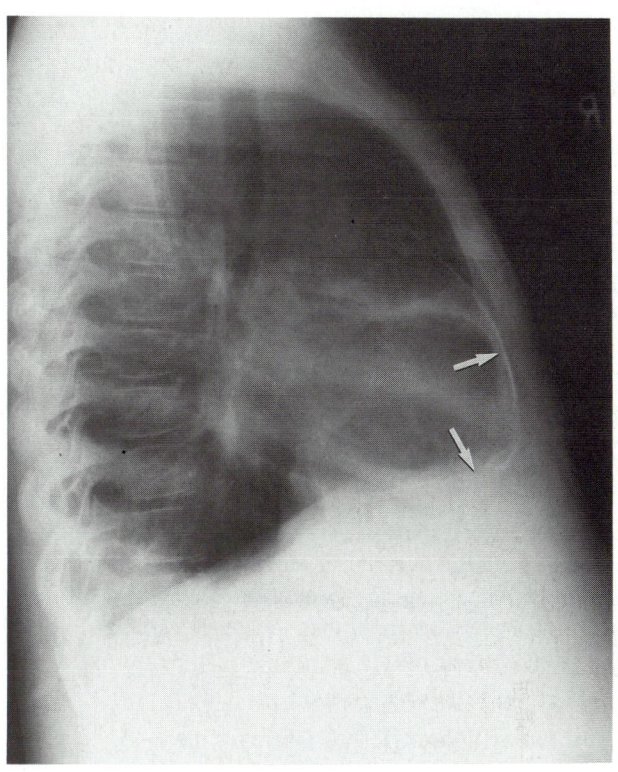

B

fibrous adhesions but diminish the ability of the pericardium to lyse fibrin.

Uremic Pericarditis

The etiology of uremic pericarditis is not known. Although initially recognized by Bright[31] in 1836, uremic toxins, fluid overload, anticoagulation, infection, and too much/too little dialysis have each been incriminated.[32] The attendant pericardial inflammation may lead to chest pain, fever, and a pericardial friction rub. Initial therapy should include non-steroidal anti-inflammatory agents and more aggressive dialysis. The timing of pericardiocentesis and/or pericardial excision has long been controversial.[33,34] Drainage has been advocated if a pericardial effusion persists following a 2-wk course of aggressive dialysis.[35] For practical purposes, a pericardial effusion is innocuous, even in uremic patients. Any evidence of hemodynamic compromise does warrant pericardiocentesis, especially in uremic patients undergoing dialysis. Similarly, recurrent pericardial effusion with hemodynamic embarrassment mandates a pericardial window with drainage either into the pleural or peritoneal space. Uremic pericardial constriction is rare and its etiology is also unclear. Surgical pericardial resection should be

contemplated only when evidence of hemodynamically significant constrictive physiology is clear.

Drug Induced Pericarditis

Procainamide (with or without an associated lupus syndrome), hydralazine, emetine, and methysergide have each been associated with pericardial inflammation, while minoxidil has been reported to induce a pericardial effusion.[36] The principles of diagnosis and surgical intervention are identical to other etiologies of pericardial effusion/tamponade/constriction.

Radiation Pericarditis

Until the 1960s, the heart was considered relatively resistant to ionizing radiation. Indeed, single cardiac doses up to 10,000 rad were well tolerated in rats.[37] In the 1960s and 1970s, a large number of patients received gratifyingly successful mediastinal radiation at Stanford for lymphomas (primarily Hodgkin's disease). Many of these patients have survived for years and continue to present for cardiac surgical evaluation. A clear dose–response is now apparent relating radiation to cardiac and pericardial disease.[37] Both an acute pericarditis and pancarditis are produced. Indeed, acceleration of coronary artery disease has also been reported.[38]

From the surgical vantage point this is a uniquely complex problem. Patients characteristically present years to decades, following their radiation therapy, with combined pericardial constriction, restrictive radiation-induced myocardial fibrosis, and a superimposed ischemic cardiomyopathy. In the large series from Stanford,[39] 20% of patients who exhibited radiation-induced "delayed pericarditis" progressed to symptomatic constriction requiring (and benefitting from) pericardiectomy.

Chylopericardium

Chylopericardium may be primary, for which no known etiologic agent is responsible, or it may occur secondary to trauma, open heart surgery, or tumor. The clinical presentation and treatment are the same as for pericardial effusion and tamponade from any other source, in addition to ligation of the thoracic duct.

Established Constrictive Pericarditis

Constrictive pericarditis is caused by marked thickening of the pericardium, dense scarring of the pericardium with pericardial sac obliteration, or calcification of the pericardium. The pathologic process commonly extends into the myocardium, causing a decrease in myocardial contractility, but the major fault in constrictive pericarditis is impairment of diastolic filling of the ventricles. Right and left ventricular diastolic pressures are elevated, leading to elevation of mean atrial pressures. The etiology of constrictive pericarditis is multiple, and virtually any of the conditions

causing acute pericarditis can lead to constriction except rheumatic fever. Two decades ago, the most common cause of chronic calcific constrictive pericarditis was tuberculosis. Today, the majority of cases are idiopathic. The specific etiology, in many cases, is not known and is ascribed to previously undetected idiopathic, viral, or tuberculous disease. The typical patient with constrictive pericarditis is often dyspneic or orthopneic, has jugular venous distention, may demonstrate ascites, and, on physical examination, frequently reveals a loud third heart sound or pericardial knock. The x-ray may show pericardial calcification, and the ECG may show low QRS voltage and, frequently, atrial fibrillation.

In recent years, two-dimensional echocardiography and CT of the chest have been helpful in confirming the diagnosis by demonstrating a thickened pericardium. Typical findings at cardiac catheterization include a rapid x and y descent in the right atrial pressure curve, equalization of mean right atrial, pulmonary wedge, RV and LV end-diastolic pressures, and the early ventricular diastolic dip and plateau or characteristic square root pattern in the RV pressure curve (Fig. 139–6).[40] Surgical resection of the diseased pericardium, as described below, generally produces dramatic improvement in symptoms of venous congestion. Removal of the visceral, as well as parietal layers, is often required for a good result. The former is more difficult and dangerous because of underlying coronary arteries and the potential for myocardial bleeding and perforation.

MALIGNANT PERICARDIAL DISEASE

Malignant tumors of breast and lung are common and metastasize to the pericardium relatively frequently. Pri-

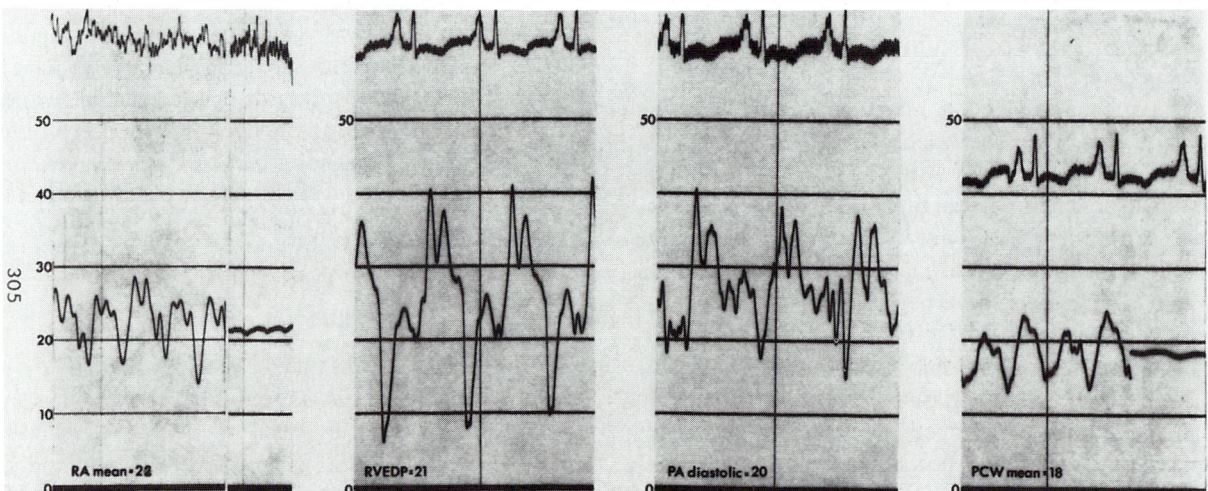

Figure 139–6. Cardiac hemodynamic findings in a patient with constrictive pericarditis. The right ventricular (RV) diastolic pressure is elevated and shows the characteristic square root pattern. The mean right atrial, RV diastolic, pulmonary diastolic, and pulmonary capillary wedge pressures approximate each other. There is a prominent y descent in the right atrial pressure tracing. (From Vanden Belt RJ, et al (eds): Cardiology, Chicago, Year Book, 1979, p 305, reprinted with permission.)

mary or contiguous pericardial malignancies include lymphomas, leukemias, thymomas, malignant mesotheliomas, teratomas, angiosarcomas, and rhabdomyosarcomas. In the therapy of these formidable clinical problems, the surgeon plays primarily a diagnostic role. When malignant tumor fills the pericardial space (with either solid tumor or malignant effusion), surgical debulking/decompression is both gratifyingly effective and astonishingly transient. It is important for the surgeon to remove a sufficient mass of malignant cells to define a diagnosis and delineate potential adjunctive therapy. In the absence of effective adjunctive chemo/radiation therapy, surgical pericardial decompression is frustratingly evanescent. Instillation of nonspecific chemotherapy (5-fluorouracil) uncommonly provides more than psychological benefit. Finally, a relatively aggressive pericardial window is typically completely invisible at autopsy weeks later. Again, surgical intervention should be directed toward finding a neoplastic process (lymphoma, seminoma) with an effective adjunctive therapy.

PERICARDIAL DECOMPRESSION AND DRAINAGE

Pericardiocentesis

The patient should be comfortably supine with electrocardiographic and blood pressure monitoring (depending upon the hemodynamic status of the patient and urgency of the procedure). No systemic analgesia is necessary. A skin weal is made over the left xiphoid–costal junction with 1% xylocaine. A 25-mL syringe containing 10 mL of xylocaine is affixed to a three-way stopcock and then to an 18-gage spinal needle. The needle is inserted (45° down and 45° to the left or right) toward the patient's left or right shoulder (Fig. 139–7A,B). Attaching this metal needle to a precordial electrocardiographic lead is to be discouraged as both confusing and unnecessary. The needle is advanced until blood or air is returned. If air is encountered, the needle should be withdrawn and reinserted with a more medial trajectory. When blood is withdrawn, 5 mL should be placed on a bed sheet to see if it clots. Defibrinated pericardial blood will not clot.[30] By manipulating the three-way stopcock, blood and fluid are removed from the pericardial space without disengaging the syringe.

Open Pericardial Drainage

The definitive treatment for cardiac tamponade is pericardial drainage. This can be accomplished temporarily by ECHO-guided pericardiocentesis with placement of a soft catheter in the pericardial space for continuing drainage. Recurrent effusion with tamponade should be treated by surgical drainage.

The subxiphoid approach to large or recurrent pericardial effusions has gained popularity in recent years (Fig.

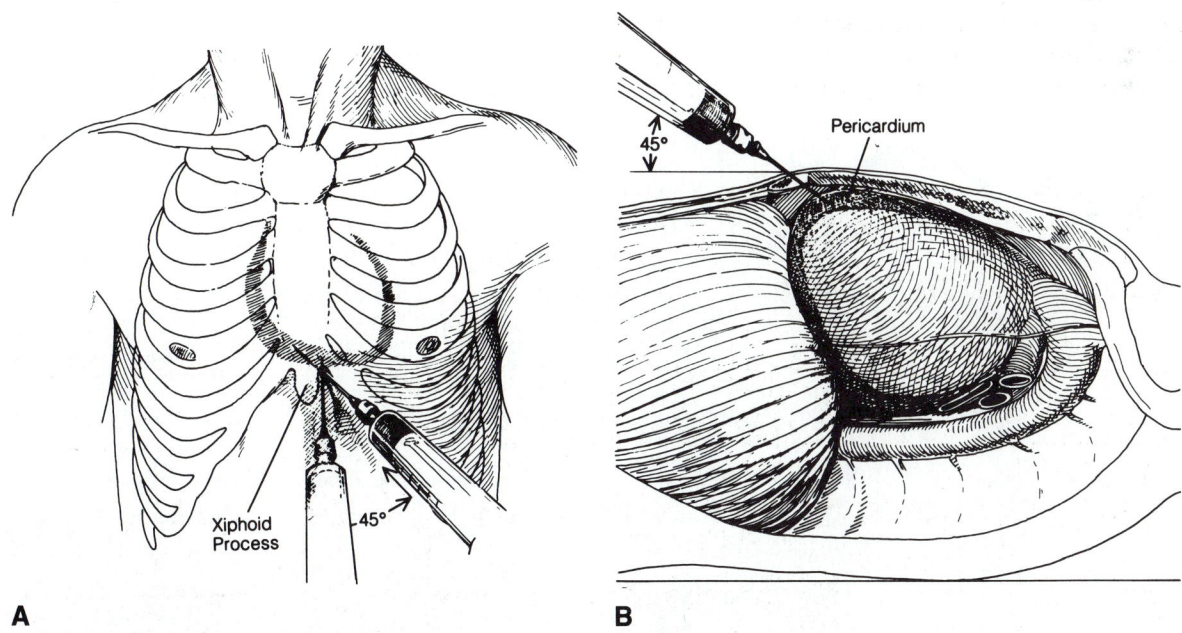

A   **B**

Figure 139–7A,B. For pericardiocentesis, an 18-gauge spinal needle is inserted at the left xiphoid–costal junction and inserted toward the inferior tip of the left scapula (angled 45° to the patient's right or left and 45° from the chest wall). The needle is advanced until blood or air is encountered; a "pop" may be appreciated as the needle tip traverses the pericardium. If air is withdrawn, the needle tip should be directed more toward the patient's midline. If blood is withdrawn, 50 mL should be aspirated and injected onto a sheet so that it can be inspected for clots. As a rule, intraventricular blood will clot, whereas debrinated pericardial blood will not clot. *(From Moore FA, Moore EE: Trauma resuscitation. In Care of the Surgical Patient, Vol. 1. Scientific American Medicine, 1994, pp 2,8.)*

139–8). It can be done under local or general anesthesia, and removal of the xiphoid process is recommended. After prepping the entire chest with betadine, 1% xylocaine is used to infiltrate the skin subcutaneously along each costal margin and over the lower portion of the sternum and then along and behind the fused ribs on each side to ensure blocking of the intercostal nerves.[41] Finally, the periosteum at the xiphisternal junction is anesthetized. A midline incision is made from the xiphisternal junction to approximately 10 cm below the tip of the xiphoid or, a 5-cm transverse incision can be made at the tip of the xiphoid. A plane is developed behind the xiphoid and the xiphoid retracted anteriorly while it is separated from the rectus sheath on either side. The xiphisternal junction is removed and, with anterior lifting of the distal portion of the sternum and downward traction on the diaphragm, a plane is developed until the pericardium appears as a fibrous membrane. The pericardium is grasped and an incision is made, allowing fluid to escape. A large chest tube is then placed in the peri-

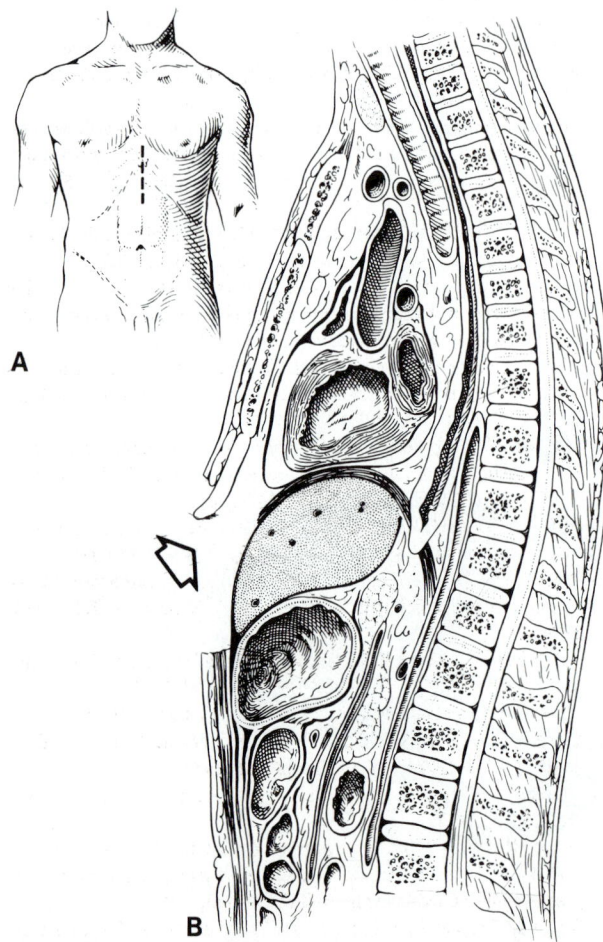

Figure 139–8. Pericardial window via the subxiphoid approach. After excising or lifting the xiphoid, the diaphragm is dissected bluntly from the sternum. This permits easy access to the pericardium. *(From Frater RW, et al: The subxiphoid approach in the treatment of pericardial effusion. Ann Thorac Surg 22:468, 1977.)*

cardial space, and the fluid is allowed to drain by gravity for several days. The fluid is sent for numerous studies, as stated in the section on pericardial aspiration. When drainage is minimal and the effusion has been adequately drained (by ECHO), the chest tube is removed. In a recent comparative trial, Naunheim et al found the subxiphoid approach to be superior to the transthoracic approach.[42] In most patients, simplicity, efficiency, and lack of pulmonary compromise characterized the subxiphoid operation (see Chap. 12).

In those patients with chronic, recurrent, bloody effusions (uremic pericarditis) or those patients with infective pericarditis, subxiphoid drainage of the effusion may not be adequate because of loculations and adhesions. We recommend, at this point, a left anterior thoracotomy, partial pericardial resection, drainage of the pericardial fluid into the left chest, and, of course, placement of a left chest tube. This is accomplished under general anesthesia. It provides adequate drainage, removal and breakage of adhesions, and evaluation of the thickened pericardium, should etiology of the underlying pericardial effusion not be known. It is an operation that is usually well-tolerated by most patients. Pericardial drainage now can also be done with the thoroscope. In those patients with infective pericarditis, where subxiphoid pericardial drainage may be less than ideal, a median sternotomy approach is recommended with, again, partial resection of the pericardium and placement of a large chest tube. In these patients, it would not be wise to perform a left thoracotomy for fear of contaminating the pleural space.

Pericardiectomy

Pericardiectomy for constrictive pericarditis corrects the hemodynamic abnormalities and produces dramatic clinical improvement. However, considerable controversy remains regarding the technique of pericardiectomy. Pericardiectomy is usually done with pump standby. Most surgeons reserve cardiopulmonary bypass for extremely difficult dissections or reoperations or if concomitant intracardiac surgery is required.

Routine monitoring of the patient is recommended, which includes an arterial line and placement of a Swan–Ganz catheter. Prior to beginning the operation, recordings of right atrial, RV, and pulmonary artery wedge pressures should be done, and cardiac output measured. The operation can be done through two incisions: either a median sternotomy or a thoracotomy (i.e., left thoracotomy or bilateral anterior thoracotomies). A median sternotomy approach provides good exposure. The operation can be safely done through that incision and has lower morbidity. The thoracotomy provides excellent exposure but is less well tolerated by the patient and adds to the morbidity of the operation.

Pericardial resection should begin with decortication of the left ventricle first to prevent the patient from going into pulmonary edema and acute right heart failure if the right ventricle was freed first. One must search for the proper plane between the thickened parietal and visceral pericardium or epicardium. The underlying fat will usually bulge through a small incision when the proper plane has been incised. The proper plane is usually avascular and superficial to the epicardium. An incision performed deeper than this plane penetrates the epicardium and can be attended by serious bleeding. Occasionally, the parietal pericardium may be extensively calcified with spicules penetrating the epicardium. These can be rongeured, but total removal is often hazardous and can result in perforation of the cardiac chambers with serious hemorrhage. As complete a pericardiectomy as possible should be accomplished, with decortication of both ventricles, both atria, and both cava. The phrenic nerves should be identified and preserved. After completion of the dissection, hemostasis is achieved and the appropriate placement of chest tubes accomplished. The adequacy of a pericardial resection can be gauged in the operating room by measuring mean right atrial pressures and RV end-diastolic pressures at the completion of the operation. There is usually prompt regression to normal values. Occasionally, in the perioperative period, there may be evidence of low cardiac output, which may respond to either inotropic support with dopamine, or, in some instances, an intra-aortic balloon pump may be required for several days.

The results of pericardiectomy have improved over the past several years, but the operation is not without risk. In a recent study from the Mayo Clinic, operative mortality was approximately 15% and a little less than one-third of their patients had evidence of low cardiac output postoperatively.[43] Median follow-up was 9 years and approximately 140 of 230 patients were in class I or class II. They recommended pericardiectomy when the diagnosis was made, because poor hemodynamic function preoperatively played an important role in the morbidity and mortality of the operation postoperatively.

REFERENCES

1. Siegel RE: Galen on surgery of the pericardium: An early record of the therapy based on anatomic and experimental studies. 26:524–527, 1974
2. Pernot C, Hoeffel JC, Henry M, et al: Partial left pericardial defect with herniation of the left atrial appendage. *Thorax* 27:246–250, 1972
3. Shapiro E, Salick AI: A clarification of the paradoxic pulse: Adolf Kussmaul's original description. *Am J Cardiol* 16:426-431, 1965
4. Churchill ED: Decortication of the heart (Delorme) for adhesive pericarditis. *Arch Surg* 19:1457, 1929
5. Delorme E: Sur un taitement chirurgical de la symphyse cardiopéricardique. Bull et mém. *Soc Chir Paris* 24:918, 1898
6. Brauer L: Über chronische adhäsive Mediastino-Perikarditis und deren Behandlung. *München med Wechnschr* 49:1072, 1902
7. Rehn L: Über pericardiale verwachsungen. *Med Klin* 16:999, 1920
8. Uglov FC: Diagnosis and surgical treatment of constrictive pericarditis. *Surgery* 47:247, 1960
9. Spodick DH: The normal and diseased peridarium: Current concepts of pericardial physiology, diagnosis and treatment. *J Amer Coll Cardiol* 1:240–251, 1983
10. Miller AJ, Pick R, Johnson PJ: The production of acute pericardial effusion. The effects of various degrees of interference with venous blood and lymph drainage from the heart muscle in the dog. 28:463–466, 1971
11. Hancock EW: Diseases of the pericardium. *Sci Am Med* 169, 1993
12. McGregor M: Pulsus paradoxus. *N Engl J Med* 301:480–482, 1979
13. Savitt MA, Tyson GS, Elbeery JR, et al: Physiology of cardiac tamponade and paradoxical pulse in conscious dogs. *Am J Physiol* 265:H1996–H2008, 1993
14. Gonzalez MS, Basnight MA, Appleton CP: Experimental cardiac tamponade: Hemodynamic and doppler echocardiographic reexamination of right and left heart ejection dynamics to the phase of respiration. *J Am Coll Cardiol* 18:243–252, 1991
15. Picard JH, Sanfilippo AJ, Newell JB, et al: Quantitative relation between increased pericardial pressure and doppler flow velocities during experimental cardiac tamponade. *J Am Coll Cardiol* 18:234–242, 1991
16. Appleton C, Hatle LK, Popp RL: Cardiac tamponade and pericardial effusion: Respiratory variation in transvalvular flow velocities studied by doppler echocardiography. *J Am Coll Cardiol* 11:1020–1030, 1988
17. Guberman B, Fowler NO, Engel PJ, et al: Cardiac tamponade in medical patients. *Circulation* 64:633–640, 1981
18. Aroney CN, Ruddy TD, Dighero H, et al: Differentiation of restrictive cardiomyopathy from pericardial constriction: Assessment of diastolic function by radionuclide angiography. *J Am Coll Cardiol* 13:1007–1014, 1989
19. Schoenfeld MH, Supple EW Jr, Dec GW Jr, et al: Restrictive cardiomyopathy versus constrictive pericarditis: Role of endomyocardial biopsy in avoiding unnecessary thoracotomy. *Circulation* 75:1012–1017, 1987
20. Engel PJ, Fowler NO, Tel CW: M-Mode echocardiography in constrictive pericarditis. *J Am Coll Cardiol* G:471–474, 1985
21. Bush CA, Stang JM, Wooley CF, Kilman JW: Occult constrictive pericardial disease: Diagnosis by rapid volume expansion and correction by pericardiectomy. *Circulation* 56:924–930, 1977
22. Risher WH, Rees AD, Ochsner JL, McFadden PM: Thoracoscopic resection of pericardium for symptomatic congenital pericardial defect. *Ann Thorac Surg* 56:1390–1391, 1993
23. VanSon JAM, Danielson GK, Callahan JA: Congenital absence of the pericardium: Displacement of the heart associated with tricuspid insufficiency. *Ann Thorac Surg* 56:1405–1406, 1993
24. Saito R, Hotta F: Congenital pericardial defect associated with cardiac incarceration: Case report. *Am Heart J* 100:866–870, 1980
25. Weder W, Klotz HP, Segesser LV, Larguader F: Thoracoscopic resection of a pericardial cyst. *J Thorac Cardiovasc Surg* 107:313–314, 1994
26. Rubin RH, Moellering RC: Clinical, microbiological and therapeutic aspects of purulent pericarditis. *Am J Med* 59:68, 1975
27. Fowler NO: Tuberculous pericarditis. *JAMA* 266:99–103, 1991
28. Quale JM, Lipschik GY, Heurich AE: Management of tuberculous pericarditis. *Ann Thorac Surg* 43:653–655, 1987
29. Dressler W: The post-myocardial infarction syndrome. *Arch Intern Med* 103:28, 1959
30. Nkere UU, Whawaell SA, Thompson EM, et al: Changes in pericardial morphology and fibrinolytic activity during cardiopulmonary bypass. *J Thorac Cardiovasc Surg* 106:339–345, 1993
31. Bright R: Tabular view of the morbid appearance in 100 cases connected with albuminous urine: With Observations. *Guys Hosp Rep* 1:380, 1836
32. Hancock EW: Diseases of the pericardium. *Sci Am Med* 176, 1993
33. Lazarus JM: Pericardial effusion. *Arch Intern Med* 144:1317, 1984
34. Leehey DJ, Daugirdas JT, Ing TS: Early drainage of pericardial effusion in patients with dialysis pericarditis. *Arch Intern Med* 143:1673–1675, 1983

35. Rutsky EA, Rostard SG: Pericarditis in end-stage renal disease: Clinical characteristics and management. *Semi Dial* **2**:25, 1989

36. Oates JA, Wilkinson GR: Principles of drug therapy. In Isselbacher KJ, Braunward E, Wilson JD, et al (eds): *Principles of Internal Medicine.* 1994, p 409

37. Stewart JR, Fajardo LF: Radiation-induced heart disease: An update. *Prog Cardiovasc Dis* **27**:173–194, 1984

38. Fajardo LF: Radiation induced coronary artery disease. *Chest* **71**:563–564, 1977

39. Fajardo LF, Stewart JR: Radiation-induced heart disease. Human and experimental observations. In Bristow MR (ed): *Drug Induced Heart Disease.* Amsterdam, Elsevier, North Holland Biomedical Press, 1980, pp 241–260

40. Vanden Belt RJ, Ronan JA, Bedynek JL: Diseases of pericardium. In *Cardiology—A Clinical Approach.* Chicago, Year Book Medical, 1979, p 291

41. Santos GH, Frater RW: The subxiphoid approach in the treatment of pericardial effusion. *Ann Thorac Surg* **23**:67, 1977

42. Naunheim KS, Kesler KA, Fiore AC, et al: Pericardial drainage: Subxiphoid vs transthoracic approach. *Eur J Cardio-thorac Surg* **5**:99–104, 1991

43. McCaughan BC, Schaff HV, Piehler JM: Early and late results of pericardiectomy for constrictive pericarditis. *J Thorac Cardiovasc Surg* **89**:340, 1985

Cardiac Tumors

Michael A. Acker and Timothy J. Gardner

Despite de Senac's assertion in 1783 that "the heart is an organ too noble to be attacked by a primary tumor,"[1] the heart has no specific immunity from neoplasia and cardiac tumors have become increasingly recognized. The prevalence of primary tumors of the heart in collected autopsy series ranges from 0.0017%[2] to 0.35%.[3] Since the advent of echocardiography, clinical experience with cardiac neoplasms has become more frequent, and most busy cardiac surgery services can expect to encounter one or two such cases per year. Because tumors represent one of the potentially curable forms of heart disease, the early diagnosis and treatment of cardiac neoplasms have assumed increasing importance.

HISTORY

The first report of a cardiac tumor appeared in 1559 and is attributed to Columbus.[4] Though tumor was distinguished from thrombus, by Hodgkin in the 1800s,[5] it was not until 1931 that the first extensive review of the literature was made of primary cardiac tumors and a useful classification system designed.[6] The first presumptive clinical diagnosis of a primary cardiac tumor was made by Barnes in 1934.[7] The first clinical diagnosis of a left atrial myxoma was made by angiography in 1952.[8] The modern era of diagnosis of cardiac tumors was ushered in in 1968 when echocardiography was first used to diagnose a left atrial myxoma, which was later confirmed at surgery and successfully removed.[9]

In 1938, Beck excised an intrapericardial cystic teratoma[10] and in 1951 Maurer successfully excised an epicardial lipoma.[11] Bahnson and Newman, in 1952, reported an early attempt to remove a myxoma from the right atrium under normothermia with caval occlusion.[12] Crafoord in 1954 was the first to remove a left atrial myxoma using car-

diopulmonary bypass.[13] This was followed shortly after by Bigelow et al, who reported a successful excision of a left atrial myxoma, encountered unexpectedly during an operation for mitral stenosis, using hypothermia and inflow occlusion.[14] The first successful removal of right atrial and ventricular myxomas was in the late 1950s by Hanlon[15] and Kay et al.[16] Biatrial myxomas were removed in 1967.[17] The first recurrence of a left atrial myxoma was reported in 1967 by Gerbode et al 4 years after its complete removal.[18]

CARDIAC TUMORS

Classification

Tumors of the heart are classified as either primary or secondary (Table 140–1). The autopsy incidence of secondary tumors ranges between 0.24 and 6.45%, or about 20 to 40 times more frequent than primary tumors in autopsy series.[19,20] Of the primary cardiac tumors, 72% were benign and 28% malignant in the largest autopsy series of 444 cases from the Armed Forces Institute of Pathology.[21] Myxoma is the most common benign tumor, and by far the most common tumor of any type, in all but the pediatric age group. Angiosarcoma followed by rhabdomyosarcoma are the most common malignant tumors of the heart.[21]

Morphology and Pathogenesis

Cardiac myxomas are benign tumors of uncertain etiology, but the concept that they are organized thrombus has been refuted.[22] Though the exact histogenesis is uncertain, it is most commonly believed that myxomas are neoplastic and that they are derived from a primitive mesenchymal cell.[23] Recent immunohistochemistry studies corroborate the concept that myxomas arise from primitive stromal cells that

TABLE 140–1. CLASSIFICATION OF HEART TUMORS

Primary
  Benign
    Myxoma
    Rhabdomyoma
    Fibroma
    Lipoma and lipomatous hypertrophy of the interatrial septum
    Papillary fibroelastoma
    Mesothelioma of the atrioventricular node
    Teratoma
    Hemangioma
    Paraganglioma and pheochromocytoma
  Malignant
    Angiosarcoma
    Rhabdomyosarcoma
    Fibrosarcoma
    Plasmacytoma
    Malignant fibrous histiocytoma
    Myxosarcoma
    Liposarcoma
    Leiomyosarcoma
    Extraskeletal osteosarcoma
    Chondrosarcoma
    Malignant schwannoma
    Carcinosarcoma
    Lymphoma
Secondary
  Metastases
  Direct extension of infradiaphragmatic tumors
    Renal cell carcinoma
    Wilms's tumor
    Intracardiac leiomyomatosis

have the capacity to differentiate along endothelial lines.[22] Supporting a neoplastic origin is the demonstration of DNA aneuploidy in a minority of myxomas[23] that are usually familial in occurrence.

Grossly, these tumors present as polypoid masses projecting into a cardiac chamber from the endocardial surface. Most commonly they are globular in shape and have a soft, gelatinous consistency (Fig. 140–1A). On cut section, they exhibit a yellow-brown or greenish hue and often contain areas of hemorrhage and necrosis (Fig. 140–1B). They most commonly have a short, broad-based attachment but can be sessile. Papillary forms may have a frond-like surface that is friable, making emboli more likely.[21]

Histologically, the diagnosis of a myxoma is based on the presence of characteristic spindle-shaped cells with an ovoid nucleus that is intimately associated with thin-walled capillaries, and these cells are embedded in a matrix of acid mucopolysaccharide.[21,22,24,25] The stroma contains variable deposits of collagen, reticular fibers, smooth muscle, lymphocytes, and plasma and mast cells (Fig. 140–2). Microscopic foci of calcium are seen in up to 20% of cases.[22] It is of surgical importance that myxomas extend almost exclusively intracavitarily, and are rarely seen deeper than the endocardium on histological sections.[26]

Myxomas can be seen in any cardiac chamber, though the majority arise in the left atrium, where they are attached to the limbus of the fossa ovalis by a short fibrovascular stalk. Rarely they may be attached to the posterior or anterior

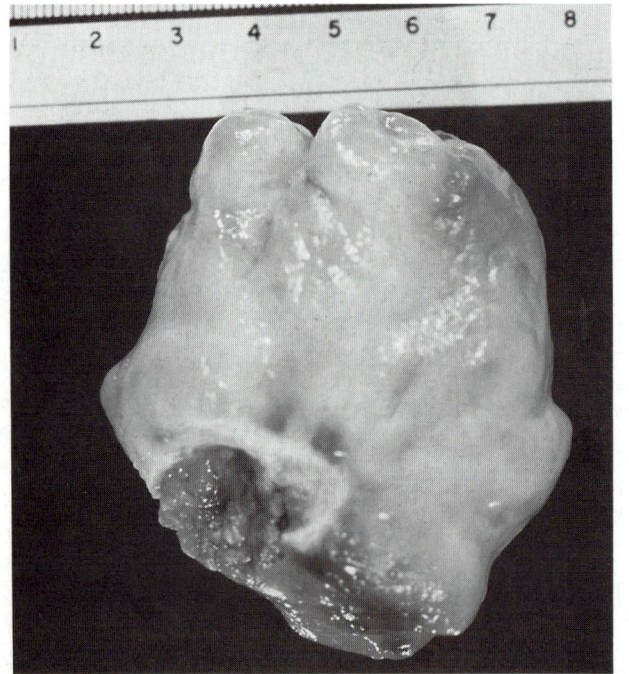

A

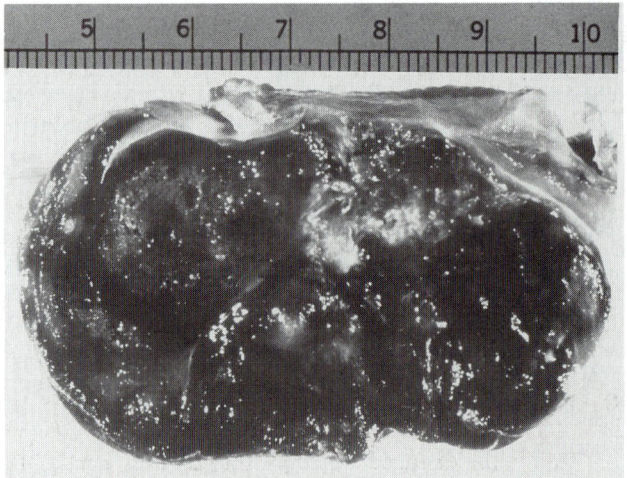

B

Figure 140–1. A. Usual macroscopic appearance of left atrial myxoma (see text). The narrow stalk, site of attachment to the interatrial septum, is visualized in the lower left corner. **B.** Histologic cross section of an atrial myxoma demonstrating heterogeneous composition of mass with myxoid, collagenous, and hemorrhagic areas seen. The pearlescent regions represent collections of ground substance or myxoid material. The capsule and point of attachment to the interatrial septum are seen at the top of the photo.

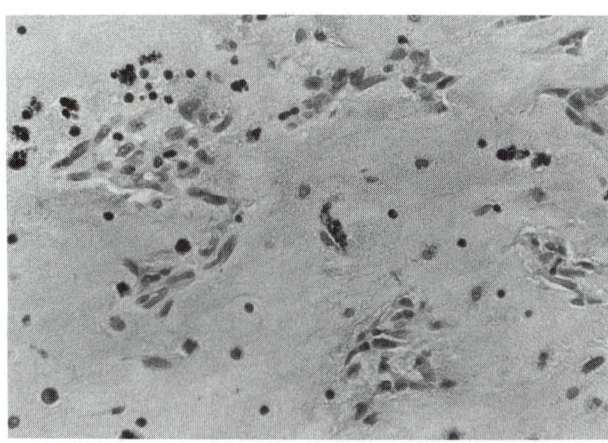

Figure 140–2. Photomicrograph of a myxoma with spindle-shaped cells representative of myxoid or connective tissue cells. The background of the photo is made up of collagenous tissue. The cells with darkly stained granules in the cytoplasm have taken up an iron stain demonstrating the presence of hemosiderin. This provides further support for the diagnosis of myxoma as opposed to other etiologies.

atrial walls.[21] Right atrial myxomas tend to be more broad-based than left atrial myxomas, with a wider attachment to the septum or atrial wall.[27] They also more often exhibit gross calcification that can be detected radiographically.

Clinical Features

Myxomas have been reported in patients of all age groups, but are most frequent in women in the fourth, fifth, and sixth decades. Between 75 and 80% of myxomas originate in the left atrium, 18% in the right atrium, and the remainder in the ventricles.[29] Biatrial myxomas have been increasingly reported[28–30]; the most common anatomic arrangement appears to be attachment of the two pedicles to opposite sides of the same region of the atrial septum.[28] Rarely right atrial myxomas may be associated with atrial septal defects.[31] Ventricular myxomas are distinctly uncommon. Left ventricular involvement is rarer than involvement of the right ventricle.[32–34] Most of these tumors are solitary growths located on the right ventricular free wall or the ventricular septum, although in some cases additional myxomas are present simultaneously in other cardiac chambers.[35] Myxomas originating from cardiac valves are rare, and only isolated cases of mitral,[36–38] tricuspid,[37,39,40] and pulmonary[41] valve involvement have been documented.

Most cardiac myxomas occur sporadically and usually are seen in middle-aged women (76%) as an isolated tumor (95%) in the left atrium (76 to 88%) without association with other conditions.[42] In 1985, however, the Mayo Clinic reported 4 of 85 patients (6%) had multiple myxomas, often involving more than one cardiac chamber.[43] Gelder et al reviewed the world's literature of familial myxomas beginning in 1971.[44] In contrast to the sporadic form, familial myxomas occur at a younger age (27 years old), more frequently in males, less commonly in the left atrium (61%), frequently multicentric (22%), and have a higher recurrence rate (10%).[42,44] Some patients with the familial myxomas may be part of a larger syndrome complex described by Carney as characterized by multicentric cardiac tumors, Sertoli cell testicular neoplasms, spotty mucocutaneous pigmentation, and primary nodular adrenocortical disease.[45] The mode of inheritance is autosomal dominant.[45] Single cardiac myxomas are seen in only a third of patients and the risk of recurrence is high (21 to 67%).[44–46] Patients who present with a myxoma at a younger age or at a location other than the right atrium or with multiple tumors probably should have their family members screened for familial cardiac myxomas and should be followed closely for recurrent disease.[44,46]

Symptoms and Signs

In the more common sporadic form of myxoma, the patient may manifest one or more of the "classic triad" of symptoms of hemodynamic obstruction, embolism, and constitutional effects.[47] Patients with left atrial myxomas often present with dyspnea, orthopnea, and paroxysmal nocturnal dyspnea, with or without hemoptysis, as in mitral stenosis. Usually, however, there is no antecedent history of rheumatic fever, and the symptoms are more rapidly progressive than in mitral stenosis. Paroxysmal dizziness or syncope is frequent, and sudden death from arrhythmia superimposed on severe pulmonary hypertension or from complete tumor obstruction of pulmonary venous return is not rare. Patients with right atrial tumors often present with symptoms and signs of inferior vena caval obstruction or right heart failure, such as hepatomegaly, ascites, and peripheral edema. Myxomas may also cause atrioventricular (A-V) valve insufficiency by preventing valve closure, or by trauma to the valve leaflets. The latter is more common in the case of right atrial neoplasms, where a calcified myxoma may destroy the tricuspid valve by a "wrecking ball" effect.[48]

Systemic embolization from left atrial myxomas is a major complication, and has been reported to occur in 25 or 50% of patients preoperatively.[49–52] The incidence of embolism from left ventricular myxomas is even higher.[53] The brain is affected in about 50% of cases, but emboli can occur to any organ, including the coronary arteries.[54,55] The neurologic deficits resulting from myxomatous embolization are usually major and infrequently resolve.[56] The presence of peripheral arterial emboli in a patient without known heart disease or atrial fibrillation should arouse the suspicion of myxoma; all such embolic material that is removed should be examined histologically.[50] The prevalence of clinical pulmonary embolism from right-sided myxomas is surprisingly low (<10%),[19] although cases of chronic pulmonary hypertension from multiple recurrent emboli[57] and massive pulmonary embolism causing death[58] have been reported.

The constitutional effects that can result from myxomas are protean. Most patients exhibit one or more of the constitutional symptoms of fever, malaise, weight loss, fatigue, myalgias, and arthralgias.[47,59] Laboratory investigations frequently reveal elevation of the erythrocyte sedimentation rate, hemolytic anemia, thrombocytopenia, and increases in the serum globulins and C-reactive protein.[47,49,60] Patients with right atrial myxomas may have polycythemia and clubbing, and hypoxemia may occur due to right-to-left shunting through a dilated foramen ovale or atrial septal defect.[47] Rarely, the patient may present with high fevers and positive blood cultures, mimicking endocarditis, due to superinfection of the myxoma with bacteria[61] or fungi.[62] Infrequently, constitutional symptoms may be the sole manifestation of myxoma, and a diagnosis of polyarteritis nodosum, collagen vascular disease, or vasculitis may be initially considered.[63]

Diagnosis

The auscultatory findings in a patient with left atrial myxoma may resemble those of rheumatic mitral valve disease. Frequently, the first heart sound as well as the pulmonary closure sound are accentuated, and a low-pitched early diastolic sound that mimics the timing of an opening snap or S3 gallop may be heard. A murmur of mitral stenosis and/or regurgitation may be present. Variation in murmurs with time and with position change has been stressed as a helpful clue to the possible presence of a myxoma.[47] In the case of a right-sided myxoma, the concurrence of an isolated tricuspid valve murmur with signs of right heart failure, in the absence of any mitral abnormality, should raise the possibility of a right atrial tumor.

The electrocardiographic findings in myxoma are diverse. With left atrial neoplasms, there may be evidence of left atrial enlargement and right ventricular hypertrophy. The majority of patients are in sinus rhythm, and atrial fibrillation is infrequent preoperatively,[59] whereas it is common following excision of the myxoma.[64] The chest x-ray may show moderate left atrial enlargement as well as evidence of pulmonary venous hypertension in cases of large left atrial tumors.[65] The ECG and radiographic findings, however, are nonspecific, and do not allow one to distinguish left atrial myxoma from moderately severe mitral stenosis.

Since the first North American application of ultrasound to visualize cardiac neoplasms in 1968,[66] echocardiography has become the most important noninvasive modality for diagnosing myxomas. Two-dimensional echocardiography is the method of choice for the primary assessment of the patient with a suspected cardiac mass.[67] Its sensitivity for the diagnosis of atrial myxomas approaches 100%.[68] The size, shape, and position of the myxoma can be defined precisely (Fig. 140–3A,B), as well as any valvular involvement. At the Mayo Clinic, the yearly incidence of cardiac tumor diagnosis has increased severalfold since the advent of two-dimensional echocardiography.[69] Recently, transesophageal echocardiography (TEE) has been compared to transthoracic echocardiography (TTE) for the evaluation of cardiac tumors. The sensitivity

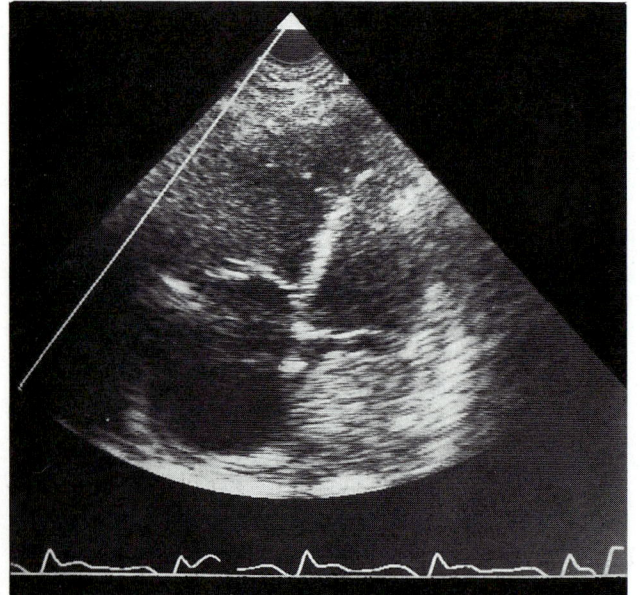

A

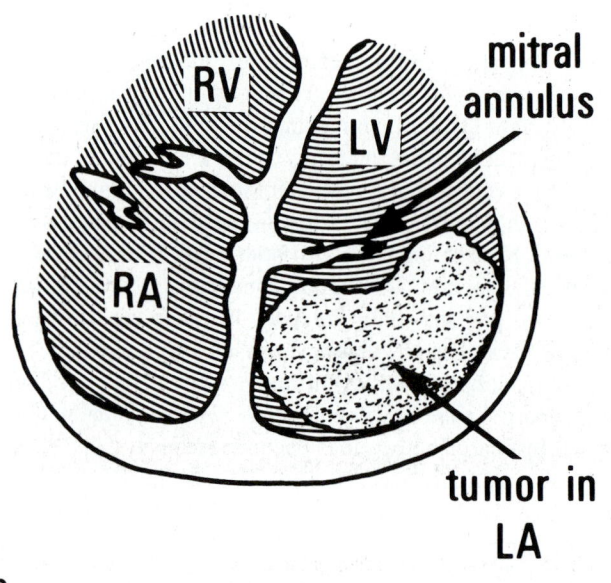

B

Figure 140–3. A. Two-dimensional echocardiogram, four-chamber view, of a large myxoma that almost completely fills the left atrial chamber. **B.** Graphic representation of **A.**

of the TEE for atrial tumors is at least equal if not superior to TTE.[70–72] TEE is superior to TTE in providing information on the exact point of tumor attachment and additional morphologic features, information that is potentially valuable for planning surgical management.[70,72] In addition, TEE has proven superior to TTE in the evaluation of intracardiac malignant tumors as well as peri- or paracardiac masses, especially when involving the right paracardiac region.[70–72] Present day two-dimensional echocardiography (TTE or TTE) has completely supplanted angiocardiography in the preoperative evaluation of patients with a suspected myxoma, avoiding the risk of systemic or pulmonary embolization.[50,73]

During the past few years there has been an increasing interest in the use of magnetic resonance imaging (MRI) and computer tomography (CT) for the diagnosis of cardiac tumor.[74,75] Though neither of these modalities is as sensitive as two-dimensional echocardiography for the diagnosis of atrial myxomas, they do provide additional specific information regarding cardiac masses (Fig. 140–4A,B). MRI in particular has proven effective in providing information regarding cardiac mural infiltration, pericardial involvement, and extracardiac tumor extension.[68] Newly developed abilities to vary MR imaging parameters permit increased specificity in the evaluation of cardiac masses and have allowed the differentiation of an atrial myxoma from thrombus as well as differentiation of various cardiac sarcomas.[76] In cases when the myxoma appears sessile or when malignancy is suspected for other reasons, information provided by MRI can be of benefit.[68,77]

In the majority of cases, however, the diagnosis of myxoma by echocardiography is straightforward. Surgery is indicated whenever the diagnosis is made, and is considered urgent since the risks of hemodynamic decompensation and embolism are ever present. In some series there is between an 8 and 10% incidence of death from embolic complications during the interval between diagnosis and surgery.[78,79]

Treatment

Surgical resection of myxomas is best carried out using cardiopulmonary bypass with separate, snared caval cannulation and under conditions of systemic hypothermia and cold cardioplegic arrest. Several principles should be adhered to to minimize the risks of perioperative embolism and myocardial infarction, the two major causes of postoperative morbidity and mortality. Gentle handling of the heart during cannulation is important. The aorta should be clamped and cardioplegia administered prior to any manipulation of the cardiac chamber harboring the myxoma. The tumor should be removed en bloc and without fragmentation. Following excisions of the myxoma, the atrium and ventricle should be irrigated profusely and aspirated with a discard sucker to wash out any residual tumor fragments.[78] The adjacent A-V valve should then be inspected for any evidence of damage to the annulus, leaflets, or chordae. If there is any question of multicentricity on the preoperative two-dimensional echocardiography, a meticulous inspection of all four cardiac chambers should be undertaken. If coronary arteriography had revealed hemodynamically significant stenoses, complete coronary revascularization should be carried out using the internal mammary artery and reversed saphenous vein grafts. There has been some controversy as to the optimal manner of approaching left atrial myxomas, since exposure is often poor due to the small size of the left atrium. Because of its flexibility, a median sternotomy inci-

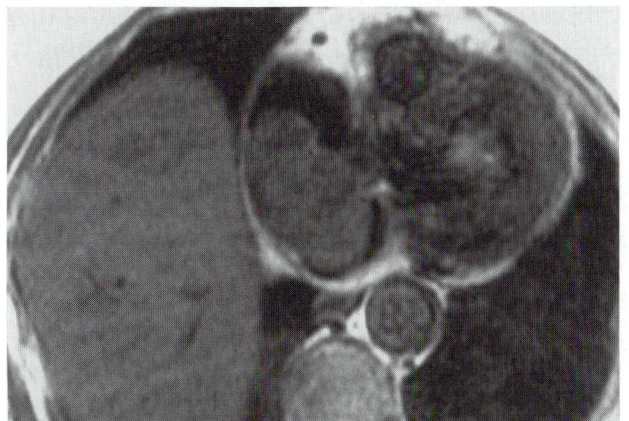

A

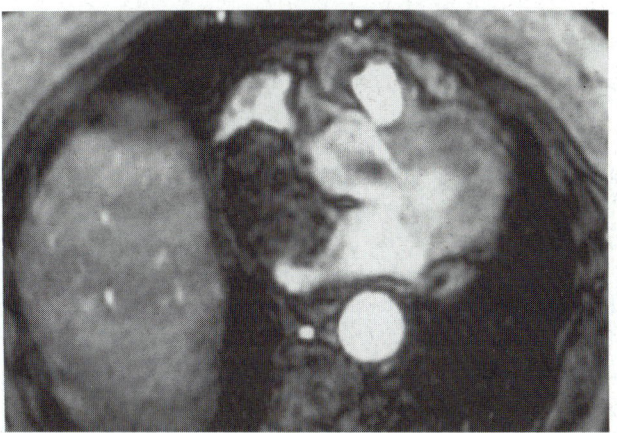

B

Figure 140–4. A. A cardiac-gated axial magnetic resonance image (MRI) using the spin-echo technique demonstrates the large right atrial mass (myxoma) and its relationship to other intracardiac structures. The left ventricle (LV) is shown and the mass appears to be contiguous with the tricuspid valve plane. **B.** A single frame from a multiple image cine-MRI loop demonstrates the large amount of hemosiderin within the mass (dark areas). Blood signal appears bright in this type of imaging and helps delineate this intracardiac abnormality.

sion is favored, although frequently the left atriotomy must be carried down around the pulmonary veins to enhance visibility. Alternatively some surgeons prefer a right thoracotomy incision, maintaining that a lateral approach gets the surgeon directly into the area of interest. A longitudinal incision in the left atrium, posterior to the interatrial groove, is first performed, and the tumor visualized. In two large series, a single left atrial incision was often sufficient to enable complete tumor resection without late recurrences.[80] Many authors, however, contend that exposure of the tumor is facilitated by a simultaneous right atriotomy, with excision of a full-thickness portion of the interatrial septum, including the fossa ovalis.[37,50,73,81–83] The myxoma, which is usually attached to the fossa ovalis, is removed through the right atrial incision if small or through the left atriotomy if larger. The created atrial septal defect is then closed by direct suture or with a pericardial or Dacron patch. This biatrial approach is particularly useful if the base of the left atrial myxoma appears sessile.[84] There is no strong evidence, however, that radical resection of the interatrial septum reduces the possibility of recurrence. In two recent series with mean follow-up of 10.5 and 17.5 years, a conservative policy of excision of the tumor and its pedicle with only a narrow rim of adjacent endocardium resulted in no recurrences in patients with the sporadic form of myxoma.[43,79]

Surgical experience with right atrial and ventricular myxomas is less common, but the same principles prevail. In the patient with a right atrial tumor, both cavae should be cannulated directly or venous drainage should be provided by superior vena caval and femoral vein cannulation. Every effort should be made to avoid tumor fragmentation during cannulation. The pulmonary artery should be clamped and an oblique right atriotomy performed. Since attachment of the myxoma to the interatrial septum may be more broad-based than in the case of a left atrial myxoma,[27] more extensive septal resection and reconstruction may be necessary. Removal of a ventricular myxoma does not require excision of full-thickness ventricular wall. Tumors in the LV outflow tract may be approached transaortically[18]; other LV myxomas may be removed via the left atrium. Right ventricular myxomas are preferentially excised through a right atriotomy, avoiding a ventriculotomy if possible.[32,35]

An important consideration at operation concerns the management of A-V valve involvement. Even if the tumor arises from valve tissue, it is often possible to avoid valve replacement.[37,40] With left atrial myxomas, mitral insufficiency due to annular dilatation is common preoperatively, and appears to be reversible on long-term follow-up even if no reparative mitral valve procedure is undertaken.[38,80] More severe mitral regurgitation can be managed successfully by annuloplasty in most instances.[59,85,86] Marked damage to the valve annulus, leaflets, and chordae is more common in the case of right atrial myxomas, perhaps because these tumors are more frequently calcified.[87] In addi-

tion, tricuspid annular dilatation caused by tumor impaction is likely to persist postoperatively.[80] Despite this, tricuspid valve repair with direct leaflet repair and annuloplasty is certainly possible,[40] and repair, or rarely replacement, is sometimes indicated during surgical intervention for right atrial myxoma.

The overall results of operative treatment for myxoma are satisfactory, and the present early mortality is less than 5%.[38,43,50,73,82,83,88] The major causes of perioperative morbidity and death relate to advanced age or to embolism and myocardial infarction, which can be prevented by meticulous technique and by a policy of simultaneously bypassing all significant coronary stenoses. The early postoperative course is frequently complicated by supraventricular tachyarrhythmia, and episodic junctional rhythms. Even complete heart block is not uncommon.[50,64,67,80,83,84,89] Although many such dysrhythmias are transient, a significant number of patients require antiarrhythmic drugs on a long-term basis and a minority need implantation of a permanent pacemaker.[64] Nevertheless, the late results following operation are usually excellent, and most patients attain New York Heart Association functional class I status.[38,43] In a long-term follow-up of 54 patients who had undergone excision of an intracardiac myxoma, Bartolotti et al reported an actuarial survival at 20 years of 91%.[50]

Local Recurrence

In a report from the Mayo Clinic, the risk of a second myxoma developing following complete resection of a sporadic, nonfamilial myxoma was between 1 and 3%[43] and in a more recent collection of 526 cases from the published literature was 4.7%.[73] Many large series report no recurrences.[26,37,38,50,73,80,90] The mean age of patients who develop a recurrence is in the early thirties,[43,73] significantly lower than the usual age group for myxoma. The time interval between initial excision and reoperation has ranged from 6 mo to 12 years, and averages $2\frac{1}{2}$ years.[43,91] Twenty-eight percent of recurrences repeat.[73,91]

The risk of local regrowth of a myxoma cannot be accurately predicted from the microscopic appearance of the primary tumor.[92] The possible causes of recurrence include inadequate resection, tumor implantation at operation, and multicentric growth.[93,73] A myxoma may recur in the atrium despite radical septal excision and patching.[92,93] At present, it is generally believed that the multigrowth potential of the tumor seems more important than inadequate surgical resection in determining recurrence.[73] The recurrent tumor may be histologically benign, resembling the primary neoplasm,[94] or may become histologically more malignant with each recurrence.[86,93] Even if benign, a recurrent myxoma may be clinically more aggressive than the primary tumor.[37,88,86] In addition, it may present in unusual locations, such as the pulmonary artery or the aorta,[92] and in a significant number of patients may occur as multiple regrowths within the same[96] or different[97] cardiac chambers.

It is now understood that multicentric recurrence of cardiac myxomas is especially frequent in patients with the dominantly inherited "myxoma complex."[43–46] Such individuals are young, tend to have a non-left atrial origin of the primary neoplasm, and have a high rate of synchronous and metachronous myxomas. There is recent evidence that myxomas from patients with multiple tumors proliferate faster than solitary tumors and have a higher incidence of DNA aneuploidy.[98,23] It is possible that in the future DNA and cytogenetic studies on myxomas might indicate more accurately the risk of recurrence, or perhaps identify a biologically unique subset of more aggressive myxomas.[23]

The recommended approach during a secondary operation in such patients includes a thorough inspection of all cardiac chambers and complete excision of all growths, with a wider and deeper margin of underlying endocardium than usual.[43] Regular follow-up with serial two-dimensional echocardiograms is particularly important in this group, who are at a high risk for the development of additional metachronous cardiac lesions. Despite careful operation for recurrent myxoma, the risk of a second recurrence is high, and has been estimated at 25%.[91] However, even if the rerecurrence is multicentric, continued aggressive surgical treatment is advised, since prolonged symptom-free survival is achievable.[91,99]

Extracardiac Recurrence

In addition to the local regrowth of myxoma, patients may rarely exhibit a distant recurrence.[92,93] Such an episode may lead to a review of the initial pathological specimen, with reclassification of cardiac tumor as sarcoma rather than a myxoma.[100] There have been a number of reports documenting the malignant potential of myxomas.[101] It has also been documented that tumor emboli from histologically benign myxomas may not only remain viable at the site of impaction, but may also displace, destroy, and invade the walls of cerebral and other arteries, leading to the formation of multiple pseudo-aneurysms[96,102–110] (Figs. 140–5 and 140–6). In at least two cases, the new appearance[104] or enlargement[102] of cerebral myxomatous aneurysms occurred some time following complete resection of the cardiac tumor, indicating that myxomatous emboli are capable of independent growth. Invasion of the media and adventitia of the pulmonary vasculature has also been described following embolism from a right atrial myxoma.[107] The existence of myxomatous mass lesions, akin to metastases, has been reported in the brain[56,108,109] and in bones and soft tissues.[56,93,108,109]

It is thus evident that patients with preoperative systemic emboli may not be rendered entirely disease-free by resection of the primary tumor alone. Such patients, especially those with cerebral emboli, should have close clinical follow-up, and the resolution or stability of lesions visualized on CT scanning, MRI, or angiography should be demonstrated. Failure of constitutional symptoms or find-

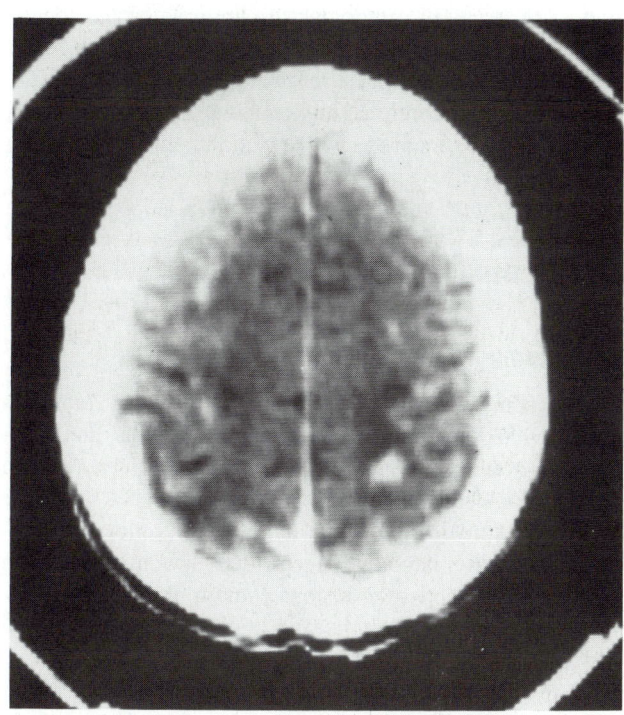

Figure 140–5. Computed tomography scan with contrast of the brain of a patient who 2 years previously underwent excision of a histologically benign left atrial myxoma. There are multiple metastases in both cerebral hemispheres. Needle biopsy revealed invasive myxoma cells.

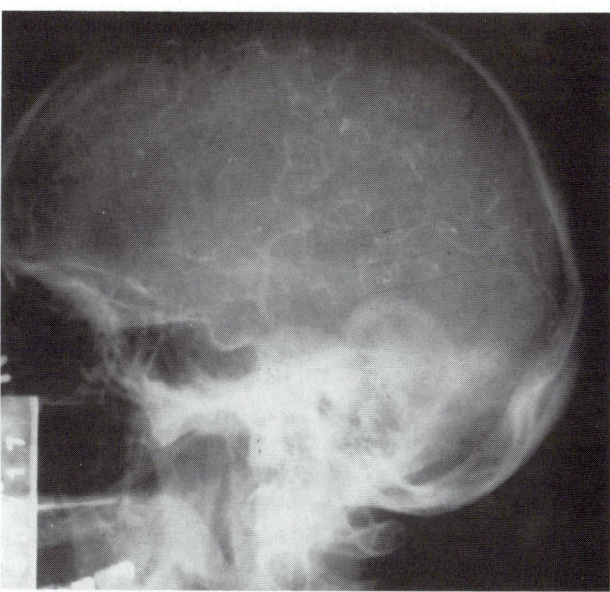

Figure 140–6. Cerebral arteriogram of the patient whose computed tomography scan is depicted in Figure 140–5.

ings of abnormal laboratory tests to improve, or the appearance of new neurologic deficits beyond the initial postoperative period, would suggest residual disease.[96] Once identified, enlarging cerebral myxomatous masses or bony lesions may be excised, with resultant clinical improvement.[56,108]

OTHER BENIGN TUMORS

Rhabdomyoma

Although myxoma is the most common cardiac tumor in adults, rhabdomyoma predominates in infants and children.[21] These benign growths present pathologically as firm grayish nodules that can easily be distinguished from the surrounding myocardium.[111] Histologically, they are composed of classic, large, glycogen-filled "spider cells."[21] On electron microscopy, the lesions contain demonstrate scattered bundles of myofibrils and appear to represent fetal hamartomas rather than true tumors.[112]

Most rhabdomyomas become manifest in the first days to weeks of life by producing hemodynamic obstruction or intractable ventricular arrhythmias.[83,111,113,114] More than half of patients with rhabdomyoma exhibit or subsequently develop the stigmata of tuberous sclerosis[111]; conversely, 50% of patients with tuberous sclerosis have recognizable intracavitary or intramyocardial rhabdomyomas on two-dimensional echocardiograms.[115] In the largest series,[112] over 90% of the rhabdomyomas were multiple, and only three patients had solitary growths. Although the left ventricle was the most frequent tumor location, 81% of patients had rhabdomyomas in the right ventricle as well, and the atria were involved in 30%. In 50% of patients, at least one tumor mass was intracavitary and obstructive.

Diagnosis of infants with rhabdomyoma is poor, with 58% of patients expiring in the first month of life and 75% by 1 year.[111] In those without severe neurologic damage from tuberous sclerosis, the prognosis appears to be favorably altered by early surgical intervention. Fifty percent of these patients, however, will later develop tuberous sclerosis.[116] The primary indication for surgery is in the rare case when the tumor appears solitary and flow is obstructed. Prior to operation, a thorough two-dimensional echocardiogram of all four cardiac chambers is essential. Since cardiac catheterization can induce severe arrhythmias and has been reported to cause a number of deaths in patients with rhabdomyoma, it is best avoided.[111] Whereas one group has recommended the radical excision of all gross lesions at operation,[117] the consensus in the recent literature is that only obstructing, intracavitary rhabdomyomas need be completely removed.[118,119] Since intramural ventricular rhabdomyomas have a limited growth potential and have been known to regress with time,[111,114] the surgical approach should be conservative, taking care to avoid damage to the ventricular septum, valvular tissue, conduction system, and

coronary arteries. However, if a serious arrhythmia is present preoperatively, endocardial mapping should be performed[113,114,82] and total resection of the lesion causing the arrhythmia should be carried out, with the expectation of cure.[113,120,121]

Fibroma

Though fibroma is the second most common cardiac neoplasm in the pediatric age group, it remains an extremely rare tumor. Less than 100 cases have been reported in the English literature and 83% have been in children.[122] Unlike rhabdomyoma, it presents as a solitary intramural tumor rather than as multiple growths. Grossly, fibromas are firm, circumscribed but nonencapsulated gray-white lesions that are occasionally calcified.[123] Although some authors consider these growths to be hamartomas,[124] the predominant view is that fibromas are true tumors of fibroblastic origin that entrap and displace segments of myocardium during their development.[21,125]

Three-fourths of pediatric patients with fibroma are diagnosed by the age of 2 years.[125] In rare cases, these tumors may be asymptomatic, which progress, presenting in adulthood.[126] There is no known sex predilection or familial incidence, although a recent report has noted the occurrence of the dominantly inherited Gorlin (multiple nevoid basal cell carcinoma) syndrome in four patients with cardiac fibroma.[127] The usual location of the neoplasm is in the ventricular septum or the LV free wall, and only rare cases have been described in the right ventricle or atria.[125,128] Clinically, the common presenting features are congestive heart failure, murmurs, and arrhythmias. Significant mitral or aortic valve dysfunction may exist, resulting from direct annular or papillary muscle involvement or interference with leaflet motion.[113,125] In addition, sudden death may occur in up to 30% of patients, presumably due to involvement of the interventricular conduction apparatus.[113,125,129]

The chest x-ray findings of cardiomegaly with an irregular left heart border and intracardiac calcification should suggest the diagnosis in the proper clinical context. Two-dimensional echocardiography has proved invaluable in localizing the tumor and in assessing valvular function preoperatively, especially in infants. In older children, angiography may reveal additional information relating to coronary artery involvement or displacement.[125]

Despite the often bulky nature of intramural fibromas, surgical intervention is indicated when feasible to obviate the risks of prolonged congestive heart failure, arrhythmias, and sudden death. As it grows, the tumor displaces but does not destroy myocardium, and there is usually enough LV muscle remaining following its excision to assure adequate contractile function. Frequently, the ventricular septal or free wall defect can be closed primarily, or if necessary, a small prosthetic patch may be used.[130] The results of surgical treatment for fibroma are favorable, and long-term survival with excellent clinical results following complete excision is possible.[113,125,122] Even incomplete resection of a very large tumor for the relief of LV outflow obstruction is worthwhile, and has been associated with asymptomatic 1- to 2-year survival, although the risk of sudden death probably remains.[113] On occasion the fibroma may be so large that conventional surgical techniques may not suffice, and an innovative approach is required. In the rare case of a large atrial fibroma, extensive reconstruction of the atrial free wall with autologous pericardium is possible following tumor excision and valvular and atrial septal repair.[130] Mustafa et al have described successful complete replacement of the interventricular septum with a large Dacron patch after removal of a biventricular fibroma in an infant.[131] The first dynamic cardiomyoplasty operation (synchronously stimulated latissimus dorsi muscle wrap) was performed by Carpentier and Chaques in 1985 following en bloc excision of a biventricular fibroma. The latissimus dorsi pedicle flap was wrapped around the heart and used not only to replace the resected myocardium, but also stimulated with a specially designed cardiomyostimulator to contribute actively to systolic function. The patient remains well today.[132] Cardiac transplantation has been performed successfully in four patients with unresectable cardiac fibromas. In the two patients where follow-up is reported, the patients are alive and well at 35 and 28 mo.[126]

Lipoma and Lipomatous Hypertrophy of the Interatrial Septum

True lipomas are encapsulated masses of adult adipose tissue that may originate in the visceral and parietal pericardium as well as throughout the heart.[21] Most reported cardiac lipomas have been diagnosed incidentally at autopsy.[133] When discovered antemortem, the lesion usually presents as a sessile subendocardial growth that bulges into a cardiac chamber and may cause obstructive signs and symptoms.[134] Less frequently, a lipoma is located within the myocardium, and produces arrhythmias and conduction disturbances.[135,136]

Although most lipomas are solitary, multiple cardiac lipomas can occur, especially in patients with tuberous sclerosis.[21] If a solitary cardiac lipoma is symptomatic, it should be excised, with anticipation of an excellent long-term result.[113] Similarly, if a large, encapsulated fatty tumor is discovered incidentally at the time of operation for another condition, it should be resected if this can be accomplished with minimal risk.[133]

Lipomatous hypertrophy of the interatrial septum refers to nonencapsulated hyperplasia of adipose tissue, which is actually more common than a true cardiac lipoma.[21] Recently, a review of 38 cases diagnosed postmortem has been reported. Most patients harboring the lesion are in the seventh and eighth decades, whereas cardiac lipomas occur in a much younger age group.[137] The mass is characteristically situated anterior to the fossa ovalis and bulges into the right atrium from beneath the atrial endocardium.[21] Although lipomatous hypertrophy of the interatrial septum is often asymptomatic, a significant number of patients have had otherwise unexplained cardiac arrhythmias[137] and some have died suddenly or following prolonged episodes of arrhythmia or congestive heart failure.[21] The lesion is now reliably diagnosed antemortem[138] as experience with two-dimensional echocardiography and other noninvasive diagnostic modalities has increased.

Papillary Fibroblastoma

Papillary fibroblastoma is a small, usually solitary neoplasm that is located primarily on the midportion of the mitral and aortic valves but can occur in addition on papillary muscles, chordae tendineae, ventricular septum, or the endocardial surface.[21,139,140] Several cases of cerebral embolism resulting from papillomas have been reported,[139–142] and sudden death due to coronary occlusion or embolism from an aortic valve fibroblastoma has occurred.[143,144] Embolization may occur from fragile papillary fronds[139] or from thrombus forming on the tumor.[142] Surgical excision of those lesions detected preoperatively by two-dimensional echocardiography has become more frequent[139–142] and is advised even in asymptomatic patients.[141]

Mesothelioma of the A-V Node

This interesting neoplasm, the so-called cardiac conduction tumor, is derived from benign mesothelial cells that are strikingly similar to the cells comprising adenomatoid tumors of the ovary and testis.[21] It appears grossly as a poorly circumscribed growth, 2 mm to 1.5 cm in diameter, located in the atrial septum superior to the septal leaflet of the tricuspid valve in the vicinity of the A-V node. It has been labeled the smallest tumor that causes sudden death[145] because of its propensity to produce complete heart block and ventricular arrhythmias. About 50 cases have been described since 1911; according to a recent report, the diagnosis has not yet been documented antemortem.[146] In several instances, placement of a permanent pacemaker for A-V block did not prevent sudden death[21,146,147] which was presumably due to ventricular fibrillation. This tumor should be considered in the differential diagnosis of complete heart block in young adults, especially in those with no prior history of cardiac disease. Confirmation of the diagnosis, in cases of larger sized mesotheliomas, may be possible by two-dimensional echocardiography or by selective coronary arteriography, with visualization of an abnormal A-V nodal artery.[148] Insertion of a permanent pacemaker followed by ablation or resection of the tumor should be curative.

Teratomas

Teratomas of the anterior mediastinum are frequent, but intrapericardial teratomas are rare, and only nine true cardiac teratomas were documented in a recent literature review.[149] They are usually benign but can occasionally be malignant. Surgical excision should be attempted since untreated tumors usually lead to early death.[150]

Cardiac Pheochromocytoma

Cardiac pheochromocytomas are extremely rare tumors, with only 30 cases reported in the literature.[151] Pheochromocytomas are functionally active chromaffin paragangliomas of the sympathetic nervous system. The mean age of presentation is 40 years, with a range from 18 to 85 years. The most common presentation is arterial hypertension, which may be associated with headache, palpitations, and sweating. Time to diagnosis after onset of clinical symptoms has ranged from months to 22 years. The diagnosis is a difficult one to make. In all patients there is an elevation of urinary catecholamines; however, localization to the heart is problematic. A negative exploratory laparotomy was performed in 17 of 32 patients.[151] Localization of the tumor to the mediastinum using a [^{131}I]metaiodobenzylguanidine scan was successful in 18 of 22 patients. Two-dimensional echocardiography, CT scan, and/or magnetic resonance imaging may be useful to localize the tumor. Coronary angiography continues to be a valuable study, for it shows the exact location of the tumor, its blood supply, and its relation to the coronary vessels.[151] Rarely, staged venous sampling to establish higher levels of catecholamines from the heart may be needed for the diagnosis. Cardiac pheochromocytomas are usually located on the roof of the left atrium, but may involve the interatrial septum and the anterior surface of the heart. The tumors are usually benign.[151–153] With modern imaging techniques, cardiac pheochromocytomas are becoming more frequently diagnosed and surgical excision usually results in relief of symptoms and total cure. This may require resection of coronary arteries or parts of the left atrial wall. Of 25 patients who underwent surgical excision, 21 survived. The four deaths were secondary to bleeding from the tumor bed, the most common surgical complication.[151]

Cardiac Hemangioma

Cardiac hemangiomas are exceedingly rare, only 23 cases having been reported in the literature.[154] The most frequent presentation is shortness of breath on exertion or arrhythmias. Diagnosis is difficult and is often delayed. Diagnosis is made and surgical resectability is determined using two-dimensional echocardiography, enhanced contrast CT scan, magnetic resonance imaging, and/or coronary angiography. The characteristic sign of angiography is a vascular blush. The tumor is usually located in the lateral wall of the left ventricle and anterior wall of the right ventricle; multiple sites are not uncommon. Surgical excision required cardiopulmonary bypass in 10 of 23 patients. Total resection

was accomplished in only about half of the other patients. Long-term prognosis for this tumor is good even if complete resection is not possible. Spontaneous regression has been reported. Thus extensive and hazardous resections should only be attempted in the patient who is symptomatic or hemodynamically compromised.[154]

PRIMARY MALIGNANT TUMORS

Primary malignant tumors of the heart are 20 to 40 times less common than metastatic cardiac lesions.[19] They are usually aggressive neoplasma that invade and displace cardiac and mediastinal structures, in addition to metastasizing. The clinical presentation may include congestive heart failure due to intracavitary obstruction or myocardial replacement by tumor, pleuritic chest pain, syncope, constitutional symptoms, refractory arrhythmias, and pericardial effusion and tamponade.[113,155–159] Diagnosis and evaluation can be done noninvasively utilizing echocardiography, CT scan, and MRI. Transthoracic echocardiography is the preferred screening test, through transesophageal echocardiography, CT with contrast, and MRI have proven better at delineation of intramyocardial and mediastinal extension. This information is invaluable to determine surgical resectability.[156] Although an occasional long-term survival has been reported following tumor resection and radiation therapy,[160] the prognosis is poor. Adjuvant chemotherapy has been attempted but has not been shown to be of benefit.[156,158,159] Survival correlates with the completeness of resection and the level of mitotic activity.[157,158] Median survival in patients who underwent complete resection was 24 mo, versus 10 mo in all other patients. Cardiac transplantation as well as cardiac autotransplantation has been performed to obtain complete local control. Incomplete resection can alleviate symptoms of heart failure in some patients even if survival is not increased.[158]

Angiosarcoma

Angiosarcoma is the most frequently identifiable primary malignant cardiac tumor.[21] Most patients with this tumor are middle-aged men. In the majority of cases, patients with angiosarcomas present with symptoms of right heart failure and chest pain. The tumor is usually a bulky mural mass in the right atrium, which protrudes into the right atrial chamber and invades the venae cavae, tricuspid valve, and pericardium.[156,161,162] Rarely the tumor may appear as a pedunculated growth in the atrium, resembling a myxoma.[160] Sixty-six to 89% of tumors will metastasize, most often to the lung, liver, and brain.[156] In patients diagnosed antemortem, usually via open pericardial biopsy or thoracotomy, the survival ranges from 3 to 15 mo.[156] Death is often by local spread, often culminating in obliteration of the pericardial space.[156] Surgical resection, the mainstay of treatment, is rarely able to yield clear margins, with complete resection possible in only 20% of cases. Cardiac transplantation has been attempted as definitive treatment for angiosarcoma in three patients. In all three, local control of the tumor was obtained, but two of the patients died 8 and 9 mo, respectively, after transplantation of multiple brain metastases.[163] The impression in the literature is that postoperative radiotherapy to the mediastinum is of value in most types of cardiac sarcoma, including angiosarcoma, and is associated with a prolonged absolute survival.[155]

Rhabdomyosarcoma

Rhabdomyosarcoma is the second most common cardiac sarcoma. The tumor arises de novo, not from malignant degeneration of rhabdomyomas. Unlike angiosarcoma, rhabdomyosarcoma does not have a predilection for any one cardiac chamber.[21,156] The tumor usually develops intramurally and often in multiple sites. In a significant number of patients, it protrudes into a cardiac chamber to produce hemodynamic obstruction. The majority of patients have constitutional symptoms of malignancy. Fifty percent present with direct pericardial extension and a third with distant metastases.[158,164] Unlike myxoma, intracavitary rhabdomyosarcoma typically invades and destroys the cardiac valves with which it comes into contact. Treatment consists of excision of the main tumor mass, followed by valve replacement if necessary. Despite postoperative radiotherapy and chemotherapy, local and distant recurrence is the rule, and the majority of patients expire within 1 year of diagnosis.[156,164]

Miscellaneous Primary Malignant Tumors

Aside from angiosarcoma and rhabdomyosarcoma, other primary malignant cardiac tumors have been described but are rare. Experience with isolated cases of plasmacytoma,[165] fibrosarcoma,[156] mesothelioma,[156] liposarcoma,[166] leiomyosarcoma,[113] extraskeletal osteosarcoma,[167] and other types of sarcoma[168–170] has confirmed that surgical treatment can result in satisfactory palliation, which is usually temporary. Occasionally, however, radical excision of the cardiac neoplasm followed by radiotherapy does produce prolonged survival.[165] Primary lymphoma of the heart is exceedingly rare[21] and if diagnosed antemortem radiotherapy and multiple agent chemotherapy are advised.[165,171,172]

SECONDARY CARDIAC TUMORS

Metastases

Metastatic tumors to the heart are the most frequent cardiac neoplasms, but are rarely encountered by the cardiac surgeon. Approximately 10 to 20% of patients who die of disseminated cancer harbor cardiac metastases,[21,173] and the frequency of secondary cardiac involvement has been in-

creasing in recent decades.[174] The most common mechanism by which tumor cells reach the heart is hematogenous spread via the coronary arteries.[174] Alternative routes include retrograde flow through cardiac lymphatics, direct extension from a contiguous intrathoracic tumor mass, and tumor spread up the inferior vena cava.[173] The pericardium and epicardium are more frequently affected by metastatic tumor than is the myocardium, which in turn is more commonly involved than the endocardium.[173] The major types of neoplasm that secondarily invade the heart include bronchogenic carcinoma, melanoma, leukemia, lymphoma, carcinoma of the breast, and soft tissue and skeletal sarcomas.[21,174,175] In most instances, cardiac involvement consists of a number of discrete tumor nodules and multiple microscopic foci of neoplastic growth; only rarely is there a solitary metastasis that can be surgically excised.[21]

The clinical presentation associated with metastases to the heart includes the emergence and relentless progression of congestive heart failure and cardiac arrhythmias that respond poorly to conventional treatment.[21,173] The chest x-ray may show rapid enlargement of the pericardial–cardiac silhouette due to the presence of a hemorrhagic pericardial effusion or myocardial replacement by tumor. Echocardiography is indicated if there is any evidence of hemodynamic obstruction, since chamber or valvular obstruction by a solitary tumor mass may be an indication for operative intervention.

The treatment of metastatic cardiac tumors depends on the number of identifiable lesions and the tumor type. Lymphomas and leukemias may respond to radiotherapy and chemotherapy,[173,176] but solid tumors that involve the heart diffusely rarely respond for a substantial period of time.[155] The creation of a subxyphoid pericardial window is frequently effective in the palliative treatment of malignant pericardial effusions large enough to cause hemodynamic compromise.[155] Up to a 1983 review, 10 known patients had undergone resection of cardiac metastases, and three intermediate-term survivors in the group had developed sarcomatous metastases after a long disease-free interval.[155] There have been additional reports documenting the successful surgical removal of intracardiac metastases from carcinoma of the testis[177,178] and uterine leiomyosarcoma.[179] En bloc resection, using cardiopulmonary bypass, of a primary pulmonary sarcoma that had invaded the left atrium has also been described.[180] Careful preoperative workup and patient selection is essential to optimize the long-term results following surgical excision of intracardiac metastases.

Direct Extension of Infradiaphragmatic Tumors

Approximately 5 to 10% of patients with renal cell carcinoma have endovascular invasion of the inferior vena cava, and up to 40% of these neoplasms extend into the right heart.[181,182] Many of these patients have no evidence of distant metastatic disease. In recent years, it has been documented that radiotherapy and chemotherapy are ineffective in managing these tumors, and that radical resection of the renal mass with concomitant removal of the caval and cardiac extension is indicated.[181–183] This technique can result in 5- and 10-year survivals of 55 and 43%, respectively, in those with venocaval invasion and no other demonstrable metastases.[184]

The surgical approach to malignant renal neoplasms that extend into the inferior vena cava and the right heart involves the use of cardiopulmonary bypass, with cannulation of the ascending aorta, superior vena cava, and either common femoral vein. The tumor thrombus is seldom densely adherent to the intima of the vena cava and atrium, and tumor extraction is usually possible by cavotomy and atriotomy alone.[183] For extensive involvement deep hypothermic total circulatory arrest, with temporary exsanguination of the patient into the pump oxygenator,[183,182] permits careful dissection within the vena cava and right atrium in a bloodless field, thus greatly facilitating the conduct of the operation. Aside from renal cell carcinoma, intravenous leiomyomatosis is an entity that may cause hemodynamic obstruction by intraluminal propagation up the inferior vena cava into the right heart.[185–188] The condition refers to the intravenous growth and extension of benign leiomyomata originating in the uterus or the walls of the large veins.[186] Fewer than 100 cases of intravenous leiomyomatosis have been documented, and as of 1986, only 14 reports of intracardiac extension had appeared in the English language literature.[187] The outcome was invariably fatal in the cases without surgical intervention; of 12 patients who had undergone operation, 11 survived. In most patients, surgical excision of the cardiac neoplasm was followed by sectioning the tumor from its stalk within the inferior vena cava. Resection of the residual abdominal growth was then performed during the same operation[185,187] or during a later, staged laparotomy.[188] Recurrence of the tumor has been noted in a significant number of cases[186,187] and frequent follow-up ultrasound examinations of the pelvis, inferior vena cava, and heart are recommended.

ACKNOWLEDGMENTS

We would like to acknowledge Drs. Vic Ferrari and John Seykora for their work in preparing the MRI and histology photographs used in this chapter.

REFERENCES

1. Whorton CM: Primary malignant tumors of the heart: Report of a case. *Cancer* 2:245, 1949
2. Straus R, Merliss R: Primary tumor of the heart. *Arch Pathol* 39:74, 1945
3. Shelburne SA: Primary tumors of the heart. *Ann Intern Med* 9:340, 1935
4. Columbus MR: *De Re Anatomica, Libri XV*. Venice, N Bevilacque, 1559, p 269
5. King TW: On simple vascular growths in the left auricle of the heart. *Lancet* 2:428, 1845
6. Yater WM: Tumors of the heart and pericardium: Pathology, symptomatology and report of nine cases. *Arch Intern Med* 48:267, 1931
7. Barnes AR, Beaver DC, Snell AMP: Primary sarcoma of the heart: Report of a case with electrocardiographic and pathological studies. *Am Heart J* 9:480, 1934
8. Goldberg HP, Glenn F, Dotter CT, Steinberg I: Myxoma of the left atrium: Diagnosis made during life with operative and post-mortem findings. *Circulation* 6:762, 1952
9. Schattenberg JT: Echocardiographic diagnoses of left atrial myxoma. *Mayo Clin Proc* 43:620, 1968
10. Beck CS: An intrapericardial teratoma and a tumor of the heart: Both removed operatively. *Ann Surg* 116:161, 1942
11. Maurer ER: Successful removal of tumor of the heart. *J Thorac Surg* 23:479, 1952
12. Bahnson HT, Newman EV: Diagnoses and surgical removal of intracavitary myxoma of the right atrium. *Bull Johns Hopkins Hosp* 93:150, 1953
13. Crafoord C: Discussion of mitral stenosis and mitral insufficiency. In CR Lam (ed): *Henry Ford Hospital International Symposium on Cardiovascular Surgery: Studies in Physiology, Diagnosis and Techniques.* Philadelphia, WB Saunders, 1955, pp 202–203
14. Bigelow WG, Dolan FG, Campbell FW: The effect of hypothermia on the risk of surgery. *Proceedings of the International Society of Surgery, Sixteenth Congress, Copenhagen*, 1955, p 631
15. Hanlon CR: Discussion of Behnson HT, Spencer FC, Andrus EC: Diagnosis and treatment of intracavitary myxomas of the heart. *Ann Surg* 145:915, 1957
16. Kay JH, Anderson RM, Meihaus J, et al: Surgical removal of an intracavitary left ventricular myxoma. *Circulation* 20:881, 1959
17. Yipintsoi T, Donauan KL, Bhamarapraquati N, et al: Bilateral atrial myxoma with successful removal. *Dis Chest* 57:828, 1967
18. Gerbode F, Kerth WJ, Hill JD: Surgical management of tumors of the heart. *Surgery* 61:94, 1967
19. Pritchard RW: Tumors of the heart: Review of the subject and report of one hundred and fifty cases. *Arch Pathol* 51:98, 1951
20. King YL, Dickens P, Chan ACL: Tumors of the heart. *Arch Pathol Lab Med* 117:1027–1031, 1993
21. McAllister HA, Fenoglio JJ: Tumors of the cardiovascular system. Fascicle 15. *Atlas of Tumor Pathology, Second Series.* Washington DC, Armed Forces Institute of Pathology, 1978
22. Burke AP, Virmani R: Cardiac myxoma: A clinicopathologic study. *Am J Clin Pathol* 100:671–680, 1993
23. Seidman JD, Berman JJ, Hitchcock CL, et al: DNA analysis of cardiac myxomas: Flow cytometry and image analysis. *Human Pathol* 22:494–500, 1991
24. Heath D: Pathology of cardiac tumors. *Am J Cardiol* 21:315, 1968
25. Tazelaar HD, Locke TJ, McGregor CG: Pathology of surgically excised primary cardiac tumors. *Mayo Clin Proc* 67:957–965, 1993
26. Silverman NA: Primary cardiac tumors. *Ann Surg* 191:127, 1980
27. O'Neill MB, Grehl TM, Hurley EJ: Cardiac myxomas: A clinical diagnostic challenge. *Am J Surg* 138:68, 1979
28. Yipintsoi T, Donavan KL, Bhamarapraquati N, et al: Bilateral atrial myxoma with successful removal. *Dis Chest* 57:828, 1967
29. Imperio J, Summers D, Krasnow N, Piccone VA: The distribution patterns of biatrial myxomas. *Ann Thorac Surg* 29:469, 1980
30. Yakirevich VS, Baliga BG, Sen G, Ionescu MI: Biatrial myxoma associated with mitral valve lesion. *Ann Thorac Surg* 39:563, 1985
31. Natarajan P, Vijayanagar RR, Eckstein PF: Right atrial myxoma with atrial defect: A case report and review of the literature. *Cathet Cardiovasc Design* 8:267, 1982
32. Viswanathan B, Luber JM, Bell-Thompson J: Right ventricular myxoma. *Ann Thorac Surg* 39:280, 1985
33. Panday S, Kotal G, Desai B, et al: Successful surgical management

of left ventricular myxoma: A case report and review of literature (letter). *J Thorac Cardiovasc Surg* **100:**146–148, 1990

34. Soma Y, Ocgwa S, Iwanager S, et al: Multiple primary left ventricular myxomas with multiple intraventricular recurrences. *Cardiovasc Surg* **33:**765–767, 1992

35. Bortolotti U, Mazzucco A, Valfre C, et al: Right ventricular myxoma: Review of the literature and report of two patients. *Ann Thorac Surg* **33:**277, 1982

36. Sandrasagra FA, Oliver WA, English TAH: Myxoma of the mitral valve. *Br Heart J* **42:**221, 1979

37. Richardson JV, Brandt B, Doty DB, Ehrenhaft JL: Surgical treatment of atrial myxomas: Early and late results of 11 operations and review of the literature. *Ann Thorac Surg* **28:**354, 1979

38. Hanson EC, Gill CC, Razavi M, Loop FD: The surgical treatment of atrial myxomas: Clinical experience and late results in 33 patients. *J Thorac Cardiovasc Surg* **89:**298, 1985

39. Suri RK. Pattankar VL, Sing H, et al: Myxoma of the tricuspid valve. *Aust NZ J Surg* **48:**429, 1978

40. El Asmar B, Acker M, Couteil JP, et al: Tricuspid valve myxoma: A rare indication for tricuspid valve repair. *Ann Thorac Surg* **52:**315–316, 1991

41. Catton RW, Gunteroth WG, Reichenbach DC: A myxoma of the pulmonary valve causing severe stenosis in infancy. *Am Heart J* **66:**248, 1963

42. Carney JA: Differences between nonfamilial and familial cardiac myxoma. *Am J Surg Pathol* **9:**53, 1985

43. McCarthy PM, Piehler JM, Schaff HV, et al: The significance of multiple, recurrent, and "complex" cardiac myxomas. *J Thorac Cardiovasc Surg* **91:**389, 1986

44. Gelder HM, O'Brian DJ, Styles ED, Alexander JA: Familial cardiac myxoma. *Ann Thorac Surg* **53:**419–424, 1992

45. Carney JA, Hruska LS, Beauchamp GD, Gordon H: Dominant inheritance of the complex of myxomas, spotty pigmentation, and endocrine overactivity. *Mayo Clin Proc* **61:**165, 1986

46. Farrah MG: Familial cardiac myxoma: A study of patients with myxoma. *Chest* **105:**65–68, 1994

47. Greenwood WF: Profile of atrial myxoma. *Am J Cardiol* **21:**367, 1968

48. Crawford FA, Selby JH, Watson D, Joransen J: Unusual aspects of atrial myxoma. *Ann Surg* **188:**240, 1978

49. Goodwin JF: The spectrum of cardiac tumors. *Am J Cardiol* **21:**307, 1968

50. Bortolotti V, Maraglino G, Rubino M, et al: Surgical excision of intracardiac myxomas: A 20-year follow-up. *Ann Thorac Surg* **49:**449–453, 1990

51. Fyke FE, Seward JB, Miller FA, et al: Primary cardiac tumors: Experience with 30 consecutive patients since introduction of two-dimensional echocardiography. *J Am Coll Cardiol* **5:**1465, 1985

52. Tipton BK, Robertson JT, Robertson JH: Embolism to the central nervous system from cardiac myxoma: Report of two cases. *J Neurosurg* **47:**937, 1977

53. Meller J, Teichholz LE, Pickard AD: Left ventricular myxoma: Echocardiographic diagnosis and review of the literature. *Am J Med* **63:**816, 1977

54. Silverman J, Olwin JS, Graettinger JS: Cardiac myxomas with systemic embolization: Review of the literature and report of a case. *Circulation* **26:**99, 1962

55. Hashimoto H, Tikahashi H, Fukiward Y, et al: Acute myocardial infarction due to coronary embolization from left atrial myxoma. *Jpn Circ J* **57:**1016–1020, 1993

56. Desousa AL, Muller J, Campbell RL, et al: Atrial myxoma: A review of the neurological complications, metastases, and recurrences. *J Neurol Neurosurg Psychiat* **41:**1119, 1978

57. Vidne B, Atsmon A, Aygen M, Levy MJ: Right atrial myxoma: Case report and review of the literature. *Isr J Med Sci* **7:**1196, 1971

58. Gonzalez A, Altieri PI, Merquez E, et al: Massive pulmonary embolism associated with a right ventricular myxoma. *Am J Med* **69:**795, 1980

59. Peters MN, Hall RJ, Cooley DA, et al: The clinical syndrome of atrial myxoma. *JAMA* **230:**695, 1974

60. Hattler BG, Fuchs JCA, Cosson R, Sabiston DC: Atrial myxoma: An evaluation of clinical and laboratory manifestations. *Ann Thorac Surg* **10:**65, 1970

61. Quinn TJ, Codini MA, Harris AA: Infected cardiac myxoma. *Am J Cardiol* **53:**381, 1984

62. Joseph P, Himmelstein DU, Mahowald JM, Stullman WS: Atrial myxoma infected with *Candida:* First survival. *Chest* **78:**340, 1980

63. Buchanan RRC, Cairns JA, Kraag G, Robinson JG: Left atrial myxoma mimicking vasculitis: Echocardiographic diagnosis. *Can Med Assoc J* **120:**1540, 1979

64. Bateman TM, Gray RJ, Raymond MJ, et al: Arrhythmias and conduction disturbances following cardiac operation for the removal of left atrial myxomas. *J Thorac Cardiovasc Surg* **86:**601, 1983

65. Steiner RE: Radiologic aspects of cardiac tumors. *Am J Cardiol* **21:**344, 1968

66. Schattenberg TT: Echocardiographic diagnosis of left atrial myxoma. *Mayo Clin Proc* **43:**620, 1968

67. Pechacek LW, Gonzalex-Camid F, Hall RJ, et al: The echocardiographic spectrum of atrial myxoma: A ten-year experience. *Tex Heart Inst J* **13:**179, 1986

68. Mundinger A, Gruber HP, Dinkel E, et al: Imaging cardiac mass lesions. *Radiol Med* **10:**135–140, 1992

69. Fyke FE, Seward JB, Edwards WD, et al: Primary cardiac tumors: Experience with 30 consecutive patients since the introduction of two-dimensional echocardiography. *J Am Coll Cardiol* **5:**1465, 1985

70. Dressler FA, Labovitz AJ: Systemic arterial emboli and cardiac masses. *Card Clin* **11:**447–460, 1993

71. Reeder GS, Khandheria BK, Senard JB, et al: Transesophageal echocardiographs and cardiac masses. *Mayo Clin Proc* **66:** 1101–1109, 1991

72. Ensberding R, Erbel DR, Kaspar W, et al: Diagnosis of heart tumors by transesophageal echocardiography. *Eur Heart J* **14:**1223–1228, 1993

73. Castells E, Ferran V, Toledo MCO, et al: Cardiac myxomas: Surgical treatment, long-term results and recurrence. *J Thorac Cardiovasc Surg* **34:**49–53, 1993

74. Tsuchiya F, Kohno A, Saitoh K, Shigeta A: CT findings of atrial myxoma. *Radiology* **151:**139, 1984

75. Seifert P, Chomka EV, Stagl R, et al: Applications of the cine computed tomographic scan for precise localization of the origin of an atrial myxoma: Surgical implications. *Ann Thorac Surg* **42:**469, 1986

76. Semelker RC, Schoenst JP, Wilson ME, et al: Cardiac masses: Signed intensity features on scin-echo, gradient-echo, gadolinium-enhanced scin-echo and turboflash images. *JMRI* **2:**415–420, 1992

77. Menegus MA, Greenberg MA, Spindola-Franco H, Fayemin A: Magnetic resonance imaging of suspected atrial tumors. *Am Heart J* **123:**1260–1268, 1992

78. Symbas PN, Hatcher CR, Gravanis MB: Myxoma of the heart: Clinical and experimental observations. *Ann Surg* **183:**470, 1976

79. Dato GMA, Benedictis M, Dato AA, et al: Long-term follow-up of cardiac myxomas (7–31 years). *J Thorac Cardiovasc Surg* **34:**114–143, 1993

80. Semb BKH: Surgical considerations in the treatment of cardiac myxoma. *J Thorac Cardiovasc Surg* **87:**251, 1984

81. Guiloff AK, Flege JB, Callard GM, et al: Surgery of left atrial myxomas: Report of eleven cases and review of the literature. *J Cardiovasc Surg* **27:**194, 1986

82. Murphy MC, Sweeney MS, Putnam JB, et al: Surgical treatment of cardiac tumors: A 25-year experience. *Ann Thorac Surg* **49:**612–618, 1990

83. Miralles A, Bracamonte L, Soncul H, et al: Cardiac tumors: Clinical experience and surgical results in 74 patients. *Ann Thorac Surg* **52:**886–895, 1991

84. Donahoo JS, Weiss JL, Gardner TJ, et al: Current management of

atrial myxoma with emphasis on a new diagnostic technique. *Ann Surg* **189:**763, 1979

85. Sasaki S, Lin YT, Redington JV, et al: Primary intracavitary heart tumors: A review of eleven surgical cases. *J Cardiovasc Surg* **18:**15, 1977

86. Cleveland DC, Westaby S, Karp RB: Treatment of Intra-atrial cardiac tumors. *JAMA* **249:**2799, 1983

87. Attar S, Lee YC, Singleton R, et al: Cardiac myxoma. *Ann Thorac Surg* **29:**397, 1980

88. St. John Sutton MG, Mercier LA, Guiliani ER, Lie JT: Atrial myxomas: A review of clinical experience in 40 patients. *Mayo Clin Proc* **55:**371, 1980

89. Poole GV, Breyer RH, Halliday RH, et al: Tumors of the heart: Surgical considerations. *J Thorac Cardiovasc Surg* **25:**5, 1984

90. Livi U, Bortolotti U, Milano A, et al: Cardiac myxomas: Results of 14 years' experience. *J Thorac Cardiovasc Surg* **32:**143, 1984

91. Gray IR, Williams WG: Recurring cardiac myxoma. *Br Heart J* **53:**645, 1985

92. Attum AA, Johnson GS, Masri Z, et al: Malignant clinical behavior of cardiac myxomas and "myxoid imitators." *Ann Thorac Surg* **44:**217, 1987

93. Read RC, White HJ, Murphy ML, et al: The malignant potentiality of left atrial myxoma. *J Thorac Cardiovasc Surg* **68:**857, 1974

94. Jugdutt BI, Rossall RE, Sterns LP: An unusual case of recurrent left atrial myxoma. *Can Med Assoc J* **112:**1099, 1975

95. Dang CR, Hurley EJ: Contralateral recurrent myxoma of the heart. *Ann Thorac Surg* **21:**59, 1976

96. Markel ML, Armstrong WF, Waller BF, Mahomed Y: Left atrial myxoma with multicentric recurrence and evidence of metastases. *Am Heart J* **111:**409, 1986

97. Hada Y, Takahashi T, Takenaka K, et al: Recurrent multiple myxomas. *Am Heart J* **107:**1280, 1984

98. McCarthy PM, Schatt HU, Winkler H, et al: Deoxyribonucleic acid ploidy pattern of cardiac myxomas. *J Thorac Cardiovasc Surg* **98:**1083, 1989

99. Waller DA, Ettles DF, Saunders NR, Williams G: Recurrent cardiac myxoma: The surgical implications of two groups of patients. *Thorac Cardiovasc Surg* **37:**226, 1989

100. Attum AA, Ogden LL, Lansing AM: Atrial myxoma: Benign and malignant. *J Ky Med Assoc* **82:**319, 1984

101. Hannah H, Eiseman G, Hisuzyskyji R, et al: Invasive atrial myxomas. *Am Heart J* **104:**881, 1982

102. Stoane L, Allen JH, Collins HA: Radiological observations in cerebral embolization from left heart myxomas. *Radiology* **87:**262, 1966

103. Burton C, Johnston J: Multiple cerebral aneurysm and cardiac myxoma. *N Engl J Med* **282:**35, 1970

104. New PFJ, Price DL, Carter B: Cerebral angiography in cardiac myxoma: Correlation of angiographic and histopathological findings. *Radiology* **96:**335, 1970

105. Price DL, Harris JL, New PFJ, Cantu RC: Cardiac myxoma: A clinicopathologic and angiographic study. *Arch Neurol* **23:**558, 1970

106. Damasio H, Seabra-Gomes R, da Silva JP, et al: Multiple cerebral aneurysms and cardiac myxoma. *Arch Neurol* **32:**269, 1975

107. Heath D, MacKinnon J: Pulmonary hypertension due to myxoma of the right atrium: With special reference to the behavior of emboli of myxoma in the lung. *Am Heart J* **68:**227, 1964

108. Seo IS, Warner TFCS, Colyer RA, Winkler RF: Metastasizing atrial myxoma. *Am J Surg Pathol* **4:**391, 1980

109. Rankin LI, Desousa AL: Metastatic atrial myxoma presenting as intracranial mass. *Chest* **74:**451, 1978

110. Budzilovich G, Aleksie S, Greco A, et al: Malignant cardiac and cerebral metastases. *Surg Neurol* **11:**461, 1979

111. Corno A, de Simone G, Catena G, Marcelletti C: Cardiac rhabdomyoma: Surgical treatment in the neonate. *J Thorac Cardiovasc Surg* **87:**725, 1984

112. Fenoglio JJ, McAllister HA, Ferrans VJ: Cardiac rhabdomyoma: A clinicopathologic and electron microscopic study. *Am J Cardiol* **38:**241, 1976

113. Reece IJ, Cooley DA, Frazier OH, et al: Cardiac tumors: Clinical spectrum and prognosis of lesions other than classic benign myxoma in 20 patients. *J Thorac Cardiovasc Surg* **88:**439, 1984

114. Garson A, Smith RJ, Moak JP, et al: Incessant ventricular tachycardia in infants: Myocardial hematomas and surgical cure. *J Am Coll Cardiol* **10:**619, 1987

115. Bass JL, Breningstall GN, Swaiman KF: Echocardiographic incidence of cardiac rhabdomyoma in tuberous sclerosis. *Am J Cardiol* **55:**1379, 1985

116. Skillington PD, Brown WJ, Eolis BD, et al: Surgical excision of primary cardiac tumors in infancy. *Aust NZ J Surg* **57:**599, 1987

117. Houser S, Forbes N, Stewart S: Rhabdomyoma of the heart: A diagnostic and therapeutic challenge. *Ann Thorac Surg* **29:**373, 1980

118. DeLoma JG, Villagra F, DeLeon JP, et al: Rhabdomyoma of the heart: Surgical treatment. *J Cardiovasc Surg* **23:**149, 1982

119. Foster ED, Spooner EW, Farina MA, et al: Cardiac rhabdomyoma in the neonate: Surgical management. *Ann Thorac Surg* **37:**249, 1984

120. Engle MA, Ebert PA, Redo SF: Recurrent ventricular tachycardia due to resectable cardiac tumor: Report of two cases in two-year-olds in heart failure. *Circulation* **50:**1052, 1974

121. Goldman S, Lortscher R, Pappas G: Surgical treatment of rhabdomyoma of the right atrium causing arrhythmias. *J Thorac Cardiovasc Surg* **89:**802, 1985

122. Yamaguchi M, Hosokowa Y, Ohasi H, et al: Cardiac fibroma: Long-term tests after excision. *J Thorac Cardiovasc Surg* **103:**140–145, 1992

123. Feldman PS, Meyer MW: Fibroelastic hamartoma (fibroma) of the heart. *Cancer* **30:**314, 1976

124. Calhoun TR, Terry EE, Best EB, Sunbury TR: Myocardial fibroma or fibrous hamartoma. *Ann Thorac Surg* **32:**406, 1981

125. Williams DB, Danielson GK, McGoon DC, et al: Cardiac fibroma: Long-term survival after excision. *J Thorac Cardiovasc Surg* **84:**230, 1982

126. Valente M, Locco P, Thiene G, et al: Cardiac fibroma and heart transplantation. *J Thorac Cardiovasc Surg* **106:**1208–1212, 1993

127. Jones KL, Wolf PL, Jensen P, et al: The Gorlin syndrome: A genetically determined disorder associated with cardiac tumor. *Am Heart J* **111:**1013, 1986

128. Geha AS, Weidman WH, Soule EH, McGoon DC: Intramural ventricular cardiac fibroma: Successful removal in two cases and review of the literature. *Circulation* **36:**427, 1967

129. Folger GM, Peters HJ: Nodular fibroelastosis (fibroelastic hamartoma): A tumorous malformation of the heart. *Am J Cardiol* **21:**420, 1968

130. Culliford AT, Isom OW, Treha NK, et al: Benign tumors of right atrium necessitating extensive resection and reconstruction. *J Thorac Cardiovasc Surg* **76:**178, 1978

131. Mustafa I, Shinebourne E, Lincoln C: Successful replacement of the interventricular septum following excision of a large intramural fibroma. *J Thorac Cardiovasc Surg* **19:**411, 1978

132. Carpentier A, Chachques JC: Myocardial substitution with a stimulated skeletal muscle: First successful clinical case. *Lancet* **1:**1267, 1985

133. Harjola PT, Ala-Kulju K, Ketonen P: Epicardial lipoma. *Scand J Thorac Cardiovasc Surg* **19:**181, 1985

134. Arciniegas E, Hakimi M, Farooki ZQ, et al: Primary cardiac tumors in children. *J Thorac Cardiovasc Surg* **79:**582, 1980

135. Reyes LH, Rubio PA, Korompai FL, Guinn GA: Lipoma of the heart. *Int Surg* **61:**179, 1976

136. Zingas AP, Carrera JD, Murray CA, Kling GA: Lipoma of the myocardium. *J Comput Assist Tomogr* **7:**1098, 1983

137. Reyes CV, Jablokow VR: Lipomatous hypertrophy of the atrial septum: A report of 38 cases and review of the literature. *Am J Clin Pathol* **72:**785, 1979

138. Simons M, Cabin HS, Jaffe CC: Lipomatous hypertrophy of the atrial septum: Diagnosis by combined echocardiography and computerized tomography. *Am J Cardiol* **54:**465, 1984

139. Edwards FH, Hale D, Cohen A, et al: Primary cardiac valve tumors. *Ann Thorac Surg* **52:**1127–1131, 1991

140. Gallo R, Kumar N, Prabhakar G, et al: Papillary fibroelastoma of mitral valve chordae. *Ann Thorac Surg* **55:**1156–1157, 1993

141. Topol EJ, Biern RO, Reitz BA: Cardiac papillary fibroelastoma and stroke: Echocardiographic diagnosis and guide to excision. *Am J Med* **80:**129, 1986

142. Fowles RE, Miller DC, Egbert BM, et al: Systemic embolization from a mitral valve papillary endocardial fibroma detected by two-dimensional echocardiography. *Am Heart J* **102:**128, 1981

143. Harris LS, Adelson L: Fatal coronary embolism from a myxomatous polyp of the aortic valve: An unusual cause of sudden death. *Am J Clin Pathol* **43:**61, 1965

144. Butterworth JS, Poindexter CA: Papilloma of cusp of the aortic valve: An unusual cause of sudden death. *Circulation* **48:**213, 1973

145. Wolf PL, Bing R: The smallest tumor which causes sudden death. *JAMA* **194:**674, 1965

146. Nishida K, Kaijima G, Nagayama T: Mesothelioma of the atrioventricular node. *Br Heart J* **53:**468, 1985

147. Lewman LV, Demany MA, Zimmerman HA: Congenital tumor of atrioventricular node with complete heart block and sudden death: Mesothelioma or lymphangio-endothelioma of atrioventricular node. *Am J Cardiol* **29:**554, 1972

148. Bharati S, Bicoff JP, Fridman JL, et al: Sudden death caused by benign tumor of the atrioventricular node. *Arch Intern Med* **136:**224, 1976

149. Cox JN, Friedl B, Mechnache R, et al: Teratoma of the heart: A case report and review of the literature. *Virchows Arch (Pathol Anat)* **402:**163, 1983

150. Costas C, Williams RL, Fortune RL: Intracardiac teratoma in an infant. *Pediatr Cardiol* **7:**179, 1986

151. Jebara VA, Sousa Uver M, Farge A, et al: Cardiac pheochromocytoma. *Ann Thorac Surg* **53:**356–361, 1991

152. Orringer MB, Sisson JC, Glazer G, et al: Surgical treatment of cardiac pheochromocytomas. *J Thorac Cardiovasc Surg* **89:**753, 1985

153. David TE, Leukei SC, Marquez-Julio A, et al: Pheochromocytoma of the heart. *Ann Thorac Surg* **41:**98, 1986

154. Brizard C, Latremoville C, Jebara VA, et al: Cardiac hemangiomas. *Ann Thorac Surg* **56:**390–394, 1993

155. Poole GV, Meredith JW, Breyer RH, Mills SA: Surgical implications in malignant cardiac disease. *Ann Thorac Surg* **36:**484, 1983

156. Thomas CR, Johnson GW, Stoddard MF, Clifford S: Primary malignant cardiac tumors: Update 1992. *Med Pediatr Oncol* **20:**519–531, 1992

157. Burke AP, Cowan D, Virmani R: Primary sarcomas of the heart. *Cancer* **69:**387–395, 1992

158. Putnam JB, Sweeney MS, Colon R, et al: Primary cardiac sarcomas. *Ann Thorac Surg* **51:**906–910, 1991

159. Turner A, Bartrick N: Primary cardiac sarcomas: A report of three cases and a review of the current literature. *Int J Cardiol* **40:**115–119, 1993

160. Sorlie D, Myhne ESP, Stalsberg H: Angiosarcoma of the heart: Unusual presentation and survival after treatment. *Br Heart J* **51:**94, 1984

161. Rettmar K, Stierle U, Sheikhzadeh A, Diedrich KW: Primary angiosarcoma of the heart: Report of a case and review of the literature. *Jpn Heart J* **34:**667–683, 1993

162. Hermann MA, Shankerman RA, Edwards WD, et al: Primary cardiac angiosarcoma: A clinicopathologic study of six cases. *J Thorac Cardiovasc Surg* **103:**655–664, 1992

163. Crespo MG, Pulpon LA, Pradas G, et al: Heart transplantation for cardiac angiosarcoma: Should its indication be questioned? *J Heart Lung Transplant* **12:**527–530, 1993

164. Schwartz JE, Schwartz GP, Judson PL, et al: Complete resection of a primary cardiac rhabdomyosarcoma: Case report, review of the lit-

erature, and management recommendations. *Cardiovasc Dis (Bull Texas Heart Inst)* **6:**413, 1979

165. Torsveit JR, Bennett WA, Hinchcliffe WA, Cornell WP: Primary plasmacytoma of the atrium: Report of a case with successful surgical management. *J Thorac Cardiovasc Surg* **74:**563, 1977

166. Nzayinambaho K, Noel H, Brohet C: Primary cardiac liposarcoma simulating a left atrial myxoma. *Thorac Cardiovasc Surg* **40:**402, 1985

167. Burke AP, Virmani R: Osteosarcomas of the heart. *Am J Surg Pathol* **15(3):**289–295, 1991

168. Winer HE, Kronzon I, Fox A, et al: Primary cardiac chondromyxosarcoma—clinical and echocardiographic manifestations: A case report. *J Thorac Cardiovasc Surg* **74:**567, 1977

169. Gelfand ET, Taylor RF, Rao S, et al: Melanotic malignant schwannoma of the right atrium. *J Thorac Cardiovasc Surg* **74:**808, 1977

170. Chen KTK: Carcinosarcoma of the heart. *J Surg Oncol* **27:**48, 1984

171. Chou ST, Arkles LB, Gill GD: Primary lymphoma of the heart: A case report. *Cancer* **52:**744, 1983

172. Takagi M, Kugimiya T, Fukii T, et al: Extensive surgery for primary malignant lymphoma of the heart. *J Thorac Cardiovasc Surg* **33:**570–571, 1992

173. Smith C: Tumors of the heart. *Arch Pathol Lab Med* **110:**371, 1986

174. Lockwood WB, Broghamer WL: The changing prevalence of secondary cardiac neoplasms as related to cancer therapy. *Cancer* **45:**2659, 1980

175. Skhvatsabaja LV: Secondary malignant lesions of the heart and pericardium in neoplastic disease. *Oncology* **43:**103, 1986

176. Miyazaki T, Yoshida T, Mori H, et al: Intractable heart failure, conduction disturbances and myocardial infarction by massive myocardial invasion of malignant lymphoma. *J Am Coll Cardiol* **6:**937, 1985

177. Melvin KN, Howard RJ, Rakowski H, et al: Embryonal carcinoma of the testis with metastases to the right atrium. *Can J Surg* **26:**86, 1983

178. O'Donnell AF, Maghur HA, Grogan L, et al: Resection of an intracardiac metastasis from malignant teratoma of the testes. *Ann Thorac Surg* **56:**1386–1387, 1993

179. Lang RM, Borow KM, Neumann A: Metastatic carcinoma involving the left atrium. *Am Heart J* **110:**884, 1985

180. Shuman RL: Primary pulmonary sarcoma with left atrial extension via left superior pulmonary vein: En bloc resection and radical pneumonectomy on cardiopulmonary bypass. *J Thorac Cardiovasc Surg* **88:**189, 1984

181. Prager RL, Dean R, Turner B: Surgical approach to intracardiac renal cell carcinoma. *Ann Thorac Surg* **33:**74, 1982

182. Marshall FF, Reitz B, Diamond DA: A new technique for management of renal cell carcinoma. *J Urol* **131:**103, 1984

183. Schecter DC: Cardiovascular surgery in the management of malignant renal tumors: Surgery of 187 cases in the literature. *Tex Heart Inst J* **10:**163, 1983

184. Skinner DG, Pfister RF, Colvin R: Extension of renal cell carcinoma into the vena cava: The rationale for aggressive surgical management. *J Urol* **107:**711, 1972

185. Iverson LIG, Lee J, Drew D, et al: Intravenous leiomyomatosis with cardiac extension. *Tex Heart Inst J* **10:**275, 1983

186. Politzer F, Kronzon I, Wieczonek R, et al: Intracardiac leiomyomatosis: Diagnosis and treatment. *J Am Coll Cardiol* **4:**629, 1984

187. Shida T, Yoshimura M, Chihara H, Nakamura K: Intravenous lieomyomatosis of the pelvis with reextension into the heart. *Ann Thorac Surg* **42:**104, 1986

188. Garcia FA, Villaneuva RA, Narciso FV, Aventura AP: Intravenous leiomyomatosis of the uterus and pelvis presenting as a cardiac tumor. *Ann Thorac Surg* **42** (Suppl):S41, 1986

Index

Page numbers followed by t or f indicate
tables or figures, respectively. CP indicates
color plates, which follow page 608 in Vol I;
page 2072 in Vol. II.

Page numbers followed by *t* or *f* indicate
tables or figures, respectively. *CP* indicates
color plates, which follow page 608 in Vol I;
page 2072 in Vol. II.

Page numbers followed by *t* or *f* indicate
tables or figures, respectively. *CP* indicates
color plates, which follow page 608 in Vol I;
page 2072 in Vol. II.

Page numbers followed by *t* or *f* indicate
tables or figures, respectively. *CP* indicates
color plates, which follow page 608 in Vol I;
page 2072 in Vol. II.

Page numbers followed by *t* or *f* indicate
tables or figures, respectively. *CP* indicates
color plates, which follow page 608 in Vol I;
page 2072 in Vol. II.

Page numbers followed by *t* or *f* indicate
tables or figures, respectively. *CP* indicates
color plates, which follow page 608 in Vol I;
page 2072 in Vol. II.

Page numbers followed by *t* or *f* indicate
tables or figures, respectively. *CP* indicates
color plates, which follow page 608 in Vol I;
page 2072 in Vol. II.

Page numbers followed by *t* or *f* indicate
tables or figures, respectively. *CP* indicates
color plates, which follow page 608 in Vol I;
page 2072 in Vol. II.

Page numbers followed by *t* or *f* indicate
tables or figures, respectively. *CP* indicates
color plates, which follow page 608 in Vol I;
page 2072 in Vol. II.

Page numbers followed by *t* or *f* indicate
tables or figures, respectively. *CP* indicates
color plates, which follow page 608 in Vol I;
page 2072 in Vol. II.

Page numbers followed by *t* or *f* indicate
tables or figures, respectively. *CP* indicates
color plates, which follow page 608 in Vol I;
page 2072 in Vol. II.

Page numbers followed by *t* or *f* indicate
tables or figures, respectively. *CP* indicates
color plates, which follow page 608 in Vol I;
page 2072 in Vol. II.

Page numbers followed by t or f indicate
tables or figures, respectively. CP indicates
color plates, which follow page 608 in Vol I;
page 2072 in Vol. II.

Page numbers followed by *t* or *f* indicate
tables or figures, respectively. *CP* indicates
color plates, which follow page 608 in Vol I;
page 2072 in Vol. II.

Page numbers followed by *t* or *f* indicate tables or figures, respectively. *CP* indicates color plates, which follow page 608 in Vol I; page 2072 in Vol. II.

Page numbers followed by t or f indicate
tables or figures, respectively. CP indicates
color plates, which follow page 608 in Vol I;
page 2072 in Vol. II.

Page numbers followed by *t* or *f* indicate
tables or figures, respectively. *CP* indicates
color plates, which follow page 608 in Vol I;
page 2072 in Vol. II.

Page numbers followed by t or f indicate
tables or figures, respectively. CP indicates
color plates, which follow page 608 in Vol I;
page 2072 in Vol. II.

Page numbers followed by *t* or *f* indicate
tables or figures, respectively. *CP* indicates
color plates, which follow page 608 in Vol I;
page 2072 in Vol. II.

Page numbers followed by *t* or *f* indicate
tables or figures, respectively. *CP* indicates
color plates, which follow page 608 in Vol I;
page 2072 in Vol. II.

Page numbers followed by *t* or *f* indicate
tables or figures, respectively. *CP* indicates
color plates, which follow page 608 in Vol I;
page 2072 in Vol. II.

Page numbers followed by *t* or *f* indicate
tables or figures, respectively. *CP* indicates
color plates, which follow page 608 in Vol I;
page 2072 in Vol. II.

Page numbers followed by t or f indicate
tables or figures, respectively. CP indicates
color plates, which follow page 608 in Vol I;
page 2072 in Vol. II.

Page numbers followed by *t* or *f* indicate
tables or figures, respectively. *CP* indicates
color plates, which follow page 608 in Vol I;
page 2072 in Vol. II.

Page numbers followed by *t* or *f* indicate
tables or figures, respectively. *CP* indicates
color plates, which follow page 608 in Vol I;
page 2072 in Vol. II.

Page numbers followed by *t* or *f* indicate
tables or figures, respectively. *CP* indicates
color plates, which follow page 608 in Vol I;
page 2072 in Vol. II.

Page numbers followed by *t* or *f* indicate
tables or figures, respectively. *CP* indicates
color plates, which follow page 608 in Vol I;
page 2072 in Vol. II.

Page numbers followed by t or f indicate
tables or figures, respectively. CP indicates
color plates, which follow page 608 in Vol I;
page 2072 in Vol. II.

Page numbers followed by t or f indicate
tables or figures, respectively. CP indicates
color plates, which follow page 608 in Vol I;
page 2072 in Vol. II.

Page numbers followed by *t* or *f* indicate
tables or figures, respectively. *CP* indicates
color plates, which follow page 608 in Vol I;
page 2072 in Vol. II.

Page numbers followed by *t* or *f* indicate
tables or figures, respectively. *CP* indicates
color plates, which follow page 608 in Vol I;
page 2072 in Vol. II.

Page numbers followed by *t* or *f* indicate
tables or figures, respectively. *CP* indicates
color plates, which follow page 608 in Vol I;
page 2072 in Vol. II.

Page numbers followed by *t* or *f* indicate
tables or figures, respectively. *CP* indicates
color plates, which follow page 608 in Vol I;
page 2072 in Vol. II.

Page numbers followed by *t* or *f* indicate tables or figures, respectively. *CP* indicates color plates, which follow page 608 in Vol I; page 2072 in Vol. II.